Medical–Surgical Nursing

Pathophysiological Concepts

With **57** Contributors

Maxine L. Patrick, R.N., Dr.P.H.

Professor

University of Washington School of Nursing

Department of Physiological Nursing

Seattle, Washington

Susan L. Woods, R.N., M.N.

Associate Professor

University of Washington School of Nursing

Department of Physiological Nursing

Seattle, Washington

Ruth F. Craven, R.N., Ed.D.

Associate Professor

University of Washington School of Nursing

Department of Physiological Nursing

Seattle, Washington

Joanne Schnaidt Rokosky, R.N., M.N.

Clinical Assistant Professor

University of Washington School of Nursing

Department of Physiological Nursing

Seattle, Washington

Pauline M. Bruno, R.N., D.N.Sc.

Professor

Intercollegiate Center for Nursing Education

Spokane, Washington

J.B. Lippincott Company

Philadelphia

London

Mexico City

New York

St. Louis

São Paulo

Sydney

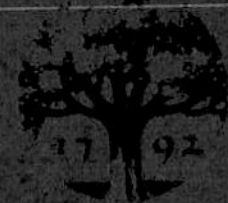

Medical–Surgical Nursing

Pathophysiological Concepts

Acquisitions and Sponsoring Editor: Diana Intenzo
Design Director: Tracy Baldwin
Interior Design: Arlene Putterman
Cover Design: Earl Gerhart
Production Supervisor: J. Corey Gray
Production Editor: Rosanne Hallowell
Indexer: Ann Cassar
Compositor: Circle Graphics
Printer/Binder: The Murray Printing Company

6 5 4 3 2 1

Library of Congress Cataloging-in-Publication Data
Main entry under title:
Medical-surgical nursing.
Includes bibliographies and index.
1. Nursing. 2. Medicine, Clinical.
3. Physiology, Pathological. I. Patrick, Maxine.
[DNLM: 1. Nursing Care. 2. Surgical Nursing.
WY 100 M4895]
RT41.M495 1986 610.73 85-24000
ISBN 0-397-54453-7

The authors and publisher have exerted every effort to ensure that drug selection and dosage set forth in this text are in accord with current recommendations and practice at the time of publication. However, in view of ongoing research, changes in government regulations, and the constant flow of information relating to drug therapy and drug reactions, the reader is urged to check the package insert for each drug for any change in indications and dosage and for added warnings and precautions. This is particularly important when the recommended agent is a new or infrequently employed drug.

Contributors

Gaylene Bouska Altman, R.N., M.N.
Lecturer
Department of Physiological Nursing
University of Washington
Seattle, Washington
Chapters 52 *Infectious Disorders of the Blood*
53 *Anemias and Related Blood Disorders*
103 *Abuse of Alcohol and Other Drugs*

Kathryn L. Anderson, R.N., M.N.
Lecturer
School of Nursing
Seattle University
Respiratory Clinical Nurse Specialist
Seattle-King County Visiting Nurse Services
Seattle, Washington
Chapters 29 *Obstructive Respiratory Disorders: Asthma, COPD, Bronchiectasis, Cystic Fibrosis*
30 *Neoplastic Disorders Related to Respiratory Function: Cancer of the Larynx and Lung Cancer*
31 *Traumatic Conditions Affecting Respiratory Function*

Carol A. Blainey, R.N., M.N.
Associate Professor
Department of Physiological Nursing
University of Washington
Seattle, Washington
Chapter 74 *Diabetes Mellitus*

Mary Boozer, R.N., M.N.
Associate Professor
Department of Physiological Nursing
University of Washington
Seattle, Washington
Chapters 42 *Assessment of Vascular Function*
43 *Nursing Strategies for Common Vascular Problems: Nursing Diagnosis, Interventions, Evaluation*

Lynda Brubacher, R.N., C.R.N., E.T.
Enterostomal Therapist
Virginia Mason Hospital
Clinical Associate
Department of Physiological Nursing
University of Washington
Seattle, Washington
Chapters 60 *Neoplastic Disorders Affecting Renal and Urinary Function*
80 *Nursing Strategies for Common Gastrointestinal Problems: Nursing Diagnosis, Interventions, Evaluation*

Margaret Auld Bruya, R.N., D.N.Sc.
Associate Professor
Intercollegiate Center for Nursing Education
Spokane, Washington
Chapter 24 *Shock*

Marci-Lee Catanzaro, R.N., Ph.D.
Assistant Professor
Department of Physiological Nursing
Clinical Assistant Professor
Department of Rehabilitation Medicine
University of Washington
Seattle, Washington
Chapters 67 *Intracranial and Spinal Cord Tumors*
68 *Infectious and Degenerative Neurological Disorders*

Terry F. Cicero, R.N., M.N., CCRN
Lecturer
Department of Physiological Nursing
University of Washington
Seattle, Washington
Chapters 89 *Musculoskeletal Inflammation and Connective Tissue Disorders*
90 *Metabolic, Structural, and Neoplastic Conditions of Musculoskeletal Origin*

Marie Cowan, R.N., Ph.D.
Associate Professor
Departments of Physiological Nursing, Pathology, and Medicine
Director, Office of Nursing Research Facilitation
University of Washington
Seattle, Washington
Chapter 22 *Atherosclerosis*

Susanna L. Cunningham, R.N., Ph.D.
Associate Professor
Department of Physiological Nursing
University of Washington
Seattle, Washington
Chapter 44 *Hypertension*

Denise Davignon, R.N., M.N.
Lecturer
Department of Physiological Nursing
University of Washington
Seattle, Washington
Chapter 84 *Gastrointestinal Structural Disorders*

Linda M. Dunn, R.N., M.N.
Critical Care Instructor
Providence Medical Center
Clinical Instructor
Department of Physiological Nursing
University of Washington
Seattle, Washington
Chapter 93 *Nursing Strategies for Common Integument Problems: Nursing Diagnosis, Interventions, Evaluation*

Mary P. Farley, R.N., M.N., CCRN
Lecturer
Department of Physiological Nursing
University of Washington
Seattle, Washington
Chapter 104 *Multiple Trauma*

Linda Felver, R.N., M.A., Ph.C.
Associate Professor
Intercollegiate Center for Nursing Education
Spokane, Washington
Chapters 13 *Fluid and Electrolyte Balance and Imbalances*
14 *Acid–Base Balance and Imbalances*

Charlene Gladney Foster, C.R.N.A., M.N., M.A.E.
Vice President
Anesthesia Northwest
Seattle, Washington
Staff Nurse Anesthetist
Eastside Group Health Hospital
Redmond, Washington
Chapters 8 *The Surgical Experience*
9 *Pain*

Betty B. Gallucci, R.N., Ph.D.
Professor
Department of Physiological Nursing
University of Washington
Seattle, Washington
Chapters 16 *Immune Responses*
19 *Neoplasia*

Sally K. Graham, C.R.N., M.S.N.
Adult Nurse Practitioner
Atlanta, Georgia
Chapter 101 *Infectious and Inflammatory Disorders Affecting Reproductive Function*

Ruth A. Gregersen, R.N., M.N., CCRN
Lecturer
Department of Physiological Nursing
University of Washington
Seattle, Washington
Chapters 21 *Hemostatic Responses*
49 *Assessment of Hematologic Function*
50 *Nursing Strategies for Common Hematologic Problems: Nursing Diagnosis, Interventions, Evaluation*
54 *Alterations in Hemostasis: Bleeding and Coagulation Disorders*

Susan Garske Halverson, C.R.N., A.N.P., M.S.
Nurse Practitioner
Planned Parenthood of Seattle—King County
Seattle, Washington
Chapter 101 *Infectious and Inflammatory Disorders Affecting Reproductive Function*

Margaret Heitkemper, R.N., Ph.D.
Assistant Professor
Department of Physiological Nursing
University of Washington
Seattle, Washington
Chapters 80 *Nursing Strategies for Common Gastrointestinal Problems: Nursing Diagnosis, Interventions, Evaluation*
82 *Infectious and Inflammatory Gastrointestinal Disorders*
83 *Ulcers of the Gastrointestinal Tract*

Constance J. Hirnle, R.N., M.N.
Lecturer
Department of Physiological Nursing
University of Washington
Seattle, Washington
Chapters 20 *Lithiasis*
61 *Urolithiasis*

Nancy Hoffart, R.N., M.S.N.
Formerly, Educational Services Manager
Northwest Kidney Center
Seattle, Washington
Chapter 58 *Acute Renal Failure*

Beverly M. Horn, R.N., Ph.D.
Associate Professor
Department of Community Health Care Services
University of Washington
Seattle, Washington
Chapters 3 *Behavioral and Emotional Responses to Illness*
4 *Cultural and Religious Considerations*

Barbara S. Innes, R.N., M.S.
Associate Professor
Seattle Pacific University
Seattle, Washington
Chapters 94 *Infectious and Inflammatory Skin Disorders*
95 *Neoplastic Skin Disorders and Related Dermatologic Conditions*

Beth Miller Kraybill, R.N., B.S.N.
Formerly, Staff Nurse
Bone Marrow Transplant/General Medicine Unit
Swedish Hospital Medical Center
Seattle, Washington
Chapter 51 *Neoplastic Disorders Affecting Hematologic Function*

Barbara R. Landau, Ph.D.
Associate Professor Emeritus
Departments of Physiology and Biophysics and of Biological Structure
University of Washington
Seattle, Washington
Chapters 12 *Dynamic Equilibrium and the Nature of Disease*
25 *Review of Anatomy and Physiology: Respiratory System*
33 *Review of Anatomy and Physiology: The Heart*
41 *Review of Anatomy and Physiology: Blood Vessels and Lymphatics*
48 *Review of Anatomy and Physiology: Blood and Blood-Forming Mechanisms*
55 *Review of Anatomy and Physiology: Renal System*
62 *Review of Anatomy and Physiology: Nervous System*
71 *Review of Anatomy and Physiology: Endocrine System*
78 *Review of Anatomy and Physiology: Gastrointestinal System*
85 *Review of Anatomy and Physiology: Musculoskeletal System*
91 *Review of Anatomy and Physiology: Integument System*
98 *Review of Anatomy and Physiology: Reproductive System*

Christine A. Larson, R.N., M.N.
Assistant Professor
Seattle Pacific University
Seattle, Washington
Chapters 72 *Assessment of Endocrine Function*
73 *Nursing Strategies for Common Endocrine Problems: Nursing Diagnosis, Interventions, Evaluation*
75 *Disorders of the Thyroid and Parathyroid Glands*
76 *Disorders of the Adrenal Glands*
77 *Disorders of the Pituitary Gland and Hypothalamus*

Debra Laurent-Bopp, R.N., M.N.
Lecturer
Department of Physiological Nursing
University of Washington
Seattle, Washington
Chapters 38 *Heart Failure*
39 *Cardiomyopathy and Infectious and Inflammatory Cardiac Disorders*

Carla A. Lee, R.N., B.S.N., M.A., Ed.S.
Assistant Professor, Chairperson, and Project Director
Nurse Clinician Program
Wichita State University
Wichita, Kansas
Chapter 103 *Abuse of Alcohol and Other Drugs*

Kathryn A. Lee, R.N., M.N.
Doctoral Candidate
School of Nursing
University of Washington
Seattle, Washington
Chapter 10 *Sensory Overload, Sensory Deprivation, and Sleep Deprivation*

Martha J. Lentz, R.N., Ph.D.
Research Assistant Professor
Department of Physiological Nursing
University of Washington
Seattle, Washington
Chapter 86 *Assessment of Musculoskeletal Function*

Anne Loustau, R.N., Ph.D.
Associate Professor
Department of Physiological Nursing
University of Washington
Seattle, Washington
Chapter 6 *Health Promotion and Patient Teaching*

Lisa L. MacGeorge, R.N., M.N.
Head Nurse
Bone Marrow Transplant
Swedish Hospital Medical Center
Seattle, Washington
Chapters 56 *Assessment of Renal Function*
57 *Nursing Strategies for Common Renal and Excretory Problems: Nursing Diagnosis, Interventions, Evaluation*
59 *Renal and Urinary Infections and Inflammatory Disorders*

Dee Malchow, R.N., B.S.N.
Limb Viability Coordinator
Harborview Medical Center
Seattle, Washington
Chapter 88 *Musculoskeletal Trauma*

Deborah Martin, R.N., M.N.
Nurse Epidemiologist
Texas Department of Health
Austin, Texas
Chapter 82 *Infectious and Inflammatory Gastrointestinal Disorders*

Janet Marvin, R.N., M.N.
Associate Professor
Department of Physiological Nursing
Department of Surgery
University of Washington
Seattle, Washington
Chapters 96 *Burn Injuries and Skin Trauma*
97 *Reconstructive Problems*

Karen Booth McCormick, R.N., M.N.
Neurological Nurse Specialist
Harborview Medical Center
Seattle, Washington
Chapters 63 *Assessment of Neurological Function*
69 *Neurological Trauma*

Thomas R. McCormick, D.Min.
Lecturer
Biomedical History
School of Medicine
University of Washington
Seattle, Washington
Chapter 11 *The Terminal Phase of Illness*

Pamela H. Mitchell, R.N., M.S., F.A.A.N.
Professor
Department of Physiological Nursing
University of Washington
Seattle, Washington
Chapters 1 *Components of Nursing Practice*
2 *Nursing Process*

Carina Knowlton Moravec, R.N., M.A., CCRN
Bone Marrow Transplant Clinical Nurse Specialist
Swedish Hospital Medical Center
Seattle, Washington
Chapter 51 *Neoplastic Disorders Affecting Hematologic Function*

Jane A. Nelson, R.N., M.N., C.A.C. II
Nurse Manager
Puget Sound Alcoholism Center
Tacoma, Washington
Chapter 103 *Abuse of Alcohol and Other Drugs*

Patricia A. Osborne, R.N., M.N., C.N.R.N.
Neuro-Science/Epilepsy Nurse Specialist
Beth Israel Hospital
Boston, Massachusetts
Chapter 66 *Cerebrovascular Disorders*

Judy Hill Ozuna, R.N., M.N.
Clinical Nurse Specialist
Veterans Administration Medical Center
Clinical Assistant Professor
Department of Physiological Nursing
University of Washington
Seattle, Washington
Chapters 64 *Nursing Strategies for Common Neurological Problems: Nursing Diagnosis, Interventions, Evaluation*
65 *Seizures*

Susan Pfister, R.N., M.N.
Instructor
Florida Junior College
Jacksonville, Florida
Chapter 92 *Assessment of Integument Function*

Christine E. Reheis, R.N., M.N.
Clinical Nurse Specialist
Oncology
Seattle, Washington
Chapters 60 *Neoplastic Disorders Affecting Renal and Urinary Function*
81 *Neoplastic and Degenerative Gastrointestinal Disorders*

Nancy L. Risser, R.N., M.N., C.A.N.P.
Respiratory Clinical Nurse Specialist
Veterans Administration Medical Center
Clinical Instructor
Department of Community Health Care Systems
University of Washington
Seattle, Washington
Chapter 28 *Respiratory Infections and Inflammatory Disorders*

Joan Shaver, R.N., Ph.D.
Associate Professor
Department of Physiological Nursing
University of Washington
Seattle, Washington
Chapters 99 *Assessment of Reproductive Function*
100 *Nursing Strategies for Common Reproductive Problems: Nursing Diagnosis, Interventions, Evaluation*

Linda M. Simmons, R.N., M.N.
Assistant Director of Nursing
Caroline Kline Galland Home
Clinical Instructor
Department of Physiological Nursing
University of Washington
Seattle, Washington
Chapters 79 *Assessment of Gastrointestinal Function*
83 *Ulcers of the Gastrointestinal Tract*

Gretchen B. Stengel, R.N., M.N.
Lecturer
Department of Physiological Nursing
University of Washington
Seattle, Washington
Chapter 70 *Alterations in Special Senses: Vision and Hearing Problems*

Martha L. Tyler, R.N., M.N., R.R.T.
Assistant Professor
Department of Physiological Nursing
Adjunct Assistant Professor
Department of Medicine
Respiratory Disease Division
University of Washington
Seattle, Washington
Chapter 32 *Acute Respiratory Failure*

Sandra L. Underhill, R.N., M.N.
Lecturer
Department of Physiological Nursing
University of Washington
Seattle, Washington
Chapters 34 *Assessment of Cardiac Function*
35 *Nursing Strategies for Common Cardiac Problems: Nursing Diagnosis, Interventions, Evaluation*
36 *Cardiac Arrhythmias and Conduction Abnormalities*
37 *Coronary Heart Disease: Myocardial Ischemia and Infarction*
40 *Valvular Heart Dysfunction*

Barbara L. Vail, R.N., M.N.
Medical–Surgical Clinical Nurse Specialist
Pacific Medical Center
Seattle, Washington
Chapter 26 *Assessment of Respiratory Function*

Candace Ann Walters, R.N., M.N.
Formerly, Lecturer
Department of Physiological Nursing
University of Washington
Seattle, Washington
Chapters 18 *Non-neoplastic Cell Changes*
102 *Neoplastic and Non-neoplastic Disorders Affecting Reproduction*

Karen A. Waxdahl, R.N., M.N.
Major, Army Nurse Corps
Chief, Nursing Education and Training Service
Silas B. Hays Army Community Hospital
Fort Ord, California
Chapter *87* *Nursing Strategies for Common Musculoskeletal Problems: Nursing Diagnosis, Interventions, Evaluation*

Margaret J. Wertz, R.N., M.N.
Research Associate
Department of Surgery
School of Medicine
University of Washington
Seattle, Washington
Chapter *17* *Infection*

Lorie R. Wild, R.N., M.N.
Medical–Surgical Clinical Nurse Specialist
University Hospital
Clinical Instructor
Department of Physiological Nursing
University of Washington
Seattle, Washington
Chapters *45* *Inflammatory Disorders Affecting Vascular Function: Phlebitis and Thrombophlebitis*
46 *Arterial Occlusion: Ischemia and Infarction Affecting Vascular Function*
47 *Vascular Structural Disorders*

Vivian C. Wolf-Wilets, R.N., Ph.D., F.A.A.N.
Professor
Department of Psychosocial Nursing
University of Washington
Seattle, Washington
Chapter *7* *Stress*

Preface

Two basic premises underlie the philosophy and framework of this text, *Medical–Surgical Nursing: Pathophysiological Concepts*. The first is a strong belief that current nursing practice must be built on application of the nursing process, with nursing diagnosis forming the cornerstone of independent nursing function. To this end, the discussion of nursing management throughout the text has been structured in such a way as to enhance assessment skills, the formulation of nursing diagnoses, the planning and implementation of nursing interventions, and the evaluation of patient outcome behaviors. Each of these steps of the nursing process is clearly delineated and identified for each of the major clinical conditions discussed.

The second premise assumes that effective and intelligent nursing care is built on a solid understanding of the pathological processes that underlie major health problems. The diverse human ailments to which we are susceptible do not occur in a mythical or magical fashion; they are, in fact, the result of pathophysiological mechanisms that disrupt homeostasis and alter normal body functions.

The text begins with an exploration of these two premises. The first unit presents our basic philosophical framework for nursing practice. In the second unit, broad nursing concepts are introduced, such as behavioral and emotional responses to illness, changes that occur with aging, and the impact of sleep deprivation and other factors on health status. Each chapter presents examples of these concepts as applied to clinical nursing practice. The third unit identifies and describes the major pathophysiological mechanisms underlying specific medical–surgical disorders. Among the pathophysiological mechanisms included are the inflammatory and immune responses, infection, disturbances in fluid–electrolyte and acid–base homeostasis, neoplastic and non-neoplastic cellular changes, ischemia and infarction, and shock. Principles upon which nursing interventions are based are presented in each of these chapters.

The pathophysiological concepts, along with associated nursing implications, serve as the unifying framework for the discussion of specific disorders that affect various body functions. Each of the remaining clinical units follows a consistent sequence of chapters, beginning with a brief review of anatomy and physiology, followed by a chapter on relevant assessment modalities. The third chapter of each unit examines the typical nursing problems or nursing diagnoses encountered in patients with disorders of the body function under discussion and provides general nursing strategies for dealing with these common problems. The remaining chapters in the unit discuss specific disorders according to the pathophysiological concepts explored in Unit III. Some disorders, such as arrhythmias, seizures, and diabetes mellitus, are handled as separate chapters because of the unique aspects of their underlying pathophysiology.

Each of the disorders discussed throughout the book is examined in a consistent manner. Information that serves as a knowledge base for nursing management consists of definition, classification, etiology, pathophysiology, clinical manifestations, and medical management (diagnosis, treatment, and prognosis). The discussion of nursing management includes assessment and nursing diagnosis, goals, interventions, and evaluation. The last unit contains nursing management for substance abuse and multiple trauma. Thus, this text moves from general philosophic and conceptual themes to increasingly specific content.

With the exception of an ethicist, the contributors to this book are nursing professionals with clinical and research expertise in the areas to which they contributed. They were selected as a reflection of our strong commitment to clinical nursing grounded in the nursing process.

This book can be used either as a textbook for nursing students or as a reference for practicing nurses. The principles of nursing management described are the bases of nursing care whether provided by the generalist or specialist.

In this book, the individual who seeks health care services is called a patient. This term is not intended to depict the person as being in a dependent relationship to the nurse; it merely refers to a recipient of nursing care. In the same vein, the pronoun *he* is used in the generic sense to mean both male and female and *she* is used to refer to nurses both male and female. The use of these pronouns in such contexts is for convenience to maintain the clarity and flow of the text.

Maxine L. Patrick, R.N., Dr. P.H.
Susan L. Woods, R.N., M.N
Ruth F. Craven, R.N., M.N., Ed.D.
Joanne Schnaidt Rokosky, R.N., M.N.
Pauline M. Bruno, R.N., D.N.Sc

Acknowledgments

A book of this magnitude cannot be produced without the contributions of a great many people. We are grateful for all the help we have received throughout this project. In particular, we wish to acknowledge the following:

The faculty, present and former, of the University of Washington School of Nursing, with whom we evolved the framework for teaching medical–surgical nursing upon which this book is based

Our sponsoring editor, Diana Intenzo, for her support, detailed guidance, and patience

Our typists, Beverly Ernst, Shirley Miller, Willow Wolfe, Joan Robinson, and others, for their long hours of typing and otherwise helping to prepare manuscripts

Our editorial consultants, Patricia Bliquez and Alison Ross, for their careful review of the manuscript

Marie Cowan, R.N., Ph.D., University of Washington School of Nursing, for contributing pathological slides from her private collection

Finally, and most importantly, we acknowledge the sustaining love and support of our families and friends and their willingness to share us with this project:

Edmund Bruno

Bill, Brent, Judy, and Kyle Craven

Signe and Deon Lambrecht

David and Juliana Rokosky

James, Jaime, and Jennifer Woods

Contents

UNIT VIII NURSING CARE OF PATIENTS WITH ALTERATIONS IN ENDOCRINE FUNCTION

UNIT IX NURSING CARE OF PATIENTS WITH ALTERATIONS IN GASTROINTESTINAL FUNCTION

UNIT XIII
NURSING MANAGEMENT OF PATIENTS IN SELECTED SITUATIONS

UNIT I

An Approach to the Nursing Process

Chapter 1

Components of Nursing Practice

Pamela H. Mitchell

I use the word nursing for want of a better. It has been limited to signify little more than the administration of medicines and the application of poultices. It ought to signify the proper use of fresh air, light, warmth, cleanliness, quiet and the proper selection and administration of diet—all at the least expense of vital power to the patient.

The same laws of health or of nursing, for they are in reality the same, obtain among the well as among the sick.

Florence Nightingale[10]

More than a century has passed since Florence Nightingale wrote these words as she described the new field of trained nursing. The components of nursing practice that she espoused sound quite contemporary: care of the ill, management of the environment to promote healing and to prevent illness, and promotion of health. The profession's goals remain much the same as they were at the inception of modern nursing. The means—the knowledge base and the environments of practice—have changed markedly. The purpose of this chapter is to provide an overview of the components of modern nursing practice (the goals, the means, and the environments) and to place these components of practice in the context of emerging nursing science—the knowledge base for achieving the goals and modifying the environments.

The Goals of Nursing

Definitions of Nursing

Even Nightingale had difficulty defining the term *nursing*. She used it as a verb (to nurse), "for want of a better." According to Webster's Third New International Dictionary, to nurse is "to nurture, to care for, to foster growth."* Professional definitions of nursing have extended the theme of nurturance and promotion of growth, and placed it in the context of health and illness. Among the varied definitions are those of Henderson, Orem, Rogers, and Roy.

Virginia Henderson. Virginia Henderson's definition of nursing is reflected in numerous definitions that followed her. She viewed nursing as "assisting the individual (sick or well) in the performance of those activities contributing to health, or its recovery (or a peaceful death) that he could perform unaided if he had the necessary strength, will or knowledge. And to do this in such a way to help him to gain independence as rapidly as possible."[6]

* By permission. From Webster's Third New International Dictionary © 1961 by G. & C. Merriam Company, publishers of the Merriam-Webster® Dictionaries.

Dorothea Orem. Dorothea Orem follows somewhat the same theme in her description of nursing as assistance of humans in providing and managing their self-care in order to "sustain life and health, recover from disease or injury and cope with their effects."[9]

Martha Rogers. In contrast, Martha Rogers saw nursing as encompassing the entirety of human existence. She views nursing primarily as a scientific endeavor describing and understanding the wholeness of humans in all aspects of their lives.[11] Nursing then is defined more by what it knows than by what it does, with a primary goal being the promotion of maximal functioning of unitary man. Her writings suggest that she believes the limiting of nursing concerns to health and illness is too narrow.

Sister Callista Roy. Sister Callista Roy also defined nursing in terms of its systematic knowledge. However, she believes that the major goal of the knowledge is that which facilitates the care of ill or potentially ill people. Nursing's major focus, in her view, is to promote adaptation (or a positive response to change) in four dimensions: physiology, self-concept, role function, and interdependence.[12]

Although these definitions are varied and tend to focus on different aspects of nursing's concern with the well-being of humans, there are common elements. These elements are

- Responses of humans to a variety of life situations (in both health and illness)
- Ability to care for oneself
- Supporting and facilitating persons to maintain and regain health

Many of these elements are reflected in the American Nurses' Association (ANA) definition of nursing: "the diagnosis and treatment of human responses to potential or actual health problems."[2] This definition was first proposed in 1976 by the New York Nurses' Association as it sought to update its nurse practice act. The definition incorporates contemporary thinking on the process of nursing (diagnosis and management) and the scope of practice (the response rather than the health problem itself). The supportive and facilitative roles of nursing, and the science underlying it are assumed as part of the skills involved in both diagnosis and management.

If understanding and treating responses to actual or potential problems of health and illness constitute the goals, or scope, of nursing practice, what are the broad categories of responses about which we are concerned? To best address this question, it is first necessary to examine what is meant by "health problem" and by "response."

Health, Illness, and Disease

Health problem as a concept cannot be readily understood without understanding the concepts of health, illness, and disease. The word *health* comes from the German language, and its early English derivations were the words "hale" and "whole." As scientific explanations began to gain prominence in Western civilization, understanding of disease predominated and health came to be viewed as primarily the absence of disease. Contemporary definitions of health, however, all emphasize optimal functioning of humans—psychologically, socially, and physically. Twentieth century conceptions of health place greater emphasis on the functioning of individuals and groups within their societies than on the presence or absence of disordered biological function alone.[3]

Although we tend to speak of disease and illness interchangeably in everyday conversation, there is a useful distinction between them. *Disease* is actually a biomedical concept and most often refers to pathology, disordered body structure, or a disordered biological state. Although we commonly think of illness as simply the reflection or consequence of disease, it is more useful to view it as a social and behavioral concept. In this view, *illness* is an impairment of role function, that is, the ability to fulfill one's functions in society.[5] Thus, illness becomes a broader concept than disease. Illness can be caused by a disease but can occur in the absence of pathology. For example, a person's injuries following an accident may have healed, but there may continue to be chronic pain that greatly impairs the person's ability to function. The person who is a paraplegic and fully independent is an example of a person with permanent pathological changes (and therefore disease) but no illness (*i.e.,* is able to carry on social functioning normally).

Since nursing's major focus is not on a person's disease or potential disease, but on the functioning of that person, the concept of illness is more central to nursing than is the concept of disease itself. Our concerns are with helping people avoid illness. Therefore, it is useful to view states of illness and health along two parallel continua. Any concept of health and illness that places these concepts at opposite ends of a pole has no place for the person who has a disease and yet is functioning quite well. Jahoda proposed a double continua for describing the function of individuals vis-à-vis both health and illness. One continuum goes from health to absence of health; the other continuum goes from illness to absence of illness.[7] Thus one could describe any individual's position along both continua. For example, the person who has just had a stroke has both disease and illness. However, as he goes through rehabilitation, he learns to compensate for the physical disabilities of functioning in his environment. Thus, he no longer has illness, although the disease (structural damage in the brain) remains.

A final element of the concept of health and illness is the environment in which we live. Halpert Dunn is credited with placing the notions of health, illness, and wellness within the context of the environment before fully describing the health status of an individual.[4] The environment can be thought of as not only the physical environment, but also the social environments of families, friends, and communities and the cultural environments of nations and races. Consider, for example, the person paralyzed from the waist down following an automobile accident. If this person is in a favorable environment, he will have access to rehabilitation facilities, have sufficient funds to pay for such services, have a supportive family, and live in a community that is accessible to persons in wheelchairs. This person would thus have a reasonably good chance of maintaining a high degree of wellness, even though he has permanent disease. Conversely, the person who is in a social and physical environment that cannot support the compensatory help he needs after such an injury may have lifelong illness and may even die from numerous long-term complications of the injury and the inability to support and maintain an independent life.

Health Problems

A health problem is anything that threatens or impairs the health of an individual, family, or group. Health problems may be diseases, such as coronary artery disease, or they may be conditions known to result in disease, such as polluted air or water. Since most definitions of health encompass both psychological and physical well-being, health problems can also arise from emotional and social states, for example, depression or inadequate financial resources. Thus, health problems can be viewed as disordered physiological, psychological, or social systems that cause or potentially cause disease, illness, or impaired well-being.

Human Response

In contrast, human responses are those physiological, psychological, or social alterations in everyday human functioning that occur because of, or secondary to, the actual or potential health problem, or that help maintain a health problem. An example of a response that occurs because of, or secondary to, a health problem is the diminished activity of a person with heart disease. The health problem, congestive heart failure, creates inefficient pumping of nutrients (oxygen and glucose) to the cells. As a result, the person experiences dyspnea (shortness of breath), diminished endurance, and perhaps edema of the extremities. The *response* to this pathophysiological state is diminished mobility and diminished activity because of the dyspnea and decreased endurance. Psychologically, the person may become depressed because of an inability to carry out usual activities; socially, that person may respond by becoming isolated from his social network.

A response that maintains a health problem can be shown in the example of the person who smokes cigarettes. Smoking and inhaling cigarettes is a potential *health problem* because it is a known risk factor for a number of diseases, such as coronary artery disease, lung cancer, and emphysema. The *behavior* of the person who either maintains or changes this risk factor (smoking or not smoking) is the human response with which nurses as well as other health workers deal. The behavior of continuing to smoke is an unhealthy response and may be due to (1) lack of knowledge of the health consequences, (2) addiction to nicotine, (3) reduction of stress response, (4) social peer pressure, or any combination of these. Thus, smoking as a risk factor for disease is the health problem; the treatable human response is the behavior of continuing or not continuing to smoke.

Types of Human Responses. Examination of the ANA Social Policy Statement and of the nursing diagnoses thus far developed by the North American Nursing Diagnosis Association suggests a typology or categorization of responses with which nurses are currently concerned. These are the following:

- Responses that promote positive health
- Responses that maintain health in the face of an unfavorable environment
- Responses that prevent illness
- Responses to existing illness (acute and chronic)
- Responses to terminal stages of illness

We must consider salient responses as occurring at three levels:

Individual
Family or other bonded group
Community or population

Table 1–1 gives examples of some of the kinds of responses that might occur in each category for each level of practice focus. In medical–surgical nursing, we work primarily with individuals and their responses, within the context of family and community. More and more, nurses working with persons who have chronic illness find that the whole family becomes the client. Nurses specializing in parent/child nursing and in community health nursing commonly have families, groups, and communities as their focus for practice.

The Environments of Nursing

Before Florence Nightingale, professional nursing did not exist. Thus the nurturing and supporting of those who were ill fell to women in the home and occurred in the home. In fact, it was not until the 20th century that significant numbers of persons began to be nursed in hospitals, in contrast to their homes. Even in the early part of this century, hospital nursing was carried out primarily by students with a cadre of graduate nurse supervisors. Most graduate nurses were employed by individual families as private duty nurses, caring for the ill in their own homes. The combination of the Great Depression and the inability of each hospital to maintain its own school of nursing in the late 1920s and 1930s served to bring graduate nurses to the hospital as their main employment setting. Today more than 60% of nurses work in hospitals or nursing homes.[1]

Today there are a number of societal and professional trends that are broadening the settings in which nursing is offered. Expanded roles for nurses include management of common and recurring disease problems (overlapping with the role of medicine) as well as the traditional nursing concern of coping with illness. Nurses practicing in expanded roles are often in outpatient clinics, nursing homes, and their community practices.

Community health nurses have traditionally worked with populations such as schoolchildren, the impoverished, or other groups with limited access to mainstream health care. Services to the homebound ill have traditionally been a small part of the practice of community health nursing. The increasing cost of hospitalization and of the technology attendant on institutional care has spurred a movement to-

TABLE 1–1
A Typology of Human Responses Relevant to Nursing from the Perspective of the Individual, Bonded Group, and Community or Population

Category of Response	*Examples of Responses*
Responses that promote positive health	*Individual* Choosing a regular exercise program Balancing work and play Seeking challenge in the environment *Family or Bonded Group* Communicating trust and love Interacting with the larger community Cohesively facing problems *Community or Population* Planning for meeting needs of the whole range of residents Promoting aesthetic features of the environment Providing adequate space
Responses that maintain health in the face of an unfavorable environment	*Individual* Learning to seek and use resources Avoidance of illness stimuli (*e.g.*, avoiding allergens) Gaining knowledge and skill in preparing nutritional meals at low cost *Family or Bonded Group* Learning to seek and use resources Recognizing and changing high-risk family behavior (*e.g.*, physical abuse, abuse of alcohol) *Community or Population* Conservation of scarce resources Public education regarding health risks
Responses that prevent illness	*Individual* Avoid smoking cigarettes Use safety devices in the workplace Manage stress response *Family or Bonded Group* Maintain immunizations Adhere to nutritious meal planning and family diet *Community or Population* Maintain facilities for treating water and sewage Financially support immunization programs
Responses to existing illness (acute and chronic)	*Individual* Decreased mobility Inability to maintain hygienic self-care Motivation to learn self-management of medical regimen *Family or Bonded Group* Social isolation Motivation to incorporate medical therapy regimen into household Potential for impaired parenting *Community or Population* Provision for home nursing services Presence or absence of financial aid for extraordinary expenses Presence or absence of agencies for specific illnesses
Responses to terminal stages of illness	*Individual* Fear of dying

(*Continued*)

TABLE 1–1
A Typology of Human Responses Relevant to Nursing from the Perspective of the Individual, Bonded Group, and Community or Population (*Continued*)

Category of Response	*Examples of Responses*
	Desire for choices regarding therapy Potential for pain
	Family or Bonded Group Anticipatory planning for reorganization of family roles Disintegration Grieving
	Community or Population Development of hospice services Bereavement counseling Presence or absence of home nursing services

ward the care of many more acutely ill persons in their own homes. Thus the settings and industry of home health care (or more accurately home illness care) are growing rapidly in the 1980s. It is likely that by the year 2000 we will find our practice settings having come full circle, with a large proportion of nursing provided in the setting of the home. However, in contrast to the early part of the century, the high technology of the modern hospital will also require highly skilled graduate nurses, sophisticated in both technological advances and in nurturing persons and families during acute illness and during acute crises of chronic illness. Thus medical–surgical nursing, in its focus on persons who have acute and chronic illness, will find the practice setting to be increasingly in the home as well as the acute care hospital.

The Means of Providing Nursing

Nursing is a service provided to both individuals and aggregates of people (*e.g.,* families, groups, populations). This service is provided both directly and indirectly. We are most familiar with the direct services, that is, the caring, comforting measures that help provide sleep, relieve pain, and reduce fear. We are also very familiar with the services that are interdependent with those of the physician, such as the administration of medical therapies and medicines and the skilled interpretation of a judgment, for example, when to give a medication. The means by which we decide if nursing is needed, what service to provide, and if the service helped is often called the nursing process. That process is described in Chap. 2.

The process of identifying and providing help is most often described and thought about in terms of individual nurses helping individual patients. However, we rarely actually provide nursing all alone to individuals outside the health care system. In reality, the means of providing nursing care derive from the skills of the individual nurses, the systems in which the care is provided, and the societal mandate for health care. These systems, which provide the context for nursing service, interact with the systems surrounding the recipient of care. The recipient may be an individual, whole family or other related group, or a community. Thus, the means of providing nursing may be influenced by the individuals being helped, by the organization that provides the care, or by the society that determines its policies and priorities regarding health.

Beginning practitioners in nursing can provide care to individuals or small groups, but they need to be cognizant of the larger systems that provide the context for the care provided. Experienced nurses who work with individuals may recognize the need to change political and care structures that impede care for individuals. Or the advanced practitioner may choose to work primarily at the system or large-group level. For example, the expert in nursing administration is working to enhance the institutional means by which nursing care is delivered. Nurses are only beginning to be highly visible at the level of influencing social policy regarding health.[8]

Throughout its history, nursing has been cognizant of the influence of the environment on the health of the recipients of nursing care. Florence Nightingale worked at both the individual and the societal level to change the environments of care to further human health. Modern practitioners of nursing will do well to recall her example of developing the profession of nursing at the individual, the group, and the societal levels.

References

1. Aiken L, Blendon R, Rogers D: The shortage of hospital nurses: A new perspective. Am J Nurs 81:1612–1618, 1981
2. American Nurses' Association: Nursing: A Social Policy Statement. Kansas City, American Nurses' Association, 1980
3. Bandman EL, Bandman B: Health and disease: A nursing perspective. In Caplan AL et al (eds): Concepts of Health and Disease: Interdisciplinary Perspectives, pp 677–692. Reading MA, Addison-Wesley, 1981
4. Dunn HL: High Level Wellness. Arlington VA. RW Beatty, 1961
5. Fabrega H: The scientific usefulness of the idea of illness. In Caplan AL et al (eds): Concepts of Health and Disease: Inter-

disciplinary Perspectives, Reading MA, pp 131–142. Addison-Wesley, 1981
6. Henderson V: The Nature of Nursing. New York, Macmillan, 1966
7. Jahoda M.: Current Concepts of Positive Mental Health. Joint Commission on Mental Health and Illness, Monograph Series, No 1. New York, Basic Books, 1958
8. Milio N: Nursing research and the study of health policy. Annual Review of Nursing Research 2:291–306,1984
9. Orem D: Nursing: Concepts of Practice, 2nd ed. New York, McGraw-Hill, 1966
10. Nightingale F: Notes on Nursing: What It Is and What It Is Not, 1860. Reprint. New York, Dover, 1969
11. Rogers M: The Theoretical Basis of Nursing. Philadelphia, FA Davis, 1970
12. Roy C: Introduction to Nursing: An Adaptation Model. Englewood Cliffs, NJ, Prentice-Hall, 1976

Bibliography

Chaska N: The Nursing Profession: A Time to Speak. New York, McGraw-Hill, 1983

Chinn P, Jacobs M: Theory and Nursing: A Systematic Approach. St Louis, CV Mosby, 1983

Fawcett J: Analysis and Evaluation of Conceptual Models of Nursing. Philadelphia, FA Davis, 1984

Sakalys J: The meaning of health and illness. In Mitchell P, Loustau A (eds): Concepts Basic to Nursing, 3rd ed, pp 3–22. New York, McGraw-Hill 1981

Chapter 2

Nursing Process

Pamela H. Mitchell

Observation tells us the fact, reflection tells us the meaning of the fact . . . reflection tells us what is to be done.

Florence Nightingale[9]

Nursing process is a shorthand term used to convey a *systematic* process of recognizing and acting on those human needs with which nurses can help. Or, in Nightingale's words, observing, interpreting, and acting on the facts.

All helping professions use this systematic process, which consists of the following steps:

Recognizing that a need for help exists	ASSESSMENT
Determining/naming the nature of the need	DIAGNOSIS
Considering how to help	PLANNING
Helping	INTERVENTION
Determining if helping has occurred	EVALUATION

The *nature of the problems* recognized, the *kind of help* provided, the *outcomes* expected, and the *criteria* by which the outcomes are evaluated vary among the helping professions. Thus these aspects constitute the *content,* or knowledge base, that underlies the *process.*

The purpose of this chapter is to provide an overview of that process within the context of the knowledge base of nursing. It is that knowledge base that distinguishes nursing from other helping disciplines. The focus of this book is on care of adults who have medical–surgical illnesses.

Components of the Nursing Process

The helping process in nursing is distinguishable from that of other disciplines by the nature of its diagnoses and therapeutics. In other words, the difference is in what the problems are called and what the nurse does about them.

The Nature of Nursing Diagnosis

Nursing diagnosis focuses on people's *responses* to the problems of health and illness.[1] In contrast, the profession of medicine focuses on the health problem itself, that is, the disease or pathology and its prevention. In making nursing diagnoses for persons with medical and surgical illnesses, the primary focus of nursing is on the person's *responses* to that state (*e.g.,* illness or potential illness).

For example, the person with congestive heart failure (CHF) has a *health problem,* arteriosclerotic heart disease, with a particular *pathophysiological state,* decreased cardiac output due to either right or left heart failure. The effect on daily living, or generalized *human response* to that health

TABLE 2–1
Contrast Between Health Problems and Human Response

Health Problem	*Human Responses*
Congestive heart failure	Decreased mobility related to decreased endurance Decreased mobility related to painful pitting edema of feet
Diabetes mellitus	High or low motivation to incorporate treatment regimen into daily acitivites Potential for alteration in sexuality Potential for injury related to delayed healing
Elective surgery	Anxiety Fear of pain Decreased mobility with risk for immobility complications
Right brain cerebrovascular accident (stroke)	Alteration in spatial orientation Decreased communication of affect Potential decreased mobility of left extremities

problem, may be decreased endurance, decreased mobility, and dependence on others for usual tasks of daily living. The medical diagnosis and plan of care for this person will be stated in terms of heart failure and treatment of the pathophysiological state. The nursing diagnosis and plan of care will be stated in terms of the effects of daily living and the means to compensate for those effects. Table 2–1 shows examples of the contrasts between the statement of the health problem and statements of responses to those problems.

The Nature of Nursing Management

Management in any helping profession is the plan of care determined to be of help in a given problem. Therapeutics are the specific activities prescribed and intended to be of help. *Medical therapeutics* are intended to alter or relieve the disease process or pathophysiological state. For example, the medication digitalis may be given to enhance the working of the failing heart muscle. Primary *nursing therapeutics* are intended to alter the person's responses to the pathology. For example, the nurse may recommend the use of a shower stool to reduce fatigue (response to the increased energy demand on the failing heart).

In the preceding example, it is obvious that there is potential for considerable overlap and blurring of boundaries between the therapeutics of medicine and nursing. The same is true between nursing and social work, occupational therapy, and a variety of other health professions. it is useful to consider the distinctions between *independent, interdependent,* and *coordinative* types of management to better understand how to distinguish those therapeutics that nurses are legally and professionally accountable for prescribing independently from those that nurses are legally and professionally accountable for implementing.

Independent Management

Independent acts are those that the nurse may initiate without consultation or prescription by other professionals. The nurse practice acts of most states and the current definition of nursing explicitly provide that nurses may diagnose and treat human responses to states of health and illness. Thus we may infer that nurses may independently recommend, prescribe, and perform those activities that affect the human response. Those areas of human response most commonly addressed in the literature on nursing therapeutics are sleep, elimination, sexuality, nutrition, comfort, mobility, self-care, orientation to health, affiliative relationships, growth and development, parenting, skin integrity, grieving, ventilation, circulation, self-concept, cognition, spirituality, health maintenance, activity, communication, and coping.[1,7,10]

Interdependent Management

Interdependent management is defined as those actions that are performed by a nurse but also require reciprocal dependence on another profession for prescription, protocol, or validation of the judgments made.[8] Some authors separate this category into interdependent (actions requiring some nursing judgments, such as prn orders) and dependent (those actions performed by the nurse but that do not allow nursing discretion).[11,13] Only the term *interdependent* will be used in this chapter because I believe that there is reciprocal dependence whenever one professional executes an act for another. This reciprocal dependence is manifested in judgments about when, whether, and how to carry out the therapeutic act.

In persons with medical and surgical diseases, it is self-evident that some portion of their health care is provided by physicians, and is directed toward treatment of the disease or pathophysiological state. Traditionally and historically, a considerable portion of nursing activity and education has been devoted to competently implementing and supporting the medical therapeutic plans. The activities of supporting, monitoring, and implementing the medical plan of care is an example of interdependent management or, in other words, of the cooperation and interdependence of two or more disciplines in the therapy of the patient. Particularly in hospitals and other institutions, the intelligent implementation of medical therapeutics is quite dependent on nursing staff. Other examples of interdependent therapeutics are those of occupational therapy and nursing in helping a disabled patient learn to dress, or the interdependent activities of respiratory therapy, medicine, and nursing in ventilation of the patient with chronic obstructive pulmonary disease.

It is important to recognize interdependent aspects of management for two reasons. First, adequate care of acutely and chronically ill persons requires that nurses be competent in implementing the delegated therapies of other professions, predominantly medicine. Second, appropriate referral of patient problems to other professions requires that the nurse who cares for persons with medical-surgical illnesses needs to know a great deal about the basis for medical therapies as well as nursing therapies.

Coordinative Management

Modern health care exposes the patient to a vast array of specialists, all intent upon helping with one specific aspect of that person's illness. The nurse is frequently the only professional who is in a position to appreciate the total impact of these disparate activities on the patient. Coordination of multiple diagnostic and treatment activities to preserve the patient's energy resources and to prevent conflicting demands is frequently an assumed but unaddressed area of nursing responsibility.

The professional nurse is also responsible for coordinating the activities of multiple levels of nursing personnel to carry out the nursing care plan for a given individual. For example, in hospitals, the professional nurse is responsible for diagnosis and management of the patient's response to his illness, but the nursing therapeutic activities may actually be carried out by nursing technicians and assistants. In home health care agencies, the professional nurse is responsible for devising the nursing care plan and subsequently coordinating its implementation by home health aides. In addition, the nurse will be coordinating the nursing plan with the plans of other professionals such as physical therapists.

The Process of Nursing

The nursing process is fundamentally both a humanistic and an intellectual activity, in which the nurse consciously or unconsciously gathers information from a variety of sources and tests it against personal and professional knowledge in an attempt to make sense of encounters with people who are in states of health and illness. Describing the process makes a complex, rather fluid process look quite orderly and linear (step by step, in one direction). Although nurses tend to carry out the process in a synthetic manner, it is possible to break it down into four steps to analyze the information stores or knowledge base necessary to do a good job of nursing acutely and chronically ill persons.

Most authors analyze or describe the nursing process in four stages:

1. Assessment/diagnosis
2. Planning
3. Intervention
4. Evaluation

Assessment/diagnosis may be described as the *diagnostic phase;* planning, intervention, and evaluation constitute the *management phases.*

Diagnostic Phase

Assessment/Diagnosis

Assessment is the act of gathering and analyzing information. Assessment implies more than just the collection of data; it includes determining the *meaning* of those data (Fig. 2–1). In the context of health care, determining the nature of the problem is the making of a diagnosis. In nursing, that diagnosis is a statement of a human response to a state of health. In general, such statements indicate a problematic human response that requires nursing help.

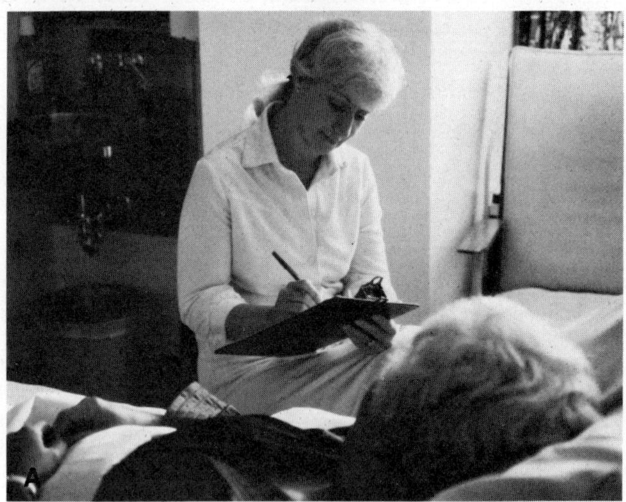

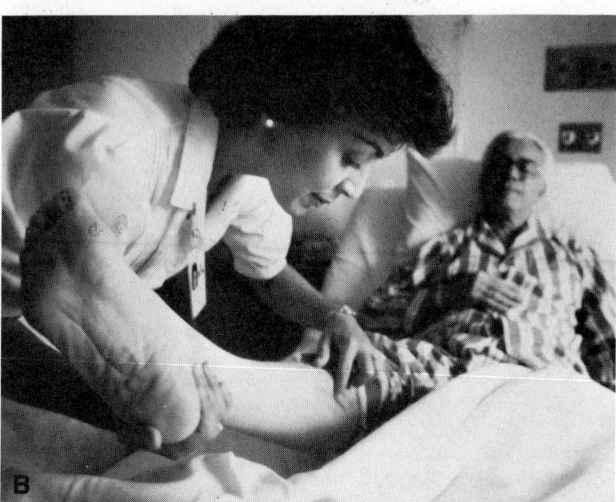

FIGURE 2–1 Assessment includes the gathering and analysis of data, both during the nursing history (*A*) and the delivery of care (*B*).

There are several components to assessment:

1. Gathering of relevant data
2. Forming hypotheses about the meaning of the data
3. Naming the conclusions

In more formal terms, one moves from

Data ⟶ Hypothesis ⟶ Diagnosis

Data Collection. Since we are interested in the ways that humans function and respond in states of health and actual or potential illness, then data should be collected about the following:

Health status	Wellness Factors maintaining wellness Illness Risk factors for illness
Responses to health status	Perceptions of health status Patterns of coping
Functional status	Current state of functioning in areas of daily living

There are a large number of assessment guides published that address these general areas of data. Table 2–2 compares the major categories used in several of these guides. Note that none of these guides uses the typical medical organization of data by organ system (cardiovascular, gastrointestinal, *etc.*). Rather, relevant data about functioning of such systems is incorporated into the appropriate functional area. For example, data about functioning of the gastrointestinal system is part of the functional area of elimination and nutrition.

The establishment of a comprehensive data base will provide information about

TABLE 2–2
Comparison of Assessment Categories by Various Authors*

Carnevali[†]	*Gordon*[‡]	*Mitchell and Loustau*[§]	*Roy*[‖]	*Yura and Walsh*[**]
Conceptual orientation				
Interrelationship between daily living and health status	Biophysical patterns of human functioning in relation to health	Coping with daily living in relation to actual/potential health problems	Modes of adaptation to stressors in the client–environment interaction	Preservation, fostering, maintenance and facilitation of integrity of the human needs of the person
Assessment categories				
Activities and patterns of daily living Demands of daily living Internal resources Breathing Circulation Cognition/emotions Elimination Mobility Nutrition Sensory abilities Sexuality Sleep External resources Personal network Housing/neighborhood Transportation/communication Needed/useable resources Health and lifestyle goals	Health perception–health management pattern Nutritional–metabolic pattern Elimination pattern Activity–exercise pattern Cognitive–perceptual pattern Sleep–rest pattern Self-perception–self-concept pattern Role-relationship pattern Sexuality–reproductive pattern Coping–stress tolerance pattern Value–belief pattern	Psychosocial status Mental and emotional status Environmental status Sensory status Motor status Nutritional status Fluid and electrolyte status Circulatory status Respiratory status Temperature status Integumentary status Comfort and rest status Sexuality status	Physiologic mode Exercise/rest Nutrition Elimination Fluid and electrolytes Oxygen and circulation Temperature regulation Regulation of senses Endocrine regulation Self-concept mode Physical self Personal self Role-Function mode Interdependence mode	Human needs of the person Acceptance of self Activity Adaptation Air Appreciation Autonomy >35 individual needs Human need for family and community Survival needs (15 needs) Closeness needs (10 needs) Freedom needs (10 needs) (*Note:* The extensive list of needs in this framework includes many areas listed in the other assessment categories in this table.)

* This comparison is representative of those found in current textbooks related to the nursing process. Data regarding aspects of health status and responses to health status and functional status are collected in each of these guides, but each is organized somewhat differently.

† Carnevali D: Nursing Care Planning: Diagnosis and Management, 3rd ed, p 114. Philadelphia, JB Lippincott, 1983

‡ Gordon M: Nursing Diagnosis: Process and Application, p 81. New York, McGraw-Hill, 1982

§ Mitchell PH, Loustau A: Concepts Basic to Nursing, 3rd ed, pp 124–130. New York, McGraw-Hill, 1981

‖ Roy C, Robert SL: Theory Construction in Nursing: An Adaptation Model. Englewood Cliffs NJ, Prentice-Hall, 1981

** Yura H, Walsh MB: The Nursing Process, 4th ed, pp 136–137. Norwalk CT, Appleton-Century-Crofts, 1983

- Risk factors for future illnesses
- Strength factors that maintain maximum wellness
- Problems that the patient may not have recognized

Thus there are two aspects to the data collection phase of diagnosis: *problem solving* and *problem seeking*. Problem-solving data are the facts collected about the primary reason the person is seeking the help of professionals, which in health care jargon is termed *presenting problem*. Appropriate information about the problem includes

- Description of the problem (patient's description)
- Duration and onset
- Precipitating exacerbating, and ameliorating factors
- What the patient thinks is happening

When the patient has fully described what he perceives as the primary problem, the nurse inquires whether there are any additional problems. When this has been completed, the nurse then does a review of functions and a history of health status and responses to health status to identify any additional actual or potential problems.

Analysis. The collection of data, however, in no way completes the process of assessment. As Nightingale noted, observation or data collection only tells us the facts. It is analysis or reflection that tells us what they mean. Studies of the reasoning processes of people solving problems in a variety of professions demonstrate that people are analyzing information even as they are collecting it. Hypotheses or "hunches" about the nature of a problem are formed very early. The more experienced the diagnostician, the earlier hypotheses are formed and confirmed by collecting additional data. Experienced clinicians quickly generate hypotheses about the problem and then focus further data collection on getting information that either confirms or refutes a particular hunch. Since all this is operating in short-term memory, which can only hold a small number of "chunks" of information, people generally have only three to five "working diagnoses" at a time.[3]

To take an example, suppose the nurse enters a patient's room and finds that the patient has hardly touched her lunchtime tray of food. She says she has no appetite. To determine if this lack of appetite represents a problem, the nurse will need to get some more information. This search for information is guided by her knowledge of a number of possible causes of loss of appetite, and her knowledge of problematic consequences of loss of appetite for overall nutritional status.

Any number of clinical problems can create a loss of appetite. These problems include loss of taste, depression, therapy that affects taste or appetite (*e.g.,* chemotherapy), nonspecific response to illness, and diseases such as hepatitis and cancer. In addition, a number of context-bound circumstances may cause loss of appetite, for example, food that is foreign to one's usual tastes, unattractively prepared food, or food served in a situation that reminds one of unpleasant circumstances.

In order to narrow all these possibilities to a manageable few, the nurse begins to ask a few questions that help guide the search for problem and cause. The most likely first question is whether this loss of appetite is new or part of an ongoing situation. It it is a constant state of affairs, it may be related to the patient's disease or clinical problem, or its therapy. Such a finding would suggest nursing diagnoses in the area of living with medical regimens. If this is a new problem, the nurse would want to determine if it is likely to persist (in which case it will need managing) or if it is likely to be transient (in which case the appropriate action would be monitoring it).

If loss of appetite is an old problem, the nurse would look beyond appetite to determine if a nutritional problem exists: are there physical-examination history and laboratory evidence of poor nutrition? Then, depending on the permanence or progression of the primary cause of poor appetite, the nurse might focus on symptom management (helping the person improve appetite or take advantage of what appetite remains to maintain or improve nutrition).

If it is a new problem and appears transient, the nurse might simply monitor intake for a period of time and discontinue concern if appetite and nutritional status remain normal. If monitoring indicates that the problem persists, the nurse would then try to find a cause and work to remedy that.

Even though the nurse has information about only one area of functioning, she has several possible causes in mind for this person's problem. If the nurse is an efficient diagnostician, she will pursue this area of nutrition before entering any others. Why, then, does she collect all that other data which appears on various data collection guides? There are two reasons to collect comprehensive data. First, there may be clues in other categories of function that help the nurse decide the etiology or source of the primary problem. For example, loss of appetite can be caused by depression, but if the nurse asks only about nutrition and eating *per se,* this important information about mood will be missed. Second, the comprehensive data base alerts the nurse to potential problems or existing problems of which the patient may not be aware.

Problem Statements and Diagnoses

The culmination of the assessment phase is the *naming* of the conclusion reached, that is, a statement of either one or more problems or diagnoses. A problem is anything that bothers the patient or any deviation from "normal" functioning that commands the attention of attending health professionals.[12] A problem within the scope of nursing practice would be a patient's response to a state of health or illness. A diagnosis is a problem plus its cause. Therefore, a nursing diagnosis is ***a response to a health or illness situation for which the patient needs help and which is within the legal scope of the nursing practice.*** This presumes that etiology is known and that independently prescribed nursing action can change the clinical state.

Carpenito makes a useful differentiation between nursing diagnoses and clinical problems. She defines clinical problems as those arising from the interdependent dimension of nursing and which nurses collaborate with physicians (or other health professionals) to treat.[4] For example, hypoglycemia is a clinical problem that may occur in relation to the medical diagnosis diabetes melitus. Although nurses may use considerable judgment in recognizing and teaching the patient to detect or prevent hypoglycemia, the management of this pathophysiological state is interdependent with the physician. However, suppose there is a person who has frequent hypoglycemia, and that this person is a teenager who neglects to monitor her diabetes and take insulin regularly. After some astute interviewing by the nurse it becomes evident that this girl is afraid of "being different" and thus does not follow her recommended regimen. A nursing diagnosis can be made: "Nonadherence to diabetic therapy related to fear of social ostracism." The problem, frequent hypoglycemic episodes, has been found to have a cause (etiology) that is within the independent range of nursing action. Thus it can be stated as a nursing diagnosis. Nursing management would then be devised to help the girl incorporate the regimen into her lifestyle as unobtrusively as possible, and to foster her self-esteem.

The terms *problem* and *diagnosis* tend to be used interchangeably in many clinical settings. Strictly speaking, they are not synonymous, since a diagnosis requires knowledge of etiology. However, the large area of interdependent practice between medical and nursing care of persons with acute illnesses makes the use of the term *problem* a pragmatic means to communicate among disciplines. In the problem-oriented recording system introduced by Weed, a problem may be anything that bothers the patient, a diagnosis, or a clinical state that needs to be followed.[12]

In this book, the term nursing diagnosis/problem is consistently used in nursing strategies and nursing care plans to name and describe the clinical phenomena addressed. A number of the problems are nursing diagnoses in the currently accepted definition (independently treated by nurses). Others are clinical problems as defined by Carpenito (problems stemming from the medical diagnosis and that require collaborative or interdependent treatment by nurse and physician).

Making Problem Statements

Currently, most authorities recommend a two-part statement: a problem and its etiology or contributing factors—for example, "Social isolation related to shame about appearance." Many authors also recommend a statement of defining signs and symptons as part of the statement. This "PES" form was introduced by Gordon.[5] The initials stand for *P*roblem; *E*tiology; *S*igns. A problem for which the cause is unknown would not have a statement of etiology, but would have a statement of manifestation in either format.

Both two-part and three-part statements are used as examples of care plans in this book. The National Conferences for the Classification of Nursing Diagnoses recommend the use of the term "related to" to link the problem and etiology statements, and this form is used in many areas. However, particularly in the western United States, a number of agencies and clinicians use the terms "secondary to" or "due to" when specifying etiology.

Examples of three-part problem statements used in this book follow. PES segments are set off from each other by brackets [ ] for illustrative purposes.

> [Potential impairment of skin integrity] [related to reduced blood flow associated with arterial occlusive disease] [and manifested by pallor on elevation of limbs and slow capillary refilling.]

> [Impaired gas exchange] [related to ventilation-perfusion mismatch associated with pulmonary embolism] [as may be evidenced by tachypnea, dyspnea, tachycardia, abnormal arterial blood gases, altered level of consciousness, anxiety, and cyanosis.]

Examples of two-part statements used in this book include

> [Ineffective airway clearance] [related to excessive or dried bracheobronchial secretions.]

> [Disturbances in self-concept] [related to loss of normal voice and facial disfigurement.]

Using Nursing Diagnoses in Medical–Surgical Settings

The movement to identify and classify nursing diagnoses is only about 10 or 12 years old at this writing. It is of tremendous importance in clarifying and codifying the scope of nursing practice, and differentiating nursing practice from that of other professions. The work is far from complete, however, and practicing nurses cannot wait for the complete and official list before naming the conclusions from their assessments. Therefore, we recommend that practicing nurses and nursing students use both nursing diagnoses and statements of clinical problems in their ongoing nursing care plans. Ideally, clinical problems should be identified as such and not be rewritten as nursing diagnoses simply because nurses participate in the treatment. A great deal of nursing practice in the medical–surgical setting is involved with skillful judgment about clinical problems. This mixture of knowledge and skill in both clinical problems and nursing diagnosis is evident throughout the chapters of this book.

Currently there are about 50 diagnostic categories with their defining characteristics accepted by the North American Nursing Diagnosis Association (NANDA). These categories are listed in Table 2–3, and the complete list of defining characteristics can be found in the proceedings of the Fifth National Conference.[7] In many institutions these categories are expected to be used by professional nurses; indeed, all assessments are expected to result in one or more categories from this list. Since this list is incomplete, it is unlikely that all clinical judgments will be found in it, unless one forces data into inappropriate categories. Therefore, we recommend that practitioners create their own statements of problem when those in the accepted list are clearly not applicable. Further, nurses should recognize that these are labels for *categories* of diagnosis, not for the complete individualized conclusion for a specific patient.

The following guidelines, adapted from Carpenito[4] and Guzzetta and Dossey,[6] are offered to help practitioners make diagnostic statements that are individualized for a specific client, and to help create a problem statement when none of the currently categorized ones fit.

- The problem statement should consist of a human response, in any of three realms: psychological, phys-

TABLE 2–3
Nursing Diagnoses Currently Approved by the North American Nursing Diagnosis Association*

Activity intolerance	Mobility, impaired physical
Activity intolerance, potential	Noncompliance (specify)
Airway clearance, ineffective	Nutrition, alteration in: less than body requirements
Anxiety	Nutrition, alteration in: more than body requirements
Bowel elimination, alteration in: constipation	Nutrition, alteration in: potential for more than body requirements
Bowel elimination, alteration in: diarrhea	Oral mucous membrane, alteration in
Bowel elimination, alteration in: incontinence	Parenting, alteration in: actual
Breathing pattern, ineffective	Parenting, alteration in: potential
Cardiac output, alteration in: decreased	Powerlessness
Comfort, alteration in: pain	Rape trauma syndrome
Communication, impaired: verbal	Self-care deficit: feeding, bathing/hygiene, dressing/ grooming, toileting
Coping, family: potential for growth	Self-concept, disturbance in: body image, self-esteem, role performance, personal identity
Coping, ineffective family: compromised	Sensory–perceptual alteration: visual, auditory, kinesthetic, gustatory, tactile olfactory
Coping, ineffective family: disabling	Sexual dysfunction
Coping, ineffective individual	Skin integrity, impairment of: actual
Diversional activity, deficit	Skin integrity, impairment of: potential
Family process, alteration in (formerly Family dynamics)	Sleep pattern disturbance
Fear	Social isolation
Fluid volume alteration in: excess	Spiritual distress (distress of the human spirit)
Fluid volume deficit, actual	Thought processes, alteration in
Fluid volume deficit, potential	Tissue perfusion, alteration in: cerebral, cardiopulmonary, renal, gastrointestinal, peripheral
Gas exchange, impaired	Urinary elimination, alteration in patterns
Grieving, anticipatory	Violence, potential for: self-directed or directed at others
Grieving, dysfunctional	
Health maintenance, alteration in	
Home maintenance management, impaired	
Injury, potential for: (Poisoning, potential for; Suffocation, potential for; Trauma, potential for)	
Knowledge deficit (specify)	

* Kim MJ et al: Classification of Nursing Diagnoses: Proceedings of the Fifth National Conference, pp 470–471. St. Louis, CV Mosby, 1984

iological, and social. These are not simply restatements of medical diagnoses or pathophysiological states.

- The problem statement is usually a two-part statement consisting of
  Problem
  Etiology or contributing factors
- or it may be a three-part statement consisting of
  Problem
  Etiology or contributing factors
  Signs and symptoms
- Problem and etiologic or symptom components are not circular, for example, anxiety related to fear of the unknown is a clearly circular statement since the second part of the statement is the definition of the first. Anxiety related to anticipation of surgery is a better statement.
- Unrelated problems should not be grouped in one statement even though they have the same etiology. For example, both decreased endurance engendered by coronary heart disease. However, each problem (decreased mobility and fear of job loss) will be managed by a different activity and therefore should be stated separately.
- Cue and symptoms (defining characteristics) are not substituted for a diagnosis. For example, excessive crying related to fear of death is not a diagnosis. Fear of death is the etiology, crying is the manifestation. Without further information we cannot tell if the diagnosis is ineffective coping, anticipatory grieving, anxiety, dysfunctional grieving, powerlessness, or spiritual distress.

Carpenito provides criteria against which to measure nursing diagnostic statements:[4]

- Is the statement a synthesis of clinical data?
- Is the problem identified within the legal and educational scope of nursing?
- Is the implied treatment within the legal and educational scope of nursing?

Any written care plan for a person with a medical or surgical illness is likely to have a combination of clinical problems for which the nurse is using judgment in implementing medical therapy, and nursing diagnoses for which the nurse is primarily responsible.

The Process of Management

The logical extension of assessment/diagnosis is management of the identified problems. In current practice, nurses are involved in management of both interdependent aspects of the medical plan (clinical problems) and nursing therapy related to the nursing diagnoses. Thus the nursing care plan represents an amalgamation of independent and interdependent activities. A recording form that incorporates the nursing data base, allows for recording of clinical problems and nursing diagnoses, and provides for ready identification of both independent and interdependent management plans is shown in Figure 2–2.

Helping patients to manage their problems of health and illness involves a series of processes, just as does the diagnosis of these problems. Once the problems or diagnoses have been identified, one needs to develop a plan for each problem, carry it out, and evaluate the results. This process of determining what seems most likely to help a given individual is called *care planning*. The carrying out of the plan is *implementation* and the determination of the match between desired and actual outcomes is termed *evaluation*. The nursing care plan (see Fig. 2–2) is a written account of that plan.

Care Planning

The plan for each problem takes the form of determining

Goals
Appropriate Strategies
Outcome

If there are multiple diagnoses and problems, one also needs to determine the priority for approaching each problem.

Goals are the objectives or hoped-for end points of the helping process. Many care planning schemes indicate both nursing goals (process behaviors of the nurse) and patient goals (expected clinical outcomes in terms of patient behavior, signs, and symptoms). The goals form the basis for evaluation of the care plan and are therefore *process criteria* and *outcome criteria*.[4] In this book, goals are frequently specified as both nursing process criteria and patient outcome criteria. For example, the standard care plan given for patients with peripheral vascular disease indicates the goal as follows:

> To prevent imbalance of tissue oxygen supply and demand as evidenced by absence of signs of ischemia and infarction.

The first part of the goal statement indicates the nursing process behavior (actions to prevent a problem); the second part indicates the outcome criteria in terms of what one would see in the patient (absence of signs and symptoms of ischemia/infarction). In contrast, the patient care-planning form in Figure 2–2 indicates only patient outcome criteria. Both forms of goal statements are currently used throughout North America.

Student Care Plan vs. Practitioner Care Plan. Care plans used in institutions are usually more condensed than those that students of nursing are expected to prepare. The use of nursing process goals as well as patient outcome goals is more common in student care plans than in practitioner plans, although they are by no means found exclusively in student plans. The most common difference between practitioner and student plans is the column labeled *rationale*. In this book most of the plans have a space for indicating the rationale for action. Such a column is rarely found in individualized plans in practice, although it is common in standardized plans. The documentation of one's rationale in planning a given action is a quite useful teaching device, and it also helps other nurses know what the primary nurse had in mind. However, with limited space for recording, most institutions have omitted that section, assuming that with most common actions, the rationale is understood by most practitioners.

Standard Care Plans. Standard care plans provide a measure of consistency and a memory guide for common and recurring problems associated with a given clinical state (*e.g.*, a particular surgery or disease). Because patients in hospitals are often grouped on a unit or otherwise identified by their medical diagnosis, such plans are usually categorized by medical diagnosis or procedure. For example, there may be standard plans for the patient with myocardial infarction and the patient with laminectomy. This type of standard care plan is indispensable in orienting the novice nurse and in providing direction for technical nursing care.

Individualized plans are those devised by the professional nurse for the range of client problems that fall outside the usual ones for any patient in a given situation. These plans rest more heavily on individually identified nursing diagnoses that are derived from the interaction of factors unique to the individual with those common to a given health problem. Any institution that uses standard care plans needs to be certain that there is space and encouragement for recording of the individualized care plan identified by the professional nurses.

Implementation

Implementation refers to the actual carrying out of the plan, with continual monitoring of the expected effects vis-à-vis what one sees happening at the moment. Cognitively, the nurse identifies from knowledge and experience those actions known or expected to affect the diagnoses in one or more ways:

Monitoring for change
Stabilizing a fluctuating situation
Promoting positive change
Maintaining a desired state

From interviews and questionnaires with over 1000 nurses, Benner identified seven major areas of nursing intervention used by nurses working in hospitals:[2]

Helping role
Teaching–coaching
Diagnostic and patient monitoring
Management of rapidly changing situations
Administering and monitoring therapeutic regimens
Monitoring and ensuring quality of health care practices
Organizational and work role competencies

From this list of domains of intervention, it is clear that modern nursing practice uses a variety of strategies to help people with their health and illness problems. It is also clear that strategies involved in managing clinical problems cannot be separated from the more independent strategies involved in treating the nursing diagnoses. The categories of managing rapidly changing situations and administering therapeutic regimens are clearly interdependent with the interventions of medicine. The helper role and the teaching–coaching actions of nurses are often quite independent.

This repertoire of actions, interventions, and strategies is what the nurse calls upon in planning care for given problems, and what is called on again as the patient situation changes while implementing the plan. Implementation is always a dynamic process, involving matching what one sees in the patient situation to what one expected to happen. The experienced nurse is able to improvise on the spot and change approaches when it is evident that things are not working out; the novice may need to get help.[2]

Evaluation

Comparing the actual outcomes to those expected (the outcome criteria on the care plan) constitutes the activity called *evaluation.* In more concrete terms, did things work out as you had hoped? If not, why not? Can it be corrected now? Sometimes what one learns from the evaluation phase can be used immediately to remedy or change an approach; other times it will help the nurse expand the repertoire of nursing actions for future patients with similar problems. The following example illustrates several aspects of evaluation.

> Mrs. A. is admitted to a neurosurgical unit for a craniotomy to remove a tumor that has affected her balance, coordination, hearing, and facial expression. In her admitting interview she has acknowledged being "scared to death," and her behavioral and verbal expressions of fear of surgery have been commented on by all who have met her. The admitting nurse makes a nursing diagnosis of "Extreme anxiety related to fear of impending surgery" and plans to reduce the manifestations of anxiety (goal and outcome criteria) through preoperative teaching about what to expect in the perioperative period (action). She also intends to reduce the incidence of postoperative complications through the preoperative teaching. Her rationale is that a number of studies have shown an overall reduction in complications and anxiety and more rapid recovery through structured preoperative teaching.
>
> During the course of describing the operating room, the preanesthetic medication, and the postoperative breathing and leg exercises, the nurse notices that Mrs. A. is becoming more and more restless, is breathing rapidly, and is looking quite fearful. At this point the nurse realizes that the patient's behavior does not match the expected outcome at all. In fact she seems to be becoming increasingly *more anxious.* She then says, "Mrs. A., you seem to be more uncomfortable than when we started talking. Tell me about what is happening to you now." Mrs. A. can not clearly identify why she is feeling even more fearful, but acknowledges that she certainly is. Finally, she says that she has always dealt with fearful events by trying hard not to think of them, and that all this detail is scaring her even more. The nurse then asks what has helped Mrs. A. get through scary times, and finds that a certainly of human presence and feeling secure in the skills of her doctor are the most helpful things. At this point, the nurse changes her approach and tells Mrs. A. who will be with her, promises to stay with her during the premedication, and arranges for Mrs. A. to meet the nurse who will be in the operating room. When all this has occurred, Mrs. A., although she is still tense, looks more relaxed and says she feels better about tomorrow.

The nurse in this example learned two important things in the process of evaluation. First, she recognized that Mrs. A. was not responding as expected to the standard preoperative nursing intervention. She was able to adapt her approach because she gathered more data and found that Mrs. A.'s personal coping style was such that the standard approach was almost guaranteed to increase rather than decrease her anxiety. The nurse realized that she had developed an ineffective plan because she had not gained enough information during the assessment phase to recognize that Mrs. A. would need a different approach. Thus, the second thing she learned was the need to identify how people usually cope with new situations in order to create individualized plans for her future preoperative patients.

This example demonstrates the dynamic nature of the care-planning process. Evaluation indicated that the approach was not working; on-the-spot data collection was instituted and a new action was generated. The reduction in the patient's anxiety behavior was taken as further evaluation. This example further illustrates what problems can arise in applying standard care plans or approaches to all patients in a class (preop patients, for example) when sufficient assessment data has not been gathered to know if the approach fits that individual.

Relationship of Nursing Process to Standards of Care

The foregoing example notwithstanding, there is a place for generalizations and standards in medical-surgical nursing. Standard care plans have been alluded to earlier. They are generalized care plans that may be applicable to most persons with a particular category of illness, under a specific medical therapeutic procedure, or at a known stage of development. They are a useful educational tool because they provide good cues to the novice about assessment criteria, common strategies, and expected outcomes. Further, their use in recording saves much repetitive writing and may allow more time for the documentation of individualized problems and plans. Their greatest danger is the stereotyping of action, as in example above, or their substitution for thinking about the needs of an individual.

Standards of care is a general term referring to a wide variety of tools developed for assuring the quality of nursing care. In general, standards refer to those approaches to care

(Text continues on page 20)

NURSING ADMISSION DATA

Patient arrived via: Amb. WC Cart

From: Home ER ECF Other

Accompanied by:

Information obtained from: (Relationship to patient)

TPR	BP	WT.	HT.

Allergies: (drug, food, other)	Reaction (describe):

VALUABLES: DESCRIPTION	LOCATION
Glasses/Contacts:	
Hearing Aid:	
Mobility Aid:	
Prosthesis:	
Dentures: Upper Lower Partial	
Wallet:	
Money:	
Watch:	
Jewelry:	

Medications	Dose	Frequency	Last Dose	Location

ORIENTATION TO HOSPITAL:
Info Booklet ☐ Call System ☐ Bed Controls ☐ Bathroom ☐ Storage ☐ TV ☐ Telephone ☐
Visiting Hours ☐ Chaplaincy Service ☐ Hospital Educational TV

Date: Time: Signature:

NURSING DATA BASE

Significant Past Health History:	Present Illness and Patient's Expectation of Hospitalization:

FUNCTIONAL AREAS: Explore Present Status, Usual Patterns, Changes, Problems, Limitations, Coping Mechanisms, Aids

SLEEP/COMFORT: i.e. pain character and relief methods, usual sleep habits, aids.

SOCIAL/EMOTIONAL: i.e. occupation, hobbies, interests, home environment, resources, support systems, feelings about illness, affect, mood.

COMMUNICATION: i.e. style, method, fluency, skills, language.

CIRCULATION: i.e. rate, rhythm, skin color/temp, peripheral pulses, edema.

RESPIRATORY: i.e. rate, rhythm, effort, smoking, lung sounds.

NEUROSENSORY: i.e. hearing, vision, neuro signs, level of consciousness, seizure disorder, sensation.

MOBILITY/SAFETY: i.e. usual activity, exercise, mobility.

HYGIENE/SKIN: i.e. general appearance, wounds, dermatitis, decubiti, bathing preference.

NUTRITION: i.e. food preferences/dislikes, special diet, appetite, recent weight changes.

ELIMINATION: i.e. normal patterns bowel and bladder, last BM, ostomies, changes.

REPRODUCTION/SEXUALITY: i.e. last exams, hernias, alterations, birth control measures, LMP.

Date: Time: RN Signature:

Room # NAME DR. CATEGORY

FIGURE 2–2 Example of recording form that incorporates nursing data base, problem list, expected outcomes, and nursing interventions. Medical therapies are indicated either in relation to nursing problems or as unincorporated orders. (Used with permission from The Swedish Hospital Medical Center, Seattle, Washington)

PATIENT CARE PLAN

Date Signature	Problems	Expected Outcomes Discharge Criteria	Nursing Actions	Date	Treatments Special Orders

UN-INCORPORATED ORDERS

Date		Date	

ROUTINES

Diet — Special Diet Instructions:

Hygiene:

Activity: I&O:

Vital Signs: Weight:

BM: Isolation:

FIGURE 2–2, cont'd.

that are expected as routine or normal for the institution or practitioner in given situations. There appear to be no rules, however, on how standards are written. Published and institutionally written nursing care standards are written in any one of three major forms:

Process
Structure
Outcome

These formats and terminology parallel those used for formal evaluation of health care, and the arguments for and against each format are similar.

Process standards generally describe what one should do to carry out proper care. Care protocols and procedure manuals tend to be written as process standards. For example, in caring for the comatose patient, a standard might be to turn the patient every 2 hours to prevent skin necrosis. Process outcomes alone only tell us if the nurse does the right thing.

Structure standards tell what the organization and physical structure of a unit or nursing service should look like to produce optimum care. Structural standards are probably more significant at the level of the institution or nursing unit rather than at the level of the individual practitioner.

Outcome standards are written primarily in terms of what the patient outcomes would be if the patient is properly nursed. For example, a standard for care of immobilized patients might be the absence of skin breakdown. Outcome standards focus only on the ends, not the means.

Many sets of institutional and published standards combine process and outcome standards, that is, both nursing actions for a given set of patients and expected outcome. Either a process or an outcome standard, if used alone, has the disadvantage that numerous variables related to the individual patient and the type of medical care may influence the patient outcome, independent of the nursing process applied. Thus, if nursing care is evaluated on the basis of outcome alone, both good and bad outcomes may be related as much to other factors as to the nursing care. The addition of process standards allow us to give our best opinion on what the prudent nurse should do as well.

Standards of care tend to be used both educationally and as standard care plans for common and recurring problems. They have legal uses as well. When a patient sues a hospital and its nurses for malpractice, standard care plans or nursing care standards from that hospital are often used as the basis to determine if the nurses acted prudently within those standards. It is in these instances that process standards become quite important, even if the outcome is less than desirable. From this standpoint, standards should reflect the minimal expectation of competent nursing for common, recurring problems. Many in-house and published standard care plans tend to look like the idea rather than the standard expectation. From the legal perspective that could be a serious problem for competent nurses.

Summary

The process of nursing is a complex, dynamic skill that involves interpersonal relationships, continual cognitive matching between the observed and the ideal, and considerable empathy with human beings who are in need of care. It all sounds rather cold and analytical when dissected for discussion. In action, it is an artistic relationship between a person or group of persons who have a need and a person or group of persons with some knowledge and skills in meeting the needs. Perhaps we should liken the process to a dance in which the dancers attempt to match their steps until they are in synchrony.

References

1. American Nurses' Association: Nursing: A Social Policy Statement. Kansas City, ANA, 1980
2. Benner P: From Novice to Expert. Menlo Park CA, Addison-Wesley, 1984
3. Carnevali D, Mitchell PH, Woods NF et al: Diagnostic Reasoning in Nursing. Philadelphia, JB Lippincott, 1984
4. Carpenito LJ: Nursing Diagnosis: Application to Clinical Practice. Philadelphia, JB Lippincott, 1983
5. Gordon M: Nursing diagnosis and the diagnostic process. Am J Nurs 76:1298-1300, 1976
6. Guzzetta CE, Dossey BM: Nursing diagnosis: Framework, process and problems. Heart Lung 12:281-291, 1983
7. Kim MJ, McFarland GK, McLane AM: Classification of Nursing Diagnoses: Proceedings of the Fifth National Conference, St Louis, CV Mosby, 1984
8. McKay PS: Interdependent decision making: Redefining professional autonomy. Nursing Administration Quarterly 7(4):21–30, 1983
9. Nightingale F: Training of nurses. In Nutting MA, Dock LL (eds): History of Nursing, Vol II, p 205. New York, GP Putnam's Sons, 1907
10. Norris C: Concept Clarification in Nursing. Rockville MD, Aspen, 1981
11. Suhyada R, Kim MJ: Documentation of nursing process in critical care. In Kim MJ, McFarland GK, McLane AM: Classification of Nursing Diagnoses, pp 166–172. St Louis, CV Mosby, 1984
12. Weed L: Medical Records, Medical Education and Patient Care. Cleveland, The Press of Case Western Reserve University, 1969
13. Wessel SL, Kim MJ: Nursing functions related to the nursing diagnosis *decreased cardiac output*. In Kim MJ, McFarland GK, McLane AM: Classification of Nursing Diagnoses, pp 192–198. St Louis, CV Mosby, 1984

UNIT II

Conceptual Themes Basic to Medical–Surgical Nursing

Chapter 3

Behavioral and Emotional Responses to Illness

Beverly M. Horn

The interaction of the biological, psychological, behavioral, and emotional systems as parts of the human system is well recognized. Von Bertalanffy defined a system as "a set of units with relationships among them."[23] However, for purposes of study, component systems of the human system are frequently presented as discrete entities, with only minor allusions being made to the complex interactions that occur. In addition, as open systems, human beings are subsystems of other larger systems. The larger systems such as family, neighborhood, and community are interrelated and interdependent, and they are in transaction with one another. Systems inside the human system are referred to as the internal environment, and those outside the human system as the external environment. Mind–body interaction is affected by internal and external interactions. According to Rogers, each individual continuously exchanges matter and energy with his environment, which is defined as the patterned wholeness of all that is external to him.[18]

Conceptual frameworks for nursing practice are based on systems theory and incorporate a holistic perspective of the human system in relation to the environment.[10,16,17,18] Consistent with the systems perspective is the definition of nursing of the American Nurses' Association as "the diagnosis and treatment of human responses to actual or potential health problems."[15] Human responses include a myriad of reactions of an individual. The diagnostic and treatment of human responses reflects the underlying assumption of numerous nursing theorists that a person is complex and that a medical diagnosis is enmeshed in complex physiological and psychological interactions within a person's self and with his environment. Rogers and Riehl and Roy affirm the wholeness of human beings, that they are open systems in interaction with the environment and that the total person—psychological, developmental, physiological, and sociocultural—is a primany focus of nursing.[17,18]

How persons respond to actual or potential health problems implies a cognitive and emotional relationship with physiological processes, or what in this chapter is referred to as mind–body interaction. Furthermore, actual or potential health problems refer to illness and disease as deviant from health. Health, illness, and disease are concepts that need to be defined and understood by nurses because their meanings are included in cognitive, emotional, and physiological responses to problems (Fig. 3–1).

Health, Disease, and Illness

Health and disease are relative states. Well-being or lack of well-being for individuals fluctuates along a continuum on a daily basis. Personal and environmental factors contribute to this state of flux. Unique internal factors within each individ-

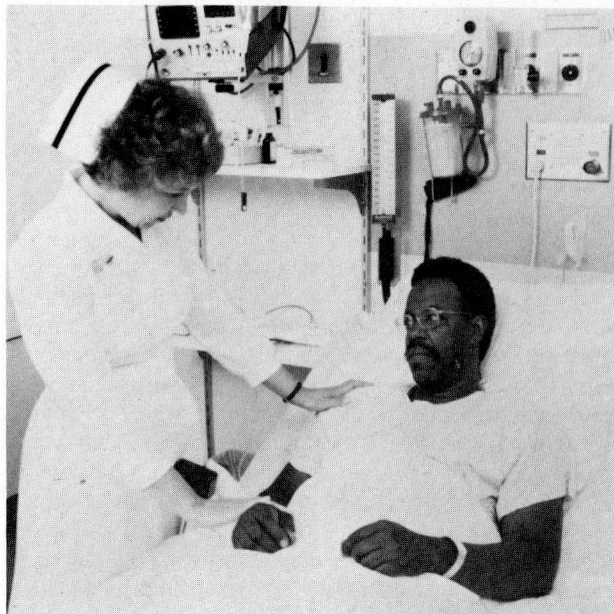

FIGURE 3–1 Understanding the emotional and physiological responses to illness is an essential component of nursing care.

ual determine how each person responds to external forces. According to Narayan and Joslin, health is more than the absence of disease or symptoms; it implies the unity of all aspects of the individual—mind, body, and spirit.[14] No one aspect can be separated from the others. Health, disease, and illness differences are identified in the following diagram:

Health	Holistic state of well-being: mind, body, and spirit
Disease	Biological and/or psychophysiological malfunction
Illness	Personal, interpersonal, and cultural reactions to disease

Although the concept of health is central to nursing theories, definitions of health vary. The variety of definitions are due to conceptualization of health as either present or absent, as a continuum, or as a holistic state. All perspectives have merit, but since the focus of this chapter is mind–body interaction in a systems framework, health will be treated as a holistic state. Winstead-Fry identified many problems associated with a precise definition of holistic health because reduction of the concept to its component parts will not convey an accurate meaning.[22] Broadly defined, the holistic perspective views the patient as an integration of body, mind, and spirit. Additional references to sources that describe problems associated with a precise definition of holistic health are found in the references at the end of this chapter.

Disease vs. Illness

Disease indicates a malfunctioning of the biological or psychological processes. The behavioral science literature distinguishes disease from illness. According to Kleinman, Eisenberg, and Good:

> That distinction holds that disease in the Western medical paradigm is malfunctioning or maladaptation of biologic and psychophysiologic process in the individual; whereas illness represents personal, interpersonal, and cultural reactions to disease or discomfort.[11]

Disease is a biomedical concept describing a condition of the patient that may be observed through objective means, such as temperature, presence of bacteria, or inability to perform social role tasks. Health care providers adhering to the biomedical concept may or may not be concerned about a holistic perspective of health because the major focus of biomedicine is to remove or ameliorate the disease process.

Illness, however, refers to how the patient perceives and responds to the state of disease. Illness may also be present when there is no observable disease process. For example, if an individual identifies certain symptoms as abnormal, he interprets the condition as illness. Illness is understood only from the patient's perspective and is a subjective phenomenon in which individuals who perceive themselves as not feeling well modify their normal behavior.[21] There is not a one-to-one relationship of illness to disease. Disease may be present when a person does not experience illness, such as in undiagnosed cancer, or in some instances of hypertension. On the other hand, a person may experience symptoms for which no disease process may be demonstrated. Because human responses to real or potential threats to health include both disease and illness, it is imperative that nurses are knowledgeable in both areas, but especially in diagnosis and treatment of illness and illness behavior.

Environmental Factors Influencing Patients' Responses To Illness

Environmental factors that influence responses are both internal and external to the patient. Separation of internal and external environments is artificial when a holistic perspective is proposed. For purposes of analysis they are treated separately in this section. The multiple interactions of internal and external environments are discussed later in the section on stress and adaptation.

Internal Factors

Internal factors include the physiological and psychological characteristics of individuals. Because the internal physiological factors are discussed throughout the text, they are not emphasized in this chapter. The major focus of this discussion is internal psychological variables influencing disease and illness. The relationship between illness and psychological factors has been identified over the years.[8,12,13,20] Cohen, in a review of the literature relating psychological factors to the development of disease, noted that two explanations are given. The first indicates that certain psychological factors predispose persons in a general way to be prey to a host of diseases. Diseases that result may be due to additional factors such as degree of exposure to pathogens, heredity, and metabolic imbalance. The general approach posits hormonal–biochemical factors affecting a general susceptibility to illness that increases the possibility of developing illnesses of many types. The second is a disease-specific explanation, namely, that certain personality types cause specific diseases.[2]

The first way of viewing personality factors as predisposing to disease in a general way is illustrated by relating disease onset to self-esteem. For example, persons with low self-esteem may perceive themselves as unable to cope with life, and they become depressed. Depression may result in lack of physical activity, either overeating or undereating with consequent poor nutrition, or possibly increased drinking or smoking. Such behaviors may predispose a person to bacterial and viral invasion or result in pulmonary, circulatory, or other systemic diseases. Figure 3–2 depicts such a relationship. Or perhaps if an individual has a genetic predisposition to a disease such as diabetes, the above-mentioned behaviors may lead to onset of diabetes mellitus.

The second way of viewing psychological factors as predisposing to disease includes the notion that a certain psychological makeup results in specific diseases such as heart disease or arthritis. This belief is documented in Friedman and Rosenman's work on type A personality and the development of heart disease.[6] Their study concluded that people who strive for achievement and perfection and are impatient and competitive have a greater chance of developing heart disease than those who take a more relaxed, unhurried approach to life.

Lazarus indicated that cognitive processes are the basis of coping activities.[13] Cognitive processes mediate emotional reactions by altering the ongoing relationship between personal and external environments in the developing emotional reactions. Thus, he believed that cognitive appraisal of any event is determined by an interplay of personality and environmental factors. Controversy exists as to the relative importance of situation vs. personal variables in predicting illness.

External Factors

Internal environmental factors or personality variables do not function in a vacuum. They are the mediators for responses to real or perceived external environmental factors, including stressors. According to Dever, environment is defined as "events external to the body over which the individual has little or no control."[3] External environments include the physical environments of air, water, soil, food, and population density. External environments also include the social environment of interpersonal relationships. Stressors are encountered in the external environment as a part of daily life and may be either biophysical or psychosocial in nature. People's ability to adapt to stressors varies. Because nursing aims to assist persons to adapt so they can attain and maintain a state of holistic health, understanding of the stressor–stress and adaptation phenomena is essential for nurses.

Stress and Adaptation

Stressors are defined as "any stimuli that effect an organismic response," with *stress* as the organismic response.[5] Stress is the nonspecific response of the body to environmental or internal demands, or both, which produce biological phenomena that tax or excel the adaptive resources of the individual.

Selye's neurophysiological theory of stress provides a framework for understanding environmental factors, both internal and external, that affect mind–body interaction and the disease–illness response. Selye's theory, based on the general adaptation syndrome (GAS), functions on the general assumption that when the organism is in a nonstress state, it is better able to mobilize resources and contend with new demands. The object of the GAS is to respond to stressors in such a way that a state of relative nonstress exists.[20]

The general adaptation syndrome as a nonspecific adaptive reaction is characterized by increased pituitary, adrenal, and cortical hormone secretions. The GAS occurs in response to an agent (stressor) producing stress. the stress response includes three phases:

Phase 1: Alarm reaction
Phase 2: Resistance
Phase 3: Exhaustion

The first phase, the *alarm reaction,* is the fight-or-flight reaction. During this phase the resources necessary to contend with the stressor are available. The individual's ability to mobilize appropriate and adequate resources determine his resultant health status.[5]

In the second phase, the *phase of resistance,* the orga-

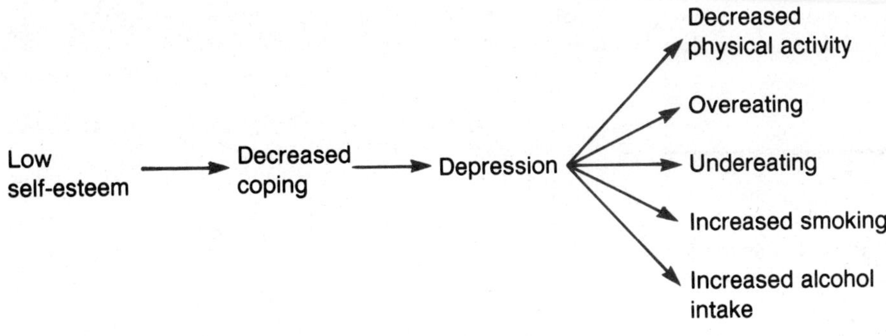

FIGURE 3–2 Interrelation of psychological factors and unhealthy behaviors.

nism actively utilizes resources. During this phase the organism may effectively adapt and not succumb to the effects of the stressor. Adaptation to one agent may be acquired at the expense of resistance to other agents.[1] However, most morphological and biochemical changes of the alarm reaction may diappear if this phase is prolonged and, in some cases, the direction of deviation from normal is reversed.

The third phase, the *phase of exhaustion,* results from prolonged exposure to the stimuli to which adaptation has developed but can no longer persist. Included in the phase of exhaustion are the stages of withdrawal and helplessness–hopelessness that place the individual at the risk of suffering the effects of the stressor.

When a stressor produces stress, *adaptation* is the adjustment that occurs. The meaning of adaptation, for this discussion, is that used by Roy and Roberts in which *adaptation* is viewed as the process of coping with stressors as well as the end state produced by this process.[19]

According to Beard, life event challenges evoke defensive physiological arousal without providing opportunities for musculoskeletal discharge of the state of arousal.[1]

An area receiving increasing attention in the nursing literature is the link between health and adaptability. Nursing intervention is directed toward assisting the patient to adapt to an ever-changing environment. The process of adaptation depends on the degree of fitness between the skills of individuals and the type of challenges with which they are confronted. To the extent that capacities are fitted well to the challenges, the flow of events is routine and ordinary.[7] Lazarus states that as environmental change is perceived, the individual cognitively appraises the situation to determine the significance of change. This appraisal will determine the quality and quantity of the emotional stress state that occurs as a result of the environmental change.

The origins of numerous disease states have been attributed to life changes. Life events require coping on the part of the individual.[9] A list of these events can be found in Chapter 7 where stress is discussed in greater detail. The relationship of life changes to illness has been strengthened by the validation of the influence of social supports as an intervening variable. For example, Beard noted that a decrease in interpersonal trust is a source of emotional stress and can be considered a factor in increasing the risk of cardiovascular disease.[1]

Compliance with treatment regimes is also attributed to the influence of psychological states. DeVon and Powers, in studying hypertension, noted that overall uncontrolled hypertensives experienced greater adjustment problems related to their illness, specifically domestic difficulties, and greater problems in extended family relationships.[4] They also experienced more psychological difficulties attributable to their illness.

Summary

In summary, the interaction of mind and body has a great influence on the development of disease and on the response to the entire phenomenon of illness. Studies in the past have supported this fact. Nurses need to consider this holistic perspective when caring for patients in a variety of settings.

References

1. Beard M: Trust, life events and risk factors among adults. Advances in Nursing Science 4:26–43,1982
2. Cohen F: Personality, stress, and the development of physical illness. In Stone C et al (eds): Health Psychology: a Handbook. San Francisco, Jossey-Bass, 1979
3. Dever AG: Epidemiology in Health Services Management. Rockville MD, Aspen Systems, 1984
4. DeVon JA, Powers MJ: Health beliefs, adjustment to illness and control of hypertension. Research in Nursing and Health 7:2–16, 1984
5. Erickson H, Swain MA: A model for assessing potential adaptation to stress. Research in Nursing and Health 5:93–101, 1982
6. Friedman N, Rosenman RH: Type A Behavior and Your Heart. New York, Knopf, 1974
7. Goosen GM, Bush HA: Adaptation: A feedback process. Advances in Nursing Science 1:51–66, 1979
8. Holmes TH, Masuda M: Life change and illness susceptibility. In Dohrenwend BS, Dohrenwend BP (eds): Stressful Life Events: The Nature and Effects. New York, Wiley, 1974
9. Holmes TH, Rahe RH: The social readjustment rating scale. J Psychosom Res 11:212–218, 1967
10. Johnson DE: The behavioral system mode for nursing. In Riehl JP, Roy C (eds): Conceptual Models for Nursing Practice, 2nd ed. Englewood Cliffs, NJ, Prentice-Hall, 1980
11. Kleinman A, Eisenberg L, Good B: Culture, illness and care. Ann Intern Med 88:251–258, 1978
12. Lazarus RS: Psychological Stress and the Coping Process. New York, McGraw-Hill, 1966
13. Lazarus RS: Cognitive and coping process in emotions. In Monat A, Lazarus RS (eds): Stress and Coping. New York, Columbia University Press. 1977
14. Narayan SM, Joslin DJ: Crisis theory and intervention: A critique of the medical mode and proposal of a holistic nursing model. Advances in Nursing Science 2:4, 1980
15. Nursing: A Social Policy Statement, Kansas City, American Nurses' Association, 1980
16. Orem DE: Nursing: Concepts of Practice, 2nd ed. New York, McGraw-Hill, 1980
17. Riehl JP, Roy C: Conceptual Models for Nursing Practice, 2nd ed. New York, Appleton-Century-Crofts, 1980
18. Rogers ME: An Introduction to the Theoretical Basis of Nursing. Philadelphia, FA Davis, 1970
19. Roy C, Roberts SL: Theory Construction in Nursing. Englewood Cliffs NJ, Prentice-Hall, 1981
20. Selye H: The Stress of Life. New York, McGraw-Hill, 1956
21. Tripp-Reimer T: Conceptualizing the construct of health integrating emic and etic perspectives. Research in Nursing and Health 7:101–109, 1984
22. Winstead-Fry P: The scientific method and its impact on holistic health. Advances in Nursing Science 2:1–7, 1980
23. von Bertalanffy L: General Systems Theory. New York, Braziller, 1968

Chapter 4

Cultural and Religious Considerations

Beverly M. Horn

Culture has many definitions, but in this chapter *culture* is defined as patterns of learned behaviors and values that are shared among members of a designated group and usually transmitted to others in the group through time. Included within the concept of culture are traditions, values, patterns of interaction, methods of economic support, and techniques for positive and negative controls on group members.[3] Everyone has a cultural background that serves as the lens through which experiences are perceived and behavioral choices made.

In working with culturally diverse patients, it is important to remember that all members of a given culture do not fit a textbook picture of the culture's typical behavior. If the nurse uses information indiscriminately, stereotyping may result. There are intracultural as well as intercultural differences in societies. Thus, individual assessments need to be made from an unbiased perspective.

Race and Ethnicity

Race and ethnicity are related terms, but they are not synonymous. *Race* refers to a system by which humans are classified into subgroups according to specific physical and structural characteristics, such as skin pigmentation, texture of hair, and features. There are three commonly recognized racial types: Caucasoid, Mongoloid, and Negroid, and their characteristics greatly overlap. *Ethnic groups* are distinguished by distinctive patterns of customs, language, and family life and may or may not have similar racial characteristics. Members of an ethnic group share a culture, whereas members of the same race frequently do not share a culture.

Cultural Relativism and Ethnocentrism

Cultural relativism is primarily an attitude that values every group as having beliefs, values, and behaviors arising out of its historical background, and its proponents believe that a group can only be understood in the light of that background. The belief in cultural relativism is a necessity for nurses working with persons of diverse cultural backgrounds. The opposite side of the coin is *ethnocentrism,* which is a characteristic of persons who feel that their way of thinking and believing is the only right and proper way.[7] Conflicting beliefs, values, and norms enter into the nurse–patient relationship and must be accounted for by the nurse. A critical need for nurses is to understand their own cultural beliefs and values relative to health and illness as well as those of other cultures, so that culturally relative assessments and interventions can be made.

Folk and Professional Health Care Systems

For many cultures, folk and professional health care systems exist side by side. The folk system is sometimes regarded by nurses as quackery, superstition, or nonscientific care. In actuality, a folk system is based on a cultural logic that has survived the test of time. The professional health care system is recognized by most cultures as having a role in the curing of disease, but it is not recognized as dealing with illness in the same meaningful way as folk systems.

Folk treatments are widespread in our society. Many Americans seek cures from naturopathic practitioners or try self-treatment. Use of over-the-counter drugs is common, as is the use of products from health food stores. Latin cultures may seek help from a curandero, and Native American Indians may use the native healing practitioner. Chinese and Southeast Asians may use herbalists and acupuncturists, or they may purchase their own medications and herbs from herbalists or the grocery store. In the South and Southeast, the root doctor and the spiritualist are often consulted. The names for curers in major ethnic groups may be found in Table 4–1.

TABLE 4–1
Curers of Selected American Ethnic Groups

Ethnic Group	*Curer*
American Indian	Medicine Man
Black American	Root Doctor Blood Doctor Voodoo man/woman
Chinese American	Acupuncturist
Ethnic Chinese Vietnamese	Herbalist Herb pharmacist
Japanese American	Herbalist
Mexican American	Curandero

Cultural Assessment

Cultural assessment is an integral part of the nursing process that leads to a nursing diagnosis. According to Tripp-Reimer, Brink, and Saunders cultural assessment has a different purpose than biological and psychological assessment.[7] The latter have generally accepted standards in which the purpose of assessment is to determine where deviations occur from the normal and then to bring the patient into conformity with the standards. On the other hand, cultural assessments are performed to identify deviations in cultural parameters, with the goal of modifying the patient's or the health care professional's belief system to increase congruence between them.[7] A culturally relativistic nurse will more frequently modify her behavior to achieve congruence.

Cultural assessment guides may be found in a number of nursing texts. Major areas to be assessed include[8]

Values	Decision making
Customs	Religion
Food	Grief/dying
Family interactions	Social structural components
Sick role	
Beliefs	

Illness vs. Disease

For many ethnic groups, illness, as defined in Chapter 3, is of greater importance than the disease, and the cure of disease can occur only when illness is considered. For these reasons persons from many cultural groups may use the professional and the folk system simultaneously when recognition is given to the fact that the professional system treats and cures disease only. Because illness is not perceived apart from disease, other curers must be sought for the person to be truly cured.

Physiological illness is also related to cultural conditioning, although direct causes of illness in specific cultures are often not known. For example, alcoholism is more prevalent among the Irish than the Jews, and blacks have a higher death rate from cardiovascular disease and cancer, particularly in the middle years, than do whites.[4,5]

Causes and Treatment of Illness

In all ethnic groups there is a cultural logic that attributes causes to illness and identifies necessary behaviors for cure. Two major systems are presented in this chapter. These systems are not mutually exclusive, that is, they are not alternative explanations, but are different logical systems that help to explain illness and cure. Explanations from one or both of these systems may exist in a given culture. The systems are harmony and balance, and the hot and cold phenomena.

Harmony and Balance

Concepts of harmony and balance are recurring themes across most groups. Harmony exists both within the person and in interrelationships among persons, as well as in interaction with the environment. These concepts relate to the need for equilibrium physiologically, socially, psychologically, and spiritually. According to Coulehan, for example, all Navajo thinking is grounded in relationships: everything is related to everything else, and the natural state of all things is harmony.[2]

According to Snow, Southern rural blacks perceive all illness as representing disharmony and conflict in some part of the person's life. Furthermore, all illness falls into the three general catgories of environmental hazards, divine punishment, and impaired social relationships.[6] These causes for illness are also common to Native American Indians, Southern Europeans, Mexican-Americans, rural midwesterners, and other cultural groups. Illness is cured by restoring the balance. To give a specific example, a Hopi man attributed the cause of his pneumonia not only to bacterial invasion, which could be treated with antibiotics, but also to an argument with an uncle, which could only be treated by reconciliation. Both would be needed for cure of the pneumonia.

Hot and Cold Phenomena

The second logical system of illness and cure relates to hot and cold phenomena. This highly complex system is based on the humoral theory of disease, which views health

TABLE 4–2
Treatment of Hot and Cold Illnesses

Illness	*Medicinals*	*Food*
Hot		
Constipation, anemia, sore throat	Aspirin, penicillin, vitamins, minerals, camphor	Alcoholic beverages, chocolate, tea, corn meal, garlic, beans
Cold		
Arthritis, asthma, diarrhea, headache	Bicarbonate of soda, chicory, barley	Fresh vegetables, dairy products, chicken, honey

as being a state of balance among the four humors of the body: blood, phlegm, black bile, and yellow bile. These humors have the characteristics of being either hot or cold. A balance between hot and cold is considered health, and if there is an imbalance between them, there is illness.

Treatment is based on the Hippocratic concept of neutralization, that is, a cold illness is treated with hot food, drugs, and herbs; and a hot illness is treated with cold food, drugs, and herbs. Qualities of hot and cold have no relationship to actual temperature but are the ascribed states of various objects or persons. In foods, for example, the categorization is based on the way they help. Fresh vegetables are "cold" because they can help in curing hot illnesses such as anemia and constipation.

A similar although different belief system is that of yin and yang found in Asian cultures. This is a folk medical system based on Eastern philosophy which holds that energy regulating the universe is composed of two opposing forces, yin and yang.[1] Yin represents the female negative force of darkness, cold, and emptiness. Yang represents the male positive force that produces light, warmth, and fullness. There must always be a balance, and imbalance causes illness. For example, an excess of yang causes fever and dehydration and must be treated with yin (cold) foods and medicines. Table 4–2 gives examples of hot and cold illnesses and their treatment with medicinals and foods.

The Family

The nuclear family consisting of a set of parents and their children is characteristic of Anglo-American culture only. For other cultures the extended family is predominant in health and illness care, especially in decision making on and carrying out health regimens. In most folk cultures grandparents are official or symbolic family leaders. The nurse may become frustrated when questions are addressed to the patient, and the grandparent answers. In Asian-American families, the parents share esteem with grandparents, uncles, and aunts. Having many family members present when health decisions are made and when care is being given is considered essential by most cultures other than Anglo-American.

Many cultures have ways of incorporating nonkin into relationships that give kin status as well as responsibility. For example, the compadre system is prevalent throughout Roman Catholic folk cultures in southern Europe, Latin America, and Puerto Rico. This refers to a relational tie established through a ritual such as baptism, and it involves special religious and social responsibilities. In Hispanic, Native American, and black families, relatives frequently consist of brothers, sisters, and stepparents who have no legal ties, but do have a formally recognized relationship.

Religion

Religion for most cultures is inextricably tied to all events of life, including health, illness, and death. Although cultures have different historical backgrounds, many cultures share the perception that illness is often caused by supernatural forces. Religious leaders become a very important part of health care. Nurses need to involve the Catholic priest, the Jewish rabbi, and the Protestant minister, as well as other religious leaders when planning care.

Nursing Implications

Nurses encounter numerous cultural and ethnic groups in the United States as well as internationally. Nurses need to learn as much as possible about the health beliefs and behaviors of the groups they work with, both from the literature and from individual informants. Because nurses cannot know about all cultural groups, including their own, it is imperative that an attitude of cultural relativism is a guiding force for nurses in approaching nursing care. Without such an attitude, knowledge of specific facts would be of little value.

References

1. Campbell T, Chang B: Health care of the Chinese in America, Nurs Outlook 21:245–249, April, 1973
2. Coulehan JL: Navajo Indian medicine: Implications for healing. J Fam Pract 10:55–61, 1980
3. French RM: Dynamics of Health Care. New York, McGraw-Hill, 1979.
4. Henderson G, Primeaux M: Transcultural Health Care. Menlo Park CA, Addison-Wesley, 1981
5. Markides KS: Mortality among minority populations: A review of recent patterns and trends. Public Health Rep 98: 252–260, May–June, 1983
6. Snow LF: Folk medical beliefs and their implications for care of patients. Ann Intern Med 81:82–96, 1974
7. Tripp-Reimer T, Brink PJ, Saunders JM: Cultural assessment: Content and process. Nurs Outlook 32:78–81, March/April, 1984

Chapter 5

Changes with Aging

Ruth F. Craven
Maxine L. Patrick
Pauline M. Bruno

Aging implies the passage of time. It is a universal property of all living plants and animals, and it applies as well to objects and to societal groupings (*e.g.*, communities, nations, populations, institutions). Human aging starts at the time of conception and progresses throughout life. The life span, the maximum age to which a human being can live, is divided into phases that extend over certain years. The commonly used categories are the following: infancy (birth to 1 yr); early childhood (1 to 6 yr); late childhood (6 to 10 yr); adolescence (10 to 18 yr); young adulthood (18 to 35 yr); early middle age (35 to 49 yr); late middle age (50 to 64 yr); young-old (65 to 79 yr); and old-old (80 yr and above).

Human aging is a broad concept that is studied from many perspectives: philosophical, religious, biological, psychological, sociological, historical, and economic. Although it is often viewed from only one of these perspectives, aging of the individual is a process that involves the *total* person in the broadest sense of that word. Physically, the aging process consists of intrinsic, subtle changes in all body systems. These changes are influenced by genetic inheritance and environmental factors. Similarly, emotional and intellectual growth are influenced by physical and environmental factors. In all stages of life, growth and development is a multifaceted process in which all aspects are interrelated.

This chapter highlights background information on aging that is essential to the nursing care of an adult population. The perspectives presented are demographic characteristics, psychosocial and physiological aspects of aging, health needs of the elderly, and special nursing considerations related to the elderly.

Demographic Characteristics

Life Expectancy

The life expectancy of human beings has been increasing over the centuries of recorded history. Life expectancy is defined as an expected number of years of life based on statistical probability. Historically, man has sought to maintain wellness throughout the life span. The search for the elixir of life appears in the writings of the Egyptians, and finding it was a goal of Christopher Columbus. However, it is not an elixir that has brought about the present expansion of life expectancy. This expansion is a phenomenon of the past century and a half, and is the result of many factors: the industrialization of society, changes in the philosophy of societal governance and human rights, sanitation engineering, and medical science.

In the middle of the 18th century, scientific data began to associate disease with filth. The first public health legislation in England combined economics with sanitation findings.

The legislation came about because it was cheaper to clean up the environment than to care for the sick and lose their economic productivity. As industrialized society developed, trade unions came into existence. They bargained for health changes in the work environment and wage increases. The increase in income contributed to improvement in living standards, including purchase of adequate food and clothing. Changes in transportation made food, clothing, and the means of sanitation improvement more readily available to most people. Governmental philosophy mandating the education of all citizens contributed to the understanding and public implementation of health practices.

Age-Related Views

Cohort groups share particular cultural traits and life experiences. The term *cohort group* refers to groups having a statistical factor in common, such as range of birth years. For instance, the 55- to 70-year-olds in today's society shared the experiences of World War II, the economic expansion and material wealth that followed in the fifties, and are now sharing the moving into their retirement phase. Such cultural traits as habits, recreational preferences, and views of the world are more similar for persons within a cohort group than between persons in this group and their children in the middle years of life. In his book *Growing Up,* Russell Baker recounts a vivid picture of the socioeconomic and cultural climate in the early part of this century and its influence on the personality and beliefs of persons growing up in that period.[1] In today's society, the baby-boom cohort group is large, and the number of persons in the group who are seeking employment is greater than the employment opportunities. The problem of employment is a shared event in the lives of the baby-boom group. Because nurses work with persons of all ages, they need to consider the historical background and life experiences of patients who are in particular age-groups. The considerations include the social, economic, and political milieu of that period.

Population Dynamics

Population dynamics are based on death rates and birth rates. Life expectancy has increased rapidly since the turn of the century, On the average, a person born in 1900 could expect to live about 50 years, whereas the average life expectancy of a person born in 1984 is 75 years. Life expectancy is one factor that influences the size of populations. A second factor is birth rate. Variability in birth rates within particular intervals of time influence the composition of a population and a particular cohort group throughout its life span. For instance, the baby boom that followed World War II has created the bulge in the present population of persons 25 to 35 years of age.

The current population in the category of 65 years old and over numbers about 22 million, or approximately 11% of the population; about 1% of this group is over 85 years of age. It is relatively common for people in their 60s to have living parents who are in their 80s. The future projection is for an increase in the number of people over age 80 (old-old category) as contrasted with young-old (65 to 79 years old).

TABLE 5–1
US Population Aged 65 Years and Over: Selected Years and Projections, 1950–2030

Year	*Number in Thousands*	*Percent of US Population*
1950	12,397	8.1
1970	20,087	9.9
1980	24,927	11.2
2000	31,822	12.2
2010	34,837	12.7
2020	45,102	15.5
2030	55,024	18.3

(US Bureau of the Census Population Report, Series P60, No. 144: Characteristics of the Population)

By the year 2010, the number of people over age 65 will increase markedly as the baby-boom generation reaches this age (see Table 5–1). Because of differences in mortality rates of males and females, women live about 10 years longer than men. Most patients in nursing homes are elderly women, many of whom are widowed. Five percent of people age 65 and over are in long-term care institutions; 20% are homebound and need health care. With the advent of Diagnostic-Related Groups (DRGs), these percentages may increase.

Geographic Locale

At the present time, about 73% of persons over age 65 reside in urban areas, which is in contrast to the general population in which the majority of people reside in the suburbs. The elderly of today often have difficulty coping with the problems caused by the changing nature of their neighborhoods. The problems they face include crime, crowding, inadequate transportation, and high living costs. Many of the elderly trying to cope with urban living are widows living alone (Fig. 5–1). Some elderly have migrated to states with warm, mild climates but, in general, migration is not a characteristic of this age-group. Therefore, states with high populations are also those with a large number of elderly. Ten states account for 56% of persons greater than 65 years old. The states with the highest percentage of elderly are New York, California, Illinois, Ohio, Florida and Massachusetts.

Economic Factors

The fact that both sexes are living longer than anticipated has created problems in the economic arrangements of society. People are receiving more money from pension funds, particularly social security, than they contributed. In the year 2010, the post–World War II baby boom will increase the number of people receiving social security, and because of the decline in birth rate in the late sixties and seventies, there will be fewer people to support this group. In 1982, there were 100 working-age adults for every 19 persons over age 65; by 2050, that ratio will be 100:38.[8]

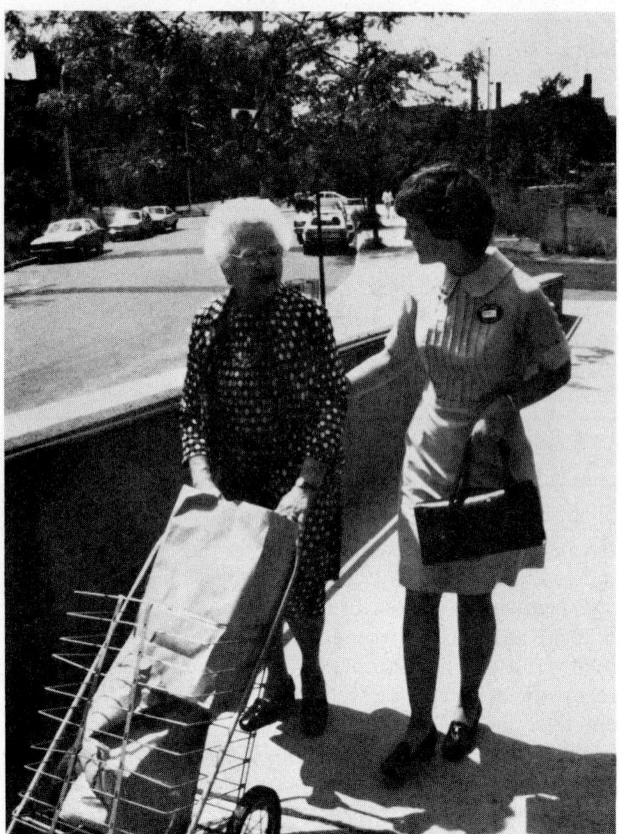

FIGURE 5-1 Elderly widows frequently face transportation problems in getting to and from the store.

Economically, retirement at age 65 usually means a lowered income. Since the 1960s, when Medicare and Medicaid were initiated, there have been changes in federally funded support programs for the elderly. In 1960, the value of benefits and services for the elderly was $17 billion. In 1981, the value was $55 billion (in 1960 terms), yet the population age 65 and over increased one and a half times. In 1961 the White House Conference on Aging found 6 million elderly to have an inadequate income; this figure decreased to 3.5 million by 1982.[11] The groups experiencing the greatest economic difficulty are minority older people and older women. These two groups are composed of persons who receive low social security benefits due to either the nature of the jobs they held in their productuve years or the fact that they were not in the labor force. The low-income elderly have difficulty paying hospital bills, buying medications, and obtaining adequate food and housing (Fig. 5–2).

Summary

In summary, the cohort groups of persons aged 65 to 79 and those age 80 and over are an increasing proportion of society as a whole. Many people in these groups are living on adequate incomes, but others exist at or below poverty level. Changes in neighborhood characteristics create coping difficulties for many elderly.

Psychosocial Aspects of Aging

Two stereotypes about the elderly picture them as being highly resistant to change and incapable of learning. To the contrary, the elderly are constantly adapting to physical changes such as decreased visual acuity and decreased muscle strength. In adapting to these changes they are also having to learn new ways of behaving. The extent of change and relearning that is required when a widow must move from her home of many years to a small apartment in a retirement home or nursing home is great. What then *is* known about the learning abilities of the elderly and their psychological growth and development?

An appreciation of the psychological aspects of aging is important for all nurses who work with the aged. A knowledge of the crises occurring in the last stage of life is useful if the nurse is to assist the elderly and their families in the attainment of developmental tasks.

These tasks are illustrated in the components of Maslow's hierarchy of needs. The five levels of human needs as defined by Maslow are dynamic, and an individual is frequently in the process of moving among the levels.[7] These levels are (1) hunger, thirst, and survival; (2) safety, self-preservation, and security; (3) belongingness and love; (4) social esteem and self-respect; and (5) self-actualization. This is particularly true of the elderly person who may be making frequent adjustments for reasons of health, loneliness, or other adaptations.

Emotional development, according to Erickson's description of the mature years, is evaluated in terms of integrity vs. despair.[4] If an individual looks back and perceives life as having been rich and fulfilling, with purpose and meaning, that individual will experience a sense of satisfaction and contentment in the remaining years. If an individual does not evaluate his life as such, he will face his final years with despair.

Cummings theorizes that the later stage of life is characterized by "disengagement," which is defined as a "mutual withdrawal" when the individual perceives the reality of being mortal.[3] Society is thought to withdraw from the elderly and the elderly to withdraw from society. This behavioral response may be initiated by the individual or by others in the social milieu, with the outcome being a movement away from involvement, achievement, and productivity on the part of the mature individual.[9]

In contrast, activity theorists suggest that social involvement, and social disengagement, facilitates successful adaptation to aging.[5] The concept involves the substitution of new social roles and activities for those that were lost (work, parenting, *etc.*) In reality, aspects of both activity and disengagement behaviors are probably apparent in all elderly persons to a greater or lesser degree as determined by their personalities throughout their life (Fig. 5–3).

Mental Function

It is commonly but incorrectly thought that older people experience a marked deterioration in mental function.[2] Men-

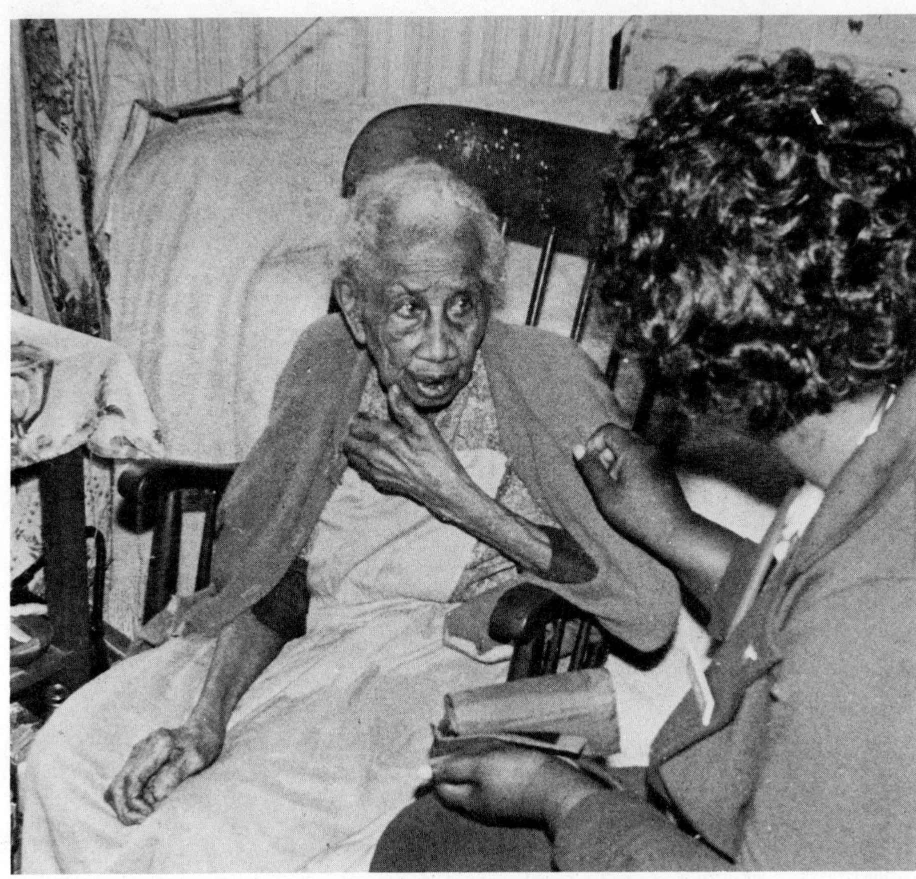

FIGURE 5–2 Low-income elderly have the greatest difficulty obtaining health care. (Courtesy of Alabama Journal, Montgomery, Alabama)

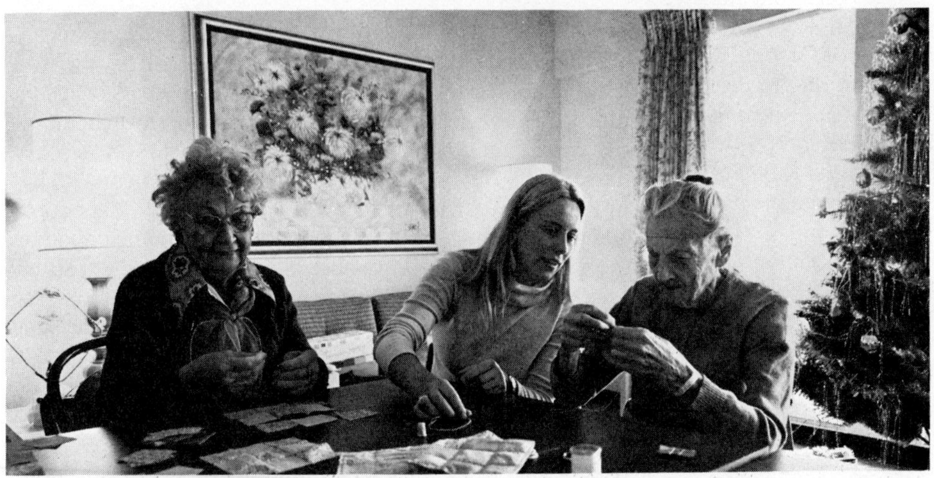

FIGURE 5–3 Remaining active and involved is an important aspect of adapting to age.

tal function is the process that occurs between stimulus perception and behavior. It includes intelligence, learning, memory, creativity, and personality. There are many problems that affect research on learning and intelligence in the elderly. These include the influence of declining health, the use of tests that were validated on young people with different educational backgrounds, the lack of motivation to do well on tests, and the use of cross-sectional data. Most old-old people in today's society have had only an eighth-grade education. Studies indicate that there may be a slight gradual decline in intelligence and learning skills, but this decline is not sufficient to interfere with an elderly person's ability to carry out the activities of daily living.

The elderly need to be taught health practices to maintain wellness and to participate in their own care when ill. The elderly learn best in a one-to-one teaching situation and a quiet environment that fosters hearing acuity (Fig. 5–4). Material should be presented in small increments, since the elderly may fatigue easily. The elderly are capable of making decisions and should be encouraged to do so. Memory is

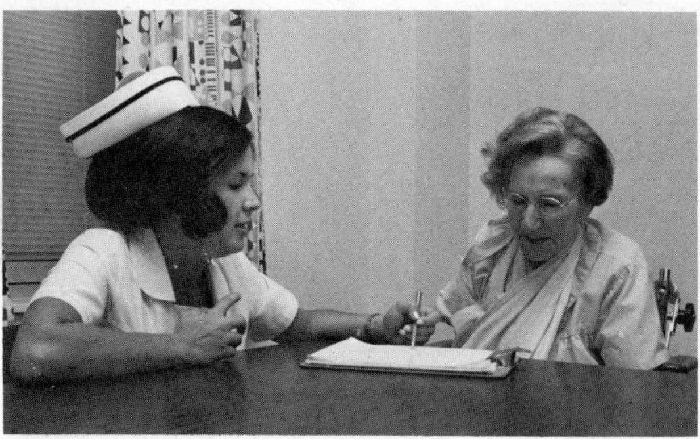

FIGURE 5–4 Teaching the elderly patient on a one-to-one basis and in a quiet atmosphere can enhance learning. (Photo by D. Atkinson)

related to learning, for one cannot learn if there is no recall of information. In general, elderly people may have a decrease in registration of new information in the brain, in storage of information, and in recall, especially of more recent events. Forgetfulness in the elderly may be related to sensory changes that decrease perception and to decreased attention to events. Memory changes in the elderly are generally not sufficient to interfere with the activities of daily living.

Mental Dysfunction

A misconception about growing old is that all people get "senile." Senility is a garbage-basket term for negative behaviors, and has no scientific basis. It is true that some elderly people lose their memory as they age, some become depressed, and others are lonesome. Some old people have physiological changes in the brain that are due to disease processes or iatrogenic effects of medications. All of these problems influence behavior, and attention should be directed toward carefully screening for physical problems before labeling aberrant behavior as due to idiopathic mental disorder.[10]

In Chapter 12 of this text, it is noted that homeostatic problems start with intracellular biochemical dysfunction. This theory is supported by recent research which indicates that the behavioral and intellectual problems of the elderly are probably rooted in biochemical, metabolic dysfunction of cerebral cells. Confusion, depression, and other behavioral changes in the elderly may be iatrogenic and reversible. These conditions should not be accepted as normal. A careful health history should be taken and a complete physical examination should be done to rule out and look for conditions that can be treated effectively.

Causes of Confusion. Stress, which arises out of the society in which the elderly person lives, can cause confusion. Sources of stress include retirement, loss or roles, relocation, death of friends and family, and institutionalization. The disruption that occurs around the event is what causes the stress. Grief, separation, rejection, loneliness, hopelessness, helplessness, powerlessness, and anxiety—all are feelings normal to an event of loss, but these feelings can produce sufficient stress to cause confusion.

Sensory changes that come with aging may result in inaccurate communication and what appears to be inappropriate behavior. Loss of or diminished senses—especially hearing and sight—can lead to feelings of paranoia. If part of a sentence or word is not heard clearly or completely, it is easy to think people are talking about you. If someone cannot see because glasses have been taken away or because there is inadequate light in the room, shadows can look like something they aren't and can be frightening. Patients who need glasses and hearing aids should always have them available.

The older person who has to leave the familiar environment of his home and go to a hospital or nursing home may become confused and disoriented. Relocation is a major source of stress for the elderly. Preventive nursing actions include spending time with the patient, using touch to convey concern, providing frequent reiteration of orienting data (time and place), and having clocks and calendars in the environment. It is essential that all actions, procedures, and routines be explained to the patient.

Other events that can precipitate confusion are disruptions of sleep (which often occur in institutions), medication problems, nutritional inadequacies, and dehydration. All these situations can occur with the elderly, especially the elderly who live alone and may be somewhat depressed. A history of events preceding the onset of the behavioral change may reveal possible causative factors. Sometimes the behavioral change is a manifestation of a serious cognitive disorder.

Alzheimer's Disease. Alzheimer's disease is a severe disorder of cognition. The onset can occur in the late middle-age years as well as in people over 65 years of age. In the older person, it is often referred to as elderly dementia of the Alzheimer's type. Severe dementia occurs in 4.4% of those over 65 years old, and mild–moderate dementia occurs in 11% to 12%.[2] With the increasing numbers of older people and the high mortality of Alzheimer's disease, it may soon be the fourth or fifth leading cause of death in the United States.

Manifestations of the disease are gradual and progressive. The family and afflicted person may not notice the changes initially. As the disease progresses, manifestations include memory loss, becoming lost in a familiar neighborhood environment, and forgetting to dress, eat, and work. Eventually, the patient loses all ability to care for himself. The patient may have problems swallowing food even when prompted, and bladder and bowel control are lost. In the final states, overall health deteriorates, with aspiration pneumonia being a usual cause of death. Patients with the disease usually live about 2 to 4 years after the diagnosis. Autopsy findings demonstrate widespread brain atrophy, with a loss of brain weight. Microscopic examination of brain tissue reveals neuritic plaques, neurofibrillary tangles, enlarged ventricles, and loss of neurons throughout the cortex.

The Alzheimer Support Group (ASIST) provides assistance to family members by giving families emotional support, information about caring techniques, and resources for respite care. The organization is also involved in research. At the present time, there is no cure or specific treatment for the disease. Since it is such a devastating disease, the National Institute on Aging gives high priority to funding research on this problem.

Summary

In summary, the basic psychological needs of the elderly are very similar to those of younger adults. Elderly persons consider good health, comfortable housing, adequate income, recognition by others, and socialization essential to their well-being. The elderly, though, typically have greater difficulty obtaining their desires than do younger adults. A primary nursing goal in caring for the elderly is to help them with the adjustments necessary to improve or maintain the quality of life. Each person has different strengths and limitations, and each person responds to stresses differently. The way an elderly person will respond is essentially the same as he has reacted to other stresses throughout his life.

Physiological Aspects of Aging

Aging is part of the developmental process in which anatomical and physiological changes occur over time. The speed with which aging changes occur varies on the basis of hereditary factors and the stresses of life. Genetic factors determine the time of onset, the course and direction, and the time sequences of the various aging processes. Life stresses can often interpose on the genetic timetable for aging.

Biological aging leads to some general responses in the older person. There is a gradual decline in functional ability, particularly where multisystem coordination is required. Age-related decrements in performance are greater in activities that require more complex functioning than in those involving individual system functions. There seems to be growing evidence that some effects of aging are related to decreased effectiveness of control mechanisms in maintaining homeostasis. These concepts undergird the readily recognized fact that the elderly have increased vulnerability to pathophysiological occurrences.

All systems of the body continue to undergo changes after reaching maturation at 20 to 30 years of age. However, biological changes progress at different rates for each person and for each body system of that person. The effects of these changes may increase the vulnerability of the elderly person to disease and disability.

Cardiovascular Changes. Changes in the cardiovascular system start during middle age and begin to present symptoms in the later years. There is a decrease in the elasticity of blood vessels and in cardiac output as cardiac muscle strength lessens, leading to a loss of cardiac reserve. In addition, diminished regional perfusion to some organs, along with the presence of atherosclerosis, may result in ischemia. Resistance in peripheral vessels increases with age as a result of diminished vascular flexibility. To overcome the increased resistance, an increase in blood pressure may be demonstrated in both systolic and diastolic measurements. The effects of these cardiac and vascular age-influenced changes are that circulatory dynamics are less efficient. With a change in body position, decreased efficiency of baroreceptors and of the valves in the veins of the lower extremities may result in inadequate cerebral perfusion, resulting in dizziness and accidents.

Respiratory Changes. Although the lungs are capable of providing adequate gas exchange throughout the life span in the absence of disease, the structures of the respiratory system do undergo changes that lead to decreased elasticity and increased rigidity. Chest wall stiffness, resulting from increased calcification of costal cartilage and decreased strength of intercostal and accessory muscles and the diaphragm, and combined with less elasticity and recoil pressure in the lungs, results in increased residual volume and decreased forced expiratory volume (FEV_1) with age. The arterial oxygen tension (Pao_2) decreases about 4 mmHg per decade whereas the arterial carbon dioxide tension (Pa_{CO_2}) and pH remain unchanged. The diminished defense mechanisms of airway clearance and immune changes combine with the previously described changes to increase the susceptibility to lung congestion and infections.

Nervous System Changes. Aging changes in the nervous system include a gradual degeneration and atrophy of neurons, leading to lessened nerve acuity and impaired sensation. Altered sensation may cause the elderly person to be unaware of tissue trauma, such as burns or pressure. Bed rest may alter cerebral perfusion and oxygenation; consequently, many elderly people become confused when they stay in bed or after they have had several hours of sleep.

Sensory Changes. The acuity of the senses declines with old age. Although the amount of decline varies with the individual, one in four persons over 65 years of age has some type of hearing problem.[10] Sound discrimination decreases with age, and there is some selective loss of hearing of the higher pitches. Such changes are usually not reversible because they are due to neurological decline (see Chap. 70 for information about the hearing-impaired person).

Twice as many elderly people have visual impairments as have hearing loss. More light is required for the aged retina to produce the same physiological sensation as was produced in the younger years, and adaptation to light and dark requires more time. Visual acuity, especially for close reading, is impaired as a result of changes in the structure of the eyeball and its muscles (see Chap. 70 for discussion of visual impairments).

The senses of taste and smell appear to decline with age. This is one explanation for the aging person's lack of appetite or loss of interest in foods that were once favorites. Since aromas often stimulate eating, the decline in the sense of smell contributes to the appetite decline in many aging persons. Decline in the senses of touch and smell present certain safety hazards that need to be discussed with the aging person and his family.

Dental Changes. With age, the gums become less elastic, and less vascular, and they recede from the remaining teeth, exposing areas of teeth not covered with enamel. These areas are sensitive to injury from brushes and coarse dentifrices. In addition, diseases of the gum, which may have been progressing symptom-free for years, may cause loss of teeth. Many elderly persons have decayed, broken, or missing teeth. The person's oral health may affect nutrition.

Changes in Kidney Function. The physiological controls of fluid and electrolyte balance provided by the kidney are altered with aging as reduced renal flow leads to a progressive decrease in the glomerular filtration rate. One major consequence of this age change is the potentiation for the half-life of many drugs that are excreted by the kidneys. Additionally, dehydration and dizziness may follow relatively short periods without food and fluid because of fluid and electrolyte imbalances. Laboratory values change with age. Assessment of the status of ill elderly should take these variations into consideration.

Musculoskeletal Changes. With aging, there is a decrease in lean muscle mass and an increase in body fat. In the musculoskeletal system, this loss of muscle fiber leads to decreased muscular strength and function. The bones lose density through demineralization. This change is particularly noticeable in the vertebral bodies by a gradual decrease in body stature and by posture changes, and the femur, which has a greater propensity for fracture. The movable joints have less mobility, with the large weight-bearing joints showing greater wear, friction, and stiffness. Maintaining activity and diet with necessary nutrients helps preserve muscle tone and decrease the rate of bone demineralization. As the body ages, muscular tone change is also seen in the gastrointestinal and genitourinary systems, contributing to increased problems of constipation and incontinence.

Integumentary Changes. The skin of an elderly person is usually thin, delicate, and sensitive to pressure and trauma. The loss of subcutaneous fat, increasing cross-linkage of collagen fibers and atrophy of elastic fiber, cause the skin to wrinkle and sag. Atrophy of sweat glands lessens the excretory function of the skin, making the skin dry, flaky, and prone to itching. Atrophy of the tiny arterioles near the epidermis impairs vasomotor homeostatic mechanisms of temperature regulation. The elderly feel cold even in warmer environments and are unable to dissipate heat in hot environments.

Health Needs of the Elderly

The nurse should be cognizant of some general concepts of aging that are useful in assessing the health needs of the elderly:

1. Age-related changes are gradual and individual and, even within individuals, different systems age at different rates.
2. Complex functions that require multisystem coordination show the most obvious decline and require the greatest compensation and support.
3. The elderly have an increased vulnerability to disease.
4. Stress situations (either physiological or psychosocial) produce a more pronounced reaction in the aged and require a longer period of time for readjustment.

The elderly frequently have an atypical presentation of an illness, such as pain being less pronounced and some typical symptoms being either missing or different than expected. Confusion, restlessness, or other altered mentation are common occurrences in the presence of illness. Obscure or unexplained deterioration of health or function should not be accepted as normal aging and needs to be carefully evaluated.

As people age they are at increased risk of becoming ill. Americans are living longer, but they are not necessarily healthier. Aging changes, both physiological and psychological, lower resistance to disease. Multiple diagnoses and chronic diseases are not uncommon among the elderly. Chronic illness has replaced terminal illness as the major health problem in America. Most older Americans have one chronic illness such as arthritis, heart condition, hearing and vision impairments, diabetes, or arteriosclerosis.

When the elderly person becomes ill he may face many adjustments that make it difficult for his basic emotional needs to be met. In addition to illness and diminished physical energy, he may have no family and few friends, or his spouse may also be ill. He may be apprehensive and worried, often fearing helplessness and physical dependence on others. Inadequate income, housing problems, and preexisting depression may further complicate his recovery.

Older women, who are more likely to be alone, often fear that if they become ill they will be placed in a nursing home or will lose their current residence and become dependent on others. Nursing homes are an important part of the health care system. They are needed as an option, but the goal of the patient on admission should be discharge and rehabilitation to independence as soon as it is possible. Home health care is available as part of Medicare. This care provides nursing assistance in the home and chore workers to do shopping, cleaning, and personal laundry. These services should be investigated and become part of the planning for discharge.

Nursing the Elderly Patient

The goal of health care to the elderly is to maintain the person's highest possible level of functioning for his age and ability. Aging should be viewed as a normal, inevitable process, one requiring adjustments in living patterns, but not withdrawal from life. An appropriate approach to aging is that of an ever changing cycle of life that eventually will end in death.

In planning nursing care for elderly patients, it is important to consider each patient's physical, social, economic, and psychological capabilities and limitations. When nursing care is given to elderly patients, a few special considerations contribute to protecting their sense of worth and their feelings of adequacy.

Communication Considerations. Demonstrating respect by remembering names and calling the person by the name they prefer being addressed with (instead of using such terms as "grandma" or "grandpa") is essential. Many people in today's society tend to refer to all people by their first name rather than by Mr. or Mrs. and the family name. This is not acceptable to some people, and it should not be done without asking permission from the individual. People who are between 70 and 80 years old were brought up in the 20s and 30s when standards of respect for their elders were different, and they have maintained these standards over the years. Using a first name may be viewed as rude, and under these circumstances, it would be difficult to establish rapport.

Since many elderly patients experience some loss of hearing, special care must be taken to ensure that the patient has heard any communication you give him. Facing an elderly patient when speaking, and speaking distinctly so the patient can lip-read inconspicuously if necessary, are useful techniques (Fig. 5–5). Shouting in an attempt to help the elderly person to hear does no good, since shouting increases the frequency of the voice pitch, moving the sound out of the range of hearing of the elderly. If a hearing aid is used, be sure that it is working properly. Written instruction as well as repetition of instructions are helpful for some elderly patients.

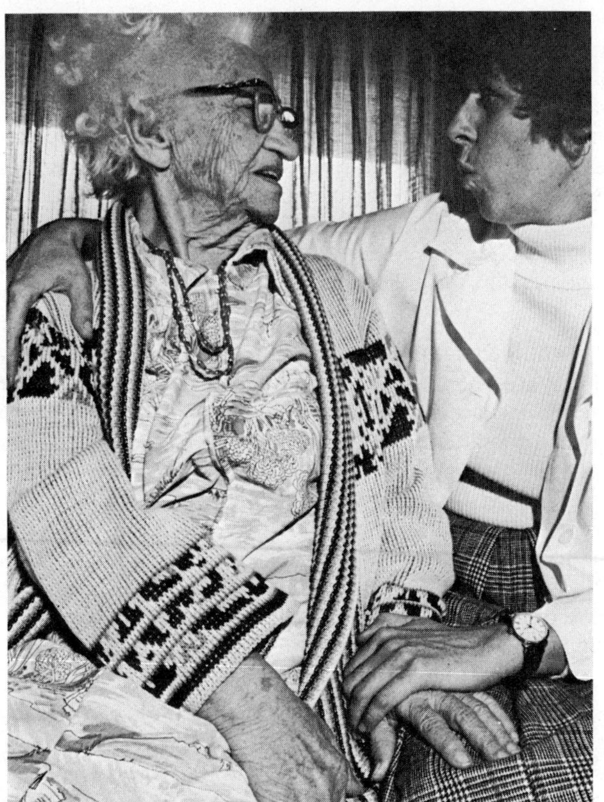

FIGURE 5–5 Since many elderly patients have difficulty hearing, take care to speak distinctly, and face the person while conversing.

Promoting Independence. Placing equipment conveniently and using self-help devices may help the elderly person maintain some degree of independence. An overbed trapeze or side rails on the bed, handrails along hallways and in the bathroom, and a walker or cane may make mobility easier. Help with personal care, such as arranging the hair, applying cosmetics, shaving, and dressing, is often appropriate, since personal appearance is important to everyone's morale.

Hygienic Practices and Skin Care. The elderly need to use somewhat different hygienic practices than a younger adult to maintain an optimum physical condition. Daily bathing is often contraindicated for the elderly because of dry skin. One or two baths a week are sufficient, although the patient who is incontinent needs local cleansing at frequent intervals and more frequent baths. Mild, superfatted soaps are preferred to regular soaps. Bath oils, lanolin, or body lotions promote water retention in the skin.

Alternating pressure mattresses, flotation pads, and flotation mattresses may be helpful in maintaining the skin intact. Most importantly, the patient's position should be changed frequently, and bony prominences and weight-bearing areas should be massaged at least every 2 hours. Sheepskin pads placed under bony prominences relieve pressure and prevent irritation of the skin. Getting the elderly out of bed as much as possible not only helps to redistribute pressure over the body, improve circulation with ventilation, and decrease bone demineralization, but it also improves the patient's psychological outlook.

Because of changes in vision and mobility, elderly persons often need assistance with foot care. Nails are often hard and scaly. Soaking the feet in warm water before cutting softens them and makes cutting easier and safer. A referral to a podiatrist may be appropriate.

Visual Aids and Denture Care. Since many people over 50 years of age wear glasses, care of glasses, particularly making certain that they are not lost or broken, is important in the nursing care of the elderly. Glasses should be kept clean, since smudged glasses rather than failing vision may be the cause of difficulty in seeing. The person should have his glasses available at all times because confusion and accidents may result if they become misplaced. Night-lights are advisable to reduce confusion of elderly patients and to prevent those who get up during the night from falling.

The loss of teeth leading to the need for dentures is common. Consequently, care of dentures and prevention of their loss are part of the general nursing care of most elderly patients. Dentures should be cleaned following each meal. Dentures are costly, therefore care should be taken that they are not lost. Dentures can also be easily mixed up, especially if the patient removes them frequently and then forgets where he puts them. Dentures should be marked to avoid confusing them with other people's dentures.

Exercise and Body Alignment. The feet and legs are often affected by disorders in peripheral circulation. It is important for aging persons to have regular exercise of the feet and legs to avoid stasis of the circulation to their lower extremities and to avoid injury and infections of their feet and legs. Precautions similar to those described for the patient who has peripheral vascular disease (see Chap. 43) should be taken by all elderly people.

As the muscles become less active and the joints less flexible with age, a posture of flexion may result. The center of gravity changes, the spine becomes rounded, and the chest and shoulders flex forward. Encouraging correct posture and deep breathing are preventive measures that are part of the daily nursing care of all elderly patients. Proper body alignment adds to the comfort of the patient when in bed as well as decreasing the need for corrective exercises later. A firm mattress is preferable and helps to make the use of supportive pillows more effective. A footboard placed at the foot of the bed helps to keep the covers off the toes and provides something against which the patient may exercise his feet and legs. Pillows may be used for support by placing them under the head, at the back, and under the arms as appropriate.

Active range-of-motion exercises should be performed several times each day by every bed patient. The patient is taught to flex, abduct, adduct, and extend each leg separately and both legs simultaneously. The heel of one foot is placed on the knee of the opposite leg and then is passed slowly down the leg to the ankle. This can be repeated, alternating the legs. Arm, hand, neck, and shoulder movements can be encouraged by having the patient first raise and lower his head, neck, and shoulders from a flat supine position without a pillow and then extend his arms in front of his chest, followed by raising them above his head. These exercises should be done in time to regular, deep respirations to encourage deep breathing in the bedfast patient. They should be taught to the patient by the nurse, and should be supervised daily by the nurse or the family member caring for the patient. The regular performance of exercises will help to prevent the loss of muscle tone and the demineralization of bones that can occur in all bed patients, regardless of age. Passive range-of-motion exercises are recommended for those people who are unable to exercise independently.

Hospitalized patients should have their shoes and should wear them when they are up. These shoes should be leather-soled, well-fitting shoes. If slippers are worn, they should also fit well and be firm, so that the person will be less likely to slip and fall.

Although rest is essential for the aged, it is undersirable for an elderly patient to be confined to bed. Even acutely ill people may be up in a chair for much of the day, and may even be encouraged to walk. Confusion, decubitus ulcers, lung congestion, increased bone demineralization, and general deterioration may result from prolonged bed rest. When the patient is being cared for by his family the great importance of keeping the patient active needs to be taught to them.

Temperature. Protective adipose tissue under the skin decreases with age, and the volume of circulating blood, particularly to the small outer arteries, may be diminished, thus affecting the ability to withstand chilling without discomfort. Decreased activity also lessens circulatory function, resulting in the lowering of skin temperature and increased sensitivity to environmental temperature changes.

The normal temperature of older persons tends to be lower than 98.6°F or 37°C. Consequently, a temperature of 99°F may be an indication of an infection. Febrile conditions in the elderly are most likely caused by bladder or respiratory disease.

Sleep Patterns and Mental Status. Elderly people usually sleep lightly and intermittently with frequent waking. Some wakefulness, therefore, can be expected in the elderly patient who is hospitalized. Having a low bed and night-light and allowing the patient to be up with adequate supervision are useful nursing actions. Although elderly patients may be unable to sleep, sedation has limited usefulness in the elderly, and other methods for inducing sleep are preferable.

Altered sleep patterns that are normal in aging need to be differentiated from depression and dementia. True dementia is characterized by a defect in memory and orientation, deterioration of intellectual functioning, and alterations in judgment and affect.[10] True dementia occurs in only about 6% of those over 65 years of age. Dementia is chronic and progressive, and may often lead to institutionalization of the person. Depression is often confused with dementia and can occur with true dementia; therefore, many elderly persons with a treatable depression are not recognized and diagnosed. Depression is a dysphoric mood, which causes loss of interest in usual activities and usually presents with a history of recent onset. Depression is characterized by at least four of the following symptoms being consistently present for about 2 weeks: altered appetite or weight; altered sleep patterns; expressions of self-reproach, guilt, and hopelessness; lack of energy; psychomotor retardation or agitation; loss of interest or pleasure in usual activities; and recurrent thoughts of suicide. If there is any possibility of the existence of depression, the elderly person should receive treatment.[10]

Nutritional Needs. Qualitative nutritional needs of the elderly are essentially the same as for other adults except that caloric needs diminish. Many elderly persons, particularly those living alone, subsist on a diet high in carbohydrates and low in vitamins, minerals, and protein. Often they think that because they are elderly they do not need much food. Increased fiber and adequate fluid intake are beneficial to the gastrointestinal system. Drinks prepared with dry skim milk supply essential protein and are useful in helping to meet the protein and calcium needs of older patients without supplying too many calories.

Gastrointestinal Function. Many elderly patients are very concerned about their bowel function. Less food and less activity contribute to reduced bowel activity. Any marked change in bowel habits, however, and any unusual reactions to normal doses of laxatives should be reported, since malignancies of the large bowel and diverticulitis are fairly common among this age-group.

Motor activity of the intestinal musculature may be decreased with age, and supportive structures in the intestinal walls become weakened. Sense perception is less acute, so that the signal for bowel elimination may be missed. Constipation may occur and in turn lead to impactions. The very elderly and somewhat confused patient should be reminded to go to the bathroom after meals. The addition of fibre, such as bran, to a person's daily food intake has been found to be helpful in preventing constipation. If the patient is constipated, it may be necessary for the nurse occasionally to carefully insert a gloved finger into the rectum to be certain impaction has not occurred.

Urinary Elimination. Frequency of voiding is common with aging, but may become a problem during illness. The glomerular filtration rate and the renal blood flow decrease gradually with age. In addition decreased muscle tone in the bladder, with resultant impairment of emptying capacity may lead to residual urine in the bladder and subsequent infection. It may be necessary to catheterize the patient to check for residual urine. One of the first signs of diminishing or failing bladder function is frequency of micturition during the night. Frequency and slight burning on urination are symptoms of bladder infection.

Unless there is a definite contraindication to high fluid intake, the elderly patient should be urged to take sufficient fluids to dilute urine and decrease its irritating properties. Fluids may be limited in the evening if nocturia is troublesome and is interfering with sleep. If the patient is quite feeble, it is good to offer a urinal, bedpan, or bedside commode during the night.

Relaxation of perineal structures in elderly women may interfere with complete emptying of the bladder and predispose to bladder infection. Because of decreased sensation, some elderly patients do not realize when the bladder must be emptied. Periodic dribbling of urine suggests that the bladder is not being emptied completely. A number of elderly men have hypertrophy of the prostate gland, which makes urination difficult. The nurse should observe the very elderly patient for distention of the bladder and consult the physician about it.

Involutional changes in the lining of the vagina lead to decreased resistance to organisms, and mild infections with troublesome discharge may result. Specific therapy may be ordered for it, and frequent local bathing followed by application of cornstarch may be helpful in allaying itching.

Sexuality. Many younger people falsely assume that older people have no interest in sex and lack the ability to perform sexually. Men and women of all ages are capable of sexual arousal and orgasm. Studies conducted at the Duke University Center for the Study of Aging revealed sexual activity in the eighth and ninth decades. Often the aged person becomes sexually inactive due only to a lack of an acceptable partner.[12]

Attitudes of health care professionals play an influential role in allowing sexual expression for old people. Sometimes professionals avoid the topic, or deny sexual needs exist by not asking about sex in health histories. They may verbally or nonverbally indicate disapproval of those who discuss sex. On the other hand, there are those who take the opposite view, that is, that all old people want to be and are sexually active—and if they aren't, something is wrong. The middle ground between the two attitudes is what the health professional should foster.

Emotional Needs. Meeting the emotional needs of the elderly is an important part of nursing care. Elderly patients often appreciate just talking with others. If possible, the nurse should plan time to visit with them daily. Volunteers may also be used to visit the elderly. Many patients appreciate visits with a clergyman.

Elderly are often comforted by being touched (Fig. 5–6). Touch conveys feelings of concern, interests, and acceptance. Older patients may respond favorably to nurses who greet them by shaking hands. Patients who are without visitors, family, or friends or who are uncomfortable may appreciate having the nurse hold their hand. "Foster grandparents" is a program in which older people care for children. There is a mutual exchange of love, thoughts, and touch that is gratifying to both the elder and the child. Touching and petting animals is another source of pleasure to the elderly. Pets in nursing homes help patients to overcome feelings of loneliness and depression.

Maintaining family contacts is a primary concern. Plans can be made for the patient to make a short visit outside the hospital or for family members to visit in the hospital. This is especially important if a husband or wife is physically unable to visit his or her spouse.

If the elderly patient likes to read, reading materials should be provided. If he is unable to see well enough to read, talking books available through public libraries may be appreciated. It is also possible to get books and magazines with large print for persons with reduced vision. Television and radio also provide diversion and stimulation.

Elderly patients are usually aware of death as an imminent possibility and sometimes see it as a welcome event. The nurse should not avoid this issue. If the nurse senses that the patient is genuinely concerned about death, she should not avoid speaking about it. The patient may wish to see and discuss his feelings with a clergyman, a family member, or the physician, or perhaps he may wish to transact some unfinished business. Being responsive to such requests is frequently more important for the patient's peace of mind than is his medical treatment. The feelings of the family of the elderly person must also be considered in dealing with the question of death since they may be very uncomfortable with the subject.

Special Nursing Considerations Related to the Elderly

Positioning and Skin Care

Elderly patients who are undergoing diagnostic tests require some special considerations. An elderly patient should never be left unattended on a treatment table. Since a person

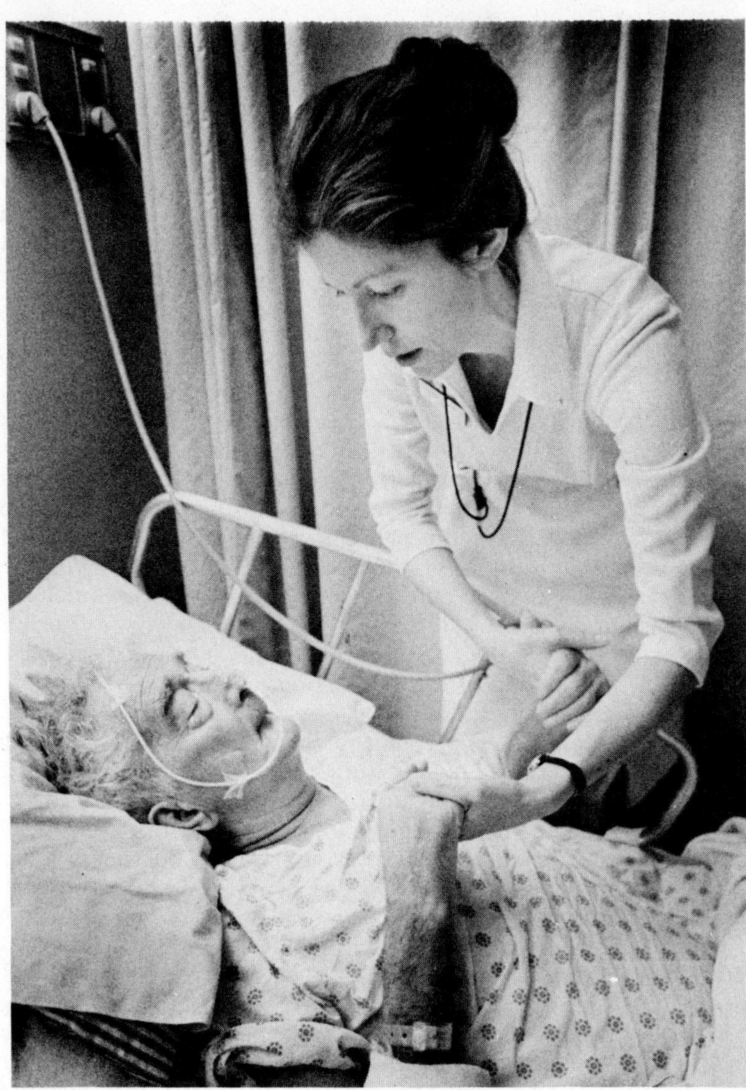

FIGURE 5–6 Touch is one means of comforting an elderly patient.

may be dizzy from postural hypotension, arising slowly and sitting on the edge of the table for a few moments before standing is advisable. Older patients with cardiovascular disease or with curvature of the spine may also be orthopneic and therefore not be able to tolerate lying flat for examinations.

Because of the rapidity with which they develop tissue trauma from pressure, elderly patients who must lie on hard surfaces such as x-ray, treatment, or operating room tables for lengthy periods of time need pressure-relieving pads placed under the normal curves of their backs and under bony prominences. The skin surrounding bony prominences should be gently massaged occasionally to improve the circulation to the area. On return to the unit the patient should always be checked for pressure areas. If possible the patient should be kept off these areas until signs of pressure disappear. If the lithotomy position is used, care must be taken to place both legs in the stirrups at the same time to prevent undue stress on less flexible muscles. The same principle applies when removing the legs from the stirrups. Care must also be taken to prevent hyperextension and hyperflexion of the joints, since many elderly patients have reduced flexibility.

Effects of Medication

Elderly persons consume disproportionately more of all kinds of medications than any other group. These medications may not be well tolerated, may result in adverse reactions and interactions, and may provoke or elicit unpredictable responses in the elderly. Age-related physiological changes contribute to altered responses to drugs in the elderly.

The *absorption* of oral drugs may be affected by the decrease of hydrochloric acid that normally occurs with aging. Drugs that depend on an acid medium may be absorbed less effectively. Absorption may also be altered by the rate of transit through the gastrointestinal system.

The *distribution* of drugs throughout the body is affected by the loss of lean body mass and the increased proportion of body fat. Fat-soluble drugs tend to be stored in fat, thereby decreasing the intensity of the reaction while increasing the duration. Within the bloodstream, the distribution of drugs is affected by the amount of serum protein, specifically the albumin, available as binding sites for drugs. In aging the serum albumin levels tend to be lower, resulting in altered concentrations of bound (inactive) and unbound (active) drugs. Unbound drugs in the circulation are active in producing the effects of the drug. Many of these drugs are excreted by the kidney in their active state. A principal mechanism of drug interaction seems to be the displacement of one drug by another from these protein-binding sites. For example, warfarin may be displaced by aspirin, indomethacin, and other drugs, causing increased anticoagulant activity.

The rate of *metabolism* of drugs in the elderly may be altered by lower levels of enzyme activity in the liver. The result of prolonged or incomplete metabolism is an increase in the half-life of some drugs, which allows the drug to exert its effective activity over a longer period of time.

The primary route of *excretion* of drugs is the kidney. Decreased renal plasma flow to the kidney, decreased glomerular filtation rate, and the decreased number of functional tubules combine to result in inefficient excretion of the active drug. This effect increases the risk of accumulation of drugs to potentially toxic levels owing to decreased renal clearance of active drug. The decreased rate of excretion along with the changes in binding sites in the blood contributes to prolonged elevation of blood level and activity of many drugs. Digoxin has a narrow margin of safety and is an example of a drug that is critically affected by the change in renal excretion.[6]

Drug treatment in the elderly has its definite place in the therapeutic regimen, but requires careful monitoring. Confusion is very often one of the earliest indications of undesirable drug effects. One principle in treatment of the elderly with medication is that the drug level should begin with the lowest dose and that the fewest possible number of drugs should be used.

In planning self-administration of drugs with the elderly patient, it is frequently helpful to determine the easiest time for him to remember to take medication. Tying it with some activity of daily living such as arising or taking meals is usually helpful. The use of a medication checksheet and the placement of the medication in an obvious place may be helpful reminders. Special care needs to be taken, however, to put the medicine where it will not accidentally be taken in place of another drug or where other family members such as small children may take it. Some elderly persons have found it helpful to use something such as an egg carton with the days marked or one of the commercially available medication reminder kits. Elderly persons should understand the medications they are taking and should be cautioned against taking extra doses of the medication in the belief that if one tablet or pill helps, two will be better.

Summary

It is most helpful when the nurse can deal with the elderly person in an emphathetic manner, demonstrating a willingness to listen, explain, and comfort and to support independent functioning. Accepting elderly individuals as they are and where they are in terms of their developmental status, as well as suspending youth-oriented attitudes and standards that may be inappropriate, are essential elements in adequately meeting the elderly person's needs and fostering a better quality of life.

References

1. Baker R: Growing Up. New York, St. Martin's Press, 1982
2. Birren J, Sloan RB: Handbook of Mental Health and Aging. Englewood Cliffs NJ, Prentice-Hall, 1980
3. Cummings E, Henry WE: Growing Old. New York, Basic Books, 1955
4. Erickson EH: Childhood and Society, 2nd ed. New York, WW Norton, 1963
5. Havighurst RJ et al: Psychology of Aging (Bethesda Conference). Public Health Rep 70:837–856, 1955
6. Ivey M: Drug use. In Carnevali D, Patrick M (eds): Nursing Management for the Elderly. Philadelphia, JB Lippincott, 1979
7. Maslow A: Motivation and Personality. New York, Harper and Row, 1954
8. Senate Aging Committee Report. Aging America: Trends and Projections. Washington DC, American Association of Retired Persons, 1984
9. Starr BD, Goldstein HS: Human Behavior and Development. New York, Springer Publishing, 1975
10. Wolanin MO, Phillips LRF: Confusion: Prevention and Care. St Louis, CV Mosby, 1981
11. Woodruff D, Buren J: Aging: Scientific Perspectives and Social Issues, 2nd ed, p 21. New York, Van Nostrand, 1983
12. Woods NF: Human Sexuality in Health and Illness, 2nd ed. St Louis, CV Mosby, 1975

Bibliography

Andres R, Bierman E, Hazard W: Principles of Geriatric Medicine. New York, McGraw-Hill, 1985

Blazer D: Depression in Late Life. St Louis, CV Mosby, 1982

Botwinick J: Aging and Behavior, 3rd ed. New York, Springer, 1984

Brocklehurst JC (ed): Textbook of Geriatric Medicine and Gerontology. Edinburg, Churchill Livingstone, 1980

Butler T, Lewis M: Aging and Mental Health, 3rd ed. St Louis, CV Mosby, 1982

Crandall R: Gerontology: A Behavioral Science Approach. Reading MA, Addison-Wesley, 1980

Eisdorfer C: Models for Clinical Psychopathology. Jamaica NY, SP Medical and Scientific Books, 1981

Eisdorfer C, Faren WE: The Psychopharmacology of Aging. Jamaica NY, SP Medical and Scientific Books, 1980

Goldberg P, Roberts J (ed): CRC Handbook on Pharmacology of Aging. Boca Raton FL, CRC Press, 1983

Hall B: Mental Health and the Elderly. New York, Grune & Stratton, 1984

Hyck M, Hoyer W: Adult Development and Aging. Belmont CA, Wadsworth, 1982

Kenney R: Physiology of Aging. Chicago, Year Book Medical Publishers, 1982

Yurick A, Spier B, Robb S, Ebert N: The Aged Person and the Nursing Process, 2nd ed. New York, Appleton-Century-Crofts, 1984

Chapter 6

Health Promotion and Patient Teaching

Anne Loustau

The Importance of Health Education

Whether ill with an acute or long-term illness or in need of information to help prevent future health problems, most people at some time are in need of health teaching. Recent research studies document the value of providing information to consumers. For example, community education programs for healthy persons have helped to change dietary patterns, with the goal of reducing the risk of cardiac disease.[10] Providing information on ways to manage minor illnesses at home has decreased unnecessary use of emergency room and ambulatory care facilities.[28] Patient education has also been shown to increase self-help skills and to assist individuals to cope more effectively with chronic illnesses such as diabetes,[19] chronic lung disease,[22] hypertension,[20] cardiac disease,[13] and cancer.[9] Teaching hospitalized patients who are scheduled for surgery about the procedures that will be done and the activities that they can perform to facilitate their recovery can reduce the discomforts that they experience and shorten their hospital stays.[8] With continued concern about the high costs of health care, teaching activities that enable patients to care for themselves and decrease the demands on the health care system will take on increased importance.[26]

The Role of the Nurse in Health Teaching

The nurse is a key person in providing educational information to patients. The American Nurses' Association defines the nurse's professional responsibility for patient teaching.[1,2] These teaching responsibilities, which are a part of each nurse's practice, include

1. Providing information to patients about the treatments they are receiving
2. Helping patients learn new skills to increase their abilities to care for themselves
3. Assisting patients in adaptations to changes in lifestyle brought about by illness

Some examples of common situations in which nurses teach patients follow. Nurses teach patients the skills for coping with the acute stages of illness and thereby reduce risks for complications. This teaching includes instruction about coughing and deep breathing and the use of assistive devices such as incentive spiromenters to support respiration, about leg exercises and early ambulation to enhance circulation, and about relaxation techniques to minimize the need for pain medicaiton (Fig. 6–1). With shortened stays and early discharge from the hospital, patients increasingly need to be able to perform technical self-care activities at home. Nurses have traditionally taught patients to care for their wounds, catheters, shunts, and stomas at home. More recently, patients have also been taught to successfully manage their own intravenous antibiotic therapy[24] and total parenteral nutrition.[29] Patients with long-term chronic illnesses such as diabetes, hypertension, and chronic lung disease also benefit from instruction on the physiology of their illness as well as self-management skills, such as when and how to take medications and strategies for adjusting the activities of daily living to correspond to the demands of illness and treatment. Nurses, as patient educators, also contribute to the risk reduction of healthy persons by encouraging good habits, such as prudent but adequate dietary intake, using seat belts when traveling in cars, increasing exercise, decreasing smoking, and discouraging unnecessary alcohol and drug use.

Although the nurse is a significant person in patient teaching, it is essential for the success of these activities that they are planned and implemented in collaboration with others, notably the patient and the patient's family or significant others. In addition to the persons in the patient's immediate environment, patient teaching is often part of a health team effort and may include planning and collaborating with health professionals such as physicians, dieticians, pharmacists, social workers, and physical and occupational therapists.

Principles of Teaching and Learning

Webster defines a principle as "a fundamental truth, an essential element—one that produces a specific effect."* In the case of patient teaching, principles serve as guidelines to help determine appropriate actions to take when the nurse is planning and implementing instructional activities. Basing one's teaching activities on principles increases the likelihood that the desired effect, successful learning, will take place. A set of patient teaching principles based on the literature from education and psychology is presented in Table 6–1. The principles are summarized and nursing implications for each of these guidelines are discussed in the following sections.

Principle #1. Meet Priority Needs First

The individual's basic needs must be met before he can be expected to be involved in learning activities. The nurse's sensitivity to the patient's physical status can provide important information about the patient's readiness to learn. Patients who are seriously ill with acute or long-term chronic illnesses will have little reserve energy to invest in learning new skills or changing valued behavior patterns. Pain associated with many illnesses as well as decreased oxygen levels and increased levels of metabolic wastes may interfere with memory and the ability to recall information. Medications, particularly pain medication, and anesthesia pose a particular problem for the surgical patient trying to remember and perform postoperative activities.[5,21,30]

Emotional factors also have an effect on the patient's ability to become involved in learning activities. Illness frequently involves some threat to a person's self-esteem. The patient must change his self-concept from one of being healthy and well to the idea of being ill with real or potential limitations on his ability to perform daily roles and activities. A person with a newly diagnosed illness may be grieving the loss of health and may be unable to consider learning the information related to the management of his disease. Cues that suggest a readiness for teaching and a willingness to

* By permission. From Webster's Third New International Dictionary © 1961 by G. & C. Merriam Company, publishers of Webster ® Dictionaries.

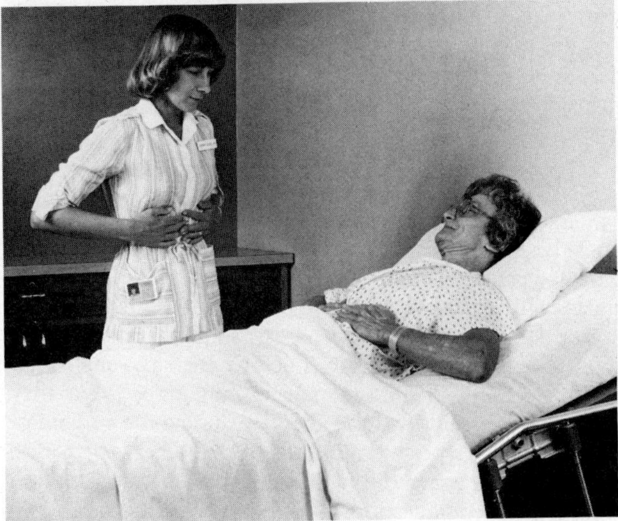

FIGURE 6–1 Health teaching includes instructing the preoperative patient in deep breathing techniques.

TABLE 6–1
Principles for Patient Teaching

1. Basic survival, comfort, and self-esteem needs must be met before patients can engage in learning new skills and behaviors.[17]
2. Patients are more likely to learn information that they consider useful and relevant to their needs.[14]
3. Patients are more likely to succeed with learning activities if goals are realistic.[4,14]
4. Patients are more likely to learn new information that corresponds to previous experience and learning.[3,7]
5. Patients are more likely to continue new behaviors if significant others are included in the planning and teaching.[6,20]
6. Data regarding the patient's intellectual and physical capabilities should guide the choice of appropriate teaching materials.[14,23]
7. The patient's learning-style preferences should guide the choice of teaching strategies.[14]
8. Practice and feedback are essential to the acquisition of new skills.[4,25]

learn include the patient's asking questions about his illness and the care he is receiving, looking at surgical wounds if they are present, and expressing concern about how he will manage at home.

Principle #2. Make Learning Relevant

Individuals are most likely to learn information that they consider to be important and relevant. Therefore, assessing what the patient considers to be a priority to know about his illness and care is essential to a successful teaching program. Meyer and Latz surveyed open-heart surgery patients about the teaching they had received before discharge and found that patients identified a number of unmet needs that they wanted specific information about, including the amount of pain to expect, types of appropriate postdischarge activities, assistance managing diet and medications, and signs and symptoms of complications.[18] A teaching plan that takes concerns such as those identified by Meyer and Latz into account will be more relevant and useful to patients.

Principle #3. Keep Learning Goals Realistic

Having patients estimate what they think they can successfully accomplish in an education program that involves behavior change has also been shown to be critical to the success of that program. Marlatt worked with individuals engaging in weight control and smoking cessation programs, and showed that people are more likely to accomplish tasks that they consider to be realistic.[16] This phenomena is referred to as self-efficacy—the importance of the individual's participation in determining changes or alterations in his behavior (Fig. 6–2).

If the patient is having to make a number of changes in his lifestyle, such as taking medications, increasing exercise, losing weight, going on a diet, and decreasing smoking, then consider the number of familiar habits to be given up and the number of new behaviors to be assumed. Consider setting priorities with this patient (one or two changes to work towards) to increase the likelihood of success. Hulka documents that too many changes at one time increase the complexity of the program and decrease the likelihood of success.[12]

Because of the relationship between the patient's perception of what he needs to know as well as his assessment of what he can successfully accomplish, the nurse will want to involve the patient in establishing goals and objectives for learning. A *goal* is a general statement about the task to be accomplished. *Objectives* are very specific, measurable statements about what the patient will do to achieve the goal. Mager describes the process for writing measurable objectives, which includes the following steps: (1) identifying the behavior to be performed, (2) defining the conditions in which the behavior is to ocurr, and (3) determining the level of acceptable performance for that behavior.[15] Examples of some common goals with specific objectives are presented in Table 6–2.

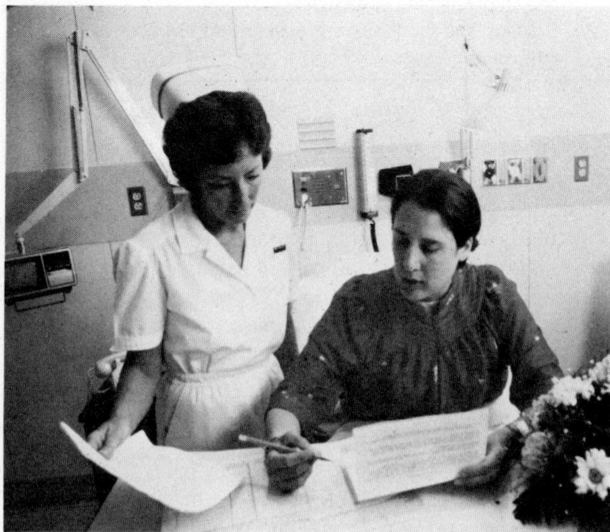

FIGURE 6–2 Maintaining realistic learning goals and involving the patient in planning the course of action enhances the learning experience.

Principle #4. Relate New Information to Previous Learning

Matching new information to familiar or previously learned material is more likely to result in successful learning. The nurse who is planning to teach a patient about his illness or how to manage his care after discharge from the hospital needs to assess what the patient has been told about his disease, whether he has had previous experience with treatment recommendations, and how well he managed this

TABLE 6–2
Patient Teaching Goals and Objectives

Goal: The patient will lose weight.
Objective: The patient will lose 5 lb (2.27 kg) in 1 month while following an 1800-calorie diet.

Goal: The patient will increase physical activity.
Objective: The patient will walk 1 mile in 20 min before dinner each evening.

Goal: The patient will plan a site-rotation plan for insulin injections.
Objective: Given anatomical drawings of possible injection sites, the patient will mark sites for self-injections of insulin for 1 month, taking into account the
1. Number of injections to be administered each day
2. Condition of the skin and underlying tissue
3. Accessibility of the site

Goal: The patient will be prepared to manage hypertensive medications at home.
Objective: The patient will state
1. The name of his hypertensive medication
2. The prescribed dose of medication to be taken
3. The times the medication is to be taken (associated with habitual behavior, such as brushing teeth, shaving, and eating, *etc.*)
4. The individual to be contacted if one or more doses are missed.

earlier regimen. Teaching should be planned to correct any misconceptions or misunderstandings the patient may hold about his illness, add new information as appropriate, and adapt the plan to correct previous difficulties and problems.

Principle #5. Include Significant Others

Including a family member or significant other in teaching sessions increases the likelihood of successful outcomes. In some instances it may be necessary to involve a helper who will share in care such as dressing changes, shunt care, catheter care and the administration of medications. A supportive person can also facilitate changes in behavior, such as decreasing or discontinuing smoking or taking on a new routine, such as an exercise program. In the situation of a patient on a special diet, including the person who does the grocery shopping and meal preparation in the instruction also increases the likelihood of a successful result.

Principle #6. Consider Individual Learning Strengths and Weaknesses

Assessing the patient's learning strengths and weaknesses will help you choose effective instructional activities and assist you in pacing your teaching to the patient's abilities. Information about the educational background of the patient is also essential to determining the complexity level of your teaching materials.

Sensory capabilities, particularly vision and hearing, are essential to learning. If these senses are compromised you will need to modify your teaching accordingly. Large-print materials will be helpful for the visually impaired. To assist the patient with hearing deficits it will be necessary to position yourself so that he can see your lips as you talk. Speaking clearly and slowly will also help patients keep pace with the information you are presenting.

The patient's reading ability is an important consideration if you are using written materials. Redman reports a number of studies which suggest that much of the material written for patient education surpasses the reading and comprehension skills of the persons for whom it was intended. Redman provides a guide to tools that can be used to evaluate the reading level of written teaching materials.[23]

Assessing the patient's comprehension of what has been presented is critical to effective teaching. The patient's verbal skill with medical terminology may not necessarily be a good indication of his comprehension. For example, Smeltzer found that patients with hypertension used common medical terms associated with their illness but did not have an understanding of what these terms meant.[27] Open-ended questions such as "What is your understanding of your illness?" or "How does your medicine help you?" will help you determine your patient's understanding of the pathophysiology and management of his illness.

Principle #7. Choose Appropriate Instructional Strategies

In addition to written material and the sharing of verbal information, today's instructional technology presents a variety of audiovisual materials from which to choose. Considering the learner's preferences in this area may serve as a guide. Age may be a key variable in this choice. A young person with experience in self-directed learning from film, slides, or audiotapes may enjoy learning from a variety of audiovisual instructional approaches, whereas another individual, an older patient perhaps, without this type of educational experience may prefer a more traditional one-to-one didactic information-sharing approach.

Considering the goals of learning may also help you choose an appropriate instructional method. If the goal requires the learning of a new skill, then one-to-one instruction including demonstration will be the method of choice. If the learning goal involves a change in behavior, then a contract—delineating what the patient will do and what the nurse will do to support this change—may be the best choice. If the patient is adjusting to a newly diagnosed illness, group meetings with individuals encountering similar experiences can provide opportunities for the patient's sharing of feelings and lead to the realization that he is not alone with his particular health problem.

Principle #8. Provide for Practice and Feedback

Patients, particularly in the learning of technical skills, will need to practice their new activities. As a teacher you will need to break the skill into its component parts, demonstrate the steps in the procedure, and allow for practice of each of the steps. The steps in teaching a patient to draw medication into a sterile syringe are shown in Table 6–3. Your positive feedback throughout the practice sessions will help to correct performance and encourage the person to master the task (Fig. 6–3).

The opportunity to practice new social skills can be critical to the successful accomplishment of lifestyle change. For example, role-playing the refusal of a food item forbidden from his diet may help a patient anticipate a difficult social situation. Choosing appropriate food items from the menu of a favorite restaurant may also help a patient adapt to a dietary change.

TABLE 6–3
Steps to be Completed to Draw Medication from Vial into Sterile Syringe

1. Identify sterile parts of the equipment (syringe, needle, and medication vial).
2. Identify the amount of medicaiton to be withdrawn.
3. Mark the level (line) on syringe that corresponds to the amount of medication to be withdrawn.
4. Fill syringe with air to appropriate mark.
5. Cleanse vial stopper with antiseptic-soaked cotton pledget.
6. Insert needle into vial stopper.
7. Inject air into vial.
8. Keeping needle tip below level of fluid, withdraw appropriate amount of medication into syringe.
9. Remove needle from vial.
10. Check to see that correct amount of medication is in syringe.
11. Expel excess air/medication from syringe.

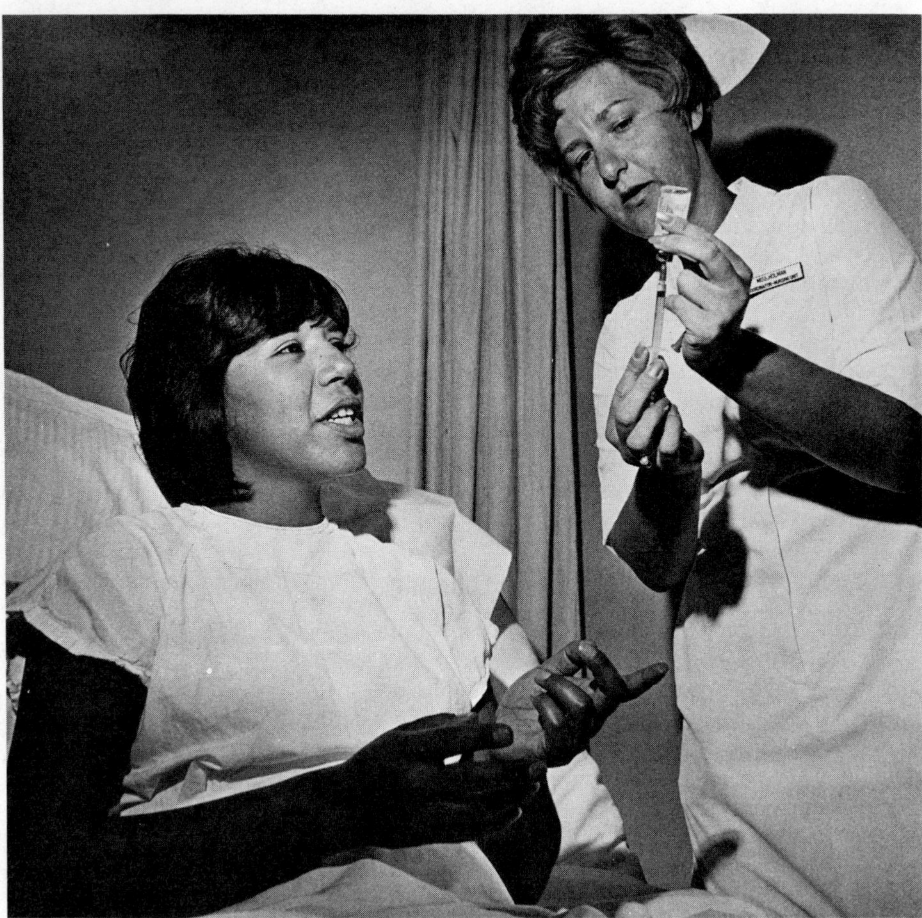

FIGURE 6–3 Demonstration is one approach to health education. In this instance, the nurse is teaching the method for preparing and giving an injection.

Haynes and Sackett suggest that long-term lifestyle changes are the hardest to maintain.[11] Some occasional failure is to be expected with patients who must follow a lifelong treatment regimen. Validating how a patient is progressing may help to identify problems and promote corrective action before serious difficulties are experienced. Questions such as "How has this new treatment helped you? What benefits are you seeing? What difficulties are you experiencing?" will help the patient to assess his progress and identify problems he may be having. If a patient is experiencing failure with a treatment plan, it is important to help that person identify what went wrong and how he might handle the situation next time. In these situations a nonjudgmental approach on the part of the nurse coupled with encouragement to continue with the program is important feedback.

Accomplishing the Task

The nurse accomplishes her role in patient education by using the steps in the nursing process described in Chapter 2. As she implements her rôle as patient teacher, the nurse assesses and diagnoses the patient's learning needs, plans and implements teaching strategies, and evaluates the results of this instruction. The following example is presented to illustrate the application of the steps in this process as well as the use of teaching principles in a patient education situation.

Ms. C.J. is a 55-year-old black female whose hypertension was first noted while she was hospitalized for a hysterectomy. She has been referred to a neighborhood clinic for further evaluation and management of her hypertension. Her blood pressure today at the clinic (average of 3 readings) is 154/98. She is given a prescription for 50 mg hydrochlorothiazide to be taken daily. Her weight is 165 lb (75 kg), height 62 inches (157 cm). You are the nurse in the clinic and Ms. C.J. is referred to you for teaching about the management of her hypertension. You learn the following information as you complete your initial interview and review her chart.

Assessment General health good, no evidence of sequelae from hypertension. Separated from husband, lives in apartment with 15-year-old daughter. Employed as a cook at a lunch counter. Completed 10th grade in high school. Mother died of a cerebrovascular accident (CVA) at age 60. Mild presbyopia, wears glasses for reading. Hearing normal. Salts food when cooking and again at the table. Cooks breakfast and dinner at home and eats a salad for lunch at the restaurant where she works. No regular exercise pattern. As you talk with her she says: "I need to take care of this high blood pressure. I don't want to have a stroke like my mother. I wonder if this problem runs in my family. Do you think my daughter will have high blood pressure too? How is this medicine going to help my blood pressure? The doctor said the salt in my diet might have something to do with all of this."

Based on your assessment data you formulate the following diagnoses:

Diagnoses (1) Ready to learn (based on verbalized questions) about management (medication and diet) of hypertension

(2) Knowledge deficit regarding

(a) Dietary management of hypertension

(b) Role of medication in the management of hypertension

(c) Role of heredity in the incidence of hypertension

(3) Fear of CVA secondary to hypertension

Plan As you consider your approach with Ms. C.J. you decide that you will want to meet her expressed concerns by providing information that answers her questions and reassures her about the positive outcomes of treatment. Her sensory abilities and educational background suggest you can use visual and written materials in a one-to-one discussion format. As you interact with Ms. C.J. you explain (using posters) what hypertension is and how it can damage her body if untreated. You reassure her that with treatment she can enjoy a normal life span. You explain how the prescribed medication and diet will help control her blood pressure. You give her pamphlets (written at the 8th-grade level) to read and suggest that she writes down questions to bring for discussion at her next clinic appointment. You talk with her about having her daughter's blood pressure checked by the nurse at the high school she attends. You want to establish realistic goals for Ms. C.J. to work towards during the next month, goals with which she is likely to experience some success. Together the two of you decide on the following plan for her to work towards.

Goal: Take medication regularly.

Objective: Ms. C.J. will take her medication at 7:00 AM each morning before she eats breakfast.

Goal: Reduce sodium intake.

Objective: Ms. C.J. will decrease the amount of salt she uses in cooking by one half and will avoid salting her food at the table.

Evaluation At her clinic appointment 1 month later Ms. C.J.'s blood pressure is 145/95 and she has lost 5 lb (2.27 kg). You provide positive feedback in the form of praise and she indicates pleasure with the progress towards her goals. She expresses interest in learning more about the management of hypertension and would like to meet others with this problem. You refer her to evening support group sessions held at the clinic for patients where films, formal presentations, and informal discussions are provided about the management of hypertension.

References

1. American Nurses' Association: The Professional Nurse and Health Education. Kansas City, American Nurses' Association, 1975
2. American Nurses' Association: Model Nurse Practice Act. Kansas City, American Nurses' Association, 1979
3. Ausubel DP: Educational Psychology: A Cognitive View. New York, Holt, Rinehart and Winston, 1968
4. Bandura A, Walters R: Social Learning and Personality Development. New York, Holt, Rinehart & Winston, 1963
5. Beauchaine DA: Memory Dysfunction Associated with Halothane Anesthesia. Unpublished Master's thesis, University of Washington, Seattle, 1979
6. Bille D. A study of patients' knowledge in relation to teaching format and compliance. Supervisor Nurse 8:55, 1977
7. Bruner JS: Toward a Theory of Instruction. Cambridge, Harvard University Press, 1966
8. Devine EC, Cook TD: A meta-analytic analysis of effects of psychoeducational intervention on length of post-surgical hospital stay. Nurs Res 5:267, 1983
9. Dodd ML: Self-care for side effects in cancer chemotherapy: An assessment of nursing interventions (Part II). Cancer Nurs 1:63, 1983
10. Fortmann SP, Williams PT, Hulley SB et al: Effect of health education on dietary behavior: The Stanford three-community study. Am J Clin Nutr 34:2030, 1981
11. Haynes RB, Taylor DW, Sackett D: Compliance in Health Care. Baltimore, The Johns Hopkins University Press, 1979
12. Hulka B, Cassel JC, Kupper LL et al: Communication, compliance and concordance between physicians and patients with prescribed medications. Am J Public Health 9:847, 1976
13. Jenkins B, Kent S, Mayberry JF et al: Patient's evaluation of a post-myocardial infarction teaching programme administered by nurses. Postgrad Med J 700:108, 1984
14. Knowles M: The Modern Practice of Adult Education. New York, Association Press, 1980
15. Mager RF: Preparing Instructional Objectives. Palo Alto, Fearon Publishers, 1962
16. Marlatt GA: Relapse prevention: A self-control program for the treatment of addictive behaviors. In Marlatt GA, Gordon JR (eds): A Self-Control Strategy for the Maintenance of Behavior Change. New York, Guilford Press, 1983
17. Maslow A: Motivation and Personality. New York, Harper & Row, 1970
18. Meyer R, Latz P: What open heart surgery patients want to know. Am J Nurs 9:158, 1979
19. Miller L, Goldstein J: More efficient care of diabetic patients in a county hospital setting. N Engl J Med 26:1388, 1972
20. Morisky DE, Levin DM, Green LW et al: Five-year blood pressure

control and mortality following health education for hypertensive patients. Am J Public Health 2:153, 1983

21. O'Neill LA: Effect of halothane anesthesia on postoperative memory. Unpublished Master's thesis, University of Washington, Seattle, 1977
22. Perry J: Effectiveness of teaching in the rehabilitation of patients with chronic bronchitis and emphysema. Nurs Res 4:219, 1981
23. Redman B: The Process of Patient Education. St Louis, CV Mosby, 1984
24. Rehm SJ, Weinstein AJ: Home intravenous antibiotic therapy: A team approach. Ann Intern Med 3:388, 1983
25. Skinner BF: The Technology of Teaching. Des Moines, The Meredith Corporation, 1968
26. Shaffer FA: A nursing perspective of the DRG world: Part I. Nursing and Health Care 1:48, 1984
27. Smeltzer C: Hypertensive patients' understanding of terminology. Heart Lung 3:498, 1980
28. Vickery DM, Kalmer H, Lowry D et al: Effect of a self-care education program on medical visits. JAMA 21:2952, 1983
29. Wesley JR: Home parenteral nutrition: Indications, principles, and cost-effectiveness. Compr Ther 4:29, 1983
30. White MJ: Effect of Halothane Anesthesia on Postoperative Memory. Unpublished Master's thesis, University of Washington, Seattle, 1975

Chapter 7

Stress

Vivian C. Wolf-Wilets

The symptoms of stress are present everywhere in our society. Toffler indicates that changes in advanced technological societies are happening so rapidly that they are exceeding our capacity for adaptation, even by those of us who grow up in technological socieities.[41] These rapid changes and their concomitant requirements for adaptation have also been associated with the increased probability of developing an illness. Holmes and Rahe developed an instrument entitled the Schedule of Recent Experiences.[18] This questionnaire asks if an individual has had changes such as the death of a spouse, a divorce, marriage, retirement from work, or detention in jail. It has been found that some of these events are much more stressful than others; for example, the death of a spouse is considered the most stressful event across a number of countries, such as Japan and the United States.[17] On the basis of previous research, each of these events is given a different weighted score (Table 7–1). As the total number of points increases, indicating that either more life changes or the more stressful life changes have occurred, the probability of illness also increases. For example, if individuals had between 150 and 200 Life Change Units (LCUs), 37% of these people had an associated health change. Those individuals with LCUs between 200 and 299 had a 51% incidence of health change; finally, persons with 300 LCUs or more had a 79% incidence of health change.[17] Because life changes can have such a powerful effect on health, Holmes has developed a list of suggestions that he feels will help anyone cope with life changes.[16] These are listed in Table 7–2.

If stress is occurring everywhere and if it can be powerful enough to cause death or health problems, then as nurses it is important that we study what stress is and its physical and psychological manifestations. This chapter will review concepts of stress and provide the background for reducing stress both in ourselves as nurses and in our patients.

History of Stress Theory

A brief history of the study of stress begins with Cannon in 1925, who was experimenting in the laboratory by exposing subjects to cold, oxygen deprivation, and blood loss. He was exploring what he termed the "fight–flight reaction." Does the organism, in the face of being under stress, "fight" to resist such forces or does it try to run away from them, termed "flight"?[6]

A few years later, another investigator began looking at other body reactions to adverse stimuli. In 1936 Hans Selye described some of the general body reactions that occurred when he injected rats with extracts of cattle ovaries.[34] The body of the animal responded in the following ways: (1) the adrenal cortex became enlarged; (2) the thymus, spleen, and

TABLE 7–1
Social Readjustment Rating Scale

Rank	Life Event	Mean Value	Rank	Life Event	Mean Value
1	Death of spouse	100	24	Trouble with in-laws	29
2	Divorce	73	25	Outstanding personal achievement	28
3	Marital separation	65	26	Wife begins or stops work	26
4	Jail term	63	27	Begin or end school	26
5	Death of close family member	63	28	Change in living conditions	25
6	Personal injury or illness	53	29	Revision of personal habits	24
7	Marriage	50	30	Trouble with boss	23
8	Fired at work	47	31	Change in work hours or conditions	20
9	Marital reconciliation	45	32	Change in residence	20
10	Retirement	45	33	Change in schools	20
11	Change in health of family member	44	34	Change in recreation	19
12	Pregnancy	40	35	Change in church activities	19
13	Sex difficulties	39	36	Change in social activities	18
14	Gain of new family member	39	37	Mortgage or loan less than $10,000	17
15	Business readjustment	39	38	Change in sleeping habits	16
16	Change in financial state	38	39	Change in number of family get-togethers	15
17	Death of close friend	37	40	Change in eating habits	15
18	Change to different line of work	36	41	Vacation	13
19	Change in number of arguments with spouse	35	42	Christmas	12
20	Mortgage over $10,000	31	43	Minor violations of the law	11
21	Foreclosure of mortgage or loan	30			
22	Change in responsibilities at work	29			
23	Son or daughter leaving home	29			

Holmes TH, Rahe RH: The social readjustment scale. Reprinted with permission from J Psychosom Res 11:213–218. Copyright 1968, Pergamon Press, Ltd.

TABLE 7–2
Suggestions to Decrease the Stress of Life Changes

- Become familiar with the life events and the amount of change they require.
- With practice you can recognize when a life event happens.
- Think about the meaning of the event for you and try to identify some of the feelings you experience.
- Think about the different ways you might best adjust to the event.
- Take your time in arriving at decisions.
- Anticipate life changes and plan for them well in advance if possible.
- Pace yourself. It can be done even if you are in a hurry.
- Look at the accomplishments of a task as a part of daily living and avoid looking at such an achievement as a "stopping point" or a time for letting down.

(Holmes T: Life situations, emotions and disease. Psychosomatics 19:754, 1978)

lymph nodes with all other lymphatic structures shrank; and (3) deep bleeding ulcers appeared in the stomach and upper intestine. These physiological changes were caused by stressors which Selye defined as agents or conditions that bring about changes requiring adaptation in the organism. He defined stress as "the rate of wear and tear caused by life."[37]

Selye described the reaction to stress as the *General Adaptation Syndrome* (GAS), which has three stages. First, there is a perception either consciously or unconsciously of a stressor and a need to act. This alerts the organism to a need to change. This first stage is called the "alarm stage." In the second stage, the pituitary gland secretes the adrenocorticotropic hormone (ACTH), which stimulates the adrenal cortex to produce corticoids. The glucocorticoids, such as cortisone, inhibit tissue inflammation; in contrast, the mineralocorticoids promote inflammation. Selye saw these hormones as "allowing the body to defend its tissues by inflammation or to surrender them by inhibiting inflammation."[36] He termed this second stage "the resistance stage."

If the demands continue or increase, the body may go into the third stage in which it becomes exhausted and is overwhelmed. This can lead to disease or death. This stage is called "exhaustion."

Stressors can be both positive and negative in that each may require adaptation. Selye called pleasant events "eustress," from the Greek prefix "eu-" meaning "good or positive."[35] An example might be going on a vacation that is pleasant but might be stressful. Negative events are called "distress." Examples might be failing a nursing course, losing your job, or becoming injured.

Selye feels that we each have a limited amount of two types of adaptive energy that are used when adapting to stress. *Superficial adaptive energy,* which is used when adapting to stress, is immediately available on demand as a bank checking account would be. It can be easily drawn upon as needed. In contrast, *deep adaptive energy* is like selling our most precious possessions; if too much of it is required, it will lead to the stage of exhaustion or death. Low adaptive energy increases the body's susceptibility to stressors such as infections.

Whereas Cannon had studied the sympathetic adrenal medullary system involved in fight–flight, Selye had studied the pituitary adrenocortical response involved in some stress reactions. These fields existed separately for many years and have now, in the last 20 years, been the subject of intensive combined research on the physiology of emotional stress. This research is leading us to answer questions such as, What are the variations in stress response to different psychological challenges and how do the brain and body respond to them?

Model of the Physiology of Emotional Stress

Henry and Ely, drawing on the work of Mason and colleagues, have provided a very interesting model for summarizing current research on emotional stress.[13,24,25] It is shown in Figure 7–1 and will be used as the basis for discussing the physiology of emotional stress.

Beginning at the top of the model (Fig. 7–1), when stimuli are perceived as stressful, the higher cortical centers can use coping patterns to keep the rest of the body from proceeding to a generalized stress reaction. For example, Mason found that in monkeys exposed to conditions such as cold, heat, and fasting, the more general adaptation response will not occur if emotional arousal is carefully avoided.[25] Bourne found that the urinary levels of 17-hydroxycorticosterone were higher in medical corpsmen on noncombat days than on combat days and were even lower than in civilian populations at home. He felt this was because the corpsmen were able to successfully rationalize, with psychological defenses, their situation; they thus avoided generalizing the stress to other parts of the body such as the adrenal cortex.[4] It should be noted, as the model indicates, that early experiences and genetics may assist an individual in having these adequate psychological defenses. Social support may also help relieve some of the effects of stress.

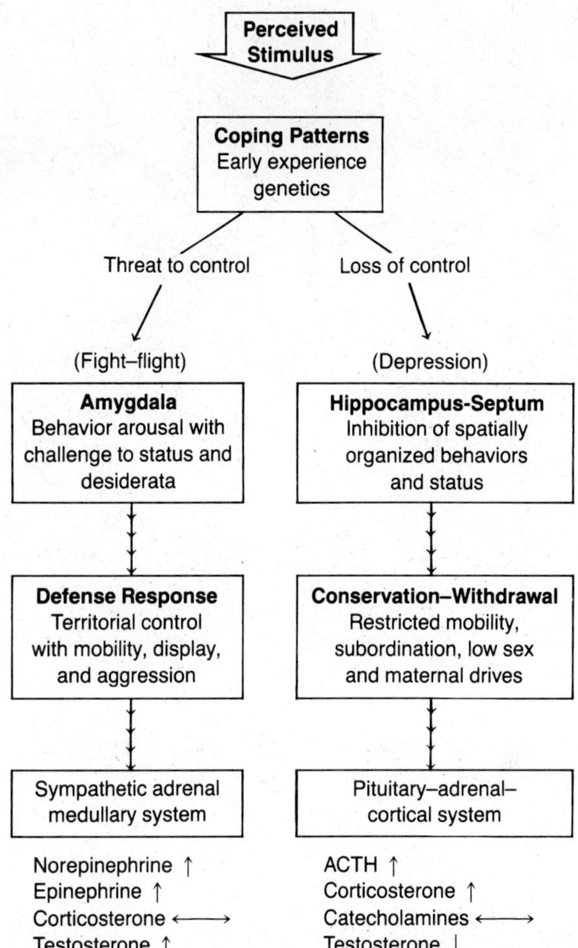

FIGURE 7–1 If the psychosocial stimulus perceived by a mammal is not inhibited at higher levels by interaction with coping patterns and social assets, a response of the limbic system will take place. The amygdala and the sympathetic adrenal–medullary system are activated when the organism is challenged in its control of the environment. But when there is loss of control and failure to meet expectations, the hippocampal pituitary–adrenal–cortical system becomes more involved as the conservation–withdrawal response is aroused. The physiological consequences of these two response patterns differ as shown; the horizontal arrow indicates no change. (Adapted from Henry JP, Stevens PM: Stress, Health, and the Social Environment, p 119. New York, Springer-Verlag, 1977)

Fight–Flight: The Amygdala and Sympathetic Adrenal Medullary System

Research is now showing that if the individual perceives a threat to his control, he will respond with a fight or flight reaction in which the amygdala is activated (Fig. 7–1, left). Figure 7–2 shows the amygdala and the hippocampus in the anatomical arrangements of the limbic system.

Animal experiments indicate that the amygdala may also be crucial in learning which stimuli are rewarding and pleasant and which are aversive and unpleasant. Kling and Steklis found that the amygdala was essential for social bonding.[20] Animal evidence also indicates that there are parts of the amygdala that may respond with different physiological patterns to fear vs. anger. In fear, the response involves vasodilation mediated by excitation of the cholinergic fibers and a modest increase in heart rate and blood pressure; pharmacologically, this is an epinephrine-related activity. In anger (a fight response), there was a sharp increase in heart rate, blood pressure, and peripheral resistance, all of which are pharmacologically related to increases in norepinephrine.[22,38] If threatened or challenged, each of us could respond in fear or anger to control a situation. Physiologically, both responses result in activation of the sympathetic nervous system and the medullary portion of the adrenal glands; levels of norepinephrine, epinephrine, and testosterone increase.

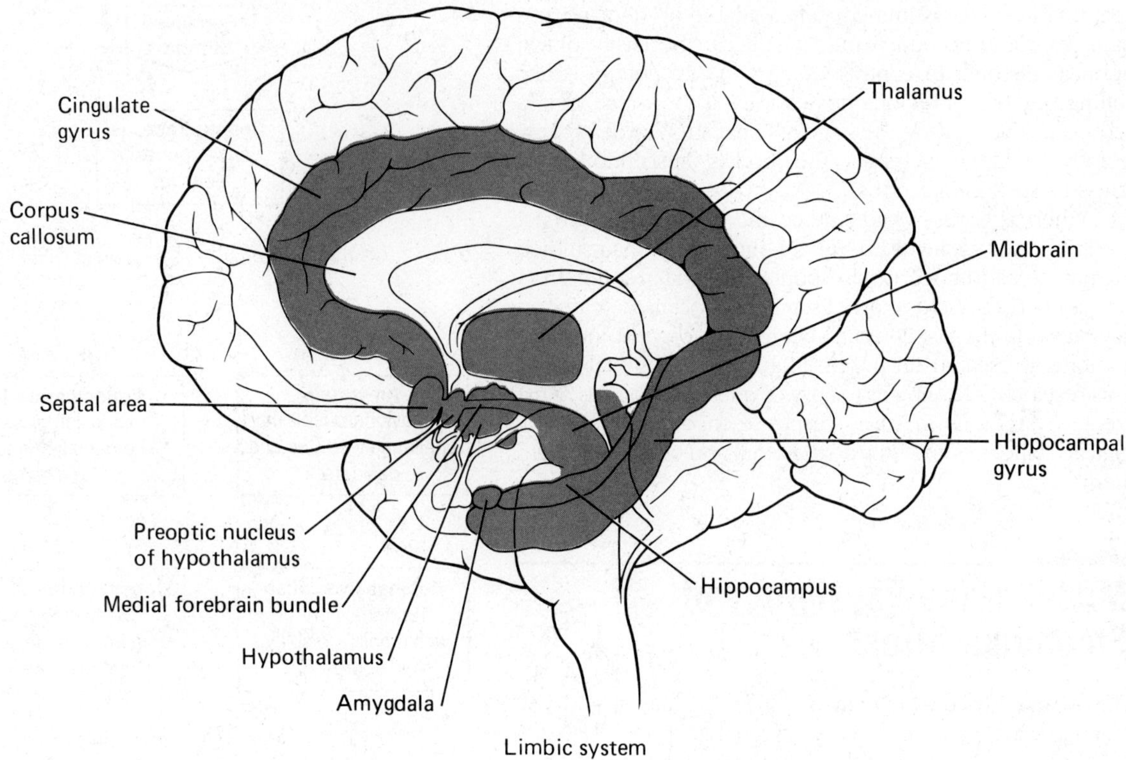

FIGURE 7–2 The limbic system, which includes the hypothalamus, governs the emotions, the viscera, and the endocrine glands. (Witherspoon JD: Human Physiology, p 112. New York, Harper & Row, 1984)

For some individuals, responding as a threat to control may also be part of their personality style. Given the same stimulus, persons with a type A behavior pattern as described by Byers and colleagues are more apt to respond with a rise in norepinephrine in the urine than are persons with a type B personality.[5] People with type A personalities speak more rapidly, use higher voice volume, are described as more competitive, and show more time urgency. They also have twice the risk of coronary heart disease.[10] People with type B personalities tend to be more relaxed, less intense, and more content.

Part of the problem of essential hypertension may be suppressed anger, guilt, and suppressed hostility.[8, 14] High renin and elevated plasma norepinephrine are also found in these essential hypertensives.[23]

Studies of monkeys indicate that impulses from the amygdala are more frequent when an animal is challenged and that they decrease when the animal engages in grooming behavior. In humans, relaxation is felt to reduce the effects of overarousal. Research by Patel and coworkers and by Benson have shown benefits from relaxation training that include decreased blood pressure, reduced cholesterol, increased skin temperature, reduced muscle tension, and decreased skin conductance (reduced perspiration).[2, 30]

Depression: The Hippocampus–Septum and the Pituitary–Adrenal–Cortical System

In contrast, a perception of loss of control as seen on the right in the model of Figure 7–1 activates the hippocampus–

septum and the pituitary–adrenal–cortical system. The hippocampus appears to have cells that can give a spatial representation. These cells can signal when a mismatch of perception vs. a former learned or known pattern occurs. It has recently been hypothesized that not only may the center be involved with physical spatial perception, but it may also be involved with learning one's place and position in a social hierarchy.[7,15]

It is hypothesized that when one becomes socially dominated or senses helplessness, impulses are transmitted from the cerebral cortex to the hippocampus, which in turn stimulates the hypothalamus. The hypothalamus then triggers the pituitary to release more adrenocorticotropic hormone (ACTH), which stimulates the adrenal cortical system. ACTH is thought to enhance learning at moderate levels, but it may also be accompanied with feelings of dejection and lack of perseverence. Overwhelming feelings of loss of control can lead to feelings of helplessness, disorientation, and depression. Seligman subjected dogs to electric shocks in situations where they cannot escape.[33] The results were that the dogs learned to be helpless and would no longer try to escape the area that was being electrically shocked when they had the opportunity. To teach them to try to escape on later trials they had to be dragged many times across a small barrier. Seligman theorizes that a similar mechanism is learned by humans and may be the underlying pattern characteristic of some depressions.[33]

In mice, ACTH has been found to decrease aggressiveness, whereas corticosterone increases submissiveness.[21] In some depressed humans there are increased daily periods of cortisol secretion and a disturbed circadian rhythm of cortisol. If these subjects are administered dexamethasone, many fail to suppress plasma cortisol; this is used as a clinical test for depression.[32]

It will be noted in Figure 7–1 that testosterone increases in the fight–flight, sympathetic adrenal–medullary reaction; in contrast, testosterone in depression (the pituitary–adrenal–cortical reaction) decreases. Some animal studies seem to indicate that testosterone may increase persistence in tasks, and focus and narrow attention.[1,40]

For the sake of differentiation an attempt has been made to define the activation of one pattern (fight–flight) vs. another (loss of control). How much either of these patterns are used will depend on the intensity of emotion felt and how frequently the events occur.

Stress Related to Disease

There are numerous instances when the two patterns both may be activated or may occur in sequence. Glass and Nixon and Bethell found that type A, coronary-prone men may start out with high norepinephrine levels, but if their struggle leads to exhaustion (loss of control) they may become depressed with an associated rise in cortisol.[12,28]

A nursing action group developed a summary chart showing some of the changes in hormones that are affected by stress and the related diseases or symptomology.[29] This chart is reproduced in Table 7–3. The list is not exhaustive but does give a broad overview of the many hormonal changes, diseases, and symptoms that may occur related to a stress reaction.

Stress reactions can be the cause of a disease or abnormal condition (primary condition) or they can result from a disease or condition (secondary condition). For example, a client who was a public health nurse came to a stress management nursing clinic. His situation was such that in order to see all his patients, he drove his car as rapidly as he could from one public health caseload family to another. He found that by ten o'clock every morning he had a severe tension headache that resulted from clenching his shoulder and neck muscles. In this case the stressors of trying to see many patients in a short time and internal worries about whether he could complete his assignment led to the development of his daily headaches. The stress reaction was the primary cause of the resulting condition. In the stress management program he was taught to plan his time differently and not to give himself negative-internal messages; he was also taught how to sense tension in his shoulder and neck muscles and how to relax these muscles even while carrying out his nursing activities. His headaches disappeared and he was able to eliminate them as long as he practiced what he had learned.

A stress reaction may also be a secondary result of another condition. Farr, Samson, and Michael studied the stress reaction that occurred in patients after surgery.[9] In this case either surgery or the condition for which the patient was having surgery could be the stressor. They found that certain circadian rhythms of the hospitalized patients were altered and uncoupled from external factors, such as time of day. For example, 17-ketosteroid excretion was elevated postoperatively. There was an elevation in the sodium–potassium excretion ratio and the timing of excretion was also disrupted. On the basis of these findings, they gave suggestions for modifying the timing of nursing care treatments or medications to help patients readjust their circadian rhythm.

Signs and Symptoms of Stress

Most of us have some symptoms of stress associated with certain activities, such as giving a speech to a group. Patients may also show signs of stress when we meet them. How can we as nurses determine what factors may act as stressors and lead to a stress reaction? One simple but very effective method is to ask the person to keep a log or diary of activities carried out in a day, what symptoms appeared at each of the recording points of the day, and how severe the symptoms were. This type of information helps determine how often symptoms occur and how severe the symptoms are. In some cases, it aids the nurse in determining the sequence and range of symptoms present in the stress reaction.

A condition that a patient might seek treatment for is Raynaud's syndrome in which the circulation in the hands may become greatly reduced, leaving the fingers and hands white and then bluish purple as the blood returns. This condition is usually made more severe by cold, but it may also occur as a psychological stress response. The activation of the sympathetic nerves reduces the diameter of the blood vessels, thus causing constriction of the circulation. In some persons this response is very pronounced. An example of a

TABLE 7–3
Diseases and Symptoms Related to Hormonal Changes from Stress

Hormonal Stress Change	*Disease/symptomatology*
↑ Gluconeogenesis (cortisol)	Diabetes mellitus Adrenal diabetes
↓ Gluconeogenesis (cortisol)	Hypoglycemia
↑ Protein catabolism (cortisol) ↓ Excretion of intracellular K^+	Muscle wasting diseases, delayed healing Hyperkalemia, cardiac arrhythmias
↑ Vasoconstriction (adrenalin, noradrenalin) ↓ Blood to kidney ↑ Renin	Hypertension Kidney disease Lactic acidosis
↑ Anti-inflammatory response (cortisol) ↓ Immunity	More infectious diseases (respiratory) Cancer (decreased surveillance of mutant neoplastic cells)
↑ Pro-inflammatory response (aldosterone)	Allergies Respiratory disease (increased inflammation) Gastrointestinal disturbance
↑ Blood clotting (adrenalin) ↑ Red blood cells	Coronary thrombosis Peripheral thrombi
↑ Myocardial contractility (adrenalin)	Raised cardiac demands
↑ Bronchial dilatation (epinephrine)	Respiratory disease (stasis of mucus leads to infection)
↑ Metabolism (adrenalin) ↓ Metabolism (noradrenalin)	Hyperthyroidism Hypothyroidism
↑ Plasma lipids (cortisol, catecholamines)	Hyperlipoproteinemia (metabolic diseases) Raised serum cholesterol, coronary artery disease Increased fat mobilization (buffalo hump, Cushing's disease)
↑ Na^+ retention, ↓ K^+ loss (aldosterone) ↑ H_2O retention ↓ Na^+ retention, ↓ K^+ loss ↓ H_2O retention	Hypertension (Cushing's disease) Cardiac arrhythmias Hypotension Muscle weakness Decreased blood volume, circulatory collapse (Addison's disease, hyperkalemia, hyponatremia, dehydration, shock)
↑ CNS stimulation (sympathetic response)	Increased confusion, depression, impulsive behavior, accident proneness, hallucinations, thought disturbances

(Nursing Action Group: Dealing with distress. Nursing Mirror, p 28, February 26, 1981)

daily log of a patient with Raynaud's syndrome is shown in Table 7–4. From this type of information the nurse can determine first that the most severe symptoms appeared when the patient fought his boss. Notice that this triggered a reaction that was even more severe than touching an extremely cold object. Dealing with customers was not stressful, but driving was. These are all very useful pieces of information when counseling this patient about stress management.

As with any problem, the history and assessment are necessary. Stressed patients might exhibit a variety of symptoms, such as cold hands or feet, tension, headache, excessive sweating, and teeth grinding. If the stress results in depression, the person may speak in a slow, hesitant voice; assume a hunched-over, tired posture; suffer from insomnia or thought disorders; and complain of subjective feelings of being down or depressed. Table 7–5 gives a quick overview of the signs and symptoms of stress.

A careful physical examination of a person showing signs of stress is particularly important if the symptoms are severe. The examination may identify or rule out possible physical causes of the symptom. For example, headaches that may appear to be stress-related could actually be caused by a brain tumor. Or a patient who appears to be depressed may have a hypothyroid condition.

TABLE 7–4
Daily Activity and Symptom Log of a Patient with Raynaud's Syndrome

Monday, August 1	*Activity*	*Symptoms*	*Rating**
10 AM	Had a knock-down-drag-out fight with my boss over my purchasing request	Both hands turned pure white and ached.	9
10:30 AM	Coffee break	Hands turned purple then pink.	2
11:30 AM	Carried frozen meat into a meat locker without gloves	Both hands turned white.	7
1–5 PM	Had appointments with several customers; sold very large meat orders	No symptoms	0
5–6 PM	Drove home in heavy freeway traffic, nearly had an accident	Hands turned white.	6

* 10 = most severe symptom; 1 = least severe symptom

TABLE 7–5
Signs and Symptoms of Stress

Fight–Flight (Threat to Control Reactions)
Cold hands and feet
Tensed muscles
Excessive sweating
Nervous movements
Tooth grinding or worn teeth
Headaches
Insomnia
Facial pain from tensing jaw muscles
Hypertension
Subjective complaints of feeling tense, nervous
Tense appearance of the jaw and facial muscles

Loss of Control (Depression Reactions)
Slowed speech
Lowered, hesitant voice
Low body mobility
Hunched-over, tired position
Subjective complaints of feeling blue, depressed, unable to concentrate
Signs of thought disorders (in severe forms)
Insomnia
Slowed metabolism
Constipation

TABLE 7–6
Tests to Diagnose Stress-Related Disease

Information	***Instruments***
Health care use	Cost of Stress (COS)
Stress symptom survey	Screening symptomatology
Affective, cognitive, behavioral and physiologic responses	Symptoms of Stress (SOS)
Life change stressor	Symptoms Checklist (SCL-90R)
Locus of control	Schedule of Recent Events (SRE)
Social networks	Personal Opinion Survey (POS)
Psychological stress response	Social Support Inventory (SSQ)
Peripheral skin temperature	Biofeedback instruments and Dinamap Blood Pressure Monitor
Muscle tension (EMG)	
Skin conductance level (SCL)	
Blood pressure/heart rate	

To help in the diagnosis of problems of stress, a variety of tests can be used. Examples of these tests are given in Table 7–6. Data from these tests frequently show that patients have had too many life changes. Counseling may help them to control or plan their lives in ways that reduce further changes. If an individual has few members in or receives little satisfaction from his social support network, ways can be explored about how he might increase the size of his network and gain more satisfaction from it. If an individual feels that others control his life, counseling can explore how he could begin to take control of his life. Many patients with problems of stress have difficulty managing their time, setting priorities, engaging in problem solving, or even understanding a good sequence of steps in problem solving. If the patient's scores show a very high level of conditions such as anger, paranoia, hostility, and depression, then intensive long-range counseling with a qualified counselor may be needed to resolve deeper conflicts appearing as a stress reaction.

In the nursing literature many conditions are being described that are basically stress reactions but are called by other names. Two conditions being described frequently in the nursing literature as occurring in nurses are termed *burnout* and *tedium.* Pines and colleagues describe burnout and tedium as characterized by physical depletion, feelings of helplessness, emotional drainage, negative self-concept, negative attitudes, and hopelessness. Burnout is the result of working with *people* who put pressure on nurses or drain their energies by being needy or creating conflicts in them.[31] Tedium is the result of *environmental* factors that create demands or conflicts. Notice that burnout is Selye's third stage of exhaustion. The nurses with more caring and giving attributes and those who are the most idealistic are the most likely to experience burnout.

Tedium is likely to occur when there is a repetitious but

demanding environment that must have your attention. If nurses and their patients can all develop mild to severe stress reactions, then we must have additional techniques to cope with our stress.

Means of Coping with or Modifying Stress

For the individual there are a number of techniques that can be used in addition to the counseling clues that have already been enumerated. As mentioned earlier, by using a *daily log* of patient activities and symptoms, the nurse may find clues as to the origin of a patient's stress-related symptoms (see Table 7–4). At times very simple solutions will bring results.

The Quieting Response

Another technique, which was developed by Charles Stroebel, is called the *quieting response.*[39] The quieting response was developed to help counteract the effects of the fight–flight reaction. When we begin tensing and notice an irritation, this increases our forehead and face muscle tension. To counteract this tension, the first step in the quieting response is to identify what is irritating us and to smile. Research has shown that smiling is associated with relaxation. By identifying the irritant we are more able to keep tension from building up unnoticed. The second step in the quieting response is to take two deep abdominal breaths. This step is designed to bring about broader body relaxation. The third step is to let the jaw go slack. Fourth, a feeling of warmth in the hands is encouraged; the purpose is to reduce sympathetic stimulation and promote warm relaxing thoughts. Finally, the phrase "Keep my body out of this" is repeated. This last step is an attempt to put a barrier between the higher centers of the brain and the rest of the body. The quieting response takes only a matter of seconds and can be used anywhere and anytime. The response should be repeated often, until it becomes a habit to relax in the face of unnecessary irritants.

Relaxation Techniques

Another set of techniques that are very useful, inexpensive to use, and relatively easy to learn are *relaxation techniques.* In 1938, Jacobson developed what he termed progressive relaxation.[19] The basic concept behind relaxation as used in stress management is that it is impossible to be tense and relaxed at the same time. In progressive relaxation an individual is taught to relax one muscle at a time. Muscle tension in the biceps, for example, can be generated by flexing the elbow. Tension should be brought to a maximum, just below the pain threshold, and then released with complete relaxation. Let the arm hang loose. Tension is then brought to a moderate level and then completely released. Finally, a barely perceived level of tension is generated and released. This same sequence is learned for every major muscle in the body, including all the facial muscles. The relaxation techniques help individuals learn to sense tension when it begins and to release it or exercise the body part. The individual who is learning relaxation must be helped to transfer his learned skills to his daily activities. Relaxation training gives the best results if it is practiced daily and if it can be done while on a break or during a large range of activities.

Many books give detailed instructions on relaxation training. Bernstein and Borkovec have even included a record in their book *Progressive Relaxation Training: A Manual for the Helping Professions.*[3] Benson has researched the effectiveness of these techniques in his book entitled *The Relaxation Response.*[2] Numerous audiotapes describe relaxation techniques. However, several notes of caution should be given to a person who is trying to learn relaxation. First, the techniques seem deceptively simple. If you can, work with an experienced group leader or teacher. He will check to see whether you are learning the techniques and are actually achieving relaxation. If you cannot afford a teacher, learning with a friend and checking each other's progress by actually feeling each other's muscle differences in tension levels and relaxation can be helpful. Second, relaxation training is only as good as the skill you achieve in it and the frequency with which it is practiced.

Biofeedback

Another major technique being used in health care is *biofeedback.* Biofeedback involves the conductance of information, by means of sensors placed on the body, about such items as muscle tension, skin temperature, and skin conductance (perspiration).[11] This information is then usually converted into a digital, auditory, or visual form. The information is seen or heard by the client on a screen or display, and can then be used by the person to change his own body state, for example, by increasing hand temperature or reducing muscle tension (Fig. 7–3). An example of a very simple biofeedback system is to hold a thermometer in your hand and learn to increase your finger temperature. In this instance, a

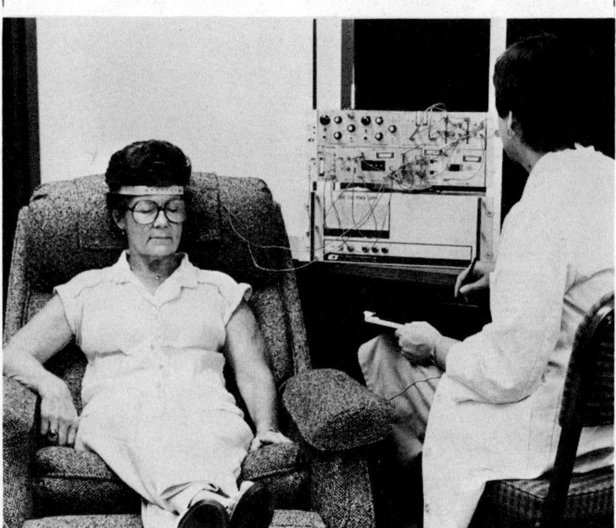

FIGURE 7–3 This patient is learning to control migraine headaches through the use of biofeedback.

thermometer is being used to give specific information that is then used cognitively by the person to change his hand temperature.

Biofeedback is used to teach subjects to control bodily functions that they might find difficult to control without precise specific information. For example, most patients with Raynaud's syndrome find it difficult to learn to control their hand temperature; with a thermistor attached to their hand and a unit that displays their digital hand temperature they can learn to increase their hand temperature at will. This control can be learned in a short time. Patients have shown significant improvement not only in their symptoms but on other psychological tests.[26, 27]

There are many types of biofeedback. Brain waves can be given as biofeedback and, through this technique, some epileptics have been taught to control their seizures. Biofeedback research data shows that some patients with hypertension who have been on medications can learn to reduce their blood pressure by using biofeedback of hand or foot temperature (monitoring of circulation). Other uses of biofeedback are still being developed. Biofeedback of nerve and muscle function is being extensively researched in rehabilitation, to help patients regain the use of body parts after a stroke.

New and exciting prospects for women's health are also emerging. For example Wolf-Wilets, Woods, and Betrus found, in a pilot study of biofeedback of skin temperature and stress management counseling, that the severity and frequency of menopausal hot flashes could be significantly reduced.[42] Dysmenorrhea has also been reduced by stress management techniques.

Summary

The most effective results in stress management are usually achieved when a combination of techniques such as counseling, relaxation training, and biofeedback are used. Stress management is an emerging form of health prevention and treatment that may improve life and may help patients avoid the necessity of taking medication. Many of the techniques can be easily learned and applied in a variety of patient care settings.

References

1. Andrew RJ, Rogers L: Testosterone, search behavior, and persistence. Nature 237:343–346, 1972
2. Benson H: The Relaxation Response. New York, William Morrow, 1975
3. Bernstein DA, Borkovec TD: Progressive Relaxation Training: A Manual for the Helping Professions. Champaign IL, Research Press, 1973
4. Bourne PG: Altered adrenal function in two combat situations in Viet Nam. In Eleftherion BE, Scott JP (eds): The Physiology of Aggression and Defeat, pp 265–290. New York, Plenum, 1971
5. Byers SO, Friedman M, Rosenman RH, Freed SC: Excretion of 3-methoxy-4-hydroxymandelic acid in men with behavior pattern associated with high incidence of coronary artery disease. Fed Proc 21(Suppl II):99–101, 1962
6. Cannon WB: Bodily Changes in Pain, Hunger, Fear and Rage: An Account of Recent Researches into the Function of Emotional Excitement, 2nd ed. New York, Appleton, 1929
7. Ely DL, Greene EG, Henry JP: Effects of hippocampal lesion on cardiovascular, adrenocortical and behavioral response patterns in mice. Physiological Behavior 18:1075–1083, 1977
8. Esler M, Julius S, Zweifler A et al: Mild high-renin essential hypertension. Neurogenic human hypertension? N Engl J Med 296:405–411, 1977
9. Farr L, Keene A, Samson D, Michael A: Alternations in circadian excretion of urinary variables and physiological indicators of stress following surgery. Nurs Res 33(3):140–146, May/June 1984
10. Friedman M, Rosenman RH: Type A Behavior and Your Heart. New York, Alfred A Knopf, 1974
11. Gaarder KR, Montgomery PS: Clinical Biofeedback: A Procedural Manual. Baltimore, Williams & Wilkins, 1977
12. Glass DC: Behavior Patterns, Stress, and Coronary Disease. Hillsdale NJ, Lawrence Erlbaum Associates, 1977
13. Henry JP, Ely DL: Physiology of emotional stress: Specific responses. J SC Med Assoc, November 1979, p 502
14. Henry JP, Meehan JP: Psychosocial stimuli, physiological specificity, and cardiovascular disease. In Weiner H, Hofer MA (eds): Brain Behavior and Bodily Disease, p 306. New York, Raven Press, 1981
15. Henry JP, Stephens PM: Stress, Health and the Social Environment: A Sociobiologic Approach to Medicine. New York, Springer-Verlag, 1977
16. Holmes T: Life situations, emotions and disease. Psychosomatics 19 (12):754, 1978
17. Holmes T, Masuda M: Life change and illness susceptibility. AAAS 94:176, 1973
18. Holmes T, Rahe R: Schedule of Recent Experiences. Copyrighted by University of Washington, School of Medicine, Department of Psychiatry, Seattle, 1967
19. Jacobson E: Progressive Relaxation. Chicago, University of Chicago Press, 1938
20. Kling A, Steklis HD: A neural substrate for affiliative behavior in nonhuman primates. Brain Behav Evol 13:216–238, 1976
21. Leshner AI, Politch JA: Hormonal control of submissiveness in mice: Irrelevance of the androgens and relevance of the pituitary-adrenal hormones. Physiological Behavior 22:531–534, 1979
22. Leyhousen P: Verhaltensstudien an Katzen. Z Tierpsychol, Suppl 2, 1960
23. McClelland DC: Inhibited power motivation and high blood pressure in men. J Abnorm Psychol 88:182–190, 1979
24. Mason JW: A review of psychoendocrine research on the pituitary-adrenal cortical system. Psychosom Med 30:576–607, 1968
25. Mason JW, Maher JT, Hartler LH et al: Selectivity of corticosteroid and catecholamine responses to various natural stimuli. In Serban G (ed): Psychopathology of Human Adaptation, pp 147–171. New York, Plenum, 1976
26. Nakagawa-Kogan H, Beaton R: Blending a conceptual model and nursing practice. In Accommodation to Self-Determination: Nursing Role in the Development of Health Care Policy, pp 28–67. Kansas City
27. Nakagawa-Kogan H, Betrus P: Self-management: A nursing mode of therapeutic influence. Advances in Nursing Science, pp 55–73, July, 1984
28. Nixon PGF, Bethell HJN: Preinfarction ill health, Am J Cardiol 33:446–449, 1974
29. Nursing Action Group: Dealing with distress. Nursing Mirror, p 28, February 26, 1981

30. Patel C, Marmot M, Terry D, Carruthers M: Coronary risk factor reduction through biofeedback-aided relaxation and mediation in patients with two or more risk factors. Circulation Abstracts 59, 60(Suppl 2):226, 1979
31. Pines A, Aronson E, Kafry D: Burnout from Tedium to Personal Growth. New York, Free Press, 1981
32. Schlesser MA, Winokur G, Sherman BM: Hypothalmic-pituitary-adrenal axis activity in depressive illness: Its relationship to classification. Arch Gen Psychiatry 37:737–743, 1980
33. Seligman MEP: Helplessness: On Depression, Development and Death. San Francisco, WH Freeman, 1975
34. Selye H: A syndrome produced by nocuous agents. Nature 138:32, 1936
35. Selye H: On the real benefits of eustress. Psychology Today Vol II (10):69, 1978
36. Selye H: Stress and Survival, p 13. Garfield C (ed). St Louis, CV Mosby, 1979
37. Selye H: The Stress of Life, revised ed, p xvi. New York, McGraw-Hill, 1976
38. Stock G, Schlor KH, Heidt H, Buss J: Psychomotor behavior and cardiovascular patterns during stimulation of the amygdala. Pflugers Arch 376:177–184, 1978
39. Stroebel C: Psychophysiological pharmacology. In Greenfield N, Sterback R (eds): Comprehensive Textbook of Psychiatry, 2nd ed. Baltimore, Williams & Wilkins, 1972
40. Thompson WR, Wright JS: Persistence in rats: Effects of testosterone. Physiological Psychology 7:291–294, 1979
41. Toffler A: Future Shock. New York, Random House, 1970
42. Wolf-Wilets V, Woods N, Betrus N: A pilot study comparing the effectiveness of skin temperature biofeedback and relaxation training for controlling menopausal hot flashes. Proceedings of the Biofeedback Society of America, 12th Annual Meeting, pp 88–91. Colorado Spring CO, 1981

Chapter 8

The Surgical Experience

Charlene Gladney Foster

Approximately 40 percent of the patients currently discharged from acute care settings have had surgery.[25] Although surgery makes some of the most valuable contributions to the health care system, it represents a substantial economic cost. To reduce this cost, short-stay or one-day surgical units are now being opened in an attempt to provide adequate surgical and postoperative care. These surgicenters may be independent or affiliated with traditional hospital settings. Although the same principles of safety and comfort apply in both settings, early recovery and adequate instruction become the central focus of concern for the short-stay patient. The scope of surgical nursing must now incorporate outpatient care along with the traditional skills of crisis intervention, asepsis, surgical assistance, life support and postoperative management.

Types of Surgery

Surgery may be done for many reasons. Usually it is performed because more conservative intervention is ineffective in achieving the desired health goals. The purposes of surgery have been listed as

- Diagnostic, such as scoping or biopsy
- Explorative, that is, determining the nature and extent of the disease, as with laparotomy
- Curative, including most dissections like cholecystectomies or appendectomy
- Constructive as in congenital deformities like cleft palate
- Reconstructive, such as cosmetic surgery or joint replacement
- Palliative, that is, to relieving symptoms, such as with gastrostomy tube placement or tracheostomy

In addition, surgeries may be classified in terms of the degree of patient risk as minor, major, or emergency surgery.

Informed Consent

Because surgery involves body intrusion and disruption beyond medical intervention, all surgical procedures require a separate informed consent. The nurse is no longer an observer in the legal arena of patients' rights. As independent professionals, nurses share the responsibility and liability for the patients' understanding and granting of permission prior to any surgical intervention. It may be argued that 'true' informed consent without influence is impossible at a time of crisis. However, the right to refuse all or part of a treatment or intervention at any point during the process should be made clear to the patient. Each separate surgical procedure requires written permission. The procedure should be stated in lay language, not medical terminology. The identity of the person who will perform the surgery must be stated. Understanding and acceptance of specifically stated risks and possible outcomes are part of the form. The signature of the patient or court-appointed guardian (except parent of a minor) is witnessed by the surgeon and one other party, frequently the nurse. In cases of emergency, the physician and institution assume the risk of no consent to save life or limb. The patient cannot have sedatives, analgesics, alcohol, or depressants prior to signing the permission. Consent for anesthesia, including technique and possible complications, may be included on the surgical permit form or on a separate form. Both surgery and anesthesia constitute legal contracts between the patient and the surgeon or anesthesiologist. Careful attention to detail will protect both the patient and the physician.[3,27,31,35]

Preparing the Patient for Surgery

The Psychological Aspects of Surgery

Surgery elicits the stress response both physiologically and emotionally. Even elective or so-called minor procedures involve an invasion and disruption of body and mind. *Fears* that are commonly associated with surgery and anesthesia are known to include the following:

1. Loss of control is associated primarily with anesthesia. General anesthesia elicits thoughts of uncontrolled actions and verbalizations. Patients frequently speak of "saying something I shouldn't." Regional or local anesthesia is stressful because it places the total responsibility or emotional reaction on the *patient* at a time when he is experiencing an extreme *threat*.
2. Fear of pain from inadequate anesthesia or postoperative analgesia is common.
3. Separation of the patient from his usual support group, such as spouse or parents, at a time when support is needed the most can be frightening. In addition, the strange attire and environment of the operating room suite makes separation from the familiar even greater.
4. Fear of disfigurement is always a factor, especially in cosmetic surgery or radical dissections.
5. Fear of death is always present and constitutes a realistic threat. Although surgery and anesthesia have progressed dramatically, the possibility of death is always present when patients are anesthetized and body integrity is broken.
6. Fear of loss of a part of the body may exist, such as in amputation and hysterectomy.

Although normal and substantiated, these fears can influence the course of anesthesia and even postoperative recovery.[32] An extremely anxious person requires greater amounts of drugs for anesthesia induction. Cardiovascular status can be affected by the increase in endogenous catecholamines elicited by the stress. Asthmatic attacks occur more frequently with increased stress. Preoperative evaluation, support, and instruction can reduce the stress level. In addition, preoperative instruction and preparation have been shown to reduce the postoperative analgesia requirements, increase compliance with postoperative instructions, and even influence the discharge date.[9,16,22,32,38]

Psychological preparation can be either supportive or informative, or a combination of the two. Determining the patient's coping method is the first step in determining the action to be taken. Many patients wish to know every detail, whereas others waive any and all explanations. Patients that seemingly have low anxiety (avoidance) may show little interest in discussing their thoughts on surgery. At the other end is the 'vigilant' patient wishing to discuss everything in great detail.[6] Factors that influence coping methods include nationality, age, and previous experiences of surgery and pain. Considering all these factors, the nursing role in preoperative preparation is to determine the patient's coping method and ability and to provide instruction based on his needs. The nurse then can provide support either openly with physical and verbal measures or subtly by reinforcing the patient's coping strengths (Fig. 8–1). Surgery is a crisis. It is imperative that the locus of control of emotion and coping remain with the patient. Emotional intervention at this time must be totally supportive and not curative. If more in-depth intervention is needed, consultation with appropriate psychiatric sources should be made. Elective surgery may need to be postponed until the patient is better able to cope.

Physiological Assessment and Preoperative History

Surgery represents a twofold threat to body integrity. Anesthesia works through neurological impairment, while at the same time cardiovascular, respiratory, and metabolic activity is usually depressed. Surgical trauma is due to tissue dissection, mechanical disruption, and histological changes during

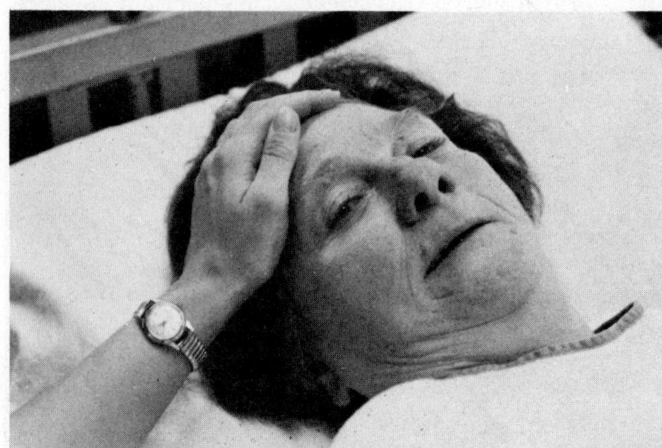

FIGURE 8–1 Some patients require psychosocial support to help reinforce their coping strengths.

the procedure. The body will respond as to any trauma of the same magnitude no matter what the setting.

Adequate preoperative preparation along with aseptic technique and better anesthesia agents and their monitoring have reduced surgical mortality. At present the operative mortality for a healthy patient having elective surgery is approximately 1 : 10,000.[10] General factors that affect mortality include the nature of the disease necessitating the operation, underlying diseases, nutritional status, urgency of the operation, and patient age.[1] Patient risk status has been roughly defined by the American Society of Anesthesiologists (ASA), and ASA classifications are given to surgical patients as follows:

I. Healthy
II. Mild systemic disease
III. Severe systemic disease
IV. Systemic disorder—imminent life threat
V. Moribund
E. Emergency placed in front of the other classifications, (*e.g.,* E.II)

Preoperative evaluation begins with patient and family history. The nurse may play a role in history taking. Many hospitals require that the operating room, recovery room, or critical care nurse see the patient before surgery whether on the unit or in a clinic setting. The preoperative visit allows for data gathering as well as for providing information and establishing rapport. Standard history forms are helpful but do not replace the need for an interview.

The preoperative history may be incorporated with the medical history or treated separately, but it should include information on the following:

- Previous anesthetic complications
- Medications
- Cardiovascular system
- Respiratory system
- Hydration and nutritional status
- Endocrine disorders
- Integumentary and skeletal status
- Oral and dental status

Previous Anesthetic Complications

Previous anesthetic complications of both the patient and any of his family should be recorded. Family response to anesthesia may reveal pertinent family traits, including pseudocholinesterase deficiencies (slow to breathe after anesthesia) or malignant hyperthermia (hypermetabolic response). A history of alcohol or drug abuse will influence the course of anesthesia.

Medications

The nurse should get information on medications currently used, both prescribed and over-the-counter, their purpose, and dose. Commonly used drugs include the following:

1. Aspirin—80% unexpected bleeding is due to aspirin use.[10]
2. Steroids, including inhalants, must be continued to prevent cardiovascular collapse.
3. Antidepressants, particularly the tricyclics, may interfere with blood pressure maintenance during anesthesia.
4. Cardiac drugs, such as digitalis preparations, calcium channel blockers, and nitroglycerine may need to be continued through the operative period.
5. Antihypertensives, such as propanalol and clonidine, must be continued up until the time of surgery to prevent rebound hypertension during surgery.
6. Diuretics may be potassium depleting. Serum potassium should be 3 to 4 meq/liter unless the patient is also on digitalis, when 3.5 meq/liter is an acceptable low level.

Cardiovascular System Assessment

Problems with cardiac status are responsible for approximately 30% of operative deaths.[10] Patients who have had a myocardial infarction in the 6 months prior to surgery are at highest risk. Patients with a history of rheumatic or valvular heart disease will need antibiotic prophylaxis to prevent myocarditis after procedures in which bacterial-containing cavities, such as the oropharyngeal/nasopharyngeal, bowel, and genitourinary tracts, are disrupted. Patients with prosthetic cardiac valves may be on anticoagulants and would need vitamin K preoperatively to prevent bleeding. Patients with angina, congestive heart failure, hypertension, dysrrhythmias, peripheral vascular disease, and pacemakers should be examined and evaluated by an internist before surgery. Any person with a suspicious medical history and, in some institutions, any one over age 40 should have had an electrocardiogram within 1 month of surgery, and cardiology consulted if indicated. Emergency surgery has four times the incidence of postoperative myocardial infarction as nonemergency surgery, and thus indicates an even more urgent need for proper preoperative evaluation.[10]

Respiratory System Assessment

When asking about respiratory status, smoking history should be obtained. If the patient has 'quit', determine how long ago. It is always advisable for patients to discontinue smoking at least 3 weeks preoperatively. Carboxyhemoglobin level is increased in smokers, causing interference with oxygen delivery while at the same time mucociliary transport is decreased, allowing for buildup of secretions that predispose to atelectasis and infection. Acute respiratory infections may require antibiotics and further evaluation (see Chap. 31 on respiratory disease). Patients with chronic disease such as emphysema, bronchitis, or asthma may require bronchodilator inhalants or medication preoperatively as well as throughout the surgical procedure. Chest x-ray studies, pulmonary screening tests, and arterial blood gas analysis may be indicated for preoperative evaluation. Instruction in and supervision of adequate pulmonary hygiene, coughing, deep breathing exercises, and incentive spirometry will aid during surgery as well as in the postoperative recovery period (Fig. 8–2). Other factors that influence pulmonary function and postoperative recovery are obesity, which reduces lung volume, and the location of the surgical site

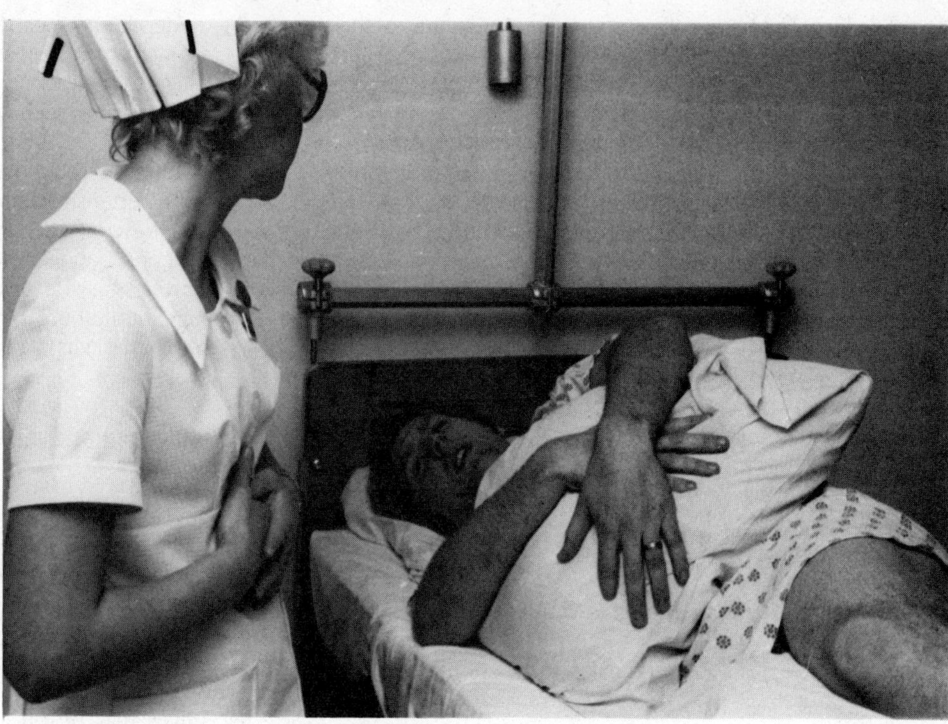

FIGURE 8–2 Teaching the techniques used in postoperative coughing is part of preoperative patient teaching.

which may cause splinting during inhalation, as can occur with thoracotomy and in an upper abdominal procedure.

Hydration and Nutritional Status

Patients often come to surgery in a volume-depleted state that is due to a number of factors, including the following:

- Gastrointestinal losses through vomiting or diarrhea
- Hemorrhage
- Third space sequestration of fluids in burns, bowel obstructions, peritonitis, and pancreatitis
- Use of diuretics
- Chronic underlying disease

Evaluation is made on clinical symptoms of postural hypotensions, loss of skin turgor, and serum electrolytes. Any patient on diuretics, with chronic disease, or who has suffered prolonged gastrointestinal losses, should undergo serum electrolyte analysis. Patients who have had nothing to eat or drink (npo) for 12 hours or more should be started on intravenous fluid infusions. Preoperative basic fluid maintenance is 4 ml/kg/hour in the absence of cardiac or renal disease. Isotonic solutions are usually ordered and nondiabetic patients should receive at least 2 liters of 5% dextrose a day.

Nutritional status plays a vital role in patient stability during surgery as well as in postoperative recovery. Preoperative malnutrition may be evaluated in the patient history by noting weight loss, low serum albumin (less than 3.5 g/100 ml) and depression of total lymphocytic count (less than 1500 per ml). Target groups include the elderly, oncology patients, renal dialysis patients, patients with metabolic disorders, patients with chronic respiratory states, and patients suffering from catabolic conditions.

Correction involves dietary supplement if time permits, feeding supplementation by nasogastric or gastrostomy tube or, if necessary, total parenteral nutrition. Total parenteral nutrition (TPN) is being used more frequently for preoperative preparation of the chronically ill.

Endocrine Disorders

Some endocrine disorders require special preoperative considerations. For patients with insulin-dependent diabetes, blood glucose levels should be above 100 mg/dl, preferably 150 to 200 mg/dl. Preoperative insulin maintenance while the patient is npo frequently requires reducing the dosage plus giving IV fluids containing dextrose. Hypothyroidism requiring emergency surgery predisposes the patient to hypotension, hypoventilation, and hyponatremia. Levothyroxine may be ordered preoperatively. Surgical stress may precipitate a thyroid storm in a patient who has hyperthyroidism. Propylthiouracil and possibly propanalol may be needed before surgery. Patients suffering adrenal suppression (Addison's disease), requiring steroid therapy for more than 2 weeks during the previous 6 months, require steroid maintenance throughout the surgical period to prevent cardiovascular collapse. Steroid maintenance is frequently required in patients suffering from asthma or ulcerative colitis. Patients with hepatic disease may require a vitamin K supplement to prevent bleeding during surgery.

Integumentary and Skeletal Status

Careful examination of the skin and skin assessment should be done on all patients, but especially on those who have vascular disease or diabetes mellitus, or those who are elderly, obese, or very thin. Pressure areas have been known to develop during surgery that lasted just 2 hours.[19] Patients should be questioned about skin conditions. For example, if a patient has eczema, skin preparation may require specific solutions. Total joint replacements and previous insertion of metal plates or pins should be documented, since this will influence the placement of cautery grounding pads during the surgical procedure. In addition, patients with an artificial eye or prior surgical placement of an intraocular lens need special treatment by surgery personnel. Patients with musculoskeletal disorders need extensive evaluation to determine the safe range of joint mobility for preventing intraoperative injury and to providing proper support. Again, careful documentation needs to be made for this information to be used by surgery personnel.

Oral and Dental Assessment

Oral and dental assessment includes noting the presence of dentures, partial dental plates, and dental caries as well as noting the general oral condition. This information is most valuable to anesthesia personnel. Dentures may be ordered left in, but this requires specific consultation with an anesthesiologist.

Preoperative Nursing Goals

Preoperative preparation usually begins the evening before surgery. Preoperative nursing goals include the following:

1. To promote rest and comfort
2. To reduce the incidence of postoperative wound infection
3. To reduce the incidence of intraoperative contamination of the lungs and the surgical field by the gastrointestinal contents
4. To prepare the patient for anesthesia

Goal 1: To Promote Rest and Comfort

Promotion of rest and comfort involves the psychological preparation discussed previously. Allowing the family or significant other to remain with the patient even after the patient is asleep and including them in preoperative instruction and teaching is considered standard practice. Providing adequate pain relief is necessary to ensure stress reduction and patient cooperation. Sedatives for sleep are usually ordered the night before surgery and frequently include the following:

- Medium and long-acting barbiturates:
  - Secobarbital (Seconal) 100 mg
  - Pentobarbital (Nembutal) 50 mg–100 mg
- Hypnotics, such as the benzodiazepines:
  - Flurazepam (Dalmane) 15 mg–30 mg
  - Diazepam (Valium) 5 mg–10 mg

Administration of sedatives should always be followed by evaluation for effectiveness and respiratory depression. Repeat doses may be ordered for these medications; however, effective analgesia and emotional support may be sufficient. Body temperature should be maintained at normothermic levels. Mild hyperthermia not only contributes to discomfort but can initiate stress responses. Sedatives and analgesics will reduce body temperature.[26,30]

Goal 2: To Reduce the Incidence of Postoperative Wound Infection

Skin preparation is a major part of preoperative care. The surgical skin preparation is frequently done the evening before surgery. Shaving the skin has been a major focus of controversy.[22] Hair follicles harbor bacteria, yet shaving the skin disrupts skin flora that can allow an increase in bacteria at the surgical site. Use of depilatory creams and electric shaving have been explored. At this time the decision remains with the surgeon. His preference should be known and specifically ordered for each procedure.

Skin preparation of various parts of the body for surgery is shown in Figure 8–3. It should be noted that the diagrams show a margin for shaving that is much wider than the surgical incision site. Good lighting, a sharp razor, and diligent care must be used to prevent knicks, cuts, or abrasions, which can also contribute to infection. In some institutions the shave preparation is done after the patient reaches the operating room area to reduce the chance of contamination from prolonged exposure preoperatively. Requiring the patient to take an early morning shower using an antibacterial soap is done in some institutions. Orthopedic patients may require a special, 10-minute scrub of the surgical area, followed by wrapping the area in a sterile towel until the patient reaches the operating room.

Goal 3: To Reduce the Incidence of Intraoperative Contamination of Lungs and Surgical Field by the Gastrointestinal Contents

Food and Fluid Restrictions. Food and fluids, including water, are withheld for 8 to 10 hours prior to the time of surgery. Patients are usually placed npo after midnight. Patients admitted the day of surgery must receive both careful verbal and detailed written instruction about withholding foods and fluids. Many patients fail to understand that failure to comply with this practice results in an increased chance for aspiration during anesthesia, which can cause chemical burn to the lungs. In addition, surgery may have to be postponed, which is costly and inconvenient. Infants under 1 year are allowed either formula feeding or sweet, clear liquids up to 4 hours before surgery. Trauma patients (including those with fractured bones) and patients requiring acute bowel resection or emergency abdominal procedures should be kept npo and placed on intravenous fluids (no matter how much time there is before surgery) because their gastrointestinal motility is reduced and gastric regurgitation is possible.

Nasogastric Tubes. Nasogastric tubes may be inserted just before surgery in patients having major abdominal pro-

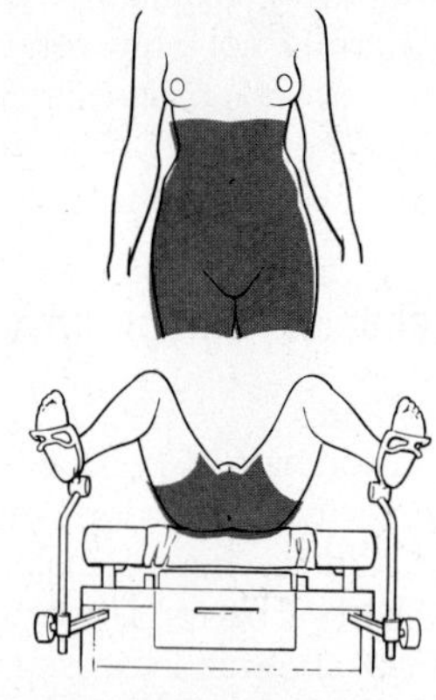

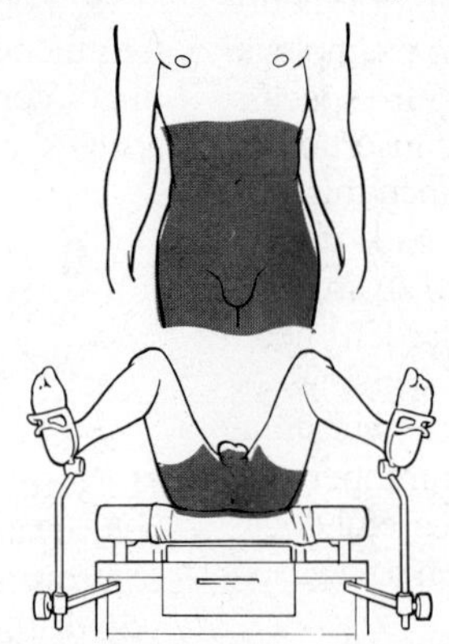

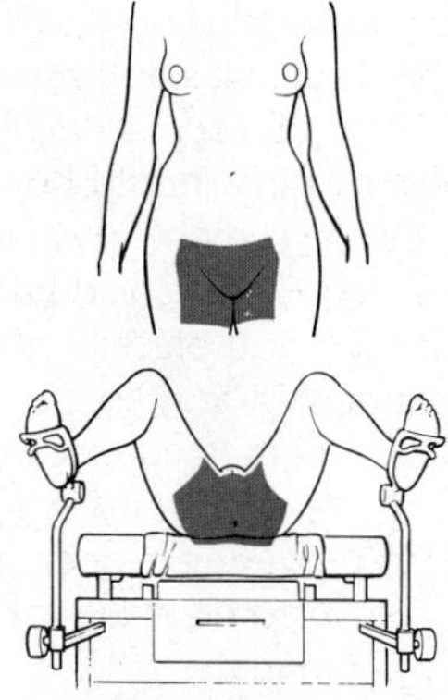

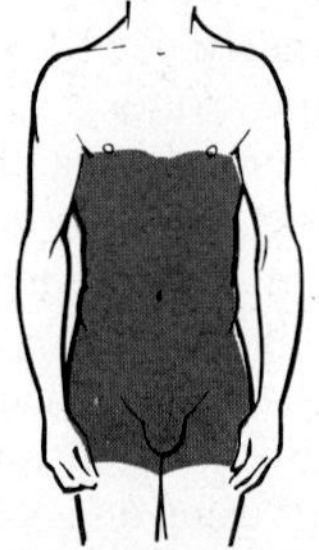

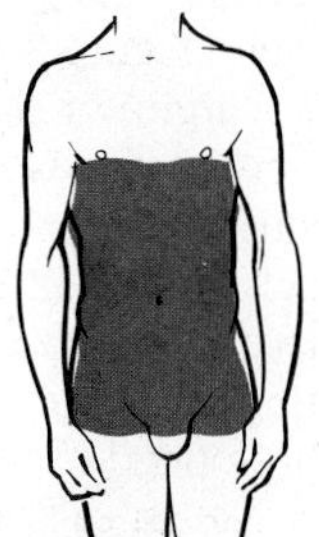

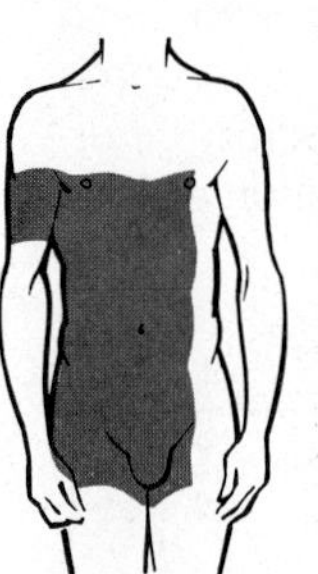

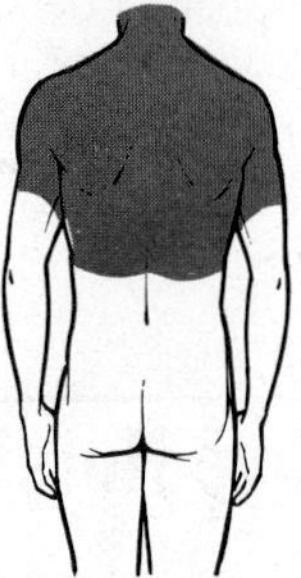

FIGURE 8–3 Skin preparation for surgery. (After Pate MO: The Preparation Manual. Long Island City, New York, Edward Weck & Co)

cedures; however, this is done more frequently after anesthesia induction. Patients who are pregnant or obese or who have a history of hiatal hernia, hyperacidity, gastric ulcer, or gastric reflux should be considered as having full stomachs. Cimetidine, 300 mg along with Maalox or Bicitra, are frequently ordered for these patients.

Laxatives and Enemas. Laxatives or enemas are ordered the evening before surgery for most abdominal surgeries, including hysterectomy and nephrectomy. In addition, enemas may be ordered the morning of surgery for operations, such as hemorrhoidectomy, that involve the gastrointestinal tract.

Preoperative Bowel Preparation. Preoperative bowel preparation is done on patients having major abdominal bowel procedures, such as bowel resection or abdominal perineal resections. Preparation to clear and clean the bowel usually begins 2 days before surgery. A typical regimen is as follows:

- Clear liquids only are allowed for 48 hours prior to surgery.
- Antibiotics such as neomycin or occasionally the cephalasporins are ordered 24 hours before surgery.
- Laxatives, enemas until clear, or three serial enemas are administered the evening before surgery or, occasionally, the morning of surgery.

During surgery, bowel activity is slowed by surgical exposure to air and manipulation, therefore reducing the bowel contents can relieve postoperative discomfort. In addition, a decompressed bowel will aid in surgical exposure and reduce the possibility of bowel perforation during the procedure.

Preparation for Surgery of Lower Extremity

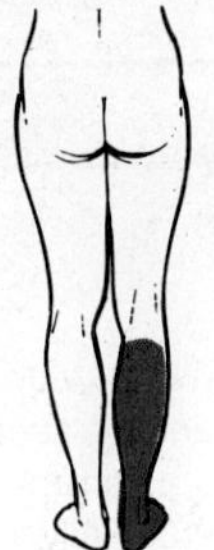

Ankle, foot, toes

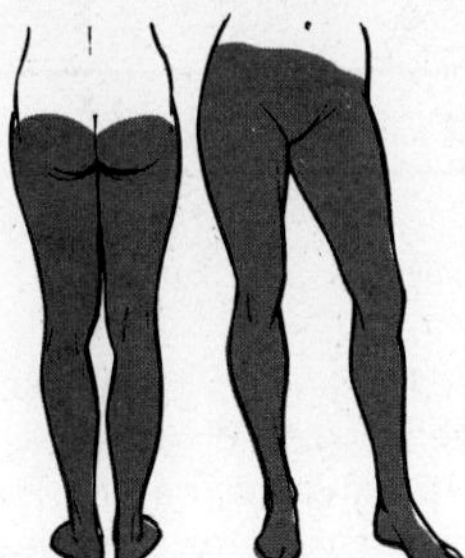

Bilateral leg surgery: varicose vein ligation, skin and bone grafts

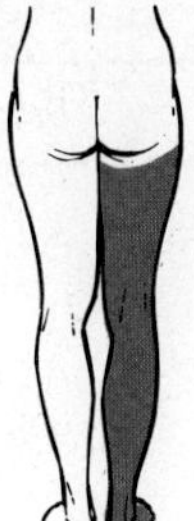

Foot, lower leg

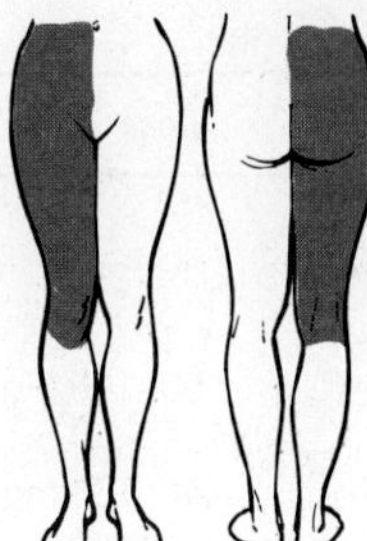

Unilateral hip operations

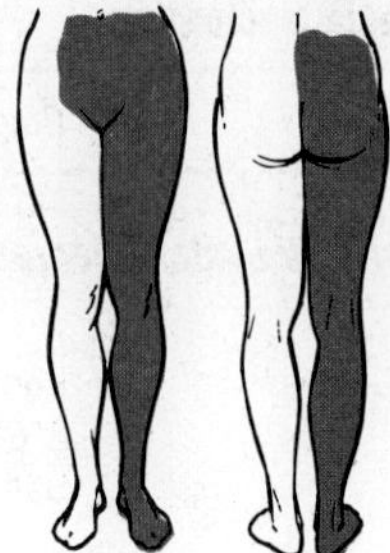

Unilateral hip and thigh operations

Preparation for Chest, Shoulder and Thoracoabdominal Operations

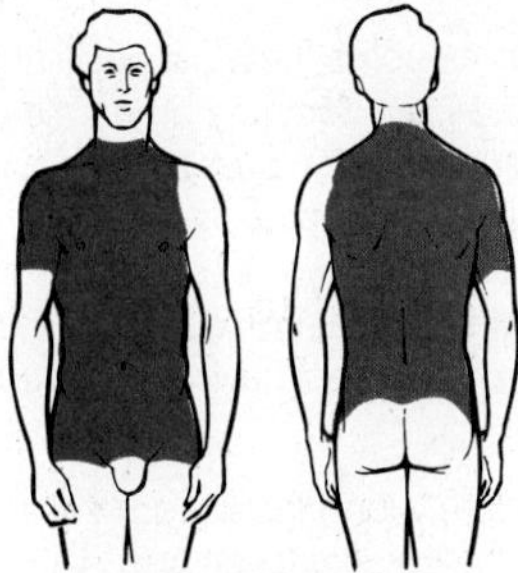

Chest, shoulders, and upper arms: for unilateral chest operations and radical mastectomies

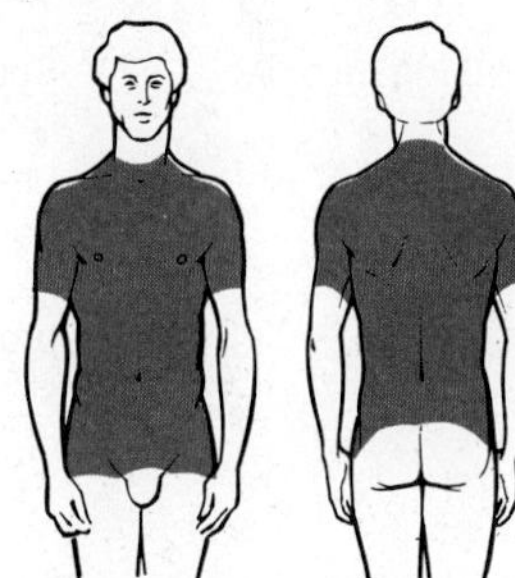

Combined thoracoabdominal operations: chest and shoulders are prepared bilaterally, anteriorly, and posteriorly

FIGURE 8–3, contd.

Goal 4: To Prepare the Patient for Anesthesia

Unless the patient is having a local anesthetic, preanesthesia medication is ordered by the anesthesia department. The objectives of preanesthesia medication are as follows:

1. To provide mental and emotional relaxation (including cortical sedation and amnesia)
2. To reduce the metabolic rate, which in turn reduces oxygen need and diminishes anesthesia requirements
3. To reduce sensory input; this may include analgesia for experienced or anticipated pain
4. To antagonize adverse autonomic nervous system stresses by lowering vagal tone, lowering catecholamine release, reducing salivary and intestinal secretions, and reducing airway irritability.

Patients who have been interviewed preoperatively and given instructions have been found to need less preanesthesia medication than patients not prepared in this manner.[32] An anesthesia "pre-med" is usually not ordered in the elderly, the very young (under 1 year), neurologically impaired patients, patients who are in shock, patients with intracranial pathology, or those suffering from pulmonary dysfunction. Premedications are not usually given to outpatients, since many of these drugs cause drowsiness for hours.

Ideally, a premedication should provide drowsiness and tranquility, yet allow the patient to be responsive and easily aroused. Drugs that are frequently used for preoperative medication can be found in Table 8–1.

IMMEDIATE PATIENT PREPARATION

1. Check the chart thoroughly for signed surgical permit, physician examination, and laboratory values.

TABLE 8–1
Preanesthesia Medication

	Drug	*Dose*	*Description*
Central Nervous System Depressants			
Sedatives			
Barbiturates	Phenobarbital (Nembutal) Secobarbital (Seconal)	50–100 mg po or IM 50–100 mg po or IM	An increased tolerance to barbiturates is seen with patients on tranquilizers or alcohol. A decreased tolerance is seen in the cachetic or elderly patient. The barbiturates provide no analgesia and may create disorientation, especially in the young or elderly.
Tranquilizers			
Butyrophenones	Droperidol (Inapsine)	2.5–5.0 mg IM	Used frequently in combination with the narcotic fentanyl (Sublimaze) for "neurolept anesthesia." In the preoperative period, by itself, it provides sedation with little cardiovascular or respiratory depression and provides excellent antiemetic action in preventing nausea. Restlessness and occasionally disorientation can occur, particularly in children.
Benzodiazepines	Diazepam (Valium)	5–10 mg po or IM	Benzodiazepines have become the most popular tranquilizers. Diazepam (Valium) is a common premedicant. Can be given intravenously although it precipitates, causes pain, and occasionally venothrombosis. Has little effect on respiration, does not cause drowsiness, allays anxiety, and produces pronounced amnesia. Postoperative instructions should not be given to the patient having received a dose of diazepam.
	Lorazepam (Ativan)	1–2 mg po	Lorazepam is an extremely long-lasting drug. Can be given intravenously without the irritation seen with diazepam. Prolonged drowsiness and amnesia has limited the use of this drug to minor operative procedures.
	Chlordiazepoxide (Librium)	5–10 mg po	Chlordiazepoxide has less amnesia effect than diazepam.
	Triazolam (Halcion)	0.25–0.5 mg po	Triazolam is a newer drug in the U.S. With a short half-life (1.5–5.0 hr), it may become popular with use for outpatient surgery.
Narcotics			
Opiods	Morphine Meperidine (Demerol)	6–10 mg IM 50–100 mg IM	Opiods' advantages include excellent analgesia with some euphoria and tranquility. Disadvantages are that they can stimulate smooth muscle spasms of bile duct and cause bronchial constriction. Therefore, they are contraindicated in patients with asthma and with biliary duct stones. Nausea and vomiting, even in the postoperative period, are common after these drugs are given. Hypotension can occur as they release histamine and frequently a reflex tachycardia occurs to compensate. The opiods are strong respiratory depressants affecting both rate and depth (rate may be decreased by half). Respiratory depression may last as long as 2–3 hr after administration.
Synthetic opiods	Fentanyl (Sublimaze)	0.05–0.1 mg IM (1–2 ml)	A much shorter acting agent than the opiods, fentanyl provides less smooth-muscle stimulation and less cardiovascular and respiratory depression. It is also not as effective for severe pain.
Anticholinergics*			
	Atropine	0.4–0.6 mg IM or IV	Produces some central nervous system effects such as blurred vision and occasionally light-headedness. Atropine depresses the sweating mechanism, causing flushing and sometimes an increase in body temperature.

(Continued)

TABLE 8–1
Preanesthesia Medication (*Continued*)

	Drug	*Dose*	*Description*
	Scopolamine	0.4–0.6 mg IM	Used more in the past especially in obstetrics for "twilight sleep." The central nervous system effecfs are much greater than with atropine, and excitement can occur, especially when used with barbiturates. Scopolamine provides more drying effects (antisialogogue) than atropine, but is less effective in treating bradycardia.
	Glycopyrrolate (Robinul)	0.2–0.4 mg IM or IV	Newer agent; no central nervous system effect and has less heart rate effect than atropine.
Antihistamines			
Histamine 1 (H_1) Antagonists	Hydroxyzine (Vistaril)	50–150 mg IM	Provides atropinelike effects such as reduced secretions and antinausea (antiemetic) while providing variable sedation. There is minimal circulatory and respiratory depression. Vistaril is painful when injected alone. It has been found that mixing it with a narcotic in the same syringe reduces the pain.
	Promethazine (Phenergan)	50 mg IM	Both promethazine and diphenhydramine provide slight sedation with some atropinelike effects.
	Diphenhydramine (Benadryl)	10–50 mg IM or IV	
Histamine 2 (H_2) Antagonists	Cimetidine (Tagamet)	300 mg po, 1–1½ hr preoperative or IV diluted to 100 ml and given slowly over 15 min	Used most frequently for reducing gastric acidity and gastric fluid volume. Cimetidine may be ordered for any patient who is pregnant or obese, or has a history of hiatal hernia, gastric reflux, or gastric ulcers. In addition it is used for patients scheduled for spinal chymopapain injection in an attempt to reduce incidence of anaphylactoid reaction.

*Earlier anesthetic agents produced profound respiratory tract secretions. The newer agents produce fewer secretions and are less irritating but still have increased vagal activity through gastrointestinal stimulation and occasionally bradycardia. Anticholinergic drugs are used to counteract these effects.

A typical preoperative order on call to the operating room is
Valium: 10 mg po at 0600 with sips of water
Morphine: 10 mg IM } on call to OR
Robinul: 0.2 mg IM }

a. Heart and lung examinations must have been done within 48 hours to 2 weeks, depending on the institution; the results must be documented and charted before the patient goes to the operating room. Some institutions also require a current chest x-ray film and electrocardiogram on all patients.
b. Laboratory values minimally include a complete blood count:
   Hemoglobin, 10 g/100 ml
   Hematocrit, 30 vol %
   White count listed
   Urinalysis
c. Bleeding times may be routine or as indicated by condition or surgery. Drawing blood must be done prior to all vascular, thyroid, kidney, or prostate surgery; it is frequently done for any major abdominal surgery for thorocotomy, and for hysterectomy patients. Blood will most likely be ordered or a sample of blood drawn for purposes of blood typing and cross-matching if needed.

   Normal bleeding time = 30 sec to 5 min
   Coagulation or clotting time = 5 to 10 min

   Check the physician's orders to see if blood is ordered and determine if it has arrived prior to surgery.
d. Check the orders for specific medications or procedures. Make sure they are done and charted.

2. Have the patient void or insert a urinary catheter if ordered.
3. Have the patient remove all jewelry, dentures, prosthetics, contact lenses, and cosmetics.
4. Provide a clean gown.
5. Administer the preoperative medication. Children must have a family member or nurse in attendance at all times after the premedication is given. THE PATIENT MUST ALWAYS BE ASSESSED FOR RESPIRATORY AND MENTAL DEPRESSION BEFORE AND AT 10 AND 20 MINUTES AFTER THE PREMEDICATION IS GIVEN. The nurse should never hesitate to withhold the preoperative medication if the patient seems

Preanesthesia Record

Directions: Fill out on all preanesthesia and pre-surgery patients. Attach to cover of patient's chart.

1. Vital Signs: T: _____ P: _____ R: _____ BP: _____ HT: _____ WT: _____
2. Consent form signed: __________ Disposal form signed: __________
3. Pre-medication: Given by: __________
4. History and physical examination date: __________
5. Laboratory work date: __________ Hgb: __________ Hct: __________
6. Skin prep completed: _____ by: __________
7. Voided: __________ Catheter in place: __________
8. Enema: __________
9. Natural teeth: __________ Denture or bridge: _____ Removed: _____
10. Contact lenses: __________ Removed: _____
11. Other prosthesis: Type: __________ Removed: _____
12. Rings taped in place: _____ Rings removed: _____
13. Pierced earrings and neck chains: __________ Removed: _____
14. Make-up removed: _____ Nail polish removed: _____
15. Clean patient gown: __________ Paper cap: _____
16. Mouth care: __________
17. Blood in Central Services: __________ Time verified: __________
    No blood ordered: __________
18. Remarks: __________
19. Signature: __________

FIGURE 8–4 Sample preanesthesia record.

unresponsive or exhibits significant respiratory or circulatory depression. If such is the case, notify the anesthesiologist immediately! Instruct the patient to remain in bed. Put up the side rails, dim the lights, provide adequate blankets, and secure the call light within the patient's reach.

6. Complete the preoperative checklist and sign your name. Attach the checklist to the chart. (A sample preanesthesia checklist is presented in Fig. 8–4.)
7. Identify the patient to whoever has come to transport the patient to surgery by matching the arm band and the chart.
8. Assist in transferring the patient to the stretcher.
9. Prepare the unit for the patient's return from surgery.

Early Postsurgery Recovery

General Postoperative Assessment

Patients in the early postoperative period are recovering from two interventions: surgical disruption of body integrity and anesthesia. Caring for patients at this vulnerable time requires knowledge of both the specific surgical procedure and the type of anesthesia and the predicted outcomes of each one. Monitoring and resuscitation skills are basic for adequate patient recovery. Patients may recover in a post-anesthesia recovery unit (PAR), an intensive care unit, or the patient's room as long as the following conditions exist:

1. A knowledgeable nurse is present at all times. The recommended ratio of nurse to patients in recovery room units is 1 : 2; with children or critically ill patients the ratio is 1 : 1.
2. The following equipment must be at the bedside:
   a. Oxygen with cannula, catheter, or mask and a means of delivering positive pressure ventilation, such as an ambu-bag and mask (Fig. 8–5)
   b. Working suction with Yankauer (tonsil) tip and catheter tip
   c. Bed with side rails
   d. IV pole
   e. Blood pressure cuff and stethoscope
   f. Emesis basin
   g. Thermometer
   h. Means for the nurse to summon help
3. The following equipment must be available on the unit (Fig. 8–6).
   a. Working laryngoscope and blades (checked monthly and dated)
   b. Variety of endotracheal tubes
   c. Emergency drugs[17]
      1. Commonly used vasopressors, such as:
         a. Ephedrine 5 mg–10 mg IV or 15 mg IM
         b. Neo-Synephrine 10 mg for IV drip

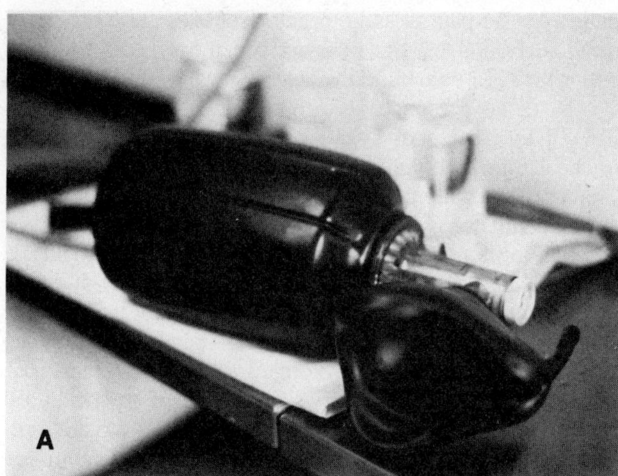

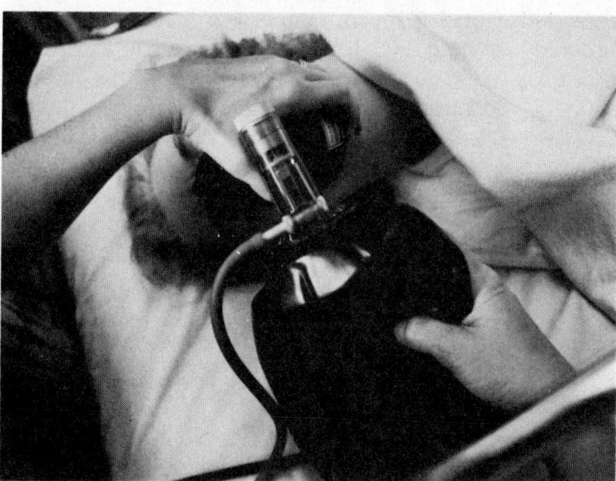

FIGURE 8–5 An Ambu bag is placed near the bedside (*A*) in case there is a need to ventilate the patient in the postoperative period (*B*).

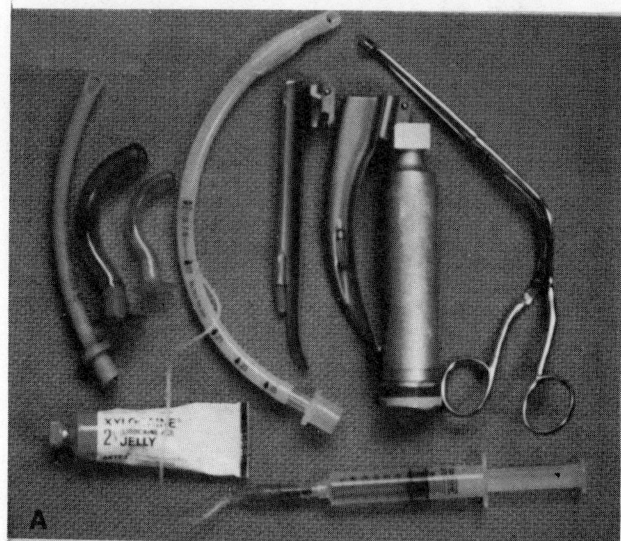

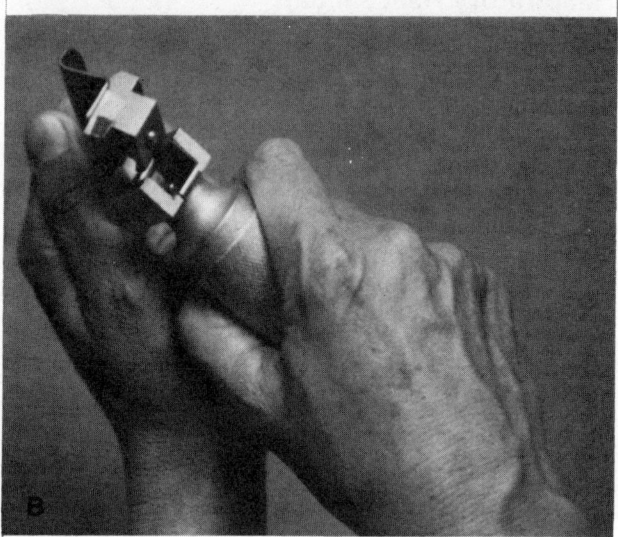

FIGURE 8–6 (*A*) Equipment necessary to maintain artificially an open airway. (*B*) Laryngoscope and blade should be checked monthly to assure they are in working order.

   c. Vasoxyl 5 mg IV bolus
2. Muscle relaxant reversal agents, such as:
   a. Edrophonium (Tensilon) 10 mg IV
   b. Neostigmine (Prostigmin) usual dose 2.5 mg IV up to 5 mg
3. Atropine, given for bradycardia, is always given with reversal agents—0.4 to 1.0 mg up to a total of 2.0 mg IV.
4. Succinylcholine (Anectine), a depolarizing muscle agent, is used for intubation, 100 mg ampules IM or IV.
5. Lidocaine, for intravenous use in cardiac arrhythmias and laryngeal irritability, 1 mg/kg IV

Patients are brought to the recovery room by the anesthetist and either the surgeon or operating room nurse. A brief report is given to the nurse in the recovery room about the surgical procedure, type of anesthesia, drugs given, intravenous fluids, blood loss, and presence of drains and catheter. The recovery room nurse immediately begins her initial patient assessment as the report is given. She then takes the initial vital signs and gives them to the anesthetist/anesthesiologist. If the patient has had a spinal block, sensory dermatome level is also checked and reported. Most recovery rooms have an anesthesiologist in charge of general PAR care. Communications regarding the patient's immediate condition are made to the anesthesiologist. The surgeon should be notified of any changes in conditions or questioned regarding general postoperative orders. Evaluation of the immediate surgical goals must be done concurrently with physical assessment; for example, pedal pulses must be taken in a patient who has had femoral artery grafts, and circulation must be checked in the extremities of patients with casts. The surgeon usually writes specific orders regarding immediate care. Antibiotics given preoperatively or during surgery should be timed from the last administration and may be required in the recovery room. Medications that the patient received preoperatively are usually resumed when the patient returns to the unit.

Postoperative Physical Assessment

Physical assessment of the patient should be done at least every 15 minutes. If drugs are given or the patient exhibits any signs of instability, more frequent evaluation is expected. Assessment is listed in the order of priority. Airway and respiratory function should always be the *first* consideration because anesthesia and adjunctive drugs can dramatically affect reflexes and respiration.

POSTOPERATIVE PHYSICAL ASSESSMENT IN ORDER OF PRIORITY

1. Respiratory assessment
2. Cardiovascular assessment
3. Body temperature assessment
4. Surgical site assessment—dressings, drains, and tubes
5. Central nervous system assessment

Respiratory Assessment

All *general* anesthetics impair respiratory function. High spinal anesthesia may also reduce respiratory effort. On entry into the recovery room, the patient's skin color should be noted.

Airway Patency

The first step of assessment is to determine airway patency. This can be done in the following ways:

1. Feeling the patient's exhaled breath against the hand or cheek remains the most reliable and easy index in determining air exchange.
2. Watching chest movements. The chest should move as a unit. Intercostal retractions or bulging, substernal retractions, abdominal breathing in opposition to the chest (rocking chair breathing) all indicate obstruction. Use of accessory respiratory muscles of the neck or nasal flaring indicate inadequate chest expansion.
3. Listening for snoring or stridor, which indicate upper airway obstruction, even if the patient "snores at home during normal sleep." Anesthetized patients are unable to change position to clear the airway as they can during normal sleep activity.
4. Checking the respiratory rate. The depth of respiration is more important than the rate. However, rates below 10 may indicate narcotic depression. Rapid rates indicate either cardiovascular compromise or increased metabolic rate and need further evaluation. Normal adult rates are between 12 to 18/minute. Children's rates decrease dramatically as they grow. For example, in an 8-lb infant the respiratory rate is about 35; in a 10-lb infant the rate is 28, until the average 1-year-old child at 20 lb has a rate of 20 and at two years old (30 lb) a rate of 18.

Airway and Endotracheal Tubes

Check the presence of a oronasal airway. The purpose of the airway is to hold the tongue forward, thus preventing upper airway obstruction (Fig. 8–7). The airway is usually expelled by the patient as he regains reflexes and consciousness. Suctioning of the pharynx can most easily be done either through or around the airway.

Note the presence of an endotracheal tube (ETT; Fig. 8–8). If the patient is breathing spontaneously, the endotracheal tube is connected to misted oxygen by way of a T-piece. If the patient is not ventilating adequately, a volume-driven ventilator is most frequently ordered. The criteria for extubation should be clearly understood: the ability to lift the head, appropriate tidal volumes (usually 10 ml/kg), and adequate blood gases. Common reasons for patients to have ETs left in place are inadequate reversal of muscle relaxants, hypothermia, major and prolonged surgical procedure, or poor preoperative respiratory status. The endotracheal tube is extremely irritating to the nasopharynx in the patient regaining consciousness. However, coughing, "hacking," or tearing from the eyes are not criteria for extubation. If the endotracheal tube is to be left in and the patient exhibits these behaviors, diazepam (Valium) or a narcotic may be ordered IV to reduce the irritation. If there are no extubation policies, specific guidelines should be given by the anesthesiologist. Most frequently, extubation is performed by the anesthesia department. IF IN DOUBT, DO NOT EXTUBATE!

A nasal endotracheal tube frequently indicates that the patient is to keep the ET tube in place. Usually nasal intubations are performed for oral or upper airway procedures or on patients with difficult oral intubations. Make certain the endotracheal tube remains secured. Hand restraints may be required for children until they can follow directions. Explaining the reason for the tube and acknowledging that the patient cannot talk reduces anxiety in many patients.

Other Respiratory Measures

Electrocardiographic monitoring should be done on all intubated patients. Auscultating for bilateral breath sounds should be done on admission to the recovery room. The tube can easily become dislodged and slip into the right mainstem bronchus, resulting in ventilation of only one lung.

Arterial blood gas analysis is indicated on all patients who require an endotracheal tube for longer than 1 hour, who have had thoracic surgery, have dusky or pale skin color, have increased agitation, or have indications of cardiovascular compromise. The nurse will order the blood gas analysis or check with the physician. After obtaining the values, she will call the results to the physician.

A *chest x-ray study* is usually done on patients who have had a thoracotomy procedure and those who are to have the endotracheal tube in place for extended periods of time, that is, hours or days. The x-ray film is checked for clarity of lung fields and tube placement.

Oxygen is administered to all new surgical patients unless otherwise indicated (such as patients with obstructive lung disease). A nasal cannula usually provides adequate delivery with a 2 liter to 4 liter flow. Additional information about oxygen therapy can be found in Chapter 27.

Respiratory Insufficiency

Respiratory insufficiency requires urgent and definitive action. The nurse should never hesitate to summon help

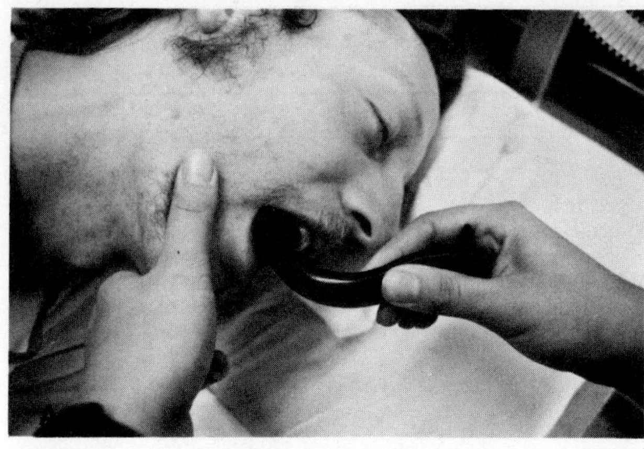

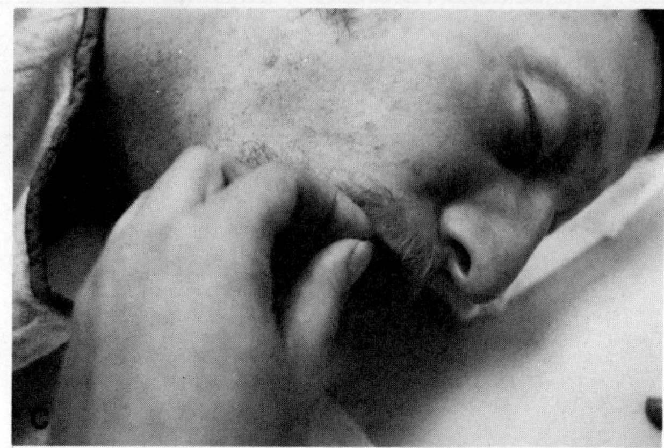

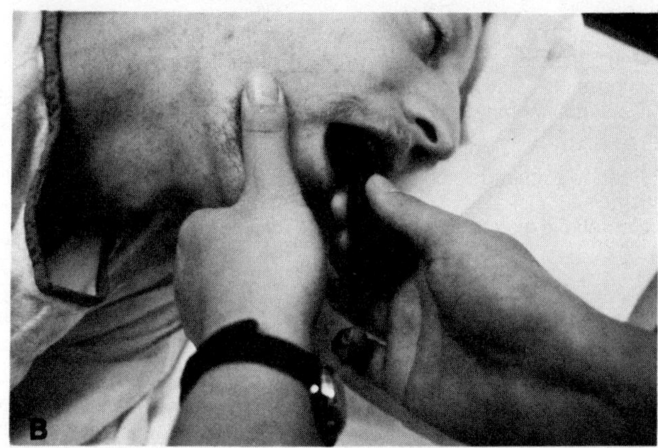

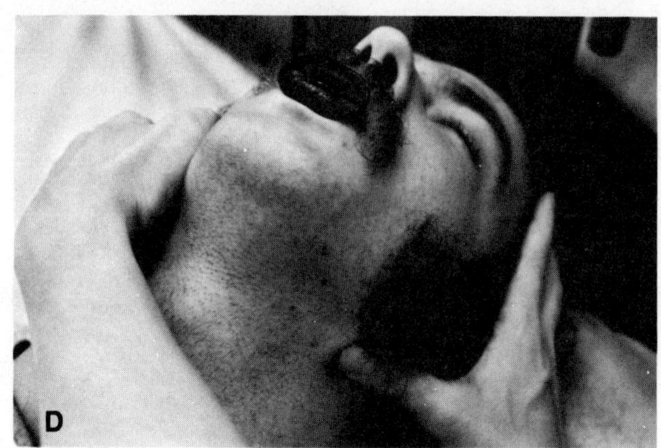

FIGURE 8–7 (*A* through *D*) Insertion of oral airway.

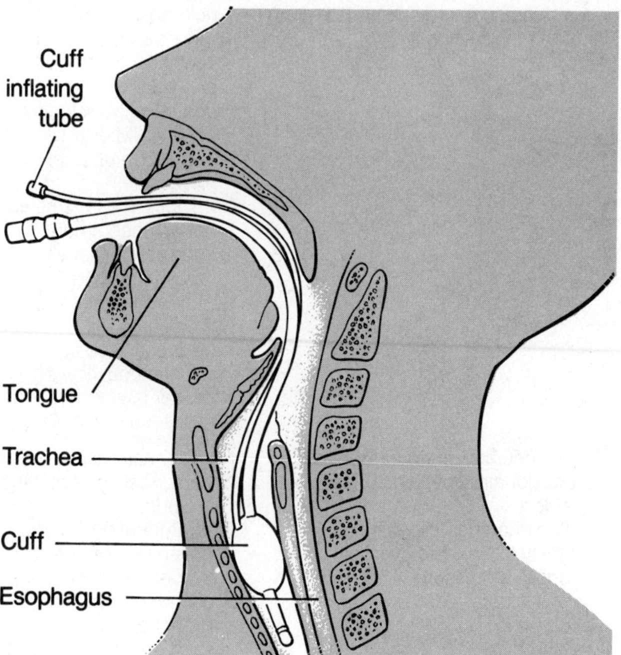

FIGURE 8–8 Diagram of endotracheal tube in position.

while continuing to maintain adequate ventilation. Table 8–2 identifies those conditions that hinder ventilation and presents the related causes, signs and actions.

Cardiovascular Assessment

The goals of cardiovascular assessment are to ensure adequate tissue perfusion and to minimize cardiac stress. Blood pressure and pulse measurements are done at least every 15 minutes in the recovery room. Sphygmomanometer blood pressure readings and radial pulse are currently considered adequate minimal measurements on most surgical patients. However, arterial lines, central venous pressure lines, and pulmonary artery wedge pressures are rapidly becoming the standard of care for many surgical patients. The recovery room nurse must possess knowledge of and skill in making these measurements to provide adequate postoperative care. Electrocardiogram monitoring is also being used more frequently in the recovery room for "routine" postoperative care and should be initiated by the nurse without hesitation or without a physician's order whenever the patient's condition is unstable.

TABLE 8–2
Respiratory Insufficiency and Management

	Cause	*Signs*	*Action*
I. **Hypoventilation** Shallow breathing resulting in inadequate exchange	Splinting from pain Narcotic or anesthetic depression Muscle weakness from "high spinal" anesthesia affecting the intercostal muscles, inadequate muscle relaxant reversal extubated too early, or recurarization	Low tidal volume (normal 10 ml/kg) Slow respiratory rate Restlessness or agitation Air hunger Low PaO_2 and high $PaCO_2$ on arterial blood gases Skin color may be pale to cyanotic.	*Determine cause* Notify anesthesiologist. Analgesia for pain Narcan if indicted for narcotic reversal Dopram (pure respiratory stimulant) occasionally used Nerve stimulator will aid in evaluating muscle paralysis. Reversal drugs or intubate, if necessary
II. **Obstruction**			
A. Tongue collapse in back of throat; commonly seen in early postoperative period	Loss of reflexes and motor tone due to anesthesia and drugs	Poor air exchange felt on hand, possibly noisy respirations Color may or may not change	Insert nasal or oral airways Hold jaw forward (Fig. 8–7).
B. Mucus or vomitus in upper airway	Accumulation of mucus in the pharynx Gastric regurgitation from full stomach (air or secretions), or patient with history of hiatal hernia	Poor air exchange with or without noise Secretions may not be seen.	Suction gently for mucus and vomitus. Be careful not to stimulate vomiting by suctioning deeply Turn patient onto right side if possible or turn head to one side. If reflexes are absent and vomitus is in the pharynx, notify the anesthesiologist *immediately* and *prepare to intubate* (Fig. 8–8).
III. **Airway Irritability**			
A. Laryngospasm: closure of vocal cords during inspiration	Laryngeal stimulation from airway or secretions on cords. Patients with history of smoking, asthma, or bronchitis are at high risk, but it can occur in all patients.	May have stridor or crowing on inspiration or may have no sound. Chest and abdomen may move in an attempt to exchange air ("rocking chair respiration").	Notify anesthesia personnel STAT. Straighten airway by holding jaw forward. Apply positive pressure ventilation with mask and bag. Prepare to give succinylcholine (IM or IV). Prepare to intubate if necessary. *Note:* Laryngospasms are not an uncommon occurrence in the recovery period. Although dangerous, the spasm will frequently subside spontaneously with proper jaw positioning and a buildup of CO_2.
B. Bronchospasm: narrowing of bronchi preventing the lungs from inflating; may be sudden, usually on induction of anesthesia, or progressive over minutes	Allergic response to drug or anesthesia. Patients with a history of asthma, pulmonary obstructive disease, or many allergies are at highest risk. Irritation of airway from suctioning or airway insertion during emergence Can occur with endotracheal tube in place (causing increased irritation)	Slight cough with no further sound Occasionally wheezing in early stage Little or no chest movement Inability to ventilate even with positive pressure	Notify anesthesia personnel immediately. Call Code. Intubate: Put on volume-driven ventilator and prepare to give aminophylline, Isuprel, bronchodilators, steroids.

Blood Pressure and Fluid Volume

Factors that affect *blood pressure* in the early postoperative period are type of anesthesia, drugs, and volume status. General anesthesia causes a reduction in vasomotor tone by centrally depressing the vital centers in the medulla. Spinal anesthesia and, to a lesser extent, epidural anesthesia lower blood pressure by direct sympathetic blockade, causing vascular dilation and peripheral pooling below the level of the block. Position alone can greatly influence blood pressure during spinal block.

Drugs such as narcotics, sedatives, and antiemetics can reduce blood pressure.

Fluid volume status of the patient frequently causes dramatic changes in blood pressure, especially in the anesthetized or medicated patient. Hypovolemia (saline deficit) can be due to a previously existing state, such as the patient having been on diuretics. Frequently it is due to inadequate fluid replacement or "third-spacing" of fluids to the extravascular space intraoperatively or to blood loss. Careful assessment is necessary before action is taken to correct the deficit. The anesthesia record will indicate the amount of intravenous fluid given intraoperatively. Most well-nourished adults come to surgery with a fluid deficit of 1000 to 1500 ml, having been npo for at least 8 hours before surgery. A more precise way of calculating fluid deficit is 1.5 to 2 ml/kg/hours npo (up to 10 hours). These calculations may have already been done by the anesthetist and may be listed on the record. The deficit is usually replaced over 3 hours, with one half given in the first hour and one quarter in the second and third hours. Fluid deficits are greater in patients who have had nasogastric suctioning, fever, bowel preps, or diuretics preoperatively.

Fluid Maintenance. In addition to making up for fluid deficit, fluid maintenance must be provided, usually at the rate of 4 ml/kg/hour during surgery. During major surgeries involving the thorax, bowel, or large vessels, the patient may have been given 10 to 15 ml/kg/hour for fluid maintenance. A patient with poor cardiac status or poor kidney function may receive as little as 2 ml/kg/hour.

Besides the fluid deficit and fluid maintenance, blood loss in the nonanemic patient is replaced with crystalloid solutions at the ratio of 1 ml blood : 3 ml crystalloid fluid. Colloids other than blood, such as plasma, 5% albumin, dextran 40, dextran 70, and hetastarch may have been used for maintaining intravascular volume instead of blood replacement or when a large amount of third-spacing is suspected in cases involving burns or the bowel, liver, or pancreas.

It is not unusual for patients to reach the recovery room still needing fluid replacement, especially in procedures lasting less than 3 hours. Intravenous fluid maintenance in the recovery room in the normovolemic patient is usually kept at 100 to 125 ml/hour for adults. Isotonic solutions such as lactated Ringer's or Polyonic R, with 1 liter of every 3 containing 5% glucose is a standard procedure. Children require much more glucose and infants should have glucose in every infusion.

Hypovolemia

Hypovolemia may be detected simply by checking urine output. The anesthesia record should indicate the half-hourly measurements during the surgical procedure. The urine collected in the bag is emptied and measured on entrance to the recovery room; half-hourly measurements should be recorded on all major surgery patients. The minimal acceptable output is 30 ml/hour. Urine output is affected by vasopressors such as dopamine and Neo-Synephrine as well as by drugs such as morphine.

A more accurate measurement of volume status is *central venous pressure* (CVP) reading. In major surgeries that may have a CVP line or a pulmonary artery catheter that has a CVP port, normal range is 5 cm to 10 cm H_2O or 6 mm Hg to 12 mm Hg. It should be kept in mind that poor cardiac function and increased pulmonary vascular resistance will give a high CVP reading.

A closing pulse pressure (a decrease in systolic and an increase in diastolic blood pressure) is frequently an early sign of hypovolemia.

Hypotension

Patients who are elderly, who have had carotid endarterectomy or a recent stroke, or who have a poor cardiac history, cannot tolerate sudden drops in blood pressure. If systolic pressure falls 20% below preoperative level (usually below 100 mmHg) or if the diastolic falls below 40 mmHg, the patient is at risk of cardiac or cerebral ischemia. If blood pressure drops below two thirds of the recognized normal levels of systolic blood pressure, a careful assessment should be made as the following steps are taken:

1. Place the patient in modified Trendelenberg position, elevating only the legs and feet. Do not place patients who have had head and neck surgery or who have increased intracranial pressure in Trendelenberg.
2. Open intravenous line at full rate.
3. Notify anesthesiologist immediately.
4. Check drains and dressing for blood loss. Consider gravity; when looking for bleeding be sure to check under the patient. Make sure all tubes are open, that is, nasogastric and chest tubes. If dressings are saturated and contain blood clots, replace them using strict aseptic technique. Estimate blood loss by weighing the saturated sponges; then weigh the dry sponges and subtract the difference. The formula is as follows:

$$1 \text{ gram adjusted sponge weight} = 1 \text{ ml blood}$$

Blood Loss

The operative and anesthesia record will indicate the amount of intraoperative blood loss. The patient's preoperative hemoglobin and hematrocrit level should be known. Healthy persons with a normal hemoglobin and hematocrit are thought to tolerate blood losses up to 20% of their blood volume. The formula for calculating the estimated blood volume is (EBV):

$$\begin{aligned} EBV &= 70 \times \text{kg body weight, adults} \\ & 80 \times \text{kg body weight, children} \\ & 65 \times \text{kg body weight, elderly (65 or older)} \end{aligned}$$

Allowable blood loss (ABL) is considered to be the amount to maintain hematocrit at 30, usually 20% loss for the healthy and 10% loss for the anemic patient. More accurate calculations may be made with the following formula:[1]

$$ABL = EBV \times \frac{\%\ Hct - 30\ (Acceptable\ Hct)}{35\ (Average\ Hct)}$$

For example, in a 70 kg man with Hct 40,

$$EBV = 70\ kg \times 70 = 4900$$

$$ABL = 4900 \times \frac{40-30}{35},\ or$$

$$4900 \times \frac{10}{35},\ or\ 1399\ ml\ ABL$$

If a *blood transfusion* is indicated, whole blood or packed red cells should be given, using a blood warmer. Transfusions should not be given through the same intravenous line as dextrose or lactated solutions. Dextrose hydrolysis cells and lactated solutions contain calcium, which can cause citrated blood to clot. The IV line should be flushed with normal saline before and after the transfusion if an existing line is used. The procedure for blood reactions should be kept in mind and the patient should be checked frequently for symptoms of hypotension, rash, chills, or fever.

Hypertension

An elevated blood pressure is frequently seen in the early postoperative period. The most frequent causes are pain, respiratory compromise, or delirium. Patients having had transurethral resections of the prostate are at risk for venous absorption of nonelectrolyte irrigating solutions at the area of resection. In these patients, central nervous system symptoms, such as a change in mental state, may precede a sudden increase in blood pressure and pulse. The condition is confirmed with low serum sodium levels, sometimes as low as 100 meq/dl. Diuretics, fluid restriction and, occasionally, hypernatremic intravenous solutions are given. An elevated blood pressure cannot be tolerated in patients with cardiac compromise, since the work of the heart is increased. Determining the cause of sudden postoperative hypertension and its early treatment is paramount.

Cardiac Monitoring

Evaluation of heart rate involves a comparison between preoperative, intraoperative, and postoperative pulse measurements. Be aware of the influence of preoperative factors such as athletic activities, medication, and anxiety state.

Bradycardia, or pulse rate less than 50, may be due to several factors. A high spinal anesthetic can cause sympathetic blockage and slow venous return with concurrent block of cardiac accelerator fibers T1–T4. Reversal of muscle relaxants used during surgery without adequate anticholinergic coverage can cause bradycardia. Reversal agents include neostigmine (Prostigmin), edrophonium (Tensilon), and pyridostigmine (Mestinon). All of the above, except edrophonium in 10-mg doses, require that atropine or glycopyrrolate (Robinul) be given to keep the pulse rate up. Vasovagal reaction is not often seen in the early postoperative period. Preoperatively, it is frequently due to anxiety. Intraoperatively, it has been associated with pain or visceral stimulation or tugging. The insertion of a nasogastric tube has been known to produce a vasovagal response. Heart block will, of course, produce bradycardia and can be associated with low blood pressure and poor cardiac output. It is hoped that a preoperative diagnosis would have been made; however, intraoperative myocardial ischemia may precipitate this condition.

NURSING INTERVENTIONS FOR BRADYCARDIA

1. Electrocardiographic monitoring is carried out for arrhythmias and continuous heart rate.
2. Frequent blood pressure measurements are taken to determine cardiac output status.
3. Atropine (0.4mg–1mg) is given intravenously or as ordered by the anesthesiologist.
4. Oxygen is administered by mask to maintain optimum delivery.

Tachycardia or a heart rate greater than 110 can be due to pain, fever, hypotension, hypoxemia, or delirium. Tachycardia increases oxygen consumption and decreases coronary artery perfusion, and it can put patients at risk for other cardiac problems. Careful evaluation is necessary to determine the cause. Nursing interventions to deal with this are the following:

1. Administer oxygen by means of a mask.
2. Take an electrocardiogram.
3. Notify anesthesiologist.

Cardiac arrhythmias are not unusual in the recovery room phase. Preventricular contractions occur frequently in the recovering patient and may be due to pain, hypoxia, or ventricular irritability. If they occur more than 5/minute, lidocaine 1 mg/kg bolus IV, may be ordered followed by a lidocaine drip if necessary. Treating the underlying cause of pain or hypoxia may alleviate the need for further drug intervention. Junctional or nodal rhythm may also frequently indicate pain. S–T changes, either elevation or depression, may indicate ischemia. Notify the anesthesiologist immediately about all arrhythmias.

Body Temperature Assessment

The goals of body temperature assessment are to prevent postoperative shivering and to maintain core body temperature within the normal range. Temperature measurements are done on all patients when admitted to PAR and every 15 minutes for patients who are shivering, have had major surgery, are children, are emaciated, are elderly, or had extremely low intraoperative temperatures. Comparisons should be made with preoperative baseline and intraoperative measurements. Core body temperature may have been measured during surgery by esophageal, tympanic membrane, rectal, or axillary probe. Comparisons are best done in the recovery room with rectal, oral, digital, or axillary (the least accurate) measurements.

Temperature monitoring in the early postoperative period can no longer be done on an occasional basis. Because of the physiological effects from deviations in body temperature, continuous temperature monitoring, both in the operating and recovery rooms, has become the standard of care.

Hypothermia

Hypothermia is a frequent intraoperative condition. Intentional intraoperative hypothermia techniques are used primarily in cardiac surgery and neurosurgery. Extracorporeal cooling of the blood and, less frequently, surface cooling with cooling blankets are used to produce temperature ranges of 24° to 28°C (75° to 83°F). Planned hypothermia allows for reduced oxygen consumption and, therefore, better tissue protection against ischemia when blood supply to major organs must be interrupted. Accidental or inadvertent hypothermia is a common occurrence during anesthesia and surgery. Loss of body temperature has been found to begin with preanesthesia medication.[26] Inactivity, lack of clothing, and vasodilating effects of the premedication all contribute to the heat loss. During surgery, all anesthesia techniques promote heat loss. General anesthesia agents obtund thermoregulatory centers in the hypothalamus and at the same time produce massive vasodilation. Spinal anesthesia produces massive vasodilation below the level of the block, thus providing a large heat gradient between the patient and the ambient air. In addition operating room temperatures usually range between 68° to 70°F (20° to 21°C) with a rapid air exchange rate. The patient is uncovered, prepped with solutions that increase the evaporative heat loss from the skin, and then has a body cavity opened or exposed that allows major heat loss directly from tissue. Patients may have core temperatures of 32°C (normal, 36.8°C) when brought to the recovery room.

There are undesirable effects associated with hypothermia. Temperatures at about 32°C can produce arrhythmias. Peripheral blood flow to extremities has been shown to correlate with body temperature, putting patients at risk of venothrombosis or thrombophlebitis. A high-risk target group includes patients with diabetes, the elderly, patients with peripheral vascular disease, and those who have had vascular surgery. Drugs metabolized at normal body temperature will have prolonged action with hypothermia. An example would be muscle relaxants used during surgery. Reversal of these drugs may be only partially effective, allowing for return of muscle paralysis, known as *recurarization*. Inhaled anesthetic agents as well as narcotics also have prolonged action in the hypothermic patient. Perhaps the greatest problem is the shivering that occurs as temperature regulatory responses return. The incidence of shivering has been estimated to occur in as many as 50% of patients. It has been documented that shivering can increase oxygen consumption by as much as 300% to 500%.[12] This increased oxygen demand can lead to hypoxia and even lactic acidosis because tissue oxygen demands may not be met. Shivering may involve large muscles, with obvious body movement, or may only affect fine muscles and be subtly seen as interference on the ECG screen.

A primary concern in the shivering patient is oxygen administration and delivery. Shivering patients with poor cardiovascular status or those who have had major surgery should have arterial blood gases drawn to determine the adequacy of tissue oxygen delivery. Attempts should be made to prevent shivering by increasing skin temperature. Providing an insulating layer of air around the body surface by means of heated bath blankets, foil-lined space blankets, or Aqua-k pads will frequently reduce shivering. Occasionally, drugs may be ordered to reduce shivering, such as antipyretics (salicylates or acetaminophen) given rectally if necessary. In extreme cases it may be necessary to administer drugs that directly depress the hypothalamus. Such drugs include chlorpromazine, Promethazine or meperidine (Demerol) in 20-mg doses.

There are measures to maintain core body temperatures. Reduce heat loss to the environment by keeping the room air above 70°F. Provide an insulating layer of air around the patient's body surface, as mentioned previously. It is important to note that extremities that feel "warm to the touch" are not an indication of core temperature. Patients who have had spinal anesthesia have peripheral vasodilation in the lower extremities, creating the warm-to-touch limb and, at the same time, allowing a large heat gradient between the extremities and the environment. For patients who are "warm and comfortable" temperature should be monitored and the extremities covered. All cold intravenous fluids, particularly blood, should be warmed through a blood warmer before being administered. Irrigating solutions for wound or bladder should also be stored in a warming cabinet before use. It is also important to prevent evaporative heat loss. The lungs are considered to be a large heat exchange unit, losing heat primarily through evaporation. Warmed, humidified, inhaled oxygen or air has been shown to be one of the most effective means of reducing heat loss.[26] Another beneficial measure is to use heat lamps directed at the patient during dressing changes and procedures that expose large body surfaces to the air, such as catheterization, and so forth. And, simply stated, the patient's skin should always be kept dry with dressing or linen changes as needed.

Hyperthermia

Hyperthermia (increase in body temperature) is seen less frequently than hypothermia in the immediate postoperative period. Patients with preoperative febrile states from dehydration, hypermetabolic conditions (*e.g.,* hyperthyroidism) or, most frequently, from inflammation caused by such conditions as appendicitis, abcesses, cysts, urinary tract infections, and cholecystitis are likely to have an elevated body temperature in the recovery room. Fever, for any reason, is cause for alarm. Sudden fever is frequently associated with bowel surgery, oral surgery, or genitourinary surgery in which a "shower" of bacteria may have been released into systemic circulation. Antibiotic prophylaxis is usually begun before surgery in these patients. The increase in temperatures may be preceded by a sudden increase in heart and respiratory rate and may be difficult to differentiate from pain in this period. Skin pallor as well as mottling may also be present. When there is a 1° increase in body temperature, metabolism increases 7% to 13%. The patient requires sugar substrate intravenously to support this increased metabolism and an increase in intravenous fluids to compensate for increased water loss.

Malignant Hyperthermia. An acute emergency condition known as malignant hyperthermia (or malignant hyperpyrexia) has been known to occur as late as 24 hours postoperatively. This is a hypermetabolic state presenting a cascade of symptoms that is triggered by many drugs used during anesthesia. Inhalation agents such as halothane and intravenous drugs such as succinylcholine or lidocaine have been implicated. Symptoms are those of a very rapid febrile state. Sudden tachycardia (rates greater than 150) may be one of the earliest signs. Muscle rigidity, most often in the jaw muscles (masseter muscle spasm), accompanies the symptoms and is due to calcium release by the skeletal muscles. Rise in body temperature is a *late* sign and when it occurs is extremely rapid, for example 2° in less than 5 minutes. It is an inherited trait with an incidence of 1 : 14,000 persons in the United States, and is seen most frequently in specific geographical areas such as the Midwest.[22]

Most facilities have developed a protocol for *malignant hyperthermia crisis* and it is advisable for a drug protocol box to be available to the recovery room for this purpose. Effective treatment and patient survival are primarily contingent on early recognition and definitive action. A "code" for malignant hyperthermia crisis should be called and the patient given 100% oxygen via positive pressure, if possible (hyperventilate to reduce the $Paco_2$). Standard protocol includes dantrolene chloride 10 mg/kg IV sodium bicarbonate 1 mg/kg massive amounts of IV fluids, and blood gases drawn on both arterial and venous samples to compare venous oxygen desaturation.

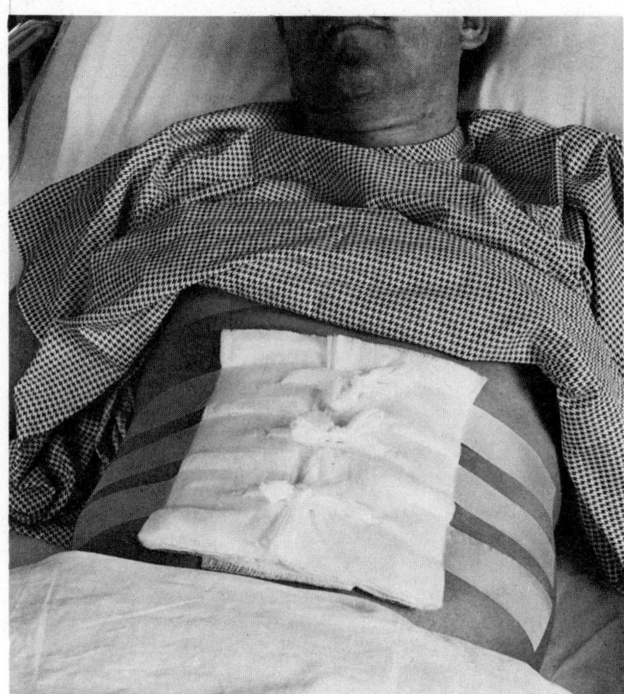

FIGURE 8–9 Montgomery straps may be used when frequent dressing changes are anticipated.

Surgical Site Assessments

The goals of assessing dressings, drains, and tubes are to maintain skin integrity; to minimize wound infection; to promote wound healing by maintaining good tissue approximation; and to adequately assess blood loss. On admission to the recovery room the patient is examined by the nurse for skin color, presence of rash, petechiae, abrasions, burns, or pressure areas. Particular attention is given to the site of the cautery grounding pad, tourniquet (noted on OR record), and to bony prominences that may have sustained undue pressure from the surgical position (noted on both OR and anesthesia records) and should have been reported by OR staff.

Dressings

Dressings are checked every 15 minutes in the recovery room. The amount and type of drainage is carefully measured and recorded. Saturated dressings should be changed using *strict aseptic technique*. Policies on the first postoperative orders refer to the frequency of dressing change. The surgeon usually does the first dressing change on the unit on the first or second postoperative day. Dressings that require frequent changing usually by nursing personnel are those that are held in place by Montgomery straps (Fig. 8–9), those that cover wound drains such as Penrose drains (noted on OR record), or those used to collect from open cavities, such as a mustache dressing for nasal surgery or perineal pad for vaginal or rectal surgery. Dressing changes that almost always require the presence of the surgeon, even if saturated, include head dressings such as those used with craniotomy or mastoidectomy procedures, orthopedic procedures, and cosmetic surgery.

Drainage Tubes

When assessing drainage it is important to remember the effects of gravity. Look for fluid pooling. For example, drainage from oral or nasal pharyngeal surgery will be swallowed (frequently causing nausea) and abdominal hysterectomy patients will have vaginal drainage.

Tissue Drains. Tissue drains such as Hemovac, Jackson-Pratt and Penrose are placed into tissue near or at the incision site (Fig. 8–10). They are usually in compartments (such as joints) that tolerate fluid accumulation poorly, in areas that have had large superficial tissue dissection, such as the breast, or in areas that receive a large blood supply, such as the kidney or neck. A Penrose drain is usually left to drain directly into the dressing. The Hemovac and Jackson-Pratt drains are connected to collection containers (Figs. 8–11 and 8–12). Frequent assessment as to type and amount of drainage in the collection bags should be made. The Hemovac drain usually requires frequent emptying and measurement of drainage.

Cavity Drainage Tubes. Cavity drainage tubes include such things as nasogastric tubes, chest tubes, urinary catheters, and T tubes. Nasogastric tubes (NG tubes) are used to relieve fluid collection on gastric or upper bowel procedures as well as to reduce gastric distention and nausea. The NG tube is usually ordered to be at low suction and will remain in place until peristalsis resumes. Patency is of prime impor-

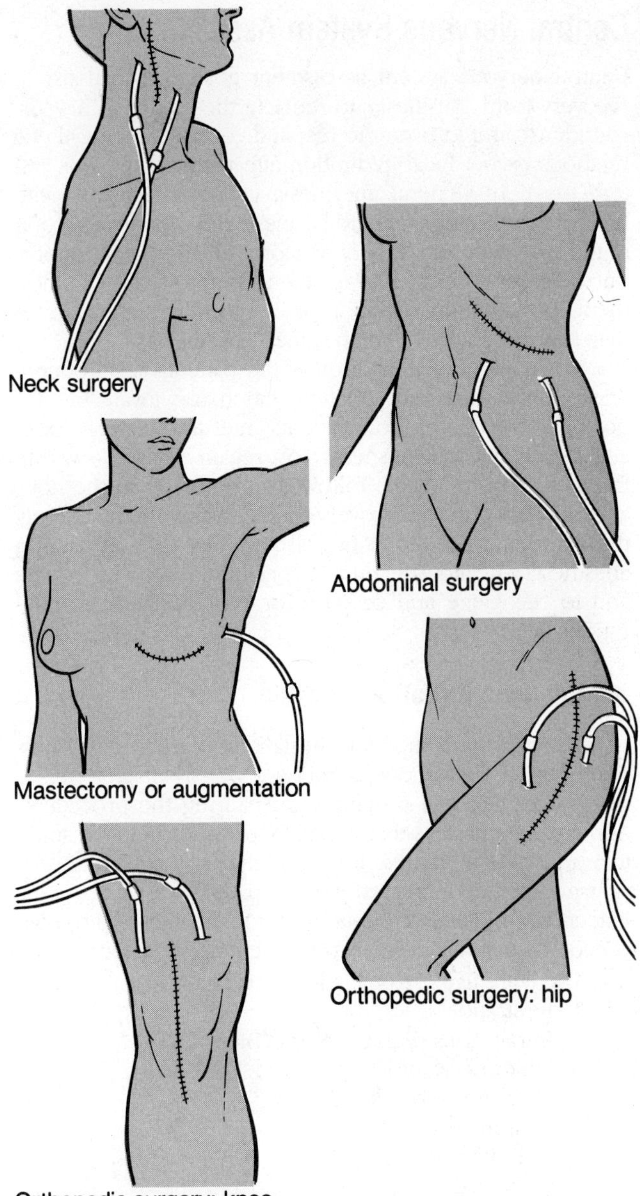

FIGURE 8–10 Typical drainage sites following specific types of surgery.

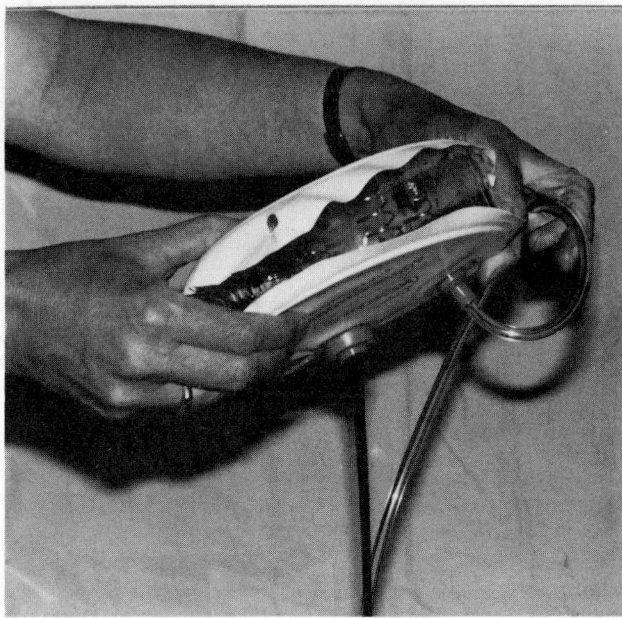

FIGURE 8–11 Hemovac drain.

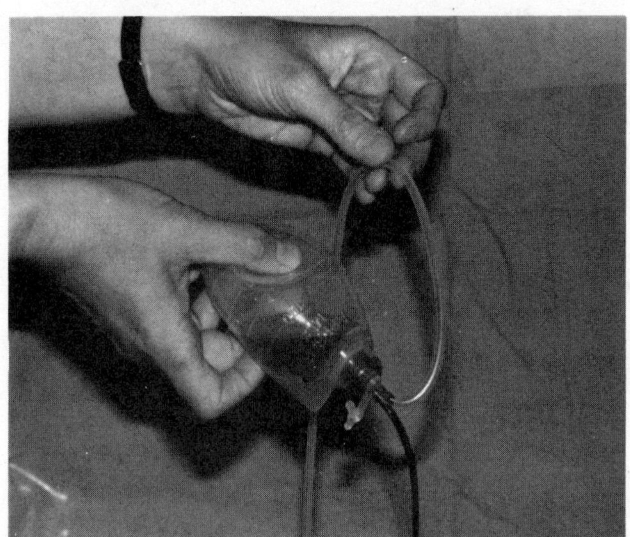

FIGURE 8–12 Jackson-Pratt drain.

tance after gastric surgery. Sterile irrigation may be ordered; careful aseptic technique should be used to protect the new surgery site. *Do not adjust the NG tube on patients having had gastric surgery*! The placement is determined during surgery and manipulation can result in dislocation of the tube or trauma to the new surgery site.

Chest Tubes. Chest tubes are used to remove air and fluid following thoractomy procedures. They are connected to a closed system either by a Pleur-Evac or traditional water seal drainage. The tubes need frequent "milking" in the early postoperative period to prevent plugging from clots. Extreme care must be used to neither dislodge or kink the tubing. *Chest tubes should never be clamped without an order* even if malfunction is suspected. Measurements of fluid drainage in the collection bottle and noting bubbling (air removal) on expiration should be done at least every 15 minutes and charted. Continuous assessment should be made of respiratory adequacy. The nurse should be familiar with the symptoms of pneumothorax, mediastinal shift, and interstitial air in order to recognize them and act immediately. Chest x-ray studies and arterial blood gas analysis are routine recovery room orders for patients with chest tubes. (Refer to Chap. 26 on assessment of the respiratory system.)

Urinary Catheters. Urinary catheters are drains for bladder, ureteral, or prostate surgery. Intermittent or continuous sterile irrigations are frequently ordered and, again, patency is of prime importance and is noted by urinary output. Collection of fluid, clots, or both at the surgical site will prevent normal vasoconstriction and potentiate active bleeding. The amount and type of urinary drainage, along with frequent palpations of the bladder margins, can indicate the patency of the drainage system. Patients who have had genitourinary surgery are frequently anesthetized by spinal block and, although alert, are unable to express usual bladder discomfort from distention.

Other Drains. Other drains placed into hollow organs include T tubes, gastrostomy, cecostomy, and cystostomy tubes. These drains are connected to separate collecting bags and are carefully secured usually by suturing into place. *Careful handling of these drains and collection bags is required*. Should the tube be accidentally pulled out, drainage leaking back into the body might result in fistula formation and infection. Aseptic technique is imperative when handling the collection tubes or dressings. The dressings are unsterile, as are the contents of the tube. They can contaminate the incision site or bacteria may travel up the tube into the body. These tubes are usually removed after 3 to 5 days when a wall of fibrous tissue has been formed.

Bleeding

Excessive bleeding is another area of surgical site assessment. There are six symptoms of excessive bleeding:

1. Continuous, excessive drainage with clots
2. Change in vital signs unexplained by other causes
3. Increase or decrease in systolic blood pressure, usually accompanied by increase in diastolic pressure ("closing pulse pressure")
4. Increase in respiratory and heart rates that may be masked by medication
5. Agitation or restlessness that may be masked by medication
6. Change in body cavity girth of abdomen or pelvis, but frequently not noticed since it requires a large volume displacement

Nursing interventions for excessive bleeding are the following:

1. Notify anesthesiologist and surgeon.
2. Increase rate of intravenous fluids.
3. Place the patient in modified Trendelenburg position if not contraindicated (*e.g.*, craniotomy, thyroidectomy, and radical neck surgery)
4. Attempt to estimate blood loss. Dressings can be weighed on a gram scale. Weigh dry dressings, then adjust scale to zero and weigh saturated dressings: 1 g = 1 ml. Blood hemoglobin and hematocrit can provide rough estimation when compared to intraoperative estimation (500 ml blood will roughly decrease hematocrit 2% to 3%). However, rapid IV infusions plus intravascular volume shifts will affect results.
5. Prepare to type and cross-match for blood transfusions if there is no blood on hand. Administer blood or colloids if needed as directed by orders. (See Chap. 50 for blood transfusions.)
6. Prepare the patient to return to surgery.

Central Nervous System Assessments

Central nervous system assessment goals are to assist in recovery from anesthesia, to reorient the patient to his surroundings, and to promote rest and comfort. All anesthetic methods except local infiltration affect central nervous system function. General anesthesia centrally depresses the level of consciousness. Regional anesthesia renders a portion of the body without sensory or motor function and can produce central depression with the absorption of local anesthetic into central circulation or by blocking a greater area than desired, such as a "high spinal" anesthesia.

A preoperative evaluation of the patient's level of consciousness and careful documentation are invaluable for postoperative comparison. Patients enter the recovery room at all levels of consciousness. Most regain awareness within minutes and are able to follow directions within the hour after admission to the recovery room. Knowledge of not only the anesthetic technique but also the agents used during anesthesia will allow the nurse to predict the recovery course and to recognize and prepare for postanesthetic complications.

Regional (Local) Anesthesia

Regional, or local, anesthesia is rendering only a portion of the body without sensation. One advantage to this is that the patient can remain awake during the procedure. Another advantage is that it usually provides better respiratory and cardiac stability for the higher risk patient. Disadvantages include increased patient anxiety and, on occasion, inadequate block. Additional sedation, analgesia and, conversion to general anesthesia is sometimes required.

There are five regional anesthesia techniques:

1. Infiltration
2. Intravenous regional block (Bier block)
3. Minor nerve block
4. Major nerve block
5. Central nerve block
   a. Epidural
   b. Caudal
   c. Spinal (subarachnoid) block

Infiltration is the technique of injecting a local anesthetic such as lidocaine into the tissue surrounding the surgical site. Conduction of all the nerves in the area is inhibited. The onset of anesthesia is rapid, and duration is related to the specific agents used, their concentration, and the addition of epinephrine. Epinephrine reduces the absorption of the local anesthetic by constricting blood vessels that normally absorb the anesthetic in the area. Local tissue infiltration is usually limited to minor, superficial procedures requiring only short duration, such as wound suturing or excision of a mole.

Intravenous regional block (Bier Block) is the administration of the local anesthetic agent into a vein of a tourniquet-occluded limb. The drug then filtrates from vascular to tissue space and eventually anesthetizes nerves in the area of the procedure. This method is used primarily for short procedures, since the the tourniquet cannot be left on for longer than an hour. Toxicity can occur on release of the tourniquet as large volumes of the local anesthetic are mobilized into systemic circulation. For this reason the tourniquet is released over a period of several minutes.

Minor nerve block is the technique used for the inhibition of small nerve conduction, such as the radial or ulnar nerve, with the injection of a drug directly around the specific nerve.

Major nerve block is the specific nerve block of large nerves, such as the sciatic, pudenal, or femoral, or the blocking of a nerve plexus, such as the brachial plexus with an axillary block. Larger volumes of more potent local anesthetics are usually needed, thus requiring longer recovery time (hours).

Central nerve block, such as lumbar epidural anesthesia, is a technique useful in procedures involving the lower abdomen, pelvis, or lower extremities, particularly for caesarian section or vaginal delivery. The local anesthetic drug is injected into the "potential" space surrounding the dura of the spinal canal. Nerve fibers are anesthetized where they leave the spinal tract. Large volumes of local anesthesia are used to obtain a desired level. It is possible for the dura to be perforated and the patient to receive a "total spinal" anesthetic. This technique provides good sensory anesthesia. Gross motor function may still be present, with the patient able to move his legs.

Caudal anesthesia is a form of epidural anesthesia in which the epidural space is entered by way of the sacral hiatus. It is used primarily in perineal and urological surgery and for vaginal delivery.

Spinal anesthesia (subarachnoid) block is the injection of a small amount of local anesthetic (lidocaine, dibucaine, or tetracaine) into the cerebrospinal fluid in the lumbar region, usually between the lumbar vertebrae at L3-4 or L2-3. Spinal anesthesia provides good analgesia and excellent muscle relaxation. Since sympathetic nerve fibers are also anesthetized, the vascular bed below the level of the block dilates and can result in profound hypotension. If the level of the block is at T-4 or above, cardiac accelerator fibers are also affected and severe bradycardia can result from a combination of reduced venous blood return and unopposed vagal stimulation. Patients receiving spinal anesthesia may be given large volumes of intravenous fluids (to increase venous return), vasopressor drugs such as ephedrine, and vagolytic drugs such as atropine to counteract the bradycardia. Block level is designated as the dermatome level at which there is a change in sensory perception. Sympathetic block is thought to be one or two dermatomes higher than motor block (one or two dermatomes below it).

Aftereffects. *Sympathetic blockade* may exist after the patient is in the recovery room. Therefore, sensory level should be assessed every 15 minutes along with other vital signs. The block will wear off in a head-to-toe manner (cephalad–caudal). Patients should remain flat until sympathetic return has been established because hypotension can occur whenever the patient's head is elevated. Sympathetic return must be evaluated indirectly by the following criteria.[13, 29]

INDICATIONS OF SYMPATHETIC INNERVATION RETURN

1. Stability of vital signs and temperatures to the preanesthesia level; the ability to vasoconstrict. (Measure body temperature return and maintain blood pressure with elevation of head and coughing—indirect method.)
2. Pinprick sensation in the perianal area, S4-5. (Complete sensory return)
3. Patient can plantar flex the foot against resistance in the supine position. (Return of motor function)
4. Patient knows whether the great toe is flexed or extended without watching. (Return of proprioception)

Other factors such as sedation or blood volume must also be considered before ambulation is attempted, just as with any new surgical patient.

Spinal headaches are thought to be due to the leakage of cerebrospinal fluid from the site of dural puncture. The use of small gauge spinal needles (22- to 25-gauge) has reduced the incidence of spinal headache in the general population. Young women of childbearing age and young men are at the highest risk for spinal headaches. Patients are no longer kept flat for hours after spinal anesthesia as a preventive measure. If a headache does occur (and this will usually happen within 24 hours), patients are then kept flat, and given fluids and analgesics. An epidural "blood patch" using the patient's own blood may be required in an attempt to seal the dural leak.

"High spinal" anesthesia can occur when the level of the block is much higher than intended. Initial symptoms usually occur soon after administration. However, high spinal symptoms have occurred as late as 1 hour after patients have received epidural anesthesia, resulting in an inadvertent dural tear. Hypotension may occur and be preceded by nausea, retching, and bradycardia (unopposed vagal stimulation). Initial treatment is atropine, vasopressors, and IV fluids. If the block continues to move up, progressive failure of intercostal muscle movement reduces chest expansion. However, the diaphgram remains functional and may increase in activity, resulting in an increase in respiratory rate and concurrent decrease in respiratory depth. Patients may become anxious and restless and require positive pressure ventilation by means of mask. Loss of sensation to hand and arms occur at thoracic levels and, if the block reaches cervical level, nasal flaring and accessory muscle activity indicate the need for intubation. Air hunger and loss of chest expansion will cause panic and then, with cervical block, loss of complete sensation will render the patient unconscious.

Treatment is supportive: maintain blood pressure with fluids and drugs and ventilate the patient until the block wears down. If conscious, the patient will need repeated reassurance that the condition is temporary and manageable.

Toxcity from Local Anesthesia. Hypersensitivity (allergy) to local anesthetics is rare, occurring in less than 1% of the population who have surgery. The incidence is highest with agents in the ester class.[20] Allergic symptoms are treated as with other allergic/anaphylactoid reactions: antihistamine, epinephrine, and cardiovascular support are given if needed. Local anesthetic toxicity can occur when there is an excessive dose, rapid absorption from a vascular site, or inadvertent intravascular injection. Toxic levels can occur with low serum proteins levels (malnutrition), an increase in PCO_2 and decrease in pH (respiratory acidosis), or liver disease, renal failure, and pseudocholinesterase deficiencies.

Symptoms of Toxicity. Local anesthetics readily cross the blood–brain barrier, causing central nervous system symptoms. Initial symptoms are excitement, numbness of tongue or mouth, general light-headedness, tinnitus, disorientation, or temporary loss of consciousness. If the blood–brain anesthetic level becomes high enough, seizure activity and possibly respiratory arrest can occur. Initially, there is an increase in heart rate and blood pressure, then hypotension and bradycardia occur from direct vasodilation and myocardial depression. Respiratory depression can occur from direct central nervous system depression or, to a much lesser extent, by depression of neuromuscular activity.

Treatment. Central nervous system excitement or seizure is treated with diazepam (Valium), 0.1 to 0.2 mg/kg or with rapidly acting barbiturate such as thiopental, 1 to 2 mg/kg. Establish an airway, ventilate and, if necessary, intubate, then hyperventilate to reduce respiratory acidosis. Hypotension is treated with vasopressors. Provide cardiac support if needed. Toxicity from bupivacaine (Marcaine) produces severe long-lasting myocardial depression that may require prolonged cardiopulmonary resuscitation.

General Anesthesia

General anesthesia causes loss of consciousness and centrally ameliorates pain perception. The degree to which the body elicits a stress response is dependent on patient condition and level of anesthesia.[5]

The agents used for general anesthesia are:

1. Induction agents
2. Inhalation agents
3. Intravenous anesthesia
   a. Narcotics
   b. Narcotic–narcotic antagonists

INDUCTION AGENTS. Induction agents are used to produce rapid hypnosis and sleep.

- *Barbiturates* (rapid-acting):
  Thiopental sodium (Pentothal)
  Sodium thiamylal (Surital)
  Methohexital sodium (Brevital)

The rapidly acting barbiturates produce unconsciousness in 15 to 20 seconds after administration. They all require respiratory support and can decrease blood pressure. The alkaline solutions can be irritating to the vein. These agents produce no analgesic properties and the short amnesia period lasts 5 to 15 minutes.

- *Etomidate (Amidate)* is a recently released drug that is very stable on the cardiovascular and respiratory systems. It has no analgesic properties. Extrapyramidal movements and pain at the injection site may be seen after administration. It provides an extremely short amnesia period of 5 minutes or less.
- *Diazepam (Valium)* does not depress the respiratory or cardiac status; however, dissociative symptoms or excitement may occur with elderly or very young patients. Pain is often experienced with intravenous injection. There is no analgesic effect, but narcotic analgesia is potentiated. Diazepam produces an extremely long amnesia, with a half-life of 24 hours, and immediate retrograde amnesia frequently occurs. Instruction given to these patients must be repeated and provided in written form.
- *Ketamine hydrochloride (Ketalar)* provides dissociative anesthesia. Reflexes remain intact and there are often roving eye movements. Heart rate, blood pressure, and intracranial pressure are increased. Respirations remain spontaneous, but there is increased salivation; therefore, ketamine is almost always given with atropine or Robinul for an antisialigogue effect. Ketamine is used most frequently in very young children or the elderly, since hallucinations are most prevalent when used in young adults. Valium is found to reduce the incidence of hallucinations seen with ketamine. Ketamine provides excellent analgesia and amnesia. A quiet, nonstimulating environment is required for recovery to prevent agitation.

INHALATION AGENTS. Inhalation agents are used for analgesia and amnesia and to maintain level of anesthesia during surgery.

- *Nitrous oxide (N_2O)* is a relatively weak agent used as an adjunct to other agents. It produces amnesia and may produce dissociation of perception and action in the adolescent and the elderly. It is rapidly eliminated by exhalation. Nitrous oxide can produce air emboli when used during procedures such as posterior fossa craniotomy, tympanoplasties or, occasionally, bowel procedures.
- *Fluothane (halothane)* is a potent primary agent used as a cardiorespiratory depressant. Cardiac arrhythmias can easily occur, especially in the patient who is anxious (endogenous catecholamines) or who has also received local injections containing epinephrine. Peripheral vasodilation can be pronounced with subsequent hypotension and loss of body heat. Flouthane is metabolized primarily by the liver. It is not used frequently in the same patient or in those with liver disease. It is used most frequently in children because of the rapid inhalation induction time. Shivering can be a frequent postoperative occurrence.
- *Enflurane (Ethane).* This is a potent primary agent with less cardiac depression than halothane. Respiratory depression can be pronounced. Systemic vascular resistance is lowered. There are many fewer metabolites than with halothane, but enflurane is used with caution in patients with kidney disease and patients with neurological or seizure disorders. It is eliminated more slowly than halothane and obese patients may "store" enflurane in fatty tissue and release it slowly for hours. Shivering due to loss of body heat is also seen.
- *Isoflurane (Forane).* Also a potent primary agent, Forane is a newly released drug. Very little cardiac depression is seen with its use, but tachycardia is a side-effect. Vasodilation occurs, but to a lesser extent than with halothane. Respiratory depression can be pronounced, especially if narcotics are also used. Isoflurane has very few metabolites, making it safer to use with the patient having kidney or liver disease.

Inhalation agents no longer used or used with restrictions include the following:

- *Diethyl ether* produced classical and dependable stages of anesthesia. Very stabilizing in the circulatory system, diethyl ether was associated with nausea and vomiting in about 57% of patients.[7] Because of its flammability properties, use of diethyl ether has been restricted to teaching hospitals.
- *Cyclopropane* is an extremely potent inhalation agent that produces profound analgesia and muscle relaxation. It is associated with cardiac arrhythmias and heavy pharyngeal secretions. Use of cyclopropane in the United States has been limited owing to its explosive nature.

INTRAVENOUS ANESTHESIA. Intravenous anesthesia includes narcotics and narcotic antagonists.

Narcotics. Narcotics may be given as either total anesthesia technique (nitrous–narcotic) or as a supplement to inhalation agents (balanced technique). All narcotics are potent respiratory depressants. Most are mildly depressing to the cardiovascular system, depending on dosage and patient condition.

Examples of two narcotics used intraoperatively are fentanyl and Innovar. Fentanyl (Sublimaze) is used extensively because of its short duration (usually 1 hour) and potent analgesia. Large doses are used for cardiac surgery. Bradycardia and muscle rigidity can occur. Innovar is a combination of fentanyl and droperidol (a sedative tranquilizer) in the ratio of 1 : 50. Innovar is a neuroleptic characterized by producing general quiescence, reduced motor activity, and profound analgesia. Respiratory depression and sedative effects may last much longer than the analgesia. Patients receiving Innovar are occasionally unable to express pain.

Narcotic antagonists. Narcan is a narcotic antagonist that provides little analgesia and is used to antagonize the respiratory depressant effects of narcotics. It may contribute to pulmonary edema in some patients. Effects of Narcan may wear off before the narcotic depression. Stadal and Talwin (pentazocine) are mild antagonists and provide good analgesia with little cardiovascular and respiratory depression (see Chap. 9 on pain).

Muscle Relaxants. Muscle relaxants are needed for intubation and to provide adequate relaxation for surgery. Succinylcholine (Anectine, Quelicin) is a commonly used depolarizing muscle relaxant that can be given as a single bolus or a drip for continuous effect. The bolus lasts no longer than 5 to 10 minutes and is rapidly broken down. Muscle fasciculation can occur after administration because the drug causes muscle depolarization before relaxation. Prior administration of small amounts of nondepolarizing agents will help prevent this; however, patients occasionally complain of muscle soreness on awakening.

Nondepolarizing muscle relaxants work by competing with acetylcholine at the motor end-plate. Although they are effective at different onset rates, all are slower and have a longer duration than succinylcholine with pancuronium, thus providing the longest duration. Nondepolarizing agents usually require reversing at the end of the procedure. Examples are the following drugs:

D-Tubocurarine (curare)
Metocurine (Metubine)
Gallamine (Flaxedil)
Pancuronium bromide (Pavulon)
Atacurium (Tracrium)
Vecuronium bromide (Norcuron)

Reversal agents such as edrophonium (Tensilon), neostigmine (Prostigmin) and pyridostigmine (Mestinon) are anticholinesterase drugs that allow buildup of acetylcholine at the motor end-plate (nicotinic activity). At the same time, muscurinic activity is also increased, which produces cholinergic effects seen as vagal stimulation, primarily in the form of severe bradycardia. Therefore, anticholinesterase drugs such as atropine and Robinul are always given with these agents.

Patients who have had muscle relaxants reversed may still be at risk for recurarization in the recovery room. Either partially or inadequately reversed patients or the hypothermic patient with slow metabolism are vulnerable. Respiratory depth, hand grip, and the ability to perform sustained head lift off the bed are gross measurements of the return of muscle strength. A peripheral nerve stimulator should be available to compare muscle twitch.

Stages of General Anesthesia. The patient recovering from general anesthesia will emerge back through the stages of anesthesia in reverse order. The excitement stage may not be observed in most adult patients; however, it still does occur, particularly in young children or the neurologically impaired. An understanding of the stages of anesthesia will allow the recovery room nurse to better provide for reflex protection. Table 8–3 presents the stages of anesthesia.

Emergence from General Anesthesia. Central nervous system assessment in the recovery room usually involves the evaluation of consciousness, motor activity, and emotional state. Patients who have had surgery affecting the central nervous system, such as craniotomy or carotidectomy, should have a more detailed neurological assessment to compare these with preoperative levels.

Historically, about 25% of patients who had received general anesthesia experienced an agitated phase during recovery; however, with the use of fluorinated anesthetics, emergence is more often quiet and tranquil. Occasionally, the patient will become restless, agitated, and disoriented; such incidence is highest in children, teenagers, and young healthy adults. Emergence delirium also occurs more frequently in patients having undergone intrathoracic and intraabdominal procedures and surgical procedures involving the neck. Careful assessment is necessary to ensure that impairment of oxygen delivery is not the cause of the symptoms.

Reorienting the patient to his environment is considerd to be part of a routine "stir-up regimen." Reorientation occurs in reverse order from anesthesia: first to person, then to place, then to time. Repetition of orientation statements is often required. When the patient remains agitated and excited in spite of reorientation, physostigmine (Antilirium)

TABLE 8–3
Stages of Anesthesia*

	Reflexes	*Respiration*	*Eyes*
I. Anagelsia amnesia	Present	Slow rate Increased depth	Some dilation Reacts to light
II. Dreams and excitement (frequently bypassed with intravenous induction agents)	Active	Irregular breathing Breath holding	Pupils widely dilated and divergent
III. Surgical Involves four planes; plane 2 and plane 3 best for surgery	In progression of loss Lid reflex Pharyngeal (swallowing) Laryngeal (can tolerate oral airway, suctioning and then intubation) Gag and corinal reflexes lost	Progressively depressed until apneic	Early plane: constricted pupils, then slightly dilated and centrally fixed
IV. Toxic Extreme depression	No reflexes	Completely flaccid	Widely dilated pupils

* Generally speaking, each stage is passed through upon induction and then reversed in sequence upon emergence from anesthesia. Intravenous induction agents have shortened the excitement stage. However, children and patients with central nervous system dysfunction may still experience the excitement stage.

may be ordered. The usual dose is 1 mg to be given slowly IV and repeated in 2 minutes, if necessary. Antilirium is an anticholinesterase and bradycardia may follow its administration. Atropine should always be available. Patients who have received ketamine (Ketalar) need a quiet area with minimal physical nursing activity. Ketamine has been associated with vivid dreams during emergence. Although the concomitant use of diazepam (Valium) has reduced this incidence, hallucinations may be triggered by loud noises or sudden abrupt movements. The patient may exhibit spontaneous randomized movement and may require one-to-one nursing for physical protection. Increased salivation may be seen, although atropine or glycopyrrolate (Robinul) is usually given to reduce this effect. Respirations remain spontaneous with no depression when ketamine is used as the primary anesthetic agent. The duration of ketamine's action is between 20 and 60 minutes.

Pain Assessment

Pain experienced in the recovery room is usually due to the cutting and retraction of tissue as well as to the intraoperative position of the patient. Assessment of pain should begin with these factors in mind. The patient may verbalize pain in addition to displaying symptoms of restlessness and agitation and an increase in blood pressure and pulse and respiratory rates. Nausea may also be a symptom of pain. Besides surgical pain, the patient may be experiencing discomfort due to distended bladder, angina pectoris, or restrictive dressings or casts.

Determining the source of pain is necessary before attempts are made to provide generalized pain relief. Before administering analgesics, other pain-relieving measures should be tried. Repositioning the patient may reduce incisional stress and gentle massage may relieve pressure area discomfort.

Evaluation of the patient's cardiovascular state, respiratory state, and level of consciousness is paramount before administering depressive analgesics. Either intravenous or intramuscular routes may be used, since the patient will remain npo until returned to the unit. The intravenous route allows for more accurate absorption of a drug and quicker relief of pain.

Narcotic doses should be reduced for the first several doses (*i.e.*, morphine, 2 mg or Demerol, 10 mg). If Innovar (droperidol and fentanyl) was used intraoperatively, the postoperative narcotic dose is usually reduced one quarter to one third of the recommended dose. Droperidol in doses greater than 0.6 mg is known to potentiate the action of narcotics, and respiratory depression can occur. Antiemetics such as promethazine hydrochloride (Phenergan), 25 mg IV, may be ordered and will reduce nausea as well as potentiate the narcotic.

Patients medicated for pain in the recovery room should be carefully observed for respiratory depression and kept in the recovery room for at least 30 minutes after the medication is given. If respiratory rate falls below 10 and is shallow, the use of Narcan, 1 mg, for narcotic antagonism may be considered. Since the narcotic may outlast the Narcan, continous observation is required in case the patient becomes renarcotized. Narcan has also been implicated in pulmonary edema in the new surgical patient.

Assessment of Nausea and Vomiting

It has been estimated that 30% to 40% of all surgical patients experience nausea, vomiting, or both.[24] The incidence is highest in women, in patients with high preoperative anxiety, and in patients having had gynecological, intra-abdominal, oral/nasal pharyngeal, eye, and vestibular procedures. Length and depth of anesthesia, mask anesthesia (air in the stomach), as well as preoperative narcotics such as Demerol are all thought to be contributing factors.

Frequently, allowing the patient to empty his stomach of air and drainage secretions is sufficient in relieving further nausea. If a nasogastric tube is in place, nausea indicates the tube is not patent. Retching cannot be tolerated in patients who have undergone craniotomy or eye procedures, because blood pressure and thus intracranial and intraocular pressure is increased. Likewise, cardiac or stroke patients cannot tolerate the stress of elevated blood pressure.

Small amounts of sedation such as droperidol, 0.6 mg or diazepam, 2.5 mg will reduce nausea. Antiemetics such as the phenothiazines (Phenergan) may be ordered, but they can cause hypotension. Again, careful assessment before and after drug intervention is extremely important during the vulnerable recovery period.

Criteria for Recovery Room Discharge

Determining when the patient can be discharged from the recovery room to the ward or short-stay unit is based on the attainment of minimum expected outcomes. A scoring system is frequently used and illustrates the need for objective evaluation in patient discharge (Fig. 8-13).

The minimum criteria are the following:

- Adequate pulmonary exchange
- Stable vital signs
- Normothermic state
- Orientation to surroundings
- Absence of surgical and anesthetic complications
- Controlled wound drainage
- Adequate urine output (20 to 30 ml/hr)
- Minimum pain and nausea

Documentation as to the extent these goals were met, along with a summarizing statement, should be made. The patient's unit is notified of the patient's return and of special equipment that is needed, and a report is made of his general condition and recovery room course.

Patients are transferred either on a recovery room bed or a stretcher. Safety straps or side rails are always used. There are no exceptions. Transferring the patient from stretcher to bed requires a minimum of two people. The bed and stretcher are stabilized by locking the wheels. Then, with one person on the outside edge of the stretcher and one person on the outside edge of the bed, the patient is gently moved onto the receiving bed. If the patient is large or unable to assist, three or four people may be needed for safe transfer. Movements should be smooth and gentle so as not to cause additonal pain or hypotension. All tubing is checked and secured, intravenous fluid rate is checked, and the patient is covered with blankets. In addition, the call light and emesis basin are placed and secured within the patient's reach; the side rails are placed in the up position. The unit nurse who is responsible must be directly notified of the patient's return to the room, and information should be exchanged regarding needed equipment, and so forth.

Postoperative Care: General Approach and Goals

Patients are returned to the surgical or short-stay unit after they have demonstrated cardiovascular and respiratory stability and have recovered major reflexes following anesthesia. A report is given to the unit nurse by the recovery room personnel. Such information as condition, vital sign trends, intravenous fluid intake and urinary output, medications given, and specific instructions are documented by the unit nurse and used as baseline data. In addition, the surgeon's postoperative orders on the chart must be checked immediately (Fig. 8–14). The first 24 hours are a particularly vulnerable time for hemorrhage and anesthesia-related problems, so that careful monitoring and assessment must be continued.

Checking the dressing and taking vital signs, including temperature, are routinely done as follows:

- Every 15 minutes × 4
- Then, every 30 minutes × 2
- Then, every hour × 4
- Then, every four hours × 24 hours

The goals for postoperative care are the following:

1. To return the patient to normal physiological function as early as possible
2. To reduce the stress of surgical trauma to a minimum
3. To promote wound healing
4. To prevent postoperative complications

Goal 1: To Return the Patient to Normal Physiological Functions as Early as Possible

Ambulation. As with all patients in acute states, safety is a major consideration with the early surgical patient. Side rails are kept up and the call light placed within reach until the patient is fully awake and can ambulate safely without assistance.

The positive effects of early movement and ambulation have long been documented.[19] Since patients undergoing surgery have most likely been immobile from anesthesia for a long period of time, position change, movement, and ambulation should begin as early as possible.[14] Criteria for ambulation most often depend on patient condition, surgical procedure, and cardiovascular and neurological stability. For patients who have had uncomplicated abdominal procedures the physician's orders may call for ambulating as early as the evening of surgery. Short-stay or outpatient surgery patients must be able to ambulate without assistance before discharge. However, ambulation may be restricted, not only by the patient's general condition, but by the amount of stress that ambulation may place on the surgical site, as may happen following many orthopedic procedures or procedures involving large areas of peripheral tissue dissection, such as radical neck surgery. The surgeon's orders dictate the amount of ambulation; however, nursing obser-

Recovery Room Score

Activity:	**Score**	**At Arrival**	**Hour 1**	**Hour 2**	**Hour 3**
Able to move 4 extremities	2	___	___	___	___
Able to move 2 extremities	1	___	___	___	___
Able to move 0 extremities	0	___	___	___	___
Respiration:					
Able to deep-breath & cough freely	2	___	___	___	___
Dyspnea or limited breathing	1	___	___	___	___
Apneic	0	___	___	___	___
Airway	0	___	___	___	___
Circulation:					
BP ± 20% of preanesthetic level	2	___	___	___	___
BP ± 20-50% of preanesthetic level	1	___	___	___	___
BP ± 50% or more of preanesthetic level	0	___	___	___	___
Consciousness:					
Fully awake	2	___	___	___	___
Arousable on calling	1	___	___	___	___
Not responding	0	___	___	___	___
Color:					
Pink	2	___	___	___	___
Pale, dusky, blotchy, jaundiced, other	1	___	___	___	___
Cyanotic	0	___	___	___	___
	Totals:	___	___	___	___

Score must be at least 7–8 for patient's release.

____
Release time

____
Nurse's signature

FIGURE 8–13 Sample recovery room scoring form for patient evaluation.

Activity level:	Bed rest tonight, then up with assistance in A.M.
Intravenous fluids: renumbering of IVs traditionally begins with first postoperative IV	#1 IV D5LR 1000 over 8 hr (125 cc/hr) #2 D5 in .45 NS 1000 over 8 hr #3 LR 1000/8 hr #4 TKO (keep open) D5LR
Diet	Sips of water tonight; clear liquids in A.M. if no nausea
Voiding:	If unable to void in 8 hr, catheterize x 1 (in & out) Intake and Output for 24 hr
Pain medication:	Demerol 50–100 mg IM every 3–4 hr prn pain
Antiemetic medication:	Phenergan 25 mg IM every 3–4 hr prn nausea
Dressing order or wound care:	Change dressings if saturated
Respiratory care:	Turn, cough, deep breath
Specific orders:	Antibiotics Irrigations Incentive spirometry Lab work (Hgb, Hct, etc.)

FIGURE 8–14 Typical postoperative physician's orders for a patient who has undergone uncomplicated surgery (hysterectomy).

vations and assessment of the patient's tolerance is vital and should be documented. *First ambulation attempts must always be done with assistance no matter what the surgical procedure and type or length of anesthesia.*

Patients who have received spinal anesthesia may be ambulated when they have demonstrated return of sympathetic function and full muscle strength. Ninety percent of patients having received tetracaine for spinal anesthesia have been shown to be fully recovered after 6 hours.[13] Because spinal anesthesia using lidocaine has a much shorter duration, recovery may be expected earlier than with tetracaine. However, patients who have had spinal anesthesia may be required to lie flat for a specified period of time if they are thought to be at greater risk for spinal headache (see earlier section in this chapter on spinal anesthesia).

Urinary Output. Urinary output is an indication of the adequacy of circulating fluids, as well as of renal and cardiac function. Patients without a urinary catheter in place should have voided within 6 to 8 hours after anesthesia. If surgery time was lengthy, greater than 2 hours, then voiding should be timed from 6 to 8 hours after the time of anesthesia induction. Evaluation of intraoperative fluid and blood replacement should allow a prediction of urinary status. Palpating the bladder margins is indicated if the patient complains of discomfort or is unable to void within the specified length of time. A full bladder may produce symptoms of restlessness or vague back pain without typical bladder discomfort. Spinal anesthesia directly blocks innervation to the bladder; distention is possible up to 24 hours after spinal anesthesia is administered. A sudden hypertensive episode in a patient recovering from spinal anesthesia while sympathetic and motor function is blocked may indicate a distended bladder.

In most cases, simply offering the bedpan/urinal or assisting the patient to the bedside commode will promote voiding. Other tactics such as running water or having the patient blow through a straw have proven beneficial. There will be difficulty in voiding if the following conditions exist:

1. The patient is cold or shivering.
2. The patient is experiencing pain.
3. The patient is unsupported. He must have support to sit up or must balance himself with his upper arms extended.
4. The patient is hypotensive.

If the bladder is distended, if the patient complains of bladder discomfort, or if the time limit is reached without voiding an adequate amount (over 100 ml), then a catheterization order should be obtained. Straight catheterization (in and out) will be sufficient for most uncomplicated surgeries. Major abdominal, perineal, and back or hip procedures require placement of an indwelling catheter. If only a small amount of urine is obtained on catheterization, the surgeon should be notified immediately.

Inadequate urine output may indicate hypovolemia, electrolyte imbalance, impending shock, or acute renal failure. The trauma of surgery (stress) has been shown to produce an antidiuretic effect, with retention of sodium, water, and potassium. In addition, anesthesia may produce changes in renal perfusion. Most general anesthetic agents depress renal function.[7] If vasopressors were used (the exception being low-dose dopamine), renal blood flow was reduced. Other intraoperative conditions that can produce renal damage include hypoxia, hypotension, multiple blood transfusions, and surgical manipulations such as aorta cross-clamping. Patients with atherosclerosis and diabetes are also at higher risk for renal failure. Evaluation for acute renal failure may include rapid infusion of intravenous fluids and may be followed by furosemide (Lasix), 10 mg IV or, occasionally, low-dose dopamine, 5 mcg/kg/min. If the cause of oliguria or anuria is determined to be acute renal failure, then fluid restriction along with dialysis are common treatment plans. Acute renal failure in the surgical patient, although not common, carries a high mortality rate.[7,22,37]

Nutritional Support. Intravenous solutions containing dextrose are usually ordered in the postoperative period until the patient experiences one of the following:

- No nausea or vomiting and the ability to retain sips of clear liquids
- Peristalsis has returned, documented by ausculating bowel sounds, palpating soft abdomen, and noting the ability to pass flatus.

Intravenous therapy will continue if the patient has had major surgery involving an open abdomen or thorax, is receiving intravenous antibiotics, or is at risk for hemorrhage.

When diet is indicated, then trial with clear liquids is ordered, followed by a progression to soft, then full diet as early as possible. Nursing responsibility is important, because timing of meals around pain medication and rest, as well as assistance with eating, may be vital to the patient's nutritional adjustment.

The effects of nutrition on wound healing and infection and defense mechanisms are known to be crucial.[24] Protein and calorie malnutrition in hospitalized patients has been documented as 35% to 50% in surgical patients and 44% in general medical patients.

Immediately after surgery, there is a sudden increase in metabolic demands, as well as an increase in urinary excretion of nitrogen. A 25% increase in oxygen consumption and calorie need is associated with elective surgical procedures. They increase by as much as 25% to 50% with multiple fractures and sepsis. At the same time, increases in cortisol and glucagon, along with decreases in insulin, impair glucose entry into the cell. This results in hyperglycemia, fatty acid mobilization, and a striking catabolism of muscle beyond that needed as a source of energy. A negative nitrogen balance develops as urinary excretion increases by as much as 30 to 50 g/day with severe trauma or major surgery (normal excretion: 11 to 17 g/day).[15]

In elective operative procedures, a negative nitrogen state is rapidly reversed, but with major trauma and surgery, the nitrogen imbalance may be prolonged. It is thought that negative nitrogen balance is reversed when the body is able to utilize carbohydrate as an energy substrate. However, the administration of moderate amounts of glucose will not reverse this process as long as the hormonal changes of stress continue.

Most patients who have had uncomplicated surgery can withstand catabolic insult if given adequate parenteral solutions containing appropriate electrolytes and a minimum of 100 g of glucose a day. However, debilitated or aged patients suffering from sepsis or multiple trauma may need early nutritional support. The administration of solutions containing amino acids have been shown to decrease urinary nitrogen excretion. Enteral and parenteral nutrition may be used to break the catabolic cycle. If the alimentary tract is functional, enteral tube feeding may be used by means of nasogastric, esophagostomy, or gastrostomy routes.[18]

When energy demands are high, nutritional support through a central venous line (frequently by way of the right subclavian vein) is utilized. Total parenteral nutrition (TPN) hyperalimentation feedings are indicated in patients who need large amounts of protein and calories, and may be given with and without lipid replacement. A greater emphasis on technical detail and strict adherence to aseptic catheter care can reduce some of the complications seen with TPN feedings.[11]

Peripheral venous nutrition is being used in some institutions for those patients who need less protein and calories. These solutions can contain fat emulsions and are isotonic.[21]

Nursing assessment of malnutrition includes general appearance and energy, wound healing progress, susceptibility to infections, weight loss, presence of triceps skin fold, and low serum albumin. Suspected malnutrition in the surgical patient 3 days or more postoperatively warrants discussion with the surgeon on nutritional supplementation.

Bowel Elimination. Immobility, pain medication, intraoperative bowel manipulation, reduced oral intake, and preoperative bowel preparation can all impede normal bowel elimination. Orthopedic patients who are limited in activity, patients having perineal procedures, those having had abdominal surgery, and the elderly are all at increased risk for developing fecal impactions postoperatively. Adequate fluid intake, as well as ambulation as much as tolerated, will reduce this risk. Mild rectal suppositories or oral agents, which provide bulk and lubrication, may be ordered. Enemas following abdominal surgery are rarely ordered, but may be indicated for the orthopedic patient if other measures fail. Loss of appetite, general discomfort and, occasionally, abdominal distention can hinder postoperative recovery. Nursing assessment and intervention can help prevent this possibility.

Paralytic ileus is a complication that may occur after abdominal and, particularly, bowel surgery. A portion of the bowel ceases normal peristalsis and either stops activity or, after a period of time, reverse peristalsis may occur. This is an extremely painful condition in which the abdomen becomes distended. Loss of appetite changes into nausea, vomiting and, occasionally, projectile vomiting of fecal matter. X-ray studies indicate distended bowel, and bowel sounds are usually absent. Treatment may begin in the early stages with return flow enemas in attempts to stimulate normal bowel activity. A nasogastric tube is indicated when vomiting is present. The need for intravenous fluids is apparent. A Miller-Abbott tube with mercury-filled balloon may be passed orally or nasally into the intestine to decompress the bowel. Once decompressed and rested, normal bowel peristalsis should occur.

Goal 2: To Reduce Surgical Stress

Pain Relief. Pain experienced by patients who have had uncomplicated major surgery is most often due to stretching of tissue and muscles during the procedure, to generalized muscle soreness from prolonged and unusual intraoperative position, and to bowel or bladder distention. Early ambulation or frequent position changes, as well as range-of-motion exercise, will reduce muscle discomfort and aid bowel and bladder function. Local incisional pain is frequently due to swelling at the suture sites and is most often noticed when stress is placed on the area during movement. Splinting the area or extremity or simply providing support during movement may be all that is needed during the first 24 hours to 48 hours postoperatively.

Outpatient surgical patients may require nothing or oral pain medication only. With all surgical patients, pain medication should be given as *often* as needed within prescribed limits to keep the patient comfortable and to promote rest. Adequate respiratory and circulatory assessment is essential to provide safety with the administration of analgesics. In addition, the use of analgesics should not interfere with movement and ambulation. (See Chapter 9 on pain.)

Promotion of Rest. Adequate time must be provided for sleep and rest. Procedures, medications, and visitors should be timed accordingly. Most patients recovering from major surgery benefit from frequent naps during the day and uninterrupted sleep at night. Occasionally, sleeping medication may be ordered. However, adequate analgesia, activity, and evening hygiene will often be all that is required.

Psychological Support. Psychological support and encouragement is based on individual needs and the surgical procedure. Most patients having surgical incisions will be concerned with their appearance. Changes in body image, lifestyle, family role, and sexuality can occur with patients who have had major dissecting surgeries.

All the fears discussed earlier in the psychological section of preoperative preparations apply to postoperative care. Patients with extreme disfigurements, particularly of the face, head, and neck, may need professional assistance to deal with their appearance. Even if the incision was small it may be of major concern to a patient. Looking at the sutures without a dressing may be difficult and often traumatic. What may be routine to a nurse is new to the patient. The patient should be told what to expect, how the skin will look when healed, and what he can do to participate in the process.

Gynecological, genitourinary, and breast surgeries produce fear of the loss of sexuality. The person is concerned about how the mate or lover may respond to these changes. Even if these concerns have been discussed preoperatively, seeing the areas and actually knowing that one is different may require additional support.

The patient may tolerate the immediate postoperative period well, but the realization of a body change will come sometime postoperatively and the patient should be prepared. Patients so often say, "If I had only known what to expect when I got home, I could have handled it." Most nurses and physicians will not have experienced the surgery personally, so it is hard to know what happens postoperatively when the patient is home. Clinical nurse specialists are good sources of referral, as are other patients.

The family, a friend, or a sibling are the best sources of support during all phases of the surgery. Patients who have a family member present may have less postoperative vomiting. These visitors should be given privileges to come and go as they please. They should be welcomed on the units as part of the health team and not made to feel they are intruding or interfering in the care of the patient.

If the family cannot be with the patient postoperatively, arrangements should be made for a telephone call to them. The nurse can talk with the family if the patient is unable to do so. Hearing the loved one's voice is most important to both parties.

Goal 3: To Promote Wound Healing

The progress of wound healing may be predicted based on presence of infection, incisional site, area of dissection, and type of surgical closure. For example, large stay or retention sutures on an abdominal incision indicate closure by secondary intention. See the discussion on wound healing in Chapter 15.

Skin Suture Removal is usually done by the surgeon or may be ordered to be done by the surgical nurse within 6 to 8 days postoperatively. Metal skin clips or staples may be used instead of silk suture and are thought to produce less tissue reaction. A nonremovable subcuticular (hidden) suture may be used and adhesive strips placed over the incision when a cosmetic closure is desirable.

Dressing Changes are indicated by the surgeon's order and must be maintained under dry aseptic conditions. Therefore, saturated dressings, no matter the source of drainage, require dressing change. The appearance of drainage should be noted and documented.

Cast Care also requires frequent observation for drainage and the presence of odor, which may indicate wound infection.

Surgical Infections continue to prolong hospitalization stay despite more than 80 years of aseptic surgery and more than 40 years or the use of antimicrobial agents.[21] Only the etiology has changed. Streptococci and pneumococci are no longer the major causes of infection and are controlled by antibiotics. However, staphylococci continue to cause nosocomial infections and the gram-negative, secondary invader bacteria (clostridia, bacteriodes, and enteric bacteria) have become major problems.[8]

Cross infection between patients and between patients and staff and autoinfections are the primary sources of transmission. In addition, frequent or prolonged supportive procedures such as urinary catheterization, tracheostomies, and ventilators are responsible for most iatrogenic infections.

Most surgical incisions are contaminated, but not infected with skin flora, and healing by primary intention is expected. Traumatic wounds are contaminated and usually result in infection.

Separation of the wound edges and sometimes of fatty layers is considered *wound dehiscence* and can result from poor tissue approximation, accumulation of fluid at the site, or infection. Wound dehiscence requires suture closure preceded by wound irrigation with antibiotic solution and may be done in the operating room or surgical ward. If all the abdominal layers have separated resulting in exposure of bowel (sometimes seen only with bulging on abdominal strain), then *wound evisceration* has taken place.

Sudden evisceration is often accompanied by severe pain and possible hypotension. The surgeon must be notified immediately and the following nursing measures should be taken:

- Place the patient on bed rest.
- Place sterile, *saline-moistened* packs on the wound to protect the bowel.
- Start intravenous administration of isotonic solution at maintenance rate (125 to 150 ml/hr) unless ordered otherwise.
- Keep the patient npo.
- Prepare the patient to return to surgery.
- Monitor vital signs.

Goal 4: To Prevent Postoperative Complications

Postoperative complications involving the renal and gastrointestinal systems, as well as those pertaining to wound healing, were discussed in the preceding sections. There can be psychological complications that will affect physiological recovery. The nurse treats the whole patient. General complications involving the respiratory and cardiovascular systems will be addressed in this section.

Respiratory Complications

Atelectasis. Atelectasis comprises approximately 90% of all postoperative complications.[34] The term *atelectasis* generally means collapse of alveoli. This collapse can occur in segments of lobes or in the entire lung. Estimates of incidence are 10% to 20% in all abdominal surgery and 20% to 30% in upper abdominal surgery.[33,34] Two major causes of atelectasis have been identified as bronchial obstruction with distal hypoventilation and a reduction in the surface-active surfactants that stabilize alveolar surface tension and allow the alveoli to stay open. Surfactant changes may occur as a result of changes in the regional blood flow during anesthesia or bed rest. In addition, an increase in mucous formation can occur. Predisposing factors that reduce ciliary action, which normally helps clear irritants from the upper airways, include anesthetic inhalation agents, smoking, obesity, and chronic obstructive disease. Other factors that inhibit respiratory effort include narcotic agents, which depress the cough reflex and immobilization and splinting of the chest, which reduces cough effectiveness and chest pain.

Atelectasis usually becomes manifest during the first 24 hours after surgery. It is usually heralded by sudden onset of fever and tachycardia. Most frequently tachycardia will precede a rise in temperature. Early findings are crackles on chest auscultation at the posterior bases and diminished breath sounds in those areas affected. Total lung capacity, residual volume, and functional residual capacity are all reduced. Diagnosis includes the above pulmonary function tests and chest x-ray studies. The latter show areas of consolidation. If atelectasis persists, clinical symptoms are those generally associated with pneumonia, such as increase in temperature, tachycardia, increase in respiratory rate and, occasionally, dyspnea and cyanosis.

TREATMENT. Treatment begins with preoperative teaching of deep breathing and coughing. Patients should be encouraged to stop smoking 3 weeks before surgery. Preoperative pulmonary function tests have been used to screen patients at higher risk.[36] Various types of apparatus to increase breathing capacity are part of preoperative preparation in some institutions.[2,20]

PREVENTION. Postoperative Prevention of atelectasis includes early ambulation, adequate hydration, and effective deep breathing with wound support for abdominal incisions. The ideal respiratory maneuver is one in which high alveolar inflation pressure is extended for a long period of time.[2] Deep breathing exercise with emphasis on sustained inspiration to total lung capacity has been consistent in effectively inflating alveoli and clearing secretions. The incentive spirometer device ensures patient participation and is known to be an effective inspiratory exercise. Whichever breathing exercise is used, nursing supervision and encouragement can make the difference between effectiveness and noneffectiveness. Chest auscultation on all high-risk patients, or those on bed rest, should be a routine nursing assessment. Studies have indicated that alveoli, once inflated, will remain inflated for at least 1 hour. Consequently, postoperative respiratory maneuvers would be done ideally every hour and at least every 2 hours during the first 24 hours.[33]

Pulmonary Embolism. Pulmonary embolism can occur after any major surgery or trauma, especially after those involving large crushing injuries of the extremities. Emboli can be caused by fat, air, amniotic fluid, or thrombus. Patients who have had vascular disease are at high risk for thromboemboli. Patients with central venous lines or pulmonary artery catheters and patients having had posterior fossa craniotomy procedures or procedures involving large venous beds such as the prostate or uterus have been known to develop air amboli by exposure of the venous beds to air. Emboli will circulate through the vascular system and may lodge in the heart, brain, or lungs. Resultant symptoms depend on the area of the emboli; for instance, pulmonary emboli result in necrosis of lung tissue. Mortality in such a case is extremely high. Symptoms include an increase in respiratory rate, shallow breathing, sharp pleural pain, fever, and hemoptysis of pink frothy sputum.

If the patient reports these symptoms, the surgeon should be notified immediately; the patient should be given oxygen by mask or cannula and placed on bed rest with the head of the bed elevated, and vital signs should be closely monitored. Arterial blood gas analysis and chest x-ray studies are standard for diagnoses, and a lung scan may also be indicated. Treatment will include anticoagulants and oxygen and respiratory support if needed. Surgery for embolectomy or venous ligation to prevent emboli migration may be indicated.

Pulmonary Edema. Pulmonary edema may occur during or immediately after circulatory overload. The most frequent cause is large intraoperative infusion volumes and is usually associated with conditions of poor cardiac function or with pulmonary damage by inhalation of noxious substances or by aspiration. Clinical symptoms include accumulation of fluid resulting in crackles (rales), reduction in lung compliance and increase in $PaCO_2$ and, frequently, bronchospasm. Scattered crackles progress to bubbling rales and rhonchi. A marked tachycardia, tachypnea (rapid respiratory rate), and cyanosis are usually present.

TREATMENT. Treatment includes immediate notification of the surgeon or anesthesiologist, placing the patient in a head-up position, respiratory support with oxygen (intubation may be required), and correction of circulatory overload with diuretics such as furosemide (Lasix) and, occasionally, reducing cardiac afterload with nitroprusside. Morphine will aid in dilating the venous bed and reducing the volume return to the lung. If the patient is intubated, intermittent positive pressure breathing with positive end-expiratory pressure (PEEP) or continuous positive airway pressure (CPAP) is indicated.

Cardiovascular Complications

Myocardial Infarction. Myocardial infarction most frequently occurs during the surgery or on the operative day. However, the first 3 postoperative days are considered a particularly vulnerable time. Patients with a history of arrhythmias, particularly premature ventricular contractions; those with a history of heart disease, particularly those with previous myocardial infarctions within the last 6 months; patients over 70 years old; and those having emergency surgery are at greatest risk for postoperative heart attack. The incidence of postoperative myocardial infarction is highest in patients who have had general anesthesia for abdominal and pelvic surgeries.[34] The most significant precipitating factor is considered to be shock during anesthesia or recovery. Chest pain may be masked by narcotics or anesthesia. However, the appearance of dyspnea, tachycardia, cyanosis, or arrhythmias should indicate the need for cardiac monitoring and immediate notification of the physician. Treatment is described in the section on coronary care and includes oxygen support, cardiac monitoring, and pain relief.

Thromboembolism. Thromboembolism usually occurs 1 to 2 weeks postoperatively. A thrombus of peripheral veins, most frequently the calf veins, may be due to direct pressure that occurred intraoperatively or from blood stasis resulting from inactivity during the postoperative period. Prevention includes elastic stockings to reduce venous stasis, adequate hydration, maintaining body temperature, and ambulation. Occasionally, low-dose anticoagulant drugs are ordered. Thromboembolism causes pain and localized warmth and swelling in the extremity involved. The clot may become dislodged and migrate to other areas of the body such as the heart, brain, or lungs, resulting in stroke, coronary occlusion, or pulmonary embolism. Treatment includes bed rest, leg elevation, and anticoagulants.

Summary

The experience of surgery, no matter what the surgical procedure, subjects the patient to psychological and physiological stress. Nursing goals and interventions are aimed at reducing and, in some cases, preventing these stresses. Knowledge of all phases of surgery is critical. Providing preoperative care and knowing what happens intraoperatively is the basis for planning and giving postoperative care. Patients are then ready for convalescence and an early discharge.

References

1. Baesl T, Buckley J: Preoperative assessment, preparation for operation, and routine postoperative care. Urol Clin North Am 10(1):3–17, 1983
2. Bartlett RH, Gazzaniga AB, Geraghty TR: Respiratory maneuvers to prevent postoperative pulmonary complications. JAMA 224(7):1017–1021, 1973
3. Berg RN: The great 'informed consent' debate: Should the disclosure of risks and alternatives be standard? J Med Assoc Ga 72(4):285–288, 1983
4. Bristain BR, Blackburn GL, Vitole J et al: Prevalence of malnutrition in general medical patients. JAMA 235:1567–1970, 1976
5. Churchill-Davidson HC (ed): A Practice of Anaesthesia, 4th ed. Philadelphia, WB Saunders, 1978
6. Cohen F, Lazarus RS: Active coping processes, coping dispositions, and recovery from surgery. Psycosom Med 35:375–389, 1973
7. Cohn I, Bornside G: Principles of Surgery. Infections, Chap. 5. New York, McGraw-Hill, 1984
8. Collins VJ (ed): Principles of Anesthesiology, 2nd ed. Philadelphia, Lea & Febiger, 1976
9. Egbert L et al: Reduction of postoperative pain by encouragement and instruction of patients. A study of doctor–patient rapport. New Engl J Med 270(16):825–827, 1964
10. Elliot D, Linz DH, Kane JA: Medical evaluation before operation. West J Med 137 (4):351–358, 1982
11. Elwyn D, Kinney JM, Askanazi J: Energy expenditure in surgical patients. Surg Clin North Am 61(3):545–555, 1981
12. Flacke J, Flacke WE: Inadvertent hypothermia: Frequent, insidious, and often serious. Semin Anesth 2(3):183–196, 1983
13. Foster CG: Relationship of Sympathetic Blockade to Blood Pressure Following Spinal Anesthesia. Unpublished Master's thesis, University of Washington, 1977
14. Foster C, Mukai G, Breckenridge, F et al: Effects of surgical positioning. AORN J 30(2):219–232, 1979
15. Gann DS: Endocrine and metabolic response to injury. In Principles of Surgery. New York, McGraw-Hill, 1984
16. George JM, Scott GS: The effects of psychological factors in recovery from surgery. J Am Dent Assoc 105:251–258, 1982

17. Goodman LS, Gilman A (eds): The Pharmacological Basis of Therapeutics, 7th ed. New York, Macmillan, 1985
18. Hensle T: Nutritional support of the surgical patient. Urol Clin North Am 10(1):109–118, 1983
19. Hick D: An incidence study of pressure sores following surgery. JANA Clinical Session, pp 49–54, 1970
20. Iverson L et al: A comparative study of IPPB, the incentive spirometer, and blow bottles: The prevention of atelectasis following cardiac surgery. Ann Thorac Surg 25(3):197–200, 1978
21. Keithy J: Infection and the malnourished patient. Heart Lung 12(1):23–27, 1983
22. Kneedler J, Dodge G: The patient's understanding of surgery. In Perioperative Patient Care. Boston, Blackwell Scientific Publications, 1983
23. Lobowitz P: Clinical Anesthesia Procedures of the Massachusetts General Hospital. Boston, Little, Brown Co., 1979
24. Mullen JL: Consequences of malnutrition in the surgical patient. Symposium on Surgical Nutrition. Surg Clin North Am 61(3): 465–486, 1981
25. National Nosocomial Infection Study Monthly Report, September, 1983. US Public Health Service, Department of Health and Human Services and Centers for Disease Control
26. Ozuna J, Foster C: Hypothermia and the surgical patient. Am J Nurs 79(4):646–648, 1979
27. Patient's Bill of Rights. Chicago, American Hospital Association, 1972
28. Peacock E: Wound healing and wound care. In Principles of Surgery. New York, McGraw-Hill, 1984
29. Pflug E, Aasheim G, Foster C: Sequence of return of neurological function and criteria for safe ambulation following subarachnoid block (spinal anesthesia). Can Anaesth Soc J 25(2):133–139, 1978
30. Pflug E, Aasheim G, Foster et al: Prevention of post-anaesthesia shivering. Can Anaesth Soc J 25(1):43–49, 1978
31. Pomorski ME: Surgical care for the aged patient: The decision-making process. Nurs Clin North Am 18(2):365–372, 1983
32. Reading AE: The short-term effects of psychological preparation for surgery. Soc Sci Med 13A:641–654, 1979
33. Risser NL: Preoperative and postoperative care to prevent pulmonary complications. Heart Lung 9:57–66, 1980
34. Schwartz S: Complications of surgery. In Principles of Surgery, 4th ed. New York, McGraw-Hill, 1984
35. Standards of Perioperative Nursing Practice. Kansas City, American Nurses Association and Association of Operating Room Nurses, 1982
36. Stein M, Cassara E: Perioperative pulmonary evaluation and therapy for surgical patients. JAMA 211(5):787–790, 1970
37. Tilney N, Lazarus M: Acute renal failure in surgical patients. Symposium on Critical Illness. Surg Clin North Am 63(2):357–375, 1983
38. Weiss O, Sriwatanatul K: Reduction of anxiety and postoperative analgesia requirement by audiovisual instruction. Lancet 1(8): 43–44, 1983

Bibliography

Alexander JW et al: The influence of hair-removal methods on wound infections. Arch Surg 118:387–350, 1983

Ballinger W, Treybal J, Vase A: Alexander's Care of the Patient in Surgery, 7th ed. St Louis, CV Mosby, 1983

Belstain BR, Blackburn GL, Hallowell E et al: Protein status of general surgical patients. JAMA 230:858–860, 1974

Cruse P, Foord R: The epidemiology of wound infection. Surg Clin North Am 60(1):27–40, 1980

Flynn M, Rovee D: Wound healing mechanisms. Am J Nurs 82: 1544–1558, 1982

Gruendemann B, Meeker MH: Alexander's Care of the Patient in Surgery, 7th ed. St Louis, CV Mosby, 1983

Guglielmo J et al: Antibiotic prophylaxis in surgical procedures. Arch Surg 118:943–955, 1983

Jung R et al: Comparison of three methods of respiratory care following upper abdominal surgery. Chest 78(1):31–34, 1980

Lederer D, Van de Water J, Indech R: Which deep breathing device should the postoperative patient use? Chest 77(5):610–613, 1980

Rhoades J: The impact of nutrition on infection. Surg Clin North Am 60(1):41–47, 1980

Schwartz S et al (ed): Principles of Surgery, 4th ed. New York, McGraw-Hill, 1984

Strauss RJ, Wise L: Operative risks of obesity. Surg Gynecol Obstet 146:286–291, 1978

Chapter 9

Pain

Charlene Gladney Foster

Defining Pain

The alleviation of pain and suffering is often viewed as the core of nursing practice. Pain is perhaps the least specific and most elusive patient problem faced by health professionals. There have been many attempts to define pain: as an unpleasant experience; an emotional experience in response to a noxious stimulus; a personal subjective state that cannot be shared; and an unexplained phenomenon. Like other subjective experiences such as anxiety and depression, the experience of pain is known only to the afflicted. Descriptive adjectives such as sharp and dull, acute and chronic, superficial and deep, and malignant and benign are often used to make the nature of pain better known.

Pain is known to exist for which it may be impossible to find the cause. If the cause is found there may be no correlation between the extent of injury and the degree of suffering. This is because of the many components of pain. There is no simple system by which pain reaches consciousness. Experimental studies in animals and man have been limited by the inability of the researcher to include the emotional component.

Carlson and Pelletteri attempted to combine the components of pain (P) in a formula.[3]

where E = Emotion, consisting of the following components:

- Social
- Psychological
- Ethnic

and N = Neurophysiological component, consisting of the following:

- Intensity
- Time

$P = E \times N$

They explained that pain may still be present if there are no noxious stimuli, but it requires the presence of emotion (E); therefore, another formula for pain is the following:

$P = E$

Mechanisms of Pain

Tissue damage or threatened tissue damage causes stimulation and firing of peripheral sensory free nerve endings known as nociceptors. These selective neurons are found in skin, adipose tissue, muscle fascia, and perivascular tissue. The nociceptors have two distinguishing features: they have a high threshold to all natural stimuli, and they have progressively augmented responses to repeated or increasingly noxious stimuli (sensitization). Sensitization has been produced by the by-products of tissue injury, such as histamine, serotonin, and bradykinin as well as by heat and chemicals, for example, hydrogen ions.

Once stimulated, the impulse is carried by either small myelinated A-delta fibers or unmyelinated C fibers. The A fibers carry sharp, localized pain as well as touch and some temperature response. The C fibers carry diffuse, dull pain and are considered polymodal because they can be activated by heat, intense mechanical pressure, or chemical mediators of inflammation. Therefore, acute tissue damage is experienced in two waves of pain: first sharp and then dull sensation. It is believed that the neurotransmitter in nociceptor transmission is substance P and is modulated by catecholamines, in particular, norepinephrine.

The afferent A-delta or C fibers pass from the dorsal root ganglia and enter the spinal cord by way of the dorsal root with a few fibers known as "second pain neurons" passing through the ventral root along with efferent motor fibers and sympathetic fibers. There is a dermatomal distribution of dorsal roots. However, overlapping of primary afferent fibers occurs within the dorsal horn. Axons in any particular dorsal root may extend over five or more spinal segments. Therefore, any point in the body may be innervated by fibers from five dorsal horns. The fibers then synapse with neurons of the dorsal horn in a layered fasion in the gray matter of the spinal cord. Cells in this region are known as *substantia gelatinosa.* This interneuron site is relevant to current pain theories. Most axons cross the midline in the anterior commissure to form the lateral spinothalamic tract that then ascends and terminates in the lateral nucleus of the thalamus. Fibers arising in the lower parts of the body are displaced laterally by fibers from the upper segments, which then occupy a medial position in the spinothalamic tracts. This laminar arrangment provides a topographical dermatome reference for sensory input to the brain. The spinothalamic tracts may be described as the most primitive paleospinothalamic tract that ascends to the brain stem transmitting dull pain and to the hypothalamus and limbic system, which add the emotional component of pain. Other fibers in the spinothalamic tracts continue by way of the neospinothalamic tract to synapse in the thalamic nuclei and relay to the cortex the conscious recognition of pain. Figure 9–1 depicts the pathways for pain and temperature impulses.

Other branches of sensory neurons that are known as second pain neurons connect with motor nerve cells and the sympathetic nervous system on the same entry side into the spinal cord. This connection with motor neurons is responsible for the withdrawal reflex in acute pain and may be responsible for chronic pain states involving increased muscle tone.

Variations in Pain Perception

Phantom Limbs. Amputation of a limb causes almost all patients to experience sensory illusions that the limb is still present. The perceived sensation is based on the dermatomal distribution of afferent neurons overlapping at the dorsal horn. A stimulus along any part of the nerve pathway is perceived as a pain at the origin of the pathway.

Referred Pain. Visceral irritation frequently produces pain that is felt not in the organ but in some somatic structure a distance away. Such pain is said to be *referred* to the somatic structure. Visceral and somatic areas that develop from the same embryonic segment have axons that converge at the same dorsal horn neurons. One theory is that somatic pain is considered much more common than visceral pain because somatic pain is a "learned signal" to noxious stimuli. Perhaps the best known example of referred pain is cardiac pain referred to the inner aspect of the left arm. Deep somatic pain may also be referred, but superficial pain is not. When visceral pain is both local and referred it is said to *radiate* from the local to the distant site.

Therapeutic Attempts at Pain Modulation

First Level: Ascending Pathway

Gate Theory

In the dorsal horn a complex interaction exists between activity originating in pain fibers and that originating from touch fibers. Spinothalamic tracts convey tactile sensation as well as nociception. Melzak and Wall suggested that the activity in large sensory nerve fibers activates an inhibitory interneuron that gives presynaptic inhibition to nerve fibers transmitting pain.[18] The mechanism is not completely understood, but may be due to a lower electrical threshold in the larger diameter touch fibers than in the smaller C-fiber nociceptors. The consequence is a reduction in pain when a touch stimulus is also given. In other words, pain sensation is not directly related to the number of impulses in the pain fibers but to a balance of activity between pain fibers and fibers that transmit other activity. This inhibitory effect is thought to explain why we do not experience pain during normal physical activities. The use of acupuncture, mustard plasters, liniments, balms, and counterirritants are all thought to be early approaches of pain modulation using this inhibition circuit. The *gate theory* has also been the basis for the development of several current methods of pain-inhibitory stimulation.

One such method is transcutaneous nerve stimulation (TNS). Surface electrodes are placed over the painful area and nonpain fibers are activated. The greatest effect is mediated by nerve fibers that have their origin in the same area as the pain. Surface electrodes are placed over the area of the spine with dermatomes supplying the area of pain, usually in the lumbar region. The ascending pain fibers travel in the anterolateral quadrant of the spinal cord by way of the spinothalamic tracts. Permanent intervention at the level of ascending pathways has been restricted to surgical lesioning: anterior cordotomy or rhizotomy. Initially, resection of the spinothalamic and spinoreticular tracts produces pain relief in 80% to 85% of cases.[15] However, in subsequent months many patients have recurrence of pain.

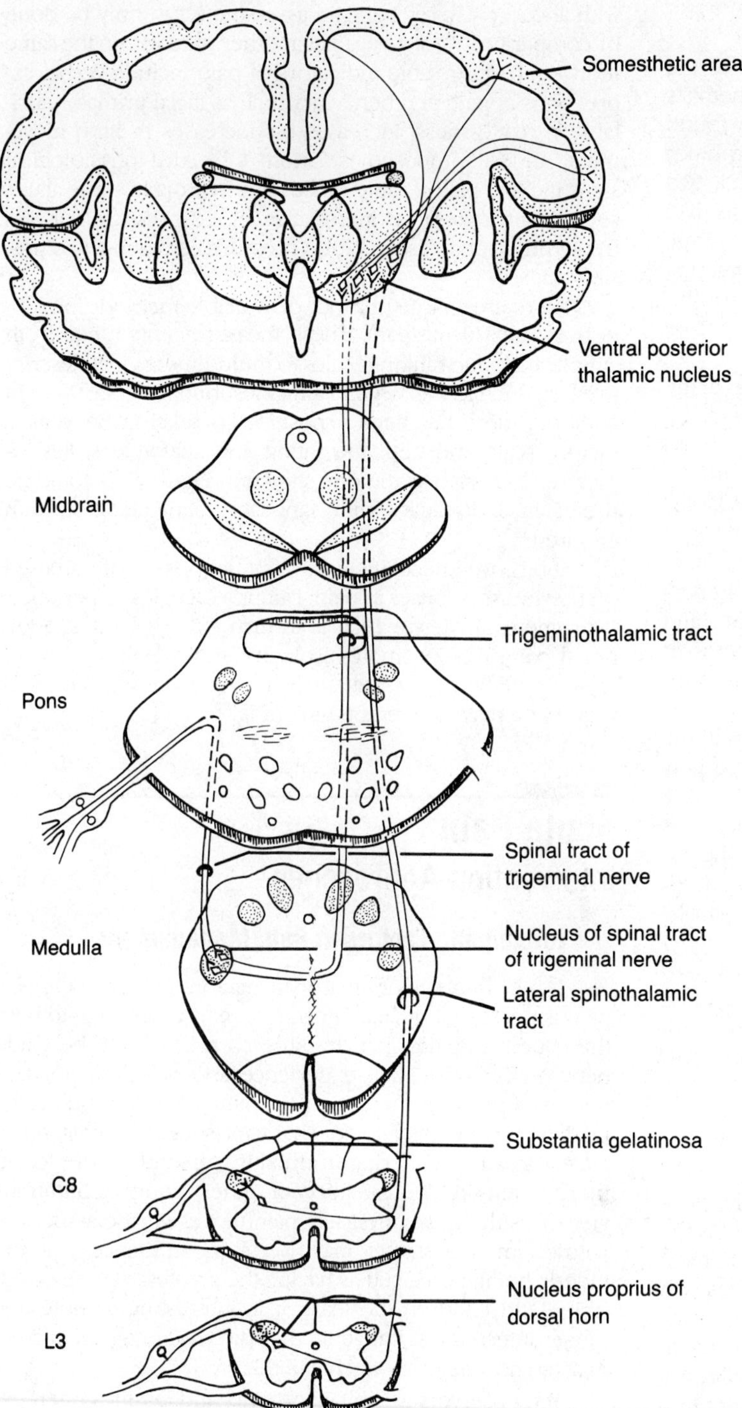

FIGURE 9–1 Pathways for pain and temperature.

Second Level: Descending Pathway

Supraspinal Brain

Research in the area of the supraspinal brain has begun only recently. Electrical stimulation of periaqueductal gray matter of the brain stem raphe and selective centers of the thalamus has been done on animals. This stimulation produces profound analgesia. Chemically implanted electrodes in the brain stem and the thalamus of patients with intolerable pain have been done on a limited basis. Success rates of around 70% have been reported;[3] however, potential risks may limit further exploration.

Opiate Receptors and Endorphins

For centuries it has been known that extract of the opium poppy provides excellent analgesia. When chemists were able to purify and make synthetic alkaloids, they found that some of the compounds (naloxone and nalorphine) could antagonize morphine. The conclusion was that two compounds (agonists like morphine and antagonists like nalorphine) compete for the same receptor site in the brain. These findings indicated the release of a naturally ocurring morphinelike substance. These endogenous opioids or *endorphins* act as neurotransmitters much as norepinephrine does on adrenergic receptors.

In 1975 Hughes and colleagues reported isolation of the first two substances of the endogenous opiate receptors: the polypeptides leu-enkephalin and met-enkephalin.[13] It has now been demonstrated that there are a variety of naturally occurring peptides that bind to these receptors. The larger peptides are called *endorphins* and the smaller ones *enkephalins.*

In the general category of endorphins, the most important ones appear to be β-endorphin, leu-enkephalin, and met-enkephalin. They are 20 to 30 times more potent than morphine. A new endorphin, dynorphin, is even more potent.[10]

Opiate receptors are present in at least three sites in the central nervous system: in the midbrain periaqueductal gray matter, in the rostroventral medulla, and in the substantia gelatinosa in the dorsal horn of the spinal cord. Enkephalins in the substantia gelatinosa presynaptically inhibit the release of substance P, which transmits pain. This interneuronal communication is known as the *endogenous opioid link.*

Endorphin activity is far from understood. In addition to endorphins outside the opioid system, neurotensin can elicit analgesia. On the other hand, pain transmission may involve somatostatin, norepinephrine, bradykinin, and prostaglandin as well as seratonin and substance P.

Third Level: Cortical

Cortical activity analyzes, integrates, and modulates the messages of pain in the intact human being. Pain threshold is the level at which pain is perceived and is fairly constant in most human beings.[31] However, pain tolerance, the point at which the individual seeks help, is highly individualized and variable. As discussed previously, pain has both a sensory (intensity) and affective (stress) component. Whereas analgesics attempt to treat the sensory component, other treatment modalities such as behavior modification, hypnosis, biofeedback, psychotherapy, and antidepressants are directed at the affective component. Clearly, the affective (subjective) component is the least measurable or understood.

Assessment of Pain

The difficulty in evaluating the intensity of pain in another individual has always existed. The subjective and behavioral components make it impossible to compare one individual with another. Therefore, pain assessment can only be done by comparing one state against another state within the same individual. Observable indicators of pain include verbal expressions of pain and behaviors such as facial grimaces, irritability, restlessness, increases or decreases in limb movement, and self-imposed isolation. Objective physiological signs include pallor, rapid pulse (bradycardia in some acute, severe pain states), an increase in blood pressure (or less frequently, a decrease in blood pressure), sweating, and possibly nausea.

There are a large number of available methods for subjectively measuring pain. These measurements range from simple analogue ranking scales to multidimensional descriptive tests such as the McGill Pain Questionnaire (Fig. 9–2). In addition, there has been a positive correlation between a picture scale and both the rating and analogue scales.[9] A picture scale such as the one shown in Figure 9–3 could be useful in individuals with language difficulties or with children.

Subjective effects include vague responses often based on previous responses to pain. Pain is a complex experience. It promotes anxiety, which is in turn experienced as additional pain. Pain promotes isolation and a feeling of helplessness. Subjective states such as anger, depression, and regression may be attempts at coping.[22]

Acute Pain

Intervention Approaches

Influencing Factors in Pain Management

It becomes evident that many factors influence the way pain is perceived by health professionals attempting to help the patient in pain. To date, little correlation can be made between the nurse's age, experience, and job satisfaction and her perception of the patient in pain. In a study done by Dudley and Holm, patient characteristics that elicit *inferences* of patient suffering in nursing personnel were found more often in the category of illness/injury. Conditions viewed as the most physically painful were those associated with trauma. Patient age may have some influence, with the elderly being perceived as having the greatest degree of suffering and children the least. It is interesting to note that nurses inferred less pain than they did psychological distress in actue hospitalized patients in this study.[6]

Yet, observers as well as patients and families often express the opinion that in many situations patients in pain were often undermedicated. Cohen found that 75.2% of postoperative patients were in moderate to severe pain, although analgesia was prescribed.[4] Weiss and colleagues found 41% of the postsurgical patients they studied to be in moderate to severe pain and 75% of the patients reported that their overall postoperative pain relief was inadequate.[29] They attempted to determine some of the influencing factors by studying the misconceptions and attitudes of physicians and nurses. They found that only 22% of both groups aimed at complete pain relief in the patient. Since the nurses and physicians were educated in different parts of the country,

McGill-Melzack
PAIN QUESTIONNAIRE

Patient's name ______________ Age ______
File No. ______________ Date ______
Clinical category (e.g. cardiac, neurological, etc.):

Diagnosis: ______________

Analgesic (if already administered):
1. Type ______________
2. Dosage ______________
3. Time given in relation to this test ______
Patient's intelligence: circle number that represents best estimate
1 (low) 2 3 4 5 (high)

This questionnaire has been designed to tell us more about your pain. Four major questions we ask are:

1. Where is your pain?
2. What does it feel like?
3. How does it change with time?
4. How strong is it?

It is important that you tell us how your pain feels now. Please follow the instructions at the beginning of each part.

Part 1. Where is Your Pain?

Please mark, on the drawings below, the areas where you feel pain. Put E if external, or I if internal, near the areas which you mark. Put EI if both external and internal.

Part 2. What Does Your Pain Feel Like?

Some of the words below describe your present pain. Circle ONLY those words that best describe it. Leave out any category that is not suitable. Use only a single word in each appropriate category—the one that applies best.

1: Flickering, Quivering, Pulsing, Throbbing, Beating, Pounding
2: Jumping, Flashing, Shooting
3: Pricking, Boring, Drilling, Stabbing, Lancinating
4: Sharp, Cutting, Lacerating
5: Pinching, Pressing, Gnawing, Cramping, Crushing
6: Tugging, Pulling, Wrenching
7: Hot, Burning, Scalding, Searing
8: Tingling, Itchy, Smarting, Stinging
9: Dull, Sore, Hurting, Aching, Heavy
10: Tender, Taut, Rasping, Splitting
11: Tiring, Exhausting
12: Sickening, Suffocating
13: Fearful, Frightful, Terrifying
14: Punishing, Gruelling, Cruel, Vicious, Killing
15: Wretched, Blinding
16: Annoying, Troublesome, Miserable, Intense, Unbearable
17: Spreading, Radiating, Penetrating, Piercing
18: Tight, Numb, Drawing, Squeezing, Tearing
19: Cool, Cold, Freezing
20: Nagging, Nauseating, Agonizing, Dreadful, Torturing

Part 3. How Does Your Pain Change With Time?

1. Which word or words would you use to describe the pattern of your pain?

1	2	3
Continuous	Rhythmic	Brief
Steady	Periodic	Momentary
Constant	Intermittent	Transient

2. What kind of things relieve your pain?

3. What kind of things increase your pain?

Part 4. How Strong Is Your Pain?

People agree that the following 5 words represent pain of increasing intensity. They are

1	2	3	4	5
Mild	Discomforting	Distressing	Horrible	Excruciating

To answer each question below, write the number of the most appropriate word in the space beside the question.

1. Which word describes your pain right now? ______
2. Which word describes it at its worst? ______
3. Which word describes it when it is least? ______
4. Which word describes the worst toothache you ever had? ______
5. Which word describes the worst headache you ever had? ______
6. Which word describes the worst stomach-ache you ever had? ______

FIGURE 9–2 The McGill-Melzack Pain Questionnaire is one method of measuring pain.

they felt that these findings were indicative of the entire United States. In addition, staff responses to questions regarding knowledge of narcotic analgesia indicated poor understanding. A major misconception was fear of addiction (although documented at less than 1% in the postsurgical population).[21] Next ranked was fear of respiratory depression, followed by lack of basic knowledge of the effects and duration of naloxone for the treatment of narcotic overdose.

Inadequate pain relief not only elicits in the patient a stress response with many physiological ramifications, but also can develop into a more complex patient–nurse conflict in which the control becomes the use of analgesics. Such conflicts can influence all other nurse–patient interactions. One approach aimed at reducing the possibility of this conflict is an on-demand system of analgesia. One study found that patients using an on-demand system were medicated more frequently, but actually used smaller doses than staff-administered analgesics. In addition, the perception of pain was considered much higher by patients in the group receiving staff-administered analgesics.[25]

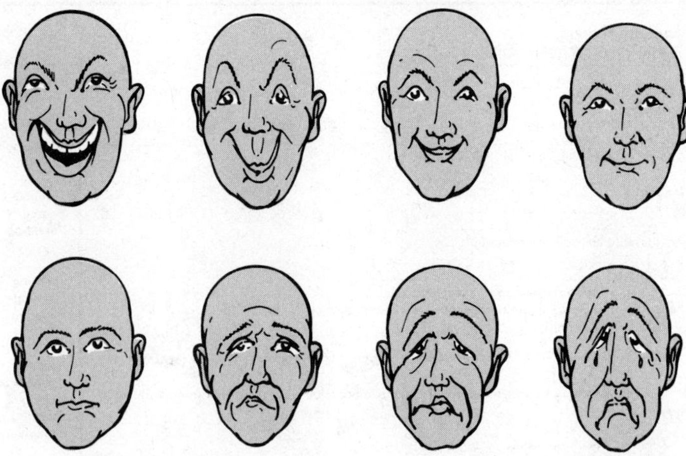

FIGURE 9–3 Eight-point picture scale of pain.

Drug Therapy

Peripheral Antialgesics

A basic understanding of the pharmacology of commonly used analgesics is primary for nurses caring for the patient in pain. As the field of knowledge grows, ongoing education for nurses in this area must be continued. Until the late 1970s pain medication consisted primarily of aspirin (and the aniline group, such as phenacetin and acetaminophen) for less severe pain and narcotic analgesics (*e.g.*, morphine, codeine, and mepheridine) for moderate to severe pain. More recently a new group of non-narcotic analgesics called *peripheral analgesics* or *antialgesics* has emerged that are more effective than aspirin. Their goal is to convert a hyperalgesic state to a normal algesic state. Centrally acting narcotics are true analgesics because they relieve pain regardless of etiology by dulling the awareness of pain on higher brain centers. The peripheral antialgesics exert their effects locally or near the point of insult. These drugs work by inhibiting prostaglandin synthesis, resulting in a reduction of prostaglandins, which lower nociception threshold at the free nerve endings. The anti-inflammatory action of these drugs is often beneficial in the treatment of inflammatory disease. However, this anti-inflammatory action is thought to be dissociated from antialgesic activity.[2] When used for analgesia alone, the new peripheral antialgesics have been shown to be more effective than aspirin, acetaminophen, or codeine in mild to moderate pain situations. Some examples of peripheral antialgesics are:

Phenylbutazone (Butazolidin)	100 mg 4 to 6 times/day
Indomethacin (Indocin)	25–50 mg 4 to 5 times/day
Ibuprofen (Motrin)	200–600 mg 4 times/day

Their most frequent side-effects are gastrointestinal disturbances, causing diarrhea, gastritis, or ulcers. All peripheral antialgesics can prolong bleeding when taken over long periods of time because they influence platelet function. Occasionally, headaches, dizziness, and changes in visual acuity have also been reported.[30] Analgesics should be taken at specific time intervals around the clock. When analgesia is time-contingent rather than symptom-contingent, less medication is usually requested and better pain relief provided.

Narcotic Analgesics (Agonists) and Antagonists

Narcotics are most often used for acute pain of limited duration or in patients with terminal disease. This general restriction is because all narcotic drugs produce increased tolerance. That is, the longer the medication is taken, the less the analgesic effect, resulting in increased dose requirements. In this set of circumstances, drug dependency can result in drug-seeking behavior. Morphine is the standard drug for comparative analgesia studies. All narcotic agents are equally potent at equivalent doses in most individuals.[7] A list of common narcotic drugs with recommended intramuscular and oral dosages is presented in Table 9–1.

Nursing Implications. The nurse must know the side effects of narcotics, and patients receiving narcotics must be carefully assessed on a routine basis. After intramuscular injection of narcotics, assessment should be made of the patient's respiratory and cardiovascular system at 15-minute, half-hour, and hour intervals. Patients with debilitating states, the elderly, children, or any patient receiving a narcotic for the first time require vigilant observation! Central nervous system effects usually include a dulling of awareness but the patient should still be arousable and able to make appropriate responses. Miosis (constricting) of the pupils will occur as sympathetic discharge is reduced. Respiratory rate and

TABLE 9–1
Narcotics Equivalent to 10 mg Morphine IM

	Dosage	
	Intramuscular (mg)	*Oral (mg)*
Morphine	10	60
Meperidine (Demerol)	50–75	200
Codeine	130	200
Alphaprodine (Nisentil)	45	
Diacetylmorphine (heroin)	3	
Fentanyl (Sublimaze)	0.1	
Hydromorphone (Dilaudid)	1.5	7.5
Methadone (Dolophine)	8	10
Oxycodone (Percodan)	15	30
Oxymorphone (Numorphan)	1.5	
Levorphanol (Levo-Dromoran)	2	4

depth are affected, with rate the best assessment for narcosis. Respiratory rates less than 10 require stimulation by patient prompting until the narcotic effect lessens. If the respiratory rate is less than 6 to 8 and associated with poor patient response or circulatory compromise, then immediate notification of the attending physician should be made. Naloxone (Narcan) 0.1 mg IV can reverse these symptoms. However, *Narcan's reversal effects may not outlast the narcotic effects.* The use of Narcan should be judicious because cases of extreme hypertension and pulmonary edema have been reported. Intubation equipment and ambu mask and bag should be standard equipment on every unit where narcotics are administered. Narcotics will lower blood pressure by venous dilation. This can be considered desirable in patients with coronary artery disease; however, extreme drops in blood pressure can occur if the patient is hypovolemic or has had anesthesia, other analgesia, or sedation. If this has occurred, depending on the individual agent, the pulse rate may increase (seen with Demerol) or decrease (seen with fentanyl). Nausea is a frequent complaint associated with narcotics, and antiemetics are often prescribed with the narcotic to reduce this effect as well as to potentiate analgesia. Sphincter of odi spasm occurs occasionally, especially in patients with gallbladder disease, and can be relieved with atropine or, if necessary, Narcan. Constipation is a long-term effect and, therefore, laxatives are often ordered on a routine basis.

Agonist–Antagonist Drugs

Drugs in this group act by binding to opioid receptor sites. These drugs vary in their effect from complete antagonism (possibly by binding at an additional antagonistic site) of narcotic activity to providing analgesia as well (agonism). If narcotics are already occupying the opioid receptor sites, then antagonism will precede any analgesia, and analgesia will be present but diminished in order of agonist activity. Table 9–2 gives the relation of antagonist to agonist activity of various narcotics.

Adjunctive Drugs

Recently, it has been shown that combining drugs that affect the central nervous system with narcotics provides better analgesia. Amphetamines have been used, particularly with patients experiencing postoperative pain, allowing the patient to remain alert for ambulation. Sedative–hypnotic drugs such as barbiturates or diazepam (Valium) are used for analgesia potentiation by mediating the "emotional component" of pain. The sedative tranquilizers, such as diphenhydramine (Benadryl) and hydroxyzine (Vistaril), are found to be just as effective without the potential for dependency or withdrawal effects.

Practical Approach to Analgesic Management

The goal of effective pain therapy should be to enable the patient to tolerate the necessary diagnostic and treatment intervention and to allow him to maintain emotional and physiological function. In acute states, such as in the post-operative or post-trauma patient, complete pain relief within the margins of physiological safety is a realistic expectation. In more chronic pain states, an expectation of functional tolerance may be more realistic. Nursing assessment and

TABLE 9–2
Narcotic Agonist/Antagonist Drugs

Narcotic antagonist activity (↑ Greatest)	Drug	Dose	Activity	Narcotic agonist activity (↓ Greatest)
	Naloxone (Narcan)	0.1–0.4 mg IM or IV *injection only*	Pure *antagonist*, no analgesia Activity lasts 3–5 hours	
	Nalorphine (Nalline)	5–10 mg IV or IM *injection only*	Primarily antagonist Analgesia equivalent to morphine 10 mg	
	Pentazocine (Talwin)	30–50 mg IM or 50 mg po	Weak antagonist Analgesia equal to morphine 10 mg	
	Nalbuphine (Nubain)	10–12 mg IM or IV *injection only*	Antagonism 10 × Pentazocine Analgesia equal to 1 to 2 × morphine 10 mg	
	Butorphanol (Stadol)	2 mg IV or IM *injection only*	Antagonism 30 × Pentazocine and 1/40 of Naloxone Analgesia 3–5 × more potent than morphine 10 mg	

Note: Antagonist action for treatment of respiratory depression due to narcotic overdose is seen within 1 to 2 min after intravenous injection but lasts only about 3 hr. Respiratory depression may outlast this reversal effect. Patients requiring narcotic antagonism *must not be left alone.*

Drugs are ranked from lowest analgesic (agonist) and greatest antagonist activity to greatest agonist and lowest antagonist activity.

approach can make the difference in the patient's attainment of his goals for therapy.

The following guidelines are directed at a systematic nursing approach for dealing with patients in pain.[25]

1. *Treat the patient, not the symptoms.* Pain is subjective. *All* complaints of pain should be treated with systematic assessment, intervention, and reassessment. Reassessment provides emotional support and assurance as well as valuable data necessary for patient safety and further intervention.
2. *Know the pharmacology of the drugs prescribed.* Know dosage, duration, how the drug is eliminated from the body, and drug interactions with other medications and food. Know the drug's side-effects and be prepared to treat them.
3. *Administer analgesics regularly,* even at night if necessary to maintain an analgesic level. If more frequent administration, a different dosage, or a different medication than ordered is needed, then notify the physician (even at home) for a change of order. Consider an "on-demand" system. As Robinson states:

   > If it is known a patient is in pain, giving the analgesic before it is requested can be most beneficial. This preserves the patient dignity. He does not have to request what is rightfully his own.[22]

4. *Know the effects of analgesics on specific patients.* For example, patients with chronic respiratory disease are at risk for severe respiratory depression after narcotic administration. The neurologically impaired may become agitated or more obtunded than is usually seen with patients receiving narcotics, making assessment difficult. Patients with cardiovascular compromise may experience intolerable drops in blood pressure or changes in heart rate.

Elderly Patients. A large group of patients requiring special attention with pain management is the *elderly.* Pain is a disorganization experience often leading to regressive behavior. Allowing the elderly patient some independence and control is often all that is needed to enable him to cope. Occasionally the older patient does not complain of pain, but behavioral changes such as agitation, irritability, isolation, and depression that may signal underlying pain.

Pain cannot be prepared for, no matter what one's previous experiences were. Learned behavioral responses may include stoicism or denial of pain.[27] Particular attention must be given to systematic assessment of pain with the patient and support of his right to expression of his pain and intervention in its management.

Administration of narcotics to the elderly requires careful titration of dosage and monitoring the effects. Kaiko and colleagues studied the effects of narcotics in the elderly and found that patients in the age range of 70 to 89 years responded as though they had received fourfold the dose given to young adults.[14] Similarly, patients in the age group of 50–69 years required less narcotics than did younger patients. In addition, clearance of plasma morphine was significantly decreased with increasing age, indicating that the frequency of administration should be lengthened. These researchers suggested that age be the criteria for choosing the initial dose and dosing frequency.

Chronic Pain

Magnitude of the Problem

Entire books have been written on the understanding and management of the patient in chronic pain. This portion of the chapter provides only an introduction to this complex and rapidly changing area. One view of the scope of the effects of chronic pain is in financial terms. In America approximately 40 to 50 billion dollars are lost annually on wages and health care costs because of pain. The financial cost of pain to each individual cannot be measured.

The Pain Clinic

The mechanisms of chronic pain are complex and may involve several causes. Patients with complaints of musculoskeletal pain involving the head, back, or extremity or patients suffering from central pain states such as tic douloureux, posthepatic neuralgia, or phantom limb are among those frequently seen as chronic pain sufferers. Patients may have difficulty obtaining adequate diagnosis and treatment, since most medical approaches are based on tissue damage as the model of pain. Inadequate or inappropriate treatment or occasionally mistreatment in the form of unnecessary surgery, ineffective medication, and protective limitations may result. The patient may suffer not only from the original pain complaint but from complications of diagnosis and ineffective therapy.[19]

The pain clinic has evolved over the last decade in response to the particular problem of chronic pain. Most pain clinics provide a multidisciplinary approach and comprise such diverse health professionals as anesthesiologists (usually in the leadership position), neurologists/neurosurgeons, orthopedic surgeons, nurses, psychiatrists/psychologists/social workers, physical therapists, and pharmacists. This multidisciplinary approach has proved most effective in evaluating and treating the individual because all environmental, social, emotional, and physical factors influence the intensity and coping mechanisms of the patient in chronic pain.

An integral part of the process of evaluation in the pain clinic is a diary of pain levels and activities kept by the patient. Comprehensive psychological and medical evaluation then helps designate appropriate intervention. Often multiple interventions are needed. Patient participation as an active member in this team approach is at the core of pain clinic treatment.

Treatment

Treatment stategies include biofeedback, acupuncture, relaxation techniques, hypnosis, assertiveness training, and role-playing. Some practitioners feel that the phenomenon of chronic pain is largely "pain behaviors."[8] Others feel that emotional, personality, or motivational components must be addressed as the major influencing factors.[26] Treatment approach is individualized. Some patients may require more physical than psychological intervention, whereas others may need more psychologically based intervention. However, treatment in the pain clinic setting almost always involves both components.

Medications

Drugs are most often prescribed for and abused by the patients suffering from chronic pain. Depending on the individual, analgesics, tranquilizers, or no medication may be tried.

Analgesics. Aspirin and acetaminophen are the most useful analgesics in the majority of chronic pain patients. Peripheral antialgesics and narcotic analgesics may be prescribed in more severe forms of pain, particularly cancer pain. It must be kept in mind that the use of analgesics, sedatives, and hypnotics for chronic pain over long periods of time has been shown to be detrimental to cognitive function and can complicate clinical management.[17]

Antidepressants. While anxiety is the experience most often associated with acute pain, chronic pain is almost always linked with depression.[23] Studies have shown that reduction of pain also brings a reduction of depression. A possible reason for the association of pain and depression is that some patients with chronic pain have been found to have lowered brain serotonin levels.[12] Lowered brain serotonin in animals increases their sensitivity to noxious stimuli. The ratio between brain serotonin and norepinephrine is associated with changes in sleep patterns. Sleep is often found to be disrupted in the chronic pain patient.

Tricyclic antidepressants are often used to increase serotonin levels by blocking its reuptake into presynaptic neurons. Two commonly used drugs are amitriptyline (Elavil, Triavil) 75 mg to 100 mg and doxepin (Sinequan) 75 mg to 100 mg, both taken at bedtime.

Sedative Hypnotics. Drug dependency in the chronic pain patient can complicate evaluation and treatment. Most patients requiring narcotics for pain control have also been using sedatives or hypnotics for analgesia potentiation as well as for depression and sleep. Ascertaining a "drug profile" may be necessary on an "in-patient" basis to provide more effective treatment. Patients begin by receiving whatever medication they wish, whenever they wish; therefore, careful documentation is necessary. Detoxification may be needed to unmask symptoms and is usually done at a reduction of 10% in dosage of drugs a day. Examples of sedative hypnotics with dosages are listed in Table 9–3.

Sedatives can hinder the patient's ability to identify and express pain. When patients become anxious, depressed, or agitated because of unrelieved pain, treatment with analgesics will often provide emotional as well as pain relief.[11]

The goal in pain medication maintenance is to provide a safe effective analgesia course without the roller coaster effects of extreme highs and lows associated with analgesia. More frequent administration of smaller amounts of medication is advocated.[12]

TABLE 9–3
Sedative Hypnotics*

Drug	*Dosage (mg)*
Secobarbital (Seconal)	100
Pentobarbital (Nembutal)	100
Chlordiazepoxide (Librium)	25
Diazepam (Valium)	10
Flurazepam (Dalmane)	30
Methaqualone (Quaalude)	300
Glutethimide (Doriden)	500
Ethchlorvynol (Placidyl)	750
Chloral hydrate (Noctec)	1000
Hydroxyzine (Vistaril)	50–100
Diaphenhydramine (Benadryl)	50–100
Meprobamate (Equanil, Miltown)	400
Liquor (100 proof)	90 ml (3 oz)

* Equivalent to phenobarbital 30 mg

The Pain Cocktail. The pain cocktail or Brompton's cocktail has been used for several years for analgesia in the patient with chronic pain. Although the ingredients may vary, a typical solution includes the following:

An analgesic	Methadone, morphine, or heroin
An antiemetic	Chlorpromazine (usually)
A stimulant	Cocaine or amphetamine
A bacteriocidal base	Ethyl alcohol or vodka
Sugared syrup	

The cocktail is given on an around-the-clock basis at every 3 to 6 hours for chronic pain associated with cancer. The roller coaster effect is minimized particularly when methadone is used since less euphoria is provided. However, several problems have been identified. The stimulant, whether cocaine or amphetamine, can cause agitation or disorientation in the elderly. On the other hand, the antiemetic, usually chlorpromazine (Thorazine), is a sedative and can produce lethargy and depression. In addition, the alcohol base can irritate mucous membranes or cause gastritis or ulcers in patients receiving radiation or chemotherapy.[11]

Nerve Blocks

When there is a specific nociception, such as with cancer or the causalgia component of chronic pain, nerve blocks have been particularly beneficial. Nerve blocks can be used diagnostically in determining the neural pathway involved. Diagnostic nerve blocks include sympathetic blocks of "differential" spinal blocks with different percentages of local anesthetic used until disappearance of symptoms has been accomplished. This information will help isolate the pain pathways involved and perhaps lead to more definitive treatment, such as denervation procedures (*e.g.,* rhizotomy) or neurolytic blocks (using phenol or alcohol).

Epidural or Subarachnoid Steroid Injections. Chronic back pain is thought to be in part due to low grade inflammation or arachnoiditis. Steroid injections of Depo-Medrol with or without local anesthetics, combined with manipulation exercises after the block have been useful. The injection is of most value when no previous surgery has been performed in that area.

Trigger Point Injections. These specific blocks are directed at the areas of localized pain. The nature of trigger points is usually myofascial, involving muscle of fascial areas expecially around the back, neck, or shoulders. Weak local anesthetics are injected. The earlier this type of intervention, the better the results in chronic pain states.

Cancer Pain

Magnitude of the Problem

Fifteen million persons a year worldwide are diagnosed as having cancer, and each year 10% of them, or 5 million, die (1979 data). Almost half (47%) of patients with all stages of cancer have pain; this increases from 78% to 87% in those with advanced disease. Lung cancer causes most of the pain reported by patients, with moderate to severe pain.[1] Pain is something that patients fear will happen to them when they are diagnosed as having cancer, and with good reason.

Causes of Cancer Pain

Pain due to cancer may have several sources. It may be caused by tumor invasion of bone with pain at the site or referred to another site. Pain may be caused by the tumor compressing nerves, obstructing shallow organs, or occluding blood supply. Secondary pain can occur as a consequence of tumor therapy with surgery, radiation, or chemotherapy. Pain can occur indirectly as a result of weakened defense mechanisms, for example, infection. Finally, pain can come from emotional factors of grief, separation, isolation, and fear.[16]

Treatment of Cancer Pain

Treatment of pain in the cancer patient must include recognition of all the causes. Fear of addiction by physician, nurses, and family often leads to undermedication. Distinction should be made between compulsive behavior addiction and physical dependence. Terminally ill patients in pain will become physically dependent on pain control. Consideration of addiction is irrelevant and inappropriate in this setting.[17] Pain medication must be given on a regular basis without the need for the patient to request it. Narcotic opioids remain the most effectively used medication in the terminally ill. Pain cocktails (described earlier) are used frequently in this setting. Two other methods of maintaining drug analgesia levels in the acute care setting are continuous intravenous infusions of opioids (particularly morphine) and epidural injection of opioids by catheter. The technique for the former requires an accurate infusion pump and careful monitoring and nursing assessment of the patient's responses. These responses are listed as follows:

1. Level of consciousness. Patients should be able to converse and move about
2. Pupils. Miosis (constriction) will occur before respiratory depression
3. Respiratory rate and depth, particularly rate
4. Blood and pulse should be stable

Epidural injections, particularly of morphine, have been used in some institutions. More widespread use of this technique has been limited in part by the need for special nursing care. Epidural morphine (requiring only small doses) is thought to diffuse through the dura into the cerebrospinal fluid and then into the spinal cord, where it acts on the dorsal horn by blocking the release of substance P. The cardiovascular system does not seem to be greatly altered. Motor function remains intact, allowing ambulation. Bladder spasm is relieved, but urination may be difficult and constipation can be noted.

An epidural catheter is placed by the anesthesiologist under strict aseptic conditions, usually in the operating room. The epidural catheter is very carefully taped in place on the patient's back. Protection of this catheter is paramount in the nursing care of these patients. Small amounts of morphine (1 mg to 5 mg) are diluted in 5 ml normal saline without a preservative and injected ***aseptically*** every 1 to 24 hours depending on the patient's needs. Alcohol should not be used to wipe the ends of the catheter because it can be very irritating and painful should a small amount of alcohol be introduced with the injection into the epidural space.

The major side-effect of epidural injections is depression. Studies have shown a depression of ventilatory function during the period of 3 to 15 hours after a morphine injection. The degree of depression comes on *very slowly over 1 to 2 hours.*[5] Narcan, 0.1 mg IV, can reverse this depression, but morphine depression may outlast the Narcan reversal.

Hourly assessment should be made of vital signs, particularly respiratory rate and depths and the pupils, in which extreme constriction (miosis) will occur before respiratory depression.

Routine assessment every 4 hours should be made of intake and output; watch for bladder distention. Examination of epidural catheter entry sites should be made for bleeding infection or possible leak of cerebrospinal fluid.

Summary

This chapter has only introduced some basic concepts of the physiology and clinical management of a complex and multidimensional phenomenon known as pain. These concepts are evolving and changing as more knowledge is gained through research and clinical practice. Pain management is a major part of nursing management for many patients. Unless pain is relieved, the patient will not benefit from his treatment and progress toward recovery will be delayed.

References

1. Bonica JJ: Management of cancer pain. Recent Results Cancer Res 89:13–27, 1984
2. Capetola R, et al: Peripheral analgesics: A Review. G. Clin Pharmacol 23:545–556, 1983
3. Carlsson CA, Pellettieri L: A clinical view on pain physiology. Acta Chir Scand 148:305–313, 1982
4. Cohen FL: Postsurgical pain relief: Patients' status and nurses' medication choices. Pain 9:265–274, 1980
5. Crawford ME et al: Pain treatment on outpatient basis utilizing extradural opiates: A Danish multicentre study comparing 105 patients. Pain 16:41–42, 1983
6. Dudley SR, Holm K: Assessment of the pain experience in relation to selected nurse characteristics. Pain 18:179–186, 1984
7. Foley K: The practical use of narcotic analgesics. Med Clin North Am 66(5):1091–1104, 1982
8. Fordyce WE: Behavioral interventions in chronic pain. J Psychosom Res 27(5):424–430, 1983
9. Frank AJM, Mall JMA, Hort JF: A comparison of three ways of measuring pain. Rheumatol Rehabil 21:211–217, 1982
10. Goodman CE: Pathophysiology of Pain. Arch Intern Med 143:527–530, 1983
11. Heidrich G, Perry S: Helping the patient in pain. ASN, pp 1818-1832, December, 1982
12. Hendler N: Depression caused by chronic pain. J Clin Psychiatry 45(3):30–36, 1984
13. Hughes J et al: Identification of two related pentapeptides from the brain with patient opiate agonist activity. Nature 258:577–580, 1975
14. Kaido R et al: Narcotics in the elderly. Med Clin North Am 66(5):1079–1089, 1982
15. Levine J: Pain and analgesia: The outlook for more rational treatment. Ann Intern Med 100:269–275, 1984
16. McGluney W, Crooks GM: The care of patients with severe chronic pain in terminal illness. JAMA 251(9):1182–1188, 1984
17. McNairy S et al: Prescriptive medication dependence and neuropsychological function. Pain 18:169–177, 1984
18. Melzak R, Wall PD: Pain mechanisms: A new theory. Science 150:971, 1965
19. Murph T: Treatment of chronic pain. In Miller R (ed): Anesthesia, Vol 2, pp 1459–1490. New York, Churchill Livingstone, 1981
20. Parkes CM: Home or hospice? Terminal care as seen by surviving spouse. J R Coll Gen Pract 28:19–30, 1978
21. Porter L, Jick H: Addiction rare in patients treated with narcotics. N Engl J Med 302:123, 1980
22. Robinson L: Psychological Aspects of the Care of the Hospitalized Patient, 2nd ed. Philadelphia, FA Davis, 1972
23. Shacham S, Revvon D, Cluland CS: The relationship of mood state to the severity of clinical pain. Pain 18:187–197, 1984
24. Skwington SM: Social cognitions, personality and chronic pain. J Psychosom Res 27(5):421–428, 1983
25. Slattery PJ: An open comparison between routine and self-administrated postoperative pain relief: Aspects of anesthesia. Ann R Coll Surg Eng 65:18–19, 1983
26. Violin A, Giurgea D: Familial models of chronic pain. Pain 18:199–205, 1984
27. Wacheter-Shikosa NL: The elderly patient in pain and the acute care setting. Nurs Clin North Am 18(2):395–401, 1983
28. Wallace K, Hays J: Nursing management of chronic pain. J Neurosurg Nurs (4):185–191
29. Weiss O et al: Attitudes of patients, housestaff and nurses toward postoperative analgesic care. Anesth Analg 62:70–74, 1983
30. Woodburg DM, Fingl E: Analgesic-antipyretics, anti-inflammatory agents. In Goodman L, Gilman A (eds): The Pharmacological Basis of Therapeutics, 5th ed. New York, Macmillan, 1975
31. Wyke BD: Neurological Aspects of Pain Theory. In Swerdlow M (ed): The Theory of Pain. Hagerstown, Harper Row, 1981

Chapter 10

Sensory Overload, Sensory Deprivation, and Sleep Deprivation

Kathryn A. Lee

All patients requiring skilled nursing care risk sensory overload, sensory deprivation, or sleep deprivation. These three states should be viewed as disorders of arousal in response to environmental stimuli. Whether patients are undergoing surgery, experiencing pain, dying of terminal illness, or having a baby, the lack of control over their environments makes them vulnerable to these disorders of arousal.

When a stimulus from either the internal or the external environment is perceived, the central nervous system (CNS) processes that incoming information and organizes it to fit with previous experiences. Any stimulus entering the CNS has the potential for being monotonous or overwhelming, ignored or perceived, or boring or enriching.

The concept of arousal is an important one for understanding how a person copes with changes in his environment. However, this concept is a complex one indeed. An identical environment can be perceived differently by different individuals. For any given person, the same stimulus can be monotonous one minute and overwhelming the next minute. One student may demand absolute quiet while preparing for an examination, whereas another can study only when music is blaring in the background. Understanding the role of CNS arousal is crucial in relation to how particular individuals perceive and process stimuli within the environment to continue to function within that environment. Whether a stimulus reaches a threshold for cortical arousal depends on how predictable it is, how intense it is, and how relevant to that individual it is.

The Arousal Mechanism

Cortical arousal, or alertness, is thought to be yet another example of the process of homeostasis. Living organisms behaving in ways necessary to maintain an optimal level of functioning also require an optimal level of sensory stimulation. In fact, the term *sensoristasis* has been suggested to describe the arousal mechanism that serves to limit incoming stimuli when an already high level of arousal is present and to enhance incoming stimuli when the arousal level is abnormally low.[27] Too much (sensory overload) or too little (sensory deprivation) stimulation from one's environment disrupts the processing of new information and interferes with the development of new strategies for coping with environmental demands. A person copes successfully with environmental demands only within an optimal range of sensory stimulation.

The reticular activating system (RAS) appears to have primary responsibility for mediating CNS arousal (Fig. 10–1) It is stimulated by visual, auditory, gustatory, olfactory, tactile, visceral, kinesthetic, somatic, and cognitive input. With its many ascending and descending connections to other areas of the brain, the RAS serves to monitor and regulate incoming sensory stimuli and thereby maintain, enhance, or inhibit cortical arousal. When the RAS is electrically stimulated in sleeping animals, arousal occurs. When the RAS is suppressed with drugs such as barbiturates, sleep results. Recent evidence points to two specific areas within the RAS as responsible for maintaining an awake, alert state. Serotonergic neurons in the raphe nuclei appear responsible for inhibiting arousal and deactivating alertness,[28] whereas noradrenergic neurons in the locus ceruleus appear responsible for maintaining an alert state.[2, 20]

Disorders in the arousal mechanism, or disrupted sensoristasis, occur when the RAS is bombarded with input as well as when the RAS fails to recognize input because the stimulus lacks relevant meaning or is of such low intensity as to be below threshold level. When stimuli are overwhelming the RAS, cortical arousal level is high and individuals experience sensory overload and feel anxiety, fear, immobility, or confusion. Persons who are placed in environments deficient in stimuli can have reduced cortical arousal and can become sensorially deprived so as to experience inactivity, boredom, depression, drowsiness, or restlessness.

Difficulty in inhibiting arousal is expressed as sleep deprivation due to difficulty in falling asleep or in maintaining sleep at appropriate times in the day–night cycle. Individuals can experience difficulty in inhibiting arousal during normal sleep periods because of either sensory overload or sensory deprivation.

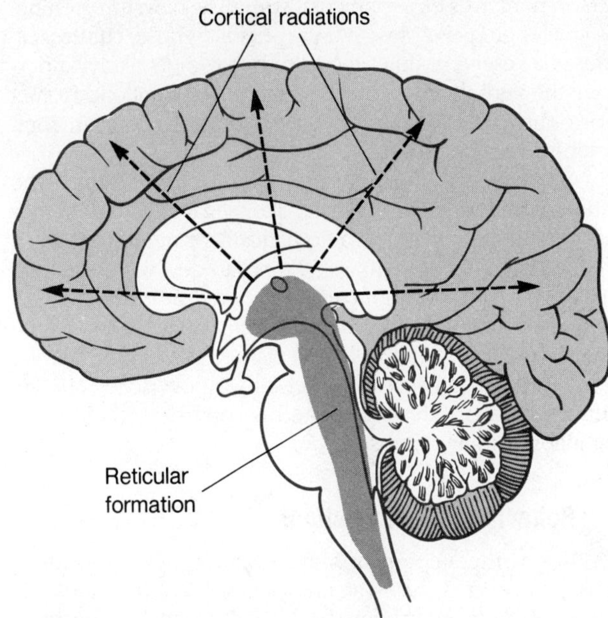

FIGURE 10–1 Reticular formation in brain stem and diencephalon with radiations to the cerebral cortex.

Sensory Overload

When sensoristasis is altered by excessive input from the environment and a person no longer feels in control, he is said to be experiencing sensory overload. Again, what constitutes excessive input for one individual is not necessarily perceived as excessive by another person. Any one source of sensation or combination of sensory input can produce a situation of sensory overload for a patient. Worrying about the outcome of a surgical procedure, listening to a physician's explanantion, and solving the problem of how to deal with a chronic illness are examples of cognitive overload. Visual overload can arise from glaring lights, adjusting to trifocal lenses, television, or colorful striped wallpaper. Noisy linen carts, a new hearing aid, and many people talking at once can contribute to auditory overload. Tactile, visceral, and somatic overload can occur as a result of pain, the excessive pressure from a cast placed too tightly on a swollen extremity, or chest restraints. Even a gentle touch can overload sensory input, depending on who is doing the touching and how the touch is perceived by the patient.

Patients at Risk

Unfamiliar environments, such as hospital rooms with cardiac monitors and noisy respirators, recovery rooms with their intense lighting and unrecognizable faces, or emergency rooms with their rapid pace of movement, are likely to expose patients to sensory overload (Fig. 10–2). This is particularly likely if the patient is also anxious, experiencing pain sensation from his internal environment, or already aroused because of medications such as caffeine that stimulate the CNS arousal mechanism.

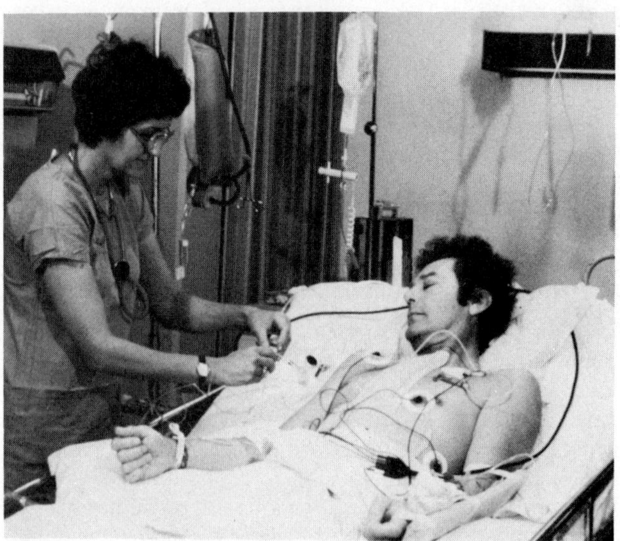

FIGURE 10–2 The intensive care unit environment may lead to sensory overload.

Infants as well as the elderly are equally at risk. The very young are continually experiencing new sensations because of their lack of life experiences. The very old are less able to process incoming stimuli as rapidly as when they were young. Culture also plays an important role in whether a person perceives environmental stimuli as new, threatening, or challenging. For instance, a person whose culture espouses a reserved, quiet mode of behavior is likely to perceive the verbal and tactile expressions of someone from a more outwardly expressive culture as intense and uncomfortably overwhelming.

One type of patient in danger of sensory overload is the patient who has had a recent stroke. Regardless of whether this person can eat a meal automatically or needs to relearn the method of feeding himself, he has to deal with olfactory, visual, and somatic input that occurs simultaneously. Although he may be able to cope well with that input, the added stimulus of talking, having visitors present, or hearing noise in the room could cause sensory overload. The resulting behavior often manifested is confusion, choking, or the inability to feed himself.

Behavioral Manifestations

Just as the amount of stimulation necessary to induce sensory overload varies among patients, so also does the behavioral response to overload.[12,22,31] Generally speaking, those who experience sensory overload attempt to move away from the source of the excess stimuli if at all possible. If the patient is restrained in any way (*e.g.,* by indwelling tubes or a fractured extremity), agitation and anxiety can occur as part of the stress of being unable to withdraw from the excessive stimuli. Elderly patients and stroke patients are more likely to experience confusion or agitation as a result of their inability to process incoming stimuli rapidly enough to organize it in a meaningful way. Young children overwhelmed by unfamiliar faces or loud, strange noises are likely to seek the comfort of their parent's embrace to block out their sensory overload.

Nursing Management

Nurses have an important role in the prevention and elimination of sensory overload. Providing a consistent, predictable pattern of stimulation will help the patient to perceive a sense of control over his environment. Without a sense of control, stimuli can be perceived as unorganized, irrelevant, and overwhelming.

Simple, reassuring explanations for procedures, tests, and examinations prepare the patient for incoming stimuli. Introducing and explaining new procedures in advance will allow time for the patient to process the information and ask questions that will make the experience more meaningful. For example, before insertion of a nasogastric tube the patient should be told who will do the procedure, why it is necessary, what the alternatives are, what is expected of him, how it will feel, and how long the procedure will take. This essential preparation is more likely to reduce sensory overload and encourage patient cooperation.

Nurses can also prevent sensory overload by working with the patient to establish a schedule for routine care such as eating, bathing, turning and coughing, and doing range-of-motion exercises. Although these activities are scheduled, preparation of the patient in advance and the patient's access to a clock will add to his sense of control. Whenever possible, patients should be given a choice in how often or when these activities are performed to promote perceived control over their environment. Speaking calmly and moving slowly within the patient's environment will reassure the patient, promote a sense of trust in his care-provider, and facilitate his control over the environment.

If you discern that your patient is already experiencing distress from sensory overload, assess his environment for possible contributing stimuli. If possible, explore with the patient what stimuli in his environment are contributing to his distress and together work out a plan to reduce or eliminate those stimuli to help the patient regain control over his environment. It may be necessary for you to restrict visitors and incoming telephone calls, provide earplugs or privacy, increase the frequency or amount of pain medication, or take any action deemed necessary to restore sensoristasis for your patient. However, in limiting sensory input caution should be taken in avoiding the opposite type of arousal disorder, that of sensory deprivation.

Sensory Deprivation

When sensoristasis is altered by a lack of a meaningful stimuli or monotonous sensory input, sensory deprivation can result. Environments with minimal or unvarying amounts of sensory stimuli place patients in danger of sensory deprivation. Yet again, what is minimal, nonmeaningful, or monotonous for one person does not necessarily have the same effect on someone else. Diffuse or dim lighting, eye patches, tube feedings, hearing loss, pulled curtains, isolation, a private room,[33] and body casts are examples of restricted environments that can predispose a patient to sensory deprivation.

Patients at Risk

Patients are at risk when there is a lack of any of the modalities of sensory input previously discussed in relation to sensory overload. As with sensory overload, all ages are equally likely to experience sensory deprivation. Cultural background also influences the perception of an environment as deficient in sensory stimulation.

Many types of patients are at risk for sensory deprivation: patients with recent spinal cord injuries[26] or brain damage;[30] patients wearing eye patches while recovering from eye surgery (Fig. 10–3) or those undergoing treatment for possible retinal detachment;[11] the elderly because of the generalized increase in threshold for all sensory modalities that occurs with advancing age;[6] patients with infected wounds who are placed in isolation; and patients in protective (reverse) isolation for immune deficiency disorders.

Patients in isolation are cared for by hospital staff who cover themselves in gowns, gloves, masks, and caps. Seeing person after person dressed the same is monotonous indeed. It leaves the patient no means of discriminating among facial characteristics, voices, and touch and provides little opportunity for social interaction between nurse and patient.

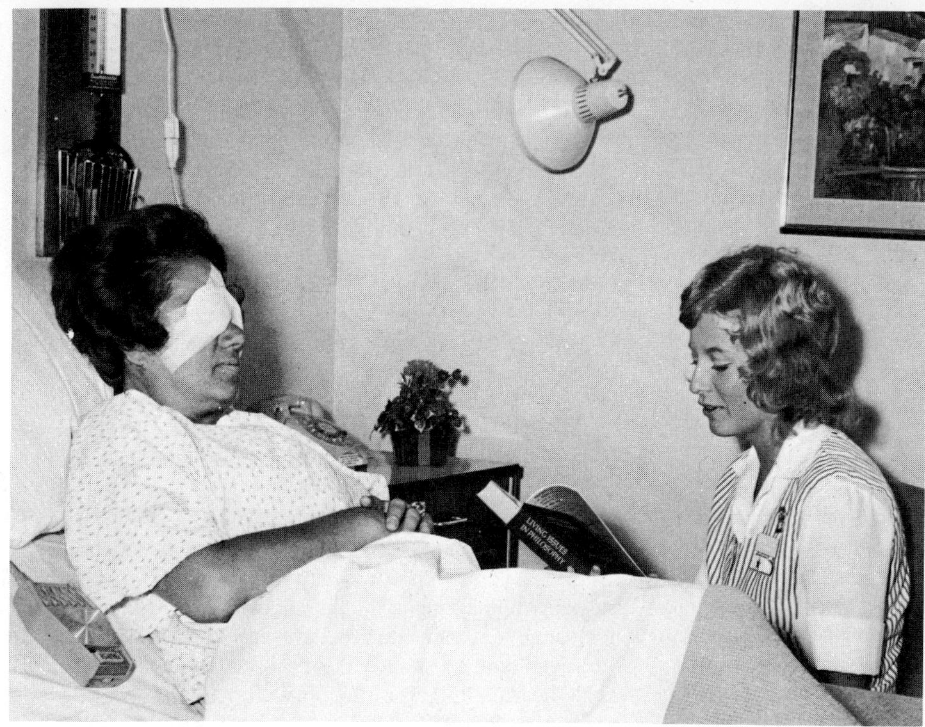

FIGURE 10–3 A patient wearing an eye patch is in danger of sensory deprivation and will benefit from having someone help to promote other types of sensory stimulation.

In addition, doors are closed, visitors are limited and, few items are permitted to flow in and out of an isolation room.

In studies of healthy volunteers undergoing sensory isolation, researchers reported that immobility can worsen an already deprived sensory environment.[10,36] The added deprivation of kinesthetic stimuli imposed by strict bed rest limits position changes and restricts movement and tension of the muscles. This form of monotony reduces stimulation of nerve endings in muscles, tendons, and joints and thereby contributes to sensory deprivation. In addition, tactile sensations are limited to the bed linen, and visual sensations are limited to the walls, ceiling, and content of a single room.

Behavioral Manifestations

Patients experiencing sensory deprivation manifest a variety of behaviors in response to a lack of input. These behaviors are just as varied as the responses to sensory overload discussed previously and can be categorized into four types.

The first type includes physical behaviors such as eating, exercising and sleeping, and running away to escape the deprived environment. When Murphy and Myers confined subjects to dark, soundproof cubicles for up to 96 hours, all subjects experienced drowsiness, excessive yawning, and sleep during the first day. By the second day, restlessness became apparent and those who were significantly more restless than the others withdrew from the study prematurely. Those who completed the study coped with the deprivation by eating and exercising.[23]

The second type of response to sensory deprivation is a change in perception. Zubek and colleagues[35] reported that deprived subjects experienced "unusual body sensations" or more preoccupation with internal sensations. Zuckerman and coworkers reported an increase in somatic complaints, such as dry mouth, heart palpitations, a warm and flushed feeling, difficulty breathing, and nausea.[37] A change in body image, such as feeling that one leg is longer than the other or feeling altogether very small, is frequently reported. Nurses often hear patients complain that the "minutes seem like hours" and this is another example of perceptual change as a result of sensory deprivation. Perceptual changes can also be severe enough to include illusions and hallucinations.

Changes in cognitive behavior also occur during periods of sensory deprivation. People who have been shipwrecked alone or who have been placed in solitary confinement report the use of mental exercises such as counting, talking to oneself, fantasizing, and keeping a diary.

The fourth type of alteration in behavior to be reported during sensory deprivation is emotional. Crying is a common response. Increased irritability and annoyance over trivial matters occurs, and feelings of confusion or panic are often expressed.

It becomes apparent from all four types of responses that the need for stimulation increases as a function of the duration of sensory deprivation and that these varied responses on the part of each individual are efforts to increase stimulation and thereby restore sensoristasis.

Nursing Management

The goal of management for sensory deprivation is to help the patient at risk achieve and maintain sensoristasis or his optimal level of arousal. Assessment of potential sources of sensory deprivation is an important first step in nursing management. With such similar behavioral responses to both sensory overload and sensory deprivation, prevention of alterations in arousal and maintenance of sensoristasis is the best strategy for patients at risk. If any of the behavioral manifestations are already present, it may be difficult to determine whether they are due to overload or deprivation. Often the planned intervention can only be based on the nurse's educated guess after a careful assessment of the patient's environment and an analysis of contributing factors. It may be helpful to imagine yourself in the patient's recumbent position perceiving some of what he may be perceiving through the bedrails and between the curtains. This insight may provide the necessary data for determining the most probable cause for the patient's behavior. After making the diagnosis of sensory deprivation it is still wise to proceed with caution and introduce more stimulation slowly. If the added stimulation appears only to increase the behavior, consider reducing the sensory input as is appropriate for the patient experiencing sensory overload.

Since sensory deprivation can result from either the absolute lack of sensory input or monotonous, unpatterned, and unmeaningful input, nursing interventions should include not only an absolute increase in sensory stimuli but also a variety of stimuli from all the sensory modalities. A person responds with a startle when a loud alarm sounds, but fails to maintain the response if the alarm continues to sound. Even though the alarm may be loud and penetrating, the lack of novelty diminishes its ability to be perceived.

In order to prevent sensory deprivation, three approaches to intervention can be considered, as follows.

1. Help the patient find ways in which he can compensate for deprivation by using self-stimulation methods such as counting, singing, reading, or reciting poetry.
2. Structure meaningful, tangible stimuli into the patient's external environment.
3. Act as a source of stimulation for the patient.

Stimuli for Patient's External Environment. An excellent example of the second approach and how the nurse can structure the external environment for patients is in a report by Carlson, in which she heightened and varied the stimuli in a six-bed orthopedic ward with immobilized elderly women.[5] She hung pictures on the walls and colorful mobiles on the doors, brought in fresh flowers daily, and even washed the windows. She added music, conversation, singing, and exercise programs. She also taught the women to make crepe paper roses for decorating their bed frames. Within 7 days she transformed a ward of bored, disoriented, apathetic-looking patients into an interacting social group of cooperating women with high morale who became physically active and shared in "each other's joys and problems."

Visual Stimulation. Other interventions for enhancing the patient's visual stimulation include the use of colorful sheets, pillow cases, pajamas, and robes. Colorful uniform tops for the nursing staff can also add stimulation. When dealing with elderly patients it is helpful to keep in mind their decreased ability to recognize colors in the shorter wavelengths (blues, greens, and violet). Red, orange, and yellow are more appropriate colors for visual stimulation in elderly groups of patients.[6] For those patients with already compromised vision, nursing management should also include placing objects within their visual field and providing them with clean prescription glasses. The use of diffuse lighting and a night-light, clocks, calendars, and functioning wristwatches can help to structure the patient's environment. A few regular daily televison or radio programs can add a variety to the patient's environment but overuse of such media soon becomes unmeaningful, monotonous stimuli. Specific interventions for the visually impaired patient are beyond the scope of this chapter. More information may be found in Chapter 70 on the discussion of nursing care for patients with alterations in special senses. There is also an excellent discussion of caring for newly blinded patients in Phillips.[25]

Auditory Stimulation. In addition to visual enhancement and variation of the external environment, other modalities need to be considered. Reading to the patient or enhancing auditory stimulation with music and conversation as was done in the Carlson study will allay sensory deprivation.[5] Identifying yourself when initiating contact with the patient, referring to the patient by his name and speaking in clear sentences when you have his attention will enhance the meaningfullness of auditory input. Patients who are already hearing-impaired must have functioning hearing aids or sounds directed at them in such a way that they can meaningfully perceive the stimulation. A complete discussion of nursing management for the hearing-impaired patient can be found in Chapter 70.

Gustatory and Olfactory Stimulation. To increase gustatory and olfactory sensory input encourage patients to smell the aroma of foods before eating and recall aromas of similar foods. Good oral hygiene and properly fitting dentures enhance taste perception. Attractive food with different textures and colors, hot foods served heated and cold foods served chilled, and different items of food eaten separately will increase taste sensations. Seasoned foods and foods brought from home add variations to taste perceptions. For the patient receiving tube feedings, increasing these sensations may be extremely difficult and other sensory modalities need to be enhanced in order to compensate.

Nurse as Source of Stimuli to Patient. In addition to these first two approaches of self-stimulation and enhancing tangible aspects of patients' visual, auditory, gustatory, and olfactory environments, the nurse can also be a source of sensory stimulation. This third approach includes the visual and auditory interventions discussed previously, such as colorful uniforms and conversations with the patient, but primarily involves tactile, cognitive, and emotional input.

Physical Interaction. The necessity for physical interaction has been evident from studies in which animals become sensory deprived when they were not permitted to touch objects placed within their visual field.[30] Not only do peole need social contact but they need physical contact as well. The need for touch increases during stress, illness, depression, and loneliness. Tactile stimulation can include such interventions as back rubs, turning or repositioning, passive range-of-motion exercises, hair brushing or comb-

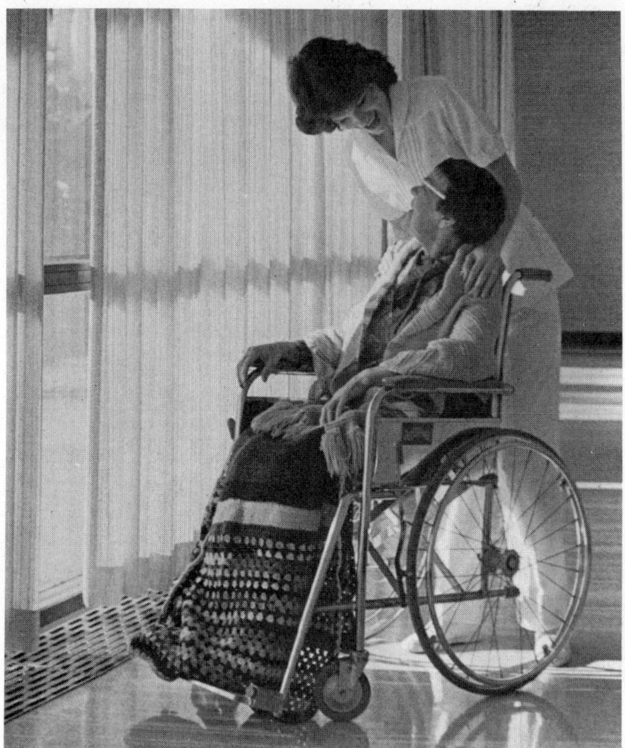

FIGURE 10–4 Exploration of the environment helps avoid sensory deficit. (Photo by Edward J. Bonner)

ing, foot soaks, hugs, and touching arms or shoulders. Since the nurse is often busy with the care and supervision of many patients, patients who are especially at risk will benefit from the nurse's arranging for family, friends, and hospital volunteers to be the source of sensory stimulation (Fig. 10–4).

Cognitive Input. Other sensory modalities that the nurse or visitor can augment include cognitive input. Including the patient in solving dilemmas such as the scheduling of his care or arranging the room to accommodate equipment can be helpful in maintaining cognitive arousal. Discussions with the patient that revolve around his hobbies or occupation can lead to the patient teaching the nurse something new. From a retired fisherman one can learn a great deal about buying fresh fish and still effectively stimulate the patient's cognitive input. Patients should be given responsibility for self-care activities and, whenever feasible, responsibility for activities on the nursing unit (such as delivering the mail or supervising another patient in the lounge) should be encouraged.

Emotional Input. The emotional responses of sensory deprivation are best managed by allowing the patient to voice his fears, concerns, and perceptions. Patients often admit feeling that they are "going crazy" or sensing the presence of someone who is not really there. Nurses should reassure patients, particularly those with patches covering their eyes, that illusions and misperceptions about their own body or their environment do occur when people are immobilized for extended periods. This reassurance, together with a release of emotional feelings, can alleviate some of the emotional responses to sensory deprivation.

Patients who are already experiencing sensory deprivation can be placed in the lounge or hallway near the nurse's station to provide opportunity for social interactions. Social interactions reinforce reality, allow reminiscences of past experiences, and provide sensory input from all modalities. With the use of all three methods for promoting and maintaining sensory input, sensory deprivation can be prevented in most cases.

Sleep Deprivation

The third type of arousal disorder to be discussed is sleep deprivation. Difficulty in inhibiting arousal at night so that sleep can occur results in complaints in insomnia and fatigue. Difficulty maintaining wakefulness during the day results in complaints of hypersomnia and fatigue.

Insomnia encompasses complaints involving difficulty getting to sleep (more than 30 minutes to fall asleep after the lights go out), difficulty in maintaining sleep (frequent awakenings during the night), and awakening too early in the morning. One or all three of these symptoms characterize someone who has difficulty inhibiting arousal during normal nocturnal sleeping hours. Insomnia can result from either sensory overload or sensory deprivation. If sensory overload is present, one's arousal level is high and input from any of the various sensory modalities (especially cognitive and emotional) can overstimulate the RAS arousal mechanism at an inappropriate time during the sleep–wake cycle. If sensory deprivation is present, one's arousal level is very low, and the RAS has not been provided with enough sensory cues to adequately discern day from night.

Hypersomnia during the day (excessive daytime sleepiness) is usually the result of nocturnal sleep disruptions that can arise for a number of reasons. In hospitalized patients the most common reasons for awakenings during the night are noise and pain. Other reasons for disrupted sleep that can lead to sleep deprivation include breathing difficulties, urinary frequency, fever,[17] anxiety and depression,[19] frequent taking of vital signs and repositioning, uncomfortable positions, and frequent feedings of newborns by new mothers.

A normal night's sleep consists of four to six cycles of nonREM (non–rapid-eye-movement) or quiet sleep alternating with REM (rapid-eye-movement) or active sleep. Each cycle spans 60 to 90 minutes. About 20% to 25% of total sleep in the young adult is REM sleep and 75% to 80% is nonREM sleep in the form of both light sleep (50% to 55%) and deep sleep (20%).[32] (See Fig. 10–5.) REM sleep appears to be necessary in order for learning and memory to occur,[14] while nonREM appears necessary for feeling well rested on awakening.

Patients at Risk

Elderly. Patients over 65 years of age are more susceptible to awakenings during the night because of noisy envi-

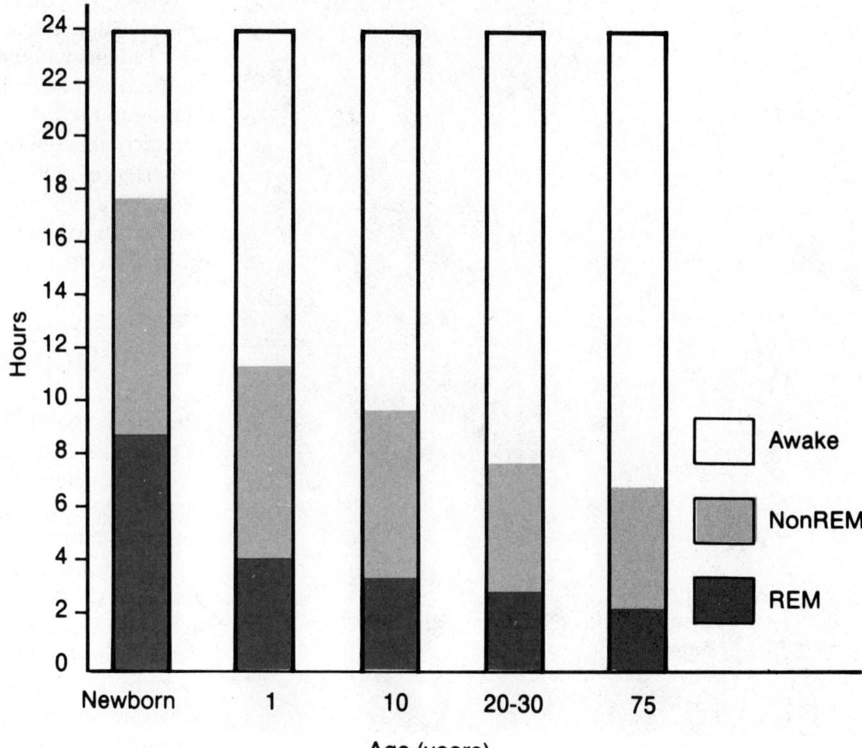

FIGURE 10–5 Alterations in the stages of sleep across the life span. (Adapted from Mitchell PH, Loustau A [eds]: Concepts Basic to Nursing, 3rd ed, p 607. New York, McGraw-Hill, 1981. Used with permission.)

ronments, since the elderly have very little or no deep sleep.[15] Their sleep is primarily light sleep (about 70% of total sleep) and REM sleep (about 20%). As much as 10% of their time in bed is distributed throughout the night as short, unconsciously perceived arousals or longer awakenings that are consciously perceived.[16, 21]

Surgical Patients. Other patients likely to suffer from fatigue or daytime hypersomnolence because of awakenings during the night are those recovering from various surgical procedures. A study of ten men on the first two nights after herniorrhaphy revealed that only one patient had any deep sleep and only five patients had any REM sleep. As a group, these patients spent 93% of their sleep period awake or in light sleep.[18] What makes these results even more important is the fact that the men were not in ward beds but in private rooms! With roommates and the accompanying increases in noise and interruptions, experiences of sleep deprivation will be even more prevalent.

Intensive Care Patients. Patients in intensive care situations risk sleep deprivation because of the lack of uninterrupted time available for sleep. Walker found that for the first 3 days in an intensive care unit the longest period of uninterrupted time was only 50 minutes.[29] On the first day the number of interactions ranged from 25 to 56, with the higher numbers occurring during changes in the nursing shifts. In addition to the interactions, lights can be on continuously, noisy monitoring devices can be aimed directly at the patient's ears, telephones can be ringing continuously, and nursing assessments or direct care can be as often as every 10 to 15 minutes. In another study, Woods found the longest period of uninterrupted sleep in an intensive care unit to range from 10 to 220 minutes.[34] She noted that most interruptions were due to monitoring devices and respiratory care measures. Dlin and his colleagues found the highest number of disruptions (eight) at shift changes between 7:00 and 8:00 in the morning and the lowest number of disruptions (four) between 12:00 and 1:00 in the morning.[9]

Respiratory Patients. A fourth group of patients in danger of sleep deprivation includes those who have disorders of the respiratory system. Although often unaware of their frequent arousals during the night, these patients are aroused by internal signals that oxygen saturation is dropping to a dangerously low level. The arousal mechanism is stimulated internally to either initiate breathing in the case of the patient with obstructive sleep apnea syndrome or initiate sighs or coughing in the case of the patient with chronic obstructive pulmonary disease (COPD) or asthma.

Apneic periods begin with an obstruction of the airway usually during nonREM sleep. As oxygen saturation declines to the point of hypoxemia, arousal occurs to a level necessary for restoring tonus to the musculature in the respiratory airway and thereby relieving the obstruction. Breathing resumes and oxygen saturation improves. These patients, usually older men who are above ideal body weight and snore heavily, are chronically sleep deprived because of continuous arousals during the night. They very rarely experience any deep sleep.[13]

The patient with COPD or asthma relies heavily on accessory muscles of respiration because of the pathologic changes in his lungs. During REM sleep all muscles of the body are extremely relaxed to the point of lacking all muscle tone. Therefore, during REM periods oxygen saturation drops precipitously and arousals or awakenings occur usually to the point of stimulating deep breaths with coughs, sighs, or bronchospasms.[8] These patients are primarily REM-sleep deprived but are also deprived of deep sleep.

Since the arousal mechanism is stimulated during periods of hypoxemia for both the patient with obstructive sleep apnea and the patient with COPD, any inhibition of that arousal can result in severe hypoxemia and death. Any medication that suppresses the CNS is also likely to inhibit arousal responses to hypoxemia. Analgesics, anesthetics, alcohol, barbiturates, and other sleeping aids do inhibit arousal and are likely to inhibit respiratory responses to lower levels of oxygen saturation in the patient with obstructive sleep apnea. These same medications also initially inhibit REM sleep, which may be of minor benefit to patients with COPD. However, on sudden withdrawal of these REM-suppressant drugs, a REM rebound effect occurs that can double the amount of REM sleep in one night. This sudden discontinuation of a CNS depressant medication exposes the patient with lung disease to severe hypoxemia.

Summary. In summary, then, any hospitalized patient is exposed to sleep deprivation for a variety of reasons. A patient can have difficulty in getting to sleep because of sensory overload and the inability to inhibit arousal or because of sensory deprivation and the inability to distinguish day and night environment cues. A patient can have difficulty in maintaining sleep because of pain, breathing difficulties, urinary frequency or incontinence, sleeping in awkward positions, or noise and other frequent interruptions.

Behavioral Manifestations

By far the most common behavior observed in someone who is experiencing sleep deprivation is the tendency to fall asleep during daytime hours. Naps during the day can successfully supplement a night of sleep disrupted by noise and interactions. However, even daytime naps in a hospital setting are often as interrupted as attempts to sleep during the night. In cases of obstructive sleep apnea or lung disease even daytime naps are interrupted by frequent arousals when hypoxemia occurs.

When sleep is prevented from occuring over a prolonged time period other behaviors and complaints arise. In addition to complaints of fatigue, attention span diminishes, coordination and fine motor skills suffer, and subjects become preoccupied with picayunish details and express difficulty with remembering new events. In experimental studies of prolonged sleep deprivation in healthy young men, irritability, hostility, misperceptions such as hypersensitive feet, confusion, lapses in memory, and illusions began to occur after about 4 days.[24] The behaviors exhibited during total sleep deprivation are similar to those experienced during sensory overload, because sensory stimuli are affecting the arousal mechanism at a time in the sleep–wake cycle when there would normally be an absence of input. Since sleep deprivation is so prevalent in patients in intensive care, any or all of these symptoms are expressed as a syndrome known as "intensive care delirium" and is often seen particularly in cardiotomy patients after about the third postoperative day.[1,3,7]

Nursing Management

When insomnia or hypersomnia is due to sensory deprivation the goal of management is to promote sleep onset. By increasing sensory stimulation during the day and reducing stimuli at night, the patient should develop or maintain a rhythmic pattern of day–night cycling in order to distinguish appropriate times for sleeping and waking. When insomnia or hypersomnia is due to sensory overload, presleep activities should have the objective of reducing anxiety and promoting relaxation. A back massage, foot soak, warm bath, comfortable position, and relief from pain will promote sleep onset.

Minimizing interruptions in sleep during the night is a monumental problem for nurses and requires careful planning and control over the patient's environment. To reduce the effects of noise, particularly for the elderly patient or the patient in intensive care, comfortable earplugs may prove invaluable. To minimize arousals and awakenings because of decreased oxygen saturation during REM sleep, low-flow oxygen therapy is sometimes prescribed.[4] If essential care necessitates awakening the patient, it should be planned so that many small tasks are completed at that time. For instance, the prn sleeping pill could be given with the scheduled evening dose of antibiotics and vital signs could be obtained, a back massage given, and extra blankets, pillows, or fluids could be provided at the same time. As is often the case, the hypnotic is given at 9:00 PM, the antibiotic at 10:00 PM or midnight, and vital signs are done by another staff member any time between 9:00 PM and midnight.

Nursing measures to promote comfort assist all patients in experiencing a better night of sleep. Wrinkle-free beds, clean and dry linen and clothing, oral care and other appropriate hygienic measures, and pain relief are essential evening activities in the nursing management of all patients. Treatments such as enemas, laxatives, or diuretics should be administered at such times that their peak effect will not be after sleep onset! It may be necessary to remind other staff to keep their voices lowered, particularly at change of shift and in the hallways outside the patients' rooms. Eliminating all but essential lighting at night is also helpful in orienting the patient to differences in day–night cycles.

Summary

The management of all three disorders of arousal involve facilitating the patient's unique level of sensoristasis. Keeping in mind that requirements for maintaining sensoristasis during waking hours are different from maintaining sensoristasis during sleep will lessen the likelihood of sleep deprivation. Acknowledging that patients are individuals who have their own unique requirements for what is an optimal level of stimulation will lessen the likelihood of sensory deprivation as well as sensory overload.

References

1. Blachy PH, Starr A: Post-cardiotomy delerium. Am J Psychiatry 121:371–375, 1964
2. Braun CMJ, Pivik RT: Effect of locus coeruleus lesions upon sleeping and waking in the rabbit. Brain Res 230:133–151, 1981
3. Broughton R, Baron R: Sleep patterns in the intensive care unit and on the ward after acute myocardial infarction. Electroencephalogr Clin Neurophysiol 45:348–360, 1978
4. Calverley PMA, Brezinova V, Douglas, NJ et al: The effect of oxygenation on the sleep quality in chronic bronchitis and emphysema. Am Rev Respir Dis 126:206–210, 1982
5. Carlson S: Selected sensory input and life satisfactions of immobilized geriatric female patients. ANA Clinical Sessions, 1968
6. Cohen S, Bunke E Sr: Sensory changes in the elderly: Programmed instruction. Am J Nurs 81:1851–1880, 1981
7. Deamer RM, Scharf M, Kales A: Sleep patterns in the coronary care unit. US Navy Medicine 59:19–23, 1972
8. DeMarco FJ, Wynne JW, Block AJ et al: Oxygen desaturation during sleep as a determinant of the "blue and bloated" syndrome. Chest 79:621–625, 1981
9. Dlin BM, Rosen H, Dickstein et al: The problems of sleep and rest in the intensive care unit. Psychosomatics 12(3):155–163, 1971
10. Downs F: Bed rest and sensory disturbances. Am J Nurs 74:434–438, 1974
11. Ellis R, Jackson CW, Rich R et al: Suggestions for the care of eye surgery patients who experience reduced sensory input. ANA Regional Clinical Conference, pp 131–137, 1967
12. Gottschalk LA, Haer JL, Bates D: Effects of sensory overload on psychological state. Arch Gen Psychiatry 27:451–457, 1972
13. Guilleminault C, Cummiskey J, Dement WC: Sleep apnea syndrome: Recent advances. Adv Intern Med 26:347–371, 1980
14. Hartmann E: The functions of sleep and memory processing. Advances in Sleep Research 6:111–124, 1981
15. Hayashi Y, Endo S: Comparison of sleep characteristics of subjects in their 70's with those in their 80's. Folia Psychiatr Neurol Jpn 36:23–32, 1982
16. Hayter J: Sleep behaviors of older persons. Nurs Res 32(4):242–246, 1983
17. Karacan I, Wolff SM, Williams RL et al: The effects of fever on sleep and dream patterns. Psychosomatics 9:331–339, 1968
18. Kavey NB, Altschuler KZ: Sleep in herniorrhaphy patients. Am J Surg 138(5):682–687, 1979
19. Lamb MA: The sleeping patterns of patients with malignant and nonmalignant diseases. Cancer Nursing, pp 389–396, October 1982
20. Leppaverori A, Putkonen PTS: Alpha-adrenoceptive influences on the control of the sleep-waking cycle in the cat. Brain Res 193:95–115, 1980
21. Lerner R: Sleep loss in the aged: Implications for nursing practice. Journal of Gerontological Nursing 8(6):323–326, 1982
22. Lindsley DB: Common factors in sensory deprivation, sensory distortion, and sensory overload. In Solomon P, Kubzansky PE, Leiderman PH et al (eds): Sensory Deprivation. Cambridge, Harvard University Press, 1961
23. Murphy DB, Myers TI: Occurrence, measurement and experimental manipulation of visual "hallucinations." Percept Mot Skills 15:47–54, 1962
24. Pasnau RO, Naitoh P, Stier S et al: The psychological effects of 205 hours of sleep deprivation. Arch Gen Psychiatry 18:496–505, 1968
25. Phillips LRF: Care of the client with sensoriperceptual problems. In Wolamin MO, Phillips LRF: Confusion: Prevention and Care. St Louis, CV Mosby, 1981
26. Richards JS, Hirt M, Melamed L: Spinal cord injury: A sensory restriction perspective. Arch Phys Med Rehabil 63:195–199, 1982
27. Schultz DP: Sensory Restriction: Effects on Behavior. New York, Academic Press, 1965
28. Trulson ME, Trulson VM: Activity of nucleus raphe pallidus neurons across the sleep-waking cycle in freely moving cats. Brain Res 237:232–237, 1982
29. Walker BB: The postsurgery heart patient: Amount of uninterrupted time for sleep and rest during the first, second and third postoperative days in a teaching hospital. Nurs Res 21:164–169, 1972
30. Walsh R: Sensory environments, brain damage, and drugs: A review of interactions and mediating mechanisms. Int J Neurosci 14:129–137, 1981
31. Walsh RN, Cummins RA: Neural responses to therapeutic environments. Advances in Behavioral Biology 17:171–200, 1976
32. Williams RL, Karacan I, Hursch CJ: Electroencephalography (EEG) of Human Sleep: Clinical Applications. New York: John Wiley & Sons, 1974
33. Wood M: Clinical sensory deprivation: A comparative study of patients in single care and two-bed rooms. J Nurs Adm 7(12):28–32, 1977
34. Woods NF: Patterns of sleep in postcardiotomy patients. Nurs Res 21:347–352, July/August 1972
35. Zubek JP, Aftanas M, Kovach K et al: Effect of severe immobilization of the body on intellectual and perceptual processes. Can J Psychol 17(1):118–133, 1963
36. Zubek JP, MacNeil M: Perceptual deprivation phenomena: Role of the recumbent position. J Abnorm Psychol 72(2):147–150, 1967
37. Zuckerman M, Albright RJ, Marks CS et al: Stress and Hallucinatory Effects of Perceptual Isolation and Confinement. Psychological Monographs, 1962

Chapter 11

The Terminal Phase of Illness

Thomas R. McCormick

This chapter examines the special issues that confront the dying patient and his family and focuses on the role of the nurse in providing care in response to the special needs of patients in the final stage of life. Most patients fear death, and many are fearful of the discomfort of pain and the indignity of increasing disability and dependence in the last days of life. In addition to the expected loss of life, there are often many smaller losses along the way: loss of health, energy, and familiar social and task-related activities. The coping needs and strategies of such patients are often intense, involving not only adaptation to the physical aspects of the terminal illness, but to the social, psychological, and spiritual issues as well.

The needs of patients and their families in facing death present special challenges and opportunities for nursing care. What is the role of the nurse caring for a patient in the terminal phase of illness? It is hoped that the nurse will formulate goals in the light of a clear and empathetic understanding of the patient, his special needs, and his family system. In the service of these goals, the nurse may also encounter some of the perplexing ethical issues surrounding death and dying such as code designations, the withholding or removal of life-prolonging instruments and devices, issues of patient autonomy and self-determination, and many more.

The Dimensions of Dying

The onset of a life-threatening or terminal illness is a critical life event, involving the physical, psychological, social, and spiritual dimensions of the patient.

Physical Dimension

Caring for the physical needs and comforts of the patient is but one aspect of the nursing process. In other chapters the issues of physical care are examined in depth. Caring for the physical aspects of the terminally ill patient has the highest nursing priority. However, in attending to physical care the nurse must respect the patient's autonomy. Patients have the right to self-determination. In most cases, patients can be consulted about their needs, and these needs should be met to the best of the nurse's ability. When a person is suffering from a recoverable illness and chooses to be treated, it is appropriate to use modern therapies to the fullest extent. However, when the patient is clearly terminally ill, the curative goal is replaced by the goals of caring, comforting, and controlling pain. Recent advances in pain control, combined with the decreasing anxiety of health professionals concerning the addiction of patients during the terminal phase of illness, have contributed immeasurably to the relief of suffering, which is the primary goal for both the patient and the nurse.

Psychological Dimension

Psychologically, the discovery of an incurable and fatal disease often brings the patient to a state of shock and numbness. This response is more commonly encountered when, in the patient's belief system, death seems premature or untimely. In such circumstances, the imminence and inevitability of death may seem unreal, and the patient may in fact deny the reality of his situation for a time. This is not at all unusual, considering the fact that it is a natural human trait to repress the fear of death most of the time. A noted psychoanalyst, Gregory Zilboorg, proposed that because most people are not in touch with their fear of death, they conclude that it is absent. The fear of death, though, is universal:

> If this fear were as constantly conscious, we should be unable to function normally. It must be properly repressed to keep us living with any modicum of comfort. We know very well that to repress means more than to put away and to forget that which was put away and the place where we put it. It means also to maintain a constant psychological effort to keep the lid on and inwardly never relax our watchfulness.[1]

Just as human beings seek to live by denying the fear of death, so many terminally ill patients use denial as a temporary defense against hopelessness and fear. Usually this is short-lived, and most patients begin to accept the reality of their prognosis. Some patients may use denial as a coping mechanism until their death. The following incident portrays an example of this more extreme form of denial.

> Mrs. S., a 52-year-old divorced woman, entered the hospital in the advanced stages of metastatic lung cancer. She had lost 45 lb, was seriously ill, and had been informed of her diagnosis. However, all of her verbalizations with staff and visitors was of the most optimistic nature. "I'm here for a few days to regain my strength, then I'm off to Sloane-Kettering for a cure. I'm hopeful that when I return my former husband and I can reconcile." She spoke these words the evening before her death, which occurred on the following morning, with no admission or acknowledgment that death was imminent.

Elisabeth Kubler-Ross, in her book entitled *On Death and Dying,* related that in addition to denial, many of her patients had feelings of intense anger and depression, and some engaged in bargaining transactions before the acceptance of their death.[5] The nurse must be careful, however, not to label or pigeonhole patients by universalizing Kubler-Ross's stages to all patients. Many patients are not angry about their illness. For some, death is accepted from the outset with calm dignity. The important distinction is that some patients do become very angry about their illness and impending death. This may be especially likely when death is untimely and when the patient has a strong sense of having much to live for. It is both healthy and natural for these angry feelings to be voiced or ventilated. In some cases, though, angry patients may not be in touch with their anger and its sources; they may project their anger onto others in their environment, whether physicians, family members, or nurses. The nurse, as the person who is usually in the patient's presence more than others, has a greater probability of being the recipient of this projected anger.

It is especially helpful if the nurse can be prepared for this anger, can refrain from reacting defensively or avoiding the patient, and can allow the patient to express his feelings. Such resilience and composure on the part of the nurse may best be developed by her examining her own feelings and attitudes about death and by moving toward a personal resolution of these feelings. Resolution of the health professional's attitudes and feelings toward death is, of course, a complex process, involving one's values, beliefs, history, and experiences pertaining to death. In the very least, it involves accepting death as a natural part of life and developing the capacity to participate gracefully in the care of patients who are involved in one of life's most important and difficult passages.

As patients experience the continuing progression of their disease, it is not unusual for them to become depressed. This is particularly true when they undergo a significant number of losses along the way. Many patients may experience loss of energy, loss of job, loss of family closeness, loss of friends, and loss of status in addition to the anticipated loss of life itself. These losses may well lead to a reactive depression. Depression may also be the result of poorly controlled pain, a reaction to pain medications, or to chemotherapy. In such times, the patient is in need of a supportive, empathetic, and caring nurse (Fig. 11–1).

The nurse, particularly one who is in the early stages of professional development, may find the terminally ill patient one of the most difficult with whom to relate. Many find it uncomfortable to be in the presence of a seriously depressed person, and when that person is also in the terminal phase of illness, is not expected to improve, and is impervious to the benefits of modern medicine, it is even more difficult. The most serious temptation for the nurse who is uncomfortable in these circumstances is to provide the physical and material aspects of care for the patient, without truly "caring for" the patient.

This pattern may also be observed in the physician who is uncomfortable with the dying patient for whom medicine has very little to offer. Rounds with the dying patient become abbreviated and doctor–patient contact minimized to the briefest extent possible. Yet, it is at just this point in the patient's pilgrimage toward death that his need for a caring and trustworthy relationship is most acute. The nurse–patient relationship at this time provides an opportunity for the nurse to care for the patient and his needs in the final stage of life, *encouraging any possibilities for growth* that may occur. This terminal stage also provides the nurse with an opportunity for growth in learning to be with patients in times of emotional intensity while at the same time maintaining personal emotional boundaries.

Social Dimension

A patient in the terminal phase of illness experiences a severe interruption of the normal social patterns and rela-

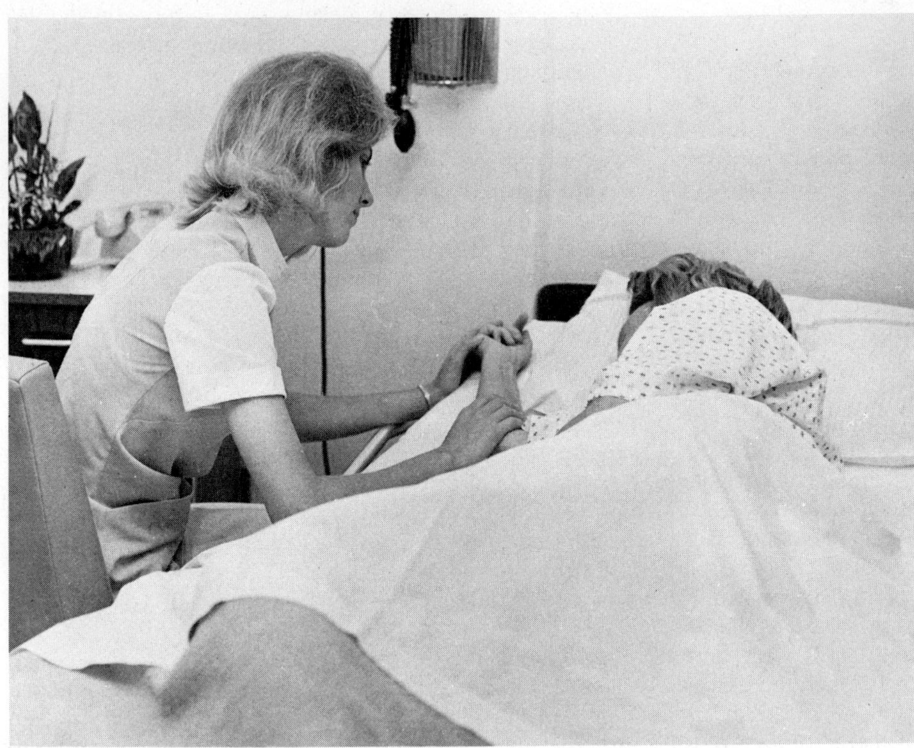

FIGURE 11–1 A supportive caring gesture on the part of the nurse can be extremely helpful to a patient who is dying.

tionships of daily life. As the patient becomes sicker, the dynamics of all his relationships may change. These changes have a significant impact on the patient's family as well, and it is usually most helpful for the nurse to become aware of the patient's "family system" to provide the care that is needed. When the husband becomes ill, the wife may suddenly be expected to fulfill many of the roles that her spouse formerly occupied. If she relied on her husband to drive the automobile, manage the family budget, and do the weekly grocery shopping, she may find it difficult to adjust to the new demands that are placed on her. She may have enjoyed depending on him as the major provider of income, the planner, and the decision maker. The changes in her behavior that are demanded by his illness may cause her to feel uncomfortable, insecure, or resentful and angry. These feelings may in turn lead to feelings of guilt for not being able to accept the adaptive changes more gracefully.

Conversely, if the wife becomes ill, the husband who has grown accustomed to having her take care of the home may suddenly find himself in the role of the homemaker. He may be uncomfortable or resentful of the fact that now it is he who cooks the meals, does the laundry, and helps the children with their homework when he would prefer relaxing with his paper at the end of a day at work.

Children, also, find that a life-threatening illness in a family member is disruptive and anxiety provoking. The normal family stability is threatened, more chores may be expected from them, and there may be financial hardships through loss of work or from the costs of treatment. The threatened loss of a parent forces children to surrender some of their dependence prematurely, and this may be very difficult and painful.

The dying patient must deal not only with the disruption of the normal patterns of family life but also with the disruption of those wider concentric circles involving relationships at work and social friends as well. The patient who becomes too sick to work is removed from the familiar social support of friends and colleagues in the workplace. Gone also is a major source of purpose, meaning, and value that most of us derive from our employment and productivity. Furthermore, many people in our society are uncomfortable in the presence of a person whose illness has been diagnosed as terminal and may go to considerable lengths to avoid social contact with a friend who is in the final stage of life. A number of patients known to have a terminal illness confided that they have observed friends and colleagues cross the street to avoid a meeting. Such friends are usually even more uncomfortable in a hospital setting, and may avoid calling or visiting the patient just when the need for support and encouragement is greatest.

Approximately 80% of the deaths in the United States occur in an institution such as a hospital, convalescent center, or nursing home. As a terminal illness progresses to the point of hospitalization, the process of social isolation often increases. The circle of social inclusion usually draws smaller and tighter in proportion to the debilitating effects of the illness. At the end of life, the social circle for the dying patient may include one or two family members, the physician, and the nurse. The nurse may thus become one of the major sources of social support in the terminal phase of illness. She may also play an important role in listening to the feelings of the patient and the family members throughout this process, helping them to understand and adapt to the changes in their circumstances. She may make a vital contribution in encouraging and facilitating communication between the patient and the family during this stressful time.

Spiritual Dimension

Most descriptions of the human being incorporate the concept of body, mind, and soul. Health professionals are encouraged to care for the whole person, although considerably more attention is usually given to the physical and mental dimensions than to the spiritual. The terminal phase of illness is, for many patients, a spiritual crisis. When death appears to be inevitable, and perhaps imminent, the patient may begin questioning, "What is to become of me? What is the meaning of my life now? Is death the end of me, or is there life after death? What are my values now as life ebbs? What are the most important tasks to attend to while life lasts?" These are typical of the spiritual questions that most patients ask themselves.

The meaning of *spiritual* is generally understood to consist of that which pertains to the spirit, the incorporeal, the sacred, or to religious values.[7] As the end of life draws near, answers to these questions may be of the greatest importance to the patient. Addressing these questions of his life's meaning becomes the task of the dying patient. To cope with his unique existential status, the patient must strive to face and understand the reality of his new status, that is, what can be changed and what must be endured. Through the discernment of these personal tasks, the individual may find the unique and singular meanings of his life in the face of his death.

Religious persons have an advantage at this point, if they have lived out their life with a belief system that provides a context for responding to and understanding these issues. For them there are rituals and sacraments in which they now find comfort, and which are administered by a priest, rabbi, minister, or chaplain of their faith, whose personal visits are often of immeasurable comfort to the devout patient. Seeking spiritual and existential solace, however, is not limited to those who come from a religious background. All patients must inevitably face the terminal stage of their illness. It is interesting to note that as society has become more secular, more persons turn to health professionals with problems that were formerly brought to the rabbi, priest, or pastor. Many patients who have developed a trusting relationship with a nurse who they perceive to truly care for them will confide in her, expressing their deepest concerns, hopes, and fears about their final hours.

As patients struggle with questions of meaning, the finite nature of life may be interpreted as a threat. Others find a spiritual perception in which death is not grounds for despair, but an impending final curtain that demands action here and now. Many patients have found the last period of their lives to be incredibly rich, as they learned to savor the moments, hours, and days. Some have let go of less important values and intensified their family relationships, knowing that time was precious. Others have taken the trip they had always postponed, reconciled unmended relationships, or simply allowed themselves to take the time to watch the sunset, to smell the flowers, or to appreciate the simple pleasures of life.

Victor Frankl, a Jewish psychiatrist who was interned in a Nazi concentration camp during much of World War II, developed a concept on the way in which one's personal values help sustain a sense of meaning and purpose in life. He described a hierarchy of values consisting of creative values, experiential values, and attitudinal values.[3]

Creative Values. Most persons find value in work, in the performance of tasks in a profession, on the job, or in a vocation as parent and partner in the care of children and family. A critical or life-threatening illness interrupts the usual patterns of work and parenthood, thus diminishing the most ordinary opportunities for the enjoyment of creative values.

Experiential Values. The experiential values are found in experiences, such as the warmth of a loving relationship, the beauty of art, the joy of learning, the pleasure of the theater, the harmony of beautiful music, and in the simple experiences of daily life. Although patients in the terminal phase of illness may find many of these experiences to be diminished, it is often the anticipation of a visit from a friend or family member that provides a sense of meaning and value in the final stage of life.

Attitudinal Values. When other sources of value are lost or diminished by the consequences of illness, a person may still find value in shaping the very attitudes that are taken toward this altered lifestyle. One may face illness and death with despair and hopelessness, or one may discover the inner strength of the resilient human spirit that allows a person to face this same condition with courage, until the very end of life. Thus, many choose to find value in life when life is threatened, even when life's limitations allow only the assertion of attitudinal values. Such is the spiritual task of coping.

The Role of the Nurse as Advocate of the Dying Patient

Nursing as it relates to patients in the terminal phase of illness will require the nurse to develop the most careful assessment of the particular needs of each patient. Such an assessment will seek an insightful understanding into the dynamics of the patient's family system. The social and cultural system of the patient must also be considered. Data gathering will require the art of skillful observation and careful listening to accurately gather a picture of the patient with his unique beliefs and values, coming from a particular family context, which is couched in its own social and cultural setting.

In recent times, more attention has been devoted to the needs of the terminally ill patient who wishes to die at home. Some nurses have specialized in providing primary care for dying patients in the home setting. When this is possible, the last days of the patient are usually more comfortable. The surroundings are familiar, family and friends have easier access, and the patient retains a larger measure of control. This is critically important. Eric Cassell said it well:

> Maintaining control over oneself is so vital to all of us that one might see all the other phenomena of illness as doing harm not only in their own right but doubly so as they reinforce the sick person's perception that he is no longer in control.[2]

In the majority of cases, the dying patient will enter the hospital at some point in the terminal phase of illness. Not all patients wish to die at home, nor do all families have the physical and emotional resources to allow this to happen. Among the many concerns of the seriously ill is the concern over helplessness in the face of a devastating or incurable illness. When the patient enters the hospital, he must surrender greater control over even the most personal aspects of living. From the moment of awakening in the morning until he falls asleep at night, the patient's schedule is dictated by someone else. Meals and medications, procedures and protocols, CT scans and chemotherapy—are all directed by persons within the health care system. More profoundly, the extension or prolongation of life itself seems to reside within the power and prerogative of the physician, upon whom the patient must depend for medical decisions and recommendations.

This dependency is quietly accepted by some patients, but in times of crisis or severe stress even the strongest of persons may regress to earlier patterns of helplessness and dependence on some figure of authority in whom there is hope for safety and comfort. Others may deeply resent this experience of powerlessness and may lash out angrily or may sullenly resist the helping efforts of the very persons who are dedicated to their care.

Nurses may respond angrily to such patients who are perceived as being uncooperative and belligerent. This is a natural reaction when one feels threatened. It is very important, therefore, for the nurse to carefully develop a concept of her role as a helping professional with patients who are terminally ill. One role for the nurse, though not advocated here, is that of *benign paternalism.* This is the concept which advocates that those in the health care environment (the physician, the nurse, and other health professionals) understand what is best for the patient and seek the patient's compliance and cooperation with the directions of the health care team. A second role concept for the nurse is that of *patient advocate.* In this role the nurse is well aware of medical recommendations for the patient, but she is also committed to learning the needs, feelings, and wishes of the patient. Frequently the nurse working in an advocacy role can provide information, act as a communications bridge between the patient and the health care system, and support the patient in a problem-solving partnership. This encourages the development of the nurse's role as patient advocate when providing care to those in the terminal stage of illness.

Coping Strategies for the Dying Patient

The patient with a terminal illness has a finite time in which to live, until death occurs. It is usually difficult to accurately predict how long the patient will live, and it is inadvisable to make specific predictions because they are usually wrong. This period between diagnosis and death is referred to by some as the dying trajectory; others have suggested that this last period of life has the potential for becoming the final stage of growth.[4] It is a period that presents many coping challenges to the dying patient. Among the dominant themes of this phase are those of loss and hope.

Loss

The idea and experience of loss is a recurrent phenomenon for the dying patient. The diagnosis of a fatal illness brings an awareness that the loss of life is inevitable. This awareness often triggers an anticipatory grief, the grief over that which is about to be lost. It is extremely painful to consider one's own demise, and the patient usually deals with these feelings for brief moments with companions in whose presence he feels comfortable doing so.

There are other losses more imminent than death for many patients. In the surgical treatment of illnesses such as cancer, the patient may lose a limb or a breast in an attempt to forestall death. In other situations the patient may lose a normal function. Patients whose treatment requires colostomy or an external urinary collection device experience, additionally, a loss of their usual body image. The need for dialysis or a ventilator represents an even more frightening loss of function. The loss of sexual function is particularly painful for some, another reminder of the intrusion of disease into the most intimate aspects of living. As the limitations of disease continue to encroach on the activities of living, the patient loses the ability to work, the companionship of friends, the comfort of health, and the dimension of "future." Adjusting to these losses demands enormous adaptive changes for the patient. The adaptation to loss is often aided by the patient's sense of hope.

Hope

Patients who are told they have a life threatening illness often cling to a strand of hope that it may not be so and that there may be a cure or a way of postponing death for a long time. Eventually, when death is near and the patient accepts death, hope has played an important role in softening the initial blow and giving him time to make his adjustments.

The nature of what the patient hopes for may change with time and changing circumstances. The patient who hoped originally for a cure, may at a later time hope for comfort and the control of pain. One who at first hoped for a cure, may later express hope for a few more days to enjoy his children or grandchildren. A patient who hoped to return to work and complete those unfinished projects may instead hope for the strength to walk around the block just once to see the colors of the fall leaves.

Coping

Hope plays a vital role in sustaining a sense of meaning and purpose for the patient in the terminal phase of illness. The nature of one's hopes can change from those held in the premorbid state. The transition toward death may be eased for the person who is able to make appropriate adaptive changes in the light of his particular situation. Most persons use the coping skills that are "in character" for them. If it is customary for them to voice their feelings, they will likely treasure the opportunity to talk about how they feel about dying. A person who has been an introvert and very private with his feelings will probably remain so in the face of death.

The patient's coping processes are enhanced by a supportive environment. Respect for the patient's self-determination and control of his situation should have priority. Effective communication is essential. However, as life and strength ebbs, there is great value in the intimacy of the "shared silence." Many patients near the end of life have expressed appreciation for the nurse or family member who could simply sit with them for a few moments, holding their hand, without expecting them to speak (Fig. 11–2). The following example shows one suggested approach.

> On entering the room of the patient, the nurse draws up a chair beside the head of the bed. The patient appears to be sleeping or even unconscious. She announces her presence by saying, "Mr. J., I am your nurse, my name is M." Touching or holding his hand she says, "I want to spend the next few minutes with you and I want you to know it's okay for us to remain in silence. You need not say a word unless you wish to."

There are occasions when the nurse is the only person present as the patient is actually dying. Assuming death is expected and there is a "no code" designation, one of the final acts of caring for the patient is simply to remain with him, offering the comforting presence of someone who cares as life ebbs away.

Ethical Issues Surrounding Death and Dying

Nurses encounter ethical dilemmas in every arena of nursing. Some of the most difficult and perplexing ethical issues arise in caring for the dying patient.

Informed Consent

It is generally accepted today, though not universally, that the patient has the right to know the truth about the diagnosis, the prognosis, and alternative courses of treatment. In former times, withholding the truth from patients concerning the diagnosis of a life-threatening illness was widely practiced. This practice was supported by several factors: (1) There was little medicine could offer of a curative nature to the dying patient. (2) It was believed that shielding the patient from the bad news, about which nothing substantive could be done, was a kind and beneficent action. (3) Physician-paternalism was generally accepted as culturally appropriate.

In more recent times the practice of candor has become the norm rather than the exception, owing to the following factors: (1) New and powerful medical interventions have a dramatic effect in arresting or altering the course of some diseases. (2) The compliance and cooperation of the patient is essential to the use of these life-prolonging interventions. (3) There is growing evidence that most patients know they are dying whether they are told or not. (4) Many patients find considerable benefit in attending to their most important agenda and bringing a close to their life and relationships when they are aware that death is near.

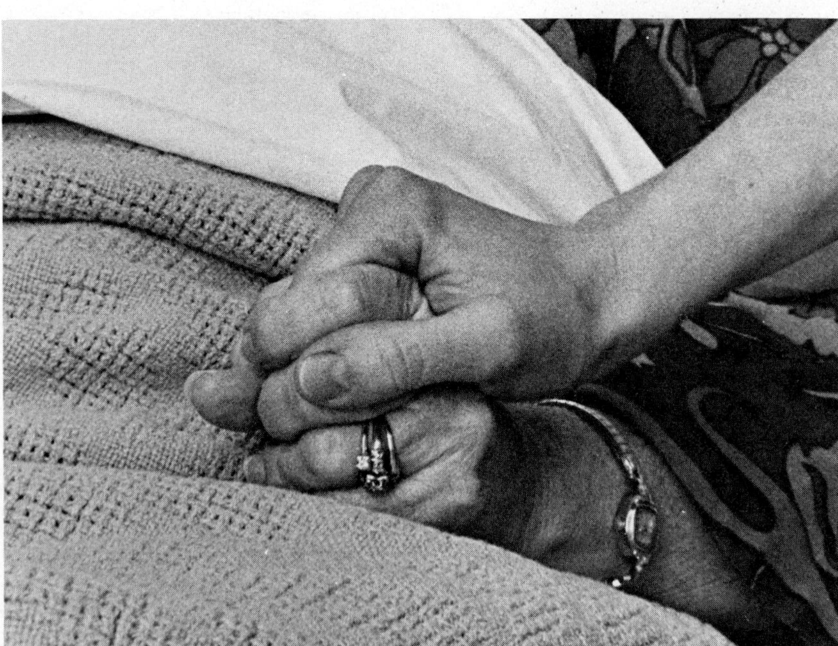

FIGURE 11–2 Holding the hand of a dying patient is frequently a source of comfort and support.

Patients have the right to information that may allow them to make informed decisions in consenting to treatment. They also have the right to refuse treatment. The health care professionals may have the greatest expertise in determining the "best" scientific management of the patient's medical problems. However, patients have the right to pursue the values that they consider "best" in terms of their own values.

An example of an ethical dilemma in nursing is seen in the following situation involving the management of information.

> The nurse is aware that the physician has avoided disclosing to the patient that her illness is fatal. As the nurse is taking her vital signs, Mrs. N. asks, "Am I going to die? I seem to feel weaker and sicker each day. What's happening to me?" The nurse then responds: "Mrs. N., what has your physician told you about your illness and what you might expect?" From this bridging intervention, the nurse then attempts to facilitate a meeting between the physician and patient in which the patient can obtain the information that she desires from the physician.

In some case the patient's mental competence may be compromised, leaving the patient incapable of granting consent for treatment. When such situations are handled informally, the closest family member may serve as surrogate decision maker. This is based on the principle of patient self-determination, because it is hypothesized that the closest kin is in the best position to know the patient's will. In formal cases, a guardian is appointed by the court to serve as surrogate decision maker, and may or may not be a family member. Some states now recognize the patient's right to appoint a person to hold durable power of attorney, meaning that the action of appointing a surrogate, when taken by a person of sound mind, remains in force when that person has lost legal competence through accident or illness, to determine his own care. The second principle that guides the surrogate is that of the best interest of the patient.[6]

Code Designations

It is increasingly the practice to give a code designation to patients in the hospital who might experience cardiac arrest. The patient has a right to participate in this decision and to express his preference as to whether or not he wishes cardiopulmonary resuscitation in the event of cardiac arrest. The following example demonstrates how the nursing role involves the nurse in potentially conflicting situations.

> Mr. O. is an 83-year-old widower in the terminal stage of illness with a metastasizing adenocarcinoma of the abdomen. His primary nurse has developed a trusting relationship with Mr. O. through his repeated hospitalizations for previous care, which included both surgery and chemotherapy. She is aware that Mr. O.'s physician has written orders for a full code in the event of a cardiac arrest. While receiving his evening medications Mr. O. takes the nurse's hand in his own and says: "Promise me that you'll let me die if anything happens to my heart, and that you won't let them do all of those heroics to keep me alive. My wife is gone, I'm getting worse each day, and I'm ready to die now."

In such a case, the nurse might see her alternatives as follows: (1) promising the patient she will fulfill his request and choosing not to report any cardiac arrest until the possibility of resuscitation would be futile, or (2) aligning herself with the physician and reinforcing the staff and institutional position on such resuscitation, or (3) listening carefully to the patient, drawing out his thoughts and feelings on the subject and reassuring him that she will quickly act to set up a meeting with his physician so that his wishes can be given the most careful consideration. In choosing one of these, or any other alternative, the nurse must consider her responsibilities to the patient, to her professional colleagues, to the institution, and to her own conscience.

At times the ethical distinction is made that the patient wishes to receive "ordinary" care, but that no "extraordinary" measures should be taken to prolong life. This language implies that the normal measures of comfort and care are appropriate, and that in the undeniable face of death, it is inappropriate to initiate procedures that would only prolong dying or extend suffering.

In former times, people signed a "living will" giving instructions for their care at the end of life. Today many state legislatures have developed a natural death act that allows persons the legal right to have entered into the chart that they do not wish life-prolonging measures to be taken when they have a terminal illness and death is imminent. This document is a useful indication of the patient's wishes when the patient has lost consciousness or competence.

It is common practice for patients to make a less formal verbal agreement with their physician about their wishes for treatment and the withholding of treatment in the terminal phase.

Some patients ask, though rarely, that the physician or nurse take measures to end their lives. Such an action is illegal in all states and is generally held to be unethical. Most moral philosophers hold that there is a significant moral difference between allowing a person to die without prolonging life and actually killing a person by a direct action.

Dicussion of ethical issues in the terminal phase of illness can be found elsewhere. Nurses interested in pursuing this subject will find a growing literature pertaining to nursing ethics. Table 11–1 lists additional ethical issues.

Hospice Movement: Alternative to Traditional Care

The locus of care and the philosophy of treatment of persons who are dying have a profound influence on nursing practice and objectives. In recent times, patients in the terminal phase of illness have with increasing frequency chosen hospice care. The hospice concept emphasizes care and comfort as the primary goals for the dying, rather than curative measures. The hospice concept may be employed within a hospital setting, within the patient's home, or in a freestanding hospice in the community. Patients who are accepting death find the hospice an acceptable alternative to traditional care.

TABLE 11-1
Ethical Issues in Caring for the Terminally Ill

1. **Disclosing the diagnosis of a fatal disease**
   Avoiding harm, *i.e.*, not depressing the patient vs. the patient's right to know
2. **Medical management**
   Physician and nurse know best through knowledge and experience; or patient's preference should take priority (patient autonomy); or when patient is incompetent, family should decide.
3. **Designations of code, or no-code status**
   The physician and nurse decide based on experience; or the patient is consulted, if competent, and determines code designation; or guardian is sought for incompetent patient.
4. **Withholding life-prolonging treatment**
   What are the patient's wishes regarding this treatment? Is the action being considered voluntary or involuntary? Is it in the "best interests" of the patient, or others? Is there agreement between patient, family, and the health care team? Is it written or verbal?
5. **Living will, or natural death act**
   Has the patient signed the document? Is it witnessed? Is it entered into the chart, and duly noted by the physician? Has the patient a terminal illness? Is death imminent?
6. **Principle of double effect**
   When one proposed action has two effects, one of which is desirable and the other foreseen but not desirable. An example is a case in which a cancer patient requires increasing quantities of morphine to alleviate pain, to the paint that respiration will be slowed, and death will be hastened; yet, not providing morphine allows great suffering.
7. **Active or passive euthanasia**
   Taking a direct action aimed at ending the life of a patient is illegal. It is almost universally unethical as well.
8. **Assisting in the suicide of a patient**
   Aiding and abetting is illegal, a felony offense. All efforts should be made to meet the patient's needs and to provide adequate management of his pain.
9. **Care vs. cure**
   Implications of nursing care for the terminally ill patient often change from "cure" to "care" orientation as death nears.
10. **Organ donation, body donation, and autopsy**
    Desire of the patient or family needs vs. research and social needs

Family members and friends have almost unlimited access to the dying person. There is an open awareness of imminent death that encourages the patient to put his affairs in order and allows him to communicate his thoughts and feelings openly. Pain relief is a major goal and is usually successfully managed, providing comfort and assurance as life nears its end.

The Family of the Dying Patient

Nursing support for the patient in the terminal phase of illness usually entails working with the family of the patient as well. Most dying patients will have some family members attending to them during this critical phase of illness. Each family has developed its own unique forms of relationships, and individuals will most likely act "in character," in keeping with the roles that have developed within the family system. Family members tend to experience the pain of anticipated separation from the dying patient in proportion to their perceived level of intimacy with or dependency on that individual or that person's dependency on them (as in the case of a dying child). The nurse must be sensitive to the needs of the family members as well as the patient, and frequently plays a key role in assisting the family through the difficult process of coming to terms with the reality of the situation and easing them through the grieving process.

The death of a child is almost universally seen as tragic. When death threatens to end life before its potential has flowered, parents especially may become extremely distraught. In most cases, the family will be in constant attendance at the bedside of the younger patient. One parent frequently remains with the younger patient all day long, and sometimes a cot is brought in so that the parent (usually the mother) may stay with the young child at night as well. It is not unusual for various family members to approach the nurse for help with their own emotional struggles in coping with such a difficult situation. They are often full of questions such as: "Could I have caught this sooner? Would it have made a difference? Could this have been inherited from us (me)? Do you think we should go for another round of chemotherapy? What would you do if this was your child? How can I get my child's physician to answer my questions?" Parents may also be critical or demanding, failing to recognize or understand that the nurse is providing care for a number of other patients at the same time. The goal of nursing care in such cases is to support the family as much as possible in coping with their own needs and concerns. After a death, particularly that of a child, family members often have a need to make one or more return visits to the hospital or office where the patient was cared for. This is to be expected, and such a visit may play an important role in bringing a close to the grieving process for family members.

Older children may pose different situations for the family members. In the case of an accident involving a teenager, parents wonder if they were too liberal in allowing social privileges. When the dying patient is an adult, the family may experience feelings of abandonment or anger at the threatened loss of a spouse, parent, wage earner, and so forth. When the course of treatment does not lead to remission, the family will frequently question the nurse about whether their loved one had the best care possible, if everything appropriately possible had been done, and if the attending physician was a good doctor. A few words of reassurance and a few moments to talk with the family at such times provides immeasurable comfort to them in their distress. The nurse does well to see the family as appropriate recipients of nursing care rather than viewing them negatively as distracters, who are interrupting nursing services.

Older patients provide still other concerns for the family. Frequently, issues arise pertaining to the intensity of treatment that should be given, especially when the dying patient is incompetent to participate in decision making, or when his mental processes are compromised. Fear of causing suffering by too aggressive intervention, and feelings of guilt for not doing enough, are commonly encountered by those in decision making. When these problems arise, the nurse may invite the next of kin to have coffee to discuss their questions and attend to their feelings in a relaxed and supportive fashion. The nurse may also allow and encourage family members to assist in the care of the patient, such as assisting with meals, but should not expect them to give all the care, or to be there at every meal. Some patients may wish to spend their final days at home, and family members who see this as unrealistic, or who do not feel capable of arranging adequate care may, nevertheless, feel quite guilty about not being able to meet this last request.

When death occurs suddenly, surviving family members find it the most difficult of situations to accept. Often it is of great benefit for surviving family members to view the body of the person who has died. They may wish to sit with the body, touch it, and speak out their thoughts and feelings in the presence of the deceased. The sensitive nurse will support this "last visit," and may even suggest such a possibility when it is deemed appropriate. Any member of the family who does not want to view the body or spend any time with the deceased will decline the invitation. Many persons have expressed the belief that the "spirit" of the dead person lingers in the room for moments or hours and that the experience of being present was, for them, a helpful and comforting part of the passage. The resolution of grief and movement toward adaptive change can be greatly enhanced by the survivors' participation and presence in the dying process and by saying good-bye when death has occurred.

Although the family is grieving from the death of their loved one, the nurse may be aware that other concerns must be resolved. The person who has died may have willed his corneas to the eye bank, and expeditious action is required. The nurse may be involved in discussions with the family if the dying patient is a suitable organ donor for heart, kidneys, skin, and so on. The nurse can be helpful to the family in discussing the need, requirement, or desirability of an autopsy in some cases. Usually the physician is involved in the resolution of these issues, and rightly so. However, the nurse is frequently much better acquainted with the family, and this relationship provides a unique opportunity for serving the emotional needs of the family at a critical juncture in their passage from death of their loved one back to normal life.

Fortunately, few individuals die alone in our society. In the great majority of cases, the family will be involved with the patient during the terminal phase of illness. The nursing implications in this situation are that the nurse will recognize that the patient is a member of a family whose needs for care and understanding are as great as the patient's, and at times, even more acute. This is particularly the case when the patient has accepted death, and the family has not. In such cases, the use of active listening by the empathic nurse can be an invaluable resource.

Summary

In conclusion, nursing is both the science and the art of caring for patients. The nurse's role eventually brings her to the bedside of a dying stranger. The expectations of her profession are that she will enter the narrowing circle of the patient's relationships in service of the personal needs of one who is in the terminal phase of illness. Thoughtful attention to one's own needs in the situation as well as to the needs of the patient can allow a nurturing and trusting relationship that may be satisfying to both parties to develop. The art of caring for the dying challenges the nurse to confront her own unfinished business and to make peace with life and death so that she may be truly present with those for whom death is imminent.

References

1. Becker E: The Denial of Death, p 17. New York, The Free Press, 1973. Also Zilboorg G: Fear of death. Psychoanalytic Quarterly, 1943, pp. 468–471
2. Cassell E: The Healer's Art. New York, Lippincott, 1976
3. Frankl V: Doctor and the Soul. New York, Alfred A Knopf, 1957
4. Kubler-Ross E: Death—The Final Stage of Growth. Englewood Cliffs NJ, Prentice-Hall, 1975
5. Kubler-Ross E: On Death and Dying. New York, Macmillan, 1969
6. President's Commission for the Study of Ethical Problems in Medicine and Biomedical and Behavioral Research: Deciding to Forego Life-Sustaining Treatment. Ethical, Medical and Legal Issues in Treatment Decisions. Report. March 1983. Washington DC: US Government Printing Office, 1983
7. Webster's New Collegiate Dictionary. Springfield, GC Merriam Company, 1973

UNIT III

Physiology and Pathophysiology Concepts and Related Principles of Nursing Management

Chapter 12

Dynamic Equilibrium and the Nature of Disease

Barbara R. Landau
Pauline M. Bruno

Health–Illness Continuum

Rather than being considered dichotomous states, health and illness should be thought of as being on a continuum extending from high-level wellness in all spheres, through absence of evident disease, to obvious disease. At one end of the continuum is health, which may be considered as the ability to adapt successfully to external and internal environmental stimuli. The healthy person is able to function effectively. At the other end of the continuum is disease; a person with a disease may be considered as unable physically to respond effectively to environmental challenges. The individual is unable to function optimally. A person in the middle area of this health–illness continuum may have some abnormal measurements but no obvious impairment of functional ability.

All living things, animals, plants, and human beings, require the maintenance of an internal environment within relatively narrow limits for normal cell function. Control and regulatory mechanisms respond to external and internal stimuli for the purpose of maintaining this internal constancy. The health state is a process of constant change within defined limits, a matter of dynamic equilibrium. Disease is a state in which the person is no longer in equilibrium. The nature of the abnormality is a quantitative variation in existing compensatory or regulatory mechanisms rather than a new or different function or structure.

Dynamic equilibrium refers to the constantly fluctuating, physiological variations within human beings. Other terms used synonymously are *steady state* and *homeostasis.* The term homeostasis is derived from Greek. Although the suffix *-stasis* means "standing," it would be a misinterpretation to think of homeostasis as a nonchanging state. Rather, it means variation within the limits required by the body for optimal function. This interpretation also holds for the phrase *steady state.* This constant fluctuation within narrow limits occurs as a response to external and internal stimuli. It encompasses all levels of physiological function from the intracellular to the whole being.

Consider the following illustration of the many challenges to dynamic equilibrium which a person may encounter in one day:

A young adult nurse, who worked until 11:30 the evening before, oversleeps and omits breakfast to keep from being late to work at the hospital. A late arrival results in the need to park some distance from the hospital. It is a cold, rainy day, and, having forgotten an umbrella, the nurse gets wet before getting to the hospital. Included in the busy day's schedule is care of a severely ill elderly person with pneumonia and an in-service education presentation to a group of nursing students. The latter is a new experience. Lunch consists of a quick snack: potato chips and a hamburger in the cafeteria prior to class. After work, a candy bar provides energy for a hair appointment. Dinner is another snack (fruit and cheese) because preparing to attend a show has a higher priority than dinner.

What are the challenges this person had to meet and the adjustments she had to make in order to maintain a steady state? Omitting breakfast required liver breakdown of glycogen and conversion to glucose to maintain energy requirement. A cold, wet environment required increased heat production by the body to maintain normal temperature range. The external environment magnified the demands on the liver and also required a vasoconstriction response to prevent loss of body heat. The hospital environment presented the challenge of bacteria. The cells lining the respiratory tract had to prevent bacteria from entering the bloodstream. The white blood cells had to respond to the foreign body stimulus of any bacteria that evaded the first line of defense. The kidney had to respond to the high sodium content of lunch and regulate the blood level by retaining water. The anxiety of teaching a class stimulated the production of adrenalin and consequently the heart rate. The liver responded to the elevated adrenalin level with breakdown of glycogen to provide the energy to cope with the stressful teaching experience. To use the glucose, the pancreas had to secrete the insulin needed for glucose metabolism. The candy bar further elevated the glucose level and increased the demand on the pancreas.

Despite all of these challenges, the healthy nurse maintained dynamic equilibrium. Most people are capable of such adjustments during much of their life span. An almost continuous response to variations in external and internal stimuli results from the activities of daily living in a complex society. The teaching of illness prevention, a function of nurses, requires an understanding of potentially harmful stimuli, the control and regulator responses, and measures to avoid excessive demands.

A person whose health status is compromised may not have adequate response mechanisms to cope with the many challenges presented in the above example. Some people in like circumstances may develop a cold, others pneumonia. A person with diabetes mellitus, a disorder of insulin secretion or utilization, might not be able to maintain a blood glucose level within normal limits and the complication of hyperglycemia may occur. And a person with a history of smoking may not have adequate protection against bacterial agents. The control and regulatory mechanisms in the young and the elderly are not always capable of adjusting to multiple, intense stimuli, and therefore these groups are particularly susceptible to disease. Figure 12–1 is a diagram showing how continuing external stress and failure of adaptive responses may result in the development of disease.

The purpose of dynamic equilibrium is maintenance of the individual in a balanced state. This is accomplished by specific body mechanisms that respond to the many potentially harmful factors constantly present in the environment. The balanced state is maintained by the following: mechanisms that respond to variations in the biochemical and physical state, neurological and neuroendocrine integrity and regulatory mechanisms, and natural defense mechanisms such as physical barriers and immune responses. Eventually,

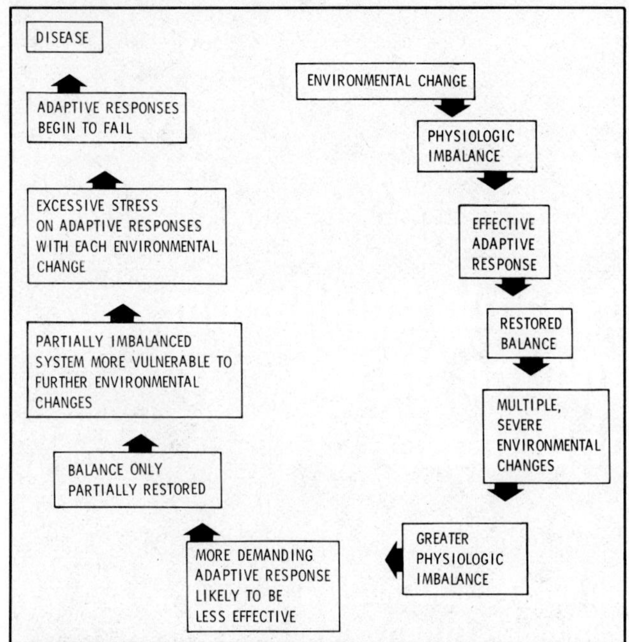

FIGURE 12–1 Concept of how unrelenting stress leads to disease. (Ramsey JM: Basic Pathophysiology: Modern Stress and the Disease Process. Menlo Park, California, Addison-Wesley Publishing Company, 1982)

these adaptive mechanisms falter and temporary illness, permanent disability, or uncontrollable disease results. Disease is manifested by alterations in control and regulatory mechanisms and by inability of the affected part to contribute to functioning of the whole being.

Nurses' responsibilities include monitoring of ill people to determine response to medical therapy and progression of disease, the making of clinical judgments based on these manifestations, and assisting people with the activities of daily living that they are unable to do for themselves. Therefore, it is essential that nurses understand the body mechanisms that respond to adverse external and internal stimuli as well as disease process and treatment. In this chapter we review the mechanisms for maintenance of dynamic equilibrium, and discuss the nature of injurious agents, etiologic factors of disease, manifestations of disease, and nursing implications.

Mechanisms of Dynamic Equilibrium

Ultimately, a state of total body balance depends on a balanced state within the cells. The maintenance of a suitable cellular environment is one of the most basic and important concepts for understanding body function. Cells are both dependent upon this regulation for their survival and responsible for carrying out this regulation. For instance, cells require a particular concentration of electrolytes, and it is the cell membrane that is responsible for this regulation.

The importance of cell function in relation to total body function governs the organization of this section. The discussion of regulatory mechanisms starts at the intracellular level (the internal solution and processes of cell activities and control mechanisms), and progresses to a consideration of intercellular communication, and then to the two main body control systems, neural and hormonal. The integration of these two systems promotes functioning of the body as a whole.

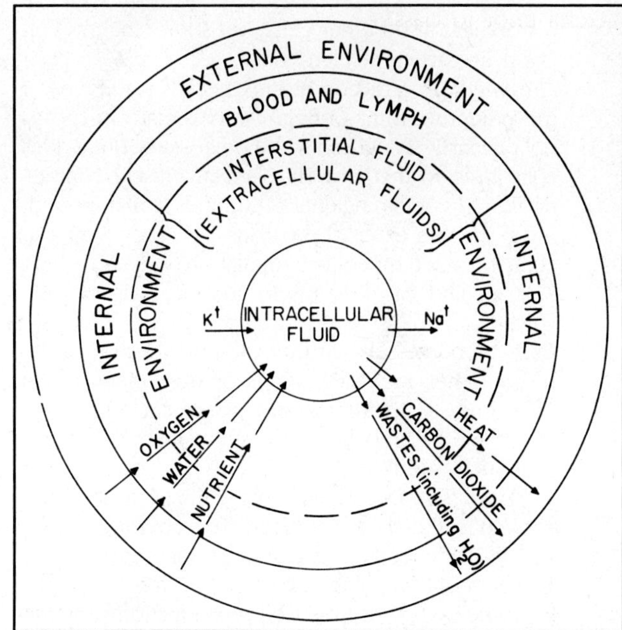

FIGURE 12–2 Functional relationship of the three body fluids. Blood, lymph, and the interstitial fluid directly bathing cells make up the internal environment of tissues and serve as the regulators of the intracellular fluid under changing conditions of the external environment. (Ramsey JM: Basic Pathophysiology: Modern Stress and the Disease Process. Menlo Park, California, Addison-Wesley Publishing Company, 1982)

Intracellular Environment

Internal Solution

As shown in Figure 12–2, the internal environment is an aqueous solution in which all chemical reactions in the body occur. Water is an ideal medium because in it many substances ionize or dissociate into their component parts and because it has excellent heat characteristics; it can take up and "store" a large amount of heat. The volume, temperature, and distribution of water, and the concentration of its many solutes must be regulated and maintained in order for cells to function optimally. The solute particles, especially inorganic ions (electrolytes), exert an osmotic effect that determines the volume and distribution of water in the body.

Cell Activities

The processes by which cells carry on their normal activities, including maintenance of their internal environment, are incredibly numerous and very complex. They fall into one of six broad categories:

1. *Transport of materials* in and out of the cell.
   a. Water and many small molecules move across cell membranes by the passive processes of diffusion and osmosis, which depend upon and are regulated by the permeability of the membrane and the concentration gradient across it, both of which may vary.
   b. The cell membrane transports many ions and molecules by active processes, which depend upon an appropriate membrane pump and a source of energy. Within limits, permeability and concentration gradients are not important for active transport.
   c. Macromolecules are transported into and out of the cell by exocytosis (fusion of membranes of substance to be secreted and cell membrane; the fused membrane opens and spills the substance into the surroundings) and endocytosis (the transfer of solid particles and fluid droplets into the cell by invagination and closure of the cell membrane). These processes differ from passive and active transport in that the materials do not actually pass through the membrane.
2. *Membrane potentials.* Maintenance of electrical gradients across the cell membrane is really a special aspect of membrane transport, because it depends upon a combination of membrane permeability (and impermeability) and passive and active transport of specific ions. The existence of suitable concentration and electrical gradients across the cell membrane are essential to normal cell function. In some disease states electrolytes may be at abnormal serum concentrations, thus interfering with the desired gradient (see Chap. 13).
3. *Metabolism.* Metabolic processes are those concerned with the breakdown, conversion, storage, and use of ingested foodstuffs, and ultimately with the management of energy obtained from them.
4. *Synthesis.* Cells synthesize many substances, both for use inside the cells and for "export." Those used in the cell include structural components of the cell. There is a continual turnover of the molecules in the cell membrane, for example, as well as in components of the organelles, and these must be replaced. Proteins are particularly important structural elements, although some lipids and polysaccharides are also used in cell structures. Enzymes, which are protein, are involved in virtually every reaction, so synthesis of protein for enzymes must also be a continuous process.

   Most cells export or secrete some of the substances they have synthesized. These include hormones (which may be peptides, amines, or steroids), neurotransmitters, a few enzymes, and other substances including prostaglandins, a variety of kinins, histamine, collagen, and others. Most of these exert a regulatory action on other cells, but some, such as collagen, are structural elements.

5. *Movement.* Contraction of muscle cells is the type of movement we think of first. It serves many purposes not primarily associated with homeostasis, but it does contribute to that as well. Skeletal muscle contractions aid in obtaining energy supplies, and in providing a suitable external environment. They may also contribute to temperature regulation (*e.g.,* shivering). Smooth and cardiac muscle are more directly involved as parts of tubular structures (*e.g.,* digestive tract, blood vessels) and the pumping action of the heart. Other important types of movement which contribute indirectly to homeostasis include ciliary action and the amoeboid movements characteristic of cells such as leukocytes.
6. *Reproduction.* During embryonic life all cells are capable of cell division by mitosis (except for gametes, which divide by meiosis), but many of them (notably nerve, muscle cells, and erythrocytes) lose the ability to divide as they mature. Cell reproduction serves to repair wounds with minimal scarring and therefore reestablishes a barrier to entrance of foreign substances.

Although responses and adjustments are carried out by the actions of individual cells, the cells do not act individually and in isolation. Many stimuli affect all cells in the vicinity, and other stimuli affect cells that are specialized to detect that particular stimulus. The response of these cells leads to an appropriate response by other, often distant, cells. Thus, although the internal environment is maintained by cell actions, it often involves a coordination of responses at the tissue, organ, and organ systems levels. Understanding homeostasis therefore involves understanding how cell processes are controlled in response to signals from within cells, from their cellular environment, and from other cells.

Intracellular Control Processes

All things cells do are regulated. Passive processes like diffusion are controlled by local conditions (membrane permeability and concentration gradients), but those which involve metabolic activities (energy) of the cells are chiefly controlled by enzyme production, action, and destruction.

Control of Enzyme Formation. The first consideration in the control of enzyme formation is the genetic aspect of enzyme production. The genetic information is contained in the deoxyribonucleic acid (DNA) molecules of chromosomes. A gene is that part of the chromosomal DNA that contains the genetic code for a particular protein, that is, an enzyme. Normally, one has genes that code for synthesis of all necessary enzymes, but occasionally there are errors or mutations during cell division and the genetic material may be inappropriately distributed. It may result in the inability to produce the enzyme for a particular reaction, or perhaps result in one incorrect amino acid in a protein molecule that will interfere with function of the enzyme. The genetic error could thereby block a whole chain of reactions and interfere with an important metabolic process, or prevent the degradation of a potentially harmful metabolite. Some such genetic alterations are incompatible with life, but others are not and become part of the genetic pool of information that may be transmitted to future generations. In recent years a rather large number of such genetic disturbances have been identified.

Assuming that cells contain the proper genes, there are two processes that must be carried out to produce an enzyme molecule. *Transcription* is the means by which the code carried on the DNA is transferred to a molecule of messenger ribonucleic acid (mRNA) as it is being synthesized. *Translation* is the process by which the code carried by the mRNA is translated into a protein molecule; it is the actual synthesis of the enzyme.

Transcription and translation are influenced by the intracellular concentration of certain substances. For example, the presence of a particular substrate may increase or induce synthesis of the enzymes needed to deal with it, or the absence of the substrate may repress the synthesis of those enzymes. Induction processes often involve inhibition of the action of a repressor protein that is blocking the formation of the necessary RNA. The repressor protein molecule binds to a specific part of the DNA molecule and blocks RNA synthesis. These and other means of influencing RNA production are also influenced by signals from outside the cell. In addition to these controls of the genetic process, synthesis of RNA and enzymes requires the availablity of the appropriate amino acids, a source of energy (ATP), and a suitable cellular environment (*e.g.,* electrolytes, pH, oxygen).

Control of Enzyme Action. Control of the action of enzymes that have been produced also requires a normal state of the internal environment. In addition, the action of enzymes depends upon the relative concentrations of substrates and products, the presence of factors that activate the enzyme, and the amount of enzyme present. The latter depends upon its rate of destruction as well as its rate of synthesis. All else being equal, when the substrate concentration is high, enzyme action is more complete, but if the products are allowed to accumulate the reaction is inhibited. Some enzymes will catalyze a reaction in either direction, and the direction and rate of the reaction are determined largely by the concentration of the reactants. It will go to the right if substrate concentration is high, but if the product concentration is high the direction will be reversed. This is important, since many chemical processes involve a series of sequential reactions.

Some enzymes require the presence of activating factors in order to bind to the substrate and change the molecule configuration. For instance, some enzymes need a *cofactor,* often a metallic ion which is tightly bound to the enzyme and aids binding with the substrate. Other enzymes require a *coenzyme.* Most coenzymes are derived from nucleotides and serve as carriers of hydrogen or of acetyl groups. They take up groups when they are released and donate them when they are needed in reactions. Many vitamins are coenzymes.

Effect of Stimuli on Intracellular Enzymes. There are many stimuli that affect the action of intracellular enzymes, and the end result produced by the stimuli depends upon which enzyme has been activated (or inactivated). It is perhaps surprising, therefore, that nearly all stimuli affect intracellular enzymes by one of only a few mechanisms. Many of them exert their action by causing the formation of *cyclic nucleotides*. Cyclic adenosine monophosphate (cAMP) is the most widely distributed of the nucleotides. AMP is derived from the ubiquitous adenosine triphosphate (ATP) found in all cells. ATP is a nucleotide composed of the nitrogenous base adenine, plus the sugar ribose, and three phosphates, two of which are attached by high-energy bonds. Removal of the two end phosphates yields AMP plus two inorganic phosphates, and the energy of the high-energy bonds. The formation of cAMP triggers a series of reactions that leads to a physiological response (see Fig. 12–3). Cyclic AMP activates one of a group of enzymes known as protein kinases. The activated protein kinases in turn activate another enzyme found in the cytoplasm by phosphorylating it, and the phosphorylated enzyme carries out the specific physiological response. For instance, there are many protein kinases, but those in each cell are specific for that cell, as are the enzymes they phosphorylate. Thus, the response elicited by formation of cAMP depends upon which protein kinases and which specific enzymes are phosphorylated in that cell. Formation of cAMP may lead to breakdown of fat in one cell, breakdown of glycogen in another, and secretion of a hormone in another.

Cyclic AMP is formed when an enzyme, *adenylate cyclase,* located in the membrane of cells is activated. Cyclic AMP is rapidly inactivated by another enzyme found in the cytoplasm of cells, *phosphodiesterase.* The rate of the final physiological process is regulated by the amount of cAMP present, and that is determined by the balance between its formation and destruction, that is, by the action of adenylate cyclase and phosphodiesterase (see Fig. 12–4).

Cyclic AMP is often referred to as a "second messenger" because it provides the connection between the initial stimulus or "first messenger" and the response mechanism. Many different stimuli cause formation of cAMP, and cAMP leads to many different physiological responses. In some cells the second messenger is believed to be cyclic guanosine monophosphate (cGMP).

A second intracellular control mechanism is the opening of calcium channels in the cell membrane, which allows calcium ions to enter the cell. Calcium is primarily an extracellular ion, and most of the calcium inside cells is located in certain organelles (such as sarcoplasmic reticulum of muscle) rather than being free in the cytoplasm. There is both a concentration gradient and an electrical gradient (calcium carries a positive charge and the inside of the cell is negative) favoring entry of calcium into the cell. The electrochemical gradient is maintained by a calcium pump that extrudes calcium ions and by the fact that the cell membrane is not very permeable to calcium.

When a stimulus (*e.g.,* a nerve impulse) causes increased permeability to calcium ions, the calcium level in the cytoplasm is raised by both movement of calcium into the cell and the release of calcium from intracellular sites. The calcium ions function as a second messenger, and in many cases bind with calmodulin, an intracellular protein, to bring about the desired action. Calmodulin is found in almost all cells, but is not very active until calcium binds to it. Binding changes the configuration of the molecule, thus enabling it to carry out its action. For example, an action potential in a muscle cell increases calcium entry into the cell and calcium release from the sarcoplasmic reticulum. In smooth muscle the calcium binds with calmodulin to trigger the contractile events. In skeletal and cardiac muscle the calcium binds to troponin (a protein which is structurally similar to calmodulin) to trigger the contractile events. In nerve endings and some secretory cells, molecules of neurotransmitter or secretion are contained in membrane-enclosed vesicles. Action potentials (see below) cause a calcium influx which enhances the fusion of vesicle membrane with the cell membrane, leading to release of the neurotransmitter or secretion. Thus, calcium often plays the role of coupler, as in excitation–contraction coupling or excitation–secretion coupling. In other cells the calcium–calmodulin complex interacts with the cAMP mechanism, sometimes inhibiting it by increasing action of the phosphodiesterase, which inactivates cAMP, and sometimes by augmenting the cAMP mechanism, enhancing adenylate cyclase action and thus increasing the formation of cAMP. Some protein kinases are also calcium dependent.

A third mechanism for controlling cell processes involves an effect upon the membrane potential. Stimulation of nerve and muscle cells results in a very brief increase in

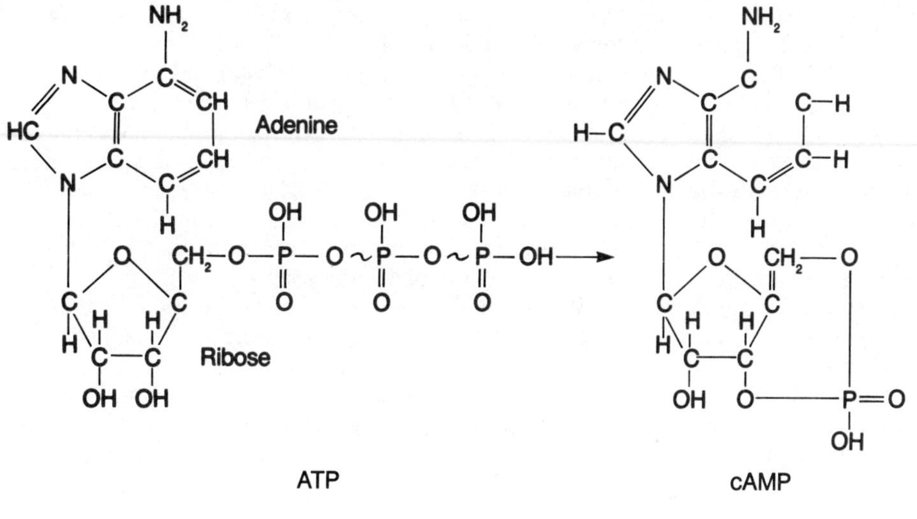

Adenine

Ribose

ATP

cAMP

FIGURE 12–3 Formation of cAMP from ATP.

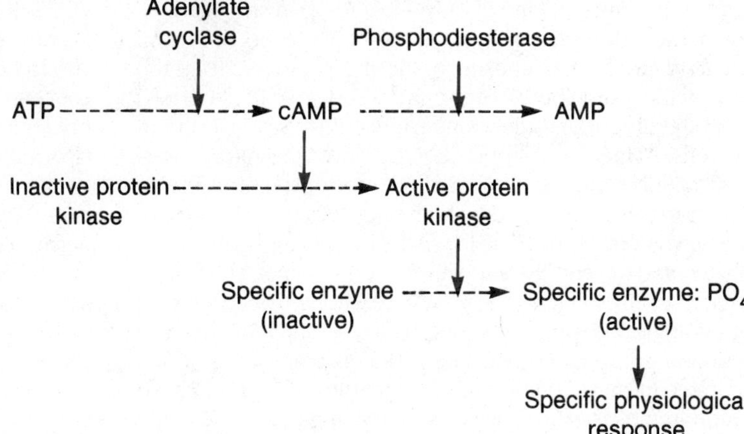

FIGURE 12–4 Activation and inactivation of cAMP. The enzyme adenylate cyclase initiates the conversion of ATP to cAMP. Subsequently, cAMP initiates the activation of other enzymes that ultimately effect cellular activity. The enzyme phosphodiesterase inactivates cAMP.

permeability to certain ions, first to sodium then to potassium, which depolarizes the membrane and produces an action potential (the change in electrical potential across the membrane of a nerve or muscle cell when it becomes active). In some nerve cells, other ion changes occur which briefly hyperpolarize the cell membrane and inhibit the development of action potentials.

A fourth possibility has been mentioned previously: the control of RNA synthesis. Steroid hormones, which are lipid soluble and hence can penetrate the lipid-containing cell membrane, and thyroid hormones, whose molecules are very small, enter the cell and exert their actions in the nucleus by affecting the synthesis of RNA.

Intercellular Communication

The next level in the hierarchy is the extracellular control of these intracellular mechanisms. Responses described above, such as the formation of cAMP, are initiated by signals from other cells, and therefore involve means by which cells communicate with each other. This leads to consideration of more complex control systems. Virtually all intercellular communication is carried out by chemicals that are released by one cell and act upon another cell.

The chemical messenger is often released very close to the cell it is to affect, but many messengers must travel some distance to reach their target cell. The messenger almost always affects or communicates with a specific cell or type of cell. The question then arises as to how the chemical messenger recognizes the cell it is to act upon.

The answer to the recognition question lies in protein molecules known as *receptors*. Receptors are located in the cell membrane, in the cytoplasm, and in the nucleus, but most are on the surface of the cell membrane. Recall that cell membranes are composed of a lipid bilayer with protein molecules distributed throughout. Some proteins are on the inner surface, some are on the outer surface, and some extend through the membrane. In some respects these proteins resemble enzymes. They differ from one another and, like enzymes, they are specific. Certain parts of the receptor molecule are exposed on the external surface of the membrane and function as binding sites to which specific molecules may bind; these are the receptor sites. When a chemical messenger, the "first messenger," comes in contact with its specific receptor and binds to it, an intracellular action is initiated. Thus, chemicals can exert their actions without ever entering the cell, which is fortunate since the cell membrane is not permeable to most of them. Only those which can penetrate the cell membrane actually enter the cell. They bind to receptors located in the cytoplasm or in the nucleus.

The chemical messengers that bind to the receptors are called *ligands*. There are many different kinds of ligands, including *neurotransmitters, hormones,* and other substances produced and released by cells such as *prostaglandins, kinins,* and *histamine*.

Since receptors are part of the cell, they are subject to the same continual turnover as other parts of the cell. Their number and distribution over the cell surface can be altered by any of several factors. Evidence suggests that a high concentration of first messenger, in many cases, tends to reduce the number of receptors for it, probably by internalization (endocytosis of receptors), and a low level of messenger tends to increase the number of receptors. The presence of some substances will increase the number of receptors for another substance. Another possibility is that a different chemical may be able to bind to the receptor, leaving no unoccupied sites for the intended chemical regulator. Changes in the *number* and availability of receptors affect the sensitivity of the cell to the substance in question. An increase in the number of receptors may lead to a hypersensitivity (*e.g.*, denervation hypersensitivity), and a lack of receptors may lead to symptoms of a deficiency condition. For example, some diabetics have normal insulin levels but insufficient membrane receptors to attain adequate intracellular levels.

Ligand–receptor binding triggers intracellular events by one of the mechanisms that have been described. It may cause one or more of the following:

- Activation of adenylate cyclase (found in the cell membrane), causing the formation of cAMP, leading to the response attributed to that ligand.
- Changes in configuration of the protein molecules in the membrane which contain calcium channels. The changes open the channels and increase calcium en-

try into the cell. Once inside, calcium may bind with calmodulin to affect certain enzyme systems.

- Changes in the membrane potential of the cell. Opening sodium, then potassium channels in nerve or muscle cells leads to depolarization and action potentials, while opening chloride channels causes hyperpolarization and inhibits action potential generation.
- Action on DNA in the cell nucleus to cause synthesis of RNA and increase protein synthesis. This mode of action is limited to those ligands that can penetrate the cell membrane.

Source of Ligands. One ordinarily thinks of nerve activity as an electrical event. The electrical response is the nerve impulse or action potential, which transmits information inside the nerve cell. However, information is transmitted to other cells by a *chemical mediator.* Normally a nerve cell is stimulated at one end. The stimulus causes development of one or more action potentials which are conducted to the other end of the neuron. Arrival of an action potential at the nerve terminal causes entry of calcium ions, which brings about release of the chemical stored in tiny vesicles in the nerve ending. The chemical, a neurotransmitter, is released into a narrow space (a neuromuscular or synaptic junction) and diffuses across it to the postjunctional or postsynaptic membrane. The postsynaptic membrane contains receptors for the particular transmitter, and the transmitter binds to them, causing changes in permeability of the membrane.

At skeletal neuromuscular junctions the transmitter is acetylcholine (ACh). It causes depolarization of the muscle cell membrane, and an action potential (impulse) occurs. The ACh is quickly destroyed or inactivated by the enzyme acetylcholinesterase (AChE), which is located on the postjunctional cell membrane, so only one action potential is produced. At junctions between nerve cells (synapses) the arrival of an action potential causes a partial depolarization. Not enough to trigger an action potential, it merely raises the excitability of the cell for a brief interval.

Other nerve cells release a different transmitter, one which causes hyperpolarization of the postsynaptic membrane and temporarily lowers its excitability. Many of the structures innervated by the autonomic nervous system (ANS), such as smooth and cardiac muscle and some glands, receive innervation from both the sympathetic and parasympathetic divisions of the ANS. The difference in the actions of the two divisions is due to the fact that ACh is released at parasympathetic neuromuscular junctions and epinephrine is released at sympathetic neuromuscular junctions. The response is related to the function of the particular type of nervous system stimulated.

Hormones are other substances that bind to ligands and initiate an intracellular response. In response to a stimulus, endocrine glands produce hormones which are carried in the bloodstream throughout the body. Hormone molecules diffuse out into the interstitial fluid where they may encounter a cell that has the "right" receptors. Hormone–receptor binding occurs and a particular response is triggered. After the hormone–receptor complex has exerted its action, the hormone typically is released, to be transported to an organ such as the liver to be inactivated and metabolized. Most hormones bind to receptors on the cell surface and do not enter the cell at all. Steroid hormones are lipid soluble and are able to cross the cell membrane and find their receptors in the cytoplasm. The hormone–receptor complex moves to the cell nucleus to stimulate the DNA to increase synthesis of RNA for a particular protein (enzyme). Thyroid hormones are also able to enter the cell, where they bind to receptors in the nucleus and increase synthesis of mRNA and rRNA.

Other chemicals are produced by cells and released into the interstitial fluid rather than into the bloodstream. As compared to hormones, these compounds differ in that they can affect cells only within diffusing distance, which may mean a rather restricted area; this is known as *paracrine action,* and these substances are called *paracrine agents.* There are quite a number of paracrine agents, and their actions are extremely varied. In some cases their true function is not actually known, but they have been indentified in areas where there are known to be receptors for them. Histamine is such a substance.

An important group of substances with paracrine actions are the prostaglandins. They are synthesized from arachidonic acid which is in most, if not all, cells. This acid is one of the essential fatty acids. There are several subgroups of prostaglandins, and their actions are quite different and often opposing. Their action usually, if not always, involves cAMP. Some prostaglandins increase cAMP content and others decrease it.

It should be noted that there may be more than one type of receptor for a particular ligand, and the response produced depends upon which sequence of events the receptor binding initiates. This explains why a ligand may have one effect on one type of cell and the opposite on another. Epinephrine is probably the best-known example. It excites smooth muscle cells in most blood vessels, but inhibits them in the vessels found in skeletal muscle and in the wall of the gastrointestinal tract. This is possible because there are two different kinds of receptors for epinephrine, known as alpha and beta receptors. These receptors are further subdivided into alpha-1 and alpha-2, and beta-1 and beta-2. Alpha receptors are excitatory (constriction) and beta receptors are inhibitory (dilation). Beta receptors exert their action through adenylate cyclase and cAMP. The mechanism of action of alpha receptors is not yet understood, but there is some evidence that they increase calcium uptake. Alpha and beta receptors were originally identified on the basis of different effects of drugs on the action of epinephrine. These differences are of importance because many drugs block or enhance actions of epinephrine at sites involving one receptor and do not affect those actions at cells that have the other receptor.

Control Systems

The final step in regulating cell function is *control or release of the chemical regulators or mediators, and coordination of their action.* It involves more complex mechanisms, often including several organs and organ systems. A control system has at least three elements: a sensor or receptor, an integration center, and an effector (plus the necessary connections). A simplified model of a control system is shown in Figure 12–5. The sensor detects a specific change (the stimulus) in a particular location and sends information to the center, which receives input from other monitors as well. Correction of the changes detected is likely to require responses that are widespread or at a distance from the stimulus. The center "considers" information received from all sensory receptors, makes a "decision," and sends messages to muscle or gland cells that will bring about the appropriate response. These cells are termed *effectors*. Most control systems operate as negative feedback systems in which the stimulus evokes a response that corrects the change. This removes the stimulus and hence the response soon diminishes. Such systems are designed to maintain a steady state and to minimize change, and thus are the basic elements of dynamic equilibrium.

The two main biological control systems are *neural* and *hormonal*. Neural control involves reflex action. The sensor or sensory receptor (which is not to be confused with a receptor site) is located at the peripheral end of a sensory nerve. The design and complexity of sensory receptors varies from simple bare nerve endings in the skin to intricate sensors in the retina or cochlea. Each receptor has a low threshold for one type of stimulus. There are sensory receptors in the skin that detect pain, touch, or temperature; receptors in the walls of some large arteries monitor pressure of the blood in the artery, and receptors in skeletal muscles respond to stretch of the muscles. Stimulation of a sensory receptor causes changes in the receptor that generate action potentials in the afferent (sensory) nerve. The nerve impulse is then conducted to a center in the central nervous system (CNS). In its simplest form a center contains a synapse, which is the connection between the afferent and efferent neurons. Excitation of the efferent (motor) neuron results in action potentials being conducted to the neuromuscular junction and transmitted to the effector. The effector, which may be

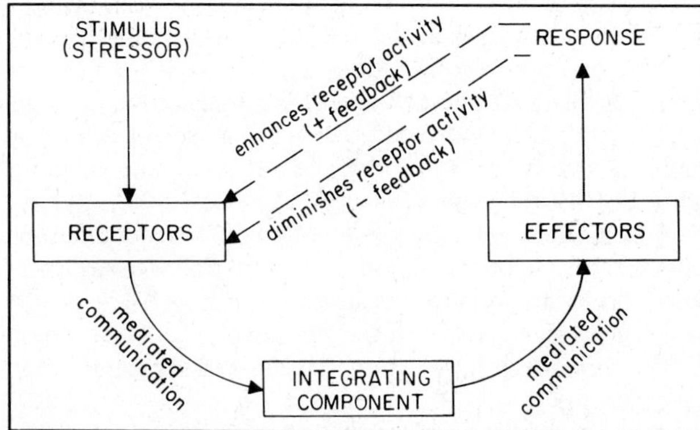

FIGURE 12–5 Simplified model of the physiological control principle. Observe that the response can either diminish (negative feedback) or enhance (positive feedback) further action throughout the system. (Ramsey JM: Basic Pathophysiology: Modern Stress and the Disease Process. Menlo Park, California, Addison-Wesley Publishing Company, 1982)

either skeletal, cardiac, or smooth muscle, or a gland, responds by contraction or secretion. The generated response should help to correct the change that initially stimulated the sensory receptor.

The *CNS center* for processing afferent impulses is usually more complicated than a simple afferent–efferent connection. There are often one or more interneurons between afferent and efferent neurons, and the afferent input to the center usually comes on neurons from different kinds of receptors and from widely separated locations. The center is a processor. It logs incoming information, weights conflicting signals, integrates and assesses all data, and then sends directives in the form of impulses in efferent nerves to some effectors and not to others.

Endocrine control systems also make use of negative feedback. When properly stimulated, the endocrine gland releases a hormone which travels to a distant effector (target organ). The stimulus may be the presence (or absence) of a substance in the cell's environment which affects it directly. For instance, the effect of the blood glucose level on insulin-secreting cells of the pancreas is one of the simplest forms of negative feedback. Elevation of the blood glucose level causes release of insulin, which lowers the glucose level and, by removing the stimulus, reduces insulin secretion.

Several feedback loops involve an additional component, the anterior pituitary gland. For example, the stimulus for secretion of thyroid hormones is thyroid stimulating hormone (TSH) from the anterior pituitary gland. The thyroid hormones inhibit release of TSH rather than acting directly on the thyroid gland. The loop is actually longer than that, because TSH release is caused by thyrotropin release hormone (TRH) produced by cells in the hypothalamus. The hypothalamus receives input from many other parts of the brain as well as from the rest of the body by way of the spinal cord. It functions as a center by integrating the incoming information, and in the thyroid hormone feedback cycle it responds by increasing or decreasing the release of TRH. Thyroid hormones circulating in the blood inhibit the release of TRH as well as TSH.

There are hypothalamic releasing hormones that control release of all pituitary hormones. The nervous system through sensory stimuli is, therefore, the initiator of the events that lead to secretion by several important endocrine glands. This action is counterbalanced by the negative feedback of these endocrine hormones acting on both the hypothalamus and the pituitary. The efferent limb of nerve reflexes and the endocrine mechanisms differ mainly in the nature of the message: action potentials which cause release of a neurotransmitter to excite effector cells, or hormones in the bloodstream that affect distant effector (target) cells.

The nervous system has a highly developed system of sensory receptors to monitor specific aspects of the environment, internal or external. Endocrine processes lack the elaborate sensing mechanisms, but when integration of many bits of information is needed, the endocrine system relies on the sensory components of the nervous system. Some endocrine glands, such as the adrenal medulla, are directly under neural control (sympathetic). There are neuroendocrine reflexes in which the afferent limb is neural and the efferent is hormonal (*e.g.,* the release of oxytocin during labor and lactation). The most important neural control, however, is the control of the anterior pituitary by hypothalamic releasing hormones, which gives the nervous system ultimate control over secretion of many hormones and many vital processes.

It is not entirely clear how the actions of paracrine agents fit into this scheme, and how their release is regulated. Their actions often modify the responses mediated by neural and hormonal mechanisms. Many of these actions occur in the brain, where it is very difficult to isolate and study events at a particular site or synapse.

When all aspects are considered, the fact emerges that these control mechanisms are quite similar and very closely related. The similarities become even more apparent when it is recognized that a number of chemical regulators may be neurotransmitters in one place, hormones in another, and have a paracrine action in yet another. There are a number of neurotransmitters in the CNS, and other chemical regulators have been identified whose actions are not specifically known. Some may affect synaptic transmission in the CNS by altering the membrane potential at nerve endings (some presynaptic endings have receptor sites to which a regulator or neutrotransmitter may bind). Increasing or decreasing the membrane potential affects the size of the arriving action potential and alters the amount of transmitter released from that nerve terminal. This is an example of what is often called a neuromodulator action. Some of the elusive chemical regulators that have been found in the brain and that have receptors there, but whose functions are not known, include aldosterone, cortisol, histamine, thyroid hormones, endorphins, several hypothalamic releasing hormones, angiotensin, estrogen and testosterone, and several gastrointestinal hormones including gastrin, secretin and cholecystokinin. Prostaglandins are also found in the brain.

Many hormones are peptides (amino acid chains composed of up to about 50 amino acids). Some of these, including nearly a dozen of those produced by the digestive tract, are present in the brain where they are transmitters, where they exert paracrine actions by modifying transmission (neuromodulators), or both. Somatostatin is produced in the pancreas, where it inhibits secretion of both insulin and glucagon by a paracrine action. It is also released from the hypothalamus as growth hormone inhibiting factor and inhibits release of growth hormone by the anterior pituitary gland.

Summary

In summary, the maintenance of dynamic equilibrium involves many regulatory and control mechanisms. These mechanisms function at all biological levels, from the intracellular to the body as a whole. The intracellular control processes, which involve metabolic activities, are controlled by enzyme production, action, and destruction. The actions of intracellular enzymes influence formation of cyclic nucleotides, movement of calcium into or out of the cell, and changes in membrane potential and RNA synthesis. Intercellular regulatory mechanisms operate by chemical messengers. The chemicals (ligands) are released by one cell and bind to receptors located on or in other cells in near proximity or some distance away. Ligand–receptor binding controls by triggering one of the above-mentioned actions of intracellular enzymes. Ligands include neurotransmitters, hormones, and paracrine agents. The final step in regulation of cell function is by means of systems that consist of a sensor, an integration center, and an effector. The two main biological control systems are neural and endocrine. These control mechanisms are similar in that a number of chemical regulators may be neurotransmitters in one place, hormones in another, and paracrine in a third instance, all of these mechanisms being important in coping with the challenges of the many potentially harmful stimuli which human beings encounter daily. When people function effectively to maintain a steady state within the range of normal, they enjoy a maximum level of wellness. Inadequacies or injuries in any area of functioning influence well being and may result in temporary illness, permanent disability, or death.

Nature of Illness

Disease may be defined as abnormal physical or mental processes, the nature of the abnormality being an alteration in normal mechanisms. Disease does not consist of new functions but rather is a modification of normal mechanisms. It is an unbalanced state which results from injury to cells. The functional change is a quantitative and qualitative variation in existing processes. Injuries may result in an increase, decrease, or absence of a substance required for balanced cell function. As discussed in the previous section, the normal control and regulatory mechanisms are at the intracellular, the intercellular, and the systemic integrative neuroendocrine levels. Likewise, injuries have their effect at these levels. Injuries may affect enzyme synthesis and action, intercellular chemical regulating mechanisms, and neuroendocrine control processes. The effect is to modify functions that normally maintain homeostasis.

Phases of Disease

Disease is classified into three phases: progressive, stable, and regressive. Initially, the dysfunction that follows from a harmful stimulus is progressive. The body's defenses, perhaps aided by medical therapy, require time to cope with this progression. Often, body defenses are successful, and the disease enters a regressive stage. In this stage the disease process is halted and the body is returned to a balanced state. At times, however, though the process is slowed and controlled the disease remains, entering a relatively stable stage. Chronic diseases are characterized by extended stable stages. Afflicted persons are usually aware of the disease and need constantly to direct efforts toward maintaining a relatively balanced state. Much of nursing and medical practice consists of helping persons with chronic illness to maintain the maximum level of wellness. In some situations, the nature of the injurious stimuli is such that the person alone or with medical assistance is unable to cope effectively and the disease continues in the progressive stage until the person dies.

Problems in Understanding Illness

Judgments about health–illness status are based on various functional indices considered in the context of the total individual. However, these indices cannot be easily categorized as normal or abnormal. Evaluation of measurements requires consideration of five relevant concepts:

- Range of normal and average values
- Consistency of a particular measurement
- Age
- Time-of-day measurement
- Potential for error

Individuals differ in the degree of response to stimuli and control of physiological parameters. Therefore, measurements of physical status such as temperature, heart rate, weight, and blood pressure reveal a range of normal and a particular average value. Few people are at the average value but most people are between some "normal" value above or below the average. A single measure of a parameter which falls outside the range of normal cannot be considered indicative of a particular disease. For instance, a single elevated blood pressure reading does not mean that the person has high blood pressure. To make this determination, the blood pressure has to be consistently outside the range of normal. Some measurements have to be taken at different times over a 24-hour period since circadian rhythms can produce variability in readings. For example, body temperature has a diurnal rhythm. It is lowest during sleep in the early morning hours and highest in the late afternoon. Other measurements, such as blood pressure and muscle strength, have characteristic changes with age. Many measurements are influenced by physical activity and nutritional intake. Lastly, the possibility of human error always exists in taking, reading, or computing a measurement. These factors are all important to consider when evaluating health–illness status. Despite the existence of highly developed methods of morphological and biochemical investigation, the normal has no precise boundaries that differentiate it from the various stages of abnormality.

Knowledge of human disease processes is also limited by experimental studies that use animals, cells *in vitro,* and autopsy findings. Animals are similar but not identical to humans, and generalizing from animal to human may be erroneous. Likewise, laboratory methods of studying cells remove the cell from its normal environment in the process and may distort its structure and change its function. Cells *in vivo* are dependent on spatial relationships with other cells and on the intercellular environment. Therefore, laboratory findings may not be an accurate indication of *in vivo* cell function and structure. Information obtained from examination of tissues following removal at surgery or autopsy is also subject to erroneous interpretation. Diseased tissue has been acted upon by body defense mechanisms and medical therapy; therefore, the changes may not accurately depict the *pathogenesis,* the cause and course of the disease. Laboratory data represents but a single point or phase in a constantly changing process, and must always be interpreted cautiously and in relation to other manifestations.

Influence of Aging

Aging consists of alterations in biological as well as sociocultural and psychological processes. As discussed in Chapter 5, biological changes are normal but for the most part involve a gradual decline in functional ability including the ability to cope with adverse stimuli. The changes occur at varying rates and are progressive. Indices of health and illness and studies of cell and tissue specimens may have different norms based on age. Sometimes aging changes appear similar to a particular disease process except for a quantitative difference.

Nature of Injurious Agents

Injurious agents are any stimuli that cause temporary or permanent disruptions of dynamic equilibrium. People have a tendency to view disease as having a single cause, perhaps because particular pathogens are associated with particular disease. However, if this were true, every person exposed to a communicable disease, such as the flu, would come down with it. The fact that some people escape the epidemic despite exposure to the organisms supports the fact that disease results not from a single cause but from the interaction of many factors related to both the host and the agent.

Classification of Injurious Agents

Classification of injurious agents is by *source of origin* and by *relationship to initiation of disease process.* Source of origin is either extrinsic or intrinsic. *Extrinsic agents* include pathogenic microorganisms, physical forces (trauma, temperature extremes, ultraviolet light), chemical forces (drugs, atmospheric contaminants), and sociocultural and psychological climates in the home, neighborhood, and community. *Intrinsic agents* may be intracellular and extracellular. Intracellular injuries are often genetic errors; these are inherent in the hereditary genetic makeup. Others may be of a congenital nature, that is, developmental errors that occur *in utero.* The intercellular environment may also be a source of harmful stimuli. For instance, the person with chronic bronchitis, a lung disorder that inhibits adequate expiration and fosters carbon dioxide retention, is vulnerable to shifts in pH of the blood to the acidotic side. An acidotic internal environment is injurious to all the cells of the body. Noxious internal environments may derive from faulty function of a particular group of cells but often affect the functioning of other parts of the body. Types of internal injurious stimuli are abnormalities of the following: physical factors such as temperature, oxygen tension, osmotic pressure, and blood flow rates; nutrients (essential amino acids, vitamins, electrolytes); products of cell function (*i.e.,* hormones and antibodies); and internal environment, resulting from the use of pharmacologic agents.

Another method of classifying injurious agents is by relationship to initiation of disease process. This classification is divided into precipitating and contributory agents. As mentioned earlier in this chapter, disease is caused not by one agent but rather by the interaction of many factors.

Precipitating agents are those that must be present for the disease to occur. They are necessary to initiate the disease process. An example of a precipitating agent is the flu virus. However, as noted earlier, the presence of the flu virus in and of itself is not sufficient for development of the disease. The presence of contributory factors is usually required for disease to occur.

Contributory or predisposing causes are often complex and may be present over a prolonged period of time. They may predispose a person to disease by weakening the person and thereby lowering the effectiveness of defense mechanisms. They may also increase the possibility of exposure to the harmful agent. Examples of contributory factors that may strengthen or weaken host resistance are nutritional status, age, biological rhythms, patterns of rest and activity, and mental/emotional status. An example of prolonged exposure to injurious stimuli is an occupation with high trauma risk.

Factors Influencing Effect of Harmful Stimuli

Factors that influence the damaging effects of injurious agents are the following:

- Quality and quantity of the harmful agents
- Location and extent of injury
- Period of time at which the injury occurs

Quality refers to the potency of the injurious agent. For instance, the potency of a small amount of poisonous snake venom may be sufficient to cause death despite excellent defense mechanisms and medical treatment. *Quantity* is the amount of injurious agent encountered. A few pathogenic microorganisms may not cause disease, whereas gross contamination of a wound would result in infection.

The *location and extent of injury* influences the ability of the person to cope with harmful agents. Injury to one of the vital organs such as the heart or brain is potentially more threatening than a fractured femur. Similarly, burns over 10% of the body are less threatening than burns over 60% of the body. A person who is exposed to sunlight almost daily over 20 or 30 years is more likely to develop skin cancer than a person who is exposed for a week or two.

Age at which one encounters an injurious agent often influences the damaging effect. As discussed in Chapter 5, elderly persons are more susceptible to adverse conditons than are young adults. The elderly have reduced resistance to the agent and decreased ability to cope with the effects of injury. All of these factors contribute to the host–agent reaction that results in the maintenance of dynamic equilibrium or in a disease process.

Mechanisms of Action of Injurious Agents

Most injuries exert their initial effect at the *molecular* and *biochemical* level. Ultimately, most forms of injury affect one or more of the following cell functions: synthesis of structural and enzymatic proteins; maintenance of electrolyte and osmotic stability; production of energy necessary for metabolic processes; and reproduction. Functional changes and resulting structural alterations are possible to determine by diagnostic procedures.

Cell Changes Following Injury. Deprivation of oxygen to cells causes a pattern of cellular injury that is often used as a model to study cell damage. The sequence of damage, as described in Chapter 23, begins with a shift from normal, aerobic cell respiration to the inefficient but oxygen-free type of metabolism called anaerobic glycolysis. The sequence of cellular events which follows culminates in impairment of DNA and RNA synthesis, rupture of lysosomes, and release of digestive enzymes that destroy cell components. The cell is no longer able to carry out its specific functions. Damage to a large number of specialized cells eventually impairs total body function.

Despite advances in knowledge, many fundamental questions concerning cell injury remain unanswered. The effect of particular harmful agents on cells and tissues, and body responses to these injuries are discussed in the following chapters.

Manifestations of Disease

Manifestations of disease are often labeled as signs or symptoms. A *sign* is objective evidence of dysfunction. Signs include such data as blood pressure, x-ray findings, blood studies, or pupil reflex. A *symptom* is subjective evidence; it is the pain which the ill person describes, or the expressed weakness and fatigue. Usually it is the body's response to the harmful agent, not the agent itself, that brings about the manifestations. Disease may be evident at any level of body organization. The intracellular disturbance is less readily discernible than alterations at the organ or system level.

Manifestations are related to the type and extent of disruption of normal function and structure and location of the injury. For instance, the manifestations of obstruction of a coronary vessel are those of heart dysfunction, but extensive injury threatens the ability of this essential organ to function effectively in distributing blood and hence oxygen to other vital organs. Therefore, signs may also include those of inadequate function of the control centers in the brain. In contrast, a localized change in the ability of a cell to control mitosis and hence cell growth (neoplasia) produces no detectable manifestations of disease until the growth overcomes the surrounding normal tissue.

Manifestations also reflect the response of control and regulatory mechanisms to adverse environments. An example of this type of manifestation is the change in respiratory effort that may be observed in a person with metabolic acidosis. The decreased pH of the blood serves as a chemical stimulus to the respiratory center. The result is an attempt to regulate the pH by expiring CO_2, which is done through prolonged expirations. Similarly, if the injurious agent is a pathogen, the manifestations are those of the infectious process. Signs and symptoms of disease result from attempts to reestablish dynamic equilibrium, and from a decrease or inability of the injured part to contribute to total body function.

Nursing Implications

Interventions to support homeostatic mechanisms are an important function of nurses. Goals of these interventions are promotion of health and care during acute and long-term illness.

Two principles relative to supporting homeostatic mechanisms are to minimize encounters with harmful agents and to maximize function of homeostatic mechanisms in threatening situations. Nurses can apply these principles by teaching persons of all ages that avoidance of harmful practices such as smoking, the use of safety devices, and proper nutrition will minimize demands on homeostatic mechanisms. To maximize ability to maintain homeostasis in threatening situations, nurses teach mentally healthy coping techniques and promote such physiological measures as immunization.

Care of both the acutely and chronically ill also calls for support of homeostatic mechanisms. The goals applicable in these situations are the same as when the goal is promotion of health: to minimize demands and maximize function. The situations, however, are more complex. Minimizing demands requires, for example, attention to a balance of rest and activity, protection from harmful environmental agents, and reduction of emotional stress. Maximizing function of homeostatic mechanisms consists of actions to promote a normal internal environment (fluid, electrolytes), nutrients, oxygen, and blood flow.

Another dimension of nursing care of the ill is to monitor disease progression and response to medical and nursing therapy, and to make clinical judgments based on data obtained. The data needed relate to mechanisms for maintenance of dynamic equilibrium and to disease process and treatment. In assessing patients, nurses should ask themselves the following questions:

- What is the normal function of the tissue that is diseased?
- What is the localized functional change resulting from the disease?
- What changes can be expected because the diseased tissue is unable to contribute to total body function?
- What regulatory control mechanisms would the body use to offset this change and reestablish a steady state?

Answers to these questions direct the nurse's observations and assist in making clinical judgments. Disease processes and treatment, and specific nursing interventions to support homeostatic measures are addressed throughout the text.

Bibliography

Adolph EF: Early concepts of physiological regulations. Physiol Rev 41:737, 1961

Bajusz E: Physiology and Pathology of Adaptation Mechanisms: Neural, Neuroendocrine, Humoral. New York, Pergamon Press, 1698

Baumann B: Diversities in conceptions of health and physical fitness. J Health Hum Behav 2(1)40–45, 1961

Cannon WB: The Wisdom of the Body. New York, Norton, 1939 (reprinted in 1963)

Capaldi RA: A dynamic model of cell membranes. Sci Am, March 1974

Dingle J: The ills of man. Sci Am 229:76–84, 1973

Engel GL: Conservation: Withdrawal—A primary regulatory process for organismic homeostasis. Ciba Found Symp 8:57–75, 1972

Exton-Smith AN: The elderly patient and multiple disease. Curr Med Res Opin (suppl)7:5–13, 1982

Ford DH, Karger B (eds): Influence of hormones on the nervous system. Proceedings of Symposium of International Society of Psychoendocrinology, Brooklyn, New York, 1970

Frohlich E: Pathophysiology: Altered Regulatory Mechanisms in Disease. Philadelphia, JB Lippincott, 1972

Goodman L: Regulation and control in physiological systems, 1960–1980. Ann Biomed Eng 8(4–6):281–290, 1980

Johnson ID: The metabolic and endocrine response to injury: A review. Br J Anesth 45:252–255, 1973

Landau B: Essential Human Anatomy and Physiology, 2nd ed. Glenview, Illinois, Scott, Foresman Company, 1980

Loewy AG, Siekevitz P: Cell Structure and Function, 2nd ed. New York, Holt, Rinehard and Winston, 1970

Ramsay JM: Basic Pathophysiology—Modern Stress and the Disease Process. Menlo Park, California, Addison-Wesley Publishing Company, 1982

Selye H: Homeostasis and heterostasis perspective. Biol Med 16:441–445, 1973

Selye H: The Stress of Life. New York, McGraw-Hill, 1956

Swanson LW: Neural mechanisms for the functional coupling of autonomic, endocrine, and somatomotor responses in adaptive behavior. Br Res 228(1):1–34, 1981

Vartanyan GA: Chemical factors in the formation of steady states in CNS. Hum Physiol 7(3):205–212, 1981

Wolf HG: A concept of disease in man. Psychosoma Med 24:25–30, 1962

Wylie CM: The definitions and measurements of health and disease. Public Health Rep 85:100–104, 1970

Chapter 13

Fluid and Electrolyte Balance and Imbalances

Linda Felver

The interior of the human body is a dynamic fluid environment. The blood that courses through the arterial vascular bed brings necessary nutrients and other chemicals to capillaries. At the capillary level, some of these substances enter the interstitial fluid and diffuse to the cells, which incorporate them into the metabolic processes that enable the cells (and ultimately the entire body) to function. Waste products formed in the process of metabolism leave the cells and pass through the interstitial fluid; they enter the capillaries and, eventually, the venous circulation, which transports them to their disposal sites. The fluid inside the cells, the fluid that surrounds the cells, and the fluid in the vascular compartment all play essential roles in this nourishment of the living cells that constitute the human body. The volume, composition, and electrolyte concentration of these fluids are of vital importance to the proper function of both individual cells and the body as a whole.

This chapter discusses both normal and abnormal aspects of this dynamic fluid environment. It begins with saline (extracellular volume) balance and imbalances, progresses to water (osmolality) balance and imbalances, discusses electrolyte balance and imbalances, and concludes with management of intravenous therapy. Because a clear understanding of the abnormal begins with knowledge of the normal, each major section opens with an explanation of the salient points of the normal situation.

Saline Balance and Imbalances

Over 50% of the weight of most adult humans is water. In young adult males, the body weight is 60% water; for young adult females the figure approximates 50%.[51] This sex difference in the percentage of body weight due to water is a reflection of the increased proportion of body fat in females. Fat tissue contains little water; muscle, on the other hand, is about 50% water. The process of normal aging causes a decrease in lean body mass with an increased proportion of body fat. As both males and females age, then, the percentage of body weight due to water decreases.

The water in the body carries many substances: gases, electrolytes, glucose, proteins, hormones—the list is seemingly endless. In this chapter, the term *fluid* will be used to denote body water and the substances within it. The term *water* will be used specifically to denote the water without including other components.

The fluid in the body is in two major compartments. The fluid that is contained within the cells is called the *intracellular fluid;* two thirds of the fluid in the body is intracellular. The other one third of the body fluid lies outside the cells; this fluid is called, appropriately enough, the *extra-*

extracellular fluid is found in two major compartments. The extracellular fluid that d vessels is in the *vascular compartment.* rrounds the cells is in the *interstitial com-* listribution of the extracellular fluid between ipartments is discussed in the edema section hapter. The vascular and interstitial compart- n the majority of the extracellular fluid. Small extracellular fluid are also contained in the ones, in dense connective tissues, and in the trans- ithelial secretions (*e.g.*, synovial, intraocular, cere- , pleural). These minor extracellular fluid compart- e not discussed further in this chapter.

cause the intracellular and extracellular fluids are ted by cell membranes, the body is able to maintain different ion concentrations in the two compartments. intracellular fluid is rich in potassium and contains little ium; the extracellular fluid, on the other hand, has a high dium concentration and a low potassium concentration. ne term *saline* is often used to refer to the extracellular luid. Saline means salt water, or more specifically, sodium chloride (NaCl) and water. When NaCl is added to the body, the cell membranes prevent the sodium ions from accumulating inside the cells. Saline added to the body, therefore, remains in the extracellular compartment.

The term *saline balance* refers to maintenance of proper volume of the extracellular fluid (vascular plus interstitial).[56] The hormone aldosterone is a major regulator of saline balance (extracellular fluid volume). Aldosterone acts on the distal tubules and collecting ducts of the kidneys to cause sodium to be reabsorbed from the renal tubular fluid into the blood. With the sodium come water and chloride ions so that aldosterone effectively causes an increase in the volume of saline in the body. As sodium ions are generally excluded from entering body cells, aldosterone secretion causes an increase in the volume of the extracellular fluid. Aldosterone is secreted by the adrenal cortex in response to a decrease in effective vascular volume (mediated by the renin–angiotensin system), to an elevation of plasma potassium, and, in a minor degree, to adrenocorticotropic hormone (ACTH).

TABLE 13–1
Terminology for Saline and Water Imbalances

Imbalance	*Synonyms*
Saline deficit	Extracellular fluid volume deficit Isotonic contraction Isosmotic dehydration Hypovolemia
Saline excess	Extracellular fluid volume excess Isotonic expansion Hypervolemia
Water deficit	Hypernatremia Water depletion Hypertonicity
Water excess	Hyponatremia Water intoxication Hypotonicity
Saline deficit and water deficit	Hypertonic dehydration Hypertonic contraction
Saline deficit and water excess	Hypotonic contraction
Saline excess and water deficit	Hypertonic expansion
Saline excess and water excess	Hypotonic expansion

Saline Deficit

A saline deficit is a deficit of salt and water isotonic to (*i.e.*, in the same concentration as) plasma. It is a decrease in the volume of the extracellular fluid. Table 13–1 gives alternate names for this imbalance.

Causes. There are numerous causes of saline deficit, as noted in Table 13–2.[51] They all involve loss of sodium-containing fluid, which may be lost by renal, gastrointestinal, or other routes. Some body fluids, such as sweat and some gastrointestinal fluids, are more dilute than the plasma (*i.e.*, they are hypotonic). If part of the water lost is replaced, but not the salts and the remainder of the water, the net result is a saline loss. Under special circumstances, a saline deficit is due to accumulation of saline in an area of the body where it is inaccessible to the normal fluid compartments. For example, saline may accumulate in the intestinal lumen as a result of intestinal obstruction or in the peritoneal cavity as a result of cirrhosis or other pathophysiological processes. Such an accumulation of fluid in an abnormal location is often called "third space fluid accumulation." A decrease in sodium *intake* will not cause a saline deficit if renal function is normal because the kidneys are very effective at conserving sodium.

TABLE 13–2
Causes of Saline Deficit

General Etiology: Loss of a Sodium-Containing Fluid
Specific Examples:
- Renal
  - Addison's disease
  - Salt-wasting disorders
  - Bedrest
  - Excessive use of diuretics
- Gastrointestinal
  - Vomiting
  - Diarrhea
  - Fistula drainage
  - Nasogastric suctioning
  - Intestinal decompression
- Other
  - Excessive diaphoresis
  - Burns
  - Blood loss
  - Third space accumulation

Knowledge of the causes of saline deficit enables a nurse to identify the persons at high risk for developing this imbalance. Once the possibility of developing saline deficit is identified, knowledge of the signs and symptoms allows careful nursing assessment.

Signs and Symptoms. Symptoms of saline deficit include:

- Weight loss (except with third space accumulation)
- Postural blood pressure drop
- Increased small vein filling time
- Neck veins flat or collapsing with inspiration
- Dizziness, syncope
- Oliguria
- Decreased central venous pressure

These manifestations are due to a decrease in both vascular and interstitial volume. A weight loss of more than 0.5 kg/day is probably a saline loss, unless a severe water (osmolality) imbalance has occurred in that time. (Water imbalance is discussed later in this chapter.) If saline accumulates in a "third space," weight loss will not occur.

The most sensitive indices of saline deficit are the signs and symptoms of inadequate circulating blood volume (hypovolemia). One sign of inadequate vascular volume is a postural blood pressure drop. To elicit this sign, the blood pressure and pulse are measured twice: first, while a person is lying supine and second, while the person is standing erect. If the blood volume is normal, there will be little change in the systolic pressure and a slight rise (5–10 mmHg) in the diastolic pressure. If the blood volume is diminished, the systolic blood pressure will decrease more than 15 mmHg, the diastolic pressure will decrease 10 mmHg or more, and the pulse will increase when the upright position is assumed. Such a postural blood pressure drop may indicate a saline deficit of 2 liters or more. Dizziness or even syncope may occur. Note that the heart rate increases with postural blood pressure drop due to saline deficit. Primary autonomic insufficiency may also cause a postural blood pressure drop but is differentiated from saline deficit by the absence of a concurrent pulse increase.[66]

Another useful clinical assessment for hypovolemia is increased filling time of the small veins in the hands or feet. A superficial vein in either of these areas can be "milked" by applying pressure with a finger at one point and running another finger up the vein, thereby pushing the blood out of the vein. Pressure is then released so that blood can again fill the vein, usually in a second or two. Figure 13–1 illustrates the technique for eliciting this sign. Small vein filling time is especially useful in assessing for hypovolemia in bedfast persons who cannot assume an upright posture. It may also serve as corroborative evidence when a postural blood pressure drop is observed. Other findings in hypovolemia may include oliguria (due to decreased blood flow to the kidneys) and flat neck veins in a person lying supine without a pillow.

Other clinical manifestations of saline deficit may indicate a severe depletion. Longitudinal furrows in the tongue, for example, develop after a loss of 3 or more liters of saline. Two frequently assessed signs are decreased skin turgor and dryness of opposing mucous membranes. Skin turgor is assessed by pinching up the skin over an area like the sternum, then releasing it to see how quickly it returns to its normal position (Fig. 13–2). If the skin remains pinched up after it is released, skin turgor is decreased and may indicate saline deficit. Other causes of decreased skin turgor are the normal aging process and recent weight loss. Dryness of mucous membranes is best detected where two mucous membranes oppose each other, such as at the gum line inside the cheek;

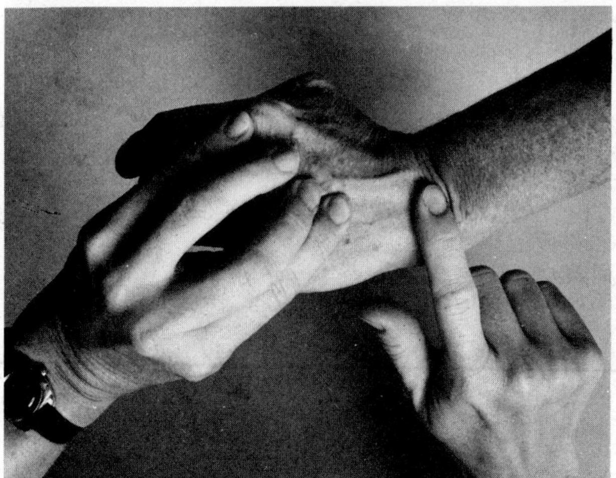

A

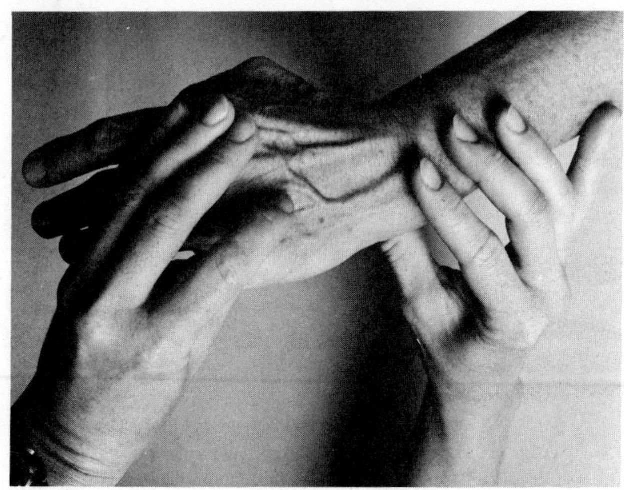

B

FIGURE 13–1 To assess small vein filling time, occlude a small vein in the hand or foot with your finger (*A*). Make sure that the extremity is below the level of the heart. While occluding the vein, milk it toward the heart so that it is flat (*B*). Release your finger and watch to see how rapidly the vein fills. If the cardiovascular system is not impaired, a small vein filling time greater than 3 to 5 seconds denotes a saline deficit.

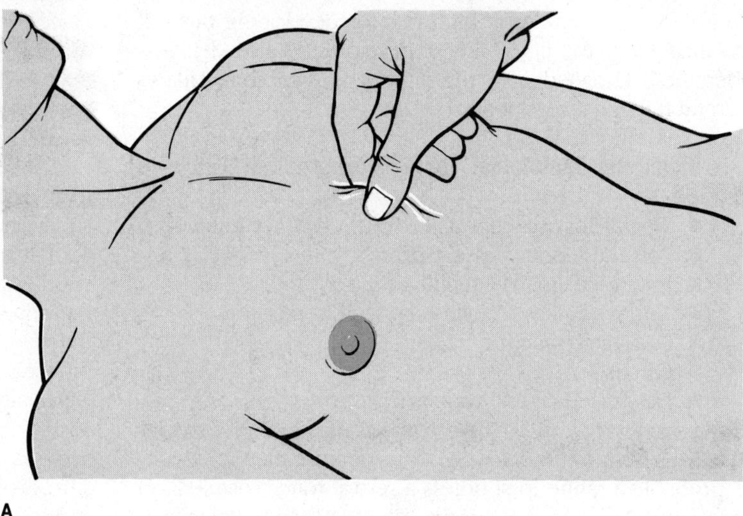

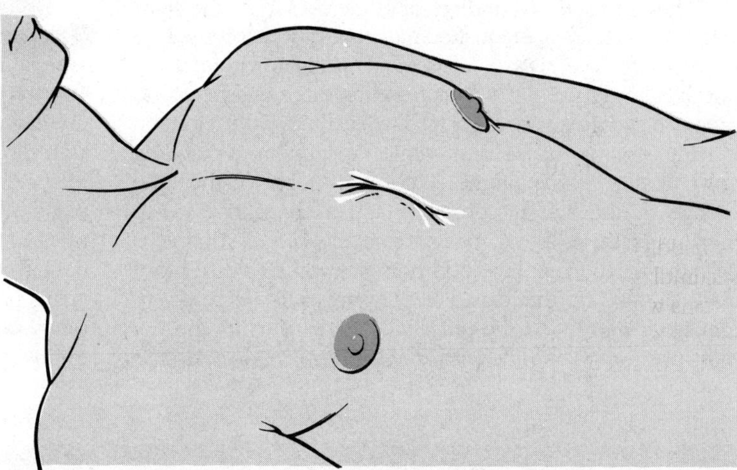

FIGURE 13–2 To assess skin turgor, pinch up the skin over the clavicle, sternum, or inner forearm (*A*). If the skin remains pinched up after it is released (*B*), skin turgor is decreased. Decreased skin turgor may occur with saline deficit, the normal aging process, or a large recent weight loss.

other situations that cause dry mouth (*e.g.,* mouth breathing) do not usually affect this area. In a prolonged severe saline deficit, the stools may be hard and dry, tears and sweat are decreased (check axillae for dryness), and the eyeballs may be soft or sunken.[50] Extreme saline deficit leads to hypovolemic shock (see Chap. 24).

An uncomplicated saline deficit is *not* accompanied by an abnormal serum sodium concentration. The serum sodium is normal because the proportion of salt and water in the blood has not changed. The amount, or *volume,* of fluid has decreased. The hematocrit, the plasma proteins, and even the BUN may rise with a saline deficit because normal amounts of these elements are contained in a smaller than normal volume of saline.

Nursing Implications. Nursing management of persons who have an actual or a potential saline deficit includes both administration of the medical therapy and independent nursing actions. Take routine postural blood pressure measurements and monitor urine output of persons at high risk for saline deficit. The medical therapy for saline deficit is saline replacement, usually intravenous. Nursing assessment for rebound saline excess caused by too vigorous saline replacement is important. Rebound saline excess may cause pulmonary edema. Listen to the lungs for crackles (rales), an indicator of pulmonary edema (see Chap. 40). If a central venous pressure monitor is in use, watch to see if the central venous pressure rises and remains above normal during saline replacement therapy. Such an increase may also indicate excessive saline replacement.

A major independent nursing action in saline deficit is the institution of safety measures to prevent falling from dizziness induced by postural hypotension. Instructing a patient to rise from bed or chair slowly may prevent a fall. Because bed rest itself promotes saline deficit, it is important for patients to exercise as much as possible within the limits of their pathophysiological conditions in order to minimize this iatrogenic deficit. Persons at risk for developing saline deficit (*e.g.,* from vomiting and diarrhea) need to be told to replace these body fluid losses with both salt and water in order to prevent saline deficit. Because overdiuresis causes saline deficit, teaching persons who take diuretics to contact a health professional if they become lightheaded is also advisable.

Saline Excess

If the volume of the extracellular fluid is abnormally increased, the disorder known as saline excess is present. The volume, but not the proportion of salt and water, is increased in both the vascular and interstitial compartments. As indicated in Table 13–1, other names for saline excess include extracellular fluid volume excess, isotonic expansion, and hypervolemia.

Excess intravenous infusion of saline-containing solutions or any clinical condition accompanied by renal retention of sodium and water may cause saline excess.[51] These etiologies are listed in Table 13–3.

TABLE 13–3
Causes of Saline Excess

General Etiology: Renal Retention of Sodium and Water
Specific Examples:
Endocrine imbalance
- Hyperaldosteronism
- Cushing's syndrome
- Glucocorticoid therapy

Secondary to a Disease Process
- Chronic renal failure
- Congestive heart failure
- Cirrhosis

Additional Etiology: Excess Intravenous Infusion of Saline Solutions (e.g. 0.9% Saline, Ringer's)

Clinical Manifestations. When a saline excess occurs, the clinical manifestations of the expanded volume may include weight gain and signs of volume expansion in both compartments of the extracellular space. A rapid weight gain (*e.g.,* more than 0.5 kg/day) is most likely due to saline excess unless correction for an osmolality disorder is necessary. Weight gain is the most sensitive index of saline excess.[45] Fluid intake and output records are a useful adjunct to evaluation of weight changes. Edema, the sign of volume expansion in the interstitial areas, may not be detectable in young or middle-aged adults until 2 or 3 liters of excess saline have accumulated.[51] Elderly adults, however, may develop ankle edema with a smaller interstitial volume increase, due to the decreased tissue elasticity of normal aging. A bedfast supine adult may gain 4 to 8 liters of saline before edema is manifested; such a saline excess could have been detected earlier as weight gain. Manifestations of saline excess in both compartments include

- Weight gain
- Edema
- Bounding pulse
- Distended neck veins
- Crackles (rales)
- Dyspnea, orthopnea
- Elevated central venous pressure

Laboratory Tests. It is important to understand that an uncomplicated saline excess is *not* characterized by an abnormal serum sodium concentration. The proportion of salt and water in the extracellular fluid remains the same; the *amount* of this fluid has increased. When saline excess develops slowly, the hematocrit is normal also because more red blood cells are produced in compensation as the amount of saline increases.

Nursing Implications. Nursing management of saline excess arises from knowledge of the causes and the clinical manifestations of the disorder. Iatrogenic saline excess can be prevented by careful monitoring of intravenous infusions of saline-containing solutions, especially those that are isotonic. (Table 13–20 lists tonicity of common intravenous solutions.) Elderly adults and persons who have mild compensated congestive heart failure are at increased risk for saline excess from overinfusion of saline-containing solutions.

Once a saline excess has developed, both administration of the medical therapy and independent nursing actions become important. Medical therapy for saline excess is usually a sodium-restricted diet, diuretics, and treatment of the underlying cause. Related nursing responsibilities include patient teaching on home management of medications and diet. Assessment of cultural dietary practices is important before initiating specific teaching about low sodium diets. Nondietary sodium sources such as softened water and many brands of antacids need to be explained.

In addition to patient teaching, initiation of fluid intake and output measurements, ongoing assessment of saline excess, and careful skin care are valuable nursing functions. Specific assessment techniques for edema and care of edematous tissue are described in the section on edema later in this chapter.

Summary of Principles of Saline Imbalances

In summary, saline imbalances are abnormalities of the amount of extracellular fluid. Since the extracellular fluid is located in two compartments, vascular and interstitial, the signs and symptoms of saline imbalances are often detected in both areas. Saline imbalances are also manifested by rapid weight changes. Nursing management of saline imbalances includes preventive measures, careful ongoing assessment, administration of the medical therapy, and independent nursing measures specific to the imbalance.

Edema

Edema is an abnormal expansion of the interstitial space. As previously discussed, edema may be a sign of saline excess. Edema is caused by mechanisms that are operative at the capillary level. These capillary mechanisms are alterations of normal capillary dynamics.[51] In the normal situation the flow of fluid from the capillaries into the interstitial space (and vice versa) is governed by the net result of several forces (Fig. 13–3). Some of these forces tend to move fluid out of the capillaries; others tend to move it into the capillaries. The *blood hydrostatic pressure* is the pressure of blood against the capillary walls in an outward direction. Analogously, the *interstitial fluid hydrostatic pressure* is the pressure of interstitial fluid against the capillary walls in an inward direction. The other two forces of importance are osmotic forces. Osmotic pressure is an inward-pulling force due to particles in a solution. The blood osmotic pressure, then, tends to pull fluid inward into the capillaries. The terms *blood colloid osmotic pressure* and *oncotic pressure* are sometimes used to denote that portion of the blood osmotic pressure due to the blood proteins. The term *blood osmotic pressure* denotes not only this colloid osmotic pressure but also the osmotic pressure due to glucose, electrolytes, and other particles. The interstitial fluid, because it has particles in it, also exerts an *interstitial fluid osmotic pressure*. This pressure, which tends to pull fluid outward from the capillaries, is weaker than the blood osmotic pressure under normal circumstances because the interstitial fluid has a very low protein content.

Normally, fluid leaves the capillaries at their arterial ends and enters the capillaries at their venous ends. This flow, which is the net result of the combination of the forces previously discussed, delivers oxygen and nutrients to cells and removes wastes products. At the arterial end of the capillary, the blood hydrostatic pressure is high; at the venous end (farther from the heart), the blood hydrostatic pressure is lower. The blood osmotic pressure also changes along the length of the capillary, rising toward the venous end as the blood becomes slightly more concentrated. Whereas the high blood hydrostatic pressure at the arterial end of the capillary predominates in moving fluid out of the capillaries, the decreasing blood hydrostatic pressure and the increased blood osmotic pressure (an inward force) at the venous end of the capillary move fluid back into the capillaries from the interstitial space. Alterations in these normal pressures may lead to accumulation of fluid in the interstitial space.

Capillary Mechanisms for Edema Formation

Four mechanisms operative at the capillary level may lead to the formation of edema, either singly or in combination. These include increased blood hydrostatic pressure, decreased blood osmotic pressure, increased interstitial fluid osmotic pressure, and impaired lymphatic drainage (Table 13–4).

Increased Blood Hydrostatic Pressure. The first mechanism that may lead to edema is increased blood hydrostatic pressure. Remember that blood hydrostatic pressure

TABLE 13–4
Capillary Mechanisms for Edema Formation

Increased Blood Hydrostatic Pressure
Increased capillary flow
Local infection
Inflammation
Venous congestion
External pressure
Venous thrombosis
Right heart failure
Decreased Blood Osmotic Pressure
Decreased serum albumin
Loss of albumin
Decreased albumin synthesis
Increased Interstitial Fluid Osmotic Pressure
Increased capillary permeability
Burns
Inflammation
Hypersensitivity reactions
Toxins
Trauma
Impaired Lymphatic Drainage
Tumor
Surgical removal of lymph nodes
Elephantiasis

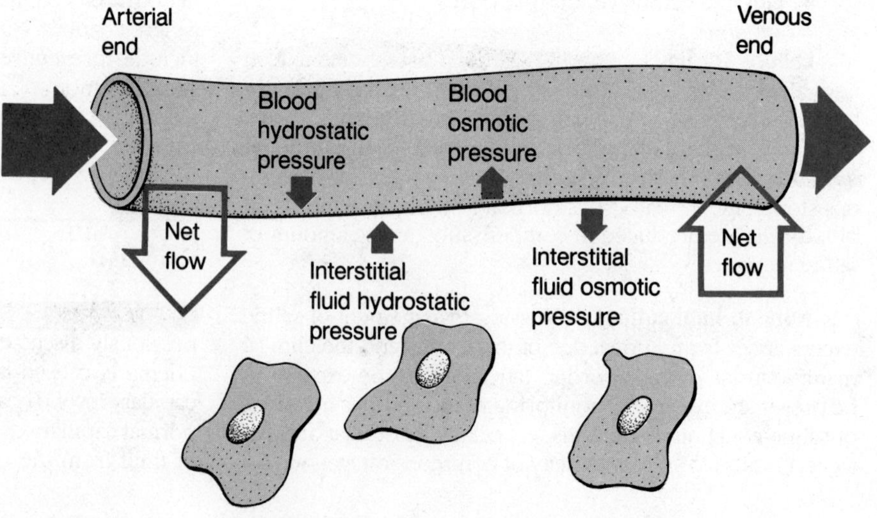

FIGURE 13–3 Normal capillary dynamics. Fluid movement into or out of capillaries is governed by the net result of four forces. Blood hydrostatic pressure and interstitial fluid osmotic pressure tend to move fluid from the capillaries into the interstitial spaces. Blood osmotic pressure and interstitial fluid hydrostatic pressure tend to move fluid from the interstitial spaces into the capillaries. Under normal conditions, the balance of these forces moves fluid out of the capillaries at their arterial end and back into the capillaries at their venous end.

tends to push fluid out of the capillaries into the interstitial spaces. If this pressure is abnormally increased, excess fluid may enter the interstitial area; edema is the result. An increase in blood flow through the capillaries increases this blood hydrostatic pressure. Such an *increased capillary flow* is seen in conditions such as local infection and inflammation. The edema thus produced is localized. *Venous congestion* also increases the blood hydrostatic pressure by back pressure. Many factors lead to venous congestion: saline excess, external pressure on veins (*e.g.,* tight garters), venous thrombosis, right heart failure, and the combination of muscle paralysis and the force of gravity when an extremity is in a dependent position. Edema due to increased hydrostatic pressure from venous congestion is often dependent edema, as in saline excess. Either increased capillary flow or venous congestion may increase the blood hydrostatic pressure enough to cause edema.

Decreased Blood Osmotic Pressure. A second capillary mechanism for edema formation is decreased blood osmotic pressure. Severe and widespread edema may occur when the serum albumin is decreased. The albumin particles normally make a major contribution to the inward pull of blood osmotic pressure. With decreased numbers of albumin particles, this inward pull diminishes and fluid leaks out into the interstitial area. Once again, edema results. The serum albumin decreases if the rate of albumin loss from the body exceeds the rate of its replacement or if there is decreased albumin synthesis. The most common route of massive *albumin loss* is through the urine in conditions such as the nephrotic syndrome. Large amounts of albumin may also be lost through the gastrointestinal tract in the less common protein-losing enteropathies. *Decreased albumin synthesis* accompanies severe protein–calorie malnutrition when the amino acids for albumin synthesis are unavailable. A decrease in albumin synthesis also occurs in liver disease (*e.g.,* cirrhosis) when the diseased liver cells are unable to function normally. Either albumin loss or decreased albumin synthesis may decrease the serum albumin to the point at which normal blood osmotic pressure is not maintained and fluid leaks into the interstitial space.

Increased Interstitial Fluid Osmotic Pressure. In the normal condition, the interstitial fluid osmotic pressure is small compared to the blood osmotic pressure, because of the absence of large amounts of protein in the interstitial fluid. If protein leaks into the interstitial fluid, the third capillary mechanism for edema formation, increased interstitial fluid osmotic pressure, occurs. The chief cause of protein entry into the interstitial space (and thus of increased interstitial fluid osmotic pressure) is *increased capillary permeability.* The increased permeability allows protein to leak out of the blood into the interstitial space. This mechanism operates systemically in conditions such as major burns and locally with inflammation and hypersensitivity reactions (*e.g.,* sprained ankle or bee sting).

Impaired Lymphatic Drainage. The fourth mechanism that contributes to the formation of edema is *impaired lymphatic drainage.* Ordinarily, slightly more fluid leaves a capillary at the arterial end than enters it at the venous end. This slight excess of fluid is drained from the interstitial area by the lymphatic system. In addition, minute amounts of protein that leave the capillaries are also removed by means of the lymphatic drainage. If the lymphatic drainage is impaired through obstruction of the lymph nodes by a tumor, by parasites (as in the filaria infestation known as elephantiasis), or through surgery, fluid and protein accumulate in the interstitial space. Once again, edema results.

Summary. In summary, edema may be caused by four capillary mechanisms: increased blood hydrostatic pressure, decreased blood osmotic pressure, increased interstitial fluid osmotic pressure, and impaired lymphatic drainage. More than one of these mechanisms may operate at the same time. The edema that accompanies local inflammation, for example, results from both increased blood hydrostatic pressure (from increased capillary flow) and increased interstitial fluid osmotic pressure (from increased capillary permeability). The edema often seen in congestive heart failure is due in part to saline excess (renal retention of salt and water) and in part to cardiac dysfunction, both of which lead to increased blood hydrostatic pressure from venous congestion.

Nursing Assessment and Management of Edema

Assessment of edema is an important nursing function. Patients whose edema is not a short-term localized occurrence need systematic daily assessment of edema. If edema is due wholly or in part to saline excess, daily weight provides a useful assessment. As previously mentioned, very rapid weight gain is a sign of saline accumulation. A 1-kg (2.2-lb) rapid weight gain denotes accumulation of a liter of excess saline, part of which will be evidenced as edema. For purposes of comparison of these daily weights, other factors that could affect weight should be controlled as much as possible. The patient should be weighed at the same time of day, on the same scale, after emptying bladder, bowel, and drainage bags, and in the same weight of clothing. The weight of bulky dressings and tubes that are discontinued should be recorded and subsequent weights corrected for this loss. Careful fluid intake and output records provide corroborative evidence for saline excess in edema patients but are not sufficient by themselves for assessment of saline balance.[45]

Another technique useful in the ongoing assessment of edema is measurement of the girth of parts. If, for example, edematous ankles are to be assessed daily, a string or tape measure placed around the ankle in the same location at the same time of day will provide data for daily comparison. Measurement in the same location can be assured through use of a reference point (*e.g.,* 1 inch above the lateral malleolus) or, if the patient agrees, by marking a spot on the skin.

Unless edema is due to a localized mechanism, check for edema in the dependent body parts: sacrum in supine patients, ankles in ambulatory ones. Be alert for the presence of periorbital edema (edema around the eyes). Question patients about shoes or rings that become too tight, a useful indication of edema. When noting the presence of edema, press gently on it with thumb or finger. If the indentation remains after the pressure is released, document the presence of *pitting edema* (Fig. 13–4).[33]

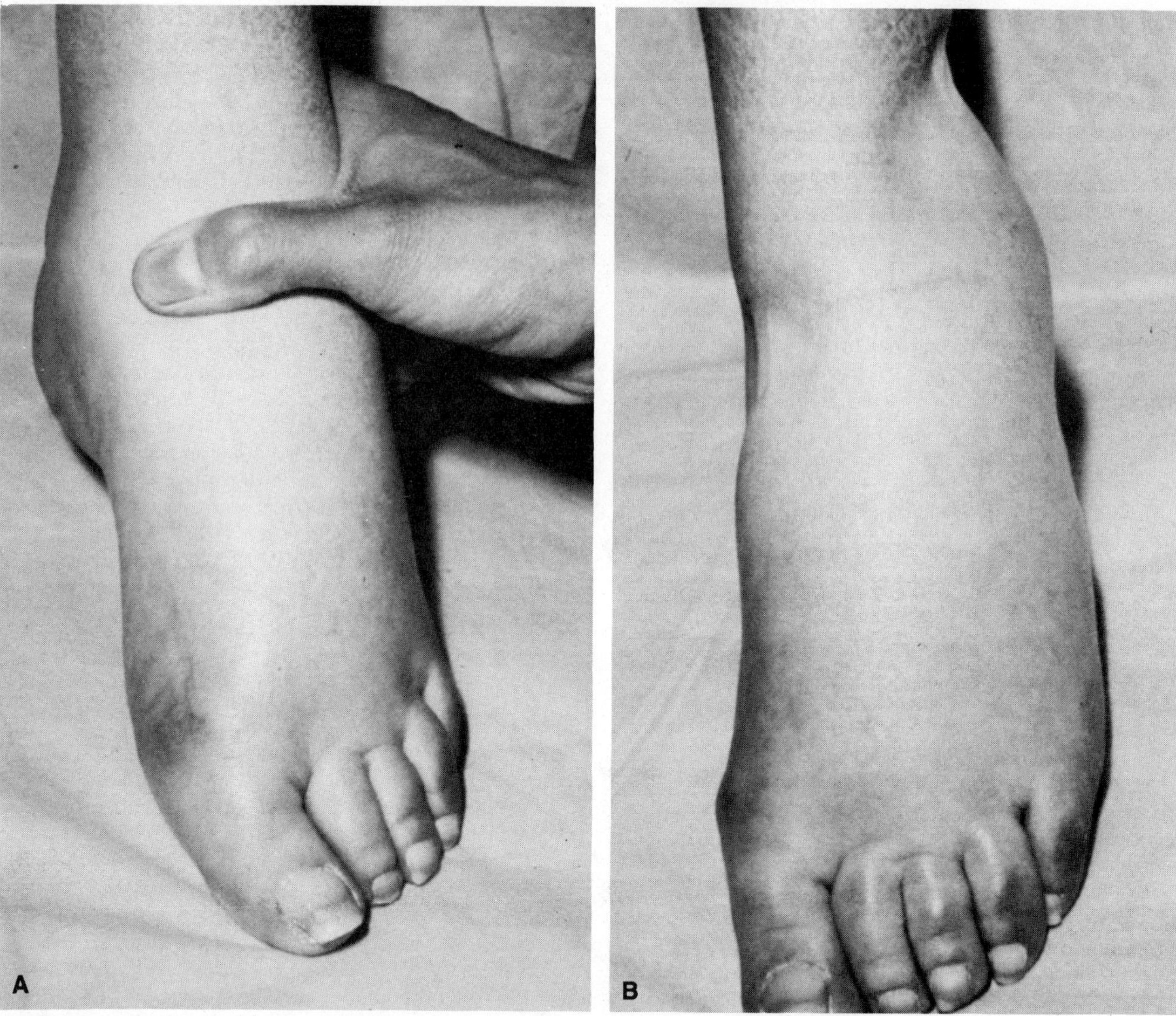

FIGURE 13–4 Pitting edema. (*A*) To check for pitting, press the edematous area firmly with the thumb; release pressure after 5 seconds. (*B*) Pitting is evident. (Reproduced with permission from Health Sciences Center for Educational Resources, University of Washington)

Nursing management of edema focuses on the prevention of tissue damage. Edematous tissue is fragile tissue. The fluid that expands the interstitial space pushes the cells farther apart from each other and farther from the capillaries, their source of nourishment. Edematous tissue is therefore especially susceptible to injury such as pressure sores or sheet burns. Careful skin care and positioning are extremely important to prevent tissue damage. Keeping the patient's fingernails short or at least smoothly manicured will help prevent tissue damage from scratching.

In addition to potential tissue damage, a second patient problem often resulting from edema is discomfort. Discomfort may range from a feeling of heaviness or puffiness to more severe unpleasant sensations of tightness or an unfamiliarity with self due to altered body image. The discomfort accompanying edema is best relieved by measures to reduce the edema. In general, if an extremity is edematous, it should be elevated to promote venous return and mobilization of the edema fluid. If arterial disease is also present, elevation of an extremity is contraindicated, as it would compromise arterial blood flow. Range of motion exercises may help to reduce edema associated with muscle paralysis. Both nursing and medical measures to relieve edema will be based on the underlying cause. Administration of the medical therapy may involve application of elastic stockings to enhance venous return or administration of diuretics or sodium-restricted diet as therapy for saline excess.

Water Balance and Imbalances

The term *water balance* refers to the maintenance of the proper proportion of salt and water in the blood. Water balance, reflected by an osmolality in the correct range, is concerned with the composition, rather than the volume, of body fluids. *Osmolality* is defined as the number of moles of particles per kilogram of water. If the osmolality is decreased, the solution has fewer particles per unit weight; it is less concentrated. If the osmolality is increased, the solution has more particles per unit weight; it is more concentrated. Thus it may be seen that the osmolality is a measure of the degree of concentration of a solution. When the concentration of the body fluids is normal, the body is in water balance.

The terms *osmolarity* and *osmolality* are often used interchangeably, although technically they are different. The osmolarity (number of moles of particles per liter of solution) varies with the temperature of the solution; the osmolality does not. Osmolality is the term used in this chapter.

The serum sodium concentration is a useful measure of water balance. The serum sodium reflects the osmolality of the blood. The normal range of the serum sodium is 135 to 145 mEq/liter in adults of all ages.[51] If the serum sodium is decreased, the osmolality of the blood has decreased; the blood is less concentrated than normal; the blood has excess water relative to the amount of salt. If the serum sodium is increased, the osmolality of the blood has increased; the blood is more concentrated than normal; the blood has a deficit of water relative to the amount of salt.

Table 13–5 lists the normal and abnormal routes of entry and exit of water that play important roles in maintenance of water balance. The term *insensible water loss* is frequently used to denote the water excreted by the lungs and by the skin as insensible perspiration. Sweat denotes visible perspiration and is not included in insensible loss. Note that salt, as well as water, is gained or lost by some of these routes; respiratory water loss, by contrast, is not accompanied by sodium loss. The major regulators of oral water intake are thirst and habit patterns. The thirst mechanism is activated by dryness of the oral mucous membranes or by an increase in the osmolality of the blood.

The excretion of water in the urine is controlled by antidiuretic hormone (ADH).[61] (Remember that aldosterone controls the excretion of saline: salt and water together. Here, the concern is with water only, without salt.) ADH is synthesized by neurons of the supraoptic and paraventricular nuclei of the hypothalamus; the axons of these neurons terminate in the posterior pituitary, from which they release ADH in response to an increase in osmolality of the blood. ADH acts on the collecting ducts of the kidney to cause reabsorption of water from the tubular fluid back into the blood—the *antidiuretic effect.* The reabsorption of water tends to dilute the blood, restoring osmolality to normal. Note that an increase in osmolality of the blood triggers both the thirst mechanism and ADH release, both of which work toward returning osmolality to normal.

The osmolality of the extracellular fluid influences the osmolality of the intracellular fluid as well. Cell membranes are freely permeable to water but not to sodium: this type of membrane is denoted a *semipermeable membrane.* If two fluids of different osmolality are separated by a semipermeable membrane, water will move through the membrane into the side that was initially more concentrated. This is the process of *osmosis.* The process of osmosis tends to equalize the osmolality (degree of concentration) of two fluids separated by a semipermeable membrane. By the movement of water through the membrane, osmosis dilutes the solution that was initially more concentrated and concentrates the solution that was initially more dilute. This process occurs in the body when osmolality imbalances occur.

TABLE 13–5
Normal and Abnormal Routes of Water Entry and Exit

Route of Entry	*Average Volume (per 24 hr)*
Gastrointestinal	
Oral	
Drink	1200 ml
Water in food	1100 ml
Metabolic water	300 ml
Rectal	—
Parenteral	—
	2600 ml average/24-hr total

Route of Exit	*Average Volume (per 24 hr)*
Renal	1500 ml
Respiratory	400 ml
Gastrointestinal	
Fecal	100 ml
Emesis	—
Fistula drainage	—
Skin	
Insensible perspiration	600 ml
Sweat	—
Drainage from lesions	—
Other	
Paracentesis procedures	—
Hemorrhage	—
	2600 ml average/24-hr total

Water Deficit

An increase in the serum sodium above 145mEq/liter, the upper limit of normal, denotes an increase in the osmolality of the blood. The blood has become too concentrated; it has a deficit of water. Water deficit is also called *hypernatremia* (see Table 13–1); this term reflects the elevation of the serum sodium that occurs with this abnormality in the relative proportion of salt and water.

The causes of water deficit are listed in Table 13–6.[13,51] Notice that there are two general etiologies: *loss of water relative to salt* and *gain of salt relative to water.* In either case, a relative water deficit is produced. Elderly adults are a high-risk group for the development of hypernatremia because the thirst sensation decreases with normal aging.[41] The incidence of water deficit (hypernatremia) in patients receiving tube feedings is especially high among elderly adults.

When the osmolality of the blood increases abnormally, osmosis occurs. Water moves from the cells into the extracellular fluid. This process tends to restore osmotic balance by diluting the extracellular fluid and concentrating the intracellular fluid, but it may cause cellular dysfunction.[46] As water leaves a cell, the cell volume diminishes; the cell essentially shrivels.

TABLE 13–6
Causes of Water Deficit

General Etiology: Loss of Water Relative to Salt
Specific Examples:
Renal
- Diabetes insipidus
- Osmotic diuresis
- Renal concentrating disorders

Other
- Prolonged diarrhea without water replacement
- Excessive sweating without water replacement
- Dysfunctional humidifier of mechanical ventilator

General Etiology: Gain of Salt Relative to Water
Specific Examples:
Decreased water intake
- No access to water
- Prolonged nausea
- Difficulty swallowing fluids (*e.g.*, advanced parkinsonism)
- Inability to respond to thirst (*e.g.*, coma, paralysis, aphasia, confusion, weakness)

Increased salt intake
- Tube feedings
- Half-and-half for ulcer diet
- Excess hypertonic NaCl or $NaHCO_3$
- Near-drowning in salt water

Clinical Manifestations. The clinical manifestations of water deficit include the following:

- Serum sodium above normal
- Thirst
- Oliguria (except with renal cause)
- Confusion
- Lethargy
- Mild muscle weakness or twitching
- Seizures
- Coma

The major clinical manifestations of water deficit are due to the shriveling and resultant dysfunction of cells in the central nervous system. These manifestations are the nonspecific signs of cerebral dysfunction: confusion, lethargy, and perhaps seizures or coma.[30,51] The severity of these manifestations varies with the extent of the water deficit and the rapidity of its development.[55] A water imbalance that develops rapidly causes more severe manifestations than an imbalance that develops gradually. When a water deficit arises slowly over a period of time, brain cells adapt to the increased intracellular osmolality; they produce extra intracellular particles (termed *idiogenic osmoles*) which diminish the amount of water that shifts out of the cells. Severe brain shrinkage in water deficit may give rise to vascular damage and intracerebral hemorrhage.

Nursing Implications. The therapy of water deficit is replacement of the water. This replacement may be oral or intravenous; in the latter case, hypotonic fluids are used. In addition to nursing management of water replacement for patients who have already developed water deficit, nursing responsibilities include preventive measures for persons at high risk for developing water deficit. Thus, water should be administered between tube feedings, to compensate for the high solute load. Use the serum sodium concentration as a guide to determine if the feedings should be diluted further. Head and neck cancer patients who administer their own feedings need teaching about water intake. So do patients who may be consuming half-and-half intermittently as prescribed for therapy of gastrointestinal ulcers (now an infrequently prescribed therapy). These persons need 8 glasses of water per day.[14] Since persons with advanced parkinsonism usually have more difficulty swallowing liquids than solids, they may need to have their fluid intake provided in fruit juice popsicles, puddings, and other semi-solids.

High-Risk Patients. Patients identified as in the high-risk category for water deficit need to be offered water frequently. Remember that a full water pitcher on a bedside table is very difficult for an ill or weak person to lift while lying in a bed with side rails. A person who is unable to move any limbs because of traction, paralysis, or body cast can still have access to water if a plastic bottle with an angled drinking straw is attached to the bedrail. Water can be frozen in the bottom of such a plastic bottle; when the bottle is then filled, the resulting ice water stays cold for hours. A modest amount of ingenuity used to make water available may avert the development of water deficit. Institute fluid intake and output measurements for persons at high risk for water deficit.

Mixed Imbalances. Water deficit often occurs clinically with saline deficit, as in a person with prolonged gastroenteritis. A person with both of these imbalances will manifest both the signs of extracellular volume deficit (*e.g.*, postural blood pressure drop) and the signs of water deficit (*e.g.*, confusion and increased serum sodium concentration). Therapy in such a mixed imbalance involves replacement of the saline plus extra water replacement to correct both the volume and osmolality imbalances. Less frequently, water deficit may accompany saline excess. This situation might occur if a person with cirrhosis who had a saline excess due to renal retention of salt and water lost access to water in a hot environment or was placed on a stringent fluid restriction. Signs of both saline excess (*e.g.*, edema) and water deficit (*e.g.*, confusion) might be present. Therapy would involve sodium restriction and water replacement.

Water Excess

When the serum sodium decreases below 135 mEq/liter, the lower limit of the normal range, the osmolality of the blood has decreased. The blood is essentially too dilute; it has a water excess relative to the number of its particles. Water excess may also be called *water intoxication,* a term that reflects the signs and symptoms of the condition, or *hyponatremia,* a term that reflects the decreased serum sodium concentration. Another term for water excess is *hypotonicity* (see Table 13–1).

Etiology. Water excess has two general etiologies: *gain of water relative to salt* and *loss of salt relative to water.* In either case, the proportion of salt to water becomes abnormal, producing a relative excess of water. Specific examples of these categories are listed in Table 13–7.[13,21,27] Hyponatremia is very common in persons who are hospitalized because antidiuretic hormone release is stimulated by surgery, trauma, nausea, and other stressors.[52] Many of the other risk factors (such as nasogastric suction) are also present in hospitalized persons.

When water excess occurs, the decreased osmolality of the blood leads to the process of osmosis. Water moves from the extracellular fluid into the cells. This process concentrates the extracellular fluid and dilutes the intracellular fluid, tending to restore osmotic balance, but cells become abnormally swollen with the excess water.[46] The clinical manifestations of water excess, including malaise, headache, confusion, lethargy, and possibly seizures and coma, are primarily due to the dysfunction of swollen cells in the central nervous system.[30,51] Notice that the signs of water excess are similar to the signs of water deficit.[55] This similarity occurs because these signs are nonspecific indicators of cerebral dysfunction. Diagnosis of these disorders is made definitively only with laboratory measurements of the serum sodium. As with water deficit, the severity of the clinical manifestations of water excess depends on the degree of the excess and on the speed with which it develops.

Nursing Implications. Although intravenous hypertonic saline may be administered to treat water excess presenting as seizures, the more usual (and safer) therapy for water excess is restriction of water intake. If water intake is restricted, to a volume less than the daily insensible losses (1000 ml), the kidneys excrete the excess water and return the osmolality of the blood to normal. Nursing management includes both measures to prevent water excess and measures to help hyponatremic persons comply with their prescribed fluid restrictions. Review of the causes of water excess (see Table 13-7) will bring to mind numerous preventive nursing measures. Some persons use frequent tap water enemas; they need to be taught safer methods of bowel management. Isotonic saline, rather than distilled water, should be used for irrigation of body cavities. Careful monitoring of flow rates of intravenous 5% dextrose in water (D5W) is important. Body fluid losses should be replaced with fruit juice and bouillon rather than water exclusively.

The use of isotonic ice chips for persons who are on nasogastric suction is another nursing measure for prevention of water excess. The intake of tap water ice chips is usually severely restricted when nasogastric suction is instituted because of the risk of developing water excess. If, however, ice is made from isotonic (0.9%) saline, no osmolality problem results, and the ice chips relieve the discomfort of dry mucous membranes from the mouth breathing associated with nasogastric tubes. Isotonic ice chips are most conveniently prepared using an ice cube tray that makes small (1 cm^3) ice cubes. Because salt water freezes unevenly, using an ice pick on large ice cubes produces ice chips with varying tonicity.

Persons who have developed severe hyponatremia may need seizure precautions. All hyponatremic persons need ongoing assessment of level of consciousness. Nursing measures such as the following can help persons comply with their prescribed fluid restrictions:[14]

- Plan the timing of fluid intake over 24 hours with the person involved.
- Have the person choose his own favorite fluids.
- Suggest eating meals dry with fluids allowed between meals.
- Provide very cold, rather than lukewarm or hot, liquids.
- Use an insulated glass to provide the illusion of volume.
- Clarify fluid restriction with the dietary department to prevent confusion.
- Have the person maintain his own intake and output records.
- Suggest moistening oral membranes with liquid before swallowing.
- Teach sham drinking.

Sham drinking, one of these measures, is appropriate for alert, cooperative persons only. It involves taking a mouthful of water, swishing it around the mouth, and then spitting it out without swallowing. This maneuver relieves the thirst associated with dry oral mucous membranes while not increasing the fluid intake.

Mixed Imbalances. In the clinical setting, water excess may be seen concurrently with saline excess or with saline deficit. For example, a person who has prolonged vomiting and diarrhea but drinks only tap water will have lost both salt and water (saline deficit) and will have lost relatively more salt than water (water excess or hyponatremia).

TABLE 13–7
Causes of Water Excess

General Etiology: Gain of Water Relative to Salt
Specific Examples:
Endocrine
- Stimulation of antidiuretic hormone

Iatrogenic
- Excessive tap water enemas
- Excessive infusion of 5% dextrose in water
- Excessive use of ultrasonic nebulizer
- Hypotonic irrigating solutions

Other
- Psychogenic polydipsia
- Near-drowning in fresh water
- Overdose of barbiturates

General Etiology: Loss of Salt Relative to Water
Specific Examples:
Renal
- Salt wasting renal disease
- Many types of diuretics, especially thiazides

Gastrointestinal
- Nasogastric suction, Vomiting, Diarrhea, Hypotonic irrigating solutions } with water but not salt replacement

Other
- Burns, Excessive sweating } with water but not salt replacement

Signs and symptoms would include postural blood pressure drop, weight loss (extracellular volume concentration), lethargy, and decreased serum sodium (decreased osmolality of extracellular fluid). As another example, both water excess and saline excess occur in persons who have severe liver failure or congestive heart failure. In these conditions, the body retains both saline and water inappropriately, through pathophysiological mechanisms that are not clearly understood. The clinical manifestations of such a state are a combination of the separate imbalances. As with any mixed saline and osmolality imbalance, both the medical therapy and the nursing management combine principles of care from the two imbalances involved.

Summary of Principles of Water Imbalances

In summary, water imbalances are abnormalities of the osmolality of the extracellular fluid. These imbalances result from factors that alter the proportion of salt and water in the extracellular fluid. Alterations in extracellular osmolality cause water to shift in or out of cells, thus altering cell volume and causing clinical manifestations of cerebral dysfunction. Nursing management of water imbalances involves preventive measures, continuing assessment of level of consciousness, administration of the medical therapy, and specific independent nursing measures.

Summary of Principles of Mixed Saline and Water Imbalances

Saline imbalances and water imbalances have been discussed separately, for the most part, in this chapter. As has been mentioned briefly, saline and water imbalances often coexist in the clinical setting. In this situation, separate the signs and symptoms of the two imbalances for ease in understanding them. Saline imbalances are extracellular volume imbalances. The signs and symptoms of saline imbalances are changes in body weight, changes in circulating blood (check neck veins and blood pressure), and alterations in interstitial volume (check skin turgor, edema). Water imbalances are osmolality imbalances. The signs and symptoms of water imbalances are cerebral dysfunction (confusion to coma) and alterations in the serum sodium concentration.

Conditions that cause loss of gastrointestinal fluids (*e.g.*, nasogastric or intestinal suction, emesis, and diarrhea) often lead to mixed saline and water imbalances. These gastrointestinal fluid losses are predominately hypotonic. Such a hypotonic fluid loss may be visualized as a saline loss plus additional water loss. If only the water (but not the salt lost) is replaced, a saline deficit and a water excess will occur. If all of the lost saline is replaced, but not the additional water, a water deficit will result. If, as is quite common, neither the saline nor the additional water lost is replaced sufficiently, saline deficit and water deficit will coexist. In any case of mixed saline and osmolality imbalance the signs and symptoms, the therapy, and the nursing management will be a combination of those for each imbalance.

Electrolyte Balance and Imbalances

Electrolytes, or salts, are found in every body fluid. In proper concentration, they enable normal body function; when electrolyte imbalances occur, cellular dysfunction or even death results. Major electrolytes considered in this chapter are potassium, calcium, phosphate, and magnesium. No matter which electrolyte is under consideration, however, certain principles apply.

In normal circumstances, electrolytes enter the body primarily through the diet. They then enter the extracellular fluid and may also be distributed into some other body electrolyte pool (such as in bones or inside cells). Electrolytes normally exit the body in the urine and also through minor routes such as feces and sweat. Electrolyte balance is a dynamic process (Fig. 13–5). In order to keep a constant electrolyte concentration in the extracellular fluid, the rates of electrolyte intake, electrolyte entry and exit into body pools, and electrolyte excretion must be finely balanced. Conditions that alter the rate of any of these processes may cause electrolyte imbalance.

Consider, for example, an *electrolyte excess* in the extracellular fluid (Fig. 13–6). Such a situation could result from an increase in the electrolyte intake, a shift of electrolytes out of the electrolyte pool into the extracellular fluid, a decrease in the rate of electrolyte excretion, or a combination of such factors. A grasp of these principles provides a framework with which to organize facts about excesses of each specific electrolyte.

Now, consider an *electrolyte deficit* in the extracellular fluid (Fig. 13-7). Such a deficit could arise from a decreased electrolyte intake, a shift of electrolytes from the extracellular fluid into some other body pool, an increase in electro-

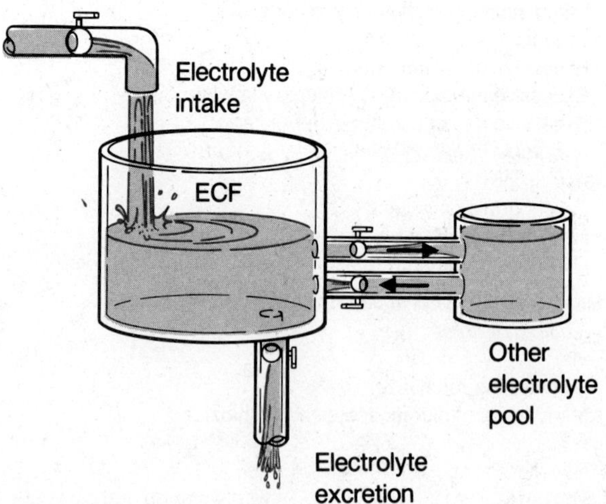

FIGURE 13–5 The dynamic process of electrolyte homeostasis. The electrolyte level in the extracellular fluid (ECF) is determined by the processes of electrolyte intake, electrolyte distribution between the extracellular fluid and other electrolyte pools, and electrolyte excretion.

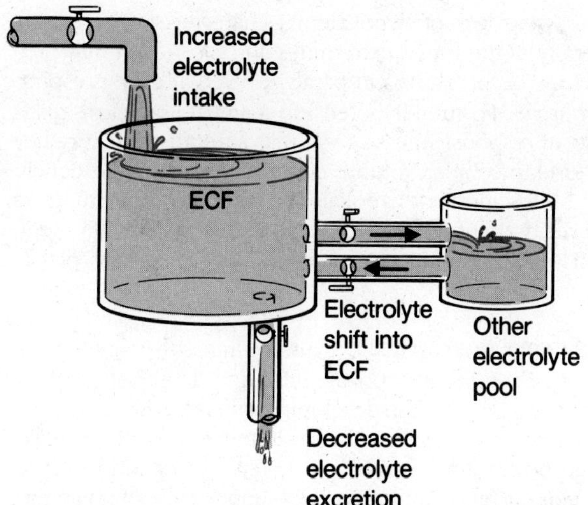

FIGURE 13–6 An extracellular electrolyte excess may be caused by increased electrolyte intake, shift of electrolytes from an electrolyte pool into the extracellular fluid, decreased electrolyte excretion, or a combination of these factors.

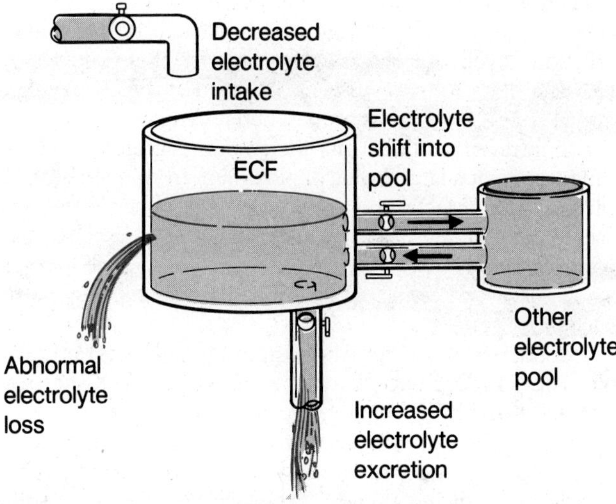

FIGURE 13–7 An extracellular electrolyte deficit may be caused by decreased electrolyte intake, shift of electrolytes from the extracellular fluid into an electrolyte pool, increased electrolyte excretion, abnormal electrolyte loss, or a combination of these factors.

lyte excretion through normal excretory routes, a loss of electrolytes through some abnormal route, or a combination of these factors. Again, an understanding of these general principles of electrolyte deficit provides the foundation upon which to build knowledge of the specific deficits.

Serum or plasma electrolyte concentrations are often measured in the clinical setting. Such measurements are useful in determining the electrolyte status of the extracellular fluid. The *serum* concentration, however, does not necessarily measure *whole body* electrolyte content, because the serum concentration may be normal when intracellular electrolyte concentration is abnormally elevated or decreased. A disturbance of either the whole body electrolyte content or solely of the serum electrolyte concentration may produce a clinical electrolyte imbalance.

The serum levels at which signs and symptoms of electrolyte imbalances occur may vary widely. Some of the factors accounting for this variation are the presence of other electrolyte imbalances, the person's degree of physiological adaptation to the electrolyte imbalance, the pH of the blood, and the rapidity of development of the imbalance. In general, rapidly developing electrolyte imbalances have more serious effects than slowly developing imbalances; however, profound physiological dysfunction, or even death, may eventually result in either case if corrective measures are not instituted.

Potassium Balance and Imbalances

Most of the potassium ions in the body are located inside the cells. Although intracellular potassium concentration averages 150 mEq/liter, the normal extracellular potassium range is 3.5 to 5 mEq/liter. Because there is a large intracellular potassium pool, measurement of the serum potassium does not necessarily provide information about whole body potassium content. Alterations in pH change the distribution of potassium ions. A decreased pH of the blood (acidemia) causes potassium ions to move out of the cellular pool into the extracellular fluid.[20] Conversely, an increase in blood pH (alkalemia) causes potassium ions to move from the extracellular fluid into cells.[59]

Many hormones affect potassium balance. The hormone aldosterone promotes the excretion of potassium in the urine. An increase of the potassium ion concentration in the blood causes increased secretion of aldosterone, which, under normal circumstances, causes the kidneys to excrete the excess. Glucocorticoid hormones also cause excretion of potassium in the urine. Both insulin and epinephrine cause potassium ions to enter the cells, of importance when determining the distribution of potassium ions in the body.[10]

The Latin word for potassium is ***kalium***: potassium imbalances are named from this root word. A deficit of extracellular potassium, for example, is termed ***hypokalemia***.

Hypokalemia

If the serum potassium drops below 3.5 mEq/liter, hypokalemia is present. Remember that hypokalemia does not necessarily signify a whole body potassium deficit, although both may be present. The four general causes of electrolyte deficits are

- Decreased electrolyte intake
- Shift of electrolytes from the extracellular fluid into an electrolyte pool
- Increased electrolyte excretion
- Abnormal electrolyte loss

These general causes provide the basis for categorizing the specific causes of hypokalemia (Table 13–8).[4, 5, 7, 47, 70]

Persons at high risk for developing hypokalemia can be identified from knowledge of the causes. Assessment and detection of the imbalance then becomes possible with knowledge of the clinical manifestations.[13]

TABLE 13–8
Causes of Hypokalemia

General Etiology: Decreased Potassium Intake
Specific Examples:
Non-iatrogenic
Anorexia
Fad diets
Fasting
Iatrogenic
NPO orders
Prolonged IV therapy without K^+
General Etiology: Entry of Potassium into Cells
Specific Examples:
Alkalosis
Familial periodic paralysis
Hypersecretion of insulin (hyperalimentation)
Transfusion of frozen RBCs (are low in K^+)
Rapid correction of acidosis during hemodialysis
Excessive beta-adrenergic stimulation
General Etiology: Increased Potassium Excretion
Specific Examples:
Urinary
Hyperaldosteronism
Cushing's syndrome
Glucocorticoid therapy
Excess black licorice ingestion (aldosterone-like effect)
Renal salt wasting
Hypomagnesemia
Diuretic therapy (potassium-sparing drugs excepted)
Carbenicillin therapy
Fecal
Diarrhea
Laxative abuse
Other
Excessive sweating without K^+ replacement
General Etiology: Potassium Loss by Abnormal Route
Specific Examples:
Emesis
Nasogastric suction
Fistula drainage

Clinical Manifestations. Signs and symptoms of hypokalemia include[51]

- Serum potassium below normal
- Abdominal distention
- Diminished bowel sounds
- Constipation
- Postural hypotension
- Skeletal muscle weakness
- Flaccid paralysis
- Polyuria, nocturia
- Cardiac arrhythmias
- Electrocardiogram changes: ST depression, flattened or inverted T waves, U waves, QT prolongation

An altered ratio of intracellular to extracellular potassium causes hyperpolarization of nerve and muscle cell resting potentials, making the cells less responsive to stimuli.

Hypokalemia is manifested in dysfunction of all three kinds of muscle: smooth, skeletal, and cardiac. The skeletal muscle weakness of hypokalemia characteristically begins bilaterally in the lower extremities and ascends. It may progress to widespread flaccid paralysis, even affecting respiratory muscles. Postural hypotension seen with hypokalemia is due to unresponsiveness of vascular smooth muscle rather than to extracellular volume depletion, as in saline deficit. The manifestations of hypokalemia may vary depending on the severity of the decrease, the rapidity of its development, the pH, the serum calcium level, and coexisting pathophysiological processes.

Nursing Implications. Nursing measures are important for prevention of hypokalemia. After identification of the persons at high risk for developing hypokalemia, appropriate teaching measures can be instituted: encouraging intake of high potassium foods (Table 13–9), instruction in bowel management, and emphasis on the importance of potassium replacement with increased secretion or abnormal route of potassium loss.[1, 11, 14] Ask for a KCl order for persons who are receiving prolonged intravenous therapy with potassium-free solutions.

The medical therapy for hypokalemia is oral or intravenous potassium replacement. Nursing management of hypokalemia includes careful monitoring of intravenous potassium replacement to prevent both cardiac arrythmias and irritation of veins. Useful guidelines are to infuse potassium no faster than 20 mEq/hr with no more than 40 mEq of potassium per liter of solution. When adding KCl to flexible plastic intravenous bags, mix the solution carefully end-to-end to prevent a large bolus of potassium from entering the infusion tube directly and providing a dangerous potassium load to the recipient. Because the body's response to a potassium load varies with the time of day, even more careful monitoring for cardiac arrhythmias is indicated when infusing KCl at night.[42]

Some people find oral potassium supplements unpalatable. The powdered agents can be mixed with fruit sherbert or mixed in while preparing gelatin. Once it has set, such gelatin can be cut into portions and eaten at medication time.[14] (Caution people to mark this high-potassium gelatin clearly as medicine.) A less expensive form of potassium supplementation is the use of prescribed amounts of potassium-containing salt substitute (*e.g.,* Neocurtasal or Morton Salt Substitute) from the grocery store.[57] Note that some salt substitutes, such as Mrs. Dash, are mixtures of herbs and are not high in potassium. Check the label for KCl.

Hypokalemia potentiates digitalis; persons who take digitalis may develop digitalis toxicity at normal therapeutic levels of digitalis if they become hypokalemic. Monitor these persons carefully for digitalis toxicity. Other nursing measures related to hypokalemia are safety measures for persons with muscle weakness and postural hypotension, positioning for adequate respiration, and frequent assessment of ability to function.

Hyperkalemia

A serum potassium concentration above 5 mEq/liter denotes the presence of hyperkalemia, an excess of potassium in the extracellular fluid. The specific causes of hyperkalemia

TABLE 13–9
Food with High Potassium Content

	Potassium		
	mg	*mEq*	*Calories*
Almonds ($\frac{1}{2}$ cup chopped; about 65)	502	12.9	387
Apricot halves in heavy syrup (1 cup)	604	15.5	220
Apricot halves (28 large dried)	1273	32.6	340
Avocado (1 10-oz California)	1303	33.4	370
Avocado (1 16-oz Florida)	1836	47	390
Banana (1)	440	11.3	100
Blackberries (1 cup)	245	6.3	85
Cantaloupe ($\frac{1}{2}$, 5-inch diameter)	682	17.5	80
Cherries (10)	129	3.3	45
Dates (10 whole)	518	13.3	220
Dates (1 cup chopped)	1153	29.6	490
Fruit cocktail in heavy syrup (1 cup canned)	411	10.5	195
Grapefruit ($\frac{1}{2}$ pink)	166	4.3	50
Grapefruit ($\frac{1}{2}$ white)	159	4.1	45
Grapefruit juice (1 cup unsweetened, white)	400	10.3	100
Molasses (1 tbsp blackstrap)	585	15	45
Orange (1)	263	6.7	65
Orange juice, fresh or canned (1 cup)	496	12.7	110–120
Orange juice, frozen reconstituted (1 cup)	503	12.9	120
Papaya (1 cup cubes)	328	8.4	55
Peaches (1 cup sliced)	343	8.8	65
Peaches (1 cup cooked dried with juice)	743	19.1	205
Potato (1 baked)	782	20.1	145
Potato (1 boiled)	556	14.3	105
Prunes (5 uncooked dried)	298	7.6	110
Raisins ($\frac{1}{2}$ cup)	553	14.2	210
Rhubarb ($\frac{1}{2}$ cup cooked with sugar)	548	14.1	380
Squash (1 cup winter, yellow)	945	24.2	130
Strawberries (1 cup)	244	6.3	55
Sunflower seeds ($\frac{1}{4}$ cup, hulled)	333	8.5	202
Turkey, dark meat (4 pieces, each $2\frac{1}{2} \times 1\frac{5}{8} \times \frac{1}{4}$ inches)	338	8.7	175
Watermelon (4 × 8-inch wedge)	426	11	110

(Data from Adams C, Richardson M: Nutritive Value of Foods. USDA Home and Garden Bulletin No. 72. Washington, DC, US Government Printing Office, 1981)

are organized in Table 13–10 under the general causes of increased potassium intake, movement of potassium out of cells, and decreased potassium excretion.[13,65,67,68] Note that increased oral potassium intake does not usually cause hyperkalemia if renal function is normal.

Clinical Manifestations. Clinical manifestions of hyperkalemia include[3,63]

- Serum potassium above normal
- Intestinal cramping
- Diarrhea
- Skeletal muscle weakness
- Flaccid paralysis
- Cardiac arrhythmias
- Cardiac arrest
- Electrocardiogram changes: peaked narrow T waves, shortened QT interval, then widened QRS, sine wave

The altered ratio of intracellular to extracellular potassium causes hypopolarization of nerve and muscle cells. The cells discharge and cannot be repolarized to fire again. Although polarized cell resting potentials are affected differently in hyperkalemia and hypokalemia, the clinical manifestations in the skeletal muscles are similar: bilateral ascending muscle weakness to paralysis, usually beginning in the lower extremities.[51] Although respiratory muscle paralysis is less common with hyperkalemia than with hypokalemia, it may occur. The chief danger of hyperkalemia is death from cardiac arrhythmias and cardiac arrest.

Nursing Implications. Nurses can prevent hyperkalemia by mixing and monitoring intravenous potassium carefully, by ascertaining that renal function is normal before administering intravenous potassium, by teaching people who use salt substitutes (KCl) to discontinue them if their urine output decreases, by requesting fresh blood for persons who will need large transfusions, and by warming blood before administering it.[54,71] (Some potassium goes back inside the erythrocytes when blood is warmed.)

If hyperkalemia develops, nursing measures include administration of the medical therapy and some independent

TABLE 13–10
Causes of Hyperkalemia

General Etiology: Increased Potassium Intake
Specific examples:
Excessive intravenous administration
Insufficiently mixed KCl in flexible plastic IV bags
Massive transfusion of blood stored longer than 3 days (K^+ leaves RBCs)
Large doses of intravenous potassium penicillin G (contains 1.6 mEq K^+/million units)
Large oral intake, only with decreased renal excretion also
General Etiology: Movement of Potassium Out of Cells
Specific examples:
Acidosis
Insulin deficiency
Massive cell death (crushing injuries, burns, cytotoxic drugs)
Arginine infusion
Large digitalis overdose
Familial periodic paralysis
General Etiology: Decreased Potassium Excretion
Specific examples:
Oliguria
Extracellular volume depletion
Renal failure
Decreased aldosterone
Addison's disease
Hyporeninism
Chronic heparin administration
Lead poisoning
Captopril administration
Other
Potassium-sparing diuretics (spironolactone, triamterene, and amiloride)

nursing measures. Medical therapy for hyperkalemia involves measures to treat the underlying cause, to move potassium into cells (insulin and glucose, bicarbonate infusion), to counteract the cardiac effects of hyperkalemia (intravenous calcium gluconate), or to remove potassium from the body (dialysis, diuretics, oral ion-exchange resins).[44,51] Independent nursing measures involve careful assessment (including use of cardiac monitor when appropriate), restriction of high potassium foods and medication, promotion of urine output, and provision of adequate dietary calories to prevent tissue breakdown with potassium release into extracellular fluid.[14]

Summary of Principles of Potassium Imbalances

Hypokalemia and hyperkalemia are imbalances of potassium concentration in the extracellular fluid. Although the pathophysiological basis is different in the two conditions, they both cause skeletal muscle weakness, flaccid paralysis, and cardiac arrhythmias. Hypokalemia causes paralytic ileus; hyperkalemia tends to cause intestinal colic. The point at which clinical manifestations appear varies not only with the degree and speed of development of the potassium imbalance but also with other factors such as the pH and calcium concentration. Informed nurses can prevent potassium imbalances, detect them early by careful assessment of the person at high risk, and institute a variety of nursing management procedures for people who have already developed these imbalances.

Calcium Balance and Imbalances

The calcium ions in the body are mostly located in the bones and teeth, with small amounts of calcium in the cells of soft tissue. The normal concentration range for calcium in the serum is 9 to 11 mg/dl (or 4.5–5.5 mEq/liter). With advancing age, the serum calcium concentration tends to increase in women and decrease in men, but it still remains within the normal range in the healthy elderly.

The serum calcium concentration is normally regulated by parathyroid hormone. The action of this hormone (which is secreted by the parathyroid glands) causes resorption of calcium from the bones, decreases the renal excretion of calcium, and facilitates the absorption of calcium from the gastrointestinal tract by promoting the activation of vitamin D. All of these actions of parathyroid hormone tend to raise the serum calcium level. As the serum calcium level falls, the secretion of parathyroid hormone is stimulated. If the serum calcium level rises too high, the secretion of parathyroid hormone is decreased by negative feedback.[32]

The major sources of calcium in most American diets are milk and other diary products (cheese, cream, sour cream, yogurt, ice cream, nonfat milk powder). In order for calcium to be absorbed from the gastrointestinal tract, an active form of vitamin D must be present. In addition to the dietary calcium, the calcium ions that are contained in the gastrointestinal secretions must also be absorbed into the body or they will be excreted in the feces.

The calcium ions in the serum are in three forms, the total of which is usually reported by the laboratory. These three forms are *ionized* (free), *bound* to protein, and *complexed* with citrate and other organic ions. Only the ionized calcium in the serum is physiologically available. Changes in pH of the extracellular fluid alter the amount of ionized calcium available and may thus cause calcium imbalances even though the amount of calcium in the body may be unchanged.

Hypocalcemia

Hypocalcemia occurs if the serum calcium falls below 9 mg/dl or if the ionized portion of the serum calcium is diminished. The causes of hypocalcemia are decreased intake or absorption of calcium, decreased physiological availability of calcium, increased calcium excretion, and calcium loss by an abnormal route. Specific examples are listed in Table 13–11 under these four categories.[6,13,34,62]

An understanding of the causes (of hypocalcemia) facilitates identification of the persons at high risk for development of hypocalcemia.

Clinical Manifestations. Early detection of hypocalcemia in high-risk persons becomes possible through knowledge of the signs and symptoms, which include the following:[48,53]

TABLE 13–11
Causes of Hypocalcemia

General Etiology: Decreased Calcium Intake or Absorption
Specific examples:
Diet lacking milk and vitamin D
Excess phytates or oxalates in diet
Steatorrhea
Malabsorption syndromes (*e.g.*, sprue)
Chronic diarrhea
Chronic laxative overuse
Pancreatitis

General Etiology: Decreased Physiological Availability of Calcium
Specific examples:
Alkalosis
Massive transfusion of citrated blood (citrate binds Ca^{++})
Rapid infusion of proteinaceous plasma expanders (bind Ca^{++})
Hypoparathyroidism
Surgical removal of parathyroids (during thyroid surgery)
Hypomagnesemia
Overuse of phosphate-containing laxatives and enemas
Excess phosphate intake (oral or intravenous)
Tumor lysis syndrome
Acute fluoride poisoning
Pancreatitis

General Etiology: Increased Calcium Excretion
Specific examples:
Chronic renal insufficiency
Pancreatitis

General Etiology: Calcium Loss by Abnormal Route
Specific example:
Wound exudate (*e.g.*, burns)

- Decreased serum calcium (or decreased ionized calcium and normal total calcium)
- Paresthesias (digital and perioral)
- Positive Chvostek's sign
- Positive Trousseau's sign
- Grimacing, muscle twitching, cramping
- Hyperactive reflexes
- Carpopedal spasm
- Tetany
- Laryngospasm
- Seizures
- Cardiac arrhythmias
- Cardiac arrest
- Electrocardiogram changes: prolonged QT interval

Note that these signs are all manifestations of increased neuromuscular excitability caused by increased cell membrane permeability.

Chvostek's and Trousseau's signs are two signs of increased neuromuscular excitability. Chvostek's sign is tested by tapping the facial nerve in front of the ear. If the corner of the mouth draws up in a grimace, the sign is positive; increased neuromuscular irritability is present. Trousseau's sign is tested by occluding arterial flow to the hand with a sphygmomanometer cuff for about 3 minutes. If the hand contorts in a carpal spasm, the sign is positive; increased neuromuscular irritability is present (Fig. 13–8). Frequent assessment of Chvostek's or Trousseau's signs in persons at high risk for hypocalcemia (*e.g.*, after thyroid surgery) may aid detection and correction of hypocalcemia before life-threatening laryngospasm or cardiac arrest occurs.

Nursing Implications. Prevention of hypocalcemia is made possible by dietary counseling, including providing a list of alternate sources of calcium for persons who do not or cannot eat dairy products (Table 13–12), and by teaching

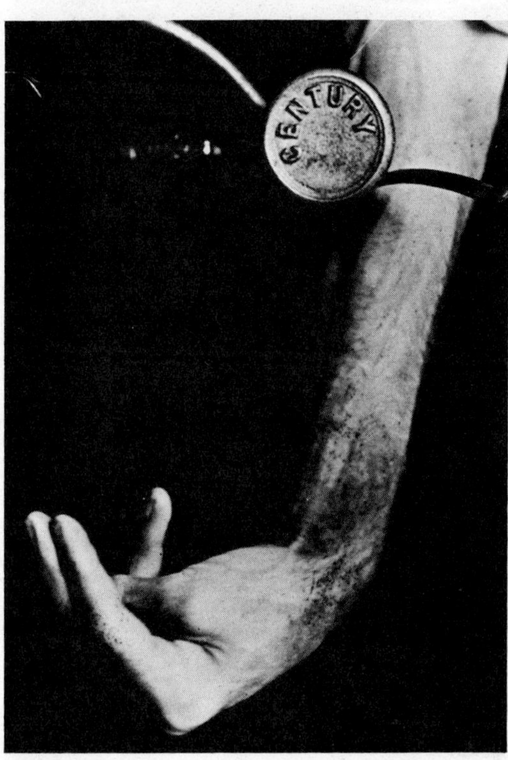

FIGURE 13–8 Manifestations of hypocalcemia. Trousseau's sign is elicited in a patient with hypoparathyroid tetany. (Ezrin C, Godden J, Volpe R, Wilson R [eds]: Systematic Endocrinology, 2nd ed, p 151. Hagerstown, Harper & Row, 1979)

TABLE 13–12
Nondairy Sources of Calcium

Almonds	Mustard greens
Beet greens	Okra
Blackstrap molasses	Oranges
Bok choy cabbage	Oysters
Broccoli	Rhubarb
Chocolate	Salmon (canned)
Collard greens	Sardines (canned)
Cream of wheat cereal	Spinach
Dandelion greens	Tofu
Farina cereal	Turnip greens
Kale	

(Data from Adams C, Richardson M: Nutritive Value of Foods. USDA Home and Garden Bulletin No. 72. Washington, DC, US Government Printing Office, 1981)

careful use of laxatives.[1] Excessive use of mineral oil will prevent absorption of fat-soluble vitamin D, thus impairing calcium absorption. Chronic diarrhea from laxative overuse also impairs calcium absorption by decreasing transit time through the bowel. Overuse of phosphate-containing laxatives and enemas may cause hypocalcemia by increasing serum phosphate.[69]

Persons who are hypocalcemic need calcium replacement. Oral calcium salts are often administered with vitamin D to increase their absorption. If intravenous calcium salts are ordered, monitor the infusion carefully. Too rapid an infusion rate may cause dangerous cardiac arrhythmias. If a calcium-containing solution infiltrates into the tissues rather than entering the vein, tissue sloughing will occur. Important nursing measures to implement while hypocalcemia is being corrected include decreasing environmental stimuli and instituting seizure precautions in cases of severe hypocalcemia. Persons who have mild hypocalcemia need to be taught to avoid hyperventilation and pressing on efferent nerves (*e.g.*, by crossing their legs), as these measures exacerbate tetany.

TABLE 13–13
Causes of Hypercalcemia

General Etiology: Increased Calcium Intake or Absorption
Specific examples:
Milk-alkali syndrome
Excessive intake of vitamin D
Sarcoidosis
General Etiology: Release of Calcium from Bone
Specific examples:
Hyperparathyroidism
Prolonged immobilization
Multiple myeloma
Leukemia
Bone tumors (primary or metastatic)
Many other malignancies (*e.g.*, breast cancer) that produce bone-resorbing substances
General Etiology: Decreased Calcium Excretion
Specific examples:
Thiazide diuretics
Familial hypocalciuric hypercalcemia

Hypercalcemia

When the serum calcium concentration exceeds 11 mg/dl, hypercalcemia is present. This condition occurs from factors that increase calcium intake or absorption, move calcium from bone into the extracellular fluid, or decrease calcium excretion (Table 13–13).[8,13,22,26]

Clinical Manifestations. The signs and symptoms of hypercalcemia, in contrast to those of hypocalcemia, are the result of *decreased* neuromuscular irritability caused by decreased cell membrane permeability. They include the following:[8,36,37]

- Increased serum calcium (or increased ionized calcium and normal total calcium)
- Anorexia
- Nausea, emesis
- Constipation
- Abdominal pain
- Polyuria
- Renal calculi
- Fatigue
- Muscle weakness
- Impaired reflexes
- Headache
- Confusion, lethargy
- Personality change
- Psychosis
- Cardiac arrest
- Electrocardiogram changes: shortened QT interval

Nursing assessment in hypercalcemia, then, includes gastrointestinal function, neuromuscular function, cognitive function, and cardiac function. Because calculi may form in the urine when excess calcium is present, straining the urine to detect calculi is another assessment technique in hypercalcemia.

Nursing Implications. The major nursing measures for prevention of hypercalcemia are directed toward increasing or maintaining mobility to prevent the withdrawal of calcium from bones that occurs with immobility. Persons who are too weak to ambulate may be placed on a tilt table for a period of erect weight bearing. People who take megadoses of vitamins need to be cautioned against huge daily doses of vitamin D (*e.g.*, 50,000 U).

A major complication in people who have hypercalcemia is renal damage from precipitation of calcium, either in minute crystals or in larger calculi. Nurses can help prevent this renal damage by encouraging 3 to 4 liters of fluid intake per day to keep the urine dilute. Dairy products should be restricted. Because an acid environment increases the solubility of calcium, measures to acidify the urine are appropriate: prune or cranberry juice, and an acid ash diet. Prevention of urinary tract infections, which tend to alkalinize the urine, is in order: careful catheter care, palpation for bladder distention, and turning immobile persons frequently to avoid stasis of urine.[14]

A person whose hypercalcemia is due to withdrawal of calcium from bones may have weakened bones as a result. Such a person will need to be turned and transferred gently, to prevent pathological fractures. Hypercalcemia potentiates digitalis; watch for digitalis toxicity. Thiazide diuretics decrease calcium excretion, so they should be withheld.[17]

Summary of Principles of Calcium Imbalances

The calcium imbalances cause abnormalities in neuromuscular function by altering neuromuscular excitability. Hypocalcemia causes increased neuromuscular excitability, which can be detected by assessment of reflexes and of Chvostek's and Trousseau's signs. Hypercalcemia causes decreased neuromuscular excitability. In addition to administration of the medical therapy, nursing care for persons who have calcium imbalances includes seizure precautions in hypocalcemia and maintaining a dilute, acid urine in hypercalcemia.

Phosphate Balance and Imbalances

In contrast to the ions already discussed, phosphate is an anion (a negatively charged ion). Phosphates are an integral part of bones and are also abundant inside cells. The normal serum phosphate concentration range is 2.5 to 4.5 mg/dl. Although serum phosphate tends to increase with age in women (still within the normal range), it tends to decrease with age in men. Some laboratories consider 2.45 mg/dl to be the low end of the normal range in elderly men.[23]

Under normal circumstances the serum phosphate and the serum calcium have an inverse relationship. Parathyroid hormone, which tends to increase the serum calcium, tends to decrease the serum phosphate by enhancing renal phosphate excretion. If serum calcium and serum phosphate both become elevated at the same time, calcium phosphate salts may precipitate in the soft tissues of the body.

Hypophosphatemia

If the serum phosphate drops below 2.5 mg/dl, hypophosphatemia has occurred. Mild hypophosphatemia is often asymptomatic. If, however, the serum phosphate falls below 1 mg/dl, severe symptomatic hypophosphatemia, a serious condition, is present.[31]

Factors that tend to decrease the serum phosphate are listed in Table 13–14. A few of these factors may cause severe symptomatic hypophosphatemia by themselves; these factors are printed in capital letters. The remaining factors may cause the severe disorder if several of them are combined.[2] The factors that move phosphate into cells are all associated with rapid cellular growth and metabolism.

TABLE 13–14
Factors that Decrease Serum Phosphate

General Etiology: Decreased Phosphate Intake or Absorption
Specific examples:
PROLONGED OR EXCESSIVE ANTACID USE*
Malabsorption syndrome
Chronic diarrhea
Chronic alcoholism

General Etiology: Movement of Phosphate into Cells
Specific examples:
HYPERALIMENTATION
REFEEDING AFTER STARVATION
RESPIRATORY ALKALOSIS (HYPERVENTILATION)
Intravenous glucose, fructose, lactate, or bicarbonate
Insulin
Epinephrine
Androgen therapy

General Etiology: Increased Phosphate Excretion
Specific examples:
DIABETIC KETOACIDOSIS
ALCOHOL WITHDRAWAL
DIURETIC PHASE AFTER SEVERE BURNS
Diuretic therapy
Corticosteroid therapy
Early chronic renal failure
Renal tubular acidosis
Hyperparathyroidism
Osteoporosis, osteomalacia
Multiple myeloma
Gout

General Etiology: Phosphate Loss by Abnormal Route
Specific examples:
Emesis
Hemodialysis

*Capitalized type denotes single causes of severe symptomatic hypophosphatemia.

Clinical Manifestations. Clinical manifestations of severe symptomatic hypophosphatemia include the following:

- Serum phosphate below 1 mg/dl
- Anorexia, nausea
- Malaise
- Decreased reflexes
- Muscle weakness, severe debility
- Myalgia
- Bone pain (with antacid overuse)
- Irritability, apprehension
- Paresthesias
- Confusion
- Stupor
- Seizures
- Coma

Depletion of erythrocyte 2,3-diphosphoglycerate impairs oxygenation, and adenosine triphosphate (ATP) depletion causes cell dysfunction.

Nursing assessment of persons at high risk for severe symptomatic hypophosphatemia is based on knowledge of these manifestations and of their usual time course. For example, during ketoacidosis, organic phosphates inside cells are decomposed; the phosphate moves out of cells and is excreted in the urine, depleting the body of phosphate. After administration of insulin, the remaining phosphates in the serum move into cells. The serum phosphate thus drops abruptly 24 to 36 hours after treatment of diabetic ketoacidosis, unless phosphates are administered. Severe symptomatic hypophosphatemia occurs 2 to 4 days after hospitalization for alcohol withdrawal and up to 10 days after initiation of hyperalimentation therapy.

Nursing Implications. In addition to careful assessment for early detection of severe symptomatic hypophosphatemia, nurses can employ preventive measures. Teaching about careful antacid use is of major importance.[25] Check to see that phosphates are being administered during hyperalimentation, alcohol withdrawal, and treatment of diabetic ketoacidosis, or that the serum phosphate concentration is being monitored during the high-risk period. Take measures to allay respiratory alkalosis (see Chap. 14).

If severe hypophosphatemia develops, assess reflexes, muscle strength, and respiratory function. Provide safety measures if muscle weakness is apparent. Profound muscle weakness in severe hypophosphatemia may necessitate mechanical ventilation.

Therapy for hypophosphatemia is oral or intravenous phosphate replacement. Since phosphate administration may decrease the serum calcium, nursing management of phosphate replacement includes assessment for the manifestations of hypocalcemia.[18] Foods with a high phosphate content are listed in Table 13–15.[1]

Hyperphosphatemia

A serum phosphate above 4.5 mg/dl indicates hyperphosphatemia. As the general principles for an electrolyte excess indicate (see Fig. 13–6), hyperphosphatemia may arise from excessive phosphate intake, movement of phosphate from cells into the blood, or impaired phosphate excretion. Specific examples of these causes are listed in Table 13–16.

Clinical Manifestations. The clinical manifestations of hyperphosphatemia vary, depending on the concurrent concentration of serum calcium. Ordinarily, the serum calcium falls as the serum phosphate rises. In this condition, the signs and symptoms observed would be the increased neuromuscular excitability of hypocalcemia. If, however, the serum calcium does not fall, calcium phosphate salts will precipitate in soft tissues of the body with signs and symptoms reflecting the location of salt formation: conjunctivitis and band keratopathy (eye), pruritus (skin), acute renal failure (kidney), or arthritis (joints).

TABLE 13–15
Foods with High Phosphate Content

Carbonated beverages (with phosphoric acid in contents)
Eggs
Meat
Milk
Processed foods (with phosphate or phosphoric acid in contents)

(Data from Adams C, Richardson M: Nutritive Value of Foods. USDA Home and Garden Bulletin No. 72. Washington, DC, US Government Printing Office, 1981)

TABLE 13–16
Causes of Hyperphosphatemia

General Etiology: Increased Phosphate Intake
Specific examples:
Excessive phosphate therapy
Overuse of phosphate-containing cathartics and enemas
General Etiology: Release of Phosphate from Cells
Specific examples:
Crushing injuries
Rhabdomyolysis
Radiation therapy
Chemotherapy of leukemia or lymphoma
General Etiology: Decreased Phosphate Excretion
Specific examples:
Oliguric renal failure
Hypoparathyroidism
Adrenal insufficiency

Nursing Implications. Since phosphate-containing cathartics and enemas are available without a prescription, teaching about bowel management is an important way of preventing hyperphosphatemia. Another preventive measure is careful monitoring of intravenous phosphate infusions.

In chronic renal failure, the risk of hyperphosphatemia is a continuous problem. Persons with this problem need to take aluminum antacids (magnesium is contraindicated) during meals. The aluminum ions bind phosphate ions in the gastrointestinal tract, preventing their absorption and thus preventing hyperphosphatemia. Explaining the reason for the antacid therapy may help people comply with it. Providing a recipe for antacid cookies may also be of benefit.

Nursing management of persons who have developed hyperphosphatemia varies with the serum calcium status. If hypocalcemia occurs, nursing care is as discussed previously. If, on the other hand, the serum calcium does not decrease, encouraging a large fluid intake to dilute the urine and retard calcium phosphate precipitation is in order (unless renal failure limits fluid intake).

Summary of Principles of Phosphate Imbalances

Phosphate is needed for metabolism and cellular growth. Rapid cell proliferation or increases in metabolism cause uptake of phosphate from the blood into the cells. If the phosphate supply is insufficient, severe symptomatic hypophosphatemia may occur. Phosphate excess, on the other hand, may occur with overuse of phosphate-containing agents or from oliguric renal failure. In addition to assessment of high-risk persons, preventive measures, and administration of the medical therapy, nursing management of persons who have developed phosphate imbalances includes safety measures in hypophosphatemia and management of hypocalcemia concurrently with hyperphosphatemia.

Magnesium Balance and Imbalances

Most of the magnesium ions in the body are located in the bones. The rest of the magnesium is inside cells, especially in liver and skeletal muscle, with only a small amount of magnesium in the blood. The normal serum magnesium range is 1.5 to 2.5 mEq/liter for adults of all ages.

Magnesium ingested in the diet is absorbed primarily from the ileum. The gastrointestinal secretions contain an appreciable amount of magnesium, much of which is normally reabsorbed, also from the ileum.

In contrast to calcium and phosphate, which are both regulated by parathyroid hormone, the serum magnesium concentration does not have a primary hormone regulator. The hormone aldosterone facilitates the renal excretion of magnesium ions.

Hypomagnesemia

Serum magnesium below 1.5 mEq/liter is known as hypomagnesemia. This condition arises from the general causes of any electrolyte deficit: decreased intake or absorption, increased excretion, or loss by an abnormal route.[13] Movement of magnesium from the serum into the bones is not

TABLE 13–17
Causes of Hypomagnesemia

General Etiology: Decreased Magnesium Intake or Absorption
Specific examples:
Chronic malnutrition
Prolonged IV therapy without Mg^{++}
Malabsorption syndromes
Chronic diarrhea
Steatorrhea
Pancreatitis
Resection of ileum
Chronic alcoholism

General Etiology: Increased Magnesium Excretion
Specific examples:
Urinary
- Diabetic ketoacidosis
- Chronic alcoholism
- Diuretic therapy
- Hyperaldosteronism
- Gentamicin toxicity
- Diuretic phase of acute renal failure

Fecal
- Steatorrhea
- Pancreatitis

General Etiology: Magnesium Loss by Abnormal Route
Specific examples:
Emesis
Nasogastric suction
Fistula drainage

usually a cause of hypomagnesemia. Specific examples of these general causes are presented in Table 13–17.[16,19,40]

Clinical Manifestations. Although the pathophysiological mechanisms are different at the cellular level, hypomagnesemia, like hypocalcemia, causes increased neuromuscular excitability. In hypomagnesemia, the cause is the increased release of acetylcholine at the neuromuscular junctions. The clinical manifestations of these two disorders are similar, although not identical. The signs and symptoms of hypomagnesemia include the following:

- Serum magnesium below normal
- Insomnia
- Hyperreflexia
- Positive Chvostek's sign
- Positive Trousseau's sign
- Leg and foot cramps
- Grimacing, twitching, tremors
- Dysphagia
- Ataxia
- Nystagmus (usually vertical)
- Tetany
- Seizures
- Extreme confusion
- Cardiac arrhythmias
- Electrocardiogram changes: ST and T wave abnormalities

Nursing assessment of hypomagnesemia includes testing Chvostek's and Trousseau's signs and monitoring reflexes.[15]

Nursing Implications. Hypomagnesemia may be prevented by inclusion of magnesium during long-term parenteral therapy and by diet counseling for persons at high risk for hypomagnesemia.[38] Foods high in magnesium include bananas, chocolate, cocoa, egg yolk, whole grain cereals, legumes (especially soybeans), meat, milk, nuts, peanut butter, and dark green vegetables.[1,35]

Nursing management of persons who have hypomagnesemia involves administration of the prescribed medical therapy (oral or parenteral magnesium replacement) as well as independent nursing actions.[14] Oral magnesium salts may have a laxative effect. Intravenous $MgSO_4$ must be administered carefully, because rapid infusion will cause flushing and sweating. Check for adequate renal function before administering parenteral $MgSO_4$. It is advisable to test the patellar reflexes before administering each dose; if these reflexes diminish or disappear, the serum magnesium should be rechecked, as it may have become elevated. Seizure precautions are appropriate in severe hypomagnesemia. As hypomagnesemia is common in persons who drink large amounts of alcohol on a chronic basis, taking a drinking history and monitoring for alcohol withdrawal are important when hypomagnesemia has no other apparent cause.[39]

Hypermagnesemia

Hypermagnesemia is elevation of the serum magnesium concentration above 2.5 mEq/liter. The major causes of hypermagnesemia are listed in Table 13–18. These causes can be categorized as increased magnesium intake or absorption and decreased magnesium excretion.[13] Magnesium release from bone into the blood may occur in hyperparathyroidism, but the initial hypermagnesemia caused by this shift is diminished by renal excretion of the excess magnesium.

Clinical Manifestations. The signs and symptoms of hypermagnesemia are manifestations of decreased neuromuscular excitability due to decreased release of acetylcholine at neuromuscular junctions, and bear some similarities to the manifestations of hypercalcemia:

- Increased serum magnesium
- Hypotension
- Flushing, diaphoresis
- Drowsiness, lethargy
- Diminished deep tendon reflexes
- Flaccid paralysis
- Respiratory depression
- Bradycardia
- Cardiac arrhythmias
- Cardiac arrest
- Electrocardiogram changes: increased T wave amplitude, prolonged P-R and QRS

Nursing Implications. Prevention of hypermagnesemia is accomplished by teaching people how to manage antacids and cathartics, and nondrug methods of bowel management.[14] Elderly persons are a high-risk population for hypermagnesemia from these preparations.[49] People who have chronic renal failure need to be instructed to avoid magnesium-containing antacids and cathartics. If hyper-

TABLE 13–18
Causes of Hypermagnesemia

General Etiology: Increased Magnesium Intake or Absorption
Specific examples:
Aspiration of sea water
Excessive use of Mg^{++}-containing cathartics
Excessive use of Mg^{++}-containing urologic irrigating solutions
Excess magnesium in dialysis fluid
Excess IV infusion of Mg^{++}
General Etiology: Decreased Magnesium Excretion
Specific examples:
Oliguric renal failure
Adrenal insufficiency

magnesemia develops, the administration of large amounts of fluid to increase renal magnesium output is important unless contraindicated by renal or cardiac disease. Hemodialysis may be necessary in renal failure.

Summary of Principles of Magnesium Imbalances

The magnesium imbalances are characterized by alterations of neuromuscular excitability. Hypomagnesemia is manifested by increased neuromuscular excitability, which is monitored by checking reflexes and Chvostek's or Trousseau's sign. In contrast, hypermagnesemia is manifested by signs of decreased neuromuscular excitability. Nurses can encourage persons at high risk for hypomagnesemia to include liberal amounts of magnesium foods in their diet. Persons who have hypermagnesemia, on the other hand, need to avoid magnesium-containing preparations, notably, many antacids and cathartics.

Principles for Understanding Mixed Saline, Water, and Electrolyte Imbalances

So far, saline, water, and the electrolyte imbalances have been discussed separately in this chapter. In the clinical setting, however, several imbalances may coexist. A quick review of the factors that cause electrolyte imbalances will bring to light some common factors. Several serum electrolyte deficits, for example, may result from vomiting, nasogastric suction, and diarrhea. These same factors may cause saline or osmolality imbalances, depending on the type of fluid or salt replacement. Several principles for understanding mixed imbalances are presented during discussion of the following clinical example.

> Susan Petersen, age 46, attended a retirement party for one of the workers in the office where she manages the advertising department. During the evening she had six martinis, which didn't concern her until she awoke in the early morning hours with epigastric pain. Soon she realized that she was experiencing something more than the gastritis she had encountered several times previously. Intense pain in her upper left abdominal quadrant radiated to her back. Nausea and vomiting were soon followed by diarrhea. Ms. Petersen was admitted to the hospital with a diagnosis of acute pancreatitis. In the hospital, an intravenous infusion of 5% dextrose in $\frac{1}{4}$ normal saline was started. A nasogastric tube was inserted and connected to suction.

With no more information than this, consider what factors place Ms. Petersen at risk for saline, osmolality, or electrolyte imbalances. Obvious factors are vomiting, diarrhea, and nasogastric suction. Ms. Petersen has lost saline, additional water, potassium, and magnesium through these routes. In addition, she has acute pancreatitis, which puts her at high risk for hypocalcemia and hypomagnesemia. Two additional risk factors are less obvious: her intravenous infusion does not contain potassium; she has had recurrent gastritis (high chronic alcohol intake?). If she overuses antacids for the gastritis, and especially if she does have a high chronic alcohol intake, she might even be at risk for severe hypophosphatemia. This process of searching for risk factors is an illustration of the first principle for understanding mixed imbalances:

1. **Look for all the risk factors.**

Is electrolyte intake altered? Is electrolyte excretion abnormally increased or decreased? Are there factors that cause electrolyte shifts? Are electrolytes being lost by abnormal routes? Is saline being gained or removed? Is some factor altering the relative concentrations of salt and water in the blood? These questions cover all of the risk factors for the imbalances presented in this chapter. Look for all the risk factors.

Once the risk factors have been delineated, a second principle is useful:

2. **Consider assessment and nursing management for each imbalance separately.**

Considering each imbalance separately is an important preliminary to developing an individualized assessment and plan of care that incorporates all of the imbalances. Attempting to formulate a plan of care without considering each imbalance separately leads to omission of important facets of care. Ms. Petersen has risk factors for saline deficit, water deficit (hypernatremia), hypokalemia, hypocalcemia, hypomagnesemia, and possibly even severe hypophosphatemia. What assessments are important for saline deficit? (postural blood pressure drop, increased small vein filling time, flat neck veins) For water deficit? (serum sodium, confusion, lethargy) For hypokalemia? (abdominal distention, skeletal muscle weakness) What denotes hypocalcemia? (increased neuromuscular excitability) Hypomagnesemia? (also increased neuromuscular excitability) Severe hypophosphatemia? (nausea, muscle weakness, bone pain) How is saline deficit prevented? Managed if it does develop? And so forth.

By itself, the principle of considering each imbalance separately leaves the user with a mass of unwieldly facts; used in conjunction with the third principle, however, it becomes a powerful tool for developing a coherent plan of care for a person with mixed imbalances:

3. **Develop an organized nursing assessment and plan of care.**

In Ms. Petersen's case, it would include daily weights, measures of blood volume, mental status, bowel sounds, skeletal muscle strength, and neuromuscular excitability. In conjunction with the above assessment, any available laboratory reports, and assessment of her ability to perform the activities of daily living, nursing diagnoses can be formulated and nursing interventions planned. For example, Ms. Petersen had abdominal distention, muscle cramps in her legs, and a positive Chvostek's sign. The standard laboratory report showed normal serum potassium and decreased serum calcium. Serum magnesium, when requested, also showed a slight decrease. An important nursing diagnosis for Ms. Petersen is potential injury from tetany or seizures due to hypocalcemia and hypomagnesemia. Nursing interventions to be instituted while these imbalances are being corrected include decreasing environmental stimuli, instituting safety measures, monitoring for alcohol withdrawal, and teaching Ms. Petersen to avoid crossing her legs, as that will exacerbate her leg cramps.

In summary, three principles, applied in order, can facilitate the understanding of and the development of organized care for persons with mixed saline, osmolality, and/or electrolyte imbalances. These principles are

1. Look for all the risk factors.
2. Consider assessment and nursing management for each imbalance separately.
3. Develop an organized nursing assessment and plan of care.

Principles of Intravenous Therapy

Intravenous therapy is frequently encountered in nursing practice. Intravenous infusions are used to replace fluid and electrolytes when an imbalance has occurred, to supply maintenance fluid and electrolytes to persons who cannot manage oral intake, to administer medications, and to supply total parenteral nutrition. (Total parenteral nutrition is discussed in Chap. 80.) Because the intravenous route provides direct access to the blood, it has advantages and disadvantages over the oral route. The intravenous route is faster than the oral route, but this very rapidity, valuable in emergency situations, makes overdosage a continual risk. Careful assessment and monitoring are thus important nursing actions for persons receiving intravenous therapy.

Nursing Implications. Nursing responsibilities for intravenous therapy include starting the infusion, managing the flow rate, monitoring for complications of intravenous therapy, and discontinuing the infusion. The technique for *starting an intravenous infusion* is outlined in Table 13–19.[9, 29, 64]

(Text continues on p 160)

TABLE 13–19
Procedure for Starting an Intravenous Infusion

Procedure	*Comments*
Prepare Equipment	
Check the order.	Order should state type and amount of solution and period over which it is to be infused.
Read label on fluid reservoir carefully.	Wrong solution may be dangerous to patient.
Check fluid reservoir for expiration date, cracks, cloudy solution.	Avoid risk of infection from contaminated solution.
Choose needle or catheter.	*Butterfly needle:* short metal needle with plastic tabs for stabilization after insertion; inserts easily; infiltrates easily. *Intracatheter:* long plastic catheter inserted through hollow metal needle which is then removed; threading catheter into vein makes insertion more difficult. *Over-the-needle catheter:* shorter plastic catheter inserted over a metal needle which is then removed; less infiltration than with metal needles but more irritating to vein.
Choose tubing; consider in-line filter or infusion pump.	Filter especially important when infusing antimicrobial agents reconstituted from powder.
Calculate infusion drip rate.	Number of drops per minute delivered by infusion set varies with the manufacturer and is printed on package.
Wash hands.	Tubing connectors and infusion port must be kept sterile.
Connect tubing to fluid reservoir and flush tubing with fluid.	All air must be removed from tubing.
Prepare the Patient	
Explain procedure.	Be alert for questions and concerns.
Position patient, raise bed to working height, adjust lighting for good visualization.	

(Continued)

TABLE 13–19
Procedure for Starting an Intravenous Infusion (*Continued*)

Procedure	Comments
Prepare the Site	
Choose hand or arm vein (Fig. 13–9).	Use nondominant side if possible to avoid interfering with daily activities. Choose most distal site available to save sites for subsequent infusions. Find straight section of vein without valves. Avoid leg veins, because of risk of thrombophlebitis.
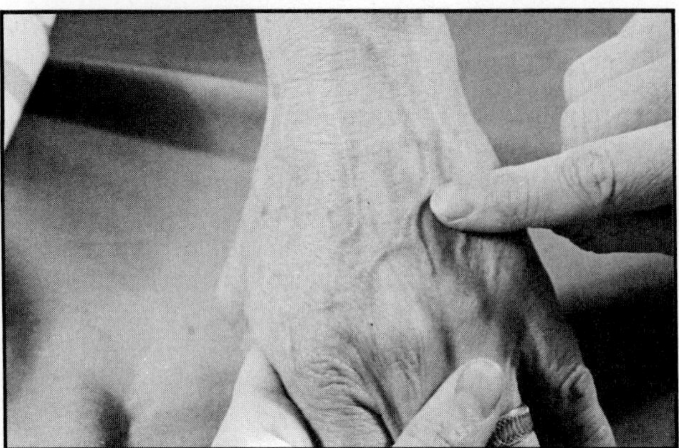 **FIGURE 13–9**	
Apply tourniquet to arm above injection site.	Occlude venous return but not arterial flow (pulse should be palpable).
Scrub injection site with iodine solution (70% alcohol if hypersensitive to iodine), using outward circular motion. Wipe off iodine with alcohol. Let dry.	Site scrubbing procedure and solution vary with institutional policy.
Perform the Venipuncture	
Hold skin taut over injection site with thumb and fingers of nondominant hand encircling the extremity from beneath (Fig. 13–10). Hold needle with bevel up at 45° angle to skin. Pierce skin. Lower needle until almost parallel to skin. Pierce vein and advance needle.	
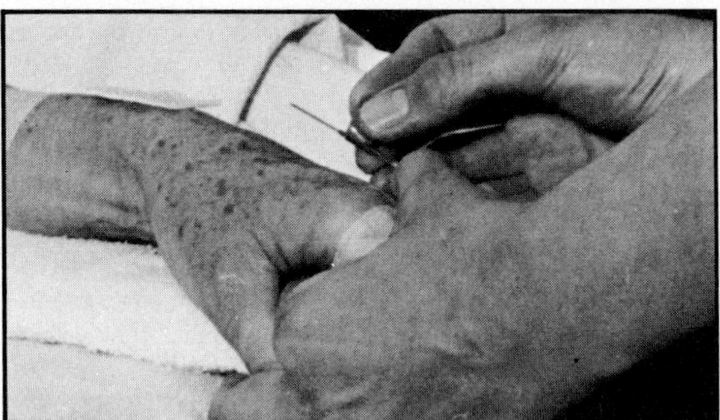 **FIGURE 13–10**	
If using over-the-needle catheter, slide catheter into vein while holding hub of needle.	To avoid breaking catheter, do not pull catheter back onto the needle or push needle back into catheter.
Release tourniquet. Quickly attach tubing and begin infusion by opening clamp. Place sterile gauze under hub.	

(*Continued*)

TABLE 13–19
Procedure for Starting an Intravenous Infusion (*Continued*)

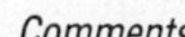

Procedure	*Comments*
Tape needle securely.	Use chevron or other taping method. Do not tape over vein where catheter or needle tip rests.
Cover site with sterile gauze, plastic bandage, or transparent dressing.	Institutional procedures vary; some use antimicrobial ointment. Do not occlude circulation by taping around limb.
Loop and tape tubing (Fig. 13–11).	Prevents dislodging if tubing is pulled.
Regulate infusion to previously calculated drip rate.	

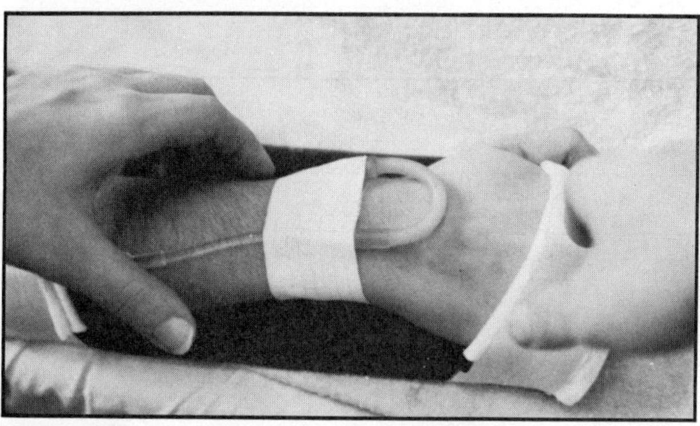

FIGURE 13–11

Procedure	*Comments*
Document the Procedure	
Label the infusion site with date, length and type of cannula, initials.	Write on tape at edge of dressing.
Apply tape label with date to tubing.	Do not write on tape over vein.
Label fluid reservoir clearly if it contains potassium (Fig. 13–12).	
Mark times and expected fluid levels on fluid reservoir.	
Record date, time, site, and type of needle or cannula in patient's chart.	

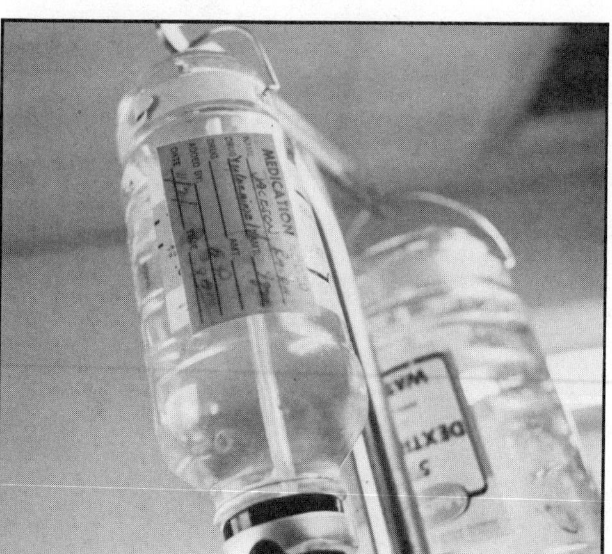

FIGURE 13–12

The procedure may be modified to meet the individual situation as long as the principles of strict asepsis are maintained.[28] As the procedure notes, care must be taken to provide the correct solution. Common types of intravenous solutions are described in Table 13–20.

Once the intravenous infusion has been started, it is necessary to *manage the flow rate* so that it will infuse over the allotted time period.[58] Too rapid infusion may cause saline excess, water excess, or an electrolyte excess, depending on the solution infusing. Too slow an infusion may deprive the patient of needed fluid and electrolytes. The drip rate for an infusion may be calculated from the following formula:

$$\frac{\text{gtt/ml delivered by equipment} \times \text{ml solution to be infused in 1 hr}}{\text{60 min/hr}} = \text{gtt/min}$$

The infusion drip rate needs to be checked frequently, as change in patient position and other factors may alter the flow rate. The flow rate of a fluid is increased by increasing the diameter of the tubing and needle or raising the height of the fluid reservoir above the infusion site.[12] Use of extension tubing decreases flow by increasing tubing length. Infusion pumps may be employed to regulate flow; they also require frequent monitoring.[24]

TABLE 13–20
Common Intravenous Solutions

Solution	*Tonicity*	*Comments*
D5W (5% dextrose in water)	Hypotonic effect after sugar enter cells	Provides water and calories (200 kcal/liter) Contains no electrolytes.
Normal saline (0.9% saline)	Isotonic	Adds saline to body Expands extracellular volume
Half-normal saline (0.45% saline)	Hypotonic	Provides water and NaCl
D5 $\frac{1}{2}$NS (5% dextrose in 0.45% saline)	Hypotonic effect after sugar enters cells	Maintenance fluid Provides water, NaCl, and calories
D5 $\frac{1}{4}$NS (5% dextrose in 0.225% saline)	Hypotonic effect after sugar enters cells	Provides water, NaCl, and calories
Balanced isotonic solution (Normosol-R, Plasma-lyte 148, Polyonic-R 148)	Isotonic	Extracellular fluid replacement Contains Na^+, K^+, Mg^{++}, Cl^-, acetate, gluconate Provides HCO_3^- by metabolism of acetate and gluconate
Ringer's solution	Isotonic	Electrolyte content (Na^+, K^+, Ca^{++}, Cl^-) similar to plasma Contains no Mg^{++} Expands extracellular volume
Lactated Ringer's solution	Isotonic	Ringer's solution with lactate (HCO_3^- source) Prevents or treats mild acidosis
Maintenance electrolyte solution (Plasma-lyte 56 in D5W, Normosol-M in D5W, Polyonic-M in D5W, Isolyte-H in D5W)	Hypotonic	Maintenance solution Contains Na^+, K^+, Mg^{++}, Cl^-, acetate Provides HCO_3^- by metabolism of acetate
Gastric replacement solution (Ionosol G with 10% dextrose, Isolyte G with 10% dextrose)	Isotonic after sugar enters cells	Replaces gastric fluid loss Contains Na^+, K^+, Cl^-, NH_4^+, sugar Provides H^+ by dissociation of NH_4^+ Low *p*H irritates veins
Duodenal replacement solution (Ionosol D-CM, Polysal, Isolyte E)	Isotonic	Replaces duodenal fluid loss Contains Na^+, K^+, Ca^{++}, Mg^{++}, Cl^-, and HCO_3^- source (acetate, citrate, or lactate)

In addition to managing infusion flow rate, nursing responsibilities include *monitoring for the complications of intravenous therapy*. These complications are infection, inflammation, infiltration, air embolism, and saline, osmolality, or electrolyte imbalances caused by excessive or inappropriate infusion.[43,60] Preventive measures, assessment, and nursing actions if these complications occur are presented in Table 13–21.

When *discontinuing an intravenous infusion*, careful technique will prevent hemorrhage and catheter embolism. Ascertain whether a plastic catheter has been inserted and, if so, what length. Untape the tubing and needle hub, being careful to stabilize the needle or catheter. Do not put pressure on the vein while withdrawing the needle (to prevent damage to the vein) but as soon as it is removed, apply firm pressure with a dry sterile gauze. Measure the length of a plastic cannula to check that it has been removed intact.

Summary

With the use of careful aseptic technique and frequent assessment and monitoring, nurses can help to minimize the hazards of intravenous therapy while maximizing the therapeutic benefits.

TABLE 13–21
Complications of IV Therapy: Prevention, Assessment, Interventions

Complication	*Prevention*	*Assessment*	*Action*
Infection			
May be localized or systemic. Piercing the skin provides entry route for microorganisms.	Use careful aseptic technique when starting infusion and when changing tubing or fluid reservoir. Examine bottle or bag for cracks and cloudiness of solution. Replace fluid reservoir and tubing every 48 hours. Discontinue infusion started during emergency under poor asepsis; replace, using aseptic technique. Use antimicrobial ointment if within institutional protocol.	Inspect infusion site daily for heat, redness, swelling, pain, discharge. Be alert for chills, elevated temperature.	Discontinue infusion. Save infusion set for possible culture.
Inflammation			
More common with acidic or hypertonic solutions. Plastic catheters are more irritating than steel needles.	Anchor cannula firmly to prevent mechanical irritation. Dilute irritating solutions as much as possible. Avoid leg veins due to risk of thrombophlebitis with subsequent pulmonary embolism.	Inspect infusion site daily for heat, redness, swelling, pain (phlebitis), and hard, cordlike vein (thrombophlebitis).	Discontinue infusion. Apply moist heat to area.
Infiltration			
Caused by infusion of fluid into subcutaneous tissue rather than into vein. Some solutions may cause sloughing of tissue.	Anchor cannula firmly to prevent tip from penetrating vein wall. Use armboard if movement might cause needle to penetrate vein wall.	Inspect area around infusion site for cold, hard swelling. Compare with opposite extremity to verify swelling. Obstruct vein proximal to infusion; infusion will continue dripping if infiltrated.	Discontinue infusion.
Air Embolism			
Caused by introduction of large quantity of air into circulation.	*Peripheral Lines:* Flush tubing with fluid before connecting.	Be alert for sudden onset of dyspnea, hypotension, chest pain, hemoptysis, cyanosis,	Clamp tubing. Turn person on left side with head down to trap air in right

(*Continued*)

TABLE 13–21
Complications of IV Therapy: Prevention, Assessment, Interventions (Continued)

Complication	*Prevention*	*Assessment*	*Action*
Air Embolism			
A common fear of hospitalized patients. More common with central lines than with regular peripheral infusions.	Check that connections are secure. Replace rigid fluid reservoir before completely empty to prevent air entry into tubing. (Flexible bags collapse and prevent this problem.) Reassure patient and explain precautions. *Central Lines:* Place patient in Trendelenburg's position and instruct to perform Valsalva maneuver during catheter insertion or removal or tubing change. Tape connections firmly.	decreasing level of consciousness, mill wheel murmur (air in right ventricle).	heart. Notify physician. Administer oxygen.
Saline, Osmolality, or Electrolyte Imbalance			
Caused by excessive or inappropriate infusion.	Calculate drip rate to deliver solution accurately. Mark fluid reservoir with time and expected fluid levels. If solution contains KCl or other additives, mark reservoir with colored sticker or tape.	Monitor drip rate frequently. Assess for signs and symptoms of likely imbalances, depending on solution being infused.	Readjust drip rate. Decrease drip rate to minimum level. Notify physician. Take independent nursing actions appropriate to the particular imbalance.

References

1. Adams C, Richardson M: Nutritive value of foods. USDA Home and Garden Bulletin No. 72. Washington, DC, US Government Printing Office, 1977
2. Aderka D et al: Life-threatening hypophosphatemia in a patient with acute myelogenous leukemia. Acta Haematol 64:117, 1980
3. Bartter F: Clinical problems of potassium metabolism. Contrib Nephrol 21:115, 1980
4. Blachley J, Knochel J: Tobacco chewer's hypokalemia: Licorice revisited. NEJM 302:784, 1980
5. Cabizuca S, Desser K: Carbenicillin-associated hypokalemic alkalosis. JAMA 236:956, 1976
6. Cohen L et al: Acute tumor lysis syndrome. Am J Med 68:486, 1980
7. Cumming AM et al: Severe hypokalemia with paralysis induced by small doses of liquorice. Postgrad Med 56:516, 1980
8. Cunningham SG: Fluid and electrolyte disturbances associated with cancer and its treatment. NCNA 17:579, 1982
9. Dailey R: Line into veins. Emerg Med 15:167, 1983
10. DeFronzo R, Felig P, Ferrannini E, Wahren J: Effects of graded doses of insulin on splanchnic and peripheral potassium metabolism in man. Am J Physiol 238:E-421, 1980
11. Delapenha RA et al: The bioavailability of potassium in bananas. West Indian Med J 29:117, 1980
12. Erickson R: Tube talk: Principles of fluid flow in tubes. Nursing 82 12:54, 1982
13. Felver L: Understanding the electrolyte maze. Am J Nurs 80:1591, 1980
14. Felver L: Electrolytes across the age continuum—implications for the practicing nurse. Wash State J Nurs 52:19, 1980
15. Felver L: Nursing assessment of hypomagnesemia in chronic alcoholism. Proceedings of the Third Annual National Conference for Nurse Educators on Alcohol and Drug Abuse. New York, National Council on Alcoholism, 1984
16. Frazier T et al: Hypomagnesemia: Higher risk using total parenteral nutrition in the treatment of patients with malignancies. J Surg Oncol 13:35, 1980
17. Gilman AG, Goodman LS, Gilman A: The Pharmacological Basis of Therapeutics, 6th ed. New York, Macmillan, 1980
18. Glimp R et al: Hypocalcemia associated with oral phosphate replacement therapy. JAMA 243:731, 1980
19. Graber T et al: Magnesium: Physiology, clinical disorders, and therapy. Ann Emerg Med 10:49, 1981
20. Halperin ML et al: Interpretation of the serum potassium concentration in metabolic acidosis. Clin Invest Med 2:55, 1979
21. Hariprased M et al: Hyponatremia in psychogenic polydipsia. Arch Intern Med 140:1639, 1980
22. Hickey RC, Samaan NA, Jackson GL: Hypercalcemia in patients with breast cancer. Arch Surg 116:545, 1981
23. Hodkinson HM: Biochemical Diagnosis of the Elderly. New York, John Wiley and Sons, 1977
24. Huey F: Setting up and troubleshooting IV pumps and controllers. Am J Nurs 83:1026, 1983
25. Insogna K et al: Osteomalacia and weakness from excessive antacid ingestion. JAMA 244:2544, 1980
26. Isaacs M: Life-threatening fluid and electrolytes in patients with cancer. Curr Probl Cancer 4:6, 1979
27. Jose CJ, Evenson R: Antecedents of self-induced water intoxication. J Nerv Ment Dis 168:498, 1980

28. Kaye W: Catheter- and infusion-related sepsis: The nature of the problem and its prevention. Heart Lung 11:227, 1982
29. Kaye W: Intravenous techniques. Heart Lung 11:306, 1982
30. Kleeman C: CNS manifestations of disordered salt and water balance. Hosp Pract 14:59, 1979
31. Knochel J: The pathophysiology and clinical characteristics of severe hypophosphatemia. Arch Intern Med 137:203, 1977
32. Knox F et al: Physiology of calcium and phosphate regulation. Physiologist 23:1, 1980
33. Kopp U, DiBona G: Diagnosis: Edema. Hosp Med 18:51, 1982
34. Kovalik SG et al: The cardiac effect of altered calcium homeostasis after albumin resuscitation. J Trauma 21:275, 1981
35. Krause MV, Mahan LK: Food, Nutrition, and Diet Therapy, 7th ed. Philadelphia, W B Saunders, 1984
36. Kukreja S: Diagnosis and management of hypercalcemia. Compr Ther 6:33, 1980
37. Lukert B: Hypercalcemia. Crit Care Q 3:11, 1980
38. Main AN et al: Magnesium status and intravenous requirements in patients with chronic inflammatory bowel disease requiring intravenous nutrition. Proc Nutr Soc 39:32-A, 1980
39. Majumdar S: Serum magnesium in delirium tremens. Am J Psychiatr 136:1343, 1979
40. Mather HM et al: Hypomagnesemia in diabetes. Clin Chim Acta 95:235, 1979
41. Miller P et al: Hypodipsia in geriatric patients. Am J Med 73:354, 1982
42. Moore-Ede M et al: Circadian variation in response to potassium infusion. Clin Pharmacol Ther 23:218, 1978
43. Ostrow LS: Air embolism and central venous lines. Am J Nurs 81:2036, 1981
44. Otrakji J: Potassium metabolism disorders. Crit Care Q 3:55, 1980
45. Pflaum SS: Investigation of intake–output as a means of assessing body fluid balance. Heart Lung 8:495, 1979
46. Pollock A, Arieff A: Abnormalities of cell volume regulation and their functional consequences. Am J Physiol 239:195, 1980
47. Rao T et al: Serum potassium levels following transfusion of frozen erythrocytes. Anesthesiology 52:170, 1980
48. Rastogi S, Arruda J: Hypocalcemia: Its clinical manifestations point to the diagnosis. Consultant 23:92, 1983
49. Ratzan R: Uncovering magnesium toxicity. Geriatrics 35:75, 1980
50. Reubi FC: Hemodynamic changes in isotonic dehydration. Contrib Nephrol 21:55, 1980
51. Rose BD: Clinical Physiology of Acid–Base and Electrolyte Disorders, 2nd ed. New York, McGraw-Hill, 1984
52. Rowe J et al: Influence of the emetic reflex on vasopressin release in man. Kidney Int 16:729, 1979
53. Rumancik W et al: The QT interval and serum ionized calcium. JAMA 240:366, 1978
54. Simon G, Boue J: The potassium load from blood transfusions. Postgrad Med 49:61, 1971
55. Simon R, Freedman D: Neurologic manifestations of osmolar disorders. Geriatrics 35:71, 1980
56. Skorecki K, Brenner B: Body fluid homeostasis in man: A contemporary overview. Am J Med 70:77, 1981
57. Sopko J, Freeman R: Salt substitutes as a source of potassium. JAMA 238:608, 1977
58. Steel J: Too fast or too slow—the erratic IV. Am J Nurs 83:898, 1983
59. Sterns RH et al: Internal potassium balance and the control of the plasma potassium concentration. Medicine 60:339, 1981
60. Stratton C: Infection related to intravenous infusions. Heart Lung 11:123, 1982
61. Sullivan L, Grantham J: Physiology of the Kidney, 2nd ed. Philadelphia, Lea & Febiger, 1982
62. Szyfelbein SK et al: Persistent ionized hypocalcemia in patient during resuscitation and recovery phases of body burns. Crit Care Med 9:454, 1981
63. Tepper D, Aronson R: Effects of potassium and calcium abnormalities. Hosp Med 20:111, 1984
64. Tully JL et al: Complications of intravenous therapy with steel needles and teflon catheters. Am J Med 70:702, 1981
65. Udezue EO, Harrold BP: Hyperkalemic paralysis due to spironolactone. Postgrad Med J 56:254, 1980
66. Underhill S et al: Cardiac Nursing. Philadelphia, J B Lippincott, 1982
67. Vilchez J et al: Hyperkalemic paralysis, neuropathy, and persistent motor neuron discharges at rest in Addison's disease. J Neurol Neurosurg Psychiatry 43:818, 1980
68. Warren S, O'Connor D: Hyperkalemia resulting from captopril administration. JAMA 244:2551, 1980
69. Wiberg J et al: Effect of phosphate or magnesium cathartics on serum calcium. Arch Intern Med 138:1114, 1978
70. Wiegand C et al: Severe hypokalemia induced by hemodialysis. Arch Intern Med 141:167, 1981
71. Williams R: Potassium overdosage: A potential hazard of nonrigid parenteral fluid containers. Br Med J 1:714, 1973

Chapter 14

Acid–Base Balance and Imbalances

Linda Felver

The degree of acidity of body fluids has a great influence on the ability of cells, and thus the body, to function. Alterations in acidity affect both metabolic processes (by altering enzyme activity) and tissue oxygenation (by altering the binding of oxygen to hemoglobin).

Acidity as measured in the clinical setting is a reflection of the hydrogen ion concentration. The more hydrogen ions present, the more acid the blood. The hydrogen ion concentration of arterial blood is 37 to 43×10^{-9} moles/liter.[19] Because the hydrogen ion concentration of body fluids is very small, pH is customarily reported instead of the hydrogen ion concentration. Technically, the pH of a solution is the negative logarithm of the hydrogen ion concentration. Practically, the pH is a straightforward concept to interpret. The pH of a solution can vary from 1 to 14, with 7.0 being neutral (neither acidic nor alkaline). A solution with a high hydrogen ion concentration is an acid solution. A pH below 7.0 denotes an acid solution. The pH of gastric fluid, for example, is around 1 or 2. A pH above 7.0 denotes an alkaline (basic) solution. The fluid in the small intestine, made alkaline by bicarbonate ions from pancreatic secretions, has a pH range of 7.0 to 8.0. If the pH of a solution decreases, the solution has become more acidic; if the pH increases, the solution has become more alkaline.

The normal pH of the blood, for adults of all ages, ranges from 7.35 to 7.45. Note that normal blood is always slightly alkaline. The body has three physiological mechanisms for maintaining pH within this normal range: buffers, lungs, and kidneys.

Buffers. Buffers are pairs of chemicals that act to neutralize small changes in pH. Important buffers are

$\frac{HCO_3^{-2}}{H_2CO_3}$	Bicarbonate buffer system (found in extracellular fluid)
$\frac{Hb^-}{HHb}$	Hemoglobin buffer system (found inside red blood cells)
$\frac{HPO_4^{-2}}{H_2PO_4}$ and $\frac{PO_4^{-3}}{HPO_4^{-2}}$	Phosphate buffer systems (most important inside cells and in the urine)
$\frac{Pr^-}{HPr}$	Protein buffer system (found in plasma and inside cells)

Buffers are the immediate defense against pH change. If there is a decrease in pH (blood too acid), then the basic portion of the buffer pair will combine with the hydrogen ion (H^+). If there is an increase in pH (blood too alkaline), the acidic portion of the buffer pair releases hydrogen ions (H^+).

Lungs. The lungs excrete carbonic acid as carbon dioxide and water. The respiratory system regulates the Pa_{CO_2} of the blood (partial pressure of carbon dioxide). When there is a decrease in pH, there is an increase in rate and depth of respiration to remove the carbonic acid from the body. When there is an increase in pH, meaning the blood is too alkaline, there is a decrease in the rate and depth of respiration to retain carbonic acid in the body.

Kidneys. The renal tubular cells excrete metabolic acids by secretion of hydrogen ions (H^+) and reabsorption of bicarbonate (HCO_3^-). Production of ammonia (NH_3) by the renal tubular cells is another acid excretion mechanism. NH_3 diffuses into the tubular fluid where it combines with H^+ to form ammonium ions (NH_4^+). NH_4^+ effectively traps H^+ and is excreted in the urine. H^+ secreted into the tubular fluid either combines with NH_3 or is buffered (principally by phosphate buffers). The kidneys regulate the HCO_3^- concentration of the blood. When the blood becomes too acidic (decrease in pH), there is increased secretion of H^+ from the extracellular fluid into the renal tubular fluid. There is also increased reabsorption of HCO_3^- from the renal tubular fluid into the extracellular fluid. Production of NH_3 also increases. When the blood becomes too alkaline (increase in pH) there is a decreased secretion of H^+, a decreased reabsorption of HCO_3^-, and a decreased production of NH_3.[2, 17, 19]

In order to maintain the normal pH of the blood, it is necessary to have 20 bicarbonate ions (HCO_3^-) for every one carbonic acid molecule (H_2CO_3). It is customary to speak of this relationship as the 20 : 1 ratio of bicarbonate to carbonic acid. If the 20 : 1 relationship is maintained, the pH of the blood is normal; if, however, the ratio is altered, then a pH imbalance has occurred.* This important relationship is the key to understanding what occurs when a pH imbalance develops. If, for example, too much HCO_3^- accumulates in the blood, the pH will be abnormal. The body can respond to this problem in two ways. First, it can take direct action through the kidneys to return the HCO_3^- concentration to normal, thus restoring the 20 : 1 ratio and the pH to normal. This is called *correction* of the problem. During correction of an acid–base imbalance, the body uses its pH-maintaining mechanisms to restore the blood chemistry to normal.

The second type of response to an acid–base imbalance is termed *compensation.* If the pH of the extracellular fluid becomes too abnormal, death will occur. A pH below 6.9 is usually fatal; at the other extreme, a pH above 7.8 has the same effect. In order to keep the pH from reaching the fatal limit when an imbalance occurs, the body's compensatory mechanisms are activated. The process of compensation works to return the pH toward normal, although it may produce a further abnormality of blood chemistry. For example, if too much HCO_3^- again accumulates in the blood, the body can take action through the lungs to increase the carbonic acid concentration of the blood as well. This action certainly does not restore the blood chemistry to normal, but it may repair the 20 : 1 ratio of HCO_3^- to H_2CO_3. (Remember, if both top and bottom numbers of a ratio are increased by the same multiple, the ratio value remains the same.) The *ratio* of bicarbonate ion to carbonic acid concentration, not the absolute concentrations themselves, determines the pH of the blood. If, through the process of compensation, the body restores this important ratio toward normal, then the pH will also return toward normal, even if the other blood values are still outside their normal ranges. The specific mechanisms of compensation are discussed with each of the four major pH imbalances: two kinds of acidosis and two kinds of alkalosis.

* The Henderson-Hasselbalch equation, an expression for computing the pH of a buffered solution, shows the relationship between pH and the $HCO_3^- : H_2CO_3$ ratio.

$$pH = pK_a + \log\frac{[HCO_3^-]}{[H_2CO_3]}$$

The pH of the blood equals the dissociation constant of carbonic acid plus the logarithm of the ratio of the bicarbonate ion concentration to the carbonic acid concentration. Substituting numbers into the equation demonstrates the importance of a 20 : 1 ratio for a normal pH.

$(pK_a - 6.1; \log 20 = 1.3)$

$$pH = 6.1 + \log\frac{20}{1} \quad \text{(note the 20 : 1 ratio)}$$

$$pH = 6.1 + 1.3$$

$$pH = 7.4$$

Acidosis

Acidosis is the presence of any process that tends to decrease the pH of the blood below the normal range. During acidosis, therefore, the pH of the blood is often abnormally low. Since the suffix *-emia* refers to the blood, such a low blood pH is known as *acidemia.* It is possible, however, to have acidosis (condition tending to decrease blood pH) without acidemia (actual low blood pH). Acidosis without acidemia occurs when the body's pH regulatory mechanisms have returned the pH to normal (full compensation) without correcting the underlying acidotic process. It may also occur with mixed pH imbalances.

There are two major kinds of acidosis: respiratory acidosis (carbonic acid excess) and metabolic acidosis (noncarbonic acid excess). Although the clinical manifestations of these two types of acidosis have some similarities, they have very different causes and different compensatory mechanisms.

Respiratory Acidosis (Carbonic Acid Excess)

The lungs normally excrete carbonic acid (H_2CO_3) from the body in the form of carbon dioxide (CO_2) and water (H_2O). The carbon dioxide, a product of cellular metabolism, is carried in the blood primarily in the form of bicarbonate ion (HCO_3^-), which is reconverted to carbonic acid (H_2CO_3) and then to carbon dioxide and water in the capillaries of the lungs. In chemical notation, this is written as follows:

$$CO_2 + H_2O \rightarrow H_2CO_3 \rightarrow H^+ + HCO_3^- \rightarrow H_2CO_3 \rightarrow CO_2 + H_2O$$

Produced by cells	Carried in the blood	Excreted by lungs

If the lungs fail to excrete the carbon dioxide that is being produced by cellular metablism, carbonic acid (H_2CO_3) accumulates in the blood. This condition of carbonic acid excess is respiratory acidosis. The normal 20 : 1 ratio of bicarbonate ion concentration to carbonic acid concentration has been disrupted.

Causes of respiratory acidosis are decreased gaseous exchange, impaired neuromuscular function of the chest, and suppression of neural ventilatory mechanisms in the brain stem. Table 14–1 presents specific examples of disorders that fall into each of these categories.[5,10,17,19] The respiratory system can be considered as a gaseous exchanger, a neuromuscular pump, and a central regulator in the brain stem. Impairment in any of these areas diminishes the ability to excrete carbon dioxide and water (carbonic acid); respiratory acidosis results.

TABLE 14–1
Causes of Respiratory Acidosis (Carbonic Acid Excess)

General Etiology: Decreased Gaseous Exchange
Specific examples:
Decreased alveolar ventilation
Chronic obstructive pulmonary disease
Emphysema
Severe asthma
Sleep apnea (obstructive type)
Atelectasis
Pneumonia
Adult respiratory distress syndrome
Pulmonary edema
Hypoventilation by way of mechanical ventilator

General Etiology: Impaired Neuromuscular Function of Chest
Specific examples:
Chest injury
Surgical incision (pain limits respirations)
Poliomyelitis
Guillain-Barré syndrome
Respiratory muscle fatigue
Myasthenia gravis
Hypokalemia
Kyphoscoliosis
Pickwickian syndrome (obesity limits chest expansion)

General Etiology: Suppression of Neural Ventilatory Mechanisms in Brain Stem (Medulla)
Specific examples:
Narcotics
Barbiturates
Sleep apnea (central type)

Clinical Manifestations. When carbon dioxide accumulates in the blood, the Pa_{CO_2} of the blood increases. The concurrent accumulation of carbonic acid decreases the pH of the blood. The resulting clinical manifestations include

Increased Pa_{CO_2}
Headache
Blurred vision
Disorientation
Tachycardia
Cardiac arrhythmias
Lethargy
Somnolence

The decreased pH of the cerebrospinal fluid alters enzyme activity, causing central nervous system depression. Increased Pa_{CO_2} causes dilation of the cerebral blood vessels, resulting in headache. As acid accumulates, hydrogen ions move from the extracellular fluid into the cells, where they are buffered. At the same time, potassium ions move in the opposite direction. Hyperkalemia, caused by this movement of potassium ions from cells into the extracellular fluid, often accompanies respiratory acidosis. The signs and symptoms of hyperkalemia are presented in Chapter 13.

When respiratory acidosis develops, the buffers have been unable to keep the pH within the normal range. The respiratory system is the cause of the problem. In respiratory acidosis, therefore, the kidneys are the remaining physiological mechanism available for compensation. In order to *correct* the imbalance, the respiratory system would need to excrete the excess carbonic acid. The kidneys cannot excrete carbonic acid but they can excrete other acids, thus moving the pH toward normal in *compensation.* As the kidneys excrete these hydrogen ions, the bicarbonate ion concentration of the blood increases. This increase of bicarbonate ion begins to restore the normal 20 : 1 ratio of bicarbonate ion to carbonic acid. As this concentration ratio approaches 20:1, the pH approaches normal. Table 14–2, which describes

TABLE 14–2
Laboratory Values in Respiratory Acidosis

	Uncompensated Respiratory Acidosis	*Partially Compensated Respiratory Acidosis*	*Fully Compensated Respiratory Acidosis*
Pa_{CO_2}	Increased	Increased	Increased
HCO_3^-	Normal	Increasing	Increased
$\frac{[HCO_3^-]}{[H_2CO_3]}$	$\frac{\text{Normal}}{\text{Increased}}$ $\left(\text{less than } \frac{20}{1}\right)$	$\frac{\text{Increasing}}{\text{Increased}}$	$\frac{\text{Increased}}{\text{Increased}}$ $\left(\text{equals } \frac{20}{1}\right)$
pH	Decreased	Moving toward normal	Normal

the laboratory values in respiratory acidosis, illustrates these changes. This renal compensation process takes several days.

Nursing Implications. Nursing care of persons who have developed respiratory acidosis is threefold in its approach: ongoing assessment, administration of the medical therapy, and nursing measures to improve alveolar ventilation. Medical therapy for respiratory acidosis involves treatment of the original cause to restore adequate ventilation or mechanical ventilation. If necessary, the excess acidity can be neutralized with intravenous sodium bicarbonate. Nursing measures to improve ventilation are vitally important for both prevention and treatment of respiratory acidosis. These measures are described in Chapter 32.

Metabolic Acidosis (Noncarbonic Acid Excess)

In contrast to respiratory acidosis (an excess of carbonic acid), metabolic acidosis occurs when there is an accumulation of any other kind of acid in the blood. The term *noncarbonic* is often used to denote all acids except carbonic acid when referring to metabolic acidosis. Examples of acids that may cause metabolic acidosis are lactic, sulfuric, citric, oxalic, acetylsalicylic, and beta-hydroxybutyric acids.

Acids such as those listed above are normally excreted by the kidneys. Impaired acid excretion is one cause of metabolic acidosis. Elderly persons are slightly more at risk for developing metabolic acidosis because it takes their kidneys longer to excrete an acid load. Other causes of metabolic acidosis are increased production of metabolic acids, utilization of abnormal or incomplete metabolic pathways, and ingestion of acids or acid precursors. These four causes of metabolic acidosis all involve accumulation of acid in the blood. It is also possible to develop metabolic acidosis by diminishing the amount of base (bicarbonate ion) in the blood, thus creating a relative acid excess. Table 14–3 gives specific examples of these five general causes of metabolic acidosis.[2,3,5,8,11,16,17,18,19,20,23]

As metabolic acidosis develops, the bicarbonate concentration of the blood decreases. This decrease is caused either directly by removal of bicarbonate from the body or indirectly when accumulating acids use up the available bicarbonate buffer. As the bicarbonate concentration decreases, the normal 20 : 1 bicarbonate ion–carbonic acid ratio is decreased and the pH of the blood decreases. A pH under 6.9 is usually fatal.

Clinical Manifestations. Clinical manifestations of metabolic acidosis arise from the decrease in cerebrospinal fluid pH, causing central nervous system depression and the following signs and symptoms:

- Decreased bicarbonate ion concentration
- Hyperventilation (compensatory mechanism)
- Headache
- Abdominal pain
- Confusion
- Drowsiness
- Lethargy
- Stupor
- Coma
- Cardiac arrhythmias

TABLE 14–3
Causes of Metabolic Acidosis (Noncarbonic Acid Excess)

General Etiology: Acid Accumulation by Ingestion of Acid or Acid Precursors
Specific examples:
Aspirin (acetylsalicylic acid)
Methanol (converted to formic acid)
Ethylene glycol (converted to oxalic acid)
Paraldehyde (converted to acetic and chloroacetic acids)
Boric acid
Elemental sulfur (sulfuric acid)
Ammonium chloride (releases H^+)

General Etiology: Acid Accumulation by Increased Production of Metabolic Acids
Specific examples:
Hyperthyroidism
Hypermetabolic state after burns or trauma
Lactic acidosis
Shock

General Etiology: Acid Accumulation by Utilization of Abnormal or Incomplete Metabolic Pathways
Specific examples:
Diabetic ketoacidosis
Alcoholic ketoacidosis
Starvation ketoacidosis

General Etiology: Acid Accumulation by Impaired Acid Excretion
Specific examples:
Oliguric renal failure
Severe hypovolemia
Shock
Hypoaldosteronism

General Etiology: Primary Decrease of Bicarbonate
Specific examples:
Urinary route: Renal tubular acidosis
Gastrointestinal route
  Severe diarrhea
  Intestinal decompression
  Ureterosigmoidostomy
  Fistula drainage
  Vomiting of intestinal contents
  Cholestyramine therapy

Neurological signs may be less pronounced in metabolic acidosis than in respiratory acidosis because the cerebrospinal fluid pH changes less rapidly in metabolic disorders (CO_2 enters cerebrospinal fluid more easily than does HCO_3^-). Hyperkalemia often accompanies metabolic acidosis.[6]

When metabolic acidosis occurs, the buffers have been unable to prevent the abnormal alteration in pH. The kidneys, which are supposed to excrete all acids except carbonic acid, are either dysfunctional or are overwhelmed. Of the three body mechanisms for maintaining pH, therefore, only the lungs are able to work effectively. Although the respiratory system is unable to excrete the metabolic acids (and thus correct the imbalance), it is able to excrete carbonic acid and compensate for the abnormally low pH. The excretion of carbonic acid is accomplished by hyperventilation (deep rapid breathing). Respiratory compensation for metabolic acidosis restores pH by restoring the

20:1 ratio of bicarbonate ions to carbonic acid. Table 14–4 illustrates the progress of respiratory compensation for metabolic acidosis. The process usually takes several hours.

Nursing Implications. Nursing care related to metabolic acidosis includes preventive measures, ongoing assessment, administration of the medical therapy, and monitoring for the complications of therapy. Knowledge of the causes of metabolic acidosis makes possible the identification of those persons at high risk who need preventive measures. Examples of such measures to prevent metabolic acidosis are diet and insulin teaching for diabetics, provision of safe weight control information (prolonged fasting leads to starvation ketoacidosis), poison prevention measures, promotion of urine output in oliguric states, and measures to avert severe hypovolemia and diarrhea.

The medical therapy for metabolic acidosis is treatment of the original cause and, if necessary, pH correction. The pH is usually kept above 7.1 to prevent fatal cardiac arrhythmias. The main agent used to elevate the pH is intravenous sodium bicarbonate.[7] Intravenous lactate, citrate, or acetate, agents that are converted to bicarbonate by the liver, may also be used. Oral bicarbonate or citrate may be administered in chronic metabolic acidosis. The major complications of this therapy are rebound metabolic alkalosis and tetany. Rebound metabolic alkalosis occurs from excess administration of bicarbonate or a bicarbonate source. The signs and symptoms of metabolic alkalosis are presented later in this chapter. Tetany may occur from hypocalcemia that arises during intravenous infusion of sodium bicarbonate when the increasing pH alters the physiological availability of calcium (see Chap. 13). Monitor Chvostek's sign during administration of bicarbonate to detect increasing neuromuscular irritability before it becomes tetany. If ampules of sodium bicarbonate are administered to combat metabolic acidosis (as during cardiopulmonary resuscitation), water deficit (gain of more salt than water) may result. The drug dichloroacetate, which increases hepatic lactate metabolism, may be administered in lactic acidosis.[21]

In addition to administration of the medical therapy and monitoring for complications of therapy, independent nursing actions are also appropriate for a person who has developed metabolic acidosis. Safety measures and frequent turning are important for persons who are stuporous. Persons who are hyperventilating may need frequent oral care to prevent discomfort from dry oral mucous membranes. Position these persons carefully to allow chest expansion, thus facilitating their respiratory compensation for metabolic acidosis.

Summary of Principles of Acidosis

Acidosis occurs when some process tends to decrease the pH of the blood (*i.e.,* make the blood more acid). Respiratory acidosis is due to impaired ability of the respiratory system to excrete carbonic acid (carbon dioxide and water). When respiratory acidosis occurs, the kidneys excrete metabolic acids, effectively raising the bicarbonate ion concentration of the blood. This compensatory mechanism restores the pH but does not correct the problem.

Metabolic acidosis is due to accumulation of any acid except carbonic acid or to decrease of bicarbonate ions. In such a case, the lungs serve as the compensatory mechanism. Hyperventilation in response to metabolic acidosis eliminates carbonic acid from the body and restores the pH, but it does not correct the original problem.

The clinical manifestations of acidosis are primarily the result of central nervous system depression, due to acidity of the cerebrospinal fluid. Medical therapy in acidosis is twofold: treatment of the underlying cause and pH correction if the pH drops too low. Nursing management of acidosis is fivefold: preventive measures, ongoing assessment, administration of medical therapy, monitoring for signs and symptoms of complications of therapy, and independent nursing actions for specific patient problems. The major focus of independent nursing actions for respiratory acidosis is improving ventilation. For metabolic acidosis, the major focus is safety and comfort measures.

Alkalosis

In contrast to acidosis, alkalosis is the presence of a process that tends to *increase* the pH of the blood above the normal range. Alkalemia, or a blood pH above the upper range of

TABLE 14–4
Laboratory Values in Metabolic Acidosis

	Uncompensated Metabolic Acidosis	*Partially Compensated Metabolic Acidosis*	*Fully Compensated Metabolic Acidosis*
Pa_{CO_2}	Normal	Decreasing	Decreased
HCO_3^-	Decreased	Decreased	Decreased
$\frac{[HCO_3^-]}{[H_2CO_3]}$	$\frac{\text{Decreased}}{\text{Normal}}$ (less than $\frac{20}{1}$)	$\frac{\text{Decreased}}{\text{Decreasing}}$	$\frac{\text{Decreased}}{\text{Decreased}}$ (equals $\frac{20}{1}$)
pH	Decreased	Moving toward normal	Normal

normal, denotes alkalosis. A fully compensated alkalosis, however, will not evidence alkalemia, as the pH has been returned to normal even while the alkalotic process continues.

Analogously with acidosis, there are two major types of alkalosis: respiratory alkalosis (carbonic acid deficit) and metabolic alkalosis (noncarbonic acid deficit). In each case, there is a compensatory mechanism to return the pH toward normal. As you might expect, the kidneys perform the compensation during respiratory alkalosis, whereas the lungs perform the compensation during metabolic alkalosis.

Respiratory Alkalosis (Carbonic Acid Deficit)

Respiratory alkalosis is a deficit of carbonic acid. Carbonic acid is normally excreted by the lungs. The excretion of carbonic acid is increased by increasing the rate and depth of respiration. If too much carbonic acid is excreted, the blood will become too alkaline; respiratory alkalosis has developed.

The primary cause of respiratory alkalosis is hyperventilation: abnormally increased rate and depth of respiration.[15] Examples of conditions causing hyperventilation leading to respiratory alkalosis are listed in Table 14–5.[5,10,17,19] Remember that hyperventilation is also the compensatory mechanism for metabolic acidosis. Indeed, the compensatory respiratory alkalosis produced in metabolic acidosis is what returns the pH toward the normal range. Hyperventilation seen clinically, then, may be the primary cause of a pH disorder (respiratory alkalosis) or it may be a compensatory mechanism for another underlying pH disorder (metabolic acidosis).

TABLE 14–5
Causes of Respiratory Alkalosis (Carbonic Acid Deficit)

General Etiology: Hyperventilation
Specific examples:
Anxiety or fear
Pain
Prolonged crying and gasping
Hypoxemia (high altitudes or pulmonary disease)
Some brain injuries
Hyperventilation by means of mechanical ventilator
Stimulation of neural ventilatory mechanisms in brain stem (medulla)
- High fever
- Meningitis
- Encephalitis
- Salicylates (overdose)
- Progesterone (high levels)
- Gram-negative septicemia

Clinical Manifestations. The signs and symptoms of respiratory alkalosis include

- Decreased Pa_{CO_2}
- Diaphoresis
- Lightheadedness
- Paresthesias (fingers, toes, circumoral)
- Muscle cramps
- Positive Chvostek's sign
- Positive Trousseau's sign
- Carpopedal spasm
- Tetany
- Syncope
- Cardiac arrhythmias

These manifestations are recognizable as due to increased neuromuscular excitability. Chvostek's sign is a useful assessment tool for increased neuromuscular excitability. (Chvostek's sign is elicited by tapping the facial nerve in front of the ear. If the corner of the mouth draws up in a grimace, the sign is positive, indicating increased neuromuscular irritability.) Respiratory alkalosis is often accompanied by severe hypophosphatemia (phosphate uptake into cells), hypokalemia (movement of potassium into cells), and effective hypocalcemia (decreased physiologically available calcium). Each of these electrolyte imbalances is discussed in detail in Chapter 13.

When respiratory alkalosis occurs, the buffers have been unable to maintain blood pH in the normal range. The respiratory system is the cause of the carbonic acid deficit. Compensation for the abnormally elevated pH will need to be performed by the kidneys. Renal compensation for a respiratory pH disorder requires several days. Many cases of respiratory alkalosis, however, are very short-lived. Thus, respiratory alkalosis may arise and be corrected (*i.e.,* original cause resolved) before full renal compensation occurs. With long-standing respiratory alkalosis, the kidneys compensate by decreasing their excretion of acid. Relatively more bicarbonate is excreted in the urine and blood bicarbonate concentration decreases, tending to restore the bicarbonate ion–carbonic acid ratio (and thus the pH) to normal. Table 14–6 depicts these changing laboratory values during compensation for respiratory alkalosis.

Nursing Interventions. Perhaps the most important nursing management technique for persons who have developed or are at risk for developing respiratory alkalosis is supportive listening to decrease the anxiety and fear that often underlie the hyperventilation. Pain control may also be valuable. Since hypoxemia may cause hyperventilation and thus respiratory alkalosis, nursing measures to improve ventilation (Chap. 27) may be important. Counting and having the person breathe with the nurse's respirations may be useful in slowing the rapid respiration rate unless it is caused by hypoxemia. In extreme cases, rebreathing the expired air by breathing into a paper bag may stop the hyperventilation by increasing the Pa_{CO_2} of the blood. Remember that it is inappropriate to attempt to stop hyperventilation if it is caused by hypoxemia; oxygenation must be improved first. Medical therapy for respiratory alkalosis centers on correction of the underlying disorder.

Metabolic Alkalosis (Noncarbonic Acid Deficit)

Metabolic alkalosis, the other type of alkalosis, is a deficit of any acid except carbonic acid. For this reason, it may be called noncarbonic acid deficit. A deficit of hydrochloric acid, for example, may result from loss of gastric acid through vomiting or nasogastric suction.

The causes of metabolic alkalosis are listed in Table 14–7.[1,4,12,17,19] Either a decrease of acid or an increase of

TABLE 14–6
Laboratory Values in Respiratory Alkalosis

	Uncompensated Respiratory Alkalosis	*Partially Compensated Respiratory Alkalosis*	*Fully Compensated Respiratory Alkalosis*
Pa_{CO_2}	Decreased	Decreased	Decreased
HCO_3^-	Normal	Decreased	Decreased
$\frac{[HCO_3^-]}{[H_2CO_3]}$	$\frac{\text{Normal}}{\text{Decreased}}\left(\text{greater than } \frac{20}{1}\right)$	$\frac{\text{Decreasing}}{\text{Decreased}}$	$\frac{\text{Decreased}}{\text{Decreased}}\left(\text{equals } \frac{20}{1}\right)$
pH	Increased	Moving toward normal	Normal

bicarbonate ions will cause the blood to be relatively too alkaline. This excessive alkalinity of the blood is manifested by an increase in the bicarbonate ion concentration and by excitation of the central nervous system in the early stages.[2,4,19]

Clinical Manifestations. An increased pH of the cerebrospinal fluid causes initial central nervous system excitation followed by central nervous system depression. The signs and symptoms are as follows:

Increased bicarbonate ion concentration
Hypoventilation (compensatory mechanism)

Initial disorder:
- Nausea, emesis
- Belligerence
- Paresthesias
- Tetany
- Seizures

Profound disorder:
- Confusion
- Lethargy
- Coma

Muscle weakness and cardiac arrhythmias with concurrent hypokalemia

Profound metabolic alkalosis causes central nervous system depression. A pH of 7.8 is considered the fatal limit. The neurological manifestations of metabolic alkalosis arise more slowly than in respiratory alkalosis.

The increased pH of metabolic alkalosis is a sign that the buffers have been overwhelmed. The kidneys have been unable to excrete the relative excess of bicarbonate. Of the mechanisms for adjusting pH, only the respiratory system is available for compensation. The lungs cannot excrete bicarbonate ions, but they can retain carbonic acid in an attempt to neutralize the excess base and return the pH toward normal. Carbonic acid (CO_2 and water) is retained in the body when the rate and depth of respiration are decreased. Such hypoventilation would be an effective compensatory mechanism for metabolic alkalosis were it not for the body's need for oxygen. Respiratory compensation for metabolic alkalosis is limited by the hypoxemia that develops with hypoventilation. Hypoxemia stimulates ventilation.[19] Of necessity, then, metabolic alkalosis is often partially, rather than fully, compensated. (See Table 14–8 for the laboratory values in metabolic alkalosis.) The compensatory mechanism may be enhanced by the administration of oxygen, which removes the hypoxic ventilatory stimulus by increasing the Pa_{O_2}.

TABLE 14–7
Causes of Metabolic Alkalosis (Noncarbonic Acid Deficit)

General Etiology: Decrease of Acid
Specific examples:
Gastrointestinal route
- Emesis
- Gastric suction

Urinary route
- Hyperaldosteronism
- Glucocorticoid excess
- Chronic excessive ingestion of black licorice (contains aldosterone-like compounds)
- Diuretic therapy

Acid movement into cells
- Hypokalemia

General Etiology: Increase of Base (Bicarbonate Ions)
Specific examples:
Excess infusion or ingestion of $NaHCO_3$
Excess administration of lactate or acetate (bicarbonate precursors)
Massive blood transfusion (citrate is a bicarbonate precursor)

Nursing Implications. The medical therapy for metabolic alkalosis is directed toward treatment of the original cause of the imbalance and toward enhancing renal bicarbonate ion excretion to correct the imbalance. The latter is usually accomplished by administering oral or intravenous saline and correcting hypokalemia with KCl. Since hypokalemia and chloride deficit may lead to metabolic alkalosis, correction of these deficits with KCl may correct the alkalosis as well. If the metabolic alkalosis is profound, dialysis may be instituted or hydrochloric acid (HCl), ammonium chloride (NH_4Cl), or arginine monohydrochloride may be administered intravenously to normalize the pH.[22,24] Persons receiving these infusions to decrease blood pH need careful monitoring for the complications of therapy: rebound metabolic acidosis (HCl, NH_4Cl, or arginine), hemolysis (NH_4Cl), ammonium encephalopathy with lethargy and coma (NH_4Cl),

TABLE 14–8
Laboratory Values in Metabolic Alkalosis

	Uncompensated Metabolic Alkalosis	*Partially Compensated Metabolic Alkalosis*	
Pa_{CO_2}	Normal	Increasing	Full compensation for metabolic akalosis is limited by the body's need for oxygen.
HCO_3^-	Increased	Increased	
$\frac{[HCO_3^-]}{[H_2CO_3]}$	$\frac{\text{Increased}}{\text{Normal}}$ (greater than $\frac{20}{1}$)	$\frac{\text{Increased}}{\text{Increasing}}$	
pH	Increased	Moving toward normal	

phlebitis (HCl or NH_4Cl), and severe hyperkalemia (arginine). Occasionally, the diuretic acetazolamide is administered to increase urinary bicarbonate excretion.

In addition to ongoing assessment, administering the prescribed medical therapy, and monitoring for complications of the therapy, independent nursing actions are possible both for prevention and for management of metabolic alkalosis. Chvostek's sign should be monitored for assessment of neuromuscular excitability. If nausea and vomiting from metabolic alkalosis are present, measures to prevent aspiration of vomitus, such as positioning on the side, are valuable. The major nursing measure to prevent the development of metabolic alkalosis is teaching proper management of antacids. Prolonged use of bicarbonate-containing antacids (baking soda, Alka-Seltzer, Bromo-Seltzer, Citrocarbonate, and Fizrin) is not advisable because excessive bicarbonate may be absorbed, giving rise to metabolic alkalosis.

Summary of Principles of Alkalosis

Alkalosis occurs when some process tends to increase the pH of the blood above the upper range of normal. Respiratory alkalosis is caused by hyperventilation, which leads to a carbonic acid deficit due to excreting too much carbon dioxide and water. If respiratory alkalosis persists for several days, the kidneys retain acid and excrete more bicarbonate to compensate for the abnormal pH.

Metabolic alkalosis is caused by a decrease of any acid other than carbonic acid (*e.g.,* loss of gastric hydrochloric acid) or an increase of bicarbonate (*e.g.,* use of baking soda as an antacid). In either case, the blood becomes too alkaline. The compensatory mechanism for metabolic alkalosis is hypoventilation, through which carbonic acid is retained to neutralize the excess bicarbonate and thus rectify the pH. The usefulness of hypoventilation as a compensatory mechanism for metabolic alkalosis is limited by the need for oxygen.

The clinical manifestations of respiratory alkalosis and of initial metabolic alkalosis are the signs and symptoms of increased neuromuscular irritability. Severe metabolic alkalosis, however, causes central nervous system depression. Medical therapy for alkalosis is directed toward treatment of the underlying cause of the disorder, with pH correction only if the pH rises dangerously high.

Preventive nursing measures are useful in persons at high risk for developing either type of alkalosis. Respiratory alkalosis is prevented by alleviating hypoxemia or relieving pain and anxiety. Metabolic alkalosis is prevented by teaching antacid management. If alkalosis develops, nursing management includes ongoing assessment, administration of the medical therapy, and independent nursing actions for specific patient problems related to alkalosis.

Acid–Base Aspects of Arterial Blood Gas Reports

The laboratory report of arterial blood gases gives the patient's values of partial pressure of oxygen (Pa_{O_2}), oxygen saturation (Sa_{O_2}), partial pressure of carbon dioxide (Pa_{CO_2}), pH, and bicarbonate ion concentration (HCO_3^-). Other measures useful in the interpretation of acid–base status, such as anion gap, base excess, or total CO_2 content, may also be reported in the electrolyte profile. The significance of alterations in Pa_{O_2} and Sa_{O_2} are described in Chapter 27, which deals with common patient problems encountered in respiratory disorders. The acid–base information provided by arterial blood gas reports is discussed here.

pH

The meaning of pH was discussed previously in this chapter. In brief, pH is a reflection of acidity, with low pH values denoting a more acidic solution and high pH values indicating a more basic (alkaline) solution. The normal pH of arterial blood is 7.35 to 7.45. A pH above the normal range is called alkalemia and denotes the presence of alkalosis. A pH below the normal range is called acidemia and denotes the presence of acidosis. It is possible to have a pH in the normal range if an acidosis and an alkalosis of nearly equal degree occur. This situation may arise with a compensated acid–base disorder or with two concurrent primary disorders. The pH represents the overall acid–base state.

Pa_{CO_2}

The Pa_{CO_2} is a measure of the pressure exerted by carbon dioxide gas in the arterial blood. Carbon dioxide is produced by cellular metabolism, and must be excreted by the lungs or it will accumulate in the blood. The normal range for Pa_{CO_2} is 36 to 44 mmHg (varies slightly from laboratory to laboratory). Any deviation from the normal Pa_{CO_2} indicates a respiratory acid–base imbalance.[13,17] Such an imbalance may be primary (*i.e.*, the original problem) or compensatory (*i.e.*, a response to another acid–base imbalance). A *rise* in the Pa_{CO_2} is due to hypoventilation and denotes respiratory acidosis: either primary respiratory acidosis or compensatory respiratory acidosis (in response to metabolic alkalosis). Analogously, a *decrease* in the Pa_{CO_2} is due to hyperventilation and denotes either primary respiratory alkalosis or compensatory respiratory alkalosis (in response to metabolic acidosis). In summary, *Pa_{CO_2} is a respiratory parameter*.

HCO_3^-

The bicarbonate ion concentration (HCO_3^-) is a metabolic parameter. It is influenced primarily by nonrespiratory causes.[13,17] The normal HCO_3^- range is 22 to 26 mEq/liter. An *increased* HCO_3^- denotes a metabolic alkalosis (noncarbonic acid deficit). Such a metabolic alkalosis may be the primary disorder or a compensatory response to respiratory acidosis. A *decreased* HCO_3^-, on the other hand, denotes metabolic acidosis, which may be either primary or compensatory (in response to respiratory alkalosis).

Base Excess (BE)

Some laboratories report base excess (BE) with arterial blood gas values. The base excess is the normal buffer base concentration of the blood subtracted from the observed buffer base concentration. The normal base excess in adults is −2 to +2 mEq/liter. If a nonrespiratory process causes a decrease of acid or a gain of bicarbonate (*i.e.*, metabolic alkalosis), the base excess exceeds +2. A large *positive base excess*, then, denotes metabolic alkalosis. If, on the other hand, bicarbonate decreases or any acid except carbonic acid accumulates (*i.e.*, metabolic acidosis occurs), the base excess is less than −2. Such a *negative base excess, or base deficit*, denotes metabolic acidosis. The base excess provides essentially the same information as the HCO_3^- concentration regarding the presence or absence of metabolic acid–base imbalances.

Total CO_2 Content

The total CO_2 content that is sometimes reported on the electrolyte profile is different from the Pa_{CO_2}, which measures gaseous carbon dioxide. Total CO_2 content is the sum of bicarbonate ion, carbonic acid, and carbon dioxide in the blood.[17] Since the bicarbonate ions are about 95% of the total CO_2 content, this value may be used as an approximation of the amount of bicarbonate present. The normal total CO_2 content averages 25.2 mEq/liter.

Anion Gap

The anion gap is reported on the electrolyte profile as an aid to discover the cause of metabolic acidosis. The anion gap is the computed difference between the serum sodium (Na^+) concentration and the sum of the concentrations of the anions chloride and bicarbonate.

$$\text{Anion gap} = [Na^+] - ([Cl^-] + [HCO_3^-])$$

The normal anion gap is 8 to 16 mEq/liter.[9] An abnormally *decreased* anion gap occurs with severe hypoalbuminemia, water excess, or multiple myeloma. An abnormally *increased* anion gap is more common. It occurs with certain types of metabolic acidosis (noncarbonic acid excess).

As has been previously explained, metabolic acidosis has two major causes: decrease of bicarbonate and accumulation of acid. Persons with metabolic acidosis due to decrease of bicarbonate have a normal anion gap. Persons who accumulate chloride-containing acids (*e.g.*, HCl, NH_4Cl) also have a normal anion gap. Persons who accumulate organic acids, however, manifest an increased anion gap. Examples of organic acids whose accumulation leads to an increased anion gap are lactic acid and the ketoacids. Table 14–9 differentiates between the etiologies of metabolic acidosis with a normal and an increased anion gap.[3,9] Occasionally, a person who has severe metabolic alkalosis will also manifest an increased anion gap due to altered charge distributions on plasma proteins in the highly alkaline blood.

Reading the Arterial Blood Gas Report

When examining an arterial blood gas report, first look at the pH. Does the pH denote acidosis or alkalosis, or is it normal (7.35–7.45)? Remember that if the pH is within the normal range, an acidosis and an alkalosis could be counteracting each other. Such a state occurs with a fully compensated acid–base imbalance or, occasionally, with two opposing primary imbalances.

Next, look at the Pa_{CO_2} (normal range 35–45 mmHg). Is there a respiratory acid–base imbalance? If so, it could be primary or compensatory. Last, look at the HCO_3^- (normal range 22–26 mEq/liter). Is there a nonrespiratory (metabolic) imbalance? If not, then the respiratory disorder is primary and no compensation has occurred yet. If there is no respiratory imbalance, then the metabolic imbalance is pri-

TABLE 14–9
Anion Gap in Metabolic Acidosis

Increased Anion Gap

Ingestion of acid or acid precursor (*e.g.*, aspirin overdose, methanol injection)
Increased metabolic acids (*e.g.*, lactic acidosis)
Abnormal or incomplete metabolism (*e.g.*, ketoacidosis)
Impaired acid excretion (*e.g.*, severe renal failure)

Normal Anion Gap

Primary decrease of bicarbonate (*e.g.*, diarrhea)
Ingestion of chloride-containing acid (*e.g.*, HCl, NH_4Cl)
Impaired acid excretion (*e.g.*, mild renal insufficiency)

mary and uncompensated. If both respiratory and metabolic acid–base imbalances are present, as indicated by abnormal Pa_{CO_2} and abnormal HCO_3^-, the value that is farther from the normal probably indicates the primary imbalance. Table 14–10 presents a method to facilitate analysis of arterial blood gas reports. If metabolic acidosis is present, use the anion gap and the patient history for clues to its cause.

It is also possible to use a nomogram or acid–base map to interpret arterial blood gas values (Fig. 14–1).[14] Plot the patient's blood gas values and read the interpretation from the chart. If metabolic acidosis is present, use the anion gap and the patient history for clues to its cause.

Notice that the acid–base map in Fig. 14–1 indicates that it is possible to have two primary acid–base imbalances at the same time. Although such occurrences are not frequent, two such disorders may cancel each other to produce a nearly normal pH with abnormal Pa_{CO_2} and HCO_3^-, or they may combine to produce a severely abnormal pH. Table 14–11

TABLE 14–10
Analysis of Arterial Blood Gases

Look at pH. For this maneuver, only a pH of 7.4 is considered to be normal, even though the range of normal is actually 7.35 to 7.45.
A pH under 7.4 indicates acidemia.
A pH over 7.4 indicates alkalemia.

Look at Pa_{CO_2} (range of normal: 35 to 45 mmHg). If Pa_{CO_2} is normal, there is no primary respiratory problem and no respiratory compensation for a metabolic problem.
Abnormal Pa_{CO_2} values are interpreted in relation to pH:
- ↑ Pa_{CO_2} plus ↓ pH: acidosis of respiratory origin
- ↑ Pa_{CO_2} plus ↑ pH: respiratory retention of CO_2 to compensate for metabolic alkalosis
- ↓ Pa_{CO_2} plus ↑ pH: alkalosis of respiratory origin
- ↓ Pa_{CO_2} plus ↓ pH: respiratory elimination of CO_2 to compensate for metabolic acidosis

Look at HCO_3^- (range of normal: 22 to 26 mEq per liter). If HCO_3^- is normal, there is no primary metabolic problem and no metabolic compensation for a respiratory problem.
Abnormal HCO_3^- values are interpreted in relation to pH:
- ↓ HCO_3^- plus ↓ pH: acidosis of metabolic origin
- ↓ HCO_3^- plus ↑ pH: renal retention of H^+ or elimination of HCO_3^- to compensate for respiratory alkalosis
- ↑ HCO_3^- plus ↑ pH: alkalosis of metabolic origin
- ↑ HCO_3^- plus ↓ pH: renal retention of HCO_3^- or elimination of H^+ to compensate for respiratory acidosis

Use above findings to diagnose acid–base status. Possible disorders include compensated or uncompensated respiratory acidosis (synonym: *hypoventilation*), compensated or uncompensated respiratory alkalosis (synonym: *hyperventilation*), compensated or uncompensated metabolic acidosis, and compensated or uncompensated metabolic alkalosis. Simultaneous respiratory and metabolic disorders are also possible. If Pa_{CO_2}, HCO_3^-, and pH are *all* within their normal ranges, acid–base status is normal.

Look at Pa_{O_2} (normal: 80 mmHg for elderly adults at sea level; 100 mmHg for young adults at sea level). A Pa_{O_2} below normal for age indicates hypoxemia.

(Rokosky JS: Assessment of the individual with altered respiratory function. Nurs Clin North Am 16:198, 1981)

TABLE 14–11
Mixed Acid–Base Imbalances

Concurrent Primary Acid–Base Imbalances	*Example of Etiology*	*Blood Gas Values*
Respiratory acidosis and Metabolic alkalosis	COPD and emesis	pH possibly near normal Pa_{CO_2} increased HCO_3^- increased
Respiratory alkalosis and Metabolic acidosis	Salicylate poisoning	pH possibly near normal Pa_{CO_2} decreased HCO_3^- decreased
Respiratory acidosis and Metabolic acidosis	COPD and diarrhea	pH greatly decreased Pa_{CO_2} increased HCO_3^- decreased
Respiratory alkalosis and Metabolic alkalosis	Hyperventilation from pain or sepsis and massive blood transfusion	pH greatly increased Pa_{CO_2} decreased HCO_3^- increased
Metabolic acidosis and Metabolic alkalosis	Renal failure and emesis	Values depend on severity and duration of the two imbalances
Two different kinds of metabolic acidosis	Diabetic ketoacidosis and lactic acidosis	pH greatly decreased Pa_{CO_2} normal or decreased (compensation) HCO_3^- decreased

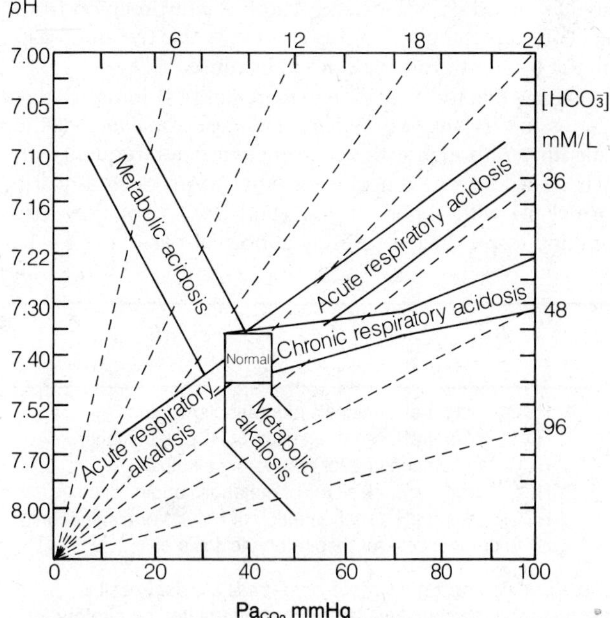

FIGURE 14–1 Diagram of acute and chronic acid–base disorders as determined by Pa_{CO_2}, bicarbonate, and pH values. (Adapted from Masoro EJ, Siegel PD: Acid–Base Regulation: Its Physiology, Pathophysiology and Interpretation of Blood Gas Analysis. Philadelphia, WB Saunders, 1977)

gives examples of mixed primary acid–base imbalances.[17] If respiratory acidosis and metabolic acidosis occur concurrently, the blood pH will be severely decreased because there will be no compensatory mechanisms operative. If, however, a primary acidosis and a primary alkalosis occur together, the pH of the blood will be the result of the two opposing imbalances.

In summary, the pH value alone does not describe a person's acid–base status. Interpretation of an arterial blood gas report is facilitated by an understanding of the mechanisms of respiratory and metabolic (nonrespiratory) acidosis and alkalosis and by a systematic approach to the laboratory report.

References

1. Barcenas C et al: Metabolic alkalosis after massive blood transfusion. JAMA 236:953, 1976
2. Cohen J, Kassirer J: Acid–base metabolism. In Maxwell M, Kleeman C (eds): Clinical Disorders of Fluid and Electrolyte Metabolism. New York, McGraw-Hill, 1980
3. Done A: The toxic emergency—Acid base disturbances: Aids to evaluation. Emerg Med 13:159, 1981
4. Dumler F: Primary metabolic alkalosis. Am Fam Physician 23:193, 1981
5. Gary N: Clinical acid–base disorders. Med Times 107:52, 1979
6. Halperin M et al: Interpretation of the serum potassium concentration in metabolic acidosis. Clin Invest Med 2:55, 1979
7. Hazard P, Griffin J: Sodium bicarbonate in the management of systemic acidosis. South Med J 73:1339, 1980
8. Hobbs J: Metabolic acidosis. Am Fam Physician 23:220, 1981
9. Hricik D, Kassirer J: Understanding and using the anion gap. Consultant 23:130, 1983
10. Kassirer J, Madias N: Respiratory acid–base disorders. Hosp Pract 15:57, 1980
11. McConnel J et al: The role of the colon in the pathogenesis of hyperchloraemic acidosis in ureterosigmoid anastomosis. Clin Sci 57:305, 1979
12. Madias N, Zelman S: What are the metabolic complications of diuretic treatment? Geriatrics 37:93, 1982
13. Mandell H: Gases and 'lytes without anguish. Postgraduate Med 69:67, 1981
14. Miller W: The ABC's of blood gases. Emerg Med 16:37, 1984
15. Missri J, Alexander S: Hyperventilation syndrome. JAMA 240:2093, 1978
16. Morris RC, Sebastian A: Disorders of the renal tubule that cause disorders of fluid, acid–base, and electrolyte metabolism. In Maxwell M, Kleeman C (eds): Clinical Disorders of Fluid and Electrolyte Metabolism. New York, McGraw-Hill, 1980
17. Narins R, Emmett M: Simple and mixed acid–base disorders: A practical approach. Medicine 59:161, 1980
18. Park R: Lactic acidosis. West J Med 133:418, 1980
19. Rose BD: Clinical Physiology of Acid–Base and Electrolyte Disorders, 2nd ed. New York, McGraw-Hill, 1984
20. Skillman T: Diabetic ketoacidosis. Heart Lung 7:594, 1978
21. Stacpoole P et al: Treatment of lactic acidosis with dichloroacetate. N Engl J Med 309:390, 1983
22. Wagner C et al: Treatment of metabolic alkalosis with intravenous hydrochloric acid. South Med J 72:1241, 1979
23. Walesky M: Diabetic ketoacidosis. Am J Nurs 78:872, 1978
24. Williams D, Lyons J: Treatment of severe metabolic alkalosis with intravenous infusion of hydrochloric acid. Surg Gynecol Obstet 150:315, 1980

Chapter 15

Injury

Inflammatory Response and Resolution

Pauline M. Bruno

The environment, both external and internal, contain substances and forces with potential for injuring or destroying human cells. Tissue injury is a relatively common occurrence throughout the life span. Fortunately, human beings and animals have the ability to localize injury and heal wounds. Survival is dependent on the orderly process of wound healing, for without this ability infection and structural defects would occur frequently.

The phrase *tissue injury* has broad connotations. It refers to situations which disrupt the normal regulatory processes of cells and tissues. As discussed in Chapter 12, the cellular environment must be maintained within rather narrow limits. In the course of daily living, cells are capable of regulating this environment as they encounter factors that threaten to disrupt or change it. These disruptive factors may destroy tissue, severely injure many of the tissue cells, or minimally interfere with cell function. Physical trauma, extrinsic chemicals, and intrinsic chemicals constitute the classification of injurious agents. The effects and examples of resulting disorders of these three categories of injuries are listed in Table 15–1.

The response of tissue to injury is a defensive one. The tissues in the area initiate processes that are directed at confining the area of injury, removing necrotic waste products, and replacing destroyed tissue with viable tissue. All of these processes are encompassed by the phrase *wound healing*.

TABLE 15–1
Injurious Agents and Resulting Disorders

Agent	*Examples of Resulting Disorders*
Physical trauma	Lacerations, fractures, burns
Blows, pressure	
Heat (causing disruption of cells or altered metabolism and release of chemical stimuli)	
Surgical incision	
Extrinsic chemicals	Allergic reactions, infections
Allergens	
Insect bites	
Toxins of pathogenic microorganisms	
Intrinsic chemicals	
Secretion of excessive hydrochloric acid by gastric cells	Gastric ulcers
Breakdown products of necrotic tissues due to inadequate circulation	Myocardial infarction, core of malignant tumors
Products of autoimmune antigen–antibody reaction	Rheumatoid arthritis

Repair of wounds is a complex, dynamic process that starts immediately after injury and may continue for a year or longer. The nature of the process is remarkably constant regardless of the nature of the injurious agent or the site of injury. Variations in the healing process result from differences in the type, extent, and location of damaged tissue and from the regenerative capacity of the tissue (Fig. 15–1).

This chapter considers the process of healing. Discussion focuses on each of the three phases of healing: inflammation (defense), reconstruction (resolution), and maturation. This is followed by a consideration of modifications of the process in long-term damage or extensive tissue destruction. The final section of the chapter discusses bone repair. The phases of healing are examined separately, although they are interdependent and overlap in time. The influence of aging changes and other factors on the healing process are integrated into the discussion. Each section concludes with a consideration of nursing implications.

Phases of the Healing Process

The phases of the healing process, inflammation, reconstruction, and maturation, overlap one another in time. The inflammatory phase is initiated at the time of injury and continues for 4 to 6 days. The reconstructive phase begins about the third or fourth day after injury and continues for 2 to 3 weeks. The final phase, maturation, is the most prolonged and may continue for over a year. Because elderly people are slower to respond to stress and to regain a steady state, their response to trauma is delayed and the time frame of the process is longer.[8]

Inflammation

The inflammatory process is a nonspecific, defensive response of the body to any type of injury. Four purposes are served by the inflammatory process:

- Control of bleeding
- Sealing the wound and protection from bacterial invasion
- Removal of debris resulting from tissue injury
- Provision of a scaffolding for deposition of collagen fiber in the reconstructive period

In medical terminology, the suffix *-itis* added to a word indicates the presence of an inflammatory process. The first element of the term indicates the site of inflammation. For instance, the term *appendicitis* means an inflammation of the appendix. The suffix indicates that inflammation is present, but does not indicate the causative agent. For example, he term appendicitis does not imply that an infection is present.

Hemostasis

The inflammatory process begins immediately after injury, with activities that arrest bleeding from damaged vessels. Hemostasis is the term for the mechanism by which bleeding is stopped; this mechanism is described in detail in Chapter 21. The initial hemostatic event is vasoconstriction, a brief period of reflex arteriolar spasm and retraction of severed blood vessels. Next, platelets accumulate and small clots form at the cut end of blood vessels. These events help to block the vessel lumen and thus control blood loss. Eventually, the blood that is lost into the tissues clots and forms a matrix of fibrin strands which later becomes a framework for repair. A scab consisting of dead tissue and clots gradually

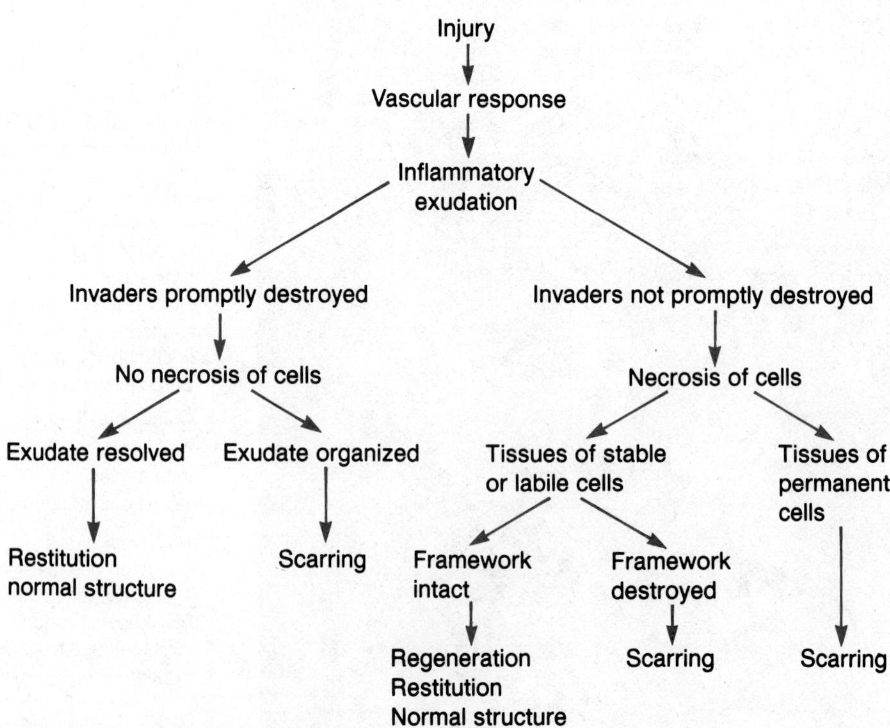

FIGURE 15–1 Pathways of reparative response. (Robbins S, Cotron RS, Kumar V: Pathologic Basis of Disease, 3rd ed. Philadelphia, WB Saunders, 1984)

forms on the surface and provides protection from microorganisms and other environmental contaminants. On a surgical wound, this hemostatic protection is usually achieved in 24 to 48 hours.

Vasodilatation and Formation of Exudate

Vessel Changes. The initial vasoconstriction is followed by dilatation of arterioles, capillaries, and venules and a resulting expansion of blood flow to the area (active hyperemia). The permeability of blood vessels then increases, permitting the movement of protein-rich plasma into the intestitial spaces. The fluid leaves the vascular compartment through openings that appear at endothelial cell junctions. This fluid, called an *exudate*, has a high protein content with a specific gravity of about 1.020.

Injury to cells apparently causes the release of intracellular chemicals that act on local microcirculation to increase permeability.[9] Some of the chemical mediators that influence vascular permability are histamine, kinins, serotonin, and prostaglandins. The extent of the inflammatory response is controlled because the mediators are enzymatically inactivated or because of the presence of inhibitors or antagonists of the mediators. Some of the mediators act immediately and others have a delayed effect. The exact mechanism of mediator action is currently unknown. The inflammatory exudate usually accumulates slowly, reaches a maximum extent in 6 to 24 hours, and then gradually subsides. Direct damage to endothelial cells destroys their mechanical integrity and functional ability; these effects sustain the inflammation.

Characteristics of Inflammatory Exudate. The characteristics of the inflammatory exudate are influenced by the *tissue affected*, the *causative agent*, and the *duration of response*. Serum, the clear liquid of blood when red blood cells are not present, is what accumulates in the interstitium when mild to moderate injuries occur. It is, for example, the fluid present in blisters. Serous exudate is also secreted from particular serous membranes such as the peritoneum and pleura. Injuries to these tissues will often result in accumulation of serous drainage in the respective cavities. Sometimes red blood cells will move out of permeable blood vessels or from lacerated vessels and create a serosanguineous exudate. Injuries to membranes that contain mucous cells produce an inflammatory exudate termed catarrhal. An example of this is the exudate from irritation of the nasal and respiratory passages and the gastrointestinal tract, which produces a clear drainage containing mucous strands.

Severe or prolonged injuries usually result in production of a fibrinous exudate. Capillary permeability increases to the extent that the large fibrinogen molecule escapes into the interstitial spaces. The fibrinogen interacts with thromboplastin substances that are present, and it is precipitated as fibrin. The fibrin may be deposited over the serous tissue surfaces, forming an opaque, grayish membrane. A fibrinous exudate may be seen over pressure lesions and burns. It also occurs internally, and, since fibrin is a sticky substance, it can cause surfaces to adhere to each other and produce fibrinous adhesions or friction rubs. Fibrinous adhesions can occur between two sections of inflammed intestines, causing kinking of the bowel and obstruction to flow of fecal contents. Friction rubs may be heard in the acute stages of inflammation of the pleural surfaces of the lungs (pleuritis).

A purulent exudate is characteristic of injuries caused by pyogenic (pus-forming) bacteria. The presence of bacteria in tissues influences the migration of leukocytes towards the site of inflammation. This process of unidirectional migration is known as *chemotaxis*. The leukocytes accumulate at the site in large numbers. They phagocytose bacteria and as they die release proteolytic enzymes that digest both dead tissue and surrounding living tissue. Pus is an inflammatory exudate that consists of numerous dead or dying leukocytes, tissue debris, live bacteria, and chemical products of the action of proteolytic enzymes. The exudate continues to accumulate, causing increasing pressure in the tissues. The site of accumulation of purulent exudate is referred to as an *abscess*. Abscesses can occur anywhere in the body. Some abscesses are absorbed and the products excreted; some become walled off by dense fibrous tissue and eventually are calcified; some abscesses rupture and create a chronic inflammatory site. When the abscess is in the skin and subcutaneous tissue, rupture of it releases the infectious material outside the body and thereby hastens repair of the damaged tissue.

Cell Movement and Action

The cellular component of the inflammatory response consists of the migration of circulating leukocytes to the interstitial spaces of the injured tissues, and phagocytosis and enzymatic digestion of dead cells and tissue elements. The leukocytes emigrate through the vessel wall into the interstitium, and by the process of chemotaxis move toward the site of injury. Chemical substances such as bacterial products (see above), complement fractions, components of the kinin system, and lymphocyte factors released at the site of injury are thought to provide chemotactic stimuli for the attraction of the leukocytes.[15] The neutrophil is the dominant cell in the exudate for the first 24 to 48 hours. Neutrophils are vulnerable to the lactic acid from dead cells that accumulates in the interstitium and therefore are relatively short-lived.

The function of the neutrophils at the injury site is phagocytosis of necrotic debris and any foreign particles such as bacteria. Phagocytosis is an energy-consuming process of ingestion and digestion. The energy is, for the most part, derived from anerobic glycolysis. The lysosomes of the neutrophils and monocytes contain hydrolytic enzymes which stimulate digestion. As the neutrophils die, monocytes migrate into the area and become dominant. The monocytes become macrophages in the tissue and persist for some time in the wound even in the absence of infection. They have a phagocytic action but also secrete products that can induce fibroblasts to enter a phase of collagen breakdown.

Lymphocytes and eosinophils may also participate in the inflammatory reaction. The eosinophils are particularly involved in allergic types of inflammation.

A few red blood cells are commonly present in the exudate as they pass through the vessel wall because of increased hydrostatic pressure (diapedesis). A hemorrhagic inflammatory exudate usually indicates severe injury to the microvasculature.

Local Manifestations

Local manifestations of inflammation depend on the severity and duration of injury. In surface wounds, inflammation is visible as redness and swelling (edema). The site is warmer to touch than surrounding tissues and is painful. Local manifestations are referred to as the cardinal signs and symptoms of inflammation and include redness, swelling, pain, and loss of movement. Table 15–2 outlines the rationale for these manifestations. Most people have observed the development of these signs and symptoms following a bruise, a mosquito bite, or perhaps a more severe injury. Although not outwardly visible, these same events occur with internal tissue damage.

Duration of Inflammatory Process

The inflammatory phase of the wound healing process is variable. In acute situations it reaches highest intensity in 24 to 48 hours and then begins to subside. The duration overlaps with the activities of the reconstruction phase. This pattern is the expected course of events with surgical wounds, soft tissue bruises, and the common cold (Fig. 15–2). At times the inflammatory phase may be more prolonged, and sometimes it is of a chronic, long-term nature.

The duration of inflammatory response is directly related to the *etiologic agent* and the *state of the body's defense mechanisms*. For instance, it is thought that immune products are the etiologic agents in rheumatoid arthritis and that this chronic inflammatory disorder is an autoimmune reaction (see Chap. 16). In rheumatoid arthritis and other autoimmune disorders, tissues are almost continuously subjected

TABLE 15–2
Explanations for Manifestations of Inflammation

Manifestation	*Rationale*
Redness	Increased blood flow (hyperemia) heightens red appearance
Heat	Increased blood flow increases heat to area Increased local metabolism
Swelling	Accumulation of inflammatory exudate in interstitial spaces, dilated blood vessels, and increased blood present
Pain	Presence of factors that stimulate nerve endings: Chemical mediators of vasodilation and chemotaxis Acidic state of exudate Distention of tissues with exudate
Loss of function	Presence of exudate Splinting to prevent pain Death of cells

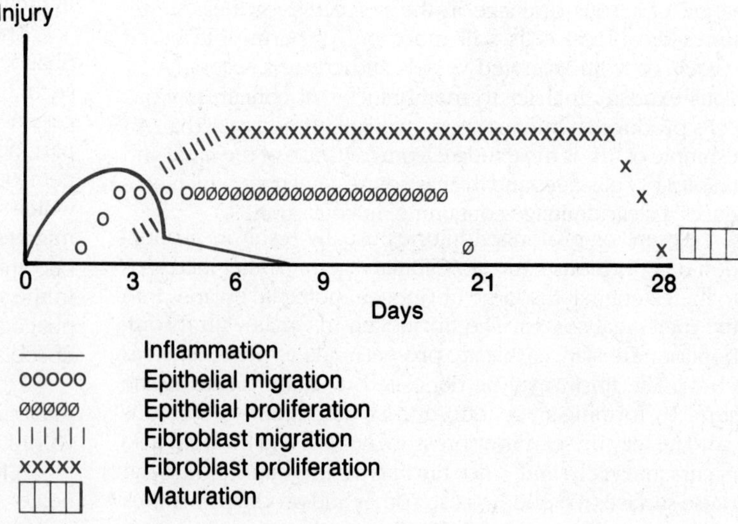

FIGURE 15–2 Time sequence of overlapping events in the repair process. (Adapted from Bruno P: The nature of wound healing. Nurs Clin North Am 14:668, 1979)

to chemical irritants that result from antigen–antibody reactions. Phagocytosis of immune complexes by neutrophils releases lysosomal enzymes capable of producing tissue injury. An example of how the state of the body's defense mechanisms influences the duration of the inflammatory response is the person with marginal nutritional status, who may not have an adequate supply of neutrophils to overcome harmful agents. These agents would then be a continuous source of injury.

The appearance of an inflammatory lesion, both gross and microscopic, provides an estimate of its duration. In prolonged inflammation, the tissue is highly vascular, soft, and granular in appearance, whereas healed tissue presents as vascular, dense scar tissue. The exudation period is prolonged in chronic inflammation. The heat, redness, and swelling are constantly present though not as intensely as in acute situations. The process of tissue reconstruction is delayed when chronic inflammation is present.

Systemic Manifestations

In addition to the above-discussed localized signs and symptoms of inflammation, the process has an adverse effect on the person as a whole. Systemically, the affected person experiences feelings of weakness, apathy, malaise, fever, increased heart rate, increased leukocytosis, and increased sedimentation rate. An explanation of these manifestations is that the soluble products of both the breakdown of damaged cells and the inflammatory reaction enter the bloodstream and lymphatics.[12] These substances are carried to other parts of the body and create an abnormal internal environment which in turn modifies the function of some tissues. When the injurious agents precipitating an inflammatory response are pathogenic microorganisms, the systemic response is usually more intense than when no infection is present. The more intense response is related to the effect of toxins on the body as a whole. Successful leukocytic action prepares the damaged tissue site for reconstruction of the damaged tissue.

Resolution

Injury is resolved when deposition of repair tissue restores continuity to the injured tissue. The process of *reconstruction* is initiated shortly after the inflammatory response commences. The ideal repair is replacement by regeneration of cells identical to those which were damaged. However, not all tissues are capable of regeneration. Thus, replacement of some of the injured tissue with connective tissue is the usual occurrence since, with the exception of minor skin trauma, few wounds are confined to one type of tissue where perfect regeneration is possible. Repair of injured multi-type tissues in an identical architectural arrangement as exists in the original tissue is also highly unlikely.

Cell types differ both in their regenerative capacity and in the time frame within they initiate regeneration following injury. Classified as *labile* are those cells which are in a constant state of loss and replacement; these include epithelial cells and blood cells. When these cells are injured, nearby, undamaged "like" cells proliferate and normal structure is restored. For instance, small, superficial skin lesions involve only epithelial cells, and these regenerate without scar formation. The majority of other cells, for example, liver and renal cells, are classified as *stable*. These cells do not routinely replace themselves but retain the potential to proliferate following injury. Cells classified as *permanent* lose the ability to proliferate at the time of birth. Nerve, skeletal muscle, and cardiac muscle cells are all believed to be permanent cells incapable of regenerating after injury. Instead, tissue repair is by connective tissue replacement.[13]

Tissue injuries are of two types: those without and those with tissue loss. Wounds without tissue loss, in which the edges are closely approximated, heal by a process known as *primary intention*, or *first intention* (Fig. 15–3). An incised, sutured wound resulting from an operative procedure illustrates this type healing. The cut edges of internal organs and skin are closely approximated by suture, and only a minimal tissue defect must be repaired. In contrast, injuries with tissue loss heal by *secondary intention* (*second intention*), which is a longer and more complex process. Because the wound edges are not approximated with sutures, new tissue must fill in the space. Examples of wounds with tissue loss are burns and other traumatic injuries, ulcerations along the gastrointestinal tract, and cell destruction that occurs with infectious, neoplastic, and degenerative processes. Whether by primary intention or by secondary intention, tissue continuity is eventually restored by the proliferation of cells with regenerative potential and deposition of connective scar tissue. The next section outlines these processes as they occur with first intention. The process of healing by second intention will be described in a later portion of the chapter.

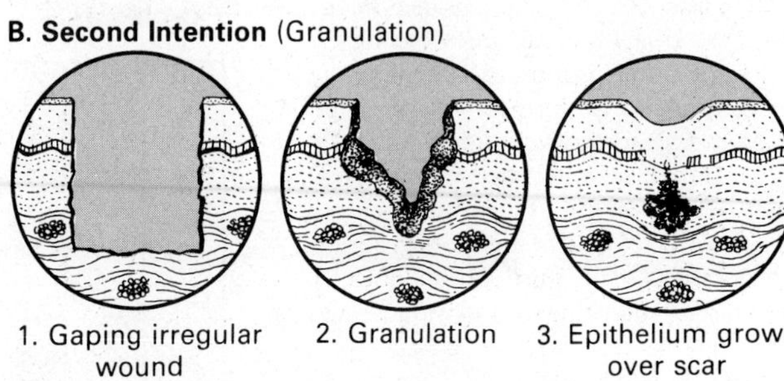

FIGURE 15–3 Wound healing. (*A*) A wound in which the edges are approximated and healing is by primary (first) intention. (*B*) A wound in which the edges are not approximated and healing is by secondary (second) intention. (Hardy JD: Hardy's Textbook of Surgery, p 109. Philadelphia, JB Lippincott, 1983)

Cell Migration and Regeneration

The phagocytosis of necrotic debris by the white blood cells prepares the injured area for the repair process. Within a few hours after injury, the undamaged cells at the margins of the damaged site start to migrate downward below the base of the clot that seals the wound.

When the injury is to epithelial tissue, that is, skin or the lining of gastrointestinal and other body tracts, the process of cell migration is termed epithelialization. These migrating cells usually meet below the clot and bridge the gap within 48 hours. Migration ends when the cells contact each other. Cell contact apparently is the signal for the cells to resume the process of growth and differentiation.[11] Epithelialization is important because this tissue serves as a barrier between the body and its environment. It covers the outer surface of the body, and lines the respiratory, gastrointestinal, and genitourinary tracts and blood vessels. Epithelial tissue halts the invasion of bacteria, toxic materials, and ultraviolet radiation, and blocks the loss of body fluids and electrolytes.

Cell proliferation is also part of the repair process of injured internal organs that are composed of parenchymal cells with regenerative potential. For instance, in a pneumococcal pneumonia involving one or more lobes of the lung, the lung tissue usually heals with complete return to normal structure and function.

Connective Tissue Deposition

Fibroblasts are the connective tissue cells responsible for synthesizing and secreting the collagen and protein polysaccharides that form scar tissue. These cells appear in the wound toward the end of the inflammatory process. The cells synthesize the collagen molecule, which consists of a polypeptide chain of amino acids. Within the extracellular space, the collagen aggregates into fibers of increasing length and diameter.[4] It provides tensile strength to the scar tissue that eventually replaces the wound defect.

Endothelial budding occurs on nearby vessels at the same time that the process of collagen synthesis and secretion is taking place. This combination of young budding capillaries and actively proliferating fibroblasts is termed *granulation tissue*. The capillaries penetrate the injured tissue, meet, and form an interconnecting network. They provide relatively large amounts of oxygen and nutrients to the cells that are actively synthesizing protein in the wound. When the continuity of the connective tissue is reestablished, the capillaries gradually recede. Figure 15–4 shows the cell populations that occupy wounds at different times.[14]

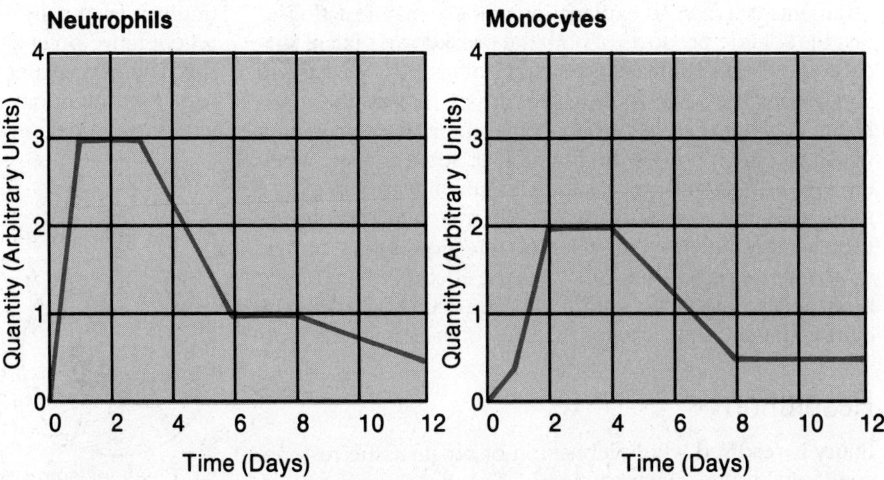

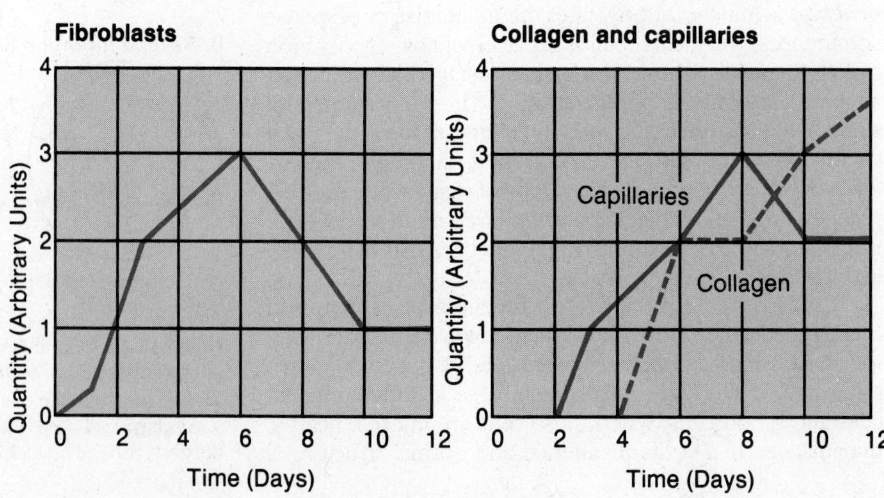

FIGURE 15–4 Cell populations that occupy the wound at different times can be divided into three groups, each with its own special task to perform. *Neutrophils* migrate rapidly to the wound but are short-lived. *Monocytes* enter the wound slightly later but persist for a longer time period. The function of both of these cell groups is phagocytosis. The third group of cells, *fibroblasts*, enters the wound within 2 days after injury and secretes the collagen precursors needed for tissue repair. The stages tend to overlap one another and may well be interdependent, since suppression of one can delay the start of the next. (Ross R: Wound healing. Sci Am 69:50, 1969. Used with permission of the author.)

Maturation

Areas of tissue damage, whether superficial or deep, undergo slow progressive change in size and shape for a number of months. Contraction, which is the movement of the full thickness of the tissue inward toward the center of the wound, shrinks the scar tissue. It is an active cellular process that depends on the action of a modified type of fibroblast, the myofibroblast. Myofibroblasts have an intracellular fibril system which is capable of contraction similar to that of smooth muscle. They also are capable of attaching themselves to adjacent tissue and exerting force on that tissue. It is thought that they provide strength to the wound.

Accompanying the process of tissue contraction is the process of reweaving and establishing a pattern of collagen fibers. After several weeks, repair tissue fibers and the adjacent original fibers interdigitate. It is thought that the laying down of repair tissue and maturation of scar tissue is the net result of simultaneous synthesis and resorption of connective tissue matrix components. As noted above, macrophases play a role in the control of simultaneous synthesis and resorption of matrix components in the damaged area. The restructuring of the collage fibers continues for a number of months, and the wound becomes pale and shrinks in size. Although the collagen content remains constant, there is a progressive increase in the tensile strength of the wound. This gain in strength is attributed to intramolecular and intermolecular cross-linking of collagen fibers and to the remodeling of fibers.[5]

During the maturational phase, some skin wounds undergo a hypertrophic change known as keloid formation. Keloid is a dense fibrous tissue that extends above the surface of the skin and beyond the original incision. The color varies from red to pink. These changes probably reflect an imbalance in the synthesis and resorption of connective tissue matrix. The incidence of keloid formation is highest in blacks and dark-skinned whites. One method of treatment is injection of corticosteroids into the scar. Another is surgical excision; however, the condition does tend to recur.

Nursing Implications During Inflammation and Repair by Primary Intention

Goals

Nursing goals are to promote the healing process and prevent complications or detect them early. To achieve these goals it is necessary to monitor the healing process; carry out interventions to minimize the extent of inflammation and ensure adequate blood flow; promote adequate nutrition, rest, and activity; and provide conditions that minimize the dangers of infection. Numerous factors, such as age, nutritional status, immune defenses, and extent of injury, modify the quality and adequacy of wound healing. A more extensive list of these factors appears in Table 15–3. It is important to assess patients for these factors and to plan care accordingly.

TABLE 15–3
Factors Modifying The Quality and Adequacy of Wound Healing

Systemic	*Local*
Age	Adequacy of blood suply
Nutritional status	Location of injury
White blood cell status	Extent of injury
Adequacy of clotting factors	Immobilization of part
Immune defenses	Presence of:
Use of corticosteroid hormones	infection
	foreign bodies

Management During the Inflammatory Process

Assessment of the person experiencing an inflammatory process due to visible injury or internal tissue damage consists of measurements and observations to determine if hemostasis has occurred and if the extent of inflammation is compromising circulation to viable surrounding tissues. An increasing heart rate and decreasing blood pressure combined with restlessness and anxiety may indicate that hemostasis has not occurred. If the injury is to external soft tissue, one may also observe increasing size of a hematoma. Application of cold will stimulate vasoconstriction and help to promote clotting. Other interventions are application of pressure, elevation of the part, and cessation of activity.

The development of inflammatory exudate is manifested as the cardinal signs and symptoms described earlier. Accumulation of inflammatory exudate can be extensive. The pressure in the interstitial spaces can compromise circulation to the injured area and also directly damage healthy tissue. Frequent observations of external wounds reveal the extent of buildup of the exudate. Dressings should be examined to assure that they do not become too tight over expanding tissues, thereby interfering with circulation. For the same reason, rings should be removed immediately if the damage is to a finger, and constricting clothing or other encircling devices loosened or removed prior to buildup of exudate. Application of cold will decrease the extent of vasodilatation and vessel permeability. However, prolonged cold applications can interfere with adequacy of the blood circulation required both for transport of neutrophils to the injured area and for maintenance of noninjured tissues.[6] The application should be on an an alternating schedule of on for 20 to 30 minutes and off for 15 minutes.

Controversy exists in the literature about the use of heat or cold applications after the initial few hours following tissue damage. Some physicians believe that heat is beneficial because it increases blood flow, bringing scavenger cells to the site and allowing for removal of waste products. Other physicians advocate the use of cold to continue control of the extent of inflammation and, hence, of pain.

A slight rise in body temperature is usually present with inflammation. This is readily apparent in patients for the first day or two following surgery. The rise may be to 38°C (100°F). A temperature rise greater than 38°C suggests the possibility of infection either as the causative agent of inflammation or as a complication of damaged tissue. Laboratory values indicative of inflammation are a slight rise in white cell count to the upper limits of normal or even to 11,000 to 12,000/cc mm. The differential would indicate an increase in the percent of monocytes and eosinophils. The sedimentation rate (measure of rate at which red cells settle to the bottom of a glass test tube) is increased, especially in chronic inflammation. The normal rates are 0 to 15 mm/hr for men and 0 to 20 mm/hr for women.

In the elderly, the slowing of homeostatic responses delays the onset and severity of the inflammatory process. This is important to consider when assessing the status of the elderly ill. The manifestations of inflammation are slow to appear and are less intense than in the young, and resolution is also slow.

Management in Reconstructive and Maturation Phases

Nutrition. Reconstruction of damaged tissue requires adequate blood flow to the injured site for delivery of oxygen and nutrients. Adequate nutrition is vital for repair of tissue. Collagen, which is synthesized by the fibroblasts, is a protein. It provides strength to the healing tissue.

Deficient nutritional status predisposes the patient to inadequate repair of tissue; the strength of the tissue is marginal and healing is delayed. The person in marginal nutritional status may be deficient in the amino acid cystine, which is essential for fibroblast synthesis of collagen. Trace minerals, for example, copper, ferrous iron, and zinc, are also necessary for collagen synthesis. In animal studies, a deficiency of zinc retarded epithelialization and the rate of gain of tensile strength.[12] Other nutrients required for healing are ascorbic acid (vitamin C) and vitamin A. Vitamin C is necessary for collagen synthesis and capillary formation. Because this vitamin is not stored in the body, it may be added to the intravenous solutions which patients receive. Vitamin A promotes formation of granulation tissue. It is also thought to promote the inflammatory response by inhibiting the anti-inflammatory action of glucocorticoids.[3] Vitamin A is stored in the liver, and the well-nourished person would have adequate stores.

In order for protein to be used for synthesis of collagen, the body must have adequate carbohydrate to meet its energy needs. If carbohydrate is not available, protein is metabolized to produce energy. In a situation of severe, extensive injury, the patient requires high caloric intake to meet energy needs as well as those of tissue repair. Persons who are at risk for delayed wound healing because of deficient nutritional states include the elderly, those with chronic illnesses, persons with severe injuries such as extensive burns, and cachectic persons (*i.e.,* those with metastatic malignancies).

Assessment of a person's nutritional status includes determination of height–weight relationship, energy level, and muscle strength. Laboratory values of serum protein level and nitrogen balance are also helpful as are skinfold measurements of the upper arm. Normal albumin level is 3.2 to 5.6 g/100 ml, and the range of normal for the albumin–globulin ratio is 1.5 : 1 to 2.5 : 1. The use of protein for energy because of inadequate carbohydrate intake contributes to a decrease in albumin levels and a change in albumin–globulin ratio. Nitrogen balance should be positive, that is, the person's nitrogen intake should exceed that which is excreted. When protein is used for energy, nitrogen is released from the protein molecule. When nitrogen is excreted in excess of intake, a state of negative nitrogen balance exists.

Nursing interventions consist of promoting adequate nutritional intake when it is possible for the patient to eat. Explanations of why certain foods are desirable may promote consumption of necessary nutrients. When patients are unable to eat, treatment may include hyperalimentation or nasogastric tube feedings (see Chap. 80).

Prior to patient discharge, the nurse teaches the importance of maintaining a nutritious diet to promote progression of tissue repair as well as to regain physical strength and energy. If no special diet has been prescribed, eating from the basic four food groups ensures adequate intake of ascorbic acid, vitamin A, protein, and trace minerals for the later reconstructive and maturational phase. Some patients may need to maintain high caloric and special nutrient intake to foster healing as well as to regain strength. Persons who live alone may need assistance with shopping in the first few weeks after hospital discharge. In these cases, the nurse would need to arrange for a chore worker or home health aide prior to discharge

Patients on Steroids. Another factor that can interfere with healing is the use of steroids. Steroids, which may be prescribed as treatment for chronic inflammatory conditions such as rheumatoid arthritis, have an anti-inflammatory effect which delays repair of tissue. Cortisone also interferes with collagen synthesis and thus predisposes to marginal strength of healing tissue.[2,3] The nurse should carefully assess the progress of wound healing in patients on steroids. Before discharge, these patients should be taught how to observe their wounds for characteristics that indicate presence or absence of healing. They should also be taught how to protect their fragile wounds and to maintain adequate nutrition for healing.

Healing of Wounds with Tissue Loss: Secondary Intention

Healing by secondary intention differs from primary healing in the duration of repair time, the extent of scarring, and the susceptibility of the wound to infection. The healing process is prolonged because of the time required for phagocytosis of necrotic tissue, proliferation of parenchymal cells, and extensive connective tissue structuring to fill in the space.

Wounds undergoing secondary healing tend to have a prolonged period of inflammation. Dominant white cells are the macrophage and lymphocytes. The inflammatory reaction is proliferative (fibroblastic) as contrasted with the exudative reaction of acute inflammation. This proliferative component involves the development and persistence of fibroplasia. Fibrin, which was formed in the initial acute inflammatory exudate, serves as a scaffolding for the movement into the area of fibroblasts and endothelial buds. The fibrin eventually is liquefied by the action of enzymes released by leukocytes. The granulation tissue, which contains fibroblasts, new capillaries, and macrophages, seals the wound and provides resistance to infection. As the capillary network develops, the tissue becomes a translucent red color. In skin and subcutaneous wounds the granulation tissue may protrude above the wound margins, and often has a mucin covering. The healing tissue is fragile and bleeds easily. As the leukocytes remove the exudate and debris, the connective tissue granulates in toward the center of the wound.

In wounds involving epithelial tissue, maturation includes migration and proliferation of epithelial cells over the connective tissue base. These epidermal cells develop contractile filament in their cytoplasm, which enables them to move over the granulation tissue and helps to contract the wound.

The extent of cell migration is limited and may not be sufficient to cover extensive tissue defects. If the wound cannot close by epithelialization, the open area becomes covered with the eschar (dried protein and dead cells). Closure is by a process of contraction. As mentioned above, contraction refers to the reduction of part or all of the defect by means of centripedal movement of the full thickness of the surrounding skin. The myofibroblasts present in granulation tissue are apparently capable of contraction. These cells also attach themselves to surrounding tissue and exert pull on it.

Wound contraction speeds and facilitates the repair of wounds. However, it can have undesirable effects, namely, the development of contractures. Contractures are deformities that result from scar remodeling and maximum skin contraction. Apparently the contracting force promotes wound closure until it is balanced by equal tension in the skin which then prevents further movement. The inelastic scar tissue pulls the tissue into a position of deformity and hence functional impairment results. The term contracture also refers to joint deformities that result from immobility. In this latter situation, muscles lose tone because of decreased use and become contracted from being held in a shortened position. Fibrosis of connective tissues surrounding joints causes the tissues to remain in a fixed position. In this situation there may be no active contraction of tissue elements, but the end result is again contracture, deformity, and loss of function.

The basic processes of wound healing with extensive tissue loss are essentially the same as in closure of primary wounds. The difference is in the duration of the events, in particular, inflammation, granulation, and contraction. Similarly, the possible effects of aging changes on healing are the same for both types of wounds.

Nursing Implications

Goals. Nursing goals for healing of open wounds are essentially the same as for those that heal by primary intention. Prevention of infection requires rigorous attention because of the high susceptibility of open wounds to this complication. The duration of healing is prolonged, and nursing attention must be attentive to needs for nutrition, ambulation, and emotional support over an extended period of time.

Assessment. Assessment of the healing process requires knowledge of the expected appearance of wounds involving skin and subcutaneous tissue. In the early period after injury, the wound may seep a serosanguineous drainage. As tissue dies it may become covered with a gray, thick, fibrinous tissue, and areas of black necrotic tissue may be present. If infection occurs, the drainage is purulent and foul smelling, and may have a color characteristic of the dominant organisms. For instance, *Pseudomonas,* a common skin organism, has a characteristic blue–green drainage. As the wound is debrided and healing progresses to establishment of granulation tissue, the appearance changes. The wound becomes red, granular looking, and often has a mucin covering. Gradually, the wound contracts and scar tissue forms.

Interventions. Early treatment of traumatic wounds may include application of ice bags over sterile dressings. The ice bags should be covered with a moisture-proof wrapper to prevent nonsterile condensation from wetting the dressings. Cold induces vasoconstriction and inhibits the extent of exudate formation, as does elevation of the injured part. This action promotes healing because it lessens the amount of exudate that must be reabsorbed. Reduction of edema helps to lessen the pain related to tissue distention and reduces the extent of cell damage from fluid compression. Cold applications must be used intermittently to prevent compromise of circulation sufficient to increase the tissue damage. They must also be used cautiously in the elderly; older persons have decreased ability to adapt to temperature change, and application of ice bags may cause chilling.

Sterile wet-to-dry dressings may be prescribed to promote debridement of the necrotic tissue. This treatment helps to clean the wound and provide a surface acceptable for epithelialization. If coarse mesh gauze is used, excessive bleeding may occur when the dried dressing is removed; therefore, fine mesh gauze, which inhibits interweaving of the granulation material into the dressing, is preferred. Because removal of dried dressings is painful, it should be coordinated with analgesic administrations to provide maximum alleviation of pain. Some physicians elect to debride with instruments to maintain cleanliness and promote epithelialization.

Controversy exists about the most desirable method of dressing wounds and achieving wound debridement. Research on superficial skin wounds of pigs (pig skin is the animal skin that most closely resembles human skin) revealed that occlusive plastic dressings increased the rate of re-epithelialization when compared with wet-to-dry dressings and air exposure.[1] This occurred with the use of both oxygen-impermeable and oxygen-permeable plastic dressings. It seems from this and other research that occlusive dressings may enhance wound healing.[10] Occlusive dressings prevent eschar formation, thereby permitting more rapid epithelial migration. A problem with some occlusive dressings is the occurrence of infection. Other occlusive dressings are nonadherent, which facilitates dressing removal and the use of topical antibiotics to decrease bacterial growth beneath the dressing.

Monitoring of the healing process is not limited to the wound itself. It requires constant attention to the person's total body functioning. To promote wound healing, interventions to achieve adequate nutritional intake and blood flow to the injured area are essential. These problems were addressed earlier.

Generalized infection and fluid and electrolyte imbalances are potential problems with open wounds. The elderly are particularly vulnerable to these conditions. Immunologic changes with age result in decreased defenses against infection. Protective isolation may be indicated for prevention of infection; however, this increases the risk of disorientation because of sensory deprivation and loneliness. Frequent nurse–patient contact may help to prevent this from happening. As noted earlier, the depressed systemic response to infection, common in the elderly, needs to be considered when assessing physical manifestations. In general, elderly people do not cope well, physically or psychologically, with the prolonged period of stress which is part of healing by secondary intention. Table 15–4 presents aging changes that influence the healing process.

Scarring is a major concern when a wound heals by secondary intention. The danger is contracture causing disfigurement and limited movement. The patient may have difficulty coping with these conditions. Initiation of physical therapy early in the course of healing may prevent these

TABLE 15–4
Aging Changes Influencing the Healing Process

Component of Healing Process	*Aging Changes**	*Possible Effects*
Inflammation	Variations in stress response	Delayed onset of inflammation Minimal intensity of inflammation Prolonged duration of inflammation Systemic response minimal
	Circulation: atrophy of dermal capillaries	Decreased blood flow to trauma site and interference with inflammatory process: exudate formation and white blood cell migration
	Inadequate clotting factors due to marginal nutrition status of elderly	Potential for prolonged bleeding and large hematoma
	Diminished response of immune system	Sluggish phagocytosis of wound debris and increased susceptibility to infection
Reconstructive events		
Cellular proliferation and differentiation	Rate of cell replication decreases with age	May slow rate of wound healing
	Decrease in slow wave sleep and hence secretion of growth hormone	Slow rate of protein anabolism and therefore wound healing
Granulation tissue	Marginal nutritional status relatively common in elderly	Inadequate collagen synthesis; marginal tensile strength of wound; danger of evisceration, dehiscence
Maturation (time dependent; scar formation)	Marginal nutritional status	Delayed wound healing, danger of wound herniation
	Sedentary tendency resulting in decreased respiration (oxygenation) and circulation	Minimal circulation to part for delivery of oxygen and nutrients
	Decreased muscle strength due to inactivity	Prolonged weakness, inability to regain previous level of well-being
Healing of wounds with tissue loss (prolonged healing process)	See above changes Maginal ability to cope with prolonged stress	Potential for loneliness, confusion, depression

* See Chapter 5.

complications. In the event prevention is not possible, the complications may be avoided by skin grafting. This is discussed further in Chapter 97. The nurse's sensitivity to the patient's feelings guides the type of emotional support given and the type of instruction provided to the patient and family.

Bone Repair

Repair of injured bone is a process of connective tissue healing. It differs from soft tissue repair in the type of cells that are active. Osteoblasts and osteoclasts are the cells that form the specialized calcified tissue of bone. These essential cells arise from the periosteum and endosteum in the injured area. As with injury to other tissues, fracture of a bone is followed by bleeding into the site and clot formation. The clot fills the region between the two bone ends and the adjacent tissues. This is followed by inflammation and cellular proliferation as in the healing of soft tissue wounds. About day 3, proliferating chondroblasts and osteoblasts are present in the wound.[7] They are responsible for synthesis of cartilage and calcified matrix in much the same way as the fibroblasts synthesize collagen.

After a week or two, the fracture site is bridged by a combination of cartilage and fibrous tissue. This bridging tissue is termed a provisonal callus. Usually some calcium is deposited in the cartilagenous material, which hardens the provisional callus. This is followed by osteoblast activity that creates new trabeculae of osteoid. Eventually the provisional callus becomes traversed by osteoid trabeculae. Progressive calcification of the osteoid callus results in replacement of the procallus with bony callus, and the fractured ends become rigidly united. Development of a bony callus usually requires about 6 weeks. Total healing is extended for months. It requires the balanced action of osteoblasts and osteoclasts, including increased calcification, to remodel the site. The final outcome is restoration of the marrow cavity and almost perfect bone repair.

Factors that are important in the healing of bone are immobilization to permit formation of calcified osteoid trabeculae, and alignment of the fracture ends. The latter is necessary to reduce the distance between the fractured ends and thereby promote union. Fracture treatment and nursing care are discussed in Chapter 87.

Summary

Healing of damaged tissues is essential for survival. It is a process that begins immediately after injury and continues for months. The process consists of three overlapping and probably interrelated phases. These phases are the inflammatory reaction, reconstruction, and maturation. The process of repair is similar for all injured tissues (*i.e.*, surgical wounds, infections, and necrosis from inadequate circulation such as myocardial infarction). Differences relate to the extent of tissue damage and the duration of time the inflammant is present. Not all injuries result in permanent damage, but usually there is some residual scarring. Sometimes the wound is so large that healing by contraction may cause permanent dysfunction. Awareness of the indicators of normal healing and a knowledge of the negative influences on wound repair are the foundation for nursing interventions aimed at promoting wound healing and preventing complications.

References

1. Alvarez OM, Mertz PM, Eaglstein WH: The effect of occlusive dressings on collagen synthesis and re-epithelialization in superficial wounds. J Surg Res 35:142–148, 1983
2. Ehrlich HP: Fibroblast contraction of collagen lattices in vitro: Inhibition by chronic inflammatory cell mediators. J Cell Physiol 116(3):345–351, 1983
3. Ehrlich HP, Hunt TK: Effect of cortisone and vitamin A on wound healing. Ann surg 167:324–328, 1968
4. Elwyn DH, Kinney JM, Askanazi J: Energy expenditure in surgical patients. Surg Clin North Am 61(3), 1981
5. Forrest L: Current concepts in soft connective tissue wond healing. Br J Surg 70(3):133–140, 1983
6. Goodwin CW: The effect of chronic hypoxia on wound healing. Adv Exp Med Biol 94:669–672, 1977
7. Greiff J: Bone fracture healing studied by 99 m Tc-Sm- polyphosphate auto radiography and scintimetry. Dan Med Bull 30(3):150–157, 1983
8. Grove GL: Age related differences in healing of superficial skin wounds in humans. Arch Dermatol Res 272(3–4):381–385, 1982
9. Hurley JV: Acute Inflammation, 2nd ed. New York, Churchill Livingstone, 1983
10. Mandy SH: A new primary wound dressing made of polyethylene oxide gel. J Dermatol Surg Oncol 9(2):153–155, 1983
11. Montandon D, D'Andiran G, Gabbinani G: The mechanism of wound contraction and epithelialization. Clin Plast Surg 4:325–346, 1977
12. Peacock E: Wound Repair, 3rd ed. Philadelphia, WB Saunders, 1984
13. Robbins SL, Cotran RS, Kumar V: Pathologic Basis of Disease, 3rd ed. Philadelphia, WB Saunders, 1984
14. Ross R: Wound healing. Sci Am 220:40, June 1969
15. Solomkin JS: Cellular and subcellular mediator of acute inflammation. Surg Clin North Am 63(2):225–243, 1983

Bibliography

Bruno P: The nature of wound healing. NCNA 14(4), 1979

Bruno P, Craven R: Age challenges to wound healing. Journal of Gerontological Nursing 8(12), 1982

Bucknall TE: Factors influencing wound complications. AR Coll Surg Engl 65(2):71–77, 1983

Hayflick L: The limited in vitro lifetime of human diploid cell strains. Exp Cell Res 37:614, 1965

Hotter AN: Physiological aspects and clinical implications of wound healing. Heart Lung 11(6):522–531, 1982

Khoury GA: Large bowel anastomoses. I. The healing process and suture anastomoses. Br J Surg 70(2):61–63, 1983

Pollack SV: Wound healing—A review. IV. Systemic medications affecting wound healing. J Dermatol Surg Oncol 8(8):667–672, 1982

Chapter 16

Immune Responses

Betty B. Gallucci
Joanne Schnaidt Rokosky

The immune system, which protects the individual against microorganisms, toxins, foreign particles, and cancer cells, is a vast network of interacting cells and plasma proteins.[3] It has been thought of as a defense system much as the alarm reaction of the neuroendocrine system is a defense reaction, but in contrast to the nervous system, in which the cells are stationary, the cells of the immune system are often migratory and can mobilize in the area of injury.

A variety of reactions, including immune reactions, are encompassed by the term *host defense reactions.* Some host defenses are general and include all those factors that are nonspecific, such as a healthy skin and mucous membrane, which are barriers to microbial colonization; mechanical factors such as sneezing and ciliary action, which expel bacteria; chemical factors such as acidic gastric secretions, which limit bacterial colonization; and the inflammatory reaction.[13, 18] (General host defenses are summarized in Table 16–1.) These reactions are considered nonspecific since the reaction tends to follow a set pattern regardless of the nature of the stimulus, that is, an inflammatory reaction follows an injury from a dirty splinter as well as from a sterile scalpel wound. Immune reactions, on the other hand, are specific reactions, that is, they are particular to the stimulus. The functions, properties, and types of immunity are outlined below:

- A. Function
  1. To recognize and destroy what is foreign
  2. To tolerate self
- B. Properties
  1. Specificity
  2. Memory
  3. Heterogeneity
- C. Effector arms
  1. Humoral immunity
  2. Cellular immunity

In this chapter, characteristics of the immune system and its defensive capabilities are described. Situations in which immune responses are inadequate or inappropriate will also be introduced, along with principles nurses can apply to enhance normal immune system behavior.

Properties of the Immune System

Specificity and *memory* are two properties that distinguish immune reactions from general host defense reactions. Immune reactions are also *heterogeneous* in that stimuli generally evoke the development of more than one immune substance.[3] These three properties are illustrated in the familiar situation of someone being vaccinated. When a person re-

TABLE 16–1
General Host Defenses

Mechanical Factors	*Chemical Factors*
Lavaging action of tears and saliva	Acidity of gastric secretion
Trapping effect of mucus-coated hairs and cilia	Acidity of vagina
Adhesive qualities of mucus lining respiratory and gastrointestinal tracts	Acidity of skin due to fatty acids
Expulsive effects of coughing, sneezing, and ciliary action	Lysozyme: an enzyme in tears, nasal secretions, saliva, urine
Cleansing effect of the flow of urine	
Desquamation of stratified epithelium from surface of skin–oral mucosa	

ceives a polio vaccine the immune system is stimulated by that particular organism and responds with a *specific* antibody response. Thus the person is protected from the polio organism but not from smallpox or other viruses. If the person is exposed to the polio organism again, he will mount a rapid and effective antibody response because of immunologic *memory*. Finally, the antibody response is *heterogeneous* in that the immune system responds by producing several different types of immune reactions to the particular polio virus even though only one of them actually provides protection.

Antigens

The immune system specifically recognizes and destroys what is foreign, but tolerates *self* (its own antigenic constituents). Not all foreign substances are capable of provoking the immune system, and some substances are better at this than others. If the foreign substance not only stimulates the immune system but also is capable of combining with the products of the immune system, then it is called an *antigen*. Foreign proteins are often good antigens, as are the complex polysaccharides found in bacterial cell walls, toxins, and microbial enzymes. Nucleoproteins can be antigens, but pure nucleic acids cannot. Fats are generally poor antigens, but lipopolysaccharides and lipoproteins can produce a reaction. Very small molecules do not stimulate the immune system but large complex molecules do, especially if they are unlike the molecules present in the individual.[29]

Allergens are antigens that provoke the production of specific immune products, especially IgE antibody, in sensitive individuals. The ability of a foreign substance to be an antigen depends not only on its chemical nature but also on host factors. A person's genetic makeup may determine which substances will be recognized by the immune system and which ones will not. This is often seen in the case of allergies. For example, not all people are allergic to such substances as ragweed pollen. The fact that allergies tend to be present in certain families also attests to the inheritability of immune reactions.[29]

Components of the Immune System

Genetic Component: Major Histocompatibility Complex (MHC)

The genetics of the immune system is probably the most well known of any system in the body. The drive to understand what controls the immune response was first prompted by kidney graft rejection.[4, 13, 29] It was noted that kidney grafts survived a longer time if the donor was a relative of the patient rather than unrelated. The major histocompatibility complex (MHC) is a multigene system called HLA (histocompatibility-linked antigens or human leukocyte antigens) in humans. Histocompatibility antigens or transplantation antigens are molecules on the surface of various cells that evoke an immune response in another person. If two people are closely matched with respect to the histocompatibility antigens, organ rejection is less likely. These genes also contain information for interactions between the cells responsible for immunologic reactions; immunoresponsiveness; susceptibility to allergic and immunologic-mediated disease; and some of the complement proteins and mediators important in immunologic reactions. Some of the diseases that have been associated with particular sets of these genes include ankylosing spondylitis, insulin-dependent diabetes mellitus, myasthenia gravis, systemic lupus erythematosus, and multiple sclerosis.

Cellular Components

In general there are two major categories of cells that are involved in immune reactions: lymphocytes that are responsible for the specific reaction with the antigen, and accessory cells that aid the lymphocytes. Both categories are necessary for an adequate immune response, and there is a great deal of interaction between the two categories. They are considered here separately for the sake of clarity.

The tissues that produce lymphocytes are collectively referred to as lymphoid organs. These organs are found throughout the body, as illustrated in Figure 16–1.

The two major classes of lymphocytes that are best understood are B lymphocytes and T lymphocytes. Other types of lymphocytes that are not as well understood are the null cells, which do not have B or T cell markers, and natural killer cells, which may be related to T cells.[17, 21, 30] Both the T lymphocytes and the B lymphocytes are composed of subpopulations of cells that have different functions. To understand how these lymphocytes received their names, a review of their origins is necessary.

B Lymphocytes. The stem cells or precursor cells of both types of lymphocytes are located in the bone marrow. It is probably here in the bone marrow that the cells destined to become functional B cells mature and develop B cell markers. (The name B cell originated from the bursa of Fabricius, a structure present only in birds. The bursa is similar in structure to the human appendix. A bursal equivalent has been sought but has not been found in humans.) After the B cells develop, they leave the bone marrow and travel by way of the cardiovascular and lymphatic systems to populate the lymphoid tissues in areas called germinal centers (Fig. 16–2). Once in the lymphoid tissue, B cells can be activated by antigens that in turn cause them to differentiate further. The mature B cell is called a *plasma* cell and it manufactures antibodies (also called immunoglobulins).[1,3,29]

FIGURE 16–1 Organs of the immune system are located throughout the body. Major lymphoid organs include the *bone marrow*, where precursor cells of both B and T lymphocytes are formed and where B cells are thought to mature; the *thymus gland*, where T cells mature; *lymph nodes*, which receive lymph circulation and have specialized compartments for B cells, T cells, and macrophages; and the *spleen*, which is the largest lymphoid organ and contains high numbers of lymphocytes. Accessory lymphoid tissues include the *tonsils* and *adenoids*, the *appendix*, and *Peyer's patches*, clumps of lymphoid tissue located in the small intestine. (Adapted from Understanding the Immune System [NIH Publication No. 84-529]. US Department of Health and Human Services, Public Health Service, October 1983)

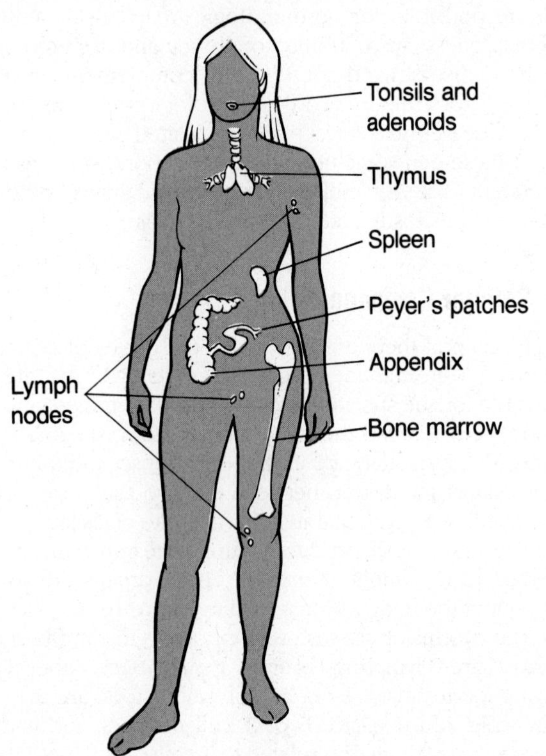

T Lymphocytes. The T cell precursors are also located in the bone marrow. The T stem cells leave the bone marrow and migrate to the thymus. In the thymus many of the T cells die, but a portion of the cells remain and mature. As they mature they acquire molecules on their cell surfaces that identify them as T cells. These cells then leave the thymus and populate the paracortical areas of lymphoid tissue, which are also known as the T cell areas (Fig. 16–2). If an appropriate antigen is presented to a T cell, it also can differentiate. The resulting subpopulations of T cells are called cytotoxic T cells, helper T cells, and suppressor T cells. Memory cells are also formed after activation of either T or B cells and they are responsible for the more rapid and heightened immunologic response on subsequent exposure to an antigen.[1,3,29]

Accessory Cells. Accessory cells cooperate with T and B cells to produce an immune reaction. The predominant accessory cells are macrophages, which are derived from the monocyte cell line. But since the inflammatory reaction is so entwined with the immune reaction, neutrophils, basophils, and mast cells and eosinophils may also be involved as accessory cells.[15]

The names given to tissue macrophages differ according to their location. In the skin and oral mucosa they are called langerhans cells; in the liver, Kupffer cells; in the connective tissue, histiocytes; in the spleen and bone marrow, free and fixed macrophages; and in the pleural cavity, pleural macrophages. Previously called the reticuloendothelial system, this system of macrophages has been renamed the mononuclear phagocyte system.[29] Since these cells are neither reticular nor endothelial cells, a name more appropriate to their structure and function was chosen.

Macrophages can bind to antigens and present the antigens to T and B cells. For some antigens this is a necessary step. Without this presentation and processing by the macrophage, the lymphocytes cannot respond to these antigens. A regulatory role has additionally been proposed for the macrophage because it can release inhibitors of the immune response. Macrophages ingest foreign particles by either phagocytosis or pinocytosis and thus process the antigen or destroy the foreign particles or dead cells. Macrophages are also important in the inflammatory response and tend to predominate late in acute infections or throughout chronic infections.[1,3,29] Figure 16–3 is an election microscopy photo showing a macrophage emigrating from a capillary.

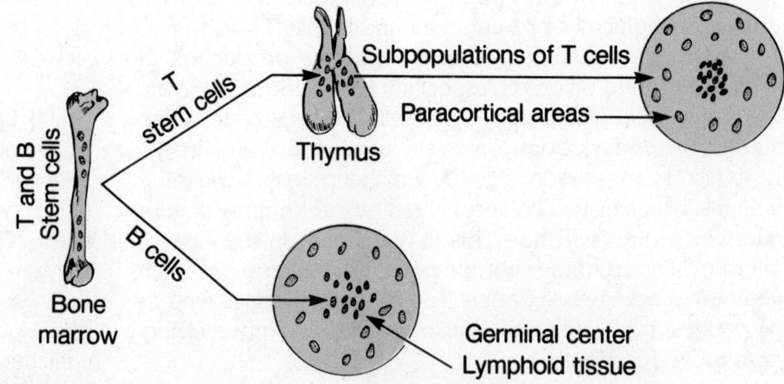

FIGURE 16–2 Lymphocyte production in bone marrow. Precursor cells of both B and T lymphocytes are located in the bone marrow. B cells further develop within the bone marrow, then migrate to germinal centers located within lymph nodes and other lymphoid organs; when stimulated by antigens, they differentiate further. T cells leave the bone marrow and mature in the thymus. Differentiation after contact with antigen occurs in the paracortical areas of lymph nodes and other lymphoid organs.

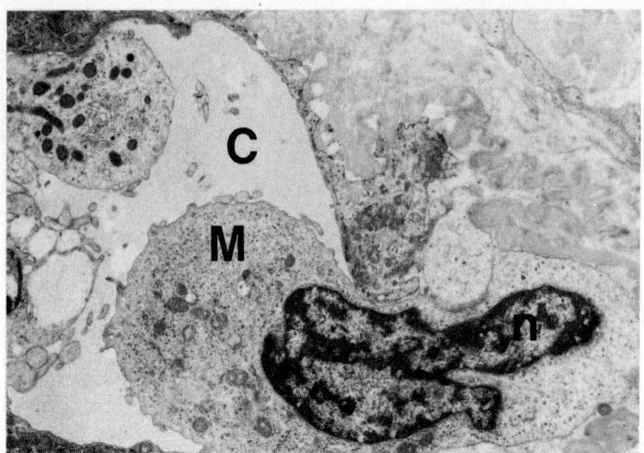

FIGURE 16–3 Electron microscopy photo shows macrophage (M) emigrating from capillary (C). After leaving vessel, macrophage will move to site of inflammation and ingest foreign particles.

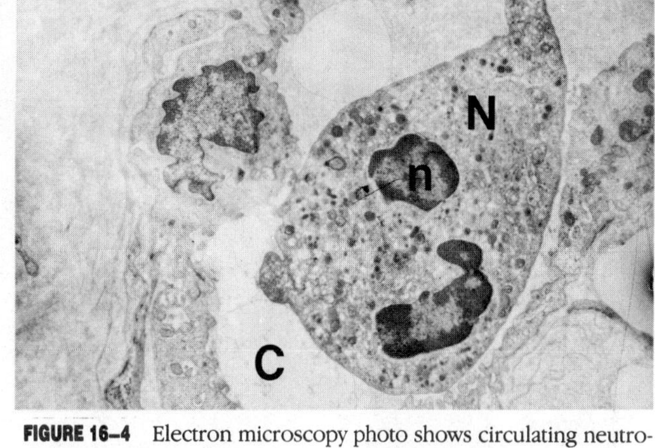

FIGURE 16–4 Electron microscopy photo shows circulating neutrophil (N) within capillary (C).

Neutrophils or *polymorphonuclear leukocytes* are phagocytes as well, and they comprise about 60% of the circulating white blood cells (Fig. 16–4). They contain many granules that are important in the digestion of microorganisms and cellular debris. Release of the granules may be partially under the control of immune factors. Neutrophils predominate early in an infectious process and release mediators of inflammation. Patients who are neutropenic, such as those receiving chemotherapy or radiation therapy for cancer, as well as bone marrow transplant patients, are at a very high risk for developing an overwhelming infection. Diabetic patients often have functionally impaired neutrophils. In all these patients the signs of inflammation may be minimal and hard to detect.[3, 29]

Basophils and *tissue mast cells* are characterized by granules that contain heparin and histamine. These cells are often found near blood vessels under the skin and near mucous membranes. In persons with allergies a particular antibody, IgE, binds to the surface of these cells. When an allergen then binds to the IgE, the granules of the mast cell or basophil are released and the allergy symptoms occur.[3, 29]

Eosinophils are important in immune reactions as regulators. Eosinophils release enzymes that can degrade histamine and other mediators of allergic reactions. In addition to their role in allergic reactions, eosinophils are also prominent in parasitic infections. They release their granules on the surface of the parasite, which causes the parasite to lyse.[1, 3, 15, 29]

Immune Reactions

An immune reaction to a specific antigen can be broken down into three major phases: afferent, central, and efferent. In the afferent phase the antigen is processed by tissue macrophages. This usually means that the foreign substance is engulfed and destroyed by the macrophage or that some of the molecules present in the antigen are attached to the cell membrane of the macrophage. The macrophage then migrates to the regional lymph node or lymphoid tissue and presents the antigen to the lymphocytes. This is the central phase. The lymphocytes are stimulated to grow and divide, that is, they become blastlike and form daughter cells. Eventually mature lymphocytes are formed. In the efferent phase the mature lymphocytes release their products, such as antibodies and lymphokines. The antibody–antigen complexes or the lymphokines can then trigger other reactions that lead to sustained inflammatory or allergic processes. The result of these reactions leads to the destruction of the foreign substance.[3]

This overall process can be further divided into two different immune reactions depending on which type of lymphocyte was stimulated. If the antigen has provoked an antibody response then the immune reaction is called *humoral immunity* (antibody reaction, immediate hypersensitivity, B cell response, or antibody-mediated hypersensitivity). If the antigen has stimulated the T cell system then the reaction is known as *cell-mediated immunity* (cellular immunity, delayed hypersensitivity, or T cell reaction). These two responses are diagrammed in Figure 16–5. If the antigen has not provoked a reaction at all it is called a *tolerogen* and the resulting state is tolerance.

One of the easiest ways to visualize these two types of immune reactions is to conduct a theoretical experiment as illustrated in Figure 16–6. The first step is to inject a rabbit with a microorganism to which it has never been exposed. The immune system will be activated; it will fight off the "bug" and protection against subsequent infections will be achieved. If blood is then drawn from this rabbit, centrifuged, and the serum separated from the cells, the protection against subsequent infections with the same organism will be located either in the serum or cellular fraction. This can be tested by injecting the serum and the organism into a second unprotected rabbit. If the animal does not get ill, then the protection was located in the humoral or serum part of the blood. This is the principle behind passive immunization of a person following exposure to hepatitis or certain other diseases. The exposed person is protected with antibodies isolated from the serum of previously exposed individuals.

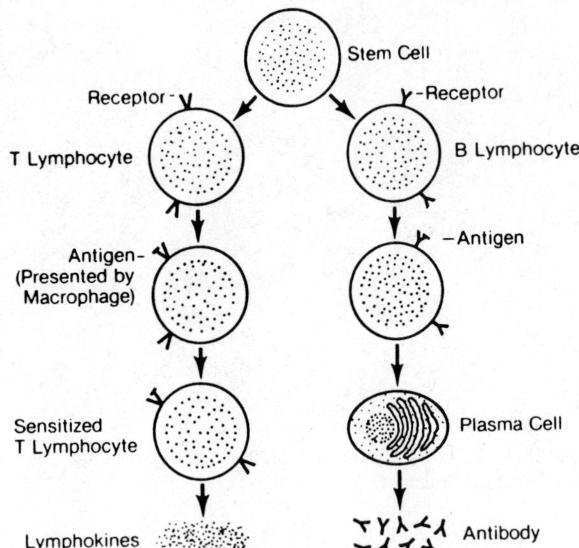

FIGURE 16–5 The immune response: cell-mediated (*left*) and humoral (*right*). (Understanding the Immune System [NIH Publication No. 84-529]. US Department of Health and Human Services, Public Health Service, October 1983)

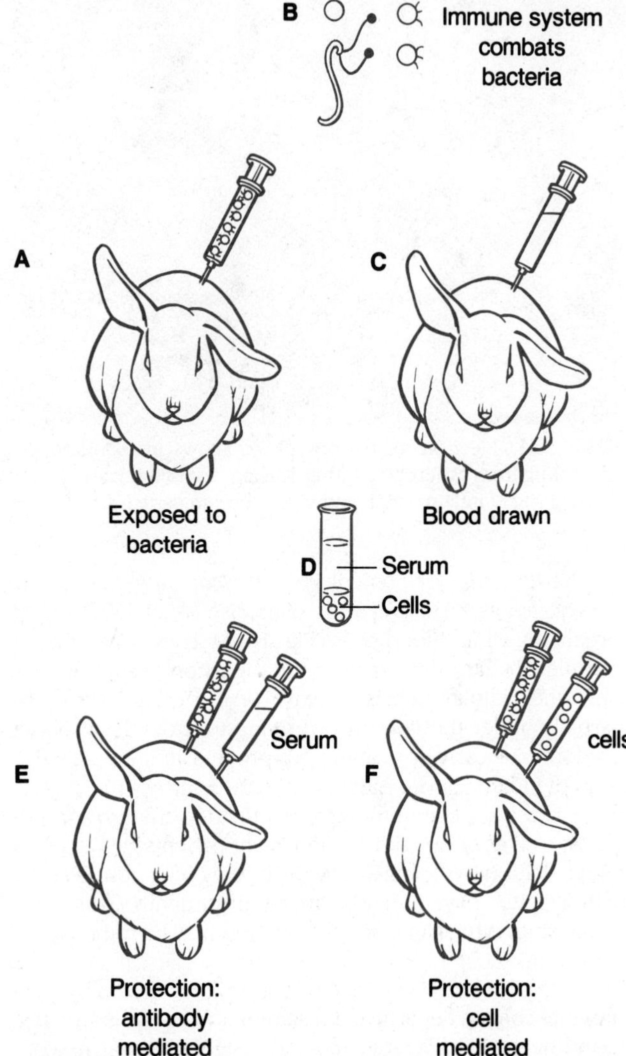

FIGURE 16–6 Experiment to show difference between cell-mediated and humoral immunity. (*A*) A rabbit is first injected with a microorganism to which it has never been exposed. After the rabbit's immune system has had time to combat the antigen (*B*), blood is drawn from the rabbit (*C*) and serum separated from cells (*D*). If the serum and organism can be injected into another rabbit and the rabbit does not become ill, the serum or humoral portion of the blood contained the immunity (*E*). Conversely, if the cells and organism are injected into another rabbit who does not become ill, the immunity was cell-mediated (*F*).

If, on the other hand, the cellular fraction of the blood protects the animal from illness, then the protection was cell mediated. Transfer of cell-mediated immunity can only occur between identical twins or, in the case of laboratory animals, in inbred lines.

Humoral Immunity

Antibodies are the protein molecules responsible for humoral immunity. These molecules are manufactured by plasma cells and are capable of antigen destruction, as shown in Fig. 16–7. Varied antibody characteristics enable them to inactivate antigen. Antibodies can be agglutinins, precipitins, complement-fixing antibodies, lysins, opsonins, or neutralizing antibodies.[13] These methods are listed and defined in Table 16–2.

Chemically, antibodies are part of a larger class of compounds called *immunoglobulines*. Immunoglobulins are proteins that may or may not have the ability to recognize and destroy antigens. Immunoglobulins constitute about 20% of the plasma proteins. The structure and chemistry of the immunoglobulins were first worked out with Bence Jones proteins. These proteins were isolated in the urine of patients with multiple myeloma (a cancer of the plasma cell line). Because these tumors result from a single cell, all the antibody manufactured is of one kind, known as *monoclonal* antibodies. Thus large quantities of a pure immunoglobin chain were available.[1,3,29]

There are five classes of immunoglobins in humans—IgG, IgA, IgM, IgD, and IgE. In addition to structural differences (shown in Fig. 16–8), there are important variations in concentration and type and location of antibody response.

TABLE 16–2
Methods by Which Antibodies Inactivate Antigen

Agglutination	Antibody links small antigen particles together into large, insoluble clumps.
Precipitation	Antibody combines with soluble antigen, resulting in precipitate formation.
Lysis	Direct antigen destruction by antibody.
Opsonization	Antibody coats antigen and renders it more vulnerable to phagocytosis.
Neutralization	Antibody combines with and thereby inactivates toxin or other biologically active product of antigen.
Complement Fixation	Antibody–antigen complex activates complement, which subsequently assists with antigen destruction.

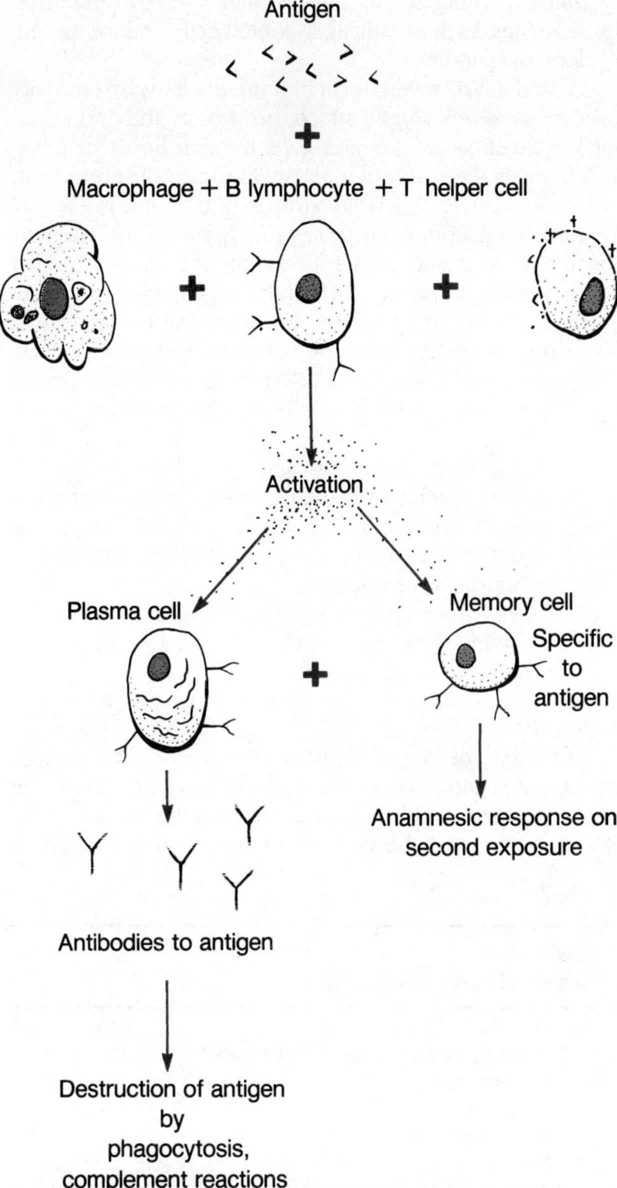

FIGURE 16–7 Humoral immune reaction. The invasion of antigen into tissues stimulates an inflammatory response in which the antigen is phagocytosed by macrophages. Macrophages, B lymphocytes, and T helper cells interact, which causes activation of the B lymphocytes. The B lymphocytes mature to form plasma cells, which subsequently produce antibodies, and memory cells, which are responsible for a secondary or anamnesic response.

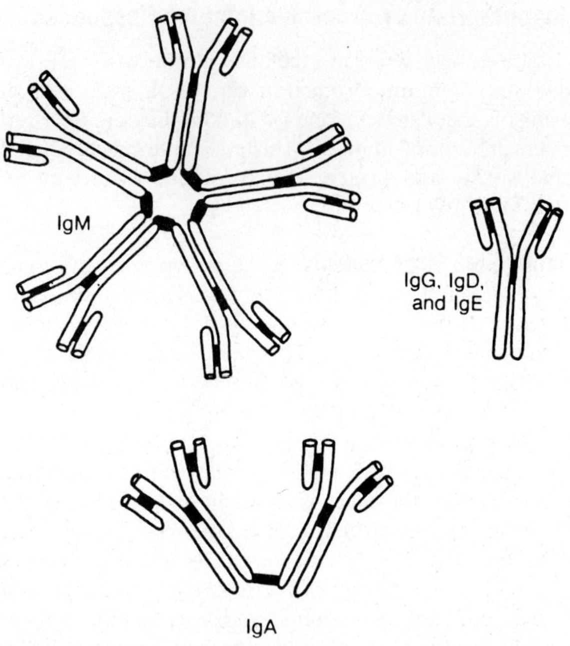

FIGURE 16–8 Immunoglobulin structure. All immunoglobulin molecules share the same basic unit in which four polypeptide chains are symmetrically arranged into two short, light chains and two longer, heavy chains. IgG, IgD, and IgE contain one such unit; IgA has two units, and IgM contains 5 units. (Understanding the Immune System [NIH Publication No. 84-529]. US Department of Health and Human Services, Public Health Service, October 1983)

These differences are summarized as follows:

- IgG (the most abundant)
  - Activates complement reactions
  - Can cross the placenta and is responsible for immunity in the newborn
- IgA (a secretory antibody)
  - Located in saliva, tears, and mucus of the respiratory, digestive, and urinary tracts
- IgM (the largest of the Igs in molecular size)
  - The second in abundance
  - The first to appear in fetal life
  - Important in a primary infection
- IgD (present in only minute amounts)
  - Possibly a regulatory antibody
- IgE (the reaginic antibody)
  - Responsible for some allergic responses (*e.g.,* ragweed, pollen, dust)
  - Also a secretory antibody

Immune reactions are a double-edged sword. In most normal situations an immune reaction protects the individual against microorganisms, toxins, and foreign particles. The other edge of the sword is that in some individuals antibody reactions are not protective but instead create tissue injury beyond what the antigen would do if there were not antibody reactions.

Protective Immune Responses

Antibodies protect us against pyogenic or pus-forming bacteria, including staphylococcus, streptococcus, *Streptococcus pneumoniae* (pneumococcus), and meningococcus. The viruses they counteract include influenza, polio, hepatitis B, and measles.

If an individual has a deficiency of humoral imunity he will be prone to pyogenic infections. For example, some infants at about 5 to 6 months of age suffer from a transitory hypogammaglobulinemia because their passively transferred maternal antibodies are degraded, and the infant has not yet made its own. Respiratory tract infections may occur at this age. There are also rare congenital hypogammaglobulinemias in which the child suffers from recurrent pyogenic infections, such as otitis media, conjunctivitis, abnormal dental decay, and eczematoid skin infections.[2,3,13,29]

Inappropriate or Excessive Immune Responses

Tissue damage from an excessive or otherwise inappropriate humoral immune reaction can result from several mechanisms that can act alone or in combination. Selected disorders of humoral immunity related to antibody-mediated hypersensitivity and proliferative B-cell-line disorders are listed in Table 16–3.

Immediate Hypersensitivity. One type of pathologic response is called an *anaphylactic reaction* or *immediate hypersensitivity* because it can occur from minutes to hours after exposure to the antigen. This type of reaction develops when antigen combines with IgE attached to mast cells and leads to the release of mast cell contents.[1,3,29]

IgE has also been called *reaginic factor* because a passive transfer of IgE from an allergic person to a nonallergic person will create the reaction in the nonallergic individual. Hay fever and asthma are primarily due to an allergen reacting with IgE on the surface of mast cells.[29] Within the mast cell granules are a variety of mediators. Histamine has already been mentioned but other mediators include heparin, which temporarily limits blood clotting in the area of injury, ECF-A or eosinophil chemotactic factor of anaphylaxis, which attracts eosinophils to the area, and leukotriene derivatives of arachidonic acid. One of the leukotrienes is called *slow-reacting substance of anaphylaxis* (*SRS-A*) and is 100 times more powerful than histamine in creating bronchospasm. This substance is the one involved in the bronchospasm of asthma. Also released from lung mast cells are a class of prostaglandins that are powerful vasodilators.

Treatment for allergies often involves desensitization injections. It is thought that these injections work by stimulating the immune system to produce IgG. If sufficient numbers of IgG molecules can reach the target tissues, the allergens can then react with the IgG and prevent the binding of the allergen to IgE on the mast cell. The IgG-antigen complex is subsequently phagocytized and destroyed by the macrophage system.[29] Another therapy for allergic reactions involves relieving the symptoms by the use of drugs. Antihistamines counteract the histamines, whereas the nonsteroid drugs, such as aspirin, indomethacin, and ibuprofen, block prostaglandins.

A particularly severe form of immediate hypersensitivity reaction is *anaphylactic shock*, in which the individual quickly develops asthma and goes into cardiovascular collapse. This is the result of a massive leakage of serum from the blood vessels which, in turn, is due to the release of chemical mediators from mast cells. Epinephrine counteracts this reaction and can be life saving. It is imperative that nurses be able to predict, recognize, and assist in the management of this life-threatening complication. Substances from drugs, foods, and stinging insects that commonly cause anaphylactic shock are listed in Table 16–4. Nursing principles related to recognizing and managing anaphylactic shock include

1. Being aware of high-risk situations
2. Applying safety measures such as assessing for a history of allergic reactions and having emergency equipment available in situations that may lead to anaphylactic reactions
3. Identifying manifestations of anaphylactic shock
4. Knowing how to initiate emergency procedures when these symptoms occur

For the details of care under each of these points refer to Table 16–5.

Another type of pathologic response is called *antibody-dependent cytotoxic hypersensitivity*. In this case, circulating IgM or IgG reacts with antigen present on the surface of the cell or tissue, and the cell or tissue is then damaged or

TABLE 16–3
Selected Disorders of Humoral Immunity

Antibody-Mediated Hypersensitivity

IgE Mediated
- Anaphylactic shock
- Hay fever
- Asthma

IgG or IgM Mediated
- Serum sickness
- Transfusion reactions

Proliferative disorders of B cell line
- Multiple myeloma
- Macroglobulinemia (Waldenström's)
- Heavy chain disease
- Non-Hodgkin's lymphoma

TABLE 16–4
Common Causes of Anaphylaxis

Drugs
- Proteins (presumably complete antigens)
  - Foreign serum
  - Vaccines
  - Allergen extracts
  - Enzymes
- Nonprotein drugs (presumably haptens)
  - Penicillin and other antibiotics
  - Sulfonamides
  - Local anesthetics
  - Salicylates

Foods
- Legumes (especially peanuts)
- Nuts
- Berries
- Seafoods
- Egg albumin

Stinging insects
- Honeybees
- Wasps
- Hornets
- Yellow jackets
- Fire ants

(Reproduced, with permission, from Stites DP et al [eds]: Basic and Clinical Immunology, 5th ed. Copyright 1984 by Lange Medical Publications, Los Altos, California)

TABLE 16–5
Nursing Responsibilities Related to Anaphylactic Shock

Prevention

Known High-Risk Situations

Second exposure or known allergies to
- Drugs (including but not limited to penicillins and other antibiotics)
- Bee or other insect venoms
- Iodine-containing contrast media (not antibody mediated)
- Foods
- Pollen extracts

Apply Safety Precautions
- Question patients regarding allergic history.
- Note allergies on patient records.
- Instruct high-risk patients about self-protective measures, such as identification bracelets, emergency kits.
- Have emergency equipment available.
- Have outpatients remain 30 min after injection of any type.
- Perform skin test before administering horse serum preparations or allergic extracts.

Management

Recognize Manifestations

Time: within minutes of injected or, less commonly, ingested antigen

Signs and symptoms:
- Itching, hives, erythema due to cutaneous involvement
- Coughing, sneezing, hoarseness, wheezing due to bronchospasm and laryngeal edema
- Hypotension, imperceptible pulse, pallor due to peripheral vascular collapse
- Nausea, vomiting, abdominal pain, diarrhea due to gastrointestinal involvement

Initiate Emergency Procedures
- Call for help.
- Maintain airway: position, insertion of oral airway or endotracheal tube, ventilation with bag and mask.
- Administer aqueous epinephrine: generally 0.2–0.5 ml of 1 : 1000 dilution subcutaneously, occasionally IV or other routes.
- Apply tourniquet proximal to injection site if antigen is injected into extremity.
- Start intravenous infusion for drug and fluid administration.
- Administer additional measures as required: oxygen, antihistamines, aminophylline, volume expanders, vasopressors.

destroyed. Complement, described later in this chapter, plays a role in this form of tissue injury. Hemolytic reactions following transfusions of incompatible blood, some forms of hemolytic anemia, and certain drug reactions are examples of a cytotoxic response.[1,3,29]

Yet another humoral immune response involves the formation of circulating antigen–antibody complexes that cause an inflammatory reaction when they become trapped in body tissues. Complement again plays a role in this *immune complex–mediated hypersensitivity*. Immune complexes have been isolated in a wide variety of human diseases, including systemic lupus erythematosis, glomerulonephritis, and rheumatoid arthritis.

Autoimmune Disease. Both immune complex formation and cytotoxic hypersensitivity have been implicated as mechanisms responsible for the tissue damage that occurs in *autoimmune disease*. In autoimmune disease it appears that the body has lost tolerance to self. There are several hypotheses about why this occurs. One scenario postulates that when self molecules resemble closely the molecules present on some microorganisms, the immune system is stimulated, causing antibodies to the microorganisms to also bind to self molecules. Another possibility is that self molecules that are usually hidden from the immune system might be released after an injury and thereby stimulate an immune response. A third possibility is that the regulatory controls of the immune response might be lost, allowing a forbidden clone of immune cells to arise. A final hypothesis suggests that a mild viral infection in a cell might be expressed as viral molecules on the cell surface. This viral infection in and of itself might cause little cell destruction, but the immune response to the viral antigen might create a great deal of cellular destruction.[3,29]

In many autoimmune diseases, autoantibodies, that is, antibodies against self molecules, have been isolated. For example, in Hashimoto's thyroiditis, antibodies are present to thyroglobulin; in systemic lupus erythematosus, antibodies against DNA, nuclear antigens, lymphocytes, and red blood cells have been isolated; and in rheumatoid arthritis, antibodies to gammaglobulin molecules are present. In many autoimmune diseases, dysfunction of cell-mediated immunity exists as well. Therefore, it is frequently unclear whether the defect leading to loss of tolerance of self originated as a humoral or a cell-mediated disorder. Examples of autoimmune diseases include

- Hashimoto's thyroiditis
- Primary biliary cirrhosis
- Systemic lupus erythematosus
- Chronic glomerulonephritis
- Rheumatoid arthritis
- Scleroderma
- Pernicious anemia
- Autoimmune hemolytic anemia
- Idiopathic thrombocytopenic purpura

Presently there are no available cures for these diseases, but often immunosuppressive agents are given to control and limit the symptoms. Subsequent chapters of this text describe the pathophysiology and nursing care specific to each of these diseases.

Proliferative B Cell Problems

Another type of immune dysfunction involves the abnormal proliferation of one or more plasma cell precursors of antibodies. The proliferating mass of cells damages normal bone marrow and other lymphoid tissue in distinctive patterns, as covered in Chapter 51. Included in these disorders are multiple myeloma, macroglobulinemia (Waldenström's), and non-Hodgkin's lymphoma.

Cell-Mediated Immunity

In a broad sense the afferent and central phases of the cellular immune response are similar to the humoral response. Macrophages process the antigens and present them to the T cell; the T lymphocytes are then activated, grow, divide, and form subpopulations of T lymphocytes. The final or efferent phase of cell-mediated immunity is, however, quite different from humoral immunity in that it depends on the activation of T lymphocyte cells rather than on the production of antibodies. Specific cell-mediated activities vary among subpopulations of T lymphocytes. T lymphocytes are good at destroying certain viruses, malignant cells, cells of a grafted organ, and cells infected with intracellular microorganisms.

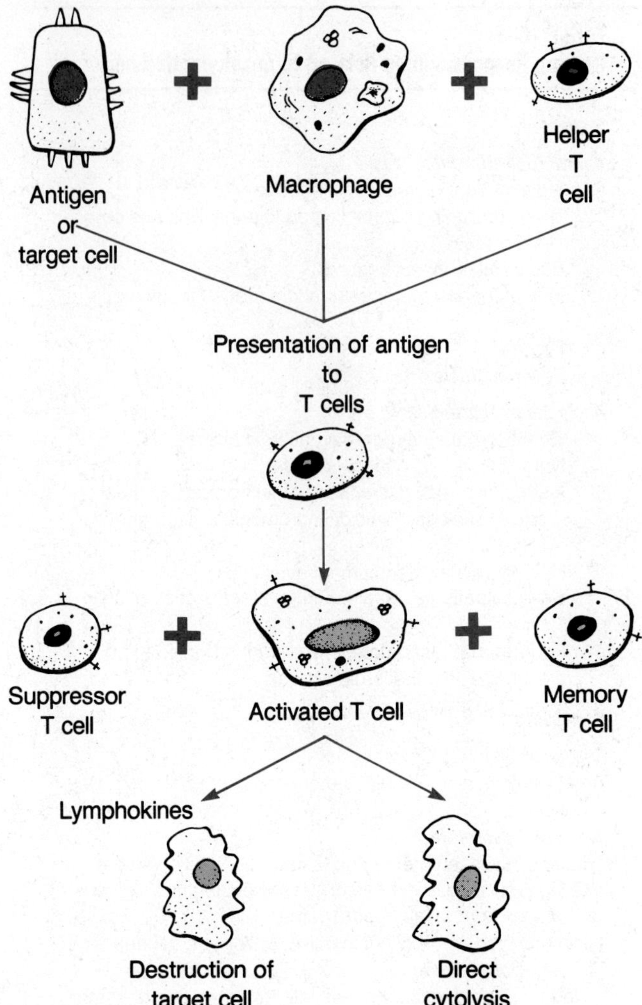

FIGURE 16–9 Cell mediated immune reaction. The interaction of antigen, macrophages, and helper T cells activates T cells. A variety of activated T cells with different functions exist: cytotoxic T cells, cells which release lymphokines, helper T cells, and suppressor T cells.

T Cell Subpopulations

One subpopulation that might result from activation is a *cytotoxic T cell line*. This line is capable of destroying target cells by direct cell to cell contact. The cytotoxic T cell comes into direct contact with the target cell. By some process that is not known, the T lymphocyte creates a change in the target cell which lyses the cell, but leaves the lymphocyte intact and capable of migrating away and reacting again with another cell. Figure 16–9 depicts this process in graphic style.

Another subpopulation of activated T lymphocytes can form and release mediators called *lymphokines*. Quite a variety of lymphokines with many different actions have been described (see Table 16–6). Even though lymphokines are described here under T cell reactions, actually whole families of similar molecules have been characterized, and some of the members can also be produced by B lymphocytes, macrophages, and other cells such as fibroblasts. Lymphokine activities include the ability to attract other white blood cells to the area, destroy target cells, inhibit viral replication, and regulate other lymphocytes.[29] Lymphokines are produced in minute quantities under normal circumstances and, therefore, until recently were difficult to study. With the development of the new genetic engineering techniques, more and purer preparations of sufficient quantities have become available for laboratory experimentation and even for therapy.

Other subpopulations that result from T cell activation are *helper T cells* and *suppressor T cells*. These cells may mediate their effect through the release of such factors as interleukins. Helper T cells help other T cells and help B cells to form antibodies to many antigens. Not only do B cells need macrophages to become activated but they also need helper T cells. Large polysaccharide molecules are among the few types of antigens that do not require T cells to generate an antibody response.[29] These antigens are called *thymus-independent antigens*. Suppressor cells function as their name suggests: they suppress both T and B cell reactions. Suppressor T cells may interfere with the helper T cells or may interfere directly with the maturation of the B lymphocytes responsible for the specific antibody production. Although humoral and cellular immunity are considered separately in this chapter, there is in reality a great deal of collaboration between T and B lymphocytes.

The immune system is self-regulated to a large extent by these populations of helper and suppressor T cells.[11,16,27,28] Perhaps an analogous system of B cells will be found in the future. Immune reactions can be potentiated by calling in granulocytes and macrophages and other lymphocytes, and can be limited through the activation of suppressor T cells to prevent extensive injury to normal tissue. Some syndromes, such as AIDS (acquired immune deficiency syndrome), are characterized by an imbalance of helper and suppressor T cells.

Memory cells are another population of cells that arises after specific activation of the T cells. These cells remain after the original antigenic stimulus is removed. If an individual is then exposed some time later to the same antigen, these cells can become quickly activated. Because these cells are an expanded population of the originally stimulated cells, at the second exposure the immunologic reaction is quicker and the quantity of antibodies or mediators released is greater.

The classic method of examining T cell reactions was to study delayed or tuberculin-type skin reactions.[1,3,13] A review of the characteristics of a positive reaction will more sharply delineate the differences between cellular and humoral immunity (see Table 16–7). A positive reaction to a tuberculin skin test, a test which evokes a cellular immune response if

TABLE 16–6
Lymphokines and Their Actions

Influencing Factors	*Action*
Macrophages	
Chemotactic factor for macrophages	Attracts macrophages to the area of injury
Macrophage activating factor (MAF)	Turns macrophages into angry killers
Macrophage inhibiting factor (MIF)	Once macrophages are attracted to an area of injury, prevents the macrophage from migrating away
Granulocytes	
Chemotactic factors for neutrophils, eosinophils, and basophils	Attract these white blood cells to the area of injury
Leukocyte inhibitory factor	Similar to MIF
Lymphocytes and Interleukins	
Mitogenic factors	Activates nonstimulated lymphocytes to grow and divide (*i.e.,* to become blasts); recruits nonsensitized lymphocytes and expands their reaction
Interleukin I (previously called leukocyte activating factor [LAF])	Derived from macrophages, promotes proliferation of T cells
Interleukin II (previously called T cell growth factor)	Derived from lymphocytes, promotes long-term proliferation of T cells
Transfer factor	Ability to transfer a specific T cell response to a nonsensitized person without transferring the immune cells
Other Cells	
Lymphotoxin	Kills cells in the immediate area
Interferon	Inhibits the replication of viral particles in infected cells and has antiproliferative capability; used in treatment of cancer
Colony stimulating factor	Stimulates stem cells of the bone marrow to differentiate

TABLE 16–7
Cell-Mediated vs. Humoral Immunity

Property	*Humoral Immunity*	*Cell-Mediated Immunity*
Time course in sensitized individual	Minutes to hours	One or more days
Histology of inflammatory lesion	Edema, polymorphonuclear neutrophils	Mononuclear cells
Transfer with	Serum (AB)	Lymphoid cells (T lymphocytes)
Specificity	Small determinants on molecules	Large molecules, usually proteins on cell surfaces

(Eisen H: Immunology: An introduction to molecular and cellular principles of the immune response. In Davis DP, Dulbecco R, Eisen HN et al: Microbiology, p 559. New York, Harper & Row, 1973)

there has been a prior exposure, develops approximately 48 to 72 hours after the injection of the antigen. In contrast, a secondary humoral immune reaction is apparent minutes to hours after the exposure (delayed vs. immediate hypersensitivity). In cell-mediated immunity, lymphocytes and macrophages predominate at the site of the injury. The histological picture of a humoral reaction instead includes edema and neutrophils. The target of a cell-mediated response is either an entire cell or large molecules, whereas antibodies bind to molecules.

Characteristics of Lymphocyte Populations

A variety of biochemical techniques are used to differentiate T cells from B cells, as discussed below. Since T and B cells and T cell subpopulations cannot be identified by their morphology, a variety of laboratory tests using biochemical techniques are performed to distinguish them. T cell subpopulations can be distinguished by monoclonal antibodies to surface markers. Immature T cells are labelled by OK3 monoclonal antibody; OKT5, OKT8 label cytotoxic and suppressor T cells. OKT4 monoclonal antibodies label helper T cells. If lymphocytes are placed into culture, the addition of certain chemicals can stimulate the cells nonspecifically to become blast cells. Phytohemagglutinin (PHA) and concanavalin A (conA) tend to stimulate T cells, and pokeweed mitogen, B cells. Another feature that distinguishes T from B cells is the ability of T cells to form rosettes with sheep red blood cells; that is, if sheep red blood cells are added to a mixture of lymphocytes then the smaller erythrocytes will bind and encircle the T cell forming something that resembles a flower. Some or all of these types of tests may be performed to characterize an immune deficiency or to diagnose such illnesses as AIDS.[3,29]

Protective Reactions

Cell-mediated immune reactions protect a person from intracelluar parasites (including the tuberculosis bacillus, the leprosy bacillus, and *Listeria*) and from fungal infections. The T cell system is also important in reactions against certain viruses such as cytomegalovirus, herpes, and mumps.[13] Protection against microorganisms such as *Toxoplasma* and *Pneumocystis* is another function of the T cell system.

Graft Rejection

Other types of reactions that are associated with the cell-mediated immune system include acute graft rejection.[1,3] This reaction occurs approximately 7 to 21 days post-transplantation of such organs as kidney, heart, and liver. It is believed that T lymphocytes initiate the reaction, although in tissue sections of the rejected organ other cell types are present and accumulate as the reaction proceeds. Eventually B lymphocytes, macrophages, and killer lymphocytes will be present besides the cytotoxic T lymphocytes. Immunologic testing is done to minimize the possibility of graft rejection and involves matching the donor and recipient for the HLA antigens on lymphocytes. If the donor and recipient are matched for the major histocompatibility antigens, then it is more likely that the organ will be accepted.

Immunosuppressive therapy, which is given after transplantation to prevent rejection, includes the use of such drugs as azathioprine, corticosteroids, and most recently Cyclosporin A. The first two drugs tend to suppress all immune responses and thereby render the patient especially vulnerable to bacterial, fungal, and viral infections.[29] On its discovery, Cyclosporin A was enthusiastically greeted because it was not as toxic as the other drugs to the hematopoietic cell lines (with the exception of the lymphocyte line). But is *is* toxic to the kidney and the liver. These immunosuppressive drugs are given before rejection phenomena occur, since it is easier to suppress a primary rejection than to inhibit the rejection once initiated. In general this is true of all immunosuppressive agents; they are more likely to prevent a primary reaction than to inhibit already established immunologic reactions.

The rejection reaction described above is called the *host-vs.-graft reaction* because the host's white blood cells reject the graft of the donor. Patients who receive a bone marrow transplantation, however, might evolve a *graft-vs.-host* reaction. In this situation, the recipient's own bone marrow is destroyed by cytotoxic chemotherapy and radiation therapy to eliminate malignant hematologic cell lines. The recipient then receives the donor's hematopoietic stem cells as the graft. Since it is impossible to match donor and recipient for all the major and minor histocompatibility antigens, the lymphocytes derived from the donor might react against the patient's cells. The common sites of this graft-vs.-host reaction include the skin, the liver, and the gastrointestinal tract (see Fig. 16–10). The tissue reaction is similar to that of host-vs.-graft reactions but the acute reaction usually starts approximately 21 to 30 days after transplantation. During this time the graft stem cells take up residence in the bone marrow and start to proliferate. Not until a period of 14 days after the transplantation can new blood cells of the graft be detected in the peripheral blood.[22,24,25]

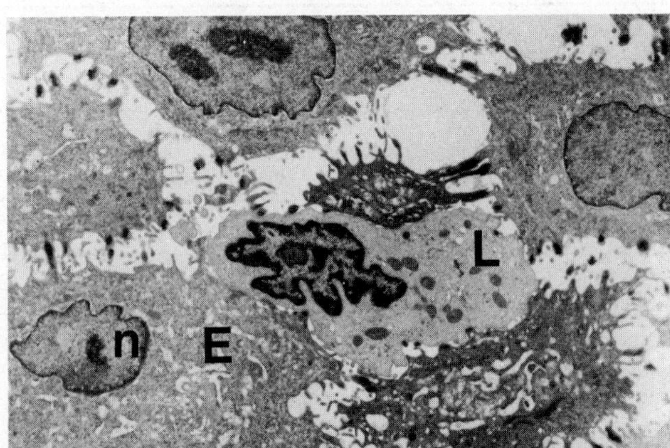

FIGURE 16–10 Graft vs. host disease. Electron microscopy photo shows T lymphocyte from graft (marked *L*) that has invaded epithelial cells (E) of the host's lip and will subsequently cause their destruction. (n = nucleus)

Immune Surveillance

Another phenomenon that involves cell-mediated immunity is immune surveillance. This theory was popularized by Burnett in the late 1950s. He proposed that the cell-mediated immune system is capable of recognizing and destroying malignant cells that arise in the individual. There is circumstantial evidence for this happening in humans: rare malignancies regress spontaneously, occasionally metastases regress after treatment of the primary tumor, and there is an increased incidence of certain tumors after immunosuppressive therapy for transplantation. In the first two cases the immune system supposedly was able to eradicate the tumor or the metastases and in the last case the lack of an immune response contributed to the development of the malignancy.[1,3,29]

However convincing these examples are, alternative explanations can be given. Spontaneous regressions are rare and usually occur in tumors that arise from embryonal tissue. Perhaps in these cases there was an alteration of the differentiation process that was self-corrected. Regression of metastases may be attributed to chemotherapy or radiation therapy. Finally, the tumors that arise in patients on immunosuppressive therapy are generally those of the lymphocyte cell line. This suggests the possibility that the immunosuppressive therapy causes an imbalance of the cell lines that allows one of the cell lines to escape the regulatory mechanisms.[3]

In general it is believed that tumors that arise are often weakly immunogenic. (Two of the more immunogenic tumors in humans are melanomas and osteosarcomas, both of which are relatively uncommon.) Therefore the tumor can escape the immune surveillance system early in the natural history of the tumor when only a few cells are present and are not in great enough number to stimulate the immune system. After the tumor progresses the number of tumor cells is too large to be controlled by the immune system.[29]

However, from laboratory and experimental animal models it is known that certain populations of lymphocytes and lymphokines can destroy tumor cells. Various immunotherapies are undergoing clinical trials to determine the extent to which these strategies can be used to control tumor growth once the primary tumor is removed by surgery, radiation therapy, or chemotherapy.[3,8,9,12,20,29] (See Chapter 19 on neoplasia.)

Cell-Mediated Tissue Injury

Many forms of injury caused by T lymphocytes are classified as *delayed hypersensitivity* because the response takes one or more days to develop.[3,13,29] The tissue injury suffered is often the outcome of T lymphocyte-mediated inflammation against a foreign antigen. Contact dermatitis is an expression of this type of response. In tuberculosis and certain other diseases, microorganisms are encased within a wall of specialized cells that sequesters them from other host tissue. Formation of this protective wall, called a *granuloma*, is stimulated by cell-mediated immunity. As described under humoral immunity, autoimmune disease is often associated with an altered functioning of the T cell system. Proliferative T cell disorders also exist. Table 16–8 lists examples of delayed hypersensitivity diseases and proliferative T cell disorders.

Expansion of Immune Reactions

Once an immune reaction is initiated, other reactions are triggered that enhance or expand the original immune response. The *complement system* is closely allied to the humoral response and the *natural killer cells* are activated in T cell reactions. Thus, specific and nonspecific reactions are closely entwined and without both of them, protective reactions are diminished.

Complement System. *Complement* plays a vital role in both immunologic and nonspecific defenses. It is a system of sequentially acting proteins contained in the globulin portion of the serum. The proteins are labelled C1 through C9 and are present in the inactive form. When C1 and an antibody–antigen complex (or plasmin, a blood clotting factor) bind together, a sequence of steps is set into motion that activates the inactive precursors until a C1–C9 complex is formed as shown in Figure 16–11. When the last step is completed a small hole is formed in the plasma membrane of the target cell. If enough holes are present then lysis of the cell ensues. In the process of converting the inactive complement proteins to active ones, small fragments of protein called *complement cleavage products* are released. These products have a wide variety of biological effects: they are responsible for anaphylactic-type reactions, they render the antigen susceptible to phagocytosis, they promote the release of histamine and other mast cell mediators, they induce leukocyte chemotaxis, and they neutralize the ability of viruses to infect cells. The first steps of complement activation may be bypassed by the alternative or properdin complement system.[3,4,13,29]

Many laboratory tests for the diagnosis of bacterial infections or autoimmune diseases detect the levels of complement proteins. Complement-fixing tests are used to detect antibody levels against a variety of bacteria and against syphillis (Wasserman test). Such autoimmune diseases as systemic

TABLE 16–8
Selected Disorders of Cell-Mediated Immunity

Delayed Hypersensitivity
Tuberculin-Type Reaction
Contact dermatitis
Graft rejection
Granuloma Formation
Tuberculosis
Sarcoidosis
Brucellosis
Proliferative Disorders of T Cell Line
Sezary syndrome
Mycosis fungoides
Some acute leukemias

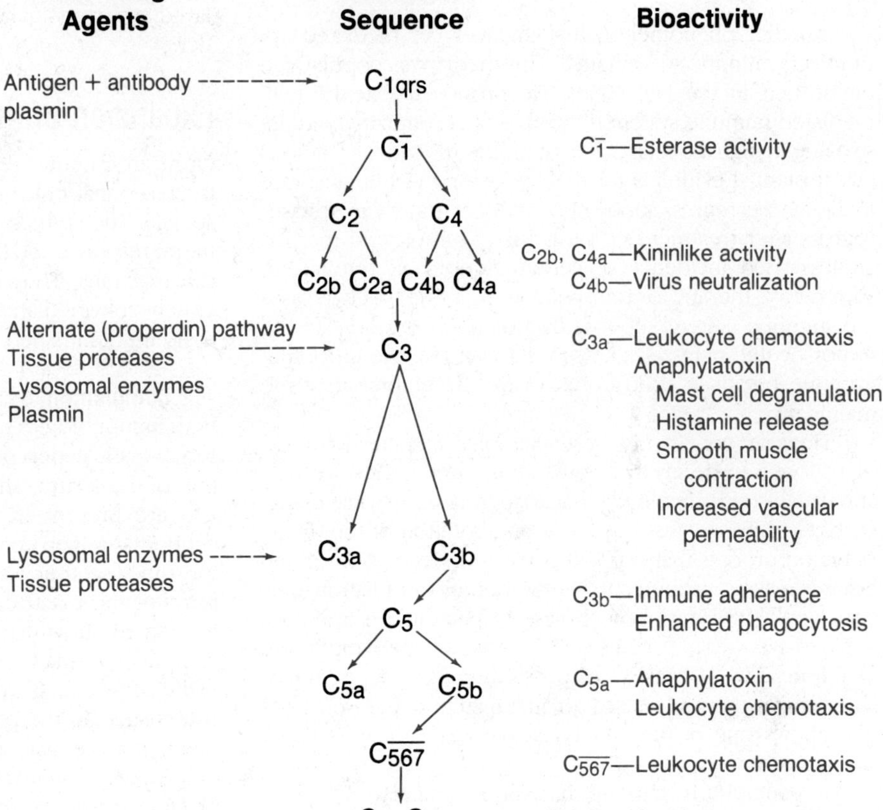

FIGURE 16–11 Classic and alternative (properdin) pathways for complement activation. The classical pathway is activated by antigen–antibody interaction; the shorter, alternative (properdin) pathway is activated by various substances such as bacterial endotoxin. Both pathways converge at C-3. Activated complement products have a wide variety of actions which enhance the immune response. (After Price SA, Wilson LM: Pathophysiology: Clinical Concepts of Disease Processes, 2nd ed. New York, McGraw-Hill, 1982)

lupus erythematosus are characterized by low levels of C1, C4, C2 and C3. It also appears that some persons with congenital deficiencies of complement proteins have a higher incidence of infectious diseases.

Natural Killer Cells. Natural killer cells are not as well characterized as T or B lymphocytes. Natural killer cells may be active in the early stages of infection along with macrophages in destroying infected cells. They also appear to be involved with the destruction of tumor cells and in graft-vs.-host disease, and are a major producer of interferon (protein produced in response to viral infection). Since natural killer cells also produce interleukin 2 (T cell growth factor), they are probably important in the regulation of T cell activity. They also appear to be important in the regulation of thymus lymphocytes and some hematopoietic cell lines. In general, these lymphocytes are capable of destroying poorly differentiated cells, such as fetal fibroblasts. Depressed natural killer cell activity is associated with active multiple sclerosis, systemic lupus erythematosus, and Chédiak-Higashi syndrome.[21,29,32]

Time Course of Immune Reactions

The time sequence is an important consideration when trying to anticipate a patient's response to a particular antigen. When the patient has been exposed to the antigen for the first time, a *primary response* ensues. If the exposure is a second or subsequent one, a *secondary response* results.

In a *primary response* (Fig. 16–12), there is a delay between the time the antigen is presented to the immune system and the period when a detectable antibody level or a T cell response to the antigen is generated. The length of this inductive phase, or latent period, depends on several factors, two of which are the quantity of the antigen presented and the chemical character of the antigen. In a humoral response, IgM is usually detected first and reaches a peak in 4 to 5 days in response to such antigens as foreign proteins, or as late as 30 to 60 days against bacterial toxoids. IgG appears somewhat later, usually within 2 weeks of the IgM peak, and in higher titers than IgM. The IgG produced usually has a higher affinity and avidity for the antigen than does IgM and therefore binds more tightly to the antigen. These IgG antibodies are actually of several types with different specificities. With this heterogeneous response there is a possibility of cross-reactivity with antigens of a similar chemical structure.[3,13]

In the *secondary response*—also called anamnestic, secondary, or booster response—there is a shorter latent period. In addition, the levels of IgG are usually higher, the antibodies that are produced have a higher affinity for the antigen, and the antibody peaks last for a longer period of time. It takes a smaller quantity of antigen to elicit a response and more memory cells are formed after a secondary response

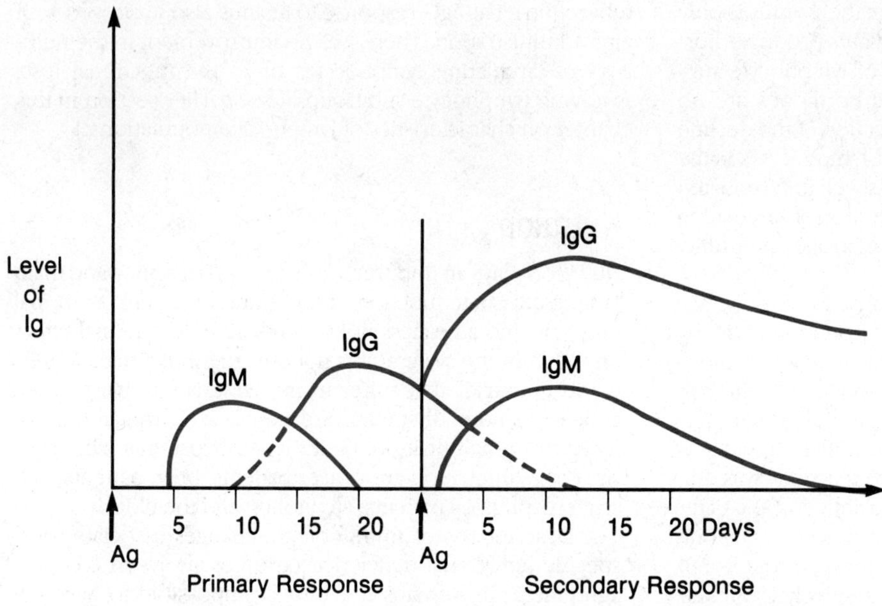

FIGURE 16-12 Primary and secondary immune responses. The primary response follows the initial exposure to an antigen. The secondary response, which is faster and greater, follows a subsequent antigen exposure.

than after a primary response. That is why the nurse should anticipate an anaphylactic response after the second or third injection of penicillin or bee venom rather than after the first exposure. The time sequence for T cell responses is similar to B cell reactions and the properties of the secondary response also hold for cell-mediated immune reactions.[3,13]

The nurse must then ask herself: "If an immune response does not protect the patient from organisms it has never seen before such as those that may be found in the hospital, what then protects the patient?" The answer lies in the first part of this chapter. General host defense mechanisms and good nursing care that maintains these defenses provide this protection. Nursing care includes all those measures that maintain the physical, chemical, and mechanical barriers to microbial colonization. Nursing care supports the inflammatory response and complement reactions. Preservation of good nutritional status is a major means of maintaining healthy skin and mucosa and assuring adequate inflammatory and immune reactions.[6,10,12,23,26]

Immunizations. Another means of protection is to stimulate the development of *active immunity* by the administration of vaccines developed from disease-producing microorganisms or their antigens. With some vaccines, periodic injections are required to maintain a sufficient immune response. The repeat immunizations evoke a secondary response. Additional information on immunizations, including a table of common active immunizations, is contained in Chapter 17.

Preformed antibodies are sometimes administered following exposure to infectious disease. The immunity conferred is passive, that is, the recipient's immune system is not induced to develop antibodies of its own. Although short-lived, this form of *passive immunization* provides important protection in some instances.

Modulation of the Immune Response

A variety of factors influence the capacity of the immune system to generate defensive responses against specific foreign stimuli. When these factors threaten the competence of the immune response, a person becomes more susceptible to infectious disease. The most obvious forms of immunoincompetence are those involving genetic failure of the immune system to develop. These congenital defects are ordinarily detected in infancy and can range from partial to total immune deficiency.[3,29] Examples include

- X-linked hypogammaglobulinemia
  Bruton's Disease
- Common variable immunodeficiency
- Congenital thymic hypoplasia
  Di George's syndrome
- Isolated IgA deficiency
- Severe combined immunodeficiency
  Swiss-type agammaglobulinemia
- Immunodeficiency with thrombocytopenia and eczema
  Wiskott-Aldrich syndrome

More common to adults are the variety of circumstances in which immune deficiency is acquired after birth. Immune responsiveness may be muted by such factors as advanced age, malnutrition, some forms of medical therapy, and by diseases involving the immune system.

Effects of Aging on the Immune Response

The thymus reaches its maximum size at puberty and undergoes a rapid involution after that.[29] Consequently, by the time an individual reaches 40 to 50 years of age the thymus is only 5% to 10% of its maximum mass. The thymus produces hormones important in the differentiation of lymphocyte subpopulations. After the age of 60 thymic hormones are no longer detectable in the serum. As a reflection of the decline of the thymic hormones, the circulating T lymphocytes in the elderly (60 to 70 years old) tend to be less well differentiated and are immature. Even though the number of circulating lymphocytes does not appear to decline with age, their functional ability does decrease.

One way to measure the T cell response in an individual is to measure the reaction of the skin to common antigens. For instance most adults will have a positive reaction to molecules unique to the fungus *Candida*. In one study, the percent of positive reactions to the antigen candidin was 73% in controls aged 19 to 75. In individuals of advanced age (that is, over 80 years), the percentage of positive reactions was only 33%. The same trend was true for mumps antigen: 80% of the controls were able to mount a positive reaction, but only 33% of the advanced age-group were able to do so. Overall, 70% of controls were able to respond positively to all antigens, but only 24% of the advanced age-group could mount positive responses.[29]

Changes in the B cell system in the elderly may be a result of the decline in the T cell system. For instance, helper T cell activity decreases; therefore, B lymphocytes are not as responsive to the antigen, and less specific antibody is formed. Generally, in the elderly the ability to mount a primary immune response is more impaired than is the ability to mount a secondary response. The quality of the response is also diminished.[31] Although the peak levels of immunoglobulins are the same in the elderly as in the young controls, the peak levels decline more rapidly and reach minimal levels more quickly in the aged. The elderly have a tendency to manufacture autoantibodies, such as antithyroglobulin antibody and rheumatoid factors. Although these changes were at first considered to be a part of the normal course of aging, recent studies demonstrate that healthy individuals over 95 years do not have high titers of autoantibodies.[29] This observation suggests that autoantibodies are not a normal part of aging and that their presence suggests slow progression of low-grade tissue damage. It has also been noted that individuals with high levels of autoantibodies generally have a shorter life expectancy than those who do not.

Will it ever be possible to intervene and correct immunodeficiencies in the elderly or prevent the decline of the immune system? Certainly there have been interesting results from animal studies. As early as 1935 it was reported that caloric restriction in mice retards the decline of some immune functions and that a high fat diet promotes autoimmunity and a decline in cell-mediated immunity. Rejuvenation experiments with immunologic cells and thymic cells have also been attempted in mice. Attempts at rejuvenation in humans are difficult because in most cases the transplanted cells will be rejected. In one experiment involving 20 aged subjects, injections of bovine thymic extract for 3 consecutive days did not alter any of the immunologic T cell tests. In another experiment involving 15 subjects over the age of 70, zinc administration improved the delayed hypersensitivity reaction to candidin and PPD (purified protein derivative of tuberculin). The IgG response to tetanus also improved with zinc administration. There was no improvement in the numbers of circulating lymphocytes or to the functional tests involving lymphocyte subgroups. (See earlier section in this chapter on characteristics of lymphocyte populations.)

Nutrition

Nutrition plays an important role in host resistance and maintaining adequate function of the immune system. Both malnutrition and an excess of nutrients have detrimental effects on the immune system. It is not only the individuals in third world countries that suffer from malnutrition. Bristian and colleagues noted that 60% of patients on a surgical unit suffered from malnutrition. Other types of patients who are at risk for malnutrition are cancer patients, burn patients, end-stage respiratory patients, alcoholics, and the elderly.[29]

Descriptions of immunologic changes associated with specific nutritional deficiencies are not always in complete agreement. In humans it is almost impossible to have one nutritional deficit without others being present. Many studies have been conducted on children with severe protein-calorie malnutrition. But this type of deficiency is also accompanied by a lack of vitamins and minerals. The age of the person at the time of the nutritional deficiency as well as whether it is a chronic or acute deficiency will influence the immune system. For instance a slowly developing chronic deficiency in children might not have as severe consequences as an acute deficiency.

The most commonly studied deficiency is known as severe protein-calorie malnutrition, of which there are two types. In kwashiorkor the diets are low in protein, fats, vitamins, and trace metals. In marasmus there is a grossly insufficient diet but the overall composition of the diet is more balanced than in kwashiorkor.[29] Severe protein-calorie malnutrition is characterized by decreased T cell responses and diminished or absent delayed cutaneous hypersensitivity reactions. These patients often have an increase in fungal, viral, and mycobacterial infections. Generally the B cell responses are preserved; often the immunoglobulin levels are normal or even elevated. Since these patients are frequently infected, an increase in immunoglobulin levels is not too surprising. The exact complex of immune deficiencies depends on the timing of the malnutrition, that is, *in utero*, in childhood, or in adulthood. Malnutrition during a primary exposure to the antigen may prevent an adequate secondary response even after the introduction of an adequate diet.[29]

Severe protein-calorie malnutrition also affects many other factors that lead to a decrease in host resistance. For instance, malnutrition delays wound healing and thereby increases the risk for infection. The neutrophils and the macrophages of patients with malnutrition are not as capable of killing phagocytized bacteria. Abnormal processing of the antigen by macrophages may also lead to a defect in the lymphocyte response. Thus, malnutrition leads to infection, which in turn leads to a hypercatabolic state and further increases the malnourished status. The cycle of malnutrition and infection must be broken to restore the individual to an optimal state.[29]

Neuroendocrine Influence

Another set of factors can modulate the immune response and the study of this field, *psychoneuroimmunology,* is one of the most rapidly growing research areas. Recent evidence suggests that life events (*e.g.,* the death of a spouse) and behavioral and psychosocial factors can all influence the immune response. These effects may be mediated through hormonal regulation or through a direct communication link between the immune system and the central nervous system.

Selye was one of the early pioneers in this field. In describing the general adaptation syndrome (GAS), he noted that the lymphoid glands atrophied when the experimental animals were constantly "stressed." In several animal species the corticosteroids can actually lyse lymphocytes. In humans, corticosteroids administered at pharmacologic doses profoundly depress the immune system. Lymphopenia and neutropenia occur several hours after the administration of steroids. The quantity of interleukins and interferons released is also reduced, and reactivity to skin antigen, as indicated by delayed hypersensitivity testing, is reduced after several weeks of steroid therapy.[5,7,19]

Selye's observations on the effect of stress on the immune system have been rediscovered recently and have led to other experiments. In one such experiment, the lymphocytes of mice subjected to inescapable shock were less capable of responding to plant mitogens. In another experiment there was more tumor growth in the mice exposed to inescapable shock as compared with those exposed to escapable shock. Comparable situations in humans, of course, are difficult to study. However, several studies have now observed that the lymphocytes of recent widowers were less capable of responding to plant mitogens as compared with their prebereavement lymphocytes. Suppression of lymphocytes was also noted in astronauts after space flights, in volunteers after 48 hours of sleep deprivation, and in runners after marathons. In the last group, the lymphocyte response returned 1 to 2 days after the event. But in the widowers the lymphocyte responses were still depressed after 14 months.[5,7,19]

The overall view is that the neuroendocrine influence is that of a modulator. When the person is exposed to events that are considered stressful, he is more at risk for the onset of illness. The opposite situation is much less studied, that is, how coping and healthy lifestyles enhance the immune response and confer resistance to illness. However, this field is rapidly expanding and new experimental results are being reported every day. When the function of the lymphocyte subpopulations and their hormonal controls are better defined and more knowledge is gained regarding the influence of the immune response on central nervous system function, then we will be able to describe the influence of stressors, and behavior and personality on the susceptibility and resistance to disease.

Summary

Nurses frequently care for patients for whom the primary disorder is a defect in the immune system. Examples include allergic disorders, such as hay fever, and systemic diseases, such as multiple myeloma and systemic lupus erythematosus. Nursing care for patients with these disorders is described in later chapters of this text. Many additional patients are at risk for decreased or inadequate immune responses that compromise the body's ability to defend against a primary disorder. Recognition of patients whose immune competence is threatened can lead the nurse to institute protective measures against infection, to improve nutrition, and to reduce environmental stressors; by so doing, complications of disease may be reduced.

References

1. Alexander JW, Good RA: Fundamentals of Clinical Immunology. Philadelphia, WB Saunders, 1977
2. Allen JC: Infection and the Compromised Host. Baltimore, Williams & Wilkins, 1976
3. Bellanti JA: Immunology III. Philadelphia, WB Saunders, 1985
4. Benacerraf B, Unane E: Textbook of Immunology. Baltimore, Williams & Wilkins, 1979
5. Besedovsky HO, Sorkin E: Immunologic-neuroendocrine circuits: Physiological approaches. Psychoneuroimmunology 545–573, 1981
6. Bodey GP: Current status of prophylaxis of infection with protected environments. Am J Med 76:678, 1984
7. Borysenko J: Psychoneuroimmunology: Behavioral factors in the immune response. Revision. 7:56, 1984
8. Broder S, Waldman T: The suppressor cell network in cancer (Part I). N Engl J Med 229:1281, 1978
9. Broder S, Waldman T: The suppressor cell network in cancer (Part II). N Engl J Med 229:1335, 1978
10. Burke IF: The Infection Prone Hospital Patient. Boston, Little, Brown & Co, 1978
11. Dorf ME, Benacerraf B: Suppressor cells and immunoregulation. Annu Rev Immunol 2:127, 1984
12. Donovan MI, Girton SE: Infection. In Cancer Care Nursing, 2nd ed. New York, Appleton-Century-Crofts, 1984
13. Eisen H: Immunology: An introduction to molecular and cellular principles of the immune response. In Davis DP, Dulbecco R, Eisen HN et al: Microbiology. New York, Harper & Row, 1973
14. Eriksson B, Hedfors E: The effect of adrenaline, insulin and hydrocortisone on human peripheral blood lymphocytes studied by cell surface markers. Scand J Haematol 18:121, 1977
15. Gleich GJ: Loegering DA: Immunobiology of eosinophils. Annu Rev Immunol 2:429, 1984
16. Green DR, Flood PM, Gershon RK: Immunoregulatory T-cell pathways. Annu Rev Immunol 1:439, 1983
17. Herberman RB: Natural killer cells. Hosp Pract 17(4):93–103, 1982
18. Larsen GL, Henson PM: Mediators of inflammation. Annu Rev Immunol 1:335, 1983
19. Locke SE, Hornig-Rohan M: Mind and Immunity: Behavioral Immunology. New York, Institute for the Advancement of Health, 1983
20. McCalla JL: Immunotherapy: Concepts and nursing implications. Nurs Clin North Am 11:59, 1976
21. Ortaldo JR, Herberman RB: Heterogeneity of natural killer cells. Annu Rev Immunol 2:359, 1984
22. Parker N, Cohen T: Acute graft-versus-host disease in allogeneic marrow transplantation. Nurs Clin North Am 18(3):569, 1983
23. Rodriguez V: Principles of supportive care in cancer treatment: Infectious complications and their treatment. In Carter SK,

Glatstein E, Livingston RB: Principles of Cancer Treatment, pp 184–197. New York, McGraw-Hill, 1984

24. Sale GE: Pathology and recent pathogenetic studies in human graft-versus-host disease. Surv Synth Pathol Res 3:235, 1984
25. Sale GE, Shulman HM (eds): The Pathology of Bone Marrow Transplantation. Masson Monographs in Diagnostic Pathology, vol 9. 1984
26. Simmons BP: Guideline for prevention of intravascular infections. Am J Infect Control 11:183, 1983
27. Singer A, Hodes RJ: Mechanisms of T cell–B cell interaction. Annu Rev Immunol 1:211, 1983
28. Smith KA: Interleukin 2. Annu Rev Immunol 2:319, 1984
29. Stites DP, Stobo JD, Fudenberg HH, Wells JV: Basic and Clinical Immunology, ed 5. Los Altos CA, Lange Medical Publications, 1984
30. Strober S: Natural suppressor (NS) cells, neonatal tolerance, and total lymphoid irradiation: Exploring obscure relationships. Annu Rev Immunol 2:219, 1984
31. Thompson JS, Wekstein DR, Rhoades JL et al: The immune status of healthy centenarians. J Am Geriatr Soc 32:274, 1984
32. Trinchieri G, Perussia B: Biology of disease human natural killer cells: Biologic and pathologic aspects. Lab Invest 50(5):489, 1984
33. Walford RL: Immunology and aging. Am Soc Clin Path 74:247, 1980

Bibliography

Alexander JW, Good RA: Fundamentals of Clinical Immunology. Philadelphia, WB Saunders, 1977

Bellanti I: Immunology II. Philadelphia, WB Saunders, 1978

Burke, IF: The Infection Prone Hospital Patient. Boston, Little, Brown & Co, 1978

Eisen, H: Immunology: An introduction to molecular and cellular principles of the immune response. In Davis DP, Dulbecco R, Eisen HN et al: Microbiology. New York, Harper & Row, 1973

Stites DP, Stobo JD, Fudenberg HH et al: Basic and Clinical Immunology, 5th ed. Los Altos, CA, Lange Medical Publications, 1984

Chapter 17

Infection

Margaret J. Wertz

The human world is teeming with microorganisms. Bacteria and other microbes abound in the external environment and thrive both on and within the body. Bacteria are normally found on the surface of the skin, in the nasopharynx, on oral mucosa, and on the epithelial surfaces of the eye. In addition, it has been estimated that over 150 viruses reside within the human being. Despite this abundance of microbial life, infection is a rare rather than commonplace occurrence. This chapter focuses on the relationship between humans and microorganisms, and those characteristics of both that tend to produce or protect against disease.

The relationship between people and microorganism is *parasitic*. A parasite is an organism that lives on or within another organism from which it obtains the environment and nutrients for growth and reproduction. If the microorganism causes the death of its host, it will also die. Thus, in a successful host–parasite relationship neither organism is harmed by the other. Such a relationship is termed *commensalism*. *Mutualism* is one step better than commensalism, and means there are advantages to both host and parasite. An example of mutualism is the synthesis of vitamin K by enteric bacteria.

Colonization is the multiplication of an organism on body surfaces without eliciting an immune response. Infection occurs when the colonizing organism produces an immune reaction. Although necessary to combat the infection, the immunologic defense can itself be harmful, increasing the injury caused by the microbe. Some bacteria are able to harm the host only under specific conditions. For example, *Escherichia coli* is a part of the normal bacterial flora of the intestine and usually causes no harm. But if *E. coli* is transported to the urinary bladder when a catheter is passed through the urethra, it becomes a pathogen capable of causing cystitis and pyelonephritis. Similarly, if *E. coli* gains access to the peritoneal cavity, peritonitis or intra-abdominal abscess can occur.

The development of infection is a result of the interplay of host defense mechanisms, microbial virulence properties, and environmental conditions. The interaction of these three determinants in the healthy person is illustrated in Figure 17–1. Here all three elements are in balance and there is no infection. In order for a microorganism to produce disease, it must be able to escape or withstand the host's defenses. If the host has compromised defenses, he may become infected by organisms that are normally considered to be nonpathogenic. Some infectious agents have the capacity to cause disease in normal people. Others are opportunistic, requiring a defect in host defenses to set up the infectious process.

The integrity of the host's defenses and the type and number of microorganisms vary from one setting to another. Hospitals typically have great impact on the elements in this scheme. Many of the usual barriers to bacteria are breached in the treatment of illness. Incisions are made in the skin, catheters are placed in the bladder, tubes are inserted into the trachea, and internal defenses are impaired by drug and radiation therapy. In addition, bacterial populations in hospitals are more resistant to antibiotics than those found in other environments.

A patient in an intensive care unit is represented in Figure 17–2. Note that there is more interaction among the components as compared with the healthy person in Figure 17–1.

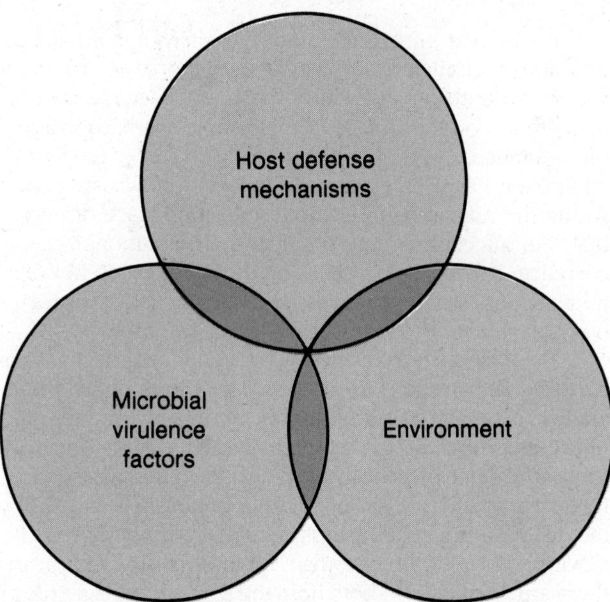

FIGURE 17–1 The risk of infection in the normal individual is near zero as represented by the point of intersection of all three factors. (Adapted from Meakins JL, Pietsch JB, Christou NV et al: Predicting surgical infection before the operation. World J Surg 4:439, 1980)

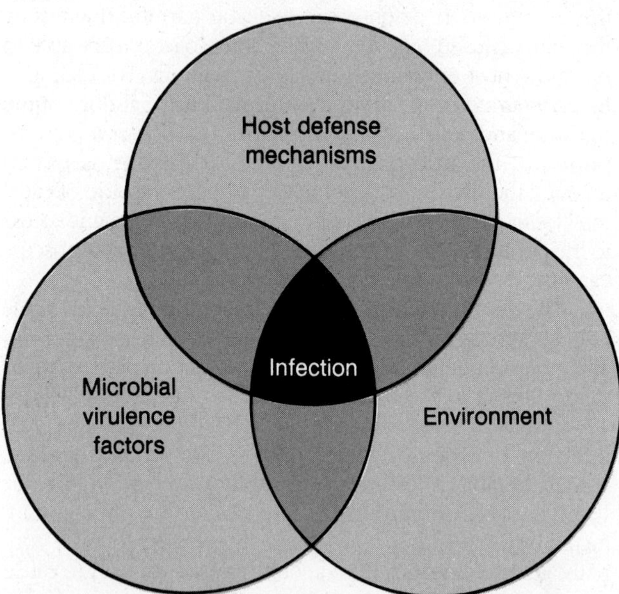

FIGURE 17–2 The patient in the intensive care unit is subject to greater interaction of these three elements. The shaded area shows the increased risk of infection. (Adapted from Meakins JL, Pietsch JB, Christou NV et al: Predicting surgical infection before the operation. World J Surg 4:439, 1980)

The greater overlap in the center indicates the increased probability of infection.

Infection Mechanisms

The term *virulence* is used to describe the disease-producing capacity of a microorganism. Bacteria have been studied more extensively than other microorganisms with respect to virulence factors. There are several methods bacteria use to elude host defense mechanisms: (1) attachment to epithelial surfaces, (2) escaping phagocytosis, (3) production of toxins, (4) causing immunologic injury, and (5) mutation.

Attachment to Epithelial Surfaces

Most infections involve or occur after damage to the skin, or to the epithelium of the respiratory, gastrointestinal, or urinary tracts. An important initial step in the development of these infections is bacterial attachment to the cells of the epithelium. This attachment allows the bacteria to escape some of the natural defenses of the host. Normal flora provide protection for the host by competing with bacteria for the specific attachment sites on the epithelial cells. Bacteria and viruses appear to have surface proteins that function as adhesive structures that are complementary to receptor sites on cells.[2] These receptors are different in different tissues. For example, influenza virus attaches to respiratory epithelial cells. *Neisseria gonorrhoeae* attaches to urethral epithelium. There are other mechanisms that allow microorganisms to attach to epithelial cells. Some bacteria have special structures such as pili that allow them to bind to host tissues. Others produce substances that help them attach to surfaces, for example, glucans and fructose are produced by *Streptococcus mutans*, which is believed to cause dental caries. Once attached, microorganisms cause disease by production of toxins and stimulation of host immune responses.

Escaping Phagocytosis

One method bacteria use to avoid phagocytosis is to impair chemotaxis. Some streptococci produce streptolysin. Because streptolysin interferes with chemotaxis, polymorphonuclear neutrophils (PMNs) are not attracted to the site of infection. Many bacteria and fungi have thick capsules that allow them to resist phagocytosis. This particular mechanism is not well understood, but the presence of the capsule itself appears to increase virulence. For example, when the capsule is removed from a strain of *Streptococcus pneumoniae*, 10,000 bacteria injected peritoneally are required to cause death in a mouse. But as few as 10 of the encapsulated bacteria are lethal.[12] Similarly, M protein of *Streptococcus pyogenes* enables it to resist phagocytosis. Only when the protein is covered by antibody can phagocytosis occur. *Staphylococcus aureus* demonstrates another mechanism used to elude PMNs. Highly virulent strains of this bacteria contain a protein (protein A) in their cell walls that blocks a portion of the IgG antibody, preventing PMNs from binding at receptor sites.

Some microbes are able to survive following phagocytosis and live within white blood cells as intracellular parasites. Microorganisms that are capable of living and multiplying within macrophages include viruses, rickettsiae, bacteria, fungi, and protozoa. *Mycobacterium tuberculosis* is readily phagocytosed but somehow prevents the lysosomes from merging with the phagosome. Other organisms are able to survive even after the lysosome and phagosome have fused. How this occurs is not known.

Toxin Production

The disease-producing ability of many bacteria involves the production of toxins and extracellular enzymes. For some microorganisms production of these substances is the most important factor in causing disease.

Extracellular Enzymes. The invasiveness of many bacteria is enhanced by enzyme production. However, the precise role that these enzymes play in determining virulence is not well understood. Hemolysins lyse red blood cells and damage white blood cells. Coagulase initiates the clotting of plasma and the formation of fibrin walls enclosing local infections. It is thought that this protects the bacteria from phagocytes and antibiotic penetration. Streptokinase, conversely, dissolves clots and is believed to help bacteria spread through tissues. Hyaluronidase and collagenases destroy intercellular proteins and also increase the spread of infection along tissue planes.

Exotoxins. The most potent poisons known are produced by bacteria. They are proteins (called exotoxins) that bind to host tissues and act as cell poisons. Their actions are diverse and include inhibition of protein synthesis, blocking of neuromuscular junctions, and hypersecretion of the small intestine. *Clostridium tetani*, *Clostridium botulinum*, *Corynebacterium diphtheriae* and *Shigella dysenteriae* all cause disease that is characterized by the action of exotoxins. *Staphylococcus aureus* is an organism that produces a potent exotoxin that is responsible for a commonly occurring food poisoning. Some strains of *E. coli* produce an enterotoxin that causes diarrhea.

Clostridium perfringens produces at least ten exotoxins. These are thought to be important in the pathogenesis of gas gangrene. They cause tissue necrosis, which decreases the oxygen content in the area and thus creates a suitable environment for anaerobic bacterial growth. One of the toxins is a collagenase that destroys the supporting matrix of muscle and other soft tissue. This allows the infection to spread along tissue planes.

The enterotoxin of *Vibrio cholerae* binds irreversibly to intestinal epithelial cells, producing diarrhea, dehydration, and electrolyte depletion. When cell-free filtrates of *V. cholerae* are administered, the clinical characteristics of cholera are observed, implicating the exotoxin as a major determinant of the disease.

Endotoxins. Endotoxins are a part of the cell wall of gram-negative bacteria. Unlike exotoxins, they are released only on the death of the bacteria. Endotoxins are large molecular complexes made up of phospholipids, polysaccharides, and proteins. The lipopolysaccharide portion is responsible for the toxic characteristics. In fact, although it is not usually dissociated from the two polysaccharides, the lipid region (lipid A) is thought to possess the toxic properties.

Small doses of endotoxin cause fever by releasing endogenous pyrogen from polymorphonuclear leukocytes and macrophages. In large doses, endotoxin causes irreversible shock and death (see Chap. 24). At less than lethal doses, endotoxin activates the complement cascade, leading to complement depletion. It also activates the coagulation system, causing intravascular coagulation and tissue injury. A profound leukopenia followed by leukocytosis is another sequela of endotoxin infection. Endotoxin causes the release of adrenocorticotropic and growth hormones from the pituitary, and causes changes in protein, carbohydrate, and lipid metabolism.

Immunologic Injury

The body has many powerful immunologic defenses against infection. However, the result of invoking these immunologic defense mechanisms can be inflammation, cell infiltration, tissue destruction, or even eventual death (see Chap. 16). A well-known example of a complication following an immunologic response is rheumatic fever, which occurs following group A streptococcal infections. There are antigens on the streptococci that are cross-reactive with heart muscle. Antibodies that are produced against these antigens form complexes not only with the streptococci but also with heart muscle and valves. These antigen–antibody complexes initiate the complement cascade and inflammatory process. This may lead to myocarditis or endocarditis and permanent damage to heart valves.

Infections by other microorganisms can also lead to formation of antigen–antibody complexes that cause further disease. For example, immune complexes can be deposited on the basement membranes of the renal glomerulus and blood vessels. The complement cascade and inflammation are then activated at these sites, resulting in immunologic damage to body tissue. This series of events causes acute glomerulonephritis and vasculitis. Immune complexes have been found in the renal tissue of patients with hepatitis B, infection with *Streptococcus pyogenes* and malaria. It is suspected that antigen–antibody complexes are involved in rashes and arthralgias caused by some adenoviruses.

Capacity for Genetic Change

Another factor that contributes to an organism's disease-producing capacity is the ability for mutation. A microorganism can continue to cause disease only as long as there is a susceptible population. Once immunity has developed the microorganism is no longer a pathogen. The influenza virus is an example of an organism that undergoes genetic change and then causes new epidemics. *Pseudomonas aeruginosa* is notorious for its ability to develop resistance to antibiotics being used to treat an infection, thus allowing it to continue to produce disease.

Host Defenses

The body has a great variety of defenses against infection. The mechanisms differ from one site to another, but local host defenses have the following characteristics:

1. An epithelial layer that acts as a biological wall (*e.g.,* skin and mucous membranes)
2. Specialized surface cell functions, *e.g.,* macrophages and cilia
3. Secretions, *e.g.,* saliva, mucus, and gastric acid
4. The normal flora that inhibits colonization by pathogens

The microbial flora can help protect against infection and may determine the specific infection that develops. Many infections are a result of changes in the host defense mechanisms that allow endogenous bacteria to gain access to sterile sites. Changes in the numbers and types of bacteria colonizing the individual can also lead to infection. When a patient is receiving antibiotic therapy, more resistant strains of bacteria replace normal flora. What follows is a discussion of specific host defenses in different areas of the body.

Skin

The skin is an inhospitable environment for many microbes. Because skin is a multilayered structure that contains closely bound epithelial cells, it is a thick mechanical barrier to the invasion of microorganisms. The cornified upper layer is constantly being shed and replaced, which helps eliminate potential pathogens. The normal dry skin lacks the necessary water for growth. Where there is more moisture, such as in skin folds, the number of bacteria is increased. The acid pH of normal skin is also incompatible with enviornmental requirements of most bacteria.

Presence of the normal resident flora is another factor that prevents the colonization of harmful bacteria. There are a great variety of organisms that can be recovered from the skin. The indigenous flora varies, as does the density of bacteria, depending on body site. Most species are gram-positive organisms. *Staphylococcus epidermidis* is present in greatest numbers. *Staphylococcus aureus* and *Streptococcus pyogenes* are found in smaller quantities. *Propionibacterium acne* is a gram-positive anaerobe that is found deep in sebaceous glands.

Respiratory Tract

The nose acts like a filter for particulate matter. The shape of the nose causes turbulence of inspired air, which allows more air to contact the mucosal epithelium; hence, the air inhaled through the nose is humidified and warmed. The mucus flow and ciliary action carry foreign matter to the epiglottis where it is swallowed. Dry air impairs ciliary action and increases the viscosity of mucus, which slows the clearance of inspired particles. In addition, there are immunoglobulins IgA and IgE in the upper airways that are important defenses against new bacteria.

Staphylococci, both *Staphylococcus aureus* and *S. epidermidis*, are the major organisms found in the nose and surrounding skin. Diphtheroids are a group of gram-positive bacilli that are also normally found in significant numbers. Because it is difficult to culture the posterior nasopharynx and sinuses owing to their anatomical structures, little is known about the normal flora of these areas; it is believed to be similar to that found in the oropharynx.

The lungs are free of microorganisms in the healthy person. Large particles that are inhaled stimulate the cough reflex and are expelled by the increased air flow of the cough. Smaller particles, including bacteria, are captured by the mucous membrane of the tracheobronchial tree, moved upward by cilia action, and then swallowed. If bacteria make it past the terminal bronchioles, they are removed by alveolar macrophages. There are also local immunity factors, including IgG, IgM, and large molecular-weight mediators providing additional protection in the lower respiratory tract. Any condition that dries the airways or causes accumulation of fluid in the alveoli interferes with the normal defense mechanisms and increases the risk of infection.

Mouth and Oropharynx

The oropharynx is lined with a thick layer of squamous epithelium that is a strong mechanical barrier to invasion by microorganisms. Saliva is produced at a rate of approximately 1 liter/day. It bathes the tissue and provides a flushing action in the mouth. Saliva also contains active elements such as mucin, lysozyme, and IgA that inhibit bacteria growth. When salivary flow is reduced, oral bacteria increase markedly. Adequate fluid intake is important for production of saliva. Postoperative patients need adequate systemic hydration and additional oral hygiene to help maintain this host defense mechanism.

The microbial flora of the mouth is dependent on the presence or absence of dental or periodontal disease. When tooth disease is present, there are increased total numbers of bacteria and increased anaerobic species. The gram-positive cocci, especially α-hemolytic streptococci, are found on the surface of teeth and mucous membranes. In the crevices between teeth, anaerobic bacteria, such as *Bacteroides melaninogenicus, Veillonella* and *Fusobacterium* sp., are numerous.

The principal organisms of the oropharynx are the α-hemolytic streptococci often referred to as *Streptococcus viridans*. Another group found in large numbers and seldom causing disease is *Neisseria* sp. *Staphylococcus aureus* and *Staphylococcus epidermidis* can also be isolated in significant quantities. A variety of anaerobic bacteria are present, similar to these found in the mouth. The flora of a normal oropharynx seldom includes Enterobacteriaceae. However, the hospitalized patient is frequently colonized by these bacteria. The precise cause is unknown, but recent work suggests that receptor sites change during the stress of severe illness.[9] Patients with chronic illness also have oropharyngeal colonization by gram-negative rods. A recent study showed increased incidence with increased levels of care.[16] Most pneumonias are preceded by the aspiration of bacteria from the oropharynx (see Chap. 28). The colonization change in hospitalized patients is thought to contribute to the development of gram-negative pneumonias.

Gastrointestinal Tract

Stomach. The normal stomach has few if any bacteria. Motility maintains low densities of intraluminal bacteria and the acid pH rapidly kills most remaining microorganisms. Some *Candida* sp. and several mycobacteria, including *Mycobacterium tuberculosis*, can survive short exposure to highly acidic conditions. During intestinal obstruction the pH of the stomach rises and the bacterial content resembles that of the oropharynx.

Small Intestine. The mucous membrane of the bowel is thin, but provides an effective barrier against most bacteria. The forward peristaltic movement keeps bacterial numbers low through most of the small intestine. There are few organisms in the first part of the small intestine. In the jejunum the indigenous flora are predominantly gram-positive bacteria. In the ileum increasing numbers of Enterobacteriaceae and anaerobic gram-negative bacteria are found. *Candida* is present in 40% of healthy individuals.

Colon. In the colon there are large numbers of bacteria. The propulsive motion is much decreased compared with the small intestine, and the quantity of bacteria is increased. The normal flora again provides one of the major defenses against pathogens. They compete for nutrients and produce compounds that are toxic to other bacteria. The largest concentration of microorganisms is found in the colon. Up to 60% of dry weight of feces is made up of bacteria.[7] Anaerobic bacteria and Enterobacteriacea predominate, but gram-positive organisms and fungal species are also found in the large intestine.

Genitourinary Tract

The mucosal lining provides an effective mechanical barrier to bacterial infection, and micturition serves as a flushing action constantly removing bacteria. Urine has a mild bacteriostatic effect itself due to its high concentration of urea, high osmolality, high ammonia content, low pH, and the presence of urinary IgA. The female genital tract is protected by mucus, which contains IgA and lysozyme.

Normally the bladder, ureters, and kidneys are sterile. Small numbers of organisms can be found in the distal portion of the urethra in both men and women. The vagina has a low pH that encourages the growth of *C. albicans* and anaerobic bacteria. Female anatomy, including a short urethra and the proximity of the urinary meatus to other structures containing large numbers of bacteria, contributes to a greater incidence of urinary tract infections in females than is seen in males.

Microorganisms in Infection

It was once thought that a relatively few organisms were able to cause infectious disease. Today it is known that essentially all microorganisms can produce infection under the right circumstances. However, the majority of infections involve only a fraction of known species. The following discussion includes the principal groups of pathogens.

Gram-Positive Cocci

Staphylococci. The genus *Staphylococcus* includes gram-positive cocci that form in irregular grapelike clusters. The most common species are *Staphylococcus aureus* (coagulase-positive) and *Staphylococcus epidermidis* (coagulase-negative), which are part of the normal flora of the skin. *S. aureus* is recognized as the more pathogenic species, and is the most common bacterial species isolated from postoperative wound infections. It is also the most common organism involved in suppurative skin infections, including furuncles, carbuncles, and minor infections (*e.g.*, acne and impetigo). The characteristic lesion is an abscess filled with liquid necrotic tissue and phagocytes surrounded by fibrous tissue. Healing usually follows quickly after the pus is drained. *S. aureus* strains produce a variety of exotoxins. Food poisoning is often the result of proliferation of *S. aureus* and its enterotoxin (an exotoxin). Another illness caused by the production of an exotoxin by *S. aureus* is toxic shock syndrome.

Less commonly associated with infectious processes, *S. epidermidis* can nevertheless be a pathogen, especially in cases of instrumentation involving the skin (such as indwelling intravenous catheters). Colonization of such a catheter can precede the development of bacteremia and endocarditis. Both species are part of the normal flora of the skin.

Streptococci. The streptococci are gram-positive cocci that occur in chains or pairs. There are three major characteristics used to describe streptococci:

1. Degree of hemolysis of red blood cells, *i.e.*, α-hemolytic (partial hemolysis), β-hemolytic (complete hemolysis), or nonhemolytic (no hemolysis)
2. Serologic groups indicating the presence of streptococcal group antigens (*e.g.*, A, B, D)
3. Biochemical and physiological characteristics

Table 17–1 lists the characteristics of the major streptococci groups.

The most common streptococci are group A, which is beta-hemolytic and comprises a single species, *Streptococcus pyogenes*. Skin or wound infections and infections of the respiratory tract are commonly caused by group A streptococci. Rheumatic fever complicates pharyngeal infection in a small percentage of cases.

Group B streptococci also comprise a single species, *S. agalactiae*. The female genitourinary tract may be colonized with group B streptococci, and neonates may develop infection, but the risk is low. In adults infections with this organism occur predominantly in diabetic and in women during the postpartum period.[1]

Enterococci constitute three of the five species of group D streptococci. They are normally found as part of bowel flora. Infection by enterococci is most often of the urinary tract or as part of a mixed infection of the intra-abdominal space. Bacteremia and endocarditis can be a serious infection of enterococci.

TABLE 17–1
Characteristics of *Streptococci*

	Hemolysis	Antigen Group	Cellular Arrangement
Group A	Beta	A	Chains
Group B	Beta	B	Chains
Enterococci	Alpha or none	D	Short chains
Viridans	Alpha or none	Not A,B, or D	Chains
Pneumococci	Alpha	None	Diplococci

The viridans streptococci comprise five species that are not β-hemolytic and are not members of groups A, B, or D. They are part of the normal flora of many body surfaces. They play their most significant role in the mouth where they contribue to tooth decay. Here also they gain access to the bloodstream and can cause bacteremia that may lead to endocarditis and brain abscess.

S. pneumoniae is similar to the viridans streptococci group but characteristically occurs in pairs called diplococci. These organisms are also called *Diplococcus pneumoniae* or commonly, pneumococci. They are reported separately because the clinical implication of the presence of pneumococci is so important (see Chap. 28). Pneumococci are often the source of infection in pneumonia, otitis media, and meningitis. Alcoholism, old age, malnutrition, and splenectomy are factors that contribute to increased susceptibility to this organism.[17]

Gram-Negative Rods

The Enterobacteriaceae are a large family of gram-negative rods that are found in the bowel as normal flora or as pathogens (see Table 17–2). The Enterobacteriaceae are faculative anaerobes, that is, they are anaerobic organisms that are able to adjust to an aerobic environment. In the Western world diseases caused by the pathogenic group are well controlled, but they still present serious public health problems in other areas of the world. These include typhoid fever (*Salmonella typhi*), bacillary dysentery (*Shigella*), cholera (*Vibrio cholerae*), and bubonic plague (*Yersinia pestis*). The gram-negative rods normally found in the intestine were once thought to have little virulence. But they have been increasingly associated with serious bacterial infections that are for the most part endogenous (caused by organisms that reside within the host) and nosocomial (hospital-acquired). The incidence of infection caused by staphylococci and streptococci has decreased, whereas infections due to enteric bacteria have increased. This may be because, while in the past debilitated patients would not have been candidates for surgery, there is now an increased use of instrumentation, and life is prolonged in both critically ill and chronically ill patients. It is in such compromised hosts that gram-negative bacteria are true pathogens.

The Enterobacteriaceae are the most frequent cause of urinary tract infections. Most often the bacteria follow the ascending route through the urethra and into the bladder. This occurs when normal defense mechanisms are not functioning. Instrumentation of the urinary tract, including catheterization, can precipitate infection by enteric bacteria.

Historically *Klebsiella* was the only coliform known to cause pneumonia. It was seen in debilitated patients such as alcoholics. Today all of the Enterobacteriaceae and *Pseudomonas aeruginosa* are common etiologic agents of nosocomially acquired pneumonias. The nasopharynx of seriously ill hospitalized patients becomes colonized with these organisms, and they may play a role in the development of later pneumonias.[8] Occasionally, inhalation therapy equipment becomes contaminated and serves as the source of pulmonary infections (see Chap. 28).

Infections of the abdomen occurring after trauma or operation often involve one or more Enterobacteriaceae. The types of infections seen include peritonitis, intra-abdominal abscess, and wound infections. These infections often occur after antibiotic therapy and therefore include more resistant bacteria. Anaerobic bacteria are often found with coliform bacteria in mixed infections of the abdomen.

Anaerobic Bacteria

Anaerobic bacteria are not able to grow at normal atmospheric concentrations of oxygen. As a group, a wide range of reduced oxygen tension is tolerated, but most anaerobic bacteria can be grown at levels between 2% and 8 percent.[15] All morphological types are represented (see Table 17–3). Anaerobes are part of the normal flora of the mouth, intestines, and female genital tract. In fact, in the colon anaerobes outnumber aerobes 1000 to 1.[7]

Anaerobic bacteria have been found to be involved in infections in virtually all body tissues. They are commonly found in combination with aerobes or multiple species of anaerobes. Most of these infections involve endogenous bac-

TABLE 17–2
Important Facultative and Aerobic Gram-Negative Rods

- Enterobacteriaceae
  - *Escherichia coli*
  - *Klebsiella* spp
  - *Enterobacter* spp
  - *Serratia* spp
  - *Proteus* spp
  - *Citrobacter* spp
- *Pseudomonas aeruginosa*
- *Haemophilus influenzae*

TABLE 17–3
Major Anaerobic Bacteria

Gram-negative bacilli
Bacteroides spp
Fusobacterium spp
Gram-positive cocci
Peptococcus spp
Peptostreptococcus spp
Gram-positive bacilli
Clostridium spp

teria, that is, the normal flora of a breached mucous epithelium. Occasionally an exogenous infection results after trauma. This is usually due to *Clostridium* sp. that are commonly found in soil.

Anaerobes require low oxygen tension and produce gases. There are clinical presentations that suggest an anaerobic component to a microbial infection. These include areas of severe tissue damage or impaired blood supply, foul odor, crepitus, infections in close proximity to breaks in mucosal barriers, infections caused by bites, infections following trauma or surgery to the gastrointestinal tract, and septic abortion. When an anaerobic infection is suspected, specimens for culture must be maintained in an environment that will preserve their viability. The difficulty is that oxygen is toxic to anaerobes and standard culture techniques do not protect the organisms from the ubiquitous oxygen. A special anaerobic container is used to hold a specimen until it is received in the laboratory. An alternative specimen container is a column of fluid in a capped syringe. Specimens must be transported immediately to the microbiology laboratory where incubation is carried out in oxygen-free containers.

Viruses

Viruses are obligate, intracellular parasites. They require the metabolic machinery of living host cells for growth. A viral particle consists of genetic material, either DNA or RNA, surrounded by protein. Some viruses have a lipid envelope that is derived from the host. Viruses produce a broad spectrum of diseases. The variation ranges from acute illnesses that resolve with viral clearing by the immune response, to dissemination throughout the body, leading to death, or to chronic disease caused by the interaction of virus and the immune system, resulting in tissue injury. The disease depends on the status of the host cell, the virus, and the environment. For example, varicella-zoster virus can cause zoster (shingles), chickenpox, or encephalitis.

There are a variety of mechanisms that viruses use to cause disease. The most common is cell lysis. The virus first infects a host cell, undergoes replication, then virions are released through lysis and death of the cell. Rhinoviruses demonstrate this type of host–virus interaction when they infect the respiratory tract. A second type of infection occurs without necessarily causing the death of the cell. The cellular function is altered as virions are produced. The viral particles are released by a budding phenomenon, and infection is transmitted from cell to cell. Some viruses enter a latent phase and reside within the cell for long periods of time without causing illness. Herpes simplex is an example of a virus that produces disease when it is reactivated.

Fungi

Yeasts are unicellular fungi occurring in abundance in soil, vegetation, and water. They require organic material to grow and, therefore, are found more commonly among decaying animal or plant material. Yeasts play an important role in man's world. The production of penicillins, corticosteroids, and organic acids is accomplished by industrial cultivation of yeasts; however, foods (cheeses and breads) and alcoholic beverages requiring the action of yeast play a more prominent role in everyday life.

Yeasts are part of the normal flora of the skin and mucous membranes of the gastrointestinal tract. Most do not injure the host under normal circumstances. When host defenses are altered, when antibiotic pressure has eliminated much of bacterial flora, or when an unusually large inoculum is encountered, an infection with yeast can occur.

The most common yeast causing infection is *Candida albicans*. It is often seen during or after antibiotic therapy and may affect a variety of tissues. Thrush (oral candidiasis) is frequently seen in infants and in terminal stages of cancer, but it can occur in immunocompetent patients receiving antibiotics. Vulvovaginal candidiasis is another complication of antibiotic administration, and it frequently occurs in diabetics and pregnant women as well. Patients may develop intertriginous candidiasis in folds of the skin. Candidiasis also occurs on the hands of those whose work requires continuous immersion in water. Other organs can become infected with *C. albicans* if there is preexisting disease or following instrumentation. Involvement of the lungs and urinary tract frequently precedes invasion of the bloodstream and systemic candidiasis.

Other yeast infections seen frequently are those involving the skin, hair, and nails. Well-known examples are athlete's feet and ringworm. More serious infections occur with subcutaneous deposition of spores, usually by thorns or splinters (*e.g.*, sporotrichosis). Another group of infections is acquired by inhalation of spores (*e.g.*, histoplasmosis, coccidiodomycosis). Pulmonary infection may then be followed by lesions at other sites. Most of these disorders occur only in immunocompromised persons and resemble the disease process of tuberculosis.

Diagnosis is usually made by culture methods similar to those used for bacteria, but because yeasts are slow growing, they may take longer to identify. The cellular structure of yeasts is more like human cells than is the structure of bacteria. Therefore drugs used to treat yeast infections are more likely to be toxic to the patient. Nystatin, which is available in a variety of forms for topical use, is the drug used to treat many local infections. Amphotericin B must be used for infections involving the bloodstream, lungs, or other organs. Adverse effects are common with amphotericin B, and patients need to be observed closely during treatment. The dosage is slowly increased, and infusion is given over 4 to 6 hours. The administration of antihistamines, antiemetics, and antipyretics is often used to minimize the nausea, vomiting, headache, and fever and chills that frequently occur. Because anemia and renal and hepatic failure can complicate long courses, more frequent blood determinations are ordered to monitor the function of bone marrow, kidneys, and liver. Other drugs used for the treatment of fungal infections include ketoconazole and flucytosine.

Parasites

Although all microorganisms of medical significance are parasites, the term parisitology refers to the study of protozoa, helminths, and arthropods that infect man. Parasites include a large number of organisms with varied and complicated life cycles. The prevalence of parasitic infestation is correlated most closely with socioeconomic conditions. In the United States the treatment of water and sewage and the use of insecticides keep parasitic infection infrequent. Travelers returning from other countries, people who have been in areas where water has been contaminated (*e.g.*, campers or skiers), patients in institutions for mental retardation, recent immigrants, and immunosuppressed patients are the groups most likely to aquire parasitic disease.

Protozoa are single-cell organisms and are often intracellular during several stages of the life cycle. Some protozoa are ubiquitous and reside within man without causing illness, while others cause a fulminating course of illness that leads to death. Various species are found in the lumen of the bowel, the genitourinary tract, the bloodstream, and other tissues, including epithelial cells, myocardium, neurons, lymph nodes, spleen, liver, and interstitial cells of the lung. Those that reside in the intestine may invade the biliary tree, liver, or pancreas through the common bile duct.

Helminths are multicellular and belong to two groups, flatworms and roundworms. Although they are extracellular, many species invade tissues, whereas others reside within the gastrointestinal tract or in the bloodstream. Like protozoa, there are several stages in the life cycle of helminths, and different hosts or different tissues may be required during maturation and reproduction.

Parasitic arthropods include mites (which cause scabies), ticks, fleas, lice, and the larvae of flies. Most produce a dermatitis that is caused by toxin introduced by a bite. Superinfection by *Staphylococcus aureus* or β-hemolytic streptococci commonly complicates the chemical dermatitis. Another significant role arthropods play is as vectors of such infectious diseases as relapsing fever, spotted fever, tularemia, bubonic plague, sleeping sickness, and malaria.

Diagnosis is made by microscopic examination of specimens. Appropriate sources are feces, abscess aspirates, duodenal contents, and blood and urogenital secretions. Specimens should be taken to the laboratory immediately after collection whenever possible. If a specimen is to be sent to another facility, shipping instructions should be obtained beforehand and closely followed. It may be necessary to obtain multiple samples over a period of time because of changing life stages of the parasites. In cases where diagnosis is difficult, serological methods are used. Many parasites induce high levels of antibody that are maintained for long periods of time. Patients with helminths also have elevated levels of IgE and high eosinophil counts.

Control of parasitic infections involves a variety of public health measures. Education, sanitation, and elimination of arthropod vectors and diseased animals are approaches that are effective in reducing these infections in man.

Patient Risk Factors

Certain characteristics make some hospitalized patients more vulnerable to infections than all other patients. Particularly important risk factors include extremes of age, and the presence of diabetes, alcoholism, or nonalcoholic drug addiction.

Age

From birth until death man must mount a defense against microorganisms. It is at either end of the continuum that he is most likely to develop an infectious disease. Both the very young and the very old have a less than optimal immune response and inadequate mechanical and chemical defenses.

The infant has not experienced a challenge to his immune system and his immune tissues are immature. Microorganisms are able to gain access to normally sterile spaces because of thin, fragile epithelial tissue. The course of disease is different in the fetus or neonate; a viral infection (*e.g.*, rubella) can cause serious damage, while in older children it is a relatively mild illness. Some infections that occur in infants are found rarely at an older age. For example, bacterial meningitis caused by gram-negative bacteria is found in infants because the enteric organisms more easily penetrate the mechanical barriers of infants and IgM-associated antibodies do not cross the placenta. After the first month of life a child is far less susceptible to this disease because of the increased synthesis of IgM immunoglobulin. The care of infants therefore requires protective measures against microorganisms that are not necessary later in life.

The elderly are also more susceptible to infectious processes. It is difficult to ascertain how much the role of aging itself plays in the lowering of resistance to infection. Alterations in the function of all aspects of the immune system have been reported. However, this seems to correlate more closely to chronic disease states rather than to aging in healthy individuals.[13] There are many chronic conditions that are associated with increased risk of infection and that are found in varying degrees and combinations in the elderly. These conditions include malnutrition, cancer, diabetes, cardiovascular disease, respiratory disease, dementia, and stroke. In addition, alterations in functional ability and changes in anatomical structures can precipitate an infection. For example, urinary tract infections occur more frequently in both older men and older women. In men, the increase can be explained by urinary stasis caused by obstruction from an enlarged prostate. Older women may become infected by increased numbers of enteric organisms near the urinary meatus owing to poor hygiene and greater adherence of these organisms to perineal cells. Older women may also experience stasis because of relaxation of the pelvic floor.

Pneumonia is one of the most serious infections afflicting the elderly. Many of the normal defenses are impaired in old age. Oropharyngeal colonization by gram-negative bacteria is more common as a person ages, as is silent aspiration of oropharyngeal secretions. These secretions are cleared less readily because of an inefficient cough and impaired mucociliary action. Macrophage function is decreased with the hypoxia and pulmonary congestion associated with heart failure, which is common in older adults. These factors acting together increase the risk of pneumonia. The most common bacterial species involved are the Enterobacteriaceae, *Staphylococcus aureus, Streptococcus pneumoniae* (pneumococcus) and *Haemophilus influenzae.* Viral infections, which can aggravate already stressed defense mechanisms, are frequently followed by bacterial pneumonia that may lead to death. For this reason the elderly, especially those with significant chronic disease, are encouraged to be vaccinated against influenza.

Nursing Implications. When caring for the elderly, nurses must always keep the possibility of infection in mind. The patient may not present with classic symptoms. He may not have fever or leukocytosis. He may not produce sputum or have a pulmonary infiltrate despite his pneumonia. He may not have abdominal pain while suffering from an abdominal source of infection. The symptoms may be vague and may include confusion, hypotension, and difficulty in breathing. A careful history, thorough physical examination, and diagnostic tests are critical in determining the site of infection.

The nursing management of infection in the elderly also presents challenges. Dehydration is almost always present. Fluid replacement must be accompanied by careful monitoring of cardiovascular status and observations for congestive heart failure. Because most antibiotics are excreted through the kidneys, renal function must also be evaluated (particularly with aminoglycoside therapy). Respiratory support may also be necessary in both pneumonia and infections at other sites. Anorexia may be especially pronounced in an elderly patient, and creativity on the part of the caregiver may be required in getting the patient to increase his protein intake.

Diabetes

The incidence of certain infections is increased in diabetic patients (see Chap. 74). Infections are potentially more serious in these patients because of the accompanying metabolic derangements, infection being the most frequent cause of ketoacidosis. The immune response has not been convincingly shown to be impaired in all diabetics. However, the neurological, vascular, and metabolic complications that occur place the patient at increased risk. For example, a neurogenic bladder causes urinary stasis and may require frequent catheterization that can result in urinary tract infection. Vascular insufficiency can lead to ischemia and gangrene in an extremity, followed by a major infection and loss of the limb. Diabetic women are predisposed to vaginitis and urinary tract infection with yeast, especially when glycosuria is present.

Nursing Implications. There is evidence that control of blood glucose may help prevent infections in the diabetic.[14] Patients should be taught proper foot care and the early signs of infection. When ketoacidosis or an unexplained change in glucose control occurs, an infection should be suspected. During an infection, urine glucose should be monitored more frequently and changes in insulin requirement expected.

Alcoholism

Chronic ethanol abuse increases the risk of experiencing an infectious disease. The role that alcohol plays in the function of immunologic defenses is unclear, but factors associated with chronic abuse are known to influence the establishment of infection. These factors include the following:

1. The altered state of consciousness during intoxication increases the possibility of aspiration and can result in trauma, which is often not treated promptly.
2. Malnutrition
3. Hepatic and pancreatic disease
4. Unsanitary environment
5. Unavailable medical care

Pulmonary infections are most closely linked with alcoholism. Incidence, recurrence rate, and mortality of pneumonia are all higher in alcoholic patients. *Streptococcus pneumoniae* (pneumococcus) is one of the most common etiologic agents. Gram-negative bacteria, especially *Klebsiella pneumoniae*, are also frequently recovered from the sputum of alcoholic patients with respiratory infection. Hepatitis, pancreatitis complicated by abscess, spontaneous bacterial peritonitis, bacteremia, and bacterial endocarditis are all more common in chronic ethanol abusers.

Nursing Implications. The diagnosis and treatment of infections are more difficult in alcoholic patients. Medical attention is often not obtained until the illness is advanced. Even in the hospital, treatment can be delayed if the patient is not able to describe his symptoms because he is intoxicated or he has delirium tremens, which often includes fever and leukocytosis. Underlying disease as well as malnutrition and dehydration need to be considered in designing care for the alcoholic. Of particular significance is discharge planning. Many alcoholics have problems with compliance to regimens of care. Since patients with infections are often discharged with antibiotics and wounds requiring care, reliable follow-up evaluations must be set up or hospital release delayed to prevent recurrence of the illness.

Nonalcoholic Drug Addiction

The most frequent medical problem drug abusers experience is infection. Most of these infections arise from microorganisms the addict injects into himself. Illicit parenteral drug abuse creates many avenues of contamination: the drug itself, the substance with which the drug is "cut," the solution used to dissolve the drug (*e.g.,* tap water or saliva), the skin, the reused or community syringe. There are similarities between the alcoholic and drug abuser. The latter often lives in an environment that increases exposure to infection;

he is often malnourished and frequently develops pneumonia. He is also more likely to develop bacteremia and consequent endocarditis, osteomyelitis, arthritis, and meningitis. Furthermore, the injection of nonsterile material causes skin and soft tissue infections. Cellulitis, subcutaneous abscess, lymphangitis, fasciitis, myositis, and thrombophlebitis are most frequently caused by *Staphylococcus aureus* and β-hemolytic streptococci, but a variety of aerobic and anaerobic bacteria, viruses, and yeasts, alone and in combination, have been reported. Tetanus occurs primarily in drug addicts and carries a mortality of almost 90% in this group.[18] By sharing needles and syringes, drug abusers transmit bloodborne infections. In the past, malaria epidemics have occurred among this population. More recently, acquired immunodeficiency syndrome (AIDS) has been found in illicit drug users. However, the most common infection associated with blood transmission is hepatitis. The majority of drug abusers have hepatitis B surface antigen. Infection by the hepatitis virus occurs early in the use of narcotics and is a common reason for hospitalization.

Nursing Implications. It is very difficult to prevent infections in drug abusers. Routine vaccination for tetanus should be encouraged. Patients at particular risk for endocarditis (those with rheumatic heart disease or prosthetic valves) should be provided with information about the consequences of parenteral drug abuse. Hospitalized patients usually require intravenous antibiotics. Because peripheral veins are often inaccessible, a central line may be placed. The patient may need to be protected from himself because the use of the intravenous line for administration of street drugs can lead to further bacteremia or to air embolism.

Response to Infection

Inflammation and Phagocytosis

The body's defenses against invading microorganisms begin with the response of inflammation at the site of injury as the body attempts to localize the infection (see Chap. 15). Inflammation occurs when there is damage to tissue, such as in the invasion of microorganisms. The signs and symptoms include redness, edema, heat, and pain. The initial effect of inflammation is the vascular response. Local arterioles and capillaries dilate, mediated by serotonin, histamine, and prostaglandins, allowing plasma to escape. In the area of injury edema fluid accumulates and fibrin forms a network that tends to limit the spread of infection. Circulating polymorphonuclear neutrophils (PMNs) begin sticking to the walls of capillaries (marginating) and then migrate toward the injured site. This migration is stimulated by chemotactic substances in the inflammatory exudate. When the PMNs reach the invading microorganisms, phagocytosis begins. The pH in the area becomes more acidic, causing lysis of PMNs by cellular proteases. Macrophages then engulf the leukocytic debris and bacteria.

Plasma proteins are normally cleared from the interstitial compartment by the lymphatics. During inflammation the lymphatic capillaries dilate to several times their normal size. Excess interstitial fluid, proteins, cells, and invading microorganisms enter the lymphatic system and are carried away. The lymph nodes act as effective filters for microorganisms by clearing lymphatic fluid before it empties into the venous system.

If the infection is not localized by the inflammatory processes, lymphangitis and lymphadenopathy occur as the infection moves into the lymphatic system. This represents the body's attempt to regionalize the infection. This can be seen in the extremities as red streaks running from the site of infection toward lymph nodes and as enlarged lymph nodes in the axilla, groin, or neck.

Thermoregulatory Response

The body has an extremely efficient mechanism for control of temperature. Alterations of the central setpoint are almost always associated with infection or inflammation. Because elevation of body temperature is such a sensitive indicator of the presence of disease, monitoring temperature is one of the most common procedures routinely performed in hospitals.

Fever can be produced by endotoxins of gram-negative bacteria as well as by other pyrogenic factors generated during bacterial growth. In addition, products of the host's own cells (endogenous pyrogens) can increase body temperature. Endogenous pyrogen does not exist stored in cells but is synthesized when an appropriate stimulus is present. Endotoxin, viruses, bacteria, antigen–antibody complexes, and specific steroids can serve as stimuli for the production and release of endogenous pyrogen by phagocytic cells (granulocytes, monocytes, and macrophages). When endogenous pyrogen is released it acts rapidly on the hypothalamus, changing the setpoint to a higher level.

Although it is customary to treat fever with antipyretics to lower body temperature, some authorities have suggested that fever may be of value in combating infection.[10] The specific role that fever plays in augmenting host defenses is not known, but several mechanisms have been suggested. Biochemical reactions are increased with heating. The rate of reaction of host defenses may be hastened at a higher temperature. The half-life of endotoxin is reduced during fever. Fever appears to increase the iron requirements of bacteria, and serum iron levels fall during infection. These two factors result in relatively less iron available for the growth of pathogenic bacteria.[5] Many bacteria are susceptible to lower levels of antibiotics at temperature levels associated with fever.

Nonetheless, increased body temperature increases catabolism and cardiac output. For each degree centigrade above normal, the biochemical reactions increase 10% to 13%. This means a greater expenditure of calories and consumption of oxygen. Heart rate increases 10 beats/minute for each one degree centigrade rise in temperature.

Nursing Implications. A patient with infection should have his temperature monitored to evaluate treatment and allow prompt intervention for excessive fever (greater than 41°C). For some patients, including those with preexisting cardiovascular, pulmonary, or central nervous system diseases and children, the temperature indicating an emergency may be lower. Ischemia may occur in patients with cardiovascular disease, respiratory distress may occur owing to increased oxygen requirements in patients with chronic pulmonary disease, and seizures may occur in children or patients with central nervous system disease. Antipyretics (aspirin or acetaminophen) are administered rectally or orally. Cooling blankets or cool baths will help lower body temperature, but they often require a drug such as chlorpromazine to block shivering.

In patients with mild to moderate fever (less than 40°C), the treatment of hyperthermia is not necessary. However, they are usually treated with antipyretics because the accompanying symptoms of headache and muscle pain are well managed with these same drugs. All patients with fever need replacement of fluids since insensible water loss is increased. Sources of glucose, protein, and electrolytes should be given. Rest is indicated for all patients with fever, but special attention is needed for patients with chronic respiratory or cardiovascular disease since their baseline functions are marginal.

Metabolic Response

Greatly increased rates of metabolism occur in response to infection. Metabolic changes begin at the onset and evolve to match the severity of the illness. Fever may account in part for the increase in metabolic rate, but with severe infection it may rise 40% to 60%, which is out of proportion to the fever.[19] Many of the alterations in metabolic control are modulated by hormones. The production of catecholamines, corticosteroids, aldosterone, thyroxine, and hormones affecting carbohydrate metabolism are all increased in response to infection. Glycogen stores are used up early in the course of an infection. Serum glucose is elevated during infection. This has been shown to be the result of gluconeogenesis rather than from an insulin deficiency. In the liver glucose is produced from amino acids, which arise from the catabolism of skeletal muscle. This action is not depressed by high levels of circulating glucose.[11] Protein and body fat are then oxidized as energy sources. The resulting metabolism is very much like that seen during long-term starvation. During the infectious process many intracellular components are lost. A state of negative nitrogen balance follows and continues until the infection is resolved. Potassium, phosphorus, magnesium, sulfur, and zinc are lost primarily through increased urinary excretion.[3]

Nursing Implications. Unfortunately the nutritional deficits caused by the infectious process cannot be reversed until the infection has been controlled. The optimal intervention can be aimed at sparing protein stores in muscle. The goal of nutritional support is to provide amino acids and moderate amounts of glucose and fat together with vitamins and trace elements. In the seriously ill patient this is usually accomplished by intravenous infusion. Patients who are able to eat are encouraged to increase their intake of protein. However, increased metabolic needs are often accompanied by anorexia. The elevation of serum glucose is exaggerated in the diabetic. A patient who has been in good control may develop a hyperglycemia requiring hospitalization for treatment. Any diabetic with an infection needs more frequent checks of his urine for glucose and may require additional insulin. Increased fluid intake is important because of almost certain osmotic diuresis.

Prevention

General Measures

The best approach to infection is prevention. Strict attention to aseptic technique, rapid treatment of traumatic injuries, gentle handling of tissues, and supporting and maintaining normal physiology are all important in preventing infection.

The nurse carries out procedures that require sterile technique and at times assists with these procedures. In the operating room it is the nurse's responsibility to assure the sterility of all individuals involved in the case. It is important to keep body areas sterile that are normally bacteria free. When procedures are performed, care must be taken to not let bacteria from surrounding areas invade sterile body spaces. Disinfection of the skin with a povidone–iodine solution and appropriate draping are designed to avoid contamination.

It is equally important to carry out procedures with accuracy and gentleness. When tissues are handled roughly damage occurs that interferes with host defenses, allowing the establishment of infection. Technique should be practiced until procedures can be accomplished without error. Repetition of such procedures as placing catheters can also damage tissue and thus destroy the body's defense mechanisms. The use of lubricants can protect mucosal surfaces.

The maintenance of normal physiology protects against invasion of microorganisms. The nurse should observe for alterations from the normal state and institute measures to approximate normal. For example, skin needs to be dry to be healthy. It should be protected from continual contact with secretions or excretions. Tissues require adequate circulation, which can be assured by avoiding prolonged pressure caused by body position.

Vaccination

The most significant management of viral infections has been with the use of vaccines. Immunizations are important components of preventive health for both the individual and the community. Many crippling or fatal diseases have been nearly eradicated since the development of immunization programs. Vaccines are available against measles, polio, smallpox, rabies, influenza, and other viral illnesses. There are also vaccines effective in preventing bacterial diseases (*e.g.*, tetanus, diphtheria, and cholera). Immunization is not without adverse effects and is recommended for groups at highest risk. Young children and the elderly are frequently involved in immunization programs. Both are at greater risk because of inadequate immune response. People traveling to foreign countries where they may come in contact with uncommon pathogens are also advised (or are required) to obtain immunizations. Population groups at risk for contracting hepatitis, such as institutionalized individuals, homosexual males, and health care professionals, may be advised to receive immunization. Table 17–4 lists the different types of immunizations available.

Many vaccines produce a local reaction (tenderness and erythema around the injection site) and fever, both of which are of short duration. If true allergic reactions including hives, wheezing, or anaphylaxis occur, the individual should not receive further injections of the vaccine. Some vaccines are prepared in animal culture, most commonly chicken or duck embryo; therefore, the patient should be questioned about egg allergy. Patients with immunoincompetence and pregnant women should not be given live virus vaccines or be intimately exposed to those receiving them.

The preparation of vaccines and recommendations for their use are constantly changing. As a nurse who is involved in the vaccination of individuals, it is necessary to obtain the latest information. The Advisory Committee on Immunization Practices of the US Public Health Service publishes this data regularly in the *Morbidity and Mortality Weekly Report,* which is gathered by the Centers for Disease Control (CDC). The product insert that is packaged with the vaccine also contains current recommendations and precautions.

Antibiotic Prophylaxis

Antibiotic prophylaxis is used to prevent infection when it is known that a person will have a high probability of exposure to specific microorganisms over a short period of time. The risk of infection must be greater than the risk of experiencing an adverse reaction to the drug. The choice of antibiotic and timing of its administration are dependent on the specific circumstances. There are few nonsurgical indications for antimicrobial prophylaxis. Patients with valvular heart disease are considered at high risk for developing endocarditis as a result of bacteremia during manipulative procedures such as dental work and are therefore treated prophylactically. The use of preventive antibiotics in surgery is routine for certain procedures. Again, the relative risk of infection is used to determine which patients will be treated with antibiotics. Operations that include the placement of prosthetic devices such as heart valves and artificial joints are performed with antibiotic coverage. Other procedures are classified as clean, clean-contaminated, contaminated, and dirty according to a system that was first reported in 1964 (see Table 17–5).[6] Prophylaxis is not indicated for clean or most clean-contaminated cases (see Chap. 8).

The time of administration of an antibiotic drug is important. In the past it was thought necessary to give antibiotics in the preoperative period and for several days postoperatively. Today it is recognized that a very short course is all that is needed, but it is important to give the drug immediately before the skin incision and to maintain blood levels during the operation when the risk of bacterial contamination is high. This concept is based on studies performed with animals, which identified the "decisive period" of antibiotic administration to be within 3 hours of bacterial contamination.[4] A drug given later has no effect in reducing wound infections. Later work confirmed these findings in humans.

TABLE 17–4
Types of Vaccines

Routine Immunizations	Special Immunizations
Tetanus	Influenza
Diphtheria	Pneumococcus
Pertussis	Hepatitis B
Poliomyelitis	
Measles	
Mumps	
Rubella	
Travel Immunizations	
Smallpox*	
Cholera	
Yellow fever	
Typhoid	
Plague	
Typhus	
Meningococcus	
Rabies	
Japanese encephalitis	
Immune globulin	

* In 1979 the World Health Organization officially announced the eradication of smallpox. Most countries no longer require travelers to present certificates of smallpox vaccination.

(Jong EC: The use of immunizations for the prevention of infectious diseases. In Altman LC (ed): Allergy and Immunology. Boston, GK Hall Medical Publishers, 1984)

Preventing the Spread of Infection

The spread of infectious disease requires a source of pathogen, a susceptible host, and a means of transporting one to the other. The source can be another person, endogenous flora, or inanimate objects. The host must be susceptible to the microorganisms or an infection will not develop. Transmission of pathogen to the host occurs primarily in four ways:

1. *Contact* with the infected individual, articles he has contaminated, or respiratory droplets
2. *Intake of vehicles of transmission,* such as water, food, drugs or blood
3. *Inhalation of airborne particles,* either droplet nuclei or dust
4. *Exposure to vector borne disease, e.g.,* mosquitoes.

In situations where little can be done to control the etiologic agent or host factors, actions to prevent infection are aimed at interrupting transmission.

Isolation Technique

The transmission of infectious disease is of special concern to those caring for the sick. The nurse must protect herself as well as her patients from acquiring an infection. Hospitals establish standards of isolation to control infections within the institution. There are, however, several problems with relying on isolation protocol. A patient must be identified as having an infectious disease before isolation

TABLE 17–5
Wound Categories

	Characteristics
Clean	No acute inflammation No break in surgical technique No entry into gastrointestinal or respiratory tract
Clean-contaminated	Minor break in surgical technique Entry into gastrointestinal or respiratory tract without gross spill Wounds involving urinary or biliary tract
Contaminated	Major break in technique Entry into gastrointestinal tract without gross spill Acute inflammation Fresh traumatic wounds
Dirty	Pus Perforated hollow viscus Old trauma Open fractures of joint spaces

procedures are instituted. The presence of the pathogen and its transmission to other individuals may occur before it is recognized that precautions are needed. Identification may be delayed because some infectious agents are capable of producing only mild symptoms or a carrier state that allows a healthy appearing person to spread the disease to innumerable contacts. Once isolation has been initiated the nurse may concentrate on the specific site of infection, forgetting or not realizing that other body secretions may be colonized by the pathogen.

To prevent the spread of infectious disease, the nurse must recognize that all body fluids, including blood, urine, sputum, saliva, pus, spinal fluid, vaginal discharge and lesion drainage, may contain pathogens. Gloves, gowns, and masks should be used appropriately whenever contact with secretions is anticipated. If unexpected exposure should occur, washing should be done as soon as possible. Likewise, materials that are soiled with body fluids should be cleansed or discarded in such a way as to prevent others from unnecessary exposure. For example, dressings from open wounds and tissues with respiratory secretions should be securely bagged so accidental spillage does not occur. Lister's counsel in 1870 is still applicable: "You must be able to see with your mental eye the septic ferments as distinctly as we see flies or other insects with the corporeal eye—if you do not see them, you will be constantly liable to relax in your precautions."

When a patient is identified as having an infection, he may be placed in isolation. Most nurses will be asked at some time to assist in the care of an isolated patient to restrict the spread of infection. The *CDC Guideline for Isolation Precautions in Hospitals* is published by the Centers for Disease Control and is the reference text for hospitals across the country. In 1983 a major revision was completed that offered an alternative to group classification of isolation requirements. The new recommendations are disease-specific, listing the isolation precautions needed for containment of pathogens in individual disease processes. This system is thought to be advantageous to the patient because it eliminates "over-isolation" and is more economical for the hospital in terms of supplies used and necessary staff time. For hospitals preferring the category-specific isolation system that has long been in use, the revision has updated these recommendations. There are seven categories in use: Strict Isolation, Contact Isolation, Respiratory Isolation, Tuberculosis (AFB) Isolation, Enteric Precautions, Drainage/Secretion Precautions, and Blood/Body Fluid Precautions. The category Protective Isolation, which was designed to reduce infections in immunocompromised patients, had not been shown to be effective and was therefore eliminated. When a patient is isolated, a card stating the precautions to be used is placed on his door. The instructions include requirements for hand washing, masks, gowns, gloves, and cleaning and disposition of patient items. The category-specific cards list on the reverse side the diseases requiring the type of isolation printed on the front. The disease-specific cards have blanks that are filled in by the hospital epidemiologist with indicated precautions. Hand washing is required of all persons entering the room. Patients may have visitors, but they must receive instruction and be supervised in the use of isolation methods. A summary of isolation requirements for selected infections is contained in Table 17–6.

Antimicrobial Agents

Antibiotic Therapy

Host defenses can be enhanced by the use of antibiotics. Antibiotics can be used either prophylactically to prevent infection or as treatment for an established infection. When an infection is caused by multiple pathogens, it may be necessary to use two or more antibiotics.

The fundamental principle of chemotherapy for infection is *selective toxicity*. This means that a substance must be harmful to the parasite while leaving the host cells intact.

TABLE 17–6
Isolation Requirements

	Private Room	*Masks*	*Gowns*	*Gloves*	*Examples of Disease*
Strict isolation	Yes	Yes	Yes	Yes	Diphtheria Varicella (chickenpox)
Contact isolation	Yes	For those close to patient	If soiling is likely	For touching infective material	Infection by multiply-resistant bacteria (*e.g., Pseudomonas, Staphylococcus aureus*) Major skin or wound infection Acute respiratory infections in young children
Respiratory isolation	Yes	For those close to patients	No	No	Measles, mumps, pertussis Meningococcal infections
AFB isolation	Yes	When patient is coughing	If soiling is likely	No	Active tuberculosis
Enteric precautions	If patient hygiene is poor	No	If soiling is likely	For touching infective material	Diarrhea with suspected infectious etiology Hepatitis A Viral meningitis Poliomyelitis
Drainage/secretion precautions	No	No	If soiling is likely	For touching infective material	Minor skin or wound infection Decubitus ulcer
Blood/body fluid precaution	If patient hygiene is poor	No	If soiling is likely	For touching blood or body fluids	Hepatitis B Hepatitis non-A, non-B Malaria AIDS

There are many substances known that will kill microorganisms, but relatively few that are not also toxic to human beings. The first agent used systemically that was selectively toxic to bacteria was sulfanilamide (one of the sulfonamides). This was followed in the same decade by penicillin. The interest in developing antibiotics has continued and new drugs are released every year (see Table 17–7).

Antibiotics alone are not sufficient to cure an infection. The phagocytes of the host act in conjunction with the drug to eliminate the pathogens. The effect of an antibiotic can be either *bacteriostatic* (slows down or prevents multiplication) or *bactericidal* (kills the organism). In either case the drug is only active against growing bacteria. Antibacterial agents curb the increasing numbers of bacteria so that the host's phagocytes are not overwhelmed and are able to clear the remaining live bacteria and cellular debris. This is why antibiotics are often continued for a period of time after the symptoms of the acute infection have resolved.

Intracellular bacteria present a more serious problem. These organisms (such as mycobacteria) are able to survive for long periods within phagocytes. There are several reasons why antibiotic therapy is inadequate for illness caused by these organisms. It is possible that the drug does not reach the bacteria or that it is inactive in the intracellular environment. The destruction of the organism is dependent primarily on the cellular defenses of the host. Recovery is slow and the general health status of the patient must be improved.

Extracellular bacteria are sometimes involved in the formation of abscesses. The conditions within the abscess cause inactivation of antibiotics and impair the function of leukocytes. Circulation is impaired, which causes decreased levels of oxygen, nutrients, and antibodies as well as the accumulation of waste products, including acids. The infection will not resolve until the pus drains either spontaneously or by surgical intervention. The presence of a foreign body will also protect bacteria against the action of chemotherapeutic agents and phagocytes. Surgical removal is required before the infection can be cured.

Empiric therapy is the administration of a drug based on what one would guess the etiologic agent to be. This method is used when it is thought to be detrimental to the patient to wait until the organism has been identified and its sensitivity pattern determined. Treatment is reevaluated when this information is available. If empiric therapy is considered necessary, the following criteria are used to determine the selection of antibiotic:

1. The site of infection (*e.g.,* skin, lung, urinary tract)
2. The age of the patient (*e.g.,* risk of childhood illnesses)

TABLE 17–7
Antibiotics

Natural penicillins	**First generation cephalosporins**
Penicillin G	Cephalothin Cephapirin
Penicillin V	Cefazolin Cephalexin
Penicillinase-resistant penicillins	Cephradine
Methicillin	**Second generation cephalosporins**
Oxacillin	Cefamandole Ceforanide
Nafcillin	Cefoxitin Cefuroxime
Dicloxacillin	Cefonicid
Penicillins with expanded spectrum	**Third generation cephalosporins**
Ampicillin	Moxalactam
Amoxycillin	Cefotaxime
Carbenicillin	Ceftizoxime
Ticarcillin	Cefoperazone
Azlocillin	Cefsulodin
Mezlocillin	Ceftazidime
Piperacillin	**Others**
Aminoglycosides	Chloramphenicol
Gentamicin	Tetracyclines
Tobramycin	Erythromycin
Amikacin	Clindamycin
Netilmycin	Vancomycin
Kanamycin	Trimethoprim/sulfisoxasole
Neomycin	

3. Where the infection was acquired (*e.g.*, hospital or community)
4. Mechanical factors (*e.g.*, biomedical instrumentation)
5. Factors affecting immunocompetence (*e.g.*, corticosteriods, transplants)
6. Potential toxicity of the antibiotic

Method of Action of Antibiotics

Antibiotics can be grouped by their method of activity against bacteria. Most antibiotics act by interfering with the synthesis or function of essential components of the microbial cell. The following is a brief discussion of the probable mechanisms responsible for the effectiveness of antimicrobial agents.

Competitive Inhibition. Sulfonamides are thought to be effective because of their similarity in structure to para-aminobenzoic acid (PABA). PABA is necessary in the enzymatic pathway that synthesizes folic acid. Sulfonamides are able to enter the reaction in place of PABA, thus inhabiting the growth of the pathogenic organism. This class of drugs has largely been replaced by more effective and less toxic antibiotics; however, they are still frequently used to treat urinary tract infections.

Inhibition of Cell Wall Synthesis. Penicillin was the first discovered antibiotic of a continually increasing number of related antibiotics. All compounds in this group act by blocking the action of an enzyme necessary for the establishment of the stable cross-linking of a polypeptide in the cell wall of bacteria. The chemical configuration of these antibiotics includes a four-membered (beta-lactam) ring.

Natural penicillins are derived from yeast cultures; thus doses are measured in biological units. They are effective against a large variety of organisms, but their most common use is in the treatment of infections caused by gram-positive cocci. Certain staphylococci and some other organisms produce the enzyme penicillinase (also called β-lactamase), which opens the beta-lactam ring and inactivates the drug. The discovery of this enzyme stimulated the development of semisynthetic penicillins that are resistant to the action of β-lactamase and are used treat staphylococcal infections. Other penicillins (such as ampicillin) have been developed that increase the spectrum of activity to include more gram-negative bacilli.

Penicillins are relatively nontoxic but do cause allergic reactions. The most frequent reaction is a skin rash with or without fever. The incidence of penicillin allergy is estimated at 1% to 5% with true anaphylactic reactions being very rare (less than 0.05%). The incidence of patients reporting past allergic reaction is, however, much higher. This discrepancy may be due to fear instilled by stories of anaphylactic shock. A careful history should be obtained before the administration of penicillins, including details of any symptoms the patient attributes to exposure in the past.

The fungus *Cephalosporium* was the source of the first of the cephalosporins. These antibiotics are similar in chemical structure to the penicillins and have a similar spectrum of activity, but they are much less likely to cause allergic reactions. Thrombophlebitis occurs frequently after intravenous administration and occasionally patients develop a maculopapular rash. The major disadvantage to the use of cephalosporins is an economic one. As a rule they are much more expensive than penicillins. New cephalosporins have been developed to expand their spectrum of activity. The subclasses have been designated as "generations." Discussions of cephalosporins may include grouping as first generation, second generation, or third generation.

Inhibition of Protein Synthesis. The aminoglycosides were also originally isolated from cultures of fungi. They act at the ribosome of the bacteria interfering with the synthesis of protein and causing cell death. Gram-positive organisms (except staphylococci and enterococci) and anaerobes are usually resistant to the aminoglycosides. They are used primarily in the treatment of infections caused by enteric gram-negative bacilli and in combination with other antibiotics to treat enterococcal and staphylococcal infections. None of the aminoglycosides is absorbed from the gastrointestinal tract. This property is used to advantage with the administration of neomycin to reduce bacterial density as a part of the preparation for surgery of the colon and to reduce the production of ammonia in cases of hepatic failure.

The aminoglycosides are relatively toxic substances. They often cause damage to the eighth cranial nerve, which occasionally results in severe hearing loss. Nephrotoxicity can also occur. The most accurate way of administering aminoglycosides is by monitoring serum levels. Two determinations are needed, one 30 minutes before the dose is given, called the *trough,* and one 30 minutes after infusion, called the *peak*. The precise time the drug is given is needed for these values to be reliable. The dose and the interval between doses may need to be adjusted.

Patients who are at high risk for developing renal damage are

1. Those with preexisting renal disease
2. Those who have periods of hypotension
3. Those with inadequate fluid intake
4. Older patients
5. Those who receive a course of therapy longer than 10 to 14 days.

Nursing interventions include administering the drug on time and infusing it over 30 to 45 minutes, maintaining an adequate fluid intake, observation of urinary output, monitoring BUN and serum creatinine, and assessment of daily weight as an indicator of fluid retention. The nurse should also observe for complaints of headache, vertigo, tinnitis, or hearing loss.

Other antibiotics that interfere with protein synthesis are chloramphenicol and the tetracyclines. Both have broad spectrums of activity covering gram-positive, gram-negative, aerobic, and anaerobic bacteria. Erythromycin is effective against most gram-positive bacteria and is often used as a substitute for penicillin in patients with penicillin allergy. It is the drug of choice against *Legionella*. Clindamycin is related to erythromycin. It is effective against most gram-positive cocci and most anaerobes.

Adverse Reactions

The most common side-effects of antibiotic therapy are gastrointestinal. Some patients may develop nausea and vomiting while taking oral antibiotics. In some cases this may be alleviated by taking the medication with food, but there are some antibiotics that are not absorbed in the presence of food or dairy products, for example, tetracycline. Diarrhea may also occur during antibiotic treatment, and patients may require additional fluids. The severity and nature of the diarrhea stools should be monitored. Usually diarrhea resolves with the cessation of antibiotic therapy, but it can lead to pseudomembranous colitis, which requires specific treatment.

Hypersensitivity reactions can also occur. These reactions usually involve fever, erythema, urticaria, and rash, but life-threatening anaphylaxis can occur. Although allergy is seen most often with penicillins and cephalosporins, it can occur with any antibiotic. A careful drug history should be taken before antibiotics are administered.

Disinfection

Disinfectants and antiseptics are different from antibiotics in that they exhibit little selective toxicity. Disinfectants are used to eliminate pathogenic organisms on inanimate objects, whereas antiseptics can be used on living tissues. The mode of action of disinfectants varies, and effectiveness is determined by concentration, duration of contact, and temperature. Warm water and the detergent action of soaps eliminates many microbes and is necessary even when further treatment is required because many disinfecting agents are inactivated by organic debris. The level of disinfection indicated or the need for destruction of all microbial life by sterilization depends on the use of an item and its exposure to pathogens. Articles to be reused should be processed in the hospital's central service department where appropriate means and expertise are available.

The use of hand-washing products containing an antimicrobial agent such as hexachlorophene, iodophors, or chlorhexidine is recommended before carrying out surgical or other invasive procedures or while caring for newborns or infected patients. At other times regular soap, running water, and friction followed by drying with a paper towel are sufficient.

Summary

Both microbial characteristics and host defensive capabilities interact to determine whether or not infections will develop. An important role of nursing is to analyze these factors for individual patients and determine their relative risk for infection. Following assessment for risk, appropriate strategies to reduce the likelihood of infection can then be identified and implemented.

References

1. Bayer AS, Chow AW, Anthony BF, Guze LB: Serious infections in adults due to group B streptococci: Clinical and serotypic characterization. Am J Med 61:498, 1976
2. Beachy E: Bacterial adherence: Adhesin-receptor interactions mediating the attachment of bacteria to mucosal surfaces. J Infect Dis 143:325, 1981
3. Beisel WR: Metabolic response to infection. Annu Rev Med 26:9, 1975
4. Burke JF: The effective period of preventative antibiotic action in experimental incisions and dermal lesions. Surgery 50:161, 1961
5. Grieger TA, Cluger MJ: Fever and survival: The role of serum iron. J Physiol 279:187, 1978
6. Howard JM, Barker WF, Culbertston WR et al: Factors influencing the incidence of wound infection. Ann Surg (Suppl) 160:32, 1964
7. Jawetz E, Melnick JL, Adelberg EA: Review of medical microbiology, 11th ed. Los Altos, CA, Lange Medical Publications, 1983
8. Johanson WG, Pierce AK, Sanford JP: Changing pharyngeal bacterial flora of hospitalized patients: Emergence of gram-negative bacilli. N Engl J Med 281:1137, 1969
9. Johanson WG, Woods DE, Chaudhuri T: Association of respiratory tract colonization with adherence of gram-negative bacilli to epithelial cells. J Infect Dis 139:667, 1979
10. Kluger MJ: The evolution and adaptive value of fever. Am Sci 66:38, 1978
11. Long CL, Spencer JL, Kinney JM, Geiger JW: Carbohydrate metabolism in man: Effect of elective operations and major injury. J Appl Physiol 31:110, 1971
12. Mims CA: The Pathogenesis of Infectious Disease. New York, Grune & Stratton, 1976
13. Phair JP: Aging and infection (review article). J Chronic Dis 32:535, 1979

14. Rayfield EJ, Ault MJ, Keusch GT et al: Infection and diabetes: The case for glucose control. Am J Med 72:439, 1982
15. Smith LDS: Anaerobic bacteria. In Lennette EH: Manual of Clinical Microbiology, 3rd ed. Washington, American Society for Microbiology, 1980
16. Valenti WM, Trudell BS, Bentley DW: Factors predisposing to oropharyngeal colonization with gram-negative bacilli in the aged. N Engl J Med 298:1108, 1978
17. Wara DW: Host defense against *Streptococcus pneumoniae:* The role of the spleen. Rev Infect Dis 3:299, 1981
18. Wilford BB: Clinical complications of drug abuse. In: A Guide for the Primary Care Physician. Chicago, AMA, 1981
19. Wilmore DW: The Metabolic Management of the Critically Ill—Support Plan. New York, Plenum, 1977

Bibliography

Adams HG, Jordan C: Infections in the alcoholic. Med Clin North Am 68:179, 1984

Bellanti JA: Immunology II. Philadelphia, WB Saunders, 1978

Cohen AG, Gold WM: Defense mechanisms of the lungs. Annu Rev Med 26:325, 1975

Cruse PJE, Foord R: The epidemiology of wound infection: A 10-year prospective study of 62,939 wounds. Surg Clin North Am 60:27, 1980

Davis BD, Dulbecco R, Eisen HN et al: Microbiology, 2nd ed. Hagerstown, Harper & Row, 1973

Dinarello CA, Wolff SM: Pathogenesis of fever in man. N Engl J Med 298:607, 1978

Ericsson CD, Kohl S, Pickering LK et al: Mechanisms of host defense in well nourished patients with chronic alcoholism. Alcoholism 4:261, 1980

Grieco MH: Infections in the Abnormal Host. USA, Yorke Medical Books, 1980

Howard JM, Barker WF, Culbertston WR et al: Factors influencing the incidence of wound infection. Ann Surg (Suppl) 160:32, 1964

Jackson MM, Lynch P: Infection control: Too much or too little? Am J Nurs 84:208, 1984

Johanson WG, Pierce AK, Sanford JP: Changing pharyngeal bacterial flora of hospitalized patients: Emergence of gram-negative bacilli. N Engl J Med 281:1137, 1969

Jong EC: The use of immunizations for the prevention of infectious diseases. In Altman LC (ed): Allergy and Immunology. Boston, GK Hall, 1984

Langslet J, Havel ML: The aminoglycoside antibiotics. Am J Nurs 81:114, 1981

Louria DB: Infectious complications of nonalcoholic drug abuse. Annu Rev Med 25:219, 1974

Mandell GL, Douglas RG, Bennett JE: Principles and Practice of Infectious Diseases. New York, John Wiley & Sons, 1979

Meakins JL, Pietsch JB, Christou NV, Maclean LD: Predicting surgical infection before the operation. World J Surg 4:439, 1980

Simmons RL, Howard RJ: Surgical Infectious Diseases. New York, Appleton-Century-Crofts, 1982

Chapter 18

Non-neoplastic Cell Changes

Candace Ann Walters

Mature living cells can respond to stressors in ways that promote cellular survival and decrease the likelihood of cellular injury. Cells can adapt by altering the cell size. An important variable determining other adaptive mechanisms of cellular response to a stressor is the cell's ability to proliferate and differentiate. Those cell types that can replicate and divide usually proliferate. Some cells may also differentiate to another cell type more capable of withstanding the altered cellular environment.

Cellular injury occurs whenever the cell's adaptive capability is exceeded. Host factors as well as characteristics of the stressor and the cell influence the point at which injury occurs. Initial injury is often reversible, but irreversible cell injury and cell death may occur at a later point.

The purpose of this chapter is to review examples of the adaptive cellular changes: atrophy, hypertrophy, hyperplasia, and metaplasia. Dysplasia, though not strictly an adaptive change, is also included. The process and morphological changes of reversible cell injury are also discussed.

Alterations in Cell Size

All cells can respond to stressors by increasing or decreasing their cell size. When the amount of work required of a mature cell increases, the likelihood of cell survival also increases if the cell surface area is enlarged. The result is that the amount of work required per unit area of cell is decreased. Alteration in cell size is the sole adaptive response available to those cells that cannot replicate and divide, for example, myocardial cells.

Atrophy

Atrophy is defined as the shrinkage in size of a mature cell because of loss of cell substance.[3] An atrophic cell has fewer mitochondria and myofilaments and less endoplasmic reticulum than a normal cell. Physiological and pathophysiological stressors are associated with the development of atrophy. Cells may atrophy when there is less need for sustained function. When the amount of work required of cells decreases, those cells atrophy. Endocrine changes that occur with aging are associated with atrophy of hormonally dependent cells.[3] Cells in the ovary, for example, shrink after menopause. Figure 18–1 shows normal breast tissue and the atrophic alteration that occurs when hormonal stimulation is lost as part of the aging process. Pathophysiological causes of atrophy include loss of normal cellular innervation, reduced blood supply, disuse, and inadequate nutrition. Figure 18–2 shows pathological atrophy of a kidney.

A positive aspect of atrophy is that as cell size and function decrease, cell survival is more likely. Another positive

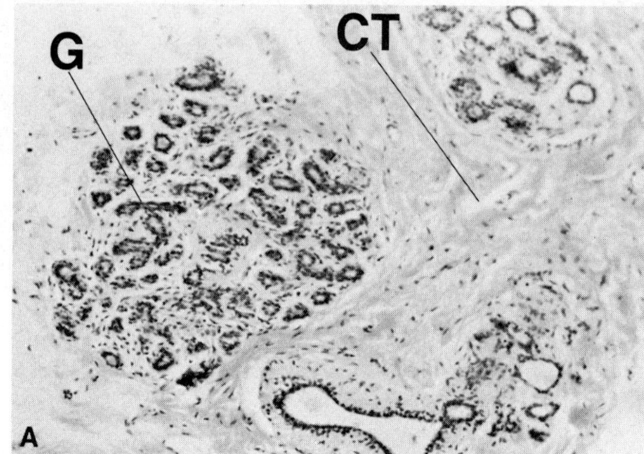

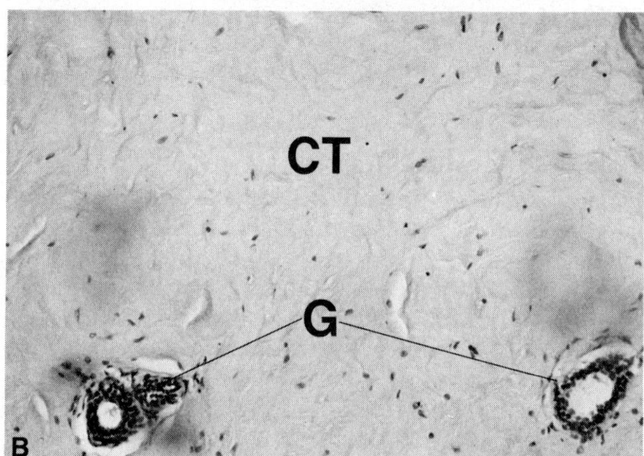

FIGURE 18–1 (*A*) Normal breast tissue contains a mixture of glandular (G) and loose connective tissue (CT). (B) In the atrophic breast, much of the glandular (G) tissue has been replaced by dense, organized connective tissue (CT). This is a normal aging change, caused by the marked reduction of estrogen stimulation. (Courtesy of Dr. Marie Cowan, University of Washington School of Nursing)

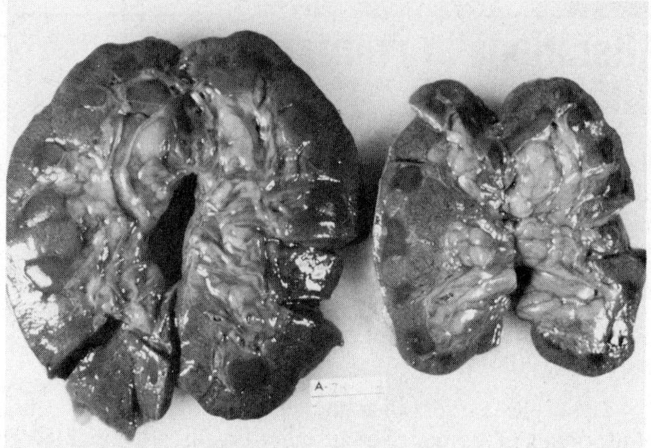

FIGURE 18–2 On the left is a normal kidney weighing 140 g. The atrophic kidney on the right weighs only 60 g. (Courtesy of Dr. Marie Cowan, University of Washington School of Nursing)

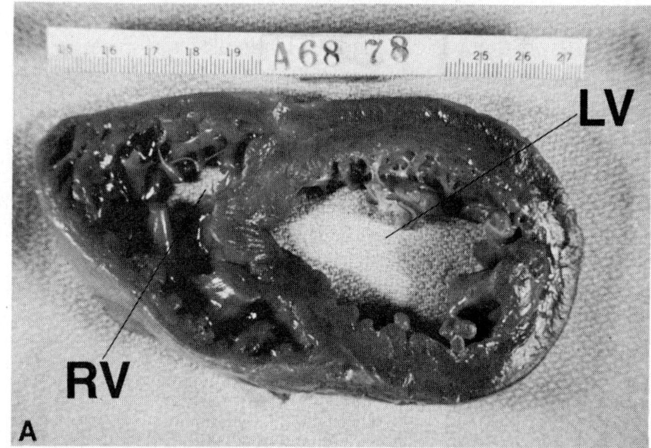

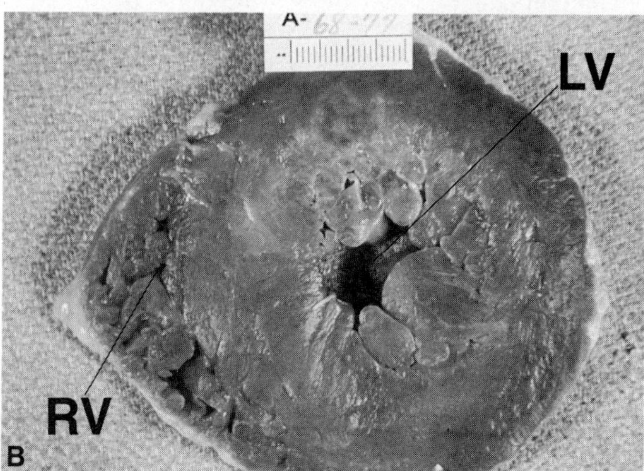

FIGURE 18–3 (*A*) A normal heart. The larger of the two chambers is the left ventricle (LV). (*B*) A hypertrophied heart. Note that the transmural tissue diameter of the left ventricle (LV) is nearly double that shown in *A*. (Courtesy of Dr. Marie Cowan, University of Washington School of Nursing)

aspect is that atrophy is reversible, and the cell may increase in size if conditions become more favorable.

Hypertrophy

Hypertrophy refers to an increase in cell size and ultimately the size of an organ caused by synthesis of more ultrastructural components.[3] Synthesis of membranes, enzymes, adenosine triphosphate (ATP), and microfilaments is increased. All cells can hypertrophy, but hypertrophy is the chief mode of adaptation of cardiac and skeletal muscle cells because of the inability of those cells to replicate and divide.[3] Hypertrophy involving cardiac muscle is shown in Figure 18–3. Increased demand for cellular function and hormonal stimulation are examples of physiological stressors producing hypertrophy. Changes in the hypertrophied cell will persist as long as the causative stimuli is applied to the cell.[5] The cell will regress toward normal if the stimulus is withdrawn.

There are limits to the degree of hypertrophy a cell can achieve. Mechanisms for this limitation are not completely understood but the limitations of normal vasculature to supply the hypertrophied cell as well as the limitations in the energy-generating capacity of the mitochondria may be important factors.[3]

Alterations in Proliferation and Differentiation

Those cells that are able to reproduce themselves have an added adaptive advantage because they increase the number of cells able to respond to the stressor. Redirection of a stem cell is another mechanism by which cells can survive situations of changed demands.

Hyperplasia

Hyperplasia refers to an increase in the number of cells in an organ or tissue.[3] Not all mature cells are capable of division. Cells that are capable of both synthesizing DNA in response to an increased demand for function and undergoing mitotic division will increase the number of cells available to share the work load. The tissue or organ will increase in volume. Table 18–1 categorizes the reproductive capacity of many body cells.

Stressors that typically induce hyperplasia in susceptible cells include hormonal stimulation, mechanical abrasion, and surgical removal of part of the liver. Age, sex, and nutritional status appear to modify the hyperplastic response. Hyperplasia can also result from endogenous hormonal manipulation. Hyperplasia resulting from a useful physiological stimulus may benefit an individual by repairing a defect in tissue or an organ, or it can prepare an organ for function, for example, hyperplasia of the breast prepares the breast for lactation. An example of breast hyperplasia is shown in Figure 18–4. Hyperplasia is a reversible cellular change. It will regress after the inducing stimulus is withdrawn.

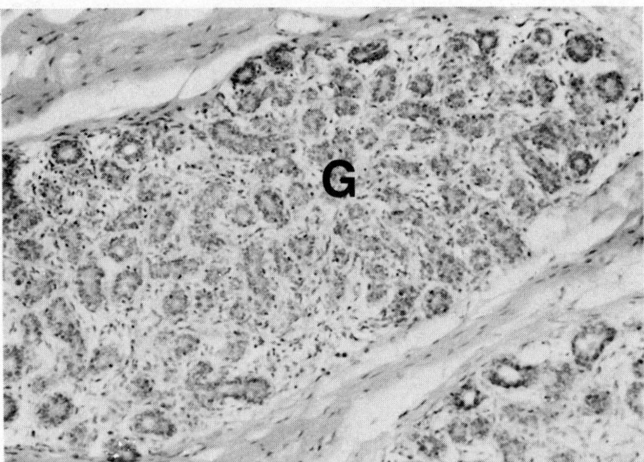

FIGURE 18–4 Breast hyperplasia. Compare the increased amount of glandular (G) tissue in this figure with the normal amount in Fig. 18–1, *A*. (Courtesy of Dr. Marie Cowan, University of Washington School of Nursing)

Metaplasia

Metaplasia is another adaptive, reversible change demonstrated by some cells. A stem cell has the normal capacity to spawn different daughter cells that then develop into distinct but related cell lines. The mature cells that populate a specific tissue are ordinarily those cells that best suit the functional demands of that tissue. As a result of a stressor, stem cells are redirected to differentiate into a different mature cell type not normally found in the area. One mature cell type, usually epithelial or mesenchymal, is replaced by another adult cell type.[3] An example of metaplasia is the replacement of normal columnar ciliated epithelial cells by stratified squamous epithelial cells as illustrated in Figure 18–5. This change occurs in the bronchi and bronchioles of habitual smokers. Though this change is protective of cell survival, in this instance an important cellular function (the ciliary activity that facilitates cleansing of the respiratory tract) is lost. Metaplasia also commonly occurs at the squamocolumnar junction of the cervix. In this instance columnar cells may be replaced by squamous cell epithelium in response to irritation.[2] Transformation of fibroblasts to osteoblasts or chondroblasts is an example of metaplasia in mesenchymal cells. This cell transformation allows the generation of new bone or cartilage.

TABLE 18–1
Capacity of Specific Cell Types for Hyperplasia

Capacity for Profound Hyperplasia	*Intermediate Capacity*	*No Capacity*
Epidermis	Bone cells	Nerve cells
Intestinal epithelium	Cartilage cells	Cardiac cells
Hepatocytes	Smooth muscle cells	Skeletal muscle cells
Fibroblasts		
Marrow cells		

Dysplasia

Dysplasia occurs in response to chronic irritation or inflammation but is not strictly an adaptive change.[1,3] A dysplastic cell differs from a normal mature cell in size, shape, and organization.[3] Figure 18–6 illustrates dysplasia of breast tissue. The cells are irregular and atypical in appearance. The number of mitoses is increased in dysplasia, but mitosis itself is not abnormal in dysplastic cells. Dysplastic cell changes are frequently found in areas of metaplasia of the bronchi, bronchioles, and cervix.

Because dysplasia has been frequently found adjacent to cancerous cells, dysplastic cell changes have been implicated as precursors of cancer. Dysplasia, however, does not always progress to cancer. Dysplasia may persist or it may reverse toward normal when the initial irritating stimulus is removed. When the causative stressor cannot be removed, cellular changes may become more severe and bizarre. Eventually, malignant changes may occur.

Reversible Cell Injuries

In some instances, internal or external forces that are applied may exceed the adaptive capacity of the cell, and cellular injury results. *Cellular injury* is defined as any adverse influence that deranges the cell's ability to maintain a steady nor-

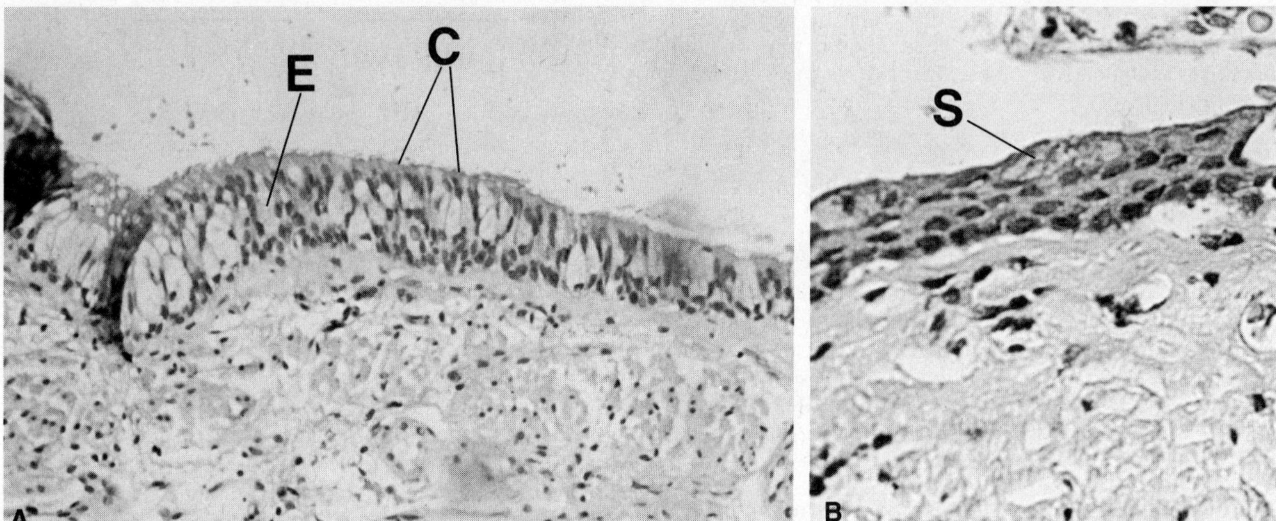

FIGURE 18–5 (*A*) The columnar epithelium (E) found in normal bronchi. These elongated cells contain rhythmically moving cilia (C), which constantly sweep foreign particles trapped in the bronchial mucus toward the oropharynx. (*B*) The ciliated columnar cells have been replaced be several rows of squamous cells (S), which are not ciliated and thus cannot contribute to lung defense. This metaplastic change is a common result of smoking. (Courtesy of Dr. Marie Cowan, University of Washington School of Nursing)

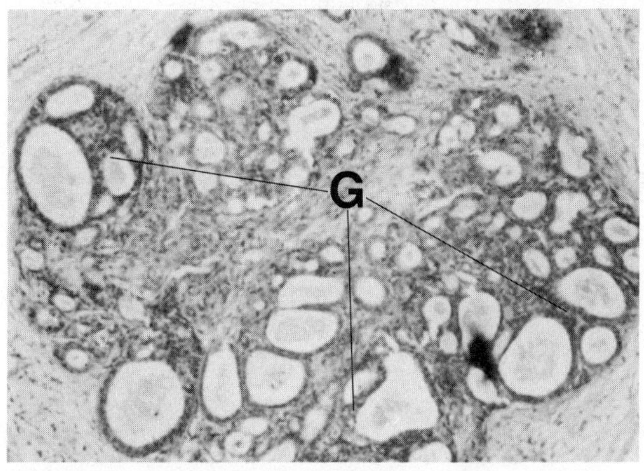

FIGURE 18–6 Dysplastic breast tissue. The cells of the glandular tissue (G) are irregular in size and shape. (Courtesy of Dr. Marie Cowan, University of Washington School of Nursing)

mal or adaptive homeostasis.[3] Cells may sustain either a reversible or irreversible injury. The degree of assault the cell can withstand without irreversible, lethal injury depends on many factors, including the characteristics of the applied force, the target cell, and the whole individual.[3] The following section of this chapter will explore the types of applied forces causing cell injury, the basic pathogenesis of reversible cell injury, and the accompanying morphological changes.

Forces Causing Cellular Injury

Forces capable of precipitating cellular injury can be characterized as *internal* or *external.*[4] Hypoxia is a common internal cause of cellular injury.[2,3,4] Cells must have a continuous supply of oxygen to maintain oxidative phosphorylation and ATP production. Inadequate blood flow, usually termed ischemia, is probably the most common cause of cellular hypoxia. (See Chapter 23) Depletion of the oxygen content in blood and interference with cellular oxidative enzyme systems are other common causes. A wide variety of other types of cell injuries are suspected of culminating in cellular hypoxia as well. Examples of these forces include nutritional deficiency, genetic errors with enzyme defects, hypersensitivity and other immune mechanisms, and abnormal accumulations of endogenous substances.[2,3,4] Cellular injury, and ultimately cellular hypoxia, can also result from external forces applied to the body, including physical trauma, infectious organisms, and chemical agents.[2,3,4] Types of physical trauma are thermal, mechanical, radiation, electrical shock, and changes in atmospheric pressure.[2,3,4] Living infectious organisms, including bacteria, fungi, and viruses, may effect cell injury by conversion of cell metabolism or elaboration of toxins.[3] Exogenous chemicals and poisons can also injure cells.[2,3]

The degree of cellular injury is influenced by the type of force applied, the duration of application, and the severity.[3] The exact amount of force a cell can sustain without irreversible injury has not been determined.

Pathogenesis of Reversible Cellular Injury

A biochemical abnormality in the affected cell is generally the first result in the process of cell injury.[2,3] This abnormality produces a change in cellular metabolism. The morphological changes detectable with a light microscope are generally later changes. It must be emphasized that not all cells will function abnormally or show changes in structure. Different cells are vulnerable in different ways to different forms of injury. For some cells the result may be adaptation, not injury.

Morphological Changes in Reversible Injury

Sublethally injured cells demonstrate some potentially reversible changes. Some texts refer to these changes as *degenerative.* These potentially reversible changes occur in all cells but are generally seen in most metabolically active cells, for instance, kidney and cardiac cells. The potentially reversible changes tend to be confined to cytoplasmic changes. Nuclear integrity is not threatened in a sublethal reversible cellular injury. Reversible changes occur relatively quickly.

Cellular Swelling. The most common morphological change first seen in cells is accumulation of water in the cytoplasm. This change happens within minutes of the injury.[3] It occurs because of disturbances of ATP production and inadequate cellular Na–K pumping. Changed ion and volume regulation result, and water accumulates in the cytoplasm. Cellular organelles and endoplasmic reticulum quickly become swollen and are converted to fluid-filled sacs. *Cytoplasmic vacuolation* (also known as hydropic change or vacuolar degeneration) occurs. Viewed microscopically, cells have an altered texture and there may be compression of the microvasculature, signaling cell enlargement.[2,3] On a gross level, an injured tissue or organ will enlarge and show an increase in weight. If all the cells of an organ are affected, the organ will be pale and have an increased weight. Reversible changes indicate mild injury and precede severe irreversible cell injury. They signal the need to direct efforts to minimize complications.

Lipid Vacuolization. A more severe, yet nonlethal reversible change in injured cells is the intracellular accumulation of lipid.[2] This change is primarily seen in cells involved in or dependent on fat metabolism.[3] Injured cardiac muscle cells and liver cells are types of cells likely to show lipid vacuolation. Under a microscope, the changes are similar to those of cellular swelling except that the cell vacuoles contain lipid.[2] As a result there will be a yellowish hue accompanying the increase in weight and swelling in the injured tissue.

Atrophy. Injured cells may also respond by reducing their mass. This process was described earlier in the chapter.

Nursing Implications

What is adaptive for the cell may or may not be adaptive for the host. Although the adaptation promotes cell survival, specialized cell function may well be altered or lost. For example, bronchial epithelial changes due to smoking will decrease ciliary function, thus impairing secretion clearance and increasing the risk of lower respiratory tract infection. Changes in vaginal epithelium with aging will decrease lubrication and may make intercourse painful. Nursing management strategies applicable to the above situations include elimination of the stressor and exogenous replacement of missing cellular function. For example, in the first instance, persons can be counseled to decrease or quit smoking. In the second situation, an elderly female could be instructed to use a water-soluble vaginal lubricant before intercourse. Other circumstances in which atrophy occurs may require strategies that stimulate cellular growth. For example, nurses can teach active range-of-motion exercises for a patient to use after removal of a cast.

The presence of reversibly injured cells signals the need to minimize exposure to the noxious force. In addition, measures that foster the health of cells should be instituted. An example of these principles applied to nursing practice is the supportive care provided in viral hepatitis. The patient is counseled to avoid alcohol and other drugs metabolized in the liver, to increase rest periods, and to eat a well balanced, high calorie diet. In this way, irreversible cell changes are minimized, and cellular adaptation is promoted.

References

1. Golden A: Pathology: Understanding Human Disease. Baltimore, Williams & Wilkins, 1982
2. Price SA, Wilson LM: Pathophysiology: Clinical Concepts of Disease Processes. New York, McGraw-Hill, 1982
3. Robbins S, Cotran RS: Pathologic Basis of Disease. 2nd ed. Philadelphia, WB Saunders, 1979
4. Walter JB: An Introduction to the Principles of Disease, 2nd ed. Philadelphia, WB Saunders, 1982
5. Walter JB, Israel MS: General Pathology, 5th ed. New York, Churchill Livingstone, 1979

Bibliography

Robbins SL, Cotran RS, Kumar V: Pathologic Basis of Disease, 3rd ed. Philadelphia, WB Saunders, 1984

Chapter 19

Neoplasia

Betty B. Gallucci
Joanne Schnaidt Rokosky

In recent years the knowledge of tumor biology has grown rapidly, thereby challenging preconceived beliefs about cancer and some of the underlying assumptions on which treatment decisions are based. Advances in knowledge have led, within the last 10 years, to the development of oncology nursing as a specialty. Professional nurses caring for patients with cancer will continue to face many changes in their practice. They will be challenged not only to keep current in their knowledge but also to help educate patients, families, and the public about new developments. In addition, the nurse will be caring for and talking with more and more families about cancer because of the greater incidence of cancer in the population over 65 years of age, which is the largest growing population sector in the United States.

Cancer is the second leading cause of death in the United States today. One of the main reasons cancer has moved to second place is the prevention of and the decline in mortality of many other diseases, so that, in relative sense, the incidence and mortality due to cancer appears to be increasing. At the very least, cancer is more noticeable and commented on by the lay public and media. In fact, mortality rates for most cancers in the last 30 years have remained the same except for pancreatic cancer, melanoma, and lung cancer, for which mortality rates are all rising (Fig. 19–1). One of the most dramatic rises has been the increase of deaths in women due to lung cancer. In several states this rate has surpassed that of breast cancer, whereas the death rate due to lung cancer in males is leveling off or declining. Other reasons that account for the apparent increase of cancer are that the risk of cancer in the older population is 10 to 100 times the risk in the younger population, and that diagnosis and reporting of cancer have improved.[2, 12]

Although 30% of Americans now living will have cancer, 5-year cure rates for cancer are now approaching 39%. If normal life expectancy is considered, then almost 50% of patients treated for cancer will be alive 5 years after diagnosis, free of this disease and with a normal life expectancy. However, these statistics are summaries and as such do not reflect the potential for an individual patient. For some can-

- *Incidence rate:* Number of new cancer cases per year per 100,000 people
- *Incidence:* Number of new cases per given population
- *Prevalence rate:* Number of all existing cases per year per 100,000 people[2]
- *Mortality rate:* Number of cancer deaths per year per 100,000 people
- *Cure rate:* Generally expressed as 5-year survival rates, the number of cases alive and symptom-free or without recurrence 5 years after the initiation of treatment.[2]

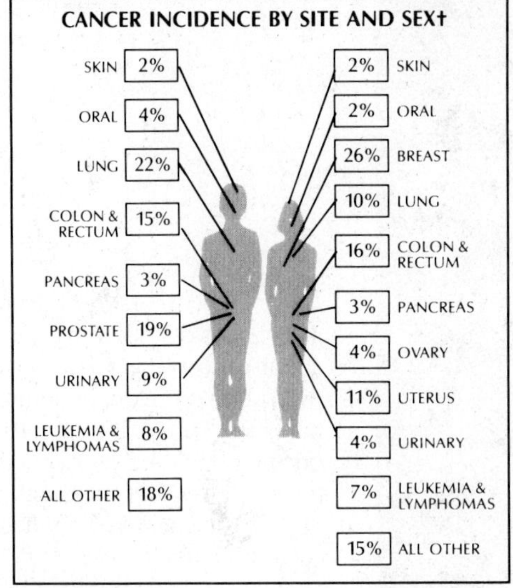

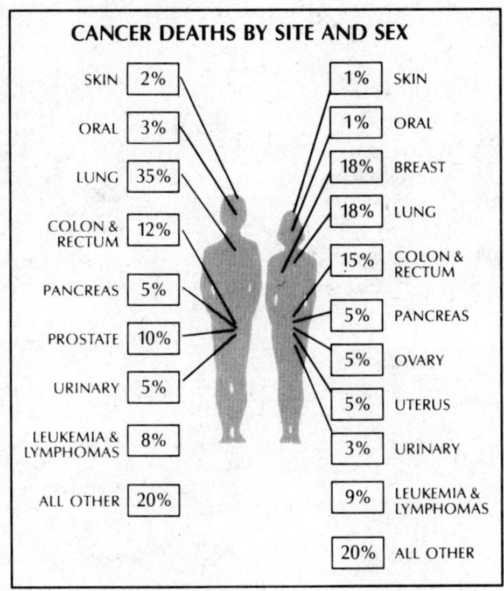

†Excluding non-melanoma skin cancer and carcinoma in situ.

FIGURE 19–1 1985 estimate of cancer deaths by site and sex. (Cancer Facts and Figures 1985. New York, American Cancer Society, 1984)

cers, such as some childhood leukemias, early stage Hodgkin's and testicular cancer, the statistics are much better, and approach 60% to 90%. For other cancers, such as lung cancer, the survival rate is only 9%. In the black population, the mortality rates tend to be higher and the survival rates lower as compared with the white population. The difference between whites and blacks has been attributed to differences in economic and social factors rather than to inherited genetic differences.[2]

If these current trends in cancer statistics hold, nurses will care for more elderly patients with cancer; cancer must be considered as a chronic illness rather than as inevitably lethal; more women will suffer from lung cancer; and, unless public education reaches the minority populations, this group will seek medical attention when the cancer is advanced and less amenable to treatment. Although these epidemiological studies provide many insights into cancer as it affects the communities in which we live, they do not prove which agents can be considered carcinogens or describe the effect of this disease on the physiological functioning of the individual. For this information we must turn to cell and tumor biology and pathophysiology. In both these fields remarkable understanding of the processes involved in cancer has occurred in the past 10 years.

Characteristics of Cancer

Benign vs. Malignant Tumors

Neoplasms or "new growths" are relatively autonomous. This means that the growth and its behavior are more or less independent of the host.[26] Neoplasms have been defined as benign or malignant; *cancer* is a common synonym used to refer to a malignant neoplasm. The difference between a benign and a malignant neoplasm depends on its behavior in the host. If the neoplasm stays localized, enlarges slowly, is homogeneous in appearance, and can be resected, then it is *benign.* On the other hand, if the neoplasm spreads or *metastasizes* to other areas of the body, infiltrates and causes the destruction of normal tissue and, if left untreated, will kill the host, then the neoplasm is considered *malignant.* It is the ability to metastasize that most distinguishes benign from malignant neoplasms, although other properties also differ between them. These properties are shown in Table 19–1. Although the word *tumor* can refer to any type of swelling, the term is conventionally used to describe both benign and malignant neoplasms.[4, 27]

> *Metastasis* is the growth of a tumor at a site not in direct anatomical connection to the primary site. The spread of the tumor from the primary to the secondary sites occurs via the lymphatics, the circulatory system, or through a coelomic cavity.

A particular cell growth can be defined as malignant only after considering its effects within the host. Nonetheless, much of the research in cancer has concentrated on cellular biology; findings from this type of research are then extrapolated to human patients. It is generally believed that a tumor begins as a single cell and that the resulting tumor in the host is a clone of cells that descended from the first cell.[35]

TABLE 19–1
Differences between Benign and Malignant Tumors

Benign	*Malignant*
Encapsulated	Invasive
Nonmetastasizing	Metastasizing
Well-differentiated	Frequently undifferentiated
Slow-growing	Often rapid-growing

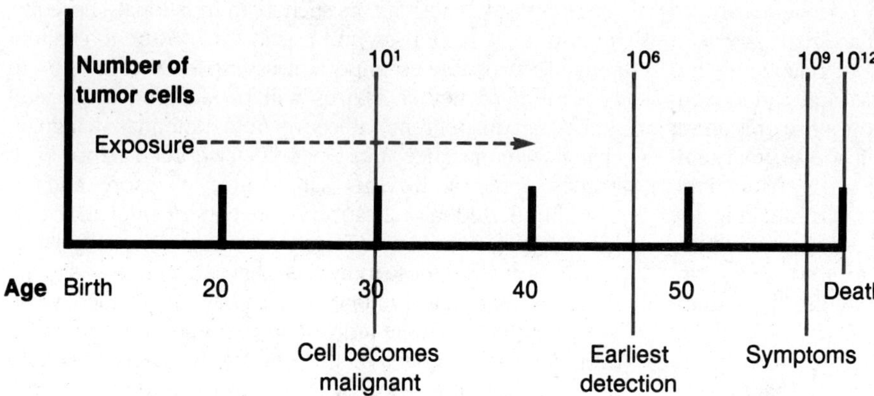

FIGURE 19–2 Model of tumor growth. Model shows that lengthy carcinogen exposure commonly precedes the development of malignancy; in this case, approximately 30 years of exposure precedes malignant change. Additional time passes before detection of the cancer is possible, in this case, over 15 years. Finally, appearance of symptoms is often late in the course of disease, when the tumor is large.

If this is the case, then by making a few assumptions a timeline projection of the tumor growth can be made. Such a projection can be seen in Figure 19–2. One of the assumptions of this type of model is that all the daughter cells survive; a second assumption is that the rate of growth or doubling time of the cell is constant. Although neither of these assumptions is entirely correct, this model can help us understand the natural history of the tumor. For example, it can be seen that the time of exposure to potential carcinogens is long. When considering the number of cells in the body exposed to carcinogens, the probability of cells actually becoming malignant is rare. In addition, the time for the first cell to divide and grow into a tumor large enough for detection is long. When tumors are small, they tend to be localized and are more likely to be successfully treated. Once tumors create symptoms they are large, the possibility of spread to distant sites is more likely, and the prognosis of the patient is worse. Therefore, early detection can save lives, but that is easier to accomplish with tumors that are located at the surface than with internal tumors.[9,28]

One example of a long natural history of a tumor is cervical cancer. Invasive cervical cancer is thought to be preceded by 10 to 20 years of premalignant lesions, such as chronic cervicitis, dysplasia, and carcinoma *in situ* (Fig. 19–3). In one study of 31 women with untreated carcinoma *in situ,* 71% of the women developed invasive cancer by the time the 12-year follow-up was completed; 80% of the women developed cancer by the 30-year follow-up. Lesions of the cervix are easily detected with a Papanicolaou (Pap) smear. Perhaps the widespread acceptance of the Pap smear has contributed to the decline in mortality due to cervical cancer. The premalignant changes can be diagnosed and surgery can be performed before the premalignant changes become malignant or the cancer becomes invasive.[1]

Carcinogenesis

Carcinogenesis is the process of inducing a malignant tumor in an animal or human. Much of the research in carcinogenesis revolves around deoxyribonucleic acid (DNA), the influence of carcinogens on DNA, and the genes that are involved in differentiation and control of cell growth. Until recently it was said that it would take a great deal of time to understand the development of tumors. Since there are histologically more than 200 tumor types, it was thought that each tumor might be initiated by a different process. The recent discovery of *oncogenes* has changed researchers' basic thinking. Oncogenes are genes, probably derived from normal growth-controlling cellular genes, which instruct the cell to behave abnormally. These oncogenes have been isolated from viruses that transform their host cells; that is, the viruses induce changes in the cells so that they resemble malignant cells. Variations of the oncogenes have been detected as normal genes, and it has been predicted that they are involved in causing normal maturation differences of the cell. At least two of the oncogenes now have been linked to growth-factors—epidermal growth factor and platelet-derived growth factor. Perhaps during carcinogenesis these genes become modified or the elements controlling the genes are lost or ineffective. These abnormal genes then in some way alter the cell so that its growth is no longer under regulatory processes.[36]

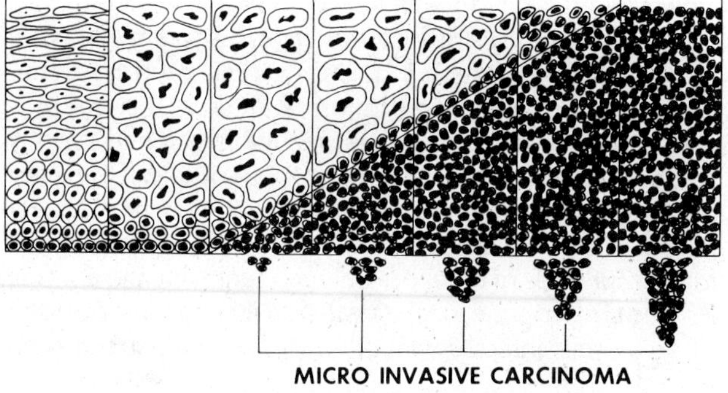

Cervical Intraepithelial Neoplasia
GRADE 1 | GRADE 2 | GRADE 3
NORMAL | CONDYLOMA | VERY MILD DYSPLASIA | MILD DYSPLASIA | MODERATE DYSPLASIA | SEVERE DYSPLASIA | IN SITU CARCINOMA
MICRO INVASIVE CARCINOMA

FIGURE 19–3 Precursors to invasive cancer of the cervix. Premalignant lesions are thought to precede the development of invasive cancer. The hypothesis represented by this figure is as follows: (1) the herpes simplex 2 virus induces development of cervical condyloma (venereal warts); (2) a clone of condyloma cells undergoes malignant transformation; (3) cells become increasingly undifferentiated, and microinvasive cancer develops. (Fenoglio CM, Ferenczy A: Etiologic factors in cervical neoplasia. Semin Oncol 9[3]:349, 1982)

An additional discovery is that many oncogenes are located at chromosomal abnormalities that are also associated with malignant tumors. Thus, the study of oncogenes has brought together several different fields: viral carcinogenesis, genetics, and immunology. In addition, since only about 20 oncogenes have been discovered and it appears that similar genes are altered in different tumors, it has changed the basic thinking of carcinogenesis. Rather than postulating that over 200 processes may initiate carcinogenesis, researchers now predict that there may be only 20 to 40 processes involved. Although it is still in the future before the clinical benefits of these discoveries will be known, it is hoped that they will lead to earlier detection methods, for, if the products of the oncogenes are characterized, then perhaps a serological test will permit detection before the tumor becomes large or metastasizes.[36]

Viral Carcinogenesis

Both *RNA and DNA viruses* have been identified as causing natural and experimental tumors in animals. The herpes viruses are DNA viruses. For almost every member of the herpes group there is some experimental or epidemiological evidence linking it to a human malignancy. For example, Epstein-Barr virus (EBV) has been associated with Burkitt's lymphoma in West African children and nasopharyngeal cancer among Asian populations. Herpes simplex virus-1 (HSV-1) has been linked to oral cancer and herpes simplex virus-2 (HSV-2) to cervical cancer. One member of the herpes group, CMV (cytomegalovirus), has not been associated with any malignancy to this date. Another DNA virus that has been linked by epidemiological evidence to human tumors is hepatitis B virus. In areas of the world where hepatitis B carriers are very common, primary cancer of the liver (hepatocellular carcinoma) is also very common. There is now available a vaccine for hepatitis B; perhaps this will be the first vaccine to prevent a human malignancy. In animals, this type of prevention has already been accomplished: a vaccine is available to prevent Marek's disease in chickens, a lymphoproliferative disease caused by a herpes virus. Vaccine trials are also ongoing to prevent feline leukemia.[9,26,30]

The RNA viruses, also called *oncoviruses* or *retroviruses,* induce leukemia, lymphoma, and mammary tumors in animals. To complete their natural cycle, these viruses must manufacture a viral DNA that is then integrated into the host cell DNA. To do this they produce an enzyme called *reverse transcriptase* (the enzyme is able to use RNA as a template to produce DNA). Since these viruses can remain latent in a cell for long periods of time, it is only by identifying the enzyme, reverse transcriptase, or the viral DNA that scientists are able to detect cells infected with these viruses. Reverse transcriptase has been identified in some human leukemia and lymphoma cells. In addition, approximately 20 oncogenes have been identified with these RNA viruses and some of these oncogenes have also been detected in human bladder cancer cells, Burkitt's lymphoma, and promyelocytic leukemia.[9,26,30]

The epidemiological and laboratory evidence is quite close to demonstrating the role of certain viruses as an etiologic agent of cancer. However, in humans, other factors besides exposure to a virus are probably involved in viral carcinogenesis. Host factors such as an individual's heredity, immunologic responses, and previous exposure to carcinogens are probably as important as exposure to a virus in determining whether a virus will produce an acute viral illness, an inapparent infection, or a potential malignant change. For instance, most people have been exposed to herpes simplex 1, the virus that produces cold sores and has been implicated in oral cancers. Ninety percent of all school age children in the United States have antibodies to this virus, which means that these individuals have been exposed to the virus and that their immune systems have responded. However, very few of all the individuals exposed to the virus will ever develop a cancer of the oral cavity. The individual's heredity, immune response, and exposure to carcinogens such as cigarette smoke are probably important in determining the outcome of a herpes viral infection.[9,26,30]

Chemical Carcinogenesis

As with any topic concerning cancer, a great deal is known about chemical carcinogenesis, but much remains to be learned. Approximately 70,000 synthetic chemicals are produced for commercial purposes every year. About 10,000 of them have been tested, and approximately one sixth of them have carcinogenic activity. Chemical carcinogenesis is not restricted only to synthetic chemicals. For example, aflatoxin B1 is one of the most powerful carcinogens known and it is a natural product, a toxin produced by the fungus *Aspergillus flavus.* This toxin has been detected in contaminated peanuts stored improperly. The high rate of hepatomas in some African populations is perhaps due to the presence of this toxin in their food. Naturally occurring low-molecular-weight organic compounds number around 100,000, but there are approximately 5 million of these types of synthetic compounds known. Although most of these synthetic compounds are produced in very small quantities, they may present a potential threat to the health of the individuals who come in contact with them. Some of the chemicals which have been investigated and linked to cancer are listed in Table 19–2.[12,26,28,30]

The process by which chemicals induce a tumor in animals has been divided into two phases, *initiation* and *promotion.* The first step, initiation, presumably occurs very rapidly. The chemical may be activated by the host tissues or enzymes and becomes the "ultimate carcinogen." Then it interacts with the cellular DNA to create a permanent change that is inherited by all daughter cells. This process of initiation then makes the cell susceptible to the effects of other chemicals called *promoters,* which subsequently induce the cell to express its malignant characteristics. Promoters administered without the initiator cannot of themselves give rise to malignancies. Some mixtures of chemicals are thought to possess both initiators and promoters and are called *complete carcinogens.* An example of a complete carcinogen is tobacco. Promoters appear to stimulate cell division and in some cases are extremely irritating to the tissue. The classic example of a promoter is croton oil. When croton oil is applied repeatedly to the skin of an experimental animal after one application of coal tar (the initiator), skin tumors develop.

TABLE 19–2
Natural and Synthetic Chemicals Linked to Carcinogenesis

Chemical	*Source*	*Site of Tumor Development*
Aflatoxins	Food	Liver
Alcohol	Food	Oral cavity, esophagus
Arsenic compounds	Occupational	Bladder
Asbestos	Occupational	Lung, pleural cavity, gastrointestinal tract
Benzene	Occupational	Hematopoietic system
Carbon tetrachloride	Occupational	Liver
Charcoal broiled foods	Food	Laboratory studies only
Cyclophosphamide	Medicinal	Bladder
Diethylstilbestrol	Medicinal	Uterus, vagina
Melphalan	Medicinal	Hematopoietic system
Phenacetin	Medicinal	Kidney
Tobacco	Environmental	Lung, oral cavity, larynx
Vinyl chloride	Occupational	Liver, lung, brain

Initiation is probably a permanent change or, at the very least, is stable over long periods of time. Promotion, on the other hand, is considered a reversible process; that is, with enough time between applications of croton oil, no effect is noted. In addition, promotion has no effect unless initiation occurs first. The exact cellular changes that occur in these two steps are not completely known. Scott and Wille propose that initiation results from defects in cell proliferation and differentiation, whereas promotion occurs when cells become unresponsive to cellular regulatory events.[26,30,31]

Although some chemicals such as tobacco smoke have been well established as etiologic agents for cancer, the evidence for such factors as fiber in the diet and the types and amount of fats is not so well understood. A study sponsored by the American Academy of Science suggests that dietary factors such as oversupply of calories act more like promoters than initiators of carcinogenesis.[7]

Even though one sixth of all the chemicals tested so far are potential carcinogens, not all chemicals deserve this label. Some chemicals have been shown to protect animals from effects of carcinogens, especially when given simultaneously with the carcinogen. These include the following: butylated hydroxyanisole (BHA), an antioxidant widely used as a food additive; disulfiram, also an antioxidant; and ethoxyquin, an antioxidant used in animal food. Some food items discovered in epidemiological studies also appear to provide protection from carcinogens. Diets that contain vitamin A and its precursors, the carotenoids, or the synthetic precursors, the retinoids, appear to protect against stomach cancer. Ingestion of diets high in cruciferous vegetables (cabbage family) appears to protect against colon cancer. Selenium and fiber have been suggested as elements in the diet that may have a role in the prevention of cancer, but the evidence for this is still quite sketchy.[7,12,17]

The testing of chemicals for their carcinogenic potential is a costly process and not a hundred percent efficient. Most authorities agree that testing involves giving approximately 50 animals of one species a low dose of chemical, giving another 50 animals a high dose, and giving a second species both the low and high doses. A third group of 50 animals receives no chemicals and serves as a control group. These animals must be housed in good conditions throughout the experiment, must be examined for tumors, must receive autopsies, and must have all tissues processed and examined for pathology. One estimate of the cost of such an experiment for one chemical in the 1970s was $250,000. Therefore, several new types of tests have been designed to serve as rapid screening devices. These rapid tests involve the testing for *mutagenesis* in bacteria (Ames test), yeasts, and mammalian cell cultures. However, because not all carcinogens are mutagens, the results of these tests must be compared with the available epidemiological evidence obtained from human populations, with knowledge of the chemical's structure, and with animal experiments.[17,30]

Radiation Carcinogenesis

By 1903, within ten years from the time radiation was discovered, skins cancers and leukemia developed in radiologists and scientists who first worked with radioactive compounds. The carcinogenic potential of radiation thus became evident. In 1972, the United Nations Committee on Radiation wrote that cancer in humans is a long-term effect of radiation. Much of the evidence for this statement was gathered from the Atomic Bomb Survivor Study of Hiroshima and Nagasaki and from patients exposed to relatively large amounts of radiation in the treatment and diagnosis of certain diseases in the 1930s and 1940s. Radiation in appropriate doses can cause cancer to arise from almost any tissue. However, host factors such as age, hormonal influences, and exposure to other carcinogens also play an important role. Children in general are more susceptible to these effects than are adults.[9,26,30]

Ionizing Radiation. Ionizing radiation, which has biological effects, produces charged particles or ions in the matter through which it passes. The units of measure or dosage that describe radiation are units of energy. Some of the more common units used in medical applications are *rad, gray,* and *rem.* A *rad* or *radiation absorbed dose* is 100 ergs of energy absorbed in 100 grams of tissue. A *gray* is equal to 100 rads and is a new term that is replacing the rad as a unit of measure. The *rem* (rad-equivalent-man) takes into account biological effects of different types of radiation. For instance, the biological effects of gamma or x-rays are different than the effects of highly accelerated neutrons. Both of these types of radiation are used in therapy and the ability to convert dosages between them allows comparisons to be drawn between different treatment regimens.[35]

Radiation that produces biological effects can be further classified as external or internal. *External radiation* is radiation from an external source passing through the body. *Internal radiation* is typically acquired through the ingestion, inhalation, or parenteral administration of radioactive compounds that are then absorbed and stored in tissue such as bone or thyroid. The biological effects of radiation are also determined by the amount of tissue irradiated. Many of the atomic bomb survivors received whole-body irradiation, whereas most medical uses of radiation are limited to small areas of the body. The direct effects of radiation are limited to the part of the body irradiated. For example, if the mediastinum were irradiated, then the direct effects of the radiation would be expressed only in the structures of the mediastinum, not elsewhere in the body.[26,30,35]

External Radiation. Leukemia was the first cancer related to radiation exposure that was seen in the atomic bomb survivors. Within 6 to 8 years after the bomb, the incidence rates of leukemia increased to levels well above those seen in the Japanese population who were not exposed. The peak risk was highest from 1950 to 1952, at which time the incidence was 116 : 100,000, as compared with 3 to 4 : 100,000 in the unexposed population. Although the risk for leukemia has declined dramatically since 1950, it still is slightly higher than the spontaneous rate. These types of statistics lead to the understanding of the concept of a *latent period* for cancer. The period for leukemia to develop was approximately 8 years; that is, the time between the initial exposure and the development of the leukemia was 8 years. Since the latent period for cancer is relatively long, it is understandable that proving the etiology of leukemia in a particular individual can be difficult if not almost impossible. Between the exposure to the agent and the development of the disease, a person is often exposed to many other agents. A person might forget an exposure and the circumstances, dosages, and time periods involved, and standards change as to types of radiation equipment in use.[30]

Within 10 to 15 years after the first atomic bomb, incidence rates increased for other cancers, including cancers of the lung, breast, thyroid, colon, and stomach. The latent period of these types of cancers, that is, cancers that originate in the epithelial tissues vs. hematopoietic or connective tissues, has been estimated to be approximately 10 to 20 years. Since many of the members of this study group were still alive in 1980, perhaps increases will be noted for other cancers as well.[30]

Internal Emitters. One of the most famous examples of internal emitters causing cancer is that of the luminescent instrument-dial painters. The paint that was used to create luminescent faces on watches and clocks contained radium. While painting, the workers licked the brushes and thus ingested the radium. (Radium, when ingested, is deposited in bone and tends to remain there.) Among this group, bone cancer or osteogenic sarcoma, a rare tumor, became prevalent. It was this type of knowledge plus laboratory experimentation that led to the limitations on surface testing of atomic weapons. Fallout from atomic weapons contains radioactive compounds that can become deposited in bone.[30]

Ultraviolet Radiation or Sunlight. One of the most ubiquitous forms of radiation that every person is exposed to is sunlight. Ultraviolet radiation is different from the radiation discussed above because it does not penetrate deeply. Even so, it is responsible for the most common cancer in people, skin cancer. Most statistics on cancer do not include skin cancer because it is highly treatable. Skin cancer has been linked to sunlight because it occurs on exposed areas of the body such as the face and arms, and because it occurs more frequently in fair-skinned people and in people whose occupations lead them to be out of doors. Recently, another more dangerous type of cancer, melanoma, has been linked to sunlight exposure. Melanoma, a cancer of the pigment-forming cells, is much more difficult to treat. With the recent rise in popularity of suntan parlors, the concern that the incidence of melanoma might rise has been expressed by many dermatologists.[30]

Tumor Biology

Cancer research spans all levels of biological organization. Many cellular components of malignant cells vary from those of normal cells. But these differences are often found to be a result of the malignancy rather than the cause of the malignant change. For instance, different antigens occur on the cell membrane of tumor cells as compared with most normal cells. These new antigens are not the causative agent that makes the cell malignant but are the result of the cell becoming malignant. Although this change cannot be used to prevent cancer, exploitation of this difference might lead to better methods of cancer detection or of chemotherapy delivery.[9,28]

Other studies of tumor cells have concentrated on changes in DNA that are more likely to be related to the development of the malignant characteristic. Tumor cells have been studied for the presence of chromosomal abnormalities. For example, gene mutations in the enzyme systems that repair ultraviolet damage to DNA occur in children with a rare inheritable disorder called xeroderma pigmentosum. Unless exposure to sunlight is prevented, these children develop multiple fatal skin cancers by the time they reach their teen years. Another example is that leukemia occurs more frequently in children with Down's syndrome as compared to children without this chromosomal abnormality.[18,30]

As important as these cellular studies are to our understanding of oncogenic processes, cancer in humans is never diagnosed on the presence of a single cell that looks malignant. The only definitive method of diagnosing cancer in patients is to look at tissue obtained from a biopsy. The pathologist examines the tissue and compares the cells and the architecture of the tissue to nearby normal tissue.

Tumor Classification

Because the study of tissues originates with the study of their development in the embryo, the classification of tumors is often based on the tissues from which the tumor is derived. In this system benign tumors are often designated by adding the suffix *-oma* to the name of the cell or tissue type. For example, a neuroma is a benign tumor of neural tissue. Malignant tumors are often named sarcoma if they are derived from the mesenchyme in embryonal development. Connective tissue comes from the mesenchymal layer, so that a malignant tumor of bone is named osteosarcoma. The general name for a malignant tumor of epithelial tissue is carcinoma. Normal epithelium, the covering and lining tissues of the body, is further classified as glandular, squamous, or transitional. Similarly, malignant tumors of the epithelium can be classified as adenocarcinomas, squamous cell carcinomas, or transitional cell carcinomas.[9,27] However, these general rules of naming tumors do not always hold. Melanoma is a malignant tumor of the pigment cells; a better term for this tumor might be malignant melanoma, but it is not commonly used. Malignant tumors derived from hematopoietic tissue are called leukemias. Further classification of the leukemias depends on which cell types are involved: erythroleukemia—malignant tumor of the red blood cell line, lymphocytic leukemia—malignant tumor of the lymphocyte cell line, and so on. Even these leukemias can be further classified to the exact cell type such as T-cell or B-cell lymphocytic leukemias.[27] Examples of tumors and the tissues from which they are derived are listed in Table 19–3.

Because epithelial tissues are constantly exposed to the environment, carcinogens interact directly with these tissues. In the elderly, whose epithelial tissues have been exposed to carcinogens for a long period of time, carcinomas are the most common types of cancers. However, in children, who have had much less exposure to carcinogens, leukemias are the most common malignant tumors.

Grading

Besides classifying the tumor according to the tissue origin, the pathologist will classify the tumor according to other characteristics. This aspect of classification is called *grading.* Grading takes into account the amount of *differentiation* exhibited by the tumor. If cells in the tumor look like the mature cells of the tissue, then the tumor is well differentiated and has a grade of 1. This type of tumor generally has a better prognosis than a tumor that is poorly differentiated or does not resemble the tissue from which it originated. Sometimes a poorly differentiated tumor is called *anaplastic.* An anaplastic tumor would have the highest grade of 4. Even though two tumors might be similarly classified and have identical grades, in two different individuals the tumors might act differently. Because each patient is unique, has a different history, different immune responses,

TABLE 19–3
Examples of Tissue and Tumor Types

	Tumor	
Tissue Type	*Benign*	*Malignant*
Epithelium		
Glandular	Adenoma	Adenocarcinoma
Squamous	Polyp, papilloma	Squamous cell carcinoma
Connective		
Bone	Osteoma	Osteosarcoma
Cartilage	Chondroma	Chondrosarcoma
Fibrous	Fibroma	Fibrosarcoma
Fat	Lipoma	Liposarcoma
Smooth muscle	Leiomyoma	Leiomyosarcoma
Striated muscle	Rhabdomyoma	Rhabdomyosarcoma
Neural	Neuroma	Sarcoma
Hematopoietic		
Lymphocytes		Lymphocytic leukemia
Lymphoid tissue		Malignant lymphoma, Hodgkin's disease
Granulocytes		Granulocytic or myelocytic leukemia
Erythrocytic		Erythroleukemia
Plasma cell		Multiple myeloma

and different reserves, similar tumors might act very differently. Talking to patients thus becomes difficult because it is not possible to give absolutes about the illness.[18, 28]

Effects of Tumor on Host

The pathophysiological responses of a patient with cancer are frequently determined by the size and extent of the tumor and by the presence or absence of metastases. If a large tumor is occupying the oral cavity, then the patients will have problems with ingestion that might lead to malnutrition. Malnutrition, in turn, will lead to an altered immunoresponsiveness. If the tumor is in the large colon, then obstruction of the lumen, changes in bowel habits, and gastrointestinal bleeding can occur. In addition, if tumors are large they often outgrow the blood supply, which leads to necrosis and bleeding. However, all the above changes are relatively late signs; the tumor would be quite large for a patient to exhibit these effects. Most small tumors are painless and symptomless. In one sense this is unfortunate. If small tumors were painful, perhaps more patients would seek earlier treatment and tumors could be treated more successfully.

Metastasis. Besides creating local effects, malignant tumors can also create effects at sites distant to the primary site. When malignant tumors metastasize, small amounts of tumor break free of the primary tumor mass and travel by way of the lymphatics or the circulatory system, or spread by way of the thoracic or abdominal cavity to other sites. At distant sites the tumor cells invade the tissue, proliferate, and create other effects. Common metastatic sites are the lymph nodes, lungs, liver, and bone. Once there is metastasis, the patient's chances of survival decrease dramatically. Metastasis to lymph nodes decreases the patient's chances for a 5-year survival by 50% as compared with survival for a patient with negative nodes. Each type of tumor tends to have its own pattern of metastases. Colon cancer frequently metastasizes to the liver, prostate cancer to the vertebral column, and breast cancer to the lymph nodes and then to bone and lungs. Leukemias, on the other hand, are systemic diseases at diagnosis because they involve the circulatory system from the start. This ability to metastasize probably accounts for most treatment failures and deaths of patients with cancer. Often the primary tumor is controlled by surgery, radiation, or chemotherapy, but the growth of the metastatic lesions leads ultimately to the death of the individual.[18, 28]

Paraneoplastic Syndromes. Malignant tumors create some systemic effects that have been named paraneoplastic syndromes. Examples of these syndromes include anorexia and cachexia, fever, hypercalcemia, inappropriate secretion of antidiuretic hormone, and clotting abnormalities. All the reasons for these effects have not yet been determined. Some effects are related to the manufacture of ectopic hormones or hormone-like substances by the tumor cells. Hormones and the tumors that produce them are listed in Table 19–4. Lung cancers often produce ectopic hormones, and a paraneoplastic syndrome might be the first sign of this tumor. Cachexia and anorexia (loss of weight and appetite that occurs in patients with cancer) have been related to profound disturbances in the metabolism of the patient. At any one time approximately 20% of patients with cancer will have symptoms of a paraneoplastic syndrome.[10]

TABLE 19–4
Paraneoplastic Hormone Activity

Hormone	*Tumors*
Parathormone	Lung (especially squamous cell), kidney, colon, parotid, lymphoma, cervix, ovary, liver, larynx, pancreas
Calcitonin	Neural crest tumors (oat cell, melanomas, bronchial carcinoids, medullary carcinoma), thyroid
ACTH*	Lung (all types including carcinoid, but usually small cell), thymus, pancreas, thyroid, stomach, ovary
ADH*	Lung (usually small cell), pancreas, prostate
Erythropoietin	Renal, cerebellum, liver, uterus, ovary
Insulin	Pancreas, liver, adrenal, sarcomas, stomach, ovary
Human chorionic gonadotropin	Liver, renal, lung, esophagus, carcinoid
Growth hormone	Lung, endometrium
Placental alkaline phosphatase	Lung, breast, colon, ovary, pancreas, stomach, cervix, lymphoma
Thyrotropin	Choriocarcinoma, moles, testis
Prolactin	Kidney

Miscellaneous "humors" (hormonelike substances) reported include glucagon, serotonin, histamine, gastrin, prostaglandins, kinins, secretin, vasopressin, catecholamines, MSH,* and renin.

*ACTH = adrenocorticotropic hormone; ADH = antidiuretic hormone; MSH = melanocyte-stimulating hormone

(DeWys WD, Killen JY: The paraneoplastic syndromes. In Rubin P, Bakemeier RF, Krackov SK [eds]: Clinical Oncology: A Multidisciplinary Approach, 6th ed. New York, American Cancer Society, 1983)

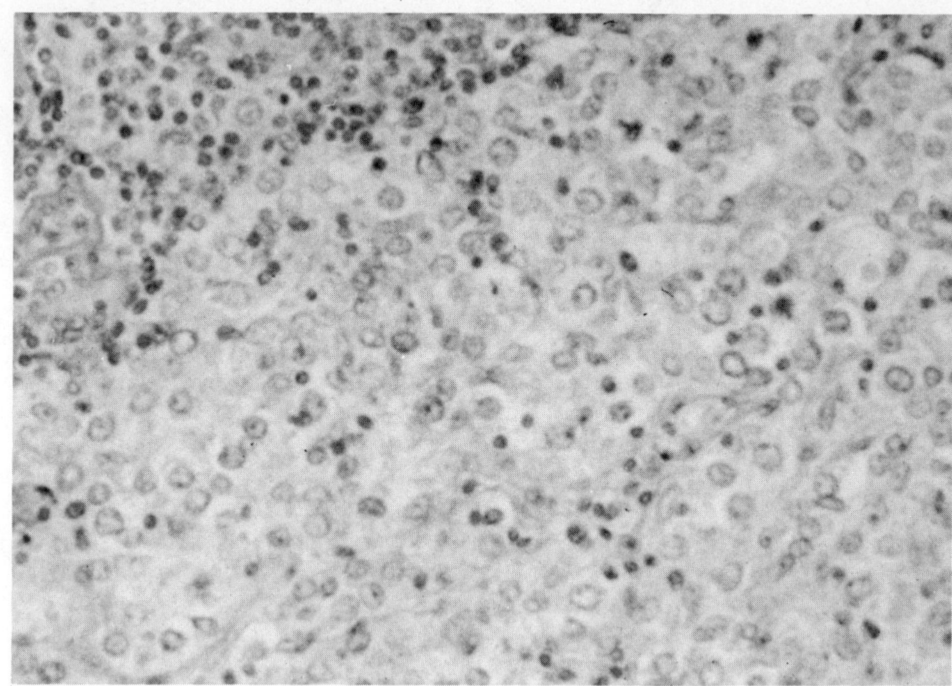

FIGURE 19–4 Microscopic view of breast cancer. The cells of the glandular tissue are abnormal: some are large pleomorphic cells with large nuclei; others are very small, pyknotic cells; still other cells show different phases of mitosis. This figure should be compared to the normal breast tissue shown in Fig. 18–1, *A*. (Courtesy of Dr. Marie Cowan, University of Washington School of Nursing)

Tumor Changes. In an attempt to account for all the effects of neoplasms, basic assumptions about the cancer cell have been reexamined. Today there is a great deal of evidence that the tumor undergoes changes as a part of its natural history. By the time of diagnosis, tumors are believed to contain a mixture of cells with different characteristics. The concept of tumor heterogeneity helps explain why certain tumor cells become resistant to chemotherapy, or why some of the cells in the same tumor are more responsive to radiation. Instead of our simple model that each daughter cell gives rise to similar daughter cells all dividing at the same rate, somatic mutations may occur in some of the tumor cells and not in others. This means that there will be some tumor cells that have a greater potential to metastasize than others, some cells in the same tumor that can produce ectopic hormones, and some cells that have different antigenic properties. Research is now ongoing to understand how this heterogeneity affects responses to therapy and what new agents might be effective, especially for treatment of metastatic disease.[9]

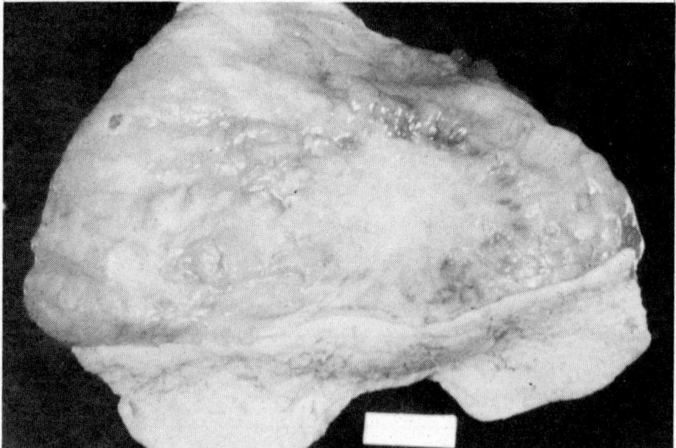

FIGURE 19–5 Carcinoma of the breast. The entire breast is made up of multiple nodules of malignant tissue. (Courtesy of Dr. Marie Cowan, University of Washington School of Nursing)

Diagnosis

A definitive diagnosis of cancer can only be made after examination of tissue obtained from a surgical procedure or *biopsy*. Biopsies may be *excisional,* meaning the whole lesion is removed, or *incisional,* in which only part of the presumptive tumor is removed. Specimens can also be obtained from a *needle* biopsy. In this case, a core of tissue is drawn up into a needle. Cytological examination of exfoliated cells, as is done in a Pap smear, can lead to a presumptive diagnosis of cancer, but often a surgical biopsy will be performed to confirm the diagnosis. In certain instances the patient with the presumptive diagnosis of cancer will be prepared at the same time for both the biopsy and the surgical procedure necessary to remove the tumor. But the general trend, especially when it comes to breast cancer, is to perform this as two separate steps. After the biopsy is performed, and a definitive diagnosis is made, then preparations for the mastectomy or other forms of treatment will be made.[9,28] Figures 19–4 and 19–5 show microscopic and gross specimens of cancer of the breast.

Often the patient will undergo many other diagnostic procedures besides the biopsy in the attempt to determine the nature and extent of the illness. These may include blood tests, diagnostic x-ray studies, and endoscopic procedures. The results from the biopsy and the other procedures are used to evaluate the extent of the disease in the patient. This process of determining the extent of tumor in an individual is called *staging*. A system of staging that is especially applicable for carcinomas is the *TNM System* (Table 19–5). T stands for primary tumor, N for regional lymph nodes, and M for metastases. If the lesion is classified as T1, then the primary tumor is localized and has not invaded surrounding tissue. A T4 lesion, on the other hand, is massive and extends beyond the borders of the organ. T2 and T3 lesions are in between these two extremes. N0 means there is no evidence for the spread of the tumor into regional lymph nodes. N1 means that there are palpable lymph nodes at the drainage site closest to the primary tumor. N4 means that lymph nodes at distant sites are involved. In M0 there is no evidence of metastases. M1 means that a single, solitary metastatic site is present. At the other extreme, M4, metastases are present in multiple organs. Staging and grading of the lesion, the gathering of clinical data, and evaluation of the patient, the family, and their resources, are all important in making decisions about therapy that will optimize the chances for recovery.[28]

Nursing Implications

In this period of time between the recognition of symptoms, if present, and the diagnostic and treatment phases, patients experience many procedures that affect them both physically and emotionally. For example, laboratory examinations often require that food be withheld from the patient, and bowel preparation for a gastrointestinal series may require the patient to have several enemas. Once the patient is finished, it is a nursing responsibility to be sure that the patient receives food and water and has time to rest. The fear of surgery and anesthesia requires the nurse to give careful and thoughtful preparation and explanations to the patient as well as the family.[34]

Surgical procedures influence the patient's metabolic status as well. The trauma of surgery can lead to a stress response (see Chap. 7). Both physical and emotional factors cause activation of the hypothalamus and pituitary–adrenal axis. As a result, corticosteroids, catecholamines, and antidiuretic hormone are released and lead to an increase in heart rate, blood pressure, and blood sugar and to water retention. Once the diagnosis of cancer is made, then further examinations and decisions about the treatment plans will also affect the patient. During this period of time patients may need help to decrease or cope with the anxieties and uncertainties that they face.[20, 34, 37]

TABLE 19–5
TNM Classification System

T Subclasses*

Tx—Tumor cannot be adequately assessed
T0—No evidence of primary tumor
TIS—Carcinoma *in situ*
T1, T2, T3, T4—Progressive increase in tumor size and involvement

***N Subclasses*†**

Nx—Regional lymph nodes cannot be assessed clinically
N0—Regional lymph nodes demonstrably normal
N1, N2, N3, N4—Increasing degrees of demonstrable abnormality of regional lymph nodes

***M Subclasses*‡**

Mx—Not assessed
M0—No (known) distant metastasis
M1—Distant metastasis present, specify site(s)

*T = Primary tumor
†N = Regional lymph nodes
‡M = Distant metastasis
(American Joint Committee on Cancer: Manual for Staging of Cancer, 2nd ed. Chicago, American Joint Committee, 1983)

Treatment

Traditionally, cancer therapy has been divided into three modalities: surgery, radiation therapy, and chemotherapy. These therapies are still the mainline treatments, but they are increasingly being used with each other or modified so as not to interfere with a second line of therapy or with reconstructive surgery. Because of the complexity of treatment, medical decisions about treatment plans, especially where there are no clear advantages to one type of therapy, are often discussed in a committee called the *tumor board.* In this committee, physicians skilled in each of the treatment areas, social workers, and nurses participate in helping to clarify the choices and determine the best approaches. The primary physician then discusses the options with the patient and family. The nurse should provide reinforcement, explanations, and further clarification for the patient.

Surgery

Surgery is one of the oldest treatments for cancer. In fact, one of the first modern-day operations was performed in 1809 by Ephraim MacDowell. He removed a 22-lb ovarian tumor from Mrs. Jane Todd Crowford who then survived for another 30 years. Today surgery is considered the major treatment modality for many types of cancer, such as colorectal cancer, and plays a role in palliation of symptoms if the tumor has become so advanced as to be unresectable. Surgery, as previously discussed, also has a major role in the diagnosis of cancer.[9, 18, 28]

If a cancer is small and localized, surgery is performed with the intent of a cure. If a tumor is of the type that the pathologist labeled *infiltrating,* then the surgery will be extensive and remove both the tumor and a wide margin of tissue that appears normal to the eye but contains malignant cells. If the tumor type is known to metastasize to the regional lymph nodes, then an *en bloc resection* is performed. In this type of resection, the tumor, the organ of origin, and the tissue that contains the regional lymph nodes are removed.[9, 18, 28]

By the time many patients are diagnosed, metastases may not be evident but micrometastases are present. *Micro-*

metastases means that small foci of tumor are present in the lymph nodes or distant organs. These foci are too small to be detected clinically at the time of first diagnosis. But a careful follow-up of a group of patients will reveal that a certain percentage will develop clinical signs of metastases within 2 to 5 years after primary therapy. In this case, surgery may be combined with radiation therapy or chemotherapy to control the primary tumor and to eradicate micrometastases.[9]

Palliative surgery, on the other hand, attempts to relieve the patient of troubling symptoms or to prevent their occurrence and prolong a comfortable life. An example might be a patient with an adenoma of the large bowel that has already metastasized to the liver. A resection of the bowel might still be performed to prevent bowel obstruction, bleeding, and painful tenesmus. A patient with a large ulcerating tumor of the breast may undergo a mastectomy not for cure, but to lead a more comfortable life.[28]

Nursing Responsibilities

The health status of the patient before the surgery will determine the risk for postoperative complications. For instance, a patient who is malnourished (has lost approximately 10% of his weight in the previous month) will be at risk for infection, delayed wound healing, and dehiscence. A patient who is obese or who has cardiovascular or respiratory disease will also have a greater likelihood for postoperative complications. The patient who undergoes palliative surgery is often compromised in a physiological sense and may be at risk not only for immediate postoperative complications but also may be at a higher risk for dying within a 30-day period after surgery. In addition to these factors, the mental status, the optimism, and the family support that a patient has will influence his outlook and ability to withstand some of the difficulties of the surgery and hospitalization.[18, 28]

After surgery the patient will be assessed for pain and for problems with the wound, including hematoma, infection, dehiscence, and evisceration. Even though surgery is considered a local or regional therapy, the entire individual is affected, including his emotional state. The respiratory system, the urinary tract, and the gastrointestinal tract all might be affected by the surgery. Careful assessment of all systems is necessary to prevent complications.

If the surgery involved the removal of the local lymph nodes, then the patient is at risk for developing lymphedema. To monitor the fluid accumulations in a limb after surgery, the patient's extremity should be measured before surgery.

Radiation Therapy

Another local–regional therapy for cancer is radiation therapy. Radiation therapy can cure certain cancers, depending on the type of tumor, the size of the tumor, the surrounding tissue, and other patient factors. Different tissues in the body as well as different tumors have different radiosensitivities. Generally speaking, tumors that arise from radiosensitive tissues are radiosensitive, and rapidly dividing tissues are more sensitive than slowly dividing tissues. Thus, the testes, ovaries, lymphoid tissues, and the bone marrow are radiosensitive, and such tissues as the bone, muscle, and nerves in the adult are radioresistant.[9, 18, 28, 35]

When used in the treatment of tumors, ionizing radiation creates its biological effects by transferring energy to the molecules present in the cell. These molecules in turn become either more energetic or ionized, which leads to reactive compounds. As these compounds react in a random fashion, then cellular damage accumulates. The presence of oxygen greatly facilitates these processes. In large tumors that have a hypoxic core, the cells in the hypoxic areas will be resistant to the radiation, whereas the cells closer to the blood supply will be sensitive. As the sensitive cells die and a new blood supply is established, the once hypoxic cells will become euoxic and thereby more sensitive. Giving the radiation over a period of time allows for this process to occur. Dividing the radiation dose, or *fractionation,* also allows time for normal tissues to recover. Most patients will receive radiation in doses of 1.8 Gy to 2.5 Gy (180 and 250 rads) per day for 4 to 6 weeks with a rest period of 2 days per week (over weekends).[28]

The effect of radiation therapy is often not immediately apparent. Because the cell can repair cytoplasmic damage, the cell may live for a time; however, as more and more damage accumulates in the DNA, it becomes less likely that daughter cells will be viable. It might take one or two cell divisions for these effects to be fully realized. Cells that are rapidly dividing have less time between divisions to repair the damage and therefore are more sensitive to radiation therapy. Because of the time gap it takes for the full effects of radiation to be seen, the patient will be monitored closely after therapy, and the full benefits of treatment might take weeks to be fully assessed.[9, 18, 28]

Radiation is also used for palliation. A patient with metastases to the bone might receive palliative radiation to control the pain or to relieve a spinal cord compression. Radiation is often used to relieve bronchial or tracheal obstruction, ulceration, or bleeding. Usually, lower dosages are used in palliation as compared with the dosages used for cure.

Radiation is delivered in two primary ways: *teletherapy,* in which the radiation is produced in a machine that is some distance from the patient, or *brachytherapy,* an implant of a radioactive substance within a cavity of the patient. Many gynecological tumors are treated with radium implants; a carcinoma of the tongue may be treated with implants of radioactive gold seeds. With respect to the implants, the amount of radiation delivered to the tumor is determined by the *inverse square law.* The intensity of the radiation is inversely related to the distance from the source. Intensity = 1/distance squared. At close distances the radiation falls off rapidly as the distance increases; at further distances the difference per unit of area becomes less of an issue. Therefore, an implant in a cavity can deliver high doses of radiation and spare nearby normal structures.[18, 28, 34]

In teletherapy, radiation can be produced by a natural radioactive source such as ^{60}Co; in this case, the resulting rays are called gamma rays. The other way to produce high-energy rays is by a machine called an *accelerator,* which uses a very high voltage electric current to deliver electrons to a target; the result of the interaction is a high-energy x-ray beam. There are other types of beams, such as the neutron beam, used in the treatment of cancer. However, most of these are currently being used on an experimental basis.

Biological Effects

The effects of radiation therapy in a patient can be estimated by knowing the dose, the volume and type of tissue irradiated, and the length of exposure. Radiation used in medicine is usually restricted to a single area of the body, and the dosage is estimated to be that which will destroy the cancer cells with the lowest probability of injuring the surrounding normal tissues. This balance between the therapeutic effect and normal tissue tolerance is estimated from previous clinical studies and experience. Because each patient is unique and has his own history, the dosages are individually adjusted.[9, 18, 28]

Tissue reactions to radiation vary according to the geographical area irradiated and the time since the treatment. For instance, if the skin is irradiated, then the first or acute reaction will be erythema; later, a dry desquamation may result or, infrequently, a moist desquamation occurs. In the irradiated area hair will be lost, but within 3 to 6 months new hair will grow. This new hair might be a different texture and a different color than the original hair. Because the underlying blood vessels are also damaged by radiation and fibrous scarring occurs, the irradiated area may always be more sensitive to injuries such as sunburn or may take longer to heal from trauma than does the surrounding tissue that was never irradiated. The skin that has been irradiated may appear as if it has undergone premature aging and in fact has less reserve and less potential for healing.[8]

This pattern of acute inflammation followed by healing and fibrous scarring occurs in other organs. The effect on the patient depends on the organ irradiated. If the esophagus is irradiated, for instance, the patient might experience dysphagia during therapy. A late effect years after therapy may be stenosis of the esophagus. If the lower gastrointestinal tract is irradiated in the course of irradiating the pelvis for a gynecological cancer, the patient may experience diarrhea and intermittent abdominal cramping during therapy. Long-term effects might be partial bowel obstruction, stenosis, or fistula formation. These long-term effects occur in a small percentage of the total patients treated.[8]

Even though the expected radiation reactions have been described as being limited to the geographical area of the radiation, it should not be forgotten that the body is an integrated whole. The radiation reaction in one organ system might influence another closely allied system. For instance, radiation damage to the lung might influence cardiac functioning. Patients undergoing radiation also might exhibit systemic effects such as fatigue, although the exact mechanisms accounting for this symptom are not known.

Nursing Responsibilities

As described previously, radiation therapy can be delivered by teletherapy, that is, by an external source, or by brachytherapy, that is, by implantation of a radioactive substance within a patient. It is important that the nurse understand similarities and differences between these two delivery systems particularly as they relate to radiation safety precautions.

External Radiation. The patient receiving *external radiation* must realize that when each treatment is over, no residual radiation persists in his body. In other words, he does not have to fear that he is "radioactive," and no radiation safety precautions are necessary outside the radiation therapy department.[19] Despite this reassurance, other aspects of external radiation may be frightening. Imagine the impact of having to lie alone in an unfamiliar treatment room, staring up at a huge, noisy machine which is delivering radiation that cannot be seen, tasted, or felt. Assisting the patient to express his concerns, acknowledging that these concerns are not unusual, and, whenever possible, altering the environment to make it more comfortable, are all important nursing interventions.[14, 29]

Side Effects. In addition, radiation therapy treatments may interrupt work and home schedules and may produce unpleasant side-effects as well. A major systemic side effect is fatigue. Patients may need help to decrease or adjust their activities around more frequent rest periods. Other generalized symptoms such as headache and nausea can be lessened by the use of analgesics and antiemetics.[6, 29]

Skin Care. It is important that patients receiving external radiation are instructed not to wash off the lines that were marked on their skin as a means of denoting the area to be treated by radiation. Patients should also be instructed in ways of protecting their irradiated skin, because some degree of skin irritation or injury is common with external radiation. The most common skin responses are erythema and extreme dryness. These reactions usually begin about the second or third week of therapy, although special skin precautions are taken from the outset of therapy. Occasionally, a moist epidermatitis reaction develops in which the skin becomes ulcerated, denuded, and resembles a second degree burn. Eventually, the skin redness gives way to a bronzed, tan appearance that may be permanent. Localized scarring can result in a variety of functional impairments.[29]

General guidelines for the protection of irradiated skin are as follows:

1. Wash treatment area with water only; use no soap, creams, or ointments without checking with the physician first.
2. Avoid rubbing skin, pat area dry after washing, and wear nonrestrictive clothing.
3. Avoid extremes of heat and cold and sun or wind exposure.[6, 29, 32]

Internal Radiation. In contrast, when patients receive *internal radiation,* they are indeed radioactive, and important safety precautions are necessary to prevent radiation exposure to people other than the patient.

Unsealed Sources. Unsealed sources of radiation are occasionally used and include isotopes such as ^{131}I and ^{32}P.

These isotopes are liquid and are frequently administered orally. The half-life of each particular radioactive isotope varies but generally is short. For example, ^{131}I has a half-life of 8.05 days. Radiation precautions are most stringent for the first 4 days; after this time the isotope is usually concentrated in the target organ and the risk of radioactive contamination of others decreases.[14] Precautions during the high-risk period (generally the first 4 days) after radioactive isotope administration are as follows:

1. If the patient vomits within the first 4 hours after isotope administration, everything touched by the vomitus is considered highly contaminated.
2. All body secretions are considered contaminated, and special disposal or decontamination procedures must be used.
3. Hospital gown and disposable dishes are used.
4. Contact with hospital personnel and visitors is limited, as described in the next section dealing with sealed radiation sources.[14]

Sealed Source. Internal radiation is more commonly administered by a *sealed source,* which means that a radioactive substance encased in a metal capsule is temporarily placed into a body cavity to deliver a high dose of radiation directly to the tumor. A variety of radioactive materials can be used this way, including radium needles, radon seeds, and ^{137}Cs. A common administration technique is afterloading, in which the container that will hold the radiation source is inserted during the time of surgery, but the actual radioactive material is inserted later in the patient's room.[6] Sealed implants are particularly common for gynecological tumors, for tumors of the head and neck, and for tumors of the rectum. They are also being used, as an alternative to surgery, for very small tumors of the breast.

Regardless of type of sealed implant, very careful precautions are necessary to prevent care-givers, and any other persons having contact with the patient, from undue radiation exposure. General safety precautions revolve around the three principles of time, distance, and shielding. The principle of *time* means that radiation exposure is proportional to the amount of time spent with the patient. Therefore, care is planned to provide the maximum amount of care in the shortest period of time.

The principle of *distance* refers to the fact that radiation intensity is inversely related to the distance from the source. The duration of safe exposure by visitor or caretaker increases as the distance from the source is increased.[14]

The principle of *shielding* refers to the use of lead shields or other equipment to reduce transmission of radiation. Figure 19–6 illustrates radiation levels in the room of a patient with a cesium implant placed in the vagina. When the nurse must make direct patient contact, she will receive the lowest radiation dosage by placing herself at the head of the bed. Note that the radiation dosage immediately behind the lead screen approximates that within the bed. However, as the distance from the shield is increased, the radiation level drops faster than it would without the shield present.[22]

Precautions. Precise precautions vary among different institutions and according to the type of implant being used. However, general guidelines are as follows:

1. Persons under 18 years of age and pregnant women are prohibited from visiting or caring for the patient with a radioactive implant.
2. Radiation badges are worn by care-givers to monitor the total amount of radiation exposure.
3. Careful observation for displacement or dislodgement of the radiation source is necessary; usually placement is checked every 4 to 6 hours.
4. A sealed, lead-lined container is kept in the patient's room in the event that accidental dislodgement occurs. In the event of dislodgement, the source is picked up with long-handled tongs and placed in the lead container; it is never picked up with the bare hands.
5. Although body wastes are not radioactive, excreta and soiled linen are often collected until it can be determined that they do not contain a dislodged radiation source.
6. The radiation source must be removed precisely at the prearranged time. When the source has been removed, the patient is no longer radioactive.[14]

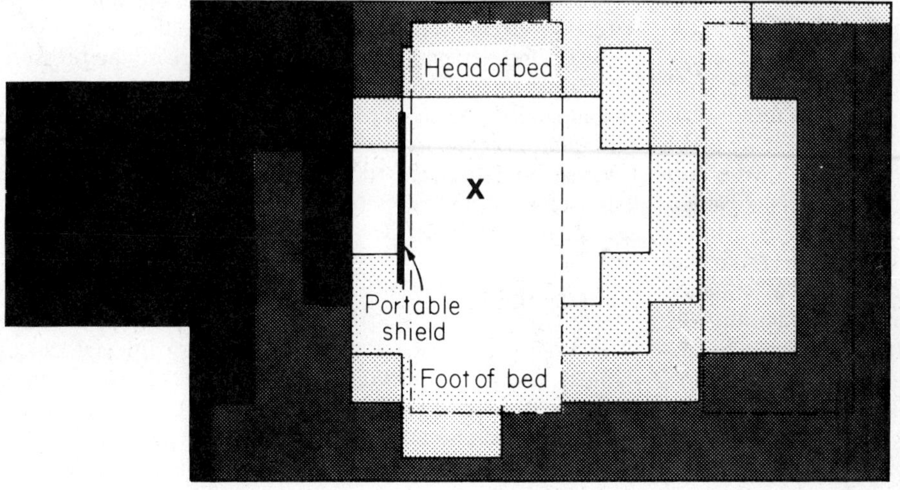

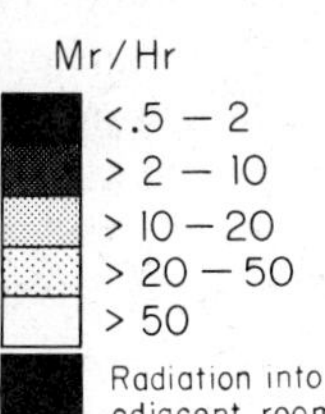

FIGURE 19–6 Cesium implant in the vagina. The head of the bed is the safest area from which to provide direct patient care. The safe area will vary according to location of the implant. For example, with an implant for head and neck cancer, the radiation intensity would be highest at the patient's head, and it would be safe to provide care from the foot of the bed.

It is important that concern for what the patient is experiencing is not overshadowed by fear of radiation exposure. As a result of the necessary safety measures, the patient will be in a private room and have limited contact with caretakers and family members. Feelings of isolation and depression may well be intensified. Complications of immobility are a risk if the patient is on bed rest to avoid dislodgement. Finally, the problems of fatigue and local irritation must be dealt with, just as for the patient receiving external radiation.

Chemotherapy

Chemotherapy is used to treat disseminated tumors and metastases. Certain tumors can be cured by chemotherapy alone. These tumors include acute lymphocytic leukemia, Hodgkin's disease, some malignant lymphomas, some testicular cancers, and choriocarcinoma. Chemotherapy is also given to patients with acute myelocytic leukemia, multiple myeloma (a cancer of the cells that form antibodies), adenocarcinoma of the breast, and ovarian cancer. In these cases, chemotherapy can cause the tumor to regress, prolong the patient's life, relieve symptoms, and in some cases, cure the patient. An additional use of chemotherapy is as an adjuvant to surgery or radiation therapy. Although micrometastases cannot be detected, it is known that there is a high probability that they exist in many cases. Surgery or radiation therapy are local therapies and cannot eliminate micrometastases, whereas chemotherapy is a systemic therapy and may be able to do so.[9, 18, 28]

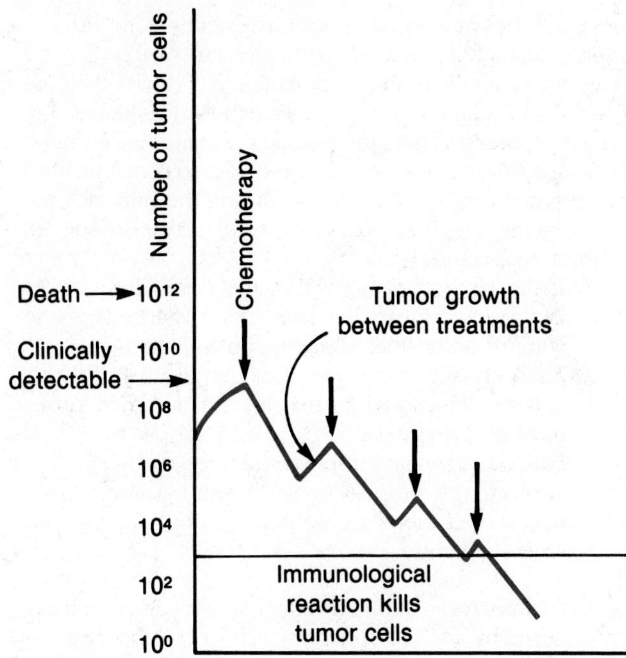

FIGURE 19–7 A malignancy is clinically detectable when it consists of approximately 10^9 cells. Chemotherapy reduces the percentage of malignant cells. If repeated at set intervals, each series of chemotherapy further reduces the tumor burden. The remaining malignant cells are believed to be destroyed by the host's own immune defenses.

Mechanism of Action

Central to understanding the rationale for chemotherapy is understanding tumor biology and cell growth. As was stated previously, a cancer can arise from a single cell, continue to divide, and eventually reach a number that will kill the patient. A tumor can be detected clinically when it reaches a size of 0.5 cm to 1 cm in diameter. This means that approximately 30 doublings have occurred and there are about 10^6 to 10^9 cells present. The cytotoxic drugs kill a set percentage of cells rather than an absolute number of cells. This concept is labeled the log cell-kill hypothesis. For instance, perhaps a single exposure to a chemotherapeutic agent can kill 99.99% of the cells present. If there are 10^9 cells present before chemotherapy, then after chemotherapy 10^5 cells will remain. In this case the chemotherapy has reduced the tumor burden by 4 logs. This also means that 100,000 tumor cells remain that are not detectable by usual clinical methods. These cells can continue to divide and eventually reach a size that will cause the death of the patient (Fig. 19–7). Therefore, chemotherapy is repeated in set intervals to further reduce the tumor cell numbers. From this example it can be seen that chemotherapy has a better chance of curing the patient if small numbers of tumor cells are present than if there is a large tumor burden. Chemotherapy might be more successful after surgery or radiation therapy when the bulk of the tumor cells has been removed.[9, 18, 28, 35]

Chemotherapy is more successful at killing rapidly dividing cells than at killing cells which have long cell-cycle times. Tumors that have short cell-cycle times, that is, short periods between mitoses, are tumors such as the acute leukemias, testicular cancers, and some of the lung cancers. These types of tumors also tend to have a high growth fraction; that is, a large percentage of the cells of the tumor is proceeding through the cell cycle. Tumors that are young or proliferating tend to be small in size, vascularized, and have a greater chance of being eradicated by chemotherapy.[9, 28]

At the time of diagnosis, tumors are composed of heterogeneous populations of cells. As the tumor growth progresses, clones of tumor cells arise through mutations that are different from the original malignant cell. As the tumor size increases, the possibility also increases that lines of cells resistant to chemotherapy will arise. In addition, exposure to the chemotherapeutic drugs tends to increase the pressure for resistant lines to appear. One method employed to overcome this resistance is to use chemotherapy early in the life of the tumor and to use *combination chemotherapy,* that is, to use multiple drugs. The use of combination chemotherapy prevents, or at the very least slows down, the rate at which resistant lines arise.[9, 28]

Drug Choice

The drugs that are chosen to treat a particular cancer must have been shown, as single agents, to have activity against that cancer. The drugs chosen for a particular combination chemotherapy regimen tend to be those with different side-effects. For example, a drug that is toxic to the bone marrow may be paired with a drug that is toxic to the gastrointestinal tract. This pairing prevents the limits of toxicity of any one normal tissue from being reached. The patient might experience more side-effects, but the effects will be less severe and the normal tissue will recover between cycles of chemotherapy.[9,28]

A huge variety of chemotherapeutic agents is currently available, and additional drugs continue to be developed. Drugs are often categorized according to their pharmacological properties, as shown in Table 19–6.

- *Alkylating agents* interfere with DNA replication in a manner similar to radiation therapy. These agents are frequently referred to as radiomimetics.[5]
- The *nitrosoureas* are a subgroup of alkylating agents that not only damage DNA but also inhibit its repair.
- The *antimetabolites* inhibit enzymes involved in nucleic acid synthesis. Because they are chemically similar to cellular metabolites, these agents are incorporated into the cell structure and block further cellular activities.
- *Vinca alkaloids* are plant extracts that arrest cell division.
- Antitumor *antibiotics* directly bind with DNA and prevent further DNA and RNA synthesis.
- *Hormones* are used to alter the growth of hormonally sensitive tumors and for additional, poorly understood, cytotoxic effects.
- *Miscellaneous* category is used for additional chemotherapeutic agents with actions different from those already described.[5] Many of these drugs are used for investigational purposes.

Drug Scheduling. Because chemotherapy is a systemic treatment and because it tends to kill cells that are proliferating, the bone marrow and the gastrointestinal tract are generally the normal tissues at highest risk for damage. However each class and each drug will have its unique toxicities. The scheduling of chemotherapy treatments revolves around giving the drugs at the shortest possible intervals while allowing normal cells to recover. It is usually bone marrow recovery that determines the treatment schedules, but the recovery of the gastrointestinal tract is also considered. Typically, the lowest blood count is reached 14 to 18 days after chemotherapy, and recovery is usually complete by 21 to 28 days. Nausea and vomiting are common side-effects of chemotherapy that are treated with antiemetics. Stomatitis or inflammation of the oral cavity resulting from chemotherapy usually resolves within 2 to 3 weeks.[9,28]

Nursing Responsibilities

While on chemotherapy, the patient usually experiences side-effects. For instance, if the patient's white blood count is low, the patient will be at risk for infection. Any symptoms of infection, such as fever, should be attended to immediately. Antibiotic therapy might be initiated without waiting for the culture results because the patient is at risk of dying from an overwhelming infection. If the patient experiences nausea and vomiting, measures should be taken to ensure the patient will receive an adequate diet. However, it should be noted that not every patient will experience these side-effects. In fact, even though patients might be experiencing symptoms from the chemotherapy they may actually feel better because their tumor is being controlled.[5,13,15,38] It is important that the nurse is aware of the side effects and toxicities that are specific for each drug being administered to her patients. (Table 19–6 summarizes the major points for numerous drugs in each category.)

Although data regarding health risks related to working with chemotherapy are by no means conclusive, there is a definite possibility that chemotherapeutic agents may be ab-

(Text continues on p 247)

TABLE 19–6
Nursing Care Chemotherapy Guide

Agent	*Route of Administration*	*Significant Side-Effects and Toxicity*	*Nursing Care*	*Major Uses*
Alkylating Agents (interfere with DNA replication; cell-cycle nonspecific)				
Mechlorethamine (Mustargen) (Nitrogen mustard) (HN_2)	Intravenous Intracavitary	Bone marrow suppression (nadir 7–12 days after 1st dose Severe nausea, vomiting, diarrhea Alopecia Sterility Birth defects	Avoid IV extravasation Assess signs and symptoms; protect against infection and bleeding Check blood counts Administer antiemetics (sedation if needed) Maintain hydration Adjust diet Assist coping with hair loss Sexual counseling Provide contraceptive information	Hodgkin's disease Lymphomas Malignant effusions

(Continued)

TABLE 19-6
Nursing Care Chemotherapy Guide (Continued)

Agent	*Route of Administration*	*Significant Side-Effects and Toxicity*	*Nursing Care*	*Major Uses*
Alkylating Agents (interfere with DNA replication; cell-cycle nonspecific)				
Melphalan (Alkeran) (L-phenylalanine mustard) (L-PAM)	Oral	Bone marrow suppression (nadir may be unpredictable) Immunosuppression Nausea Sterility	Assess signs and symptoms; protect against infection and bleeding Check blood counts Administer antiemetics Sexual counseling	Multiple myeloma Ovarian cancer Breast cancer
Busulfan (Myleran)	Oral	Bone marrow suppression Pulmonary toxicity	Assess signs and symptoms; protect against infection and bleeding Check blood counts (especially platelet count and granulocyte level) Assess signs and symptoms of pulmonary dysfunction	Chronic myelocytic leukemia
Chlorambucil (Leukeran)	Oral	Minimal; prolonged use; immunosuppression, bone marrow suppression	Assess signs and symptoms; protect against infection and bleeding Check blood counts	Chronic lymphocytic leukemia
Cyclophosphamide (Cytoxan) (Ctx)	Oral Intravenous	Bone marrow suppression, immunosuppression Nausea, vomiting Alopecia Hemorrhagic cystitis Sterility Birth defects	Assess signs and symptoms; protect against infection and bleeding Check blood counts Administer antiemetics Assist in coping with hair loss Maintain hydration; must have high fluid output (genitourinary irrigation may be given for patients receiving high dose) Watch for signs and symptoms of cystitis Sexual counseling Provide contraceptive information	Multiple myeloma Lymphomas Small-cell lung cancer Breast cancer
Triethylene thiophosphoramide (Thiotepa)	Intracavitary	Bone marrow suppression	Turn patient every 15 min for 1 hr to distribute drug Assess signs and symptoms; protect against infection and bleeding Check blood counts	Malignant effusions
Nitrosoureas Agents (alkylating agents; inhibit DNA replication)				
Carmustine (BCNU)	Intravenous	Severe nausea, vomiting Bone marrow suppression (nadir 4–6 wk after dose)	Administer antiemetics Assess signs and symptoms; protect against infection and bleeding Check blood counts (especially platelets and granulocytes)	Brain tumors Gastrointestinal cancer Melanoma

(*Continued*)

TABLE 19–6
Nursing Care Chemotherapy Guide (Continued)

Agent	*Route of Administration*	*Significant Side-Effects and Toxicity*	*Nursing Care*	*Major Uses*
Nitrosoureas Agents (alkylating agents; inhibit DNA replication)				
Lomustine (CCNU)	Oral	Same as carmustine	Same as carmustine	Lymphomas Lung cancer
Vinca Alkaloids (bind to microtubular proteins; necessary for cell division during mitosis; cell-cycle phase specific)				
Vinblastine (Velban)	Intravenous	Bone marrow suppression (nadir 5–10 wk after dose) Nausea, vomiting Alopecia Neuropathy (rare)	Avoid IV extravasation Assess signs and symptoms; protect against infection and bleeding Check blood counts (especially granulocyte count) Administer antiemetics Assist in coping with hair loss	Hodgkin's disease Testicular tumors
Vincristine (Oncovin) (VCR)	Intravenous	Peripheral neuropathy Autonomic neuropathy: severe constipation, paralytic ileus	Avoid IV extravasation Assess signs and symptoms of neurotoxicity: depression of Achilles tendon reflex (earliest sign), parasthesias in fingers and toes, inability to perform fine motor skills, weakness Assess bowel habits: adminster stool softeners, cathartics, and enemas as needed	Acute lymphoblastic leukemia Hodgkin's disease Lymphomas
Antimetabolites (inhibit enzymes of nucleic acid synthesis, generally cell-cycle phase specific)				
Cytarabine (Cytosar) (Cytosine arabinoside) (Ara-C)	Intravenous Intrathecal	Bone marrow suppression (nadir 12–14 days after dose) Nausea, vomiting, diarrhea Stomatitis Hepatitis (may occur within 1 wk after dose) Birth defects	Assess signs and symptoms; protect against infection and bleeding Check blood counts Administer antidiarrheal agents, antiemetics Maintain hydration Adjust diet Frequent mouth care and assessment Assess signs and symptoms of hepatitic dysfunction Provide contraceptive information	Acute leukemia
5-Fluorouracil (Fluorouracil) (5-FU)	Intravenous	Severe bone marrow suppression Severe nausea, vomiting, diarrhea Alopecia (rare) Hyperpigmentation (enhanced photosensitivity)	Assess signs and symptoms; protect against infection and bleeding Check blood counts Administer antiemetics, antidiarrheal agents Maintain hydration Adjust diet Frequent mouth care and assessment Advise patient to avoid sunlight	Breast cancer Gastrointestinal tract

(Continued)

TABLE 19-6
Nursing Care Chemotherapy Guide (Continued)

Agent	Route of Administration	Significant Side-Effects and Toxicity	Nursing Care	Major Uses
Antimetabolites (inhibit enzymes of nucleic acid synthesis, generally cell-cycle phase specific)				
Methotrexate (MTX)	Intravenous Oral Intrathecal	Bone marrow suppression Stomatitis Severe diarrhea Hepatic toxicity Birth defects Renal toxicity with high doses Neurotoxicity (acute and chronic) with intrathecal administration	Assess signs and symptoms; protect against infection and bleeding Check blood counts Administer antidiarrheal agents Maintain hydration Adjust diet Assess signs and symptoms of hepatic dysfunction Frequent mouth care and assessment Provide contraceptive information For high doses: make sure citrovorum factor ("rescue") has been given Maintain intravenous hydration (3000 ml/m^2/day) Monitor intake and output Check that drug levels and renal function tests are taken Keep urine alkaline to augment renal clearance (acetazolamide, sodium bicarbonate) For intrathecal administration: assess signs and symptoms of neurotoxicity (nausea, vomiting, headache, dementia)	Acute leukemia Choriocarcinoma Breast cancer Head and neck cancer Testicular cancer Lung cancer High doses: Osteosarcoma
6-Mercaptopurine (Purinethol) (6-MP)	Oral	Bone marrow suppression Nausea, vomiting Hepatic dysfunction	Assess signs and symptoms; protect against infection and bleeding Check blood counts Administer antiemetics Adjust diet Assess signs and symptoms of hepatic dysfunction: jaundice	Acute leukemia
6-Thioguanine (Thioguanine) (6-T6)	Oral	Bone marrow suppression (may be delayed) Nausea, vomiting Hepatic dysfunction Stomatitis	Assess signs and symptoms; protect against infection and bleeding Check blood counts Administer antiemetics Adjust diet Assess signs and symptoms of hepatic dysfunction Frequent mouth care and assessment	Acute leukemia
5-Azacytidine	Intravenous	Severe nausea, vomiting (reduced when given drug as continuous infusion)	Administer antiemetics, antidiarrheal agents Adjust diet	Acute granulocytic leukemia

(Continued)

TABLE 19–6
Nursing Care Chemotherapy Guide (Continued)

Agent	*Route of Administration*	*Significant Side-Effects and Toxicity*	*Nursing Care*	*Major Uses*
Antimetabolites ***(inhibit enzymes of nucleic acid synthesis, generally cell-cycle phase specific)***				
		Diarrhea Bone marrow suppression Hepatic toxicity	Maintain hydration Assess signs and symptoms; protect against infection and bleeding Check blood counts Assess signs and symptoms of hepatic dysfunction	
Hydroxyurea (Hydrea) (OH-urea)	Oral	Bone marrow suppression Nausea, vomiting Stomatitis Skin reactions Alopecia	Assess signs and symptoms; protect against infection and bleeding Check blood counts Administer antiemetics Frequent mouth care and assessment Observe skin closely Assist coping with hair loss	Chronic granulocytic leukemia Prostate cancer High leukocyte count in acute leukemia
Antibiotics ***(natural products of soil fungi; inhibit DNA and RNA synthesis, generally cell-cycle phase nonspecific)***				
Dactinomycin (Cosmegen) (Actinomycin-D)	Intravenous	Bone marrow suppression Nausea, vomiting Diarrhea Alopecia Stomatitis "Recall phenomenon" Birth defects	Avoid IV extravasation Assess signs and symptoms; protect against infection and bleeding Check blood counts Administer antiemetics, antidiarrheal agents Adjust diet Maintain hydration Assist coping with hair loss Frequent mouth care and assessment Assess skin in previously radiated sites Provide contraceptive information	Wilms' tumor Rhabdomyosarcomas Choriocarcinoma Testicular cancer
Doxorubicin (Adriamycin)	Intravenous	Severe bone marrow suppression Alopecia Nausea, vomiting Stomatitis Cardiac toxicity Red-colored urine (harmless) "Recall phenomenon"	Avoid IV extravasation Assess signs and symptoms; protect against infection and bleeding Check blood counts Assist coping with hair loss Administer antiemetics Adjust diet Frequent mouth care and assessment Assess signs and symptoms of cardiac toxicity: arrhythmias, dyspnea, edema Inform patient of urine change Assess skin in previously radiated sites	Lymphomas Leukemia Sarcomas Breast cancer
Daunomycin (Daunorubicin)	Intravenous	Similar to doxorubicin	Same as doxorubicin	Acute leukemia

(*Continued*)

TABLE 19–6
Nursing Care Chemotherapy Guide (Continued)

Agent	Route of Administration	Significant Side-Effects and Toxicity	Nursing Care	Major Uses
Antibiotics ***(natural products of soil fungi; inhibit DNA and RNA synthesis, generally cell-cycle phase nonspecific)***				
Bleomycin (Blenoxane)	Intravenous Intramuscular Subcutaneous	Pulmonary toxicity (pneumonitis, pulmonary fibrosis) Skin reactions (hyperpigmentation, ulceration, erythema) Stomatitis Alopecia Nausea, vomiting Anaphylaxis Fever	Assess signs and symptoms of respiratory distress (especially dyspnea, crackles) Assess skin carefully Frequent mouth care and assessment Assist coping with hair loss Administer antiemetics Adjust diet Give test dose (1 mg), and observe for anaphylaxis: fever, hypotension, wheezing Take temperature Administer antipyretics	Head and neck cancer Testicular cancer Lymphomas
Mithramycin (Mithracin)	Intravenous	Severe bleeding Arterial clotting Hepatic toxicity Renal toxicity Nausea, vomiting Stomatitis Central nervous system reactions (headache, weakness, fatigue) Fever Hypocalcemia	Assess signs and symptoms of bleeding Check platelet count and coagulation studies Assess signs and symptoms of hepatic, renal dysfunction Administer antiemetics Frequent mouth care and assessment Frequent signs and symptoms of central nervous system dysfunction Observe signs and symptoms of hypocalcemia Monitor temperature	Testicular cancer Hypercalcemia associated with malignancy
Mitomycin-C (Mutamycin)	Intravenous	Bone marrow suppression (delayed, serious) Nausea, vomiting Diarrhea Stomatitis Alopecia Fever	Avoid IV extravasation Assess signs and symptoms; protect against infection and bleeding Check blood counts (especially WBC and platelet count) Administer antiemetics, antidiarrheal agents Adjust diet Frequent mouth care and assessment Assist coping with hair loss Monitor fever	Breast cancer Head and neck cancer Gastrointestinal tumors
Hormones ***(affect the growth pattern of hormonally responsive tumors)***				
Estrogen				
Diethylstilbesterol (DES)	Oral	Nausea, vomiting Fluid retention Gynecomastia in males Uterine bleeding Alterations in libido, impotence	Administer antiemetics Adjust diet Monitor daily weight Intake and output Note edema; observe for uterine bleeding	Prostate cancer Breast cancer (postmenopausal)

(Continued)

TABLE 19–6
Nursing Care Chemotherapy Guide (Continued)

Agent	*Route of Administration*	*Significant Side-Effects and Toxicity*	*Nursing Care*	*Major Uses*
Hormones (affect the growth pattern of hormonally responsive tumors)				
		Hypercalcemia Hepatic toxicity (high doses)	Check radiation to male breast tissue prior to dose Sexual counseling Assess coping with body changes Assess signs and symptoms of hypercalcemia: confusion, polyuria, constipation Assess signs and symptoms of liver dysfunction	
Antiestrogen				
Tamoxifen (Nolvadex) (TAM)	Oral	Nausea, vomiting Uterine bleeding Hot flashes Thrombocytopenia (mild) Blurred vision	Administer antiemetics Asess signs and symptoms of bleeding Check platelet count Assess visual changes	Breast cancer
Progestins				
Megestrol acetate (Megace) (MEG)	Oral	Minimal	Observe for side-effects	Endometrial cancer Breast cancer
Medroxyprogesterone acetate (Depo-Provera)	Intramuscular	Fluid retention (minimal)	Daily weights Note edema	Endometrial cancer Breast cancer Renal cell cancer
Androgens				
Testosterone propionate (Neo-Hombreol)	Intramuscular	Fluid retention Masculinization in women Altered libido	Daily weights Note edema Sexual counseling Assist coping with body changes	Breast cancer (post-menopausal)
Fluoxymesterone (Halotestin)	Oral	Fluid retention Masculinization in women Hepatic toxicity	Daily weights Note edema Sexual counseling Assist coping with body changes Assess signs and symptoms of hepatic dysfunction	Breast cancer (post-menopausal)
Adrenocorticosteroids				
Prednisone (PRED)	Oral	ALL STEROIDS (prolonged, high doses) Fluid retention, hypertension Hypokalemia Diabetes Immunosuppression Gastrointestinal bleeding Potassium loss Mood swing, psychosis Cushingoid changes Osteoporosis	ALL STEROIDS Daily weights Note edema Monitor blood pressure Assess signs and symptoms: hypokalemia Give potassium replacement (*e.g.*, bananas) Assess signs and symptoms of diabetes: polyuria, polydipsia, check urine for sugar/acetone	Leukemia Lymphomas multiple myeloma CNS metastases Hypercalcemia

(*Continued*)

TABLE 19–6
Nursing Care Chemotherapy Guide (Continued)

Agent	Route of Administration	Significant Side-Effects and Toxicity	Nursing Care	Major Uses
Adrenocorticosteroids				
			Assess signs and symptoms: protect against infection Assist coping with body changes and emotional lability	
Dexamethasone (Decadron)	Oral	See prednisone	See prednisone	See prednisone
Methylprednisolone sodium succinate (Solu-Medrol)	Intravenous	See prednisone	See prednisone	See prednisone
Podophyllotoxins				
Etoposide (VP-16)	Intravenous Oral	Bone marrow suppression Nausea, vomiting Diarrhea Alopecia Hypotension after rapid IV infusion, fever, anaphylactic reactions	Assess signs and symptoms; protect against infection and bleeding Check blood counts Administer antiemetics, antidiarrheal agents Adjust diet Maintain hydration Assist coping with hair loss Monitor temperature Observe for signs and symptoms of anaphylaxis	Small-cell lung cancer Testicular cancer
Teniposide VM-26	Same as Etoposide	Same as Etoposide	See Etoposide	Brain tumors
Miscellaneous Agents				
L-Asparaginase (L-ASP) (Elspar)	Intravenous Intramuscular	Anaphylaxis Hepatic toxicity Pancreatitis Coagulopathy CNS disturbances: hallucinations, depression	Observe carefully for anaphylaxis (be prepared with emergency supplies) Test dose in patient with prior exposure to drug Assess signs and symptoms of hepatic dysfunction: pancreatitis Check mental status	Acute lymphoblastic leukemia
Procarbazine (Matulane) (PROC)	Oral	Bone marrow suppression, immunosuppression Nausea, vomiting Central nervous system toxicity: depression, restlessness, psychosis, somnolence, ataxia, convulsions Birth defects Hemolytic anemia	Assess signs and symptoms; protect against bleeding and infection Check blood counts Administer antiemetics Assess mental status for confusion, depression, and drowsiness Inform patient to avoid barbiturates, antihistamines, alcohol, narcotics, sedatives, antihypertensive agents, sympathomimetics, tricyclic antidepressant drugs, ripe bananas, and cheese Provide information for contraception	Lymphomas Hodgkin's disease Lung cancer

(Continued)

TABLE 19–6
Nursing Care Chemotherapy Guide (Continued)

Agent	Route of Administration	Significant Side-Effects and Toxicity	Nursing Care	Major Uses
Miscellaneous Agents				
Dacarbazine (DTIC-Dome)	Intravenous	Bone marrow suppression Nausea, vomiting	Assess signs and symptoms; protect against infection and bleeding Check blood counts Administer antiemetics	Malignant melanoma Sarcomas Lymphomas
Experimental Drugs				
Hexamethylmelamine (HMM)	Oral	Nausea Bone marrow suppression (mild) Neurotoxicity (with prolonged use)	Administer antiemetics Assess signs and symptoms; protect against infection and bleeding Check blood counts Assess signs and symptoms of neurological dysfunction	Ovarian cancer Lung cancer Lymphomas
Cis-dichlorodiamine dichloroplatinum (II) (DDP) (Cisplatin) (Platinol)	Intravenous	Nausea, vomiting Renal toxicity Hearing loss Anaphylaxis	Administer antiemetics Hydrate patient: begin IV 12 hr prior to therapy and continue at 100 ml/hr Assess signs and symptoms of renal dysfunction: monitor intake and output Check for daily serum creatinine, and creatinine clearance tests Assess hearing frequently (audiograph prior to dose) Observe for signs of anaphylaxis	Testicular tumors Ovarian cancer Bladder cancer Head and neck cancer
Mitotane (Lysodren) (0, P′-DDD)	Oral	Nausea, vomiting Diarrhea Central nervous system effects: depression, lethargy, vertigo Adrenal insufficiency, proteinuria	Administer antiemetics, antidiarrheal agents Adjust diet Assess behavioral, neurological changes Caution patient to avoid tasks requiring mental alertness Stop drug and administer steroids if severe trauma or shock	Inoperable adrenal cortical carcinoma

(Adapted from Sarna LP: Concepts in the nursing management of patients receiving cancer chemotherapy and immunotherapy. In Vredevoe DL, Derdiarian A, Sarna LP et al [eds]: Concepts of Oncology Nursing, pp 88–114. Englewood Cliffs NJ, Prentice-Hall, 1981)

sorbed into the skin or inhaled. Therefore, careful precautions are essential for any person who prepares or administers chemotherapeutic agents.[5] The National Cancer Institute has published safety guidelines for preparation and administration of chemotherapeutic agents. These are presented in Table 19–7.

Biological Response Modifiers

Compounds, vaccines, and drugs that tend to enhance the patient's own responses, particularly those of the immune system, are known as biological response modifiers. In the late 1970s only a few members of this class of compounds that assist the body to destroy tumor cells were known. At that time, the approach was called immunotherapy. Vaccines such as BCG vaccine, *Corynebacterium parvum,* mixed bacterial vaccines, immune RNAs, and vaccines made of tumor cell extracts were tried in patients. There were some successes in very select patient populations but the results were not as great as was desired. Within this same time frame a whole new biotechnology evolved that made it possible to manufacture, on a large scale, monoclonal antibodies by means of a method called hybridoma technique. Products can also be manufactured by recombinant DNA technique.

TABLE 19–7
Guidelines for the Safe Preparation and Administration of Chemotherapeutic Agents

During Agent Preparation

- Prepare the agent under a vertical laminar airflow hood that vents exhaust air outdoors.
- Wear surgical gloves and a closed-front gown with knit cuffs.
- Thoroughly wash skin with soap and water if contact with the agent occurs. If the agent comes in contact with the eye, hold the eyelid open, flush with water for at least 15 minutes, and contact the physician.
- Vent vials containing reconstituted agents to avoid spraying and spillage when the needle is withdrawn.
- Place a cotton ball dampened with alcohol around the needle and vial top during needle withdrawal and around the neck of an ampule while breaking. A dampened cotton ball should also be placed at the tip of the needle when ejecting air bubbles from a filled syringe. Use a new sterile needle for administration.
- Avoid self-inoculation.
- Cleanse the interior of the vertical hood with 70% alcohol after completion of agent preparation.
- Dispose of intact needle and syringe, gloves, and other waste products in a leak-and-puncture-proof container and incinerate. Waste bags should be labled CANCER CHEMOTHERAPY WASTE.
- Wash hands after removing gloves.
- Gowns should be laundered in the usual manner.

During Agent Administration

- Wear a closed-front gown with knit cuffs and disposable surgical gloves.
- Place a sterile cotton ball dampened with alcohol on the tip of the needle when removing air bubbles, then change needles and use a sterile one to inject medication.
- Dispose of intact needle and syringe, gloves, and other waste products in a leak-and-puncture-proof container and incinerate. Gowns should be laundered in the usual manner.
- Wash hands after removing gowns.

(Brager BL, Yasko JM: Care of the Client Receiving Chemotherapy. Reston, Virginia, Reston Publishing, Co, 1984)

These two new biotechnologies are making compounds such as interferon, macrophage activating factor, tumor necrosis factor, and anti–T lymphocyte antibody available for treatment of cancer. Some of these compounds are currently being examined by clinical trials in which their efficacy is being tested in patients. Other compounds are being discovered; it will be several years before these compounds will become available for testing.[16,24,25,33]

Because these compounds are new and still undergoing testing, their potential for curing certain cancers and their toxicities are not known. From the early trials it can be predicted that side-effects of fever, malaise, anorexia, and flulike symptoms will commonly occur. Because many of these compounds are proteins, allergic and anaphylactic reactions might also develop. In the first trials of the monoclonal antibodies it was noted that anti-antibodies were formed by the patient. This finding is not too surprising since the monoclonal antibodies are mouse proteins. Different schedules for the administration of the monoclonal antibodies are being tried to minimize this effect. Attempts are also being made to link monoclonal antibodies to chemotherapeutic agents so that the chemotherapy can be delivered more selectively to the tumor cells and thereby decrease the toxicity to normal tissues.[11,21,24,25]

A *hybridoma* cell is a cell that results from the fusion of two different cell lines. In the case of monoclonal antibodies, a mouse lymphocyte capable of manufacturing a particular antibody, for example, to a cancer cell, is fused to a myeloma cell. The myeloma cell contributes the potential for unlimited cell division. As a result, the hybridoma cell can form many colonies, each manufacturing the antibody of interest.

In the *recombinant DNA technique,* a foreign gene such as the mammalian gene for interferon is inserted into an organism such as E. coli or yeast. The microorganism then manufactures the gene product, such as interferon. Almost unlimited quantities can be manufactured, whereas in the human, only minute amounts are produced.

The rationale for using immunotherapy or biological response modifiers comes predominantly from animal experiments. In animals, tumor antigens can be recognized by the animal immune system and a response is then initiated. In humans, there is some evidence that tumor-associated antigens do exist and that an immunologic response can be initiated. Burkitt's lymphoma, neuroblastoma, and malignant melanoma are several tumors in which the evidence is the strongest. It has also been suggested that chemotherapeutic cures may be partially due to an immune response. As discussed in the chemotherapy section, the drug regimens kill a percentage of the tumor cells; therefore, it may be improbable that the last tumor cell is killed by drugs. However, cures with chemotherapy are possible, perhaps because the last tumor cells are killed by the patient's own immune reaction. From animal experiments it is known that the immune reaction can kill small numbers of tumor cells but it is overwhelmed by large numbers. In the case of humans it is postulated that surgery or radiation therapy eliminates the bulk of the cancer cells, the chemotherapy reduces the number of tumor cells further, and then the patient's own immune system completes the process. In this very broad sense then surgery, radiation therapy, and chemotherapy can all be considered as a form of immunotherapy.

Prevention

Perhaps no discussion of cancer can be considered complete without a review of prevention. Prevention can be divided into primary, secondary, and tertiary prevention.

Primary Prevention

In primary prevention, cancer is prevented because the etiologic agents are removed from the environment or a premalignant lesion is removed from the patient. For instance, if individuals could be convinced to stop smoking, one third of all cancer deaths in men and approximately one tenth of the cancer deaths in women could be prevented. Alcohol is an important cocarcinogen or promoter of cancers of the oral cavity and liver. Diets that are high in fats have been linked to breast, colorectal, and prostate cancers. On the basis of current evidence that dietary factors contribute to cancer, the American Cancer Society has recently recommended that Americans should decrease their intake of saturated fats, increase their dietary fiber intake, and include vitamin C and vitamin A from fresh fruits and vegetables in the diets. Everyone, especially people with fair skin, should consider limiting their exposure to sunlight or use lotions with ultraviolet-screening properties. People working in industries that use carcinogens should take proper precautions to limit their exposure; an example is the wearing of respirators while working around asbestos.[23,24] Table 19–8 summarizes predisposing conditions for cancers of various body sites.

TABLE 19–8
Examples of High-Risk Patients for Specific Cancers

Site	*Predisposing Condition*
Cervix	Women who start sexual activity early, have multiple partners and pregnancies.
Colon and rectum	Multiple polyposis, long-standing ulcerative colitis
Intraoral	Cigarette smokers, tobacco chewers
Lung	Cigarette smokers, asbestos and uranium workers
Skin	Farmers and other outdoor workers, fair-skinned persons who sunburn easily
Stomach	Pernicious anemia, atrophic gastritis
Thyroid	Exposure to ionizing radiation

(Patterson WB: Principles of surgical oncology. In Rubin P, Bakemeier RF, Krackov SK [ed]: Clinical Oncology: A Multidisciplinary Approach, 6th ed. New York, American Cancer Society, 1983)

Secondary Prevention

Secondary prevention is the attempt to identify individuals with cancer before signs or symptoms develop. Early detection and screening are other terms for secondary prevention. Cancers that are detected early are believed more amenable to therapy; hence, lives will be saved. In this regard, the American Cancer Society has published guidelines on the types of examinations and when these exams are to be performed. These guidelines were formulated after examining the evidence of the efficacy of the tests, an estimate of the cost/benefit ratio, and the knowledge of the natural history of the cancer. The summary is included in this text (see Table 19–9); however, a careful reading of the ACS pamphlet *Guidelines of the Cancer-Related Checkup: Recommendations and Rationale* is recommended for better understanding.[1] These guidelines are also available in a format suitable for lay people.[3] As the study of oncogenes progresses it is hoped that someday it might be possible to detect products of these genes by a serological test. If this ever becomes feasible, then perhaps cancers can be identified and eradicated at even earlier stages.[1,9,30]

TABLE 19–9
Guidelines for the Early Detection of Cancer in People Without Symptoms

Age 20–40	**Age 40 and Over**
Cancer-Related Checkup Every 3 Years Should include the procedures listed below plus health counseling (such as tips on quitting cigarettes) and examinations for cancers of the thyroid, testes, prostate, mouth, ovaries, skin, and lymph nodes. Some people are at higher risk for certain cancers and may need to have tests more frequently.	***Cancer-Related Checkup Every Year*** Should include the procedures listed below plus health counseling (such as tips on quitting cigarettes) and examinations for cancers of the thyroid, testes, prostate, mouth, ovaries, skin, and lymph nodes. Some people are at higher risk for certain cancers and may need to have tests more frequently.
Breast	***Breast***
• Exam by doctor every 3 yrs	• Exam by doctor every year
• Self-exam every month	• Self-exam every month
• One baseline breast x-ray study between ages 35–40	• Breast x-ray study every year after 50 (between ages 40–50, ask your doctor)
• Higher risk group: Personal or family history of breast cancer, never had children, first child after 30	• Higher risk group: Personal or family history of breast cancer, never had children, first child after 30
Uterus	***Uterus***
• Pelvic exam every 3 yr	• Pelvic exam every year
Cervix	***Cervix***
• Pap test—after 2 initial negative tests 1 yr apart—at least every 3 yr; includes women under age 20 if sexually active	• Pap test—after 2 initial negative tests 1 yr apart—at least every 3 yr
• Higher risk group: Early age at first intercourse, multiple sex partners	• Higher risk group: Early age at first intercourse, multiple sex partners

(*Continued*)

TABLE 19-9
Guidelines for the Early Detection of Cancer in People Without Symptoms (*Continued*)

	Age 40 and Over
	Endometrium
	• Endometrial tissue sample at menopause if at risk
	• Higher risk group: Infertility, obesity, failure of ovulation, abnormal uterine bleeding, estrogen therapy
	Colon and Rectum
	• Digital rectal exam every year
	• Guaiac slide test every year after age 50
	• Proctological exam—after 2 initial negative tests 1 yr apart—every 3 to 5 yr after age 50
	• Higher risk group: Personal or family history of colon or rectal cancer, personal or family history of polyps in the colon or rectum, ulcerative colitis

(Cancer-Related Checkups. Publication No. 2070-LE. New York, American Cancer Society, 1980)

Tertiary Prevention

In tertiary prevention, the emphasis is on the expedient treatment of those individuals with symptoms and the prevention of disabilities that might arise because of therapy. The warning signals listed by the American Cancer Society are as follows:

- Change in bowel or bladder habits
- A sore that does not heal
- Unusual bleeding or discharge
- Thickening or lump in breast or elsewhere
- Indigestion or difficulty in swallowing
- Obvious change in wart or mole
- Nagging cough or hoarseness

These signals do not necessarily mean cancer, but they should be checked.

Summary

The diagnosis of cancer no longer means a death sentence for the patient; approximately 50% of all patients with cancer will live their normal life span. For this reason it is imperative that all those who care for the patient with cancer practice the principles of rehabilitation from the first day the patient enters the health-care setting. Often it is easier to prevent the disabilities that might arise than to correct them. For the half of the patients that will eventually die with this chronic disease, the practice of rehabilitative principles will ensure that they lead as comfortable lives as possible. The nurse provides a safe and therapeutic environment and recognizes and helps to prevent those complications that result from inactivity or disuse. The nurse can help the patient maintain his independence as long as possible by helping him to manage pain and by teaching him to use adaptive devices, to communicate, to eat, and to move. Specific problems the patient may encounter are determined by the type of cancer, the therapy, and the age and health status of the patient. The nurse can help the patient and the family adjust to the illness by providing accurate information tempered by an understanding of the patient's heritage, psychological state, and resources. A commitment to continuing education means that the nurse will be able to translate the latest scientific findings to the patient and the family and ensure that the best possible nursing care is given to the patient.[15,34,38]

References

1. ACS report on the cancer-related health checkup. Ca-A Cancer Journal for Clinicians 30(4):194, 1980
2. American Cancer Society: Cancer Facts and Figures 1984. New York, American Cancer Society, 1983
3. American Cancer Society: Cancer-Related Checkups. Publication Number 2070-LE, New York, ACS, 1980
4. Bonfiglio TA, Terry R: The pathology of cancer. In Rubin P, Bakemeier RF, Krackov SK (eds): Clinical Oncology: A Multidisciplinary Approach, 6th ed. New York, American Cancer Society, 1983
5. Brager BL, Yasko JM: Care of the Client Receiving Chemotherapy. Reston VA, Reston Publishing Company, 1984
6. Burns N: Nursing and Cancer. Philadelphia, WB Saunders, 1982
7. Committee on Diet, Nutrition, and Cancer/Assembly of Life Sciences/National Research Council: Diet, Nutrition, and Cancer. Washington DC, National Academy Press, 1982
8. Del Regato JA, Spjut HJ: Ackerman and del Regato's Cancer Diagnosis, Treatment and Prognosis, 5th ed. St Louis, CV Mosby, 1977
9. DeVita VT, Hellman S, Rosenberg SA (eds): Cancer Principles and Practice of Oncology. Philadelphia, JB Lippincott, 1982
10. DeWys WD, Killen JY: The paraneoplastic syndromes. In Rubin P, Bakemeier RF, Krackov SK (eds): Clinical Oncology: A Multidisciplinary Approach, 6th ed. New York, American Cancer Society, 1983
11. Di Julio JE, Bedigian JS: Hybridoma monoclonal antibody treatment of T-cell lymphomas: Clinical experience and nursing management. Oncology Nursing Forum 10(2):22, 1983
12. Doll R, Peto R: The Causes of Cancer: Quantitative Estimates of Avoidable Risks of Cancer in the United States Today. New York, Oxford Press, 1981

13. Donoghue M, Nunnally C, Yasko J: Nutritional Aspects of Cancer Care. Reston VA, Reston Publishing Company, 1980
14. Donovan MI: Cancer Care: A Guide for Patient Education. New York, Appleton-Century-Crofts, 1981
15. Donovan MI, Girton SE: Cancer Care Nursing, 2nd ed. New York, Appleton-Century-Crofts, 1984
16. Engleberg NC, Eisenstein BI: The impact of new cloning techniques on the diagnosis and treatment of infectious diseases. N Engl J Med 311(14):892, 1984
17. Hiatt HH, Watson JD, Winsten JN: Origins of Human Cancer: Book A, Incidence of Cancer in Humans; Book B, Mechanism of Carcinogenesis; Book C, Human Risk Assessment. Cold Spring Harbor Conferences on Cell Proliferation, Vol 4. Cold Spring Harbor Laboratory, 1979
18. Kahn SB, Love RR, Sherman C, Chakravorty R: Concepts in Cancer Medicine. New York, Grune & Stratton, 1983
19. Leaky I: Nursing care of the cancer patient: Radiation therapy. In Bouchard-Kurtz R, Speese-Owens N: Nursing Care of the Cancer Patient, 4th ed. St Louis, CV Mosby 1981
20. Marino LB (ed): Cancer Nursing. St Louis, CV Mosby, 1981
21. Mayer D, Hetrick K, Riggs C, Sherwin S: Weight loss in patients receiving recombinant leukocyte A interferon (IFLrA): A brief report. Cancer Nursing 7 (1):53, 1984
22. Molbo DM: Cancer. In Carnevali DL, Patrick M: Nursing Management for the Elderly. Philadelphia, JB Lippincott, 1979
23. Nutrition and Cancer: Cause and Prevention. American Cancer Society Special Report. Ca-A Cancer Journal for Clinicians 34(2):121, 1984
24. Oldham RK: Biologicals and biological response modifiers: Fourth modality of cancer treatment. Cancer Treat Rep 68 (1):221, 1984
25. Oldham RK: Monoclonal antibodies in cancer therapy. J of Clinical Oncology 1(a):582, 1983
26. Pitot HC: Fundamentals of Oncology, 2nd ed. New York, Marcel Dekker, 1981
27. Robbins SL, Cotran RS: Pathologic Basis of Disease, 2nd ed. Philadelphia, WB Saunders, 1979
28. Rubin P. Bakemeier RF, Krackov SK (eds): Clinical Oncology: A Multidisciplinary Approach, 6th ed. New York, American Cancer Society, 1983
29. Sarna LP: Concepts of nursing care for patients receiving radiation therapy. In Vredevoe DL, Deriarian A, Sarna LP: Concepts of Oncology Nursing. Englewood Cliffs NJ, Prentice-Hall, 1981
30. Schottenfeld D, Fraumeni JF Jr: Cancer Epidemiology and Prevention. Philadelphia, WB Saunders, 1982
31. Scott RE, Wille JJ: Research review mechanisms for the initiation and promotion of carcinogenesis: A review and a new concept. Mayo Clin Proc 59:107, 1984
32. Strohl RA, Hogan CM: The nurse and cancer care. In Rubin P, Bakemeier RF, Krackov SK (eds): Clincal Oncology: A Multidisciplinary Approach, 6th ed. New York, American Cancer Society, 1983
33. Vitetta ES et al: Immunotoxins: A new approach to cancer therapy. Science 219 (4585):644, 1983
34. Vredevoe D, Derdiarian A. Sarna LP et al: Concepts in Oncology Nursing. Englewood Cliffs NJ, Prentice-Hall, 1981
35. Walter J: Cancer and Radiotherapy: A Short Guide for Nurses and Medical Students, 2nd ed. New York, Churchill Livingstone, 1977
36. Weinberg RA: A molecular basis of cancer. Sci Am 249(5):126, 1984
37. Weisman AV: Coping with Cancer. New York, McGraw-Hill, 1979
38. Yasko JM: Guidelines for Cancer Care: Symptom Management. Reston VA, Reston Publishing Company, 1983.

Bibliography

Suggested Readings

Alt J: Selected Abstracts on Oncology Nursing. International Cancer Research Data Bank Program of the National Cancer Institute, NIH Publication Number PB83-922804. Washington, US Department of Health and Human Services, 1983

Cancer Chemotherapy Guidelines and Recommendations for Nursing Guidelines and Practice. Oncology Nursing Society, 1984

Jones RB, Frank R, Mass T: Safe Handling of Chemotherapeutic Agents: A Report from the Mount Sinai Medical Center. American Cancer Society Professional Education Publication. New York, American Cancer Society, 1983

Kreamer K, Aquila K, Haller M et al: Information about radiation therapy. Oncology Nursing Forum 11(4):67, 1984

Longman AJ, Rogers BP: Altered cell growth in cancer and the nursing implications. Cancer Nursing 7(5):405, 1984

Shimkin MB: Contrary to Nature. NIH Publication No. 76-720. Washington, Department of Health, Education, and Welfare, 1977

Periodicals for Nursing Care of Patients with Cancer

Ca-A Cancer Journal for Clinicians, New York, American Cancer Society, Inc

Cancer Nursing: An International Journal for Cancer Care. Official publication of the International Society of Nurses in Cancer Care and the European Oncology Nursing Society. New York, Masson Publishing USA, Inc.

Cancer Nursing News. American Cancer Society Newsletter for Nurses. New York, American Cancer Society

Oncology Nursing Forum. Official publication of the Oncology Nursing Society, 3111 Banksville Road, Pittsburgh PA 15216

Chapter 20

Lithiasis

Constance J. Hirnle

Human disease resulting from stone formation is not peculiar to our industrialized society. Evidence of lithiasis can be traced back 7000 years, to the age of an Egyptian pharaoh from whom a stone was extracted. Greek writings of Hippocrates (400 BC) and Galen (AD 200) document stone disease, postulate causes for stone formation, and discuss the medical and surgical treatment of the time. More recent medical literature continues to document the occurrence and treatment of stone-related illness.

Calculus means "pebble" in Latin. A calculus is a mass of precipitated material usually derived from mineral salts. Frequently this concretion is deposited in excretory ducts. A condition in which a person has a calculus is referred to as *lithiasis* (from a Greek word meaning "stone formation"). Lithiasis can be described more definitely by the addition of prefixes to the root. Such prefixes often note the location of the stone. For example, cholelithiasis refers to stones in the gallbladder, whereas nephrolithiasis refers to a stone in the kidney.

Calcification, the deposition of calcium salts in body tissues, is a process which often accompanies cardiac valve disease or metastatic cancer. This process is distinct from calculus formation and is discussed in Chapter 22.

The purpose of this chapter is to explain the process of calculus formation, those factors that affect calculus formation, and the physiological effects of calculi once they occur. Specific types of calculi are briefly introduced. More detailed information describing urinary and biliary stones can be found in Chapters 61 and 82.

Factors Promoting Stone Formation

Supersaturation of Crystalloid Content of the Secretion

Stones are formed when crystalloids (substances capable of forming crystals) precipitate out of solution to form solid material. An important factor in determining whether this precipitation will occur is the number of particles per volume of liquid. When a solution contains all the particles that it can hold it is said to be *saturated*. Calculi cannot form in solutions that have not reached this saturation point. An illustration of this principle would be adding salt to a beaker of water. At a specific point, when no more salt can be added and still remain in solution, the solution is said to be saturated. Beyond this point, if more salt is added, precipitation will occur. *Supersaturation* is the term given to this solution. The more supersaturated the solution, the more likely calculi will form.

Specific crystalloids responsible for stone formation can vary greatly. Urinary stones are most commonly composed of calcium oxalate or calcium phosphate, but they can also be composed of magnesium ammonium phosphate, uric acid, or cystine. When any of these substances are present in the urine in abnormally large amounts, the likelihood of stone formation from this material is greatly enhanced. The increased concentration of the stone's constituent in the urine is the most important factor in the predisposition to stone development.[5] Although supersaturation is necessary for crystals to precipitate out of solution, supersaturated urines do not always cause this to happen.[3] When research finds the answer to why certain individuals do not form stones, even in the presence of supersaturated urine, we may be able to use this information to prevent stone formation in susceptible individuals. Figure 20–1 shows multiple calculi located throughout the kidney.

Gallstone formation is also related to saturation levels, in this case within bile. Supersaturation of cholesterol or a decreased amount of bile salts or lecithin can promote cholesterol stone formation, whereas pigment stones appear to be related to supersaturated levels of unconjugated bilirubin.

Nidus

In addition to supersaturation, a nidus, or nucleus around which layers can be deposited, is important in the development of a calculus. A solid mass acting as a nidus can be composed of a variety of materials, such as fibrin, necrotic epithelial cells, or a foreign body. In supersaturated solutions, substances themselves may crystallize out of solution, providing a nidus upon which further deposition may occur.[1]

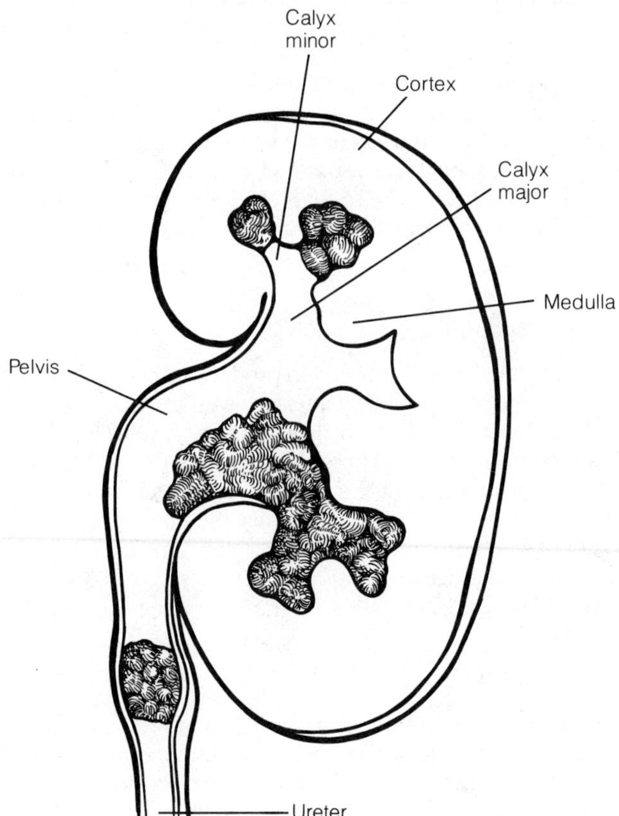

FIGURE 20–1 Sites of kidney stone formation.

Inhibitors of Stone Formation

Certain factors present in urine are thought to inhibit stone formation. Pyrophosphate is the most significant urinary stone inhibitor. It suppresses nucleation and retards the growth of nuclei already formed.[1] Other inhibitors found in urine are mucopolysaccharides, diphosphonates, urea, citrate, magnesium, certain amino acids, and trace metals.[5] Inhibitors of biliary stone formation have also been hypothesized but they are less well understood.[6]

Stasis

Stasis of the supersaturated solution further promotes calculi formation since crystals precipitate more readily from a fluid that is stagnant. Urinary stasis can result from immobility, urinary obstruction, or neurological impairment to the bladder. Biliary stasis can be the result of spasms of the sphincter of Oddi, faulty gallbladder emptying, obstructions in the duct of or malformation of the gallbladder itself. Delayed emptying of the gallbladder may be related to hormonal factors.

Infection

Inflammatory damage that results from the infectious process can predispose an individual to calculus formation. Urea-splitting organisms have been directly linked with renal calculi composed of struvite. Bacteria in the urine can also serve as particulate nidi to further enhance stone formation. The inflammatory process often increases capillary permeability , which can foster increasing saturation levels of substances linked to calculi formation. Inflammation also promotes stasis by decreasing lumen size within the urinary system.

Cholelithiasis is directly linked to infection and inflammation of the gallbladder or bile ducts. Inflamed mucosa permits increased absorption of bile salts which decreases the solubility of cholesterol. *Escherischia coli* is commonly found to occur in conjunction with pigment stones, whereas streptococcus is more commonly associated with cholesterol stones.[4]

pH of Solution

The pH of a solution can affect the solubility of many stone-forming compounds, thus increasing or decreasing the saturation level of the element within the solution. For example, uric acid salts are insoluble in an acid urine, but as the pH increases above 5.5, more uric acid salts will remain in solution. Renal tubular necrosis and the administration of carbonic anhydrous inhibitors foster stone development by altering urinary pH.

Process of Calculus Formation

Even though the exact interplay of etiologic factors is unclear in stone formation, the physical process of calculi formation is a simple building process containing two phases—*nucleation* and *aggregation*. Nucleation is the formation of a nidus either heterogeneously or homogeneously. Aggregation is a layering process during which the stone increases in size.

Nucleation

In the process of nucleation, crystallites are formed from supersaturated solutions. Most nucleation is heterogeneous, in that it depends on a solid particle similar in crystal structure from which the nucleus can form. Homogeneous nucleation occurs when supersaturation of the solution is great enough for crystallites to adhere to each other to form a nucleus.[2]

Aggregation

Once a homogeneous or heterogeneous nucleus is formed, aggregation can occur as long as the solution remains supersaturated. This is a building process in which the nucleus gradually increases in size because of the addition of more crystallites. The interplay of factors such as saturation level, stasis, infection, pH, and inhibiting factors will determine the amount of aggregation occurring around any given nucleus.

TABLE 20–1
Types of Calculi

Name	*Location*	*Composition*
Urolithiasis	Urinary tract (kidney, ureters, bladder)	Calcium, 65% Struvite, 15% Uric acid, 10% Cystine, 10%
Cholelithiasis	Gallbladder Common bile duct	Cholesterol Pigment Mixed composition
Prostate calculi	Prostate	Calcium phosphate Calcium oxalate Struvite
Salivary calculi	Salivary gland	Carbonic apatite Hydroxyapatite
Pancreatic calculi	Pancreas	Calcite Brushite
Broncholithiasis	Bronchus	Calcium phosphate Calcium carbonate
Articular calculi	Joint	Sodium urate Calcium urate
Lacrimal calculi	Tear duct	

Physiological Alterations Caused by Calculi

Calculi are often found on postmortem examination in individuals who have been symptom-free and never sought medical assistance. The size and location of the calculi are important in determining the physiological alterations and the onset of symptoms. Urinary and biliary tract stones are most common and for that reason are the most significant clinically. The specific pathophysiology of each type of urolithiasis is discussed in detail in Chapter 61. Biliary stones are covered in Chapter 82. Stones have also been found to form in other areas of the body, including the prostate, pancreas, salivary glands, and tear ducts (Table 20–1). Regardless of location, if the calculus grows large enough to interfere with physiological functioning, symptoms become apparent and removal is warranted. The most common signs and symptoms are pain, obstruction, infection, and hemorrhage.

Pain

Pain is a common symptom in lithiasis. The sudden distention of tissue or spasm of a duct can result in excruciating pain. Renal colic is caused when hydrostatic pressure distends the renal pelvis and proximal ureter. Intermittent episodes of intense pain occur in which the pain often radiates from the kidney to the abdomen, genitalia, and legs. Biliary colic results from the lodging of stones in the cystic duct, causing the gallbladder to spasm as it attempts to empty bile into the duodenum. The result is severe, intermittent upper right abdominal pain that radiates to the back and right shoulder.

Obstruction

As stones migrate, they often produce obstruction when they partially or completely interfere with the flow of urine or bile. In renal calculi, hydronephrosis results from the obstruction and can lead to renal damage. In the gallbladder, calculus obstruction of the cystic duct interferes with the flow of bile into the duodenum so that the bile is unavailable to aid in fat digestion. Obstruction of the common bile duct results in obstructive jaundice. Figure 20–2 shows stones deposited in various locations of the biliary duct system.

Infection

Stasis, resulting from obstruction, often predisposes the individual to the growth of microorganisms, causing infection. Under normal conditions, due to the cleansing action of the moving fluids, microorganisms have little opportunity to colonize in hollow organs and their ducts. When fluid mobility is decreased, the cleansing action is lost. Pyelonephritis is

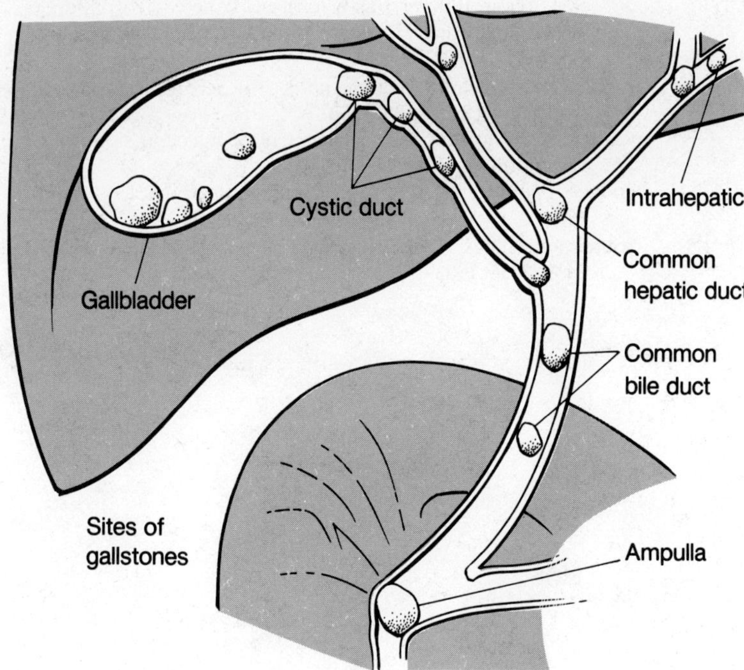

FIGURE 20–2 Gallstones are located in multiple sites, where they may cause pain, obstruction, infection, or bleeding.

a common infectious complication of urolithiasis, whereas ascending cholangitis frequently accompanies gallstones. Symptoms of infection, such as fever, chills, elevated white blood count, and positive cultures for bacteria, are often found in the individual with a calculus.

Hemorrhage

Presence or movement of calculi in ducts or hollow organs can cause trauma to the delicate mucosal lining. This trauma can cause bleeding as surface capillaries are scraped and broken. Hemorrhage is more frequent if the stone is irregularly shaped and rough in texture. Microscopic or gross hematuria is often associated with urolithiasis. Hemorrhage associated with cholelithiasis is more difficult to detect.

Nursing Implications

Knowledge of factors promoting calculus formation may sometimes permit nurses to initiate preventive strategies. Prevention is particularly applicable for nephrolithiasis and may include changes in diet and increases in fluid intake. These measures are described in detail in Chapter 61. Prevention of cholelithiasis is more difficult because reversible predisposing factors have not yet been clearly identified.

When a patient presents with a clinical picture suggestive of lithiasis, nursing interventions focus on the relief of symptoms. As previously described, intense pain is characteristically associated with both urolithiasis and cholelithiasis. Narcotic administration and nursing techniques to minimize the pain are therefore of great importance. Additionally, bleeding and manifestations of obstruction or infection may be present. Interventions specific to these problems are discussed in later chapters.

References

1. Brenner B, Rector F: The Kidney, 2nd ed. Philadelphia, WB Saunders, 1981
2. Coe F: Nephrolithiasis: Pathogenesis and Treatment. Chicago, Year Book Medical Publishers, 1978
3. Londsdal K: Human Stones. Sci Am 219(6):104, 1968
4. Maki T: Pathogenesis of calcium bilirubinate gallstones: Role of E. coli, β-glucuronidase and coagulation by inorganic ions, polyelectrolytes and agitation. Ann Surg 164:90, 1966
5. Robbins S, Angell M, Kumar V: Basic Pathology. Philadelphia, WB Saunders, 1981
6. Sodeman W, Sodeman T: Pathologic Physiology: Mechanisms of Disease, 6th ed. Philadelpia, WB Saunders, 1979

Bibliography

Banner MP, Pollack HM: Urolithiasis in the lower urinary tract. Semin Roentgenol 17(2):140–148, 1982

Coe F, Parks J: Hyperuricosuria and calcium nephrolithiasis. Urol Clin North Am (8)2:227–244, 1981

Derrick F, Carter WC: Kidney stone disease: Evaluation and management. Postgrad Med 66(4):115–125, 1979

Fleisch H et al: Urolithiasis Research. New York, Plenum Press, 1976

Gault P: How to break the kidney stone cycle. Nursing 78 8:24–31, 1978

Gracie WA, Ransohoff DF: The natural history of silent gallstones. N Engl J Med 307(13):798–800, 1982

Kinney AB, Bount M: Effect of cranberry juice on urinary pH. Nurs Res 28:287–290, 1979

Lyles K, Drezner M: An overview of calcium homeostasis in humans. Urol Clin North Am 8(2):209–226, 1981

Menon M, Krishnan CS: Evaluation and medical management of the patient with calcium stone disease. Urol Clin North Am 10(4):595–615, 1983

Metheny N: Renal stones and urinary pH. Am J Nurs 82:1372–1375, 1982

Nemoy NJ: Axioms on renal calculi. Hospital Medicine 15(2):8–19, 1979

Netter F: Ciba Collection of Medical Illustrations, Vol 3 Digestive System; Part III Liver, biliary tract, and pancreas. Vol 6 Kidneys, Ureters and Urinary bladder. Summit, NJ, CIBA Pharmaceutical Co, 1964

Pak C: The spectrum of pathogenesis of hypercalciuria. Urol Clin North Am 8(2):245–252, 1981

Resnick M: Evaluation and management of infection stones. Urol Clin North Am 8(2):265–276, 1981

Rodgers A, Spector M: Human stones. Endeavour 5(3):119–126, 1981

Sound and shock waves shatter kidney stones. JAMA 249(18): 2433–2435, 1983

Chapter 21

Hemostatic Responses

Ruth A. Gregersen

Normal Hemostasis

The normal hemostatic mechanism is designed to protect against bleeding from blood vessels that have developed a break in their integrity.[9] Hemostasis is usually accomplished by a combination of three interrelated processes:

1. Rapid contraction of involved and adjacent blood vessels
2. Formation of a platelet plug and release of substances that enhance vasoconstriction and coagulation
3. Blood coagulation by way of both the intrinsic and extrinsic systems

The first two responses occur immediately, whereas the third acts over a longer period to maintain hemostasis. These three processes are balanced by the complex mechanism of fibrinolysis, which slowly breaks down formed clots and maintains the fluid nature of blood. The balance between these processes is vital. Imbalance in one direction leads to excessive bleeding and shock, while imbalance in the other direction leads to excessive clotting or thrombosis.

This chapter reviews the normal hemostatic mechanism, then introduces alterations in the system that lead to abnormal bleeding or clotting. Lastly, an overview of nursing measures related to hemostatic disorders is presented.

The Hemostatic Mechanism

Vascular Contribution to Hemostasis. All blood vessels are lined with a continuous single layer of endothelial cells. One of the basic functions of normal intact endothelium is its nonreactivity to platelets and coagulation factors by a variety of passive and active mechanisms.[9]

Rapid vasoconstriction is a direct response following vessel injury. This vasoconstriction is probably due to the release of serotonin and other substances from platelets.[2] The relative importance of vasoconstriction varies with vessel size. In small vessels, platelet plug formation alone can halt bleeding. The larger vessels, veins, and arteries are more dependent on vasoconstriction along with the activation of the other hemostatic components.

Platelet Contributions to Hemostasis. Thrombocytes (platelets) are small, non-nucleated cell fragments formed in the bone marrow. About 80% are found circulating in the blood and 20% are in the spleen. Platelets have multiple functions. They continuously maintain vascular integrity. Without platelets, red cells move through the vessel walls and may appear as red spots (petechiae) in the skin. Platelets initially arrest bleeding by platelet plug formation and later help stabilize the plug. Platelets may also promote vascular healing by stimulating the growth of arterial smooth muscle and skin fibroblasts through the release of platelet-derived growth factor (PDGF).[3]

The formation of a hemostatic plug begins within seconds of vessel injury by the adhesion of platelets to the exposed connective tissue (particularly collagen) in the vessel wall (Fig 21–1).[3] The adhesion involves the interaction of platelet surface glycoproteins ($GP1_b$) with the connective tissue. A coagulation factor is required as a plasma cofactor.[9] In addition, the adhesion is accompanied by a platelet shape change from discoid to irregular spheres with spine pseudopods.[4]

The initial adhesion of platelets to connective tissue is followed by adherence of platelets to each other, a process known as *aggregation*. Platelet aggregation is accomplished by the release of adenosine diphosphate (ADP), which is a substance that promotes platelet aggregation by binding to specific platelet receptors.[3] Other substances, such as collagen, thrombin, epinephrine, platelet activating factor, and vasopressin also stimulate aggregation. All of these substances require the presence of extracellular calcium ions for aggregation. Contact of platelets with collagen fibers or the action upon them by other aggregating agents stimulates the synthesis within the platelets of prostaglandins and thromboxane A_2 (a potent platelet aggregating and vasoconstricting agent.)[3]

To stimulate further aggregation and hemostatic processes, the platelets secrete substances from storage granules (see Table 21–1). This *release reaction* is stimulated by many substances, including ADP, epinephrine, collagen, and

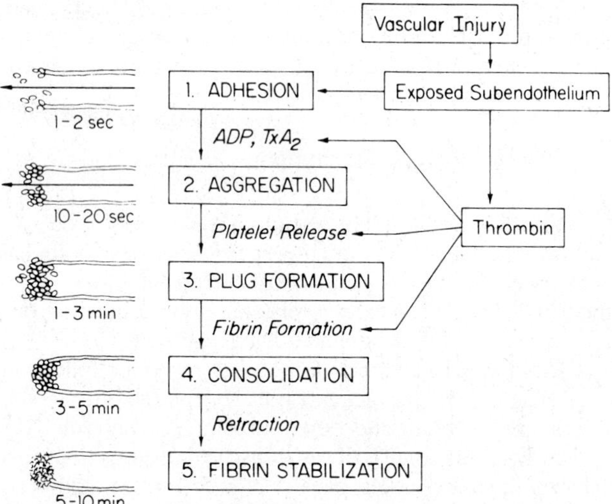

FIGURE 21–1 Hemostatic plug formation. The formation of a platelet plug proceeds through the following sequence: (1) platelet adhesion to exposed subendothelial connective tissue structures; (2) platelet aggregation by ADP, thromboxane A_2, and thrombin recruitment through transformation of discoid platelets into reactive spiny spheres that interact with one another through calcium-dependent fibrinogen bridges; (3) contribution of platelet coagulant activity to the coagulation process which stabilizes the plug with a fibrin mesh; and (4) retraction of the platelet mass to provide a dense thrombus. (Thompson AR, Harker LA: Manual of Hemostasis and Thrombosis, 3rd ed, p 11. Philadelphia, FA Davis, 1983)

TABLE 21–1
Selected Substances Found in Platelet Storage Granules

Alpha granules (readily released)	Platelet factor 4 (PF_4) Low affinity PF_4 Beta thromboglobulin Fibrinogen Growth factor(s) Factor V Factor VIII/von Willebrand factor
Dense bodies (require greater platelet stimulation for release)	ATP, ADP (storage pool) Serotonin

(Adapted from Hardisty RM: Platelets, blood vessels and hemostasis: Disorders of platelet and vascular function. In Hardisty RM, Weatherall DJ [eds]: Blood and Its Disorders, 2nd ed. Oxford, Blackwell Scientific Publications, 1982

thrombin. Platelet adhesion, aggregation, and release reaction all work together to form the temporary platelet plug, soon to be bound together and converted into the stable clot by fibrin.

Blood Coagulation. Table 21–2 lists the 12 coagulation factors and their synonyms as designated by the International Committee on Nomenclature of Blood Clotting Factors. The numerals are assigned in order of discovery and indicate nothing about the sequence of reaction. The substance previously labeled factor VI has since been identified as a component of one of the other coagulation factors; therefore, it has been eliminated. The most recently described factors have not been assigned roman numerals.

All coagulation factors (with the exception of factor IV, calcium) are proteins. They all circulate inactively in the plasma (except factor III, tissue factor, which is released from damaged cells). The major site of synthesis of the coagulation proteins (with the exception of factor VIII) is the liver.[10] Vitamin K is essential for the synthesis of the prothrombin factors (II, VII, IX, and X).

The active forms of each factor are indicated by the lower case "a" following the roman number (with the exception of factor I, fibrinogen, which is converted to fibrin, and factor II, prothrombin, in which the active form is called thrombin).

The goal of all the interactions of the coagulation proteins is the formation of thrombin, which stabilizes the platelet plug and produces the desired change of fibrinogen to fibrin. The fibrin forms a gel that we recognize as the clot.

Clotting of blood can be initiated in two ways (see Fig. 21–2). One requires factor III (tissue factor), which is released at the site of injury, possibly from the intima of blood vessels.[9,12] Since tissue factor is not found in the blood, it is an extrinsic substance in coagulation, therefore the name *extrinsic pathway*. Tissue factor reacts with factor VII and factor IV (calcium) to convert factor X to its active form.

The second way blood clotting is initiated is by way of the *intrinsic pathway*. This pathway is initiated when factor

TABLE 21–2
International Nomenclature for Blood Coagulation Factors

Factor	*Synonyms*	*Function*
I*	Fibrinogen	Converted by thrombin to fibrin, which stabilizes blood clot
II†	Prothrombin, prethrombin	Precursor of thrombin, which converts fibrinogen to fibrin
III	Tissue factor, tissue thromboplastin	Tissue lipoprotein, which initiates the extrinsic pathway
IV	Calcium	Necessary for interaction of all clotting factors except XI, XII, and IIa
V*	Proaccelerin, labile factor, accelerator globulin (AcG)	Accelerates the conversion of prothrombin to thrombin in the common pathway
VI	Number is not now used	
VII†	Proconvertin, serum prothrombin conversion accelerator (SPCA), stable factor, autoprothrombin I	Activates factor X in the extrinsic pathway
VIII*	Antihemophilic globulin (AHG), antihemophilic factor (AHF), antihemophilic factor A, platelet cofactor I	Assists factor IXa in activating factor X in the intrinsic pathway
IX†	Plasma thromboplastin component (PTC), Christmas factor, antihemophilic factor B, autoprothrombin II, platelet cofactor II	Activates factor X in the intrinsic pathway
XI	Plasma thromboplastin antecedent PTA), antihemophilic factor C	Activated by factor XII; accelerates thrombin formation
XII	Hageman factor	Activated by "foreign" surface in intrinsic pathway
XIII*	Fibrin-stabilizing factor (FSF), fibrinase, Laki-Lorand factor	Produces a stronger fibrin clot
Pre-kallikrein	Fletcher factor	Contact activating factor
High-molecular weight kininogen		Contact activating factor

* Activity is destroyed during the coagulation process.
† Vitamin K dependent for production

XII is exposed to a "foreign" surface such as collagen, skin, or glass outside the body. (This is why blood clots in glass blood collection tubes unless an anticoagulant is added.) All of the elements of the intrinsic pathway are found within the plasma.

The intrinsic pathway proceeds as a cascade of enzymatic reactions, with the active form of each factor activating the next. Factors XII, XI, and IX must be activated in sequence before factor X is converted to factor Xa. Factor VIII, platelet lipoprotein (platelet factor 3), prekallikrein, and high-molecular-weight kininogen (HMWK) are additional requirements in various stages of the cascade.

Both of these systems culminate in the *common pathway*. Activated factor X (Xa) is responsible for the conversion of prothrombin to thrombin. Factor V, platelet factor 3 (pF_3), and calcium are involved in the reaction.[12] Thrombin then acts as an enzyme to split the fibrinogen molecule to produce fibrin monomers that polymerize to form a loose fibrin mesh.[5] Through the interaction of factor XIIIa and calcium, a tough, insoluble fibrin polymer (stable clot) is formed. This holds the adherent, aggregated platelets onto the disrupted vascular surface, which prevents or minimizes blood loss. Platelet contraction then draws the fibrin polymers tightly over the exposed vascular wall (clot retraction) and away from blood flow within the vessel lumen.[5]

It is important to remember that the intrinsic and extrinsic systems act interdependently. The extrinsic system may accelerate coagulation by rapidly producing small amounts of thrombin which can (1) convert factors V and VIII to more rapidly reactive forms, (2) enhance platelet aggregation, (3) activate factor XIII, as well as (4) institute fibrin formation.[12]

The Fibrinolytic Mechanism and Inhibition of Coagulation

Several mechanisms exist in the circulation for maintaining blood in a fluid state. Flowing blood reduces the chance of focal fibrin formation by removing procoagulant material before activation is completed.[9] The liver and reticuloendothelial system remove activated clotting factors and fibrin.[6] Several proteins, including antithrombin III, which is found in blood, inactivate the activated coagulation factors. Antithrombin III reacts with thrombin and other activated clotting factors to form an inactive complex. Heparin, a substance found in the liver, lungs, and other tissues, reacts with antithrombin III to increase its rate of activity several thousandfold. The mechanism for this activation is hypothesized to result from a conformation change in antithrombin III.[11]

The fibrinolytic mechanism for dissolving fibrin is produced by the action of plasmin. Plasmin is formed from a precursor, plasminogen, normally abundant in plasma. The complex mechanism of fibrinolysis, diagrammed in Figure 21–3, is a physiological process of removing unwanted insoluble fibrin deposits by plasmin, a specific protease that digests stabilized fibrin polymers within the thrombus.[3] The fibrinolytic process produces several products termed *fibrin degradation products* (FDPs) or fibrin split products. These products act as anticoagulants by delaying the polymerization of fibrin.

Disorders of Hemostasis and Coagulation

The hemostatic mechanism is very complex with many different but interrelated components. A disorder in any one of these areas will lead to abnormal bleeding or clotting. Bleeding disorders can be caused by abnormalities of blood vessels, platelets, or plasma coagulation factors, or a combination of these. The bleeding may be a fairly minor manifestation, such as easy bruising of the skin, or major, with massive hemorrhage leading to shock and possible death.

Abnormal clotting can occur in arteries or veins. The

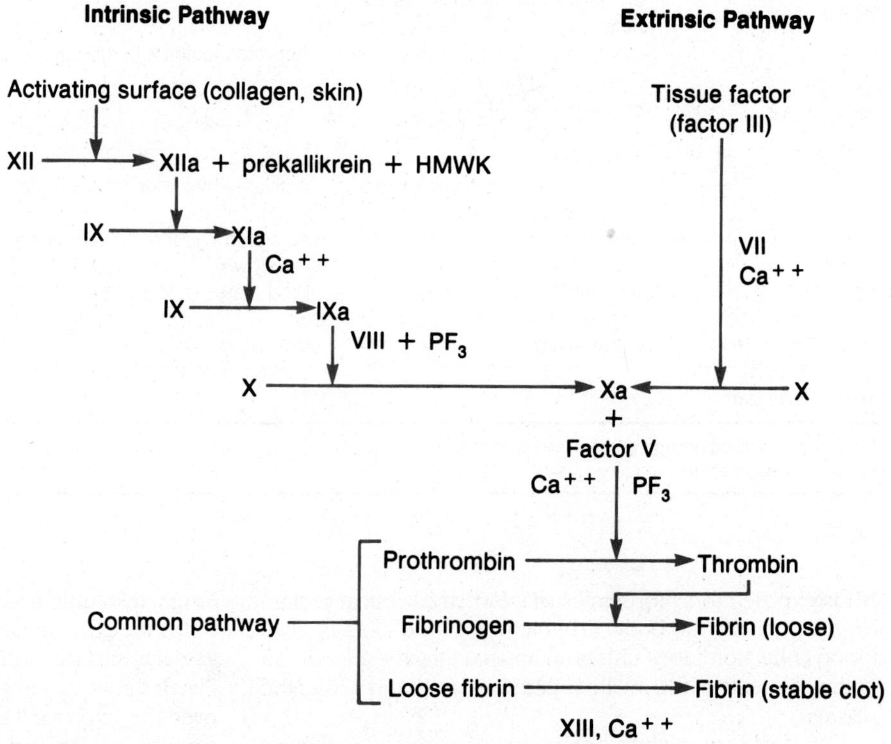

Intrinsic Pathway

Extrinsic Pathway

Activating surface (collagen, skin)

XII → XIIa + prekallikrein + HMWK

IX → XIa

Ca++

IX → IXa

VIII + PF_3

X → Xa ← X

Tissue factor (factor III)

VII

Ca++

Xa + Factor V

Ca++ PF_3

Common pathway

Prothrombin → Thrombin

Fibrinogen → Fibrin (loose)

Loose fibrin → Fibrin (stable clot)

XIII, Ca++

FIGURE 21–2 The intrinsic and extrinsic pathways lead to activation of factor X. Activated factor X plus factor V are essential to the activation of the common pathway which leads to the formation of a stable blood clot.

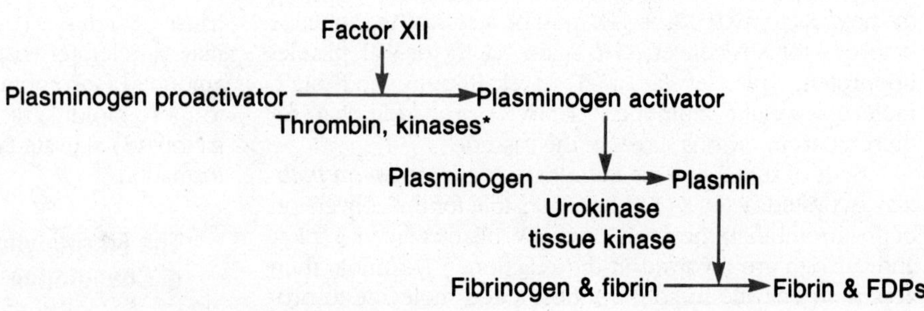

FIGURE 21–3 The fibrinolytic system causes lysis of blood clots. Plasmin splits fibrin into degradation products (FDPs).

manifestations depend on the location of the clot. Fairly minor problems such as inflammation, swelling, and pain occur with superficial thrombophlebitis, whereas death can occur from infarcted brain tissue due to a clot in a cerebral artery. The most commonly encountered disorders are briefly addressed in this chapter and more thoroughly discussed in Chapter 54.

Clinical Assessment of Hemostasis

A careful patient history is essential to direct nursing as well as medical assessment of hemostatic abnormalities. An in-depth history will often point toward an accurate diagnosis that can then be corroborated by physical examination and laboratory studies.

To clinically assess bleeding, historical data should be obtained that includes the type of bleeding (petechiae, bruising, single or multiple bleeding sites), pattern of bleeding (spontaneous vs. postinjury or surgery), family history of bleeding problems, previous or current therapy (drugs, over the counter as well as prescription), and associated diseases (*e.g.,* liver disease, kidney disease, cancer). Table 21–3 lists various types of bleeding that may be found on physical examination and suggests possible causes. Included in this list are petechiae (Fig. 21–4), purpura (Fig. 21–5), ecchymoses (Fig. 21–6), telangiectases, and hermarthroses. The ultimate diagnosis of bleeding problems depends on laboratory testing.[9] Laboratory tests are presented in Chapter 49.

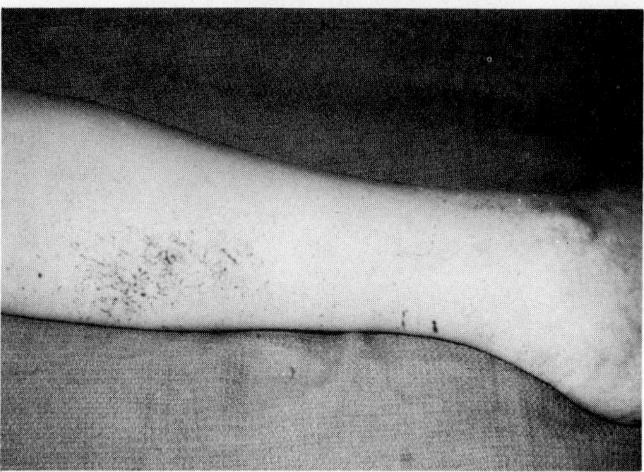

FIGURE 21–4 Petechiae. Small capillary hemorrhages resulting from vessel or platelet abnormalities. (Reproduced with permission from Health Sciences Center for Educational Resources, University of Washington)

The clinical assessment of clotting disorders depends on whether the clot formation is arterial or venous. In addition, manifestations vary according to the tissue affected (such as the heart, brain, or lungs) and will be discussed elsewhere. Distinctive characteristics between arterial vs. venous clot formation are covered later in this chapter. Laboratory tests

TABLE 21–3
Physical Findings in Bleeding Disorders

	Description	*Probable Cause*
Petechiae	Small capillary hemorrhages, flat, 1–3 mm in diameter, do not blanch with pressure, deep red or reddish purple in color; most common in dependent areas	Vessel or platelet abnormalities
Purpura	Petechiae that have grown together to form larger lesion	Vessel or platelet abnormalities
Ecchymoses (bruises)	Large macular areas, blue-black initially, fading to brownish green, then yellow; due to blood in the subcutaneous tissues and skin	Usually from veins Common with disorders of platelet and vessels as well as coagulation defects
Telangiectases	2–3 mm purple or red purple flat macular spots; blanch with pressure, bleed easily; common on face, lips and mucous membranes, hands and feet	Spider telangiectasis due to liver disease and pregnancy Hemorrhagic telangiectasis due to a hereditary bleeding disorder of blood vessels
Hemarthrosis	Hemorrhage into synovial joints. May be no external evidence of bleeding, only complaints of severe joint pain	Severe hereditary coagulation disorders

(Wintrobe MM, Lee GR, Boggs DR et al: Clinical Hematology, 8th ed. Philadelphia, Lea & Febiger, 1981)

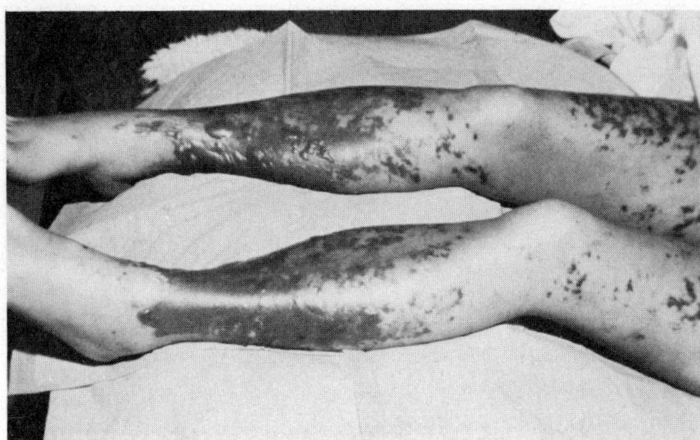

FIGURE 21–5 Purpura. Petechiae which have coalesced to form larger lesions, due to vessel or platelet abnormalities. (Reproduced with permission from Health Sciences Center for Educational Resources, University of Washington)

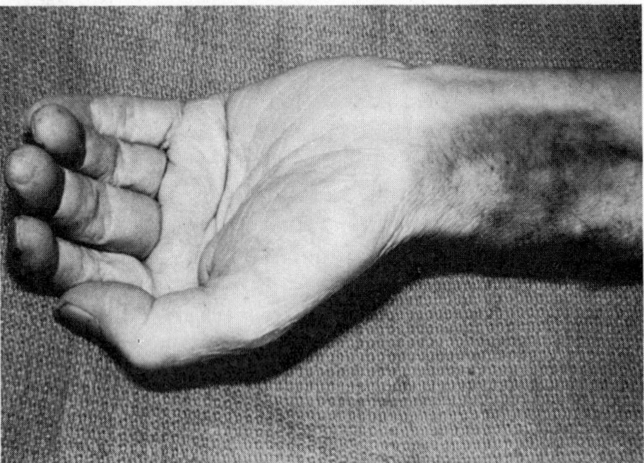

FIGURE 21–6 Ecchymosis. Large blue-black area due to extravasation of blood into skin and subcutaneous tissue; caused by vessel, platelet, or coagulation abnormality. (Reproduced with permission from Health Sciences Center for Educational Resources, University of Washington)

are fairly nonspecific and are generally used for monitoring anticoagulant therapy rather than for diagnosis.

Abnormal Bleeding

Vascular Disorders. The presence of purpura (see Table 21–3), without platelet or blood coagulation abnormalities, implies a vascular disorder. The diseases associated with vascular abnormalities are commonly termed nonthrombocytopenic purpuras.

The basic pathophysiology of bleeding due to vascular abnormalities is not well known; however, a feature common to all of these conditions is the loss of vascular integrity with an increase in vascular permeability and fragility.[14] Vascular disorders can be caused by a wide variety of mechanisms, such as systemic diseases, drugs, allergic disorders, and infections. The manifestations vary from local skin eruptions and bleeding from mucous membranes to serious, widespread bleeding. Purpuric skin lesions are common to many of the vascular disorders. Platelet function and coagulation factors are normal.

Platelet Disorders. The major classifications of platelet disorders are (1) thrombocytopenia: insufficient number of platelets; (2) thrombocytopathy: functionally abnormal platelets; and (3) thrombocytosis: excessive platelets. These disorders may be further classified into distinct diagnoses as discussed in Chapter 54.

Petechial bleeding commonly occurs with platelet abnormalities. Petechial lesions of severe thrombocytopenia are not elevated and frequently will first appear over the ankles. They may later become widespread.[1] Minor cuts bleed for a long time because platelet plugs do not form. Post-traumatic or postsurgical bleeding usually has an immediate onset and responds to local measures such as pressure over the area. Mucosal, renal, and gastrointestinal bleeding are also common in thrombocytopenia.

Coagulation Disorders. Many blood coagulation disorders are congenital, for example, the hemophilias. Other disorders, such as disseminated intravascular coagulation, are acquired. The bleeding manifestations of congenital coagulation disorders may be mild, with skin and mucosal bleeding, or severe, with hemarthroses and intramuscular hematomas. Petechiae are rare, but gastrointestinal bleeding, epistaxis (nosebleed) and menorrhagia (excessive menstrual bleeding) are common. Serious bleeding following trauma or surgery is a hazard. The bleeding of acquired coagulation disorders manifests in a variety of ways. Petechiae and ecchymoses are very common along with bleeding from around sites of injury and every body orifice.

Thrombosis and Thromboembolism

"The formation of a clotted mass of blood in the noninterrupted cardiovascular system is known as a thrombosis, and the mass itself is termed a *thrombus.*"[7] A thrombus that breaks loose and travels within the blood vessel is termed an *embolus,* thus the term *thromboembolism.* The potential outcome from either thrombosis or embolism is infarction, which causes the necrosis of cells and tissue.[7] Infarction of the heart and brain is the most important cause of illness and death in the developed countries of the world.[14]

The development of a thrombus is caused when the normal process of hemostasis is inappropriately activated. Endothelial injury, stasis or turbulence of blood flow, and hypercoagulability of the blood are the three major factors involved in the pathophysiology of thrombosis. These three factors, known as the triad of Virchow, were first described by Rudolf Virchow in 1846.[14] It is important to remember that a combination of these factors is frequently responsible for thrombus formation.

The pathophysiology of thrombosis seems to be somewhat different in veins as opposed to arteries (Table 21–4). Some factors identified as causing vessel wall abnormalities in veins are direct trauma, venous disease, and chemical irritation from intravenous solutions or drugs.[8] Atherosclerosis is often the process that damages the vessel wall in

TABLE 21–4
Conditions Associated with Increased Risk of Thrombosis

Venous Thrombosis	*Arterial Thrombosis*
Vessel Wall Abnormalities	*Abnormal Vascular Surface*
Trauma or surgery	Atherosclerotic cardiovascular disease
Venous disease	Hypertension
Chemical irritation from intravenous drugs	Cigarette smoking
	Hyperlipidemia
Increased Venous Stasis	Diabetes
Immobilization	Lack of physical exercise
Surgery	
Pregnancy	*Altered Blood Flow*
Congestive heart failure	Atrial fibrillation
Varicosities	Arterial aneurysms
Obesity	Mitral stenosis (atrial dilatation)
Advanced age	Dyskinetic contraction of myocardium
Hypercoagulability	
Pregnancy	*Hypercoagulability*
Nephrotic syndrome	Same as listed under venous thrombosis
Disseminated cancer	
Oral contraceptives	
Antithrombin III deficiency	
Thrombocytosis	
Liver disease	
Polycythemia	

(Adapted from Thompson AR, Harker LA: Manual of Hemostasis and Thrombosis, 3rd ed, p 141. Philadelphia, FA Davis, 1983)

arteries.[14] Anything that causes exposure of collagen fibers in the vessel wall of both arteries and veins may cause rapid platelet adhesion, aggregation, and thrombus formation.

Stasis is the most important change in blood flow in veins leading to thrombus formation. Stasis may result from reduced cardiac output due to heart failure or shock, venous return impairment due to shallow respirations or pressure on veins, or lack of muscular activity as occurs during bed rest. Alteration in blood flow causing arterial thrombosis may be due to an aneurysm or turbulent flow at points of arterial bifurcation or stenosis.[13] It should be emphasized, however, that the rapid blood flow in arteries tends to discourage thrombus formation.

Changes in the blood leading to increased coagulability may occur during pregnancy or in women taking oral contraceptive drugs. These changes are due to elevated levels of coagulation factors.[13] Increased numbers of platelets may also predispose to thrombus formation. Deficiencies in antithrombin III and reduced hepatic function may be thrombogenic factors in patients with liver disease and in premature infants.

The type of thrombus formed is usually different in arteries as opposed to veins. *Arterial thrombi* usually begin at the site of endothelial injury or turbulence.[7] The arterial thrombus is a dry, friable, tangled mass that is composed of layers of platelets and coagulated fibrin. Arterial thrombi are termed *white thrombi* because they are primarily composed of platelets and fibrin and lack red blood cells.

An arterial thrombus that adheres to the inner surface of the heart or artery (most commonly the aorta) is known as a *mural thrombus.* In arteries smaller than the aorta the thrombus usually builds rapidly until it completely obstructs the lumen. Although any artery can be affected, the following sites are involved most frequently: coronary, cerebral, femoral, iliac, popliteal, and mesenteric arteries. Embolization of an arterial thrombus is usually the result of the entire thrombus being detached.[7]

Venous thrombosis, also termed *phlebothrombosis,* is almost always occlusive. In the slower moving blood of the veins, the thrombus frequently creates a long cast in the lumen of the vessel. The venous thrombi, which have a rich admixture of red blood cells to the tangled strands of pale gray fibrin, are thus termed *red thrombi.*[7] Figures 21–7 and 21–8 show renal vein thrombosis and its outcome.

Venous thrombi most commonly affect the veins of the lower extremities (90%) in the following order of frequency: deep calf, femoral, popliteal, and iliac veins. Venous thrombi are usually attached to the vessel at the point of origin; however, the tail that builds up behind the occluding head may or

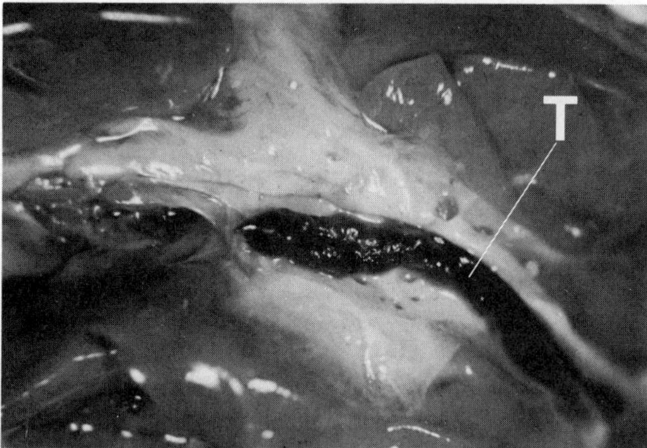

FIGURE 21–7 A thrombus (T) is located in the renal vein. (Courtesy of Dr. Marie Cowan, University of Washington School of Nursing)

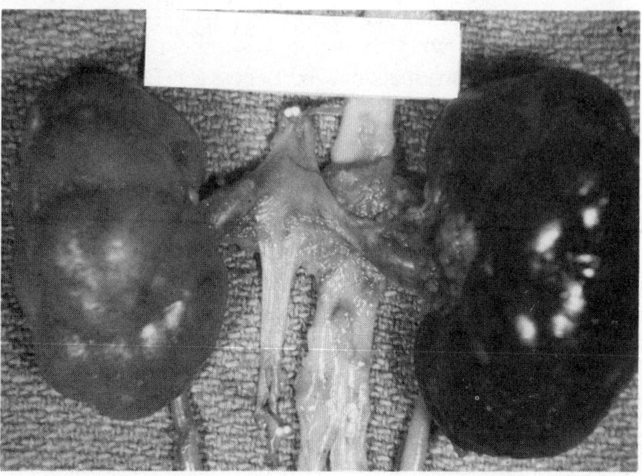

FIGURE 21–8 The kidney on the right is distended and hyperemic as the consequence of a thrombus obstructing its renal vein. (Courtesy of Dr. Marie Cowan, University of Washington School of Nursing)

may not be attached. This tail is most likely to break off and create an embolus. The resulting embolus frequently lodges in a pulmonary artery, causing the signs and symptoms of a pulmonary embolus (see Chap. 46).

If the patient survives the initial effects of thrombosis, one or more of the following sequences evolves: (1) the thrombus may propagate and cause obstruction of a critical vessel, (2) it may embolize, (3) it may be removed by fibrinolysis, or (4) it may undergo organization and become incorporated within the vessel wall. The first three eventualities have been discussed earlier in this chapter. The third eventuality rarely happens spontaneously. The fourth occurrence happens when a thrombus persists *in situ* for a few days. A series of events occurs, resulting in organization and recanalization of the thrombus that reestablishes to some extent the continuity of the lumen of the vessel.[7]

Principles of Nursing Management

A major nursing goal in all hospitalized patients is to identify patients at risk for hemostatic disorders. It is important for the nurse to be familiar with events, illnesses, and drugs that predispose to bleeding or clotting. Once patients at risk are identified, efforts must be made toward early detection of bleeding or clotting problems (see Tables 46–1 and 50–1).

Bleeding. Prevention of injury that may cause bleeding in a patient at risk is important. These patients must be handled gently. Measures such as using a soft toothbrush and protecting the feet with sturdy slippers or shoes will decrease the possibility of injury. Teaching patients to avoid injury by carefully handling sharp objects, using an electric razor, and wearing protective gloves are all ways that can prevent bleeding episodes. Patients must also be taught to avoid aspirin and aspirin-containing products because aspirin increases the possibility of bleeding in patients at risk.

If bleeding does occur, nursing responsibilities include measures to halt or control the bleeding, such as direct pressure over the bleeding site or application of cold to promote vasoconstriction. When bleeding is severe, replacement of blood or blood products may be necessary. Table 50–2 lists the nursing responsibilities associated with blood transfusion therapy.

Thrombosis. Prevention of thrombus formation in patients at risk is vital. Nursing measures such as early ambulation, active and passive range-of-motion exercises, deep breathing, and use of antiembolism stockings (TEDS) will all improve venous return and thus minimize venous stasis. Risk factors such as smoking, hypertension, and sedentary lifestyle are associated with coronary artery and peripheral vascular disease. Both assessment for presence of risk factors and assistance to patients who are attempting to reduce their risks are important nursing functions to decrease the likelihood of arterial thrombosis.

Medications such as aspirin and dipyridamole are oral agents that prevent platelet aggregation. These drugs may be prescribed for patients at risk for arterial thrombosis. Low doses of heparin are frequently administered parenterally to hospitalized patients at risk of venous thromboembolism. Teaching patients about these drugs is a major nursing responsibility.

When thrombosis has occurred, the focus of nursing care enlarges to include prevention and recognition of embolization, tissue infarction, and untoward effects of medications used to combat clot formation. Heparin, in larger doses, and oral anticoagulants such as the coumarin derivatives are commonly used to reduce additional growth of the thrombus. Fibrinolytic drugs may be adminisered to actually dissolve formed clots. Guidelines for administration of each of these drugs is covered in Chapter 46. Thromboembolic problems specific to various body systems will be addressed in later units of this text.

References

1. Aster RH: Thrombocytopenia due to enhanced platelet destruction. In Williams WJ, Beutler E, Erslev AJ, Lichtman MA (eds): Hematology, 3rd ed. New York, McGraw-Hill, 1983
2. Ganong WF: Review of Medical Physiology, 11th ed. Los Altos, Lange Medical Publications, 1983
3. Hardisty RM: Platelets, blood vessels and hemostasis: Disorders of platelet and vascular function. In Hardisty RM, Weatherall DJ (eds): Blood and Its Disorders, 2nd ed. Oxford, Blackwell Scientific Publications, 1982
4. Miale JB: Laboratory Medicine—Hematology, 6th ed. St Louis, CV Mosby, 1982
5. Moake JL, Funicella T: Common bleeding problems. Clin Symp 35:3, 1983
6. Nossel HL: Bleeding. In Petersdorf RG, Adams RD, Braunwald E et al: (eds): Harrison's Principles of Internal Medicine, 10th ed. New York, McGraw-Hill, 1983
7. Robbins SL, Angell M, Kumar V: Basic Pathology, 3rd ed. Philadelphia, WB Saunders, 1981
8. Roberts W: Thromboembolic complications in patients with cardiac disease. In Underhill SL, Woods SL, Sivarajan ES, Halpenny CJ (eds): Cardiac Nursing. Philadelphia, JB Lippincott, 1982
9. Thompson AR, Harker LA: Manual of Hemostasis and Thrombosis, 3rd ed. Philadelphia, FA Davis, 1983
10. Williams WJ: Biochemistry of plasma coagulation factors. In Williams WJ, Beutler E, Erslev AJ, Lichtman MA (eds): Hematology, 3rd ed. New York, McGraw-Hill, 1983
11. Williams WJ: Control of coagulation reactions. In Williams WJ, Beutler E, Erslev AJ, Lichtman MA (eds): Hematology, 3rd ed. New York, McGraw-Hill, 1983
12. Williams WJ: Sequence of coagulation reactions. In Williams WJ, Beutler E, Erslev AJ, Lichtman MA (eds): Hematology, 3rd ed. New York, McGraw-Hill, 1983
13. Williams WJ: Thrombosis. In Williams WJ, Beutler E, Erslev AJ, Lichtman MA (eds): Hematology, 3rd ed. New York, McGraw-Hill, 1983
14. Wintrobe MM, Lee GR, Boggs DR et al: Clinical Hematology, 8th ed. Philadelphia, Lea & Febiger, 1981

Chapter 22

Atherosclerosis

Marie Cowan

The purpose of this chapter is to provide an understanding of the pathological process that leads to progressive atherosclerotic plaques in the coronary arteries. The process has been found to be multifaceted in its origins. The pathogenesis of atherosclerosis is unknown, but several hypotheses will be presented. In this chapter, the major emphasis is on the arterial wall.

Arteriosclerosis

Atherosclerosis should not be confused with other forms of arteriosclerosis. Arteriosclerosis literally means "hardening of the arteries," and refers to three disorders that have in common thickening and loss of elasticity of arterial walls. These disorders are atherosclerosis, medial calcific sclerosis, and arteriolar sclerosis.

Atherosclerosis. Atherosclerosis refers to the accumulation of smooth muscle cells, lipids, and connective tissue in the intima of large and middle-sized muscular arteries, such as the aorta, coronary, carotid, vertebral, femoral, and iliac arteries. It accounts for a large proportion of myocardial infarctions, cases of ischemic heart disease associated with sudden death (usually as a result of acute onset of ventricular fibrillation), and chronic angina pectoris. It also accounts for many strokes (those due to cerebral ischemia and infarction); numerous cases of peripheral vascular disease; and most aneurysms of the lower abdominal aorta, which can rupture and cause sudden fatal hemorrhage. Atherosclerosis is the most frequent cause of death in the United States and Western Europe.

Medial Calcific Sclerosis. Medial calcific sclerosis, or Mönckeberg's sclerosis, is characterized by a ringlike accumulation of calcium deposits in the media of medium-sized muscular arteries, such as the femoral, tibial, radial, and ulnar arteries, and in the arterial supply of the genital tract in both sexes. Although atherosclerosis and medial calcific sclerosis can occur in the same person, the two disorders are totally distinctive anatomically, clinically, and etiologically. Medial calcific sclerosis does not produce narrowing or occlusion of the arterial lumen and does not produce significant clinical signs or symptoms.[21]

Arteriolar Sclerosis. Arteriolar sclerosis (or arteriolosclerosis) is marked by proliferative or hyaline thickening of all the walls of small arteries and arterioles, particularly those of the kidney. The narrowing of the arteriolar lumina causes impairment of blood supply to affected organs. The disorder is generally related to acute or severe elevations of blood pressure and is therefore characteristic of hypertension. The condition is also seen in diabetes mellitus.[21]

Normal Arterial Wall

The walls of arteries contain three layers: the intima, the media, and the adventitia. As the diameter of the vessels decrease in size, the three separable coats become progressively indistinct and eventually are no longer identifiable at the level of the arteriole.

Intima. The intima consists of a layer of endothelial cells lining the lumen. Beneath the endothelium is the subendothelial layer, consisting of delicate loose connective tissue that may contain an occasional smooth muscle cell. The intima is separated from the media by a continuous boundary of elastic fibers, the internal elastic lamina. The endothelial cell barrier normally is impermeable to proteins in the blood.

Media. The media consists mostly of circumferentially arranged smooth muscle cells. Variable amounts of elastin, collagen, and proteoglycans are interposed among the smooth muscle cells.

Adventitia. The adventitia consists mostly of connective tissue with elastic fibers. The predominant cell of the adventitia is the fibroblast. In larger vessels, vasa vasorum branch profusely in the adventitia. The vasa vasorum provide nutrition to the adventitia and the media in larger vessels since the layers are too thick to be nourished by diffusion from the bloodstream. The intima and the most internal portion of media are avascular and receive metabolites by diffusion from the bloodstream (Fig. 22–1).

Atherosclerotic Lesion

The intima of the arterial wall is the principal involvement site of atherosclerosis, although secondary changes are occasionally found in the media resulting from arterial dilatation and localized aneurysm formation. The lesions associated with atherosclerosis can be classified into three morphological types: the fatty streak, the fibrous plaque, and the complicated lesion.

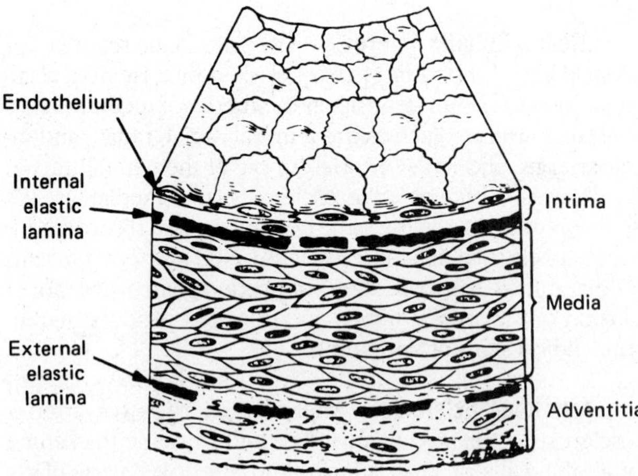

FIGURE 22–1 Structure of normal muscular artery. (Ross R, Glomset JA: N Engl J Med 295:370, 1976. Reprinted by permission from the New England Journal of Medicine.)

Fatty Streak

The fatty streak is a yellowish, smooth lesion. It does not obstruct blood flow and is not associated with any clinical signs and symptoms. The lesion is characterized histologically by the presence of lipid deposits within the smooth muscle cells and macrophages in the intima of the artery. These cells "balloon out" because of the lipid in them and are commonly referred to as foam cells. The lipid is mostly cholesterol and cholesterol esters.

Fatty streaks have been observed in people of all ages from infancy to old age. Fatty streaks have been commonly seen, post mortem, in infants, young children, and young adults.[29,37] Whether these lesions are irreversible and, also, whether the fatty streak is the precursor of the fibrous plaque, are controversial.

Raised Fibrous Plaque

The characteristic lesion of atherosclerosis is the raised fibrous plaque. The fibrous plaque is a yellowish gray elevated lump on the inner surface of the artery (Fig. 22–2). It protrudes in varying degrees into the arterial lumen, sometimes completely obstructing arterial blood flow. There may be more than one atherosclerotic plaque on an artery.

There are three major histological characteristics of the fibrous plaque:

1. Proliferation of smooth muscle cells and macrophages
2. Intracellular and extracellular lipid deposits
3. An accumulation of connective tissue, including collagen, elastic fibers, and proteoglycans

The plaques are localized in the intima of the artery. Smooth muscle cells ordinarily are located in the media and give the artery its contractility. The smooth muscle cells in the intima of the plaque probably are derived from those in the media. The smooth muscle cells secrete collagen, elastin, and glycosaminoglycans.[21,22,23,35]

Typically the plaques consist of a fibrous cap, made of mostly collagen and smooth muscle cells, and a deeper, central part in which there is a disorganized mass of lipid material (mostly cholesterol and cholesterol esters), cellular debris, and plasma proteins. The center of larger plaques may exude a thick, yellow liquid at autopsy, from which the name *atheroma,* the Greek word for gruel, is derived.[21]

Complicated Plaques

The complicated lesion is a fibrous plaque with calcification, rupture of the plaque, hemorrhage into the plaque, or thrombus formation. The complicated lesion is most often associated with important clinical signs and symptoms caused by complete occlusion of blood flow to an organ.

Although atherosclerosis occurs universally in most populations, complicated plaques are seen only in individu-

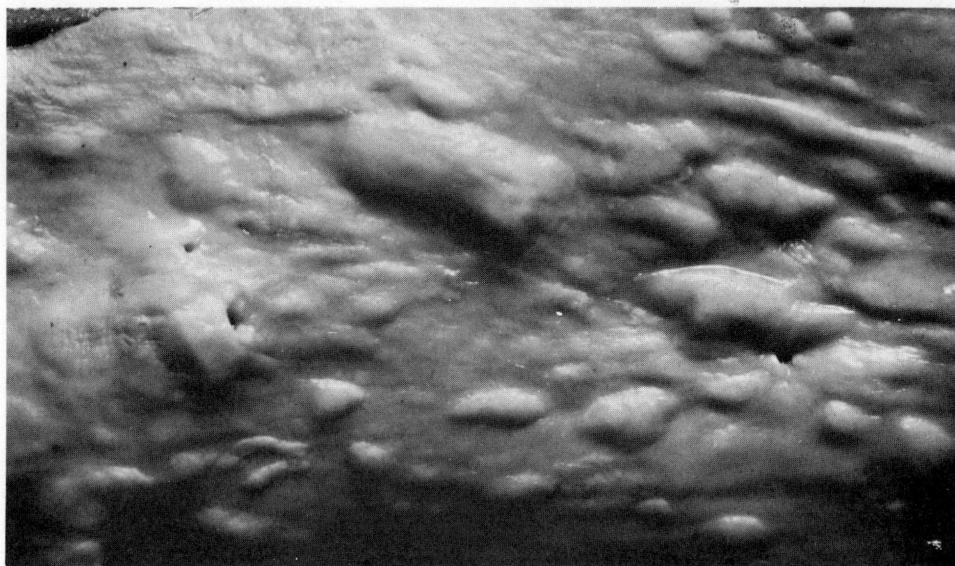

FIGURE 22–2 Atherosclerotic inner surface of an artery. (Original magnification × 2.5. Benditt E: Sci Am 236:75, 1977. Courtesy of E. P. Benditt)

als with advanced disease. For example, in some individuals with advanced coronary artery disease, all three major coronary arteries of the heart may have calcification; significant atherosclerotic stenosis of greater than 75% occlusion may be present at multiple arterial sites, and an occlusive thrombus may have formed in one of the arteries, resulting in an acute myocardial infarction. As another example, in some individuals the entire abdominal aorta may resemble a very large, continuous complicated lesion. In these cases, although atherosclerosis is basically an intimal disease, the underlying media undergoes considerable pressure atrophy and loss of elastic tissue, causing sufficient weakness to permit an arterial dilatation, called an *aneurysm.* The untreated aneurysm can result in fatal rupture and hemorrhage. In the aorta, the important complications resulting from the plaques are aneurysm or large mural thrombi that may dislodge and yield emboli. Occlusion of the aorta by a thrombus is unusual. However, in smaller arteries, especially those of the heart or the brain, the narrowing caused by the atheromatous plaques accompanied by thrombosis will lead to occlusion and is the event that causes myocardial infarction or stroke, respectively.[21]

Pathogenesis

The pathogenesis, or cause, of atherosclerosis is unknown. This chapter will present an overview of the major hypotheses of the pathogenesis of atherosclerosis. The major hypotheses are six: lipid insudation, encrustation, hemodynamic, clonal senescence, monoclonal, and response-to-injury. For more detailed information, reference should be made to various reviews or books.[6,8,15,21,24,25,34,36]

For any concept of the cause of atherosclerosis, the following factors should be taken into consideration:

1. The role of the important risk factors
2. The mechanisms of smooth muscle cell proliferation within the intima
3. The presence of lipid in the lesion
4. The localization of the lesions in certain areas of the artery.

Because no single theory adequately explains all these observations, the hypotheses are not to be considered mutually exclusive. They have all been combined, modified, and extended with the result that the current dominant hypothesis is the response-to-injury hypothesis.

Lipid Insudation Hypothesis. This first hypothesis, defined by Virchow in 1856,[8] held that cellular proliferation in the intima was a form of inflammation caused by infiltration of lipids and plasma proteins from the blood. As shall be discussed later, this hypothesis has been incorporated into the more modern response-to-injury hypothesis.[7,12,27,31]

Encrustation (Thrombogenic) Hypothesis. The second hypothesis, thought to be originally defined by Rokitansky, held that the fibrous plaque begins as a mural thrombus that is converted or organized into a mass of dense connective tissue.[8] Few investigators believe that thrombus formation is the sole cause of atherosclerosis, but parts of the theory still prevail. It is currently thought that endothelial injury, with platelet deposition, plays a role in the formation of plaques.

Hemodynamic Hypothesis. Hemodynamic factors such as turbulence, shearing stresses, and pressures tangential to the vessel circumference have been used to explain why plaques are more often situated near arterial branches, and why some arteries or arterial segments are regularly more severely involved by atherosclerosis than others.[11,13] The abdominal aorta is much more involved than the thoracic aorta, and aortic lesions tend to occur more frequently at the opening of the major arterial branches. The most heavily involved vessels (after the abdominal aorta) are the coronary arteries, the popliteal arteries, the descending thoracic aorta, the internal carotids, and the vessels of the circle of Willis. Arteries of the upper extremity are usually spared.[21,38]

Hemodynamic factors may play a part in endothelial injury, and thus parts of this hypothesis have been incorporated into the response-to-injury hypothesis. For example, in the experimental animal, a shear force applied for a long time results in the formation of connective tissue in the intima of the artery. The tissue is characterized by dense collagen, a few smooth muscle cells, and accumulation of lipid.[11] This type of lesion, mediated by shear stress, is thought to be one of the cellular mechanisms of hypertension, which is known to be one of the risk factors of atherosclerosis.

Clonal Senescence Hypothesis. The clonal senescence hypothesis relates atherosclerosis to age, which is one of its risk factors. This hypothesis accounts for smooth muscle proliferation in the intima because of "loss of growth control" of the cells in the media due, perhaps, to either old age or injury.[10,14,16,17,18] These concepts are relatively new and speculative.

Monoclonal Hypothesis. The monoclonal hypothesis holds that the atherosclerotic plaque is due to a proliferation of smooth muscle cells that are monoclonal.[1,2,3,20] In other words, each atherosclerotic lesion is started by a single smooth muscle cell and the rest of the proliferative cells are the progeny or descendants or clones of that cell. Benditt[1,2,3] proposed that some mutagenic event (such as hydrocarbons from cigarette smoking), endogenous metabolite (such as cholesterol), or virus[5,9] provides the single cell with a selective advantage. The result of this advantage is that the progeny of that altered cell have increased capacity for growth (Fig. 22–3).

The monoclonal hypothesis represents a departure from the traditional viewpoint of atherogenesis. This proposal suggests that plaques may be equivalent to benign monoclonal neoplastic growths.[33] The scientific significance of this hypothesis is that consideration is given to factors that transform cells.[32]

Response-to-Injury Hypothesis. This theory states that the lesions of atherosclerosis are started as a response to some kind of injury to the endothelial wall of the artery.[24,25] The injury could be due to one of many factors: mechanical, chemical, hormonal, or immunologic.[19] Permeability changes of the intimal membrane would occur at the sites of injury so that platelets, lipoproteins, and other substances of the blood could diffuse into or come in contact with the intimal layer.

Supporters of this hypothesis suggest that humans can suffer endothelial injury, for example, from the increased shear stress in hypertension, from hydrocarbons in cigarette smoking, and from carbon monoxide, plasma cholesterol catecholamines, angiotensin,[30] or hormones (Fig. 22–4).

Injury to the arterial endothelium causes an immediate platelet response with platelet adherence to the subendothelial connective tissue, aggregation, and release of the contents of platelet granules (Fig. 22–5). Growth stimulating factors released from platelets,[26,28] macrophages[4] or, perhaps some other plasma constituent lead to the migration of the smooth muscle cells from the media to the intima, followed by their proliferation (Fig. 22–6). The smooth muscle cells normally would be protected from growth stimulating factors by the endothelial cell barrier. The smooth muscle cells secrete collagen, elastin, and proteoglycans resulting in large amounts of connective tissue matrix in the intima. Increased amounts of lipids accumulate because of the increased permeability of the endothelial wall. There is some evidence that hypercholesteremia itself leads to increased endothelial permeability and endothelial damage.[4,27,36]

Single or short-lived injurious events are followed by regeneration of endothelial cells, which is an adaptation of the tissue to recover the hole made by the injury, resulting in restoration of the endothelial barrier and, perhaps, regression of the lesion. However if the injury is chronic or repeated, the balance between reendothelialization and smooth muscle cell proliferation may be tipped, resulting in the development of an atheromatous plaque.[24,25] This balance, possibly affected by risk factors, may determine whether the lesion progresses or stays the same size. Thus continuous hyperlipidemia, high blood pressure, smoking, and other risk factors may cause continued injury and progression of the lesion (Fig. 22–7).

Summary

In summary, although much more research needs to be done, it now appears likely that the previous divergent theories are in the process of combining into a unified concept that atherosclerosis is a continuous response to injury of multiple origins. It is very likely that there is no one cause of

FIGURE 22–3 Genesis of a plaque as proposed by the monoclonal hypothesis. The process begins in the inner media. There are two cell types. (1) A single cell (*dark color*) has undergone mutation that gives it a selective advantage, and some stimulus causes the mutated cell to divide. (2) Its daughter cell migrates into the intima. (3, 4) The progeny of the mutated cell, having a selective advantage and perhaps somehow freed of some curb on proliferation, continue to multiply, thickening the intima and (5) eventually forming a lumpy plaque, all of whose cells are progeny of the original cell that mutated. The last drawing (6) shows, by way of contrast, a polyclonal plaque, which is the kind that would arise from the migration and proliferation of many cells of both cell types. (Benditt E: Sci Am 236:80, 1977. Copyright 1977 by Scientific American, Inc. All rights reserved.)

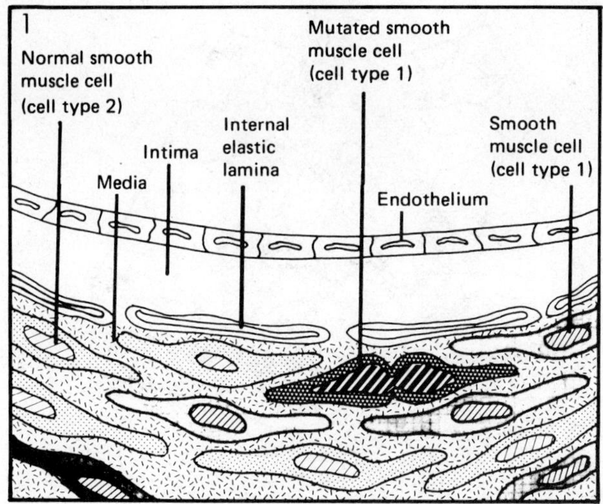
1
Normal smooth muscle cell (cell type 2)
Mutated smooth muscle cell (cell type 1)
Intima
Media
Internal elastic lamina
Smooth muscle cell (cell type 1)
Endothelium

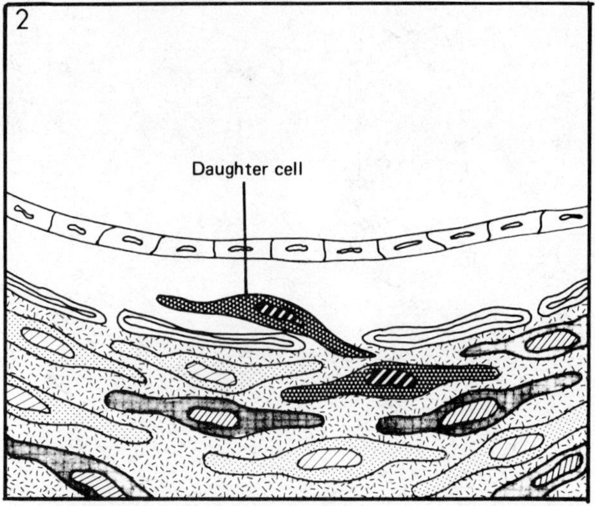
2
Daughter cell

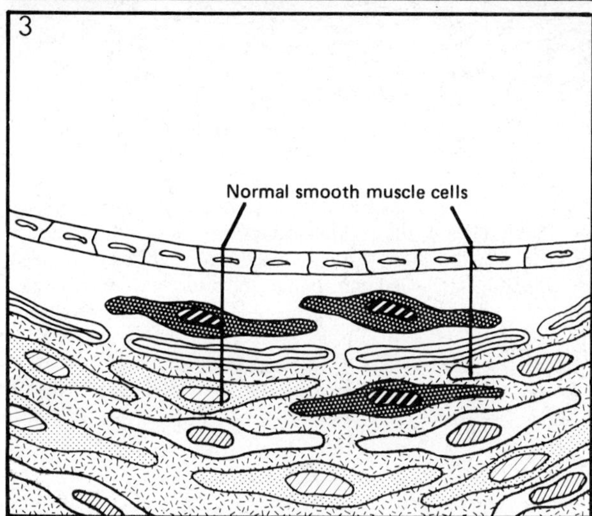
3
Normal smooth muscle cells

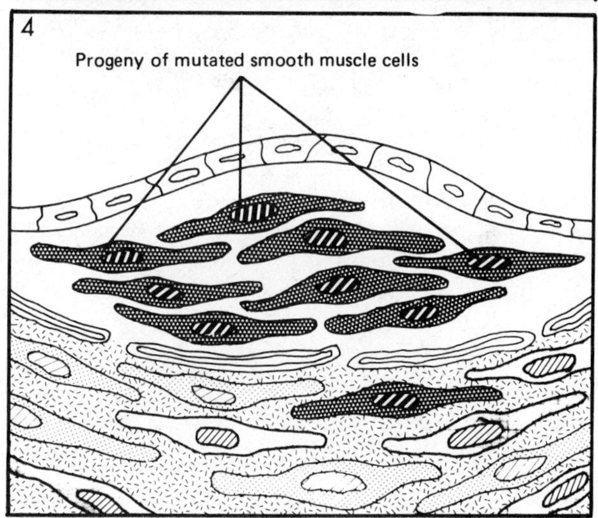
4
Progeny of mutated smooth muscle cells

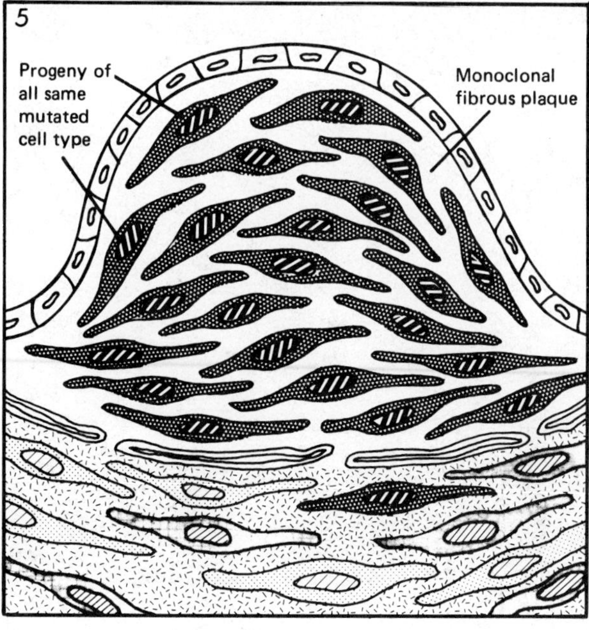
5
Progeny of all same mutated cell type
Monoclonal fibrous plaque

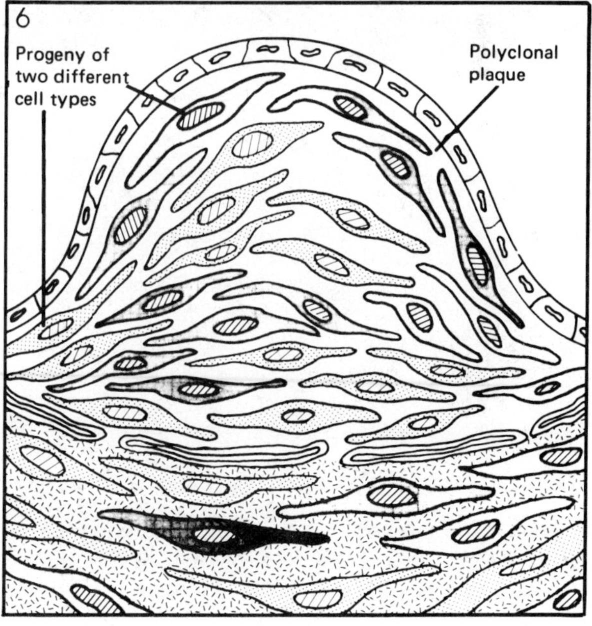
6
Progeny of two different cell types
Polyclonal plaque

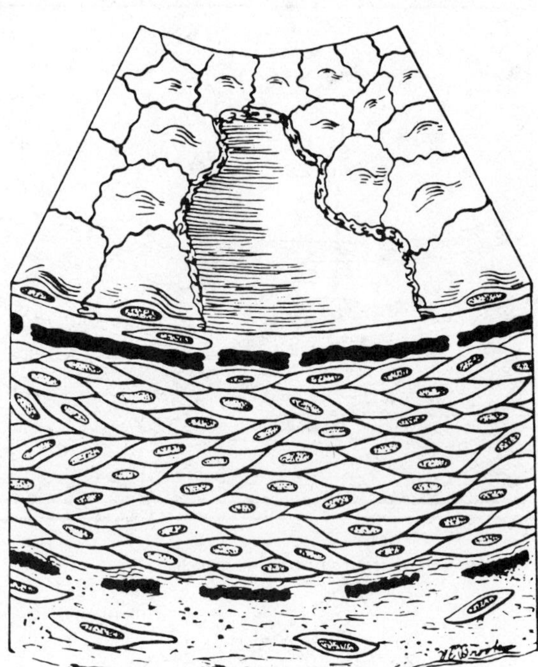

FIGURE 22–4 Endothelial desquamation caused by several different forms of injury, possibly resulting in exposure of the underlying intimal connective tissue. (Ross R, Glomset JA: N Engl J Med 295:420, 1976. Reprinted by permission from the New England Journal of Medicine.)

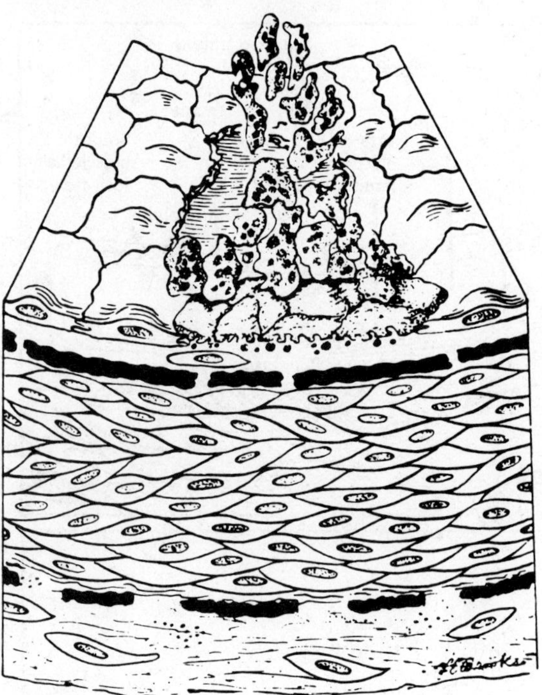

FIGURE 22–5 Platelet aggregates, or microthrombi, may form as a result of adherence of the platelets to the exposed subendothelial tissue. Platelets that adhere to the connective tissue release granules whose constituents may gain entry into the artery wall. Platelet factors thus may interact with plasma constituents in the artery wall and stimulate intimal smooth muscle proliferation and formation of new connective tissue. (Ross R, Glomset JA: N Engl J Med 295:421, 1976. Reprinted by permission from the New England Journal of Medicine.)

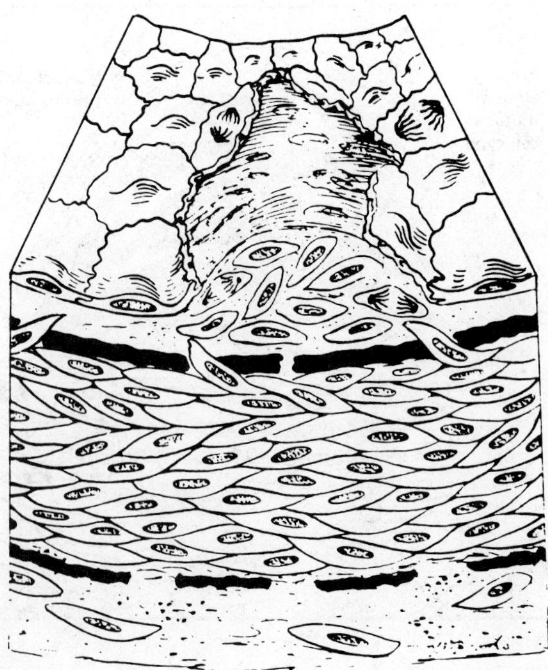

FIGURE 22–6 Smooth muscle cells migrating from the media into the intima through fenestrae in the internal elastic lamina and actively multiplying within the intima. Endothelial cells regenerate in an attempt to recover the exposed intima, which thickens rapidly owing to smooth muscle cell proliferation and formation of new connective tissue. (Ross R, Glomset JA: N Engl J Med 295:421, 1976. Reprinted by permission from the New England Journal of Medicine.)

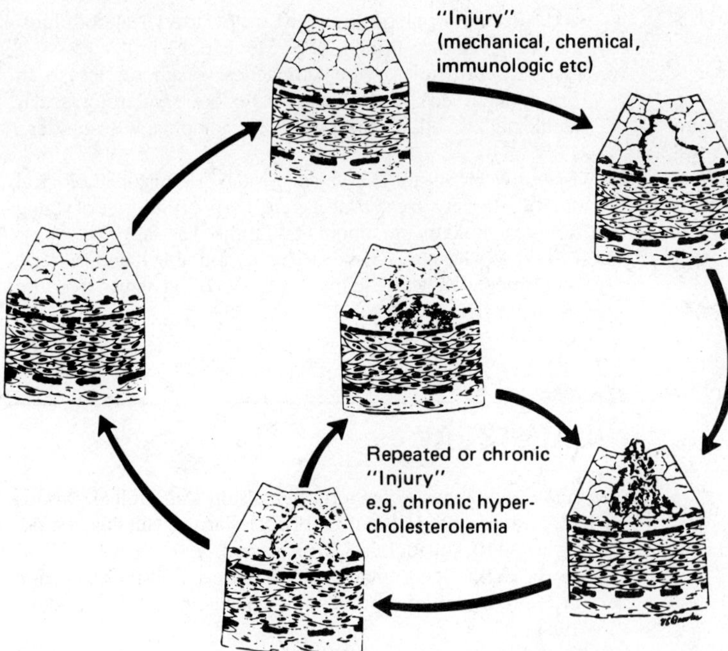

FIGURE 22–7 Two possible cycles of events in the response-to-injury hypothesis. The large cycle may represent what occurs in all persons at varying times. Endothelial injury may lead to desquamation, platelet adherence, aggregation, and release, followed by smooth muscle proliferation and connective tissue formation. If the injury is a single event, the lesions may go on to heal and regress, leaving a slightly thickened intima. The smaller, inner cycle demonstrates the possible consequences of repeated or chronic injury to the endothelium; lipid deposition may occur and smooth muscle proliferation may continue after a sequence of proliferation, regression, proliferation, and regression. This leads to a complicated lesion, containing newly formed connective tissue and lipids, which may eventually calcify. This sequence of events could lead to a complicated lesion that goes on to produce clinical sequelae, such as thrombosis and infarction. (Ross R, Glomset JA: N Engl J Med 295:423, 1976. Reprinted by permission of the New England Journal of Medicine.)

atherosclerosis, no single initiating event, and no exclusive pathogenetic mechanism. Perhaps the cumulative effect of many factors is involved. Note that the atherosclerotic plaques themselves do not cause signs or symptoms. These plaques result in clinical disease only by narrowing the arterial lumen to cause ischemia; sudden occlusion of the lumen by thrombosis, causing infarction; providing a site for thrombosis and then embolism; and formation of aneurysm and rupture. Although theoretically any organ in the body may be involved, symptomatic atherosclerotic disease occurs most frequently in the heart, brain, kidneys, lower extremities, and small intestine. The pathophysiology of the most frequent outcomes, ischemia and infarction, is described in Chapter 23, which follows. Nursing interventions will be introduced in that chapter and expanded in later chapters of the book.

References

1. Benditt E: The origin of atherosclerosis. Sci Am 236:74–85, 1977
2. Benditt E, Benditt JJ: Evidence for a monoclonal origin of human atherosclerotic plaques. Proc Natl Acad Sci USA 70:1753–1756, 1973
3. Benditt EP, Gown AM: Atheroma: The artery wall and the environment. Int Rev Exp Pathol 21:115–118, 1980
4. Brown MS, Goldstein JL: Lipoprotein metabolism in the macrophage: Implications for cholesterol deposition in atherosclerosis. Annu Rev Biochem 52:223–261, 1983
5. Burch JE: Viruses and arterosclerosis. Am Heart J 87:407, 1974
6. Cowan MJ: Pathogenesis of atherosclerosis. In Underhill SL, Woods SL, Sivarajan ES, Halpenny CJ (eds): Cardiac Nursing, 1st ed, pp 103–110. Philadelphia, JB Lippincott, 1982
7. Davignon J: The lipid hypothesis. Arch Surg 113:28–34, 1978
8. Duguid JB: Pathogenesis of atherosclerosis. Lancet 2:925–927, 1949
9. Fabricant CG et al: Virus-induced atherosclerosis. J Exp Med 148:335–340, 1978
10. Florentin RA, Nam SC, Jana Kideui K et al: Population dynamics of arterial smooth muscle cells. II. In vivo inhibition of entry into mitosis of swine arterial smooth muscle cells by aortic tissue extracts. Arch Pathol 95:317–320, 1973
11. Glagov S: Mechanical stresses on vessels and the non-uniform distribution of atherosclerosis. Med Clin North Am 57:63–77, 1973
12. Goldstein J, Brown M: Lipoprotein receptors, cholesterol metabolism and atherosclerosis. Arch Pathol 99:181–184, 1975
13. Haimovici H, Mailer N: Role of arterial tissue susceptibility in experimental canine atherosclerosis. Journal Atherosclerosis Research 6:62–74, 1966
14. Hayflick L: The cell biology of human aging. Sci Am 242:58–65, 1980
15. Kolata G: Atherosclerotic plaques: Competing theories guide research. Science 194:592–594, 1976
16. Martin GM: Cellular aging—clonal senescence. Am J Pathol 89:484–512, 1977
17. Martin GM: Cellular aging—post replicative cells. Am J Pathol 89:513–530, 1977
18. Martin GM: Sprague CA: Symposium on in vitro studies related to atherogenesis: Life histories of hyperplastoid cell lines from aorta and skin. Exp Mol Pathol 18:125–141, 1973
19. Minick CR: Immunologic arterial injury in atherogenesis. Ann N Y Acad Sci 275:210–227, 1976
20. Pearson TA, Wang A, Salezo K et al: Clonal characteristics of fibrous plaques and fatty streaks from human aortas. Am J Pathol 81:379–387, 1975
21. Robbins SL, Cotran RS, Kumar V: Blood vessels. In Pathologic Basis of Disease, 3rd ed, pp 502–519. Philadelphia, WB Saunders, 1984
22. Ross R, Riebanoff SJ: The smooth muscle cell. I. In vivo synthesis of connective tissue proteins. J Cell Biol 50:159–171, 1971
23. Ross R: The smooth muscle cell. II. Growth of smooth muscle in culture and formation of elastic fibers. J Cell Biol 50:172–186, 1971

24. Ross R, Glomset JA: The pathogenesis of atherosclerosis, Part I. N Engl J Med 295:369–377, 1976
25. Ross R, Glomset JA: The pathogenesis of atherosclerosis, Part 2. N Engl J Med 295:420–425, 1976
26. Ross R, Glomset J, Karuja B et al: A platelet-dependent serum factor that stimulates the proliferation of arterial smooth muscle cells in vitro. Proc Natl Acad Sci USA 71:1207–1210, 1974
27. Ross R, Harker L: Hyperlipidemia and atherosclerosis. Science 193:1094–1100, 1976
28. Ross R, Vogel A: The platelet-derived growth factor. Cell 14:203–210, 1978
29. Schwartz CJ: Gross aortic sudanophilia and hemosideria deposition: A study on infants, children, young adults. Arch Pathol 83:325–332, 1967
30. Schwartz SM: Assessment of angiotensin endothelial injury by incident light microscopy. Fed Proc 35:208, 1976
31. Stein V, Stein O: Lipid synthesis and degradation and lipoprotein transport in mammalian aorta. Ciba Found Symp 12:165–184, 1973
32. Thomas WA, Florentin RA, Reiner JM et al: Alterations in population dynamics of arterial smooth muscle cells during atherogenesis. Exp Mol Pathol 24:244–260, 1976
33. Thomas WA, Kim DN: Atherosclerosis as a hyperplastic and neoplastic process. Lab Invest 48:245–255, 1983
34. Watts H: Basic aspects of the pathogenesis of human atherosclerosis. Hum Pathol 2:31–55, 1971
35. Wight TN, Ross R: Proteoglycans in primate arteries. II. Synthesis and secretion of glycosaminoglycans by arterial smooth muscle cells in culture. J Cell Biol 67:675–686, 1975
36. Wissler RW: Principles of the pathogenesis of atherosclerosis. In Braunwald E (ed): Heart Disease: A Textbook of Cardiovascular Medicine, 2nd ed, pp 1183–1204. Philadelphia, WB Saunders, 1984
37. Wissler RW, McAllister HA, Vesselinovitch D: A histopathological study of the fatty streak in aortas and coronary arteries of young American military personnel. Am J Pathol 78:64a, 1975
38. Wolinsky H, Glasgov S: Comparison of abdominal and thoracic aortic medial structure in mammals. Deviation of man from the usual pattern. Circ Res 25:677–686, 1969

Bibliography

Cowan MJ: Pathogenesis of atherosclerosis. In Underhill SL, Woods SL, Sivarajan ES, Halpenny CJ (eds): Cardiac Nursing, 1st ed, pp 103–110. Philadelphia, JB Lippincott, 1982

Robbins SL, Cotran RS, Kumar V: Blood vessels. In Pathologic Basis of Disease, 3rd ed, pp 502–519. Philadelphia, WB Saunders, 1984

Wissler RW, McAllister HA, Vesselinovitch D: A histopathological study of the fatty streak in aortas and coronary arteries of young American military personnel. Am J Pathol 78:64a, 1975

Chapter 23

Ischemia and Infarction

Joanne Schnaidt Rokosky

A frequent cause of cellular injury is deprivation of oxygen. Insufficient oxygen to cells, regardless of the underlying cause, is called *hypoxia*. Because a major function of the circulatory system is to deliver oxygen to cells, hypoxic injury is often the consequence of a reduction in arterial blood flow, a process known as ischemia. Specifically, *ischemia* is defined as a reduction in arterial flow so that the oxygen supply to a tissue is insufficient to meet its oxygen demand.[5,15] Tissues deprived of adequate blood flow for their metabolic needs are referred to as ischemic and undergo a progression of events that, if not reversed, culminate in the death of the tissue. Death of tissue due to inadequate blood flow is called *infarction*.[2,11,15]

Causes of Ischemia

Many processes can impair blood flow to tissues and result in ischemia. Arteries can be narrowed by the development of atherosclerotic plaque, a process which is often the cause of ischemic injury to the heart and brain. Narrowing of an artery by clot formation produces identical effects. Intermittent arterial spasms, as occur in Raynaud's phenomenon and disease, may also cause ischemic damage.[12] In these instances, the ischemia is localized and affects only the tissues supplied by the involved artery. Ischemia may also be a generalized phenomenon, as in shock, when systemic arterial flow is inadequate to meet tissue demands throughout the body (see Chap. 24).

The obstruction of venous blood flow can indirectly impair arterial perfusion of tissues. When such an obstruction is sufficient to cause rise in venous pressure, local capillary dynamics are altered (see Chap. 13), and arterial blood flow is reduced. Injuries involving the extremities pose a particularly high risk because bony and fascial compartments within the limb contain fluid accumulations inside a rigid space.[14] Casts or circumferentially tight dressings can lead to the same result.

Sequence of Cellular Events with Ischemic Injury

To a varying degree all human cells use oxygen to produce the energy required for their many life-sustaining activities. When cells are deprived of oxygen by ischemia, the rate of cellular metabolism is slowed or stopped, the cell volume is altered, and structural changes eventually occur within the cell. Although these changes have been studied most comprehensively in myocardial cells, they are believed to occur in all cells in a predictable fashion.

Normal Production of Energy by Aerobic Metabolism

Cells require energy to transport substances across their membranes, to synthesize materials, and to perform specialized physiological activities, such as muscle contraction and glandular secretion. Energy for these activities is derived from the breakdown of foodstuffs and stored in the form of the compound adenosine triphosphate (ATP). To fuel metabolic processes, phosphate compounds are then released from ATP and energy is liberated. Because of its important role in storing and releasing energy, ATP is often described as energy currency.

Within each cell, the mitochondria function as power plants for the generation of ATP. Ingested carbohydrate, fat, or protein can be used for this energy source after their degradation to glucose, fatty acids, or amino acids, respectively. Because protein is essential for cell synthesis, it is usually spared whenever another substrate is available.

When oxygen is present, the final derivation of energy from all foodstuffs is accomplished through a complicated series of reactions known as the citric acid or Krebs cycle (see Fig. 23–1). The breakdown of glucose is often used to illustrate this sequence, although the steps are different for each foodstuff. By a series of complex chemical reactions catalized by mitochondrial enzymes, glucose molecules are split into pyruvic acid. the pyruvic acid is then converted to acetylcoenzyme A (acetyl-CoA), which enters the citric acid cycle and is degraded to carbon dioxide and hydrogen atoms. The quantity of ATP formed during these processes is not large. Most of the body's ATP is generated during a subsequent process called oxidative phosphorylation in which the previously formed hydrogen atoms and dissolved oxygen combine to form water. By this oxygen-dependent process, 38 mol of ATP, in contrast to 2 mol each in the first two reactions, are formed for every mole of glucose expended.[4] Thus, a large source of energy is made available for future biochemical reactions.

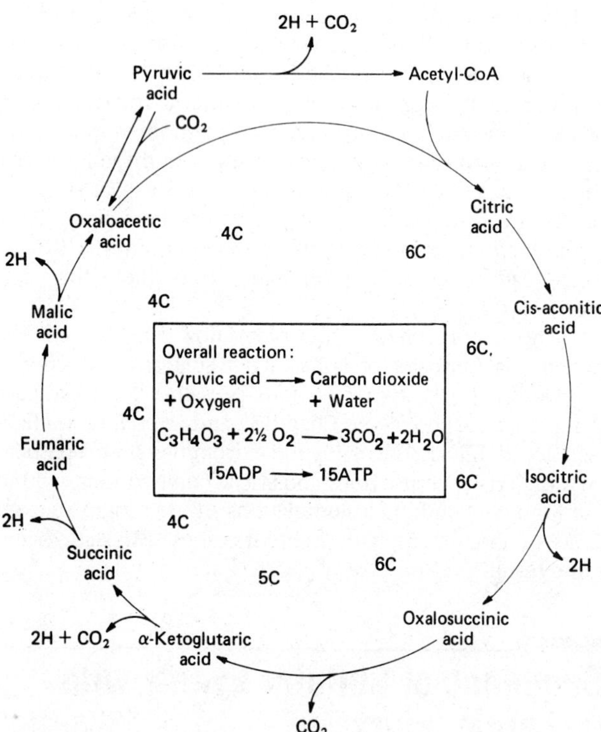

FIGURE 23–1 Citric acid cycle. The numbers in the circle (6C, 5C, 4C) indicate the number of carbon atoms in each of the acid intermediates. Note that two H atoms are transferred for each turn of the cycle proper, generating by oxidative phosphorylation a total of 15 ATP. (Ganong WF: Review of Medical Physiology, 11th ed. Los Altos, California, Lange Medical Publications, 1983. Copyright 1983 by Lange Medical Publications. Reproduced wth permission.)

Effects of Oxygen Deficiency on Cellular Metabolism

When ischemia deprives cells of adequate oxygen, aerobic metabolism is replaced by a less efficient *anaerobic* system. Because glycolysis is not oxygen driven, glucose continues to be degraded into pyruvic acid. Without oxygen, however, pyruvic acid is unable to enter the Krebs cycle and, along with hydrogen atoms, begins to accumulate. The hydrogen and pyruvic acid then react with the molecule nicotinamide adenine dinucleotide (NAD^+), a metabolic cofactor, to form lactic acid. The lactic acid thus allows continued but minimal ATP production at the expense of acid accumulation in and around cells. The consumption of one molecule of glucose for anaerobic metabolism yields only 2 mol of ATP in contrast to the 38 mol produced by aerobic metabolism.

Results of Anaerobic Metabolism

The decrease in energy production resulting from ischemia profoundly impairs cellular function. The changes that occur are sequential and, initially, are all reversible. These changes are diagrammed in Figure 23–2.

Loss of Active Transport and Cell Swelling. One of the earliest effects of ischemia is on the active transport systems that move materials to and from the interiors of cells. These active transport systems operate by means of an ATP-dependent enzyme, ATPase, and permit concentrations of substances to differ on either side of the cell membrane. Within all cells, active transport maintains the electrolyte composition of the intracellular fluid. Sodium ions are actively extruded from cells in a 3 : 2 ratio for potassium ions that are pumped in. As a result, the interior of the cell is high in potassium ions but low in sodium ions, a state opposite to that of the surrounding extracellular fluid. When the quantity of ATP, and hence ATPase, is decreased as a result of ischemia, sodium–potassium pumping ceases. Because random diffusion is no longer opposed by active transport, positively charged sodium and its negatively charged partner, chloride, begin to accumulate within the ischemic cells. Simultaneously, potassium ions accumulate in the extracellular fluid. Water passively accompanies the movement of sodium and chloride into cells, so as to keep the concentration of particles equal on both sides of the cell membrane. The result of this influx of water is cell swelling. The manufacturing appa-

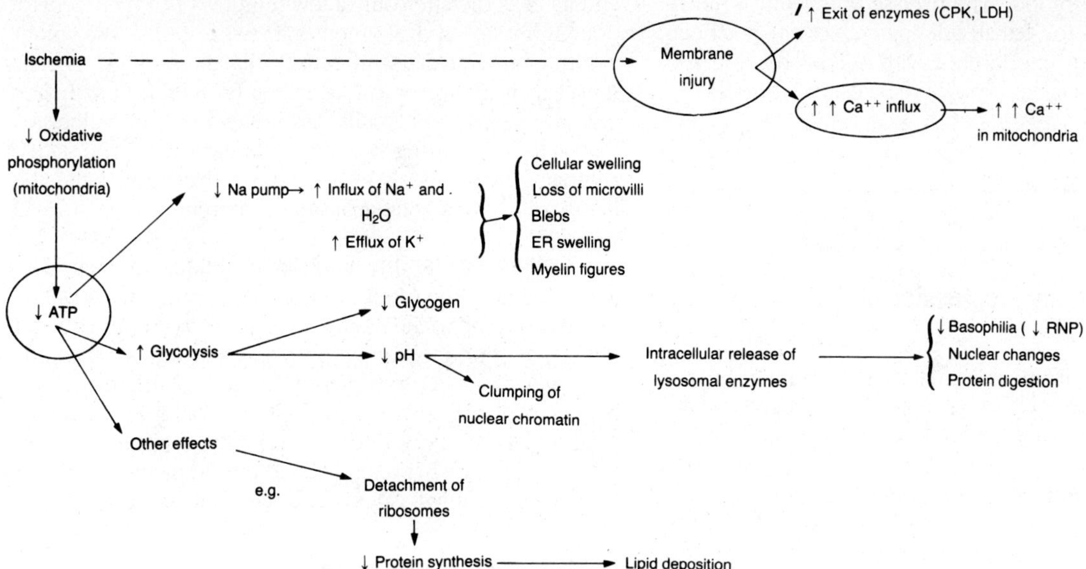

FIGURE 23–2 Postulated sequence of events in ischemic injury. Note that while the reduced ATP levels have a central role, ischemia may directly cause membrane damage, by currently uncertain mechanisms discussed in the text. The circled events appear to be the three most critical phenomena. (Adapted from Robbins SL, Cotran RS, Kumar V: Pathologic Basis of Disease, 3rd ed, p 5. Philadelphia, WB Saunders, 1984)

ratus of the cell, called the endoplasmic reticulum, is affected first.[12] As the ischemia continues, additional structural alterations develop, such as continued disruption of the endoplasmic reticulum and formation of water-filled blebs at the cell surface. The mitochondria now swell, and defects in the cell membrane also occur.[5,12] Calcium and lipids accumulate as a consequence of abnormal ATP production.[12] The overall effect of this cellular swelling is gradual deterioration in all aspects of cell function.

Effects on Action Potentials. The deterioration of active transport mechanisms interferes with nerve and muscle cell capability for transmitting electrochemical information. Impulses are propagated by means of cellular action potentials that involve the rapid, temporary exchange of sodium for potassium ions across the cell membrane. One of the active transport systems affected by ischemia is the previously described sodium pump that permits levels of sodium and potassium to accumulate against their concentration gradients. As active sodium and potassium pumping ceases and concentrations equalize on the two sides of the cell membrane, the capacity to develop action potentials gradually slows. Ultimately, cell firing stops. Specific consequences depend on the tissue affected. For example, ischemia of myocardial tissue contributes to the development of cardiac arrhythmias.

Development of Cellular Acidosis. The decrease in cellular ATP stimulates the rate of anaerobic glycolysis to increase. As a result, cellular glycogen is rapidly depleted, and lactic acid accumulates within the cells. An early consequence of cellular acidosis is clumping of chromatin, the DNA-containing material located within the cell's nucleus.[12] As the ischemia progresses, both cellular acidosis and cell swelling contribute to injury of the membrane-bound sacs containing various intracellular enzymes. These lysozomal enzymes are the digestive apparatus of the cell and are normally sequestered from other cell contents. When released by damage to their membranes, the lysozomal enzymes digest structural components of the cell and may damage neighboring cells and organs as well.[1] Furthermore, leakage of these enzymes into the blood plasma is a clinical parameter of cell death.

Severity of Ischemia

The extent of ischemic injury depends on the degree to which cellular energy production is impaired by the limitation in arterial blood flow. Either a high tissue demand for oxygen or a sharp reduction in arterial flow can increase the likelihood of ischemic damage. Tissues with only mild ischemia retain sufficient blood flow to sustain a mixture of aerobic and anaerobic metabolism and the continued removal of metabolic end products. As ischemia progresses in severity so that tissue demands for oxygen increasingly outweigh oxygen supply, anaerobic metabolism predominates and end products begin to accumulate. The complete absence of arterial flow leads to total ischemia, a state in which metabolism is exclusively anaerobic, and no metabolic end products can diffuse from the ischemic site.[5] If the extent and duration of ischemia are sufficient, the affected cells may become irreversibly injured, that is, the cells will die despite reperfusion with arterial blood.[5] The precise biochemical mechanism responsible for lethal cell injury has not yet been elucidated; however, interference with ATP production and cell membrane damage are known to be critical factors.[12]

Infarction

Factors Promoting Progression of Ischemia to Infarction

The transition from ischemia to infarction is by no means inevitable. Several factors must be considered when assessing the risk of infarction for a particular tissue.

Rate of Development. Slowly developing ischemia is better tolerated than ischemia of sudden onset. When the development has been gradual, channels for collateral blood supply may open up, and affected cells may adapt to the decreased blood supply by undergoing atrophy.[12] With rapid onset, these compensatory maneuvers are less possible.

Ability of Tissue to Compensate for Decreased Blood Supply. Several patterns exist by which tissues can receive blood from alternative sources. For example, the lungs and the liver have dual blood supplies. In the lungs, the bronchial circulation provides a backup source of blood that can compensate for a reduction in pulmonary artery flow. The liver is supplied by both the portal circulation and the hepatic artery. The arterial circulation to other tissues is arranged in parallel. For example, the radial and ulnar areries form parallel routes to the forearm. So long as one artery is intact, infarction is unlikely. Similarly, the area of brain within the circle of Willis is protected by the parallel linkage of anterior and posterior cerebral arteries. Some tissues with a single blood supply have small, interconnecting anastomoses that can continue to provide blood if a large artery is occluded. The small intestine is an example of a tissue with many such anastomoses. Collateral channels are somewhat less prevalent within the heart but do provide some protection. The kidney, however, has very few such anastomoses, and occlusion of a major renal artery nearly always leads to infarction. In sum, tissues that receive blood by more than one route are far more able to compensate for a reduced blood supply than are tissues that receive blood from a single source.[12]

Tissues can also compensate for a reduction in arterial flow by increasing the amount of oxygen they remove or extract from the blood delivered to them. The lungs and kidneys are examples of tissues that are well perfused and normally extract only a small percentage of their available oxygen. When blood flow decreases, they can compensate by increasing oxygen extraction. In contrast, the heart has nearly maximal oxygen extraction at rest and cannot increase its oxygen supply in this manner.

Oxygen Requirements of Affected Tissue. The outcome of ischemia is heavily influenced by the degree to which the involved tissue needs oxygen to sustain its metabolic activities. The brain is critically dependent on oxygen and its cells die after only a few minutes of oxygen deprivation. Although survival time is somewhat longer, the vulnerability of myocardial and renal cells is also high. Skeletal muscle cells, however, can usually survive for hours.[9] In general, the parenchymal cells of a tissue are more vulnerable than is the supporting structural framework.[12,13] The state of cellular activities is also important in that actively metabolizing cells have a greater oxygen requirement.

Oxygen Availability in Arterial Blood. A final factor that influences the likelihood of infarction is the quality of blood delivered to the tissues. Anemia decreases the quantity of oxygen bound to hemoglobin and thus limits the amount of oxygen that can be delivered. Because of the relationship between dissolved oxygen and hemoglobin saturation, hypoxemia similarly reduces potential oxygen delivery. When anemia or hypoxemia is severe, lung and other relatively invulnerable tissues may undergo infarction.

Sequelae of Infarction

When cells are irreversibly injured, lysozomal enzymes that contribute to cell destruction are released. Within a short time, the dead cells evoke an inflammatory reaction. Leukocytes accumulate at the site and begin to phagocytize cell debris. As in other areas involving extensive tissue destruction, this process culminates in the formation of a fibrous tissue scar (see Chap. 15).

Cell Necrosis. Cells that have succumbed to lethal ischemia undergo the various morphological changes known as necrosis. Of the various patterns of necrosis, coagulation necrosis is most common after an infarction. The cellular architecture is preserved for several days before degenerating. An exception is found in brain tissue, which quickly undergoes liquefaction as a result of infarction. Regardless of the pattern of necrosis, the end result is the total dissolution of the cell.[12]

Appearance of Infarcted Tissue. Immediately after an infarction, the involved tissue is dark in color, and the margins between infarcted and noninfarcted tissue are poorly defined. During the next 24 hours, the distinction between dead and viable tissue becomes clearer and there is often a rim of hyperemia indicating extensive inflammation at the border between dead and living tissue. With time, the color of the infarcted tissue either remains dark red or becomes pale. Pale or *white infarcts* are most common after arterial occlusion of solid tissues. For example, they are commonly seen in the heart and kidney. The reason is that little adjacent or collateral circulation enters the area to compensate for the loss of the primary arterial circulation. As a result, the infarcted tissue soon becomes bloodless and takes on a white appearance. Infarction involving the heart is shown in Figure 23–3. *Red infarcts* are most common in well-perfused, loose tissue such as lung or small intestine. The generous blood

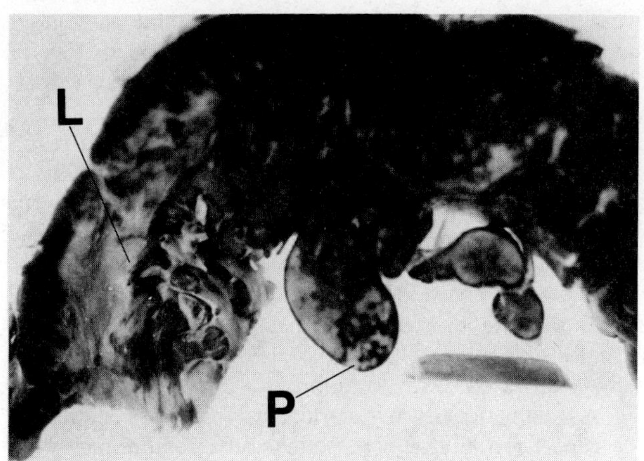

FIGURE 23–3 Myocardial infarction. The tissue section was incubated in nitroblue tetrazolium, a special stain to detect lactic dehydrogenase enzyme loss. Because necrotic areas have lost the enzyme, they do not take up the stain and therefore are white in appearance. Areas of infarction can be noted along the lateral left ventricle (L) and the posterior papillary muscles (P). (Courtesy of Dr. Marie Cowan, University of Washington School of Nursing)

supply helps to delay infarction. The extravasation of blood, due to injury to the vascular endothelial cells, contributes to a red, congested appearance.

If bacterial infection accompanies or develops in the infarcted tissue, it is known as *septic infarction*. Abscess formation commonly complicates this type of infarct. Septic infarction is also referred to as *gangrene*. In dry gangrene, the coagulative pattern of necrosis predominates; in wet gangrene, areas of liquefaction predominate, and the infarcted tissue appears swollen.

Recognition of Ischemia and Strategies to Prevent Infarction

The opportunity to reverse ischemia and prevent infarction is greatest when the ischemic process is detected soon after its onset. Strategies to prevent infarction are best determined after assessing the vulnerability of the affected tissue to infarction and the consequences of infarction for the person as a whole. Such an assessment requires analysis of the factors promoting infarction, recognition of manifestations, and evaluation of the individual's overall physiological and psychological condition.

Recognition of Ischemia

Pain. Pain is an important indication of ischemia in many tissues. In the heart, myocardial ischemia gives rise to angina pectoris. Deprivation of oxygen to skeletal muscles is also associated with pain. Gradual occlusion of the arterial supply to skeletal muscles, as with atherosclerosis involving the lower extremities, often leads to cramping sensations during exercise. This type of pain is known as intermittent claudication. If the ischemia of skeletal muscles is somewhat greater, pain may occur at rest and be accompanied by paresthesias or numbness. Acute obstruction of a major artery to an extremity causes initially intense pain, which is followed by numbness and absence of sensation.[17] Pain also results from ischemia affecting the abdominal viscera. For example, acute ischemia involving the small intestine leads to severe abdominal pain. If the ischemic process is of a milder, chronic nature, the pain is duller and may occur only after meals.[6]

The mechanisms by which ischemia leads to pain are not fully understood. It is possible that peripheral nerve endings are stimulated by increased pressure from cell swelling and other factors.[8] Another possibility is that the release of kinins and other chemical mediators within the ischemic area causes the pain.[16]

Elevated Serum Enzymes. Enzymes, the essential catalysts for cellular metabolism, are contained within all body cells. Damage to cells causes release of these enzymes and subsequent increases in their serum concentration. With some tissues, measurements of enzymes in the serum are useful for diagnosing lethal cell damage caused by ischemia. They are particularly important in helping to establish the diagnosis of myocardial infarction. Of the many serum enzymes, only those that can be used to decipher the location and extent of infarction are included here.

The two transaminase enzymes catalyze amino group transfer in the Krebs cycle and thus enhance energy production.[3,19] One of the transaminase enzymes is known as *SGOT* (serum glutamic-oxaloacetic transaminase) or, more accurately, as *AST* (aspartate aminotransferase). Heart and liver tissue are its chief sources, followed by skeletal muscle, kidney, and pancreas. Because it is found in so many tissues, an elevated SGOT level is not diagnostically conclusive but instead may reflect cellular necrosis from a variety of causes and in a variety of tissues. The other transaminase is *SGPT* (serum glutamic-pyruvic transaminase), also known as *ALT* (alanine aminotransferase). Concentrations are high in the liver, kidney, heart, and skeletal muscle. Renal infarction may cause a rise in SGPT.[18] However, as with SGOT, increased levels of this enzyme are nonspecific.

Lactic dehydrogenase, usually called *LDH,* catalyzes the reaction between pyruvate and lactate during glycolysis.[7] Although the enzyme is present in nearly all cells, slight variations in molecular structure exist, which can be identified by serum protein electrophoresis. These subtypes are known as isoenzymes and are relatively tissue-specific. LDH_1 predominates in heart muscle and erythrocytes. LDH_2 has a high serum concentration and is believed to originate from reticuloendothelial cells. LDH_3 is prevalent in brain and kidney tissue. The kidneys, skeletal muscle, and liver all contain LDH_4, and LDH_5 is found in the liver, skeletal muscle, and ileum.[19] An increase in LDH_1 and LDH_2, with the concentration of LDH_1 greater than LDH_2, is highly suggestive of myocardial infarction. LDH levels also increase with renal and pulmonary infarction.[18,19]

Creatine phosphokinase, also called creatine kinase, is usually abbreviated as *CPK* or *CK*. The heart, brain, and skeletal muscle are major sources of this enzyme.[19] Like LDH, it can be fractionated into isoenzymes by electrophoresis.

Brain tissue produces primarily the BB isoenzyme. Skeletal muscle predominantly contains the isoenzyme known as MM. Although heart muscle contains significant quantities of CPK-MM, it produces large quantities of the MB isoenzyme as well. A rise in serum level of CPK-MB isoenzyme occurs solely with myocardial damage; it is therefore an important, although not conclusive, diagnostic indicator of myocardial infarction.[19] Total CPK levels may increase with muscle or brain infarction.[18]

Additional Manifestations in Selected Tissues. In addition to the presence of pain or elevated serum enzymes, signs and symptoms may appear that are specific to the affected tissue or organ. Many of these manifestations of ischemia can also reflect organ dysfunction from a variety of other causes. When risk factors for ischemia are present, however, evidence of these signs and symptoms may help to confirm the diagnosis and to gauge the severity of the ischemic process.

Myocardial ischemia causes mechanical and electrical changes in heart function. Ischemia impairs both the ability of myocardial muscle fibers to shorten (contractility) and the ability of the heart to generate adequate pressure to eject blood (compliance). As a result, stroke vo me falls.[16] Electrical changes stem from altered cellular action potentials. A wide variety of cardiac arrhythmias can develop, depending on the location and severity of the ischemia. These arrhythmias and their consequences for the patient are described in Chapter 36.

The electroencephalogram pattern shows abnormalities within seconds after brain tissue becomes severely ischemic. Patients suffering from brain ischemia exhibit many changes in cerebral function. These changes vary from impaired judgment in the case of mild or chronic ischemia to loss of consciousness if cerebral blood flow has been extensively or acutely reduced.[13]

Kidney function also suffers from ischemia. As a result of decreased renal blood flow, the glomerular filtration rate decreases, and urine output drops. If arterial flow to the kidneys is not rapidly increased, renal failure may develop.[1,13]

Inadequate blood flow to the extremities can affect the skin, subcutaneous tissue, and even skeletal muscles. Manifestations of sudden, complete arterial occlusion include pain, pallor, coldness, numbness, and loss of arterial pulses.[17] If the occlusion is gradual or incomplete, manifestations are more subtle. Increased venous pressure may compress the arterioles without obliterating the arterial pulse. In this situation, pain and paresthesias are the primary manifestations of ischemia.[8,10]

Strategies to Reduce Ischemia and Limit Infarction

Because restoration of arterial flow can only help cells that remain viable, the major goal in managing ischemia is to reduce ischemia and prevent infarction. In general, strategies either increase the oxygen supply to an ischemic tissue or decrease its oxygen needs. If infarction has already occurred, these strategies are continued to prevent its extension to the surrounding tissues. The techniques briefly outlined below will be described more fully elsewhere in the text where they are applicable to the management of specific disorders. Examples of nursing interventions are listed in Table 23–1.

TABLE 23–1
Nursing Interventions to Limit Infarction

Data	*Significance*	*Possible Nursing Interventions*
Assessment of Ischemic Tissue for Vulnerability to Infarction		
Rate of ischemia development	Rapid onset provides little time for tissue to compensate for decreased blood supply	Analyze all assessment data to determine risk of infarction and need for nursing measures to protect ischemic tissue. Examples of protective measures include
Pattern of blood supply to affected tissue	Anatomical pattern of single blood supply and few anastamoses increases risk of infarction	• Positioning affected tissue flat or slightly dependent to prevent gravity from impeding arterial flow • Positioning to avoid kinking or compressing arteries • Resting affected part (may require bed rest) • Decreasing environmental stress • Relieving pain with analgesia
Oxygen requirements of affected tissue	High oxygen requirement increases infarction risk	
Presence of pain	Continued or increased pain may indicate extension of ischemic process Pain increases metabolic demands	
Elevated serum enzyme values	Confirm infarction	

(*Continued*)

TABLE 23–1
Nursing Interventions to Limit Infarction (Continued)

Data	*Significance*	*Possible Nursing Interventions*
Assessment of Other Body Systems for Additional Factors Contributing to Risk of Infarction		
Respiratory System		
Severe hypoxemia $Pa_{O_2} < 60$ mmHg)	Decreases oxygen delivery to tissues	Provide supplemental oxygen
Shallow breathing	Contributes to development of hypoxemia, acidosis	Position for maximal respiratory muscle excursion Coach to increase depth of breathing
Airway obstruction	Contributes to development of hypoxemia, acidosis	Position to maintain airway patency Remove secretions by cough, tracheal suction, chest physiotherapy
Cardiovascular System		
Hypotension	Decreases organ perfusion	Administer isotonic fluid, vasopressors as ordered Position to maximize available arterial flow
Anemia	Decreases oxygen delivery to tissues	*Mild:* Dietary replacement for anemias caused by nutritional deficiency, iron supplements as ordered *Severe:* Blood transfusions as ordered, oxygen administration, activity reduction
Arrhythmias	May reduce cardiac output and thus decrease organ perfusion	Assess effect on cardiac output Determine etiology of arrhythmia and appropriate intervention
Atherosclerosis	Decreases oxygen perfusion	*Short term:* Position to maximize available arterial flow *Long term:* Teach methods to reduce risk factors for atherosclerosis
Renal System	Decreases elimination of anaerobic metabolism end products Increases acidosis (metabolic)	Avoid nephrotoxic drugs Restrict diet as needed (*e.g.*, K^+, protein)
Neurological System		
Decreased or altered level of consciousness	May limit ability to comply with therapy May increase risk of self-injury	Protective measures as needed
Increased temperature	Increases metabolic needs	Avoid application of local heat to ischemic tissue Lower body temperature without inducing shivering: antipyretics, cool sponges, cool environment
Anxiety	Increases metabolic needs	Reduce anxiety by explaining procedures, allowing expression of feelings, administering anti-anxiety drugs
Pain (from any cause)	Increases metabolic needs	Relieve pain by analgesia, positioning, distraction
Endocrine System		
Diabetes mellitus	Decreases organ perfusion due to increased atherosclerosis Delays recognition of ischemia due to sensory impairment	*Short term:* Inspect extremities for ischemia *Long term:* Teach inspection and self-care for feet
Hyperthyroidism	Increases metabolic demands	Provide adequate nutrition to meet increased caloric needs Decrease environmental stress
Adrenal cortical insufficiency	Decreases ability to compensate for decreased blood flow by stress response	Administer isotonic fluid and corticosteroids as ordered

(Continued)

TABLE 23–1
Nursing Interventions to Limit Infarction (Continued)

Data	*Significance*	*Possible Nursing Interventions*
Assessment of Other Body Systems for Additional Factors Contributing to Risk of Infarction		
Gastrointestinal System		
Anorexia	Decreases metabolic substrate available for tissue repair	Provide small, nourishing meals Administer antiemetics as needed
Large meals	Temporarily divert blood supply from vital organs to gut	Provide small, frequent meals
Musculoskeletal System		
Muscular activity	Increases metabolic needs	Rest involved tissue (may require bed rest)
Integumentary System		
Lesions or breakdown	Increases likelihood of septic infarction	Inspect for evidence of skin breakdown Use aseptic technique for dressing changes involving ischemic subcutaneous tissue
Reproductive System		
Sexual intercourse	Temporarily increases metabolic demands	*Long term:* Discuss resumption of sexual activity and, if necessary, adaptations to reduce metabolic demands (particularly relevant for myocardial ischemia

Methods of Increasing Oxygen Supply. The arterial flow to an ischemic area can be increased by numerous methods. Physician-directed measures include administration of drugs to dissolve arterial clots or retard their formation and surgical procedures to revascularize ischemic areas or remove arterial obstructions. Arterial flow can also be maximized by nursing interventions. For example, patients can be positioned to avoid kinking or compressing the arteries supplying an ischemic limb. When hypovolemia exists, arterial flow can be increased by restoring blood volume with normal saline or plasma expanders.

Maintenance of the oxygen content of arterial blood is equally important. Severe anemia may require treatment with blood transfusions. Hypoxemia is managed by increasing the amount of oxygen that is inspired.

Methods of Decreasing Oxygen Needs. A major principle guiding the care that a nurse provides for a patient with ischemia is to minimize the metabolic needs of the affected tissue. When an extremity is ischemic, for example, active and passive exercise should be curtailed until the risk of infarction subsides. The gastrointestinal system is rested by withholding oral intake. Bed rest is indicated if myocardial infarction is believed imminent.

Fever increases the metabolic rate of the body approximately 13% for every 1°C that the temperature is elevated over normal.[2] Fever must be controlled without inducing shivering, which also increases the metabolic rate. Because local application of heat also increases metabolic demands and the danger of thermal injury, it should be avoided whenever a tissue is ischemic.

Stress, from any cause, likewise increases the metabolic demands of tissues. Stressors can be of a biochemical nature, as in infection, or can have a psychological basis. Control of the environment to reduce stress is an important aspect of nursing care to prevent infarction.

Summary

Nurses have an important role in the recognition of ischemia and prevention or limitation of infarction. One aspect of this role involves the recognition of clinical situations in which ischemia is possible. In such a circumstance, both careful assessment of tissues at risk and interventions to optimize their oxygen supply are necessary. Another aspect of the nursing role is the recognition of situations in which ischemic change has not yet occurred but is possible in either the short or long term. In this type of situation the interventions often involve teaching preventive strategies directly to patients or clients. Subsequent chapters of this text will provide detailed interventions pertinent to ischemia and infarction involving specific body systems.

References

1. Baue AE: Metabolic abnormalities of shock. Sug Clin North Am 56:1059–1071, 1976
2. Beland IL, Passos JY: Clinical Nursing: Pathophysiological and Psychosocial Approaches, 4th ed. New York, Macmillan, 1981

3. Corbett JV: Laboratory Tests in Nursing Practice. Norwalk CT, Appleton-Century-Crofts, 1982
4. Ganong WF: Review of Medical Physiology, 11th ed. Los Altos, Lange Medical Publications, 1983
5. Jennings RB, Ganote CE, Reimer KA: Ischemic tissue injury. Am J Pathol 81:179–198, 1975
6. LaMont JT, Isselbacher KJ: Diseases of the small and large intestine. In Petersdorf RG, Adams RD, Braunwald E et al (eds): Harrison's Principles of Internal Medicine, 10th ed, pp 1752–1765. New York, McGraw-Hill, 1983
7. Lehninger AL: Bioenergetics, 2nd ed. Menlo Park CA, WA Benjamin, 1973
8. Martinez AC et al: Effect of ischaemia on sensory evoked potentials. Electromyogr Clin Neurophysiol 20:183–192, 1980
9. Matsen FA: Compartmental syndrome. Clin Orthop 113:8–14, 1975
10. Matsen FA: Compartmental syndromes. Hosp Pract 15:113–117, 1980
11. Price SA, Wilson LM: Pathophysiology, 2nd ed. New York, McGraw-Hill, 1982
12. Robbins SL, Cotran RS: Pathologic Basis of Disease, 2nd ed. Philadelphia, WB Saunders, 1979
13. Robin ED, Simon LM: Oxygen transport and cellular respiration. In Frohlich ED (ed): Pathophysiology: Altered Regulatory Mechanisms in Disease, 3rd ed, pp 163–182. Philadelphia, JB Lippincott, 1984
14. Sheridan GW: Compartment syndromes. Bulletin of the Mason Clinic 34:93–98, 1980
15. Smith LH, Thier SD: Pathophysiology: The Biological Basis of Disease. Philadelphia, WB Saunders, 1981
16. Solack SD: Pathophysiology of myocardial ischemia and infarction. In Underhill SL et al (eds): Cardiac Nursing, pp 111–123. Philadelphia, JB Lippincott, 1982
17. Strandness DE: Vascular diseases of the extremities. In Petersdorf RG, Adams RD, Braunwald E et al (eds): Harrison's Principles of Internal Medicine, 10th ed, pp 1491–1498. New York, McGraw-Hill, 1983
18. Wallach J: Interpretation of Diagnostic Tests, 3rd ed. Boston, Little, Brown & Co, 1978
19. Widmann FK: Clinical Interpretation of Laboratory Tests, 9th ed. Philadelphia, FA Davis, 1983

Bibliography

Chaudrey IH, Clemens MG, Baue AE: Alterations in cell function with ischemia and shock and their correction. Arch Surg 116:1309, 1981

Chaudrey IH: Cellular mechanisms in shock and ischemia and their correction. Am J Physiol 245:R-134, 1983

Hinkle PC, McCarty RE: How cells make ATP. Sci Am 123:104, 1978

Robbins SL, Cotran RS, Kumar V: Pathologic Basis of Disease, 3rd ed, pp 5–9, 108–112. Philadelphia, WB Saunders, 1984

Chapter 24

Shock

Margaret Auld Bruya

Shock has been defined in many ways but essentially may be viewed as a generalized state of severe circulatory inadequacy. This inadequacy causes a disproportion between circulating blood volume and the capacity of the vascular beds. As a result of this disproportionate distribution, tissue perfusion is inadequate and cellular hypoxia, cellular destruction, and ultimately, multiple organ failure may occur.

Shock is most frequently seen in patients in emergency rooms or critical care units but is not limited to any specific nursing care area. Nurses need to know predisposing factors, causative events, and clinical manifestations.

Although reduced blood flow to tissues is a common denominator of shock, each type of shock that is discussed in this chapter has distinct physiological properties and abnormalities that require nursing and medical therapies appropriate to the diagnosis. Conceptualizing the cellular level at which shock occurs will allow the nurse to recall the origin of clinical manifestations, the basis for complications, and the rationale for therapy.

Circulatory homeostasis is essential to the maintenance of the body. The three mechanisms through which circulatory homeostasis is maintained are

1. *Volume:* a sufficient circulating blood volume
2. *Pump:* a healthy heart to pump and circulate the volume
3. *Resistance:* the vascular system capable of accommodating blood flow to the capillaries and its return to the right side of the heart

Without these three components acting in concert, the body will be unable to compensate for the failure of any one or more of the mechanisms. As a result, shock will be clinically evident.

Compensatory mechanisms will allow for minor variations in the three components, but unless appropriate treatment is instituted, the compensatory mechanisms will ultimately fail. Failure of compensatory mechanisms or lack of appropriate treatment leads to the patient's death.

The degree of protection afforded by these temporary mechanisms reflects the degree to which the manifestations of shock can be delayed or averted. For example, certain mechanisms compensate for low or decreasing blood volume, some mechanisms compensate for a failing heart, and others compensate for excessive peripheral vascular bed dilation. Many of the signs and symptoms presented by the patient are a direct result of these compensatory mechanisms.

Classification

Numerous classifications of the shock syndrome have been offered. These various means of labeling shock can be very confusing (Table 24–1).

TABLE 24–1
Labels for Shock Commonly Found in the Literature

Allergic shock	Insulin shock
Anaphylactic shock	Neurogenic shock
Bacterial shock	Oligemic shock
Burn shock	Peptone shock
Cardiogenic shock	Septic shock
Diabetic shock	Spinal shock
Endotoxic shock	Surgical shock
Hematogenic shock	Tourniquet shock
Hemorrhagic shock	Toxic shock
Histamine shock	Traumatic shock
Hypovolemic shock	Vasogenic shock
Iatrogenic shock	Vasovagal shock

This text presents four basic types of shock:

1. *Hypovolemic shock,* caused by loss of circulating vascular volume
2. *Cardiogenic shock,* caused by failure of the cardiac muscle as a pump either through trauma or ischemia and infarction
3. *Septic shock,* caused by infection
4. *Vasogenic or neurogenic shock,* caused by a sudden, severe vasodilation of the vascular bed, resulting in relative hypovolemia

Although shock occurs in a wide variety of conditions and presents as a result of a multitude of different clinical situations, the very young and the elderly are more likely to develop hypovolemic and septic shock following surgery or trauma than is the young and healthy adult. Persons with chronic or debilitating diseases such as diabetes mellitus, atherosclerosis, or congestive heart failure respond less favorably to therapies.

Hypovolemic Shock

Failure of, or a significant reduction in, venous return to the right heart results when the intravascular volume of blood fails to fill the vascular capacity. This may be caused by excessive loss of blood from hemorrhage, from excessive loss of plasma as a result of burns or inflammation, or from the fluid losses caused by prolonged vomiting or diarrhea. On rare occasions heat prostration and insufficient antidiuretic hormone release will cause hypovolemic shock.

Many conditions that cause shifts in the intracellular, intravascular, and extracellular fluid compartments can lead to vascular hypovolemia and ultimately to shock. Conditions such as inflammation, intestinal obstruction, trauma, and anaphylaxis may cause shock.

Probably the most common form of hypovolemic shock results from the loss of circulating blood volume. Symptoms of blood loss, such as thirst, weakness, pallor, cool or clammy skin, and apprehension, do not occur until about 30% of the blood volume is lost. (See Table 24–2 for comparative signs that occur in the various stages of shock.) If bleeding can be controlled, blood replacement should avert progression to *refractory shock,* which is resistant to treatment. When cessation of bleeding and blood replacement do not improve the patient's condition, other factors are to be considered, for example, plasma loss, increased vascular capacity, and inability of the heart to pump.

If volume loss continues, compensatory mechanisms no longer can protect the vital centers from the irreversible cell damage caused by inadequate perfusion. Clinically, the depressed function of cells, tissues, and organs becomes progressively worse, and a vicious cycle of deterioration towards death occurs.

Prevention. Early detection and treatment of fluid losses should prevent hypovolemic shock from occurring. In emergency situations, such as trauma involving crush or penetrating injuries, or open, bleeding sites, control of bleeding becomes paramount. Concurrently, blood or blood-product replacement is essential. During surgical procedures, adequate volume replacement should be carefully monitored. Surgical wounds should be checked postoperatively for leakage which, if undetected, could contribute to a shock state.[5] Some bleeding sites, such as gastric ulcers, are not always amenable to wound closure. Whole blood is then administered to provide support until healing can occur.

Cardiogenic Shock

Cardiogenic shock includes shock due primarily to ineffective cardiac pumping and subsequent myocardial ineffectiveness.[7] It occurs in instances of myocardial insufficiency, structural abnormalities, and cardiac arrhythmias. Cardiac tamponade, pulmonary embolism, congestive heart failure, and papillary muscle rupture may all contribute to the development of cardiogenic shock. Two terms are frequently used in cardiogenic shock: pump failure and power failure. The term *pump failure* is used to describe inadequate contractility of the heart muscle, and *power failure* describes deficiencies of the heart's electrical conduction system (see Chap. 36). Either condition may lead to shock and ultimately death. Patients in cardiogenic shock have a mortality rate ranging from 60% to 85%.[8]

Characteristic of cardiogenic shock is a markedly depressed cardiac output. Because of this loss of cardiac output, adequate tissue perfusion cannot be maintained because too little blood is forced into the arteries. The other compensatory mechanisms, such as increased heart rate, increased sympathetic mediated vasoconstriction, and increased contractility of the heart muscle, are ineffective in combating the deleterious effects of the reduced cardiac output unless the basic disorder is corrected by therapeutic measures. Cardiogenic shock is self-perpetuating: as the heart fails to perfuse the cells in all organs, irreversible injury and death of the patient result.

Septic Shock

Septic shock generally means a shock secondary to serious systemic infections and bacteremia, with an incidence between 25% and 40% of patients with gram-negative bacteremia.[6] Despite the use of antibiotics and highly sophisticated nursing care units, septic shock has an excess of 50% mortality.[9] Organ dysfunction, as in other forms of shock, is

TABLE 24–2
Comparison of Events Occurring in Stages of Hemorrhagic Shock

Response to Hemorrhage	*Compensated Shock (Early stage)*	*Impending Shock*	*Refractory Shock (Late Stage)*
Blood loss	Minimal (15%)	Moderate (30%)	Severe (45%)
Vascular response	Recruitment of extracellular fluid; contraction great veins	Arteriolar constriction, reduced flow to skin, bone, and muscle. Tachycardia, reduced cardiac output	Cardiac output markedly reduced; hypotension; blood flow to viscera impaired
Signs and symptoms	Transient, increased respiratory rate, pupillary dilation, increased sweat gland activity	Thirst, orthostatic hypotension, apprehension, weakness and pallor, skin cool and pale	Air hunger, altered state of consciousness
Metabolic response	Slight	Increased glycolysis and lipolysis; increased glucose, fatty acids, lactate in blood. Respiratory alkalosis. Decreased urinary sodium and volume	Severe lactic acidosis; severe oliguria Mixed venous P_{O_2} approaching 20 mmHg
Nervous	Increase in blood pressure	Receptors in aorta and carotid arteries sense fall in blood pressure and stimulate sympathetic branch of autonomic nervous system	

due to cellular hypoxia. Depletion of high-energy phosphates, depression of mitochondrial function, anaerobic metabolism with intracellular acidosis, cellular swelling, rupture of lysosomal membranes, and disintegration of cellular walls due to perfusion pressure failure collectively result in widespread changes in body tissues.[11] In septic shock, the primary etiologic agent is an endotoxin, a part of the bacterial cell wall released into circulating blood when the bacteria are destroyed.

Clinically, the incidence of shock associated with infections is high. Patients at high risk for development of septic shock include the elderly, the debilitated, the cirrhotic, and those with altered immune mechanisms. Characteristically, persons resuscitated from hypovolemic traumatic shock who incur multisystem trauma are also in a a high-risk category for septic shock. Those persons, particularly the elderly or debilitated, who have surgery or instrumentation involving the genitourinary, gastrointestinal, and biliary tracts are also at risk. For an overview of leading factors predisposing to the development of septic shock, see Table 24–3.

Extensive experimental and clinical studies have delineated the hemodynamic changes in septic shock.[4] As bacteremia progresses, the body's protective mechanisms are overwhelmed owing to immune suppression, overwhelming numbers of microorganisms, or resistance of bacteria to antibiotics.

Following the initial phase of hyperdynamic cardiovascular and metabolic states, the loss of peripheral vascular tone and splanchnic pooling effectively reduce blood volume returning to the heart, consequently decreasing arterial

TABLE 24–3
Factors Predisposing to the Development of Septic Shock

Increasing Number of Invasive Procedures
Genitourinary instrumentation, *e.g.*, urinary catheters
Indwelling catheters in blood vessels, *e.g.*, IVs, CVP, hyperalimentation
Blood transfusions
Pacemaker insertions
Abortions
Surgery, especially genitourinary, gastrointestinal

Increasing Number of Compromised Hosts
Elderly
Very young, *e.g.*, very low birth weight infants
Transplantation patients
Burned patients
Alcoholics
Liver disease patients
Patients with dysfunctional spleens
Drug abusers
Traumatized patients
Hospitalized patients with open wounds

Reservoir of Antibiotic Resistance
Overuse of antibiotics

Pharmacological Therapies Altering Host Response
Corticosteroids
Chemotherapy
Nonsteroidal anti-inflammatory drugs
Bone marrow suppression

pressure, central venous pressure, and cardiac output. Disturbances in gas exchange in the lung occur because of arteriovenous shunting and increased extravascular lung water. Stasis in the circulating blood volume decreases oxygen availability and utilization by tissues. Development of cellular hypoxia contributes to myocardial depression and increased capillary permeability. Intravascular clotting occurs, further compromising the flow of blood and subsequent venous return. As this type of shock progresses, it closely resembles other types of shock.

Neurogenic/Vasogenic Shock

Massive peripheral vasodilatation causes shock because the blood volume, although adequate for a normal vascular bed, is insufficient to fill a markedly enlarged vascular compartment. Primary vasodilatation that results from sympathetic nervous system blockage is called *neurogenic shock*. Fainting is a transient episode of this type of shock. Spinal anesthesia and, much less commonly, general anesthesia can result in more severe forms of neurogenic shock. The neurogenic shock that can accompany spinal anesthesia is a consequence of sympathetic blockade by the anesthetic agent and resultant peripheral vasodilatation.[1] Because the anesthesia-induced vasodilatation is predictable, careful precautions are taken that prevent the development of shock in a majority of cases. These precautions are described in Chapter 8. Primary vasodilatation can also be a component of anaphylactic shock. In this case, the vasodilatation is due to antigen–antibody mediated release of vasodilator substances (see Chap. 16). Shock caused by the presence of vasodilator substances is often referred to as *vasogenic shock*.

Sequence of Events

Although shock has many diverse causes, all causes will eventually lead to generalized cellular dysfunction from inadequate tissue perfusion. Shock symptoms begin in the microcirculation and affect all cell structures and functions. Although this presentation implies a sequence of events, it is rather a simultaneous and overlapping process that occurs.

Compensation

To accurately observe and initiate therapy for the potential shock patient, the nurse must recall both the normal compensatory mechanisms and the pathophysiological mechanisms associated with shock. The total body effectively responds to periods of stress, such as blood loss or serious injury, for short periods of time. This response, generally termed *homeostatic control mechanism,* is an attempt of the body at self-preservation.

The major physiological responses to a stressor such as shock occur in the major maintenance organs: the cardiovascular, renal, pulmonary, and central nervous systems. Other systems, particularly the gastrointestinal and musculoskeletal systems, are also affected.

Cellular events occur before the clinical changes become evident. The findings may be grouped into three stages (see Table 24–2). The three stages are

Stage 1: Compensated shock
Stage 2: Impending shock
Stage 3: Refractory shock

Although these stages—compensated, impending, and refractory shock—are not clearly defined in the clinical setting, these categories do provide a general framework for the nurse to understand the complex occurrences in shock. Specific responses to shock are influenced by the severity and duration of the shock state, the specific tissues involved and their needs, and the previous state of health as well as the age of the patient. Responses thus vary with the stage of shock and the individual patient.

Compensated Shock

In stage 1, or compensated shock, blood loss has been minimal (less than 15%), and the cardiac output may be decreased as a result of any of the multiple causes of shock. Nonspecific changes occurring at the cellular level are recruitment of extracellular fluid and contraction of the great veins. The signs and symptoms of compensated shock seem to be transient (*e.g.,* increased respiratory rate and pupillary dilation), and the metabolic response is quite slight.

Impending Shock

In stage 2, or impending shock, the cardiac output is decreased and compensatory mechanisms are fully activated. For short time periods, these compensatory mechanisms may be successful in restoring cardiac output and blood pressure. Without support and treatment, however, impending shock will progress to refractory shock. Regardless of the type of shock, compensation can be divided into three interrelated categories of homeostatic mechanisms: nervous, hormonal, and chemical.

Compensatory Homeostatic Mechanisms

Nervous System Compensation. When cardiac output diminishes, receptors in the aorta and carotid arteries recognize a fall in blood pressure. The messages that are sent to the vasomotor center in the medulla of the brain result in the stimulation of the sympathetic branch of the autonomic nervous system. This stimulation causes the body to prepare for a stress state. Heart rate is increased, and heartbeat is more forceful; as a result, cardiac output is increased, and blood pressure is raised. Blood vessels vasodilate to provide more oxygen to the myocardium. In addition, blood vessels to the skin, gastrointestinal tract, and kidneys vasoconstrict to shunt blood to the priority organs: the heart and the brain. Because of the decreased peripheral blood flow, the skin appears cool and pale. Urinary output decreases because of reduced renal blood flow. Vasoconstriction of the vessels of the gastrointestinal tract produces decreased activity and slowed or impaired peristalsis. Bowel tones are hypoactive or absent. The results of the vasoconstriction include elevation of blood pressure and increased venous return to the heart. Other sympathetic responses include the following: pupillary dilation, vasodilation of vessels to the skeletal muscles, an increase in respiratory rate and depth, and an increase in sweat gland activity, producing clammy, moist skin.

Hormonal Compensation. The hormonal effects that occur in a stress response caused by shock are the result of the sympathetic nervous system response previously described. When the sympathetic vasoconstriction shunts blood away from the kidneys, the juxtaglomerular apparatus (JGA) releases renin. In the circulation, renin reacts with the substrate angiotensinogen, to produce angiotensin I. In the lungs, angiotensin I is altered to form angiotensin II, which is a potent vasoconstrictor of both arteries and veins. The result of this potent vasoconstriction is to further increase blood pressure and facilitate venous return to the right side of the heart. Simultaneously, angiotensin II activates the adrenal cortex to release the mineralocorticoid, aldosterone. This hormone increases reabsorption of both sodium and water (see Chap. 13).

The sympathetic response further activates the anterior pituitary gland to release adrenocorticotropic hormone (ACTH). This ACTH acts on the adrenal cortex to increase the release of glucocorticoids, which elevate the serum glucose concentration. The adrenal medulla also causes the release of an increased amount of the catecholamines, epinephrine and norepinephrine. The catecholamines increase serum glucose concentrations by stimulating glycogenolysis in the liver.

Chemical Compensation. The third type of compensation, chemical compensation, occurs following the reduction of cardiac output and reduced blood flow to the lungs.[10] As a result of this reduced blood flow to the lungs, the physiological dead space is increased and ventilation/perfusion imbalances occur, so that ventilated alveoli no longer have adequate blood flow through the capillary bed. With this resultant decreased oxygen tension in the blood, the chemoreceptors, which are sensitive to low oxygen tension, cause an increase in the rate and depth of ventilation. Because of this hyperventilation, there is a decrease in the carbon dioxide tension in the blood, and respiratory alkalosis develops. As a result of this reduction in carbon dioxide tension, cerebral blood vessels vasoconstrict. Cerebral vasoconstriction leads to cerebral ischemia, or hypoxia. Impairment of cerebral function is further compounded by reduced oxygen tension secondary to decreased cardiac output and ventilation/perfusion imbalances. Cerebral dysfunction may be manifested by restlessness, agitation, confusion, drowsiness, lethargy, and a decreasing level of consciousness.

Clinical Findings

The clinical findings in this state of impending shock include the following:

Blood Pressure. The blood pressure is adequate to perfuse the vital organs. Systolic blood pressure is increased because of increased stroke volume, whereas diastolic blood pressure is elevated because of systemic arterial vasoconstriction. If the shock is due to a blood loss, this system will ultimately fail.

Heart Rate. The heart rate is increased due to sympathetic stimulation. One would observe a sinus tachycardia with an atrial rate of over 100 beats/minute.

Skin. The skin is cool, pale, and clammy as a result of the peripheral vasoconstriction and increased sweat gland activity.

Urine. The urinary output is decreased as a result of the reduced blood flow to the kidneys. Urine osmolarity is high, and the urinary sodium concentration is low because of the increased sodium reabsorption.

Respirations. The respiratory pattern is typically rapid and deep. Tachypnea, with a respiratory rate greater than 20 breaths/minute, is very common.

Bowel Sounds. Bowel sounds are diminished because blood vessels in the gastrointestinal tract have vasoconstricted in an attempt to shunt blood to the heart and brain. Gastric motility is diminished, and bowel sounds are hypoactive or absent.

Pupils. Pupils may be dilated because of sympathetic stimulation, but they do react to light stimulation.

Level of Consciousness. The person who is in this impending shock stage will have a varied sensorium because of the hypoxia and hypocapnia. The patient may appear to be restless, agitated, anxious, or confused. Memory and judgment are typically impaired. As shock continues and as the vital organs of the heart and brain are put in greater jeopardy, lethargy, depression, or coma may ensue because of the brain cell hypoxia.

Refractory Shock

All the physiological changes that occur in the impending shock stage of shock will be present in the refractory stage. The refractory stage of shock occurs if the cause of shock is not corrected and compensatory mechanisms fail or if the treatment instituted is too little or too late. In this stage, when the compensatory mechanisms fail in maintaining cardiac output, the other body systems die.

Sequence of Events

While it may serve a purpose for a period of time, prolonged capillary vasoconstriction results in oxygen deficit. This oxygen deficit causes decreased ATP production, and anaerobic metabolism occurs. The cells are then functionally impaired and release toxic substances. Because capillary blood flow is reduced, these toxic substances accumulate in the tissues and alter the local tissue environment. With these changes in tissue environment, the environment becomes more acid. The acid pH causes precapillary sphincters to relax and allows blood to flow into the capillary bed. This flow of blood is occurring while the precapillary sphincters are open and while the postcapillary vessels are more resistant and remain vasoconstricted.[2] As a result, while blood flows freely into the capillary bed, blood flow from the capillary bed is impeded. Capillary hydrostatic pressure increases, so that fluid is pushed from the capillary bed into the tissues. Local factors (such as histamine) may simultaneously increase capillary permeability and facilitate this fluid shift. Increased capillary permeability additionally causes protein to leak from the vessels. Serum colloid osmotic pressure is lowered, and more and more fluid leaves the capillary bed and moves into the tissues, or interstitial space.

The leakage of fluid from capillaries into the tissue bed further reduces the intravascular circulating blood volume. Because the viscosity of blood is increased as the fluid is lost through the capillaries, the blood flow is reduced, causing capillary sludging. Sludging of red cells, platelets, and other large proteins diminishes the circulatory volume and further reduces circulating blood flow. In addition, the accumulation of excess fluid in the interstitial fluid creates edema, which causes further cell dysfunction.

The loss of circulating blood volume and impaired capillary flow result in reduced venous return and reduced cardiac output. With this reduced cardiac output and subsequent decreased blood pressure, perfusion of coronary arteries may be decreased. The heart may become ischemic. Ischemic myocardium is prone to arrhythmias, and the myocardium functions less and less effectively as a pump. Infarction may also occur. With this continued vasoconstriction, peripheral or cutaneous blood flow is diminished. Ischemia of distal parts, such as toes, fingers, tip of the nose, and ear lobes, will be reflected in weak or absent pulses and cold extremities. Obviously, when inadequate blood flow to these distal parts has occurred for a long period of time, necrosis may occur secondary to local ischemia. The body's defense against microbial injury is reduced or eliminated, both locally and systemically, as these areas of necrosis occur.

Body System Effects

Continued vasoconstriction affects specific body organ systems in specific ways.

Brain. In the brain, with the cerebral blood flow diminished, the patient's sensorium and level of consciousness also diminish. The patient may act in a bizarre manner; he may have personality changes, or altered or decreased response to painful stimuli.

Kidneys. In the kidneys, because of the prolonged vasoconstriction, oxygen delivery to the nephrons is inadequate. With the lack of oxygenation, the nephrons are unable to do their work of filtration, secretion, and reabsorption. As the tubular cells of the nephron suffer from ischemia, the cells themselves may die, slough off into the urine, and impair further blood flow by blocking the tubules. A condition known as acute tubular necrosis (ATN) may occur as a result of this prolonged vasoconstriction. Acute tubular nephrosis will lead to acute renal failure and, if not reversed in a short period of time, may cause permanent renal damage.

Gastrointestinal Tract. In the gastrointestinal tract, the prolonged vasoconstriction results in superficial alterations of the wall of the gastrointestinal tract. This local damage will result in edema, hemorrhage, and congestion of the intestinal wall. The intestinal tract, which had previously been a line of defense against bacteria, no longer functions in this manner when edema, hemorrhage, and ulceration occur. Ulceration of the wall also increases the incidence of stress ulcers and precipitates episodes of gastrointestinal bleeding. This bleeding from the ulcers further diminishes the circulating blood volume. The patient may complain of nausea, anorexia, and vomiting because of the reduced blood flow and congestion of the gastrointestinal circulatory vessels.

Liver. In the liver, the function is reduced because of the vasoconstriction. Blood from the gastrointestinal tract is no longer effectively filtered before it returns to the right heart. With impaired circulation to the liver, metabolic activities, such as gluconeogenesis and fat metabolism, are impaired. Drugs detoxified by the liver will accumulate in the body, and adjustments in dosage need to be considered. Waste products, such as ammonia and lactic acid, are not metabolized. Liver cells themselves eventually become ischemic and die. Elevation of the liver enzymes is seen in laboratory values.

Pancreas. When the pancreas is affected by vasoconstriction, pancreatic ischemia, which causes an increase in amylase and lipase levels in the blood, may occur. Pancreatic cells also become ischemic and release proteolytic enzymes, resulting in formation of myocardial depressant factor (MDF). This polypeptide is thought to interfere with the role of calcium in coupling electrical excitation with mechanical contraction of the heart.

Lungs. In the lungs, vasoconstriction results in ischemic or damaged cells, which release toxic products, such as histamine, serotonin, or hydrogen ions. These toxic products act to increase pulmonary arteriovasoconstriction and increase capillary permeability. Dramatic fluid shifts occur in the pulmonary capillaries and in the pulmonary interstitial space. Prolonged arterial vasoconstriction can lead to pulmonary capillary hydrostatic pressure exceeding that of the interstitial space. This great fluid loss into the interstitial space leads to interstitial edema. As this edema increases, fluid moves from the alveoli, producing alveolar edema. The lungs then can no longer perfuse or ventilate. Arterial blood gases now reflect hypoventilation, with increased carbon dioxide tension and decreased pH. Decreased diffusion and perfusion are indicated by low oxygen tension in the arterial blood. Clinically, this is called shock lung, adult respiratory distress syndrome, or primary pulmonary edema (see Chap. 31).

In this final stage of shock, the body does not respond favorably to any form of therapy. The combined failure of multiple organ systems overwhelms the body's attempts at compensation, and the term *irreversible* is used to imply that death is inevitable. During this stage, the blood pressure may show an elevation or a turn towards normal for short periods of time, but the cellular biochemical dysfunction has resulted in so many destructive enzymes and toxins that the patient does not recover. Irreversible organ system failure is evidenced by manifestations of cardiac failure, acidosis, blood clotting aberrations, and inadequate cerebral blood flow.

Clinical Course

Cardiac Failure. Coronary perfusion of the myocardium decreases because of the fast heart rate, decreasing stroke volume, low blood pressure, and lack of oxygen perfusion pressure. As a result, contractility of the myocardium is impaired. Acidosis and toxins further reduce contractility, and the heart is increasingly less effective as a pump. Cardiac output thus falls even further, diminishing cardiac perfusion. As the cycle perpetuates itself, the heart eventually fails, leading to death.

Acidosis. Acidosis is present for several reasons, including impaired cellular function secondary to poor tissue perfusion, reduced renal function (which allows retention of metabolic products), and respiratory failure. Acidosis contributes to decreased contractility of the heart and to the loss of vasomotor tone. These effects of acidosis further impair tissue perfusion, renal function, and respiratory function.

Aberrations in Blood Clotting. The syndrome of disseminated intravascular coagulation (DIC) is an additional feature of irreversible shock. This syndrome begins with a state of hypercoagulability initiated by sluggish capillary flow and the presence of acidosis, bacterial endotoxins, and thromboplastins. Platelets and red blood cells aggregate and become fibrous clots that occlude small vessels and perpetuate additional clot formation. Massive microagglutination ensues. As a result, platelet and clotting factors are consumed, with the end result being an increase in fibrinolytic activity and the presence of fibrin split products (FSP) in the circulation. Diffuse bleeding, often seen on mucosal surfaces such as in the gastrointestinal tract, the trachea, and the urinary tract, then occurs. Massive bleeding may occur from these sites, leading to further loss of intravascular circulating blood volume.

Inadequate Cerebral Blood Flow. As cardiac output and blood pressure fall below levels essential for vital organ function, the cerebral blood flow diminishes. Severe cerebral ischemia occurs, causing a depression of vital centers in the brain. Specifically, the vasomotor center of the medulla fails to function, leading to loss of sympathetic tone. The result is a drop in blood pressure, a very slow heart rate, and a lethal drop in tissue perfusion. As cerebral blood flow is further diminished, the brain becomes further anoxic, and death occurs.

Nursing Implications

Prevention

The major goal in shock is that of prevention. In general, the purpose of strategies that nurses use should be to identify any patients at risk for any types of shock and initiate treatment early, before the point at which signs and symptoms reflect the body's response to the shock state. The nurse is responsible for a thorough history and accurate, repeated observations in order to identify those patients who are potential shock victims.

Cardiogenic Shock. Patients who have acute myocardial infarction, especially anterior wall involvement, are at particular risk of developing cardiogenic shock. The nurse's responsibility in the prevention of cardiogenic shock in a patient with acute myocardial infarction is aimed primarily at diminishing or minimizing the work load of the heart. The infarction size influences the potential development of cardiogenic shock. The nurse is responsible for implementing measures to reduce further myocardial injury by administering drugs to block sympathetic stimulation, by administering glucose and potassium to increase aerobic metabolism and energy production, and by judicious use of drugs to increase the force of contraction and reduce myocardial oxygen needs. The maintenance of physical and emotional rest, sodium restriction, and oxygen administration may also aid in reducing infarction size (see Chap. 37).

Hypovolemic Shock. Patients who have multiple trauma, have sustained burns, have severe vomiting, or are undergoing extensive surgical procedures may develop hypovolemic shock. The nurse should be careful to observe for fluid balance status. Accurate and complete intake and output records are essential for a patient who has undergone surgery, suffered multiple long bone fractures, or been involved in a motor vehicle accident in which multiple contusions are present. The nurse also needs to take into account unmeasured fluid losses that might occur through the respiratory tract, through perspiration, and through drainage from surgical wounds.

If the patient has frank bleeding, which might occur with postoperative patients, direct pressure applied on or above the site will prevent or reduce the amount of blood loss. In some instances, an emergency procedure such as the use of the military "antishock trousers" is applied to the lower extremities and abdomen. This suit is designed to compress the veins, which provides autotransfusion up to 1 liter from the capacitance vessels to the right heart (Fig. 24–1).

Septic Shock. Septic shock may occur in patients with impaired or altered host defenses as well as in those patients who may have tube placement in body orifices, particularly instrumentation of the urinary bladder. Prevention of contamination of the patient may be improved by the use of strict aseptic technique and frequent, careful hand washing. Debilitated elderly or chronically ill patients have weakened, impaired host defenses, and they are candidates to develop sepsis.

Neurogenic/Vasogenic Shock. Patients who undergo spinal anesthesia are at risk for neurogenic shock as a result of temporarily blocked sympathetic nervous system impulses. Careful positioning and fluid replacement are necessary during both the surgical procedure and immediate postoperative period, as described in Chapter 8. Vasogenic shock is most commonly associated with systemic anaphylaxis; methods of prevention and treatment are described in Chapter 16.

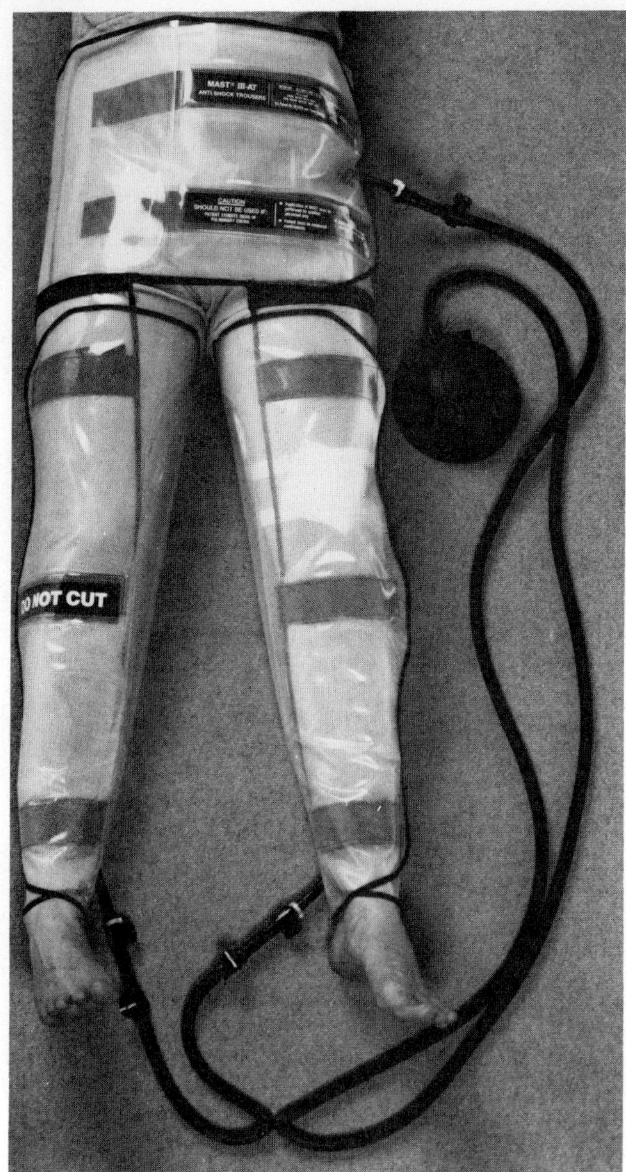

FIGURE 24–1 Antishock trousers are designed to apply counterpressure to the lower extremities and abdomen in order to redirect blood flow from the lower part of the body to the heart, the brain, and other vital organs.

Patient Assessment

One of the most important aspects of the nursing process in shock is the assessment. For all patients, the integration of subjective, objective, and technical data about the patient is essential. Early detection of subtle changes that occur in the patient is essential. The nurse needs to take into account the clinical findings, the information from invasive hemodynamic monitoring (if available), and laboratory data to assess and establish baseline data on these patients. Such baseline data should be continually assessed and reassessed throughout the clinical course of the patient. Table 24–4 will help the nurse compare signs and symptoms and assessment primaries in hypovolemic, cardiogenic, and septic/neurogenic shock.

To highlight the important clinical findings of shock, the nurse needs to be alert to the following factors.

Level of Consciousness. Because the level of consciousness is diminished when inadequate cerebral blood flow exists, the nurse needs to be alert to early changes in the patient's behavior. Changes such as restlessness or anxiety, confusion, agitation, and irritability, if not previously present in a patient, should alert the nurse to assess the patient's condition more fully. The family may alert the nurse to subtle changes in personality and judgment as well as changes in skin or altered sleep patterns. These clues are important in helping the nurse detect that brain cells are suffering from prolonged lack of oxygen. The patient may become less and less responsive to verbal stimuli as well as to pain-causing stimuli. If the signs and symptoms of shock are ignored or untreated, coma and death may ensue.

Blood Pressure. Changes in blood pressure are dependent on the rate of volume loss and on the amount of stimulation to the sympathetic adrenal/medullary mechanism. Often, in early shock, the blood pressure may be normal or even elevated. The diastolic pressure is increased because of arteriovasoconstriction. As the shock state progresses, blood pressure falls and pulse pressure narrows. It is important to note that a decrease in blood pressure is a late sign of shock

Pulse. The pulse rate usually increases in all types of shock. Whereas the amplitude is weak and thready in hypovolemic and cardiogenic shock, it is full and bounding in septic or neurogenic shock. There is regularity to the pulse rate except in the case of cardiogenic shock where arrhythmias occur.

Cardiac Output. The cardiac output in most shock states is normal up to the point at which blood loss approximates 30%.

Vasoconstriction. Vasoconstriction occurs with all types of shock but is seen less with the septic, vasogenic, and neurogenic forms because of the direct action of toxic products on the vascular smooth muscle. In severe hypovolemic and cardiogenic shock, the veins will collapse on digital pressure. In septic or neurogenic shock, however, veins are full and do not collapse under pressure.

Respiratory System. Hyperventilation is present in all types of shock. Blood gases initially show a diminished Pa_{CO_2} and diminished Pa_{O_2}. As the shock progresses, Pa_{CO_2} rises and Pa_{O_2} falls. Subjectively, the patient may experience air hunger, shortness of breath, or dyspnea.

Renal System. The urinary output depends on the volume of blood and plasma delivered to the kidneys. Because decreasing urinary output reflects a diminution of fluid circulating to the kidneys, determination of hourly urines is essential in a patient suspected of shock. Less than

TABLE 24–4
Shock Classification, Comparison of Signs and Symptoms, and Assessment Parameters

	Hypovolemic Shock	*Cardiogenic Shock*	*Septic/Neurogenic/Vasogenic Shock*
	Goal: To restore circulating blood volume	*Goal:* To restore effective heart action	*Goal:* To restore vasoconstrictive mechanisms, thereby decreasing vascular bed size
Circulatory System			
Blood pressure			
Systolic	Decrease dependent on the rate of volume loss and/or amount of stimulation of sympathetic adrenal medullary mechanism	Decreases	Decreases
Diastolic	May increase because of early arteriole vasoconstriction Orthostatic hypotension present in moderate (30%) fluid loss	May increase because of early arteriole vasoconstriction, then fall	Decreases
Pulse pressure	Narrowing pulse pressure due to arteriole vasoconstriction	Narrowing	Narrowing
Pulse			
Rate	Increases (tachycardia)	Increases (tachycardia)	Increases (tachycardia)
Amplitude	Weak, thready	Weak, thready	Full, bounding
Regularity	Usually regular	Irregular	Regular
Cardiac output	Normal until blood loss passes into moderate (30%) stage	Diminished due to failure of pump	Normal until vascular bed dilates beyond compensatory mechanisms
Vasoconstriction	Mild until refractory shock	Mild until refractory stage	Vasodilation of arterioles and precapillary sphincters because of interference with sympathetic nervous system or because of direct action of toxic products on vascular smooth muscles
Veins	Collapse on digital pressure in severe fluid loss	Full, if severe and sudden	Full, without collapse
Respiratory System			
Rate	Hyperventilation Minute volume is 1.5 to 2 times normal	Hyperventilation	Hyperventilation
Blood gases	Decreased Pa_{CO_2} normal Pa_{O_2}, then increased Pa_{CO_2} and decreased Pa_{O_2} as shock progresses		
Subjective	Air hunger	Short of breath	Dyspnea
Renal System			
Urine output	Normal to slightly depressed as blood loss occurs, then becomes oliguric (<25 ml/hr)	Dependent on volume of plasma/blood delivered to kidneys	Decreases as fluid shifts from intravascular to interstitial and intracellular spaces
Urine osmolality	Increased	Increased	Increased
Urine sodium	Decreased	Decreased	Decreased
Acid–Base Balance	Respiratory alkalosis, then metabolic and respiratory acidosis	Respiratory alkalosis, then metabolic and respiratory acidosis	Respiratory alkalosis, then metabolic and respiratory acidosis
Integument			
Skin	Minimal to little change in compensated shock. Cool and clammy as shock progresses	Minimal if compensated. Cool, pale, and ashen as shock progresses	Flushed in early shock; cool, cyanotic and mottled in neurogenic and vasogenic. Cool and clammy in septic shock

(*Continued*)

TABLE 24–4
Shock Classification, Comparison of Signs and Symptoms, and Assessment Parameters (*Continued*)

	Hypovolemic Shock	*Cardiogenic Shock*	*Septic/Neurogenic/Vasogenic Shock*
	Goal: To restore circulating blood volume	*Goal:* To restore effective heart action	*Goal:* To restore vasoconstrictive mechanisms, thereby decreasing vascular bed size
Integument			
Lips	Progress to cyanotic	Progress to cyanotic	Progress to cyanotic
Nail beds	Normal to cyanotic Capillary filling time extended	Cyanotic. Extended capillary filling time	Normal until progress to refractory stage
Neuroregulatory System			
Sensorium/orientation	Early: hyper, alert, apprehensive. Then confusion vagueness, lethargy, and unconsciousness	Early: anxiety, vagueness, and apprehension. Unconsciousness ensues as pump fails.	Anxiety, dizziness, progresses to unconsciousness
Motor	Restless until unconsciousness, weakness, and fatigue due to cellular hypoxia	Restless until unconsciousness, weakness, and fatigue due to cellular hypoxia	Restless until unconsciousness, weakness, and fatigue due to cellular hypoxia
Pupils	Dilated	Dilated	Dilated
Temperature	Varies with cause; decreases with blood loss, increases with burns	May rise slowly in response to myocardial damage	With toxic shock, fever often present
Hematologic System	Release of RBCs from bone marrow to increase vascular volume Platelet sluggishness; platelet aggregation to promote wound healing Late stages of disseminated intravascular coagulation (DIC)		
Gastrointestinal–Hepatic System			
Mouth, mucous membranes	No obvious changes early, then thirst due to high sodium levels and cellular dehydration	No obvious changes early, then thirst due to high sodium levels and cellular dehydration	May be dry due to fever
Nausea, vomiting		Often present	Often present
Bowel sounds	As perfusion decreases, bowel sounds may be diminished.	As perfusion decreases, bowel sounds may be diminished	Fluid shifts may cause edema and diminishing bowel sounds.

25 ml/hr of urine indicates oliguria. In shock, urinary osmolarity is consistently increased, and urinary sodium is decreased.

Integument. In hypovolemic shock, cool and clammy skin is observable only as shock progresses. In cardiogenic shock, cool, pale, and ashen skin is more commonly found. In neurogenic or septic shock, the patient is flushed initially, then becomes cool or cyanotic as compensatory mechanisms fail. The lips are easy to assess, because of their accessibility as well as their normal color. As the shock progresses, they become more cyanotic. The nail beds, as a reflection of reduced circulation to the distal extremities, are cyanotic. Capillary filling time is extended as the body attempts more and more to shunt blood from the extremities by peripheral vasoconstriction.

Neuroregulatory System. In the neuroregulatory system the sensorium, motor function, and temperature are to be assessed. Assessment of the sensorium is the same as for level of consciousness, discussed above. The motor system is assessed by determining whether muscle use is appropriate. Weakness and fatigue, due to cellular hypoxia and buildup of toxic substances within the skeletal muscles, contribute to deviations in normal muscle functioning. The temperature varies with the cause of shock but, typically, the temperature may decrease with blood loss or may increase with burns. If the shock is due to a toxin, fever is often present.

Gastrointestinal–Hepatic System. The mouth and mucous membranes may show no obvious early changes, yet the patient may complain of a great deal of thirst, which is due to water deficit (see Chap. 13). Dry mucous membranes may be caused by fever and septic shock. Nausea and vomiting are often present because the gastrointestinal tract has the blood shunted away from it.

Bowel sounds are also diminished because of the shunting of blood away from the gastrointestinal tract and the resultant lack of peristalsis.

Nursing Interventions

Nursing interventions for the patient in shock depend both on definitive care and supportive measures.

Outcome criteria for a patient in shock are the following:

- Return to the normal state of consciousness
- Blood pressure within 20 mmHg of the preshock level
- Strong regular pulse rate and regular respirations
- Normal temperature and warm, dry skin
- Urinary output between 30 and 60 ml/hour

Definitive Care. The nursing care needs to be specific for the different types of shock. For patients who have cardiogenic shock, definitive care includes increasing coronary perfusion to minimize myocardial ischemia, which may be accomplished either by surgical revascularization or provided through rest and pharmacological therapy. For patients who have hypovolemic shock, the site of fluid loss must be identified and, if possible, the loss must be quickly controlled. Other definitive measures include identification of internal injuries and surgical repair of hemorrhaging vessels. Other losses, such as fluid losses through vomiting, must be identified and prevented. Nursing care may be directed toward preventing massive diarrhea, reducing vomiting, or decreasing unwarranted diuresis. For patients who have anaphylactic or toxic shock, the definitive care is to neutralize the effects of the toxin and to restore vascular tone.

Supportive Measures. Until definitive treatment is effected, the goals of supportive nursing measures are to maintain adequate tissue perfusion by restoration and maintenance of effective ventilation, maintaining an optimum state of hydration with adequate circulating blood volume, and maximizing the effectiveness of the heart as a pump.

To restore and maintain effective ventilation, a patent airway must be maintained. This may be established by tilting the head backward and clearing the air passages of mucous or foreign bodies. Removal of secretions can be accomplished through suctioning, postural drainage, or chest physiotherapy.

To maintain an optimum state of hydration with adequate circulating blood volume, fluids are replaced. Specific types of fluid volume replacement include whole blood or blood products, plasma expanders, and crystalloid solutions. The type of fluid volume replaced will be highly dependent on the kind of fluid lost.[3]

To maximize the effectiveness of the heart as a pump, drugs are administered to improve the ability of the heart to deal with preload or afterload, as well as to improve the force of the myocardial contraction.

In order to preserve vital organ functioning, pharmacological agents are administered to maintain an adequate blood pressure (minimum: 80 to 90 mmHg systolic); steroids are administered to preserve blood vessel integrity; and measures are taken to maintain an optimum acid–base environment.[10] Adequate nutrition is essential to cellular integrity and organ function. Caloric requirements may range from 2000 to 5000 calories/day to meet the maintenance and restorative needs of the body.

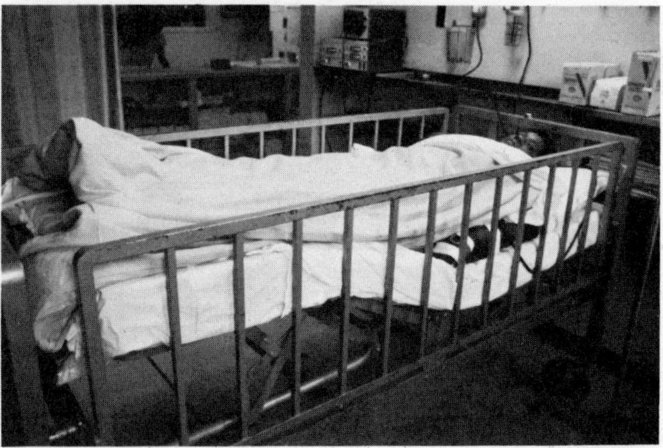

FIGURE 24–2 Correct positioning for a patient in shock. Legs are elevated to encourage venous return.

Supportive measures for patients in shock are essential, and include a body position of comfort, when possible, and a position to facilitate venous return. Lowering the head in relation to the body (Trendelenburg position) is contraindicated. Studies have shown that the Trendelenburg position causes, among other things, the diaphragm to ascend, which reduces total lung volume and ventilation.[1] Instead, the head is kept flat, but the legs are often elevated (modified Trendelenburg) (Fig. 24–2).

The patient and family members must receive psychological support. Both the patient and family members may use ineffective defense mechanisms to attempt to cope with the physiological and psychological state of shock.

Summary

The patient who is in a state of shock presents a complex challenge to a nurse. These patients may appear in any situation in which nurses work, and they may be of any age. Aspects of nursing care include identification of patients at risk, assessment of every body system for the signs and symptoms of shock, and interventions to maintain tissue perfusion and eliminate the initiating cause.

References

1. Bordicks KJ: Patterns of Shock, 2nd ed. New York, Macmillan, 1980
2. Collins JA: The pathophysiology of hemorrhagic shock. Prog Clin Biol Res 108:5–29, 1982

3. Drake RE, Gabel JC: Role of colloid osmotic pressure in shock resuscitation: Fluid and blood therapy in anesthesia. Contemp Anesth Pract 6:101–117, 1983
4. Hathaway R: Hemodynamic monitoring in shock. Journal of Emergency Nursing 3:37–42, 1977
5. Houston MC, Thompson WL, Robertson D: Shock: Diagnosis and management. Arch Intern Med 144:1433–1439, 1984
6. McCabe WR: Gram-negative bacteremia. Adv Intern Med 19:135–138, 1974
7. McGurn WC: Cardiogenic shock. In McGurn WC: People with Cardiac Problems: Nursing Concepts. Philadelphia, JB Lippincott, 1981
8. Niles NA, Wills RE: Heart failure. In Underhill SL, Woods SL, Sivarajan ES, Halpenny CJ: Cardiac Nursing, Philadelphia, JB Lippincott, 1982
9. Puri VK, Vincent JL: The pathophysiology of septic shock. Int Surg 67:5–8, 1982
10. Rice V: Shock: A clinical syndrome. Critical Care Nurse, 1982
11. Schumer W: Shock as a syndrome of metabolic failure. In Weil MH, Shubin H (eds): Critical Care Medical Handbook. New York, John H Kolen, 1974

Bibliography

Adams CW: Recognition and evaluation of cardiogenic shock. Heart Lung 2:893–895, 1973

Armstrong P, Baigrie R: Hemodynamic monitoring in critically ill patients. Heart Lung 9:1060–1062, 1980

Bastiaans JC, Vleeming W: The effect of compensation of acidosis on survival in endotoxin shock. Adv Shock Res 6:163–174, 1981

Bordicks KJ: Patterns of Shock, 2nd ed. New York, Macmillan, 1980

Carrico CJ, Maier RV: Balanced salt solutions in massive trauma. Contemp Anesth Pract 6:57–83, 1983

Clough DH, Higgins P: Discrepancies in estimating blood loss. Am J Nurs 81:331–333, 1981

Davidson I: Hemodilution, oxygen consumption, and recovery from surgical shock: A study on the efficacy of different plasma substitutes. Ann Clin Res 13:44–47, 1981

Dietzman RH, Beckman CB, Lillehei RC: Pharmacologic and mechanical support for managing cardiogenic shock. Geriatrics 28:69–79, 1973

Frazie S, Nail L: New challenge in cardiac nursing: The intra-aortic balloon. Heart Lung 2:526–532, 1973

Goldfarb RD: Cardiac mechanical performance in circulatory shock: A critical review of methods and results (review article). Circ Shock 9:633–653, 1982

Grove L: The microcirculation and shock. Journal of American Association of Nurse Anesthetists 40:185–192, 1972

Guntheroth WG, Abel FL, Mullins GL: The effect of Trendelenburg's position on blood pressure and carotid flow. Surg Gynecol Obstet 119:345–348, 1964

Guthrie MM (ed): Shock. New York, Churchill Livingstone, 1982

Harke H, Rehman S: Coagulation disorders in massively injured patients. Prog Clin Biol Res 108:213–224, 1982

Hassett J, Cerra FB, Siegel J et al: Multiple systems organ failure—A very brief summary (symposium paper). Injury 14:93–97, 1982

Lucas CE, Harrigan E, Denis R, Ledgerwood AM: Impaired renal concentrating ability during resuscitation from shock. Arch Surg 118:642–645, 1983

Monafo WW: Volume replacement in hemorrhage, shock, and burns. Adv Shock Res 3:47–56, 1980

Moss G, Saletta J: Traumatic shock in man. N Engl J Med 290:724–729, 1974

Munro H: Hormones and the metabolic response to injury. N Engl J Med 300:41–42, 1972

Nagy S, Hantos Z, Kiebniczki J et al: Increase of functional residual capacity in hemorrhagic shock. Circ Shock 9:579–587, 1982

Nursing care of patients in shock, Part 1: Pharmacotherapy. Am J Nurs 82:943–964, 1982

Nursing care of patients in shock, Part 2: Fluids, oxygen, and the intra-aortic balloon pump. Am J Nurs 82:1401–1422, 1982

Nursing care of patients in shock, Part 3: Evaluating the patient. Am J Nurs 82:1723–1746, 1982

O'Rourke MF: Cardiogenic shock following myocardial infarction. Heart Lung 3:252–257, 1974

Perry AG, Potter PA (eds): Shock: Comprehensive Nursing Management. St Louis, CV Mosby, 1983

Pinsky MR: Cause-specific management of shock. Postgrad Med 73:127–139, 1983

Purcell JA: Shock drugs: Standardized guidelines. Am J Nurs 82:965–973, 1982

Riede U, Sandritter W, Mittermayer C: Circulatory shock: A review. Pathology 13:299–311, 1981

Rutherford RB, Buerk CA: The pathophysiology of trauma and shock. In Quidema GO, Rutherford RB, Ballinger WF (eds): The Management of Trauma, 3rd ed. Philadelphia, WB Saunders, 1979

Schwartz RA, Cerra FB: Shock: A practical approach. Symposium on Perioperative Care of the Urologic Patient. Urol Clin North Am 10:89–100, 1983

Shumer W: Metabolism during shock and sepsis. Heart Lung 5:416–421, 1976

Stein AP, Baughman DC: Nursing implications of toxic shock syndrome. Critical Care Update, 17–19, 1981

Stude C: Cardiogenic shock. Am J Nurs 74:1636–1640, 1974

Taylor J, Weil MH: Failure of the Trendelenburg position to improve circulation during clinical shock. Surg Gynecol Obstet 21:1005–1010, 1967

Tripp A: Basic pathophysiological mechanisms of shock. New York, McGraw-Hill, 1979

Trunkey DD, Sheldon GF, Collins JA: The treatment of shock. In Quidema GD, Rutherford RB, Ballinger WF (eds): The Management of Trauma, 3rd ed. Philadelphia, WB Saunders, 1979

UNIT IV

Nursing Care of Patients with Alterations in Respiratory Function

Chapter 25

Review of Anatomy and Physiology
Respiratory System

Barbara R. Landau

In the following pages, *respiratory function* is discussed in the physiological sense as the exchange of oxygen and carbon dioxide between the external environment and the cells, rather than in the biochemical sense as the intracellular processes by which oxygen is "used" and carbon dioxide is produced. The organs and structures that make up the respiratory system provide for movement of gases between the external environment and the blood, but the transport of these gases to and from the cells is a function of the cardiovascular system.

Structure of the Respiratory Tract

Upper Respiratory Tract

The upper portion of the respiratory tract consists of the nasal cavity, the pharynx, and the larynx (Fig. 25–1). Air entering the nasal cavity is warmed, moistened, and filtered before coming in contact with the delicate respiratory membranes. The nasal cavity is a small space with a large surface area due to the presence of conchae (turbinates). The paranasal sinuses (frontal, maxillary, sphenoid, and ethmoid) and nasolacrimal duct open into the nasal cavity.

The pharynx consists of the nasopharynx, oropharynx, and laryngopharynx. The nasopharynx lies posterior to the nasal cavity. The auditory (eustachian) tube opens into it, and the pharyngeal tonsils (adenoids) are on its posterior wall. The oropharynx is posterior to the oral cavity and serves digestive as well as respiratory functions. The laryngopharynx lies behind the larynx and opens into it and into the esophagus and oropharynx.

The larynx is the superior end of the series of airways leading to the lungs; it functions as the voice box. The larynx consists of several cartilages, fibrous membranes, and skeletal muscles and is connected to the hyoid bone by a fibrous membrane.

The vocal cords are parallel bands of elastic fibers and skeletal muscle fibers that extend from the thyroid cartilage anteriorly to the arytenoid cartilages posteriorly. The space between the vocal cords is the glottis. Air moving through the glottis passes between the vocal cords and causes them to vibrate and produce sound.

Lower Respiratory Tract

No gas exchange occurs in the trachea, bronchi, or bronchioles, which constitute the conducting airways of the lower respiratory tract (see Fig. 25–1). Because the pressure of the air in these structures may be less than atmospheric pres-

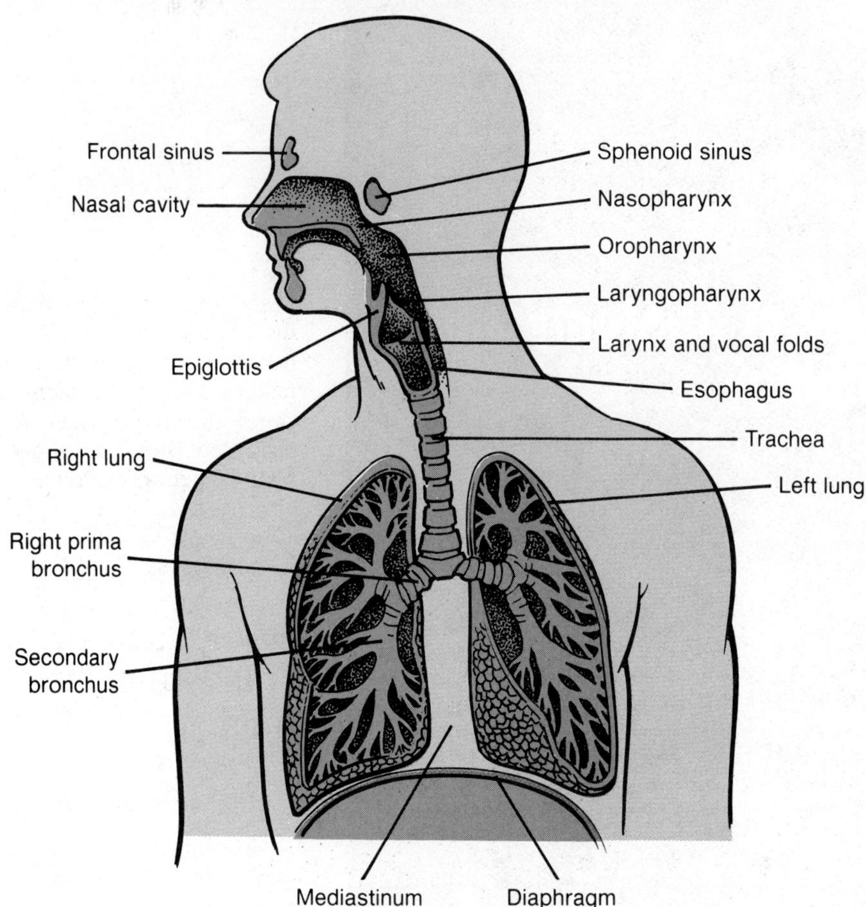

FIGURE 25–1 The respiratory system.

sure, they would probably collapse without the cartilage in their walls. The cartilage rings are incomplete in bronchi and decrease progressively in size and number to the terminal bronchioles, which contain no cartilage. Cilia in the lower respiratory tract beat toward the pharynx, a movement that facilitates removal of mucus from these airways. Contraction of the smooth muscle, which constricts the airways (especially the bronchioles), is caused by parasympathetic (vagal) stimulation. Stimulation of sympathetic (β-adrenergic) fibers inhibits the muscle and dilates these passages.

The respiratory portions of the respiratory tree, namely, the respiratory bronchioles, alveolar ducts, and alveoli (Fig. 25–2), are those portions in which gas exchange occurs. Alveoli are quantitatively and functionally the major elements of lung tissue. All gas exchange occurs across alveolar walls and into the adjacent capillaries.

Lungs and Thoracic Cavity

The lungs fill most of the thoracic cavity (see Fig. 25–1). The apex reaches up under the sternal end of the clavicle, and the edges of the broad base extend far down between the ribs

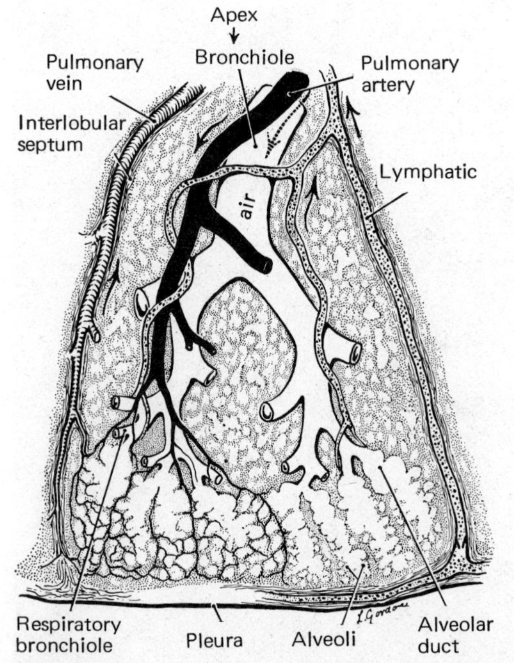

FIGURE 25–2 Schematic drawing of a lobule of the lung.

and the diaphragm. Airways and blood vessels enter the lungs at the hilus on the medial surface. The right lung has three lobes, the superior, middle, and inferior, and the left lung has two lobes, the superior and inferior.

At about the level of the fifth or sixth thoracic vertebra the trachea bifurcates into right and left primary bronchi, which enter the right and left lungs, respectively. The right bronchus divides into three secondary bronchi, one to each lobe, and the left bronchus forms two secondary bronchi, one to each lobe. Secondary bronchi divide into from two to five tertiary bronchi, each of which supplies a segment of that lobe, forming units known as bronchopulmonary segments. The pulmonary arteries branch, and the pulmonary veins converge in a similar fashion.

The lungs are also supplied by bronchial vessels, nerves, and lymphatics. The bronchial arteries are several tiny branches from the thoracic aorta that supply tissue of the larger airways. The deep bronchial veins that drain lung tissue empty into a pulmonary vein, and superficial bronchial veins empty into the azygos system. The nerves are autonomic fibers to smooth muscle of the bronchi and bronchioles and to vascular smooth muscle.

The thoracic cavity is bounded on all sides and above by the "rib cage" (ribs, vertebral column, and sternum) and by the diaphragm below. It is a sealed cavity (except for the tracheal opening) filled by the right and left lungs and by the midline structures of the mediastinum, which effectively separate the right and left portions of the thoracic cavity (Fig. 25–3). Mediastinal structures include the heart, esophagus, trachea, and primary bronchi, and the aorta, venae cavae and azygos veins, pulmonary arteries and veins, nerves, and lymphatics.

The Pleura

The inner surface of the thoracic wall and the superior surface of the diaphragm are covered by a serous membrane, the parietal pleura. At the hilus it is reflected back over the surface of the lungs as the visceral pleura (see Fig. 25–3). The pleura does not enclose mediastinal structures individually, but it covers them and with the pericardium forms a medial wall for the right and left portions of the thoracic cavity.

Lung Volumes

The volume of air that is or may be in the lungs can be divided into several fractions (Fig. 25–4). The *total lung capacity* (TLC) is made up of the *vital capacity* (VC), which is the air that can be moved in and out, and the *residual volume,* which cannot be expelled from the lungs. In normal quiet breathing, a *tidal volume* (TV) of about 0.5 liter is moved in and out with each breath—roughly 10% of the VC. Air that can be exhaled beyond a normal expiration is the *expiratory reserve volume,* and air that can be inhaled beyond a normal inspiration is the *inspiratory reserve volume.* The *inspiratory capacity* is the inspiratory reserve volume plus TV. At the end of a normal expiration the lungs still contain 2.5 liters to 3 liters of air (the residual volume and expiratory reserve volume), known as the *functional residual capacity* (FRC). Therefore, with each breath the 500 ml of inspired air is "diluted" by the 2.5 liters to 3 liters of the FRC already present.

The differences in lung volume between male and female are due primarily to differences in size of the thoracic cavity. The most dramatic change that occurs with aging is the

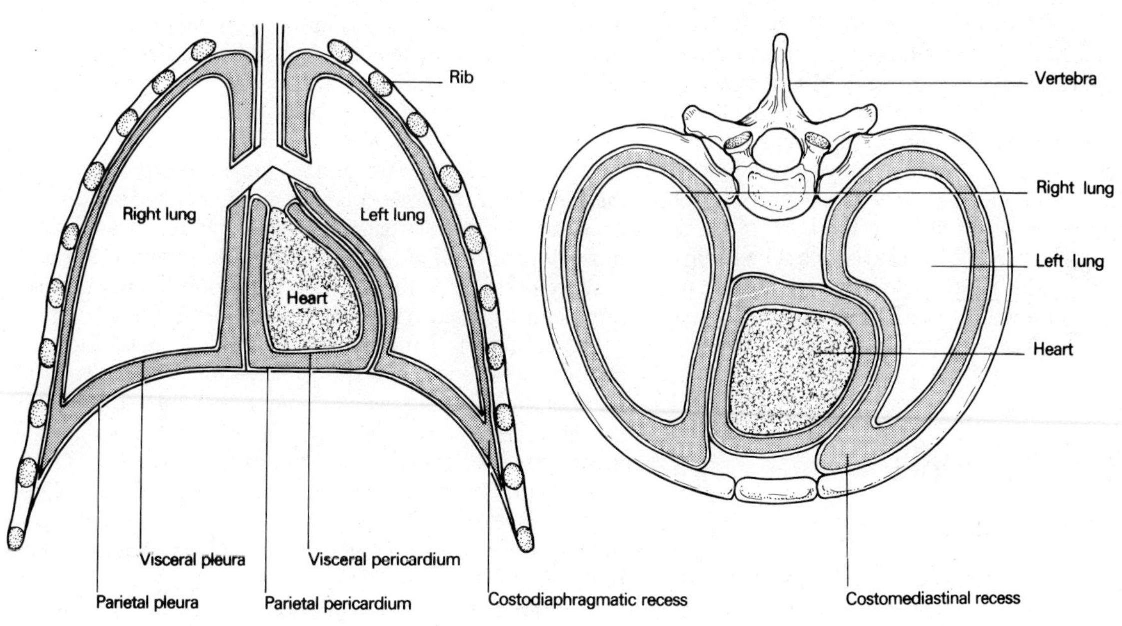

FIGURE 25–3 Pleura and pericardial cavities. (*A*) Coronal section. (*B*) Transverse section. (Thompson JS: Core Textbook of Anatomy: Philadelphia, JB Lippincott, 1977)

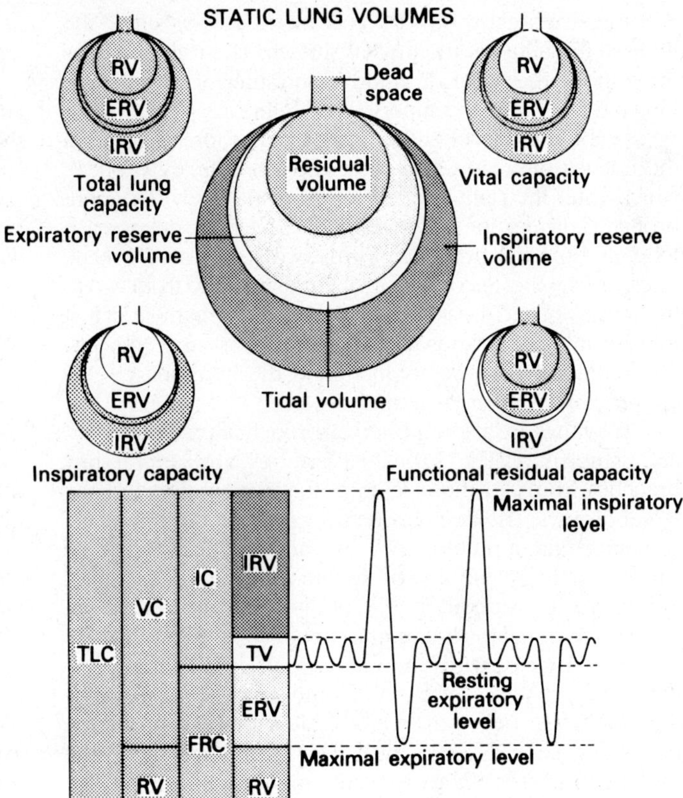

FIGURE 25-4 Division of total lung capacity into lung volumes and lung capacities. In the small diagrams surrounding the large central one, the shaded areas outline the volumes that constitute the various lung capacities. (Adapted from Comroe JH Jr et al: The Lung: Clinical Physiology and Pulmonary Function Tests, 2nd ed. Chicago, Year Book Medical Publishers, 1962)

increase in residual volume and FRC, with corresponding decreases in VC and inspiratory reserve volume. The chief factor in these changes is the loss of elastic recoil of the lungs.

Air left in the airways at the end of an expiration does not reach the outside and is first to enter the alveoli with the next inspiration. This is the *dead space* air, and amounts to about 150 ml. With a tidal volume of 500 ml, only 350 ml of atmospheric ("fresh") air enters the alveoli. Alveolar ventilation is therefore less effective when breathing is rapid and shallow.

Pulmonary ventilation (also called minute ventilation) is the volume of air breathed per minute. It is the product of TV and breathing rate, which is about 6 liters to 7.5 liters/minute. *Alveolar ventilation* (TV − dead space × breathing rate) is the important value, but pulmonary ventilation is much easier to measure and is commonly used to assess delivery of air to the lungs.

Ventilation of the Lungs

Mechanics of Breathing

Air is moved in and out of the lungs by the pressure gradients caused by changes in size of the thoracic cavity. The pressures that exist in the thorax at end-expiration when the respiratory muscles are relaxed provide a baseline for considering changes that cause air to move. The intrapulmonary pressure is the same as that of the atmosphere; if it were not, air would move, since the airways are open. The intrapleural pressure, however, is about 4 mm Hg below that of the atmosphere. Because there is no real "space" in the intrapleural cavity and the parietal and visceral layers of pleura are in contact, the lungs are forced to expand whenever the thorax expands. The cohesion between the pleural layers is similar to that of two pieces of glass the adjacent surfaces of which have been moistened; the glass pieces slide about freely but are very difficult to pull apart.

Inspiration occurs when the thoracic cavity is enlarged, intrapleural pressure falls, and the lungs are expanded. Air in the lungs now occupies a larger space, and intrapulmonary pressure falls below that in the atmosphere, causing air to move into the lungs. At the end of inspiration, intrapulmonary pressure is the same as atmospheric pressure, but intrapleural pressure remains lower.

Contraction of the diaphragm (and decreased tone of abdominal muscles) is responsible for most of the enlargement of the thoracic cavity in quiet breathing. Movement of the rib cage becomes more prominent when ventilation is increased, as in exercise, and the external intercostal muscles may be assisted by other muscles of inspiration. Maximal inspiratory effort with a closed glottis can produce intrapulmonary pressures nearing 100 mm Hg below atmospheric pressure.

In quiet breathing, expiration is a passive process that occurs when the inspiratory effort ceases. The diaphragm relaxes, tone returns to the abdominal muscles, and the diaphragm rises. As inspiratory muscles relax, gravity and the elastic recoil of the lung cause the rib cage to return to the end-expiratory position. Reducing the thoracic volume compresses the air in the lungs, raises intrapulmonary pressure, and air moves out until intrapulmonary pressure is again the same as atmospheric pressure. The muscles of expiration become involved when ventilation is increased, during forced expiration, or during straining (forced expiration with the glottis closed). With a maximal expiratory effort, intrapulmonary pressure may be more than 100 mm Hg above atmospheric pressure.

Compliance and Ventilation

The effect of changes in intrapulmonary pressure on ventilation depends upon the compliance of the lungs and thorax. Compliance is a measure of the distensibility of these tissues and is measured in terms of lung volume change per unit of pressure change (milliliters of air per centimeter of water). Greater compliance means greater distensibility and less pressure required to inflate the lungs. Compliance is reduced by fibrosis or other conditions that reduce the flexibility of thoracic structures, and it is also reduced when the volume of fluid in the lungs is raised, as by pulmonary edema, congestion, or increased pulmonary blood volume.

The ventilatory problems of reduced compliance are associated with the inability to move enough air and the greater effort required to do so. Increased compliance may also cause problems, often associated with difficulty in expelling air from the lungs. Loss of elasticity, for example, removes the recoil, which is so important in expiration. A certain amount of such loss occurs with aging, which alters the balance between lung recoil and the tendency of the rib cage to expand; the result is an increase in the FRC.

Airway Resistance

Movement of a gas (air) or liquid (blood) through a tube (airway or blood vessel) is directly proportional to the pressure drop along the tube and inversely proportional to the resistance. The resistance to flow is related to the viscosity of the gas or fluid, the length of the tube, and its diameter. Several physiological factors can alter airway resistance. One of these is lung volume; resistance decreases as the lungs inflate, chiefly because lung expansion applies some traction to airway walls. Contraction of bronchiolar muscle increases airway resistance. Parasympathetic (vagal) stimulation and acetylcholine cause constriction, as does histamine. Sympathetic stimulation, epinephrine, and norepinephrine are bronchodilators.

Pulmonary Circulation and Perfusion of the Lungs

Gas exchange is as dependent upon perfusion of alveoli with blood as it is upon alveolar ventilation. Since the output of the right ventricle equals that of the left ventricle, the flow through the pulmonary and systemic circuits is the same. There are important differences, however, since the pulmonary circuit is shorter and the vessels are generally of greater diameter and have thinner walls and very little smooth muscle. As a result, the intrapulmonary circuit is a low-resistance and low-pressure pathway. Pulmonary pressures are roughly one sixth those in the systemic circuit.

Although the entire cardiac output (5 liters/min) flows through the pulmonary circuit, only about 1 liter of blood is in the thoracic cavity at any given instant, and about half of that is actually in the lungs. About one half of the thoracic blood volume (400 ml–500 ml) is displaced to the lower extremities (the systemic circuit) upon assuming the upright position and shifts back to the thorax in a supine position. The lungs and thorax are therefore a potential blood reservoir.

Exchange and Transport of Gases

Partial Pressure of a Gas

The atmosphere is a mixture of gases, each of which contributes to the total pressure in proportion to its concentration (the number of its molecules) in the mixture. Nitrogen accounts for 600 mmHg, oxygen 159 + mmHg, and carbon dioxide and other gases for less than 1 mmHg of the total atmospheric pressure of 760 mmHg. The pressure exerted by each gas is its partial pressure, or tension. Slightly more than one fifth of the air is oxygen (159/760 = 20.94%), while four fifths is nitrogen (79.03%). These percentages change as the air enters the lungs, is moistened, reaches the alveoli, and eventually enters the circulatory system (Table 25–1).

Diffusion of Gases

Gases move among the alveoli, the bloodstream, and the tissues by diffusion, a passive process that depends upon the concentration gradient. Both oxygen and carbon dioxide are lipid-soluble and therefore can pass through cell membranes and diffuse through the cell.

Transport of Oxygen

Because of their limited solubility in blood plasma, the amount of oxygen or carbon dioxide dissolved is not sufficient to meet the body's needs. Hemoglobin (Hgb) is the major constituent of red blood cells and is the means by which most oxygen is transported in the blood. The percentage of Hgb bound to oxygen is referred to as Hgb saturation. Even though nearly all of the oxygen is transported bound to Hgb, the amount of dissolved oxygen (P_{O_2}) remains a vital element in transport because it determines the amount of oxygen bound to Hgb. Diffusion of oxygen from alveoli to plasma to red cells to Hgb depends upon the P_{O_2} gradients. The relationship between P_{O_2} and oxygen binding by Hgb is shown in the oxygen dissociation curve (Fig. 25–5).

The relationship between oxygen uptake and release is not a linear one. At the normal arterial P_{O_2}, Hgb is about 97% to 98% saturated and the dissociation curve is relatively flat. A further increase in arterial (or alveolar) P_{O_2} would have little effect on saturation. Arterial P_{O_2} can be reduced quite a bit

TABLE 25–1
Partial Pressures of Oxygen and Carbon Dioxide in Air and Blood (at Sea Level)*

	Dry Air	*Moist Air (Tracheal)*	*Alveolar Air*	*Arterial Blood*	*Venous Blood*
Oxygen	159.1	149.2	104	100	40
Carbon dioxide	0.3	0.3	40	40	46
Water vapor	0.0	47.0	47	47	47
Nitrogen	600.6	563.5	569	573	573
Total pressure	760.0	760.0	760	760	760

* All measurements in millimeters of mercury (mmHg).
(Modified from Comroe JH, Jr: Physiology of Respiration, 2nd ed, p 9. Chicago, Year Book Medical Publishers, 1979. Reproduced with permission.)

before saturation is seriously impaired, since when arterial P_{O_2} is 60 mmHg, the Hgb is still nearly 90% saturated. As plasma P_{O_2} falls further, the slope of the dissociation curve becomes steeper, and a small change in P_{O_2} causes a marked change in Hgb saturation.

Transport of Carbon Dioxide

Carbon dioxide is transported in the blood in three forms: dissolved in the plasma, as carbamino compounds, and as bicarbonate. About 5% of the carbon dioxide is carried in solution in the plasma, another 5% as carbamino Hgb, and the remaining 90% is carried as bicarbonate.

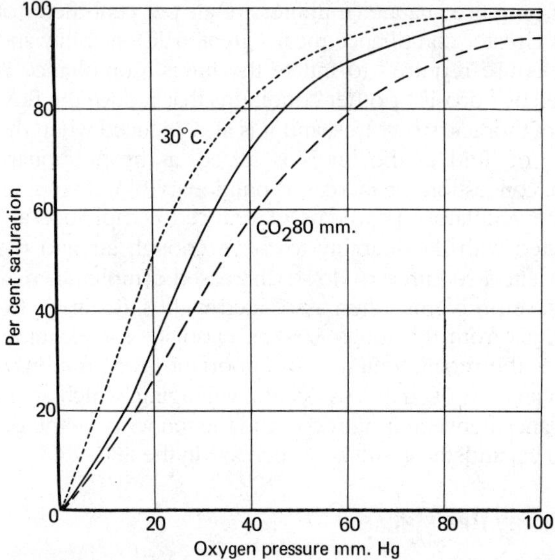

FIGURE 25–5 Graph showing oxygen dissociation curves. Note that when the carbon dioxide is increased, the normal curve (*solid line*) is shifted to the right (*dashed line*); thus, for any partial pressure of oxygen the hemoglobin binds less oxygen. Also note that a decreased temperature causes the curve to shift to the left (*dotted line*), so for any partial pressure of oxygen the hemoglobin binds more oxygen.

Control of Ventilation

There are two aspects to the control of ventilation: a mechanism to produce rhythmically alternating inspiration and expiration, and a mechanism to adjust pulmonary ventilation to meet changing needs. In the heart, automaticity is an inherent property, but rhythmicity of the breathing cycle is of neural origin and the effectors are totally dependent upon their innervation. The level of pulmonary ventilation is determined by factors that modify the basic neural control mechanism.

The Generation of Rhythmic Breathing

Rhythmic breathing movements are initiated in a respiratory center located in the medullary portion of the reticular formation of the brain (Fig. 25–6). Inspiration occurs upon stimulation of inspiratory neurons that synapse with motor neurons to the muscles of inspiration. The most important are the phrenic nerve to the diaphragm and fibers of the intercostal nerves to the external intercostal muscles. The phrenic nerve arises mainly from C4, and the intercostal nerves from the thoracic spinal nerves. Stimulation of expiratory neurons excites motor neurons to muscles of expiration and inhibits inspiratory neurons by reciprocal innervation. The latter effect is more important in quiet breathing because expiration is passive and occurs whenever inspiratory activity is interrupted. The reciprocal connections in the respiratory center between inspiratory and expiratory neurons ensure that excitation of one is accompanied by inhibition of the other.

If the medullary respiratory center and its connections with respiratory muscles are the only parts functioning, rhythmic breathing still occurs—it may not be regular, but the lungs will be ventilated. Two additional centers provide for a "fine" adjustment to this "coarse" breathing mechanism. One of these, called the apneustic center, is located in the lower pons. The other center is the pneumotaxic center, located in the upper pons.

An additional mechanism for interrupting inspiration is the inflation reflex (Hering–Breuer reflex). Inflation of the lungs stimulates stretch receptors in the airways and interrupts inspiration. In humans the reflex is believed to be a protection against overinflation of the lungs rather than an important regulator of the breathing cycle.

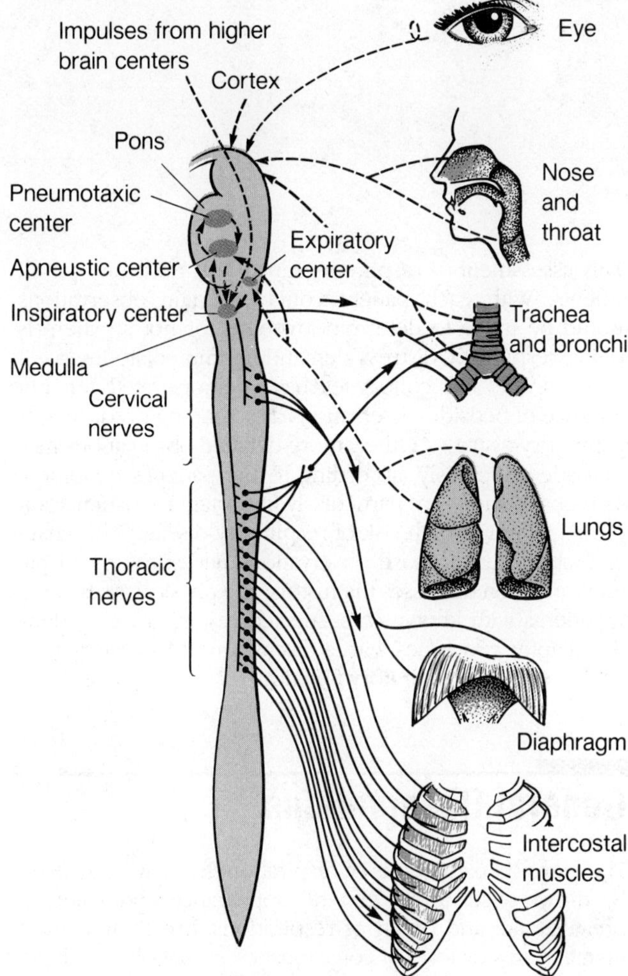

FIGURE 25–6 Schematic representation of activity in the respiratory center. Impulses traveling over afferent neurons activate central neurons, which in turn activate efferent neurons that supply the muscles of respiration. Thus, respiratory movements may be altered by a variety of stimuli.

Regulation of Pulmonary Ventilation

The respiratory system controls levels of oxygen, carbon dioxide, and hydrogen ions, and the important stimuli that affect pulmonary ventilation are associated with changes in these chemicals.

Central Chemical Control. Central control mechanisms involve responses to stimuli that arise centrally, that is, within the body. Carbon dioxide, the production of which is the result of metabolic activity, is said to be the most potent known stimulus to respiration and arterial P_{CO_2} is probably the most important factor in the minute-to-minute regulation of pulmonary ventilation. As an uncharged molecule, carbon dioxide can diffuse through membranes and is not blocked by the blood–brain barrier; thus, it enters both the brain interstitial fluid and the cerebrospinal fluid (CSF). When carbon dioxide diffuses into the CSF it combines with water to form carbonic acid (H_2CO_3). Hydrogen ions are subsequently released and cause an increase in pulmonary ventilation. The increase in ventilation reduces the alveolar P_{CO_2}, and, by excreting more carbon dioxide, a fall in pH is avoided. Hyperventilation can produce alkalosis by "blowing off" carbon dioxide. Thus, as it regulates ventilation, carbon dioxide also regulates or maintains acid–base balance.

Peripheral Chemical Control. Peripheral chemical regulation involves receptors in the carotid and aortic bodies located at the bifurcation of the internal and external carotid arteries and in the arch of the aorta. The chemoreceptors respond to a fall in P_{O_2}, a fall in pH, and a rise in P_{CO_2} in the arterial blood flowing through them; the most sensitive response, however, is to a fall in P_{O_2}.

Low oxygen causes little increase in ventilation until the P_{O_2} of inspired air reaches about 60 mmHg (and Hgb saturation about 90%), which occurs when oxygen content of the air is reduced by about half, to 10% (from 21%). The arterial chemoreceptors, therefore, do not exert important control of normal respiration, but they become important when the P_{O_2} of inspired air is reduced.

Nonchemical Effects of Respiratory Movements. Of the nonchemical effects on respiration, the most important are exerted by the brain. There is voluntary (cortical) control over respiratory activity—within limits, however, since chemical drives will eventually override voluntary control. A number of receptors located throughout the body can have an effect on ventilation and respiratory movements. Among them are receptors in airways of the lung, which, when stimulated by irritants such as smoke, noxious gases, or dust, cause bronchoconstriction as well as hyperventilation.

Bibliography

Comroe JH: Physiology of Respiration, 2nd ed. Chicago, Year Book Medical Publishers, 1974

Comroe JH, Forster RE II, Dubois AB et al: The Lung: Clinical Physiology and Pulmonary Function Tests, 2nd ed. Chicago, Year Book Medical Publishers, 1962

Crouch JE: Functional Human Anatomy, 3rd ed, chap 22, pp 516–538. Philadelphia, Lea & Febiger, 1978

Ganong WF: Review of Medical Physiology, 11th ed, chaps 34–37, pp 520–562. Los Altos, Lange Medical Publications, 1983

Junqueira LC, Carneiro J: Basic Histology, 4th ed, chap 18. Los Altos, Lange Medical Publications, 1983

Landau BR: Essential Human Anatomy and Physiology, 2nd ed, chaps 19–21, pp 495–538. Glenview, Scott, Foresman Company, 1980

Leeson TA, Leeson CR: Histology, 4th ed, chap 12, pp 401–426. Philadelphia, WB Saunders, 1981

Slonim NB, Hamilton LH: Respiratory Physiology, 3rd ed. St Louis, CV Mosby, 1976

Tortora GJ: Principles of Human Anatomy, 3rd ed, chap 20, pp 522–552. New York, Harper & Row, 1983

Vander AJ, Sherman JS, Luciano DS: Human Physiology: The Mechanisms of Body Function, 3rd ed, chap 12, pp 327–365. New York, McGraw–Hill, 1980

West JB: Respiratory Physiology: The Essentials, 3rd ed. Baltimore, Williams & Wilkins, 1985

Chapter 26

Assessment of Respiratory Function

Barbara L. Vail

Daily assessment of respiratory function is necessary for all patients. With each patient contact, certain observations should be made to determine whether or not a patient is having respiratory distress demanding immediate interventions. Pardee and colleagues have demonstrated the importance of bedside observations as screening predictors of respiratory distress.[9] Other, more detailed observations may be made judiciously, according to the patient's condition. Such observations are particularly important for patients suffering from or at high risk of respiratory disease. This chapter first addresses those observations necessary for all patients and then discusses the history and physical assessment of patients with known or suspected respiratory disorders. The chapter concludes with a discussion of laboratory tests used to evaluate respiratory function.

General Observations

There are six parameters of respiration that may be assessed by direct observation: general appearance and ability to breathe, rate and depth of respirations, breathing pattern, mental status or level of consciousness, skin color, and general body size.

A great deal of information can be gathered immediately about a patient's respiratory function by observing his general appearance. Observations can be made as one first meets the patient who has been newly admitted to the hospital or as one walks into the room of a patient having respiratory difficulty. The nurse should observe whether the patient appears comfortable and is able to breathe easily without effort or is visibly concentrating on each breath. She should note his ability to move about and change positions as he is breathing and whether he can lie flat or is able to lie only on one side. The nurse should note whether the head of the bed must be elevated in order for the patient to breathe. Postures that indicate difficulty breathing include having to sit up in bed, leaning forward hunched over a bedside table, or needing a pillow for support (orthopneic position).

While greeting him, the nurse should notice the patient's ability to breathe while he speaks. Must he speak only in short phrases or take a breath with each word? The person who is having difficulty may appear tense and anxious or he may appear fatigued and lethargic. It is also important to observe the use of accessory muscles of breathing. Normally, quiet breathing does not require the use of neck, chest, or shoulder muscles.

Respiratory rate and depth should also be noted immediately. Normally the respiratory rate ranges between 14 breaths and 20 breaths per minute, but with disease, respiratory rate may increase to as high as 40 breaths to 50 breaths/

TABLE 26–1
Altered Patterns of Respiration

Pattern	*Characteristics*	*Causes*
Tachypnea	Rapid, shallow	Fever Restrictive lung disease Pleuritic chest pain
Bradypnea	Slow but regular	Increased intracranial pressure Brain tumors Sleep Drugs
Hyperpnea	Increased depth, rate normal	
Hyperventilation	Increased depth and rate	Exercise, anxiety Metabolic acidosis
Kussmaul	Deep breathing; fast, normal, or slow rate	Metabolic acidosis Diabetic ketoacidosis
Cheyne–Stokes	Gradually deep and fast, then shallower and slower alternating with periods of apnea	Sleep Heart failure Renal failure Cerebral vascular accident Drug overdose Brain damage
Ataxic (Biot's breathing)	Short bursts of irregular breathing interspersed with periods of apnea	Spinal meningitis Brain damage Respiratory depression, medullary level
Apneustic	Prolonged gasping-type of breath	Brain damage in respiratory center

min.[11] The patient's breathing pattern can be noted as his vital signs are checked. Altered patterns of respiration include tachypnea, bradypnea, hyperpnea, hyperventilation, Kussmaul, Cheyne–Stokes, ataxic, and apneustic. The description and causes of each of these breathing patterns are described in Table 26–1.

A most important indication of respiratory function is the patient's mental status or level of consciousness. Patients who are confused and disoriented may be hypoxemic.

Another immediate clue to the patient's respiratory condition is skin color. However, since there are many skin colors among people and colors vary according to the lighting of the room, this data should be interpreted cautiously. The patient should be observed in bright daylight if possible. Variations in skin color include pallor, ruddiness, flushed appearance, and cyanosis. These variations and their implications are listed in Table 26–2. Peripheral cyanosis, often noted at ear lobes and fingertips, is not a reliable indicator of inadequate oxygenation, since it may be caused by vasoconstriction resulting from cold or nervousness. Cyanosis can be better evaluated by inspecting the inside of the mouth and tongue. For cyanosis to appear here, at least 5 g/dl of reduced hemoglobin must be present; this level approximates the oxygen saturation of venous blood.[10] Even the presence or absence of central cyanosis does not always reflect the status of tissue oxygenation. For instance, in the anemic patient, tissues may be hypoxic even in the absence of cyanosis, and in the polycythemic patient, cyanosis may be present even with adequate oxygenation.

General body size may also give a clue to problems with respiratory function. Obese patients are vulnerable to hypoventilation, which may be a particularly severe problem postoperatively. A cachectic body may be an indication of chronic disease and can be explored more in the history.

TABLE 26–2
Assessment of Skin Color

Appearance	*Possible Significance*
Pallor	Chronic disease
Ruddiness	Polycythemia, chronic bronchitis
Flushed skin	Fever, infection
Cyanosis	
Peripheral	Vasoconstriction due to cold, nervousness
Central	Decreased tissue oxygenation

Current Status

Assessment of current status may be brief for the patient in obvious respiratory distress, or it may be made in more detail when interviewing the newly admitted patient. Regardless of the length of the assessment, aspects of all the following should be included: chief complaint; presence of dyspnea, coughing, or pain; and vital signs.

Chief complaint should be explored with the person by asking about present concerns, including the reason for seeking treatment. Events leading up to his present condition and the duration of symptoms should be explored. The patient's interpretation of the cause of his present condition may give insight into his feelings and his knowledge of his disease.

Dyspnea related by the patient should be examined by asking him to describe his current breathing and how it relates to his normal state. The relationship of the dyspnea to activities of daily living can be assessed by asking the homemaker how her breathing affects such strenuous tasks as vacuuming and making beds. Men may be asked about activities such as mowing the lawn, putting up storm windows, or taking out the trash. Whether or not the dyspnea interferes with sexual performance may be relevant.[1]

Coughing is another important element to determine in evaluating current status. The person should be asked whether he coughs or whether his cough has recently changed. Whether or not the cough is productive and the frequency, amount, and appearance of sputum are important.

Pain with breathing should be investigated, and the location, intensity, and duration of any pain should be described. Pain due to fractured ribs, muscle strain, or pleural involvement often occurs with deep inspiration.

Changes in vital signs indicative of respiratory dysfunction include hypotension, tachycardia, and fever, as well as respiratory rate, depth, and pattern.

History

Medical History

Chronic illnesses, either respiratory or other types, are important to be noted in a respiratory history. Many cardiac, neurologic, or peripheral vascular problems may affect respiratory status adversely.

Past respiratory diseases, such as tuberculosis, pneumonia, or bronchitis, can signal the need for nursing alert. The patient should be questioned about the presence of emphysema, bronchitis, or pneumonia, as well as any past chest surgery.

Recent or frequent respiratory infections may be significant and may suggest nursing interventions to prevent or minimize infection as well as the need to teach the patient steps for prevention of infection. Recent respiratory infection can signal the possibility of postoperative complications.

Medications currently in use, including the use of oxygen at home, should be ascertained. Drugs that may adversely affect respiration, such as sedatives, narcotics, propranolol (causes bronchoconstriction), and alcohol, should be particularly noted. Use of bronchodilators, antituberculosis drugs, and corticosteroids also should be investigated further.

Allergies are significant, since patients with allergies may also have respiratory problems. The person should be asked to describe his specific reaction and questioned as to whether or not he has ever had an anaphylactic reaction. A patient with asthma should be questioned about known allergens, and steps should be taken to eliminate any possible exposure to allergens in the hospital.

A smoking history is important, since cigarette smoke affects mucus production and ciliary action and is a significant risk factor for lung cancer and chronic obstructive pulmonary disease (COPD). Present and past smoking habits need to be included, and the type of device used (*e.g.*, cigarettes, pipe) should be identified. The number of packs smoked per day multiplied by the number of years the patient smoked yields the "pack years." The greater the pack years, the higher the association with respiratory dysfunction. If the person states that he has quit smoking, he should be asked the reason, since many people quit as a result of respiratory symptoms or disease.

Family and Social History

The ages and health status of family members may provide significant information about inherited respiratory disease and the patient's family situation. The present living situation may provide additional clues to the patient's support systems and sources of stress. Questions concerning the patient's financial status may shed light on his ability to purchase needed medications and special food. Questions about recreational interests and usual types of exercise help in assessing current activity level and the extent to which respiratory problems affect the patient's lifestyle.

The patient's present or past occupation may give clues of exposure to toxic substances, such as asbestos, that affect the respiratory system. Exposure to toxic substances or diseases may also occur through travel. For example, travel to Africa, India, or Asia increases the likelihood of exposure to tuberculosis, and travel to the Ohio Valley may expose one to histoplasmosis.

The patient's understanding of his illness or treatment has important implications for formation of learning objectives. Closely related to the patient's understanding of his illness are his emotional responses and coping mechanisms. Questions about how the patient feels his lifestyle has been affected by the illness may help to uncover some of these factors. Patients with chronic respiratory diseases often feel a sense of loss of power and prestige as well as fear and anxiety and may exhibit dependence or withdrawal behaviors. Knowledge of the patient's educational level may help in planning specific teaching strategies.

Physical Examination

Before beginning the physical examination of the respiratory patient, the nurse should make sure that the patient knows what to expect. There should be as much light as possible, and the room should be quiet. In addition, adequate privacy and warmth must be considered, since the patient will be partially disrobed for the examination.

The examination begins with the patient in the sitting position, if possible. The posterior chest is examined by inspection, palpation, percussion, and auscultation. One side is compared with the other for variations, proceeding from the top downward. The patient may lie down after inspection of the anterior chest, and palpation, percussion, and auscultation of the anterior chest can be done in the supine position.

While examining the lungs, it is important to keep in mind the location of the underlying lobes of the lungs in relation to the patient's anatomy. Remember that the right lung consists of three lobes, the upper, middle, and lower lobes, while the left lung consists of upper and lower lobes only. There are two approaches to locating respiratory findings: through lobal localization and through visualization of imaginary lines on the chest wall.

Lobar localization consists of dividing the lungs into lobes, using the patient's anatomy to indicate dividing points of the lobes. This technique is shown in Figure 26–1.

For the front of the chest (anterior):

- The dividing line (horizontal fissure) for the right upper and middle lobe is at the fourth rib (nipple line in males).
- The line dividing the right middle lobe and lower lobe (oblique fissure) curves from the armpit at the fourth rib down to the sixth rib at the midclavicular line.
- The division of the left upper and lower lobes is also at this level on the left side.
- The apex or top of the lung is 2 cm to 4 cm above the inner third of the clavicle.
- The lungs extend down to the sixth rib at the midclavicular line and to the eighth rib at the midaxillary line.

For the back of the chest (posterior):

- Only the upper and lower lobes are accessible.
- The division between the upper and lower lobes is approximately at the level of the scapula.
- The lower edge of the posterior lung is normally at the level of the tenth rib and may descend to the twelfth rib on deep inspiration.
- Note that the seventh rib is usually immediately below the border of the scapula.
- Also note that in order to examine the middle lobe, one must examine the lateral chest.

Visualizing imaginary lines over the chest wall is an-

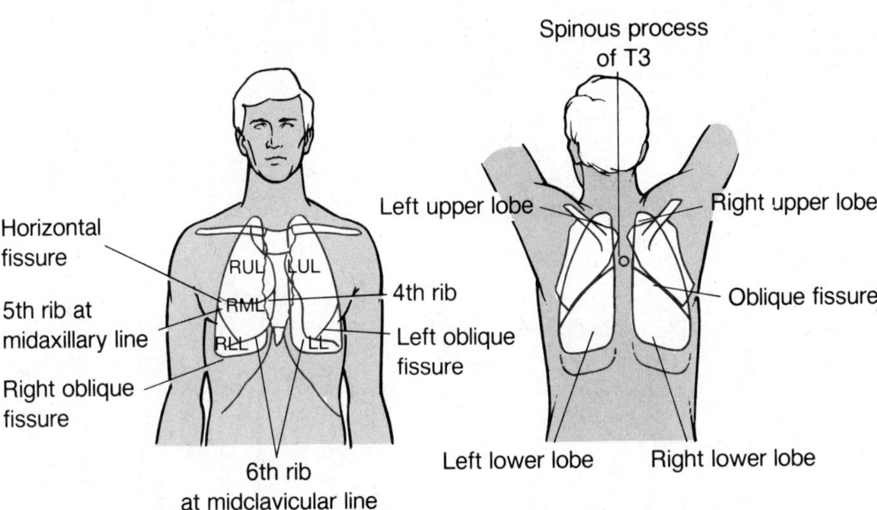

FIGURE 26–1 Examining the lungs by lobar localization. Each lung is divided approximately in half by an oblique or major fissure. (*A*) *Anterior chest:* The right lung is divided by the horizontal or minor fissure into the right upper and right middle lobes. This fissure runs from the right midaxillary line at the level of the 5th rib across anteriorly at the level of the 4th rib. The right lung is further divided by the oblique fissure into the right middle and right lower lobes. This fissure curves from the armpit at the 4th rib down to the 6th rib at the midclavicular line. The left oblique fissure similarly divides the left upper and lower lobes. (*B*) *Posterior chest:* The locations of the oblique fissures are approximated by lines drawn from the 3rd thoracic spinous process obliquely down and laterally. These lines are close to the vertebral borders of the scapulae when a person's hands are placed on top of his head. They divide upper from lower lobes.

other way to locate findings. This method is illustrated in Figure 26–2. The anterior chest can be divided by the right and left midclavicular lines and by the midsternal line. Under the arm, laterally, are the anterior axillary, midaxillary, and posterior axillary lines. The posterior chest is divided by the right and left scapular lines and midline by the vertebral line. The ribs serve as horizontal lines both anteriorly and posteriorly. Posteriorly, the ribs are identified in relation to the scapula and vertebrae or by tracing the rib from front to back.

Sequence of Physical Examination

Physical examination is done best in an orderly sequence, proceeding from inspection to palpation, percussion, and auscultation.

Inspection

In addition to the items under general observation, which are noted in all patients, it is possible to differentiate between those items one must observe during a brief examination of a patient in respiratory distress and those additional items that can be examined during a more leisurely examination. The latter can be done on the initial admission of a patient not in respiratory distress.

The Patient in Respiratory Distress. In addition to noting the breathing rate and pattern on first observation, the nurse should note the length of inspiration compared with that of expiration. Normally, the length of expiration is slightly longer than that of inspiration. In patients whose airway resistance is increased, expiration commonly is prolonged. Patients with prolonged expiration may be using pursed-lip breathing, in which exhalation occurs slowly, with lips pursed together. Many patients with COPD adopt this pattern naturally. In restrictive diseases, the pattern is often one of rapid, shallow breaths.[3]

Nasal flaring on inspiration, in an effort to increase air intake, may be observed in patients in distress. Patients working hard to expel air from their lungs may exhibit a pattern of intercostal space retraction on inspiration and bulging on expiration; this pattern indicates an obstruction to airflow and is often seen in laryngeal or tracheal obstruction or asthma attacks.

The nurse should note whether accessory muscles of breathing (scaleni, trapezii, and sternocleidomastoid) are used in inspiration, expiration, or both. These muscles are shown in Figure 26–3. *En bloc movement* refers to movement of the entire chest up and down, which is typical of patients with COPD or asthma. Noisy respirations such as wheezing, inspiratory stridor (high-pitched wheeze), or gurgling are signs of upper-airway obstruction and require immediate actions such as suctioning, repositioning, or intubating.

The Nonacute Patient. The chest configuration is usually first noted on inspection. The anteroposterior (AP) diameter is compared with the lateral diameter of the chest and is best visualized from the side of the patient. Normally the AP diameter is approximately one half the lateral diameter. If the AP diameter is increased such that the two diameters are about equal, giving the chest a rounded appearance, the condition is known as barrel chest. This is

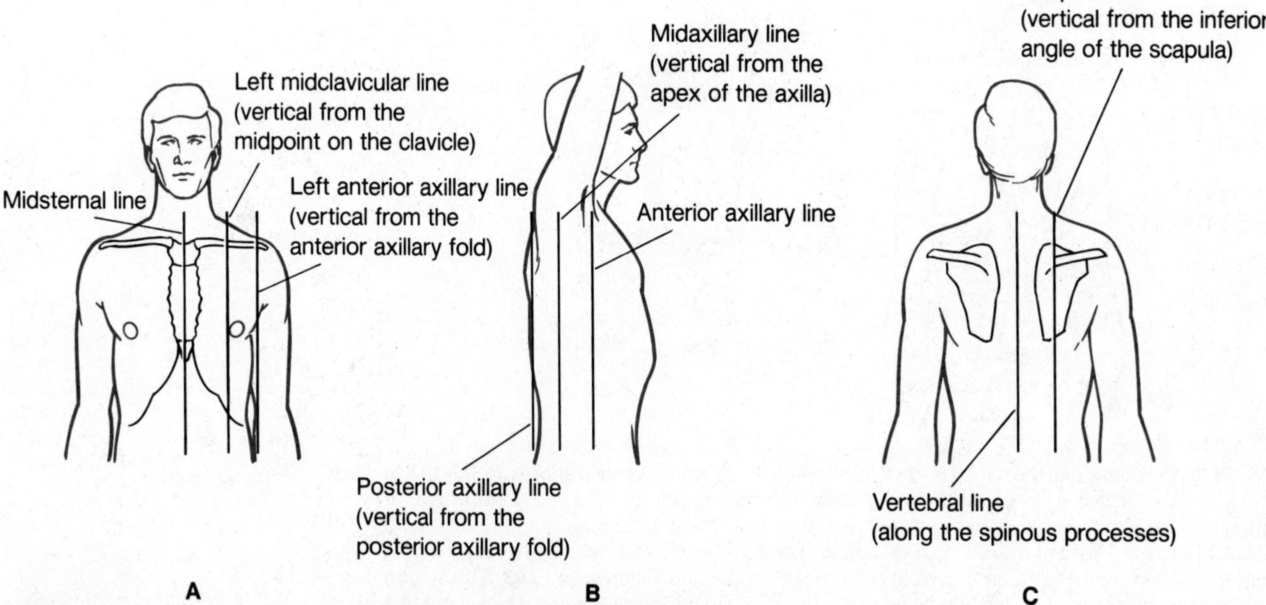

FIGURE 26–2 Imaginary lines. (*A*) The anterior chest is divided by the right and left midclavicular lines and midsternal line. (*B*) The lateral chest is divided by the right and left anterior axillary lines, midaxillary lines, and posterior axillary lines. (*C*) The posterior chest is divided, midline, by the vertebral line and by the right and left scapular lines.

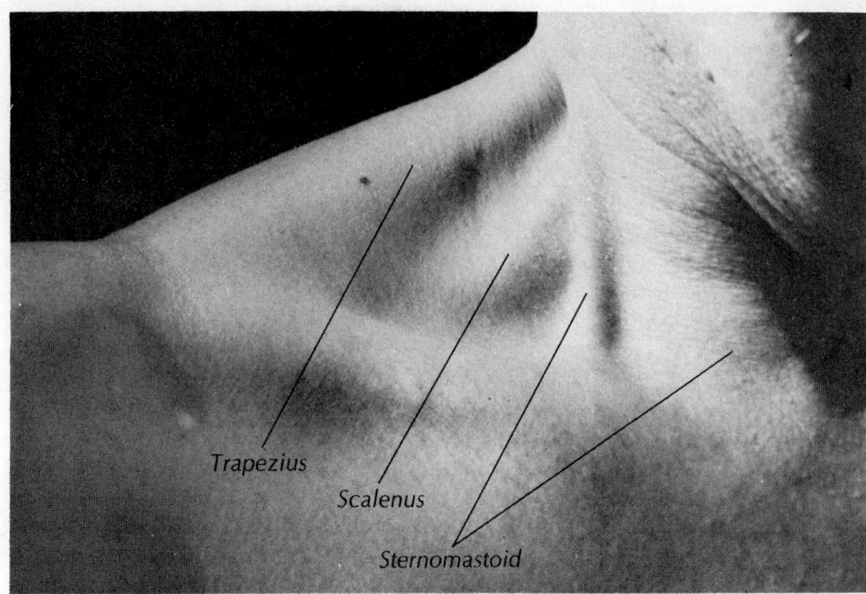

FIGURE 26–3 Accessory muscles of breathing. These muscles are used when breathing is labored. The trapezius, scalenus, and sternomastoid muscles in the neck are generally used during inspiration, and the abdominal muscles are used during expiration.

often a result of emphysema but can also occur normally with aging. Other deformities that may interfere with respiratory function include kyphosis, scoliosis, and other deformities of the spine. These deformities are shown in Figure 26–4. In kyphosis the spine is bent outward, giving a hunchback appearance. This may occur in older persons and in those with bone disease. Scoliosis is a lateral S-shaped curve of the spine that often causes one shoulder to be higher than the other. If severe, either of these conditions may cause distortion of underlying lungs and restrict the movement of the thoracic cage. Two other deformities of the thorax that might be observed are pigeon or chicken breast (pectus carinatum) and funnel chest (pectus excavatum). Pigeon breast is not usually associated with respiratory dysfunction; however, funnel chest, if the depression is deep, may interfere with both respiratory and cardiac function.

Symmetry of chest movement is noted by combining inspection and palpation, since it may be difficult to assess using inspection alone. Asymmetry, or one-sided chest expansion, may indicate a problem such as fractured ribs, pneumothorax, atelectasis, phrenic nerve disorder, malfunctioning endotracheal tube, or simply splinting due to pleuritic pain. In order to evaluate symmetry posteriorly, the nurse should place her hands under the scapula on each side with palms flat against the chest and thumbs opposite each other (Fig. 26–5). As the chest expands, the hands should separate simultaneously with the thumbs separating an equal distance apart. To assess anteriorly, hands should be placed on each side of the sternum and under the nipples with thumbs meeting at the xiphoid process.

Clubbing of the fingers may be observed on inspection. If present, the angle between the nail and finger is about 20°. Clubbing may be associated with cardiorespiratory diseases such as bronchiectasis, lung cancer, congenital heart disease, and polycythemia.[5] The mechanism of development is unclear. Clubbing is shown in Figure 26–6.

Palpation

Palpation may usually be done at the same time as inspection and is used to assess symmetry as mentioned above. In addition, thoracic expansion, tracheal position, and vocal or tactile fremitus may be assessed.

The Nonacute Patient. Note the presence of pain or any bulges or masses felt on the chest, then assess for fremitus, a vibration felt by palpating the chest wall. Fremitus occurs normally in all persons, but the quality of the sound changes according to the condition of the patient (Table 26–3). Fremitus is usually assessed posteriorly, since there is less muscle tissue and no breast tissue to interfere with transmission. The palm of the hand is placed on the chest while the patient says "ninety-nine" (creates large vibrations). Fremitus is felt over the posterior, anterior, and lateral portions of the chest systematically from top to bottom and compared left with right.

The Patient in Respiratory Distress. The soft tissues, ribs, and intercostal spaces may quickly be palpated to detect areas of pain or tenderness. Sensitive areas may indicate trauma with rib fractures.

Crepitus is identified by a crackling feeling or popping sound and may be felt either at the neck or near the top of the chest. It is caused by small air bubbles in the subcutaneous tissue and occurs as a result of air leaking into tissue from a tear in the lung after neck or chest surgery or when a fractured rib punctures the pleura.[5]

Intercostal bulging may also be noted by palpation as well as by inspection.

Tracheal deviation should be assessed by palpation. Deviation results from thyroid gland enlargement, lymph node enlargement, or displacement of the mediastinum by pleural effusion, tumor, pneumothorax, or atelectasis.[10] When the

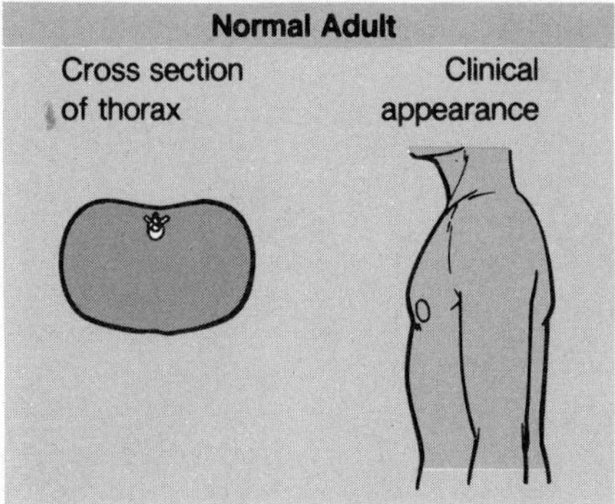

In the normal adult the ratio of anteroposterior to lateral diameter ranges from 1:2 to 5:7.

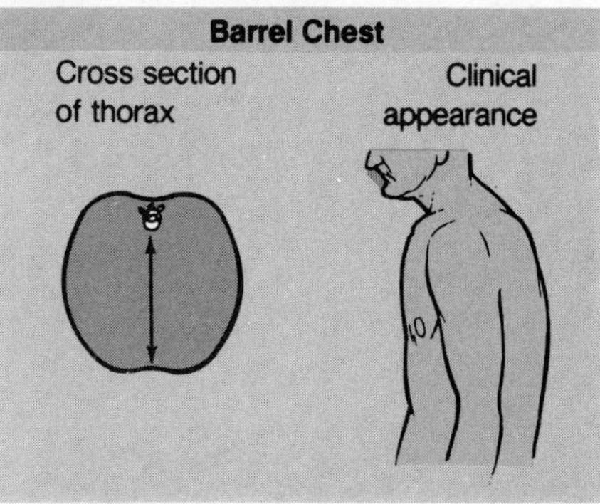

A barrel chest is associated with pulmonary emphysema or normal aging. The ratio of anteroposterior to lateral diameter approximates 1:1.

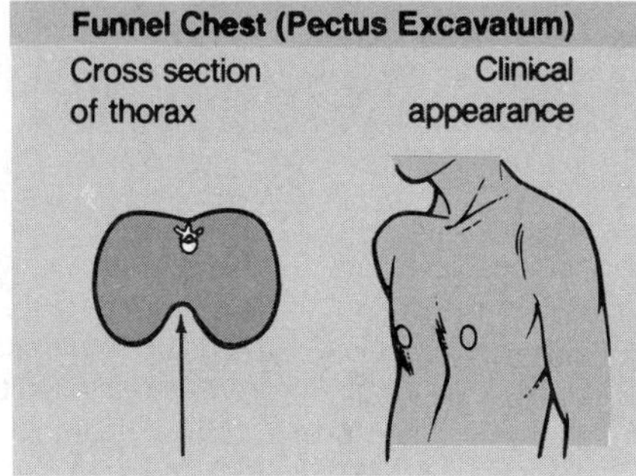

A funnel chest is characterized by a depression in the lower portion of the sternum. Compression of the heart and great vessels may cause murmurs.

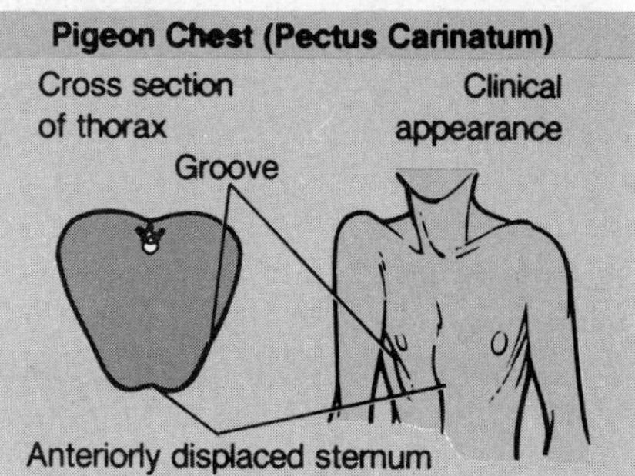

In a pigeon chest the sternum is displaced anteriorly, increasing the anteroposterior diameter. Grooves in the chest wall accentuate the deformity.

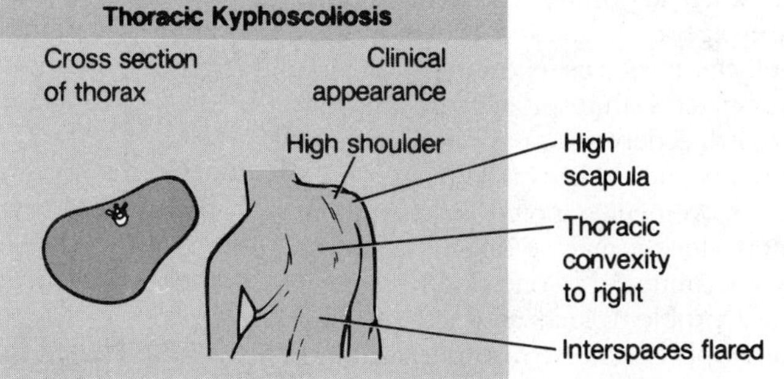

In thoracic kyphoscoliosis the spine is curved and the thorax shows corresponding deformities. Distortion of the underlying lungs may make interpretation of lung findings very difficult.

FIGURE 26–4 Deformities of the thorax. (Bates B: A Guide to Physical Examination, 3rd ed, p 150. Philadelphia, JB Lippincott, 1983)

nurse palpates the suprasternal notch, the tracheal rings will be felt directly above it if the trachea is midline. Another method is to stand behind the patient, place a finger on each side of the trachea at the suprasternal notch and compare the size of the space felt on each side. Normally it should feel equal. Conditions that collapse or compress tissue pull the trachea toward the affected side. Conditions in which there is increased intrathoracic pressure on the affected side push the trachea to the opposite side. These abnormal findings on palpation are summarized in Table 26–4.

Percussion

Percussion is used to assess the density or aeration of the lungs by tapping over various parts of the chest wall to differentiate the sounds heard, which vary over air, fluid, or consolidation. The technique is usually used to confirm findings from other methods. The five major types of percussion sounds are resonance, hyperresonance, tympany, flatness, and dullness. The characteristics and examples of each are described further in Table 26–5.

While percussion is being performed, the patient should preferably be sitting up. The nurse should tap with the distal portion of one of her fingers and keep all other fingers off the chest wall. She should begin at the apices of the lung and progress downward, alternating sides to compare findings. Anteriorly, she should percuss between rib interspaces. The entire chest should be resonant except in the area of the heart tissue, where it should be dull. The technique requires practice and is perhaps best used in the patient not in respiratory distress.

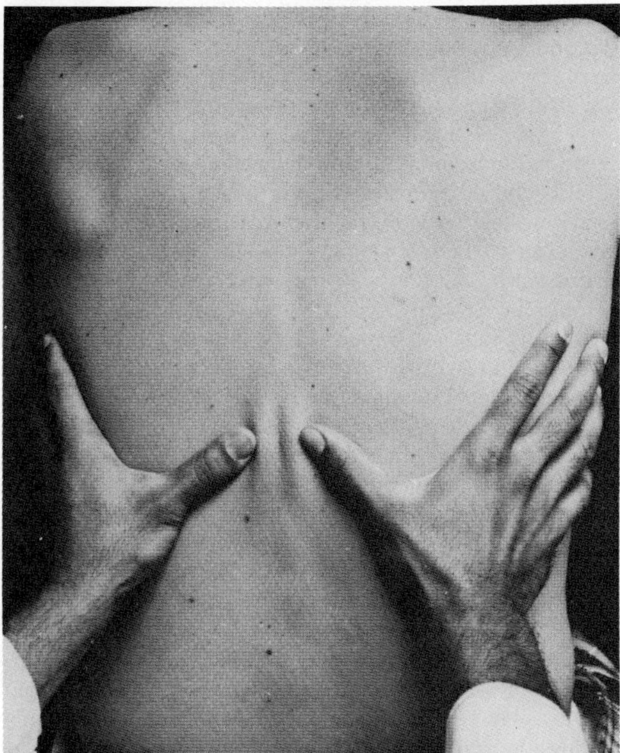

FIGURE 26–5 Assessment for symmetry chest movement. The palms are placed under the patient's scapulae with the thumbs next to each other. As the chest expands during inspiration, the thumbs should separate equally.

Diaphragmatic excursion can also be assessed in the nonacute patient using percussion. The patient should breathe normally as the nurse percusses posteriorly along the midscapula line to the spot where resonance changes to a dull note. This is the level of the diaphragm on expiration. Next, the patient should inspire deeply and hold his breath as the nurse continues to percuss from the previous dullness until dullness is reached again. Normally this is approximately 4 cm to 6 cm down and is known as diaphragmatic excursion.[3] Excursion may be decreased in states of hyperinflation such as emphysema, in which the diaphragm position usually stays lower.[10] Normally the diaphragm should be slightly higher on the right side as a result of the liver pushing against the lung. Elevation of the diaphragm results from liver enlargement, ascites, or paralysis of the diaphragm. Diaphragmatic excursion, however, should be equal on both sides.

Auscultation

Lung auscultation is performed in patients with or without respiratory distress. During auscultation, the patient should be in a sitting position if at all possible. The anterior,

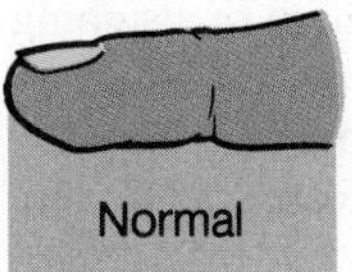

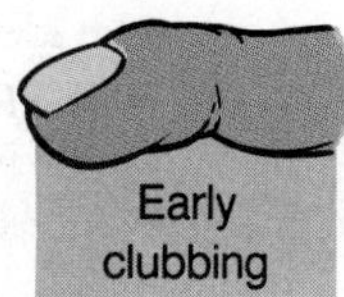

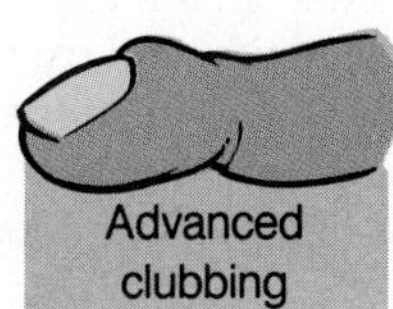

FIGURE 26–6 Clubbing. (*Left*) The angle between the nail and digit is about 20°. (*Center*) Flattened angle represents early stage of clubbing. (*Right*) In advanced clubbing, the nail is rounded over the end of the finger. Note also that the distal phalanx is bulbous and of greater depth than the proximal portion of the finger (interphalangeal depth). (After Buckingham WB: A Primer of Clinical Diagnosis, 2nd ed. New York, Harper & Row, 1979)

TABLE 26–3
Summary of Fremitus Findings

Type	*Significance*	*Characteristics*
Normal	Vibrations secondary to transmission of vibration from vocal cords to chest	Strong over trachea, weaker over periphery, equal bilaterally
Increased fremitus	Accumulation of secretions or solid tissue causes increased transmission	Strong vibrations palpable in distinct area
Decreased fremitus	Pleural thickening or increased air causes interference with vibration transmission	Little or no vibrations felt in all or specific areas

TABLE 26–4
Abnormal Palpation Findings

Finding	*Associated Conditions*
Crepitus	After neck or chest surgery Fractured rib Chest tube insertion
Intercostal bulging and retraction	Laryngeal or tracheal obstruction Tumor
Tracheal deviation	Thyroid gland enlargement Lymph node enlargement Pleural effusion Tumor Pneumothorax Atelectasis
Increased fremitus	Pneumonia Fibrosis Atelectasis
Decreased fremitus	Pleural effusion Pneumothorax Emphysema

the posterior, and the lateral portions of the chest are examined from top to bottom and compared right with left. Both inspiration and expiration should be identified by listening with the flat diaphragm of the stethoscope placed firmly on the chest. The patient can be instructed to breathe normally or slightly more deeply than normal, but through the mouth.

Lung Sounds. Compare the length of sound on inspiration and expiration to determine whether normal vesicular lung sounds are present over lung fields. The American College of Chest Physicians and the American Thoracic Society Joint Committee on Pulmonary Nomenclature recommend describing the intensity and quality of breath sounds according to two classifications: normal vesicular breath sounds and bronchial breath sounds. *Bronchial sounds* are heard normally over the larger air passages; heard elsewhere, they indicate disease. In abnormal states, breath sounds may also be absent or decreased in intensity.[12] *Adventitious sounds* (not normally occurring) include gurgles, wheezes, crackles, and pleural friction rubs. According to the American Thoracic Society, the classification of sounds can be divided into discontinuous and continuous sounds.[12] *Crackles,* more traditionally described as rales, are described as crackling, discontinuous bubbling sounds. They are thought to be the result of sudden equalization of differing pressures within the airways and may reflect the popping open of small airways or alveoli that have deflated. Another theory is that they represent movement of fluid in small airways.[5] Continuous sounds, the other major category, have a longer duration than crackles. They are divided into high-pitched wheezes and lower-pitched snoring sounds called gurgles or rhonchi. *Rhonchi* are rumbling, snoring sounds caused by the movement of air through airways that are partially obstructed by secretions, tumors, or mucosal swelling. High-pitched, continuous sounds, called *wheezes,* are associated with the airway narrowing found in asthma or airway obstruction.

Another adventitious sound is the *pleural friction rub,* a grating sound or vibration associated with breathing, heard when absence of pleural fluid causes the pleura to rub together. It may be heard over a relatively confined area of the chest, often the anterolateral chest, where the greatest thoracic movement occurs. Table 26–6 describes the characteristics of these sounds in more detail.

The Patient In Respiratory Distress. Auscultation provides information about airflow and thus is extremely helpful in the assessment of respiratory distress. In addition to identifying abnormal sounds, it is important to listen for absent or diminished breath sounds. Decreased breath sounds are

TABLE 26–5
Percussion Sounds

Sound	*Characteristics*	*Example*
Normal resonant	Slightly hollow, low-pitched	Normal lung tissue
Hyperresonance	Very loud, hollow, low-pitched	Emphysema (air-filled lung)
Tympany	Loud, drumlike	Large pneumothorax Normal over stomach
Dull	Thud; intermediate between flat and resonant	Pneumonia Atelectasis Pulmonary edema Tumor Pleural effusion Normal over liver
Flat	Short, dull tone	Pneumonectomy Massive atelectasis

heard in patients with emphysema or pleural effusion or over atelectatic areas.[2] They also occur normally in obese persons and during hypoventilation.

The Nonacute Patient. Changes in voice transmission can also be assessed using the stethoscope for auscultation. These changes can indicate consolidation much in the same way as does palpation for fremitus. Findings identified as egophony, whispered pectoriloquy, and bronchophony are described in Table 26–7. Both pneumonia and pleural effusion can cause changes in voice transmission.[2] Vocal sounds may be decreased when breath sounds are absent or decreased, as in pneumothorax, pleural effusion, obesity, and bronchial obstruction.

TABLE 26–6
Breath Sounds

Term	*Etiology*	*Inspiration/Expiration*	*Common Clinical Association*
Quality of Breath Sounds			
Vesicular breath sounds	Air moving through normal lung tissue	Inspiration longer than expiration; expiration softer	Normal lung tissue
Bronchial breath sounds	Air moving through large airways or in periphery; caused by lack of peripheral airflow or increased turbulence in smaller airways	Expiration equal to or longer than inspiration; expiration louder	Pneumonia Atelectasis
Diminished or absent breath sounds	Caused by greater thickness between lungs and stethoscope, or by decreased or absent airflow	Inspiration and expiration diminished or absent	Obesity Emphysema Pneumonectomy Pleural effusion Pneumothorax
Adventitious Breath Sounds			
Crackles (coarse or fine)	Reopening of peripheral airways previously closed as a result of obstruction or restrictive disease	Discontinuous sound that is intermittent, crackling, or bubbling sound of short duration Heard more commonly on inspiration May or may not change after cough Late inspiration indicates restrictive disease Early inspiration indicates airway obstruction	Congestive failure Chronic bronchitis Fibrosis Resolving pneumonia Shallow breathing
Gurgle	Air moving through airways that are narrowed or partially obstructed from secretions, tumors, or mucosal swelling	Continuous low-pitched snoring sound Heard predominantly on expiration	Sputum
Wheeze	Same as gurgle	Continuous high-pitched musical sound heard on expiration, inspiration, or both	Bronchial asthma Bronchitis Pulmonary edema (extensive)
Pleural friction rub	Inflamed pleural surfaces rubbing together	Grating sound or vibration associated with breathing Heard on both inspiration and expiration	Pneumonia Tuberculosis Cancer Pleurisy

Laboratory Data

Chest X-ray

Purpose and Types

Chest x-rays are used as screening tests, for diagnosis, for measuring progress of therapy and extent of disease process, and for determining placement of various types of tubes and catheters. X-rays are produced from an x-ray tube that is directed so that the rays pass through the chest and are recorded on photographic film. To avoid causing a shadow on the x-ray film, the patient should remove any clothes with buttons or metal clasps and all jewelry or other metal objects above the waist.

Chest films may be taken in either a posterior-to-anterior (PA) position or an anterior-to-posterior position (AP). The standard chest film is usually taken PA, indicating that the x-ray beam entered the posterior chest and the film plate is against the anterior chest. In this type of film the heart will be less magnified, since it is closest to the film, and thus the cardiac outline can be seen distinctly.

Portable chest films are usually taken either AP or supine, with the film behind the patient's back and the x-ray beam entering the anterior chest first. In this type of film the heart will appear magnified, since it is further away from the film.[7] The AP portable film is obtained at a closer distance from the patient (generally about 3 feet, as opposed to 6 feet); this distance further magnifies the heart and makes its outline less distinct. It is for these reasons that a film taken in the radiology department is generally preferable to a portable film, if the patient can be moved.

Chest films are generally taken upright. When taken supine, lung volumes decrease and infiltrates are highlighted. Usually the film is taken at full inspiration, since fully aerated lungs are visualized best.[7] It is important to be sure that the patient is as straight as possible against the film and not rotated, since this will alter the position of structures on the film and interfere with interpretation. Motion of the patient will also interfere, and all tubes should be away from the chest if possible.

Other types of chest films include the lateral, lordotic, lateral decubitus, and right and left anterior oblique films. *Lung tomography,* a technique that scans various planes of lung and films these sections, is used to study cavities, neoplasms, and densities of the lung. This is accomplished by simultaneously moving the x-ray tube and film about the patient so that some planes are in focus while others are blurred.

Interpretation

Knowledge of some aspects of x-ray film interpretation can be helpful to the nurse because information about the location and extent of abnormalities indicates where to focus interventions such as chest percussion. In addition, the location of tubes can be ascertained by reading x-ray films. Correct positioning of endotracheal tubes, nasogastric tubes, central venous pressure catheters, pulmonary artery catheters, pacemakers, and chest tubes can be verified.

A chest film is usually read as though the reader were looking at the patient; when a film is on the viewbox, the patient's right side is to one's left. An x-ray picture is like a photographic negative, with white indicating lack of exposure and black indicating intense exposure. Different densities cast different shades on the film and form the basis for identification and outlines of structures. The lungs, stomach, and trachea are largely air, are less dense, and therefore appear black. Soft tissues and blood are mostly water and appear gray. Bone is very dense and appears white. An object or structure can be distinguished on the film only by looking at its edges and *only* if the edge contrasts with the surrounding density. Thus, bronchi, which are air-filled and next to air-filled lung tissue, are normally not visible. However, if the lung tissue surrounding an airway becomes filled with fluid, making it denser, bronchi may be visible. This is called an air bronchogram and is an abnormal finding.[4]

Normal chest x-ray films reveal the lungs, heart in midposition of the chest, trachea, and major bronchi. The aorta, pulmonary arteries, and some pulmonary veins are visible at the hilum. The lung parenchyma usually is not visible.

In chest films indicative of consolidation (alveoli filled with fluid or inflammatory cells from pneumonia or pulmonary edema), the areas of consolidation appear white. Fluid-filled airways may be visible, or air-filled airways in consolidated tissue may appear as air bronchograms. Figure

TABLE 26-7
Changes in Voice Transmission

Finding	*Characteristics*	*Cause*
Egophony	"E" changes to "ay"	Consolidation of lung tissue (pneumonia) or Compression of lung tissue (pleural effusion)
Whispered pectoriloquy	Whispered sounds louder and more distinct than usual	
Bronchophony	Voice heard louder and more distinctly than usual	

26–7 is a chest film showing consolidation. Atelectasis (alveolar collapse) may resemble consolidation or may appear as linear streaks at the lung bases.[4]

Arterial Blood Gases

Arterial blood-gas measurements are taken in order to assess gas exchange. Serial measurements help to determine the effectiveness of both nursing and medical interventions to improve oxygenation and gas exchange.

Arterial blood samples are most commonly drawn from the radial, brachial, or femoral artery. The sample may also be obtained through an arterial line. The radial artery is usually the preferred site for arterial puncture because it is easily located on the inner aspect below the thumb and it is close to the surface of the skin. A radial artery puncture is shown in Figure 26–8. An Allen test is performed prior to using the radial artery in order to determine the adequacy of ulnar blood flow when the radial artery is blocked. This test is performed by occluding both the radial and ulnar pulses momentarily and then releasing the ulnar side while maintaining pressure on the radial pulse. The fingers and hand are assessed for return of color, indicating adequate circulation from the ulnar artery. The skin is then cleansed with a cleansing agent such as povidone–iodine prior to the puncture. A local anesthetic may be used prior to the puncture if the patient is extremely apprehensive or if arterial vasospasm is known to occur and cause difficulty in obtaining the sample. A heparinized syringe is used to obtain the sample, and it will automatically fill as the needle is inserted into the artery. Approximately 3 ml to 5 ml of blood is needed. After withdrawing the needle, pressure is immediately applied to the site with a gauze pad and maintained for at least 5 minutes. Patients taking anticoagulants and those with bleeding disorders will require a longer time until the bleeding has stopped. Since they affect oxygen and carbon dioxide findings, air bubbles in the sample are removed immediately by gently tapping on the syringe. The syringe is then capped, placed on ice to slow chemical activity in the blood, and sent immediately to the lab.

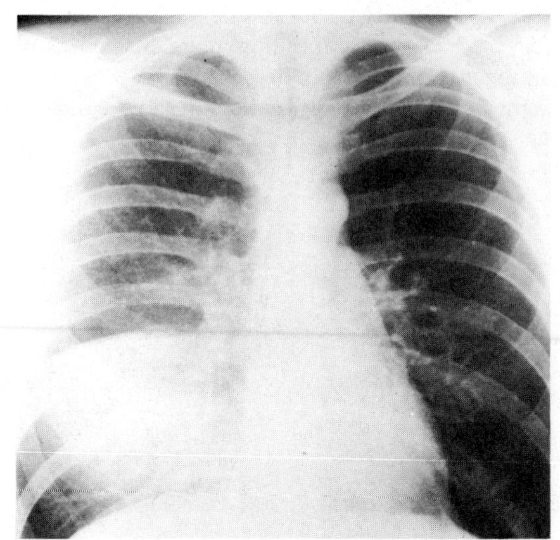

FIGURE 26–7 PA chest radiograph indicating consolidation in the right middle lobe. The cause is pneumonia. (Lillingten GA: Roentgenographic patterns of worsening pulmonary function. In Burton GG, Hodgkin JE [eds]: Respiratory Care: A Guide to Clinical Practice, 2nd ed, p 312. Philadelphia, JB Lippincott, 1984)

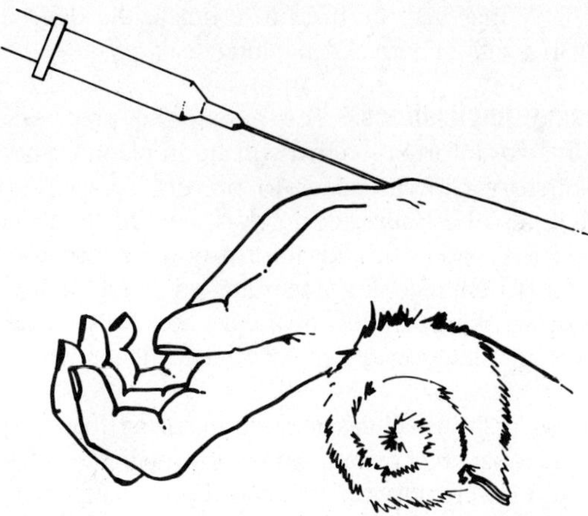

FIGURE 26–8 Optimal position for radial artery puncture. Note the extension of the wrist and the angle of entry of the needle. (Guenter CA: Respiratory function of the lungs and blood. In Guenter CA, Welch MH [eds]: Pulmonary Medicine, 2nd ed, p 154. Philadelphia, JB Lippincott, 1982)

Nursing responsibilities include maintaining the client at room air or on the prescribed supplemental oxygen for at least 20 minutes prior to the blood gas and preventing complications. Respiratory rate, temperature, and patient tolerance and activity should be measured and recorded at the time of the test. Observation for complications such as hematomas and infection is also important. The femoral site in the inguinal area is particularly vulnerable to these complications.

Measurements obtained by this sample include the following:

- Pa_{O_2}, or oxygen tension, which indicates the amount of oxygen dissolved in the arterial blood
- $Paco_2$, or carbon dioxide tension of arterial blood, which gives information about the adequacy of ventilation, namely, whether hyperventilation or hypoventilation is occurring
- blood pH, which measures the hydrogen ion concentration of the arterial blood
- HCO_3^-, or bicarbonate, a measurement of the base ratio combined with oxygen

For a more detailed interpretation of the results of arterial blood gases, see Chapter 14.

Pulmonary Function Tests

Pulmonary function tests provide valuable information about pulmonary function abnormalities. They are used to evaluate the reason for dyspnea, to evaluate preoperatively patients with potential lung disease, to detect at an early stage pulmonary disease in patients at risk, to evaluate the effects of medications, and to follow the progression of pulmonary disease. They may also be used to estimate the degree of disability in a patient with chronic lung disease.

Nursing Implications. For nurses the preoperative evaluation gives information that will aid in planning necessary respiratory care in order to prevent complciations. Nurses will also be interested in tests used to help detect early signs of disease, since this information may provide the impetus for patient teaching (including encouraging the patient to stop smoking). Evaluating the degree of disability will aid nurses in planning activities of daily living with the patient.

Nursing responsibilities include ensuring that the patient gets adequate rest prior to and following the test. A light meal should be encouraged prior to the test, and medications are often withheld. The general test procedure and the fact that it is not painful should be explained to the patient. The most recent culture results should be checked for infection with communicable organisms and the lab advised if there is a possibility of equipment contamination.

Lung Volumes

A spirometer is the equipment used for tests of lung volumes and capacities. The patient is instructed to breathe only through the mouth into a mouthpiece; noseclips are usually used.

Lung volumes are measured in order to determine the amount of air that can be inhaled and exhaled. They are compared with measurements of normal persons who are of the same age, height, sex, and race as the patient. Lung volumes and capacities are illustrated in Figure 25–4 and include the following:

Tidal volume: air moved in and out of the lung in quiet breathing (usually 10% of vital capacity)
Inspiratory reserve volume: air inhaled beyond normal inspiration
Inspiratory capacity: tidal volume plus inspiratory reserve
Vital capacity: air that can be moved in and out of lungs
Expiratory reserve volume: air that can be exhaled beyond normal exhalation

The residual volume (RV), or amount of air remaining in the lungs after a maximal expiration, and the functional residual capacity (FRC), the amount of air remaining in the lungs at the end of a normal expiration, must be determined by gas-dilution methods, such as the helium-dilution method or the nitrogen-washout technique. Body plethysmography is another means of testing RV and FRC in which the entire body is enclosed in a capsulelike unit. This test is particularly useful for patients with lung disease, since gas-dilution methods may result in underestimation of the FRC.

Flow Rates

Flow-rate measurements are used to evaluate the performance of the lungs in moving air in and out and are useful for detecting obstructive airway disease. These measurements include the following:

FVC: Forced vital capacity
FEV_1: Forced expiratory volume in 1 second
FEV/FVC: Ratio of forced expiratory volume to the forced vital capacity
$FEF_{25-75\%}$: Forced expiratory flow over the midportion of the forced vital capacity
MVV: Maximal voluntary ventilation

The FVC is one of the most common flow rates determined. The patient takes the deepest breath possible and blows it out of his lungs as fast as he can. The volume of air expelled during the first second is known as the forced expiratory volume in 1 second (FEV_1). This measurement is illustrated in Figure 26–9. The volume in 2 seconds ($FEV_{2.0}$) and in 3 seconds ($FEV_{3.0}$) can also be determined. The volume is then expressed as a percentage of the total gas exhaled (FEV/FVC). Healthy persons usually exhale at least 75% of their vital capacity flow rate in 1 second, and almost all of it in 3 seconds.[5] Prolonged expiration greater than 5 seconds in duration usually indicates obstructive airway disease.[3]

The middle part of the FVC, or the flow rate between 25% and 75% of the FVC, can also be measured and is called the $FEF_{25-75\%}$. The expiratory flow rates during this portion are thought to be least dependent on patient effort and more truly a measure of the ability of the lungs to recoil and of the thoracic cage to exert pressure. This test is most sensitive to

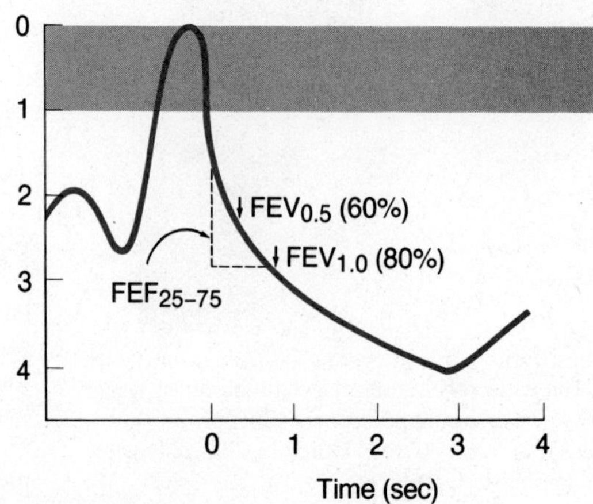

FIGURE 26–9 Determination of flow rate measurements from a normal spirometric tracing. The first portion of the forced expiratory vital capacity is most effort-dependent. The middle portion of the FVC, the FEF_{25-75}, is least dependent on patient effort and is believed to be more accurate. In this tracing 60% of the FVC is exhaled in the first half second, and 80% by the end of the first second.

disease affecting the caliber of small airways and thus reflects the development of small-airway obstruction.[5]

Another timed test is the MVV, which measures the maximum amount of air that can be breathed out in one minute. The rate and depth of respiration are measured as the patient breathes in and out as rapidly and as deeply as possible for 15 seconds, after which the volume for one minute is calculated. The results vary, depending on the patient's endurance, motivation, and cooperation.

Interpretation

Test results are interpreted on the basis of degree of deviation from normal. Tables of norms are based on age, sex, weight, and height, However, there is no separation of smokers and nonsmokers. The range of normal values is wide, since predicted values are based on averages. A patient may initially have a vital capacity greater than his predicted normal. If he then loses part of his vital capacity in the early stages of disease, it may still lie within the normal range. For this reason pulmonary function tests are most valuable when serial tests are done and each can be compared with the previous one.

Test results that are abnormal and indicate disease are generally classified into three patterns: obstructive, restrictive, or mixed.

Obstructive Pattern. Obstructive disorders are those that narrow air passages, creating turbulence and increased resistance to air flow. Examples are emphysema, chronic bronchitis, bronchiectasis, and cystic fibrosis.

Lung volumes are usually normal or increased. Air trapping occurs as a result of the difficulty of exhaling air through narrowed airways; thus, residual volume is often increased along with FRC. In patients with intermittent obstruction such as asthma, the air trapping will be temporary. Total lung capacity (TLC) may also increase, particularly in conditions such as emphysema in which alveolar walls are weakened and lungs lose elastic recoil. The residual volume/total lung capacity (RV/TLC) ratio may also increase in severe to moderate disease.[6] Vital capacity may decrease in severe obstruction because the greatly increased residual volume interferes with the vital capacity. In addition, blocked airways may prevent the patient from exhaling maximally and further contribute to a diminished vital capacity.

Forced expiratory values are usually reduced. The FEV_1 may not be reduced in early disease, but the ratio of FEV_1/FVC is usually reduced. Decreased flow rates are also reflected by a reduction in the $FEF_{25-75\%}$, which is sensitive to even early stages of disease (Table 26–8).

Restrictive Pattern. Lung expansion is restricted in patients with restrictive diseases. Thus, volumes and capacities tend to be decreased, but RV/TLC will be normal. Examples of restrictive diseases are interstitial fibrosis, pulmonary edema, pneumonia, and kyphoscoliosis. Flow rates may be reduced, normal, or even increased. If flow rates are decreased, it is due to the overall reduction in FVC. Therefore, FEV_1/FVC may be normal, and it is best to compare this ratio when interpretation suggests a restrictive pattern (see Table 26–8).

Mixed Pattern. Patients may have more than one disorder, such as emphysema and mild congestive heart failure, which results in combined obstructive and restrictive patterns. The vital capacity is reduced in combined disorders, and flow rates are reduced out of proportion to the reduced vital capacity. The FEV_1/FVC is reduced. MVV is normal or decreased. A reduced TLC is also present, indicating restriction along with obstruction (see Table 26–8).[6]

Interpreting Response to Bronchodilator Drug Dosages. Pulmonary function tests may be used to determine the effectiveness of drug therapy and the patient's response to various dosages. In this case the drug is given to the patient in the lab. After waiting a few minutes to allow the drug to begin work, timed vital capacities are made and compared with previous measurements made without the drug. If the person has no response, obstructive disease probably involves the lower airways. If there is improvement in upper airways such as the bronchi, asthma may be involved.

Bedside Pulmonary Function Tests

Pulmonary function tests at the bedside may be useful for simple screening before or after surgery, as mass screen-

TABLE 26–8
Patterns of Pulmonary Function Abnormality

Function	*Normal**	*Obstructive*	*Restrictive*	*Combined*
FVC	≥ 80	N to ↓	↓	↓
FEV_1	≥ 80	N to ↓	↓	↓
FEV_1 × 100/observed FVC	≥ 75	↓	N to ↑	↓
$FEF_{25-75\%}$	≥ 80	↓	↑, N, or ↓	↓
TLC	80–120	N to ↑	↓	↓
RV × 100/TLC	25–40	↑	N	↑

*Normal (N) values represent the percentage of predicted value except for FEV_1 × 100/FVC and RV × 100/TLC, which are absolute percentages. ↓, decreased; ↑, increased. (Burton GG, Gee GN, Hodgkin JE: Respiratory Care, p 212. Philadelphia, JB Lippincott, 1977)

ing tests, as indicators of the adequacy of therapy, and for monitoring patient progress. Portable electronic spirometers are used with either digital displays or graphic readouts. The patient is asked to breathe as deeply as possible and to blow out hard and fast as long as possible into a mouthpiece attached to the machine. The patient needs much verbal encouragement to continue blowing out as long as possible. The curve of the FVC that is produced is used to measure FEV_1 and $FEF_{25-75\%}$. These data can be used to indicate the need for further studies or to indicate the adequacy of postoperative therapy. For example, measurements can be made at the bedside to determine the effectiveness of bronchodilators given to patients.

Bronchoscopy and Bronchography

Bronchoscopy is performed by passing either a rigid or flexible fiberoptic bronchoscope into the trachea and bronchi in order to directly inspect and observe the pharynx, larynx, trachea, and bronchi. The procedure may be performed at the patient's bedside, in the operating room, or in a special procedure room. Its purposes can be either diagnostic or therapeutic. Diagnostically, it may be performed in order to examine tissues or collect specimens, to determine the location and extent of a pathologic process, and to detect tracheobronchial damage after prolonged intubation. Therapeutic purposes include removal of a foreign body, removal of mucus plugs from lower airways (saline may be administered through the bronchoscope to aid in removal of secretions), and drainage of abscesses.

A bronchogram is performed to inspect the bronchial tree by x-ray film after the introduction of a radiopaque liquid that may be instilled by means of a catheter through the nose and into the trachea through the bronchoscope tube. The patient is tilted into various positions to distribute the dye to the bronchi and bronchioles, and a series of radiographs is then taken.

Nursing Implications. Patient preparation for both bronchoscopy and bronchogram is the same. An informed consent is obtained prior to the procedure. Food and fluids are withheld, usually 6 hours before the test. Preoperative medications such as atropine and a sedative or narcotic may be ordered. Patients with respiratory insufficiency must be observed closely for respiratory depression following administration of these drugs. Patients should be assessed for loose teeth, and dentures and contact lenses should be removed.

If the procedure is to be done at the bedside, oxygen, oral suction, and an emergency cart should be properly set up. A local anesthetic is used to spray on the throat and nasal cavity and then to anesthetize vocal cords before the bronchoscope is inserted into the patient's airway.

Throughout the procedure the patient must breathe through his nose and try not to cough. The nurse should monitor for changes in skin color and vital signs, since this procedure may cause hypoxemia. Respiratory distress may occur from an adverse reaction to the anesthetic agent or from a pneumothorax. Infection and hemorrhage (more likely after bronchoscopy) are other possible complications.

Following bronchoscopy the patient should be kept in a semi-Fowler's position and vital signs monitored. Some blood-tinged sputum may be normal after the procedures, but frankly bloody sputum may signal hemorrhage and should be reported immediately. Copious sputum may be produced afterwards, and usually all sputum is collected for 24 hours for cytology studies and culture. The patient may complain of sore throat and hoarseness. He should be advised to refrain from smoking or straining his voice and reassured that the throat soreness is temporary. Cool mist may be given prophylactically to prevent laryngeal edema, which may cause airway obstruction.

Following a bronchogram, the patient should be encouraged to cough in order to expectorate the contrast material. In some cases, postural drainage may be required. Because the contrast material can obstruct distal bronchioles, the patient's temperature is monitored for 24 hours in order to detect atelectasis.

After both procedures, food and fluids are restricted until after the gag reflex returns (usually in 1½ to 2 hours). To test for the presence of a gag reflex, the nurse should touch the back of the throat with a cotton-tipped swab or tongue blade.

Mediastinoscopy

Mediastinoscopy involves use of a mediastinoscope, which is inserted through a small incision in the suprasternal notch and into the mediastinum, where inspection and biopsy of lymph nodes are performed. Mediastinoscopy is a surgical procedure and can detect lymphoma or sarcoidosis and aids in staging lung cancer.

After the test, the nurse should monitor vital signs and check the dressing for bleeding or fluid drainage. It is also important to observe for fever, crepitus, and pneumothorax.

Lung Biopsy

Biopsy specimens of any tracheobronchial structures may be obtained through a bronchoscope. In addition, needle biopsy specimens of lung or pleural tissue are obtained by inserting a needle tip into the pleural space. These biopsies are most often performed to determine whether a tumor is benign or malignant. Pneumothorax is the most common complication of this procedure, and hemorrhage, although rare, is another possible complication. A third method, used when a diagnosis cannot be made by other procedures, is the open-lung biopsy. This may also be done if a large specimen is required for pathological analysis. Open-lung biopsy requires anesthesia and a thoracotomy surgical procedure.

Thoracentesis

Aspiration of air or fluid from the pleural space is achieved by thoracentesis, in which a needle is inserted into the pleural space. This procedure may be performed for diagnostic purposes, to relieve pulmonary congestion, or to instill medication into the pleural space.

The procedure should be explained to the patient ahead of time and a consent form obtained. The nurse should prepare the patient for the pressure sensations that may be felt and emphasize the importance of not moving during the procedure. Vital signs are obtained prior to the procedure, and a sedative may be ordered. The patient is positioned seated on the edge of the bed and leaning over the bed table (Fig. 26–10), or straddling a chair backwards, or turned on the unaffected side with the head elevated 30° to 40°. Usually a local anesthetic is used at the site of needle insertion. The thoracentesis needle is advanced to the pleural space, the stylet removed, and suction applied with a three-way stopcock and syringe or drainage receptacle attached to the needle. The stopcock is turned to prevent air from entering the pleural space during the aspiration procedure. During this time, vital signs are taken frequently, and the patient is observed for signs of distress. Pneumothorax, subcutaneous emphysema, hypovolemic shock, pulmonary edema, or cardiac distress can occur when large amounts of fluid are removed quickly. Pyogenic infection can result from contamination during the procedure. Following a thoracentesis, specimens are sent for examination as ordered by the physician, and the patient's vital signs and dressing over the puncture site are checked frequently. The nurse should observe the patient for coughing or expectoration of blood, which indicates lung trauma from the procedure. A chest film is usually ordered to detect pneumothorax and to evaluate the results of the procedure.

Pulmonary Angiography

Pulmonary angiography is a radiographic examination of the pulmonary circulation following injection of a radiopaque iodine contrast agent. The dye is injected through a catheter inserted into a systemic vein and threaded into the pulmonary artery. Usually the purpose is to confirm pulmonary emboli when scans prove nondiagnostic.[7] It may also be used to evaluate congenital or acquired lesions of pulmonary vessels.

Possible complications include arterial occlusion, myocardial perforation or rupture, and ventricular arrhythmias. Following the procedure, the nurse observes for hematoma or inflammation at the site, for signs of myocardial perforation or rupture, and for arterial occlusion (check temperature, sensation, color, presence of pulse in extremity).

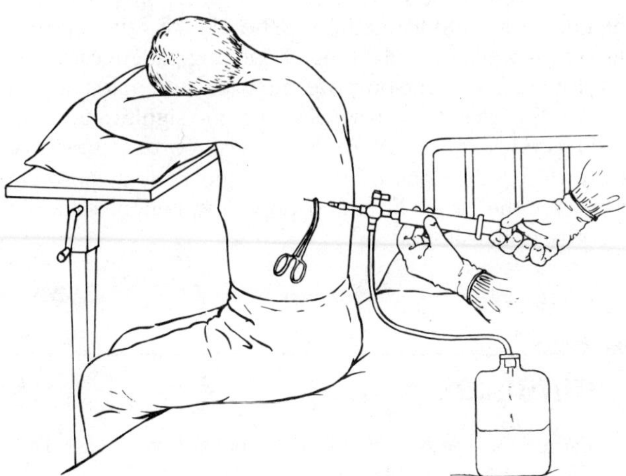

FIGURE 26–10 Technique for thoracentesis. (Gazzaniga AB: Surgical considerations in pulmonary disease. In Burton GG, Hodgkin JE [eds]: Respiratory Care: A Guide to Clinical Practice, 2nd ed, p 892. Philadelphia, JB Lippincott, 1984)

Lung Scan

Perfusion Scan. A perfusion scan produces a visual image of blood perfusion through the lung and is used to confirm pulmonary emboli or other blood-flow abnormalities.

A radioactive contrast agent is injected into a vein in the arm, and a scanning device records the pattern of pulmonary radioactivity. A normal lung shows a uniform uptake pattern, whereas areas of decreased blood flow show low radioactive uptake (Fig. 26–11).

Ventilation Scan. A ventilation scan, which is performed after the perfusion scan, detects ventilation abnormalities and thus distinguishes parenchymal diseases (such as emphysema, sarcoidosis, and tuberculosis) from vascular abnormalities such as pulmonary emboli.

During the procedure, the patient is asked to hold his breath for a short time after inhaling a mixture of oxygen and radioactive xenon gas (^{133}Xe), which diffuses through the lungs. A scanning device then records the pattern.

In case of vascular obstruction, such as that caused by pulmonary embolism, the perfusion to embolized areas is decreased but ventilation is maintained. In parenchymal disease, ventilation is abnormal in areas of consolidation.

Sputum Studies

Sputum studies are the most common tests ordered for all patients in whom chest disease is suspected. A culture gives information about the specific organisms present in the sputum and also may be collected to determine the response to treatment; it should be obtained prior to beginning antibiotic therapy. Sensitivity studies guide antibiotic selection.

Gram stains are a quick way to determine whether bacteria are gram-negative or gram-positive and can guide therapy until culture and sensitivity results are obtained. A cytologic examination is performed to determine the presence of abnormal cells that might indicate malignancy.

The nurse is usually responsible for collecting sputum, either by helping the patient to expectorate or by endotracheal aspiration. The patient should be instructed to take a few deep breaths, then cough after a forced expiration. Because the first sputum raised in the morning is generally the most productive of organisms, the patient should be given a covered, sterile sputum container at night and instructed to cough immediately after awakening if possible. Other measures, such as increasing fluid intake, ultrasonic nebulizer, and aerosolized bronchodilator treatment, may be helpful if a specimen cannot be obtained. Tracheal suction may be performed and a sputum trap used to collect specimens when other measures fail or when the patient is intu-

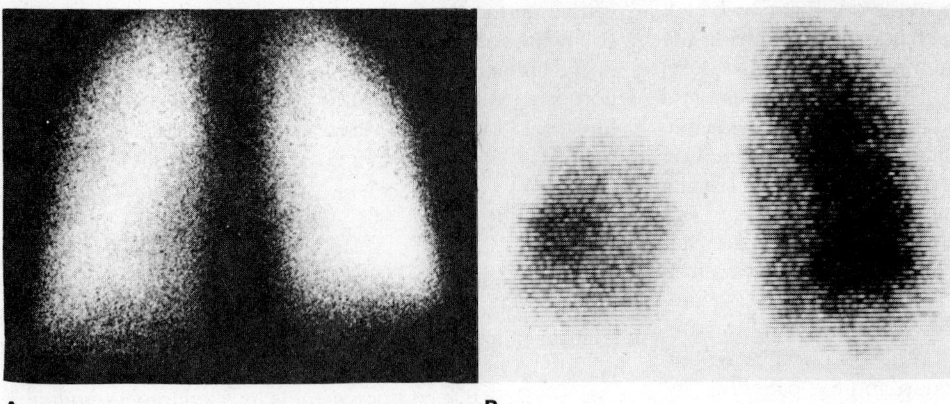

FIGURE 26–11 Perfusion scans (posterior view). (*A*) Normal perfusion scan. (*B*) Perfusion scan showing a lobar defect involving the right upper lobe, consistent with pulmonary embolism but caused by a bronchogenic carcinoma. (Burton GG, Hodgkin JE [eds]: Respiratory Care: A Guide to Clinical Practice, 2nd ed, p 823. Philadelphia, JB Lippincott, 1984)

bated. Unless a 24-hour collection has been ordered, the specimens should be covered and sent immediately to the laboratory, since standing sometimes causes overgrowth of contaminant organisms.

Pleural Fluid Studies

Samples of pleural fluid are obtained by thoracentesis. The specimen is examined for color, consistency, glucose and protein content, culture and sensitivity, acid-fast staining, differential cell count, cytology, and the enzymes lactic dehydrogenase (LDH) and amylase.

Blood that appears in the pleural fluid as the result of a traumatic tap should clear as aspiration continues. Positive bacterial cultures of pleural fluid indicate empyema. A high percentage of neutrophils suggest septic inflammation, and predominating lymphocytes may mean tuberculosis or fungal or viral effusions. Serosanguineous fluid may be associated with malignancies. An elevated level of LDH also may be associated with malignancy. Pleural fluid amylase levels are elevated in pleural effusions associated with pancreatitis. Pleural fluid glucose levels, if 30 mg to 40 mg/dl lower than blood glucose levels, may indicate malignancy, bacterial infection, nonseptic inflammation, or metastases.[8]

Ear Oximetry

The ear oximeter is a noninvasive means of monitoring arterial oxyhemoglobin saturation. It can be used in evaluation of sleep disorders, in regulating oxygen therapy in some patients, and in clinical exercise testing. The device has a specially designed earpiece that fits on the pinna of the ear, warms it, transmits wavelengths of light through the ear, and returns the signals to the oximeter. An internal computer calculates oxyhemoglobin saturation based on the fact that red light is more easily transmitted through oxygenated than deoxygenated blood. The measured value corresponds to the arterial hemoglobin saturation. The device is most useful as a monitoring tool for patients whose Pa_{O_2} values are below about 65 mmHg. Above this Pa_{O_2}, because of the flat shape of the hemoglobin dissociation curve, the ear oximeter is less useful. It also is inaccurate in low cardiac-output states, since peripheral perfusion is altered and readings from the ear are then inaccurate.

Conclusion

Knowledge and practice of respiratory history and physical examination skills are essential for all nurses. The information obtained is used to make critical decisions concerning the need for immediate actions to be taken for the patient in distress as well as for planning of ongoing patient care.

Knowledge of the purpose, methods, and potential complications of diagnostic tests as well as the significance of the findings is also necessary for all nurses in order to carry out the nursing functions of preparing the patient, observing him after the procedure, and providing patient education and emotional support.

References

1. Barbee RA: The medical history in pulmonary disease. Respir Care 29, No. 1:68, 1984
2. Bates B: A Guide to Physical Examination, 3rd ed, p 136. Philadelphia, JB Lippincott, 1983
3. Burton GG: Practical physical diagnosis in respiratory care. In

Burton GG, Hodgkin JE (eds): Respiratory Care: A Guide to Clinical Practice, 2nd ed. Philadelphia, JB Lippincott, 1984

4. Felson B, Weinstein A, Spitz H: Principles of Chest Roentgenology: A Programmed Text. Philadelphia, WB Saunders, 1965
5. Harper R: A Guide to Respiratory Care: Physiology and Clinical Applications. Philadelphia, JB Lippincott, 1981
6. Hodgkin JE: Routine pulmonary function tests. In Burton GG, Hodgkin JE (eds): Respiratory Care: A Guide to Clinical Practice, 2nd ed. Philadelphia, JB Lippincott, 1984
7. Lillingten GA: Roentgenographic patterns of worsening pulmonary function. In Burton GG, Hodgkin JE (eds): Respiratory Care: A Guide to Clinical Practice, 2nd ed. Philadelphia, JB Lippincott, 1984
8. Nurse's Reference Library: Diagnostics. Springhouse, PA, Intermed Communications, 1981
9. Pardee NE, Winterbauer RH, Allen JD: Bedside evaluation of respiratory distress. Chest 85:203, 1984
10. Smith S: Clinical assessment of the pulmonary patient. In Traver G (ed): Respiratory Nursing: The Science and the Art. New York, John Wiley & Sons, 1982
11. Tobin MJ, Chadha TS, Jenouri G et al: Breathing patterns 1. Normal subjects. Chest 84:202, 1983
12. Updated Nomenclature for Membership Reaction. Reports from the ATS Ad Hoc Committee on Pulmonary Nomenclature. ATS News 7:8, 1981

Bibliography

Guenter CA: Respiratory function of the lungs and blood. In Guenter CA, Welch MH, Hogg JC (eds): Clinical Aspects of Respiratory Physiology. Philadelphia, JB Lippincott, 1978

Hunter PM: Bedside monitoring. Nursing Clin North Am 16:211, 1981

King RC: Examining the thorax and respiratory system. RN 45:54, 1982

Malasanos L, Barkauskas V, Moss M et al: Health Assessment, 1st ed. St Louis, CV Mosby, 1977

Mechanical ventilation: Patient assessment and nursing care. Am J Nurs 80:2191, 1980

Nurse's Reference Library: Assessment. Springhouse, PA, Intermed Communications, 1982

Rokosky JS: Assessment of the individual with altered respiratory function. Nursing Clin North Am 16, No. 2:195, 1981

Tinker J: Understanding chest x-rays. Am J Nurs 76:54, 1976

Wade J: Respiratory Nursing Care: Physiology and Technique, 2nd ed. St Louis, CV Mosby, 1977

West JB: Pulmonary Pathology: The Essentials, 2nd ed. Baltimore, Williams & Wilkens, 1982

Chapter 27

Nursing Strategies for Common Respiratory Problems

Nursing Diagnosis
Interventions
Evaluation

Joanne Schnaidt Rokosky

Ineffective Airway Clearance
Impaired Gas Exchange
Pleural Disruption
Dyspnea
Ineffective Breathing Patterns

The focus of this chapter is interventions for common physiological disturbances of respiratory function. For persons with acute, self-limiting respiratory illnesses, the most important type of intervention may be health teaching to enable self-management of symptoms and prompt recognition of complications. Often it is the nurse who can provide this instruction best. For patients with severe respiratory disease, whether acute or chronic, collaborative interventions by nurses, physicians, and respiratory therapists are necessary to correct the underlying problem, provide supportive care, and monitor the progress of the disease or its therapy. Although the interventions in this chapter are described under Nursing Diagnoses, they are not restricted to the nurse and might just as appropriately be called respiratory-care strategies.

Ineffective Airway Clearance

Nursing Diagnosis

Ineffective airway clearance related to altered or excessive tracheobronchial secretions, ciliary stasis, ineffective or absent cough as manifested by auscultation of rhonchi or wheezes, cough with or without sputum production, and dyspnea.

Physiological Basis of Airway Clearance

Because the act of breathing continually exposes the lungs to inhaled microbes, dusts, and noxious gases, numerous protective defense mechanisms have evolved. A particularly important component of this defense system is the mucociliary escalator, a combination of mucous layer and cilia that helps defend the airways from the larynx to the terminal bronchioles. These airways are lined with columnar epithelium containing cilia that beat rhythmically at a rate of over 1000 beats per minute. Tracheobronchial mucus and other fluids produced within the lungs form a mucous blanket consisting of an underlying watery layer (sol layer) and an upper, gelatinous layer (gel layer).[36] The cilia beat freely in the sol layer and stimulate a wavelike motion in the gel layer; as a result, the gel layer is gradually propelled up the respiratory tract and carries deposited particles out of the lung and back to the oropharynx.

Multiple factors, many of them poorly understood, control the consistency of the mucous blanket and the rhythmic beating of cilia. Stimulation by the parasympathetic nervous system and response to irritation by infection, allergy,

Appreciation is expressed to Martha L. Tyler, M.N., R.R.T. for her critical review of the content of this chapter.

noxious vapors, and other factors play a role in increasing secretion.[8,36,63] The normal pattern of rapid, rhythmic ciliary beating is impaired by factors such as cigarette smoking, inhalation of noxious gases and irritating dusts, local and general anesthetics, high concentrations of sedative agents and narcotics, altered bronchial mucus consistency, high inspired oxygen concentrations, and cuffed endotracheal tubes.[38,63] Mucociliary defenses are known to be impaired in diseases such as chronic bronchitis, asthma, cystic fibrosis, and bronchiectasis. It remains unclear whether the dysfunction results from abnormal mucus, abnormal cilia, or both.[36]

Mucokinesis is the term used to describe the overall process of mucus clearance. In addition to being influenced by mucus characteristics and by ciliary activity, adequate mucokinesis requires airway patency and the ability to generate an effective cough. Despite the fact that production and movement of bronchial mucus is a continuous process, one is normally unaware of the presence of tracheobronchial secretions. The tiny amounts of mucus that reach the oropharynx are swallowed without conscious awareness. Only when the secretions are excessive is one aware of sputum that must be expectorated or swallowed. Thus, sputum production is, by definition, abnormal.[63]

When secretions are abnormally retained, an initial effect is an increased resistance to airflow. If some airways are obstructed completely, lung compliance will fail, portions of the lung will be underventilated, and inadequate oxygenation may result. In addition, the alterations in airway resistance and compliance may produce the sensation of dyspnea.[38]

Interventions

The goal of all nursing interventions is to clear the airways of excessive secretions. Interventions can focus on either changing the character of tracheobronchial secretions or on increasing their clearance from the airways. Frequently, both types of efforts are required and are performed in conjunction with each other.

Establishing strategies to remove secretions first requires assessment of the factors that are impairing clearance.

- Is the quantity of mucus production excessive, as may be the case in chronic bronchitis?
- Has infection or water deficit possibly increased secretion viscosity?
- Is muscle weakness limiting the ability to generate an effective cough?

The interventions that are chosen should address these etiologic factors specifically. In addition, the interventions that are initially attempted should be those that are the least invasive and most free of side-effects. Interventions that are commonly initiated or performed by nurses include supervised coughing, chest physical therapy (CPT), delivery of humidity or aerosol therapy, and tracheal suction.

Coughing Measures

Supervised coughing is the least invasive method of helping patients clear secretions and is also a fundamental component of many other methods of bronchial hygiene such as postural drainage. Many patients do not cough effectively and will benefit from nursing interventions to improve their technique. By understanding the mechanism of a normal cough, the nurse can identify the specific assistance a patient needs. The sequence of a normal cough includes a deep inspiration to provide a bolus of air behind the retained secretions, glottic closure to trap the inspired air in the lungs, forceful contraction of the abdominal muscles to force the diaphragm upward and increase intrathoracic pressure, and sudden reopening of the glottis and expulsion of air at a velocity of 75 mi to 100 miles/hour.[3,37]

Teaching Effective Cough. A basic requirement for effective coughing is a body position that allows for both a deep inspiration and a forceful expiration using the abdominal muscles. The ideal position is for a patient to sit up in a chair or at the edge of the bed with his head and spine flexed slightly and the feet planted on the floor or otherwise supported. Although a patient may be unable to assume this ideal position, it should be remembered that there is no possible way to cough well when lying flat in bed. An alternative to having the patient sit is to elevate the head of the bed and have the patient flex his knees toward his chin and brace his feet on the bed mattress. Yet another alternative is for the patient to turn on his side to cough, keeping the upper body flexed forward and knees flexed toward the chin.

Once the patient is positioned properly, the cough technique can be altered to compensate for the patient's disability. For example, inspiratory capacity is limited in patients with restrictive pulmonary disease. Interventions should focus on helping such patients inspire more deeply before coughing. The patient with retained secretions who has had abdominal or thoracic surgery may have difficulty achieving both deep enough inspiration and sufficient abdominal contraction. Because pain is often a significant limiting factor, analgesics should be given approximately one half hour before assisting the postoperative patient to cough. Patients should be taught to keep efforts deliberate in order to lessen the pain that may accompany sudden movement. Splinting the abdomen with a pillow, the nurse's hands, or the patient's own hands will stabilize the incision and further decrease the pain of coughing (Fig. 27–1). Staging the actual cough into two or three expiratory blasts may also be less fatiguing and more productive. Quadriplegics or other patients who have lost control of their abdominal muscles need assistance to achieve the high flow rate needed for an explosive cough. They can be assisted by manually forcing the diaphragm upward following a deep inspiration.

In patients with obstructive disease, the act of coughing tends to precipitate airway collapse. Such patients may find the following technique of staged, controlled coughing beneficial:

1. Take a deep breath through the nose and hold it for 2 seconds.
2. Leaning forward, cough gently three times.
3. Repeat as needed.

An alternative technique is "huff" coughing or coughing with an open glottis. In this technique, the patient whispers the word "huff" as he coughs and thus avoids closing the glottis. This maneuver is believed to generate higher flow

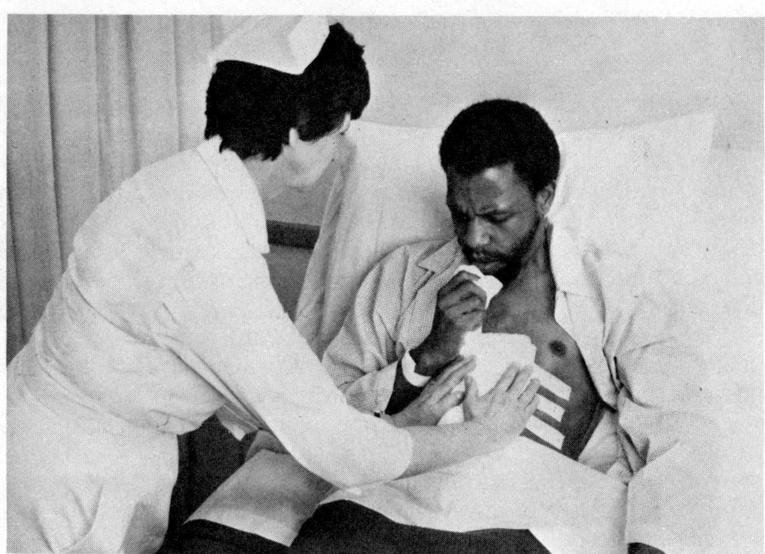

FIGURE 27–1 Staged coughing with wound support is designed to help produce an effective cough without excessive increases in airway pressure or pain. (Respiratory Care: Concepts and Techniques, an audiovisual publication of JB Lippincott, 1980)

rates by preventing the collapse of unstable bronchial walls and is recommended for use by patients with chronic obstructive pulmonary disease.[28,38]

Chest Physical Therapy

When cough alone is ineffective, additional measures may be employed to loosen sputum and to aid in its clearance from the tracheobronchial tree. Among these measures is chest physical therapy (CPT), a group of airway clearance maneuvers that includes postural drainage, percussion, and vibration.

Postural drainage is a method of using gravity to aid in the removal of secretions. Specific positions are chosen that drain the particular segments of the lung in which secretions have accumulated. Commonly used positions are illustrated in Figure 27–2.

Percussion consists of rhythmic clapping of the chest wall with cupped hands over the lung segment to be drained. This technique is illustrated in Figure 27–3. The percussive force is thought to change mucus from a gel to a more fluid state and to physically dislodge the mucus from airway walls. It is known to increase tracheal transport velocity.[38]

Vibration is a repetitive, shaking pressure of the hands that is applied to the chest wall during exhalation. It is believed to facilitate expiration, loosen mucus, and, perhaps, induce cough. In order to be effective, these maneuvers must be accompanied by coughing. If the patient is unable to cough productively after CPT, he may require tracheal suction.

Indication. The clinical effectiveness of CPT is controversial and has been the subject of numerous investigations. Although studies have demonstrated increased sputum clearance, the relative effectiveness of postural drainage versus percussion versus cough has been subject to debate.[2,39,42,64] There is also controversy regarding the effects on gas exchange following this therapy.[30,39] Pulmonary function values have generally been shown to improve when CPT achieves clearance in patients with copious tracheobronchial secretions.[56] It is generally agreed that CPT is a technique that should be reserved for patients with excessive secretions that cannot be cleared by coughing.[29] Patients with chronic obstructive pulmonary disease, bronchiectasis, cystic fibrosis, neuromuscular dysfunction, or decreased level of consciousness or those who are intubated are particularly vulnerable to episodes of inadequate clearance. CPT on a long-term, prophylactic basis is not usually justified. Two exceptions are for young children with cystic fibrosis and for patients with bronchiectasis.[38] Both conditions are characterized by production of voluminous quantities of thick sputum that may require routine CPT to achieve adequate clearance.

Complications. Although complications are infrequent, serious complications of CPT have been reported. These complications include massive pulmonary hemorrhage, hypoxemia, rib fractures, increased intracranial pressure, and a decrease in cardiac output.[58] As a consequence, CPT is generally contraindicated in the following situations[38,58]

Active or recent hemoptysis
Lung abscess
Rib fractures
Uncontrolled hypoxemia
Increased intracranial pressure
Cardiovascular or hemodynamic instability
Severe bronchospasm

Guidelines. When the need for CPT has been established, certain guidelines should be followed including the frequency of instituting the procedures, the choice of postural drainage positions, and the length of time the position is maintained. These guidelines are outlined in Table 27–1.

Tracheal Suction

Indications. Some patients may require tracheal suction to remove accumulated secretions. Because improper suctioning can have lethal consequences, patients should not

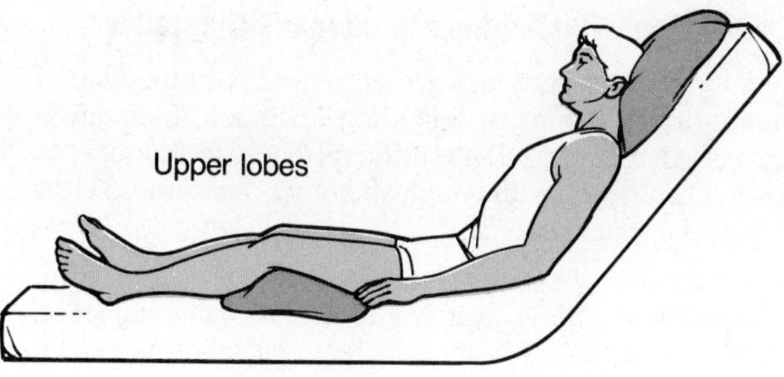

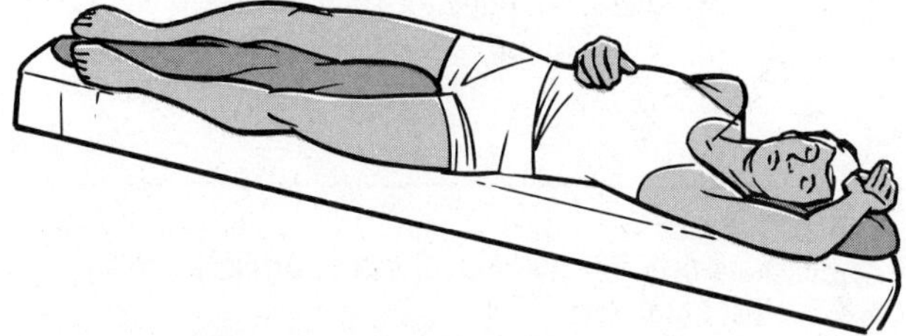

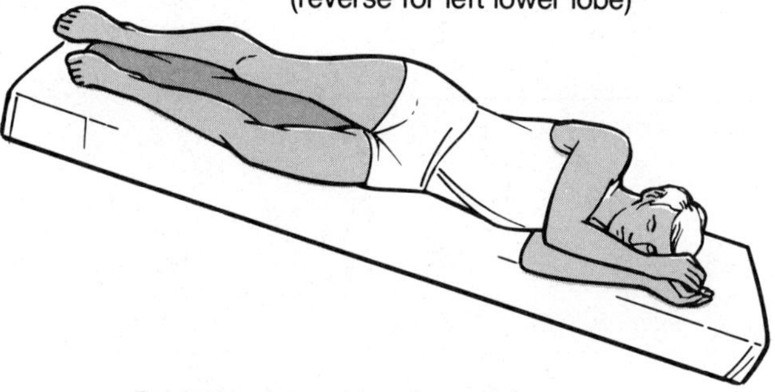

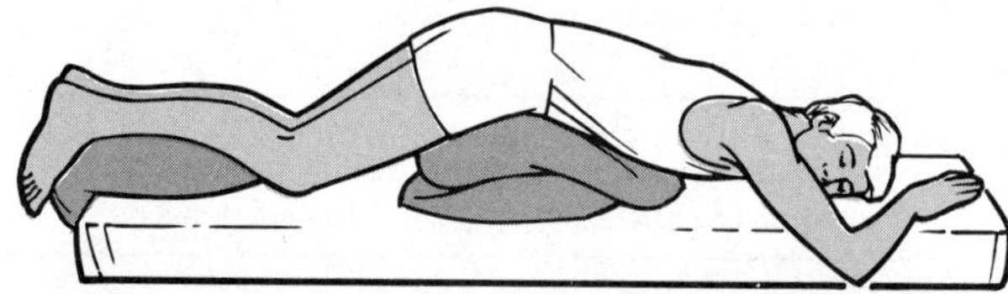

FIGURE 27–2 Frequently used postural drainage positions. The drainage angle is adjusted by raising the foot of the bed 12 inches for the middle lobes and 18 inches for the lower lobes or by using pillows under the hips. (After Luce JM, Tyler ML, Pierson DJ: Intensive Respiratory Care, p 140. Philadelphia, JB Lippincott, 1984)

be suctioned when a less invasive procedure such as supervised coughing may suffice. Even when it has been determined that tracheal suction is appropriate, as is usually the case with intubated patients, suctioning on a routine basis is unjustified. Instead, the need for suctioning should be determined by careful assessment of the patient. Secretions may be seen bubbling within an endotracheal or tracheostomy tube, or rhonchi may be auscultated over the central airways.

Equipment. Once the need for suction has been determined, the proper equipment must be chosen. Of particular importance is the choice of suction catheter. If the diameter of the suction catheter is very small, it will suction mucus less

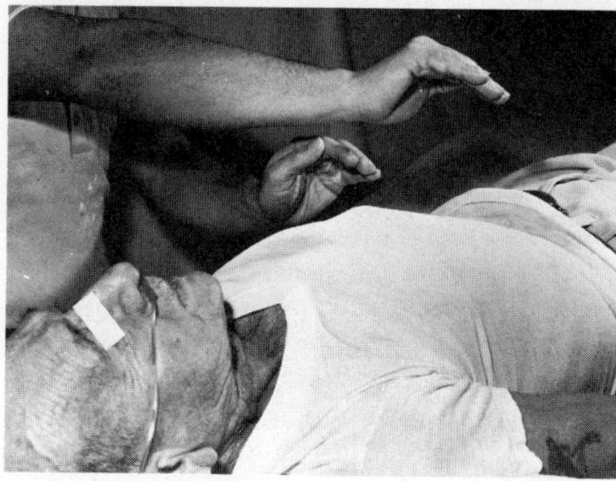

FIGURE 27–3 Hand positioning for chest percussion. (Barrascout JR: Chest physical therapy and related procedures. In Burton GG, Hodgkin JE: Respiratory Care: A Guide to Clinical Practice, 2nd ed, p 670. Philadelphia, JB Lippincott, 1984)

TABLE 27–1
Guidelines for Chest Physical Therapy

Frequency

1. Frequency of CPT varies according to the patient's condition.
2. If done twice daily, the usual times are in the morning before breakfast and just before bedtime. If done more often, the best additional times are before lunch and dinner.
3. Regardless of the specific time chosen, CPT must be done before meals or 2 hours afterwards, in order to reduce the risk of vomiting and subsequent aspiration.
4. If a bronchodilator has been ordered, it should be used 20 minutes prior to CPT.

Postural Drainage

1. Each postural drainage position should be maintained for 10 to 15 minutes.
2. Ordinarily, no more than three positions are used; the positions chosen are those that will drain regions of the lung in which secretions have accumulated (see Fig. 27–2).
3. Upper regions of the lung are drained first.
4. Modifications in the positions may be necessary for patients who are extremely weak.

Percussion and Vibration

1. Percussion and vibration are performed while the patient is in each drainage position.
2. Percussion is contained for 2 minutes, followed by several vibrations.
3. The strength of percussion and vibration must be adjusted to the condition of the patient. For example, gentle pressure is necessary for a person with osteoporosis.
4. Percussion and vibration should not be done over the spine, sternum, breasts, or beneath the rib cage.
5. The techniques should be curtailed if they cause pain.

Coughing

1. The patient should cough in each bronchial drainage position.
2. The amount, color, and consistency of sputum produced in each position should be recorded.
3. For patients unable to cough effectively, tracheal suction may be substituted for coughing.[26,38]

effectively. However, as the catheter diameter increases, the space available for air flow between the catheter and endotracheal tube decreases, and negative pressure is created, which can result in areas of atelectasis. Studies have established that the outside diameter of a suction catheter should be no larger than half the inside diameter of the endotracheal or tracheostomy tube being entered.[50,51]

Clinically, choosing the proper catheter can be difficult because suction catheters are usually sized in French gauge, but tracheostomy and endotracheal tubes can be sized according to French, millimeter, or Jackson gauge. Relationships among various gauges and recommended suction catheter sizes are given in Table 27–2. By having a general idea of these relationships, the nurse can choose a suction catheter size that is both safe and effective.

Complications. Intubation causes bacterial colonization within the trachea, normally a sterile environment, and predisposes to respiratory *infection.* The debilitated status of most patients who require tracheal suction further contributes to the infection risk. Therefore, efforts should be taken to minimize bacterial contamination during suctioning by using a sterile catheter, gloving the hand manipulating the catheter, and rinsing the catheter in a solution free of contaminants.

The major immediate risk of tracheal suction is *hypoxemia.* This complication has been well documented in the literature, as have numerous techniques for its prevention.[5,7,11,54] The current recommendation is to preoxygenate patients before and following every pass of the suction catheter.[20,24,55] An anesthesia bag is used to deliver 100% oxygen at a lung volume approximately 1.5 times the patient's tidal volume. By hyperinflating the lungs before suction, the normal gas mixture is rapidly replaced by oxygen. Following passage of the suction catheter, hyperinflation reverses the microatelectasis resulting from the negative pressure generated by suction.

Procedure. The sample suction procedure outlined in Table 27–3 contains specific guidelines to minimize the likelihood of complications. See also Fig. 27–4.

Additional Techniques to Increase Clearance

A variety of techniques are employed with the goal of thinning tracheal mucus, including hydration, humidification, aerosol therapy, and medications. These techniques are used in conjunction with cough and other measures to clear the tracheobronchial tree.

Hydration. Because it is known that water depletion impairs mucociliary clearance, increasing oral or parenteral fluid intake is often an initial step for patients with thick secretions. However, it is not known whether increased hydration can thin tracheobronchial secretions once they have formed.[35] Nevertheless, an intake of 1.5 liters to 2.0 liters per day is generally recommended unless the patient has an-

TABLE 27–2
Approximate Size Relationships Between Artificial Airways and Suction Catheters

Airway Gauge: Internal Diameter (mm)	Airway Gauge: French	Airway Gauge: Jackson	Maximum Size Suction Catheter to Use (French)
2.5	13	00	6
3.0	15	0	
3.5	16.5	1	8
4.0	18	2	
4.5–5.0	21	3	10
5.5	24	4	
6.0–6.5	27	5	12
7.0	30	6	14
7.5–8.0	33	7	16
8.5	36	8	18
9.0–9.5	39	9	
10.0	42	10	20

(Adapted from Caldwell SL, Sullivan KN: Artificial airways. In Burton GG, Hodgkin JE [eds]: Respiratory Care: A Guide to Clinical Practice, 2nd ed, p 513. Philadelphia, JB Lippincott, 1984)

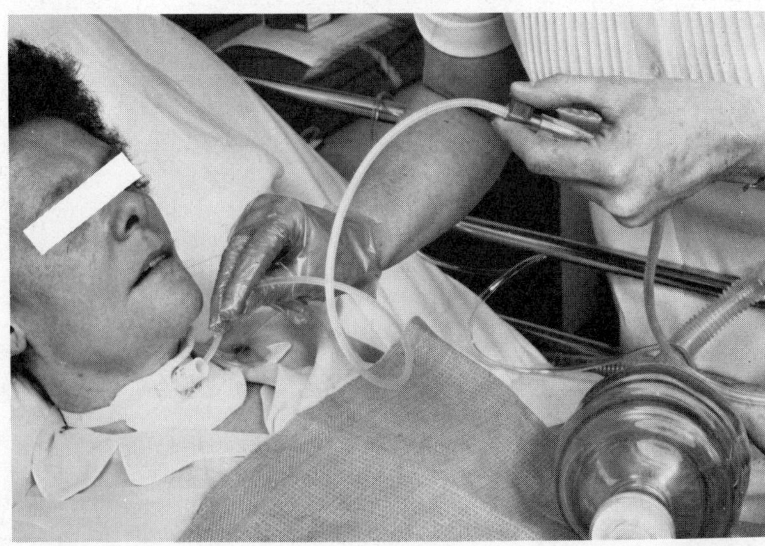

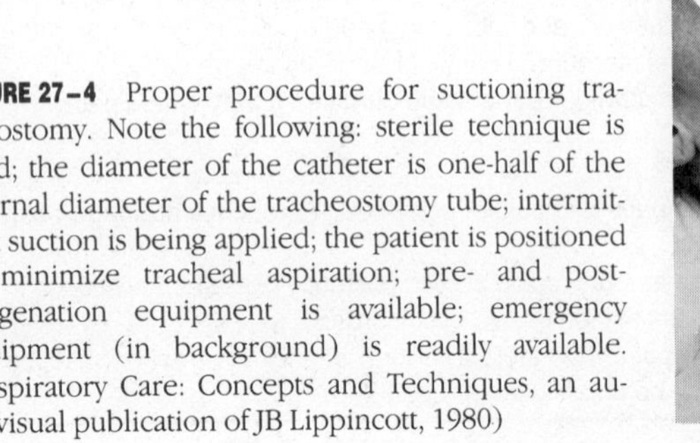

FIGURE 27–4 Proper procedure for suctioning tracheostomy. Note the following: sterile technique is used; the diameter of the catheter is one-half of the internal diameter of the tracheostomy tube; intermittent suction is being applied; the patient is positioned to minimize tracheal aspiration; pre- and post-oxygenation equipment is available; emergency equipment (in background) is readily available. (Respiratory Care: Concepts and Techniques, an audiovisual publication of JB Lippincott, 1980)

TABLE 27–3
Tracheal Suction

Equipment Needed
Anesthesia bag attached to oxygen flowmeter
Gloves
Sterile saline (less than 24 hours old); or, in some hospitals, midstream tap water
Container for saline: sterile container packaged with suction catheter or nonsterile paper cup
Suction catheter: ½ internal diameter of tracheal tube, with Y connector or constructed with suction control valve

Procedure	***Rationale***
1. Turn on oxygen liter flow to anesthesia bag (8–10 liters); exact flow depends on filling of particular bag.	1. Use of anethesia bag allows delivery of 100% oxygen at a hyperinflation volume.
2. Pour saline (or tap water) into cup.	2. To rinse secretions from catheter.
3. Glove.	3. Gloving decreases transmission of the nurse's own or other patients' bacteria.
4. Attach suction catheter to suction. Start with low suction (100–150 mmHg). Increase as necessary.	4. Pressure needed will vary with amount, consistency of secretions, and catheter size.
5. Lubricate catheter with saline.	5. To facilitate passage of catheter.
6. Give 3 to 4 deep breaths with 100% oxygen from bag. Follow patient's respirations, if possible.	6. To prevent hypoxemia.
7. Insert catheter quickly past end of tracheostomy or endotracheal tube (until resistance is felt); keep suction off (finger off control valve or Y connector).	7. Breathing is restricted while suction catheter is in tracheal tube; keeping suction off decreases trauma to mucosa.
8. Withdraw catheter slightly. Apply suction. Slowly remove catheter with continuous rotating motion (Fig. 27–4).	8. Slight space between bronchus and catheter decreases potential for atelectasis and mucosal damage.
Limit total suction time to 15 seconds (from insertion to removal).	Longer time periods more likely to cause hypoxemia.
Observe individual patient's tolerance: color, heart rate and rhythm.	Some patients cannot tolerate even 15 seconds of suction.
9. Give 3 to 4 deep breaths with 100% oxygen from bag. Follow patient's respirations if possible.	9. Reverses microatelectasis and prevents hypoxemia.
10. Rinse catheter with saline.	10. Removes adhered mucus and prevents reintroduction into trachea.
11. Repeat steps 6 through 9 until airway is clear. Bag at end of procedure.	
12. *For tube with inflated cuff:* While second nurse applies positive pressure by means of the anesthesia bag, deflate cuff and immediately suction oropharynx. Reinflate cuff.	12. Positive pressure pushes secretions that have pooled just above the cuff into the mouth where they can be coughed out or removed by suction.
13. Suction oropharynx after completing tracheal suction.	13. Prevents contamination of trachea with oropharyngeal flora.
14. Discard catheter, glove, and cup.	14. Reuse of equipment would introduce bacteria into trachea.

other condition, such as renal or cardiovascular disease, that mandates a limited fluid intake.

Liquids may also be delivered to the tracheobronchial tree by humidification or by aerosolization. *Humidity* refers to the water vapor content of the air. By contrast, an *aerosol* consists of particles of liquid suspended in a gas.

Humidification Therapy. Part of the function of the upper respiratory tract is to warm and humidify the air flowing through the upper respiratory tract, so that by the time inhaled air reaches the alveoli it has reached body temperature and is fully saturated with water vapor. Patients with artificial airways require external humidification to substitute for the function of the upper respiratory tract that is being bypassed. Patients receiving oxygen at high flow rates also need external humidification to compensate for the irritating effects of inhaling a dry gas.

Water vapor may soothe airways and help loosen adhered secretions. Patients frequently report improved clearance after additional humidity is added to their immediate environment. However, objective patient studies showing that humidification decreases sputum viscosity are lacking.[38] The most common humidifiers are "bubble diffusion humidifiers," which break down the gas (air or oxygen) into tiny bubbles and thereby increase the surface area exposed to the liquid contained in the humidifier (Fig. 27–5). Because warm air can contain more water vapor before becoming saturated, these devices are often heated.

Aerosol Therapy. As with humidification, the clinical efficacy of aerosol therapy has been questioned. It has not yet been established that inhaled water or saline will alter secretions that are already thick and dried or even that these aerosols are deposited in the lower airways.[45,63] Nevertheless, this form of therapy is exceedingly common in hospital practice, and many patients report subjective improvement.

Clinically, many types of equipment are used to generate an aerosol. Most aerosol generators provide humidity as well. In a jet nebulizer (Fig. 27–6), gas is forced into a water reservoir through a narrow tube, and the velocity of the gas is thereby increased. The high-speed gas causes water to be siphoned up a tube and sprayed against a baffle, then broken up into fine particles that are visible as a mist. With an ultrasonic nebulizer, electrical energy is converted to high-frequency vibrations, which in turn break up water into tiny particles. The mist produced is extremely dense. Complications of ultrasonic nebulizer therapy include fluid overload in infants and production of bronchospasm. As a result, this piece of equipment is used less commonly today than in the past. Patients for whom it is used must be monitored very carefully. Because of its irritating effects on the tracheobronchial tree, the ultrasonic nebulizer is an effective means of stimulating the production of a sputum sample when a patient is unable to cough productively on his own.

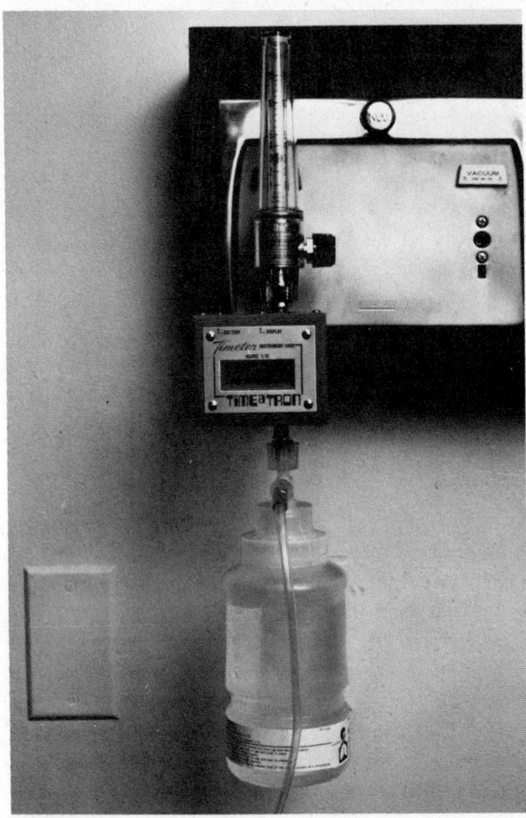

FIGURE 27–5 Disposable bubble diffusion humidifier attached to timer and flowmeter. (Respiratory Care: Concepts and Techniques, an audiovisual publication of JB Lippincott, 1980)

Measures to Reduce Nosocomial Infection. Nosocomial infection has been associated with the use of respiratory equipment. Bubble humidifiers do not cause infection because bacteria are too large to be transmitted by water vapor. However, because aerosol generators form droplets of water, bacteria can become suspended in the mist and can be transmitted from the nebulizer to the patient's lungs.[31] As a consequence, careful techniques are essential to minimize contamination of this equipment. Usual recommendations are as follows:[26,38]

- Wash hands before handling equipment and avoid touching the insides of masks, tubing, or other equipment.
- Change respiratory equipment every 24 hours.
- Use sterile water to fill nebulizers. The container of sterile water should be discarded after 24 hours.
- Empty fluid that has condensed in the tubing into a receptable, never back into the nebulizer reservoir.
- Do not allow tubing to touch the floor.

Medications. In addition to providing a water mist, aerosol generators are also often used to deliver respiratory medications directly to the airways. The medications most often delivered in this manner are bronchodilator drugs and mucokinetic drugs.

Bronchodilators. Bronchodilators are discussed in detail in Chapter 29, in the section on asthma. When given by the inhaled route, they are rapidly effective and thus are extremely useful for the emergency relief of bronchospasm. For patients subject to bronchospasm, bronchodilators may also aid in secretion removal by keeping the airways open so that secretions can be coughed or drained out.

Mucokinetic Agents. Mucokinetic agents are drugs that alter the consistency and clearance of tracheal bronchial

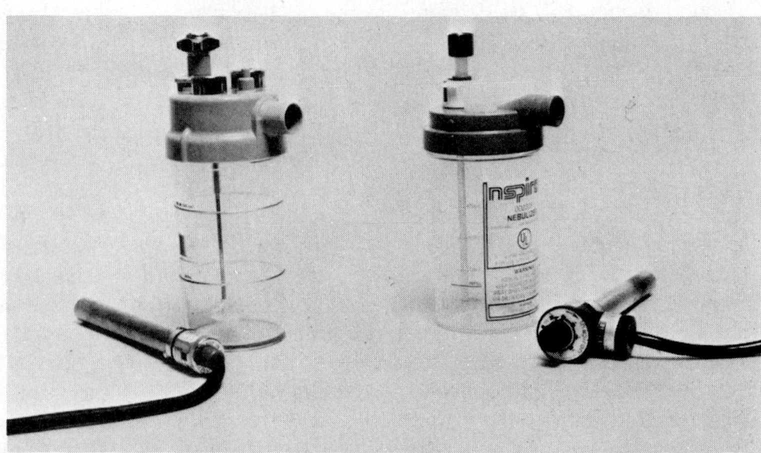

FIGURE 27–6 Jet nebulizers. (*Left*) Nondisposable model with reusable heater. (*Right*) Disposable type with reusable heater. (Respiratory Care: Concepts and Techniques, an audiovisual publication of JB Lippincott, 1980)

secretions. A wide range of drugs fits into this category—diluents, expectorants, and mucolytics. Water and saline are classified as *diluents,* and their use has been discussed above.

Expectorants, or bronchomucotrophic drugs, are substances that increase the volume of tracheobronchial secretions. The efficacy of these drugs has not been documented objectively.[19,43] Expectorants in current use include guaifenesin, terpin hydrate, and potassium iodide. Specific guidelines for their use are given in Table 28-2.

Mucolytics are substances believed to change the structural integrity of mucoid airway secretions. The mucolytic drug currently marketed in the United States is *N*-acetylcysteine (Mucomyst).

Many other drugs, most notably the sympathomimetic bronchodilators, are known to affect various aspects of mucociliary clearance.[53] Further study is needed to determine the clinical usefulness of mucokinetic drug therapy.

Evaluation

Just as the diagnosis of ineffective airway clearance is established by assessing the patient for the presence of retained secretions, so is the effectiveness of nursing interventions determined by assessment for secretions. When interventions have been effective, lung auscultation will reveal an absence of or reduction in rhonchi. Additionally, the patient may report decreased dyspnea following bronchial hygiene maneuvers.

Impaired Gas Exchange

Nursing Diagnosis

Impaired gas exchange related to restrictive or obstructive lung disease as manifested by decreased Pa_{O_2}, increased Pa_{CO_2}, signs of impaired gas exchange such as irritability, decreased mental acuity, fatigue, and somnolence.

Physiological Basis: Hypoxemia and Hypercapnia

Many specific respiratory conditions can become so severe that they impair the gas-exchange function of the lungs. The result is *hypoxemia,* an inadequate level of oxygen in the arterial blood, with or without *hypercapnia* (carbon dioxide retention in the arterial blood). When the disease progresses slowly, hypoxemia is a gradual development, and hypercapnia, if present, is associated with a normal arterial pH. An acute condition or a sudden exacerbation of a chronic lung disease can cause an abrupt deterioration in gas exchange that is referred to as acute respiratory failure. Specific lung conditions that may chronically or acutely impair gas exchange are discussed in subsequent chapters of this unit. The problem of acute respiratory failure is addressed in Chapter 32. This chapter presents an overview of therapies used to manage both hypoxemia and hypercapnia and is a basis for the discussion in succeeding chapters.

Intervention: Oxygen Therapy

Oxygen Equipment

The goal of any form of oxygen therapy is to achieve a Pa_{O_2} of at least 60 mmHg. An alternative to measuring the Pa_{O_2} is to monitor hemoglobin saturation with an ear oximeter. In that case, the hemoglobin saturation should be at least 90%.

Oxygen can be delivered by either a low-flow or high-flow system. In a low-flow system, the oxygen that is delivered provides only part of the patient's inspired gas. As the patient breathes, he sucks in room air to mix with the oxygen and provide an adequate amount of inspired air. A high-flow oxygen delivery system is self-contained, that is, the premixed air and oxygen provides all the inspired gas that the patient breathes.[26,44] Examples of oxygen delivery systems are pictured in Figure 27–7.

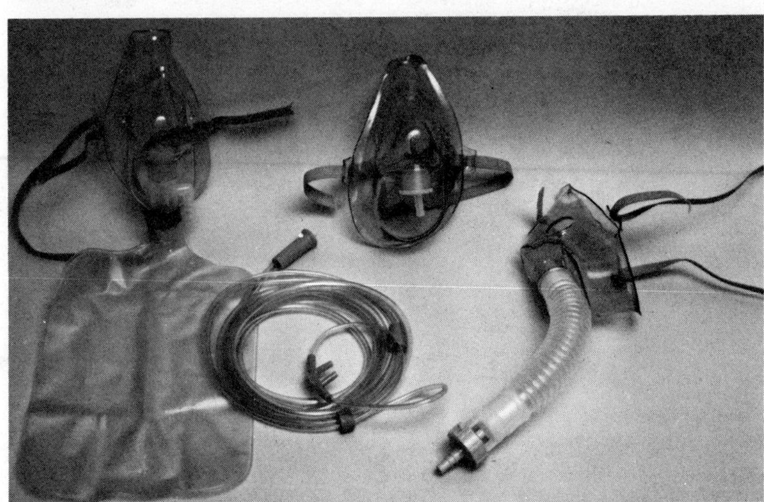

FIGURE 27–7 Oxygen therapy devices to deliver moderate to low oxygen concentrations. Clockwise from bottom center: nasal cannula, partial rebreathing mask, simple face mask, and venturi mask. The first three are low flow devices; the venturi mask is a high flow device.

Low-Flow Systems. The most common low-flow oxygen delivery systems are the nasal cannula and the simple mask. The nasal cannula, also called nasal prongs, consists of a tubing with two small prongs that fit into a patient's nostrils (Fig. 27–8). Cannulas are inexpensive, disposable, relatively comfortable, and do not need to be removed for eating or other activities. Because nothing fits around the mouth, they do not interfere with coughing and do not give the patient a feeling of claustrophobia. Soreness of the nares and over the ears may result from long-term uses. Nasal cannulas can be used with an oxygen flow rate of 1 liter to 6 liters/min; a flow rate beyond 6 liters is drying to the nasal mucosa and uncomfortable for the patient. It is important to keep the nasal prongs correctly inserted into both nares, since displacement of one prong has been shown to cause a drop in Pa_{O_2}.[27] Humidification is probably unnecessary with flow rates under 4 liters/min.[18]

The other common low-flow oxygen system is the simple mask, which fits over the mouth and nose (Fig. 27–9). As the patient breathes in, room air is drawn in through small holes on the side of the mask and mixes with the oxygen. Disadvantages of this system are that patients may feel claustrophobic and that the mask must be removed for eating, coughing, and taking medications. The mask must be run at a flow rate of at least 5 liters/min in order to flush out exhaled air and prevent a buildup of carbon dioxide.[44]

With any low-flow system, the amount of room air that is entrained and mixes with the delivered oxygen varies with the patient's breathing pattern. When a patient's breaths are shallow, little room air is entrained and higher inspired oxygen concentrations result. Conversely, when a patient takes deep or rapid breaths, he pulls in more room air and the inspired oxygen concentration falls.[52] Therefore, the oxygen liter flow setting is not a guarantee of the amount of oxygen a patient is actually receiving. Depending on the patient's ventilatory pattern and liter flow, patients can receive approximately 24% to 40% oxygen.

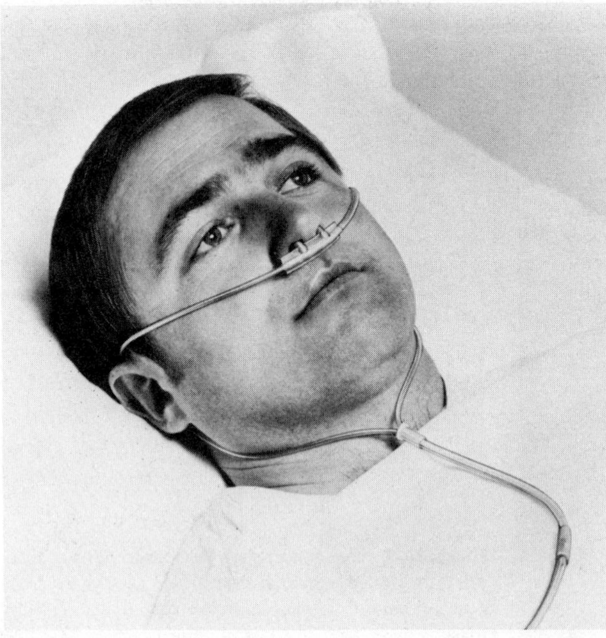

FIGURE 27–8 Nasal cannula. (Courtesy of Hudson Oxygen Company)

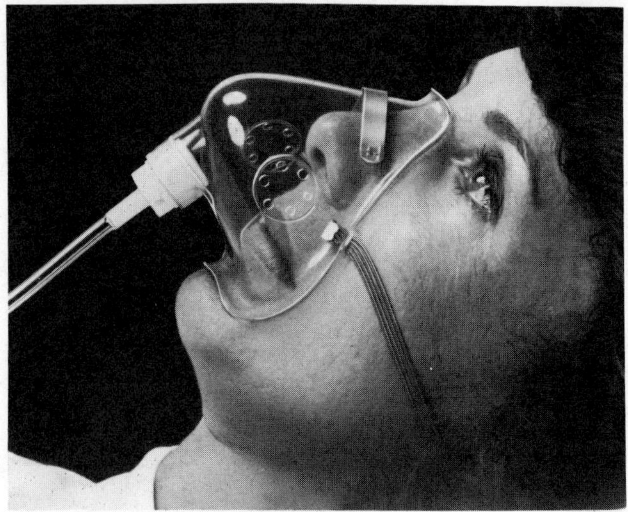

FIGURE 27–9 Simple mask. (Courtesy of Hudson Oxygen Company)

High-Flow Systems. Most high-flow oxygen systems are masks. Theoretically, all inspired gas is provided by the high-flow system, and oxygen delivery can be regulated precisely. The ability to guarantee the precise percentage of oxygen being delivered is a major advantage when caring for unstable patients. However, this guarantee assumes that the mask is kept in place. As described earlier, a mask intereferes with activities such as eating, taking medications, and coughing and can cause claustrophobia. Therefore, masks are often removed, especially by extremely hypoxemic patients who are often restless and confused but need the oxygen most.

In a nonrebreathing mask (Fig. 27–10), oxygen is delivered into a reservoir bag, then, through a one-way valve, into the mask and to the patient. When the patient breathes out, the valve closes and exhaled air flows out into the atmosphere through holes in the side of the mask. These masks can provide close to 100% oxygen if they fit snugly, but they are very uncomfortable to wear. The flow rate must be high enough to prevent the reservoir bag from collapsing. Nonrebreathing masks are generally used only for short periods of time.[26,44]

A partial rebreathing mask is the same as a nonrebreathing mask except that exhaled air is not prevented from entering the reservoir bag. The first third of the exhaled gas, which did not participate in gas exchange and is roughly the same as the gas that was inhaled, is recycled. From 60% to 90% oxygen can be delivered.[44]

The venturi mask (Fig. 27–11) was designed to limit oxygen delivery to a set percentage between 24% and 50%. As oxygen flows in, the opening through which it flows narrows, pressure drops, and a specific amount of room air is entrained to mix with the oxygen. The size of the opening can be altered to adjust the amount of air entrained and the

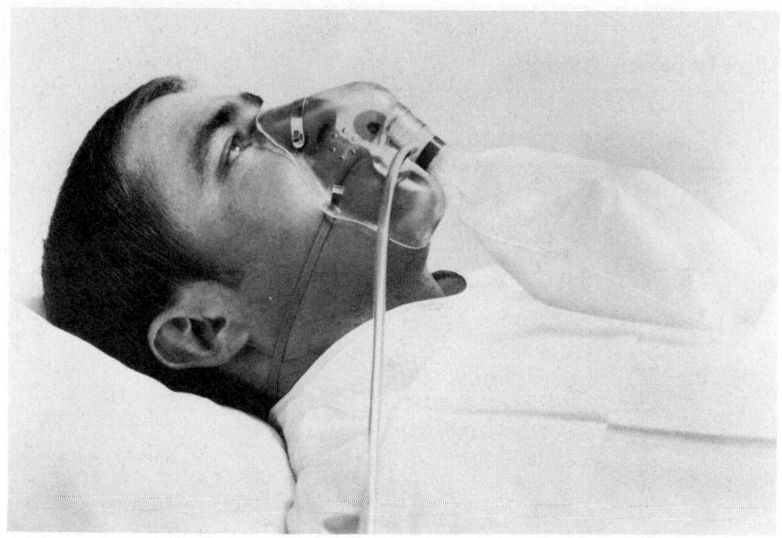

FIGURE 27-10 Nonrebreathing mask. (Courtesy of Hudson Oxygen Company)

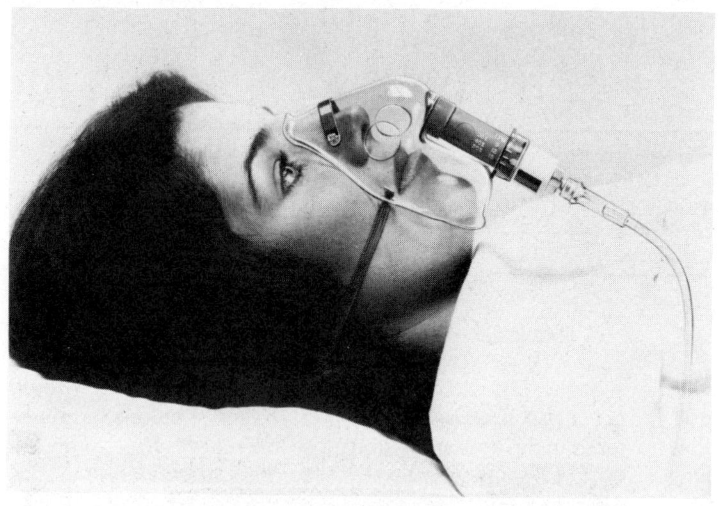

FIGURE 27-11 Venturi mask. (Courtesy of Hudson Oxygen Company)

percentage of oxygen subsequently delivered. The venturi system allows precise limitation of oxygen delivery. However, the mask is usually not tight enough to prevent a hyperventilating patient from entraining additional room air with breathing. In this event, the oxygen delivery will be less than the set percentage. In addition, the general disadvantages of masks are retained.

Nursing Care of Patients Receiving Oxygen

Predicting Effects of Supplemental Oxygen. When caring for a patient receiving oxygen therapy, it is important to gauge the effect of supplemental oxygen upon the patient's blood-gas status. This type of analysis requires knowledge of the oxygen dose and of the patient's arterial blood-gas values. Oxygen dose is often abbreviated as FI_{O_2}, meaning *fraction of inspired oxygen.* FI_{O_2} can be roughly predicted from the oxygen liter flow, as shown in Table 27–4. From this information, the expected effect of supplemental oxygen on the Pa_{O_2} can be determined. A quick but only approximate method is to multiply the FI_{O_2} by five. The value obtained is the predicted arterial blood oxygen that would result if a patient with normal lungs received that percentage of oxygen. For example, the predicted minimal Pa_{O_2} for a patient breathing 30% oxygen is 150 mmHg. When a patient's Pa_{O_2} is less than this value, it can be assumed that he would be hypoxemic if breathing room air. A comparison of the predicted and actual Pa_{O_2} will show the degree of hypoxemia. A more precise but considerably more complicated method is shown in Table 27–5. The advantage of this method is that the effects on oxygenation of hypoventilation (as measured by Pa_{CO_2}) can be calculated.

Supportive Care. Although it seems obvious that patients who require oxygen therapy need to keep the delivery constant, clinically this is often not the case. A patient able to sit in a chair or ambulate needs a tubing long enough to accommodate these activities. Similarly, patients receiving oxygen by mask need an alternate nasal cannula system for mealtime. Nasal cannulas and masks should not be removed to check oral temperature.[13, 21]

TABLE 27–4
Oxygen Concentrations for Delivery Systems*

System	*Oxygen Flow Rate (liters/min)*	FI_{O_2} *Range*
Nasal cannula	1	0.21–0.24
	2	0.23–0.28
	3	0.27–0.34
	4	0.31–0.38
	5–6	0.32–0.44
Venturi masks	4–6 (total flow = 105)†	0.24
	4–6 (total flow = 45)	0.28
	8–10 (total flow = 45)	0.35
	8–10 (total flow = 33)	0.40
	8–12 (total flow = 33)	0.50
Simple masks	5–6	0.30–0.45
	7–8	0.40–0.60
Masks with reservoirs	5	0.35–0.50
Partial rebreathing	7	0.35–0.75
	10	0.65–1.00
Nonrebreathing	4–10	0.40–1.00

*Values listed in this table are approximate.
† Values for total gas delivered are for the Accurox Venturi Mask.
(Ryerson GG, Block AJ: Oxygen as a drug: Chemical properties, benefits, and hazards of administration. In Burton GG, Hodgkin JE [eds]: Respiratory Care: A Guide to Clinical Practice, 2nd ed, p 407. Philadelphia, JB Lippincott, 1984)

Careful patient positioning is a supportive measure that can maximize the benefits of oxygen therapy. In general, hypoxemic patients should be positioned so that blood flow in the lung is directed by gravity toward the areas of the lung that are most normal. The Pa_{O_2} has been found to decrease when patients are positioned so that the greatest blood flow is to areas with atelectasis or consolidation. In patients of middle age and beyond, the horizontal position causes the Pa_{O_2} to drop in a similar fashion. For patients with disease affecting only one lung, the good lung should be positioned down.[41, 57]

Complications of Oxygen Therapy. Patients receiving oxygen therapy are subject to complications caused by the therapy itself. Oxygen toxicity is an extremely serious complication of oxygen therapy. The mildest form of oxygen toxicity is tracheobronchitis, an entirely reversible syndrome in which substernal pain and nonproductive cough develop within 12 to 24 hours of breathing 100% oxygen. Longer exposures to 100% oxygen can result in acute parenchymal lung injury that involves primarily the pulmonary capillaries. The damage is very similar to that found in adult respiratory distress syndrome, discussed in Chapter 31. Chronic parenchymal lung injury, culminating in fibrotic changes termed *bronchopulmonary dysplasia,* is a problem affecting principally newborns.

The potential development of oxygen toxicity should never preclude its use. Hovever, oxygen should be administered in the lowest possible dose that relieves hypoxemia. An FI_{O_2} under 60% is generally considered safe for long periods. Whenever possible, delivery of 100% oxygen should be limited to 24 hours.[4, 46]

Fire is another potential hazard of oxygen therapy. Oxygen is itself neither combustible nor explosive. However, flammable materials ignite more readily and burn more vigorously in an oxygen-enriched atmosphere. A major hazard is ignition of the oxygen administration set and direct burn injury to the patient or nearby surroundings. Patients should never smoke while receiving oxygen, and, ideally, there should be no smoking in the same room. It is easier to enforce these rules in a hospital than in the home.

Suppression of the hypoxic ventilatory drive is a complication of importance to patients with chronic obstructive pulmonary disease. Patients with chronic carbon dioxide retention do not respond to CO_2 as a ventilatory stimulus and require hypoxia to trigger their breathing. Because the hypoxic drive is stimulated at a Pa_{O_2} of 60 mmHg to 65 mmHg, elevation of the Pa_{O_2} beyond this level with supplemental oxygen results in decreased ventilation and hypercapnia. By administering oxygen at a low flow rate and monitoring arterial blood-gas values for significant effects on Pa_{CO_2} and pH, this complication can be prevented.

TABLE 27–5
Calculation of Expected Effect of Increased F_{IO_2}

Use alveolar gas equation:

$P_{AO_2} = (F_{IO_2} \times 713) - (Pa_{CO_2}/0.8)$

Components include

P_{AO_2} = Partial pressure of alveolar oxygen (to be calculated)
F_{IO_2} = Fraction of inspired oxygen
Pa_{CO_2} = Value from patient's arterial blood gas
713 = Barometric pressure of 760 mmHg minus water vapor pressure of 47 mmHg
0.8 = Factor to estimate rate at which oxygen is being removed from alveolus (based on ratio of oxygen consumption and carbon dioxide production)

Example:

F_{IO_2} = 40%; patient's Pa_{CO_2} = 40 mmHg and Pa_{O_2} = 80 mmHg

$P_{AO_2} = (.40 \times 713) - (40/0.8)$
(Note: the product of F_{IO_2} × barometric pressure is called P_{IO_2})
$P_{AO_2} = 285 - 50$
P_{AO_2} = 235 mmHg
Expected Pa_{O_2} for patient (alveolar to arterial oxygen difference):
$Pa_{O_2} = P_{AO_2} - 10$ mmHg
In this case, expected Pa_{O_2} = 225 mmHg

Significance:

A comparison of the expected Pa_{O_2} value of 225 mmHg and the patient's actual Pa_{O_2} value of only 80 mmHg indicates that the patient has significant lung disease. Oxygen therapy has raised the patient's Pa_{O_2} to 80 mmHg, a value that is much lower than predicted for the given F_{IO_2} but adequate for tissue needs. Removal of the oxygen should be expected to cause a significant drop in Pa_{O_2}, perhaps to life threatening levels.

Intervention: Intubation and Mechanical Ventilation

Airway Intubation

An open airway is an obvious requirement for effective ventilation. Loss of airway patency may be a consequence of soft tissue or foreign body obstruction and may complicate a variety of interrelated patient situations, such as trauma, cardiac arrest, and unconsciousness. Airway patency can often be restored by tilting the head back or thrusting the jaw forward. An additional technique is the insertion of an oral or nasopharyngeal airway to relieve soft tissue obstruction and permit clearance of secretions. A detailed description of these methods can be found in Chapter 35, in the section on cardiopulmonary resuscitation.

When these methods prove ineffective or when mechanical ventilation is planned, intubation of the trachea is required. Access to the trachea can be achieved through the mouth (oral endotracheal tube), through the nose (nasal endotracheal tube), or directly through an incision into the trachea (tracheostomy or cricothyroidotomy, an emergency alternative to tracheostomy). Advantanges and disadvantages of these routes to the trachea are compared in Table 27–6.

Mechanical Ventilation

The most common purpose of intubation is to establish a route for mechanical ventilation. The decision to mechanically ventilate a patient is made by the physician on the basis of clinical and arterial blood-gas data as well as knowledge of the patient's underlying pathophysiology. Acute, severe respiratory acidosis (elevated Pa_{CO_2} with pH less than 7.25) and hypoxemia that is unrelieved by nasal cannula or mask are major criteria.

The ventilators currently used in hospital settings deliver a gas mixture (air and oxygen) to the lungs by means of positive pressure; that is, they operate by blowing gas into the lungs (Fig. 27–12). These machines can be divided into two main categories: pressure-cycled ventilators, in which inspiratory gas flow stops when a preset pressure is reached, and volume-cycled ventilators, in which a preset volume is deliverd regardless of the pressure generated. Because their effectiveness is much less limited by changes in a patient's lung compliance or airway resistance, volume ventilators are the usual choice for prolonged mechanical ventilation. When a volume ventilator is used, it can be set to control the patient's ventilation completely or to allow him to set his own breathing rate.

A ventilator is set for a variety of parameters, including the F_{IO_2}, tidal volume, rate, and degree to which the patient can control his ventilatory pattern. These parameters are described in Table 27–7. It is necessary to check ventilator settings routinely to make sure they are correct. However, it is of the utmost importance to keep in mind that it is the patient, and not the machine, who is the focus of nursing assessment and care. Care of the intubated and mechanically ventilated patient is a shared responsibility of the nurse, respiratory therapist, and physician that is outlined in the following paragraphs. More detailed information can be found in specialized books on critical care.

Assessment and Maintenance of Patent Airway

Tube Location. Assessment of tube location is essential immediately following placement and periodically thereafter. Auscultation of the lungs for bilaterally equal breath sounds can be followed by chest-film confirmation of accurate placement. Inadvertent insertion of an endotracheal tube into the right (or rarely, left) main stem bronchus will limit ventilation to one lung and cause hypoxemia. Accidental insertion of a tracheostomy tube into the soft tissues of the neck will similarly preclude adequate ventilation.

Fixation. Adequate fixation of the artificial airway is necessary to maintain proper tube position within the tra-

TABLE 27–6
Tracheal Airways

	Translaryngeal		*Tracheostomy*
	Endotracheal Tube	*Nasotracheal Tube*	
Insertion	Through mouth	Through nose	Through incision in neck
Advantages	Rapidly inserted with minimal tissue trauma; appropriate for emergencies	More comfortable for long-term use Easy to stabilize Oral feeding possible	Most comfortable for long-term use Oral feeding well tolerated
Disadvantages	Causes gag reflex in conscious patients Requires bite block to prevent biting and occluding tube Increases salivation Hard to stabilize Precludes oral feeding Can cause tracheal–esophageal fistula Not recommended for long-term use	Requires expert for insertion Not appropriate in emergencies Can cause acute sinusitis, nasal necrosis, otitis media, tracheal–esophageal fistula	Requires surgery Not appropriate in emergencies Can cause stoma infection, bleeding, airway obstruction, tracheal–esophageal fistula
Nursing care	Perform frequent oral hygiene Assess mouth for lesions from pressure or infection Monitor intracuff pressure Allow patient to suction oral cavity ad lib, if alert	Perform frequent nose care Assess for nasal necrosis and other complications Monitor intracuff pressure	Clean and inspect stoma frequently If tracheostomy has inner cannula, remove and clean Monitor intracuff pressure

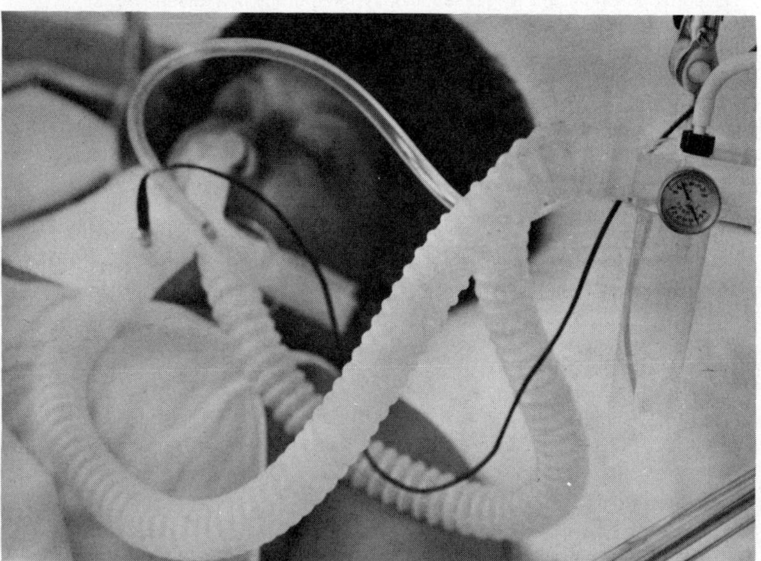

FIGURE 27–12 Intubated patient being mechanically ventilated. (Respiratory Care: Concepts and Techniques, an audiovisual publication of JB Lippincott, 1980)

chea and to prevent complications of excessive tube movement. Endotracheal tubes are secured with tape, and tracheostomy tubes are tied in place. The hands of a confused or agitated patient may need to be restrained to prevent him from extubating himself prematurely. An endotracheal tube that is not securely taped will slide back and forth against surrounding structures. Some laryngeal irritation is unavoidable and characteristically causes temporary hoarseness after extubation. However, severe laryngeal irritation may produce respiratory obstruction, either from massive laryngeal edema or from the formation of granulation tissue as the inflamed area heals.[14]

TABLE 27–7
Common Settings on Volume Ventilators

Parameter	*Description*
Mode	
Assist	Patient initiates *all* breaths
Control	Ventilator initiates *all* breaths
Assist/control	Basic ventilator rate set; patient can trigger additional breaths but cannot decrease rate below that set
Intermittent mechanical ventilation (IMV)	Patient breathes spontaneously; also receives machine-delivered breaths at preset volume and frequency
Tidal volume	Volume of air delivered by machine Commonly set at 10 ml–12 ml/kg
Respiratory rate	Rate of machine-delivered breaths Varies according to mode and patient's breathing pattern but must be high enough initially to supply adequate minute ventilation for patient who may not trigger machine
FI_{O_2}	Percentage of oxygen delivered Often initiated at 100% then decreased according to results of arterial blood-gas analyses
Peak or inspiratory flow rate	Rate at which tidal volume of air is delivered Initial setting usually 50–80 liters/min Alert patients and those with obstructive disease may prefer faster rate
Sigh	Larger volume breath given to prevent microatelectasis Unnecessary if large (10–12 ml/kg) tidal volume used If required, 10 sigh breaths/min at two times tidal volume is a common setting
Positive end-expiratory pressure (PEEP) (also called continuous positive pressure ventilation [CPPV])	Positive pressure maintained in lungs throughout ventilatory cycle Used to increase functional residual capacity, reduce alveolar collapse, and improve oxygenation
Alarms	
High pressure	Triggered by exceeding preset pressure limit during delivery of tidal or sigh volume
Disconnect	Triggered by patient disconnection from ventilator or leak in system
Electrical	Triggered by electrical failure
	(Additional alarms on some ventilators)

Humidification. Because an artificial airway bypasses the natural humidification provided by the upper respiratory tract, external humidification is necessary to prevent drying of tracheobronchial secretions and irritation of the airways. A heated nebulizer will provide humidity equivalent to that achieved by breathing through the nose. Condensed water that accumulates within the tubing should be removed by emptying it into a wastebasket or other container.

Suction. Intubated patients nearly always require tracheal suction to remove tracheobronchial secretions that may accumulate and obstruct the airway. Suctioning is indicated when secretions are seen within the artificial airway or auscultated as rhonchi. For a patient ventilated with a volume-cycled ventilator, a sudden increase in the machine's pressure requirement is an additional clue to the need for suctioning. Increasing the oxygen delivery by the ventilator to 100% for 1 to 2 minutes before initiating suctioning is an alternative to preoxygenation and hyperventilation with an anesthesia bag.[24]

Providing for Communication. It is extremely frustrating for a patient with an artificial airway to be unable to talk to his caretakers or loved ones. Helping the patient communicate by writing on a tablet or pointing to letters or words mounted on cardboard is an important part of supportive nursing care. Use of speaking devices such as the Olympic Trach-Talk or Pitt Speaking Tracheostomy Tube also facilitates communication for tracheostomized patients. If the patient does not have an inflated tracheostomy cuff (see below), occluding the tube opening temporarily will allow the patient to speak.

Assessment and Care of the Mechanically Ventilated Patient

In addition to the care required to maintain his artificial airway, the mechanically ventilated patient requires additional measures to prevent complications related specifically to the use of the mechanical respirator.

Fighting the Ventilator. A patient may breathe out of phase with or "fight" the ventilator as a result of an acute change in his physiological condition, ventilator malfunction, inappropriate ventilator settings for his metabolic or psychological needs, anxiety, or pain. Careful assessment of both the patient's condition and the machine settings is therefore needed as a basis for determining appropriate interventions. Pain relief, adjustment of ventilator settings, and sedation are examples of possible solutions.

Barotrauma. Another possible complication is the development of barotrauma, that is, injury caused when alveoli are overdistended and ruptured by excessive volume or when the underlying disease process causes alveolar necrosis. The most common types of injury include pneumothorax, pneumomediastinum, and subcutaneous emphysema. Patients at highest risk are those ventilated at high tidal volumes. By frequently monitoring breath sounds and vital signs, nurses may be able to detect these complications at an early stage.[6,33,38] Management of these complications is discussed in a later section of the chapter.

Tracheal Ischemia. An inflated cuff near the distal end of the endotracheal or tracheostomy tube is used to prevent air from escaping around the artificial airway during mechanical ventilation. The hazard of providing this necessary seal is that excessive pressure exerted against the tracheal wall can cause necrosis of the tracheal mucosa. The risk of this complication can be reduced by using low-pressure, high-volume cuffs and by routinely monitoring intracuff pressure to make certain that it remains under 25 cm H_2O (30 mmHg).[25]

Infection. Nosocomial infection is a complication that is discussed in an earlier section of this chapter. Ventilator tubing is generally changed every 24 hours, although there is some evidence that changing at 48-hour intervals may be acceptable.[9]

The patient on a mechanical ventilator is usually critically ill and deserves ongoing assessment of every body system and careful supportive nursing care to prevent systemic complications from arising during this therapy. Table 27–8 summarizes major complications.

The criteria for discontinuing or *weaning* from mechanical ventilation are essentially the converse of those that led to its initiation. In patients with borderline respiratory function or decreased strength of their respiratory muscles, weaning can be a complicated process that requires the cooperative efforts of all members of the respiratory-care team.

Evaluation

The most important tool for evaluating interventions to improve gas exchange is arterial blood-gas measurement. The effectiveness of both medical therapies, such as mechanical ventilation, and nursing therapies, such as positioning, can be determined by monitoring for changes in arterial blood-gas measurements. Arterial blood-gas values consistent with effective interventions include a pH between 7.35 and 7.45 and a Pa_{O_2} that is within normal limits for the patient's age and lung function: 95 mmHg to 100 mmHg for young adults, 75 mmHg to 80 mmHg for the elderly, and 60 mmHg for patients with chronic obstructive pulmonary disease.

Pleural Disruption*

Nursing Diagnosis

Impaired gas exchange related to the presence of air or fluid in the pleural space with loss of normal ventilatory mechanics, as manifested by shortness of breath, chest or shoulder pain, anxiety or changes in mental status, tachycardia, and tachypnea.

Alteration in comfort related to rib fracture, penetrating wound, or surgical incision, as manifested by verbalization of pain or dyspnea or both, tachycardia, tachypnea, and increased blood pressure.

Physiological Basis

The pleural "space" is really a potential space. The chest wall is lined with the parietal pleura, and the lung is covered by the visceral pleura. A very thin layer of pleural fluid allows

*This section was written by Kathryn L. Anderson, M.N.

TABLE 27-8
Complications of Mechanical Ventilation

Complications According to Body System	*Nursing Assessment and Interventions*
Respiratory	
Irritation, necrosis of airway mucosa	Monitor intracuff pressure. Ensure adequate humidity. Secure airway to prevent tube motion.
Barotrauma	Monitor for decreased breath sounds and other evidence of pneumothorax.
Oxygen toxicity	Monitor for increasing ventilator pressure requirements, dry cough, substernal chest pain. Administer lowest possible FI_{O_2} to maintain safe Pa_{O_2}.*
Infection	Change ventilator tubings every 24–28 hours and prevent contamination. Use aseptic technique for suctioning.
Cardiovascular	
Decreased cardiac output	Monitor blood pressure, pulse, invasive hemodynamic measurements, and peripheral perfusion.
Cardiac arrhythmias	Monitor cardiac rhythm. Adjust ventilator settings to maintain safe values for Pa_{O_2} and pH.* Treat life-threatening arrhythmias.*
Water excess	Monitor serum sodium values.
Saline excess	Monitor weights, peripheral edema.
Gastrointestinal	
Stress ulcers	Monitor nasogastric aspirate and stools for occult blood. Monitor pH of gastric fluid. Maintain pH over 4.0 with antacids, cimetidine.*
Gastric dilatation	Monitor bowel sounds, abdominal distention.
Paralytic ileus	Insert nasogastric tube if patient develops ileus.*
Malnutrition	Monitor weight, serum albumin levels, skin fold measurements. Initiate enteral or intravenous alimentation.*
Acid–base disturbances	
(Major effects on respiratory, cardiovascular, renal, neurologic function)	
Respiratory acidosis Respiratory alkalosis Metabolic alkalosis	Monitor pH of arterial blood Adjust ventilator settings to achieve patient's normal range and/or normalize pH.* Monitor serum potassium and chloride values and sources of electrolyte loss. Replace saline, KCl losses.*

(Continued)

TABLE 27–8
Complications of Mechanical Ventilation (*Continued*)

Complications According to Body System	*Nursing Assessment and Interventions*
Immobility (affects all body systems)	
	Monitor skin condition. Turn frequently; monitor effect of position on Pa_{O_2}. Initiate active or passive bed exercises. Sit patient in chair or walk as soon as feasible (mechanical ventilation does not preclude).

* Physician order required.

these two membranes to slide over each other during normal respiration. Negative intrapleural pressure is created because the chest wall always tends to spring outward and the lungs tend to recoil inward. This negative pressure is required for the lungs to remain expanded throughout the respiratory cycle. Between breaths, it maintains the lungs at a resting lung volume (functional residual capacity), which keeps the majority of airways open.

Disruption of the pleural space causes loss of negative intrapleural pressure, allowing partial or total lung collapse, decrease in the resting lung volume, ventilation impairment, and alteration in arterial blood gases. Potential causes of such a disruption are many: internally, a fractured rib, ruptured bleb or bulla, or growth of a tumor with rupture into the pleural space may be responsible; external and iatrogenic causes include stab, gunshot, or other penetrating wounds of the chest, the surgeon's scalpel, and thoracentesis or biopsy needles. Air (pneumothorax), blood (hemothorax), chyle (chylothorax), or other fluid (pleural effusion) may leak into and create an actual pleural pace. Thoracostomy, or chest, tubes are placed into the pleural space to drain the air or fluid, reexpand the lung, and restore negative intrapleural pressure. Restoration of normal ventilatory mechanics results in the reestablishment of the resting lung volume and correction of arterial blood gases (unless complicated by other illness or injury).

Intervention: Water-Seal Drainage

Principles

In order to provide care for a patient with chest tubes, the nurse must first have a basic understanding of the mechanics of ventilation as well as an understanding of how the drainage system works. Knowledge of the former is assumed (refer to Chapter 25 for a review); the latter is the focus of this discussion.

The classic apparatus for chest drainage is a three-bottle drainage system. When this basic system is understood, mastery of the many disposable devices, which incorporate all the functions of the three-bottle system into a single unit, should easily follow. This system is illustrated in Figure 27–13.

Water-Seal Bottle. The water-seal bottle acts as a one-way valve through which air or fluids can leave the patient's chest but cannot return. The bottle has an airtight stopper, through which two glass stems, or straws, pass. One end of the longer stem is connected to the chest drainage tube; the other is submerged 2 cm to 3 cm beneath the surface of sterile water or saline, which has been added to the bottle. The second, shorter stem acts as a vent and allows air to escape from the bottle. When the patient exhales, positive pressure in the lung forces air out of the pleural space, through the chest tube, and into the bottle; the air then bubbles out through the water and is vented to the atmosphere. When the patient inhales, negative pressure in the chest pulls water up into the stem or chest tube to a height equal to the pressure in the thorax. Pressure in the chest with normal respiration rarely exceeds −20 cm H_2O. Therefore, as long as the bottle is more than 20 cm below the patient's

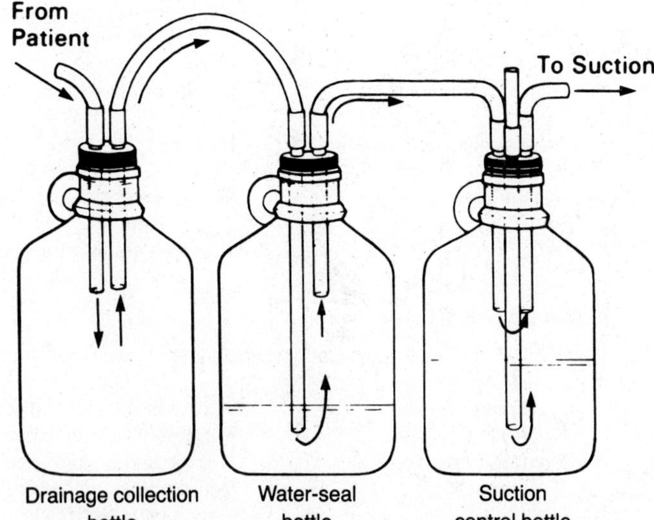

FIGURE 27–13 Three-bottle system for water-seal drainage. (After Brannin PK: Management modalities: Respiratory system. In Hudak CM, Lohr TS, Gallo BM: Critical Care Nursing, 3rd ed, p 205. Philadelphia, JB Lippincott, 1982)

chest there is no danger of water entering the pleural space. Usual recommendations for bottle placement are 60 cm to 90 cm below the patient's chest.

The stem to which the chest tube is connected must not be submerged more than a few centimeters beneath the water surface because resistance to the expulsion of air or fluids from the chest during expiration is equal to the length of tubing under water.[22] The intrathoracic pressure must therefore be greater than the length of tubing under the surface of the water in order for drainage to occur. Since intrathoracic pressure is normally about 5 cm H_2O on expiration, the depth of the tube must be less.

Drainage Collection Bottle. The water-seal bottle alone is sufficient for drainage of a pneumothorax when air is the only substance being evacuated from the pleural space. However, when blood or other fluid is to be removed, a second bottle is required. If fluids were allowed to drain into the water-seal bottle, the liquid level would rise, causing the situation described above; that is, a high intrathoracic pressure would be required to force the expulsion of air or fluid from the pleural space.

The drainage collection bottle is inserted into the system between the patient and the water-seal bottle. Two short glass stems pass through the bottle's airtight stopper. Fluid from the patient drains into the bottle through one stem, and displaced air is vented through the second stem to the long stem in the water-seal bottle by means of a connecting tubing.

Suction Control Bottle. When the patient has a large air leak into the pleural space or when large amounts of fluid need to be drained (such as post-thoracotomy), suction may be applied to the system to hasten the process. Suction is generated from an external source such as a suction pump or wall outlet, but the amount of suction applied to the chest drainage tubing is determined by the third bottle in the drainage system. This bottle has an airtight stopper through which two short glass stems and one long stem pass. The short stems are connected to the water-seal bottle and to the suction source. The long stem is submerged in water or saline, and the depth of submersion determines the amount of suction applied to the system. When the suction is turned on, air enters the long stem from the atmosphere. If the stem is submerged to a depth of 20 cm, the amount of suction required to displace all of the water from the tube and cause atmospheric air to bubble through the water is -20 cm H_2O. If the suction pressure is turned up, more atmospheric air will enter the suction control bottle and cause more vigorous bubbling through the water, but the amount of suction applied to the drainage system will not change. Gentle, continuous bubbling indicates that the suction pressure is set at an effective but not excessive level.

If the suction source is turned off but is not disconnected from the drainage system, there are no air vents in the system. If the patient has a persistent air leak into the pleural space, the air can no longer escape, pressure will build within the system, and a tension pneumothorax may result. Therefore, whenever suction is discontinued, the suction bottle should be disconnected from the suction pump or wall outlet. Some single-unit drainage systems have a built-in safety vent that opens and allows air to escape should pressure in the system reach an excessive level.

Patient Assessment

Of necessity, assessment of the patient with chest tubes includes those findings that are associated with the underlying condition as well as those related to the chest drainage itself. Patients with chest tubes in place may include otherwise healthy young persons who have experienced spontaneous pneumothorax, post–cardiac-surgery patients, cancer victims with tumors that have invaded the pleural space, and many other patients with conditions of varying complexity. The reader is referred to the appropriate chapters in this book for nursing care relating to the underlying illness. The following section is limited to the ventilatory dysfunction requiring chest tube placement.

The patient who is admitted to the hospital primarily because of symptoms related to impairment of ventilatory mechanics, whether spontaneous or due to penetrating chest trauma, is likely to be short of breath. The degree of dyspnea will vary with the size of the pneumothorax or hemothorax as well as with the presence or absence of underlying lung disease.[40] Collapse of one lung is likely to be fairly well tolerated by a healthy young person but could be catastrophic in a person with severe emphysema. Cyanosis, an unreliable but widely reported sign, may be present. Apprehension or mental status changes associated with hypoxemia may occur. Patients with spontaneous pneumothorax may describe the sudden onset of unilateral, sharp, stabbing chest pain that increases in severity with coughing or deep breathing and may splint the affected side.[40]

Physical assessment, as in all acutely ill patients, should be rapid in the initial phase and should be repeated as time progresses. Vital signs, while markedly affected by concomitant conditions, will likely show an increased heart and respiratory rate. Breath sounds and chest excursion will be decreased or absent on the affected side. In pneumothorax the chest is hyperresonant to percussion, and tactile fremitus is diminished. When fluid is present in the pleural space, breath sounds are diminished, the chest is dull to percussion, and tactile fremitus is decreased. A chest film will usually reveal the presence of air or fluid in the pleural space. In uncomplicated cases of lung collapse arterial blood-gas analysis will reveal modest hypoxemia, hypocapnia, and an increased pH.

Drainage of the pleural space should result in rapid resolution of the majority of symptoms and signs described. However, ongoing assessment by the nurse is important to evaluate effects of therapy, recurrence of symptoms due to malfunctioning of the drainage system, and recurrence of symptoms after chest drainage has been discontinued.

Maintaining the Drainage System

Following placement of the chest tube, the physician sutures the tube site and tapes it securely. The nurse should check the dressing for drainage at regular intervals following tube placement. When the drainage system is set up in anticipation of tube insertion, all connections should be taped securely. Bottles should be placed well below the chest to facilitate drainage and prevent backflow. Extra tubing can be coiled on the bed and taped or pinned to the sheet to prevent formation of dependent loops (Fig. 27–14); care should be taken to allow the patient enough slack for turning and other position changes.

Observation of the Drainage System. Each bottle or compartment in the single-unit system should be inspected carefully at regular intervals appropriate to the patient's condition, at least once per shift. The water level in the water-seal bottle should be checked and, if necessary, sterile water added. When there is no suction in use, the air vent should be open; gentle fluctuations in the level of fluid in the glass stem can be observed with the patient's respirations. The fluid level should rise in the tube during inspiration and fall during expiration. This excursion, or tidaling, reflects changes in intrapleural pressure during respiration and should be no greater than 2 cm to 6 cm H_2O.[32] Greater fluctuations indicate an increase in the work of breathing, and the nurse should assess the patient for causes.

Fluctuations in the water-seal stem will be reversed (that is, the fluid level falls with inspiration and rises with expiration) when the patient is being mechanically ventilated, since ventilation occurs in response to positive, not negative, pressure. Chest tubes placed in the mediastinum or pericardium following cardiac surgery will not fluctuate with respiration (because there is less variation in pleural pressure), nor will tubes that are kinked or obstructed. When no fluctuations are seen, the patient should be asked to take a deep breath, and the suction can be briefly discontinued. If fluctuations still are not apparent, the chest tube may be obstructed by a blood clot or the lung may be reexpanded and pressing against the chest tube eyelets. The probable cause is determined by clinical assessment of the patient's condition and chest-film findings.

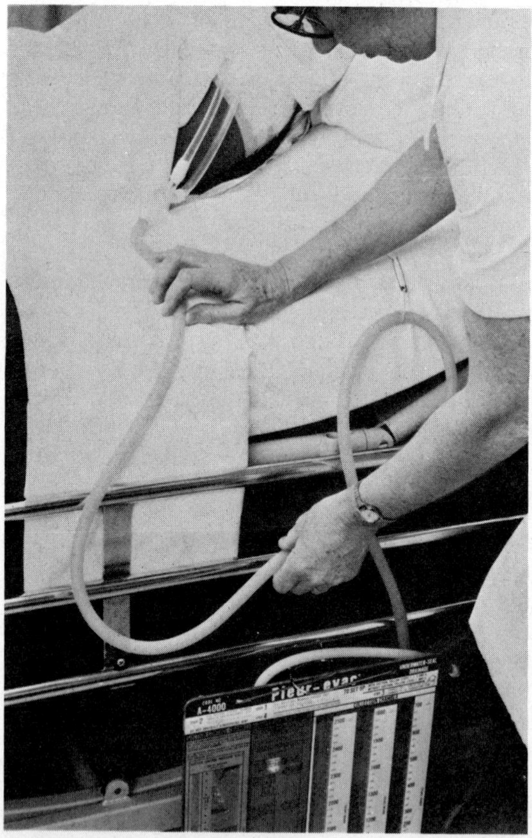

FIGURE 27–14 Dependent loops in the drainage tubing should be avoided because they can create back pressure and impair evacuation of air and fluid. (Respiratory Care: Concepts and Techniques, an audiovisual publication of JB Lippincott, 1980)

Water in the water-seal bottle should not bubble. Bubbling in this bottle indicates an air leak somewhere in the drainage system or in the patient. Figure 27–15 explains how to systematically locate the cause of this development.

The drainage collection bottle is observed for the amount, color, and character of drainage with a frequency appropriate to the patient's condition. The level of drainage should be marked on the bottle at specified intervals or at least every 8 hours.

When a suction control bottle is used, the water level must be checked regularly to ensure that the ordered amount of suction is being applied. The suction regulator should be set at a level that provides continuous, gentle bubbling in the suction control bottle. Bubbling in the suction control bottle may stop if the patient has an increasing air leak. In this case, the suction source must be opened wider until bubbling recurs, so as to keep up with the air leak. When the suction is discontinued, the system must be opened by disconnecting the tubing to the suction source.

Clamping. Mythology surrounding chest tube care in the past stated that all patients with such tubes in place must have a set of clamps at the bedside in case accidental disconnection should occur. However, when the principles of chest drainage are clearly understood, it is obvious that clamping of chest tubes is almost always a bad idea. If the patient has an air leak from the lung into the pleural space, clamping the tube can cause recurrence of the pneumothorax or, worse, tension pneumothorax. With a tension pneumothorax, air that enters the pleural space is trapped and builds up, exerts pressure against surrounding lung tissue and mediastinal structures, reduces cardiac output, and, ultimately, may cause death. Therefore, chest tubes should be clamped for no more than a few seconds, for the purpose of troubleshooting an air leak in the system or for changing the bottles.[16] The clamps should be left in plain view so that the nurse will not forget to remove them. Chest tubes may also be clamped according to the physician's order for a short period immediately prior to their removal. During this period, the patient must be closely observed for recurrence of symptoms and reconnected to drainage should symptoms develop.

Disconnection. If chest tubes become disconnected, both ends should be cleaned and the tubes then reconnected. If the bottle is cracked or broken, the end of the chest tube may be submerged in any container of sterile water to provide a water seal until the tube can be reconnected. If the chest tube itself comes out of the patient's chest, petrolatum gauze should be applied to the entry site and the physician notified.

Stripping. Another aspect of care of the patient with chest tubes that is currently being reexamined is the procedure of stripping, or milking, the tubes. The goal of stripping is to mechanically dislodge clots or debris and move them toward the drainage collection bottle.[17]

Tubes are stripped in one of several ways. In the first method, the tube is grasped with one hand just below the connection of the drainage tube to the thoracostomy tube. The second hand then slides along the tubing, squeezing it so that the contents are moved along (Fig. 27–16). The first hand is released and placed above the sliding hand. The second hand repeats its sliding motion, and this process is continued until the entire tube has been stripped. Two other methods of chest tube stripping are hand-over-hand squeezing from patient to drainage bottle, with complete release of the tubing after each compression, and fanfolding of the tubing followed by squeezing and release.

The efficacy as well as possible adverse effects of stripping are largely unknown. It is known that continuous low levels (−20 cm H_2O) can cause delay of closure of pleural air leaks and trap tissue in catheter eyelets.[17] Recent research has demonstrated that very high (−400 cm H_2O or more) transient pressures can be generated by chest tube stripping, suggesting that until more is known about its effects, stripping should be undertaken with some degree of caution.[15]

The nurse must rely on her own good judgment in deciding whether or not to strip chest tubes. If air is the only substance being drained, the tubes clearly do not need to be stripped. Serous or serosanguineous drainage is unlikely to clot; fresh blood is somewhat more likely to do so. However, drainage may be maintained by keeping the tubing in a straight line with no dependent sections. If necessary, the tubing can be squeezed gently and released completely to prod the drainage along.[17] This method of stripping (squeeze and release) is likely to generate only −30 cm H_2O of suction, compared with the −90 cm to −400 cm H_2O caused by the grip-and-slide method.[15]

Supportive Care

In addition to maintenance of the drainage system, other nursing measures in the care of the patient with chest tubes include providing relief of discomfort and prevention of complications of immobility.

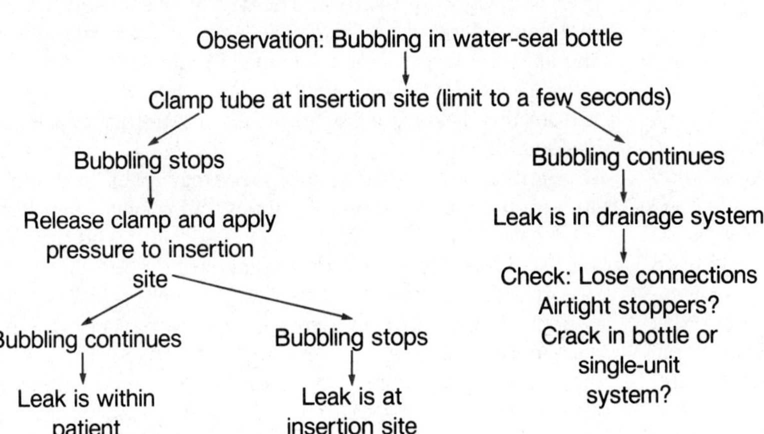

FIGURE 27–15 Locating source of air leak in chest drainage system.

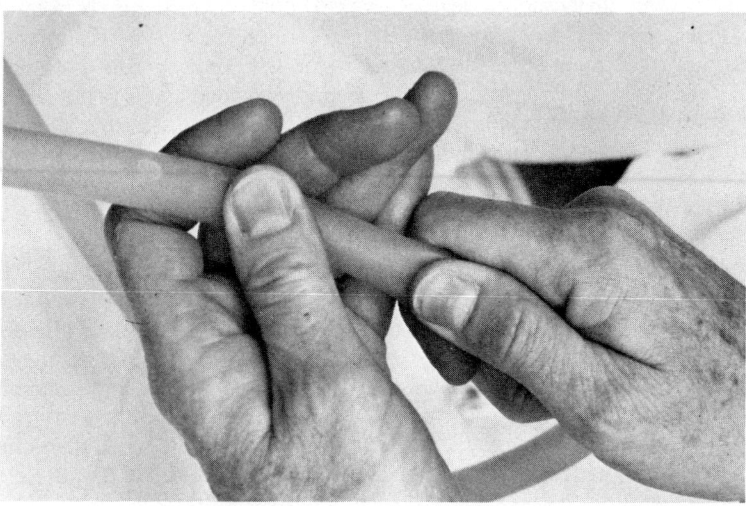

FIGURE 27–16 Technique for grasping the drainage tubing when "stripping" it. (Respiratory Care: Concepts and Techniques, an audiovisual publication of JB Lippincott Co, 1980)

Patients with spontaneous pneumothorax, fractured ribs, or penetrating or blunt chest trauma, as well as post-thoracotomy patients, are likely to experience pain. Adequate pain relief is important in facilitating good respiratory care and maintaining mobility. Unless contraindicated by the type of surgery or existence of other injuries, patients with chest tubes in place may be up as much as they can tolerate. Care should be taken to avoid tension on the tubes when the patient is sitting or walking.

Deep breathing facilitates drainage of the pleural space and should be encouraged. When blood gases are deranged, oxygen is administered to relieve hypoxemia. Trauma patients and postoperative patients may be receiving mechanical ventilation; care of the ventilator patient is discussed earlier in this chapter.

Finally, patients who are short of breath or in pain are likely to be anxious and fearful. Hypoxemia may add the complications of agitation, apprehension, and restlessness. Expert technical care to provide relief of pain and hypoxemia delivered with a calm, patient, and understanding approach will go far in relieving these most distressing symptoms. Whenever possible, the nurse should provide information in anticipation of chest tube insertion, removal, or other aspects of therapy. Understanding what is happening to oneself removes much of the fear associated with strange and uncomfortable procedures.

Chest Tube Removal

Chest tubes are usually removed at the bedside by the physician. The patient performs a Valsalva maneuver to increase pressure in the pleural space and to prevent air entry as the physician pulls the tube out. The wound is covered immediately with petrolatum gauze. Sterile 4 × 4 = inch gauze pads are applied and the dressing is taped tightly. A chest film is ordered to ensure that lung expansion is maintained without the drainage tube. The dressing is checked at regular intervals; a small amount of serous drainage is expected. The nurse observes the patient for any signs of recurrent lung collapse.[61] Before discharge, the patient is instructed in how to dress the chest tube site and is told the signs and symptoms he should promptly report to the physician.[16]

Evaluation

The goals of nursing care of the chest tube patient have been achieved when a number of objective and subjective data are measured or observed.

Adequate gas exchange has been restored when arterial blood-gas values have returned to normal on room air: Pa_{O_2} 60 mmHg or greater; Pa_{CO_2} 40 mmHg; pH 7.35 to 7.45. Restoration of normal lung mechanics has been achieved when the lung remains inflated after the chest tube has been removed and when normal breath sounds are auscultated. Vital signs, specifically heart and respiratory rate, are normal. The patient verbalizes relief of shortness of breath and anxiety and appears to be comfortable.

Relief of pain has been achieved when the patient verbalizes that he is comfortable and he appears restful. The patient does not splint the affected side and can perform pulmonary hygiene maneuvers comfortably. Heart rate, respiratory rate, and blood pressure are normal.

Dyspnea

Nursing Diagnosis

Dyspnea related to acute or chronic lung or cardiovascular dysfunction, as manifested by subjective report of shortness of breath, and, possibly, by observations of interrupted speech pattern, use of accessory muscles of respiration, and anxious facial expression.

Physiological Basis

The term *dyspnea* implies difficult or uncomfortable breathing. As defined by the American Thoracic Society, dyspnea is "an unpleasant 'subjective' feeling of difficult or labored breathing."[1]

The presence of dyspnea does not necessarily indicate disease. In fact, normal persons commonly experience dyspnea with vigorous exertion. The degree of exertion leading to dyspnea depends on such factors as age, physical training, and altitude. Some authorities refer to this expected type of dyspnea as "physiologic breathlessness," in order to separate it from the dyspnea associated with respiratory or cardiac dysfunction.

Among the many conditions that may result in dyspnea are emphysema, pulmonary fibrosis, pulmonary embolism, and heart failure. Conditions often associated with dyspnea are listed in Table 27–9. The sensation of dyspnea is known to correlate better with a disturbance of the ventilatory component of lung function than with a disturbance in gas exchange. Normal ventilation is required in order to provide the ongoing flow of air needed for gas exchange. The maximum volume of air that can be inspired and expired is referred to as the ventilatory capacity and reflects the ability of the chest to function as a bellows. It is generally agreed that dyspnea develops when there is an imbalance between a person's ventilatory capacity (supply) and his need for ventilation (demand).[47,59] However, the precise means by which this discrepancy between supply and demand is perceived as dyspnea is unclear. One theory with considerable support suggests that dyspnea develops whenever the force required for the respiratory muscles to achieve a particular length is excessive. This so-called length–tension inappropriateness is relayed to the brain, and the sensation of dyspnea results.[10,47] It is as if the person has to work too hard for the volume of air he gets. Many components of the ventilatory apparatus can be specifically affected by respiratory or cardiac disease, including the ribs, spine, respiratory muscles, peripheral and central nervous control, extrapulmonary and intrapulmonary airways, alveolar tissue, pleura, and pulmonary vessels.[23] For this reason it is conceivable that more than one mechanism is responsible for the production of dyspnea.

TABLE 27–9
Selected Pathologic Conditions Associated with Dyspnea

Condition	*Characteristic Pattern of Dyspnea*
Respiratory	
Emphysema	Insidious onset; progressive
Asthma	Intermittent; often very severe, life threatening during attack; dyspnea absent between asthma attacks
Interstitial fibrosis	Initially only with exercise; later at rest
Adult respiratory distress syndrome (ARDS)	May precede other signs and symptoms
Lung cancer	Usually insidious but may be sudden if acute airway obstruction occurs
Aspiration	Severe and sudden, often associated with severe coughing, sometimes with complete obstruction and apnea
Upper airway obstruction	Often history of previous endotracheal intubation; usually worse on inspiration; inspiratory stridor may be present only during exercise
Cardiovascular	
Left ventricular failure (coronary heart disease, mitral stenosis, aortic insufficiency, severe hypertension)	May begin with progressive, exertional dyspnea Frequently associated with paroxysmal nocturnal dyspnea, orthopnea May be associated with angina, weakness, intermittent claudication, pulmonary or peripheral edema
Pulmonary embolism	Should be suspected when sudden, not readily explained dyspnea occurs
Congenital heart disease	Often associated with inadequate cardiac output, for example, during exercise
Anemia	Only when hemoglobin level is under 8 g/ml
Neurological	
Neuromuscular disease (muscular dystrophy, multiple sclerosis, spinal cord injury, amyotrophic lateral sclerosis)	Often insidious; aspiration is common cause of sudden intermittent episodes
Severe anxiety	Usually occurs at rest Patients often complain that they cannot get a deep enough breath May be associated with hyperventilation and symptoms of respiratory alkalosis, complaints of dizziness, fatigue, unsteady legs, and chest pain

Interventions

The symptom of dyspnea can be acute or chronic. When it arises suddenly and unexpectedly, dyspnea is usually an indication that something is seriously wrong and the situation demands emergency actions. However, dyspnea can also be a long-term manifestation associated with chronic lung disease. In these cases, interventions focus on helping the patient cope with this uncomfortable sensation. Thus, rapid assessment is essential to distinguish between dyspnea that signals an acute change in a patient's condition and dyspnea that is a long-term aspect of chronic lung or cardiac disease. When dyspnea represents a life-threatening emergency, the nursing goal is to maintain ventilation and gas exchange. When dyspnea has been established to be of a long-standing nature, the goal of nursing interventions is to help the patient manage his life despite this disabling symptom.

Assessment

The first step in the assessment of dyspnea is to recognize it. Patients may report the symptom or there may be outward signs that lead the nurse to suspect that the patient is dyspneic. It is important to keep in mind that dyspnea is a symptom, just as pain is a symptom. It is the patient who perceives and reports dyspnea, and, as is true with pain, the patient's word must be believed. Since the term dyspnea is foreign to most lay persons, a patient can be asked, "How does your breathing feel?" or "Are you getting enough air?" A patient may say that he feels short of breath, is out of breath, cannot get enough air, cannot catch his breath, is aware of his breathing, or that his chest feels tight.

Signs that suggest that a person is experiencing dyspnea include the following:

Interrupted speech pattern
Use of accessory muscles
Anxious facial expression

Acute Unexplained Dyspnea. Once it has been established that a person is experiencing dyspnea, it is necessary to clarify the onset and establish whether the sensation of breathlessness is acute or chronic. An abrupt and unanticipated onset of severe dyspnea requires little additional data for the nurse to recognize it as a potentially life threatening emergency.

Interventions must be immediate and must focus on maintaining pulmonary ventilation and gas exchange while the cause is established and definitive care initiated. Because the sensation of breathlessness is very frightening and is aggravated by anxiety, the nurse should leave the patient only as necessary to summon help. Specific interventions are as follows:

1. Make certain that the patient's upper airway is not obstructed, a condition that could be the cause of or a contributing factor to the dyspnea.
2. Start oxygen if there are signs of impaired gas exchange. Although it would be ideal to have arterial blood-gas values first, in this situation guaranteeing an adequate oxygen supply is the priority. A starting flow rate of 4 liters/min is usually appropriate.[48]
3. Position the patient upright. If the patient prefers and can tolerate dangling, this position will diminish venous return to the heart and reduce pulmonary congestion, which may be a contributing factor. If the patient is weak, a high-Fowler's position should be used instead. Regardless, the patient will benefit from having his arms supported.

Chronic Dyspnea. When the onset of dyspnea has been gradual, detailed historical data can be collected. Such data may help to establish whether the dyspnea is respiratory or cardiac in nature and whether there are reversible mechanisms contributing to the dyspnea, such as bronchospasm, infection, or pulmonary edema. Historical data also provide extremely important information about how dyspnea has affected the patient's life.

Data Analysis. This in-depth evaluation of dyspnea is a responsibility shared by the physician and the nurse, with the primary focus of the physician being to establish the cause, and the primary focus of the nurse being to assist the patient to deal with the symptom. The physician will use findings from the history and physical examination, chest film, pulmonary function tests, and arterial blood-gas values to separate respiratory from cardiac causes of dyspnea and to determine reversibility. The nurse can use these findings to plan and evaluate the effectiveness of nursing interventions. In addition, it is extremely important for the nurse to obtain specific data that describe how dyspnea is affecting the patient's life and what the patient does to control dyspnea. Questions that may be asked to elicit this information are listed in Table 27–10.

Interventions for Chronic Dyspnea

Efforts should begin with the identification of any contributing factors that are potentially reversible. Nurses work collaboratively with physicians to identify and reverse causes such as infection, pulmonary edema, bronchospasm, and anxiety.

Patient Education. An important area of independent nursing intervention is patient education. Patients often need considerable instruction to learn how to identify possible factors that may be increasing their dyspnea on a given day and how to decide when medical assistance is necessary. This kind of decision making is complex and will be beyond the capacity of some patients or their caregivers. In those instances, other types of help may be needed, such as the ongoing evaluation by a visiting nurse.

Another extremely important intervention is to help the patient with chronic dyspnea understand that in this situation *oxygen therapy is not necessarily warranted.* Patients often want oxygen desperately because they believe it will relieve their dyspnea. However, as explained above, dyspnea correlates better with ventilatory rather than gas-exchange impairment. Although it is appropriate to supply oxygen in an emergency on the empirical basis that there may also be impaired gas exchange, it is not appropriate to use oxygen in this manner for chronic forms of dyspnea not associated with

TABLE 27–10
Assessment of Dyspnea

Current History

1. Describe what happens when you get short of breath.

2. Do you get short of breath when you are
   ____ lying down and resting?
   ____ sitting and resting?
   ____ walking up an incline or upstairs?
   ____ walking at a slow pace on level ground?
   ____ doing daily hygiene (brushing hair, shaving, showering, dressing)?
   ____ doing household tasks (washing dishes, vacuuming, mowing the lawn, straightening up the house)?
   ____ eating?
   ____ doing something else? List:

3. Which of the following symptoms do you have?
   ____ Cough? When?
   ____ Sputum production? When?
   Amount/day?
   Color: White/Clear? Other (describe):
   Consistency: Thin/Saliva-like? Thick?
   ____ Wheezing? When?
   ____ Ankle swelling? When?
4. How often do you get short of breath?
   ____ infrequently ____ once/day
   ____ intermittently ____ once/week
   ____ continuously
5. What actions help you get over your shortness of breath?
   ____ rest, or stopping activity
   ____ changing position: lying down? sitting up?
   ____ coughing up mucus
   ____ medication; specify:
   ____ breathing exercise; specify:
6. Do you smoke now? ____ Yes ____ No
   If yes, do you smoke: ____ cigars ____ cigarettes ____ pipe
   How many cigars, packs, or pipefulls per day?
   How many years?
7. Have you ever smoked? ____ Yes ____ No
   If yes, when did you quit?
   Did you smoke: ____ cigars ____ cigarettes ____ pipe
   How many cigars, packs, or pipefuls per day?
   How many years?
8. Are there any stresses (job, family) in your life? ____ Yes ____ No
   If yes, describe:
9. What medications are you currently taking? (include dosage)

(Adapted from Rifas EM: How You and Your Patient Can Manage Dyspnea. Nursing 80, 10:38, 1980)

hypoxemia. Instead, the patient needs to learn that the feeling of breathlessness does not in itself represent a threat to life.

Activity Tolerance. A patient needs to learn ways of altering activities in order to reduce the demands on his crippled ventilatory apparatus. Examples of energy-conservation techniques such as sitting in a chair to take a shower are listed in Table 27–11. Learning a variety of body positions to use during periods of extreme breathlessness is another strategy. Sitting forward in a chair with the elbows supported on the thighs is a classic posture. Similar benefits can be achieved by leaning over the back of a chair or by supporting the back against a wall. These positions are illustrated in Figure 27–17. Progressive relaxation training may help to reduce anxiety that can be contributing to dyspnea. Pursed-lip breathing is a valuable technique for patients with obstructive disease and is described in Chapter 29.

TABLE 27–11
Energy-Conservation Techniques

General Principles:
Plan ahead.
Sit to work whenever possible.
Rest before onset of fatigue.
Avoid rushing.

Examples of Specific Techniques for Self-Care Activities

Bathing
Choose time of day when energy is highest.
Sit on bath bench or shower chair.
Use hand-held shower.
Use warm rather than hot water.
Put on terry robe to dry rather than using towel.

Dressing
Lay out clothes night before.
Sit to dress.
Dress lower body first.
Avoid heavy or tight clothes (women may prefer T-shirt instead of brassiere).

Meals
Plan frequent, light meals.
Store food and utensils at waist level.
Keep frequently used items in one place.
Sit to prepare foods.
Air dry dishes rather than wipe.

Exercise. An important aspect of helping a patient with chronic dyspnea is to *increase exercise tolerance.* As they automatically reduce activities that produce breathlessness, dyspneic patients become deconditioned, and their lack of fitness further exacerbates the dyspnea. A safe level of activity can be estimated by monitoring blood pressure and heart rate during exercise, and the patient can be instructed in a gradually increasing program of walking and conditioning exercises.

Techniques to increase the strength and endurance of the inspiratory muscles are currently under investigation. Inspiring through a device such as the Pflex or a specially adapted incentive spirometer increases the resistance to breathing. A program of systematic exercise using such devices has been shown to increase strength of the diaphragm and other muscles of inspiration. However, conclusions regarding its effectiveness in decreasing dyspnea or improving exercise tolerance and ability to perform activities of daily living have not yet been drawn.[34]

Physicians sometimes prescribe narcotics to help reduce extreme dyspnea that is curtailing activity. Oral or sublingual morphine is recommended for patients with terminal lung cancer, and codeine has recently been used for patients with chronic obstructive pulmonary disease.[12,60]

Evaluation

Because dyspnea is a subjective sensation, the patient's report of how his breathing feels is a major factor in evaluating all interventions. Patients may state that they feel less breathless or that they are better able to accomplish daily activities. In the case of sudden, acute dyspnea, maintenance of adequate gas exchange is critical and can be evaluated by arterial blood-gas measurements. Psychological factors sometimes affect the patient's perception of shortness of breath. In this case, objective measures such as pulmonary function tests may help to validate the effectiveness of interventions.

Ineffective Breathing Patterns

Patients with lung disease often change their breathing patterns unconsciously to adapt to changed ventilatory requirements. For example, patients with restrictive lung disorders such as pneumonia or fibrosis generally adopt a pattern of rapid, shallow breathing that allows their stiff lungs to breathe at a lower energy cost.[59] In patients with severe chronic obstructive pulmonary disease, inspiration also tends to be rapid and shallow but is accompanied by a prolonged expiratory phase. Altered patterns such as these are physiologically useful and should not be classified as ineffective. There may be instances in which a patient adopts a breathing pattern that is not of physiological benefit. These are discussed below under two diagnostic statements. Although these problems may occur simultaneously, the diagnosis, interventions, and evaluation for each are different.

Nursing Diagnosis: Hyperventilation

Ineffective breathing pattern related to hyperventilation, as manifested by subjective complaints of numbness or tingling, observation of deep or rapid breathing, or both, and confirmation by blood-gas analysis showing a marked decrease in Pa_{CO_2} associated with normal Pa_{O_2} and increased pH.

Interventions

Anxiety may cause patients to hyperventilate and develop respiratory alkalosis. Because respiratory alkalosis is a normal compensatory mechanism for metabolic acidosis and for hypoxemia, it is very important to rule out these causes before initiating any interventions to slow the rate and depth of ventilation. When determined to be appropriate, measures to decrease the rate and depth of ventilation include coaching the patient to slow his breathing, breathing into and out of a paper bag, and administering medications to relieve pain and anxiety. Respiratory alkalosis and measures for controlling hyperventilation are discussed in more detail in Chapter 14.

Evaluation

When interventions to control psychologically induced hyperventilation have been successful, the patient will verbalize a decrease in sensations of numbness and tingling and may verbalize that pain and anxiety have decreased as well. Observation will indicate a decrease in the patient's respiratory rate and depth, and the patient should appear calmer.

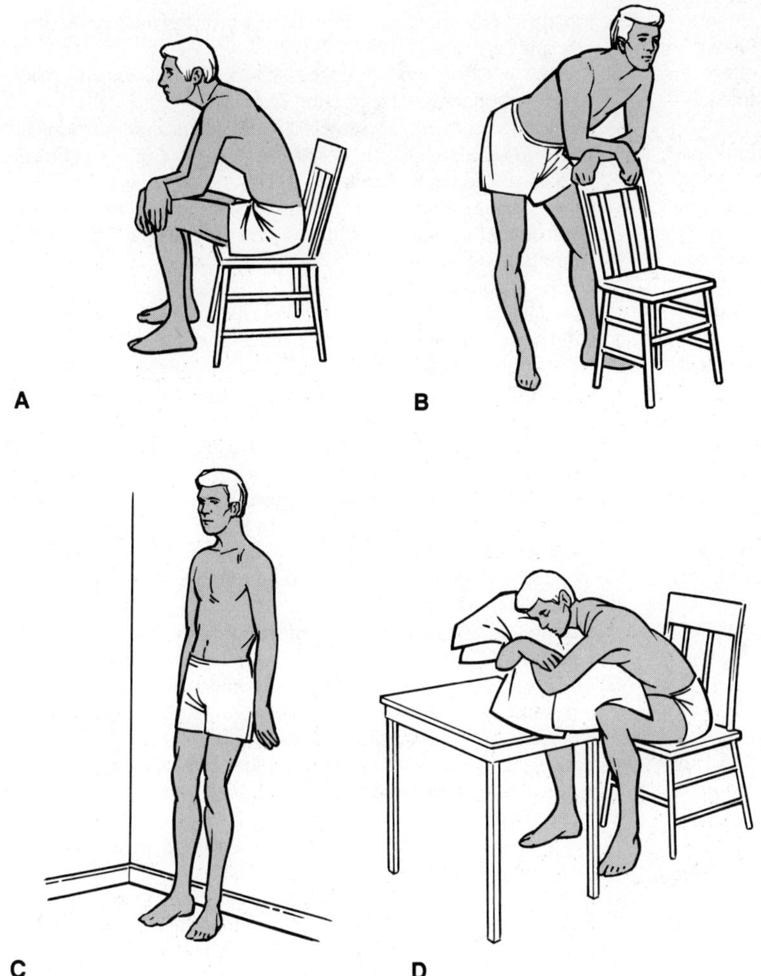

FIGURE 27–17 Body positions to facilitate breathing during periods of dyspnea. (*A*) Sitting forward in a chair with elbows supported. (*B*) Leaning over back of chair. (*C*) Supporting back against wall. (*D*) Leaning over stack of pillows or overbed table, with arms supported.

Conclusive evidence would be provided by arterial blood-gas values within normal limits.

Nursing Diagnosis: Absence of Sighing

Ineffective breathing pattern related to postoperative absence of normal sighing, as manifested by auscultation of shallow breath sounds or basilar crackles, fever, and atelectasis on chest film.

Interventions

Periodic sighing is important to reexpand alveoli that have collapsed during tidal breathing. Following surgery on the chest or upper abdomen, patients temporarily lose the normal pattern of unconsciously interposing deeper, or sigh, breaths onto their normal breathing pattern.[62] As a result, patients with other risk factors for respiratory problems, including those who smoke cigarettes, are obese, or have chronic lung disease, are at postoperative risk of developing atelectasis and clinically significant hypoxemia. Nurses can monitor for postoperative atelectasis by frequently auscultating the chest for decreased breath sounds and crackles and by checking for fever over 38 C°. Just as important as assessment are interventions to decrease atelectasis and the possibility of hypoxemia. Research to date has shown a deep breath held for 3 seconds to be the most effective technique.[49] This technique can be accomplished by teaching the patient to take, and hold, five to ten deep breaths several times each hour. An incentive spirometer is an inexpensive device that gives visual reinforcement of properly practiced technique.

Evaluation

Bedside criteria that indicate that interventions have been successful include auscultation of normal breath sounds and absence of fever. These findings can be confirmed by a normal chest film.

References

1. ATS Pulmonary Nomenclature Subcommittee on Respiratory Physiology: Updated Nomenclature for Membership Reaction. ATS News 4:12, 1978
2. Barrascout JR: Chest physical therapy and related procedures. In

Burton GG, Hodgkin JE (eds): Respiratory Care: A Guide to Clinical Practice, 2nd ed. Philadelphia, JB Lippincott, 1984

3. Bateman JRM, Newman SP, Daunt KM et al: Is cough as effective as chest physiotherapy in the removal of excessive tracheobronchial secretions? Thorax 36:683, 1981
4. Block ER: Oxygen therapy. In Fishman AP: Update: Pulmonary Diseases and Disorders. New York, McGraw-Hill, 1982
5. Boba A, Cincotti JJ, Piazza TE et al: The effects of apnea, endotracheal suction, and oxygen insufflation, alone and in combination, upon arterial oxygen saturation in anesthetized patients. J Lab Clin Med 53:680, 1959
6. Bone RC: Complications of mechanical ventilation and positive end-expiratory pressure. Respir Care 27:402, 1982
7. Boutros AR: Arterial blood oxygen during and after endotracheal suctioning in the apneic patient. Anesthesiology 32:114,. 1970
8. Comroe JH: Physiology of Respiration. Chicago, Year Book Medical Publishers, 1965
9. Craven DE, Connolly MG, Lichtenberg DA et al.: Contamination of mechanical ventilators with tubing changes every 24 or 48 hours. N Engl J Med 306:1505, 1982
10. Derenne J-PH, Macklem, Roussos C: The respiratory muscles: Mechanics, control and pathophysiology, Part II. Am Rev Respir Dis 118:373, 1978
11. Downes JJ, Wilson JF, Goodson D: Apnea, suction, and hyperventilation: Effect on arterial oxygen saturation. Anesthesiology 22:29, 1961
12. Doyle D (ed): Palliative Care: The Management of Far-advanced Illness. London, Croom Helm, 1984
13. Dressler DK, Smejkal C, Ruffolo ML: A comparison of oral and rectal temperature measurement on patients receiving oxygen by mask. Nurs Res 32:373, 1983
14. Dubick MN, Wright BD: Comparison of laryngeal pathology following long-term oral and nasal endotracheal intubations. Anesth Analg 57:663, 1978
15. Duncan C, Erickson R: Pressures associated with chest tube stripping. Heart Lung 11:166, 1982
16. Erickson R: Chest tubes: They're really not that complicated. Nursing 11:34, 1981
17 Erickson R: Consultation. Nursing 13:96, 1983
18. Estey W: Subjective effects of dry versus humidified low flow oxygen. Respir Care 25:1143, 1980
19. Facts and Comparisions. Philadelphia, JB Lippincott, 1984
20. Fell T, Cheney FW: Prevention of hypoxia during endotracheal suction. Ann Surg 174:24, 1971
21. Felton CL: Hypoxemia and oral temperatures. Am J Nurs 78:56. 1978
22. Fishman NH: Thoracic Drainage: A Manual of Procedures, 1st ed. Chicago, Year Book Medical Publishers, 1983
23. Gold WM: Dyspnea. In Blacklow RS: MacBryde's Signs and Symptoms. 6th ed. Philadelphia, JB Lippincott, 1983
24. Goodnough SKC: The effects of oxygen and hyperinflation on arterial oxygen tension after endotracheal suctioning. Heart Lung 14:11, 1985
25. Guzman L, Norton LC: Minimizing cuff-related laryngeal-tracheal complications. Focus 9:23, 1982
26. Harper RW: A Guide to Respiratory Care. Philadelphia, JB Lippincott, 1981
27. Hess D, D'Agostino D, Magrosky S et al: Effect of nasal cannula displacement on arterial oxygen tension. Respir Care 29:21, 1984
28. Hietpas BG, Roth RD, Jensen WM: Huff coughing and airway patency. Respir Care 24:710, 1979
29. Hodgkin JE: The scientific status of chest physiotherapy. Respir Care 26:657, 1981
30. Holody B, Goldberg HS: The effect of mechanical vibration physiotherapy on arterial oxygenation in acutely ill patients with atelectasis or pneumonia. Am Rev Respir Dis 124:372, 1981
31. Johanson WG: Infectious complications of respiratory therapy. Respir Care 27:445, 1982
32. Kersten L: Chest tube drainage system: Indications and principles of operation. Heart Lung 3:97, 1974
33. Kirby RR, Smith RA, Desautels DA: Mechanical ventilation. In Burton GG, Hodgkin JE: Respiratory Care: A Guide to Clinical Practice, 2nd ed. Philadelphia, JB Lippincott, 1984
34. Larson M, Kim MJ: Respiratory muscle training with the incentive spirometer resistive breathing device. Heart Lung 13:341, 1984
35. Lehnert BE, Schachter EN: The Pharmacology of Respiratory Care. St Louis, CV Mosby, 1980
36. Lopez–Vidriero MT: Lung secretions. In Clarke SW, Pavia D (eds): Aerosols and the Lung: Clinical and Experimental Aspects. London, Butterworths, 1984
37. Loudon RG: Cough: A symptom and a sign. Basics of Respir Dis 9:1, 1981
38. Luce JM, Tyler ML, Pierson DJ: Intensive Respiratory Care. Philadelphia, WB Saunders, 1984
39. May DB, Munt PW: Physiologic effects of chest percussion and postural drainage in patients with stable chronic bronchitis. Chest 75:29, 1979
40. Meador B: Pneumothorax: Providing emergency and long-term care. Nursing 8:43, 1978
41. Norton LC, Conforti CG: The effects of body position on oxygenation. Heart Lung 14:45, 1985
42. Oldenburg FA, Dolovich MB, Montgomery JM et al: Effects of postural drainage, exercise, and cough on mucus clearance in chronic bronchitis. Am Rev Respir Dis 120:739, 1979
43. Pavia D: Lung mucociliary clearance. In Clarke SW, Pavia D (eds): Aerosols and the Lung: Clinical and Experimental Aspects. London, Butterworths, 1984
44. Peterson GM: Application and assessment of oxygen therapy devices. Nurs Clin North Am 16:241, 1981
45. Pierce AK, Saltzman HA: Conference on the Scientific Basis of Respiratory Therapy: Final reports: Summaries and recommendations. Am Rev Respir Dis 110:7, 1974
46. Pierson DJ: The toxicity of low-flow oxygen therapy. Respir Care 28:889, 1983
47. Rapaport E: Dyspnea: Pathophysiology and differential diagnosis. Prog Cardiovasc Dis 3:532, 1971
48. Rifas EM: How you and your patient can manage dyspnea. Nursing 10:34, 1980
49. Risser NL: Preoperative and postoperative care to prevent pulmonary complications. Heart Lung 9:57, 1980
50. Rosen M, Hillard EK: The use of suction in clinical medicine. Br J Anaesth 32:486, 1960
51. Rosen M, Hillard EK: Further consideration on tracheal suction catheters, Br J Anaesth 36:124, 1963
52. Ryerson GG, Block AJ: Oxygen as a drug: Chemical properties, benefits, and hazards of administration. In Burton GG, Hodgkin JE (eds): Respiratory Care: A Guide to Clinical Practice, 2nd ed. Philadelphia, JB Lippincott, 1984
53. Sackner MA: Effect of respiratory drugs on mucociliary clearance. Chest (suppl) 73:958, 1978
54. Shim C, Fine N, Fernandez R et al.: Cardiac arrhythmias resulting from tracheal suctioning. Ann Intern Med 71:1449, 1969
55. Skelley BFH, Deeren SM, Powaser MM: The effectiveness of two preoxygenation methods to prevent endotracheal suction-induced hypoxemia. Heart Lung 9:316, 1980
56. Sutton PP: Chest physiotherapy and cough. In Clarke SW, Pavia D (eds): Aerosols and the Lung: Clinical and Experimental Aspects. London, Butterworths, 1984
57. Tyler ML: Complications of positioning and chest physiotherapy. Respir Care 27:458, 1982
58. Tyler ML: The respiratory effects of body positioning and immobilization. Respir Care 29:472, 1984

59. West JB: Pulmonary Pathophysiology: The Essentials, 2nd ed. Baltimore, Williams & Wilkins, 1982
60. Woodcock AA, Gross ER, Gellert A et al: Effects of dihydrocodeine, alcohol, and caffeine on breathlessness and exercise tolerance in patients with chronic obstructive disease and normal blood gases. New Engl J Med 305:1611, 1981
61. Woodin LM: Your patient with a pneumothorax. Nursing 12:50, 1982
62. Zikria BA, Spencer JL, Kinney JM et al: Alterations in ventilatory function and breathing patterns following surgical trauma. Ann Surg 179:1, 1974
63. Ziment I: Respiratory Pharmacology and Therapeutics. Philadelphia, WB Saunders, 1978
64. Zinman R: Cough versus chest physiotherapy. Am Rev Respir Dis 129:182, 1984

Bibliography

Brannin PK: Management modalities: Respiratory system. In Hudak CM, Lohr TS, Gallo BM (eds): Critical Care Nursing, 3rd ed. Philadelphia, JB Lippincott, 1982

Caldwell SL, Sullivan KN: Artificial airways. In Burton GG, Hodgkin JE (eds): Respiratory Care: A Guide to Clinical Practice, 2nd ed. Philadelphia, JB Lippincott, 1984

Demers RR: Complications of endotracheal suctioning procedures. Respir Care 27:453, 1982

Fairman RP, Glauser FL: Dyspnea. In Glauser FL (ed): Signs and Symptoms in Pulmonary Medicine. Philadelphia, JB Lippincott, 1983

Fuchs PL: Streamlining your suctioning techniques, Part 1: Nasotracheal suctioning; Part 2: Endotracheal suctioning; Part 3: Tracheostomy suctioning. Nursing 14:39, 46, 55, 1984

Fulmer JD, Snider GL: ACCP-NHLBI National Conference on Oxygen Therapy. Chest 86:234, 1984

Harris RB, Hyman RB: Clean vs. sterile tracheotomy care and level of pulmonary infection. Nurs Res 33:80, 1984

Irwin MM, Openbrier DR: A delicate balance: Strategies for feeding ventilated COPD Patients. Am J Nurs 85:275, 1985

Landis K, Smith S: The mechanically ventilated patient: A comprehensive nursing care plan. Crit Care Q 6:43, 1983

Marini JJ: Postoperative atelectasis: Pathophysiology, clinical importance, and principles of management. Respir Care 29:516, 1984

Vincent JE: Medical problems in the patient on a ventilator. Crit Care Q 6:33, 1983

West GA, Primeau P: Nonmedical hazards of long-term oxygen therapy. Respir Care 28:906, 1983

Chapter 28

Respiratory Infections and Inflammatory Disorders

Nancy L. Risser

The respiratory tract, both the upper and lower portions, can be affected by a wide variety of inflammatory conditions. The first part of this chapter considers those inflammatory conditions that affect the upper airway. Many of these disorders are common and are frequently managed by the person himself on an outpatient basis. For this reason, it is of utmost importance that nurses provide health teaching that will enable persons to manage symptoms safely and to recognize complications that require the intervention of a health-care provider.

The second part of the chapter covers problems of the lower airway that are inflammatory or restrictive in nature. In many cases, inflammation is the cause of a restrictive disorder that develops subsequently.

Inflammatory Disorders of the Upper Airway

Common Cold (Acute Rhinitis)

Definition and Etiology

The common cold, referred to technically as acute rhinitis or coryza, is a mild, self-limiting syndrome of the upper respiratory tract caused by one of a number of viruses and characterized by mucous membrane inflammation and discharge. It is the leading cause of visits to a physician and is a major cause of industrial absenteeism.

In adults the highly contagious common cold may be caused by a variety of viruses including rhinoviruses, coronavirus, parainfluenza viruses, and mycoplasmal organisms. Adenovirus and influenza viruses also produce the common cold, but the syndrome is more severe and often involves the lower respiratory tract as well.[41] Traditionally environmental exposure to cold and damp has been implicated to influence susceptibility, but its actual role is unproven. Annual epidemics occur in cold months (September to May). Reinfection may occur with the same type of virus.

Pathophysiology and Clinical Manifestations

The specific events following viral invasion of the upper respiratory tract are not well understood. Immunologic mechanisms may play a role in the development of the respiratory epithelial damage that occurs.

The incubation period varies with different viruses but is usually 48 to 72 hours. Cold symptoms include cough, sore throat, pain, fever, nasal discharge, sneezing, and other symptoms, as listed in Table 28–1. Examination of the nasal mucosa may reveal redness and edema. The pharynx and tonsils usually are without edema or exudate but may be mildly to moderately reddened. Cervical lymph nodes may be enlarged and mildly tender to palpation.

Colds usually progress gradually for the first 1 or 2 days, followed by maximal symptoms for 2 or 3 days and then gradual subsiding of symptoms. Cigarette smokers have a prolonged duration of symptoms up to 2 weeks or longer.[6]

As a result of changes in bacterial flora that reside in the upper respiratory tract, a small percentage of colds are complicated by secondary bacterial infections. These infections include pneumonia, tonsillitis, purulent sinusitis, and otitis media. Patients who are already debilitated or have underlying bronchopulmonary disease may have their balance of control tipped by a cold that would hardly make a younger, healthier person uncomfortable.

Medical Management

Diagnosis of the specific virus causing a cold is usually not possible. Diagnostic laboratory tests are not necessary unless another disease process or complication is suspected.

Because antimicrobial therapy neither shortens the course of the acute illness nor prevents development of secondary infections, antibiotics are prescribed only when secondary bacterial infection is present.[62,64] Instead, medical management is symptomatic and nonspecific. General measures include rest, fluids, a balanced diet as tolerated, and use of aspirin. Decongestants may be prescribed to afford relief of rhinorrhea and nasal obstruction (Table 28–2). Unless there is also an allergic component to the symptoms, antihistamines contribute little more to congestion control than what is provided by decongestant administration.[99]

Nursing Management

Assessment and Nursing Diagnosis

Although self-diagnosis by the patient is usually correct, it is important to distinguish the uncomplicated common cold from the fewer than 5% that are accompanied by secondary bacterial complications.[41] A history of frequent colds suggests a need to search for correctable conditions that may contribute to recurrent colds. These include allergic or vasomotor rhinitis, nasal deformities, and cigarette smoking.

TABLE 28–1
Comparison of Usual Clinical Manifestations of Inflammatory Conditions of the Upper Respiratory Tract

	Common Cold Rhinovirus	*Allergic Rhinitis*	*Influenza*	*Streptococcal Pharyngitis*	*Acute Sinusitis*
Duration of illness	3–7 days	Weeks, months	Worst 1–5 days, symptoms for 10–14 days	Usually clears in about 3 days	Days, months if not treated
Cough	Dry, clear mucus if any	None, unless caused by postnasal drip	Severe, nonproductive	None or dry hacking	Usually from postnasal discharge
Sore throat	Dry throat, mild soreness; should disappear in 2–3 days	None	Present	Red, inflamed, may be exudate	Sometimes
Pain	General aches	None	Prominent general muscle aches, headaches	Throat and cervical glands	Over sinuses; worse in morning
Fever	Low-grade, if present	None	Over 100°F, up to 104°F	Variable, over 100°F	Variable, over 100°F
Nasal discharge	Watery, copious, followed by purulent discharge, nasal obstruction	Copious watery discharge, nasal stuffiness, itchy	Rhinorrhea	None	Purulent, yellow thick discharge if total obstruction not present
Other	Sneezing, hoarseness, nasal smear has polymorphonuclear leukocytes	Snoring; sneezing; itching, redness, tearing of eyes; eosinophils on nasal smear	May have vomiting, diarrhea, abdominal pain	Headache, rash, abdominal pain	Nausea, malaise sometimes present

TABLE 28-2
Common Drugs Prescribed for Upper Respiratory Tract Infections

Type of Drug	*Indications*	*Drug Name*	*Adult Dosage*	*Common Side-Effects*	*Nursing Considerations*
Antibiotics	Sinusitis, bronchitis	Ampicillin	250–500 mg PO q6h × 10 days	GI symptoms, skin rash, fever	Take allergy history
		Trimethoprim (TMP)–sulfamethoxazole (SMZ)	2 tablets bid (80 mg TMP, 400 mg SMZ/tablet) × 10 days	Rash, GI symptoms, headache	
	Group A β-hemolytic streptococcal pharyngitis, tonsillitis	Benzathine penicillin G	1–2 million units IM		Drug of choice
		Penicillin V	250–500 mg PO q6h × 10 days		Take on empty stomach
		Erythromycin	250–500 mg PO q6h × 10 days		Used for patients with penicillin sensitivity
	Mycoplasma pneumoniae	Tetracycline	250–500 mg PO q6h	Skin rashes, GI symptoms	
		Erythromycin	400–500 mg q6h PO	Hepatic dysfunction, GI symptoms, skin rash	May increase theophylline level
Analgesics Antipyretics	Fever, muscle aches, sore throat, symptom relief	Acetaminophen (Tylenol)	650 mg q4h PRN up to 4000 mg/24 hr maximum		Drug interaction with warfarin sodium
		Acetylsalicylic acid	650 mg q4h PRN up to 3500 mg/24 hr maximum	Gastric irritation, nausea, diarrhea, skin eruptions	Avoid in asthma, hay fever, nasal polyp syndrome *Contraindications:* hypersensitivity, bleeding ulcer Discontinue if dizziness, reduced hearing, or tinnitus ensues
Decongestants (sympathomimetic amines)	Symptomatic relief of rhinorrhea or nasal obstruction in common cold, rhinitis, influenza syndrome, sinusitis	(Multiple products available) *Topical* Phenylephrine 0.25%–0.5% (Neo-Synephrine) Oxymetazoline 0.05% (Afrin)	2–3 drops or spray in each nostril	Rhinitis medicamentosa (rebound nasal congestion) Increased blood pressure Drying of nasal mucosa	Administer with patient seated with head tilted back. Use drops or spray for only 5 days and never more than 2 weeks. Longer use may damage nasal membranes.
		Oral Phenylpropanolamine: Regular Long-acting Pseudoephedrine (Sudafed)	 25–50 mg orally q4–8h 75 mg q12h 60 mg q4–6h	Tremor, restlessness, headache, insomnia, urinary retention, nausea, tachycardia, palpitations	Avoid or use cautiously in patients with diabetes mellitus, peripheral vascular disease, hypertension. Drug interactions: MAO inhibitors, beta-blockers, methyldopa, indomethacin
Antihistamines	Allergic rhinitis (hay fever)	Chlorpheniramine maleate: Regular Sustained-release	 4 mg q4–6h up to 24 mg/24 hr maximum 8 mg q8–12 h up to 24 mg/24 hr maximum	Drowsiness, dizziness, sedation, hypotension in elderly Blurred vision, thickened bronchial secretions, urinary retention, nasal stuffiness	Conraindicated in lower respiratory tract conditions Usually combined with decongestants Cautious use in hyperthyroidism, glaucoma, cardiovascular disease, prostatic hypertrophy, hypertension, pyloroduodenal obstruction

(*Continued*)

TABLE 28–2
Common Drugs Prescribed for Upper Respiratory Tract Infections (*Continued*)

Type of Drug	*Indications*	*Drug Name*	*Adult Dosage*	*Common Side-Effects*	*Nursing Considerations*
Antihistamines		Diphenhydramine	25–50 mg q4h up to 150 mg/24 hr maximum	Dry mouth or throat, disturbed coordination, fatigue, tremor, epigastric distress	Drug interactions: alcohol, MAO inhibitors, sedatives, and other central nervous system depressants
Antitussives	Cough suppressant	Codeine	10–20 mg q3–4h up to 120 mg/24 hr maximum	Respiratory depression, drowsiness, gastric upset	*Contraindications:* Reduced ventilatory function Rarely used unless cough is totally nonproductive or severely-fatiguing
		Dextromethorphan	10–20 mg q4h up to 120 mg/24 hr maximum		
Expectorants	Productive cough to thin secretions and promote their clearance	Guaifenesin (Robitussin) 100 mg/5 ml	200–400 mg q4h up to 2400 mg/24 hr maximum	Mild, uncommon; gastric upset	Adequate hydration is best expectorant Effectiveness controversial
		Terpin hydrate elixir	200 mg q4h up to 1200 mg/24 hr maximum		
		Potassium iodide (saturated solution) 750–1500 mg/ml	10–15 drops (1–1.5 g) tid with meals	Side-effects occur frequently: dyspnea, diarrhea, skin reactions, burning feeling in mouth, gum soreness, sneezing, nausea, increased salivation	*Contraindicated* in pregnancy and in patients with impaired renal function or iodide hypersensitivity
Corticosteroids	Allergic rhinitis (hay fever); perennial	Beclomethasone dipropionate	Intranasal spray 1 spray bid–qid (42 μg/spray)	Intranasal bleeding, burning, sneezing	
	Eosinophilic nonallergic rhinitis	Dexamethasone	2 sprays bid–tid (0.08 mg/spray)		
		Prednisone	20–40 mg PO qd × 1–3 weeks and then gradual reduction of dosage	Multiple, including hyperglycemia, hypersensitivity, ulcer, and psychological effects	Systemic corticosteroids rarely necessary

GI, gastrointestinal tract; MAO, monoamine oxidase

Questions about life stresses and coping mechanisms may also be appropriate.

Frequent nursing diagnoses are as follows:

- Alteration in comfort related to inflammation of the upper respiratory tract by cold virus
- Knowledge deficit related to cold transmission, symptom relief, or signs of complications

Goals. Most colds are managed by the patient at home, usually without consulting a health-care provider. Therefore a primary nursing goal is that the patient and family learn to prevent transmission of the virus to others and to relieve symptoms.

Interventions

Prevention of Transmission. Although viruses responsible for causing a cold may be ubiquitous, direct exposure to larger numbers of organisms such as droplet nuclei from a sneeze greatly increases the chances of development of an infection after exposure. People with colds should therefore be cautioned to avoid crowded places, infants, very young children, and elderly or chronically ill persons during the 3 to 6 days they are usually shedding viruses.[42] Frequent hand washing, covering the mouth for coughing or sneezing, and careful disposal of waste tissue are general measures that reduce the spread of the causative virus.

Symptom Management. Patients may be as active as their feeling of well-being and energy allows. During the peak of illness when the patient is most contagious to others, restricted activity is advisable. There are no specific dietary limitations. Eight ounces of water or other fluid should be taken every hour or two unless contraindicated by another condition such as renal failure or congestive heart disease.

A sore throat can be treated symptomatically by gargling with salt water (½ tsp table salt in 8 oz warm water). Topical analgesics such as lozenges, gargles, and sprays are often used for sore throat without much documented effectiveness. However, a patient can be advised to try these and to evaluate their effectiveness in his situation. Painful nasal maceration can be relieved by applying a petroleum-based ointment.

When a client has a cold, he will probably have reduced the frequency of his smoking. This is a good time to advise the patient to quit smoking completely, referring him to self-help resources or community programs for the skills to accomplish this change in lifestyle. The patient should be aware of the risks and side-effects as well as the proper uses of any over-the-counter medications he uses or plans to use for cold symptoms. Patients on prescribed medications should be instructed to inform or consult with a health-care provider before using any over-the-counter medications. If antihistamines or decongestants have been prescribed, the nurse should teach the patient to monitor for side-effects such as drowsiness or urinary obstruction (see Table 28–2). The effectiveness of large doses of ascorbic acid (vitamin C) to prevent or speed recovery from a cold remains unproven.[21] If prescribed medications are to be administered by nose drops or spray, the patient should correctly demonstrate the procedure to use and state the date after which he will stop using them. Patient instructions for the use of nasal sprays are given in Table 28–3. Similar instructions can be used for nose drops.

Since retained secretions increase the chances of bacterial complications and a prolonged course of the disease, cough suppressants should generally be avoided, particularly if the patient has any sputum production or previous underlying condition affecting mucociliary function, such as chronic bronchitis or a history of smoking. In the few persons in whom cough, often due to postnasal discharge, interferes with rest or creates symptoms such as chest wall pain, a cough suppressant may be prescribed or taken as part of an over-the-counter preparation.

TABLE 28–3
Instructions to Patients for Use of Nasal Sprays

1. Sit upright with your head tilted backwards.
2. Spray deeply into each nostril and sniff at the same time.
3. Use two squeezes in each nostril followed by a pause of at least 1 minute.
4. Remain in a position with the head tilted backwards during this period to facilitate the medication movement to the affected areas.
5. If the nose remains congested, the process may be repeated once again to open more proximal parts of the nasal passages.
6. Under no circumstances should nasal spray be used for more than 2 consecutive weeks.

Recognition of Complications. Patients should be taught symptoms of complications that should be reported to a health-care provider:

- A temperature over 101° F.
- Throat pain or white spots on the throat or tonsils
- Cough that produces thick yellow or gray sputum (phlegm, mucus)
- Shaking chills
- Chest pain
- Earache
- Shortness of breath
- Skin rash
- Pain in the teeth, face, or head over sinuses

To prevent the spread of infected materials up the eustachian tubes, patients should be instructed to use only gentle force for nose blowing by blowing as infrequently as possible through both nostrils at the same time and with the mouth slightly open.

Evaluation

The person with a cold should be able to

- Describe ways to prevent spreading the cold and being exposed in the future
- Recognize symptoms of complications to report to the health-care provider
- Describe safe methods for obtaining symptom relief

Allergic and Nonallergic Rhinitis (Hay Fever)

Definition and Etiology

The term *allergic rhinitis* refers to any reaction of nasal mucosa to foreign antigen. The episodes of rhinitis are seasonal when associated with sensitizing allergens, such as pollens, that occur intermittently; acute and intermittent when associated with allergens such as cigarette smoke and air pollution; and perennial when associated with ubiquitous substances such as dust, animal dander, or mold spores. Chronic allergic rhinitis affects up to 20% of the population.[100] *Chronic nonallergic rhinitis* is less common and refers to a nasal reaction to factors such as changes in air temperature, odors, and changes in head position.[79] Chronic sinus or nasopharyngeal infections also may cause chronic rhinitis. Another category of chronic nonallergic rhinitis involves a combination of nasal eosinophilia and nasal polyps; this condition is called *eosinophilic nonallergic rhinitis.*[79]

Pathophysiology and Clinical Manifestations

In persons with allergic rhinitis, inhaled allergens react with IgE antibody and cause the release of chemical mediators. This results in vasodilation of nasal blood vessels and increased mucus secretion (rhinorrhea). Responses of the nasal mucosa are the same in chronic rhinitis but do not follow contact with an allergen. Obstruction of the eustachian tube and sinus orifice may complicate rhinitis and lead to serous otitis media and sinusitis.

An important form of chronic nonallergic rhinitis is *rhinitis medicamentosa.* In this condition, overuse of topical sympathomimetics (including cocaine) causes rebound vasodilation and α-adrenergic blockage and leads to nasal obstruction. Systemic α-adrenergic blockers (*e.g.,* reserpine), beta agonists (*e.g.,* terbutaline sulfate), and (rarely) oral sympathomimetics may also cause rhinitis medicamentosa.

Clinical manifestations are localized to the mucosa directly contacted, usually the nose and eyes (see Table 28–1). The nasal mucosa appears pale red or gray, swollen, and boggy with a thin clear discharge. Polyps or enlarged nasal turbinates may be observed. The conjunctiva may be reddened and edematous.

Medical Management

Historical and physical data along with nasal cytology assist diagnosis of the type of rhinitis. In normal persons nasal secretions contain few eosinophils, but in persons with allergic or eosinophilic nonallergic rhinitis, abundant eosinophils are observed. Skin tests are misleading in many patients but may be helpful to confirm a diagnosis in persons with an allergy history and nasal eosinophilia.[100]

Symptomatic medical treatment includes maintenance of an allergen-free atmosphere and use of antihistamine and sympathomimetic drugs to control symptoms. Antihistamines block histamine effects at receptor sites. Although most are effective initially, their relief of symptoms often diminishes with regular use. Sympathomimetics may be given alone or in combination with antihistamines for their decongestant effects. (see Table 28–2.)

In cases of severe hay fever uncontrolled by the above measures, intranasal corticosteroids are used. Inhalation usually results in improvement within 2 weeks; after that time the dosage is tapered. Oral prednisone is rarely necessary for allergic rhinitis.

Immunotherapy (hyposensitization or desensitization) is sometimes helpful for allergic rhinitis. The allergen, such as pollen, is administered subcutaneously in gradually increasing doses for at least 2 to 3 years. Therapy may be started 3 to 6 months before the beginning of seasonal symptoms.

Surgical correction of a deviated nasal septum or polyps may relieve some cases of chronic rhinitis. Polyps often recur.

Nursing Management

Assessment and Nursing Diagnosis

The combination of watery nasal discharge, sneezing, and itching eyes in people with a personal or family history of allergy suggests allergic rhinitis rather than a common upper respiratory tract infection. The health history should include details on timing of symptoms and exposure as well as medication history. Often symptoms of chronic rhinitis are aggravated during pregnancy.[100]

Although nursing diagnoses must be established individually, after assessment, frequently encountered diagnoses include:

- Alteration in comfort related to allergic response of nasal mucosa to foreign antigen
- Knowledge deficit related to factors precipitating rhinitis episodes

Goals. The goals of nursing interventions are to reduce the frequency of episodes and to relieve or control symptoms with a minimum of side-effects and cost.

Interventions

Prevention. The initial approach taken for anyone with allergic rhinitis involves separation of the person from sensitizing allergens. When pollen or dust is the allergen, an air conditioner with an electrostatic precipitating filter, car air conditioners, or even dust-proof respiratory masks are of value. To decrease dust in the bedroom, the mattress and pillow are covered with an airtight nonantigenic material such as plastic; carpets, drapes, bedspreads, and other lint-producing materials are removed; and blankets made of synthetic material are used. Damp dusting and vacuuming should occur daily while the patient is not present. Household pets, often sources of allergens, may need to move outdoors. Patients may need assistance balancing the need for symptom relief with the upheaval in usual lifestyle these measures require.

Situations that lead to exaggerated parasympathetic (cholinergic) stimulation should be avoided in both allergic and nonallergic rhinitis. These situations include lying down, alcohol ingestion, temperature and humidity changes, and other nonspecific irritants such as fumes, smoke, dust, strong odors, and aerosols.[100] Cigarette smoking is a lifestyle that is difficult yet important to change. Exposure to passive smoke is also a problem for some. Elevation of the head when in a supine position may counteract the increased airway resistance that occurs in recumbency. Since vigorous exercise induces sympathetic discharge, vasoconstriction, and nasal patency, a regular exercise program may be effective for symptom relief of chronic rhinitis.[100]

Symptom Relief. Methods of administration and side-effects of decongestants and antihistamines are similar to those discussed for the common cold. Antihistamines should be taken regularly for best therapeutic results.[100] Patients using antihistamines can be counselled that initial sedative side-effects diminish with long-term use and can be minimized by beginning with bedtime doses. Antihistamine and decongestant combinations and long-acting preparations are expensive but convenient and result in regimens that are better adhered to.

If the patient requires corticosteroid therapy, he needs to be aware of its side-effects and of the advantages of discontinuing its use as soon as possible. Since the abrupt discontinuation of corticosteroids may exacerbate symptoms, patients must not run out of medications and must follow a prescribed schedule of gradually tapering when the medication is discontinued.

Injections for desensitization must be administered following a strict schedule to gradually increase the antigen exposure. Epinephrine 1 : 1000 must be ready for immediate injection if an anaphylactic reaction occurs. The patient should understand that a realistic goal is reduction in symptoms and amount of medications needed, not elimination of symptoms.

When a patient overuses local decongestants and develops rhinitis medicamentosa, his rebound congestion is refractory to the pharmacologic decongestant action. All local decongestants must be discontinued. Until nasal congestion symptoms clear in a week or two, saline lavages and corticosteroids or oral decongestants may be used. Warm irrigation of nasal tissue with saline is soothing, augments mucociliary flow, and reduces forceful nose blowing. Some patients are instructed to perform this technique themselves by using a special right-angled rubber-tipped nasal adaptor placed on a Water Pik device.[100]

A well-recognized syndrome of perennial nonallergic eosinophilia rhinitis, nasal polyps, and aspirin idiosyncrasy exists.[100] These patients should be advised to avoid over-the-counter drugs that contain aspirin.[94]

Patients should be instructed to contact their health-care provider if the medications fail to control symptoms or if they experience any symptoms of complications (see Acute Rhinitis).

Evaluation

Following nursing interventions to decrease patient symptoms, the patient with allergic rhinitis should

- Report reduced frequency, duration, and severity of episodes of allergic rhinitis
- Report the use of decongestant and antihistamine drugs at appropriate intervals without the development of side-effects

Influenza

Definition and Etiology

Influenza is an acute disease of the respiratory tract accompanied by fever and systemic symptoms. It is caused by one of three types of influenza virus (types A, B, C) that cause recurring winter epidemics in temperate climates. The virus antigen undergoes changes over time, accounting for cyclic widespread epidemics. Epidemics in a community last 3 to 6 weeks, usually affecting school children first and then spreading to adults.[20]

Pathophysiology and Clinical Manifestations

Transmission of influenza is usually airborne but can be by direct contact. During the 1- to 5-day incubation period, the virus invades the tracheobronchial mucosa. Desquamation and cell death of the ciliated columnar epithelium result.

The illness has a sudden onset with prominent respiratory tract symptoms (see Table 28–1). With type B influenza gastrointestinal tract symptoms are present as well. The throat may not appear inflamed but tender cervical lymph nodes are usually present. The chest examination is usually normal or reveals only a few crackles. Most adults with influenza do not have the complete severe syndrome, but one or another type of symptom predominates.

Persons with influenza should begin to experience improvement in symptoms in 1 to 5 days and continue to improve progressively. The total duration of illness rarely exceeds 10 days, although patients may experience 1 or 2 weeks of lassitude.[20]

In persons with underlying heart or lung disease, the virus may extend to the lung parenchyma, causing influenzal pneumonia. Other complications of influenza include bacterial pneumonia, neurologic syndromes such as Guillain–Barré or encephalitis, exacerbation of underlying respiratory insufficiency, or acute sinusitis.

Medical Management

Influenza is diagnosed on the basis of the clinical picture when a community epidemic exists. A throat culture may be obtained to exclude streptococcal cause of symptoms.

Treatment is supportive to relieve symptoms and may include decongestants, expectorants, antitussives, or analgesics as well as rest and fluids. Amantadine hydrochloride will speed symptom resolution and, if given prophylactically, will prevent about 50% of type A influenza virus infections.[20]

Nursing Management

Assessment and Nursing Diagnosis

A health history should note the presence of chronic diseases such as chronic obstructive pulmonary disease (COPD) or heart disease, since they predispose to the most common influenza complication, bacterial pneumonia. It is also important to be aware of the course of the illness. Any recurrence of cough, chest pain, purulent sputum, or fever after symptoms and fever have initially remitted suggests the onset of a superimposed bacterial complication.

Examples of possible nursing diagnoses include

- Alteration in comfort related to respiratory tract and systemic inflammation caused by influenza viruses
- Potential impaired gas exchange related to secondary development of influenzal or bacterial pneumonia
- Fluid balance disturbance related to diarrhea and vomiting
- Alteration in nutrition, less than body requirements, related to nausea and gastrointestinal discomfort

Goals. Goals of nursing interventions are to prevent development of influenza in high risk persons and to relieve symptoms and prevent complications in those who have influenza.

Interventions

Annual vaccination is recommended for persons who have chronic diseases that increase the chance of influenza complications. Persons over 65 and those with cancer; diabetes; chronic renal, heart, or lung disease; chronic anemia; or neuromuscular disorders should be advised to receive an annual injection of influenza virus vaccine. When an influenza epidemic exists, unvaccinated persons at high risk of influenza complications should consult their physician regarding the prophylactic use of 4 to 6 weeks of amantadine.

Supportive nursing care for influenza is similar to that for other viral upper respiratory tract infections. Because the person with influenza tends to be sicker, bed rest and a more prolonged convalescence may be necessary.

Evaluation

Persons at risk for influenza should be able to

- State why the vaccine is important
- Verbalize plans to obtain annual vaccination

Patients with influenza should be able to

- Report an appropriate plan to use measures including over-the-counter medications for symptomatic relief
- List symptoms of complications to report

Sinusitis

Definition and Incidence

The paranasal sinuses are a group of air-containing spaces situated around the nasal cavity and adjoining the orbits and anterior cranial fossa. The frontal and maxillary sinuses are shown in Figure 28–1. Sinusitis occurs when their mucosal lining becomes inflamed. Sinusitis may be purulent or nonpurulent, acute or chronic, and is identified by the individual sinuses involved (*e.g.,* frontal sinusitis or sphenoid sinusitis). Pansinusitis refers to involvement of all sinuses. The maxillary sinus is most often involved, and the posterior ethmoid and sphenoid sinuses least often affected by acute sinusitis. Approximately 0.5% of common colds are complicated by sinus infection, making it one of the most common problems seen in outpatient medical practice.[62]

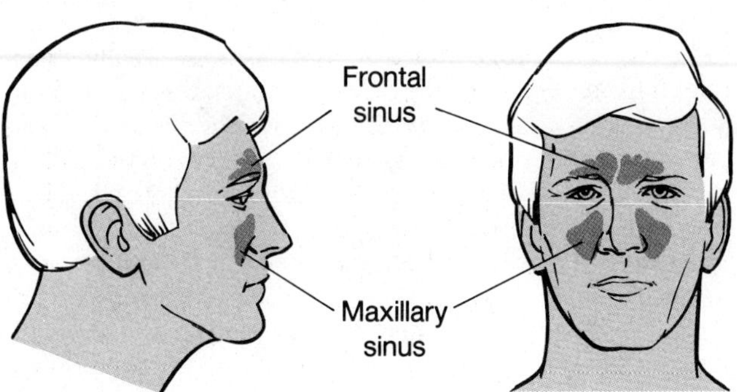

FIGURE 28–1 Frontal and maxillary sinuses.

Etiology and Pathophysiology

Acute sinusitis infections usually result from either the bacterium *Streptococcus pneumoniae* (30%) or *Hemophilus influenza* (20%).[60] Repeated or prolonged episodes of acute sinusitis that are untreated or treated inadequately may progress to *chronic sinusitis.* Anaerobes play a more significant role in the etiology of chronic than of acute sinusitis. *Pseudomonas aeruginosa* causes some cases of hospital-acquired sinusitis.

Most cases of acute sinusitis result from obstruction of the sinus openings following a viral upper respiratory tract infection. Normally cilia on the epithelial cells lining the sinuses propel mucus out through these openings into the nasal cavity. When sinus openings are occluded, exudate accumulates within the sinus cavities. Occasionally sinusitis is the result of direct extension from a dental infection. Prolonged or untreated infections produce irreversible changes in the sinus mucosal lining so that sinus sterility can no longer be maintained.

Chronic sinusitis is the most common complication of acute sinusitis. Rare but serious complications include orbital cellulitis, brain abscess, and meningitis.[82]

Clinical Manifestations

Symptoms of acute sinusitis resemble those of acute rhinitis but are more severe (Table 28–1). Patients may complain of constant severe pain in the forehead, cheek and upper teeth, base of skull, or behind the eyes. Systemic symptoms such as fever, nausea, and malaise vary with the severity of the infection and host resistance and are often absent.

Palpation over the involved sinus produces tenderness even when pain may not be a symptom. Redness or swelling may occur over the involved sinus. Nasal congestion and mucopurulent or purulent discharge is noted if total obstruction of sinus drainage has not occurred. Sinus dullness or opacity is usually present when sinuses are transilluminated.

Chronic sinusitis may produce no symptoms or only a mild postnasal discharge, a fetid musty odor, or a nonproductive cough. Nasal obstruction and profuse purulent nasal and postnasal discharge may occur. When headache is present, it often improves later in the day as draining occurs.

Medical Management

Diagnosis is based on the history, presence of sinus tenderness, and at times on transillumination and sinus-film findings. In otherwise healthy persons with uncomplicated paranasal sinus infection, routine microbiologic studies are not usually necessary.[23,60] When bacteriologic studies are required, direct puncture and aspiration of the sinus cavity is necessary, since nasal discharge or throat cultures do not identify responsible bacteria accurately.[43]

Goals of medical therapy include control of bacterial pathogens and drainage of the infected sinuses. Because the sinuses are so close to the central nervous system and the orbit, prompt elimination of pathogens is desirable. Although the effectiveness of antibiotic therapy compared with that of local measures and decongestants alone remains controversial for acute sinusitis, most physicians believe antibiotics shorten the disease course and prevent complications.[28, 63] Drugs commonly used in acute sinusitis include ampicillin and trimethoprim–sulfamethoxazole (see Table 28–2).[60] Chronic sinusitis is generally treated with penicillin G or ampicillin.

To reduce mucosal edema and facilitate sinus drainage, decongestants are prescribed orally or topically. Analgesics such as acetylsalicylic acid or acetaminophen usually relieve pain adequately.

The purposes of sinus aspiration or sinus surgical procedures are to relieve pressure, to drain purulent material, and to obtain material for accurate Gram stain and culture. Surgical treatment is more often indicated for chronic sinusitis than for acute sinusitis. A submucous resection of an obstructing septum, removal of nasal polyps, or an intranasal antrotomy (trocar insertion through maxillary sinus wall) may be performed to promote drainage. Sinus irrigations of the antra (maxillary sinuses) with sterile warm normal saline or a Praetz displacement procedure (ethmoid and sphenoid sinuses) may also facilitate drainage.[23] If these more conservative treatments are ineffective, radical sinus surgery by the external approach, such as a Caldwell-Luc operation, may be considered, but infection usually complicates this surgery.[67]

Clinical symptoms, with the exception of cough, improve within 5 days and resolve in 10 to 15 days with appropriate antibiotics and drainage procedures. Radiographic changes and cough resolve more slowly over 3 to 6 weeks.[8]

Nursing Management

Assessment and Nursing Diagnosis

The health history should elicit information on allergies and other conditions that predispose to development of multiple episodes of acute or chronic sinusitis, such as nasal septal deviation or polyps, irritation from cocaine abuse, cigarette smoking, or prolonged nasogastric or nasotracheal intubation.[60]

The nursing diagnosis most frequently associated with sinusitis is alteration in comfort secondary to inflammation of the mucosa lining the paranasal sinuses. A less common diagnosis is potential for infection secondary to extension of sinus infection into the central nervous system.

Interventions

The goals of nursing interventions are to relieve pain and to prevent or recognize complications.

Persons with sinusitis are advised to reduce their normal activities until acute symptoms have subsided. There are no particular dietary restrictions, although persons with moderate to severe infections may be anorexic or nauseated and may benefit from easily digested high-calorie high-carbohydrate foods. Analgesics provide pain relief.

Nurses need to monitor hospitalized patients for signs of complications, and outpatients need to be taught to recognize these signs and symptoms. Indications for consulting a physician include the following: temperature over 102° F; severe headache not relieved by prescribed drugs or aspirin; chills; vomiting; any new or increased swelling over the face, especially the forehead, eyes, side of the nose or cheek; blurred vision; or a nose bleed.[37, 61]

Patients should know that no over-the-counter drugs should be combined with prescription medications. Irritants such as pollution, occupational dusts, and cigarette smoke should be avoided. Principles of drainage facilitation employing local warmth, adequate fluids, and proper use of medications and steam must be understood. Topical decongestants should be discontinued as soon as possible, preferably in less than 5 days.[57] The patient should be taught the proper way to blow his nose. The purpose and importance of keeping referral appointments for surgery to correct problems such as nasal polyps or deviated septum should also be understood.

Evaluation

Expected outcomes are that patients with sinusitis can

- Describe complications that should be reported to a health-care provider
- Report reduction in symptoms

Pharyngitis, Tonsillitis, and Laryngitis

Definitions

Pharyngitis is a general term that refers to inflammation of the pharynx. *Tonsillitis* refers to an inflammation of the tonsils, particularly the palatine tonsils on either side of the oropharynx. These tonsils are illustrated in Figure 28–2. *Laryngitis* refers to an inflammation of the laryngeal mucosa. Because the three problems frequently coexist, they are discussed together in this chapter.

Etiology

Acute pharyngitis often accompanies other viral upper respiratory tract disorders affecting the nose, sinuses, larynx, or trachea. A relatively common and important bacterial pharyngitis is caused by a group A β-hemolytic streptococci (*Streptococcus pyogenes*). The organism is usually transmitted from person to person and is much less common in adults than in children. *Chronic pharyngitis* may result from chronic nose or sinus infection or local irritation by alcohol, tobacco, or spicy foods. *Acute tonsillitis* is usually caused by a bacterial infection, often streptococci. *Acute laryngitis* may be produced by viral or bacterial infection; by irritants such as smoke, alcohol, or hot liquids; or by excessive use of the voice. *Chronic laryngitis* may follow repeated infections, allergic episodes, chronic irritant inhalation, or long-term vocal abuse.[23]

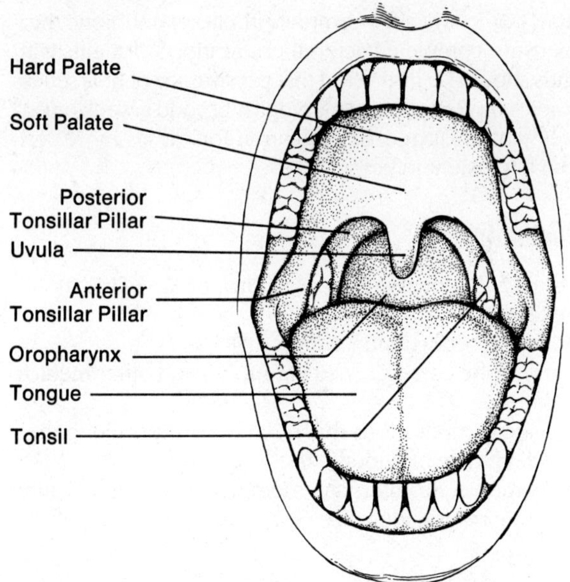

FIGURE 28–2 Anatomy of the mouth, as seen by intraoral examination. When inspecting the oropharynx, the patient should be asked to say, "Ah," which causes the soft palate to elevate; thus the pharynx can be better seen.

Pathophysiology

A wide range of inflammatory changes is possible. Viral infection frequently is characterized by a milder response than is bacterial infection.

Complications of bacterial pharyngitis and tonsillitis include extension to the middle ear (otitis media) or adjacent lymph nodes, acute sinusitits, peritonsillar abscess, or cervical lymph node extension and abscess. Less commonly, blood-borne extensions such as meningitis and pneumonia may occur.

Streptococcal infections may trigger poststreptococcal autoimmune phenomena, most commonly rheumatic fever or acute glomerulonephritis. Symptoms begin 1 to 4 weeks after the onset of infection. One streptococcal infection does not provide immunity from the development of a future one.

Laryngeal edema in small airways produces obstruction that is termed "croup." Because adults have larger airways, laryngeal edema in adults does not cause inspiratory stridor, dyspnea, or croup. Rarely, swelling of the epiglottis (epiglottitis), usually caused by infection with *H. influenzae,* may produce severe airway obstruction and necessitate immediate tracheotomy.

Clinical Manifestations

The clinical presentation of acute pharyngitis can vary from a minimal sore throat, low-grade fever, and slight hyperemia on examination in viral pharyngitis to the rapid onset of severe sore throat with high fever, malaise, tender cervical lymph nodes, and a red, slightly swollen mucus-covered pharyngeal wall in streptococcal infection.[95] When tonsillitis is present, the tonsils are red, swollen, and covered with pus. *S. pyogenes* releases an erythrogenic toxin that produces a generalized red sandpaper-like rash, which is called "scarlet fever." Chronic pharyngitis may produce a dry throat with mucus production and cough. Laryngitis is usually characterized by hoarseness, cough, dysphagia, and a dry sore throat.

Medical Management

Pharyngitis and tonsillitis are diagnosed by the clinical picture. When streptococci or other bacteria are suspected, throat cultures for these organisms are obtained. In viral infections the white blood cell count remains normal, whereas it may be elevated in bacterial infections. Examination of the larynx requires use of either a mirror, for indirect laryngoscopy, or a laryngoscope. In acute laryngitis the vocal cords are edematous and inflamed. With chronic inflammation, a thickened dull edematous mucosa is present.

Medical therapy is symptomatic unless antibiotics are needed for a bacterial infection. Streptococcal infection is treated with penicillin (see Table 28–2.) Although untreated streptococcal pharyngotonsillitis resolves spontaneously in 5 to 7 days, prompt antibiotic therapy prevents rheumatic fever, shortens the course of the disease, and reduces the chances of suppurative complications.[62] Beginning antibiotic therapy during the first week after infection will prevent the development of rheumatic fever.[60]

When chronic tonsillitis results from repeated or unresolved infection, surgical excision is considered. The mere presence of enlarged palatine tonsils and adenoids is not an indication for surgery. Although the value of and indications for adenotonsillectomy remain controversial, most surgeons agree that recurrent acute ear infections, recurrent or chronic infections of tonsils and adenoids despite adequate antibiotic therapy, or peritonsillar abscess necessitates removal of tonsils.

Nursing Management

Assessment and Nursing Diagnosis

In addition to assessing for physical manifestations of pharyngitis and tonsillitis, the nurse must be alert to indications of streptococcal infection.

When patients are assessed for laryngitis, it should be recognized that hoarseness occasionally is a manifestation of a more serious abnormality such as cancer of the larynx, vocal cord polyp, or noncarcinomatous ulceration. Careful determination of the length of symptoms is therefore important. Another condition that must be recognized is acute epiglottitis. Although this medical emergency is more common in children, it can occur in adults and should be suspected when there is severe sore throat along with drooling saliva. Because examination can induce complete airway occlusion from bronchospasm, the throat should not be examined *in any manner* when epiglottitis is suspected unless facilities for immediate intubation or tracheostomy are available.

Possible nursing diagnoses include

- Alteration in comfort related to sore throat
- Potential impaired verbal communication due to sore throat or vocal cord inflammation
- Fluid volume depletion (saline deficit and water deficit) secondary to fever and painful swallowing
- Potential cardiac and renal dysfunction secondary to poststreptococcal autoimmune disease

Goals. Nursing-care goals are to recognize group A streptococcal pharyngotonsillitis, to reduce complications, and to relieve discomfort.

Interventions

Recognition of Streptococcal Infection. Although the distinction between viral and streptococcal pharyngitis can sometimes be made by the greater severity of symptoms of streptococcal infection, there are so many exceptions that a definite diagnosis of streptococcal infection is possible only by throat culture. Throat cultures should also be obtained from all symptomatic family members and close contacts of patients with known streptococcal pharyngitis and from all asymptomatic contacts who have a history of rheumatic fever or who live in a community where a rheumatic fever outbreak exists.[50]

When antibiotics are prescribed for streptococcal infection, the patient needs to be counselled to use the full 10-day course to prevent rheumatic fever, even if his symptoms subside sooner. Patients should be advised to use measures to reduce disease spread (see Common Cold).

Symptom Relief. As long as a fever over 100° F is present, rest in a chair or bed is advisable. Return to activity is allowed within the limits of what the patient can comfortably tolerate. Foods or fluids that are chemically, thermally, or mechanically irritating should be avoided. High-protein high-calorie liquids such as soups or milk shakes are advisable, with solids added when they can be tolerated.

Analgesics such as aspirin or acetaminophen may be used to relieve the sore throat and fever. Local relief may be obtained with frequent gargles or throat irrigations using warm nonirritating liquids such as normal saline or 30% glucose. Oral aspirin as a gargle or aspirin-containing gum or an anesthetic spray may be prescribed to temporarily decrease pain. Adequate fluid intake and most inhalations may help relieve dryness. Oral hygiene measures and an ice collar to the neck may also provide symptomatic relief.

Complications. Patients should report a fever over 101° to 102° F or one that does not normalize in 1 to 2 days. Any new symptoms such as red painful joints, vomiting, earache, cough, skin rash, severe headache, or chest pain should be reported. Fever persisting more than 4 days after beginning antibiotic treatment for streptococcal pharyngitis, difficulty in swallowing, extreme tonsillar enlargement, or asymmetric tonsils or uvula suggests the complication of peritonsillar abscess. If an initial throat culture was positive for group A β-hemolytic streptococcus, a repeat culture may be taken 3 to 5 days after completion of oral antibiotic therapy to ensure complete bacterial eradication.[50] Patients with laryngitis should be instructed that persistence of hoarseness and other symptoms of acute laryngitis beyond a week or two requires further diagnostic evaluation for causes more serious than a transient infection.

Evaluation

Patients with pharyngitis, tonsillitis, or laryngitis should be able to

- Report reduction in symptoms
- Describe correct use of antibiotics and other medications
- State complications that need to be reported to their health-care provider
- Demonstrate alternate methods of communicating while resting the voice

Diphtheria

Definition and Etiology

Diptheria is an acute infection caused by the gram-positive bacillus *Corynebacterium diphtheriae.* It usually affects the respiratory tract but may involve any mucous membrane or skin. Diphtheria is usually transmitted by aerosolized droplets from carriers or persons with disease or by direct contact with infected skin. The disease remains communicable for 1 to 2 days after antibiotic therapy is initiated and for 2 to 4 weeks if untreated.

Now that diphtheria toxoid is available for immunization, the disease rate has declined to less than 100 cases/year in the United States.[49] The disease occurs more commonly in crowded conditions, explaining the higher prevalence in the winter. Native Americans, Mexican Americans, and blacks experience attack rates ten times higher than the rest of the population.[68]

Pathophysiology

C. diphtheriae colonizes and multiplies on mucosal and epithelial surfaces. Most commonly the upper respiratory tract is invaded (called tonsillar diphtheria), producing membrane inflammation and formation of a fibrous exudate. The potent toxin produced by the bacilli spreads throughout the body and produces complications such as peripheral neuritis, myocarditis, and respiratory failure.

The usual incubation period of diphtheria is 2 to 4 days. Pathology and clinical manifestations vary with the potency of toxin produced by the organism, the site of infection, and the host's immune function. Diphtheria that occurs in previously immunized persons is usually mild.

Clinical Manifestations

The onset of tonsillar diphtheria is sudden. A sore throat, which is almost always present, is usually the patient's main reason for seeking health care. The sore throat, fever, and malaise are followed rapidly by prostration and severe signs of toxemia. Cough, hoarseness, and dysphagia are present in about one fourth of patients.

Examination of the oropharynx reveals marked local inflammation with a thin, patchy, removable red exudate that is replaced within hours by a firmly adherent thick gray membrane. When diphtheria extends into cervical lymph glands and adjacent soft tissue, a "bull neck" appearance occurs.

Diphtheria can affect the skin without involving other areas. It presents as nonhealing ulcers on the face and extremities. These ulcers have raised margins, often involve underlying tissues, and may have a superimposed bacterial infection. If the nasal area is involved, a serosanguineous crusty discharge appears. Systemic, cardiac, and neurologic symptoms are rare when only the skin is involved.

Medical Management

A definite diagnosis of diphtheria depends upon culture of the organism and demonstration of toxin production using a gel-diffusion test. An elevated white blood cell count and proteinuria may be present if the toxin has caused systemic complications.

Because of the severity of untreated disease, treatment is often started based on suspicion of disease from history of exposure and immunization status, symptoms, and physical examination findings. When diphtheria is suspected, diphtheria antitoxin is administered after obtaining material for cultures. Since the antitoxin is effective only against free toxin and not against intracellular toxin, prompt antitoxin administration is essential. Prior to administering the antitoxin, patients must have skin or conjunctival tests with diluted antitoxin to detect allergy to horse serum. Antibiotics such as penicillin or erythromycin are also administered to prevent multiplication of the *C. diphtheriae* organisms at the infection site, to eliminate the carrier state, and to treat the frequent secondary infections with hemolytic streptococci.[39]

The prognosis in diphtheria varies with the age of the patient, the severity of the disease, and the promptness of antitoxin administration. The mortality rate of 10% to 30% is higher in older persons, more severe disease, and with delay in antitoxin administration.[68]

Nursing Management

Assessment and Nursing Diagnosis

Because patients with diphtheria are at risk for airway obstruction and for systemic damage caused by toxins, repeated assessment is essential.

Potential nursing diagnoses are many and include, in particular,

- Ineffective airway clearance secondary to obstruction by fibrous diphtherial membrane
- Decreased cardiac ouput secondary to myocarditis
- Alteration in comfort secondary to pharyngitis

Goals. Goals of nursing interventions are to prevent diphtheria by effective immunization, to prevent spread of the disease, and to maximize comfort and prevent complications in patients with the disease.

Interventions

Prevention. For continuous protection from diphtheria, adults should receive boosters of diphtheria–tetanus (Td) toxoid every 10 years after receiving an initial childhood series of five diphtheria–pertussis–tetanus (DPT) vaccinations. Prior to administration of a Td booster, the nurse should take a history of previous adverse reactions to diphtheria-tetanus immunizations. Since adults tend to have more severe, often systemic, reactions to the larger diphtheria doses in usual childhood toxoid (DPT, DT), only "adult-type" absorbed purified Td toxoid should be used for persons over 12 years of age. At the time of administration of toxoid, patients should be instructed in the duration of protection provided by booster immunization and side-effects to expect (sore arm for several days). Information on immunization dosage and date should be recorded on the patient's immunization record or on a wallet medical identification card. When tetanus toxoid is needed as a result of an injury, diphtheria–tetanus toxoid rather than tetanus toxoid alone should be administered if the patient's last Td booster was more than 10 years ago.

Care of Patients with Diphtheria. During antitoxin administration, the patient must be observed for symptoms of anaphylaxis, and epinephrine must be immediately available at the bedside. To prevent transmission of the disease, diphtheria patients are placed in strict isolation until antibiotic therapy is complete and three negative cultures of the lesion are reported. Contacts need to be identified, screened, and immunized or treated.

Patient activity is limited to absolute bed rest for at least 3 weeks until the danger of myocarditis has passed. A liquid to soft diet as tolerated, throat irrigations with hot saline or 30% glucose, and analgesics are often used. Fluids are encouraged. Oxygen and cool mist may be administered, and supportive care to prevent aspiration pneumonia is carried out.

Since diphtheria can rapidly progress to airway obstruction or other serious complications, careful nursing monitoring for disease progression or toxin effects is essential. Half of diphtheria deaths result from myocarditis. Patients with symptoms of this complication (hypotension and arrhythmias) require transfer to an intensive care unit for continuous cardiac monitoring and may need oxygen, as well as drugs to treat arrhythmias and shock.

Toxic involvement of the cranial nerves may produce signs such as nasal speech, strabismus, or inability to move the eyes. The toxin may progress to involve the motor intercostals and extremities.

Respiratory status monitoring is especially important for pharyngeal or laryngeal diphtheria. Suction equipment should be at the bedside and used as necessary. Because infection can progress to airway obstruction so rapidly, a tracheostomy may be done when either the clinical picture or indirect laryngoscopy suggest laryngeal involvement. Mechanical respiratory support may also be needed.

Evaluation

When nursing goals relative to diphtheria have been met, people at risk for diphtheria will report plans to obtain current diphtheria vaccination. Patients with diphtheria will

- Be free of respiratory, cardiovascular, and other complications as manifested by patent airway, heart rate and blood pressure within normal limits, and normal neurological findings
- Report a decrease in pharyngitis and other symptoms.

Inflammatory and Other Restrictive Disorders of the Lower Airway

It is important for the nurse to understand whether the nature of a patient's pulmonary disease is restrictive, obstructive, or mixed, because the patient problems and nursing interventions will differ accordingly. In restrictive respiratory tract disorders, the total lung capacity is reduced. The volumes measured by pulmonary function tests may be less than those normally predicted for a person of the patient's age, sex, and height. The characteristic differences in pulmonary function test findings between restrictive versus obstructive disease are described more fully in Chapter 26.

Table 28–4 lists examples of restrictive lung disease according to etiologic category. In most cases the elastic properties of lung tissue are intrinsically altered such that the lungs become abnormally stiff (lower compliance) and an increased work of breathing results. Severe inflammatory conditions involving the gas-exchange region of the lung commonly produce this type of restrictive disease. A small group of patients have extrinsic rather than intrinsic lung disease. In these cases the disease affects the chest wall respiratory muscles or pleura and results in a lowered lung capacity. In the remainder of this chapter some of the more common causes of restrictive lung disease are discussed.

The first lower-airway disorder to be discussed, acute bronchitis, is an exception to the other lower-airway disorders that are discussed in the remainder of this chapter. Acute bronchitis affects only the airways and does not reduce the elasticity of lung tissue. As a result, it causes an obstructive rather than restrictive pattern of disease.

TABLE 28–4
Examples of Restrictive Lung Disease According to Etiologic Category

Extrinsic

- Skeletal
  - Kyphoscoliosis
  - Ankylosing spondylitis
  - Pectus excavatum
  - Crush chest
- Pleural
  - Pleural effusion
  - Fibrothorax
  - Pneumothorax
- Neuromuscular
  - Cord transection
  - Diaphragmatic paralysis
  - Myasthenia gravis, muscular dystrophy, amyotrophic lateral sclerosis

Intrinsic

- Interstitial alveolar
  - Infectious: pneumonias, tuberculosis, fungal infections
  - Neoplastic: Hodgkin's disease, bronchioalveolar carcinoma
  - Thromboembolic: fat embolism, pulmonary embolism
  - Cardiovascular: pulmonary edema
  - Mixed connective tissue: lupus erythematosus, scleroderma, rheumatoid lung
- Inhalational
  - Organic dusts: farmer's lung (hay fungus), pigeon breeder's disease, bagassosis (sugarcane or hemp fibers), byssinosis (cotton dust)
  - Inorganic dusts: silicosis, asbestosis, coal worker's pneumoconiosis, berylliosis, siderosis
  - Toxic: smoke inhalation, oxygen toxicity, aspiration pneumonia
- Airway disease: small airway disease
- Idiopathic granuloma: sarcoidosis, eosinophilic granuloma, Wegener's granuloma, Goodpasture's syndrome
- Drug toxicity: methotrexate, busulfan
- Idiopathic interstitial fibrosis: interstitial pneumonia

Acute Bronchitis

Etiology and Pathophysiology

Acute bronchitis is an inflammation of the bronchi. Most episodes of bronchitis are caused by viral infection, although secondary bacterial infection may exacerbate or prolong the symptoms. Other causes include inhalation of smoke, dust, or chemical irritants; high levels of air pollution; and, in young adults, *Mycoplasma pneumoniae*.[40, 59] In hosts with impaired defenses or, more rarely, in normal hosts with especially virulent organisms, acute bronchitis can be complicated by progression to bronchopneumonia.

Clinical Manifestations

A person with acute bronchitis usually has a cough and muscular-type chest pain. Mucoid or purulent sputum production may occur along with fever and chills. Unless there is preexisting underlying disease, dyspnea does not usually accompany bronchitis. The severity of symptoms is influenced by the causative agent. Fever is usually under 101° F. Physical examination may reveal normal breath sounds or scattered rhonchi and wheezes that reflect bronchial secretions and spasm.

Medical Management

The clinical distinction between bronchitis and pneumonia is based mainly on the physical examination. Sputum cultures usually yield common mouth organisms without a predominant pathogen. Chest films are usually unnecessary unless the clinical assessment is unclear, in which case the chest film does not show the parenchymal involvement that is found in pneumonia.

Since bacteria are rarely primary causes of bronchitis, antibiotics are usually unnecessary.[63] However, in certain debilitated patients or those with impaired respiratory function, antibiotics may be administered to prevent secondary bacterial infections.

Patients with underlying asthma may need bronchodilator medication during the course of an acute bronchitis episode. Antitussive or expectorant medications may be prescribed.

Nursing Management

Assessment and Nursing Diagnosis

While bronchitis may be a minor disorder for most persons, it can be life-threatening for those with underlying cardiopulmonary problems. The health history and patient examination need to include information on underlying health problems as well as documentation of the presence or absence of signs and symptoms of bronchitis or its complication of pneumonia. The amount and character of sputum can give a clue to viral (mucopurulent; less than 2 tbsp/day) or bacterial bronchitis (purulent; more than 2 tbsp/day).[50]

Nursing diagnoses that may apply in this condition include

- Alteration in comfort related to bronchial inflammation
- Potential impaired gas exchange related to secondary development of pneumonia
- Knowledge deficit related to symptom relief or recognition of complications

Goals. Goals of nursing interventions are to prevent further bronchial irritation, to relieve symptoms, and to prevent extension of the infection.

Interventions

Because most patients with bronchitis are treated on an ambulatory basis, a primary nursing intervention is patient education regarding appropriate self-care measures for the current disease and measures to prevent its recurrence. Smokers should be advised to quit. Symptomatic relief is provided using measures similar to those for the common cold and pharyngitis. Rest, a well-balanced diet, avoiding exposure to further irritants or infections, and measures to promote secretion clearance are advised.

If antibiotics are prescribed, patients need to understand the purpose and dosage of the medicine, side-effects to report, and the importance of completing the entire course of the antibiotic even if symptoms have cleared.

Patients and family should be instructed not to delay seeking further health care for worsening symptoms such as unremitting fever, dyspnea, or drowsiness.

Evaluation

Patients should be able to

- State components of self-care including clearance of secretions, use of prescription and over-the-counter medications
- List symptoms to report to a health-care provider
- Describe preventive measures to avoid recurrent infection

Pneumonia

Definition

Pneumonia is an inflammatory process affecting the lung parenchyma. Despite medical advances, pneumonia is the fifth most common cause of death in the United States. Pneumococcal pneumonia alone accounts for 30,000 annual deaths.[53] Bacterial pneumonia, with a 20% to 30% mortality rate, remains the most common infectious cause of death in the United States.

Etiology

Lung infections are labeled by their etiologic agent, the host reaction (*e.g.*, classic or atypical), and the extent of anatomical involvement. Infections involving only the alveoli in contact with bronchioles are labeled *bronchopneumonia,* whereas infections affecting entire lobes are labeled *lobar pneumonia* (Fig. 28–3). Although pneumonia, like bronchitis, may be caused by inhaled noxious chemical irritants, most often it is caused by microorganisms that are inhaled or aspirated. Causative organisms can be fungal, viral, protozoal, or bacterial. Bacterial agents are further classified as anaerobic or aerobic, and gram-positive or gram-negative.

Much of the pneumonia in adults is caused by bacteria. Up to 80% of community-acquired pneumonia is caused by *Streptococcus pneumoniae* (the pneumococcus), while gram-negative bacteria, often antibiotic-resistant, cause most pneumonia in hospitalized patients.[14, 53] In aspiration pneumonia, the organisms are usually the mixed anaerobic and aerobic flora of the upper respiratory tract. Influenza and varicella are the most common viral causes of pneumonia in adults.

Organisms that do not cause pneumonia in persons with normal lung defenses may often cause life-threatening infections in immunosuppressed hosts. For example, patients with COPD are at risk of pneumonia from *H. influenzae* and *Legionella pneumophilia* (Legionnaire's disease). Fungal and protozoal infections also can cause pneumonia in compromised hosts.

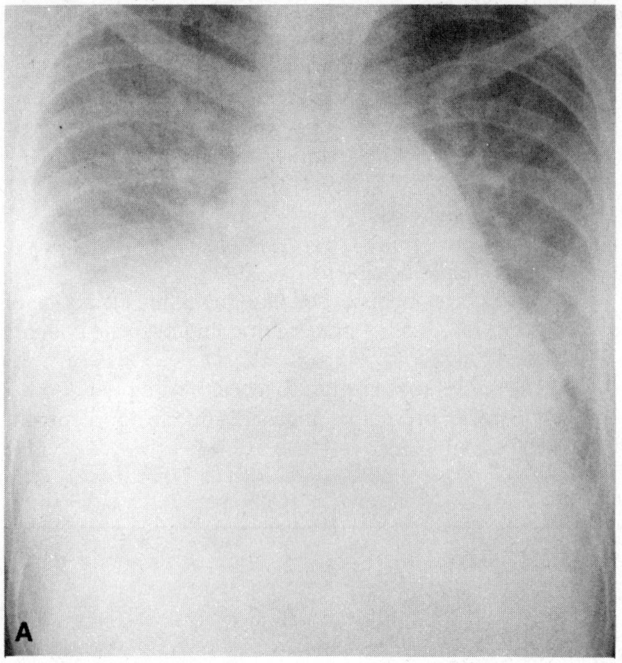

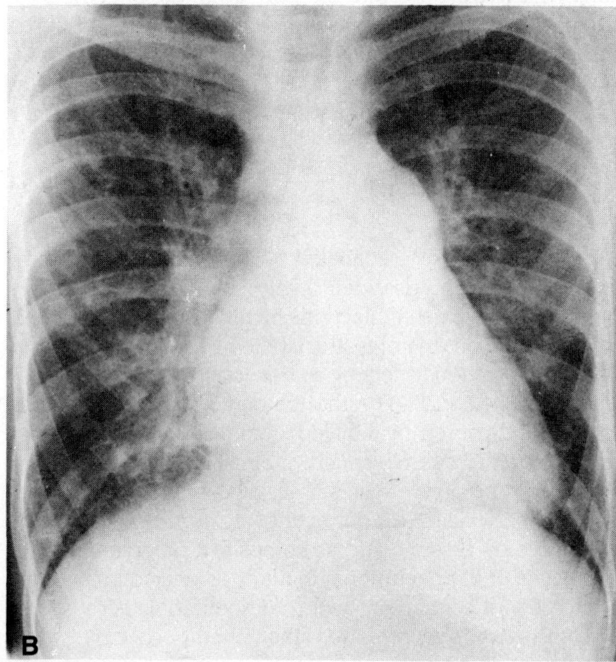

FIGURE 28–3 (*A*) Right lobar pneumonia. Note the consolidation of the right lower lobe. The left lung field is essentially normal. (*B*) Complete resolution of the pneumonia after 2 weeks of antibiotic therapy. (Department of Radiology, Methodist Hospital of Brooklyn)

Pathophysiology

When normal lung-clearance mechanisms are overwhelmed by an inoculum of bacteria, a classic inflammatory response occurs (see Chap. 15). An exudate of fibrin-containing fluid, bacteria, polymorphonuclear leukocytes, and erythrocytes fills the alveoli and may enhance further bacterial growth and spread.

The extent of pulmonary dysfunction caused by pneumonia varies according to the severity of the disease and the person's previous lung function. In pneumonia, some alveoli are underventilated while others are collapsed or fluid-filled. Although pulmonary vessels constrict in areas of alveolar hypoxemia, some blood flow continues and returns to the heart unoxygenated. Most but not all pneumonias are accompanied by hypoxemia, which is due to this shunt effect and to the increased work of breathing that accompanies reduced lung compliance from fluid-filled alveoli.

Normally hyperventilation accompanies pneumonia, resulting in a lowered blood carbon dioxide level Pa_{CO_2}. However, mucus plugs, pleuritic pain, and fatigue can all contribute to reduced ventilation and result in elevated Pa_{CO_2} levels in persons with preexisting lung disease.

Bacteremia occurs in over 25% of patients with pneumococcal pneumonia. Other, less common, complications include meningitis, pleural effusion, empyema, endocarditis, and pericarditis.

Aspiration of material into the lower airways produces varying results, depending upon the substance aspirated. Aspiration of even small amounts of gastric acid causes an immediate severe reaction consisting of bronchospasm, interstitial and alveolar edema, and hypoxemia. Aspiration of large amounts of inert liquids such as water, barium, or tube-feeding liquids causes little chemical injury but may obstruct the airways.

If the invading bacteria contain no virulence factors that cause tissue necrosis or ischemia, healing after pneumonia is generally accompanied by restoration of interalveolar septa and airways to their normal states. Pneumonias caused by organisms such as staphylococcus or *Klebsiella* are accompanied by tissue necrosis, which may progress to abscess formation or heal with scarring or fibrosis.

Untreated pneumococcal pneumonia has a mortality rate of 20% to 40%, and untreated *Klebsiella* pneumonia 40% to 60%. With adequate early antimicrobial therapy, the fatality rate of pneumococcal pneumonia is 5% to 10% and of *Klebsiella* near 30%. The most frequent causes of death are shock and pulmonary edema.[53]

Clinical Manifestations

Typical Pneumonia. The clinical manifestations of pneumonia vary with the infecting organism and the host's condition. The classic or "typical" presentation of bacterial pneumonia involves a sudden onset of shaking chills, high fever, pleuritic chest pain, and cough productive of greenish or rusty purulent spututm. The pain is worse with respiration and is sometimes referred to the shoulder or abdomen. To splint the pain, the patient may lie on his affected side. Abdominal distention, nausea, and vomiting may occur.

On examination the patient has fever, tachycardia, shallow respirations (30–40/min), and possibly nasal flaring, accessory muscle use, and cyanosis. Orthopnea is usually not present. Auscultation of the affected area reveals diminished breath sounds and fine crackles initially but later reveals signs of consolidation as indicated by bronchial breath sounds.

Organisms causing this classic presentation in adults include *S. pneumoniae, H. influenzae, Staphylococcus aureus,* and *Klebsiella pneumoniae.*

Atypical Pneumonia. Pneumonia caused by organisms such as viruses or *mycoplasma pneumoniae* (organism intermediate between bacterium and virus) often presents in a different manner. The onset of this atypical pneumonia syndrome is gradual, with 3 to 4 days of general malaise, headache, sore throat, earache, rash, and dry nonproductive cough. Later, the cough may become productive of mucoid sputum. Chest soreness from coughing occurs more commonly than does pleuritic pain. Lung examination may reveal crackles but not evidence of consolidation. Fever, shaking chills, and respiratory distress may be present. Pneumonia caused by *L. pneumophilia* has features of an atypical syndrome, often with nausea, vomiting, diarrhea, and confusion.[90]

Even when the infecting organisms are bacteria that usually produce a classic syndrome, a blunted response may occur in elderly, debilitated, immunosuppressed, or alcohol-addicted persons. The presentation in these patients resembles an atypical pneumonia or may evidence even fewer clues to the underlying pneumonia. At times, lethargy or agitation, with or without fever, may be the only sign of infection.

Aspiration Pneumonia. Aspiration pneumonia often results in an indolent, localized anaerobic bacterial process with a gradual onset of low-grade fever and cough over several days to weeks. Later, copious foul-smelling sputum is expectorated. Because more virulent organisms are present in hospitals, aspiration pneumonia in this setting often begins more abruptly and has a more severe course.[32]

Medical Management

Diagnosis. The single most useful diagnostic test in pneumonia is the sputum Gram stain, which must be obtained before antibiotic therapy is started.[13] It requires obtaining a true sputum (*not spit*) specimen, a difficult task at times. Expectoration, the traditional method of obtaining sputum, is often unreliable because the specimen is contaminated with multiple normal flora during passage through the oropharynx, and cultures yield "mixed flora overgrowth," obscuring the real pathogen. If the patient is unable to produce sputum by supervised coughing, induction of sputum with an ultrasonic nebulizer or nasotracheal suctioning is attempted.

A chest film that shows evidence of consolidation is considered diagnostic of pneumonia. However, a normal film may be present early in the disease course or in dehydrated patients. Additional diagnostic tests are performed as indicated by the patient's condition. Arterial blood-gas measurements are obtained if severe pneumonia or bronchospasm is present. The white blood cell count is usually elevated to a greater degree in bacterial than in atypical pneumonia. A rapid direct-staining immunofluorescent technique may be used to search for *L. pneumophilia* in sputum.

Blood samples for culture are important in the elderly or in persons with signs of sepsis or other complications. If pleural fluid is present, thoracentesis is performed.

Medical Treatment. Pneumonia is usually treated with antimicrobial drugs (Table 28–5). The decision regarding choice of drug is based on knowledge of the likely organism, Gram stain results, the clinical severity of infection, the presence of underlying disease in the patient, and the presence of complications.[19]

Except where mixed organisms or overwhelming infection of unknown etiology is present, combination antibiotic therapy is avoided. Drugs such as trimethoprim–sulfamethoxazole or pentamidine are used for protozoal infections such as *Pneumocystis carinii,* amphotericin B is used for fungal pneumonia, and antiviral agents such as amantadine are used for viral pneumonias. The antibiotic choice is reevaluated when culture and sensitivity results are available. The patient's condition is then monitored for improvement, toxicity, or need for therapy reevaluation. Other therapeutic measures such as oxygen administration, analgesia, and hydration are discussed under nursing interventions.

Prognosis. The course of recovery varies with the etiologic agent, the host's condition, and the therapy provided. If untreated, the symptoms persist until a "crisis" (time temperature begins to fall rapidly) occurs, usually in 7 to 10 days. Response to therapy usually occurs within 24 to 48 hours and is accompanied by gradual reduction in clinical manifestations as the pneumonia resolves. In atypical pneumonias, fever and cough may persist for up to 6 weeks. Clearance of the infiltrate shown on the chest film often occurs weeks after clinical recovery.

Nursing Management

Assessment and Nursing Diagnosis

Nurses must identify patients at high risk for pneumonia so that aggressive measures to prevent its development can be used.

Conditions that interfere with major lung defenses and therefore predispose to pneumonia are listed in Table 28–6. The normal protective flora of the upper respiratory tract changes in sick and hospitalized patients, increasing their risk of infection.[54, 71] Hospitalized patients are also exposed to more virulent and antibiotic-resistant microbes. Patients with extended stays in the intensive care unit, laryngeal or pharyngeal surgery, or endotracheal intubation are at highest risk for nosocomial pneumonia. Bacterial aspiration pneumonia is often not accompanied by observed aspiration but is known to occur in the elderly, in debilitated persons with impaired cough or swallowing mechanisms, or in patients with any disorder of consciousness.

Characteristics of sputum affect its ease of clearance. Dry sputum moves with more difficulty. Purulent sputum is more

TABLE 28–5
Initial Antibiotic Therapy of Pneumonia in Adults

Infectious Agent	*Drug(s) of Choice*
Classic syndrome	
Streptococcus pneumoniae, uncomplicated	Penicillin G procaine, 300,000 units IM q8h; aqueous crystalline penicillin G 400,000 units IV q6h; penicillin V 250 mg PO q6h
S. pneumoniae, complicated (empyema), metastatic infection	Penicillin G, 3–4 million units IV q4–6h
Hemophilus influenzae	Ampicillin, 1–2 g IV q4–6h
Staphylococcus aureus	Nafcillin, 1.5 g IV q4h
S. aureus, "methicillin-resistant"	Vancomycin, 1 g IV q12h
Klebsiella pneumoniae	Cefazolin, 1 g IV q6h plus aminoglycoside (gentamicin or tobramycin 1.7 mg/kg/8 hr)
Atypical syndrome	
Mycoplasma pneumoniae	Erythromycin, 500 mg q6h
Legionella pneumophilia	Erythromycin, 500–1000 mg q6h
Aspiration syndromes	
Mixed anaerobic/aerobic pharyngeal flora, uncomplicated	Penicillin G, 1 million units IV q4–6h
Mixed anaerobic/aerobic flora with empyema or abscess	Penicillin G, 3–4 million units IV q4–6h
Anaerobic with suspected gram-negative aerobe	Penicillin G, as above, plus gentamicin or tobramycin
Anaerobic with *S. aureus*	Clindamycin, 600 mg IV q6h
Hematogenous syndromes	
S. aureus	Nafcillin as above
Escherichia coli	Ampicillin, 1.5 g IV q4h plus gentamicin or tobramycin
Septic emboli from pelvic or enteric source	Clindamycin, 600 mg IV q6h plus gentamicin or tobramycin

(Adapted from Frame PT: Acute infectious pneumonia in the adult. Basics Respir Dis 10:7, 1982)

viscous and less elastic. Situations characterized by ineffective cough, such as postoperative pain, endotracheal tubes, tracheostomies, and debility predispose to aspiration pneumonia.

Patients with immunologic defects are at increased risk of pneumonia for a number of reasons. Use of corticosteroids reduces bacterial clearance from the lungs, reducing the number and phagocytic ability of macrophages. In cancer, both cell-mediated immunity and the absolute number of granulocytes are reduced by malnutrition, chemotherapy, and radiation therapy. This reduces the support that macrophages receive from white blood cells to combat infectious organisms, especially increasing the risk of viral, fungal, and parasitic infections.

Both alcoholics and smokers have impaired ciliary function and macrophage function. Alcoholics have abnormal pharyngeal flora and an increased aspiration risk related to the episodic neurological depression from alcohol.

Respiratory viral infections damage ciliated epithelium and paralyze intracellular bacteriocidal capabilities of macrophages. About half of the patients who develop the two most common adult pneumonias, pneumococcal and *Hemo-*

TABLE 28-6
Conditions that Predispose to Pneumonia Development

Excessive sputum
Ineffective cough
Altered level of consciousness
Primary or acquired immune deficiency
Debility or chronic disease
Smoking
Alcoholism
Malnutrition
Hospitalization (altered oropharyngeal flora)
Upper respiratory tract infection
Old age

philus influenzae, have viral infections before they develop the bacterial pneumonia.

Nurses must also be alert for early signs of pneumonia so that specific therapy can be initiated early.

Nursing Diagnoses. A possible nursing diagnosis for a patient at risk of pneumonia is potential for parenchymal lung infection (pneumonia) related to aspiration of oropharyngeal or gastric secretions, contamination of respiratory equipment, or impaired host defenses. Many nursing diagnoses might be applicable for patients with pneumonia, such as

- Alteration in comfort: pain, dyspnea related to inflammation of lung parenchyma and pleura
- Ineffective airway clearance related to excessive tracheobronchial secretions, pleuritic pain
- Impaired gas exchange related to shunt
- Potential bacteremia or other systemic infection related to spread of infection beyond lung parenchyma
- Fluid volume deficit (water deficit and saline deficit) related to increased insensible and respiratory fluid loss

See the accompanying Nursing Care Plan for the Patient with Pneumonia.

Goals. In a susceptible patient, the goal of nursing care is to prevent the development of pneumonia. For patients with pneumonia, nursing goals are to relieve symptoms and to prevent deterioration in the patient's health status.

Interventions

Health Promotion. Prevention of pneumonia is accomplished by activities directed toward reducing acquisition of organisms, suppressing colonizing organisms, and improving host defenses. Since respiratory equipment is a frequent source of gram-negative bacilli such as *Pseudomonas aeruginosa,* equipment with reservoir nebulizers such as home humidifiers and cool-mist nebulizers should be cleaned periodically and used only when clinically essential. In hospitals, careful handwashing and elimination of solutions in open containers are essential to prevent the spread of virulent, often antibiotic-resistant, organisms. Screening of visitors and personnel with respiratory tract infections will also reduce exposure to organisms. Invasive procedures such as suctioning should be done only as a last resort.

Once present, colonizing organisms are suppressed by several activities. Good oral hygiene, including brushing and flossing the teeth, reduces the number of microbes in the oropharynx. Measures to prevent aspiration in high-risk patients must be applied, such as correct positioning, monitoring ability to swallow and handle secretions, and feeding and administering nasogastric tube feedings using correct procedures and with the head of the bed elevated. Antacids or hydrochloric acid antagonists (cimetidine) may be prescribed to neutralize gastric acidity and reduce the severity of potential aspiration of stomach contents. If aspiration is observed, suctioning or bronchoscopy should be performed, but it does not remove all aspirate.

Host defenses can be improved by adequate nutrition, vaccination with influenza and pneumococcal vaccines, smoking cessation, and prudent use of drugs, such as alcohol, corticosteroids, oxygen, narcotics, and cough suppressants that depress bronchopulmonary defenses.[7] Since many pneumonias are preceded by viral infections such as influenza, persons with chronic disease or those older than 65 should receive annual influenza vaccination. A vaccine containing polysaccharides from 23 types of pneumococcal pneumonia common in the United States is also available, but its indications for use remain controversial.[18,48,66] Current recommendations from the Centers for Disease Control (CDC) and manufacturers include immunizing healthy adults over 65 years old and younger adults with chronic conditions such as sickle cell anemia, chronic bronchopulmonary, cardiac, or renal disease, and those whose spleens have been removed. Revaccination is not recommended.

Supportive Interventions. Supportive care interventions for patients with pneumonia include those appropriate for persons with a fever. Pharmacologic and physical measures may be used to lower a fever. However, phagocytosis seems to be favored at high temperatures, and there is a trend toward less aggressive fever control. Rest is needed to reduce oxygen demand, but regular deep breathing, active and passive leg exercises, and frequent position changes (every 1–2 hours at least) to reduce the risk of pulmonary embolism and to prevent further atelectasis must be carried out. Depending upon the lung areas involved, positioning with the good lung down or in the prone or high-semi Fowler's position can improve oxygenation compared with that achieved with the supine position.[38] When one lung is affected, turning from the unaffected side to the back with the involved side up can allow more equal ventilation/perfusion matching and thus reduce shunt and hypoxemia.

To improve gas exchange and facilitate resolution of the infection, secretions are cleared from the airway using the components of bronchial hygiene discussed in Chapter 27. In pneumonia, fluid losses occur through diaphoresis and increased metabolic and respiratory rates. Adequate hydration is best achieved by encouraging oral fluids within the limits of the patient's cardiac and renal function. Fluid intake;

(*Text continues on page 371*)

NURSING CARE PLAN FOR THE PATIENT WITH PNEUMONIA

NURSING DIAGNOSIS 1: Impaired gas exchange related to shunt
Manifested by decreared Pa_{O_2}, decreased arterial pH, and signs of impaired gas exchange such as irritability, decreased mental acuity, tachycardia, tachypnea, fatigue, and somnolence

GOAL 1.1: To maximize gas exchange and maintain oxygenation of vital organs

Nursing Interventions	Rationale	Outcome Criteria
1. During acute illness, keep patient on bed rest.	1. Rest reduces oxygen needs of vital organs.	1–8. Pa_{O_2} within normal limits for the patient's age and baseline lung function: a. 95–100 mmHg for young adults b. 75–80 mmHg for elderly adults c. 60 mmHg for patients with chronic obstructive pulmonary disease Pa_{CO_2} 35–45 mmHg or at patient's baseline Arterial pH betveen 7.35 and 7.45
a. Assist patient to exercise legs.	a. Leg exercises reduce venous stasis and risk of thromboembolism, which would aggravate hypoxemia.	
b. Turn patient frequently.	b. Movement in bed reduces complications of immobility such as atelectaris, which could worsen gas exchange.	
c. Position patient to maximize ventilation and blood flow to healthy lung tissue.	c. Pa_{O_2} usually best when patient positioned with healthy lung down.	
d. Monitor effect of position change on ABGs.	d. Depending on location and extent of disease, patient may not be able to tolerate some positions.	
2. During convalescence, assist patient to gradually increase ambulation and other activities.	2. Activity reduces cardiovascular deconditioning and promotes return of strength.	
3. Assist patient to take, and hold, 5–10 deep breaths hourly (can be done with incentive spirometer).	3. Sustained deep breaths, to total lung capacity, help re-expand collapsed alveoli.	
4. Assist patient to clear tracheobronchial secretions (see Nursing Diagnosis 2).	4. Accumulated secretions reduce alveolar ventilation and contribute to hypoxemia and increased work of breathing.	
5. Reduce fever over 101° F with antipyretics, tepid sponging.	5. High fever increases oxygen demands of body tissues.	
6. Administer prescribed antibiotics at correct dose and interval.	6. Antibiotic therapy speeds resolution of bacterial pneumonia, thereby leading to improved gas exchange.	
7. Maintain delivery of oxygen at correct liter flow.	7. Removal of oxygen cannula or mark can caure hypoxemia.	
8. Monitor patient for signs of worsened hypoxemia, hypercapnia (acute respiratory failure).	8. Clinical signs suggest need for change in treatment (confirm with ABGs).	

(*Continued*)

NURSING CARE PLAN FOR THE PATIENT WITH PNEUMONIA *(Continued)*

NURSING DIAGNOSIS 2: Ineffective airway clearance related to excessive tracheobronchial secretions, pleuritic pain
Manifested by rhonchi, wheezes, increased tactile fremitus, or change in color or amount of sputum

GOAL 2.1: To maintain clear airway

Nursing Interventions	Rationale	Outcome Criteria
1. Assist patient to cough effectively.	1. Coughing clears airways of excessive secretions.	1–4. Absence of or reduction in rhonchi, wheezes, tactile fremitus; normalization of sputum color, amount
a. Administer analgesic before having patient cough.	a. Pain limits ability to generate effective cough.	
b. Help patient to sit or lie on side with knees flexed.	b. Effective cough requires a body position that allows deep inspiration and forceful abdominal contraction.	
2. Encourage fluids, 2000–3000 cc daily (ree Nursing Diagnosis 5).	2. Hydration is believed to reduce sputum viscosity.	
3. Administer chest physical therapy to patient with retained secretions and weak cough.	3. Gravity and other mechanical factors may help to dislodge secretions and make them easier to cough out.	
4. Remove secretions by tracheal suction if patient is unable to clear them by coughing.	4. Tracheal suction removes secretion in central airways but should be a last resort because of risks of hypoxemia and infection.	

NURSING DIAGNOSIS 3: Alteration in comfort: pain, dyspnea, related to inflammation of lung parenchyma and pleura
Manifested by subjective reports of pain and breathlessness and by observations of strained expression, reluctance to cough and move, or interrupted speech pattern

GOAL 3.1: To relieve pain

Nursing Interventions	Rationale	Outcome Criteria
1. Administer prescribed analgesics for pain.	1. Pain control is necessary so that patient can rest and comply with treatment measures.	1. Patient reports decreased pain.
2. Administer prercribed ethyl chloride spray to painful areas on chest.	2. Local pain relief may permit patient to deep breathe, cough, and move.	2. Patient can cooperate with coughing, turning, and other therapy.
3. Use nonpharmacologic means of pain control: distraction, positioning.	3. Nonpharmacologic measures can block transmission of pain impulses.	

GOAL 3.2: To relieve dyspnea

Nursing Interventions	Rationale	Outcome Criteria
1. Allow patient to choose position of comfort; monitor effects of position on ABGs.	1. Work of breathing is reduced in certain positions.	1. Patient reports decreased dyspnea. Patient can cooperate with coughing, turning, and other therapy.
2. If patient is hypoxemic, administer oxygen at prescribed liter flow.	2. Hypoxemia may cause tachypnea and aggravate sensation of breathlessness.	
3. Assist with feeding, bathing, and other personal care when patient is acutely ill.	3. Reducing work for patient reduces dyspnea.	

(Continued)

NURSING CARE PLAN FOR THE PATIENT WITH PNEUMONIA (*Continued*)

NURSING DIAGNOSIS 4: Potential bacteremia or other systemic infection related to spread of infection beyond lung parenchyma
Manifested by tachycardia, hypotension, decreased urine output, altered level of consciousness, sustained high fever, or chills

GOAL 4.1: To contain infection within lungs and prevent dissemination to other body systems

Nursing Interventions	Rationale	Outcome Criteria
1. Administer prescribed antibiotics at correct dose and interval.	1. Antibiotics speed resolution of bacterial pneumonia and decrease likelihood of organism spread.	1–6. Chest x-ray reveals resolution of pneumonia. Vital signs and urine output are within normal limits.
2. Assist patient to clear tracheobronchial secretions (see Nursing Diagnosis 2).	2. Retained secretions may provide medium for continued microorganism growth.	
3. Provide frequent mouth care.	3. Mouth care reduces the number of microorganisms that can be aspirated.	
4. Position to prevent aspiration.	4. Aspiration of oropharyngeal bacteria is associated with development of pneumonia.	
5. Encourage well-balanced diet of at least 1800 cal (liquids, solids, or total parenteral nutrition).	5. Good nutritional status enhances ability of body defenses to fight infection.	
6. Monitor patient for early evidence of systemic infection and report signs promptly so that blood cultures can be obtained.	6. Systemic infection may be more readily treated if detected early.	

NURSING DIAGNOSIS 5: Fluid volume deficit (water deficit and saline deficit) related to increased insensible and respiratory fluid loss
Manifested by increased serum sodium (water deficit) and postural hypotension (saline deficit)

GOAL 5.1: To maintain normal body fluid osmolality and circulating blood volume

Nursing Interventions	Rationale	Outcome Criteria
1. Monitor fluid status. a. *Water balance:* Increased serum sodium value and weight loss indicate water deficit. b. *Saline balance:* Postural blood pressure drop, weight loss, decreased urine output indicate saline deficit.	1. Correct fluid replacement is based on assessment of type and extent of loss.	1–2. Serum sodium value within normal range; absence of postural blood pressure drop.
2. Administer fluid replacement (oral or intravenous) as needed to replace water and saline loss. a. *Water deficit:* Oral "free" water, intravenous 5% dextrose in water b. *Saline deficit:* Oral or intravenous saline-containing solutions	2. Increased fluid intake is needed to replace insensible and respiratory fluid losses.	

urine color, specific gravity, and amount (over 1000 ml–1500 ml/24 hr); skin turgor; weight; and secretion consistency can be monitored to assess the need for intravenous or supplemental fluids.

Chest physiotherapy and intermittent positive pressure breathing (IPPB) are unproven adjuncts to secretion clearance.[36] Chest physiotherapy does continue to have advocates because antibiotics cannot combat infections unless the area is drained, and gravity may be necessary to raise secretions to a level at which cough can be effective.

When pleuritic pain is present, it may be relieved using local ethyl chloride spray or injected analgesia. Since cough promotes clearance of airway secretions, it is usually not suppressed. If abdominal distention is present because of air swallowing, a rectal tube or neostigmine methylsulfate may be ordered to provide decompression.

Initially the dyspneic patient with pneumonia is often anorexic, and a liquid diet is preferred. With improvement a normal diet will be tolerated. Enough calories are needed daily to offset the catabolic effect of the infection.

When hypoxemia is present ($Pa_{O_2} < 60$ mmHg), oxygen is administered to correct arterial oxygen levels to 60 mmHg to 70 mmHg. Oral temperatures can usually be taken accurately without removing the mask or nasal cannula.[26, 46]

Patients with pneumonia require careful and continuous monitoring until their clinical condition improves. In addition to monitoring for response to therapy and drug allergies or side-effects, the nurse must be alert to signs and symptoms of complications. For example, antibiotic treatment of a primary bacterial pneumonia often changes normal flora and facilitates the development of serious secondary gram-negative pulmonary infections.[19] Regardless of the cause, pneumonia, if severe enough, can result in acute respiratory failure (see Chap 32). It is important to monitor vital signs, breath sounds, and observe for signs of hypoxemia or hypercarbia frequently. Increased pulse rate, altered thinking, fall in blood pressure, and oliguria may herald septic shock. Mental or neurological symptoms such as delirium or nuchal rigidity may suggest meningitis.

Evaluation

The goal of preventing pneumonia in susceptible patients is measured by outcome criteria. These must be individualized and also should include a time frame for achievement:

- Patient's lungs are clear to auscultation and percussion
- Patient's chest film reveals no areas of consolidation

Examples of outcome criteria to evaluate the goal of relieving symptoms and preventing complications of pneumonia are listed below. Again, these criteria must be individualized and include a time frame for achievement.

- Patient's arterial blood-gas values and vital signs are within acceptable range
- Chest film reveals resolution of pneumonia
- Patient verbalizes a decrease in pain, breathlessness, and other symptoms
- Patient describes components of self-care necessary to prevent, reduce, or recognize complications:
  - Plans for taking medications as prescribed
  - Plans for follow-up medical appointments
  - Plans for rest and gradual resumption of activities
  - Deep breathing and bronchial hygiene techniques
  - Complications to report

Tuberculosis

Definition and Epidemiology

Tuberculosis is a reportable infectious disease that most commonly affects the lung. In tuberculosis the distinction between infection and disease is important. Up to 50% of the world's population may currently be infected with *Mycobacterium tuberculosis,* the organism causing most of the tuberculosis that occurs in humans.[86] However, fewer than 5% of persons exposed and infected will ever develop clinical disease.[73]

Before the introduction of antituberculosis chemotherapy in the late 1940s, tuberculosis was the leading cause of death in the United States. Improved living standards, public health measures, and more effective drugs have resulted in a markedly lower disease rate in economically developed countries such as the United States.

Although new tuberculosis infections in the United States are infrequent, deaths from tuberculosis continue to occur, and tuberculosis remains the leading cause of death among communicable diseases about which the CDC receives mortality data.[17] Active tuberculosis occurs more frequently in males, the economically disadvantaged, and inner city residents. Previously a disease of children and young adults, 75% of active cases in the United States are now associated with reactivation of the disease later in life. Certain occupational groups such as health workers have an incidence of tuberculosis greater than that in the general population. Alcoholics, people using corticosteroids, and patients with gastrectomies, ileal bypass surgery for obesity, and debilitating diseases are predisposed to develop tuberculous disease.[30, 31, 86] Immigrants from areas such as Southeast Asia with high tuberculosis case rates and Americans who have lived for prolonged periods in these countries also have a higher risk of becoming infected with tubercle bacillus.[65] Cases in foreign-born persons now account for about 20% of the total number of cases in the United States.[25]

Etiology

Tubercle bacilli are transmitted worldwide by person to person transmission and by drinking infected milk. Usual spread is by inhalation of airborne organisms coughed or sneezed into the environment by persons with active pulmonary tuberculosis. These droplet nuclei are so small ($2\ \mu$–$10\ \mu$) that they remain airborne and viable for hours.[11] When inhaled they can pass through usual nasal filtering and mucociliary airway defenses directly into alveoli.

M. tuberculosis is an acid-fast, weakly gram-positive, aerobic bacillus that grows in proportion to the oxygen tension of the environment. *Mycobacterium bovis,* the other mammalian tubercle bacillus, has been eliminated as a cause of tuberculosis in the United States through milk pasteurization and cattle tuberculin testing programs.[84]

Pathophysiology

Primary tuberculosis respresents an initial infection by the bacilli, whereas secondary or reactivation tuberculosis results from reactivation of a primary infection.

Primary Infection. Once deposited on the alveoli surface, the tubercle bacilli begin to multiply and an inflammatory response ensues. Macrophages phagocytize the tubercle bacilli, but the bacilli remain viable inside the macrophages and continue to replicate.

Three to eight weeks after implantation of the original tubercle bacillus, the development of cellular immunity facilitates intracellular killing of the tubercle bacillus by sensitized T lymphocytes. A tuberculin skin test becomes positive at this time (see Chap 16.)[63]

The development of cellular immunity somehow stimulates the formation of a granuloma at the site at which the infectious organisms were initially deposited. A granuloma is a collection of modified macrophages that encircles the infectious organisms and walls them off from adjacent tissue. Granulomas that form in tuberculosis are often referred to as tubercles.

Over time, the center of the tubercle undergoes necrosis, becoming soft and cheesy (termed caseous necrosis). In most cases, the tubercle bacilli growth is eventually contained inside the tubercle, probably as a result of low oxygen concentrations and acidosis within the caseous lesions. Usually the host remains asymptomatic, and after about 3 months the tubercle is replaced with fibrosis, calcification, and even ossification. Even after healing and fibrosis of the tubercle, significant numbers of tubercle bacilli remain alive but dormant in untreated persons.[11]

During the weeks that the nonimmune host is developing immunity, the tubercle bacilli spread to distant body parts through lymphatic channels and the bloodstream. Usually host defense processes control further spread of the infection and the person does not become clinically ill.

In about 5% of newly infected person, tuberculous infection progresses to disease within a few years. In persons unable to limit bacilli replication, the lungs are the most common site of tuberculous disease. Massive tissue damage occurs, with progressive inflammation and tissue necrosis, termed liquefaction. Cavity formation occurs. Surrounding structures are compressed and blood vessels erode. The person has moved from the infected state to the diseased state, and symptoms and chest-film abnormalities appear.

Hemorrhage, pneumonia, or pleural effusion may complicate tuberculosis. The serious condition of miliary tuberculosis occurs when caseous material spreads through an eroded blood vessel and forms numerous small foci in the lungs and other body organs.

Secondary Infection. Secondary infection is the phase of tuberculous infection following reactivation of primary infection or reinfection of a previously exposed host.

The usual cause of secondary infection is reactivation and growth of dormant bacilli that have persisted in an old infected focus. Inhaled tubercle bacilli rarely cause secondary infection, since initial infection with tubercle bacilli provides strong immunity.[11,63] When reactivation occurs, the pathological sequence parallels that of primary disease development: softening of the tubercle caseous focus, liquefaction, disintegration of local structures including bronchial walls, local drainage, and development of cavitary lesions.

When tuberculosis causes extensive damage to lung tissue, the vital capacity and other lung volumes are decreased. Quite often arterial oxygen tension is preserved despite extensive lung destruction, indicating that perfusion is decreased to match the decreased ventilation.

Extrapulmonary Tuberculosis. When tuberculous infection occurs outside the lungs, a similar process of tubercle formation and caseous necrosis occurs. In the kidney, initial lesions occur in the cortex. Central nervous system lesions are either well circumscribed (tuberculoma) or present as meningitis. Skeletal tuberculosis produces arthritis and osteomyelitis.

Clinical Manifestations

Persons with tuberculosis *infection* do not have clinical symptoms, chest-film findings, or positive bacterial cultures. Infection is detected by the presence of a positive reaction to a tuberculin skin test (see Diagnosis).

Persons with tuberculous *disease* often appear well and may be asymptomatic. Tuberculous disease is diagnosed by skin tests and by sputum Gram stain and culture, not by the clinical picture. Symptoms that do occur are usually generalized and mild, such as easy fatigability, anorexia, low-grade afternoon fevers, mild weight loss, and, in women, irregular menses. Pulmonary symptoms are less often initital symptoms of tuberculosis.[9] A chronic nonproductive or productive cough is the most common pulmonary symptom, but pleuritic or dull, recurring chest pain may also occur.

Physical examination findings may or may not be present and are not diagnostic of tuberculosis. Fever, erythema nodosum (painful nodules, usually on legs), or swollen cervical glands may appear. Fine crackles may be heard over the involved lung. If pleural effusion is present, dullness to percussion and reduced or absent breath sounds may overlie the effusion.

Medical Management

Diagnosis

Determination of which classification category accurately describes a person's tuberculosis status depends upon the interpretation of the results of the tuberculin skin test, chest film and sputum Gram stain and culture results.

Skin Test. The tuberculin skin test is the most useful test for the diagnosis of past or present tuberculous infection. When antigen is injected into persons sensitized by mycobacterial infection, induration (swelling) occurs several days later at the site. Persons for whom tuberculin skin testing is indicated include the following:

- Persons with signs (*e.g.,* radiographic abnormality) and/or symptoms (cough, hemoptysis, weight loss) suggestive of current tuberculosis disease
- Recent contacts with persons with known tuberculosis or persons suspected of having tuberculosis
- Persons with abnormal chest films compatible with past tuberculosis
- Persons with medical conditions that increase the risk of tuberculosis (*e.g.,* silicosis, gastrectomy, diabetes, immunosuppressive therapy, lymphomas)
- Groups at high risk of recent infection with *M. tuberculosis,* such as immigrants from Asia, Africa, Latin America, and Oceania; some inner city and skid row populations; personnel and long-term residents in some hospitals, nursing homes, mental institutions, and prisons[3]

Tuberculin can be administered intradermally (Mantoux) or by multiple puncture tests (Tine, Mono-Vac). Although the multiple puncture tests are used for screening, only a Mantoux test should determine diagnosis and treatment decisions.[2]

Purified protein derivative (PPD) tuberculin stabilized with Tween 80, intermediate strength, is the standard test material.[3] An intradermal injection of 0.1 ml PPD tuberculin is administered to cause a wheal on the volar surface of the left arm. The correct angle for intradermal injection is shown in Figure 28–4. To ensure a standard dosage, tuberculin should never be transferred from one container to another, and skin tests should be given immediately after the syringe is filled.

Tuberculin skin tests are read 48 to 72 hours after injection, the time when the greatest induration is usually present. The skin is inspected under a good light and by palpation for the presence or absence of induration. No induration is correctly recorded as "0 mm induration" (not "negative"). Standard categories of reaction are labeled negative (0 mm–4 mm), doubtful (5 mm–9 mm), and positive (10 mm or more). A significant tuberculin test reaction represents infection but does not prove disease.

Absence of a reaction to the tuberculin skin test does not exclude tuberculous disease. Negative reactions have been documented in up to 20% of patients with tuberculosis, particularly in persons with advanced disease, malnutrition, or debility.[3]

A doubtful reaction (5 mm–9 mm induration) may be due to recent infection, cross sensitivity with other mycobacteria, or partial anergy. The test is usually repeated within a week.

In persons who developed tuberculous infection several years previously, the tuberculosis hypersensitivity may wane so that an initial tuberculin skin test produces a nonsignificant reaction. Repeated testing of uninfected persons will not sensitize them to tuberculosis, but the stimulus of a skin test in previously sensitized persons may increase the size of reaction so that a second test causes an apparent "conversion." Therefore, in settings in which adults are skin tested on a routine basis, a two-stage testing process is recommended. All reactions with less than 10 mm of induration are retested a week later to minimize the chance of later interpreting a boosted reaction as a conversion. If the second of the two initial tests is 10 mm or greater, it probably represents a boosted reaction.

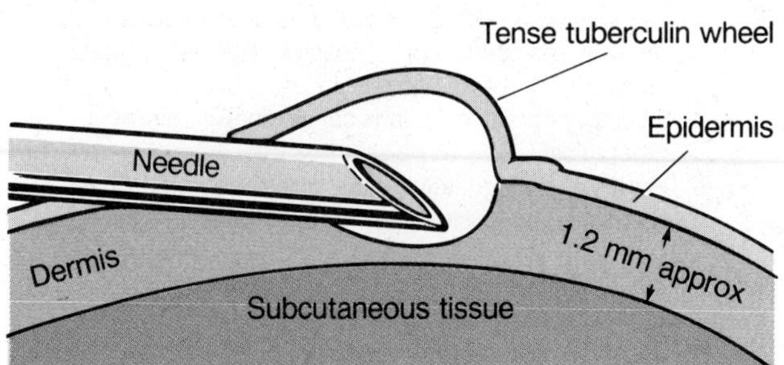

FIGURE 28–4 Mantoux test for administration of PPD tuberculin. The subject's skin should be stretched taut and the needle, bevel up, inserted just beneath the skin surface. When the tuberculin is injected, a tense white wheal should appear. (Audio Visual Medical Marketing, Inc, 1984. Produced under an educational grant from Parke-Davis)

Additional Tests. Tuberculosis may produce almost any form of pulmonary abnormality on *chest x-ray films.* However, many persons with positive tuberculin skin test reactions have no abnormalities on films and no tuberculous disease.

Growth of *M. tuberculosis* from the appropriate specimen is needed to confirm a diagnosis of tuberculosis. Antituberculous drug therapy cannot begin until adequate specimens for bacteriologic study are collected. Generally, three early morning sputum specimens are collected on successive days.[2] Because tuberculosis can localize in almost any anatomical site, other clinical specimens such as urine, pleural fluid, or biopsy material may also be collected for bacteriologic study. Microscopic examination of a specimen smear is used to guide therapy until culture results are available.

Treatment

Medical treatment of tuberculosis depends upon the extent of tubercle bacilli exposure, infection, or disease. The American Lung Association and the American Thoracic Society have jointly developed a system by which the entire population is classified according to tuberculosis exposure and infection. This classification system is summarized in Table 28–7. Drug chemotherapy is administered with goals of preventing development of active disease or treating active tuberculosis.

Preventive Medical Chemotherapy. Clinical tuberculous infection is prevented by administering bacille Calmette–Guérin (BCG) vaccine to uninfected persons or by prescribing isoniazid (INH) to recently infected or selected high-risk persons. BCG vaccine is a live attenuated strain of *M. bovis* with little virulence in humans. It gives vaccinated persons uncertain protection from tuberculous disease and is used to prevent primary tuberculous infection in parts of the world where tuberculosis is common.[5,85] It is not rou-

TABLE 28–7
Classification of Tuberculosis

0. *No Tuberculosis exposure, not infected*
   No history of exposure, reaction to tuberculin skin test not significant
1. *Tuberculosis exposure, no evidence of infection*
   History of exposure, reaction to tuberculin skin test not significant
2. *Tuberculous infection, no disease*
   Significant reaction to tuberculin skin test, negative bacteriologic studies (if done), no clinical and/or roentgenographic evidence of tuberculosis
   Chemotherapy Status: preventive
3. *Tuberculosis: Current disease*
   M. Tuberculosis cultured (if done), otherwise *both* a significant reaction to tuberculin skin test *and* clinical and/or roentgenographic evidence of current disease
   Location of Disease
   The predominant site shall be listed. Other sites may also be listed. Anatomical sites may be specified more precisely.
   Bacteriologic status
   Chemotherapy status

   The following data are necessary in certain circumstances:
   Roentgenogram findings
   Tuberculin skin test reaction
4. *Tuberculosis: No current disease*
   History of previous episode(s) of tuberculosis, or abnormal stable roentgenographic findings in a person with a significant reaction to tuberculin skin test, negative bacteriologic studies (if done), no clinical and/or roentgenographic evidence of current disease
   Chemotherapy status
5. *Tuberculosis suspect* (Diagnosis pending)
   Chemotherapy status

(Summarized from Diagnostic Standards and Classification of Tuberculosis and Other Mycobacterial Diseases. American Thoracic Society, 1981)

tinely recommended in the United States, since its use converts tuberculin skin tests to positive and thus eliminates subsequent ability for early discovery and treatment of tuberculous infections. BCG should not be administered to persons already tuberculin skin test–positive.

INH is administered prophylactically to persons without proven infection who have been recently exposed to active tuberculosis but have not yet had time to develop an immune response to the tuberculin test. All household contacts, especially children under 5 years of age, are considered for 3 months of INH chemoprophylaxis unless the patient's skin test becomes positive, requiring more aggressive therapy.

INH reduces the relatively small tubercle bacilli population in newly infected and healed lesions and can prevent active clinical disease in almost all infected persons who take it as prescribed.[30] A decision of whether or not to prescribe INH prophylactically is made on an individual basis by weighing the lifetime risk of developing tuberculosis and the opportunity for infecting others against the risk of serious adverse reactions that can result from one year of INH therapy. Since the risk of progressive disease is greatest soon after infection, recent tuberculin skin test converters are most likely to benefit from chemoprophylaxis. Table 28–8 summarizes the recommendations for chemoprophylaxis.

Treatment of Active Tuberculosis. To break the chain of infection transmission, antituberculous drug therapy is started as soon as specimens for bacteriologic examination are obtained and a presumptive diagnosis of tuberculosis is made. Long-term drug therapy is administered on an outpatient basis, although patients with clinically active pulmonary tuberculosis may be hospitalized initially. Because patients with extrapulmonary tuberculosis are much less infectious, they are often managed entirely as outpatients.[84] Drugs used for the treatment of tuberculosis are summarized in Table 28–9. Chemotherapy of tuberculosis differs from other antimicrobial therapy programs in several ways:

- The use of multiple drugs is necessary to prevent the emergence of drug-resistant organisms. Interrupted drug therapy or doses that are too low also foster development of resistant organisms.
- Rather than divided doses, a single daily drug dosage is preferred to achieve peak serum concentrations and minimize side-effects.
- Since no drug is capable of killing dormant bacilli, prolonged chemotherapy is necessary to kill the slow or intermittently growing tubercle bacilli population within macrophages and solid caseous areas.[5,27]
- No matter which regimen is used, follow-up of patients is essential to ensure adherence to the prescribed regimen and to monitor drug effectiveness and side-effects.

The current standard drug regimen to treat active tuberculosis is INH and rifampin for 9 months.[5,56] When resistant organisms are suspected or the person has traveled outside the country, ethambutol or streptomycin may be

TABLE 28–8
Isoniazid Prophylaxis for Tuberculosis

Indications

Persons under 35 years of age (some authorities say 20) with skin test conversion to positive within last 2 years
Persons over 35 years of age
1. Roentgenographic findings consistent with dormant tuberculosis
2. Previous inadequately treated active tuberculosis
3. Special high-risk situations

Contraindications

History of adverse reaction to INH
Evidence of progressive disease
Previous course of adequate INH therapy
Active liver disease
Pregnancy

Dosage: 300 mg PO in single daily dosage for one year

INH, isoniazid.

TABLE 28–9
Drug Treatment for Tuberculosis

	Abbrev.	*Dosage** Daily Dose	Twice Weekly Dosage	Most Common Side-Effects*	Tests for Side-Effects*	Drug Intractions†	Remarks*
Commonly used drugs							
Isoniazid	INH	5–10 mg/kg up to 300 mg PO or IM	15 mg/kg PO or IM	Peripheral neuritis, hepatitis, hypersensitivity.	SGOT/SGPT (not as a routine).	Phenytoin—synergistic Antabuse	Bactericidal to both extracellular and intracellular organisms. Pyridoxine 10 mg as prophylaxis for neuritis; 50–100 mg as treatment.
Rifampin	RMP	10 mg/kg up to 600 mg PO	10 mg/kg up to 600 mg PO	Hepatitis, febrile reaction, purpura (rare).	SGOT/SGPT (not as a routine).	Rifampin inhibits the effect of oral contraceptives, quinidine, corticosteroids. Coumarin drugs and methadone, digoxin, oral hypoglycemics; PAS may interfere with absorption of rifampin.	Bactericidal to all populations of organisms. Orange urine and other body secretions. Discoloring of contact lens.
Streptomycin	SM	15–20 mg/kg up to 1 g IM	25–30 mg/kg	Eighth nerve damage, nephrotoxicity.	Vestibular function, audiograms;‡ BUN and creatinine.	Neuromuscular blocking agents—may be potentiated to cause prolonged paralysis.	Bactericidal to extracellular organisms. Use with caution in older patients or those with renal disease.
Pyrazinamide	PZA	15–30 mg/kg up to 2 g PO	50–70 mg/kg	Hyperuricemia, hepatotoxicity.	Uric acid, SGOT/SGPT.		Bactericidal to intracellular organisms. Combination with an aminoglycoside is bactericidal.
Ethambutol	EMB	15–25 mg/kg	50 mg/kg PO	Optic neuritis (reversible with discontinuation of drug; very rare at 15 mg/kg), skin rash.	Red-green color discrimination and visual acuity.‡ Difficult to test in a child under 3 years.		Bacteriostatic to both intracellular and extracellular organisms, primarily used to inhibit development of resistant mutants. Use with caution with renal disease or when eye testing is not feasible.
Less commonly used agents							
Capreomycin	CM	15–30 mg/kg up to 1 g IM		Eighth nerve damage, nephrotoxicity.	Vestibular function, audiograms;‡ BUN and creatinine.	Neuromuscular blocking agents—may be potentiated to cause prolonged paralysis.	Bactericidal to extracellular organisms in cavities. Use with caution in older patients. Rarely used with renal disease.
Kanamycin	KM	15–30 mg/kg up to 1 g IM		Auditory toxicity nephrotoxicity, vestibular toxicity (rare).	Vestibular function, audiograms;‡ BUN and creatinine.	Neuromuscular blocking agents—may be potentiated to cause prolonged paralysis.	Bactericidal to extracellular organisms. Use wlth caution in older patients. Rarely used with renal disease.

(Continued)

TABLE 28–9
Drug Treatment for Tuberculosis (Continued)

	Abbrev.	Dosage* Daily Dose	Twice Weekly Dosage	Most Common Side-Effects*	Tests for Side-Effects*	Drug Intractions†	Remarks*
Less commonly used agents							
Ethionamide	ETA	15–30 mg/kg up to 1 g PO		GI disturbance, hepatotoxicity, hypersensitivity.	SGOT/SGPT		Bacteriostatic to both intracellular and extracellular organisms. Divided doses may help GI side-effects; has a metallic taste. Avoid use during pregnancy.
Para-amino-salicylic acid (amino-salicylic acid)	PAS	150 mg/kg up to 12 g PO		GI disturbance, hypersensitivity, hepatotoxicity, sodium load.	SGOT/SGPT		Bacteriostatic to extracellular organisms only. GI side-effects very frequent, making cooperation difficult.
Cycloserine	CS	10–20 mg/kg up to 1 g PO		Psychosis, personality changes, convulsions, rash.	Psychological testing.	Alcohol—may aggravate or precipitate psychiatric problems.	Bacteriostatic to both intracellular and extracellular organisms. Alcohol may aggravate psychiatric problems. Very difficult drug to use. Side-effects may be blocked by pyridoxine, ataractic agents, or anticonvulsant drugs.

*Check product labeling for detailed information on dose, contraindications, drug interaction, adverse reactions, and monitoring.
†Reference should be made to current literature, particularly on rifampin, because it induces hepatic microenzymes and therefore interacts with many drugs.
‡Initial examination should be done at start of treatment.
SGOT, serum glutamic-oxaloacetic transaminase; SGPT, serum glutamic-pyruvic transaminase; GI, gastrointestinal; BUN, blood urea nitrogen.
(Adapted from American Thoracic Society: Treatment of tuberculosis and other mycobacterial diseases. Am Rev Respir Dis 127:790–796, 1983)

added during the first 2 to 8 weeks. Larger doses of INH and rifampin given twice weekly have success rates similar to those of standard treatment.

When drug resistance or intolerance prevents use of INH or rifampin, 18 months or more of less effective and more toxic drug combinations is necessary (see Table 28–9). Tubercle bacilli, recovered prior to antituberculous drug therapy, are cultured and tested in the laboratory for susceptibility to the major antituberculous drugs. Because this sensitivity testing takes 4 to 6 weeks, results guide long-term but not initial drug decisions.

Surgery. In the past, collapse therapy surgical procedures and pulmonary resection were often used to treat tuberculosis. Because chemotherapy now effectively controls the tubercle bacilli, pulmonary resection or thoracoplasty is rarely needed.

Prognosis. In active disease a favorable response to therapy usually occurs within 2 to 3 weeks. Often sputum cultures and chest films are repeated monthly initially and then less often when improvement is established. A persistently positive sputum culture beyond 3 months after treatment suggests the failure to take prescribed drugs or the development of drug-resistant organisms.

Nursing Management

Assessment and Nursing Diagnosis

Data Analysis. Before tuberculosis is diagnosed, it must be suspected. If a diagnosis of tuberculosis is considered only when classic symptoms are reported in a person with recent exposure to tuberculosis infection, only about 5% of cases will be detected. Since most pulmonary tuberculosis today develops as a late recrudescence of a dormant infection, nurses must be alert to risk factors of tuberculous disease.

All patients coughing and raising sputum should be considered as possibly having tuberculosis. Chest films should be obtained and history reviewed to determine previous disease, tuberculin skin test reaction, and therapy with drugs. The clinical situation is assessed with knowledge of the patient's exposure to tuberculosis, the presence or absence of conditions predisposing to tuberculosis, and the current tuberculosis situation in the local community. When a diagnosis of tuberculosis has been tentatively established, the patient's close contacts within the community must also be evaluated for presence of tuberculous infection or disease.

Information about alcohol consumption and other medication use can alert the nurse to the potential for drug interactions or increased risk of drug side-effects. For example, the risk of severe liver toxicity with INH increases with alcohol use and age.[5] Persons with nutritional deficits are at increased risk of INH-associated vitamin B_6 deficiency and deserve prophylactic pyridoxine therapy. It is also important to assess the patient's likelihood of compliance with long-term drug therapy.

Nursing Diagnoses. Based on the results of individual patient assessment, nursing diagnoses can be formulated. An example of a nursing diagnosis for a person at risk of tuberculosis infection is as follows: potential for developing tuberculosis infection related to the transmission of bacilli by persons with active, untreated disease.

Numerous diagnoses and problem statements are possible for persons who have tuberculosis infection or disease. Examples are listed below, but these must be modified to fit individual patients:

- Potential for infecting contacts secondary to transmission of tubercle bacilli
- Alteration in comfort related to infection of lung parenchyma by *M. tuberculosis*
- Potential noncompliance with antituberculosis drug therapy related to inadequate knowledge, inadequate social or family support, prolonged length of therapy, or unpleasant side-effects of medication
- Body image disturbance related to perceived stigma of having tuberculosis

Goals. The goals of nursing intervention are to prevent tuberculosis transmission, prevent disease development in persons who are infected, and to decrease symptoms in persons with disease.

Intervention: Preventing Spread of Infection

Transmission of tuberculosis is prevented by the identification and treatment of persons with active disease. Diagnosed and suspected cases must be reported to the local health department. The nurse can aid the health department's investigation of contacts by obtaining family information during the patient's health history and encouraging the patient's close contacts to be evaluated and take preventive treatment. Young children exposed to tuberculosis are especially susceptible to disease and require conscientious attention.

Tuberculosis control is based on principles of surveillance (searching out each case) and containment (proper treatment of case and contacts). Surveillance in the United States, an area of low tuberculosis incidence, is difficult because random repetitive mass screening is not appropriate.[4] Containment comprises examination and treatment of contacts, preventive therapy of infected persons, and assuring that persons with tuberculosis disease obtain and continue correct therapy.

A person with active pulmonary tuberculosis is prevented from contaminating the air with tubercle bacilli by several means, including taking antituberculous drug therapy and covering his nose and mouth. Antituberculous chemotherapy is the most effective way to prevent microbial contamination of the air because it reduces coughing caused by tuberculosis, as well as the amount of sputum and the tubercle bacilli concentration in the sputum.

Covering the nose and mouth decreases the likelihood of atomized secretions becoming airborne. Generally a patient should be required to submit to the continual discomfort of masks only when he leaves the room or, if a high transmitter, when hospital personnel or visitors are in the room. To be effective, masks must filter out particles as small as 1 μ, fit snugly, cover the nose and mouth, and be discarded or sterilized after each use. Having a patient wear a mask when a visitor is in his room may reduce the addition of bacilli to the air during coughing, but transmission will not be prevented since the room air has already been contaminated.

Microbial contamination of room air can be eliminated by air control that introduces fresh air into a room and exhausts air outside without recirculation. Alternately, tubercle bacilli in room air can be destroyed by ultraviolet light or a high-efficiency filter before circulation.[75]

Sputum should be expectorated into tissues or a covered sputum container and discarded in the toilet or collected in a bag to burn. The bacilli are destroyed by 1 to 2 hours of sunlight, 5 minutes at boiling temperature, or by autoclaving. The danger of infection from contaminated surfaces is negligible, making gowns and gloves unnecessary as long as careful handwashing is practiced.

Patients differ in the speed at which they become noninfectious. Effective chemotherapy actually taken by a patient without advanced cavitary disease usually controls infectiousness within days, although positive cultures or smears persist longer.[4,77] A decreasing or negative smear bacillary count supports an assessment that the patient is a nontransmitter. Even patients with cavitary disease who have taken antituberculosis drugs for at least 2 weeks, who cover their mouths when coughing, and who are unlikely to have resistant organisms present no risk of contagion.[53] The rare patient with large numbers of bacilli who must take drugs less effective than INH or rifampin may remain contagious 1 or 2 months.

Home Care Considerations. Precautionary measures to prevent bacilli transmission are less aggressive at home than for the hospitalized patient who may expose other patients who are likely to develop serious complications if infected. Visitors may be limited during the first few weeks at home, and a room alone is preferable initially.

No special precautions are necessary for extrapulmonary tuberculosis except following usual handwashing and good housekeeping practices and usual sanitary procedures for care of dressings and urine.

Intervention: Monitoring Drug Therapy

Toxicity of the major antituberculous drugs is low, with side-effects occurring in 3% to 4% of patients.[53] Table 28–9 lists common side-effects and drug interactions for which patients should be monitored.

The nurse has an important role in ensuring the success of antituberculosis chemotherapy. Activities include monitoring and promoting adherence to the therapeutic regimen, monitoring drug toxicity, and educating the patient and family.

Although more than 95% of patients can be treated successfully the first time, this rate of success is rarely achieved because many patients fail to take their medications as prescribed. Although demographic variables do not completely predict compliance, the profile of a person at risk for nonadherence is a single, unemployed, inner city, male alcoholic.[1,4]

A nonjudgmental question, such as, "People often have difficulty remembering to take pills regularly; do you?" will detect a significant number of persons with medication regimen adherence problems. A therapeutic regimen characterized by a shorter duration of therapy, fewer drugs, and less frequent dosage schedules, as well as a quality relationship with the patient, may improve compliance.

Perhaps a third of tuberculosis patients require alternatives to self-medication such as direct professional administration of drugs daily or twice weekly.[77] The twice-weekly administration in a clinic, at home, or at work by a public health nurse is currently the most cost-effective solution to the problem of patients who do not adhere to the prescribed regimen. This twice-weekly regimen is preceded by 1 or 2 months of daily drugs with conventional dosages, usually in the hospital.[4]

Intervention: General Supportive Measures

Activity restrictions such as bed rest are no longer warranted unless the patient has other problems such as fever or hemoptysis. There is little evidence that climate has any significant role in the management of tuberculosis. Patients should resume normal activities as soon as possible depending on their response to treatment, the nature of usual activities, and who will be exposed to them during normal activities. No special diet is beneficial in tuberculosis, although normal weight should be maintained by a well-balanced nutritious diet.

When the cough is productive it should be encouraged and not suppressed with drugs. It is important that the patient be taught to cough with minimal effort.

There is still a stigma attached to persons with tuberculosis, especially among the elderly and in certain cultural groups. When a person is diagnosed as having tuberculous infection or disease, it is important for the nurse to determine the meaning of this information to the patient. The emotional response to tuberculosis by many people is still that of "being unclean" or "sinful" and may connote a dire prognosis. The felt stigma of tuberculosis may prevent open communication between patient and friends and relatives, even hampering detection of those contacts of active cases who need treatment.

Like any new diagnosis of a serious disease, patient reactions may vary from anger to denial to depression. Reassurance can be provided by educating patients about the meaning of the disease today, explaining the difference between infection and active disease, and assuring the patient that tuberculosis occurs in all social and economic classes, that modern chemotherapy is truly curative, and that prolonged periods of hospitalization and isolation are no longer necessary.

Evaluation

A person with or at risk for tuberculosis infection should be able to

- Distinguish between infection and disease in tuberculosis
- State that he has a significant (positive) reaction to a tuberculin skin test
- List symptoms that suggest active disease

If given prophylactic chemotherapy with INH, the person should be able to

- State the drug name, purpose, and dosage
- State signs and symptoms of side-effects to report
- State when and how often he will take the medication
- State when and where to get a new medication supply
- Explain the importance of full compliance and completion of the drug regimen

A person with active tuberculosis should be able to

- Explain how tuberculosis is spread
- Describe and implement measures to take to prevent spread
- State drug names, purpose, dosage, and side-effects
- Adhere to drug therapy and state when he will take medications
- Describe and implement actions to be taken for side-effects
- List symptoms that indicate a relapse or worsening
- State where to get a new medication supply
- Report how long the medications need to be continued and what will happen if they are discontinued earlier
- Describe symptoms indicating the need for care after completion of the drug course

Atypical Mycobacterial Disease

Atypical mycobacteria are found worldwide in the environment, most commonly in soil. Despite the exposure and infection of many persons with these organisms of low virulence, disease is uncommon and poorly understood.[22]

In humans the pathophysiology of disease with atypical

mycobacteria, such as the most common *Mycobacterium kansasii* or *Mycobacterium intracellulare-avium* is similar to that of *M. tuberculosis* except the disease may progress more slowly. Microscopically these bacteria are identical to *M. tuberculosis* bacilli but can be distinguished on culture.

Treatment. Drug treatment differs depending on the strain involved. Success from drug treatment of *M. kansasii* approaches 100% using the same two- or three-drug regimens used for *M. tuberculosis. M. intracellulare-avium* is a more serious disease that is often highly resistant to antituberculosis drugs. The administration of up to six drugs for a treatment period of several years and, where possible, surgical excision of involved areas are needed. Even if treated successfully, as many as one third of patients with *M. intracellulare-avium* may die of underlying pulmonary disease within a few years.[22]

Nursing Management. Nursing management for patients with disease from atypical mycobacterium is similar to that for *M. tuberculosis* but requires knowledge of differences in prognosis, therapy, and severity among the atypical strains. Since human to human transmission has not been reported, isolation of these patients is not required.[53]

Fungal Lung Infections

The spores of fungi (yeasts and mold) are omnipresent in the air we breathe. They may reach the airways without causing disease. Many common fungi such as the *Candida* and *Aspergillus* genera normally do not cause disease but can cause life-threatening pneumonia in persons with impaired defense systems (such as those receiving corticosteroid or cancer chemotherapy). A few fungi produce chronic granulomatous lung disease that resembles tuberculosis. Histoplasmosis and coccidioidomyocosis, the two most common and important causes of fungal pulmonary disease, are geographic in distribution, grow in the soil, and are transmitted by dust rather than by person to person contact. They are discussed in detail below. These and other less common fungal lung diseases are also outlined in Table 28–10.

TABLE 28–10
Fungal Infections of the Lung

Infection	*Organism*	*Characteristics*	*Medical Therapy*
Coccidioidomycoses	*Coccidioides immitis*	Soil fungus growing in southwestern United States Infects ⅔ of persons who breathe spores; 40% of infected persons develop cold or flu like symptoms Chronic pulmonary disease or disseminated disease rarely occurs, usually in immunosuppressed hosts Diagnosed by sputum culture, skin testing, serum complement titers, and chest films.	No drug therapy for asymptomatic or primary pneumonitis Amphotericin B for disseminated disease Ketoconazole is suppressive but not curative Meningeal infection treated with IV and intrathecal amphotericin B
Histoplasmosis	*Histoplasma capsulatum*	Worldwide distribution, more common in eastern and midwest United States river valleys Grows in soil enriched by bird or bat excreta 40% of persons who inhale spores develop mild illness after 2-week incubation time 1%–5% of infections cause clinical syndromes of influenzalike illness, disseminated disease, or pneumonia	No therapy for acute primary form Amphotericin B for disseminated disease or persistent positive cultures and active lung disease Ketoconazole
Candidiasis	*Candida* species	Pneumonia results from hematogenous spread from distant sites in immunocompromised hosts Diagnosis by lung biopsy, blood and skin biopsy cultures	Amphotericin B 5-Fluorocytosine

(Continued)

TABLE 28–10
Fungal Infections of the Lung (*Continued*)

Infection	*Organism*	*Characteristics*	*Medical Therapy*
Cryptococcus	*Cryptococcus neoformans*	Worldwide distribution Infection of lungs and meninges after inhaling yeast from excreta of birds	Usually monitored using cultures and x-ray films without therapy Amphotericin B if host is immunosuppressed or meninges are infected
Blastomycosis	*Blastomyces dermatitidis*	Found in Mississippi Valley and northern Midwest Inhalation causes chronic granulomatous infection of lungs, skin, and bone May be self-limited illness	Often monitored without treatment unless extending beyond lungs Amphotericin B Ketoconazole (long-term effectiveness not known)
Actinomycosis	*Actinomyces israelii*	*Not a fungus;* an anaerobic gram-positive bacterium; present in cervicofacial or dental infections, causing disease in humans when aspirated	Penicillin G, 10–20 million units IV daily for 4–6 weeks followed by 6–12 months of oral penicillin
Nocardiosis	Soil-borne aerobic *Actinomyces* species	Infection from inhalation of soil-borne organisms Bronchopneumonia in immunosuppressed hosts may progress to heart, central nervous system, or subcutaneous involvement	Surgical drainage and sulfadiazine continued for 6 weeks
Aspergillosis	Several species of mold *Aspergillus*	Causes a variety of clinical pictures including allergic aspergillosis, invasive or disseminated infection, or fungus ball Clinical symptoms of lung infection plus wheezing and expectorating brown sputum plugs	Amphotericin B Corticosteroids Bronchodilator medications

Histoplasmosis and Coccidioidomycosis

Epidemiology and Pathophysiology

More than 50 million persons in the United States have been infected with *Histoplasma capsulatum,* an organism prevalent in the Mississippi, Ohio, and Missouri River valleys.[76] Inhaled spores multiply in lung alveoli, then are engulfed by phagocytes and transported to lymphoid tissue, where a granulomatous reaction occurs similar to that in tuberculosis. Solitary round granulomas or apical lung scarring and cavitation remain after the infection is contained. Localized ulcerative lesions in the larynx, skin, or abdominal organs or a progressive systemic illness may develop in very young or in immunosuppressed hosts.

The soil fungus causing coccidioidomycosis grows in well-defined areas of southern California, western Texas, Arizona, and New Mexico. Inhaled fungus arthrospores cause an inflammatory reaction in lung alveoli. The arthrospores convert to spherules, which mature and release endospores that are phagocytosed and produce granulomas wherever they are deposited. A few infected persons develop a secondary disease with chronic pulmonary disease or dissemination. General dissemination may result in granulomatous lesions of the brain, bone, skin, or other organs and anemia or phlebitis. In the cavitary form of the disease, rupture into the pleura may produce empyema or pneumothorax. The risk of local progression or dissemination outside the lung is highest in males, members of dark-skinned races, pregnant women, diabetics, and immunosuppressed hosts.[76]

Clinical Manifestations

Symptoms of primary histoplasmosis usually are mild and resolve completely after a few days to weeks, leaving no residual damage to lung structure.[35] A severe pneumonia can develop when a large number of organisms have been inhaled from a heavily contaminated source.[12] In certain hosts, such as middle-aged smokers, the fungi proliferate more rapidly and lead to a chronic, cavitary form of the disease. Disseminated disease with sustained fever, anemia, and hepatic and splenic enlargement may occur in immunosuppressed hosts.

Fewer than one half of persons infected with coccidioidomycosis develop symptoms varying from those of the common cold to more severe, influenzalike symptoms. Physical examination of the chest occasionally shows signs of apical consolidation or a one-sided pleural effusion. Some patients develop hypersensitivity manifestations such as nodules of the skin (erythema nodosum), a measleslike rash (erythema multiforme), and joint pain.

Medical Management

For all fungal infections, a definitive diagnosis is made by finding the microscopic organism in stained sections of body secretions or tissues and by finding specific host responses in serologic or skin test reactions.

No treatment is necessary for the common acute primary forms of either histoplasmosis or coccidioidomycosis. For chronic, progressive, or disseminated disease, patients are hospitalized for administration of the fungicidal antibiotic, amphotericin B.[12] Ketoconazole is a less toxic alternative to amphotericin B that can be administered orally; it is so new that it is unknown if patients who respond initially may relapse later.[76] In chronic cases, surgical therapy may be necessary.[12]

Nursing Management

Assessment and Nursing Diagnosis

Since clinical manifestations of fungal lung diseases resemble those caused by viruses or *M. tuberculosis,* a careful health history aids assessment. Geographic location, travel history, occupational history, and information about common daily activities can provide exposure data important in suggesting the causative organism.

Nursing Diagnoses. For persons at risk of exposure, a possible nursing diagnosis is potential lung or systemic infection related to inhalation of fungal spores.

Many nursing diagnoses are possible for persons who have developed histoplasmosis or coccidioidomycosis. Among them are the following:

- Potential impairment in gas exchange secondary to development of fungal pneumonia
- Potential alteration in comfort related to fungal invasion of lung parenchyma and possible joint pain

Goals. Goals of nursing interventions are to minimize exposure of persons to dust contaminated with histoplasmosis or coccidioidomycosis spores and to eradicate the spores in infected persons.

Interventions

Prevention of exposure to high inocula of histoplasmosis requires recognition and avoidance of high-risk areas where *H. capsulatum* are likely to grow (*e.g.,* bat-infested caves and mushroom cellars). People raising chickens, pigeons, or other birds should be advised to wet-down bird areas before cleaning to prevent raising dust that could be inhaled. The prevention of widespread infection of the population in endemic areas is not currently feasible.

Prevention of coccidioidomycosis consists of avoidance of the exposure that occurs by visiting endemic areas. Infection is most likely to occur toward the end of the wet season in the desert when the subsoil is still damp and the surface is dry.[12] Air conditioned cars or rooms may provide some protection during a visit.

When hospitalized, patients with histoplasmosis or coccidioidomycosis do not need to be placed in isolation, since fungal infections are not transmitted person to person. If amphotericin B is prescribed, the nurse may be responsible for administration and should monitor for toxicity. Side-effects of common antifungal drugs are listed in Table 28–11. Drug dosage is reduced daily if blood urea nitrogen (BUN) or creatinine values rise progressively. Potassium supplementation may be needed.

Amphotericin B is usually infused with heparin or hydrocortisone to reduce thrombophlebitis, which has a 70% incidence.[93] Patients often require premedication with aspirin, acetaminophen, antihistamine, narcotics, or antiemetics to reduce the acute reaction during infusion. Timing of infusion at bedtime may minimize side-effects. If ketoconazole is prescribed, the nurse must be aware that antacids or cimetidine blocks its absorption.[74]

Evaluation

When interventions have been successful, persons at risk of contracting histoplasmosis or coccicioidomycosis should be able to state means by which they can decrease their exposure to the fungi. Persons with mild histoplasmosis or coccidioidomycosis should be able to describe complications that should be reported to a health-care provider.

For persons with severe disease requiring hospitalization, outcome criteria include the following:

- Patient's arterial blood-gas values and vital signs are within acceptable range.
- Patient's laboratory values show normal renal function
- Patient's chest film reveals resolution.
- Patient verbalizes decrease in respiratory or systemic symptoms.

Pneumoconioses: Silicosis and Asbestosis (Fibrotic Lung Disease)

Definition and Etiology

Pulmonary fibrosis is a general term applied to all types and causes of interstitial fibrous change. *Pneumoconioses* are a specific group of lung diseases caused by inhaled dusts. They account for a major portion of the various types of interstitial and alveolar fibrotic conditions that result in restrictive lung disease.

TABLE 28–11
Antifungal Drugs

Drug	*Dosage**	*Side-Effects*	*Tests for Side-Effects*
Amphotericin B	10 mg IV initially, increasing 10 mg/day to 0.5 mg/kg daily dose Then 1.0–1.2 mg/kg IV on alternate days to reach cumulative dosage of 1.5–2.5 g over 2–10 weeks Infuse over 4–6 hours (some settings use 1–2 hours)	Acute toxicity Common: fever, chills, nausea, vomiting, malaise, myalgia, sweats. Less common: hypotension, seizures, bronchospasm Chronic toxicity Nephrotoxicity Reduced red blood cell production Local thrombophlebitis (70% incidence)	1 mg IV test dosage for hypersensitivity initially Serum BUN, creatinine, and potassium and urinary sediment monitored
Ketoconazole	400 mg/day PO with meals, increasing to 800 mg–1200 mg qd continued for about 6 months	Nausea, vomiting, abdominal pain, pruritus	
5-Fluorocytosine	50–150 mg/kg daily for 1–3 months	Abdominal discomfort, diarrhea, hepatotoxicity, bone marrow suppression, skin rash	Liver function test, blood counts

* Dosage and schedule varies with organism and disease site.

In many cases inhalation of the damaging substances is work-related, as shown in Table 28–12, which lists occupational pneumoconioses. The two most common pneumoconioses, silicosis and asbestosis, are described in the text that follows.

Silicosis and Asbestosis. Silicosis usually results from long-term inhalation of minute crystalline silica particles during exposure in mining, sandblasting, and many other manufacturing processes. Silicosis increases the risk of active pulmonary tuberculosis, since tubercle bacilli multiply more easily when silica has damaged macrophages.[58, 102]

Exposure to asbestos has been widespread, occurring in asbestos mining, milling and manufacturing processes, construction and insulation work, and during use of finished products with asbestos. In addition to causing fibrosis, asbestos exposure is associated with pleural mesothelioma, bronchogenic cancer, and cancers of the larynx, throat, colon, and kidney. The risk of cancer for smokers exposed to asbestos is 55 times the risk for exposed nonsmokers.[80]

Pathophysiology

Diffuse fibrosis of the interstitial lung layer produces lung stiffness and reduced compliance. Consequences of reduced pulmonary elasticity are reduced lung volumes and capacities, ventilation maldistribution, and increased work of breathing.

Inhaled silica particles initiate a sequence of macrophage death, liberation of enzymes destructive to cells, additional macrophage production, inflammation, collagen formation, and then fibrosis. Avascular nodules form in the lung and eventually enlarge to a size visible on chest films.

Deposition of asbestos fibers in the alveloi causes a process similar to that of silicosis. The fibrotic process obliterates the alveolus and involves adjacent air spaces.[81] The asbestos fibers also penetrate the peribronchial spaces and spread to other parts of the body.

Clinical Manifestations

Persons with silicosis or asbestosis are asymptomatic initially. Breathlessness with exertion is the initial symptom, progressing over time to dyspnea at rest. Cough may be present, especially in smokers.

Initially, arterial oxygen decreases only with activity. Later, arterial blood gases show hypoxemia at rest, and clubbing, cyanosis, and pulmonary heart disease may develop. Unlike in obstructive lung disease, effective carbon dioxide exchange is usually maintained. In the late stages of disease, repeated respiratory infections, nonpleuritic chest pain, cough, and wheezing may be present.

The respiratory pattern is one of rapid ($>$30/min) shallow ($<$400 ml tidal volume) breaths. Crackles that do not clear with coughing may be present on lung auscultation and are most evident at the axillary and posterior lung bases.

Medical Management

Diagnosis. In addition to a history of exposure, clinical disease features, chest films, and pulmonary function tests aid medical diagnosis. In silicosis there are no specific

TABLE 28–12
Occupational Pneumoconioses

Disease	*Causative Particles*	*Examples of Occupations at Increased Risk*
Silicosis	Crystalline silica or silicon dioxide	Ceramics worker, brick maker, coal miner, sandblaster, stone cutter
Asbestosis	Asbestos fibers, especially crocidolite fiber	Asbestos mining, brake or clutch manufacturer, insulator, shipbuilder, roofer
Baritosis	Barium	Barite miner, glassmaker, missile worker, x-ray tube maker
Beryllium disease	Pure beryllium metal and its salts	Ceramics worker, foundry worker, grinder, metal worker
Aluminum pneumoconiosis	Aluminum	Ammunition maker
Coalworker's pneumoconiosis	Coal dust	Coal miner
Siderosis	Iron	Welder, ship breaker
Talcosis	Certain talcs (hydrate magnesium silicate) fibers	Cosmetics worker, paper maker

laboratory findings. In asbestosis, sputum examination for asbestos bodies or, more rarely, biopsy may be done to demonstrate fibrosis and asbestos bodies in the walls of respiratory bronchioles.[97] When the patient is experiencing severe dyspnea on activity, arterial blood-gas values are obtained at rest and after exercise to evaluate the need for oxygen therapy.

The chest radiograph pattern characteristic of silicosis consists of rounded regular opacities in middle and upper fields, whereas asbestos produces a pattern of irregular lower-lobe linear opacities.[15]

Treatment. There is no specific treatment for pulmonary fibrosis of any type. The real hope for the future control of these diseases is prevention. Many pneumoconioses are irreversible, and ending exposure to the offending substance does not always delay progression.[102] Supplementary oxygen and airway support may be needed during acute respiratory crisis or in extensive disease. Antibiotics, bronchodilators, and expectorants may be prescribed in appropriate situations to treat disease complications. Corticosteroids are not beneficial unless an autoimmune disease is also present.[47]

Nursing Management

Assessment and Nursing Diagnosis

Data Analysis. A comprehensive carefully obtained occupational history is the first step to the detection of all pneumoconioses. Key information to collect includes the presence of symptoms and their relation to past or present work, the type of hazardous exposure, the level and duration of exposure, and the presence of similar illness in coworkers with similar jobs.[88]

In addition to gathering data about a person's past history, the nurse, in assessing patients with fibrotic restrictive lung disease, determines their current degree of breathlessness, daily living patterns, exercise ability, and sleep patterns. To identify factors that may exacerbate illness, recent infections or exposures should be reviewed, as well as smoking history, exposure to dust or fumes, adequacy of hydration, and any changes in cough or sputum.

The patient's and family's perceptions of the meaning and prognosis of the disease should be determined. Understanding of the disease process and anticipation of the future as it relates to symptoms, marriage, sexuality, and employment should be explored.[44]

In some situations, discontinuing exposure to the offending substance will allow healing of the lung injury to occur. When the fibrosis is permanent, however, it can be expected that the nurse will be in contact with a patient who has severe, basically untreatable lung disability. The impact on his life can be profound.

Nursing Diagnoses. Although nursing diagnoses must be formulated individually on the basis of assessment data, some probable diagnoses are as follows:

- Dyspnea related to disturbed ventilatory mechanics as a result of severe lung scarring
- Activity intolerance related to severe breathlessness

- Impaired gas exchange related to permanent scarring involving alveolar–capillary membrane
- Sexual dysfunction related to breathlessness (SOB), hypoxemia, or psychological factors
- Ineffective individual or family coping related to irreversible, progressive disability

Goals. A basic goal is to present exposure to dusts that cause pneumoconiosis. For those with pneumoconiosis, goals are to prevent further disease and balance activity with lung functional capability.

Interventions

Prevention. Prevention of pneumoconioses is a public health challenge that will require a cooperative effort of health-care and other professionals. Difficulties include underdeveloped methodology for prevention, a long latent disease period between exposure and appearance of disease, nonspecific pulmonary symptoms that make linking disease with a specific agent difficult, and exposure of many persons to substances before their toxicity is recognized.

Changes in industry products, automation, dust control, ventilator use, and preemployment and periodic screening to counsel high-risk workers away from exposure are measures currently used to reduce occupational risks.[45] Persons with risk factors such as smoking that predispose to disease development should be counselled to avoid exposure or to eliminate the risk factors.

Respirators to protect workers from dust vary from simple surgical masks to self-contained breathing devices. Since they change breathing patterns by increasing resistance and dead space, many workers opt not to use them. Teaching workers the importance of finding and using acceptable effective respirators is an important preventive nursing action.

Supportive Nursing Care. Nursing interventions vary with the degree of functional impairment present. Principles of intervention similar to those used for rehabilitation of other chronic diseases apply.[89] Persons with severe fibrosis are often dyspneic, and management of scarce energy is a major problem. When dyspnea on exertion is significant, life becomes a slow-paced schedule with few moments when energy is not consumed by activities of daily living or the therapeutic regime. The pursed-lip breathing pattern that helps patients with obstructive disease is not useful in purely restrictive lung disease (see Chap 29). Because tidal volumes are so small, an increased respiratory rate is necessary to maintain blood oxygenation. Many patients require oxygen at high flow rates continuously or during activity. Like patients with COPD, these patients benefit from adequately paced and regular activity, relaxation training, nutritional support, time and energy management, and work simplification techniques. In pneumoconioses such as coal worker's pneumoconiosis in which both obstructive disease and restrictive disease are present, measures of breathing retraining and secretion clearance are appropriately applied.[91]

Education about the mechanisms and effects of the disease as well as therapies can help the patient cope with the disease. If the patient has home oxygen or other equipment, he and his family need to be able to explain its purpose and demonstrate its proper use. Patients need to understand measures to use to prevent respiratory infections, such as influenza vaccines, and need to recognize infections early and take appropriate action.

Persons with asbestosis who have higher cancer risks deserve regular stool examinations for occult blood and sigmoidoscopy screening for gastrointestinal tract cancers.[16] They should be aware of early symptoms of cancers to report.

Like patients with COPD, persons with chronic restrictive lung disease probably judge therapeutic effectiveness by how well they can mobilize resources to live within their limitations.[29] Unfortunately, adherence to the therapeutic regime does not always guarantee a good outcome. If complications occur, patients and family may feel discouraged if they have adhered diligently to their self-care regime or guilty if they have been lax.

Evaluation

Caring for patients with irreversible pneumoconioses is a difficult challenge because of the progressive nature of the disease and the relatively few therapeutic options that can be offered to the patient. Nevertheless, patients can be assisted to live more comfortably within the limitations posed by the disease. When goals related to nursing care for patients with pneumoconioses have been met, the patient should be able to

- Maintain arterial blood-gas values within acceptable limits
- State the reason for oxygen or other forms of therapy
- Demonstrate safe oxygen use
- State a plan for a realistic daily activity schedule, with time for rest between activities
- Describe measures to prevent and recognize respiratory infection
- Identify support systems that can assist him or his family to cope with the effects of the disease upon his life

Sarcoidosis

Etiology and Pathophysiology

Sarcoidosis is a chronic progressive disease of unknown etiology that most frequently involves the lung. It can affect multiple tissues including the skin, spleen, eyes, lymph nodes, liver, and small bones of the hands and feet. The disease most commonly begins between the ages of 20 and 40 and is more frequent in blacks than in whites and more common in women than in men.

All affected tissues contain granulomas that heal by scar formation and, in some cases, result in significant restrictive lung disease. Characteristic immunologic abnormalities are present, but it is uncertain whether these cause the condition or result from the disease process.

Clinical Manifestations

Although most persons with sarcoid have no symptoms, a wide variety of symptoms can occur depending upon the site of granulomatous inflammation and disease type. The acute type of sarcoid, which usually occurs in younger persons, has an abrupt onset and high spontaneous remission rate, whereas the chronic form, insidious in onset, is more often progressive.

Erythema nodosum, red watery eyes (uveitis), and pulmonary symptoms of cough, shortness of breath, wheezing, or chest discomfort may accompany systemic manifestations of fever, weight loss, malaise, and fatigue.

Along with the skin lesions, enlargement of lymph nodes, the parotid gland, the liver, and the spleen may be observed. Lung examination is usually normal. Complications of the progressive form of the disease include hemoptysis, respiratory failure, and blindness.

Medical Management

Diagnosis. The diagnosis of sarcoidosis is made by excluding other possible causes of the clinical findings, since no test provides a definitive diagnosis. Chest films show enlargement of hilar lymph nodes (adenopathy) in 50% of the cases. Mediastinoscopy, fiberoptic bronchoscopy with transtracheal biopsy, or biopsy of other tissue involved such as salivary or lymph glands is performed when a tissue specimen is necessary for diagnosis.

Treatment. Because of the variable natural disease history, indications for medical therapy are often debated. Persons without clinical symptoms are not treated. In severe or systemic disease, corticosteroids are prescribed in order to reduce the inflammatory changes that lead to irreversible fibrosis. Because tuberculosis reactivation often occurs in association with sarcoidosis, INH prophylaxis may be used when the patient has a significant reaction to the tuberculin skin test.[55,83]

Prognosis. Remission usually occurs within 2 years of diagnosis, especially in patients with clear lungs.[83] In some of the remaining patients, severe fibrosis progresses and results in respiratory failure. The overall mortality rate for sarcoidosis is 5% to 10%.

Nursing Management

Assessment and Nursing Diagnosis

Data Analysis. In addition to the health history and examination usually collected for persons with pulmonary problems, it is important to obtain data on the meaning of the condition to the patient and his family. Patients are often young, and the disease has an impact on career and other family decisions. The presence of other correctable respiratory disease risk factors, such as smoking or occupational dust or fume exposure, should be sought.

Nursing Diagnosis. Nursing diagnoses for the patient with sarcoidosis will vary according to the extent of pulmonary and other involvement and must be individualized following patient assessment. Several examples of possible nursing diagnoses for a patient with respiratory symptoms are as follows:

- Dyspnea related to widespread granuloma formation throughout lung parenchyma
- Potential impairment in gas exchange related to granulomatous involvement of lung tissue
- Alteration in skin integrity related to presence of erythema nodosum or cutaneous granulomas
- Ineffective individual or family coping related to the diagnosis of a potentially chronic disease

Goals. Nursing goals are to relieve symptoms, to prevent disease complications, and to assist the patient and family to successfully adjust to the diagnosis of a chronic disease.

Interventions

Since diagnosis of sarcoidosis is often difficult, patients and family need caring support during the often frustrating and prolonged diagnostic phase. Nursing interventions vary widely depending upon the stage of the disease and the severity of clinical symptoms. Patients and family deserve counseling about the nature of the disease, the need for ongoing medical care and regular eye examinations, correct use of corticosteroid medications, and symptoms that should be reported to a physician (red or painful eyes, blurred vision, and dyspnea on exertion). Patients with more serious impairment of pulmonary function require nursing care appropriate for restrictive chronic lung disease. These interventions were discussed previously, under the pneumoconioses.

Evaluation

When nursing goals related to sarcoidosis have been achieved, the patient will be able to

- Describe measures needed for self-care, including medication regimen and routine, follow-up appointments
- State signs and symptoms of complications to report to health-care provider
- Identify sources of support, if needed, to help him cope with the effects of the disease.

Suppurative Lung Disease

Empyema and Lung Abscess

Etiology and Pathophysiology

The term *empyema* is usually used to refer to an accumulation of pus in the thoracic cavity. Anaerobes and aerobes each cause about half the cases of empyema.[78] Most commonly, empyema results from a primary pulmonary disease such as pneumonia, tuberculosis, pulmonary infarction, or lung abscess. Mediastinal infection or infections below the diaphragm may also spread to the pleural space. A pH below 7.3 in pleural effusions has been suggested as a predisposing factor.[72]

A *lung abscess* is a fluid- and air-filled cavity that is formed when a suppurative (pus-forming) lung infection destroys lung parenchymal tissue. The majority of primary lung abscesses result from the aspiration of oral secretions.[78] Rarely, blood-borne septic materials after bowel surgery, septic abortion, or intravenous drug injection are responsible. Anaerobic bacteria are most common, but some cultures yield aerobic bacteria as well.[10]

Initially a lung abscess is isolated, but eventually it erodes and ruptures into a bronchus. If the abscess can drain freely, healing eventually occurs. When drainage is incomplete, the abscess walls become fibrotic and lined with epithelial cells, preventing complete healing. Empyema, brain abscess, and bronchiectasis can complicate lung abscess.

Clinical Manifestations

Empyema. The clinical picture of empyema varies. In acute illness, cough, high fever, unilateral chest pain, and malaise may occur. Weight loss, general malaise, and low-grade fevers may be symptoms of chronic empyema. Physical findings vary with the amount of pleural fluid. When sufficient fluid is present, unequal chest expansion, dullness to percussion, and decreased or absent breath sounds over the involved area are present.

Lung Abscess. A patient with an abscess may have a gradual or an abrupt onset of manifestations that includes sweats, fever, cough, and chest pain. When the abscess erodes and ruptures into a bronchus, large amounts of blood-streaked sputum may suddenly be expectorated. If the cause of the abscess is anaerobic organisms, the sputum is gray or brown and foul-smelling. If the abscess becomes chronic (lasting 2 or more months), weight loss and anemia may be present.

Medical Management

Diagnosis. Accurate antimicrobial treatment of suppurative lung diseases depends upon reliable identification of the bacteria causing the abscess or empyema. Sputum specimens obtained by transtracheal aspiration or percutaneous lung aspiration are more reliable than are secretions expectorated or obtained by bronchoscopy.[78] Empyema fluid is collected by thoracentesis.

Treatment

Empyema. For empyema, treatment involves combating infection with antibiotics and providing prompt drainage to minimize the development of fibrosis. Antibiotics are administered systemically and, occasionally, locally into the pleural space. Although thoracentesis is sometimes adequate to establish drainage, closed drainage with chest tubes or open drainage is usually necessary.[78] Pus is drained using a chest tube inserted into the involved area and connected to water-seal drainage with suction (see Chap 27).

When empyema is chronic and the lung is fibrosed to the chest wall, a surgical rib resection with open drainage may be necessary. If persistent massive fibrous entrapment of the underlying lung (termed *fibrothorax*) complicates the disease course, the fibrous lung tissue is removed surgically (decortication).

Lung Abscess. Because lung abscesses usually involve several organisms, two or more antibiotics may be ordered concurrently. Penicillin is commonly included in the regimen and continued for 4 to 8 weeks. Measures to improve local tissue oxygenation and promote drainage are necessary to assist antibiotic action. Percutaneous catheter insertion or aspiration through bronchoscopy may be used to drain secretions. Surgery may be necessary for severe hemoptysis and for the few abscesses that fail to respond to antimicrobial drug therapy.

Nursing Management

Nursing Diagnosis

Although nursing diagnoses must be established individually following patient assessment, probable nursing diagnoses include

- Alteration in comfort, pain, and cough, related to suppurative infection of lung tissue
- Potential for infection related to spread of infection within the lungs or to other organs

Goals. The major goals of nursing interventions are to eliminate the infection and relieve symptoms.

Interventions

The patient with empyema will usually have one or more closed chest tube drainage systems. Frequent observation of patency is necessary because the purulent drainage can cause blockage. When the empyema space is sealed, gravity drainage is possible without lung collapse and allows the patient better mobility.

Postural drainage may be used to achieve drainage of the purulent material contained in a lung abscess. The nurse administering this therapy needs to be aware of the location of the abscess and postural drainage positions required. Patients may need instruction and supervision to cough effectively and raise secretions. Additional supportive nursing measures include positioning for maximal oxygenation and drainage (abscess area up), hydration, deep breathing, and leg exercises to prevent complications such as thrombosis. Patients need to be monitored for evidence of complications such as hemorrhage, infection of other organs, and development of empyema.

Discharged patients need to understand their antibiotic regimen, the importance of good oral hygiene, symptoms of worsening or complications to report, and the importance of follow-up care.

Evaluation

For hospitalized patients, outcome criteria indicating goal achievement include the following:

- Patient verbalizes that pain is decreased
- Decreased frequency of cough and volume of sputum production
- Absence of fever, leukocytosis, and other signs of infection
- Arterial blood-gas values within normal limits
- Patient's lung examination reveals normal breath sounds, resonance to percussion, and symmetric chest expansion

Patients who will convalesce at home should be able to

- State medication regimen to be followed
- Describe complications that should be reported to health-care provider

In either case, outcomes need to be tailored to the individual patient and include a time frame for achievement.

Spontaneous Pneumothorax*

Definition and Etiology

Spontaneous pneumothorax is a sudden, often idiopathic collection of air within the pleural cavity that occurs in the absence of external trauma. When idiopathic, spontaneous pneumothorax is most typically found in tall, thin males under the age of 40. The specific cause underlying the development of most cases of spontaneous pneumothorax is obscure. Among older persons, spontaneous pneumothorax can be a complication of emphysema or cancer, or can be associated with inflammatory diseases, connective tissue or immunologic-based diseases, and localized disruptions such as fibrosis. In women, the development of spontaneous pneumothorax is sometimes attributed to pleural endometriosis and is timed with menstruation. A high percentage of those persons who develop spontaneous pneumothorax are smokers.[24,34]

Pathophysiology

Spontaneous pneumothorax usually results from the rupture of an air-filled bleb (blister) within or adjacent to the visceral pleura. Blebs are believed to form when air from a ruptured alveolus dissects through interstitial tissue and into the visceral pleura where it accumulates as a cyst. In the case of idiopathic pneumothoraces, these blebs are most frequently located at the lung apex. The cause of the initial alveolar rupture is not well understood but has been related to infection. A congenital origin for the cysts is also postulated.[34]

*Section on spontaneous pneumothorax written by Joanne Rokosky.

Clinical Manifestations

Sudden onset of sharp, pleuritic chest pain is an almost invariable complaint of patients with spontaneous pneumothorax. The pain may follow coughing, sneezing, or other exertion or may appear at a time of complete rest and is often accompanied by dyspnea. Findings on physical examination consistent with spontaneous pneumothorax include tachypnea, asymmetric chest expansion, decreased tactile fremitus, hyperresonance to percussion, decreased breath sounds, and, possibly, evidence of mediastinal shift.[24,52]

Medical Management

A tentative diagnosis of spontaneous pneumothorax is corroborated by the identification of a pneumothorax on chest film. A small pneumothorax in a mildly symptomatic, otherwise healthy patient may only be observed for evidence of continued resolution.[52] More frequently, however, the insertion of chest tubes is required for treatment. When closed chest drainage does not resolve the pneumothorax or if the pneumothorax is recurrent, surgical resection of the blebs or pleural abrasion is considered. The prognosis for recovery from spontaneous pneumothorax is highly dependent on the patient's underlying condition. Young patients with idiopathic pneumothoraces generally recover well from the episode. However, recurrence rates average 50%. In patients whose pulmonary reserve has been limited by other respiratory disease, the prognosis is much worse.[24,34]

Nursing Management

Nursing Diagnosis

The problems for a patient that result from spontaneous pneumothorax are dependent both on the size of the pneumothorax and on the patient's baseline lung function. Nursing diagnoses are thus highly dependent on the findings from the history and physical assessment. Among the nursing diagnoses that may be established are those related to the immediate problems posed by the pneumothorax. Two potential nursing diagnoses are as follows:

- Impaired gas exchange related to the presence of air in the pleural space with loss of normal ventilatory mechanics
- Alteration in comfort, pain, related to lung collapse

These two diagnoses were discussed fully in Chapter 27 and are not addressed further here. A third potential diagnostic statement relates to prevention of recurrence:

- Knowledge deficit related to prevention and recognition of recurrent pneumothorax

Interventions

If knowledge deficit is established, the goal of nursing interventions is to reduce the chances of recurrence. Patients with idiopathic spontaneous pneumothorax should be instructed to avoid those situations and activities that may predispose to pneumothorax as a result of alterations in atmospheric pressure. Occupations and activities to avoid include scuba diving and piloting aircraft.[52] Because a high percentage of those persons who develop spontaneous pneumothorax are smokers, they should be strongly encouraged to stop smoking as well. When the development of pneumothorax is related to the presence of a severe underlying lung disease, the focus of nursing interventions should be to ascertain that the patient knows how to recognize this complication and can summon appropriate assistance. In either case, patients need to understand that recurrence is very possible and that more definitive medical therapy may prove necessary.

Evaluation

Outcomes to evaluate goal achievement related to ensuring adequate knowledge are as follows:

- The patient can state signs and symptoms that may indicate recurrence and a plan for getting assistance
- The patient can state factors, such as continued smoking, that may increase the risk of recurrence.

Pleurisy and Pleural Effusion

Etiology and Pathophysiology

Pleurisy refers to an acute or chronic inflammation of the pleura with exudation into its cavity and onto its surface. When liquid is present within the pleura, it is called *pleural effusion.*

The etiology may be chemical or infectious in nature. Pleurisy, often with pleural effusion, occurs in association with a wide variety of pulmonary and cardiac diseases: chest wall infections, pericarditis, pulmonary embolism, connective tissue diseases, malignancy, chest trauma, pneumonia, and tuberculosis.

In acute pleurisy, the pleura becomes reddened, then covered with an exudate of fibrin, lymph, and cellular elements (dry stage). Extensively inflamed pleural surfaces tend to adhere, sometimes resulting in permanent adhesions.

When inflammation progresses beyond the dry state, copious exudate of serum creates a pleural effusion. Depending on its protein content, the effusion is classified as an exudate (high content of protein, cells, or solid material derived from cells) or a transudate (high fluidity and low protein and cells).

Both pleuritic chest pain and pleural fluid accumulation restrict lung expansion, resulting in reduced volumes and predisposition to atelectasis and infection.[96] Large pleural effusions can create hypoxemia from a shunt that occurs when lung portions are compressed by the fluid and do not ventilate despite continued blood flow.

Clinical Manifestations

Symptoms of pleurisy are a "stitch" in the side, chills followed by fever, cough, and pain, usually worse with cough and inspiration. Pain may be mild or severe, sharp, and knife-like. If a large pleural effusion develops, dyspnea and a nonproductive cough may occur.

Chest wall motion is often reduced on the affected side. Intercostal tenderness may be present. The patient may press the affected side with his hand or lie on it to reduce pain. In pleurisy, auscultation will detect a pleural friction rub. Physical findings of reduced or absent breath sounds and a dull percussion note over the affected area are present with pleural effusion.

Medical Management

Therapy of dry pleurisy (without effusion) involves identifying and treating the underlying disease. Antitussive medications for a hacking nonproductive cough and analgesics for pain relief may be prescribed.

Pleural effusion is diagnosed by clinical findings and chest films. Although more than 200 ml of fluid must be present for detection on usual anteroposterior and lateral chest films, as little as 5 ml can be detected if a lateral decubitus view is taken after the patient remains in the correct position 5 minutes.[96]

Pleural effusions are also treated by identifying and treating the underlying cause. This may involve antibiotic treatment for infection, drug therapy for congestive heart failure, or radiation treatment for malignancy.

For emergency relief, fluid may be removed during a thoracentesis, but it usually recurs unless the underlying cause is treated. Effusions from malignancy may be treated using chemical sclerosing agents or surgical methods to obliterate the pleural space. Improvement in pleurisy or pleural effusion can be expected with improvement in the underlying disease.

Nursing Management

Assessment and Nursing Diagnosis

Because pleurisy is associated with many conditions, some of them serious, effort should be made to determine the cause of the pleuritic symptoms. For example, patients with pulmonary emboli often complain of pleuritic chest pain.

Following assessment, specific nursing diagnoses can be established. Two possible examples of nursing diagnoses follow:

- Potential impairment in gas exchange related to presence of large pleural effusion or shallow breathing
- Alteration in comfort, pain, and shortness of breath, related to inflammation of pleural space

Goals of nursing care are to relieve pain and to prevent further complications such as atelectasis or pneumonia that may result from hypoventilation.

Interventions

Respiratory function should be monitored. To prevent atelectasis, the patient needs to be repositioned and asked to take sustained deep breaths every hour or two. A high Fowler's position facilitates chest expansion.

Although tight chest binders were used in the past to reduce pleuritic pain, this is uncommon today because it contributes to the development of atelectasis. Adequate analgesia combined with frequent deep breathing and perhaps chest splinting during coughing is used. If no secretions are present, antitussives may be used. If secretions are present, cough suppressants should be avoided while bronchial hygiene measures to clear secretions are employed.

The patient should be monitored for fever, increased dyspnea, and reduced breath sounds or other changes that suggest a complication.

Evaluation

Outcomes indicating achievement of goals related to nursing interventions include the following:

- Patient verbalizes a decrease in pain, shortness of breath, and other symptoms
- Patient's arterial blood-gas values are within acceptable range
- Patient's lung examination reveals normal breath sounds and resonance to percussion

Special Conditions

This chapter closes with a discussion of conditions that, although not predominately respiratory in nature, may severely impair respiratory function. The primary defect for most of these disorders involves either the thoracic cage or the nervous system. When severe, each condition can cause restrictive lung disease that is similar in many respects to the respiratory disorders described above.

Thoracic Cage Disorders

Kyphosis and Scoliosis

Kyphosis refers to a posterior curvature of the spine that may be associated with poor posture, chronic arthritis, tuberculosis, or growth disturbances of the vertebral epiphysis.

Scoliosis refers to a lateral curvature of the spine. In most cases its cause is unknown, although tuberculosis or neuromuscular disease can lead to the condition. Although mild cases have no physiological impact on the lungs, severe scoliosis can result in serious consequences.[98] Deformities severe enough to lead to respiratory impairment are obvious on physical examination and chest radiographs.

Early in these diseases, patients may have dyspnea associated with a uniform reduction of all lung volumes.[92] The chest wall is stiff and muscles operate inefficiently. Patients experience frequent respiratory infections that may lead to progressive ventilation and perfusion mismatching, arterial hypoxemia, pulmonary hypertension, and eventually respiratory failure. The increased work of breathing may also be associated with a reduced ventilatory response to carbon dioxide and carbon dioxide retention.[98]

Ankylosing Spondylitis

Ankylosing spondylitis is a disease of unknown etiology that is characterized by gradual systemic scarring within joints and immobility of vertebral joints with fixation of the ribs. Chest movement becomes markedly reduced, but the vital capacity is usually reduced only minimally.[92] Airway resistance is normal. Since this disease affects the chest wall and not the lung or diaphragm, pulmonary compliance, ventilation distribution, and blood-gas values are usually normal.[92] Respiratory failure rarely occurs.

Rib Fractures

Rib fractures from thoracic trauma result in abnormal lung bellows function. Tidal volume may be severely reduced with maldistributed ventilation and severe hypercapnia and hypoxemia. Chapter 31 discusses the assessment and care of patients with chest trauma.

Obesity

Obesity can be associated with a restrictive lung impairment. More often obese persons do not have the reduced total lung capacity that is required for a strict definition of restrictive lung disease.[33] However, their reduced expiratory reserve volume often results in preferential ventilation of upper rather than lower lobes and closure of some lung alveoli before the end of tidal breathing. The hypoventilation or lack of ventilation, especially in lower lobes, results in ventilation/perfusion mismatching and hypoxemia.[92]

Obesity often creates pulmonary problems by encroachment of the posterior pharyngeal airway, resulting in intermittent upper-airway obstruction occurring during sleep (labeled obstructive sleep apnea).[51]

Nursing Management

Specific nursing diagnoses, goals, interventions, and evaluation criteria for patients with thoracic cage disorders that create restrictive lung disease depend upon the extent of the lung pathophysiology. They are generally similar to those for patients with other chronic restrictive conditions. Measures to prevent respiratory infection, or at least to recognize infections and institute prompt care, are important. Patients and family should be counselled about adjustments required by the physiological limitations and self-care requirements of a chronic condition. The reader is referred to the appropriate chapters for management of the underlying condition.

Neurological and Neuromuscular Disorders

As Chapter 25 discussed, the control of ventilation in humans is a highly complex process that integrates respiratory neural centers, muscles, and bellows (chest wall and lungs). An abnormality in any one of these components interferes with the ability to regulate alveolar ventilation. The hallmark of these alveolar regulation disturbances is an increase or descrease in the arterial carbon dioxide tension.

Neuromuscular Disorders

Many neurological disorders that affect respiratory motor nerves or myoneural junctions interfere with the ability to take deep breaths, creating reduced lung volumes and alveolar hypoventilation. Depending upon the disease stage and degree of motor neuron loss, multiple sclerosis, myasthenia gravis, and polio (see Chap 67 and 68) can limit lung function. When these diseases involve the most important muscle of respiration, the diaphragm, dyspnea results. Respiratory infection is a frequent complication that results from ineffective coughing. The effects of progressive disease on lung function are monitored by vital capacity and arterial blood-gas results.

Cervical spine injuries (see Chap 69) above the level of the third to fifth cervical roots produce respiratory paralysis requiring ventilator respiration.

Primary muscular disorders such as muscular dystrophy (see Chap 67) may affect respiratory muscles, leading to reduced lung volumes, and eventually to hypoventilatory respiratory failure.

Depression of Medulla Respiratory Center

When brain lesions such as tumors or infarctions affect areas associated with respiratory control, changes in the respiratory pattern can be observed. If the diencephalon is affected, sighs, yawns, and a Cheyne–Stokes respiratory pattern can be observed. Midbrain involvement is associated with an increased rate and depth of breathing, whereas lesions of the pons result in rapid, shallow, regular breaths. When the respiratory center in the medulla is involved, ataxic respirations precede death.[70]

The central chemoreceptors located in the medulla can have their ventilatory sensitivity to blood and spinal fluid carbon dioxide tension suppressed by a wide variety of drugs including sedatives, hypnotics, narcotics, and anesthetics.[87] The magnitude of the depression is related to drug dosage.[69]

Nursing Management

Nursing management for the various neuromuscular disorders is contained in other sections of this text. Assessment of a patient with any of these disorders should include careful observation for respiratory dysfunction caused by the primary neuromuscular problem. Appropriate nursing diagnoses can then be established.

Whenever a drug with respiratory depressant properties is prescribed, particularly to an elderly patient or one with obstructive lung disease, the smallest effective dose should be given initially. Any increase in dosage must be made cautiously with appropriate monitoring. Antipsychotic, antidepressant, and nonnarcotic analgesic drugs, which generally do not cause respiratory depression, should be substituted where possible in high-risk patients.[101]

Nurses have an important responsibility to monitor reactions to drugs with respiratory depressant properties and to report observations of depressant side-effects, withholding ordered dosages where appropriate. Patients who use these drugs, especially the elderly and those with preexisting respiratory conditions, need to understand their dangerous side-effects.

References

1. American Thoracic Society: Treatment of tuberculosis in alcoholic patients. Am Rev Respir Dis 116:559–564, 1977
2. American Thoracic Society: Diagnostic standards and classification of tuberculosis and other mycobacterial diseases, 14th ed. Am Rev Respir Dis 123:343–358, 1981
3. American Thoracic Society: The tuberculin skin test. Am Rev Respir Dis 124:356–363, 1981
4. American Thoracic Society: Control of tuberculosis. Am Rev Respir Dis 128:336–342, 1983
5. American Thoracic Society: Treatment of tuberculosis and other mycobacterial diseases. Am Rev Respir Dis 127:790–796, 1983
6. Aronson MD, Weiss St, Ben RL et al: Association between cigarette smoking and acute respiratory tract illness in young adults. JAMA 248:181–183, 1982
7. Austrian R: Pneumococcal vaccine: Development and prospects. Am J Med 67:547, 1979
8. Axelson A, Runze U: Comparison of subjective and radiologic findings during the course of acute maxillary sinusitis. Ann Otol Rhinol Laryngol 92:75, 1982
9. Bailey WC: Diagnosis of tuberculosis. Clin Chest Med 1:209–217, 1980
10. Bartlett JG, Finegold SM: Anaerobic infections of the lung and pleural space. Am Rev Respir Dis 110:56–77, 1974
11. Bates JH: Transmission and pathogenesis of tuberculosis. Clin Chest Med 1:167–173, 1980
12. Bindschadler DD: Pulmonary fungus diseases. In Mitchell RS, petty TL (eds): Synopsis of Clinical Pulmonary Disease, 3rd ed. St Louis, CV Mosby, 1982
13. Boerner DF, Zwadyk P: The value of the sputum Gram's stain in community-acquired pneumonia. JAMA 247:642–645, 1982
14. Bradsher RW Jr: Overwhelming pneumonia. Postgrad Med 74:201–217, 1983
15. Brooks SM: An approach to patients suspected of having an occupational pulmonary disease. Clin Chest Med 2:171–178, 1981
16. Casey KF, Rom WN, Moatemed F: Asbestos related disease. Clin Chest Med 2:179–202, 1981
17. Centers for Disease Control: Tuberculosis: United States, 1983. MMWR 33:77–78, 1984
18. Centers for Disease Control: Update: Pneumococcal polysaccharide vaccine usage: United States. MMWR 33:3071, 1984
19. Cole RB: Drug Treatment Respiratory Disease. Nw York, Churchill Livingstone, 1981
20. Couch RB: Orthomyxoviruses: Influenza. In Stein JH: Internal Medicine. Boston, Little, Brown & Co, 1983
21. Coulehan JL: Ascorbic acid and the common cold. Postgrad Med 66:153, 1979
22. Davidson PT: The management of disease with atypical mycobacteria. Clin Notes Respir Dis 18:3–13, 1979
23. Deatsch WW: Ear, nose and throat. In Krupp MA, Chatton MJ (eds): Medical Diagnosis and Treatment, 1983, pp 93–110. Los Altos, Lange Medical Publications, 1983
24. DeVries WC, Wolfe WG: The management of spontaneous pneumothorax and bullous emphysema. Surg Clin North Am 60:851, 1980

25. Dowdle WR: Surveillance and control of infectious diseases: Progress toward the 1990 objectives. Public Health Rep 98:210–218, 1983
26. Dressler DK, Smejkal C, Ruffolo ML: A comparison of oral and rectal temperature measurement on patients receiving oxygen by mask. Nurs Res 32:373–375, 1983
27. Dutt AK, Stead WW: Chemotherapy of tuberculosis for the 1980s. Clin Chest Med 1:243–251, 1980
28. Evans FO Jr, Snyder JB, Moore WEC et al: Sinusitis of the maxillary antrum. N Engl J Med 298:413–416, 1978
29. Fagerhaugh S: Getting around with emphysema. In Strauss AL, Glaser BG (eds): Chronic Illness and the Quality of Life. St Louis, CV Mosby 1975
30. Farer LS: Chemoprophylaxis against tuberculosis. Clin Chest Med 1:203–208, 1980
31. Farer LS: The public health aspects of tuberculosis. Semin Respir Med 2:175, 1981
32. Frame PT: Acute infectious pneumonia in the adult. Basics Respir Dis 10:1–8, 1982
33. Gazioglu K, Israel RH: The pulmonary function test. In Poe RH, Israel RH (eds): Problems in Pulmonary Medicine for the Primary Physician. Philadelphia, Lea & Febiger, 1982
34. Getz SB, Beasley WE: Spontaneous pneumothorax. Am J Surg 6:823, 1983
35. Goodwin RZ, Loyd JE, Des Pres RM: Histoplasmosis in normal hosts. Medicine 60:231–266, 1981
36. Graham WGB, Bradley DA: Efficacy of chest physiotherapy and intermittent positive pressure breathing in the resolution of pneumonia. N Engl J Med 299:624–677, 1978
37. Griffith HW: Instructions for Patients, 3rd ed. Philadelphia, WB Saunders, 1982
38. Grosmaire EK: Use of patient positioning to improve PaO_2: A review. Heart Lung 12:650–653, 1983
39. Grossman M, Jawetz E: Infectious diseases: Bacterial. In Krupp MA, Chatton MJ (eds): Current Medical Diagnosis and Treatment, pp 836–861. Los Altos, Lange Medical Publications, 1983
40. Guidoth TL, Goldsmith JR: Air pollution and family health. Am Fam Phys 27:165–172, 1983
41. Gwaltney JM Jr: The common cold. In Mandell GL, Douglas RG Jr, Bennett JE (eds): Principles and Practices of Infectious Diseases. New York, John Wiley & Sons, 1979
42. Hall CB: Respiratory syncitial virus. In Madell GL, Douglas RG, Bennett JE (eds): Principles and Practices of Infectious Disease. New York, John Wiley & Sons, 1979
43. Hamory GH, Sande MA, Sydnor A Jr et al: Etiology and antimicrobial therapy of acute maxillary sinusitis. J Infect Dis 139:197–202, 1979
44. Hanson EI: Effects of chronic lung disease on life in general and on sexuality: Perceptions of adult patients. Heart Lung 11:435–441, 1982
45. Harber P: Prevention and control of occupational lung disease. Clin Chest Med 2:343–355, 1981
46. Hasler ME, Cohen JA: The effect of oxygen administration on oral temperature assessment. Nurs Res 31:265–268, 1982
47. Hinshaw HC, Murray JF: Diseases of the Chest, 4th ed. Philadelphia, WB Saunders 1980
48. Hirschmann JV, Lipsky BA: Pneumococcal vaccine in the United States: A critical analysis. JAMA 246:1428–1432, 1981
49. Hoeprich PD: Diphtheria. In Hoeprich PD (ed): Infectious Diseases, 3rd ed. Philadelphia, Harper & Row, 1983
50. Hoole AJ, Greenberg RA, Pickard CG Jr: Patient Care Guidelines for Nurse Practitioners, 2nd ed. Boston, Little, Brown & Co, 1982
51. Hyde RW: Dyspnea. In Poe RH, Israel RH (eds): Problems in Pulmonary Medicine for the Primary Physician. Philadelphia, Lea & Febiger, 1982
52. Ingram RH Jr: Diseases of the pleura, mediastinum, and diaphragm. In Petersdorf RG, Adams RD, Braunwald E et al (eds): Harrison's Principles of Internal Medicine, 10th ed. New York, McGraw–Hill, 1983
53. Jawetz E: Infections in the lung. In Krupp MA, Chatton MJ (eds): Current Medical Diagnosis and Treatment, p 123. Los Altos, Lange Medical Publications, 1983
54. Johanson WG, Pierce AK, Sanford JP et al: Nosocomial respiratory infections with gram negative bacilli: The significance of colonization of the respiratory tract. Ann Intern Med 77:701, 1972
55. Johns CJ, Macgregor MI, Zachary JB et al: Extended experience in the long term corticosteroid treatment of pulmonary sarcoidosis. Ann NY Acad Sci 278:722, 1976
56. Kasik JE: Tuberculosis and other mycobacterial diseases. In Rakel RE (ed): Current Therapy, pp 125–132. Philadelphia, WB Saunders, 1984
57. Kelley HW: Respiratory diseases. In Katcher BS, Young LY, Koda-Kimble MA (eds): Applied Therapeutics: The Clinical Use of Drugs, 3rd ed. San Francisco, Applied Therapeutics, 1983
58. Lapp NL: Lung disease secondary to inhalation of nonfibrous minerals. Clin Chest Med 2:219–233, 1981
59. Levin S: The atypical pneumonia syndrome. JAMA 251:945–948, 1984
60. Levy ML, Ericsson CD, Pickering LK: Infection of the upper respiratory tract. Med Clin North Am 67:153, 1983
61. Liu C: Sinusitis. In Hoeprick PD (ed): Infectious Diseases, 3rd ed. Philadelphia, Harper & Row, 1983
62. McHenry MC, Weinstein AJ: Antimicrobial drugs and infections. Med Clin North Am 67:5–16, 1983
63. Manson RM, Rushing JL: Respiratory tract and mediastinum. In Krupp MA, Chatton MJ (eds): Current Medical Diagnosis and Treatment, pp 111–163. Los Altos, Lange Medical Publications, 1983
64. Monto AS, Ullman BM: Acute respiratory illness in an American community: The Tecumseh Study. JAMA 227:164–169, 1974
65. Morse DL, Hansen RE, Swalbach G et al: High rate of tuberculin conversion in Indochinese refugees. JAMA 248:2983–2986, 1982
66. Moss JM: Pneumococcus infection in diabetes mellitus: Is this justification for immunization? JAMA 243:3301–3303, 1980
67. Murray JP: Complications after treatment of chronic maxillary sinus disease with Caldwell–Luc procedure. Laryngoscope 93:282-284, 1983
68. Pape JW, Johnson WD Jr: Gram-positive aerobic bacilli infections: Corynebacteria and listeria. In Stein JH (ed): Internal Medicine, Boston, Little, Brown & Co, 1983
69. Pavlin EG, Hornbein: The control of breathing. Basics Respir Dis 7:1–6, 1978
70. Plum F, Posner JB: The Diagnosis of Stupor and Coma, 3rd ed. Philadelphia, FA Davis, 1980
71. Podjasek JH: Respiratory infection in the mechanically ventilated patient: An overview. Heart Lung 12:5–10, 1983
72. Potts DE, Levin DC, Sahn SA: Pleural fluid in parapneumonia effusions. Chest 70:328–331, 1976
73. Robbins SL, Cotran RS: Pathologic Basis of Disease, 2nd ed. Philadelphia, WB Saunders, 1979
74. Sanford JP: Guide to Antibiotic Therapy. West Bethesda, MD, 1984
75. Sanford JP, Pierce AK: Lower respiratory tract infections. In Bennet JV, Brachman PS (eds): Hospital Infections. Boston, Little, Brown & Co, 1979
76. Sarosi GA: Management of fungal diseases. Am Rev Respir Dis 127:250–253, 1983
77. Sbarbaro JA, Davidson PT: Pulmonary tuberculosis. In Mitchell RS, Petty TL (eds): Synopsis of Clinical Pulmonary Disease, 3rd ed, pp 136–150. St Louis, CV Mosby, 1982

78. Schachter EN: Suppurative lung disease: Old problems revisited. Clin Chest Med 2:41–49, 1981
79. Seebohm PM: Allergic and nonallergic rhinitis. In English GM (ed): Otolaryngology, Vol 2. Philadelphia, Harper & Row, 1984
80. Selikoff IJ, Hammond ED: Asbestos and smoking. JAMA 242:458, 1979
81. Selikoff IJ, Lee DHK: Asbestos and disease. New York, Academic Press, 1978
82. Sheffield RW, Cassisi NJ, Karlan MS: Complications of sinusitis: What to watch for. Postgrad Med 63:93–96, 99–101, 1978
83. Simon HB: Management of sarcoidosis. In Goroll AH, May LA, Mulley AG (eds): Primary Care Medicine. Philadelphia, JB Lippincott, 1981
84. Simon HB: Management of tuberculosis. In Goroll AH, May LA, Mulley AG (eds): Primary Care Medicine. Philadelphia, JB Lippincott, 1981
85. Simon HB: Screening for and prophylaxis of tuberculosis. In Goroll AH, May LA, Mulley AG (eds): Primary Care Medicine, pp 148–150. Philadelphia, JB Lippincott, 1981
86. Simon HB: Mycobacteria. In Rubenstein E, Tederman DD (eds): Scientific American Medicine. New York, Scientific American, 1984
87. Steen SN: The effects of psychotropic drugs on respiration. Pharmacol Ther B 2:717–741, 1976
88. Stoeckle JD: Screening for occupational respiratory disease. In Goroll AH, May LA, Mulley AG (eds): Primary Care Medicine, pp 151–154. Philadelphia, JB Lippincott, 1981
89. Strauss AL, Glaser BG (eds): Chronic Illness and the Quality of Life. St Louis, CV Mosby, 1975
90. Swartz MN: Clinical aspects of Legionnaire's disease. Ann Intern Med 90:492, 1979
91. Thomson PS, Willis JC: Compliance challenges in a black lung clinic. Nurs Clin North Am 17:513–521, 1982
92. Tisi G: Restrictive lung disease. In Pulmonary Physiology in Clinical Medicine, pp 175–188. Baltimore, Williams & Wilkins, 1980
93. Utz J: Chemotherapy of the systemic mycosis. Med Clin North Am 66:221–234, 1982
94. Van Tyle WK: Internal analgesic products. In Handbook of Non Prescription Drugs, 7th ed. Washington, DC, American Pharmaceutical Association, 1982
95. Walsh BT et al: Recognition of streptococcal pharyngitis in adults. Arch Intern Med 135:1493, 1975
96. Wegmann JA, Forshee T: Malignant pleural effusion: Pertinent issues. Heart Lung 12:533–543, 1983
97. Weill H: Asbestos-associated disease: Science, public policy, and litigation. Chest 84:601–608, 1983
98. West JB: Pulmonary Pathophysiology: The Essentials, 2nd ed. Baltimore, Williams & Wilkins, 1982
99. West S, Branden B, Stolley P et al: A review of antihistamines and the common cold. Pediatrics 56:100, 1975
100. Zeiger RS, Schatz M: Rhinitis. In Stein JH (ed): Internal Medicine. Boston, Little, Brown & Co, 1983
101. Ziment I: Respiratory Pharmacology and Therapeutics. Philadelphia, WB Saunders, 1978
102. Ziskind M. Jones RN, Weill H: Silicosis. Am Rev Respir Dis 113:643, 1976

Bibliography

Occupational and Environmental Health Committee of the American Lung Association of San Diego and Imperial Counties: Taking the occupational history. Ann intern Med 99:641–651, 1983

Wade JF: Comprehensive Respiratory Care: Physiology and Technique, 3rd ed. St Louis, CV Mosby, 1982

Wilson WR: Antimicrobial chemoprophylaxis. Med Clin North Am 67:99–112, 1983

Chapter 29

Obstructive Respiratory Disorders

Asthma
COPD
Bronchiectasis
Cystic Fibrosis

Kathryn L. Anderson

Asthma

Definition and Etiology

Asthma is defined as a syndrome of reversible obstructive airway diseases that is characterized by contraction of the smooth muscles of the airway, hypersecretion of mucus, and inflammation.[20] Episodes of airway obstruction are recurrent but are separated by asymptomatic periods. Although asthma is usually associated with children or allergies, it can in fact begin at any age, can occur in the absence of allergies, and can be disabling. Asthma may occur in adults who have no other respiratory disease but is more often found as a reversible component of chronic obstructive pulmonary disease (COPD).[31]

In the past, asthma was classified as either extrinsic or intrinsic according to the presence or absence of identifiable precipitating stimuli and a history of allergy. "Allergic" asthma was classified as extrinsic, and nonallergic asthma was known as intrinsic. However, because it is now recognized that characteristics of both extrinsic and intrinsic asthma may be present in a single person, this classification is less popular now than it once was.[33] A more useful way of categorizing asthma is according to specific etiologic factors such as allergy-causing substances, infections, drugs, and psychological factors. Table 29–1 lists many factors that can precipitate episodes of asthma.

Pathophysiology

Two mechanisms that produce bronchospasm in asthma have been identified: anaphylactic reaction and autonomic imbalance.

Immediate Hypersensitivity or Anaphylactic Reaction. There is a relatively high concentration of mast cells in the respiratory tract. Exposure to an antigen to which the host has been sensitized results in the release of numerous chemical mediators from the mast cells. These mediators affect the lung by causing the following: dilatation and increased permeability of small blood vessels, producing inflammation; contraction of bronchial smooth muscle, producing bronchospasm; and increased secretion from mucous membranes.

Autonomic Imbalance. The degree to which bronchial smooth muscles contract at any moment is determined to a lesser extent by the balance of cholinergic (parasympathetic) and adrenergic (sympathetic) stimulation. Cholinergic stimulation causes contraction of bronchial smooth muscle and bronchoconstriction, whereas adrenergic stimulation causes relaxation and bronchodilation. There is thought to be an imbalance of these two stimuli in asthmatics; thus, there may be a hyperactive cholinergic system and a hypoactive adrenergic system, resulting in bronchoconstriction. The abnormality is illustrated by the fact that β-adrenergic blocking agents (*e.g.*, propranolol) cause bronchospasm in asthmatics but not in nonasthmatics.[12,13,20,44]

Effects of Acute Airway Obstruction. The result of acute bronchoconstriction (bronchospasm), mucosal edema, and increased airway secretions is obstruction of the airways and a subsequent decrease in expiratory flow rates. Because expiratory air flow is reduced, air becomes trapped and the lungs hyperinflate. Some airways may become plugged with mucus, resulting in areas of atelectasis. Overall ventilation decreases because of the obstruction, and hypoxemia can occur if ventilation and perfusion are no longer matched. Hypercapnia is usually a later development and results from the severe obstruction, the high work of breathing, and, eventually, from exhaustion. The effects of acute airway obstruction are illustrated in Figure 29–1.

Medical Management

Diagnosis. As stated in the definition, asthma is a syndrome characterized by periods of quiescence, which may be of long duration, punctuated by intermittent "paroxysmal" attacks.[37] One of the major difficulties in diagnosing asthma in adults who are not experiencing an acute attack is the lack of obvious signs and symptoms.[35] The patient may complain of such vague symptoms as cough, dyspnea on exertion, or weakness. The arterial blood gases and chest film may be normal. However, baseline pulmonary function tests may reveal signs of obstruction to airflow even when the patient is asymptomatic. The forced expiratory volume in one second (FEV_1) may be reduced by as much as 50% below baseline before symptoms appear. $FEF_{25-75\%}$, or forced expiratory flow between 25% and 75% of the forced vital capacity (FVC), a measurement of small-airway obstruction, may also be reduced.[33]

The diagnosis of asthma is made after ruling out other possible causes for the patients symptoms and after documenting reversible airway obstruction. Other potential diagnoses in adults whose symptoms may resemble those of asthma are

- Foreign body aspiration
- Anatomical abnormality of upper airway
- Cardiac asthma
- Pulmonary embolus
- Anaphylactic shock
- Carcinoid syndrome
- Extrinsic allergic alveolitis
- COPD without reversibility
- Acute bronchitis

The most important factor in the diagnosis of asthma is the demonstration of significant improvement in expiratory flow rates (*i.e.*, FEV_1, $FEF_{25-75\%}$) following administration of an inhaled bronchodilator.[31] An increase of 15% or more in FEV_1 and 25% or more in $FEF_{25-75\%}$ is considered to be significant improvement and therefore evidence of reversible airway obstruction. Other criteria used for diagnosis include a history of episodic respiratory distress, demonstrated allergy by a positive skin test, blood or sputum eosinophilia, or antigen-specific IgE in the blood. The latter three findings are particularly useful in detecting allergic asthma.[31,33]

TABLE 29–1
Factors Known to Precipitate Asthmatic Episodes

Allergic factors
Usually pollen, mold spores, animal dander
Occupational irritants including inorganic and organic chemicals, dusts, and grains
Autonomic imbalance
Infection, usually viral
Pharmacological factors
β-adrenergic blockers (*e.g.*, propranolol)
Prostaglandin inhibitors
Aspirin, in association with nasal polyps and sinusitis
Nonsteroidal anti-inflammatory drugs (*e.g.*, ibuprofen, indomethacin)
Ethanol
Anticholinesterase drugs (*e.g.*, neostigmine, edrophonium chloride)
Yellow food coloring
Psychological factors
Respiratory heat loss (exercise-induced asthma)
Cold air
Exercise

(Data from Hodgkin JE: Chronic Obstructive Pulmonary Disease: Current Concepts in Diagnosis and Comprehensive Care, 1st ed. Park Ridge, American College of Chest Physicians, 1979; Hudgel DW, Madsen LA: Acute and chronic asthma. A guide to intervention. Am J Nurs 80:1971, 1980; Leff A: Pathophysiology of asthmatic bronchoconstriction. Chest 82, 13s, 1982)

Treatment. The goals of medical therapy in asthma are prevention of acute attacks and relief of the symptoms.

First, the patient's baseline respiratory function is evaluated and other respiratory tract diseases (*e.g.*, sinusitis, nasal polyps, rhinitis, postnasal drip) are treated. Treatment of these conditions is important because nasal mucosal edema and postnasal drip may induce bronchospasm. Antihistamines and decongestants may be sufficient therapy, or antibiotics may be required if infection is present.[15,37]

Chronic wheezing requires therapy with oral bronchodilators. The first drug prescribed is a long-acting theophylline preparation, such as Theo-Dur. If wheezing persists, an oral or inhaled β_2-adrenergic agonist, such as albuterol or metaproterenol sulfate, is added.[15,34,37] Finally, oral corticosteroids (prednisone, prednisolone) may be added to the regimen if the patient has not responded to therapeutic doses of the other drugs and if a 2-week trial results in significant improvement in expiratory flow rates.[31] In some patients, an inhaled corticosteroid (beclomethasone dipropionate) may be substituted for the oral drug.

Episodic wheezing, such as that experienced in

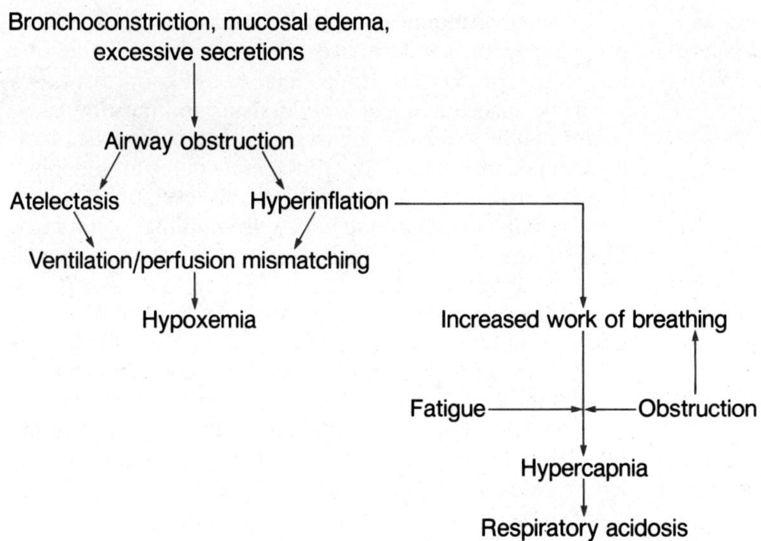

FIGURE 29–1 Pathophysiology of acute asthma. (Adapted from Ghory AC, Patterson R: Treating Asthma in the Elderly. Geriatrics, 35:32, 1980)

exercise-induced asthma, may be prevented with the inhalation of a β_2-adrenergic agonist (*e.g.,* metaproterenol) or cromolyn sodium prior to the precipitating activity. However, cromolyn is rarely useful in bronchospasm associated with COPD.[15,34,37]

Nursing Management: Nonacute Asthma

Nursing interventions during asymptomatic periods are different than those during an acute asthma attack. Historical information is particularly important for planning interventions that may minimize future acute episodes. Physical assessment is of less importance and is discussed later in the section on acute asthma.

Assessment and Nursing Diagnosis

Data Analysis. The nurse should question the patient closely, although not intrusively, as to any pattern there might be to his acute episodes. This information may lead to the identification of specific precipitating factors.[15] A family history of asthma or patient history of allergies may also lead to the identification of precipitating factors, which may then be eliminated or avoided. Because lack of understanding of the prescribed medication regimen may lead to poor compliance, the nurse must assess the patient's knowledge of the purpose, use, and side-effects of each medication. The patient should also be asked about other medical problems for which he is being treated. In some instances, medications used to treat other problems may induce bronchospasm, including β-adrenergic blocking agents such as propranolol and timolol maleate (Timoptic Solution).

During the patient interview, the nurse can gather information regarding the patient's attitude toward his illness and how the disease has affected his life. Denial of the illness may result in poor adherence to the therapeutic regimen and failure to monitor symptoms, whereas anxiety may lead to panic and overmedication.[15] It is important to determine whether the patient feels he has control over his disease or whether the disease controls his life.[35] The patient who feels responsible for control of what happens to him is more likely to comply with prescribed therapy than is the person who feels helpless in the face of unpredictable or unpleasant symptoms.

The number of stressors being experienced by the patient may influence the ability to prevent acute attacks. Although psychological factors are rarely the sole cause of attacks, stress and change may play a part in inducing bronchospasm.

The attitude of the patient's family may also be important. A supportive family may have a positive influence on the patient's attitude, acceptance, and adherence to the therapeutic regimen, whereas a nonsupportive, denying, or anxiety-producing family may be a factor that precipitates asthmatic episodes.[15]

Finally, a reasonable search of the patient's home or work environment may be made in an effort to identify respiratory irritants.[31] The presence of several pets in the home, family members or co-workers who smoke cigarettes, or known occupational causes of asthma are a few of the obvious possible causes of bronchial irritation. Elimination of the irritant must also involve reasonable measures. The improvement in health status that may result from major changes in the patient's lifestyle, such as moving or changing jobs, may not be worth the trauma associated with such changes.

Nursing Diagnoses. After analyzing the indepth history as well as other assessment parameters, the nurse can formulate diagnoses. Among the many potential nursing diagnoses for the patient with nonacute asthma are the following:

- Ineffective individual or family coping related to insufficient knowledge of asthma and its management, inadequate support system, negative body image, disruption of personal or family lifestyle by disease
- Noncompliance related to knowledge deficit, denial of illness, or perceived lack of control over symptoms

Goals. The desired outcome of nursing interventions in nonacute asthma is that the patient accepts responsibility for control of his disease, and, as a result, the frequency and severity of acute attacks are decreased. In order to achieve this goal, the patient must have sufficient knowledge of his disease and treatment to make good decisions.

Interventions: Health Teaching

Patient education begins with an explanation of the pathophysiology of asthma, adjusted to a level appropriate to the patient's learning abilities. Once the mechanisms of the disease process are understood, the patient can then understand how his prescribed medications can help relieve his symptoms.

Pharmacotherapy. The common side-effects of asthmatic medications that should be included in patient teaching are listed in Table 29–2. In general, the patient should be able to explain the reason he is taking each medication and the correct dosage and time he should take it. He should know the common side-effects of each drug and when to notify his physician or nurse if side-effects appear.

TABLE 29–2
Common Side-Effects of Frequently Used Prescription Medications for Asthma

Methylxanthines (theophylline, aminophylline)
- Central nervous system: headache, irritability, restlessness, insomnia, muscle twitching, convulsions
- Cardiovascular: tachycardia, palpitations, extrasystoles, flushing, hypotension
- Gastrointestinal: nausea, vomiting, diarrhea, epigastric pain, hematemesis

Sympathomimetics (metaproterenol, albuterol, terbutaline)
- Central nervous system: tremors
- Cardiovascular: tachycardia

Oral adrenal corticosteroids (prednisone, prednisolone)
- Central nervous system: euphoria or depression
- Cardiovascular: petechiae, bruising, edema, hypertension
- Metabolic/endocrine: hypokelamia, hypocalcemia, diabetes, hypothalamic–pituitary–adrenal axis suppression
- Gastrointestinal: nausea, vomiting, increased appetite, peptic ulcer
- Immunologic: immune suppression, increased susceptibility to infection
- Muscoloskeletal: weakness, osteoporosis
- Appearance: fat deposition (moon face, buffalo hump, truncal obesity)

Inhaled adrenal corticosteroids (beclomethasone)
- Gastrointestinal: oral *Candida* infection

Cromolyn sodium
- Respiratory: bronchospasm, throat irritation
- Skin: rash

(Data from Kirilloff LH, Tibbals SC: Drugs for asthma: A complete guide. Am J Nurs 83:55, 1983; Ziment I: Respiratory Pharmacology and Therapeutics, 1st ed. Philadelphia, WB Saunders, 1978)

A methylxanthine, usually a long-acting theophylline preparation or its derivative, aminophylline, is the first medication prescribed. The patient should know that doses are to be spaced at equal time intervals and must be taken even when he feels well so that a constant therapeutic blood level can be maintained. The therapeutic range for theophylline is narrow: 10 μg to 20 μg/ml. At this level, bronchodilation is optimal and adverse effects are minimal. A level less than 10 μg/ml indicates inadequate bronchodilation, while above 20 μg/ml, adverse or toxic effects are common.[18]

Maintenance of a therapeutic blood level of theophylline is complicated by the fact that the half-life of the drug is affected by many factors. Because cigarette smoking decreases the half-life of theophylline, relatively higher doses are needed. Cimetidine and some antibiotics increase the half-life of theophylline, as do liver disease, congestive heart failure, and fever.[18,44]

Sympathomimetics such as metaproterenol, terbutaline sulfate, or albuterol may be prescribed in oral or inhaled forms. Inhaled bronchodilators have the advantage of producing fewer systemic side-effects than oral medications, but many older patients have difficulty using the metered-dose devices properly. A recent development in the use of metered-dose devices is the use of "spacers," which makes it easier for patients to use the devices effectively (Fig. 29–2). Another option is the use of an electrically powered nebulizer, such as a PulmoAide, which allows the drug to be inhaled over approximately 10 minutes. When inhaled drugs are used, the patient should be able to demonstrate proper use of the metered-dose inhaler or nebulizer. He should also be able to demonstrate how to clean and care for his equipment (Table 29–3).

Oral adrenal corticosteroids should be taken with food or an antacid to minimize gastric irritation by the drug. The entire daily dose should be taken at one time in the early morning to coincide with the body's release of adrenal hormones. They should never be discontinued suddenly, since an Addisonian crisis may be precipitated (Table 29–4).

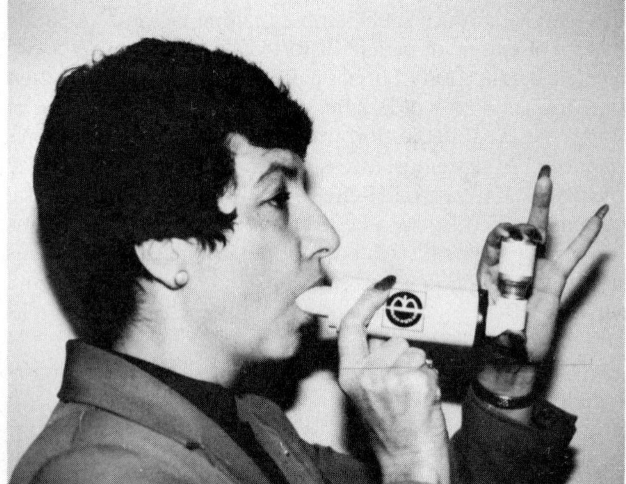

FIGURE 29–2 Use of metered-dose device with spacer. Insertion of a metered-dose device into a spacer allows the medication to be inhaled over several breaths rather than during one inspiration.

TABLE 29–3
Cleaning of Home Inhalation Therapy Equipment*

1. Each night, wash tubing, mouthpiece, nebulizer, *etc.*, in mild detergent, such as Joy, Lux, or Ivory; scrub thoroughly.
2. Rinse equipment well, making sure all soap is removed.
3. Soak equipment in solution of 2 parts white distilled vinegar and 3 parts distilled water for 20 minutes.
4. Rinse. Air dry on a clean towel. Be sure to remove all water from the tubing.
5. When dry, store in a plastic bag or dust-free area.

* Specific instructions vary among medical centers. The above are the recommendations of the American Thoracic Society.

(Data from American Thoracic Society: Statement for the committee on therapy. Am Rev Respir Dis 98:521, 1968; Hodgkin JE: Chronic Obstructure Pulmonary Disease: Current Concepts in Diagnosis and Comprehensive Care, 1st ed. Park Ridge, American College of Chest Physicians, 1979)

TABLE 29–4
Symptoms of Addisonian Crisis, or Glucocorticoid Withdrawal Syndrome

Emotional letdown, depression
Malaise, headache, fatigue, lethargy, weakness
Orthostatic hypotension, dizziness, fainting
Anorexia, nausea
Hypoglycemia
Weight loss
Conjunctivitis, rhinitis
Arthralgias, myalgias, stiffness
Desquamation of skin
Exacerbation of primary disease
Exacerbation of secondary disease (*e.g.*, dermatitis, conjunctivitis, rhinitis)

(Adapted from Ziment I: Respiratory Pharmacology and Therapeutics. Philadelphia, WB Saunders, 1978)

Inhaled corticosteroids should be used following an inhaled bronchodilator to optimize delivery of the aerosol to the airways. The patient should gargle with mouthwash afterward in order to prevent oral infection by *Candida albicans*. The nurse should emphasize that this drug is not intended for use during an acute episode of wheezing or as a "prn" (as needed) medication. Instead, it is a long-acting, maintenance form of therapy for the control of symptoms of chronic asthma.

Cromolyn sodium is a drug used primarily in patients with allergic asthma. When used prior to exposure to an allergen, it can prevent or minimize the symptoms of an attack.[40] However, the nurse must stress to the patient that this drug is of no use *during* an acute attack. The drug has been administered by a Spinhaler, a device that produces a powder for inhalation by puncturing a medication-filled capsule. Cromolyn has recently become available in the United States in a solution for nebulization. The patient should be able to demonstrate proper use and cleaning of either device.

Antibiotics may be used during episodes of acute respiratory infection. As with all antibiotics, the patient should take the entire course regardless of how well he feels. Most forms of tetracycline, a commonly used broad-spectrum antibiotic, should not be taken with milk or antacids, since these substances can decrease absorption of the drug.

Over the Counter Drugs. Owing perhaps to the nature of the disease (*i.e.*, paroxysmal, frightening attacks of severe dyspnea), asthmatics are often tempted to try nonprescription medications for relief of their symptoms. There is a wide variety of well-advertised over-the-counter (OTC) medications available to them. Unfortunately, most of these medications contain methylxanthines (theophylline) or sympathomimetics (epinephrine, ephedrine), which can have adverse effects, especially when used in combination with prescription drugs (Table 29–5). They may interfere with the action of prescribed medications and may predispose to side-effects. For example, use of OTC theophylline in addition to prescription theophylline can increase the likelihood of toxicity. Because most of the inhalant drugs, such as epinephrine, are extremely short acting, there is a high potential for overuse and tachyphylaxis (rebound bronchospasm).

TABLE 29–5
Constituents of Commonly Used Over-the-Counter Antiasthmatic Medications

Sympathomimetics	
Epinephrine:	Commonly used as inhalant. Patients like its rapid onset, but duration is short (1 hour). *Adverse effects:* tachycardia, headache, anxiety, tremor, nausea, dizziness, tachyphylaxis (acute tolerance), bronchial irritation and edema, dried secretions, rebound bronchospasm. Can exacerbate other health problems and alter effectiveness of other medications.
Ephedrine:	Commonly used in tablets. *Adverse effects:* same as epinephrine. When used in combination with theophylline can increase toxicity.
Methylxanthines	
Theophylline:	Oral (see Table 29–2). *Adverse effects:* headache, irritability, restlessness, insomnia, muscle twitching, convulsions, tachycardia, palpitations, extrasystoles, flushing, hypotension, nausea, vomiting, diarrhea, epigastric pain, hematemesis.
Expectorants	
Guaifenesin:	Oral. Efficacy in doubt. *Adverse effects:* gastric irritation, emesis.

(Data from Webber–Jones JE, Bryant MK: Over-the-counter bronchodilators. Nursing 10:34, 1980; Ziment I: Respiratory Pharmacology and Therapeutics, 1st ed. Philadelphia, WB Saunders, 1978)

The nurse can minimize the likelihood of use of OTC medications by educating the patient in the use of his prescribed medications; when his therapeutic regimen is optimized, he will no longer need the other drugs.[41] Increased knowledge of the potentially adverse effects of these medications may also lead to a decrease in their use.

Environmental Irritants. In addition to medication teaching, the nurse can assist the patient in identifying and avoiding irritants that can cause bronchospasm. The person with allergic asthma should maintain as dust-free an environment as possible; rugs, drapes, bedding, and furniture should be cleaned regularly. If a single pollen has been identified as the causative agent, hyposensitization by serial injections may be given. Patients who are allergic to food or food additives may need a dietary consult.[15] The patient should know the importance of early treatment of any respiratory infection.[15,37] In general, these patients should avoid such irritants as cigarette smoke, spray cleaners, and hair sprays. Temperature and humidity controls in the home environment may be of benefit to some patients.[37]

Anxiety-Reducing Measures. For patients who tend to be anxious or in whom anxiety exacerbates bronchospasm, relaxation exercises may be helpful.[37] Controlled breathing techniques, such as pursed-lip breathing, should be taught during asymptomatic periods, so that they may be used when an acute attack begins. Pursed-lip breathing can slow the rate of respiration, prevent airway collapse, and may decrease anxiety by giving the patient something on which to concentrate[10,37] If a patient has a problem with retained pulmonary secretions, postural drainage and chest physical therapy may be taught. (see Chap 27).[10,15]

Evaluation

Examples of outcome criteria indicating achievement of goals related to asymptomatic periods of asthma are that the patient

- Verbalizes personal responsibility for managing symptoms
- Describes, in lay terms, what asthma is and how it can be controlled
- Identifies factors that precipitate episodes of bronchospasm
- States techniques to reduce airway irritation
- Describes correctly the actions, side-effects, and administration techniques for all medications
- Adheres to medication regimen to avoid acute attacks

Outcome criteria must be specifically designed for individual patients and should include a time frame for achievement.

Nursing Management: Acute Asthma

Nursing care during an acute asthmatic attack is much different than that for nonacute asthma. Nursing assessment is rapid and ongoing, so that the effects of treatment are being evaluated constantly.[10] As contrasted to assessment in nonacute asthma, in the acute situation history taking is minimized and the primary focus is physical examination and interpretation of laboratory tests. Interventions are intensive and aggressive and are aimed at alleviating symptoms.

Assessment and Nursing Diagnosis

Nursing History. The nursing history is kept to a minimum. If the patient is able to answer, the nurse should try to ascertain which, if any, medications the patient normally takes or has taken during the attack. If he has tried to treat himself at home prior to seeking professional assistance, he may have ingested or inhaled large amounts of medications that can complicate therapy. If the patient cannot provide the information, careful monitoring for signs of drug toxicity is essential.

Physical Assessment. Physical assessment techniques are extremely important in evaluating seriousness of the attack. The patient with severe, acute bronchospasm presents as a fearful, diaphoretic person who assumes an orthopneic posture when sitting. Wheezing may be audible without a stethoscope. The patient may be using the accessory muscles of respiration to breathe, and supraclavicular and intercostal retractions may be noted. The anteroposterior chest diameter may be increased because of air trapping and subsequent hyperinflation. The neck veins may be distended as a result of an increase in intrathoracic pressure.

During an acute asthma attack, the patient is likely to be tachycardic, particularly if he is hypoxemic. As treatment progresses, the cardiac effects of bronchodilators, tachycardia and arrhythmias, may also be noted. The blood pressure is often elevated, and a pulsus paradoxus may be heard. Pulsus paradoxus means that the systolic blood pressure is at least 15 mmHg lower during inspiration than during expiration and is the result of fluctuations in intrathoracic pressures with inspiration and expiration. Respirations are usually rapid and shallow.

Auscultation of the chest may reveal crackles and varying degrees of wheezing. Expiratory wheezing is expected; inspiratory wheezing indicates worsening bronchospasm. The absence of wheezing following initiation of therapy may indicate relief of the bronchospasm. However, cessation of wheezing may also indicate a further decrease in air movement due to increasing bronchospasm. The nurse must distinguish between these two possibilities by evaluating other clinical signs and laboratory data.

Arterial Blood-Gas Analysis. Arterial blood gases provide the most accurate data: the Pa_{O_2} and Pa_{CO_2} reflect the adequacy of oxygenation and ventilation, respectively. As an asthma attack worsens, hypoxemia develops as a result of decreased movement of air through obstructed airways. Respiratory alkalosis (low Pa_{CO_2} with an increased pH) indicates that the patient is hyperventilating as a compensatory maneuver to bring in more oxygen (see Chap 14). A normal or increasing Pa_{CO_2} is a sign of impending ventilatory failure and demands immediate action.

In the absence of arterial blood values, the nurse should observe for signs of both hypoxemia and hypercapnia: confusion, fatigue, headache, dizziness, sedation. The nurse must not mistake apprehension or restlessness for anxiety, since it is just as likely to be a sign of hypoxemia or hypercapnia. An alert patient will probably be extremely anxious, but this justifiable response to a terrifying situation must be distinguished from the cardinal mental status changes of acute respiratory failure (see Chap 32).

Nursing Diagnoses. Nursing diagnoses that can be anticipated during an acute episode of asthma include the following:

- Ineffective airway clearance related to bronchoconstriction
- Potential impaired gas exchange secondary to bronchospasm-induced ventilation/perfusion mismatch
- Anxiety related to dyspnea

Goals. At this time, the primary goals of nursing intervention are to reduce bronchospasm and to prevent hypoxemia and hypercapnia.

Interventions

Continuing assessment for changes in the patient's condition is essential to gauge the effectiveness and safety of medication therapy used to reduce bronchospasm. Additional nursing measures are instituted to improve secretion clearance and patient comfort.

Medications are usually administered parenterally, either intravenously (IV) or subcutaneously (SC). Intravenous aminophylline must be administered with caution because of the narrow therapeutic range and the possibility of toxicity, particularly when the patient has been on maintenance therapy. Corticosteroids may also be given intravenously. β-Adrenergic agonists may be given subcutaneously or by nebulizer. The nurse must observe the patient for side-effects, particularly tachycardia.

When β-adrenergic agonists are inhaled through a nebulizer, the patient should be coached to take slow, deep inspirations and to hold his breath with each inspiration if possible. The patient is encouraged to cough, and if he is unable to do so, suctioning may be required for removal of retained secretions. Postural drainage may help to clear secretions if the patient is able to tolerate changes in position.[10,15,34,37]

Oxygen is administered at high flow rates unless the patient is a chronic CO_2 retainer. (The concept of CO_2 retention is discussed later in this chapter.) A nasal cannula is preferred; a face mask may cause a sensation of suffocation and must be removed for talking or coughing.

The nurse should assist the patient into a position of comfort that he chooses. The patient may be too anxious to follow instructions to use learned breathing or relaxation techniques, and the nurse may find that the best way to help him is by providing comfort and reassurance through touch and physical presence.[10]

Although the efficacy of systemic hydration in liquefying bronchial secretions is subject to debate, it is generally recommended as part of any bronchial hygiene effort. Because of the high insensible water loss in acute asthma, intravenous and oral hydration is important. The nurse is responsible for monitoring intake and output and is also in the best position to observe the patient for extreme diaphoresis, rapid respiratory rate, and signs and symptoms of water deficit.

The patient with acute asthma is likely to remain anxious until his symptoms are controlled. However, the nurse can do much to decrease external causes of anxiety brought about by the unfamiliar, often chaotic, hospital environment. First, the nurse must project a calm attitude while caring for the patient and be careful not to communicate the anxiety that she may be feeling in the situation. Because the anxious patient is less able to follow instructions, the nurse must repeat them patiently as needed. The nurse should stay with the patient as much as possible, and the patient's call bell should be answered promptly. The immediate environment can be modified to provide a sense of personal space. Nighttime lighting and elimination of unnecessary talking and intrusions may also help to provide a calm atmosphere.[10]

Status Asthmaticus. Most acute asthmatic episodes can be resolved with maximum therapy. An episode of asthma that fails to respond to treatment is known as *status asthmaticus*. When respiratory failure and ventilatory failure are impending as indicated by a falling Pa_{O_2} and rising Pa_{CO_2}, the patient may require intubation and mechanical ventilation. Nursing care of the mechanically ventilated patient is discussed in Chapter 27; all other aspects of care for acute asthma remain the same.

Evaluation

Successful goal achievement during an acute asthma exacerbation can be measured by outcome criteria in which the patient

- Has normal breath sounds by auscultation
- Has arterial blood-gas values within normal range
- Maintains normal mental status as evidenced by alert state, lucid conversation, orientation to person, place, and time

Chronic Obstructive Pulmonary Disease (COPD): Emphysema and Chronic Bronchitis

Definition

COPD is a syndrome of chronic airflow obstruction and includes at least two (and sometimes three) distinct disease entities. The interrelationship of these disease entities is illustrated in Figure 29–3. Emphysema and chronic bronchitis are obstructive lung diseases that can occur alone but most often are seen in combination in a single patient. For purposes of treatment, it is helpful to determine which disease is predominant in an individual patient.[3] In addition, there is often an asthmatic or reversible component to the

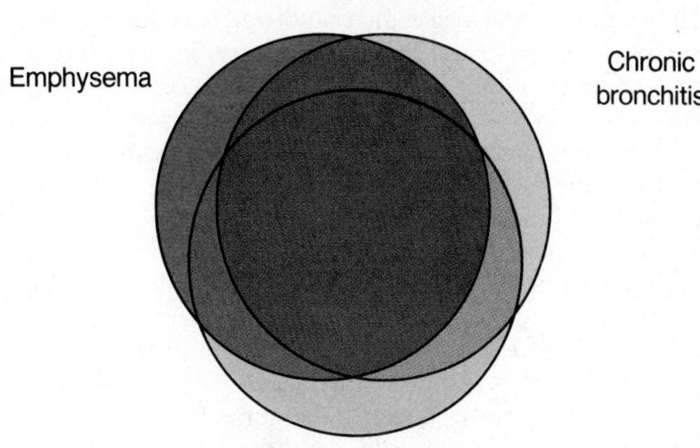

FIGURE 29–3 COPD is a syndrome of three separate diseases: emphysema, chronic bronchitis, and asthma. To varying degrees, all three disease components are present in most patients.

obstruction.[31] Because asthma has already been discussed in detail above, it is described here only as it relates to management for the person with COPD.

Epidemiology and Etiology

COPD is the second most common cause of disability compensation under the Social Security Administration, costing approximately 1.5 billion dollars annually and accounting for more than 20,000 deaths each year in the United States.[14] Clearly, COPD is a major public health problem, as well as a cause of tremendous suffering; yet the tragedy of the disease is magnified by the fact that its cause is known, and therefore it is largely preventable. Numerous scientific studies have demonstrated an association of cigarette smoking with COPD, but to date, far less money, time, and effort have been spent on prevention of smoking than on treating the illnesses smoking causes.

A few factors other than cigarette smoking may be involved in the etiology of COPD. Air pollution may play a role in its development, since there is a higher incidence of the disease in urban areas than in rural areas. Occupational exposure to some dusts and gases may also contribute to development of COPD. Finally, a genetic abnormality known as alpha$_1$-antitrypsin deficiency causes emphysema in a small number of persons, and there may also be a genetic predisposition to the development of chronic bronchitis.

Emphysema

Definition and Pathology. Emphysema is defined anatomically, meaning that the disease is described by the changes that occur in the structure of the lung. Emphysema is characterized by enlargement of the air spaces distal to the terminal bronchiole and destruction of alveolar walls.[42] There is some loss of the airways as well. The changes in emphysema are illustrated in Figure 29–4.

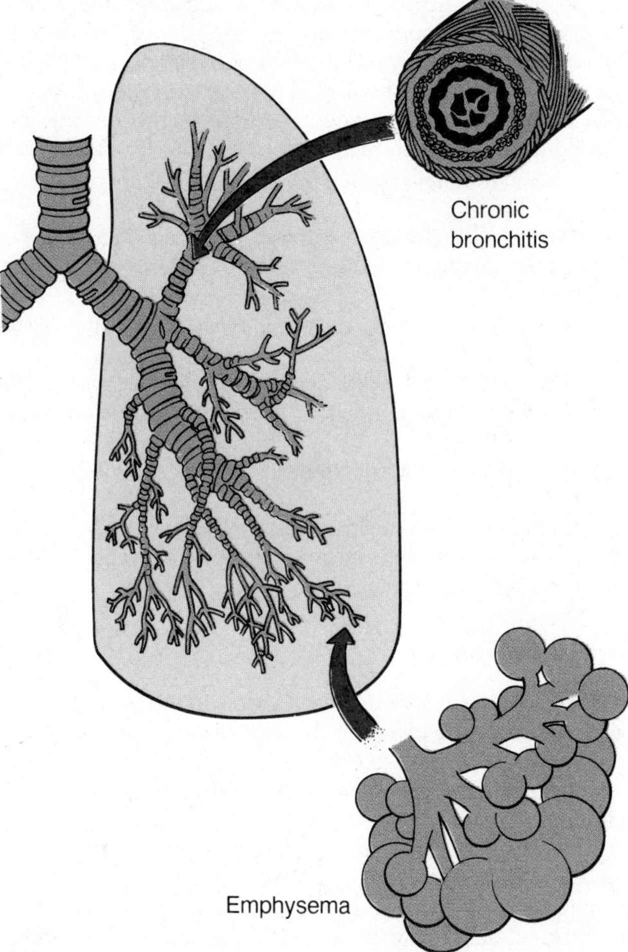

FIGURE 29–4 Comparison of the pathology of emphysema versus chronic bronchitis. In emphysema, the alveolar walls are destroyed and air spaces are permanently enlarged. Airway obstruction results from the loss of radial traction on small airways. In chronic bronchitis, hyperplasia and hypertrophy of mucus-producing cells cause excessive mucus secretions and lead to airway obstruction.

The tissue destruction may be further characterized by the location of the lung damage. In centrilobular emphysema, the central part of the lobule is destroyed. This type of emphysema usually begins in the apex of the lung and spreads downward. In panlobular emphysema, the entire lobule is affected, and the damage can occur anywhere in the lung. Emphysema resulting from alpha$_1$-antitrypsin deficiency is severe, panlobular, and begins in the lower lobes of the lung.

Pathophysiology. Airway obstruction in emphysema results from the loss of elastic recoil of the lung due to destruction of tissue. Airways tend to collapse because the radial traction normally exerted by lung tissue to keep them open has been lost. Although the patient may have little difficulty getting air into his lungs, he may find it hard to get air out; the lungs no longer "spring back" to their normal volume on exhalation, and the airways collapse as the patient tries to force air out. Inability to exhale the normal tidal volume and loss of elasticity result in air trapping and subsequent hyperinflation of the lungs.

Because pulmonary capillaries are destroyed at the same time that alveolar walls are lost, ventilation and perfusion remain fairly well-matched in emphysema. As a result, gas exchange is not impaired, and arterial blood-gas values may remain in the normal range. The effect of emphysema on arterial blood gases is shown in Figure 29–5. In end-stage disease with extensive loss of the pulmonary capillary bed, pulmonary vascular resistance will eventually rise, and the right ventricle will hypertrophy in response. Alteration in the structure or function of the right ventricle as the result of lung disease is called *pulmonary heart disease (PHD)* and is discussed in more detail later in this chapter. An older but still frequently encountered synonym for PHD is cor pulmonale.

Clinical Manifestations. The patient with "pure" or predominant emphysema is often referred to as a "pink puffer." The term "pink" refers to the fact that, until late in the disease, the person with emphysema is generally not hypoxemic. The term "puffer" derives from the fact that the predominant symptom in emphysema is dyspnea, which is often present at rest and becomes severe with exertion. Because the primary damage caused by the disease does not involve the airways themselves, cough and sputum production are minimal.

The emphysematous patient is thin, with decreased muscle mass and signs of weight loss. Chronic hyperinflation causes an increase in anteroposterior chest diameter, resulting in what is known as a "barrel chest." Use of accessory muscles of respiration, including the sternocleidomastoid and scalene muscles, is marked. The patient often assumes a characteristic orthopneic or "three-point" posture and may be observed using pursed-lip breathing in order to prolong exhalation and prevent airway collapse (Fig. 29–6).

On examination, the chest is hyperresonant to percussion, and there may be limited movement of the diaphragm. Breath sounds are diminished on auscultation.[17,24,32,42]

Chronic Bronchitis

Definition. Chronic bronchitis is described according to its symptomatology and is defined as a daily cough productive of sputum for at least 3 months of the year for 2 consecutive years.[12]

Pathology and Pathophysiology. Pulmonary damage in chronic bronchitis occurs in the airways as shown in Figure 29–4. The mucus-producing glands of the large airways hypertrophy and produce excessive secretions. The small airways show chronic inflammatory changes, peribronchial fibrosis, mucus plugging, and an increase in bronchial smooth muscle.

Airway obstruction and air trapping are the results of mucus plugging and inflammation. Retained secretions predispose the patient to repeated respiratory tract infections.

Ventilation and perfusion mismatching occurs as blood flow continues to alveoli that are no longer being ventilated

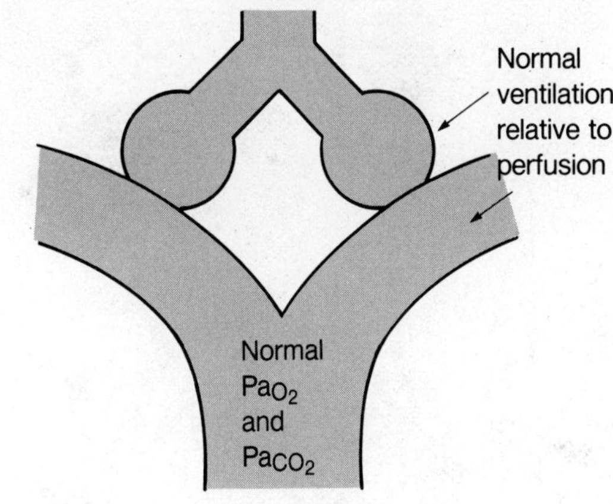

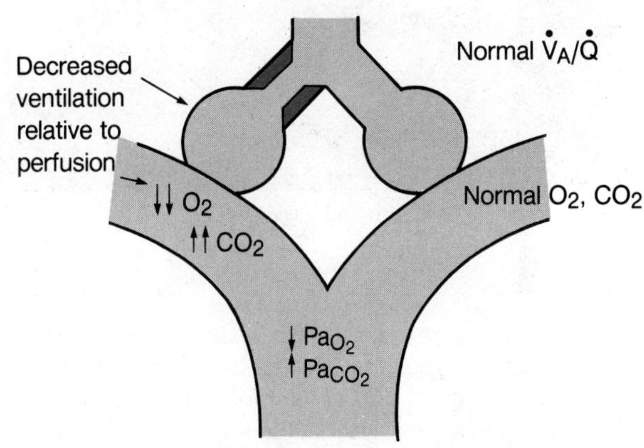

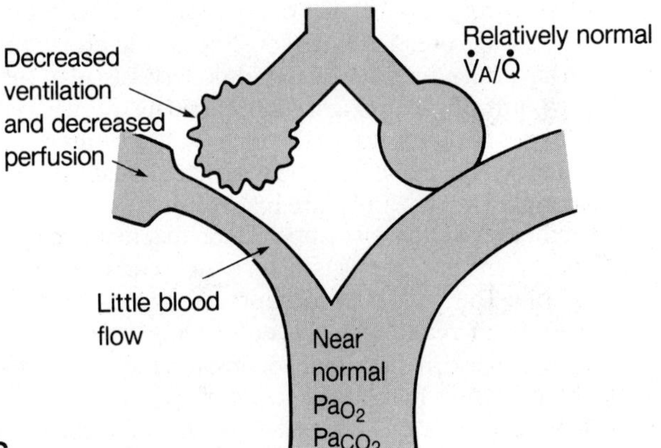

FIGURE 29–5 Comparative effects of emphysema and chronic bronchitis on arterial blood gases. (*A*) Normal alveolus. Ventilation ($\dot{V}_A$) and perfusion ($\dot{Q}$) to the alveolus are equally balanced, and the ABGs are normal. (*B*) Change characteristic of chronic bronchitis. Airway obstruction decreases ventilation relative to perfusion ($\downarrow \dot{V}_A/\dot{Q}$); the results are hypoxemia and hypercapnia. (*C*) Changes characteristic of emphysema. Alveolar walls and pulmonary capillaries are destroyed together and disease ventilation and perfusion remain balanced. As a result, until the final stages of the disease, the ABGs remain close to normal. (Adapted from Culver BH [ed]: The respiratory system: Syllabus for human biology 540 [lecture notes]. Seattle, University of Washington, 1982)

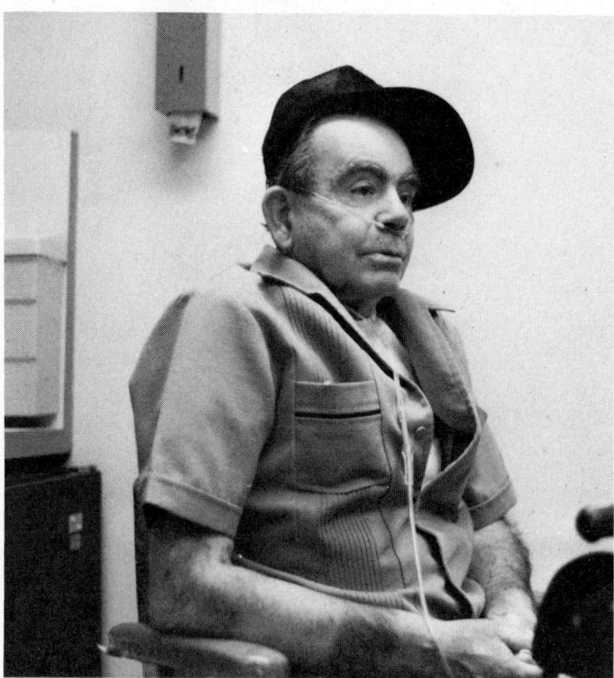

FIGURE 29–6 Patient with end-stage COPD.

because of airway obstruction. Failure to oxygenate the blood leads to hypoxemia, and failure to ventilate the alveoli causes a buildup of CO_2 in the blood (hypercapnia). Figure 29–5 compares these arterial blood-gas changes to those in emphysema.

Alveolar hypoxia (*i.e.,* a low partial pressure of oxygen in the alveoli secondary to inadequate ventilation) causes a physiological response of pulmonary capillary vasoconstriction. When widespread, this response results in elevation of pulmonary artery pressure and pulmonary vascular resistance. Hypertrophy of the right ventricle (PHD) occurs as the ventricle tries to pump against the increased pressures. If the elevated pressures persist and the ventricle is unable to compensate, right-sided heart failure may result.[8,39]

Another physiological compensation that may occur as a result of chronic hypoxemia is an increase in hematocrit and hemoglobin. The body tries to improve oxygen delivery to the tissues by increasing the oxygen-carrying capacity of the blood. An increase in the amount of unsaturated hemoglobin in the blood results in the appearance of cyanosis.

Hypercapnia, or CO_2 retention, may become chronic as the patient apparently "chooses" a high Pa_{CO_2} over the high work of breathing required to maintain a normal Pa_{O_2}. The kidneys compensate for the respiratory acidosis by retaining bicarbonate, and the pH remains normal.

Clinical Manifestations. The patient with "pure" or predominant chronic bronchitis is often referred to as a "blue bloater," for reasons described below. The major complaint of these patients is of a productive cough for many years. There is usually a history of heavy cigarette smoking and of frequent respiratory infections.[3] Dyspnea is a late development in the course of chronic bronchitis.

The patient with chronic bronchitis is usually well-nourished and may even be overweight; if severe PHD is present, he may be edematous as well (hence, the term "bloater"). He may appear cyanotic because the hemoglobin is not fully saturated with oxygen (hence, the term "blue"). In the presence of severe blood-gas abnormalities, he may be drowsy or confused. Dyspnea is usually not marked.

The chest is resonant to percussion, and coarse rhonchi and wheezing may be heard on auscultation. In the presence of PHD with enlargement of the right ventricle, a sternal lift or epigastric pulsations may be palpated. In right ventricular failure, the liver may be enlarged and tender to palpation secondary to venous congestion.

Medical Management

Diagnosis of COPD

Emphysema. Diagnosis of COPD is based on the patient history, clinical findings as described above, and laboratory findings. In emphysema, signs of hyperinflation will be seen on the chest film. Pulmonary function tests will show the effects of air trapping, with increases in total lung capacity (TLC) and residual volume (RV). Expiratory flow rates (FEV_1, FVC, $FEF_{25-75\%}$) will be decreased because of airway collapse on exhalation.

Arterial blood gases may show mild to moderate hypoxemia and normal hemoglobin saturation. The Pa_{CO_2} is usually normal or low. This value reflects a difference in respiratory drive between the patient with emphysema and the patient with chronic bronchitis. For reasons that are not yet known, the emphysematous patient works very hard to maintain a normal Pa_{O_2}; the Pa_{CO_2} is low or normal because he must hyperventilate to do so.

Chronic Bronchitis. In chronic bronchitis, the chest film may be unremarkable except for an increase in lung markings and, in the presence of PHD, an enlarged cardiac silhouette. Pulmonary function tests may show an increase in RV due to air trapping behind plugged or inflamed airways; expiratory flow rates are decreased because of the airway obstruction. Arterial blood gases reveal severe hypoxemia and some degree of hypercapnia. The pH is normal because of renal compensation for the respiratory acidosis. The hematocrit and hemoglobin values may be elevated.

Treatment of COPD

Treatment is aimed at those aspects of the disease that have the potential for reversibility in the individual patient. Reversible components are those associated with the asthmatic and bronchitic components of COPD; these include airflow obstruction due to bronchospasm, excessive airway secretions, PHD, and acute exacerbations.[16] Those aspects of the disease that are associated with emphysema, particularly dyspnea, are less likely to respond to medical therapy. Specific measures for dealing with the problem of dyspnea are discussed below in the section on nursing interventions.

Treatment of Bronchospasm. Asthma has been described earlier in this chapter as the reversible component of COPD. The treatment of bronchospasm in COPD is much the same as it is for asthma; oral long-acting theophylline, oral or inhaled β-adrenergic agonists (albuterol, metaproterenol, isoetharine, terbutaline), and oral or inhaled corticosteroids are the mainstays of therapy. The reader is referred to the discussion of asthma for details.

Another drug that is sometimes used to reverse bronchospasm in COPD is atropine. As discussed above, some bronchospasm may be the result of a hyperactive cholinergic (bronchoconstrictive) nervous system. Atropine is an anticholinergic drug that when given as an aerosol, causes bronchodilation.[21,44]

Treatment of Excessive Secretions. There are two approaches to the management of excessive airway secretions. First, an effort is made to decrease the production of mucus by removing any airway irritants such as cigarette smoke or air pollution. Second, retained secretions are removed by a variety of bronchial hygiene measures, such as systemic hydration, bronchodilator inhalation, and chest physical therapy. One or more of these measures may be successful for an individual patient.

Systemic hydration with a fluid intake of up to 2500 ml to 3000 ml per day is thought to liquefy airway secretions so that they are more easily coughed out by the patient.[3] Although there is little or no scientific evidence to support this hypothesis, it continues to be recommended as a bronchial hygiene measure.[16]

The second component of a bronchial hygiene program is the use of an inhaled bronchodilator, usually a β-adrenergic agonist such as metaproterenol or isoetharine. Bronchodilation improves airflow and allows for maximum cough effectiveness. These drugs may also stimulate the mucociliary escalator, thus enhancing secretion removal. Inhalation of heated moisture or "bland" aerosols such as normal saline may also be used, but their benefits in secretion removal have not been substantiated by research.

The use of postural drainage and other components of chest physical therapy in COPD is controversial. Some studies suggest that such therapy is indicated primarily for those patients who do not have an effective cough.[27] Others feel that most patients with retained secretions deserve a trial of therapy.[16] Whether the therapy is used or not will likely be determined by the philosophy of the particular physician or medical center and the needs of the individual patient.

Mucolytic drugs such as *N*-acetylcysteine (Mucomyst) may be administered as aerosols. These agents lyse the proteins in mucus and thereby liquefy secretions.[44] However, the efficacy of mucolytic agents is unproven, and they are not without adverse effects. For example, *N*-acetylcysteine can induce bronchospasm because it is a hypertonic solution.

Other agents that are often used but for which evidence of therapeutic efficacy is lacking are expectorants such as guaifenesin and saturated solution of potassium iodide (SSKI). The risks involved in the use of these drugs possibly outweigh the benefits gained. SSKI can cause a hypersensitivity reaction and hyperthyroidism. Guaifenesin causes gastric irritation and may cause emesis.[12,16,44]

Treatment of Pulmonary Heart Disease

Management of PHD is an essential aspect of therapy. As discussed above, the etiology of PHD is alveolar hypoxia. The therapeutic measures described above, such as bronchodilation and secretion removal, may improve alveolar ventilation to the point that alveolar hypoxia is relieved. If alveolar hypoxia, and therefore hypoxemia, persist, continuous oxygen therapy is prescribed. Diuretics may provide symptomatic relief of edema and may remove excess water from the lungs.[8,16] The use of digitalis in PHD is controversial, since the risks of therapy may outweigh the benefits. Digitalis can improve cardiac output (a desirable effect), but it may also increase pulmonary artery pressure (an undesirable effect).[3] There is a high risk of digitalis toxicity when hypoxia, hypokalemia, and acid-base disturbances are present.[8]

Treatment of Acute Exacerbations

Acute exacerbations of COPD are usually associated with an acute bronchial infection. Signs and symptoms of infection are an increase in sputum volume or consistency, a change in sputum color, fever, or increased fatigue or dyspnea. Exacerbations can often be managed successfully without hospitalization by administration of a broad-spectrum antibiotic (ampicillin, tetracycline), intensification of the bronchial hygiene regimen, and an increase in corticosteroid dosage. Fever increases CO_2 production and thus increases the need for alveolar ventilation. Rest and control of fever are important in decreasing the need for alveolar ventilation.

If the patient is unable to receive or perform the appropriate therapy at home, or if he does not improve with home therapy, he will need to be hospitalized for more intensive treatment. Unless complications occur, intravenous medications, intensive pulmonary hygiene, and continuous oxygen therapy will produce a successful outcome.

In advanced COPD with exacerbation, a common complication is acute respiratory failure (ARF). ARF occurs when the patient is no longer able to maintain adequate gas exchange and is reflected by seriously abnormal arterial blood gases. ARF is characterized by a Pa_{O_2} under 50 mmHg, with or without a pH less than 7.30 and a Pa_{CO_2} greater than 50 mmHg.

The signs and symptoms of ARF are those of the precipitating event (such as infection), those of the underlying COPD, and those of the blood-gas abnormalities. The signs include restlessness, confusion, tachycardia, headache, diaphoresis, cyanosis, loss of consciousness, hypotension, tremors and depressed respirations (Table 29–6).

Treatment is aimed at reversing the precipitating event (*i.e.*, treating infection), improving ventilation with bronchodilators and bronchial hygiene measures, and correcting hypoxemia with controlled oxygen therapy.

If the patient fails to improve with maximal therapy or appears to be approaching exhaustion, mechanical ventilation may be indicated. Because COPD patients are difficult to wean, this decision must be made thoughtfully (except in the case of cardiopulmonary arrest, when intubation is mandatory). The decision to mechanically ventilate the COPD pa-

TABLE 29-6
Signs and Symptoms of Blood-Gas Abnormalities in ARF*

Restlessness
Confusion
Tachycardia
Headache
Diaphoresis
Unconsciousness
Central cyanosis
Hypotension
Tremors or asterixis
Depressed respirations
Miosis

* $Pa_{CO_2} > 50$ mmHg; $Pa_{O_2} < 50$ mmHg; pH < 7.30.

tient is based primarily upon the potential to reverse the precipitating event and the age of the patient. The goal of treatment is to buy time while the underlying event is treated and to rest a fatigued patient. The weaning process should be begun as early as possible to optimize the chances of success.[29]

Acute respiratory failure is discussed in detail in Chapter 32.

Course and Prognosis

Both chronic bronchitis and emphysema are diseases of many years' duration. Their course is slowly progressive, particularly when the patient continues to smoke cigarettes. The onset of chronic bronchitis occurs in the 20s and 30s with a cigarette smoker's cough, with progression of the disease to disability in middle age.[32] The course is punctuated by frequent exacerbations. PHD is a late development, and death is the eventual outcome.[1,30]

Symptoms of emphysema are usually first noted in the 40s and 50s, and there is a slowly progressive course of dyspnea, muscle wasting, and decreasing activity tolerance over 20 or more years. Acute respiratory failure and PHD occur in the terminal phases of the disease.[3]

Nursing Management

As with asthma, there are acute and chronic aspects of nursing care in COPD. The discussion is divided into two sections: nursing care in chronic airway obstruction, and nursing care in acute exacerbation of COPD.

Most persons with COPD are diagnosed late in the course of their disease, when there is relatively little that can be done for them. With a change in focus toward early diagnosis and routine screening of high-risk populations (*i.e.,* smokers), more could be done to help them. For example, patients could be encouraged to stop smoking and helped to do so, and they could be taught the importance of avoiding infection. Early detection would also provide more meaning to the concept of pulmonary rehabilitation, the goal of which is to optimize patient functioning and improve quality of life for the COPD patient.[30]

Nursing Care in Chronic Airway Obstruction

Assessment and Nursing Diagnosis

Nursing History. The nursing history in COPD is an important source of information for determining patient needs, problems, and strengths. By eliciting from the patient what his primary symptoms are, the nurse can determine whether his disease is predominantly emphysema, bronchitis, or asthma, and nursing care can be planned appropriately.

Another important component of the history pertaining to the COPD itself is identification of factors that precipitate acute exacerbations for the individual patient. The nurse should try to determine which symptoms characterize an exacerbation for that patient so that they can be recognized and treated early in their course.

Other information pertinent to the nursing data base includes other medical or surgical conditions or treatment that may influence the plan of care. For example, the nurse would not advise vigorous systemic hydration as a bronchial hygiene measure in a COPD patient who also had cardiac or renal insufficiency.

A family history, including other family members who smoke or have pulmonary disease, may be important for counseling both the patient and family members. The smoking history is of interest, particularly if the patient is still smoking, and may be useful for counseling him to stop. The amount of smoking the patient has done is measured in "pack-years," and is equal to the number of packs smoked per day times the number of years of smoking. An allergic history may be important in the patient with a significant asthmatic component to his disease. An occupational history is most useful if the patient is still working in an environment in which he is exposed to potentially harmful dusts or pollution.

The patient should be asked whether he has ever had a pneumococcal vaccination, and if so, when. The nurse should also ask whether the patient receives a flu shot each year. These vaccinations are recommended for all persons over the age of 65 and for anyone with chronic lung disease.[4]

Finally, the nurse should assess the patient's knowledge regarding the medications or treatments he is taking, including the reason he is taking them, the correct dosage and time he should take them, and common side-effects of the drugs.

Physical Assessment. The nurse should be able to elicit the information related to physical assessment of the COPD patient that was described above. Knowledge of the patient's symptoms and how they affect his life is essential for appropriate nursing care planning. In addition, the ability to interpret arterial blood-gas values is mandatory for the nurse working with chronic respiratory patients. The nurse uses this knowledge in planning patient teaching and in assessing the appropriateness and effectiveness of therapy.

Psychosocial Assessment. The psychosocial assessment may provide clues as to how well the patient is coping with his disease and how the disease has affected his life. The patient's belief system, past coping patterns, and emotional response to his disease should be explored. His self-perception and feelings of self-worth can be determined by verbal and nonverbal clues, including such factors as neatness of dress, degree of eye contact, and posture.[23]

The nurse should be aware of stressors that are affecting the patient, including the illness itself, marital or other family problems, and financial difficulties. Equally important are the patient's coping assets, which may include the presence of family or friends, knowledge of community resources, adequate financial resources, and adequate housing. Even persons who are highly stressed can cope well in the presence of adequate emotional, financial, and environmental resources.

Nursing Diagnoses

Several nursing diagnoses may be drawn from the nursing data base. Nursing standards and diagnoses for COPD that have been developed by the American Thoracic Society Section on Nursing are listed in Table 29–7 and include dyspnea, ineffective airway clearance, impaired gas exchange, self-care deficit, impaired mobility, alteration in nutrition, and others. The discussion that follows is based on those diagnoses, although some modifications have been made. It should be remembered that not all of these diagnoses are relevant for every COPD patient. Instead, after thorough assessment of an individual patient, the nurse should determine which of these, or possibly other, diagnoses are appropriate. See the accompanying Nursing Care Plan for the Patient with Chronic Obstructive Pulmonary Disease.

The overall goals of all nursing interventions are to maximize gas exchange, to minimize symptoms, and to assist the patient to cope with chronic disease.

TABLE 29–7
Nursing Diagnoses for Patients with COPD

Dyspnea	
Etiology:	Physiological alterations, airway irritants
Airway clearance ineffective	
Etiology:	Tracheobronchial secretions, airway infection, ineffective cough, bronchoconstriction
Gas exchange impaired	
Etiology:	Ventilation/perfusion mismatch, bronchoconstriction, shunt, diffusion impairment, pulmonary congestion
Self-care deficit	
Etiology:	Lowered energy level, hypoxemia, depression
Mobility impaired	
Etiology:	Lowered energy level, hypoxemia
Nutritional alteration, less than body requirements	
Etiology:	Lowered energy level, shortness of breath, poor appetite, gastric distention, depression
Nutritional alteration, more than body requirements	
Etiology:	Lowered activity level, depression, excessive calorie intake
Fluid volume, alterations in excess (saline excess)	
Etiology:	Fluid retention secondary to pulmonary heart disease
Sleep-pattern disturbance	
Etiology:	Anxiety, depression, hypoxemia and/or hypercapnia, shortness of breath
Noncompliance with therapy	
Etiology:	Lack of knowledge or understanding; complexity of therapy; memory deficit; psychosocial, cultural, economic conflicts; other physical disabilities
Sexual dysfunction	
Etiology:	Physiological alterations, hypoxemia, shortness of breath, effect of medications, psychological factors
Self-concept, disturbance in body image, self-esteem, role performance	
Etiology:	Changes in body appearance, function, personal and societal role; increased physical and psychological dependence

(Adapted from Abraham M, Atkinson M, Boyce B et al: Standards for nursing care of patients with COPD. ATS News 7:31, 1981)

Interventions

Dyspnea

The diagnosis of dyspnea is particularly relevant for patients in whom emphysema is a major component of their COPD. As was discussed earlier, destruction of lung tissue in emphysema results in difficulty moving air in and out of the lungs, primarily due to loss of elasticity and airway collapse on exhalation. Pursed-lip breathing can slow the rate of exhalation and maintain positive airway pressure so that airways remain open during exhalation.[37] Pursed-lip breathing consists of a normal inspiration followed by a slow exhalation through pursed lips.

Because of the hard work of breathing and chronic hyperinflation of the lungs in emphysema, the patient recruits the accessory muscles of respiration and tends to lose the use of the diaphragm. Breathing retraining to restore use of the diaphragm as the primary muscle of respiration can increase respiratory efficiency and decrease the work of breathing. The patient is instructed in abdominal–diaphragmatic breathing by resting a hand on the upper abdomen while he is positioned comfortably in a supine or sitting position. The abdominal muscles should relax and the abdomen protrude on inspiration. Muscle contraction occurs on exhalation, and the abdomen returns to a resting position.[37] Both pursed-lip and abdominal–diaphragmatic breathing techniques can be coordinated with such activities as walking, stair climbing, and exercise.

Impaired Airway Clearance

Impairment of airway clearance related to bronchoconstriction and excessive mucus secretions results from both the asthmatic and bronchitic components of COPD. These two aspects of airway clearance will be discussed separately.

(*Text continues on page 409*)

NURSING CARE PLAN FOR THE PATIENT WITH CHRONIC OBSTRUCTIVE PULMONARY DISEASE

NURSING DIAGNOSIS 1: Ineffective airway clearance related to excessive tracheobronchial secretions, lower respiratory infection, ineffective cough, or bronchoconstriction
Manifested by rhonchi, wheezes, increased tactile fremitus, dyspnea, cough, or sputum production
GOAL 1.1: To maintain clear airways

Nursing Interventions	Rationale	Outcome Criteria
1. Instruct patient a. To cough effectively.	1. a. Effective cough reduces airway collapse and is more energy efficient.	1–5. Absence of or reduction in rhonchi, wheezes, tactile fremitus, cough, and sputum production. Patient reports decreased dyspnea.
b. To increase hydration by drinking 8–10 glasses of liquid and increasing environmental humidity.	b. Hydration may decrease sputum viscosity.	
c. In use of prescribed medications: bronchodilators, steroids, antibiotics.	c. Bronchodilators open airways so that secretions can be coughed out; steroids reduce airway inflammation, thus increasing airway diameter; antibiotics treat airway infection, leading to decreased sputum production.	
2. If use of above measure does not eliminate retained sputum, instruct patient in chest physical therapy.	2. Chest physical therapy enhances sputum clearance by mechanical factors and gravity.	
3. Assist patient to identify potential signs of infection.	3. Early recognition and treatment decreases severity of infection and likelihood of complications.	
4. Encourage patient to obtain influenza and pneumococcal vaccines and to avoid contact with people with respiratory infection.	4. These measures decrease risk of contracting lower respiratory infection.	
5. Assist patient to identify and avoid airway irritants.	5. Irritants may cause bronchospasm and decrease airway clearance.	

NURSING DIAGNOSIS 2: Dyspnea related to chronic ventilatory dysfunction and airway irritants
Manifested by subjective report of shortness of breath and observations of orthopnea, interrupted speech pattern, use of accessory muscles of respiration, tachypnea, or anxious facial expression
GOAL 2.1: To reduce reversible factors contributing to dyspnea and to promote continued activities of daily living despite presence of dyspnea

Nursing Interventions	Rationale	Outcome Criteria
1. Instruct/assist patient a. In energy conservation techniques.	1. a. Energy conservation decreases demands on limited ventilatory apparatus.	1–2. Patient reports decreased dyspnea. Patient continues daily activities.
b. To coordinate pursed lip breathing with activities of daily living.	b. Slow, controlled exhalation decreases airway collapse and may decrease dyspnea.	
c. In positions to adopt during periods of dyspnea.	c. Positions that give support but minimize restriction on thorax may reduce dyspnea.	
d. In abdominal–diaphragmatic breathing.	d. Breathing retraining may restore use of diaphragm and may reduce work of breathing.	
2. Assist patient to identify and control reversible causes of dyspnea, such as bronchospasm, infection, and heart failure.	2. Elimination of reversible factors may reduce dyspnea.	

(*Continued*)

NURSING CARE PLAN FOR THE PATIENT WITH CHRONIC OBSTRUCTIVE PULMONARY DISEASE (*Continued*)

NURSING DIAGNOSIS 3: Impaired gas exchange related to decreased ventilation in relation to perfusion
Manifested by decreased Pa_{O_2} and increased Pa_{CO_2} and by signs of impaired gas exchange such as irritability, decreased mental acuity, fatigue, or somnolence

GOAL 3.1: To maintain acceptable blood gas values

Nursing Interventions	Rationale	Outcome Criteria
1. Administer continuous, low-flow oxygen therapy.	1. Continuous low-flow oxygen decreases mortality in hypoxemic COPD patients.	1–5. Pa_{O_2} of 60 mmHg or slightly above (hemoglobin saturation of 90%); arterial pH within normal range; Pa_{CO_2} at patient's baseline. Absence of signs such as fatigue, confusion, and somnolence.
2. Instruct patient in safe oxygen use.	2. Improper oxygen use can lead to hazards such as fire, elimination of hypoxic drive to breathe.	
3. Assist patient to identify and reduce bronchospasm and retained secretions.	3. Bronchospasm and retained secretions narrow airways and can contribute to hypoxemia.	
4. Teach patient and family to recognize signs and symptoms of hypoxemia and hypercarbia.	4. Prompt recognition of hypoxemia and hypercapnia reduces risk of complications.	
5. Avoid use of medications that depress respiratory drive.	5. Respiratory depressant medications may cause hypoventilation and subsequent hypercapnia and hypoxemia.	

NURSING DIAGNOSIS 4: Excess fluid volume (saline excess) related to pulmonary heart disease
Manifested by peripheral edema, weight gain, hepatic congestion, or jugular venous distention

GOAL 4.1: To maintain normal fluid volume status

Nursing Interventions	Rationale	Outcome Criteria
1. Have patient wear continuous low-flow oxygen.	1. Oxygen reverses pulmonary vasoconstriction due to alveolar hypoxia and reduces right-sided heart failure (pulmonary heart disease).	1–4. Weight within patient's baseline range; absence of peripheral edema, hepatic congestion, jugular venous distention.
2. Instruct patient to monitor weight and check feet for edema.	2. Weight gain and edema indicate weight fluid retention.	
3. Assist patient to reduce sodium intake.	3. Dietary sodium increases water retention in susceptible individuals.	
4. Teach patient safe use of prescribed diuretics.	4. Diuretics cause excretion of saline, potassium, and other electrolytes.	

NURSING DIAGNOSIS 5: Self-care deficit or impaired mobility related to hypoxemia, dyspnea, and depression
Manifested by inadequate personal hygiene, muscle wasting, decreased exercise tolerance

GOAL 5.1: To maintain self-care and desired activities

Nursing Interventions	Rationale	Outcome Criteria
1. Have hypoxemic patient use oxygen during activities.	1. Hypoxemia increases fatigue and reduces energy to perform tasks.	1–4. Normal oxygen level is maintained during activity. Patient reports increased ability to complete self-care activities.
2. Instruct patient in energy conservation techniques.	2. Energy conservation increases what can be done with limited energy.	
3. Schedule gradually increasing exercise program.	3. Routine exercise improves cardiovascular conditioning and may increase ability to perform desired activities.	
4. Establish an exercise program using an inspiratory resistive device.	4. Inspiratory muscle training may improve efficiency of respiratory muscles.	

(*Continued*)

NURSING CARE PLAN FOR THE PATIENT WITH CHRONIC OBSTRUCTIVE PULMONARY DISEASE (*Continued*)

NURSING DIAGNOSIS 6: Altered nutrition, less than body requirements, related to low energy level, dyspnea, anorexia, GI distention, and depression

Manifested by history of recent weight loss, present weight under 90% of minimal acceptable weight, abnormal serum albumin, or skin-fold measurements

GOAL 6.1: To maintain body weight within normal limits for height and sex

Nursing Interventions	Rationale	Outcome Criteria
1. Instruct patient a. To determine caloric needs.	1. a. Hard work of breathing may increase caloric needs beyond that expected by patient.	1–3. Patient maintains or gains weight. Improvement is shown in values for serum albumin, skin-fold measurements.
b. To eat frequent small meals.	b. Hyperinflated lungs limit stomach capacity.	
c. To take high-protein, high-calorie liquids.	c. Liquid supplements contain high calories in relatively small volume.	
d. To avoid gas-producing foods.	d. Avoidance of bloating foods leaves more room to ingest nutrients.	
2. Have hypoxemic patients wear oxygen during meals.	2. Hypoxemia reduces energy to eat.	
3. Refer patient for outside assistance such as Meals on Wheels.	3. Convenient foods reduce energy expenditure for meal preparation.	

NURSING DIAGNOSIS 7: Sleep pattern disturbance related to anxiety, depression, hypoxemia and/or hypercapnia, or shortness of breath

Manifested by insomnia, fatigue, or decreased ability to perform activities of daily living

GOAL 7.1: Promote normal sleep pattern

Nursing Interventions	Rationale	Outcome Criteria
1. Assist patient to identify and reduce sources of anxiety.	1. Anxiety may contribute to difficulty in sleeping.	1–3. Patient reports feeling rested upon arising.
2. Instruct patient to a. Use inhaled bronchodilator at bedtime.	2. a. Bronchospasm and retained secretions may interrupt sleep.	
b. Avoid daytime naps.	b. Naps decrease nighttime sleepiness.	
c. Increase daytime activity.	c. Inactivity decreases need for sleep.	
d. Reduce alcohol and caffeine intake.	d. Drugs alter sleep patterns.	
3. Instruct hypoxemic patients to use oxygen during sleeping hours.	3. Nocturnal hypoxemia contributes to sleep disturbances and daytime fatigue.	

NURSING DIAGNOSIS 8: Sexual dysfunction related to physiologic alterations, hypoxemia, shortness of breath, effect of medications, or psychological factors

Manifested by report of impotence, decreased social interaction, changes in relationships

GOAL 8.1: To achieve sexual relationship that is satisfactory for patient and partner

Nursing Interventions	Rationale	Outcome Criteria
1. Provide opportunity for patient to verbalize concerns.	1. Expression of concerns leads to constructive problem-solving.	1–3. Patient reports increased satisfaction with sexual function.
2. Identify causes of dysfunction (physical, psychological, medications) and modify reversible factors.	2. Identification of causes enables modification of potentially treatable factors.	
3. Instruct patient to perform bronchial hygiene measures before trying to have intercourse, to use alternate positions, and to wear oxygen if hypoxemic.	3. Maximizing bronchial hygiene and oxygenation and conserving energy may lead to successful sexual functioning.	

Bronchoconstriction. Most of the medications used for COPD are aimed at relief of bronchoconstriction, and they are identical to those used for asthma. The reader is referred to the section Nursing Care in Nonacute Asthma for applicable information on medication teaching.

Avoidance of airway irritants may be important in prevention of bronchospasm in COPD. The major irritant is, of course, cigarette smoke. If the patient continues to smoke, the nurse must evaluate why he does so and whether he has any desire to stop. The nurse can offer encouragement to the patient who is trying to stop smoking and can provide information on smoking cessation programs.[6]

Another major irritant is infection, which is often frequent and repeated in chronic bronchitis. The patient should be taught ways to avoid respiratory tract infection, such as avoidance of crowds and persons with colds or flu. The importance of pneumococcal pneumonia and influenza vaccinations should be taught. The patient and family must know the signs and symptoms of a respiratory infection and what to do should symptoms appear. An increase in shortness of breath, increased cough or sputum production, and change in color or consistency of sputum are symptoms that the patient should report promptly to his physician.

Other irritants that may produce bronchospasm include occupational and environmental pollutants, such as dusts, gases, and air pollution, and household pollutants such as sprays or aerosols. These substances should be avoided whenever possible.

Retained Secretions. Bronchial hygiene measures aimed at removal of retained secretions have been discussed above. These may include oral or systemic hydration and, occasionally, inhalation of moisture such as steam or bland aerosols. When inhaled bronchodilators or corticosteroids are used, the nurse instructs the patient in the proper use and cleaning of the metered-dose inhaler or nebulizer. The nurse can help to identify patients who are likely to benefit from postural drainage and chest physical therapy and can assess the patient's response to the therapy.

Some patients are unable to cough effectively and waste energy trying to raise thick, sticky secretions. The nurse can teach these patients a controlled cough technique, which saves energy by increasing the efficiency of the coughing effort. Sometimes called a "staged" or "cascade" cough, the effect of the controlled cough is to first move secretions from the smaller to the larger airways and then to expectorate them. Initially, the patient takes several deep breaths, using pursed-lip breathing. He then takes a maximal inspiration, followed by a series of coughs at successively lower lung volumes. Bending forward while coughing may be helpful.[6]

Impaired Gas Exchange

Gas exchange is impaired when excessive secretions plug airways and bronchoconstriction limits airflow. If medications and bronchial hygiene measures are maximized and the patient remains hypoxemic, continuous oxygen therapy will be prescribed. It should be emphasized that documented hypoxemia is the *only* justification for oxygen administration to COPD patients.

Oxygen is administered at low flow rates in COPD. In normal persons the primary ventilatory drive is hypercapnia. However, in the chronically hypercapnic, bronchitic patient, a rising Pa_{CO_2} is no longer a stimulus to respiration, and hypoxemia becomes the primary ventilatory drive. If too high an oxygen concentration (FI_{O_2}) is delivered to a chronic CO_2 retainer, the hypoxic drive is abolished, and the patient may stop breathing. Therefore, an oxygen concentration is chosen that maintains normal oxygen saturation of the hemoglobin (90% or greater), *not* that which maintains a normal Pa_{O_2} (greater than 60 mmHg).

The implication for nursing care is obvious. The patient should be instructed that he should use his oxygen as many hours in the day as possible, but he must never increase the flow of oxygen above the prescribed level. Continuous oxygen use (that is, more than 20 hours per day) is optimal because the mortality rate decreases inversely with the number of hours of oxygen use per day.[9, 26]

The desired method of delivery is usually a nasal cannula. Although the FI_{O_2} delivered by cannula is less precise than that of a venturi mask, the cannula has several advantages. These include patient comfort and the fact that the cannula need not be removed for talking, eating, or coughing. Masks may produce a sensation of suffocation, which is particularly frightening for a dyspneic patient.[38]

The patient must be instructed in the safety aspects of oxygen therapy. Although oxygen does not burn spontaneously, it will support combustion. Therefore, cigarette smoking should be strictly prohibited within 10 feet of the oxygen source, as should any source of a spark or flame.

Home Care Considerations. The hospital staff nurse may be called upon to order home oxygen for the patient. The nurse should be familiar with the various systems available and should know that costs are extremely high but can vary widely. Attempts should be made to ensure delivery of the most economical yet appropriate system for the patient's lifestyle.

Finally, the nurse should instruct the patient and his family in the signs and symptoms of hypoxemia and hypercapnia (see Table 29–7). Because these signs can be vague and often involve a change in mental status, they can easily be misinterpreted as psychological disturbances. The family should know how to seek help should these signs appear.

Excess Fluid Volume

Excess fluid volume (saline excess) results from PHD. As described above, alveolar hypoxia leads to constriction of the pulmonary vascular bed, increased pulmonary vascular resistance, right ventricular hypertrophy, and eventually, right ventricular failure. Fluid retention due to right ventricular failure results in peripheral edema and weight gain. Continuous oxygen therapy is the best treatment for PHD, but diuretics and potassium supplements may also be prescribed. The patient should know the reason he is taking the medications, the correct dosage, timing, and the common side-effects of the medications. The nurse should instruct the patient in the symptoms of hypokalemia, as well as dietary sources of potassium. If digitalis is prescribed, the patient should know the signs and symptoms of toxicity.

The patient is instructed to weigh himself daily at the

same time, wearing the same amount of clothing. If his weight increases by 2 pounds in one day or 5 pounds in one week, he should notify his nurse or physician. A weight gain of this degree represents fluid retention. The patient should be instructed in a low-sodium diet and given the rationale for decreasing sodium intake. Compliance with the prescribed diet is likely to be better if the patient understands why it is important to avoid sodium.

Self-Care Deficit and Impaired Mobility

As dyspnea and hypoxemia worsen over the years, persons with COPD may gradually become dependent upon others for many activities of daily living. Self-care deficit and impaired mobility are frequent nursing diagnoses for these persons. The patient may become depressed because of the chronic illness itself or because of the limitations it has imposed upon his life. The nurse and occupational and physical therapists can help the patient to regain independence in many activities by teaching him how to use energy efficiently.

The patient can be taught how to coordinate his breathing with activities so that he becomes less short of breath with exertion. Energy-conservation measures such as modification of the home environment so that the patient can reach needed objects more easily, the use of assistive devices for reaching and carrying objects, pacing of activities, and planned periods of rest can all help decrease energy expenditures. A planned exercise program may improve the efficiency with which muscles utilize oxygen. If it has been demonstrated that the patient's hemoglobin becomes desaturated with exercise, he should be instructed to use oxygen with activity.[2]

Alterations in Nutrition

Alterations in nutrition can be either less or more than body requirements. Shortness of breath, a low energy level, and depression can all result in a diminished appetite in the patient with COPD. Many patients become more short of breath during and immediately after meals, and many quickly experience a feeling of fullness when gastric distention exerts upward pressure against hyperinflated lungs. Frequent, small meals may help to decrease these sensations. High-calorie, high-protein supplements such as milk shakes and commercially prepared supplements (Ensure, Sustacal, Isocal) can add calories and nutrients to the diet. Gas is another cause of gastric distention, and the patient should be instructed to avoid gas-forming foods. OTC preparations containing simethicone may be used to decrease gas. If the patient is hypoxemic, oxgyen may help to relieve dyspnea during and after meals.

The patient who is overweight should be instructed in the importance of weight control. The more he weighs, the harder he will have to work to breathe. The patient's daily intake can be evaluated by having him keep a diary or record of everything he eats and drinks in a 24-hour period. Using this information, the nurse can identify ways in which the patient can decrease his intake and yet maintain good nutrition. An exercise program can help to increase the patient's energy expenditure.

If meal preparation is difficult for the patient, he should be referred to community agencies that provide easy-to-prepare meals for homebound persons. A dietary consult may be helpful for both the under-weight and over-weight COPD patient.

Disturbed Sleep Patterns

Anxiety, depression, inactivity, and medications that are nervous system stimulants (*e.g.,* theophylline) may all contribute to disturbance of sleep patterns in COPD patients. The first step in improving sleep is to identify factors that are affecting the individual patient. Then, usual or desired sleep habits can be identified and worked toward.

The nurse can explore sources of anxiety with the patient. Once identified, practical steps can be taken to decrease or eliminate the anxiety. For example, a patient who is afraid of waking up at night unable to breathe can be taught to maximize his bronchial hygiene routine before bedtime, or to have an inhaled bronchodilator available at the bedside should he awaken short of breath. Relaxation techniques can be taught for use at bedtime, and panic routines can be practiced for use during the night.

Antidepressants and antianxiety agents must be used with caution in persons with COPD because of their depressant effect on respiration. However, some drugs, particularly the tricyclic antidepressants, can be used safely. The nurse can assess the effects of these drugs for benefits and potential hazards.

Finally, many persons have difficulty sleeping at night because they are not tired. Many patients engage in minimal activity during the day, or they may nap frequently. By increasing daytime activity and minimizing naps, the patient may feel more tired when bedtime arrives.

Nonadherence

Noncompliance with therapy is a problem that is not limited to the COPD patient, and so is mentioned only briefly here. A specific factor important in COPD that may lead to failure to adhere to the prescribed therapeutic regimen is a poor memory or diminished cerebral functioning due to hypoxemia. If the problem persists with maximal therapy and correction of the hypoxemia, direct supervision of the therapy by a home nursing service or friends or family may be required.

Sexual Dysfunction

Difficulty with sexual function in the COPD patient may be due to a number of factors, including physiological alterations, shortness of breath, depression, hypoxemia, or medication.[2] A prerequisite for discussion of this subject with the patient and his partner is an open, accepting atmosphere in which concerns can be expressed freely.

The nurse must first assess whether either the patient or partner perceives that a problem exists. If one or the other feels that there is a problem, efforts are made to determine whether the dysfunction is physiological or psychological. If the male can obtain an erection or the female can become sexually aroused, the dysfunction is probably psychological.

The nurse should assess whether the patient's medications may be causing a decrease in sexual desire or function. If the medications are known to inhibit sexual function, the nurse can consult with the physician regarding modifications that can be made in the drug regimen. If changes are not possible, the patient may feel better just knowing that the medications are the cause of the dysfunction.

If no apparent reversible reason can be found for the sexual dysfunction, other measures to enhance sexual function may be tried. The patient and partner may be encouraged to use expressions of intimacy other than intercourse, such as touch, which can be satisfying for many people. The chances for "successful" sexual functioning can be maximized by trying to have intercourse at the time of day that the patient feels best and by optimizing pulmonary function before trying (by using inhaled bronchodilators or oxygen, for example). The couple may be taught alternative positions so that the healthy partner does most of the "work."

If none of these measures improves sexual functioning and the patient or his partner remains dissatisfied, they may be referred for sexual counselling.

Altered Self-Concept

As with noncompliance, disturbances in self-concept, self-esteem, body image, and family and societal roles may occur in the patient with any chronic disease. The major strategies for dealing with these changes include the following: identifying factors that lead to the problem; assisting the patient in finding and optimizing his psychological strengths; fostering independence as much as is possible; and supporting the patient even when he may be coping well.[2]

Evaluation

Specific outcome criteria must be set for each patient individually, based on knowledge of the underlying physiological and psychological status. However, general guidelines for outcome criteria are as follows:

- Patient maintains arterial blood-gas values within acceptable range (baseline values are determined individually but include Pa_{O_2} of at least 60 mmHg)
- Patient demonstrates techniques to decrease breathlessness and other symptoms
- Patient identifies support systems that can assist him and his family to cope with the effects of COPD upon his life

Nursing Care In Acute Exacerbation of COPD

Assessment and Nursing Diagnosis

As with an acute asthmatic attack, the nursing assessment of the COPD patient with acute exacerbation is much less extensive than it is in a nonacute situation. Questioning of the patient is limited to information about the current exacerbation and the medications the patient has taken. The nurse can also assess the patient's mental status during the initial interview and note signs of hypoxemia and hypercapnia.

The vital signs are likely to show tachycardia or arrhythmias, particularly if the patient is hypoxemic. The temperature may be elevated if infection is present, but immunosuppression due to chronic corticosteroid therapy or the effects of aging may diminish this response. Pulsus paradoxus may be heard if severe airway obstruction is present.

Chest auscultation may reveal crackles, rhonchi, or wheezes, depending on the etiology of the exacerbation. Sputum should be examined for color and thickness, and a specimen should be obtained for culture. Peripheral edema should be noted.

Nursing diagnoses in acute exacerbation of COPD are the same as for chronic care. However, the emphasis is placed on physiological disturbances rather than on the rehabilitative aspects of care. The primary goal of all nursing interventions is to maintain gas exchange within acceptable limits for that patient.

Interventions for Specific Nursing Diagnoses

Ineffective Airway Clearance. Bronchial hygiene measures to treat ineffective airway clearance are intensified. Postural drainage and chest physical therapy may be performed if the patient is able to tolerate position changes. Following these treatments, the patient is encouraged to cough. If he cannot cough effectively, suctioning may be required.[7]

The maintenance medication regimen is intensified when a patient enters the hospital with an acute exacerbation. Aminophylline, corticosteroids, and antibiotics are administered intravenously. The nurse monitors the patient for signs and symptoms of aminophylline toxicity, including nausea, vomiting, and, in extreme cases, seizures. β-Adrenergic agonists are given by oral, subcutaneous, or inhaled routes, and the nurse must assess the patient for side-effects, particularly tachycardia and arrhythmias.

The nurse ensures adequate hydration by administration of oral and intravenous fluids and by keeping accurate records of intake and output. The patient should be weighed daily and observed for signs of fluid retention.

Impaired Gas Exchange. Impaired gas exchange is often a problem during an exacerbation. As in chronic care of COPD, hypoxemia is treated with controlled low-flow oxygen therapy. The goal of therapy is an oxygen saturation of at least 90%, and the nurse monitors the adequacy of therapy by evaluation of the arterial blood gases. The nurse is responsible for ensuring the constant, uninterrupted delivery of the correct concentration of oxygen.

Hypercapnia is treated by indirect methods. The nurse ensures that the liter flow of oxygen is at the level prescribed and is never increased. The restless patient should not be sedated because most sedatives are respiratory depressants. Occasionally, the nurse may be called upon to keep the patient awake through the night in order to avoid the hypoventilation and hypercapnia induced by sleep, thus avoiding intubation.[7]

The criteria for intubation and mechanical ventilation of the COPD patient are discussed above. Care of the mechanically ventilated patient is discussed in Chapter 27. Otherwise, nursing care of the mechanically ventilated COPD patient is the same as for the nonventilated patient, with emphasis on maintenance of nutrition and activity.

Excess Fluid Volume. Excess fluid volume (saline excess) results if the exacerbation induces a temporary episode of PHD. The best therapy for PHD is continuous oxygen therapy, and again, the nurse ensures the constant delivery of the prescribed F_{IO_2}. When fluid retention is severe, diuretics and potassium supplements may be given. The nurse accurately records the intake and output and daily weight and monitors the patient for signs and symptoms of hypokalemia. The nurse should also be aware of the potential for hypokalemic hypochloremic alkalosis in the COPD patient (see Chap 13). The sodium intake is restricted. The patient is assessed for cardiac arrhythmias, particularly if digitalis is given.

Self-Care Deficit and Impaired Mobility. Problems relating to self-care deficit and impaired mobility generally increase during an exacerbation. Except in severe heart failure, the patient should be as active as possible, even when he is intubated and on a ventilator. He should be out of bed, walking with assistance and oxygen whenever possible. If the patient must remain in bed, active or passive range of motion exercises should be performed several times a day. Periods of activity should be alternated with planned rest periods.

Alteration in Nutrition. Nutritional intake is often inadequate during an exacerbation of COPD. The importance of adequate nutrition cannot be overemphasized. The work of breathing is extremely high in the COPD patient in exacerbation, and an adequate nutritional intake is mandatory. Lack of adequate nutrition in the mechanically ventilated patient results in muscle wasting and inability to wean the patient from the machine.

The principles of nutrition in acute exacerbation are the same as they are in chronic care. Frequent, small feedings with high-calorie, high-protein supplements are given. The intubated patient may receive tube feedings or total parenteral nutrition.

Sleep Disturbance. A sleep pattern disturbance is probable during an exacerbation, yet the acutely ill COPD patient requires adequate rest in order to carry on the high work of breathing. Otherwise, he will become exhausted. The nurse can promote rest by providing an environment that is conducive to sleep. Low-level lighting and minimal disturbances may help, as may comfort measures such as a back rub at bedtime. Sedation is used with extreme caution because of the potential for respiratory depression.

Evaluation

Attainment of the primary goal of maintaining gas exchange can be evaluated by measuring arterial blood-gas values. If they fall within the patient's normal, compensated range, the goal has been achieved. Examples of desirable blood-gas values include

- pH within normal range (7.35–7.45)
- Pa_{CO_2} at patient's normal baseline
- Pa_{O_2} of 60 mmHg or slightly above (with or without supplemental oxygen)

Bronchiectasis

Definition and Etiology

Bronchiectasis is defined as an abnormal dilatation of the bronchi due to destruction of the elastic and muscular components of the bronchial wall, usually caused by infection.[19,25,37]

In the past, the onset of bronchiectasis usually occurred in childhood. Measles, pertussis, or other viral infections were often followed by pneumonia, which led to temporary or permanent lung injury. More recently, immunization for childhood diseases, as well as the development of antibiotics to treat pneumonia, has resulted in a declining incidence of childhood bronchiectasis.

Today, the onset of bronchiectasis generally occurs later in life and is associated with a variety of infectious and congenital and acquired disorders. Infectious causes include tuberculosis and other granulomatous infections and bacterial pneumonias. Cystic fibrosis and Kartagener's syndrome are the most common congenital causes of bronchiectasis. Other conditions associated with bronchiectasis include atopic asthma and congenital or acquired immune deficiency states.

Two major morphologic classifications of bronchiectasis have been identified. Cylindrical bronchiectasis may occur following an episode of pneumonia and usually resolves within a few months. In this type of bronchiectasis, the airways do not taper in diameter as they normally should, and fewer generations of bronchioles are present. In the second type of bronchiectasis, saccular bronchiectasis, outpouching or ballooning of the bronchial walls causes an increase in diameter of the airways as well as a loss of generations of airways. Figure 29–7 illustrates these changes. Saccular bronchiectasis is usually irreversible.[11] It is this permanent type of change that is discussed below.

Pathophysiology

In the case of childhood onset of bronchiectasis, a single episode of infection may be identified as the cause of lung damage. In later-onset bronchiectasis, recurrent infection may be the culprit. In both cases, infection damages the bronchial mucosa and underlying cartilage and muscle tissue, which is then replaced by fibrous scar tissue. The normal bronchial epithelium is replaced by nonciliated low cuboidal or squamous epithelium. The normally elastic bronchial tube is thus replaced by a flabby sac.[19]

Obliteration of the smaller airways causes a loss of compliance in the affected area; thus, coughing may be ineffective in removing secretions. Inflammatory changes in bronchial wall mucosa cause an increase in secretions, which may then pool in the dilated bronchioles and increase the likelihood of infection. Retained secretions and bronchiolar obliteration, if severe, cause mismatching of ventilation and perfusion with subsequent hypoxemia and PHD.

Clinical Manifestations

The patient with bronchiectasis presents with a chronic cough productive of a large amount of sputum. There is often

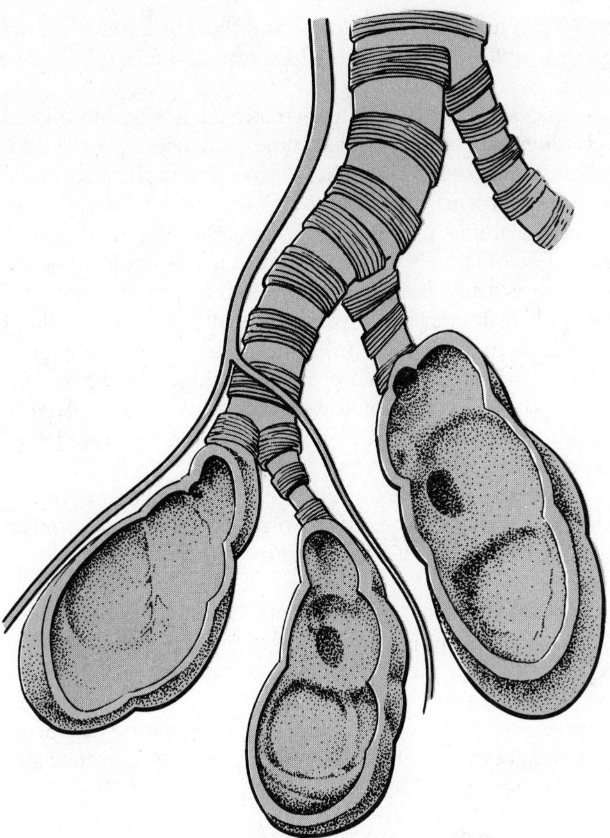

FIGURE 29–7 Saccular bronchiectasis. The bronchial walls are permanently dilated.

a history of recurrent pneumonia, although the onset of symptoms may be traced to a specific episode of infection. Hemoptysis is common, and may range from blood streaking to frank hemorrhage.

Many persons with bronchiectasis have no symptoms at all. In the presence of localized disease (*e.g.,* affecting only one segment of a lung), symptoms may be mild. However, with extensive bronchial damage, the symptoms may resemble those of COPD and may be incapacitating.[37] The patient with severe bronchiectasis may appear weak, with muscle wasting and digital clubbing.

Chest auscultation may reveal persistent localized inspiratory crackles and generalized rhonchi, which may clear with coughing.

Medical Management

Diagnosis. The diagnosis of bronchiectasis is often presumptive, based on the elimination of other potential causes of chronic cough and recurrent infection. Standard diagnostic tests include a chest film, sputum cultures, pulmonary function tests, bronchoscopy, and a sweat test.

The chest film may show nonspecific abnormalities, including increased lung markings, a honeycomb appearance, and atelectasis. Pulmonary function tests may be normal if bronchiectasis is mild or localized. In severe or diffuse disease, an obstructive pattern similar to that of COPD will be found. Arterial blood-gas measurements may show hypoxemia because of ventilation/perfusion mismatching.

In a few cases, bilateral bronchograms may be done. A bronchogram involves visualization of the bronchi on film following instillation of a radiopaque dye. Because of hazards associated with this procedure (including bronchospasm, pneumonia, and allergic reaction to the dye or medication), its use is restricted to patients who are being considered for surgery, and it is performed only when the patient is medically stable.

Treatment. When a diagnosis of bronchiectasis has been made, an aggressive program of medical management is instituted. Postural drainage and chest physical therapy are the mainstays of therapy. Positioning for treatment may be tailored to the location of the patient's disease. Antibiotic therapy is chosen empirically or by sputum culture and should be begun immediately when symptoms of infection appear.

If the patient does not improve with medical management, surgery may be indicated. Only patients with localized disease and adequate pulmonary function are candidates for surgery. In diffuse disease, surgery is not indicated for removal of the worst areas of bronchiectasis because there is no long-term improvement in symptoms following operation.[19]

Prognosis. The availability of preventive vaccines and antibiotic therapy has dramatically improved the prognosis for bronchiectasis over the last 40 years. With the exception of the congenital causes of the disease, the etiologies of which are unknown, bronchiectasis should now be regarded as preventable.

Nursing Management

Nursing care in bronchiectasis is the same as that in chronic bronchitis, with particular emphasis on bronchial hygiene measures to treat the most common nursing diagnosis: ineffective airway clearance. These measures include adequate hydration, inhaled moisture or bronchodilators, controlled coughing, and postural drainage and chest physical therapy. Airway irritants such as cigarette smoke, fumes, and air pollution should be avoided. Influenza and pneumonia vaccinations should be given to prevent infection. Adequate nutrition is important for maintaining resistance to infection.

Cystic Fibrosis

Cystic fibrosis is usually thought of as a disease of childhood, and indeed, many persons with cystic fibrosis do not survive into adulthood. However, with better methods of diagnosis and the comprehensive care provided by major treatment centers, life expectancy for cystic fibrosis has improved over the last 4 decades. As of 1976, the national 50%-survival rate was 16 years of age.[43] With the improved survival into young adulthood, persons with cystic fibrosis will be seen on the adult medicine unit with increasing frequency. This discussion is limited as much as possible to the care of the adult patient.

Definition and Etiology

Cystic fibrosis is a genetic disease that is thought to be transmitted in an autosomal recessive pattern. Because the specific genetic defect is not yet known, the disease is described in terms of its pathology. Abnormalities of most or all of the exocrine glands of the body are involved. The three most important organ systems involved are the lungs, the pancreas, and the sweat glands. Other structures affected include the sinuses, salivary glands, small intestine, biliary system, uterine cervix, and male genital tract.[28,37]

Among the white population in the United States, 1 in every 20 persons is a carrier of the cystic fibrosis gene. The disease occurs in approximately 1 in 2000 live births in this group. Cystic fibrosis is much less common among other population groups, occurring once in every 17,000 births among blacks in the United States, and even more rarely among those of Asian descent.

Pathophysiology and Clinical Manifestations

Pulmonary. Except for cases of meconium ileus, an intestinal obstruction presenting at or shortly after birth, the pulmonary disease in cystic fibrosis determines the life span of almost all patients. While other effects of the disease may not be found in all patients, obstructive lung disease is universal and most likely will be the cause of admission to the hospital.

The sequence of events in development of the lung disease is not known, but persons seem to be susceptible to pulmonary infection in infancy, and pathologic lung changes occur at an early age. Initial changes are dilatation and hypertrophy of the mucus-producing glands, followed by mucus plugging of small airways. Chronic or recurrent infection results, which in turn leads to bronchitis, bronchiolitis, and bronchiectasis. Progressive destruction of lung tissue results in hypoxemia, PHD, and eventually, death.

The clinical picture of cystic fibrosis is that of COPD, particularly chronic bronchitis. The primary symptom is a productive cough, and with progression of the disease there is increasing shortness of breath and decreasing exercise tolerance.

Pulmonary function tests initially reveal obstruction of small airways, with progression to the large airways over time. RV and FRC increase as a result of air trapping and hyperinflation. The chest film shows hyperinflation, patches of atelectasis or infiltration, bronchiectasis, and, possibly, pneumothorax. Sputum cultures typically grow two predominant organisms: *Staphylococcus aureus* and *Pseudomonas aeruginosa.* The *Pseudomonas* organism is a rare strain found almost exclusively in cystic fibrosis, and it is extremely difficult to eradicate.[36,43]

Pancreas and Gastrointestinal Tract. The degree of pancreatic involvement varies among patients. Some patients have few pancreatic symptoms, and there is a tendency for these symptoms to become less severe as the person grows older.

In cystic fibrosis, the pancreatic ducts become dilated and plugged with secretions; some structures become atrophied or fibrosed.[36] The tissue destruction causes pancreatic insufficiency and an inability to absorb fats and the fat-soluble vitamins A, D, E, and K. The fat maldigestion results in the loss of up to 70% of ingested fat in the stool. Stools are characteristically frequent, bulky, loose, greasy, and foul-smelling. Maldigestion and abnormal intestinal mucus gland secretions may result in intestinal obstruction (sometimes referred to as "meconium ileus equivalent"). Signs and symptoms include right lower quadrant abdominal pain, nausea or vomiting, and a palpable mass in the right lower quadrant.[5]

Extensive pancreatic damage with obliteration of the islets of Langerhans results in diabetes. This complication occurs in about 8% of adult patients.[5]

Sweat Glands. Chloride and sodium content of sweat is markedly higher than normal in persons with cystic fibrosis. Although the abnormality causes few problems for the patient, it is important because it provides the basis for diagnosis (see below). The only symptoms may be heat prostration on hot days and a susceptibility to hypochloremia and hyponatremia (see Chap 13).

Genitourinary Tract. Males with cystic fibrosis have a markedly abnormal genital tract. The vas deferens, seminal vesicles, and epididymis may be atrophied or absent, resulting in a decreased semen volume or aspermia. There is a high incidence of inguinal hernia, hydrocele, and undescended testicles. Ninety-seven percent to 98% of males with cystic fibrosis are sterile.

Low fertility in females is believed to result from tenacious cervical mucus that can plug the cervical os. However, children have been conceived by women with cystic fibrosis. Menarche is often delayed, usually by about 2 years. Secondary amenorrhea often occurs when severe nutritional deficits or pulmonary disease is present.

Medical Management

Diagnosis

The diagnosis of cystic fibrosis is based on the presence of two of the four following criteria: a positive sweat test; the presence of chronic obstructive lung disease; pancreatic insufficiency; family history of the disease.[43]

Sweat Test. Quantitative pilocarpine iontophoresis, or sweat testing, is the only reliable diagnostic test available. The procedure involves local stimulation of the sweat glands of the forearm, collection of the sweat, and analysis for chloride and sodium. Persons with cystic fibrosis have two to five times the concentrations of chloride and sodium in their sweat compared with normal persons. The test may be repeated to ensure a correct diagnosis.[36]

Treatment

Treatment for cystic fibrosis is based on the concept of comprehensive care, involving many disciplines including medicine, nursing, respiratory and physical therapy, and social work. Medical treatment tends to be aggressive and is aimed primarily at the pulmonary and pancreatic aspects of the disease.

Because repeated pulmonary infection is one of the hallmarks of cystic fibrosis, antibiotics play a major role in treatment. The regimen may vary: specific antibiotic therapy may be given based on sputum cultures, or continuous antibiotic therapy may be given as prophylaxis or in the presence of continuous bacterial colonization of the lungs. In general, the maximum therapeutic dose is given for long treatment periods. If the patient does not improve with oral antibiotics, intravenous antibiotics will be given either at home or in the hospital.

Bronchial hygiene measures are important and are similar to those used for COPD. Aerosols are used to deliver bronchodilators, mucolytics, and, occasionally, antibiotics. Postural drainage and chest physical therapy have long been mainstays of therapy, but their use for all patients has been questioned in recent years. In the future, alternatives to postural drainage such as physical exercise may become increasingly common. Efforts may be made to identify those persons who are likely to benefit most from chest physical therapy.

Pancreatic insufficiency is relieved by the administration of pancreatic enzymes (Pancrease, Cotazym) with each meal or snack. Simethicone may relieve flatus. Adequate nutrition can often be maintained with an unrestricted, well-balanced diet. Despite malabsorption of fat-soluble vitamins, deficiencies of vitamins A, D, and K are rare. Vitamin E deficiency is common, and a supplement is given.[5] Insulin may be required when the patient is hyperglycemic.

Prognosis

The course of the disease is variable among individuals, but cystic fibrosis is inevitably progressive and fatal. Common pulmonary complications that increase in frequency with advancing disease include atelectasis, pneumothorax, and hemoptysis. Complications are treated aggressively in the majority of cases; however, as in end-stage COPD, mechanical ventilation is avoided whenever possible unless a potentially reversible process is occurring. The development of respiratory failure and PHD signals the onset of the final stages of the disease. Death results from overwhelming pulmonary secretions and resultant airway obstruction and its complications.

Nursing Management

Assessment

In addition to severe physical limitations, persons with cystic fibrosis face almost overwhelming psychosocial problems. The nursing assessment includes information that indicates how well the person is coping with his illness and how it has affected his life.

History. The nursing history includes information related to the disease itself (*e.g.*, how frequently the patient experiences respiratory infections) as well as identification of illnesses other than cystic fibrosis that may influence care. In order to assess compliance with the prescribed medical regimen, it is important to determine the amount of knowledge the patient has about the disease and its treatment. The presence of other family members with cystic fibrosis or the previous death of a family member as the result of the disease may provide clues about the patient's outlook or attitude toward his illness. Educational and occupational data may indicate how well the adult with cystic fibrosis has adjusted to independent living and may provide clues to his self-concept and self-esteem. Social factors, such as marital status and who the patient lives with (such as parents), also provide clues to the patient's ability to manage independently.

Psychosocial Assessment. Some of the coping mechanisms commonly used by patients with cystic fibrosis include denial, depression, withdrawal, and, particularly in adolescents, rebellion. Coping assets that should be assessed may include family and spousal support, financial resources (including insurance), religion, friends, access to health-care professionals, and cystic fibrosis support groups.

Physical Assessment. The person with cystic fibrosis is often small for his age, may show delayed sexual development, and often has digital clubbing. The patient will complain of a frequent, productive cough, and the nurse determines the usual quantity of sputum expectorated in a day and the color and viscosity of the sputum. The number and quality of stools per day should be assessed. Greasy or floating stools indicate that the patient is not taking enough pancreatic enzyme replacement. If the patient complains of abdominal pain, the location, quality, onset, and duration of the pain should be assessed.

The vital signs may reveal tachycardia, especially if the patient is febrile or hypoxemic. The temperature is elevated during acute infection. The respiratory rate is often rapid, particularly when the patient is febrile.

Examination of the chest reveals hyperinflation with an increase in anteroposterior chest diameter and use of accessory muscles of respiration. The chest is hyperresonant to percussion, and crackles, rhonchi, or wheezing may be heard on auscultation. Peripheral edema is a sign of PHD. Fluid and nutritional status can be evaluated by measurement of intake and output, assessment of skin turgor, moistness of mucous membranes, and evidence of muscle wasting.

Nursing Diagnoses and Interventions

For the most part, nursing care for the pulmonary component of cystic fibrosis is the same as that for chronic bronchitis. The reader is referred to the sections in this chapter for discussion of interventions related to these nursing diagnoses: ineffective airway clearance; impaired gas exchange; excess fluid volume; and alteration in nutrition. Other interventions specific to cystic fibrosis are discussed below. The overall goal of all interventions is to assist the patient in managing the symptoms and dealing with the personal and family upheaval caused by cystic fibrosis.

Vitamin Deficiency. Vitamin deficiency results from malabsorption of fat-soluble vitamins A, D, E, and K. Vitamin E deficiency is the most common deficiency and results in decreased survival for erythrocytes and, possibly, neuropathy. The patient should be instructed in the rationale for the replacement therapy; that is, prevention of anemia and neuropathy. Vitamin K deficiency may occur, and the patient should be instructed to notify his physician if signs of bleeding occur.

Fluid Imbalance. High sweat electrolyte loss may lead to fluid and electrolyte imbalance. The nurse monitors the serum chloride and sodium levels, as well as intake and output. The nurse observes the patient for signs of saline and water depletion. The patient should be instructed in the importance of a fluid intake of 2000 ml per day. It may be important for the patient to avoid extreme heat in order to prevent heat prostration.

Noncompliance. Noncompliance with the prescribed regimen may occur secondary to lack of knowledge, denial, insufficient financial resources, or other reasons. The nurse can explore with the patient the reasons for noncompliance and can develop alternative plans based on the stated reasons. Patient education is essential, since compliance is likely to improve if the patient understands the rationale for the therapy.

Some patients may not perform prescribed therapies such as chest physical therapy because they have no one available to assist them with it. The nurse can help to identify family, friends, or community resources that may be able to assist with therapy or can instruct the patient in self-care using a mechanical vibrator.

The most important factor in ensuring compliance is the setting of patient goals with the active participation of the patient. Modifications in the plan of care should be made whenever possible to make it easier to incorporate therapy into the patient's everyday life.

Self-Concept Disturbance. Physical dependence or altered appearance may result in disturbance in self-concept, body image, self-esteem, and role performance. For a number of reasons, the patient with cystic fibrosis may have had difficulty with the adolescent developmental task of acquiring a positive self-image. As an adolescent, he lagged behind peers in development at a time when being different is something to be avoided at all costs. Development of secondary sex characteristics may have been delayed, or he may have been smaller, thinner, or paler than his peers. He may have been unable to keep up with his peers in physical activities, or he may have been isolated because of treatment schedules or frequent illness.

The adult with cystic fibrosis may have difficulty establishing independence from his parents. He may have been treated as a "sick child" all his life and thus may act like one. He may be forced to remain dependent on his parents for money or treatments. He may be unable to find a job because of physical limitations, reluctance of employers to hire him, or inability to obtain required insurance.

The best way to help the adult patient with cystic fibrosis to accept himself is by communicating acceptance of him. The nurse can help the patient to explore these issues and can provide information on community resources that can assist him toward independence and acceptance. The patient can be instructed in self-care and independent decision making so that even though he may remain financially or otherwise dependent on others, his self-esteem will be enhanced. Support groups for adults with cystic fibrosis can provide role models and emotional support for the patient.

Sexual Dysfunction. Most men with cystic fibrosis are sterile, but the individual patient should not be counseled until his sterility is proven by semen analysis. If the patient is sterile, he and his spouse may be encouraged to adopt children, keeping in mind the patient's ability to care for a growing child. It is important for the patient and spouse to consider the possiblity that the child will be raised by a single parent.

Women with cystic fibrosis are relatively infertile compared with normal women, and the nurse can help to foster realistic expectations regarding the likelihood of becoming pregnant. The nurse can help the patient to make good decisions regarding child-bearing by providing information on the possible outcomes of pregnancy. Pregnancy places severe physiological stress on the woman with cystic fibrosis and may shorten her life span. The chances that a cystic fibrosis mother will bear a child with cystic fibrosis are relatively high. Finally, the patient must consider the effect of her shortened life span on the child and her ability to care for an active, growing child.[22]

Ineffective Coping. Depression or anxiety may occur in the face of the fatal prognosis. The fatal prognosis may precipitate an anxiety reaction even in the healthiest patient with cystic fibrosis. Depression is another likely response to having a chronic, fatal illness. The nurse can help to foster acceptance of the disease and prognosis without hopelessness by providing an atmosphere for open discussion and acknowledgment of feeling. A social work referral may be appropriate. During the terminal phase of the illness, expression of feelings and the presence of loved ones can smooth the transition from life to death.

Evaluation

Although outcome criteria for patients must be designed individually based on the specific nursing diagnoses that have been established, examples are as follows:

- Patient demonstrates methods of reducing predominant manifestations and complications of disease, including
  - Techniques for clearing secretions
  - Ability to recognize early signs of infection or other exacerbation
  - Dietary measures to achieve nutritional and fluid and electrolyte balance

- Patient reports decrease in symptoms that interfere with lifestyle
- Patient and family express concerns regarding effects of disease and its outcome
- Patient identifies sources of additional individual and family support during crisis periods

References

1. Abraham AS: The management of patients with chronic bronchitis and cor pulmonale. Heart Lung 6:104, 1977
2. American Thoracic Society: Statement by the committee on therapy. Am Rev Respir Dis 98:521, 1968
3. Bordow RA, Moser KM: COPD: Clinical and laboratory manifestations, pathophysiology and prognosis. In Bordow RA, Stool EW, Moser KM (eds): Manual of Clinical Problems in Pulmonary Medicine, 1st ed. Boston, Little, Brown & Co, 1980
4. Centers for Disease Control: Recommendation of the Public Health Service advisory committee on immunization practices. MMWR 27:25, 1978
5. Davis PB: Cystic fibrosis: Clinical manifestations in older patients. Clin Notes Respir Dis 21:3, 1983
6. Feldman J: Chronic obstructive pulmonary diseases: Chronic care. In Traver GA (ed): Respiratory Nursing: The Science and the Art, 1st ed. New York, John Wiley & Sons, 1982
7. Feldman J: Chronic obstructive pulmonary diseases: Acute care. In Traver GA (ed): Respiratory Nursing: The Science and the Art, 1st ed. New York, John Wiley & Sons, 1982
8. Fishman AP: Chronic cor pulmonale. Am Rev Respir Dis 114:775, 1976
9. Flenley DC: Long-term oxygen therapy: State of the art. Respir Care 28:876, 1983
10. Gorringe–Moore R: Asthma. In Traver GA (ed): Respiratory Nursing: The Science and the Art, 1st ed. New York, John Wiley & Sons, 1982
11. Guenter CA, Welch MH: Pulmonary Medicine, 2nd ed. Philadelphia, JB Lippincott, 1982
12. Hodgkin JE: Chronic Obstructive Pulmonary Disease: Current Concepts in Diagnosis and Comprehensive Care, 1st ed. Park Ridge, American College of Chest Physicians, 1979
13. Hogg JC: The pathophysiology of asthma. Chest 82:8s, 1982
14. Hoidal JR, Niewoehner DE: Pathogenesis of emphysema. Chest 83:679, 1983
15. Hudgel DW, Madsen LA: Acute and chronic asthma: A guide to intervention. Am J Nurs 80:1791, 1980
16. Hudson LD, Pierson DJ: Comprehensive respiratory care for patients with chronic obstructive pulmonary disease. Med Clin North Am 65:629, 1981
17. Ingram RH Jr: Chronic bronchitis, emphysema, and airways obstruction. In Petersdorf RG, Adams RD, Braunwald E et al (eds): Principles of Internal Medicine, 10th ed. New York, McGraw–Hill, 1983
18. Kirilloff LH, Tibbals SC: Drugs for asthma: A complete guide. Am J Nurs 83:55, 1983
19. Kremsdorf R: Bronchiectasis. In Bordow RA, Stool EW, Moser KM (eds): Manual of Clinical Problems in Pulmonary Medicine, 1st ed. Boston, Little, Brown & Co, 1980
20. Leff A: Pathophysiology of asthmatic bronchoconstriction. Chest 82:13s, 1982
21. Marini J, Lakshminarayan S: The effect of atropine inhalation in "irreversible" chronic bronchitis. Chest 77:591, 1980
22. Matson JA, Capen CV: Pregnancy in the cystic fibrosis patient. J Reprod Med 27:373, 1982
23. Moeckly M, Kile M: The psychosocial assessment. In Traver GA (ed): Respiratory Nursing: The Science and the Art, 1st ed. New York, John Wiley & Sons, 1982
24. Moser KM, Bordow RA: Chronic obstructive pulmonary disease: Definition, epidemiology, and pathology. In Bordow RA, Stool EW, Moser KM (eds): Manual of Clinical Problems in Pulmonary Medicine, 1st ed. Boston, Little, Brown & Co, 1980
25. Murray JF: Bronchiectasis and broncholithiasis. In Petersdorf RG, Adams RD, Braunwald E et al (eds): Principles of Internal Medicine, 10th ed. New York, McGraw–Hill, 1983
26. Nocturnal Oxygen Therapy Trial Group: Continuous or nocturnal oxygen therapy in hypoxemic chronic obstructive lung disease. Ann Intern Med 93:391, 1980
27. Oldenburg FA, Dolovich MB, Montgomery JM et al: Effects of postural drainage, exercise, and cough on mucus clearance in chronic bronchitis. Am Rev Respir Dis 120:739, 1979
28. O'Neill E: Cystic fibrosis. In Sexton DL (ed): Chronic Obstructive Pulmonary Disease: Care of the Child and Adult, 1st ed. St Louis, CV Mosby, 1981
29. Petty TL: Critical care for chronic air-flow limitation: Emphysema, chronic bronchitis, and cystic fibrosis. Semin Respir Med 3:263, 1982
30. Petty TL, Cherniack RM: Comprehensive care of COPD. Clin Notes Respir Dis 20:3, 1981
31. Pierson DJ: Asthma in the elderly: Special challenge. Geriatrics 37:87, 1982
32. Price SA, Wilson LM: Pathophysiology: Clinical Concepts of Disease Processes, 2nd ed. New York, McGraw–Hill, 1982
33. Ramsdell JW: Asthma: Clinical presentation and diagnosis. In Bordow RA, Stool EW, Moser KM (eds): Manual of Clinical Problems in Pulmonary Medicine, 1st ed. Boston, Little, Brown & Co, 1980
34. Ramsdell JW: Asthma: Management. In Bordow RA, Stool EW, Moser KM (eds): Manual of Clinical Problems in Pulmonary Medicine, 1st ed. Boston, Little, Brown & Co, 1980
35. Rogers TR: Clinical problems in the adult with asthma. Nurs Clin North Am 16:293, 1981
36. Schwachman H: Cystic fibrosis. Curr Probl Pediatr 8:5, 1978
37. Sexton DL: Chronic Obstructive Pulmonary Disease: Care of the Child and Adult, 1st ed. St Louis, CV Mosby, 1981
38. Traver GA: Respiratory Nursing: The Science and the Art, 1st ed. New York, John Wiley & Sons, 1982
39. Tyler M: Pulmonary heart disease. In Underhill SL, Woods SL, Sivarajan ES et al (eds): Cardiac Nursing, 1st ed. Philadelphia, JB Lippincott, 1982
40. Ward J: Cromolyn sodium: A new approach to treatment of asthma. Heart Lung 4:415, 1975
41. Webber–Jones JE, Bryant MK: Over-the-counter bronchodilators. Nursing 10:34, 1980
42. West JB: Pulmonary Pathophysiology: The Essentials, 2nd ed. Baltimore, Williams & Wilkins, 1982
43. Wood RE, Boat TF, Doershuk CF: Cystic fibrosis: State of the art. Am Rev Respir Dis 113:833, 1976
44. Ziment I: Respiratory Pharmacology and Therapeutics, 1st ed. Philadelphia, WB Saunders, 1978

Bibliography

Abraham M, Atkinson M, Boyce B et al: Standards for nursing care of patients with COPD. ATS News 7:31, 1981

Ghory AC, Patterson R: Treating asthma in the elderly. Geriatrics 35:32, 1980

Hudson LD: The acute management of the chronic airway obstruction patient. Heart Lung 3:93, 1974

Jacobs JW: Cystic fibrosis as it affects the patient and his family. Respir Ther 7:52, 1977

Liggins MR: Cystic fibrosis into the teens and beyond. Patient Care 9:120, 1976

McDonald GJ: A home care program for patients with chronic lung disease. Nurs Clin North Am 16:259, 1981

Maxwell M: Review of literature of physiotherapy in cystic fibrosis. Physiotherapy 66:245, 1980

Morrison ML: Respiratory Intensive Care Nursing, 2nd ed. Boston, Little, Brown & Co, 1979

Orenstein DM, Franklin BA, Doershuk CF et al: Exercise conditioning and cardiopulmonary fitness in cystic fibrosis. Chest 80:392, 1981

Passero MA, Remor B, Salomon J: Patient-reported compliance with cystic fibrosis therapy. Clin Pediatr 20:264, 1981

Rossman CM, Waldes R, Sampson D et al: Effect of chest physiotherapy on the removal of mucus in patients with cystic fibrosis. Am Rev Respir Dis 126:131, 1982

Sjoberg EL: Nursing diagnosis and the COPD patient. Am J Nurs 83:245, 1983

Stanley L: You really can teach COPD patients to breathe better. RN 41:43, 1978

Stockdale–Woolley R: Sexual dysfunction and COPD: Problems and management. The Nurse Pract 8:16, 1983

Chapter 30

Neoplastic Disorders Related to Respiratory Function

Cancer of the Larynx
Lung Cancer

Kathryn L. Anderson

A discussion of neoplasms of the respiratory system, that is, laryngeal and lung cancers, is a study of contrasts. Although these two diseases share a common etiology (cigarette smoking), affect similar patient populations, and cause some of the same symptoms, there are distinct differences in prevalence, treatment, and prognosis. All head and neck tumors combined account for fewer than 5% of cancers, while lung cancer is the second most common type of cancer in the United States. Treatment in laryngeal cancer is often curative, even in advanced stages, but treatment for lung cancer is likely to be palliative even when it is detected early. Finally, the prognosis for cancer of the larynx is often good (with 5-year survival greater than 50%), but the outlook even for lung cancer that is detected early is extremely poor (with 5-year survival of only 5%).

Cancer of the Larynx

Incidence and Etiology

The relative incidence of laryngeal cancer is low, accounting for about 2% of all cancers in the United States, with 80% to 90% of laryngeal cancers occurring in males.[11] However, disproportionate attention has been paid to the disease because of the potentially disfiguring and disabling effects of treatment. While early tumors may be treated with simple surgical procedures or radiation, advanced or metastasized tumors require extensive surgery, which may radically alter a patient's appearance, permanently abolish his ability to speak and smell, and alter the way he breathes. All of these potential traumas demand a skilled, knowledgeable, and compassionate team approach to care, involving the surgeon, nurse, radiotherapist, speech therapist, nutritionist, social worker, and volunteers.

Considerable evidence attributes the etiology of laryngeal cancer to heavy cigarette smoking. Although alcohol abuse is implicated in the cause of many head and neck cancers, its role in cancer of the larynx is not clear.[11] As with chronic obstructive pulmonary disease (COPD), the known relationship between smoking and disease emphasizes the importance of prevention through education about the hazards of smoking and ways to stop smoking.

Classification

As with all neoplasms, laryngeal cancer is described according to anatomical location and presence and extent of metastasis. Such a classification system, based on the type of primary tumor, nodal involvement, and extent of metastasis, helps to determine appropriate treatment (Table 30–1).

TABLE 30-1
TNM Classification for Cancers of the Larynx

Primary Tumor (T)

TIS—Carcinoma in situ
T1 — Tumor confined to one site
T2 — Involving more than one site in region of origin
T3 — Extension beyond region or fixation of cord
T4 — Massive tumor involving bone, cartilage, deep muscle, or skin

Nodal Involvement (N)

N0 — No clinically positive node
N1 — Single clinically positive node ≤ 3 cm in diameter, same side of midline as tumor (homolateral) only
N2 — Single clinically positive node 3 cm–6 cm in diameter; multiple homolateral clinically positive nodes none > 6 cm diameter
N3 — Massive nodes: homolateral, bilateral, or contralateral nodes

Distant Metastasis (M)

M0 — No known distant metastasis
M1 — Distant metastasis present

Stage Grouping

I— T1 N0 M0
II— T2 N0 M0
III— T3 N0 M0; T1 or T2 or T3, N1, M0
IV— T4, N0, M0
Any T, N2 or N3, M0
Any T, any N, M1

(Adapted from Zagars G, Norante JD: Head and neck tumors. In Rubin P, Bakemeier RF, Krackov SK (eds): Clinical Oncology for Medical Students and Physicians: A Multidisciplinary Approach, 6th ed, p 236. Rochester, American Cancer Society, 1983)

The anatomical location of the tumor is important in determining both treatment and prognosis. Tumors confined to the vocal cords are called *glottic* cancers, while those involving structures above the cords are called *supraglottic* cancers. Tumors of structures below the vocal cords are called *infraglottic* or *subglottic* tumors. These divisions are shown in Figure 30–1.

The primary tumor is also described according to size and extent. An *in situ* lesion is a tumor that has affected only the top layer of cells of the cord, with no invasion of the underlying tissue. As the tumor increases in size, it is described according to the mobility or immobility (fixation) of the cord, confinement of the tumor to the larynx, or extension of the tumor beyond the larynx.[19]

The degree of local lymph node involvement is described according to location and size of affected nodes. The presence or absence of distant metastases and their locations are also determined. The vocal cords themselves have little lymphatic drainage, and cord tumors are unlikely to metastasize early. However, other laryngeal structures have rich lymphatic drainage, and these tumors will readily metastasize.[15]

Pathophysiology

Chronic irritation of the larynx from cigarette smoke is believed to lead to cell changes that precede the development of cancer. These changes may be epithelial hyperplasia (keratosis) or leukoplakia, the formation of white patches on the vocal cords.

Carcinoma *in situ* describes a full-thickness replacement of the epithelium by malignant cells, without invasion of underlying cells.[13] The growth of the tumor eventually leads to invasion and fixation of the vocal cord. However, this squamous cell–type cancer tends to remain localized and metastasizes slowly because of the sparse lymphatic drainage.[13, 15] The tumor cells are well differentiated, indicating a good prognosis.

Clinical Manifestations

In addition to the tendency to remain localized, glottic tumors carry a good prognosis because they produce an early symptom: hoarseness. If heeded, this symptom leads to early diagnosis and prompt treatment.

Because the vocal cords are not involved directly in supraglottic cancer, there may not be any early symptoms of this type of tumor. The first symptom may be painful or difficult swallowing due to obstruction. The cancer may first be detected by palpation of an enlarged cervical lymph node, indicating that metastasis has already occurred. Dyspnea and stridor are signs of significant airway obstruction and indicate the presence of a large tumor.

Medical Management

Diagnosis. In general, any person who complains of hoarseness for 2 weeks should be examined for cancer.[13, 15] Inspection of the larynx by laryngoscope may reveal a tumor. Palpation of the neck may reveal lymph node enlargement; tenderness may indicate invasion of other tissues.[13]

A number of diagnostic radiologic studies may be done in order to determine the extent of the primary tumor and metastasis. These may include chest or neck films, computed tomography (CT) or laryngogram.

Treatment. The treatment of laryngeal cancer is determined by the site of the primary tumor and the presence and location of metastases. A variety of treatment options are available, including radiation therapy and surgery. Chemotherapy, so far, plays little role in the treatment of laryngeal cancer.

Radiation may be the treatment of choice for early, nonmetastatic glottic and supraglottic tumors because it is associated with a lower incidence of complications in comparison with surgery. If the tumor recurs, surgery may be performed later. Radiation therapy may also be used as an adjunct to surgery.

Surgical Treatment. A number of surgical procedures are available for the treatment of laryngeal cancer.

The simplest way to remove a localized glottic tumor is

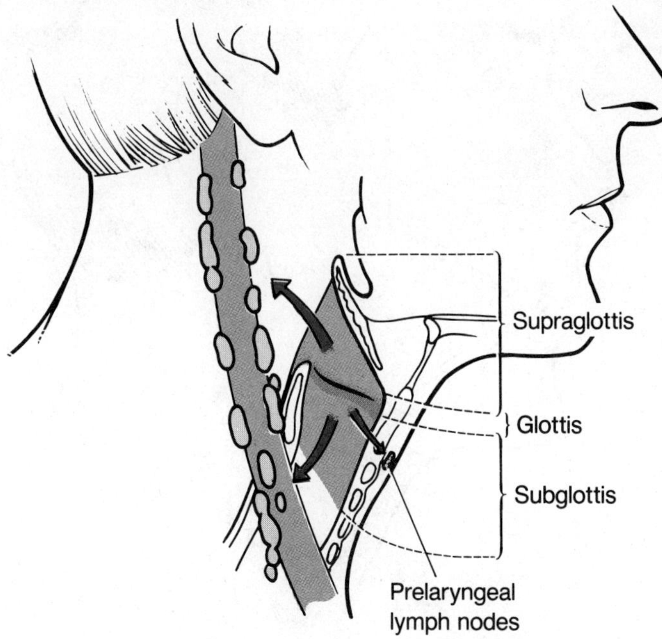

FIGURE 30–1 Classification of laryngeal tumors by anatomical location. Glottic tumors are confined to the vocal cords; because the vocal cords have sparse lymphatic drainage, these tumors metastasize slowly. Tumors of the supraglottis and subglottis involve structures above and below the vocal cords, respectively. Because of the rich lymphatic drainage of these areas, tumors at these sites metastasize readily. The diagram shows the principal lymph drainage of the endolarynx and its direction toward the deep jugular chain. (After Nauman HH: Surgery of malignant tumors of the larynx. In Nauman HH [ed]: Head and Neck Surgery, Vol 4, Neck, p 147. Philadelphia, WB Saunders, 1984)

by *laryngoscopy.*[8] No incision is required, and there is little change in the patient's voice following the procedure.

A second procedure for removal of a localized glottic tumor is a *laryngofissure.* A midline (vertical) neck incision is made, the thyroid cartilage is opened, and the affected vocal cord is removed. A temporary tracheostomy is performed to ensure a patent airway immediately following surgery.[15] A *hemilaryngectomy* may be done through the same incision. The incision for a hemilaryngectomy is shown in Figure 30–2. In this procedure, the thyroid cartilage, arytenoid cartilage, false vocal cord, and true vocal cord are removed. Postoperatively, the patient may have difficulty swallowing, and tube feedings or total parenteral nutrition may be required for the first 3 or 4 postoperative days. The long-term effect of laryngofissure is hoarseness. The airway and swallowing will be normal.

A *supraglottic laryngectomy* is performed when the patient has a large supraglottic tumor. A horizontal neck incision is made, and the epiglottis, false vocal cords, and hyoid bone are removed. The true vocal cords are left intact. The major postoperative problems are difficulty in swallowing and aspiration secondary to removal of the epiglottis. In the long term, aspiration occurs only occasionally, and the patient has a normal voice and airway. A supraglottic laryngectomy is often performed in conjunction with a unilateral radical neck dissection (see below).

For a large glottic or supraglottic tumor with fixation of the vocal cords, *total laryngectomy* will be performed. Figure 30–3 illustrates a total laryngectomy. This procedure involves removal of the true and false vocal cords, epiglottis, hyoid bone, cricoid cartilage, and two or three rings of the trachea. A permanent tracheostomy is performed. The implications of this procedure are profound. The patient loses his voice and has a permanent artificial airway. Swallowing is normal. Figure 30–4 shows the alteration in upper-airway structure and function following total laryngectomy.

A radical neck dissection is indicated when there are known metastases to cervical lymph nodes or as prophylaxis for metastasis. This procedure involves removal of the cervical lymph nodes and the surrounding tissue. The postoperative condition and long-term effects are determined largely by other procedures performed at the same time. Radical neck dissection may be done in conjunction with surgery for any tumor of the head or neck. Regardless of the primary tumor involved, this type of surgery is always disfiguring.[15,16]

Prognosis. The prognosis for laryngeal cancer is generally good, although as with any cancer, it is related to the extent of disease at the time of diagnosis. For lesions without fixation of the vocal cord, the 5-year survival rate is 80% to 90% following radiation or surgery. Tumors with cord fixation have a 5-year survival rate of 75% after total laryngectomy. For tumors with metastasis to cervical lymph nodes, the 5-year survival rate is 50%.[19]

Nursing Management: Preventive Measures for Health Promotion

Although the majority of nursing interventions to be described focus on the treatment phase of illness, it should be remembered that the nurse's role in prevention of laryngeal cancer is equally, if not more, important. The nursing history for any patient hospitalized for any reason should include assessment of the patient's smoking habits. If a patient is currently a smoker, the nurse should try to elicit, in a nonthreatening way, the reasons why the patient smokes and whether he has any desire to stop. Patients who express an interest in stopping can be provided with information regarding smoking-cessation programs. A list of such programs can usually be obtained from the local chapter of the Ameri-

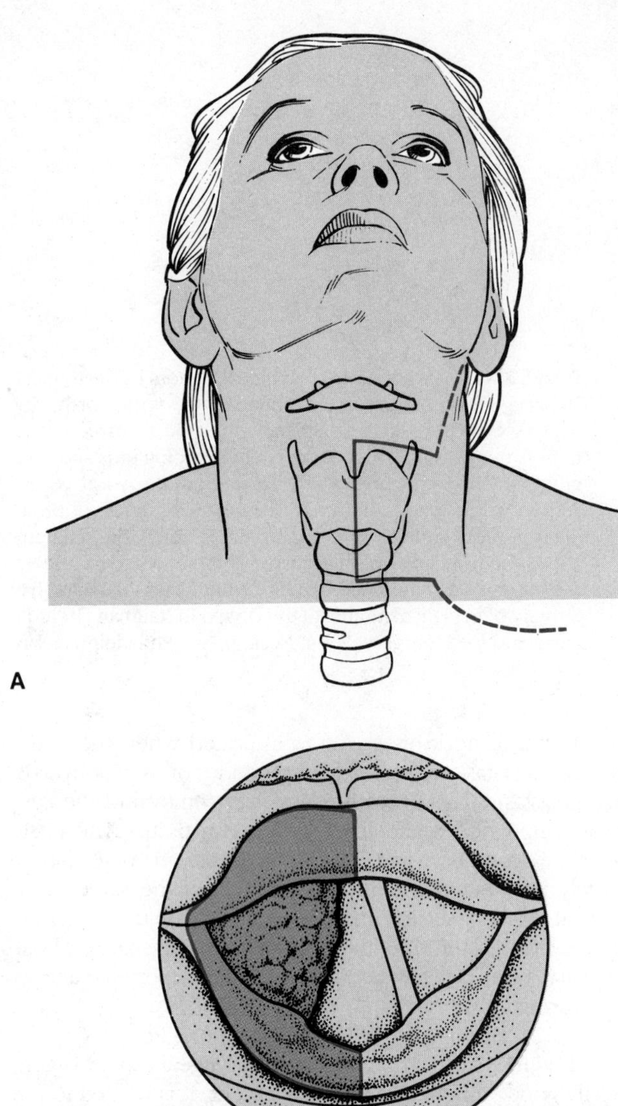

FIGURE 30–2 Hemilaryngectomy. One half of larynx and corresponding half of cricoid cartilage is removed. (*A*) Incision for hemilaryngectomy; the dotted line shows an extension for radical neck dissection. (*B*) Portion of larynx that is excised. (After Nauman HH: Surgery of malignant tumors of the larynx. In Nauman HH [ed]: Head and Neck Surgery, Vol 4, Neck, pp 186, 188. Philadelphia, WB Saunders, 1984)

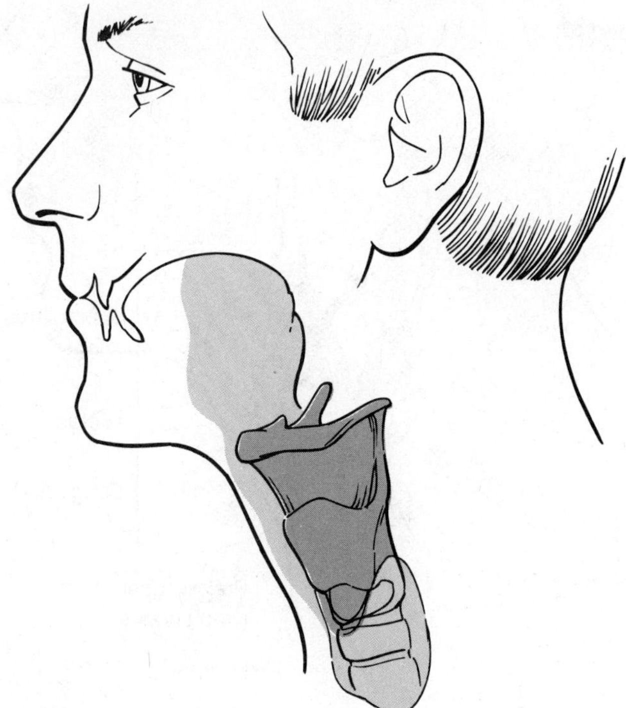

FIGURE 30–3 Diagram of total laryngectomy. Depending on the extent of the tumor, neighboring structures are removed (*gray area*). (After Nauman HH: Surgery of malignant tumors of the larynx. In Nauman HH [ed]: Head and Neck Surgery, Vol 4, Neck, p 209. Philadelphia, WB Saunders, 1984)

can Lung Association. Patients who are trying to stop smoking need support and encouragement and should be given positive reinforcement for successful efforts. Finally, nurses should serve as role models for their patients by abstaining from cigarette smoking. Patient education regarding the importance of smoking cessation for health will have little credibility when the patient observes health-care personnel practicing the very habit they are condemning.

When the diagnosis of laryngeal cancer has been established, the medical treatment varies with the location and extent of tumor involvement. As described above, surgical excision or radiation therapy is the usual mode of treatment. Nursing management related to surgical excision is described first, followed by a discussion of nursing management related to radiation therapy

Preoperative Nursing Management

Assessment and Nursing Diagnosis

Preoperative assessment consists of evaluation of the patient's knowledge of and feelings about what is going to happen to him during and after surgery. The nurse can determine how much of what the surgeon has told the patient and his family has been absorbed. In addition, the patient's fears regarding the diagnosis of cancer, the surgery itself, and life after surgery can be assessed. The meaning of the illness to the patient and his family, particularly as it affects family roles, is important. The nurse should also determine what the patient and family strengths are, including such coping assets as family, friends, religious faith, and adequate financial resources.

Examples of nursing diagnoses that might be established are the following:

- Knowledge deficit related to surgery for laryngeal cancer
- Ineffective personal or family coping related to knowledge deficit, anxiety, or deficient support systems.

During the preoperative period, the major goals of

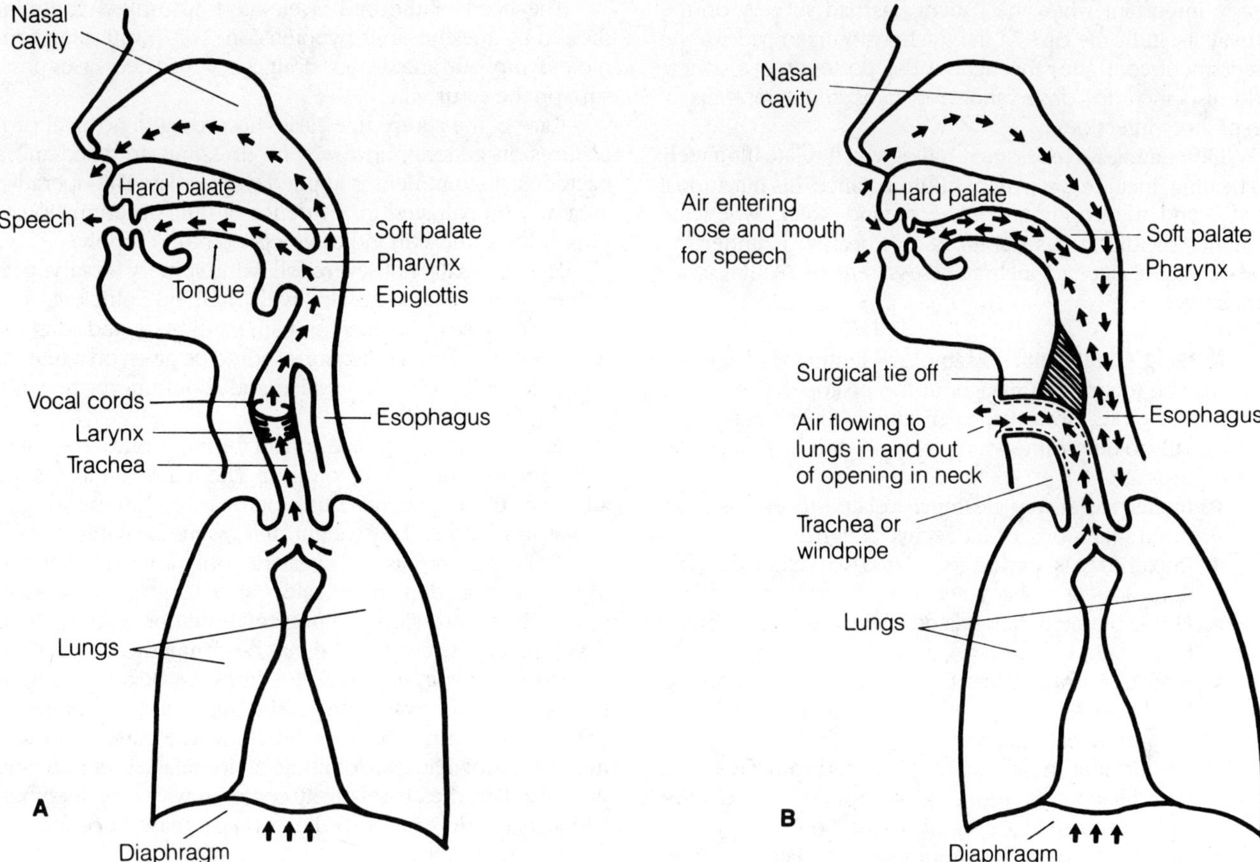

FIGURE 30–4 Direction of air flow (*A*) before and (*B*) after a total laryngectomy. (American Cancer Society)

nursing interventions are to facilitate optimum coping by the patient and his family and to ensure adequate preparation for the surgical procedure.

Interventions

The nurse provides information about the surgery as the patient shows readiness to accept it. If possible, the nurse should be present when the surgeon describes the procedure to the patient, so that the correct information can be reinforced. The nurse can tell the patient what he can expect after surgery, particularly which tubes he will have in place and what they are for. If a tracheostomy will be performed, a method of communication must be established before surgery. A magic slate, flash cards, or hand signals are methods that are frequently used. A visit from the speech therapist or a laryngectomee who speaks well can be arranged for the prelaryngectomy patient. (A laryngectomee is a person who has undergone total laryngectomy.)

In order to smooth the postoperative course, the nurse establishes a trusting relationship with the patient and his family. The nurse can emphasize the importance of coping assets for recovery after surgery. For example, the patient should be encouraged to continue normal contact with friends after his operation, rather than withdrawing from them. The nurse can facilitate the constructive use of defense mechanisms by recognizing their legitimacy (*e.g.,* the use of denial after hearing the diagnosis of cancer). The nurse can promote patient acceptance of his new "self" by projecting acceptance of him both before and after surgery.

Evaluation

Prior to surgery, the patient will

- Describe, in lay terms, the surgical procedure and expected postoperative course
- Express concerns regarding his disease, its treatment, and the effects upon his life

Postoperative Nursing Management

Assessment and Nursing Diagnosis

Nursing assessment and interventions throughout the postoperative period are important in identifying potential problems early in their course so that they may be treated promptly. In the early postoperative period, the focus of assessment is on recognition of problems that are potentially life threatening or may impair healing. All postoperative patients should be assessed immediately for airway patency and signs of hypoxemia (See Chap 27). This assessment is particularly important when the patient has had surgery on the airway itself. In the case of the tracheostomized patient, the assessment continues throughout the postoperative course and also includes observation for signs and symptoms of respiratory infection.

Other areas for assessment, all of which relate ultimately to healing, include the patient's fluid balance, his nutritional status, and the condition of the wound. Later, when the patient's condition has stabilized and healing is underway, the focus enlarges to include assessment of readiness for discharge.

Nursing Diagnoses. Examples of nursing diagnoses that may be identified throughout the postoperative period are listed below. However, each patient must be assessed individually to determine which of these, or other, diagnoses are appropriate.

- Ineffective airway clearance related to excessive or dried secretions, or ineffective cough
- Impaired gas exchange related to retained secretions, loss of airway patency, or respiratory infection
- Fluid volume deficit related to postoperative hemorrhage
- Altered nutrition, less than body requirements, related to dysphagia, incisional pain, nausea, anorexia, aspiration, or fistula formation
- Impairment in skin integrity related to delayed surgical healing as a result of infection, excessive saliva, or inadequate blood supply to incision.
- Impaired verbal communication related to total laryngectomy
- Self-care deficit (feeding, airway management) related to lack of knowledge, anxiety, or arm and shoulder weakness
- Disturbance in self-concept related to loss of normal voice and facial disfigurement

The primary goals of nursing intervention are to achieve healing without complications and to achieve readiness to manage self-care at home.

Early Postoperative Interventions

The patient with a tracheostomy is suctioned as frequently as needed to remove retained secretions. If the tracheostomy tube has an inner cannula, it is removed and cleaned under cool running water with a nylon brush at frequent intervals and as needed. Air or oxygen going to the tracheostomy is humidified to prevent drying of secretions and respiratory tract mucosa. The nurse can assist with frequent turning by supporting the patient's head to avoid stress on suture lines. The patient is also encouraged to cough and deep breathe and should be out of bed on the first postoperative day.

The vital signs are checked frequently in the immediate postoperative period, and signs of hemorrhage (hypotension, tachycardia) and infection (fever, tachycardia) are reported. Wound drainage is measured, and the character of the drainage is noted. A marked increase in drainage may indicate hemorrhage; a decrease or cessation of drainage may mean that the drains are not patent. If the drains are connected to suction, the nurse ensures that it is maintained.

The head of the bed is elevated 30° unless contraindicated by anesthesia or hypotension. This positioning promotes lymphatic and venous drainage, which decreases pressure on the suture line.

Care of the suture line varies according to hospital procedures. In general, however, no dressings are used and a bacteriostatic ointment is applied twice a day. The operative area may be palpated for evidence of fluid accumulation. A pink color to the skin indicates a good blood supply.

Pain is usually not severe following surgery for laryngeal cancer, and mild analgesics will often be sufficient. The nurse must assess the need for pain medication and administer as needed. Pain medications should be given on a regular schedule while they are needed and should never be withheld for fear of addiction.

Adequate nutrition is essential for the surgical patient in order for wound healing to occur. The nurse can assess the adequacy of the patient's nutrition by careful monitoring of intake and output, daily weight, and wound healing.

If the patient has a nasogastric tube, it is connected to intermittent suction immediately after surgery to maintain gastric decompression and prevent aspiration. One to three days postoperatively the tube may be clamped, and if there is no nausea or vomiting, tube feedings are begun. Feedings may begin with water and skim milk and, if tolerated, progress to commercial tube feedings. The patient must be monitored for nausea, vomiting, abdominal distention, and diarrhea. Diarrhea is relatively common with tube feedings, and a change in type of feeding or a decrease in concentration may be required.

Not all postoperative patients will have a nasogastric tube in place. However, these patients may have difficulty with eating because of dysphagia, pain, nausea, or anorexia. Small, frequent portions of foods the patient likes may help to improve nutrition. The patient with a supraglottic laryngectomy may aspirate food. He should be taught to flex his neck forward and hold his breath while swallowing, then forcefully exhale to blow away food debris.[10]

Later Postoperative Interventions

Several days postoperatively the wound edges may appear necrotic, indicating that the blood supply to the skin has been lost and cell death has occurred. Flap necrosis may lead to erosion of the carotid artery. If any bleeding appears at the suture line, the physician must be notified immediately. If hemorrhage ("blowout") occurs, pressure is applied and help is summoned without leaving the patient.

Another serious, but not life threatening, complication that may occur several days postoperatively is fistula formation. This complication occurs when there is breakdown along the suture line in the pharynx, causing saliva to leak out through the skin, with eventual formation of a fistula tract. Signs of fistula formation are redness and swelling of the neck, and fever.

The patient with a fistula must have a nasogastric tube for feeding because food ingested normally will come out through the fistula tract. A large amount of fluid may be lost, and the nurse must observe for signs of saline and water deficit and accurately record intake and output. Skin care must be meticulous in order to prevent maceration from the flow of saliva. The fistula itself is packed with sterile gauze every 4 to 6 hours. Healing will eventually take place but may be very slow. If the patient is to be sent home with a nasogastric tube in place, he must be taught self-care and feeding as early as possible.

Patient Teaching for Home Care

When the patient's condition has stabilized following the immediate postoperative period, nursing care focuses on preparing the patient for discharge. The nurse continues to monitor the patient for potential problems as well.

If the patient has a permanent tracheostomy, as following total laryngectomy, he is taught self-care as early as possible. He and his family should learn to suction using clean technique, to remove and clean the inner cannula, and to clean the tracheostomy site itself. At home, a vaporizer or kettle of boiling water may be used to increase humidity in the air. A moist 4 × 4-inch gauze pad may be used to cover the stoma.

Resection of the cranial nerves can cause motor degeneration and atrophy of the trapezius muscle. The result is shoulder drop and pain or aching. When wound healing is adequate, the patient should be taught exercises to strengthen the muscle. Range of motion exercises for the neck and shoulder and wall-climbing exercises with the fingers can be taught. The nurse can encourage the patient to maintain good posture. The patient should not lie on the affected side and should not carry more than 2 pounds on that side.

Long-Term Postoperative Interventions

Although the patient may have had preoperative instruction in ways to communicate following surgery, nothing can adequately prepare him for the trauma associated with the permanent loss of his voice. The nurse can help the patient by preparing him for the depression and grief that is normal following such a loss, and by providing support to him and his family as he experiences these feelings.

Speech Therapy and Communication Techniques. Esophageal speech is a technique of speaking that utilizes the regurgitation of swallowed air to produce sound. The patient may receive some preoperative teaching in this technique and will be seen by a speech therapist after surgery. With continual encouragement by the staff and constant practice by the patient, many laryngectomy patients learn to communicate using esophageal speech. However, the nurse must recognize that not all patients will develop adequate speech. She can help the individual patient to cope with the frustrations and disappointment that may follow.

Patients who are unable to learn esophageal speech may use an artificial or electronic larynx to help them communicate. The artificial larynx may also be used to maintain communication while esophageal speech is being learned.

For outpatient support and teaching, the patient may be referred for home care to be provided by a nurse, physical therapist, speech therapist, or social worker. The patient may also be encouraged to join the local "Lost Cord" Club, a group of laryngectomees who provide help with speech, emotional support, and practical information for everyday living. The patient should get a medical identification bracelet stating that he breathes through a tracheostomy.

Coping Strategies. The laryngectomy or radical neck dissection patient has many reasons to feel depressed or to wish to withdraw from family and social contacts. To help the patient accept his "new" self and thereby help him to maintain social contacts and return to work, the nurse can communicate acceptance of the patient. The nurse can encourage expression of feelings regarding the patient's self-image and perceived changes in his lifestyle caused by the surgery. Independence can be fostered by teaching and encouraging self-care as early as possible in the postoperative course. The patient's communication can be facilitated by the means described above.

Evaluation

Evidence that goals related to postoperative management of the laryngeal cancer have been achieved includes observations that

- The surgical incision is clean and healing
- The patient demonstrates self-care techniques related to feeding and removal of tracheobronchial secretions
- The patient demonstrates successful methods for communicating his needs
- The patient demonstrates a positive self-image

More specific outcomes must be designed individually depending on the type of surgery performed and the patient's preoperative status.

Nursing Care of the Patient Receiving Radiation Therapy

Assessment and Nursing Diagnosis

Some patients with cancer of the larynx will receive radiation therapy either alone or as an adjunct to surgical treatment. Assessment for integrity of the skin and oral mucosa and assessment of nutritional status are extremely important throughout the course of the radiation treatments.

Expected nursing diagnoses include

- Alteration in skin or mucosal integrity related to radiation therapy damage to tissues adjacent to the tumor
- Alterations in nutrition, less than body requirements, related to the effects of radiation on the mouth and esophagus

Goals. The primary goal of all nursing interventions is to prevent radiation-induced complications. Thus, nursing care for the patient is concerned primarily with prevention of and managing the side-effects of the therapy. If the radiation therapy is to be done on an outpatient basis, the patient or family members must be taught appropriate observations and interventions to carry out at home.

Interventions

Dryness of the mouth due to thick or absent secretions is known as xerostomia and is a common problem during radiation therapy. In order to maintain integrity of the oral mucosa, good, frequent oral hygiene is essential. The mouth may be irrigated with mouthwash, saline, or prescribed solutions. Lemon drops may be used to stimulate salivation, or artificial saliva may be used to moisten the mouth.

Radiation therapy may cause anorexia and, along with xerostomia, can lead to inadequate nutrition and hydration. Good nutrition and hydration help to maintain healthy tissues, and the nurse monitors the patient for weight loss related to anorexia, dysphagia, or malaise. Small, frequent feedings or use of nutritional supplements may be required to maintain adequate nutrition.

Radiation therapy can cause ulceration or irritation of the skin at the therapy site. The nurse observes the skin for evidence of breakdown and instructs the patient to do the same at home. The patient is instructed not to use any creams, lotions, or powders on the skin and to protect the skin from exposure to sunlight. The patient should not wash off the markings made by the radiologist.

Evaluation

The patient who is undergoing radiation therapy for cancer of the larynx will

- Maintain weight within ______ pounds of baseline (weight established individually)
- Maintain intact oral mucosa and skin

Cancer of the Lung

Etiology and Epidemiology

Lung cancer is the second most common type of cancer in the United States, and its incidence is increasing. The typical victim has been a male, aged 50 to 70 years, with a long history of cigarette smoking. However, more women are being diagnosed with lung cancer as more and more women smoke cigarettes. This increase among women has made lung cancer the leading cause of cancer deaths in this country. One hundred thousand people died of lung cancer in the United States in 1980.[1,7,12]

As with laryngeal cancer and COPD, these statistics are all the more tragic because the primary etiology of lung cancer is known, and the disease is largely preventable. Numerous scientific studies have demonstrated a strong association between cigarette smoking and lung cancer. Cigarette smokers are 8 to 20 times more likely to develop lung cancer than nonsmokers, and the chance of getting lung cancer increases proportionately with the number of cigarettes smoked.

Another factor that may contribute to the development of lung cancer is occupational exposure to asbestos, uranium, and possibly some other irritants. However, cigarette smoking also plays a role in increasing the risk of lung cancer with occupational exposure to irritants. Asbestos and smoking act synergistically; thus, an asbestos worker who smokes is 92 times more likely to develop lung cancer than a nonsmoker not exposed to asbestos.[1]

There is a 1.3 to 2.3 times greater risk of developing lung cancer in an urban environment than in a rural one. However, this increase is relatively minor in comparison with the increased risk caused by smoking.

Classification

Cancer of the lung is classified according to the type of cell involved—epidermoid (squamous), small cell (oat cell), adenocarcinoma, and large cell (anaplastic). These cell types are described in Table 30–2. Non–small cell disease is staged according to the TNM system—size and location of the primary *t*umor, lymph *n*ode involvement, and *m*etastatic spread (Table 30–3).

Small cell cancers are not staged according to the TNM system but rather as limited-stage disease or extensive-stage disease. Limited stage disease is defined as disease confined to one hemithorax and to regional lymph nodes (mediastinal and contralateral hilar, ipsilateral supraclavicular). Extensive stage disease is defined as disease beyond that described, including distant metastasis.

Staging is important in determining medical treatment, but because it does not directly affect nursing care, it is not discussed here. It is important to remember, however, that the lungs have both a rich blood supply and lymphatic drainage system, so that lung tumors tend to metastasize early. At the time of diagnosis, it is likely that local nodal involvement and distant metastasis have already occurred. Figure 30–5 shows a large tumor in the hilar region of the lung.

Clinical Manifestations

The diagnosis of lung cancer may be difficult because the symptoms may be nonspecific and may not be pulmonary. Pulmonary symptoms, such as a productive cough, may mimic other lung conditions. Nonpulmonary symptoms may be as vague as loss of appetite or may be a systemic syndrome not often associated with the lung. For simplicity, this discussion focuses on only the most common and primarily pulmonary symptoms. A list of common extrapulmonary syndromes is provided in Table 30–4.

Dyspnea, development of a cough, or a change in the person's typical cough may be symptoms of lung cancer. Hemoptysis is uncommon but is very frightening when it occurs. A slowly resolving pneumonia may result from bronchial obstruction by a tumor.

Arm and shoulder pain may occur when the tumor affects the brachial plexus, and hoarseness may result from pressure on the recurrent laryngeal nerve. Phrenic nerve involvement results in paralysis of one side of the diaphragm. Horner's syndrome may result from involvement of the cervical sympathetic nerves. This syndrome includes unilateral miosis, partial ptosis, enophthalmos, and loss of sweating. Swelling of the face or eyelids results from pressure on the superior vena cava.

TABLE 30–2
Lung Cancer Cell Types

Cell	*Location*	*Intrathoracic Metastasis*	*Extrathoracic Metastasis*	*Other*
Epidermoid (squamous) 30%–50% of lung tumors	Arise from epithelium of bronchial tree	Hilar, mediastinal lymph nodes; pleura; diaphragm; opposite lung; cardiovascular system	Liver, kidney	
Small cell (oat cell) 25%	Bronchial tree	Bronchial, hilar, mediastinal nodes; soft tissues	Bone marrow, regional nodes, pancreas, liver, adrenal glands, CNS, endocrine organs	Early metastasis, usually metastasized to bone at time of diagnosis
Adenocarcinoma 25%	Arise from bronchial surface epithelium or underlying mucous glands, but tend to be more peripheral than epidermoid and small cell carcinomas		Regional lymph nodes, adrenal glands, bone, kidney, CNS	Most common tumor found in nonsmokers
Large cell (anaplastic) 15%	Peripheral	Mediastinal nodes, pleura, cardiovascular system	Liver, adrenal glands, CNS, bone, GI tract	Primary tumor may be very large; late metastasis

CNS, central nervous system; GI, gastrointestinal

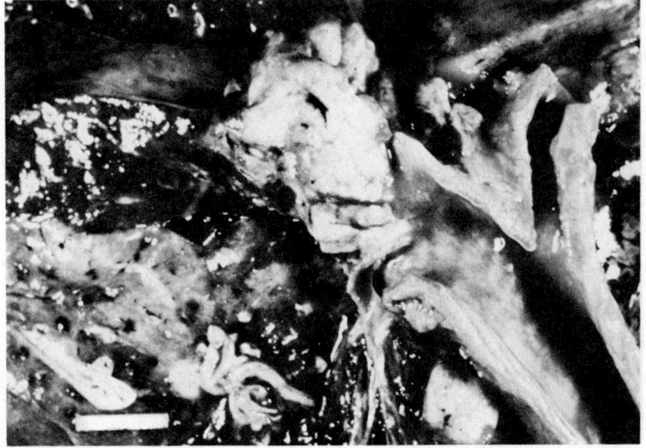

FIGURE 30–5 Bronchogenic carcinoma. Large tumor is obstructing a bronchus. (Courtesy of Dr. Marie Cowan, University of Washington School of Nursing)

Some nonspecific systemic signs of lung cancer include weight loss, anorexia, nausea, vomiting, and weakness.

Medical Management

Diagnosis. A diagnosis of lung cancer may be suspected when a patient presents with any of the signs and symptoms described above, or when a routine chest film reveals an abnormality. A careful history may reveal heavy cigarette smoking or exposure to occupational hazards such as asbestos.

In early stages of lung cancer, there may be no significant physical findings, and even in advanced disease they may be subtle. The patient may have digital clubbing on inspection. Palpation may reveal enlarged cervical, supraclavicular, or axillary lymph nodes. A localized wheeze may be heard when the tumor obstructs a bronchus. The breath sounds will be diminished if a pleural effusion or pneumothorax is present.

The chest film is most helpful when it is compared with previously obtained films. Sputum cytology may show malignant cells.

A number of diagnostic tests may be used to establish the diagnosis and determine the extent of metastasis. A biopsy done by bronchoscopy is helpful for centrally located tumors. Peripheral tumors may require a closed-needle biopsy. A mediastinoscopy or open-lung biopsy may also be done.

The history and physical examination will guide the search for distant metastases. Liver, brain, or bone scans may be performed if the outcome of these tests will affect treatment.

Treatment. Surgical removal for cure is the treatment of choice for localized non–small cell cancers. However, only one third of lung cancer patients have tumors that can

TABLE 30–3
Staging of Lung Cancer (Non–Small Cell)*

Primary Tumors	
T	— Primary tumor.
T0	— No evidence of primary tumor.
TX	— Tumor proven by presence of malignant cells in bronchopulmonary secretions but not visualized roentgenographically or bronchoscopically.
TIS	— Carcinoma in situ.
T1	— Tumor that is 3.0 cm or less in greatest diameter, surrounded by lung or visceral pleura and without evidence of invasion proximal to a lobar bronchus at bronchoscopy.
T2	— Tumor more than 3.0 cm in greatest diameter, or tumor of any size that invades the visceral pleura or is associated with atelectasis or obstructive pneumonitis and extends to the hilar region. At bronchoscopy, the proximal extent of demonstrable tumor must be within a lobar bronchus or at least 2.0 cm distal to the carina. Any associated atelectasis or obstructive pneumonitis must involve less than an entire lung, and there must be no pleural effusion.
T3	— Tumor of any size with direct extension into an adjacent structure, such as chest wall, diaphragm, or mediastinum and its contents, or tumor demonstrated bronchoscopically to involve a main bronchus less than 2.0 cm distal to the carina; any tumor associated with atelectasis or obstructive pneumonitis of an entire lung or pleural effusion.
Regional Lymph Nodes	
N	— Regional lymph nodes.
N0	— No demonstrable metastasis to regional lymph nodes.
N1	— Metastasis to lymph nodes in peribronchial and/or ipsilateral hilar region (including direct extension).
N2	— Metastasis to lymph nodes in the mediastinum.
Distant Metastasis	
M	— Distant metastasis.
M0	— No distant metastasis
M1	— Distant metastasis, such as in scalene, cervical, or contralateral hilar lymph nodes, brain, bones, lung, liver.
These categories of T, N, and M may be combined into the following groups or stages:	
Occult Carcinoma	
TX N0 M0	— Occult carcinoma with bronchopulmonary secretions containing malignant cells but without other evidence of the primary tumor or evidence of metastasis.
Stage I	
TIS N0 M0	— Carcinoma in situ.
T1 N0 M0	— Tumor that can be classified T1 without any metastasis to the regional lymph nodes.
T1 N1 M0	— Tumor that can be classified T1 with metastasis to the lymph nodes in the ipsilateral hilar region only.
T2 N0 M0	— Tumor that can be classified T2 without any metastasis to nodes or distant metastasis.
NOTE:	TX N1 M0 and T0 N1 M0 are also theoretically possible, but such a clinical diagnosis would be difficult if not impossible to make. If such a diagnosis is made, it should be included in Stage I.
Stage II	
T2 N1 M0	— Tumor classified as T2 with metastasis to the lymph nodes in the ipsilateral hilar region only.
Stage III	
T3 with any N or M	— Any tumor more extensive than T2.
N2 with any T or M	— Any tumor with metastasis to the lymph nodes in the mediastinum.
M1 with any T or N	— Any tumor with distant metastasis.

* AJC definitions of TNM categories.
(Carr DT, Mountain CF: Staging of lung cancer. Semin Respir Med 3:154–163, 1982)

TABLE 30–4
Common Extrapulmonary Syndromes Associated with Lung Cancer

Metabolic	
Hypercalcemia (especially with epidermoid or anaplastic tumors)	
Inappropriate ADH	(almost always with small cell tumors)
Cushing's syndrome	(almost always with small cell tumors)
Carcinoid syndrome	
Neuromuscular	
Peripheral neuritis	
Cortical or cerebellar degeneration	
Myopathy	
Dermatologic	
Acanthosis nigricans	
Dermatomyositis	
Skeletal	
Pulmonary hypertrophic osteoarthropathy, including clubbing	
Vascular	
Migratory thrombophlebitis	
Nonbacterial verrucous endocarditis	
Hematologic	
Anemia	
Disseminated intravascular coagulopathy	

be considered eligible for surgical resection.[18] Whenever possible, lobectomy is preferred over pneumonectomy because of the lower morbidity following surgery.

The most radical surgery is a pneumonectomy, or removal of the entire lung. This procedure is avoided if possible because of the high risk of complications associated with it. A more desirable procedure is a lobectomy, in which only the affected lobe is removed. A segmentectomy, or removal of a single lung segment, removes even less lung tissue. A wedge resection, or removal of a small amount of tissue without regard for the anatomical divisions of the lung, may be used to remove a very small tumor.

Surgery is not performed as a palliative measure in lung cancer and is contraindicated unless the tumor is localized. Other contraindications include the following: a diagnosis of small cell cancer, because metastasis is assumed at time of diagnosis; metastasis to the opposite lung, or outside of the thorax; tumor invasion or metastasis to the pulmonary artery, vena cava, vertebrae or ribs, major nerves, contralateral thoracic lymph nodes, pleura, or carina; the presence of malignant pleural effusion; and poor medical condition.

Radiation therapy for lung cancer may be definitive (curative) or palliative. Definitive therapy is given for an unresectable intrathoracic tumor or for a resectable tumor when the patient cannot be operated on because of an underlying medical condition.

Palliative radiation may be given for relief of symptoms such as hemoptysis, obstruction of a bronchus or major vein, esophageal compression, or cough pain. Radiation may shrink bone or brain metastases and cause a reduction in symptoms.

Chemotherapy may be used in up to 50% of patients because of the frequency of metastasis. Small cell tumors are the most responsive to chemotherapy, whereas there is little response in epidermoid or adenocarcinoma. Immunotherapy using bacille Calmette–Guérin (BCG) vaccine may be helpful in early tumors.

Prognosis. Little progress has been made toward prevention, early detection, or treatment of lung cancer. No change is expected in the rising incidence as large numbers of people continue to smoke cigarettes. Mass screening of susceptible populations by chest film has not resulted in improvement in prognosis. Finally, attempts to establish effective treatment regimens have not yet produced an improvement in survival rate.

Therefore, the prognosis for lung cancer remains exceedingly poor, with a 20% 1-year survival rate and only 5% of patients alive after 5 years. Virtually all of those who survive for 5 years have localized, resectable tumors at the time of diagnosis. The average overall survival time is only 6 to 9 months from diagnosis.

Nursing Management

As has been the case with nearly all of the diseases discussed in the last two chapters, the role of nurses in the prevention of lung cancer is of the utmost importance. Smoking cessation is discussed above, and it is even more relevant here. The nurse has a responsibility to instruct all patients in the health consequences of smoking and to be a role model for patients by abstaining from smoking.

Nursing care in lung cancer may be divided into three phases, a classification that recognizes the stages through which the patient will pass. These are the diagnostic, treatment, and terminal phases.[5] Although they can be expected to overlap, nursing diagnoses are provided for each phase. This list of nursing diagnoses is by no means all-inclusive. Rather, the diagnoses presented are meant to serve as examples; based on the assessment data, they must be modified to fit individual patients.

Nursing Management: Diagnostic Phase

Assessment and Nursing Diagnosis

A thorough nursing assessment is important during all phases of cancer care but is discussed in detail here.

The nursing history may include information regarding smoking habits and occupational exposures to known carcinogens. The history of the current illness itself may be important in understanding the patient's response to his illness because he may have been feeling fine when confronted with a catastrophic diagnosis.

The physical assessment potentially includes many body systems because of the relatively frequent involvement of extrapulmonary sites. Some selected elements of physical assessment are discussed below.

Cerebral metastasis may cause a change in the level of consciousness or behavior, as well as motor deficits. Apathy, depression, malaise, fatigue, or muscle weakness may result from hypercalcemia.[5] Cardiovascular assessment may reveal tachycardia and hypotension if the patient is saline depleted. Hypercalcemia may cause bradycardia and electrocardiographic (ECG) changes, including a widened T wave. Nutritional status and hydration are assessed by weight, intake and output, skin turgor, and moistness of mucous membranes.

The psychosocial assessment includes recognition of the fear and anxiety associated with the potential diagnosis of cancer. The nurse must also recognize the impact the illness may have on the patient and family, since the patient is likely to be the primary wage earner. Coping mechanisms that have been used successfully in past crises should be identified, as should social supports available to the family.

Nursing diagnoses depend on the results of assessment. A frequent diagnosis is ineffective individual or family coping related to a fear of or inadequate knowledge about cancer.

Interventions

Nursing interventions during the diagnostic workup for lung cancer are directed at the goal of relieving the anxiety and fear the patient is experiencing. The nurse can provide support and empathy for both the patient and family members. Anxiety surrounding diagnostic procedures can be relieved by explaining them to the patient in terms he can understand and by reinforcing information given by the physician. Successful goal achievement can be evaluated by observations that indicate decreased patient or family anxiety.

Nursing Management: Treatment Phase

Assessment and Nursing Diagnosis

Once the diagnosis of lung cancer has been made, treatment is chosen based on stage of the disease. Nursing care is tied closely to the type of medical therapy that is chosen. Nursing care for the three major modes of therapy—surgery, radiation, and chemotherapy—is discussed separately. The history and physical assessment information presented earlier in the diagnostic phase is applicable to all three modes of treatment. Additional assessment parameters specifically related to each of these methods of treatment are included in the following discussion.

Nursing Diagnoses. Among the many nursing diagnoses that can be established as a result of ongoing assessment are the following:

- Ineffective airway clearance related to pain, weakness, postoperative decreased lung volumes, or decreased cough reflex
- Impaired gas exchange related to retained secretions, atelectasis, or pneumonia
- Alteration in nutrition, less than body requirements, related to postoperative pain, anorexia, weakness, or chemotherapy or radiation effects on the gastrointestinal tract
- Potential for infection related to surgical disruption of skin integrity, chemotherapy-induced leukopenia, retained tracheobronchial secretions, or atelectasis
- Alteration in comfort, pain related to surgical incision or tumor mass
- Anxiety related to fear of lung cancer or lack of knowledge regarding treatment procedures

Goals. The primary goals of nursing interventions are to prevent treatment-related complications and to maximize remaining lung function. Nursing interventions to achieve these overall goals are addressed in the sections dealing with surgical excision, radiation therapy, and chemotherapy.

Preoperative Interventions

In order to provide useful information for the patient, the nurse must first know what type of surgery is planned. As a rule, the surgeon will remove the smallest amount of lung tissue possible in order to preserve the maximum amount of lung function. This principle is particularly important for the patient who already has impaired lung function and cannot tolerate loss of a large amount of lung tissue.

Preoperative nursing assessment includes historical information such as smoking and occupational history, the presence of preexisting lung disease such as COPD, and other medical conditions that may complicate care. The amount of dyspnea and coughing, as well as preoperative activity tolerance, may help to predict potential postoperative pulmonary complications. There is a strong correlation between abnormal pulmonary function tests, especially forced expiratory volume in one second (FEV_1), forced vital capacity (FVC), and maximal voluntary ventilation (MVV), and postoperative complications.[14] Arterial blood-gas analysis provides baseline data that may be used for later comparison.

If the patient has preexisting lung disease that will increase the risk of surgical complications, efforts are made to optimize lung function preoperatively. The patient is instructed to stop smoking as long as possible before surgery, although the benefit of doing so may be marginal.[14] Bronchial hygiene measures (including inhaled, oral, or intravenous bronchodilators; systemic hydration; postural drainage; and chest physical therapy) may be instituted.

All patients are taught respiratory-care maneuvers that they will be expected to perform postoperatively. These include deep breathing and use of the incentive spirometer and effective cough techniques. A maximal inspiration that is held for at least 3 seconds may be the most effective method for prevention of postoperative atelectasis, and the incentive spirometer is an inexpensive and simple way to facilitate it.[14] Coughing is also important, particuarly when the patient has preexisting lung disease.[14] Staged or controlled coughing techniques may be taught, since they may cause less pain for the postoperative patient. A "huff" cough, or forceful exhalation with an open glottis, may also be taught.[6]

The patient is taught arm exercises that he will perform postoperatively to prevent a "frozen" shoulder. Simple arm exercises include arm circles and lifting the affected arm to shoulder level.[3] Passive and active leg exercises for prevention of thrombus formation and subsequent embolus are also taught.

Based on the type of surgery to be performed, the patient is prepared for the tubes and dressings he will have postoperatively. These may include chest tubes, Foley catheter, endotracheal tube, nasogastric tube, and intravenous lines (IVs). The patient should also be prepared for incisional pain and reassured that he will receive adequate pain medication.

Postoperative Interventions

Immediate postoperative concerns include maintenance of a patent airway and frequent monitoring of vital signs. Suctioning may be necessary to remove airway secretions, but it is contraindicated in the pneumonectomy patient because of the risk of traumatizing the suture line of the bronchial stump.[3] High-flow oxygen therapy may be given if not contraindicated by preoperative carbon dioxide retention. The patient is monitored closely for signs and symptoms of hypoxemia, and frequent arterial blood-gas analysis may be performed.[3]

The vital signs are checked frequently. Postoperative tachycardia due to pain, hypoxemia, hypovolemia, and acid–base imbalance is common, but other arrhythmias require prompt treatment.[3] Central venous pressure or pulmonary artery pressures may be monitored, particularly in the pneumonectomy patient. Pulmonary artery pressures will be elevated in this patient as the cardiovascular system compensates for the loss of a large amount of lung tissue. A temperature elevation immediately after surgery indicates atelectasis. Later in the postoperative course, a fever indicates infection.

Most thoracotomy patients may be positioned on either side or on their backs. However, the pneumonectomy patient cannot be positioned with the nonoperative side down. Positioning with the unoperated side down may cause a mediastinal shift to that side, or drowning if the bronchial stump suture line ruptures.[4]

With the exception of the pneumonectomy patient, thoracotomy patients will return from surgery with one or two chest tubes in place. When the chest is opened during surgery, some degree of lung collapse occurs. In order to provide drainage of fluid and escape of air from the intrapleural space, chest tubes are inserted (see Chap 27). When the tubes are functioning properly, the lung reinflates. The nurse ensures patency of the tubing and checks for kinks or dependent loops. The amount and character of drainage is noted, and any abnormalities, such as excessive drainage, are reported. "Stripping" of chest tubes should probably be avoided when possible because the procedure tends to generate large negative pressures that can injure lung tissue.[9]

Pneumonectomy patients will most likely not have chest tubes in place so that the pleural space can fill with fluid. The fluid accumulation prevents overexpansion of the remaining lung and a mediastinal shift, as well as reducing the risk of infection.[3]

Intravenous fluids are administered cautiously after thoracic surgery. Pulmonary edema may develop quickly, particularly in the pneumonectomy patient because of loss of half of the pulmonary capillary bed. A central venous pressure line or Swan–Ganz catheter may be required to accurately monitor fluid balance.[3]

Pain medication should be administered as needed in order to facilitate turning, coughing, deep breathing, and early ambulation. The patient is monitored for adequacy of analgesia and for signs of respiratory depression. Should these signs appear, the patient should be aroused by stimulation. A narcotic antagonist and emergency equipment should be readily available should the patient not respond.[3]

The most common complications that occur following any surgery are atelectasis, pneumonia, acute respiratory failure, and pulmonary embolism.[15] Following anesthesia, lung volumes are decreased, leading to collapse of alveoli and, eventually, atelectasis. In addition, airway secretions are retained because of a decrease in mucociliary transport, a diminished cough reflex, and drying of the airways by preoperative medications and anesthetic gases. The thoracotomy patient runs a particularly high risk of these complications. In order to prevent pulmonary complications, the patient is encouraged to turn frequently while in bed, and ambulation may be begun on the first postoperative day. Deep breathing and coughing techniques that were taught preoperatively are performed regularly, ideally at one-hour intervals. The incision should be splinted with a pillow during coughing maneuvers. If the patient has a preexisting lung impairment or if early atelectasis or secretion retention occurs, aggressive bronchial hygiene measures are instituted. Leg exercises are begun while the patient is still in bed, and mini-dose anticoagulation therapy may be given to prevent thrombus formation.

Other less frequent complications include hemorrhage, wound infection, and cardiac arrhythmias. A bronchopleural fistula, an air leak into the pleural space, may occur following pneumonectomy. Air may leak into the subcutaneous tissue, causing subcutaneous emphysema, or into the pleural space, causing a mediastinal shift to the unoperated side (see Chap 31).[3]

Radiation Therapy Interventions

Radiation therapy for lung cancer is often done on an outpatient basis, although it may be begun while the patient is in the hospital. If the patient is to be discharged, the hospital nurse should evaluate the need for home nursing care or for a social work referral. The patient may be referred to the American Cancer Society for assistance with transportation to his radiation treatments.

Potential complications of radiation therapy for lung cancer include pneumonitis and pulmonary fibrosis, gastrointestinal tract upset, dry mouth, and skin breakdown. Nursing interventions for dry mouth and skin breakdown are discussed above. Nursing observations to detect pneumonitis include monitoring for signs and symptoms of infection, such as cough and sputum production, fever, rhonchi or wheezing, and shortness of breath. The patient should be instructed to report any of these symptoms should they occur at home.

Nausea, vomiting, and diarrhea due to radiation therapy

may exacerbate an already poor nutritional state. Antidiarrheal and antiemetic medications may be given. Good nutrition, including binding foods, should be emphasized. A dietary consultation may be appropriate.

Chemotherapy Interventions

The specific chemotherapy to be given will be determined by the individual physician. Some of the commonly used chemotherapeutic agents for lung cancer are listed in Table 30–5.

The patient and family may be anxious or fearful about the therapy because they do not understand it. The nurse can help by providing information about the expected benefits and potential adverse effects of the drugs. Chemotherapy may prevent metastasis, shrink the primary tumor or metastases, relieve symptoms caused by the tumor(s), and improve survival.[17] However, because the drugs affect all the body cells, not just the cancer cells, other less desirable effects may occur. Most of the adverse effects result from the drug's effects on rapidly dividing cells, such as those of the bone marrow, gastrointestinal tract, and hair.

Cancer chemotherapy may cause suppression of the bone marrow, resulting in leukopenia or thrombocytopenia. The nurse observes the patient for signs and symptoms of infection, such as fever, chills, or flulike symptoms. Signs of bleeding, such as hemorrhage, hematoma, hematuria, or bleeding gums, are also monitored. The patient and family members are instructed to report these symptoms should they occur at home. The nurse also interprets results of blood tests for the family.[17]

Nausea and vomiting are common effects of chemotherapy, and the patient should be prepared for their occurrence. Antiemetic medications may be given, and good hydration is maintained. The patient is observed for signs of saline and water depletion and electrolyte imbalance.

The patient should also be prepared for alopecia, or loss of the hair. He may be reassured that the hair will grow back, but it may be a different color or texture than it was before.

Anorexia and lethargy may also occur. Nasogastric or parenteral feeding may be required in order to maintain adequate nutrition. If the patient will use parenteral feeding at home, he and the family must be instructed in self-care. A dietary consultation may be needed, and a high-calorie, high-protein diet may be prescribed.

TABLE 30–5
Chemotherapy Drugs Commonly Used to Treat Lung Cancer

Type of Cancer	*Drug*
Non–small cell carcinoma	CAMP
	Cyclophosphamide
	Doxorubicin (Adriamycin)
	Methotrexate
	Procarbazine
	FAM
	5-Fluorouracil
	Doxorubicin (Adriamycin)
	Mitomycin C
	CAP
	Cyclophosphamide
	Doxorubicin (Adriamycin)
	Cis-platinum
Small cell carcinoma	CMC
	Cyclophosphamide
	Methotrexate
	Lomustine (CCNU)
	VAP
	Vincristine
	Adriamycin
	Procarbazine

(Adapted from Van Houtle P, Salazar OM, Philips CE et al: Lung cancer. In Rubin P, Bakemeier RF, Krackov SK (eds): Clinical Oncology for Medical Students and Physicians: A Multidisciplinary Approach, 6th ed, p 236. Rochester, American Cancer Society, 1983)

Evaluation

Specific parameters to evaluate the overall goals of preventing treatment-related complications and maximizing remaining lung function must be designed individually on the basis of the patient's condition and the type of medical treatment. General examples from which to establish individual outcome criteria are listed below:

- Successful clearance of tracheobronchial secretions
- Arterial blood-gas values within normal or acceptable range for that patient
- Weight within ________ pounds (established individually)
- Absence of wound, respiratory, or other infection
- Pulmonary function test values within guidelines considered acceptable for that patient

Nursing Management: Terminal Phase

Assessment and Nursing Diagnosis

When the patient's disease becomes so advanced that medical therapy can no longer affect the prognosis, the patient enters the terminal phase of his illness. Medical therapy is now aimed at palliation of symptoms, and nursing care is of the utmost importance. The major nursing diagnoses include

- Grieving related to anticipated death
- Alteration in comfort, pain and dyspnea, related to enlarging tumor mass
- Ineffective coping by the family related to impending death

Goals. The goals of nursing care are to promote patient comfort, to facilitate passage through the dying process, to promote family acceptance, and to promote maintenance of the family unit.[2,5]

Interventions

The physical symptoms of pain and discomfort from coughing or dyspnea are evaluated continually. Pain medications are administered on a regular schedule, not as needed. Tolerance to toxic effects of narcotics will increase with tolerance to analgesia, so the dose must be increased as needed. Side-effects of narcotics, such as respiratory depression, constipation, and decreased level of consciousness, are monitored, and dosages adjusted if necessary. A bowel program can decrease the likelihood of constipation.

The patient is positioned for his own comfort. Oxygen may be administered if indicated by blood-gas analysis or, occasionally, by symptoms of dyspnea. Atropine may be given to dry upper airway secretions if they are troublesome to the patient.

The patient may express fear of his impending death and grief over separation from his loved ones. The nurse must carefully assess his readiness to accept preparation for death and facilitate his passage when he is ready. An open, accepting attitude encourages expression of feelings and fears. The nurse can facilitate the presence of family members so that the dying experience is not a lonely one. Finally, the nurse encourages the patient and family to make plans for the survivors so that the patient does not worry what will happen to a spouse or other loved one when he is gone.

See the accompanying Nursing Care Plan for the Patient with Terminal Lung Cancer.

Evaluation

Examples of successful goal achievement include the patient's ability to

- Express grief
- Share grief with family members
- Report decreased pain, dyspnea

NURSING CARE PLAN FOR THE PATIENT WITH TERMINAL LUNG CANCER

NURSING DIAGNOSIS 1: Alteration in comfort, pain, and dyspnea, related to enlarging tumor mass and metastatic spread Manifested by subjective reports of breathlessness and pain (bone, chest) and by observations of tachypnea, tachycardia, restlessness, or strained expression

GOAL 1.1: To promote comfort

Nursing Interventions	Rationale	Outcome Criteria
1. Administer analgesics, such as nonsteroidal anti-inflammatory agents and narcotics, on scheduled basis.	1. Scheduled versus prn use decreases emphasis on symptoms, may reassure patient that pain agents will be adequately controlled.	1–2. Patient reports decreased pain, and there is evidence of decrease in tachycardia, restlessness, and other possible indicators of pain.
2. If patient finds them acceptable, use nonpharmacologic measures for pain relief; measures include imagery, distraction, and progressive relaxation.	2. Nonpharmacologic measures can temporarily reduce awareness of pain.	

GOAL 1.2: To relieve dyspnea

Nursing Interventions	Rationale	Outcome Criteria
1. Reduce reversible causes of dyspnea such as heart failure, bronchospasm, infection.	1. Elimination of reversible factors may reduce dyspnea.	1–4. Patient reports decreased dyspnea and continues activities of daily living.
2. Assist patient to use energy conservation techniques.	2. Energy conservation decreases ventilatory demands.	
3. Administer prescribed oral or sublingual morphine sulfate.*	3. Morphine is believed to decrease dyspnea by reducing tachypnea.	
4. Assist patient with feeding, bathing, and other personal care.	4. Reducing work for patient reduces dyspnea.	

(Continued)

NURSING CARE PLAN FOR THE PATIENT WITH TERMINAL LUNG CANCER (*Continued*)

NURSING DIAGNOSIS 2: Ineffective airway clearance related to pain, weakness, excessive tracheobronchial secretions, lower respiratory infection, or decreased cough reflex
Manifested by increased tactile fremitus, auscultation of rhonchi, or altered sputum characteristics

GOAL 2.1: To improve secretion clearance

Nursing Interventions	Rationale	Outcome Criteria
1. Instruct patient, if he is able a. To cough effectively.	1. a. Effective cough reduces wasted energy.	1–3. Chest examination reveals decreased rhonchi and other evidence of secretions. Patient reports decreased dyspnea.
b. To increase hydration.	b. Hydration may decrease viscosity of sputum.	
c. To increase humidity of environment.	c. Increased ambient humidity may decrease sputum viscosity.	
d. In correct use of prescribed bronchodilators, antibiotics, steroids.	d. Bronchodilators open airways so that secretions can be coughed out; antibiotics treat airway infection and reduce sputum production; steroids reduce airway inflammation, thus increasing airway diameter.	
2. Relieve pain (see Nursing Diagnosis 1).	2. Pain limits ability to generate effective cough.	
3. Assist patient and family to recognize potential signs of infection.	3. Lower respiratory infection increases tracheobronchial secretion production and may further compromise clearance.	

GOAL 2.2: To reduce discomfort from copious secretions

Nursing Interventions	Rationale	Outcome Criteria
1. Instruct alert patient to suction his mouth using Yankauer device.	1. Oral suction causes less discomfort when the patient does it for himself.	1–4. Patient verbally reports decreased dyspnea or appears to be breathing easily. Family members appear less concerned by sound of tracheal secretions in dying patient.
2. Position patient to maintain open airway and prevent aspiration.	2. Aspiration may cause pneumonia and increase discomfort.	
3. Prepare family members in advance for gurgling sound of tracheal secretions (death rattle) when death is imminent.	3. Knowledge that tracheal secretions are normal and do not usually cause discomfort for a dying patient may decrease family distress.	
4. Administer prescribed atropine if patient or family is uncomfortable as a result of airway secretions.	4. Anticholinergic action dries secretions in oral pharynx.	

NURSING DIAGNOSIS 3: Impaired gas exchange related to retained secretions, atelectasis, pleural effusion, or pneumonia
Manifested by Pa_{O_2} under 60 mmHg

GOAL 3.1: To maintain adequate oxygenation of body organs

Nursing Interventions	Rationale	Outcome Criteria
1. Administer continuous oxygen by nasal cannula.	1. Increasing the FI_{O_2} may reverse hypoxemia and decrease tissue hypoxia.	1–2. Pa_{O_2} of greater than 60 mmHg (or hemoglobin saturation greater than 90%)
2. Eliminate reversible causes of hypoxemia, such as lower respiratory infection, pleural effusion.	2. Reversible factors may further limit already compromised lung function.	

(*Continued*)

NURSING CARE PLAN FOR THE PATIENT WITH TERMINAL LUNG CANCER (*Continued*)

NURSING DIAGNOSIS 4: Alteration in nutrition, less than body requirements, related to pain, anorexia, weakness, or to effects of chemotherapy and radiation
Manifested by progressive weight loss, decreased serum albumin level, abnormal skin fold measurements

GOAL 4.1: To reduce rate of weight loss

Nursing Interventions	Rationale	Outcome Criteria
1. Instruct patient a. To eat small, frequent meals.	1. a. Small meals cause less stomach distention and are better tolerated by anorexic patients.	1–3. Patient maintains weight or reduces rate of loss.
b. To take high protein, high calorie supplements.	b. Liquid supplements contain high calories in small volume.	
c. To avoid gas-producing foods.	c. Avoiding bloating foods leaves more room to ingest nutrients.	
2. Refer patient to outside assistance, such as Meals on Wheels.	2. Convenience foods reduce energy expenditure for meal preparation and may make patient more likely to eat.	
3. Explain to family that loss of appetite is a normal consequence of terminal illness.	3. Knowledge that anorexia is normal when death is imminent may help family tolerate patient's reduced food intake.	

NURSING DIAGNOSIS 5: Grieving related to multiple role changes, loss of personal control, or anticipated death
Manifested by sorrow, denial, anger, or depression

GOAL 5.1: To promote quality of life for patient

Nursing Interventions	Rationale	Outcome Criteria
1. Foster expression of feelings by patient and family.	1. Providing open atmosphere encourages expression of feelings.	1–7. Patient and family express feelings of grief. Patient and family verbalize wishes related to life closure.
2. Facilitate patient's attempts to make decisions and retain all possible control over life.	2. Maintenance of personal choice reduces feelings of frustration and helplessness.	
3. Assist patient and family to identify and complete unfinished business.	3. Resolution of unfinished agenda may help patient and family to be ready for death.	
4. Assist patient and family to formulate a plan for life closure that is compatible with their value systems.	4. Patient and family should be helped to express their wishes and meet their needs as they identify them.	
5. Include family in plan of care for patient.	5. Family members feel less helpless when they can participate in care.	
6. Prepare family members for feelings and experiences they may have after patient dies.	6. Knowing feelings are normal promotes acceptance of grieving process.	
7. Identify resources for family to use during bereavement period.	7. Outside resources may help family in resolution of grief.	

Twycross RG, Lack SA: Therapeutics in Advanced Cancer, pp 180–181. London, Pitman Publishing Limited, 1984

(Appreciation is expressed to Johanna Surla, RN, MN, Clinical Supervisor, Transition Services, Visiting Nurse Services, for her assistance with this care plan.)

References

1. Bordow RA: Lung cancer: Classification, pathology, and epidemiology. In Bordow RA, Stool EW, Moser KM (eds): Manual of Clinical Problems in Pulmonary Medicine, 1st ed. Boston, Little, Brown & Co, 1980
2. Boyer MW: Treating invasive lung cancer. Am J Nurs 77:1916, 1977
3. Burkhart C: After pneumonectomy. Am J Nurs 83:1562, 1983
4. Cameron MI: What patients need most before and after thoracotomy. Nursing 8:28, 1978
5. Chaffin P, Reininger S: Bronchogenic carcinoma: A review and study. Nurse Pract 6:14, 1981
6. Cimprich B, Gaydos D, Largan R: A preoperative teaching program for the thoracotomy patient. Cancer Nurs 1:35, 1978
7. Cooper JS, Pizzarello DJ: Concepts in Cancer Care, 1st ed. Philadelphia, Lea & Febiger, 1980
8. DeSanto LW: The options in early laryngeal carcinoma. N Engl J Med 306:910, 1982
9. Duncan C, Erickson R: Pressures associated with chest tube stripping. Heart Lung 11:166, 1982
10. Larsen GL: Rehabilitation for the patient with head and neck cancer. Am J Nurs 82:119, 1982
11. Million RR, Cassisi NJ, Wittes RE: Cancer in the head and neck. In DeVita VT, Hellman S, Rosenberg SA (eds): Cancer: Principles and Practice of Oncology, 1st ed. Philadelphia, JB Lippincott, 1982
12. Minna JD, Higgins GA, Glatstein EJ: Cancer of the lung. In DeVita VT, Hellman S, Rosenberg SA (eds): Cancer: Principles and Practice of Oncology, 1st ed. Philadelphia, JB Lippincott, 1982
13. Ogura JH, Thawley SE: Cysts and tumors of the larynx. In Paparella MM, Shumrick DA: Otolaryngology, vol 3, 2nd ed. Philadelphia, WB Saunders, 1980
14. Risser NL: Preoperative and postoperative care to prevent pulmonary complications. Heart Lung 9:57, 1980
15. Saunders WH, Havener WH, Keith CF et al: Nursing Care in Eye, Ear, Nose, and Throat Disorders, 4th ed. St Louis, CV Mosby, 1979
16. Shumrick DA: Neck dissection. In Paparella MM, Shumrick DA: Otolaryngology, vol 3, 2nd ed. Philadelphia, WB Saunders, 1980
17. Sovik C: The nursing care of lung cancer patients: Emphasizing chemotherapy. Nurs Clin North Am 13:301, 1978
18. Van Houtle P, Salazar OM, Phillips C et al: Lung cancer. In Rubin P, Bakemeier RF, Krackov SK (eds): Clinical Oncology for Medical Students and Physicians: A Multidisciplinary Approach, 6th ed. Rochester, American Cancer Society, 1983
19. Zagars G, Norante JD: Head and neck tumors. In Rubin P, Bakemeier RF, Krackov SK (eds): Clinical Onocology for Medical Students and Physicians: A Multidisciplinary Approach, 6th ed. Rochester, American Cancer Society, 1983

Bibliography

Ahana DN, Kunishi MM: Cancer Care Protocols for Hospital and Home Care Use, 1st ed. New York, Springer, 1981

Auerback O: Natural history of carcinoma of the lung. In Fishman AP (ed): Pulmonary Diseases and Disorders, vol 2, 1st ed. p 1388. New York, McGraw–Hill, 1980

Carr DT, Mountain CF: Staging of lung cancer. Semin Respir Med 3:154–163, 1982

Cook S: Bronchogenic carcinoma: Pre-op and post-op care. RN 41:83, 1978

Early lung cancer detection: Summary and conclusions. Am Rev Respir Dis 130:565, 1984

Gardner WH: Problems of laryngectomees. Rehab Rec 2:15, 1961

Hande KR, Des Prez RM: Current perspectives in small cell lung cancer. Chest 85:669, 1984

Jett JR, Cortese DA, Fontana RS: Lung cancer: Current concepts and prospects. CA, A Cancer Journal for Clinicians 33:74, 1983

McConnell EA: How to truly help the patient with a radical neck dissection. Nursing 6:58, 1976

Matthews MJ: Morphologic aspects of malignant tumors of the lung. In Fishman AP (ed): Pulmonary Diseases and Disorders, vol 2, 1st ed. New York, McGraw–Hill, 1980

Nauman HH: Surgery of malignant tumors of the larynx. In Nauman HH (ed): Head and Neck Surgery, Vol 4, Neck. Philadelphia, WB Saunders, 1984

Ogura JH, Thawley SE: Surgery of the larynx. In Paparella MM, Shumrick DA: Otolaryngology, vol 3, 2nd ed. Philadelphia, WB Saunders, 1980

Searcy L: Nursing care of the laryngectomy patient. RN 35:35, 1972

Selawry OS, Hansen HH: Lung cancer. In Holland JF, Frei E (eds): Cancer Medicine, 2nd ed. Philadelphia, Lea & Febiger, 1982

Shedd DP: Cancer of the head and neck. In Holland JF, Frei E (eds): Cancer Medicine, 2nd ed. Philadelphia, Lea & Febiger, 1982

Sturgis KB: Clinical picture of lung cancer. In Fishman AP (ed): Pulmonary Diseases and Disorders, vol 2, 1st ed. New York, McGraw–Hill, 1980

Thomas BJ: Coping with the devastation of head and neck cancer. RN 37:10, 1974

Chapter 31

Traumatic Conditions Affecting Respiratory Function

Joanne Schnaidt Rokosky
Kathryn L. Anderson

Trauma to the respiratory system can involve structures of either the upper or lower respiratory tract. Injuries to the midportion of the face or to the structures of the upper respiratory tract directly (nasal cavity, pharynx, larynx) can compromise airway patency and result in airway obstruction. Maxillofacial and nasal injuries are covered in the first portion of this chapter. Laryngeal trauma is discussed along with tracheobronchial injuries later in this chapter.

Lower respiratory tract injuries are more commonly referred to as chest trauma and may involve injury to virtually all structures and organs in the thorax: bone, lung, heart, great and other blood vessels, trachea, esophagus, spinal cord, and diaphragm. Nursing care of the patient with spinal cord injury and myocardial injury is discussed in Chapter 69 and Chapter 104, respectively. The other injuries listed above are covered in the second portion of this chapter.

Upper Respiratory Tract Injuries

Epistaxis

Epistaxis, or nosebleed, is a frightening but rarely life threatening result of injury to the rich network of nasal vessels or their thin mucosal covering. The type of trauma that can induce epistaxis varies from direct and severe injury, such as might occur with a fist fight, to less obvious forms of trauma such as excessive nose blowing, infection, or exposure to harsh winds. Epistaxis can also be a manifestation of underlying disease, such as platelet or coagulation disorders. In addition to having nasal bleeding, patients with epistaxis may cough and spit up blood that has drained into the throat.

Medical Management

The initial diagnosis of epistaxis is generally obvious, although the extent of blood loss may not be apparent if the patient is swallowing blood. Following emergency management to arrest the bleeding, a careful history and physical examination are important to establish the underlying cause.

For treatment, epistaxis is often categorized as anterior, ethmoidal, or posterior hemorrhage. Anterior hemorrhages, which arise from a junction of vessels at the anterior nasal septum, are controlled by applying pressure, clearing blood

Appreciation is given to Mary Farley, RN, MN, for her critical review of the content in this chapter.

and clots from the nasal passages, then cauterizing the bleeding agent with an electrical device or with a chemical such as silver nitrate. An ethmoidal hemorrhage is a sudden, massive bleed of the ethmoidal arteries; surgical ligation may be required for control. Posterior hemorrhages originate from the artery supplying the lateral nose and posterior septum. The hemorrhage may be stopped by use of tight nasal packing (Fig. 31–1), a Foley catheter, or a special balloon to compress bleeding points. If packing or balloons fail to arrest the bleeding, surgery may be required to ligate the bleeding vessel.[9,11,16]

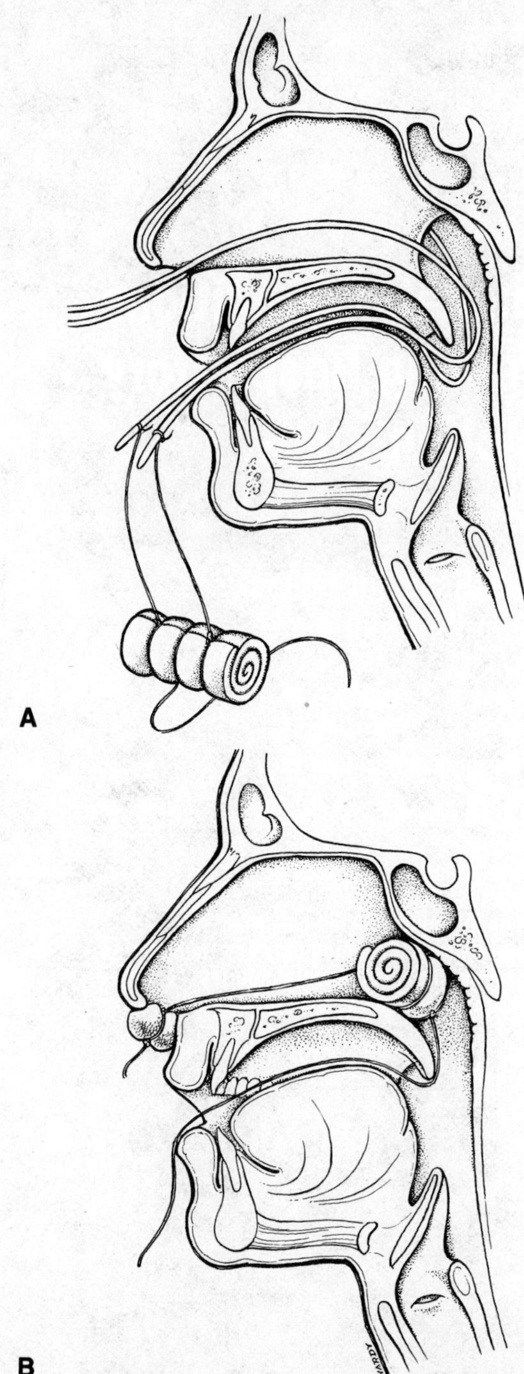

FIGURE 31–1 Placing of the posterior nasal pack. (*A*) The catheters are brought out through the mouth and tied with the lateral sutures on the pack; then the catheters are withdrawn through the nose. These sutures are then tied over a small piece of sponge at the columella. (*B*) The middle suture is brought out through the mouth and taped to the cheek.

Nursing Management

Assessment and Nursing Diagnosis

The nurse in an acute care setting is most likely to encounter patients with severe, sustained epistaxis. In this situation, careful assessment is necessary to ensure airway patency and avoid complications of nasal packing. In addition, patients often require instructions for first-aid management of repeat episodes. Possible nursing diagnoses are as follows:

- Ineffective airway clearance related to accumulated bloody drainage
- Alteration in comfort related to nasal and sinus obstruction caused by nasal packing or balloons
- Knowledge deficit related to first-aid management or recognition of complications
- Anxiety related to the bleeding episode

Interventions

The goals of nursing interventions are to minimize discomfort and prevent complications.

Because patients with severe epistaxis are usually frightened, it is important for the nurse to try to allay fears. Some people may be concerned that the bleeding means impending stroke. The patient should be kept in a Fowler's position and assisted to lean forward and expectorate blood. There is a risk that accumulated blood in the throat may be aspirated and, when swallowed, may cause nausea and vomiting. The presence of packing or a balloon in the nose is extremely uncomfortable because it obstructs nasal, sinus, and lacrimal drainage. If eating is difficult, a liquid diet may be preferable to solid foods. Mouth care should be performed frequently.

Patients need careful observation for complications such as local or generalized infection, otitis media, sinusitis, and aspiration. If a nasal balloon is used, the nurse should be aware that it may cause necrosis of the tip of the nose. The balloon pressure is usually released temporarily every 20 minutes, and nasal tissues must be observed for evidence of pressure necrosis. Placement of the balloon must also be carefully monitored; airway obstruction is possible should it become dislodged. Patients with packing or balloons are vulnerable to hypoxemia and are generally given supplemental oxygen. Arterial blood gases should be checked in elderly patients or patients with underlying cardiovascular or respiratory disease.

Before discharge, patients should be taught to avoid factors that may predispose to recurrence. For example, they should not pick the nose or blow it hard. If dry air is a predisposing factor, the patient may benefit from increased humidity in the home. The patient should be taught to stop a nose bleed by pinching the nostrils together and leaning forward so that blood does not drain into the throat.[9,16]

Evaluation

When nursing goals related to management of epistaxis have been achieved, the patient will

- Maintain a patent airway
- Be free of infection and other complications
- Report reduced discomfort
- Demonstrate correct techniques for blowing the nose and for arresting nasal bleeding
- Describe measures to prevent recurrence

Nasal and Maxillofacial Fractures

Nasal fractures may be isolated injuries or may be associated with other facial fractures. Characteristic manifestations include epistaxis, pain, swelling, and hematoma of the nose and lower eyelids. The nasal septum may be deviated or shattered.

Maxillofacial fractures usually result from motor vehicle accidents or from direct trauma to the face. Because significant force is required to produce a maxillary fracture, these fractures are categorized as severe trauma. Maxillary fractures are grouped into three categories, according to increasing severity—LeFort I, II, and III. These categories are illustrated in Figure 31–2.

- A LeFort I fracture is a low, transverse fracture involving the floor of the nose and the lower maxilla.
- A LeFort II fracture involves the middle portion of the maxilla and the floor of the orbit. This fracture is the most common of the three.
- A LeFort III fracture involves a high maxillary fracture in association with extensive damage to adjacent bones, with the result that the facial bones are separated from the skull. This, the most serious of maxillofacial fractures, is also referred to as craniofacial dysjunction.[7]

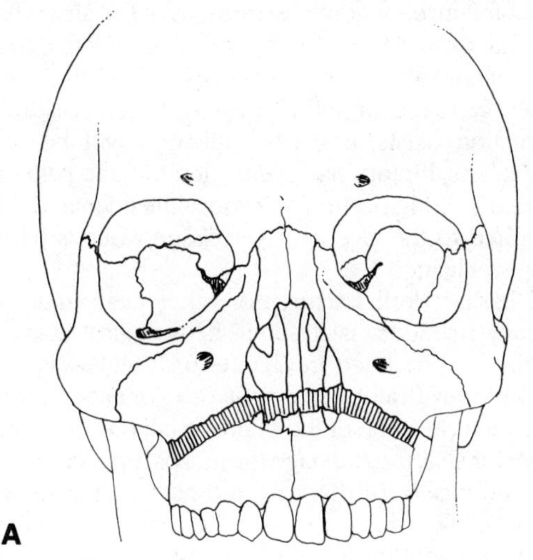

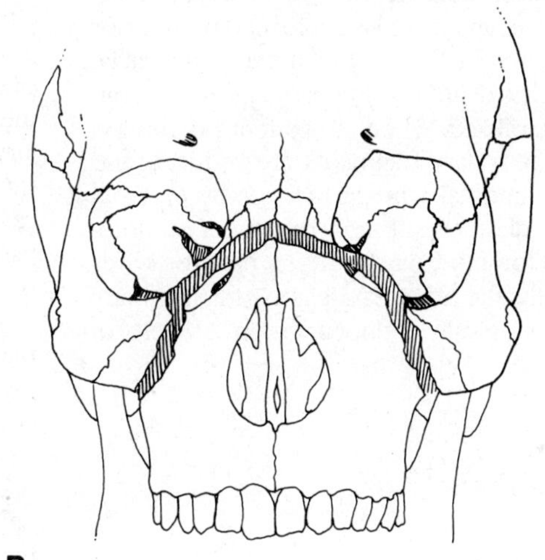

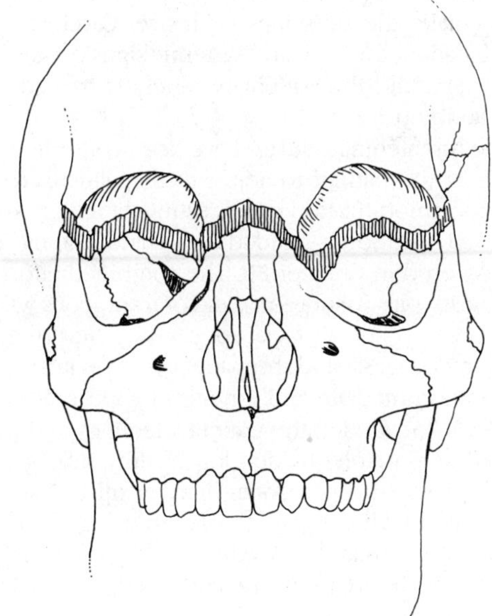

FIGURE 31–2 LeFort classification of midfacial fractures. (*A*) A LeFort I fracture is low, transverse, and involves the floor of the nose and the lower maxilla. (*B*) A LeFort II fracture involves the middle portion of the maxilla and the floor of the orbit. (*C*) A LeFort III fracture is a serious injury of the upper maxilla in which the facial bones are separated from the skull. (Grossman JA: Minor Injuries and Disorders: Surgical and Medical Care, p 229. Philadelphia, JB Lippincott, 1984)

All these fractures are frequently accompanied by extensive soft tissue trauma.

When a frontal injury to the face occurs, the facial bones absorb some of the impact that would otherwise be directed at the brain. Although the facial injury is, in a sense, protective of deeper structures, simultaneous injuries are common, especially to the spinal cord.[5]

Patients with maxillofacial fractures may have severe pain. Other common signs include epistaxis, jaw malocclusion, mobility of the facial bones, conjunctival hemorrhages, and bruising of the soft palate.[11,20]

Medical Management

An uncomplicated nasal fracture can generally be diagnosed on the basis of history and clinical findings. Within the first few hours of injury, simple, nonoperative reduction is usually possible. If several hours elapse before the patient is seen or if the injury is extensive, surgical correction is required. This treatment is delayed for several days until swelling subsides.

The diagnosis of maxillofacial fracture is suspected on the basis of clinical presentation and is confirmed by anterior lateral facial films.[7] Often, definitive treatment of the facial fractures must be delayed until accompanying, life threatening injuries have stabilized. When the patient's condition permits surgery, the maxillary fragments are reduced and then immobilized by internal wire fixation or by external traction with a halo or plaster head cap. The patient is immobilized in this fashion for 4 to 6 weeks, after which the wires are removed. Generally, the prognosis is good for maxillary fractures that can be surgically reduced within 2 weeks of injury.[1]

Nursing Management

Assessment and Nursing Diagnosis

Prevention of airway obstruction must be the initial priority with any facial injury. With maxillofacial injuries, both the fractures and the soft tissue swelling contribute to a high risk of airway obstruction. In addition, maxillofacial fractures are often accompanied by other life threatening problems such as spinal cord injury.

Nursing Diagnoses. Among the possible nursing diagnoses for patients with facial fractures are the following:

- Potential airway obstruction related to fracture deformity and soft tissue swelling
- Body image disturbance related to altered facial appearance
- Alteration in nutrition, less than body requirements, related to facial immobilization
- Potential for infection related to extensive soft tissue injury or to cerebrospinal fluid (CSF) leakage when associated with basilar skull fracture
- Alteration in comfort, pain, related to fracture of facial bones and swelling of adjacent soft tissues

Goals. The immediate goal of all nursing interventions is to detect, or ideally prevent, life threatening complications. Later goals are to maximize healing and minimize discomfort.

Interventions

Nasal Fracture. Although airway obstruction is an infrequent complication of simple nasal fracture, the nurse must be alert to this possibility when caring for a patient with a broken nose. Prior to reduction of the nasal fracture, the patient is kept in a sitting position and ice packs are applied to reduce swelling. The patient should be encouraged to expectorate, rather than swallow, any blood. Before discharge, the patient should be taught about complications to report, such as hematoma of the nasal septum. He should be aware that he will be able to breathe through his nose after the swelling subsides, but that loss of smell (anosmia), sinusitis, and atrophic rhinitis may be long-term complications.

Maxillofacial Fracture. When caring for a patient with a maxillofacial fracture, ongoing assessment of the airway is essential. Airway obstruction could result from edema, the presence of clots or other foreign material, or the displacement of bones, cartilage, or soft tissues. When high risk for airway obstruction exists, tracheal intubation will be required. If spinal cord injury has been ruled out, the patient can be placed in a sitting position to reduce the edema. Cold packs are applied to the face after soft tissue wounds have been thoroughly cleaned.

Because basilar skull fractures or other head injuries may accompany maxillofacial trauma, neurological assessment is required, as outlined in Chapter 63. CSF leakage is common, and bloody drainage from the nose or ears should be analyzed by letting some of the drainage fall onto a gauze pad. If positive for CSF, the drainage forms a pale pink ring or halo around the blood. In this case the patient should be instructed not to blow his nose, and the draining orifices should be covered lightly with sterile dressings. It is important not to obstruct the flow of drainage, and care must be taken not to make the dressings occlusive. Careful examination of the patient for local and systemic signs of infection is also important, and the patient is generally treated with intravenous antibiotics.

Once life threatening injuries have been controlled, the nurse can assist the patient to adjust to the difficult repair process. Facial immobilization makes eating difficult at a time when increased nutrition is needed for wound healing. This problem is covered in Chapter 80. The combined efforts of otolaryngologists, plastic surgeons, and oral surgeons will do much to restore the patient's facial appearance. Nevertheless, this is a lengthy process, and the patient may be justly worried about both immediate and long-term appearance. The nurse should acknowledge the patient's feelings and assist him, as much as possible, to develop healthy strategies to cope with his changed appearance. High maxillary fractures may be associated with diplopia.[20] Safety measures, such as the use of a walker, may be needed. If the patient is discharged before these problems are corrected, he should be advised not to drive a car. If the patient has halo traction, pin sites are inspected and cleaned as for other types of skeletal traction. Once the immobilizing devices are removed, the patient should be encouraged to exercise his jaw. Chewing gum is a good method.[1]

Nurses can play a role in prevention of facial injuries by urging persons to wear the shoulder harness when riding in an automobile or to wear a helmet when riding a motorcycle. Naturally, nurses should heed their own advice.

Evaluation

When goals related to management of facial fractures have been achieved, the patient will

- Maintain a patent airway
- Be free of infection or other complications
- Report reduced discomfort
- Describe medical follow-up and self-care measures needed for successful recovery

Chest Trauma

Approximately 25% of all traumatic deaths in the United States are directly attributable to chest injuries, and such injuries contribute significantly to mortality in another 25% to 50% of trauma victims.[8] Chest trauma is classified into two categories: blunt and penetrating trauma. Blunt trauma is usually the result of deceleration or compression due to a motor vehicle accident or fall. Penetrating injuries occur most commonly as the result of gunshots and stabbings, although other projectiles may occasionally cause penetrating wounds.

Chest Wall Injuries

Etiology and Pathophysiology

Injuries to the chest wall include injuries of the soft tissue, bone fractures, and subcutaneous emphysema. Because it is the fractures that are associated with respiratory disturbance, they are the focus of this section.

Rib, sternal, and clavicular fractures are the result of blunt chest trauma. Fractures of the first and second ribs are caused by very severe trauma and are indicative of potentially serious injury to the heart, aorta, tracheobronchial tree, lungs, or brachial plexus. Similarly, clavicular fractures may cause multiple injuries to the brachial plexus, subclavian vessels, or other structures.

Fractures of two or more adjacent ribs or the sternum may cause a condition known as *flail chest.* Such fractures create an area of instability in the chest wall, which is characterized by paradoxical chest movement; that is, the unstable or flail segment moves inward during inspiration and outward during expiration (Fig. 31–3). Respiratory insufficiency associated with flail chest is due primarily to underlying pulmonary contusion, in addition to the impaired ventilatory mechanics resulting from the flail.[10] Fracture of the sternum may be associated with severe intrathoracic injuries, particularly myocardial contusion, and may also cause a flail chest.

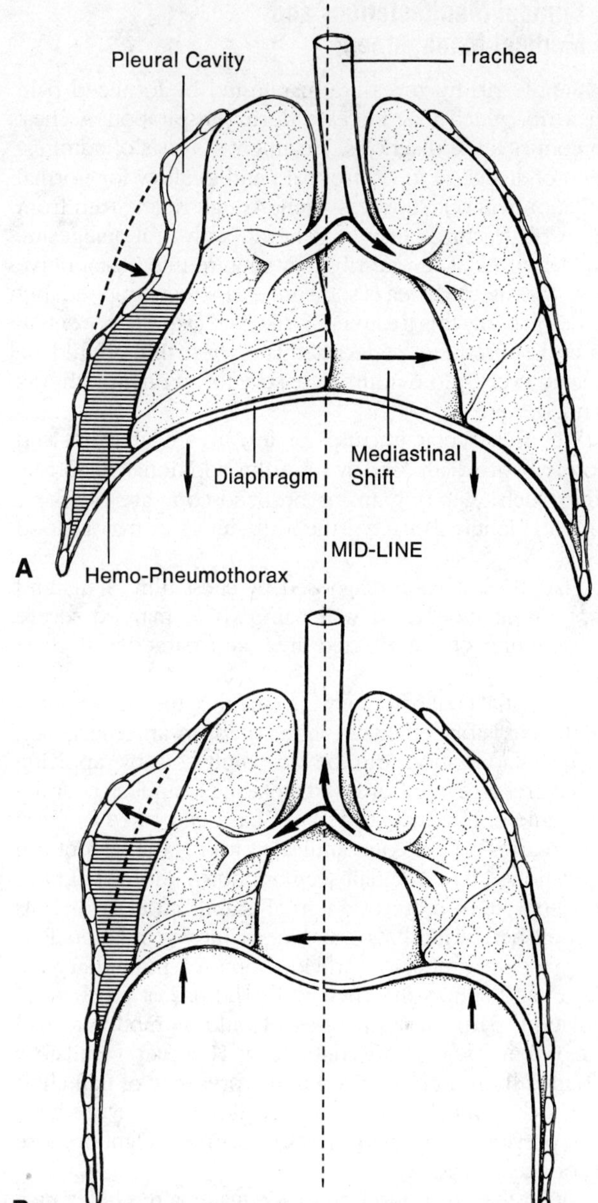

FIGURE 31–3 Respiration in a flail chest. (*A*) Flail area of right chest wall, which moves in with inspiration. Air moves into the left (normal) lung from the right bronchial tree as well as by normal tracheal inflow. Ventilation of the right lung is compromised. The mediastinum shifts to the uninjured side. (*B*) On expiration, air is driven out through the trachea and into the right (injured) side. This movement of air from one lung to the other is known as "pendulum movement." Movement of the flail segments extends the area of lung contusion. In addition, if the mediastinal shift is great enough, the pendulum movement can cause significant deoxygenation. Hemopneumothorax further compromises oxygen exchange.

Clinical Manifestations and Medical Management

Simple rib fractures are manifested by localized pain over a rib, which may increase during inspiration. A chest film confirms the diagnosis. Treatment consists of administration of analgesia to control pain and to allow for normal ventilation without suppressing the cough reflex. Pain from simple rib fractures may be relieved with oral analgesics, while fractures of several ribs may require intercostal nerve block. The affected area is sometimes taped or strapped, but in older patients this treatment is likely to cause hypoventilation and subsequent atelectasis. The chest film should be repeated every 4 to 6 hours to ensure that a pneumothorax has not developed.

When clavicular fractures or fractures of the first and second ribs are diagnosed by x-ray film, additional diagnostic studies such as aortogram or bronchoscopy are often required to identify damage to the heart, lungs, or major blood vessels.

Flail chest can be diagnosed by chest film. Signs and symptoms include chest wall pain, which may be severe with splinting of the affected area, and paradoxical chest movement.

The initial goal of therapy is to stabilize the flail segment so that ventilatory efficiency is restored. In an emergency, external stabilization can be accomplished by applying manual pressure to the area or by placing a sandbag over the flail segment. If spinal cord injury has been ruled out and other injuries do not contraindicate turning, the patient can be positioned with the flail segment down. More definitive treatment often requires internal stabilization, which is accomplished by intubation and mechanical ventilation. Positive pressure ventilation provides optimal pulmonary expansion and splints the chest wall. The use of mechanical ventilation, particularly in cases of mild to moderate flail chest, is a matter of some controversy. However, ventilatory assistance should be provided in the presence of flail chest plus shock, three or more associated injuries, severe head injury, previous pulmonary disease, fracture of eight or more ribs, or age over 68 years.[22]

Other therapy is directed to adequate pain relief, which may require administration of intercostal nerve blocks. Chest physical therapy, including coughing and deep breathing in the nonintubated patient, is often indicated for treatment of the underlying pulmonary contusion. Other treatment for pulmonary contusion is described below.

The diagnosis of fractured sternum is established by chest film. Severe pain, splinting, and paradoxical chest motion will be present. Medical management includes analgesia, treatment of other injuries, and mechanical ventilation if required for stabilization and adequate ventilation.

Nursing Management

Assessment and Nursing Diagnosis

The severity of chest wall injuries ranges from uncomplicated rib fractures to multiple bone fractures associated with life threatening lacerations of the heart and blood vessels. Nonetheless, the first priority is always to assess the adequacy of ventilation, gas exchange, and circulating blood volume. Based on this assessment a variety of nursing diagnoses are possible. Some of these diagnoses may involve independent interventions by the nurse, and others may demand the urgent collaborative efforts of the physician and other members of the health care team.

Examples of nursing diagnoses are as follows:

- Impaired gas exchange related to pulmonary contusion and disturbed ventilatory mechanics
- Decreased cardiac output related to injuries of the heart and major blood vessels
- Alteration in comfort, pain, related to rib fractures and soft tissue injury

Goals. The overall goal of nursing interventions is to ensure adequate tissue oxygenation. Related goals are to maintain cardiac output and relieve discomfort.

Interventions

Nursing interventions vary according to the severity of injury to the chest wall and the extent to which underlying structures are involved. Lung injuries are discussed in a later section of this chapter, while injuries to the heart and major blood vessels are discussed in Chapter 104.

Simple Rib Fracture. Pain is the major problem associated with simple rib fractures. To compensate for the severe pain associated with moving or breathing, the patient tends to develop a shallow breathing pattern and avoids taking deep or sigh breaths.[14] The purpose of pain relief is to interrupt this pattern of shallow breathing, which can result in the development of atelectasis, pneumonia, and hypoxemia. Elderly patients or those with chronic cardiorespiratory disease are usually hospitalized until it is certain that their condition is stable. Prior to discharge, patients should understand the need for continued mobility and frequent deep breathing. They should be instructed to report signs of atelectasis or pneumonia such as fever, productive cough, or increased dyspnea.[20]

Flail Chest. Patients with flail chest are at high risk of developing hypoxemia with or without hypercapnia. The impairment in gas exchange may not be present originally but may develop later as a result of fatigue and pain.[14] Interventions, including mechanical ventilation, for the nursing diagnosis of impaired gas exchange are described in detail in Chapter 27. Currently, intermittent mechanical ventilation (IMV) is the recommended mode of ventilation. With this ventilator setting, patients are able to breathe spontaneously in addition to receiving mechanically delivered breaths and are often better able to tolerate mechanical ventilation. Positive end-expiratory pressure (PEEP), which maintains positive pressure in the lungs throughout the entire respiratory cycle, is used to increase the resting lung volume, prevent alveolar collapse, and improve arterial oxygenation.

Whether or not they are mechanically ventilated, pain relief is an important component of care for patients with flail chest. Severe pain, accompanied by tachycardia and tachypnea, increases tissue oxygen demands and increases the risk of hypoxia in vital organs.

Evaluation

When nursing goals have been achieved, the patient will have the following:

- Adequate circulating blood volume to vital organs, as evidenced by systolic blood pressure over 80 mmHg, urine output over 25 ml/hour
- Adequate ventilation and gas exchange, as evidenced by arterial blood gases within normal limits:
  - pH 7.35–7.45
  - Pa_{O_2} of 95 mmHg–100 mmHg for young adults, 75 mmHg–80 mmHg for elderly adults, 60 mmHg for patients with chronic obstructive pulmonary disease (COPD)
- Increased comfort, as evidenced by ability to tolerate turning and other respiratory care maneuvers

Lung Injuries

Pulmonary Contusion and Laceration

In pulmonary contusion, deceleration injury secondary to blunt trauma or shock-wave effects from high-velocity missiles (*i.e.,* bullets) cause the formation of interstitial edema and intra-alveolar hemorrhage. Failure to adequately ventilate the affected area causes increased shunt and hypoxemia. Pulmonary contusion is suspected whenever flail chest is present, although it is not always associated with rib fractures. Other signs and symptoms include respiratory distress, abrasions or ecchymoses over the affected area, and bloody bronchial secretions with cough or suctioning. The chest film may be normal or show patchy infiltrates initially, but within hours may show consolidation. The onset of hypoxemia may be delayed but develops as edema increases in the area of contusion.

In contrast to pulmonary contusion, pulmonary laceration usually occurs with penetrating chest trauma. Occasionally, a fractured rib due to blunt trauma causes this injury.

When an injury is at or below the nipple line, rupture of the diaphragm should be suspected. In addition to interfering with normal chest excursion, this injury may allow the herniation of bowel contents into the chest cavity.[3]

Medical Management

The goal of therapy for pulmonary contusion is to support the patient while the edema resolves. How to achieve this goal is a matter of some debate. Aggressive therapy utilizes mechanical ventilation to stabilize the chest wall and maintain adequate ventilation and oxygenation. IMV with PEEP is the treatment of choice.

More conservative therapy utilizes mechanical ventilation only when the Pa_{O_2} cannot be maintained at or above 60 mmHg with supplemental oxygen supplied by mask or cannula. Since some studies indicate that pulmonary contusion is increased by overhydration, fluid is restricted to 50 ml/hour if not contraindicated by hypovolemia.[19] In the past, some clinicians preferred colloid fluids to crystalloid for fluid resuscitation because it was thought that excessive crystalloid infusion resulted in a decrease in colloid osmotic pressure (COP) with subsequent extravasation into alveoli and interstitium. However, recent evidence suggests that COP is not a significant posttraumatic factor in lung edema. Rather, increased capillary hydrostatic pressure and arterial capillary permeability due to the lung contusion itself, or to sepsis, appear to be the determining factors.[18]

Other therapeutic measures for pulmonary contusion include vigorous pulmonary toilet, supplemental oxygen therapy, and pain control with intercostal blocks and narcotics. The use of corticosteroids is controversial.[6] Diuretics may be used to treat fluid overload.

Fifty percent to 70% of persons with pulmonary contusion will develop pneumonia, while 35% will develop pulmonary abscess, empyema, or both. Other complications include chronic pulmonary insufficiency and pneumothorax.[8]

Most pulmonary lacerations require only chest tube drainage for an accompanying hemothorax or pneumothorax (see below). Only about 4% of lacerations are associated with massive hemorrhage, requiring thoracotomy for removal of a lung segment, lobe, or entire lung. In contrast, surgical repair of diaphragmatic rupture is generally required.[8]

Nursing Management

Assessment and Nursing Diagnosis

Pulmonary contusion can be associated with other injuries such as flail chest or it can exist independently. Regardless, the major threat is that the lung damage will be sufficient to impair gas exchange. Among possible nursing diagnoses are the following:

- Impaired gas exchange related to traumatic hemorrhage and edema of the lung parenchyma
- Alteration in comfort, pain, related to soft tissue injury

Interventions

The major goals of nursing interventions are to ensure adequate tissue oxygenation, maintain gas exchange, and relieve discomfort. Ongoing assessment of gas exchange and overall tissue perfusion is achieved by frequent arterial blood gas and vital-sign measurement and by clinical assessment for evidence of hypoxemia, hypercarbia, and shock.

A patient with lung contusion also requires considerable supportive care. Pain relief must be sufficient to allow deep breathing and cooperation with chest physical therapy. When there is evidence of retained secretions, the patient should be helped to cough more effectively. Because damaged lung tissue is highly susceptible to infection, the appearance of any sputum that is produced should be checked carefully. Purulent sputum should be cultured as a basis for antibiotic prescription. Supplemental oxygen may be provided by mask or in conjunction with mechanical ventilation. Unless contraindicated by other associated injuries, the patient should be turned frequently. The effect of any position change on the Pa_{O_2} values should be monitored. It can be expected that oxygenation will be optimal when the patient is positioned with the healthy lung down.

Evaluation

Nursing goals have been achieved when gas exchange is maintained and when the patient is comfortable. Specific outcomes include the following:

- Arterial blood-gas values within acceptable limits
- Patient verbalizes that he is more comfortable and demonstrates ability to cooperate with turning, coughing, and other procedures

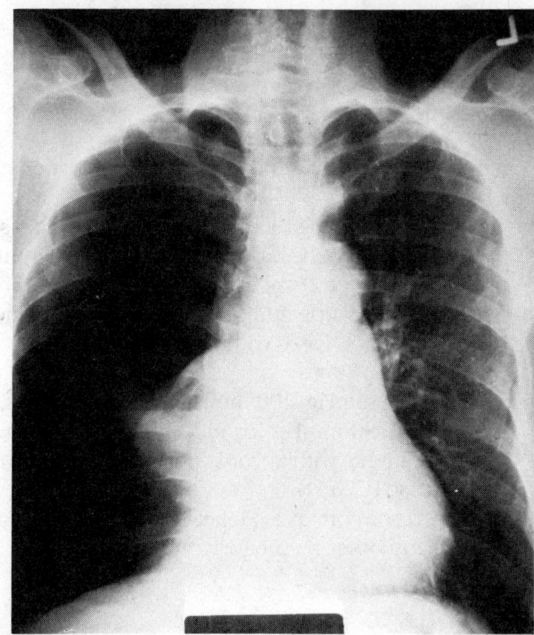

FIGURE 31–4 Pneumothorax with some tension on the right as demonstrated by tracheal shift to the left. (Wolcott MW: Ambulatory Surgery and the Basics of Emergency Surgical Care, p 280. Philadelphia, JB Lippincott, 1981)

Pleural Injuries: Pneumothorax and Hemothorax

Etiology and Pathophysiology

Accumulation of air in the pleural space, or pneumothorax, usually occurs following chest wall laceration, gunshot wounds, fractured ribs, alveolar disruption, bronchial disruption, or esophageal injury.[4] A pneumothorax may be open or closed, and either type may lead to a tension pneumothorax (Fig. 31–4).

An open pneumothorax or sucking chest wound allows atmospheric air to enter the pleural space during inspiration. Equilibration of atmospheric and intrapleural pressures occurs rapidly, with resulting ipsilateral lung collapse, shift of the mediastinum to the contralateral side, and incomplete expansion of the contralateral lung. Increased intrathoracic pressure on both sides of the chest impairs venous return.

A closed pneumothorax may occur following blunt trauma, when the pleura has been punctured by fractured ribs or when alveolar, bronchial, or esophageal injuries cause leakage of air into the pleural space. If air continues to enter the pleural space, the same pathophysiological events will occur as in open pneumothorax; that is, collapse of the lung, mediastinal shift, impingement on ventilation of the opposite lung, and decreased venous return.

Tension pneumothorax represents the progresson of either of the above conditions to the point that the cardiopulmonary embarrassment becomes life threatening. The open chest wound may act as a one-way valve, allowing air to enter the pleural space on inspiration, but closing to prevent escape of air on expiration. Similarly, air leaks from within the chest may occur in only one direction, causing an increasing pneumothorax. In either case, pressure within the chest builds until decreased venous return causes a fall in cardiac output, and ventilation is severely impaired. If not treated immediately, tension pneumothorax can be rapidly fatal.

Like pneumothorax, hemothorax, or blood in the pleural space, may occur as a result of blunt or penetrating chest trauma. Hemothorax is often accompanied by pneumothorax following chest trauma. Most hemothoraces are caused by bleeding from the parenchyma of the lung. This bleeding is slow and sometimes self-limited as a result of low pressure in the pulmonary vascular system, the presence of clotting factors in the lungs, and the compression of the injured area by the accumulated blood.[22] Continued significant bleeding indicates injury to pulmonary or systemic vessels.

Clinical Manifestations

Physical examination in simple pneumothorax may or may not reveal chest wall injury such as an open chest wound or contusion. Breath sounds on the affected side are diminished, and the chest is hyperresonant to percussion. Tachypnea and respiratory distress may be noted. Subcutaneous emphysema may be observed or palpated under the skin. An upright chest film should readily confirm the diagnosis.

When tension pneumothorax occurs, an alert patient may complain of dyspnea and chest pain. Tachypnea and tachycardia are observed. Hypotension results from the decrease in cardiac output. Tracheal deviation is observed or palpated. Impaired venous return causes distention of neck veins. Breath sounds are diminished, and hyperresonance is noted on the affected side. Arterial blood-gas analysis reveals hypoxemia as a result of intrapulmonary shunting and decreased cardiac output. On chest film, the ipsilateral lung is collapsed and the heart and mediastinum are displaced to the contralateral side. The ipsilateral hemidiaphragm is depressed and the intercostal spaces are widened.

There may be no symptoms with a small hemothorax. In larger accumulations of blood, the breath sounds are diminished on the affected side, and the chest is dull to percussion. In cases of severe bleeding, respiratory distress, mediastinal shift, and shock may be present. The diagnosis may be confirmed by upright chest film.

Medical Management

Treatment of an open chest wound with pneumothorax includes covering of the wound with a sterile, airtight dressing and placement of a chest tube high in the chest to remove the accumulated air (Fig. 31–5). Closed pneumothorax is also treated with chest tube placement, which should result in cessation of the air leak. If the air leak persists after chest tube placement, bronchoscopy is performed to look for tracheal or bronchial tears. Such injuries require surgical repair.

Emergency treatment of tension pneumothorax can proceed prior to obtaining a chest film, since the delay in therapy can be fatal. A large-bore needle is inserted into the second or third anterior intercostal space to relieve the intrathoracic pressure by converting the injury to an open pneumothorax. A chest tube is then inserted as soon as possible.

Very small, uncomplicated hemothoraces may be observed by serial chest films. In most hemothoraces, chest tube drainage is necessary and sufficient treatment. The chest tube is placed low to facilitate drainage of fluid; if pneumothorax is present, a second, higher tube may be required. As the lung reexpands, tamponade of the parenchyma causes cessation of bleeding. If bleeding continues after chest tube insertion, an injured blood vessel is probably the source. When drainage exceeds 200 ml/hr for 4 hours, if blood loss totals 1000 ml to 1500 ml, or if bleeding is unceasing, thoracotomy is indicated.[4,22] In some cases, blood drained from the chest may be filtered and reinfused into the hypovolemic patient. This autotransfusion eliminates the possibility of complications associated with homologous blood transfusions.

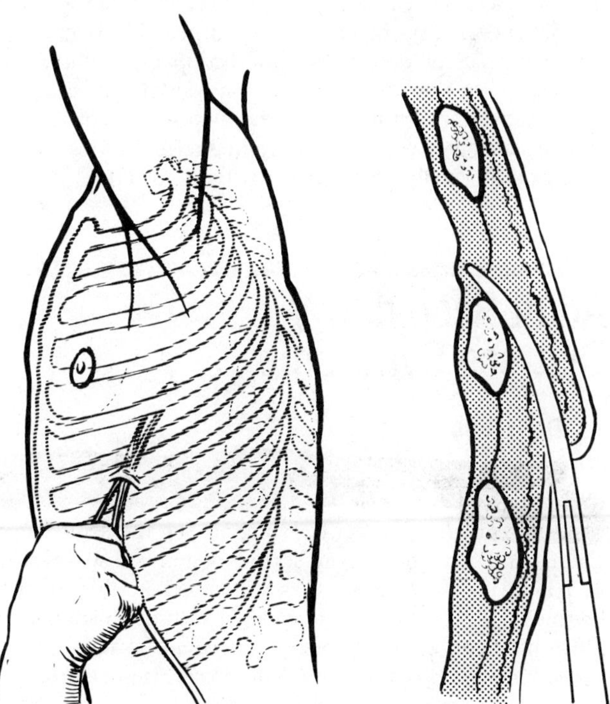

FIGURE 31–5 Placement of tube high in chest to remove accumulated air in pneumothorax. (Wolcott MW: Ambulatory Surgery and the Basics of Emergency Surgical Care. Philadelphia, JB Lippincott, 1981)

Nursing Management

Assessment and Nursing Diagnosis

As described in the section on pathophysiology, there is a wide variation in the initial severity of pleural injury and the likelihood of an injury progressing to serious complications. Nursing interventions must simultaneously include supportive care and assessment for life threatening complications. The relative importance initially assigned to each aspect of care depends on the presenting injury. However, ongoing assessment may suggest changes in the nursing care focus later.

Several examples of nursing diagnoses follow. These are listed, in increasing order, according to threat to life.

- Alteration in comfort related to lung collapse, penetrating wounds, rib fracture
- Impaired gas exchange related to the presence of air or blood in the pleural space with loss of normal ventilatory mechanics
- Fluid-volume deficit related to accumulation of blood in pleural space
- Potential decreased cardiac output related to impairment of venous return by greatly increased intrapleural pressure (tension pneumothorax)

Interventions

The ultimate goal of all nursing interventions is to maintain oxygenation of vital organs. Maintaining normal gas exchange is a closely related goal. The basic management of water-seal drainage is covered in Chapter 27 and is not repeated here. Instead, this discussion focuses on the recognition of complications specific to traumatic pleural injury.

Ultimately, a significant air leak will manifest itself as a tension pneumothorax. Agitation, tachycardia, and an initial rise in blood pressure followed by hypotension are among signs alerting the nurse to this possibility.[2] Clamping the chest tubes of a patient whose trauma has caused an air leak may precipitate tension pneumothorax and is strictly contraindicated. Emergency management of this complication is described above.

With hemothorax, significant bleeding due to a torn pulmonary or systemic vessel may lead to hypovolemic shock. In addition to carefully monitoring the amount of chest tube drainage, the patient must be monitored for hypotension and other signs of fluid volume (saline) deficit. Although stripping of chest tubes is controversial, it may be a required procedure in the case of hemothorax, in which clots can obstruct the chest drainage tubes.

The risk of infection is particularly high when pneumothorax is caused by penetrating trauma such as a stab or gunshot wound. Empyema may develop within 24 to 48 hours of injury, and the patient should be observed carefully for fever and unilateral chest pain.[6] (See Chapter 28.)

Evaluation

When goals related to the nursing care of patients with traumatic pleural disruption have been achieved, the patient will

- Have arterial blood-gas values within acceptable limits
- Have adequate circulating blood volume to vital organs
- Maintain normal lung mechanics after chest tube removal, as evidenced by chest film and auscultation of normal breath sounds
- Verbalize comfort or appear to be comfortable, as evidenced by ability to tolerate coughing, deep breathing, turning, and other respiratory-care maneuvers

Laryngeal and Tracheobronchial Injuries

Traumatic injuries to the larynx, trachea, and major bronchi may be the result of blunt or penetrating trauma. A large percentage of injuries to the larynx or cervical trachea are attributed to automobile accidents in which the person is thrown forward and strikes the hyperextended neck against the dashboard. Injuries to the distal trachea or bronchi frequently occur near the carina and involve shearing of the distal portion of the bronchial tree away from the fixed proximal portion.

Physical findings suggestive of laryngeal or tracheobronchial injury include the following: massive subcutaneous emphysema; mediastinal emphysema; hemoptysis with respiratory distress; and continued massive air leak from a pneumothorax or failure of the lung to reexpand after chest tube placement. Studies used for diagnostic confirmation may include laryngoscopy, x-ray film, computer tomography (CT), bronchoscopy, or bronchography. Concomitant esophageal injury must be established or ruled out, usually by having the patient swallow a water-soluble, radiopaque dye.[17]

Medical Management

Emergency treatment of laryngeal and tracheobronchial injuries starts with guaranteeing a patent airway. Tracheostomy is usually required for laryngeal or high tracheal injuries. Lower injuries may be managed initially with intubation. If ventilation is difficult, the uninjured bronchus may be selectively intubated. If a pneumothorax is present, a chest tube is placed for drainage. Injuries to the cervical spine must be suspected and either ruled out or treated.

Tears of less than one third the circumference of the airway and tears high in the trachea may be managed without thoracotomy as long as ventilation is adequate and the lung has reexpanded. All other tears require surgical repair as soon as possible, since delay in treatment increases morbidity and mortality significantly. Late diagnosis may result in the proliferation of granulation tissue into the lumen of the airway. Tracheal or laryngeal stenosis will result if the granulation tissue is not removed.

Nursing Management

Assessment, Nursing Diagnosis, and Interventions

The key to management of laryngeal and tracheobronchial injuries is recognition. When assessing a patient soon after thoracic injury, the nurse should be suspicious whenever signs of airway obstruction are seen in conjunction with massive subcutaneous emphysema or continuing air leak, despite chest tube placement. In this case, the nursing diagnosis of ineffective airway clearance related to obstruction of airway by injured bone or soft tissue demands immediate medical intervention to restore airway patency. Signs of airway obstruction may also develop later if the injury was small enough to escape earlier detection. Again, surgical treatment to restore airway patency is usually required.

Whenever a bronchial or tracheal tear has been diagnosed, the patient, even if awake and cooperative, should be restrained, and all other precautions should be taken to avoid inadvertent extubation. The only possible entry to the patient's airway may be the indwelling tube, and loss of the tube would probably result in the patient's death.

Adult Respiratory Distress Syndrome

Definition

Adult respiratory distress syndrome (ARDS) is a serious respiratory complication of trauma to the lungs or other body systems. In addition to being among the sequelae of trauma, ARDS can arise from serious systemic diseases such as pancreatitis. However, it is described in this chapter because it is so frequently associated with traumatic injury. ARDS has been known by many other names, among them shock lung and post-traumatic pulmonary insufficiency.

Pathophysiology

The varied pathologic conditions that can give rise to ARDS culminate in the breakdown of the lung's structural integrity. How individual factors precipitate this syndrome continues to be the subject of considerable research. Pulmonary hypoperfusion is believed by many to be a major initiating factor. Initial damage is believed to involve the pulmonary capillaries and the cells that make up the alveolar lining, with the result that capillary permeability increases and alveoli become flooded with protein-containing fluid. Surfactant production is impaired by the alveolar edema, and massive atelectasis develops. The full-blown syndrome of ARDS is characterized by severe hypoxemia, dyspnea, a marked reduction in lung compliance, and the presence of extensive lung infiltrates.[10] Pathologically, the lungs are hemorrhagic, congested, and airless.[12]

Clinical Manifestations

The onset of ARDS is usually within 1 to 3 days after the precipitating injury.[13] The patient becomes dyspneic, tachypneic, and confused, and arterial blood gases show a decrease in both the Pa_{O_2} and Pa_{CO_2}.[21] Diffuse infiltrates can be seen on the chest film.

Medical Management

Hypoxemia is profound and unresponsive to oxygen therapy with a cannula or mask. In addition, the stiff, noncompliant lungs are difficult to expand with spontaneous breathing. For these reasons, patients require mechanical ventilation, usually with PEEP. Because of the extensive lung edema, intravenous fluids are administered cautiously and only as necessary to maintain systemic tissue perfusion. High doses of corticosteroids are sometimes administered to reduce the inflammatory process within the lung, but the effectiveness of this practice is controversial.[10, 15] ARDS is, by definition, a form of acute respiratory failure, and management is addressed further in Chapter 32.

Nursing Management

Assessment and Nursing Diagnosis

Identification of patients at risk is a first priority. Disorders associated with ARDS are listed in Table 31–1. A recent study shows that persons with three simultaneous risk factors have an 85% probability of developing ARDS.[13] These persons should be frequently and systematically assessed for the signs and symptoms of hypoxemia. Unexplained dyspnea and clouding of mental status are particularly important early clues. The suspicion of hypoxemia must always be corroborated by arterial blood-gas analysis.

The major nursing diagnosis for a patient with ARDS is as follows: impaired gas exchange related to interstitial and alveolar lung edema.

Interventions

The primary goals of nursing interventions are to maintain pulmonary gas exchange and systemic tissue oxygenation and to minimize additional lung damage.

The general management of a patient with any form of acute respiratory failure is discussed in the next chapter.

TABLE 31–1
Disorders Associated with Adult Respiratory Distress Syndrome

Shock
Infection (gram-negative sepsis, pneumonia)
Trauma (fat emboli, lung contusion, nonthoracic trauma)
Liquid aspiration (gastric juice, fresh or salt water drowning, hydrocarbon fluids)
Drug overdose (heroin, methadone, barbiturates)
Inhaled toxins (smoke, corrosive chemicals, high concentrations of oxygen)
Hematologic disorders (disseminated intravascular coagulation, massive blood transfusion)
Metabolic disorders (pancreatitis, uremia)
Miscellaneous (increased intracranial pressure, eclampsia, air emboli, radiation pneumonitis)

(Adapted from Hopewell PC: Adult respiratory distress syndrome. Basics Respir Dis 7:1, 1979)

Some aspects of nursing care are peculiar to ARDS. Because the patient is highly vulnerable to fluid overload, hemodynamic monitoring is usually indicated. In addition to regulating intravenous fluids so that hemodynamic variables, such as the pulmonary capillary wedge pressure, remain low-normal, the patient must be observed carefully for other indications of adequate tissue perfusion.

Mechanical ventilation with PEEP generally reduces the FI_{O_2} required for the patient to have an acceptable arterial oxygen level. Regardless, the nurse should be aware that oxygen toxicity is possible and may contribute to the lung pathology. For this reason, the FI_{O_2} is kept at the lowest possible level required to maintain the Pa_{O_2} slightly over 60 mmHg.[15, 21]

Because sepsis can either cause or complicate ARDS, efforts to prevent and to identify infecting organisms must be vigorous. Any suspicious secretions or drainage must be cultured, and the patient must be monitored carefully for fever and other signs of infection.

Evaluation

When nursing goals related to the management of ARDS have been achieved, the patient will

- Have arterial blood-gas values within acceptable limits
- Maintain adequate circulating blood volume to vital organs

References

1. Bernstein L: Intermediate and high transverse fractures of the maxilla. In Mathog RH: Maxillofacial Trauma. Baltimore, Williams & Wilkins, 1984
2. Brannin PK: Management modalities: Respiratory system. In Hudak CM, Lohr TS, Gallo BM: Critical Care Nursing, 3rd ed. Philadelphia, JB Lippincott, 1982
3. Budassi SA (ed): Chest Trauma. J Emerg Nurs 9:356, 1983

4. Cowley RA, Dunham CM (eds): Shock Trauma/Critical Care Manual: Initial Assessment and Management. Baltimore, University Park Press, 1982
5. Dawson RLG: Injuries of the facial skeleton. In Ballantyne J, Groves J (eds): Diseases of the Ear, Nose and Throat, Vol 3, The Nose and Sinuses. London, Butterworths, 1979
6. Glennon SA, Matus VW, Bryan–Brown CW: Respiratory disorders. In Kinney MR, Dear CB, Packa DR et al (eds): AACN's Clinical Reference for Critical-Care Nursing. New York, McGraw-Hill, 1981
7. Helfrick J: Pathogenesis and evaluation of maxillary fractures. In Mathog RH: Maxillofacial Trauma. Baltimore, Williams & Wilkins, 1984
8. Jones KW: Thoracic Trauma. Surg Clin North Am. 60:957, 1980
9. Lamb C: Coping with special nasal problems. Patient Care. 17:111, 1983
10. Luce JM, Tyler ML, Pierson DJ: Intensive Respiratory Care. Philadelphia, WB Saunders, 1984
11. Lucente FE, Sobol SM: Essentials of Otolaryngology. New York, Raven Press, 1983
12. Pare JA, Fraser RG: Synopsis of Diseases of the Chest. Philadelphia, WB Saunders, 1983
13. Pepe PE, Potkin RT, Reus DH et al: Clinical predictors of the adult respiratory distress syndrome. Am J Surg, 1982
14. Peters RM: Chest trauma. In Shibel EM, Moser KM (eds): Respiratory Emergencies. St Louis, CV Mosby, 1977
15. Petty TL: Adult respiratory distress syndrome (ARDS). In Mitchell RG, Petty TL (eds): Synopsis of Clinical Pulmonary Disease. St Louis, CV Mosby, 1982
16. Rosnagle R: Epistaxis. In English GM (ed): Otolaryngology, vol 2, Diseases of the Nose and Sinuses. Philadelphia, Harper & Row, 1984
17. Snow JB, Jr: Diagnosis and therapy for acute laryngeal and tracheal trauma. Otolaryngol Clin North Am 17:101, 1984
18. Tranbaugh RF, Elings VB, Christensen J et al: Determinants of Pulmonary Interstitial Fluid Accumulation After Trauma. J Trauma 22:820, 1982
19. Trinkle JK, Richard JD, Franz JL: Management of flail chest without mechanical ventilation. Ann Thorac Surg 19:355, 1975
20. Wells–Mackie JJ: Facial trauma. In Parker JG (ed): Emergency Nursing: A Guide to Comprehensive Care. New York, John Wiley & Sons, 1984
21. West JB: Pulmonary Pathophysiology: The Essentials, 2nd ed. Baltimore, Williams & Wilkins, 1982
22. Wilson RF: Trauma. In Shoemaker WC, Thompson WL, Holbrook PR: The Society of Critical Care Medicine: Textbook of Critical Care. Philadelphia, WB Saunders, 1984

Bibliography

Corpening J: Cardiothoracic trauma. In Mann JK, Oakes AR: Critical Care Nursing of the Multi-Injured Patient. American Association of Critical-Care Nurses. Philadelphia, WB Saunders, 1980

Furgurson JE, Meislin HW: Airway problems in the trauma victim. Topics Emerg Med 1:9, 1979

Hopewell PC: Adult respiratory distress syndrome. Basics Respir Dis 7:1, 1979

Hoyt KS: Chest trauma. Nursing 83 13:34, 1983

Jurkovich GJ, Moore EE: Thoracic trauma. Trauma Q 1:37, 1984

Kohn MS: Management of chest injuries. Topics Emerg Med 1:79, 1979

Krause C: Nasal fractures: Evaluation and repair. In Mathog RH: Maxillofacial Trauma. Baltimore, Williams & Wilkins, 1984

Landercasper J, Cogbill TH, Lindesmith LA: Long-term disability after flail chest injury. J Trauma, 24:410, 1984

Tammelin BR: Respiratory management of the trauma patient. Topics Emerg Med 6:25, 1984

Chapter 32

Acute Respiratory Failure

Martha L. Tyler

Definition

Acute Respiratory Failure (ARF) is defined as a sudden impairment in the respiratory system that results in a failure to take up sufficient oxygen and/or a failure of sufficient carbon dioxide elimination to meet the metabolic requirements of the body. The nature and degree of failure in meeting metabolic demand is reflected by the arterial blood-gas values. While recognizing that circumstances such as altitude and the patient's age alter the range of normal, most clinicians agree that respiratory failure is present when the arterial oxygen tension (Pa_{O_2}) is 50 mmHg or less when breathing room air.[2,5,16,18,22]

Depending on the degree of carbon dioxide elimination, respiratory failure may be described as normocapneic, hypocapneic, or hypercapneic. A failure of arterial oxygenation can occur without a concurrent failure of carbon dioxide elimination. In this type of respiratory failure, carbon dioxide elimination can be either normal (normocapneic respiratory failure) or greater than normal (hypocapneic respiratory failure).[3] In the latter case, the Pa_{O_2} is abnormally low while the arterial carbon dioxide tension (Pa_{CO_2}) remains either within the normal range or is low, indicating increased carbon dioxide elimination.

Hypercapneic respiratory failure, also called ventilatory failure, is present when carbon dioxide elimination is below normal, resulting in a Pa_{CO_2} that is 50 mmHg or more and a pH of less than 7.30. The presence of the pH abnormality confirms the acute nature of the condition and differentiates it from chronic respiratory failure.

Chronic respiratory failure occurs slowly over a period of time, usually in patients with chronic obstructive pulmonary disease (COPD). In this type of failure, the Pa_{O_2} and Pa_{CO_2} worsen gradually, allowing time for the kidneys to retain bicarbonate and buffer the respiratory acidosis that occurs when carbon dioxide elimination is impaired.[16,22]

Etiology

Patients with chronic respiratory failure are those most at risk for ARF.[3] They often have an acute hypercapneic respiratory failure superimposed on their chronic dysfunction as a result of a lung infection or cardiac decompensation; these conditions tip the precarious balance the patient maintains between metabolic demands, supply of oxygen, and carbon dioxide elimination.

Other categories of diseases or conditions frequently associated with ARF include[31]

- Central nervous system depression (drug overdose, cerebral vascular accidents, head injury)
- Chest wall or diaphragm dysfunction (trauma, thoracic, or upper abdominal surgery)
- Defects in neuromuscular transmission (myesthenia gravis, spinal cord injury)
- Restrictive conditions (interstitial fibrosis, adult respiratory distress syndrome [ARDS], kyphoscoliosis, obesity)
- Obstructive defects (laryngeal edema, prolapsed tongue, aspiration of foreign objects, bronchospasm, COPD, retained secretions)
- Cardiovascular disease (congestive heart failure, pulmonary embolism)

This list is not exhaustive but does indicate the wide variety of patients that are at risk for ARF.

ARF must be recognized and treated immediately, since it is a potentially fatal condition that progresses rapidly. Although it is not immediately fatal, chronic respiratory failure is associated with organ damage and changes in function that leave the patient with little or no reserve to meet sudden increases in metabolic demand. Examples of arterial blood-gas values typical of ARF (normocapneic, hypocapneic, and hypercapneic) and chronic respiratory failure are shown in Table 32–1.

Pathogenesis: Hypoxemia

Low Inspired Oxygen Tension

A low oxygen tension in the inspired gas (P_{IO_2}) is a common cause of hypoxemia and a potential cause of ARF at high altitudes, where the total barometric pressure, and therefore the partial pressure, of oxygen is low. A low P_{IO_2} also occurs during fires in enclosed areas. The oxygen in the room is rapidly consumed by the process of combustion. This often results in asphyxia of persons trapped in the area before the fire itself is an immediate threat. Another example of a low P_{IO_2} occurs in hospitalized patients when the inadvertent closure of valves that control the supply of oxygen to ventilators and anesthesia machines results in iatrogenic ARF.

Alveolar Hypoventilation

Alveolar hypoventilation results in a decrease in Pa_{O_2} because an insufficient volume of oxygen-containing air reaches the gas-exchange surfaces of the lung. The degree of alveolar hypoventilation is assessed by measuring the Pa_{CO_2}. Ordinarily, alveolar ventilation is directly proportional to carbon dioxide production; however, if the lung bellows or lung parenchyma is grossly disordered, carbon dioxide elimination is compromised and the Pa_{CO_2} will rise. Assessing alveolar hypoventilation by clinical means, such as observing the breathing pattern, is often misleading. This is because overall ventilation, often measured as minute ventilation, may be normal or even increased but may not be reaching alveoli that are perfused. The amount of ventilation that is wasted is called dead-space ventilation since it does not participate in either carbon dioxide elimination or oxygen uptake.

Alveolar Gas Equation. The degree of hypoxemia is in proportion to the decrease in alveolar ventilation and the concomitant increase in Pa_{CO_2}. The amount of hypoxemia attributable to alveolar hypoventilation can be calculated using the alveolar gas equation. This equation shows that the alveolar oxygen tension (P_{AO_2}) and ultimately the Pa_{O_2} are equal to the P_{IO_2} minus the alveolar carbon dioxide tension (P_{ACO_2}) divided by the respiratory exchange ratio. Because the P_{ACO_2} is difficult to determine directly, the measured Pa_{CO_2} is substituted. The respiratory-exchange ratio adjusts the Pa_{CO_2} so that its value more nearly approximates the known metabolic relationship between carbon dioxide production and oxygen consumption. Although this relationship varies with the fuel being metabolized and can be measured, a value of 0.8 is customarily used. The equation when breathing room air is :

$$P_{AO_2} = P_{IO_2} - Pa_{CO_2}/0.8$$

At sea level, and if the Pa_{CO_2} is normal at 40 mmHg:

$$\begin{aligned} P_{AO_2} &= 150 - 40/0.8 \\ &= 150 - 50 \\ &= 100 \text{ mmHg} \end{aligned}$$

When the Pa_{CO_2} is high, for instance double the normal value, or 80 mmHg, the P_{AO_2} is reduced as follows:

$$\begin{aligned} P_{AO_2} &= 150 - 80/0.8 \\ &= 150 - 100 \\ &= 50 \text{ mmHg} \end{aligned}$$

The Pa_{O_2} will be approximately 40 mmHg, since there is a normal difference of 10 mmHg between the P_{AO_2} and Pa_{O_2}. The P_{AO_2} and Pa_{O_2} are never equal because a small amount of blood always circulates through the lung without passing through gas-exchange areas of the lung. However, if the Pa_{O_2} is more than 10 mmHg to 15 mmHg below the calculated P_{AO_2}, hypoxemia from other causes is present in addition to

TABLE 32–1
Arterial Blood Gases in Acute Respiratory Failure and Chronic Respiratory Failure

	pH	Pa_{O_2}	Pa_{CO_2}	HCO_3^-
ARF (normocapneic)	7.38	50	41	24
ARF (hypocapneic)	7.60	25	25	24
ARF (hypercapneic)	7.15	50	80	28
Chronic respiratory failure	7.35	50	80	44

any hypoxemia caused by alveolar hypoventilation. These other causes include intrapulmonary rhunt, ventilation/perfusion ($\dot{V}_A/\dot{Q}$) mismatch, and, rarely, diffusion impairment, all of which are described below.

As can be seen from the alveolar gas equation, the Pa_{CO_2} must nearly double before ARF (as defined by a Pa_{O_2} of 50 mmHg or less) occurs when alveolar hypoventilation is the only gas-exchange derangement.

Acidemia. Often of equal and sometimes greater concern is the acidemia that occurs when Pa_{CO_2} elimination decreases acutely. For example, a sudden rise in Pa_{CO_2} from 40 mmHg to 50 mmHg (10 mmHg) will cause a decrease in PA_{O_2} from 100 mmHg to 87 mmHg, and assuming a normal alveolar to arterial oxygen difference, the Pa_{O_2} will fall from a normal of 90 mmHg to 77 mmHg. While a Pa_{O_2} of 77 mmHg is below normal, it does not represent ARF and vill not cause tissue hypoxia. On the other hand, that same acute increase in Pa_{CO_2} of 10 mmHg will result in a change in pH from 7.4 to 7.3 or less.

- Acute acidemia causes cardiac dysfunction and arrhythmias[12]
- The increase in Pa_{CO_2} causes cerebrovascular dilatation and neurological problems varying from confusion and restlessness to lethargy and coma.

Causes. Alveolar hypoventilation is often caused by disorders outside the lung itself. Examples of such conditions include drug overdoses, trauma to the rib cage or diaphragm (flail chest and ruptured diaphragm), and respiratory or generalized muscular disorders. In advanced COPD the work of breathing may become so great (due to hyperinflation of the lungs and obstructed airways) that the respiratory muscles are unable to keep up with the demand and become fatigued, and the Pa_{CO_2} gradually rises.[7,27,29] The respiratory muscles are at a disadvantage because the diaphragm is pushed down and flattened by the air trapped in the lungs. When a muscle must contract from an already shortened position, it cannot develop the same force, and its endurance is markedly reduced.[25]

Ventilation-Perfusion Mismatch

$\dot{V}_A/\dot{Q}$ mismatching is the most common cause of hypoxemia. It results in a greater than normal difference in the alveolar to arterial oxygen difference but little change in Pa_{CO_2}—unless alveolar hypoventilation is also present. $\dot{V}_A/\dot{Q}$ relationships in the lung can vary from areas of zero ventilation with normal perfusion (called intrapulmonary shunt, see below) to areas of ventilation in excess of perfusion (called wasted or dead-space ventilation).

Hypoxemia due to $\dot{V}_A/\dot{Q}$ mismatch occurs when the $\dot{V}_A/\dot{Q}$ ratio is *low*. In this situation, ventilation is unevenly distributed and is *less* (but not absent) than perfusion in many areas of the lung. In low $\dot{V}_A/\dot{Q}$ areas, the venous blood, which reaches only the level of oxygen that is present in the poorly ventilated alveoli, returns to the left side of the heart incompletely oxygenated. In the left atrium, the poorly oxygenated blood mixes with blood returning from areas of lung with good $\dot{V}_A/\dot{Q}$ matching. The overall result, the Pa_{O_2}, ir determined by the proportion of well-oxygenated to poorly-oxygenated blood. The degree of obstruction to air flow in the low $\dot{V}_A/\dot{Q}$ areas in turn determines how low the oxygen will be in the blood that comes from those areas.

Because there is still some air flow to the low $\dot{V}_A/\dot{Q}$ areas, it is possible to raise the PA_{O_2} in those areas by giving the patient supplemental oxygen to breathe. Only small increases in the oxygen (FI_{O_2}) are required to return the Pa_{O_2} to a safe range, which is a Pa_{O_2} between 50 mmHg and 60 mmHg. A large increase in saturation of the hemoglobin with oxygen occurs between those values, resulting in a substantial increase in the oxygen content of the blood. In contrast to alveolar hypoventilation, $\dot{V}_A/\dot{Q}$ mismatching most commonly occurs in disorders of the lung itself: asthma and COPD, for example.

Intrapulmonary Shunt

Intrapulmonary shunt occurs when alveoli are collapsed in conditions such as atelectasis, or full of pus as in pneumonia, or flooded with edema fluid from left ventricular failure or from ARDS or neonatal respiratory distress syndrome (NRDS). The pathogenesis of hypoxemia differs from that of low $\dot{V}_A/\dot{Q}$ areas in that *no* ventilation occurs in the abnormal areas of the lung. Blood perfusing these areas remains at the partial pressure of venous oxygen, which provides a hemoglobin saturation of 75% or less. Oxygen therapy cannot increase the alveolar oxygen in the abnormal areas of lung because there is no ventilation at all to these abnormal areas. The increase in hemoglobin saturation in the areas of normal ventilation and $\dot{V}_A/\dot{Q}$ matching will be only from the usual value of 97% to 100%. This is insufficient to overcome the major deficit in oxygen saturation in the blood from the areas of shunt, and the oxygen content of the arterial blood improves little if at all.

Shunt can be differentiated from low $\dot{V}_A/\dot{Q}$ by giving the patient 100% oxygen to breathe. If shunt is present, there is little or no improvement in Pa_{O_2}, whereas in low $\dot{V}_A/\dot{Q}$ conditions, the Pa_{O_2} improves substantially.

- It is important to differentiate between those two causes because the measures necessary to treat the hypoxemia associated with intrapulmonary shunt are different than those used to treat the hypoxemia associated with $\dot{V}_A/\dot{Q}$ mismatching.

Diffusion Limitation

Because the transfer of oxygen from the alveolus to the blood occurs by the process of diffusion, conditions causing diffusion limitation are a possible cause of hypoxemia. However, gas transfer from alveolus to blood is very fast and appears to overcome diffusion barriers in most cases. Red blood cells traverse an alveolar capillary in about 0.75 second while equilibration of oxygen between alveolus and blood takes only 0.25 second. Even when conditions causing interstitial scarring or edema increase the diffusion distance, it is felt that the reserve time (0.5 second) for equilibration makes diffusion limitation an unlikely cause of ARF.

Clinical Manifestations

The clinical manifestations of ARF include both adaptive or compensatory responses to the physiological stress of hypoxemia and the specific pathophysiological effects of tissue hypoxia in organs or body systems.[14,24] The changes in function due to hypoxemia in major organs and systems and the associated clinical signs and symptoms are listed in Table 32–2. These signs do not appear until the Pa_{O_2} is 55 mmHg to 60 mmHg because significant desaturation of the blood does not occur above these values. Without desaturation the blood oxygen content does not fall and the organs are not oxygen-deprived unless there are other diseases or conditions that result in marked anemia or decreased cardiac output. As the Pa_{O_2} falls below 60 mmHg, compensatory mechanisms are called into play to maintain oxygen delivery.

Cardiovascular Effects

Usually the first sign to appear is an increase in heart rate (cardiac output). This increase occurs because the heart is so metabolically active that it requires more oxygen per minute than any other organ. If the blood is hypoxemic, the heart must increase the rate at which the blood is delivered to the coronary arteries to meet its oxygen demands. A faster rate increases the cardiac oxygen demands even further, and this compensatory mechanism is reasonably successful only until hypoxemia is very severe, usually around a Pa_{O_2} of 30 mmHg. At this point pathophysiological changes in function begin to develop in the heart and other organs. Arrhythmias occur as cellular metabolism fails and cells of the conductive tissues die.[12]

Respiratory Effects

Compensatory changes in respiratory system function are not especially marked or early in the course of hypoxemia. Respiratory rate usually increases but may not be able to increase if the hypoxemia is associated with severe lung disease, respiratory muscle paralysis or fatigue, or central nervous system depression. Shallow breaths and slow respiratory rates are associated with the latter condition.[34] With prolonged alveolar hypoxia, the pulmonary artery pressure increases and observable systemic changes due to increased venous congestion occur.[15] Signs such as liver enlargement and lower-extremity edema are visible when the right ventricle can no longer overcome the increased pulmonary artery pressure. Decreased function of the kidney for sodium and water excretion may add to the edema of right ventricular failure. Right ventricular failure due to pulmonary disease is called pulmonary heart disease or cor pulmonale.[10] This condition is a frequent complication of COPD (See Chap 29).

Dyspnea is not a specific symptom of hypoxemia. However, because ventilation is often increased to compensate for increased dead space, or the work of breathing is often increased in diseases that cause hypoxemia due to V_A/Q mismatching, dyspnea is often present with hypoxemia.[6] On the other hand, the absence of dyspnea does not mean that hypoxemia is not present. Both dyspnea and respiratory drive vary from person to person.[34] Many patients become severely hypoxemic without complaining of shortness of breath.

TABLE 32–2
Clinical Manifestations and Pathophysiological Effects of Hypoxemia

Organ or System	*Change in Function*	*Clinical Signs and Symptoms*
Brain	Impaired mentation	Decreased cognitive ability, somnolence
	Increased perfusion and CSF pressure	Headache, confusion, restlessness, pinpoint pupils, coma
Heart	Increased cardiac output, heart rate; arrhythmias, decreased cardiac output	Bounding pulses, tachycardia; cyanosis, bradycardia
	Cardiac arrest ($Pa_{O_2} < 30$ mmHg)	Absent pulse and blood pressure
Respiratory	Increased ventilation	Increased respiratory rate, or depth, or both; dyspnea
	Increased pulmonary artery pressure	Increased systemic venous pressure, enlarged liver, peripheral edema, peristernal heave and gallop (pulmonary heart disease)
Metabolism	Increased lactic acid production	Increased respiratory rate, somnolence
Kidneys	Decreased sodium and water excretion	Edema
Bone marrow	Increased red blood cell mass	Plethora, headache, decreased cognitive ability, cyanosis

CSF = cerebrospinal fluid.

Cerebral Effects

Brain function is particularly sensitive to hypoxemia because brain tissue is capable of only very limited anaerobic metabolism. In hypoxemia, autoregulatory mechanisms increase blood flow to the brain; when these mechanisms are inadequate, mentation is impaired. If increased cerebral blood flow causes an increase in intracranial pressure, headache is a frequent symptom. Cognitive deficits are seen with moderate hypoxemia and are usually reversible with oxygen administration.[19] Severe hypoxemia results in confusion, restlessness, and eventually coma.

Acid–Base Effects

When severe hypoxemia overstresses cardiac compensatory mechanisms, lactic acid is produced in tissues forced to resort to anaerobic metabolism. Interestingly, lactic acidosis causes a more consistent increase in respiratory rate than does hypoxemia alone. In order to maintain a normal pH, respiratory rate increases, thereby eliminating more carbon dioxide, which, in turn, decreases the overall acid load of the blood.

Hematologic Effects

Polycythemia, an increase in the red blood cell mass, occurs as the bone marrow reacts to stimulation by erythropoietin. The erythropoietin is turned on by hypoxemia in an attempt to improve the oxygen content of the blood. This is an effective compensation until the blood becomes hyperviscous. The increased hemoglobin makes the skin plethoric and sometimes cyanotic-appearing even when hypoxemia is mild. Cyanosis appears when 5% of the hemoglobin is desaturated. If excess hemoglobin is present, desaturation of the required 5% of the hemoglobin occurs more easily while, conversely, anemic patients very seldom appear cyanotic. Cyanosis may also appear when the blood is well oxygenated but the cardiac output is low or there is a regional decrease in blood flow. An example of this situation is the desaturation and cyanosis of the fingertips that occurs when the hands are cold and vasoconstricted. Overall, the presence of cyanosis indicates desaturation of the blood in the tissues where it is present, but the absence of cyanosis does not eliminate the possibility of hypoxemia.

Medical Management

Diagnosis

The diagnosis of ARF is suspected by recognizing the signs and symptoms described above; confirmation of the diagnosis is made on the basis of arterial blood-gas values.[13] Many other tests, such as pulmonary function tests and chest roentgenograms, may also be performed to determine the exact nature and degree of the condition causing the hypoxemia. Unfortunately, the signs and symptoms of ARF do not present until the patient is already close to respiratory failure (Pa_{O_2} 55 mmHg–60 mmHg), making a high index of suspicion for this condition particularly important. Failure to oxygenate tissues not only changes organ function, it also results in damage that may be irreversible, particularly within the central nervous system.

Treatment

Oxygen Therapy. The primary treatment of ARF is to give oxygen. Because tissue hypoxia is life threatening, it is always best to err on the side of too much oxygen in an emergency situation.[3] On the other hand, excessive oxygen is itself toxic to some tissues, especially the alveoli, or can reduce the drive to breathe in certain patients.[23] Therefore the overall goal of oxygen therapy is to achieve a satisfactory level of hemoglobin saturation (around 90% or a Pa_{O_2} of 60 mmHg) at the lowest possible dose of oxygen.[19]

This dose, or concentration, varies widely depending on the cause of the hypoxemia.[16] In hypoxemia caused by ventilatory failure, oxygen may not be needed at all after ventilation is restored. However, oxygen must be used until adequate ventilation is ensured because the goal is to have all the air, no matter how little reaches the alveoli, be high in oxygen. When hypoxemia is caused by intrapulmonary shunt, it usually is severe and is not very responsive to increased oxygen concentrations. An example of this situation is ARDS discussed in Chapter 31. Other conditions causing intrapulmonary shunt and requiring high oxygen doses are pneumonia and atelectasis. $\dot{V}_A/\dot{Q}$ mismatch is the most frequent cause of hypoxemia. The dose of oxygen required usually is rather small, on the order of 2 liters per minute or 25% to 28%.

Under all circumstances the efficacy of a selected dose of oxygen must be determined by an arterial blood-gas measurement. In order to allow time for areas of low ventilation to fill with the new oxygen concentration, the blood for follow-up blood-gas determinations is not drawn until 20 minutes after the oxygen therapy is initiated or changed.

Other Therapies. Many other therapies are used to try to cure or improve the underlying cause or causes of hypoxemia and hypercapnea, if they coexist. For example, antibiotics are used to treat an infectious cause, and bronchodilators are used to treat bronchospasm. These therapies are described in the other chapters in this section and are not discussed here.

However, there are two other important factors that often negate or diminish the effectiveness of the ultimate goal of treatment of hypoxemia, which is to provide adequate oxygen to the tissues.[8] These other factors are the amount of hemogloblin available and the adequacy of the cardiac output. Therefore, supportive therapies for these conditions, such as blood or packed-cell transfusions and intravenous fluids, or cardiotonic drugs, or both, are often administered concurrently with oxygen. In addition, because acidemia often adds to the organ dysfunction accompanying ARF, close watch is kept on the acid–base status of the patient. Sodium bicarbonate may be given intravenously to treat severe acidemia until the underlying cause is determined and treated.

Prognosis

ARF can almost always be treated successfully if it is recognized early enough. Unfortunately, the signs and symptoms of ARF are not specific. Restlessness and confusion and tachycardia all have a variety of possible causes; however, because hypoxemia is potentially lethal it should be confirmed or eliminated as a cause first by obtaining an arterial blood-gas measurement. Once hypoxemia has been eliminated, other causes of confusion (*e.g.,* stroke, metabolic derangements), restlessness, and tachycardia (*e.g.,* anxiety) can be investigated.

Nursing Management

Assessment and Nursing Diagnosis

Assessing patients for ARF means watching for the clinical signs and symptoms listed in Table 32–2. The goal of the assessment is the prevention of ARF. However, not all patients can be, or need to be, assessed for ARF. Developing a high-risk profile is helpful in determining which patient should be assessed frequently.

Assessing Risk Factors. Patients at high risk for developing ARF are those with conditions resulting in one or more of the causes of hypoxemia. All persons living at high altitude are at greater risk for ARF than those living at sea level because for the former, "normal" Pa_{O_2} is lower than that for persons living at sea level. They will reach ARF sooner or with less lung disease or with milder hypoventilation than will sea level patients. Nurses working at high altitudes (*e.g.,* Denver, Colorado, which is one mile high) should be familiar with the normal barometric pressure for their area (630 mmHg for Denver versus 760 mmHg for sea level) and adjust all Pa_{O_2} examples in text books downward as indicated (*e.g.,* in Denver the normal Pa_{O_2} for a young person is 70 mmHg–75 mmHg).

Age is also a risk factor, since it is known that Pa_{O_2} declines with age even in persons with normal lungs.[32] The normal Pa_{O_2} in a person 70 years of age is around 80 mmHg, 20 mmHg closer to respiratory failure (Pa_{O_2} 50 mmHg) than a young normal person whose Pa_{O_2} is 95 mmHg to 100 mmHg. The older person living at a high altitude appears to be at a significant disadvantage. Actually, in most persons there is a mild hyperventilation that "turns on" when the Pa_{O_2} reaches 60 mmHg and maintains the Pa_{O_2} close to that value unless other causes of hypoxemia overwhelm this compensatory hyperventilation.

Another risk factor is any condition leading to alveolar hypoventilation. Chest wall injuries, neuromuscular diseases, drugs or toxic agents, brain and spinal injuries, respiratory center depression, and severe obstructive and restrictive lung diseases are all possible causes of alveolar hypoventilation and therefore of ARF.

Because $\dot{V}_A/\dot{Q}$ mismatch is caused by partially obstructed airways such as might occur in chronic bronchitis, asthma, or emphysema, patients with these diseases should be included in the high-risk category. Patients who smoke often have chronic bronchitis, which is sometimes dismissed as just a smoker's cough. If something occurs that makes these patients reluctant to cough, such as abdominal surgery, excessive secretions may collect in the airways, leading to partial obstruction or complete airway plugging and a $\dot{V}_A/\dot{Q}$ mismatch or intrapulmonary shunt, respectively. With these concepts in mind, a nurse on a busy postoperative floor should give highest priority to deep-breathing and secretion-clearance therapies for those patients known to have productive coughs (for whatever reason) prior to surgery.[16,17] Those with thoracic or abdominal surgery, especially upper abdominal incisions, would have priority over patients with lower abdominal or extremity surgery.[11]

Nursing Diagnoses. When it is determined that patients are at risk, the nursing diagnoses include

- Potential impaired gas exchange related to decreased ventilation relative to perfusion, shunt, hypoventilation, low inspired oxygen tension, or diffusion limitation
- Potential ineffective breathing pattern related to respiratory muscle fatigue

Interventions

The goals of all nursing interventions are to maximize alveolar gas exchange and maintain perfusion and oxygenation of vital organs.

When ARF has already been diagnosed, ongoing nursing assessment is an extremely important feature of nursing care. By observing for the signs and symptoms of hypoxemia listed in Table 32–2 and by monitoring arterial blood-gas values, the patient's progress and the effectiveness of medical and nursing interventions can be followed.

In addition to assessing patients for the pathophysiological changes that occur during ARF, a unique nursing function is to assess the patient's response to the effects of ARF. The information obtained can be used to plan supportive nursing interventions that maximize gas exchange and minimize the demands on already-stressed vital tissues.

One common patient response is acute anxiety, which usually accompanies severe hypoxemia just as it does any life threatening condition.[9] Anxiety is of special concern for the patient with hypoxemia because anxiety causes increased catecholamine excretion, which in turn increases metabolism and oxygen demand, just when oxygen supply is most compromised. In addition, the patient may have an increased respiratory rate or be dyspneic or have a prolonged expiratory phase, which interferes with speech and the expression of specific fears or concerns. Interventions to reduce anxiety include the following: questions to the patient should be framed so that single-word answers can be given; the patient's questions should be anticipated and answered before they are asked; stimulation from the environment should be minimal; the patient's previous coping strategies should be ascertained and maximized if the ARF is a complication of long-standing COPD.

Careful positioning of the patient is another supportive nursing intervention. When acutely distressed, the patient

NURSING CARE PLAN FOR THE PATIENT WITH ACUTE RESPIRATORY FAILURE

NURSING DIAGNOSIS: Inadequate gas exchange related to decreased ventilation relative to perfusion (low $\dot{V}_A/\dot{Q}$), shunt, hypoventilation, low inspired oxygen tension, or diffusion limitation

GOAL: To maximize gas exchange and maintain perfusion of vital organs

Nursing Interventions	Rationale	Outcome Criteria
1. Monitor patient for signs of worsened hypoxemia, hypercapnia, acidosis	1. Clinical symptoms suggest need for change in treatment (confirm with ABGs)	1–11. ABGs within safe limits: ▪ Pa_{O_2} at least 60 mmHg (desirable level dependent upon patient's underlying disease) ▪ Pa_{CO_2} at patient's baseline ▪ pH within normal range
2. Maintain placement of oxygen delivery system; monitor correct liter flow	2. Displacement associated with decreased Pa_{O_2}; excessive O_2 can decrease respiratory drive in patients with chronic CO_2 retention	2. Adequate systemic perfusion evidenced by ▪ Normal vital signs ▪ Normal mentation ▪ Normal urine output
3. Position to maintain open airway, prevent aspiration	3. Aspiration may cause pneumonia and exacerbate ARF	
4. Monitor breath sounds indicating: ▪ Need for cough or suction ▪ Increased wheezing ▪ Sudden decrease or absence of breath sounds ▪ Change in crackles	4. Secretions or bronchospasm may aggravate hypoxemia; decreased breath sounds may indicate pneumothorax; crackles may indicate atelectasis or left-sided heart failure	
5. Position patient to maximize ventilation and blood flow to healthy lung tissue	5. Pa_{O_2} best when patient is positioned with healthy lung down	
6. Turn frequently and monitor effect of position change on ABGs	6. Inadequate movement may lead to complications of immobility	
7. Assist patient to maintain but not exceed safe levels of activity by passive or active bed exercise, positioning in chair, ambulation	7. Immobility will compromise every body system	
8. Monitor nutritional status (weight, skin folds, serum albumin)	8. Malnutrition weakens respiratory muscles[1,21]	
9. Institute nutritional support (supplemental feedings, enteral or parenteral hyperalimentation)		
10. Maintain hydration	10. Water deficit may impair secretion clearance	
11. Decrease patient anxiety	11. Anxiety increases metabolic oxygen demands	

ABGs = arterial blood gases.

should be assisted to a position of comfort, almost always a sitting position.[20] As the patient becomes able to tolerate repositioning, the position of choice is one that maximizes blood flow to healthy lung tissue.[33]

It is generally inadvisable to attempt to slow or otherwise change a patient's breathing pattern. The respiratory rate may be very fast and look very abnormal, but patients automatically use a pattern that causes them the least work. Aside from suggesting pursing the lips on exhalation to those patients who do not spontaneously use this breathing pattern, no attempt should be made to slow or otherwise change the patient's breathing pattern. Attempts to change the breathing patterns of patients with COPD has recently been shown to cause them more dyspnea and move them closer to respiratory muscle fatigue.[4]

Respiratory muscle fatigue may occur during ARF for

several reasons. The work of breathing may be greatly increased by the condition causing the hypoxemia; severe asthma is an example.[27] In addition, hyperinflation of the lung with trapped air pushes the diaphragm down, limiting its ability to generate force and increase the volume of the lung, leaving the intercostal and accessory muscles to carry most of the work.[25,27] The concurrent hypoxemia may lead to anaerobic metabolism causing a greater demand for ventilation while decreasing the oxygen supply to the respiratory muscles.

Respiratory muscle fatigue has been associated with an increase in respiratory rate, respiratory paradox, and respiratory alternans.[7,13,29] Respiratory paradox is a pattern in which only the chest rises during inspiration; the abdomen sinks in instead of rising. This is a sign that the diaphragm is not participating in ventilation (contracting and descending). Rather, it is being sucked up into the chest by the negative pressure created in the thoracic cavity as the inspiratory muscles contract. Respiratory alternans occurs as the intercostals and the diaphragm take turns in contracting during inspiration, apparently to spell each other. Several breaths of "intercostal" breathing (chest only rises) occur, followed by several diaphragmatic breaths (abdomen only rises).[7] Observing any of these patterns would lead to a nursing diagnosis of ineffective breathing pattern due to respiratory muscle fatigue. Further assessment would be necessary before the cause of the respiratory muscle fatigue could be determined and specific interventions planned.

A general nursing care plan for the patient with ARF is presented here. Additional specific nursing interventions will be determined by the type of underlying condition that has led to the development of ARF and may include strategies to clear secretions, reduce bronchospasm, or eliminate infection.[16,17,26,28,30] Principles for caring for patients who are receiving oxygen therapy or who are being mechanically ventilated are discussed in Chapter 27.

Evaluation

Regardless of its cause, nursing interventions for ARF are ultimately determined by their impact on the patient's arterial blood gases and systemic perfusion and oxygenation. Specific outcomes include the following:

- Patient's arterial blood gases show
  - pH within normal range
  - Pa_{CO_2} at patient's usual baseline
  - Pa_{O_2} of at least 60 mmHg (desirable level dependent upon patient's underlying disease)
- Adequate systemic perfusion as evidenced by vital signs, mentation, and urine output within normal levels

References

1. Arora NS, Rochester DF: Respiratory muscle strength and maximal voluntary ventilation in undernourished patients. Am Rev Respir Dis 126:5, 1982
2. Balk R, Bone RC: Classification of acute respiratory failure. Med Clin North Am 67:551, 1983
3. Beck B: Oxygen therapy in acute and chronic pulmonary disease. In Ziment I (ed): Practical Pulmonary Disease. New York, John Wiley & Sons, 1983
4. Bellemare F, Grassino A: Force reserve of the diaphragm in patients with chronic obstructive pulmonary disease. J Appl Physiol 55:8, 1983
5. Bone RC: Acute respiratory failure: Classification, differential diagnosis, and introduction to management of respiratory failure. In Burton GG, Hodgkin JE (eds): Respiratory Care: A Guide to Clinical Practice, 2nd ed. Philadelphia, JB Lippincott, 1984
6. Burki NK: Dyspnea. Clin Chest Med 1:47, 1980
7. Cohen CA, Zagelbaum G, Gross D, et al: Clinical manifestations of inspiratory muscle fatigue. Am J Med 73:308, 1982
8. D'Alonzo GE, Dantzker DR: Respiratory failure, mechanisms of abnormal gas exchange, and oxygen delivery. Med Clin North Am 67:557, 1983
9. Dudley DL, Sitzman J: Psychosocial and psychophysiologic approach to the patient. Sem Respir Med 1:59, 1979
10. Fishman AP: Cor pulmonale: General aspects. In Fishman AP (ed): Pulmonary Diseases and Disorders. New York, McGraw-Hill, 1980
11. Ford GT, Whitelaw WA, Rosenal TW, et al: Diaphragm function after upper abdominal surgery in humans. Am Rev Respir Dis 127:431, 1983
12. Hudson LD: Cardiovascular complications in acute respiratory failure. Respir Care 28:627, 1983
13. Hudson LD: Evaluation of the patient with acute respiratory failure. Respir Care 28:542, 1983
14. Hudson LD: Prognosis: Immediate and long-term sequelae of acute respiratory failure. Respir Care 28:663, 1983
15. Lloyd TC, Jr: Effect of alveolar hypoxemia on pulmonary vascular resistance. J Appl Physiol 19:1086, 1964
16. Luce JM, Tyler ML, Pierson DJ: Intensive Respiratory Care. Philadelphia, WB Saunders, 1984
17. Mackenzie CF (ed), Ciesla N, Imle PC et al: Chest Physiotherapy in the Intensive Care Unit. Baltimore, Williams & Wilkins, 1981
18. Moser KM, Spragg RG (eds): Respiratory Emergencies, 2nd ed. St Louis, CV Mosby, 1982
19. Nocturnal Oxygen Therapy Trial Group: Continuous or noctural oxygen therapy in hypoxemic chronic obstructive lung disease: A clinical trial. Ann Intern Med 93:391, 1980
20. O'Neill S, McCarthy DS: Postural relief of dyspnea in severe chronic airflow limitations: Relationship to respiratory muscle strength. Thorax 38:595, 1983
21. Openbrier DR, Irwin MM, Rogers RM et al: Nutritional status and lung function in patients with emphysema and chronic bronchitis. Chest 83:17, 1983
22. Petty TL: Intensive and Rehabilitative Respiratory Care, 3rd ed. Philadelphia, Lea & Febiger, 1982
23. Pierson DJ: The toxicity of low-flow oxygen therapy. Respir Care 28:889, 1983
24. Pingleton SK: Complications of acute respiratory failure. Med Clin North Am 67:725, 1983
25. Rochester DF, Arora NS: Respiratory muscle failure. Med Clin North Am 67:573, 1983
26. Sexton DL: Chronic Obstructive Pulmonary Disease: Care of the Child and Adult. St Louis, CV Mosby, 1981
27. Sharp JT, Danon J, Druz WS et al: Respiratory muscle function in patients with chronic obstructive pulmonary disease: Its relationship to disability and to respiratory therapy. Am Rev Respir Dis 110 (part 2):154, 1974
28. Standards for nursing care of patient with COPD: A report of the nursing standards subcommittee of the ATS Section of Nursing—Scientific Assembly on Clinical Problems. ATS News 7:31, 1981

29. Tobin MJ, Chadha TS, Jenouri G et al: Breathing patterns: II. Diseased subjects. Chest 84:286, 1983
30. Traver GA (ed): Respiratory Nursing: The Science and the Art. New York, John Wiley & Sons, 1982
31. Tyler ML: Acute respiratory failure: The patient with chronic obstructive lung disease. In Kenner C, Guzetta C, Dossey B (eds): Critical Care Nursing: Body, Mind, Spirit, 2nd ed. Boston, Little, Brown & Co, 1985
32. West JB: Pulmonary Pathophysiology: The Essentials, 2nd ed. Baltimore, Williams & Wilkins, 1982
33. Zack MB, Pontoppidan H, Kasemi H: The effect of lateral positions on gas exchange in pulmonary disease: A prospective evaluation. Am Rev Respir Dis 110:49, 1974
34. Zwillich C: The control of breathing in clinical practice: Its significance and assessment. Sem Respir Med 4:247, 1983

UNIT V

Nursing Care of Patients with Alterations in Cardiovascular Function

Heart Function Vascular Function Hematologic Function

Section 1

Heart Function

Chapter 33

Review of Anatomy and Physiology

The Heart

Barbara R. Landau

The cardiovascular system is the link between cells and the external environment. It consists of a pump that forces a fluid, in which essential materials are dissolved, through a series of ducts and conduits. The pump is considered in this chapter and the vessels and fluid in Chapters 41 and 48.

The cardiovascular system is truly a circulatory system, for the blood travels in one direction around a circular course, and it is a closed system, except for capillary exchange. It is generally considered as two circuits (systemic and pulmonary) with one pump, but it may also be considered as one circuit with two pumps which happen to be joined (Fig. 33–1). The right part of the heart pumps blood through the pulmonary part of the circuit and the left pumps it through the systemic portion. Each pump has a receiving chamber (atrium) and an ejection chamber (ventricle), and each receives blood from one circuit and delivers it to the other. The blood flows because each ventricular pump generates enough pressure (but only enough) to overcome resistance in the circuit and force blood through it and back to the other pump. Pressure is highest in the contracting ventricles, and it falls progressively as it passes through arteries, capillaries, and veins, to the atria. The ventricles must be strong enough to develop sufficient pressure, and the vessel walls sturdy enough to withstand it. Accordingly, ventricle walls are thicker than atrial walls, arteries are thicker than veins, and the left ventricle and systemic vessels are, in general, thicker than those of the right ventricle and pulmonary circuit.

Because the circuit is continuous, the two ventricles must pump equal amounts of blood (except during the few beats when the heart is adjusting its output). Each ventricle must pump as much blood as comes to it, and conversely, it cannot pump more blood than it receives.

Because the needs of the tissues are not equal or constant, the system must be able to adjust the amount of blood delivered to them. Blood flow can be raised by increasing the rate at which blood is circulated throughout the entire system, or by increasing the fraction of the total flow that is delivered to a particular organ.

Anatomy of the Heart

Heart Structure

The heart appears to rest on the diaphragm, and is oriented with the tip or apex to the left, and the base above and mostly behind the sternum. The inner surface of the heart is covered by endocardium, a single layer of epithelium and underlying connective tissue, which is continuous with the endothelial lining of arteries and veins. The outer surface of the heart is covered by a thin epithelial and connective tissue

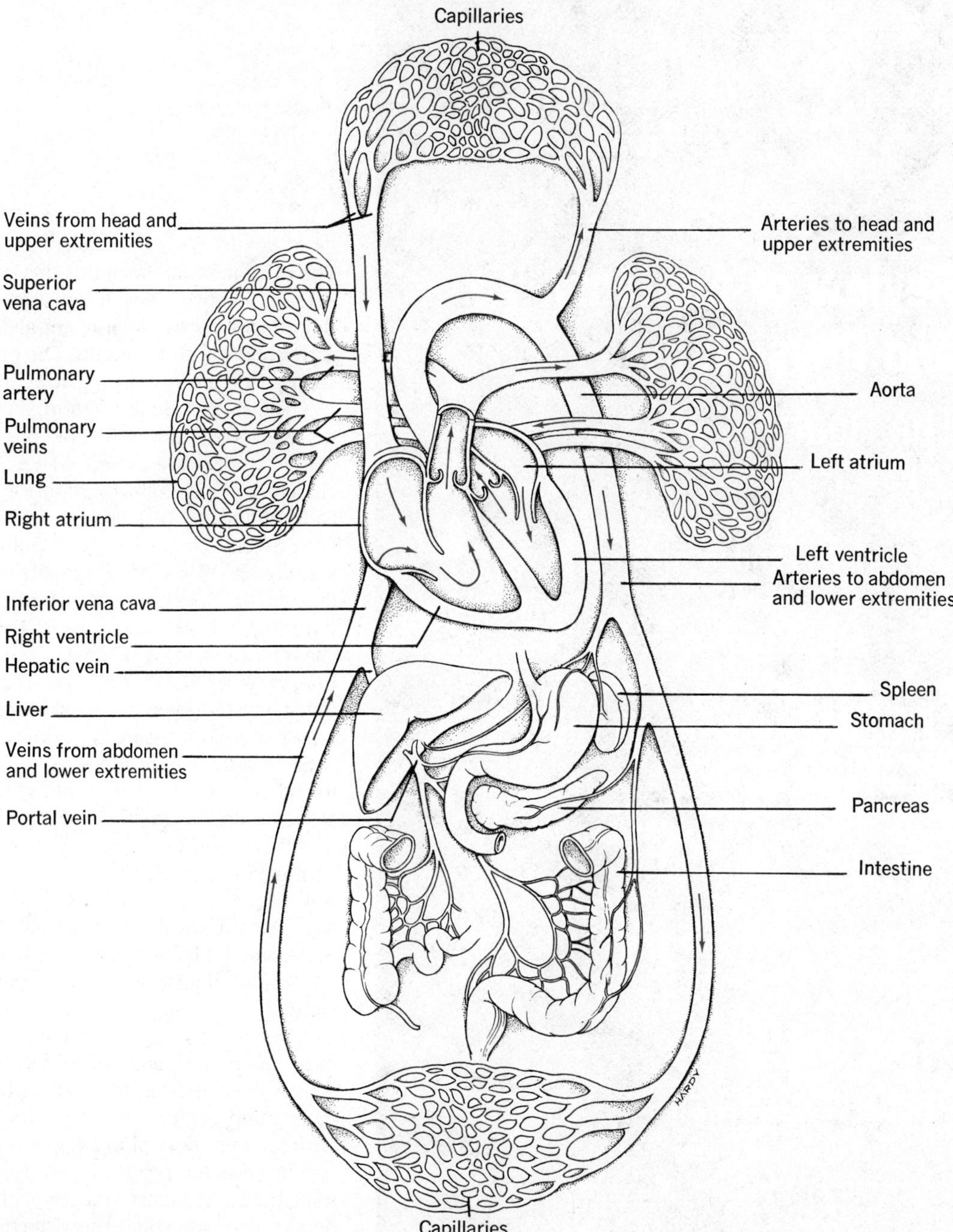

FIGURE 33–1 Diagram of the pulmonary and systemic circulations.

layer, the epicardium. It extends a short distance over the great vessels, then is reflected back, forming a sturdy sac, the pericardium, that encloses the entire heart (Fig. 33–2). The heart fills most of the enclosed pericardial sac, but fat may accumulate in the epicardium and encroach on space available.

The right and left sides of the heart are separated by the interatrial and interventricular septa. The boundary between the atria and ventricles is marked externally by the atrioventricular (AV) groove. Internally there is a plate of dense collagenous connective tissue known as the fibrous skeleton of the heart, which forms four rings that encircle the openings of the AV and semilunar (aortic and pulmonary) valves, and also anchors cardiac muscle fibers.

Bundles of cardiac muscle arise from the fibrous skeleton, and wrap around the ventricles in a winding and spiraling manner. Contraction is a wringing and squeezing action which reduces the capacity of the chambers and raises the pressure in them. There are bands of muscle, the trabeculae carneae, on the inner surface, and papillary muscles protrude into the lumen.

The artia receive blood from veins (the venae cavae or

the pulmonary veins), and they send it to the right or left ventricle, from which it is forced into the pulmonary artery or the aorta. There is a valve at the exit from each chamber, but there are no valves at the entrance to the atria, and consequently blood can flow into them continuously (Fig. 33–3).

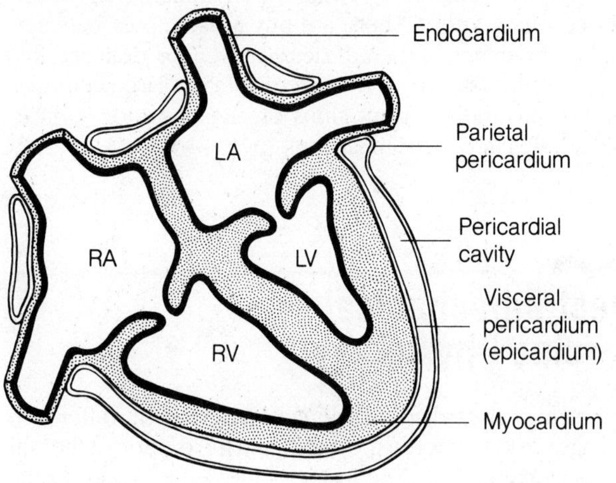

FIGURE 33–2 Diagram of the layers of the heart that shows the visceral pericardium, the pericardial cavity, and the parietal pericardium.

HEART VALVES. The AV valves consist of small flaps or cusps attached around the opening in the fibrous skeleton (Fig 33–3). The right AV valve, with three cusps, is the tricuspid valve, and the left, with but two cusps, is the bicuspid or mitral valve. The valve cusps are connective tissue and lack muscle fibers; they do not contract, but are moved passively by the pressure of the blood on either side of them. When the ventricles contract they are carried upward, blocking the opening into the atria. Tiny threads, the chordae tendineae, extend from papillary muscles to the free edge of each cusp. The papillary muscles contract with the rest of the ventricular muscle and place tension on the chordae tendineae that prevents the valves from turning "inside out."

Blood Circulation Through the Heart

Blood leaves the ventricles through the semilunar valves, which consist of three tiny crescent-shaped patch pockets on the inside of the artery. These valves also are controlled by the pressure of the blood on the two sides of them. During diastole, pressure is higher in the arteries; blood pushing back toward the ventricles fills the pockets, and their free edges abut, sealing the opening. During systole, the blood forced through the valve neatly folds the pockets back against the vessel wall, where they do not interfere with the flow of blood.

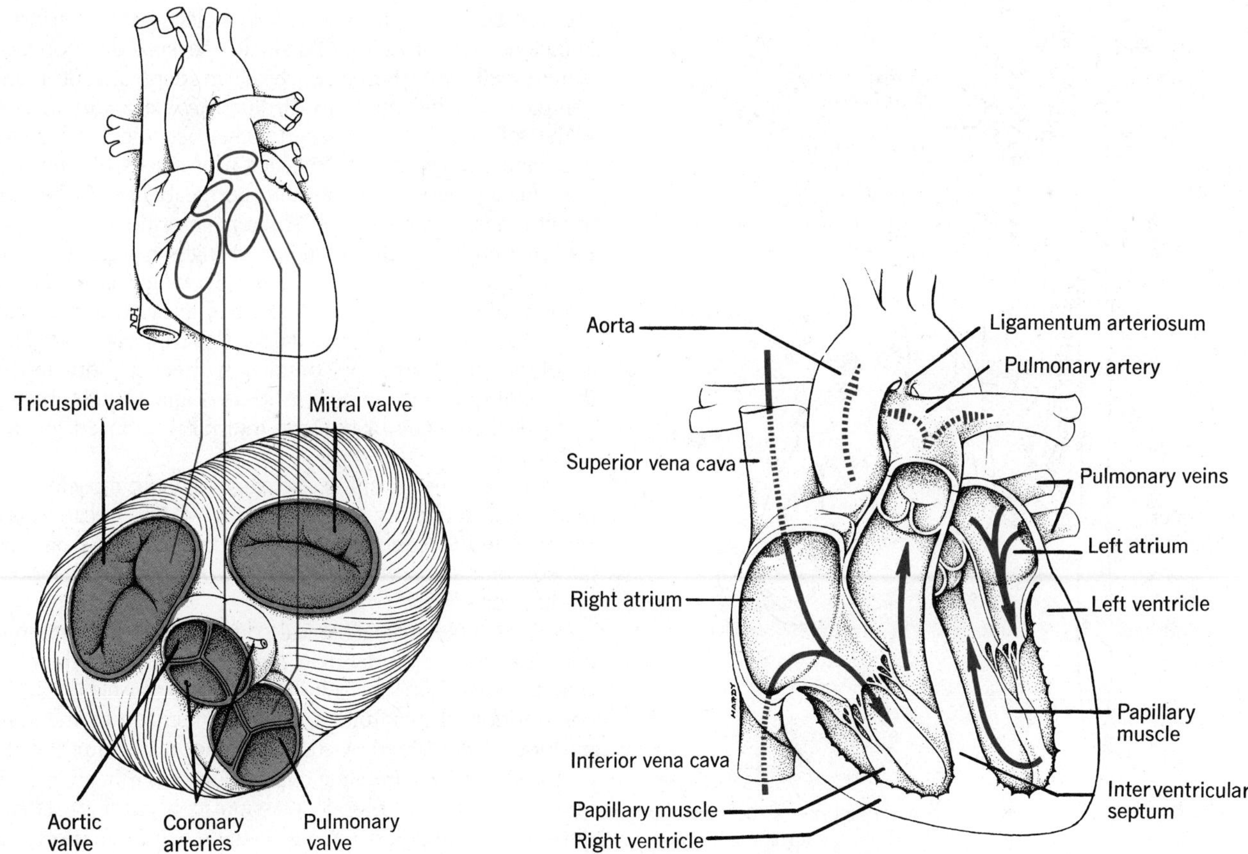

FIGURE 33–3 (*A*) Valves of the heart. In the lower drawing the atria have been removed and the heart tilted forward; thus the valves are seen from above. (*B*) Direction of blood flow within the heart.

Nerve Supply to the Heart

The heart is innervated by the autonomic nervous system. The sympathetic component arises from the upper thoracic region of the cord and passes to the sympathetic chain (Fig. 33–4). Cardiac nerves arise from the superior, middle, and stellate ganglia, and form plexuses about the aorta and pulmonary vessels. The fibers terminate in the region of the pacemaker and conducting system (sinoatrial and atrioventricular nodes) and the ventricular muscle. The parasympathetic innervation is carried in the vagus nerves. The fibers enter the cardiac plexuses with sympathetic fibers (but with no functional connection) and end in the region of the sinoatrial (SA) and atrioventricular (AV) nodes, with few if any fibers to the ventricular myocardium. Impulses in these fibers are controlled from the cardiac center in the medulla.

Blood Supply to the Heart

The myocardium receives its blood supply from the right and left coronary arteries which arise from the aorta just beyond the aortic valve (Fig. 33–5). They encircle the heart in the AV groove and anastomose on the posterior surface, giving off numerous branches to the musculature along the way. The right coronary artery supplies mainly the right ventricle. The left coronary is larger and forms two main branches, the left anterior descending branch along the interventricular septum and the circumflex artery, which continues around the heart. A posterior descending artery may be supplied mainly by either the circumflex (left) or the right coronary artery. There are tiny anastomoses between terminal branches of the arteries. The venous drainage follows a similar pattern, and converges into a large vein that empties into the coronary sinus on the posterior surface, which drains into the right atrium.

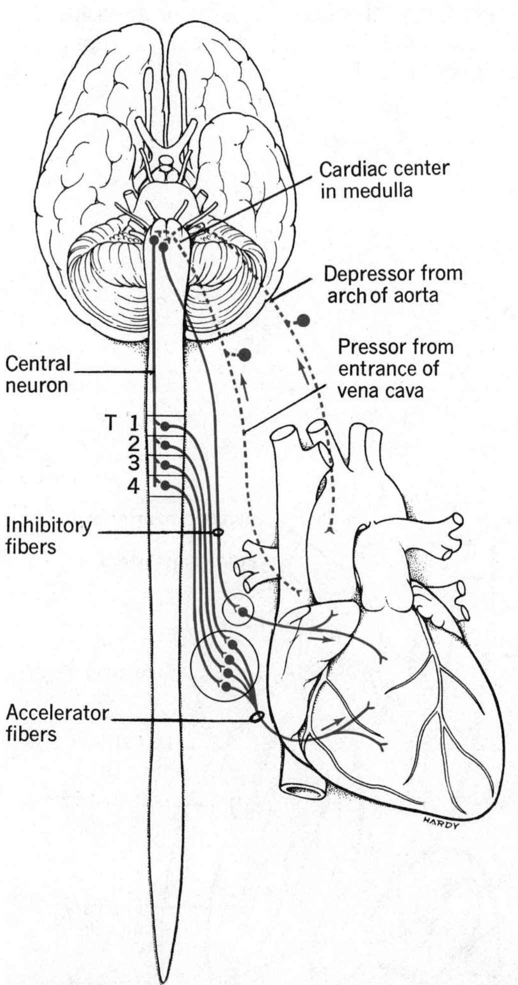

FIGURE 33–4 Diagram showing the nerve supply of the heart. Afferent pathways are indicated by dashed lines, efferent pathways by solid lines.

Electromechanical Cardiac Physiology

In the normal cardiac muscle cell, an electrical difference (voltage) exists between the inside and the outside of the cell across its membrane. The inside of the cell is negative relative to the outside of the cell. When the magnitude of this difference is reduced (the inside of the cell becomes less negative), *depolarization* has occurred and contraction of muscle cell results. A cardiac muscle cell is normally depolarized when a neighboring cell is depolarized (although it can also be depolarized by external electrical stimulation). Sufficient depolarization of a single specialized conduction system cell will therefore result in depolarization and contraction of the entire myocardium. *Repolarization* occurs as the cell returns to its baseline state (becomes more negative), and corresponds to relaxation of myocardial muscle.

During depolarization the permeability of the cell membranes to certain ions (sodium, chloride, calcium, potassium) changes. One of those changes results in an increased permeability to calcium, allowing for uptake of calcium into the cell. This increase in intracellular calcium concentration leads to shortening of the muscle fibers and development of tension (contraction). After a short period, the membrane voltage returns to its original value, the calcium that had accumulated in its interior is removed, and the cell relaxes.

Cardiac muscle, unlike skeletal or smooth muscle, has a prolonged refractory period during which it cannot be restimulated to contract. This protects the heart from sustained contraction (tetany), which would result in sudden cardiac death.

Normal electromechanical coupling and contraction of the heart are dependent on the composition of the fluid (extracellular fluid) surrounding the heart muscle cells. The composition of this fluid is in turn influenced by the composition of the blood. A change in blood calcium concentration may therefore alter contraction of the heart muscle fibers. A change in blood potassium concentration is also important since potassium affects the normal electrical voltage of the cell.

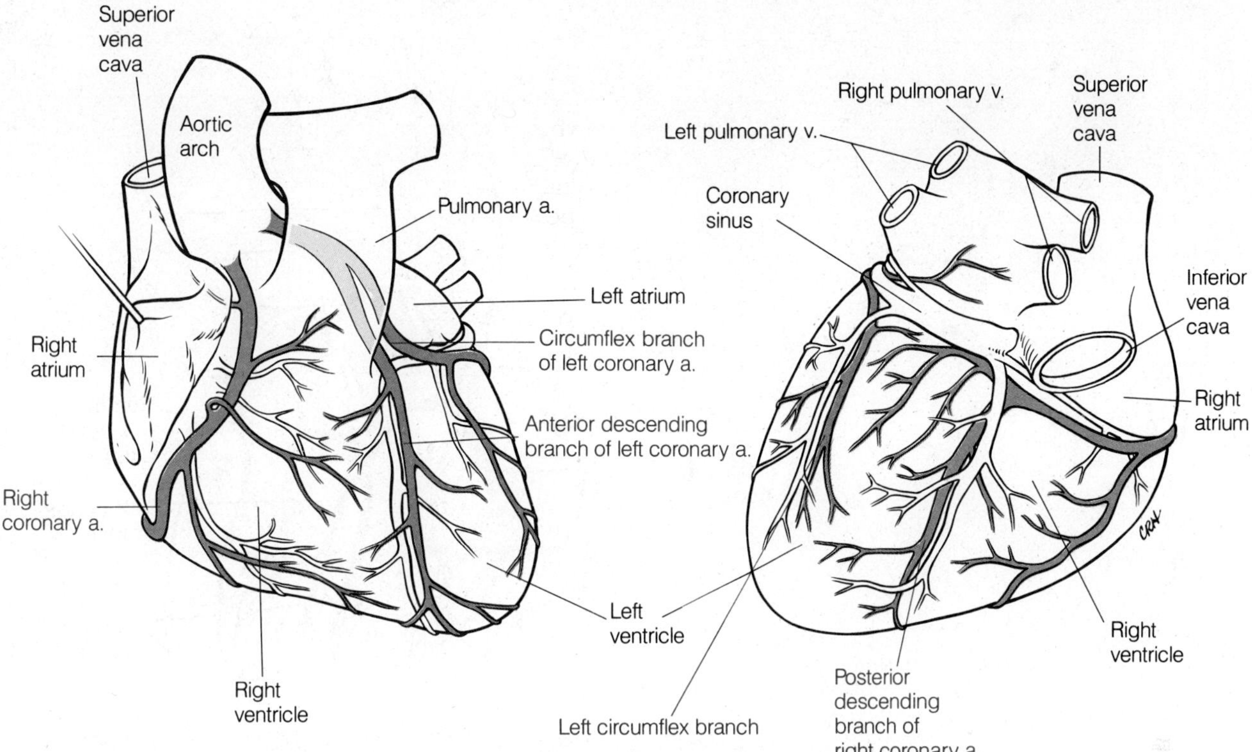

FIGURE 33–5 Diagram of the coronary arteries that arise from the aorta and some of the coronary veins.

Excitation of the Heart: The Conducting System

It is almost axiomatic that the heart possesses automaticity, as evidenced by the fact that a heart removed from the body can continue to contract. Impulse conduction in muscle is not very rapid, however, and there is a special mechanism to initiate impulses and rapidly deliver them to the entire muscle. This system of specialized tissue, known as the conducting system of the heart, is located just under the endocardium. It consists of modified muscle tissue which is striated and contracts but does not develop much tension. It is, however, capable of conducting impulses much more rapidly than ordinary cardiac muscle.

The conducting system is made up of several components: the SA node, the AV node, the AV bundle (bundle of His), with its right and left branches, and terminal branches or Purkinje fibers (Fig. 33–6). The SA node is located in the right atrium just below the entry of the superior vena cava and is the pacemaker of the heart. The vagal and sympathetic fibers that affect heart rate end in the vicinity of pacemaker cells in the SA node. Acetylcholine from vagal endings slows the heart rate; epinephrine and norepinephrine from the sympathetic nerve endings increase the heart rate.

An impulse generated in the SA node is conducted through atrial muscle to the AV node. The AV node is located on the right side of the interatrial septum. Conduction over the atria to the AV node is relatively slow, and it is also rather slow within the AV node. Once the AV node is excited, however, the impulse is rapidly conducted over the AV bundle to the ventricle.

The AV bundle arises from the AV node and passes down the interventricular septum a short distance before it divides into right and left bundle branches. The bundle branches descend on either side of the septum toward the apex and continue up the right and left sides of the heart, giving off numerous branches to the myocardium (including papillary muscles). The terminal Purkinje fibers ramify throughout the subendocardial surface and penetrate to reach deeper muscle fibers. The last portion of the heart to be depolarized is along the AV groove. Conduction through this system is rapid, and the entire ventricular myocardium is depolarized within about 0.08 to 0.1 sec, which causes virtually simultaneous contraction of all fibers.

Repolarization begins at the SA node and rapidly spreads over atria, which are repolarized by the time ventricular contraction begins. The sequence of ventricular repolarization is the same as that of depolarization, with surface repolarization appearing first at the apex, and last on the sides near the AV groove.

All parts of the conducting system are capable of initiating beats, but the SA node is the pacemaker because it depolarizes most rapidly. If it were destroyed the AV node may become the pacemaker, but the rate would be slower and the usual delay between atrial and ventricular contractions would be absent. If the more terminal portions of

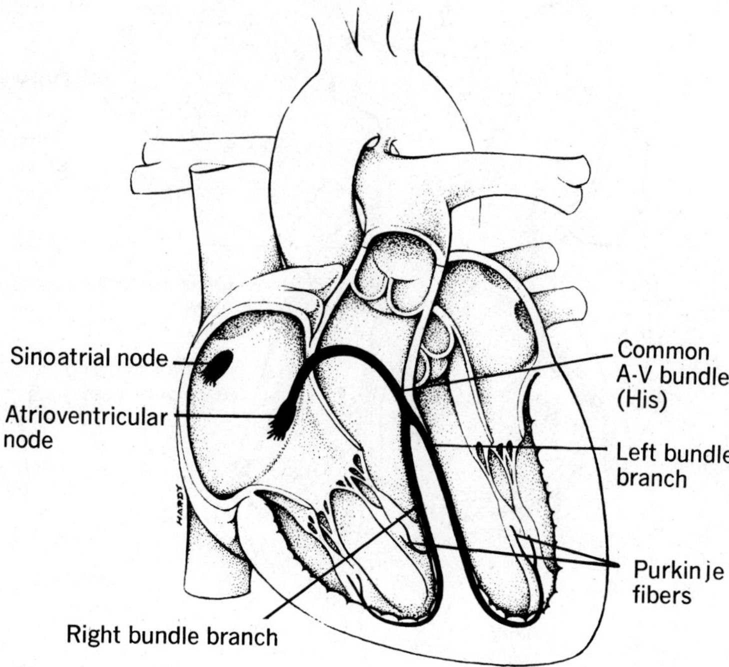

FIGURE 33–6 Conducting system. Diagram showing relations of the sinoatrial node, the atrioventricular node, the common atrioventricular bundle and its branches.

the conducting system were to begin rhythmic initiation of beats, the rate would be still slower. Although it is unlikely, the terminal portions are capable of becoming hyperirritable and initiating a single impulse or a series of impulses. The conduction pathway from such ectopic foci, of course, is not normal.

Cardiac Cycle

Cardiac events during a single beat are known as the cardiac cycle. Blood enters the atria at low pressure and leaves the ventricles at high enough pressure to drive it through the pulmonary and systemic circuits. Diastolic pressure in the left atrium and ventricle are only 1 to 2 mm higher than those on the right, but systolic pressure in the pulmonary artery is only about one sixth that in the aorta. The timing of pressure changes and of valve operations is essentially the same on the two sides.

During diastole, the AV valves are open and the semilunar (aortic and pulmonary) valves are closed. The pressure is relatively high in the arteries but is only a few mmHg in the right atrium and very slightly less in the ventricle. Blood from the venae cavae flows continuously into the right atrium and on into the right ventricle, and blood from the pulmonary veins flows continuously into the left atrium and ventricle.

The atria contract, causing a slight increase in atrial and ventricular pressure. The increase is small because most of the blood has already moved into the ventricles, and since there are no valves at the entrance to the atria, some blood tends to move back toward the veins when they contract.

Ventricular contraction begins, and ventricular pressures almost immediately exceed those in the atria. Blood moving back toward the atria closes the AV valves abruptly, and blocks that avenue of escape. The sudden closure of the AV valves (both tricuspid and mitral) sets off a series of low-frequency vibrations that cause the first heart sound. The chordae tendineae, and the papillary muscles to which they are attached, hold the valve cusps securely in position and prevent regurgitation of blood into the atria. The force of ventricular contraction and the slight bulging of the floor of the atria cause a tiny brief rise in atrial pressure.

As soon as the AV valves close, the ventricles are completely closed off. Continued contraction produces no change in ventricular volume, but the pressure within the chambers rises sharply; this is an isovolumetric (isometric) contraction. The pressure changes in the left and right ventricles operate the aortic and pulmonary valves in unison. When intraventricular pressure exceeds that in the aorta, the aortic valve is forced open. The pressure routinely measured as diastolic pressure is the pressure in the systemic artery just before the valve opens. As soon as the aortic valve opens, blood is forced into the aorta, and the arterial pressure rises to a peak, which is measured as systolic pressure. As the ventricle begins to relax, its pressure falls below that in the aorta, and blood tends to flow back into the ventricle. It catches in the pockets of the semilunar valve, closing it suddenly and firmly, and causing a momentary rise in the arterial pressure (the dicrotic notch). Sudden closure of the semilunar valves sets off oscillations in the column of blood in the artery that produce the second heart sound, which marks the end of systole and the beginning of diastole. When the semilunar valves snap shut, the ventricles are again closed off and pressure in the ventricles falls (isovolumetric relaxation). When it falls below that in the atria, the AV valves open and blood flows into the ventricles.

Blood continues to enter the atria while the AV valves are closed, and atrial pressure and volume rise slowly throughout systole. When the AV valves open, the accumulated blood enters the ventricle. It fills most rapidly during the early part of diastole, then more slowly, and with relatively little added by atrial contraction. Ventricular volume falls most rapidly at the beginning of ejection and tapers off as its volume and the force of contraction decline, and the opposing arterial pressure rises.

The beat takes about 0.8 sec, for a heart rate of 75 beats/min. Systole occupies about 0.3 sec and diastole 0.5 sec. At a heart rate of 120 beats/min, each cycle must be completed in 0.5 sec. Systole and diastole are both shortened, but diastole more so. If the heart rate reaches 180 beats/min, each cycle lasts only 0.33 sec, and the need for faster contraction and shorter systole is obvious, but filling time is seriously reduced. For many adults, maximum heart rates are in the range of 160 beats/min; beyond that, cardiac output begins to fall because of insufficient ventricular filling.

Pressure in the atria is always low, and pressure in the artery (aorta or pulmonary) is always high, while ventricular pressure varies from lower than in the atria during diastole to higher than in the artery during systole. After the semilunar valves close, pressure in the artery falls continually until the next ventricular contraction. The slope of the decline is determined by the rate at which blood flows from the arterial system into capillaries, and that is determined by the peripheral resistance. The diastolic pressure in the artery is a measure of the resistance each ventricle must overcome to fulfill its role as a pump; the left ventricular pressure must exceed the pressure in the aorta before any blood can be ejected. The systolic pressure represents the additional force that ejects blood against that pressure. The difference between them, the pulse pressure, indicates how well the ventricle has succeeded. An increase of either diastolic or systolic pressure forces the heart to develop more pressure or to pump less blood, or both, and thus increases the work of the heart.

Cardiac Output

The effectiveness of the heart is determined by the cardiac output, which is the volume of blood pumped by each ventricle in a minute. It is determined by the number of beats per minute, the heart rate, and the volume of blood pumped with each beat (the stroke volume). Based on average values of a resting heart rate of about 70 beats/min, and a stroke volume in the range of 70 ml/beat, the cardiac output would be about 5 liters/min. The total blood volume is also about 5 liters, so at rest the heart pumps all the blood each minute, and an average blood cell would make a complete circuit from right atrium to right atrium in a minute. The total blood flow required by the tissues ultimately depends upon their metabolic activity; in a resting adult it is about 70 ml/kg/min. An average-sized individual of 70 kg therefore requires a cardiac output in the range of 5 liters/min. Cardiac output correlates more closely with body surface area than with body weight, however, and is often expressed in terms of the cardiac index. For the 70 kg individual, this would be about 3.2 liters/min/m^2 body surface area.

Bibliography

Berne RM, Levy MN: Cardiovascular Physiology, 4th ed. St Louis, CV Mosby, 1981

Crouch JE: Functional Human Anatomy, 3rd ed, pp 402–426. Philadelphia, Lea & Febiger, 1978

Ganong WF: Review of Medical Physiology, 11th ed, pp 414–506. Los Altos, California, Lange Medical Publications, 1983

Landau BR: Essential Human Anatomy and Physiology, 2nd ed, pp 409–432; 477–492. Glenview, Illinois, Scott, Foresman & Company, 1980

Ross G: Essentials of Human Physiology, 2nd ed, pp 121–286. Chicago, Year Book Medical Publishers, 1982

Schmidt RF, Thews G: Human Physiology, pp 358–396. New York, Springer-Verlag, 1982

Tortora GJ: Principles of Human Anatomy, 3rd ed, pp 293–354. New York, Harper & Row, 1983

Vander AJ, Sherman JS, Luciano DS: Human Physiology: The Mechanisms of Body Function, 3rd ed, pp 253–326. New York, McGraw-Hill, 1980

Chapter 34

Assessment of Cardiac Function

Sandra L. Underhill

Nursing care is based on data obtained from assessment. A nursing assessment of a patient with heart disease includes taking a history, performing a physical examination, and interpreting basic tests that reflect cardiac function. In addition, nurses must be able to incorporate medical history data into the nursing assessment so that the interdependent nursing and medical responsibilities are completed in the correct priority sequence.[17,18]

Cardiovascular History

Cardiac patients who are acutely ill require a different initial history than do cardiac patients with stable or chronic problems. A patient experiencing an acute myocardial infarction (MI) requires immediate and possibly lifesaving medical and nursing interventions (*e.g.,* relief of chest discomfort and treatment of arrhythmias) rather than an extensive interview. For this patient, a few well-chosen questions regarding chest discomfort*, associated symptoms (such as shortness of breath or palpitations), drug allergies and reactions, current medications, history of other major illnesses, and smoking history should be asked at the same time one is assessing vital signs (heart rate and rhythm, and blood pressure) and starting an intravenous line. When the patient is more stable, a more extensive history should be obtained.[18]

It is important that nurses working in acute care facilities understand how to obtain both medical and nursing histories. The medical history does not necessarily need to be complete, but must provide enough data to make informed clinical judgments. When the physician takes the medical history during the patient's hospital admission, the nurse's responsibilities are to be aware of the data collected, validate her own findings, and compare episodes of the same symptoms that occur during hospitalization with the patient's previous experiences.[18]

Medical History

Medical history taking is divided into three main areas: the patient's chief complaint, the history of the present illness, and the personal and family medical history.

* Patients do not always admit to having chest "pain"; therefore, "pain equivalents" should be used when eliciting the quality of discomfort. Common descriptions used by patients include strangling, constriction, tightness, aching, squeezing, pressure, heaviness, expansion, choking in the throat, indigestion, and burning.

Chief Complaint

The chief complaint is the reason why the patient came to the hospital and represents his priority for treatment. It should be recorded within quotation marks exactly as stated. The chief complaint should also indicate duration, for example, "shortness of breath for 1 week."

Occasionally, a patient may have more than one chief complaint. These should be listed in the order of importance to the patient. If the patient has more than three chief complaints, they should be recorded with the history of present illness.

History of Present Illness

To describe history taking, a sample symptom, chest discomfort, will be used throughout this explanation. Obtaining the history of the present illness starts with a more detailed discussion of the chief complaint, for example, "Tell me more about your chest discomfort." There is a wide range in patients' abilities to express thoughts accurately, logically, and succinctly. Some patients need guidance more than others. Listen to the patient. It is best to let him tell his story in the most comfortable manner. However, patients who appear to be rambling need to be redirected by clarifying or leading questions.

The information that must be obtained when describing any symptom is the time and manner of onset, duration, frequency, location, quality, quantity, setting, associated phenomena, and alleviating or aggravating factors. Pertinent negative answers should also be listed.

The time of onset should also be recorded when possible with both the date and time, for example, "9 PM on December 22nd." The manner of onset is the factor or factors that usually precipitate the symptom, for instance, "chest pain brought on by an unusually heavy meal." Frequency and duration should be stated specifically rather than generally. Statements such as "I have chest pain a lot of the time" has meaning only to the patient. Descriptions such as "once a week," "once a day," or "more than three times a day" provide much more information. Likewise, a response that the pain lasts just a "short time" is subjective and should be restated as, for example, "2 minutes," "15 minutes," or "1 hour."

The patient describes the exact location of the symptom by pointing to it with one finger. If the pain radiates, the patient should trace its path with a fingertip. The unique qualities of a symptom should be noted, such as color, appearance, and texture. Pain, the most common symptom of cardiovascular disease, is so subjective that its quality is particularly difficult to describe. Thus, whenever possible, it is important to use the patient's own words (in quotation marks). Terms such as dull, sharp, stabbing, burning, aching, crushing, or throbbing are frequently used. To better understand the meaning of the symptoms to the patient, his response to it should be recorded, for example, "It makes me stop what I'm doing and sit down," or "I can continue my activities without stopping."

Quantity refers to the size, extent, or number of the symptoms. The quantity of the chest discomfort is described in terms of its severity. Again, this is extremely subjective and might best be rated on a ten-point scale, ranging from "barely noticeable" (1) to "the worst pain I've ever had" (10). The severity of the pain should be charted as a fraction, for example 2/10 or 10/10.

Ask the patient to describe the setting and if he was alone or with someone else when the symptoms occurred. If the symptom has occurred before, ascertain if the setting, the circumstances, or the presence of another person is consistent during symptom onset. This information may be useful later in counseling or teaching a patient insight into the development of his symptoms.

The patient should be asked if any other symptoms are associated with the chief complaint. For example, palpitations and dizziness might always precede the chest pain. If the patient mentions associated symptoms, these should be described in the same manner as the chief complaint. It is also important to note whether associated symptoms also occur independently.

Factors that improve the symptom, for instance, resting, changing position, or taking medication, should be noted. Likewise, conditions that make the chief complaint worse, such as eating, exercising, or being in a cold climate, must also be recorded. These factors can provide helpful diagnostic information. To complete the present illness history, it is also important to record any negative responses to the interviewer's questions, for example, "The chest pain is not made worse by strenuous exercise."

Personal and Family Medical History

The medical history is divided into two sections: personal and family. The personal history includes past illnesses, allergies, immunizations, habits, social history, and medications taken regularly. Usual childhood diseases, injuries, operations, or other major illnesses should be recorded under past illnesses. When discussing childhood diseases, the nurse should specifically question the patient about streptococcal infection, and the possibility of rheumatic fever. The major illnesses that should be specifically asked about are previous chest discomfort or heart attack, high blood pressure, chronic obstructive airway disease, diabetes mellitus, or bleeding disorders.

Any allergic reaction, for example, to drugs, food, environmental agents, or animals, should also be noted. The examiner should always ask if the patient has an allergy to penicillin and, if so, what the reaction consists of. The nurse should also inquire about allergic reactions to commonly used emergency drugs, such as lidocaine hydrochloride and morphine sulfate. Both the allergen and the reaction should always be noted, because some patients confuse an allergic reaction with a drug's side-effect. Alcohol, drug, and tobacco habits must also be recorded. The smoking history should always be known prior to oxygen administration and recorded as the number of pack-years (packs per day multiplied by the number of years) the patient has smoked.

Social history includes marital status, number of children, occupation, and hobbies. Any other pertinent lifestyle pattern can also be noted, for example, particular dietary habits. It is important that all prescription and over-the-counter drugs, and home remedies that the patient takes be known. If the patient has brought his medication with him, it should be sent home or to the pharmacy for verification and safekeeping.

A family history is taken to determine the health status of the patient's immediate family. Notations about the age and health status of each family member are made, both for those who are living and those who are deceased, with the possible or confirmed diagnosis now or at death. This information can be written into the health record or diagrammed on a family tree.

Nursing History

When caring for an acutely ill cardiac patient, one must focus first on assessment of the heart and cardiac output. Patients with atherosclerotic coronary heart disease (CHD) commonly experience chest discomfort, shortness of breath, fatigue, reduced urine output, changes in mentation, palpitations, loss of consciousness, edema and weight gain, and postural hypotension with dizziness and light-headedness. Patients with valvular heart disease may also have symptoms of right or left heart failure, arrhythmias, or chest discomfort.

Chest Pain

Not all chest discomfort is related to myocardial ischemia. Guidelines are useful in differentiating chest discomfort due to serious, life threatening conditions from that due to less serious conditions or to conditions that would be treated in a different manner. However, there are four important points to remember when evaluating chest discomfort[17]:

1. In a patient who has a history of or who is at risk for developing coronary heart disease, always assume that the chest discomfort is secondary to ischemia until proven otherwise. This is because unrelieved myocardial ischemia is immediately life threatening and can extend the size of the infarcted area of the heart, resulting in serious complications such as lethal arrhythmias or cardiogenic shock. Chest discomfort related to other conditions, such as pulmonary emboli, usually is not as *immediately* life threatening.
2. There may be little correlation between the severity of the chest discomfort and the gravity of its cause. That is, pain is subjective and depends in part on a lifetime of experiences. A stoic individual may not admit to having much discomfort and yet may be having a large MI. Another individual may express extreme pain and yet may be experiencing stable angina rather than an acute MI. Stress can increase pain. Taking into account the patient's usual response to pain (often obtained from a family member) and the patient's sociocultural heritage will assist the nurse to better interpret the patient's pain response. Positive objective signs such as changes in the electrocardiogram (ECG) are, however, clear indicators of the importance of the subjective symptom. It is important to realize that negative electrocardiographic criteria do not rule out the clinical significance of the chest pain.
3. There is often poor correlation between the location of chest discomfort and its source because of "referred pain"—pain originating in one location but being interpreted by the patient as occurring in another location. Commonly with cardiac pain, the discomfort is perceived as being in the arm, jaw, neck, or epigastric area rather than in the chest, when in fact it is due to myocardial ischemia.
4. The patient may have more than one clinical problem occurring simultaneously, particularly in light of the economy, which has caused many patients not to seek medical assistance until a crisis arises. Problems that would ordinarily have been detected and treated during clinic visits have not been, because many patients cannot afford elective medical care. The hospitalized patient of the 1980s is far sicker than the hospitalized patient of the 1970s.

Assessment of Cardiac Function

For the acutely ill cardiac patient, the areas that reflect cardiac function are assessed first. To facilitate the gathering of subjective information for a cardiac nursing history, examples of questions, using the sample symptom of chest discomfort, follow. However, it is important to phrase the questions according to the appropriateness of the situation and to pursue logically areas where further clarification is necessary. When the patient's condition permits, all other functional areas should be assessed.[17,18]

1. Circulation

   Chest discomfort (use the same format for additional symptoms)

   Do you ever have any chest discomfort?
   When exactly do you get the discomfort?
   What were you doing when the chest discomfort occurred?
   Exactly how often does the chest discomfort occur?
   How many minutes does it usually last?
   Can you point to the exact location where it starts?
   Does the discomfort move anywhere else?
   If so, can you trace its path with your fingertip?
   What words would you use to describe how the discomfort feels?
   What do you do when you have the chest discomfort?
   Quantify your pain on a 1-to-10 scale.
   Where were you when the pain occurred?
   If the chest discomfort has occurred before, has the setting been the same?
   Were you alone at the time or with someone else?
   Did you notice any other symptoms that occurred at the same time?
   If yes, does this other symptom ever occur by itself?
   What can you do to make the chest pain better?
   What can you do to make it worse?
   What activities are necessary for you to do that you are no longer able to do because of your chest discomfort?

Are you on any medication to improve your chest discomfort?
Does any medication you are taking affect your chest If yes, what is the medication?
Does any medication you are taking affect your chest discomfort?
What time of day do you prefer to take your medication?

Additional symptoms related to circulation
Weight gain or loss
Swelling in the hands, feet, or legs (or, if bedridden, the sacrum)
Dizziness
Fatigue
Lightheadedness
Palpitations
Manifestations of high blood pressure (such as headaches)
Coldness of hands or feet

2. Breathing
Are you ever short of breath?
When do you become short of breath?
How do you make your breathing better?
What makes it worse?
How long has breathing been a problem?
What activities are necessary for you to do that you are no longer able to do because of your breathing?
Are you taking any medication to improve your breathing?
If yes, what is the medication?
Does any medication that you are on affect your breathing?
If yes, what is the medication?
What time of day do your prefer to take your medication?

3. Urination
Is the amount of your urine output normal for you?
Do you ever get up at night to use the bathroom?
How many times?
When did you notice the change?
Do you take a diuretic?
When do you take it?

4. Mentation?
Do you think as fast as you used to? as clearly?
Do you laugh or cry more easily than before?
When did you notice the change?
Are you taking any medication that might affect your thinking?

Other Data

Information obtained from the nursing history is necessary to formulate nursing diagnoses, to plan individualized care while the patient is hospitalized, and to aid in discharge planning, including appropriate teaching. Knowledge of the patient's perceptions of the effects of the disease process on activities of daily living will enable you to identify specific aims for cardiac rehabilitation, or to devise strategies for modifying certain activities. Since dietary modification (reduction of sodium, saturated and total fats, and calories) will probably be prescribed, assess the following:

Food preferences (including cultural or ethnic favorites)
Eating habits (canned or commercially prepared foods versus fresh foods; restaurant or fast-food dining versus home cooking)
Who shops for groceries?
Who prepares the meals?

Knowledge of the patient's health insurance and financial status assists the nurse in advocating an affordable therapeutic regimen, for example, avoiding expensive combination or sustained-release medications when drugs that are as effective and less costly are available. Knowing the patient's risk for coronary heart disease enables the nurse to help the patient identify behaviors that may be contributing to the progression of his heart disease, and to devise a realistic plan for modifying those behaviors.

Cardiac Status and Prognosis

After the history is completed, it may be possible to categorize the patient according to the New York Heart Association's Cardiac Status and Prognosis Classification.[13] This classification, which replaces the New York Heart Association's Functional and Therapeutic Classification, may be helpful in the management of the patient's activities. The classification of cardiac status includes etiologic, anatomic, and physiologic diagnoses. The classification of prognosis is based on the potential efforts of optimal current medical and surgical care. The four subdivisions of each classification are

Cardiac Status	*Prognosis*
1. Uncompromised	1. Good
2. Slightly compromised	2. Good with therapy
3. Moderately compromised	3. Fair with therapy
4. Severely compromised	4. Guarded despite therapy

However, the New York Heart Association's Functional and Therapeutic Classification is still being used in the clinical setting (Table 34–1).[13a] According to the functional part of this classification system, the person may be classified as I, II, III, or IV, depending on the degree to which activities of daily living are affected by the heart disease. The therapeutic aspects of classification are categorized as A, B, C, D, or E, depending on the amount of activity restrictions called for.

Physical Assessment

Assessment of physical findings should confirm data obtained in the medical and nursing histories. Baseline information is obtained on admission. Until the examiner becomes skilled in physical assessment, the initial findings should be validated by an experienced clinician. In the acutely ill cardiac patient, physical examination includes routine vital signs taken every 4 hours, or more frequently if indicated. As the patient improves, assessments are done once per shift, and progress to once per day until discharge. Because they spend 24 hours a day with the patient, nurses are in the best position to identify any changes that may

TABLE 34–1
Functional and Therapeutic Classifications of Patients with Diseases of the Heart

Functional Classification		*Therapeutic Classification*	
Class I	Patients with cardiac disease but without resulting limitations of physical activity. Ordinary physical activity does not cause undue fatigue, palpitation, dyspnea, or anginal pain.	Class A	Patients with cardiac disease whose physical activity need not be restricted in any way.
		Class B	Patients with cardiac disease whose ordinary physical activity need not be restricted, but who should be advised against severe or competitive efforts.
Class II	Patients with cardiac disease resulting in slight limitation of physical activity. They are comfortable at rest. Ordinary physical activity results in fatigue, palpitation, dyspnea, or anginal pain.	Class C	Patients with cardiac disease whose ordinary physical activity should be moderately restricted, and whose more strenuous efforts should be discontinued.
Class III	Patients with cardiac disease resulting in marked limitation of physical activity. They are comfortable at rest. Less than ordinary physical activity causes fatigue, palpitation, dyspnea, or anginal pain.	Class D	Patients with cardiac disease whose ordinary physical activity should be markedly restricted.
Class IV	Patients with cardiac disease resulting in inability to carry on any physical activity without discomfort. Symptoms of cardiac insufficiency or of the anginal syndrome may be present even at rest. If any physical activity is undertaken, discomfort is increased.	Class E	Patients with cardiac disease who should be at complete rest, confined to bed or chair.

(New York Heart Association)

occur. It is to the patient's benefit for the nurse to detect changes early, before serious complications develop. The cardiac care unit nurse who telephones the physician to report that the patient "just does not look good" lacks the credibility of the nurse who identifies "a new S_3 gallop, bilateral crackles halfway up the posterior lung fields, and jugular venous distension of 14 cm." Any changes observed in the assessment should be recorded in the patient's record and reported to the physician.

A cardiac physical assessment should include an evaluation of the following:

- The heart as a pump: reduced pulse pressure, cardiac enlargement, and presence of murmurs and gallop rhythms
- Filling volumes and pressures: the degree of jugular vein distention, and the presence or absence of crackles, peripheral edema, and postural changes in blood pressure
- Cardiac output: heart rate, pulse pressure, systemic vascular resistance, urine output, and central nervous system manifestations.
- Compensatory mechanisms: increased filling volumes, peripheral vasoconstriction, and elevated heart rate

The examination proceeds logically from head to toe, and with practice can be done in approximately 10 minutes. The areas examined include general appearance, blood pressure, radial pulse, the hands, the head and neck, the heart, the lungs, the abdomen, and the feet and legs.

General Appearance

Observe the patient's level of distress. Level of consciousness should be noted and described. Appropriateness of thought content, reflecting the adequacy of cerebral perfusion, is particularly important to evaluate. Family members who are most familiar with the patient can be of help in alerting the examiner to subtle behavior changes. The nurse should also be aware of the patient's anxiety level, not only to attempt to put him more at ease, but to realize its effect upon the cardiovascular system.

Blood Pressure

The technique of blood pressure measurement is described in Chapter 44. Important points to remember are as follows[10]:

- The cuff size must be appropriate for the patient.
- The sphygmomanometer should be calibrated correctly.

- The patient's arm should be at heart level.
- Initial recordings should be made on both arms, and subsequent measurements should be taken on the arm with the highest pressure.
- The position of the patient and the site of blood pressure measurement should be recorded.
- The presence of an auscultatory gap (see Chap. 44) should be considered, especially in patients with high blood pressure. To avoid obtaining falsely low systolic blood pressures, palpate prior to auscultating the systolic pressure.

Evaluate the patient's current blood pressure. If it differs greatly from usual, immediate intervention may be required. Blood pressures greater than 140/90 mmHg increase the heart's work and oxygen consumption. Blood pressures less than 90/60 mmHg may further reduce blood and oxygen delivery to an already compromised myocardium. Taking into account symptoms of myocardial ischemia and adequacy of cerebral and peripheral perfusion may enable the examiner to judge more accurately the clinical significance of blood pressure changes in the cardiac patient.

Pulse Pressure

Pulse pressure is the difference between the systolic and diastolic blood pressures, expressed in mmHg. For example, if the blood pressure is 110/70 mmHg, the pulse pressure is 40 mmHg. Pulse pressure reflects stroke volume, ejection velocity, and systemic vascular resistance. Use pulse pressure as a noninvasive indicator of the patient's ability to maintain cardiac output. If the pulse pressure in the cardiac patient falls below 30 mmHg, further assessment of the patient's cardiovascular status may be indicated.

Postural Blood Pressure Changes

Postural (orthostatic) hypotension occurs when the blood pressure drops after an upright posture is assumed, and is usually accompanied by dizziness, lightheadedness, or syncope. Although there are many causes of postural hypotension, the three most commonly seen in the cardiac patient are saline depletion; inadequate vasoconstrictor mechanism, which prevents the blood vessels from constricting properly; and autonomic insufficiency, which interferes with nervous system control of heart rate. Postural changes in blood pressure, along with appropriate history, can help the clinician determine the cause. Important points to remember are as follows[18]:

- Position the patient supine and as flat as symptoms permit for 10 minutes prior to the initial measurement of blood pressure and heart rate.
- Always check supine measurements prior to upright measurements.
- Always record both heart rate and blood pressure at each postural change (lying, sitting, standing).
- Do not remove the blood pressure cuff between position changes, but do check to see that it remains placed correctly.
- Assess postural blood pressure changes with the patient sitting on the edge of the bed with feet dangling. If an anticipated fall in blood pressure does not occur, or if you are assessing the patient for safety in ambulation, check the blood pressure again with the patient standing. Carefully monitor the patient while he is standing to prevent a fall.
- Wait 1 to 3 minutes after each postural change prior to measuring blood pressure and heart rate. (This wait provides a convenient time to auscultate the posterior lung fields with the patient in the sitting position.)
- Be alert for any signs or symptoms of patient distress, and if necessary return the patient to bed prior to test completion.
- Record any signs or symptoms that accompany the postural change.

Normal responses to postural changes include increased heart rate (to offset reduced stroke volume and to maintain cardiac output); a slight-to-15 mmHg drop in systolic pressure; and a slight drop to an increase of 5 to 10 mmHg in diastolic pressure.[4,5,16]

In the presence of a history of saline loss (such as with diuretic therapy), saline depletion should be suspected when, in response to sitting or standing, the heart rate increases, and *either* the systolic pressure decreases by 15 mmHg *or* the diastolic blood pressure drops by 10 mmHg.[14] It is difficult to differentiate saline depletion from inadequate vasoconstrictor mechanisms by postural changes in vital signs alone. With saline depletion, reflexes to maintain cardiac output (increased heart rate and peripheral vasoconstriction) function correctly, but because of lost extracellular fluid volume, these reflexes are not adequate to maintain systemic arterial pressure, and the blood pressure falls. With inadequate vasoconstrictor mechanisms, the heart rate again responds appropriately, but because of diminished peripheral vasoconstriction, blood pressure drops. Differentiation, therefore, depends in part on the history. However, it is important to note that saline depletion and inadequate vasoconstrictor mechanisms are not mutually exclusive.

In autonomic insufficiency, the heart rate is unable to increase to compensate for the gravitational effects of upright posture. Autonomic insufficiency may be due to primary dysfunction of the reflexes controlled by the autonomic nervous system. More commonly, however, it is due to the actions of drugs such as digoxin, β-adrenergic blocking agents, or calcium channel blockers that prevent the heart rate from responding to a reduction in cardiac output. Peripheral vasoconstriction may be absent or diminished. The presence of autonomic insufficiency does not rule out concurrent saline depletion.

Radial Pulse

Rate and Rhythm. Each pulse wave is indicative of a cardiac contraction. However, each cardiac contraction does not necessarily result in a peripheral pulse. (Extremely fast heart rates or premature beats have shortened diastolic filling times, resulting in an inadequate stroke volume and, therefore, diminished or absent pulses.) The radial artery is the most common site for counting the pulse rate. For cardiac patients who are not acutely ill, if the pulse rhythm is regular, the rate can be counted radially for 15 seconds and multiplied by four to determine the pulse rate per minutes. For any patient, if the pulse rhythm is irregular, the pulse should be counted simultaneously both apically and radially for one full minute, and any discrepancy between contractions heard and pulses felt should be noted. Apical–radial differences commonly occur with atrial fibrillation and premature beats, such as premature ventricular contractions. It is important that the apical–radial rates be counted during the *same* minute. If the apical–radial difference is very large, if the rate is very fast, or if the examiner is not yet very skilled, it may be helpful to have two people count for the same minute.

Quality. Normally, the upstroke of the pulse wave is smooth and rapid. Small, weak pulses indicate a diminished pulse pressure. Large, bounding pulses indicate increased pulse pressure. Because the radial artery is small and peripheral, subtle qualities of the pulse wave will not be detected as easily as in larger, more central arteries (such as the carotid or femoral).

Hand

In the cardiac patient, the following are the most important findings to note when examining the hands:

- *Peripheral cyanosis.* Peripheral cyanosis implies decreased blood flow rate in the periphery, which allows more time for the hemoglobin molecule to become desaturated. This may occur normally with peripheral vasoconstriction associated with a cold environment, or pathologically in conditions that reduce blood flow, for example, cardiogenic shock.
- *Pallor.* Pallor can denote anemia (with concomitant decreased oxygen-carrying capacity) or an increased systemic vascular resistance.
- *Capillary refill time.* Capillary refill time provides an estimate of the rate of peripheral blood flow. Capillary refill time is assessed by pinching the finger or toe and then releasing the pressure, noting how long it takes for a normal color to return. Normally, reperfusion occurs almost instantaneously. More sluggish reperfusion indicates a slower peripheral rate, for example, in heart failure.
- *Hand temperature and moistness.* Hand temperature and moistness are controlled by the autonomic nervous system. Normally, hands are warm and dry. Under stress, they may be cool and moist: In cardiogenic shock, hands become cold and clammy.
- *Skin mobility.* Skin mobility is decreased by edema.
- *Skin turgor.* Skin turgor is reduced in dehydration and aging.
- *Clubbing.* Clubbing of the fingers (and toes) implies chronic hemoglobin desaturation, as in congenital heart disease, but rarely may be a normal variant.

Head and Neck

Head. In examining the head, the cardiac nurse needs to be concerned primarily with checking the lips and earlobes for peripheral cyanosis, and the buccal mucosa for central cyanosis. In central cyanosis, hemoglobin never becomes fully saturated with oxygen. It implies serious heart or lung disease and is accompanied by peripheral cyanosis. In severe heart disease, a right-to-left shunt exists in which blood passes through the lungs without being oxygenated, as happens in severe congestive heart failure with interstitial pulmonary edema. In severe lung disease, changes produced by chronic obstruction airway disease or fibrosis prevent oxygenation.

Jugular Vein Distention (Neck). Jugular vein distention is caused by filling volume and pressure on the right side of the heart. Jugular veins act like manometers: blood in the jugular veins assumes the level that corresponds to the central venous pressure (CVP). Central venous pressure reflects right atrial or right ventricular end-diastolic pressure. The normal jugular vein distention is 4 to 10 cm. Jugular venous distention greater than 10 cm reflects right ventricular failure and is a late finding in left ventricular failure. To measure jugular vein distention,

1. Begin with the patient supine, although the backrest can be elevated for patient comfort.
2. Visualize the neck veins (either the internal or external jugular veins can be used).
3. Position the patient's backrest so that the meniscus in the neck vein can be seen below the angle of the patient's jaw.
4. Determine heart level by finding the phlebostatic axis (fourth intercostal space at the sternum, intersecting the mid anterior–posterior line; Fig. 34–1, *A*).
5. Occlude the neck vein at the angle of the jaw and observe the level of the meniscus. (Do not strip the vein, because backfilling of blood may be prevented by a venous valve.)
6. Measure the *vertical* distance between the phlebostatic axis and the meniscus with a centimeter ruler. The distance in centimeters corresponds to the CVP (Fig. 34–1, *B*).

Lungs

Respiratory findings frequently exhibited by cardiac patients include the following:

- *Tachypnea.* Rapid, shallow breathing may be noted in patients who have heart failure or pain, or who are extremely anxious.
- *Cheyne-Stokes Respirations.* Patients in severe left ventricular failure may exhibit Cheyne-Stokes breathing. Of particular importance is the duration of the apneic period.
- *Hemoptysis.* Pink, frothy sputum is indicative of pulmonary edema.
- *Cough.* A dry, hacking cough from irritation of small airways is common in patients with pulmonary congestion from heart failure.
- *Crackles.* Heart failure, or atelectasis associated with bed rest, splinting from ischemic pain, or the effects of pain medicine and sedatives, often result in development of crackles. Typically, crackles are first noted at the bases (because of gravity's effect on fluid accu-

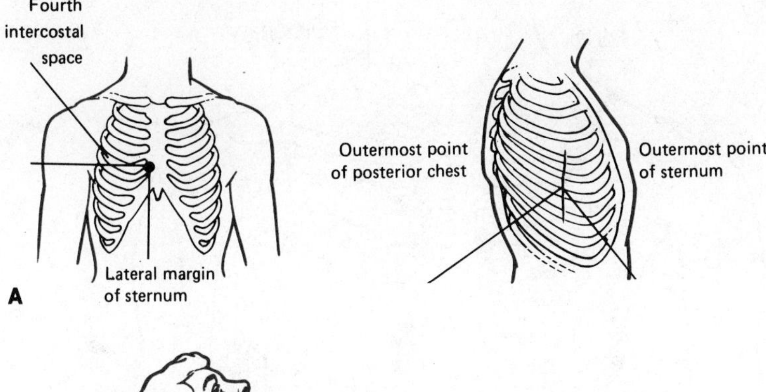

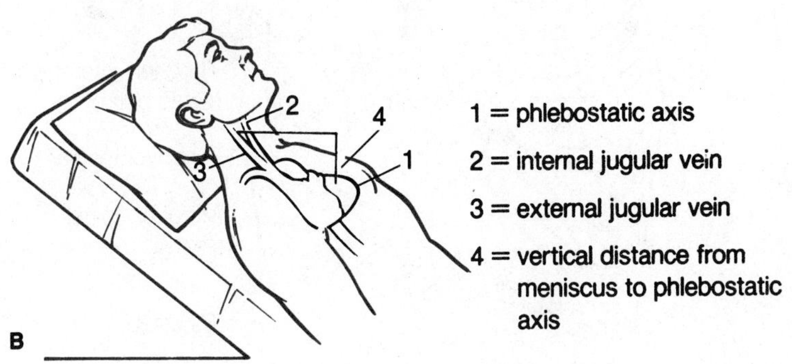

FIGURE 34–1 Assessment of jugular vein distension. (*A*) The phlebostatic axis is the crossing of two reference lines: a line from the fourth intercostal space at a point where it joins the sternum, drawn out to the side beneath the axilla; and a line midpoint between the anterior and posterior surfaces of the chest. (*B*) The reference point used in assessing jugular distension: (*1*) the phlebostatic axis, (*2* and *3*) the internal and external jugular veins, and (*4*) the vertical distance from the meniscus to the phlebostatic axis.

mulation and decreased ventilation of basilar tissue), but may progress to all portions of the lung fields.

- *Wheezes.* Compression of small airways by interstitial pulmonary edema may cause wheezing. Beta-blocking agents, such as propranolol, may precipitate airway narrowing, especially in patients with underlying pulmonary disease.

Abdomen

For the cardiac patient, two components of the abdominal examination are frequently performed:

- *Determination of liver size.* Liver engorgement occurs because of decreased venous return secondary to right ventricular failure. The liver will be enlarged, firm, nontender, and smooth. *Hepatojugular reflux* may be demonstrated by pressing firmly over the liver for 30 to 60 seconds and noting a 1-cm rise in jugular vein distention.
- *Assessment of bladder distention.* Urine output is an important indicator of cardiac output. In a patient who is unable to void (*i.e.,* secondary to strict bed rest or following atropine sulfate administration) or who has not voided in spite of adequate fluid intake, always assess for bladder distention prior to initiating other measures.

Feet and Legs

Many patients with heart disease have associated peripheral vascular disease or peripheral edema secondary to heart failure. In addition, many cardiac patients undergo cardiac catheterization, which can compromise arterial circulation. Also, thrombophlebitis is a complication associated with bed rest and requires careful monitoring. Therefore, adequacy of peripheral arterial circulation and venous return should be assessed in all cardiac patients.

Cardiac Assessment

The precordium should be assessed in an orderly fashion. The precordial areas that are named for the heart valves are actually located over the valvular outflow tracts rather than over the valves themselves. Seven precordial areas should be examined (Fig. 34–2):

1. The aortic valve area is the second right intercostal space.
2. The pulmonic valve area is the second left intercostal space.
3. The tricuspid valve area is at the lower left sternal border.
4. The mitral valve area is at the apex of the heart.
5. The right ventricular area is over the lower half of the sternum and the left parasternal area.
6. The third left intercostal space, Erb's point, is where selected abnormalities of the aortic or pulmonic valves may be detected.
7. The epigastric area is where aortic or right ventricular pulsations can be detected.

The techniques of inspection, palpation, percussion, and auscultation should be used, in that order, when performing a cardiac examination. The patient's room should be quiet and permit privacy. For the cardiac nurse, it is most important to establish a baseline so that change can be documented rather than to diagnose a particular problem.

Inspection

For proper inspection of the precordium, the patient should be supine and flat, with chest exposed. Tangential lighting, or light shone from the side (*e.g.,* a gooseneck lamp or a penlight), rather than overhead lighting, should be used

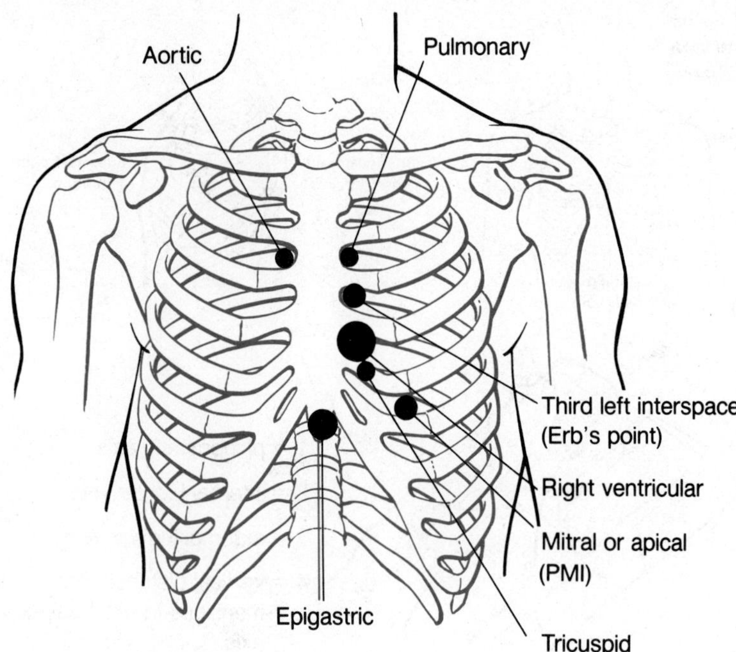

FIGURE 34–2 Areas to be assessed in the precordial examination.

so that shadows are cast on the anterior chest wall, allowing the examiner to detect more easily any movement. It may also be helpful for the examiner to crouch down so that the chest wall is at eye level. Any pulsating movement over any of the seven areas should be noted.

Except at the mitral area, movement over any of the valvular outflow tracts is abnormal. For example, pulsation over the second right intercostal space may represent an aortic aneurysm, and pulsation over the second left intercostal space could represent increased filling pressure or flow in the pulmonary artery. Slight movement over the sternum can be normal in thin individuals and in those with fever or anemia who may have hyperdynamic heartbeats. However, a sternal rise which is sustained after cardiac contraction indicates right ventricular enlargement.

Normally, the point of maximum impulse (PMI) or apical impulse can be seen at the apex. It should lie within the fifth intercostal space, medial to the midclavicular line, and should have a rapid upstroke and downstroke. The PMI cannot be seen in every patient. In thin patients it is easily detected, whereas in those who have large breasts or barrel chests, or who are obese, it may not be visible. A PMI that is below the fifth intercostal space, lateral to the midclavicular line, or seen in more than one intercostal space represents left ventricular enlargement.

Paradoxical movement of the left anterior precordium is suggestive of a left ventricular aneurysm. With paradoxical movement, as the apex contracts, the aneurysmic area bulges. This ectopic impulse is usually seen above the PMI. Pulsations in the epigastric area may be normal in very thin individuals, but may also represent an abnormality.

Palpation

Abnormal movement that was not visible on inspection may be detected by palpation. However, some movement is more easily seen than felt. All seven areas should be palpated, using either the heel of the hand (the palmar surface of the hand at the wrist), the ulnar surface of the hand, or the fingers. The heel or ulnar surfaces are more sensitive to thrills (vibrations), whereas the fingers are more sensitive to pulsations. Thrills indicate turbulence of blood blow and are associated with murmurs.

First, examine the sternal area for a right ventricular lift or heave. Next, palpate the four valvular outflow tract areas and Erb's point, starting with the aortic area, then moving to the pulmonic area, Erb's point, the tricuspid area, and last, the mitral area.

Assess the PMI for location, size, amplitude, and duration. The normal PMI is felt as a light tap, extending over 1 to 2 cm or less. The PMI is felt immediately following the first heart sound, and lasts halfway through systole. An impulse that is diffuse (felt over two intercostal spaces) or sustained throughout systole represents left ventricular enlargement. Palpate for paradoxical movement. If the PMI cannot be felt with the patient lying supine, examine the patient while he lies on his left side, which will bring the apex of the heart against the chest wall; the quality of the apex beat can still be determined even though its size and position cannot.

Aortic or right ventricular pulsations can be felt in the epigastric area. By placing the palmar surface of the hand over the epigastrum and sliding the fingers under the rib cage, the examiner can differentiate these pulsations. Pulsations beating downward against the fingertips indicate right ventricular movement, whereas those pushing forward originate in the aorta. An increased aortic pulse could indicate abdominal aortic aneurysm or aortic regurgitation.

Percussion

Percussion is used to evaluate the size of the heart. The technique of mediate percussion involves the examiner placing the passive hand firmly over the area to be percussed and striking the distal interphalangeal joint of the middle finger of that hand (the pleximeter) with the middle finger of the opposite hand (the plexor; Fig. 34–3).

Five sounds are identifiable through percussion: resonance, hyperresonance, tympany, dullness, and flatness (Table 34–2). Resonance is a sustained moderate pitch, elicited over lung tissue. Hyperresonance is a moderate to high-pitched sound that is sustained longer than resonance and is heard over air-filled lungs. Tympany is a musical, higher-pitched tone than heard in resonance and is sustained the longest. It reflects air in closed structures (such as the stomach and intestines) which vibrates with the surrounding tissue. Dullness is a short, high-pitched sound heard over relatively airless solid tissue such as the heart and liver. Flatness is another short high-pitched sound that is elicited from percussing solid tissue with the least amount of trapped air, such as the arms and leg muscles.

Determination of heart size is not thought to be as accurate with percussion as with palpation.[1] More accurate information can be obtained from a good posterior–anterior chest film.

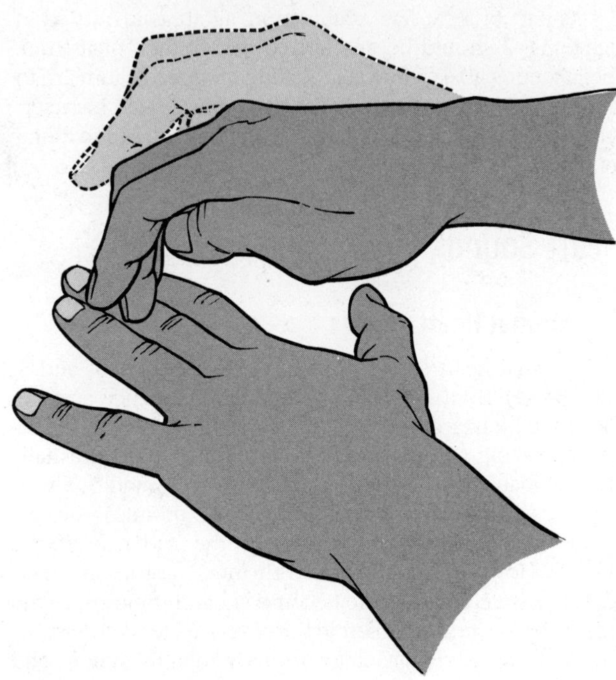

FIGURE 34–3 The technique of percussion.

Auscultation

A good-quality stethoscope is required for cardiac auscultation. Although the human ear is able to hear sounds ranging in frequency from 20 cycles per second or hertz (Hz) to 20,000 Hz, it is most sensitive to 1000 to 5000 Hz. The frequency of most heart sounds is less than 1000 Hz. The stethoscope must transmit these low-frequency sounds to the ear.

The parts of the stethoscope are the earpieces, tubing, and chest pieces. The earpieces should fit comfortably into the ear canal and should be snug enough so that extraneous sound cannot enter. They must also be kept free of ear wax. Double tubing with a small internal diameter (3mm) should extend from the earpieces to the chest pieces. Additionally, the tubing should be reasonably short (25–30 cm) so that sound is not "diluted," and should be thick to minimize room noise.[11]

There are two basic types of chest pieces: the diaphragm and the bell. The diaphragm, which brings out higher frequencies and filters out the lower ones, is useful for listening to the first and second heart sounds (S_1 and S_2) and to high-frequency murmurs. It should be pressed firmly against the skin. The bell filters out high-frequency sounds and accentuates low-frequency sounds. Diastolic filling sounds and low-frequency murmurs are heard best with the bell. It should rest lightly on the chest; if firm pressure is applied, the skin becomes taut and acts like a diaphragm. When auscultating heart sounds, stand on the patient's right side so that as you place the bell of your stethoscope on the patient's chest, the chest piece is balanced. Because the bell does not have to be held in place, the possibilities of creating extraneous sounds and filtering out low frequencies are reduced.

TABLE 34–2
Sounds Produced by Percussion

Record of Finding	*Intensity*	*Pitch*	*Duration*	*Quality*	*Anatomical Region Where Sounds May Be Encountered*
Tympany	Loud	High	Moderate	Drumlike	Air in closed structure vibrates in concert with tissue surrounding it; the gastric air bubble; air in intestine
Hyperresonance	Very loud	Very low	Long	Booming	Air-filled lungs, as in emphysema
Resonance	Moderate to loud	Low	Long	Hollow	Normal lung
Dullness	Soft to moderate	High	Moderate	Thudlike	Liver
Flatness	Soft	High	Short	Flat	Muscle

(Reproduced by permission from Malasanos et al: Health Assessment, 2nd ed. St Louis, The CV Mosby Co, 1981)

As part of a cardiac examination, all areas identified in Figure 34–2 should be auscultated except the epigastrum. The listener's goals when auscultating the precordium are to identify normal heart sounds, the heart rate and its characteristics; murmurs; extrasystolic sounds; and the diastolic filling sounds.

Heart Sounds

Normal Heart Sounds

Normal heart sounds consist of two sounds: S_1 and S_2 (Fig. 34–4). Both are of relatively high frequency and can therefore be heard clearly with the diaphragm of the stethoscope. Systole (the period between S_1 and S_2) is normally shorter than diastole (the period between S_2 and S_1); with slow heart rates (less than 100 beats per minute), the two sounds are easily distinguished by the cadence of the rhythm. However, in more rapid rhythms diastole shortens, so that systole and diastole become equal in time or, as the rate increases further, diastole becomes shorter than systole. In this instance, in order to properly identify systole and diastole, the examiner should palpate the carotid artery while listening to the heart; the carotid upstroke immediately precedes S_2.

The S_1 is primarily due to closure of the mitral and tricuspid valves, and is therefore heard loudest at the apex of the heart. Phonetically, if the heart sounds are "lub-dup," S_1 is the "lub." Usually, mitral and tricuspid closure is heard as a single sound.

The S_2 results primarily from closure of the aortic and pulmonic valves, and is loudest at the base of the heart. Phonetically, the "dup" of the "lub-dup" is the S_2. Physiological (normal) splitting of the S_2 occurs during inspiration. During inspiration, an increased amount of blood is returned to the right side of the heart. Pulmonic valve closure (P_2) is delayed because of the extra time needed for the increased blood volume to pass through the pulmonic valve. On expiration the split sounds merge (see Fig. 34–4). Abnormal (paradoxical) splitting of the S_2 can also occur. Paradoxical splitting is due to any mechanism that causes late aortic valve closure (A_2), such as electrical delays (left bundle branch block, right ventricular pacing, or right ventricular ectopy), or mechanical delays (aortic stenosis, systolic hypertension, left ventricular failure, or left ventricular ischemia; see Fig. 34–4). Because P_2 is soft, and A_2 is comparably loud and easily transmitted, a split S_2 is heard best in the second right intercostal space (aortic valve outflow tract).

Diastolic Filling Sounds

Diastolic filling sounds (S_3 and S_4) occur as blood enters a noncompliant or nonresiliant ventricle during the two phases of rapid ventricular filling: protodiastole, the early rapid filling (S_3); and, with atrial contraction, the active, rapid filling (S_4). Blood entering a noncompliant ventricle causes vibrations of the valves and supporting structures, resulting in sounds of very low frequency. They can arise from either or both ventricles.

A physiologic S_3, or S_3 sound, can be heard in healthy children or young adults, but disappears by age 30. In people over the age of 30, it is called an S_3 gallop (or ventricular gallop) and signals loss of ventricular compliance. It is one of the first clinical findings associated with cardiac decompensation, such as left ventricular heart failure (left ventricular S_3 gallop), or primary pulmonary hyptertension and cor pulmonale (right ventricular S_3 gallop). An S_3 gallop follows the S_2 in a "lub-dup-*ta*" cadence (see Fig. 34–4). Using the bell of the stethoscope, listen for a left ventricular S_3 gallop over the apex of the heart; for a right ventricular S_3 gallop, listen over the lower left sternal border. By having the patient lie on his left side, the apex is brought forward against the chest wall, making the left ventricular S_3 louder and therefore easier to hear.

The S_4, or atrial, gallop is commonly heard in older people. It occurs following atrial contraction as the blood is ejected into the noncompliant ventricle. Even though this is the fourth heart sound, because it occurs at the end of diastole, it is heard immediately before S_1, and sounds like "*ta*-lub-dup" (see Fig. 34–4). Atrial gallops are heard in the majority of patients who have had a myocardial infarction, and in a large number of patients experiencing angina pectoris (chest pain). It may also be detected in patients with coronary heart disease, hypertensive cardiovascular disease, cardiomyopathy, and aortic stenosis. Unlike the S_3 gallop, an S_4 gallop does not necessarily imply cardiac failure. As with the S_3, listen using the bell of the stethoscope. A left ventricular S_4 gallop is heard best at the apex, with the patient lying in the left lateral position; right ventricular S_4 gallops are loudest over the lower left sternal border.

Patients with severe cardiac failure can have both S_3 and S_4 gallops. If the heart rate is slow enough, four distinct heart sounds can be heard (quadruple rhythm; see Fig 34–4). However, if a patient is sick enough to have a quadruple rhythm, he usually also has tachycardia. In this case, the S_3 and S_4 fuse in mid-diastole to one loud diastolic sound, a summation gallop, which resembles the sound of a galloping horse (see Fig. 34–4).

In a noncompliant ventricle, it stands to reason that there should be more resistance to active ventricular filling than to passive ventricular filling; therefore, an S_4 gallop should be generated more easily than an S_3 gallop. It follows that one would expect all patients in normal sinus rhythm (on ECG) who have an S_3 gallop to also have an S_4 gallop. However, this is frequently not the case. The cause for this is unknown, although one possibility may be an absence of actual mechanical atrial contraction in spite of electrical atrial activity.

Heart Murmurs

Heart murmurs are sounds produced in the heart or great vessels by turbulent blood flow. Murmurs are classified according to systolic or diastolic timing; intensity; location; radiation, such as to the back, neck, or axilla; configuration, such as crescendo or decrescendo; and quality, such as harsh, rough, rumbling, blowing, squeaking, or musical.

The nurse must be particularly concerned with changes in murmurs rather than in the diagnosis of them; the one

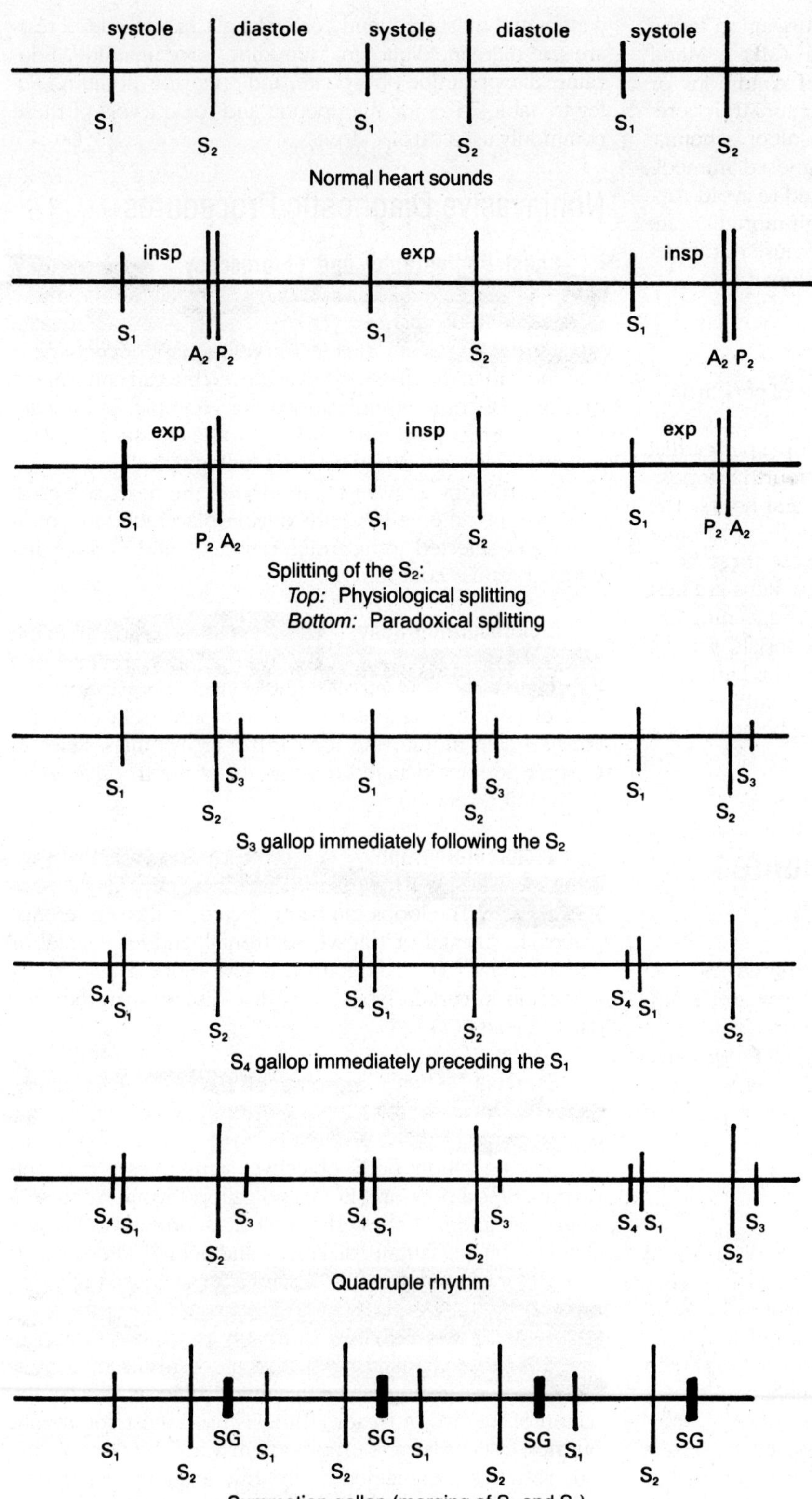

FIGURE 34–4 Normal and abnormal heart sounds.

exception is the new murmur of mitral regurgitation in the patient with acute myocardial infarction (MI).[19] Mitral regurgitation can result from a number of conditions or disease processes, but in the patient with acute MI, it is related to papillary muscle dysfunction as a result of ischemia. The murmur must be recognized and diagnosed immediately because interventions must be instituted to avoid rupture of the papillary muscle. There is a high mortality rate associated with papillary muscle rupture because of the development of sudden and profound heart failure.

Pericardial Friction Rub

Pericardial friction rubs are characteristic of pericarditis, which occurs in more than 15% of patients with acute MI. Approximately 7% of patients with MI develop a pericardial friction rub; it commonly occurs within the fourth day post-MI.[7] Rubs may be transient, lasting only several hours. The rub occurs with heart movement: atrial systole, ventricular systole, and ventricular diastole. Each of these three components creates its own short, scratchy sound. Rubs are best heard either with the patient sitting upright and leaning forward with the breath expelled (most appropriate for the patient with an acute MI) or with the patient on his hands and knees in bed or on the examination table (useful in a nonacute situation). A pericardial friction rub can be heard with or without a pericardial effusion.

Diagnostic Tests and Procedures Related to Cardiac Function

Diagnostic tests and procedures are ordered by the physician to confirm data obtained by interview and examination. Some tests are relatively easy to interpret, while others must be interpreted by expert clinicians. All require that basic explanation be given to the patients. Some necessitate special orders prior to the test and special monitoring by the nurse following the procedure.

Laboratory Tests

Laboratory tests may be ordered to assist in the diagnosis of acute MI (angina pectoris cannot be confirmed by either blood or urine studies); to measure abnormalities in blood chemistries which could affect prognosis of a cardiac patient; to assess the degree of the inflammatory process; to screen for risk factors associated with the development of coronary heart disease; to determine baseline values prior to therapeutic intervention; to assess drug levels; and to screen generally for any abnormalities.[22] The function of cardiac enzymes and their role in diagnosing myocardial infarction is covered in detail in Chapter 37.

Plasma Drug Levels. Plasma drug level tests enable the clinician to determine if prescribed medications are in therapeutic, subtherapeutic, or toxic ranges, and to screen for drugs that have not been prescribed. For the cardiac patient, the most frequently ordered plasma drug level tests are for digoxin, digitoxin, quinidine, procainamide, lidocaine, disopyramide phosphate, and phenytoin sodium.[2] Refer to Table 34–3 for therapeutic and toxic levels of these commonly used cardiac drugs.

Noninvasive Diagnostic Procedures

Chest Radiographs and Fluoroscopy. A chest radiograph, or chest x-ray film, allows the clinician to determine the size, contour, and position of the heart, and to appreciate any physiologic alterations in the pulmonary circulation. It does not aid in the diagnosis of acute MI, but can confirm the presence of some complications, for example, pulmonary edema. Correct placement of heart catheters, such as pacemakers, is also confirmed by chest radiographs.[8]

Fluoroscopy allows visualization of the heart and great vessels over time. It is useful during placement and positioning of selected intracardiac catheters, and in assessing unusual cardiac contours.

Electrocardiography. The 12-lead electrocardiograph assists in the diagnosis of many diseases and provides vital information about a patient's condition and progress. Single-lead electrocardiographs (most commonly MCL_1 or MCL_6) are useful in monitoring for cardiac arrhythmias. Refer to Chapter 36 for a detailed description of electrocardiogram (ECG) interpretation.

Vectorcardiography. The vectorcardiogram is a two-dimensional view of the cardiac electrical forces displayed in vector loops. The loops can be projected on three reference planes; horizontal or transverse; frontal; and left sagittal or lateral. The vectorcardiogram may give more diagnostic information in certain types of cardiac disease than the standard 12-lead ECG.[21]

Exercise Testing. Exercise testing is defined as the observation, measurement, and recording of the physiologic responses to a known amount of work. These physiologic responses include both objective signs (heart rate and rhythm, blood pressure, ECG, and gallop rhythms) and subjective symptoms (chest discomfort, shortness of breath, claudication, leg fatigue, dizziness, and lightheadedness).

There are two major indications for exercise testing: to measure exercise capacity in order to assess fitness for work, sports, and other activities in health and disease[3]; and to assess functional impairment and mechanisms of impairment. Exercise testing can be dynamic, isometric, or a combination of the two. A treadmill test is used most commonly, but step tests or bicycle ergometry may also be done.[15] Specific results are explained by the physician; the nurse uses the information when implementing or explaining the exercise prescription.

Instructions to the patient should include the following[15]:

- Get adequate sleep and rest the night before the test.
- Have a light breakfast or lunch (without coffee or tea, or alcohol) at least 2 hours before the test.

TABLE 34–3
Plasma Levels of Commonly Used Cardiac Medications

Drug	*Therapeutic Level*	*Toxic Level*
Digoxin	0.8–1.6 ng/ml	>2.4 ng/ml (Renal excretion of digoxin diminished by quinidine, reduce maintenance digoxin doses by 30–50%.)
Digitoxin	14–26 ng/ml	>34 ng/ml
Quinidine sulfate	2.3–5 μg/ml (double extraction method)[9]	>5 μg/ml
Procainamide hydrochloride	4–8 μg/ml	>8 μg/ml
NAPA (N-acetylprocainamide, active metabolite of procainamide)	2–22 μg/ml	>22 μg/ml
Lidocaine hydrochloride	1.6–5 μg/ml	>5–10 μg/ml
Disopyramide phosphate	2–4 μg/ml	Not established
Phenytoin sodium	10–20 μg/ml	>30 μg/ml (Toxic symptoms appear at lower plasma levels in uremia, hypoalbuminuria, some forms of liver disease, and hyperkalemia.[20, 25])

- Wear loose-fitting, absorbent clothing (shorts or pants) which are not made of nylon (*Women:* wear a bra and a short-sleeved, loose-fitting blouse that buttons down the front.) Wear well-fitting, comfortable shoes (not slippers) with rubber soles. This is extremely important for stability, comfort, and ease of walking on a moving, inclined surface.
- Discontinue medications only as directed by the physician.
- Avoid hot baths or showers for at least 2 hours after the test, because this may result in further vasodilatation with potentially serious hypotension.

Echocardiography. In echocardiography, ultrasound (1 million Hz) is sent into the heart through the chest wall and recorded as it returns. An ECG is recorded simultaneously to time events in relation to the cardiac cycle. Motions of these echoes are traced on an oscilloscope and recorded on film. Echocardiography is particularly useful in the diagnosis of chest structual abnormalities, such as ventricular wall dilatation or hypertrophy, septal thickening, and valvular stenosis or insufficiency. Prior to the advent of echocardiography, this information could only be obtained through invasive procedures, such as cardiac catheterization.[6]

Phonocardiography. Because heart sounds are of such low intensity and occur within milliseconds of one another, heart sounds are not always heard on auscultation; even when heard, their origins are not always clear. The phonocardiogram allows the clinician to validate these heart sounds. A graphic, simultaneous recording of heart sounds, pulse waves, and the ECG is made. Timing of the sounds and pulse waves is then correlated to events in the cardiac cycle.[6]

Radioisotope Studies. Radioisotope studies are useful for detecting MI and decreased myocardial blood flow, and for evaluating left ventricular function. The radioisotopes are injected intravenously and scans are done using a gamma scintillation camera.[6]

Technetium pyrophosphate (^{99m}Tc) is taken up into areas of infarction. This technique of myocardial infarction imaging (or "hot spot" identification) is most reliable when the infarction is large.

Thallium-201 is used to evaluate myocardial blood flow through vessels too small to visualize with coronary arteriography. Often this is paired with an exercise test to compare changes in myocardial perfusion during exercise and at rest. In this technique, "cold spots" representing areas with a lack of myocardial perfusion correlate to ischemic areas.

Gate blood pool scanning utilizes a computer to analyze ventricular function. By comparing the difference in the amount of the radioactive tracer in the end-diastolic volume, the ejection fraction can be calculated. This test can also be used to assess the differences in ventricular function during rest and exercises.

Invasive Diagnostic Tests

Hemodynamic Monitoring

Hemodynamic monitoring can be done at the bedside as well as in the cardiac catheterization laboratory. Bedside hemodynamic monitoring includes measurement of central venous pressure (CVP), pulmonary artery and pulmonary artery wedge pressures (PAP and PAWP), and systemic intra-arterial pressures. Refer to Table 34–4 for a complete list of normal hemodynamic pressures.

Central Venous Pressure. Central venous pressure is the pressure within the right atrium or superior vena cava, and reflects right ventricular end-diastolic pressure or right ventricular filling pressure (preload). The normal CVP is 4 to 10 cm H_2O, or 3 to 7 mmHg. The CVP is determined by fluid volume, vascular tone, and contractility. Causes of increased CVP are increased blood volume, vasoconstriction, and decreased contractility. The CVP is usually elevated in right heart failure, tricuspid regurgitation, and cardiac tamponade. In patients with acute left ventricular MI, right ventricular failure is usually secondary to left ventricular failure; therefore, in this patient population, elevated CVP is usually a late sign indicative of left ventricular failure. The CVP may be lowered by saline depletion, vasodilatation, or enhanced cardiac contractility.

The CVP catheter site should be prepped by shaving and cleansing the skin with an antiseptic solution. A local anesthetic may be used. The catheter is threaded through the arm or neck vein into the superior vena cava, just above or within the right atrium. Once the CVP catheter is inserted, antiseptic ointment and a dry, sterile dressing are applied. The dressing, intravenous bag, manometer, and tubing are changed every 24 hours.

Vascular pressure is measured by the height of a column of water in a manometer. When measuring CVP, it is crucial that the zero mark on the manometer be placed at the correct position, the phlebostatic axis (see Fig. 34–1). Once this position is located, the chest should be marked with ink. When the phlebostatic axis is used, the CVP can be measured correctly with the patient supine at a backrest position up to 20°. The most common complications of CVP monitoring are infection and air embolism.[23]

Wedge Pressures. Pulmonary artery pressure (PAP) and pulmonary artery wedge pressures (PAWP) reflect left-sided heart pressures, and are, therefore, more useful in assessing left ventricular failure than is the CVP. Pulmonary artery pressures are monitored only in cardiac intensive care units and not on general medical–surgical units.

A balloon-tipped floating catheter is inserted into a large vein which leads into the superior vena cava and right atrium. The balloon is inflated, and the catheter is carried rapidly by the flow of blood through the tricuspid valve, into the right ventricle, out the pulmonic valve, and into a branch of the pulmonary artery. When the catheter tip reaches a small pulmonary artery, the balloon is deflated, and the catheter is secured with sutures.

TABLE 34–4
Normal Adult Values for Data Collected During Cardiac Catheterization

Pressures (mmHg)	
Systemic arterial	
Peak-systolic	100–140
End-systolic	60–90
Mean	70–105
Left ventricular	
Peak-systolic	100–140
End-diastolic	3–12
Left atrial	
Left atrial mean (or PAWP)	1–10
"a" wave	3–15
"v" wave	3–15
Pulmonary artery	
Peak-systolic	15–30
End-diastolic	4–12
Systolic mean	10–20
Right ventricular	
Peak-systolic	15–30
End-diastolic	0–8
Right atrial	
Mean	0–8
"a" wave	2–10
"v" wave	2–10
Left Ventricular Volume	***(biplane angiography)***
End-systolic volume (ml/m^2)	24–36
End-systolic volume (ml/m^2)	70–104
Ejection fraction (%)	58–70
Resistance (dynes-sec-cm^{-5})	
Total systemic resistance	770–1500
Total pulmonary resistance	100–300
Pulmonary arterial (vascular) resistance	20–120
Flow	
Cardiac output (l/min)	4.0–8.0
Cardiac index (l/min/m^2)	2.8–4.0
Stroke index (ml/beat/m^2)	35–70
Stroke volume (ml/min/m^2)	60–130
Oxygen consumption (ml/min/m^2)	125
Oxygen Saturation (%)	
Right atrium	60–75
Right ventricle	60–75
Pulmonary artery	60–75
Left atrium	95–100
Left ventricle	95–100
Aorta	95–100

(After Yang SS, Bentivoglio LG, Maranhao V et al: From cardiac catheterization data to hemodynamic parameters, 2nd ed, p 269. Philadelphia, FA Davis, 1978)

Pulmonary artery systolic (PAS) and diastolic (PAD) pressures are obtained by means of a transducer and blood pressure monitor. Normal PAP is 25/9 mmHg, with a mean pressure (PAM) of 15 mmHg. When the balloon is inflated, the catheter is "wedged" in the pulmonary artery. Pressures transmitted to the catheter reflect left ventricular end-diastolic pressure (LVEDP). At end-diastole, when the mitral valve is open, PAP is the same as left atrial pressure (LAP) and left ventricular pressure (LVP), unless the patient has mitral valve disease or pulmonary hypertension. The PAWP is a mean pressure, and is normally 4.5 to 13 mmHg.[26]

Catheter site care is the same as that of a CVP. The catheter flush solution is heparinized normal saline, delivered in small amounts using a pressure bag and flush device. As with the CVP, it is essential to place the transducer at the phlebostatic axis to ensure reproducible readings in backrest positions up to 20°.[24] (With some pulmonary artery catheters, the CVP can also be measured.) Complications of PAP monitoring include infection, pulmonary artery rupture, pulmonary thromboembolism, pulmonary infarction, catheter kinking, arrhythmias, and air embolism.[23]

Cardiac Output. Cardiac output can also be measured using the pulmonary artery catheter, the cardiac output computer, and the technique of thermodilution. Five to ten milliliters of iced or room-temperature solution is injected into the proximal lumen, and the cardiac output is then displayed on the computer. It is recommended that three cardiac output measurements be taken and an average computed. Normal cardiac output ranges from 4 to 8 liters/min.[23]

Cardiac Index. Cardiac index more accurately reflects cardiac output, because body size is taken into account. (Cardiac index equals cardiac output divided by total body surface area.) Normal cardiac index ranges from 2.8 to 4.0 liters/min/m^2. Once cardiac index is known, one can follow the patient's hemodynamic status by creating a cardiac function curve (Frank-Starling curve), plotting the PAWP on the horizontal axis, and the cardiac index on the vertical axis.[23]

Systemic Intra-arterial Pressure Monitoring. Systemic intra-arterial pressure monitoring is used to obtain direct and continuous blood pressures in critically ill patients with severe high blood pressure or hypotension, who are on potent vasoactive drugs, or who are at high risk of developing cardiogenic shock. Arterial catheters are also helpful when obtaining arterial blood gas samples and serial blood samples. Intra-arterial monitoring is restricted to patients in critical care units.

Once an arterial site is selected (radial, brachial, femoral, or dorsalis pedis), collateral circulation to the area must be confirmed prior to catheter placement. Confirmation of collateral circulation can be done by either the Allen's test or the ultrasonic Doppler test.[23] (If no collateral circulation existed, and the cannulated artery became occluded, ischemia and infarction of the area distal to the cannulated site could occur.)

Site preparation and care is the same as for CVP catheter insertion. The catheter flush solution is the same as for pulmonary artery catheters. A transducer is attached to the catheter, and pressures are obtained in mmHg. Complications of intra-arterial pressure monitoring include local obstruction with distal infarction, external hemorrhage, massive ecchymosis, dissection, air embolism, blood loss, pain, arteriospasm, or infection.[23]

Cardiac Catheterization

Cardiac catheterization is a diagnostic procedure in which one or more catheters are inserted into the heart or great vessels, under fluoroscopy, using either a transarterial or transvenous approach. Indications for cardiac catheterization include the following[12]:

- Known or suspected cardiac disease severe enough to require percutaneous transluminal coronary angioplasty or aortocoronary bypass surgery
- Chest discomfort of unknown etiology for which coronary heart disease cannot be ruled out
- Stable but severe angina pectoris, with or without previous MI and unresponsive to medical management
- Unstable angina pectoris
- Uncontrolled heart failure, ventricular arrhythmias, or cardiogenic shock associated with acute MI, septal perforation, ventricular aneurysm, or papillary muscle dysfunction
- Abnormal ECG in apparently healthy individuals whose occupations involve public safety, such as airline pilots
- When the suspected cardiovascular impact would have a major impact on the patient's lifestyle, or when there is a reasonable doubt as to the accuracy of the medical diagnosis
- History of MI in previously asymptomatic patients 50 years of age or less
- Strongly positive indications of coronary heart disease from exercise-test ECG in individuals with mild or no angina pectoris
- Evaluation of percutaneous transluminal coronary angioplasty or aortocoronary bypass graft patency.

Angiography is the technique of injecting dye into the vascular system to outline the cardiac chambers and the coronary arteries. It is accompanied by cineangiograms (rapidly changing films or movies) which record the passage of the contrast media. Angiography is particularly useful in identifying obstructive lesions in the coronary arteries.

Right heart catheterization is performed for the purposes of measuring right heart pressures; evaluating the pulmonic and tricuspid valves; sampling blood oxygen content of right heart chambers for detection of left-to-right shunt; determining cardiac output by the direct Fick method; and evaluating mitral valve stenosis or insufficiency by transseptal approach. The right heart can be approached through the basilic vein and superior vena cava, or through the femoral vein and inferior vena cava.[12]

Left heart catheterization is performed for the purposes of pressure measurement to evaluate left ventricular, and mitral and aortic valve functioning (see Table 34–4); angiography to evaluate mitral and aortic valve disease; and left heart ventriculography. The two main approaches to the left heart are retrograde entry through the aortic valve or transseptal entry through the right atrium.[12]

Ventriculography is performed by opacification of the ventricular cavity with contrast medium and, using cineangiocardiography, filming ventricular motion. Ventriculography can be performed to evaluate valve structure or function, to define ventricular anatomy, and to evaluate ventricular function.[12]

Coronary arteriography is performed to determine the presence of coronary obstructions and to define coronary anatomy. Cineangiograms can then be carefully reviewed following the procedure.

Nursing Considerations. Precatheterization nursing responsibilites include preparing the patient to[12]

- Remain fasting after midnight prior to the procedure.
- Expect the procedure to last approximately 2 hours, and that the room may be cold and the table hard.
- Expect certain temporary sensations during catheterization, such as palpitations (as the catheter is passed and its tip touches the myocardium); a desire to cough (as the dye is injected into the right heart); and a feeling of heat (particularly in the head as contrast medium is injected into either side of the heart).

Postcatheterization nursing responsibilities include[12]

- Watching the puncture (or cutdown sites) for hematoma formation, and checking the peripheral pulses in the affected extremity (dorsalis pedis, posterior tibial pulse in the lower extremity; radial pulse in the upper extremity) for arterial insufficienty (every 15 minutes for 1 to 2 hours, then every 1 to 2 hours until stable).
- Evaluating extremity temperature and color, and any complaints of pain, numbness, or tingling sensations in the affected extremity to determine signs of arterial insufficiency, and reporting any changes promptly.
- Watching for arrhythmias by observing the cardiac monitor, listening to the apical heart sounds, and evaluating the pulse for rhythm changes.
- Having the patient remain in bed with little movement of the involved extremity, per unit protocol.
- Reporting any complaint of chest discomfort immediately.
- Administering pain medication for site discomfort, as ordered.

References

1. Bates B: A Guide to Physical Examination, 2nd ed. Philadelphia, JB Lippincott, 1979
2. Bond EF, Underhill SL: Antiarrhythmic and cardiotonic drugs. In Underhill SL, Woods SL, Sivarajan ES, Halpenny CJ (eds): Cardiac Nursing. Philadelphia, JB Lippincott, 1982
3. Bruce RA: Exercise testing of patients with coronary heart disease. Ann Clin Res 3:323–332, 1971
4. Dustin HP, Tarazi RC, Hinshaw LB: Mechanisms controlling arterial pressure. In Frolich ED (ed): Pathophysiology, 2nd ed. Philadelphia, JB Lippincott, 1976
5. Frank MJ, Alvarez-Mena SV: Cardiovascular Physical Disease. Chicago, Year Book Medical Publishers, 1973
6. Hall M: Echocardiography, radioisotope studies, and phonocardiography. In Underhill SL, Woods SL, Sivarajan ES, Halpenny CJ (eds): Cardiac Nursing. Philadelphia, JB Lippincott, 1982
7. Hurst JW, Logue RB, Walter PF: The clinical recognition and medical management of coronary atherosclerotic heart disease. In Hurst JW, Logue RB, Schlant RC et al (eds): The Heart, 4th ed. New York, McGraw-Hill, 1978
8. Huseby JS: Radiologic examination of the chest. In Underhill SL, Woods SL, Sivarajan ES, Halpenny CJ (eds): Cardiac Nursing. Philadelphia, JB Lippincott, 1982
9. Kessler KM, Lowenthal DT, Warner H et al: Quinidine elimination in patients with congestive heart failure or poor renal function. N Engl J Med 290:706–709, 1974
10. Kirkendall WM, Feinleib MD, Freis ED et al: Recommendations for Human Blood Pressure Determination by Sphygmomanometers. Dallas, American Heart Association, 1980
11. Leatham A, Leech GJ: The Principles of Auscultation. In Hurst JW, Logue RB, Rackley CE et al (eds): The Heart, 5th ed. New York, McGraw-Hill, 1982
12. Newton KM: Cardiac catheterization. In Underhill SL, Woods SL, Sivarajan ES, Halpenny CJ (eds): Cardiac Nursing. Philadelphia, JB Lippincott, 1982
13. New York Heart Association Criteria Committee: Major changes made by Criteria Committee of the New York Heart Association. Circulation 49:390, 1974

13a. New York Heart Association Criteria Committee: Diseases of the Heart and Blood Vessels: Nomenclature and Criteria for Diagnosis, 6th ed. Boston, Little, Brown & Co, 1964

14. Scribner BH: Fluid and Electrolyte Balance, 7th ed. Seattle, University of Washington Press, 1969
15. Sivarajan ES: Exercise testing. In Underhill SL, Woods SL, Sivarajan ES, Halpenny CJ (eds): Cardiac Nursing. Philadelphia, JB Lippincott, 1982
16. Tarazi RC, Gifford RW Jr: Systemic arterial pressure. In Sodeman WA Jr, Sodeman WA (eds): Pathologic Physiology, 5th ed. Philadelphia, WB Saunders, 1974
17. Underhill SL: Assessment of cardiovascular function. In Brunner LS, Suddarth DS (eds): Textbook of Medical–Surgical Nursing, 5th ed. Philadelphia, JB Lippincott, 1984
18. Underhill SL: History-taking and physical examination of the patient with cardiovascular disease. In Underhill SL, Woods SL, Sivarajan ES, Halpenny CJ (eds): Cardiac Nursing. Philadelphia, JB Lippincott, 1982
19. Underhill SL: Diagnosis and treatment of the patient with coronary artery disease and myocardial ischemia. In Underhill SL, Woods SL, Sivarajan ES, Halpenny CJ (eds): Cardiac Nursing. Philadelphia, JB Lippincott, 1982
20. Wit AL, Rosen MR, Hoffman BF: Electrophysiology and pharmacology of cardiac arrhythmias. VIII. Cardiac effects of diphenylhydantoin Br Heart J 90:397–404, 1975
21. Woods SL: Electrocardiography, vectorcardiography, and polarcardiography. In Underhill SL, Woods SL, Sivarajan ES, Halpenny CJ (eds): Cardiac Nursing. Philadelphia, JB Lippincott, 1982

22. Woods SL, Laurent-Bopp D: Laboratory tests using blood and urine. In Underhill SL, Woods SL, Sivarajan ES, Halpenny CJ (eds): Cardiac Nursing. Philadelphia, JB Lippincott, 1982
23. Woods SL, Grose BL: Hemodynamic monitoring in patients with acute myocardial infarction. In Underhill SL, Woods SL, Sivarajan ES, Halpenny CJ (eds): Cardiac Nursing. Philadelphia, JB Lippincott, 1982
24. Woods SL, Grose BL, Laurent-Bopp D: Effect of backrest position on pulmonary artery pressures in critically ill patients. Cardiovascular nursing 18(4):19–24, 1982
25. Woosley RL, Shand DG: Pharmacokinetics of antiarrhythmic drugs. Am J Cardiol 41:986–995, 1978
26. Yang SS, Bentivoglio LG, Maranhao V et al: From Cardiac Catheterization Data to Hemodynamic Parameters, 2nd ed. Philadelphia, FA Davis, 1978

Chapter 35

Nursing Strategies for Common Cardiac Problems

Nursing Diagnosis Interventions Evaluation

Sandra L. Underhill
Susan L. Woods

The *Standards of Cardiovascular Nursing Practice* (1981)[4] provide a framework for utilizing the nursing process for patients with altered cardiovascular function. People with cardiac disorders commonly have problems such as chest discomfort, decreased or absent cardiac output, shortness of breath, and anxiety. Most of these problems are presented in this chapter as nursing diagnoses as defined by Kim.[2] The assessment portion of the nursing process as it relates to patients with cardiac disease can be found in Chapter 34. Goals, interventions, and evaluation of these diagnoses are presented in this chapter.

Alteration in Comfort: Pain

Nursing Diagnosis

Alteration in comfort is related to myocardial ischemia or infarction, or inflammatory heart disease manifested by complaints of chest discomfort/pain; increased blood pressure, heart rate, and respiratory rate; or fear and anxiety. Classically, the symptom associated with myocardial ischemia is precordial chest pain. However, many patients experience chest discomfort which they do not describe as pain, such as a pressure or burning sensation. Furthermore, not all discomfort from ischemia is located in the chest, but may radiate to the arms, neck, or back. In addition, patients with inferior ventricular wall ischemia may only have symptoms of vagal stimulation, such as nausea, or an urge to belch or to defecate. Therefore, in the patient with coronary heart disease, one needs to treat rapidly these symptoms of ischemia. (Refer to Chap 37 for a more complete discussion of ischemic pain.)

Myocardial ischemia can be caused by any process that decreases myocardial blood flow or increases myocardial oxygen demand. Examples of pathologic processes that decrease myocardial blood flow are coronary heart disease, coronary spasm, hemorrhage or other saline depletion, anemia, aortic valve disease with calcific occlusion of the coronary ostia, left heart thrombus formation with embolization to the coronary arteries, decreased left ventricular filling time (tachyarrhythmias), and increased blood viscosity (polycythemia). Examples of pathologic processes that increase myocardial oxygen use include tachycardia; increased left ventricular wall tension due to congestive heart failure, aortic stenosis, or cardiomyopathy; and increased impedance to left ventricular ejection of blood (increased afterload). Afterload can be increased by high blood pressure, by aortic stenosis, or by an increase in systemic vascular resistance from any cause. Myocardial oxygen use is increased by any process that increases catecholamine release, such as pain, stress, exercise, anxiety, or fear.

Interventions

The goals of nursing interventions are (1) to relieve chest discomfort and other symptoms of myocardial ischemia (diaphoresis, nausea, and other gastrointestinal complaints); (2) to detect early the recurrence of chest discomfort; and (3) to prevent chest discomfort.

General comfort measures may be helpful in relieving chest discomfort. However, knowledge of the specific etiology of the discomfort enables the nurse to prescribe more definitive interventions. For example, when caring for the patient with chest discomfort related to myocardial ischemia, interventions are based on restoring the balance between myocardial oxygen supply and demand as described in Chapter 37. For patients with chest discomfort from inflammatory heart disease, nursing interventions include assisting the patient to find a position of comfort (usually sitting) and reducing physical activity (bed rest).

Evaluation

Outcome criteria reflect goal attainment of the three stated goals. Outcome criteria for relief of chest discomfort are as follows:

- Patient reports reduction or relief of chest discomfort, or other symptoms of ischemia are reduced or relieved. (Symptoms need to be specifically stated.)
- Heart rate, blood pressure, and respiratory rate return to patient's baseline levels. (Specific ranges need to be stated for each individual.)
- Patient's skin is warm and dry.
- Patient appears restful.
- Patient expresses that he is physically comfortable.
- Patient expresses less fear and anxiety.

The time frame for goal attainment should be stated but may vary depending upon etiology and acuity of the problem. For example, chest discomfort related to myocardial ischemia must be reduced within 5 minutes, whereas chest pain related to pericarditis need not be relieved within 5 minutes.

Outcome criteria for early detection of the recurrence of chest discomfort are as follows:

- Patient reports chest discomfort at its onset.
- Patient follows prescribed therapy.

Outcome criteria for prevention of chest discomfort are as follows:

- Patient reports that chest pain/discomfort has not recurred.
- Heart rate, blood pressure, and respiratory rate remain at baseline level.
- Patient's skin is warm and dry.
- Patient expresses continued physical comfort.
- Patient appears restful.

Decreased Cardiac Output

Nursing Diagnosis

Decreased cardiac output is related to right or left ventricular failure, arrhythmias and conduction abnormalities, saline deficit (reduced preload), or increased impedance to left ventricular ejection (increased afterload). The manifestations are decreased systemic arterial blood pressure (with compensatory increase in heart rate), angina, arrhythmias, alteration in mentation, fatigability, decreased urine output, cool and clammy skin, anorexia, or cachexia. These manifestations are the result of decreased tissue perfusion. Alteration in tissue perfusion can occur for other reasons as well. Since cardiac output is the product of stroke volume and heart rate, a reduction in either factor without compensatory changes in the other factor will result in a decrease in cardiac output and thus tissue perfusion.

Interventions

Goals for nursing interventions are (1) to allow for as much independence as possible in activities of daily living by maximizing cardiac output to eliminate signs and symptoms of inadequate tissue perfusion; (2) to reduce the demands of daily living to be compatible with the patient's reduced cardiac output; and (3) to prevent the recurrence of decreased cardiac output.

General nursing measures may be helpful in improving the manifestation of decreased cardiac output. However, knowledge of the specific etiology enables the nurse to describe more definitive interventions. For example, when caring for the patient who has left ventricular failure as a result of increased preload, interventions are based on decreasing venous return to the heart. As discussed in Chapter 40, positioning the patient in a semi-Fowler's position or sitting position is a nursing intervention that decreases venous return to the heart.

The patient may need assistance in determining activities and demands of daily living that are incompatible with his hemodynamic state. He may need others to assist him in usual activities such as bathing, shaving, and eating. The patient should be allowed as much independence as possible in activities of daily living.

If the patient has decreased cardiac output due to saline deficit, nursing interventions are aimed at increasing preload, such as positioning the patient flat, and at increasing intravascular volume with oral fluids (milk, broth, tomato juice). The nurse should also question the use of drugs that decrease intravascular volume (*i.e.,* diuretics).

Evaluation

The patient carrying out as much independent activity as possible will do so without manifestations of reduced tissue perfusion. Manifestations of adequate tissue perfusion include unchanged or increased blood pressure compared to the patient's baseline (range in mmHg must be stated for each patient); unchanged or decreased pulse compared to the patient's baseline (range in beats per minute must be stated for each patient); absence of chest discomfort or other symptoms of myocardial ischemia (specific for each patient); absence of arrhythmias or complaints of palpitations; alert and oriented behavior without changes in mentation; activities of daily living completed without complaint of fatigue; urine output greater than 30 ml/hour; warm and dry skin; no complaints of loss of appetite; and no loss in muscle mass. If the demands of daily living must be reduced to be compatible with the patient's reduced cardiac output, the outcome criteria should reflect that the manifestations of decreased cardiac output are not worsened during activities of daily living. Manifestations and activities need to be specifically stated.

Outcome criteria for preventing the recurrence of decreased cardiac output are as follows:

- Patient reports that chest discomfort or other symptoms of myocardial ischemia, palpitations, fatigability, anorexia, and reduced urine output have not recurred.
- Blood pressure, heart rate, and rhythm remain within patient's normal range. (Specific ranges for each need to be stated.)
- Skin remains warm and dry.
- Patient continues to be alert and oriented with no changes in mentation.

Alteration in Breathing Pattern

Nursing Diagnosis

Shortness of breath is related to heart failure, hypoxemia, pain, fear, and anxiety. It is manifested by rapid, shallow breathing, anxiety, decreased involvement in activities of daily living, sleep disturbances, and difficulty in verbal communication.

Cardiac causes of hypoxemia include congenital heart disease, heart failure, and pulmonary embolism due to right heart mural thrombosis.

Interventions

Goals for nursing interventions include the reduction, relief, or prevention of shortness of breath and, if necessary, the reduction of the demands of daily living to be compatible with the patient's shortness of breath. General measures to facilitate respiration, such as allowing the patient to assume an upright position of comfort, help not only to decrease venous return to the heart, but also to increase tidal volume. Thus, heart congestion is reduced (decreased preload) and gas exchange is improved.

Because shortness of breath can be extremely frightening to the patient, particular attention needs to be directed toward decreasing fear and anxiety. Fear and anxiety can be somewhat alleviated by a supportive, calm, competent manner. The patient's activities and demands of daily living need to be determined and if necessary altered to be compatible with the patient's shortness of breath.

Evaluation

Outcome criteria for reducing, relieving, or preventing shortness of breath are as follows:

- Patient reports that shortness of breath is reduced, relieved, or prevented.
- Respiratory rate, rhythm, and depth return to acceptable levels. (Specific description of each is needed.)
- Patient appears more restful.
- Patient expresses less fear and anxiety.
- Patient reports less difficulty sleeping.
- Patient speaks more freely.
- Patient participates in activities of daily living without becoming short of breath.

Cardiac Arrest

Absence of cardiac output is related to lethal ventricular arrhythmias, cardiac rupture, cardiac tamponade, or anything that obstructs blood flow through the heart or great vessels, such as obstruction of an artificial valve. This event is manifested by absence of blood pressure, pulse, and respiration; unconsciousness; and ventricular tachycardia, flutter or fibrillation, asystole, marked bradycardia, or electromechanical dissociation.

Cardiopulmonary Resuscitation

Because in most instances irreversible brain damage occurs within 4 minutes of cardiac arrest, basic life support must be instituted immediately. Basic life support according to the American Heart Association Standards consists of cardiopulmonary resuscitation (CPR).[3] The goal, to provide effective CPR until definitive therapy can be instituted, is shared by all members of the health team.

The ABCs of CPR consist of
A—airway
B—breathing
C—circulation

Unresponsiveness is established by shaking the patient's shoulder and asking him if he is all right.

Airway

An airway must be established in order to ensure adequate ventilation. If the patient does not respond, call for help. The tongue is the most common cause of airway obstruction; lifting the jaw forward (chin lift) and tilting the head back lifts the tongue away from the back of the throat (Fig. 35–1, *A*). Another technique is the jaw thrust method, in which the entire jaw is forced forward by placing the fingers of both hands behind the angles of the jaw or by grasping the jaw (holding the mandible and lower teeth) and tilting the head backward at the same time (Fig. 35–1, *B*). You should not use the head tilt method for patients with cervical spine injuries; instead, with your index fingers displace the mandible forward without moving the patient's head. If the airway is obstructed, apply suction to the area of obstruction, or roll the patient onto his side and with two fingers clear his mouth.

While keeping the airway open, place your ear over the victim's mouth and nose and look toward his chest (Fig. 35–2). For 3 to 5 seconds, look for any rise and fall of the chest, listen for the escape of air during exhalation, and feel for the flow of air on your cheek.

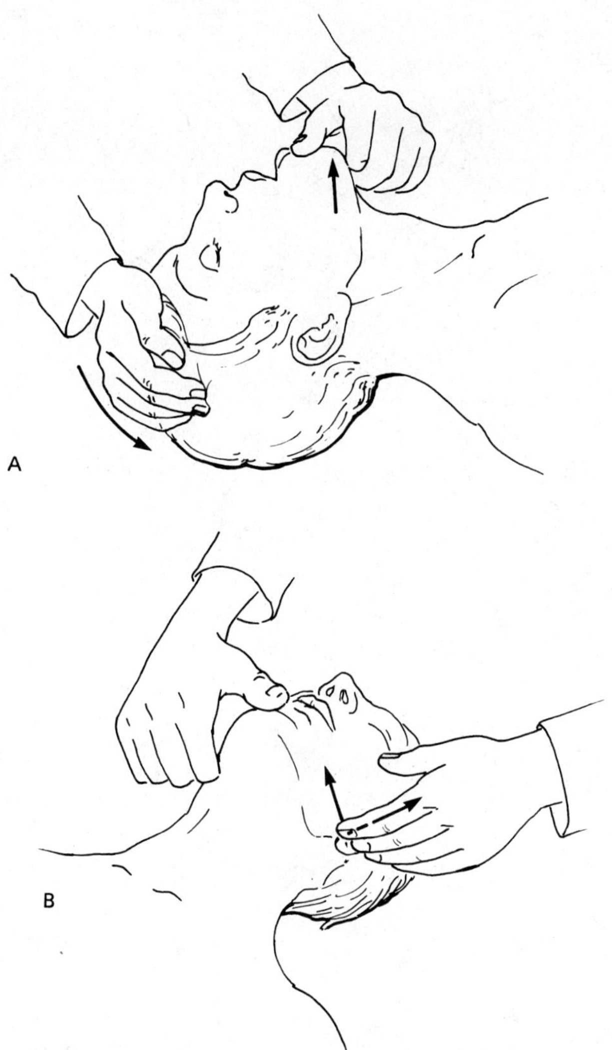

FIGURE 35–1 (*A*) Head tilt, chin lift method of opening the airway. (*B*) Jaw thrust method of opening the airway. The entire jaw is forced forward by placing the fingers of both hands behind the angles of the victim's jaw or by grasping the jaw holding the mandible and lower teeth and tilting the head backward.

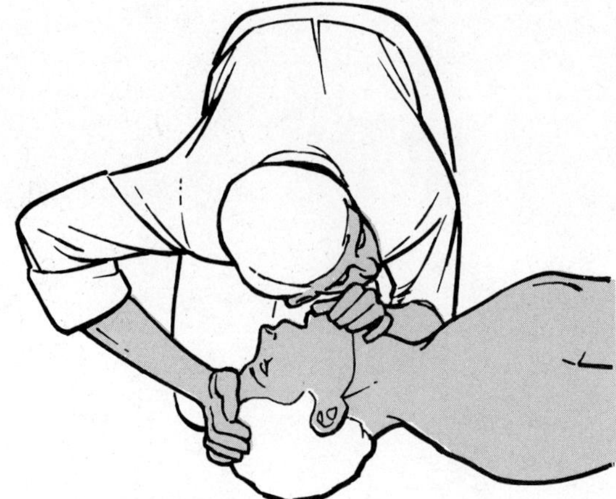

FIGURE 35–2 Method for determining if a person is breathing. Place your ear over the victim's mouth and nose, and look toward the chest for signs of movement and for sound of air escaping from the nose or mouth during exhalation.

Back Blow and Chest Thrust. If the airway is completely obstructed by a foreign body, the patient will be unable to speak, breathe, or cough. Back blows and chest thrusts may be necessary.

In order to clear a completely obstructed airway in the patient with an adequate cardiac output, the following procedures should be initiated. If the patient is standing or sitting, (1) position yourself at the side and slightly behind the victim; (2) place your other hand on his chest to support him; and (3) deliver four sharp blows to the back with the heel of your hand over the victim's spine between the shoulder blades (Fig. 35–3). Then (1) stand behind him, placing your arms directly under his chest; (2) place the thumb side of your fist on his breastbone, but not on the xiphoid process or the margins of the rib cage; and (3) grasp your fist with your other hand and exert four quick compressions (Fig. 35–4).[1]

If the patient is lying down or has inadequate or absent cardiac output, kneel and roll him onto his side, facing you, with his chest against your thighs, and deliver four sharp blows to the back as described above. Then place him on his back and kneel close beside him, open his airway, and turn his head to one side. The position of the hands for the application of chest thrust is the same as that for applying closed-chest heart compression (heel of hand on lower half of sternum). Exert four quick downward thrusts that will compress the chest cavity.[1]

Back blows produce an instantaneous increase in pressure in the respiratory passages, which may dislodge the foreign body either completely or partly. The manual thrusts produce a more sustained increase in pressure in the respiratory passages and may help to dislodge the foreign body. Combination of the two techniques clears the upper airway better than either one separately.[1]

Breathing

If the patient does not begin to breathe spontaneously, artificial ventilation must be begun immediately. There are several methods: mouth-to-mouth, mouth-to-stoma, and mouth-to-artificial airway. There are also various devices for assisting ventilation.

Mouth-to-mouth breathing is accomplished by pinching the patient's nose closed with your thumb and index finger of one hand while exerting pressure on his forehead to maintain the backward tilt of the head. After taking a deep breath, make a tight seal around the patient's mouth and blow into his mouth. Give four quick full breaths without allowing time for full lung deflation between breaths, then two breaths after each cycle of 15 compressions (Fig. 35–5). If there are two people doing CPR, one breath every 5 seconds is needed. Ventilation is adequate if the chest rises and falls, and if air can be felt and heard leaving the lungs. Artificial ventilation should not be interrupted for more than 5 seconds.

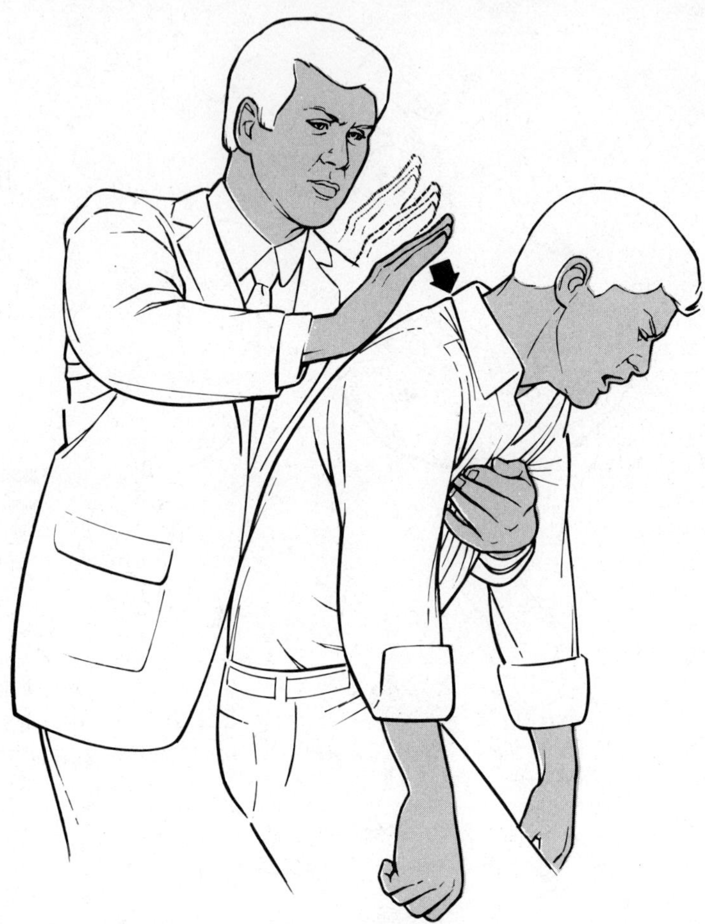

FIGURE 35–3 Technique for delivering a back blow in a standing position to clear an object from an obstructed airway. Position yourself at the side slightly behind the victim. Place your hand on his chest to support him. Deliver four sharp blows to the back with the heel of your other hand over the spine between the shoulder blades.

In mouth-to-nose ventilation, tilt the patient's head back, placing one hand on his forehead while using the other hand to lift his lower jaw. Take a deep breath, make a seal between your mouth and the victim's nose, and blow air into his lungs. With mouth-to-stoma ventilation (for patients with a laryngectomy), the head tilt and jaw thrust maneuvers are unnecessary.

An S-tube artificial airway can be used, but maintaining a tight seal around the mouth is difficult. An oropharyngeal airway should be used whenever a breathing device with a mask is used. Artificial airways should be lubricated with sterile water-soluble jelly or water prior to insertion. The tip of an upside-down airway is directed toward the palate while the jaw is pulled forward and downward. When the tip of the airway hits the back of the throat, the airway is rotated so that the tip is in the direction of the trachea and is advanced until the flange is flush with the lips. Ventilation should begin immediately, either mouth-to-airway or ventilation-assisting device-to-airway. The trachea may be intubated with an endotracheal tube to create an airway or to improve the existing airway.

Indications for endotracheal intubation include the following:

- Cardiac arrest
- Respiratory arrest
- Inability of rescuer to artificially ventilate the unconscious patient by conventional methods
- Inability of the patient to protect his own airway (coma, areflexia)
- Prolonged artificial ventilation

During artificial ventilation, air can distend the stomach, thereby promoting regurgitation and reducing lung volume by elevating the diaphragm. With the patient's head turned to the side, moderate pressure over the stomach will force air out of the mouth. Insertion of a nasogastric tube will maintain deflation of the stomach.

Circulation

If cardiac arrest occurs, the patient will be pulseless. He will either have electrical–mechanical dissociation, marked bradycardia, ventricular tachycardia or fibrillation, or asystole. If the carotid pulse is absent, artificial circulation should be started immediately. Five to ten seconds is required to establish pulselessness by feeling for the pulse in the neck. For an adult, the precordial thump is worthwhile if the arrest is both witnessed and monitored. A sharp blow delivered within 1 minute of the arrest, with the fist to the midsternum of the patient from a distance of 8 to 12 inches, may convert the arrhythmia to a normal rhythm (Fig. 35–6).

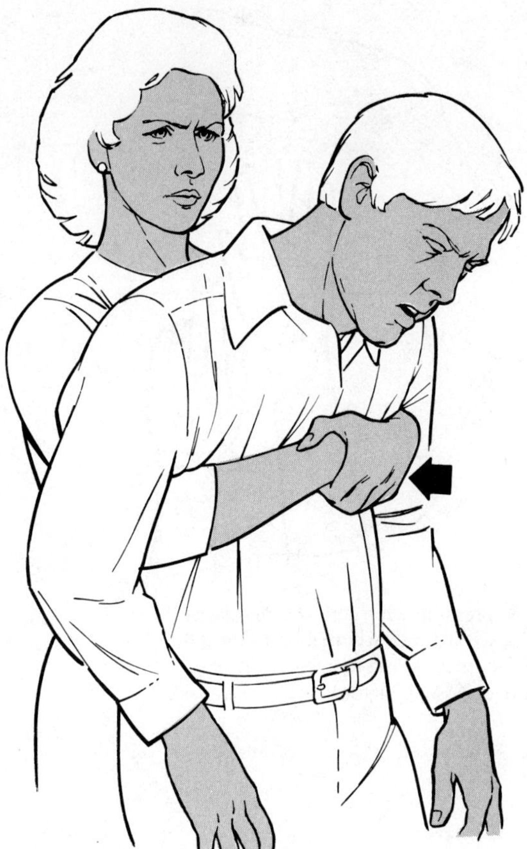

FIGURE 35–4 Technique for chest thrust. Stand behind the victim, placing your arms directly under his chest. Make a fist with one hand and place the thumb side of your fist on the breastbone (not on the xiphoid process or margins of the rib cage). Grasp your fist with the other hand and exert four quick compressions.

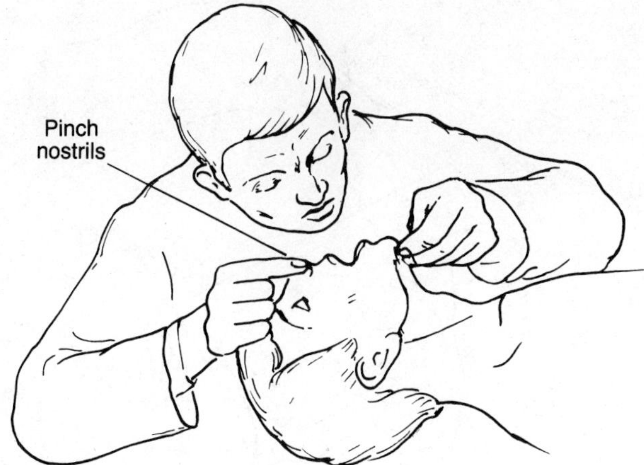

FIGURE 35–5 Mouth-to-mouth breathing. Pinch the person's nose closed with your thumb and index finger of one hand while exerting pressure on his forehead to maintain a backward tilt of the head. Blow four quick full breaths into patient's mouth. Follow with two breaths after each cycle of 15 compressions.

Adequate circulation may be established by external cardiac compression. External cardiac compressions are rhythmic applications of pressure over the lower half of the sternum resulting in pulsatile artificial circulation. Properly performed cardiac compressions result in a systolic blood pressure of over 100 mmHg. With the adult patient in a horizontal position (to ensure flow to the brain) on a firm surface, cardiac compression is achieved by exerting 80 to 120 pounds of pressure over the lower half of the sternum (about 1 inch above the xiphoid process). The sternum is compressed vertically 1½ to 2 inches at a regular rate of 60/min. The heel of one hand is on top of the other hand (Fig. 35–7). The rescuer's shoulders are directly over the patient's sternum and the rescuer's arms are straight. The heel of the hand should not be removed from the patient's chest between compressions, but the pressure exerted should be released. A ratio of five chest compressions to one interposed breath is maintained if two rescuers are present (Fig. 35–8, *A*). Interposed breathing prevents a drop in blood flow. If there is only one rescuer, the ratio is two breaths to fifteen chest compressions (Fig. 35–8, *B*).

Complications of CPR include gastric distention, rib fractures, laceration of the liver, fat emboli, and costochondral separation.

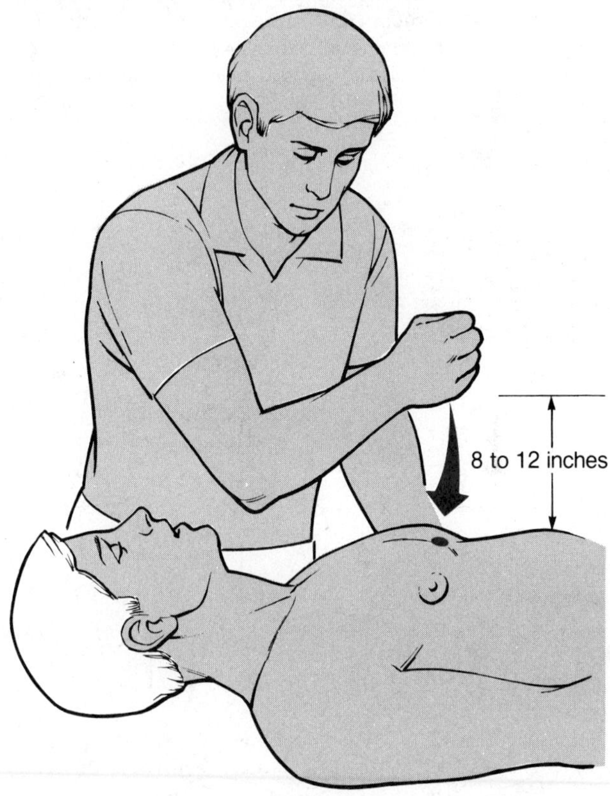

FIGURE 35–6 Precordial thump for a witnessed and monitored cardiac arrest. A sharp blow is delivered (within 1 minute of the arrest) to the midsternum from a distance of 8–12 inches.

Evaluation

Effectiveness of CPR that is initiated before irreversible brain damage occurs is determined by pupils that constrict when exposed to light, which is an indication of adequate

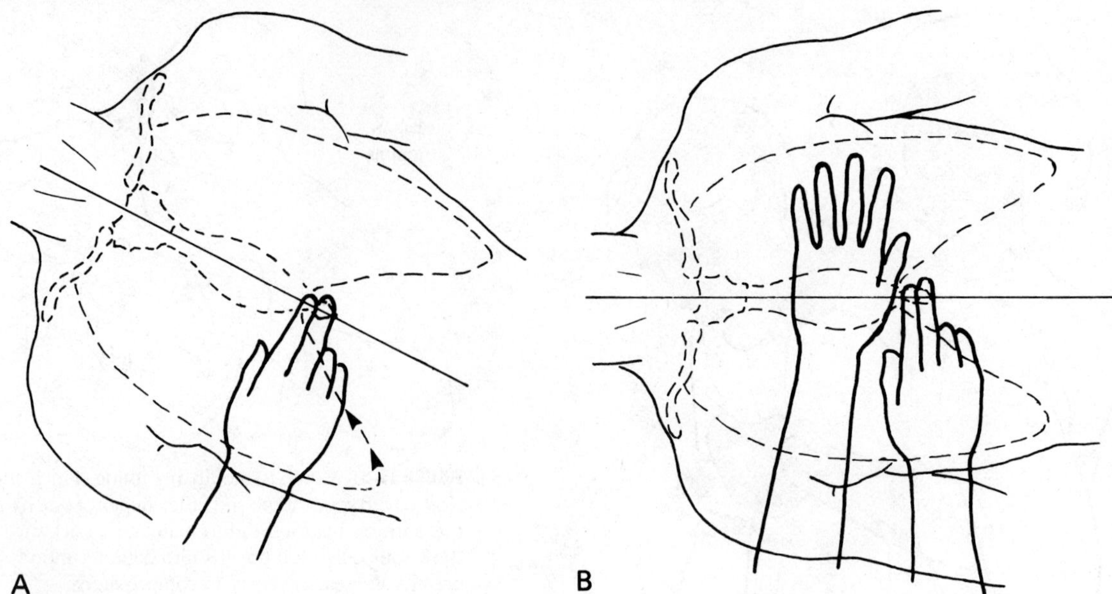

FIGURE 35–7 Placement of the hands for closed chest cardiac compression. (*A*) With the middle and index fingers of the lower hand, follow the lower edge of the rib cage to the notch where the ribs meet the sternum. (*B*) With the middle finger on the notch and the index finger placed next to it, place the heel of the other hand on the lower half of the sternum, next to the index finger. (A Manual for Instructors in Basic Cardiac Life Support, American Heart Association, 1980)

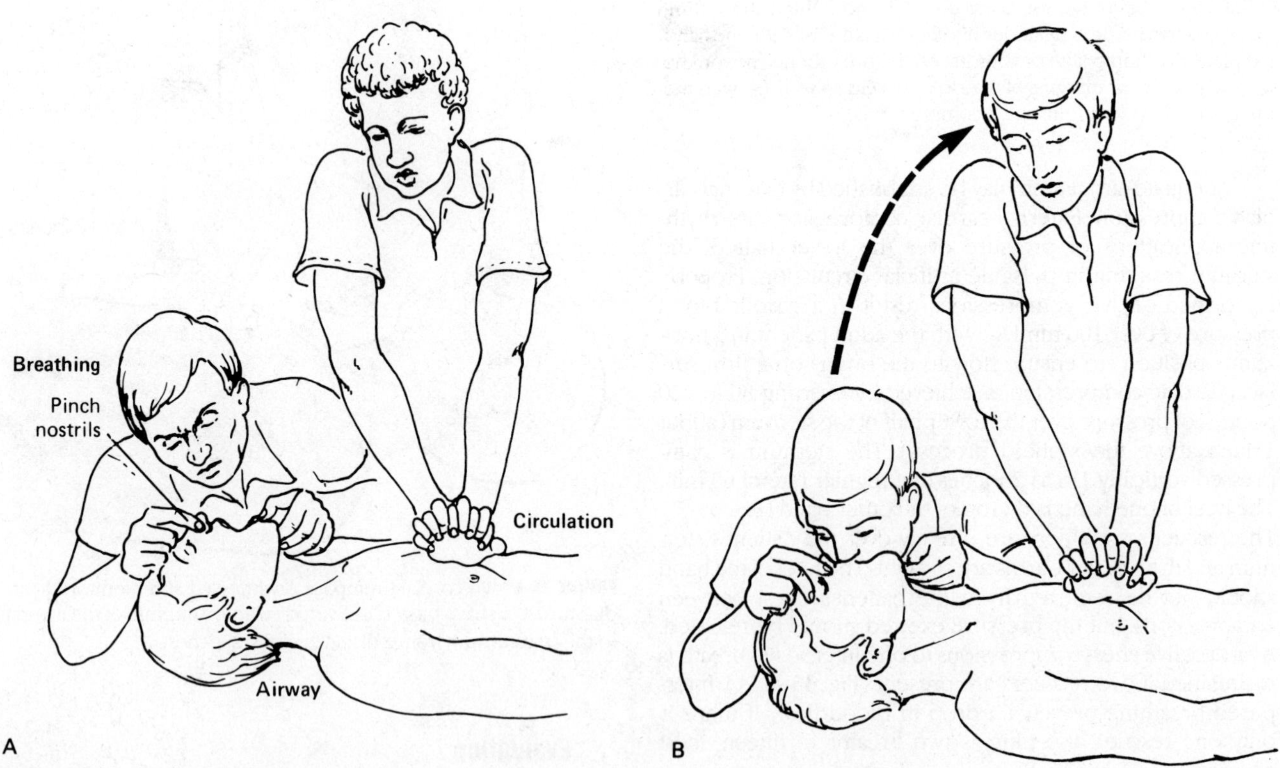

FIGURE 35–8 One and two rescuer methods for CPR. (*A*) In two rescuer CPR, a ratio of five chest compressions to one interposed breath is maintained. (*B*) For one rescuer, the ratio is two breaths to fifteen chest compressions.

oxygenation and blood flow to the brain; and a palpable pulse during cardiac compression. Unfortunately, all patients do not respond to competent CPR.

Advanced Cardiac Life Support

Advanced cardiac life support includes (1) use of adjunctive equipment and special techniques for establishing and maintaining effective ventilation and circulation; (2) cardiac monitoring and rhythm recognition; (3) establishing and maintaining an intravenous infusion route; and (4) use of drugs and defibrillation.[5] In addition, basic cardiac life support may be necessary to support the patient prior to and during this definitive therapy. Responsibility for advanced cardiac life support is shared with other members of the health care team.

Drugs used during advanced cardiac life support include oxygen, sodium bicarbonate, epinephrine, atropine, lidocaine, procainamide, bretylium, verapamil, calcium chloride, morphine sulfate, norepinephrine, dopamine, dobutamine, and isoproterenol. See Table 35–1 for the purposes, dosages, comments, and side-effects of each of these drugs.

Defibrillation

Defibrillation is used immediately after onset of ventricular fibrillation or ventribular tachycardia without a peripheral pulse. Defibrillation completely and simultaneously depolarizes all the myocardial cells. This terminates the chaotic electrical activity, allowing the sinus node to regain control of the heart rhythm. Successful defibrillation may not be possible if the myocardium is anoxic or acidotic.

(*Text continues on page 498*)

TABLE 35–1
Drugs Used During Cardiopulmonary Arrest

Drug	*Purpose*	*Dosage*	*Side-Effects and Comments*
Oxygen	To correct hypoxemia	4–10 liters/min	The rescuer's exhaled breath will deliver only 16% to 17% oxygen. Bag-mask or bag-tube systems should have supplemental oxygen attached. There is no lung damage when 100% oxygen is used for less than 24 hours (in adults). It is also important to adequately ventilate the patient in order to prevent or correct respiratory acidosis.
Sodium bicarbonate ($NaHCO_3$)	To correct metabolic acidosis	1 mEq/kg IV initially. One half (0.5 mEq/kg) of initial dose given IV every 10–15 min. Analysis of arterial blood gases should guide treatment.	$HCO_3^- + H^+ \leftrightarrows H_2CO_3 \leftrightarrows CO_2 + H_2O$ Since CO_2 production is increased, adequate ventilation is required. Excessive $NaHCO_3$ leads to metabolic alkalosis with displacement of oxyhemaglobin dissociation curve and consequent impairment of oxygen release to tissues. Hyperosmolality may also develop. Catecholamines and calcium salts should not be added to bicarbonate infusions, because inactivation results. Since bicarbonate has a high pH, avoid mixing any drugs with it.
Epinephrine	To increase perfusion pressure during cardiac compressions To improve the myocardial contractile state To stimulate spontaneous contractions (*e.g.*, in asystole) To increase the vigor of ventricular fibrillation	0.5–1 mg IV or intratracheally (5–10 ml of a 1 : 10,000 solution). Repeat every 5 min as needed. If tracheal and venous routes are not available, the drug may be administered carefully by the intracardiac route.	Epinephrine should not be added directly to a bicarbonate infusion, since catecholamines may be inactivated by alkaline solution.

(*Continued*)

TABLE 35–1
Drugs Used During Cardiopulmonary Arrest (*Continued*)

Drug	*Purpose*	*Dosage*	*Side-Effects and Comments*
Atropine	To accelerate cardiac rate by creating a positive chronotrophic effect due to parasympatholytic action (reduces vagal tone); by creating a positive dromotropic effect that accelerates AV conduction	0.5 mg IV; repeat every 5 min as needed, up to a total of 2 mg	Increased heart rate may be deleterious in patients with acute MI. Atropine should be given to patients with acute MI only if the bradycardia results in hemodynamic changes. Effects are less in older patients (decreased vagal tone). Use with caution in patients with narrow-angle glaucoma. Be aware of the possibility of acute urinary retention.
Lidocaine	To suppress ventricular arrhythmias To elevate the threshold for VF	1 mg/kg followed by an infusion of 1–4 mg/min	Myocardial and circulatory depression CNS changes: drowsiness, disorientation, decreased hearing ability, paresthesias, muscle twitching, and agitation Focal and grand mal seizures
Procainamide	To suppress ventricular arrhythmias May be effective when lidocaine is not	100 mg IV every 5 min at a rate of 20 mg/min up to 1 g, as needed to control arrhythmia; infusion at 1 to 4 mg/min	Hypotension Widening of QRS complex and lengthening of the PR and QT intervals AV block and cardiac arrest
Bretylium tosylate	To eliminate VF To suppress ventricular arrhythmias	For VF, 5 mg/kg undiluted is given rapidly IV. Then defibrillation is attempted. If VF persists, the dose is increased to 10 mg/kg and the shock is repeated. For VF, mix 500 mg in 50 ml and give 5–10 mg/kg IV over 8–10 min. The second dose of 5–10 mg/kg can be given in 1–2 hr if arrhythmia persists, and if necessary every 6–8 hr. Alternatively, the drug can be administered as a continuous infusion at a rate of 2 mg/min.	Initial transient increase in arterial pressure and cardiac rate is followed by a decrease in both. Cardiac output and preload remain unchanged. In the alert patient, vomiting may occur after rapid injection. Postural hypotension may occur. Contraindicated in digitalis toxicity, except with intractable VF.
Verapamil	To suppress some supraventricular tachyarrhythmias and to slow the ventricular responses in atrial flutter and atrial fibrillation To slow conduction through the AV node	0.075–0.15 mg/kg (maximum: 10 mg) IV over 1–3 min, then 0.15 mg/kg (maximum: 10 mg) over 30 min after first dose if necessary. (Total cumulative dose within 30 min should not exceed 15 mg.)	Transient hypotension Negative inotropic effect Coronary and peripheral vasodilator Contraindicated with concurrent use of IV beta-blocking drug
Calcium	To stimulate spontaneous or more forceful myocardial contractions by creating a positive inotropic effect; enhancing ventricular excitability; and prolonging systole	5–7 mg/kg of 10% calcium (Ca) chloride solution (3.4–6.8 mEq); may be repeated every 10 min Ca gluceptate 5–7 ml (4.5–6.3 mEq) Ca gluconate 10–15 ml (4.8–7.2 mEq)	Calcium and digoxin are synergistic. Calcium and bicarbonate when mixed form a precipitate. Each should be given separately. Use of calcium in cardiac arrest is controversial.

(*Continued*)

TABLE 35–1
Drugs Used During Cardiopulmonary Arrest (Continued)

Drug	*Purpose*	*Dosage*	*Side-Effects and Comments*
Morphine sulfate	To relieve pain and to treat pulmonary edema (decreases venous return to the heart)	2–5 mg IV every 5–30 min (15 mg in 15 ml IV solution)	Respiratory depression Hypotension May depress heart rate Incompatible with heparin sodium
Norepinephrine	To elevate arterial blood pressure (alpha effect) and to improve myocardial contractility (beta effect)	4 mg in 500 ml D5W by continuous infusion (16 μg/ml). After observing the response to initial dose of 2–3 ml/min, adjust rate of flow to maintain systolic blood pressure above 90 mmHg	Intra-arterial pressure monitoring may be needed for accurate measurement of pressure. Markedly increases myocardial oxygen requirements, which can increase ischemia and infarct size. Decreases renal blood flow. Ischemic necrosis and sloughing of superficial tissues occur if solution infiltrates. Phentolamine 5–10 mg in 10–15 ml saline injected into area of infiltration prevents necrosis and sloughing of tissue.
Dopamine HCl	To elevate blood pressure and to improve cardiac output, and at low doses to improve renal and mesenteric blood flow	200 mg in 250 ml D5W by continuous infusion 2–10 μg/kg/min (dopaminergic and beta effects) > 10 μg/kg/min (beta and alpha effects; beginning loss of dopaminergic effect) > 20 μg/kg/min (alpha effect reverses dopaminergic effect)	Most common adverse effects are ectopic beats, nausea, and vomiting. Tachyarrhythmias may result. Undesirable degree of vasoconstriction (increased afterload) may result with doses greater than 20 μg/kg/min. Cutaneous necrosis and sloughing of tissue can occur with infiltration and should be treated with phentolamine as described above. This drug is contraindicated in patients with pheochromocytoma, and is inactivated in alkaline solutions. Discontinue gradually instead of abruptly.
Dobutamine HCl	To increase cardiac output (beta effect) by increasing contractility in refractory congestive heart failure	250 mg in 1000 ml D5W by continuous infusion 0.5 μg/kg/min may be effective, but the usual range is 2.5–10 μg/kg/min	Increases myocardial oxygen need, and thus can cause further myocardial ischemia and infarction Causes tachyarrhythmias in doses greater than 20 μg/kg/min
Isoproterenol HCl	To increase cardiac output by increasing heart rate (beta effect) in symptomatic atropine-refractory complete heart block	1 mg in 500 D5W by continuous infusion; 2–20 μg/min titrated to maintain heart rate of 60 beats/min	Substantial increase in myocardial oxygen need, resulting in myocardial ischemia and extension of myocardial infarction. Can result in a lethal arrhythmia, ventricular fibrillation. Use with extreme caution in patients who have digitalis toxicity or hypokalemia.

(McIntyre KM: Cardiovascular pharmacology: Part 2. In McIntyre KM, Lewis AJ (eds): Textbook of Advanced Cardiac Life Support, pp 117–132. Dallas, American Heart Association, 1983; White RD: Cardiovascular pharmacology: Part 1. In McIntyre KM, Lewis AJ (eds): Textbook of Advanced Cardiac Life Support, pp 99–114. Dallas, American Heart Association, 1983)

In defibrillation, the electrode paddles are applied to the anterior chest. The standard electrode paddle position for the closed-chest procedure is one paddle just to the right of the upper sternum below the right clavicle and the other paddle just to the left of the cardiac apex (Fig. 35–9). In order to reduce skin resistance to current flow and to prevent skin burns, one of the following must be placed between the electrodes and the chest wall: saline-soaked 4-by-4 gauze pads, electrode paste, or defibrillator pads (adhesive pads with electrode gel). Care should be taken to prevent contact between the two areas of conductive material because electrical bridging may occur. If saline-soaked gauze pads or commercial defibrillator pads are used, cardiac compressions can be resumed after defibrillation without the hands slipping on the chest, a problem that occurs with electrode paste.

Pressure (20 to 25 pounds) is exerted on each paddle in order to ensure good skin contact. No one should be touching the patient or the bed when the defibrillator is fired. The defibrillator is then discharged at 200 to 360 watt-seconds (joules). Defibrillation can occur only if the synchronizer switch is in the *off* position. Successful defibrillation will result in the return of a pulse. Check the cardiac monitor to diagnose the rhythm.

Cardioversion

Cardioversion is used to terminate arrhythmias that have QRS complexes. It may be necessary to terminate ventricular tachycardia with a pulse, or supraventricular tachycardias. It may be an elective procedure. If the patient is alert, informed consent is obtained. The patient is usually given diazepam intravenously prior to cardioversion to promote anesthesia.

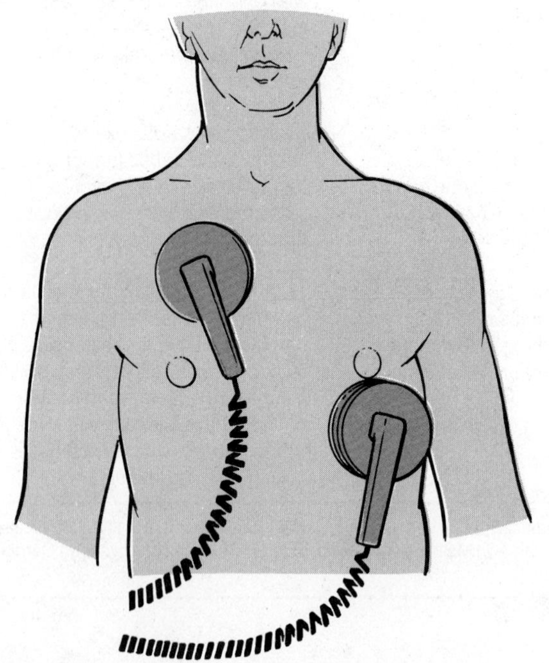

FIGURE 35–9 Proper positioning of defibrillator paddles.

The amount of voltage used varies from 25 to 360 watt-seconds. Digoxin is usually withheld for 48 hours prior to elective cardioversion to prevent postcardioversion arrhythmas. The synchronizer switch is turned to *on*. The defibrillator is synchronized with a cardiac monitor such that an electrical impulse is discharged during ventricular depolarization (the QRS complex). If the discharge were not synchronized, the electrical impulse could be delivered during the vulnerable period of the cardiac cycle (the last half of the T wave), and result in ventricular tachycardia or fibrillation. The synchronizer switch is therefore turned *on* so that when fired the unit discharges immediately after the onset of the next QRS complex. The discharge buttons should be held until the synchronizer fires the defibrillator. If ventricular fibrillation occurs after cardioversion, the defibrillator must be immediately recharged, the synchronizer turned to *off*, and defibrillation repeated. After use, the defibrillator should be turned to *off* to prevent accidental discharge of the paddles. Oxygen flow should be stopped during precordial shock, if possible, to avoid the hazard of fire.

The most successful response would include conversion to sinus rhythm, strong peripheral pulses, and adequate blood pressure. However, not all patients return to sinus rhythm after cardioversion, but may have an improved cardiac output and blood pressure due to a change in cardiac rhythm. Airway patency should be maintained, oxygen therapy reinstituted, and the patient's state of consciousness assessed. Vital signs should be obtained at least every 15 minutes for 1 hour, every 30 minutes for 2 hours, then every 4 hours.

Evaluation

Even when advanced cardiac life support is performed according to the guidelines of the American Heart Association, not all patients can be successfully resuscitated. Outcome criteria used to determine effective resuscitation are adequate cardiac output and return to baseline level of consciousness. Not all patients who have successful cardiac resuscitation have complete cerebral resuscitation.

Anxiety

Nursing Diagnosis

Anxiety may be related to a myriad of factors including fear of death, chest pain or discomfort, diagnosis of heart disease, the nature of chronic illness, role change, activity limitation, sensory overload, sensory deprivation, lack of personal resources, a knowledge deficit, and sleep disturbance. Anxiety may be manifested by increased pulse rate, arrhythmias, increased blood pressure, increased respiratory rate, shortness of breath, diaphoresis, chest pain, changes in the patient's normal behavior patterns (increased complaints, talkativeness, forgetfulness, short attention span, inability to concentrate, and restlessness), complaints of feeling anxious, and changes in facial expression.

Interventions

The main goals of nursing interventions related to anxiety in the cardiac patient are to detect early the signs and symptoms of anxiety, as anxiety can increase myocardial oxygen need; to reduce or eliminate anxiety; and to prevent, when possible, anxiety from occurring.

Nursing interventions to detect anxiety include monitoring for the patient's manifestations of anxiety. Note the patient's complaints of feeling anxious. Monitor heart rate and rhythm, blood pressure, respiratory rate and rhythm, changes in patient's normal behavior patterns, and changes in facial expressions. Explore with the patient and family their perceptions about behaviors, thoughts, and feelings.

If possible, nursing interventions to reduce or eliminate anxiety should be based on the etiology of the anxiety. Some interventions are supportive in nature since the etiology cannot be identified, eliminated, or changed. Other interventions are aimed at altering the cause of the distress. For example, as discussed in Chapter 11, some patients and families have realistic fears about dying and need assistance directed toward helping them with their feelings about death and their preparation for the patient's death. On the other hand, some patients may have anxiety associated with chest pain, and the intervention is primarily to relieve the pain and to provide reassurance.

Nursing interventions to prevent occurrence or recurrence of anxiety include measures that control the environment, for example, controlling lighting and noise. As discussed in Chapter 10, providing a consistent, predictable pattern of stimulation will help the patient feel control over his environment. If possible, determine what stimuli in the patient's environment contribute to his distress and together work out a plan to reduce or eliminate stimuli.

Further discussion of these common problems can be found in this unit in the chapters that follow.

References

1. A Manual for Instructors of Basic Cardiac Life Support. Dallas, American Heart Association, 1981
2. Kim MJ, McFarland GK, McLane AM: Classification of Nursing Diagnoses. Proceedings of the Fifth National Conference, pp 470–471. St Louis, CV Mosby, 1984
3. Standards and guidelines for cardiopulmonary resuscitation (CPR) and emergency cardiac care (ECC). JAMA 244:453–509, 1980
4. Standards of Cardiovascular Nursing Practice. Kansas City, American Nurses Association, 1981
5. Textbook of Advanced Cardiac Life Support. Dallas, American Heart Association, 1983

Bibliography

Woods SL: Arrhythmias complicating myocardial infarction. In Underhill SL, Woods SL, Sivarajan ES, Halpenny CJ (eds): Cardiac Nursing, pp 363–377. Philadelphia, JB Lippincott, 1982

Chapter 36

Cardiac Arrhythmias and Conduction Abnormalities

Susan L. Woods
Sandra L. Underhill

Principles of Electrocardiography

Electrical Conduction Through the Heart

The electrical impulse of the heart results in a series of cardiac events that cause the heart to contract. The impulse begins in the sinoatrial (SA) node, which is located in the upper or superior portion of the right atrium. The impulse travels from the SA node across the atria, resulting in atrial contraction. The impulse then moves to the atrioventricular (AV) node. There is a slight delay in the impulse at the AV node before it continues down the right and left bundle branches and the Purkinje fibers to the ventricular muscle, at which time the ventricles contract (Fig. 36–1).

The SA and AV nodes are controlled by the sympathetic and parasympathetic nervous systems, which thereby control the rate at which the heart beats. The sympathetic nerves cause the heart rate to increase; the parasympathetic system (by way of the vagus nerve) slows the heart rate.

Electrocardiography

The electrocardiogram (ECG) is a graphic record of the electrical activity of the heart. Impulse formation and conduction throughout the heart produce weak electrical currents through the entire body. The difference in potential between a positive and a negative area within the body can be measured by a galvanometer, an instrument with a wire between the poles of an electromagnet. As current passes through the wire, the instrument is controlled by the magnetic field. The ECG machine or electrocardiograph, contains a galvanometer that detects changes in surface potential, amplifies the signal, and records these body surface potential changes over time on calibrated moving paper. By convention, if a positive electrode is placed on the side facing the advancing wave of depolarization, a positive deflection will be produced (Fig. 36–2, *A*). If the poles of the galvanometer are reversed, however, a negative deflection will be produced. The magnitude of the deflection represents the thickness of the muscle involved. If a positive electrode is placed on the side from which the wave of depolarization is receding, a negative deflection will result (Fig. 36–2, *B*). If an electrode is placed at right angles (perpendicular) to the wave of depolarization, a biphasic deflection or no deflection (isoelectric) will occur (Fig. 36–2, *C*).[11]

Normally, the ECG consists of 12 leads: three bipolar standard leads (I, II, and III); three unipolar leads (aVR, aVL, aVF); and six unipolar chest leads. The three bipolar leads

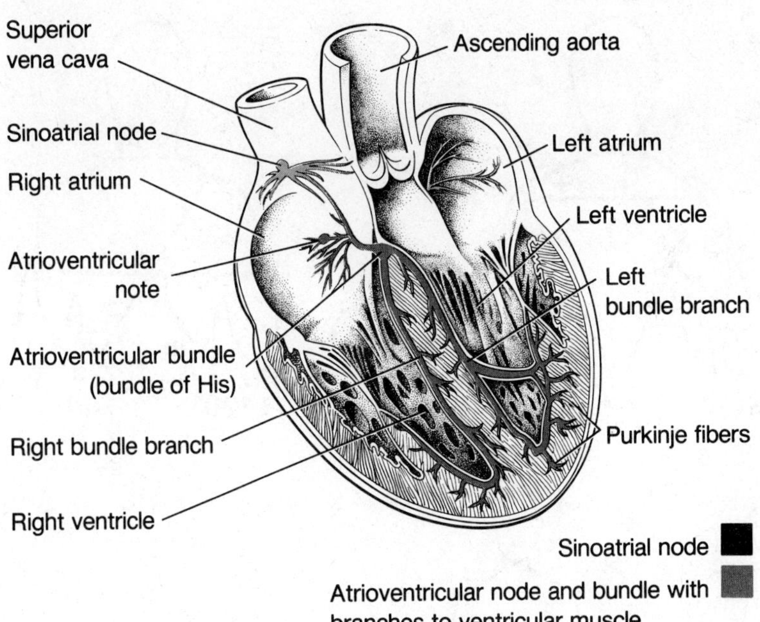

FIGURE 36–1 Internal conduction system of the heart.

represent a difference of electrical potential between two selected sites. Lead I is the difference of potential between the left arm (LA) and the right arm (RA). Lead II is the difference of potential between the left leg (LL) and the right arm (RA). Lead III is the difference of potential between the left leg (LL) and the left arm (LA). Einthoven's triangle is based on the equation, lead II = lead I + III. If leads I, II, and III are bisected by each other, the triaxial reference is produced (Fig. 36–3). Each of these three leads is 60° apart.[3]

Electrocardiographic Apparatus. In addition to obtaining the standard 12-lead ECG, the electrocardiograph can be used in other ways. One lead can be continuously monitored on an oscilloscope (a fluorescent screen). The waveform from this lead can be written out to provide a permanent record. Continuous electrocardiographic monitoring is especially useful in the intensive care unit, cardiac care unit, or telemetry floor to detect arrhythmias.

One lead of the electrocardiograph can be monitored by a small tape recorder (Holter recorder) and recorded on a continuous (1–24 hr) magnetic tape recording. The patient can then be monitored during the day or night to detect arrhythmias or evidence of myocardial ischemia during activities of daily living. The tape recorder weights approximately 2 pounds and can be carried over the shoulder. The patient keeps a diary of his activity, noting the time of any symptoms, experiences, or any unusual activities performed. The tape recording is then examined using a specialized instrument called a scanner, analyzed, and interpreted. Evidence obtained in this way is helpful in diagnosing arrhythmias and myocardial ischemia and in evaluating therapy such as antiarrhythmic and antianginal drugs or pacemaker function.

The ECG can also be transmitted by telemetry (telephone lines), thus freeing a patient from a cable connected to the oscilloscope. The ECG signal can then be monitored miles away.

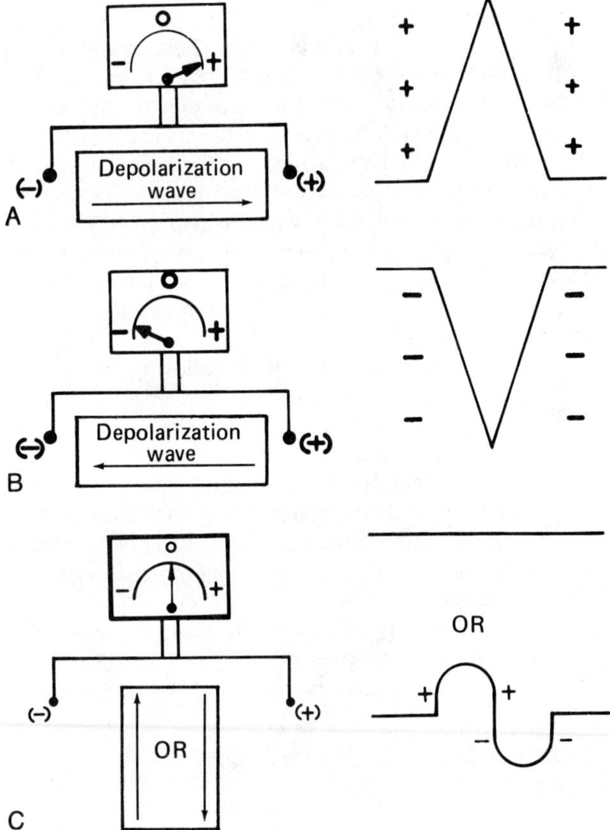

FIGURE 36–2 (*A*) Wave of depolarization toward a positive electrode. Any electrical activity that moves in the direction of a positive electrode is written upright by the ECG machine. (*B*) Wave of depolarization away from a positive electrode. Any electrical activity that moves away from a positive electrode is written downward. (*C*) Wave of depolarization perpendicular to a positive electrode. Any electrical current that moves perpendicular to a positive electrode is written biphasically or isoelectrically.

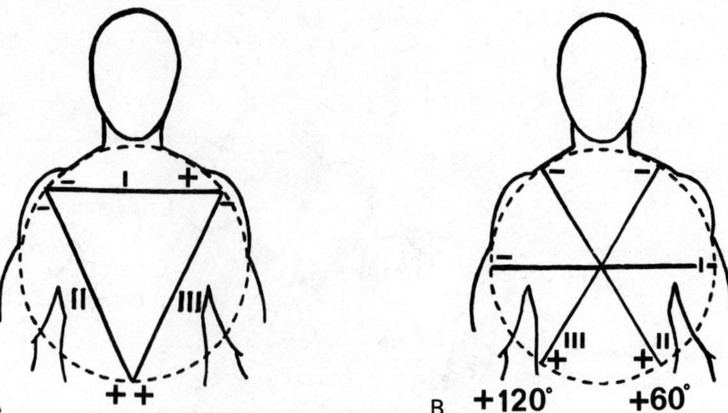

FIGURE 36–3 (*A*) Bipolar leads (Einthoven's triangle). (*B*) Triaxial reference figure for bipolar leads.

Procedure for Obtaining a 12-Lead ECG

To obtain a 12-lead ECG, the electrodes are placed on the patient as shown in Fig. 36–4. With the electrodes in these positions, the first six leads can be obtained. To ensure good contact between the skin and the electrode, the electrodes are first placed on a flat surface just above the wrists and ankles, and electrode paste or an alcohol sponge is placed under each electrode. The limb straps are adjusted firmly, to hold the electrodes in place. These straps should not pinch the patient's skin or be so tight as to decrease circulation distal to the strap. The lead selector on the machine is then turned to record each of the six leads. Next, the six V leads are obtained by placing the chest electrodes in the six precordial positions shown in Figure 36–5. These electrodes are secured to the skin with a suction cup. The lead selector switch is turned to V to record these leads. The arm and leg electrodes must be attached to the patient in order to obtain the V leads. Some ECG machines record three or six leads simultaneously.[11]

Each ECG form should include the following identifying information:

1. Patient's name and identification number
2. Location, date, and time of the recording
3. Patient age, gender, and cardiac medication
4. Race, body build (weight and height measurements), blood pressure, tentative clinical diagnosis, clinical status, and noncardiac medications, such as phenothiazines
5. Any unusual position of the patient during the recording, or the presence of thoracic deformities, amputation, respiratory distress, or muscle tremor.[8]

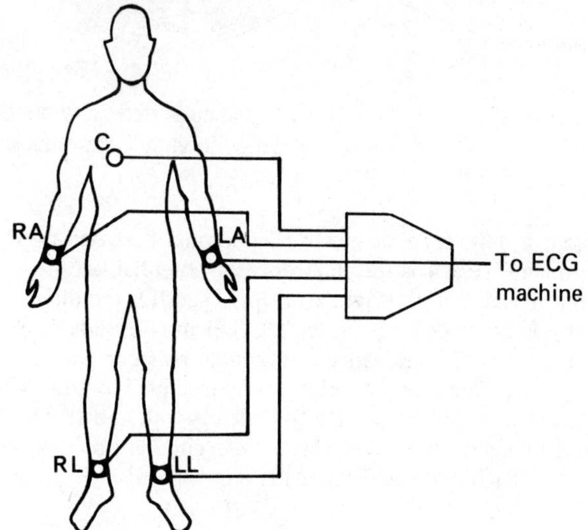

FIGURE 36–4 Twelve-lead ECG electrode placement.

Procedure for Attaching a Patient to a Cardiac Monitor

The positive, negative, and ground electrodes are placed on the chest according to the lead selected for monitoring. Commonly used leads are lead II, lead III, MCL_1 (modified left arm lead in the V_1 position), and MCL_6 (modified left arm lead in the V_6 position; Fig. 36–6).[7] For leads MCL_1 and MCL_6, the negative and ground electrodes are placed on the back of the shoulder rather than on the chest to prevent skin breakdown over potential subclavian intravenous or pacemaker

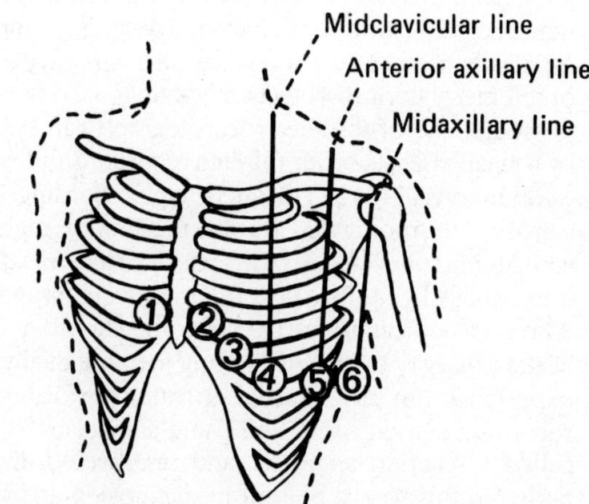

FIGURE 36–5 Six standard precordial leads: electrode placement. (*1*) Fourth intercostal space, at right side of sternum. (*2*) Fourth intercostal space, at left side of sternum. (*3*) Midway between positions *2* and *4*. (*4*) Fifth intercostal space, midclavicular line. (*5*) Same level as *4* in the anterior axillary line. (*6*) Same as *4* and *5* in the midaxillary line.

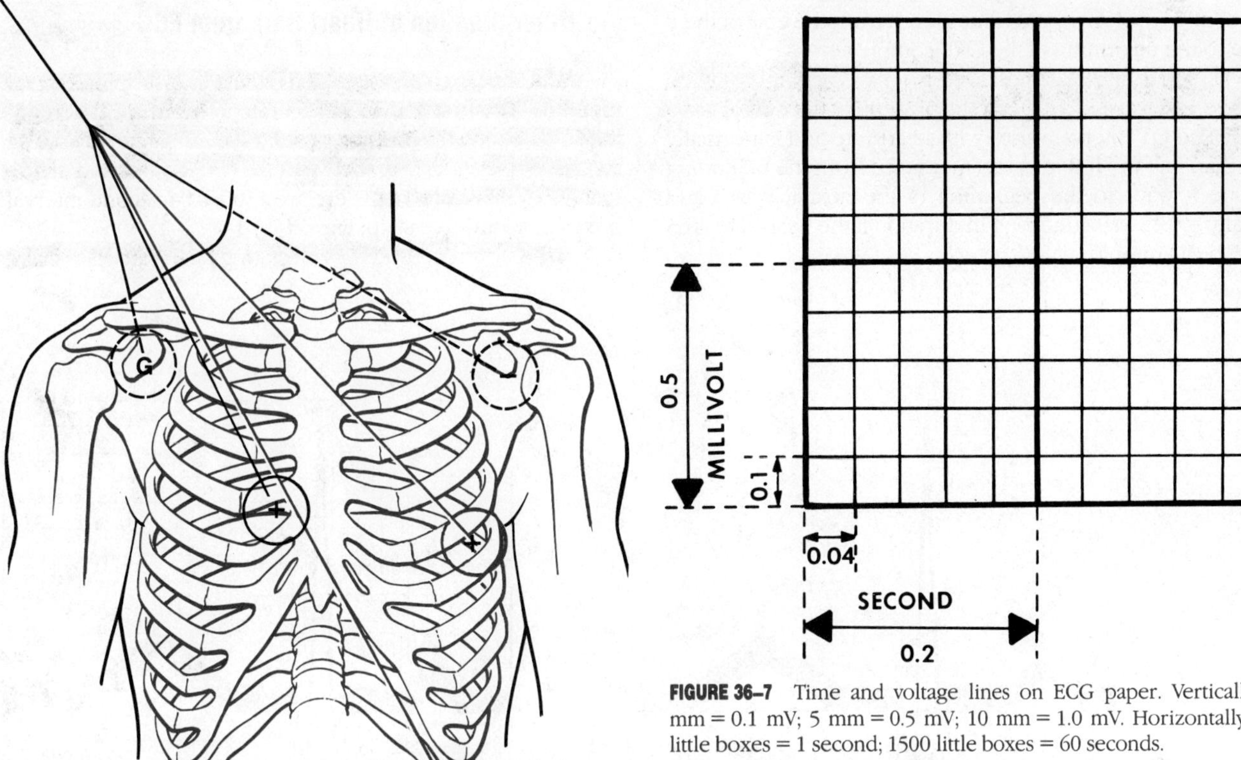

FIGURE 36–6 Hookup for constant monitoring with MCL_1 (black lines). The positive electrode is placed in the V_1 position; the negative electrode is placed on the outer one fourth of the left posterior shoulder; and the ground is placed on the right posterior shoulder. Red lines show alternative temporary placement of the positive electrode to obtain MCL_6: the positive electrode is placed in the V_6 position. To obtain M3, the positive electrode is placed on the left upper abdomen.

FIGURE 36–7 Time and voltage lines on ECG paper. Vertically: 1 mm = 0.1 mV; 5 mm = 0.5 mV; 10 mm = 1.0 mV. Horizontally: 25 little boxes = 1 second; 1500 little boxes = 60 seconds.

sites. The electrode site on the skin should be clean (use alcohol), dry (use gauze), and relatively flat. Hair should be shaved and the skin mildly abraded to reduce skin resistance. The pre-jelled electrodes are applied to the chest, the alarm for heart rate are set (30% above and below the patient's heart rate), and the alarm system is activated. Electrodes should be changed often enough (usually about every 1 to 3 days) to prevent skin breakdown and to provide artifact-free tracings. The patient should be given an explanation of the purpose of ECG monitoring and his questions should be answered.

Interpretation of a Rhythm Strip

Generally, ECG paper moves at speed of 25 mm/second. Each small box horizontally is equal to 0.04 second. One large box (5 small boxes) horizontally equals 0.20 second; one large box (5 small boxes) vertically is equal to 5 mm. Ten millimeters equal 1 millivolt (mV). The ECG is calibrated to 1 mV vertically in order to standardize the ECG (Fig. 36–7).

Waves, Complexes, and Intervals

The ECG is composed of several components or waves: the P wave, the QRS complex, the T wave, the ST segment, the PR and QT intervals, and possibly a U wave. The *P wave* represents atrial muscle depolarization (Fig. 36–8). It is normally 2.5 mm or less in height and 0.11 second in duration.

The *QRS complex* represents ventricular muscle depolarization. The first negative deflection after the P wave is the Q wave, which is less than 0.03 second in duration and less than 25% of the R-wave amplitude. The first positive deflection after the P wave is the R wave; the S wave is the first negative deflection after the R wave. The QRS complex is measured from the beginning of the Q wave, or the R wave if no Q wave is present, to the end of the S wave. The QRS complex is normally 0.04 to 0.10 second in duration.

The *T wave* represents ventricular muscle repolarization. It follows the QRS complex and is usually of the same deflection as the QRS complex. If a U wave is present, it will follow the T wave. The presence of a U wave may indicate an electrolyte abnormality.

The *ST segment,* which represents early ventricular repolarization, is from the end of the S wave (J point) to the beginning of the T wave.

The *PR interval* is measured from the beginning of the P wave to the beginning of the Q wave, or to the beginning of the R wave if no Q wave is present, and represents the time required for the impulse to travel through the atria, conduction system, and Purkinje fibers. Normally in adults, the PR interval ranges from 0.12 to 0.20 second in duration. The PR segment is isoelectric and is measured from the end of the P wave to the beginning of the QRS complex.

The *QT interval* is measured from the beginning of the Q wave, or R wave if no Q wave is present, to the end of the T wave. The QT interval varies with heart rate and is normally less than half the R-R interval (measured from the beginning of one R wave to the beginning of the next R wave) and usually is 0.32 to 0.40 second in duration if the heart rate is 65 to 95 beats/minute.

Determination of Heart Rate from ECG

Heart rate can be obtained from the ECG strip by several methods. The first and most accurate, if the rhythm is regular, is to count the number of 0.04-second intervals (0.04 second is one small box) between the two R waves and divide that number into 1500. (There are 1500, 0.04-second interval boxes in a 1-minute strip; Fig. 36–9, *A*.)

The second method for computing heart rate, especially

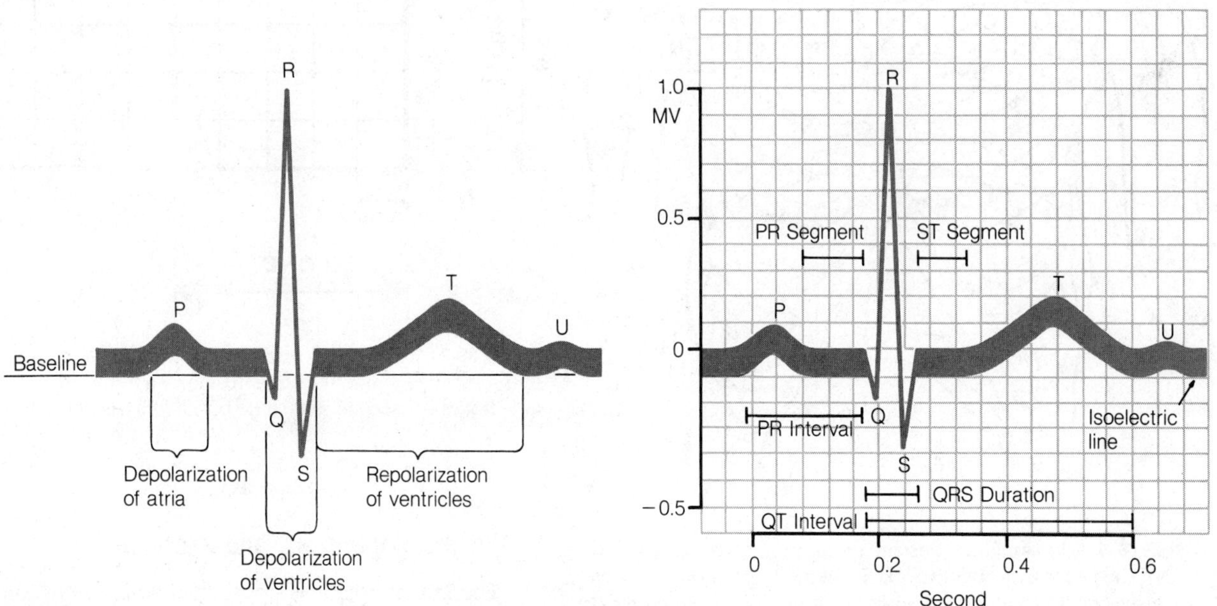

FIGURE 36–8 Diagram of the electrocardiogram (lead II) and representative depolarization and repolarization of the atria and ventricle. The P wave represents atrial depolarization; the QRS complex, ventricular depolarization; and the T wave, ventricular repolarization. Atrial repolarization occurs during ventricular depolarization and is hidden under the QRS complex.

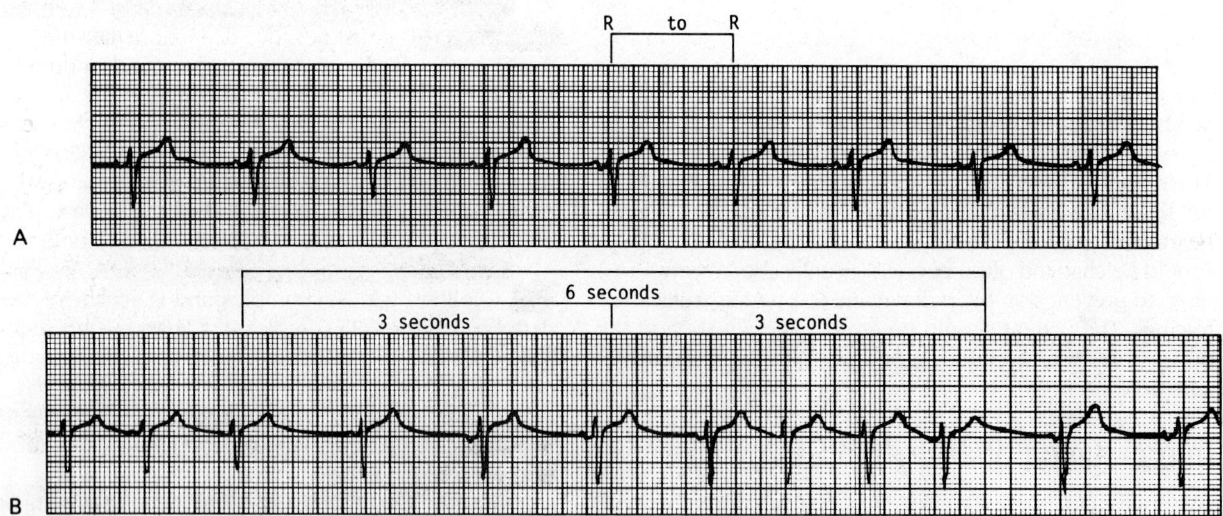

FIGURE 36–9 (*A*) Heart rate determination for a regular rhythm. There are approximately 25 little boxes between two R waves. This number divided into 1500 equals 60. The heart rate is 60. There are five large boxes between R waves; thus the rate is approximately 60 per minute. (*B*) Heart rate determination if the rhythm is irregular. There are approximately seven R–R intervals in 6 seconds; 7 times 10 equals 70. The heart rate is 70.

useful when the rhythm is irregular, is to count the number of R-R intervals in 6 seconds and multiply that number by 10. The ECG paper is usually marked at 3-second intervals (15 large boxes horizontally) by a vertical line at the top of the paper (Fig. 36–9, *B*). The R-R intervals rather than each QRS complex are counted. If QRS complexes were counted, the computed heart rate would be too high.

Arrhythmias

Cardiac arrhythmias are disturbances in rate, rhythm, or conduction of the heart's electrical impulses and are diagnosed from the ECG. Altered impulse formation or conduction can result in an irregularity of heart rhythm. Arrhythmias can be due to myocardial ischemia, overstretching of the myocardium, digitalis intoxication, hypoxia, hyperkalemia or hypokalemia, fever, acidosis or alkalosis, exercise, or increased circulatory catecholamines.[11]

Arrhythmias can be classified by heart rate, anatomic origin, blocks, or the manner in which the impulse is formed. Classically, arrhythmias have been classified by anatomic origin and by heart rate. Various conduction abnormalities are described here according to the anatomy involved and the degree of block manifested.

Arrhythmias Originating in the Sinus Node

Arrhythmias originating in the sinus node are sinus bradycardia, sinus tachycardia, sinus arrhythmia, and sinus arrest.

Normal Sinus Rhythm

Normal sinus rhythm (NSR; Fig. 36–10) has the following characteristics:

- *Rate:* 60 to 100 beats/minute
- *P waves:* Precede each QRS complex; PR interval is normal (0.12 second to 0.20 second)
- *QRS complex:* Usually has a normal interval (0.04 second to 0.10 second)
- *Conduction:* Through the atria, AV node, and ventricles usually normal

Sinus Bradycardia

Sinus bradycardia (Fig. 36–11) may be a normal finding; it is commonly seen in trained atheletes. Other causes of sinus bradycardia include myocardial infarction (MI) involving the sinus node, severe pain, administration of drugs (propranolol, reserpine, and methyldopa), hypoendocrine states (myxedema, Addison's disease, panhypopituitarism), anorexia nervosa, hypothermia, surgical damage to the sinus node, and vagal stimulation.[2] Vagal stimulation may be caused by high blood pressure; Valsalva maneuver; glossopharyngeal or oculocardiac reflex; carotid sinus stimulation; stimulation of receptors in left ventricle or coronary sinus when the heart is distended; fear, despair, isolation, hopelessness; morphine sulfate administration; digitalis intoxication; or increased intracranial pressure.

The following are characteristics of this arrhythmia:

- *Rate:* 40 to 60 beats/minute
- *P waves:* Precede each QRS complex; PR interval normal
- *QRS complex:* Usually normal
- *Conduction:* Usually normal
- *Rhythm:* Regular

All aspects of sinus bradycardia should be the same as those of normal sinus rhythm, except for the rate. If slow heart rate is causing significant hemodynamic changes with resultant syncope (fainting from insufficient flow of blood to the brain), angina, or ectopic arrhythmias, then treatment is directed toward increasing heart rate. If the decrease in heart rate is due to vagal stimulation, attempts should be made to prevent further vagal stimulation. If the patient has digitalis intoxication, then digitalis should be withheld. If atropine does not increase heart rate, then the slow rate is not caused by vagal stimulation.

Sinus Tachycardia

Sinus tachycardia (Fig 36–12) may be caused by fever, acute blood loss, anemia, shock, exercise, heart failure, pain, hypermetabolic states, anxiety, or sympthomimetic or parasympatholytic drugs. The ECG pattern is as follows:

- *Rate:* 100 to 180 beats/minute
- *P waves:* Precede each QRS complex; may be buried in the preceding T wave; PR interval normal
- *QRS complex:* Usually has a normal interval
- *Conduction:* Usually normal
- *Rhythm:* Regular

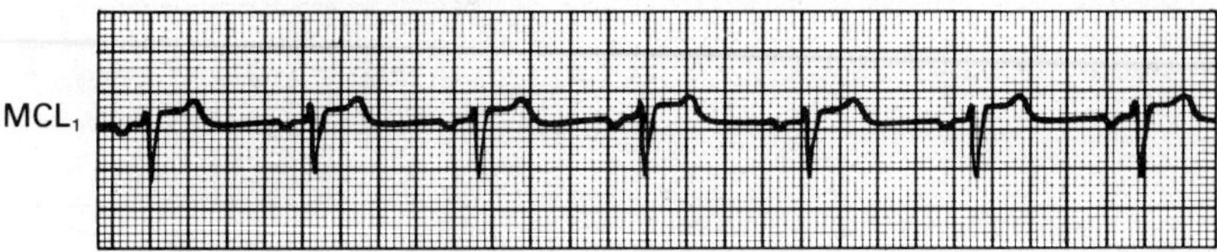

FIGURE 36–10 Normal sinus rhythm.

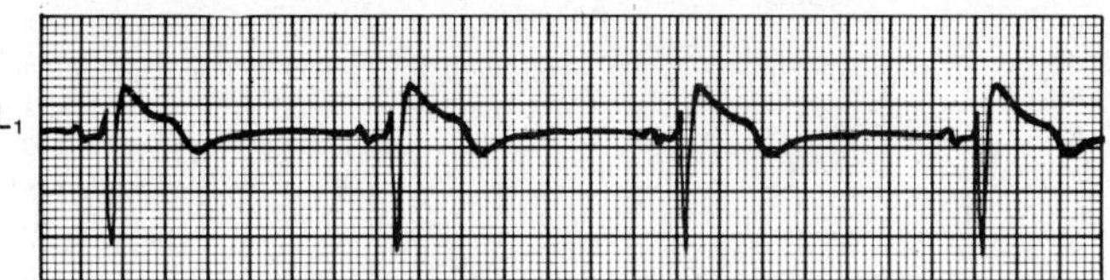

FIGURE 36–11. Sinus bradycardia.

All aspects of sinus tachycardia should be the same as those of normal sinus rhythm, except for the rate.

Treatment is usually directed at the primary cause. Carotid sinus pressure may be effective in slowing the rate temporarily, and thereby help to rule out other arrhythmias. As heart rate increases, diastolic filling time decreases, resulting in reduced coronary artery filling and less ventricular diastolic filling (decreased preload).

Sinus Arrhythmia

Sinus arrhythmia (Fig. 36–13) is a common variant of normal sinus rhythm and occurs as a normal phenomenon. Normally, with inspiration there is a degree in left ventricular stroke volume, resulting in a compensatory increase in heart rate to maintain cardiac output. Sinus arrhythmia commonly occurs in the young or aged, especially with slower heart rates or following enhanced vagal tone from digitalis or morphine. It is absent in the neonate and is commonly found in patients with Cheyne-Stokes respiration. The sinus impulse may vary reflexly with respiration. Afferent impulses from the lungs travel to the medulla, and efferent impulses travel over the vagus nerve to the sinus node.[2]

This arrhythmia is characterized by the following ECG changes:

- *Rate:* 60 to 100 beats/minute
- *P waves:* Precede each QRS; PR interval normal
- *QRS complex:* Usually normal
- *Conduction:* Usually normal
- *Rhythm:* May be related to breathing (rate increases with inspiration and decreases with expiration), or the irregularity may be unrelated to respiration. The irregularity can best be seen by measuring R-R intervals

Treatment is usually not necessary, but increasing the heart rate with exercise or sympathomimetic drugs will in many cases abolish this arrhythmia.

Sinus Node Arrest

Sinus node arrest (Fig. 36–14) can result from excessive carotid sinus pressure or other forms of vagal stimulation, involvement of the sinus node or sinus node artery in acute MI, or degenerative forms of fibrosis.

Sinus arrest within normal sinus rhythm has the following characteristics:

- *Rate:* Usually 60 to 100 beats/minute, but frequently in the bradycardia range (fewer then 60 beats/minute)
- *P waves:* When P waves are present, the PR interval is usually normal. If escape beats from the junction or ventricle occur, the P wave may be absent or inverted before or after the QRS complex.
- *QRS complex:* Not present during sinus arrest unless escape beats occur
- *Ventricular conduction:* Usually normal when it occurs
- *Rhythm:* Irregular. Escape beats from the junctional and ventricular areas are common. The variation will be found by measuring the R-R intervals. The P-P intervals will be variable.

Treatment is directed toward normalizing heart rate and eliminating the cause.

Arrhythmias Originating in the Atrial Muscle

Arrhythmias originating in the atrial muscle are the following: premature atrial contractions (PACs); wandering atrial pacemaker (WAP); multifocal atrial tachycardia (MAT); par-

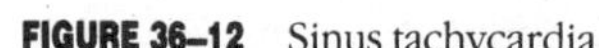

FIGURE 36–12 Sinus tachycardia.

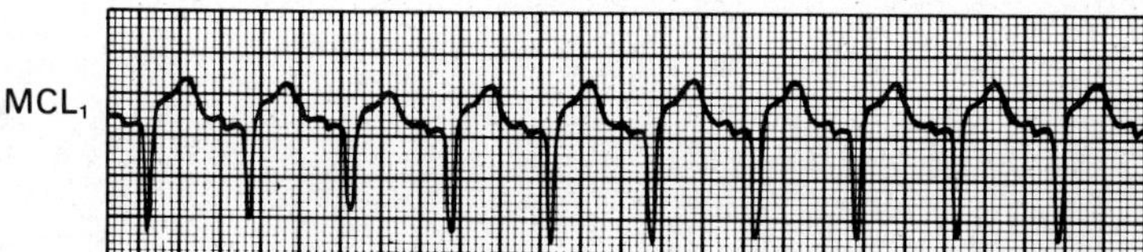

FIGURE 36–13 Sinus arrhythmia.

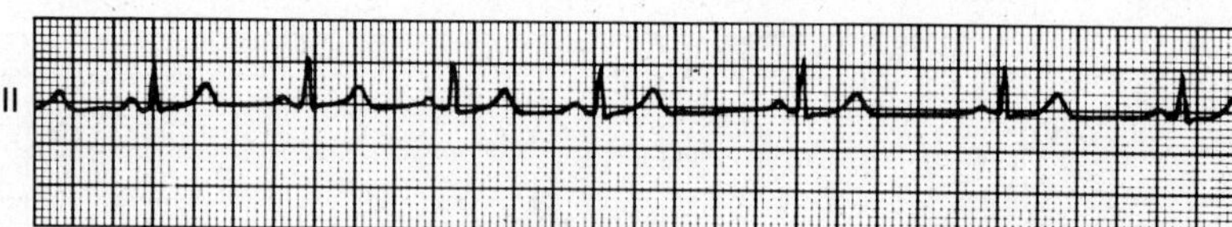

FIGURE 36–14 Sinus node arrest.

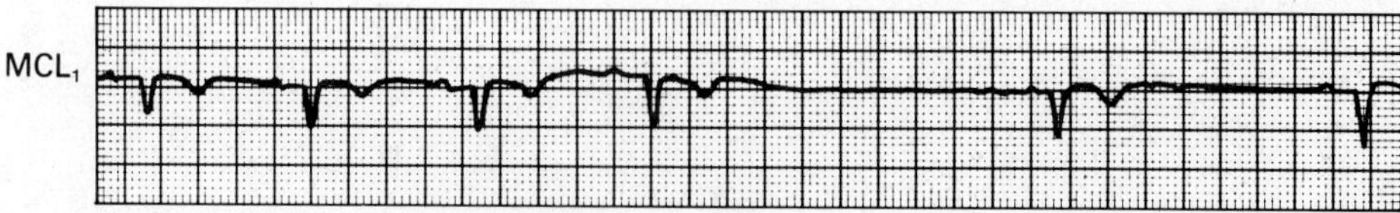

oxysmal atrial tachycardia (PAT); atrial flutter; and atrial fibrillation.

Premature Atrial Contractions

Premature atrial contractions (PACs; Fig. 36–15) may be seen in normal hearts or may be caused by atrial muscle irritability due to caffeine; alcohol; nicotine; stretched atrial myocardium as in heart failure; stress or anxiety; hypokalemia; atrial ischemia, injury or infarction; hypoxia; or hypermetabolic states. The patient may say that his heart skipped a beat. A pulse deficit (difference between apical and radial pulse rate) may exist if the impulse occurred so prematurely that the ventricles did not have time to fill adequately. If PACs are frequent (more than six per minute) a more serious arrhythmia, such as atrial fibrillation, could occur.

Premature atrial contractions have the following characteristics:

- *Rate:* 60 to 100 beats/minute
- *P waves:* Usually have a configuration different from that of the P waves that originate in the SA node. Another site in the atria has become irritable (enhanced automaticity) and fires before the normal firing time of the SA node. PR interval may vary from the PR intervals of impulses originating in the SA node.
- *QRS complex:* May be normal, aberrant, or absent. If the ventricles have completed their repolarization phase, they can respond to this early stimulus from the atria.
- *Conduction:* Usually normal
- *Rhythm:* Regular, except vhen the PACs occur. The P wave will be early in the cycle and usually will not have a complete compensatory pause. (Time between the preceding complex and the following complex is less than the time for two R-R intervals.)

If PACs are infrequent, no treatment is necessary. If they are frequent (more than six per minute) or occur during atrial repolarization, treatment is directed toward the cause.

Wandering Atrial Pacemaker

Wandering atrial pacemaker (WAP; Fig. 36–16) occurs when there is variation in the vagal tone at the sinus node or when there are changes in sympathetic stimulation. This arrhythmia is commonly seen in patients with digitalis intoxication. The patient is usually unaware of the arrhythmia.

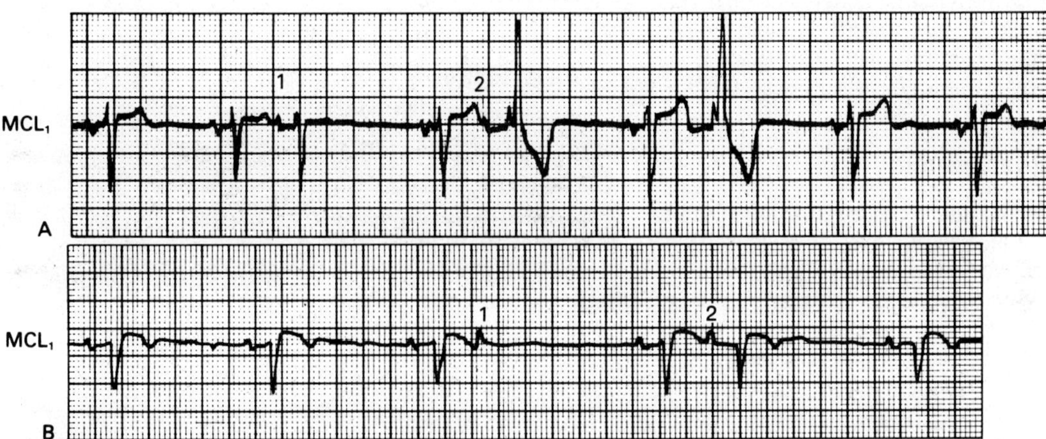

FIGURE 36–15 (*A*) Premature atrial contractions. Beat labeled *1* is a PAC with normal ventricular conduction, and beat labeled *2* is a PAC with aberrant ventricular conduction. (*B*) Premature atrial contractions. Beat labeled *1* is a PAC without ventricular conduction, and beat labeled *2* is a PAC with normal ventricular conduction.

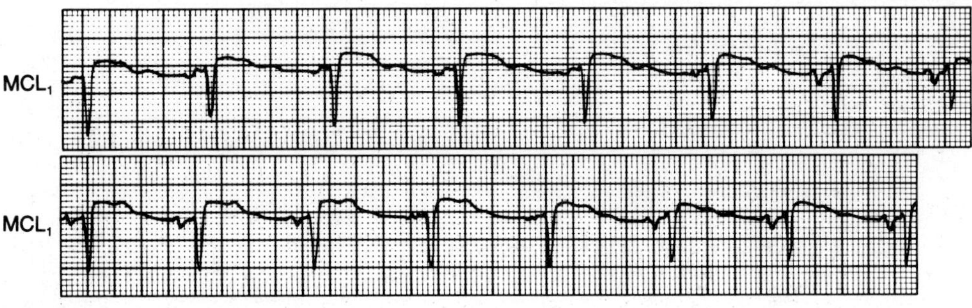

FIGURE 36–16 Wandering atrial pacemaker.

Wandering atrial pacemaker is characterized by the following:

- *Rate:* 60 to 100 beats/minute (If the rate is greater than 100, it is called multifocal atrial tachycardia.)
- *P waves:* Will vary from impulse to impulse in size and configuration. Stimulus coming from the SA node or close to it will produce normal-looking P waves. As the pacemaker wanders closer to the AV node, the P waves will become flatter or even inverted. The PR interval varies, depending on the closeness of the pacemaker to the AV node. At least three different P wave configurations must be seen.
- *QRS complex:* Usually normal
- *Conduction:* Conduction from the AV node through the ventricles will usually be normal.
- *Rhythm:* The R-R intervals may vary because of the variations in the PR intervals.

There usually is no need for treatment. Observe for digitalis intoxication. If decreases in heart rate alter cardiac output significantly, then sympathomimetic or parasympatholytic drugs can be used.

Multifocal Atrial Tachycardia

Multifocal atrial tachycardia (MAT; Fig. 36–17) is most commonly associated with severe pulmonary disease. It is similar to WAP except that the atrial rate is greater than 100 beats/minute. Treatment is directed toward eliminating the cause and decreasing the heart rate with a drug such as propranolol. Digitalis may worsen the rhythm.

Paroxysmal Atrial Tachycardia

Paroxysmal atrial tachycardia is characterized by abrupt onset and abrupt cessation. Rhythm may be triggered by emotions, tobacco, caffeine, fatigue, sympathomimetic drugs, or alcohol. Paroxysmal atrial tachycardia is not usually associated with organic heart disease. The rapid rate may produce angina owing to decreased coronary artery filling. Cardiac output is reduced and heart failure may occur. The patient frequently does not tolerate this rhythm for long periods.

Paroxysmal atrial tachycardia (Fig. 36–18) is characterized by the following:

- *Rate:* 150 to 250 beats/minute
- *P waves:* Ectopic and slightly to grossly normal; may be found in the preceding T wave; PR interval shortened (less than 0.12 second)
- *QRS complex:* Usually normal, but may be distorted if aberrant conduction is present
- *Conduction:* Usually normal
- *Rhythm:* Regular

The patient may not be aware of paroxysmal atrial tachycardia. Treatment is directed toward eliminating the cause and decreasing the heart rate. Morphine sedation slows the rate without further treatment. Carotid sinus pressure usually slows the rate or stops the attack and is usually more effective after digitalis or pressors. The use of vasopressors has a reflex effect on the carotid sinus by elevating the blood pressure and thus slowing the heart rate. Short-acting digitalis preparations may be used. Propranolol may be tried if digitalis is unsuccessful. Quinidine may be effective. Cardioversion may be necessary if the patient does not tolerate the fast heart rate.

Atrial Flutter

Atrial flutter (rapid, regular "fluttering" of the atria) is usually associated with rheumatic heart disease, atherosclerotic heart disease, thyrotoxicosis, acute cor pulmonale, congestive heart failure, and MI. Any ventricular response of 150 should be suspect for atrial flutter with a 2 : 1 block.

Atrial flutter (Fig. 36–19) is characterized by the following:

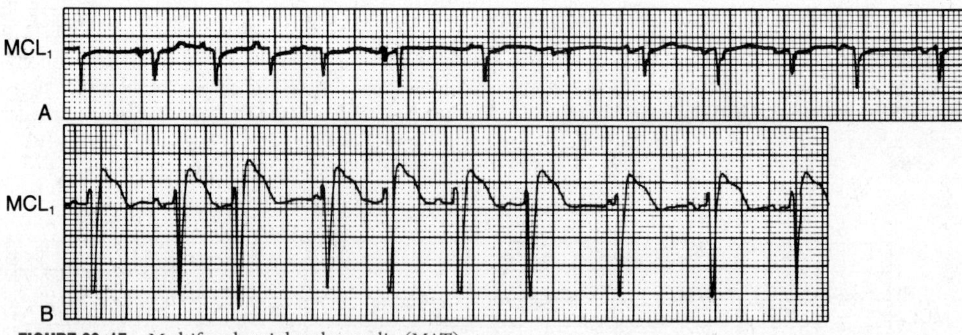

FIGURE 36–17 Multifocal atrial tachycardia (MAT).

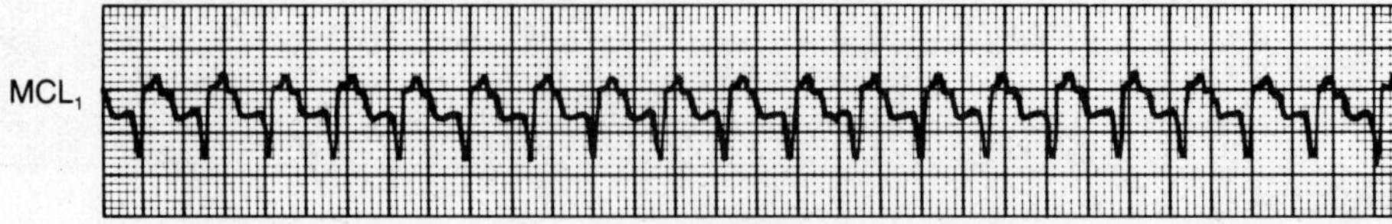

FIGURE 36–18 Paroxysmal atrial tachycardia.

- *Rate:* Atrial rate 250 to 350 beats/minute; most commonly 300. The ventricular rate will usually show some degree of block with the ventricle responding in a 2:1 or 4:1 pattern, rarely 3:1. There may be variations in the block pattern, particularly if treatment has been started.
- *P waves:* Characterized by the F waves (flutter waves seen between R waves) occurring in a regular fashion and in a sawtooth or picket-fence pattern. One F wave usually falls within the QRS-T complex.
- *QRS complex:* Usually normal, except where aberrant conduction is present
- *Conduction:* Usually normal
- *Rhythm:* Usually regular, but irregularities in the block pattern are not uncommon.

Treatment is directed toward eliminating the cause, decreasing the rate of ventricular response, and decreasing arrhythmias myocardial irritability. If quinidine is administered, 1:1 conduction could occur unless a negative dromotropic effect is present. Carotid sinus massage may unmask the flutter waves and increase the flutter rate. Cardioversion can usually be achieved with low, direct current shock (10–50 watt-seconds)

Cardioversion

Cardioversion is used to terminate arrhythmias that have QRS complexes and is usually an elective procedure. The patient is alert, and informed consent is obtained. The patient is usually given diazepam intravenously prior to cardioversion to promote anesthesia. The amount of voltage used varies from 25 to 400 watt-seconds. Digoxin is usually withheld for 48 hours prior to cardioversion to prevent postcardioversion arrhythmias.

The synchronizer is turned on. The defibrillator is synchronized with a cardiac monitor so that an electrical impulse is discharged during ventricular depolarization (the QRS complex). If the defibrillator were not synchronized, it could discharge during the vulnerable period (T wave) and result in ventricular tachycardia or fibrillation. The synchronizer switch is therefore turned *on* so that the unit discharges immediately after the onset of the next QRS complex. The discharge buttons should be held until the synchronizer fires the defibrillator.

If ventricular fibrillation occurs after cardioversion, the defibrillator must be immediately recharged, the synchronizer turned *off*, and defibrillation repeated. After use, the defibrillator should be turned *off* to prevent accidental discharge of the paddles. Oxygen flow should be stopped during precordial shock, if possible, to avoid the hazard of fire.

Indications of a successful response are conversion to sinus rhythm, strong peripheral pulses, and adequate blood pressure. Airway patency should be maintained and the patient's state of consciousness assessed. Vital signs should be obtained at least every 15 minutes for 1 hour, every 30 minutes for 2 hours, then every 4 hours.

Atrial Fibrillation

Atrial fibrillation (disorganized and uncoordinated twitching of atrial musculature) is usually associated with atherosclerotic heart disease, rheumatic heart disease, heart failure, thyrotoxicosis, cor pulmonale, and congenital heart disease.

Atrial fibrillation (Fig 36–20) is characterized by the following:

- *Rate:* An atrial rate of 350 to 600 beats/minute; ventricular response usually 120 to 200 beats/minute
- *P waves:* No discernible P waves; irregular undulation, termed fibrillary or "f" waves, is seen; PR interval cannot be measured.
- *QRS complex:* Usually normal
- *Conduction:* Usually normal through the ventricles. Characterized by an irregular ventricular response, because the AV node is incapable of responding to the rapid atrial rate. Impulses that are transmitted cause the ventricles to respond irregularly.
- *Rhythm:* Irregular and usually rapid, unless controlled. Irregularity of rhythm is due to concealed conduction within the AV node.

A rapid ventricular response reduces the time for ventricular filling and hence the stroke volume. The atrial kick, which is 25% to 30% of the cardiac output, is also lost. Heart failure frequently follows. Coarse atrial fibrillation (slower atrial rate) is more easily converted than fine atrial fibrillation (faster atrial rate). There is usually a pulse deficit. Treatment is directed toward eliminating the cause, decreasing the atrial irritability, and decreasing the rate of the ventricular response. In patients with chronic atrial fibrillation, anticoagulant therapy may be used to prevent thromboemboli from forming in the atria.

Sometimes a mixture of atrial flutter and atrial fibril-

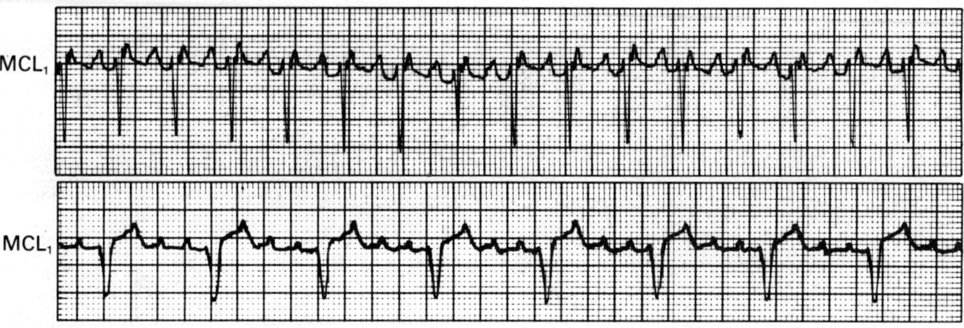

FIGURE 36–19 (*A*) Atrial flutter with 2:1 conduction. (*B*) Atrial flutter with 4:1 conduction.

lation is seen, and some call this atrial flutter–fibrillation. Others refer to this as coarse atrial fibrillation. Such an arrhythmia is best classified as a atrial fibrillation when the criteria for atrial flutter are not satisfied.

Tachycardia–Bradycardia Syndrome

Tachycardia–bradycardia syndrome is characterized by tachyarrhythmias (paroxysmal atrial fibrillation, flutter, or tachycardia) followed by SA block or sinus arrest, resulting in Stokes-Adams attacks. Clinical correlation with this syndrome has been found with coronary atherosclerosis, amyloidosis, renal insufficiency with azotemia, and trauma following open heart surgery. Some have used the tachycardia–bradycardia syndrome and sick sinus syndrome interchangeably, but this is not totally accurate, because the sick sinus syndrome includes a variety of sinus and atrial arrhythmias and only indicates a "sick" sinus node. In tachycardia–bradycardia syndrome, not only is the sinus node sick, but the impulse formation at the AV node is depressed as well.[5]

Marked bradycardia (heart rate of fewer than 20 beats/minute or prolonged asystole, exceeding 10 seconds) results in cerebral ischemia. Hence, lightheadedness, dizziness, syncope, or convulsions may occur. The tachycardia may cause such symptoms as palpitations, weakness, or chest pain. Treatment is directed toward suppressing the tachycardia with medications (quinidine, procainamide, digitalis, and propranolol) and maintaining an adequate heart rate with a pacemaker.

Arrhythmias Originating in the Junction

Arrhythmias originating in the junction (area between the atria and ventricles around the AV node) are as follows: junctional rhythm, premature junctional contraction, accelerated junctional tachycardia, and paroxysmal junctional tachycardia.

Junctional Rhythm

A junctional rhythm may occur if there is digitalis intoxication or sinus node disease resulting in a decreased ratc of the sinus node. Because the sinus rate is so slow, the junction may complete to be the pacemaker. Junctional rhythm (Fig. 36–21) has the following characteristics:

- *Rate:* 40 to 60 beats/minute
- *P waves:* Usually inverted and may occur before, during, or after the QRS complex, depending on the location of the pacemaker in the junctional tissue. The junctional tissue delays antegrade and retrogarde conduction.
- *QRS complex:* Normal
- *Conduction:* The atria are usually stimulated by the junctional tissue, resulting in an inverted P wave (called retrograde conduction). The conduction from the junctional tissue through the ventricles is usually normal (called antegrade conduction).
- *Rhythm:* Usually regular

There is usually no need for treatment, unless a reduction in the heart rate alters cardiac output markedly. If cardiac output decreases so that chest pain, syncope, or arrhyth-

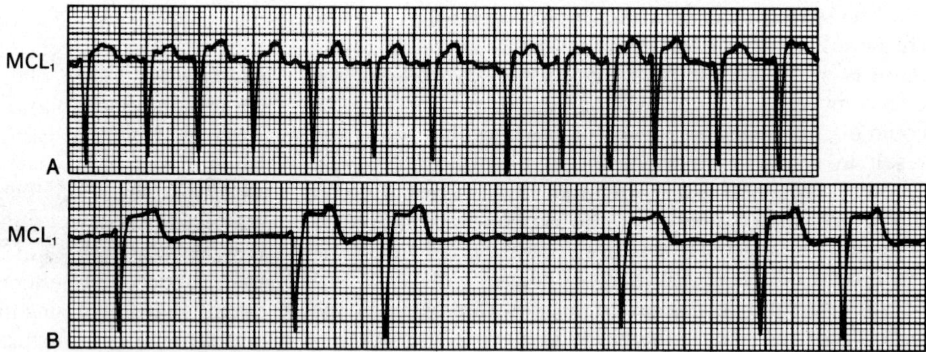

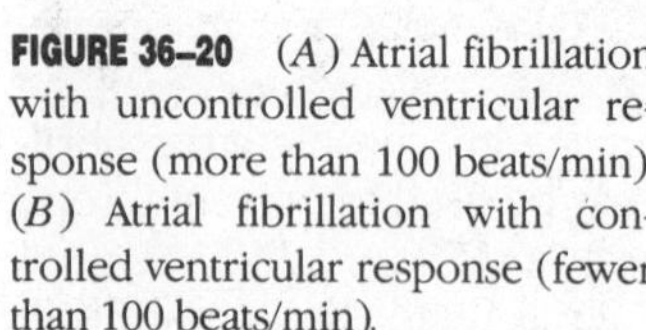

FIGURE 36–20 (*A*) Atrial fibrillation with uncontrolled ventricular response (more than 100 beats/min). (*B*) Atrial fibrillation with controlled ventricular response (fewer than 100 beats/min).

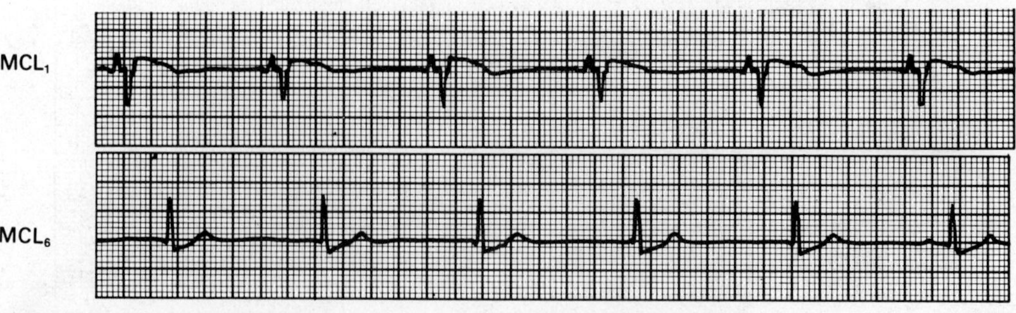

FIGURE 36–21 Junctional rhythm.

mias occur, sympathomimetic or parasympatholytic drugs may be used. Digitalis should be withheld. Quinidine, procainamide, phenytoin, propranolol, hyperkalemia, vagal stimulation depress junctional escape centers.

Premature Junctional Contractions

Premature junctional contractions (PJCs) occur because of increased irritability of the junctional tissue. Irritability can be due to digitalis intoxication or to coronary heart disease, resulting in decreased flow through the AV nodal artery. PJCs (Fig. 36–22) have the following characteristics:

- *Rate:* 60 to 100 beats/minute if the basic rhythm is normal sinus rhythm
- *P waves:* May occur before, during, or after the QRS complex, depending on the location of the pacemaker in the junctional tissue. The PR intervals vary and are shorter than normal (less than 0.12 second).
- *QRS complex:* May be normal or aberrant
- *Conduction:* The atria are stimulated in a retrograde fashion. The ventricular conduction is usually normal.
- *Rhythm:* Regular, except for the premature contraction. The compensatory pause is usually incomplete. Usually, no treatment is indicated. Digitalis should be withheld. If PJCs occur more frequently than six per minute, an antiarrhythmic drug may be prescribed.

Accelerated Junctional Rhythm and Paroxysmal Junctional Tachycardia

In accelerated junctional rhythm and paroxysmal junctional tachycardia, irritability in the junctional area has increased, resulting in a faster rate. Characteristics of these rhythms (Fig. 36–23) are as follows:

- *Rate:* Accelerated junctional rhythm, 60 to 100 beats/minute; paroxysmal junctional tachycardia, 100 to 250 beats/minute.
- *P waves:* The positive of the P wave in relation to the QRS complex will vary according to the location of the pacemaker in the junctional tissue. The configuration of the P wave will also vary accordingly. If the P wave is seen, it is usually inverted.
- *QRS complex:* May be normal or aberrant
- *Conduction:* Retrograde to the atria; normal through the ventricles
- *Rhythm:* Regular

Ventricular rate is less than 100 beats/minute for accelerated junctional rhythm and over 100 beats/minute for paroxysmal junctional tachycardia.

If the patient is on digitalis, it should be withheld until digitalis intoxication is ruled out, since this is a very common arrhythmia associated with digitalis intoxication. If the patient is not on digitalis, it may be given to increase AV conduction time. If the patient does not tolerate the rate, as demonstrated by signs and symptoms of a decreased cardiac output, then cardioversion may be necessary. This arrhythmia must be documented on the ECG to differentiate from sinus tachycardia or paroxysmal atrial tachycardia. When a rapid junctional rhythm occurs with a bundle branch conduction defect, it is difficult to distinguish this rhythm from ventricular tachycardia.

Arrhythmias Originating in the Ventricular Muscle

Arrhythmias originating in the ventricular muscle are the following: premature ventricular contractions, ventricular bigeminy, accelerated ventricular rhythm, ventricular tachy-

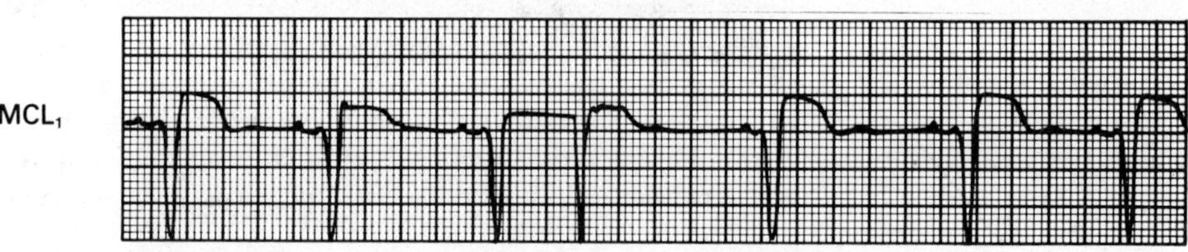

FIGURE 36–22 Premature junctional contractions.

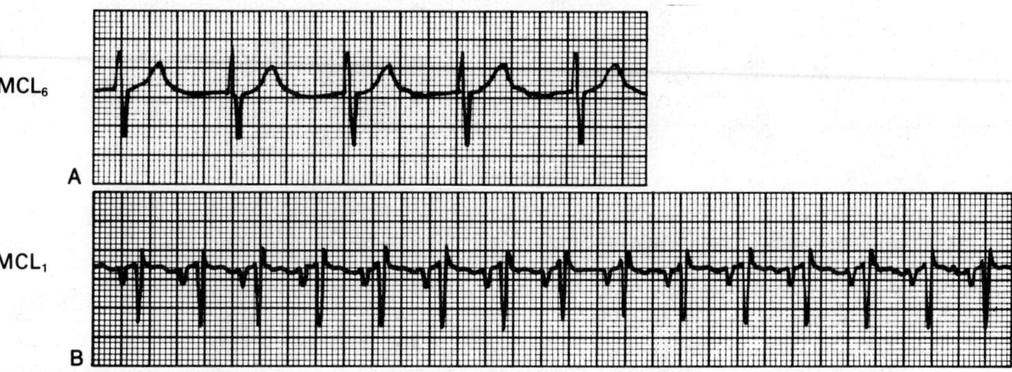

FIGURE 36–23 (*A*) Accelerated junctional rhythm. (*B*) Junctional tachycardia.

cardia, ventricular flutter, ventricular fibrillation, and ventricular asystole.

Premature Ventricular Contractions

Premature ventricular contractions (PVCs; Fig. 36–24) are considered serious precursors of ventricular tachycardia and ventricular fibrillation when they occur in increasing number (more than six a minute), are multiformed, occur in pairs or triplets, or come on the T wave (R-on-T). Premature ventricular contractions can be caused by hypoxia, hyperkalemia or hypokalemia, myocardial stretch from heart failure, myocardial irritation caused by an intracardiac catheter or pacemaker electrode, increased circulating catecholamines, or acidosis or alkalosis. If PVCs are frequent and so premature as to result in a pulse deficit, they could result in a decrease in cardiac output. Infrequent PVCs are usually not serious in themselves. Usually the patient will feel a palpitating sensation, but will have no other complaints. However, the seriousness lies in the fact that these PVCs may lead to more serious ventricular arrhythmias.

PVCs have the following characteristics:

- *Rate:* 60 to 100 beats/minute
- *P wave:* May be completely obscured, hidden in the QRS complex of the premature beat. The sinus rhythm is usually uninterrupted, resulting in a complete compensatory pause. If a premature P wave is seen before the wide QRS complex, the impulse is probably a premature supraventricular beat (an impulse that originates in the atria or junction) with aberration and not a PVC.
- *QRS complex:* Usually wide and bizarre; usually longer than 0.10 second in duration; may have the same focus in the ventricle, or may have a wide variety of configurations if occurring from multiple foci in the ventricles
- *Conduction:* Occasionally retrograde through the junctional tissue and atria
- *Rhythm:* Irregular when the premature beat occurs.

In order to decrease the myocardial irritability, the cause must be determined and, if possible, corrected. An anti-arrhythmic drug may be useful for immediate and possibly long-term therapy.

Ventricular Bigeminy

Ventricular bigeminy is frequently associated with digitalis excess, coronary heart disease, acute MI, and heart failure. The term *bigeminy* refers to a condition in which every other beat is premature. Atrial and junctional bigeminy can also occur; therefore, the origin of the bigeminy must be stated. If the PVCs or normal beat occurs every third beat, it is termed ventricular trigeminy; if it occurs every fourth beat, ventricular quadrigeminy.

Ventricular bigeminy (Fig. 36–25) has the following characteristics:

- *Rate:* May occur at any heart rate, but rate is usually less than 90 beats/minute
- *P waves:* The same as described for PVCs; may be hidden within the QRS complex
- *QRS complex:* Every other beat is a PVC with a wide, bizarre QRS complex and a complete compensatory pause.
- *Conduction:* The sinus beats are conducted from the sinus node in a normal fashion; the PVCs start in the ventricles and may have retrograde conduction through the junctional tissue and atria.
- *Rhythm:* Regularly irregular

The treatment for ventricular bigeminy is the same as for PVCs. Since the underlying cause of ventricular bigeminy is frequently digitalis toxicity, this should be ruled out or treated if present.

Accelerated Ventricular Rhythm and Ventricular Tachycardia

Accelerated ventricular rhythm and ventricular tachycardia (Fig. 36–26) are caused by the same mechanism as are PVCs. Ventricular rates less than 100 beats/minute are termed accelerated ventricular rhythm, and ventricular rates greater than 100 beats/minute are termed ventricular tachycardia. These rhythms can be associated with coronary heart disease and may precede ventricular fibrillation. Ventricular tachycardia is extremely dangerous and usually is considered an emergency. The patient is generally aware of this rapid rhythm and is quite anxious. The rapid heart rate compromises cardiac output, because the time for diastolic filling of

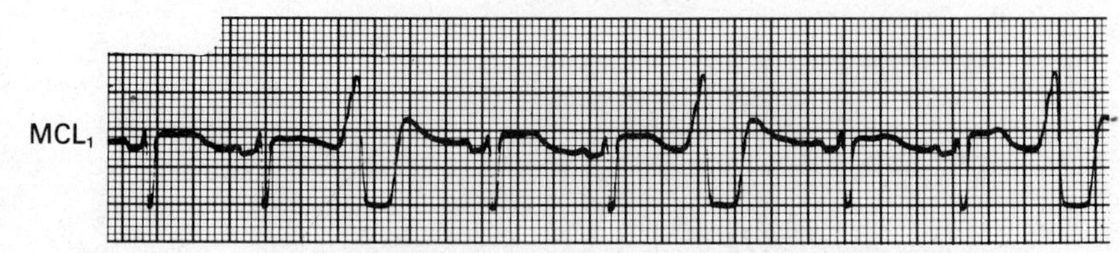

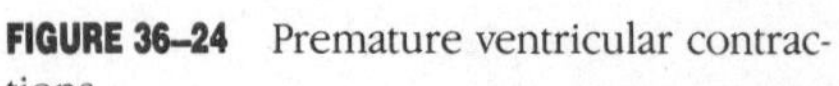

FIGURE 36–24 Premature ventricular contractions.

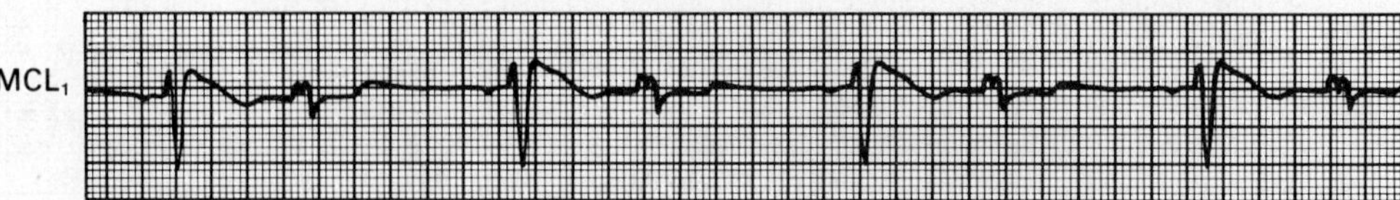

FIGURE 36–25 Ventricular bigeminy.

the heart is reduced (decreased preload) and stroke volume is reduced. Coronary artery filling is also reduced because of the shortened diastolic time. In patients with myocardial ischemia, this arrhythmia can further compromise myocardial blood supply. During ventricular tachycardia, AV dissociation usually occurs. The loss of synchrony between the atria and the ventricles during diastole results in the loss of atrial contraction and active filling of the ventricles, which in turn leads to further reduction in stroke volume; cardiac output decreases. The reduced cardiac output could reduce blood pressure such that the patient exhibits signs of decreased perfusion to vital organs.

Accelerated ventricular rhythm and ventricular tachycardia have the following characteristics:

- *Rate:* Accelerated ventricular rhythm 40 to 100 beats/minute; ventricular tachycardia 150 to 200 beats/minute
- *P waves:* Usually buried in the QRS complex complex; if seen, they do not necessarily fall in the normal pattern with the QRS. The ventricular contractions are dissociated from the atrial contractions.
- *QRS complex:* Have the same configurations as those of a PVC: wide and bizarre, with T waves in the opposite direction. A ventricular beat may fuse with a normal QRS, resulting in a fusion beat. Three or more PVCs in a row constitute ventricular tachycardia.
- *Conduction:* Rhythm originates in the ventricle, with possible retrograde conduction to the junctional tissue and atria
- *Rhythm:* Usually regular, but irregular ventricular tachycardia is also seen. The ventricular rhythm is rapid. The P waves, if seen, are at a slower rate and are regular. There is no association between the atrial rhythm and the ventricular rhythm (AV dissociation).

The patient's tolerance or lack of tolerance of this rapid rhythm will dictate the therapy to be given. The cause of the myocardial irritability must be determined and corrected, if possible. Antiarrhythmic drugs may be used. Cardioversion may be indicated if the reduction in cardiac output is marked.

Ventricular Flutter

Ventricular flutter has all the characteristics of ventricular tachycardia, but the rate is even faster. The clinical picture is exactly the same as ventricular standstill: the patient may be cyanotic and convulsing; there is not audible heartbeat and no palpable pulse; and the patient is not breathing. This arrhythmia is usually fatal without immediate treatment.

Ventricular flutter has the following characteristics:

- *Rate:* 200 to 400 beats/minute
- *P waves:* No visible P waves are seen.
- *QRS complex:* Rapid, bizarre, picket-fencelike complexes. T waves are not visible.
- *Conduction:* Rhythm originates in ventricles. There may be retrograde conduction through the AV node and atria.
- *Rhythm:* Not precisely regular

The treatment for ventricular flutter is similar to that for ventricular tachycardia. However, ventricular flutter is a far more acute emergency because the patient is without circulation. This arrhythmia will be fatal unless converted immediately; therefore, no initial attempts are made to convert this arrhythmia with drugs. Precordial shock is the first action to be taken and, in the absence of a physician, may be given immediately by the nursing staff. If a defibrillator is not readily available, external cardiac massage, assisted ventilation, and intravenous supportive drugs should be initiated at once. If the nurse present is having trouble discerning if the arrhythmia is ventricular tachycardia or ventricular flutter, her main concern should be the patient's tolerance of the arrhythmia, and she should treat the arrhythmia as the patient's tolerance indicates.

Ventricular Fibrillation

Ventricular fibrillation is a rapid, ineffective quivering of the ventricles. With this arrhythmia, there is no audible heartbeat, no palpable pulse, and no respirations. This pattern is so grossly irregular it can hardly be mistaken for another type of arrhythmia. Malfunction of the monitor may produce such a pattern, but in that case, the clinical picture of the patient would rule out the diagnosis of ventricular fibrillation. Ventricular fibrillation is usually fatal without immediate treatment, since only 5% convert spontaneously.

Ventricular fibrillation (Fig. 36–27) has the following characteristics:

- *Rate:* Rapid, uncoordinated, ineffective
- *P waves:* Usually not seen
- *QRS complex:* Rapid, irregular undulation without

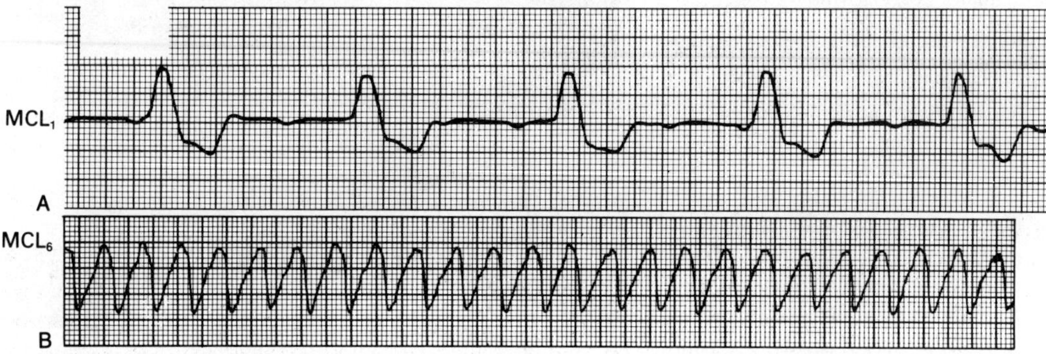

FIGURE 36–26 (*A*) Accelerated ventricular rhythm. (*B*) Ventricular tachycardia.

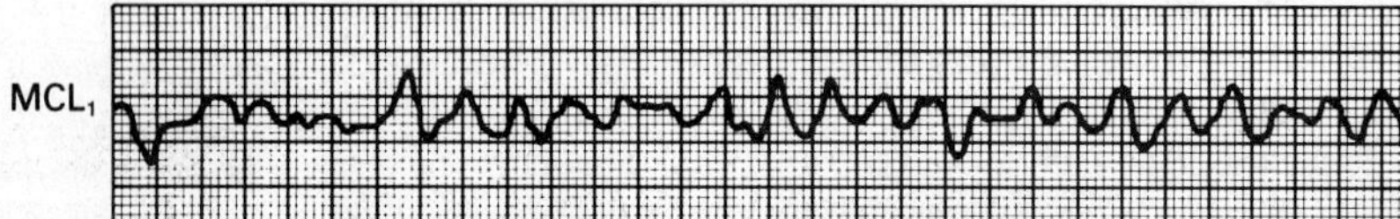

FIGURE 36–27 Ventricular fibrillation.

specific pattern (multifocal). The ventricles have only a quivering motion.

- *Conduction:* Foci are located in the ventricles, but so many foci are firing at one time that there is no organized conduction: no ventricular contractions occur.
- *Rhythm:* Extremely irregular and uncoordinated, without specific pattern

Defibrillation. Immediate treatment is defibrillation with 200 to 400 watt-seconds. A synchronized machine will not fire on this disorganized rhythm because there are no predominant waves it can recognize. Defibrillation is used immediately after onset of ventricular fibrillation or of ventricular tachycardia without a peripheral pulse. Defibrillation completely depolarizes all the myocardial cells and terminates the chaotic electrical activity, allowing the SA node to regain control of the heart rhythm unless the myocardium is anoxic or acidotic, in which case this may not be possible.

In defibrillation the electrode paddles are applied to the anterior chest. The standard electrode paddle position for the closed-chest procedure is as follows: one paddle just to the right of the upper sternum below the right clavicle and the other paddle just to the left of the cardiac apex (Fig. 36–28).

In order the reduce skin resistance to current flow and to prevent skin burns, one of the following may be placed between the electrodes and the chest wall: saline-soaked 4-by-4 gauze pads; electrode paste; or defibrillator pads (adhesive pads with electrode gel). Care should be taken to prevent contact between the two areas of conductive material because electrical bridging may occur. If saline-soaked gauze pads are used, cardiac compression can be resumed after defibrillation without the hands slipping on the chest, a problem that occurs with electrode paste.

- Exert 20 to 25 pounds of pressure on each paddle in order to ensure good skin contact.
- Do not let anyone touch the patient or the bed when the defibrillator is fired.
- Discharge the defibrillator at 200 to 400 watt-seconds, depending on the weight of the patient.

It is suggested that 3.5 to 6 watt-seconds per kg of body weight be used.[6] Defibrillation can occur only if the synchronizer switch is off, because a QRS complex is required for synchronized defibrillation, and ventricular fibrillation has no QRS complexes. After defibrillation, the cardiac monitor and pulse are checked for signs of restored sinus rhythm.

If defibrillation has been unsuccessful, cardiopulmonary resuscitation should be started immediately. Epinephrine and sodium bicarbonate may be used if fibrillation is fine. Epinephrine may make the fibrillation coarser and thus easier to convert with defibrillation. Blood pressure should be supported, using vasopressors. At no time during the resuscitation should the external cardiac message and the assisted ventilation be stopped for longer than 5 seconds.

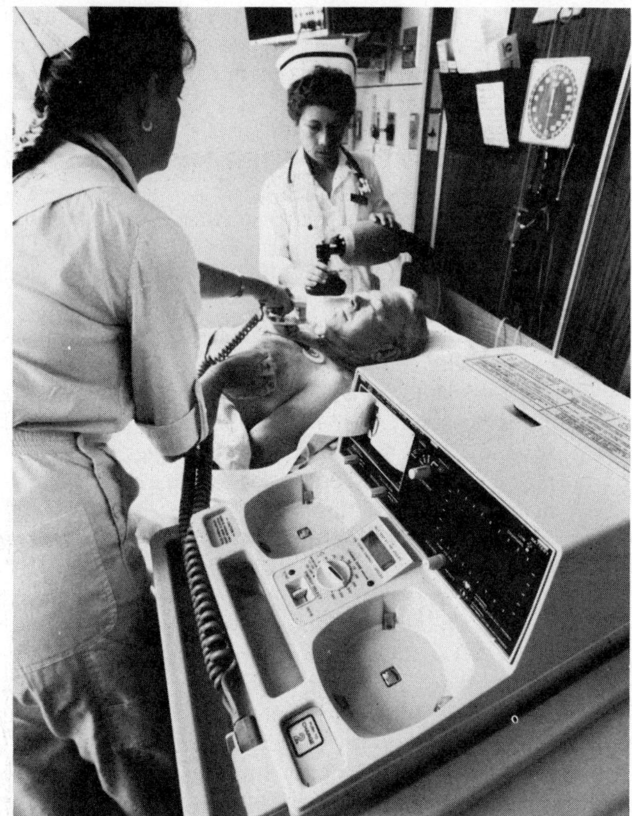

FIGURE 36–28 Technique for defibrillating patient.

Ventricular Asystole

In ventricular asystole there are no QRS complexes. There is no heartbeat, no palpable pulse, and no respiration. Ventricular asystole is fatal without immediate treatment. Ventricular asystole (Fig. 36–29) has the following characteristics:

- *Rate:* None
- *P waves:* May be evident, but they do not conduct through the AV node and ventricles
- *QRS complex:* None
- *Conduction:* Possibly, through the atria only
- *Rhythm:* None

Cardiopulmonary resuscitation is necessary to keep the patient alive. To decrease any vagal stimuli, 0.5 mg of atropine should be administered intravenously. Epinephrine should be administered and repeated at 5-minute intervals. Sodium bicarbonate should be given. Epinephrine and sodium bicarbonate are not compatible and may not be mixed together. Insertion of a transthoracic or transvenous pacemaker may be necessary.

Conduction Abnormalities

There are three types of heart block that result from a decreased conduction, usually between the junctional tissue and the Purkinje fibers: first-degree, second-degree (Mobitz I and Mobitz II), and third-degree block.

First-Degree Heart Block

First-degree heart block is usually associated with organic heart disease or may be due to the effect of digitalis. It is seen frequently in patients with inferior MIs (if the AV nodal artery is involved).

First-degree heart block (Fig. 36–30) has the following characteristics:

- *Rate:* Variable, usually 60 to 100 beat/minute
- *P waves:* Precede each QRS complex. The PR interval is greater than 0.20 second in duration.
- *QRS complexes:* Follow each P wave; usually normal
- *Conduction:* Delayed conduction, usually anywhere between the junctional tissue and the Purkinje network, produces a prolonged PR interval. Ventricular conduction is usually normal.
- *Rhythm:* Usually regular

This arrhythmia is important, since it may lead to more serious forms of heart block. If is often a warning signal. The patient should be monitored closely for any advancing block.

Second-Degree Heart Block, Mobitz Type I

Second-degree heart block, Mobitz type I (Wenckebach phenomenon), is usually associated with organic heart disease and is frequently due to digitalis intoxication. This block is frequently seen in association with MI that involves the AV nodal artery.

Second-degree heart block type I (Fig. 36–31) has the following characteristics:

- *Rate:* Variable, usually 60 to 100 beats/minute
- *P waves:* Precede each QRS complex. The PR interval becomes increasingly longer until finally a QRS complex is dropped and then the cycle is repeated.
- *QRS complex:* Follows most P waves, except when QRS complex is dropped
- *Conduction:* The PR interval becomes increasingly longer until an impulse is not conducted through the ventricles because it is blocked somewhere between the junctional tissue and the Purkinje network.
- *Rhythm:* Irregular, since the R-R interval becomes progressively shorter until a QRS complex is dropped.

Digitalis intoxication should be ruled out. Depending on the hemodynamic changes produced, efforts to normalize the heart rate may be necessary.

Second-Degree Heart Block, Mobitz Type II

Second-degree heart block, Mobitz type II, is also caused by organic heart disease, by MIs involving the AV nodal artery, and by digitalis intoxication. This type of block results in a reduced heart rate and usually a reduced cardiac output. (Cardiac output is the product of stroke volume and heart rate.)

Second-degree heart block type II (Fig. 36–32) has the following characteristics:

- *Rate:* 30 to 55 beats/minute. The atrial rate may be two, three, or four times faster than the ventricular rate.
- *P waves:* There are two, three, four P waves for each QRS complex. The PR interval of the conducted beat is usually normal in duration.

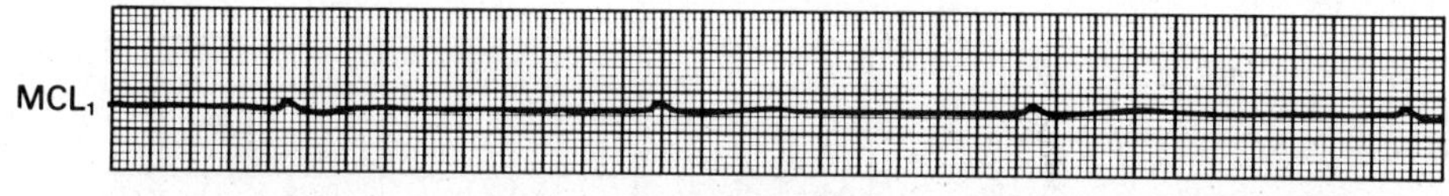

FIGURE 36–29 Ventricular asystole.

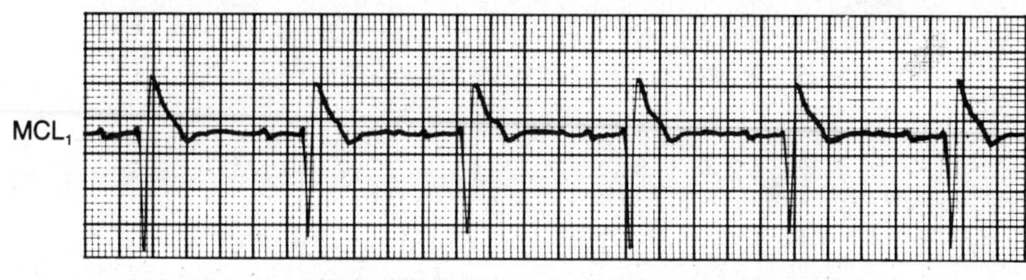

FIGURE 36–30 First degree heart block.

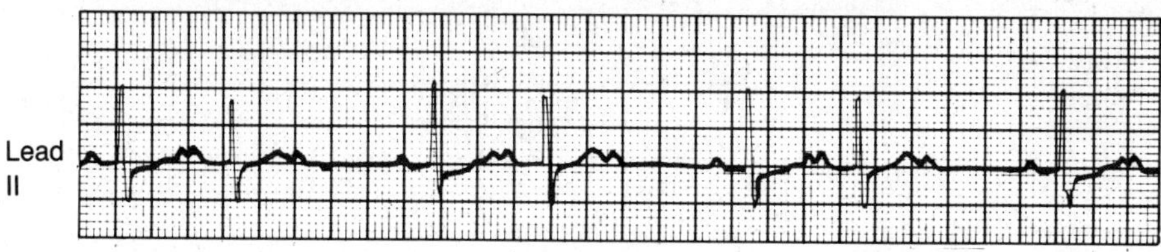

FIGURE 36–31 Second degree heart block, Mobitz type I.

- *QRS complex:* Usually prolonged
- *Conduction:* One or more of the impulses are not conducted through the ventricles
- *Rhythm:* Usually slow and regular. When an irregularity is seen, it is due to the fact that the block is varying from 2 : 1 to 3 : 1 or to some other combination.

Treatment is directed toward increasing the heart rate to maintain a normal cardiac output. Digitalis intoxication should be ruled out and myocardial depressant drugs withheld.

Third-Degree Heart Block

Third-degree heart block (complete heart block) is also associated with organic heart disease, digitalis intoxication, and MI. The heart rate may be markedly decreased, resulting in a decrease in perfusion to organs, such as the brain, heart, kidneys, lungs, and skin.

Complete block (Fig. 36–33) has the following characteristics:

- *Rate:* Atrial rate 60 to 100 beats/minute; venticular rate 40 to 60 beats/minute if the escape rhythm originated in the junction, 20 to 40 beats/minute if the escape rhythm originated in the ventricle
- *P waves:* The P waves originating from the SA node are seen regularly throughout the rhythm, but they have no association with the QRS complexes.
- *QRS complex:* If the escape rhythm originated in the junction, the QRS complexes have a normal supraventricular configuration, but have no association with the P waves. QRS complexes occur regularly. If the escape rhythm originated in the ventricle, the QRS complex is longer than 0.10 second in duration, usually broad and slurred. These QRS complexes have the same configuration as the QRS complex of a PVC.
- *Conduction:* The SA node is firing, and P waves can be seen. They are all blocked and not conducted to the ventricles. Escape rhythms originating in the junction are usually conducted normally through the ventricles. Escape rhythms from the ventricles are ectopic with aberrant configuration.
- *Rhythm:* Usually slow but regular.

Treatment is directed toward increasing perfusion to vital organs. This may include increasing the rate of the escape rhythm; a junctional rhythm can be increased by use of a parasympatholytic (anticholinergic) agent; a ventricular rhythm can be increased by use of a sympathomimetic agent. It may also include insertion of a temporary transvenous pacemaker.

Cardiac Pacemaker

A cardiac pacemaker may be required to maintain an effective heart rate. A pacemaker provides artificial electrical stimulus to the heart muscle when either the impulse initiation or the intrinsic conduction system is defective. Temporary and permanent pacemaker units may be used depending on etiology and prognosis of the arrhythmia. Basically, the component parts of both temporary and permanent pacemakers are the same and consist of a pulse generator (electrical supply source, usually lithium-salt batteries) and a catheter with electrodes (delivers the electrical stimulus to the myocardium). Pacemakers are generally identified according to the location and mode of action. Location refers to the area of the heart where the stimulating or pacing electrode is placed, for example, in the atrium or ventricle. Therefore, if the stimulating electrode is in the ventricle, the pacemaker is classified ventricular. Mode of action is described as a preprogrammed type of delivery from the circuitry in the pulse generator. Classification is based on the presence or absence of a sensing mechanism. The presence of a sensing mechanism would allow the pacemaker to respond only when needed. Figure 36–34 illustrates pacemaker rhythms.[4]

The electrode for temporary pacing is usually inserted transvenously into the right ventricle using the antecubital, femoral, jugular, or subclavian approach. Temporary epicar-

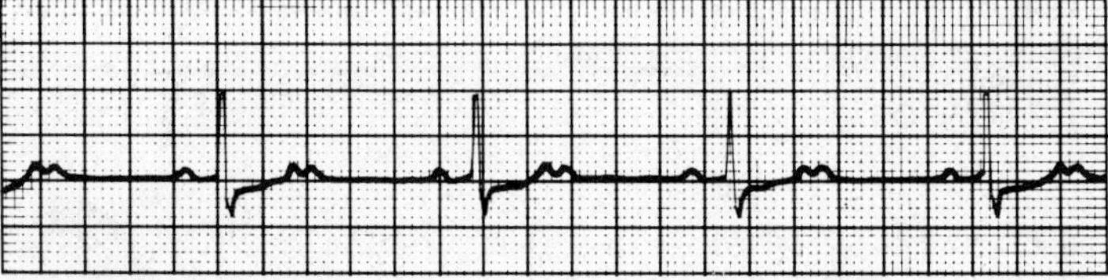

FIGURE 36–32 Second degree heart block, Mobitz II (2 : 1 pattern).

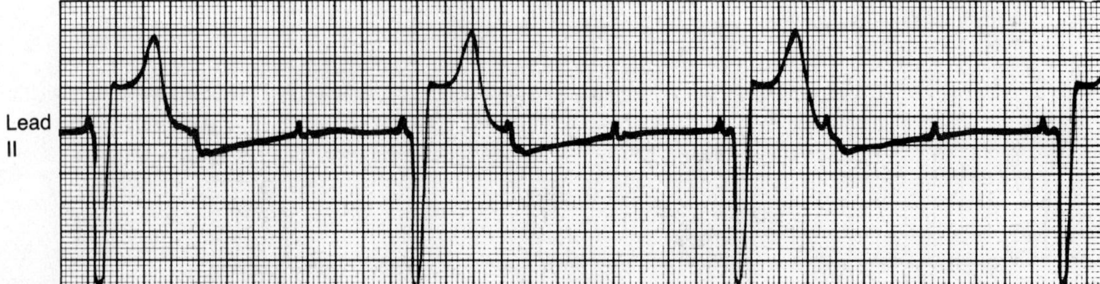

FIGURE 36–33 Complete heart block, third degree.

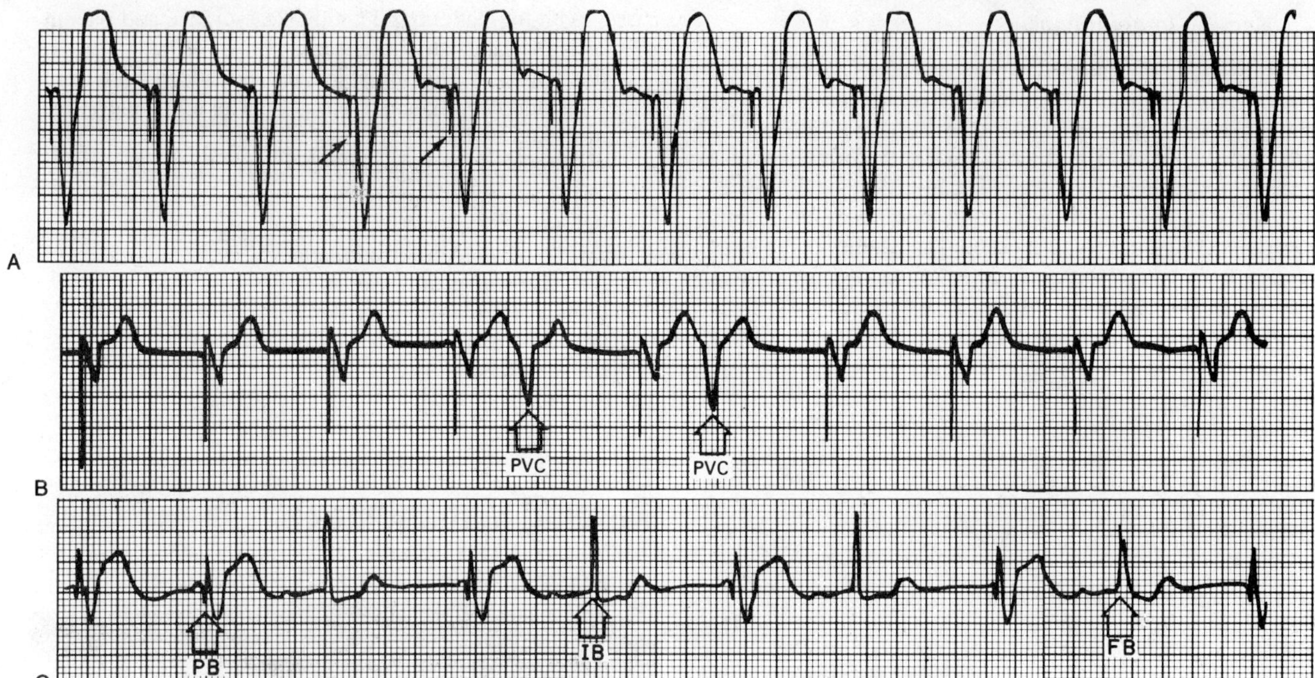

FIGURE 36–34 (*A*) Fixed rate pacemaker: ventricular, lead MCL_1. The pacemaker delivers stimuli continuously at a constant rate to the ventricles regardless of the intrinsic rhythm. A pacemaker spike (*arrows*) precedes each ventricular depolarization. A wide QRS complex follows (left bundle branch block pattern) due to late depolarization of the left ventricle. (*B*) Demand pacemaker. The pacer sensed PVCs (beats 5 and 7) and delayed firing approximately. (*C*) Demand pacemaker: paced beats (PB), intrinsic beats (IB), and a fusion beat (FB).

dial pacing may be used after cardiac surgery. The electrodes are loosely sutured on the epicardial surface of the heart and the electrode terminals are brought through the chest wall; these terminals are attached to a pulse generator if needed. Transthoracic pacing is used in emergencies and involves inserting an electrode through the chest wall into the myocardium. The terminals are attached to the pulse generator.

Permanent pacing may be required in some cases. Direct myocardial stimulation for permanent cardiac pacing can be either epicardial by thoracotomy (transthoracic or mediastinal), or endocardial by way of the transvenous approach. By far the majority of permanent pacemakers are implanted transvenously. There are several advantages to this method. The procedure is a relatively minor one, can be performed under local anesthesia, and has a low morbidity and mortality rate. A thoracotomy, which could be contraindicated in aged or debilitated patients, is not necessary. The cephalic, external jugular, or internal jugular veins are the most commonly used. A small incision is made just above the clavicle, usually on the right but sometimes on the left side of the neck, and the electrode is threaded into the vein. The catheter is advanced to the right ventricle and lodged beneath the trabeculae in the apex area. A separate incision is made below the clavicle and a tunnel is burrowed beneath the subcutaneous fat up to the neck vein incision. The electrode catheter is passed down through the tunnel to the battery-powered generator. A subcutaneous pocket is formed to place the pulse generator (sometimes encased in a Dacron pouch; Fig. 36–35). Connective tissue eventually grows into the Dacron fibers of the pouch and firmly anchors it to the chest wall. The generator is tested and the incision is closed. The skin layer over the pulse generator protrudes about ½ inch above the normal skin surface.[4]

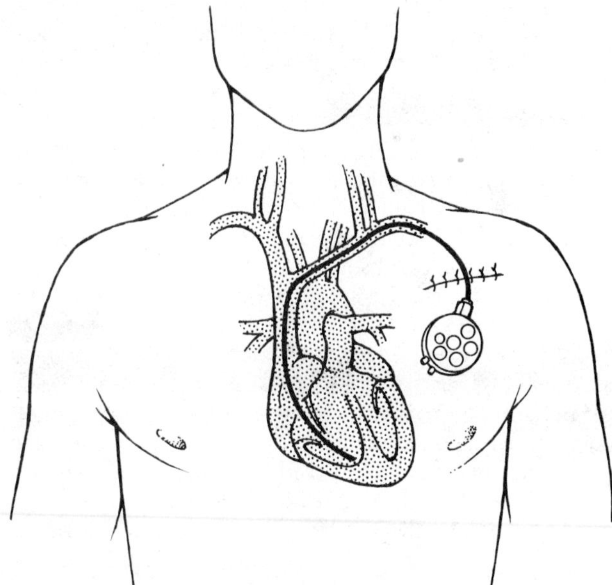

FIGURE 36–35 Transvenous insertion of a permanent pacemaker.

Nursing Interventions

For *temporary pacing,* the nurse prepares the patient for the procedure. As time permits, in conjunction with the physician, the nurse explains the procedure to the patient and family and answers their questions. Informed written consent is obtained. The pacemaker insertion site is washed and shaved. The pacemaker equipment and emergency equipment is gathered and checked. The patency of the intravenous line is assessed and the ECG machine or cardiac monitor is attached to patient. The pacemaker electrode can be inserted with or without the use of fluoroscopy. During catheter insertion, the nurse assists the physician as needed, monitors the cardiac rhythm, frequently assesses the effectiveness of local anesthesia, and provides physical and emotional support to the patient. After pacemaker insertion the physician's orders are implemented. Pacemaker function is assessed and its effect on hemodynamics is evaluated every 2 to 4 hours. Activity limitations are based on site of pacemaker insertion. With electrode insertion in the antecubital site, the arm is immobilized to prevent electrode dislodgment. Unit policy and physician orders vary regarding activity. The dressing at the site of insertion is changed daily and the site is assessed for signs of infection. The patient should be assessed for potential complications, which include phlebitis, thrombosis, and perforation of the myocardium by the electrode.

The nurse must be aware of electrical safety precautions because of the possibility of leakage current flowing through the pacemaker electrode into the heart, resulting in ventricular fibrillation. Some of these precautions include not touching exposed pacemaker wires unless wearing rubber gloves; properly grounding all electrical equipment; and not attaching the patient simultaneously to two pieces of electrical equipment that are not on a common ground.

For *permanent pacing,* the nurse provides routine preoperative care, including teaching. Postoperative care involves implementing the physician's orders (vital signs, 12-lead ECG, bed rest, pain medications); preventing postoperative atelectasis; checking the operative site for bleeding, swelling, or drainage; observing for pacemaker function and its effect on cardiac output; observing for cardiac arrhythmias; and observing for potential complications. Potential complications include electrode breakage, right ventricular perforation by the electrode tip, pacemaker unit rejection, and pressure necrosis of the skin overlying the pulse generator. The date and time of insertion, type of pacemaker, and the selected rate should be noted on patient's care plan and nursing notes. Usually the dressing will be removed on the first postoperative day by the surgeon; sutures will be removed in approximately 1 week, usually after the patient's discharge.[4]

The nurse has the opportunity and the responsibility to help patients and families understand pacemakers. The first introduction to a pacemaker for many patients may be during an emergency situation when the patient is symptomatic. Fear of the unknown and fear of dying are commonly experienced by patients, and therefore learning and retention are minimal. Fears of pacemaker failure and dependency on a life-support system are expressed verbally and nonverbally by many patients. These fears must be identified and discussed with the patient and family. Reassurance and patient education may alleviate these fears.[4]

The teaching plan must be individualized and reinforced the medical management plan. The following information should be included[4]:

Anatomy and physiology of the heart
Basic pacemaker function
Signs and symptoms of pacemaker failure
Electromagnetic interference
Care of the insertion site
Timing of battery replacement
Medications
Physical activity
Follow-up care

Nursing Management

Assessment and Nursing Diagnosis

Based on the subjective and objective data obtained, the following nursing diagnoses are frequently derived for patients with arrhythmias and conduction disturbances:

- Decreased cardiac output related to any arrhythmia, conduction disturbance, pharmacologic effects, or pacemaker failure, manifested by loss of consciousness, hypotension, decreased pulse pressure, chest discomfort, or dyspnea
- Alteration in tissue perfusion (cerebral, cardiopulmonary, renal, peripheral) related to decreased blood pressure, thromboemboli, or pharmacologic effects, manifested by change in mentation, chest discomfort, dyspnea, oliguria, cool, clammy skin, or fatique
- Alteration in comfort: pain related to an imbalance between myocardial oxygen supply and demand, thromboemboli, and therapeutic procedures (pacemaker insertion, cardioversion, defibrillation, surgery), manifested by complaints of chest discomfort or operative site discomfort; increase in blood pressure, pulse, and respiration; facial grimacing; restlessness
- Fear related to possibility of death, the therapeutic interventions, possibility of change in lifestyle and employment, or financial obligations, manifested by complaints of loss of control and feeling emotionally unstable; increase blood pressure, pulse, and respiration; restlessness; increased ectopic activity; increase in attention-getting behaviors; and increase in information-seeking behaviors
- Activity tolerance related to hypotension, pulmonary congestion, invasive procedures, pharmacologic effects, sleep deprivation, or stress, manifested by dyspnea on exertion, complaints of inability to perform activities of daily living, fatigue, failure of blood pressure to increase with activity, and failure of heart rate to return to baseline 5 minutes after activity
- Knowledge deficit about cause of arrhythmias, purposes of procedures, and therapeutic interventions, medications, pacemaker, and follow-up care

related to arrhythmias and treatment, manifested by information-seeking behavior, expressions of inaccurate perceptions of concepts, and inadequate performance of prescribed behavior

Interventions

Goals. General goals for nursing interventions include early detection, treatment, and prevention of the nursing diagnoses related to the patient with arrhythmias and conduction disturbances.

Lethal Ventricular Arrhythmias. For the patient with lethal arrhythmias, treatment is directed toward eliminating the arrhythmia and when possible the cause. Lethal arrhythmias may be preceded by warning arrhythmias, such as PVCs. Treatment of warning arrhythmias depends on etiology of coexisting conditions. For example, PVCs during acute myocardial ischemia are treated very aggressively, whereas PVCs in a patient without myocardial ischemia may be evaluated to determine hemodynamic effect prior to treatment. Not only is it necessary to be able to recognize arrhythmias, but the nurse must also be aware of the threat each poses for the individual patient. This includes knowing which arrhythmias warn of impending lethal arrhythmias and being prepared to treat them—and treat them aggressively.[10]

Constant ECG monitoring is required for all hospitalized patients at risk for having new or recurrent arrhythmias. It is important to determine if the arrhythmia occurs in association with, or is related to, any activity. Laboratory tests should be checked to determine the presence of hypokalemia or hypoxemia. Lungs should be auscultated frequently (every 4 hours) to determine the presence of crackling rales, which may indicate heart failure. If the patient has a heart catheter or electrode, the presence of PVCs may indicate mechanical irritation to the myocardium. If the etiology of the arrhythmia is myocardial ischemia, then nursing measures are directed towards restoring the balance between myocardial oxygen supply and demand. The patient must be assessed frequently (every 2–4 hours) to determine the effect of the arrhythmia and the treatment of the arrhythmia on the patient's cardiac output. Routine nursing care should also include emotional support during this life-threatening period. The nurse can recognize problems, help the patient solve them, and help the patient and family cope with present limitations.[10]

Antiarrhythmic drugs are frequently prescribed. Apical–radial heart rates and blood pressures should be obtained on all patients receiving antiarrhythmic medications. If the heart rate or rhythm has changed and if an arrhythmia is suspected, an electrocardiographic rhythm strip and then a full 12-lead ECG should be obtained. Exercise tolerance testing or 24-hour ECG recordings during the patient's normal activities may help document the presence or absence of arrhythmias.[1] Extreme caution should be exercised when administering any antiarrhythmic agent in the face of heart block with recent MI or digitalis toxicity. The antiarrhythmic drug may suppress lower pacemaker foci, which are necessary if the heart block becomes more advanced, whether or not the worsening of the heart block is related to the drug administered.[1]

Patients and their families need to have an understanding of the antiarrhythmic drug or drugs, and the importance of adhering to the therapy as prescribed by the physician. A dosage schedule should be implemented that will provide optimal antiarrhythmic protection for the patient without interfering with his lifestyle or disturbing his sleep any more than necessary. A patient who states his unwillingness to take a drug every 4 hours around the clock should discuss the possibility with this physician of switching to a long-acting (and usually more expensive) preparation. (Long-acting preparations are not available for all antiarrhythmic drugs.) Patients who are able to detect the symptoms of arrhythmia (*e.g.,* palpitations, dizziness, lightheadedness, fatigue) should be advised to notify the nurse or physician when arrhythmias increase.[1]

Bradyarrhythmias. In bradyarrhythmias, the nurse maximizes the patient cardiac output by interventions to increase preload and thus stroke volume, and to increase heart rate. Preload can be immediately increased by either lowering the head of the patient's bed or by elevating the patient's legs. Drugs that reduce preload, such as venodilators, should be withheld. The physician must be notified immediately. Heart rate can be increased by gently waking a sleeping patient, by having the patient move in bed, and by withholding medications that have a negative chronotropic effect. The nurse must be aware of the hemodynamic effects of all the medication the patient is currently taking so that, in consultation with the physician, appropriate judgments about administration of these medications can be made.[9]

Tachyarrhythmias. Assessment and treatment of patients with tachyarrhythmias is similar to that of patients with lethal ventricular arrhythmias. Patients with tachyarrhythmia are at risk for decreased cardiac output due to decreased diastolic filling time with resultant decreased tissue perfusion. With some tachyarrhythmias, that is, atrial fibrillation with or without a controlled ventricular response, stasis of blood in the atria and atrial appendages predisposes the patient to thrombus formation and possible embolization.

Nursing measures for patients with decreased cardiac output include interventions that decrease myocardial oxygen need and increase myocardial oxygen supply. If the cause of the arrhythmia is known, nursing interventions when possible are directed toward eliminating the cause. For example, patients with left atrial myocardial stretch from heart failure that results in atrial fibrillation would benefit from any intervention to improve heart failure. For patients with caffeine-induced tachycardia, interventions would include dietary instruction.[9]

Evaluation

Specific outcome criteria are developed for the plan of care. When possible outcomes should be measurable, and should be individualized for each patient. In addition, an appropriate and realistic time frame should be included as part of the outcome criteria.

To detect early the manifestations of problems of arrhythmias and conduction disturbances. If problems are not detected in a timely manner complications of that problem would arise. It may be necessary to modify the prescribed interventions, including increasing the frequency of evaluation of specific assessment parameters, reassessing accepted ranges in parameters, adding additional evaluation parameters, or to change the intervention.

To reduce or eliminate problems of arrhythmias and conduction disturbances and their manifestations with nursing and delegated medical interventions. Criteria used to evaluate successful reduction or elimination of the identified problems and their manifestations are both subjective and objective data. These data are specific to the particular problem.

To prevent when possible the occurrence of problems associated with arrhythmias and conduction disturbances. Outcome criteria used to evaluate interventions to meet this goal are subjective and objective data that reflect absence of identified or potential problems.

References

1. Bond L, Underhill SL: Antiarrhythmic and cardiotonic drugs. In Underhill SL et al (eds): Cardiac Nursing, pp 442–465. Philadelphia, JB Lippincott, 1982
2. Foster WT: Principles of Acute Coronary Care. New York, Appleton-Century-Crofts, 1976
3. Goldman MJ: Principles of Clinical Electrocardiography, 11th ed. California, Lange Medical Publications, 1979
4. Haskin JB: Pacemakers. In Underhill SL et al (eds): Cardiac Nursing, pp 518–541. Philadelphia, JB Lippincott, 1982
5. Kaplan BM, Langendorf R, Levi M et al: The tachycardia–bradycardia syndrome. Med Clin North Am 60:81–99, 1976
6. Instructor's Manual for Advanced Cardiac Life Support. American Heart Association, 1982
7. Marriott HJL, Fogg E: Constant monitoring for cardiac dysrhythmias and block. Mod Concepts Cardiovasc Dis 39(6):103–108, 1970
8. Surawicz B, Uhley H, Borun R et al: Task force I. Standardization of terminology and interpretation. Am J Cardiol 41:130–145, 1978
9. Woods SL: Arrhythmias complicating myocardial infarction. In Underhill SL et al (eds): Cardiac Nursing, pp 363–377. Philadelphia, JB Lippincott, 1982
10. Woods SL: Diagnosis and treatment of the patient with an uncomplicated myocardial infarction. In Underhill SL et al (eds): Cardiac Nursing, pp 326–337. Philadelphia, JB Lippincott, 1982
11. Woods SL: Electrocardiography, vectorcardiography, and polarcardiography. In Underhill SL et al (eds): Cardiac Nursing, pp 196–247. Philadelphia, JB Lippincott, 1982

Chapter 37

Coronary Heart Disease

Myocardial Ischemia and Infarction

Susan L. Woods
Sandra L. Underhill

Definition

Three major coronary arteries (the right, the left anterior descending, and the left circumflex) provide the blood supply to the myocardium. When blood flow through these arteries decreases, myocardial ischemia, infarction, or both can occur. Myocardial ischemia is a result of an imbalance between myocardial oxygen supply and demand. Ischemia is reversible, but if myocardial blood flow is not increased or if myocardial oxygen demands are not reduced, then the ischemia can progress to cell death or necrosis, known as myocardial infarction (MI).

Incidence

Even though there has been as 32% decrease in mortality from coronary heart disease from 1968 to 1981, heart and blood vessel disease is still the leading cause of death in the United States. There are 42,750,000 Americans who have one or more forms of heart or blood vessel disease. Of these, 4,600,000 have coronary heart disease. Over one fifth of all persons killed by cardiovascular disease are under age 65. Myocardial infarction is the leading cause of death in the United States. There are 350,000 people per year who die of MI before reaching the hospital. The average victim waits 3 hours before deciding to seek medical help. Approximately 1.5 million Americans had an MI in 1984, and about 550,000 died.[16]

Pathophysiology

Decreased oxygenated blood flow to the myocardium, increased myocardial need for oxygen, or a combination of both can result in myocardial ischemia and infarction. The epicardial arteries that lie on the surface of the heart are large. As they branch and penetrate through the myocardium to the endocardium, they become smaller and thus perfusion is reduced. Normally, myocardial tissue perfusion occurs during diastole rather than systole, which maximizes coronary blood flow. During myocardial contraction, coronary blood flow is reduced because of the tremendous transmural pressure that is capable of constricting the small, endocardial arteries and arterioles. In coronary heart disease, coronary arteries are narrowed and endocardial blood flow is further reduced. Therefore, ischemia and infarction classically progress from the endocardium to the epicardium. If all three layers of the heart are infarcted, the infarction is termed *transmural*. If only the epicardial surface is ischemic or infarcted, spasm of the epicardial arteries is usually involved.

Beyond the area of infarction, there are the areas of injury and ischemia, which contain many viable muscle cells. Figure 37–1 illustrates these zones. Thus, the infarcted area

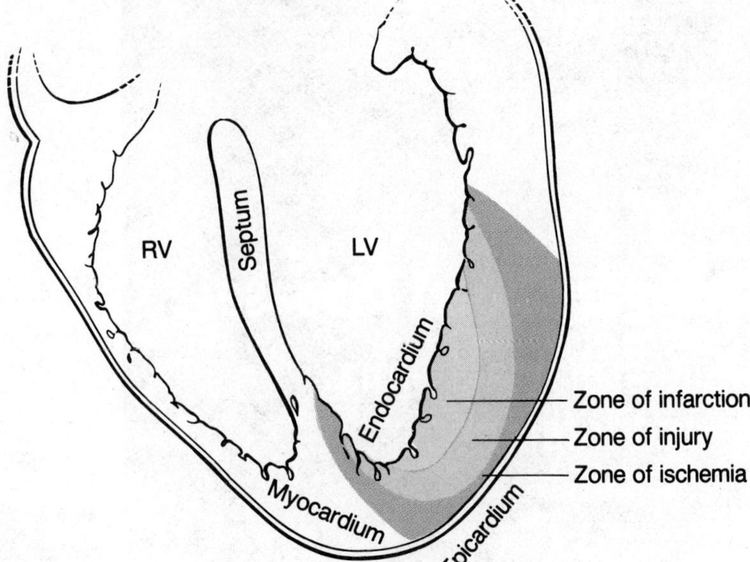

FIGURE 37–1 Tissue damage following myocardial infarction. The area around the infarction (necrosis) is the zone of injury, and the area around the injury is the zone of ischemia.

could expand if there were a large demand placed on the infarcted heart. The eventual size of the infarct is dependent on the extent of collateral circulation, the degree of anaerobic metabolism, and the demand placed on the heart.[52]

Factors that decrease blood supply to the myocardium are atherosclerosis of the coronary arteries and other nonatherosclerotic causes such as circulatory disorders (*e.g.*, hypovolemia, anemia, polycythemia, hypotension, and valvular abnormalities) or other conditions affecting the coronary arteries.

The most common cause of ischemic heart disease is coronary artery atherosclerosis. Atherosclerosis is a degenerative process of the arterial wall that eventually narrows the coronary arteries and can reduce blood flow to the myocardium. As discussed in Chapter 22, atherosclerosis is a complex disease and there are many hypotheses as to its origin.

Another cause is coronary artery spasm, which commonly occurs. The smooth muscle fibers in the coronary arterial walls contract and therefore temporarily narrow the vessel lumen. Spasm results in myocardial ischemia, and it may contribute to the development and size of the myocardial infarction. It has been proposed that coronary artery spasm is due to the enhanced sensitivity of the alpha receptors of the autonomic nervous system. Certain vasoactive substances may also contribute to the development of coronary spasm, for example, catecholamines, and prostaglandins.[2]

At rest, the myocardial cells normally extract a large amount of oxygen from the coronary blood flow. A near maximal amount of oxygen is already extracted by the myocardium during rest, yet the oxygen requirement of the heart can increase manyfold. This additional oxygen can only be supplied by increasing the coronary blood flow. Coronary blood flow increases proportionately to myocardial metabolism and oxygen consumption.[5] Factors that can increase myocardial oxygen need are enhanced catecholamine release (*e.g.*, from emotional stress), tachycardia (*e.g.*, from stress, anemia, heavy lifting, and eating large meals), myocardial hypertrophy (*e.g.*, from chronic high blood pressure, congestive heart failure), and increased cardiac work (*e.g.*, from high blood pressure, aortic valve disease, heart failure).

Risk Factors

The specific etiology of coronary heart disease is unknown. However, many risk factors have been identified. The four major coronary heart disease risk factors are cigarette smoking, high blood pressure, hyperlipoproteinemia, and emotional stress. Table 37–1 categorizes risk factors for coronary heart disease.

Unavoidable Risk Factors

Unavoidable risk factors include age, gender, family history of coronary heart disease, and ethnic background. However, in the presence of unavoidable risk factors, the risk of coronary heart disease can be modified to some degree by controlling other risk factors known to be modifiable. Age is associated with an increasing incidence of coronary heart disease. In men, the occurrence increases steadily with age, but in women its incidence increases sharply after menopause. For unknown reasons, the incidence of coronary heart disease in postmenopausal women still remains less than for men.[26] Family history of coronary heart disease is important in predicting the occurrence and prognosis of this disease. Ethnic background may also be a risk factor. For example, high blood pressure is more prevalent in blacks than whites. However, ethnicity in a broader sense implies lifestyle as well as ethnic origin. Although ethnic origin is not modifiable, the lifestyles associated with particular cultures can be altered.[56]

Atherogenic Personal Attributes

Modifiable risk factors for coronary heart disease include elevated serum lipoproteins, elevated arterial blood pressure, and glucose intolerance. These personal attributes can be modified to reduce risk.

TABLE 37–1
Risk Factors for Coronary Heart Disease

Unavoidable risk factors
Age
Gender
Family history of coronary heart disease
Ethnic background
Atherogenic personal attributes
Elevated serum lipoproteins
Elevated blood pressure
Glucose intolerance
Lifestyle habits
Cigarette smoking
Physical inactivity
Obesity and weight change
Emotional stress
Estrogen as contraceptive or as therapy

(Blackburn H: Risk factors and cardiovascular disease. In American Heart Association, pp 2–20. New York, EP Dutton, 1980)

Elevated serum lipoproteins are considered to be a major risk factor of coronary heart disease. Lipids are naturally occurring organic substances that include triglycerides, phospholipids, and plant and animal sterols. Fatty acids are the building blocks of triglycerides and phospholipids. Cholesterol is a sterol found in animal tissues. Lipids bound to protein are known as lipoproteins. Lipids that circulate in the blood as part of lipoprotein complexes are triglycerides, cholesterol, and phospholipids. The larger the lipoprotein particle size, the greater is the ratio of fat to protein, and, therefore, the lower the density. High concentrations of high-density lipoprotein (HDL) in the serum seem to have a protective effect against atherosclerosis development.[22,35] Conversely, low HDL levels (below 35 mg/dl) are associated with increased risk of coronary heart disease.

Elevated serum cholesterol greatly increases the risk of coronary heart disease.[22,27] In both men and younger women (under 50 years of age), serum triglyceride alone does not constitute a risk, but appears to be implicated only when serum cholesterol is also elevated.[14] However, in women over 50 years of age, serum triglyceride is superior to serum cholesterol in predicting risk of coronary heart disease.[23]

High blood pressure is also a major risk factor of coronary heart disease. Elevated systolic and diastolic arterial blood pressures (greater than 140/90 mmHg) are major contributors to the development of cardiovascular disease, particularly stroke and heart failure.[25,38]

Glucose intolerance doubles cardiovascular mortality. The impact of diabetes mellitus is substantially greater in women than in men, tends to diminish with age, and varies widely with the number of coexisting risk factors.[39]

Lifestyle Habits

Lifestyle habits include cigarette smoking, physical inactivity, obesity and weight change, emotional stress, and estrogen as either contraception or replacement therapy. Each of these risk factors can be eliminated or modified.

Cigarette smoking is a major risk factor of coronary heart disease and has been shown to cause more deaths from myocardial infarction and sudden cardiac death than from either lung cancer or chronic obstructive lung disease. Three compounds in cigarette smoke have been implicated as causative agents in coronary heart disease development: "tar," nicotine, and carbon monoxide. Related factors include

1. The number of cigarettes smoked
2. How long the person has smoked, expressed simply as pack-year history (packs/day multiplied by number of smoking years), *e.g.,* 2 packs/day × 10 smoking years = 20 pack-years
3. The age at which the person started to smoke
4. The pattern of inhaling

A typical high-risk individual has smoked several packs per day for many years, began smoking at a young age, and inhales. Male cigarette smokers, regardless of the number of cigarettes smoked, have a 70% higher mortality rate than male nonsmokers.[51] In young women (under age 50) who smoke 35 cigarettes or more per day, the rate of myocardial infarction is 20 times that of young women who never smoked.[49] Women who smoke and use oral contraceptive agents or estrogens for other reasons are at increased risks.[20,21] Pipe and cigar smokers, although at greater risk than nonsmokers, run less risk of developing coronary heart disease than cigarette smokers, probably because they inhale less smoke. The risk of death from coronary heart disease is reduced when cigarette smoking is stopped. After 10 years of not smoking cigarettes, the risk of mortality from coronary heart disease approaches that of a nonsmoker.[51]

Physical activity is associated with an increased risk of myocardial infarction. Rigorous physical activity may confer some protection from the complications of coronary heart disease and may lower blood pressure in mild hypertension,[39] but it has also been associated with sudden death in asymptomatic persons who have coronary heart disease.

Obesity is associated with increased risk of developing coronary heart disease. Obesity is defined as body-mass index (weight/height^2) greater than 20% above the ideal value. A controversy exists regarding the risk of obesity alone vs. other known risk factors that frequently accompany obesity, such as advancing age, elevated blood pressure, and elevated serum cholesterol.[28]

Weight change, that is frequent and in large amounts is also associated with an increased risk.[1]

Emotional stress has direct effects on the cardiovascular system, including an increased need for oxygen by the heart. Stress also influences the risk of coronary heart disease through its effect on lifestyle in general (*i.e.,* Type A personalities), including the kinds and amounts of food eaten, cigarette and alcohol use, and exercise.[39]

Alcohol use by itself is not a risk factor of coronary heart disease, although in excessive amounts it creates other health problems. Alcohol raises the heart rate and increases myocardial oxygen consumption. The setting in which alcohol is consumed should be considered. A quiet, relaxing drink at home may have very little consequence, whereas multiple drinks with friends in a smoke-filled room following a heavy meal may increase myocardial stress.[36,50]

Estrogen as contraception or replacement therapy is also a risk factor for the development of coronary heart disease in women. Myocardial infarction among young, healthy women is rare. Use of oral contraceptive agents (estrogen and progestin) is associated with an increased risk of nonfatal and fatal myocardial infarction in young women. In women ages 30–39, the incidence of nonfatal MI among oral contraceptive users is 2.7 times greater than in nonusers. The incidence of fatal MI is similar: 2.8 times greater risk for women aged 30–39 who use oral contraceptives than for those who do not, and 4.7 times greater risk for women aged 40–44 who use oral contraceptive agents than for those who do not. The risk from cigarette smoking acts synergistically with the risk from oral contraceptive agents. In conjunction with estrogen use, other major risk factors such as hyperlipoproteinemia, high blood pressure, and glucose intolerance also appear to have additive effects.[32,33] For oral contraceptive users, the death rate from all types of circulatory disease increases with age, duration of oral contraceptive use, and cigarette smoking.[3]

The incidence of acute MI in women under age 46 taking supplementary estrogens is similar to the incidence of MI from oral contraceptive agents.[20,21] However, no positive relationship between acute MI and estrogen therapy in older women (over age 50) has been found.[43]

Risk Factor Combination

Combination of risk factors have a synergistic effect. The greater the number of risk factors, the greater is the risk of developing coronary heart disease.[24]

Related Disorders

There are four clinical manifestations of coronary heart disease: angina pectoris, myocardial infarction, heart failure, and cardiac arrest. Our discussion will concentrate on angina and MI.

Angina Pectoris

Clinical Manifestations

Symptoms of angina, literally "strangling of the chest," result from myocardial ischemia due to an imbalance in myocardial oxygen supply and demand. Angina is a subjective symptom that usually lasts 2 to 5 minutes if the precipitating factor is relieved, occasionally lasts 5 to 15 minutes, and rarely endures 15 to 30 minutes. Patients do not always admit to having chest "pain" and, therefore, pain-equivalents should be used when eliciting the quality of discomfort. Common descriptions used by the patient include strangling, constriction, tightness, aching, squeezing, pressing, heaviness, expanding sensation, choking in the throat, indigestion, and burning. Some patients clench their fist over the sternum when describing the discomfort (Levine's sign). It is unusual for patients to experience no chest discomfort as a result of myocardial ischemia.[55]

Location of the discomfort is usually in the retrosternal region, although it may occur anywhere in the chest. It may radiate down both arms, but it usually radiates down the left arm; sometimes the pain radiates up to the mandible, maxilla, and teeth, to the tongue or hard palate, or to the front or back of the neck. The patient may complain of aching in the left interscapular region or of an aching shoulder, wrist, elbow, or forearm, which is more significant when it is not related to effort involving the shoulder or the arm. Sometimes patients experience discomfort only in an area of radiated pain without any discomfort in the chest itself. The location of the discomfort can change with the natural history of the disease, probably as a result of a new ischemic area.

Effort angina is associated with increased myocardial oxygen consumption, such as physical exertion or emotional stress. Spontaneous angina occurs without apparent relation to increased myocardial oxygen consumption, such as coronary artery spasm. It usually occurs at rest.[40]

Assessment

Physical examination of the patient with angina is usually normal. On inspection there may be alteration in appearance, or the patient may exhibit transient signs of dyspnea, pallor, or cold, clammy skin. Heart rate and blood pressure may increase at the onset of the ischemic episode. Pulsus alternans may be present. On auscultation an S_3 or S_4 gallop may be noted, and the murmur of mitral regurgitation secondary to ischemia of the papillary muscle may be present. A paradoxically split S_2 wave may be heard.[57] These terms are explained in Chapter 34 on cardiac assessment.

Diagnosis of angina pectoris is made by history, ECG recordings taken at rest and during exercise, radionuclide imaging, and cardiac catheterization. Routine chest radiography, echocardiography, and serum enzyme determinations are not useful in assessing the presence of angina. The resting electrocardiogram is not helpful in diagnosing ischemic heart disease unless it is taken during an ischemic episode when characteristic signs can be recorded.[55]

Medical Management

Treatment of the patient with angina depends on whether the symptoms of ischemia are acute (and therefore apt to progress to a myocardial infarction) or chronic in nature, or are stable or unstable (based on previous symptoms). For any patient experiencing myocardial pain, pain management is a priority, not only for patient comfort but also to decrease myocardial oxygen consumption.

Treatment of angina is based on decreasing myocardial oxygen demand and increasing myocardial blood and oxygen supply, or both. Rest, diet, drugs, and lifestyle changes constitute basic therapeutic approaches. Table 37–2 presents a summary of selected therapies that either decrease myocardial oxygen demand or increase coronary blood and oxygen supply.

Pharmacotherapy

Medications used in the treatment of angina include nitrates, beta-blocking agents, calcium-channel blocking agents, antilipid agents, and platelet behavior modifying drugs.

TABLE 37–2
Selected Therapies to Reduce Ischemia and Infarction

Decrease Myocardial O_2 Consumption	*Increase Coronary Blood and O_2 Supply*
Rest	Oxygen
Selected diet (small, frequent, easily digested meals; no caffeine)	Nitroglycerin
Nitroglycerin and long-acting nitrates	Ca^{2+} channel blocking agents
Narcotic analgesics	Revascularization
Beta-blocking agents	Streptokinase therapy
Ca^{2+} channel blocking agents	Percutaneous transluminal coronary angioplasty (PTCA)
Vasodilators	Coronary artery bypass graft surgery
Sedatives and tranquilizers	Antiplatelet agents (long-term)
Stool softeners and laxatives	Antilipid agents (long-term)
Diuretics	Exercise program
Antihypertensive agents	Risk factor modification
Stress management	

Nitrates such as nitrogylcerin are commonly used to reduce the pain associated with angina. Nitroglycerin is a vasodilator, which acts primarily to reduce venous return to the heart (preload) and, therefore, decrease myocardial oxygen consumption. Vasodilatation of the coronary artery may also help improve myocardial blood flow. In addition, nitroglycerin reduces coronary artery spasm.

Beta-blocking agents are used alone and in combination with other drugs to treat angina. Beta-blocking agents decrease heart rate and myocardial contractility, thereby decreasing myocardial oxygen consumption.

Calcium-channel blocking agents are used to increase myocardial blood flow and to decrease the work of the heart.[30] Blood flow is increased by coronary artery vasodilatation, and heart work is decreased by systemic arterial vasodilatation.

Antilipid agents are used in certain types of hyperlipoproteinemia as an adjunct to dietary management. These agents are used long-term to decrease serum cholesterol and triglycerides, thus reducing the risk of coronary heart disease.

Drugs that modify *platelet behavior* are useful in the treatment of coronary heart disease. Platelet adhesion and aggregation are initially involved in arterial thrombosis formation. Therefore, inhibiting platelet function may prevent myocardial infarction or other arterial thromboembolic events. Sulfinpyrazone, acetylsalicylic acid, and dipyridamole are used to inhibit platelet function.

Nursing Interventions

Interventions for the patient with angina focus on relieving discomfort, preventing myocardial infarction, and teaching the patient how to prevent and treat angina.[55] A careful assessment is necessary to determine the degree and location of pain based on the patient's description and vital signs. The patient should be placed at rest and given any antianginal medication as prescribed. A supportive, calm approach will help allay fear and anxiety that can create added stress. The physician should be informed that the patient has experienced angina, and an ECG may need to be obtained if the pain persists for 30 minutes or more.

The teaching program underscores the need for rest and relaxation and adherence to the medication regimen (taking nitroglycerin as prescribed), as well as the absolute necessity of seeking medical attention if the pain lasts more than 30 minutes. The patient should be aware of the factors that can precipitate a myocardial infarction and the measures to take to offset these factors. Overall adherence to diet, medications, and activity level is emphasized. A list of nursing interventions for the patient with angina is presented in Table 37–3.

Myocardial Infarction (MI)

Myocardial infarction occurs after prolonged ischemia over a period of 4 to 6 hours.

Clinical Manifestations

Symptoms of MI are the same as those of ischemia, but they may not be transient in nature. Of all patients with MI, 75% to 85% of patients with acute MI have chest discomfort. The history is typical of MI if severe and prolonged chest discomfort is present. The onset of chest discomfort is abrupt and lasts longer than 15 to 30 minutes. This chest discomfort may be associated with indigestion, nausea and vomiting, diaphoresis, syncope, palpitations, or dyspnea. However, sometimes the history is atypical and the chest discomfort is mild or even absent in 15% to 25% of all patients with MI.

Assessment

Physical examination of the patient with acute MI is usually unremarkable, but provides baseline data. An S_3 gallop reflecting decreased compliance of the infarcted area may be present. Findings are nonspecific for diagnosis of MI; positive findings may be indicative of complications or coexisting disease.

Diagnosis of MI is made by history, ECG, and serum enzyme values. Classification of MI is based on location of the infarction and the layers of the heart involved. Although MIs

TABLE 37–3
Nursing Interventions for the Hospitalized Patient with Angina

1. Assess, document, and report to the physician the following:
   a. The patient's description of the chest discomfort including location, radiation, duration, and the factors that affect it
   b. The effect of the myocardial ischemia on cardiovascular hemodynamics (perfusion to the heart, brain, kidneys, and periphery)
2. Immediately reduce patient's physical activity to the level of activity before occurrence of chest discomfort.
3. Administer nitroglycerin or other antianginal medications as ordered, and continuously evaluate the patient's response to therapy.
4. Provide restful environment and allay fear and anxiety by being supportive, calm, and competent.
5. For patients experiencing chest discomfort that is either prolonged (greater than 30 minutes) or unrelieved (after the prescribed amount of nitroglycerin), obtain a 12-lead ECG, and if MI is suspected, draw baseline and serial cardiac enzymes.
6. Promote the patient's physical comfort by providing individualized, basic nursing care.
7. Teach the patient to do the following when angina pectoris occurs:
   a. Rest and relax.
   b. Take nitroglyerin as prescribed, and if no relief of chest discomfort has occurred within 30 minutes, immediately seek medical attention.
   c. Call the physician if a change in the pattern of angina pectoris has occurred.
8. Teach the patient to do the following to prevent myocardial ischemia with potential MI from occurring:
   a. Be aware of precipitating factors:
      1. Physiological, such as activity during cold weather or after a heavy meal
      2. Psychological, such as anger or grief
   b. Reduce precipitating factors by, for example:
      1. Taking prophylactic nitroglycerin
      2. Reducing physical activity and psychological stress that usually results in chest discomfort
      3. Countering emotional stress by regular physical exercise
      4. Practicing a stress-reduction technique of choice
   c. Be aware of specific risk factors, and in collaboration with the health care team, establish a plan to reduce or eliminate these risk factors.
   d. Adhere to the therapeutic plan (such as diet, medications, and activity level) prescribed for control of myocardial ischemia, or any other disease processes.

can occur in any heart chamber, most MIs occur in the left ventricle because its oxygen need is greatest. Left ventricular infarctions are generally classified as anterior, inferior, posterior, or lateral. Myocardial infarction can occur in the subendocardium or epicardium, or can be transmural, involving all three layers of the heart.

ECG Changes. Typical ECG changes are seen in 88% of patients with acute MI. Unequivocal ECG changes are the development of abnormal, persistent Q waves, and evolving ST-segment changes lasting longer than 1 day (Fig. 37–2). If these unequivocal changes are present, the diagnosis may be made from the ECG alone. The ECG may show equivocal changes, consisting of ST-segment elevation, a symmetrical inversion of the T wave, a pathological Q wave in a single ECG record, or conduction disturbances.[40] If the MI is small, subendocardial, or in the lateral or posterior wall in the presence of an old MI or left bundle branch block, the ECG provides little or no information. Also, when there is a balanced loss of myocardial forces, such as infarction in both anterior and posterior walls, there are minimal ECG changes.

Cardiac Enzymes and Isoenzymes. Acute MI can be confirmed by the presence of abnormally high levels of enzymes or isoenzymes in the serum. Enzymes used in the diagnosis of acute MI are creatine kinase (CK) and its isoenzyme CK-MB or CK-2, and lactic dehydrogenase (LDH) and its isoenzymes. Enzymes are released from all cells as they die, and are, therefore, nonspecific in relation to the particular organ that has been damaged. Certain isoenzymes, however, come only from myocardial cells, and reflect death of cardiac muscle specifically. Because different enzymes are released into the blood at varying periods following acute MI, it is crucial to perform blood samplings in relation to the time of onset of chest discomfort. If drawn too early, enzymes may not yet be elevated; if drawn too late, enzymes may already have returned to baseline values. Refer to Table 37–4 for normal values and to Table 37–5 and Figure 37–3 for the time course of cardiac enzymes.

Creatine kinase is regarded as the most sensitive and reliable indicator of all cardiac enzymes. There are three CK isoenzymes: CK-MM (specific to skeletal muscle), CK-MB (specific to heart muscle), and CK-BB (specific to brain tissue). Normally, CK-MB is not present in the serum. When total CK is elevated and CK-MB is present, it is indicative of acute myocardial damage (such as acute MI, multiple defibrillations, or following cardiac surgery). The rise of CK begins within 3 hours and peaks within 24 hours of myocardial damage. Therefore, blood samples should be drawn on admission and at 12, 24, and 36 hours after onset of chest

TABLE 37–4
Normal Values of Cardiac Enzymes and Isoenzymes

Creatinine Kinase		
Total CK	***CK-MB***	
Female: ≤2.5 U, or 5–35 mU/ml	None	
Male: ≤4.3 U, or 5–55 mU/ml	None	
Lactic Dehydrogenase		
Total LDH	***LDH Isoenzymes and Activity***	
80–120 Wacker Units, or	LDH_1	17–27%
71–207 IU/liter, or 150–450	LDH_2	28–38%
Wroblewski Units, or	LDH_3	19–27%
63–155 U (male), or 62–131	LDH_4	5–16%
U (female)	LDH_5	5–16%

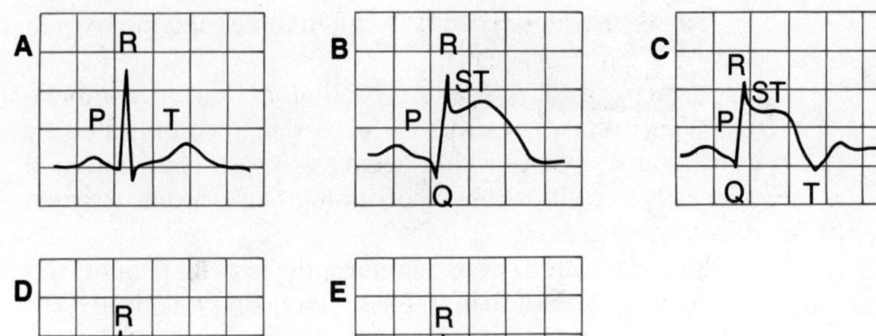

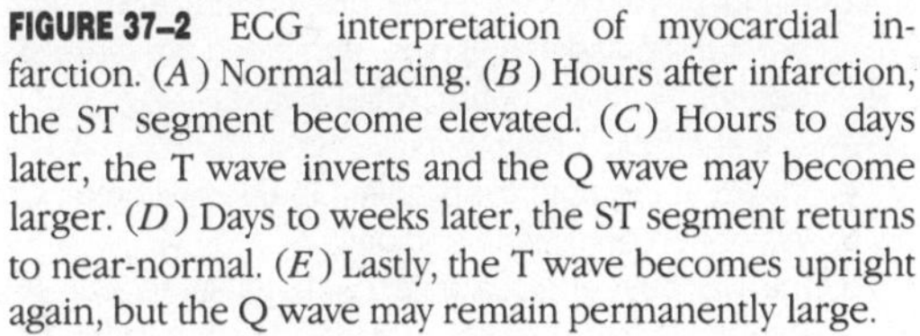

FIGURE 37–2 ECG interpretation of myocardial infarction. (*A*) Normal tracing. (*B*) Hours after infarction, the ST segment become elevated. (*C*) Hours to days later, the T wave inverts and the Q wave may become larger. (*D*) Days to weeks later, the ST segment returns to near-normal. (*E*) Lastly, the T wave becomes upright again, but the Q wave may remain permanently large.

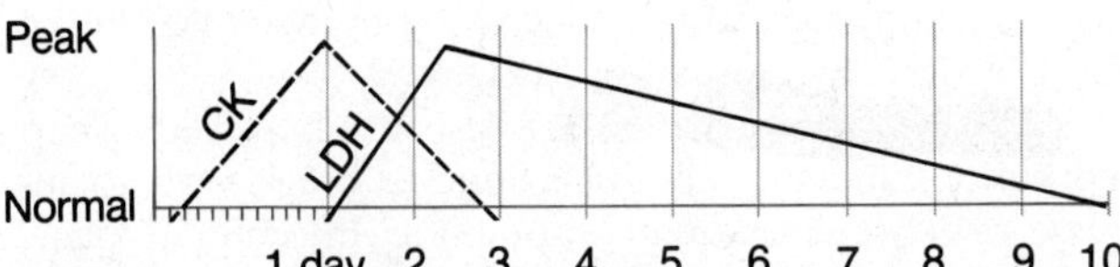

FIGURE 37–3 Time course of cardiac enzyme rise following myocardial infarction. CK elevation (broken line) occurs 3 to 6 hours after onset of MI and returns to normal after about 3 days. LDH (solid line) reaches a peak between 48 to 72 hours and may take 7 to 10 days to return to baseline.

TABLE 37–5
Time Course of Cardiac Enzyme Rise

Enzyme	*Onset*	*Peak*	*Return to Normal*
Creatinine kinase	3–6 hr	24 hr	72–96 hr
Lactic dehydrogenase	24 hr	48–72 hr	7–10 days

discomfort. Acute MI can be confirmed or ruled out within 24 hours.

Lactic dehydrogenase is not as reliable an indicator of acute myocardial damage as is CK. However, because total LDH peaks later and is elevated longer than other cardiac enzymes, total LDH and LDH isoenzymes are useful diagnostic tests in patients who may have sustained acute MI, but who do not seek medical assistance for 24 hours or longer after onset of chest discomfort. There are five LDH isoenzymes, but only two (LDH_1 and LDH_2) are important in the diagnosis of acute MI. Both LDH_1 and LDH_2 predominate in heart, kidney, and brain, but normally the percentage of LDH_2 compared to LDH_1 is greater. When the percentage of LDH_1 exceeds that of LDH_2, the pattern is said to have "flipped," and indicates acute myocardial damage.

Medical Management

Treatment of infarction includes restoration of myocardial blood flow, reduction in infarct size, and prevention of complications. For the patient experiencing worsening effort or spontaneous angina, angina for the first time, or angina of a different nature (prolonged or in a different location), a preliminary diagnosis of acute MI is made, until proven otherwise. Because over 60% of all deaths from MI occur within the first 2 hours of symptom onset and because half of those who die do so prior to reaching the hospital, it is imperative that the patient receive medical attention as soon as possible. This can be achieved by having a prehospital community system of cardiac life support. Basic to this community-wide system is an informed public, an efficient communication center, trained medical and paramedical teams, and appropriate vehicles and equipment. This system provides for basic and advanced cardiac life support at the site of the attack in order to stabilize the patient, and to transport the patient directly to a hospital cardiac care unit (CCU) under immediate cardiac monitoring conditions.[60]

CCU Care. The CCU is an area in a hospital that is equipped with special electronic devices used in monitoring patient with actual or potential heart problems. It is staffed by nurses with clinical expertise in cardiovascular nursing. Since the advent of the CCU in the early 1960s, mortality of cardiac patients has dramatically decreased. Some authorities suggest that in MI patients, this decreased mortality ranges from 10% to 24%. The main objective of the CCU is to prevent, detect, and treat cardiac arrhythmias, which were originally the leading cause of death of the patient with MI. Additional objectives are to prevent, detect, and treat other complications that occur because of MI.[60]

In order to meet these objectives, the CCU is generally a confined area with limited access from other parts of the hospital. It affords a quiet, temperature-controlled environment, often with private rooms. Resuscitative equipment and electrocardiographic monitoring devices with automatic alarm systems are provided. The basic equipment includes individual oscilloscopes at each patient's bed and a base oscilloscope with multiple channels at the nurse's station that displays the individual patient's ECG. The most important aspect of the CCU, however, is not the equipment but the special nurses who care for the patients in this unusual environment.[60]

Treatment of MI is based on decreasing myocardial oxygen demand and increasing myocardial blood and oxygen supply, or both. Table 37–6 presents an example of care parameters of a patient with an acute, uncomplicated MI, based on the physician's orders.

TABLE 37–6
Care of the Patient with an Acute, Uncomplicated MI (Based on Physician's Orders)

1. Bed rest with bedside commode for 24 hours. Activity according to stated protocol
2. If the patient's vital signs are normal and stable, temperature, pulse, respiration, and blood pressure should be obtained every 4 hours (while awake)
3. Constant ECG monitoring
4. Intake and output every shift. Guaiac testing all stools
5. Weight on admission and daily
6. Intravenous angiocatheter with injection cap. Heparin, 0.15 ml (1000 U/ml), or 10 U (10 U/ml) heparin IV every 8 hours and prn to maintain patency of IV catheter
7. Oxygen, 2 to 5 liters/minute by nasal prongs
8. Diet: Full liquid diet (1 g sodium) for three meals; no coffee or tea; decaffeinated coffee and salt substitute permitted; no extremely hot or cold foods. Advance diet to 3 g-sodium diet, low cholesterol as tolerated. ______ calorie restriction
9. Chest pain medication: (*appropriate analgesia order*)
10. Minor pain medication: (*appropriate analgesia order*)
11. Colace, 100 mg orally twice a day; milk of magnesia, 30 ml orally as needed
12. Sleeping medication: (*appropriate order*)
13. 12-lead ECG on admission and daily for 3 days, and with chest pain or with a new arrhythmia. Place copy on the-patient's chart.
14. SGOT, CK, LDH, and LDH isoenzymes on admission and daily for 3 days, and with sudden onset of chest. CK isoenzymes on admission and every 12 hours (after the onset of symptoms) times three. M-12, complete blood count, sedimentation rate, prothrombin time, partial thromboplastin time, VDRL, urinalysis, and portable chest film on admission.
15. The qualified CCU nurse is authorized according to stated policy to give complete resuscitation to this patient, including defibrillation and administration of intravenous medications as required.

Pharmacotherapy

Medications used in the treatment of MI include nitrates, narcotic analgesics, oxygen, beta-blocking agents, calcium antagonists, sedatives, hypnotics, and laxatives, anticoagulants, and thrombolytic agents.

Nitroglycerin can be given sublingually, intravenously, or topically and is commonly given to reduce pain associated with MI.

Narcotic analgesics are used with acute MI to relieve pain that is unrelieved with nitroglycerin. Morphine sulfate intravenously is the drug of choice for acute MI not only because it relieves pain, but because it reduces both anxiety and preload. Because morphine is vagotonic, it may reduce heart rate. Meperidine hydrochloride has an atropinelike effect and therefore tends to increase heart rate. Thus in patient with bradycardia, meperidine may be the drug of choice. Contraindications include patients with known sensitivity, acute head injury, or other acute neurological dysfunction. It should be used with caution in patients who have severely reduced respiratory reserve.[6]

Supplemental oxygen is useful in increasing the oxygen supply to the myocardium.

Beta-blocking agents are used alone and in combination with other drugs to treat acute MI uncomplicated by heart failure. Beta-blocking agents decrease heart rate and myocardial contractility, decreasing myocardial oxygen consumption.

Mortality after MI is significantly less in patients receiving propranolol than in those not taking this drug. Current recommendations are that patients with recent MI without contraindications to beta blockade receive propranolol for at least 3 years after MI.[4]

Calcium-channel blocking agents are used during MI to increase myocardial blood flow and to decrease the work of the heart.[30] Blood flow is increased by coronary artery vasodilatation, and heart work is decreased by systemic arterial vasodilatation (decreased afterload).

Hypnotics and laxatives are also used. Anxiety, sleep deprivation, and the Valsalva manuever are known to increase myocardial oxygen consumption. In acute MI, pharmacological agents are used to promote sleep and rest and to prevent straining with bowel movements.

Anticoagulants are used in the management of patients with infarction. *Heparin* inhibits blood clotting by interfering with the conversion of prothrombin to thrombin and by inhibiting platelet aggregation. Therapeutic doses of heparin do not dissolve clots but prevent new thrombus formation. Heparin is used in the prevention and treatment of a variety of arterial and venous thromboembolic disorders. It is most effective in the treatment of venous thrombosis that may occur with physical immobility. Low-dose heparin is used in the prophylaxis of deep vein thrombosis. Small doses of heparin neutralize thrombin precursors but not thrombin itself.

Coumarin competes with vitamin K, which is essential for the manufacture of clotting factors II, VII, IX, and X in the liver. Thus the pharmacological effect of coumarin is due to competitive inhibition of the hepatic synthesis of vitamin K–dependent clotting factors. Coumarin is highly bound to albumin in the blood (99%) with very little drug remaining in a free state. The small amount that is free provides the therapeutic effect of the drug. Thus any substance that will displace oral anticoagulants from albumin binding sites raises the level of the free drug in the blood and increases the therapeutic effect. Changes in the availability of vitamin K also alter the therapeutic responses to oral anticoagulants. There is considerable lag time between peak plasma concentrations and therapeutic response (24 to 72 hours). This lag time coincides with the gradual decrease in these clotting factors. Coumarin is metabolized by the liver, with negligible amounts being excreted in the urine. The major side-effect of coumarin is hemorrhage. When it occurs, vitamin K is usually administered intravenously. Because vitamin K antagonizes oral anticoagulants, the patients are refractory to all oral anticoagulants for several days after its administration.

The indications for oral anticoagulant therapy are very similar to those for heparin. Since this drug can be given orally, it is prescribed for patients requiring long-term anticoagulation. As with heparin, the use of oral anticoagulants after MI is variable. Some physicians advocate the use of oral anticoagulants for 2 or 3 months after the infarction to decrease the incidence of deep vein thrombosis and thromboembolism. Coumarin is also given for 3 months to patients after streptokinase therapy.

Streptokinase Therapy. Streptokinase is a thrombolytic agent used to dissolve thrombi in the coronary arteries, thus restoring myocardial blood flow. Once the clots are dissolved, reperfusion of the myocardium occurs, and chest pain is often relieved.

Streptokinase may be infused by way of intravenous or intracoronary routes. Currently, intravenous streptokinase is administered to the patient in the CCU. Intracoronary infusion is performed in the cardiac catheterization laboratory using the same access techniques as for coronary angiography. With intracoronary injection, the success rate is 75%; with intravenous infusion, the success rate is 50%.

Prior to intracoronary streptokinase administration, intracoronary nitroglycerin and/or nifedipine is give to eliminate coronary artery spasm, which contributes to vessel narrowing. Spasm is the cause of occlusion in approximately 3% of the cases. If coronary artery spasm is not the cause of the occlusion, streptokinase therapy is begun.[37] An example of one protocol of intracoronary streptokinase dosage is 10,000 to 20,000 U, followed by 1,000 to 4,000 U/minute for two hours until the clot lysis and perfusion is restored. The infusion is continued for 15 minutes to 1 hours after lysis to maintain patency. Total dose ranges from 150,000 to 500,000 U. An example of the dosage of intravenous streptokinase is 500,000 U of streptokinase over 20 minutes, followed by an additional 500,000 over 40 minutes up to 1.5 million U. Regardless of the route of administration, patients usually receive a continuous heparin infusion when the fibrinogen level is greater than 100 mg/100 ml. (Normal fibrinogen level is 200 to 400 mg/100 ml.)

After either intracoronary or intravenous streptokinase therapy when the fibrinogen level reaches 100 mg/100 ml, heparin is administered by continuous infusion at a rate to maintain partial thromboplastin time between two and two-and-a-half times the patient's control.[37] Heparin is continued until the patient is converted to oral anticoagulants (usually 2 to 4 days). The prothrombin time is maintained at two times the patient's control for 3 months.

Streptokinase is most effective if administered as soon as possible after a thrombosis has occurred, preferably within 3 to 6 hours of the event. Since it creates a systemic lytic state, streptokinase will lyse all clots in the body, including those at needle puncture and biopsy sites. Its half-life is 93 minutes. Contraindications to streptokinase are as follows: recent or active gastrointestinal or genitourinary bleeding; intracranial malignancy or hemorrhage; recent surgery or trauma, including traumatic cardiopulmonary resuscitation; early pregnancy (first 18 weeks); any other condition in which bleeding would be particularly dangerous or difficult to manage; recent streptococcal infection; allergy to streptokinase; and having received streptokinase within the past 6 to 12 months.[46] However, antibodies to streptokinase do not develop for up to 7 days; therefore patients can receive streptokinase again during that time.

Coagulation studies are used to evaluate the effects of streptokinase (thrombin time, partial thromboplastin time, prothrombin time, fibrinogen, fibrin degradation products, and platelet count), heparin (partial thromboplastin time), and coumarin (prothrombin time). Hematocrit is assessed to detect blood loss.

Nursing Interventions

Care of the patient receiving streptokinase therapy includes preparing the patient for cardiac catheterization if the intracoronary route is used, providing direct care during the procedure, and monitoring the patient following streptokinase infusion. Patients who receive streptokinase are at risk for bleeding, reperfusion arrhythmias, recurrent thrombosis, allergic reactions, and extreme anxiety. Therefore, priority goals for nursing interventions include early detection, treatment, and prevention of the above risks.

Prior to the procedure, the nurse collects baseline assessment data, including

1. History of any contraindications to streptokinase
2. Current medications (prescribed and over-the-counter)
3. Cardiovascular physical examination
4. Temperature
5. Laboratory studies, including complete blood count, cardiac enzymes and isoenzymes, electrolytes, blood urea nitrogen, creatinine, liver enzymes, coagulation studies (fibrinogen, fibrin degradation products, thrombin time, prothrombin time, partial thromboplastin time, and plasminogen)
6. Electrocardiogram

In addition, before streptokinase therapy is begun all intravascular lines need to be started. Four lines are usually started if the patient is to receive IV streptokinase (one for streptokinase and then heparin, one for lidocaine, one for nitroglycerin or other emergency drug, and one for blood drawing). If the intracoronary route is used, intracoronary streptokinase is administered during cardiac catheterization. Measures must be taken to prevent bleeding in the patient who has received thrombolytic therapy. The femoral arterial sheath used in the cardiac catheterization is left in place for 24 hours. Since patients who receive streptokinase cannot form clots for several hours, the sheath provides the hemostasis. While the sheath is in place, the patient is kept nearly flat to prevent flexion of the leg and potential disruption of hemostasis and distal blood flow.

Complications of Streptokinase Therapy

Bleeding, arrhythmias, allergic reactions, fever, and anxiety may occur as a result of streptokinase therapy. *Bleeding* is one of the major complications following streptokinase administration. Bleeding can be overt or internal and can occur anywhere in the body. In addition to hemorrhage at the femoral arterial or any other puncture sites, signs and symptoms of bleeding may include the following: neurological changes, flank or abdominal pain, decreased hemoglobin, hematuria, hematemesis, or guaiac-positive stools. With excessive blood loss, patients may also experience hypovolemic shock and may require reversal of streptokinase with aminocaproic acid (Amicar). Platelet and blood transfusion may also be necessary. When the sheath is removed, direct pressure is applied over the puncture site for a minimum of 10 minutes. Once bleeding has stopped, a pressure dressing is applied over the site; a sandbag may provide additional pressure if needed.

In addition to the routine precautions taken to prevent bleeding, patients receiving streptokinase require the following interventions:

1. Minimize needle punctures by using previously started intravenous lines for blood specimen withdrawal and substituting oral for parenteral medications, when possible.
2. Minimize physical handling of the patient.
3. Eliminate objects in the environment that could cause physical trauma to the patient (*e.g.*, objects left in bed).
4. Avoid concurrent use of platelet-active drugs (*e.g.*, aspirin or Persantine).[46]
5. If the patient is restless, protect him from bruising. If IV infiltration or dislodgment occurs, the IV line should be left in place for 8 hours after streptokinase administration.

Reperfusion Arrhythmias. When streptokinase therapy results in reperfusion in the myocardium, most patient experience reperfusion ventricular arrhythmias. These arrhythmias must be treated aggressively if a lethal arrhythmia is to be prevented. Some unit protocols include prophylactic use of lidocaine for patients with acute MI with or without streptokinase therapy.

Allergic Responses. Allergic responses to streptokinase are minimized by determining which patients are at risk for an antigen–antibody reaction. Patients at high risk include those who have had streptokinase in the recent past (6 to 12 months), or those who have streptococcal infections. These patients might receive a different thrombolytic agent, or they might receive prophylactic steroids or antihistamines prior to therapy. Allergic reactions range from mild fever and urticaria to anaphylactic shock. Mild reactions are treated with antihistamine and acetaminophen. Signs and symptoms of anaphylaxis need to be detected and treated aggressively (see Chap. 24).

Recurrent Thrombosis. Recurrent thrombosis can occur and should be suspected in these patients following streptokinase treatment if chest pain returns. Clinical manifestations and treatment are the same as for the patient with acute MI. Heparin infusion and oral anticoagulants are given to prevent recurrent thrombosis and infarction.

Anxiety. The patient and family often experience extreme anxiety because of the life threatening nature of acute MI and because therapy must be initiated as soon as possible after the symptom onset (preferably within 4 hours). The scenario of streptokinase therapy frequently includes hurried movement of patients, rapid explanations, and quick decision making during a time when the patient is experiencing pain, anxiety, and fear.[37] Anxiety needs to be detected and treated early and prevented as much as possible. A calm, competent manner, simple explanations of procedures and sequence of events, and answering questions as they arise may help to allay fear and anxiety.

Major Complications of Myocardial Infarction

Incidence and Risk

Major complications of MI include arrhythmias, heart failure, cardiogenic shock, pulmonary embolism, and structural heart problems. The most commonly occurring complications are arrhythmias and heart failure. Physical immobility and recumbency predispose the patient with MI to other complications related to sleep deprivation, sensory deprivation, and sensory overload.

Arrhythmias

Arrhythmias occur in the patient with MI for a variety of reasons. The normal initiation and conduction of impulses may be altered because of ischemic and infarcted myocardial cells. Necrotic cells are electrically silent and neither initiate nor conduct impulses. Ischemia can cause normal pacemaker cells to increase their firing rate or can allow nonpacemaker cells to initiate ectopic impulses (increased automatically). Other causes of increased automaticity in patients with acute MI are hypoxemia, disturbances of acid–base balance, disturbances of electrolyte balances (K^+, Ca^{2+}, Mg^{2+}), myocardial-cell stretch related to heart failure, fever, and stress resulting in increases in circulating catecholamines. The rate of pacemaker cell firing and conduction through the heart can be decreased owing to vagal stimulation related to the site of the MI, the Valsalva maneuver, or the nausea and vomiting that may be associated with acute MI. Ischemic or injured myocardial cells and normal adjacent cells may conduct impulses at different rates, thus allowing abnormal initiation and conduction of impulses (reentry).[59]

Heart Failure

Ischemic myocardium does not contract normally, and necrotic tissue does not contract at all. In addition, there may be areas of the ventricles that bulge during systole (ventricular aneurysms), resulting in asynchronous contraction. Because of the decrease in contractility the heart's pumping ability is impaired. When the heart can no longer keep up with the body's demand for oxygenated blood, heart failure ensues. If more than 40% of the left ventricle is infarcted, severe heart failure or cardiogenic shock develops. Cardiogenic shock is associated with an 80% to 90% mortality rate.

Pulmonary Embolism

Pulmonary embolism occurs as a consequence of prolonged bed rest. Patients with uncomplicated MI ambulate early and usually are not at risk for complications of physical immobility and recumbency.[58] Patients who are physically immobilized because of complications of MI are prone to thrombus formation because blood viscosity is increased, which leads to hypercoagulability; venous stasis occurs, and external pressure is exerted against the veins.[41] The saphenous vein is the most common site of superficial vein thrombosis. The ileofemoral veins, popliteal segments, or small veins of the calf are the common sites of deep vein thrombosis. Fragments of deep vein thrombus can dislodge and result in potentially lethal pulmonary emboli. Fragmentation can occur as part of the natural dissolution process or from mechanical forces that change pressure in the vessels. Activities that can change the pressure within a vessel include standing, sudden muscle activity after prolonged bed rest, or the Valsalva maneuver.[12]

Structural Heart Problems

Structural problems caused by acute MI include papillary muscle rupture, ventricular aneurysm, ventricular rupture, and rupture of the interventricular septum.[47] Any of these structural problems can result in mild to severe heart failure or angina. Pericarditis can also occur.

Papillary muscle rupture can occur with papillary muscle necrosis. Mitral insufficiency is the result of left ventricular papillary muscle rupture.

Ventricular aneurysms occur due to bulging necrotic areas following transmural MI.

Ventricular rupture is most common during the second week following transmural MI because the removal of necrotic tissue (phagocytosis) occurs more rapidly than collagen formation, resulting in a thin, weak ventricular wall.

Ventricular septal rupture is rare but can occur within the first week after septal MI. If the septum is necrotic from the MI, the septum becomes thin and weak and cannot withstand the left ventricular pressure.

Pericarditis can occur early or late in the course of MI. With epicardial and transmural MI, the pericardium can become inflamed.

Early pericarditis results in a serous, or less commonly sanguineous, exudate from the inflamed pericardium, leading to an accumulation of fluid in the pericardial sac. This accumulation if rapid can result in pericardial tamponade and shock due to compression of the heart.

Late pericarditis (Dressler's syndrome) can occur up to 28 months after MI. The etiology is unknown, but current research suggests an autoimmune response.

Nursing Management

Assessment and Nursing Diagnoses

Although the data obtained from the patient and his family could support most of the accepted nursing diagnoses, the most common nursing diagnoses for the patients with coronary heart disease follow. The diagnostic statements are written utilizing problem–etiology–symptom (P-E-S) format. The examples of etiologies and manifestations are common but not inclusive.

1. *Decrease in myocardial tissue perfusion* related to an imbalance between myocardial oxygen supply and demand manifested by chest discomfort, arrhythmias and conduction disturbances, and/or heart failure
2. *Alteration in comfort: pain* related to an imbalance between myocardial oxygen supply and demand manifested by patient complaints of chest discomfort with or without radiation to arms, neck, or jaw and by nonverbal expressions of discomfort (*e.g.,* facial grimacing, clutching chest). Other common etiologies of pain are surgical incisions, pericarditis, and pulmonary emboli.
3. *Decreased cardiac output* related to arrhythmias and conduction disturbances, heart failure, cardiogenic shock, or hemorrhage manifested by abnormal pulse rate and rhythm, deterioration in other hemodynamic parameters, decreased mentation, decreased urine output, moist, cool skin, peripheral edema, or abnormal respiratory rate and rhythm.
4. *Fear and anxiety* related to diagnosis, treatment, or prognosis of myocardial ischemia and infarction manifested by subjective complaints of fear and anxiety from patient and family, restlessness, abnormal rate and rhythm of pulse and respiration, or abnormal blood pressure
5. *Knowledge deficit* about the disease process, medical or surgical management plan, risk factor modification, or return to usual activities of daily living, related to lack of recall, nonuse of information, misinterpretation, cognitive limitations, disinterest, lack of familiarity with available resources, or denial of disease, manifested by the patient being unable to describe the disease process; unable to explain the rationale behind the diagnosis, treatment, and prognosis of myocardial ischemia and infarction; unaware of activity limitations and prescribed medications; or unaware of cardiac risk factors and how to modify them.

Goals. The basic goals of cardiac nursing care are (1) to detect early the manifestations of problems, (2) to reduce or eliminate these problems and their manifestations with nursing and delegated medical interventions, (3) to prevent when possible the occurrence of these problems and their manifestations, and (4) to promote and reinforce good health practices.

Interventions

Interventions are related to the specific etiology of the problem.

CCU Care

The patient suspected of having an acute MI is admitted directly to the CCU. Most CCUs have standing admission orders, but it is up to the nurse to implement these orders in correct priority sequence using sound clinical judgment. In the acute phase, goals of treatment are shared by medicine and nursing:

1. Rapid management of existing problems (*i.e.,* relief of chest discomfort, nausea or vomiting, dyspnea)
2. Prevention or early detection of arrhythmias and other complications of MI
3. Beginning rehabilitation

These goals are achieved while attempting to restore and maintain the balance between myocardial oxygen supply and demand.[60]

Early assessment of the patient not only serves to establish priorities of needs and provide baseline data for further nursing plans, but also initiates a relationship between the patient and the nurse that can promote confidence in the CCU nursing staff. Initial priorities of care include rhythm recognition and treatment, starting an intravenous line, and relieving chest discomfort and dyspnea.[60]

Rhythm Recognition and Treatment. This is the first priority in the care of a patient with acute MI. The patient is usually transported to the CCU with continuous ECG monitoring. The patient must remain on this monitor until the CCU monitoring system is attached. An appropriate lead is selected for monitoring, and the electrodes are placed on the chest accordingly.

The electrode site on the skin should be clean (use alcohol), dry (use gauze), and relatively flat. Hair should be shaved, and the skin should be mildly abraded to reduce the resistance. The electrode is then applied to the chest, the alarm limits for heart rate are set (30% above and below the patient's heart rate), the beeper in the patient's room is turned off, and the alarm system is activated. Electrodes should be changed often enough (usually about 1 to 3 days) to prevent skin breakdown and to provide artifact-free tracings. The patient should be given a brief explanation of the purpose of ECG monitoring; his questions should be answered.

The patient's heart rate, rhythm, and conduction must be continuously assessed, since most arrhythmias occur within the first 2 to 3 days after acute MI; 95% of these patients will have arrhythmias. Intervention must be directed toward prevention by recognizing and controlling conditions that predispose the patient to arrhythmias. Some of these conditions are hypokalemia, acidosis, hypoxemia, pain, anxiety, fever, and myocardial stretch (caused by heart failure).

Early identification of arrhythmias and prompt, aggressive treatment are necessary if mortality from MI is to be reduced. Arrhythmias can result in reduced cardiac output and coronary blood flow, increased myocardial oxygen need, and predisposition to a lethal arrhythmia. The cardiac monitor must be under constant surveillance if arrhythmias are to be detected and treated early, to prevent further problems for the patient.

Vital Signs. Vital signs, including blood pressure, pulse, respiration, and temperature (oral or rectal) should be obtained on admission and every 2 to 4 hours as needed.[34]

Intravenous Line. An intravenous line (angiocatheter) is established. Since scalp-vein needles are easily dislodged, they should be used only temporarily until a more stable intravenous line can be established. This intravenous line is used to give pain medications and emergency cardiac drugs. The intravenous line can be capped or an intravenous solution of 5% dextrose and water can be attached and infused at a rate to keep the vein open. If the intravenous line is capped, 10 U to 100 U of heparin in 1 ml of saline should be injected every 8 hours and following injection of medication in order to maintain patency. A simple explanation of procedures is useful to the patients.[60]

Chest Discomfort. Chest discomfort, dyspnea, and anxiety are common complaints. If the patient complains of chest discomfort, he should be given analgesic medication. The anxiety associated with pain increases myocardial oxygen demand. In order to decrease myocardial oxygen need, morphine sulfate is given intravenously in small increments of 1 mg to 5 mg. Morphine should not be given to patients who have advanced atrioventricular block or sinus bradycardia since it has a vagotonic effect. Morphine decreases blood pressure, heart rate, and respiratory rate.[42] If the heart rate is less than 70, meperidine may be the drug of choice.[31] Oxygen at 2 to 4 liters/minute by nasal prongs may decrease chest discomfort by increasing oxygen supply to the myocardium.[13,18] Dyspnea can also cause anxiety and can be relieved by the administration of oxygen. Also, the administration of oxygen may diminish the conversion of ischemic myocardium to necrotic tissue. The magnitude of this benefit is not clear, and the primary physiological mechanisms remain obscure.[8] Arterial blood gases should be used to evaluate the effectiveness of oxygen therapy and to assess acid–base balance.[60]

Physical rest in bed with the backrest elevated, or in a cardiac chair, will assist in decreasing chest discomfort and dyspnea. The head-up position is beneficial for the following reasons: tidal volume is improved, since there is reduced pressure from abdominal contents on the diaphragm, and thus oxygen exchange is improved; drainage of the upper lobes of the lungs is improved;[18] and venous return to the heart (preload) and cardiac output are reduced, thus the work of the heart is reduced.[60]

The nurse assesses and documents the patient's cardiovascular, renal, respiratory, neurological (level of consciousness) and psychological status. These data provide baseline values. If the patient is anxious, myocardial oxygen demand is increased. Explanations of all the activities and equipment will assist in relieving the patient's anxiety. The patient's visiting with family or friends may either reduce or create anxiety. Assessment of the effect of visitors and appropriate intervention is a nursing responsibility. Unit policies should be flexible to provide individual care.[60]

Myocardial Oxygen Needs. Nursing management of the patient with MI focuses on restoring the *balance between myocardial oxygen supply and demand.* The size of the infarction is determined by the demand and supply of oxygen to the ischemic and injured zones. Some ways to decrease the patient's myocardial oxygen need are to promote bed rest with progressive mobilization, assist the patient with activities of daily living, and control the environment to minimize stress.[60]

Bed Rest. Bed rest is important to the healing heart, but it is not without complications. Immobility has many adverse effects. For the patient with an uncomplicated myocardial infarction activity usually progresses as follows:[60]

CCU day 1 Bed rest with use of bedside commode

CCU day 2 With assistance, sitting on the bed with legs

dangling for three times a day (at times other than mealtime) for 5 minutes

CCU day 3 Sitting in chair three times a day (at times other than mealtime), for 5 to 15 minutes, as tolerated

CCU day 4 Length of time sitting in chair increased as tolerated by patient

CCU day 5 Walking in room for 5 minutes, or as tolerated

Activities of Daily Living. Activities of daily living can pose a problem to the independent person because he is now dependent on the nurse for assistance. Most CCU staff allow the patients to feed themselves. The diet selected should minimize myocardial work, maintain normal extracellular volume, and minimize patient pain and discomfort.[10] Digestion requires increased cardiac output, which increases the myocardial oxygen consumption. Full liquid diet for 24 hours facilitates digestion: the need to chew has been eliminated, and thus there is less cardiac demand than a regular diet.[60] Table 37–7 presents dietary principles during the acute phase of MI.

The patient's arms should be supported on the overbed table during meals to prevent an unconscious Valsalva maneuver. In a Valsalva maneuver, air is forced over a closed glottis, resulting in increased intrathoracic pressure. This increased intrathoracic pressure may be as high as 80 mmHg and causes a decreased venous return to the heart (decreased preload) and vagal stimulation, resulting in decreased cardiac output.[45] When the force air is released, the intrathoracic pressure is decreased, and preload is increased, resulting in an increased work load for the heart. The Valsalva maneuver can occur with activities such as turning or moving up in bed, reaching, vomiting, pulling, defecating, or coughing. Therefore, the patient should be instructed to avoid breath holding, and to breathe in and out with the mouth open while engaging in these activities.[17]

TABLE 37–7
Dietary Principles During the Acute Phase of MI

1. Avoid large meals, which potentially increase demand for splanchnic blood flow and thereby increase postprandial cardiac work.
2. Minimize volume of gastric contents in order to decrease the chance of vomiting and aspiration in the event of cardiac emergencies.
3. Avoid ingestion of myocardial stimulants, such as caffeine or theobromine (tea).
4. Avoid swallowing exceptionally cold or hot food and drink, to help decrease the possibility of cardiac arrhythmias.
5. Avoid as much as possible foods that contribute to constipation and resultant straining with bowel movements, which may predispose a patient to vagal cardiac rhythm changes.
6. Limit foods known to commonly produce excessive gas during the digestive process, such as dried beans, legumes, and apple juice.
7. Offer a diet ample in potassium for all patients except those in renal failure. Most patients on potassium-wasting diuretic therapy will also require supplemental potassium treatment. (Most salt substitutes contain potassium chloride.)

(Diet and Coronary Heart Disease. Dallas, American Heart Association, 1978)

The use of a bedside commode with assistance is less work than the use of a bedpan. The position one assumes when using a commode is more natural and allows for appropriate and optimum utilization of the muscles of defecation (abdominal and rectal). Sufficient fluid intake is necessary to prevent constipation. Stool softeners will decrease the need for straining and possibly prevent a Valsalva maneuver.

Hygiene Care. Initially, the patient will need to be bathed (day 1) and then assisted with the bath (days 2 to 5). The patient with an uncomplicated MI usually can take a warm shower after he is discharged from the CCU. A warm shower is preferred over a hot shower, since a hot shower could result in vasodilatation and markedly reduced preload and cardiac output. The patient may need to use a chair in the shower or may need assistance with washing. Discussion of these activities with the patient and physician is necessary to determine their preferences and to develop a workable care plan.[60]

The intravenous site should be inspected daily for signs of inflammation (*i.e.,* redness, swelling, and heat). Findings should be documented in the patient's chart. Unless an occlusive, transparent dressing is used, the site should be cleaned with an antiseptic, and an antibiotic ointment and a dry sterile dressing should be applied. If the site is inflamed, a new intravenous line should be placed in a different site prior to discontinuing the old line. The intravenous site should be changed at least every 3 days. Also, electrode sites on the chest should be assessed daily for skin irritation. When electrodes are changed, the site should be washed with soap and water. Different areas of the chest should be selected for application or new electrodes.[60]

It is important to allow the patient as much independence as possible to promote his self-confidence, which in turn facilities psychological and physiological recovery.[42] All activities are modified to meet individual needs.

Psychological Problems. Psychological problems that are apt to occur early in the hospitalization can be recognized and in some instances prevented.[54] The nurse helps the patient and his family cope with these problems. Typically, the patient reacts to an MI with the following behavioral responses: anxiety, denial, depression, anger, or aggressive sexual behavior.

To maintain an environment that reduces stress, one must ensure a calm, quiet, optimistic atmosphere. The staff must demonstrate efficiency and competence in their care. In addition, what is stressful to one individual may not be stressful to another. Thus, each patient must be assessed to determine a suitable environment that reduces stress. Antianxiety drugs such as diazepam may also be useful.[6, 18]

The accompanying care plan, Nursing Care Plan of the Patient in the CCU (uncomplicated myocardial infarction), delineates major problems. This suggested plan of care must be individualized for each patient and is not meant as a

(Text continues on page 538)

NURSING CARE PLAN FOR THE PATIENT IN THE CCU (UNCOMPLICATED MYOCARDIAL INFARCTION)

NURSING DIAGNOSIS/PROBLEM 1: Chest discomfort related to an imbalance between myocardial oxygen supply and demand
GOAL 1.1: To detect early and to relieve chest discomfort

Nursing Interventions	Rationale	Outcome Criteria
1. Initially assess, document, and report to the physician the following: a. The patient's description of chest discomfort, including location, radiation, duration of pain, and factors that affect it. b. The effect of chest discomfort on cardiovascular hemodynamic perfusion; to the heart, to the brain, to the kidneys, and to the skin.	1. These data assist in determining the cause and effect of the chest discomfort and provide a baseline so that posttherapy symptoms can be compared. a. There are many conditions associated with chest discomfort. There are characteristic clinical findings of ischemic pain. b. Myocardial infarction decreases myocardial contractility and ventricular compliance and may produce arrhythmias by promoting reentry and increased automaticity. Cardiac output is reduced, resulting in reduced blood pressure and decreased organ perfusion. The heart rate may increase as a compensatory mechanism to maintain cardiac output.	1–6. Patient reports relief of chest discomfort within 15 to 30 minutes. Patient appears comfortable: a. Seems restful b. Respiratory rate, cardiac rate, and blood pressure return to prediscomfort level c. Skin warm and dry Effects of chest discomfort on cardiovascular hemodynamics detected to maintain within normal limits: a. Heart rate, rhythm, and conduction b. Blood pressure c. Mentation d. Urine output e. Serum BUN and creatinine f. Skin color, temperature, and moisture
2. Obtain a 12-lead ECG recording during pain, as prescribed, to determine extension of infarction or variant angina.	2. An ECG during pain may be useful in the diagnosis of an extension of myocardial ischemia, injury, and infarction, and of variant angina.	
3. Administer oxygen as prescribed.	3. Oxygen may increase the oxygen supply to the myocardium is actual oxygen saturation is less than normal.	
4. Administer narcotic or analgesic medications as prescribed and evaluate the patient's response continuously.	4. Narcotics are useful in alleviating chest discomfort, decreasing anxiety, and increasing sense of well-being. The side-effects of these medications can be dangerous and the patient's status must be asessed.	
5. Ensure physical rest; use of the bedside commode with assistance; backrest elevated to comfort; full liquid diet as tolerated; arms supported during upper extremity activity; use of stool softener to prevent staining at stool. Teach patient to exhale with physical movement to avoid a Valsalva maneuver, and to practice the relaxation response. Visitor privileges are individualized, based on patient response. Provide a restful environment, and allay fears and anxiety by being supportive, calm, and competent.	5. Physical rest reduces myocardial oxygen consumption. Fear and anxiety precipitate the stress response; this results in increased levels of endogenous catecholamines, which increase myocardial oxygen consumption. Also, with increased epinephrine the pain threshold is decreased and pain increases the myocardial oxygen consumption.	
6. Promote the patient's physical comfort by providing individualized basic nursing care.	6. Physical comfort promotes the patient's sense of well-being and reduces anxiety.	

(Continued)

NURSING CARE PLAN FOR THE PATIENT IN THE CCU (UNCOMPLICATED MYOCARDIAL INFARCTION) (*Continued*)

NURSING DIAGNOSIS/PROBLEM 2: Potential arrhythmias and conduction disturbances related to reduced coronary blood flow

GOAL 2.1: To detect early and to prevent the occurrence of arrhythmias and conduction disturbances by restoring the balance between myocardial oxygen supply and demand

Nursing Interventions	Rationale	Outcome Criteria
1. Administer prophylactic antiarrhythmic medications as prescribed.		1. Ideally, normal sinus rhythm without arrhythmia is maintained or restored, or the patient's baseline heart rate, rhythm, and conduction are maintained or restored.
2. Using a cardiac monitor, continuously assess heart rate, rhythm, and conduction, and document every 4 hours and prior to administration of medications that have a cardiovascular effect. Determine the effect of the arrhythmia on the patient's blood pressure and perfusion to the heart, brain, and kidneys, and report marked changes to the physician.	2. Early detection of arrhythmia allows initiation of therapy and may prevent a lethal arrhythmia. Arrhythmias can result in reduced cardiac output, hypotension, and reduced perfusion to vital organs.	2–4. Previous heart rate, rhythm, and conduction restored. All arrhythmias and conduction disturbances are detected as they occur and do not progress to ventricular fibrillation or asystole.
3. Administer antiarrhytmic and other medications as prescribed or according to hospital policy, and evaluate continuously the patient's response to therapy.		
4. Obtain a 12-lead ECG with any marked change in heart rhythm.	4. A 12-lead ECG assists in the diagnosis of arrhythmias and conduction disturbances and of further myocardial damage.	
5. Assess patient's status to determine other causes of the arrhythmias or conduction disturbances: a. Perform a cardiovascular assessment. b. Obtain a chest x-ray film.	5a,b. Data obtained from the history and physical examination and from laboratory studies can assist in the diagnosis of the disease processes (such as left ventricular failure or pulmonary embolism) that can cause arrhythmias by the mechanisms of hypoxemia or myocardial stretch. Also, a chest x-ray film provides information regarding the placement of catheters within the heart. Abnormal placement of the catheter within the heart can cause mechanical irritation of the myocardium and result in arrhythmias.	5a,b,c. Normal heart and breath sounds without adventitious sounds. Serum potassium remains between 3.6 mEq/liter and 5.5 mEq/liter. Calcium remains between 4.6 mEq/liter and 5.5 mEq/liter. Hemoglobin remains between 12 g/100 ml and 18 g/100 ml. Serum drug levels are within the therapeutic range. Arterial blood gases on room air remain within the normal limits. Chest x-ray film remains within normal limits. Incorrect position of heart catheters is detected early.
c. Obtain venous blood (for electrolytes, hemoglobin, appropriate drug levels) and arterial blood (for blood gases) as prescribed.	c. Electrolyte imbalance (especially potassium or calcium) can cause arrhythmias and conduction disturbances. Reduced hemoglobin decreases the oxygen-carrying capacity of the blood. Hypoxemia, acidosis, alkalosis, and concurrent drug toxicity or subtherapeutic drug levels can cause arrhythmias and conduction disturbances.	

(*Continued*)

NURSING CARE PLAN FOR THE PATIENT IN THE CCU (UNCOMPLICATED MYOCARDIAL INFARCTION) *(Continued)*

NURSING DIAGNOSIS/PROBLEM 3: Respiratory difficulties (shortness of breath, dyspnea, orthopnea) related to reduced cardiac output

GOAL 3.1: To detect early and to prevent respiratory difficulty

Nursing Interventions	Rationale	Outcome Criteria
1. Initially and every 4 hours, and with chest discomfort, assess, document, and report to the physician abnormal heart sounds (particularly S_3 and S_4 gallops and the holosystolic murmur of left ventricular papillary muscle dysfunction), abnormal breath sounds (particularly crackles), and patient intolerance to specific activities.	1. These data are useful in diagnosing left ventricular failure. Diastolic filling sounds (S_3–S_4 gallop) result from decreased left ventricular compliance associated with myocardial infarction. Papillary muscles dysfunction (from infarction of the papillary muscle) can result in mitral regurgitation and a reduction in stroke volume, leading to left ventricular failure. The presence of crackles (usually at the lung bases) may indicate pulmonary congestion from increased left heart pressures. The association of symptoms and activity can be used as a guide for activity prescription and a basis for patient teaching.	1–4. Patient does not complain of shortness of breath, dyspnea on exertion, orthopnea, or paroxysmal nocturnal dyspnea. Respiratory rate remains less than 20 breaths per minute with physical activity and 16 breaths per minute with rest. Skin color is normal. Pa_{O_2} and Pa_{CO_2} are within normal range. Heart rate is less than 100 beats per minute with blood pressure within normal limits for this patient. Normal chest film.
2. Ensure physical rest and comfort.	2. Rest decreases myocardial oxygen need.	
3. Full liquid diet for 24 hours as prescribed	3. Digestion requires increased cardiac output, which increases the myocardial oxygen consumption. Full liquid diet facilitates digestion because the need to chew has been eliminated, thus requiring less cardiac demand than eating a regular diet.	
4. Teach patient: a. To adhere to the diet prescribed (*e.g.,* explain low sodium, low calories)	4. a. Low-sodium diet may reduce extracellular volume, thus reducing preload and afterload, and thus myocardial oxygen consumption. In the obese patient, weight reduction may decrease cardiac work and improve tidal volume.	
b. To adhere to activity prescription	b. The activity prescription is determined individually to maintain the heart rate and blood pressure within safe limits.	

NURSING DIAGNOSIS/PROBLEM 4: Reduced perfusion to vital organs related to reduced cardiac output

GOAL 4.1: To detect early and to prevent decreased systemic tissue perfusion by restoring the balance between myocardial oxygen supply and demand

Nursing Interventions	Rationale	Outcome Criteria
1. Initially and every 4 hours, and with chest discomfort, assess, document, and report to the physician the following:	1. These data are useful in determining a low cardiac output state.	1. Signs and symptoms of reduced tissue perfusion are detected within 4 hours.

(Continued)

NURSING CARE PLAN FOR THE PATIENT IN THE CCU (UNCOMPLICATED MYOCARDIAL INFARCTION) (*Continued*)

Nursing Interventions	Rationale	Outcome Criteria
a. Hypotension b. Tachycardia and other arrhythmia c. Fatigability d. Mentation changes (use family input) e. Reduced urine output (less than 250 ml/8 hours) f. Cool, moist, cyanotic extremities		
2. Provide rest and comfort.	2. Rest decreases myocardial oxygen need. Physical comfort promotes the patient's sense of well-being and reduces anxiety.	2. Blood pressure remains within the individual's normal range. Ideally, normal sinus rhythm without arrhythmia is maintained or patient's baseline rhythm is maintained between 60 and 100 beats per minute without further arrhythmia. No complaints of fatigue with prescribed activity. Remains fully alert and oriented and without personality change. Urine output is greater than 250 ml/8 hours. Extremities remain warm and dry with normal color.

NURSING DIAGNOSIS/PROBLEM 5: Anxiety and fear of death

GOAL 5.1: To detect early and reduce signs and symptoms of anxiety and fear

Nursing Interventions	Rationale	Outcome Criteria
1. Assess, document, and report to the physician the patient's and family's level of anxiety and coping mechanisms.	1. These data provide information about the psychological well-being and a baseline so that posttherapy symptoms can be compared. Causes of anxiety are variable and individual, and may include acute illness, hospitalization, pain, disruption of activities of daily living at home and at work, changes in role and self-image owing to chronic illness, and lack of financial support. Because anxious to the patient, the nurse must also reduce the family's fear and anxiety.	1–7. Patient reports less anxiety. Patient and family discuss their activities and fears about death. Patient and family appear less anxious. Patient is restful, respiratory rate less than 16 per minute, heart rate less than 100 per minute without ectopic beats, blood pressure within his normal limits, skin warm and dry. Patient participates actively in a progressive rehabilitation program. Patient practices stress-reduction techniques.
2. Provide rest and comfort.	2. Rest and comfort decrease myocardial oxygen needs.	
3. Assess the need for spiritual counseling and refer as appropriate.	3. If a patient finds support in a religion, religious counseling may assist in reducing anxiety and fear.	

(*Continued*)

NURSING CARE PLAN FOR THE PATIENT IN THE CCU (UNCOMPLICATED MYOCARDIAL INFARCTION) *(Continued)*

Nursing Interventions	Rationale
4. Allow patient (and family) to express anxiety and fear: a. By showing a genuine interest and concern b. By providing a conducive atmosphere c. By facilitating communication (listening, reflecting, guiding) d. By answering questions	4. Unresolved anxiety (the stress response) increases myocardial oxygen consumption.
5. Use of flexible visiting hours allows the presence of a supportive family to assist in reducing the patient's level of anxiety.	5. The presence of supportive family members may reduce both patient's and family's anxiety.
6. Encourage active participation in a hospital cardiac rehabilitation program.	6. Prescribed cardiac rehabilitation may help to eliminate fear of death, may reduce anxiety, and may enhance feelings of well-being.
7. Teach stress reduction techniques.	7. Stress reduction techniques may help to reduce myocardial oxygen consumption and may enhance feelings of well-being.

(Adapted from Underhill SL et al: Cardiac Nursing. Philadelphia, JB Lippincott, 1982)

standard care plan to be used on all patients. It is meant to demonstrate the use of the nursing process with a patient with this disease and to provide a guideline for developing an individual plan of care.

Patient Teaching

Patient and family teaching is begun as soon as readiness to learn is apparent.

Content to be included in these teaching sessions is as follows:

Risk factors
The normal heart and circulation
The coronary arteries
The disease process
Diagnosis of a heart attack
The healing process
Progression of activity
Suggested progression of activity during the acute stage
Suggested progression of activity during the subacute stage
Suggested progression of activity during the convalescent stage
The first 1 to 2 weeks after discharge from the hospital
A walking program at home
Activity guidelines
Sexual intercourse after a heart attack
Psychological factors
Dietary suggestions
Smoking
Alcohol
Medication
Community resources

The patient without complications is usually discharged from the CCU after 3 to 5 days. The nasal oxygen and intravenous line may be discontinued, and the patient transferred by means of a wheelchair to an intermediate care unit or to a medical floor. This transfer should be anticipated and the rationale explained to the patient and family. The anticipation of transfer may reassure the patient. To provide continuity of care, the unit to which the patient is being transferred should be notified of the patient's transfer, and the written plan of care, physician orders, and patient's progress should be shared.[60]

Post-CCU Care

During the post-CCU phase the risk of complications from MI is markedly reduced. The difference between the intermediate care unit and the medical unit is the intensity and constancy of assessment of cardiac function and potential complications. For example, in the intermediate care area the patient's heart rhythm should be continuously monitored by telemetry; on the medical floor the patient may be monitored, but less frequently. During this phase the patient is allowed to be more independent in activities of daily living. The area designed for intermediate care should be adjacent to or in continuity with the CCU, thus permitting efficient utilization of manpower and physical resources and facilitating patient transfer. Monitoring and resuscitation capability for intermediate care should be identical with that of the CCU. In some institutions the intermediate care unit is not restricted to patients discharged from the CCU, but is a place for any patient with cardiovascular disease who may benefit from the monitoring or resuscitative capability of this unit.[60]

Cardiac Rehabilitation

Cardiac rehabilitation is a process of actively assisting the cardiac patient to achieve and maintain optimum health.[9] Components of cardiac rehabilitation are education of the patient and family, and prescription for activity and exercise. Cardiac rehabilitation is divided into three phases. Phase one begins with the acute illness and ends with hospital discharge. Phase two begins after the hospital discharge and continues through convalescence at home. Phase three is long-term conditioning.

Education of the patient and family cannot begin until readiness to learn has been determined. When it has been established that the patient and family are ready to learn, a teaching plan should be developed, including an explanation of the pathophysiology of a heart attack, the risk factors involved, the dietary changes that are required, the activity and exercise protocols advised, and the means of dealing with the psychological reactions to a myocardial infarction and learning to return to a more meaningful life.

Modification of risk factors includes changing dietary habits, controlling high blood pressure, stopping smoking, exercising regularly, and reducing stress. Dietary changes that should be made include reducing total fat intake and substituting polyunsaturated fats for saturated fats, reducing calories to maintain ideal body weight, and reducing sodium intake for patients who have high blood pressure or heart failure. In addition, alcohol consumption should be modified since alcohol increases myocardial oxygen consumption. When designing strategies for prevention and cessation of smoking, assessment of the psychological aspects of smoking behavior is important. Psychological needs are met by smoking for the following reasons: smoking reduces tension, provides sensory stimulation, enhances self-image (especially in the young), and is a social act. Many formal programs that help adults to stop smoking are available, but of the 29 million smokers who have stopped since 1964, 95% have done so on their own.[57]

Patients who have never exercised regularly may have difficulty incorporating regular exercise into their normal activities. Joining a formal exercise program may provide the motivation needed. Awareness of the effects of stress on the body and the heart and of the types of situations that induce stress may provide an incentive to avoid emotional stressors when possible. Unfortunately, many stress-inducing situations cannot be avoided, but responses to these situations may be altered through stress-reduction techniques. In addition, regular physical activity such as running, swimming, or bicycling and more leisure-time activity may help to dispel some of the effects of emotional stress on the cardiovascular system.[57]

Activity and exercise prescriptions are given as guidelines. Activity includes movements that are accomplished in the course of meeting human physiological needs. Exercise refers to physical exertion.[48]

Goals of long-term conditioning include (1) retaining a physical working capacity commensurate with the occupational needs and leisure time interests of the patient, and (2) obtaining and maintaining optimal cardiovascular functional capacity.[48] Exercise prescriptions are based on isotonic exercises that raise the heart rate to 60% to 80% of the maximal heart rate (obtained from an exercise tolerance test).

Evaluation

Specific outcome criteria are developed for the plan of care. When possible, these outcomes should be measurable and should be individualized for each patient. In addition, an appropriate and realistic time frame should be included as part of the outcome criteria. The major outcome criteria are as follows:

To detect early the manifestations of problems of coronary heart disease (CHD). If problems are not detected in a timely manner, complications of that problem will arise. It may be necessary to modify the prescribed interventions, including increasing the frequency of evaluation of specific assessment parameters, reassessing accepted ranges in parameters, adding additional evaluation parameters, or changing the intervention.

To reduce or eliminate problems of CHD and their manifestations with nursing and delegated medical interventions. Criteria used to evaluate successful reduction or elimination of the identified problems and their manifestations are both subjective and objective data. These data are specific to the particular problem.

To prevent when possible the occurrence of problems associated with CHD. Outcome criteria used to evaluate interventions to meet this goal are subjective and objective data that reflect absence of identified or potential problems.

To promote and reinforce good health practices. The outcome of interventions that reflect promoting and reinforcing good health practices are subjective and objective measures of a healthy lifestyle.

Invasive Therapy

Angioplasty

Angioplasty, or percutaneous transluminal coronary angioplasty (PTCA) is a procedure that can be of benefit to selected patients with coronary heart disease. Performed under fluoroscopy in the cardiac catheterization laboratory, PTCA is done by introducing a balloon-tipped catheter into the femoral artery and advancing it retrograde in the aorta, into the coronary artery. The balloon is inflated at the point of stenosis in an attempt to reduce or eliminate the occluding lesion (Fig. 37–4). Continuous intravenous heparin infusion is used to prevent thrombus formation. Intracoronary streptokinase

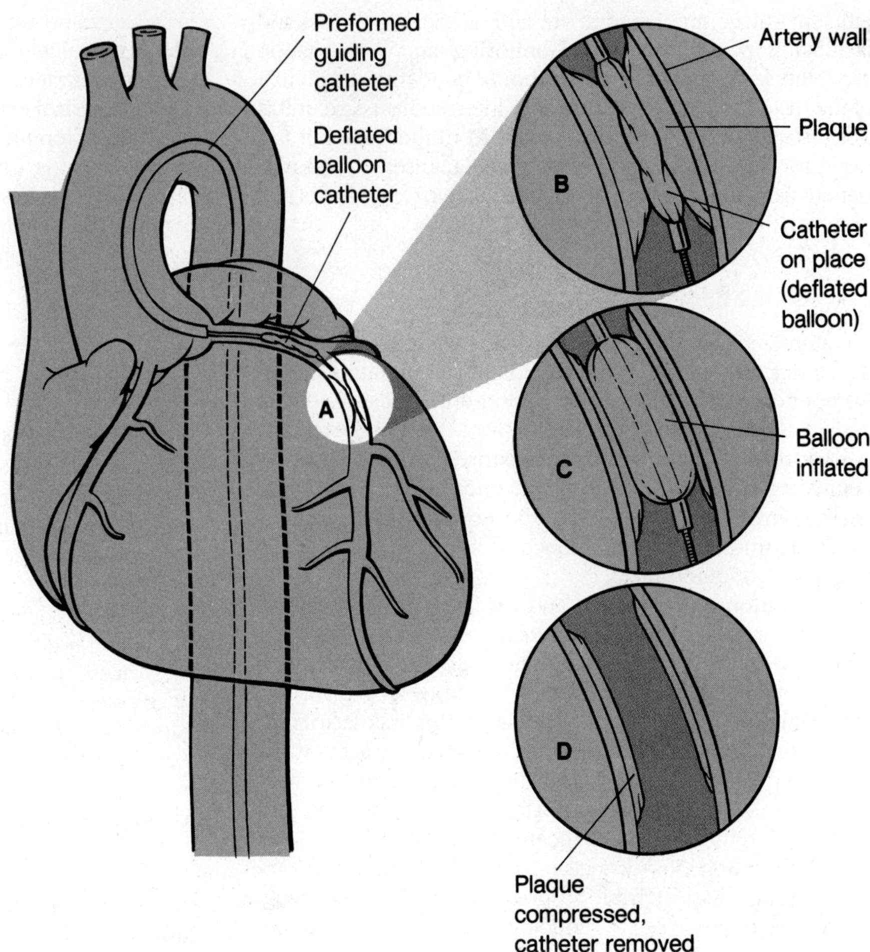

FIGURE 37-4 (*A*) A guiding catheter is advanced under fluoroscopy by way of the femoral artery into the ascending aorta and positioned here within the opening of the left anterior descending branch of the left coronary artery. (*B*) The balloon dilatation catheter is then advanced into the coronary artery and manipulated until the balloon portion is positioned within the artherosclerotic lesion. The gold markers on either side of the balloon, visualized under fluoroscopy, identify the position of the balloon. (*C*) Once in position, the balloon is quickly inflated by a small hydraulic pump (commonly to 4 atmospheres) for 4 or 5 seconds with a mixture of saline and contrast media. Repeated inflations are performed, if necessary, and pressure measurements proximal and distal to the lesion are made to determine if successful dilatation can be produced. The "controlled injury" to the intimal layer produced by the balloon dilatation causes the release of thrombogenic factors. Anticoagulants, dextran, and aspirin (administered pre-PTCA) help prevent thrombus formation. (*D*) The balloon catheter is pulled back, and contrast media is injected through the guiding catheter to confirm that the atherosclerotic lesion has been sufficiently compressed to permit significant improvement in coronary blood flow. (After Am J Nurs, Sept 1981)

infusion may be combined with PTCA for thrombolysis under certain conditions.

Care of the patient undergoing PTCA is similar to the care given to a patient who has had a cardiac catheterization. Risks connected with the procedure include acute occlusion of the coronary artery due to spasm or thrombus formation, acute arterial dissection or rupture, and myocardial infarction. Because of the risks, angioplasty is currently performed in a facility where the cardiac surgery team in on standby. The mortality for PTCA is about 1%, and the chances of having emergency (coronary artery bypass graft) surgery is about 6%.

In contrast to coronary artery bypass graft surgery, PTCA is done under local anesthesia and, if successful, requires a convalescence of only 2 to 4 days with no limitations caused by prolonged debilitation or incisional pain. However, as with bypass surgery, the disease process that caused the lesion is not altered, and therefore discharge teaching must stress the need to modify the risk factors.

Nursing Interventions

Nursing care of the angioplasty patient is similar to any patient undergoing cardiac catheterization. Patients are usually unstable and may be experiencing an acute MI. Because angioplasty is only performed in a hospital that has a cardiac surgical team on standby, patients may need to be transferred from their hospital to an institution with cardiac surgery capabilities. This transfer to a new environment with a different health care team may contribute to anxiety.

Vasoactive drugs (*i.e.*, nitroglycerin and calcium-channel blocking agents) may be administered before, during, and after the angioplasty, contributing to alterations in blood pressure and heart rate. Patients must be closely monitored for the recurrence of angina and for changing cardiac rate and rhythm. Activity is restricted to bed rest for 12 to 24 hours. The patient may be in the CCU for only 24 hours; hospital discharge depends on clinical signs and symptoms. Anticoagulation is used to prevent thrombi from developing on the newly disturbed atherosclerotic lesion.[29]

Coronary Bypass Surgery

Coronary artery bypass surgery is commonly used today to restore coronary artery blood flow to myocardium distal to a coronary artery stenosis or occlusion. It is estimated that more than 100,000 persons undergo coronary bypass surgery each year in the United States, making it the most often performed of all surgical operations.

After the induction of suitable anesthesia, segments of

the saphenous vein are harvested. A median sternotomy is performed. The patient is placed on cardiopulmonary bypass, and cardioplegia (paralysis of the heart) is induced with hypothermia and injection of potassium chloride. The vein segments are checked for patency and valve location and direction, are trimmed to fit, and are anastomosed to the aorta just distal to the aortic valve. The graft is then anastomosed to the coronary artery just distal to the occlusion (Fig. 37–5). Flow through the graft is checked using a Doppler probe. As many as seven grafts may be placed, but three or four is most common. The heart is warmed, flushed with fluid, and countershocked, if necessary, to restore cardiac rhythm. Bypass is weaned and discontinued. The operative field is observed for adequacy of hemostasis, and the pericardium is left open or removed to prevent tamponade in the event of excessive postoperative bleeding. The incision is closed using wire sutures to approximate the sternum. One or two mediastinal drainage tubes are placed; in some institutions the left pleura is opened, and a chest tube is inserted.

Mortality for this surgery is estimated at about 3%. Patients at increased risk for perioperative (within 30 postoperative days) mortality are those in whom the number of grafts is less than the number of diseased vessels, and those with obstruction of the left main coronary artery. Other risk factors include poor general condition and presence of other diseases, especially pulmonary and renal. Operative risk is reduced by optimizing the patient's condition.

Revascularization is not a permanent cure. The atherosclerotic process that affected the coronary arteries is not arrested; some studies show that up to 30% of grafts are occluded within 6 months. Although angina may be eliminated or decreased by bypass surgery, it may return, and myocardial infarction may occur or reoccur. Modification of lifestyle by reduction of risk factors is imperative.

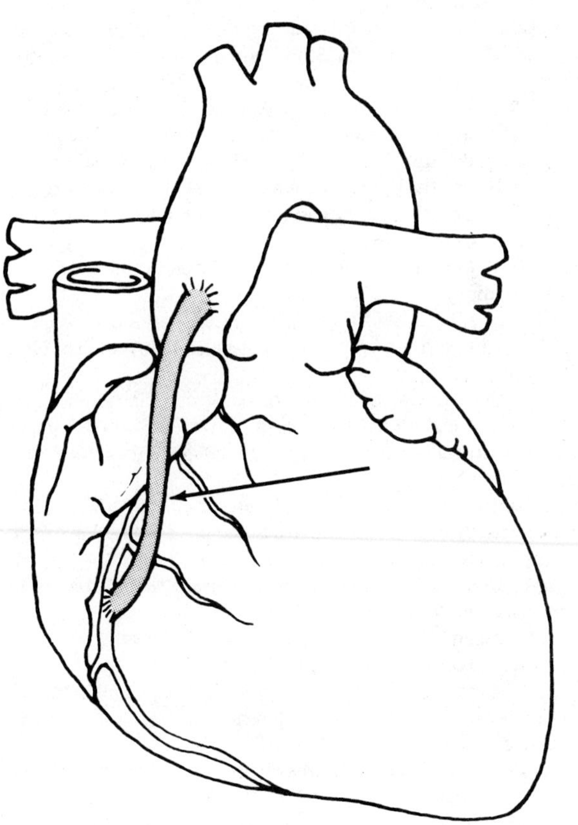

FIGURE 37–5 A section of saphenous vein is used to bypass a coronary artery.

Nursing Interventions

Nursing care of the patient undergoing coronary bypass surgery begins on admission with a complete nursing assessment that is used to formulate the patient's plan of care. In addition to routine preoperative teaching, specific information about coronary artery bypass surgery and the anticipated sequence of events from admission to discharge should be shared with both the patient and his family. Other preoperative teaching includes information about:[61]

- Hospital routines, including ICU visiting policies
- The ICU, including meeting the staff and touring the unit
- Respiratory therapy, including equipment and patient participation
- Physical preparation for surgery
- Routine postoperative care, including intravascular catheters, chest tubes, and pain management
- Communication while intubated

Time should be allowed for patient and family to assimilate this information, to express concerns, and to ask questions.

Postoperative Nursing Management. Postoperative nursing management of the patient who has had bypass surgery includes a general assessment with emphasis on cardiovascular and pulmonary function. Data from a variety of sources are integrated.

Following bypass surgery, the cardiovascular parameters monitored include heart rate and rhythm, blood pressure, central venous and pulmonary pressures, heart sounds, and cardiac output.

Ventricular ectopic rhythms may develop in the initial 24 hours following surgery, possibly from the trauma of surgery, or from potassium imbalance and ventricular distention due to failure. Some physicians initiate a continuous lidocaine infusion for 24 to 48 hours postoperatively as a preventive measure. The nurse is responsible for continually checking for the effectiveness of the therapy and for noting and reporting any recurrence or worsening of the problem. Another possible arrhythmia following bypass surgery is sinus bradycardia or junctional rhythm that may occur as a result of metabolic problems secondary to extracorporeal circulation. The condition usually reverses itself spontaneously in a day or two. But if the rhythm results in low systemic pressures, the patient may be placed at increased rates or given medication to increase heart rate and therefore improve cardiac output and prevent other complications.

Hypertension or hypotension are other problems that may occur. Hypertension may occur from peripheral vasoconstriction and increased catecholamine release. It is important that the patient be medicated to control mean arterial pressure at less than 110 mmHg to lessen the risk of postoperative hemorrhage and possible rupture of the bypass graft suture line.

Hypotension may be treated with IV therapy if hemorrhage or saline depletion is the cause. If a slow heart rate is the blame, then the patient should be paced or medicated to increase heart rate. Antiarrhythmic drugs may be given to control irregular heart rhythm.

The respiratory parameters that need to be monitored include respiratory rate, chest excursions, breath sounds, arterial blood gases, vital capacity, and inspiratory effort (while the patient is intubated). Because decreased respiration is a common side-effect of anesthesia and surgery involving the thorax, the patient will be on mechanical ventilation for 6 to 48 hours after surgery. Frequent monitoring of arterial blood gases is important as is intermittent hyperinflation and endotracheal suctioning. When the patient is alert enough to understand the need to cough and demonstrates good respiratory parameters, he should be weaned from the ventilator. Once weaned, the patient may receive humidified oxygen by mask and should be encouraged to cough and breathe deeply. An incentive spirometer or intermittent positive pressure breathing (IPPB) may be used every 1 to 3 hours.

Prior to being discharged from the ICU, the patient will be extubated (usually within 6 to 24 hours), taking foods and fluids by mouth, sitting up in a chair, and be able to walk short distances. Patient and family anxiety should be anticipated at the time of ICU discharge. Transfer of the patient from the ICU to an intermediate care unit is similar to the transfer from the CCU.

Hospital discharge is usually 3 to 7 days after transfer from the ICU. Preparing the patient and his family for discharge from the hospital is similar to the preparation for discharge of a patient following acute myocardial infarction.

References

1. Ashley FW, Kannel WB: Relation of weight change to changes in atherogenic traits: The Framingham Study, J Chronic Dis 27:103–144, 1974
2. Baim DS, Harrison DC: Nonatherosclerotic coronary heart disease (including coronary artery spasm). In Hurst JW, Logue RB, Rackley CE et al (eds): The Heart, 5th ed, pp 1158–1170. New York, McGraw-Hill, 1982
3. Beral V, Kay CR: Mortality among oral contraceptive users. Lancet ii:727–731, 1977
4. Beta-Blocker Heart Attack Trial Research Group: A randomized trial of propranolol in patients with acute myocardial infarction. 1. Mortality results. JAMA 247:1707–1714, 1982
5. Bond EF: Physiology of the heart. In Underhill SL et al (eds): Cardiac Nursing, pp 13–26. Philadelphia, JB Lippincott, 1982
6. Burke LE: Common noncardiac drugs used in the cardiac care unit. In Underhill SL et al (eds): Cardiac Nursing, pp 431–441. Philadelphia, JB Lippincott, 1982
7. Burke LE: Nitrates. In Underhill SL et al (eds): Cardiac Nursing, pp 478–483. Philadelphia, JB Lippincott, 1982
8. Coglman MM: Effects of oxygen on ischemic myocardium. Heart Lung 7(4):635–640, 1978
9. Comoss PM, Burke EAS, Swails SH: Cardiac Rehabilitation: A Comprehensive Nursing Approach. Philadelphia, JB Lippincott, 1979
10. Diet and Coronary Heart Disease. Dallas, American Heart Association, 1978
11. Feldman EB: Saturated fats. In Feldman EB (ed): Nutrition and Cardiovascular Disease, pp 30–58. New York, Appleton-Century-Crofts, 1976
12. Fitzmaurice J: Venous thromboembolic disease: Current thoughts. Cardiovasc Nurs 14(1):1–4, 1978
13. Foster WT: Principles of Acute Coronary Care. New York, Appleton-Century-Crofts, 1976
14 Gordon T, Castelli WP, Hjortland MC et al: High density lipoprotein as a protective factor against coronary heart disease. The Framingham Study, Am J Med 62:707–714, 1977
15. Healy BB, Becker LC, Flaherty JT: Myocardial infarction. In Harvey AM, Johns RJ, McKusick VA et al (eds): The Principles and Practice of Medicine, 21st ed. Norwalk, Appleton-Century-Crofts, 1984
16. Heart Facts 1984. Dallas, American Heart Association, 1984
17. Holland JM: Cardiovascular Nursing: Prevention, Intervention, and Rehabilitation. Boston, Little, Brown & Co, 1977
18. Holloway NM: Nursing the Critically Ill Adult. Menlo Park CA, Addison-Wesley Publishing Co, 1979
19. Inter-Society Commission for Heart Disease Resources: Report of primary prevention of atherosclerotic diseases. Circulation 42:A55–A95, 1970
20. Jick H, Dinan B, Rothman KJ: Noncontraceptive estrogens and nonfatal myocardial infarction. JAMA 239(14):1407–1408, 1978
21. Jick H, Dinan B, Rothman KJ: Oral contraceptives and nonfatal myocardial infarction. JAMA 239(14):1403–1406
22. Kannel WB: Recent findings of the Framingham Study. Resident and Staff Physician 24:56–71, 1978
23. Kannel WB, Castelli WP, Gordon T et al: Serum cholesterol, lipoproteins, and the risk of coronary heart disease. Ann Intern Med 75(1):1–12, 1971
24. Kannel WB, McGee D. Gordon T: A general cardiovascular risk profile: The Framingham Study. Am J Cardiol 38(1):46–51, 1976
25. Kannel WB, Gordon T, Schwartz MJ: Systolic versus diastolic blood pressure and risk of coronary heart disease. The Framingham Study. Am J Cardiol 27(4):335–345, 1971
26. Kannel WB, Hjortland MC, McNamara PM et al: Menopause and risk of cardioavascular disease. The Framingham Study. Ann Intern Med 85:447–452, 1976
27. Keys A (ed): Coronary Heart Disease in Seven Countries. Circulation (suppl I) 41:1–211, 1970
28. Keys A, Aravanis C, Blackburn H et al: Coronary heart disease: Overweight and obesity as risk factors. Ann Intern Med 77:15–27, 1972
29. Killpack AK: The use of intracoronary streptokinase and percutaneous transluminal angioplasty. In Woods SL (ed): Cardiovascular Critical Care Nursing, pp 15–29. New York, Churchill Livingstone 1983
30. Laurent-Bopp D: Calcium-channel blockers. In Woods SL (ed): Cardiovascular Critical Care Nursing, pp 31–49. New York, Churchill Livingstone, 1983
31. Lown B, Vassaux C, Hood WB et al: Unresolved problems in coronary care. Am J Cardiol 20:494–508, 1967
32. Mann JI, Inman WHW: Oral contraceptives and death from myocardial infarction. Br Med 2:245–248, 1975
33. Mann JI, Vessey MP, Thorogood M et al: Myocardial infarction in young women with special reference to oral contraceptive practice. Br Med J 2:241–245, 1975
34. McNeal GJ: Rectal temperatures in the patient with an acute myocardial infarction. Image 10(1):18–23, 1978
35. Miller NE, Forde OH, Thelle DS et al: The Thromso Heart Study. High density lipoprotein and coronary heart disease: A prospective case control study. Lancet i:965–967, 1977

36. Newton K: Cardiac rehabilitation: Lifestyle adjustments. In Underhill SL et al (eds): Cardiac Nursing. Philadelphia, JB Lippincott, pp 562–570, 1982
37. Nissen MB: Streptokinase therapy in acute myocardial infarction. Heart Lung 13(3):223–229, 1984
38. Relationship of blood pressure, serum cholesterol, smoking habits, relative weight and ECG abnormalities to incidence of major coronary events: Final report of the Pooling Project. J Chronic Dis 31(4):201–306, 1978
39. Report of Intra-Society Commission for Heart Disease Resources. Circulation 70:157A–205A, July, 1984
40. Report of the Joint International Society and Federation of Cardiology/WHO Task Force on Standardization of Clinical Nomenclature. Nomenclature and criteria for diagnosis of ischemic heart disease. Circulation 59(3):607–609, 1979
41. Roberts W: Thromboembolic complications in patients with cardiac disease. In Underhill SL et al (eds): Cardiac Nursing, pp 393–403. Philadelphia, JB Lippincott, 1982
42. Rogers DJ, Branyon ME, Kinney MR: Care of the cardiac patient. In Andreoli et al (eds): Comprehensive Cardiac Care, pp 280–334, 1979
43. Rosenberg L, Armstrong B, Jick H: Myocardial infarction and estrogen therapy in post-menopasual women. N Engl J Med 294:1256–1259, 1976
44. Scheidt S, Ascheim R, Killip T III: Shock after myocardial infarction. Am J Cardiol 26:556, 1970
45. Secor J: Coronary Care, A Nursing Specialty. New York, Appleton-Century-Crofts, 1971
46 Sharma GVRK, Cella G, Parisi AF et al: Thrombolytic therapy. N Engl J Med 306(21):1268–1275, 1982
47. Siewicki BJ: Complications involving heart structures. In Underhill SL et al (eds): Cardiac Nursing, pp 404–411 Philadelphia, JB Lippincott, 1982
48. Sivarajan ES: Cardiac rehabilitation: Activity and exercise program. In Underhill SL et al (eds): Cardiac Nursing, pp 551–561. Philadelphia, JB Lippincott, 1982
49. Slone D, Shapiro S, Rosenberg L et al: Relation of cigarette smoking to myocardial infarction in young women. N Engl J Med 298(23):1273–1276, 1978
50. Smith JW: Alcohol and disorders of the heart and skeletal muscles. In Estes RJ, Heinemann ME (eds): Alcoholism: Development, Consequences and Interventions, pp 176–184. St Louis, CV Mosby, 1977
51. Smoking and Health, A Report of the Surgeon General. DHEW Publication No. (PHS) 79-50066. Washington DC, US Department of Health, Education and Welfare, 1979
52. Sollack SD: Pathophysiology of myocardial ischemia and infarction. In Underhill SL et al (eds): Cardiac Nursing, pp 111–123. Philadelphia, JB Lippincott, 1982
53. Status of fat in food and nutrition (Symposium). J Am Oil Chem Soc 51:244–264, 1974
54. Stern MJ: Psychosocial rehabilitation following myocardial infarcton and coronary artery bypass surgery. In Wenger NK, Hellerstein HK (eds): Rehabilitation of the Coronary Patient, pp 453–471. New York, John Wiley, 1984
55. Underhill SL: Diagnosis and treatment of the patient with coronary artery disease and myocardial ischemia. In Underhill SL et al (eds): Cardiac Nursing, pp 311–325. Philadelphia, JB Lippincott, 1982
56. Underhill SL: Coronary artery disease risk factors. In Underhill SL et al (eds): Cardiac Nursing, pp 132–148. Philadelphia, JB Lippincott, 1982
57. Underhill SL: History-taking and physical examination of the patient with cardiovascular disease. In Underhill SL et al (eds): Cardiac Nursing, pp 150–172. Philadelphia, JB Lippincott, 1982
58. Underhill SL: Physical immobility and recumbency. In Underhill SL et al (eds): Cardiac Nursing, pp 412–418. Philadelphia, JB Lippincott, 1982
59. Woods SL: Arrhythmias complicating myocardial infarction. In Underhill SL et al (eds): Cardiac Nursing, pp 363–377. Philadelphia, JB Lippincott, 1982
60. Woods SL: Diagnosis and treatment of the patient with uncomplicated myocardial infarction. Underhill SL et al (eds): Cardiac Nursing, pp 326–337. Philadelphia, JB Lippincott, 1982
61. Wulff KS, Hong PA: Surgical intervention for coronary artery disease. In Underhill SL et al (eds): Cardiac Nursing, pp 338–354. Philadelphia, JB Lippincott, 1982

Bibliography

Allen JA, Throm LA: Percutaneous transluminal coronary angioplasty: A new alternative for ischmemic heart disease. Critical Care Nurse 2(1):24–29, 1982

Aronow WS: Clinical use of nitrates. Modern Concepts of Cardiovascular Disease XLVIII(6):31–35, 1979

Cowley MJ, Block PC: Percutaneous transluminal coronary angioplasty. Modern Concepts of Cardiovascular Disease 59(5):25–29, 1981

Cowley MJ, Gold HK: Use of intracoronary streptokinase in acute myocardial infarction. Modern Concepts of Cardiovascular Disease 51(5):97–102, 1982

Das Gupta DS: Principles and Practice of Acute Cardiac Care. Chicago, Year Book Medical Publishers, 1984

Guzzetta CE, Dossey BM: Cardiovascular Nursing: Bodymind Tapestry. St Louis, CV Mosby, 1984

Hackett TP, Cassem NH: Psychologic aspects of rehabilitation after myocardial infarction and coronary artery bypass surgery. In Wenger NK, Hellerstein HK (eds): Rehabilitation of the Coronary Patient, pp 437–451. New York, John Wiley, 1984

Hillard S: Intracoronary streptokinase infusion. Nursing 82 12(5):58–65, 1982

Horvath PT: Care of the Adult Cardiac Surgery Patient. New York, John Wiley & Sons, 1984

Kulbertus HE, Wellens HJJ: The First Year After a Myocardial Infarction. Mount Kisco, Futura Publishing, 1983

Kuller L: Risk factor reduction in coronary heart disease. Modern Concepts of Cardiovascular Disease 53(2):7–11, 1984

Nemens E: Beta-blocker drugs. In Woods SL (ed): Cardiovascular Critical Care Nursing, pp 221–247. New York, Churchill Livingstone, 1983

Newton KM: Coronary artery disease risk factors. In Woods SL (ed): Cardiovascular Critical Care Nursing, pp 51–72. New York, Churchill Livingstone, 1983

Rossi LP, Haines VM: Nursing diagnosis related to acute myocardial infarction. Cardiovascular Nursing 15(3):11–15, 1979

Schettler G, Rapaport E, Pyorala K et al: Joint Recommendations on secondary prevention of persons with clinical heart disease. Heartbeat 1:1–10, 1984

Scordo KA: This procedure called PTCA. Nursing 82 12(2):50–55, 1982

Wenger NK, Hellerstein HK: Rehabilitation of the Coronary Patient. New York, John Wiley & Sons, 1984

Woods SL (ed): Cardiovascular Critical Care Nursing. Contemporary Issues In Critical Care Nursing, vol 5. New York, Churchill Livingstone, 1983

Chapter 38

Heart Failure

Debra Laurent-Bopp

Heart failure is a general term used to describe a pathophysiological state in which abnormal cardiac function results in the heart that can no longer pump an adequate supply of blood in relation to the venous return and to the metabolic needs of the tissues. Heart failure is not a diagnosis and its etiology should be carefully sought. The composite of clinical manifestations that result from circulatory congestion in congestive heart failure (CHF) usually develops because of decreased myocardial contractility.

For nurses to provide care for patients with heart failure, basic physiological mechanisms must be understood. In addition, heart failure must be understood from the standpoint of etiology, pathophysiology (including compensatory mechanisms), and the hemodynamics of the cardiovascular system. With this knowledge the nurse will be able to implement a nursing care plan, which may include restriction of activity and diet, hemodynamic monitoring, medications, and assistance to patients and families to effectively cope with an acute or chronic illness.

Etiology and Pathophysiology

Heart failure may result from conditions causing abnormal volume overload, abnormal pressure overload, myocardial dysfunction, filling disorders, or increased metabolism (Table 38–1).[27,29] All these conditions may be included in the following categories:

1. Increase in cardiac work, taxing myocardial reserve beyond its limits
2. Anatomical or functional abnormalities of the myocardium that prevent adequate handling of a normal work load
3. Interference with the capacity to pump blood that does not involve myocardial function directly.

Basic cardiac physiological mechanisms such as stroke volume, heart rate, cardiac output, preload, afterload, and contractility are altered in heart failure.

Cardiac output is dependent on the relationship between heart rate and stroke volume; it is the product of these two variables. The stroke volume is the amount of blood ejected by a ventricle during each systolic contraction. Several factors influence cardiac output and stroke volume, the first being heart rate.

Heart rate is defined as the number of times the ventricles contract per minute, and it is extrinsically controlled by the autonomic nervous system. Preload, the second factor, is the volume of blood in the ventricles at the end of diastole, immediately before the onset of ventricular contraction. According to the *Frank-Starling law of the heart,* stretching of the myocardial fibers during diastole increases the force

TABLE 38–1
Conditions Causing Heart Failure

Abnormal Volume Load	*Abnormal Pressure Load*	*Myocardial Dysfunction*	*Filling Disorders*	*Increased Metabolic Demand*
Aortic incompetence	Aortic stenosis	Cardiomyopathy	Mitral stenosis	Anemias
Mitral incompetence	Idiopathic hypertrophic subaortic stenosis	Myocarditis	Tricuspid stenosis	Thyrotoxicosis
Tricuspid incompetence	Coarctation of the aorta	Coronary artery disease	Cardiac tamponade	Fever
Overtransfusion	Hypertension	Ischemia	Restrictive pericarditis	Beriberi
Left-to-right shunts	Primary	Infarction		Paget's disease
Secondary hypervolemia	Secondary	Arrhythmias		Arteriovenous fistulas
		Toxic disorders		

(Michaelson CR (ed): Congestive Heart Failure, p 45. St Louis, CV Mosby, 1983)

of contraction during systole: this in turn increases stroke volume or cardiac output. However, there is a point where no further myocardial fiber stretch will improve cardiac output and will actually depress it. An index of left ventricular preload is the left ventricular end-diastolic pressure (LVEDP) or the pulmonary artery wedge pressure; the central venous pressure or right atrial pressure is an index of right ventricular preload.[6, 19, 35]

The third factor is afterload, or the resistance against which the ventricles must pump. Afterload is primarily determined by aortic impedance and systemic vascular resistance.[29, 30]

The property of contractility is the last variable affecting ventricular function. Contractility is the force of contractions generated by the myocardium under given loading conditions. The myocardium has its own inherent property to alter its contractile force and velocity.[19, 35]

The basic function of the heart is to transfer blood coming to the ventricles from the low pressure venous system into the higher pressure arterial system. Impaired cardiac function results in failure to empty venous reservoirs and in reduced delivery of blood into the arterial circulation. Systemic and pulmonary venous volumes are elevated, and the amount of blood ejected into the pulmonary artery and aorta is depressed. Hemodynamically, these alterations appear as elevated ventricular end-diastolic pressure, elevated systemic and pulmonary venous pressures, and a decreased cardiac output.[6] Clinical indicators are due to activated compensatory mechanisms, reduced cardiac reserve, accumulation of extracellular fluid, and impaired organ perfusion.[5, 6, 10]

Compensatory Mechanisms

When the heart is presented with an increased work load, a number of physiological alterations are evoked in an attempt to maintain normal cardiac pumping function. These include[6, 19]

1. Sympathetic nervous system response to baroreceptors or chemoreceptors
2. Renal-mediated fluid retention and peripheral vasoconstriction
3. Stretching of cardiac muscle and dilatation to accommodate increased volume (Frank-Starling response)
4. Myocardial hypertrophy

In heart failure, stimulation of the *sympathetic nervous system* represents the most immediately responsive mechanism of compensation. Stimulation of the β-adrenergic receptors in the heart causes an elevation in heart rate and contractility to raise stroke volume and cardiac output. Sympathetic effects on the peripheral vascular system increase vascular tone to raise systemic vascular resistance (SVR) and mean systemic filling pressure, thereby augmenting venous return, preload, and afterload (the amount of resistance to blood flow). The next stage of compensation occurs as a result of partial recovery of the heart and renal conservation of fluid.[6]

Renal compensation is initially triggered by a drop in kidney perfusion that decreases glomerular filtration and activates the renin, angiotensin, and aldosterone mechanisms and results in increased SVR and increased salt and water absorption, which augments blood volume and increases systemic filling pressure and venous return. Again, this results in enhanced preload, afterload, and contractility.[28, 35]

The relationship between preload and stroke volume or cardiac output has been explained by the Frank-Starling law of the heart. As discussed previously, sympathetic stimulation will increase venous return, and expansion of blood volume from renal compensatory mechanisms will occur, thus increasing the end-diastolic volume or preload. Increased preload in turn augments contractility.[6, 19, 35]

Myocardial hypertrophy with or without chamber dilatation is a compensatory mechanism whereby the heart increases its muscle mass and alters its geometrical configuration in response to a sustained elevated work load. This mechanism is self-limiting.[6, 35]

All mechanisms of compensation act primarily to restore cardiac output to normal or near normal levels. However, during the course of heart failure these cardiac and peripheral circulatory adjustments may eventually cause deleterious effects to pump function since all of them contribute to an increase in myocardial oxygen consumption. If pump function remains depressed in spite of maximal activities of all compensatory mechanisms, severe systemic and pulmonary congestion results and the heart is no longer able to meet tissue metabolic demands.[6,28,35] Table 38–2 presents the pathophysiological findings that directly and indirectly produce signs and symptoms of heart failure.

Types of Heart Failure

There are various terms purported to describe the pathology of heart failure, with each system of classification revealing a theory about the causes of heart failure. Each is discussed here briefly.[6,20,27]

Backward and Forward Failure. As the ventricle fails to pump its volume, blood accumulates and pressure rises in the ventricles, atria, and venous systems. A primary etiology of backward failure is mechanical cardiac obstruction.

The term *forward failure* is applied to a situation in which the primary pathology is decreased cardiac output, which subsequently leads to a decrease in vital organ perfusion. Eventually there is an increase in extracellular fluid volume that leads to symptoms of systemic congestion.

Both of these pathologies are seen in the majority of patients with chronic heart failure.

Acute and Chronic Failure. The clinical manifestations of acute and chronic heart failure depend on how rapidly the syndrome develops. Acute heart failure may be the initial manifestation of heart disease or may indicate exacerbation of a chronic cardiac condition. The marked decrease in left ventricular function may be due to acute myocardial infarction, acute valvular dysfunction, or hypertensive crises. The events occur so rapidly that the sympathetic nervous system compensation is ineffective, resulting in the rapid development of pulmonary edema and circulatory collapse (cardiogenic shock). Chronic heart failure develops over a period of time and is usually the end result of an increasing inability of physiological mechanisms to compensate. It can be caused by valvular disease, high blood pressure, or chronic obstructive pulmonary disease.

Left-Sided and Right-Sided Failure. Right ventricular failure is associated with failure to empty the systemic venous reservoirs, causing elevated systemic venous pressure. Left ventricular failure exists when left ventricular stroke volume is reduced and there is failure to empty the pulmonary venous reservoirs, which causes elevated pulmonary venous pressure and reduced cardiac output. Left ventricular failure is by far the most frequent of the two instances in which only one side of the heart is affected. It can be caused by arterial high blood pressure, myocardial ischemia or infarction, aortic valve incompetence or stenosis, or mitral valve incompetency or stenosis. Persons with chronic volume overload, high output states, cardiomyopathies, or arrhythmias demonstrate signs of left heart failure prior to those of right heart failure.

Left ventricular failure is the most common cause of right ventricular failure. Right ventricular failure develops most frequently as a result of sustained pulmonary hypertension. This condition includes persons with congenital anomalies (tetralogy of Fallot or ventricular septal defect), severe pulmonary infections, or massive pulmonary embolization. In addition, patients suffer pulmonary hypertension secondary to mitral or aortic stenosis.

Although in clinical practice reference is made to right and left ventricular failure, pure unilateral heart failure is rare. Therefore, over time an isolated abnormal ventricular work load will be responsible for total heart failure.

Low Output and High Output Syndrome. In response to high blood pressure and hypovolemia, low output syndrome appears. It is evidenced by impaired peripheral circulation and peripheral vasoconstriction. The word *syndrome,* however, makes it clear that the failure represents a reaction rather than a primary pathology.

Any condition that causes the heart to work harder to supply blood may be categorized as high output syndrome. High output states require an increased oxygen supply to the peripheral tissues, which can only occur with an increased cardiac output. Reduced systemic vascular resistance (afterload) is characteristic of this condition, and augments peripheral circulation and venous return, which in turn increases stroke volume and cardiac output. It may be caused by increased metabolic requirements as seen in hyperthyroidism, fever, and pregnancy, or it may be triggered by hyperkinetic conditions such as arteriovenous fistulas, anemia, and beriberi.

Intractable and Refractory Failure. This type of failure implies persistent heart failure in spite of all known pharmacological, mechanical, and dietary efforts to improve myocardial contractility, control heart rate, and manipulate preload and afterload.[6] Those patients affected show persistent pulmonary and systemic congestion with a low cardiac output at rest.

Clinical Manifestations

The signs and symptoms that characterize heart failure can be considered in the context of the four components of the syndrome: failure of the right ventricle as a pump, failure of the left ventricle as a pump, pulmonary venous congestion, and systemic venous congestion. Symptoms are often described as those due to left-sided or right-sided heart failure, and although the symptoms of both types overlap, each has been separated here for discussion.[5,39]

Right-sided heart failure, associated with increased systemic venous pressures, gives rise to the clinical signs of jugular vein distention, hepatomegaly, dependent peripheral edema, and ascites.

Left-sided heart failure, associated with elevated pulmonary venous pressure and decreased cardiac output, appears clinically as breathlessness, weakness, fatigue, dizziness, confusion, pulmonary congestion, hypotension, and death. Table 38–3 lists the various objective and subjective indicators for right and left ventricular failure.

TABLE 38-2
Pathophysiological Findings in Heart Failure

Abnormality Directly Producing Signs and Symptoms	*Promoted By*	*Opposed By*
Decrease in arterial flow to brain and heart	Decrease in left ventricular output	Increase in total blood volume (↑ preload) Local decrease in arteriolar resistance (↓ afterload)
Decrease in arterial flow to skin, skeletal muscles, and abdominal viscera	Decrease in left ventricular output Local increase in arteriolar resistance (↑ afterload)	Increase in total blood volume
Decrease in systemic arterial pressure	Decrease in left ventricular output	Increase in total blood volume (↑ preload) Overall increase in arteriolar resistance (↑ afterload)
Increase in myocardial oxygen demand	Increase in myocardial wall tension, itself promoted by increases in afterload, preload, and radius of each ventricle Increase in pulse rate	
Increase in pulmonary capillary pressure	Increase in left ventricular preload Increase in total blood volume	Decrease in right ventricular output
Increase in systemic venous pressure	Increase in right ventricular preload Increase in total blood volume	Decrease in systemic capillary outflow
Decrease in cardiac output (of left or right ventricle)	Decrease in stroke volume	Increase in pulse rate
Decrease in resistance of arterioles to brain and heart	Decrease in local oxygen tension	Increase in adrenergic stimulation
Increase in resistance of most arterioles, including those to skin, skeletal muscles, and abdominal viscera	Increase in adrenergic stimulation	Decrease in local oxygen tension
Increase in preload and radius of each ventricle	Increase in end-diastolic volume of each ventricle, itself promoted by increases in residual volume, venous return, and total blood volume	
Increase in total blood volume	Increase in total body sodium, itself the result of a decrease in renal sodium excretion, prompted by a decrease in renal blood flow	

(Adapted from Cohen S: New concepts in understanding congestive heart failure. Part I: How the clinical features arise. AJN, January 1981, p 135)

TABLE 38–3
Clinical Indicators of Left and Right Ventricular Failure

Left Ventricular Failure	Right Ventricular Failure
Objective Findings	
Tachycardia	Neck vein pulsations and distention
Decreased S_1	Increased jugular venous pressure
S_3 and S_4 gallops	Edema
Crackles (rales)	Hepatomegaly
Pleural effusion	Positive hepatojugular reflux
Diaphoresis	Ascites
Pulsus alternans	
Subjective Findings	
Breathlessness	Weight gain
Cough	Transient ankle swelling
Fatigue and weakness	Abdominal distention
Memory loss and confusion	Gastric distress
Diaphoresis	Anorexia, nausea
Palpitations	
Anorexia	
Insomnia	

Acute pulmonary edema can develop suddenly and the clinical manifestations include marked dyspnea and orthopnea; expectoration of frothy, pinked-tinged sputum; pallor and cyanosis; hypotension; obtundation; and confusion.[23]

Cardiogenic shock represents circulatory failure due to severe depression of myocardial contractility in which cardiac output is markedly depressed. This clinical syndrome is characterized by hypotension, tachycardia, impaired mentation, oliguria, and peripheral vascular collapse.

Medical Management

Diagnosis

The diagnosis of heart failure is made by the history taking, physical examination, and collection of data from diagnostic adjunctive studies.[39]

Cardiovascular findings may be very subtle and often occur before secondary congestive phenomena are noted in the lungs, liver, kidneys, or tissues. Cardiomegaly is usually present, and the x-ray film is the most reliable method of detecting this condition. However, there is no way to judge the degree to which cardiomegaly represents hypertrophy or enlargement. The cardiothoracic ratio and heart volume seen on x-ray film are helpful in determining the left ventricular end-diastolic volume. The x-ray film appearance of the lungs can reflect the varying degrees of heart failure, from prominent pulmonary veins to interstitial pulmonary edema.[20]

The electrocardiogram is not helpful in assessing the presence or degree of heart failure, but it will demonstrate patterns of ventricular hypertrophy, arrhythmias, and any degree of myocardial ischemia, injury, or infarction.[38,39]

The echocardiogram is useful in diagnosing cardiac valvular changes, pericardial effusion, chamber enlargement, and ventricular hypertrophy. Radionuclide studies (Tc pyrophosphate imaging or thallium scintigraphy) have also become important in providing clues as to the presence and etiology of cardiac failure.[39]

Right-side heart catheterization with a pulmonary artery quadruple-lumen thermodilution catheter can aid in the diagnosis and assessment of severity of heart failure. The various hemodynamic variables measured by this catheter are cardiac output by thermodilution, right atrial pressure, and pulmonary artery systolic, diastolic, and wedge pressures. The cardiac output would be decreased in heart failure, whereas the right atrial pressure or central venous pressure (CVP) is either normal in left heart failure or elevated in right heart failure. The pulmonary artery wedge pressure (PAWP) indirectly measures the left ventricular end-diastolic pressure, which is a measure of end-diastolic volume or preload and is elevated in heart failure.[28]

Laboratory tests include blood chemistries, hematological screen, and urinalysis. Electrolyte imbalances in heart failure reflect complications of failure as well as the use of diuretics and other drug therapy. Disturbances in sodium and potassium are particularly significant. In patients with severe heart failure, an increase in total body water dilutes body fluid and is reflected by a decrease in the serum sodium. Diuretics may also contribute to this low serum sodium if fluid intake is not restricted. Hypokalemia, or low serum potassium level, may complicate heart failure as the result of the use of diuretics such as thiazides and furosemides, since these diuretics may lead to excessive excretion of potassium. Hyperkalemia, or elevated potassium level, may occur secondary to depressed effective renal blood flow and lower glomerular filtration rate.[20,39]

Any impairment of kidney function may be reflected by elevated blood urea nitrogen (BUN), creatinine, and uric acid. Elevated bilirubin, serum glutamic-oxaloacetic transaminase, and lactate dehydrogenase result from hepatic congestion. Urinalysis may reveal proteinuria and high specific gravity.[20]

The arterial blood gases usually show a drop in Pa_{O_2} (hypoxemia) and a low Pa_{CO_2}. In the clinical situation of heart failure the alveoli become filled with fluid, causing a decrease in Pa_{O_2}, whereas the compensatory attempt to increase the Pa_{O_2} by hyperventilating causes a decrease in the Pa_{CO_2}, resulting in a mild respiratory alkalosis.[6,39]

In seriously ill patients, direct determination by means of an arterial line of intra-arterial pressure is necessary, since systemic arterial pressure determines the perfusion pressure of various organ systems and is predominantly a product of the cardiac output and the systemic vascular resistance. In heart failure a drop in cardiac output is compensated by an increased systemic vascular resistance in an attempt to maintain the arterial blood pressure in normal range.[6,39]

Treatment

There are three major approaches to treating patients with heart failure.[38,39] The first is removal of the underlying cause, which may include surgical correction of structural abnormalities, and medical treatment of such conditions as infective endocarditis and hypertension. The second approach is the removal of the precipitating cause, such as infections, arrhythmias, and pulmonary emboli. The third is the treatment or control of heart failure. Therapy for heart failure is directed at reducing the work load of the heart and manipulating the various factors that determine cardiac performance, such as contractility, heart rate, preload, and afterload.[11,21,24]

Improvement of pump performance or enhancement of myocardial contractility can be achieved by the use of inotropic agents. The various agents used for a positive inotropic effect are (1) digitalis glycosides, (2) sympathomimetic agents such as dopamine or dobutamine, and (3) phosphodiesterase inhibitors such as amrinone.[4]

Digitalis is given to improve contractility and increase cardiac output, which results in reduction of pulmonary vascular congestion and central venous pressure.[36,37] *Sympathomimetic agents* are most effective in cases where the β-adrenergic receptors are fully responsive. In severe chronic heart failure where a β-receptor response is lost, phosphodiesterase inhibitors may have a limited role.[4]

Severe bradycardia, or atrial or ventricular arrhythmias that do not respond to appropriate drug therapy may respond to the use of a temporary pacemaker to restore a normal heart rate.

Reduction of cardiac work load in both acute and chronic failure requires physical and emotional rest. Conjunctive measures such as mild sedation and sleep/activity pattern modifications may be necessary. In addition, weight reduction in obese patients will decrease the work load on the heart.

The relief of excessive preload can be obtained by the use of diuretics and vasodilator therapy. Diuretics can reduce the ventricular filling pressure and eliminate pulmonary congestion. Nitrates are primarily reducers of the preload since they dilate the systemic veins, and by reducing venous return they ultimately reduce the left ventricular filling pressure.[2,3,18,33]

The aim of vasodilator therapy is the reduction of afterload as reflected by systemic vascular resistance.[7,8,33,34,40] As a direct arteriolar dilator with direct inotropic effects, hydralazine can improve left ventricular function by reducing afterload and myocardial oxygen consumption, augment stroke volume, and improve cardiac output.[9,31] Nifedipine, a calcium-channel blocking agent, is a potent peripheral vasodilator that can be given sublingually in acute left ventricular failure with pulmonary edema.[32]

Other vasodilators that provide combined preload and afterload reduction include nitroprusside, prazosin, and captopril or enalapril. Intravenous nitroprusside remains the drug of choice for severe low-output, left-sided heart failure since it acts rapidly and has a balanced effect, dilating both veins and arterioles.[17] It is particularly useful in severe refractory heart failure caused by aortic or mitral valve incompetence.[12]

Prazosin, an α-adrenergic blocking agent established for hypertension, has been tried in refractory heart failure. Acting as an "oral nitroprusside," prazosin dilates both peripheral arterial and venous systems.[13]

The use of angiotensin inhibitors such as captopril or enalapril may be the most effective vasodilator for the treatment of advanced congestive heart failure since it blocks the formation of angiotensin II (reducing afterload), inhibits the release of aldosterone, thus inhibiting sodium retention,and in addition, produces venodilatation (thus reducing preload).[1,14,15]

Table 38–4 compares the effects of selected agents that unload the heart and are utilized in heart failure.

The *mechanical support of circulation* may be tried for the patient with intractable heart failure after all medical approaches have been exhausted. The intra-aortic balloon pump is used to reduce afterload at the time of systolic contraction and to increase myocardial perfusion during diastole. The heart transplant procedure is reserved for patients with congestive heart failure that is refractory to medical therapy and cannot be helped by traditional cardiac surgery.[22] The totally artificial heart is a more recent development.

Control of excessive sodium and water retention can be achieved with careful use of diuretics and a low sodium diet of 1.6 to 2.8 g/day. Mechanical removal of fluid is usually not required in acute heart failure, but it may be required in chronic failure. If fluid collects in serous cavities, thoracentesis, paracentesis, or dialysis may be necessary. Phlebotomy is a technique rarely used.

Acute pulmonary edema is the catastrophic and dramatic indicator of heart failure. The therapeutic goal to increase oxygenation and ventilation includes placing the patient in a high Fowler's position and administering a high concentration of oxygen, usually assisted by mechanical ventilation. Morphine sulfate is also used for its narcotic effect, and it decreases venous and arterial vasoconstriction, thereby reducing preload and afterload.

The use of rapid-acting diuretics such as furosemide or ethacrynic acid are measures taken to decrease venous return to the heart. Application of rotating tourniquets may be necessary. Nitroglycerin orally or intravenously may also be used to reduce preload by inducing vasodilatation.

The use of inotropic, sympathomimetic, and vasodilating agents are used to increase peripheral perfusion. These include digoxin, dopamine or dobutamine, and nitroprusside.

Prognosis. The prognosis of patients with heart failure can no longer be stated in a meaningful way because today the clinical course can be modified by many forms of treatment.

Nursing Management

Assessment

In whatever setting a nurse is working, whether it is a clinic, a nursing home, or the patient's home, she will care for patients in some phase of heart failure. The nurse may be the first person to assess its presence. One must know what to assess and the significance of the findings, provide appro-

TABLE 38–4
Comparative Effects of Agents for Unloading the Heart and for Heart Failure

Agent	*Preload (Peripheral Veins)**	*Afterload (Peripheral Arteries)**	*Direct Inotropic Effect*	*Heart Rate†*	*Proposed Indication*
Nitrates	+++	+	0	↑ or 0	Backward left ventricular failure; pulmonary edema
Hydralazine (Apresoline)	0	+++	+	↑ or 0 (↑ ↑ if no failure)	Chronic forward failure (except valvular stenosis)
Nifedipine (Procardia)	0	++	0	↑ or 0	Acute left ventricular failure with pulmonary edema (except valvular stenosis)
Nitroprusside (Nipride)	+++	+++	0	0	Heart failure of acute myocardial infarction or regurgitant valves
Captopril (Capoten)	+	++	0	↑	Left ventricular failure
Prazosin (Minipress)	++	++	0	↓ or 0	Forward and backward failure (except valvular stenosis)

* + = dilatation; † ↑ = increase; ↓ = decrease
(Adapted from Opie LH, Harrison DC: Vasodilating drugs. In Opie LH (ed): Drugs for the Heart, pp 135–137. Orlando, Grune & Stratton, 1984)

priate intervention, and teach the patient lifestyle modifications to prevent its recurrence. In achieving these functions the nurse has an essential role in patient care.

The best means of controlling heart failure is through early detection and treatment of the predisposing factors. Early detection of high blood pressure, arteriosclerosis and atherosclerosis, valvular disorders, and congenital anomalies may ensure the client early treatment and prevention of complications.

A major goal of assessing the patient in heart failure is to determine the type and severity of the underlying disease and the extent of the syndrome. Identification of the early onset of cardiac failure may allow therapeutic means to be instituted on an ambulatory basis. When the client is admitted to the hospital the problems associated with heart failure may have become more advanced and required supervised administration of medications, as well as other measures to reduce the edema and improve myocardial performance. The nurse should be aware of key manifestations and specifically search for them in each phase of the nursing history and physical examination.[16, 25, 26]

Left-Sided Failure. Major clinical indicators of left-sided heart failure include shortness of breath, cough, weakness or fatigue, change in mental status, diaphoresis, pallor or cyanosis, alterations in heart rhythm, and S_3 and S_4 gallops.

Dyspnea, or abnormally uncomfortable breathing, is a cardinal manifestation of left-sided failure. The failing left ventricle causes the pulmonary venous pressure to rise, which results in pulmonary congestion. The patient may refer to dyspnea as breathlessness, difficulty in breathing, or trouble in catching one's breath. The classic progression in heart failure is exertional dyspnea, orthopnea, paroxysmal nocturnal dyspnea, dyspnea at rest, and acute pulmonary edema.

The nurse must carefully question the patient regarding the presence of dyspnea and the sequence in which it developed. In *exertional dyspnea* the patient becomes aware of the inability to continue previously tolerated levels of activity. Dyspnea at rest in the recumbent position is known as *orthopnea.* Patients usually use a number of pillows in order to sleep.

Patients who describe sudden awakening with a feeling of smothering 2 to 5 hours after falling asleep have *paroxysmal nocturnal dyspnea.* This condition is usually relieved by sitting upright, dangling the feet, or by walking. Quantifying how long it takes for relief helps determine the extent of nocturnal pulmonary congestion.

With increasing severity of heart failure the patient may experience *dyspnea at rest,* and he will not be able to carry out most activities. The most severe form of dyspnea, *acute pulmonary edema,* develops spontaneously, with the patient exhibiting anxiety, agitation, tachycardia, diaphoresis, and pallor or cyanosis.

Another key finding associated with dyspnea is *cough.* It is usually an irritating, periodic, nocturnal, nonproductive cough. The patient may expectorate scant amounts of clear mucus; in severe pulmonary edema, frothy sputum and hemoptysis may occur as a result of an intra-alveolar mixture of fluids, air, and red blood cells.

As the third manifestation of left-sided heart failure,

weakness or fatigue is precipitated by decreased perfusion to the muscles. Patients will describe a feeling of heaviness in their arms and legs.

Decreased cerebral perfusion due to low cardiac output will lead to *changes in mental status,* such as restlessness, insomnia, nightmares, or memory loss. Anxiety agitation, paranoia, and fear of impending doom may develop as the syndrome progresses.

Altered heart rhythm and sounds may also be noted. Over time an increasing heart rate may be seen even though the patient is at rest. Premature atrial and ventricular contractions and atrial fibrillation are common. Extra heart sounds, such as S_3 and S_4, may be heard over the apical area.

Right-Sided Failure. Major clinical indicators of right-sided heart failure include peripheral edema, weight gain, gastrointestinal complaints (*e.g.,* nausea, abdominal distention), and diuresis at rest.

Dependent ascending *peripheral edema* is a manifestation in which edema begins in the lower legs and ascends to the thigh, genitalia, and abdominal wall. Patients may notice shoes fitting tightly or marks left on the feet from their shoes or socks. *Weight gain* is what most patients recognize, and consistent morning daily weights will help to detect any sudden weight gain. An adult may retain 10 to 15 lb (4 to 7 liters of fluid) before pitting edema occurs.

Congestive hepatomegaly, which is characterized by a large, tender, pulsating liver, and ascites also occur. Liver engorgement is caused by venous engorgement, whereas ascites results from transudation of fluid from the capillaries into the abdominal cavity. *Gastrointestinal complaints* of nausea and anorexia may be a direct consequence of the increased intra-abdominal pressure.

Another finding related to fluid retention is *diuresis at rest.* When at rest the body's metabolic requirements are decreased and cardiac function improves. This decreases systemic venous pressure, allowing edema fluid to be mobilized and excreted.

Classification. The knowledge of the manifestations of right- and left-sided heart failure allows the nurse to evaluate the patient's current level of involvement. A method of summarizing clinical indicators, following the course of illness, and assisting in communication among health care professionals is to use the classification of cardiac status devised by the New York Heart Association (see Chap 34).[14]

Nursing Diagnoses

Nursing diagnoses of acute and chronic heart failure are derived from the specific areas of patient assessment previously discussed. These diagnoses may include the following:

1. Decreased cardiac output related to mechanical factors (preload, afterload, or inotropic state of the heart) and electrical factors (conduction, rhythm, and rate).
2. Potential excess of fluid volume related to ineffective contractility, increased afterload and hypertrophy, and decreased glomerular filtration rate.
3. Potential deficit in fluid volume with electrolyte depletion related to diuretic therapy used in heart failure.
4. Impaired gas exchange related to altered oxygen supply and blood flow in pulmonary congestion.
5. Potential impairment of skin integrity related to decreased tissue perfusion (circulation) and alteration in skin turgor (edema).
6. Knowledge deficit about disease/treatment/drug therapy related to misunderstanding of interdependence of cardiac function/disease/stress, influence of risk factors, and necessary lifestyle modifications.
7. Self-care deficit related to decreased activity tolerance.
8. Anxiety related to change in health status (acute or chronic illness) and threat of death.

Goals

The goals for these diagnoses include prevention of symptoms of decreased output by restoring the balance between myocardial oxygen supply and demand, and early detection of the signs and symptoms of decreased cardiac output. Fluid volume and electrolyte balance should be stabilized and maintained. Early detection and prevention of the signs and symptoms of pulmonary venous congestion and skin breakdown are essential. Knowledge needs to be provided regarding cardiac function, treatment regimens, and necessary lifestyle modifications (diet and activity). Detection and reduction of anxiety is also indicated.

Interventions

The nursing priorities in caring for a patient with heart failure are to assist in determination of the underlying cause, decrease cardiac work load and improve pump performance, provide information about the disease and its treatment and reoccurrences, and provide support for psychosocial concerns.

The nurse and physician have three common goals in the intervention for decreased cardiac output: (1) to improve pump performance, (2) to reduce cardiac work load, and (3) to control excessive sodium and water retention. General nursing interventions include monitoring of vital signs, and monitoring and documentation of arrhythmias. Assessment for hypotension, tachycardia, decreased peripheral pulses, and signs of decreased peripheral perfusion such as cool, diaphoretic skin is made.

Improvement of pump performance through the use of inotropic agents and digoxin involves the nurse in observing for side-effects such as anorexia, nausea, vomiting, blurred vision, headache, and arrhythmias. The nurse must also be aware of factors that predispose a client to digitalis intoxication, including age (especially the elderly), renal dysfunction, electrolyte abnormalities (hypokalemia and hypercalcemia), and acid-base disturbances (acidosis and alkalosis). Periodically monitoring serum digoxin levels is important.

Reduction in cardiac work load includes initial bed rest, assessment of anxiety, and maintenance of a quiet, relaxed environment with frequent rest periods. With the use of vasodilating agents in acute heart failure, the nurse will accurately monitor the blood pressure (usually through intra-arterial monitoring), pulmonary artery pressures, and cardiac outputs. Detailed interventions can be found in the accompanying Nursing Care Plan for the Patient with Heart Failure.

The control of excessive sodium and water output are usually controlled through a low sodium diet and diuretics. Nutritional and medication instructions must be provided. Nursing interventions for patients include accurate determination of intake, output, and daily weights and measuring and monitoring electrolytes daily.

Interventions for fluid volume alteration (excess or deficit) are similar to those already discussed, such as vital signs assessment, intake and output, and electrolyte monitoring. Additional interventions include evaluation of breath sounds, observations for anasarca, and frequent mouth care.

Monitoring of arterial blood gases with documentation of Pa_{O_2} and Pa_{CO_2} levels are needed in patients with impaired gas exchange. Assessment of vital signs, breath sounds, and the use of accessory muscles are also noted and documented. The patient should be placed in an elevated position. If the patient is in acute pulmonary edema, rotating tourniquets may be used, and further nursing interventions will include checking of peripheral pulses, and the color and temperature of extremities.

Interventions for the impairment of skin integrity include observation for reddened, excoriated areas, the use of sheepskin or an alternating pressure mattress, frequent massages and position change, and initiation of decubitus care.

For knowledge deficit and self-care deficit, interventions begin with assessment of the patient's and family's level of knowledge. Discussions could include normal heart function, the disease process, treatment regimen, medications, and signs and symptoms.

Evaluation

For the patient with a decreased cardiac output, the outcome criteria are that the patient will demonstrate hemodynamic stability, an absence of arrhythmias, and an understanding of measures to reduce the work load of the heart.

Excess fluid volume criteria are that the fluid volume will be stabilized as evidenced by normal heart and breath sounds, respiratory rate, clearing lung fields, and absence of tissue edema. Skin integrity will be maintained by the absence of reddened or ulcerated skin areas. Fluid deficit criteria are that the serum electrolytes are maintained within normal limits and no postural hypotension occurs.

The patient with impaired gas exchange will demonstrate absence or resolution of pulmonary venous congestion and will demonstrate normal gas exchange, as demonstrated by the absence of dyspnea, orthopnea, cough, tachypnea; by the presence of normal blood gases, heart rate, wedge, and cardiac output; and by response to oxygen administration, drug intervention, and/or rotating tourniquets.

The patient with a knowledge deficit and self-care deficit will verbalize signs and symptoms of decompensation that require immediate intervention. He will identify stress factors and some techniques for handling them, and will also identify the relationship of the treatment regimen to recurring episodes and complications. The patient will also restrict his activity to below failure threshold and not experience any complications of decreased activity.

Patients with anxiety will verbalize their anxiety and show a reduction in anxiety state. These patients therapeutically respond to a quiet environment and will use effective coping mechanisms. The patient will also demonstrate an understanding of the meaning of heart failure to include its etiology, signs and symptoms, and the acute and chronic nature of heart failure specific to him.

NURSING CARE PLAN FOR THE PATIENT WITH HEART FAILURE

NURSING DIAGNOSIS/PROBLEM 1: Decreased cardiac output related to mechanical factors (preload, afterload, or inotropic state of the heart) and electrical factors (conduction, rhythm, and rate)

GOAL 1.1: To prevent symptoms of decreased cardiac output by restoring balance between myocardial oxygen supply and demand

Nursing Interventions	Rationale	Outcome Criteria
1. Initially, keep on bed rest and eliminate activities eliciting a Valsalva response. Note response to activities.	1. Valsalva maneuvers increase myocardial oxygen consumption; already stressed heart may be unable to respond adequately; cardiac output falls sharply.	1–5. Absence of signs and symptoms of cardiac decompensation. The following measurements will return towards patient's optimal level:
2. Maintain a quiet, relaxed environment with frequent rest periods.	2. Emotional excitement stimulates the sympathetic nervous system, producing cardiovascular effects. Rest allows for decreased myocardial workload and full rest of the body.	▪ Hemodynamic measures (*e.g.*, blood pressure, heart rate, central venous pressure, pulmonary artery wedge pressure) ▪ Electrical conduction of the

(Continued)

NURSING CARE PLAN FOR THE PATIENT WITH HEART FAILURE (*Continued*)

Nursing Interventions	Rationale	Outcome Criteria
3. Place in Fowler's or semi-Fowler's position.	3. Reclining position favors venous return (↑ preload), overloading an already inefficient myocardium. The upright positions favor expansion of lungs by gravity and decrease abdominal organ pressure on diaphragm.	heart: ideally normal sinus rhythm ▪ Respiratory status: respiratory rate, lung fields, ABGs ▪ Urinary output ▪ Mental status
4. Institute measures to prevent thromboembolic phenomena.	4. Prolonged bed rest and decreased circulation time predispose to formation of clots and emboli.	
5. Administer cardiac glycosides as ordered (digitalis).	5. Glycosides increase myocardial contractility, improve cardiac output, slow heart rate.	
a. Monitor serum digitalis levels periodically.	a. Liver congestion and decreased glomerular filtration rate may interfere with metabolism and excretion.	
b. Monitor for side-effects of drug therapy.	b. Increased contractility (inotropic state of heart) increases myocardial oxygen requirements and thereby may compromise cardiac function.	
c. Withold digitalis and notify physician if marked changes occur in cardiac rate and/or rhythm or signs of toxicity.	c. Rate of occurrence of toxicity is high because of narrow margin between therapeutic and toxic ranges. Digitalis toxicity produces arrhythmias similar to those being treated with digitalis therapy.	

GOAL 1.2: To detect early signs and symptoms of decreased cardiac output due to heart failure

Nursing Interventions	Rationale	Outcome Criteria
1. Assess for hypotension, pulses alternas, tachycardia, regularity of pulse, decreased peripheral pulses, and signs of decreased perfusion such as cool, diaphoretic skin.	1. These signs are indicative of decreased and inadequate cardiac output. Decreased blood pressure, increased pulse may indicate worsening heart failure.	1–3. Signs and symptoms of decreased cardiac output are detected within 4 hours of onset.
2. Monitor/document cardiac rate and rhythm.	2. Arrhythmias and conduction disturbances often occur because of hypoxia.	
3. Determine baseline ABGs, BUN and creatinine; record accurately intake and output.	3. Decreased perfusion to lungs may be reflected in decreased Pa_{O_2} and increased Pa_{CO_2}. Metabolic acidosis results from anaerobic metabolism, secondary to decreased tissue perfusion. Decreased urine output and an increase in BUN and creatinine reflect decreased renal perfusion.	

References

1. Awan NA, Massie BM: New strategies in the management of severe chronic heart failure: Captopril. Am Heart J 104:1125–1228, 1982
2. Armstrong PW, Armstrong JA, Marks GS: Pharmacokinetic-hemodynamic studies of intravenous nitroglycerin in congestive heart failure. Circulation 62:160–166, 1980
3. Armstrong PW, Armstrong JA, Marks GS: Pharmacokinetic-hemodynamic studies of nitroglycerin ointment in congestive heart failure. Am J Cardiol 46:670–676, 1980
4. Benotti JR, Grossman W, Braunwald E: Hemodynamic assessment of Amrinone—a new inotropic agent. N Engl J Med 299:1373–1378, 1978
5. Braunwald E: Clinical manifestations of heart failure. In Braunwald E (ed): Heart Disease: A Textbook of Cardiovascular Medicine, pp 488–502. Philadelphia, WB Saunders, 1984
6. Braunwald E: Pathophysiology of heart failure. In Braunwald E (ed): Heart Disease: A Textbook of Cardiovascular Medicine, pp 447–466. Philadelphia, WB Saunders, 1984
7. Chatterjee K, Massie B, Rubin S et al: Long-term out-patient vasodilator therapy of congestive heart failure. Am J Med 65:134–145, 1978
8. Chatterjee K, Parmley WW: Vasodilator therapy for acute myocardial infarction and chronic congestive heart failure. J Am Coll Cardiol 1:133–153, 1983
9. Chatterjee K, Parmley WW, Massie B et al: Oral hydralazine therapy for chronic refractory heart failure. Circulation 54:879, 1978
10. Cohen S: New concepts in understanding congestive heart failure. Part I: How the clinical features arise. AJN, pp 119–142, January 1981
11. Cohen S: New concepts in understanding congestive heart failure. Part II: How the therapeutic approaches work. AJN, pp 357–380, February 1981
12. Cohen JM, Burk L: Nitroprusside. Ann Intern Med 91:752, 1979
13. Colucci WS: Alpha-adrenergic receptor blockade with prazosin. Ann Intern Med 97:67–77, 1982
14. Criteria Committee of the New York Heart Association: Nomenclature and Criteria for Diagnosis of Diseases of the Heart and Great Vessels, 8th ed. New York, New York Heart Association, 1979
15. Davis R, Ribner HS, Keung E et al: Treatment of chronic congestive heart failure with captopril, an oral inhibitor of angiotensin-converting enzyme. N Engl J Med 301:117–121, 1979
16. Duncklee JE: Protocol: Congestive heart failure. Nurse Pract 9(9):15–21, 1984
17. Franciosa JA, Dunkman WB, Wilen W et al: Optimal left ventricular filling pressure during nitroprusside infusion for congestive heart failure. Am J Med 74:457–464, 1983
18. Franciosa JA, Nordstrom LA, Cohn JN: Nitrate therapy for congestive heart failure. JAMA 240:443–446, 1978
19. Ganong WF: Preview of medical physiology. Los Altos CA, Lange Medical Publications, 1977
20. Gazes PC: Cardiac failure in adults. In Gazes PC (ed): Clinical Cardiology, 2nd ed, pp 429–480. Chicago, Year Book Medical Publishers, 1983
21. Gazes PC: The management of congestive heart failure. Curr Probl Cardiol 8(11)1–70, 1984
22. Jamieson SW, Stinson EG, Shumway NE: Cardiac transplantation in 150 patients at Stanford University. Br Med J 1:93–98, 1979
23. Kusumi RK, Walker SS, Fulkerson PK et al: Unilateral pulmonary edema associated with left ventricular failure. Heart Lung 13(3):263–266, 1984
24. Mason DT: Symposium on vasodilator and inotropic therapy of heart failure. Am J Med 65:101, 1978
25. McCauley: Probing the ins and outs of congestive heart failure. Nursing 12(11):60–65, 1982
26. McGurn WC: Congestive heart failure. In McGurn WC (ed): People with Cardiac Problems: Nursing Concepts, pp 317–339. Philadelphia, JB Lippincott, 1981
27. Michaelson CR: Pathophysiology of heart failure: A conceptual framework for understanding clinical indicators and therapeutic modalities. In Michaelson CR (ed): Congestive Heart Failure, pp 44–83. St Louis, CV Mosby, 1983
28. Niles NA, Wills RE: Heart failure. In Underhill SL et al (eds): Cardiac Nursing, pp 378–392. Philadelphia, JB Lippincott, 1982
29. Opie L: The Heart, pp 301–313. London, Grune & Stratton, 1984
30. O'Rourke MK: Vascular impedance in studies of arterial and cardiac function. Physiol Rev 62:570–623, 1982
31. Packer M, Meller J, Medina N et al: Hemodynamic characterization of tolerance to long-term hydralazine therapy in severe chronic heart failure. N Engl J Med 306:57–62, 1982
32. Polese A, Fiorentini C, Olivari MT et al: Clinical use of a calcium antagonistic agent (nifedipine) in acute dyspnea edema. Am J Med 66:825–830, 1979
33. Ribner HS, Bresnaham D, Hsieh AM et al: Acute hemodynamic responses to vasodilator therapy in congestive heart failure. Prog Cardiovasc Dis 25:1–42, 1982
34. Ross J: Effects of afterload or impedance on the heart: Afterload reduction in the treatment of cardiac failure. Cardiovasc Med 2:1115, 1977
35. Schlant RC, Sonnenblick EH: Pathophysiology of heart failure. In Hurst JW et al (eds): The Heart, 5th ed, pp 382–407. New York, McGraw-Hill, 1982
36. Selzer A: Digitalis in cardiac failure. Arch Intern Med 141:18, 1981
37. Smith TW: Digitalis in the management of heart failure. Hosp Pract 19(3):67–92, 1984
38. Smith TW, Braunwald E: The management of heart failure. In Braunwald E (ed): Heart Disease: A Textbook of Cardiovascular Medicine, pp 503–559. Philadelphia, WB Saunders, 1984
39. Spann JF, Hurst JW: The recognition and management of heart failure. In Hurst JW et al (eds): The Heart, 5th ed, pp 407–457. New York, McGraw-Hill, 1982
40. Zellis R, Flaim SF, MosKowitz RM et al: How much can we expect from vasodilator therapy in congestive heart failure? Circulation 59:1092–1097, 1979

Chapter 39

Cardiomyopathy and Infectious and Inflammatory Cardiac Disorders

Debra Laurent-Bopp

Cardiomyopathy describes a group of diseases that affect the myocardium without affecting other cardiovascular structures such as heart valves or the coronary arteries. Many cases of heart failure are now known to result from cardiomyopathy rather than from coronary heart disease.

Myocarditis, endocarditis, and pericarditis are all examples of infectious or inflammatory cardiac disorders. These diseases are not limited to the myocardium; they also involve other cardiovascular structures and surrounding tissues.

Cardiomyopathies

Cardiomyopathy connotes any structural or functional abnormality of the ventricular myocardium. In this text, cardiomyopathy is used to denote a condition affecting primarily the myocardium. By describing diseases in which pathological processes primarily involve the heart muscle, it is possible to distinguish cardiomyopathies from a similar pathological condition that results from coronary heart disease, congestive heart failure, high blood pressure, or valvular disease.

Etiology

The cardiomyopathies are subclassified etiologically as primary (idiopathic, heart muscle disease of unknown cause) and as secondary (rare specific heart disease).[31] Secondary cardiomyopathies are those in which the heart muscle is affected as part of a generalized or systemic process, and they include the following:[44]

1. Infective or inflammatory myocarditis
2. Infiltrative diseases such as amyloidosis (a disease characterized by accumulation of an abnormal protein in various organs and tissues) and systemic lupus erythematosis
3. Nutritional cardiomyopathies such as beriberi (thiamine deficiency) or potassium deficiency
4. Neurological and neuromuscular diseases such as progressive muscular dystrophy

Pathophysiology

Cardiomyopathies are now considered in three major groups based on abnormalities of function and structure: (1) dilated congestive, (2) hypertrophic, and (3) restrictive/obliterative.[28,29] The major characteristics of each group are presented in Figure 39–1.

Dilated Congestive Cardiomyopathy. Dilated congestive cardiomyopathy is probably the most common cardiomyopathy. The striking features are cardiomegaly with dilata-

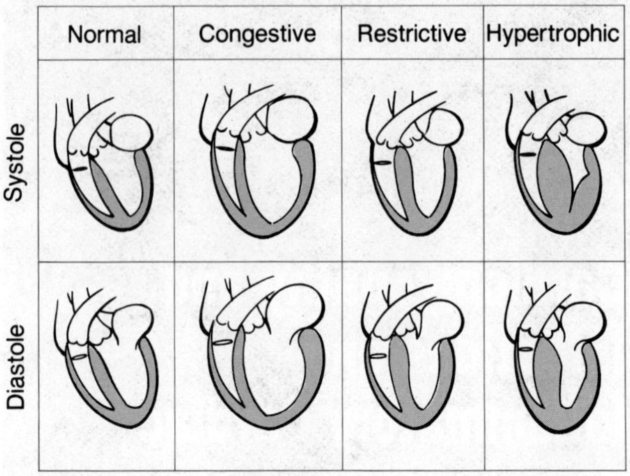

	Normal	Congestive	Restrictive	Hypertrophic
Systole				
Diastole				

FIGURE 39–1 Diagram of the heart with different types of cardiomyopathy at end-systole and end-diastole. (Goldman MR, Boucher CA: Value of radionuclide imaging techniques in possessing cardiomyopathy. Am J Cardiol 46:1232, 1980. Reproduced with permission.)

tion of the ventricles, impairment of systolic function, and increased myocardial mass. A number of conditions appear to be related to this cardiomyopathy, including alcohol abuse, immunologic disorders, high blood pressure, viral infections, pregnancy and the puerperium, and a number of chemical and physical agents that produce toxic effects on the myocardium.[29]

Hypertrophic Cardiomyopathy. Hypertrophic cardiomyopathy is usually genetically transmitted and is characterized by a marked disorganization of myocardial fibers, particularly in the septum. The cardinal feature is a marked increase in myocardial mass with small ventricular cavities.

Hypertrophic cardiomyopathy may cause obstruction to the ventricular outflow tract, which is due to a hypertrophic septum bulging into the outflow tract. If this occurs, systolic movement of the anterior mitral valve leaflet may cause mitral regurgitation. This condition is also called idiopathic hypertrophic subaortic stenosis (IHSS) or hypertrophic obstructive cardiomyopathy (HOCM).[65]

Restrictive/Obliterative Cardiomyopathy. This type of cardiomyopathy denotes restriction of filling of the ventricles caused by endocardial or myocardial disease or both, producing hemodynamic and clinical responses similar to constrictive pericarditis, such as precordial pain, pericardial friction rub, and dyspnea. The most common cause worldwide is endomyocardial fibrosis. When the endocardial disease becomes extensive, the ventricular cavity may become reduced in size. This is known as the "obliterative" phase.[12,27] In the Western world the restrictive form is the least prevalent of the cardiomyopathies, and amyloidosis is its most common cause.[32,56]

Characteristics of the three main types of cardiomyopathy in relation to pathophysiology are presented in Table 39–1.

Secondary cardiomyopathies, despite the implications of the disease or syndrome underlying it, have the same pathophysiology as the primary forms. Several diseases have both primary and secondary effects on the heart. An example is amyloidosis in which there are direct effects from the primary disease and secondary effects of increased work load of the heart because of the effects of the disease on other organs.

Clinical Manifestations

The degree of clinical manifestations presented by patients with primary cardiomyopathy depends on the variations in pathophysiology described above.

Dilated Congestive Cardiomyopathy. The excessive chamber enlargement found in dilated congestive cardiomyopathy results in gross impairment of the heart's contractile function. Cardiac decompensation results and is accompanied by either pulmonary or systemic congestion. Pulmonary arterial hypertension is usually present if right ventricular failure is secondary to left ventricular failure.[56] Thus the physical signs are those of congestive heart failure, with the onset of left ventricular failure manifested by dyspnea, initially on exertion and then at rest, a nocturnal dry cough, and at times pulmonary edema followed by symptoms of right ventricular failure.[32] Both ventricular and supraventricular arrhythmias, including atrial fibrillation, may be observed in these patients.[59] Premature ventricular contractions are the most common arrhythmia.[58]

Hypertrophic Cardiomyopathy. The wide clinical spectrum of hypertrophic cardiomyopathy depends on the extent and severity of the disease (nonobstructive vs. the obstructive type or IHSS), the rate of progression, and the age of the patient. The major symptoms are dyspnea and chest pain. Dyspnea is caused by the increased pulmonary venous pressure from the high left ventricular end-diastolic pressure.[32] These pressure abnormalities result from impaired ventricular filling and increased wall thickness as a result of hypertrophy.[53] The greatly hypertrophied myocardium due to diminished diastolic blood flow may result in angina. Potentially contributing to ischemia is the narrowing of the small coronary arteries as a result of elevated intramyocardial wall tension.

A high incidence of ventricular arrhythmias is associated

TABLE 39–1
Primary Cardiomyopathies

		Hypertrophic			
	Dilated Congestive	*Nonobstructed*	*Obstructed (IHSS)*	*Restrictive / Obliterative*	
Pathophysiological features	Fibrosis of myocardium and endocardium Dilated chambers Mural thrombi prevalent	Primary hypertrophy of all walls Disproportionately hypertrophied septum Relatively small chamber size	Same as nonobstructed with obstruction of the left ventricular outflow tract associated with the hypertrophied septum and mitral valve incompetence	Mimics constrictive pericarditis Fibrosed walls can neither expand nor contract effectively Chambers normal to moderately enlarged	Fibrosis affects endocardium primarily; may involve chordae tendinae Chambers narrowed, emboli are common; outflow tracts are preserved until relatively late
Clinical signs and symptoms	Fatigue and weakness Heart failure mainly left-sided Arrhythmia or heart block Systemic or pulmonary emboli Moderate to severe cardiomegaly, S_3 and S_4 gallops Atrioventricular valve regurgitation	Dyspnea Angina Fatigue, syncope, palpitations Mild cardiomegaly S_4 gallop common Atrial fibrillation Ventricular arrhythmias Sudden death is common. Heart failure (late sign)	Same as nonobstructed with mitral regurgitation murmur that increases with Valsalva maneuver Atrial fibrillation	For both types: Dyspnea and fatigue Right-sided heart failure Mild to moderate cardiomegaly S_3 and S_4 gallops Atrioventricular valve regurgitation Heart block Emboli	
Medical management	Symptomatic treatment of heart failure Vasodilators Control of arrhythmias	For both types: Symptomatic treatment β-adrenergic blockade Conversion from atrial fibrillation *Surgery:* Ventriculomyotomy or muscle resection with mitral valve replacement Digitalis, nitrates, and other vasodilators are usually contraindicated		For both types: Supportive treatment of symptoms Treatment of hypertension if present Conversion from arrhythmia Exercise restrictions Emergency treatment for acute pulmonary edema should be planned	

(Compiled from information in Heuter DC: Diseases of the pericardium, myocardium, and endocardium. In Wilkins RW, Levinsky NG (eds): Medicine, Essentials of Practice, 2nd ed. Boston, Little, Brown & Co, 1978 and from Wynne J, Braunwald E: The cardiomyopathies and myocarditis. In Braunwald E (ed): Heart Disease. Philadelphia, WB Saunders, 1981)

with this cardiomyopathy.[11,45] Supraventricular arrhythmias are another frequent complication, with atrial fibrillation reported in approximately 10% of patients.[6,11,45]

In patients with obstruction (IHSS), peripheral pulses have a characteristic double impulse (pulsus bisferiens).[7]

Restrictive/Obliterative Cardiomyopathy. The earliest clinical finding in restrictive/obliterative cardiomyopathy is exertional dyspnea, progressing to paroxysmal noctural dyspnea.[53] The capacity of the ventricles to dilate is greatly limited in restrictive cardiomyopathy, and ventricular filling is largely diminished. Biventricular contractile dysfunction usually develops and leads to pulmonary and systemic congestion and diminished perfusion.[53] A history of chest pain is common.[32] Table 39–1 highlights the clinical manifestations of the above primary cardiomyopathies.

Much greater variation of the signs and symptoms is noted in those with the secondary form of cardiomyopathy.

Medical Management

Primary cardiomyopathy requires conservation of the myocardium. The mode of therapy depends on the pathological changes and the extent of cardiac involvement. Secondary cardiomyopathy requires that the medical management is relevant to the patient's underlying condition. Infections are a common cause of the disease. Primary prevention becomes a key factor.

Diagnosis. For *dilated congestive cardiomyopathy,* the chest x-ray film reveals cardiomegaly and biventricular dilatation, which is further confirmed by radionuclide blood pool imaging, angiocardiography, and echocardiography. The echocardiogram also shows poor movement of the posterior free wall of the ventricle and paradoxical movement of the septum.[35,59]

The ECG in *hypertrophic cardiomyopathy* shows left ventricular hypertrophy. In radionuclide imaging techniques, a technetium scan confirms decreased left ventricular volume, and myocardial imaging with thallium (^{201}Tl) defines the increased myocardial mass and configuration.[26] Angiocardiography is an important diagnostic tool and is often definitive.[32]

Cardiomegaly is evidenced on the chest x-ray film in *restrictive/obliterative cardiomyopathy.* Radionuclide imaging techniques using ^{201}Tl may differentiate this cardiomyopathy from constrictive pericarditis and dilated congestive cardiomyopathy.[54] Angiocardiography reveals marked trabeculation of the left ventricle, and an endomyocardial biopsy will disclose amyloid disease.[32,49,53,56]

Treatment. For both *dilated congestive* and *restrictive/obliterative cardiomyopathy,* the therapeutic goals and management are the same as for congestive heart failure. Of primary consideration is the conservation of energy through rest, and oxygen administration. Increasing cardiac output and enhancing contractility are done through the use of vasodilating agents, diuretics, and cardiac glycosides.[37,58,59,64] A sodium-restricted diet is also prescribed. Antiarrhythmic drugs should be used to control heart rate and to provide maximum cardiac output.[8]

Because thrombus formation is common in patients with dilated congestive cardiomyopathy, long-term anticoagulant therapy is recommended, especially for those who have gross cardiac enlargement, congestive heart failure, or atrial fibrillation.[58,59] Surgical treatment for dilated congestive cardiomyopathy is heart transplantation.[65]

Early symptomatic treatment of angina and dyspnea, and control of tachycardia in patients with *hypertrophic cardiomyopathy* result in a fairly good prognosis. Beta-adrenergic blockers such as propranolol are used to control heart rate by reducing sympathetic stimulation of the heart and enhancing ventricular filling.[32,59] Most recently, calcium-channel blocking agents such as verapamil have been used with symptomatic and hemodynamic improvement.[34] Vasodilators and long-acting nitrates may also be used for control of angina. When the degree of heart work is controlled, dyspnea and angina subside.

Antiarrhythmic drugs or pacemaker therapy may be needed to control arrhythmias. Atrial arrhythmias need to be treated aggressively to prevent further compromise of ventricular filling; electrical cardioversion may be required.[32] Episodes of ventricular arrhythmias should also be treated, and although it is not known which drug is most helpful, amiodarone has proved helpful.[27]

IHSS, the obstructive form of hypertrophic cardiomyopathy, is managed somewhat differently. Although β-adrenergic blockers and verapamil[23] are used, nitrates, vasodilators, and digitalis are contraindicated when there is an obstruction because the vasodilating and positive inotropic effects may augment the obstruction.[48]

People with IHSS who have symptoms of right-sided failure are in danger of developing sudden episodes of pulmonary edema since their disease is relatively far advanced.

Surgical treatment for hypertrophic cardiomyopathy includes ventriculomyotomy (area of mitral outflow tract) or partial septal resection in selected patients. Mitral valve replacement is rarely indicated.[6,10,32,41,50]

Prognosis. The course of *dilated congestive cardiomyopathy* is usually downhill, and death commonly ensues within 6 months to several years after the onset of symptoms. The mean survival time is 5 years.[3,32]

The natural history of *hypertrophic cardiomyopathy* is extremely variable, ranging from a long life with few symptoms, to a rapidly progressive disease that is fatal in a few years.[14] Most deaths associated with this cardiomyopathy are sudden and unrelated to functional status. Sudden death may be precipitated by arrhythmias, myocardial ischemia, or a severe increase in left-ventricular inflow resistance or outflow tract obstruction.[11,30]

Attempts to treat amyloidosis in *restrictive/obliterative cardiomyopathy* are highly unsatisfactory; most patients die within a few years.[32]

Nursing Management

Nursing management of patients with cardiomyopathy focuses on the promotion of rest in acute situations and on screening and counseling about health maintenance when patients are not hospitalized.[44] Secondary cardiomyopathy requires the nurse to superimpose the care relevant to the patient's underlying condition onto the care specific to the cardiac pathophysiology and individual needs. Primary prevention broadens the nurse's role in the care of these patients.

Nursing Diagnoses and Interventions. Common problems related to the cardiomyopathies are:[20]

1. Dyspnea related to congestive heart failure
2. Fatigue related to inadequate cardiac output or congestive heart failure
3. Chest pain (angina) related to low cardiac output (mainly hypertrophic cardiomyopathies)
4. Syncope related to obstruction of the ventricular outflow tract (low cardiac output)
5. Anxiety (fear of sudden death)
6. Depression
7. Noncompliance with prescribed treatment

Nursing care of patients with dilated congestive cardiomyopathy and restrictive/obliterative cardiomyopathy are the same as nursing management for heart failure as described in Chapter 38. The nursing management of patients with hypertrophic cardiomyopathy parallels that of myocardial ischemia as discussed in Chapter 37. The major nursing diagnosis for these patients relates to decreased cardiac output and chest pain resulting from myocardial ischemia. To detect early signs of decreased cardiac output, vital signs are monitored every 4 hours along with urine output, skin temperature, and levels of consciousness. Bed rest is maintained to reduce myocardial oxygen consumption, and the patient is instructed to avoid activities that elicit a Valsalva response. The nurse should also administer the prescribed medication such as propranolol or other β-adrenergic blocking agents and verapamil, a calcium-channel blocking agent. The nursing interventions to relieve chest discomfort include reducing the patient's physical activities, encouraging bed rest, and ascertaining with the patient those activities that precipitate pain.

In addition to the continuing disease process associated with the cardiomyopathies, the patient must learn to cope with the uncertain prognosis of his disease. Problems may arise with the patient's self-perception and role relationship pattern.

The Nursing Care Plan for the Patient with Hypertrophic Cardiomyopathy is a general plan that must be individualized to meet specific patient needs.

NURSING CARE PLAN FOR THE PATIENT WITH HYPERTROPHIC CARDIOMYOPATHY

NURSING DIAGNOSIS/PROBLEM 1: Decreased cardiac output related to cardiac dysfunction secondary to left ventricular failure

GOAL 1.1: Prevent symptoms of decreased cardiac output by restoring balance between myocardial oxygen supply and demand

Nursing Interventions	Rationale	Outcome Criteria
1. Initially keep on bed rest and eliminate activities eliciting a Valsalva response. Note response to activities.	1. Valsalva maneuvers increase myocardial oxygen consumption; already stressed heart may be unable to respond adequately; cardiac output falls sharply.	1–4. Absence of signs of cardiac decompensation as evidenced by: a. Blood pressure remains within individual's normal range. b. Ideally, normal sinus rhythm without arrhythmias c. No complaints of fatigue with prescribed activity d. Remains fully alert and oriented e. Extremities warm and dry with normal color f. Urine output greater than 250 ml/8 hr shift
2. Administer propranolol or other β-adrenergic blocking agents as ordered.	2. Propranolol or other β-blocking agents prevents the increase in outflow obstruction found with exercise. Allows more time for diastolic filling, thus improving ventricular volume needed by hypertrophic cardiomyopathy patients.	
3. Administer verapamil, a calcium channel blocking agent, as ordered.	3. Used if patient fails to respond to β-blocking agents. Controls ventricular response in atrial fibrillation. May cause a decrease in the left ventricular outflow obstruction.	
4. Avoid the following drugs: a. Vasodilators b. Inotropic agents c. Digoxin d. Diuretics	4 a. Vasodilators may worsen the obstruction; thus avoid with hypertrophic patients to treat chest pain. b–c. Inotropic agents and digoxin increase myocardial contractivity and degree of obstruction. d. Diuretics can decrease the circulating blood volume and may aggravate the symptoms of hypertrophic cardiomyopathy.	

(Continued)

NURSING CARE PLAN FOR THE PATIENT WITH HYPERTROPHIC CARDIOMYOPATHY (*Continued*)

GOAL 1.2: To detect early signs and symptoms of decreased cardiac output

Nursing Interventions	Rationale	Outcome Criteria
1. Every 4 hours assess for hypotension, tachycardia, regularity of pulse, decreased peripheral pulses, and signs of decreased peripheral perfusion, such as cool skin, diaphoresis and decreased urine output.	1. Data obtained are indicative of decreased and inadequate cardiac output.	1–2. Signs and symptoms of decreased cardiac output are detected within 4 hours of onset.
2. Assess changes in sensorium every 4 hours.	2. May signify inadequate cerebral perfusion secondary to decreased cardiac output	

NURSING DIAGNOSIS/PROBLEM 2: Alteration in comfort related to myocardial ischemia secondary to reduced coronary blood flow resulting in chest discomfort

GOAL 2: To relieve chest discomfort by restoring the balance between myocardial oxygen supply and demand

Nursing Interventions	Rationale	Outcome Criteria
1. Decrease physical activity during anginal attacks. Keep supine or in semi-Fowler's position.	1. Rest decreases the demand on the ischemic heart.	1–3. Absence of signs of chest discomfort as evidenced by: a. Patient reporting relief of chest discomfort, if present b. Effect of chest discomfort on detected hemodynamics maintained within normal limits
2. Assess for occurrence of pain with verbal/nonverbal cues.	2. Pain can be expressed verbally and nonverbally.	
3. Assist patient to identify precipitating events and discuss changes that may be necessary in daily activities.	3. Prevent angina attacks that may progress to myocardial damage.	
a. Patient should not stand or sit up suddenly.	a. Sudden sitting or standing transiently reduces venous return and increases ventricular outflow tract obstruction.	
b. Patient can squat or raise legs.	b. Squatting or raising legs can increase blood flow.	

Inflammation and Infection of the Heart and Surrounding Tissues

Myocarditis

Myocarditis is focal or diffuse inflammation of the myocardium. It may be acute or chronic and can occur at any age. Frequently myocarditis is asymptomatic, and recovery is usually spontaneous without residual effects. Diffuse myocarditis may lead to profound congestive heart failure.[41]

Etiology and Pathophysiology

The most common cause of myocarditis in the United States is idiopathic; however, it may also result from an infection.[54] The viral, bacterial, and parasitic infections as well as the hypersensitive immune reactions and other causes of myocarditis are listed in Table 39–2.

Acute myocarditis has been commonly associated with viral infections, which for the majority are self-limiting. Microscopically, the picture is of an edematous myocardium infiltrated with lymphocytes and macrophages but essentially undamaged.[21,35]

Bacterial myocarditis is still an important cause of disability and mortality. Its occurrence may be a result of streptococcal invasion of the myocardium, endocardium, and pericardium in addition to the autoimmune response of rheumatic fever. The antigenic code of the host cells (heart fibers) is altered, and the patient's immune mechanism takes over, unselectively killing the causative agent and host cells; thus it is an autoimmune response.[21] Diphtheria may also affect the heart in the autoimmune (indirect) and direct pathological forms. An outcome of necrosis (diffuse, focal, or both) of cardiac tissue is congestive heart failure (CHF) after the underlying infection is gone. Hypertrophy results from the combination of increased cardiac work load and decreased muscle fiber capacity. Scar formation (fibrosis) after the inflammatory stage in conjunction with hypertrophy leads to the increased risk of CHF. Permanent myopathy may occur after the active infective stage is over.

TABLE 39–2
Causes of Myocarditis

Viral infections
Coxsackie A and B viruses
Influenza
Adenoviruses
Echoviruses
Rubeola
Rubella
Bacterial infections
Tuberculosis
Tetanus
Staphylococcal infections
Pneumococcal infections
Gonococcal infections
Diphtheria
Hypersensitive immune reactions
Postcardiotomy syndrome
Rheumatic fever
Radiation therapy
Chemical poisons
Parasitic infections
Toxoplasmosis
Chagas' disease

Clinical Manifestations

Myocarditis usually causes nonspecific symptoms such as fatigue, dyspnea, palpitations, and fever. If myofibril degeneration occurs, it may result in right and left heart failure, with cardiomegaly, neck-vein distention, resting or exertional tachycardia, and arrhythmias. Increased amplitude of S_1, S_3, and S_4 gallops, or systolic ejection murmurs may be present. A pericardial friction rub is heard if pericarditis is present.[40]

Patients may manifest the signs of infection in addition to the signs and symptoms of cardiac pathophysiology that lead to heart failure, or else the course may remain subclinical until the stage of heart failure.[21, 44]

Medical Management

A patient's history may reveal recent febrile upper respiratory infection, viral pharyngitis, or other systemic infection. Although laboratory tests cannot confirm the myocarditis, cardiac enzymes, increased white blood cell count, and elevated antibody titers support the diagnosis. Blood, stool, and throat cultures may identify bacteria or isolate the virus. The most reliable diagnostic aid is ECG changes, typically showing diffuse ST-segment and T-wave abnormalities, conduction defects, and other supraventricular arrhythmias.[40]

The goals of therapy include cure of the infection if possible and protection of the myocardium through the conservation of energy. Treatment includes antibiotics for bacterial infection and bed rest to decrease cardiac work load. Heart failure requires restriction of activity to decrease myocardial oxygen comsumption, oxygen therapy, diuretics, sodium restriction, and digitalis. Caution should be exercised when administering digitalis because some patients show a sensitivity to even small doses.[40] Pericardiocentesis may be performed if a pericardial effusion is further compromising the cardiac output. Antiarrhythmics, such as procainamide and quinidine, should also be used with caution since they depress myocardial contractility. Anticoagulation therapy is used for thromboembolism.

The vast majority of patients recover spontaneously; myocarditis caused by Chagas' disease (a parasitic protozoa) and diphtheria are the major exceptions to the generally favorable prognosis.[35]

Nursing Management

Nursing management of patients with myocarditis focuses on the promotion of rest in acute situations and on screening and counseling about health maintenance when patients are not hospitalized.

The major nursing diagnosis of decreased cardiac output is managed by promoting bed rest, administering antibiotics and corticosteroids as prescribed, and continuously monitoring pulse rate and rhythm, electrolyte levels, and cardiac function. ECG changes may herald arrhythmias, necessitating changes in treatment. Progressive or life-threatening arrhythmias require immediate intervention. Evaluation criteria indicate that the patient has achieved hemodynamic and electrophysiological stability as reflected in a return to previous heart rate, rhythm, and conduction and in a positive response to aggressive medical therapy if needed.

Infective Endocarditis

Endocarditis implies an inflammatory process involving the endocardial surface of the heart, which includes the valves. It may be an inflammatory lesion, as seen in rheumatic fever, or an infectious process with direct bacterial, rickettsial, or fungal invasion.

Etiology

Infective (previously called bacterial) endocarditis is currently categorized according to the virulence of the infecting organism. In acute infective endocarditis, the organism is extremely pathogenic and virulent. *Staphylococcus aureus* causes most cases of acute infective endocarditis, generally infecting normal heart valves and causing rapid and debilitating valvular damage.[42] The β-hemolytic streptococcus is also extremely virulent and a causative agent of acute infective endocarditis.

Subacute infective endocarditis usually is caused by organisms relatively low in virulence and normally present in the body. As the organism responsible for most cases of subacute infective endocarditis, *Streptococcus viridans* is a group of α-hemolytic bacteria commonly found in the oral cavity. Classically this organism becomes engrafted on deformed or damaged heart valves, such as rheumatic, congenital, or insufficient valves of any cause. Other causative agents of subacute infective endocarditis include the nonhemolytic and microaerophilic streptococci commonly found in the oral cavity and respiratory, gastrointestinal, and female genitourinary tracts.[2]

Other types of agents that may result in endocarditis include such gram-negative organisms as *Escherichia coli, Klebsiella, Proteus, Pseudomonas,* and *Salmonella.*[15] Fungal infections include *Aspergillus, Candida,* and *Histoplasma* organisms.[18]

Pathogenesis. Fifty to sixty percent of the acute infective endocarditis occurs in patients without any previous cardiac deformities.[22,62,63] The reason for the localization of infection on normal heart valves is not clearly understood. One theory states that the highly virulent organisms exhibit a unique property that permits adherence to the endothelial surface of the heart valve.[10,11,14]

Four mechanisms appear to be involved with the selectivity and localization of subacute infective endocarditis:[62,63]

1. Preexisting valvular damage or cardiac defects
2. Presence of bacteremia
3. Formation of sterile platelet-fibrin thrombi
4. Development of a high titer of agglutinating antibodies specific to the infecting organism

Pathophysiology

Infections forming on heart valves produce endothelial lesions that are called vegetations. The active vegetations are composed of three layers: (1) an inner layer of platelets, fibrin, and white and red blood cells, which is the largest layer; (2) the middle layer, which is composed primarily of the infectious organism; and (3) an outer layer that is composed of fibrin and microorganisms.[62] The infectious organism finds a protective sanctuary in the platelet-fibrin vegetation, necessitating prolonged courses of antibiotic therapy.

The vegetations have irregular edges and are easily torn away. They tend to occur where blood flows through a narrow orifice and usually grow on the low pressure side of a defect or injury. The mitral valve is the site most frequently involved, followed by the aortic, tricuspid, and pulmonic valves, in that order.[62]

Acute infective endocarditis causes sloughing of tissue early in its course. Erosion of a valve leaflet or myocardial damage may very quickly give rise to heart failure. The vegetations tend to be softer, larger, and more easily torn away, causing major emobolic complications. There is a greater incidence of predominating right-sided failure in acute infective endocarditis, as evidenced by peripheral edema, weight gain, and anorexia, although the vast majority of patients still exhibit signs of left-sided heart failure, as evidenced by fatigue, shortness of breath, and pulmonary edema.

Subacute infective endocarditis is much more commonly found on the left rather than the right side of the heart.[4] An estimated 75% of people with subacute infective endocarditis have previously had rheumatic fever and an additional 10% have congenital defects.[24] The danger posed to the untreated patient is (1) congestive heart failure due to valve erosion leading to regurgitation, and (2) embolization due to irregular vegetations that are torn away traveling to the brain, kidney, spleen, or mesentery.

Clinical Manifestations

Patients may present with (1) an acute clinical course with sudden fever, septicemia, valvular insufficiency, heart failure, and perhaps stroke or splenic infarction or (2) an indolent course lasting several months of chronic low-grade fever, anemia, weight loss, splenomegaly, and a heart murmur. Sudden deterioration may occur at any time from systemic embolization or valve rupture.[43,57]

Peripheral manifestations include petechiae, splinter hemorrhages in the nailbeds, Roth spots (hemorrhagic spots with white centers in the fundi), and Osler's nodes (painful lesions on the pads of fingers or toes). Although still controversial, the peripheral manifestations are now believed to be caused by an allergic vasculitis of the arterioles rather than microemboli.[36,52] In addition, there are a number of immunologic disorders including rheumatoid factor (IgM and anti-IgG antibodies), reduced complement levels, hypergammaglobulinemia, and cryoglobulinemia.[9,52]

Medical Management

Several conditions predispose to endocarditis including congenital heart disease, rheumatic heart disease, mitral valve prolapse, cardiac defects, and other problems as outlined in Table 39–3. Possible ports of entry for infecting organisms include the oral cavity (recent dental procedures within 3 to 6 months); skin rashes, lesions or abscesses; infections (skin, gastrointestinal, genitourinary or central nervous system); and surgery or invasive procedures or therapies such as tonsillectomy, bronchoscopy, endoscopy, cystoscopy, and prosthetic valve replacement. Patients who are at risk for developing infective endocarditis must be carefully assessed in the history.[33] The history is particularly important in terms of duration of symptoms and preexisting pathology. Initial assessment for the presence and intensity of heart murmurs is also important.

A positive blood culture is of prime diagnostic and therapeutic importance. Both aerobic and anaerobic cultures should be obtained. Laboratory studies generally reflect a leukocytosis and, in subacute cases, normochromic, normocytic anemia. Although a nonspecific test, the sedimentation rate is elevated in 98% of cases. The ECG may reveal conduction abnormalities.

TABLE 39–3
Conditions Predisposing to Endocarditis

Congenital heart disease
Rheumatic heart disease
Cardiac surgery
Mitral valve prolapse
Cardiac defects
Intravenous drug abuse
Intravascular foreign bodies such as:
- Pacemaker electrodes
- Intravenous catheters
- Dialysis shunts
- Hyperalimentation catheters

Immunosuppression related to:
- Burn injury
- Cancer
- Diabetes
- Hepatitis

Treatment. Treatment goals include the eradication of the infectious organism and the prevention of sequelae. Frequently, the severity of this disease requires initiation of therapy before bacteriological confirmation is obtained. Broad-spectrum coverage, with drugs such as high-dose intravenous penicillin or a semisynthetic penicillin, plus gentamicin, streptomycin, or vancomycin, usually is recommended.[43] Once the results of cultures and sensitivity tests are reported, therapy can be appropriately altered and must continue for 4 to 6 weeks.

Supportive therapy such as rest is the major preventive measure against development of heart failure. Emergency valvular replacement surgery becomes necessary in those patients with intractable heart failure due to valvular insufficiency. People who develop infection at the site of a prosthetic valve may also require valve replacement.[4]

For persons with valvular or congenital heart disease, the American Heart Association recommends prophylactic antibiotic treatment.[1,16] Table 39–4 illustrates the antibiotic

TABLE 39–4
Antibiotic Prophylaxis in Heart Disease Patients

Procedure	*Standard Regimen*	*For Patients Allergic to Penicillin*
Dental procedures and surgery of the upper respiratory tract	Penicillin alone Parenteral–oral combined: Aqueous crystalline penicillin G (1,000,000 U IM) mixed with procaine penicillin G (600,000 U IM). Give 30 min to 1 hr prior to procedure and then give penicillin V (formerly called phenoxymethyl penicillin) 500 mg orally every 6 hr for 8 doses. Oral: Penicillin V (2 g orally 30 min to 1 hr prior to procedure and then 500 mg orally every 6 hr for 8 doses)	Erythromycin (1 g orally 1½–2 hr prior to procedure)
For patients with prosthetic heart valves	Penicillin plus streptomycin: Aqueous crystalline penicillin G (1,000,000 U IM) mixed with procaine penicillin G (600,000 U IM) plus streptomycin (1 g IM). Give 30 min to 1 hr prior to procedure; then penicillin V 500 mg orally every 6 hr for 8 doses.	Vancomycin (1 g IV over 30 min to 1 hr). Start initial vancomycin infusion ½–1 hr prior to procedure; then erythromycin 500 mg orally every 6 hr for 8 doses
Genitourinary tract and gastrointestinal tract surgery or instrumentation*	Aqueous crystalline penicillin G (2,000,000 U IM or IV) or ampicillin (1 g IM or IV) plus gentamicin (1.5 mg/kg—not to exceed 80 mg—IM or IV) or streptomycin (1 g IM). Give initial doses 30 min to 1 hr prior to procedure. If gentamicin is used, then give a similar dose of gentamicin and penicillin (or ampicillin) every 8 hr for two additional doses.† If streptomycin is used, then give a similar dose of streptomycin and penicillin (or ampicillin) every 12 hr for 2 additional doses.†	Vancomycin (1 g IV given over 30 min to 1 hr) plus streptomycin (1 g IM). A single dose of these antibiotics begun 30 min to 1 hr prior to procedure is probably sufficient, but same dose may be repeated in 12 hr.†

* In patients with significantly compromised renal function, it may be necessary to modify the dose of antibiotics used. Some of these doses may exceed the manufacturer's recommendations for a 24-hr period. Since they are recommended only for a 24-hr period in most cases, however, it is unlikely that toxicity will occur.

† During prolonged procedures, or in case of delayed healing, it may be necessary to provide additional doses of antibiotics. For brief outpatient procedures such as uncomplicated catheterization of the bladder, one dose may be sufficient.

(From Committee on Rheumatic Fever and Bacterial Endocarditis, Council on Cardiovascular Disease in the Young, American Heart Association: Prevention of bacterial endocarditis. Circulation 56:2, 1977) prophylaxis to be used when such patients undergo dental procedures, surgery of the upper respiratory tract, and surgery or invasive procedures of the genitourinary and gastrointestinal tracts.

Infective endocarditis has a 25% to 35% mortality rate even with treatment.[13] Involvement of the left side of the heart (particularly the aortic valve), heart failure, gram-negative bacteria and fungal infections, and endocarditis developing after replacement with a prosthetic valve are associated with a poor prognosis.[51] The mortality rate for prosthetic valve endocarditis is significantly higher because it is difficult to cure the infection without reoperating.[47]

Nursing Management

Nursing management includes all levels of prevention as well as the general care of persons with active disease.

Primary prevention should focus on prevention of the disease through education of the population at risk. Included in the health teaching program is information on the disease process, the importance of good daily oral hygiene, and the importance of carrying emergency identification if the need for immediate care is necessary.

Secondary prevention is the specific preventive care in the hospitalized population at risk. Patients at risk are those with a history of congenital or rheumatic heart disease, those who have had cardiac surgery, patients who are parenteral drug abusers, or patients with intravascular devices such as IV catheters, dialysis shunts, hyperalimentation catheters, or pacemakers.

Detecting early signs and symptoms of infection involves ongoing assessment such as recording temperatures at least twice daily in graph form to identify any patterns of elevation, taking vital signs at least twice daily to detect widening pulse pressures as an indication of increasing aortic incompetence, and checking for heart murmurs through cardiac auscultation. A new or changed murmur may indicate a regurgitant heart valve.

To prevent infection in these patients the nurse would observe basic general principles of asepsis such as thorough hand washing, which is the single, most important infection control measure. Maintain strict aseptic technique, including the wearing of masks, gowns, and gloves, when changing dressings or attending to any intravascular catheter. The rationale for these measures is to prevent airborne and contact organisms from entering the sterile field. If at all possible, the same person should perform these procedures to allow for continuity of observation and the detection of day-to-day changes. An added measure would be to develop a policy of routine changes in peripheral intravenous sites to prevent thrombophlebitis and reduce the opportunity for organisms to grow in one site. A patient who responds effectively to all these care measures should remain free of any signs of endocarditis.

When endocarditis is suspected, blood cultures are done to detect the infecting organism, and antimicrobial therapy is instituted as prescribed. Periodic blood samples are drawn to determine if the infection is abating, and temperature checks are done every 4 hours to monitor progress. The patient is also observed for any signs of drug reaction such as the presence of a rash, urticaria, diarrhea, anaphylactic reactions, or other adverse responses to the antimicrobial therapy.

One critical complication for a patient with endocarditis is the development of venous or arterial embolization related to the presence of valvular vegetation and the predisposing risk of thrombi formation. Measures to prevent this complication include range-of-motion exercises and frequent change of position to decrease the risk of thrombi formation, having the patient wear antiembolism hose to promote venous return, administering anticoagulants as prescribed, and providing meticulous care of IV sites to diminish the chances of irritation and infection.

Ongoing assessment to detect early signs of embolization is essential. Peripheral pulses should be recorded every 4 hours or as necessary, and the calf muscle area in the leg should be checked for tenderness (Homan's sign), swelling, and redness. Additional signs of embolization depend on the area affected. They include a decrease in level of consciousness, visual changes, severe headache, upper left abdominal pain radiating to the left shoulder, shortness of breath, chest pain, reduced urine output, hematuria, increased serum creatinine and BUN, and possibly arrhythmias and pericarditis. Any such signs should be reported immediately because embolization is a serious, life-threatening occurrence.

For an overview of the nursing management of endocarditis, see the accompanying Nursing Care Plan for Preventing and Managing Endocarditis.

NURSING CARE PLAN FOR PREVENTING AND MANAGING ENDOCARDITIS

NURSING DIAGNOSIS/PROBLEM 1: Potential for the hospital patient to develop nosocomial infection
GOAL 1.1: To prevent infection

Nursing Interventions	Rationale	Outcome Criteria
1. Observe basic general principles of asepsis and thorough hand washing when nursing the patient at risk.	1. Hand washing is the single most important infection control measure.	1–5. Patients at risk remain free of endocarditis.

(Continued)

NURSING CARE PLAN FOR PREVENTING AND MANAGING ENDOCARDITIS (*Continued*)

Nursing Interventions	Rationale
2. Maintain strict aseptic technique in the care and dressing changes of all intravascular catheters, pacemakers (wear mask, gown, gloves).	2. Airborne and contact organisms are prevented from entering sterile field.
3. Develop protocols for aseptic technique so that with change of personnel, procedure is the same every day.	3. Scientifically based protocol for procedures establishes standards for nursing procedures. These standards can be used to maintain the quality of patient care.
4. Plan staffing so that the procedure is performed by the same person, if possible, for continuity of observation.	4. It is easier to note day-to-day changes if all personnel use the same techniques.
5. Develop policy for routine changes in peripheral intravenous sites.	5. Prevents thrombophlebitis and allows the vein to be used more than once. Allows greater opportunity for isolation and growth of organisms.

GOAL 1.2: To detect early the signs and symptoms of infection

Nursing Interventions	Rationale	Outcome Criteria
1. Graph temperature recordings daily; take temperature at least twice day.	1. To detect elevations early and recognize patterns.	1–2. The signs and symptoms of infection are detected within 12 hours: a. Elevated temperature greater than 98.6° b. Presence of new murmur
2. Take vital signs accurately at least twice daily and note changes in cardiac auscultation such as new or changed murmurs.	2. A widened pulse pressure indicates increasing aortic incompetence. New or changed murmurs indicate a regurgitant heart valve.	

NURSING DIAGNOSIS/PROBLEM 2.1: Cardiac valve infection (infective endocarditis) related to causative agent (name organism when identified)

GOAL 2.1: To identify infecting organism from blood culture studies without complications from the procedure

Nursing Interventions	Rationale	Outcome Criteria
1. Obtain blood cultures by aseptic technique. a. Recommend venipuncture technique for obtaining blood for cultures: 1. Prepare the skin with 2% iodine followed by 70% alcohol. Obtain at least three tubes of blood for culture, label them #1, #2, #3, in the order draw.	1. With the large numbers of bacteria residing on the skin, correct skin preparation to prevent contamination is crucial. If the organism is present in tube #1, skin contamination must be suspected. If present in all three samples, endocarditis is confirmed.	1–2. Aseptic technique is maintained throughout venipuncture for blood cultures. Causitive agent is identified. The patient will not experience any complications such as: a. Redness b. Swelling c. Discomfort
2. Incubate the blood specimens in both aerobic and anaerobic media.	2. To detect both types of organisms	

(*Continued*)

NURSING CARE PLAN FOR PREVENTING AND MANAGING ENDOCARDITIS (*Continued*)

Nursing Interventions	Rationale	Outcome Criteria
3. Explain purpose of frequent blood cultures and how often they will be drawn.	3. Unresolved anxiety increases myocardial oxygen consumption.	3. The patient will not exhibit high level of anxiety related to blood culture procedure and will verbalize the need for and general description of the procedure.

GOAL 2.2: To prevent complications

Nursing Interventions	Rationale	Outcome Criteria
1. Administer antipyretics/analgesics and antimicrobial therapy as ordered. a. Check history for allergies. b. Maintain IV. c. Check for drug reaction, *e.g.,* toxicity, rash, fever.	1. Analgesics are useful in alleviating discomfort. Antipyretics decrease temperature. Antimicrobial therapy will be specific to causative agent of endocarditis.	1–3. The patient will demonstrate symptomatic improvement without complications by: a. Temperature returns to normal in 4 to 5 days. b. The patient's blood culture studies are negative in 1 week. c. Complaints of malaise and fatigue will decrease. d. Patient will participate in ROM exercise. e. No presence of rash, urticaria, diarrhea, anaphylactic reactions, or other adverse reactions to antimicrobial therapy.
2. Check temperature every 4 hours or as indicated.	2. Indicates active inflammatory process.	
3. Evaluate extent of malaise related to immobility vs. chronic infection vs. anemia. a. Monitor serial Hb, Hct. b. Monitor blood cultures and assess for signs and symptoms of abating infection. c. Assist with active or passive ROM exercises.	3. Cause of malaise must be differentiated because nursing and medical interventions need to be specific to cause.	

NURSING DIAGNOSIS/PROBLEM 3.1: Potential for injury from venous or arterial embolization related to presence of valvular vegetations and thrombi predisposing to risk of embolization

GOAL 3.1: To detect early venous or arterial embolization

Nursing Interventions	Rationale	Outcome Criteria
1. Assess and document every hour or as needed: a. Level of consciousness b. Visual changes c. Splenic pain d. Auscultate lung fields e. Shortness of breath f. Urine output g. Presence of blood in urine h. Heart rate, blood pressure, and heart sounds i. Peripheral pulses	1. These data are useful in diagnosing embolization in the cardiac, pulmonary, cerebral, splenic, and renal areas.	1. Any signs and symptoms of embolization to be detected within 1 hour

Pericarditis

The heart is enclosed by a pericardial sac that is composed of two surfaces. The inner surface encasing the heart is called the visceral pericardium (or epicardium), and the outer surface attached to different structures in the chest is called the parietal pericardium. Normally there is 10 ml to 20 ml of pericardial fluid between the contracting surfaces of the visceral and parietal pericardium, serving as a lubricant to allow the heart to move freely within the pericardial sac.

Etiology and Pathophysiology

Pericarditis refers to an alteration of the pericardium regardless of etiology, and it may produce clinical and pathological changes of acute pericarditis, pericarditis with effusion with or without cardiac tamponade, and chronic constrictive pericarditis. Pericarditis may be caused by idiopathic, infectious, inflammatory, autoimmune, and metabolic factors as well as by trauma, drugs, and the presence of a tumor (see Table 39–5).[25,43]

In pericarditis the specific changes and alterations of the pericardium depend on the specific etiology. Inflammation of the pericardium may result in localized or generalized deposition of fibrin. This deposition of fibrin can produce constrictive pericarditis whereby the pericardium becomes rigid and unable to stretch. More commonly, the potential space between the parietal and visceral layers of the pericardium may fill with sufficient fluid to produce pericardial restriction (effusion or tamponade).[60] The nature of the effusion may be serous, bloody, or purulent depending on whether the process is primarily inflammatory or includes infection.[39] Compression of the heart either by fibrosis or pericardial fluid results in the heart not being able to fill completely.

In pericardial effusion, mainly the rate and not the volume of fluid accumulation determines whether cardiac tamponade will ensue. Severe tamponade may occur with as little as 100 ml to 250 ml if the fluid accumulates rapidly, whereas in the chronic states the pericardium has stretched and adapted to the effusion, and 1000 ml of fluid may accumulate before hemodynamic changes occur.[24]

TABLE 39–5
Etiology of Pericarditis

- Idiopathic (nonspecific)
- Infectious
  - Bacterial
  - Viral
  - Tuberculosis
  - Fungal
  - Parasitic
- Inflammatory
  - Collagen disease (SLE and scleroderma)
  - Rheumatoid arthritis
  - Rheumatic fever
- Hypersensitivity or autoimmune
  - Postpericardectomy
  - Postmyocardial infarction (Dressler's syndrome)
- Metabolic
  - Uremia
  - Myxedema
- Trauma
- Tumor
- Drugs
- Miscellaneous
  - Dissecting aneurysm
  - Pulmonary disease

Clinical Manifestations

Acute pericarditis usually has three signs and symptoms: precordial pain, a pericardial friction rub, and dyspnea.[25] The precordial pain is usually aggravated by breathing, turning in bed, or lying on the left side; it is relieved by sitting up. A pericardial friction rub is heard when the pericardial surfaces lose their lubricating fluid because of inflammation. Dyspnea results from compression of the bronchi or the lung parenchyma by the distended pericardium.[19] General symptoms of infection, fever, chills, fatigue, and malaise may also be present.

In cardiac tamponade, reduction in cardiac output leads to tachycardia, hypotension, and decreased pulse pressure. The rapid accumulation of pericardial fluid and decreased circulating volume result in pulsus paradoxus, increased central venous pressure, and ECG changes. Kussmaul's sign is noted owing to impaired right-sided cardiac filling.[55]

Signs of chronic right-sided heart failure are seen in patients with constrictive pericarditis, including dyspnea, exertional fatigue, hepatomegaly, orthopnea, and pericardial edema.[5]

Medical Management

The diagnosis of pericarditis is made, in part, by history and clinical signs and symptoms. The chest x-ray film will detect significant pericardial effusion. In acute pericarditis, distinct ECG changes can be found in 80% of patients.[17] Echocardiography is helpful in establishing specific types of pericardial disease.[38]

Treatment of pericarditis is usually achieved by appropriate analgesics for pain and/or anti-inflammatory agents. Some patients require steroid therapy. Control of infection by appropriate antibiotic therapy may be necessary. If the cardiac function becomes seriously impaired, a pericardiocentesis is performed to remove fluid from the pericardial sac.

A complete pericardiectomy involving removal of both the parietal and visceral layers of the pericardium is indicated for patients with constrictive pericarditis.[66]

The prognosis of pericarditis is dependent on the causative disease and/or the occurrence of complications of cardiac tamponade or constrictive pericarditis.

Nursing Management

Nurses must understand the nature of pericarditis, its causes, its therapeutic modalities, and the specific nursing care to help patients tolerate an anxiety-producing and painful process with potential for major complications.

Nursing Diagnoses and Interventions. Major nursing diagnoses include (1) alteration in comfort related to pericardial inflammation as evidenced by chest pain, elevated temperature, and diaphoresis and chills and (2) decreased cardiac output related to pericardial changes, possibly resulting in cardiac effusion and tamponade.

Assessing for pain, administering analgesics and anti-inflammatory agents as prescribed, maintaining bed rest and assuring a comfortable position are basic comfort measures. If fluid begins to accumulate in the pericardial sac, leading to cardiac effusion or tamponade, the signs to watch for are increased venous pressure (jugular vein distention and dyspnea), a decrease in blood pressure, and a quickened heart rate resulting from decreased stroke volume. Any such signs should be reported immediately.

The patient should be placed in a low Fowler's position to decrease cardiac pressure, and oxygen should be administered as prescribed. A pericardiocentesis may be necessary to remove fluid, thereby relieving intrapericardial pressure. Nursing responsibilities during the procedure include continuing assessment of the patient's status and monitoring of ECG and central venous pressure. Emergency equipment for defibrillation and resuscitation should be on hand if severe life-threatening complications arise. A more detailed overview of nursing care is presented in the accompanying Nursing Care Plan for the Patient with Pericarditis.

NURSING CARE PLAN FOR THE PATIENT WITH PERICARDITIS

NURSING DIAGNOSIS/PROBLEM 1: Alteration in comfort related to pericardial inflammation as evidenced by chest pain, temperature elevation, diaphoresis, and chills

GOAL 1.1: To relieve chest pain, chills, and diaphoresis

Nursing Interventions	Rationale	Outcome Criteria
1. Assess for presence of pain. a. Observe patient for verbal/nonverbal cues. b. Obtain clear description of pain. c. Record and report occurrences and description of pain and response to interventions.	1. Timing and characteristics help differentiate cardiac inflammatory process from other conditions that also cause chest pain, *e.g.,* MI, dissecting aortic aneurysm and/or pulmonary embolus.	1–4. Absence of chest pain: a. Patient reports relief of chest pain. b. Patient appears comfortable: 1) Seems restful 2) Respiratory rate, heart rate, and blood pressure are within acceptable range. 3) Tolerates passive ROM exercises Absence of chills and diaphoresis
2. Allow patient position most comfortable to alleviate pain.	2. Patient may be more comfortable in upright position and leaning forward, since heart is suspended from great vessels.	
3. Administer analgesics and anti-inflammatory agents as ordered.	3. Analgesics are useful in alleviating chest discomfort. Anti-inflammatory agents help to decrease the inflammation of the pericardial surfaces, decrease temperature, and reduce the effusion to decrease compromised function.	
4. Maintain bed rest while chest pain, fever, and/or friction rub are present.	4. Physical rest reduces myocardial oxygen consumption.	

GOAL 1.2: To detect early signs and symptoms of inflammation

Nursing Interventions	Rationale	Outcome Criteria
1. Observe and record: a. Temperature every 4 hours or as indicated b. Signs and symptoms of infection c. For pericardial friction rub every 2 hours	1. Indicates active inflammatory process.	1–2. Signs and symptoms of inflammation detected: a. Abnormal temperature b. Diaphoresis and/or chills c. Signs and symptoms of infection

(Continued)

NURSING CARE PLAN FOR THE PATIENT WITH PERICARDITIS (*Continued*)

Nursing Interventions	Rationale	Outcome Criteria
2. Monitor 12-led ECGs serially for characteristic changes of pericarditis if suspicious of presence and/or documented.	2. Data obtained from ECG can assist in the diagnosis of pericarditis and indicate resolution of the disease process.	d. Friction rub, if present e. ECG changes

NURSING DIAGNOSIS/PROBLEM 2: Decreased cardiac output related to structural factors: changes in the pericardium
GOAL 2: To detect early the signs and symptoms of cardiac effusion or tamponade

Nursing Interventions	Rationale	Outcome Criteria
1. Monitor carefully for changes in hemodynamic status and record: a. Increased venous pressure 1. Jugular vein distention 2. Elevated CVP (right atrial pressure) 3. Complaints of dyspnea b. Decreased or altered BP 1. Narrowing pulse pressures 2. Pulsus paradoxus c. Sinus tachycardia d. Anxiety	1. Speed and amount of fluid accumulation in the pericardial sac related to pericardial effusion determines onset of symptoms. These data are useful in diagnosing cardiac effusion or tamponade. Increased venous pressure indicates pericardial restriction. Decreased BP and sinus tachycardia result from decreased stroke volume.	1–3. Signs and symptoms of cardiac effusion and tamponade are detected at onset. a. Distended neck veins b. Increased CVP c. Dyspnea d. Hypotension (100 mmHg) and decreased pulse pressure (20 mmHg) e. Pulsus pardoxus (10 mmHg) f. Sinus tachycardia (heart rate, 100 beats/minute) g. Anxiety
2. If cardiac tamponade should develop, monitor: a. Venous pressure, BP, and heart rate every 15–30 minutes b Rhythm strips continuously c. 12-lead ECG every 30 minutes or as indicated	2. Same as #1 above	
3. Place patient in low Fowler's position, administer O_2 as ordered.	3. Increased oxygen to myocardium will promote aerobic metabolism. Fowler's position decreases cardiac pressure by increasing thoracic space.	
4. Assist with pericardiocentesis (usually removal of 100–200 ml). Results are dramatic.	4. Increased intrapericardial pressure impairs diastolic filling. When heart is surrounded by positive pressure, left ventricular filling is reduced, causing stroke volume and arterial BP to decline. Removal of fluid decreases intrapericardial pressure.	4. The patient will demonstrate resolution of cardiac tamponade by: a. Responding to pericardiocentesis b. Responding to rapidly infused saline to increase venous pressure

References

1. American Heart Association: Prevention of bacterial endocarditis. Dallas, American Heart Association, 1980
2. Barry J, Gump DW: Endocarditis: An overview. Heart Lung 11:138, 1982
3. Beahrs MM, Tajik AJ, Seward JB: Hypertrophic obstructive cardiomyopathy: Ten to 21 year follow-up after portal septal myectomy. Am J Cardiol 51:1160–1165, 1983
4. Beeson PB: Bacterial endocarditis. In Beeson PB, McDermott W (eds): Cecil-Loeb Textbook of Medicine, 14 ed. Philadelphia, WB Saunders, 1975
5. Blake SA: Etiology of chronic constrictive pericarditis. Br Heart J 50(3):273–276, 1983
6. Bohachick P, Rongaus AM: Hypertrophic cardiomyopathy. Am J Nurs 84(3):320–326, 1984
7. Borggrefe M, Breithardt G, Ostermeyer J et al: Arrhythmias in hypertrophic obstructive and nonobstructive cardiomyopathy. Eur Heart J Suppl F:345–351, 1983
8. Brev CS, Lindenmuth JE, Tillisch JH: Treatment of patients with

congestive cardiomyopathy during hospitalization: A case study. Heart Lung 11(3):229–234, 1982

9. Cabane J, Godeau P, Herreman G et al: Fate of circulatory immune complexes in infective endocarditis. Am J Med 66:277–282, 1979
10. Cain T, Campbell D, Paton B, Clarke D: Operation for discrete subvalvular aortic stenosis. J Thorac Cardiovasc Surg 87(3):366–370, 1984
11. Canedo MI, Frank MJ, Abdulla AM: Rhythm disturbances in hypertrophic cardiomyopathy: Prevalence, relation to symptoms and management. Am J Cardiol 45:848–855, 1980
12. Chew CY, Ziady GM, Raphael MJ et al: Primary restrictive cardiomyopathy. Non-tropical endomyocardial fibrosis and hypereosinophilic heart disease. Br Heart J 39:399–413, 1977
13. Christopherson DJ, Sivarajan ES: Infective endocarditis. In Underhill S, Woods S, Sivarajan ES, Halpenny CJ (eds): Cardiac Nursing. Philadelphia, JB Lippincott, 1982
14. Ciro E, Maron BJ, Bonow RO et al: Relation between marked changes in left ventricular outflow tract gradient and disease progression in hypertrophic cardiomyopathy. Am J Cardiol 53(8):1103–1109, 1984
15. Cohen PS, Maguire JH, Weinstein L: Infective endocarditis caused by gram-negative bacteria: A review of the literature, 1945–1977. Prog Cardiovasc Dis 22:205, 1980
16. Committee on Rheumatic Fever and Bacterial Endocarditis, Council on Cardiovascular Disease in the Young, American Heart Association: Prevention of bacterial endocarditis. Circulation 56:2, 1977
17. Darsee J, Braunwald E: Diseases of the pericardium. In Braunwald E (ed): Heart Disease. Philadelphia, WB Saunders, 1980
18. Dorney ER: Endocarditis. In Hurst JW (ed): The Heart, 5th ed. New York, McGraw-Hill, 1982
19. Dossey BM: The person with pericarditis, pericardial effusion, and cardiac tamponade. In Guzetta CE, Dossey BM (eds): Cardiovascular Nursing: Bodymind Tapestry. St Louis, CV Mosby, 1984
20. Dracup K: Unraveling the mysteries of cardiomyopathy. Nursing 79 9:84–87, 1979
21. Duffy K, Roewer MK, Goding CM: A severe case of viral myocarditis. Am J Nurs 6:1148–1151, 1981
22. Durak DT, Petersdorf RG: Changes on epidemiology of endocarditis. In Kaplan E, Taranta A (eds): Infective Endocarditis. American Heart Association Monograph #52. Dallas, American Heart Association, 1977
23. Eldar M, Hod H, Battler A: Obstructive hypertrophic cardiomyopathy with left-sided cardiac failure: Improvement after verapamil treatment. Am J Cardiol 53:644–645, 1984
24. Fowler N: The recognition and management of pericardial disease and its complications. In Hurst JW (ed): The Heart, 5th ed. New York, McGraw-Hill, 1982
25. Gazes PC: Pericardial diseases. In Gazes PC (ed): Clinical Cardiology, 2nd ed. Chicago, Year Book Medical Publishers, 1983
26. Goldman MR, Boucher CA: Valve of radionuclide imaging techniques in assessing cardiomyopathy. Am J Cardiol 46:1232, 1980
27. Goodwin JF: Cardiomyopathy: An interface between fundamental and clinical cardiology. In Hayase S, Morao S (eds): Cardiology. Exerpta Medica, 1979
28. Goodwin JF: Congestive and hypertrophic cardiomyopathies. A decade of study. Lancet 1:731, 1970
29. Goodwin JF: Prospects and predictions for the cardiomyopathies. Circulation 50:210, 1974
30. Goodwin JF: Kirkler DM: Sudden death in cardiomyopathy. Adv Cardiol 25:98–106, 1978
31. Goodwin JF, Oakley CM: The Cardiomyopathies. Br Heart J 34:545, 1972
32. Goodwin JF, Roberts WC, Wenger NK: Cardiomyopathy. In Hurst JW (ed): The Heart, 5th ed, pp 1299–1362. New York, McGraw-Hill, 1982
33. Guzetta CE: The person with infective endocarditis. In Guzetta CE, Dossley BM (eds): Cardiovascular Nursing: Bodymind Tapestry, St Louis, CV Mosby, 1984
34. Hanrath P, Schluter M, Sonntag F: Influence of verapamil therapy on left ventricular performance at rest and during exercise in hypertrophic cardiomyopathy. Am J Cardiol 52:544–548, 1983
35. Hayakawa M et al: A long term follow-up study of acute viral and idiopathic myocarditis. Jpn Circ J 47(11):1304–1309, 1983
36. Heffner JE: Extracardiac manifestations of bacterial endocarditis. West J Med 131:85, 1979
37. Hueter DC: Diseases of the pericardium, myocardium, and endocardium. In Wilkins RW, Levinsky NG (eds): Medicine: Essentials of Practice, 2nd ed, pp 389–399. Boston, Little, Brown, & Co, 1978
38. Janas AG, Arjunan K, Meyer RA et al: Differentiation of constrictive pericarditis and restrictive cardiomyopathy using digitalized echocardiography. J Am Coll Cardiol 1(2):541–549, 1983
39. Johanson BD, Dungca CV, Hoffmeister D et al: Standards for Critical Care. St Louis, CV Mosby, 1981
40. Long GD: Myocarditis. Nursing 82, 12:59, 1982
41. Maron BJ, Koch JP, Kent KM et al: Results of surgery for idiopathic hypertrophic subaortic stenosis. J Cardiovasc Med 5:145, 1980
42. May JM: S. aureus endocarditis: A review and plea for early surgery. Virol Med 106:829, 1979
43. McCarty RJ: The medical cardiac patient. In Sanderson RG, Kurth CL (eds): The Cardiac Patient, 2nd ed. Philadelphia, WB Saunders, 1983
44. McGurn WC: Miscellaneous cardiac pathology. In McGurn WC (ed): People with Cardiac Problems: Nursing Concepts, pp 373–387. Philadelphia, JB Lippincott, 1981
45. McKenna WJ: Arrhythmia in hypertrophic cardiomyopathy: Exercise and 48-hour ambulatory electrocardiographic assessment with and without beta-adrenergic blocking therapy. Am J Cardiol 45:1–5, 1980
46. Miller MH, Cassey JI: Infective endocarditis: New diagnostic techniques. Am Heart J 96:123, 1978
47. Mills SA: Surgical management of infective endocarditis. Am Surg 195:364–367, 1982
48. Mookherjee S, Henion W, Warner R et al: Sodium nitroprusside therapy in congestive cardiomyopathy—Variability in hemodynamic response. J Clin Pharmacol 18:67, 1978
49. Mortensen SA, Egeblad H: Endomyocardial biopsy guided by cross-sectional echocardiography. Br Heart J 50:246–251, 1983
50. O'Connell JB, Fowles RE, Robinson JA: Clinical and pathological findings of myocarditis in two families with dilated cardiomyopathy. Am Heart J 107(1):127–135, 1984
51. Pelletier LL, Petersdorf RG: Infective endocarditis: A review of 125 cases from the University of Washington Hospitals, 1963–1972. Medicine 56(4):287–313, 1977
52. Phair JP, Clarke J: Immunology of infective endocarditis. Prog Cardiovasc Dis 22:137, 1979
53. Przybojewski JZ, Daniels AR, Van der Walt JJ: Primary cardiac amyloidosis. A review of the literature. S Afr Med J 57:831, 1980
54. Pura LS, Conchita SS: Underlying causes and precipitating factors in heart failure. In Michaelson CR (ed): Congestive Heart Failure, pp 108–110. St Louis, CV Mosby, 1983
55. Pursley P: Acute cardiac tamponade. Am J Nurs 83(10):1414–1418, 1983
56. Roberts WC, Waller BF: Cardiac amyloidosis causing cardiac dysfunction: Analysis of 54 necropsy patients. Am J Cardiol 52:137–146, 1983

57. Santoro J, Kaye D: Axions of infective endocarditis. Hosp Med 2(1):8–21, 1977
58. Segal JP, Stapleton MF, McClellan JR: Idiopathic cardiomyopathy: Clinical features, prognosis, and therapy. In Harvey WP (ed): Current Problems in Cardiology, pp 1–49. Chicago, Year Book Medical Publishers, 1978
59. Shabetai R: Cardiomyopathy: How far have we come in 25 years, how far yet to go? J Am Coll Cardiol 1:252–263, 1983
60. Spodick DH: The normal and diseased pericardium: Current concepts of pericardial physiology, diagnosis, and treatment. J Am Coll Cardiol 1:240–251, 1983
61. Timmis AD, Daly K, Monaghan M et al: Pericardiocentesis in myocarditis: The protective role of the pericardium in severe heart failure. Br Med J 287(6402):1348, 1983
62. Weinstein L, Schlessinger JJ: Pathoanatomic, pathophysiologic, and clinical correlations in endocarditis, Part I. N Engl J Med 291:832, 1974
63. Weinstein L, Schlessinger JJ: Pathoanatomic, pathophysiologic, and clinical correlations in endocarditis, Part II. N Engl J Med 291:1132, 1974
64. Wold B: Dilated (congestive) cardiomyopathy: Considerations for the coronary care unit nurse. Heart Lung 12(5):544–551, 1983
65. Wynne J, Braunwald E: The Cardiomyopathies and Myocarditis. In Braunwald E (ed): Heart Disease: A Textbook of Cardiovascular Medicine. Philadelphia, WB Saunders, 1981
66. Zucherman J: Rational use of operation in pericardial constriction. Int Surg 62:204, 1977

Chapter 40

Valvular Heart Dysfunction

Sandra L. Underhill

Valvular heart dysfunction is a common health problem. It occurs when the heart valves are unable to fully open (a condition called stenosis) or fully close (a condition called insufficiency or regurgitation). In valvular stenosis, the failure of the valves to open completely causes a decrease in the forward flow of blood from one heart chamber to another. In valvular insufficiency, the inability of the valves to close completely causes some of the blood to flow backward or to regurgitate into the chamber from which it is being propelled.

Valvular heart disease is classified on the basis of four components:

1. The etiology of the lesion, which also includes whether it is acute or chronic
2. The valve or valves involved (mitral, aortic, tricuspid, or pulmonic)
3. The nature of the problem (stenosis, insufficiency, or a combination of the two)
4. The degree of dysfunction as defined by the New York Heart Association (NYHA) Functional and Therapeutic Classification, as described in Chapter 34 (Table 34–2).

Etiology

Rheumatic carditis, resulting from acute rheumatic fever is the most common cause of acquired valvular dysfunction. Rheumatic heart disease primarily involves the left heart valves, especially the mitral valve. However, isolated involvement of one valve is rare. Rheumatic valvular lesions in rank order of occurrence are mitral stenosis, mitral insufficiency, aortic stenosis, and aortic insufficiency. The tricuspid valve is involved infrequently, and the pulmonic valve is affected rarely. The order of frequency of involvement correlates with the hemodynamic stress placed upon each of the valves. The closed mitral valve is subjected to a higher stress by systemic arterial systolic pressure than the closed aortic valve, which is subjected to the systemic diastolic pressures. The right heart is subjected to the low pressures of the pulmonary circulation.[8]

Tests in the diagnosis of valvular heart disease are cardiac catheterization, radionuclide imaging, echocardiography, electrocardiography, exercise testing, and chest radiography.

Mitral Stenosis

Pathophysiology. In response to recurrent rheumatic endocarditis, the valvular leaflets and chordae tendineae become fibrous, and the commissures fuse and the chordae tendineae shorten, narrowing the valvular outflow tract.

Because the velocity of blood flow through the stenotic mitral valve cannot be increased, left atrial pressure (LAP) rises, the left atrium dilates, pulmonary artery pressure (PAP) increases, and the right ventricle hypertrophies.

Pulmonary vascular changes may occur in patients with severe mitral stenosis as a result of structural changes in the aterioles and arteries, and of vasoconstriction in the small arteries. This increase in vascular resistance protects the pulmonary arteries from large increases in right ventricular output, and it protects the patient from resultant symptoms of pulmonary congestion. Pulmonary vasoconstriction is usually reversible following surgical correction of the stenosis.[19]

Clinical Manifestations. Patients with mild mitral stenosis are generally asymptomatic. As the valvular orifice narrows, symptoms appear insidiously and are initially precipitated by exercise. The increased venous return that occurs with exercise causes left atrial pressure to rise because the increased blood volume is unable to move through the stenotic valve.[19]

Patients can be divided into two groups: younger patients with elevated left atrial pressure, a normal cardiac output, and pulmonary congestion; and older patients with high pulmonary vascular resistance, variable degrees of right heart failure, and low cardiac output. Patients in the younger group usually manifest respiratory symptoms such as paroxysmal dyspnea, hemoptysis, or pulmonary edema. The older patients most likely demonstrate findings consistent with low cardiac output, for instance dyspnea, fatigue and weakness. Dyspnea is the most important symptom associated with mitral stenosis; it occurs in both patient groups.[17]

Chronic right ventricular failure produces peripheral edema and hepatic engorgement. Atrial fibrillation from dilatation of the left atrium occurs in 40% of patients with mitral stenosis, usually older patients with long-standing valvular disease. Once atrial fibrillation occurs, left ventricular filling is reduced, the heart rate increases, and blood tends to stagnate in the atria. Because of this movement of blood, mural thrombi are likely to form on the walls of the atria and in the atrial appendages, resulting in pulmonary or systemic embolization.[19]

Physical Assessment. Blood pressure is usually not affected unless the disease process has progressed to the point of causing low cardiac output. The pulse is usually normal on palpation, although the amplitude may be diminished in long-standing disease. The cardiac rhythm may be regular or rapidly irregular, as in atrial fibrillation.

On auscultation, the principal finding is a rumbling, apical diastolic murmur (blood flowing with difficulty and under increased pressure through the stenotic valve). The intensity of the murmur changes with blood flow and may disappear altogether in end-stage disease. With exercise, which increases return, the intensity of the murmur increases.

Cardiac catheterization is the definitive diagnostic test of mitral stenosis. The cross sectional area of the mitral valve and intra-cardiac pressures can be determined. The most important finding is a pressure gradient across the mitral valve, with elevated left atrial pressure or pulmonary artery wedge pressure.

Medical Management. Mitral stenosis, if untreated, has a gradual downhill course that may be accelerated if atrial fibrillation develops. It may also be adversely affected by pregnancy, bacterial endocarditis, or embolization. Definitive therapy for mitral stenosis is surgical, but management by medical therapy is often required to control some aspects of the disease process.

The medical care of rheumatic mitral valvular disease focuses on treating acute pulmonary edema or heart failure, controlling atrial fibrillation, and treating or preventing embolization, bronchopulmonary infection, bacterial endocarditis, and recurrences of rheumatic fever.[15,17] Normal sinus rhythm should be reestablished by electrical cardioversion or by pharmacological agents and maintained with antiarrhythmic therapy. For patients in atrial fibrillation, anticoagulants are necessary for the prevention of thromboemboli.[9]

Mitral Insufficiency

Nonrheumatic Etiology. The common nonrheumatic causes of mitral insufficiency seen in the acute care setting are coronary heart disease, resulting in papillary muscle dysfunction or rupture, and acute bacterial endocarditis, causing rupture of a valve leaflet or the chordae tendineae. Heart failure from any cause may result in ventricular enlargement to such a degree that the atrial annulus becomes dilated and the mitral valve is no longer able to cover the enlarged orifice. Congenital abnormalities can also result in insufficiency.

Pathophysiology. The pathology of mitral insufficiency is the same as mitral stenosis, but the fibrotic and calcific changes occur in such a way that the valve leaflets are prevented from closing rather than opening.

Mitral insufficiency is the result of inadequate valve closure and regurgitant flow from the left ventricle back into the left atrium during ventricular systole. Therefore, the output of the left ventricle is divided into systemic (forward) and regurgitant (backward) flow. The amount of forward vs. backward flow depends on the severity of the insufficiency and the degree of resistance to outflow through the aortic valve (afterload).

Mitral insufficiency results in increased preload of both left-sided chambers. Regurgitant output is returned from the left atrium to the left ventricle during diastole, so that both the normal amount of blood plus the additional regurgitant volume must be ejected during ventricular systole. This high volume forces the heart to work harder and causes both the left atrium and left ventricle to dilate and hypertrophy. When the onset of mitral insufficiency is gradual (rheumatic), usually only a slight rise in ventricular diastolic pressure accompanies the increase in diastolic volume because the left ventricle is able to increase its compliance (ability to distend). However, if the onset is sudden (such as with papillary muscle or chordal rupture), compensatory mechanisms (increased ventricular compliance) do not have time to develop, left ventricular end-diastolic pressures (LVEDP) rapidly increase, heart failure and shock ensue, and death occurs unless the insufficiency is reduced.[19]

When mitral insufficiency is a result of rheumatic heart disease, it usually coexists with some degree of mitral stenosis. A calcified mitral valve that is immobile or "fixed" may produce an insignificant degree of stenosis but a considerable amount of insufficiency.

Clinical Manifestations. Mitral insufficiency usually progresses slowly; patients may remain symptom-free for decades or their entire lives. Early symptoms of mitral insufficiency are exertional dyspnea, palpitations, and fatigue, which are characteristically relieved by rest. They are usually insidious, but they may be precipitated by acute illness such as systemic embolization, atrial fibrillation, pulmonary edema from other causes, pulmonary infection, pulmonary emboli, bacterial endocarditis, spontaneously ruptured chordae, or systemic hypertension. Pulmonary edema and hemoptysis are not as common as in mitral stenosis. In chronic mitral insufficiency, right heart failure is a late development, and it is usually progressive and intractable.[19]

Physical Assessment. On auscultation a loud, systolic murmur can be heard, which is loudest at the apex; it may radiate to the axilla and the back. It is usually high-pitched and blowing, but if very loud, it becomes harsh. In severe mitral insufficiency an S_3 gallop may be heard.

Cardiac catheterization is the definitive diagnostic test for mitral insufficiency. Intra-cardiac pressures can be obtained, the percentage of insufficiency can be assessed, and the mitral valve area can be calculated.

Medical Management. Selection of patients who will benefit from surgical treatment of mitral regurgitation is difficult because postoperative left ventricular function is variable and cannot be predicted easily. If the left ventricle is already compromised, valvular failure can result in left ventricular failure.[3] For this reason and because of postoperative complications, replacement of the mitral valve is usually performed before irreversible left ventricular dysfunction occurs.[15]

Mitral Valve Prolapse

Mitral valve prolapse is more common in females, with a peak incidence in the fourth decade. Etiology of this abnormality is variable and may be seen with myxomatous degeneration of the mitral leaflet tissue, in acute or chronic rheumatic heart disease, in coronary heart disease, and in otherwise apparently healthy individuals.[11] Familial occurrence has been well established.[2]

Mitral valve prolapse occurs as a result of the valvular leaflets enlarging, and the valve billowing and prolapsing into the left atrium during systole. With continuing ballooning of the valve, the supporting structures (chordae tendineae and papillary muscles) are stressed, contraction of the papillary muscles is reduced, and mitral insufficiency occurs.[1]

Clinical Manifestations. Atypical chest pain is common, even in mild cases, and it is usually the presenting symptom. The pain is sharp, localized to the left chest, and may resemble ischemic pain. The pain usually is of short duration, although it may last several hours. This pain is not necessarily associated with electrocardiographic abnormalities or exertion, but it is frequently precipitated by fatigue. Chest pain may be secondary to papillary muscle ischemia (from the stress placed on the papillary muscles during prolapse) or coronary artery spasm (from focal trauma).[5,10] Fatigue, palpitations, and syncope may be associated with arrhythmias, which can be atrial or ventricular in origin; focal trauma has also been implicated as their cause. Chest pain, fatigue, and activity intolerance may be cyclic in nature, improving for long periods for no apparent reason.

Rupture of the chordae tendineae can occur, producing sudden mitral regurgitation. Sudden cardiac death is actually quite uncommon, but it has been widely associated with mitral valve prolapse in the past; it is probably secondary to ventricular fibrillation.

Physical Assessment. Heart rate and blood pressure are usually normal. Inspection and palpation of the precordium reveal no abnormality except in extreme cases of mitral insufficiency.

Auscultatory findings are usually sufficient to diagnose mitral valve prolapse. The first heart sound is followed by a nonejection or mitral click, and by a crescendo–decrescendo murmur that continues to, and sometimes through, the second sound. The click is thought to be due to tensing of the prolapsed leaflet with gradual "give" in the supporting structures. The late systolic murmur is indicative of regurgitant flow through the prolapsed mitral valve. The murmur is heard best at the apex, and it is high-pitched and musical.

Medical Management. Medical management is directed toward relief of symptoms. Chest pain does not always respond to drug therapy, although nitroglycerin provides relief for some patients. Results with propranolol are variable.[2,7] When explaining the atypical chest pain to the patient, it may be helpful to compare it to a headache, which is bothersome but usually of little physiological consequence.[7] Arrhythmias should be treated. Long-term prognosis is generally good. All patients with prolapsed mitral valve should have prophylaxis against bacterial endocarditis. If mitral insufficiency develops, the mitral valve should be replaced.

Aortic Stenosis

Etiology. Nonrheumatic aortic stenosis almost always is a result of a congenitally bicuspid valve. In persons older than 70 years of age calcification of the aortic valve is common and usually nonsignificant.

Rheumatic causes lead to fusion of the commissures with thickening and fibrosis of the cusps, eventually resulting in valve calcification. If all three commissures are affected, the valve becomes immobile, and aortic insufficiency also results.

Pathophysiology. Aortic stenosis results in increased afterload, forcing the left ventricle to hypertrophy with little or no dilatation. This tremendous concentric hypertrophy may allow left ventricular output to remain essentially normal for many years. Ventricular systolic pressures are elevated and may reach 200 to 300 mmHg. These high pressures can only be sustained for short periods, for instance during mild exertion. A marked reduction in cardiac output can result in pulmonary edema. Eventually right heart failure can result.

Clinical Manifestations. Symptoms of aortic stenosis occur because of reduced cardiac output, increased cardiac work load, and increased end-diastolic pressures.

The classic symptoms are syncope that occurs with exertion, angina pectoris, and dyspnea. Significantly reduced cardiac output resulting in reduced cerebral and coronary perfusion also contributes to syncope on exertion. The reduced cardiac perfusion can cause either tachyarrhythmias or bradyarrhythmias, which further diminish cerebral and coronary blood flow. Rarely, syncope may be due to advanced atrioventricular block from conduction system disease.

Angina pectoris may occur even in the absence of significant coronary heart disease, precipitated by the very high myocardial oxygen consumption of the hypertrophied left ventricle and by reduced coronary blood flow. However, angina may be the result of coexisting coronary heart disease. Survival time is approximately 2 years following the appearance of syncope and angina that is not related to coronary heart disease.

Dyspnea is caused by left heart failure and the inability to maintain forward flow. Heart failure and pulmonary edema in the patient with aortic stenosis are ominous.

Sudden death occurs in 14% to 18% of all patients with aortic stenosis, including those who are asymptomatic. Sudden death usually occurs during periods of strenous exercise; it is probably due to ventricular fibrillation.[19]

Physical Assessment. Blood pressure is usually normal in patients with aortic stenosis. An indication of the severity of the stenosis may be reflected by pulse pressure, which decreases to 30 mmHg or less in patients with severe disease. Atrial fibrillation usually does not occur unless there is coexisting mitral stenosis. In advanced disease the carotid pulse characteristically is small, slow-rising, and sometimes prolonged. The pulse may be normalized if aortic insufficiency is also present. The apex impulse is relatively quiet in patients with aortic stenosis. The point of maximal impulse (PMI) is not necessarily displaced (unless there is left heart failure) but is sustained. A presystolic heave may be present.[19] A diamond-shaped systolic murmur is characteristically noted on auscultation.

Cardiac catheterization provides a definitive diagnosis of aortic stenosis by demonstrating a systolic pressure gradient between the left ventricle and the aorta. A pressure gradient of 50 mmHg or more is considered to be significant.

Medical Management. Surgical therapy is the only definitive treatment for aortic stenosis; it is recommended when left ventricular failure, syncope, or angina develop. Because of the risk of sudden death, surgery is recommended in patients who have pressure gradients greater than 50 mmHg, and even in those who are asymptomatic.[14,17] In order to reduce the possibility of sudden death, strenuous physical activity must be stopped in all patients with significant disease until the stenosis can be surgically corrected.

Medical treatment is used to manage the symptoms until surgery can be performed. Heart failure and angina are treated as they occur. Asymptomatic patients with pressure gradients less than 50 mmHg do not require therapy. As with mitral valve disease, prophylaxis against recurrent rheumatic fever and bacterial endocarditis is necessary for patients with aortic stenosis.

Aortic Insufficiency

Nonrheumatic causes of aortic insufficiency include bacterial endocarditis, syphilitic aortitis, cystic medial necrosis, dissecting aortic aneurysms, traumatic tears of the aorta, and congenitally defective bicuspid valves.[8,17]

In rheumatic disease, scarring, rolling, retraction, stiffness, and eventual calcification of the leaflets prevent closure of the cusps. Calcification may result in an immobile valve and a fixed orifice, and therefore combined stenosis and insufficiency.

Pathophysiology. An overload of blood volume into the left ventricle occurs during aortic insufficiency from the combination of blood entering normally from the left atrium and regurgitant blood reentering through the incompetent aortic valve. Retrograde flow occurs during diastole when ventricular pressure is low and aortic pressure is high. The left ventricle dilates and hypertrophies as a result of this volume overload. In total aortic insufficiency, the heart becomes so enlarged that it is termed *ox heart* or *cor bovinum*.

Several compensatory mechanisms exist to maintain normal cardiac function despite valvular incompetence. In long-standing aortic insufficiency, the left ventricle remains compliant, allowing a large increase in volume. A more forceful contraction and a prolonged ejection time result in an increased stroke volume, which commonly may be twice normal. This increased stroke volume allows cardiac output to remain normal. Interestingly, exercise produces beneficial results in these patients by decreasing diastolic reflux. In order to maintain cardiac perfusion, which can be compromised by the increased cardiac work load and the decreased diastolic perfusion pressure, coronary blood flow shifts from diastole to systole. Early in the course of the disease, forward flow is maximized by a lowered systemic vascular resistance. In more advanced stages, the systemic vascular resistance increases, causing retrograde flow to increase as well.

In acute aortic insufficiency with sudden increases in left ventricular volume there is not sufficient time for compensatory mechanisms to develop. Large influxes into a relatively indistensible left ventricle leads to a decrease in the forward flow of blood, and heart failure quickly ensues. Death results unless the pressure gradient can be quickly reduced.[19]

Clinical Manifestations. Significant aortic insufficiency may be present for many years or even a lifetime without the development of symptoms. The first symptom likely to be noted is an awareness of a hyperactive heart and pulse, for example, visible throbbing in the neck and palpitations, especially while lying on the left side. Dizziness, especially when standing up quickly, occurs often and is thought to result from pronounced pressure changes in the cerebral vessels. Dyspnea from moderate exertion occurs commonly but is not necessarily progressive. However, when the patient reaches the point that dyspnea is precipitated by normal activity, a rapid downhill course follows.

More than 50% of patients with aortic insufficiency eventually develop angina pectoris. As an isolated symptom angina does not necessarily represent a poor prognostic sign. When angina becomes atypical, prolonged, or worse at night, and is accompanied by congestive heart failure, the situation becomes serious. Coronary heart disease may be totally or partially responsible for chest pain in the older age-group. Once heart failure clearly develops, the chances of sudden death are increased. A distinctive syndrome has been noted in advanced cases when death appears imminent: tachycardia, sweating, flushing, paroxysmal hypertension, and severe chest pain develop. It is thought that heart failure develops at night because of mobilization of edema fluid. Additional stress is placed upon the system: myocardial oxygen consumption increases, as does systemic vascular resistance. Consequently, as the reflux worsens, angina develops and pulmonary congestion becomes more severe.[19]

Physical Assessment. There are many peripheral signs apparent with moderate to severe aortic insufficiency. A rapidly rising and collapsing pulse ("water-hammer" or Corrigan's pulse) is characteristic with significant aortic insufficiency. The forceful ventricular contraction causes a rapid upstroke, while the retrograde flow and peripheral vasodilatation result in diastolic collapse. Systolic hypertension, decreased diastolic pressure (sometimes as low as 40 mmHg), and a widened pulse pressure are numerical indicators of the bounding pulse. Visible pulsations may be seen in the carotid, subclavian, and brachial arteries. Occasionally, a double systolic peak (pulsus bisferiens) can be felt if firmer than usual pressure is exerted over the carotid pulse. In severe aortic insufficiency, systolic blood pressure may range from 20 to 60 mmHg higher in the legs than in the arms (Hill's sign), probably because of an accentuation of the normal blood pressure response in the lower extremities. Capillary pulsation, representing peripheral vasodilatation, can be observed as alternating flushing and paling of the nailbeds. When large arteries are auscultated, pistol-shot sounds can be heard; a to-and-fro murmur (systolic and diastolic) can be elicited with slight compression by the stethoscope. Head bobbing with each aortic pulsation is also characteristic of hemodynamically significant aortic insufficiency.[19]

On auscultation there is a high-pitched, blowing, decrescendo, diastolic murmur that starts with the second sound; its intensity varies with the pressure gradient.

Cardiac catheterization may be performed prior to surgery for visualization and quantification of the extent of regurgitation. However, physical findings and noninvasive tests are sufficient to establish the diagnosis of aortic insufficiency.

Medical Management. Once symptoms of aortic insufficiency have developed, the aortic valve should be surgically replaced. It is recommended that surgery be performed on patients regardless of symptoms if left ventricular hypertrophy can be documented by chest radiography and electrocardiography and if the systolic blood pressure is 140 mmHg or more with a diastolic blood pressure of 30 mmHg or less. Until that time no treatment may be needed, although the patient should be examined at regular intervals. Heart failure and angina should be managed medically until surgery is performed. Prophylactic measures to prevent recurrence of rheumatic fever and bacterial endocarditis are necessary.

Surgical Management

Repair or replacement of heart valves has had a major effect on the prognosis of valvular heart disease. Correct timing, however, is crucial. If intervention is too early, the patient is denied years of prosthetic-free living; if intervention is too late, irreversible myocardial damage has already occurred.[9]

Reparative Procedures

Repair of a valve, when feasible, is always preferred to replacement. Surgical repair allows the patient to retain his native valve for many years, thus avoiding late complications of prosthetic valves.[9] In selected patients, mitral valve repair can be performed with great success. The aortic valve is rarely repaired, except in aortic stenosis in children; in this instance an aortic commissurotomy may be performed.

Mitral Commissurotomy. Mitral commissurotomy, the procedure of choice in pure mitral stenosis, can be performed closed (without cardiopulmonary bypass) or open. In the United States, with certain exceptions, open mitral commissurotomy is favored. Mitral commissurotomy is offered to patients with symptoms such as dyspnea, activity intolerance, fluid retention, orthopnea, paroxysmal dyspnea, and weight loss that interfere with productivity and enjoyment of life. Establishment or recurrence of atrial fibrillation, or occurrence of arterial thromboemboli are also indications for mitral commissurotomy. Feasibility of this procedure is based on preoperative assessment of a pliable mitral valve: loud, delayed S_1, opening snap, and absence of radiographic evidence of valve calcification.[15]

After a median sternotomy is performed, the heart and the patient are cooled at the start of the cardiopulmonary bypass. The aorta is cross-clamped, multidose, hypothermic potassium cardioplegia is used to protect the heart, and the left atrium is opened. After final evaluation of the feasibility for repair, incisions are made into the anterior lateral and posterior medial commissures. If the chordae are also fused, they may be separated carefully by sharp dissection. The degree of residual insufficiency is assessed. Any thrombi in the left atrium are removed, and the left atrial appendage is oversewn prior to discontinuing bypass. As the cross-clamp is removed and the heart is filled with blood, strict precautions are taken to avoid air emboli.[15]

The postoperative course of patients undergong mitral commissurotomy is similar to that of any patient undergoing heart surgery. Mean left atrial pressure should be maintained at about 14 mmHg using blood transfusions as necessary. If arterial blood pressure is higher than the patient's normal pressure, left ventricular afterload reduction is accomplished by continuous nitroprusside infusion. When possible, sinus rhythm should be maintained, if necessary including the use of atrial pacing at a rate up to 110 impulses/minute. If these measures fail to optimize cardiac performance (based on thermodilution cardiac output measurements), small doses of inotropic agents (*e.g.,* dopamine, dobutamine, isoproterenol, or epinephrine) may be required. If the patient's hemodynamic status is good, he is usually extubated a few hours after surgery.[20]

Hospital mortality is low (approximately 1%) following mitral commissurotomy. Morbidity is minimal, and it may include both atrial and ventricular arrhythmias. Optimal return of function may not be fully achieved for 3 to 6 months following surgery. Most patients have marked clinical improvement. Reoperation may be necessary for some patients after 5 to 20 years.[15]

Mitral Annuloplasty. Mitral annuloplasty is the reparative procedure for an insufficient mitral valve. Mitral annuloplasty involves reconstruction of the leaflets and the annulus. Only about 20% of patients with mitral insufficiency requiring surgery meet the criterion for annuloplasty: a mobile, noncalcified valve.[15]

Timing of surgery (either annuloplasty or replacement) to correct mitral insufficiency is crucial. Rather than delaying surgery as may be recommended for correction of mitral stenosis, early surgery is recommended for correction of mitral insufficiency. Surgery performed early in the course of mitral insufficiency, prior to the onset of symptoms, improves long-term patient survival because left ventricular function is still good. The left ventricle must be capable of enduring an increase in myocardial work, or low cardiac output and congestive heart failure will ensue. If surgery is delayed until left ventricular dysfunction is advanced and irreversible, left ventricular function may worsen, decreasing long-term survival.[15]

The surgical technique of mitral annuloplasty is the same as that described for mitral commissurotomy, except that instead of the mitral orifice being widened, the leaflets and annulus are reconstructured in such a way as to narrow the orifice. Combined mitral commissurotomy and annuloplasty may be done for coexisting mitral stenosis and insufficiency.[15] Operative mortality is related to the patient's preoperative clinical condition.

Replacement Procedures

Mitral Valve Replacement. Mitral valve replacement is indicated if the leaflets are calcified and immobile. Surgical technique is similar to that described for mitral commissurotomy. The valve is excised, leaving sufficient residual valvular tissue for valve seating. The new valve, either biological or prosthetic, is sutured into place (Fig. 40–1). If there is associated coronary heart disease, saphenous vein grafts are used to bypass the lesion. Valve replacement is associated with more late complications than is repair, and it is related to the degree of disability prior to surgery.[15]

Aortic Valve Replacement. Aortic valve replacement is indicated for both aortic stenosis and aortic insufficiency. A median sternotomy is performed, and the patient is placed on cardiopulmonary bypass as described for mitral commissurotomy. The aortic valve is removed, and the replacement valve is sutured into place. Coronary artery bypass grafting can be done if there is associated coronary heart disease.

Immediate postoperative care is the same as described for patients following valve surgery. Most patients have good hemodynamic status after aortic valve replacement. Many patients have arterial hypertension, which stresses the aortotomy and increases left ventricular afterload; nitroprusside is used to decrease the high blood pressure by reducing afterload. Premature ventricular contractions are treated aggressively with antiarrhythmic agents. Atrial pacing between 90 and 100 impulses/minute also effectively suppresses the ventricular arrhythmias, but without the complications frequently associated with pharmacological therapy.[14]

The current operative mortality for isolated aortic valve replacement is between 2% and 3%. If coronary artery bypass grafting is added, operative mortality increases to 3% to 5%. Hemorrhage is an important cause of early postoperative mortality.[14]

Following valve replacement for aortic stenosis, ventricular function is fairly stable. These patients attain near normal indices of cardiac function. Even severely symptomatic patients with aortic stenosis have good recovery and long-term survival following surgery. There is slightly less favorable long-term prognosis in patients whose aortic valves were replaced because of insufficiency. This poorer prognosis is related to left ventricular dysfunction seen in aortic insufficiency, even among those who are asymptomatic. For this reason surgery is now recommended earlier in patients with significant left ventricular volume overload from aortic regurgitation.[14]

Prosthetic and Biological Valves. Recent advances in the surgical therapy and prognosis of valvular heart disease are due in part to the development of prosthetic (synthetic) and biological (tissue) valves. The selection of a particular valve is based on several factors: the design of the valve, durability, the potential for thrombosis, and hemodynamic properties. The factors are weighed against the size of the annulus and certain clinical conditions, such as the desirability of long-term anticoagulation. Prosthetic valves are categorized according to the pattern of blood flow (central or lateral) through the valve.

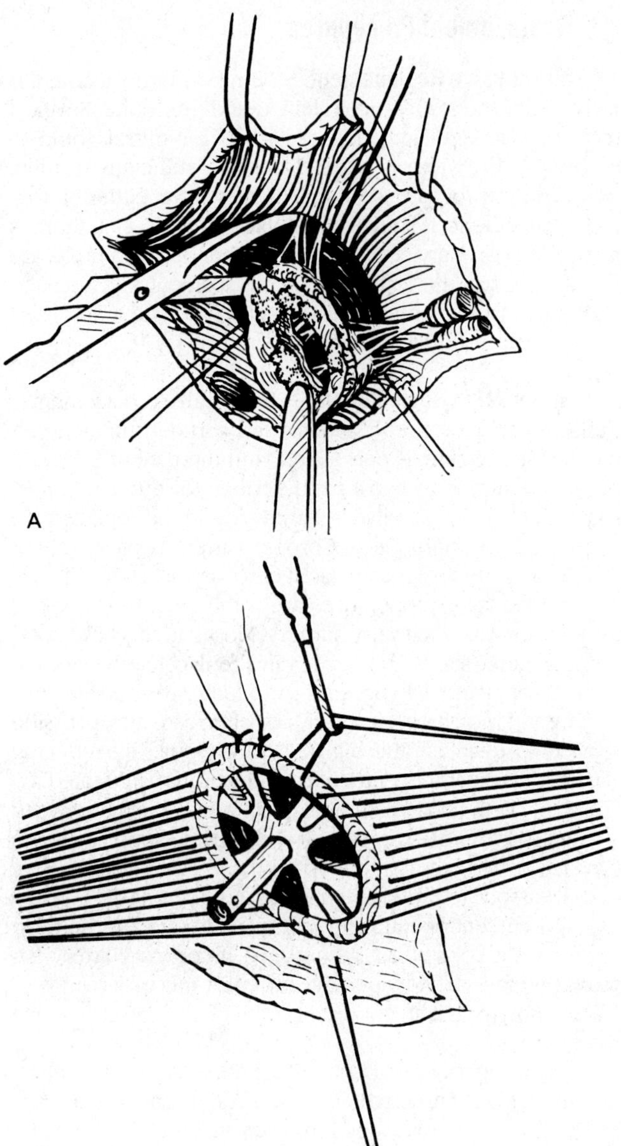

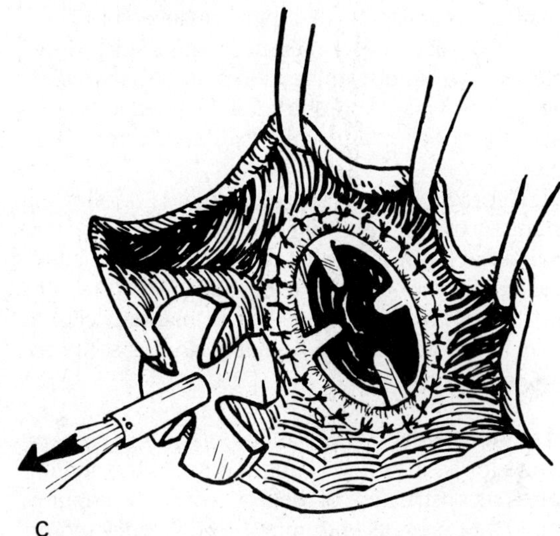

FIGURE 40–1 Mitral valve replacement. The diseased valve is excised (*A*) and replaced by a prosthesis sutured into the annulus (*B, C*)

Central flow valves nearly simulate normal blood flow. At present, only biological valves achieve this pattern. An example is the Hancock stent-mounted porcine xenograft (Fig. 40–2, *A*).

A major advantage to biological valves is that they are essentially nonthrombogenic. Patients who are in normal sinus rhythm do not require long-term anticoagulation. The reduced threat of thrombosis with these valves is particularly important for those patients in whom long-term anticoagulation should be avoided, such as children, young adult females, patients over 70 years old, or persons with a history of bleeding peptic ulcer disease.[14] However, biological valves are not as durable as prosthetic valves, and they usually require replacement every 7 to 10 years.

Lateral flow valves are synthetic protheses which direct blood away from the normal central flow. The Starr-Edwards ball valve (Fig. 40–2, *B*) consists of a metal cage with three struts and an enclosed hollow stellite ball. Changes in chamber pressure cause the ball to move back and forth in its cage, opening and closing the valvular orifice. Disk valves have a flat lens suspended in an abbreviated cage; the disk opens and closes in response to differences in chamber pressure (Fig. 40–2, *C*). Although improvements have helped reduce the possibility of thrombosis, at the present time it is recommended that all patients with prosthetic valves have long-term oral anticoagulation.

Complications. Complications of prosthetic or biological valves include thromboembolism, infection, prosthesis malfunction, paravalvular leak, and hemolytic anemia.

Emboli usually occur because patients have not achieved adequate anticoagulation (prothrombin time is two to two-and-a-half times normal). Dipyridamole may be added to coumarin to lower the incidence of thromboemboli.[9]

Because a prosthetic or biological valve is susceptible to harboring blood-borne bacteria, all patients should be given prophylactic antibiotics during dental and other minor surgical procedures, or at the earliest indication of infection. Prosthetic valve endocarditis is a serious complication, which may lead to valve dehiscence, heart failure, and emboli. Treatment consists of antibiotic therapy alone, or it may require replacement of the prosthetic valve.[9]

Malfunction of the prosthetic valve may occur as a consequence of thrombus formation, alteration in the structure of the valve (wear and tear over time), the ball or disk sticking in the cage, or improper surgical technique (incorrect placement or size).[9] Valvular replacement is usually indicated.

Paravalvular leaks between the prosthetic ring and the annulus occur because of spontaneous tears of the suture line or because of infection. The patient's clinical course should be followed; when the leak becomes significant, surgical repair or replacement is indicated.[9]

Hemolytic anemia is a consequence of shortened red cell survival time in all patients with prosthetic valves. Move-

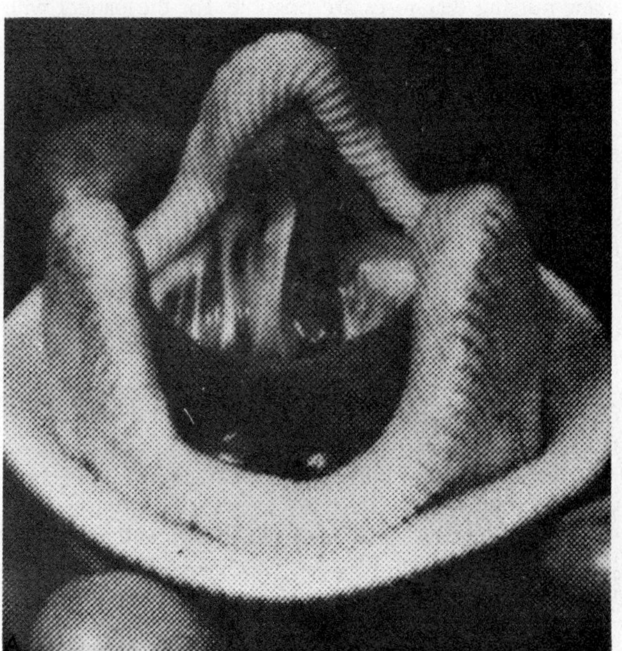

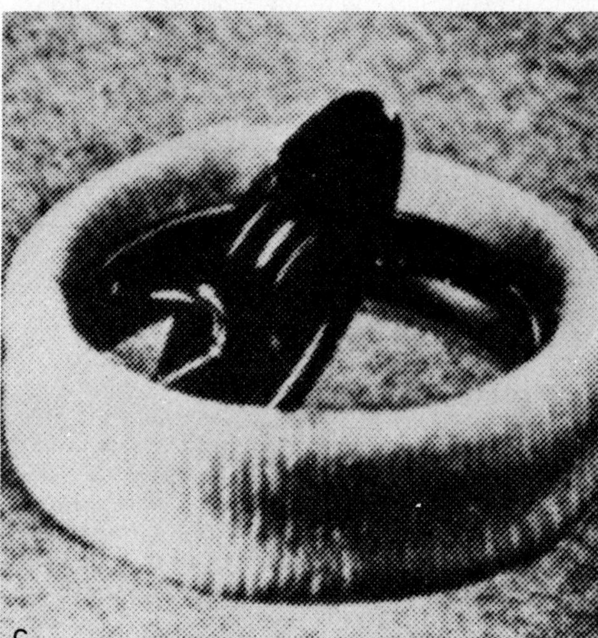

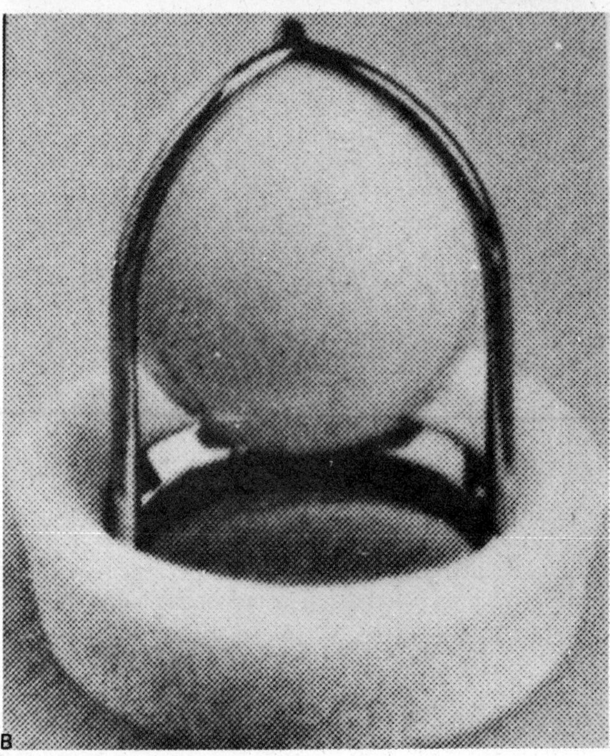

FIGURE 40–2 Examples of prosthetic valves. (*A*) A Hancock stent-mounted porcine xenograft. (*B*) Starr-Edwards ball valve. (*C*) Björk-Shiley disk valve. (Cohn LH, Collins JJ: Primary Cardiology 4(4):15, 1978)

ment of the valve ball or disk causes varying degrees of destruction of the red blood cells. Commonly, hemolysis is mild and the patient can compensate by increasing red blood cell production. Rarely, hemolytic anemia occurs. Chronic intravascular hemolysis causes loss of iron in the urine; iron deficiency anemia may result after several years.[19]

Postoperative Management

Generally, these patients are given anticoagulants (*e.g.*, coumarin) starting 48 hours postoperatively for a duration of 10 days to 6 weeks. If the valve was replaced rather than repaired, depending on the type of replacement valve and the patient's rhythm, oral anticoagulants may be required for life.[15] If atrial fibrillation persists despite pharmacological or electrical attempts to cardiovert the rhythm, chronic digitalis or propranolol therapy is indicated to control ventricular response rate. Prophylactic antibiotics against bacterial endocarditis should continue for life.

Nursing Management

Assessment and Nursing Diagnosis

Nursing management of the patient with valvular heart disease may involve caring for the patient in varying stages of the disease process: as the diagnosis is made; when severe symptoms interfere with the ability to perform daily functions; immediately before, during, or after surgery; or during a stable period. Nursing responsibilities differ for each stage.

Nursing History. The nursing history of a patient with valvular heart disease provides important information pertaining to current symptoms and their effects on the patient's activities of daily living; the usual response to a stressful situation, such as a new diagnosis; the patterns of previous adherence to prescribed therapy; lifestyle habits; and underlying knowledge base of health in general and valvular heart disease in particular.

Physical Assessment. In valvular heart disease, symptoms (such as shortness of breath, fatigue, and chest pain) are nonspecific, and complications (such as infection, heart failure, and thromboemboli) have multiple etiologies. Information obtained from physical assessment assists the clinician to diagnose the specific etiology of the symptom and to evaluate the course of prescribed therapy.

Most nurses are not expected to diagnose the etiologies of murmurs. Acquired valvular heart disease usually develops insidiously; the physician confirms the diagnosis of chronic, rheumatic valvular heart disease and follows the patient in a clinic setting. When these patients are admitted to the hospital, it is with a diagnosis of known valvular disease. In these instances, the nurse is provided with baseline data on which to compare initial and subsequent findings. If the patient's condition deteriorates, a change in the murmur should be reported to the physician.

All nurses working in cardiac care units should be able to diagnose the murmur of papillary dysfunction. The patient with acute myocardial infarction is at risk for developing papillary muscle dysfunction as a result of papillary muscle ischemia. In this instance, a new murmur of mitral regurgitation would be evident. It is imperative that the diagnosis be made as soon as possible so that appropriate therapy to reduce myocardial oxygen demand be instituted. If unrecognized, papillary muscle ischemia could progress to infarction and rupture, usually at the site of chordal attachment.

Nursing Diagnoses. With individualized patient care, many nursing diagnoses are possible. For the patient with valvular heart disease, the most frequently encountered, currently accepted nursing diagnoses follow.[13]

Alteration in breathing pattern related to the hemodynamics associated with mitral or aortic stenosis or insufficiency, or pulmonary embolism as a consequence of atrial fibrillation, manifested by dyspnea at rest or with exertion

Decreased cardiac output related to the hemodynamics associated with mitral or aortic stenosis or insufficiency, manifested by fatigue, dizziness, or syncope

Activity intolerance related to the hemodynamics of mitral or aortic stenosis or insufficiency, or reduction in coronary, cerebral, or skeletal muscle perfusion as a result of decreased cardiac output, manifested by exertional dyspnea, effort angina, effort syncope, exertional palpitations, or fatigue

Alteration in comfort: pain, related to increased myocardial oxygen consumption associated with aortic stenosis, or reduced coronary blood flow associated with the hemodynamics of mitral or aortic stenosis or insufficiency, manifested by angina pectoris

Absence of cardiac output related to cardiac arrest as a consequence of severe aortic stenosis or mitral valve prolapse, manifested by unconsciousness and absence of pulse and respiration

Alteration in comfort: pain, related to invasive procedures or valvular surgery, manifested by incisional pain

Extracellular fluid volume excess related to primary right ventricular failure associated with mitral stenosis, or biventricular failure associated with mitral insufficiency, or aortic stenosis or insufficiency, manifested by peripheral, dependent edema, weight gain, loss of appetite, or ascites

Anxiety related to newly diagnosed valvular heart disease with associated implications for lifesytle change, or fear of cardiac arrest as a consequence of aortic stenosis or mitral valve prolapse, manifested by changes in normal behavior patterns, increased heart and respiratory rate, increased blood pressure, diaphoresis, or changes in facial expression

Increased cardiac output related to the hemodynamics associated with mitral and aortic insufficiency, manifested by a hyperdynamic heart and pulse, and signs of left ventricular dilatation and hypertrophy

Noncompliance related to knowledge deficit, the complexity of the prescribed regimen, lack of communication, or a variety of personal factors (to be determined from the nursing history), manifested by missed appointments, partially used or unused medications, behavior that deviates from that which is prescribed, persistence of symptoms, or progression of the disease process[6]

Alteration in cerebral tissue perfusion related to thromboemboli as a consequence of inadequate anticoagulation, manifested by signs and symptoms of a stroke

Potential for infection as a result of surgery, dental procedures, intravenous drug abuse, or noncompliance with prophylactic antibiotics, resulting in signs and symptoms of bacterial endocarditis or recurrent rheumatic fever

Knowledge deficit related to new diagnosis, lack of motivation, denial of problem, inability to learn (lack of readiness to learn, language problem, decreased cerebral perfusion, or other personal priorities, such as relief of chest pain or dyspnea), manifested by verbalizing knowledge deficit, expressing inaccurate perceptions, or incorrectly performing or not complying with a prescribed behavior.[6]

Interventions and Evaluation

Symptoms and complications of valvular heart disease are nonspecific. Nursing care of patients with valvular heart disease focuses on symptom management: early detection, treatment, and prevention. Goals, interventions, and evaluations of goal achievement for each of the above nursing diagnoses have been described elsewhere in this text.

References

1. Barlow JB, Bosman CK, Pocock WA et al: Late systolic murmurs and non-ejection ("mid-late") systolic clicks. Br Heart J 30:203–218, 1968
2. Barlow JB, Pocock WA: The problem of nonejection systolic clicks and associated mitral systolic murmurs: Emphasis on the billowing mitral leaf syndrome. Am Heart J 90(5):636–655, 1975
3. Brockman SK: Surgery of the cardiac patient. In Silber EN, Katz LN (eds): Heart Disease, pp 1301–1390. New York, Macmillan, 1975
4. Buda AJ, Levene DL, Myers MG et al: Coronary artery spasm and mitral valve prolapse. Am Heart J 95(4):457–462, 1978
5. Carpenito LJ: Handbook of Nursing Diagnosis. Philadelphia, JB Lippincott, 1984
6. Cobbs BW Jr: Clinical recognition and medical management of rheumatic heart disease and other acquired valvular disease. In Hurst JW, Logue RB, Schlant RC et al (eds): The Heart, 3rd ed, pp 826–971. New York, McGraw-Hill, 1974
7. Eliot RS, Edwards JE: Pathology of rheumatic fever and chronic valvular disease. In Hurst JW, Logue RB, Schlant RC et al (eds): The Heart, 4th ed, pp 952–965. New York, McGraw-Hill, 1978
8. Fortuin NJ: Cardiac murmurs and other manifestations of valvular heart disease. In Harvey AM, Johns RJ, McKusick VA et al (eds): The Principles and Practice of Medicine, 21st ed, pp 203–221. Norwalk, Appleton-Century-Crofts, 1984
9. Gottlieb R, Chung EK: Mitral valve prolapse–click syndrome. In Chung EK (ed): Quick Reference to Cardiovascular Disease, pp 87–94. Philadelphia, JB Lippincott, 1977
10. Hall M: Echocardiography, radioisotope studies, and phonocardiography. In Underhill SL, Woods SL, Sivarajan ES, and Halpenny CJ (eds): Cardiac Nursing, pp 276–287. Philadelphia, JB Lippincott, 1982
11. Kim MJ, McFarland GK, McLane AM: Classification of Nursing Diagnoses. Proceedings of the Fifth National Conference. St. Louis, CV Mosby, 1984
12. Rackley CE, Edwards JE, Karp RB et al: Aortic valve disease. In Hurst JW, Logue RB, Rackley CE et al (eds): The Heart, 5th ed, pp 863–892. New York, McGraw-Hill, 1982
13. Rackley CE, Edwards JE, Karp RB et al: Mitral valve disease. In Hurst JW, Logue RB, Rackley CE et al (eds): The Heart, 5th ed, pp 892–927. New York, McGraw-Hill, 1982
14. Shaffer AB, Silber EN: Rheumatic fever and rheumatic heart disease. In Silber EN, Katz LN (eds): Heart Disease, pp 697–758. New York, Macmillan, 1975
15. Underhill SL: Valvular disorders. In Underhill SL, Woods SL, Sivarajan ES, Halpenny CJ (eds): Cardiac Nursing, pp 635–650. Philadelphia, JB Lippincott, 1982
16. Winkle RA, Lopes MG, Popp RL et al: Life threatening arrhythmias in the mitral valve prolapse syndrome. Am J Med 60(7):961–967, 1976

Section 2

Vascular Function

Chapter 41

Review of Anatomy and Physiology
Blood Vessels and Lymphatics

Barbara R. Landau

The vascular system carries the blood to and from the cells in arteries, arterioles, capillaries, venules, and veins. The exchange between blood and interstitial fluid occurs only in capillaries; the other vessels are for transport. Arterial vessels deliver blood rapidly under high pressure, and venous vessels collect and return it to the heart at low pressure. Their structure reflects their different roles.

Structure of Blood Vessels

Three layers of tissue are recognized in blood vessel walls, but all layers are not present in each vessel (Fig. 41–1). The *tunica intima,* the innermost layer, consists of a single layer of squamous epithelium—the endothelium—plus a minimal amount of subendothelial connective tissue. The *tunica media,* which is often quite thick, may be predominantly smooth muscle, elastic or collagenous fibers, or a combination. The *tunica adventitia* is mostly collagenous connective tissue and blends into the surrounding fascia or subcutaneous tissue. Large vessels may contain vasa vasorum, the small blood vessels that supply vascular tissue.

Arteries and Arterioles. The largest arteries are called elastic arteries because of the large amount of elastic tissue in the tunica media. It enables them to distend and accommodate the blood forced into them during systole, and to recoil and maintain pressure during diastole. In more peripheral arteries the proportion of elastic tissue declines and smooth muscle increases as the vessels become smaller and their walls thinner. Muscular arteries are small arteries with a considerable amount of smooth muscle. Smooth muscle is also the outstanding feature of arterioles, but the smallest arterioles have only a single layer of smooth muscle cells spiraling around them. Because the small muscular arteries and arterioles can change diameter, they are the resistance vessels, and are responsible for changes in the peripheral resistance.

Capillaries. Capillaries are the smallest vessels; they are about 1 to 2 mm in length and their diameter is about that of an erythrocyte. The capillary wall is only endothelial cells and a basement membrane, with a few connective tissue fibers and perivascular cells along the outer surface. Almost all of the exchange across capillary walls is passive transfer through the intercellular junctions. Lipid-soluble substances, including oxygen and carbon dioxide, can diffuse through the cells, and some large molecules are taken in by pinocytosis on one side, transported across the cell, and extruded from the other side by exocytosis.

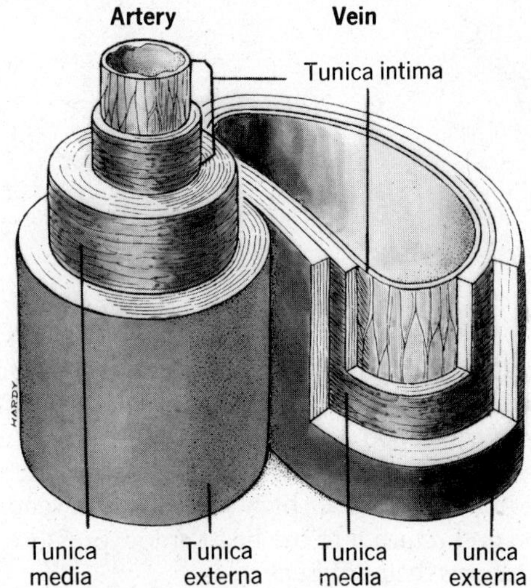

FIGURE 41-1 Medium-sized artery and vein showing relative size and thickness of the three coats, or tunics.

Veins and Venules. In general, the lumens of venules and veins are much larger than those of corresponding arteries. The walls are much thinner and collapse readily; there is little elastic tissue, and only a limited amount of smooth muscle. Because of their great capacity, veins are a potential blood reservoir and are known as capacitance vessels.

Hemodynamics

The distribution of blood throughout the vascular system is governed by several components. Flow, pressure, and resistance are the primary factors. The volume and capacity of the system, velocity of flow, and elasticity of the vessels modify the effects of the primary factors.

Flow

Flow is the volume of fluid flowing past a given point per unit time, and is usually measured as milliliters or liters per minute. In the systemic circuit, flow means the cardiac output, but flow can also refer to the blood flow to an organ or part. Maintenance of an adequate blood flow through the entire circuit and to individual organs is the function of the cardiovascular system. Like any fluid, blood flows from a region of high pressure to one of low pressure. The volume of flow is proportional to that pressure gradient, but is impeded by any resistance along the way.

Pressure

Two aspects of pressure are important: the pressure inside the vessel and the pressure gradient along its length. The actual distending force is the transmural pressure, which is the difference between the pressure inside the vessel (the hydrostatic pressure) and that outside the vessel (the tissue pressure). The distending force is resisted by the tension within the wall of the vessel. The law of Laplace, as applied to blood vessels, states that

$$P = T/R$$

where P = transmural pressure, T = wall tension, and R = radius. Thus in small-diameter vessels, less wall tension is needed to withstand a distending pressure, which explains why thin-walled capillaries are able to withstand moderately high pressures. The tension required in the wall of the aorta is several thousand times that needed for capillaries. A weak spot in a vessel wall is less able to withstand the internal pressure.

The other important aspect of pressure is the pressure gradient from one end of the vessel to the other; it is the driving force that causes the blood to flow. If pressure were the same everywhere, there would be no flow no matter how great that pressure. In the circulatory system, blood is pumped into the arteries at a high pressure and it returns to the heart at a pressure near 0, so the pressure gradient in the circuit is virtually equal to the arterial (aortic) pressure.

Resistance

A rather high pressure is required to move blood through the vascular system because of several types of resistance to flow, namely, the viscosity of the blood, and the length and diameter of the vessel (and vascular bed). Viscosity is the internal resistance of the fluid to changing its shape (as occurs when it flows). The greater the viscosity, the more pressure is required to cause flow. Viscosity of blood varies with the hematocrit and plasma protein concentration, and is increased when either is raised.

The frictional resistance caused by fluid sliding along vessel walls is proportional to the area of contact, and therefore is related to the length and diameter of the vessel. In a large vessel, the outermost layer of blood is slowed by contact with the stationary wall, but inner layers are slowed less and in the center there is little frictional drag. In small-diameter vessels, especially capillaries, relatively more of the blood is in contact with the vessel wall, and frictional resistance is greatest in these vessels. Any roughness of the internal surface of the vessel also increases resistance.

The relationship between the factors that contribute to the resistance to flow as derived from Poiseuille's law is

$$R = 8\eta L/\pi r^4$$

where R = total resistance, η = viscosity, L = vessel length, and r = radius of the vessel. The most significant feature is the great effect of the radius of the vessel: flow is doubled by an increase in radius of less than 20%. This is physiologically important because vessel radius is the only readily variable component of resistance. Although frictional resistance is greatest in capillaries, the smooth muscle in resistance vessels (arterioles and small muscular arteries) is the variable resistance needed to regulate pressure and flow.

The curve of pressures in the systemic circuit shows the same contour, with pressure highest in the arteries and falling continually to the right atrium. The drop is greatest where the resistance is greatest—across the variable diameter arterioles and small muscular arteries and the very small diameter capillaries—leaving a low pressure in the veins. Increasing peripheral resistance by arteriolar constriction raises arterial (upstream) pressure and is a major mechanism for controlling mean arterial pressure. Vasodilatation lowers peripheral resistance and arterial pressure, and raises pressure downstream in the capillaries and small veins.

In summary, flow of blood, or any other fluid, is directly proportional to the pressure gradient, and inversely related to the resistance:

$$F = P/R, \text{ or } P = F \times R$$

When applied to the circulatory system, flow is the cardiac output, the pressure gradient may be taken as the mean arterial pressure, and the resistance is the total peripheral resistance, especially that of the resistance vessels and capillaries. Thus, if flow is to remain constant, an increase in resistance must be accompanied by an increase in pressure. Likewise, arterial pressure is determined by flow (cardiac output) and resistance to flow (peripheral resistance).

Although these relationships are more often applied to the systemic circuit, they apply to the pulmonary circuit as well. The flow (cardiac output) is the same in both, but the resistance is much lower in the pulmonary circuit, and the pressure is correspondingly less.

Volume and Capacity

It is apparent that without enough fluid to fill the system, there will be no pressure. It has been estimated that the blood volume is sufficient to cause a pressure of 7 mmHg throughout the entire circulatory system. (The pumping action of the heart transfers blood from the venous side to the arterial side, creating a pressure gradient.) A reduction in blood volume (due either to loss of fluid from the body or from the vascular system) makes it difficult for compensatory mechanisms to maintain pressure and flow.

The total blood volume of 4 to 6 liters is distributed unevenly throughout the vascular system. At a given instant, approximately 20% of the blood in the systemic circuit is in the arteries, 5% is in the capillaries, and 75% is in the venules and veins. (The *flow* through them is the same, however.) The pressure is relatively high in arteries, and the elastic arteries can be further distended, though the increase in their capacity is not great. Blood is under low pressure in veins, and under ordinary conditions many veins are partially collapsed (flattened), but a very small pressure increase will round them out and greatly increase their content. It is because of their great capacity and the ease of increasing it that the venous system is a potential reservoir for blood, and veins are known as capacitance vessels.

Velocity of Flow

The velocity at which fluid moves through a tube is determined by the flow and the size of the tube. (It is important to distinguish between *velocity,* as measured by distance per unit time, mm/sec, and *flow,* which is volume per unit time, ml/min). When flow is constant, the velocity varies inversely with the cross-sectional area of the channel. The cross-sectional area to be considered, however, is not that or each vessel but the area of the vascular bed at the level. The aorta is the largest artery, but as all of the blood flows through the aorta, its cross-sectional area is that of the entire vascular bed. As the aorta branches into smaller vessels, the total cross-sectional area of the vascular bed increases considerably.

The cross-sectional area of a single capillary is less than 0.05 cm^2, but there are so many capillaries that the total cross-sectional area of capillaries is in the range of 4000 cm^2. Accordingly, the average velocity in the aorta is approximately 30 to 35 cm/sec, but only about 0.03 cm/sec in capillaries, roughly a 1000-fold difference. Velocity increases again as blood moves into progressively larger veins, but does not reach that in the aorta because the cross-sectional area of the two venae cavae is greater than that of the aorta.

Pulsatile Flow

The preceding descriptions were based on a continuous flow of blood, but the heart ejects blood intermittently. It forces about 70 to 80 ml of blood into the aorta in about 0.3 sec, followed by about 0.5 sec during which no blood enters the aorta. Because of the peripheral resistance, blood forced into it does not simply flow through to the capillaries. When a pulsatile pump forces fluid into a rigid tube with some resistance at its outlet, pressure in the tube rises sharply with each stroke and fluid spurts from the open end with great force, but the pressure drops suddenly at the end of the stroke and flow abruptly declines. In an elastic tube such as the aorta and other elastic arteries, much of the pressure energy imparted to the ejected blood is transferred to the vessel walls as a distending force which increases their capacity and allows them to accommodate more of the just-ejected blood. The pressure in the artery rises, giving added impetus to the movement of blood, but neither the pressure nor the velocity increases as much as in a rigid-walled vessel. At the end of systole there is no more ventricular force to cause movement of the blood, but with the elastic recoil of the arteries, the energy that distended them is applied to the blood and maintains a pressure on it to drive it through the resistance offered by the arterioles and capillaries. Pressure in the arterial system slowly declines throughout diastole because the volume of blood in them steadily decreases.

In order for there to be pressure in a duct or vessel between strokes of a pulsatile pump, there must be both a resistance at the outflow and elasticity of the vessel wall. Without the resistance, fluid rapidly flows through with little pressure rise. Without elasticity, the wall is not distended, and pressure rises sharply during ejection, but there is no elastic recoil to maintain pressure between strokes.

The pressure increase during systole is rapidly transmitted through the arterial blood as a pressure wave. It travels over the arterial tree, causing the distension (the pulse) that can be palpated in any artery. The contour of the pressure wave changes slightly as it moves peripherally, and is damped considerably at the arterioles; pulsations have usually been extinguished at capillaries and veins. To a certain extent, the pressure wave is reflected back from the smaller vessels to sum with the pulse wave of the next heart beat. As a result, systolic pressure is higher and diastolic pressure is lower in more distal arteries (abdominal aorta, femoral artery) than in the ascending aorta. The mean arterial pressure, however, always declines further from the heart.

Pressure and Flow in Systemic Arteries

The arterial pressure is a primary concern because it is the driving force that causes the flow of blood through the tissues. It is also a resisting force which the left ventricle must overcome in order to pump blood, and a pressure blood vessels must withstand. The pressure and flow of blood in arteries (either the whole arterial system or the arteries to a particular organ) are regulated by mechanisms that bring about adjustments in those hemodynamic factors just described.

The pressure in arteries is determined by the flow of blood into them from the heart and the resistance to flow out of them into the capillaries. The other significant factor is that of volume and capacity: the blood volume must be sufficient to cause some pressure. The two mechanisms of the minute-to-minute regulation of mean arterial pressure are the cardiac output and the variable aspect of arteriolar vasoconstriction.

Cardiac Output

Cardiac output is determined by heart rate and stroke volume. The heartbeat is initiated by pacemaker cells in the sinoatrial node, whose discharge frequency is altered mainly by autonomic nerves that end near them. Inhibitory parasympathetic (vagal) and excitatory sympathetic fibers are both tonically active, but the vagal effects are dominant. These fibers are the efferent limb of reflexes whose afferents influence both cardiac and vasomotor centers. That is, most stimuli that alter heart rate also alter arteriolar resistance. The presence of certain hormones (*e.g.,* epinephrine), drugs, or ion changes in the environment of pacemaker cells also affects heart rate.

Stroke volume is determined by the pressure in the aorta and the contractility of the myocardium. The arterial pressure, as a resistance to ejection of blood, is an afterload which must be overcome in order to pump blood into the artery. Contractility refers to the force or tension developed by contraction of the myocardial fibers. It is affected primarily by the venous return and diastolic filling (and distension or stretch of the muscle fibers) which has the effect of a preload. An adequate venous return depends to a great extent on factors which prevent pooling in the large-capacity venous system. Sympathetic stimulation and epinephrine also increase the force of ventricular contraction at a given diastolic volume.

Peripheral Resistance

All forms of resistance affect arterial pressure, but it is the resistance offered by smooth muscle in arterioles and small arteries that alters peripheral resistance to regulate mean arterial pressure. The peripheral resistance is increased by vasoconstriction and reduced by vasodilatation. The amount of constriction is determined by neural effects and by local chemical changes.

The innervation of vascular smooth muscle is almost entirely sympathetic. Vascular smooth muscle in most organs (including skin and viscera) have α-adrenergic receptors which cause contraction (constriction). The vascular beds of the abdominal viscera and skin are large enough that resistance changes in them can markedly change mean arterial pressure, and the net effect of sympathetic stimulation is an increase in peripheral resistance and mean arterial pressure.

Sympathetic discharge of vasomotor neurons is mediated through a vasomotor center of the medulla. Constrictor or pressor (sympathetic) neurons, and dilator or depressor (parasympathetic) neurons are intermingled with cardiac accelerator and inhibitory neurons, and most inputs that affect one affect all. That is, a stimulus that causes cardiac acceleration also increases vasoconstriction, and reduces tone of cardiac inhibitors and the few parasympathetic vasodilators. Thus, the input to vasomotor centers is the same as to the cardiac centers, and includes the baroreceptors in the carotid and aortic sinuses, which provide what is probably the most important minute-to-minute regulation of arterial pressure. Other input comes from the low-pressure receptors in the atria and great veins, arterial chemoreceptors, and a wide variety of sensory receptors (*e.g.,* pain receptors). A number of centers in the brain, including several areas of the cortex, also influence the medullary centers. The hypothalamus, in its temperature regulating role and as a channel for input from various areas of the cortex, exerts important controls over these cardiovascular centers.

Control of skeletal muscle blood vessels is more complex. They are not highly innervated, but the smooth muscle cells have α- and β-adrenergic, as well as cholinergic receptors. The α receptors cause constriction; the β receptors have a dilator action. A few sympathetic neurons release acetylchloine which also causes dilatation when it binds to cholinergic receptors. In skeletal muscle, the usual effect of sympathetic stimulation is a decrease in resistance because the dilatation brought about by binding β and cholinergic receptors overrides the vasoconstrictor effects of binding α receptors. Thus, sympathetic stimulation increases peripheral resistance in most vascular beds, but lowers it in skeletal muscle vessels.

In addition to neural controls, peripheral vessels are affected by local conditions, which are particularly important for skeletal muscle vessels. Skeletal muscle is capable of great increases in metabolic rate, which causes changes in the composition of the interstitial fluid around the muscle cells and their blood vessels. These include increases in carbon dioxide, lactic acid, and perhaps other metabolities, and in H^+ and K^+, osmolality, and temperature, as well as a decrease in oxygen. All of these changes have a dilator effect on the vessels in that region. Thus, skeletal muscle activity causes local changes that dilate muscle vessels and markedly reduce resistance in those vessels, and increase blood flow to the active muscles.

Among other chemicals that are vasodilators are histamine, kinins, and some prostaglandins. Chemicals with a constrictor action include serotonin, some prostaglandins, and angiotensin.

Renin–Angiotensin System. Angiotensin, one of the most powerful vasoconstrictors known, is derived from angiotensinogen (renin substrate) which is present in the blood. Renin, an enzyme produced by juxtaglomerular cells in the kidney, activates angiotensinogen to angiotensin I, which becomes angiotensin II by the action of a converting enzyme chiefly in the lungs (Fig. 41–2). Angiotensin II has a half-life of only 1 to 2 min, as it is rapidly inactivated in the lungs and several other tissues. During this brief time it exerts two important actions: arteriolar vasoconstriction with the accompanying increase in mean arterial pressure, and stimulation of aldosterone secretion by the adrenal cortex. Aldosterone increases sodium reabsorption and potassium excretion by the distal and collecting tubules in the kidney.

The presence and action of angiotensin II depends primarily on renin, which also has a short half-life. A number of factors cause renin release, and most of them decrease the extracellular fluid (ECF) volume or arterial pressure (especially in the renal arteries), or cause sympathetic discharge. The juxtaglomerular cells, which are located in the walls of the afferent arterioles, also function as baroreceptors and release renin in response to a fall in pressure in these vessels. Adjacent to the juxtaglomerular cells is the macula densa, a modified portion of the distal tubule. It contains cells that are stimulated by some aspect of ion transport, probably a decreased rate of transport of Na^+ (or Cl^-) from the lumen of the distal tubule. A reduction in ion transport in the distal tubule causes release of renin from the juxtaglomerular cells. The renin–angiotensin system, therefore, is activated by a reduction of ECF volume or arterial pressure (which is associated with reduced ECF volume), and by reduced Na^+ reabsorption, due either to low Na^+ availability or reduced tubular reabsorption. The effect is vasoconstriction which raises the arterial pressure, and secretion of aldosterone which increases sodium reabsorption. The sodium retention helps to raise the fluid volume and blood pressure as well.

Pressure and Flow in Systemic Veins

Veins are downstream from the resistance vessels. The pressure of blood entering the veins is relatively low, and since they are often partially collapsed, their capacity can be greatly increased by "rounding up" a somewhat flattened vessel. A vein that is flattened or collapsed is not totally occluded, however, for channels remain along the edges of the collapsed portion; collapse does increase their resistance, however. Since veins contain about 75% of the blood in the systemic circuit, a small change in this fraction will have a marked effect on pressure and flow in the entire circuit by its effect on venous return. The small amount of smooth muscle in veins is not important in regulating peripheral resistance, but does help to control storage in them.

The effect of gravity on the reservoir action, and hence on venous return, is one of the most important aspects of venous function. In the reclining position the pressure gradient from distal veins to the heart is slight. In the upright position pressure is much greater in the feet because the hydrostatic pressure of the column of fluid from the feet to the heart must be added to the basic pressure gradient in the systemic circuit. This pressure affects arteries as well as veins, but the effect is more noticeable in veins because the pressure is so much less in them. In a simple U-tube manometer,

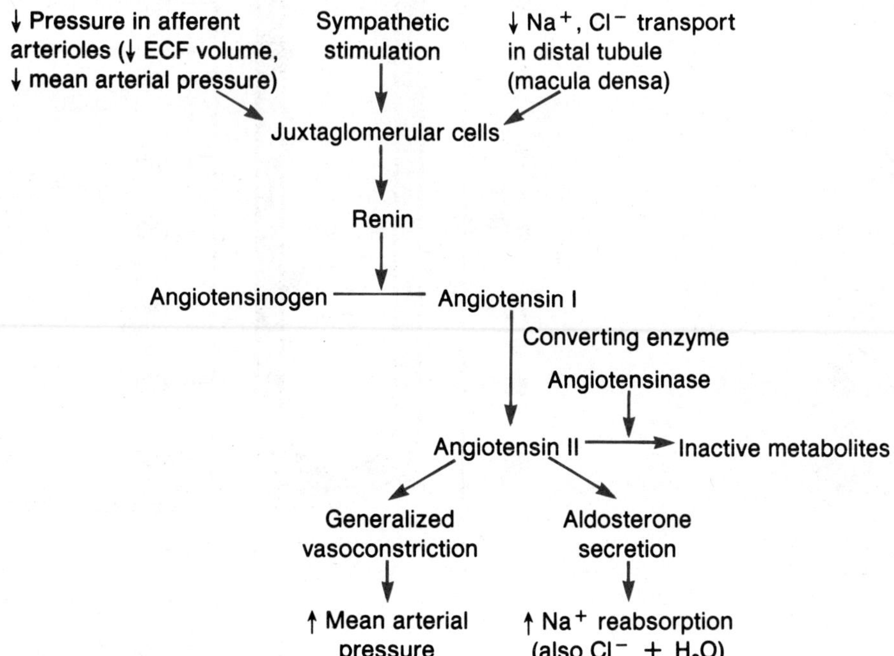

FIGURE 41–2 The renin-angiotensin

the pressure of fluid in the two limbs increases from top to bottom but is the same in the two limbs at any given level. When fluid is poured into one limb the level rises equally in both; the pressure required to raise the fluid in the "other" limb was provided by the increased hydrostatic pressure at the bottom of the first limb. The same is true of the systemic vessels in the lower extremities (Fig. 41–3), for if arteries are considered to be one limb of the manometer and veins the other, the hydrostatic pressure in one limb balances that in the other, and is highest in the feet. In the circulatory system, however, there is a marked pressure difference between arteries and veins. The effect of the pressure gradient caused by the heart's action and the peripheral resistance between arteries and veins must be added to the hydrostatic effect of the columns of blood. If the mean pressure of blood leaving the heart is 95 mmHg, and that entering the right atrium is 5 mmHg, a pressure difference reasonably close to 90 mmHg would exist between arteries and veins at all distances below the heart, with pressures in both being highest in the feet. As in a U-tube manometer, blood moving down the arterial limb is balanced by the blood up in the venous limb.

There is a problem, however, because the pressure in the lower parts is high enough to distend the veins and fill them to capacity. More blood remaining in the veins results in less blood returning to the heart, and the reduced venous return soon will be reflected in a fall in cardiac output and mean arterial pressure. Reduced arterial pressure stimulates arterial baroreceptors, which increases heart rate and peripheral resistance. The latter may help to raise arterial pressure, but an increased heart rate will not help unless venous return is also increased. The effect of gravity is also critical for arteries and veins above the heart (cerebral vessels), for the pressure decreases in both arteries and veins. (It does not become negative in veins, however, for partial collapse raises resistance in them.)

Venous return can be improved by reducing venous pooling, which can be achieved by applying external pressure to the veins. Contraction of skeletal muscles in the ex-

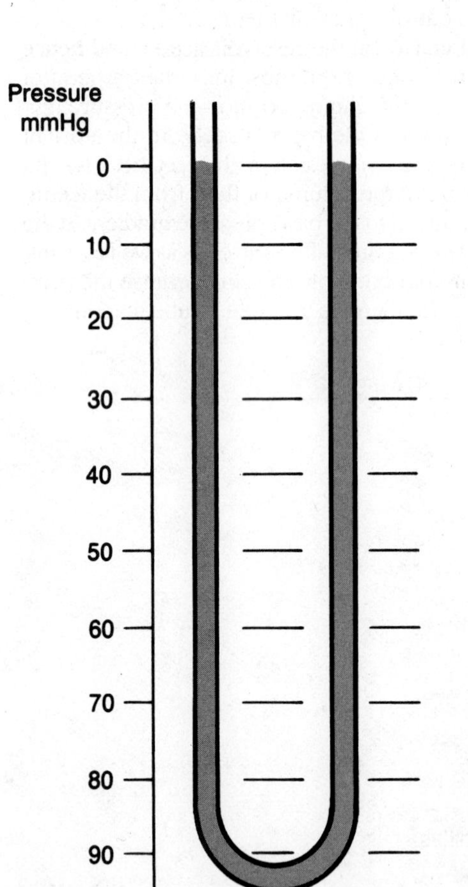

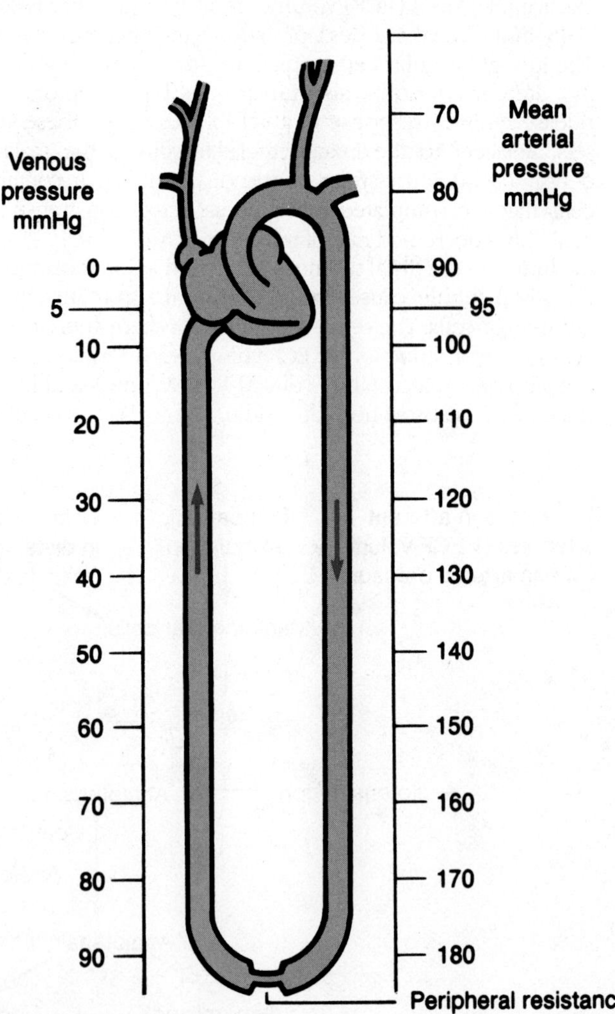

FIGURE 41–3 Comparison of pressures in systemic arteries and veins with pressures in a U-tube manometer. In the manometer, pressures are equal in the two limbs at any given level. In the circulatory system, pressures are higher in the arterial limb (because of ventricular contraction and peripheral resistance), but the hydrostatic effects are the same in the arterial and venous limbs. Veins above the heart are flattened.

tremities collapses nearby veins and forces blood upward. When the muscles relax, valves in the veins prevent backflow and allow the veins to refill from upstream vessels. Repeated rhythmic contractions, as in walking, markedly reduce venous pressure in the lower extremity and improve venous return. Venous return can also be increased by lowering pressure in the venae cavae, thereby improving the pressure gradient. The subatmospheric intrapleural pressure is a distending force on the vessels in the thorax, especially veins because of their low pressure. Deep breathing, a sigh, or even a normal inspiraton further lowers the intrapleural pressure and aids return of blood into the thoracic cavity.

The Microcirculation

The capillaries are the only blood vessels whose walls permit ready passage of ions, molecules, and fluid. They are the sites of the vital exchange of nutrients, gases, wastes, hormones, and other substances required to meet the needs of the cells, and the transfer of fluid and electrolytes necessary to maintain the volume and composition of the extracellular fluid.

Capillaries are not simply parallel channels between arterioles and venules; they branch and anastomose, forming a network of minute channels (Fig. 41–4). The specific organization of capillary beds differs slightly from one organ to another, but in a typical bed tiny vessels known as metarterioles (or preferential or thoroughfare channels) arise from arterioles and empty into venules. They have a few scattered smooth muscle cells in their walls. True capillaries (no smooth muscle) arise from metarterioles as well as arterioles. A thin ring of muscle, the precapillary sphincter, surrounds the origin of each true capillary and controls the flow of blood into it. If the sphincters are constricted, blood flow is restricted to the metarterioles, and capillary exchange is reduced. When the sphincters are open, the blood flow in the true capillaries increases and the diffusion distance from capillary to tissue cells decreases. (In resting skeletal muscle, only 5% to 10% of the capillaries are open.) Precapillary sphincters are subject to the same neural and local controls as arteriolar smooth muscle. They are also affected by the transmural pressure (capillary pressure minus tissue pressure).

Capillary exchange is a passive process which depends upon the surface area, the permeability of the capillary wall (which *permits* movement), and the gradients (which *cause* movement). As noted earlier, lipid soluble materials (O_2, CO_2) diffuse directly through the endothelial cells, and small amounts of material are moved by vesicular transport (pinocytosis and exocytosis), but most exchange involves passage at junctions between endothelial cells or through their fenestrations (pores).

The osmotic and hydrostatic pressure gradients are the major forces that determine the movement of fluid (and solutes) in and out of the bloodstream. The osmotic pressure is the colloid osmotic pressure (COP) due to the presence of nondiffusible solutes (protein). Other osmotically active particles present can diffuse, so do not contribute to the osmotic pressure gradient. The COP gradient, or effective COP, is the difference between the plasma COP of about 27–28 mmHg and the tissue COP of 2–3 mmHg (higher around discontinuous capillaries). It favors inward movement of fluid (which carries diffusible solutes). The hydrostatic pressure gradient, or effective filtration pressure, is the difference between the pressure in the capillary and that in the tissues, and favors the outward movement of fluid and diffusible solutes. It is about 32 mmHg at the venous end. At the arterial end of the capillary effective filtration pressure is greater than the COP and

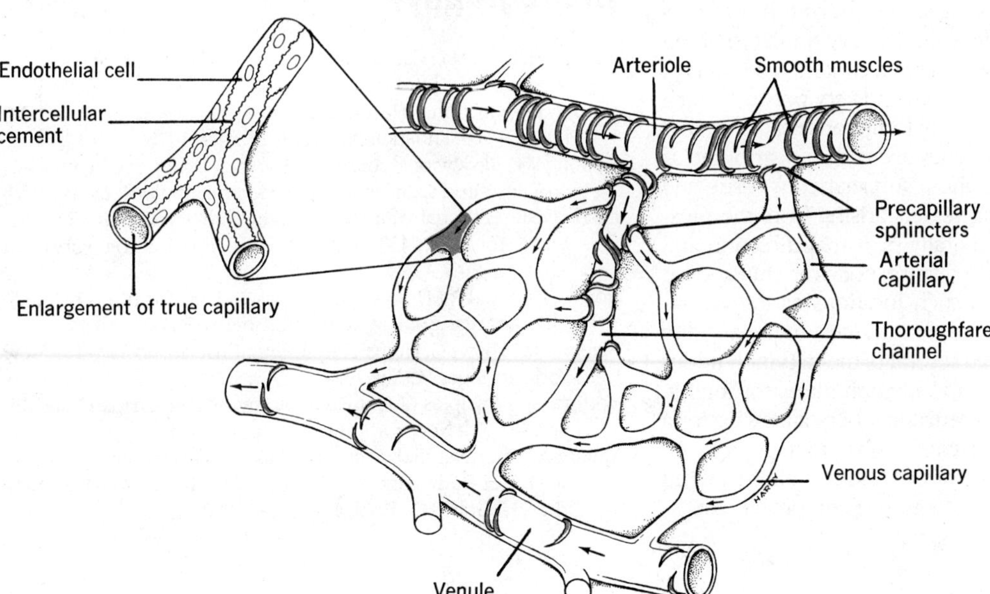

FIGURE 41–4 Diagram of a capillary bed. Precapillary sphincters are relaxed, thus permitting flow of blood through the capillary network. A greatly magnified portion of capillary wall is shown in the inset (*upper left*).

there is a net movement of fluid and solute *out* of the capillary, but at the venous end the gradient is reversed and there is a net movement of fluid *into* the capillary.

Any conditions which alter these gradients will affect the fluid balance. The COP gradiant could be reduced by low plasma protein or increased capillary permeability (allowing protein to diffuse out) and it could be increased by dehydration. Capillary pressure could be raised by an increase in arterial pressure, by arteriolar dilatation (so more of the force of the arterial pressure would reach the capillaries), or by increased venous pressure (back-up). It could be reduced by a fall in arterial pressure, arteriolar constriction, or reduced blood volume. Conditions which increase effective filtration pressure, reduce effective COP, or increase capillary permeability lead to edema. Even under optimal conditions, however, filtration from capillaries is usually slightly greater than return, but accumulation of fluid in the tissues is prevented by the lymphatic system.

The Lymphatic System

The lymphatic system serves as an auxiliary venous system. Its capillaries and collecting channels transport fluid from the tissue spaces back to the bloodstream. Its main function, therefore, is to maintain the volume of the extracellular fluid (both interstitial fluid and plasma) by taking up excess fluid as well as any protein that has leaked into the tissues, and returning it to the circulation. Other important functions are the transport of lipids and perhaps some large molecule hormones into the circulation. The lymphatic system also serves an important protective function because the lymph nodes contain macrophages which are phagocytes, and lymphocytes which are basic to immune responses.

The fluid in lymphatic vessels is known as lymph, the name given to tissue fluid that has entered a lymph vessel. Its composition is that of tissue fluid, and is very similar to blood plasma except for a much lower protein content. The walls of lymph capillaries are extremely thin and very porous, which enables large particles such as chylomicrons, bacteria, and even blood cells to penetrate. They are widely distributed as networks and plexuses throughout subcutaneous tissue and in and around organs. Lymph vessels arising from the plexuses carry the lymph in a generally proximal direction and toward lymph nodes. Clusters of lymph nodes are interposed along the lymph channels in such locations as the elbow, axilla, knee, inguinal region, neck, and mesentery, and the lymph typically passes through several of them. Lymph nodes contain a reticular network, and as lymph filters through it, the macrophages among the reticular fibers attack bacteria and other "undesirable" substances that may have been picked up in the lymph. Lymph nodes also contain lymphoid nodules where lymphocytes come to rest and proliferate.

Lymph vessels from the lower half of the body (including the abdominal cavity) converge and empty into the cisterna chyli, a saclike chamber which lies anterior to the vertebral column at about the L1–L2 level. The thoracic duct, the largest lymph vessel, arises from the cisterna chyli and ascends along the posterior body wall, passes behind the heart, and enters the left subclavian vein near its junction with the left internal jugular. Before it enters the vein, it receives lymph vessels from the left arm, left side of the head, neck, and upper trunk. Lymph channels that drain the right upper quadrant (right side of head, neck, trunk, and right arm) converge into the right lymphatic duct which enters the right subclavian vein.

The importance of the lymphatic system is indicated by the fact that it returns 2 to 4 liters of fluid to the bloodstream in 24 hours, a volume approximately equal to the total plasma volume. The amount of protein returned to the bloodstream in this fluid is equal to about one fourth to one half of the circulating plasma protein. Failure to return either the fluid or the protein would have disastrous effects on cardiovascular function.

The forces that propel lymph back to the circulation are not entirely clear. There is no driving force from behind as in the circulatory system, and the pressure in lymph vessels is very low. Numerous valves to prevent backflow, and since it is a low pressure system, external pressures including contraction of adjacent skeletal or smooth muscle, or even pulsation in nearby arteries, and the subatmospheric intrathoracic pressure all contribute to the movement of lymph. Smooth muscle in the walls of larger lymphatic vessels becomes more active when lymph flow increases, and may also be a significant factor.

Bibliography

Berne RM, Levy, MN: Cardiovascular Physiology, 4th ed. St Louis, CV Mosby, 1981

Crouch JE: Functional Human Anatomy, 3rd ed, Chaps 19 and 20, pp 427–469. Philadelphia, Lea & Febiger, 1978

Ganong WF: Review of Medical Physiology, 11th ed, Sec VI, pp 414–506. Los Altos, California, Lange Medical Publications, 1983

Landau BR: Essential Human Anatomy and Physiology, 2nd ed, Chaps 16–18, pp 433–492. Glenview, Illinois, Scott, Foresman and Company, 1980

Ross G: Essentials of Human Physiology, 2nd ed, Part IV, pp 121–286. Chicago, Year Book Medical Publishers, 1982

Schmidt RF, Thews G: Human Physiology, Chap 18, pp 397–455. New York, Springer-Verlag, 1982

Tortora GJ: Principles of Human Anatomy, 3rd ed, Chaps 12 and 13, pp 298–374. New York, Harper & Row, 1983

Vander AJ, Sherman JS, Luciano DS: Human Physiology: The Mechanisms of Body Function, 3rd ed, Chap 11, pp 253–326. New York, McGraw-Hill Book Company, 1980

Chapter 42

Assessment of Vascular Function

Mary Boozer
Ruth F. Craven

A peripheral vascular assessment includes examining both the arterial and venous circulation while obtaining a history from the patient. The history should include the identifying data such as name, age, height, and weight, as well as occupation, religious preference, and support systems. These will be used in evaluation of the patient and in planning subsequent patient care.

Let the patient tell you what the problem is. A person with peripheral vascular disease will often complain of pain, cramps, and swelling of the affected extremity. It is important to get a thorough description of the pain, because the type of pain experienced by the patient can often help determine the diagnosis and the severity of the problem.

Many patients with peripheral vascular problems are older and have other medical problems that will need to be considered in planning care. Since many medications affect circulation, a list of the medications that the patient is taking will be necessary. The current diagnosis on the presenting problem will assist in the assessment of the patient. It may be necessary to obtain some of the above information from records and family members if the patient is not able to provide it.

Occlusive Arterial Disease

Occlusive arterial disease may be manifested by a variety of characteristics including pain; edema; diminished pulses and blood pressure; changes in skin color, temperature, and turgor; reduced sensations; itching; tingling; numbness; thickened nails; and possible loss of muscle bulk. A complete list of the characteristics of occlusive arterial disease can be found in Table 42–1.

Pain: Intermittent Claudication

Intermittent claudication refers to the ischemia and pain that is present in a patient with peripheral vascular disease. Strictly speaking, claudication means limping, which may or may not occur in intermittent claudication. A careful history of intermittent claudication can be useful in making the diagnosis and determining the extent of the problem. In venous disease the pain is often localized and the involved area is warm and tender to the touch. The patient may complain of some tenderness, aching, or cramping. This complaint is usually of recent origin and often involves the calf muscles or the foot.

Intermittent claudication is as characteristic of peripheral artery disease as angina pectoris is of coronary heart disease. The description of the pain will vary from patient to patient, but usually includes fatigue, weakness, aching, cramping, numbness, limping, or a combination of these.

TABLE 42–1
Characteristics of Occlusive Arterial Disease

Pain, intermittent claudication, cramping, severe fatigue
Edema
Pulses: diminished to absent
Blood pressure: diminished
Arteriosclerosis present
Skin
  Color: pallor, cyanosis, telangiectasis, mottling, pigmentation
  Temperature: diminished
  Sensation: diminished, itching, tingling, numbness
  Loss of turgor: thin, shiny, atrophic, dry
  Absence of hair
Thick hardened nails, loss of nail bed angle
Motion may be compromised
Gait: stumbling
Ulcers may be present
Muscles: may be loss of muscle bulk
Symmetry: compare to other extremity

However the pain is described, it is usually relieved with rest and increases on exertion. This exercise–pain–rest cycle is the same from day to day and is aggravated in general by walking and in particular by walking up a hill or stairs. The amount of exercise that produces the intermittent claudication is relatively constant and helps determine the severity of the problem. It is important to document the amount of exercise it takes to produce the pain and discomfort.

The pain is due to inadequate oxygenation of the tissues distal to an occlusive process. If the occlusion increases, the person is able to do even less exercise without having pain. When occlusive arterial disease progresses and produces more severe ischemia, pain at rest occurs. Rest pain due to ischemia is a severe and rather constant pain which is often worse at night. The increasing ischemia affects the nerves as well as the other tissues and produces *lancinating,* shooting pain which is most severe in the toes and feet, even at rest. Elevation of the limb aggravates the pain as it further decreases the blood flow.

Edema

Edema is an abnormal accumulation of fluid in the interstial spaces. Often the patient with venous or arterial disease will have edema associated with impaired circulation. The edema that occurs is often dependent edema and is relieved by rest. One or both of the lower extremities may be involved. Dependent edema often begins with a swelling of the ankles and feet. It progresses upward as it becomes more severe. Edema is often less in the morning and increases as the legs remain in a dependent position.

In assessing edema, the circumference of each calf is measured at the site of the edema. This is done to establish a baseline and for comparison of one limb to the other. The extent of the edema is documented for future reference. Gently press the edematous area with your finger. If the indentation of your finger remains in the tissue, this is called pitting edema (Fig. 42–1). Fluid will gradually refill the indentation made by your fingers. If pitting edema is present, this is documented.

General Physical Examination

Skin and General Observations

The general physical examination of the person with peripheral vascular problems includes inspection, palpation, and auscultation. Make a general inspection of hands, arms, legs, and feet. Note any wounds, ulcerations, rashes, or breaks in skin continuity. Feel the blood vessel as you take the pulse and note presence of any arteriosclerosis/atherosclerosis. If arteriosclerosis is present the vessel will feel firm. Atherosclerosis is characterized by lipid deposits on the intimal wall of an artery. As the disease progresses with more and more plaque building up, the arterial lumen is narrowed, and this leads to diminished oxygenation of tissue beyond the occlusion. Arteriosclerosis includes any process causing thickening and hardening of the arterial wall.

Note the color of each limb. In occlusive peripheral vascular disease there is often pigmentation of the skin and telangiectasia (spider angioma). The involved limb may be white (pallor) or blue (cyanosis) but is often discolored in occlusive arterial disease. Sometimes mottling of the limb will occur.

The temperature of the limb may be diminished, but an inflammatory process can cause the limb to feel warm to the touch. Ischemia can affect the nerves, causing diminished sensation. Motion may be compromised.

Note the texture of the skin. There is often a loss of turgor in arterial disease and skin becomes thin, shiny, and atrophic. In occlusive disease, the hair on the limb is often absent. The nails are often thick and hardened. There may be clubbing present with the loss of nail bed angle.

Check for loss of muscle bulk and muscle tone. If possible have the patient walk and check the gait, noting any limping, shuffling, or stumbling. Check for symmetry by comparing the findings on one limb with the other and note any differences.

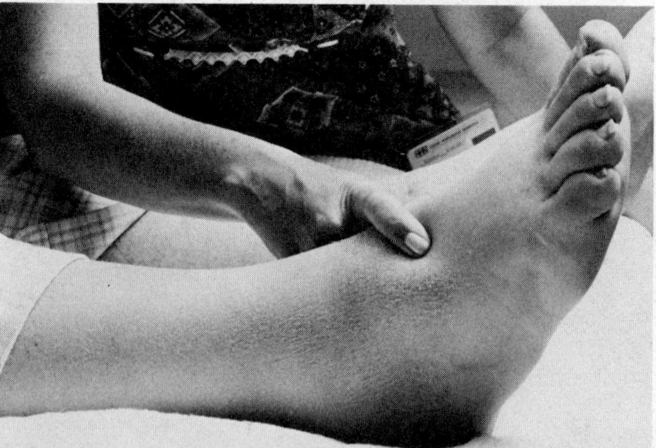

FIGURE 42–1 Pitting edema is evidenced by a clearcut impression of the finger after pressure is released.

Pulse

Evaluation of the radial pulse is done as a part of any physical examination, sometimes without thought given to anything but rate. A pulse can be taken wherever an arterial vessel can be compressed to feel the pressure wave transmitted from the aorta. The arteries where a pulse can be palpated in the lower extremiteis are the dorsal artery of the foot, and the posterior tibial, anterior tibial, popliteal, and femoral artery. In the upper extremities, the arteries that can be palpated are the radial, ulnar, and brachial (Fig. 42–2).

The pulses commonly assessed in the routine physical examination of the upper extremities are the radial, ulnar, temporal, and common carotid. Those routinely assessed in the lower extremities are the dorsalis pedis, posterior tibial, popliteal, and femoral. Pulses should be assessed from the most distal pulses first, proceeding to the proximal pulses; this will help detect the level of the obstructive disease. Note the absence of any pulse. Using a scale for grading the volume of the pulse helps to communicate to others the status of the pulse precisely and provides more reliability from one person to another.

A scale that may be useful is the following:

0—Pulse is not palpable.

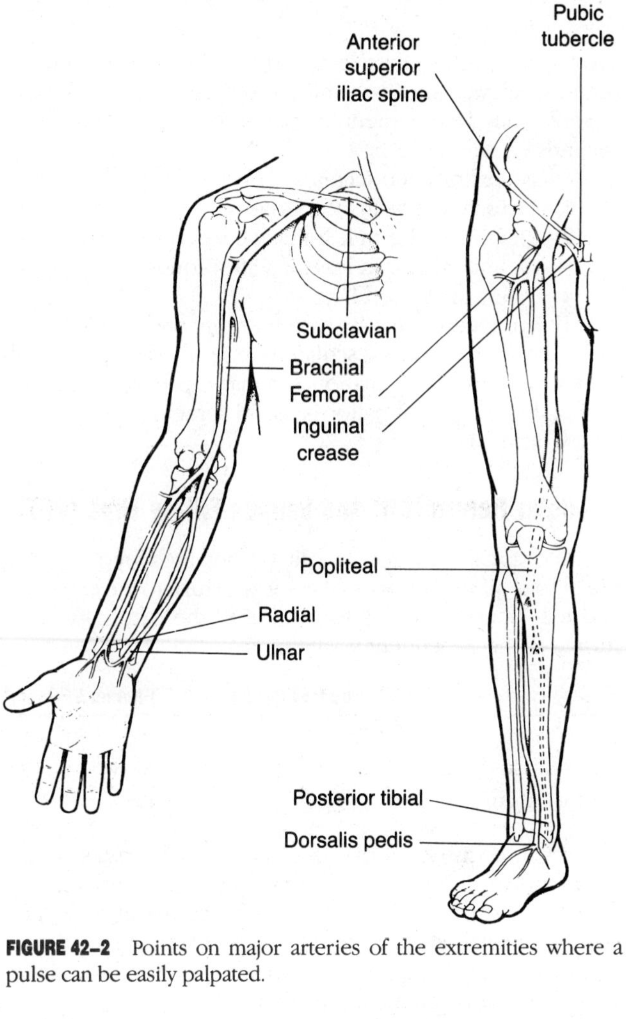

+1—Pulse is thready, weak, and difficult to palpate; it may be obliterated by pressure.

+2—Pulse is difficult to palpate, so light palpation is necessary. Once it is located it is palpable.

+3—Pulse is easily palpable, does not fade in and out, and is not obliterated by pressure. This pulse is considered to have normal volume.

+4—Pulse is strong, bounding, hyperactive, easily palpated, and not obliterated with pressure. In some cases, such as aortic regurgitation, it may be pathological.[5]

In recording, a number system similar to that used in grading heart murmurs can be used. The first number represents the volume of the pulse and the second the maximum number in the scale being used. Using this scale and recording a +2/4 indicates that the pulse is difficult to palpate, so light palpation is necessary, but once it is located it is palpable. A recording of 0/4 would indicate that the pulse is not palpable. Using a scale like this removes the need to chart the quality of the pulse and clearly indicates to all the quality of the pulse. The scale being used needs to be recorded in the record so that all health team members are using the same scale. Bilateral comparisons can be made to determine any difference that may exist. If pulses are difficult to detect, the site should be marked so that it can be more easily found on subsequent examinations of the patient.

If the pulses are difficult to detect, a Doppler probe can be used to more closely assess the circulation in a patient with extensive peripheral vascular disease (Fig. 42–3). A simple portable Doppler will let you check weak pulses and detect diminished flow undetectable by palpation, auscultation, or any other noninvasive method. This ultrasound instrument can be directed at the involved area. The beam is reflected off red blood cells moving through the area. The reflection will vary according to the velocity of blood flow in the vessel. A small transducer in the probe receives and transmits a narrow beam of ultrahigh frequency sound. The frequency, or pitch, changes in proportion to the velocity of the blood flow. The typical sound produced by an artery is pulsating and multiphasic. The sound produced by a vein is intermittent, resembles a windstorm, and varies with the respirations.

FIGURE 42–2 Points on major arteries of the extremities where a pulse can be easily palpated.

Blood Pressure

The blood pressure is taken on the brachial artery and is considered elevated if it is above 140/90. Obtain proper size cuffs and take segmental limb pressures at the level of thigh, calf, and ankle. A cuff that is too small relative to the width of the limb will produce falsely elevated pressure. (Details of blood pressure measurement are presented in Chaps. 34 and 44.) Normally the supine pressure at the ankle is equal to or greater than the systolic level at the brachial site. Blood pressures are taken at the most distal site first. Comparisons of blood pressure on both the right and left sides are done to detect any differences. If possible, blood pressures are taken before and after exercise. Abnormalities not apparent before exercise become readily apparent after exercise.

The Doppler probe can be used to obtain the systolic pressure by placing the cuffs in the manner described above.

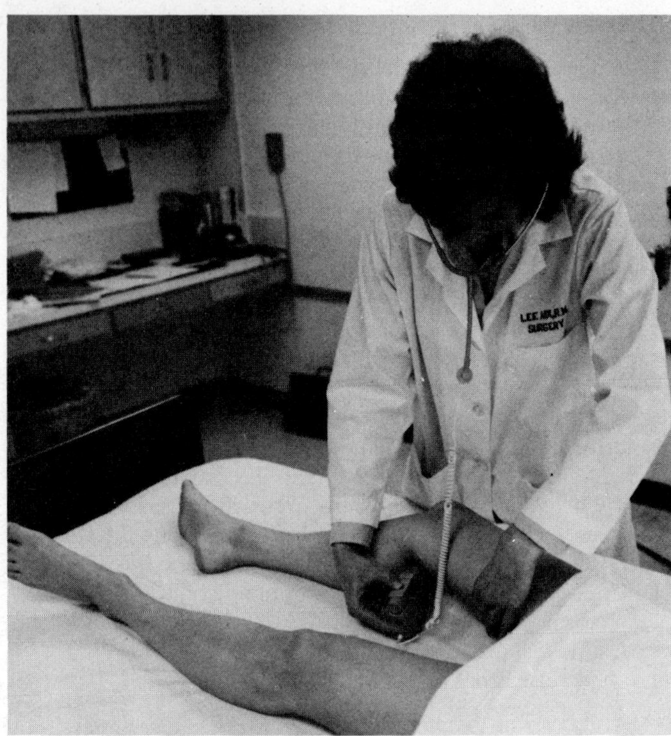

FIGURE 42-3 Use of the Doppler probe to examine peripheral circulation. (Hardy JD: Hardy's Textbook of Surgery, p 973. Philadelphia, JB Lippincott, 1983)

Inflate the cuff above the patient's systolic pressure, place the probe over the artery, and listen for the arterial signal as you deflate the cuff. Record the pressure at the time you heard the first sound.

Bruit

Check for the presence of bruits (sounds or murmurs heard over an artery during auscultation). A partially occluded artery sometimes will produce a swishing sound. It is especially important to auscultate the carotid, abdominal, and femoral arteries for bruits that indicate a partial occlusion.

Capillary Refill Time

The capillary bed is part of the vascular network that is most distal from the heart. Capillary refill time is an indication of peripheral perfusion and cardiac output, and can be checked while checking pulses. Depress the nail bed of a finger or toe until the skin blanches. Release pressure and note the amount of time required for preexisting color to return. Normally capillary vessels refill in a fraction of a second. It can be considered normal if they refill within 3 seconds. More than 3 seconds is considered sluggish. Noting the seconds is more meaningful than "good blanching." Assessing the skin temperature is important. In a cold environment low body temperature can affect the refill time.

Grading Elevation Pallor (Leg Raising)

When arterial insufficiency is present a grayish pallor of the foot comes on shortly after the leg is raised. Dependency produces a dusky rubor to appear gradually over 30 to 60 seconds. Elevate the extremity at 60° above the level and observe the development of pallor over a period of 60 seconds.

0—No pallor in 60 seconds
1—Definite pallor in 60 seconds
2—Definite pallor in less than 60 seconds
3—Definite pallor in less than 30 seconds
4—Pallor on the level[6]

This procedure may be extremely uncomfortable for the patient with occlusive vascular disease. Elevating the limb further diminishes circulation and may cause pain. Observation of the location of pallor is useful sometimes in locating severe ischemia.

Color Return (CR) and Venous Filling Time (VFT)

Additional information can be obtained by observing the time required for normal color to return to the extremity and for superficial veins to refill after the extremity is returned to the dependent position.

	Time for CR(sec)	Time for VFT(sec)[6]
Normal	10	15
Moderate ischemia	15–25	20–30
Severe ischemia	40+	40+

In occlusive disease there is some loss of sensation, and neurological deficits occur. These deficits often affect the patient's gait and stance. The loss of sensation can be dangerous. A physical assessment for peripheral vascular disease includes at least a partial neurological assessment to determine the extent of deficit. (See Chap 63.)

Occlusive Arterial Disease Involving the Arms

Since the majority of the occlusive arterial disease occurs in the lower extremities the previous discussions have been primarily about the lower extremities. However, occlusive arterial disease can involve the arm or hand. When the upper extremities are involved the procedures and general assessment are essentially the same as for the lower extremities. An additional bedside evaluation, the Allen test, is done to determine the patency of the ulnar artery distal to the wrist and is useful in demonstrating occlusive disease at the wrist or in the palmar arch. Compress the radial artery to determine the patency of the ulnar artery (Fig. 42–4). Ask the patient to clench his fist, which will cause the hand to blanch. Then have him relax his hand. If there is a prompt return of color to the hand while the radial artery is still compressed, the ulnar artery is patent. If pallor of the hand presists as long as the radial artery is compressed, the ulnar artery is probably occluded.[6]

Occlusive arterial disease of the subclavian artery, usually the left, is not uncommon. It is often identified by a lower blood pressure in the opposite arm. At first there may be no symptoms in occlusive disease of the arm; when symptoms begin to occur they are the same as for the leg. Pain and swelling are often the first symptoms noted by the patient.

Venous Problems

Varicose veins and thrombophlebitis are two of the most common venous problems.

Varicose Veins

Varicose veins are readily identified as dilated, tortuous, sacculated veins. Often present in both lower extremities, these veins become more prominent after long periods of standing. There is usually a history of edema, cramps of the legs and feet, and a heavy feeling in the legs at the end of the day. Nocturnal cramping especially of calves and feet is common.

In veins there are a series of valves that hold the blood until compression of the vein occurs. Normal activity of the muscles causes compression of veins and moves the blood back to the heart. In varicose veins these valves are absent or defective and the blood is not transported back to the heart as rapidly as it should be. Blood is pooled in the veins, accounting for the distended veins. The Trendelenberg test can further confirm the malfunctioning of the veins. Have the patient lie down with the leg elevated until the vein empties, then have the patient stand. A normal vein fills from below, a varicose vein fills from above.

Thrombophlebitis

Thrombophlebitis is an inflammation of the vein associated with clot formation. Superficial veins are hard, thready, and sensitive to pressure and they are warm to the touch, reddened, and engorged. Edema is often present and muscle cramping frequently occurs. The patient often has systemic symptoms such as an elevated temperature, fatigue, and general malaise.

Deep vein thrombosis may have no symptoms at all but edema is usually present. There often is pain, warmth, and mottling of the leg. If edema is severe, the leg may be cool and cyanotic. Thrombophlebitis can threaten the life of the patient because a clot can become dislodged. This embolus, which can travel and cause damage to vital organs, is frequently the source of pulmonary embolism.

Thrombophlebitis can be assessed by testing for *Homans' sign* or *cuff sign.* Homans' sign can be elicited by having the patient dorsiflex the foot; if this causes pain in the calf or foot, thrombophlebitis may be present. To elicit the cuff sign, place a blood pressure cuff over the limb and measure the point at which inflation of the cuff causes pain.

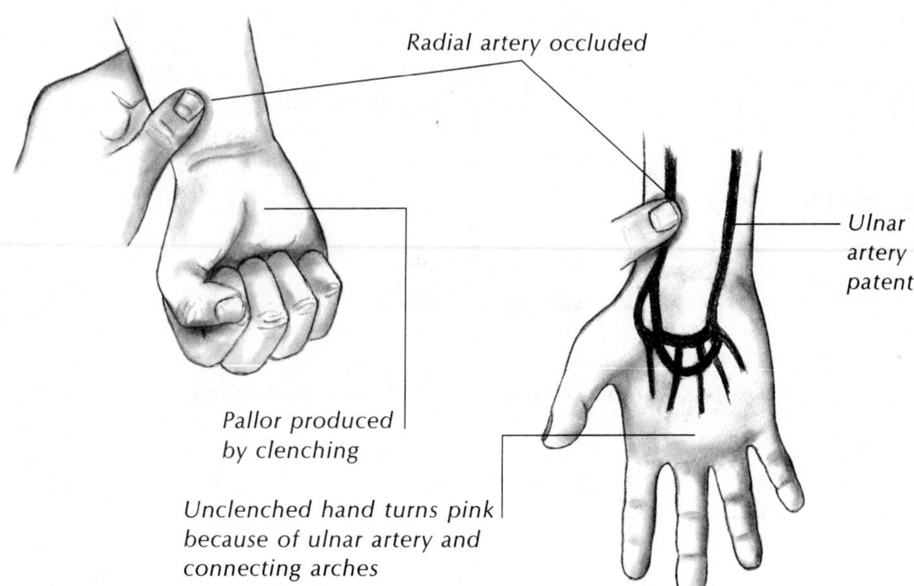

FIGURE 42–4 The Allen test to determine patency of ulnar artery.

Do the same on the other legs and then make comparisons. The cuff sign is an objective way of measuring the tenderness and of following the resolution or progression of phlebitis.

When edema is present, measuring the circumference with a tape measure on admission and periodically can yield information as to the resolution and progression of the disease. The chosen site should be marked so that the same site is measured each time in order to be accurate.

Table 42–2 presents a summary of the characteristics of venous problems.

Lymphedema

Lymphedema occurs when more fluid is being transferred from the circulation than can be reabsorbed by the venous system. Lymphedema may be a primary disorder or obstruction of the lymphatic system but more commonly is secondary to some other disorder. It is common in all patients with peripheral vascular disorders. Primary lymphedema is usually either congenital or caused by some inflammation or obstruction of the lymphatic system. Lymphedema usually increases during the day and decreases at night when the patient is resting. The cause of the edema needs to be determined and then appropriate treatment can be prescribed. If the lymphedema is congenital in origin or caused by an inflammation or obstruction of the lymphatics, treatment may be difficult. As the disease progresses the skin becomes thickened and rough, and discoloration occurs. Because nutrition to the tissues is impaired, infections and ulcerations are common.

Additional Diagnostic Tests

Noninvasive Diagnostic Tests

More diagnostic tests are usually done in patients with cardiovascular disease. These are usually carried out in a vascular laboratory and are not a part of the routine bedside assessment of the peripheral vascular system. Usually, the nurse explains these tests to the patient and the family. Clear, simple explanations are necessary.

TABLE 42–2
Characteristics of Venous Problems

Pain: exercise may relieve
Edema: worse at end of day, relieved with rest
Veins: dilated, tortuous, sacculated; often bilateral; may be hard and thready to the touch
Cramps: nocturnal common
Heavy feeling at the end of the day
Skin: may be warm, reddened, mottled, pigmented
Homans' sign: positive

Treadmill Tests. Prior to the treadmill test, pressures are taken. The patient then walks on a treadmill at a 10% grade, 2 miles per hour for approximately 5 minutes. Following the exercise the patient returns to the examining table, where ankle pressures, pulse volume recording, and brachial systolic pressures are obtained. With a major occlusive disease, there is a pronounced decrease in the ankle pressure index and a change in the pulse volume waveform following exercise.

Skin Temperature Studies. Skin temperature tests have to be done in a carefully controlled environment in order to yield accurate data. They are useful in comparing one extremity to the other. Skin temperature studies are influenced by many factors and are never used as the only diagnostic technique.

Plethysmography. Plethysmography, which measures volume changes that occur with changes in the cardiac cycle, is useful in evaluating both arterial and venous problems. Blood pressure cuffs of the appropriate size are applied to each segment of the leg (ankle, calf, and thigh). The most distal cuff is inflated first to 65 mmHg. Changes in leg volume produce proportional changes in the inflated cuff. A pressure transducer in the instrument records the changes on graph paper. The cuff is deflated and the process repeated on the other segments. Venous plethysmography combined with Doppler evaluation is a noninvasive, portable, reliable test for deep venous thrombosis.

Velocity Waveform Analysis. Velocity waveform analysis is often done using a hand-held Doppler probe. A tracing is obtained for velocity waveform analysis using a recording device connected to the Doppler amplifier. Segmental (ankle, calf, and thigh) pressure changes during the cardiac cycle are recorded on graph paper. Analysis of these recordings will help to determine whether an artery is patent or occluded.

^{125}I-Fibrinogen Leg Scanning. Fibrinogen leg scanning sometimes helps to detect thrombi. Leg scanning should not be used alone since falsely positive results can occur over a hematoma, a large wound, or a large area of inflammation. Scans also may fail to detect thrombi, particularly in the iliac vein. Also, it can take as long as 72 hours for enough radioactivity to accumulate in the thrombus to show a positive result.

Invasive Diagnostic Tests

Any test that requires entering an artery or vein has some risk attached to it. Therefore these tests, when employed, require caution on the part of the whole medical team. The patient may be sensitive to the contrast media used. The possibility of an anaphylactic reaction, vagal reaction, renal failure, and death exists. In most instances these complications do not occur but being aware that they may occur is imperative.

Angiography. Angiography is used to visualize the internal heart and blood vessels. A radiopaque dye is injected into an artery and a series of x-ray films are taken. The dye permits the viewing of the size and shape of the arteries. Any abnormalities can be demonstrated. A cutdown may be necessary in some instances in order to inject the dye. The dye used contains iodide and may cause a severe allergic reaction. Watch respirations closely for any signs of dyspnea or wheezing, gasping inspiration (crowing), which indicates an allergic response affecting the respirations. Check for nausea, vomiting, numbness of extremities, diaphoresis, and tachycardia; these usually occur immediately but can occur later. In addition, observe for urticaria, flushed skin, and decreased urinary output. Check the site of injection for irritation, inflammation, or hematoma formation since the dye is irritating to the surrounding tissues. Carefully monitor the patient for hemorrhage and shock secondary to the artery being entered.

Venography. Venography is the best test for diagnosing deep vein thrombosis, but is used sparingly because of the associated risks. It is an invasive procedure and involves the injection of a dye into the patient's bloodstream. X-ray films are taken and filling defects in the veins can be evaluated. The patient is watched closely for the same reactions to the dye as discussed under angiography. In addition, close observation for the development of thrombophlebitis is essential. Check the site of injection for any irritation, hematoma, or bleeding.

Summary

As indicated earlier, many patients with peripheral vascular disorders are older and often have many medical problems. A thorough systematic peripheral vascular assessment provides a great deal of information on the general health of the total person.

References

1. Argondizzo NT, Adler J: Programmed instruction: Patient assessment: Pulses. Am J Nurs 79:115–132, 1979
2. Bastarache MM: Assessing peripheral vascular disease: Noninvasive testing. Am J Nurs 83:1552–1556, 1983
3. Hudson B: Doppler ultrasound stethoscope. Nursing 83 5:55–57, 1983
4. Hull R: Current approach to diagnosis of deep vein thrombosis. Modern Concepts of Cardiovascular Disease 51:129–132, 1982
5. Miller KM: Assessing peripheral perfusion. Am J Nurs 78:1673–1674, 1978
6. Spittell JA: Recognition and management of chronic atherosclerotic occlusive peripheral arterial disease. Modern Concepts of Cardiovascular Disease 50:19–23, 1981

Bibliography

Boozer M, Craven R: Nursing care of the patient with chronic occlusive peripheral artery disease. Cardiovasc Nurs 15:4, 1981

Craven R, Boozer M: Disorders of the peripheral vascular system. In Underhill SL et al (eds): Cardiac Nursing. Philadelphia, JB Lippincott, 1982

Fahey VA: Deep vein thrombosis. Nursing 84 3:34–41, 1984

Peterson FY: Assessing peripheral vascular disease at the bedside. AJN 83:1549–1551 1983

Phipps WJ, Long VC, Woods NF: Medical-Surgical Nursing, 2nd ed, pp 1142–1163. St Louis, CV Mosby, 1983

Price S, Wilson L: Pathophysiology: Clinical Concepts of Disease Processes, pp. 384–392. 2nd ed, New York, McGraw-Hill 1982

Chapter 43

Nursing Strategies for Common Vascular Problems

Nursing Diagnosis
Interventions
Evaluation

Mary Boozer
Ruth F. Craven

People with peripheral vascular disorders have many of the same problems whether the location of the problem is in the veins or in the arteries. In order to provide proper intervention, the nursing diagnosis needs to establish whether the veins or the arteries are the source of the problem. Many of the patients are elderly and may have problems in both the veins and arteries. The problems that are discussed in this chapter that are related to vascular problems in the extremities are

Alteration in comfort: pain
Decreased tissue perfusion
Inflammation

Alteration in Comfort: Pain

Nursing Diagnosis

Painful extremities related to inadequate oxygenation of the tissue distal to the site of an occlusion are manifested by the symptoms of intermittent cramping pain, numbness, aching, and severe fatigue when the ischemic muscles are active. These symptoms are promptly relieved by rest. Since the major part of the work of walking is done by the calf muscles, they are the most common sites of intermittent claudication for occlusive lesions above the level of the knee.

Rest pain, which is worse at night, clearly indicates the flow of blood to the area has been severely diminished and is inadequate to meet the oxygen demands of tissues at rest. The increasing occlusion or inadequacy of the collateral circulation produces ischemia to the nerves as well as to the other tissues. This ischemia of the nerves produces lancinating, shooting pain which is most severe in the toes and foot, even at rest. Elevation of the limb always aggravates the pain as gravitational pull further decreases blood flow, and conversely, in the early stages, pain may be relieved by having the limb in a dependent position.

Interventions

The major goal is for the patient to be able to manage the activities of daily living without the occurrence of pain. The other goals are to reduce the pain of the intermittent claudication, numbness, aching, and severe fatigue due to the ischemia, and to improve circulation in the compromised vessels.

General comfort measures such as regular exercise and rest periods along with warm baths may be useful in relieving pain. The specific etiology for the cause of the pain and the diminished circulation needs to be determined in order for the most beneficial nursing strategies to be employed. For example, arteriosclerosis obliterans involves the medium and larger arteries, while thromboangiitis obliterans involves small arteries and arterioles. Different nursing therapies may be employed specifically depending on the medical diagnosis (see Chap 46).

Careful documentation of the pain and other symptoms is needed in order to determine the extent of the problem and the success of the treatment.

Evaluation

After successful intervention, the patient should report a decrease in the amount of intermittent claudication. The extremity should be warm to the touch. The color of the limb should reflect no pallor, cyanosis, or rubor. Peripheral pulses should be present and equal. The patient should be resting and comfortable.

Decreased Tissue Perfusion

Nursing Diagnosis

Other symptoms resulting from progressive distal occlusion occur. The affected limb is often cool compared to its counterpart and to the skin proximal to the affected area. Color changes may also occur such as pallor due to the decreased flow; cyanosis due to diminished, inadequate blood flow; and reddish blue discoloration due to capillary and venular responses to anoxia. The skin becomes dry, shiny, and devoid of hair in response to the chronic severe ischemia. The toenails become brittle, thickened, and deformed. When collateral blood flow to areas of the limb is severely compromised, inflammation, ulcerations, and areas of gangrene may develop, often in the lower portion of the affected limb. Any sudden changes in color, temperature, or pain must be treated as an emergency situation.

Edema is often present in patients with either venous or arterial disease associated with the impaired circulation. The edema that occurs is often dependent and improves with rest.

Insufficient circulation and tissue hypoxia in the upper extremities has many manifestations similar to those in the lower extremities. Color and temperature changes accompany pain and swelling. Documentation of these symptoms and of ways in which the person obtains relief are a necessary first step. Definitive diagnosis is needed in order to determine whether vascular occlusion or vasospasm is the etiologic factor (see Chap 46). Careful documentation of the vital signs including the peripheral pulses along with the change in symptoms will help to determine success or failure of the treatment. The goal is to improve the tissue perfusion of oxygenated blood which would be evidenced by the decrease of pain, improved color, warm extremities, and absence of edema.

Interventions

It is important to document the pain and other symptoms in order to determine the extent of the problem and the amount of care needed. Early in the course of the occlusive process, the person should exercise some measures to control and stabilize the process for as long as possible. Losing excess weight in order to reduce the workload on the lower extremity is recommended if the person is overweight. Restricting the use of tobacco which causes peripheral vasoconstriction is essential. These two measures alone may be immediately helpful. In conjunction with this, a daily exercise program in which the person walks on a flat surface for a distance short of the onset of claudication followed by a rest period is thought to help promote the development of collateral circulation. If the symptoms become progressively worse, as evidenced by paresthesias, unrelenting pain at rest, and advanced ischemic changes, surgery should be considered.

The person with an occlusive disease usually has a chronic progressive disease and needs understanding, supportive nursing care. Patient teaching is an important feature of nursing therapy. Reinforcing the need for weight reduction and restricting the use of tobacco is an essential element in controlling the progress of the disease. Instruction includes meticulous foot care, proper-fitting shoes, immediate attention to blisters and cuts, and careful nail trimming. The ischemia increases susceptibility to inflammation and often causes delayed wound healing. The person should also avoid restrictive clothing such as tight stockings or garters, and should not cross the legs, because both of these practices mechanically impede the blood flow in already compromised arteries. Adherence to a daily exercise program should be encouraged in an effort to stimulate the development of collateral circulation. Exercise helps the person's mental outlook as well as improving physical progress. For the person who has developed minor ulcerations or other tissue breakdown, a diet with adequate protein and vitamin C for wound healing, and reestablishing and maintaining integrity is needed.

The person with arterial insufficiency soon learns that having his legs in a dependent position lower than the heart relieves some of his symptoms; however, keeping the legs dependent increases the venous pressure and promotes dependent edema. The medical treatment of most peripheral vascular disease is palliative and involves the use of vasodilators and analgesics. Surgical treatment may be appropriate in some cases (see Chap 46). Careful documentation of the vital signs including the peripheral pulses along with the change in symptoms will help to determine success or failure of the treatment.

Evaluation

Outcome criteria reflect attainment of the stated goals. Outcome criteria for relief of pain and for improved circulation are as follows:

- Patient reports decreased occurrence of intermittent claudication.
- Patient reports improved sensation in the affected extremity.
- Activity tolerance for walking distance will improve and the fatigue will be less.
- Skin color will appear more consistent with skin of unaffected areas.

- Skin will not have unhealed ulcerations or unresolved inflammation.
- Temperature of affected extremity will be comparable to unaffected areas of the extremities.

Inflammation of the Extremities

Nursing Diagnosis

Edema and pain related to an inflammatory process in the veins can cause the limb to be warm to the touch, reddened, and engorged. In addition, the patient often has systemic symptoms such as an elevated temperature, fatigue, and general malaise. Pain and edema are often prominent symptoms of the inflammatory process (see Chap 47).

The physiological interruption in this situation is due to incompetent blood return from the periphery to the central circulation. Blood pools in the affected extremity, causing edema, redness, elevated local temperature, and pain.

Interventions

The goal is to reduce patient discomfort due to a venous inflammatory process. Knowledge of the cause of the inflammatory process and the exact location which is affected is essential for guiding the more specific nursing strategies. For example, the management of thrombophlebitis will vary depending on whether it is a superficial or a deep vein thrombosis.

To promote improved circulatory competency, nursing strategies must focus on improving the blood return. The affected limb should be kept at the level of the heart or slightly elevated. Having the limb in a dependent position only increases the problem caused by venous incompetency. The affected limb should not be massaged because of the possibility of dislodging an embolus.

Much of the management centers around prevention. High-risk patients are managed by the use of active and passive exercises, early ambulation, and antiembolic stockings.

While hereditary factors are an important consideration, other factors toward which patient education can be focused are avoiding obesity; proper application of support hose; limiting long periods of standing or sitting; and avoiding crossing legs when seated.

Evaluation

Outcome criteria for reducing patient discomfort due to venous inflammation are as follows:

- Patient will have absence of symptoms of inflammation (redness, heat, pain, and swelling) in the affected extremity and an absence of Homans' sign.
- Patient will demonstrate no complications, such as thromboembolus.
- Extremity will return to normal size and shape without complaint of tenderness or aching.
- Patient has a regular program of exercises and rest.

Much of the nursing care of patients with peripheral vascular disorders centers around prevention. This is accomplished through patient teaching; regular programs of exercise and rest; and meticulous care of the involved extremities.

Bibliography

Argondizzo NT, Adler J: Programmed instruction—patient assessment: Pulses. Am J Nurs 79(1):115–132, 1979

Boozer M, Craven R: Nursing care of the patient with chronic occlusive peripheral artery disease. Cardiovasc Nurs 15:4, 1981

Craven R, Boozer M: Disorders of the peripheral vascular system. In Underhill SL et al (eds): Cardiac Nursing. Philadelphia, JB Lippincott, 1982

Eddy ME: Teaching patient with peripheral vascular disease. Nurs Clin North Am 12(6):151–159, 1977

Hudson MF: Safeguard your elderly patients' health through accurate physical assessment. Nursing 83:58–64, 1983

Hull R: Current approach to diagnosis of deep vein thrombosis. Modern Concepts of Cardiovascular Disease 51(11):129–132, 1981

Miller KM: Assessing peripheral perfusion. Am J Nurs 78:1673–1674, 1978

Peterson FY: Assessing peripheral vascular disease at the bedside. Am J Nurs 83(11):1549–1551, 1983

Phipps WJ, Long B, Woods NF: Medical-Surgical Nursing: Concepts and Clinical Practice, 2nd ed. St Louis, CV Mosby, 1983

Price S, Wilson L: Pathophysiology: Clinical Concepts of Disease Processes, 2nd ed. New York, McGraw-Hill, 1982

Ryzewski J: Factors in the Rehabilitation of Patients with Peripheral Vascular Disease. Nurs Clin North Am 12(1):161–168, 1977

Taggart E: The physical assessment of the patient with arterial disease. Nurs Clin North Am 12(1):109–118, 1977

Chapter 44

Hypertension

Susanna L. Cunningham

High blood pressure (hypertension) is a significant problem for nursing because of the high percentage of the population affected and the serious consequences of uncontrolled high blood pressure. As discussed throughout this chapter, nursing has a vital role in all phases of blood pressure control. The key elements of a high blood pressure control program for any individual or group are education, screening, referral, diagnosis, treatment, long-term monitoring, and evaluation. Nursing has a variety of roles in all these areas of control, from independent practitioner to collaborator to interdependent co-worker.

Epidemiology

Approximately 58 million Americans between 6 and 74 years of age have high blood pressure, making it the most common type of heart or blood vessel disorder.[27] Despite the fact that high blood pressure is often considered as a cardiovascular disease entity, it is important to remember that high blood pressure is only a sign, *not* a disease. In some ways it is analagous to fever in that frequently it is recognized and treated even though an underlying cause cannot be found. High blood pressure is often considered as a disease entity because in 90% to 95% of cases of elevated blood pressure an underlying etiology cannot be identified. A vast amount of research is currently focused on determining the cause or causes of high blood pressure.

In addition to the fact that it is the most common cardiovascular problem in America, high blood pressure is extremely important because it is one of the major modifiable risk factors for atherosclerosis, myocardial infarction, and cerebrovascular accident. Smoking, elevated serum cholesterol levels, and diabetes mellitus are the other major modifiable risk factors for heart disease. Even though the underlying cause or causes are not known, almost all forms of elevated blood pressure can now be controlled by nonpharmacologic or pharmacologic therapy, or a combination of the two. The ability to treat high blood pressure effectively is one of the major cardiovascular advances of this century.

The importance of controlling high blood pressure can be appreciated by examining the relationships between diastolic blood pressure and either mortality or morbidity. In Figure 44–1 the relationship between diastolic blood pressure and the probability of dying in a 12-year period following the blood pressure measurement is shown. This graph reveals that there is a curvilinear relationship between diastolic blood pressure and the probability of dying. Quite simply, the higher the diastolic pressure the higher the probability of dying. In fact, the probability of dying doubles if one goes from a diastolic pressure of 60 mmHg to a pressure of 85 mmHg. For morbidity, similar curves can be drawn for the

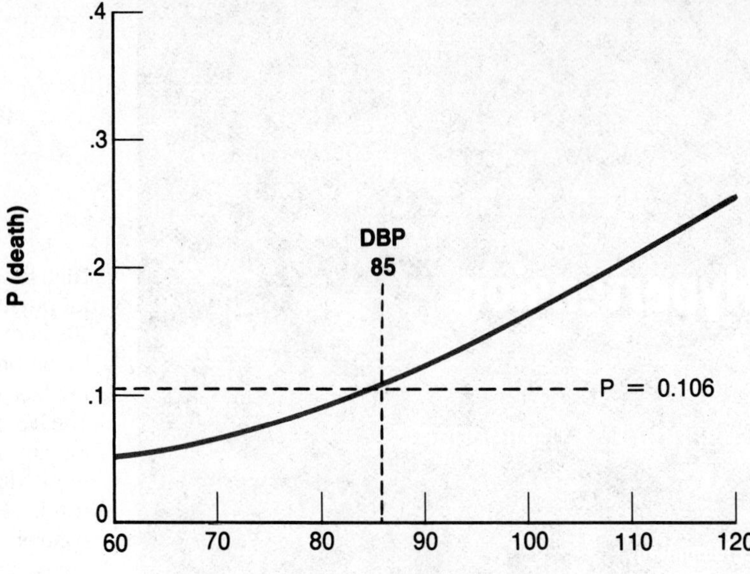

FIGURE 44–1 The probability of death from all causes in 12-year follow-up by baseline diastolic blood pressure for men 40 to 54 years of age from the US National Pooling Project.[37] The dotted lines show that an increase in diastolic blood pressure from 60 to 85 mmHg doubles the probability of death. (Adapted from Labarthe DR, Blaufox MD, Carey RM, Gifford RW et al: Recommendations for a revised approach to defining high blood pressure: Final report of the working group. National High Blood Pressure Education Program, NIH-LBI, 1982)

relationships between diastolic blood pressure and the probability of suffering a cerebrovascular accident or myocardial infarction in a period of years after the blood pressure was taken. Although most of the epidemiology for high blood pressure and its consequences is currently done in reference to the diastolic blood pressure, similar curves can be drawn for systolic blood pressure.

The prevalence of high blood pressure in the American population varies markedly with race and sex. The hypertension prevalence rate among black Americans is 38.2% as compared with a rate of 28.8% among whites. The prevalence rate of hypertension in men is 33%, compared with 26.8% in women. When both age and sex are considered, black women have the highest prevalence rate, followed in descending order by black men, white men, and then white women. In addition, hypertension is more severe in blacks, who have two times more moderate hypertension and three times more severe hypertension than whites.

In recent years there has been a movement away from the term *hypertension* to the phrase *high blood pressure.* The use of the word hypertension has led to the misconception that a person must be "hyper" or tense in order to have the problem of an elevated pressure. Since persons who are calm in manner and who are not "hyper" can and do have increased levels of blood pressure, practitioners are encouraged to use the term high blood pressure, particularly when communicating with the lay public. The word hypertension is still used in communication between health care professionals.

Classification

One of the challenges in understanding the problem of high blood pressure is making sense of the many different terms, definitions, and classifications of high blood pressure that have evolved over the years. It is helpful to consider that the three main systems for classifying blood pressure are based on the etiology, the level of the blood pressure, or the prognosis.

The classification system that is based on etiology designates blood pressure as *primary* or *essential* if an underlying disease process cannot be identified. As noted above, in approximately 90% to 95% of individuals with elevated pressures, a cause cannot be determined. The main theories about the cause or causes of essential hypertension and the most common causes of secondary hypertension are discussed in the following section on the etiology of hypertension.

The actual levels of an individual's blood pressure and the known risk associated with those pressure levels are the basis for the classification system published by the Third Joint National Committee on the Detection, Evaluation, and Treatment of High Blood Pressure.[33] As shown in Figure 44–2, the Third Joint National Committee classification system divides high blood pressure into several categories depending on an individual's diastolic and systolic blood pressures. In this system diastolic pressure is the main criterion for designating elevated levels of pressure, with systolic pressure considered only when it is 140 mmHg or greater and diastolic pressure is less than 85 mmHg. If diastolic pressure is greater than 90 mmHg, then it is the sole criterion for designating an individual as having mild, moderate, or severe blood pressure.

The 1984 classification differs from those of previous Joint National Committee Reports in several ways. First, a new category, *high normal blood pressure,* which is defined as a systolic pressure less than 140 mmHg and a diastolic pressure of 86 to 89 mmHg, was established. This category was created so that persons with higher levels of diastolic pressure could be identified and followed more closely with yearly blood pressure checks and lifestyle counseling in an effort to retard or prevent the development of established

Diastolic Blood Pressure (mmHg)	Systolic Blood Pressure (mmHg)		
	Less than 140	140 to 159	160 or greater
Less than 85	Normal blood pressure	Borderline isolated systolic hypertension	Isolated systolic hypertension
85 to 89	High normal blood pressure		
90 to 104	Mild hypertension		
105 to 114	Moderate hypertension		
115 or greater	Severe hypertension		

FIGURE 44–2 Blood pressure classification based on confirmed* diastolic and systolic pressures in the same individual 18 years and older.
(* The average of two or more measurements on two or more occasions. From 1984 Report of the Joint National Committee on Detection, Evaluation, and Treatment of High Blood Pressure.)

hypertension. Another change was the abolition of different levels of acceptable pressure for persons over 36 years of age. The last significant change was the establishment of another new category of high blood pressure, *borderline isolated systolic hypertension,* which refers to persons with diastolic pressures less than 90 mmHg and systolic pressures between 140 and 159 mmHg.

Isolated systolic hypertension refers to a systolic pressure of 160 mmHg or greater with a diastolic pressure of less than 90 mmHg. This type of hypertension is found most commonly in the elderly, although it can occur in younger persons as well. Since relatively little is known about this kind of hypertension, a large multi-center double-blind placebo controlled trial known as the Systolic Hypertension in the Elderly Program (SHEP) is currently being conducted.

The blood pressure classification system that is based on prognosis defines blood pressure as either *benign* or *malignant.* The term *benign hypertension* indicates that the condition is progressing very slowly with relatively little change from year to year. *Malignant* or *accelerated hypertension* indicates a disease process that it is progressing very rapidly with a high likelihood of death within a year unless therapy is initiated.

Two other terms, *labile* and *borderline hypertension* are frequently encountered in the literature. Although there is some confusion over the exact meaning of the terms, the word labile is usually used to indicate fluctuation of an individual's blood pressure between normotension and hypertension. That is, on some occasions the person's pressure is found to be elevated and other occasions it is not. Since every person's pressure varies throughout the day there is no clear definition of how great the fluctuation must be for a person to be considered to have labile hypertension. Borderline high blood pressure is a term used to indicate pressures that are between normotension and hypertension. In the 1984 Joint National Committee classification system the term borderline is used only in relation to isolated systolic hypertension. Other classification systems based on actual pressure levels have sometimes used borderline hypertension to indicate persons who have diastolic pressures between 90 and 95 mmHg. In addition some authors use the terms labile and borderline hypertension interchangeably.

Etiology

Primary Hypertension

Primary or essential hypertension is persistent elevated blood pressure for which there is no apparent cause or associated underlying disease. The adjective *essential* was used because it was previously thought that higher arterial pressures were essential to force the blood through diseased blood vessels and provide adequate organ perfusion. Treatment studies have demonstrated this belief to be false, and it is now known that treatment is effective in reducing the morbidity and mortality associated with untreated hypertension.[13,28,37,38]

Although the cause or causes of primary or essential hypertension are unknown, there are many theories which attempt to explain it. Despite the multiple theories, none of them is widely accepted among researchers in the field. Some of the theories that are currently being investigated are as follows:

- There is an increased concentration of circulating vasoconstrictor substances such as angiotensin II; a decreased concentration of vasodilator substances such as prostaglandins or kinins; or both.
- Sympathetic nervous system activity is increased, resulting in increased vasoconstriction.
- There is a fundamental defect in membrane perme-

ability, resulting in a decrease in the efflux of sodium ion out of cells. As a result of the increase in intracellular sodium and therefore decreased gradient between intracellular and extracellular sodium concentrations, there is a decrease in sodium-linked calcium transport out of cells. The increase in intracellular calcium in vascular smooth muscle cell causes increased muscle contraction and raises systemic vascular resistance and blood pressure.[4]

More than one of these theories may be correct or ultimately none of them may be found to explain the cause or causes of hypertension. Despite the existance of many animal models, research in the area has been hampered by the lack of a model which truly represents human essential hypertension. The animal models have, however, made a significant contribution to the understanding of the effects of persistent elevated pressure on tissue structure and function.

Secondary Hypertension

Secondary hypertension refers to an elevated blood pressure for which an underlying disease or condition can be identified. Despite the fact that the underlying problem may be known, it is not always possible to explain the relationship between the problem and the development of hypertension. Neither is it always possible to treat the hypertension by correcting the underlying disorder.

Even though secondary hypertension accounts for only 5% to 10% of all cases of hypertension and thus is relatively uncommon, there are many underlying conditions which have been identified. The 1984 Joint National Committee Report recommends that additional diagnostic investigation for potential causes of secondary hypertension be limited to the following situations:

- Persons in whom the age, history, physical examination, degree of elevated pressure, or initial laboratory findings suggest secondary hypertension
- When there is a poor response to pharmacologic therapy
- A sudden increase in pressure in an individual whose pressure has previously been well controlled
- When the person has malignant hypertension

The most common causes of secondary hypertension are chronic renal failure and renovascular disease. Because of the implications for prevention and early recognition, nurses should be aware of the exogenous causes of secondary hypertension such as lead poisoning, use of birth control pills, and excess ingestion of licorice, which contains a mineralocorticoid.

Pathophysiology

Hemodynamic Patterns in Hypertension

There are at least two hemodynamic patterns seen in individuals with high blood pressure. One pattern is seen in those with borderline high blood pressure and the other in persons with established essential hypertension. Since blood pressure is the product of cardiac output and systemic vascular resistance, it is reasonable to expect that there will be changes in one or both of these parameters. An additional factor to remember is that cardiac output is the product of stroke volume and heart rate, which means that changes in vascular volume may be related to the development of hypertension.

In borderline or mildly elevated blood pressure, elevations in cardiac output and heart rate have sometimes been found with normal or low systemic vascular resistance. These elevations have not been found by all researchers, however, and there is some discussion as to whether the increases in rate and cardiac output may be caused by an exaggerated response to the invasive studies used to measure output and peripheral resistance. The range of cardiac index (cardiac output divided by body surface area) does seem to be wider in persons with mild or borderline high blood pressure, with more high values than seen in normal people.[8]

In established essential high blood pressure there is general agreement that cardiac output and index are within normal limits and the main hemodynamic change is an increased systemic vascular resistance.

Influence of High Blood Pressure on the Body

Cardiovascular Effects. With persistent elevated blood pressure, the heart progressively develops concentric hypertrophy. Although it has long been believed that the hypertrophy developed as a result of prolonged exposure to an elevated total peripheral resistance (afterload), it has recently been suggested that the myocardial hypertrophy may also be part of the disease process of essential hypertension.[11] Hypertensive individuals in whom cardiac hypertrophy has become clinically apparent are also found to have other abnormalities of myocardial structure and function, including left atrial enlargement, decreased cardiac index, decreased ejection fraction, left ventricular dilatation, and increased heart rate. Although individuals with cardiac hypertrophy may be asymptomatic for many years, eventually myocardial decompensation occurs, resulting in the clinical signs of congestive heart failure (see Chap 40).

Current evidence indicates that some forms of antihypertensive therapy result in a reduction in left ventricular hypertrophy. Studies of rats with inherited forms of hypertension indicate that treatment with methyldopa, β-adrenergic receptor blocking agents, and converting enzyme inhibitors causes regression of left ventricular hypertrophy, while vasodilators such as minoxidil and hydralazine do not cause any regression. Further research will show whether the same results can be found in humans.[11]

There is a circular relationship between hypertension and atherosclerosis in that hypertension is a risk factor for atherosclerosis, and atherosclerosis, particularly of the renal arteries, can promote the development of hypertension. Since hypertension is one of the major modifiable risk factors for atherosclerosis, particularly coronary heart disease, a clear understanding of the management of high blood pressure is critical for nurses interested in preventive health and promotion of optimal life styles.

Ophthalmic Effects. Ophthalmoscopic examination of the retina provides an opportunity to assess the effects of high blood pressure on the microcirculation. In mild high blood pressure the only changes that may be seen in the microvasculature are focal and generalized narrowing, and straightening of the vessels. With accelerated hypertension, more extensive damage is seen. Linear hemorrhages, cotton wool spots (patchy white areas with indefinite edges), and papilledema are seen in the retina itself. The smaller retinal blood vessels show continued narrowing, while the larger arteries become wider, tortuous, and irregular. If papilledema is seen, the prognosis for client recovery is poor. Successful treatment and control of the hypertension can result in resolution of the linear hemorrhages, cotton wool spots, and papilledema, but not of the vascular changes.

Cerebrovascular Effects. A significant increase in cerebrovascular disease is seen in conjunction with hypertension, and the risk is intensified if there is coexisting diabetes mellitus, electrocardiographic evidence of left ventricular hypertrophy or elevated blood lipids. Post-mortem examination of the brains of persons who had hypertension reveals atherosclerosis of the larger arteries and fibrinoid necrosis (a form of vascular degeneration) or the smaller arteries and arterioles. These arterial lesions can result in large and small intracerebral hemorrhages due to rupture of the vessel walls, and also small areas of infarction (lacunar infarctions) due to obliteration of the arterial lumen. In addition, persons with elevated blood pressures are at risk for transient ischemic attacks (TIAs, see Chap 66). During assessment of clients with elevated pressures, it is important to determine whether they have experienced any of the symptoms that are associated with TIA, because some people who have these symptoms do subsequently have cerebrovascular accidents.

Renal Effects. The most significant effect of high blood pressure on the kidney is seen in individuals with malignant or accelerated hypertension. In uncomplicated essential hypertension only minor vascular changes with little influence on renal function have been noted. In malignant hypertension the main lesion is severe narrowing of some of the interlobular arteries, resulting in ischemia and atrophy of the nephrons distal to the lesion. Areas whose arterial blood supply is not decreased may hypertrophy. Overall there is a net loss of kidney tissue, and ultimately signs of renal failure may become apparent (see Chap 58).

Clinical Manifestations

Signs of High Blood Pressure

The best indicator of high blood pressure is an elevated blood pressure as measured by sphygmomanometer. The definitions of various levels of high blood pressure are given in the beginning of this chapter. It is, however, important to recognize that one elevated reading does not necessarily mean that an individual has hypertension. First, two or more measurements of blood pressure are obtained on any client visit, and these readings are averaged to obtain the blood pressure for that visit. Accurate blood pressure measurement technique is obviously critical since several different types of errors can be made which have significant effects on the recorded pressure.

Once an average blood pressure has been obtained for a client visit, the person is either referred to a physician for diagnosis or is asked to return for a repeat measurement, depending on how elevated the first average pressure was. The recommended criteria for client referral are shown in Figure 44–3.

Other signs of hypertension occur as a result of target organ damage. Cardiac hypertrophy, especially left ventricular hypertrophy, can be evaluated by electrocardiogram or by x-ray examination of the chest. Elevations in serum creatinine concentration or blood urea nitrogen (BUN) may signal kidney damage. An elevated BUN is a less reliable indicator because it can also be elevated by an increase in protein intake or by a decrease in blood volume. A history of TIAs may indicate central nervous system dysfunction. As previously discussed in the section on pathophysiology, ophthalmoscopic examination of the optic fundus of the eye may reveal vascular changes which are thought to be indicative of changes in other blood vessels.

Symptoms of High Blood Pressure

There are no symptoms that are reliably correlated with an elevated blood pressure. It is for this reason that hypertension has become known as "the silent killer." This lack of apparent symptoms can make it difficult to convince clients that they have a serious health problem requiring lifelong attention. Nurses play a key role in educating clients about the increased mortality and morbidity associated with high pressure.

The two symptoms that have long been associated with high blood pressure are headaches and nosebleeds (epistaxis). Although the majority of studies have not found positive relationships between these two problems and hypertension, the blood pressure of clients with these symptoms should always be measured as part of the routine physical examination. One study of the records of 2051 individuals with epistaxis found that the people with hypertension had an increase in the severity but not the incidence of nosebleeds.[31]

Important Factors in Blood Pressure Measurement

Since critical diagnostic and therapeutic decisions are based on the measurement of a single variable—blood pressure—it is imperative that the measurement be as accurate as possible. The national standards are in the American Heart Association pamphlet, "Recommendations for Human Blood Pressure Determination by Sphygmomanometers," which can be obtained from your local American Heart Association

<table>
<tr><th rowspan="2">Diastolic Blood Pressure (mmHg)</th><th colspan="3">Systolic Blood Pressure (mmHg)</th></tr>
<tr><th>Less than 140</th><th>140 to 199</th><th>200 or greater</th></tr>
<tr><td>Less than 85</td><td>Recheck within 2 years**</td><td rowspan="2">1st Occasion
Confirm within 2 months

2nd Occasion
Evaluate or refer promptly to a source of care</td><td rowspan="2">Evaluate or refer to a source of care within 2 weeks</td></tr>
<tr><td>85 to 89</td><td>Recheck within 1 year</td></tr>
<tr><td>90 to 104</td><td colspan="3">1st Occasion
Confirm within 2 months
2nd Occasion
Evaluate or refer promptly to a source of care</td></tr>
<tr><td>105 to 114</td><td colspan="3">Evaluate or refer to a source of care within 2 weeks</td></tr>
<tr><td>115 or greater</td><td colspan="3">Evaluate or refer immediately to a source of care</td></tr>
</table>

Two or more measurements should be taken on each occasion and the average used as the value for that visit.
****Rechecking within one year is recommended for individuals at increased risk (*i.e.*, family history, obesity, blacks, oral contraceptive use, and high alcohol intake.)**

FIGURE 44–3 Follow-up criteria based on diastolic and systolic measurements on two occasions in asymptomatic individuals 18 years and older. (From 1984 Report of the Joint National Committee on Detection, Evaluation, and Treatment of High Blood Pressure.)

office. Some of the key points and potential sources of error are reviewed here.[14]

Cuff Size. One of the most common sources of error in the measurement of blood pressure is the use of a cuff containing an inflatable bladder which is the improper size for the client's arm or limb. Use of a bladder which is too narrow will result in an erroneously high blood pressure reading, while too wide a cuff will result in an erroneously low reading. The American Heart Association recommends that the width of the inflatable bladder should be 40% of the circumference of the mid-point of the arm or limb, or 20% wider than the limb's diameter (Fig. 44–4). The length of the inflatable bladder should be twice its width.

Check to determine that the site where you are practicing has an appropriate variety of cuff sizes for its expected clientele. Some institutions have only a few very large and very small cuffs, and it is important to know where these are located. If your client's upper arm is too large for the available cuff, check to see if that cuff would be the correct size for the forearm. If it is, then place that cuff around the lower arm and auscultate the Korotkoff sounds over the radial artery.

Pressure Gauge. A second cause of inaccurate blood pressure measurement is an inaccurate pressure gauge or manometer. Before using either an aneroid or mercury manometer, check to see that the gauge reads zero when no pressure has been applied to the cuff. With no pressure applied, the meniscus of the mercury column should be opposite zero and the needle of the aneroid gauge should be pointing to zero. If the zero is correct then a mercury manometer will usually be accurate.

For an aneroid manometer, one further check on accuracy is required: *calibration* or systematic standardization against a mercury manometer. Figure 44–5 is a diagram of how to connect an aneroid gauge to a mercury manometer. The mercury manometer should be pumped up to approximately 250 mmHg and then stopped at 50 mmHg intervals as the pressure is released. The pressure on the aneroid gauge should equal the pressure on the mercury column at every interval, that is, at 250, 200, 150, 100, and 50 mmHg. If the aneroid gauge is found to be inaccurate it should be returned to the manufacturer or to the institution's medical instrument facility. The accuracy of aneroid sphygmomanometers should be checked every 2 to 3 months, or more often if they are heavily used or subjected to rough treatment.

Auscultatory Gap. A third potential error in blood pressure measurement is the presence of an auscultatory gap, which is the temporary disappearance of the Korotkoff sounds after phase I and during part of phase II. The sounds associated with the phases of the Korotkoff sounds are as follows:

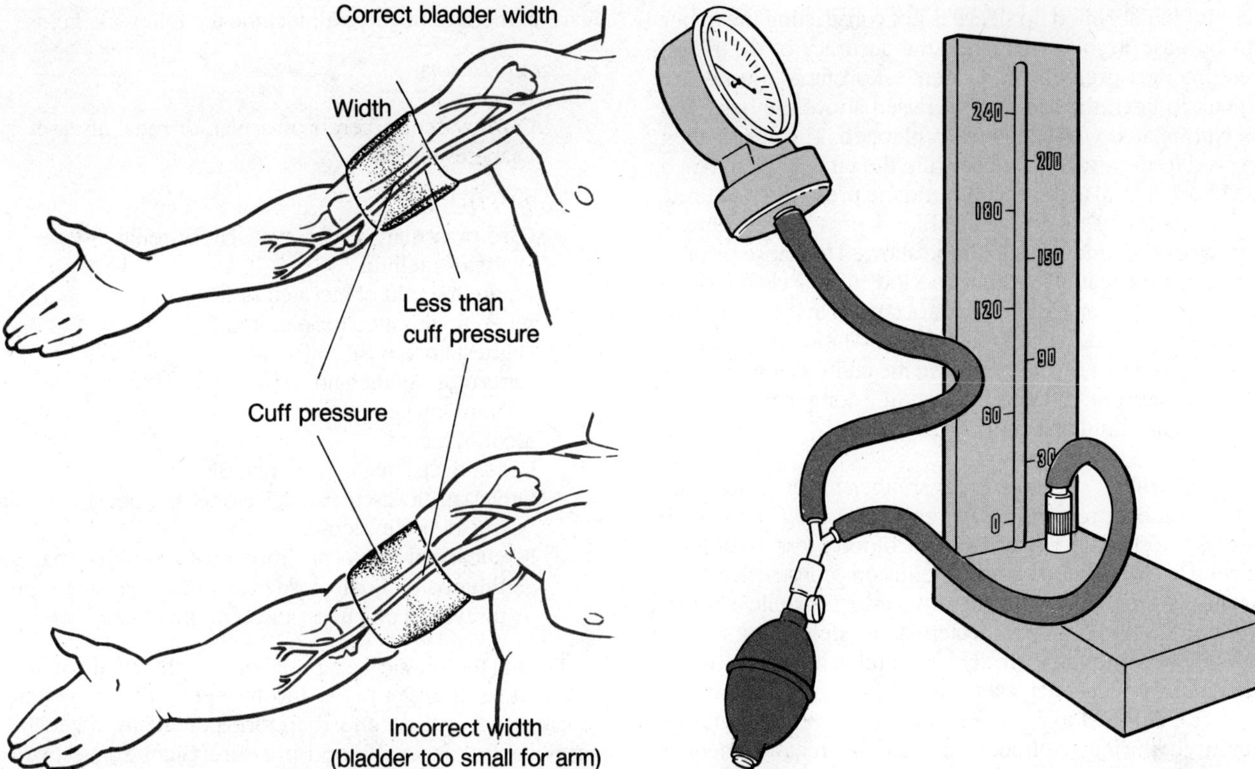

FIGURE 44–4 Cuff bladder and arm relationships. On the bottom the bladder width is small for the arm and the artery never has full cuff pressure applied. An erroneously high pressure results. On the top the bladder width is adequate for the arm, and full cuff pressure is applied to the brachial artery.

FIGURE 44–5 Use of a Y connector to calibrate an aneroid sphygmomanometer. The reference mercury manometer must be functioning perfectly to obtain reliable results.

Phase I
Sound: First appearance of faint, clear tapping sounds that gradually increase in intensity
Recorded as systolic BP
Phase II
Sound: A swishing or murmurlike quality
Phase III
Sound: Becomes crisper and increases in intensity
Phase IV
Sound: Distinct muffling occurs; sounds become soft and blowing
Phase V
Sounds disappear
Recorded as diastolic BP[36]

In some clients, particularly those with elevated pressures, as the pressure in the cuff is reduced the first Korotkoff sounds will be heard, then the sounds will disappear briefly and then be heard again at a pressure up to 40 mmHg lower than the initial sounds. Failure to appreciate the existence of an auscultatory gap results in a potentially serious underestimate of the person's systolic blood pressure.

To avoid this problem the true systolic pressure should be first evaluated by palpation. To palpate the systolic pressure, apply the cuff to the client's arm as usual, then inflate the bladder while palpating the radial pulse. Inflate to approximately 30 mmHg above the pressure when the pulse can no longer be palpated. Then deflate the cuff until the radial pulse can again first be felt. This pressure is a good estimation of systolic pressure. The cuff should be inflated to approximately 30 mmHg above this estimated systolic pressure during auscultatory measurement of blood pressure. For repeated measurements of blood pressure, as would be done for a hospitalized client, it is not necessary to repeat the palpation every time.

Diastolic pressure in the adult is most closely correlated with the disappearance of the Korotkoff sounds (phase V). In children it correlates more closely with the fourth Korotkoff sound, commonly known as "muffling." In some adults there is no disappearance of sound until the pressure is at or near zero. In this case the systolic pressure and the fourth and fifth Korotkoff sounds, muffling and disappearance, should be recorded in the format: 115/74/0. In addition, the position of the client at the time the pressure was recorded and the arm or limb in which it was measured should be recorded, at least at the time of the initial assessment of the client.

Arm Position. For screening and routine blood pressure measurements, the client should be comfortably seated with the forearm supported at heart level. If the client is supine or standing, the limb and blood pressure cuff must be at heart level for the reading to be accurate. The clothing should be removed or loosely folded out of the way so that the majority of the upper arm is bare. Care should be taken that a folded or rolled up sleeve is not constricting the upper arm because it could influence the accuracy of the blood pressure measurement. If a client's Korotkoff sounds are difficult to hear, the arm can be raised above the head and the cuff inflated while the arm is elevated. The arm is then lowered to the usual position while the cuff is deflated at a rate of 2 to 3 mmHg per second, and the pressure measured. If it is necessary to repeat the blood pressure reading, a period of 1 to 2 minutes should be allowed to elapse prior to reinflating the cuff. This time period allows clearance of vascular congestion that may have occurred in the lower arm during the period the cuff was inflated. The time that needs to be allowed varies with how long the cuff was inflated; that is, the longer the cuff was inflated, the longer the interval until the cuff should be reinflated.

Respiration. Respiration is another factor that can influence blood pressure measurement. During inspiration there is a normal decrease in systolic blood pressure of up to 12 mmHg. In tense pericardial effusion, constrictive pericarditis, restrictive cardiomyopathy, severe chronic obstructive lung diseases, and hypovolemia, the decline in systolic pressure becomes abnormally large and is known as pulsus paradoxus.[23] In clients with any of the above conditions or at risk of developing them, systolic pressure should be measured during expiration so that the measurement is standardized.

Orthostatic Hypotension. Blood pressure is measured in the lying, sitting, and standing positions to assess for the presence of orthostatic hypotension. Normally, when an individual goes from a supine to an upright position, there is a fall in systolic pressure of approximately 10 mmHg, a rise in diastolic pressure of 5 mmHg, and a 5 to 20 beat per minute increase in heart rate.[29] There is, however, considerable individual variation in these values. Whenever possible, postural blood pressure should be measured on routine contacts with the health care system so that each individual's normal response is known. If there is a fall of more than 10 to 15 mmHg in systolic pressure or any fall in diastolic pressure that is accompanied by symptoms of inadequate cerebral perfusion such as dizziness, visual dimming, or head and neck discomfort, then the person has orthostatic hypotension.[29] Assessment for orthostatic hypotension should begin with the client resting in the supine position for at least 10 minutes. After the blood pressure and apical heart rate have been measured, the client is assisted to the sitting and then standing positions, where the blood pressure and heart rate are remeasured after 1 to 3 minutes in each position.[36]

Diagnosis

A client is referred to a physician for evaluation and diagnosis if his blood pressure is found to be elevated. The physician's evaluation will be focused on determining whether the client has any other risk factors for cardiovascular disease; whether there is any evidence of damage to the major target organs for hypertension, that is, heart, kidneys, brain, and eyes; and whether it is primary or secondary hypertension.[33]

A careful medical history will include the following items:

Family History

Elevated BP
Cardiovascular, cerebrovascular, or renal disease
Diabetes mellitus

Patient History

Cardiovascular, cerebrovascular, or renal disease
Diabetes mellitus
When first told of elevated BP
When first treated for elevated BP
Highest known BP
Pattern of weight gain
Sodium intake
Alcohol intake
Use of drugs that may elevate BP
Other cardiovascular risk factors (*e.g.,* obesity, smoking, hyperlipidemia)
Psychosocial and environmental factors that may influence BP control, such as emotional stress, cultural food practices, and economic status

During the physical examination the physician will look for evidence of target organ involvement and for evidence indicating secondary, and therefore potentially reversible, causes of the elevated blood pressure. Signs suggestive of secondary hypertension include the following:

- Abdominal or flank masses (polycystic kidneys)
- Abdominal bruits, those that lateralize or have a diastolic component (renovascular disease)
- Delayed or absent femoral or arterial pulses (coarctation of the aorta)
- Truncal obesity with pigmented striae (Cushing's syndrome)
- Tachycardia, sweating, and pallor (pheochromocytoma)

During the physical examination the blood pressure will be taken several times and averaged to obtain a value for the visit. In addition, the pressure will be measured in the supine or flat, sitting, and standing positions as well as in both arms. A significant fall in systolic or diastolic pressure, or in both, with assumption of the upright posture can indicate either sympathetic nervous system disease or saline deficit. Blood pressure may be lower in one arm because of constriction of the arterial blood supply to the arm by a blood vessel malformation or because of external pressure on the vessel.

Laboratory tests including hemoglobin, hematocrit, serum potassium and creatinine levels, electrocardiogram, and complete urinalysis will provide additional information for diagnosis and determination of target organ damage. Because some pharmacologic therapies for hypertension can result in potentially adverse biochemical changes, baseline levels of glucose, uric acid, cholesterol, and total and high density lipoproteins are determined. Some of these results also provide data about current cardiovascular risk factors.

If the data from the initial evaluation indicate the possibility of secondary hypertension, further diagnostic tests will be ordered as indicated. Extensive diagnostic testing is not recommended for every client because of the relative rarity of secondary hypertension and because of the need to limit unnecessary costs and client risk.

Although not routine at this time, 24-hour ambulatory blood pressure monitoring is currently being investigated as a further tool in evaluating clients with high blood pressure. For some individuals, blood pressure is highest at the doctor's office and lowest at home. Values at work are usually somewhere between these two extremes. For 24-hour monitoring the client wears a cuff connected to a miniature recording device while going about usual daily activities. The cuff inflates at regular intervals and the pressure and time are recorded. The physician then can obtain a read-out of the client's blood pressure over an entire day. The cost-effectiveness, reliability, and diagnostic usefulness of this technique are not yet clearly established.

Treatment

Tremendous advances in the treatment of high blood pressure have occurred since the early part of this century when all that was available was the Kempner rice diet, which consisted primarily of rice, fresh fruit, and fresh vegetables. Today an array of effective treatments allows the client and practitioner to tailor a therapeutic program to match the needs and preferences of the individual client. While this choice improves the ability to control elevated pressure, it also requires that the nurse be informed about the various modes of therapy, and their advantages and disadvantages. The two major categories of antihypertensive treatment are *nonpharmacologic* and *pharmacologic*—treatment with and without drugs.

Lifestyle Changes

Nonpharmacologic approaches to the control of high blood pressure can be described as lifestyle or behavior changes. The lifestyle changes that have been clearly demonstrated to result in a decrease in blood pressure include weight reduction, sodium restriction, exercise, and biofeedback techniques. For each client it is necessary to determine which of these lifestyle changes are appropriate and acceptable. For some clients, lifestyle alterations alone will result in blood pressure control, whereas other clients will also require drug therapy. Investigation on nondrug therapy is in its infancy, and new developments in this area should be anticipated during the next decade.

Dietary Considerations. The two most effective nonpharmacologic modalities for the reduction of elevated blood pressure are *weight reduction* and *sodium restriction.*[16] Other dietary interventions for blood pressure control have been proposed, but there is not yet sufficient data available to evaluate their effectiveness. Maintenance of *potassium intake* is important for patients on some types of diuretic therapy and may also have a role in reducing blood pressure.

There is a significant, positive relationship between body weight and blood pressure in that risk of developing hypertension increases as the body weight increases. Research has clearly demonstrated that for most overweight individuals with high blood pressure, weight loss will result in a fall in pressure.[16,26,34] In addition, it is not always necessary for the person to achieve "ideal body weight" in order to achieve pressure control. The scientific basis for the relationship between body weight and blood pressure has not yet been determined.

Despite many years of research on the nature of the relationship between sodium intake and high blood pressure, the link between the two is not well understood. It is known, however, that in some populations there is a positive relationship between dietary sodium intake and the incidence of high blood pressure, and also that restriction of sodium intake in persons with elevated pressure results in a fall in pressure. Specific information on how to help patients achieve and maintain a low sodium diet is presented in the Nursing Management section under Knowledge Deficit.

Since diuretic therapy, particularly with the thiazide and loop diuretics, frequently results in potassium depletion, a high potassium diet is recommended for hypertensive patients. In addition, a recent study by Parfrey and co-workers found that adding 100 mEq potassium per day to the normal diet of persons with essential hypertension resulted in a significant fall of 8.9 mmHg in blood diastolic pressure after 6 weeks.[24] There have also been reports about the influence of calcium, magnesium, and other ions on arterial blood pressure; however, these results are still controversial, and practical recommendations for patient care cannot be made at this time.[19]

Exercise. Exercise training consisting of at least 30 minutes of exercise 2 to 3 times per week has been demonstrated to have a blood pressure-lowering effect in some individuals.[5,30] One study by Roman and co-workers showed that in a group of middle-aged women, blood pressure was reduced during training but returned to higher levels when the exercise was stopped.[30] Regular isotonic exercise is recommended for individuals with elevated pressures, both for its pressure-lowering effects and as an adjunct to dieting for weight reduction.[35]

Relaxation Techniques. Biofeedback of physiological variables such as pulse-wave velocity, and various relaxation techniques have been demonstrated to be effective methods of lowering blood pressure for periods up to 1 year.[2,10,25] These strategies can be offered as alternative methods of therapy for persons who are interested or who are unable to tolerate other forms of treatment. The requirement of a therapist trained in biofeedback techniques and of 10 or more training sessions requires both commitment of the client and closeness to a center with the necessary therapists and equipment.

Other Factors. Smoking cessation and reduction of saturated fat intake are recommended for persons with high blood pressure to decrease their overall cardiovascular risk, even though these two measures do not directly influence blood pressure. In addition, since an alcohol intake of more than four drinks per day has been associated with elevated blood pressure, persons with a history of excessive intake should be informed of this relationship and counseled to seek help to control their drinking.[15] Despite a popular be-

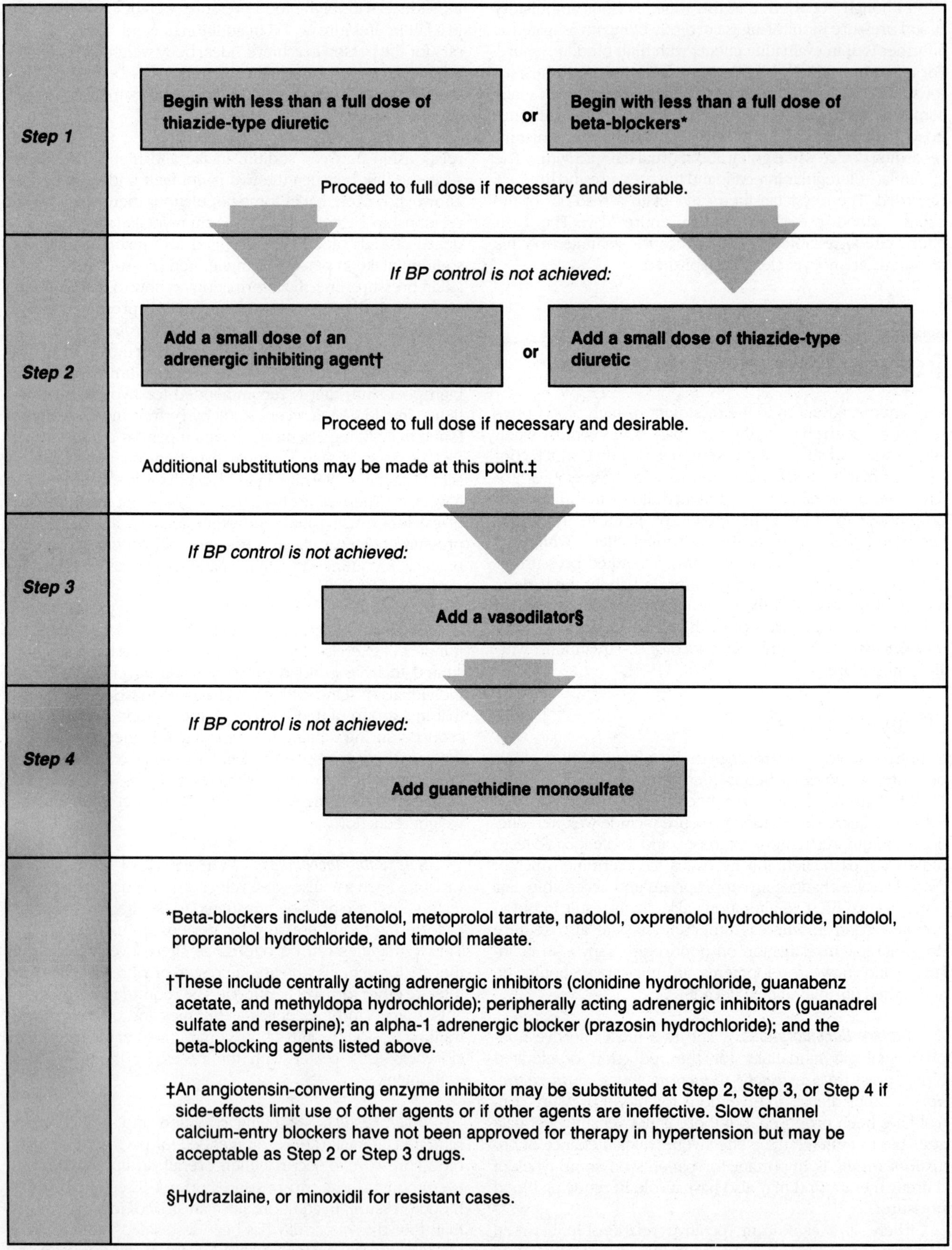

Step 1

Begin with less than a full dose of thiazide-type diuretic

or

Begin with less than a full dose of beta-blockers*

Proceed to full dose if necessary and desirable.

Step 2

If BP control is not achieved:

Add a small dose of an adrenergic inhibiting agent†

or

Add a small dose of thiazide-type diuretic

Proceed to full dose if necessary and desirable.

Additional substitutions may be made at this point.‡

Step 3

If BP control is not achieved:

Add a vasodilator§

Step 4

If BP control is not achieved:

Add guanethidine monosulfate

*Beta-blockers include atenolol, metoprolol tartrate, nadolol, oxprenolol hydrochloride, pindolol, propranolol hydrochloride, and timolol maleate.

†These include centrally acting adrenergic inhibitors (clonidine hydrochloride, guanabenz acetate, and methyldopa hydrochloride); peripherally acting adrenergic inhibitors (guanadrel sulfate and reserpine); an alpha-1 adrenergic blocker (prazosin hydrochloride); and the beta-blocking agents listed above.

‡An angiotensin-converting enzyme inhibitor may be substituted at Step 2, Step 3, or Step 4 if side-effects limit use of other agents or if other agents are ineffective. Slow channel calcium-entry blockers have not been approved for therapy in hypertension but may be acceptable as Step 2 or Step 3 drugs.

§Hydrazlaine, or minoxidil for resistant cases.

FIGURE 44–6 Stepped-care approach to drug therapy. (1984 Report of the Joint National Committee on Detection, Evaluation, and Treatment of High Blood Pressure)

lief that coffee drinking is associated with high blood pressure, there is no scientific data indicating such a relationship.

Pharmacotherapy

Evidence that the reduction of blood pressure by pharmacologic treatment is effective in reducing the morbidity and mortality associated with hypertension has been collecting since the early 1960s. It has now been demonstrated that overall mortality, cardiovascular mortality, and the incidence of cerebrovascular accident is decreased by the pharmacologic therapy.[12, 28, 38, 39] The data, however, do not yet indicate any decrease in the incidence of myocardial infarction. The benefits of treatment have been most apparent in middle-aged men and least apparent in white women.[32]

Stepped Care

For mild, moderate, and severe hypertension, if nonpharmacologic approaches to blood pressure management are not effective in lowering an individual's diastolic pressure below 90 mmHg or if the individual is unwilling or unable to alter his lifestyle, pharmacologic therapy is recommended. The current standard for the pharmacologic treatment of hypertension as outlined in the Third Joint National Committee Report on Detection, Evaluation, and Treatment of High Blood Pressure is known as stepped care (Fig. 44–6). For stepped care the person is started out on small doses of a drug, either a thiazide-type diuretic or a β-adrenergic blocking agent, and then the dose is increased and other medications are added or substituted sequentially until the diastolic pressure is less than 90 mmHg or the side-effects of drug therapy become intolerable. This approach allows care to be tailored to the individual and allows some flexibility within the guidelines. It is recommended that 2 to 3 months be allowed to elapse between medication changes to let the medications achieve their full effect. The medications in each level of stepped care and their recommended dosages are shown in Table 44–1. Table 44–2 contains a listing of the most common adverse effects for each drug.

Although the stepped care approach to the care of individuals with hypertension was developed by a panel of national experts, not all medical practitioners agree with it. Another protocol for the management of clients with hypertension has been proposed by Laragh and Sealey. Their diagnostic and treatment schema is based on their *vasoconstriction-volume model* of hypertension.[17] This approach to patient care uses the same medications as stepped care, but has different criteria on which to base the decision about which drug should be used for a particular client.

A key nursing function when caring for clients on antihypertensive medications is patient education. In addition to the usual information that should be given to any patient placed on medications, the importance of continuing to take the pills must be stressed. The person should know that if adverse effects are encountered, these should be reported to the doctor so that the medication or dosage can be altered. One great challenge for people with high blood pressure is to keep taking their pills for long periods of time. The support that is needed to stay on medications is discussed under Nursing Management. Persons on β-adrenergic block-

TABLE 44–1
Antihypertensive Agents*

	Dosage Range⁺ *(mg/day)* *(Initial–Maximum**)*
Diuretics	
Thiazides and Related Sulfonamide Diuretics	
Bendroflumethiazide	2.5–5
Benzthiazide	25.0–50
Chlorothiazide sodium	250.0–500
Chlorthalidone	25.0–50
Cylcothiazide	1.0–2
Hydrochlorothiazide	25.0–50
Hydroflumethiazide	25.0–50
Indapamide	2.5–5
Metolazone	2.5–5
Methyclothiazide	2.5–5
Polythiazide	2.0–4
Quinethazone	50.0–100
Trichlormethiazide	2.0–4
Loop Diuretics	
Bumetanide†	0.5–10‡
Ethacrynic acid	50.0–200‡
Furosemide	80.0–480‡
Potassium-Sparing Agents	
Amiloride hydrochloride	5.0–10
Spironolactone	50.0–100
Triamterene	50.0–100
Adrenergic Inhibitors	
β-Adrenergic Blockers¶	
Atenolol	25.0–100
Metoprolol tartrate	50.0–300
Nadolol	20.0–120
Oxprenolol hydrochloride	160.0–480
Pindolol	20.0–60‡
Propranolol hydrochloride	40.0–480‡
Propranolol long-acting (LA)	80.0–480
Timolol meleate	20.0–60‡
Central Adrenergic Inhibitors	
Clonidine hydrochloride	0.2–1.2‡
Guanabenz acetate	8.0–32‡
Methyldopa	500.0–2000‡
Peripheral Adrenergic Antagonists	
Guanadrel sulfate	10.0–150‡
Guanethidine monosulfate	10.0–300
Rauwolfia alkaloids	
Rauwolfia (whole root)	50.0–100
Reserpine	0.05–0.25 (additional derivatives available)
α-1 Adrenergic Blocker	
Prazosin hydrochloride	1.0–20‡
Combined α- and β-Adrenergic Blocker	
Labetalol hydrochloride#	200.0–1200
Vasodilators	
Hydralazine hydrochloride	50.0–300‡
Minoxidil	5.0–100‡

(Continued)

TABLE 44–1
Antihypertensive Agents* (Continued)

	*Dosage Range⁺ (mg/day) (Initial–Maximum**)*
Angiotensin-Converting Enzyme Inhibitors	
Captopril	37.5–150‡
Enalapril maleate#	10.0–40
Slow Channel Calcium-Entry Blocking Agents†	
Diltiazem hydrochloride	120.0–240***
Nifedipine	30.0–180***
Verapamil hydrochloride	240.0–480***

* All drugs are listed by generic name. If more specific information is desired, consult the *Physicians' Desk Reference*, 38th Edition, 1984.
⁺ The dosage range may differ slightly from recommended dosage in the *Physicians' Desk Reference* or package insert.
** The maximum suggested dosage may be exceeded in resistant cases.
† These drugs have not been approved for the treatment of high blood pressure by the Food and Drug Administration (FDA).
‡ This drug is usually given in divided doses twice daily.
¶ Atenolol and metoprolol are cardioselective; oxprenolol and pindolol have partial agonist activity.
# This drug has not been approved by the FDA.
*** This drug is usually given in divided doses three or four times daily.
(The 1984 Report of the Joint National Committee on Detection, Evaluation, and Treatment of High Blood Pressure, p 18)

ing agents particularly need to know that adverse effects can occur if they abruptly stop taking their pills.

Step Down Program

Once blood pressure control has been established on antihypertensive medications for a 6- to 12-month period, it may be possible to begin to decrease or "step down" the dosage or amount of medication that a client is taking. There will be an increased chance for success in stepping down if the client has been able to implement some of the nonpharmacologic or lifestyle changes during this period. This step down should be done under careful supervision, with periods of several months between medication changes. If a client is finally able to cease medication, he should continue to have his blood pressure monitored regularly for the remainder of his life.

Since data on the efficacy of treating borderline isolated systolic hypertension will not be available until the completion of the multi-center Systolic Hypertension in the Elderly Program, current recommendations for treatment represent a consensus opinion from leaders in the area in blood pressure control. If the decision is made to treat the client with borderline isolated systolic hypertension, salt restriction and weight reduction are recommended. Use of reduced doses of diuretics or centrally acting adrenergic inhibitors is recommended for treatment of isolated systolic hypertension. Because guanethidine, guanadrel sulfate, and prazosin sometimes cause orthostatic hypotension, they

TABLE 44–2
Adverse Drug Effects

Drugs	*Side-Effects*	*Precautions and Special Considerations*
Diuretics		
Thiazides and related sulfonamide diuretics	Hypokalemia, hyperuricemia, glucose intolerance, hypercholesterolemia, hypertriglyceridemia, sexual dysfunction	May be ineffective in renal failure. Hypokalemia increases digitalis toxicity. Hyperuricemia may precipitate acute gout.
Loop diuretics Bumetanide** Ethacrynic acid Furosemide	Same as for thiazides	Effective in chronic renal failure. Cautions regarding hypokalemia and hypeuricemia as above. Hyponatremia may be found, especially in the elderly.
Potassium-sparing agents	Hyperkalemia	Danger of hyperkalemia in patients with renal failure.
Amiloride hydrochloride	Sexual dysfunction	
Spironolactone	Gynecomastia, mastodynia, sexual dysfunction	
Triamterene		

(*Continued*)

TABLE 44–2
Adverse Drug Effects (Continued)

Drugs	*Side-Effects*	*Precautions and Special Considerations*
Adrenergic Antagonists		
Beta-adrenergic blockers* Atenolol Metoprolol tartrate Nadolol Oxprenolol hydrochloride Pindolol Propranolol hydrochloride Timolol maleate	Bradycardia, fatigue, insomnia, bizarre dreams, sexual dysfunction, hypertriglyceridemia, decreased HDL cholesterol	Should not be used in patients with asthma, chronic obstructive pulmonary disease (COPD), congestive heart failure, heat block (> first degree) and sick sinus syndrome. Use with caution in patients with diabetes mellitus and peripheral vascular disease.
Central-acting adrenergic inhibitors	Drowsiness, dry mouth, fatigue, sexual dysfunction	
Clonidine hydrochloride		Rebound hypertension may occur with abrupt discontinuance.
Guanabenz acetate		Same as for clonidine.
Methyldopa		May cause liver damage, and positive direct Coombs' test result.
Peripheral-acting adrenergic inhibitors	Sexual dysfunction, nasal congestion	
Guanadrel sulfate	Orthostatic hypotension, diarrhea	Use cautiously in elderly patients because of orthostatic hypotension
Guanethidine monosulfate	Same as for guanadrel sulfate	Same as for guanadrel sulfate.
Rauwolfia alkaloids	Lethargy	Contraindicated in patients with history of mental depression.
Reserpine	Same as for Rauwolfia alkaloids	Same as for Rauwolfia alkaloids.
α-1 adrenergic blocker		
Prazosin hydrochloride	"First doser" syncope, orthostatic hypotension, weakness, palpitations	Use cautiously in elderly patients because of orthostatic hypotension.
Combined α- and β-adrenergic blockers		
Labetalol hydrochloride⁺	Nausea, fatigue, dizziness, asthma, headache (rare)	Contraindicated in sick sinus syndrome, in heart block (> first degree); use with caution in cardiac failure, bronchial asthma, COPD, diabetes mellitus.
Vasodilators		
In general:	Headache, tachycardia, fluid retention	May precipitate angina in patients with coronary heart disease.
Hydralazine hydrochloride	Positive antinuclear antibody (without other changes)	Lupus syndrome may occur (rare at recommended doses).

(Continued)

TABLE 44–2
Adverse Drug Effects (Continued)

Drugs	*Side-Effects*	*Precautions and Special Considerations*
Vasodilators		
Minoxidil	Hypertrichosis, ascites (rare)	May cause or aggravate pleural and pericardial effusions.
Angiotensin-Converting Enzyme Inhibitors**		
Captopril	Rash and dysgeusia (rare at recommended doses)	Can cause reversible, acute renal failure in patients with bilateral renal arterial stenosis. Neutropenia may occur in patients with autoimmune collagen disorders. Proteinuria (rare at recommended doses).
Enalapril maleate⁺	Same as for captopril	Same as for captopril.
Slow Channel Calcium-Entry Blocking Agents**		
In general:	Headache, hypotension, dizziness	
Diltiazem hydrochloride	Nausea	Use with caution in patients with congestive failure or heart block.
Nifedipine		
Verapamil hydrochloride	Flushing, edema, and constipation	Same as for diltiazem hydrochloride.

* Sudden withdrawal has been reported to be hazardous in patients with heart disease.
+ Not yet approved by the FDA.
** These drugs have not been approved by the FDA for the treatment of high blood pressure.
(The 1984 Report of the Joint National Committee on Detection, Evaluation, and Treatment of High Blood Pressure, pp 20–21)

should be avoided in the elderly to prevent adding to their already increased risk of falling.[33]

Hypertensive Emergencies

There are situations in which blood pressure needs to be reduced rapidly. The Third Joint National Committee has defined hypertensive emergencies as those situations in which blood pressure must be lowered within 1 hour, while hypertensive urgencies are those in which blood pressure must be lowered within 24 hours. The difference between these two situations is the speed with which end-organ damage or death would be expected to occur. Examples of hypertensive emergencies include hypertensive encephalopathy, intracranial hemorrhage, acute left-ventricular failure with pulmonary edema, dissecting aortic aneurysm, and severe hypertension associated with other medical conditions. Examples of hypertensive urgencies include perioperative hypertension and accelerated hypertension without apparent impending complications. Medications and dosages recommended for use in hypertensive urgencies and emergencies are listed in Table 44–3.[33]

Nursing Management

Nursing's role in the management of high blood pressure takes many forms depending on the clinical setting, the type of client population, and the level of expertise of the nurse. In the following section, nursing's role is discussed in two broad categories: first, in relation to screening activities designed to detect unknown or uncontrolled high blood pressure; and second, in relation to the care of persons under treatment for hypertension.

Screening Assessment

Blood pressure screening activities are designed to find persons unaware of their elevated pressure, and those aware of their problem but not currently under active care. Early experience with screening programs that had no provision for follow-up or tracking found that such programs were ineffective in getting detected cases into care and under control. Screening programs, therefore, should not be undertaken

TABLE 44–3
Drugs for Managing Hypertensive Emergencies and Urgencies

Drugs	Intramuscular, mg*	Intravenous (IV) Single Dose, mg	Intravenous (IV) Continuous Infusion§	Onset of Action	Adverse effects
Direct Vasodilators					
Diazoxide		50–100 IV bolus**	15–30 mg/min over 20–30 min	3–5 min	Nausea, vomiting, hyperglycemia, hyperuricemia, hypotension, flushing, tachycardia, chest pain
Sodium nitroprusside			50–100 mg/liter	Instantaneous	Nausea, vomiting, muscle twitching, sweating, thiocyanate intoxication, apprehension
Hydralazine hydrochloride	10–50	10–20†	200 mg/liter	Intramuscularly 20–30 min; IV 10–12 min	Tachycardia, palpitations, flushing, headache, vomiting, aggravation of angina
Nitroglycerin			0.5–10 μg/kg/min	2–5 min	Bradycardia, tachycardia, flushing, headache, vomiting, methemoglobinemia
Sympathetic Blocking Agents					
Reserpine	1–5			2–3 hr	Drowsiness, stupor, bradycardia, hypotension, activation of peptic ulcer
Labetalol hydrochloride		20–80 IV bolus	2 mg/min; 300 mg max	5–10 min	Vomiting, nausea, scalp tingling, burning in throat and groin, pain at injection site, postural hypotension, dizziness
Methyldopate hydrochloride		250–500¶		2–3 hr	Drowsiness
Trimethaphan camsylate			1000 mg/liter	5–10 min	Paresis of bowel and bladder, orthostatic hypotension, blurred vision, dry mouth
α-Receptor Blocking Agents					
Phentolamine	5–15	5–15 (rapid injection essential)	200–400 mg/liter	Instantaneous	Tachycardia, flushing

* Start with the smallest dose shown. Subsequent doses and intervals of administration should be adjusted according to the response of blood pressure.

§ Start infusion slowly and adjust rate according to response of blood pressure. Constant surveillance is mandatory. Concentration of solution can be adjusted to patient's fluid requirements.

*** To be given at intervals of 5–10 min.

† The total dosage should be contained in a volume of at least 20 ml and the solution should be administered from a 20- or 50-ml syringe. Blood pressure should be monitored continuously while the injection is being made. Rate of injection should not exceed 0.5 ml/min. To avoid hypotension, the injection should be stopped frequently when the blood pressure is falling.

¶ Diluted up to 100 ml and injected during a 30- to 60-min period.

(The 1984 Report of the Joint National Committee on Detection, Evaluation, and Treatment of High Blood Pressure, p 25) unless provision for follow-up care is included. Additionally, because many Americans now have their pressure checked during routine contact with members of the health care team, the National High Blood Pressure Education Program recommends that screening activities be focused on high-risk groups and on those with limited access to the health care system.[33] Groups at higher risk include blacks, working-age men, obese individuals, and blood relatives of persons with known high blood pressure.

When planning or participating in screening activities, nurses need to be cognizant of the educational opportunity afforded. Exposure to such large groups provides the chance to inform or ask all participants about

- The blood pressure reading and what the numbers mean
- The necessity for regular blood pressure rechecks
- The potential consequences of uncontrolled high blood pressure and the importance and benefits of blood pressure control
- Lifestyle habits that may help to prevent the development of high blood pressure (limit sodium intake, avoidance of being overweight, and regular exercise)
- Previous treatment for high blood pressure
- Other risk factors for cardiovascular disease

For persons whose first pressure reading is elevated, two or more pressure measurements should be taken and averaged to obtain the blood pressure for that occasion. Individuals whose averaged pressure is elevated (diastolic pressure > 90 mmHg or systolic pressure > 140 mmHg) should be asked to return for follow-up blood pressure measurements or should be referred directly to a source of care according to the guidelines in Figure 44–3. It is important to remember that these values are intended as guidelines, and clients can be referred at lower pressures or can be asked to return for repeat measurements sooner if there are signs or symptoms of end-organ disease or if the nurse's clinical judgment is that they should be seen earlier. Since the number of clients who return for follow-up or make appointments to see their health care practitioner will be influenced by the screener, it is critical that effective use be made of the relatively brief screening period.

Management of Known High Blood Pressure

Assessment

The nursing assessment of clients known to have hypertension includes measurement of blood pressure in the lying, sitting, and standing positions. Repeated measurements of pressure during the visit are then usually made in the sitting position. A basic assessment of cardiac and vascular function should be done if this is the first visit to the care situation or if indicated by the history or client condition on a follow-up visit. As stated previously, two or more blood pressure measurements are made during the visit, and the pressures are averaged to get the value for that visit. Other data to be collected include the following:

- A brief description of the client's experiences since the last visit to the care facility or prior to admission
- Client knowledge about blood pressure and hypertension
- Knowledge about prescribed treatments, both lifestyle modification and medications
- Presence of other cardiovascular risk factors
- Duration of the elevated blood pressure
- The occurrence of any side-effects of therapy

Nursing Diagnoses

The two nursing diagnoses that will occur most frequently in clients with elevated pressures are inadequate knowledge about high blood pressure and its causes, consequences, and treatment related to a lack of effective teaching; and noncompliance with the treatment plan related to factors such as insufficient knowledge, inability to follow therapeutic regimen, lack of social support, or lack of involvement in development of the care plan. In addition, clients may develop a variety of other problems which would lead to nursing diagnoses in areas such as fluid balance and circulation.

Knowledge Deficit

A client with high blood pressure may lack information about any or all aspects of high blood pressure control. The magnitude of the client's knowledge deficit will be determined during the nursing assessment. Before developing teaching goals and a care plan, the nurse should carry out further discussion with the client to learn his level of knowledge, his emotional readiness for learning, and the level of teaching best suited to his capabilities.

If the client's knowledge deficit is in the area of the nature of high blood pressure and its causes, consequences, and treatment, a teaching plan should be developed accordingly. Be sure that the level is appropriate for the client. Teaching aids such as pamphlets, brochures, and movies are often available through the local offices of the American Heart Association or American Red Cross, from state departments of chronic disease control, from the National High Blood Pressure Education Program, and from many pharmaceutical companies.

Reducing Sodium Intake. Helping clients overcome a lack of knowledge about the low sodium diet includes the following goals and interventions.

Goals. The goals for the clients related to lack of knowledge about low sodium diet would be

1. To be able to state the rationale for sodium restriction in the treatment of high blood pressure
2. To recognize significant sources of sodium in foods
3. To achieve and maintain a sodium intake of no more than 2 grams (2000 mg) per day

Interventions. Interventions to increase a client's knowledge of low sodium diets must begin with the nurse and client understanding the underlying rationale. A sodium-restricted diet is prescribed for people with high blood pressure, heart failure, renal disease, idiopathic edema, or other conditions in which fluid retention is a problem. In the initial encounter the nurse should ask if the client has had any previous experience with a low-sodium diet and, if so, what instructions were given, how successful was the client with the diet, and how does he feel about returning to the diet. The responses to these questions will give a background for developing a teaching plan.

Next, it is important to determine the client's understanding of why a sodium-restricted diet is important as part, or all, of therapy. The most important concept is that excess sodium intake often causes body fluid retention, which then contributes to high blood pressure and edema. The client on diuretic therapy needs to know that diuretic drugs are more effective when the person is on a sodium-restricted diet.[9]

Once the nurse has determined the client's previous experience with low sodium diets and his knowledge about why the diet is important, she can provide, or reinforce and supplement, the following information:

- Sodium is 40% of table salt, which is sodium chloride
- Salt and sodium, although related, are not synonymous
- Sodium is in foods in a variety of forms including sodium bicarbonate (baking soda), sodium benzoate (a preservative), sodium saccharin (a sweetening agent), and other chemical compounds. All these forms of sodium must be counted in the prescribed daily amount of sodium.
- Even though it does not taste "salty," a food may contain significant amounts of sodium. For example, hot cakes, butter, and syrup at a fast food restaurant may contain more than 1 gram of sodium.
- The following food groups are arranged in descending order from those containing the most naturally occurring sodium to those containing the least: grain and cereal products; meats, fish, and poultry; milk and cheese products; oils and fats; and fresh legumes, garden fruits, and vegetables.[3]

The next step is to plan how to modify the client's usual diet so that it contains only the prescribed amount of sodium. Ideally, the client should keep a diary of all food eaten over a given time period, such as a week, and then the client, nurse, and dietician if available can analyze it to determine which diet patterns need to be changed and which do not. If the situation does not allow this kind of analysis, then one can ask the client to recall what foods have been eaten over the past couple of days. Taking the food history allows tailoring of the instructions to the individual situation and prevents telling the client to avoid foods that would never be eaten anyway.[12] It is also important to ask which meals are eaten out, which are eaten at home, and who prepares the meals eaten at home. To include the food preparer in the dietary teaching, ask the client to bring that person in on the next clinic visit.

Although the level of sodium intake that is prescribed may vary, a 2-gram sodium diet is what is commonly recommended for persons with high blood pressure. Two grams of sodium is equal to five grams of salt or 43.5 mEq of sodium. Since most food product labels give sodium amounts in milligrams, it is helpful to tell the client that he is allowed 2000 mg per day. Reading product labels is one of the most useful skills that the client and food preparer can acquire. All foods that carry nutrition labels are now required by the Food and Drug Administration to list the sodium content.

Lowering the sodium content in the diet can be done by taking four steps:

1. Remove the salt shaker from the table.
2. Do not use salt in cooking.
3. Avoid canned or processed convenience foods that are high in sodium.
4. Use low sodium seasoning such as herbs and spices instead of salty flavorings.[6]

A handout or publication listing the sodium content of common foods should be provided so that, at least during the initial weeks, food eaten can be recorded daily and the daily sodium intake can be estimated each evening. This type of exercise is a valuable learning tool. In fact, each nursing student should consider doing it to become familiar with obvious and hidden sources of sodium in the diet.

Evaluation. Evaluation of goal achievement can take several approaches. Food diaries for 3 or more days can again be used to calculate the amount of dietary sodium. The client's self-report of adherence to the diet, including ways found to adapt favorite recipes or foods to the low-sodium requirement, will provide additional information. Twenty-four-hour urine collection for sodium analysis will give the most exact data about how much sodium the client is actually ingesting. This measurement can be very useful in providing feedback to a client about his success in lowering sodium intake. If the 24-hour sodium intake is not near the therapeutic goal, remember to use a nonjudgmental approach in discussing problems with following the diet. The results can be used as a basis for problem solving with the client.

Compliance/Noncompliance

Compliance can be defined as the degree to which the client follows the prescribed therapeutic regimen. *Adherence* and *acceptance* are sometimes used as alternate terms for compliance. Although compliance is frequently discussed in relation to hypertension, it can be an issue in any aspect of patient care. Poor compliance may indicate a problem on the part of the provider as well as the client. Some of the ways that the provider can fail include not giving clear instructions, not giving any instructions, or not assessing the client's readiness or primary concerns.

Assessment. To determine if there is or may be a problem with compliance to the therapeutic regimen, the nursing assessment will include questions about concerns or difficulties in managing health problems. Has the client been treated for high blood pressure previously, and what was the outcome? Has the client ever had any problems with following treatments prescribed for other conditions? What have been his experiences with medication-taking and altering lifestyle? Answers to questions like these will offer clues about how the client may respond to the treatment prescribed for his high blood pressure. In addition, if the client's blood pressure does not decrease in response to the regimen within a reasonable period of time, the nurse should reassess for any indication of noncompliance so that some of the strategies mentioned below can be utilized or reinforced.

A nursing diagnosis in this area might be poor compliance to the prescribed low sodium/low calorie diet related to lack of social support, or too confusing instructions.

Goals. Client goals related to poor compliance to the prescribed low sodium/low calorie diet would be

1. To have a family member be involved to support the client in following diet
2. To be able to restate clear and simple diet instructions
3. To state a specific goal for sodium and calorie intake

Interventions. Interventions to improve compliance are most effective when two or more are used in combination. Used alone, these strategies have not been effective. The nursing assessment will provide a basis for deciding which of the following approaches will be appropriate for the individual.

Clear and simple instructions are critical for ensuring compliance. Statements such as "cut down on your salt intake" or "try increasing your exercise" leave the client uncertain about what to do and may result in confusion, frustration, and worry. A better instruction would be "decrease your sodium intake to 2000 mg a day," followed by instruction on facts about sodium and salt, label reading, and low-sodium cooking as described in thc previous section, Knowledge Deficit. Simple instructions as well as simple therapeutic regimens increase compliance. It is much easier to take one or two medications once or twice daily than multiple medications three to four times daily.

It is not necessary to teach clients all about high blood pressure on one visit, or to try to have them change several behaviors at a time. Begin with basic and simple information, then add more gradually over the time you have available (1 or 2 days in a hospital or weeks to months in a home or clinic). If you only have a brief period, such as during a hospitalization, perhaps a teaching plan can be developed with the hospital discharge planner, using resources available to the client in the community.

Another critical factor in compliance is involving clients as active partners in their care plans. Clients are ultimately in charge of their own care, and early recognition of this fact will engage clients as participants. Four critical patient behaviors necessary in achieving blood pressure control have been identified by a working group of the National High Blood Pressure Education Program. These critical behaviors are as follows:

1. Make the decision to control blood pressure.
2. Take medication as prescribed (or follow treatment plan as prescribed).
3. Monitor progress toward blood pressure goal.
4. Resolve problems which block achieving blood pressure control.[39]

Recognition of these behaviors and their sequential nature will guide assessment and care planning. If the client has not yet decided that blood pressure control is important, then a care plan that focuses on teaching him how to take his medications would be unlikely to be very beneficial. The plan should be directed towards determining why blood pressure is not seen as important by the client and toward teaching about the consequences of uncontrolled high blood pressure. Not everyone decides to control blood pressure for the same reasons, so it will be important to get to know the client well enough to know what might be a motivating factor.

Having the person measure his own blood pressure and setting a specific goal pressure for him to achieve are two strategies that have been used successfully. Blood pressure measurement can be taught to clients individually, or they can be referred to the American Red Cross classes if they are available in your area. Home monitoring of blood pressure can provide the team treating the client with valuable information about the effectiveness of treatment and how the client's pressure varies through the day. It is also very useful for clients whose pressures are always highest at the health care facility. The concept of goal blood pressures was used extremely successfully in a large multicenter study known as the Hypertension Detection and Follow-up Program. In this study the client's goal was a diastolic pressure less than 90 mmHg if the diastolic blood pressure was greater than 100 mmHg, or a decrease of 10 mmHg if the original pressure was between 90 and 100 mmHg.[13]

Involvement of a family member has been demonstrated to be very effective in helping individuals to achieve blood pressure control.[18] The family member can be reached by having him or her come to clinic visits with the client or, if the situation allows, by visiting the client and family at home. Involvement of the family member provides the client with a support and reminder system. In addition, it helps to ensure that the family understands the therapeutic regimen, which may affect the whole family. For example, putting an individual on a low calorie and low sodium diet may mean changes for everyone in the family. If the food preparer does not understand the diet or considers it an unnecessary bother, then it is very unlikely that the client will be successful in losing weight or reducing sodium intake. Family members can also be taught blood pressure measurement with the client.

For some clients, knowing that they can buy life insurance at a lower premium if their blood pressure is under control may be a motivating factor. The client will need to consult with the insurance companies to see which ones offer this arrangement.[21]

Evaluation. Evaluation of goal achievement is based on whether the client has achieved goal blood pressure. Another method that has been used is counting the client's pills on each visit to determine how many have been taken. This method seems to imply a lack of trust in the client and may be best saved for persons of limited ability who need to be more closely monitored. In addition, one can monitor the client's progress in making lifestyle changes such as losing weight. Client logs of home blood pressure readings will offer valuable information about pressures between clinic or hospital visits.

Summary

This chapter points out the many ways that nurses can be involved in the direct care of people with high blood pressure. Nurses can in addition have a critical role in other blood pressure control activities. These opportunities include community planning, coordination of community blood pressure control activities, political activity to ensure adequate funding for community programs, public education, and research into client problems with achieving blood pressure control.

References

1. Amery A, Bulpitt C, Fagard R, Staessen J: Does diet matter in hypertension? Eur Heart J 1:299, 1980
2. Benson H: Systemic relaxation and the relaxation response. N Engl J Med 296:1152, 1977
3. Blackburn H, Prineas R: Diet and hypertension: Anthropology, epidemiology, and public health implications. Prog Biochem Pharmacol 19:31, 1983
4. Blaustein MP: Sodium ions, calcium ions, blood pressure regulation, and hypertension: A reassessment and a hypothesis. Am J Physiol 232:C165, 1977
5. Choquette G, Ferguson RJ: Blood pressure reduction in "borderline" hypertensives following physical training. Can Med Assoc J 108:699, 1973
6. Controlling sodium and calories. Seattle, American Heart Association, Washington Affiliate, 1983
7. Coordinating Committee of the National High Blood Pressure Education Program: Collaboration in high blood pressure control: Among professionals and with the patient. Ann Intern Med 101:393, 1984
8. Conway J: Hemodynamic aspects of essential hypertension in humans. Physiol Rev 64:617, 1984
9. Dustan HR, Tarazi RC, Bravo EL: Diuretic and diet treatment of hypertension. Arch Intern Med 133:1007, 1974
10. Engel BT, Glasgow MS, Garader KR: Behavioral treatment of high blood prssure. III. Follow-up results and treatment recommendations. Psychosom Med 45:23, 1983
11. Frohlich, ED: The heart in hypertension. In Genest J, Kuchel O, Hamet P, and Cantin M (eds): Hypertension: Physiopathology and Treatment, 2nd ed, pp 791–810. New York, McGraw-Hill, 1983
12. Hill M: Helping the hypertensive patient control sodium intake. Am J Nurs 79:906, 1979
13. Hypertension Detection and Follow-up Program Cooperative Group: The effect of treatment on mortality in mild hypertension. N Engl J Med 307:976, 1983
14. Kirkendall WM, Feinleib M, Freis ED, Mark AL: American Heart Association recommendations for human blood pressure determination by sphygmomanometer. Circulation 62:1145A, 1980
15. Klatsky AL: The relationship of alcohol and the cardiovascular system. Annu Rev Nutr 2:51, 1982
16. Langford HG, Blaufox MD, Oberman A, Hawkins M et al: Dietary therapy slows the return of hypertension after stopping prolonged medication. JAMA 253:657, 1985
17. Laragh JH, Sealey JE: Renin–sodium profiling: Why, how, and when in clinical practice. Cardiovasc Med 2:1053, 1977
18. Levine DM, Green JW, Deeds SG, Chwalox J, Russell RP, Finlay S: Health education for hypertensive patients. JAMA 241:1700, 1979
19. McCarron DA: Low serum concentrations of ionized calcium in patients with hypertension. N Engl J Med 307:226, 1982
20. Messerli FH, Frohlich ED: High blood pressure: A common side effect of drugs, poisons, and food. Arch Intern Med 139:682, 1979
21. Moser M, Rafter J, Gajewski J: Insurance premium reductions: A motivating factor in long-term hypertensive treatment. JAMA 251:756, 1984
22. Multiple Risk Factor Intervention Trial Research Group: Multiple risk factor intervention trial: Risk factor changes and mortality results. JAMA 248:465, 1982
23. Nutter DD: Measurement of the systemic blood pressure. In Hurse JW, Logue RB, Rackley CE, Schlant RC et al (eds): The Heart, Arteries and Veins, 5th ed, pp 182–187. New York, McGraw-Hill, 1982
24. Parfrey PS, Wright P, Goodwin FJ, Vandenburg MJ et al: Blood pressure and hormonal changes following alteration in dietary sodium and potassium in mild essential hypertension. Lancet 1:59, 1981
25. Patel C, Marmot MG, Terry DJ: Controlled trial of biofeedback-aided behavioral methods in reducing mild hypertension. Br Med J 282:2005, 1981
26. Reisin E, Abel R, Modan M, Silverberg D, et al: Effects of weight loss without salt restriction on the reduction of blood pressure in overweight hypertension patients. N Engl J Med 289:1, 1978
27. Report of the Subcommittee on Definition and Prevalence of the Joint National Committee on Detection, Evaluation, and Treatment of High Blood Pressure: Hypertension prevalence and the status of awareness, treatment, and control in the United States. Approved by the National High Blood Pressure Education Committee, January 1985
28. Report by the Management Committee: The Australian therapeutic trial in mild hypertension. Lancet 1:1261, 1980
29. Robertson D, Robertson RM: Orthostatic hypotension—diagnosis and therapy. Modern Concepts of Cardiovascular Disease 54:2, 1985
30. Roman O, Camuzzi AL, Villalon E, Klenner C: Physical training program in arterial hypertension. Cardiology 67:320, 1981
31. Shaheen OH: Arterial epistaxis. J Laryngol Otol 89:17, 1975
32. Staessen J, Cattaert A, Fagard R, Lijnen P et al: Epidemiology of treated, compared to untreated, hypertension. In Genest J, Kuchel O, Hamet P, Cantin M (eds): Hypertension Physiopathology and Treatment, 2nd ed, pp 1069–1093. New York, McGraw-Hill, 1983
33. The 1984 Report of the Joint National Committee on Detection, Evaluation, and Treatment of High Blood Pressure. Arch Intern Med 144:1045, 1984
34. Tuck ML, Sowers J, Dornfeld L, Kledzik G, Maxwell M: The effect of weight reduction on blood pressure, plasma renin activity, and plasma aldosterone levels in obese patients. N Engl J Med 304:930, 1981
35. US Department of Health, Education, and Welfare: The Framingham study: An epidemiological investigation of cardiovascular diseases. Section 31. The results of the Framingham study applied to four other US-based epidemiological studies of cardiovascular disease. DHEW Publication No. (NIH) 7a6a,1083, Washington DC, US Government Printing Office, 1976
36. Underhill SL: History-taking and physical examination of the patient with cardiovascular disease. In Underhill SL, Woods SL, Sivarajan ES, Halpenny CJ (eds): Cardiac Nursing. Philadelphia, JB Lippincott, 1982
37. Veterans Administration Cooperative Study Group on Antihypertensive Agents. Effects of treatment on morbidity in hypertension. I. Results in patients with diastolic blood pressure averaging 115 through 129 mmHg. JAMA 202:1028, 1967
38. Veterans Administration Cooperative Study Group on Antihypertensive Agents. Effects of treatment on morbidity in hypertension. II. Results in patients with diastolic blood pressure averaging 90 through 114 mmHg. JAMA 213:1143, 1970
39. Working Group to Define Critical Patient Behaviors in High Blood Pressure Control. Patient behavior for blood pressure control. JAMA 241:2534, 1979

Chapter 45

Inflammatory Disorders Affecting Vascular Function

Phlebitis
Thrombophlebitis

Lorie R. Wild

Phlebitis
Deep Vein Thrombophlebitis
Lymphangitis and Lymphadenitis

This chapter discusses the care of the patient with inflammatory disorders which affect peripheral vascular function. Conditions frequently associated with these types of disorders include phlebitis, deep vein thrombophlebitis, lymphangitis, and lymphadenitis.

Phlebitis

Phlebitis is the inflammation of a vein. Phlebitis affecting a superficial vein is a frequent complication in patients undergoing intravenous (IV) therapy. The overall incidence of phlebitis is estimated to be between 11% and 70%.[7]

Etiology

Several risk factors for developing infusion-related phlebitis have been identified. The major risk factor for developing phlebitis is the duration of IV therapy, particularly the duration of the IV access device.[7,10,13] Infusion-related phlebitis is lowest when IV cannulae are in place less than 24 hours. The most dramatic increase in the incidence of phlebitis occurs when cannulae remain in place beyond 72 hours.[7,13,15]

The type and size of the IV access device used also relate to the risk for developing phlebitis. Plastic catheters are associated with a higher incidence of phlebitis than are stainless steel needles.[6,7,13] Large bore cannulae are more likely to cause a phlebitis, especially when placed in a small vein.[15]

Other associated risk factors for phlebitis related to IV therapy are the location of the insertion site and the types of fluids being infused. The veins of the hand, wrist, or forearm are less likely to become phlebitic than veins in the lower extremities. Fluids and IV drugs high in either osmolality or particulate matter are associated with an increased incidence of phlebitis.[7,13,15]

Pathophysiology

Mechanical and chemical irritation of the vein leads to phlebitis. Causes of this irritation include the indwelling IV cannula itself, especially a plastic catheter, and the fluids infusing through it. The variable pH and the particulate matter of infusates and drugs can injure the delicate lining of the venous wall.

The inflammatory process stimulated by vessel injury or microbial contamination causes further changes in blood flow through that vein. The localized inflammation accounts for the signs and symptoms associated with phlebitis.

Clinical Manifestations

Superficial phlebitis presents as a linear area of redness following the involved vein. The affected vein may feel cord-like with palpation. The inflamed area may feel warm to the touch, indurated, or swollen. The swelling may not be pronounced with phlebitis of the superficial veins since blood flow is easily shunted to other, deeper vessels. However, if a deep vein is involved, venous congestion and swelling are likely to occur because of impaired collateral blood flow.[13]

The patient typically complains of tenderness in the affected area. The tenderness is usually accentuated with palpation of the phlebitic vessel or with direct pressure. Movement of the affected extremity may also be impaired.

The clinical manifestations of phlebitis may be blunted or delayed in some patients. The inflammatory response is inhibited in immunosuppressed patients. The localized tenderness associated with phlebitis may not be reported by patients who have diminished sensation or movement in a cannulated extremity.

Medical Management

The diagnosis of phlebitis is made on the basis of the patient's complaint and the physical examination since the clinical manifestations of the disorder are generally readily apparent. Other diagnostic studies are seldom used unless deep vein involvement is suspected. Several scales are available for grading the severity of phlebitis using criteria such as the degree of pain, erythema, swelling, and induration as well as the condition of the vein as determined by palpation.[6,7,15]

Nursing Management

Management of phlebitis is twofold. First, prophylactic measures are used to prevent phlebitis. The single most effective prophylaxis is in IV therapy maintenance. Rotating IV sites every 48 to 72 hours is essential to minimize the risk of phlebitis.[7,10] The choice of an IV access device (size, and steel needle vs. plastic catheter), and where and how it is inserted can also help prevent phlebitis. The smallest possible cannula (length and gauge) should be inserted into the distal arm veins whenever possible. Meticulous site care prevents localized wound infection which could lead to phlebitis.[10,13,15] To reduce chemical irritation, drugs administered by the IV route should be as dilute as possible to retain efficacy and comply with any fluid restrictions.

Definitive treatment for phlebitis is primarily symptomatic. The application of moist heat promotes blood flow in the affected extremity. Elevating the extremity assists venous return and reduces swelling. Analgesics and nonsteroidal, anti-inflammatory agents may be prescribed.

In the event of infectious complications resulting from phlebitis, appropriate antibiotic therapy is indicated. Heparin therapy may also be started to prevent thrombus formation. In rare cases, venectomy may be necessary.

Although phlebitis is a frequent complication of IV therapy, the inflammation present is generally mild and time-limited. Severe infectious complications such as septic thrombophlebitis and bacteremia are infrequent.[13] Immunosuppressed and burned patients are at greatest risk for infectious complications, necessitating meticulous surveillance of IV therapy in these groups.

The nursing care of the patient with phlebitis is outlined in the accompanying sample Nursing Care Plan for the Patient with Phlebitis. While nursing management focuses primarily on promoting circulation in the affected extremity as well as providing comfort measures to relieve symptoms, it must be reemphasized that the key to the problem of phlebitis is its prevention. Identification of patients at risk and careful monitoring of IV therapy are essential to avoid infusion-related phlebitis.

Deep Vein Thrombophlebitis

A thrombus is a clot or solid mass formed by blood components. *Thrombosis* refers to the formation or presence of blood clots within a vessel. The term *phlebitis* refers to an inflammation of a vein. Thus, the condition thrombophlebitis occurs when there is a clot with concurrent venous inflammation. Thrombophlebitis must be differentiated from the condition known as phlebothrombosis. Phlebothrombosis, a blood clot in the absence of venous inflammation, occurs less frequently but has a greater risk of embolization (the clot moving within the bloodstream) because the thrombus is loosely attached to the vessel wall. In thrombophlebitis the by-products of the inflammatory process help the clot to adhere to the vessel wall. Thrombophlebitis occurs most frequently within the extremities and may affect either a superficial or a deep vein. Often deep vein thrombophlebitis is difficult to detect since the clinical signs of inflammation may be discrete. Deep vein thrombosis is thought to occur in approximately 35% of hospitalized patients and is associated with additional complications such as embolization.[9]

Etiology and Pathophysiology

There are three factors which, when all present, predispose a patient to thrombosis and subsequent thrombophlebitis. These three factors are commonly known as Virchow's triad (Fig. 45–1). First, the vessel involved must have suffered some type of injury, particularly damage to the endothelial layer. Research has shown that microscopic endo-

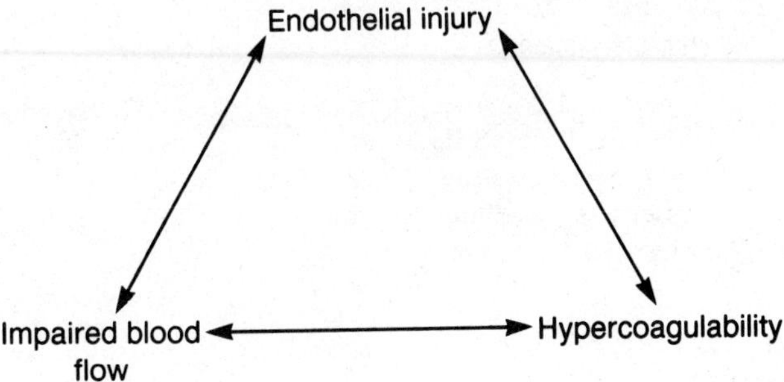

FIGURE 45–1 Virchow's triad: factors that predispose a patient to thrombosis and thrombophlebitis.

NURSING CARE PLAN FOR THE PATIENT WITH PHLEBITIS

NURSING DIAGNOSIS/PROBLEM 1: Alteration in peripheral tissue perfusion related to reduced venous blood flow.

GOAL 1.1: To prevent inflammation associated with IV therapy.

Nursing Interventions	Rationale	Outcome Criteria
1. Rotate IV sites every 48 to 72 hours.	1. The incidence of phlebitis dramatically increases with infusion devices left in place beyond 48 to 72 hours.[6, 7, 10, 13]	1–3. IV site free of a. Redness b. Warmth c. Induration d. Swelling Venous cord not palpable.
a. Use smallest gauge and length cannula possible.	a. Small bore, short cannulae produce less mechanical trauma to the vessel.	
b. Whenever possible, use stainless steel needles for IV access.	b. Stainless steel needles cause less tissue trauma and less chemical irritation than do plastic catheters.[15]	
c. Use veins in upper extremities, with preference to those in the distal forearm or hand.	c. Veins in the upper extremities are less likely to become phlebitic.[13, 15]	
d. Use strict aseptic technique during IV insertion.	d. Proper skin preparation and aseptic insertion technique minimizes amount of bacterial seeding of the IV access device which could lead to phlebitis.[10, 13]	
2. Maintain IV site.	2.	
a. Anchor cannula and tubing securely.	a. Securely anchoring the cannula and tubing reduces intravascular movement and mechanical trauma.	
b. Apply sterile dressing following site care every 48 to 72 hours and prn.	b. Dressing changes and site care prevents infection and possible seeding of the cannula by microorganisms.[10, 13]	
c. Change IV tubing sets every 24 to 48 hours.	c. Tubing changes minimize chance for infection resulting from a contaminated tubing apparatus.[10]	
3. Dilute IV push medications as much as possible.	3. Adequate dilution of medication reduces chemical irritation.	

GOAL 1.2: To detect early inflammation/phlebitis.

Nursing Interventions	Rationale	Outcome Criteria
1. Inspect and document appearance of IV sites every 8 hours, assessing for redness, warmth, induration, tenderness, swelling, palpable venous cord.	1. The signs and symptoms listed indicate inflammation.	1. Signs and symptoms of phlebitis, as outlined under Nursing Interventions, detected within 8 hours of occurrence.

(Continued)

NURSING CARE PLAN FOR THE PATIENT WITH PHLEBITIS (*Continued*)

GOAL 1.3: To minimize inflammation associated with phlebitis.

Nursing Interventions	Rationale	Outcome Criteria
1. Apply warm, moist heat to affected extremity.	1. Warm, moist heat increases blood flow in affected area.	1–3. Signs and symptoms of inflammation subside within 24 hours.
2. Elevate affected extremity.	2. Elevating affected extremity above heart level promotes venous return and reduces swelling.	
3. Administer anti-inflammatory agents as ordered by the physician.	3. Anti-inflammatory agents help reduce degree of inflammation pharmacologically.	

NURSING DIAGNOSIS/PROBLEM 2: Alteration in comfort related to phlebitis.
GOAL 2.1: To relieve discomfort in affected extremity.

Nursing Interventions	Rationale	Outcome Criteria
1. Apply warm, moist heat to affected extremity.	1. Increasing blood flow to affected extremity and promoting venous return help minimize discomfort associated with inflammation.	1–2. Discomfort relieved, demonstrated both verbally and nonverbally by patient. No signs of wincing with movement, guarding, or tensing of extremity.
2. Administer analgesics as ordered by physician.	2. Analgesics help to relieve discomfort pharmacologically.	

thelial damage is present prior to the development of venous thrombosis when associated with tissue trauma and reduced blood flow.[11] Injury may be the result of sustained pressure on the vessel or surrounding tissue as might occur from prolonged immobility of an extremity, or pressure points caused by plaster casts, crossed legs, elastic topped knee socks, or a bed where the knee gatch is raised too high. As discussed above, vessel injury can result directly from IV cannulae, and IV solutions and drugs infused through them. Injury to the vessel activates an inflammatory response which can be seen both histogically and, in most cases, clinically.

The second factor in the triad is impaired blood flow within the involved vessel. Normally, the pumping action of muscles against the venous vasculature assists venous return and is seen most vividly within the lower extremities. When an extremity remains immobile for any period of time, this pumping action is lost, resulting in venous stasis and pooling of blood, especially within the soleal sinuses. Decreased muscle pumping action and a reduction in venous velocity from prolonged standing results in the exertion of backward pressure on the venous valves, complicating venous pooling. Postoperative patients have been shown to have a decrease in total limb blood flow.[12] Any condition which acts to slow blood flow or decrease venous return to the right side of the heart places a patient at risk for developing thrombophlebitis.

The final predisposing factor of the triad involves hypercoagulability of the blood itself. Changes in blood constituents may occur as a result of polycythemia, severe anemia, or circulating endotoxins from systemic infections.[9] A deficiency in the amount of antithrombin III present has been proposed as a causative factor for thrombosis; however, a common coagulation abnormality has yet to be identified.[12]

Risk Factors

Certain patient populations are a greater risk for the development of deep vein thrombophlebitis. Several risk factors have been identified which all relate to the three etiological factors discussed previously. The major clinical risk factor is age. The relative risk of developing venous thrombosis is dramatically increased for patients over 40 years of age. For every 20 years, the relative risk for developing venous thrombosis more than triples.[8] For example, a 60-year-old patient is about three times more likely to develop thrombosis than is a 40-year-old patient and ten times more likely than a 20-year-old. The reasons behind the elderly patient's increased risk for thrombosis remains speculative, at best. The mechanisms involved are multifactorial but may include reductions in antithrombin III levels, increased factor VII, or direct changes in the vascular structures.[12] Changes in activity levels and decreased muscle tone may also predispose elderly patients to deep vein thrombophlebitis.

The postoperative patient's risk for developing deep vein thrombophlebitis also depends on the type of surgery performed. Orthopedic surgery is associated with a high risk for thrombosis; hip surgery constitutes the highest risk, with an incidence of 50% to 70%. Surgery following traumatic injury is also related to a higher incidence of thrombosis, primarily because prophylaxis is not possible and the coagulation cascade may already be activated. General surgery and neurosurgery are associated with 20% to 30% incidence of thrombosis; urological surgery is associated with a 10% to 40% incidence, depending on the procedure performed.[2]

Persons with a history of varicose veins or previous thrombosis are also at a higher risk for thrombosis. In both cases the venous capacitance is altered and venous pooling may result, thus predisposing the patient to development of thrombophlebitis.

The incidence of thrombosis is higher in patients with infections or malignancies. The higher risk is suspected to be due to alterations in the coagulation system.

Patients with cardiac disease are also at a higher risk for the development of thrombosis. The mechanisms predisposing these patients include general cardiac insufficiency along with alterations in blood flow and hemodynamic pressures, which may decrease venous return and subsequently cause venous stasis and pooling. In addition, patients with cardiac disease may be less active and are more prone to the hazards of stasis associated with immobility.[2,8,12]

Finally, patients who are undergoing estrogen therapy are at greater risk for the developmetn of thrombosis.[2,5,8] Estrogens are believed to induce distention of peripheral veins and changes in the coagulation and fibrinolytic systems. Because estrogen levels are elevated during pregnancy and puerperium, these patients are also at greater risk.[9]

Clinical Manifestations

The clinical manifestations of deep vein thrombophlebitis include the signs and symptoms associated with the inflammatory response: redness, swelling, heat, and pain. The clinical manifestations of deep vein thrombophlebitis may be somewhat elusive. It is estimated that approximately 50% of all patients who develop deep vein thrombophlebitis exhibit no signs or symptoms.[14] The patient may complain of some tenderness or aching in the extremity, most commonly in the calf, which is the most frequent site of the thrombosis. Some degree of cramping may be present with movement or at rest. One of the classic signs of deep vein thrombosis is a positive Homans' sign, which can be described as pain occuring in the affected calf with forceful dorsiflexion of the foot. The symptom probably occurs as a result of compression of the thrombosed vessel against peripheral nerves located near the calf muscles.[1] Caution must be taken, however, when interpreting Homans' sign because any inflammation near the calf muscles may also elicit pain with dorsiflexion. A false positive diagnosis of thrombosis can occur up to 50% of the time.[14]

While a positive Homans' sign may signal thrombosis in the lower extremities, a positive cuff sign may indicate thrombosis in the upper or lower extremities. The cuff sign is elicited by inflating the blood pressure cuff until pain is caused.

Other signs of deep vein thrombophlebitis may include warmth and redness of the affected extremity. Asymmetry between two extremities may also be present, with the affected limb being slightly larger owing to the congestion and edema associated with the inflammatory process.

Medical Management

When thrombosis is suspected in a patient, perhaps by the presence of clinical signs and symptoms, further diagnostic studies are indicated. These diagnostic studies include phlebography, nuclear venography, plethysmography, ultrasound, thermography, and ^{125}I-fibrinogen tests.[2,12]

Medical treatment of thrombophlebitis centers around prophylaxis. Preventive measures include mechanical methods to improve venous flow and prophylactic anticoagulation. The approach to treatment evolves from the triad of factors which predispose patients to the development of thrombosis.

Mechanical measures to deter venous stasis include antiembolism stockings, passive and active leg exercises, and early ambulation. Pneumatic cuffs and calf muscle stimulators may also be used.

The use of prophylactic anticoagulants has become a standard of practice for many hospitalized patients, particularly for those at highest risk for the development of thrombosis as previously discussed. The use of low dose heparin has been shown to decrease the incidence of deep vein thrombosis, and its use prophylactically has been recommended by the American Heart Association. The regimen utilizes 5000 units of subcutaneous heparin given two to three times daily, for the duration of bed rest and up to 1 week afterward. Larger doses do not appear to correlate with a lowered incidence of thrombosis and tend to increase the chance of bleeding.[1,2,3,12]

Agents other than heparin are also used for prophylaxis of thrombosis. Dextran is often employed as a prophylactic anticoagulant, especially with patients for whom any bleeding would be detrimental, such as neurosurgical patients. Dextran has been shown to be more effective than heparin for thromboprophylaxis in hip surgery patients.[2] Other agents used include oral anticoagulants such as sodium warfarin (Coumadin) and platelet influencing agents (aspirin, dipyridamole, sulfinpyrazone, flurbiprofen, ticlopidine). Combination therapies may also be implemented.

Definitive treatment for deep vein thrombophlebitis centers around symptom management and prevention of embolization. Pulmonary embolus is a serious sequel to thrombosis and is associated with a high mortality rate. (Refer to Chap 46 for further discussion of pulmonary embolism.) Anticoagulation with heparin and Coumadin are initiated to prevent further thrombus formation.[3] Occasionally thrombolytic agents such as streptokinase or urokinase may be employed in an attempt to dissolve the clot, particularly if it is totally occlusive. There remains a debate over activity limitations and elevation of the affected limb in persons with documented deep vein thrombophlebitis. Proponents suggest that the risk of embolization with activity and movement is too high, while opponents propose that immobility and limbs in dependent positions only serve to further increase venous stasis and its complications.

Surgical intervention for venous thrombosis is seldom necessary and is used only when other methods of treatment are contraindicated and the patient is at high risk for pulmonary emboli. In these cases a thrombectomy or a caval interruption may be performed in order to prevent the passage of emboli. Caval interruption can be accomplished by the transvenous placement of an umbrella filter into the inferior vena cava or by partial ligation of the caval segment. The umbrella filter traps emboli traveling from distal sites toward the pulmonary vasculature. Because caval interruption with an umbrella filter traps clots, vena caval occlusion can occur postoperatively, necessitating its removal.[4]

The prognosis for patients with deep vein thrombophlebitis is favorable. For most patients the problem resolves quickly without complications or residual morbidity. Unfortunately, in some patients deep vein thrombophlebitis is a recurrent problem. These patients are especially at risk for pulmonary emboli. Recurrent deep vein thrombophlebitis can also lead to postphlebitic syndrome, where affected veins become chronically scarred and dilated with marked venous insufficiency.[12] The problems associated with postphlebitic syndrome are similar to those encountered in varicose veins (Chap 47).

Nursing Management

The primary approach to nursing management of the patient at risk for the development of deep vein thrombophlebitis includes identifying the high-risk patient and implementing vigorous attempts to prevent its occurrence. Such attempts include encouraging leg exercises and early ambulation to increase muscle activity in the legs, and thereby improving venous return and avoiding venous stasis. For patients on bed rest, turning, coughing and deep-breathing at least every 2 hours will help reduce the risk of vessel injury and will promote venous return. In addition, antiembolism stockings may be used to improve venous return and flow rate in the legs. Other measures to improve venous return include elevating the foot of the bed 6 to 8 inches and making sure that the knee gatch on the bed is not raised to avoid exerting prolonged pressure on the popliteal area.

To detect signs of thrombophlebitis, the nurse should assess the patient at regular intervals for any evidence of inflammation such as redness, swelling, asymmetry, tenderness, aching, and Homans' sign. Any such signs must be documented and reported to the physician immediately.

Should thrombophlebitis occur, the nursing interventions would be based on the treatment prescribed by the physician, including the administration of anticoagulants, analgesics, and anti-inflammatory agents. Some physicians prefer to have the extremity elevated; others prefer that the leg be left flat to prevent embolization. There are also varied opinions about activity; some will insist on bed rest; others will prescribe moderate activity. Warm moist heat will help increase blood flow and antiembolism stockings will help prevent venous stasis. The area of the affected extremity should not be rubbed to avoid the danger of embolization.

To detect embolization, it is important to assess the patient every 2 hours. The signs to look for include sudden onset of dyspnea, chest pain, and tachypnea, alterations on levels of consciousness, abnormal arterial blood gases, and altered ECGs. An overview of nursing care with nursing diagnoses, goals, and outcomes is presented in the accompanying Nursing Care Plan for the Patient with Deep Vein Thrombophlebitis.

Lymphangitis and Lymphadenitis

Lymphangitis is the inflammation of lymphatic channels. Lymphadenitis is the inflammation of lymph nodes and is commonly referred to as "swollen glands." Any type of bacterial or viral infective process could lead to lymphangitis or lymphadenitis, or both. Lymphadenitis is seen more commonly in children than in adults.[1]

Pathophysiology

The lymphatic vessels travel adjacent to arteries and veins and ultimately empty by way of the thoracic duct and the right lymphatic duct into the venous system by means of the left innominate and right subclavian veins, respectively. The lymphatic system is important in maintaining fluid homeostasis within the vasculature and processing by-products of the immune response. Local inflammation of lymphatic channels or nodes can impair lymphatic flow. Diminished or obstructed lymphatic flow alters both fluid balance and blood flow.

Clinical Manifestations

The clinical manifestations of lymphangitis include the cardinal signs of inflammation: redness, tenderness, swelling, and warmth in the affected extremity. Red streaks following the lymphatic channels and fever may be present.

In lymphadenitis, tenderness and swelling may be noted in lymph nodes, especially those in the neck. The patient may experience fever and chills, in addition to the localized discomfort.

Medical Management

The diagnoses of lymphangitis and lymphadenitis are made by history and physical examination. Other types of diagnostic testing to assess lymphatic structures are unnecessary. Routine microbiology studies and cultures from any infected sites (throat, sputum, urine, blood) may be done to help isolate the infecting organism.

Medical treatment for both lymphangitis and lymphadenitis is primarily symptomatic. Analgesic, antipyretic, or anti-inflammatory agents may be prescribed. Generally, appropriate antibiotic coverage is also initiated.

Lymphangitis and lymphadenitis are usually mild, time-limited inflammattions lasting from 4 to 14 days.[1] Infective complications can occur, however, leading to lymphatic obstruction and lymphedema. Prompt resolution of the inflammation and the offending organism helps circumvent more serious complications.

Nursing Management

Nursing care of the patient with lymphangitis or lymphadenitis is similar to the care required for patients with phlebitis and deep vein thrombophlebitis as elucidated in the accompanying Nursing Care Plans. Application of a warm, moist compress over the affected area not only enhances perfusion, but also helps promote patient comfort. Encouraging rest and fluids are other comfort measures which are especially important for the febrile patient.

NURSING CARE PLAN FOR THE PATIENT WITH DEEP VEIN THROMBOPHLEBITIS

NURSING DIAGNOSIS/PROBLEM 1: Alteration in peripheral tissue perfusion related to inflammatory process.

GOAL 1.1: To prevent the formation of thrombi and inflammation.

Nursing Interventions	Rationale	Outcome Criteria
1. Encourage movement of lower limbs. a. Leg exercises b. Early ambulation	1. Increased muscle activity in lower extremities improves venous return by muscle pumping action, thereby reducing venous stasis.	1–6. Absence of signs and symptoms of inflammation: redness, warmth, swelling, positive Homans' sign, tenderness and aching in affected limb.
2. Encourage turning, coughing, and deep breathing at least every 2 hours.	2. Turning helps to alleviate pressure points to tissues, thereby decreasing risk for vessel injury and venous stasis. Deep breathing increases negative intrathoracic pressure, thus promoting improved venous return.	
3. Apply antiembolism stockings as ordered.	3. Antiembolism stockings improve venous flow rate in the lower limbs.[2]	
4. Administer anticoagulants as ordered by physician.	4. Anticoagulants deter thrombus formation. See discussion above.	
5. Elevate foot of bed 6 to 8 inches.	5. Foot elevation to this level improves venous return and helps reduce venous stasis.[1]	
6. Do not engage knee gatch of patient's bed.	6. A raised knee gatch exerts prolonged pressure on the popliteal area and vessels which may induce vessel injury and inhibit venous return by compression.	

GOAL 1.2: To detect early and to treat thrombophlebitis, should it occur.

Nursing Interventions	Rationale	Outcome Criteria
1. Assess patient every 8 hours; document and report the presence of signs and symptoms of inflammation: redness, swelling, asymmetry, tenderness, aching, Homans' sign.	1. Presence of any signs and symptoms of inflammation may signal thrombosis.	1. Thrombophlebitis detected within a 4-hour time span.

(Continued)

NURSING CARE PLAN FOR THE PATIENT WITH DEEP VEIN THROMBOPHLEBITIS (*Continued*)

Nursing Interventions	Rationale	Outcome Criteria
2. Implement treatment of thrombophlebitis as ordered by physician.	2.	2. Treatment of affected area within 1 hour of detection.
a. Administration of anticoagulants	a. Anticoagulants help prevent further clot formation and may help prevent embolization.	
b. Positioning of extremity	b. Extremity may be elevated to promote venous return, or left flat to prevent embolization of thrombi.	
c. Activity restrictions	c. Some physicians require bed rest for their patients to reduce risk of embolization; others suggest moderate activity restrictions and encourage sitting for short periods to prevent further stasis and other complications of prolonged immobility.	
d. Application of warm, moist heat	d. Application of warm, moist heat increases blood flow to affected area.	
e. Application of anti-embolism stockings	e. Antiembolism stockings improve venous flow rate.	
f. Administration of analgesics	f. Analgesics help to reduce discomfort experienced by patient.	
g. Administration of anti-inflammatory agents	g. Anti-inflammatory agents help reduce the degree of inflammation present and may also aid in promoting venous flow.[2]	
3. Avoid rubbing or massaging the affected area.	3. Rubbing or massaging increases the danger of the thrombus breaking off and embolizing.	3. No signs and symptoms of pulmonary embolism evident. Normal breathing pattern (no dyspnea). No complaints of chest pain. Normal heart rate and ECG. Normal mentation and awareness. Normal blood gas.
4. Assess, document, and report any signs and symptoms of pulmonary embolus every 2 hours, and as necessary. a. Sudden onset of dyspnea, chest pain, tachypnea b. Alterations in level of consciousness c. Abnormal arterial blood gases d. Electrocardiographic alterations	4. Pulmonary embolism is the most common and serious sequel to thrombisis and may occur rapidly.	4. Signs and symptoms of pulmonary embolism detected within a 2-hour time span.

References

1. Abramson DL: Circulatory Diseases of the Limbs. New York, Grune & Stratton, 1978
2. Bergqvist D: Postoperative Thromboembolism. Berlin, Springer-Verlag, 1983
3. Deykin D: Current status of anticoagulant therapy. Am J Med 72:659–664, 1982
4. Fernsebner B, Baum PL, Bartlett C: Surgical prevention of pulmonary emboli: Vena caval interruption. AORN J 29(1):56–70, 1984
5. Kaplan NM: Cardiovascular complications of oral contraceptives. Annu Rev Med 29:31, 1978
6. Larson E, Hargiss C: A decentralized approach to maintenance of intravenous therapy. Am J Infect Control 12(3):177–186, 1984
7. Larson E, Lunche S, Tran JT: Correlates of IV phlebitis. NITA 7:203–205, 1984
8. Nicolaides AN, Irving D: Clinical factors and the risk of deep venous thrombosis. In Nicolaides AN (ed): Thromboembolism. Baltimore, University Park Press, 1975
9. Rose AD: Diseases of the veins. In Silver MD (ed): Cardiovascular Pathology, Vol 2. New York, Churchill Livingstone, 1983
10. Simmons BP: Guideline for prevention of intravascular infections. Guideline for prevention of intravenous therapy-related infections. In National Nosocomial Infections Study Report, Annual Summary, 1979. Atlanta, Centers for Disease Control, 1982
11. Stewart CJ: The role of the vessel wall in deep venous thrombosis. In Nicolaides AN (ed): Thromboembolism. Baltimore, University Park Press, 1975
12. Strandness DE, Thiele BL: Selected Topics in Venous Disorders. Mount Kisco, New York, Futura Publishing Company, 1981
13. Stratton CW: Infection related to intravenous infusion. Heart Lung 11:123–135, 1982
14. Sutton GC: Venous thrombosis and pulmonary embolism. Medicine SA 24:91, 1978
15. Turco SJ: Infusion phlebitis. Crit Care Monitor 2(6):1,4–5, 1982

Bibliography

Fahey VA: An in-depth look at deep vein thrombosis. Nursing 14(3):35–41, 1984

Friedman SA: Vascular Diseases. Littletown, Massachusetts, John Wright-PSG Inc, 1982

McCarthy ST: Peripheral Vascular Disease in the Elderly. Edinburg, Churchill Livingstone, 1983

Nichols EG, Barstow RE, Cooper D: Relationship between incidence of phlebitis and frequency of changing IV tubing and percutaneous site. Nurs Res 30:247–252, 1983

Nursing diagnoses: Direct routes to your patient's vascular problems. Nursing 14(9):64D, 1984

Taylor DL: Thrombophlebitis: Physiology, signs, and symptoms. Nursing 13(7):52–53, 1983

Wilson JE, Bynum LJ, Parkey RW: Heparin therapy in venous thromboembolism. Am J Med 70:808–816, 1981

Chapter 46

Arterial Occlusion

Ischemia and Infarction Affecting Vascular Function

Lorie R. Wild

The focus of this chapter is the management of patients with vascular disorders leading to ischemia and infarction of the extremities. These severely debilitating disorders not only jeopardize limb viability but are also potentially fatal. Vascular disorders can be divided into two categories: arterial occlusive disorders and functional arterial or vasomotor disorders. Chronic arterial occlusive problems include arteriosclerosis obliterans and thromboangiitis obliterans (Buerger's disease). Arterial embolism and pulmonary embolism are examples of acute arterial occlusive disorders. Raynaud's disease is an example of a functional disorder in that it is vasospastic and no pathological changes are evident within the vessels. Each of the disorders mentioned above is discussed with regard to etiology, pathophysiology, clinical manifestations, and treatment modalities, with a special focus on the nursing care of afflicted patients.

Arteriosclerosis Obliterans

Arteriosclerosis is a general term associated with a loss of elasticity and the hardening within the medial layer of the walls of small arteries. Atherosclerosis, a type of arteriosclerosis, affects primarily the intimal layer of the medium- and large-sized arteries. Atherosclerotic plaques containing lipids, fatty acids, cholesterol esters, and crystals are also found. Arteriosclerosis obliterans is the partial or complete obliteration of the arterial vessels, particularly within the extremities. The obstruction results from atheromatous plaques which effectively reduce the diameter of the vessel. The irregular surface of the vessel wall created by the plaque promotes thrombus formation, which can further reduce lumen diameter. The obstructed vessel thus impedes blood flow to the extremities, leading to ischemia and infarction.

The onset of arteriosclerosis obliterans generally occurs between the ages of 45 and 70 years with a mean age of 56 years.[1] The disorder is seen more frequently in men than in women and usually occurs at a later age in women. Persons who also have diabetes mellitus are at greater risk for developing the disease.

Etiology

Several causes for the development of arteriosclerosis obliterans have been advanced, but no one cause has been conclusively identified. Some of the theories proposed include errors in fat or lipid metabolism, coagulation defects, and genetic predisposition.[1] Alterations in blood supply to the arterial wall as a result of hemodynamic forces, catecholamine release related to stress, chemicals such as carbon monoxide and nicotine from cigarette smoke, mechanical trauma, or viruses may also contribute to the development of the disorder.[18]

Pathophysiology

The pathology associated with arteriosclerosis obliterans involves the atherosclerotic plaque which is seen as a proliferation of endothelial cells, a necrotic core, and a fibrous cap. The necrotic core contains cholesterol esters, cholesterol crystals, and calcium deposits. The fibrous cap contains arterial smooth muscle cells, collagen, and lipid filled cells (foam cells). There is also evidence of intimal thickening as well as degenerative changes within the medial layer involving atrophy of vascular smooth muscle cells in addition to collagen and calcium deposits. Platelet aggregation and thrombus formation at the site of the atheromatous lesion are also common.[1,18]

Compensatory mechanisms may come into play to preserve blood flow to the tissues of the extremities. A network of collateral circulation may develop, thus allowing vessels below the obstruction to fill. Symptomatology may be less severe when the disease is segmentalized and adequate collateral circulation exists.

Clinical Manifestations

The clinical manifestations of arteriosclerosis obliterans result from decreased oxygen delivery to the peripheral tissues and may include intermittent claudication, resting pain, alterations in skin color and temperature, trophic changes, and diminished or absent peripheral pulses. The severity of the observed signs and symptoms relates to the extent of the disorder. In diffuse disease, fewer collaterals are formed; thus, signs and symptoms are generally more severe. When obstructed vessels are more segmentalized, collateral circulation may adequately supply vessels distal to the obstructed area, thus minimizing signs and symptoms.

Intermittent Claudication. The symptom most commonly found in arteriosclerosis obliterans is intermittent claudication. Typically, the patient will describe the onset of a cramplike pain after walking a certain distance, which will disappear if he rests at that point. The area where the patient experiences the pain relates to the level of the obstructed vessel (Fig. 46–1). The cramping pain results from the buildup of metabolic wastes within the muscle tissue.[1,18] An exercising muscle demands more oxygen, and because arterial flow is decreased, less oxygenated blood reaches the tissues. Waste products from both aerobic and anaerobic metabolism build up in the muscle. The local irritation of peripheral nerves by these toxic wastes causes the ischemic pain. When the patient rests, the metabolites are washed out of the tissue and the pain dissipates. Figure 46–2 summarizes the mechanisms of intermittent claudication.

Resting Pain. In advanced chronic arterial occlusive disease the patient may experience pain in the affected extremities while at rest. The pain will frequently occur at night and may interfere with sleep. The pain is often described as a burning, numbness, or tingling in the toes.[18] The resting pain results from ischemic neuritis and is often alleviated by standing or walking. The mechanisms of resting pain differ from those associated with intermittent claudication. When the patient assumes a recumbent position both hydrostatic and systemic pressures decrease. As a result, blood flow to the tissues is reduced and tissue ischemia follows. When the patient stands, hydrostatic and systemic blood pressures increase, thus restoring flow to the tissues.

Impaired blood flow may also cause impotence. Impotence is usually seen in advanced arterial occlusive disease, especially with aorto-iliac obstruction.[18]

Pallor and Mottling. Pallor and mottling of the extremities are common findings in arteriosclerosis obliterans. When the patient ambulates, pallor of the feet can be intensified as the active muscle "steals" blood flow from skin. Redness may also be present when the extremity is in a dependent position as a result of reactive hyperemia within the arterioles. Extremities may appear reddened and swollen in long-standing arteriosclerosis obliterans because patients

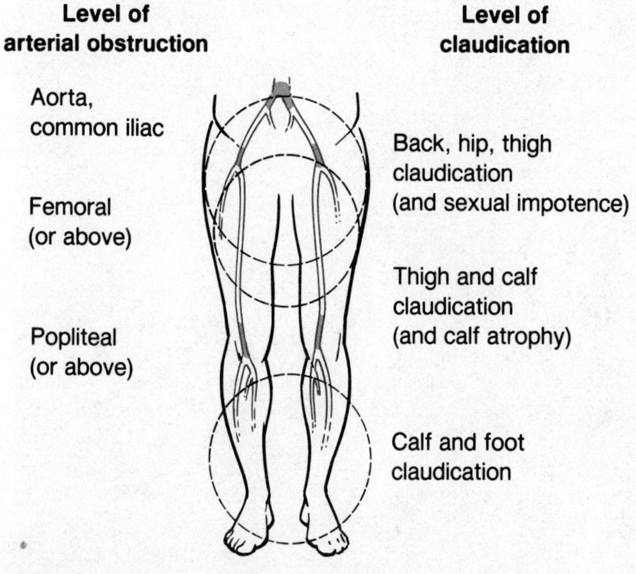

FIGURE 46–1 Approximate levels of ischemic symptoms. The distribution of symptoms suggests the level of arterial occlusion. (After Hardy JD: Surgery of the Aorta and Its Branches. Philadelphia, JB Lippincott, 1960)

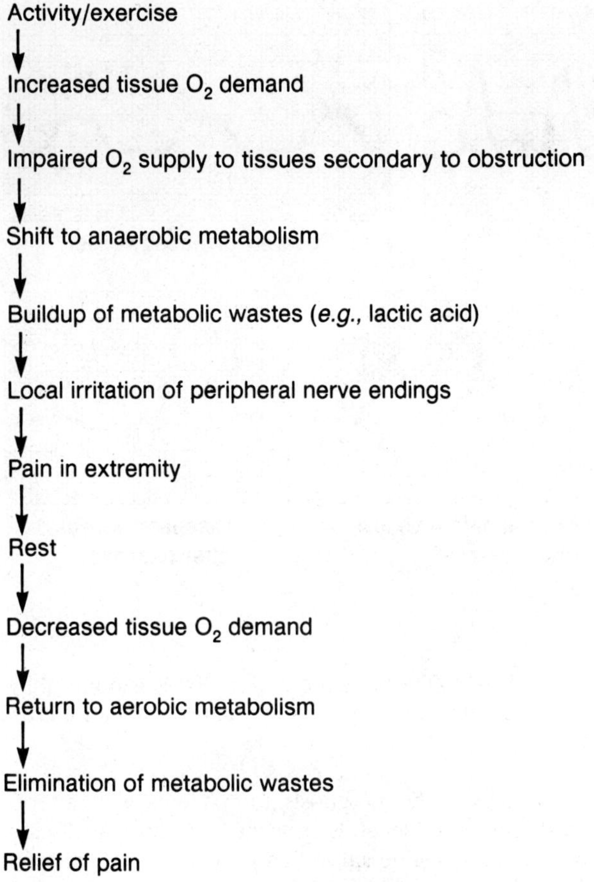

FIGURE 46–2 Mechanisms of intermittent claudication.

keep the affected extremities in dependent positions to alleviate discomfort.[18]

Gangrene. Gangrene can develop in an extremity where complete occlusion has been present for several days. A pregangrenous extremity appears deep purple in color and is unaffected by position or pressure changes. A necrotic, gangrenous extremity, or portion of an extremity, appears black, shriveled, and hard.

An extremity can potentially become gangrenous without the patient's knowledge as sensation may be severely diminished or absent in arteriosclerosis obliterans. The decreased sensation evolves from long-standing reduction in blood flow to the tissues. The patient with diabetes mellitus is at greater risk for undetected tissue necrosis because of peripheral neuropathies complicating the disease.

Skin Changes. Usually, the skin of affected extremities feels cool and dry in a patient with arteriosclerosis obliterans. Skin temperature may be uneven between extremities. The patient may also subjectively complain of a "cold foot" which does not change when exposed to warmer temperatures. The coolness is a result of reduced skin blood flow. If adequate collateral blood flow is present, alterations in skin temperature may not be as pronounced.

Trophic changes also accompany chronic arterial occlusive disease. These changes are a result of inadequate tissue nourishment due to diminished arterial blood flow through the extremity. The patient with arteriosclerosis obliterans often exhibits skin which is thin, smooth, and shiny. Sparsity or absence of hair growth on affected limbs is common. Nail thickening may also be present. Often muscle bulk and tone may be reduced or asymmetric between the extremities.

Peripheral Pulses. Peripheral pulses may be diminished or absent in affected extremities of patients with arteriosclerosis obliterans. Alterations in the quality of peripheral pulses are frequently encountered and occur distal to the occluded artery. Assessment of peripheral pulses assists in locating occluded vessels. Capillary refill time may also be prolonged (greater than 3 seconds) as a result of peripheral occlusion.

Medical Management

Diagnostic Studies. Diagnostic studies which determine the quality of blood flow are useful in the assessment of arteriosclerosis obliterans. These studies utilize directional Doppler ultrasound for velocity waveform analysis, and plethysmography for pulse volume waveform analysis and segmental limb pressures.

Tracings from velocity waveform analysis are shown in Figure 46–3. The normal patent vessel typically has a triphasic complex: upward deflection due to forward flow of systole; downward deflection due to reverse flow in late systole and early diastole; and upward deflection due to forward flow in late diastole.[3] Variations of normal will be present depending on the location of the artery, the degree of vasodilatation, and the extent of any stenosis. Tracings from diseased vessels typically have no second or third deflections and are more widened, which a rounded systolic peak with becomes more pronounced as the severity of the obstruction increases.

The duplex scan is a more sophisticated diagnostic tool used to evaluate arterial occlusive disease. Duplex scanning using pulsed Doppler ultrasound allows ultrasonic imaging in addition to qualitative flow studies.

Pulse volume waveform analysis, by means of plethysmography, records changes in extremity blood volume during the events of the cardiac cycle. Examples of pulse volume waveform tracings before and after exercise are shown in Figure 46–3. Normally, a rapid upstroke is followed by an immediate downstroke which is interrupted by a diastolic widening and notch. In a diseased vessel, the diastolic notch is lost and the entire waveform is widened.[3] In severe disease, a few changes in pulse volume occur, thus creating a damped tracing.

Segmental limb pressures are used most frequently in assessment of arterial occlusive disease. Systolic pressures are measured, using a pneumatic cuff, in each arm, each thigh, each calf, and each ankle. A difference of 20 mmHg or more between limb segments indicates occlusive disease. An ankle-to-arm index (ankle systolic pressure divided by brachial systolic pressure) is also calculated. Arterial disease is suspected if the ankle-to-arm index is less than 1.[3]

Angiography may also be utilized in the diagnosis of arterial occlusive disorders. This invasive procedure aids

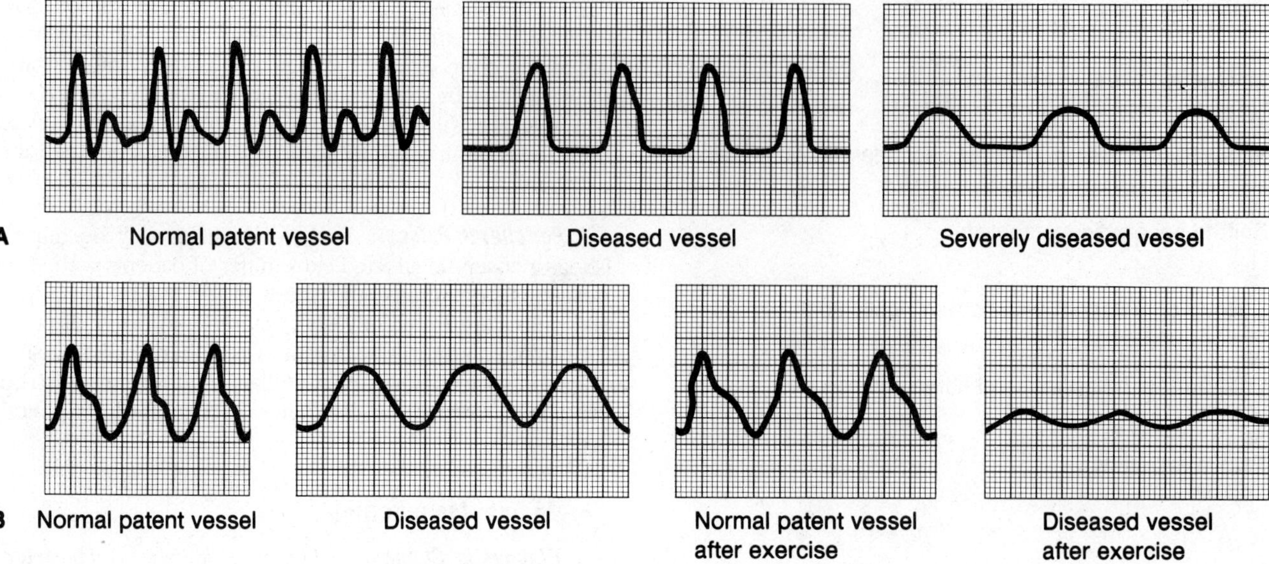

FIGURE 46–3 (*A*) Velocity waveform analysis. (*B*) Pulse volume waveform analysis.

in precisely locating vessel stenosis and the degree of obstruction.

Treatment. Treatment of arteriosclerosis obliterans is palliative at best. Patients are encouraged to stop smoking if this has been a past habit. Exercise programs such as Buerger-Allen exercises (Fig. 46–4) and walking are commonly prescribed.

Specific successful medical regimens are not yet available. Beta-stimulating drugs (nylidrin, isoproterenol, isoxsuprine) have been tried but are not of great value in providing adequate vasodilatation without other undesired side-effects.[1] Nifedipine, a calcium antagonist, may be used in arteriosclerosis obliterans for the peripheral vasodilatation associated with its actions. Antilipemic agents may also be utilized in an attempt to retard the atherosclerotic process.

An emphasis on safety and hygiene is essential in order to prevent injury and infection in extremities with compromised blood flow. If infections do occur, aggressive treatment with local and systemic antibiotics is mandatory. If the infectious process within the wound progresses, surgical debridement may be necessary.

For patients with segmental, localized disease, surgical revascularization is possible. Candidates for revascularization include patients who are in general good health, young patients, those who are able to conduct activities of daily living but have a rapidly deteriorating ability to walk, and those with impending ulceration or gangrene.[1] In revascularization surgery, a synthetic graft is used to bypass the occluded vessel. The Dacron graft is anastomosed to a patent arterial source both proximal and distal to the lesion. Typical bypass sites include aorto-femoral, ilio-femoral, and femoro-popliteal (Fig. 46–5). An extra-anatomic bypass may also be performed in patients for whom traditional bypass surgery is not possible or recommended. In the extra-anatomical bypass, the synthetic graft is anastomosed to the patent artery, tunneled throught the subcutaneous tissues, and anastomosed distal to the occluded region. Extra-anatomical bypass sites include axillofemoral and femoral–femoral cross over.

Prognosis. The prognosis for patients with arteriosclerosis obliterans depends upon the severity of the disease. If the disease is segmentalized and not associated with underlying diabetes mellitus or hypertension, the prognosis is good, especially for the affected limb. Nonsegmental, diffuse disease is associated with more complications such as necrosis and gangrene. Nonsegmental disease is more common in conjunction with other underlying disorders as mentioned above. It is important to remember that arterial occlusive disorders such as arteriosclerosis obliterans are chronic and progressive due to the atherosclerotic process. The key to a successful prognosis is in the prevention of the disorder by the modification of risk factors identified as atherogenic and contributing to the disease process.

Nursing Management

Patients with arterial occlusive disorders require keen nursing management to minimize sequellae associated with the disorders and to prevent ischemia and infarction of the peripheral tissues. It should be remembered that arterial occlusive disorders such as arteriosclerosis obliterans and thromboangiitis obliterans are chronic and progressively debilitating.

As previously indicated, the basic problem or nursing diagnosis for a patient with an arterial occlusive disorder is inadequate tissue perfusion resulting from an imbalance in the demand and supply of oxygen to the affected tissues. Possible complications that can result include ischemia and infarction, skin breakdown, and the threat of wound infection. The nursing interventions are therefore aimed at improving oxygen supply to the tissues by developing an exer-

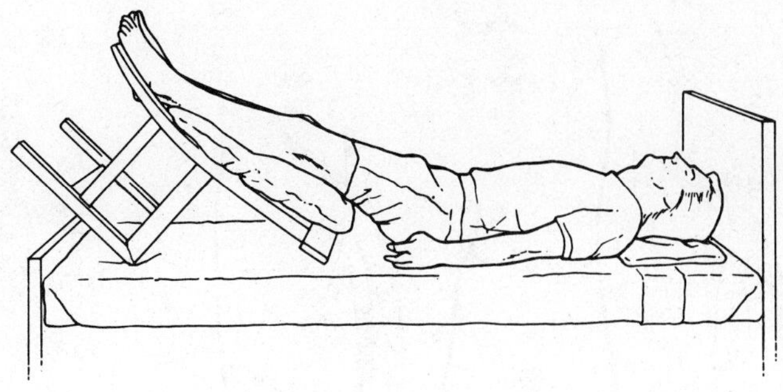

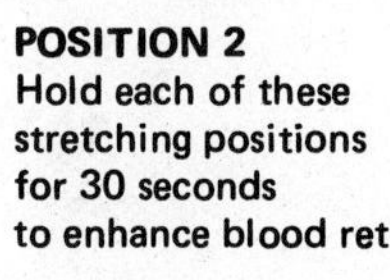

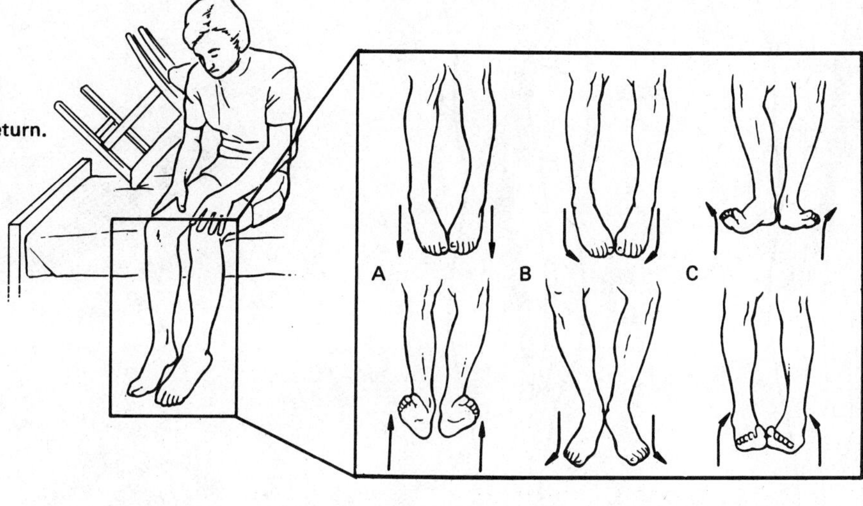

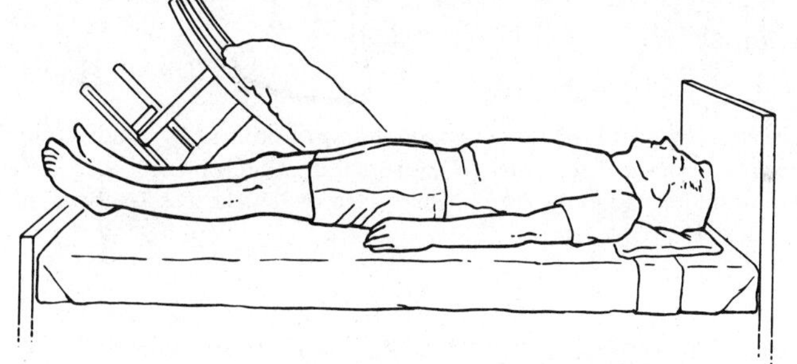

FIGURE 46–4 Buerger-Allen exercises. Do exercise series 6 times, 4 times a day. (Forshee T, Minckley B: Lumbar sympathectomy. RN, July 1976)

cising program with the patient; advocating health practices to avoid restrictive clothing, exposure to cold, smoking, and stress; and administering the medications prescribed. Careful monitoring of peripheral pulses, capillary refilling time, skin conditions, and evidence of intermittent claudication are intended to detect signs of ischemia and infarction. The nurse is also involved in teaching the patient about foot care, temperature control, safety measures to avoid injury to the feet and hands, and daily inspection of the skin of the affected extremities or body part. The details for these interventions, with rationale and expected outcomes, are spelled out in the accompanying Nursing Care Plan for Patient with Ischemia and Infarction Affecting Peripheral Vascular Function. The care plan is designed to be a framework; the nursing diagnoses/problems, goals, interventions, and outcome criteria for goal achievement must be individualized in order to meet each patient's unique needs.

Nursing Care Following Revascularization

Some patients with arterial occlusive disorders may be candidates for revascularization surgery. Beyond the routine postoperative care for patients undergoing peripheral vascular bypass surgery, there are some specialized needs and assessment criteria. The primary concern postoperatively is to prevent or detect occlusion of the graft. Nursing interventions include assessing peripheral pulses, capillary refilling time, and skin temperature every 15 minutes for the first

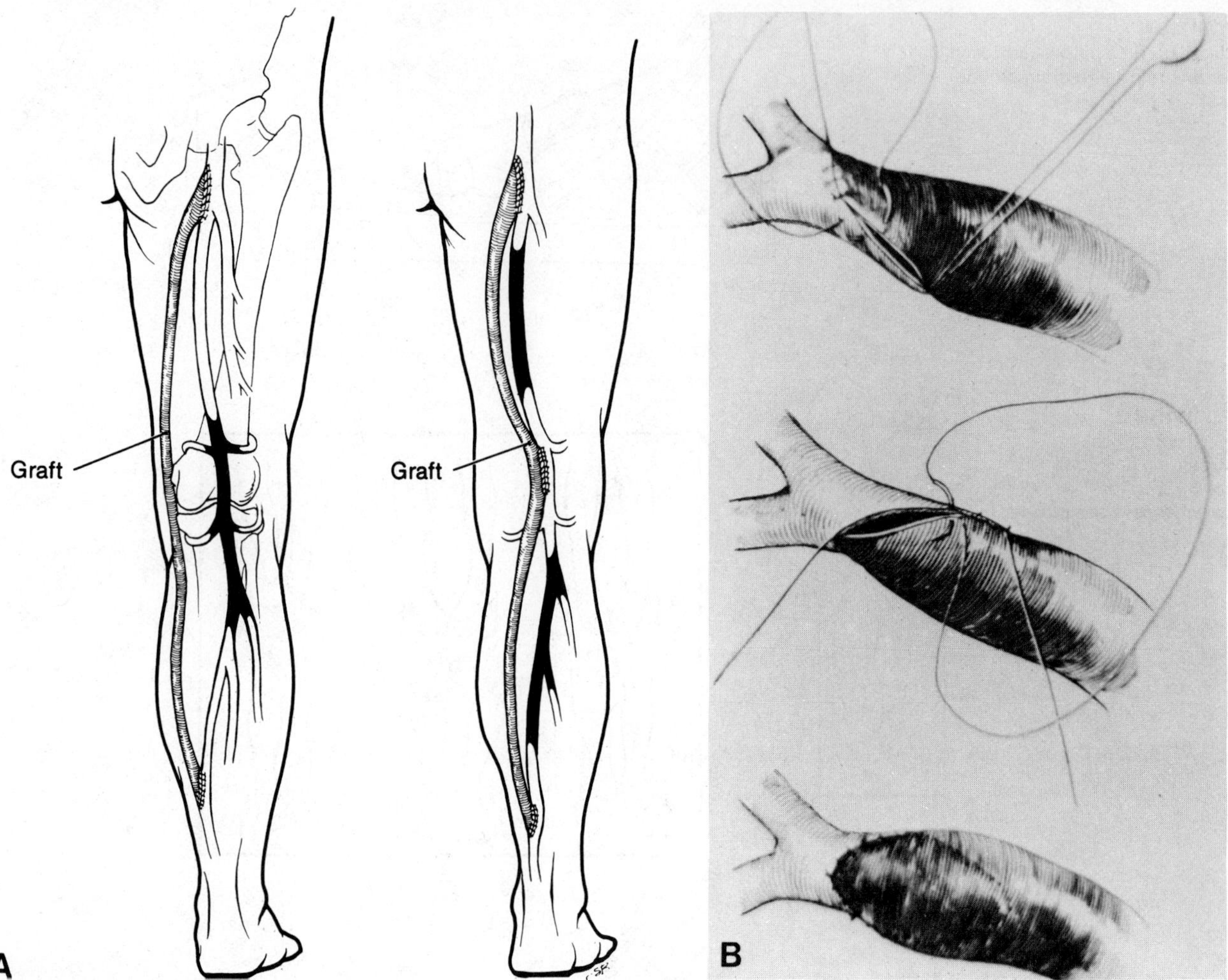

FIGURE 46–5 (*A*) Standard (*left*) and sequential (*right*) femoropopliteal bypasses. Note the side-to-side anastomosis to the isolated popliteal segment. (*B*) Spatulated end-to-end anastomosis with continuous suture technique, important for use in the distal bypass. (Hardy JD: Hardy's Textbook of Surgery, p 910. Philadelphia, JB Lippincott, 1983).

hour postoperatively and then every hour thereafter. It is also important to assess for any signs of severe cramplike pain in the operated extremity which may occur with occlusion. Pressure from blankets can be avoided by using a bed cradle. To prevent the graft from kinking, the patient should be instructed not to flex hips or knees (depending on the site of surgery). Adequate fluid balance should be maintained to prevent contracture of the vascular bed with resultant decrease in blood flow and possible clot formation. A more detailed plan of care is presented in the Nursing Care Plan for the Patient Undergoing Revascularization Surgery. However, as previously mentioned, this care plan is only a guideline, and must be individualized to meet specific patient needs.

Nursing Care Following Amputation

If necrosis of peripheral tissues results from ischemia and infarction with arterial occlusive disorders, surgical amputation of the affected limb may be necessary. The new amputee has unique nursing care needs. In addition to the continuing disease process associated with arterial occlusive disease, the patient must learn to cope with the loss of a limb. For more detailed discussion of amputation, see Chapter 88.

Possible nursing diagnoses related to the loss of a limb include grieving, ineffective individual or family coping, alterations in comfort, potential or actual self-care deficit, and impaired physical mobility. Alterations in sensory perceptions may also occur as a result of "phantom limb." In phantom limb, the patient experiences pain, tingling, or other types of sensation which is perceived to be within the limb which was amputated.

Patient goals relate to the identified problems and nursing diagnoses. General patient goals include independent completion of activities of daily living, improved mobility with the aid of a prosthesis, crutches, walker, or wheelchair, acceptance of limb loss, and coping with related lifestyle changes which could result from loss of a limb.

One intervention is to provide supportive environments for patients who have undergone amputation of a limb. The

NURSING CARE PLAN FOR THE PATIENT WITH ISCHEMIA AND INFARCTION AFFECTING PERIPHERAL VASCULAR FUNCTION

NURSING DIAGNOSIS/PROBLEM 1: Imbalance of tissue oxygen supply and demand related to arterial occlusive disease.

GOAL 1.1: To prevent imbalance of tissue oxygen supply and demand.

Nursing Interventions	Rationale	Outcome Criteria
1. Develop exercise plan (Buerger-Allen exercises) with the patient; set realistic goals, weekly.	1. Exercise helps to increase blood flow to tissues, thereby improving muscle tone and size.	1–7. Absence of the signs and symptoms of ischemia and infarction: a. No pain in affected extremities b. Extremities warm to touch c. Absence of pallor, rubor, or cyanosis in extremities. d. Adequate muscle bulk in extremities e. Peripheral pulses equal in all extremities f. No ulcerated and necrotic tissue
2. Instruct patient to avoid wearing restrictive garments (girdles, elastic-topped knee socks, and tight shoes).	2. Restrictive garments may inhibit blood flow to the extremities.	
3. Instruct patient to avoid exposure to cold temperatures.	3. Exposure to cold temperatures increases metabolic demand by the tissues and may also induce further vasconstriction in an extremity where blood flow is already compromised.[6]	
4. Elevate head of bed (approximately 8 inches).	4. Arterial blood supply can be increased to the lower extremities by positioning them lower than the heart and allowing gravity to assist.	
5. Encourage patient to stop smoking.	5. Smoking is strongly related to the development of vascular diseases. Nicotine may induce further vasoconstriction of the blood vessels.	
6. Administer prescribed medications (vasodilators, antilipemics).	6. Vasodilators may help to increase blood flow in diseased vessels. Antilipemics may aid in arresting or retarding plaque formation and growth.	
7. Assist patient in identifying stressors and developing methods to cope with them.	7. Stress responses may further increase vasoconstriction and metabolic demands.	

GOAL 1.2: To detect early signs and symptoms of ischemia and infarction

Nursing Interventions	Rationale	Outcome Criteria
1. Assess peripheral pulses, quantitatively, every 4 hours or as necessary and document. Report to physician any changes in pulse characteristics, especially any new inequalities.	1. Assists in locating partial or complete vessel occlusion. The sudden disappearance of a peripheral pulse where previously present may signal acute occlusion necessitating immediate medical intervention.	1–5. Signs and symptoms of ischemia and infarction detected within 4 hours of occurrence. — Resting pain — Altered skin color (pallor, rubor, cyanosis) — Cool skin temperature — Muscle atrophy — Unequal peripheral pulses — Tissue necrosis
2. Assess and document capillary refill time.	2. Normal capillary refill time is less than 3 seconds. Capillary refill time is strongly influenced by environmental conditions and is not diagnostic in and of itself.	
3. Assess and document the skin of the extremities for color, temperature, and absence/presence of hair, nail thickening, ulcerations, or necrosis.	3. Trophic changes appear in the extremities of patients with arterial occlusive disease.	

(Continued)

NURSING CARE PLAN FOR THE PATIENT WITH ISCHEMIA AND INFARCTION AFFECTING PERIPHERAL VASCULAR FUNCTION (*Continued*)

Nursing Interventions	Rationale
4. Assess and document incidence and distance of intermittent claudication and resting pain; report any changes in frequency or severity of pain.	4. Decreasing claudication distance and resting pain may represent progression of disease. Severe pain of sudden onset may indicate acute arterial occlusion or embolism.
5. Assess and document muscle size and symmetry in order to monitor trends of muscle changes.	5. Muscles will atrophy as a result of decreasing nourishment from decreased blood flow to the muscle tissues.

NURSING DIAGNOSIS/PROBLEM 2: Potential/actual impairment of skin integrity related to reduced blood flow.

GOAL 2.1: To prevent injury and the subsequent formation of ulcers in extremities with compromised blood flow.

Nursing Interventions	Rationale	Outcome Criteria
1. Maintain warm, properly humidified environment.	1. A properly humidified environment helps prevent skin from becoming too dry, thus avoiding chafing and cracking.	1–2. Integument of extremities is clean and intact, without signs of ulceration or necrosis.
2. Teach patient to complete daily foot care.	2. Daily foot care allows the patient to inspect his feet as well as cleanse the extremities.	

GOAL 2.2: To detect early and to treat ulcerations, should they occur.

Nursing Interventions	Rationale	Outcome Criteria
1. Inspect extremities daily for small cracks and open areas. Teach patient to also perform daily inspection.	1. Decreased sensation in the affected extremities may limit the patient's ability to detect small breaks in the integument.	1–2. Integumentary breaks detected within 24 hours of occurrence.
2. Document presence of arterial ulcers if detected. — Location — Size — Characteristics — Drainage	2. Arterial ulcers can occur between toes, at tips of toes, on heels, above lateral malleolus, over metatarsal heads, on side or sole of foot.	
3. Document, daily, the condition of the ulcer.	3. The healing process can be monitored closely with daily documentation of wound appearance.	3–4. Arterial ulcer shows evidence of healing during hospitalization: — Absence of purulent drainage — Presence of granulation tissue — Closure of ulcer
4. Implement treatment of ulcer as ordered by physician, which may include — Wet-to-dry dressings — Bed rest — Topical or systemic antibiotics — Immobilization of extremity	4. Wet-to-dry saline dressings help to promote tissue granulation and wound healing. Bed rest helps to decrease metabolic demands, especially to the affected extremity. Antibiotics may be necessary if the wound is infected. Immobilization of the extremity may help to support and preserve new tissue growth.	

NURSING CARE PLAN FOR THE PATIENT UNDERGOING PERIPHERAL REVASCULARIZATION SURGERY

NURSING DIAGNOSIS/PROBLEM 1: Potential decrease in tissue perfusion related to graft occlusion.
GOAL 1.1: To prevent graft occlusion.

Nursing Interventions	Rationale	Outcome Criteria
1. Instruct patient not to flex at the hips (for aorto-femoral bypass) or knees (for femoral–popliteal bypass).	1. Flexion at these joints could cause the graft to kink, thereby reducing blood flow to the extremity.[2]	1–4. Patent operative graft evidenced by — Palpable peripheral pulses distal to operative site — Extremity warm (subjectively and objectively) — Absence of ischemic pain, *i.e.,* pain other than incisional pain — Skin color without pallor or cyanosis
2. Maintain fluid (saline) balance.	2. Saline deficit induces contracture of the vascular beds which may decrease blood flow to the extremities, promoting clot formation and possible graft collapse.[2]	
3. Use blanket cradle at foot of bed.	3. Blanket cradle helps to decrease pressure from blankets on extremities.	
4. Administer anticoagulants and antiplatelet medications as ordered.	4. Anticoagulants and antiplatelet agents help reduce incidence of clot formation and embolization (refer to Chap 47).	

GOAL 1.2: To detect early and to treat graft occlusion should it occur.

Nursing Interventions	Rationale	Outcome Criteria
1. Assess and document evidence of adequate blood flow to the extremity, every 15 minutes for the first hour postoperatively, then every hour. a. Peripheral pulses (quantitatively) b. Capillary refill time c. Skin temperature	1. It is important to note that peripheral pulses may not be palpable for the first 6 to 12 hours postoperatively because of vasospasm or trapped air bubbles from graft closure.[2] Pulses may be detectable by Doppler ultrasound.	1–3. Graft occlusion detected within 1 hour of occurrence and may be seen as — Sudden disappearance of pulses distal to graft. — Cold extremity distal to operative site — Cramplike pain in operative extremity — Pallor or cyanosis distal to operative site.
2. Assess patient for the presence of pain in operative extremity.	2. A severe, cramplike pain may accompany acute graft occlusion. Burning or stinging sensations often characterize incisional pain.	
3. Report to physician any aberrations of above assessment criteria.	3. Graft occlusion requires immediate medical attention.	

patient must be assisted in relearning many activities of daily living. Physical and occupational therapy may be of some assistance in helping the patient adapt to any limitations in mobility.

Goal achievement can be assessed by observation of the patient's ability to complete activities of daily living as well as accepting assistance if necessary. Patients may report a sense of well-being and acceptance of any limitations to activity which they may be experiencing.

Thromboangiitis Obliterans

Thromboangiitis obliterans, also known as Buerger's disease, is an inflammatory vascular disorder involving digital vascular occlusions. The disorder is generally localized with segmental obstructions of small arteries. Buerger's disease is a chronic disorder and may progress to affect major arteries.[11]

Etiology

Buerger's disease is usually seen in young males whose ages range between 16 and 40 years.[1] The disease rarely strikes women. The disorder is directly related to cigarette smoking and a smoking history must be present for positive diagnosis.[15] The precise etiology of the disease has not been determined.

Pathophysiology

Inflammatory changes within the small arteries are the hallmark of Buerger's disease. There is a proliferation of polymorphonuclear leukocytes and histiocytes, which are later replaced by macrophages. A large grayish or yellow mass fills the lumen of the involved artery but there are no signs of plaque formation. Intimal proliferation is also present but there are no medial changes as seen in arteriosclerosis obliterans. In the advanced chronic stages, connective tissue becomes more dense and thrombi become fibrous tissue which occlude vessel lumens.[1]

Clinical Manifestations

The signs and symptoms accompanying thromboangiitis obliterans are similar to those of arteriosclerosis obliterans, including pain, changes in color and temperature, and trophic changes. Intermittent claudication, however, is noticeably absent in Buerger's disease. Lesions on the tips of the fingers are commonly seen with the the disorder (Fig. 46–6).[1]

Smoking greatly enhances the symptomology of Buerger's disease. The pain associated with ulceration or gangrene in thromboangiitis obliterans is thought to be of greater intensity than in arteriosclerosis obliterans and is strongly exacerbated by smoking. Cessation of smoking often helps relieve the painful symptoms of Buerger's disease.[1,15]

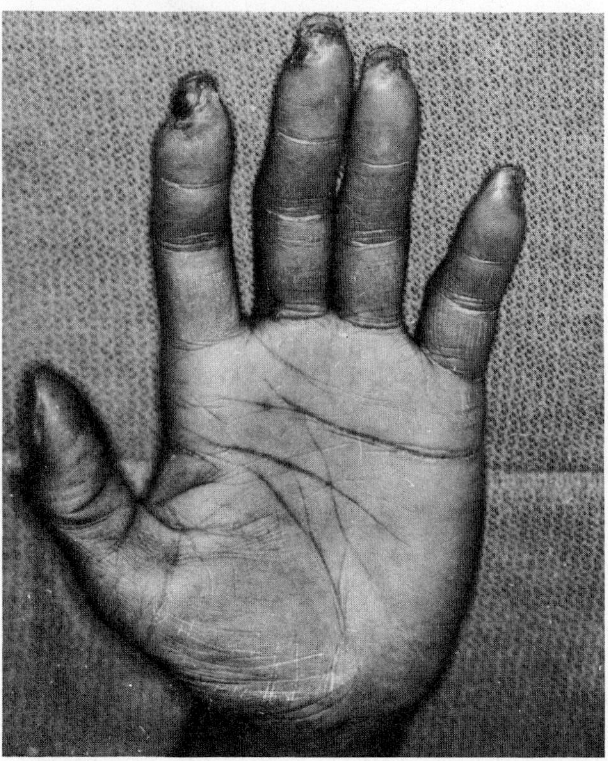

FIGURE 46–6 Ischemic ulcers of left second, third, and fourth fingers of a 40-year-old patient with thromboangiitis obliterans. The patient was a heavy smoker and had involvement of all four extremities. The arteriogram disclosed occlusion of the radial and ulnar arteries just proximal to the wrist joint and involvement of the distal portions of the digital arteries. A left upper thoracic sympathectomy was carried out, followed later by amputation of the distal phalanx of the index finger. Microscopic study of the small vessels of the digit showed narrowed lumina by proliferative endothelial lesions. (Haimovici H: Diseases of small arteries of the extremities. In Hardy JD [ed]: Rhoads Textbook of Surgery, 5th ed. Philadelphia, JB Lippincott, 1977)

Medical Management

The diagnosis of thromboangiitis obliterans can be made by history and physical examination. As previously mentioned, a smoking history must be present for diagnosis of Buerger's disease. Peripheral arteriography offers the most conclusive diagnosis. Arteriographic findings in Buerger's disease are different from those seen in arteriosclerosis obliterans in that the artery is smooth and filling defects are absent both above and below the blocked portion of the vessel.[1]

Definitive treatment for thromboangiitis obliterans is limited. Cessation of smoking offers the best treatment as it relieves many of the symptoms and retards the progression of the disease.[15] Ulcerated extremities require aggressive treatment with antibiotic agents and proper wound care in order to prevent necrosis. Amputation of necrotic extremities may be necessary in advanced disease.

Although the prevalence of thromboangiitis obliterans is still somewhat low, for those who are afflicted it remains a chronic and debilitating disorder. Only hygienic measures appear to be of value in preventing the progression of the disease.

Nursing Management

Nursing care of the patient with thromboangiitis obliterans parallels the care of the patients with arteriosclerosis obliterans and is directed at improving tissue perfusion, preventing ischemia and infarction, and avoiding skin breakdown with possible wound infection. The Nursing Care Plan for the Patient with Ischemia and Infarction gives general guidelines for nursing care. Special emphasis should be placed on the prevention of infection, a common complication of Buerger's disease. For patients with severity of infection, ischemia, or necrosis of the extremities, amputation may be performed. In addition, an important nursing diagnosis is knowledge deficit with regard to smoking. Patients should understand the relationship between smoking habits and progression of the disorder.

Raynaud's Disease

Raynaud's disease is a functional, vasospastic disorder which afflicts primarily young women. The onset of the disorder generally occurs between the ages of 18 and 40 years and is seen most frequently in teenagers and women in their twenties.[1] Raynaud's disease is associated with arterial vasospasm following some type of cold or emotional stimuli. The vasospasm occurs independent of vessel pathology and occurs most frequently in the arteries of the hands and digits, although the feet and toes may also be affected.[1,8] Primary Raynaud's disease must be differentiated from Raynaud's "phenomena." Raynaud's phenomena may occur in other arterial occlusive disorders when vasospasm complicates underlying pathological disease.

Etiology

The intense vasospasms seen in Raynaud's disease are precipitated by noxious stimuli such as cold or emotional stress. The pathogenesis of the vasospasm is unclear. Several theories have been proposed to explain the apparent hyperreactivity of the arteries to such noxious stimuli. Some suggest that there may be inherent defects in the arteries themselves or defects in basal heat production which would limit the ability of cutaneous vessels to dilate. Another possibility may be an excess of locally produced norepinephrine at the alpha receptors in the arteries of the hands and digits. Sympathetic nerve involvement has also been suggested; however, vasospasm has been shown to persist following sympathetic denervation.[1,8]

Pathophysiology

Generally, there are no pathological changes within the vasculature associated with Raynaud's disease. In extremely advanced cases some intimal hyperplasia and medial fibrosis may be present in affected arteries. Telangiectasis appearing on the hands, forearms, and face may also be present in advanced Raynaud's disease; these lesions have been shown to consist of dilated venules within the subcapillary venous plexus.[1]

Clinical Manifestations

Color changes within the hands and fingers in response to cold or emotional stimuli best characterize Raynaud's disease. The color changes are consistent and occur bilaterally and symmetrically.[8] The fingers often change color first, followed by the hands and sometimes the forearms.[1]

In long-standing Raynaud's disease with frequent vasospastic episodes, trophic and sensory changes may occur. Skin may become pale, shiny, and taut. Nail thickening and clubbing may also be present. Joints may also be affected, in which case stiffness and deformities may occur. Ulceration and necrosis can also occur but are more uncommonly seen.[1,8]

Medical Management

The diagnosis of Raynaud's disease is made, in part, by history. Plethysmographic studies may also be used. Patients with primary Raynaud's disease show normal pulse waveforms prior to exposure to cold stimuli. Following a 30-second immersion of the hand in ice water, plethysmographic tracings are obtained at 1-minute intervals. If normal waveform and pressure do not return after 10 minutes, a diagnosis of pathological vasospasm, or Raynaud's disease, can be made. If abnormal plethysmographic tracings were present prior to cold stimuli, underlying arterial occlusive disease is likely present and is the cause of Raynaud's phenomena.[16]

Medical treatments used in Raynaud's disease are aimed at relieving vasoconstriction and promoting vasodilatation in the extremities. Alpha blocking agents such as phenoxybenzamine and tolazoline hydrochloride help to relax vasospasm and promote vasodilatation. The rauwolfia alkaloids (reserpine) may help reduce vasoconstriction. Nitroglycerin ointment, histamine preparations, nylidrin, cyclandelate, and nifedipine may help relax vascular smooth muscle and promote arterial flow. While all of these agents may help alleviate symptoms, other systemic side-effects limit their use.[1,8]

Surgical intervention may be implemented. Sympathectomy may be performed, but results are unpredictable.[8]

Primary treatment for Raynaud's disease involves adaptation to the disorder and avoidance of situations and stimuli which precipitate vasospastic episodes. Avoiding exposure to cold and reducing emotional stress may be the best interventions. Patients are commonly instructed to stop smoking because this may induce further vasoconstriction.

When vasospasm does occur, relief may be evoked by submerging the patient's hands in warm water. Water temperature should not exceed 90°F (32°C) to avoid possible thermal injury. Some patients report relief of symptoms by drinking a warm beverage or by applying warmth to the upper thoracic area where the sympathetic ganglion lie.[8]

Most patients suffering from Raynaud's disease experience mild to moderate symptoms and related disability. As a result, the overall prognosis is good and patients are able to cope with the inconveniences associated with the disorder. However, in more severe cases ischemia and permanent damage to the extremities can result.

Nursing Management

A functional arterial occlusive disorder such as Raynaud's disease, can be severly disabling for patients who are afflicted. These patients have special nursing care needs, many of which include teaching.

Assessment and Nursing Diagnosis

An example of a nursing diagnosis for a patient with a functional arterial occlusive disorder such as Raynaud's disease is *potential for alteration in peripheral tissue perfusion resulting from a vasospastic arterial occlusive disorder*. Peripheral ischemia would be evidenced in the affected extremity by pain, alteration in skin color (pallor, cyanosis, rubor) and temperature (coolness), reduced movement, diminished or absent pulses, or delayed capillary refill time.

Goals. The primary goal of the patient with a functional arterial occlusive disorder is the prevention of vasoconstriction. A secondary goal would be prompt relief of vasoconstriction and subsequent pain, should it occur.

Interventions

Patients suffering from functional arterial occlusive disorders need extensive teaching about methods to avoid cold temperatures and subsequent vasoconstriction. Patients can be encouraged to wear gloves when handling cold objects from refrigerators or freezers as well as when they are out of doors in colder weather. Warm clothing such as socks, shoes, hats, and sweaters may also help prevent chills.

Another method to reduce vasoconstriction may involve stress reduction. Peripheral vasospasms associated with a disorder such as Raynaud's disease are often the result of emotional stress. Relaxation techniques, massage, or biofeedback may benefit the patient.

If vasoconstriction does occur despite preventive measures, methods to relieve the vasoconstriction should be employed. Immersing the extremities in warm water, taking a warm bath, or drinking a warm beverage may help bring relief. With these measures caution must be taken to avoid temperatures which are too hot, as sensation may be diminished in conjunction with vasoconstriction. Some patients report relief of symptoms when warmth is applied to the upper back in the area of the sympathetic ganglion.[8]

Evaluation

Outcome criteria would involve signs and symptoms of adequate peripheral tissue perfusion. Patients may subjectively state the absence of vasospasm by reporting that their hands feel warm and that they have not experienced pain or discomfort. Signs of adequate tissue perfusion would include skin which is of baseline color and temperature, full peripheral pulses, and capillary refill times of less than 3 seconds.

If vasoconstriction does occur, interventions would be made immediately. Relief of vasoconstriction should be achieved within one-half hour.

Acute Arterial Occlusion

Acute arterial occlusion is a vascular emergency. The ischemic consequences of a sudden block to arterial blood flow may be severe. Limb viability is threatened because profound tissue necrosis may occur within 6 to 12 hours.[4,17]

Etiology

One of the most common causes of acute arterial occlusion is arterial embolism. Arterial emboli result from the dislodgement of a more proximal thrombus which is carried through the bloodstream until it eventually lodges in a smaller arterial branch. Approximately 94% of arterial emboli originate within the heart. Figure 46–7 summarizes the sources of emboli as well as their ultimate distribution. Over 90% of arterial emboli lodge within the distal aorta or lower extremities; only 3% to 11% lodge within branch arteries of the upper extremities.[7]

Acute arterial occlusion could result from conditions other than embolization, such as acute arterial thrombosis, dissecting aneurysms, arterial trauma, hematoma formation, or iatrogenic causes such as postarterial catheterization.[4] Acute occlusion from any of these causes presents in a similar fashion to embolization.

Clinical Manifestations

Acute arterial occlusion typically presents as the "six Ps": pain, pallor, paresthesias, paralysis, pulselessness, and polar (coldness).[4] Differentiation between acute arterial thrombosis and embolism can often be made from the clinical history. Signs and symptoms accompanying embolization are of sudden onset without prior symptoms of arterial insufficiency. Acute thrombosis has a more gradual onset with prior symptoms of peripheral vascular insufficiency. A history of atrial fibrillation strongly suggests embolism. The appearance of the affected limb also differs somewhat between embolism and thrombosis. In embolism, the extremity has more of a yellowish, waxy appearance, whereas in thrombosis the extremity appears more mottled or cyanotic with less cadaveric pallor.[4,17] The patient with thrombosis may also have bruits and pulse deficits in unaffected extremities; pulses in unaffected extremities are usually normal in patients with acute arterial embolization.[4]

Arterial Doppler studies are helpful in the diagnosis of acute arterial occlusion. Definitive diagnosis of arterial occlusion is made by arteriography. (See Chap. 42 for details on these diagnostic tests.)

Treatment. Initial treatment of acute arterial occlusion by embolism involves anticoagulation with heparin. A loading dose of 5,000 to 10,000 units is given intravenously followed by a continuous infusion drip, titrated to prolong partial thromboplastin time (PTT) to twice normal. Usual dosage ranges between 1,000 to 5,000 units per hour.[17]

Surgical intervention, by embolization, is the treatment of choice for acute arterial occlusion once the patient has been stabilized. An arterial embolectomy is performed. A small incision is made in the proximal artery followed by the insertion of a Fogarty balloon catheter. The balloon catheter is then passed through the embolus; the balloon is inflated

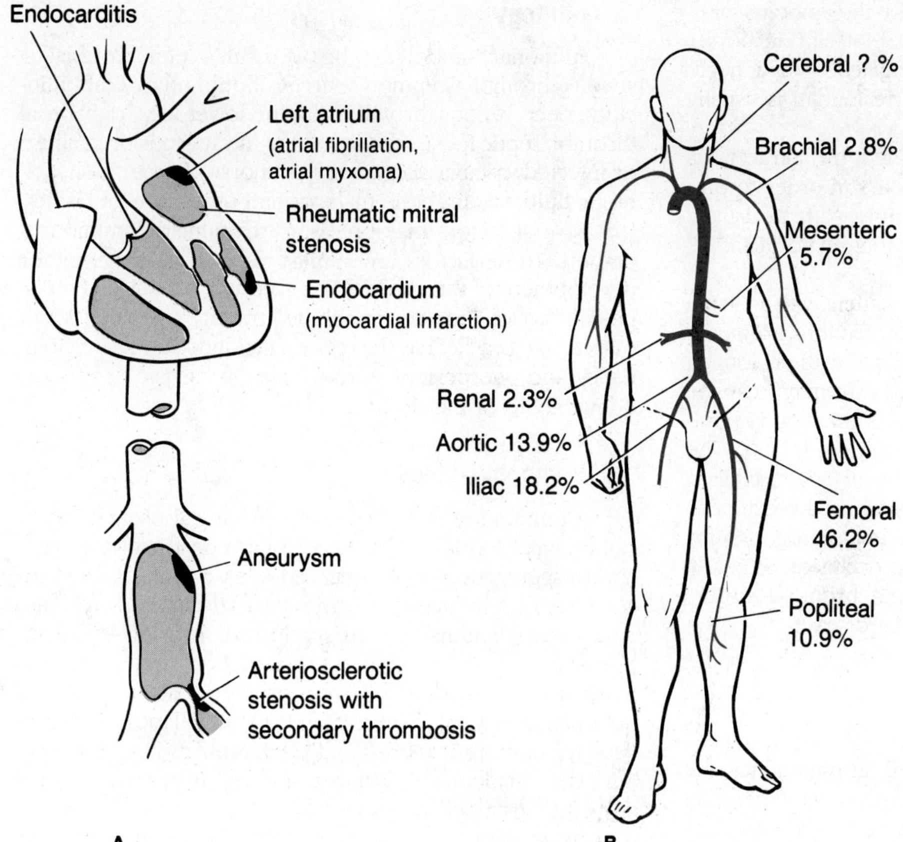

FIGURE 46–7 (*A*) Sources and (*B*) distribution of emboli.

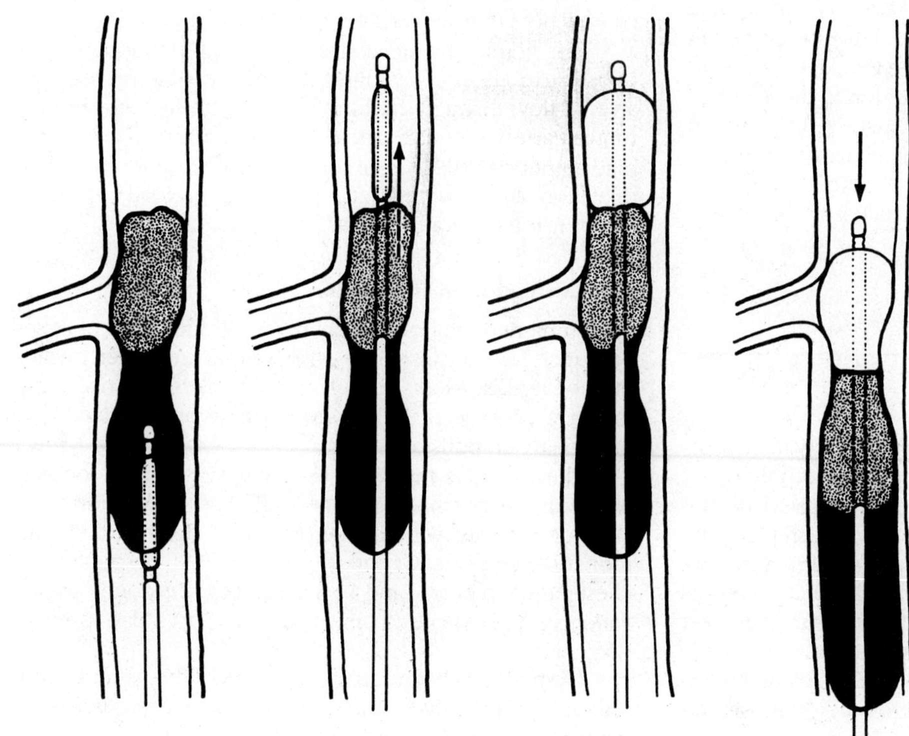

FIGURE 46–8 Technique for extraction of embolus with balloon catheter. (Hardy JD: Hardy's Textbook of Surgery, p 939. Philadelphia, JB Lippincott, 1983)

and gently withdrawn in order to remove the embolus without incurring further damage to the vessel itself (Fig. 46–8). Following extraction the vessel is irrigated with a heparinized saline solution. An operative arteriogram is usually obtained to ensure arterial patency.[4,17]

The patient is generally maintained on intravenous heparin postoperatively for 12 to 24 hours in order to prevent recurrent embolization. After this time, patients usually begin oral anticoagulant agents such as sodium warfarin.[4]

Prognosis. The prognosis for the patient with an acute arterial occlusion is good provided interventions are made quickly. Limb viability is severely threatened with prolonged ischemia. Amputation of the affected extremity may be necessary if tissue necrosis ensues. The amputation rate following embolectomy is low, approximately 5% to 20%. The overall mortality rate associated with acute arterial occlusion ranges between 10% and 40% depending on the extent of any underlying atherosclerosis.[4] The ultimate prognosis for these patients is unsure because acute occlusion is nearly always associated with other underlying chronic disorders such as myocardial or peripheral vascular disease.

Nursing Management

Since acute arterial occlusion is a medical emergency, the goals of prevention, early detection, and prompt intervention are essential in order to maintain limb viability. Revascularization will be attempted surgically. If necrosis is severe, amputation of the extremity will be necessary. Guidelines for the nursing care of the patient recovering from revascularization surgery have already been discussed and are summarized in the Nursing Care Plan for Patients Undergoing Peripheral Revascularization Surgery. Preoperatively, an appropriate nursing diagnosis to include is anxiety related to the abrupt onset of the disorder in addition to the threat to the affected limb and the emergency surgery necessary to correct the problem. Astute assessment, explanation of procedures, and caring reassurance to the patient are critical interventions to relieve anxiety experienced by the patient.

Pulmonary Embolism

Pulmonary embolism is an acute pulmonary vascular disorder. In the event of pulmonary embolism the pulmonary vasculature may be partially or completely occluded; pulmonary infarction and necrosis may follow complete obstruction. The incidence of symptomatic pulmonary embolism is estimated to be in excess of 650,000 occurrences annually and is thought to be the leading nonsurgical cause of death in hospitalized patients.[5,19] Pulmonary embolism is fatal in approximately 38% of symptomatic patients.[5] Mortality is even higher in patients for whom the diagnosis was missed.

Etiology

Pulmonary emboli may be the result of either arterial or venous thrombi. Common sources of pulmonary emboli include deep venous thrombi from the lower legs, right atrial thrombi, septic foci (often related to intravenous drug abuse or infected vascular access sites), tumors, atheroemboli, amniotic fluid, fat, air, bone marrow, and other foreign bodies.

Several factors may predispose patients to pulmonary emboli. These factors are similar to those risk factors for development of thrombi as discussed in Chapter 45. Predisposing factors include immobility, trauma, age (the 50- to 65-year age bracket has the highest incidence), obesity, pregnancy and puerperium, and co-existing cardiac neoplastic, hematologic, or metabolic disease.[5]

Pathophysiology

A pulmonary embolism is a mechanical obstruction to pulmonary blood flow. As a result of this obstruction there is a local aggregation of platelets and release of vasoactive substances which induce vasoconstriction. Histamine, serotonin, and prostaglandins are also released, causing bronchoconstriction.[12] The persistent obstruction and associated vasoconstriction and bronchoconstriction act together to produce a ventilation–perfusion (VQ) imbalance. With pulmonary embolism there is adquate ventilation in conjunction with inadequate perfusion. Arterial hypoxemia results from any sustained VQ mismatch.

In an attempt to compensate for the ventilation–perfusion imbalance, respiratory rate increases. Consequently, arterial P_{CO_2} levels drop as carbon dioxide is blown off. However, instead of correcting the VQ mismatch, the reduction in arterial P_{CO_2} induces even further broncho- and vasoconstriction, thus perpetuating the problem.

The hemodynamic consequences of pulmonary embolism can also be profound. Because of the decrease in arterial flow through the lungs, there is an increase in pulmonary artery pressures and right ventricular pressures. Cardiac output eventually decreases because of right ventricular dilatation and lowered left ventricular preload. Systemic hypotension generally follows.[5,12]

Clinical Manifestations

Pulmonary embolism may have a sudden, abrupt onset or it may have an insidious onset mimicking other cardiopulmonary disorders. Keen assessment skills are necessary for early detection of the signs and symptoms associated with pulmonary embolism.

Chest pain is the most common symptom associated with pulmonary embolism. Chest pain has been reported by 88% of patients with angiographically documented pulmonary embolism. Of those patients, 74% described the chest pain as pleuritic and 14% described it as nonpleuritic.[5] Patients reported chest pain as much as 3 to 4 days prior to diagnosis.

Dyspnea has been reported by 85% of the patients studied with pulmonary embolism.[5] The dyspnea was generally experienced more acutely than was chest pain.

Apprehension and cough have been reported by 59% and 53% of patients, respectively. Other symptoms of pulmonary embolism included diaphoresis, palpitations, hemoptysis, nausea, vomiting, chills, and syncope. Clinical signs of pulmonary embolism involve several body systems. A key respiratory sign is tachypnea; a respiratory rate greater than 16 per minute has been observed in 92% of patients with documented pulmonary embolism.[5] Often, crackles can be auscultated over the affected lung.

Heart rate may be elevated in patients with pulmonary embolism; however, 44% of patients studied had heart rates within normal limits (60 to 100 beats/min). Fever, which may also be present with pulmonary embolism, could also account for an increase in heart rate. Other cardiac signs may include the development of a cardiac gallop or murmur located in the pulmonic valve area, and an increase in the intensity of the pulmonic component of the second heart sound.

Medical Management

Diagnosis. If a pulmonary embolism is suspected in any patient, immediate diagnostic studies are indicated. Arterial blood gas determination, electrocardiogram (ECG), and chest roentgenogram are three tests which can be done quickly and are able to provide preliminary information about the patient's condition. Generally, patients with pulmonary embolism have profound hypoxemia with arterial P_{O_2} levels ranging between 60 and 65 mmHg.[5] Arterial P_{CO_2} may be normal or decreased from normal as a result of tachypnea associated with pulmonary embolism. However, if normal arterial blood gases are found, a diagnosis of pulmonary embolism cannot be ruled out.

An ECG may be abnormal in patients with pulmonary embolism, although it is nonspecific in approximately 80% of those patients. The ECG is of greatest diagnostic value in massive pulmonary embolism where 87% of patients show consistent ECG changes. The most common ECG finding is a pattern of right ventricular strain which is related to alterations in right ventricular and pulmonary artery pressures.[5,12]

Chest roentgenogram is usually abnormal in pulmonary embolism. Most frequently abnormalities are seen in the lower lobes. An elevated diaphragm and pleural effusions may also be evident. Chest roentgenographic abnormalities are more common in patients who also have underlying cardiopulmonary disorders.

Laboratory studies such as blood cell counts, coagulation studies, and serum enzyme determinations are generally nonspecific and are of limited value in the diagnosis of pulmonary embolism.[5] However, these laboratory studies may be helpful in differentiating pulmonary embolism from other disorders such as myocardial infarction or pneumonia.[5,12]

More definitive diagnosis can be made by means of a noninvasive lung VQ scan. In pulmonary embolism, a defect will be evident in the perfusion portion of the scan in conjunction with a normal ventilation scan. An abnormal VQ scan suggests pulmonary embolism. If the VQ scan is normal, the liklihood of pulmonary embolism is low. A definitive diagnosis of pulmonary embolism can best be made by means of pulmonary angiography. While the time and costs involved with the invasive pulmonary angiography could preclude its routine use in the diagnosis of pulmonary embolism, it remains the most reliable clinical study available.[5,12]

Treatment. The first goal of treatment for pulmonary embolism is to maintain cardiopulmonary function. Intensive respiratory and cardiac support may be necessary.

Anticoagulation with intravenous heparin is used in the initial treatment of pulmonary embolism in order to prevent recurrence. Dosage is regulated to keep activated partial thromboplastin time (APTT) between 60 and 80 seconds. Heparin therapy is continued for 7 to 10 days, followed by warfarin therapy for at least 12 weeks.[5]

Thrombolysis by means of either streptokinase or urokinase may also be instituted. Streptokinase and urokinase act to boost endogenous thrombolysis in order to dissolve the clot.[5,12] Streptokinase is usually given for 24 hours; urokinase is usually given for 12 to 24 hours. Thrombin time should be kept at two to seven times baseline.[5] Thrombolytic therapy is generally followed by heparin therapy in an attempt to prevent recurrence.

Patients for whom anticoagulation or thrombolysis is contraindicated may be surgically treated by means of a vena caval interruption. Caval interruption helps prevent passage of emboli to the lung. Pulmonary embolectomy may also be performed in conjunction with cardiopulmonary bypass; however, mortality rates with this procedure are in excess of 50%.

Only 10% of all pulmonary emboli is considered to be incurable. With prompt identification and treatment, prognosis is good for patients with pulmonary embolism. Successful treatment results in little long-term morbidity. Long-term sequellae such as pulmonary hypertension and cor pulmonale may be seen in patients with underlying cardiopulmonary disease or those with massive emboli.[5,12]

Nursing Management

Because pulmonary embolism can be a life-threatening event, the emphasis of nursing management is its prevention. As discussed in Chapter 45, prevention of thrombus formation and thrombophlebitis is also the first step for the prevention of pulmonary embolism. Early detection of pulmonary embolism is essential. Fifty percent of those patients who die of pulmonary embolism do so within the first hour and 75% do so within 2 hours.[5]

Supporting ventilatory function with oxygen therapy and administering anticoagulants are a critical part of nursing management, as is the close monitoring of vital signs and levels of consciousness to determine adequate gas exchange and cardiac output. The specific details of this care are spelled out in the Nursing Care Plan for the Patient with Pulmonary Embolism. Again, this plan is a general one and must be individualized to meet specific patient needs.

NURSING CARE PLAN FOR THE PATIENT WITH PULMONARY EMBOLISM

NURSING DIAGNOSIS/PROBLEM 1: Impaired gas exchange related to ventilation–perfusion mismatch associated with pulmonary embolism.
GOAL 1: To normalize gas exchange.

Nursing Interventions	Rationale	Outcome Criteria
1. Support respiratory function. a. Supplemental oxygen by face mask or, if necessary, endotracheal intubation and mechanical ventilation b. Elevate head of bed as tolerated by patient.	1. Profound arterial hypoxemia often accompanies pulmonary embolism. Supplemental oxygen may help in decreasing the degree of hypoxemia and the alveolar–arterial oxygen difference. Elevating the head of the bed allows for better chest expansion with respiration.	1–6. Arterial blood gases within normal limits. Heart rate between 60 and 100 beats/min. Respiratory rate ≤ 20/min. Patient denies dyspnea. Patient alert and oriented or at baseline level of conscousness. No cyanosis evident.
2. Administer analgesics or sedatives as necessary and as ordered.	2. Analgesia may help relieve the patient's discomfort; sedation may help relieve the patient's anxiety. By reducing the level of discomfort and anxiety, respiratory rate may also decrease, thus reducing additional vaso- and bronchoconstriction caused by lowered P_{CO_2} levels.	
3. Administer anticoagulants as ordered by the physician.	3. Anticoagulants help decrease the recurrence of emboli.	
4. Administer thrombolytic agents as ordered by the physician.	4. Thrombolytic agents boost endogenous thrombolysis and may help to dissolve the emboli, thus restoring blood flow through the pulmonary vasculature.	
5. Assess and document vital signs hourly and as needed.	5. Vital signs which are within normal limits may indicate improved gas exchange, particularly respiratory rate and heart rate.	
6. Obtain arterial blood gas samples every 2 to 4 hours as needed.	6. Arterial blood gas analysis offers a quantitative assessment of gas exchange.	

NURSING DIAGNOSIS/PROBLEM 2: Potential decrease in cardiac output related to pulmonary embolism.
GOAL 1: To detect early and to treat decreased cardiac output, should it occur.

Nursing Interventions	Rationale	Outcome Criteria
1. Assess vital signs and document every hour or as needed. — Heart rate — Blood pressure	1. Cardiac output can decrease as a result of pulmonary embolism. An increase in heart rate is the first compensatory mechanism for reduction in cardiac output. Systemic hypotension results from decreases in cardiac output.	1–4. Any signs of decreased cardiac output detected within 1 hour or less: — Heart rate 100 beats/min — Blood pressure (systolic) <90 mmHg — Decreased level of consciousness — Agitation — Urine output ≤30 ml/hr
2. Assess level of consciousness every hour or as needed, and document.	2. As cardiac output is decreased, brain blood flow is compromised, resulting in agitation, anxiety, and decreased level of consciousness.	

(Continued)

NURSING CARE PLAN FOR THE PATIENT WITH PULMONARY EMBOLISM (*Continued*)

Nursing Interventions	Rationale
3. Measure and record urine output every hour.	3. Renal blood flow is decreased with a reduction in cardiac output. Less than 30 ml/hr signals a reduction in renal blood flow most probably due to a reduction in cardiac output.
4. Report to physician any alterations in the above assessment criteria.	4. Decreases in cardiac output require prompt medical attention.

References

1. Abramson DI: Circulatory Diseases of the Limbs: A Primer. New York, Grune & Stratton, 1978
2. Atchison JS, Murray J: Post-vascular surgery: When happiness can be a warm foot. Nursing 8:36–39, 1978
3. Barnes RW: Peripheral vascular disease and thrombosis. In Joist JH, Sherman LA (eds): Venous and Arterial Thrombosis. New York, Grune & Stratton, 1979
4. Bastarache MM, Giuca J, Horowitz LM et al: Assessing peripheral vascular disease: Noninvasive testing. Am J Nurs 83:1552–1556, 1983
5. Bell WR, Simon TL: Current status of pulmonary thromboembolic disease: Pathophysiology, diagnosis, prevention, and treatment. Am Heart J 103:239–261, 1982
6. Brunner LS, Suddarth DS: Lippincott Manual of Nursing Practice, 2nd ed. Philadelphia, JB Lippincott, 1978
7. Buch WS, Fogarty TJ: Arterial embolism. In Hardy JS (ed): Rhoads Textbook of Surgery, 5th ed. Philadelphia, JB Lippincott, 1977
8. Craven R, Curry TD: When the diagnosis is Raynaud's. Am J Nurs 81:1007–1009, 1981
9. Doyle JE: All leg ulcers are not alike: Managing and preventing arterial and venous ulcers. Nursing 13:58–63, 1983
10. Ekers MA, Bhagwan S: EAB: A new route for vascular rehabilitation. Nursing 12:34–41, 1982
11. Guthaner DF, Wexler L: Peripheral arteriography and therapeutic arteriographic techniques. In Miller DC, Roon AJ (eds): Diagnosis and Management of Peripheral Vascular Disease. Menlo Park, California, Addison-Wesley Publishing Company, 1982
12. McFadden ER, Braunwald E: Cor pulmonale and pulmonary embolism. In Braunwald E (ed): Heart Disease, 2nd ed. Philadelphia, WB Saunders, 1984
13. Miller KM: Assessing peripheral perfusion. Am J Nurs 78:1673–1674, 1978
14. Peterson FY: Assessing peripheral vascular disease: At the bedside. Am J Nurs 83:1549–1551, 1983
15. Roon AJ: The history and physical examination of the patient with peripheral vascular disease. In Miller DC, Roon AJ (eds): Diagnosis and Management of Peripheral Vascular Disease. Menlo Park, California, Addison-Wesley Publishing Company, 1982
16. Rutherford RB: Noninvasive evaluation of peripheral vascular disease. In Miller DC, Roon AJ (eds): Diagnosis and Management of Peripheral Vascular Disease. Menlo Park, California, Addison-Wesley Publishing Company, 1982
17. Shoor PM, Fogarty TJ: Acute arterial insufficiency. In Miller DC, Roon AJ (eds): Diagnosis and Management of Peripheral Vascular Disease. Menlo Park, California, Addison-Wesley Publishing Company, 1982
18. Taggert E: The physical assessment of the patient with arterial disease. Nurs Clin North Am 12:109–115, 1977
19. Wenger NK: Pulmonary embolism: Recognition and management. Consultant 20:85–96, 1980
20. Wissler RW: Principles of the pathogenesis of atherosclerosis. In Braunwald E (ed): Heart Disease, 2nd ed. Philadelphia, WB Saunders, 1984

Bibliography

Bernstein EF: Noninvasive Diagnostic Techniques in Vascular Disease. St Louis, CV Mosby, 1978

Coffman JD: Intermittent claudication, rest pain, physiologic concepts and therapeutic approaches. Prog Cardiovasc Dis 22:53–72, 1979

Coffman JD, Davies WT: Vasospastic diseases: A review. Prog Cardiovasc Dis 18:123–146, 1977

Craven RF, Boozer M: Disorders of the peripheral vascular system. In Underhill SL, Woods SL, Sivarajan ES, Halpenny CJ (eds): Cardiac Nursing. Philadelphia, JB Lippincott, 1982

Datta PK: The last resort. Nursing Mirror 154:41–43, 1982

DeWolfe V: Intermittent claudication. American Family Physician Monograph, American Academy of Family Physicians, June, 1979

Doyle JE: Arterial insufficiency. Nursing 11:74–79, 1981

Eddy ME: Teaching patients with peripheral vascular disease. Nurs Clin North Am 12:151–159, 1977

Fagin-Dubin L: Atherosclerosis: A major cause of peripheral vascular disease. Nurs Clin North Am 12:101–107, 1977

Nicolaides AN: Thromboembolism. Baltimore, University Park Press, 1975

Quinless F: P.V.D.: Physiology, signs, and symptoms. Nursing 14:52–53, 1984

Raab D: Peripheral vascular disease: How to recognize it, how to treat it. Canadian Nursing 78:30–33, 1982

Ream I: Counseling patients with leg pain. Nursing 7:54–57, 1977

Sexton DL: The patient with peripheral arterial occlusive disease. Nurs Clin North Am 12:89–99, 1977

Sparks C: Peripheral pulses. Am J Nurs 75:1132–1133, 1975

Chapter 47

Vascular Structural Disorders

Lorie R. Wild

This chapter discusses management strategies for patients with disorders involving vascular structures, including aortic aneurysms, varicose veins, and lymphedema. Disorders of vascular structure may be either acute or chronic. Acute disorders may be life threatening, while chronic disorders may be extremely debilitating.

Aortic Aneurysm

An aneurysm is a ballooning and weakening within the wall of an artery. Changes in the integrity of the elastic fibers of the medial layer lead to stretching and segmental dilatation of the arterial wall.[8] An aneurysm can develop in any artery but is frequently seen in the ascending or descending aorta. The abdominal aorta is most commonly involved. Nearly 98% of all abdominal aneurysms are located in the infrarenal aorta.[8, 15, 18] The descending thoracic aorta is the second most common site, with the ascending and transverse portions following in frequency of occurrence.[24]

One of the greatest risk factors associated with aortic aneurysm formation is the presence of generalized cardiovascular disease, such as arteriosclerosis or atherosclerosis, and high blood pressure. Patients with aortic aneurysm are most commonly over 60 years of age and more likely to be men. The incidence is approximately seven times higher in men than in women.[1]

Classification

Aortic aneurysms can be classified as three types: true, false, or dissecting.[24] True aneurysms are either fusiform or saccular (Fig. 47–1,*A*). In a fusiform aneurysm the entire circumference of the aortic segment balloons. In a saccular aneurysm a unilateral, saclike dilatation of the aorta occurs. While most true aneurysms are the fusiform type, a saccular aneurysm is most prone to rupture as a result of increased lateral pressures.[18]

In a false aneurysm, the vessel ruptures and although blood leaks out, it is confined by surrounding muscle tissue and fascia (Fig. 47–1,*B*). Ultimately, a thrombus forms at the rupture site and seals the damaged vessel wall.[24] False aneurysms can result from trauma to the vessel or from graft rupture; vessel disease is seldom the cause.[24]

A dissecting aneurysm, or aortic dissection, occurs when blood leaks into and accumulates between the intimal and medial layers of the vessel wall (Fig. 47–1, *C*).[10, 18, 24] An intimal tear is present in nearly 95% of patients with aortic dissection.[10] The hematoma formed by the accumulated blood usually extends in an antegrade fashion (with the flow of blood).[10, 13]

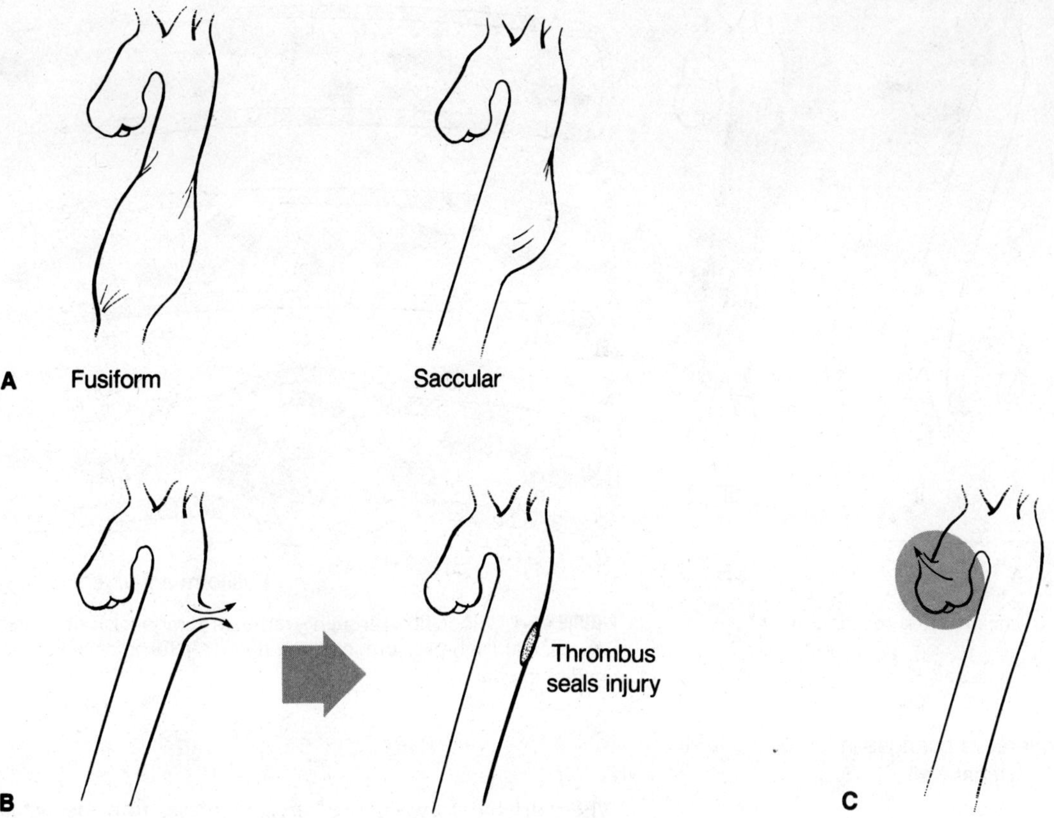

FIGURE 47–1 Types of aneurysms. (*A*) True aneurysms. (*B*) False aneurysm. (*C*) Aortic dissection.

Aortic dissections can be further classified by the location of the tear and the extent of the hematoma. The traditional DeBakey classification (types I, II, and III) is widely used (Fig. 47–2). The tear is in the ascending aorta in both type I and II. The difference between types I and II is the extent of the hematoma. In type I, the hematoma extends the length of the aorta to the iliac bifurcation. The hematoma seen in type II is limited to the ascending portion of the aorta. A DeBakey type III is a dissection in the descending aorta, distal to the left subclavian artery. Recently, a Stanford group introduced a simplified classification scheme (Fig. 47–2), in which all dissections involving the ascending aorta are classified as type A. Type B dissections are those occurring in the descending aorta.[5]

Aortic dissections can be further classified as acute or chronic. A dissection is considered acute if less than 2 weeks elapse between injury and the initiation of treatment. If more than 2 weeks separate injury and therapy, the dissection is considered chronic.[13]

Etiology

High pressure and pulsatile flow as seen with high blood pressure markedly contribute to aneurysm formation. Pulsatile flow increases the mechanical stress upon the vessel wall and has been shown to be the primary offender in aneurysm formation, particularly in aortic dissection.[22] Pregnancy may also predispose to aneurysm formation secondary to both circulatory and hormonal changes present in the perinatal period.[10]

Degenerative changes in the arterial wall also lead to aneurysm formation. Disorders such as arteriosclerosis, and to a lesser extent atherosclerosis, cause structural weakening within the vessel walls (see Chap. 22). Some congenital conditions also cause weakening of the vessel walls leading to aneurysm.[10,18]

Infections causing aortitis can also induce aneurysm formation. Historically, syphilis has been associated with the development of aortic aneurysm but is not often the infecting organism today.[1,8]

Finally, aortic injury may result in aneurysm formation. Aortic dissection and false aneurysm are frequently associated with chest trauma.[10]

Pathophysiology

The pathogenesis and the compensatory responses seen in aortic aneurysm result from arterial wall changes and altered hemodynamics (Fig. 47–3). The arterial wall weakens in response to degenerative changes within the medial elastic layers. The elastic tissue becomes fragmented with muscle cell loss and medial necrosis. The loss of elastic segments allows segmental widening. Tension within the aortic wall increases with this segmental widening. The tension in-

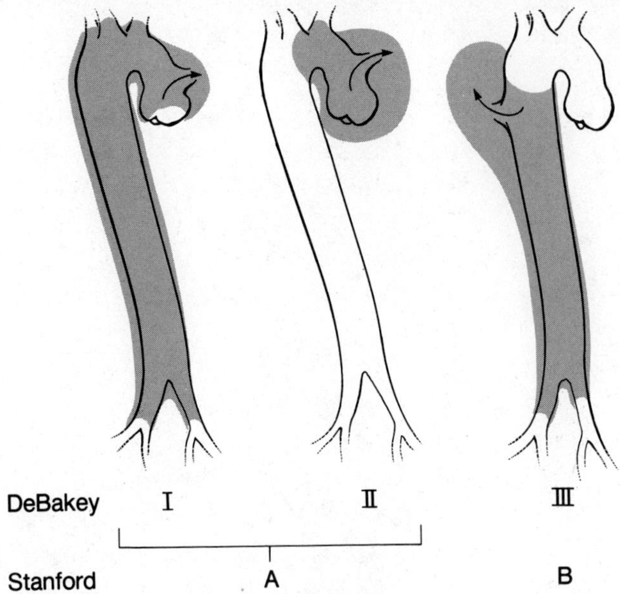

FIGURE 47–2 Classification schemes for aortic dissections.

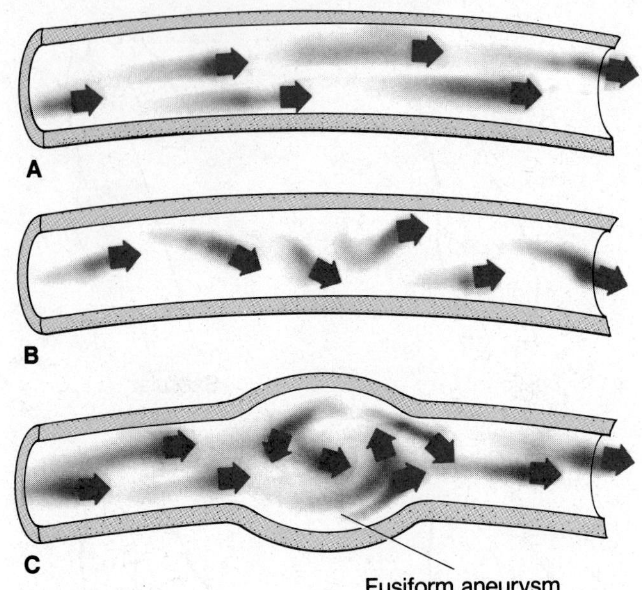

FIGURE 47–4 Blood flow through arteries. (*A*) Smooth laminar flow, normal. (*B*) High pressure, pulsatile flow. (*C*) Turbulence in widened segment.

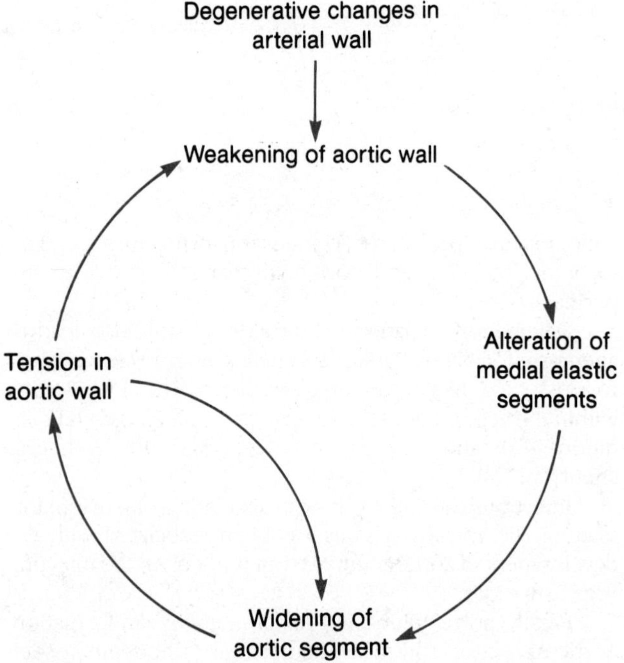

FIGURE 47–3 Etiology and pathophysiology of aneurysm formation.

creases because it is proportional to the product of pressure and the radius of the segment. Increased wall tension causes further weakening and widening of that aortic segment, creating a viscious cycle.

Complicating the arterial wall changes is the alteration in blood flow. Normally, pulsatile blood flow through arteries is considered to be laminar, or smooth (Fig. 47–4,*A*). When driving forward pressures increase, flow becomes more turbulent (Fig. 47–4,*B*). The turbulence places additional stress on the arterial wall, leading to structural changes and segmental weakening. As the aneurysm develops, blood flow through the affected segment becomes even more turbulent, perpetuating the cycle (Fig. 47–4,*C*).

Thrombi can also form in stagnant areas of the aneurysm and at sites of intimal injury. These thrombi can embolize and compromise distal arterial blood flow.

The aneurysm will rupture if the vessel wall is unable to expand further and pressures within the weakened segment exceed what the vessel wall is able to withstand. Aortic aneurysm rupture is a vascular emergency. Of those abdominal aneurysms which rupture, 80% to 90% will rupture into the retroperitoneal space. The remaining 10% to 20% rupture into the peritoneal cavity.[18] Death is certain without surgical repair.

The pathogenesis of aortic dissection differs somewhat from that of true aneurysm formation. Degenerative changes within the medial elastic layer of the artery not only weaken the arterial wall, but also reduce the cohesiveness between the medial and intimal layers.[22] The reduced cohesiveness in the presence of high pressures and pulsatile flow through the aorta increases the risk of intimal tearing and subsequent dissection. Lateral movement of the aorta within the mediastinum during systole is another factor contributing to aortic dissection.[22] Lateral movement of the vessel places additional stress on the aortic wall which can result in dissection, especially when subjected to high intravascular pressures.[22]

If the intimal layer of the arterial wall does tear, blood flows between the intimal and medial layers, creating a hematoma. The hematoma can propagate throughout the aorta.

Typically, the hematoma expands proximally with the flow of blood.

The expanding hematoma seen in dissection causes narrowing of the arterial lumen and increases intravascular pressures. Since increased pressures place additional stress on the weakened arterial wall, more blood flows into the medial space. Thus the hematoma continues to expand and another viscious cycle begins.

If the intimal tear is in the ascending aorta (DeBakey type I or II, Stanford type A), the hematoma may extend into the pericardium, resulting in cardiac tamponade. Cardiac tamponade is the leading cause of death for patients with aortic dissection.[13] As the hematoma expands throughout the pericardium, the ventricles are compressed, and cardiac output decreases severely.

Occasionally, a thrombus may form at the tear site in aortic dissection, "sealing" the injured intima. However, in the presence of sustained high intravascular pressures and turbulent blood flow, the clot may easily dislodge, reactivating the dissection and hematoma growth.

Clinical Manifestations

The clinical manifestations of aortic aneurysm vary depending on the location of the aneurysm and whether it is intact or has ruptured. The clinical manifestations of aortic dissection are similar to those seen with ruptured aortic aneurysm.

Intact Aneurysm. Many patients with aortic aneurysms, whether thoracic or abdominal, are asymptomatic. The intact aneurysm is commonly detected following a routine chest or abdominal x-ray.

With an *abdominal aortic aneurysm,* patients typically experience generalized, steady, or gnawing abdominal or low back pain which is unaffected by movement.[1,18] The pain is due to compression of nerves by the aneurysm and may last from hours to days. A sensation of gastric or abdominal fullness is also common and is the result of pressure on intestinal structures, especially the duodenum.[1,18,24] Intermittent claudication may also be reported by patients and is associated with decreased blood flow to the extremities. If the aneurysm places pressure on abdominal veins, such as the iliac veins or the inferior vena cava, venous congestion may result, causing lower extremity edema. Altered renal function may be present if the aneurysm is suprarenal. However, since most aneurysms of the abdominal aorta are infrarenal, altered renal function is not common prior to aneurysm rupture.

Pain associated with a *thoracic aneurysm* is usually referred to the scapular region and results from pressures exerted on the musculoskeletal structures of the thorax. The aneurysm can cause erosion of bony and soft tissues within the thorax.[18] Other symptoms reported by patients may include hoarseness, dysphagia, or dyspnea secondary to pressure upon the laryngeal nerve, the esophagus, and the lungs, respectively. Respiratory signs are most frequently associated with thoracic aortic aneurysm growth. A cough, stridor, or wheezing may be present. The expanding mass within the mediastinum may cause tracheal deviation. Recurrent pneumonitis is also common in patients with thoracic aortic aneurysm and is related to compression of the tracheobronchial tree.[18,24]

Depending on the location of the aneurysm, disparity of pulses and blood pressure between the extremities may be present. Changes such as these occur when the aneurysm is located on the aortic arch or at arterial bifurcations.

Rupture of Aortic Aneurysm. Sudden onset of severe abdominal or low back pain signals rapid expansion and rupture of an *abdominal aortic aneurysm.* The severe pain experienced by patients with aneurysmal rupture is due to the stretching and stripping of retroperitoneal tissues by free blood within the abdominal cavity.[1]

The signs of hemorrhagic shock quickly follow aneurysm rupture. Tachycardia and hypotension occur rapidly. Other associated signs include marked vasoconstriction leading to skin mottling, decreased level of consciousness, diaphoresis, and oliguria. Abdominal distension with ecchymosis or hematoma in the flank or groin regions may also follow aneurysm rupture.[1,18] Pulses distal to the ruptured portion of the aorta may be absent. Paraplegia may develop due to the absence of spinal blood flow.[24] Other systemic signs might include fever and leukocytosis.[1]

If the aneurysm ruptures into the duodenum, massive gastrointestinal bleeding ensues with hematemesis and melena.[18] An abdominal aortic aneurysm can also rupture into the inferior vena cava, creating a large arteriovenous fistula and high output cardiac failure.[13,18]

The patient with a rupture of a *thoracic aortic aneurysm* presents with signs and symptoms similar to those seen with the abdominal counterpart. The pain is of equal intensity but usually is experienced in the intrascapular area. This area has often been the site of previous discomfort for the patient.[18] Signs of hemorrhagic shock predominate. Pulse deficits and paraplegia may also be present.

If the thoracic aneurysm ruptures into the lungs, intrapulmonary hemorrhage results and the patient can experience massive hemoptysis.[18,24] The thoracic aneurysm could also rupture into the superior vena cava and cause high output cardiac failure.

Aortic Dissection. The clinical manifestations of aortic dissection vary according to the location of the injury and the progression of the dissecting hematoma through the aorta. However, one symptom reported by 79% to 90% of all patients is severe chest pain.[18,19] A "painless" aortic dissection is the exception rather than the rule. Patients generally describe their chest pain as a ripping, tearing, or stabbing sensation of sudden onset.[18] Unlike the chest pain associated with myocardial infarction, which may have a gradual onset or buildup, the pain of aortic dissection is immediately at its fullest intensity.[18] Pain in the anterior thorax suggests proximal dissection; pain in the interscapular region suggests distal dissection.[18,19] If the dissection occurs in the proximal ascending aorta, myocardial blood flow can be compromised, compounding ischemic myocardial pain with the pain of dissection.[13]

Other signs and symptoms of aortic dissection result from the propagating hematoma. As previously mentioned, myocardial ischemia may cause heart failure. Acute aortic valve insufficiency frequently accompanies proximal dissection as evidenced by a high-grade aortic regurgitation murmur.[13,18,19]

Absent or unequal pulses may be present in the extremities following dissection due to either compression of the arterial lumen or reduced arterial blood flow. Pulse deficits in the upper extremities are common with proximal dissections, whereas disparity in lower extremity pulses are seen in distal dissection.[13,19]

As described previously, pericardial tamponade can develop secondary to aortic dissection. Signs and symptoms associated with cardiac tamponade include pulsus paradoxus, hypotension, and a sudden elevation of central venous (right atrial) pressure. Eventually, hemodynamic pressures equalize (right atrial pressure = left atrial pressure).

Syncope and changes in level of consciousness result from compromised cerebral blood flow. Reduction in cerebral blood flow can be the result of carotid artery compression by a proximal expanding hematoma, hypovolemia, or pericardial tamponade.

Spinal, gastrointestinal, or renal arterial flow may also be reduced with aortic dissection, either directly or as a result of vasoconstriction and shunting in response to the dissection. Paraplegia, bowel infarction, anuria, and acute tubular necrosis leading to renal failure may follow.[13]

Medical Management

Diagnosis

Several diagnostic modalities may be employed in the detection of aortic aneurysm or dissection. The patient's history and physical examination can be very helpful, especially in aortic dissection. The onset of signs and symptoms associated with aortic aneurysm or dissection, as discussed above, may be insidious, but are generally considered to be classic for the disorders.

Most aortic aneurysms are detected on routine chest or abdominal x-ray films. A widened mediastinum usually signals thoracic aneurysm formation or growth. Approximately 75% of abdominal aortic aneurysms can be visualized by a lateral x-ray film of the lumbar spine, especially if the aneurysm wall is calcified. Chest x-ray films are also helpful in the diagnosis of aortic dissection, particularly with proximal dissections. An abnormally widened aortic silhouette is characteristic of proximal dissection. Pleural effusion and tracheal deviation may also be evident.[18]

Echocardiographic and abdominal ultrasound are other noninvasive tests which can detect aortic aneurysms or dissection. Ultrasound is most helpful in detecting aneurysms of the abdominal aorta. Ultrasound can accurately assess the contour and diameter of the vessel such that future studies can be done to evaluate aneurysmal growth.[1,18] Unfortunately, ultrasound is a less reliable tool for detecting and tracking aortic dissection.[13]

Computerized tomography (CT) is gaining acceptance as a reliable diagnostic tool in screening for aortic aneurysm and dissection.[13] The CT scan is also a noninvasive study and can give additional information unobtainable by ultrasound. The CT scan allows visualization of the aneurysm's effect on other organs, particularly the position of the renal arteries in reference to an abdominal aneurysm. In addition, retroperitoneal hemorrhage can be detected by CT scanning.[18]

The CT scan is also more reliable in detecting descending aortic aneurysms than is ultrasound.[18] The use of CT scanning with injection of contrast dyes has been shown to be an effective, reliable method for diagnosing both ascending and descending aortic dissections.[18,21]

Aortic angiography, or aortography, continues to be the most definitive diagnostic technique for detecting aortic aneurysm or dissection.[13,18] A contrast dye is injected into the femoral or axillary artery. If an aneurysm is present, it can be localized and outlined by fluoroscopy. Aortography is most helpful in the diagnosis of aortic dissection because the origin and extent of the dissection can be localized. Arterial flow to distal organs will also be shown with angiography. The drawbacks to angiography are cost and the invasive nature of the study. Also, if a thrombus is present in the aneurysm or at the site of dissection, the diagnosis may be missed. Even so, angiography remains the mainstay of diagnostic evaluation for aneurysm or dissection and is typically performed prior to any surgical intervention.

Treatment

Aortic aneurysm or dissection can be treated either medically or surgically, or a combination of both. Patients with aortic aneurysms less than 6 cm in diameter are typically treated by medical interventions alone. Patients are encouraged to lose weight, exercise, and stop smoking. Such measures modify risk factors of disease progression and may help to reduce blood pressure. Blood pressure may also be controlled by diuretics and antihypertensives. Patients with aortic aneurysm require frequent follow-up, at least yearly, to track aneurysm growth or changes.

In the case of aortic dissection, prompt accurate diagnosis is essential for successful therapeutic management.[13,22] The treatment for aortic dissection is similar to that for aortic aneurysm. A blend of medical and surgical interventions is often necessary.

Surgery. Surgical intervention to correct aortic aneurysm is generally indicated by symptomatic aneurysms, or those larger than 6 cm.[14,15,18] In these cases, an elective aneurysmectomy is usually done. The surgical procedure involves cross-clamping of the aorta and iliac arteries, resection of the aneurysm, and replacement with a knitted or woven Dacron graft.[17,18] In some instances, with large aneurysms, an intrasaccular approach may be used. The aneurysmal sac is opened, and the graft is anastomosed within it; finally, the aneurysmal sac is sewn around the graft.[17] This intrasaccular approach is generally associated with shorter cross-clamp times.[18]

Recently, surgeons report the success of a total exclusion technique. In this procedure, the aorta is ligated directly above and below the aneurysm. Extra-anatomical, right axillofemoral, and femoral–femoral bypass graft are also placed. This new technique may be beneficial for patients with high operative risks. Other operative nonresective procedures, such as aneurysm thrombosis, have met with limited success.[11]

In the event of aneurysm leakage or rupture, emergency operative intervention is necessary. Aneurysm rupture without surgical repair is a lethal event.[8, 18]

Operative procedures may include either placing a "patch" graft over the injured vessel, or placing a Dacron graft, as with aneurysmectomy. In type A dissections (*i.e.,* tear in proximal ascending aorta) the aortic valve, or tissue supporting the valve, may also be involved; these procedures require the placement of an aortic valve prosthesis (Fig. 47–5).

PREOPERATIVE MEASURES. Patients experiencing acute aortic dissection require drug therapy preoperatively to achieve hemodynamic stabilization. The patient will usually have an arterial line and urinary catheter placed to monitor blood pressure and urine output. A pulmonary artery catheter may also be inserted. Propranolol hydrochloride, an adrenergic beta-blocker, is typically given intravenously to reduce myocardial contractility. Sodium nitroprusside is also given to reduce and maintain blood pressure (systolic ranging 100 to 120 mmHg; mean ranging 55 to 70 mmHg). Trimethaphan is sometimes used in lieu of sodium nitroprusside, although the latter is the agent of choice.[22] Analgesic and anxiolytic agents may also be administered to promote comfort. Relief of pain by the combination of these drugs suggests stabilization of the dissection. Once stabilized, the patient is ready for surgical repair.

POSTOPERATIVE MANAGEMENT. Postoperative management of aortic aneurysm and dissection are similar. Drug therapies used include continuing sodium nitroprusside (or trimethaphan) and propranolol and administration of broad-spectrum antibiotics.[13] The overall incidence of postoperative complications is 5% to 10%.[13] Postoperative complications of aortic aneurysm or dissection repair include hemorrhage from graft rupture or leaking at the anastamosis and acute renal failure secondary to decreased renal blood flow pre- and intraoperatively. Paralytic ileus may result from both anesthesia and the manipulation of the bowel during surgery. Bowel infarction can also occur owing to prolonged ischemia or ligation of the mesenteric or hypogastric arteries. Paraplegia can result from reduced spinal artery blood flow and cord ischemia; approximately 5% of patients experience postoperative paraplegia lasting from weeks to years.[9, 13, 15, 24] Fluid and electrolyte imbalances frequently occur as a result of blood loss, hemodilution, and renal insufficiency.[24] Wound graft infections are also a threat and are seen most commonly following abdominal aortic aneurysm repair. Graft infections account for 20% to 50% of postoperative deaths.[24]

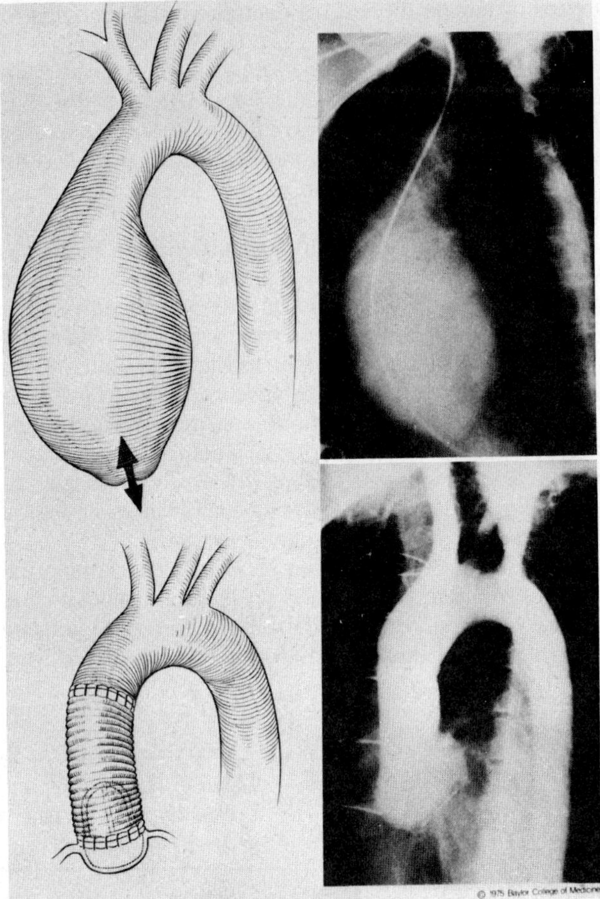

FIGURE 47–5 (*Top*) Drawing and preoperative aortogram illustrate a fusiform aneurysm of the ascending aorta with aortic valvular insufficiency. (*Bottom*) Drawing and postoperative aortogram demonstrate a satisfactory appearance following resection of the aneurysm of the ascending aorta and aortic valve, and replacement with a prosthetic aortic valve and Dacron graft. Cardiopulmonary bypass is required for replacement of the aortic valve and ascending aorta. (DeBakey ME, Noon GP: Aneurysms of the ascending aorta and transverse arch. In Hardy JD [ed]: Rhoads Textbook of Surgery, 5th ed. Philadelphia, JB Lippincott, 1977)

Prognosis

The prognosis for patients with aortic aneurysm or dissection varies depending on the location and the size of the lesion. Other risk factors affecting prognosis include age and underlying medical problems such as myocardial infarction and pulmonary disease.[14, 16] Often, patients succumb to other complications of arteriosclerosis and athersclerosis before aneurysm rupture or dissection.[18]

The prognosis for a patient with an abdominal aortic aneurysm is directly related to its size. More than 50% of all aneurysms larger than 6 cm rupture within 1 year, whereas only 15% to 20% of those less than 6 cm rupture within that time frame.[18] Darling and co-workers reported a 25% incidence of rupture for abdominal aneurysms measuring 4 to 7 cm, 45% for those between 7 and 10 cm, and 60% for those larger than 10 cm.[6] The mean survival time for untreated abdominal aortic aneurysms less than 6 cm in diameter is approximately 34 months, in contrast with 17 months for aneurysms larger than 6 cm.[20]

If an abdominal aneurysm is resected electively, operative mortality ranges between 1.7% and 16%.[3,16] If the aneurysm ruptures, mortality increases to 40% to 60%, even with surgery.[3,15,16] These figures emphasize the need for close monitoring of aneurysm growth in order to prevent rupture.

Patients with thoracic aortic aneurysm have an 80% to 85% survival with elective surgical correction. Patients who are asymptomatic with a thoracic aneurysm have a higher 5-year survival rate than do those with symptoms. The risk of thoracic aneurysm rupture increases with size, similar to the abdominal version, as does operative mortality.[18]

In aortic dissection, overall prognosis is related to the type of dissection (type A or B), whether it is acute or chronic, and how it was treated (medically, surgically, or both). The best prognosis follows a combination of medical stabilization followed by surgical correction.[13,22]

In general, it must be emphasized that the surgical repair of either aortic aneurysm or dissection is not a cure. Surgical repair and other medical treatments only eliminate a major cause of death for these patients. The underlying disease process of arteriosclerosis or atherosclerosis continues. Long-term follow-up is mandatory for these patients to monitor their cardiovascular disease.

Nursing Management

Preoperative Care

Patients with aortic aneurysm or acute dissection require expert nursing care with continual assessment of vascular integrity to detect early changes in their condition. Astute assessment and nursing care must be maintained throughout the perioperative period to prevent serious complications associated with altered tissue perfusion. The clinical manifestations of altered tissue perfusion are summarized in Table 47–1.

For patients experiencing acute aortic dissection or impending aneurysm rupture, nursing care is typically delivered in the critical care setting. Most patients are surrounded by an array of equipment and monitoring devices. Such devices assist in detecting early changes in tissue perfusion resulting from aortic dissection or aneurysm rupture. Patients will be placed on a cardiac monitor and have an arterial

TABLE 47–1
Clinical Manifestations of Altered Tissue Perfusion Related to Aortic Dissection or Aneurysm Rupture

System	*Manifestations*	*Assessment*
Renal	Urine output < 30 ml/hr	Check hourly urine output.
	Hematuria	Urine "dipstick" for blood.
Gastrointestinal	Hematemesis Melena	Check for guaiac in all emesis and stools.
	Absent bowel sounds	Auscultate bowel sounds in each quadrant hourly.
	Abdominal pain	Assess presence and character of any abdominal discomfort.
Peripheral vascular	Absent or unequal peripheral pulses	Palpate or Doppler peripheral pulses hourly. Mark pulse points on extremities.
	Cool, mottled, or cyanotic extremities	Assess color, temperature, and sensation in extremities, hourly.
	Unequal blood pressures in extremities (differences > 10 mmHg)	Check blood pressure in all extremities, hourly.
Coronary	Chest pain	Assess presence and character of chest pain. Obtain ECG with chest pain.
	Tachycardia (HR > 100/min), arrhythmias	Continuously monitor heart rate and rhythm.
Cerebral	Anxiety Decreased level of consciousness (LOC)	Assess LOC, hourly.

line placed to closely follow blood pressures. A pulmonary artery catheter might also be placed to monitor pulmonary artery wedge pressures and cardiac output. A urinary catheter is inserted to enable close hourly monitoring of urine output. The amount of monitoring equipment and the fast-paced environment of the critical care unit, in addition to the potential threat of death, is anxiety producing for both the patient and his family or those close to him. It is important that the nurse explain equipment, unit routines, and all procedures to both the patient and his family to allay some of their anxiety. Sedatives may be ordered for the patient to reduce physiological responses to stress.

Often the patient experiences acute pain related to the aortic dissection or impending aneurysm rupture. Antihypertensive medications and beta-blockers are administered to control the hemodynamic forces contributing to the propagation of the hematoma or aneurysm, and to subsequently reduce pain. Oxygen and analgesics are also given for pain relief.

Postoperative Care

If the patient does undergo surgery, he would again be monitored in the critical care unit during the initial postoperative period. A potential for alteration in tissue perfusion persists into the postoperative period and relates to the risks of the operative procedure itself (aortic clamp or cardiopulmonary bypass times), acute changes in aortic graft integrity (leakage, rupture, occlusion), or hypovolemia. Nursing interventions focus on the prevention of graft rupture or occlusion.

Antihypertensive and beta-blocker medications are administered to reduce hemodynamic stressors on the vessel wall and to preserve the graft anastomosis. Intravenous fluid replacement helps correct hypovolemia and prevents graft collapse. The backrest elevation of the patient should not exceed 30° to 45° since sharp hip flexion could cause the aortic graft to kink. Likewise, the knee gatch should not be engaged because this compresses popliteal vessels and restricts venous return. Antiembolism hose will promote venous return.

Tissue Perfusion. Frequent assessment of tissue perfusion as outlined in Table 47–1 must continue throughout the postoperative period to allow early detection of any changes. An abrupt increase in wound drainage or deterioration of vital signs suggest graft rupture, a surgical emergency. An aortic graft which is leaking may cause a slow accumulation of blood within the abdomen, seen as increasing abdominal girth measurements. Also, if renal blood flow is compromised, serum potassium, blood urea nitrogen, and creatinine may rise.

Fluid Balance. Another problem in the postoperative period is that of fluid balance. A saline deficit can occur as a result of intravascular volume loss. Fluid shifts into interstitial spaces ("third spacing") may also occur, causing a functional saline deficit and reduced circulating volume. Assessment of fluid balance should include hourly monitoring of urine output, vital signs, central venous pressure and pulmonary artery wedge pressure, edema formation, wound drainage, and level of consciousness. Laboratory values (serum electrolytes, albumin, proteins, and hematocrit), weight, abdominal girth, and skin turgor should initially be assessed on a daily basis. Postural blood pressure and pulse should be checked whenever possible since a postural drop in blood pressure is indicative of saline deficit.

Respiratory Support. Patients are usually endotracheally intubated with their breathing supported, in part, by a mechanical ventilator. It is important to explain to the patient and family the purpose of the ventilator and that the patient will be unable to talk as long as the endotracheal tube is in place. Also, such patients are at risk for ineffective airway clearance related to both intubation and discomfort from their large surgical wound. Nursing interventions to maintain the patient's airway, keep it free of secretions, include assessing patency and status of airways and lung fields, assisting the patient in airway clearance (endotracheal suction or cough and deep-breathing), frequent turning, and providing adequate hydration. Positioning the patient and assisting him in "splinting" his incision with pillows prior to suctioning or coughing will help reduce any associated discomfort.

Impaired Skin Integrity. Another nursing diagnosis for the patient with aortic aneurysm or dissection repair is that of impaired skin integrity with potential for infection related to a large surgical wound and artificial graft. In order to prevent wound and graft infection, strict aseptic techniques are mandatory for all dressing changes. The wound, dressing, and surrounding skin must be kept clean and dry. Wound drainage contained within saturated dressings provides an optimum medium for bacterial growth. Moisture associated with saturated dressings not only macerates healthy skin around the wound, but may also lead to bacterial seeding of the wound by a wicking action. Administration of broad spectrum antibiotics also helps prevent postoperative infections. Such preventive measures combined with vigilant assessment of vital signs, wound drainage characteristics, and degree of healing help reduce the morbidity and mortality from infections associated with aortic aneurysm/dissection repair. Fever (temperature > 38.5°C or 101.3°F), tachycardia, elevated white blood cell count, incisional tenderness and erythema, and purulent wound drainage are early signs of wound/graft infections requiring prompt medical intervention.

Other Nursing Diagnoses. Additional nursing diagnoses which may be applicable to patients recovering from surgical repair of aortic dissection of aneurysm may include alteration in nutrition (less than body requirements); impaired physical mobility; alteration in comfort; and knowledge deficit about risk factors of cardiovascular disease. This final nursing diagnosis holds extra importance in that aortic dissection or aneurysm is an overt sign of underlying cardiovascular disease. Repair of the aneurysm or dissection does not arrest the underlying disease. Risk factor modification is important for these patients.

Varicose Veins

Structural alterations within either the venous walls or valves result in a nonocclusive venous disorder known as varicose veins. The disorder usually affects the superficial veins of the lower extremities. Varicosities are most common in the saphenous vein and its tributaries (Fig. 47–6) but can also develop elsewhere, such as in the esophageal and hemorrhoidal veins.[1]

Varicose veins are a common problem occurring in approximately 10% of the general population and most frequently in women.[1] Risk factors include a family history of varicose veins and advanced age. Any condition which impedes venous return from the lower extremities, including prolonged standing or sitting, obesity, pregnancy, or constricting garments, predisposes a person to varicose formation.

Etiology

Varicose veins result from inherent structural weaknesses in either the walls or valves of the veins. Since veins are normally distensible, there may be a hereditary component to account for the degree of weakness present and the development of varicose veins.[1] Primary varicosities usually have an insidious onset, while secondary varicosities may be a result of deep vein insufficiency or thrombosis.[7]

Pathophysiology

Any situation which hinders venous return from the lower extremities initiates the mechanism responsible for varicose vein formation. Blood pools in the lower extremities and veins dilate, stretching the venous walls. When the veins stretch and dilate, the valve leaflets no longer *approximate,* allowing retrograde flow. This retrograde flow and resultant back pressure causes further dilatation, and the cycle continues. Structurally, venous walls are thin and somewhat elastic, and have little vascular smooth muscle.[23] As hydrostatic pressures increase, the veins stretch; the walls stiffen and are not able to recoil effectively.[23] Ultimately, the veins become chronically enlarged and tortuous.

Clinical Manifestations

Because the superficial veins are most frequently affected, patients with varicose veins often have prominent, enlarged, and tortuous veins visible in their legs. The veins may appear purplish in color and feel hard or rope-like when palpated.[1]

A common symptom reported by patients with varicose veins is a sensation of heaviness or fullness in the legs, especially after prolonged standing. Patients may also complain

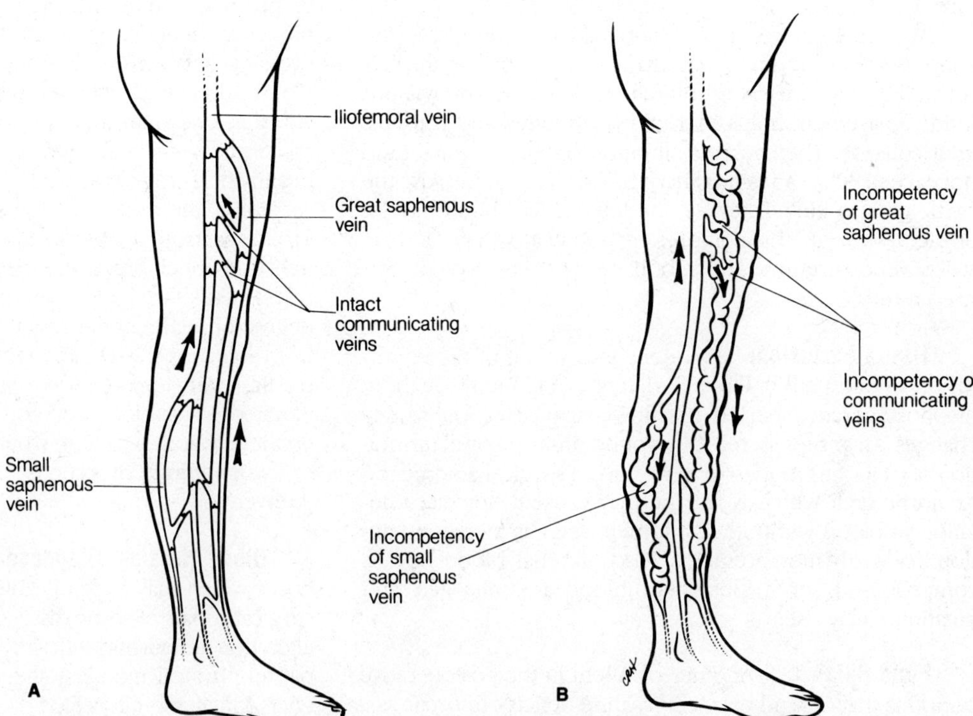

FIGURE 47–6 The superficial and deep venous channels of the leg. (*A*) Normal venous structures and flow patterns. (*B*) Varicosities in the superficial venous system that are the result of incompetent valves in the communicating veins. The arrows in both views indicate the direction of blood flow. (Modified from Abramson DI: Vascular Disorders of the Extremities, 2nd ed. New York, Harper & Row, 1974)

of leg fatigue and muscle cramping, which can become sharp and stabbing.[1] Such discomfort is due to reduced blood supply to tissues from venous stasis. Leg fatigue and cramping may be intensified at night. Many women also report exacerbation of discomfort in the premenstrual period and during pregnancy.

If varicosities have been long-standing, the impaired circulation resulting may lead to skin color changes and the formation of venous stasis ulcers. Skin of the lower extremities that is brownish in color or that has a rusty pigmentation is suggestive of chronic venous stasis.

Medical Management

Diagnosis. The Trendelenburg test is a noninvasive diagnostic tool for assessing valvular competence in the veins of the lower legs.[1,7] The patient lies down with legs elevated to 65° in order to facilitate venous emptying. A tourniquet is placed on the upper thigh to occlude only the superficial veins. The patient then stands and both the direction and speed with which the veins fill are recorded (Fig 47–7). The tourniquet is removed and again the direction and velocity of venous refill is noted. When varicosities and incompetent valves are present, the veins fill rapidly from below; when the tourniquet is released, there is a rapid flow of blood downward.[1,7]

Other noninvasive diagnostic tests may be performed to evaluate varicose veins. Impedence plethysmography, Doppler ultrasound, and computerized tomography may each be helpful in differentiating varicose veins from other deep venous problems.[7]

Another diagnostic modality which may be used in phlebography, or venogram. Radiopaque dye is injected into the dorsel vein of the foot. Venous blood flow and valvular competence can then be evaluated by x-ray film.[1,7]

Treatment. Treatment incorporates general hygienic measures, sclerosing therapy, surgical intervention, or combinations thereof. Hygienic measures include weight loss and avoiding situations which decrease venous return, such as standing or sitting for prolonged periods of time, crossing the legs at the knees, and wearing contstricting garments. Patients are also instructed to elevate the foot of the bed approximately 6 to 8 inches and to wear full leg elastic support stockings.[1,7]

More aggressive therapies are indicated when vari-

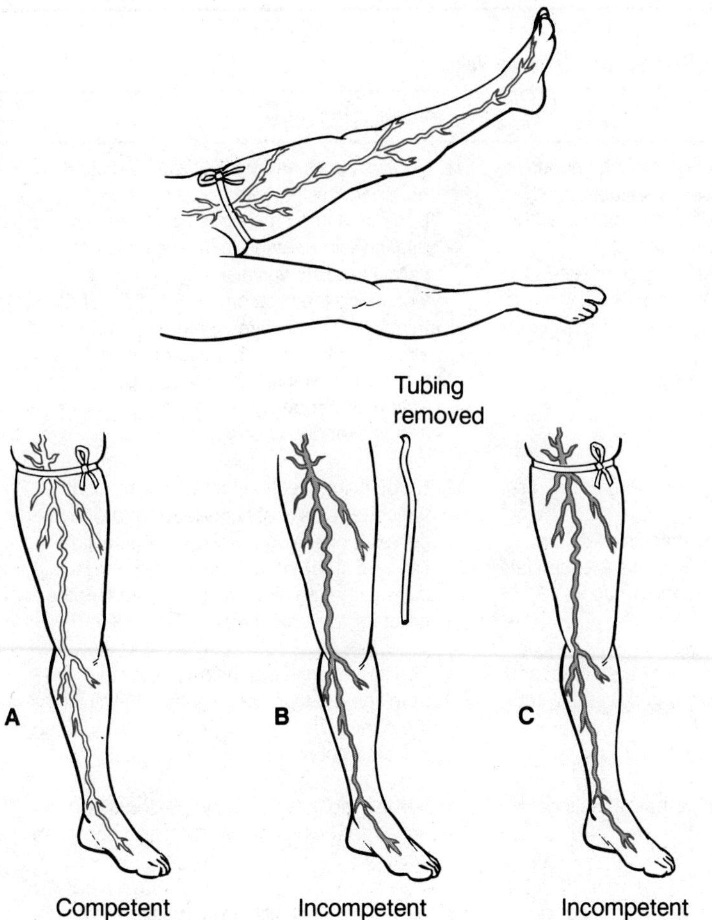

FIGURE 47–7 Trendelenburg test. Leg is elevated to empty veins and tourniquet applied. (*A*) Leg dependent, tourniquet in place with slow filling of veins, *i.e.,* competent short saphenous and communicating veins. (*B*) Tourniquet off and veins fill rapidly, *i.e.,* incompetent long saphenous system. (*C*) Similar test, but when leg is dependent and tourniquet in place there is rapid filling of veins, *i.e.,* incompetent short saphenous vein or communicating veins, or both.

cosities are advanced and the patient is at risk for developing venous ulcers. Sclerosing therapy involves the injection of a chemical, sodium tetradecyl sulfate or sodium morrhuate, into the varicose vein. This produces a type of local chemical thrombophlebitis, causing the endothelial walls of the vein to adhere to each other, obliterating the vessel. This therapy is used infrequently and has limited clinical value.[1]

A surgical ligation and stripping of the effected vein is the treatment of choice for advanced varicose veins. The vein involved is first ligated at the proximal and distal ends and then removed. Ligation alone is less effective than the combination of ligation and "stripping."

Varicose veins are a chronic problem. Although the disorder is not life-threatening, it can be debilitating, and complications can arise. Venous stasis ulcers and cellulitis may result from altered blood flow. Bleeding and hemorrhage can occur if the varicosity erodes through the skin.

Recurrence of varicose veins following surgical treatment is also common. The recurrence is due, in part, to the added stress placed on remaining veins following removal of the primary varicosities.[1,7] Because of the rate of recurrence, proper hygienic precautions must be taken by the patient.

Nursing Management

Patients with varicose veins require supportive and educative nursing care. Some patients may have a lack of knowledge or exposure to information about varicose veins, their cause and their treatment. Others may misinterpret information or not follow through with instructions. Thus, the focus of nursing care and teaching should be the prevention of situations leading to venous stasis. Use of prophylactic measures can markedly reduce the morbidity associated with this chronic disorder. Often, patients are motivated to institute such measures because of body image changes and the cosmetic aspects of varicose veins. Table 47–2 summarizes key teaching points for patients with varicose veins.

Lymphedema

Lymphedema is an occlusive disorder of lymphatic structures. Lymphedema may be disabling for affected patients as a result of cosmetic disfigurement and functional loss.

TABLE 47–2
Health Teaching for the Patient with Varicose Veins

Teaching Point	*Rationale*
1. Instruct patient about promoting venous return and preventing venous stasis. a. Avoid long periods of standing or sitting. b. Do not sit with legs crossed. c. Do not wear constricting garments. d. Elevate feet when sitting. e. Exercise regularly; walking is especially good. f. Wear support stockings.	1. Venous stasis and pooling cause distention of superficial leg veins, placing excessive back pressure on venous valves. Prolonged dilation and pressure of the vessel and valves leads to valvular incompetence, worsening the problem. Any activity or clothing restricting venous return must be avoided. Measures to enhance venous return must be taken. The muscle-pumping action accompanying exercise greatly enhances venous return.
2. Explain to patient the chronicity of the disorder. a. Only palliative treatment is available. b. Prevention of venous stasis is essential to maintain comfort and function.	2. Surgical intervention for the treatment of varicose veins is only palliative and primarily serves a cosmetic purpose. Surgical ligation and stripping actually places additional stress on remaining veins, heightening the need for hygienic measures as outlined.
3. Explain to patient need for careful foot and leg care to avoid injury and possible infection in extremities.	3. The alteration in blood flow in the lower extremities reduces tissue nutrition. Any injury there may heal slowly and has an increased risk of infection.
4. Encourage patient to verbalize feelings about appearance.	4. Verbalizing feelings about personal appearance may help in clarification and decrease anxiety.
5. Discuss ways to minimize visibility of varicosities: wearing slacks, opaque hose, longer skirts or dresses.	5. Minimizing visibiilty of varicosities may help shift focus from that body part to another.

Etiology

Lymphedema is considered to be primary or secondary, based on etiology. Primary lymphedema is generally considered to be the result of errors in the development of lymphatic structures.[1] Clinical conditions subsumed under primary lymphedema include congenital lymphedema, Milroy's disease (congenital familial lymphedema), and lymphedema praecox. The cause of congenital lymphedema is unknown, although genetic factors do seem to have a role in its development. Unlike congenital lymphedema, where there are no familial tendencies, the swelling seen in Milroy's disease is usually present in more than one family member. Lymphedema praecox, seen most commonly in girls and young women, results from problems in lymphatic drainage of the lower limbs; its cause is unknown.[1,14]

Secondary lymphedema can result from infection, direct injury, or obstruction. Inflammatory lymphedema may follow recurrent cellulitis or may be due to direct invasion of the lymphatics by organisms.[1] Trauma to lymphatic structures may follow surgery or limb injury. Some degree of lymphedema is evident in up to 30% of postoperative radical mastectomy patients.[12] Often, tumor cells invade lymphatic structures, causing blockage and subsequent swelling.

Pathophysiology

Normally, highly permeable lymphatic vessels filter and drain interstitial fluids. The main trunks of lymphatic vessels have tricuspid, one-way valves similar to veins. As the pale yellow lymph fluid travels proximally, small lymph channels converge to form larger channels. Ultimately, lymph fluid empties into the vena cava by way of the thoracic duct.

In primary lymphedema, lymph channels are notably absent or hypoplastic.[1] In both primary and secondary lymphedema, the lymphatic structures may widen and dilate, leading to lymphatic valvular incompentence. Surgical procedures and tumor cell invasion are other ways in which lymphatic structures are mechanically interrupted.

Since lymph is a protein-rich fluid, obstruction of drainage channels allows interstitial fluid to accumulate. The resultant increased interstitial oncotic pressure leads to further fluid accumulation and swelling.

One distinguishing characteristic of lymphedema is the visible fibrosis of lymph channels, interstitium, and skin.[1] Fibrotic changes ultimately occur in both primary and secondary lymphedema.

Clinical Manifestations

Clinical signs and symptoms of lymphedema are similar in both the primary and secondary types. Swelling, either diffuse or localized, in one or more limbs is always seen in lymphedema (Fig. 47–8). The area of swelling depends on which lymph channels are affected. The swelling may be pitting and is generally painless in primary lymphedema.[1,4]

Inflammatory lymphedema (secondary) is often associated with lymphangitis and cellulitis. The patient may present with fever, aching, and malaise. The affected limb is swollen, warm, and tender. Red streaking ascending the affected limb may also be evident and indicates lymph channel involvement.

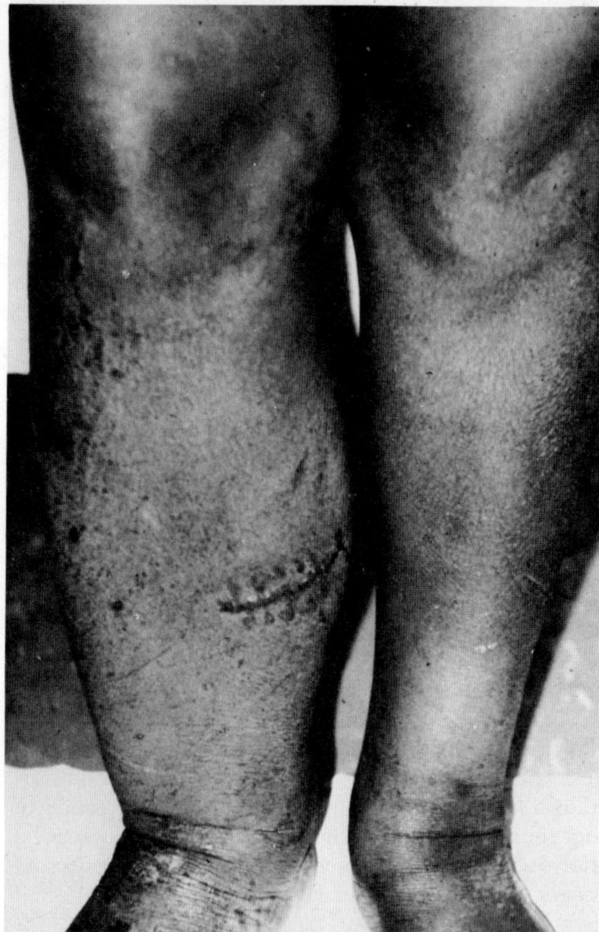

FIGURE 47–8 Primary lymphedema in a 17-year-old girl. Note the swelling in both legs, which is more marked on the right. Repeated episodes of cellulitis aggravated the edema. (Hardy JD: Hardy's Textbook of Surgery, p 993. Philadelphia, JB Lippincott, 1983)

If attacks of inflammatory lymphedema are recurrent, each attack tends to leave more residual edema. The swelling may become permanent and is evidenced by thickening of the skin and fibrosis of the subcutaneous tissues (fibroedema). Such a progression is known as elephantiasis, and the structural changes seen further impair lymphatic drainage, worsening the condition of the extremity.[1]

Medical Management

The diagnosis of lymphedema is usually made by careful patient history and may be verified by lymphangiography. Lymphangiography is most helpful in differentiating primary and secondary lymphedema because of the structural aberrancies seen in the primary types.

The medical treatment for lymphedema lies primarily in its prevention. In primary lymphedema, where alterations in lymphatic structures are inborn, conditions which promote excess lymph fluid formation must be averted.

Prophylactic measures include meticulous hygiene of the affected limb. Clothing, hose, or accessories worn on the affected limb must be loose and nonrestrictive.

Injury to the skin or tissue of an affected body part will ultimately lead to increased lymph formation as the body's defenses act to repair the injured portion. The lymphatic channels normally serve as exit routes for the by-products of the inflammatory response. Such drainage is impaired in lymphedema.

Active medical measures to treat lymphedema include a low sodium diet and bed rest with the affected limb elevated.[1] Diuretics may also be used to assist in the mobilization of fluids.

Once swelling is controlled, many patients are fitted with special rubberized support stockings (or sleeve, if the arm is affected). Some patients with severe recurring lymphedema require a 100% pararubber bandage to wrap the affected extremity.[1] Such a bandage is stronger than standard elastic types (*e.g.,* Ace wraps) and renders greater support in the control of swelling.[1]

Pneumatic compression pumps may also be used in cases of severe swelling. Such devices intermittently inflate and deflate, delivering a uniform pressure wave and mobilizing excess fluid in a proximal direction.[1,2]

Surgical intervention for severe lymphedema is rarely performed and is not considered to be efficacious. In drastic cases, when a patient is severely handicapped by the disorder, as a last resort, procedures which involve removal of either subcutaneous tissue or superficial lymphatics may be performed.[1] Such surgical procedures produce marked cosmetic effects which can also be disabling to affected patients.

Lymphedema is not associated with high mortality. The degree of morbidity depends on the extent and chronicity of the disorder. Physical activity may be curtailed as a result of large, heavy limbs. Psychological disturbances may result from the profound cosmetic changes associated with the disorder.

Nursing Management

The approach to nursing care of patients with lymphedema is similar to that of varicose veins. Both conditions are chronic and pose cosmetic problems. The focus is, again, on prevention. Although lymphedema often is the consequence of other underlying problems, the prevention of swelling is possible by relatively simple measures, such as elevating the affected extremity, wearing elastic stockings or an arm support, and exercising the extremity regularly through range of motion movement. Such measures assist in promoting lymphatic–venous flow and in draining any excess fluid accumulation. It is equally important to alert the patient to wear protective clothing or shoes, to avoid moving heavy objects, and to walk carefully in order to avoid injury to the affected extremity. Injury increases blood and lymphatic flow in the extremity. If lymphatic channels cannot compensate, swelling from fluid accumulation will result. To offset any self-consciousness over appearance, the patient can wear long flowing garments to hide the swollen extremity.

References

1. Abramson DI: Circulatory Diseases of the Limbs: A Primer. New York, Grune & Stratton, 1978
2. Alexander MA, Wright ES, Wright JB et al: Lymphedema treated with a linear pump: Pediatric case report. Arch Phys Med Rehabil 64:132–133, 1983
3. Botta GC, Contini S, Adorni A: Abdominal aortic aneurysms: Some controversial points. J Cardiovasc Surg 24:481–487, 1983
4. Cowie V: Yellow nail syndrome: Zellweger syndrome. Nurs Mir 1958 (inside back cover), 1984
5. Daily PO, Trueblood HW, Stinson EB et al: Management of acute aortic dissections. Ann Thorac Surg 10:237, 1970
6. Darling RC, Messina CR, Brewster DC et al: Autopsy study of unoperated abdominal aortic aneurysms. The case study for early resection. Circulation (Suppl II) 56:161, 1977
7. Fitzgerald FT, Graor R, Lofgren EP et al: When the complaint is varicose veins. Patient Care 18:22–54, 1984
8. Friedman SA: The evaluation and treatment of patients with arterial aneurysms. Med Clin North Am 65:83–103, 1981
9. Gornick CC, Kjellstrand CM: Acute renal failure complicating aortic aneurysm surgery. Nephron 35:145–157, 1983
10. Hirst AE, Gore I: The etiology and pathology of aortic dissection. In Doroghazi RM, Slater EE (eds): Aortic Dissection. New York, McGraw-Hill, 1983
11. Kwaan JHM, Khan RM, Connolly JE: Total exclusion technique for the management of abdominal aortic aneurysms. Am J Surg 146:93–97, 1983
12. Markowski J, Wilcox JP, Helm PA: Lymphedema incidence after specific post mastectomy therapy. Arch Phys Med Rehabil 62:449–451, 1981
13. Miller DC, Stinson EB: Acute and chronic aortic dissections. In Miller DC, Roon AJ (eds): Diagnosis and Management of Peripheral Vascular Disease. Menlo Park, California, Addison-Wesley, 1982
14. Nash T, Gold J: Surgery for abdominal aortic aneurysms. Med J Aust 2:434-436, 1983
15. Olcott C, Mehigan JT: Aneurysms of the abdominal aorta and peripheral arteries. In Miller DC, Roon AJ (eds): Diagnosis and Management of Peripheral Vascular Disease. Menlo Park, CA, Addison-Wesley, 1982
16. Ranakokko V, Havia T, Inberg MV et al: Abdominal aortic aneurysms: A clinical and autopsy study of 408 patients. Acta Chir Scand 149:151–155, 1983
17. Sheiner NM: Technical aspects in the management of abdominal aortic aneurysms. Can J Surg 26:523–526, 1983
18. Slater EE, DeSanctis RW: Diseases of the aorta. In Braunwald E (ed): Heart Disease, 2nd ed. Philadelphia, WB Saunders, 1984
19. Sutton MSJ, Oldershaw PJ, Miller GAH et al: Dissection of the thoracic aorta. J Cardiovasc Surg 22:195–202, 1981
20. Szilagy DE, Smith RF, DeRusso FJ et al: Contribution of abdominal aortic aneurysmectomy to prolongation of life. Ann Surg 164:678, 1966
21. Thorsen MK, San Dretto MA, Lawson TL et al: Dissecting aortic aneurysms: Accuracy of computed tomographic diagnosis. Radiology 148:773–777, 1983
22. Wheat MW: Pathogenesis of aortic dissection. In Doroghazi RM, Slater EE (eds): Aortic Dissection. New York, McGraw-Hill, 1983
23. Wiederhelm C: The capillaries, veins, and lymphatics. In Ruch TC, Patton HD (eds): Physiology and Biophysics, Vol II. Philadelphia, WB Saunders, 1974
24. Zimmerman TA, Ruplinger J: Thoracoabdominal aortic an-

eurysms: Treatment and nursing interventions. Crit Care Nurs 3:54–63, 1983

Bibliography

Acosta J, Khan F, Chitkara R: Trepopnea resulting from large aneurysm of sinus of valsalva and descending aorta. Heart & Lung 11:342–344, 1982

Baum PL: Abdominal aortic aneurysm? This patient takes AAA care. Nursing 12:34–41, 1982

Czapinski N, Antig P, Beloria D et al: Nursing plan for abdominal aortic aneurysms. AORN 37:205–210, 1983

Kluge RM: Infections of prosthetic cardiac valves and arterial grafts. Heart & Lung 11:146–151, 1982

Pokrovsky AV: Classification and surgical treatment of dissecting aortic aneurysms. J Cardiovasc Surg 24:89–94, 1983

Quinlan M: Edema: What really causes it, how to control it, RN (April), pp 55-57, 1984

Section 3

Hematologic Function

Chapter 48

Review of Anatomy and Physiology
Blood and Blood-Forming Mechanisms

Barbara R. Landau

The blood provides communication between the external and internal environments. Its most obvious role is transport, which makes it part of the digestive, respiratory, excretory, and endocrine systems. In carrying out the transport role, blood contributes to such regulatory mechanisms as fluid and acid–base balance, and temperature regulation. Leukocytes are important for body defenses.

The amount of blood necessary to meet these needs is about 70 to 75 ml/kg body weight. This is about 5 liters in a 70-kg man, and varies between 4 and 6 liters in most individuals (5–6 + liters in men and 4–5.5 liters in women). Blood volume is controlled by mechanisms designed to maintain a constant volume or to restore it when other factors change it. Compensatory mechanisms include adjusting the capacity of the circulatory system to maintain the mean arterial pressure when the volume changes, and restoration of the volume by changes in fluid intake or urine output. Resulting changes in hydrostatic and osmotic pressure gradients across capillary walls may either relieve or worsen the problem.

Blood is a connective tissue with a fluid matrix. This vital, multipurpose matrix is red, sticky, about five times as viscous as water, and capable of clotting. It consists of plasma, the fluid portion, in which numerous inorganic and organic ions and molecules are dissolved, and in which cellular (formed) elements are suspended. The cellular elements are red blood cells (RBCs) or erythrocytes, white blood cells (WBCs) or leukocytes and platelets, which are cell fragments.

The fluid and cellular components can be separated by centrifugation. The cells, which pack at the bottom of the tube, occupy roughly 45% of the volume, and the upper 55% is plasma. The cellular volume, or hematocrit, is about 47% in men and 42% in women. The cellular mass is almost entirely erythrocytes, but a thin film of leukocytes and platelets, called the buffy coat, can be detected at the surface. The hematocrit increases as the number of cells increases (polycythemia) or the fluid volume decreases (dehydration), and vice versa. Drawn blood will form a clot, which is a red gelatinous mass in which blood cells are trapped. The clot later retracts and squeezes the fluid from it; this fluid is serum. It differs from plasma in that it lacks the clotting elements: plasma will clot; serum will not.

Plasma

At 55% of total blood volume, the plasma varies between about 2.5 and 3.5 liters (or 5% of body weight). By weight, it is 90% to 93% water, 6% to 8% protein, 1% to 2% other organic compounds, and 0.9% to 1% inorganic ions (Table 48–1). The protein content is higher in plasma than in other extracellular fluids, but the water and electrolyte concentrations are virtually the same. The importance of the electrolytes lies not only in specific roles of individual ions, but in the total ion concentration, for it determines the tonicity of the extracellular fluid. Organic substances in plasma other than proteins include nutrients, metabolites (wastes), hormones, and enzymes.

The many different proteins in plasma can be electrophoretically separated into albumin, globulins, and fibrinogen. Albumin is the most abundant and has the smallest molecules, so it is the major contributor to the plasma colloid osmotic pressure (COP) and the protein most likely to leave the circulation. Albumin is also a carrier protein for several substances. The globulins have been subdivided into $\alpha 1$, $\alpha 2$, $\beta 1$, $\beta 2$, and γ globulins. Based on their structure and function they are also classified as glycoproteins and lipoproteins. Glycoproteins are mostly α globulins, and many of them are carriers. Most lipoproteins are β globulins and are the primary carrier molecules for lipid and lipid-soluble substances. Other β globulins are metal-binding proteins. Most of the albumins and α and β globulins are produced in the liver, but the γ globulins, as immunoglobulins or antibodies, are produced by plasma cells in lymphoid tissues and released into the circulation. Fibrinogen is a large molecule which, as the precursor to fibrin, is the basis of blood clotting.

TABLE 48–1
Composition of Human Plasma

Constituent	*Concentration*
Water	91–93 g/dl (91–93% by weight)
Total Protein	6–8 g/dl
Albumin	3.2–4.5 g/dl
Globulins	2.3–3.6 g/dl
Fibrinogen	0.2–0.4 g/dl
Electrolytes (Inorganic Ions)	0.9 g/dl (0.9% by weight)
Na^+	136–145 mEq/liter
K^+	3.5–5.0 mEq/liter
Ca^{2+}	4.6–5.5 mEq/liter
Mg^{2+}	1.5–2.0 mEq/liter
Cl^-	100–106 mEq/liter
HCO_3^-	27 mEq/liter
Phosphate	2 mEq/liter
Sulfate	0.5–1.5 mEq/liter
Organic Compounds	
Glucose	70–110 mg/dl
Total amino acids	40 mg/dl
Total lipids	400–1000 mg/dl
Cholesterol	150–350 mg/dl
Blood urea nitrogen (BUN)	10–25 mg/dl
Nonprotein nitrogen (NPN)	20–45 mg/dl
Creatinine	0.7–1.5 mg/dl
Uric acid	3–7 mg/dl

Cellular Elements

Erythrocytes

Erythrocytes (red blood cells, RBCs) are important for their content of hemoglobin (Hb), the oxygen-binding protein. Circulating RBCs consist of a plasma membrane, a lipoprotein stroma (framework), and the cytosol which contains the hemoglobin, but they have no nucleus or organelles. In an isotonic environment, the cells are biconcave discs about 7 to 8 μ in diameter (Fig. 48–1). The shape provides flexibility for passage through narrow capillaries and a large surface area for diffusion of gases, and also permits a sizable increase in cell volume without destroying the cell. In a hypertonic environment RBCs lose fluid and shrink (crenation), and in a hypotonic environment they gain fluid and swell. These changes are reversible within limits, for an excessive volume increase will rupture the membrane (hemolysis), allowing hemoglobin to escape into the plasma. Other substances including some drugs, snake venoms, and some infections also destroy RBC membranes.

Under certain conditions, including a sluggish circulation, RBCs tend to stick together like a stack of coins (rouleaux: see Fig 48–1, *A*) or they may clump or agglutinate (as in transfusion reactions). These responses reduce the surface area available for gas exchange and interfere with their passage through small blood vessels.

Without a nucleus, the cells are unable to reproduce or renew their protein (enzyme) complement, but they withstand the buffeting of travel through the vascular system quite well, and have an average life span of about 120 days. This means that about 2.5 to 3 million cells are destroyed each second, which obviously requires RBCs to be produced at the same rate.

Erythropoiesis

In adults, red blood cells are produced in the red bone marrow of the verbetrae, sternum, ribs, iliac crest, and ends of some long bones. Red marrow is much more extensive in the fetus, for it has not yet been replaced by yellow marrow. The fetal spleen and liver also produce RBCs, and under certain conditions can regain their erythropoietic capacity in adults.

Red cells arise from an undifferentiated stem cell (sometimes called a hemocytoblast) which has potential to develop along one of several pathways (Fig. 48–2). Some of its daughter cells become committed to the erythrocytic pathway, and become erythroblasts. In a series of mitoses, successive generations of cells become progressively smaller and contain fewer organelles, but more and more hemoglobin. Finally, the nucleus is extruded and phagocytized. The resulting cells resemble mature RBCs except for a few remaining strands of RNA which stain as a network, and the cells are called reticulocytes. When the RNA disappears the cells are no longer able to synthesize hemoglobin or enzymes, and are now mature erythrocytes. The whole process takes approximately 7 days, with roughly 3 days accounted for as reticulocytes. Typically, about 1% of circulating RBCs are reticulocytes, but that fraction may be greater when erythropoiesis is accelerated.

Control of Erythropoiesis. The rate of RBC formation is controlled largely by erythropoietin, a glycoprotein hor-

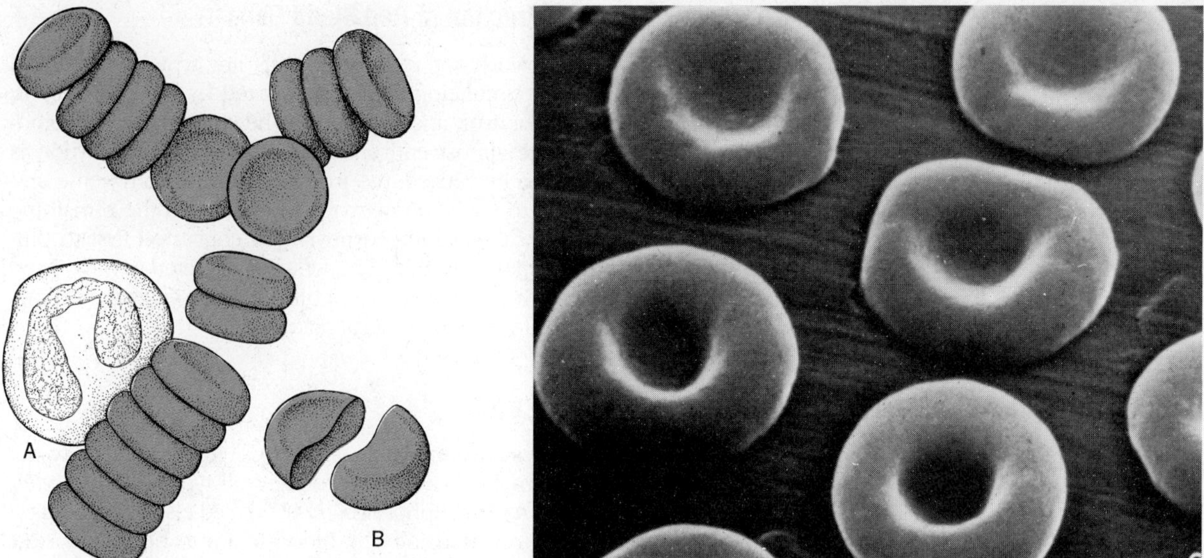

FIGURE 48–1 (*Left*) Red blood cells grouped in rouleaux (like a stack of coins). One white blood cell (*A*) also is shown. (*B*) A red cell split to show its biconcave shape. (*Right*) Scanning electron micrograph of normal red blood cells. Original magnification ×5000. The normal biconcave disk shape of these cells is apparent. (Courtesy of STEM Laboratories, Inc and Fisher Scientific Co)

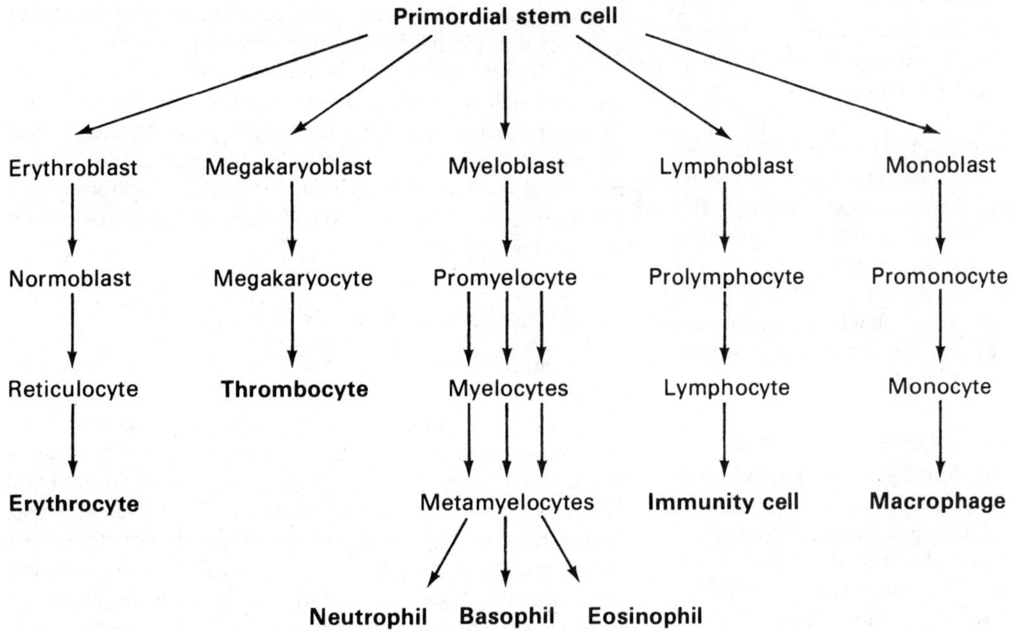

FIGURE 48–2 Diagrammatic summary illustrating orderly development of erythrocytes, thombocytes, and leukocytes from a primary cell, or forefather, called a primordial stem cell.

mone that stimulates the conversion of erythrocytic stem cells to erythroblasts. Much of the erythropoietin comes from the kidney, but some also comes from other organs, especially the fetal liver. There is some question as to whether the kidney actually releases erythropoietin, or produces a substance (renal erythropoietic factor, REF) which activates a protein in the blood to form erythropoietin. In any case, the hormone is essential for normal erythropoiesis. The chief stimulus for increased production of erythropoietin is tissue hypoxia brought about by a reduced Pa_{O_2} or a lack of hemoglobin (loss of blood or RBCs), The number of circulating red cells increases 2 or 3 days after an increase in erythropoietin, even though the hormone has a half-life of only about 5 hours. It is inactivated mainly in the liver.

Hemoglobin

Synthesis of hemoglobin is a major part of erythropoiesis. Hemoglobin (Hb) is made up of a protein (a globin) and a pigment (heme). One heme is attached to each of four chains, and each heme contains iron (Fe^{2+}), which binds the oxygen. If the iron is oxidized (Fe^{3+}), methemoglobin is formed, which does not bind oxygen. Hemoglobin has a high affinity for oxygen, and binds it in a loose reversible association.

$$\underset{\text{deoxyHb}}{Hb} + O_2 \rightleftharpoons \underset{\text{oxyHb}}{HbO_2}$$

In arterial blood, 97% to 98% of the hemoglobin is in the form of oxyhemoglobin; in venous blood about 75% is oxyhemoglobin and 25% deoxyhemoglobin.

Factors Essential for Normal Erythropoiesis

Iron. Iron is needed for normal red cell formation, because it is necessary for synthesis of hemoglobin. It is also found in myoglobin and several important enzymes. The metabolism of iron is unique, for there is no mechanism for excreting it. The body recycles iron and regulates its iron content by controlling its absorption. Iron is absorbed from the upper small intestine by active transport. In mucosal cells most of the iron binds to a protein (apoferritin), forming the storage form, ferritin. Normally, only a small portion of ingested iron is absorbed, the actual amount being determined largely by the ferritin content of the mucosal cells. Some iron is released into the plasma, binds to a carrier protein (transferrin), and is carried to the liver and other cells to be stored as ferritin.

About two thirds of the iron in the body is in hemoglobin, some is in myoglobin in muscle, and much of the remainder is stored as ferritin. The iron is used in hemoglobin synthesis comes from these ferritin stores and from iron released by destroyed red cells, and is transported to the bone marrow by transferrin. A small amount of iron is lost from the body in the feces in conjunction with desquamation of intestinal mucosal cells. Women, however, lose a significant amount of iron in menstrual blood.

Vitamin B_{12} and Intrinsic Factor. Vitamin B_{12} is a cobalt-containing vitamin needed for normal production and maturation of red blood cells. It affects certain reactions necessary for DNA synthesis, and a lack is associated with the presence of large primitive red cells (megaloblasts). Lack of vitamin B_{12} is usually due to inadequate absorption from the digestive tract, which is most often due to lack of glycoprotein, called intrinsic factor. It is produced by the parietal (HCl-producing) cells of the gastric mucosa, and binds the vitamin, making possible its absorption from the ileum. Following absorption, the vitamin is released into the bloodstream and carried to the liver for storage until it is released for transport to the bone marrow, where it promotes produciton of normal red cells.

Folic Acid. Folic acid is another B vitamin necessary for normal red cell formation. Its actions are somewhat related to those of vitamin B_{12} in that both involve reactions needed for DNA synthesis, and a lack of folic acid also contributes to megaloblastic anemias.

Destruction of Red Blood Cells

Old worn-out red blood cells are typically removed from the circulation and phagocytized by macrophages in the spleen, liver, and elsewhere. The components of hemoglobin are almost entirely recycled. The globin portion is split off to be reused; the iron is removed from heme and returned to the bone marrow for reuse; and the remaining portion of the heme (porphyrin) is converted first to biliverdin and then to bilirubin, which is excreted in the bile by the liver. It is the presence of bilirubin that gives the yellowish color to bile and to fecal material.

Leukocytes

Leukocytes (white blood cells, WBCs) function in body defenses. The bone marrow produces all types of leukocytes, although most lymphocytes are produced elsewhere. Leukocytes are released into the bloodstream to be transported, and leave it to carry out their actions. Although RBCs outnumber WBCs in the circulation by about 500:1, about 75% of the developing cells in the bone marrow are WBCs. This is because most leukocytes have a short life span, and most leave the circulation after a few hours. WBCs are found in connective tissue, in many organs, and particularly in lymphoid organs. They arise from committed stem cells and develop along individual pathways (see Fig. 48–2).

White blood cells are classified as granulocytes (or polymorphonuclear leukocytes), monocytes, and lymphocytes. The granulocytes are characterized by the presence of cytoplasmic granules and a nucleus that becomes multilobed as the cell ages. Even though monocytes and lymphocytes are known as agranulocytes, a few cytoplasmic granules can be detected with special stains.

Granulocytes

Granular leukocytes are identified as neutrophils, eosinophils, and basophils by the staining characteristics of their granules. Neutrophils are the most abundant, and in practice "polymorphonuclear leukocyte" usually refers to neutrophils. Their numerous tiny granules take a neutral stain and are, in fact, lysosomes. Neutrophils are extremely phagocytic, and with the proper chemotactic stimulus, demonstrate their ameboid activity by passing between cells of the capillary wall into the tissues to attack invading bacteria. Their life span is very short, and the entire neutrophil population is replaced about 2½ times each day. Neutrophils respond very quickly and are the first line of defense for bacterial invasion. The material phagocytized by neutrophils is enclosed in vesicles whose membranes then fuse with those of the neutrophilic granules (lysosomes), and the lysosomal enzymes proceed to destroy it.

Eosinophils are characterized by their acid-staining granules. They phagocytize antigen–antibody complexes and release enzymes that alleviate some symptoms of allergic responses (*e.g.,* a histaminase to break down histamine). Their granules apparently contain a protein that can damage certain parasites. The number of eosinophils increases markedly in certain allergic and parasitic conditions, but

ACTH and glucocorticoids (cortisol) reduce the eosinophils count by causing them to be sequestered in the spleen and lungs.

Basophils have only a few large basic-staining granules, which contain histamine and heparin. In some respects these cells resemble mast cells (whose granules also contain histamine and heparin). Their function is not clear.

Monocytes

Monocytes are large cells which arise from the same committed stem cells as granulocytes, but by a different pathway. They usually leave the circulation within about 24 hours to become the tissue macrophages that make up the reticuloendothelial system. Many macrophages remain in the connective tissue, but others come to rest in specific organs (such as the liver, the respiratory alveoli). Monocytes respond to chemotactic signals of bacterial invasion. They respond more slowly than neutrophils, but carry on for a longer period of time. They demonstrate ameboid activity, especially after leaving the circulation. Monocytes are "voracious eaters," and will phagocytize tumor cells, viruses, dead cells, and even other macrophages.

Lymphocytes

The original stem cells for lymphocytes are in the bone marrow, but during embryonic life developing lymphocyte precursor cells migrate from the bone marrow, some going to the thymus and some to a tissue that is very likely the fetal liver and maybe the fetal spleen. At these sites the cells undergo conditioning and become transformed in the special environments, and then migrate to lymphoid tissue in other parts of the body, especially the spleen and lymph nodes. Cells from the thymus become T lymphocytes and are responsible for cellular immunity. Cells from the other tissues become B lymphocytes; they can become plasma cells which produce immunoglobulins (antibodies). Immune mechanisms are further discussed in Chapter 16.

Platelets

Platelets are tiny fragments broken off from very large cells in the bone marrow called megakaryocytes. Platelets have no nucleus but contain, among other things, actin and myosin, phospholipids, and granules, some of which contain ADP, ATP, serotonin, and some clotting factors. They are involved in virtually every aspect of hemostasis, especially clot formation, largely by releasing the contents of their granules.

Hemostasis

The need for a quick and effective means to prevent loss of blood from the vascular system is obvious, but it is equally important to guard against inappropriate clot formation. To accomplish this dual role, the clotting factors are normally present in the plasma, but in inactive form. The formation of a clot, however, is only the final step in hemostasis. For a complete discussion of hemostasis, see Chapter 21.

Blood Groups and Blood Typing

A number of antigens are linked to protein molecules in the plasma membrane of red blood cells; well over 100 distinct antigens have been identified. Antibodies to some of them are naturally occurring, and other antibodies are formed following exposure to another person's red blood cells. Antigens are present in the gamma globulin (immunoglobulin) fraction of the plasma proteins.

The antibodies have two binding sites, and apparently act by forming a bridge between red blood cells, causing clumping or agglutination of the cells. The antigens on the red blood cells are therefore called agglutinogens, and the antibodies are known as agglutinins. There are numerous possibilities for forming such antigen–antibody complexes, but only two are common enough to be clinically significant: the ABO system and the Rh system.

The ABO System

Blood is grouped or typed according to the presence of absence of A and B antigens on the red cell membrane. An individual's red cells may have one, both, or neither, and the blood type is designated as A, B, AB, or O, accordingly. Two forms of A agglutinogens have been identified, A_1 and A_2, but their reactions are similar. The agglutinogens are determined genetically, with their presence being dominant, that is, an individual who inherits an O gene from one parent and an A from the other has type A blood (OA).

Agglutinins (antibodies) against A and B agglutinogens are naturally occurring. Within the first few months of life agglutinins are developed against the agglutinogens *not* present on the red cells (Table 48–2). Agglutination following blood transfusion is due to the effect of the recipient's plasma on the donor's erythrocytes. The transfused plasma is usually diluted enough by the recipient's plasma that its agglutinins do not affect the recipient's cells.

Since type O blood contains no agglutinogens, its cells would not be agglutinated by any plasma. Those with Type O blood are said to be "universal donors" because their blood can be given to anyone. Type AB blood contains no aggluti-

TABLE 48–2
The ABO Blood System

Blood Type	*Agglutinogen (On Cells)*	*Agglutinin (In Plasma)*	*Plasma Agglutinates Cells of Blood Type*	*Occurrence in USA (%)*
O	none	anti-A, anti-B	A, B, AB	45
A	A	anti-B	B, AB	41
B	B	anti-A	A, AB	10
AB	AB	none	none	4

nins, so cannot agglutinate any type cells; those with Type AB blood are sometimes known as "universal recipients."

Rh Antigens

The Rh antigens, named for the rhesus monkeys in which they were first studied, have many subgroups but are generally described simply as presence or absence of the antigen: Rh-positive or Rh-negative. About 85% of whites, 95% of blacks, and 99% of Orientals have the antigen and are Rh-positive. Antibodies against the Rh antigen are not naturally occurring. They are produced in Rh-negative blood upon exposure to agglutinogens of Rh-positive cells, and a reaction (agglutination) occurs upon subsequent exposure to the Rh antigen. This may occur upon a second transfusion of Rh-positive blood into an Rh-negative individual. It may also occur during pregnancy when an Rh-negative mother has an Rh-positive fetus. If any Rh-negative red cells should cross the placenta during pregnancy or, as is more likely, if there is any mixing of blood during delivery, antibodies will be formed in the mother's blood. In a subsequent pregnancy, if the fetus is Rh-positive, the Rh agglutinogens may enter the fetal circulation and cause a reaction, hemolytic disease of the newborn or erythroblastosis fetalis. This condition can also be caused by other antigen–antibody reactions, but occurs rarely.

Cross-Matching

A quick test of compatibility can be obtained by adding a few donor red blood cells to recipient plasma on a slide. Agglutination is a sign of incompatibility of the two bloods. Such a test provides a check against possible error, as well as for the possibility of incompatibility of some of the other less common antigen–antibody systems. Further assurance would come from a second test of adding recipient cells to donor plasma.

Blood in Acid–Base Regulation

The blood contributes to the maintenance of acid–base balance because of the presence of buffers which make it possible for acidic or alkaline substances to be transported with but minimal changes in the blood pH. For a complete discussion of acid–base balance, see Chapter 14.

Bibliography

Ganong WF: Review of Medical Physiology, 11th ed, Chap 27, pp 414–433. Los Altos, California, Lange Medical Publications, 1983

Landau BR: Essential Human Anatomy and Physiology, 2nd ed, Chap 14, pp 385–408. Glenview, Illinois, Scott, Foresman and Company, 1980

Ross G: Essentials of Human Physiology, 2nd ed, Chap 5, pp 123–136. Chicago, Year Book Medical Publishers, 1982

Schmidt RF, Thews G: Human Physiology, Chap 16, pp 331–357. New York, Springer-Verlag, 1982

Vander AJ, Sherman JS, Luciano DS: Human Physiology: The Mechanisms of Body Function, 3rd ed, Chap 11, 17, pp 253–326, 521–556. New York, McGraw-Hill, 1980

Chapter 49

Assessment of Hematologic Function

Ruth A. Gregersen

History
Physical Examination
Diagnostic Studies

Assessment of hematologic function involves taking a thorough history, physical examination, and laboratory tests. The nurse must be knowledgeable about each aspect of the assessment, as subtle clues may be valuable in the diagnosis of the problem. The information gained from the assessment is vital in planning nursing care.

History

A thorough history is essential in the assessment of hematologic function. It should include the following: history of the present illness; past medical history, including ingestion of drugs and exposure to chemicals; family history; and a review of systems.

History of the Present Illness

Many hematololgic disorders are associated with vague general symptoms. For example, fatigue, malaise, lassitude, and general weakness are common symptoms associated with anemia. These symptoms may interfere with the patient's ability to perform activities of daily living. In addition to noting these vague symptoms, the nurse should look for more specific indications of hematologic disorders. Fever is a common manifestation of lymphomas or leukemias. Night sweats suggest the presence of a low-grade fever. Weight loss should be evaluated. Bruising and unusual or excessive bleeding may be signs of hemostatic deficiences. Specifics of the present illness should be evaluated in association with other relevant findings from the history and physical examination.

Medical and Drug History

Previous hematologic problems may be a clue to the present illness. The patient should be carefully questioned as to previous problems such as anemia, poor wound healing, excessive bleeding (for example, when associated with dental extraction), previous blood transfusions (the number and possible complications), and any recurring infections. It should be determined whether there has been a previous diagnosis of liver problems such as hepatitis or cirrhosis or if there have been past surgeries such as splenectomy, tumor removal, replacement of a prosthetic heart valve, and excision of the duodenum.

Iron, vitamin B_{12}, and folic acid are necassary for the development of red blood cells; therefore, a careful dietary history is important. Many drugs, such as those listed in Table 49–1, interfere with normal hematologic function. It is important to remember that over-the-counter drugs, as well as prescription drugs taken regularly, are often forgotten or not recognized as "drugs." Agents such as mild analgesics, birth control pills, laxatives, tranquilizers, and sedatives are often in this category. Alcohol use should be included in the drug history and dietary history, as chronic alcohol abusers frequently have vitamin deficiencies with or without damaged livers.

In addition to chemical exposure through drug use, many people are exposed to a variety of chemicals, which may be potentially harmful, through the environment, particularly in the work setting. Exposure to radiation, as a treatment modality or as the result of an accident, increases the incidence of some hematologic problems and should be investigated.

Family History

A carefully obtained family history can be of great importance in patients with hemostatic disorders. Particular attention must be given to bleeding disorders in family members. Other features to be investigated in a family history are jaundice, anemia, malignancies, and congenital red blood cell dyscrasias such as sickle cell disease.

Review of Systems

In hematologic disorders almost every system can be involved. Therefore, careful questioning regarding each system must be included in the history. A long list of common hematologic findings associated with each system and sug-

TABLE 49–1
Partial List of Drugs that May Affect Hematologic Function

Drug	*Clinical Use*	*Hematologic Effect*
Alcohol		Decreases platelet production
Amphotericin B	Antifungal agent	Anemia
Acetylsalicylic acid	Analgesic, antipyretic, anti-inflammatory agent	Inhibits platelet aggregation Prolongs bleeding time
Amitriptyline	Antidepressant	Agranulocytosis, leukopenia, thrombocytopenia
Azathioprine	Immunosupressant	Anemia, leukopenia
Carbamazepine	Pain of trigeminal neuralgia	Anemia, leukopenia, thrombocytopenia
Chloramphenicol	Antibiotic	Anemia, neutropenia, thrombocytopenia
Chlorothiazide	Diuretic	Decreases platelet production, provokes formation of platelet antibodies
Colchicine	Reduce inflammation of gout	Inhibits platelet function
Corticosteroids	Anti-inflammatory agents	Lymphopenia, neutrophilia, inhibits platelet function
Diphenylhydantoin	Anticonvulsant	Provokes formation of platelet antibodies, anemia, bone marrow depression
Dipyridamole	Vasodilator	Inhibits platelet function, leukocytosis
Epinephrine	Sympathomimetic	Leukocytosis
Estrogens	Birth control Menopausal symptoms Uterine bleeding Prostatic cancer	Suppress platelet production; increase factors V, VII, VIII, and X[12]; increase the frequency of thromboses[11]

(Continued)

TABLE 49–1
Partial List of Drugs that May Affect Hematologic Function (*Continued*)

Drug	*Clinical Use*	*Hematologic Effect*
Furosemide	Diuretic	Inhibits platelet function
Gentamycin	Antibiotic	Inhibits platelet function
Hydralazine	Antihypertensive	Inhibits platelet function
Indomethacin	Anti-inflammatory	Inhibits platelet function, leukopenia, anemia
Lithium	Antipsychotic	Leukocytosis, inhibits platelet function
Methyldopa	Antihypertensive	Hemolytic anemia, provokes formation of platelet antibodies
Phenothiazines	Antipsychotic	Leukopenia, leukocytosis, anemia, thrombocytopenia
Phenylbutazone	Anti-inflammatory	Anemia, leukopenia, neuropenia, thrombocytopenia
Propranolol	Beta-blocker	Inhibits platelet function, agranulocytosis
Quinidine	Antiarrhythmic	Anemia, thrombocytopenia, leukopenia, agranulocytosis
Quinine	Antimalarial	Anemia, thrombocytopenia, agranulocytosis[5]
Trimethoprim-sulfamethoxazole	Antibacterial	Anemia, leukopenia, neutropenia, thrombocytopenia

(Adapted from Jennings BM: Nursing assessment: Hematologic system. In Louis SM, Collier IC [eds]: Medical Surgical Nursing: Assessment and Management of Clinical Problems. New York, McGraw-Hill, 1983; and Wintrobe MM, Lee GR, Boggs DR et al: Clinical Hematology, 8th ed. Philadelphia, Lea & Febiger, 1981)

gested possible causes for each finding are presented in Table 49–2. A review of this table will indicate the wide range of symptomatology related to hematologic disorders.

Physical Examination

The physical examination should be performed on every patient, paying sufficient attention to *all* systems to obtain a full evaluation of the person's general health. Certain areas, however, are especially pertinent to hematologic disorders and therefore will be given particular attention in this chapter. They include the skin, eyes, mouth, lymph nodes, spleen, liver, and nervous system.[10]

Skin. The color and texture of the skin may indicate the presence of hematologic dysfunction. Dry, coarse skin, jaundice, pallor, cyanosis, itching, petechiae, purpura, and ecchymosis are all possible indications of hematologic disorders. The specific disorder for each of these signs is listed in Table 49–2. The patient should be examined in daylight rather than incandescent light, as the yellow color of this kind of light masks the yellow color of the patient. The skin must also be examined for petechiae, ecchymoses, and other signs of hemostatic disorders.

Eyes. Jaundice and pallor may be detected from examination of the eyes. A yellowish tinge to the sclera indicates an accumulation of bile pigment from excessive hemolysis. Conjunctival pallor indicates reduced quantity of hemoglobin. The physician or a skilled nurse must perform an ophthalmoscopic examination of the eyes, as retinal hemorrhages and exudates occur in patients with severe anemia and thrombocytopenia.

Mouth. The mucosa of the mouth may reveal ulcerations that are common in neutropenic clients. Swelling, redness, and bleeding of the gums may occur with leukemia. Hemorrhagic disease may cause bleeding from the mucosa. The tongue may be totally smooth in patients with pernicious

(*Text continues on page 676*)

TABLE 49–2
Assessment of Hematologic Function: Review of Systems

System	*Finding*	*Possible Etiology*
Nervous system	Headache	Anemia or polycythemia; invasion or compression of brain by leukemia, lymphoma or infection; hemorrhage into brain due to thrombocytopenia or other bleeding disorders
	Parasthesias	Peripheral neuropathy in pernicious anemia or secondary to hematologic maligiancy, therapy with vincristine
	Confusion	Malignant or infectious process involving the brain or severe anemia
	Impairment of consciousness	Increased intracranial pressure secondary to hemorrhage or tumor, severe anemia, or polycythemia
Eyes	Visual disturbances	Anemia or polycythemia
	Blindness	Retinal hemorrhages due to anemia or thrombocytopenia
	Jaundiced sclera	Accumulation of bile pigment because of excessive hemolysis
	Conjunctival pallor	Reduced quantity of hemoglobin
Ears	Vertigo, tinnitus, "roaring"	Marked anemia
Nose	Epistaxis (nose bleed)	Any bleeding disorder
	Anosmia (olfactory hallucinations)	Pernicious anemia
Mouth	Smooth, sore tongue	Pernicious anemia, iron or vitamin deficiencies
	Bleeding gums or oral mucosa	Any bleeding disorder, thrombocytopenia
	Ulceration of tongue or oral mucosa	Leukemia, neutropenia
	Pallor	Reduced quantity of hemoglobin
Neck, chest, and heart	Painless swelling	Lymphoma (may be painful with secondary infection)
	Dyspnea	Anemia (usually with effort)
	Tachycardia with or without palpitations	Anemia (compensatory mechanism to increase cardiac output)
	Angina pectoris	Anemia (due to decreased oxygen supply to the heart, can depend on rapidity with which anemia develops)
	Tenderness of the sternum	Leukemia, multiple myeloma
	Murmurs (usually systolic)	Anemia (due to increased quantity and speed of blood through valves)

(*Continued*)

TABLE 49–2
Assessment of Hematologic Function: Review of Systems (*Continued*)

System	*Finding*	*Possible Etiology*
Gastrointestinal system	Dysphagia	Mucous membrane atrophy associated with chronic iron-deficiency anemia
	Anorexia	No specific significance
	Abdominal pain	Intestinal obstruction by lymphoma, retroperitoneal bleeding, acute hemolysis, allergic purpura, sickle cell disease
	Diarrhea	Malabsorption secondary to small-bowel lymphoma, pernicious anemia (infrequent)
	Gastrointestinal bleeding (hematemesis or melena)	Thrombocytopenia or other bleeding disorder
Genitourinary system	Hematuria	Any bleeding disorder
	Red urine	Intravascular hemolysis. Ingestion of beets in iron-deficient patients
	Impotence or bladder dysfunction	Spinal cord or peripheral nerve damage due to hematologic malignancies or pernicious anemia
	Amenorrhea	No specific significance, may accompany any serious disease
	Menorrhagia	Iron deficiency or any bleeding disorder
Back and extremities	Back pain	Hemolytic reactions
	Arthritis or arthralgia (joint pain)	Acute leukemia, sickle cell disease, gout secondary to increased uric acid production due to hematologic malignancies or hemolytic anemia; hemarthroses in patients with bleeding disorders
	Bone pain	Hematologic malignancies, congenital hemolytic anemias (sickle cell)
	Edema of lower extremities	Obstruction to veins or lymphatics by enlarged lymph nodes
	Leg ulcers	Sickle cell anemia
Skin	Dry, coarse texture	Iron deficiency anemia
	Jaundice	Pernicious or hemolytic anemias, liver involvement
	Pallor	Reduced quantity of hemoglobin
	Cyanosis	Methemoglobinemia, polycythemia
	Itching	Hodgkin's disease, lymphomas
	Petechiae, purpura	Blood vessel or platelet abnormalities
	Ecchymosis	Coagulation defects

(Adapted from Williams WJ: Clinical evaluation of the patient. In Williams WJ, Beutler E, Ersley AJ, Lichtman MA [eds]: Hematology, 3rd ed. New York, McGraw-Hill, 1983)

anemia and iron-deficiency anemia, or it may be ulcerated in patients with leukemia or neutropenia.

Lymph Nodes. Lymph nodes are widely distributed in the body and any node or group of nodes can be involved. The detection of enlarged or tender nodes in the cervical, axillary, epitrochlear, inguinal, or femoral regions may indicate hematologic disease. Enlarged lymph nodes are usually detected in superficial parts of the body by palpation, although they are sometimes large enough to be seen.[10] Palpation should be gentle and is best performed with a circular motion of the fingertips, watching the patient's face for signs of discomfort.

Spleen and Liver. The spleen and liver should be gently palpated and percussed to detect enlargement. The liver may be enlarged in leukemia. Lymphomas, mononucleosis, and leukemia may cause enlargement of the spleen.

Nervous System. A thorough examination of neurologic function is necessary in many patients with hematologic disease. Vitamin B_{12} deficiency can impair cerebral, olfactory, spinal cord, and peripheral nerve function. Tumor growth in the brain or spinal-cord compression may be due to a malignant lymphoma. A variety of neurologic abnormalities may develop in patients with various leukemias and lymphomas.

Diagnostic Studies

The role of the nurse in diagnostic studies can vary depending on the setting. The nurse, whenever possible, should explain thoroughly any diagnostic procedure in simple, clear language. Written instructions facilitate compliance when the procedure requires preparatory protocols.

Hematologic dysfunctions frequently require repeated acquisition of blood specimens. Although one reseach study has shown loss of blood volume to be minor in most cases,[4] the nurse should keep a record of blood loss due to specimen collection in severely compromised patients. Combining blood draws and using a indwelling intravascular catheter whenever possible can reduce volume loss and discomfort to the patient. This is especially important when withdrawing blood for coagulation studies in patients with bleeding tendencies.[2]

Laboratory Blood Studies

Composition of Blood. The average person has 5 liters of blood divided into 3 liters of plasma and 2 liters of blood cells. The cells, produced in the bone marrow, are the focus of laboratory study in hematologic dysfunction. The blood cells are classified as follows:[1]

1. Erythrocytes (red blood cells)
2. Leukocytes (white blood cells)
   a. Granulocytes (granular leukocytes)
      1) Neutrophils
      2) Eosinophils
      3) Basophils
   b. Agranulocytes (agranular leukocytes)
      1) Lymphocytes
      2) Monocytes
3. Thrombocytes (platelets)

Blood Cell Disorders. Red blood cell (RBC) disorders are of two types—anemias and polycythemias. Anemias are severe reductions in circulating red cells; polycythemias are abnormal increases in red cells.

White blood cell (WBC) disorders are termed leukocytosis (increased number of cells) or leukopenia (a decreased number of cells). There are many types of white blood cells, each with a different function. Variations in the counts of the different types of cells may be indicative of a wide range of problems, including infection, leukemia, agranulocytosis, or granulocytopenia.[1]

The most common platelet disorder is thrombocytopenia (decreased platelets). However, thrombocytosis (increased platelets) may also occur

Blood Collection Procedures. Capillary blood is preferred for a peripheral blood smear and may also be used for other tests when large quantities of blood are not needed. Capillary blood withdrawal is done by a skin puncture in the tip of a finger or earlobe in an adult. In young infants, the great toe or heel is used, while in infants over 1 year old, the tip of the finger is used.

Venipuncture is necessary for most tests that require large quantities of blood or require the blood to be anticoagulated (unclotted). Hematomas can be prevented by using a quick needle stick, releasing the tourniquet before the needle is withdrawn, and applying sufficient pressure over the puncture site after the needle is withdrawn. Drawing blood for any laboratory test from the same extremity that is being used for intravenous medication or fluid should be avoided.[7]

Bone Marrow Aspiration. Bone marrow aspiration is performed by the physician, but the nurse usually assists with the procedure. After a local anesthetic is injected, a short, rigid, sharp needle with a stylet is introduced through the periosteum into the marrow cavity of the posterior iliac crest (preferred site in all patients over 12–18 months of age), anterior iliac crest, sternum, spinous vertebral process, ribs, or tibia (children). The stylet is removed and 0.2 to 0.5 ml of marrow fluid is aspirated. After removal of the needle, pressure is applied over the puncture site until bleeding, if any, ceases and a small sterile dressing is applied.

Patient preparation is extremely important. The nurse must explain the procedure as well as the purpose of the test. The patient must be reassured that it is normal to be anxious about this procedure especially if the person has had it done before. Moderate-to-severe discomfort lasting only a few seconds may be felt when the aspiration is done, especially if the iliac crest is used.[1] The patient should be positioned on his back or side according to the site selected. If the iliac crest site is used, the patient may be prepared for pain by being told to hold a pillow and bite into it if pain is experienced.[1] Bed rest for 30 minutes after the procedure is recommended. A slight soreness over the puncture site for 3 to 4 days is normal.

The nurse should watch for bleeding at the puncture site, signs of shock, and continued pain, which may indicate fracture (especially if the sternal site is used). Analgesics or sedatives may be necessary for some patients before and after the procedure.

Blood Tests. The complete blood count (CBC) is a basic screening test in hematologic function. The CBC includes: WBC and differential, RBC, hematocrit (Hct), hemoglobin (Hgb), the peripheral smear, and the platelet count. Table 49–3 lists each test and presents the normal

TABLE 49–3
Complete Blood Count Tests

Test	*Normal Ranges*		*Comments*
White blood cell count (WBC)	5,000–10,000 mm^3		Leukocytosis is usually due to an increase of only one type of white cell (see differential below) and frequently occurs in acute infections. Marked leukopenia is extremely dangerous as it leaves the body unprotected against invading agents.
Differential white blood cell count (Diff)	*Absolute Values (no./mm^3)*	*Relative Values (% of total WBCs)*	*Cells function to combat:*
Neutrophils	3000–7000	60–70%	Bacterial infections, inflammatory disorders
Eosinophils	50–400	1–4%	Allergic disorders, parasitic infections
Basophils	25–100	0.5–1%	Blood dyscrasias, myeloproliferative diseases
Lymphocytes	1000–4000	20–40%	Viral infections, bacterial infection
Monocytes	100–600	2–6%	Chronic infections
Red blood cell count (RBC)	Men: 4.2–5.4 × 10^6/liter Women: 3.6–5.0 × 10^6/liter		The main value of the RBC count lies in the gross evaluation of the indices (see below) as it aids in differentiating anemias.
Hematocrit (Hct)	Men: 40–54% Women: 37–47%		The volume of RBCs in 100 ml of blood $\left(i.e., \frac{\text{Volume of RBCs}}{\text{Total Blood Volume}}\right)$
Hemoglobin (Hgb)	Men: 14–16.5 g/dl Women: 12.0–15.0 g/dl		Oxygen-carrying pigment of the RBCs
Red blood cell indices (peripheral smear)			
Mean corpuscular volume (MCV)	87–103 μm^3		Indicates size of the RBC; decreased values in iron-deficiency and pernicious anemia; increased values in liver disease, alcoholism, deficiency of folate or vitamin B_{12}
Mean corpuscular hemoglobin concentration (MCHC)	32–36%		Measures the average concentration of Hgb in the RBCs
Mean corpuscular hemoglobin (MCH)	27–32 picograms (pg)		Measure of the average weight of Hgb in RBC
Platelet count	150,000–350,000/mm^3		Decreased levels predispose patient to bleeding, increased levels predispose patient to thrombosis.

(Adapted from Fischbach FT: A Manual of Laboratory Diagnostic Tests, 2nd ed. Philadelphia, JB Lippincott, 1984; and Tilkian SM, Conover MB, Tilkian AG: Clinical Implications of Laboratory Tests, 3rd ed. St. Louis, CV Mosby, 1983)

TABLE 49–4
Tests of Hemostasis and Blood Coagulation

Test	*Normal Range*	*Rationale*	*Common Causes of Abnormalities*
Bleeding time			
Duke method (earlobe)	1–6 min	Detects vascular and platelet abnormalities	Thrombocytopenia, von Willebrand's disease; platelet dysfunction; vascular defects; prolonged in disseminated intravascular coagulation (DIC)
Ivy method (forearm)	1–9 min		
Coagulation time			
Whole blood clotting time	5–10 min	Assists in monitoring and regulating heparin therapy (partial thromboplastin time is more sensitive and more widely used, see below).	Severe deficiencies of coagulation factors in the intrinsic and common pathways; presence of circulating heparin
Lee-White clotting time	5–10 min		
Recalcification time	90–120 sec		
Fibrinogen	160–415 mg/dl	Detects fibrinogen levels. Increased fibronogen indicates hypercoagulability; decreased fibrinogen suggests a bleeding tendency.[6]	Inhibitors of thrombin or of fibrin polymerization; decreased in DIC
Fibrin split products (FSPs) or fibrin degradation products (FDPs)	Negative	Determines the degree of consumptive coagulopathy	DIC; fibrinogenolysis; liver disease; thromboembolic disorders
Partial thromboplastin time (PTT)	30–45 sec	Assists in monitoring and regulating heparin therapy; screening test for coagulation abnormalities; assesses intrinsic coagulation system	Hemophilia, vitamin K deficiency; liver disease; prolonged in DIC; in the presence of heparin
Activated partial thromboplastin time (aPTT)	16–25 sec	Same as PTT	Same as PTT
Platelet count	150,000–350,000/mm³	Detects abnormal levels of platelets	Thrombocytopenia (idiopathic thrombocytopenia purpura, anemias, infection, toxic drugs). Thrombocytosis (cancer, leukemia, trauma, acute infections); decreased in DIC
Prothrombin time (PT)	11–16 sec	Screens for coagulation abnormalities; assesses extrinsic coagulation system; used to monitor and regulate oral anticoagulant therapy	Prothrombin deficiency, vitamin K deficiency; liver disease; prolonged in DIC; presence of coumarin derivatives
Thrombin time	13–17 sec (normals vary widely)	Reflects adequacy of thrombin; detects fibrinogen abnormalities; useful to screen for heparin contamination of blood specimens[11]	Inhibitors of thrombin or fibrin polymerization; prolonged in DIC

(Adapted from Wintrobe MM, Lee GR, Boggs DR, Bithell TC, Forster J, Athens JW, Lukens JN: Clinical Hematology, 8th ed. Philadelphia, Lea & Febiger, 1981)

TABLE 49-5
Other Blood Tests that Assess Hematologic Function

Test	*Normal Range*	*Comments*
Erythrocyte sedimentation rate (ESR)	Men: 0–15 mm/hr* Women: 0–20 mm/hr*	Measures the rate at which RBCs settle out of unclotted blood in 1 hr. Most often used as a gauge for determining the progress of an inflammatory disease.
Reticulocyte count	Men: 0.5–1.5% of total RBCs Women: 0.5–2.5% of total RBCs	Used to differentiate anemias due to bone marrow failure from those due to hemorrhage or hemolysis. Reticulocytes are immature red blood cells.
Bilirubin Total Direct Indirect	 0.3–1.3 mg/dl 0.1–0.4 mg/dl 0.2–0.18 mg/dl	As a byproduct of hemolysis, the bilirubin will rise with excessive destruction of RBCs or inability of the liver to excrete normal amounts. An increase in indirect levels is associated with the former, an increase in direct with the latter.
Iron Serum iron Total iron-binding capacity (TIBC)	 42–135 mg/dl 250–450 mg/dl	Serum iron refers to bound iron. TIBC refers to the saturation of transferrin, a protein which binds iron; TIBC is decreased when the body has excess iron and increased when a deficiency exists.
Coombs' test Direct Indirect	 negative negative	Used to differentiate between types of hemolytic anemias. Direct done on RBCs. Indirect done on serum.

* Values vary according to the method used.
(Adapted from Fischbach FT: A Manual of Laboratory Diagnostic Tests, 2nd ed. Philadelphia, JB Lippincott, 1984)

values. The coagulation (blood clotting) profile is essential in determining the client's hemostatic function. The most common coagulation tests are: bleeding time, coagulation time, fibrinogen, fibrin split products, partial thromboplastin time (PTT), platelet count, prothrombin time (PT), and thrombin time. Table 49–4 presents these coagulation studies, normal values, rationales, and the common causes of abnormalities.

Other blood tests which may be important in the assessment of hematologic function include sedimentation rate, reticulocyte count, bilirubin, iron, and Coombs' test (Table 49–5). Many clients with hematologic dysfunction require blood transfusions. Prior to blood administration, a blood type and cross-match must be performed.

Other Diagnostic Studies

Radioisotope and radiologic studies and biopsies may be performed to further evaluate hematologic function. Radioisotope studies include spleen scans and bone scans to evaluate the structure of the spleen or bone. These tests are done in the nuclear medicine department and should be fully explained to the patient. An example of a radiologic study is lymphangiography which involves the infusion of radiopaque dye into the lymph vessels in the dorsum of both feet. X-ray films are taken immediately and on the following day. The nursing interventions include explaining the procedure to the patient, watching for iodine sensitivity, and instructing the patient that his or her urine will be blue for 1 or 2 days as the dye is excreted. There may also be periods of transient fever, general malaise, and diffuse muscle aches for the first 12 to 24 hours. See Table 49–6 for an overview of these and other tests.

Summary

Hematologic disorders occur for a variety of reasons. Patients who are hospitalized may develop hematologic problems related to medical therapy. It is essential that the nurse be aware of patients who are at high risk and assess for the development of problems.

TABLE 49–6
Diagnostic Studies of Hematologic Function

Study	Description and Purpose	Nursing Responsibility
Radioisotope Studies		
Spleen scan	Evaluates the structure of the spleen. Radioactive isotope is injected IV.	Explain procedure to patient. Test is done in the nuclear medicine department. Patient does not require radioactive precautions.
Bone scan	Evaluates the structure of the bone. Radioactive isotope is injected IV.	Same as for spleen scan.
Radiologic Studies		
Lymphangiography	Evaluates deep lymph nodes. Radiopaque dye is infused into lymph vessels in the dorsum of both feet. X-ray films are done immediately and on the following day.	Explain procedure to patient. Watch for iodine sensitivity. Instruct patient that urine will be blue from dye excretion for 1–2 days. Transient fever, general malaise, and diffuse muscle aches are common for 12–24 hr.
Biopsies		
Bone marrow	Diagnoses multiple myeloma, leukemia, and some lymphomas. Also used to evaluate efficacy of leukemic therapy.	See text.
Lymph node	Done to obtain lymph tissue for histologic examination to determine diagnosis and therapy.	Explain procedure to patient. Change dressing daily and inspect wound for healing. Watch for bleeding.
Open	Done in surgery with direct visualization of area.	
Closed (needle)	Done at bedside.	

References

1. Fischbach FT: A Manual of Laboratory Diagnostic Tests, 2nd ed. Philadelphlia, JB Lippincott, 1984
2. Gregersen RA, Underhill SL, Detter JC, Schmere G: Withdrawal of blood specimens from heparinized radial artery catheters for coagulation studies. (abstract) Circulation 68(III): 223, 1983
3. Jennings BM: Nursing assessment: Hematologic system. In Louis SM, Collier IC (eds): Medical Surgical Nursing: Assessment and Management of Clinical Problems. New York, McGraw-Hill, 1983
4. Lanuza DM, Jennrick JA: The amount of blood withdrawn for diagnostic test in critically ill patients. Heart and Lung 5:933, 1976
5. Malseed RT: Pharmacology: Drug Therapy and Nursing Considerations. Philadelphia, JB Lippincott, 1982
6. Miale JB: Laboratory Medicine: Hematology, 6th ed. St Louis, CV Mosby, 1982
7. Russo LT, Coombes DL, Underhill SL, Detter JC: Reliable measurements of serum potassium and glucose from radial artery lines. (abstract) Heart and Lung 13:310, 1984
8. Tilkian SM, Conover MB, Tilkian AG: Clinical Implications of Laboratory Tests, 3rd ed. St Louis, CV Mosby, 1983
9. Thompson AR, Harker LA: Manual of Hemostasis and Thrombosis, 3rd ed. Philadelphia, FA Davis, 1983
10. Williams WJ: Clinical evaluation of the patient. In Williams WJ, Beutler E, Erslev AJ, Lichtman MA (eds): Hematology, 3rd ed. New York, McGraw-Hill, 1983
11. Williams WJ: Disorders of hemostasis-thrombosis. In Williams WJ, Beutler E, Erslev AJ, Lichtman MA (eds): Hematology, 3rd ed. New York, McGraw-Hill, 1983
12. Wintrobe MM, Lee GR, Boggs DR, Bithell TC, Forster J, Athens JW, Lukens JN: Clinical Hematology, 8th ed. Philadelphia, Lea & Febiger, 1981

Chapter 50

Nursing Strategies for Common Hematologic Problems

Nursing Diagnosis Interventions Evaluation

Ruth A. Gregersen

Patients with hematologic problems can experience a wide variety of symptoms which have the potential to affect all areas of their lives. Bleeding, infection, weakness, and fatigue, problems that commonly affect patients with hematological disorders, are discussed in this chapter.

Bleeding Related to Hematologic Dysfunction

Actual bleeding or the potential for bleeding results from disruption of the processes that accomplish hemostasis: vasoconstriction, platelet plug formation, and blood coagulation. As discussed in Chapter 54, many pathologic processes can lead to disturbed hemostatic function. See the accompanying Nursing Care Plan for the Patient with Actual Bleeding or the Potential for Bleeding.

Assessment and Nursing Diagnosis

Bleeding from hemostatic dysfunction can result in decreased tissue perfusion as evidenced by postural hypotension, tachycardia, tachypnea, decreased urine output, cool clammy skin, and altered levels of consciousness.

The major nursing goals are early detection, treatment, and prevention of bleeding.

To detect for early signs of bleeding, the nurse should check the skin for petechiae, purpura, and ecchymosis, and observe for epistaxis, bleeding from the gums, blood in the stools, and any bleeding from wounds or puncture sites. All body excreta such as emesis, nasogastric drainage, feces, urine, and wound drainage should be checked for signs of occult blood. Other possible means of measuring blood loss include weighing blood-soaked linen and dressings. Signs of internal bleeding may be evident in complaints of flank pain, swelling of the joints, and decreased level of consciousness. Continual monitoring of vital signs is also important. Any signs of chest pain, decreased urine output, cool clammy skin and pallor should be reported immediately.

Interventions

To prevent bleeding episodes, protect the patient from injury, provide gentle oral care, use padded side rails and assist the patient from a lying to a sitting position. Nursing measures which may precipitate bleeding should be modified if possible to avoid unnecessary bleeding. For example, use alternate arms when taking blood pressure readings, avoid unnecessary IM or subcutaneous injections or use a

(*Text continues on page 684*)

NURSING CARE PLAN FOR THE PATIENT WITH POTENTIAL FOR BLEEDING RELATED TO HEMATOLOGIC DYSFUNCTION

NURSING DIAGNOSIS/PROBLEM: Potential for decreased tissue perfusion related to bleeding.
GOAL 1.1: To detect early the signs and symptoms of bleeding.

Nursing Interventions	Rationale	Outcome Criteria
1. Observe for bleeding from the following areas: skin, mucous membranes, wound and puncture sites.	1, 2, 4. The signs of bleeding vary according to the site and cause.	1–5. Any abnormal or excessive bleeding will be detected, documented, and reported to the physician.
2. Test all body excreta (emesis, nasogastric drainage, sputum, feces, urine, wound drainage) for occult blood.		
3. Measure and record blood loss by any route: (*e.g.,* blood-soaked linen and dressings; sanitary napkins).	3. One liter of fluid weighs about 1 kg.	
4. Observe for signs of internal bleeding: abdominal/flank pain; swelling of joints; decreased level of consciousness; headache.		
5. Monitor and record the following vital signs every hour and prn during bleeding episodes every two to four hours thereafter: a. Postural BP and pulse b. Respirations c. CVP (if available) or neck veins d. Pulmonary artery pressure (PAP) and pulmonary wedge pressure (PWP) (if available).	5. a. Inability to maintain postural adjustments in BP and pulse will occur in volume depletion before overt shock is present.[9] Saline depletion (includes blood) should be suspected when, in response to sitting or standing, the heart rate increases and either the diastolic BP drops by 10 mm Hg or the systolic pressure decreases by 15 mm Hg.[14]	
6. Assess for signs of decreased tissue perfusion as evidenced by: a. ↓ level of consciousness—restlessness, agitation, apprehension b. Chest pain c. Decreased urine output d. Cool, clammy skin e. Pale skin and mucous membranes.	6. Increasing restlessness, agitation, and anxiety frequently accomany early shock and reflect mild hypoxia.[7] Within seconds after bleeding begins the fall in arterial pressure will activate baroreceptors causing compensatory changes. General constriction of vessels of the skin (producing marked pallor), splanchnic area, skeletal muscles, and kidney (leading to decreased urine output).[11]	6. Signs and symptoms of decreased tissue perfusion will be detected, documented, and reported as they occur.
7. Monitor the following laboratory tests: a. Hemoglobin (Hbg) and hematocrit (Hct) b. Coagulation studies c. Platelets.	7. Abnormal laboratory values may indicate bleeding.	7. Abnormal laboratory tests will be detected and reported.

(Continued)

NURSING CARE PLAN FOR THE PATIENT WITH POTENTIAL FOR BLEEDING RELATED TO HEMATOLOGIC DYSFUNCTION (*Continued*)

GOAL 1.2: To minimize blood loss and to replace blood volume as necessary.

Nursing Interventions	Rationale	Outcome Criteria
1. Control active bleeding by a. Applying direct pressure for 5–10 minutes b. Applying ice or cold compresses over the site of bleeding c. Resting the affected part and elevating above the level of the heart if possible d. Lavaging stomach with iced saline to control bleeding from GI tract.	1. Direct pressure will stop bleeding and allow a clot to form if appropriate coagulation factors are present. Cold causes vasoconstriction which will assist in the control of bleeding.[11]	1–2. Intravascular volume will be maintained as evidenced by maintenance of vital signs. Tissue perfusion will be maintained as evidenced by lack of signs and symptoms of hypoperfusion. Overt bleeding will cease or lessen.
2. Administer blood and blood products as ordered.		

GOAL 1.3: To prevent bleeding episodes.

Nursing Interventions	Rationale	Outcome Criteria
1. Protect patient from injury by the following: a. Be gentle in turning patient, changing dressings, and providing oral care. b. Pad side rails and other sharp surfaces.	1. Patients with acute hematologic disorders bleed very easily, therefore, they must be protected from trauma.	1–2. Absence of active bleeding. Vital signs are within normal limits for that patient. Laboratory test within normal limits (Hgb, Hct).
c. Remove unnecessary clutter from the bedside.	c. Prevents patient from falling or tripping.	
d. Wipe up spills immediately.	d. Avoids slipping.	
e. Assist the patient upon rising from a recumbent position (especially if postural hypotension is a problem).		
2. Modify nursing interventions which may precipitate bleeding. a. Intramuscular or subcutaneous injection should be avoided. If injection cannot be avoided, use small-gauge needle.	2. a. Any interruption of the skin integrity will cause bleeding in patients with hemostatic dysfunction.	
b. Frequent BP monitoring. (Alternate extremities used for readings.)	b. The pressure of the blood pressure cuff may cause petechiae in patients with vascular or platelet disorders.	
c. Avoid the use of nasogastric (NG) or oxygen tubes which may irritate mucous membranes.	c. The friction of tubes rubbing on mucous membranes may cause bleeding in these patients.	

(*Continued*)

NURSING CARE PLAN FOR THE PATIENT WITH POTENTIAL FOR BLEEDING RELATED TO HEMATOLOGIC DYSFUNCTION (*Continued*)

Nursing Interventions	Rationale
d. Avoiding the use of aspirin and aspirin-containing products.	d. Aspirin interferes with the function of platelets by inhibiting the release reaction (see Chapters 21 and 54); thus, aspirin may enhance bleeding.[13]

GOAL 1.4: Patient practices preventive measures to minimize bleeding.

Nursing Interventions	Rationale	Outcome Criteria
1. Teach patient the following safety precautions to prevent injury: a. Use a soft-bristle toothbrush or cotton swabs for oral care. b. Use an electric razor for shaving. c. Wear sturdy slippers or shoes when ambulating. d. Do not over-exert or strain as it may precipitate further bleeding. Avoid: ▪ Using force to blow nose ▪ Straining with bowel movements ▪ Forceful coughing	1. Prevention of injury will reduce bleeding episodes.	1–5. Patient can state measures to minimize bleeding. Absence of active bleeding.

small gauge needle and apply pressure after removing the needle. It is also important to avoid using aspirin which could precipitate bleeding.

When bleeding occurs the immediate goal is to minimize blood loss and replace blood volume as necessary. Bleeding is controlled by applying direct pressure for 5 to 10 minutes and by applying ice or cold compresses over the bleeding site. For bleeding from the GI tract, lavaging the stomach with iced saline may be ordered. Blood and blood products are administered as ordered.

Blood Transfusion Therapy

There are different types of blood replacement components that may be ordered:

Whole blood	Consists of red blood cells (RBCs), plasma, white blood cells (WBCs), and platelets
Red blood cells	Composed of RBCs, reduced plasma, WBCs, and platelets
Platelets	Composed of platelets, some WBCs, plasma, some RBCs
Plasma (fresh frozen)	Composed of plasma, all coagulant factors, no platelets
Granulocyte concentrates	Composed of granulocytes, lymphocytes, platelets, some RBCs

The timing and administration of these blood replacement components vary as do the nursing responsibilities for each. The details of these differences are outlined in Table 50–1.

Every hospital should have a procedure for the administration of blood and blood products. However, there are some general protocols to observe prior to administration.

Two responsible persons should

1. Check the order on the chart
2. Compare the blood type and unit number on the compatibility record and the unit of blood or blood product
3. Compare the patient's blood type and the unit blood type.
4. Compare the patient's name and hospital number listed on the compatibility record with the patient's arm band
5. If there are any contradictions, do not give the blood or blood products

Adverse Reactions to Blood Transfusions. Patients may have adverse reactions to blood transfusions and should be monitored closely for any such responses. The most serious response is an acute hemolytic reaction characterized by increased pulse and respirations, hypotension, chills, fever, flushing, headache, chest discomfort, dyspnea, and shock.

TABLE 50-1
Administration of Blood and Blood Components

Component	*Composition*	*Nursing Responsibilities During Administration**
Whole blood	Red blood cells (RBCs), plasma, white blood cells (WBCs), platelets	Store at 1–6° C until time of administration; record baseline vital signs (VS) prior to transfusion; administer through a filter (170 micron); filter may be used for 2–3 units but not for more than 6 hr; infuse only with normal saline (NS); infuse first 50 ml slowly and observe patient for signs of a reaction; if no reaction, one unit may be infused (in patients without circulatory failure) in 1–1½ hr; maximum infusion time is 6 hr. Record VS at end of transfusion and during the transfusion if there is concern about a reaction.
Red blood cells	RBCs, reduced plasma, WBCs, and platelets	Nursing responsibilities are the same as administration of whole blood. In addition: squeeze bag to mix cells every 20–30 min during administration, may add 50–100 ml of NS if necessary to assist infusion.
Platelets	Platelets, some WBCs, plasma, some RBCs	Do not refrigerate, record baseline VS, administer through a 170-micron filter that has not been used for other blood products. Administer only with NS; administer rapidly (20–30 min for 6 units); do not use pressure cuffs to speed administration.
Plasma (fresh frozen)	Plasma, all coagulation factors, no platelets	Use within 60 min of thawing; record baseline VS; administer through a filter; administer as rapidly as the patient tolerates (250 ml over 30–45 min in patients without circulatory failure).
Granulocyte concentrate	Granulocytes, lymphocytes, platelets, some RBCs	Must be infused within 24 hr of collection; record baseline VS; administer through a 170-micron filter; infuse only with NS; may be administered 1–2 hr (usually 200–600 ml).
Cryoprecipitate	Fibrinogen; Factors VIII and XIII, von Willebrand's factor	Do not refrigerate; must be administered within 6 hr of thawing; record baseline VS; administer through a filter (any filter can be used); infuse only with normal saline; administer rapidly (10–12 units in 20–30 min).

* Prior to administration, two responsible persons should: (1) check the order in the chart, (2) compare the blood type and unit number on the compatibility record and the unit of blood or blood product; (3) compare the patient's blood type and the unit blood type; (4) compare the patient's name and hospital number listed on the compatibility record with the patient's arm band; (5) if there are any contradictions, do not give the blood or blood product. (Platelets and plasma are ABO specific but are not cross-matched; cryoprecipitate need not be made from the same type of blood as the patient's.)

When such signs occur, the transfusion should be stopped immediately, the physician notified, along with the blood bank, and the patient monitored for vital signs, urine output and ECG irregularities. To prevent or treat renal failure, diuretics should be administered to maintain urine flow. Blood and urine specimens should be collected, and the blood unit, tubing, and filter should be sent to the lab.

Other possible reactions may be classified as febrile, allergic (mild), anaphylactic, and hypervolemic. Table 50–2 reviews the potential adverse effects of blood transfusions and lists steps which should be followed to prevent or minimize their occurrence. It also proposes a management plan which may be followed if these adverse effects occur.

Infection Related to Hematologic Dysfunction

All hospitalized patients have the potential to develop infections; however, the potential is increased in patients with hematologic disorders. Diseases or drugs that alter white blood cells (WBCs) decrease the patient's normal defenses and ability to fight infection.

Nursing Diagnosis

The major nursing diagnosis/problem is infection related to abnormal increased production of immature white blood cells (WBCs) or reduced WBC counts. The abnormal WBC count may be secondary to the disease process itself or medical treatment such as chemotherapy and radiotherapy. Signs and symptoms of infection in these patients are: excessively high or low WBC counts, fever, chills, recurrent upper respiratory tract infections, cuts and abrasions that do not heal, dysphagia, and lesions in the mouth, throat, groin, perirectal and vaginal areas. Exudates, heat, and swelling of local infection may not be present if the patient is neutropenic.[4]

Interventions

When the body's normal ability to fight infection is compromised, one of the major nursing goals is to prevent infec-

(*Text continues on page 688*)

TABLE 50–2
Reactions to Blood Transfusions*

Reaction	*Clinical Manifestations*	*Prevention*	*Management*
Acute Hemolytic Reaction (most severe)			
1. Interaction of recipient antibodies with donor red blood cell (RBC) antigen 2. Severity of reaction is dose related. 3. Hemolysis may occur if red blood cells (RBC) strike filter, are overheated, or mixed with solutions other than normal saline (NS). 4. Usually due to clerical errors	1. Increased pulse and respiration; hypotension 2. Chills, fever, flushing 3. Low back or thigh pain 4. Headache or feeling of fullness in the head 5. Feeling of chest constriction, pleuritic chest pain, dyspnea 6. Hemoglobinuria (red urine) 7. Abnormal bleeding 8. Shock	1. Carefully follow identification procedures when; • Type and cross blood sample is drawn • Signing units out of blood bank • At the bedside before administration with two-person check of patient and blood 2. Follow check-out procedures: • Check ABO group and Rh label with compatibility record. • Check unit label numbers with compatibilty number. • Verify compatibility record with patient's full name and hospital number. • Examine blood for brown, red, or pink plasma, clots and gas bubbles. 3. Assess patient: • Obtain baseline vital signs (VS). • Stay with patient for first 15–30 min of the transfusion. • Assess patient at least every hour during the transfusion. 4. Administration • Use a 19-gauge needle. • Only infuse with normal saline. DO NOT piggyback medications. • Change blood filter every 2–3 units. • Infuse first 50 ml slowly (15 drops/min).	1. Stop transfusion immediately. Keep vein open with normal saline. 2. Notify physician. 3. Notify blood bank. 4. Monitor vital signs, urine output, and electrocardiogram. 5. Maintain intravascular volume with crystalloids or colloids. 6. Prevent or treat renal failure with diuretics (furosemide) to maintain urine flow. 7. Send unit, tubing, and filter to lab. 8. Collect urine and blood specimens.
Delayed Hemolytic Reaction			
	1. Subtle; most signs and symptoms go unnoticed 2. Usually occurs 10–14 days posttransfusion	Same as for acute hemolytic reaction	Most cases require no treatment because RBC destruction is gradual.
Febrile (most common)			
1. Usually due to recipient antibodies directed against donor platelets, lymphocytes, and granulocytes	1. Fever with or without chills 2. Headache, flushing, tachycardia, palpitations	1. Premedicate with antipyretic. 2. Keep patient warm.	1. Stop transfusion and keep vein open with NS.

(*Continued*)

TABLE 50–2
Reactions to Blood Transfusions* (*Continued*)

Reaction	*Clinical Manifestations*	*Prevention*	*Management*
Febrile (most common)			
2. Most common in multiparous and multitransfused patients	3. Malaise, myalgia	3. Transfuse leukopoor blood to patients who have had two prior reactions. 4. Filter blood through a 20–40-micron microaggregrate filter	2. Assess patient for acute hemolytic reaction. 3. May give antipyretic. 4. Keep patient warm. 5. Monitor VS. 6. May simply decrease rate of transfusion if acute hemolytic reaction has been ruled out.
Allergic (mild)			
1. Etiology unknown but probably caused by antibodies against plasma proteins. 2. Second most common reaction 3. Symptoms dose related	1. No fever 2. Itching, hives, urticaria, erythemia, rash 3. Anxiety	1. Administer diphenhydramine (Benadryl) 15–20 min prior to transfusion to patients with allergies.	1. Stop transfusion and keep vein open with NS. 2. If no other symptoms develop, resume transfusion slowly. 3. Administer antihistamines.
Allergic (anaphylaxis)			
1. May be caused by IgG anti-IgA antibodies in patients who are IgA deficient 2. Very rare 3. Rapid onset within minutes of starting transfusions	1. Flushing, dyspnea, wheezing 2. Hypotension, shock 3. Vomiting, cramping, diarrhea 4. No fever 5. Chest tightening 6. Itching 7. Anxiety 8. Arrest/death	1. Give only IgA deficient blood to patients with anti-IgA antibodies 2. May use washed RBCs	1. Stop transfusion and keep vein open. 2. Maintain intravascular volume with crystalloids. 3. Give epinephrine. 4. May need vasopressors. 5. Monitor VS.
Hypervolemic			
1. Due to administration of excessive volume or at a rate faster than the heart can accept 2. More common in: • Children and elderly • Patients with amputation (decreased vascular space) • Chronic anemia • Patients with compromised cardiac status • Use of whole blood rather than RBCs in patients with normal blood volume	1. Dry cough, dyspnea 2. Crackles at base of lungs 3. Distended neck veins 4. Bounding pulse, increased blood pressure 5. Feeling of tightness in chest	1. Do not give whole blood unless volume is needed. 2. Give at a rate within the circulatory reserve of the patient. 3. Monitor venous pressure and lung sounds of patients prone to circulatory overload.	1. Stop or slow transfusion and keep vein open. 2. Elevate head of bed. 3. Monitor VS and venous pressure. 4. Administer diuretics, oxygen, morphine, vasodilators, and aminophylline as necessary.

*Blood transfusions carry a risk of disease transmission. Serum hepatitis, malaria, cytomegalovirus, sphillis (rare), infectious mononucleosis, toxoplasmosis, Epstein-Barr virus, acquired immune deficiency syndrome (AIDS), and other infections carried in the blood may be transmitted from the donor to the transfusion recipient. To prevent disease transmission, donors and their blood must be carefully screened. In addition, the benefits of transfusion and the risk of potential infection must be weighed.

tion by reducing exposure to pathogens in the hospital environment. The patient should be placed in a private room with an attached bathroom to protect him or her from other patients or objects that are infected. Because handwashing is considered the most important barrier to transmission of infection,[7] all hospital personnel must use meticulous handwashing technique. Visitors must also be taught to wash their hands before entering the patient's room. The number of visitors may need to be limited. It is important not to assign staff with colds or other communicable illnesses to care for the patient.

Common sources of contamination such as the sink, bathtub, and respiratory therapy equipment may need to be cultured. Flowers and plants should not be allowed in the patient's room. Fresh produce should be eliminated from the diet of patients who are severely neutropenic (500 WBCs/mm^3 or less).[4] Members of the health-care team, including the nurse, the physician, and the infection control nurse should assess the need for protective or reverse isolation. Protective isolation is intended to more fully protect the patient from the environment.[5] A laminar air-flow room is an unidirectional air-flow barrier that establishes an air environment in which the infection-prone patient is free from contact with exogenous microorganisms.[3] If a laminar air-flow room is available, the need for this high level protection should be assessed.

Infections may also be prevented by reducing the number of normal endogenous organisms. Indwelling urinary catheters, one of the major sources of infection in the hospitalized patient, should be avoided. Providing or teaching the patient good personal hygiene is extremely important. Personal hygiene includes handwashing, especially before meals and after urination or defecation, hair washing, bathing, oral care, nail care, and perineal care. In addition, respiratory hygiene techniques, such as coughing and deep breathing and turning in bed should be taught.

Any break in the skin could provide an entry for organisms.[4] Common entry routes include the respiratory and urinary tracts, the mouth, and breaks in the skin.[7] To prevent infection by maintenance of skin integrity, venipunctures and injections should be avoided when possible. The patient should be ambulated or turned every 1 to 2 hours if on bed rest to prevent decubitus formation.

Another major nursing goal is early detection of developing or existing infections. The nurse should assess for signs and symptoms of infection such as fever (above 38°C), chills, persistent cough or sore throat, and burning on urination. The nose, mouth, and perineal area should be inspected daily for open sores. In addition, the results of cultures from blood, urine, pharynx, rectum, and wounds should be monitored and reported to the physician.

Existing infections are usually treated with antibiotic therapy. It is the responsibility of the nurse to administer antibiotics on time to maintain therapeutic blood levels. Granulocyte transfusions may be given if infection fails to respond to appropriate antibiotic therapy.[1] The nurse must observe for and report any adverse reactions such as fever, chills, shortness of breath, hypotension, tachycardia, and hypoxia. Because these patients have the potential to develop sepsis, the temperature, pulse, and blood pressure should be monitored every 4 hours. Low blood pressure, tachycardia, subnormal temperature, or temperature spikes may be indicative of sepsis.

Evaluation

The specific outcome criteria used to evaluate the effectiveness of nursing interventions designed to prevent infection are a normal body temperature, absence of chills, mucous membranes free of lesions and negative cultures (blood, urine, sputum, and wounds). Thorough nursing assessment will detect any signs and symptoms of infection so that the physician can begin treatment early.

Weakness and Fatigue Related to Hematologic Dysfunction

A marked decrease in red blood cells (RBCs) commonly leads to weakness and fatigue. These complaints alter the patient's ability to perform activities of daily living, decreasing power to contend with normal life occurrences. With the added stress of hospitalization, the patient may benefit from strategies designed to maximize coping mechanisms.

Nursing Diagnosis

A decrease in hematocrit and hemoglobin, complaints of decreased exercise and activity tolerance (as evidenced by dyspnea on exertion, excessive heart rate, and blood pressure rise with only minor exertion), irritability, inability to concentrate, and depression are all signs and symptoms which lead to the nursing diagnosis/problem of weakness and fatigue related to insufficient RBCs. The decreased RBCs may be secondary to a disease process or chemotherapy and radiotherapy. The two major nursing goals are to enable the patient to complete activities of daily living without undue fatigue and to prevent the signs of stress often associated with fatigue.

Interventions

Nursing care should be planned to conserve the patient's strength by alternating rest periods and activity. Allow the patient to set a time schedule so that daily tasks can be spaced to coincide with times when energy level is at its peak.[6] The nurse may need to assist with activities such as bathing, eating, hair brushing, and oral hygiene to allow the patient to use limited energy for ambulation, coughing and deep breathing, and other activities designed to prevent the complications of bed rest. Instruct the patient to stop an activity if palpitations or shortness of breath occurs.

Provide a quiet environment, relocating the patient if necessary to avoid disturbing noises. Plan at least 2 hours or more of undisturbed sleep at night to allow a complete sleep cycle.

Signs of stress such as irritablility, inability to concentrate, depression, and tearfulness are often associated with fatigue. The characteristics of fatigue should be described to the patient and family. Awareness that fatigue results from depleted energy reserves and that fatigue requires a period of restoration, promotes an understanding of the resultant signs of stress. Discourage communication and avoid patient teaching during periods of excessive fatigue. Messages received during a state of fatigue are poorly perceived.[3] Teach family members that important messages should be delayed if the patient feels fatigued as the potential for stress is increased by fatigue.

To provide comfort and safety, it may be necessary to assist the patient in getting out of bed and ambulating. Because chronic fatigue tends to preclude muscular exercise as a heat-producing mechanism, the patient may complain of feeling cold.[6] Provide warmth by using warmed blankets, cotton socks, and flannel gowns or pajamas.

Evaluation

Because the diagnosis of fatigue is subjective, it is important to use the patient's feelings as well as our observations as an evaluation tool. Subjective outcome criteria may be that the patient expresses a feeling of well-being after rest periods and activities of daily living are completed without feelings of exhaustion, shortness of breath, or palpitations. Objective outcome criteria are patient interest in and initiation of activities, ability to concentrate, and minimal rise in heart rate and blood pressure during an activity.

The patient and family should be able to identify the signs and symptoms of stress which may accompany fatigue. In addition, the patient and family will demonstrate appropriate techniques for coping with the signs and symptoms of stress.

Summary

The nursing strategies and care plan presented in this chapter can be used to treat patients with hematologic disorders experiencing the problems of bleeding, infection, or fatigue. These nursing strategies may also be generalized to patients with other disorders experiencing similar problems. For example, the patient with heart failure may also experience fatigue. Additional nursing strategies for patients with specific hematologic problems can be found in the chapters dealing with these disorders.

References

1. Brunner LS, Suddarth DS: The Lippincott Manual of Nursing Practice, 3rd ed. Philadelphia, JB Lippincott, 1982
2. Clements MJ, Mattson A: Prevention of Social and Emotional Problems in Boys with Hemophilia. New York, The National Hemophilia Foundation, 1983
3. Campbell C: Nursing Diagnosis and Intervention in Nursing Practice, 2nd ed. New York, John Wiley, 1984
4. Crane LR, Emmer DR, Grguras A: Prevention of infection on the oncology unit. In Arking LM, McArthur BJ (eds): The Nursing Clinics of North America, 15(4), 1980, pp. 843–855.
5. Doenges ME, Jeffries MF, Moorhouse MF: Nursing Care Plans: Nursing Diagnosis in Planning Patient Care. Philadelphia, FA Davis, 1984
6. McGurn WC: People with Cardiac Problems: Nursing Concepts. Philadelphia, JB Lippincott, 1981
7. Mitchell PH, Loustau A: Concepts Basic to Nursing, 2nd ed. New York, McGraw-Hill, 1981
8. Nossel HL: Disorders of blood coagulation factors. In Petersdorf RG, Adams RD, Braunwald E, Isselbacher KJ, Martin JB, Wilson JD (eds): Harrison's Principles of Internal Medicine, 10th ed. New York, McGraw-Hill, 1983
9. Scribner BH (ed): A Teaching Syllabus for the Course on Fluid and Electrolyte Balance, 7th rev. Seattle, University of Washington, School of Medicine, 1969
10. Smith L: Reactions to transfusions. Am J Nurs, 84(9): 1096–1101, 1984
11. Smith JJ, Kompine JP: Circulatory Physiology. Baltimore, Williams & Wilkins, 1980
12. Snyder EL: Blood Transfusion Therapy. Arlington, VA. American Association of Blood Banks, 1983
13. Thompson AR, Harker LA: Manual of Hemostasis and Thrombosis, 3rd ed. Philadelphia, FA Davis, 1983
14. Underhill SL: History taking and physical examination of the patient with cardiovascular disease. In Underhill SL, Woods SL, Sivarajan ES, Halpenny CJ (eds): Cardiac Nursing. Philadelphia, JB Lippincott, 1982

Chapter 51

Neoplastic Disorders Affecting Hematologic Function

Carina Knowlton Moravec
Beth Miller Kraybill

Leukemia

Definition and Classification

Leukemia refers to a group of neoplastic diseases of the blood-forming tissues. The bone marrow is the organ primarily affected, but the spleen and lymph nodes are also often involved. Leukemia is characterized by the abnormal, uncontrolled proliferation of one type of hematopoietic cell (*i.e.,* lymphocyte, granulocyte, or monocyte) or the precursors of those cells. Figure 51–1 diagrams the probably origin of hematopoietic malignancies. The abnormal cells that are produced in leukemia are impaired in their maturation and in their functional capabilities.

Leukemia is the second leading cause of death among children between the ages of 4 and 14 years. It is second only to congenital abnormalities. However, leukemia is not solely a children's disease. In 1982, 23,500 new cases were reported in the United States. Of those, 21,000 new cases occurred in adults and 2,500 in children.

Leukemias are generally classified into four types: acute or chronic, and lymphoid or myeloid in origin. The terms acute or chronic refer to rapidity of onset and progression of the disease as well as the maturity of the cell line involved. Chronic leukemias are not a chronic phase of the acute leukemias. Acute leukemia is rapid in onset and progresses rapidly. Untreated, a patient with acute leukemia may only have a life expectancy of days to months. In acute leukemia, the cellular morphology consists of very immature, undifferentiated cells. Chronic leukemias have a gradual onset and a prolonged clinical course. Life expectancy may be greater than 5 years in some cases. However, with modern therapy the life expectancy of patients with acute leukemia often exceeds that of the chronic leukemias. The predominant cells produced in chronic leukemias are relatively mature. Thus, the functional capabilities of chronic leukemia cells are generally better than those of the cells involved in acute leukemia.

Acute leukemias tend to occur most frequently in children 2 to 4 years of age. The incidence decreases by age 8 and remains low until age 65 when it starts to increase again. Chronic leukemias are more common in people over 20 years of age with the incidence increasing up to a peak, high incidence in the sixties. Chronic lymphocytic leukemia is uncommon under the age of 45.

Leukemias are also classified according to the cellular origin of the proliferating cells (*i.e.* myeloid or lymphoid). Thus leukemias are classified into four major types:

- Acute myeloid leukemia (myelocytic, granulocytic, myelogenous, myeloblastic) or AML
- Acute lymphocytic leukemia (lymphoblastic) or ALL

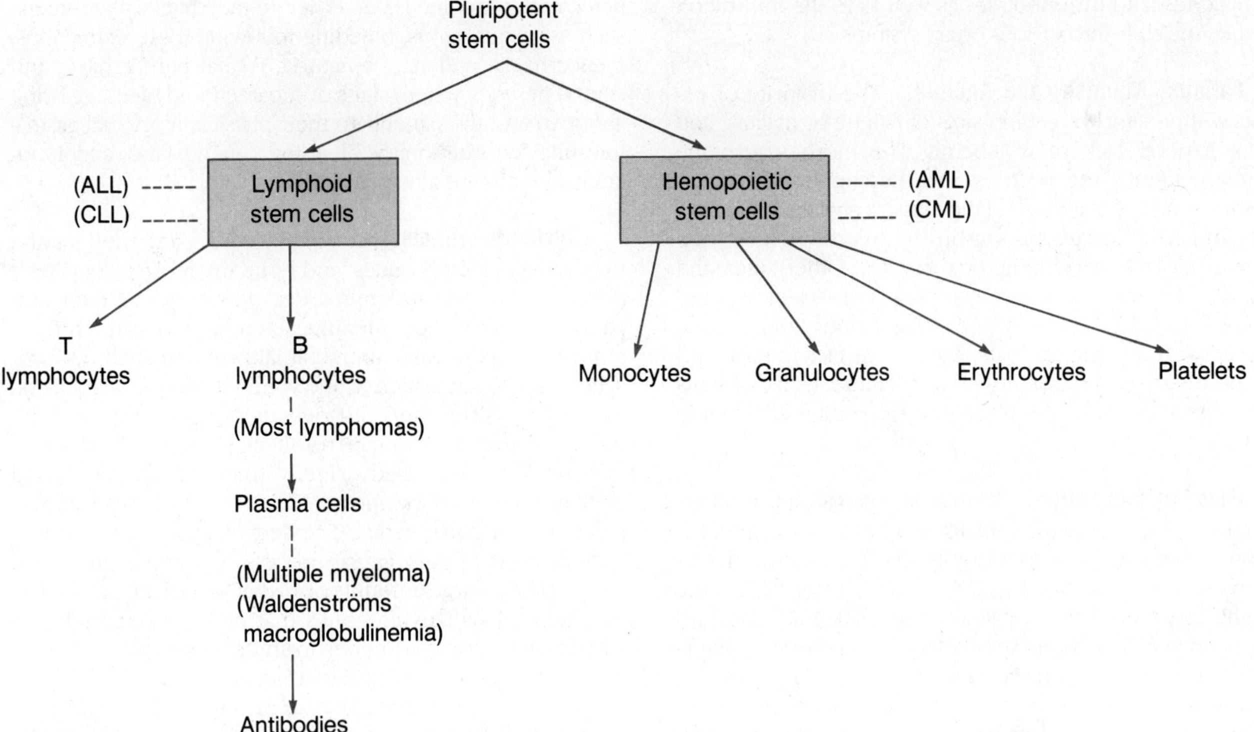

FIGURE 51-1 Probable origin of hematopoietic malignancies. The myelogenous leukemias (AML and CML) are believed to originate from the hemopoietic stem cell that differentiates into monocytes, granulocytes, erythrocytes, and platelets. The lymphocytic leukemias (ALL and CLL) are believed to originate from lymphoid stem cells that differentiate into T lymphocytes and B lymphocytes. Most lymphomas are thought to involve B lymphocytes. Both multiple myeloma and Waldenström's macroglobulinemia affect plasma cells. The origin of Hodgkin's disease remains uncertain, although the malignant Reed-Sternberg cell is believed to be derived from monocyte-macrophage cells.[12,13]

- Chronic myeloid leukemia (myelogenous, granulocytic, myelocytic) or CML
- Chronic lymphocytic leukemia (lymphoid) or CLL.

The terms of lymphoblastic and myeloblastic are used in association with the acute leukemias because the cells produced in these two forms of the disease are usually immature blasts. The term acute nonlymphocytic leukemia (ANL) is often used to describe all the various sub-types of acute myeloid leukemia which include acute myeloblastic leukemia without maturation (M_1), acute myeloblastic leukemia with maturation (M_2), acute promyelocytic leukemia (M_3), acute myelomonocytic leukemia (M_4), acute monocytic leukemia (M_5), and acute erythroleukemia (M_6).

Etiology

The exact etiology of leukemia is unknown. However, in a few cases, the following factors have been found to be associated with leukemia: (1) exposure to large doses of ionizing radiation; (2) exposure to benzene and other chemicals. Both of these factors are associated with an increased incidence of acute myeloid leukemia (AML) and chronic myeloid leukemia (CML); (3) congenital conditions such as Down's syndrome which is associated with an increased incidence of acute lymphocytic leukemia (ALL) and acute myeloid leukemia (AML).

A positive Philadelphia chromosome (Ph^1) is found in approximately 90% of cases of chronic myeloid leukemia. Many believe this is evidence that supports a genetic abnormality as the cause of CML. However, because there does not seem to be concordance of CML among identical twins, many other believe that the disease is acquired. In animals, viral causes of leukemia have been well established. However, evidence supporting viral causes of leukemia in humans is not consistent or convincing.

Pathophysiology

The primary problems in leukemia generally stem from the increased production of immature or abnormal leukocytes. Regardless of their maturity, these abnormal cells do not function correctly. As a result of the massive proliferation of these cells in the marrow, other cell lines such as erythrocytes and thrombocytes do not develop normal amounts of red blood cells and platelets. Leukemic cells can infiltrate the bone marrow, the blood, and various other body organs such as tonsils, lymph nodes, spleen, kidneys, gingivae, skin, and the central nervous system.

Clinical Manifestations

The manifestations of leukemia are related to the impaired function of the immature or abnormal leukocytes, erythrocytes, and thrombocytes as well as to the infiltration of leukemic cells into various organ systems.

Fatigue, Malaise, and Anemia. The majority of patients will present with complaints of fatigue or malaise and just a general lack of well-being. The more severe the anemia, generally, the more severe is the fatigue and malaise. Anemia develops as a result of the massive amounts of leukocytes and lymphocytes present in the marrow which then "crowd out" the developing erythrocytes. Other signs and symptoms of anemia include complaints of weakness, lethargy, headache, tinnitus, dyspnea, palpitations, and edema. Patients with anemia are pale, often have tachycardia, and may have signs and symptoms of heart failure. (A list of signs and symptoms at the time of diagnosis is presented in Table 51–1.)

Fever and Infection. Fever with or without an overt infection is the primary complaint in 15%–10% of patients.[7] Night sweats usually accompany fevers. Infection is not as common a presenting complaint as fevers, however, it is the leading cause of death in patients with leukemia. The preponderance to infections results from immature or abnormally functioning leukocytes and in particular, granulocytopenia. Infections may manifest as ulcerations of the mouth and throat, sinusitis, largynitis, bronchitis, pneumonia, urinary tract infections, infections of the skin and nails, peritonsillar and perirectal abscesses, as well as septicemia. Although fungal infections are not common at diagnosis, they become more prominent later in the course of the disease.

Bleeding Tendencies. Abnormal bleeding tendencies and actual hemorrhage are related to the decreased production and increased destruction of platelets. Easy bruising, petechiae, nosebleeds, or other hemorrhagic phenomena such as oozing gums, bleeding following tooth extractions, menorrhagia, melena, hematuria, retinal hemorrhage, and central nervous system signs of subarachnoid bleeding bring about 10% of the patients to their physician.[17] Actual gastrointestinal or pulmonary bleeding can be fatal, and intracranial bleeds are almost always fatal.

TABLE 51–1
Common Signs and Symptoms at Time of Diagnosis with Leukemia

Symptoms
Fatigue
Bone or joint pain
Fever without infection
Weight loss
Abnormal masses
Purpura
Other hemorrhage
Infection
Abdominal fullness
Abdominal pain
Easy bruising or bleeding
Signs
Splenomegaly
Hepatomegaly
Lymphadenopathy
Sternal tenderness
Petechiae and/or ecchymosis
Retinal hemorrhage
Fever

Systemic Effects. Leukemia cells infiltration of the liver, spleen, lymph nodes, and bone marrow presents with symptoms such as abdominal discomfort, sternal pain, and pain in other bones. Meningeal infiltration can produce symptoms of increased intracranial pressure such as headaches, papilledema, nausea and vomiting, double vision, cranial nerve palsies, and disorientation. Leukemic cell infiltration of the kidneys can result in renal insufficiency as evidenced by decreased urine output and elevated blood urea nitrogen and creatinine. Renal insufficiency can also result from hyperuricemia. The destruction of large amount of leukocytes in the disease process or antileukemic treatment releases large amounts or uric acid into the blood. The uric acid crystallizes in stones that obstruct renal tubules. Patients with uric acid nephropathy may complain of renal pain and have frequent urinary tract infections.

Patients with leukemia may present with weight loss, tachycardia, dyspnea on exertion, and intolerance to heat secondary to an increase in metabolism.

Medical Management

Diagnosis

Typically patients will present with fatigue, pallor, fever, malaise, and purpura. These signs and symptoms will alert the physician to the possibility of leukemia. The final diagnosis is based on the results of bone marrow aspirate for cellular identification of the type of leukemia and a marrow biopsy to determine the architecture and degree of cellularity of the marrow. A peripheral blood count will show an elevated leukocyte count in most patients but even when the count is normal or low, a large number of blasts will be present. One type of leukocyte will predominate over the other. The patient may also have anemia (low red blood cell count), bleeding tendencies, and liver or spleen enlargement. Common laboratory findings in leukemia are listed in Table 51–2.

Treatment

Acute Forms. In acute forms (ALL and AML), the ultimate goals of antileukemic therapy is to cure the patient. However, this is more realistic in acute lymphocytic leukemia than acute myeloid leukemia. Thus, treatment is geared toward inducing a complete remission and maintaining it for as long as possible. Complete remission is defined as the absence of any leukemia-related symptoms and signs; normal laboratory findings, including the differential count, platelets, and hematocrit; and most important, a normalization of the marrow.

The principles of treatment for acute lymphocytic leukemia (ALL) and acute myeloid leukemia (AML) generally involve four phases:

TABLE 51–2
Common Laboratory Findings in Leukemia

Laboratory Test	*ALL*	*AML*	*CML*	*CLL*
WBC	▲↓↔	↑↓↔	▲▲▲	▲▲▲
Neutrophils	↓	↓	↑	↔
Lymphocytes			↑↑	▲▲
Blasts	+	+	+ (especially in blast crisis)	
Hematocrit	↓	↓↓	↓	↓
Platelets	↓↓	↓↓	▲▲▲↔	↓↔
Auer rods	−	+	+ (blast crisis)	−
Uric acid	▲↔	▲↔	▲↔	↔
Serum albumin	↘	↘	↔	↔
Serum calcium	↑ (rare)			
Potassium		↓	↑	
Copper	↑			
Philadelphia chromosome			+	
Leukocyte alkaline phosphatase			↓↓	

▲ indicates common finding
↑, ↓ indicates slightly elevated or decreased value, respectively
↑↑, ↓↓ indicates moderately elevated or decreased values, respectively
↑↑↑ indicates extremely elevated values
↔ indicates normal values
↘ indicates values that consistently decrease over time
\+ indicates a positive finding
− indicates a negative finding

1. Induction of complete remission
2. Prevention of central nervous system relapse (meningeal leukemia)
3. Maintenance therapy
4. Determination of when to discontinue maintenance therapy

Currently, combination drug therapy (Table 51–3) is used to achieve complete remission as combining agents are more likely to result in a complete remission than using single agents alone. Intrathecal methotrexate and craniospinal irradiation is used for central nervous system prophylaxis. Maintenance therapy usually also includes a combination of agents give for 1 to 5 days at 3- to 4-week intervals.

Bone marrow transplantation is currently being used with increasing frequency and with increasingly improving results in the treatment of patients with acute leukemia. The chances of maintaining a prolonged remission in patients with AML in second or subsequent remissions and those with AML in first remission are slim. Achieving and then maintaining a prolonged remission in patients with ALL in second or subsequent relapse or AML in first relapse are uncommon. Bone marrow transplantation has been shown to prolong life expectancy in patients who fall into these categories. The principle of marrow transplantation is to eradicate the leukemia and immunosuppress the patient with high doses of chemotherapy and total body irradiation. Because these high doses also eradicate all the normal stem cells in the bone marrow, it must be replaced by infusing marrow from a human leukocyte antigen-matched donor. The transplanted stem cells migrate to the patients marrow where they begin to produce healthy leukocytes, erythrocytes, and thrombocytes.

Chronic Forms. Complete remission is rarely achieved or even attempted in the chronic forms of leukemia (myeloid and lymphocytic), and survival is rarely prolonged by the use of chemotherapy in these diseases. Instead, the goal of therapy for chronic myeloid leukemia is (1) to normalize the leukocyte count and (2) to treat the symptoms of leukemia such as bleeding or infections. Generally, platelet counts and hematocrit normalize concurrently with the leukocyte count. Leukopheresis is occasionally used to remove large numbers of leukocytes. Splenectomy has been attempted, but has not been found to increase survival or to prevent blast crisis, the terminal event in CML.

The disease course of chronic lymphocytic leukemia is generally benign. Many patients remain asymptomatic for years. Because antileukemic therapy for CLL has no or very little effect on survival, often patients are not treated until they begin to develop complications.

Prognosis

Prognosis depends on several factors, including type of leukemia, age at diagnosis, presenting symptoms, and presence or absence of central nervous system or other organ involvement. With the development of effective chemo-

TABLE 51–3
Example of Medications Used in the Treatment of Leukemias and Lymphomas

Medications	
Acute Lymphoblastic Leukemia	
Induction	
prednisone + vincristine	
prednisone + 6-mercaptopurine	
prednisone + methotrexate	
prednisone + cyclophosphamide	
prednisone + vincristine + aspariginase	
prednisone + vincristine + daunomycin	
prednisone + vincristine + cyclophosphamide + aspariginase	
Maintenance Therapy	
6-mercaptopurine + methotrexate	
6-mercaptopurine + methotrexate + cyclophosphamide	
6-mercaptopurine + methotrexate + cyclophosphamide + vincristine	
6-mercaptopurine + cyclophosphamide + vincristine	
Acute Myeloid Leukemia	
Induction	
"7 & 3": cytosine arabinoside + daunomycin (or adriamycin)	
"TRAP": 6-thioguanine + daunomycin + cytosine arabinoside + prednisone	
"7 & 3 + PV": Cytosine arabinoside + daunomycin + prednisone + vincristine	
"TAD": cytosine arabinoside + 6-thioguanine + daunomycin	
"POMP": prednisone + vincristine + methotrexate + 6-mercaptopurine	
Maintenance Therapy	
daunomycin × 1 day cytosine arabinoside × 5 days	4 times at 3–4-week intervals
cytosine arabinoside × 5 days 6-thioguanine × 5 days	repeated every 4 weeks
Chronic Myelogeneous Leukemia	
busulfan (Myleran) (This is the mainstay of treatment for CML.)	
hydroxyurea	
chlorambucil	
6-mercaptopurine	
melphalan	
Chronic Lymphocytic Leukemia	
steroids	
chlorambucil	
total body irradiation	

therapy, the use of combination drug therapy and bone marrow transplantation, the prognosis of leukemia has improved.

Acute Lymphocytic Leukemia. Without therapy, life expectancy of a patient with ALL can be measured in days or months, with the terminal event usually being overwhelming infection or massive hemorrhage. Modern therapy, including induction, maintenance, and central nervous system prophylaxis as well as supportive therapy for complications has improved life expectancy considerably since the introduction of antileukemic therapy in 1948. Currently, approximately 90% of children and 65% of adults can be put into complete first remission.[20] Age has been found to be a significant prognostic indicator. In ALL age 15 seems to be the dividing line between children and adults for prognostic purposes.[17]

Unfortunately, many patients who achieve a complete remission relapse, with relapse being more common in adults than in children. Relapse can occur in the bone marrow, the central nervous system, or in the testes despite maintenance therapy, central nervous system prophylaxis, and testicular irradiation. The incidence of central nervous system and testicular relapse is now increasing as the length of remission is increasing. Once the patient has relapsed, complete remission is still possible but in a smaller percentage of patients and usually for shorter period of time than for first remission. Despite the problems with frequent relapse in ALL, approximately 50% of children are cured of the disease. The definition of cure is vague, but one can say that the child who has been in complete remission for 2 years following a 2.5-year maintenance course has less than a 10% chance of relapse.[17]

Multiple factors have been found to influence the ultimate prognosis. As discussed above, age influences survival, with those children between the ages of 3 and 7 having the best chance of survival. Obesity is an adverse prognosticator. A high initial white count ($>100{,}000/mm^3$) predisposes to cerebrovascular occlusion or hemorrhage. Females have a higher survival rate than males. Central nervous system disease at the time of diagnosis reflects a poor prognosis. Black and non-Caucasian patients as well as those who are bleeding or infected at time of diagnosis have a worse prognosis. Patients with T cell or B cell acute lymphocytic leukemia have poorer prognosis than those with the common ALL antibodies (CALLA) or with null cells. It is important to remember that although all these factors help predict the final outcome, the most critical factor for survival is the achievement of complete remission.

Overall, the median survival for children is 36 to 42 months and 18 months for adults. Marrow transplantation has been found to increase survival in patients transplanted in second or subsequent remissions. Children in second remission tend not to survive beyond 3.5 years. However, 35% of children in second remission who are transplanted with a matched sibling are still alive 4 years later.*

Acute Myeloid Leukemia. Again, without therapy, life expectancy is very short for patients with AML. Median survival is 2 to 2.5 months. As with acute lymphocytic leukemia, the achievement of complete remission is the single best prognostic indicator because patient who are treated with standard chemotherapy but who do not achieve complete remission have the same life expectancy as those who do not receive treatment. Although acute myeloid leukemia is less common in children than in adults, children with AML tend to have a higher occurrence of complete remission than do adults. Overall, complete remission is achieved in approximately 70% of patients.[15] Relapse, however, is common and although second and subsequent remissions can be achieved

* Thomas ED: Personal communication, 1984

they are usually of short duration. Overall, cure is rare in AML. The median survival is 1 year and even for those who achieve complete remission, it does not exceed 18 to 24 months. As with acute lymphocytic leukemia, marrow transplantation has been found to increase survival in patients with AML in first remission. On conventional chemotherapy only 20% of these patients are still alive in 5 years, whereas with a marrow transplant from a matched sibling, the 5-year survival rate is 50%.[†]

There are a few factors that influence prognosis in AML. The presence of Auer rods predicts a longer period of remission. Patients who develop AML after a period of preleukemia or after cytotoxic therapy for other illnesses tend to respond poorly to therapy.

Chronic Myeloid Leukemia. Complete remission is rarely achieved in CML, thus the goal of therapy if focused on alleviating symptoms and normalizing laboratory values. Chemotherapy has not been found to increase survival appreciably. Median survival is 3 to 3.5 years.[9] Conversion to blast crisis is usually the terminal event, and death ensues within 10 weeks if the patient does not respond to therapy and within 27 weeks if the patient does respond.[9] Death is usually due to infection or hemorrhage. Blast crisis is defined as a change in the course of CML into an AML-type picture with massive proliferation of blasts and promyelocytes in the blood and bone marrow. Fever, anemia, splenomegally, thrombocytopenia, or thrombocytosis, enlargement of the lymph nodes, or a sudden increase in the leukocyte count may herald the onset of blast crisis. The onset of blast crisis is still a random, unpredictable event and occurs with a frequency of about 25% per year in those patients who have been diagnosed for over 2 years. Bone marrow transplantation has improved survival significantly, such that patients transplanted in the chronic phase of the disease have a 40% to 50% 2-year survival rate. Those patients transplanted in blast crisis have a 15% to 20% 2-year survival rate with transplantation.[‡]

Prognostic indicators for patients with chronic myeloid leukemia include the following: Younger patients survive longer. Patients with asthenia, weight loss, bone pain, fever, night sweats, and gastrointestinal disturbances at the time of diagnosis have shorter survival times than those without these symptoms. A leukocyte count less than 100,000/mm^3, normal liver function, and a negative Philadelphia chromosome all predict improved survival. Patients with very high or very low platelet counts have a poor prognosis.[5]

Chronic Lymphocytic Leukemia. As CLL generally runs a fairly benign course and occurs late in life, treatment is generally aimed at symptomatic relief and treatment of complications. Nearly one third of patients die of unrelated, concurrent diseases. The average life expectancy after diagnosis is 3 to 6 years, but may be as long as 20 years. The most common cause of death in patients with CLL is infection. The best prognostic indicators are how well a patient responds to therapy and the severity of the disease as judged by the presence or absence of fatigue, infection, masses, organ enlargement, lymphadenopathy, sternal tenderness, and abnormal blood values such as a high lymphocyte count, anemia, thrombocytopenia, and neutropenia.

† Thomas ED: Personal communication, 1984
‡ Sanders JE: Personal communication, 1984

Nursing Management

Management of the patient with leukemia is similar to the management of the patient with Hodgkin's disease, with non-Hodgkin's lymphomas, and with multiple myeloma. Because of the similarity in care, general nursing management for patients with these disorders will be discussed toward the end of the chapter.

Hodgkin's Disease

Definition and Classification

Hodgkin's disease is one of a group of neoplastic tumors that affect the lymphoid tissue and as such are termed lymphomas. It is characterized by a progressive, painless enlargement of the lymph nodes and can also affect the spleen and liver. Eventually, tissues and organs throughout the body can be involved.

Two systems of classification are employed with each patient: histological classification and clinical staging. Histologic classification and prognosis are based on the cellular composition of the infiltrate in the lymph nodes. Hodgkin's disease is distinguished by the presence of Reed-Sternberg cells, atypical, giant histiocytes, in addition to other abnormal cells in the infiltrate. The Ann Arbor Clinical Staging Classification was adapted in 1971 to provide some uniformity in reporting[3] (Table 51–4). There are four stages (I, II, III, and IV) based on the number, location, and degree of involved lymph nodes.

Hodgkin's disease tends to occur in young adults between the ages of 15 and 35. There is also an increased incidence between the ages of 55 and 75. It tends to occur more frequently in men than in women, in those who have had infectious mononucleosis or tonsillectomy, and in those taking hydantoin derivatives such as Dilantin. There does tend to be an increased risk for developing Hodgkin's disease when one member of the family has it. Perhaps a familial immunological deficiency predisposes family members to Hodgkin's disease.

Etiology

Various factors have been studied as possible etiological factors for Hodgkin's disease. These include viral, genetic, ethnic, and immunologic factors, and exposure to gamma radiation, in addition to many others. No conclusive evidence has been found to support these as etiological factors with the exception that there is some tendency for clustering of Hodgkin's disease in families, and there is a higher incidence of it in Hiroshima survivors.

TABLE 51–4
Ann Arbor Clinical Staging Classification[3,8]

Stage	Definition
I	Involvement of a single lymph node region (I) or of a single extralymphatic organ or site (I_E)
II	Involvement of two or more lymph node reigons on the same side of the diaphragm (II) or localized involvement of an extralymphatic organ or site and of one or more lymph node regions on the same side of the diaphragm (II_E).
III	Involvement of lymph node regions on both sides of the diaphragm (III), which may also be accompanied by involvement of the spleen (III_S) or by localized involvement of an extralymphatic organ or site (III_E) or both (III_{SE}).
IV	Diffuse or disseminated involvement of one or more extralymphatic organs or tissues, with or without associated lymph node involvement.

The presence or absence of fever, night sweats and/or unexplained loss of 10% or more of body weight in the 6 months preceding admission are denoted by the suffix letters B and A, respectively.

Biopsy-documented involvement of stage IV sites is also denoted by letter suffixes: marrow = M+; lung = L+; liver = H+; pleura = P+; bone = O+; skin and subcutaneous tissue = D+.

Adopted at the workshop on the Staging of Hodgkin's Disease held at Ann Arbor, Michigan, April 1971.

(From Kaplan HS, Rosenberg SA: Hodgkin's disease: Current recommendations for management. CA 25:306–319, 1975)

Pathophysiology

As in other neoplastic blood disorders, Hodgkin's disease is characterized by the proliferation of one type of cell, in this case the Reed-Sternberg cell. These cells and other lymphocytes, histiocytes, eosinophils, plasma cells, and neutrophils completely or partially replace the normal architecture of lymph nodes affected by Hodgkin's disease.

Typically, Hodgkin's disease begins in one lymph node then spreads to other lymph nodes and to the spleen by the lymphatic channels. Hodgkin's disease can also spread by the vascular system to the marrow or the liver. Vertebrae may also be invaded, as well as the ureters and bronchi because of their proximity to lymph nodes. Nodes may grow slowly and then enlarge rapidly during fever, only to subside again when the temperature returns to normal. Symptoms occur from either pressure exerted by large nodes or infiltration of the lymphoma into vital organs. Treatment of lymphoma reduces or eradicates the lymph nodes but occasionally the disease cannot be controlled and death results.

In the terminal stage, many small nodules are a more common finding than a few large nodules, and the patient usually has fever, weight loss, and cachexia. Pleural and peritoneal effusions can occur as a result of lymphomatous infiltration. Liver or pulmonary failure from invasion by the lymphoma can be a cause of death. Neutropenia (reduced numbers of neutrophils) and immune suppression secondary to therapy predisposes some patients to systemic herpes virus infections, tuberculosis, toxoplasmosis, or bacterial infections. Pancytopenia (reduction of all blood cells) from bone marrow suppression by chemotherapy or from fibrosis of the marrow is seen late in the course of the disease. Multifocal leukoencephalopathy has also been a cause of death. Fortunately, many patients who never achieve a full remission live for more than 20 years without any of the above complications.

Clinical Manifestations

The most common presenting feature in Hodgkin's disease is an enlarged, painless cervical node. The left side is involved more frequently than the right, predisposing the person to spread of the disease to the abdomen by the thoracic duct. Periodic fevers are common following many different patterns. Other signs and symptoms that occur commonly, some that occur only with advanced disease, and some less common ones are listed in Table 51–5.

Medical Management

Diagnosis

The typical patient will present with cervical lymph node enlargement, pruritis, alcohol-induced pain, fevers, lymphopenia, and neutrophilia. Although this is the typical picture of Hodgkin's disease, a lymph node biopsy to determine the presence of Reed-Sternberg cells is necessary for a definitive diagnosis. Other characteristic histologic features can also be identified with a lymph node biopsy. The physical examination of a patient suspected of having Hodgkin's disease should emphasize lymph node chains, liver, spleen, and bony tenderness.[8] Occasionally, a mediastinal or hilar mass may be noted on a routine chest x-ray film, or an x-ray film taken to determine the cause of symptoms related to the mass. Some of these patients will not have accompanying enlarged peripheral nodes. In such cases whole lung tomography should be performed to identify other involved nodes. A mediastinoscopy may also be performed to determine mediastinal node involvement.

If a patient develops symptoms typical of Hodgkin's disease but without peripheral lymph node enlargement and with a normal chest x-ray film, bilateral pedal lymphangiography should be performed. Inguinal, iliac, and paraaortic nodes will be visible within 24 hours of dye injection. The procedure should be performed with caution in those patients with significant pulmonary disease because the dye may precipitate pulmonary symptoms.

Laboratory tests for Hodgkin's disease include a complete blood count, platelet count, alkaline phosphatase as a measure of liver function, sedimentation rate, and serum copper. Common laboratory findings include the following: In most patients the leukocyte count will be elevated, and neutrophil, eosinophil, monocyte, and basophil count may be elevated or normal; lymphocyte count is often decreased; platelet count may be normal or elevated and the red cell count may be normal or low; Reed-Sternberg cells may or may not be present in the peripheral blood; serum calcium is often elevated, but can be normal; if the kidneys are involved, the blood urea nitrogen may be elevated; and if the liver is involved, alkaline phosphatase will be elevated.

TABLE 51–5
Signs and Symptoms of Hodgkin's Disease

Symptoms	*Cause*
Common	
Enlarged, painless cervical node	HD infiltration
Periodic fevers without other symptoms of infection and with night sweats	HD involvement of internal nodes or viscera
Generalized pruritis	Unknown
Weight loss	Cachexia, increased metabolism
Alcohol-associated pain in area of HD infiltration	Unknown
Common with Progressive Involvement	
Cough, dyspnea, chest pain	Pulmonary infiltration or mediastinal node involvement
Fatigue, malaise, anorexia	Anemia secondary to increased erythrocyte destruction and chemotherapy
Less Common	
Paraplegia	Compression of spinal cord by enlarged nodes
Bone pain, fractures	Infiltration of bones
Brachial, lumbar, sacral neuralgias	Compression of nerve roots by enlarged nodes
Laryngeal paralysis	Pressure on laryngeal nerve
Dysphagia	Pressure on esophagus
Signs	*Cause*
Common	
Enlarged cervical or supraclavicular lymph nodes, more common on left than right	HD infiltration
Mediastinal node involvement	HD infiltration
Edema and cyanosis of the face and neck	Enlarged nodes impede the venous return to the heart via the superior vena cava
Common with Progressive Involvement	
Jaundice	Pressure on hepatic duct
Increased susceptibility to infection	Impairment of immune system from the disease process and treatment
Pleural effusion	Pleural infiltration
Less Common	
Generalized lymphadenopathy	HD infiltration
Splenomegaly, hepatomegaly	HD infiltration
Cyanosis	Pulmonary infiltration
Renal, gastrointestinal disorders	Infiltration

A marrow biopsy is often performed to determine whether there is any infiltration of abnormal cells in the marrow. A scan of the liver and spleen will be performed to determine involvement if liver function tests are abnormal or there is hepatomegaly. If the scan is positive for liver involvement, a liver biopsy or a laparotomy will be done for staging purposes. A splenectomy, liver biopsy, and multiple lymph node biopsies can be performed at the same time. X-ray films of vertebrae, pelvis, proximal long bones, and the areas of bony tenderness can aid in determining involvement in these areas.

Treatment

Treatment is based on the clinical staging and is aimed at curing the patient. Cure is defined as being disease free for 10 years following diagnosis. It is generally accepted that patients in stage I or II-A receive extended field radiotherapy and those in stage III-B or IV received combination chemotherapy with the possible addition of radiotherapy. There is, however, disagreement regarding the optimal treatment for the other stages, thus various combinations of chemotherapy and radiotherapy may be used for these stages. Use of radiotherapy at doses of 4,000 rads over a 6-week period and allowing a 2-week rest period in the middle has demonstrated a high rate of cure with less morbidity due to the rest period.[18] Combination chemotherapy has been found to have more promising results than using single agents alone. The "gold standard" in the treatment of Hodgkin's disease is MOPP, a regimen of mechlorethamine (nitrogen mustard), vincristine (Oncovin), procarbazine, and prednisone. It is given six times at 28-day intervals. MOPP therapy as well as radiotherapy causes many side-effects, the nursing care of which is be discussed later in the chapter.

Prognosis

Overall, there is a 50% 10-year survival or permanent cure rate for Hodgkin's disease when therapy includes careful staging and the use of intensive radiotherapy or combination chemotherapy plus radiotherapy.[8] The most favorable prognosis is for patients diagnosed in stage I or II who are treated with intensive radiotherapy. Patients diagnosed in stage III and treated with MOPP chemotherapy with or without radiotherapy have a survival rate close to that of stages I and II. Patients diagnosed in stage IV have a comparably poorer prognosis, although their 5-year survival is close to 40%. Patients over 40 years of age have a poorer prognosis than younger patients, as do those patients presenting with symptoms of fever, weight loss, and night sweats.

Nursing Management

The plan of care for the patient with Hodgkin's disease is similar to the plan of care of patients with leukemia, with non-Hodgkin's lymphomas, and with multiple myeloma. This plan of care is discussed later in this chapter.

Non-Hodgkin's Lymphomas

Definition and Classification

Non-Hodgkin's lymphomas are a group of neoplastic tumors that affect the lymphoid tissue with exception of Hodgkin's disease. According to Rappoport, they can be classified by cell type as lymphocytic, well differentiated; lymphocytic, poorly differentiated; histiocytic; or mixed cell. They may also be classified as nodular or diffuse. There are various other classifications used and thus other terms may be used in reference to one of the above classifications.

The Ann Arbor clinical staging for Hodgkin's disease can be adapted for use in non-Hodgkin's lymphoma. Stages I and II indicate involvement of one or more lymph nodes, respectively, on the same side of the diaphragm. Stage III denotes disease on both sides of the diaphragm but limited to the lymph nodes. Stage IV denotes lymph node and visceral involvement (*i.e.,* marrow or liver). Stage I_E indicates involvement of only one organ such as the stomach or bowel without lymph involvement.[12]

Non-Hodgkin's lymphomas are fairly uncommon in the United States, comprising only approximately 2% of all cancers.[6] They tend to occur more commonly in males than in females. Incidence of the disease shows an early preadolescent peak, a decrease in the late teens, and an increase again in the early twenties which continues to rise with increasing age. As with Hodgkin's disease some familial patterns have been found. Some association has been found between non-Hodgkin's lymphoma and primary immunodeficiency syndromes, therapeutic immunosuppression for bone marrow and heart transplantation, acquired immune disorders, skin cancer, lung cancer, and some chromosomal abnormalities. Occupational factors that may add to the risk of developing non-Hodgkin's lymphoma include working as a chemist or veterinarian, or working in the rubber industry, working with petroleum refining, herbicides, or arsenic.

Etiology

As with leukemias and Hodgkin's disease, the etiology of non-Hodgkin's lymphoma is unknown. Factors that seem to increase the risk of developing the disease are discussed above.

Pathophysiology

Nodular or follicular lymphomas are neoplastic transformations of follicular B lymphocytes. Patients with nodular lymphoma usually present with stage III or IV disseminated disease. The clinical course may be indolent with or without aggressive therapy. Well-differentiated lymphocytic lymphomas are neoplastic transformations of the secretory B-cell system. Poorly differentiated lymphocytic lymphomas represent neoplasms of thymic lymphoblasts. Histiocytic and mixed cell lymphomas represent neoplasms of various cell origins.[7]

The first lymph nodes to enlarge in non-Hodgkin's lymphomas are usually those of the neck, although axillary or inguinal nodes may enlarge first. As in Hodgkin's disease, as the disease progresses, the lymphoma spreads to other lymph nodes and various organs by lymphatic channels and blood. Pressure on organs or structures by enlarged lymph nodes or lymphomatous infiltration of organs causes the symptoms and complications seen in non-Hodgkin's lymphomas. Eventually, the bone marrow is infiltrated, causing symptoms similar to leukemia.

Death generally occurs from bacterial infection, although fungal infections can also be fatal in these patients. Infection results from a deficient antibody production, infiltration and destruction of normal tissue in vital organs, or secondary to neutropenia from bone marrow infiltration. Severe hemorrhage secondary to thrombocytopenia is a cause of death in some patients. In other patients, death occurs from gastrointestinal or renal failure secondary to lymphomatous infiltration. Central nervous system involvement can occur in the form of meningeal infiltration, intracerebral tumors, and spinal cord compression. Treatment of central nervous system disease can usually reduce morbidity.

Clinical Manifestations

The earliest sign of non-Hodgkin's lymphoma is generally painless cervical or supraclavicular lymph node enlargement. The nodes are usually freely movable, distinct, and rubbery. Most patients are diagnosed in stage III or IV. Fatigue, malaise, weight loss, fever, or night sweats bring some patients to their physician, but these symptoms are more common in patients with widespread disease. Pruritis, gastrointestinal symptoms, and bone pain occur but are uncommon. Few patients have generalized lymphadenopathy early in the course of the disease. Chest x-ray films may reveal enlarged hilar or mediastinal nodes. Bone marrow infiltration is a common finding in advanced non-Hodgkin's lymphoma and is indicative of stage IV disease.

Medical Management

Diagnosis. The physician is usually alerted to the possibility of non-Hodgkin's lymphomas by a history of a lump or other mass, recurrent infections, an episode of herpes zoster, or unexplained anemia or bleeding. The diagnosis of non-Hodgkin's lymphoma is based on biopsy results on the excised lymph nodes. The differential diagnosis depends on the histologic findings specific for non-Hodgkin's lymphoma. Once the diagnosis is made, staging is determined using the same techniques as are used for Hodgkin's disease.

Treatment. Treatment of non-Hodgkin's lymphoma depends on the extent or stage of the disease. Overall, a goal of curing the disease is only realistic in patients with localized disease. Patients with stage I or II disease receive radiation at doses of 3,500 to 4,000 rads at a rate of 1,000 rads per week. The radiation is given to the primary site as well as to a large area of surrounding tissue. Unfortunately, few patients present this early in the course of the disease.

Patients in stage III may be treated with radiotherapy if the disease is limited to the lymph nodes. Patients who have diffuse lymphoma in stage III are usually treated with combination chemotherapy. COPP and CVP regimens are frequently used. COPP consists of cyclophosphamide, vincristine (Oncovin), procarbazine, and prednisone and is given every 28 days. CVP consists of the same drugs excluding procarbazine and is repeated every 21 days.[14] Patients in stage IV are generally treated with combination chemotherapy, with the addition of radiotherapy if needed to relieve symptoms. Nursing care of the side-effects of chemo- and radiotherapy is discussed later in the chapter. Bone marrow transplantation for non-Hodgkin's lymphoma is currently being performed in certain centers, but results are generally poor.

Prognosis. The prognosis of non-Hodgkin's lymphoma is generally poor. Important factors that influence survival are the histologic type, clinical stage of the disease, and the response to therapy. Overall, approximately 50% of patients survive for 26 months and 28% survive 5 years or more.[19] Those with diffuse disease have a poorer prognosis than those with disease limited to one lymph node. Patients with nodular disease live longer than those with diffuse disease. Those with nodular lymphocytic, well-differentiated lymphoma have the best prognosis and those with undifferentiated lymphocytic lymphoma, the worst prognosis. In one large group of patients the following median survival times were found: lymphocytic, poorly differentiated, and mixed cellularity, diffuse types, 2 years; nodular types, 7 to 8 years; histiocytic, diffuse, 1 year; nodular, 3 to 4 years.[17]

General Nursing Management of Patients with Neoplastic Hematologic Disorders

Patients with neoplastic hematologic disorders face a multitude of problems, both actual and potential, which require extensive nursing interventions. Included in the list of possible nursing diagnoses are fatigue, potential for infection, potential for bleeding, nutrient insufficiency, side-effects of chemotherapy or radiation therapy (mucositis, nausea, vomiting, diarrhea), pain, and other alterations in comfort. Body image problems and coping difficulties and general knowledge deficit of the disease process, its treatment and prognosis are other problem areas that require nursing interventions.

Fatigue

Assessment and Nursing Diagnosis

The proliferation of leukemic, lymphoma, or plasma cells in these patients and the effects of therapy lead to reduced red blood cell production with less oxygen available for activity and energy needs. Decreased hematocrit and hemoglobin levels are noted, and the patient complains of decreased tolerance for exercise and general activities as evidenced by dyspnea, excessive heart rate, increased blood pressure, and possible chest pain on exertion.

Interventions

The nursing goals to deal with the problem of fatigue related to reduced red blood cell production are aimed at reducing tissue demand for oxygen and increasing oxygen supply.

Because the overproduction of the affected blood cells results in increased metabolism, causing chronic fatigue and malaise, the patient should be encouraged to sleep at least 8 hours a night with naps and frequent rest periods during the day. The same rest patterns should be provided during hospitalization by organizing and consolidating care to allow for uninterrupted sleep. Fever will also increase metabolic demands. Therefore monitoring temperature every 4 hours is a means of detecting early signs of fever. If the temperature rises above 38.5°C, the physician may prescribe acetaminophen or the use of alcohol or tepid sponge baths, ice packs, or a hypothermia blanket.

To increase oxygen supply to the tissues, oxygen therapy may be instituted as prescribed, especially during daily activities or if dyspnea occurs on exertion. Decreased hemoglobin results in diminished oxygen-carrying capacity with potential for hypoxia and resultant fatigue. Therefore, hemoglobin and hematocrit levels should be monitored and transfusion therapy with red blood cells or leukocyte-poor RBCs given as ordered. Adverse reactions appear to be reduced when leukocyte-poor RBCs are used in transfusion-dependent patients.[14] It is also important to monitor intake and output and vital signs carefully for indications of possible circulatory overload and congestive heart failure (CHF). Anemia can predispose to CHF, especially in those patients receiving concomitant blood, antibiotics, and chemotherapies.[14] CHF reduces the amount of oxygenated blood available to tissues, resulting in fatigue and activity intolerance.

Evaluation

The patient should be able to perform ADLs independently or with minimal assistance. Such activities should result in a minimal rise in heart rate and blood pressure with no complaints of fatigue or signs of dyspnea. The hematocrit will be maintained at greater than or equal to 30% and arterial Pa_{O_2} will be in the range of 70 to 100 mmHg. Other outcome criteria include maintenance of baseline weight and clear lung sounds on auscultation and a CVP of 4 to 8 cm H_2O.

Potential for Infection

Assessment and Nursing Diagnosis

The increased production of immature white blood cells or the reduction in WBC secondary to the disease process, chemotherapy, or radiation therapy predisposes the patient to infection. The patient will have excessively high or low white blood cell counts and may complain of fever, chills, recurrent upper respiratory tract infections, dysphagia, cuts and abrasions that do not heal, as well as lesions in the mouth, throat, groin, perirectal, and vaginal areas that do not heal.

Interventions

To assist the patient with low resistance, the nurse establishes goals to prevent infection, detect early signs and symptoms of infection, implement the prescribed therapy, and identify any toxic effects that may occur in response to antibiotic therapy.

To minimize the spread of infection, meticulous handwashing must be carried out by all persons who come in contact with the patient. The patient in turn should avoid contact with anyone who has had a cold or other infections. Invasive procedures that can provide a portal of entry to organisms should be avoided, including injections, urinary catheterizations, and rectal procedures. If such procedures are deemed necessary, then any sites of entry must receive meticulous care. Antibiotics may be prescribed as a prophylactic measure or as direct treatment for documented infection. Administering these medications at prescribed intervals is necessary to maintain therapeutic blood levels.

Monitoring white blood cell (WBC) counts, vital signs (every 4 hours), and other system functions is essential to detect early signs and symptoms of infection. Initially WBCs may be increased or in the normal range. However, these cells are immature and not able to combat infection. WBCs may also be decreased on diagnosis. Thus the number of infection-fighting cells are reduced. The usual manifestations of infection may be altered in the leukemia patient. Either subnormal temperature or temperature spikes with chilling may be indicative of sepsis.[14] Tachypnea, low arterial Pa_{O_2}, tachycardia, and changes in the patient's level of consciousness may also be early signs of sepsis. Low blood pressure is generally a later sign. Assessment of the mouth, nose, axilla, groin, perirectal, and vaginal areas is part of daily care. Mucosal tissues are especially susceptible to breakdown and infection as a result of damage from chemotherapy or radiation therapy in combination with a warm, moist environment. Any deviations from normal in these areas should be documented and reported.

Specific antibiotic therapy may be initiated on the basis of cultures that identify a causative organism. It is important to monitor the patient to evaluate the effects of this therapy. Early detection of continual or recurrent infection can allow for prompt changes in antibiotic therapy. Any toxic effects of a specific drug, such as tinnitus, loss of hearing, or progressive renal failure (oliguria, and rising serum creatinine and BUN) must also be noted so that the dosage may be adjusted or a less toxic antibiotic may be substituted.

Evaluation

The patient's vital signs and temperature are key indicators in evaluating the response to therapy and nursing care. The temperature, blood pressure, and pulse rates should remain within normal range for the patient. Any deviations from these baseline values should be detected early and reported, as should urinary, perianal, pulmonary, or skin infections. Antibiotic therapy specific for the causative organism is instituted as prescribed. The nurse should continue to observe the patient for continued signs and symptoms of infection, indications that the antibiotic therapy is not effective.

Potential for Bleeding

Assessment and Nursing Diagnosis

Decreased platelet production may occur as part of the disease process or result from the chemotherapy and radiation treatment. Platelet counts of less than 50,000 indicate a definite bleeding risk. At platelet counts of less than 15,000 almost all patients will bleed spontaneously. However, the count at which a given patient will experience abnormal bleeding is highly individualized.[14] Continued monitoring of platelet counts and assessment for possible signs of bleeding such as tachycardia, increased pulse rate, hypotension, diaphoresis, and changes in levels of consciousness are essential elements in caring for these patients.

Interventions

Because patients with leukemia, lymphoma, and multiple myeloma are at risk for bleeding, the nurse caring for such a patient has major goals of preventing bleeding, detecting any indications of bleeding, initiating measures to control or counter bleeding when it occurs, and being alert for any adverse reactions to therapeutic measures such as blood component transfusions.

Nursing measures to prevent bleeding are based on efforts to avoid injury. The use of invasive objects such as rectal thermometers, suppositories, enemas, vaginal suppositories or tampons, and intramuscular or subcutaneous injections should be avoided. Invasive procedures such as liver biopsy, lumbar puncture, and open lung biopsy should not be carried out in patients with platelet counts of less than 50,000. Invasive procedures increase the risk of tissue injury and secondary bleeding. If arterial blood gases (ABGs) are required, apply consistent firm pressure for at least 10 to 20 minutes or until the oozing stops. Consistent firm pressure helps to promote hemostasis and clot formation.

Careful oral hygiene should be followed because treatment measures for leukemia, lymphoma, and multiple myeloma can cause the gums and mucous membranes to become thin and dry, thereby making them more susceptible to damage, bleeding, and infection. Using a soft toothbrush and encouraging the patient to rinse his or her mouth with normal saline every 2 to 4 hours can assure cleanliness and provide comfort as well as lubricating the mouth to avoid drying and possible injury. Applying petroleum jelly to the lips is another protective measure that can be used.

Bleeding in noncompressible areas such as the lungs, esophagus, stomach, and intestines can be dangerous. The patient should be instructed not to strain during bowel movements and to avoid strong coughing and retching because these actions can promote bleeding episodes. Because bleeding from the rectum can result from excessive straining the patient should be encouraged to maintain an adequate fluid intake as well as to take stool softeners or bulk laxatives as ordered. Nose bleeds are common in these patients, and they should be instructed to avoid blowing their nose forcefully or picking at it. If the patient is nauseated, the nurse should provide antiemetics as ordered to prevent retching.

Protecting the patient from injury should also be part of the nursing plan, especially if the patient goes through periods of confusion from fever or other causes. Special precautionary measures should be followed to avoid injury including using padded bed rails during bedrest and assisting the patient when up. Injuries from falls or other environmental hazards can result in bleeding and hematoma formation. If fever is the cause of altered mentation, aggressive measures to reduce body temperatures should be initiated. However, acetaminophen (Tylenol) not aspirin, should be administered because aspirin increases bleeding time by reducing platelet adhesion and aggregation.[1] It can also cause gastric irritation and possible bleeding. Fevers may also accelerate platelet consumption, thus reducing already low platelet counts.

Measures to detect early bleeding include monitoring platelet counts regularly and obtaining and documenting vital signs and mentation every 4 hours. Tachycardia, hypotension, pallor, and diaphoresis may be indicative of internal hemorrhage. Changes in the level of consciousness (LOC), increasing restlessness, and tachycardia may indicate cerebral bleeding. Stools, urine, and emesis should be checked for signs of occult as well as frank bleeding, because internal bleeding may occur without evidence of frank blood.

When bleeding is detected or when blood counts are extremely low, transfusion therapy with red blood cells, platelets, or fresh whole blood may be prescribed. An important nursing function is to monitor the patient for signs of a hemolytic transfusion reaction such as fever, chills, flushing, itching, hypotension, tachycardia, and chest tightness. Fever and chills may be indicative of a reaction to leukocytes. The use of leukocyte-poor RBCs generally reduces the incidence of these reactions. Such reactions can easily be treated with acetamenophen and diphenhydramine. However, if the patient develops hypotension, tachycardia, and chest tightness, the transfusion should be stopped immediately and the physician contacted for an order of fluids and epinephrine. Platelet reactions are similar to leukocyte reactions, and the treatment is the same. Once the patient has begun to react to platelets, premedicate with diphenhydramine intravenously immediately prior to starting the transfusion.

Evaluation

Platelet counts should be maintained above 15,000 to 20,000 or above the level the individual patient needs to prevent spontaneous bleeding episodes. If platelet counts are adequate, the patient should not develop hematomas, hemoptysis, or rectal, GI, urinary tract, or vaginal bleeding, and will be able to carry out oral hygiene without signs of mucous membrane breakdown or bleeding. However, invasive procedures and injuries of any sort should be avoided until the platelet count reaches 50,000. For those who experience bleeding, early detection of the signs and symptoms such as tachycardia, hypotension, pallor, restlessness, diaphoresis, and altered mentation allows for the early initiation of therapeutic measures. Transfusion therapy should enable the patient to regain normal blood values, heart rate, blood pressure, and level of consciousness. Prompt treatment of any adverse reactions to transfusion therapy such as chills and fever or hypotension helps establish a normal body temperature, promote hemostasis, and prevent serious side-effects.

Inadequate Nutrition

Assessment and Nursing Diagnosis

The rapid proliferation of leukemic, lymphoma, or plasma cells in affected patients leads to increased metabolism which deprives the normal body cells of nutrients. This deficit is evidenced by signs of muscle wasting and weight loss and complaints of fatigue. Assessing the patient's nutritional status by monitoring weight and calorie intake can help reverse these signs and promote patient well-being.

Interventions

Providing adequate nutritional intake and rest to meet the body's increased metabolic needs becomes the nurse's goal for these patients. One way to achieve this goal is to offer high-protein, high-calorie foods in frequent small amounts. Small meals are often better tolerated than large quantities of food at one sitting. In addition to providing nutrients, it is important to monitor fluid intake and encourage the patient to drink approximately 5 liters of fluid daily to offset insensible fluid loss that is caused by increased metabolic rates. For patients who cannot eat sufficient amounts of food to meet nutritional needs, hyperalimentation and lipids may be prescribed. Hyperalimentation provides highly concentrated calories, vitamins, and minerals. Lipids provide the necessary fat components of the diet as well as extra calories.

In addition to increased nutritional intake, patients should be encouraged to avoid overactivity that could stress their systems and reduce their already low metabolic reserves. Signs of overexertion include increased heart rate, dyspnea, diaphoresis, and fatigue.

Evaluation

Adequate calorie intake and protein intake will be reflected in a stable weight, normal muscle mass, normal skin turgor, and normal neck veins. Fluid intake should be at least 500 ml greater than output daily. If the patient is diaphoretic, even more intake should be allowed. A balanced activity and rest schedule conserves energy and enables the patient to be active without experiencing dyspnea, tachycardia, or fatigue.

Central Nervous System Alterations

Assessment and Nursing Diagnosis

Leukemic or lymphomatous cell infiltration in the central nervous system (CNS) can cause the affected patient to develop cranial nerve abnormalities, convulsions, or even coma. The patient may complain of prolonged headaches and frequent vomiting.

Interventions

Nursing care of the patient with CNS involvement from these hematologic disorders is aimed toward the prevention of and early detection of the signs and symptoms of such involvement. One nursing function is to assist the physician with the administration of chemotherapeutic agents by lumbar puncture (intrathecally) or other procedures. These agents must be administered directly into the cerebral spinal fluid (CSF) to achieve therapeutic levels, as they do not cross the blood–brain barrier easily. Such procedures can be frightening to patients and should be explained thoroughly prior to starting. Some patients prefer to prepare mentally for the procedure for at least a full day, some require less time. Acknowledgment and respect of such requests help to promote patient cooperation.

Despite the use of intrathecal chemotherapy and cranial irradiation, some patients will develop CNS involvement. Early recognition of cranial nerve abnormalities, including being alert to complaints of prolonged headaches and frequent vomiting, allows for prompt diagnosis and initiation of therapy, thus enhancing the outcome. Patients should be assessed daily for these signs and symptoms. Changes in the patient's baseline behavior should be reported and followed up with a neurological examination if indicated.

Laboratory exam of the cerebrospinal fluid will verify the presence of leukemia or lymphoma cells, thus a diagnostic lumbar puncture is performed when CNS infiltration is suspected. The procedure may also be performed to verify the absence of CNS infiltration. Again, the nurse should provide the patient with a thorough explanation of the procedure, the reasons it is being performed, and the answers it will provide.

Evaluation

Careful assessment of the patient at risk may allow for early detection of the signs and symptoms of CNS infiltration prior to the development of seizures or coma. If diagnostic or therapeutic lumbar punctures are necessary, the patient should be cooperative during the procedure.

Side-Effects of Chemotherapy or Radiation Therapy

Assessment and Nursing Diagnosis

The goal of chemotherapy and radiation therapy is to destroy the rapidly dividing tumor cells. The side-effects of chemotherapy and radiation therapy are generally seen in those parts of the body that are composed of rapidly dividing cells such as the bone marrow, the gastrointestinal tract, the reproductive system, and hair follicles. Thus, the side-effects seen include: pancytopenia, mucositis, nausea, vomiting, diarrhea, hyperuricemia, alopecia, and sterility.

Interventions

Early recognition, documentation, and treatment of the side-effects of chemotherapy and radiotherapy are the major nursing goals in the care of these patients.

Interventions for pancytopenia and the resultant complications include monitoring the patient's WBC and platelet counts and hematocrit to detect pancytopenia early in its development. If these counts begin to drop abnormally low levels, the nurse should report these values to the physician who will usually discontinue therapy until the counts begin to rise. Blood component replacement and antibiotics will probably be ordered to help the patient through this critical time.

Mucositis. The mouth can be a major source of discomfort for these patients as mucositis is a common side-effect. The nurse should assess the mouth daily for areas of breakdown. Special attention should be given to the buccal region, the throat, gums, and under the tongue. Oral candida and herpes simplex virus (HSV) are common pathogens in oral infections and should be reported and cultured as soon as they are noted. Herpes simplex lesions are generally raised, red, or pustulant, whereas candida manifests as a generalized whitish coating and white plaques in the mouth. These infections usually occur in the neutropenic patient or the patient on antibiotics. Usually, the patient already has some mucositis, and the development of these infections can make their mouths quite painful. Thus, early recognition and treatment is well appreciated.

As always, prevention is the best cure, and patients should be encouraged to rinse their mouth with saline every 4 hours early in the treatment phase and increase the frequency to every 2 hours as mucositis begins to develop. Patients should be diligent about brushing their teeth with a soft toothbrush or sponge to prevent decay. Topical antifungal agents such as mycostatin may be ordered to prevent or treat candida infections. Topical anesthetics such as Diclomine or Zylocaine may be necessary to promote the aggressive mouth care that is so necessary for these patients. Dry, cracked lips are often a problem after radiotherapy, and petroleum jelly or other such ointments should be applied to lips as needed. Besides adding to patient discomfort, cracked lips easily become infected and so should be avoided. Mucositis and the oral infections that often accompany it can be very painful. The patient may require pain medication to promote comfort as well as to allow the patient to comply with the mouth-care regimen. Treatment may include topical anesthesia, narcotic boluses, or narcotic infusion.

Nausea, Vomiting, Diarrhea. The nausea, vomiting, and diarrhea experienced by these patients can be very distressing. The degree of nausea should be assessed every 2 hours during therapy and treated liberally both to promote patient comfort and to prevent retching which can cause esophageal tears. Commonly used antiemetics include: prochlorperazine maleate (Compazine), chlorpromazine hydrochloride (Thorazine), diphenylhydramine (Benadryl), droperidol (Inapsine), dexamethasone (Decadron), and metoclopramide (Reglan). The nurse should be aware of the side-effects of each antiemetic that is administered to the patient. For example, phenothiazines can cause hypotension and lethargy, making the patient more susceptible to falls and injury. When multiple antiemetics are administered, blood pressure should be monitored closely and safety measures such as assisting the patient when up, keeping siderails up, and frequent checks of mentation and level of consciousness should be employed. Metoclopramide and droperidol may cause extrapyramidal symptoms. These symptoms, which present as tongue swelling, dysphagia, dystonia, or hyperexcitability, are uncomfortable and potentially dangerous. They should be treated promptly with diphenhydramine 25 to 50 mg IV. Often, relaxation can potentiate antiemetic therapy. Thus, comfort measures such as cool cloths, reduction of environmental stimulation, frequent mouth care, massages, and relaxation tapes or other relaxation techniques should be employed by the nurse.

Antidiarrheals such as diphenoxylate hydrochloride (Lomotil), loperamide hydrochloride (Imodium), and tincture of opium should be administered liberally, within limits of the physician's order. If, despite such medications, diarrhea continues, perianal care should be given following each bowel movement to prevent skin breakdown and infection. Perianal abscess is a serious complication of frequent diarrhea and skin breakdown. Towelettes, soft cloths, or facial tissue are softer than toilet tissue and should be used instead of it. Sitz baths and local heat may be ordered to promote healing. Topical anesthetics may be used if the irritation becomes painful. Hypovolemia and electrolyte imbalance can result from frequent vomiting and diarrhea. The nurse should maintain a strict intake and output, and the patient should be weighed daily. If the patient cannot maintain an oral fluid intake to equal the loss, fluid replacement may be necessary. Large amounts of emesis can result in alkalosis and hypochloremia; large amounts of diarrhea can result in acidosis and hypokalemia. Thus, the nurse should monitor electrolytes and acid–base status as available and report abnormal values. All stools and emesis should be tested for guaiac because the mucosal damage from chemotherapy or radiotherapy makes these tissues more susceptible to trauma from emesis and diarrhea.

Renal Problems. Uric acid is released from the cells that are destroyed, serum uric acid levels can become elevated. The nursing goals related to the resultant hyperuricemia center around the prevention of renal damage. The renal damage results from the accumulation of uric acid crystals in the renal tubules. Large amounts of urine output prevent this accumulation by diluting and enhancing the excretion of uric acid crystals. The nurse should provide the patient with 3 to 4 liters of oral or IV hydration daily, as prescribed. Uric acid crystals can be prevented from forming by Allopurinol or alkalinization of the urine with sodium bicarbonate or acetazolamide (Diamox).[14] The nurse should administer these agents as prescribed. If renal damage does occur, it will be evidenced by elevated serum creatinine and BUN levels. They should be monitored as available, and abnormal values reported to the physician.

Alopecia. Alopecia is another common side-effect of therapy. The goal of care is aimed at preparing the patient for the potential loss of hair and thus allow the patient to begin coping with this problem early. The nurse should discuss some of the options the patient has to provide him or her with some control over this situation. Because hair does not fall out evenly, the patient may choose to shave it off once it starts falling out. Whether or not the head is shaved, the patient may use head coverings such as wigs, scarves, or hats to improve appearance. The patient should also be assured that the hair loss is not permanent, but that the texture and color of the regrowth hair may be different.

Sexual Function. Radiation and certain chemotherapy medications have the potential of causing sterility. The goal of the nurses caring for a patient who is just beginning treatment should be to inform the patient and family of this potential, thus allowing them to begin planning strategies to cope with sterility. Males approaching their reproductive years should be provided information about sperm banks if one is available in the area. During therapy, however, sexually active men and women should be encouraged to use birth control measures. Sterility does not occur in everyone, and radiotherapy and some chemotherapy can be detrimental to the developing fetus.

Evaluation

Potential side-effects of chemotherapy and radiotherapy should be observed for and detected early, thus allowing for prompt intervention, reducing the severity of the symptoms. Anemia, neutropenia, and thrombocytopenia should be detected and treated as soon as these counts become abnormal. The patient should report only minimal discomfort from mucositis and oral infections after the appropriate interventions have been taken. Treatment should result in a regression of oral lesions.

The patient who develops vomiting or diarrhea should be maintained at a normal intravascular volume with the appropriate crystalloid solution as evidenced by a balance intake and output, stable weight, normal neck veins and skin turgor, and the absence of orthostatic blood pressure and heart rate changes. Serum potassium, CO_2, and chloride should also remain within the normal limits. The patient should report complete relief of nausea from antiemetics, experience no retching, and be able to eat 100% of daily caloric and nutritional needs.

Protective measures instituted for the patient who becomes drowsy should be effective enough to prevent all falls or other injuries. If extrapyramidal symptoms occur (swelling of tongue, dysphagia, dystonia or hyperexcitability) they will be recognized and treated immediately. Gastrointestinal bleeding will be recognized as soon as it develops. The patient who still has diarrhea despite antidiarrheal treatment will not develop perianal excoriation, breakdown, or infection.

If alkalinization of urine is the goal, the urine pH will be maintained at greater than 7.0. Creatinine and BUN should remain normal during treatment, but if any elevations of these values occur, they will be reported immediately.

Patients should prepare feasible plans of action to cope with alopecia and with sterility prior to the occurrence of either of these side-effects of therapy.

Alterations in Comfort

Assessment and Nursing Diagnosis

Leukemic cell infiltrates and the side-effects of antileukemic therapy can potentially cause alterations in patient comfort. Leukemic infiltration of bones and joints can cause arthralgias and complaints of pain in these areas. Infiltrations in the spleen and liver result in abdominal pain. The patient who develops CNS infiltrations will complain of headache and photophobia. Chemotherapy and radiotherapy can cause mucositis and dysphagia. The severity of pain ranges from mild to severe.

Interventions

The goal of the nurse caring for the patient who is in pain is to control it effectively enough that the patient is able to perform activities of daily living (ADLs) independently. This should be accomplished with the minimum of side-effects such as hypotension, respiratory depression, constipation, and narcotic tolerance. Measures such as relaxation, diversion, massage, bathing, or the application of heat or cold can be used to enhance the effects of analgesics, possibly reducing the amount of medication necessary to control the pain. However, the use of tranquilizers should be avoided because they tend to only increase the sedative effect, but not the analgesic effect of pain medications, such as morphine.[4] The level of pain a patient is experiencing should be assessed daily. Early treatment of pain is generally more successful and requires less analgesia than pain that has been allowed to escalate. The location, character, and duration of pain should be documented to aid in the diagnosis of specific areas of infiltration. Precipitating factors such as coughing, retching, hiccups, movement, noise, or light should also be documented. This information can be used to determine if certain physical or environmental manipulations will reduce the frequency of pain episodes.

Initial drug treatment should be with mild analgesia such as acetaminophen (Tylenol) or propoxyphene (Darvon) to reduce the chances of side-effects or narcotic tolerance. If more potent analgesics become necessary, morphine sulfate is the narcotic of choice, although meperidine hydrochloride (Demerol) and hydromorphone hydrochloride (Dilaudid) are also used. During periods of acute or prolonged severe pain, analgesics should be administered routinely within the limits of the prescription, rather than on a prn basis. Intervals of pain and of pain relief are inherent in prn scheduling. The patient is conditioned to seek analgesia after a specific period of time, reinforcing drug-dependent behavior. In addition, higher doses of narcotics are necessary for pain relief once the pain becomes severe than are needed for the relief of pain that is kept at tolerable levels.[2] The use of morphine infusion should be considered if the patient requires morphine intravenous injections every 1 to 2 hours. Often, less morphine is required over a 24-hour period once a constant infusion is begun.[2] Respiratory rate and blood pressure should be monitored in any patient receiving narcotic analgesia. Respiratory rate less than 10 bpm may not be sufficient for proper oxygenation and ventilation. Depending on the patient, a systolic blood pressure drop of 10% or more may compromise peripheral or vital organ perfusion. If blood pressure drops to less than 90 mmHg systolic, measures such as fluids, raising the foot of the bed, and lowering the narcotic dose should be employed. Nalaxone (Narcon), a narcotic antagonist, should only be used if absolutely necessary because the pain will return as soon as it is given. Patients receiving narcotics should be encouraged to take up to 3 liters of fluid daily, eat a high bulk diet, and take stool softeners if prescribed to prevent the constipation that is often a problem with these drugs. The nurse should monitor the frequency of bowel movements.

Pain is a highly individual and subjective perception. Establishing trust with the patient by attempting to understand the patient's perceptions can help to decrease anxiety and in turn reduce pain. The nurse should verbally and nonverbally convey to the patient that his or her pain is understood and efforts will be made to control it, and should avoid being judgmental about the patient's pain.

Evaluation

The patient who has been experiencing pain should get sufficient relief from pain management interventions that he or she is able to perform ADLs independently without major discomfort. If narcotic analgesia is necessary, the patient's respiratory rate should remain above 9 bpm and blood pressure should remain within 90% of baseline. Level of consciousness and mentation should remain unimpaired. The bowel program should result in a soft, formed bowel movement daily or every other day.

Ineffective Coping

Assessment and Nursing Diagnosis

The diagnosis and treatment of a life-threatening disease usually results in changes in the person's body image. This can lead to alterations in the emotional well-being of the patient and may be evidenced by changes in relationships with significant others. Often, communication is strained because family members are attempting to protect each other's emotions. Many times, the patient or other family members are unable to express feelings of frustration, anger, pain, or fear of loss, because they feel guilty that they even have these feelings.

Interventions

The goal of nurses caring for patients and families facing a life-threatening disease and its treatment is to encourage them to verbalize their questions, expectations, and desires related to the disease and treatment plan. They should be encouraged to do this both with the nurse and with each other.

Numerous factors determine the patient's and the family's response to illness and treatment. These include physical, psychological, emotional, cultural, spiritual, and social factors. The nurse's assessment shall include all these factors to ensure that nursing interventions will be well-received by the patient and family. The establishment of a trusting relationship between the nurse, the patient, and the family helps to reduce patient anxiety and promote well-being and compliance with the treatment regimen. This can be accomplished through consistent patient assignments, primary nursing, open communication, supportive care, and by spending nontask-oriented time with the patient and family.

Once a trusting relationship has been established, the nurse can identify and document the coping mechanisms that the patient and family members are using. Nurses may not agree with the coping mechanisms employed by some patients and families, but must remember that their coping mechanisms are helping to reduce their anxiety. Even anger and denial may be important coping mechanisms and may need to be supported or worked through. Referrals to other health-care team workers, such as social workers, clergy, support groups, home health nurse, and psychosocial clinical nurse specialists should be initiated when appropriate.

As the patient moves through the health care system, it is important to provide consistent and thorough information so other health-team workers are prepared to care for the patient as an individual. The care plan is an ideal medium for the communication of individualized information.

During the patient's hospitalization, the family can sense the patient's feelings of helplessness and isolation. They should be encouraged to become involved in the care of the patient, doing things such as bathing the patient, preparing some foods, assisting with turning or ambulating, and doing dressing changes.

Often, patients and families have either unrealistic goals or have a sense of utter hopelessness. The nurse should elicit the expectations they have of treatment and in turn reiterate consistent information about the probable outcomes for the individual. Often, the family and patient have set such long-term and high goals that they lose sight of the progress the patient may be making. The nurse should assist the patient and family in setting and adhering to realistic goals throughout the treatment course. Achievement of these goals will foster hope which will permit the patient and family to plan for the future.[14]

There will always be patients who fail the treatment regimens. The nurse must be able to recognize the time to change the focus of care from cure to palliation, and support the family and patient through this difficult time. If discussions about the possibility of death have not already occurred, the family should be encouraged to do so at this time, both among themselves and with the patient.

Evaluation

With the encouragement of the nurse and other health-care team workers, the patient and family should be able to verbalize feelings of anger, denial, frustration, fear, or hope. Members of the family should be active participants during the course of treatment, helping the patient through daily routines and difficult times. They should have hope for success if that is appropriate for the patient, but if treatment is unsuccessful and the patient dies, they should be ready to accept the death when it occurs.

Knowledge Deficit

Assessment and Nursing Diagnosis

The patient and family who do not cooperate with lab tests, treatments, or in learning skills in preparation for discharge home usually behave so out of lack of understanding of the disease or its treatment. Fear often results from lack of knowledge, hence their unwillingness to cooperate with procedures or medications that seems strange to them or that they think will harm them.

Interventions

The goal of the nurse is to provide the family and patient with information on the disease, treatment, and related procedures in language they can understand. The learning atmosphere should be such that they feel comfortable asking questions. The information provided should be thorough enough that the patient or family can give informed consent for and actively participate in the therapeutic regimen.

Patient education on the disease process and treatment should begin at the time of admission to the hospital or with the first contact in an outpatient setting, giving ample opportunity for repetition. This helps the patient and family assimilate the information over time.[14] All tests and procedures must be explained prior to initiating them, especially those associated with discomfort such as lumbar punctures and bone marrow aspirations. This allows the patient time to prepare and to mobilize coping mechanisms. Relaxation techniques for use in stressful or painful situations can provide the patient with a sense of control. Some techniques may be more successful than others for an individual patient, thus several should be taught. These include rhythmic breathing, guided imagery, progressive muscle relaxation, and massage. The patient should be encouraged to practice these techniques in nonstressful situations.

Because infections can progress so rapidly with disastrous consequences, families should be instructed in the prevention and detection of infection. Instruction should include the importance of thorough and frequent handwashing, avoiding crowds and anyone with colds, flu, or other communicable diseases, and reporting any such exposure to the physician. The patient should keep regular dental appointments. Infections can still occur despite measures to prevent them. The family and patient must be taught to recognize deviations from normal temperature, bowel or bladder habits, energy level, respiratory function, and general appearance.

Bleeding may still be a potential complication once the patient is discharged. The patient and family must be taught to apply the measures used to prevent bleeding to their own habits and lifestyle. These measures include: avoidance of aggressive exercise of contact sports when the platelet count is less than 50,000. Patients should not use straight-edge razors to shave. They should not take rectal temperatures, use suppositories, enemas, vaginal suppositories, or tampons. Patients should be given a bowel program to help them avoid constipation. For dental hygiene, they should use a soft toothbrush. Dental floss should only be used if they can avoid trauma to their gums.

Teaching should always be done in a comfortable, quiet environment with adequate time given for return demonstrations, repetitions, and questions. The teaching plan should be adjusted toward the patient's and family's individual learning styles, including techniques most useful to them, such as reading, visual aids, demonstration/return demonstration, or verbal discussion.

Evaluation

The patient and family should be able to state in their own words what the disease process and treatment involve and how this will influence their lifestyle. An understanding of the pending procedures, the reasons for it, and the expected outcomes should lead to cooperation during the procedure. The patient should be able to perform relaxation techniques without coaching during stressful or painful procedures or other situations.

Once the patient is ready to be discharged, the family and patient should be able to perform the necessary motor skills independently. The patient and family must be able to repeat how they can best avoid infections and bleeding and how to detect the symptoms if these complications do occur.

Multiple Myeloma

Definition and Classification

Multiple myeloma is a neoplastic disease of plasma cells in which mature and immature plasma cells proliferate progressively and uncontrollably. Symptoms result from their infiltration in the bone marrow, lymph nodes, liver, spleen, and kidneys as well as the destruction of bone tissue. Incidence in the United States is about one to two per 100,000 in Caucasians and two to four per 100,000 in blacks. The mean age at time of diagnosis is 62 years.

Etiology

The cause of multiple myeloma is not known. As with leukemia and the lymphomas, there is an increased incidence of myeloma in Hiroshima survivors.

Pathophysiology

A widespread proliferation of the malignant plasma cells occurs in the bone marrow, with ensuing destruction of bone. Anemia, leukopenia, and thrombocytopenia result as marrow is progressively involved. Products of the myeloma cells suppress immune function, thus predisposing the patient to infection. Myeloma cells overproduce certain proteins and their constituent polypeptide chains (M-components). The overproduction of M-components is responsible for the hyperviscosity syndrome, cryoglobulinemia, amyloidosis, and other hemostatic abnormalities. Renal failure results from an excretion of monoclonal light chains by the myeloma cells.

Clinical Manifestations

The onset of multiple myeloma is usually gradual and insidious and is usually preceded by an asymptomatic period that may last from 5 to 20 years. During the asymptomatic period, the only manifestations of the disease may be an elevated sedimentation rate, unexplained proteinuria, or an M-component on serum electrophoresis. Recurrent infections, weakness, and weight loss herald progression of the disease. Ultimately, the skeletal system is involved and chronic renal disease develops. Skeletal system involvement classically produces low back pain as well as swelling, tenderness, unrelenting pain, and pathologic fractures. Height may decrease by several inches due to recurrent compression fractures of the thoracic and lumbar vertebrae. Characteristic osteolytic changes may show up on x-ray films. Early in the disease, a picture of diffuse osteoporosis may be seen.

The major cause of death and common initial finding is an increased susceptibility to infection. A substance released from the myeloma cell indirectly suppresses normal B-cell function. This factor combined with granulocytopenia due to either marrow involvement or chemotherapy produce the susceptibility to infection.

Chronic renal failure is common in the later stages of the disease. It is caused by a number of factors, but primarily by the filtration of large amounts of Bence Jones proteins through the glomeruli into the proximal renal tubules. Eventually, tubular function is impaired by the accumulation of these proteinaceous bodies. Hypercalcemia due to bone destruction predisposes to hypercalcinuria and the development of renal stones. Hyperuricemia from increased cellular turnover results in uric acid crystallization and subsequently obstruction in the renal tubules, adding to renal failure. Neurologic involvement is manifested as compression of the spinal cord causing paraplegia or as direct involvement of nerve tissue causing neuropathies and cranial nerve abnormalities. Confusion, delirium, and coma may result from hypercalcemic encephalopathy.

Patients with multiple myeloma may complain of undue sensitivity to cold. The hyperviscosity syndrome from a high concentration of blood proteins interferes with circulation to the brain, eyes, kidneys, and digits. Confusion and other central nervous system symptoms may develop suddenly as a result of this syndrome.

Most patients with multiple myeloma develop anemia and leukopenia secondary to chemotherapy. Platelet counts are usually normal but platelet function may be abnormal leading to bleeding tendencies.

Medical Management

Diagnosis. Diagnosis of multiple myeloma is based on marrow aspiration and biopsy in which plasma cells or myeloma cells can be identified. Bone or tissue biopsies with plasmocytoma are also diagnostic for multiple myeloma. Myeloma protein may be demonstrable in the plasma or urine. X-ray films show osteolytic lesions or osteoporosis. Multiple myeloma may be present in peripheral blood smears.

Treatment. Treatment of multiple myeloma is aimed at relieving symptoms, reducing tumor mass, controlling pain, and treating the complications. Cure of multiple myeloma is not a realistic goal. Chemotherapy is the treatment of choice and generally consists of melphalan or cyclophosphamide. Some combination regimens that include vincristine have been found to induce remission better than single drug therapy. Localized radiotherapy is used in multiple myeloma in the setting of painful bone lesions with subsequent prompt relief of pain, healing of fractures, and at times, prevention of cord compression.

Relief of pain is often difficult in myeloma patients but can sometimes be achieved with aspirin or codeine, although frequently meperidine or morphine is necessary. Mobilization of these patients is necessary to prevent further bone demineralization, hypercalcemia, hypercalciuria, renal stones, and potential renal damage. However mobilization is a major challenge as the patient is usually afraid of the ensuing pain and possible pathological fractures. These are very real concerns which can be diminished by providing the patient with an analgesic prior to ambulation and always accompanying the patient when he or she is out of bed. Sodium fluoride therapy causes positive calcium balance, increased bone mineralization, and some patients have reported a decrease in pain. Patients treated with dichloromethylene diphosphate (CL_2MDP) have shown a dramatic decrease in bone demineralization and a decrease in the urinary excretion of calcium. Both treatments have side-effects that the patient may not be able to tolerate.

Patients with multiple myeloma also require large amounts of hydrating fluid to prevent calcium, uric acid, and protein accumulation in the renal tubules. Hypercalcemia may also be treated with 1) saline infusions which promote calcium excretion, 2) prednisone, 3) phosphate, 4) furosemide, and 5) mithromycin if the hypercalcemia is accompanied by nausea and vomiting.

Renal failure can be prevented or its onset delayed if the hyperuricemia and hyperuricosuria are treated with adequate fluids and allopurinol to prevent uric acid crystallization. Hemo or peritoneal dialysis may be necessary as renal function decreases. Anemia and infections are treated with blood transfusions and antibiotics, respectively. Spinal cord compression is a medical emergency and requires immediate surgical decompression, followed by local radiotherapy.

Prognosis. Chemotherapy and radiotherapy can induce at least partial remission of multiple myeloma and may prolong life. Median survival is now 2 to 4 years with the treatment described above. The prognosis of multiple myeloma has shown a marked improvement since the introduction of alkylating agents to the treatment plan. Cause of death in multiple myeloma is generally due to infection.

Nursing Management

Assessment and Nursing Diagnosis

Patients with multiple myeloma suffer from severe bone pain, especially with movement. Because of this, the tendency is for them to stay in bed, immobilized. As a result, patients with multiple myeloma are at an increased risk for pulmonary atelectasis and infections. Also, immobility adds to the tendency toward osteoporosis already present in patients with this disorder. Thus, already brittle bones are further weakened and the potential for spontaneous bone fractures is increased. Osteoporosis also results in an increased calcium reabsorption from the bones into the blood and urine. Hypercalciuria enhances the formation of renal stones and potentially severe renal damage.

The formal nursing diagnoses can therefore be summarized as pain; activity intolerance, immobilization, ineffective breathing patterns, potential for injury from spontaneous fractures or falls, altered urinary elimination patterns, and potential for infection.

Pancytopenia is also a problem in patients with multiple myeloma as the proliferating plasma cells infiltrate the marrow and suppress other marrow functions. Thus, the potential for infections, bleeding, and anemia is present and should be managed as discussed earlier.

Goals. The major goal of medical therapy is to reduce the tumor mass. The potential problems and nursing interventions of chemo- and radiotherapy have been discussed earlier in this chapter.

A major goal in the nursing management of these patients is the control of pain. Chemo- and radiotherapy can reduce pain by reducing the tumor burden. However, pain is often very severe and other measures are often necessary to prevent or control the pain.

Mobilization of the patient is essential for the prevention of complications such as advanced osteoporosis and renal failure. Only the possibility of spinal cord compression from spinal fractures should prevent these patients from walking.

Large amounts of fluid intake are necessary to keep the kidneys flushed and prevent renal calculi and renal failure. Patients should maintain a urine output of at least 1500 ml every 24 hours.

Intervention

Control of pain in the patient with multiple myeloma can be very challenging. Morphine infusion is the drug of choice in the hospital because it has fewer side-effects than other analgesics. Morphine infusions are maintained at the level the patient requires to prevent pain or keep it a tolerable level for performing activities of daily living. The patient may also be placed on oral analgesics consisting of methadone, morphine, or codeine. It is important to remember to ask the patient when admitted to the hospital how much medication he or she has been taking at home. The nurse should attempt to provide an equivalent amount of the pain medication ordered in the hospital. Many of these patients are on massive amounts of pain medication at home, and as such will not suffer from respiratory depression and hypotension at doses that would depress other patients.

Ambulation of these patients is also a real challenge as it is very painful for the patient. In addition to pain, they often also have a great fear of falling and breaking brittle bones as they are usually unsteady on their feet. Analgesics can be administered in advance so that the peak effect occurs during the ambulation. It usually takes oral medications one-half hour and intravenous medications a few minutes to begin to exert their analgesic effects. Orthopedic braces can be used to support the patient if needed. It is important to accompany the patient any time he or she is up out of bed to prevent accidents or falls.

Hydration can be achieved orally or with intravenous fluids. A patient with multiple myeloma may require up to 3 to 4 liters of fluid per day to prevent renal calculi from developing. Corticosteroids and mithramycin are administered to patients with severe hypercalcemia associated with nausea and vomiting. The nurse should be aware of changes in the blood urea nitrogen and creatinine if they are ordered.

In the hospital, the patient should be assessed at least daily for signs of increasing tumor mass, especially around the spinal area. The development of paraplegia in these patients is a medical emergency. The patient's tumor must be resected and the patient treated with chemo- and radiotherapy.

Patient teaching and emotional support are extremely important. Patients must be aware of the signs and symptoms of infection, spontaneous bone fractures, renal failure, and increasing tumor mass.

Evaluation

The patient should be pain free or the pain should be controlled enough so the patient can carry on activities of daily living. Pain control should be achieved without signs of oversedation such as respiratory rate lower than 10 per minute. Blood pressure should not drop by more than 10% of the patient's normal pressure.

The patient should ambulate at least twice a day and be up in a chair at least twice in addition. This should be accomplished without excessive pain to the patient and without injury.

Hydration should be kept at a sufficient level to maintain a urine output of at least 1500 ml per 24 hours. Creatinine and BUN should remain within normal values.

Signs of increasing tumor mass will be identified early and medical help sought promptly, thus preventing permanent paraplegia or other problems.

Patients should be allowed to go through the grieving process and then accept their disease and work to improve the quality of their life with family and friends.

Splenic Disorders

Definition and Classification

Splenic enlargement or splenomegaly may be idiopathic or it may be the first and only sign of a disease process. Thus, although patients with splenomegaly should be examined to determine the cause of enlargement, in some cases no known ill effects result from it. The term hypersplenism has been used in the past to identify disorders linked with splenomegaly such as anemia, leukopenia, or thrombocytopenia. Lacking any other cause for these disorders, it was thought that the spleen was responsible for destroying or sequestering one or more of the cellular elements of the blood in large quantities. However, with increasing knowledge, it has been found that most disorders that were once attributed to hypersplenism are in fact due to another organ or tissue. Thus, the term hypersplenism is not used as often now as it once was since it is not specific enough in most cases.

Etiology

The causes of splenomegaly are varied. Infections, metabolic, circulatory, endocrine, neoplastic, and mechanical disorders can all cause splenomegaly. During an infectious or inflammatory process the spleen may enlarge due to increasing numbers of reticuloendothelial cells which clear bacteria, protozoa, and damaged cells from the blood. Increasing antibody production during an infectious process may enlarge the spleen as well. Many chronic infections are associated with splenomegaly. All of the following may be associated with an enlarged spleen: tuberculosis, syphilis, rheumatoid arthritis, malaria, and some fungal and protozoal infections.

The spleen may enlarge secondary to removing large quantities of abnormal blood cells from the circulation. This enlargement can be considered a hypertrophy due to an increased workload. Some causes of the so-called hyperplastic splenomegaly include: various forms of anemia, myelofibrosis, primary splenic neutropenia and pancytopenia, hereditary spherocytosis, idiopathic thrombocytopenic purpura, and tropical splenomegaly. In certain conditions, such as Gaucher's disease, lipedema, gargoylism, and others, splenomegaly may be the result of macrophage engorgement by indigestible materials.

Cysts and neoplasms may enlarge the spleen. Sarcomas of the spleen are usually associated with lymphosarcoma, follicular sarcoma, reticulum cell sarcoma, or Hodgkin's sarcoma. Lung, breast, skin, and cervical carcinomas may metastasize to the spleen.

Portal hypertension can be associated with a chronic congestive splenomegaly and ensuing anemia and leukopenia. Cirrhosis of the liver, thrombosis, or stenosis of the portal vein or splenic vein can all cause chronic congestive splenomegaly.

Pathophysiology

The functions of the spleen include: 1) purifying the blood of bacteria; 2) purifying the blood of antigens and developing antibodies to them; 3) hematopoiesis in the fetus; in adults, hematopoiesis in the spleen is abnormal and only occurs in persons with bone marrow suppression and pancytopenia; 4) destroying red blood cells when they reach the end of their 120-day life span; 5) destroys fragile or defective RBCs; 6) some iron metabolism; 7) removing particulate inclusions from red blood cells without destroying the cell itself.

An enlarged spleen can sequester or destroy large numbers of red cells, white cells, and platelets. Splenomegaly does not necessarily cause a reduction in red cell survival time. Rather, the anemia seen is most probably due to an increase in the total plasma volume resulting in a dilutional anemia. However, the leukopenia and neutropenia associated with splenomegaly are probably due to an increased destruction of white blood cells as well as to increased sequestration. Thrombocytopenia associated with splenomegaly is probably due to sequestration more than destruction.

Clinical Manifestations

Leukopenia, anemia, and thrombocytopenia are the most common laboratory findings in splenomegaly. The low white cell, red cell, and platelet counts are most often due to the underlying disease process causing the splenomegaly but may also be due to sequestration or destruction of these blood cells by the spleen.

The patient may complain of abdominal pain or fullness due to the pressure of the enlarged spleen on surrounding organs. A mass in the left upper quadrant may be palpated. Patients may also complain of lassitude, weakness, and malaise due to the reduction of red blood cells. Leukopenia predisposes patients to infections. Thus, the patient may note an increased number of infections, and slow-healing, easily infected cuts. Thrombocytopenia below 50,000/mm^3 increases the risk for bleeding. The patient may notice that an unusually long time is required for cuts to stop bleeding, that he or she bruises easily, and may even develop bloody stools, oozing gums, heavy menstrual bleeding, and other unusual bleeding tendencies. Laboratory bleeding times may or may not be prolonged, depending on the level of thrombocytopenia. Other signs and symptoms of leukopenia, anemia, and thrombocytopenia are discussed in the section on Leukemia. Other laboratory studies may be abnormal but are related to the underlying cause of the splenomegaly rather than splenomegaly alone, and thus are not discussed here.

Medical Management

Diagnosis. A palpable mass in the left upper quadrant may be due to an enlarged spleen or cysts or tumors on other organs in close proximity. An enlarge spleen is not always palpable so other diagnostic studies should be performed rather than relying solely on palpation.

Angiography may be used to distinguish between splenic cysts and tumors and nonsplenic tumors. Scans of the spleen, including ultrasound and CT scans are very accurate in determining spleen size. X-ray films are often misleading because the spleen may not be visible even when enlarged.

To determine the amount of splenic sequestration or cell destruction ^{51}Cr-labeled red cells or platelets are used. To assess the degree of red cell pooling a ratio of total body to venous blood hematocrit may be determined. Splenic mixing curves are also used to assess the degree of red cell pooling.

Splenic puncture may or may not be included in the diagnostic testing. Although, the findings can help confirm the results of other tests, in many instances they are nondiagnostic or misleading.

Treatment. As discussed above, splenomegaly is generally due to an underlying disease process. Thus, treating the underlying disease process will often result in a reduction of spleen size. In some instances splenectomy may be indicated. Using the broadest of terms, splenectomy is indicated when the spleen is destroying blood cells and not indicated when it is producing antibodies or acting as a hematopoietic organ. Specifically, splenectomy is generally beneficial in patients with hereditary spherocytosis, idiopathic thrombocytopenic purpura, acquired hemolytic disease, and in some patients with congestive splenomegaly. It can be useful in staging for Hodgkin's disease and non-Hodgkin's lymphomas. In cases where the cause of the splenomegaly was unclear and neutropenia or pancytopenia was part of the picture, splenectomy has shown favorable results as well as helping in the diagnosis of the disease process. In other diseases of the blood, splenectomy may or may not be useful, thus the indications are not clearly defined.

Traumatic splenic rupture is a common indication for splenectomy. However, few physicians are using rupture as an automatic indication for splenectomy because of the increased chance for fulminant sepsis following the splenectomy.

If possible, splenectomy should be avoided in children as the spleen is the major source of antibody formation in children. If the splenectomy is absolutely necessary, the child may be placed on prophylactic antibiotics to prevent infection. Some centers are avoiding the complications associated with chronic antibiotic use by sending children home without antibiotics and instructing parents to bring the child to the Emergency Department if the child's temperature rises to 102°F or higher.[11]

Prognosis. The prognosis of splenic disorders generally depends on the underlying disease process. The prognosis of those patients who receive a splenectomy depends not only on the underlying disease process, but on the risks associated with the splenectomy itself. Until recently the spleen was considered to be a nonessential organ. Since the mid-1950s, however, it has become obvious the patients of all ages who have their spleen removed are at risk for developing the postsplenectomy syndrome. Infants and young children have a particularly high incidence of this syndrome.

The postsplenectomy syndrome is characterized by septicemic infection, frequently with meningeal involvement. Fever is usually 104°F or higher. The infection is often fulminant, and death can ensue within 12 to 24 hours of onset. The most common pathogen is pneumococci, although hemophilus influenzae and meningococci may be found in some cases. Those patients at greatest risk for developing the postsplenectomy syndrome are children under 3 to 4 years of age and those patients who have underlying immunodeficiency disorders. The immune system of children under 3 to 4 years is not mature enough to make large amounts of antibodies against encapsulated organisms such as the pneumococcus. However, unlike macrophages from the liver, splenic macrophages can phagocytize these organisms and thus compensate for the lack of antibody. Without a spleen these organisms proliferate rapidly and cause overwhelming infections. Adults who are immunodeficient from the underlying disease or its treatment such as Hodgkin's disease are also at higher risk for developing the postsplenectomy syndrome. There may also be an increased risk for myocardial infarction following splenectomy in men. It is thought that the increased numbers of platelets found in patients following a splenectomy may predispose them to myocardial infarction.

Patients who have had a splenectomy secondary to traumatic rupture or laceration seem to be at a lower risk of complications. Small, functional spleens have been found in some of these patients years later. The spleen is known to regenerate itself if it is only partially resected and it is thought that in traumatic splenectomies some pieces of splenic tissue may be left behind. If these pieces of tissue receive a blood supply they can regenerate.

Nursing Management

Assessment and Nursing Diagnosis

The patient with splenic disorders is usually neutropenic, thrombocytopenic, anemic, or pancytopenic. These patients are at high risk for the development of infections, bleeding, lethargy, and other signs and symptoms described in the general nursing management section in this chapter. If a splenectomy is performed, the patient is at high risk for developing the postsplenectomy syndrome characterized by high fevers, shocklike state with a low blood pressure and frequently accompanied by a meningeal infection. This syndrome can occur early or late following splenectomy. Immediately following the surgery, patients are at high risk for bleeding due to low platelet counts at the time of surgery. Occasionally, the thrombocytopenia persists following the splenectomy, though in most patients it is resolved by surgery. Patients may, on the other hand, develop high platelet counts that predispose them to thrombosis. The patient who has a splenectomy secondary to trauma may also have other foci of internal bleeding and should be observed closely for hemorrhagic shock. Other problems common in surgical patients can also occur in these patients.

Abdominal distention can be a problem as other organs such as the stomach or intestines move to fill the space left by the spleen.

Goals. The major goal of care following a splenectomy is early recognition of the postsplenectomy syndrome. Patients and families should be instructed on how to recognize these symptoms and what they should do about them. The goal for patients with a low platelet count is early recognition and prevention of bleeding. Patients with high platelet counts should be observed for signs of thrombosis such as cold mottled extremities; strokes, with changes in level of consciousness and hemiplegia; myocardial infarction accompanied by chest pain, arrhythmias, and drop in blood pressure; abdominal pain or discomfort or postprandial cramping secondary to mesenteric thrombosis. Early recognition of these signs of thrombosis allows for early intervention and may reduce the severity of the residual impairment. Early recognition of internal bleeding in the patient with a splenectomy secondary to trauma may prevent the development of hemorrhagic shock. The nurse should observe the patient for a drop in blood pressure; elevation in the heart rate; cool, clammy skin; abdominal distention; and abdominal pain. Early recognition of abdominal distention due to other organs filling in the upper quadrant allows the nurse to intervene early and to prevent patient discomfort.

Interventions

If the patient begins to demonstrate signs of the postsplenectomy syndrome, the physician should be contacted for antibiotic therapy. The nurse should obtain blood, urine, sputum, and other cultures as ordered. Antibiotics should be initiated as soon as they are ordered, on a STAT basis, but after the cultures are obtained. Steroids may be ordered, but their use is still controversial in septic shock. If they are ordered, doses of 10 to 15 mg/kg of Solu-Medrol or the equivalent are not uncommon. The patient and family should be instructed to be suspicious of any high fever and contact the physician immediately. In some centers, patients are taught to come into the Emergency Department to be evaluated for any fever over 102°F.

Internal bleeding can be treated by whole blood administration, and if platelets are low, platelet infusions. A patient who continues to bleed should be taken to surgery to correct the source of bleeding.

The patient who develops signs and symptoms of thrombosis should be placed on heparin therapy and then observed for bleeding or oozing. Some patients may be placed on prophylactic low-dose heparin. They, also, should be observed for signs of bleeding or oozing and partial thromboplastin times or bleeding times watched carefully. If mesenteric thrombosis occurs, small bowel resection is usually necessary.

An abdominal binder can help relieve abdominal distention as can neostigmine 0.5 to 1.0 mg subcutaneous or intramuscular every 4 to 6 hours for 2 to 3 days.

Evaluation

The patient should remain afebrile and free of temperature spikes. If antibiotics are needed for high fevers, the patient should improve with their administration. Blood pressure should remain within the patient's normal limits. Patients should be free of the signs and symptoms of bleeding (*i.e.,* blood pressure and heart rate should be within normal limits and there should not be any abdominal distention or pain). The patient should be free of any signs or symptoms of thrombosis, such as abdominal pain or discomfort, or postprandial cramping, level of consciousness should be stable, and the patient should be able to move all four extremities without problems. The patient should be free of any chest pain or discomfort, arrhythmias and blood pressure and heart rate should be within the patient's normal limits. Extremities should be warm and pink. If the patient is on heparin therapy there should not be any oozing present. If the heparin therapy is for treatment of thrombosis rather than prevention, the partial thromboplastin time should be at 1½ to 2½ times normal for a therapeutic effect.

Patients should have a stable abdominal girth and be free of pain and discomfort.

References

1. Brunner LS, Suddarth DS: Blood disorders. In The Lippincott Manual of Nursing Practice, 3rd ed, pp 231–262. Philadelphia, JB Lippincott, 1982
2. Burnakis T: Treatment of severe, chronic pain by continuous parenteral infusion of morphine. Hospital Pharmacy 18:618–624, 1983
3. Carbone PP, Kaplan HS, Musshoff K, et al: Report of the committee on Hodgkin's disease staging classification. Cancer Res 31:1860–1861, 1971
4. Foley KM: The practical use of narcotic analgesics. Med Clin North Am 66:1091–1103, 1982
5. Goldman JM, Lu D: New approaches in chronic granulocytic leukemia—origin, prognosis, and treatment. Semin Hematol 19:241–256, 1982
6. Greene MH: Clinical and environmental predisposing factors. In Berard CW, moderator: A multidisciplinary approach to non-Hodgkin's lymphomas. Ann Intern Med 94:218–235, 1980
7. Jaffe ES: Non-Hodgkin's lymphomas as neoplasms of the immune system, pp 222–230. In Berard CW, moderator: A multidisciplinary approach to non-Hodgkin's lymphomas. Ann Intern Med 94:218–235, 1980
8. Kaplan HS, Rosenberg SA: Hodgkin's disease: Current recommendations for management. CA 25:306–319, 1975
9. Koeffler HP, Golde DW: Chronic myelogenous leukemia—new concepts (second of two parts). N Engl J Med 304:1269–1274, 1981
10. Luckmann J, Sorensen KC: Nursing persons with other major disturbances of the blood and blood-forming organs. In Medical-Surgical Nursing: A Psychophysiological Approach, 2nd ed, pp 1056–1084. Philadelphia, WB Saunders, 1980
11. Pearson HA: Splenectomy: Its risks and its roles. Hosp Prac 15:85–94, 1980
12. Rubin P: Clinical Oncology, 6th ed. ACS, 1983
13. Ultmann JE, DeVita VT: Hodgkin's disease and other lymphomas. In Petersdorf RG, Adams RD, Braunwald E, et al: Harrison's Principles of Internal Medicine, 10th ed. New York, McGraw-Hill, 1983
14. Ultmann JE, Stein RS: Non-Hodgkin's lymphoma: An approach to staging and therapy. CA 25:320–333, 1975
15. Weinstein HJ, Mayer RJ, Rosenthal DS, et al: Treatment of acute myelogenous leukemia in children and adults. N Engl J Med 303:473–478, 1980
16. Wessler RM: Care of the hospitalized adult patient with leukemia. Nurs Clin North Am 17:649–663, 1982
17. Wintrobe MM: Acute lymphoblastic leukemia. In Clinical Hematology, 8th ed, pp 1507–1535. Philadelphia, Lea & Febiger, 1981
18. Wintrobe MM: Hodgkin's disease. In Clinical Hematology, 8th ed, pp 1648–1680. Philadelphia, Lea & Febiger, 1981
19. Wintrobe MM: Lymphomas other than Hodgkin's disease. In Clinical Hematology, 8th ed, pp 1681–1725. Philadelphia, Lea & Febiger, 1981
20. Zighelboim J: Treatment of acute lymphoblastic leukemia, pp 762–765. In Cline MJ, moderator: Acute leukemia: Biology and treatment. Ann Intern Med 91:758–773, 1979

Bibliography

Acute Leukemia Progress, a film. Burchenal JH, consultant. American Cancer Society, 1984

Aur RJA, Simone JV, Verzosa MS, et al: Childhood acute lymphocytic leukemia: Study VIII. Cancer 42:2123–2134, 1978

Baccarani M, Corbelli G, Tura S: The Italian Cooperative Study Group on chronic myeloid leukemia: Early splenectomy and polychemotherapy versus polychemotherapy alone in chronic myeloid leukemia. Leukemia Research 5:149–157, 1981

Blume KG, Forman SJ: Bone marrow transplantation for hematologic malignancies. J Cell Physiol Suppl 1:99–102, 1982

Bolin RW, Robinson WA, Sutherland J, et al: Busulfan versus hydroxyurea in long-term therapy of chronic myelogenous leukemia. Cancer 50:1683–1686, 1982

Bortin MM, Gale RP, Kay HEM, Rim AA, for the Advisory Committee of the International Bone Marrow Transplant Registry: Bone marrow transplantation for acute myelogenous leukemia: Factors associated with early mortality. JAMA 249:1166–1175, 1983

Clift RA, Thomas ED, Fefer A, et al: Treatment of chronic granulocytic leukemia in chronic phase by allogeneic marrow transplantation. Lancet 620–623, 1982

Cooper RA: Diseases of the spleen. In Cohn HF, Conn RB, (eds): Current Diagnosis 6. Philadelphia, WB Saunders, 1980

Dearth JC, Fountain KS, Smithson WA, et al: Extreme leukemic leukocytosis (blast crisis) in childhood. Mayo Clin Proc 53:207–211, 1978

Durant J, Omura GA: Leukemia. In Nealon RF (ed): Management of the Patient with Cancer, 2nd ed. Philadelphia, WB Saunders, 1976

Hoagland HC: Acute leukemia and its complications. Mayo Clin Proc 53:260–261, 1978

Johnson FL, Thomas ED, Clark BS, et al: A comparison of marrow transplantation with chemotherapy for children with acute lymphoblastic leukemia in second or subsequent remission. N Engl J Med 305:846–851, 1981

Koeffler HP, Golde DW: Chronic myelogenous leukemia—new concepts (first of two parts). N Engl J Med 304:1201–1209, 1981

Lange B, Littman P, Schnaufer L, et al: Treatment of advanced Hodgkin's disease in pediatric patients. Cancer 42:1141–1145, 1978

Le Blanc DH: People with Hodgkin's disease: The nursing challenge. Nurs Clin North Am 13:281–300, 1978

Marx JL: Tumors: A mixed bag of cells. Science 215:275–277, 1982

Mayer RJ: More than MOPP for advanced Hodgkin's disease? N Engl J Med 306:800–802, 1982

Miller RA, Maloney DG, Warnke R, et al: Treatment of B-cell lymphoma with monoclonal anti-idiotype antibody. N Engl J Med 306:517–522, 1982

Moloney WC, Rosenthal DS: Treatment of early acute nonlymphatic leukemia with low dose cystosine arabinoside. Haematology and Blood Transfusion 26:59–62, 1981

Nossel HL: Bleeding. In Petersdorf RG, Adams RD, Braunwald E, Isselbacker KJ, Martin JB, Wilson JD (eds): Harrison's Principles of Internal Medicine, 10th ed. New York, McGraw-Hill, 1983

Preisler HD, Raza A: Chronic myelocytic leukemia: Comments on new approaches to therapy. Cancer Treat Rep 66:1073–1076, 1982

Prosnitz LR, Kapp DS, Weissberg JB: Radiotherapy (first of two parts). N Engl J Med 309:771–777, 1983

Prosnitz LR, Kapp DS, Weissberg JB: Radiotherapy (second of two parts). N Engl J Med 309:834–840, 1983

Storb R, Thomas ED: Allogeneic bone-marrow transplantation. Immunol Rev 71:77–102, 1983

Yunis JJ: The chromosomal basis of human neoplasia. Science 221:227–236, 1983

Chapter 52

Infectious Disorders of the Blood

Gaylene Bouska Altman

Certain infectious diseases affect the blood system in various ways and can be discussed as infectious blood disorders. These diseases are transmissible, and care needs to be taken to avoid contamination. Infectious mononucleosis, septicemia, and acquired immune deficiency syndrome (AIDS) will be discussed in this chapter.

Infectious Mononucleosis

Infectious mononucleosis is an acute self-limiting infectious disease caused by a herpeslike virus, the Epstein-Barr virus (EBV). It is most common among young people between 15 and 25 years of age, especially among college-age students. Both sporadic and epidemic forms of the disease are seen. The disease is mildly contagious and transmission is believed to be by intimate contact, especially kissing. The incubation period is anywhere from 2 to 6 weeks following exposure. The disease is generally characterized by an increase in mononuclear elements of the blood. The course of the disease is generally mild with a good prognosis.

Clinical Manifestations

The signs and symptoms are those of a general infectious process. Malaise is the usual early complaint, often accompanied by gradual onset of fever, sore throat, headache, enlarged lymph nodes, generalized aches and pains, and anorexia. Moderate enlargement of the spleen and liver may be present with jaundice and some abdominal discomfort. A petechial rash with diffuse redness may appear. Rarely, serious complications accompany the disease (*e.g.,* encephalitis and rupture of the spleen). Periodically, extensive mononuclear infiltration produces symptoms related to any body tissue so that the clinical picture can resemble other conditions, including neurological or cardiac manifestations. Recurrences are rare.

Medical Management

Diagnosis. The diagnosis is established on the basis of clinical manifestation of fever, lymphadenopathy, sore throat and splenomegaly, a stained blood smear of atypical lymphocytes, and a positive heterophil agglutination test. The rising titer in the serum agglutinin usually appears in the second week. This test is based on the fact that the infectious patient's blood causes clumping, or agglutination of the erythrocytes of another animal. A titer of 1 : 160 is considered diagnostic even though a rising titer during the early stage is highly suggestive. The monospot or "Spot Test" has been developed for early detection of infectious mononucleosis, because agglutinins can be identified at lower levels. The leukocyte count may be normal or low but usually leukocytosis, somewhere between 10,000 and 20,000 cells/mm^3, develops with approximately 10% of large, immature, vacuolated lymphocytes.

Treatment. No specific measures are available. The disease is usually self-limiting with a good prognosis. Acute symptoms usually last about a week, and fatigue may persist 2 to 4 weeks. Symptoms are usually relieved by analgesics and bed rest, especially until the febrile state is terminated. Activity is usually regulated according to tolerance levels unless complicating factors are present. Antibiotics may be ordered for sore throat especially if B-hemolytic streptococcal sore throat is present. Warm saline or analgesic gargles may help relieve symptoms of pharyngitis.

Hepatitis is benign and requires no special treatment even when laboratory abnormalities persist. In severe cases of infectious mononucleosis, steroids may be used. Complications are uncommon but can be serious and require the appropriate management. Pneumonitis, myocarditis, hemolytic anemia, thrombocytopenia, or ruptured spleen may occur. Abdominal pain and shock may be indicative of a ruptured spleen. Neurological complications appear in some outbreaks. There is some evidence to indicate depressed cellular immunity during the disease and for some time after the main course. Live vaccines should therefore be avoided for several months and until complete recovery.

Nursing Management

Nursing Diagnoses

Common nursing diagnoses for the patient with infectious mononucleosis are activity intolerance, alterations in comfort, alterations in oral mucous membrane, social isolation, especially in school and university-age patients requiring long-term rest, and possibly situational depression.

Goals. Common goals include teaching the patient about the need for rest, adequate nutrition, and watching for signs of complications. In the patient requiring long-term decrease in activity, prevention of psychological isolation and depression should be part of the nursing goals.

Interventions

Nursing responsibilities are directed toward the relief of symptoms and the promotion of rest and comfort. Bed rest may be used until fever, malaise, and headache lessen. Cool sponge baths, salicylates, and large fluid intake are used for reducing fever. Warm saline gargles may lessen symptoms of pharyngitis. Liquid or a soft diet may be necessary until the sore throat lessens. Excessive activity should be limited to avoid splenic rupture. The patient should be protected against secondary infections especially in the acute phase. Depression may result from chronic fatigue and weakness. If infectious mononucleosis occurs in an adolescent or child, adequate nutrition for normal growth and development is of concern as well as depression and resentment of a normally active child.

Evaluation

The disease is self-limiting if care is taken for rest and general health care. The patient will complain less of fatigue and be able to tolerate normal activities. The patient will not complain of mouth and throat soreness, and the mucosa will return to normal color.

Septicemia

Etiology and Clinical Manifestations

Sepsis or septicemia refers to a generalized bacterial infection in the bloodstream. Bursts of bacteria may enter the bloodstream in patients with infections and is called *bacteremia.* However, if the lymphatic system or medical therapy is not effective in terminating the spread of infectious agents, the bacteria may continuously invade the bloodstream. Generally, the macrophages of the reticuloendothelial system avert the further multiplication of the bacteria. However, if the macrophage system is overwhelmed, these organisms will persist and multiply in the bloodstream and cause the clinical picture of septicemia. In this circumstance the patient experiences fever, chills, malaise, and finally prostration. If untreated, the patient may progress to cardiovascular collapse. Sometimes in the presence of severe infections, "clumps" of organisms may lodge in the small vessels of organs causing microabscesses and tissue damage.

Some patients admitted to acute care hospitals acquire infections. Most of these are gram-negative bacteria (*e.g., Escherichia coli, Klebsiella, Enterobacter, Serratia, Pseudomonas aeruginosa,* and *Proteus*). Some gram-positive bacteria are responsible for bacteremia. The patients especially susceptible are patients who have been burned; those on immunosuppressive therapy; those with invasive diagnostic procedures, indwelling catheters, or ventilatory equipment; those with chronic underlying diseases; and patients with severe trauma, blood dyscrasias, poorly controlled diabetes; and the elderly. Any patients with extensive tissue damage (*e.g.,* trauma, or major surgery) or in whom a foreign body has been implanted (*e.g.,* a valve prosthesis) are at risk.

If septicemia is not arrested, it can progress to septic shock. As discussed in Chapter 24, the patient may first experience fever and a rapid and strong pulse, and a normal or slightly decreased blood pressure. The patient breathes rapidly and may even hyperventilate. The skin initially stays flushed, warm, and dry. At this stage, the patient has hyperdynamic shock with a decrease in systematic vascular resistance, an increase in cardiac output with little or no change in oxygen consumption and pulmonary artery wedge pressure. If the septic shock continues, the systematic vascular resistance increases, cardiac output decreases, and oxygen consumption decreases. The cardiac function is inadequate and the vessels are unable to compensate for the depressed function.

Medical Management

The treatment is dependent on the organism invading the bloodstream and on the underlying medical problem. Treatment is directed toward eliminating the cause.

Nursing Management

Nursing Diagnoses

Common nursing problems associated with septicemia are the potential for spread of infection and fluid volume deficit due to an elevated temperature. If shock ensues, alteration in systemic tissue perfusion becomes a problem.

Goals. Common goals include preventing or arresting the spread and severity of the infectious process; providing rest and comfort, and adequate nutrition to assist the patient in maintaining the ability to resist the spread of infection; and providing adequate hydration. If septic shock ensues, goals would include maintaining systemic tissue perfusion.

Interventions

Many of the nursing interventions are dependent upon the cause and the underlying problems. First, prevention should be the primary concern. Any patient with an infection can be a candidate for the development of septicemia. The nurse needs to use caution in caring for these patients; strict aseptic techniques should be used. As discussed in Chapter 17, patients at risk should be isolated from infected patients. The patient should be monitored for signs of impending infections and treated.

Once the patient has septicemia, high doses of antibiotics will be used. Because side-effects are possible, the nurse should be alerted to these. In addition, it is important to assess the patient's renal function. Fluid deficit is a problem; therefore, adequate hydration should be maintained.

Rest becomes essential for the patient because the body is in an extremely compromised state. Scheduling of activities and rest periods is important.

Mortality from septic shock is in excess of 50%. Assessment of the patient to identify early the signs and symptoms of shock is of utmost importance. Signs of mental changes (*e.g.,* agitation and anxiety) may be early clues. Once shock has occurred, nursing management centers mainly around maintaining tissue perfusion and promoting comfort of the patient.

Evaluation

The main goal is to prevent septic shock; therefore signs and symptoms of septic shock would be absent. Otherwise outcome criteria would be that the patient no longer has an increased temperature or other signs and symptoms of the infectious process and does not have the presence of bacteria in the blood.

Acquired Immune Deficiency Syndrome (AIDS)

Acquired immune deficiency syndrome (AIDS) is a disorder characterized by a profound defect in cellular immunity weakening the body's ability to fight diseases and hence making the patient highly susceptible to certain opportunistic infections. AIDS is associated with one or more of the following: *Pneumocystis carinii* pneumonia and certain other opportunistic infections such as Kaposi's sarcoma or lymphomas. There is no preexisting cause of immunodeficiency.

AIDS resembles other recognized immune deficiencies; however, it is unique in its complexity and viral etiology. The Human T-cell lymphotropic virus (HTLV III) of the D-type has been identified as the probably etiologic cause of AIDS. Other viruses may be causative and are being investigated.

AIDS was first identified in the United States in 1979. Since its identification the disease has been constantly on the rise with limited information available on its cause and treatment. As of June 1981, the Centers for Disease Control (CDC)* has maintained national surveillance for the syndrome. As of August 1985, over 12,400 cases had been reported. The number of cases has doubled every 6 to 9 months with the CDC reporting about 130 new cases each week. In late 1984, a slowing trend in new cases was reported but only temporarily. The mortality rate is steadily increasing with no known cure. AIDS victimizes mainly homosexual men (73% of cases), intravenous drug users (17%), persons receiving transfusions (2%), heterosexual contacts (1%), and others (7%).[8†] Some cases in patients with only heterosexual contact have been reported. Most patients are about 15 to 35 years of age.

The spread is thought to be mainly by blood and body fluids. Specifically, the two major means of transmission of the infectious agent are through sexual contact and blood transfusion. In sexually transmitted disease the patients have usually reported multiple sexual contacts with vigorous or traumatic anogenital techniques causing mucosa traumatization and rupture of small blood vessels. The incubation for AIDS by sexual transmission has been reported at 7 to 24 months. Blood transfusions are another method for the transfer of the disease. This includes blood and specialized blood products, such as factor VIII used in treating hemophilia. Besides hemophiliacs, a few cases in other patients receiving blood have been reported, thus causing great concerns over available blood products and intensive investiga-

*The Centers for Disease Control in Atlanta, Georgia, is a national center to which state health departments forward information gathered from local health departments. Data about communicable and chronic diseases, including information about epidemiology, trends, and care, are compiled and published weekly.

† Personal Communication, CDC

tions. Indeed, this has recently led to a serologic test for use in blood banks to screen donors for the presence of antibodies to HTLV-III. This test is expected to allow blood banks to screen out donors whose blood products might carry infectious HTLV-III virus. One study using such a serologic test found positive results in 22% to 65% of gay males with AIDS or pre-AIDS, 87% of IV drug users, 52% to 72% of Hemophilia A patients, 37% of female sex partners of AIDS males, and less than 1% of persons with no known risk factors.[1] These patients with positive serological tests are asymptomatic carriers, making identification and prevention of AIDS difficult.

In May 1983, the US Public Health Service requested that high risk groups refrain from donating blood, specifically homosexuals, bisexual men with multiple sex partners, IV drug users, hemophiliacs, and recent Haitian immigrants. In February 1985 new tests were found to detect antibodies to the HTLV-III virus in the blood allowing for more careful screening of blood supplies.

Legal and ethical difficulties have been identified because a positive result does not necessarily mean that the person will develop AIDS. It may indicate exposure to the virus and development of antibodies. Even with the use of the serologic test, it is still imperative that high-risk groups avoid blood donation because after exposure it may take time before the antibodies develop. Thus, it is possible for blood donors to be carriers of the virus and to be negative by serologic screening.

Clinical Manifestations

It may take months to years for symptoms to develop. A pre-AIDS syndrome may first be noted that is characterized by malaise, weight loss, and unexplained lymphadenopathy at two or more sites for more than 4 months with no apparent etiology. In the pre-AIDS state, fewer helper T cells are present. As the disease progresses the symptoms are those of recurrent infections, persistent fever, extreme fatigue, progressive weight loss, anorexia, dry cough unrelated to smoking or a cold, persistent diarrhea, thick whitish coating on the tongue and throat, skin rash and pallor, and swollen lymph glands.[6]

Many patients with AIDS present with severe recurrent infections of many types. Because of the suppressed immune system they are unable to fight the infections. Other patients develop Kaposi's sarcoma. Kaposi's sarcoma without the presence of AIDS is rare in the United States. Patients with Kaposi's sarcoma have sudden dark-blue or purple-brown nodules or plaques (Fig. 52–1). The lesions begin on the feet and ankles then may progress proximally and may also be found on the hands and arms. Lesions may occur in the gastrointestinal tract, thereby causing bleeding. Lesions may occur in the respiratory tract. Lymphedema is associated with and commonly precedes lesions.

Mortality is high with deaths caused by severe infections and metastatic tumors. The CDC reported the overall mortality in 1984 as 40%, but with 80% mortality 2 years after diagnosis and 100% 3 years after diagnosis. Patients with Kaposi's sarcoma and no other opportunistic infections had slightly better survival rates.[5]

Medical Management

Treatment is very limited because much is not understood about the disease. The underlying infections are treated with appropriate antibiotics. Some experimental drugs (*e.g.,* suramin and interferon) have been used with limited success. Otherwise most of thé treatment is monitoring of symptoms and supportive care.

Nursing Management

Nursing Diagnoses

Common nursing diagnoses for these patients are the potential for spread of infection, anxiety due to poor prognosis, disturbances in self-concept related to lifestyle, and possible guilt for contracting and/or spreading disease.

Goals. Common nursing goals for the patient with

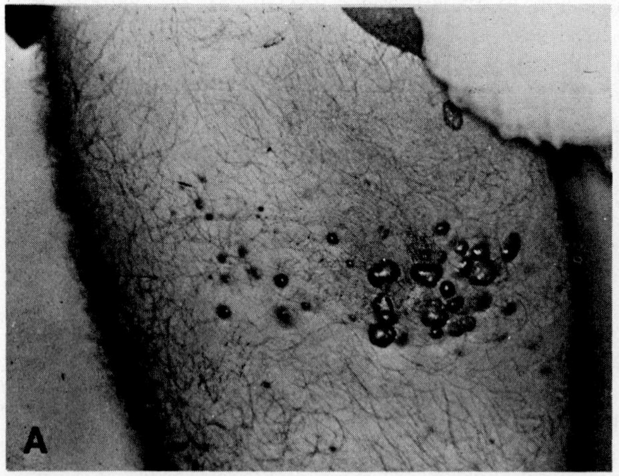

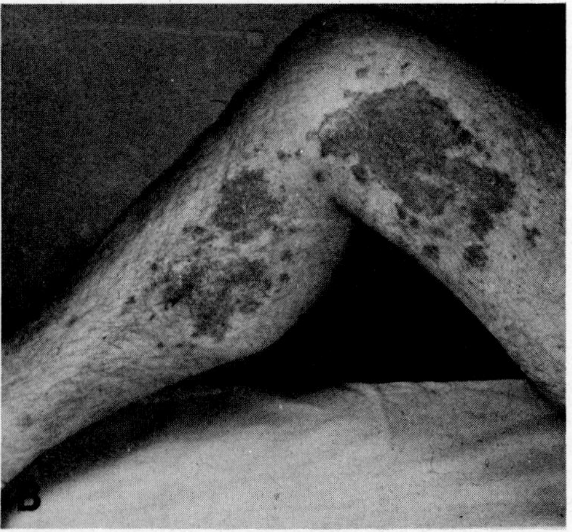

FIGURE 52–1 Kaposi's sarcoma. (*A*) Nodules. (*B*) Plaque lesions. (Wolcott MW: Ambulatory Surgery and the Basics of Emergency Surgical Care, p 223, Philadelphia, JB Lippincott, 1981)

AIDS are to avoid the spread of the infection and to assist the patient in dealing with the prognosis, anxiety, alteration in self-concept, and depression.

Interventions

The nursing care required depends on the patient's underlying condition. Patients will require considerable supportive care for both physiological problems and psychological problems. This will include supportive care for a patient with extreme fatigue, fever, and anorexia. Schedule activities to allow for rest periods. Plan small frequent meals and encourage high-protein, high-calorie foods. Most patients have severe weight loss. If a fever is present, cool baths may help. Some patients may be on chemotherapy and require oral care and antiemetics. Psychological support is critical. Patients may be extremely depressed because of the poor prognosis. Guilt, anger, and confusion may be present because of contact of the disease and lifestyle. The patient may become isolated from friends because of their fear of contracting the disease. Staff may experience fear in caring for these patients because so much is unknown about the disease. Nursing staff should examine their own feelings regarding their fears and the patient's lifestyle.

AIDS is an infectious disease and a reportable disease. Because much is not known about the transmission of the disease, guidelines have been developed. Hospital personnel because of their contact with blood and body fluids from AIDS patients may be at increased risk and should therefore take special precautions. These precautions are listed in Table 52–1.

All patients with AIDS should be taught that potentially infectious agents which could be transmitted to other people are present in their blood and other body substances. The patients should also be taught that they are susceptible to infections from others. Handwashing and good personal hygiene should be emphasized for the patients with AIDS for their protection and for the protection of others. Data indicate that most people remain infected. Although patients may remain asymptomatic they can transmit HTLV-III to others. There is a risk of infecting others by sexual intercourse, sharing of needles, and possibly exposure of others through oral–genital contact, or intimate kissing. Recommendations developed by the Centers for Disease Control that should be

TABLE 52–1
Precaution Guidelines for Nursing the AIDS Patient

- Gloves are worn for anticipated contact with any patient's blood, pus, feces, urine, or oral secretions. Gloves are not necessary for contact with unsoiled articles or intact skin.
- Gowns are worn when it is likely that personnel's clothing will be soiled by any patient's blood, pus, feces, urine, or oral secretions. Gowns are not necessary for other contact.
- Hands should be carefully washed before and after removing gowns and gloves and before leaving the room.
- Masks are worn for anticipated respiratory contact with droplet secretions (*e.g*, coughing patient who does not cover mouth and nose), suctioning patient, or AIDS patients who also have untreated tuberculosis. Masks are otherwise unnecessary. A coughing patient may need to be masked for transport outside the room.
- Protective eyewear may be useful in situations in which splatter with blood or body fluid such as sputum is anticipated.
- Extreme care should be taken to avoid accidental wounds with sharp instruments contaminated with potentially infectious material. If punctures occur report to the appropriate health-care area for venipuncture for future study.
- Personnel with open lesions should avoid contact with materials from AIDS patients.
- Laboratory specimens from all patients are handled with equal care. Specimens from AIDS patients may be labeled "Blood and Body Fluids Precautions" to remind laboratory personnel to exercise proper care. After specimens are taken to the laboratory, personnel need to wash their hands.
- Linen soiled with blood or body substances from patients are to be bagged to prevent leakage and color coded to alert laundry personnel of its contents. Laundry personnel will use gloves to handle it.
- Reusable articles soiled with blood or body substances are specially bagged for isolation to prevent leakage and identified so that Central Supply personnel will glove to handle them.
- (Specific to Operating Room) Soiled instruments are washed in a suitable microbiocide, then processed through normal sterilization procedures.
- Syringes, needles, and other sharp objects are placed in a heavy plastic needle container in the patient's room. Used needles should not be broken off or recapped before disposal (due to increased injury incidence when needles are recapped).
- Trash and disposable articles soiled with blood or body substances are placed in separate, labeled plastic bags to prevent leakage.
- Although the infection precautions described previously should be used for all patients, the use of cards on patients' doors to remind personnel is common. The most appropriate card for AIDS is *Blood and Body Fluid Precautions*. AIDS patients may also need other reminder cards if they have additional infectious diseases, such as tuberculosis.
- AIDS patients may be transported to other departments as necessary, with care taken to prevent soilage with blood or body substances. AIDS patients with good personal hygiene may eat in the cafeteria, but should not handle or prepare food or drinks which may be used by other people while in the hospital.
- Pregnant women should not care for patients who are diagnosed as having AIDS.
- Patients with AIDS do not necessarily require a separate room; however, they should not come in contact with patients with infections. If the patient is too ill to use good hygiene (*e.g.*, those with diarrhea, incontinence, or behavioral changes from neurological involvement), a private room may be necessary.
- Discharge cleaning of the patient's room is performed in the usual fashion. Concurrent cleaning should include prompt clean-up of blood and body substances by gloved personnel using bleach.[2,4,7]

relayed to the patient with the HTLV-III virus include the following:

- The efficacy of condoms in preventing infection of HTLV-III is unproven, but consistent use of them may reduce transmission.
- Toothbrushes, razors, or other implements should not be shared.
- Women with a seropositive test, or women whose sexual partner is seropositive, are themselves at increased risk of acquiring AIDS. If they become pregnant, their offspring are also at increased risk of acquiring AIDS.
- After accidents resulting in bleeding, contaminated surfaces should be cleaned with household bleach freshly diluted 1 : 10 in water.
- Devices that have punctured the skin, such as hypodermic and acupuncture needles, should be steam sterilized by autoclave before reuse or safely discarded. Whenever possible, disposable needles and equipment should be used.
- When seeking medical or dental care for intercurrent illness, these persons should inform those responsible for their care of their positive antibody status so that appropriate evaluation can be undertaken and precautions taken to prevent transmission to others.
- If sexual contact has occurred or needles have been shared with an infected person, a test for HTLV-III antibodies should be done.
- Persons infected with HTLV-III should refrain from giving blood, plasma, body organs, or other tissues, or sperm.
- Regular medical evaluations and follow-up are essential.[3]

Evaluation

Examples of subjective and objective data that would demonstrate goal achievement are as follows:

1. Patient expresses a sense of well-being and has some sense of hope now and for the future.
2. The disease is not spread to others.
3. The patient expresses less anxiety.
4. Nonverbal expressions of anxiety and depression are reduced.

References

1. Abstract HTLV-III in the semen and blood of a healthy homosexual man. Science 226:451–453, 1984
2. Centers for Disease Control: Acquired immune deficiency syndrome (AIDS): Precautions for clinical and laboratory staff. Morbidity and Mortality Weekly Report 31(43):577–580, 1982
3. Centers for Disease Control provisional public health service inter-agency recommendations for screening donated blood and plasma for antibody to the virus causing acquired immunodeficiency syndrome. Morbidity and Mortality Weekly Report 34:(1):5–7, 1985
4. Conte JE, Hadley WK, Sande M: Infection control guidelines for patients with acquired immuno-deficiency syndrome (AIDS). New Engl J Med 309(12):740–744, 1983
5. Medical Staff Conference. The acquired immune deficiency syndrome (AIDS)—a multidisciplinary enigma. West J Med 140(1):66–81, 1984
6. Memon AS: Acquired immunodeficiency: A diagnostic update. Resident and Staff Physician 30(2):35–43, 1984
7. Nursing Department and Infection Control Committee, Harborview Medical Center, Seattle, Washington, 1984
8. Wolfsy CB: The infectious diseases. In Rackel RE (ed): Current Therapy, pp 1–9. Philadelphia, WB Saunders, 1985

Bibliography

Abstract HTLV-III in saliva of people with AIDS-related complex and healthy homosexual men at risk for AIDS. Science 226 (4673):447–448, 1984

Centers for Disease Control: Morbidity and Mortality Weekly Report 34(1):1–3, 1985

Centers for Disease Control: Morbidity and Mortality Weekly Report 34(2):21–31, 1985

Chamherlard ME, Castro KG, Haverkos HW, et al: Acquired immunodeficiency syndrome in the United States: An analysis of cases outside high incidence groups. Ann Intern Med 101:617–623, 1984

Hirsch MS, Wormser GP, Schooley RT, et al: Risk of nosocomial infections with human T-cell lymphotropic virus III (HTLV-III). New Engl J Med 312(1):1–4, 1985

Hirsch MS, Schooley RT, Ho DD, et al: Possible viral interactions in the acquired immunodeficiency syndrome (AIDS). Reviews of Infectious Disease 6(5):726–731, 1984

Kotler D, Gaetz HP, Lange M, et al: Enteropathy associated with the acquired immunodeficiency syndrome. Ann Intern Med 101(4)421–428, 1984

Pardo V, Martin A, Colton RM, et al: Glomerular lesions in the acquired immunodeficiency syndrome. Ann Intern Med 101(4)429–434, 1984

Petersdorf RG, Adams RD, Braunwald E, et al: Harrison's Principles of Internal Medicine, 10th ed. New York, McGraw-Hill, 1983

Sinkovics JG, Gyorkey F, Melnick JL, et al: Acquired immune deficiency syndrome (AIDS): Speculation about its etiology and comparative immunology. Reviews of Infectious Diseases 6(5):745–760, 1984

Chapter 53

Anemias and Related Blood Disorders

Gaylene Bouska Altman

Classification and General Assessment

Anemias can be categorized into those with primary and secondary causes; that is, diseases in which abnormalities in the number of erythrocytes are due either to a disease process within the hematopoietic system or to a disease outside the hematopoietic system which secondarily affects red cell production or longevity. Furthermore the primary anemias can be divided into those that are due to blood loss, those due to defective or decreased formation of erythrocytes (erythropoiesis), and those resulting from premature destruction of erythrocytes. Table 53–1 illustrates this categorization of the anemias and lists some common examples of each.

Although the diagnosis of anemia is based largely on laboratory studies, one should not fail to perform a nursing history and physical examination because information obtained by these methods can often expedite making the correct diagnosis. For example, the symptoms of fatigue, weakness, and general malaise although nonspecific are common in patients with most chronic anemias. Historical data regarding the magnitude and frequency of menstrual flow and any evidence of blood in the stools, either readily apparent fresh blood or melena are obviously helpful. Information regarding drug use or chemical exposure can also be important. For example, patients with seizure disorders taking drugs such as phenytoin, primidone, or phenobarbital may occasionally develop folate deficiency and a megaloblastic anemia, while aplastic anemia can be caused by ingestion of chloramphenicol, phenylbutazone, and exposure to chemicals such as benzene and some insecticides. Because certain anemias are inherited, a family history can be useful. For example, hereditary spherocytosis is an autosomal dominant disease seen in all races while glucose-6-phosphate dehydrogenase deficiency (G6,PD) is an x-linked disorder of intermediate dominance common in black and certain Mediterranean ethnic groups, especially Sicilians, Greeks, Arabs, and Sephardic Jews. Hence, inquiries into a patient's ethnic background and family history of anemia may yield diagnostically useful information.

The physical examination may also be helpful although rarely are any physical signs diagnostic of anemia. Nonetheless, pallor of the skin and mucous membranes is usually present in patients with anemia. Jaundice may be seen in pernicious anemia or some hemolytic processes, and dry skin and hair and spooning or koilonychia of the nails may occur in iron deficiency anemia. In pernicious anemia neurologic manifestations may develop and indeed are more worrisome than the anemia itself because these abnormal-

TABLE 53–1
Classification of the Anemias

Type	Examples
I. Primary	
A. Blood loss	Acute blood loss anemia, chronic (iron deficiency)
B. Defective erythropoiesis	Vitamin B_{12} deficiency, folate deficiency, aplastic anemia
C. Preurative erythrocyte destruction	Hereditary spherocytosis and elliptocytosis, glucose-6-phosphate dehydrogenase deficiency, hemoglobin disorders—sickle cell anemia, thalassemias
II. Secondary	Infection, azotemia, cirrhosis, acquired hemolytic anemias

ities may not reverse with treatment. Symptoms include numbness and paresthesias of the extremities, ataxia, poor position sense, and abnormal mentation. With this information as a background, we will now discuss certain selected anemias.

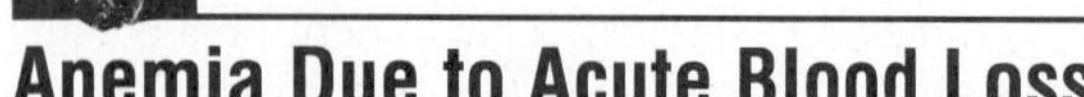

Anemia Due to Acute Blood Loss

Definition and Pathophysiology

Posthemorrhagic anemia can result from acute blood loss. Some causes are severed blood vessels due to trauma, spontaneous rupture of an aneurysm or erosion of an artery from an ulcerative lesion, necrosis, or cancerous growths. A large number of erythrocytes are lost resulting in a normocytic and normochromic anemia. The red cells are normal, but movement of fluid into the vascular compartment causes hemodilution and a fall in the red blood cell count and hemoglobin. There is a rapid decrease in blood volume and, therefore, reduced oxygen-carrying capacity of the blood. The hypoxia due to blood loss stimulates red cell production by the bone marrow. If iron stores are normal, the red blood cells that were lost are soon replaced. The severity of the patient's condition will be determined by the rate of bleeding, the site of the hemorrhage, and the total volume of blood lost.

An adult of average build has a total blood volume of 6000 ml. Usually an adult can lose as much as 500 ml without any serious effects. If over 1000 ml is lost, the patient will experience symptoms.

Clinical Manifestations

Clinical manifestations are related to both hypovolemia and hypoxemia and may initially be restlessness or irritability. The patient may become weak, dizzy, and experience syncope. Other findings are cool moist skin, diaphoresis, pallor, rapid thready pulse, rapid respirations, severe headache, thirst, and eventually disorientation. The disorientation indicates cerebral anoxia. Other internal organs become affected by the hypoxia. If untreated or uncontrolled, the blood pressure continues to drop, and shock ensues. Hypovolemic shock occurs when there is a blood loss of 10% to 15% of the circulating blood. It can be due to reasons other than blood loss (*e.g.*, plasma loss or extracellular fluid loss).

Initially the blood loss may not be severe enough to cause serious effects and compensatory mechanisms are able to maintain an adequate blood pressure and tissue perfusion to prevent cell damage. As the blood loss continues, a stage of decompensated shock occurs, blood pressure falls, blood flow to the heart and brain is impaired, fluid begins to leave the capillaries and blood flow becomes sluggish, and there is cell damage. Even with blood replacement, if vital signs cannot be stabilized, irreversible shock occurs and death ensues. (See Chapter 24.)

Laboratory findings may not be evident until several hours after the blood loss after which hemoglobin and hematocrit are eventually decreased. If iron stores are normal the red cells that were lost will be eventually replaced. However, in the first 24 hours after the blood loss it may be difficult to assess the patient's laboratory findings. Vasoconstriction and loss of plasma volume result in a pooling of blood in a smaller space and cause the hematocrit, hemoglobin, and erythrocyte count to be deceptively high. Finally, after the first day, depending on the severity of blood loss, and after treatment, extracellular volume enters the intravascular compartment and decreased laboratory findings reflect the anemia.

Medical Management

Treatment usually involves emergency treatment to stop and control the hemorrhage, to rapidly restore blood volume with blood transfusions, and to treat the shock. Most often the patient receives intravenous infusions, especially plasma, until blood can be typed and cross matched. If the blood loss is not severe, oral fluids may be tolerated. Iron stores will need to be replaced. If the hypovolemic shock is not controlled, other medical measures may be needed. (See Chapter 24 on shock.)

Nursing Management

Nursing Diagnoses

Common nursing diagnoses for the patient experiencing acute blood loss are as follows: Decreased cardiac output related to decreased intravascular volume; decreased systemic tissue perfusion related to decreased blood pressure and increased systemic vascular resistance; and alteration in nutrition related to nausea and vomiting.

Goals. Goals for nursing interventions are to detect early signs and symptoms of blood loss, to prevent or reduce blood loss, and to reduce the demands and activities of daily living to be compatible with the patient's cardiac output.

Interventions

As discussed in Chapter 24, acute blood loss will require immediate treatment to control bleeding and restore blood volume. Abdominal bleeding may cause nausea and eventually vomiting. Stool and emesis should be checked for occult blood. Observation of symptoms, time of day of symptoms, relation to food, location of discomfort can help locate the site of bleeding. Aspirin or any gastric irritants need to be avoided. Patient may be on antacids which need to be carefully spaced and given at times to protect the gastric mucosa from irritating foods. Tension of the abdomen may indicate a worsening state. If the patient has increased nausea, vomiting, and abdominal discomfort, a decision to stop all oral intake may be made.

Other causes of blood loss can be from an operative site. Incisions should be checked and signs of internal hemorrhage elicited. Accident patients who become anemic should be monitored for internal hemorrhage.

Whatever the cause of blood loss some basic nursing action is necessary. Carefully observe for pale conjunctiva, mucous membranes, nail beds, and palms. Monitor vital signs. Low-grade fevers may occur with blood loss. Measure urinary intake and output. Dyspnea can occur and in more severe blood loss, oxygen may be required. Patient may chill easily; a warm room and warm blankets may provide comfort. Pain, precordial spasms, and headaches can occur and require comfort measures. Fatigue is usually present, and activities should be grouped to allow time for the patient to have periods of uninterrupted rest. Complications (*e.g.*, shock, angina pectoris, myocardial infarction, prostration, and thrombocytopenic purpura) can occur and need to be detected early.

Evaluation

Signs and symptoms of bleeding should be detected at onset. If blood loss has been prevented, then vital signs, hemoglobin, and hematocrit will be normal. There will be no evidence of bleeding. Stools and urine will be guaiac negative. The patient will report less fatigue and no dyspnea.

Anemia Due to Chronic Blood Loss

Chronic blood loss results from the continuous loss of a small number of erythrocytes. In the adult a blood loss of 2 to 4 ml per day is sufficient to cause an iron deficiency anemia. It can be the result of blood loss from peptic ulcers, intestinal polyps, hemorrhoids, diverticulosis, or a malignancy in the gastrointestinal tract. Excessive aspirin intake may cause undetected gastrointestinal bleeding. Prolonged or excessive menses may cause chronic blood loss. Each ml of blood contains 0.5 mg of iron and the average menstrual flow is about 44 ml with a loss of 22 mg of iron. Chronic blood loss does not affect the blood volume but rather leads to iron deficiency anemia (discussed later). The bleeding must be located, controlled, and corrected with diet and iron supplement.

Iron Deficiency Anemia

Definition and Pathophysiology

Iron deficiency anemia in adult patients is often due to chronic blood loss. In contrast to acute blood loss which produces anemia because of rapid and large loss of erythrocytes, chronic blood loss leads to anemia because of the slow depletion of total body iron stores. In general the loss is occult. The most common causes of chronic blood loss have previously been mentioned. Less common reasons for iron deficiency anemia are pregnancy, because the fetus takes about 500 mg of iron from the mother during gestation; inadequate dietary intake which is most common in young children, the elderly, and indigent; and decreased iron absorption which can occur in patients with gastrectomies, achlorhydria (absence of hydrochloric acid production), and chronic diarrhea or malabsorption.

Normally the metabolism of iron is very precisely regulated. Daily losses are small and average about 0.5 mg per day. The daily American diet contains 10 to 20 mg of iron, however only 5% to 10% (0.5–2.0 mg) of this is absorbed. Thus iron metabolism is normally a closed system and only under the circumstances mentioned above does iron deficiency develop.

Clinical Manifestations

Some unique signs and symptoms are diagnostically useful. One of these is pica or the desire to eat unusual solid substances. Those commonly reported are the ingestion of clay, cornstarch, and ice. Another unusual but characteristic complication of iron deficiency anemia is Plummer-Vinson syndrome which is the development of thin membranous webs in the esophagus. When this occurs patients usually complain of dysphagia. Other physical findings which are characteristic of iron deficiency anemia are stomatitis at the edges of the lips, atrophy or tenderness of the tongue known as glossitis, and the aforementioned concave irregularity of the nails known as koilonychia.

The typical laboratory findings of iron deficiency anemia are a reduction in hematocrit and hemoglobin with microcytic and hypochromic red cells. The platelet and leukocyte counts are usually normal. Serum iron levels are low, while serum iron-binding capacity is elevated, hence iron saturation is low, usually 10% or less. However, the most specific test for iron deficiency is a bone marrow stain for hemosiderin; iron in the marrow should always be absent in this condition. In fact, absent iron stores are the earliest findings in patients with chronic iron depletion and only later does microcytosis, hypochromia, and finally anemia, develop. Bone marrow aspirates also show increased numbers of nucleated red cells.

Finally another sensitive laboratory test for iron deficiency is the serum ferritin level. This level is generally quite low (less than 12 μg/liter) in these patients compared to mean values of 120 μg/liter in males and 56 μg/liter in females. In contrast, in the anemia of chronic disease which can be confused with iron deficiency, ferritin levels are normal or high.

Initially a differential diagnosis is made. Iron deficiency anemia is the only anemia in which bone marrow hemosiderin is absent, hence if a bone marrow aspirate is performed a definite diagnosis can be made.

Medical Management

Management includes two important aspects: iron replacement and identifying the source of the iron loss. In general the latter requires evaluation of the gastrointestinal tract for a source of occult bleeding. Iron replacement is best and most inexpensively achieved with ferrous sulfate therapy 300 mg three times a day. Treatment for about 6 months is usually required to replenish total body stores. Response is usually evident in about 10 days manifested as a reticulocytosis and a gradual increase in hemoglobin and red cell indexes. Parenteral iron is only indicated for patients who fail to absorb iron normally such as those who have undergone gastrectomy or those with sprue.

Nursing Management

Nursing Diagnoses

Common nursing diagnoses for the patient with iron deficiency anemia are as follows: Alteration in nutrition related to inadequate iron intake, excessive iron depletion, or decreased absorption of iron; knowledge deficit about adequate iron intake; alteration in comfort; and stomatitis of the lips and glossitis related to inadequate iron stores.

Goals. Common goals of nursing interventions include early detection of the signs and symptoms of occult bleeding, teaching the patient and family about adequate iron intake and medical therapy, assisting the patient to reduce activities and demands of daily living to be compatible with symptoms, and reducing mouth discomfort.

Interventions

Urine and stool should be checked for occult blood. Encourage adequate nutrition and hydration. Oral and parenteral iron therapy may change stool formation requiring diet changes. Oral care should be frequent, and irritating foods and beverages should be avoided. Explain the importance of a diet high in iron and give the patient a list of foods that are high in iron. Explain the importance of taking the prescribed iron. Long-standing anemia can lead to heart failure, hypochromia, microcythemia, and severe dysphagia. Thus the patient will need continued medical supervision. Because of symptoms of fatigue, lassitude, possibly dyspnea, palpitations, and even at times angina, nursing care should be organized to provide rest periods.

Evaluation

Signs and symptoms of occult urinary and gastrointestinal bleeding are detected early. Patient and family can list foods that are high in iron and can describe how the patient's diet will be improved as a result. The patient can explain the need for adequate iron intake. Patient will complain of less fatigue if reduction in activity and demands of daily living is adequate. The patient complains less of mouth soreness and the mouth is less red and swollen.

Vitamin B_{12} Deficiency Anemia (Pernicious Anemia)

Definition and Pathophysiology

Vitamin B_{12} deficiency anemia can occur for two major reasons: (1) absence of intrinsic factor, a 50,000 molecular weight glycogen secreted by the parietal cells of the gastric mucosa which is required for vitamin B_{12} absorption, or (2) some disease process of the distal ileum, the site at which B_{12} absorption occurs. Autoimmune processes such as antibodies to intrinsic factor or gastric parietal cells are present in most patients with pernicious anemia. Other causes of this disorder include gastrectomy, which removes the vitamin B_{12}-producing cells, or regional ileitis and resection of the ileum which interfere with vitamin B_{12} absorption even when intrinsic factor synthesis is normal.

Pernicious anemia is rare before age 35, increases in incidence with age, and is most common in Scandinavian, English, and Irish people, while rare in Oriental people. Total body stores of vitamin B_{12} are about 5 mg; daily loss is approximately 2.5 μg and clinical signs of pernicious anemia do not develop until levels have been reduced to about 10% of normal.

Clinical Manifestations

Manifestations include the signs and symptoms of any chronic anemia (fatigue, weakness, general malaise), although mild icterus may occur giving the patient a characteristic pale yellow appearance. In contrast to other chronic anemias, this disease can affect other organ systems most notably the central and peripheral nervous systems. The signs and symptoms of neurologic involvement include numbness and paresthesias of the extremities, weakness, ataxia, poor coordination, loss of vibration sense and deep reflexes, and ultimately mental disturbance.

The characteristic laboratory findings in the peripheral blood are large oval erythrocytes (macrocytes) with some irregularity of shape (poikilocytosis), hyperpigmentation of the nuclei of granulocytes, and reductions in red cell numbers, leukocytes, and platelets. The reason for these findings is that vitamin B_{12} is necessary for normal cellular DNA synthesis; when it is deficient cells having relatively rapid turnover experience slow DNA synthesis but normal cytoplasmic development. Hence these cells tend to enlarge. Other rapidly dividing cells which are commonly affected when vitamin B_{12} is deficient are those of the gastrointestinal tract; therefore megaloblastosis of the intestinal epithelium may occur resulting in malabsorption, glossitis (inflammation of the tongue), and anorexia.

The bone marrow shows a hyperactive picture with megaloblastic changes. Marrow hemosiderin is increased. Other diagnostic findings include a low serum B_{12} level (<100 mg/ml), abnormal absorption of radiolabeled vitamin B_{12} as measured by the Schilling test, and increased serum lactic dehydrogenase activity due to release of the enzyme into the circulation from abnormal red cell precursors.

The only common entity that mimics pernicious anemia is folate deficiency anemia which will be discussed subsequently. Other rare diseases that can present similarly are acquired sideroblastic anemia, acute erythroleukemia, and orotic aciduria, an unusual hereditary syndrome of defective pyrimidine metabolism.

Medical Management

Management of pernicious anemia includes treatment with intramuscular vitamin B_{12} (cyanocobalamin) 100 μg, one to three times a week, until serum levels have normalized. Thereafter 100 μg per month is sufficient. Patients must be continued on this therapy for a lifetime.

Nursing Management

Nursing Diagnoses

Common nursing diagnoses for the patient with pernicious anemia are as follows: Alteration in nutrition related to inability to absorb vitamin B_{12}; alteration in comfort; glossitis; lack of information about medical management plan, specifically lifetime B_{12} injections; and potential for injury from accident related to peripheral neuropathy, poor coordination, and weakness.

Goals. Goals of nursing interventions are as follows: To reduce the demands and activities of daily living to be compatible with symptoms; to relieve mouth discomfort; and to provide information about medical management.

Nursing Interventions

As with any anemia, patients with pernicious anemia experience fatigue, dyspnea, palpitations, or angina, and require rest periods. Patients may experience tingling and numbness of feet, weakness, ataxia, and poor coordination. Care should be taken to prevent falls and injury to the extremities. Pernicious anemia can also cause dyspepsia and anorexia. Encourage adequate nutrition and hydration and teach the patient about a healthy diet. Special oral care is required, before eating and usually every 2 hours, for a sore or burning tongue. A soft diet can help to decrease oral irritation. Complaints of a sore tongue should be documented.

Administer vitamin B_{12} medications and instruct the patient in self-administration of injections. Encourage progressive ambulation because the patients with long-standing pernicious anemia may have become sedentary.

Evaluation

The patient's signs and symptoms should be reduced or eliminated. Hemoglobin should be normal. Nutritional status should be improved. Patient can describe rationale for medical management. Accidents and falls are prevented.

Folate Deficiency Anemia

Definition and Pathophysiology

Folic acid is a vitamin required for the transfer of one-carbon moieties such as methyl and formyl groups to various organic compounds. The acceptors of these one carbon moieties are ultimately necessary for the synthesis of methionine purines, and deoxythymidylate and deoxyuridylate monophosphates, which are required for cellular and particularly nuclear maturation. For this reason folic acid deficiency causes a nuclear-cytoplasmic abnormality analogous to that produced by vitamin B_{12} deficiency, and hence, a hematologic picture identical to that of pernicious anemia.

Like vitamin B_{12}, folate is normally obtained by absorption through the intestine, but unlike B_{12} the body stores are small (5–20 mg) and sufficient to last only 1 to 2 months in situations of deprivation. The principal dietary sources of folic acid are fruits and vegetables. The minimum daily requirement is 50 μg and this may increase several fold during times of high demand such as pregnancy. Hence, the most common cause of folic acid deficiency is malnutrition especially in the setting of alcohol abuse. Other causes of deficiency include sprue, chronic hemolytic anemias because they markedly increase folate utilization as a result of ineffective erythropoiesis, and the use of drugs which either interfere with folate absorption such as primidone, phenytoin, phenobarbital, or agents such as methotrexate, pyrimethamine, or triamterene which block the reduction of folic acid to its metabolically active product, folinic acid.

Another frequent cause of folic acid deficiency is pregnancy. Indeed about 20% of pregnant women are found to have low serum folate levels. Furthermore in twin pregnancies and those complicated by toxemia or abruptio placentae the incidence of deficiency is even higher. Nonetheless only a small percentage of folate-deficient pregnant women actually develop megaloblastic anemia.

Clinical Manifestations

Manifestations are the already mentioned signs and symptoms of any chronic anemia (fatigue, weakness, malaise). Of importance and in contrast to vitamin B_{12} deficiency, central and peripheral nervous system abnormalities do not occur in folate deficiency.

The hematologic findings of folate deficiency anemia are very similar to those outlined above for pernicious anemia. In brief these are a peripheral smear showing macrocytosis, hypersegmented polymorphonuclear leukocytes, and reduced numbers of total leukocytes and platelets. The marrow reveals a decreased myeloid to erythroid ratio, hypercellularity, and abundant iron stores. However in contrast to pernicious anemia, folate deficiency anemia is characterized by normal vitamin B_{12} absorption (Schilling test), and normal gastric acidity. The diagnosis of folate deficiency anemia is confirmed by a serum folate level less than 3 ng/ml, normal being greater than 7 ng/ml.

Obviously the most important task is to differentiate vitamin B_{12} deficiency from folate deficiency. Other conditions which can cause a peripheral macrocytosis are liver disease, alcoholism (independent of its common association with folate deficiency), hypothyroidism, aplastic anemia, and hemolysis. However if the degree of macrocytosis is marked (*i.e.* a mean corpuscular volume (MCV) greater than 110) these diagnoses are unlikely and one is probably dealing with either folate or vitamin B_{12} deficiency.

Medical Management

Treatment includes folate 1 mg per day. In patients with malabsorption 5 mg per day may be required. Following the initiation of treatment a reticulocytosis is usually seen in 4 to 7 days with the anemia correcting in 1 to 2 months. It is important to remember that folate therapy may correct the megaloblastic anemia of vitamin B_{12} deficiency while having no effect on ever-worsening neurologic manifestations of this disease. For this reason one must be certain of the diagnosis and not use a hematologic response to folate therapy to rule out vitamin B_{12} deficiency.

Nursing Management

Nursing care for the patient with folate deficiency is similar to that for the patient with pernicious anemia, except that the patient with folate deficiency does not have any central or peripheral nervous system abnormalities. Nursing care is organized to prevent fatigue and includes measures to optimize the patient's nutritional status.

Sickle Cell Anemia

Definition and Pathophysiology

This anemia is a severe multisystem disease caused by a single substitution of the amino acid valine for glutamic acid at the sixth residue of the beta chain of the hemoglobin molecule. It affects black persons and in the United States 0.15% of black children are affected. Adults have a lower prevalence because they die at early ages. The pathogenesis of this disorder is the direct result of the change in the structure of sickle hemoglobin. Sickle hemoglobin alters its shape when it is deoxygenated, producing crescent or sickle-shaped red cells (Fig. 53–1) which obstruct the capillary blood flow and produce increased blood viscosity and local tissue hypoxia. Furthermore, these rigid and obstructing

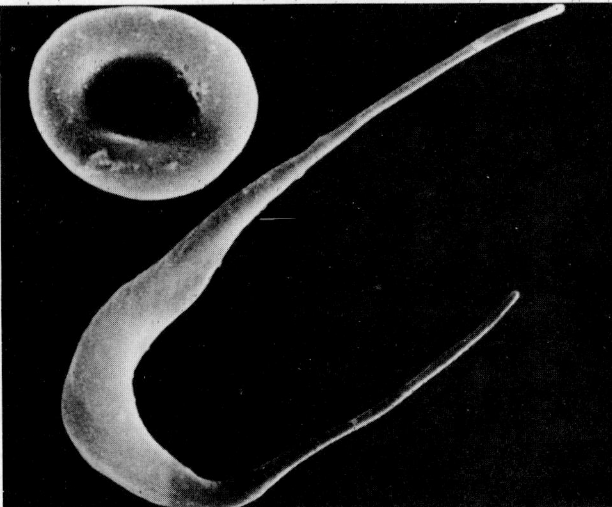

FIGURE 53–1 This photo of a sickled and a normal red blood cell was taken under the auspices of the Comprehensive Sickle Cell Center, University of Miami.

cells may initiate small vessel occlusions and local tissue infarction.

Clinical Manifestations

Manifestations of sickle cell anemia do not usually appear until about age 6 months because the fetal hemoglobin, which carries over from *in utero* development, is not adversely affected by oxygen desaturation as is sickle hemoglobin. By 6 months of age most fetal hemoglobin has been replaced by sickle hemoglobin. Constitutional symptoms of sickle cell anemia are growth impairment, failure to thrive, and increased infections especially with streptococcus pneumoniae.

The anemia of sickle disease is severe with hematocrit values usually less than 30%. The symptoms produced by this are those common to any chronic anemia. During episodes of severe infection or if folic acid deprivation occurs these patients may experience "aplastic crisis" with a rapid drop in hematocrit. The reason for this complication is that at all times sickle cell patients are experiencing accelerated red cell destruction with compensatory erythroid hyperplasia and increased red cell synthesis. If something like a serious infection or folate deficiency impairs the capacity to maintain this high level of erythrocyte production, the hemocrit drops because the rapid destruction of erythrocytes continues.

The major morbidity and mortality of sickle cell disease results from recurrent vaso-occlusive events. These can be either acute causing localized painful crises, or chronic, resulting in chronic end organ damage. Acute crises occur episodically, often associated with acute infections and most often affect the abdomen, chest, and joints. Acute crisis may mimic acute abdominal processes such as appendicitis or visceral perforation, acute thoracic events such as pneumonia or pulmonary infarcts, or acute arthritis such as gout or rheumatoid arthritis. Sickle crises can also affect the central nervous system and present as a seizure, stroke, or coma.

After many acute crises the patient usually develops signs of chronic end organ damage due to the cumulative effects of many years of vaso-occlusive episodes. The organs damaged by these events are the lung, heart (congestive failure), liver (infarcts and fibrosis), gallbladder (gallstones due to increased red cell lysis and bilirubin production), kidney (failure to concentrate urine due to repeated infarcts), penis (priapism), bones (sclerosis, aseptic necrosis, osteomyelitis), eyes (retinal detachment, vitreous hemorrhage), skin (ulcers), and central nervous system (cerebral thrombosis).

The peripheral blood smear shows normochromic, normocytic red cell, target cells, and some sickle cells. The metabisulfite test produces sickling in the majority of the cells and hemoglobin electrophoresis confirms the diagnosis.

Sickle cell anemia must be differentiated from heterozygous sickle entities such as sickle thalassemia, and sickle-hemoglobin C disease. Patients with sickle-thalassemia can be distinguished because they have hypochromic microcytic cells and fewer sickle cells. Sickle C disease is distinguished from homozygous sickle disease by hemoglobin electrophoresis.

Medical Management

Management is supportive since no cure or prevention exists. Infections should be treated promptly to prevent serious complications or aplastic crises. Polyvalent pneumococcal vaccine should be given to reduce the risk of pneumococcal infection. Folic acid should be given to keep up with the heightened demand. Painful crises are treated with fluids, oxygen, and analgesics although the high risk of opiate dependence must be recognized.

Nursing Management

Nursing Diagnoses

Common nursing diagnoses for the patient with sickle cell anemia are as follows: alteration in systemic tissue perfusion related to clumping of sickle-shaped red blood cells; alteration in comfort: pain related to tissue ischemia and infarction; and knowledge deficit about medical management.

Goals. Goals of nursing intervention include early detection and treatment of the signs and symptoms of sickle cell anemia. Also it is important to prevent infarction and folic acid deprivation.

Interventions

Signs and symptoms of decreased systemic perfusion need to be detected early and reported to the physician. Pain can be relieved or reduced with general comfort measures and analgesics. Joint immobilization may relieve some pain. Hot or cold compresses may be helpful. Because any pressure on the area of discomfort can augment the pain, measures to relieve pressure should be provided. A cradle can be used to keep linen off the painful joint areas. The patient may need information about the deficiency and its management. Infection and folic acid deprivation can result in "aplastic crisis." Thus measures to prevent infection are necessary, and encouraging a diet adequate in folic acid is essential.

Evaluation

The outcome criteria for goal achievement include early detection, relief, and reduction of the signs and symptoms of sickle cell anemia. The patient should be able to describe medical therapy and relate the therapy to the disease process.

Aplastic Anemia

Aplastic anemia is an anemia from severe hypoplasia of the bone marrow. This anemia is an uncommon condition with an incidence of approximately 4 people per million in the United States. It is characterized by severe hypoplasia of the bone marrow usually affecting erythroid, myeloid, and thrombopoietic cell lines or in some cases only red cell precursors. In over half of the cases an etiology is not found. Among the known causes are a number of drugs and chemicals, most notably chloramphenicol, phenylbutazene, benzene, and some insecticides. Other associated causes are hepatitis virus and irradiation.

Clinical Manifestations

Manifestations of aplastic anemia are those common to all chronic anemias. However, the fact that these patients can develop severe thrombocytopenia ($<20,000$ platelets/mm^3) and neutropenia (<500 polymorphonuclear leukocytes/mm^3) also places them at risk of developing purpura, bleeding, and serious infection.

The peripheral blood reveals a severe anemia often with a red cell count below 1×10^6/ml. The cells are usually normal in appearance or slightly macrocytic; the leukocyte and platelet counts may be depressed as already noted. The bone marrow shows very few erythroid, myeloid, and platelet precursors; instead fat cells are abundant.

Aplastic anemia can be confused with hypersplenism, myelofibrosis, and a number of malignancies (*i.e.,* lymphoma, Hodgkin's disease, and aleukemic leukemia). In hypersplenism the marrow is hyperactive and the spleen is enlarged. Neither of these finding is characteristic of aplastic anemia. A myelofibrosis hepatosplenomegaly occurs; peripheral erythrocytes showed marked changes in size and shape especially tear-drop shaped cells and the marrow is fibrotic rather than fatty. Finally the malignant disorders can be distinguished from aplastic anemia by many features, one of these being the characteristic bone marrow findings of each.

Medical Management

A careful historical search should be made to identify an etiologic agent. If a drug or chemical known to cause aplastic anemia is identified it must be discontinued or avoided. Beyond this the two major forms of therapy are: androgenic steroids and bone marrow transplantation. Adrogenic steroids are the only currently available agents that are effective in stimulating remaining bone marrow precursor cells to proliferate. The most commonly used agents are fluoxymesterone, oxymetholone, methandrosterolone, testerone, and nandrolone. These agents have many potential side-effects such as virilization, hepatic toxicity, amenorrhea, and salt and water retention. Bone marrow transplantation is a means of replacing the destroyed marrow with that from a normal donor. To be successful the donor must be human lymphocyte antigen (HLA) compatible. The main side-effect of bone marrow transplantation is graft versus host disease. Lastly when necessary transfusion therapy with red cells and platelets should be offered.

The prognosis of aplastic anemia is poor; greater than 50% of patients with complete marrow failure die usually within a year of diagnosis. The main causes of death are hemorrhage and overwhelming infection.

Nursing Management

The patient with aplastic anemia frequently has the following problems: bleeding, infection, and fatigue. (These problems are discussed in depth in Chapters 50 and 51.)

Patients with aplastic anemia require some investigative work in finding the cause. Attempts should be made to identify possible toxic agents in the patient's personal and work environment. This can include medications, exposure to radiation, hair dyes, plant spray insecticides, volatile solvents, or large doses of antileukemic drugs. Meticulous attention should be given to avoid exposure to infections. Reverse isolation may be necessary. Explain the procedure, duration, and the need for isolation. Good skin hygiene is essential. Decubitus ulcers can occur. If a urinary catheter is needed, extra precaution should be used to avoid urinary tract infections. Assist the patient in coughing and deep breathing to prevent stasis of secretions and hypoventilation. Provide a restful environment and organize care to provide periods of uninterrupted rest. Observe carefully for any signs of bleeding.

Because of therapy with androgenic steroids observe for side-effects of virilism, sodium retention, hepatic changes, and muscle cramps and leukoagglutinins manifested by chills and fever following a transfusion. Because of poor prognosis of the disease emotional support is essential and lifestyle must change to conserve energy.

Immunohemolytic Anemia

Definition and Pathophysiology

Immunohemolytic anemia, also called acquired autoimmune hemolytic anemia, is a disease process in which immune reactants become attached to the surface of circulating erythrocytes and in so doing lead to the increased removal of these cells from the circulation and their subsequent destruction. Two immune components derived from plasma are commonly involved in this process—immunoglobulin G and the C3 component of complement. Immune hemolytic anemias can be subdivided into two major categories, those in which the abnormal anti-red cell antibodies are reactive at body temperature and those which are reactive in the cold. Table 53–2 presents a categorization of common diseases in which warm- and cold-induced immune hemolytic anemias occur. It is evident from the information in this table that immune mediated hemolytic anemia is not a specific disease but in fact an immunologic complication associated with a number of recognized diseases or the result of a reaction to certain drugs. In some cases this form of anemia has no apparent etiology, as is the case in two-thirds of warm-antibody cases.

Diagnosis: Coombs' Test. The direct Coombs' test, used to diagnose immune hemolytic anemia of any cause, relies on the ability of antibodies, prepared in animals against specific components in the human serum, to agglutinate red blood cells if those components are present on the membrane of erythrocytes. As mentioned previously the components of concern are IgG and C3; antisera which react with IgG produce a so-called gamma Coombs' reaction and those reacting with C3 produce a nongamma Coombs'. As routinely performed a direct Coombs' test will be positive when more than 500 molecules of IgG are bound to the surface of each red cell.

The indirect Coombs' test, used in the diagnosis of autoimmune hemolytic anemia, measures circulating anti-red cell antibody in the circulation. In other words this is excess antibody not bound to the surface of the red cell; hence the indirect Coombs' test is only positive when the direct test is also positive.

Drug-Induced Causes. Although it is impossible to discuss all the diseases which can present with autoimmune anemia, drug-induced causes deserve special attention. In drug-induced hemolytic disease three specific mechanisms are recognized. The first is that caused by the antihyperten-

TABLE 53–2
Classification of Immunohemolytic Anemia

A. Warm antibody type
   1. Idiopathic
   2. Lymphomas—chronic lymphocytic leukemia, non-Hodgkin's lymphoma
   3. Systemic lupus erythematosus
   4. Drug-induced
      alpha methyldopa
      penicillin
      quinidine

B. Cold antibody type
   Cold agglutinin disease
      Acute—mycoplasma infection, infectious mononucleosus
      Chronic—idiopathic, lymphoma

sive agent alpha methyldopa. This drug produces a positive Coombs' test in 20% of patients who take it but in only 0.3% does hemolytic anemia develop. The mechanism of this effect is uncertain but it is known that the drug does not directly play a role in the reaction. Probably this agent produces a change in red cell membrane structure, producing new antigens which promote the production of antibodies which then bind to the altered red cells.

The second mechanism is that of penicillin-induced hemolytic anemia. This drug when used in high doses can act as a hapten combining with the membrane of red cells and thereby stimulate the production of anti-red cell antibodies.

Thirdly a number of drugs, of which quinidine is the best recognized example, can stimulate anti-red cell antibodies by an "innocent bystander" reaction. These agents do not bind to the red cell membrane as does penicillin, but first stimulate antibody formation; antigen (drug)–antibody reaction occurs; and the drug–antibody complex then binds to the red cells and produces injury.

Clinical Manifestations

Signs and symptoms are identical to the findings of any chronic anemia. In addition hemolysis may express itself with additional findings, specifically fever, jaundice, hepatomegaly, and splenomegaly. When hemolysis is acute, shock, abdominal pain, and thrombocytopenic purpura may occur.

The peripheral smear shows normochromic normocytic red cells; however spherocytes and nucleated red cells may be present. The reticulocyte is usually elevated, often very high (>50%). The bone marrow shows erythroid hyperplasia and large amounts of hemosiderin. The serum bilirubin is often elevated with the indirect fraction being predominant. Serum haptoglobin is low or absent. As already mentioned, a positive Coombs' test is essential to the diagnosis.

The various hemoglobinopathies can present a similar picture; however they can be diagnosed by hemoglobin electrophoresis, and the Coombs' test is negative in these disorders. Similarly in hereditary spherocytosis and congenital nonspherocytic hemolytic anemia, two nonimmune hemolytic diseases, the Coombs' test is negative.

Medical Management

Treatment of the underlying disease, when it is known, is the first measure. When no primary diagnosis is known or its treatment is insufficient, prednisone therapy 10- to 20 mg four times a day is usually initiated. The dose is reduced to the smallest needed to maintain normal hemoglobin levels. When corticosteroids are insufficient or large doses are required on a chronic basis, splenectomy is usually necessary.

Nursing Management

The nursing management of a patient with immunohemolytic anemia is the same as for any patient with chronic anemia. In addition, the patient may have a fever. Cool application either with sponging or compresses can be useful depending on the degree of the fever. A cool environment or cooling blankets facilitate decreasing the temperature. The patient may be in a state of fluid deficit and need increased fluid intake. Antipyretic agents may be prescribed.

Polycythemia Vera

Definition and Pathophysiology

Polycythemia vera is a malignant disease of the bone marrow which usually presents in middle to late life. It is slightly more common in men than women, rare in children, uncommon in blacks, and occurs with increased frequency in Jews of European heritage. The deficiency takes a progressive course leading to death in an average of 2 years without therapy and 10 to 12 years with appropriate therapy. The disease is a myeloproliferative syndrome which leads to an increase in production of erythrocytes, leukocytes, and platelets. In early stages of the disease, red cell production may be the only abnormality; but as the disease progresses pathologically, increased white cell and platelet production always occurs.

Clinical Manifestations

There are increased numbers of circulating red cells, white cells, and platelets and they are generally plethoric, hypermetabolic, and have splenomegaly often of massive proportion. Due to the increased viscosity of the blood, patients may experience venous and arterial insufficiency expressed as painful extremities. Increased viscosity can also produce central nervous system abnormalities such as dizziness, vertigo, tinnitus, and visual abnormalities. These patients are also at risk of both bleeding (usually nose bleeds and gastrointestinal bleeds from peptic ulcers) and thromboses. About 5% to 10% of patients may develop gout due to the hyperuricemia of increased cell turnover.

This disease is characterized by the following laboratory findings: elevated hemoglobin values, an increased red cell mass ranging from 35 to 60 ml/kg, a very low sedimentation rate, an elevated (>12,000) leukocyte count in about 60% of patients, an increased absolute basophil count, and an increase in total platelets in about 50% of patients. Transcobalamin I and III, which are vitamin B_{12}-binding proteins, are elevated in most patients. Serum and urinary erythropoietin levels are decreased in these patients in marked distinction to the levels in secondary polycythemia.

Polycythemia vera must be differentiated from secondary polycythemias (to be discussed shortly) and relative polycythemia which is a condition in which the plasma volume is contracted producing a spurious elevation of the hemotocrit.

Medical Management

Management of polycythemia vera is controversial. Phlebotomy alone is successful in extending the average survival of patients from 2 to 12 years. Phlebotomy should be performed when the hemotocrit reaches 60, and the aim should be to maintain the level at 40% to 45%. Adjunctive radioactive phosphorus(^{32}P) and chlorambucil therapy appears to promote the development of acute leukemia and should probably only be considered in patients who cannot be managed with phlebotomy alone. Hydroxyurea can also be used in difficult cases.

Nursing Management

Nursing Diagnoses

Common nursing diagnoses for the patient with polycythemia vera are as follows: decreased systemic tissue perfusion related to increased blood viscosity; alteration in comfort; pain related to ischemia; and bleeding related to ulcers and thrombosis.

Goals. Goals for nursing interventions include early detection of signs and symptoms of arterial insufficiency, bleeding, and pain; and relief of pain and bleeding.

Interventions

Signs and symptoms of arterial insufficiency, such as painful extremities, angina, dizziness, vertigo, tinnitus, and visual abnormalities, should be detected and reported to the physician. Any signs of bleeding such as nosebleeds and gastrointestinal bleeds should also be detected and reported. (Measures to control bleeding are discussed elsewhere in this text.)

Evaluation

Outcome criteria include: signs and symptoms of arterial insufficiency and bleeding are detected at onset and reported to the physican; pain is relieved; bleeding is stopped.

Secondary Polycythemia

Definition and Pathophysiology

These are disorders of increased red cell mass which result from increased erythropoietin production and can occur appropriately as a consequence of systemic hypoxia or renal ischemia, or may occur inappropriately by neoplastic production of this hormone. Erythropoietin synthesis normally occurs in the kidney and is stimulated by blood oxygen concentrations. Normal levels are 10 to 20 mU/ml. Causes of secondary polycythemia are chronic lung disease, congenital heart disease producing right to left shunts, renal ischemia, and high altitude exposure. Other causes are tumors which can produce erythropoietin. These are renal cell carcinoma, hepatoma, cerebellar hemaryoblastoma, pheochromocytoma, ovarian carcinoma, adrenal carcinoma, and uterine leiomyoma. In addition, certain rare hemoglobin abnormalities cause secondary polycythemia because these structurally abnormal hemoglobins have an unusually high affinity for oxygen and therefore cause relative tissue hypoxia.

Clinical Manifestations

Manifestations are similar to polycythemia vera except that splenomegaly, bleeding and thrombolic complications, and secondary gout are uncommon. Signs and symptoms of the primary disorder such as chronic lung disease should also be evident. Patients with secondary polycythemia secondary to abnormal hemoglobins are usually normal even with hematocrits as high as 65%.

Laboratory findings include an elevated hematocrit and red cell mass. Patients generally do not have elevated leukocytes or platelet counts but do have elevated erythropoietin levels while patients with polycythemia vera have reduced levels. Other laboratory findings are those related to the primary disease, such as arterial hypoxemia in chronic lung disease.

Medical Management

Management must be appropriate to the primary disease. According to patients with chronic lung disease increasing lung function and reducing hypoxemia are essential. If this is not possible and the increased red cell mass is causing hyperviscosity, then phlebotomy may be required. The same is true of cardiac disease causing right to left shunts. Secondary polycythemia due to renal disease (cyst, hyrdonephrosis, renal vascular disease) and that due to neoplasms is treated by surgical correction of the primary disease.

Nursing Management

Nursing care for patients with secondary polycythemia is dependent upon the etiology of the polycythemia. For example, nursing care of the patient with chronic lung disease, which is a common cause of polycythemia, is aimed at reducing hypoxemia and improving lung function. It may also be necessary to assist the patient to reduce the demands and activities of daily living to be compatible with symptoms. (See Chapter 27.)

Bibliography

Adamson JW: The polycythemias: Diagnosis and treatment. Hosp Pract 18(12):49–57, 1983

Bullock B, Rosendahl P: Pathophysiology: Adaptations and Alterations in Function. Boston, Little, Brown & Co., 1984

Emes JH, Nowak TJ: Introduction to Pathophysiology: Basic Principles of the Disease Process. Baltimore, University Park Press, 1983

Hathaway G: The child with sickle cell anemia: Implications and management. Nurse Pract 9(10):16–22, 1984

Hutchison MM: Aplastic anemia: Care of the bone marrow transplant patient. Nurs Clin North Am 18(3):543–546, 1983

Kellermeyer RW: General principles of the evaluation and therapy of anemias. Med Clin North Am 68(3):533–543, 1984

Lenzer JM: Hematologic aspects of alcoholism. Physician Assistant 8(8):83–88, 109–112, 1984

Lubkin I: Evaluating iron-deficiency anemia. Nurse Pract 7(9):34–37, 1982

Nicolle LS: Anemia of chronic disorders. Nurs Pract 9(11):19–22, 1984

Porth C: Pathophysiology Concepts of Altered Health State. Philadelphia, JB Lippincott, 1982

Robbins SL, Angell M, Kumar V: Basic Pathology, 3rd ed. Philadelphia, WB Saunders, 1983

Rooks Y, Pack B: A profile of sickle cell disease. Nurs Clin North Am 18(1):131–139, 1983

Spiltell JA: Clinical Medicine, vol 5. Philadelphia, Harper & Row, 1982

Thomas ED, Storb R: Acquired severe aplastic anemia: Progress and perplexity. Blood 64(2):325–328, 1984

Vichinsky EP, Hurst D, Lubin B: Sickle cell disease: Basic concepts. Hosp Med 19(9):128–130, 1983

Walters I, Baysinger M, Buchanan I, et al: Complications of sickle cell disease. Nurs Clin North Am 18(1):139–143, 1983

Chapter 54

Alterations in Hemostasis

Bleeding and Coagulation Disorders

Ruth A. Gregersen

Disorders of hemostasis can occur at all levels of the hemostatic mechanism. These disorders are usually categorized as vascular, platelet, or coagulation abnormalities. In each case, bleeding is the primary manifestation. The bleeding may be minor, such as petechiae and easy bruising of the skin, or major, with massive hemorhage. Occasionally, a defect may exist in more than one area. Liver disease, for example, may affect both platelets and some coagulation factors. This chapter will focus on the medical and nursing management of the more common abnormalities in each category.

Bleeding Due to Vascular Dysfunction

In the absence of platelet or blood coagulation abnormalities, the presence of purpura (purplish patches due to extravasation of blood into the skin) implies a vascular disorder.[7] The diseases associated with vascular abnormalities, listed in Table 54–1, are commonly termed nonthrombocytopenic purpuras. These diseases are diverse and include autoimmune problems such as allergic purpura and drug-induced purpura as well as nonallergic purpuras caused by infections (bacterial, viral, rickettsial, and protozoal), vitamin C deficiency (scurvy), inheritable disorders (hereditary hemorrhagic telangiectasia, Ehlers-Danlos syndrome), connective tissue disorders (senile purpura, Cushing's disease, corticosteroid purpura), and others.[20]

Etiology/Pathology/Clinical Manifestations

A feature common to all these conditions is the loss of vascular integrity with an increase in vascular permeability and fragility.[7] The bleeding associated with nonthrombocytopenic purpuras occurs primarily from mucous membranes or under the skin in the form of petechiae, purpura, and ecchymosis and is rarely serious.[12]

Medical Management

The etiology of many of these disorders is incompletely understood. The diagnosis is usually made from the appearance of the lesions and the clinical findings which are often characteristic. Laboratory test results of platelet function and blood coagulation are usually normal.[20] Management to a large extent is limited to treatment of the underlying disease. Supportive measures such as blood transfusions occasionally may be required.

TABLE 54–1
Bleeding Disorders Due to Vascular Abnormalities

I. Autoimmune Vascular Purpuras

Allergic purpuras
Drug-induced (atropine, quinine, penicillin, aspirin, some sedatives, sulfonamides, others)
Purpura fulminans

II. Infections

Bacterial (scarlet fever, diphtheria, endocarditis, others)
Viral (smallpox, measles, other)
Rickettsial (typhus, Rocky mountain spotted fever, others)
Protozoal (malaria, toxoplasmosis)

III. Structural Malformations

Hereditary hemorrhagic telangiectasia
Hereditary disorders of connective tissue
Acquired disorders of connective tissue (scurvy, senile purpura, Cushing's disease, others)

IV. Miscellaneous

Purpura simplex
Purpura associated with skin disease
Autoerythrocyte sensitization
Paraproteinemias

(Adapted from Wintrobe MM, Lee GR, Boggs DR, Bithell TC, Forster J, Athens JW, Lukens JN: Clinical Hematology, 8th ed. Philadelphia, Lea & Febiger, 1981)

Bleeding Due to Deficient or Defective Platelets

Platelet disorders may be due to altered number or function of platelets. Platelet disorders are probably the most common hemostatic abnormality found in hospitalized patients and thrombocytopenia (decreased platelets) is the most common cause of abnormal bleeding.[20]

Thrombocytopenia

Thrombocytopenia is defined as a platelet count of less than 100,000/mm^3.[13] The normal platelet count ranges from 150,000 to 350,000/mm^3. If the platelet count is decreased but above 40,000/mm^3, spontaneous bleeding is uncommon. However, bleeding may occur after injury or surgery. With platelet counts between 10,000 and 20,000/mm^3, spontaneous bleeding occurs commonly.[13] Platelet counts below 10,000/mm^3 usually cause severe bleeding.[13]

Etiology and Pathophysiology

A low platelet count may result from one or a combination of mechanisms. These include disorders of platelet production, distribution and dilution, or destruction.[17] (See Table 54–2.)

TABLE 54–2
Classification of Thrombocytopenia

Mechanism	***Specific Disorder***
Disturbances in platelet production	
Megakaryocytic hypoplasia	Congenital (Francon's anemia, prematurity, intrauterine drugs, infection) Acquired (radiation, chemicals and drugs, alcohol, insecticides, infections, lupus erythematosus, heroin, neoplastic marrow replacement)
Ineffective platelet production	Hereditary (autosomal or sex-linked types, May-Hegglin anomaly, Wiskott-Aldrich syndrome) Acquired (vitamin B_{12} or folate deficiency, paroxysmal nocturnal hemoglobinuria, preleukemia)
Disturbance in platelet distribution or dilution	Splenic pooling (splenomegaly) Vascular pooling (hypothermia) Dilution (massive transfusions)
Disturbance in platelet destruction	Combined consumption of DIC (snake venoms, tissue injury, obstetrical complications, neoplasms, infections) Isolated platelet consumption (thrombotic thrombocytopenic purpura, hemolytic-uremic syndrome, purpura fulminans, vasculitis, prosthetic valves, extracorporeal circulation) Immune platelet destruction (idiopathic thrombocytopenic purpura; post-transfusion purpura; isoimmune neonatal purpura; drugs (*i.e.,* quinidine, digoxin, chlorothiazides, sulfonamides); infections and solid tumor-induced antibodies)

(Adapted from Thompson AR, Harker LA: Manual of Hemostasis and Thrombosis, 3rd ed. Philadelphia, FA Davis, 1983)

Decreased platelet production, verified by bone marrow aspiration and biopsy, may be a result of decreased production or defective maturation of platelets. The bone marrow aspirate usually shows a decreased number of visible megakaryocytes (the cells that give rise to platelets) when platelet production is extremely diminished. Decreased production may be a result of drugs used in cancer chemotherapy, ethanol, and irradiation of the bone marrow. Disease, such as aplastic anemia, lupus erythematosis, leukemia, and congenital deficiencies, may also decrease platelet production. With defective maturation, the number of megakaryocytes in the bone marrow is normal or increased; however, thrombopoiesis is "ineffective." Defective maturation may result from vitamin B_{12} or folate deficiency, hereditary disorders, or disorders in which myeloid tissue proliferates.[13]

Disturbances in platelet distribution are due to splenomegaly (splenic pooling) or hypothermia (vascular pooling). Normally the spleen holds about 20% of the platelets. This pooling increases proportionately with the size of the spleen. Hypothermia (lowering the body temperature to less than 25°C) causes platelet pooling in the liver. The treatment of thrombocytopenia secondary to splenic pooling is directed to the underlying disease while thrombocytopenia due to hypothermia responds to rewarming.[17] Treatment of massive blood loss by transfusion of large volumes of stored blood, in which the viability of platelets is impaired, dilutes the platelet count. Excessive bleeding due to dilutional thrombocytopenia can be prevented by transfusing platelet concentrates when the platelet count is less than 100,000/mm^3.[17]

Accelerated destruction of platelets (a decrease in the survival time from 10 days to less than 1 day) is a frequent cause of thrombocytopenia. The most common causes of this destruction are antibody-mediated platelet injury and increased utilization in disseminated intravascular coagulation (DIC). Autoantibodies in idiopathic thrombocytopenic purpura, systemic lupus erythematosus, chronic lymphocytic leukemia, and autoimmune hemolytic anemia may cause platelet destruction. In addition, alloantibodies associated with pregnancy or transfusions and antibodies associated with certain drugs (*i.e.,* quinidine, quinine, and sulfonamides) are known to cause antibody-mediated thrombocytopenia.[13] The medical management is based upon identifying and removing the cause or treating the underlying disease. Corticosteroids may be given to enhance capillary integrity, and platelet transfusions are used if hemorrhage develops. (Thrombocytopenia associated with DIC will be discussed later in this chapter.)

Thrombocytopenia may be due to more than one cause. Alcoholic liver disease causes decreased production of platelets by the direct toxic effect of alcohol as well as ineffective production due to folate deficiency. Splenomegaly secondary to cirrhosis with portal hypertension increases platelet pooling. In addition, platelet survival is decreased due to direct effects of alcohol.[17] Abstaining from alcohol and administration of folate will usually allow the platelet count to return to normal in 1 to 2 weeks.[17]

Extracorporeal circulation as used in cardiac surgery produces thrombocytopenia.[17] Platelet counts are decreased for several days after bypass due to platelet utilization in the injured tissues. Platelet transfusions are admdinistered if excessive bleeding occurs.

Clinical Manifestations

Clinical manifestation of spontaneous bleeding under the skin due to thrombocytopenia are petechiae, purpura, or ecchymosis. Petechial lesions of severe thrombocytopenia are not elevated and frequently first appear over the ankles although they may become widespread. Minor cuts bleed for a long time because platelet plugs do not form. Post-traumatic or post-surgical bleeding usually has an immediate onset and responds to local measures such as pressure over the area. Mucous membrane surfaces such as the mouth, nose, uterus, and gastrointestinal, urinary, or respiratory tracts are common sites of bleeding.[13] Central nervous system bleeding is the most serious site for spontaneous bleeding and may be fatal.[13]

Idiopathic Thrombocytopenic Purpura

Idiodpathic thrombocytopenic purpura (ITP) may be considered the prototype thrombocytopenic state.[13]

The definition of this disorder is a low platelet count due to accelerated destruction of platelets.[20] This disorder can be acute or chronic; however, it usually has a sudden onset. Acute ITP occurs most frequently in children from 2 to 6 years old and over 80% recover within 6 months without treatment. Chronic ITP occurs commonly in women from 20 to 40 years old. Over 90% of adults with ITP fail to undergo spontaneous remission.[17]

Etiology and Patholophysiology

Platelets are coated with antibodies made by B lymphocytes, although platelet function is preserved. When platelets pass into the spleen, with their surface altered by antibodies, macrophages sequester and destroy them.[21] In the process, the platelet antigens are exposed to more B lymphocytes in the spleen, and additional antibodies are made by splenic lymphocytes.[21]

Clinical Manifestations

The major clinical manifestation of ITP is purpura over the limbs, upper chest, and neck. In young children a viral illness often precedes the purpura. The absence of an enlarged spleen, a low platelet count, and large numbers of megakaryocytes in the bone marrow are hallmarks of the disease.[20]

Medical Management

Medical management includes treatment with corticosteroids, splenectomy, and vincristine. Corticosteroids are used in the treatment of chronic ITP and may induce a clinical cure. Corticosteroids interfere with the phagocytosis of platelets in the spleen and may displace the antibodies from the platelet. Because the spleen is the site of destruction of platelets as well as the site of antibody production, removal of the spleen often affects a clinical remission or cure if steroids are ineffective.[21] Vincristine may be used to stimulate the production of platelets, although the mechanism of action is unclear.[21]

Thrombocytopathy

A prolonged bleeding time associated with a normal platelet count suggests a disturbance of platelet function. These disorders are classified according to defects in adhesion, primary aggregation, and release reaction.

Etiology and Pathophysiology

A defect in platelet adhesion is found in von Willebrand's disease and will be discussed later. Thrombasthenia is a congenital disease which has a defect in the primary aggregation response.[13]

Drugs may impair platelet function by inhibiting the release reaction which impairs platelet aggregation.[13] A single 200-mg dose of aspirin inhibits release by blocking the production of thromboxane A_2, which mediates the release reaction.[17] The effect persists for the life span of the platelet (7–10 days). Many other anti-inflammatory drugs such as phenylbutazone and indomethacin also inhibit platelet release reaction. These drugs do not cause bleeding by themselves but may aggravate an underlying disorder of hemostasis.[13]

Uremia, cirrhosis, dysproteinemia, and myeloproliferative syndromes may also cause a deficit of platelet function. These defects are not completely understood.

Clinical Manifestations/Medical Management

Clinical manifestations of thrombocytopathy are the same signs and symptoms associated with thrombocytopenia.

Medical management is directed toward removing or treating the underlying cause.

Thrombocytosis

Thrombocytosis is a platelet count greater than normal.

Etiology and Pathophysiology

Thrombocytosis has been reported in association with many pathological conditions (Table 54–3). In essential thrombocytosis (thrombocythemia) platelet production appears to be autonomous. Megakaryocyte numbers and volume are both increased.[17]

Clinical Manifestations

Clinical manifestations of thrombocytosis are as follows: platelet counts frequently over one million, enlarged spleen, bleeding, and thromboembolism.

Medical Management

Medical management includes alkylating agents to lower platelet counts when symptoms of bleeding or thromboembolism occur.

In secondary thrombocytosis, megakaryocyte number is increased but volume is decreased. Because there is little evidence that secondary thrombocytosis results in clinical sequelae, therapy is directed toward the underlying illness.[17]

Nursing Management of Platelet Disorders

Assessment and Nursing Diagnosis

Regardless of the cause of platelet disorders, the nursing diagnosis is: potential for bleeding related to platelet disorders leading to petechiae, purpura, and ecchymosis of the skin or signs and symptoms of bleeding from any mucous membrane.

Goals. The nursing goals are the early detection, and prevention or control of bleeding.

Interventions

Because many platelet disorders are associated with drug therapy and other diseases, the nurse must continually assess those clients at risk for signs of bleeding. Bleeding associated with platelet disorders is usually from superficial

TABLE 54–3
Classification of Thrombocytosis

I. Primary (autonomous)
    A. Essential thrombocythemia
    B. Other myeloproliferative disorders

II. Secondary (reactive)
    A. Inflammatory disorders
        1. Acute rheumatic fever
        2. Rheumatoid arthritis
        3. Ulcerative colitis
        4. Tuberculosis
        5. Cirrhosis
        6. Osteomyelitis
    B. Blood disorders
        1. Chronic granulocytic leukemia
        2. Acute hemorrhage
        3. Hemolytic anemia
        4. Iron deficiency anemia
    C. Malignancy
        1. Carcinoma
        2. Hodgkin's disease
    D. Postoperative
    E. Response to drugs
    F. Response to exercise

(Adapted from Williams WJ: Classification of disorders of hemostasis. In Williams WJ, Beutler E, Erslev AJ, Lichtman MA (eds): Hematology, 3rd ed. New York, McGraw-Hill, 1983)

sites; however, the evaluation of emesis, urine, and stool for overt or occult bleeding is vital.

Teaching clients to carefully read the labels and avoid over-the-counter drugs that may contain aspirin, which may aggravate bleeding associated with platelet disorders, is very important. Avoidance of injury should also be stressed in teaching these clients. In addition the nurse should encourage clients to have a complete medical evaluation when prolonged epistaxis, petechiae, easy bruising, and other signs of bleeding tendencies develop.

Administration of platelets may be required for some clients with platelet dysfunction. Because one unit of platelets will increase the platelet count by 5,000 to 10,000 mm,[3] 6 to 10 units are usually transfused at one time.[17] Proper administration techniques are important to preserve platelet function. Platelets are provided ABO specific but are not crossmatched so only knowledge of the client's blood type is needed. Platelet concentrates may be stored for 72 hours at 20°C to 24°C with constant and gentle agitation. Concentrates may be pooled (several units mixed) before administration; however they must be transfused within 6 hours after pooling.[16]

Platelet concentrates must be administered at room temperature through a standard (170-micron) filter (microfilters must not be used). A new filter must be used each time because using a filter that already contains debris from other blood products will impair flow and substantially reduce the number of platelets administered. Administer platelets by intravenous drip infusion or by direct push method at a rate of 6 units over 20 to 30 minutes.[2] Normal saline is the only fluid that can be used with platelets. Pressure cuffs or infusion pumps must not be used during administration because they may damage the platelets.

Chills, fever, and allergic reactions may occur. Fever must not be treated with antipyretics containing aspirin because they will inhibit platelet function.

TABLE 54–4
Common Blood Coagulation Disorders

I. Congenital
   A. Abnormalities of plasma factors
      1. Hemophilia A (factor VIII deficiency)
      2. Hemophilia B (factor IX deficiency, Christmas disease)
      3. Factor XI deficiency (plasma thromboplastin antecedent)
      4. Factor XII deficiency (Hageman factor)
      5. Fibrinogen deficiency
   B. Abnormality of plasma factors involved in platelet function
      1. von Willebrand's disease

II. Acquired
   A. Vitamin K deficiency
   B. Liver disease
   C. Amyloidosis
   D. Nephrotic syndrome
   E. Gaucher's disease
   F. Sytemic lupus erythematosus
   G. Circulating anticoagulants
   H. Disseminated intravascular coagulation

(Adapted from Williams WJ: Classification of disorders of hemostasis. In Williams WJ, Beutler E, Erslev AJ, Lichtman MA (eds): Hematology, 3rd ed. New York, McGraw-Hill, 1983)

Bleeding Due to Deficient or Defective Clotting Factors

Bleeding due to coagulation disorders results from either congenital or acquired defects or deficiencies of the clotting factors, including hemophilia, von Willebrand's disease, vitamin K deficiency, liver disease, and nephrotic syndrome, to name a few. A partial list of these disorders is presented in Table 54–4.

Congenital Coagulation Disorders

Inherited coagulation deficiencies are rare, affecting approximately 1 in 10,000 persons.[17] Bleeding disorders due to congenital defects may be caused by a defect or deficiency of any of the plasma coagulation factors except factor XII, prekallikrein, and high molecular weight kininogen. The absence of these factors does not cause bleeding.

The most common congenital bleeding disorders are hemophilia A (factor VIII deficiency), hemophilia B (factor IX deficiency, also termed Christmas disease), and von Willebrand's disease (factor VIII/von Willebrand's deficiency). Eighty percent of hemophiliacs have hemophilia A while the other 20% have hemophilia B. The true prevalence of von Willebrand's disease is not known but it may be one of the most common congenital bleeding disorders.[14] The other clotting deficiencies are extremely rare.

Hemophilia

Both hemophilia A and B are sex (X chromosome)-linked recessive disorders (Fig. 54–1), which means that a female carrier of hemophilia will transmit the defective X chromosome to one half of her sons, who will be hemophiliacs and to one half of her daughters, who will be carriers. A male hemophiliac will transmit the X chromosome to all of his daughters, who will be carriers. Female carriers do not commonly manifest any bleeding tendency.[14]

Etiology and Pathophysiology

Two proteins, antihemophilic and von Willebrand factors, (together termed factor VIII complex) circulate in plasma apparently bound to one another.[14] The function of the antihemophilic factor is to act as a cofactor for factor IXa in the activation of factor X. (See Chapter 21 for a more

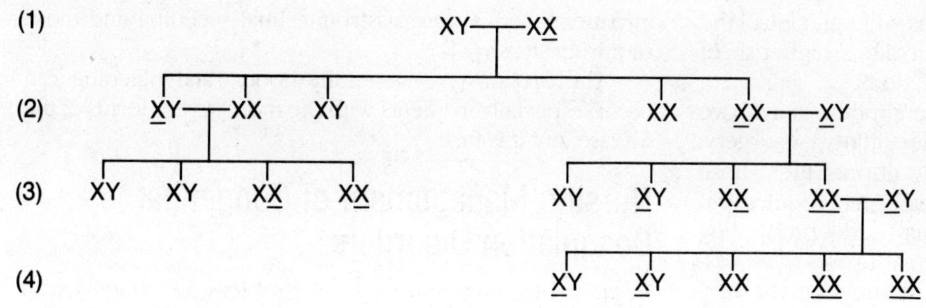

FIGURE 54-1 The heredity pattern of hemophilia. The defect is carried by the X chromosome. The offspring of a female carrier (XX) and a normal male (XY) may be normal (XY, XX) a female carrier (XX) or a hemophiliac male (XY). Mating of two individuals who each possess the defect may result in exclusively hemophiliac offspring (generation 4).

detailed description of blood coagulation.) Defective activity of this molecule, refered to as factor VIII coagulant activity (VIII:C), is responsible for hemophilia A. The von Willebrand protein (factor VIII:svWF), which constitutes most of the protein of the factor VIII complex, binds to the surface of platelets and is essential for the normal formation of platelet plugs.[14] An abnormality of factor VIII:vWF accounts for the impaired hemostasis in clients with von Willebrand's disease. Hemophilia B occurs as a result of factor IX deficiency.

Pathology of hemophilia A and B (deficiencies of factor VIII:C and IX) will be discussed together because they are clinically indistinguishable. The bleeding manifestations of hemophilia are related to the client's clotting factor activity level (Table 54–5). Because platelet plug formation, the first line of defense against bleeding, is normal in both hemophilia A and B, the onset of bleeding is characteristically delayed for several minutes or hours after injury.

Clinical Manifestations

Clinical manifestations of hemophilia are bruises, ecchymosis, and deep subcutaneous and intramuscular hematomas. Petechiae and purpura do not occur in hemophilia. Frequent hemarthroses (extravasation of blood into joints) are a characteristic symptom in moderate and severe hemophilia and often result in permanent joint damage.[14] Bleeding may occur at any site of the body. However it is potentially fatal due to the effects of local pressure when it is intracranial or laryngeal in location or near vital organs such as the heart or lungs.[14]

Medical Management

The medical management of hemophilia includes laboratory tests to establish the definitive diagnosis of hemophilia in those clients giving a history of bleeding with or without a familial pattern. The platelet count and function and bleeding time are normal. The whole blood clotting time is prolonged in severe hemophilia, whereas in mild hemophilia it may be normal. The prothrombin time is normal while the partial thromboplastin time is prolonged. Low factor VIII:C is diagnostic for hemophilia A, while low factor IX is diagnostic of hemophilia B.

Medical therapy of bleeding episodes consists of the transfusion of material containing the defective or missing factor. This temporarily corrects the specific defect. Cryoprecipitate, containing about 120 factor VIII units and 150 to 200 mg of fibrinogen per bag, is used to treat bleeding episodes in clients with hemophilia A. Plasma is used to treat mild bleeding edpisodes in hemophilia B while factor IX

TABLE 54-5
Relationship of Clotting Factor Activity Levels to Severity of Bleeding in Hemophilia

Factor VIII:C Activity Level (% of Normal)	*Classification*	*Bleeding Manifestation*
50–100		None
25–50		Bleeding may be excessive after major trauma
5–25	mild	Severe bleeding after surgery or major trauma; some bleeding after minor trauma; no spontaneous bleeding
1–5	moderate	Severe bleeding after minor injury; occasional spontaneous hemorrhages
<1	severe	Frequent spontaneous bleeding into muscles and joints

(Adapted from Nossel HL: Disorders of blood coagulation factors. In Petersdorf RG, Adams RD, Braunwald E, Isselbacher KJ, Martin JB, Wilson JD (eds): Harrison's Principles of Internal Medicine, 10th ed. New York, McGraw-Hill, 1983)

concentrates are used only when plasma will not control the bleeding as factor IX concentrates contain a high risk of hepatitis and thromboembolic complications.[4]

Clients with milder forms of hemophilia may have severe hemorrhage after dental extraction, injury, or surgery; however, they are able to live a fairly normal life. Those clients with a severe form of the disease may require frequent admission to the hospital and may develop crippling joint deformities from repeated hemarthroses. Life expectancy has been greatly prolonged by replacement therapy. However, severe hemorrhage causing death still occurs quite frequently.[14]

Von Willebrand's Disease

Von Willebrand's disease is a congenital bleeding disorder transmitted as an autosomal (nonsex-determining chromosomal) dominant or recessive trait. Therefore the disease occurs in both sexes. The impaired hemostasis is due to a quantitative or qualitative abnormality of factor VIII:vWF.[18]

Etiology and Pathophysiology

As discussed earlier, the von Willebrand factor constitutes most of the protein of the factor VIII complex. This protein can bind to both platelets and the subendothelium thereby promoting the accumulation of platelets at sites of blood vessel injury.[18] It is therefore responsible for the initial arrest of bleeding. There are several different types of the disease with mild to severe bleeding disorders. The exact structural defects of the protein in von Willebrand's disease have not been identified.[14] Reduction in factor VIII:C (antihemophilic factor) activity is often present, apparently as a secondary phenomenon.[17]

Clinical Manifestations

Clinical manifestations usually begin in childhood and tend to decrease with age.[18] The most common bleeding sites are the mucous membranes and the skin. Clients bruise easily and have frequent nose bleeds.[14] Petechiae are rare.[14] Recurrent gastrointestinal bleeding and menorrhagia occur, but hemarthroses occur only in clients with very low levels of factor VIII:C.[14]

Medical Management

The bleeding time and the antihemophilic factor assay are the most useful tests in the initial evaluation of von Willebrand's disease. However, they both may fluctuate widely in an individual on repeated testing.[14] Due to the heterogeneity of the disorder, no single normal test is sufficient to exclude the diagnosis. The bleeding time is usually prolonged and the concentration of von Willebrand protein is usually low.

Mild bleeding in von Willebrand's disease may respond to local measures such as application of cold and gentle pressure. Transfusion of normal plasma has a more lasting effect on the factor VIII level in most patients. A cryoprecipitate rich in factor VIII will usually correct the prolonged bleeding time and increase the factor VIII levels and is used in patients with severe gastrointestinal bleeding and those requiring surgery.

The prognosis is generally good. Fatal bleeding can occur, especially in clients with the more severe forms of the disease, but it is rare.[18]

Nursing Management of Congenital Coagulation Disorders

Because bleeding is a common problem for patients with hematologic disorders, the nursing care has been discussed in Chapter 50. Clients with congenital coagulation disorders have some special problems and concerns in addition to the problem of hemorrhage. The diagnosis of congenital coagulation disorders is usually made in infancy. Learning that a child has a lifelong medical problem is obviously stressful to parents and may cause ineffective coping patterns in both the parents and the child as he or she matures and understands the disorder. In addition, teaching parents to cope with bleeding episodes is vital. Effective counseling and teaching cannot be done in a single session in the hospital or clinic setting. Periodic sessions, preferrably in the client's home, are best for teaching the parents and allowing them to discuss their feelings. The types of interventions suggested for providing psychosocial support is presented in the accompanying Nursing Care Plan for the Family and Client with Hemophilia. A health-team member experienced in dealing with the problems of hemophilia can best provide this teaching and counseling. The teaching program can begin with an assessment of the parents' understanding of the disease and how it has affected family living. The teaching interventions address such issues as how to recognize and treat bleeding episodes; how to deal with such problems as hemarthroses, minor skin lacerations, and serious head injuries; what options exist for obtaining transfusion therapy; how to prevent and minimize bleeding episodes and what kinds of common problems and concerns are associated with the disease. An example of a teaching plan, adapted from a booklet published by the National Hemophilia Foundation, can be found in Table 54–6.

Acquired Coagulation Disorders

Acquired coagulation defects are much more common than congenital coagulation disorders. These defects may be mild and present as somewhat increased operative bleeding or as acute generalized bleeding from several sites.

Vitamin K Deficiency

Vitamin K is essential for the synthesis of prothrombin and clotting factors VII, IX and X. Therefore, associated coagulation defect may be severe.[15] These factors contain γ-carboxyglutamic acid and their completed synthesis requires vitamin K as a cofactor for the vitamin K-dependent carboxylase.[6] In the abrence of vitamin K, these blood clotting proteins contain decreased γ-carboxyglutamic acid and are functionally inert.[6]

One natural source of vitamin K, a fat-soluble vitamin, is

TABLE 54–6
Health Teaching for the Family of Patient with Hemophilia

Assessment

1. Elicit and discuss answers to the following questions with the parents:
   a. What do they know about the congenital coagulation disorder?
   b. Was the condition initially misdiagnosed (*e.g.*, as leukemia or child abuse)?
   c. Is there a family history of the disease? If so, how was the parent related?
   d. Have any relatives with the disease died of bleeding?
   e. Did the parents suspect that they might have a child with a bleeding disorder?
   f. Was the baby planned?
   g. What are the parent's plans for future child bearing?
   h. Are finances currently a problem or likely to become one?
   i. Are supportive family members or friends nearby?
   j. What aspects of the disease worry the family?
2. Assess the impact of the illness upon the marital relationship.
   a. Are the parents supportive of each other?
   b. Is blame being placed?
3. Assess the effects of the diagnosis on siblings.
   a. Is there regressive behavior, anger toward, or excessive concern for the hemophiliac infant?
   b. Is there a lack of parental attention toward the siblings?

Teaching Interventions to Assist Parents to Recognize Bleeding Episodes

1. Teach parents the common kinds of bleeding episodes to expect and how to recognize and treat them (may need to present the information several times).

Hemarthrosis

a. Joints commonly affected are knees, elbows, and ankles.
b. Manifestations are pain followed by limitation of motion and, finally, swelling.
c. Treatment
   Rest the joint totally; pack the joint in ice; infusion of factor replacement; and range of motion exercises without weight bearing

Minor Skin Lacerations

a. Apply local pressure, cold, or thrombin.
b. Infusion of factor replacement if bleeding does not respond to local measures.
c. Lacerations should be cleaned and sutured as necessary.
d. Follow-up care should be sought.

Head Injuries

a. Intracerebral bleeding is a major cause of death and requires immediate treatment.
b. Signs and symptoms: Lethargy, confusion, unequal pupils
c. Immediate infusion of factor replacement
d. Observation for 1–2 days frequently in the hospital

Transufusion Therapy Teaching

1. Offer parents several alternative ways to obtain transfusion therapy for child.
   a. Home transfusion therapy
   b. Outpatient transfusions at local hospital emergency room or physician's office
   c. Transfusions at a hemophilia care center.
   e. Reassure parents that proper treatment can control bleeding and allow their child to lead a nearly normal life.

Preventive Measures to Minimize Bleeding Episodes

1. Teach parents/clients to avoid aspirin and aspirin-containing products because aspirin interferes with the function of platelets by inhibiting the release reaction. Provide the generic name and teach parents or client to read labels of over-the-counter drugs.
2. Teach the importance of wearing an emergency medical tag. In case of injury, it is vital that medical personnel be aware of the bleeding disorder.
3. Encourage patents/client to seek medical care from a physician knowledgeable in the treatment of the disease.
4. Teach parents and client activities which are safe and those to avoid
   Encourage: swimming, bicycling, hiking, tennis, golf, etc.
   Avoid: contact sports such as football, boxing, soccer, etc.

Common Chronic Problems Associated with Disease

Chronic Joint Disease

1. Provide the parents with information regarding chronic joint disease.
   a. Prevent damage by regular maintenance transfusions, exercise, and judicious use of protective splints.
   b. Avoid aspirin in all forms for the relief of joint pain.

Dental Care

1. Encourage the parents/child to seek regular prophylactic dental care to avoid the need for extensive extractions later in life.
2. Teach parents/client how to provide regular gentle oral care.

food, particularly green leafy vegetables. The intestinal bacterial flora is another source. Oral administration of antibiotics may cause decreased intestinal flora leading to vitamin K deficiency in the absence of dietary intake.[14] Obstructive jaundice or biliary fistulas cause lack of bile salts which impairs absorption of vitamin K. Intestinal malabsorption syndromes may also cause vitamin K deficiency.

Clinical manifestations associated with the disorder may vary from only laboratory evidence of the deficient state to serious spontaneous hemorrhage.[6] The type of bleeding is similar to that occurring with other coagulation defects. Symptoms of vitamin K deficiency can develop in 1 to 3 weeks if intake of the vitamin is stopped.[6]

Medical management involves correction of the underlying cause. Vitamin K deficiency is characterized by a prolonged prothrombin time (PT) and often a prolonged partial thromboplastin time (PTT). The diagnosis is confirmed if the PT and PTT are rapidly (within 8–12 hours), completely corrected by administration of vitamin K.[6]

(*Text continues on page 740*)

NURSING CARE PLAN FOR THE FAMILY AND CLIENT WITH HEMOPHILIA[3]

NURSING DIAGNOSIS/PROBLEM 1: Potential ineffective family coping related to learning that their child has a congenital coagulation disorder.

GOAL 1: To assist parents to discuss and accept their feelings regarding the diagnosis and to develop a trusting relationship between the family and providers of care.

Nursing Interventions	Rationale	Outcome Criteria
1. Encourage parents to express their feelings and fears.	1. In helping clients cope directly with anxiety or stress, the source of the feelings must be identified.[10]	1–6. Parents will: ▪ Discuss feelings openly. ▪ Support each other and not place blame. ▪ Ask questions. ▪ Seek help from family and friends. ▪ Appear relaxed and comfortable with care givers.
2. Reassure parents that feelings of anxiety, sadness, anger or guilt are normal.	2. Knowing that others have experienced the same feelings in similar circumstances may help alleviate the feelings.	
3. Answer questions.	3. The initial shock of learning the diagnosis may prevent parents from fully understanding specific information. Answers to questions may need repeating.[3]	
4. Encourage parents to use the emotional and practical support available from others (family members, friends, neighbors).	4. Support from family and friends decreases fears and anxiety.	
5. Instruct the parents in normal child development, and how their reactions will influence their child's personality development.	5. Knowledge about what to anticipate facilitates effective coping behaviors.	
6. Reassure that the family can call the hemophilia center staff at any time.	6. Reassurance that the parents can obtain help at any time will alleviate anxiety and develop trust in the providers of care.	

NURSING DIAGNOSIS/PROBLEM 2: Potential social and emotional problems related to the diagnosis of congenital coagulation disorder leading to behavior problems, psychological disorders, poor school attendance, and unemployment.

GOAL 2: To maintain normal social and emotional development.

Nursing Interventions	Rationale	Outcome Criteria
Toddler age		
1. Offers parents counseling and support as bleeding episodes increase.	1. The mobility and exploratory behavior associated with the toddler age usually cause an increase in bleeding episodes.	1–5. The toddler develops a sense of autonomy and independence.
2. Encourage parents to join a support group of other parents of children who have bleeding disorders.	2. The counsel of other parents is often particularly valuable because they speak from experience.	
3. Discuss safety measures: suitable toys, car seats, and avoidance of falls from high places.	3. Safety measures that are appropriate for all young children are generally sufficient.	
4. Caution against subtle overprotection such as repeated cautions to "be careful."	4. Overprotection interferes with the development of normal assertiveness and independence.	
5. Encourage parents to use the same disciplinary methods with all siblings and encourage age-appropriate chores.	5. Overindulgence and lack of responsibility may severely handicap the child in later life.	

(Continued)

NURSING CARE PLAN FOR THE FAMILY AND CLIENT WITH HEMOPHILIA[3] (*Continued*)

Nursing Interventions	Rationale	Outcome Criteria
Childhood		
1. Encourage parents to participate in some appropriate exercise with their child such as swimming, bicycling, or hiking, and encourage the child to exercise regularly.	1. Exercise is important for normal motor development and the strengthening of muscles that protect joints. The child with a bleeding disorder may need the parents' encouragement to try new activities.	1–7. The child participates in regular exercise. The child develops normal social skills. Absences from school are minimal.
2. Encourage nursery school attendance.	2. Nursery school attendance helps the child develop social skills early and offers reassurance that he or she can survive without a parent's constant attention.	Academic progress continues as appropriate for age and abilities. The child provides self-care and seeks assistance from parents, teachers, and health-care providers as appropriate.
3. Encourage regular school attendance rather than one for handicapped children.	3. Regular school enhances the child's sense of being normal and provides daily experience in dealing with the regular world.	
4. Educate teachers and school administrators about the bleeding disorder.	4. Education of the teachers will dispel unrealistic fears about the disorder and assist them to recognize common bleeding problems.	
5. Encourage the parents to expect the child to perform on the same level as other children of the same age.	5. The success in school performance provides the foundation for later academic and occupational success.	
6. Assist the child in answering peers' questions about the disease.	6. Effforts to normalize social experience are vital to the child's self-image.	
7. Begin to teach the child about the disease and necessary treatment.	7. The child must learn independence in all areas of life.	
Adolescence		
1. Help the family to anticipate the difficult period of adolescence.	1. Attempts of the adolescent to gain independence may lead to conflict with parents, teachers, doctor, or other authority figures.	1–5. Normal adolescent emotional upheaval will not interfere with the client's reliable self-care and protection. Reckless behavior and medical noncompliance will not occur. An appropriate career will be chosen.
2. Encourage the parents to allow the adolescent to make most of the decisions regarding activities and encourage self-care of the disease.	2. Independent decision making helps keep the adolescent out of the field of combat with authority figures.	
3. Encourage attendance at group meetings with other teenagers with bleeding disorders.	3. Group meetings allow discussion of concerns about illness and its effect on peer relationships.	
4. Encourage discussion of sexual concerns.	4. Due to the influence of the disorder on masculine self-esteem, the teen may be afraid that masturbation or sexual intercourse will cause hemorrhage.	
5. Encourage that vocational guidance be started in junior high school.	5. The preoccupation with becoming an independent person may take precedence over career planning.	

Vitamin K administration will correct the hemostatic defect within 8 to 12 hours. Clients with marked bleeding may be treated with fresh frozen plasma.

Nursing Management

Nursing Diagnosis. The nursing diagnosis for patients with vitamin K deficiency is: Potential for bleeding related to clotting factor defects manifested by prolonged PT and PTT, bruises, ecchymosis, and deep subcutaneous and intramuscular hematomas (or signs and symptoms of bleeding from any site).

The *goals* are to prevent bleeding episodes by identifying those patients at risk and to prevent complications associated with medical therapy.

Interventions. A common setting of vitamin K deficiency is the postsurgical client who has developed an infection. The absence of dietary intake and the presence of antibiotic therapy often leads to vitamin K deficiency unless supplemental vitamin K is administered. Evaluation of the PT and PTT results to detect this defect and administration of vitamin K to prevent bleeding are essential.

Vitamin K is frequently administered parenterally if bleeding is active because absorption of the oral preparation is unreliable.[6] Due to the risk of hematoma formation with intramuscular injection, intravenous (IV) infusion may be necessary. Rapid IV injection of vitamin K has been associated with anaphylactic reactions; thus the infusion must be given slowly, at a rate of 1 mg or fraction thereof over 1 minute or longer. Dilution with at least 10 ml of diluent is recommended to facilitate the prescribed rate of administration. The patient must be constantly assessed during and immediately following IV administration for indications of shock.

Evaluation. Evaluation is accomplished by obtaining subjective and objective data. Examples of these data are: (1) absence of bleeding in those clients at risk for developing vitamin K deficiency, (2) absence of complications (hematoma formation and anaphylactic reaction) in those clients receiving vitamin K therapy, and (3) normal PT and PTT laboratory values.

Impaired Hepatic Synthesis of Clotting Factors

Liver disease is one of the most common causes of coagulation defects.[14] Because the liver is the major site of synthesis of all of the coagulation proteins except factor VIII, severe liver impairment will alter hemostatic response.

In obstructive liver disease, only vitamin K-dependent coagulation factors, which require bile salt for absorption from the gut, are affected.[11] In contrast, cirrhosis, and other diseases which affect liver cells, impair synthesis of nearly all coagulation proteins.[11] Thrombocytopenia is commonly associated with portal hypertension and may increase the chances and severity of bleeding.[11] Decreased synthesis of coagulation inhibitor proteins, such as antithrombin, and ineffective clearance of activated coagulation factors predispose clients with hepatic disease to venous thromboembolism.[11]

The major *clinical manifestation* of severe liver disease is massive hemorrhage. Bleeding from esophageal varices is common; however, bleeding may occur from any site.

Medical Management

Laboratory test abnormalities in liver disease often include prolonged PT and PTT, moderate decreases in platelet and fibrinogen levels, and elevated levels of fibrin degradation fragments.

Bleeding episodes are treated by the infusion of plasma which also contains antithrombin III.[14] An associated vitamin K deficiency should be treated with vitamin K. Unfortunately, unless liver cell function improves, the bleeding due to liver failure does not respond well to therapy.

Nursing Management

The nursing care of clients with bleeding disorders due to liver disease is a challenge. Frequently the bleeding disorder is severe and associated with end-stage liver disease. In addition to management of the bleeding problem, which, if severe, requires admission to the intensive care unit, the nurse must assist the client and family in dealing with the possibility of death.

Disseminated Intravascular Coagulation

Disseminated intravascular coagulation (DIC) is a "pathological syndrome resulting from the formation of thrombin, subsequent activation and consumption of certain coagulation proteins, and production of fibrin thrombi."[9] The result is diffuse bleeding from depletion of clotting factors and platelets.[15]

Etiology and Pathophysiology

Intravascular coagulation may result from any of the following mechanisms that stimulate clotting: (1) release of tissue thromboplastin into the circulation (extrinsic pathway), (2) activation of the intrinsic pathway, (3) stasis, (4) defective clearing of activated clotting factors, (5) defective fibrinolysis.[15] About 50% of clients with DIC have obstetric problems, while another 33% have cancer.[15] Table 54–7 lists these and other disorders associated with DIC.

The two major consequences of DIC are bleeding and organ ischemia.[15] Widespread deposition of fibrin within the microcirculation leads to ischemia in organs such as the kidney. The red blood cells hemolyze due to trauma while passing through the fibrin strands.[15] Bleeding ensues as the platelets and clotting factors are consumed. The intravascular clotting activates fibrinolysis which yields circulating fibrin

TABLE 54-7
Disorders Associated with Disseminated Intravascular Coagulation (DIC)

Direct Release of Tissue Thromboplastin into Circulation (extrinsic pathway)

I. Obstetric Complications
  A. Abrupto placenta
  B. Abortions
    1. Septic
    2. Saline-induced
  C. Retained placental tissue
  D. Amniotic fluid embolism
  E. Placental previa
  F. Eclampsia

II. Neoplasms
  A. Acute leukemia
  B. Lymphomas
  C. Carcinomas
  D. Others

III. Tissue Injury
  A. Massive trauma
  B. Extensive burns
  C. Dissecting aneurysm of aorta
  D. Extensive surgery
  E. Fat embolism
  F. Extracorporal circulation
  G. Head trauma

IV. Snake Bites

Pathogenesis Uncertain or Mixed (endothelial damage, vasculitis, stasis, hemolysis)

I. Infections
  A. Bacterial (particularly due to gram-negative organisms)
    1. Septicemia and septic shock
    2. Meningococcemia
  B. Mycotic
    1. Histoplasmosis
    2. Aspergillosis
  C. Rickettsial
  D. Viral
    1. Herpes
    2. Rubella
    3. Smallpox
    4. Hepatitis
    5. Reye's syndrome

II. Autoimmune Disease and Hypersensitivity Reactions
  A. Drug reactions
  B. Renal homograft rejection
  C. Graft vs host disease
  D. Anaphylaxis

III. Miscellaneous
  A. Liver disease
  B. Heat stroke
  C. Adult respiratory distress syndrome
  D. Hypoxia and hypoperfusion

(Adapted from Wintrobe MM, Lee GR, Boggs DR, Bithell TC, Forster J, Athens JW, Lukens JN: Clinical Hematology, 8th ed. Philadelphia, Lea & Febiger, 1981)

split products (FSP). Fibrin split products aggravate bleeding because they inhibit platelet aggregation, act as anticoagulants, and impair fibrin polymerization.[15] (See Figure 54–2.)

Clinical Manifestations

Clinical manifestations range from prolonged bleeding from a venipuncture site to spontaneous massive hemorrhage.[15] In massive hemorrhage, bleeding occurs from mucous membranes, sites of injury (including venipuncture and injection sites), and every orifice. Deep tissue bleeding may also occur. Petechiae, purpura, and ecchymosis are very common.[14]

Medical Management

The diagnosis of DIC should be suspected whenever abnormal bleeding occurs in association with certain disorders. Multiple coagulation test abnormalities found in DIC include prolonged PT, PTT, and bleeding time; decreased fibrinogen and platelet count; increased fibrinolysin test; positive fibrin split products; and decreased levels of factors II, V, VIII, and X.[5]

The treatment of DIC is directed toward removal of the underlying disorder. For example, infection requires the use of antibiotics. Fetal death or retained placenta requires the removal of the uterine contents and cancer may respond to chemotherapeutic agents.[14] General support measures, such as fluid and blood replacement, and maintenance of adequate oxygenation and tissue perfusion are also essential.[9]

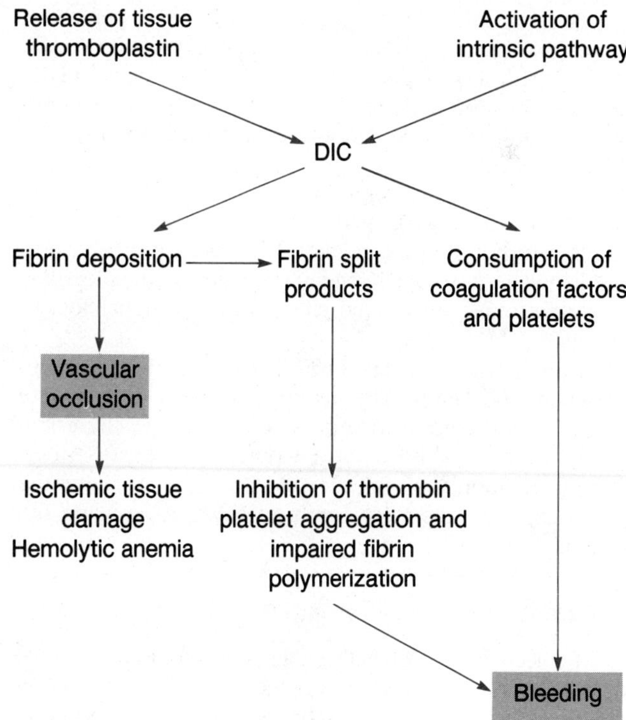

FIGURE 54–2 Schematic illustration of the major consequences of DIC. (Adapted from Robbins SL, Angell M, Kumar V: Basic Pathology, 3rd ed. Philadelphia, WB Saunders, 1981)

Transfusions of platelets and cryoprecipitate for factors V and VIII and fibrinogen replacement may be necessary. The use of heparin a potent anticoagulant, to inactivate the intravascular clotting thus inhibiting consumption of the coagulation factors, is very controversial.[9,14,17] Bleeding is enhanced by heparin; therefore, platelets and clotting factors must also be given.[9]

The prognosis of DIC varies markedly depending on the underlying cause and the amount of intravascular clotting.[15] Disseminated intravascular coagulation may cease spontaneously or it may respond to prompt and aggressive treatment.[15] In other cases, the organ ischemia and bleeding lead to death.

Nursing Management

Assessment and Nursing Diagnosis

The primary nursing diagnosis for the patient who has developed DIC is: Potential for bleeding related to increased utilization of platelets and clotting factors manifested by petechiae, purpura, and ecchymosis (or signs and symptoms of bleeding from any site). The second nursing diagnosis is: Anxiety related to the fear of death leading to ineffective coping.

Goals. The primary nursing goals in the management of DIC are to identify those clients at risk, to detect bleeding problems early, and to reduce fear and anxiety.

Interventions

Prolonged bleeding from an injection site, petechiae, occult blood from body excreta, or other signs of bleeding in clients at risk should alert the nurse to the possibility of DIC. Because 50% of persons with DIC are obstetric clients, nurses working in this area must be particularly astute in their assessments.

Because the bleeding from DIC may be massive, these clients are usually managed in the intensive care unit. In addition to fulfilling the nursing responsibilities related to resolving the cause of DIC and management of the bleeding, the nurse must protect the client from additional foci of bleeding.

Hemorrhage associated with DIC is very frightening to the client and family. The nursing staff must demonstrate efficiency and competence in patient care. The client and family must be allowed and encouraged to express their fears. In addition, the use of flexible visiting hours allows the presence of a supportive family to assist in reducing the patient's anxiety.

Evaluation

Subjective and objective data used to evaluate goal achievement are: (1) absence of bleeding in those patients at risk for developing DIC, (2) normal coagulation laboratory values, (3) control of bleeding in those patients who develop DIC, (4) reduced fear and anxiety in patients (and their families) experiencing hemorrhage due to DIC.

References

1. Beiersdorfer WA, Clements MJ, Weisman C: The Student with Hemophilia: A Resource for the Educator. New York, National Hemophilia Foundation, 1982
2. Blood and Blood Components. Seattle, Puget Sound Blood Center, 1982
3. Clements MJ, Mattsson A: Prevention of Social and Emotional Problems in Boys with Hemophilia. New York, National Hemophilia Foundation, 1983
4. Counts RB, Clements MJ, Thompson AR: Hemophilia Care Syllabus. Seattle, Puget Sound Blood Center, 1978
5. Fischbach F: A Manual of Laboratory Diagnostic Tests, 2nd ed. Philadelphia, JB Lippincott, 1984
6. Furie B: Disorders of the vitamin K dependent coagulation factors. In Williams WJ, Beutler E, Erslev AJ, Lichtman MA (eds): Hematology, 3rd ed. New York, McGraw-Hill, 1983
7. Gottlieb AJ: Disorders of hemostasis—nonthrombocytopenic purpuras. In Williams WJ, Beutler E, Erslev AJ, Lichtman MA (eds): Hematology, 3rd ed. New York, McGraw-Hill, 1983
8. Hedlin A: Hemostasis and the nature of its defect in hemophilia. Canadian Nurse 76:15, 1980
9. Marder VJ: Consumptive thrombohemorrhagic disorders. In Williams WJ, Beutler E, Erslev AJ, Lichtman MA (eds): Hematology, 3rd ed. New York, McGraw-Hill, 1983
10. Mitchell PH, Loustau A: Concepts Basic to Nursing, 3rd ed. New York, McGraw-Hill, 1981
11. Moake JL, Funicella T: Common bleeding problems. Clin Symp 35:3, 1983
12. Nossel HL: Bleeding disorders due to vessel wall abnormalities. In Petersdorf RG, Adams RD, Braunwald E, Isselbacher KJ, Martin JB, Wilson JD (eds): Harrison's Principles of Internal Medicine, 10th ed. New York, McGraw-Hill, 1983
13. Nossel HL: Platelet disorders. In Petersdorf RG, Adams RD, Braunwald E, Isselbacher KJ, Martin JB, Wilson JD (eds): Harrison's Principles of Internal Medicine, 10th ed. New York, McGraw-Hill, 1983
14. Nossel HL: Disorders of blood coagulation factors. In Petersdorf RG, Adams RD, Braunwald E, Isselbacher KJ, Martin JB, Wilson JD (eds): Harrison's Principles of Internal Medicine, 10th ed. New York, McGraw-Hill, 1983
15. Robbins SL, Angell M, Kumar V: Basic Pathology, 3rd ed. Philadelphia, WB Saunders, 1981
16. Snyder EL, Kennedy MS: Blood Transfusion Therapy. Arlington, American Association of Blood Banks, 1983
17. Thompson AR, Harker LA: Manual of Hemostasis and Thrombosis, 3rd ed. Philadelphia, FA Davis, 1983
18. Weiss HJ: Disorders of hemostasis—congenital disorders of uncertain pathogenesis—von Willebrand's disease. In Williams WJ, Beutler E, Erslev AJ, Lichtman MA (eds): Hematology 3rd ed. New York, McGraw-Hill, 1983
19. Williams WJ: Classification of disorders of hemostasis. In Williams WJ, Beutler E, Erslev AJ, Lichtman MA (eds): Hematology, 3rd ed. New York, McGraw-Hill, 1983
20. Wintrobe MM, Lee GR, Boggs DR, Bithell TC, Forster J, Athens JW, Lukens JN: Clinical Hematology, 8th ed. Philadelphia, Lea & Febiger, 1981
21. Zeluff GW, Natelson EA, Jackson D: Thrombocytopenic purpura—idiopathic and thrombotic. Heart Lung 7:327, 1978

UNIT VI

Nursing Care of Patients with Alterations in Renal and Urinary Function

Chapter 55

Review of Anatomy and Physiology
Renal System

Barbara R. Landau

The kidney is the major excretory organ because it controls excretion of many substances. The lungs excrete carbon dioxide and the skin excretes water, small amounts of electrolytes, and some wastes such as urea. The renal function of the kidney, however, is to maintain the volume and composition of the extracellular fluid (ECF). By excreting or retaining individual constituents of the plasma, the kidney is able to regulate the composition, tonicity, volume, and pH of the plasma, and hence of the tissue fluid. By producing urine, the kidney is able to excrete wastes and other substances in solution. The regulatory role of the kidney also includes some endocrine functions: the secretion of renin and erythropoietin (or a precursor) and the final activation of vitamin D.

Anatomy of the Kidney

The kidneys are located on the posterior abdominal wall, roughly between the 12th thoracic and 3rd lumbar vertebrae (Fig. 55–1, *A*), with an adrenal gland atop each kidney. They are retroperitoneal, and each is enclosed by a fibrous capsule and often embedded in a mass of adipose tissue. The hilus on the medial surface is the site of entry or exit of the renal blood vessels, nerves, and lymphatics, and the renal pelvis, which funnels urine into the ureter.

The outer portion of the kidney is the cortex and the inner portion is the medulla, which consists of about a dozen renal pyramids (Fig. 55–1, *B*). The renal sinus is the open area occupied by the renal pelvis, vessels, and nerves, with any remaining space filled with adipose tissue. The tip of each pyramid (the papilla) is enclosed by a minor calix that fits over it rather like a suction cup. Several minor calices join to form the major calices, which converge to form the renal pelvis.

The renal artery abruptly divides into interlobar arteries that pass between pyramids and branch into arcuate arteries, which ramify along the boundary between medulla and cortex. Interlobular arteries arise from the arcuates and pass through the cortex toward the surface, giving rise to the afferent arterioles that enter the glomerular capsules. The veins, which have a corresponding pattern, converge to renal veins that drain into the inferior vena cava (not the portal system).

Structure of the Nephron

The nephron is the functional unit of the kidney, and there are over a million of them in each kidney. A nephron consists of a glomerular (Bowman's) capsule and a tubule (Fig. 55–1, *C* and *D*). The glomerular capsule contains the glomerulus, which is a tuft of capillaries that arises from an afferent arteriole; together they make up the renal corpuscle.

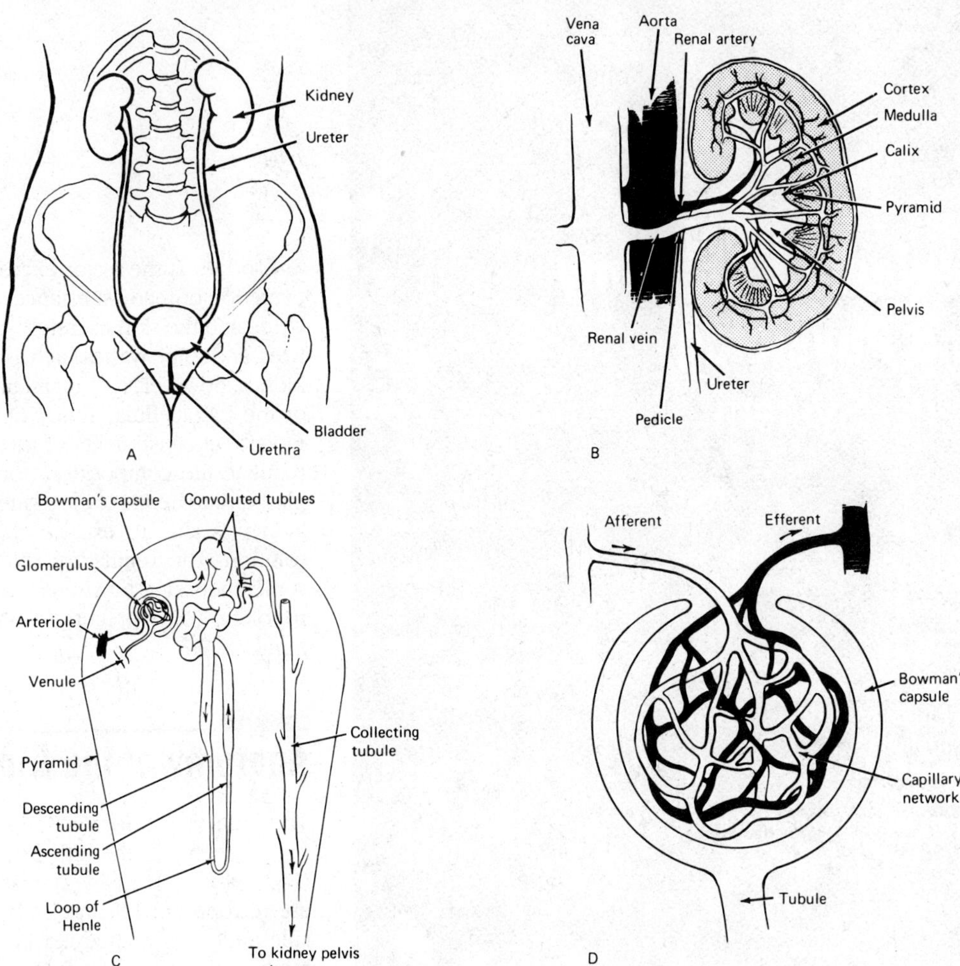

FIGURE 55–1 Structures of the urinary system. (*A*) The urinary tract. (*B*) Interior of kidney. (*C*) A nephron. (*D*) Bowman's capsule.

The capsule is a double-walled sphere that completely encloses the glomerulus. The tubule arises from the capsule and follows a tortuous but predictable course. Its various segments differ in structure, function, and location. Distal convoluted tubules empty into collecting ducts or tubules. The cortical portions of collecting ducts carry on functions similar to those of the distal convoluted tubules, but the medullary portions have different and specific roles. Collecting ducts empty their contents (urine) into a calyx at the papilla of a medullary pyramid.

All glomerular capsules and convoluted tubules (both proximal and distal) are in the cortex. Nephrons whose glomerular capsules are near the medulla (juxtamedullary nephrons) have very long loops of Henle that extend far into the pyramid, and nephrons whose glomerular capsules are further from the medulla (cortical nephrons) have shorter loops of Henle that extend only a short distance into the medulla.

Innervation. There is no firm evidence of innervation of renal tissue *per se,* but renal blood vessels receive a sympathetic vasoconstrictor innervation. There is little tonic vasoconstriction, however, and sympathetic action is not essential for normal function—a transplanted kidney functions very well without nerve supply. The juxtaglomerular cells also receive sympathetic innervation, which causes renin secretion. There are some sensory fibers from the kidney, and especially from the renal pelvis and ureter, as is evidenced by the pain caused by kidney stones.

The Formation of Urine

In carrying out its regulatory and excretory roles, the nephron must be selective in what it creates or retains, and it must be reasonably economical in terms of energy expenditure. The processes involved in urine formation—filtration, reabsorption, and secretion—effectively meet these requirements. Filtration is a passive process by which plasma is transferred from the glomerular capillaries to the glomerular capsule. The driving force is the blood pressure. Reabsorption is a tubular function by which filtered fluid and solutes are returned to the bloodstream. Secretion involves transfer of solutes from peritubular capillaries into the tubule for excretion. Thus, a fraction of the plasma delivered to the glomerulus is filtered, most of the filtrate is reabsorbed, and a small amount of solute is added by secretion. What remains in the tubule is excreted as urine.

Filtration

Filtration depends on the permeability characteristics of the membrane and on a suitable pressure gradient. The term *glomerular filtrate* applies to fluid that has passed from the glomerulus into the capsule; as soon as the fluid begins to move down the tubule its composition is altered by tubular processes, and it becomes tubular fluid rather than glomerular filtrate. Although this very porous membrane permits rapid transfer, the size of particles that can pass is about the same as other capillaries. Thus the filtrate contains no blood cells and virtually no plasma protein. The filtrate concentration of other solutes is the same as, and varies with, their plasma concentrations. Exceptions are substances bound to protein that is not filtered, and the slight effect of nonfilterable protein molecules in the plasma on the movement of some ions (Donnan effect).

Renal arteries are short and branch abruptly; therefore, the pressure of blood in the glomerulus is higher than in most capillaries. It is opposed by a small pressure in the capsule and by the colloid osmotic pressure (COP) of the plasma. The net result is a filtration pressure about twice that in other capillaries. In typical capillaries pressure falls sharply as blood traverses the capillary bed, but pressure falls very little along glomerular capillaries because, unlike other capillaries, there is a variable resistance at the downstream end (smooth muscle of the efferent arterioles) that helps to maintain the pressure. Because of the great porosity of the membrane, filtration occurs rapidly, but since proteins are not filtered the COP rises as blood moves along the glomerular capillaries. An equilibrium is usually reached somewhere along the capillary, and there is no filtration beyond that point.

The kidney receives approximately one fourth of the cardiac output, and a cardiac output of 5 liters/minute brings about 600 ml to 750 ml of plasma to the kidneys each minutes. Between 16% and 20% of this plasma is filtered, resulting in a glomerular filtration rate (GFR) of about 125 ml/minute, or about 7.5 liters/hour, and nearly 180 liters in a 24-hour period. Yet only 1 liter to 1.5 liters of urine are excreted in a 24-hour period, all the remaining filtrate being reabsorbed.

The amount of any solute filtered in a minute (mg/min) is the filtered load. It depends on the plasma concentration of that solute and the GFR. There is a linear relationship between amount filtered and GFR.

Since urine is formed from the glomerular filtrate, the rate of filtration must be maintained, and this can be achieved by controlling renal blood flow and glomerular filtration pressure. When a greater volume of blood flows through each glomerular capillary, it travels more rapidly and a greater part of the capillary loop becomes involved in the filtration process, so that more filtrate is formed. A major factor in controlling renal blood flow is the degree of constriction in afferent arterioles, because the constriction determines how much blood gets into the glomerulus. Afferent arterioles also help to protect glomerular capillary pressure against marked changes in the mean systemic arterial pressure. Pressure in the glomerulus is also controlled by constriction of the efferent arterioles. Vasoconstriction raises the capillary pressure, and vasodilation lowers it. Because resistance can be controlled at either end of the glomerular capillaries, filtration pressure is well controlled.

Renal vascular smooth muscle responds to local conditions as well as to sympathetic stimulation. A denervated perfused kidney (such as a transplanted kidney) can maintain a reasonably constant filtration rate at arterial pressures between about 80 and 180 mmHg. Such regulation, termed *autoregulation,* occurs in many organs, but is particularly well developed in the kidney. The mechanism is not well understood, but it is believed to be a direct response of the vascular smooth muscle (especially of afferent arteriole) to stretch.

Reabsorption

Reabsorption involves transfer of filtered fluid or solutes through tubular cells into surrounding tissue fluid, from which it diffuses into peritubular capillaries (or vasa recta). Transport may be by passive processes, which depend upon an osmotic, chemical (concentration), or electrical gradient, or by active transport, which involves the expenditure of energy and transport against a gradient.

In general, transport in the proximal tubule is a large scale operation, involving both active and passive means: most of the water, Na^+, K^+, Cl^-, and HCO_3^-, and usually all of the glucose and amino acids are reabsorbed from it. The distal and collecting tubules deal with smaller quantities, but the transport of water and several ions is regulated directly or indirectly by hormones. Regulation of reabsorption in the proximal tubules is a "coarse adjustment," and regulation in the distal and collecting tubules is the "fine adjustment."

All water reabsorption is passive. The major driving force for removal of such large volumes of water is the osmotic gradient created by active reabsorption of solutes. Small nonpolar molecules such as urea are reabsorbed passively with the water (bulk transfer), and some electrolytes may be transported passively in response to electrical or concentration gradients.

Active transport is a pumping process that moves solute against a gradient. Sodium is reabsorbed by active transport from most of the tubule. Sodium enters tubular cells by diffusion down its electrochemical gradient, and it is pumped out of the cell.

The mechanism known as secondary active transport is quite effective because normally only traces of glucose are excreted. However, if the plasma glucose concentration is high enough, glucose will appear in the urine. Glucose is said to be a threshold substance because it is not normally excreted unless the threshold is exceeded. The threshold is the plasma level at which glucose begins to appear in the urine. Note that insulin does not regulate transport of glucose across tubular (or intestinal) cells.

Reabsorption of water raises the solute concentration in the tubules, which favors their reabsorption, and reabsorption of the positively charged sodium ions creates an electrical gradient for reabsorption of negatively charged ions such as chloride. Several ions, including lactate, citrate, phosphate, and chloride are reabsorbed with sodium. Potassium reabsorption is more complex because most of it is reabsorbed in proximal tubules, probably by both active and passive mechanisms, and then some is secreted into distal tubules. Almost all filtered calcium is reabsorbed by passive and active transport, part of it linked to sodium transport. Phosphate is actively reabsorbed, but only partially.

Although it is a waste product, urea is a small molecule

that diffuses readily, and about half of it is reabsorbed. Amino acids are actively transported in a manner similar to that of glucose; they bind to molecules that operate with sodium. Any traces of protein that may be filtered are usually reabsorbed, probably by pinocytosis or perhaps by active transport. Transport is limited, so that an increase in filtration generally results in excretion of protein. Other actively reabsorbed substances include ascorbic acid, creatine, uric acid, and ketone bodies.

Secretion

Tubular secretion is the process by which ions or molecules are transferred from peritubular capillaries into the tubular lumen by active or passive transport. These substances may also be filtered (unless protein-bound), but the secreted particles are from the peritubular capillaries.

Two physiologically important ions that are secreted are H^+ and K^+. Ammonia is synthesized in tubular cells and then secreted. Other physiological substances that are secreted include creatinine, hippuric acid, and some metabolites. Nonphysiological secreted substances include several dyes (some used for diagnostic or quantitative studies) and a number of drugs, notably penicillin.

Urinary Passages and Micturition

Urine from the collecting ducts enters the renal pelvis and is funneled into the ureter to be carried to the urinary bladder, where it accumulates until an appropriate stimulus causes the bladder to contract and expel the urine through the urethra. The ureters, which are retroperitoneal, descend along the posterior wall of the abdominal cavity and enter the bladder on its posterior inferior surface. The urethra leaves from the inferior surface of the bladder. The volume and composition of the urine do not change after it leaves the kidney.

The smooth muscle of the ureters consists of generally spiralling fibers which initiate several peristaltic contractions per minute that move urine toward the bladder. The ureters penetrate the muscle obliquely, and with no sphincter at the orifice, the bladder muscle tends to keep the entrance closed, thus preventing reflux of urine into the ureters.

The muscle of the bladder, the detrusor muscle, is quite thick, and its fibers wrap around in a rather random fashion; the three layers often described are distinct only near the urethral orifice. The trigone is the region in the floor of the bladder defined by the urethral and two ureteral openings. An internal urethral sphincter is often described, which consists of bands of smooth muscle on either side of the urethral orifice. The external sphincter is formed by skeletal muscle that surrounds the urethra a short distance below the bladder. These muscles are part of the floor of the pelvic cavity through which the urethra must pass to leave the body cavity (the urogenital diaphragm surrounding the membranous urethra in men).

The bladder is innervated by

1. Parasympathetic fibers from S1–S3, which run in the pelvic nerve and synapse in the bladder wall. They are excitatory to the detrusor muscle.
2. Sympathetic fibers from L2–L4, which pass through the sympathetic chain and synapse in the inferior mesenteric ganglion. They supply blood vessels and some smooth muscle fibers in the region of the internal sphincter.
3. Somatic efferent fibers from S1–S3, which run in the pudendal nerve to the skeletal muscles of the external urethral sphincter.
4. Sensory fibers, especially from stretch receptors in the detrusor muscle, which travel with the pelvic nerve to the sacral cord to synapse with ascending fibers.

The bladder maintains a certain amount of tone, but also exhibits plasticity. As its volume increases, the bladder distends to accommodate the additional fluid with imperceptible pressure increases. In humans, the first sensation or urge to void occurs at about 150 ml. A volume of about 400 ml triggers reflex contraction of the detrusor muscle, and intravesicular pressure rises sharply. The response is a spinal cord reflex initiated by stimulation of the stretch receptors in the muscle. In addition to contraction of the detrusor muscle, other muscles involved include the skeletal muscles of the pelvic floor (relaxation) and possibly abdominal muscles (contraction). The internal sphincter does not seem to be involved in micturition, but it is believed that, in men, sympathetic stimulation may cause its contraction to prevent semen from entering the bladder during ejaculation.

The reflex response is also modified by centers in the brain with connections to the sacral reflex center. There are regions in the pons and hypothalamus that facilitate contraction, and one in the midbrain that inhibits contraction. The cerebral cortex contains centers that inhibit, facilitate, and also provide an element of voluntary control. Voluntary control of smooth muscle may seem contradictory, but it is believed that voluntary relaxation of the skeletal muscles of the pelvic floor and external sphincter may tend to pull down on the bladder and trigger contraction of the detrusor muscle.

Suggested Readings

Crouch JE: Functional Human Anatomy, 3rd ed, pp 540–559. Philadelphia, Lea & Febiger, 1978

Ganong WF: Review of Medical Physiology, 11th ed, pp 563–597. Los Altos CA, Lange Medical Publications, 1983

Junqueira LC, Carneiro J: Basic Histology, 4th ed, Chap 20. Los Altos CA, Lange Medical Publications, 1983

Landau BR: Essential Human Anatomy and Physiology, 2nd ed, pp 649–678. Glenview IL, Scott, Foresman and Company, 1980

Leeson TS, Leeson CR: Histology, 4th ed, pp 429–455. Philadelphia, WB Saunders, 1981

Marsh DJ: Renal Physiology. New York, Raven Press, 1983

Pitts RF: Physiology of the Kidney and Body Fluids, 3rd ed. Chicago, Year Book Medical Publishers, 1974

Tortora GJ: Principles of Human Anatomy, 3rd ed, pp 604–623. New York, Harper & Row, 1983

Vander AJ: Renal Physiology. New York, McGraw-Hill, 1975

Vander AJ, Sherman JS, Luciano DS: Human Physiology: The Mechanisms of Body Function, 3rd ed. New York, 1980

Chapter 56

Assessment of Renal Function

Lisa L. MacGeorge

The regulatory function of the kidney is to maintain the volume and composition of the extracellular fluid. In so doing, it has a major role in controlling the environment of all body cells and organs and hence in maintaining dynamic equilibrium. Kidney function affects all systems of the body.

Assessment of renal excretory function consists of history taking, physical examination, determination of plasma and urine composition, tonicity volume and pH, radiological studies, and examination of renal biopsy tissue.

Nursing care of persons with renal dysfunction requires independent management of problems of elimination as well as interdependent management of problems of renal excretory function. Nursing assessment includes the need to obtain data about elimination in relation to its effect on the ability to carry out activities of daily living. These data are obtained when taking a history and doing a physical assessment.

History

Nursing History

The nursing history should include questions about elimination problems and what methods have been used to cope with these problems. The person may or may not have a history of difficulty with control of urinary elimination. If a problem of control is identified, then data need to be obtained as to the satisfactory and unsatisfactory methods used to cope with this problem. It is necessary to determine the person's feelings about the situation and the effects the problem may have on marital relationships and social activities. These data would be used in deriving nursing diagnoses.

Many disease states and lifestyle factors may predispose patients to renal dysfunction. The presence of any of these factors in a patient's past health history should arouse suspicions about potential renal dysfunction. The most common disease states in which renal dysfunction may be a sequela are diabetes mellitus, high blood pressure, gout, neoplasms, systemic lupus erythematosus, leukemia, multiple myeloma, and connective tissue disorders. Other disease conditions and lifestyle factors that may contribute to eventual renal disease include the use of nephrotoxic substances (see Table 56–1), excessive use (abuse) of over-the-counter analgesics, recent bacterial infections (particularly skin and respiratory), urinary tract infection, stones or trauma, manipulation of the urinary tract for diagnostic procedures, and past pregnancies. Additional information that may indicate underlying renal dysfunction include general malaise, unexplained illness, and changes in urinary excretion patterns.

Certain medications may mask the signs of infection, change the appearance or volume of the urine, or cause other physiological changes that may complicate the assessment of renal function. Therefore, it is essential that the history include a thorough and accurate list of all medications and dosages that the patient has recently taken or is currently taking.

Occasionally severe loss of renal function occurs without symptoms, and it is discovered on a routine physical examination. Generally, these patients do not have any preexisting disease. Idiopathic renal failure is the term given to this type of renal disease (see Chap. 59).

Any information that can be collected regarding earlier workups for similar problems may be helpful in dating the onset and progression of renal dysfunction. Records can probably be obtained from the previous health care providers.

Elderly patients have a decreased number of functioning nephrons and therefore a reduced glomerular filtration rate as part of the normal aging process. This physiological change needs to be considered when assessing and providing care for the older person.

TABLE 56-1
Nephrotoxic Substances

Nephrotoxic Substances
Aminoglycosides
Penicillins
Tetracyclines
X-ray contrast media
Diphenylhydantoin
Phenylbutazone
Uric acid
Calcium
Carbon tetrachloride
Methyl alcohol
Ethylene glycol
Phenols
Heavy metals (mercury, arsenic, gold, or lead)
Some analgesics
Pesticides, fungicides
Hemoglobulinuria due to incompatible blood transfusion
Myoglobulinuria due to crushing injury, burns, or alcoholic myopathy
Cyclosporin A
Amphotericin
Methotrexate

Family History

Certain conditions or diseases may be familial in that their presence in a family may increase the risk of another family member having the same problem. A significant family history would include polycystic kidney disease, hereditary nephritis, adult renal disease, chronic urinary tract infection, urinary calculi, diabetes mellitus, systemic lupus erythematosus, high blood pressure, and gout. The presence of any of these conditions in a family should be a clue to the possibility of potential renal disease.

Physical Assessment

Questions related to renal function include those regarding voiding patterns, both normal and abnormal, the appearance of the urine, complaints of pain or discomfort over the kidney area, along the course of the ureters and when voiding, the presence of edema, and general well-being.

Voiding Patterns

Deviations from normal voiding patterns include frequency, urgency, hesitancy (difficulty initiating urination), dysuria, incontinence, retention (difficulty emptying the bladder), and nocturia. All of these manifestations of renal dysfunction influence the patient's functional status. For instance, incontinence requires the use of special protective devices that can be costly, may cause skin irritation and even excoriation, and force the person to withdraw from social contacts because of fear of accidents in public. Nocturia may interfere with sleep and may be a potential accident hazard when the person gets out of bed to go to the bathroom.

Urine Volume and Appearance

Changes in urinary volume should be determined and evaluated in relation to intake. The person should be questioned about volume of daily fluid intake. Urine output volumes that are disproportionate to intake volume are generally referred to as *polyuria* (excessive urine volume), *oliguria* (diminished urine volume), and *anuria* (cessation of urine output). It is most informative to reinforce these labels with actual documentation of estimated volumes for both intake and output. In order to confirm and quantify the problem the nurse should independently initiate intake and output recordings making sure the patient, family, and other nurses are well informed and aware of the necessity for accurate quantification and documentation.

Appearance of the urine is generally reported in terms of color and clarity. Normal urine color ranges from colorless to dark amber, reflecting changes in both content (*e.g.,* bilirubin) and concentration, and is clear (free of sediment). Abnormalities in the appearance of the urine include discoloration such as red or brown urine, frank hematuria (blood in the urine), cloudiness, and the presence of red cells, casts, and sediment. The color of urine is influenced by drugs, presence of blood, protein, casts, and the degree of concentration. Drugs that influence urine color are phenazopyridine (Pyridium) and riboflavin which cause the urine to appear orange, phenacetin which causes the urine to be brownish gray, and the phenothiazines which give a reddish brown appearance.[3]

Pain and Edema

Complaints of pain or discomfort related to renal problems include dysuria (pain on urination), flank pain, pain at the costovertebral angle, and groin pain. Male patients with renal stones may have pain that radiates to the testes.

Decreased ability of the kidney to filter and to regulate sodium excretion can result in edema. Edema may adversely affect the person's functional ability. For instance, swollen feet and ankles may interfere with wearing shoes and hence with mobility. Fluid retention may also increase circulating fluid volume and the work of the heart, thereby causing fatigue and decreased functional capacity. The presence of periorbital edema, pedal edema, sacral edema, or anasarca (generalized edema) is important contributory data for the diagnosis of renal insufficiency or failure. Because edema is related to many pathophysiological states and is not specific to renal problems, it should be evaluated in relation to all the abnormal findings.

Vital Signs, Weight, and Other Signs

As always, a baseline temperature, pulse, blood pressure, respiratory rate, and weight should be obtained. Of these, blood pressure and weight are the most obvious indicators of renal dysfunction. When renal function is decreased, the body is unable to adequately eliminate the fluid that is ingested or formed as a result of body metabolism. An increase in weight and blood pressure reflect an increase in body fluid volume. The temperature, pulse, and respiratory rate are more general indicators of physiological status.

Azotemia (condition of a buildup of nitrogenous wastes in the blood) secondary to the kidneys' inability to excrete nitrogenous wastes may cause changes in the skin and mucous membranes. These changes include a yellowish brown cast to the skin (may resemble a sun tan), skin excoriation and infections, the presence of uremic crystals, stomatitis, and an acetone breath odor. These signs are very diagnostic of end-stage renal failure. Depending on the etiology and course of the renal disease and the subsequent fluid and electrolyte imbalances, the patient may be very edematous. With advanced renal disease or end-stage renal failure there is multiple organ involvement and failure at which time all physical assessment parameters are extremely important for the nurse to monitor (see Chap. 59).

As part of the physical assessment, the nurse observes the appearance of the abdomen since renal tumors or large polycystic kidneys may distort abdominal contour. Auscultation of the midline of the abdomen can reveal a bruit or murmur if aortic or renal stenosis is present. The normal adult kidney is not palpable. The urinary bladder is palpable when distended. The nurse needs to palpate the lower abdomen and determine if bladder distention exists before performing a catheterization.

Degrees of Renal Dysfunction

Every organ system in the body depends on the kidneys for proper function. However, there are many degrees of renal failure, ranging from mild renal insufficiency to end-stage renal failure. A patient with mild renal insufficiency may present with complaints of alteration in well-being, "just not feeling well," tired, and so on. In contrast, a patient with severe renal failure may have marked multisystem involvement. The person with advanced renal failure often is too weak to carry out activities of daily living; the level of functional ability must be determined because this is necessary data for making nursing diagnoses.

Laboratory Tests

Laboratory studies consist of analysis of blood and urine samples. The urine analysis indicates the adequacy of renal function and the possibility of system infection. Inadequate renal function is also reflected in the blood level of substances that should be filtered, secreted, and excreted.

Urine Studies

Many urine tests are performed in an effort to diagnose renal disease. Some tests are convenient for nurses to perform on the nursing units. These tests include volume, specific gravity, and osmolarity. Twenty-four hour volume should be evaluated in relation to intake.

The *specific gravity* and *osmolarity* are indications of the kidneys' concentrating ability. Urine that is most concentrated in the early morning and less concentrated later in the day suggests normal concentrating ability.[2] A specific gravity that is constantly at 1.010 can indicate the kidneys' inability to either concentrate or dilute the urine. The presence of osmotically active substances such as protein and sugar in the urine will raise both specific gravity and urine osmolarity because of an increased number of molecules in the urine. Nurses generally use the specific gravity more than urine osmolarity because the equipment to perform the test is less costly and more convenient to use on the nursing units.

Further urine tests include creatinine clearance, urea, urine pH, urine electrolytes (sodium, chloride, potassium), ketones, protein, blood, and glucose. The laboratory technicians usually perform some of these tests; however, it is often a nursing responsibility to check urine for protein, glucose, and ketones. The normal values for these tests are listed in Table 56–2.

The urine test used most often clinically to monitor the progression and severity of renal failure is the *24-hour creatinine clearance.* Creatinine is a product of muscle metabolism and remains fairly constant with normal physical activity. Because creatinine is freely filtered and is neither reabsorbed nor secreted by the renal tubules, it is a fairly accurate indication of the glomerular filtration rate. Table 56–3 explains the procedure for obtaining a 24-hour urine collection for creatinine clearance.

Twenty-four hour urine collection is also used to evaluate the amount of *protein* being lost in the urine of patient with nephrotic syndrome. The nephrotic syndrome is a term applied to renal disorders that are characterized by massive edema, proteinuria, and unusually elevated serum cholesterol and lipids.[2]

The remainder of the urine tests provide contributory data as to the type of renal failure, electrolyte balance problems, and to detect bleeding. These findings in turn guide subsequent intervention.

Blood Studies

The laboratory blood tests most commonly used to evaluate renal function are creatinine, blood urea nitrogen

(*Text continues on page 754*)

TABLE 56–2
Renal Excretory Function Studies

Test	Normal Value*	Abnormal Trends Consistent with Renal Dysfunction	Significance Related to Renal Function	Nursing Considerations
Routine Urinalysis				
Volume	1–2 liters/24 hr	Decreased	Indicates renal tissues' ability to excrete water	Evaluate volume in relation to intake. 30 ml/hr urine output is minimal physiological baseline Necessitates accurate measurement and documentation. Anticipate and look for physiological signs and symptoms of volume overload.
Specific gravity	1.005–1.025	Decreased	Indicates renal tissues' ability to concentrate urine	Evaluate in relation to other physiological signs and symptoms of body water status
Osmolality	100 mOsm 1000 mOsm/L	Decreased	Indicates body water status	Note trends vs. isolated values
Protein	Absent	Present	Can be benign sign in athletes Indicates glomerular dysfunction in renal disease Always present with the nephrotic syndrome	Quantify the amount of protein as small, moderate, or large as indicated on color change analysis charts. Important to quantify, document, and note changes especially for patients with nephrotic syndrome. Also watch for degree of edema and hypoalbuminemia.
Blood	Absent	Present	Indicates trauma, infection, or dysfunction anywhere in the renal or urinary system	Quantify blood as small, moderate, or large. R/O other sources of blood such as vaginal or rectal.
Bacteria	Absent	Present	Indicates infection, generally pyelonephritis or infection of the urinary tract	Important to teach patients how to obtain a clean urine specimen to facilitate accurate culture and sensitivity.
RBC, WBC, red cell casts	Absent	Present	Is a nonspecific indication of renal trauma, infection, or pathological condition	
Crystals	Absent	Present	Indicate the potential for renal or urinary stones	
Glucose and ketones	Absent	Present	Indicate metabolic status more than renal dysfunction	Use these values as contributory to the overall physiological assessment.
Creatinine clearance	60–120 ml/min	Decreased	Indicates filtration ability of kidney	Evaluate in relation to age. With aging, value may be slightly decreased because older people have decreased number of functioning nephrons. Watch for trends to determine changes in status. Accurate values depend on correctly performed collection procedure.

(Continued)

TABLE 56–2
Renal Excretory Function Studies (continued)

Test	Normal Value*	Abnormal Trends Consistent with Renal Dysfunction	Significance Related to Renal Function	Nursing Considerations
Serum Studies				
Creatinine	0.4–1.2 mg/dl	Increased	Specifically indicates status of renal function	Must always evaluate in relation to the baseline and trends Generally a very constant value; if increased even 0.1 mg/dl, it is significant.
Blood urea nitrogen (BUN)	5–25 mg/dl	Increased	Indicates status of renal function but is less specific than creatinine	BUN is affected by fluid balance, nutritional status, medications, and other disease processes.
Potassium	3.5–5.0 mEq/liter	Usually increased	Indicates renal tubular ability to excrete	With certain pathophysiological conditions or use of potassium wasting diuretics the potassium may actually be low and is not an indication of improving renal function. Hyperkalemia can cause serious, even fatal cardiac arrhythmias.
Ratio (blood urea nitrogen to creatinine)	20 : 1	Increased	Probably volume deficit, catabolic state. Loss of lean body mass. Rise in creatinine out of proportion to BUN indicates problem is renal. The kidney is unable to filter and excrete creatinine.	Evidence of decreased renal blood flow, inadequate circulating volume. Need to consider fluid intake Evidence of renal dysfunction. Need to monitor urine output and urine characteristics
Osmolarity	280–300 mOsm/liter	Increased or decreased	Indicates body water balance; imbalances may be water excess (decreased osmolarity) or water deficit (increased osmolarity).	Water imbalances are often iatrogenically caused and may not be from a renal disorder.
Albumin	3.2–5.5 g/dl	Decreased	Degree of hypoalbuminuria depends on the degree of glomerular capillary leakage, disease process, and nutritional status.	Important to understand the relationship of albumin levels to fluid status, serum Ca^{2+} measurements (see Chaps. 13, 14, 72), wound healing, and general physiological function
Calcium	4.0–5.0 mEq/liter or 9.0–11.0 mg/dl	Decreased	In renal failure, vitamin D is not converted to its active form which is necessary for calcium absorption from the gut.	Many renal failure patients take routine calcium supplements and an activated form of vitamin D. It is important to remember that the calcium may remain at normal levels if the parathyroid gland is secreting extra PTH, which causes calcium to be released from bone-termed secondary hyperparathyroidism.

(Continued)

TABLE 56–2
Renal Excretory Function Studies (*Continued*)

Test	*Normal Value**	*Abnormal Trends Consistent with Renal Dysfunction*	*Significance Related to Renal Function*	*Nursing Considerations*
Serum Studies				
Phosphorus	3.5–5.5 mEq/liter	Increased	In renal disease, the kidney tubules are unable to excrete phosphate	Most patients with renal failure take some form of aluminum hydroxide (either liquid or capsule), which binds phosphorus in the intestine where it is excreted as fecal matter. Nurses play a major role in teaching patients the importance of this medication.
Magnesium	1.4–2.2 mEq/liter or 1.7–2.7 mg/dl	Increased	In renal failure, magnesium is not excreted by the renal tubules.	Nurses must be aware of magnesium-containing medications and substances (in some antacids) and attempt to find alternative solutions to meet patient's needs. Elevated magnesium levels can cause severe neurological side-effects and may lead to seizures. Hemodialysis is the most efficient method of lowering serum magnesium in an anuric individual.
Hematocrit	Female: 36–47/dl Male: 40–54/dl	Decreased	In renal failure, the kidneys do not secrete erythropoietin in normal amounts; erythropoietin stimulates the bone marrow to make red blood cells.	Many renal failure patients acclimate and function adequately with hematocrit of approximately 20/dl.
pH	7.35–7.45	Decreased	Metabolic acidosis occurs in renal failure because of the renal tubule cells' inability to buffer H^+ ions.	

*University Hospital Laboratory Manual. Seattle, University of Washington, 1980

(BUN), potassium osmolarity, albumin, calcium, magnesium, phosphorus, arterial blood gases, and hematocrit. The normal values for all of these tests are listed in Table 56–2.

As renal function begins to decline, the glomeruli become unable to filter the *creatinine,* which is then reflected in an increased serum creatinine. A decrease in urine creatinine clearance with a simultaneous rise in serum creatinine is an indication of worsening renal function. The serum creatinine value is used in calculating creatinine clearance. It is extremely important to assess trends in the serum creatinine vs. an isolated value because differences in the amount of muscle mass for each person may alter the baseline value from one individual to another. It is also important to know the rate of rise by noting trends in creatinine values.

As one ages, atrophy of nephrons occurs resulting in a decrease in functional units of the kidney. This suggests that creatinine clearance may be decreased because of a decrease in the number of functioning nephrons. However, the serum creatinine is generally not elevated because muscle mass decreases with age. The decreased amount of creatinine produced offsets the decrease in the number of functioning nephrons, and therefore creatinine clearance does not change.

The *blood urea nitrogen* (BUN), a product of protein metabolism, is also used as an indication of renal function

TABLE 56–3
Procedure for Collecting 24-Hour Urine for Creatinine Clearance

1. Explain procedure to patient and, if appropriate, ask patient to repeat the procedure to ensure that he understands the protocol and will comply with it.
2. Instruct the patient to empty bladder and note exact time. Discard urine.
3. Collect and save all urine for the next 24 hours in a clean bottle or carton. Preservatives and refrigeration are not required.
4. At exactly 24 hours, make last collection. Save last sample.
5. Be sure that the exact starting and ending time are recorded.
   Note: If patient is not able to void exactly 24 hours later, just record the exact time he does void and notify laboratory that it was not exactly 24 hours. The laboratory can adjust their equation.
6. Draw blood sample for serum creatinine during this 24-hour period.

but this is not as accurate as the creatinine clearance because BUN is affected by many other conditions such as body fluid status, cellular metabolism, medications, nutritional status, and other disease processes.

Serum *osmolarity, sodium,* and *chloride* may be lowered or elevated depending on the particular type of renal disease.

Serum *potassium* is generally elevated with renal disease and reflects renal tubule dysfunction. Hyperkalemia is a very significant indication of renal dysfunction and can cause fatal cardiac arrhythmias (see Chaps. 39 and 57).

Serum *calcium* is generally low in renal disease. The health kidney changes vitamin D to its active from which is necessary for the absorption of calcium from the intestine. In renal disease the kidney is not able to transform vitamin D to its activated form, thereby preventing calcium absorption from the intestine.

Serum *phosphorus* may be elevated because it is not excreted by a dysfunctional kidney. In addition, serum phosphorus always maintains a reciprocal relationship with calcium. *Parathyroid hormone* (PTH) is secreted in response to a low calcium and high phosphorus level. Parathyroid hormone causes calcium to be released from already formed bone in an effort to increase serum calcium. When renal disease is present, the kidneys are not able to excrete phosphate adequately; therefore, both calcium and phosphate may become elevated. Elevated levels signal the possibility of calcium deposition into soft tissue and major organs.

Serum *magnesium* is elevated by the kidneys' inability to excrete magnesium. A high serum magnesium value is often aggravated by the fact that many medications and antacids given to patients in renal failure contain magnesium. Nurses must be aware of magnesium-containing medications and other substances and must attempt to find alternate solutions to meet patients' needs.

Diseases affecting glomerular cell function may be manifested by a *low serum albumin* if the diseased glomerular basement membrane becomes more permeable. Albumin is then filtered and excreted in the urine. The degree of hypoalbuminemia will depend on many factors, such as the specific disease process and level of glomerular insufficiency as well as the nutritional status. Loss of albumin lowers serum osmolarity. A lowered serum osmolarity interferes with normal reabsorption of interstitial fluid into blood vessels, and edema results.

Metabolic acidosis occurs in renal disease because the renal tubules are unable to buffer H^+ ion. Both the *pH* and *serum bicarbonate* values obtained from analysis of an arterial blood sample would be low. A low hematocrit occurs when renal disease interferes with erythropoietin production and secretion. Erythropoietin normally stimulates the bone marrow to produce red blood cells.

Diagnostic and Radiological Tests

Many radiological tests are performed in an effort to reach a correct diagnosis, to ascertain the severity of the problem, and to direct intervention. Such tests include cystoscopy, abdominal x-ray film (KUB), excretory urogram (intravenous pyelogram—IVP), retrograde pyelogram, voiding cystourethrogram, renal arteriogram, renogram, computed tomography, and ultrasound (Fig. 56–1). Table 56–4 lists and describes the various tests most often performed. The nurse has a tremendous responsibility concerning radiological tests. The patient must be adequately prepared both physically and psychologically for these procedures. It is important that the nurse be knowledgeable about the procedures in order to prepare the patient for the test. This preparation includes teaching the patient what is involved in the procedure and his role in the success of the procedure. It is also a nursing responsibility to support the patient through any anxiety or discomfort he may experience, and to provide

(*Text continues on page 758*)

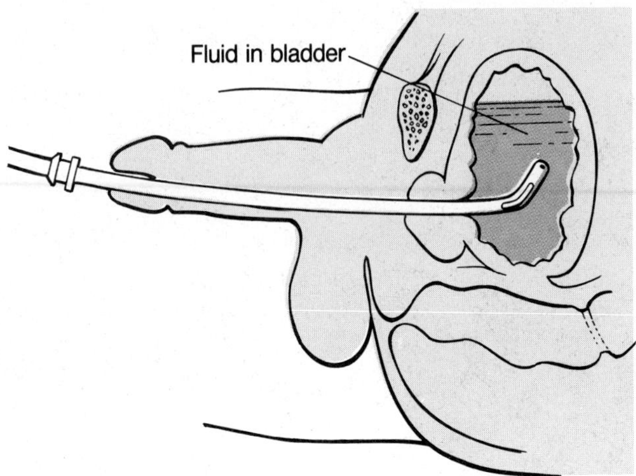

FIGURE 56–1 Cystoscopic examination of a male bladder.

TABLE 56–4
Diagnostic Studies of Renal Excretory System

	Purpose	*Procedure*	*Nursing Considerations*
Cystoscopy	• Allows visualization of the ureteral opening, bladder wall, trigone, and urethra • Structural abnormalities can be visualized and tissue biopsies obtained. • Urine flow from both ureters can be seen.	Cystoscope with a light is inserted through the urethra and into the bladder.	• Patient encouraged to drink fluids or intravenous is used to assure urine flow. • Explain to patient that it may be an uncomfortable procedure. Passage of the instrument and distention of bladder with fluid precipitate a desire to void. • Due to tissue irritation, patient may experience dysuria, frequency, and hematuria after the procedure. • Watch for urine retention, signs of infection, and prolonged or excessive hematuria after the procedure. • Monitor output and vital signs.
Abdominal x-ray film (KUB)	Reveals calcific deposits or gross renal abnormalities such as marked changes in kidney size	Flat x-ray plate is placed over abdomen and x-ray film is taken.	• Assure patient that procedure is painless. • Bowel prep may be done to avoid gas or fecal interference with visualization.
Excretory Urogram (intravenous pyelogram—IVP)	Assists in the evaluation of the function, filling, and emptying of urinary tract	• Contrast material is injected intravenously. • As the kidney filters and excretes the dye, x-ray films are taken at specific intervals.	• Bowel prep to avoid gas or fecal interference with visualization • Determine if the patient has a known allergy to iodine. • Explain that there will be a sense of warmth with injection of dye. • Watch for anaphylaxis; have emergency epinephrine available. • Fluids will usually be withheld by mouth after midnight. The resulting slight dehydration will help to concentrate the dye. *Note:* This is not done if the patient has multiple myeloma since hypercalcemia and increased urinary proteins are usually present, and dehydration may cause intrarenal obstruction by calcium crystals. • Observe for any changes in renal function after completion of the procedure; contrast medium is nephrotoxic. • Observe for volume depletion arising from the osmotic diuresis effect of the contrast medium.
Retrograde pyelogram	Outlines the renal pelvis and ureters	Contrast media is injected into each ureter through a cystoscope.	• Explain to patient that it may be an uncomfortable procedure. • Patient may experience dysuria, frequency, and hematuria following the procedure. • Determine if the patient has a known allergy to iodine.

(*Continued*)

TABLE 56–4
Diagnostic Studies of Renal Excretory System (*Continued*)

	Purpose	*Procedure*	*Nursing Considerations*
			▪ Watch for anaphylaxis; have emergency epinephrine available. ▪ Observe for urinary retention, infection, and prolonged or excessive hematuria after the procedure.
Voiding cystourethrogram	▪ Film before voiding outlines the bladder wall. ▪ Film during voiding outlines urethra and reflux of urine into ureters. ▪ Film after voiding demonstrates if bladder has emptied completely.	Contrast medium is instilled into the bladder through a cystoscope and films are taken before, during, and after voiding.	The same as outlined for retrograde pyelogram above.
Renal arteriogram	Allows visualization of the renal circulation	▪ In the *translumbar* approach, a needle is inserted through the soft tissue in the lumbar region into the aorta. The dye is injected into the aorta. ▪ In the *femoral approach,* the femoral artery is punctured, and a catheter is threaded up to the renal artery. Contrast medium is injected into the aorta or renal artery. ▪ Films are taken as the contrast medium passes through the renal circulation. ▪ Contrast media may also be injected intravenously. If so, the timing of x-rays depends on circulation time.	▪ Preparation of skin site in groin, and skin scrub and shave ▪ Bowel prep to prevent gas or fecal interference with visualization ▪ Determine if the patient has a known allergy to iodine. ▪ Watch for anaphylaxis; have emergency epinephrine available. ▪ Fluids will be withheld by mouth after midnight. ▪ Explain that sensation of warmth may occur along a vessel when contrast medium is injected. ▪ Observe for any changes in renal function, because contrast medium is nephrotoxic. ▪ Observe for volume (saline) depletion secondary to the osmotic diuretic effect of the contrast medium. ▪ Check peripheral pulses to detect problems with circulation due to trauma of vessels. ▪ Examine puncture site frequently to detect possible bleeding and hematoma. ▪ Cold applications and pressure dressings may be used at puncture site to prevent bleeding and decrease pain.
Renogram	▪ Records the radioactive patterns that mark the outline of the kidney and allows visualization of intrarenal masses and the amount of renal blood flow ▪ Records the appearance and disappearance of radioactivity over both kidneys, which demonstrates the relative function of each kidney	▪ Radioactive isotope with contrast medium is injected intravenously. ▪ A nuclear medicine scanning machine or photography is used to follow the radioactive isotopes. ▪ The tracer dose used negates the need for precautions against radioactivity.	▪ Teach the patient that diagnostic doses of radioactive substances are not harmful. ▪ There is no need for special precautions in handling excreta. ▪ There is no discomfort with the test except for patient's being positioned on an x-ray table.

(*Continued*)

TABLE 56–4
Diagnostic Studies of Renal Excretory System (*Continued*)

	Purpose	*Procedure*	*Nursing Considerations*
	▪ Used to detect vascular disease, obstructions, tumors, and malfunctioning kidneys ▪ Used frequently to detect rejection in renal transplant patients		
Computed tomography	▪ CT scanners permit visualization of kidney and blood vessels. ▪ Used to detect tumors, cysts, and change in size of kidney	Placement on machine table	▪ Positional discomfort: patient must not move while pictures are being taken. ▪ Not painful
Ultrasound	▪ Permits differentiation of solid masses and fluid collections. ▪ Detects tumors, cysts, obstructions, abscesses.	▪ Machine passes sound waves into internal body structures. ▪ Computer inteprets tissue density based on sound waves and prints out in picture form.	▪ Explain procedure. ▪ Not painful

adequate subsequent follow-up care. Often the nurse is the only person available to provide information and reassurance for the patient.

Renal Biopsy

The renal biopsy is an invasive procedure that is not routinely performed on every patient with renal disease and is not without considerable risk to the patient. It is used specifically to determine (1) the specific histological diagnosis if this is essential for deciding on the appropriate treatment, (2) the severity of the disease process and potential for recovery of function, and (3) the potential of functional recovery of a transplanted kidney that is currently not functioning.

A renal biopsy produces a sample of renal tissue for histological examination. The biopsy, performed by a nephrologist, is obtained by percutaneous needle puncture or by a surgical incision. Often, ultrasound is used to assist in percutaneous needle biopsies. Because it is a procedure that has potential serious complications such as hemorrhage and infection, it is reserved for patients to whom the results are essential for appropriate management.

A biopsy is contraindicated in patients who

1. Are uncooperative or unconscious (the biopsy is actually performed on inspiration, so that the patient must be able to take a breath on command)
2. Have only one kidney
3. Have polycystic kidneys
4. Have septicemia
5. Have severe hypertension
6. Have bleeding coagulopathies
7. Are on dialysis and have received heparin within the last 4 to 6 hours

Histological changes that may be seen as a result of a renal biopsy are (1) swelling, proliferation, and necrosis of the epithelium, (2) deposits and crescentic formations (loops) on the basement membrane, (3) proliferation, necrosis, and scarring of the mesangial cells, and (4) thrombosis and inflammation of glomerular capillaries.[1]

Nursing Considerations. It is important that the nurse prepare the patient for a renal biopsy so as to ensure cooperation and to alleviate anxiety and fear. The nursing care after a renal biopsy is extremely important. Bleeding complications must be prevented, and observations must be made to detect indications of infection or decreased renal function secondary to the procedure. The exact protocol used by different institutions may vary but generally it includes the following: (1) a sterile pressure dressing and external pressure for a short time if requested by the physician (can be applied with a sandbag), and (2) bed rest for 24 hours.[1] The biopsy area, the external dressing, and vital signs should be assessed frequently for signs of bleeding. Urine output should also be closely followed to detect any untoward changes in renal function secondary to renal tissue damage during the biopsy.

Inadequate renal function results from various pathological disorders such as infection, tumors, congenital malformations, familial diseases, vascular disorders, and obstructive conditions. Regardless of the etiology, renal disease presents pathophysiological problems that require similar nursing strategies. Chapter 57 discusses common nursing strategies for patients with renal dysfunction.

References

1. Brundage D: Nursing Management of Renal Problems, 2nd ed, pp 35–40. St Louis, CV Mosby, 1982
2. Uldall R: Renal Nursing, 2nd ed, pp 25–26. Oxford, Blackwell Scientific Publications, 1977

3. Underhill S et al: Cardiac Nursing. Philadelphia, JB Lippincott, 1982

Bibliography

Billings DM, Stokes LG: Medical Surgical Nursing: Common Health Problems of Adults and Children Across the Life Span. St Louis, CV Mosby, 1982

Brundage DL: Nursing Management of Renal Problems, 2nd ed, St Louis, CV Mosby, 1982

Brenner BM, Rector FC (eds): The Kidney, Vols 1 and 2. Phildelphia, WB Saunders, 1981

Hekelman FP, Ostendarp CA: Nephrology Nursing: Perspectives of Care. New York, McGraw-Hill, 1979

ˉarson E, Lindbloom L, Davis KB: Development of the Nephrology Nursing Practitioner: A Focus on Independent Learning. St Louis, CV Mosby, 1982

Roberts S: Renal assessment: A nursing point of view. Heart Lung 8:105–115, 1979

Strand MN, Elmer LA: Clincal Laboratory Tests, 2nd ed. St Louis, CV Mosby, 1980

Uldall R: Renal Nursing, 2nd ed. Oxford, Blackwell Publications, 1977

Chapter 57

Nursing Strategies for Common Renal and Excretory Problems

Nursing Diagnosis Interventions Evaluation

Lisa L. MacGeorge
Pauline M. Bruno

Following a thorough assessment of the patient with potential or existing renal dysfunction, a nursing care plan is developed, implemented, and evaluated. Nursing management of these patients requires knowledge of the causes of renal and excretory disorders, the degree of dysfunction, the pathophysiological course and its sequelae, the medical treatment modalities, and the nurse's role in assisting the patient and family. The patient and family require nursing interventions and instruction in learning to cope with functional disabilities that may result from renal disease, and in early detection or prevention of potential complications.

The renal system is responsible for and involved in many essential body functions. Knowledge of these functions allows the nurse to more easily anticipate potential nursing problems that may occur secondary to renal/excretory dysfunction. Kidneys are directly responsible for the volume and composition of the extracellular fluid, regulation of fluids and electrolytes, elimination of metabolic waste products, erythropoietin production, vitamin D activation, calcium absorption, and the metabolic portion of acid–base regulation. Renal dysfunction may result from disturbances of blood flow, intrarenal cell damage, tumors, and obstruction to urine flow.

Nursing problems related to renal inability to carry out its functions are numerous. The severity of the problem will vary directly with the extent of renal dysfunction. These problems are grouped under headings of alterations in fluid and electrolyte balance, inadequate elimination of metabolic waste products, and alterations in patterns of urinary elimination—incontinence and retention. Because of the vital nature of renal function relative to maintenance of homeostasis, the nursing problems are numerous and increase in complexity with increasing severity of dysfunction.

Alterations in Fluid and Electrolyte Balance

Fluid Volume Excess

Nursing Diagnosis/Problem. Potential for fluid volume excess (saline excess) is related to renal insufficiency of an acute or chronic nature and is manifested by increasing blood pressure, increased weight, and decreased functional ability. With renal damage the nephrons lose their ability to filter sodium and to excrete water. Sodium is osmotically active and therefore holds water in the extracellular compartment. Sodium and water excesses precipitate volume overload with the potential for high blood pressure, congestive heart failure, and pulmonary edema.

Interventions. The goals of nursing interventions are the following: to maintain sodium intake within a prescribed level; to detect evidence of impending complications of hypervolemia; and to promote maximum self-care within the tolerance limits of the individual.

Important nursing functions when the kidney is unable to adequately excrete sodium include quantifying, observing, and documenting the intake of sodium and loss of sodium-containing fluids (*i.e.,* urine, gastrointestinal tract, wound drainage, *etc.*) and replacing or restricting sodium-containing fluids when indicated. Monitoring serum electrolyte levels provides evidence of renal function. Patients and families need explanations of why sodium intake is restricted and of foods to avoid in the diet. (A list of these foods can be found in Table 57–1.)

The essential assessment parameters for volume status include daily weight, postural blood pressure measurements, pulse rate and quality, auscultation of lungs, presence or absence of pedal and sacral edema, and the status of neck veins.[4] Diuretics and antihypertensives are generally prescribed together to prevent the cardiovascular complications of sodium excess. Urine output measurements compared with measurements of fluid intake provide evidence of the effectiveness of this therapy. Patients may need instruction about the action of the medications, the possible side-effects, and the importance of following the prescribed schedule for taking them. The patient may need assistance in arranging a daily schedule to accommodate the need for frequent voidings after taking a diuretic. Patients on antihypertensives should be instructed in the technique of stimulating circulation by moving their legs before changing position (in order to avoid sudden drops in blood pressure).

Excess fluid volume increases the work load of the heart; therefore, nursing interventions should include assisting the person to establish activity–rest schedules. The patient should be encouraged to maximize self-care activities within the level of tolerance. This level will vary with the severity of the disease.

TABLE 57–1
Foods High in Sodium and Potassium

Sodium	*Potassium*
Tomato juice	Raw vegetables
Potato chips	Winter squash
Pretzels	Greens
Relishes	Potato
Pickles	Nuts
Condiments containing salt, baking powder, baking soda, monosodium glutamate	Dried fruits
	Bananas
	Oranges
	Honeydew melon
Any processed foods: TV dinners, sandwich spreads, soup, bouillon, cheese, cheese spreads, casserole mixes	Cantaloupe
	Grapefruit
	Apricot juice
	Apricots
Celery	
Milk	
Peanut butter	
Butter	
Soft drinks	

Evaluation. The outcome criteria for maintaining sodium level within prescribed limits are the following:

1. Serum sodium levels are within normal range.
2. Patient reports nutritional intake that is within prescribed limits.
3. Patient can identify foods that should be avoided in the diet.

The extent of renal damage may be such that medications are needed to control serum sodium levels and prevent complications of volume excess. The outcome criteria for prevention of complications are the following:

1. Patient adheres to the prescribed drug therapy.
2. There is minimal (+1) or no evidence of pedal or sacral edema.
3. Increased urine output is noted after patient takes a diuretic.
4. Patient weighs self daily. No increase in weight is noted
5. Lungs are clear to auscultation.
6. Blood pressure is within desired baseline for the particular patient.
7. Fluid intake volume is equal to urine output volume.
8. No distention of neck veins is observed.
9. Patient can state actions of medications and necessary safety precautions.

The outcome criteria for promoting maximum self-care activities include the following:

1. Patient participation in activities of daily living does not result in fatigue.
2. Patient adheres to a daily routine that does not result in fatigue.

Potassium Excess

Nursing Diagnosis/Problem. Potential for potassium excess is related to alteration in tubular secretory function. Potassium imbalances are common in renal failure and may be severe and life threatening. Hyperkalemia is the most common potassium imbalance. It was a frequent cause of death before the advent of dialysis and other methods of controlling it. Hyperkalemia causes cardiac muscle irritability and eventually ventricular fibrillation. Any level above 6.0 mEq/liter is potentially dangerous, although cardiac arrest seldom occurs at levels below 7.5 mEq/liter. In addition to primary renal failure, some other conditions may cause hyperkalemia. In situations where there is extensive tissue damage (trauma), the fast rise in serum potassium may exceed the ability of the kidney to excrete it. Trauma to tissue, hemolysis, and administration of whole blood or packed red blood cells cause increased release of potassium into the bloodstream. Other causes of increased serum potassium levels include acidosis and increased intake of potassium-containing substances (see Chap. 13).

Interventions. The goals are to maintain the patient's serum potassium within normal limits and to take prompt action to either increase or decrease the potassium should it be outside normal limits. The patient who has severe renal dysfunction should be frequently monitored for serial serum potassium levels (usually daily unless serum potassium is rising rapidly and then measurements are indicated more often) and, if the level is over 6.0 mEq/liter, the patient should be placed on a cardiac monitor. Electrocardiogram changes that occur specifically with hyperkalemia include peaked T waves, widening of the QRS complex, a prolonged Q-T interval, and eventually cardiac arrest. Symptoms of a high potassium level may include nausea, vomiting, weakness, paresthesia of the extremities, mental confusion, and restlessness.

A low potassium diet and regular renal dialysis are usually adequate measures to control serum potassium. However, if dialysis has not been initiated and the potassium reaches critical levels (>6.0 mEq/liter) the following emergency measures may be used temporarily until dialysis can be started:

1. Calcium gluconate is administered intravenously to counteract the toxic effects of potassium on the cardiac muscle.
2. Insulin and glucose are given intravenously to drive the potassium from the vascular space into the cells.
3. Sodium bicarbonate is administered intravenously if acidosis is present: it reduces the serum potassium as the acidosis is reversed (be cognizant of the amount of sodium that is being given and its effect on fluid balance).
4. Cation exchange resins are given orally or as an enema; they exchange potassium for another cation in the gastrointestinal tract.
5. Dialysis, either hemodialysis or peritoneal dialysis, is the most efficient means of lowering the serum potassium.

Evaluation. Goal achievement can be determined by the following:

1. Patient adheres to a potassium diet.
2. Patient states he has no nausea, vomiting, weakness, or paresthesia of extremities.
3. Serum potassium is within normal limits.
4. An elevated serum potassium level is brought down to normal limits by the emergency methods listed above.

Magnesium Imbalance

Nursing Disgnosis/Problem. Magnesium imbalance is related to an alteration in renal tubular function. Serum magnesium levels are increased during oliguria but generally are not a problem unless magnesium-containing medications have been given. Serum magnesium levels are decreased during diuresis or polyuric states, during prolonged gastrointestinal loss, and in the patient with burns.

Interventions. The goals are to maintain the serum magnesium within normal limits and to take action to return serum levels to normal should they be outside normal limits.

Nurses should be aware of serum serial magnesium levels and signs and symptoms that may indicate an imbalance. Signs and symptoms of hypermagnesemia include hypotension (magnesium has a vasodilating effect), nausea, vomiting, drowsiness, hyperreflexia, and muscular weakness. These manifestations usually occur when serum magnesium is over 5.0 mEq/liter. Symptoms of hypomagnesemia include weakness, tremors, personality changes, vertigo, convulsions, confusion, and hyperreactive reflexes and are usually seen when serum magnesium is less than 0.8 mEq/liter. Hypomagnesemia results in increased neuromuscular irritability.

The most important nursing intervention in the prevention of hypermagnesemia is to avoid giving any magnesium-containing substances. All medications, especially antacids, should be closely checked to be certain they do not contain magnesium. Patients should be taught about this danger. In some situations, avoidance of magnesium intake will not be sufficient to prevent hypermagnesemia. In these situations the magnesium level will be lowered with the use of dialysis.

Dietary teaching is the most important nursing intervention for persons with magnesium deficits. Magnesium-containing foods include green vegetables, fruits, milk, and nuts. In acute situations, magnesium salts are given orally or parenterally.

Evaluation. Goal achievement is attained if the patient states he does not have any of the above listed symptoms of hypermagnesemia or hypomagnesemia and if the serum magnesium is within normal limits.

Calcium and Phosphate Imbalance

Nursing Diagnosis/Problem. Calcium and phosphate imbalance is related to the inability of the kidney to activate vitamin D within the body and to prevent renal excretion of phosphate, and to the interrelationship of the serum level of the two electrolytes. As previously mentioned in Chapter 56, calcium absorption from the intestine is dependent on the activated form of vitamin D. The kidneys are responsible for activating exogenous vitamin D within the body. With renal disease, this activation of vitamin D is greatly decreased and subsequently there is a decrease in calcium absorption from the intestine. Parathormone, which is secreted from the parathyroid gland in response to a low serum calcium level and a high phosphate level, causes calcium release from already formed bone. This loss of calcium from bone causes profound bone porosity and predisposition to pathological fractures.

Renal dysfunction inhibits excretion of phosphate; hence the serum level rises. A high serum phosphate level causes increased parathormone output and further aggravates bone resorption. Another serious complication of an elevated phosphate level is that a Ca^{2+}/PO_4 product of more than 60 mg/dl predisposes to calcium deposition in major organs such as the heart, liver, and spleen. Secondary hyperparathyroidism may occur if the imbalances continue without intervention. This is reversible if serum calcium and phosphate levels are brought within normal limits. Secondary hyperparathyroidism can be considered a physiological compensatory mechanism for a pathophysiological condition.

Interventions. The goal is to maintain serum calcium and phosphate levels within normal limits without overactivating the parathyroid gland. Nursing interventions consist of monitoring serum calcium and phosphorus levels and administering the appropriate medications. Usually a pharmacological form of activated vitamin D (active metabolite 12.5, dihydrotachysterol) and a phosphate binder is prescribed. Calcium supplements such as calcium gluconate, calcium carbonate, or calcium lactate may be administered in conjunction with vitamin D preparations.

Phosphate binders such as aluminum hydroxide come in capsule or liquid form and are given to bind phosphate in the intestine; this bound phosphate is then eliminated in the feces. Because aluminum hydroxide is very constipating, nurses need to encourage the person using this binder to be physically active and to ingest foods high in fiber. A stool softener is usually an accompanying prescription. Patient teaching regarding the importance of these medications is a fundamental part of nursing care.

The physician may periodically order a serum parathormone level to assess parathyroid function. The nurse should monitor this level and assess for signs and symptoms of hyperparathyroidism (see Chap. 75).

Additional nursing management includes protection of the patient from activity that may potentiate a pathological fracture. Daily weight bearing is also essential for prevention of calcium loss from bone. Nursing interventions should ensure that patients engage in daily activity that includes weight bearing whenever possible.

Evaluation. Goal achievement is evidenced by normal serum calcium, phosphorus, and parathormone levels. Other criteria include the following:

1. Patient demonstrates the ability to state the reason for medications.
2. Patient adheres to the medication regimen.
3. Patient participates in physical activity on a daily basis.
4. Patient reports adequate bowel function.

Inadequate Elimination of Metabolic Waste Products (Uremic Toxicity)

Renal dysfunction results in inadequate elimination of electrolytes and metabolic waste products. Renal disease may progress slowly to eventual renal failure. The early symptoms of impaired function may be treated, but cure is often not possible. Some renal diseases are incurable. As the disease progresses, the disturbance in renal function becomes increasingly severe as does the consequence relative to maintenance of body homeostasis. Periodic lowering of high blood levels of nitrogenous waste products, electrolytes, and other substances by hemodialysis or peritoneal dialysis will prolong the life of the afflicted person. Dialysis is the process of diffusion across a semipermeable membrane. When possible a kidney transplant may be performed.

Uremic toxicity is a term used to describe a toxic condition caused by the retention of nitrogenous wastes and biochemical alterations that occur with untreated renal failure. All of the following nursing diagnoses/problems relate to the care of patients with acute and chronic (end-stage) renal disease, including patients receiving hemodialysis, peritoneal dialysis, and renal transplantation. Nurses are intensely involved in independent, interdependent, and coordinative types of nursing care for these patients. The specifics of dialysis treatment are presented in Chapter 58.

Alteration in Mental Status

Nursing Diagnosis/Problem. Alteration in mental/neurological status is related to inadequate elimination of metabolic waste products. As the BUN level rises the patient may exhibit signs of disorientation, confusion, restlessness, delirium, psychosis, and may even progress to convulsion or coma. This is sometimes referred to as *uremic encephalopathy*.

Urea readily crosses the blood–brain barrier and once into the central nervous system (CNS) does not easily reenter the systemic circulation. In addition urea is an osmotically active substance that attracts abnormal amounts of body water into the CNS. Eventually, the cells of the CNS swell and predispose the patients to seizures.

As previously discussed in the preceding chapter on assessment, the best indicators of changes in renal function are the serum creatinine and the 24-hour creatinine clearance. The best indicator, however, of the toxic effects of decreased renal function on the rest of the body is the blood urea nitrogen (BUN) level. The higher the BUN the more the uremic symptomatology that will be evident. A patient who is treated appropriately for renal failure may avoid or be rescued from this toxic symptomatology. Uremic toxicity affects many body systems and if not treated may be very serious and eventually life threatening.

Interventions. The primary goal is to maintain the BUN level at which the patient does not exhibit signs and symptoms of uremic encephalopathy. This level is not absolute and will vary for each patient. However, most patients will exhibit encephalopathic symptomatology with a BUN level greater than 120 mg/dl.

The nursing intervention consists of assessment of changes in mental status and orientation. It is extremely important that the nurse document clearly in behavioral terms the ongoing status changes and characteristics of patients during this time. Generally a neurological checklist is an ideal documentation tool. It is important that the patient have an orienting and safe environment. Clocks and calendars in the room may help the patient with orientation to time and place. The room should be free of safety hazards and seizure precautions should be initiated, as discussed in Chapter 65.

Evaluation. Goal accomplishment can be assessed by observing for changes in the mental/neurological status of the patient in conjunction with changes or a rise in the BUN level. Achievement is attained when the patient does not evidence restlessness, disorientation, or delirium and the BUN is maintained at less than 120 mg/dl.

Alteration in Sensory/Neurological Status

Nursing Diagnosis/Problem. Alteration in sensory/neurological status is related to inadequate elimination of metabolic waste products and uremic toxicity. Uremia may lead eventually to the development of a symmetrical *peripheral neuritis* that affects the feet and legs. "Pins and needles" and loss of sensation are followed later by loss of power and foot drop. Because loss of vibration sense occurs early, conduction studies are used in the diagnosis of peripheral neuritis. With the initiation of dialysis, the neuritis gradually improves. The condition also improves with renal transplantation.

Interventions. The primary goal is to initiate appropriate treatment for renal failure before manifestations of peripheral neuritis develops. The secondary goal is to provide symptomatic relief and safety measures if the neuritis already exists or is not eliminated with the institution of treatment.

It is essential that nurses assess for and document change in peripheral neurological status. It is also important to explain to patients what may be happening and that this disturbing condition will improve with treatment. Safety of the patient is a nursing responsibility. It is important to protect against injury during periods of decreased sensitivity. The patient should be made aware of heat-related dangers. Before bathing, the patient should have someone else test the water temperature, and the patient should handle heated objects with protective devices. Ataxia increases the risk of falls, especially if hazards exist in the environment. Assistance with mobility may be necessary.

Evaluation. Outcomes are achieved if assessment reveals no signs and symptoms of sensory/neurological changes, and the patient reports an absence or decrease in sensation of "pins and needles" and the presence of vibratory sensation. The nurse's own observations would indicate a hazard free environment, and the patient would report adherence to prescribed safety measures.

Metabolic Acidosis

Nursing Diagnosis/Problem. Metabolic acidosis is related to retention of acidic waste products of metabolism. Patients with renal failure are usually in metabolic acidosis. This state is signaled by a low serum bicarbonate and low CO_2 combining power. Acidosis predisposes to hyperventilation, which reduces the amount of CO_2 available to form carbonic acid (respiratory compensation), and cardiac arrhythmias. Patients are usually not symptomatic until the bicarbonate level is less than 12 mEq/liter at which point respiratory compensation is not sufficient (see Chap. 14). The acidosis causes potassium to be released from the cells and further aggravates any previous problem with hyperkalemia.

Interventions. The goal is to prevent or reverse metabolic acidosis by the initiation of dialysis or by renal transplantation and to maintain bicarbonate or CO_2 combining power within normal limits. Intravenous sodium bicarbonate will temporarily control the acidosis, but when this treatment is used, thought must be given to the amount of sodium the patient is receiving. Nurses need to promptly record administration of this medication. Regular dialysis, once initiated, is usually sufficient to control the acidosis. Nurses should be aware of the caveat that when acidosis is reversed too rapidly there is potential for both rebound hypocalcemia and hypokalemia.

Evaluation. The criteria for evaluating goal achievement are the serum bicarbonate level, by means of an arterial blood gas, or the CO_2 combining power, by means of a venipuncture blood sample and the extent of hyperventilation. The normal blood values for both serum bicarbonate and CO_2 are approximately 24 mEq/liter. However, renal failure patients usually adjust to and function at a lower value and always have some degree of respiratory compensation (increased respiratory rate). The outcome criteria are specific to the individual patient and depend on baseline data and the severity of the disease.

Potential for Inadequate Cardiac Output

Nursing Diagnosis/Problem. Potential for inadequate cardiac output is related to pericarditis associated with inadequate excretion of nitrogenous waste products of metabolism. Pericarditis, an inflammation of the pericardial sac, is a serious complication for uremic patients and does not seem to be closely related to BUN level. It does generally occur with long-standing uremia but does not correlate well with a particular degree of uremia. The hallmark sign of pericarditis is a pericardial friction rub, a scratching sound that can be heard upon auscultation of the heart. Detection of this sound when assessing patients with renal dysfunction requires immediate notification of a physician. The greatest danger associated with pericarditis is subsequent cardiac tamponade (inability of the heart to contract because of compression by a large pericardial inflammatory effusion. The manifestations of tamponade are distant heart sounds and hypotension. The hypotension results from compression of the heart and hence inadequate cardiac muscle contraction and cardiac output.

Interventions. The goals are to prevent pericarditis by the treatment of renal failure, which promotes elimination of nitrogenous wastes, and by early detection of a pericardial friction rub with rapid initiation of treatment measures. It is extremely important that auscultation for a potential pericardial friction rub be a regular part of the nursing assessment. Any suspicion of a friction rub warrants notification of the physician. Assistance with dialysis is a nursing responsibility (see Chap. 58). Because cardiac tamponade can result from bleeding into the pericardiac sac, all potential risks for bleeding should be minimized, that is, minimal heparinization if the patient is on dialysis.

Evaluation. The outcome of preventive measures is the absence of a pericardial friction rub either prior to or after treatment to remove nitrogenous waste products has been initiated. The outcome criteria in the event a pericardial friction rub is detected is nonoccurrence of cardiac tamponade.

Potential for Bleeding

Nursing Diagnosis/Problem. Potential for bleeding is related to inadequate platelet function. Uremia causes platelets to become dysfunctional and subsequently bleeding coagulopathies present. Though total numbers of platlets may be normal there is a qualitative defect that renders them less efficient in stopping bleeding. As the uremia is reversed the platelets become more functional. Bleeding is less of a problem with frequent regular dialysis.

Interventions. The nurse's goal is to protect patients with renal dysfunction from activities that predispose to bleeding and to promote platelet function by controlling the uremic environment. Nursing management includes protecting the patient from unnecessary invasive procedures such as as intramuscular injection, providing a safe environment to protect against injury, and patient teaching to avoid, or exercise extreme caution in performing, those activities that may predispose to bleeding, that is, shaving, brushing teeth, doing household chores, and falling. Once treatment is initiated and uremia controlled, platelet function will improve greatly.

Evaluation. The goal can be considered accomplished when bleeding episodes due to preventable causes are avoided. The platelet count is not an accurate assessment parameter because even though the absolute number may be within normal limits, the platelets may be dysfunctional.

Activity Intolerance

Nursing Diagnosis/Problem. Decreased ability to perform activities of daily living is related to renal failure and uremia. Generally, anemia develops gradually with chronic renal failure. The manifestations of anemia are fatigue, weakness, and inability to perform activities of daily living. The pathophysiological basis for this type of anemia is inability of the kidneys to produce erythropoietin. Erythropoietin normally stimulates the bone marrow to make erythrocytes. In addition, red blood cells have a decreased life span in a uremic environment. This anemia is not cured by iron or other hematinic factors and may have to be treated with transfusion if the hematocrit falls too low. It is not uncommon for renal failure patients to function with a hematocrit of around 20.

Intervention. The primary goal is to help the patient conserve energy to accomplish priority activities for daily living with a minimum of fatigue. A second goal is to detect and report extremely low hematocrit levels so that treatment with blood transfusions may be initiated.

Nurses may need to assist the patient with activities for daily living. The nurse teaches the patient and family signs of low energy and intolerance to activity and methods of scheduling activities to allow for rest periods. The family is also taught how to assist the patient with personal hygiene and mobility.

Folate and anabolic steroids are both administered as part of the treatment for the anemia seen with renal failure. The mechanism of this therapy is not entirely clear and its effectiveness varies among individuals. The objective for this therapy is to promote erythropoiesis. Masculinization, acne, sodium retention, and possible hepatocellular carcinoma are disturbing side-effects and may contraindicate the use of anabolic steroids. Initiation of this therapy must be carefully thought through in terms of the physiological benefit vs. the liver damage and altered body image (particularly for the female patient) it may cause for the patient. Nurses play a critical role in evaluating the effect of medication therapy, in assessing the energy level of the patient, and in teaching the patient and family. Folate (iron) is sometimes prescribed in an attempt to overcome the iron deficiency component of anemia. Because both antacid therapy and food delay the absorption of iron the effectiveness of this therapy is questionable. Unnecessary blood loss should be avoided and blood losses during dialysis minimized as much as possible.

Evaluation. Outcome criteria include the following:

1. Patient expression of ability to accomplish some degree of personal self-care without excessive fatigue
2. Family members demonstrate ability to provide assistance with personal care and mobility.
3. Patient adheres to prescribed medication therapy.
4. A maintenance of hematocrit level that is maximum for the individual (will vary with degree of renal dysfunction)

Potential for Infection

Nursing Diagnosis/Problem. Potential for infection is related to inadequate elimination of waste products (uremic toxicity). One complication of uremia that affects all body systems and functional areas is infection. For reasons that are poorly understood uremia predisposes to infection. The most common infections are those of the skin, mouth, salivary glands, urinary tract, and lungs. Septicemia is common among uremic patients.

Interventions. The primary goal is to prevent infection. Other goals are early detection of existing infection, facilitation of treatment by notifying the physician promptly, and carry out prescribed interdependent therapy.

Nursing management to prevent or treat infection includes the following: performance of frequent, regular dialysis for optimal control of uremia (as ordered by the physician); culture of all infected or potentially infected sites (including blood cultures) if the patient develops a fever; sputum cultures at the earliest sign of a respiratory infection; routine throat and urine cultures; good oral hygiene; avoidance of long-term use of urinary catheters; meticulous intravenous site care; and prompt observation, communication, and documentation of manifestations of the development of infection so that therapy can be initiated. It should be noted that once an infection is active, it increases the BUN by causing tissue breakdown that aggravates the uremic syndrome even further. As always, prevention is the ideal.

Evaluation. Goal achievement can be evaluated by the absence of infection or by evidence that a present infection is resolving with treatment. Signs of recovery from infection include absence of fever, negative cultures or decreasing bacterial counts in cultures, absence of signs of inflammation at intravenous injection sites, wound healing without purulent drainage, improvement in general state of well-being, and resolution of initial symptoms.

Inadequate Wound Healing

Nursing Diagnosis/Problem. Inadequate wound healing is related to uremic toxicity. Wound healing is delayed during severe renal dysfunction because of decreased collagen synthesis. The relationship between renal dysfunction and decreased collagen synthesis is not entirely clear. However, the most recent wound healing research, relative to the cellular physiology and pathophysiology of the wound, is exciting and may add new insight into delayed wound healing secondary to uremia.[2]

Interventions. The goals of nurses are to prevent delayed wound healing by controlling uremic toxicity and to promote optimal healing. The best interventions for the problem of inadequate wound healing are to decrease the BUN level by regular frequent dialysis or successful renal transplantation and to promote wound healing by provision of an oxygen-rich environment and adequate nutrition. By the avoidance of hypotension or hypovolemia, blood flow and oxygenation to all tissues is facilitated. Adequate or supplemental nutrition is necessary to promote optimal healing. (See the following section Inadequate Nutrition.)

Evaluation. Goal achievement can be evaluated by frequent assessment of wounds and the status of healing. An adequately healing wound is evidenced by decreasing extent of inflammation over the first few days, absence of drainage, approximation of wound edges, and shrinkage in size of wound. Discomfort at the wound site should be minimal after the first few days.

Inadequate Nutrition

Nursing Diagnosis/Problem. Inadequate nutrition is related to uremic toxicity. Nutritional status is profoundly affected by renal function. As the BUN level rises and metabolic acidosis ensues, the patient may became very anorexic. In addition, the conservative treatment of renal failure includes many dietary restrictions and may make it difficult to find foods that are palatable. With an elevated BUN, protein often doesn't taste palatable to patients. Fresh fruits may be appealing to the patient but may be restricted owing to their high potassium content and the kidneys' decreased ability to excrete potassium.

Often fluids are severely restricted and patients may feel very dry and thirsty. Thirst is a function of both physiological thirst and cultural norms. Many of the pathophysiological processes and treatments involved in renal failure predispose to thirst, that is, increased BUN level, fluid restriction, possible water deficit, and so on. In addition, eating and drinking have traditionally been social activities in our society. This may make restricting fluids particularly difficult for patients. To make the patient more comfortable, hard candies or gum may be provided. These may help to decrease the feeling of a dry mouth and to decrease the desire for fluids.

Interventions. The goals are to maintain body weight within normal range for the individual, prevent muscle wasting, and prevent problems of fluid and electrolyte imbalance. Nursing has a critical role in helping to maintain nutritional status. Most hospitals have dieticians who work with nurses and patients in providing nutritional needs and meeting personal preferences. By consulting with dieticians, nurses can help to develop a successful nutritional plan for patients with renal failure.

The major dietary restrictions for a patient include fluids, sodium, potassium, magnesium, and protein. Fluids are restricted due to inadequate renal excretion with the potential for the effects of volume overload. Sodium is retained in the body with renal failure and further aggravates the problem of volume overload. Knowledge of serum electrolyte and protein levels are a necessary part of the nurse's assessment. Generally, a renal diet is restricted to 2 g of sodium/day. In addition to table salt, other foods and fluids to avoid are listed in Table 57–1. Nurses should also be cognizant of the amount of sodium contained in medications that patients are required to take. Serum potassium levels may become quite high when the kidneys fail. High potassium levels are particularly toxic to the cardiac muscle. Table 57–1 also contains a list of food high in potassium. Salt substitute, which is potassium chloride, should be avoided. Potassium is lost during cooking; therefore, all fruits and vegetables should be cooked before eating, making certain all the liquid is removed.

As mentioned earlier, hypermagnesemia generally occurs only with an increased intake of magnesium-containing compounds. One of the biggest and most often forgotten sources of magnesium are antacids. Be sure to check the contents of all antacids prior to giving them to a patient in renal failure. Because the excretion of nitrogenous wastes is decreased in renal failure, protein is usually restricted, particularly prior to the initiation of dialysis. The protein that is allowed should be of high quality, such as eggs, meat, poultry, and fish. Once dialysis is initiated, the protein restriction may be liberalized. More protein is removed with peritoneal dialysis than with hemodialysis and those patients may actually require high protein diets.

Muscle wasting may become a problem owing to nutritional deficiencies in protein that leads to breakdown of lean body mass. Lack of exercise may contribute to muscle atrophy. Nurses, in conjunction with the dietician and physical therapist, should devise a plan of care that will assist in avoiding or minimizing these complications.

Evaluation. Goal accomplishment is successful when problems secondary to inadequate nutrition are avoided, and nutrition is provided to promote optimal function for all body systems. Evidence of goal achievement includes the maintenance of serum electrolyte and protein levels and body weight (evidence of fluid retention) within acceptable limits for the individual. Muscle strength is maintained. The patient should report adherence to the prescribed dietary regime.

Sexual Dysfunction

Nursing Diagnosis/Problem. Sexual dysfunction is related to uremic toxicity. Problems related to severe renal dysfunction are increased libido and potency in men, and suppression of libido, ovulation, and menstruation in women. In addition to the effects of uremia, certain medications such as some of the antihypertensives cause impotence in men and questionable sexual dysfunction in women.

Interventions. The goal is to assist the patient and family to understand and cope with changes in sexuality related to the impact of renal dysfunction on the reproductive system. Patients need a comfortable, open rapport with someone to be able to express their concerns about the effect of renal dysfunction on their sexual relationships. Patients often feel that this is a problem unique to themselves and feel as though they cannot discuss it with anyone else. The nurse should assess the patient's emotional status and knowledge level regarding sexual dysfunction. By explaining the side-effects of the disease process or medications on sexual/reproductive function, the nurse may provide an opportunity for the patient to discuss his concerns. It may be appropriate to suggest sexual counseling for the patient and family after assessing their readiness.

Evaluation. A successful outcome is achieved if the patient and family are able to discuss the problem and seek counseling if this is necessary. Patient and family reports of the use of successful coping actions is another measure of goal achievement.

Alteration in Skin Integrity: Uremic Dermatitis

Nursing Diagnosis/Problem. Alteration in integument is related to uremic toxicity. The integument is greatly affected by the uremic syndrome. Uremic dermatitis is common and consists of dryness, scaliness, pruritis. A characteristic coloration is present that consists of pale mucous membranes and nail beds, and shallow yellowish brown skin (appears as a washed-out suntan). Numerous petechiae may be present owing to alterations in the coagulation system. In untreated advanced uremia, uremic crystals may actually develop on the skin.

Interventions. The nurse's aims are to prevent alterations in integument by controlling uremic toxicity and to assist the patient to develop coping mechanisms for skin discoloration. Nursing management of these problems should be directed toward comfort measures and participation in the treatment chosen to reverse the uremic process. Regular, frequent dialysis to decrease and control the level of blood urea nitrogen or renal transplantation ultimately will be required. Prior to initiation of definitive treatment, alterations in integument can be partially controlled with symptomatic management. The tannish coloration will remain except after renal transplantation.

Evaluation. The goals are achieved if the skin is free of dryness, scaliness, and pruritis. The patient will express freedom from discomfort.

Ineffective Coping

Nursing Diagnosis/Problem. Potential for problems in adapting to a change in lifestyle is related to long-term dialysis treatment. Many physical, financial, and psychological limitations are imposed on patients and families who receive hemodialysis or peritoneal dialysis over an extended period of time. The treatment restricts mobility for a period of time every 2 to 3 days. Although the cost of the equipment has decreased over the time period that long-term dialysis treatment has been available, it continues to be a major financial expenditure. To carry out the treatment in the home setting usually requires assistance from another person. The person receiving the treatment is thus placed in a dependent position.

Interventions. The goals of nursing are to teach the patient and family how to perform the dialysis treatment and assist them in adapting to the changes the treatments make in their lifestyle.

Each patient and family situation is individual, and a recipe for helping patients and families to cope does not exist. Many resources are available to help patients and families to cope specifically with dialysis and transplantation. It is important that nurses know what resources are available and how to optimally utilize them. Nurses have the best opportunity to assess the psychosocial needs of patients and families and to determine the appropriate timing for various types of assistance. Social workers, patient support groups, financial counselors, and community groups may all be helpful at different times during the process from diagnosis and treatment to long-term adaptation. Nurses must draw on their knowledge of and skills in dealing with anxiety, stress, and the coping process during hospitalization. For a primary care-taker and a professional nurse, experiencing this process with patients and families requires maturity, commitment, emotional energy, and dedication. It is also necessary that nurses who work in this area recognize the importance of their own mental health and develop adequate coping mechanisms to enable themselves to maintain an accurate perspective regarding their own life and mortality.

Evaluation. Criteria for evaluating goal achievement are the following:

1. The patient and family accurately perform the dialysis procedure in the treatment center and later in the home setting.

2. Patient and family report confidence in their ability to perform the procedure and take necessary actions in an emergency situation.
3. Patient and family report feeling comfortable in the newly established lifestyle.
4. Financial problems are resolved such that the family report having adequate income for essentials of life and some nonessentials.

Alteration in Patterns of Urinary Elimination

Alteration in patterns of urinary elimination are related to functional disorders or to obstructions. The functional disorders are usually of nervous system origin. They may be a disturbance of central nervous system integrative function or of motor control. Obstructions may occur along the course of the ureters, within the bladder or the urethra, or may result from external pressure. The nature of the obstruction may be a tumor, severe inflammation and infection, or calculus. Externally, the pressure of an enlarging uterus with pregnancy or a tumor in the pelvic cavity may compress the bladder, ureters, or urethra and interfere with elimination. The effect of functional or obstructive disorders is either urinary retention or incontinence. Patients experiencing either type of alteration in urinary excretion often share three problems in common, namely, emotional stress, increased potential for infection, and difficulty with appropriate use of drainage devices. These latter three problems will be addressed first followed by a discussion of retention and incontinence.

Emotional Stress

Nursing Diagnosis/Problem. Alteration in emotional comfort is related to inability to meet the socially accepted standard of voluntary control of micturition. Feelings of embarrassment and guilt may be expressed. Sometimes the feelings are not expressed but rather the person may avoid talking about the problem and even deny some symptoms. A second reason for emotional discomfort is the embarrassment some people experience with the physical examination and treatment associated with the external genitalia. Manifestations of discomfort include generalized muscle tension, and the fact that sometimes the person may either withdraw or become hyperactive and talkative.

Interventions. The goal of nursing is to promote patient comfort. It will often help the patient to relax if the nurse explains the procedures to be performed in a matter-of-fact manner accompanied by a touch. The nurse can open the topic for discussion by statements to the effect that some people are embarrassed when they have problems of urinary elimination. A discussion of feelings may relieve some of the discomfort. It is also important to provide privacy for treatments and to carry out procedure quickly. The patient may need frequent reassurance and support.

Evaluation. Criteria for goal achievement are the following:

1. The patient discusses his feelings about the situation.
2. The patient reports a decrease in discomfort.
3. Generalized muscle tension and behavioral manifestations of discomfort are decreased.

Problems Related to Catheterization

Potential for Infection from Catheterization

Nursing Diagnosis/Problem. High risk for bladder and urinary tract infection is related to the use of invasive devices to obtain urine flow and to the stasis of urine that may attend the underlying pathology. The manifestations of bladder infection are urgency, dysuria, frequency, hematuria, fever, positive urine cultures, and bacteriuria. There is danger of infection whenever invasive techniques are used; catheterization, however, seems to be particularly hazardous. Catheterization is the major cause of hospital-acquired infections. There are two sources of bacterial entry with catheterization: (1) use of nonsterile equipment or contamination of the equipment when carrying out the procedure, and (2) irritation of the urethral or bladder mucosa with instrumentation. This latter is especially likely when the tissues are inflamed. There is always bacteria along the lumen of the urethra and around the urinary meatus; therefore, trauma to mucous membrane may permit entry of bacteria.

The longer the catheter is is place, the greater the danger of infection. Indwelling catheters must be connected to a closed drainage system that prevents the entrance of bacteria by migration along the lumen of the catheter, but it is possible for bacteria to migrate inward from the meatus along the outer wall of the catheter. Indwelling catheters are used in many different situations in order to reestablish urine flow or obtain accurate intake and output record (often on an hourly basis) or to allow tissue time to heal. Some of the situations in which indwelling catheters are used are the following:

1. When the patient is critically ill and frequent data is needed to maintain electrolyte and acid–base balance.
2. Postoperatively when the patient is most apt to have difficulty voiding for a few days.
3. Following trauma to the spinal cord and hence interference with motor control.
4. Following cerebral trauma when the patient may be unconscious.
5. To permit bladder irrigation especially after bladder surgery.

Interventions for Catheter Care

The goals of nursing are to prevent occurrence of bladder infection with the use of catheters, and if infection occurs to detect it promptly so that treatment may be instituted. The care of patients presenting with lower urinary tract infections is discussed in Chapter 59.

Catheter Selection. Interventions to prevent occurrence center around the procedure of catheterization and management of an indwelling catheter. Selection of the proper size and type of catheter contributes to preventing tissue trauma. Catheter size depends on the age and size of the patient. Tissues atrophy with age and urethral openings may narrow. Catheters for adults range in size from 14 to 22. The average size for an adult female is 16 or 18, whereas it is 18 or 20 for the adult male. The catheter selected should be smaller than the external meatus to prevent trauma to the muscosa.

Urethral catheters are usually made of rubber, nylon, or plastic although sometimes metal of glass catheters may be used. Ureteral catheters are usually made of silk. An in-and-out catheterization is done with a straight catheter, which usually has an opening at the end of the catheter as well as along the side. Indwelling catheters are used when continuous drainage is required. The most commonly used indwelling catheter is the Foley. This catheter has a double lumen with an inflatable balloon near the tip. The balloon is inflated after the catheter is in the bladder and thus prevents the catheter from slipping out of the bladder (Fig. 57–1). The balloon is either 5 ml or 30 ml in size. The 5-ml balloon is the one usually used. The 30-ml balloon is used for applying pressure when there is bleeding.

Procedure for Catheterization. After selection of the proper catheter, the procedure is carried out using aseptic technique that starts with careful cleansing of the meatus. Adequate lighting and exposure is necessary to assure identification of the meatus and skillful, gentle insertion of the well lubricated catheter. The catheter should be advanced steadily until urine starts to flow. Control of the catheter has to be maintained in order that it does not slip out of the bladder. Gentle pressure just superior to the symphysis will help to assure adequate urine drainage. The catheter should be removed promptly as urine drainage ceases. If resistance is encountered in inserting the catheter, the catheter is held steady, the patient is asked to take a deep breath and try to relax, and the nurse then attempts to advance the catheter. If resistance continues the procedure is discontinued and the physician notified in order to avoid trauma. Persons who have obstructions or strictures or who are very tense are ones in whom resistance is likely to be encountered. An instance in which nurses should not do a catheterization is in the postoperative period following surgery of the urethra or bladder.

If an indwelling catheter is being inserted, the balloon should be inflated after the urine has ceased draining. The end of the Foley is then attached to the closed drainage system, maintaining asepsis (Fig. 57–2). The system should

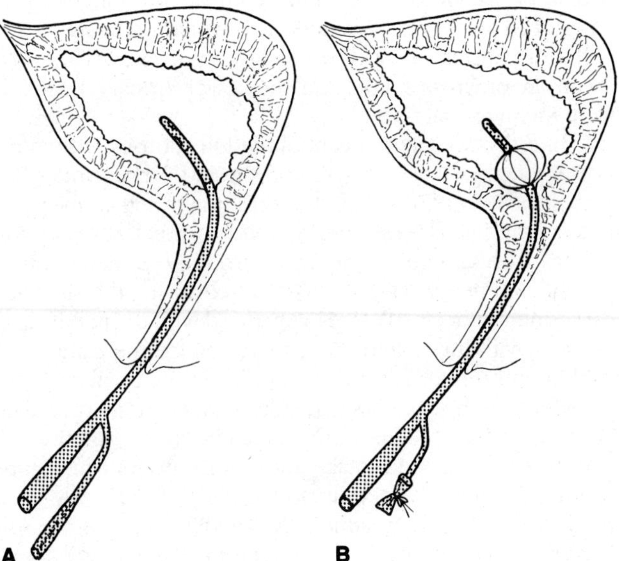

FIGURE 57–1 (*A*) An indwelling (Foley) catheter has been inserted into the urinary bladder. (*B*) The bag is inflated to prevent the catheter from slipping from the urinary bladder.

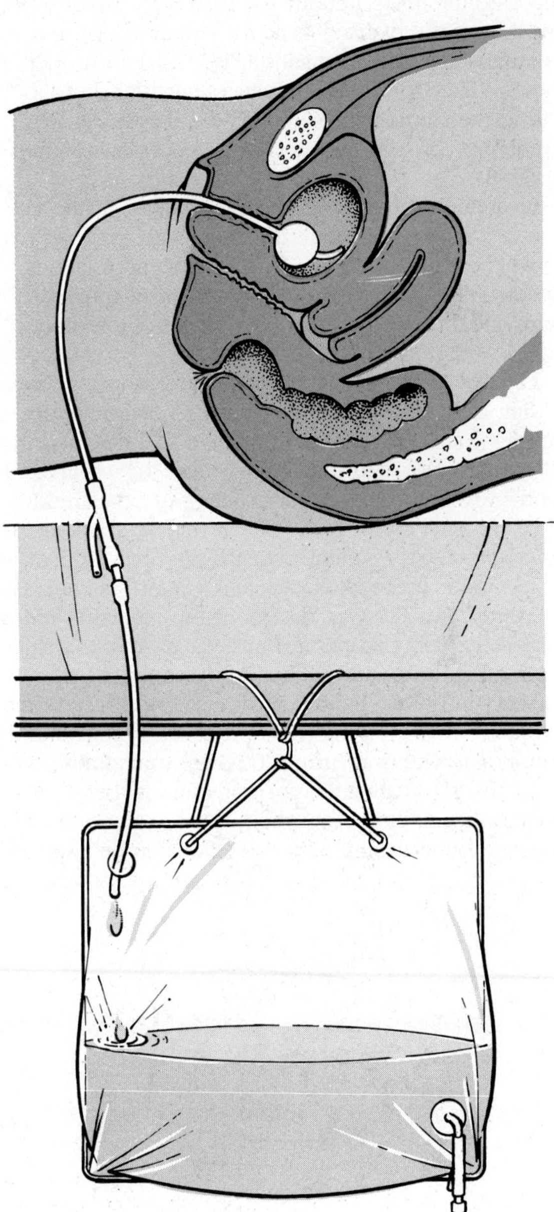

FIGURE 57–2 Illustration of a closed urinary drainage system. Notice the inflated balloon on the catheter within the bladder.

not be disconnected except to change to a new system. It should be emptied every 8 hours to minimize the danger of bacterial growth. To prevent bacterial migration up the tubing, the drainage bag is kept below the level of the tubing, and the system should hang free and not rest on the floor. There is usually a one-way valve at the insertion of the tubing into the drainage bag but this should not negate the use of the latter two techniques for keeping the drainage bag at the lowest level. The tubing must be kept straight so that the urine will drain downward and not remain pooled along the tubing.

The Foley catheter should be taped securely to the body to prevent back and foward movement of the catheter at the meatus. Movement would traumatize the meatus and urethra and increase the danger of infection. In men, the catheter is taped onto the lower abdomen for the purpose of straightening the penoscrotal angle and thus minimizing the danger of trauma and fistula formation (Fig. 57–3). In women, the catheter is fixed to the inner aspect of the thigh, but a loop is made in the catheter proximal to the fixation in order to prevent pull on the catheter with movement of the leg (Fig. 57–4).

Cleanliness of the meatus and catheter at the site of entrance is achieved by daily cleansing with soap and water. This will help to prevent accumulation of encrustations. The procedure should be done gently to avoid trauma to the meatus and thereby increasing the danger of infection.

Patency of Catheter System. The purpose of the indwelling catheter is to maintain urine flow; therefore, patency of the system must be maintained. The flow of urine as well as the color and consistency must be observed frequently. External causes of obstruction of flow are kinking and dependent looping of the tubing, and internal causes are clots and excessive sediment. If the problem is clots, irrigations may be ordered. The usual irrigation solution is normal saline. The Foley is disconnected from the drainage equipement, using aseptic technique. An Asepto syringe is used to gently insert the solution, and it should be allowed to drain back by gravity. If drainage does not occur, suction may be applied by depressing the bulb of the syringe and then attempting to withdraw urine. This will sometimes pull out the clot that is plugging the opening of the catheter tip. If no drainage occurs, the system should be reconnected and the physician notified. Continuous irrigation may be instituted. If the problem is excessive sediment, the best solution is to change the catheter and drainage system.

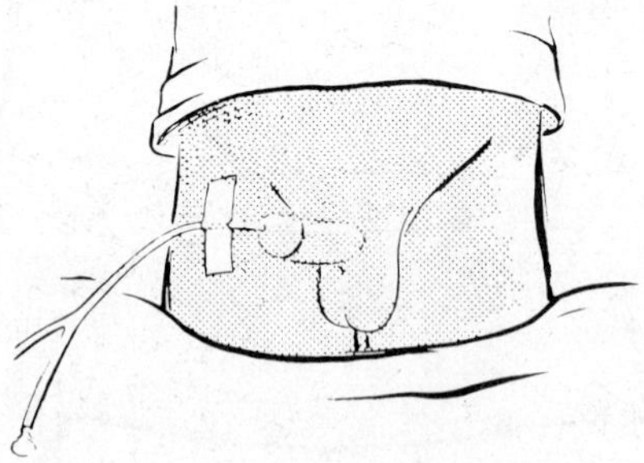

FIGURE 57–3 In men, the catheter is taped in such a way as to eliminate pressure and irritation at the penoscrotal angle.

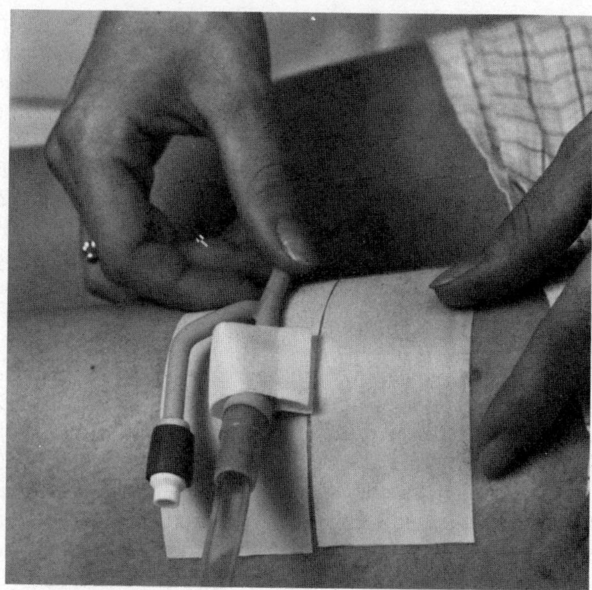

FIGURE 57–4 Method for securing an indwelling catheter on a woman's leg. The securing device is Cath-Secure, a disposable product that eliminates the use of repeat applications of adhesive. Notice the point at which the catheter is secured. There is no chance of constriction of the catheter or of contamination, because the device cannot slide past the catheter lumen. A similar device for securing a catheter could be made with strips of adhesive. (Photo courtesy of the MC Johnson Company, Inc., Leominster, Massachusetts)

Interventions to Avoid Infection. Interventions to prevent infections were discussed earlier in this chapter. They included such measures as ensuring a high fluid intake and maintenance of an acid urine. These measures are also relevant to prevention of bladder infections. In addition, women should be taught to dry the perineum after voiding with an anterior to posterior movement. This will avoid bringing the rectal organisms forward to the urinary meatus. The most common organisms infecting the lower urinary tract are from the intestinal tract.

Interventions to detect possible infection include monitoring for the signs and symptoms noted earlier under Potential for Infection from Catheterization. Another measure is to obtain a urine sample to send to the laboratory for culture. The sample can be drawn from the catheter with a syringe and needle (Fig. 57–5). After cleansing the site with povidone-iodine, the Foley is punctured with the needle and urine is withdrawn into the catheter. Since the catheter is rubber and rubber is elastic, the puncture will seal off itself.

If infection should occur, culture and sensitivity studies are usually done to identify the infectious agent. The preventive measures of fluid intake and acidification of urine are instituted if they are not already in effect. Commonly used medications for the treatment of bladder infection are sulfisoxazole (Gantrisin) or nitrofurantoin (Furadantin). These medications do not promote the development of resistant strains of organisms as is relatively common with some other antibiotics, yet they are effective in inhibiting the growth of the organisms that usually infect the lower urinary tract. Another antiseptic medication with analgesic properties, sulfamethoxazole (Bactrim) is also used frequently.

Evaluation

Criteria for determining achievement of the goal of prevention of infection associated with catheter use are the following:

1. Bacterial counts from urine cultures are within normal limits (less than 1×10^4).
2. Patient reports that he does not experience frequency, urgency, or dysuria.
3. Temperature is within normal limits.
4. Urine flows freely in drainage.
5. Urine output and fluid intake balance.
6. Urine pH is acid (pH 6.5).
7. Urine drainage equipment is clean.
8. Urine drainage equipment is correctly anchored.
9. Drainage tubing is free of kinks and loops.

Criteria for determining the achievement of detection of infection and treatment are the following:

1. The patient reports that urgency, frequency, and dysuria are no longer present.
2. Bacterial counts from culture are approaching normal limits (less than 1×10^5).
3. Patient reports a daily fluid intake of 2.5–3 ml.
4. Patient reports a dietary intake of acid-ash foods.

Knowledge Deficit: Home Care of Catheter

Nursing Diagnosis/Problem. Knowledge deficit of patient and family is related to self-care ability with an indwelling catheter. The knowledge deficit is manifested by the patient and family in their inability to describe the specifics of necessary care to maintain urine flow and prevent infection. This inability results in expressions of anxiety and concern about home care. Patients may need an indwelling catheter on a temporary or permanent basis. Some of the reasons for this need are terminal illness with mental clouding, severe discomfort with movement onto the bedpan, obstructions awaiting surgical treatment, and following genitourinary surgery.

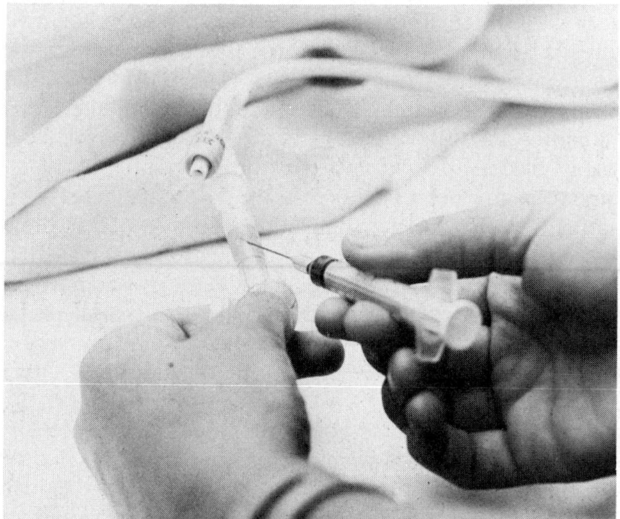

FIGURE 57–5 Method of obtaining a urine sample from a closed urinary drainage system.

Interventions. The goal is patient or family ability to provide safe self-care in the home setting. Safe care consists of prevention of trauma and infection and maintenance of urine flow. Both the patient and family member should be taught the elements of care unless the patient is mentally incapable of comprehending, in which case more than one family member should be taught. It is essential to refer the patient to a visiting nurse service for follow-up care in the home and to provide written instructions as part of the take-home material.

The same interventions to prevent infection as the nurse carries out in the institution are taught the patient and family for use at home. These were discussed in the previous section. Instruction should stress the need for cleanliness in the home environment, hand washing before and after handling the equipment, and the need to wash around the meatus and the catheter daily with soap. Other instructions include avoidance of separation of catheter and drainage system except for application of a leg drainage bag in the morning if the patient is mobile and reattachment to the closed drainage system at night. Before disconnecting the closed drainage system to attach the leg bag, the site of attachment can be cleansed with soap and water or an alcohol sponge. The loose end of the closed drainage system can then be covered with a sterile gauze or a plastic cap that is washed with soap and water prior to each use.

In the home setting it is possible to reuse the drainage equipment, providing that it is sterilized. It can be washed with soap and water and soaked in a half-strength vinegar solution for 15 minutes. It is advisable *not* to reuse the Foley catheter when this item needs to be changed. Supplies are provided on discharge and the person is instructed as to where further supplies can be obtained. The visiting nurse will also assist with this need.

Instruction about observations of urine flow and actions to maintain a dilute urine with an acid pH are also provided. The patient and family should be instructed to contact the physician or go to the hospital emergency room if urine flow should diminish or cease and if manifestations of infection are present.

Evaluation. Goals are achieved if the patient or family member can

1. Demonstrate accurately how to clean the equipment, disconnect the catheter from the drainage system, attach the leg bag, and reverse the procedure.
2. State the observations to make relative to urine flow and the action to take if flow diminishes or ceases.
3. Report adherence to a regimen to maintain a dilute urine with an acid pH.
4. Report an absence of manifestations of the presence of infection.

Bladder Control Problems Following Catheterization

Nursing Diagnosis/Problem. Occurrence and manifestation of problems in reestablishing control of urine elimination after catheter removal depends on the length of time the catheter has been in place, the age and muscle tone of the patient, and the reason for catheter use. Catheters that have been in place for days or longer tend to dilate tissues, especially sphincter muscles. If the catheter was placed following surgery in the pelvic region, edema may still be present contributing to decreased muscle tone. Muscle weakness to varying degrees is part of the normal aging process, and this contributes to problems of regaining urine control in the older age-group. The presence of bladder infection makes reestablishment of control difficult. When catheters are used following surgical procedures, such as bladder fulguration and prostatectomy, specific problems related to these conditions (*e.g.,* hematuria) may occur. Also the possibility of sphincter damage is highest in patients who have had genitourinary surgery.

Interventions. The goals of intervention are to prepare the patient for possible problems and to assist the patient in regaining control of urinary elimination. Without alarming the patient, the nurse should discuss the possibility that dribbling may occur for a few hours to a few days following catheter removal. The reason for this is explained. If the problem occurs, the patient is provided with protective devices for this temporary period. The device could be perineal pads for the female patient and perhaps a condom attached to a drainage bag for the male patient. Dribbling that persists for more than a few days may be due to sphincter damage and may be expected in some postoperative patients.

To differentiate dribbling due to muscle weakness from that due to sphincter damage, the nurse needs to obtain specific information. Desired information includes if the dribbling is constant (incontinence) or occurs only with urgency or stress. In the latter situation it is usually due to muscle weakness. Incontinence due to muscle weakness usually occurs when the person is standing or walking and is usually not experienced in the prone position, whereas it occurs in all positions if it is due to sphincter damage. If the problem is one of muscle weakness, the patient should be taught perineal exercises because these may help in regaining control. These exercises consist of tightening and relaxing perineal and gluteal muscles. One exercise is to practice stopping the urine stream for 5 seconds two or three times with each voiding. Another exercise is to tighten the perineal muscles as if to prevent voiding and hold for 5 seconds. This exercise can be done frequently throughout the day. A third is to periodically tighten the gluteal muscles—squeezing the buttocks together and adducting the thighs.

Following catheter removal, the patient should be encouraged to drink fluids to distend the bladder. It is necessary to record the time the catheter was removed and the volume of intake. The nurse must be certain the person voids within 8 hours. The bladder needs to be assessed for distention during that time. The volume of intake may indicate a need to consult with the physician prior to 8 hours if the patient does not void. Sometimes it is necessary to do an in-and-out catheterization once or twice before the patient progresses to self-control of elimination. Records of intake and output must be maintained until adequate output is achieved. The patient should receive full explanation of problems and of their role in providing accurate data about voiding, and assurances that the problem is not uncommon if this is certain.

Potential for bladder infection (cystitis) exists after catheter removal especially if the patient has muscle weakness and the bladder is not completely emptied, leading to stasis. The signs and symptoms of bladder infection have been discussed in this section.

Evaluation. Outcome criteria are the following:

1. Patient provides necessary information about the amount of fluid intake and output.
2. Patient reestablishes voluntary control of urine elimination.
3. There is an absence of signs and symptoms of cystitis.

Urinary Retention

Nursing Diagnosis/Problem. Retention, the inability to void, could be related to one of several factors, including postoperative complications, neurological trauma and infection, obstruction, or critical illness. Retention is usually a short-term problem in the postoperative patient, the critically ill person, or the person with an obstruction that can be successfully treated. In other situations, such as neurological disease or trauma, there may be damage to the cauda equina or sacral segments of the cord. The problem in such situations is long-term. Retention problems may occur when a person needs to take selected medications for prolonged periods of time. These are medications that have β-adrenergic blocker action, such as propranolol; antispasmotic–anticholinergic action, such as atropine; and antidepressant–antipsychotic agents, such as phenothiazines.

Manifestations of acute retention from obstruction are voiding a small quantity of urine with decreased intensity of urinary stream, anuria, suprapubic pain, and distended palpable bladder. In chronic situations, the intensity of the stream is also decreased unless anuria occurs. Other manifestations are overflow incontinence (the loss of small amounts of urine with a high volume bladder residual), difficulty in starting the stream, frequency, urgency, and nocturia. Complications of urinary retention are infection, calculi formation, and potential renal damage from the pressure of urine accumulation in the ureters and renal pelvis.

Interventions. The goals are to reestablish voluntary control of micturition when this is physically possible, reestablish urine flow, prevent overdistention of the bladder, prevent infection, and prepare the patient and family for long-term management. If the retention is of an acute nature, such as postoperative retention, interventions to promote relaxation of the sphincter muscles are used. These interventions include the standing position for the male, the sitting position for the female, privacy, running water at the sink in the room, pouring water over the labia of the female, placing the hands in water, and sitting in a sitz bath. The physician may prescribe bethanechol chloride (Urecholine), which will stimulate the bladder detrusor muscle. If these measures fail, catheterization is performed. The importance of maintaining an intake and output record to assist in evaluating the possible need for catheterization is most important. Voidings or catheterizations should not exceed 400 ml to 500 ml. If the bladder is distended beyond this amount, the blood vessels in the bladder wall are compressed and blood flow is diminished. Removal of amounts greater than 500 ml allows the blood vessels to dilate and fill with blood. As the vessels in the bladder wall fill with blood, the circulating blood volume decreases, and the patient may feel faint.

In situations where the person needs to be on medications that inhibit bladder contraction, the person should be taught to measure intake and output in order to detect beginning chronic distention due to incomplete emptying of the bladder, and to use the Credé method of assisting the bladder to empty (application of manual pressure over the bladder). The importance of maintaining adequate fluid intake needs to be stressed. The person should be aware of the manifestations of the problem (*e.g.,* frequency, urgency, dribbling) and should report changes to the physician at routine follow-up visits.

The person who is physically unable to regain voluntary control of micturition but who is alert and capable of learning self-care may be taught to do intermittent self-catheterization as contrasted with establishing indwelling catheter drainage. These are usually patients who have sustained spinal cord injury or have a neurological disorder with an atonic (lower motor neuron lesion) neurogenic bladder. Nursing interventions in the rehabilitation of these patients are discussed in Chapters 64 and 69. The interventions relative to preparing patients and families for managing the bladder problem with an indwelling catheter, including prevention of infection, were discussed in the preceding section.

Evaluation. Criteria for evaluating goal achievement are the following:

1. The patient has voluntary control of elimination when this is physically possible.
2. When catheterization is necessary, the volume obtained does not exceed 500 ml.
3. The patient with a long-term retention problem reports carrying out the practices recommended to prevent infection.
4. The patient with a long-term retention problem can state the manifestations of retention and reports if these have occurred.

Incontinence

Incontinence is related to urologic pathology or neurological disorders that interfere with integrative or control functions. The manifestations of uncontrolled voiding often occurs when the bladder reaches 150 ml to 200 ml of urine. This amount of urine in the bladder usually stimulates the parasympathetic stretch receptors in the bladder wall and initiates stimuli to the reflex center in the S_2–S_4 segments of the spinal cord. The impulses are carried through the reflex arc and back to the detrusor muscle, which responds by contracting.

Urologic disorders that are associated with incontinence are damage to the sphincter (*i.e.,* surgeries for malignancies where it is sometimes impossible to avoid external sphincter damage), infection causing severe irritation to the bladder mucosa that in turn triggers the urethrobladder reflex, and weakness of the perineal structures. Damage to the external sphincter prevents it from contracting under the stimulus of voluntary impulses. It is this contraction with the assistance of contraction of the perineal muscles that enables people to control voiding. If the sphincter damage cannot be repaired surgically, then incontinence becomes a lifelong problem. Incontinence of infectious origin or weakness of perineal muscles is usually a short-term problem.

Incontinence associated with neurological deficits is often a long-term problem. Pathology of the central or peripheral nervous system such as cerebral vascular accident, multiple sclerosis, tumor, and spinal cord trauma may cause permanent tissue damage. Incontinence resulting from these conditions is discussed in the Unit that addresses alterations in neurological function, Unit VII, Chapters 64, 66, 67, and 69.

Stress Incontinence

Nursing Diagnosis/Problem. Incontinence associated with relaxation of perineal structures is referred to as stress incontinence. The manifestation of this disorder is involuntary loss of urine in situations that cause a sudden increase in intra-abdominal pressure. The situation may be sudden sneezing, coughing, or laughing. The condition is usually seen in women and may be related to obstetrical injury, muscle atrophy with aging, lesions of the bladder neck, and other conditions. It may also be seen in men following prostatic surgery.

Interventions. The goal of nursing interventions for persons experiencing stress incontinence is patient control of urine flow. The patient who seeks assistance with the problem is taught perineal exercises. Strengthening of the muscles may result in control especially if the stress incontinence is mild.

If control is not achieved with muscle strengthening through practice of perineal exercises, surgical intervention may be recommended. The surgical treatment is a vesicourethropexy, which consists of suturing the urethra to the fascia of the rectus muscle of the abdomen and providing support to the neck of the bladder (Marshall-Marchetti procedure). The patient has an indwelling catheter placed for a few days postoperatively. The amount and color of the urine must be recorded. The urine will be pink in the immediate postoperative period but this should gradually clear. If bleeding persists beyond a couple of days, the physician should be consulted. Observations should also be made for vaginal bleeding.

The patient may have difficulty voiding when the catheter is removed, and the practices recommended in the previous section should be instituted. The patient should be taught not to use the Valsalva maneuver since this would put strain on the sutures and could also restart bleeding. Stool softeners may be used to prevent straining.

Evaluation. Goal achievement is attained if the following occurs:

1. Patient reports practicing perineal exercises.
2. Patient reports no involuntary loss of urine with coughing or sneezing.
3. Patient who has surgery reports a return to normal control of urine with stress.

Temporary Incontinence

Nursing Diagnosis/Problem. Temporary incontinence may occur in acutely ill, unconscious, and elderly patients. At times, especially in the acutely ill, the patient becomes confused, is unable to think clearly and may have sensory depression, all of which contribute to incontinence. The unconscious person is unable to exercise voluntary control. Elderly patients often become temporarily confused when hospitalized and may not be aware of the need to void especially if they are receiving medications. Disorders of cerebral function that can occur in the late middle or older age-groups (*e.g.,* Alzheimer's disease) may result in incontinence.

Interventions. The goals of nursing interventions for the patient with temporary incontinence associated with acuteness of illness, confusion, or decreased level of consciousness are to prevent bladder distention and keep the patient dry. The patient may have an indwelling catheter in place if physiological problems require accurate intake and output measurements. If the indwelling catheter is not indicated, then nursing intervention is a scheduled toileting. The toileting schedule should be planned with consideration of fluid intake, including the type of fluid. For instance, if the patient has coffee for breakfast, the caffeine may act as a diuretic. The bedpan or commode should be offered about an hour after breakfast. A second consideration is the pattern of daily activities; most people void on arising in the morning and just before retiring at night. A toileting schedule of every 2 hours will usually keep the patient dry. As the patient's health status improves, he should regain voluntary control.

Sometimes elderly persons are slow to regain control. The toileting schedule must be maintained for a longer period of time. As the patient regains strength, he may be walked to the bathroom, the normal environment for toileting. This action may assist the patient in gaining control. The measures cited earlier for prevention of infection should be instituted. The toileting schedule may need to be continued after discharge. The patient or family member should be taught the schedule and the importance of continuing with it. The family needs encouragement and support in maintaining the schedule. They also need instruction about protective devices since these may need to be used in conjunction with toileting.

Evaluation. Goal achievement is attained if the following occur:

1. Patient is kept dry.
2. Patient voids on a planned schedule.
3. Patient regains voluntary control.
4. Patient goes home on a training schedule, and the patient and family report continuance of the schedule and the results.

The Patient Unable to Regain Control of Voiding

Interventions. The nursing goals for the patient who is unable to regain control of voiding are to keep the patient dry, clean, and free of odors and keep the skin intact. Examples of patients who will need this kind of care are those who are unconscious for a prolonged period of time, elderly persons with cognitive dysfunction, and some patients with progressive weakness or terminal illness.

External urinary drainage systems may be used with male patients. This consists of a condom that is secured to the penis and attached to a drainage system that goes to a leg bag or a closed drainage system. The leg bag is used in the daytime if the patient is mobile. Precautions need to be taken to avoid constricting circulation when the condom is attached to the penis. External urinary systems are readily available from hospital supply agencies. The directions for application should be followed carefully. The appliance should be changed daily and the penis cleaned. The skin should be checked for signs of excoriation and for edema. This device usually is effective for the male patient who is capable of self-care as well as the person dependent on the nurse for care.

Female patients usually use protective pants (Fig. 57–6). These waterproof pants are lined with disposable, absorbent pants and are closed with Velcro, which facilitates changing them when the patient has mobility problems. The pants need to be changed frequently to prevent odors and skin irritation. Daily sitz baths help to keep the skin clean and intact. The perineum should be washed whenever wet pants are changed. Skin observations are made with each change.

The use of waterproof pants may provide the patient with assurance that accidents will not occur in public. The patient may then feel comfortable in participating in social events.

If the patient is to be discharged home, the patient and family need instruction about application of the external drainage system, the use of protective pants, skin care, and where to obtain supplies. Referral to visiting nurses will provide a source for consultation when problems arise.

Evaluation. Criteria for goal achievement are the following:

1. Patient is odor free.
2. Skin of the patient is clean, dry, and free of excoriations.

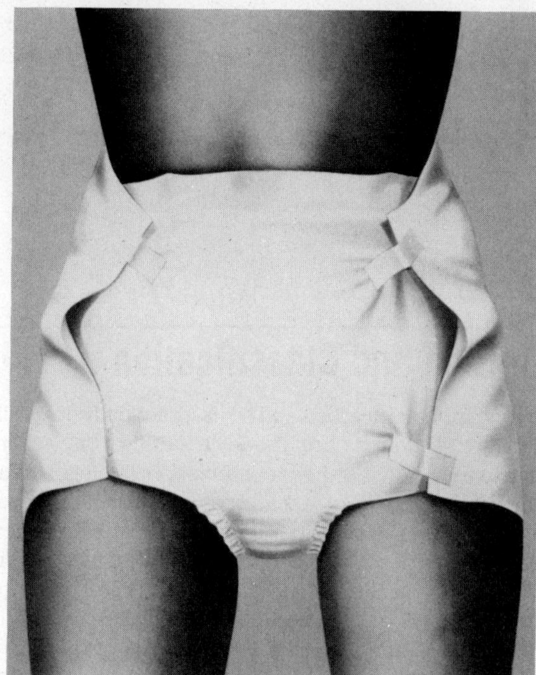

FIGURE 57–6 "Attends" incontinent brief.

3. When cognitively possible, the female patient reports daily bathing of the perineal area and frequent changing of protective pants. The male patient attaches the external drainage system correctly. The penis is clean and the skin is free of edema and excoriation.
4. The patient or family seeks consultation if problems arise in coping with the incontinence.

References

1. Brundage D: Nursing management of Renal Problems, 2nd ed. St Louis, CV Mosby, 1980
2. Hunt, G: Physiology of wound healing (verbal communication). Seattle, Continuing Medical Education Conference, University of Washington, School of Medicine, July 27, 1983
3. Larson E, Lindbloom L, Davis KB: Development of the Nephrology Nurse Practitioner: A Focus on Independent Learning, pp 110–116. St Louis, CV Mosby, 1982
4. Scribner BH: Teaching syllabus for course Fluid and Electrolyte Balance, 7th revision. Seattle, University of Washington, School of Medicine, 1969

Bibliography

Bennett WM, Porter GA, Bagley SP: Drugs and renal disease. New York, Churchill Livingston, 1978

Brundage D: Nursing Management of Renal Problems, 2nd ed. St Louis, CV Mosby, 1980

Freedman P, Smith EC: Acute renal failure. Heart Lung 4:6, 1975

Groer M, Shekleton M: Basic Pathophysiology. St Louis, CV Mosby, 1983

Larson E, Lindbloom L, David KB: Development of the Nephrology Nurse Practitioner: A Focus on Independent Learning. St Louis, CV Mosby, 1982

Miller TR, Anderson RJ, Linas SL et al: Urinary diagnostic indices in acute renal failure: A prospective study. Ann Intern Med 89(1):47–50, 1978

Schrier RW: Acute renal failure: Pathogenesis, diagnosis, and management. Hosp Pract 16(3):93–98, 101–105, 1981

Schrier RW: Renal and electrolyte disorders, 2nd ed. Boston, Little, Brown, & Co, 1980

Chapter 58

Acute Renal Failure

Nancy Hoffart

Definition and Classification

Acute tubular necrosis (ATN) is potentially reversible renal failure of sudden onset usually resulting from ischemic damage to the tubular segment of the nephron. It constitutes two thirds of the cases of acute renal failure, with an occurrence rate of 20 to 40 cases per million population per year.[8] (Table 58–1 lists other categories of acute renal failure.) Most often it is a complication of other serious medical or surgical conditions. Terms used synonymously with acute tubular necrosis are acute tubulointerstitial nephritis, vasomotor nephropathy, reversible intrinsic renal failure, renal parenchymal failure and, in some cases, acute renal failure.

Individuals particularly likely to develop acute tubular necrosis as a complication of ischemia are people with underlying intrinsic renal disease and people with vascular disease such as high blood pressure, diabetes mellitus, or atherosclerosis. Those over 60 years of age are at risk because atrophy of nephrons occurs as part of the normal aging process, and this decreases reserve renal function when renal damage occurs. Dehydration at the time of renal insult and obstetrical complications such as severe preeclampsia and septic abortion predispose the patient to the development of ATN.[8,12]

Etiology and Pathophysiology

Ischemic acute tubular necrosis is caused by decreased blood volume or redistribution of blood away from the kidneys, both of which result in decreased renal blood flow. As the blood flow to the kidneys falls, oxygen and other nutrients are not available for cellular metabolism. Cells are damaged and the kidneys' ability to function is affected. The ischemic period required to sustain renal damage is variable; it may be as short as 30 minutes or as long as several hours. There are other situations that result in acute damage to the renal tubules, including shock, severe muscle injury, burns, hemorrhage, and severe toxemia. A general list of causes is presented in Table 58–2. Toxic- and pigment-induced ATN have a course and treatment similar to ischemic ATN. Toxic damage causes necrosis of the cells of the proximal tubules and obstruction of the tubules.

Four pathophysiological events are thought to contribute to the renal dysfunction of acute tubular necrosis. These are backleak of glomerular filtrate through the damaged epithelial cells of the tubule, tubular obstruction from cellular debris, decreased blood flow through the glomerulus, and decreased permeability of the glomerular basement membrane. Currently the relative importance of each of these

TABLE 58–1
Categories of Acute Renal Failure

Prerenal Azotemia

Prerenal azotemia results from decreased renal blood flow.

Causes:

Some causative examples are decreased cardiac output due to cardiogenic shock or cardiac tamponade and decreased intravascular volume due to hemorrhage, gastrointestinal loss, or burns.

Treatment:

Prerenal azotemia is treated by improving the cardiac output and replacing fluid losses.

Postrenal Azotemia

Postrenal azotemia results from obstructed urine outflow.

Causes:

The obstruction may occur within the urinary tract itself, because of stones, ureteral stricture, bladder lesions, *etc.*, or the obstruction may be from surrounding organs or tissues, such as prostatic hypertrophy or a pelvic tumor.

Treatment:

Postrenal azotemia is treated by relieving the obstruction.

Intrinsic Renal Damage

Intrinsic renal damage results from injury to the renal parenchyma.

Causes:

Causes include acute episodes of glomerulonephritis, renal artery or vein occlusion, emboli, acute pyelonephritis, crystal or protein deposition, an acute tubular necrosis.

Treatment:

Treatment of the specific cause is required.

events in the development and progression of ATN is uncertain, but experimental studies verify their occurrence. The result of these pathological changes is a decrease in the glomerular filtration rate, and when this occurs the removal of solutes, wastes, and water by the kidneys is impaired.

Clinical Manifestations

The clinical signs and symptoms of acute tubular necrosis vary among patients. Some individuals may be critically ill; others will have few or mild symptoms. This variability is attributed to the degree of renal impairment and concurrent insult to other organ systems.

Urine Production

Anuric ATN is rare; approximately 50% of ATN is oliguric; the remainder is nonoliguric.[11] Regardless of the amount of urine produced, biochemical abnormalities and clinical manifestations are similar, but in nonoliguric ATN the manifestations are usually less severe.

Oliguric ATN has three states. During the first phase urine production is less than 400 ml/day. The oliguric phase may last a few days to weeks, with a mean of 10 to 12 days. The second phase is diuresis. In this phase increasing amounts of urine are produced, indicating recovery of renal function. Clinical symptoms and biochemical abnormalities improve as this phase progresses. The diuretic phase may last as long as the oliguric phase. As renal function continues to improve, the individual enters the recovery phase, which is noted by a returning ability of the kidneys to concentrate urine. Fluid and electrolyte status returns to normal and clinical symptoms abate. The average length of this phase is 17 days, although it may take months or years for renal function to return to pre-ATN levels.

Distinct phases based on changes in urine volume cannot be defined for nonoliguric ATN because the quality of urine remains in the normal or near normal range throughout the disease process. The progression from failure to recovery of function follows a course similar to but shorter in duration than that of oliguric ATN.

In both oliguric and nonoliguric ATN patients experience many clinical manifestations. The most frequent abnormalities are fluid and electrolyte imbalances, acid–base disorders, retention of metabolic wastes, gastrointestinal bleeding, anemia, and infection.

Fluid and Electrolyte Imbalances

Volume excess can occur in anuric and oliguric ATN. Excessive sodium intake may lead to peripheral and pulmonary edema and high blood pressure, which in turn causes circulatory dysfunction. Normal or excessive water intake may lead to hyponatremia with associated central nervous system disorders. Hyperkalemia is a frequent occurrence because of the kidneys' inability to excrete potassium. Elevated serum potassium may be a result of dietary intake, increased catabolism associated with stress and cell damage, or internal bleeding. If serum potassium levels exceed 6 mEq/liter, ventricular fibrillation or asystole may ensue. Elevated serum potassium prolongs intraventricular conduction and may be manifested by electrocardiographic changes such as depressed P waves, peaked T waves, lengthened PR intervals, wide QRS complexes, and frequent premature ventricular contractions. Other electrolyte disorders include hyperphosphatemia and hypocalcemia. Phosphorus rises because it is not excreted by the damaged kidneys. In an attempt to maintain normal serum Ca PO_4 ratios there is an inverse fall in calcium that is sustained by alterations in parathyroid hormone and vitamin D functions (see Chaps. 13 and 14).

In nonoliguric ATN, with normal fluid intake and urine output, fluid balance is maintained. Hyperkalemia is less likely to occur in nonoliguric ATN because the kidneys retain some of their ability to excrete potassium. Hyperphosphatemia and hypocalcemia occur as in oliguric ATN.

Other Manifestations

Acid–Base Disorders. Metabolic acidosis occurs early in the course of acute tubular necrosis because acids produced during normal metabolism are not excreted by the kidneys. The respiratory center may compensate for the acidosis by increasing the respiratory rate, resulting in a normal serum pH and a low serum bicarbonate level. Acidosis contributes to hyperkalemia by shifting potassium from the intracellular to the extracellular space.

Retention of Metabolic Wastes. As renal failure progresses, waste products such as urea nitrogen and creatinine accumulate in the blood, producing a constellation of symptoms termed the uremic syndrome (discussed in detail in Chap. 57). Symptoms of this syndrome are anorexia, nausea, vomiting, diarrhea, hiccups, headache, drowsiness, mental slowing, stupor, coma, agitation, asterixis, muscle twitching, and seizures. Coagulopathy occurs because uremia decreases platelet adhesiveness and makes the individual prone to excessive bleeding, particularly from the mucous membranes.

Gastrointestinal Bleeding. Gastritis has long been one of the complications of uremia, although the exact reason is unknown. Gastritis along with nausea, vomiting, coagulopathy, and stress contribute to gastrointestinal bleeding. Bleeding in most cases is mild, but if continuous, it causes significant blood loss. It occurs anywhere along the length of the gastrointestinal tracts.

Anemia. Anemia is a frequent complication of acute tubular necrosis and is due to a combination of factors. In many cases ATN is caused by a condition associated with blood loss or hemolysis. This is compounded by coagulopathy and poor nutrition. A hematocrit of 20% to 30% is common. Symptoms of anemia are a decreased tolerance for activity, lethargy, fatigue, weakness, tachycardia, and shortness of breath.

Infection. The person with ATN is predisposed to infection. Uremia compromises both the cellular and humoral immune systems. Poor nutrition, stress, and breaks in body integument provide further opportunity for infection to develop. Common sites include infection of the urinary tract, respiratory tract, wounds, and bloodstream and dialysis access.

TABLE 58–2
Causes of Acute Tubular Necrosis

Ischemic Causes

- Shock
  - Septic
  - Cardiogenic
- Aortic cross-clamping
  - Abdominal aortic aneurysm repair
- Muscle injury
  - Rhabdomyolysis
  - Crush injury
- Dehydration and blood loss
  - Burns
  - Hemorrhage
    - Traumatic
    - Surgical
    - Postpartal
  - Uncompensated water and electrolyte losses
- Severe toxemia
- Intravascular hemolysis
  - Transfusion reaction
- Pericardial tamponade
- Acute pancreatitis

Toxic Causes

- Antibiotics
  - Aminoglycosides
  - Cephalosporins
  - Amphotericin B
  - Colistin
- Fluorinated anesthetics
- Heavy metals
  - Mercury
  - Arsenic
  - Platinum
  - Lead
- Radiographic contrast media
- Organic solvents
  - Carbon tetrachloride
  - Ethylene glycol

Pigment

- Hemoglobin
- Myoglobin
- Methemoglobin

Medical Management

Diagnosis

When an individual has azotemia or other symptoms of renal dysfunction, a diagnosis of ischemic acute tubular necrosis will require ruling out other renal problems. The first step is review of the medical history; a history of any of the events listed in Table 58–2 will suggest ATN. The diagnosis is confirmed by laboratory studies and physical examination. Laboratory studies that aid in differentiation are urinalysis and serum chemistries. Physical examination to determine hydration, presence of urinary tract obstruction, and presence and severity of uremic symptoms is necessary. Noninvasive radiographic studies such as abdominal x-ray films, ultrasonography, and computed tomography may be necessary. Because of the risk of hemorrhage, renal biopsy is not indicated if history and examination are suggestive of ATN. If, however, there is no obvious cause of renal failure or if renal dysfunction persists 3 or more weeks a biopsy is warranted.

Treatment

The goals of medical treatment for the individual with acute tubular necrosis are to prevent further damage to the kidneys, to promote recovery of renal function, and to prevent complications.

To reverse the renal damage or alter its progression, volume status must be corrected. For the patient with prerenal azotemia, this necessitates correction of hypoperfusion by administering fluids and may be coupled with administration of loop diuretics, such as mannitol or furosemide

(Lasix). Diuretics are effective only when used early in the course of ATN. The results achieved from diuretic therapy have been mixed. In some instances it has had no effect; in others oliguric ATN has been converted to nonoliguric ATN. Often diuretics shorten the course of the illness.[2,9]

If renal failure progresses despite preventive measures, fluid and electrolyte disorders must be managed. Fluid restrictions will be ordered. Potassium will be closely monitored. A cation exchange resin, sodium polystyrene sulfonate (Kayexalate), administered orally or as a retention enema, may be ordered to control serum potassium. If hyperkalemia develops, treatment will depend on the severity. When the condition is life threatening, intravenous administration of calcium to counteract the effects of potassium on the myocardium and an infusion of glucose and regular insulin or sodium bicarbonate to force the potassium into the cells is necessary. Rapid removal of potassium is achieved by instituting dialysis.

Anemia and blood loss must be treated. Administration of aluminum hydroxide antacids (Amphojel, Basaljel) or cimetidine (Tagamet) is usually sufficient to prevent and control gastrointestinal bleeding. If bleeding is severe, iced lavage, gastroscopy, or surgical intervention may be necessary (see Chaps. 80 and 83).

Blood transfusions are indicated when there is a significant drop in hematocrit or when the patient becomes symptomatic of anemia. Packed red blood cells are preferred because they are less likely than whole blood to cause fluid overload.

Drug Precautions

When drugs are prescribed for the individual with acute tubular necrosis many factors must be considered because most drugs and drug metabolites are excreted by the kidneys. First, the half-life of many drugs is extended, predisposing the patient to drug overdose, toxicity, and interaction. This is common with antibiotics and cardiac glycosides. Second, potentially nephrotoxic drugs such as aminoglycosides, cephalosporins, and antifungal agents can cause further renal damage; thus, dose and frequency of administration require adjustment. Third, some drugs such as meperidine (Demerol) have an active metabolite that is renally excreted. With renal damage the metabolite remains in the system and causes toxicity. Fourth, antibiotics that are sodium or potassium salts must be administered with caution to prevent development of hypernatremia or hyperkalemia. Last, selected drugs are contraindicated for the patient with ATN. For example, aspirin compounds the risk of bleeding. Magnesium-containing antacids are others, since the damaged kidneys will not excrete the excessive magnesium and it can accumulate to toxic levels. This list is not exhaustive of medications requiring modification; it serves only to illustrate the need for careful medication prescribing. Frequently updated guidelines for drug administration in renal failure supply useful information.[3]

Dialysis

Dialysis is begun before or at the first appearance of uremic symptoms. The goal is to prevent uremic complications and to keep the BUN below 80 to 100 mg/dl and serum creatinine below 8 to 10 mg/dl. Dialysis is urgently required if the patient is in severe pulmonary edema or congestive heart failure, hyperkalemic (potassium over 7 mEq/liter), severely acidotic (plasma bicarbonate under 15 mEq/liter), or experiencing symptoms of uremia. Both hemodialysis and peritoneal dialysis are successful in treating acute tubular necrosis, especially when instituted early. Advantages, disadvantages, and contraindications for each mode are identified in Table 58–3. The mode chosen will depend on the clinical status of the patient, concurrent disease conditions, urgency

TABLE 58–3
Comparison of Hemodialysis and Peritoneal Dialysis

	Advantages	*Disadvantages*	*Contraindications*
Hemodialysis	Short treatment (3–5 hr) Efficient removal of metabolic wastes and fluid	Requires specialized staff and equipment Requires systemic heparinization Hypotension and disequilibrium occur frequently	Marked cardiovascular instability Extreme hypotension Uncontrolled hemorrhage (of nonuremic origin)
Peritoneal dialysis	Can be performed manually Requires no heparinization Few episodes of hypotension or disequilibrium	Long treatment (10–14 hr) High risk for peritonitis Fluid in abdomen may cause respiratory impairment Protein loss	Open abdominal wounds or stomas Recent bowel surgery Extensive scarring or abdominal adhesions Hypercatabolic state Respiratory impairment

of treatment, and availability. Every-other-day dialysis is most common, but in hypercatabolic or life-threatenting states daily dialysis is necessary. Dialysis is discontinued when the renal system recovers sufficiently to maintain function without it or when other organ systems sustain irreversible damage.

Hemodialysis

Hemodialysis is the removal of waste products and excess water from the body by circulating the blood through a dialyzer (artificial kidney) outside the body. Waste products are removed by diffusion across an artificial membrane into the dialysis fluid (Fig. 58–1). Ultrafiltration, a hydrostatic pressure gradient, is used to remove fluid.

A semipermeable artificial membrane (dialyzer) is utilized to mimic the filtering capabilities of the human kidney. Substances are exchanged across the membrane according to pressure, concentration, or osmotic gradients. Only those substances that are small enough to pass through the semipermeable membrane are exchanged. Larger particles such as albumin molecules and red blood cells do not pass through and are not lost from blood circulation. For example, when a patient's potassium is high, the concentration of potassium is lower in the dialysate, so that the potassium that

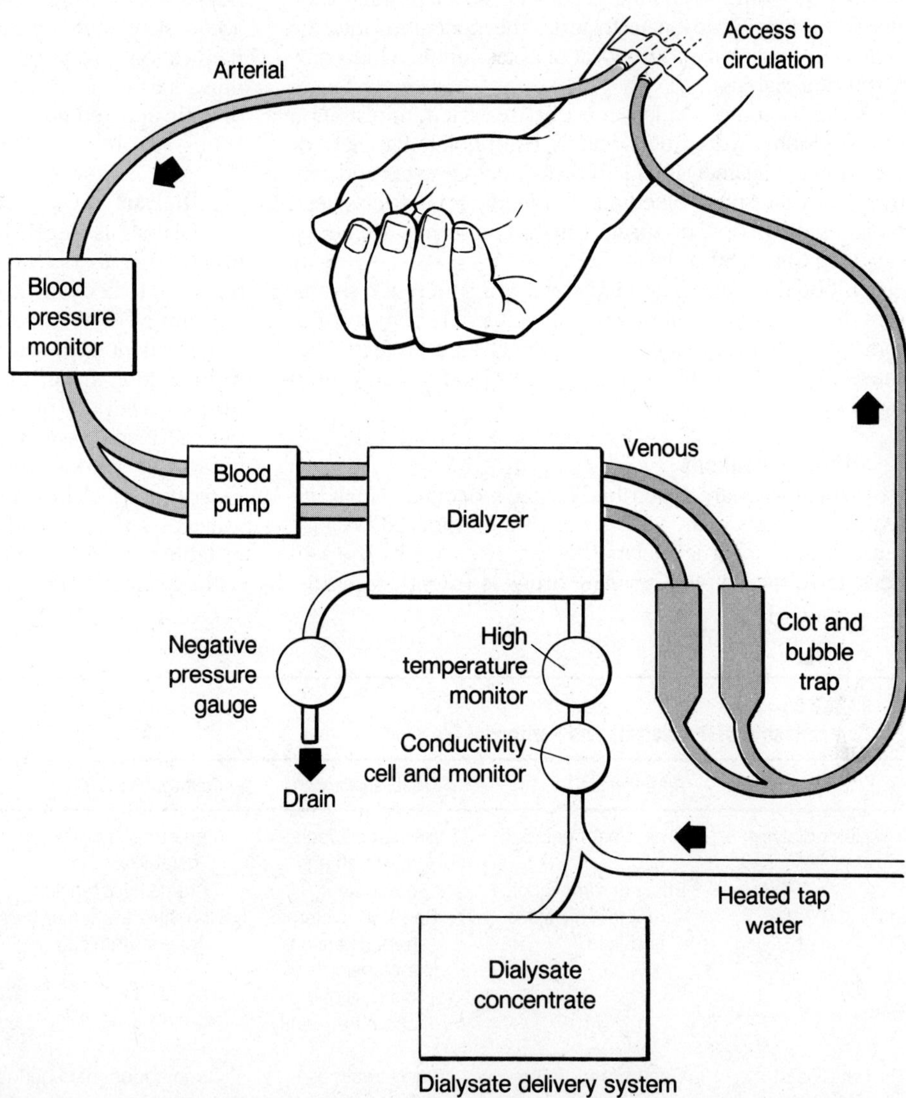

FIGURE 58–1 In hemodialysis, blood from an artery is pumped into a dialyzer, where it flows through coils of cellophane tubing which serve as a semipermeable membrane. Blood circulates through the coils which are bathed by a special dialysis solution. This solution has approximately the same chemical composition as the blood, except for urea and other substances ordinarily removed by the kidneys. Thus, the movement of waste products from the blood into the dialysis solution occurs by simple diffusion and filtration. The dialysis solution is changed at frequent intervals to maintain the proper concentration gradients for the substances that are to be removed. After passing through the tubing, dialyzed blood is returned to the body by way of a vein.

is high in the blood will diffuse across the membrane to the area of lower concentration (the dialysate).

Hemodialysis utilizes an artificial membrane that has the same permeability as the renal tubules and glomerular capillaries. By use of a blood pump and an extracorporeal (outside the body) set of tubing, blood flows on one side of the semipermeable membrane and dialysate flows on the other. Manipulating the concentration of substances in the dialysate and the hydrostatic pressure on both sides of the membrane allows certain amounts of water, electrolytes, and toxins to be removed from the body in order to achieve a predetermined fluid and electrolyte balance.

Hemodialysis necessitates access to the bloodstream. In acute dialysis three means are available. The external arteriovenous (AV) shunt is the most common access for acute dialysis. Access may also be achieved by percutaneous puncture of either the femoral or subclavian vein. These catheters can be inserted at the bedside but require skill for ease of placement. Both can be left in place for repeated dialyses. Between treatments the catheter is injected with a heparinized normal saline solution, capped, and covered with an occlusive dressing. Care is needed to prevent infection, clotting, or dislodgement. A femoral catheter is generally left in place 24 to 72 hours. Its position inhibits mobility and may cause discomfort because of inability to flex at the hip. Its location near the perineum increases the possibility of infection. The subclavian catheter can be left in place for many weeks if properly cared for. Its position produces minimal discomfort or immobility. The methods of caring for the various access devices can be found in Table 58–4.

Hemodialysis requires systemic anticoagulation to prevent clotting of the blood as it circulates through the dialyzer. Anticoagulation is achieved by administering small amounts of heparin into the blood as it enters the dialysate. For the person who is actively bleeding or likely to hemorrhage this poses problems. To lessen the risk, heparin doses as low as 1000 units to 2500 units may be adequate. In some cases an antagonist, protamine sulfate, may be given as the blood reenters the body to neutralize the heparin or as a single dose on completion of dialysis.

Peritoneal Dialysis

Peritoneal dialysis is the removal of waste products and excess water from the body by cycling sterile dialysis fluid into the peritoneal cavity (Fig. 58–2). Waste products in the blood circulating through the peritoneal capillaries diffuse across the peritoneal membrane into the dialysate. Excess body water is removed by osmosis that is created by adding solutes to the dialysis fluid. Peritoneal dialysis is performed manually or with automated or semiautomated equipment and may be intermittent or continuous.

Peritoneal dialysis requires access to the peritoneal cavity to instill and drain the dialysis fluid. Two devices are available, a Teflon catheter and a soft Silastic catheter. Both are introduced, under local anesthetic, through the abdominal wall. The Teflon catheter is a rigid device used for only one dialysis. The Silastic catheter is softer and is tunneled through the abdominal wall; it can be used for repeated treatments. It requires more skill and time for insertion and careful cleaning and dressing between treatments to prevent infection (see Table 58–4).

Systemic anticoagulation is unnecessary in peritoneal dialysis. Heparin may be added to the dialysis fluid to prevent the formation of fibrin clots that could plug the catheter.

TABLE 58–4
Care of Access Devices in Dialysis

	AV Shunt	*Femoral or Subvlavian Catheter*	*Peritoneal Catheter*
Frequency of cleansing	Daily Whenever dressing becomes wet or exit site is exposed.	Every other day Whenever dressing becomes wet or exit site is exposed.	Daily Whenever dressing becomes wet or exit site is exposed.
Procedure for cleansing	Clean exit sites and tubing with antiseptic agent. Dress with 4″ × 4″ sponges and Kling, without kinking or compressing cannula tubing. Secure cannula clamps to dressing.	Clean exit site with antiseptic agent. Apply topical anti-infective ointment to exit site. Cover with 4″ × 4″ sponges. Secure with occlusive dressing.	Clean exit site with antiseptic agent. Paint area around exit site with iodophor. Cover with 4″ × 4″ sponges. Secure with nonocclusive dressing.
Watch for complications	Clotting: dark blood, separation of cells and serum in shunt tubing, and cool to touch. Infection: exit sites red, tender, swollen, or draining	Clotting: inability to asirate or inject solution through catheter. Infection: exit site red, tender, swollen, or draining, and fever.	Infection: exit site red, tender, swollen, or draining, and fever.

Special reminders:

When cleaning use cotton-tipped applicators and clean from the exit site out (clean to dirty). Each applicator should be used only once.
Care must be taken to prevent a confused patient from dislodging the wound access.
To decrease the risk of infection wear gloves and mask when exit site is exposed.

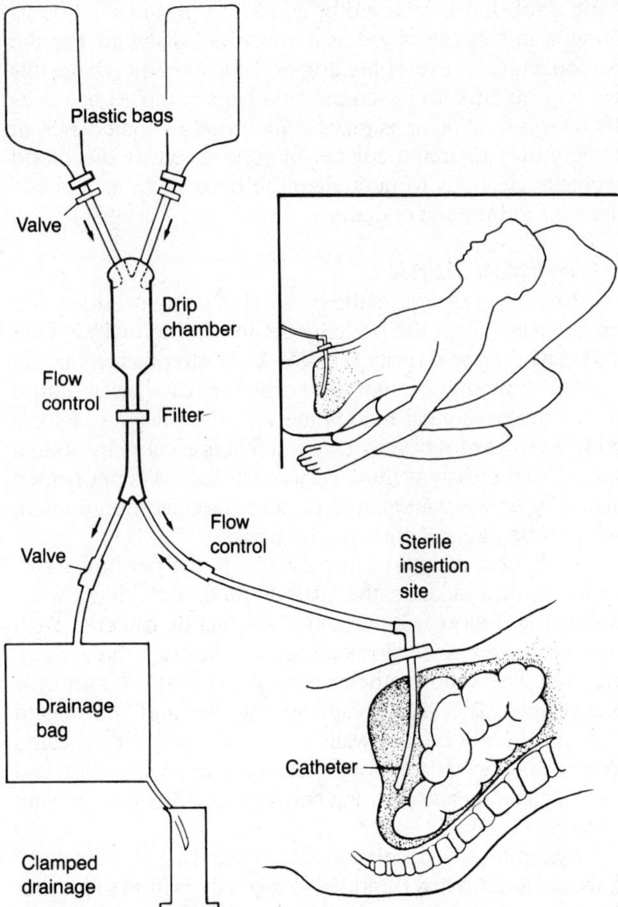

FIGURE 58–2 The usual equipment arrangement for the performance of peritoneal dialysis. (Flamenbaum W, Hamburger R J: Nephrology: An Approach to the Patient with Renal Disease, p 573. Philadelphia, JB Lippincott, 1982)

When instilled in this manner, the heparin is not systemically absorbed.

Nursing Interventions

PATIENT TEACHING. If dialysis is necessary, both the patient and family will need an explanation of the procedure in order to prepare for the treatment sessions and to allay anxiety about what to expect. The teaching plan should include information on when, where, and how the treatment will be carried out, what sensations may be experienced (possible light-headedness, dizziness, nausea, vomiting and sweating); and what to expect if postdialysis symptoms occur. For hemodialysis this may include weakness, lethargy, and headache. A sample teaching plan for the dialysis patient is presented in Table 58–5.

CARE DURING DIALYSIS. A nurse caring for a patient undergoing dialysis should plan general nursing measures so as not to interrupt the patient while dialysis is underway and should implement comfort strategies to promote rest during treatment. During treatment it is important to observe hourly for possible dialysis disequilibrium such as headache, increased blood pressure, decreasing pulse rate, stupor, seizures, or coma (Fig. 58–3). Any such signs should be reported immediately. The interventions for these selected problems are presented in Nursing Care Plan for the Patient Undergoing Dialysis.

Prognosis

Acute tubular necrosis carries a poor prognosis. Mortality rates ranging from 30% to 80% have been reported.[2,6,13] Because the individual being treated for ATN often has serious and extensive underlying disease the survival rate has not improved during the past 20 to 30 years. Nonuremic factors that significantly affect prognosis are age and cause of ATN. The prognosis is worse for the person over 60 years of age.[2,10] Acute tubular necrosis that develops after cardiovascular or gastrointestinal surgery has the highest mortality rates.[6,8] Uremic factors that affect prognosis are presence of prior renal dysfunction and urine production. Those with a history of renal dysfunction are more likely to suffer permanent damage. Oliguric ATN has a higher mortality rate than nonoliguric.[1,5] The most frequent cause of death is infection, followed closely by cardiovascular complications and gastrointestinal bleeding.[9,13] Malnutrition contributes to the high mortality rate.

Nursing Management

Nursing care of the individual with acute tubular necrosis will vary with the severity of the illness and the cause of renal insult. Many of these people are suffering from other conditions, such as cardiovascular surgery and septicemia, which complicate their care and compound their potential for problems. More than one problem requires comprehensive

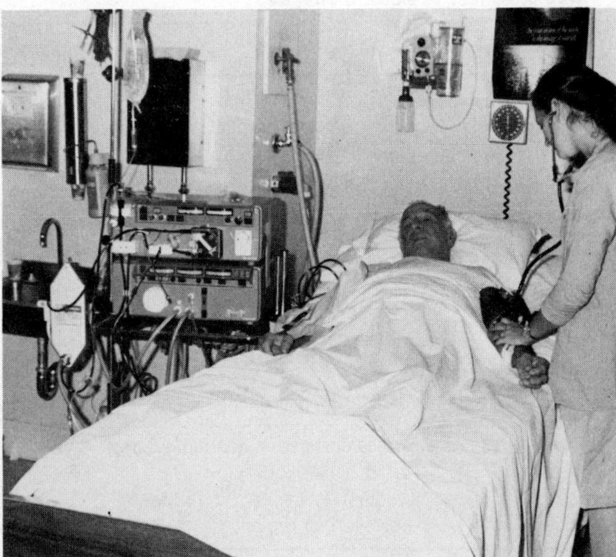

FIGURE 58–3 Nurse monitoring the patient undergoing hemodialysis in the hospital. (Courtesy of Georgetown University Medical Center)

TABLE 58–5
Teaching Plan for the Patient on Dialysis

Nursing Intervention	*Rationale*
Teach the patient that dialysis for acute tubular necrosis is a temporary measure.	In most cases of acute tubular necrosis, renal function returns within 3–6 weeks.
Explain the dialysis procedure to the patient, including when, where, and how it will be done.	Allows patient to prepare for the treatment.
Explain the typical sensations experienced during dialysis.	Knowing that these sensations may occur will minimize anxiety in the event that they do occur.
During *hemodialysis* these may include light-headedness, dizziness, nausea, vomiting, sweating, and feeling faint. Generally the treatment is painless.	Related to drops in blood pressure that occur as a result of changes in blood volume.
During *peritoneal dialysis* these may include coolness and pressure as the dialysis fluid enters the peritoneal cavity, abdominal tightness, and shortness of breath.	Related to the amount of dialysis fluid in peritoneal cavity
Instruct patient to notify nurse should any of these symptoms occur.	Gives the patient some control and will allow the nurse to treat the cause of the symptoms.
Explain to patient and family that he may not feel better after the first treatment.	Multiple dialysis may be required before the paitent notices subjective improvement. If he expects to feel better immediately he may be extremely disappointed or feel the treatment is not working.
Explain the possible postdialysis symptoms.	
Following hemodialysis treatment the patient may be weak, lethargic, and have a headache.	Symptoms are related to rapid changes in fluid and electrolyte status.
Postdialysis symptoms rarely occur after peritoneal dialysis.	Fluid and electrolyte changes occur slowly and over a longer period of time, allowing accommodation.

nursing care for the patient and family, particularly during the early course of the disease. Other aspects of nursing care are discussed in the following sections. These serve as a framework that must be tailored to a particular patient's unique needs.

Fluid and Electrolyte Status

Nursing Diagnosis. Possible nursing diagnoses related to fluid and electrolyte status are fluid volume excess, alterations in respiratory function related to pulmonary edema, impairment of skin integrity related to poor perfusion and skin breakdown in edematous areas, and alterations in cardiac output due to elevated serum potassium and congestive heart failure. Volume excess may be manifested as pulmonary edema, peripheral edema, or congestive heart failure.

Goals. The focus of nursing care is to prevent volume excess. If excess occurs the goal of care is preventing attendant complications, especially prevention of hyperkalemia.

Interventions. Intervention begins with evaluation of fluid status. Accurate intake and output, daily weights, measurement of blood pressure, assessment of lung sounds, status of mucous membranes, and examination for peripheral edema are the components of this assessment. A prime nursing action to prevent volume excess is to control the administration of both oral and parenteral fluids (see Chap. 57).

If *pulmonary edema* develops, nursing care must ensure adequate ventilation. It is imperative that the patient's position allows for maximum ease in respiratory effort. Constrictive clothing should be relieved. Reassurance to decrease anxiety that might increase respiratory rate is necessary. Consultation with the physician regarding the probable need for *dialysis* to remove fluid becomes a necessary nursing action. Frequent suctioning of the ventilated patient and encouragement of the nonventilated patient to expectorate secretions is required. Prevention of skin breakdown if peripheral edema occurs includes measures such as elevation of the extremities, relief of pressure points and constrictions, and keeping the skin clean and dry (see Chap. 43).

The primary role for the nurse caring for the person in danger of developing *hyperkalemia* is control of potassium intake, both oral and intravenous. Hyperkalmia can also be prevented by administering sodium polystyrene sulfonate (Kayexalate) orally or as a retention enema as ordered. In the intestine this will exchange sodium ions for potassium ions that are then excreted in the stool. Because hyperkalemia may develop despite preventive measures, a second important role is monitoring. Signs and symptoms of hyperkalemia

NURSING CARE PLAN FOR THE PATIENT UNDERGOING DIALYSIS

NURSING DIAGNOSIS/PROBLEM 1: Potential for inadequate removal of fluid during dialysis.
GOAL 1: Assist in determining the amount and adequacy of fluid removal during dialysis.

Nursing Interventions	Rationale	Outcome Criteria
1. Obtain predialysis and postdialysis weights using the same scale and with the same amount of bedding.	1. Makes possible accurate determination of fluid removal	1–2. Postdialysis weight loss will be evident. Usually approximately equivalent to weight gain since previous dialysis
2. If patient is weighed during a peritoneal dialysis treatment, drain the dialysis fluid from the abdomen.	2. Weight measured should not include the weight of the dialysis fluid.	

NURSING DIAGNOSIS/PROBLEM 2: Potential for dialysis disequilibrium.
GOAL 2: Minimize symptoms and potential for injury during and after dialysis.

Nursing Interventions	Rationale	Outcome Criteria
1. Avoid giving general care measures and special procedures during dialysis.	1. Positional changes and movement may potentiate the possibility of hypotension and other dialysis complications such as blood line separation.	1. Patient will have no or few symptoms of complications. That is, after dialysis he will be normotensive, have no change in heart rate, no headache, seizures, and no change in mental status.
2. Hold meals 1 hr before and during dialysis.	2. The presence of food in the stomach will shunt blood flow to the visceral organs and contribute to hypotension, nausea, and vomiting.	2. Early detection and reporting of impending complications.
3. Allow the patient to rest after dialysis.	3. Patient may be tired and lethargic after the dialysis procedure. Rest minimizes symptoms of dialysis disequilibrium (see below).	3. Patient regains strength and engages in ADLs.
4. After dialysis, encourage the patient to move from lying to standing gradually and assist with ambulation.	4. Orthostatic blood pressure changes are common postdialysis due to fluid removal during the treatment. gradual position changes and assistance will help prevent blood pressure drops and falls that might lead to injury.	4. Patient is able to stand without any feeling of dizziness or fainting due to orthostatic hypotension.
5. Every hour throughout dialysis, more often if adverse signs occur, observe for and document dialysis disequilibrium. a. Headache b. Increasing BP c. Decreasing pulse rate d. Stupor e. Seizures f. Coma	5. Dialysis disequilibrium is cerebral edema that results from migration of extracellular water into the brain cells as the osmolality of blood and cerebrospinal fluid change. It occurs more frequently in severely uremic patients, during the first few treatments, and in individuals having hemodialysis. The symptoms may present during dialysis and if they do the treatment is slowed or discontinued. As the osmolality of the blood and cerebrospinal fluid equilibrate the symptoms will abate.	5. The patient will be as follows: a. Free from signs of cerebral edema b. Have no complaints of headache c. BP will remain within normal limits d. Pulse rate steady e. Alert and oriented

are muscle weakness and flaccidity, irregular pulse rate, and ECG changes as outlined previously in this chapter. If noted, these findings should be brought to the physician's attention immediately and treatment initiated. If blood transfusions are ordered, the nurse must watch for hyperkalemia since blood products can contain a significant amount of free potassium.

Evaluation. Maintenance of a stable weight, normal blood pressure, and absence of edema will indicate normal fluid status. Clear lungs, normal oxygen–carbon dioxide exchange, and normal skin color and turgor are further signs of adequate volume status. Serum potassium of 3.5–5.3 mEq/liter and a normal ECG will indicate adequate control of potassium intake.

Nutrition

Nursing Diagnosis. Alteration in nutrition, less than body requirements, occurs because the patient is critically ill and experiences stress and catabolism. In addition the gastrointestinal symptoms experienced by the uremic patient as discussed previously compounded with necessary diet modifications make ensuring adequate nutrition a challenge. In many cases oral feedings are not possible, so that tube feedings through a nasogastric, gastrostomy, or ileostomy tube are indicated. Many of these patients are too ill to receive enteral feedings; thus, intravenous hyperalimentation is necessary.

Goals. The goal is to provide adequate nutrition by whatever route possible to promote healing and to prevent infection.

Interventions. The diet should provide enough protein to prevent negative nitrogen balance (1.5 g/kg body weight/day), be high in calories, (35–50 kcal/kg body weight/day), and restrict fluid, sodium, and potassium.[4] For the patient receiving oral feedings, timing and presentation of meals is important. The uremic person usually experiences more nausea and vomiting in the morning; thus a small breakfast and larger meals later in the day are advantageous. Serving meals as soon as they are transported to the nursing unit is a must; this allows them to be presented in the most appealing manner. Eating less than an hour before hemodialysis treatment predisposes the patient to hypotensive episodes, nausea, and vomiting during the treatment. If the patient does miss a meal because of dialysis, the meal must be served afterwards to maintain caloric intake.

The benefits of hyperalimentation (see Chap. 80) to the person with acute tubular necrosis are the same as to any seriously ill person, but the risk of infection from the catheter and the chances of fluid overload and electrolyte imbalance are higher. The nurse must thus use strict sterile technique during catheter care and bag and tubing changes and must be alert for signs and symptoms of infection and fluid and electrolyte imbalances. When the patient with ATN is receiving hyperalimentation he will often require daily dialysis to prevent fluid overload.

Anxiety

Nursing Diagnosis. Anxiety related to fear and the physiological and psychological stress of the illness and hospitalization may occur in the patient with acute tubular necrosis. Manifestations are tachycardia, elevated blood pressure, palpitations, insomnia, tension, apprehension, helplessness, loss of control, irritability, anger, crying, inability to concentrate, confusion, or disorientation. The patient's anxiety may be focused on one aspect of his disease. In many cases this focus is the dialysis access, for it is a visual representation of the illness.

Goals. The nursing goals are to alleviate stressors, thereby enabling the patient (and family) to express concerns and to cope with the illness, and to provide comfort and security.

Interventions. Since many of these patients will be in an intensive care unit, their circadian rhythms will be interrupted. When possible, normal sleep and meal patterns should be maintained. Stress may be decreased by respecting the individual's privacy and encouraging his participation in decisions regarding care and activities. Family members must also be included in these considerations. If the patient is agitated, stuporous, confused, or comatose, the family's anxiety may be the focus for nursing intervention. Facilitating family cohesiveness and support through visitation privileges and assistance in care are valuable means of alleviating stress.

An aid for reducing anxiety is an explanation of and preparation for medical and nursing procedures. When preparing patients and their families for new experiences, an explanation of the procedure along with a description of the typical sensations experienced during the procedure or treatment leads to more accurate expectations. Understanding of sensations decreases anxiety.[7] The sensory information includes telling the patient what he might feel, see, hear, smell, or taste. When the patient has an altered mental status, the nurse must explain to the family the pathophysiological and psychological basis for this and when possible give reassurance that this will clear.

Evaluation. Goal achievement will be verified if the patient and family are able to express fears and communicate their needs, express an understanding of the treatment process, and participate in decisions and implementation of care.

Drug Side-Effects

Nursing Diagnosis. Potential problems with management of medications relate to renal dysfunction and the subsequent dangers of overdose and toxicity. Nurses share responsibility in providing safe drug therapy.

Goals. The goal is to monitor the patient for manifestations of undesirable side-effects of drugs.

Interventions. One of the interdependent nursing functions is participation in drug therapy. As discussed earlier in this chapter, drug modifications are required for the patient in renal failure. The nurse must be knowledgeable and alert to the symptoms of drug reaction and toxicity. When a drug reaction or drug toxicity is suspected the medication must be held and the physician notified. Care must be given when administering drugs near the time of dialysis. Some medications are removed during dialysis; thus administration schedules should be adjusted to maintain drug efficiency. Antihypertensive medications may need adjustment so they don't predispose the patient to hypotension during dialysis. Guidelines that recommend modification of specific drugs are available.[3]

Evaluation. The goal is achieved if any adverse reactions to drugs are detected promptly and severe complications are avoided.

The Elderly Patient with ATN

Some special considerations must be given when caring for the elderly patient with acute tubular necrosis. Ensuring adequate nutrition will be a challenge, for frequently the elderly patient has fewer nutritional reserves, will resist diet modifications, and may already have a poor appetite. Careful assessment of food likes and dislikes plus offering frequent nourishment will be important. The aluminum hydroxide antacids administered to prevent gastrointestinal bleeding combined with inactivity and fluid restrictions make constipation a problem in the geriatric patient who may already be prone to constipation. High-fiber foods plus adherence to the patient's normal toilet routines may help minimize this. Frequently stool softeners or laxatives are necessary.

Skin dryness and breakdown will be more common in the elderly because of edema, bed rest, and the decreased production of skin oils and loss of elasticity due to aging. Preventive measures discussed earlier in the chapter will be necessary. If the elderly patient has cardiovascular impairment and requires hemodialysis, certain considerations are important. Vascular changes will make establishment of the hemodialysis access a challenge and will require careful observation for potential access problems. Cardiovascular instability may lead to intradialytic complications such as hypotension, angina, and arrhythmias.

Mental and behavioral changes occur with greater frequency in the critically ill and dialyzed geriatric patient because of the stress, environmental changes, uremia, and dialysis. These problems may be prevented or lessened by providing a consistent daily routine for the patient, encouraging family and friends to visit, adding some personal belongings to the hospital environment, and explaining procedures in advance.

Recovery of Renal Function and Discharge Planning

As renal function improves the intensity of nursing care lessens. Continuing care to prevent late complications is coupled with increased emphasis on recovery and return to normal activities. The patient and his family must be made aware of improvements in his condition and changes in care that result. When discharge nears, education regarding self-care activities and the necessity of follow-up care is important. Since acute tubular necrosis is generally a complication of another condition, the discharge planning will include special instructions regarding the precipitating problem. On occasion an individual is discharged from the hospital before dialysis is discontinued. In this case, the patient and family must be taught about the renal diet, dialysis access care, and prescribed medications. Arrangements must be made with the outpatient dialysis unit for scheduling treatments. For the elderly patient still receiving dialysis at the time of discharge a home health aide, temporary nursing home placement, or transportation assistance may be necessary.

Death

Nursing Diagnosis. Because the patient with acute tubular necrosis is often critically ill and death rates are high, a possible nursing diagnosis is grieving on the part of the patient and family related to anticipated loss. Symptoms include anger, denial, fear, guilt, depression, crying, withdrawal, insomnia, fatigue, gastrointestinal disturbances, and weight loss.

Goals. The nursing goal is to help the patient and family express their grief.

Intervention. Encourage the patient and family to share concerns. Promote family cohesiveness so that they can obtain support from each other and make necessary decisions surrounding the death. Assist the family to identify grief reactions and complete the grief work associated with each reaction.

Evaluation. The patient and family will be able to express their grief, participate in decision making for the future, and share feelings and concerns with each other.

Conclusion

Providing nursing care to the person with acute tubular necrosis requires knowledge of the disease and thoughtful application of the nursing process. The several physical manifestations of ATN are coupled with the anxiety and stress that accompany any serious illness. Comprehensive nursing care will require attention to the emotional needs of the patient and family as well as to the complexities of the physical care.

References

1. Anderson RJ, Linas SL, Berns AS et al: Nonoliguric acute renal failure. N Engl J Med 296:1134, 1977
2. Arbeit LA, Weinstein SW: Acute tubular necrosis: Pathophysiology and management. Med Clin North Am 65:147, 1981
3. Bennett WM, Aronoff GR, Morrison G et al: Drug prescribing in

renal failure: Dosing guidelines for adults. Am J Kidney Dis 3:155, 1983

4. Brown RO: Nutritional support in acute renal failure. American Association of Nephrology Nurses and Technicians Journal 10:25, 1983
5. Diamond JR, Yoburn DC: Nonoliguric acute renal failure. Arch Intern Med 142:1882, 1982
6. Gornick CC, Kjellstrand CM: Acute renal failure complicating aortic aneurysm surgery. Nephron 35:145, 1983
7. Johnson JE, Kirchhoff KT, Endress MP: Altering children's distress behavior during orthopedic cast removal. Nurs Res 24:404, 1975
8. Kjellstrand CM, Ebben J, Davin T: Hemodialysis in patients with acute tubular necrosis. Trans Am Soc Artif Intern Organs 27:45, 1981
9. Kjellstrand CM, Pru CE, Jahnke WR, Davin TD: Acute renal failure. In Drukker W, Parsons FM, Maher JF (eds): Replacement of Renal Function by Dialysis, 2nd ed. Boston, Martinus Nijhoff, 1983
10. McMurray SD, Luft FC, Maxwell DR et al: Prevailing patterns and predictor variables in patients with acute tubular necrosis. Arch Intern Med 138:950, 1978
11. Myers, BD: Pathogenesis of postischemic acute renal failure in man. Kidney 16:37, 1983
12. Schrier RW: Manual of Nephrology: Diagnosis and Therapy. Boston, Little, Brown & Co, 1981
13. Tilney NL, Morgan AP, Lazarus JM: Acute renal failure in surgical patients. In Tilney NL, Lazarus JM (eds): Surgical Care of the Patient with Renal Failure. Philadelphia, WB Saunders, 1982

Chapter 59

Renal and Urinary Infections and Inflammatory Disorders

Lisa L. MacGeorge
Pauline M. Bruno

Glomerulonephritis

Definition/Classification

Glomerulonephritis is a nonbacterial inflammation of the glomeruli of both kidneys. It has many causes and presents in many different forms. The basic underlying pathology in all forms is an antigen/antibody reaction in some portion of the glomeruli, and for this reason it is generally termed an immunologic disease.

The classification is either acute glomerulonephritis or chronic glomerulonephritis. Often the acute form never resolves but rather progresses to the chronic disease. However, chronic disease can develop without being preceded by the acute disorder.

Glomerulonephritis may also be classified into four major categories according to the type of glomerular membrane change. These categories are (1) minimal cell change, (2) proliferative, (3) membranous, and (4) menbranoproliferative. Minimal cell change suggests that the glomerular defect is very minor and thus the prognosis is good. Proliferative suggests multiplication of a particular cell in the glomeruli. The change may be either diffuse or localized and may range from mild to severe. Membranous glomerulonephritis refers to a thickening of the glomerular capillary wall and subsequent narrowing of the capillar lumen (Fig. 59–1). Membranoproliferative suggests that both changes are occurring in the same glomeruli simultaneously. The basis for the classification is examination of tissue taken by biopsy.

Acute Glomerulonephritis

Etiology and Pathophysiology

The most common etiologic factor of acute glomerulonephritis is the group A hemolytic streptococci. The disease frequently follows an acute respiratory infection or skin infection. It has a latent period of up to a month after the onset of the infection. The age-groups most often affected are children and young adults.

The immune process consists of the deposition of antigen–antibody complexes in the glomerular wall. The immune reaction activates the inflammatory response (see Chaps. 15 and 16). The lysosomes released during the inflammatory response damage the glomerular basement membrane. Proliferation of glomerular cells then occurs and, based on examination of biopsied tissue, the glomerulonephritis is categorized as described above.

The damaged glomeruli lose the ability to filter selectively. Permeability is increased; therefore, protein mole-

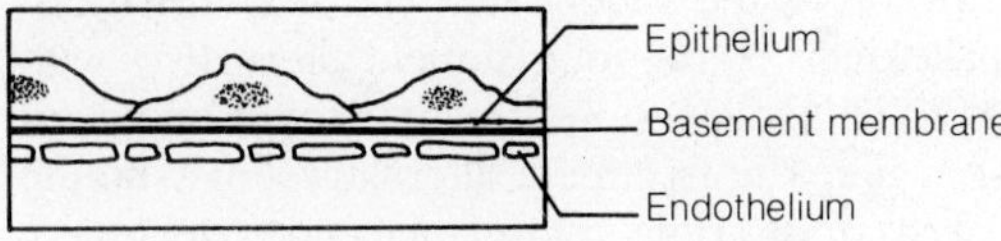

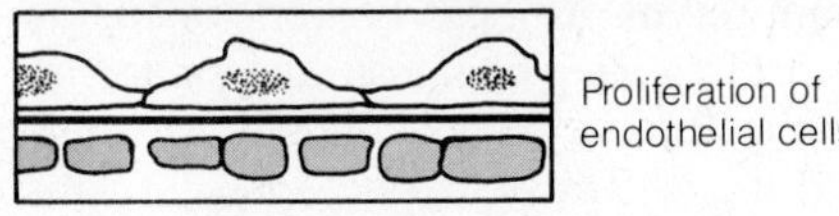

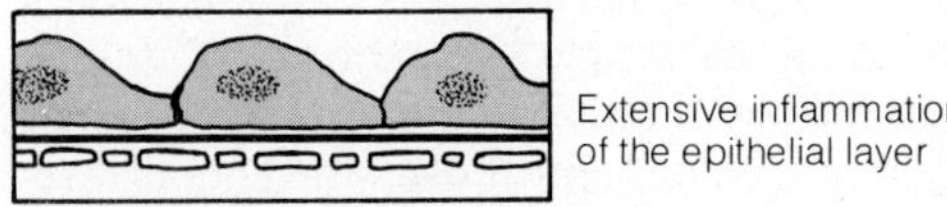

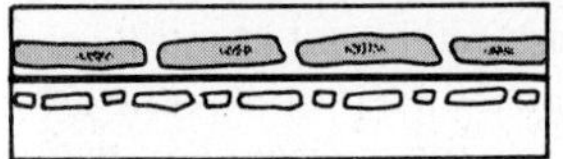

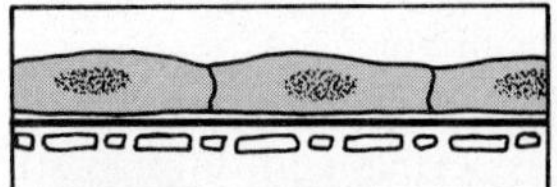

FIGURE 59–1 Changes in the glomerular membrane that occur with acute proliferative glomerulonephritis, rapidly progressive glomerulonephritis, minimal change nephrosis, and membranous glomerulonephritis.

cules and red blood cells are filtered from the plasma to the urine. Glomerular damage also decreases the functional surface area. The result of these changes is a reduction in the glomerular filtration rate (GFR).

Clinical Manifestations

Signs and symptoms include increased specific gravity with a smoky appearance to the urine, hematuria with red cell casts, proteinuria, oliguria, edema, high blood pressure, headache, and elevated creatinine and blood urea nitrogen (BUN). Serum complement levels may be normal or decreased and the antistreptolysin O titer may be elevated, which may indicate the presence of antibodies to streptococcal organisms. The fluid retention resulting from the reduction in GFR causes circulating volume overload.

Medical Management

Treatment is symptomatic and aimed at preventing the complications of fluid overload. Sodium and fluid restrictions depend on the degree of edema and the extent of blood pressure elevation. Diuretics and antihypertensive medications may be necessary. Protein restrictions, if any, depend on the BUN level and the amount of protein losses in the urine. Bed rest is prescribed until the edema and elevated blood pressure return to near normalcy. The infection is treated if it is still present, and usually penicillin is prescribed for months as prophylaxis against recurrence. Dialysis may be started if signs of renal failure appear.

The prognosis for adults with acute glomerulonephritis is guarded. Approximately 60% to 70% of the adult patients recover completely. Of the remainder, some die from complications (*e.g.*, heart disease) of the initial disease and some experience worsening of the disease and are diagnosed as having rapidly progressive glomerulonephritis (RPGN).

Rapidly Progressive Glomerulonephritis

RPGN is a devastating form of proliferative glomerulonephritis. It is named for its very rapid progression with subsequent renal failure within days to months vs. months to years. The hallmark sign of RPGN is a crescent-shaped proliferation of epithelial cells on the glomerular basement membrane that literally strangles the surrounding glomerular cells.

The clinical manifestations generally include varying degrees of high fevers, oliguria, hematuria, proteinuria, hypoalbuminemia, and uremic toxicity as renal failure progresses. The treatment consists of steroids, plasmapheresis which removes the lethal antibody, or a combination of both. This treatment has variable success rates. Most patients eventually require treatment with dialysis or transplantation.

Nursing Management

Nursing Diagnosis/Problem. The problems associated with the care of patients with acute glomerulonephritis include alterations in fluid, electrolyte, and acid–base balance, potential for recurrence of infection, and decreased level of self-care.

Goals. The goals are to minimize the fluid, electrolyte, and acid–base imbalances, to assist in the treatment of infection and prevent a recurrence, and to promote self-care to the maximum possible extent consistent with the course of the disease.

Interventions. Nursing management consists of monitoring the clinical signs and symptoms and providing supportive care. The complications to anticipate and assess for are increasing blood pressure and/or hypertensive crisis, cardiac failure due to volume overload, and acute renal failure.

Antibiotics must be administered at the desired intervals to assure maintenance of a consistent blood level. The patient and family need instruction about the reason for the medication and the importance of preventing further infection. Environmental conditions that may be hazardous (*e.g.*, crowds) are discussed as preventive measures in addition to prophylactic antibiotics. In the acute hospital setting, the patient may need to be in protective isolation.

Activity is limited while the blood pressure is elevated, while edema exists, and while the BUN is elevated. The patient needs an explanation of the importance of not stressing the kidney in order to promote tissue healing. However, self-care, to the extent possible without fatigue or an increase in heart rate or blood pressure, should be encouraged. Since the proteinuria may persist for months and even years, the patient needs follow-up care. This includes planning a daily routine that is not fatiguing, daily weights, nutrition planning, and emphasis on adherence to antibiotic therapy.

Evaluation. Signs of clinical improvement include an increasing urine output, decreasing weight, decreasing hematuria, decreasing blood pressure, and improving sense of well-being. The patient reports continuance of antibiotic therapy and the ability to do activities of daily living without an increase in proteinuria or hematuria and without fatigue. The patient reports no occurrences of infection.

Chronic Glomerulonephritis

Etiology and Pathophysiology

Chronic glomerulonephritis may be an outcome of the acute form of the disease or it may occur with no history of previous renal disease or infection. In the latter situation, the patient is usually in the middle adult years.

The course of chronic glomerulonephritis is variable. In some patients, it progresses slowly and the loss of renal function is gradual. In other patients, severe high blood pressure develops, which in turn hastens renal damage. The renal changes consist of a thinning of the cortex, arteriosclerotic thickening of the renal arteries, and a progressive destruction of the glomeruli. The kidney atrophies and renal function progressively decreases.

Clinical Manifestation

The signs and symptoms of chronic glomerulonephritis are similar to those described above for the acute form except that they are not as severe until the damage becomes extensive. An exception is the chronic type that follows from an initial acute disease. In this situation, the person's condition worsens rapidly.

In the chronic-from-acute type of glomerulonephritis, the patient may experience dependent edema in the morning, and mild headaches and moderate elevation of blood pressure. The onset of dyspnea on exertion and orthopnea are signs of worsening of the condition. Urinalysis would reveal the presence of hematuria, proteinuria, and casts. As the disease progresses, the patient begins to have signs and symptoms of curtailed renal function.

Medical Mangement

There are two types of definitive medical management of end stage renal disease: *dialysis* and *renal transplantation*. Dialysis was discussed in the preceding chapter as a temporary procedure which is part of the treatment for acute renal failure. However, the patient with end stage renal disease has to make decisions about treatment alternatives with the recognition that some form of treatment will be necessary throughout life. The treatment alternatives may be (1) temporary dialysis until a renal transplant can be performed; (2) long-term hemodialysis or peritoneal dialysis; (3) a return to long-term dialysis if renal transplant should fail or to temporary dialysis until retransplant can be performed; (4) selection of renal transplant after being on dialysis for an extended period of time. The overall goal of definitive therapy is to maintain fluid and electrolyte balance, prevent signs and symptoms of uremia, and sustain life for patients with end stage renal disease.

Maintenance dialysis is that which is performed on a regular basis either in the patient's home or on a routine schedule in a hospital-based center or a special clinic. It may be either hemodialysis or peritoneal dialysis. Hemodialysis for the patient with end stage disease is usually through a surgically created internal arteriovenous fistula. An artery, usually in the upper extremity, is anastomosed side to side to a nearby vein. The direct flow of arterial blood into the vein causes enlargement of the vein, which then permits repeated venipuncture access for connection to the dialyzer. For maintenance hemodialysis, the internal arteriovenous fistula is superior to the external cannula (described in the preceding chapter) because the incidence of clotting and infection is decreased, activity is not restricted, and there are no problems with accidental cannula displacement.

Maintenance *peritoneal dialysis* may also be accomplished by means of a catheter that is permanently implanted into the cavity through an incision below the umbilicus. The catheter has two internal cuffs which serve as barriers to infection. Tissues grow around these cuffs and thereby prevent infection from traveling inward from the exit site of the catheter. Delivery of the dialysate to the peritoneal cavity and removal after a set period of time can be accomplished by closed systems using one of the machines currently available. The machine delivers the sterile water and concentrate in a ratio that produces the desired dialysate solution. Timers on the machine can be set to deliver the desired amount of dialysate, maintain it in the peritoneal cavity for a certain period, and drain it for a designated time. A newer method not requiring machines is also available. These are discussed under the nursing management section.

Renal transplantation is the other form of treatment that may be available to the patient with end stage renal disease. Renal transplantation is the implantation of a kidney from one human to another. Donors are generally histocompatible relatives or cadaveric donors. The greatest threat to a successful transplant is rejection of the transplant kidney.

Histocompatibility studies are carried out prior to transplant to determine the possibility of an immune response. Histocompatibility or tissue typing is the identification of antigens on the leukocytes which are coded genetically on the sixth chromosome followed by the matching of two people with the same antigenic makeup. Matching is done in an attempt to decrease the possibility of the recipient's body recognizing the new kidney as foreign. Because not all antigens have been identified, even an apparently perfect antigenic match does not ensure that a rejection of the transplanted kidney will not occur. Donors and recipients without any histocompatible antigens have virtually no chance of a successful transplant.

Immunosuppressive therapy is a highly important component of the transplant procedure. It is essentially a state of drug-induced immunological tolerance in which the body's ability to recognize and attack foreign material is reduced. Presently, the most common immunosuppressive therapy includes a combination of azathioprine (Imuran), corticosteroids (prednisone), occasionally antilymphocyte globulin (ALG), and most recently Cyclosporin-A.

Another technique being used to prevent rejection is donor-specific transfusions. This procedure consists of spaced transfusions of the kidney donor's blood into the person who is to receive the kidney. Three transfusions are given, each 2 weeks apart. The purpose is to determine if the recipient is likely to reject the donated kidney and to desensitize the recipient to the donor's tissues. The transplantation is carried out if a cross matching of blood from the donor and recipient is compatible.

The donor is carefully assessed for both physical and emotional health. The donor will be functioning with only one kidney after the surgery; therefore, the person must be highly motivated to donate and must be in good health.

The prognosis for patients with end-stage renal disease who receive dialysis is favorable. Patients learn to do the treatment at home and life expectancy is extended for years. The patient who has a transplant will have a favorable prognosis providing the transplanted kidney is not rejected. In the event of rejection, the patient returns to the dialysis treatment.

Nursing Management: Patient on Maintenance Dialysis

Nursing Diagnosis/Problem. The success of dialysis as a treatment modality for patients with end stage renal disease depends strongly on the involvement of the patient, and in many cases the family, in the treatment. Nursing diagnoses are knowledge and psychomotor deficits related to self management of dialysis treatment and possibly ineffective coping with the lifestyle changes demanded by the treatment regimen. The chronic nature of the illness creates many problems for the patient or family, including problems in interpersonal relationships, financial burdens, and lifestyle changes.

Goals. The goal of nursing is to achieve patient and family understanding of the disease, the treatment regimen, and the necessary changes in lifestyle. The ability of the patient and the family to successfully cope with the changes required is dependent upon understanding and acceptance of the situation.

Intervention: Hemodialysis. Hemodialysis is a complicated procedure, and some patients or their families may be unable to learn how to carry it out in a home setting. Therefore, three options are usually available: (1) in-center dialysis where nurses do the dialysis; (2) self care, but at dialysis centers where the patient does most of the treatment with some assistance from the nurse; and (3) home dialysis conducted by the patient or a family member, or another assistant. Patient teaching is essential regardless of the option selected. Dialysis is only one aspect of treatment. Other aspects are diet restrictions and medications, which were discussed in previous chapters.

All dialysis procedures have four phases: predialysis, initiation of the treatment, treatment, and postdialysis. The *predialysis* process includes preparation of the dialyzer and assessment of patient status. The dialyzer tubings must be flushed with the dialysate solution to be certain all the air is removed from the system. Likewise, the channels for blood flow from the patient through the machine must be flushed with normal saline.

Assessment of the patient consists of weights, vital signs, observing for edema, and listening to the lungs to detect abnormalities. These measurements are compared to findings at the previous treatment. The patient or family member needs to carry out this assessment in the home setting, and should be taught the significance of findings and when to seek consultation with the nurse at the treatment center.

Initiation of dialysis consists of cleaning the skin and placement of the large bore needles into the internal fistula. Cleanliness of the skin is essential to prevent infection. Proper management of the fistula is essential to maintain patency, and prevent clotting and infection. The patient and family need to develop the ability to initiate dialysis and to care for the site of insertion.

Monitoring during dialysis consists of taking vital signs and observing for possible clotting of blood, and for adverse reactions to the treatment such as hypotension from loss of blood into the machine. To prevent hypotension, the blood flow is started slowly and increased gradually. Other possible adverse responses are discussed in the previous chapter. Patients and families need to understand why these responses might occur, and how to determine if the reaction is such that the treatment center should be contacted. Patients and their families also need to understand how the equipment functions, and what to check and do if alarm systems indicate occurrence of a problem.

Prior to disconnecting the patient from the system, a bottle of normal saline is attached in order to flush the system and return as much blood as possible to the patient. Insertion site care is given after disconnecting the patient, and vital signs are taken. The patient or family member must learn how to disconnect the system, and also needs to know how to care for the equipment. Patient teaching of hemodialysis treatment requires an extended period of time and is individualized. Nurses who function in this specialty receive advanced training for the role.

Intervention: Peritoneal Dialysis. Maintenance peritoneal dialysis may be recommended for persons with cardiovascular problems, individuals living alone who want to do home dialysis, persons with learning difficulties, and those who no longer have patent vascular sites for hemodialysis. It is a more time consuming process than hemodialysis but is simpler to carry out and less costly. The use of peritoneal dialysis for acute renal failure was discussed in the preceding chapter.

The person on peritoneal dialysis may elect one of three methods. One method, intermittent peritoneal dialysis (IPD), is carried out on a routine basis of three to five times a week for 8 to 12 hours each time. This procedure may be done at a treatment center or at home. It requires the use of a machine to deliver and drain the dialysate solution. The treatment can be performed while the patient is sleeping.

A second method is continuous ambulatory peritoneal dialysis (CAPD). As the name implies, the treatment is ongoing, all day, every day. The dialysate solution is in a plastic bag which is connected to the indwelling peritoneal catheter. The solution is allowed to flow into the peritoneal cavity, the tubing is clamped, and the bag is then collapsed and carried in a pocket. After a period of 4 to 8 hours the tubing is unclamped, the dialysate flows by gravity back into the original bag which is discarded, and another bag of fresh solution is attached to the peritoneal line. This process does not require the use of any machines; therefore, the patient can be ambulatory. The major problems with the system is the danger of peritonitis and the need for continuous treatment. However, the continuous treatment does have the physiological advantage of a continuous movement of waste solutes out of the blood and therefore the achievement of balanced blood chemistries.

The third method is continuous cycling of peritoneal dialysis (CCPD). In this method, the patient is dialyzed on a cycler machine at night, obtaining three to four exchanges. The final exchange is left in the peritoneal cavity for the day. This system does allow the patient to be active during the day. The number of entries into the peritoneal line are fewer than with CAPD, thereby reducing the danger of peritonitis.

The patient can usually learn to do peritoneal dialysis in less time than is required to learn hemodialysis. The categories of information to be taught are similar. The patient must learn how to (1) care for the indwelling catheter and the skin at the insertion site; (2) connect up the type of equipment being used; (3) care for the equipment; and (4) monitor responses to treatment and evaluate the significance of these responses. Patient understanding of the reasons for a specific method of care is essential. The ability to carry out aseptic technique is essential. Monitoring of response to treatment includes self-weights, taking vital signs, and listening to heart sounds. These need to be recorded and followed closely in order to determine if excessive fluid is being retained. The patient may need to make adjustments in the dialysate solution or contact the treatment center nurse for consultation.

Evaluation. Goal achievement for teaching either hemodialysis or peritoneal dialysis is evidenced by the ablity of the patient or family to

1. Explain why dialysis is necessary and the effect it has on the body
2. Explain the procedure for monitoring body responses to the treatment, the significance of adverse responses, and the action to take in the event of such responses.
3. Adhere to the dietary restrictions.
4. Adhere to medication therapy.
5. Demonstrate accurate initiation and discontinuance of treatment.
6. Demonstrate action to take if the monitoring system of the machine should indicate malfunctioning.
7. Demonstrate how to care for the equipment.
8. Demonstrate how to care for the insertion site (peritoneal or circulatory).
9. Plan a schedule that will permit activities of interest and work.

Nursing Management: Patient Having Renal Transplant

Nursing Diagnoses/Problems. Many of the problems of patients experiencing renal transplant are similar to those of other people having surgery. However, the need for a donor who will lose a body organ and the recipient's potential for failure of the transplanted organ are problems specific to people having this type of surgery. These problems generate particular fears and anxieties which may be decreased when the patient and family acquire knowledge about the procedure and postoperative care. Other problems are the potential for adverse reactions to medications, for infection, and for rejection of the transplanted kidney.

Goals. The goals of nursing management are for prevention or early detection of adverse reactions to the transplanted organ, the surgery, or the medications; prevention of infection; education of patient and family about the procedure and postoperative care; and decreasing patient and family anxiety.

Intervention: Preoperative. The donor may not have had any previous contact with the health care system and will need explanations of preoperative laboratory studies and explanations of preoperative and postoperative care. Specifically, the person needs an opportunity to express concerns about the procedure and even to reverse the decision to donate a kidney.

The recipient will most likely be familiar with hospital routines. The nurse needs to discuss with the patient and family the transplant procedure and some pre- and postoperative treatments. The recipient may need to be on dialysis prior to surgery to obtain the best possible blood chemistries. After surgery, dialysis may need to be used for a few days until the transplanted kidney is functioning. The patient will have a Foley catheter in the urinary bladder, since hourly monitoring of output will be necessary postoperatively. The catheter drainage also enables detection of postoperative bleeding.

Usually it is not necessary to remove the recipient's kidneys since the primary disease has no effect on the transplant. Nephrectomy may be necessary if recurrent kidney infections are present since this could damage the transplanted kidney. The transplanted kidney is usually placed in the anterior iliac fossa. The renal artery and vein are anastomosed to either the iliac or hypogastric artery and vein. The ureter is transplanted into the bladder.

Interventions: Postoperative. The postoperative care of the patient having a renal transplant is basically the same as for any surgical patient. The differing problems are the impaired wound healing and defense mechanisms which result from the need for immunosuppressive therapy. The immunosuppressive therapy may be started preoperatively.

The Foley catheter allows for accurate urine measurement and keeps the bladder empty, thereby allowing for healing of the ureterovesical anastomosis. Bladder irrigations may be ordered to keep the urine pink tinged and to prevent clot formation. Catheter care is essential to prevent infection.

Position changes should be done carefully to protect the transplanted kidney. The physician may order particular positions. Sitting for long peirods may be discouraged as this may foster kinking of the ureter.

Technical complications that can occur postoperatively are (1) clotting, bleeding, or stenosis of the renal artery at the anastomosis site; (2) wound infection, which is a complication related to immunosuppressive drugs; and (3) obstruction or leakage at the anastomosis site. Clinical complications are rejection and adverse drug reactions.

Rejection may mimic infection, or its symptoms may be masked by the effect of immunosuppressive drugs; therefore detection may be delayed. Rejection is of three types: hyperacute, acute, and chronic. *Hyperacute rejection* occurs immediately after implant. The flow of recipient blood into the donor kidney brings antibodies that attack the foreign tissue and cause infarction. The donor kidney must be removed as there is no treatment for this irreversible rejection. However, the occurrence of hyperactive rejection is relatively rare because of advances in tissue typing and cross matching.

Acute rejection can occur as soon as a week and as long as a year or two after transplant. Many recipients experience one or two acute rejection episodes. The antigen–antibody reaction causes acute tubular necrosis. The manifestations of rejection include fluid retention and hypertension; oliguria and perhaps anuria; temperature elevation above 37.8° C, although this maybe masked by the action of the steroids; weight gain; malaise; elevations of serum creatinine, and electrolytes and blood urea nitrogen (BUN). Treatment usually consists of large doses of intravenous prednisolone (Solu-Medrol) and is effective if initiated promptly. Dialysis may be necessary during a rejection episode.

Chronic rejection occurs over a period of months or years. It is usually caused by antibody destruction of the donor kidney. There is no treatment to reverse the process and eventually the patient has to return to maintenance dialysis. Manifestations include gradual increases in weight, serum creatinine, and blood urea nitrogen, and fluid retention. The patient usually needs special assistance and support in coping with the need to return to dialysis treatment.

The nurse who works with patients having renal transplant needs an understanding of the commonly used *immunosuppressive drugs*. Azathioprine, which is used in immunosuppressive therapy, blocks the normal antigen–antibody response and platelet function, and therefore predisposes the patient to infection and bleeding. If the dose is too large it may depress bone marrow function. Nursing implications include preventing unnecessary exposure to infection, astute observation for signs and symptoms of infection, and protection from unnecessary trauma that may cause bleeding. Nurses, in conjunction with physicians, should monitor the white blood cell counts to detect potential bone marrow suppression.

Adrenocorticosteroids in therapeutic doses suppress the inflammatory response and have many side-effects, such as increased susceptibility to infection, gastrointestinal ulceration and bleeding, sodium and water retention, hyperglycemia, emotional lability, blurred vision, muscle wasting, acne, and Addison's symptoms with rapid steroid withdrawal. The nursing interventions include protection from infection; antacid administration; guaiacing all stools to monitor for bleeding; monitoring weight carefully; determining postural blood pressures; monitoring serum sodium and distention of neck veins; monitoring blood sugar; supporting the patient with reassurance of the reversibility of emotional lability with reduced dosage; initiating regular physical therapy; providing medicated soap for acne; and making sure steroids are always tapered before discontinuation to avoid Addison's symptoms.

An important aspect of the nursing care required for patients receiving corticosteroids is patient teaching. Patients should be taught self-care for the purpose of avoiding infections, to take antacids routinely to prevent gastrointestinal ulceration, to perform daily skin care for acne, and to participate in regular exercise to maintain muscle tone. A plan for outpatient follow-up by community nurses is initiated prior to discharge.

Antilymphocyte globulin (ALG) is horse serum that contains anitbodies against human lymphocytes. The side-effects are mainly those of serum sickness from the horse serum and include fever, chills, pruritis, hematuria, joint pains, and anaphylaxis. The nursing interventions include prior skin testing with horse serum to test for a reaction; premedication of the patient with diphenhydramine hydrochloride (Benadryl) ½ hour prior to ALG administration to minimize histamine-medicated reactions; discontinuation of infusion if any symptoms of serum sickness develop; and treatment of symptoms.

Cyclosporin-A is a relatively new drug being used for the treatment of organ rejection. Its more worrisome side-effect is nephrotoxicity (renal damage). The major nursing intervention is to monitor the serum creatinine daily and communicate any increasing trends immediately. Generally, any signs of renal damage warrant reduction of dosage or temporary discontinuation of the drug.

The patient who has had a transplant needs to know the manifestations of rejection as discussed above and the action to take if they should occur. The patient needs to contact the physician immediately. Rehospitalization will probably be necessary. The other teachings are concerned with prevention of infection, adequate nutrition and dietary modifications, and activity. The instruction is similar to that given patients in the early phase of chronic glomerulonephritis. In addition, nurses need to realize the psychosocial effects of renal disease and then to assist patients and families in their adaptation to the physical and financial limitations on their pattern of living.

Evaluation. Evidence of goal achievement is as follows:

1. The patient does not have any untoward reactions to medications.
2. If medication reactions occur, the manifestations are detected early and corrective treatment is initiated promptly.
3. Patient does not develop an infection.
4. Manifestations of rejection, if they occur, are detected early and treatment is initiated promptly.
5. The patient accurately describes manifestations of rejection and action to take if these occur.
6. Patient accurately describes necessary precautions to take to avoid infections and maintain adequate nutrition.

Nephrotic Syndrome

The nephrotic syndrome is a term applied to a group of signs and symptoms associated with severe renal disorders. The signs and symptoms are proteinuria, hypoalbuminemia, and edema.

Etiology and Pathophysiology

The proteinuria results from increased permeability of glomeruli. Causative factors are diseases that damage the glomerular membrane. The most common offender is glomerulonephritis. Other diseases are collagen disorders such as systemic erythematosus, diabetes mellitus, and circulatory disease.

The event that controls the severity of the syndrome is the extent of protein loss. Protein loss lowers the serum colloidal osmotic pressure of the blood. The loss of protein deprives the liver of its source for synthesis of albumin. A low serum albumin leads to reduced serum oncotic pressure and hence to retention of fluid in the interstitial spaces, that is, edema. One of the first manifestations of the problem is periorbital edema, especially in the morning. The edema gradually becomes generalized. The retention of fluid in the interstitial spaces lowers the circulating plasma volume, which stimulates sodium retention.

Since the serum albumin levels are low, the high molecular weight proteins remain in the serum. These are the lipoproteins. The result is hyperlipidemia and hypercholesterolemia. Some of the smaller lipoproteins move through the porous glomerular membrane. Lipoproteinuria causes the urine to appear foamy.

Clinical Manifestations

As identified above, the manifestations associated with this syndrome are proteinuria, hypoalbuminemia, edema, and hyperlipidemia. As the disease progresses, the patient becomes nauseated and may vomit. Anorexia and abdominal pain may occur. When glomerulonephritis is the underlying disease, the patient also has hematuria and an elevated blood pressure.

Medical Management

Diagnosis is based on the signs and symptoms. The serum levels give an indication of the severity of the disease.

Treatment aims at reducing the extent of the edema, improving the serum albumin level, and treating the underlying problem when possible. Dietary intake of protein supplements will provide the substances needed for synthesis of albumin. Corticosteroids may be prescribed to decrease the extent of the inflammation and glomeruli damage. Steroids are used when the nephrotic syndrome is associated with lupus erythematosus. Cyclophosphamide (Cytoxan), an immunosuppressive and cytotoxic drug, is used as an alternative to steroid therapy. The adverse effects of cyclophosphamide are bone marrow suppression (especially of the white cells), hemorrhagic cystitis, amenorrhea, aspermatogenesis, and alopecia. The therapeutic and adverse effects are dose dependent. Fortunately, a low dose is usually effective and few of the adverse effects are experienced. With prolonged treatment the alopecia may occur regardless of the dose. The hair will grow back as soon as the treatment is discontinued. Even if a complete remission is not achieved, the glomerular lesion will usually be controlled. However, the nephrotic syndrome and its complications may continue.

The prognosis for the nephrotic syndrome depends on the underlying etiology. The syndrome may persist for a prolonged period of time and may eventually become a chronic renal failure.

Nursing Management

Nursing Diagnosis/Problem. The nursing diagnoses include potential for infection, alterations in nutritional intake, potential for adverse effects of medication, and self-care deficits. The use of corticosteroids increases the danger of infection but does help to control inflammation of the glomeruli. Dietary intake of increased amount of protein to replace the severe loss through glomerular permeability is essential. Other medications, such as cyclophosphamide (Cytoxan) have undesirable side-effects, that is, nausea and vomiting. The alteration in renal function disrupts the dynamic equilibrium of the body. The decreased albumin level and loss of red blood cells predispose the patient to weakness and fatigue.

Goals. The goals of nursing care are to prevent infection, obtain adequate nutritional intake, detect signs of adverse drug reactions, and maintain self-care to the maximum extent possible.

Interventions. The nurse must help the patient protect himself against infection. Actions will include protective isolation during hospitalization. Avoidance of crowds and people with obvious infection when at home is essential. The need to seek immediate treatment for infection if it occurs is emphasized in the teaching program.

Loss of appetite is usual. The diet needs to be palatable to the patient. Extra protein is highly desirable. Proteinuria should be monitored for quantity of loss. Usually sodium intake is limited to some extent. Not adding salt to food and avoiding foods high in sodium may be all that is necessary. Diuretics may be used. If so, the patient needs to be instructed about intake of foods containing potassium if the diuretic fosters potassium excretion.

The nurse needs to monitor the effects of prednisone and cyclophosphamide. Even though hemorrhagic cystitis is rare with low doses of cyclophosphamide, nurses should routinely check for blood in the urine. The white blood count should be monitored for a trend of decreasing count. Patients will need emotional support as they face changes in body image due to steroid therapy, such as hair loss and possible sterility.

In the hospital environment, the activities of daily living are planned according to the tolerance level of the patient. The patient is helped to plan a regimen to follow at home that will maximize activity and self-care without precipitating fatigue and weakness. The need for nursing care extends beyond the hospital. Community nurse referrals are usually necessary. The patient and family often need assistance in adjusting to the chronic nature of the disease. The nurse will need to follow up on the teaching done in the hospital and will need to provide long-term support to the patient and family. Patients and families should be offered the option of participating in support groups.

Evaluation. The goals of care are achieved if infections are prevented, the dietary intake of protein is adequate to maintain serum albumin level, sodium intake is within prescribed amount and serum sodium is within normal limits, adverse side-effects of drug therapy are detected, and the patient performs self-care without fatigue.

Urinary Tract Infection

Infections of the urinary tract are divided into upper and lower tract infections. The upper tract infections are *pyelonephritis* and *ureteritis*. Those in the lower tract are *cystitis* and *urethritis*. The urinary tract is the second most common site of infection, the first being the respiratory tract. Urinary tract infections may result in chronic renal failure.

Etiology and Pathophysiology

Urinary tract infections endanger kidney function by causing pyelonephritis, which is a bacterial invasion of the kidneys. *Escherichia coli* of the Enterobacteriaceae species is the most common cause of urinary tract infection. Other organisms may include other enterobacteria, *Klebsiella,* and *Proteus.* All of these organisms are part of the fecal flora and gain access to the urinary tract through the perineal area. Predisposing factors include urologic instrumentation, obstruction, suppressing the urge to void, and alkaline urine. Patients at high risk for urinary tract infections include pregnant women, diabetics, men over age 50 with prostatitis, catheterized patients, the elderly, and immunosuppressed or debilitated patients.[2]

According to Cunha,[1] nosocomial urinary tract infections are the most common type of hospital-acquired infections in the United States. More than 90% of nosocomial urinary tract infections are related to the use of indwelling catheters. Catheter infections account for nearly one half of all infections acquired in the hospital. The majority of patients with catheter-associated bacteriuria are at little or no risk for developing ascending pyelonephritis.

The remainder of this chapter will present the clinical manifestations of various infections along the urinary tract. Because nursing management of patients with urinary tract infections is similar regardless of infectious site, the section on nursing management will follow the discussion of specific infections.

Clinical Manifestations: Pyelonephritis

Pyelonephritis is a bacterial invasion of the renal calices, parenchyma, and renal pelvis. It is usually an ascending infection from the lower urinary tract, but it may be of blood-borne origin. This condition may be acute or chronic and symptomatic or asymptomatic. It may affect one or both kidneys.

The main signs and symptoms of acute symptomatic pyelonephritis are flank pain, fever (often in excess of 102° F), chills, general malaise, anorexia, and foul-smelling, cloudy urine. Diagnosis may be difficult in the elderly in which the presenting symptoms may be confusion, deterioration of general health, and incontinence. The findings of numerous white cells and bacteria in the urine confirms a diagnosis of pyelonephritis.

Clean-catch urine specimens are sent to the laboratory for culture and sensitivity. However, the physician may start the patient on a broad-spectrum antibiotic before the sensitivities have come back. Bacteremia associated with pyelonephritis is transient, and random blood cultures are often negative.

Chronic pyelonephritis is caused by bacterial inflammation of the kidney and subsequent scarring, fibrosis, and tubular dilation. High blood pressure and at least some degree of renal failure are present. There may be no bacterial or white cells in the urine at this time; therefore, the diagnosis is usually made by an intravenous pyelogram. Renal biopsy may be unreliable because the infection may be localized and missed by the biopsy puncture. Other tests of renal function, such as BUN and creatinine, are also performed. Treatment is much the same as with acute pyelonephritis but attention should also be paid to controlling high blood pressure to prevent further renal damage.

Clinical Manifestations: Cystitis

Cystitis is an inflammation of the bladder from any cause, but it is most often secondary to bacterial infection (*i.e.,* Escherischia coli). The symptoms are generally very bothersome and include frequency, urgency, dysuria, and a feeling of incomplete emptying of the bladder. Women have a higher incidence of cystitis than men. Several reasons exist for the increased incidence of cystitis in women: (1) sexual intercourse may actually manipulate the urethra so as to allow bacteria to enter, (2) a shorter urethra in women increases the introduction of perineal bacteria, (3) pregnancy and childbirth distort the anatomy of the urethra and bladder neck and allow bacterial entry, and (4) damage to the pelvic floor muscles and ligaments may lead to a degree of prolapse with further distortion of the urethral opening and introduction of bacteria. In addition, men may not be as susceptible as women to cystitis because of the bactericidal properties of prostatic secretions. Cystitis in men is infrequent unless a precipitating problem exists, such as enlargement of the prostrate in middle-aged and elderly men. The diagnosis of cystitis is made by a combination of patient symptoms (as stated above) and a white cell count of greater than 20 cells/cm in the urine. Cystitis is usually not accompanied by a fever and if a fever is present it generally is low grade.

Clinical Manifestations: Urethritis

Urethritis is an inflammation of the urethra. It may be acute or chronic. The etiology includes bacterial infection, sexually transmitted diseases such as gonorrhea, and chemical irritation secondary to the use of bath powders, spermicidal jellies, and bubble bath. The symptoms are nocturia, frequency, and burning on urination. Generally, men have a discharge, whereas women do not. The urinary meatus may be red and swollen.

Medical Management

Medical management of urinary tract infections consist primarily of prescribing the appropriate antibiotic medications and encouraging patient or community education to prevent those problems that can be avoided with modifications in behavior or lifestyle.

Medications. Pyridium (phenazopyridine HCl) is the medication most often used for the symptomatic relief of cystitis and urethritis. It is a weak antiseptic but is used for lower urinary tract infections because it is thought to have a soothing "topical anesthetic effect" on the urinary tract mucosa when excreted in the urine. It tends to relieve the burning pain and feeling of urgency.

Sulfonamide antibiotics are the most commonly prescribed urinary antibacterials. *Escherichia coli,* the gram-negative organism responsible for about 85% of acute cases, can often be controlled by treatment with sulfonamides.[3] However, physicians will require a urine culture and sensitivity to check whether that particular organism causing the infection will be susceptible to a sulfonamide preparation. The sulfonamide derivatives preferred for treating acute, chronic, and recurrent urinary tract infections caused by susceptible bacteria are those that quickly reach high levels in the urine as the derivatives are rapidly being excreted by the kidneys. Their usefulnesss is limited by (1) the emergence of resistant strains of previously susceptible bacteria, and (2) the development of sensitization and subsequent allergic or idosyncratic reactions that require withdrawal of these drugs. In the case of an allergy to sulfonamides, other antibiotics with acceptable action against urinary tract infections (that is, penicillin derivatives) are substituted.

Methenamine mandelate, a synthetic sulfonamide substitute, may be used as a broad-spectrum antibacterial agent in the continued treatment of chronic or recurrent urinary tract infections.

During infection, urea-splitting pathogens that produce ammonia cause the urine to be alkaline. Medications such as ascorbic acid (vitamin C), methenamine, and sodium biphosphate may be administered to acidify the urine.

Education and Prevention. Physicians, in conjunction with other health professionals, play an important role in the education of patients at risk for urinary tract infections. Although most often nurses actually initiate and evaluate patient teaching, it requires support from the physician in terms of time and a commitment to facilitate and reenforce the teaching.

Nursing Management

Nursing Diagnosis. Nursing diagnoses include discomfort related to irritation of the mucous membrane from the infectious process, decreased energy related to the body response to the infectious process, potential for extension of infection, and knowledge deficit related to methods for preventing urinary tract infections.

Goals. The goals are to relieve discomfort and promote rest, teach practices to prevent further infections, and monitor the response to medications.

Interventions. Prevention of discomfort may include administration of analgesics; promotion of fluid intake to dilute the urine and thereby decrease the mucosal irritation; and promotion of an acid-ash diet to acidify the urine, which inhibits bacterial growth. Sitz baths may be soothing when the infection site is the bladder or urethra.

The infectious process demands energy expenditure; consequently the patient may be tired and weak. Bed rest may be desirable for a few days. Assistance with activities of daily living may be necessary.

Nurses are responsible for administration of the medications and the evaluation of patient responses. They must also educate patients about their medications so that the patient may participate in his own care.

When administering Pyridium the nurse must tell the patient that this medication will cause orange-colored urine. This will disappear as soon as the medication is discontinued. Pyridium has no antimicrobial action and is administered for relief of urgency and burning pain.

Patients should always be questioned regarding previous reactions to specific antibiotics. If patients have experienced previous reactions to a certain antibiotic, that medication and those medications in the same class should be avoided. Any medication allergies should be documented and communicated to the physician. Patients who have a history of previous treatment with a particular antibiotic are potentially at risk for an allergic reaction when the antibiotic is prescribed at a later time.

The first dose of an antibiotic that is a repeat for the patient should be given under the supervision of a nurse, or if given on an outpatient basis, the patient should be taught signs and symptoms of an allergic reaction (see Chap. 24). Antibiotics may have other side-effects such as diarrhea and gastric upset. Some antibiotics may be taken with food and others should be taken on an empty stomach. The pharmacist is a good resource for information on medication administration. Nurses should teach patients that blood levels of antibiotics need to be constant and that the dosing schedule is important. Also, patients need to know that it is necessary to complete the full course of medication prescribed.

If medication is prescribed to acidify the urine, nurses need to check the effectiveness of the drug by determining the urine pH (which should be less than 6). If the patient is being treated at home, he needs to be taught to check the urine pH.

The nurse needs to teach measures to prevent recurrence of urinary tract infections. Female patients should be taught to wipe front to back after elimination, urinate after sexual intercourse, maintain adequate hydration, and practice good perineal hygiene. Maintenance of general health and well-being contribute to overall prevention of problems such as urinary tract infections.

Bacteriuria associated with an indwelling catheter cannot be eliminated by present techniques and methods but its incidence may be reduced to acceptable levels by the use of aseptic technique at the time of catheter insertion, continual cleanliness of the insertion site and catheter, and maintenance of a *closed* drainage system. Because bacteremias may arise secondary to urinary catheters, it is important that nurses identify those patients who are at risk and assess the significance a bacteremia may have for the particular patient. Prophylactic antibiotics may be prescribed for immunosuppressed patients or patients with a prior history of endocarditis. Catheterization may be completely avoided in some cases.

Evaluation. A successful outcome is such that the patient is free of urinary tract infection and symptomatology and is educated regarding the risk factors and prevention of urinary tract infections. Goal achievement would consist of the patient reporting a decrease in discomfort, including discomfort with voiding, a fluid intake of at least 2500 ml, and an increased energy level. Other signs of effective interventions are decreased bacterial count in the urine to less than 100,000/ml (which indicates the normal bacterial flora and bacteria are not multiplying), no fever, and increased appetite. The patient would be able to describe necessary actions to prevent recurrence of the infection.

References

1. Cunha BA: Nosocomial urinary tract infections. Heart Lung, 11(6):545–551, 1982
2. Sheehan SL et al: Understanding urinary tract infection in women: The first step to controlling it. Nursing 82, 12(11):68–71, 1982
3. Uldall R: Renal Nursing, 2nd ed, p 65. Oxford, Blackwell Publications, 1977

Bibliography

Brundage DL: Nursing Management of Renal Problems, 2nd ed. St Louis, CV Mosby, 1982

Clifford CM: Urinary tract infection—a brief selective review. Int J Nurs Stud 19(4):213–222, 1982

Goodman L, Gilman A (eds): The Pharmacological Basis of Therapeutics, 6th ed. New York, Macmillan, 1980

Kennedy AP: The nursing management of patients with long term indwelling catheters (research). J Adv Nurs 7(5):411–417, 1982

Larson E, Lindbloom L, Davis KB: Development of the Nephrology Nurse Practitioner: A Focus on Independent Learning. St Louis, CV Mosby, 1982

Rodman MJ, Smith DW: Clinical Pharmacology in Nursing. Philadelphia, JB Lippincott, 1985

Schrier RW: Renal and Electrolyte Disorders, 2nd ed. Boston, Little, Brown Co, 1980

Uldall R: Renal Nursing, 2nd ed. Oxford, Blackwell Publications, 1977

Wong ES: Guideline for prevention of catheter associated urinary tract infections. Am J Infect Control 11(1):28–36, 1983

Chapter 60

Neoplastic Disorders Affecting Renal and Urinary Function

Christine E. Reheis
Lynda Brubacher

Renal Adenocarcinoma

Renal adenocarcinoma (renal cell carcinoma or hypernephroma) is the most common cancer arising in the kidney.[7] The tumor arises in the renal parenchymal cells and accounts for 80% to 85% of all primary renal neoplasms.[5,16] Although it is a relatively rare tumor, it accounts for approximately 2% to 3% or 18,000 new cases of cancer annually.[7,20]

The incidence in the United States is 7.5 per 100,000 population per year.[16] Twice as common in men, renal adenocarcinoma accounts for 2.1% of male cancer deaths and 1.6% of female cancer deaths per year.[7,20] The average age at diagnosis is 55 to 60 years.[7,16] The tumor is rarely seen before the age of 20.

Familial cases of renal cell adenocarcinoma have been reported, and may occur in association with Hippel-Lindau's disease.[16] Geographic distribution of patients with this tumor is diverse. Although there seems to be little variation in incidences among racial and ethnic groups, the disease is more prevalent in Scandinavians and North Americans and less so in Asians and Africans.[7,16] There also seems to be an increased incidence in individuals living in urban as opposed to rural environments.

Etiology

No specific cause has been found for renal cell carcinoma. There has been no definite relationship found between hormonal, viral, or chemical carcinogens and the development of this cancer.[16] Likewise, no specific occupational exposures have been directly associated with the development of renal adenocarcinoma.[16] However, dimethylamine, or lead acetate, has been shown experimentally to induce renal tumors.[2] Tobacco use has also been implicated as an etiologic agent. The carcinogen dimethyl nitrosamine, found in tobacco smoke, has been suggested as an explanation for the statistically increasing incidence of renal cell carcinoma in persons using various forms of tobacco.[1]

Pathophysiology

The natural history of renal cell carcinoma is unpredictable. The disease may progress rapidly, with death ensuing, or patients may live for years with unresected primary tumor and known metastatic disease.[16] Renal cell carcinoma is one of the most common malignancies to undergo spontaneous regression. Regression of the disease should, however, not be equated with a cure, since a majority of patients will have recurrence of tumor within several years.[4,16]

The tumor locally infiltrates the kidney capsule. It is

highly angioinvasive, spreading into the renal vein and vena cava, and resulting in widespread hematogenous metastasis, especially to lung and bone.[5] With further progression of disease, additional sites of metastasis include brain, thyroid, adrenals, colon, spleen, diaphragm, and liver.[6,18]

Clinical Manifestations

Renal cell carcinoma is often called the "internist's tumor" because of the challenging nature of its diverse and often obscure presenting signs and symptoms. Earliest complaints of weakness, weight loss, and anemia occur in one third of patients presenting with this disease.[7] The classic triad of signs and symptoms of renal cell carcinoma is described as flank pain, hematuria, and palpable tumor mass.[5,7,16] Unfortunately, the presence of these three symptoms is only seen in 5% to 10% of patients at presentation and generally is a manifestation of far-advanced disease.[16] Renal tumors are more often found incidentally during the course of various diagnostic tests.

Pain associated with renal carcinoma is described as a constant, dull ache confined to the flank or abdomen. If bleeding is present within the tumor the pain may be increased or acute. Significant bleeding may result in the passage of clots in the urine, thus leading to clot colic. Diffuse pain may also signify the local extension of disease and the presence of distant metastases.[16]

The second sign associated with the triad, gross or microscopic hematuria, usually occurs only when tumor has invaded the renal pelvis. If bleeding is present, it is generally only intermittent.

Palpation of an abdominal or flank mass is the least commonly encountered third sign of the triad. When detectable, the mass is generally firm, homogeneous, nontender, and found to move with respiration. If a hemorrage into the tumor has occurred, pain may be associated with palpation of the mass.[16]

The lack of characteristic early signs and symptoms of renal cell carcinoma prevents early diagnosis. Early disease may remain clinically silent for a long time. In the early states, renal damage is not sufficient to cause signs and symptoms of fluid and electrolyte and acid–base imbalance. Renal cell carcinoma may disguise itself with a variety of symptom patterns suggestive of other diseases. Many systemic and hormonal manifestations are associated with renal cell carcinoma. They are known collectively as paraneoplastic syndromes and include such common clinical manifestations as fever, anemia, erythrocytosis, hepatic dysfunction, hypercalcemia, and amyloidosis.[16]

Medical Management

Diagnosis. Radiologic procedures are of primary importance in diagnosing renal cell carcinoma. The following tests are commonly performed in an attempt to diagnose this tumor:[5,16]

Excretory urography, or *intravenous pyelogram* (IVP). This test, which shows alterations of the kidney, is the first step toward diagnosis of most renal tumors.

Nephrotomography is a safe procedure that is useful in differentiating between renal cysts and tumors.

Ultrasonography is useful in differentiating cystic vs. solid renal lesions.

Retrograde pyelography aids in opacificating portions of the collecting system that are not visualized by IVP.

Selective renal arteriography is a highly accurate means of diagnosing renal cell carcinoma. It provides evidence of the extent of the tumor and defines the renal blood supply preoperatively.

Computed tomography (CT) scans define the nature of the lesions and show the relationship of tumor to the structures surrounding the kidneys (*i.e.,* renal vein, vena cava, and lymph nodes).

Venacavography is useful in determining the extent of the tumor. The presence of filling defects or obstructions in the vena cava or renal vein helps define the type of surgery required.

In addition to the clinical diagnostic workup, the staging workup for renal cell carcinoma involves a surgical evaluation. Staging decision is based on findings at surgical exploration, biopsy, pathological evaluation of the totally resected kidney, its tumor and nodes.[5] The pathological staging of renal cell carcinoma is as follows:

Stage I	Tumor is confined within the kidney capsule.
Stage II	Tumor invades through the renal capsule but is confined within Gerota's fascia.
Stage III	There is local spread. Tumor has invaded regional lymph nodes, ipsilateral renal vein, or inferior vena cava.
Stage IV	There is tumor extension to adjacent organs other than the ipsilateral adrenal gland or documentation of distant metastasis.

The workup for metastatic disease should include chest tomography, bone scan, liver function studies and liver/spleen scans, since these are sites of early metastasis.

Treatment. The treatment of choice for renal cell carcinoma is total surgical excision or radical nephrectomy. This procedure involves ligation of the tumor vasculature as early as possible during surgery to prevent dissemination of tumor cells. The surgery involves removal of the kidney without opening its surrounding fascia (Gerota's fascia) and removal of the corresponding adrenal gland, which is encompassed by the same fascia. With involvement of regional lymphatics and periaortic lymph nodes, regional lymphadenectomy should be performed in conjunction with radical nephrectomy.[16]

Tumor invasion of the renal vein and inferior vena cava usually occurs as a well-vascularized thrombus. When this is present, and identifiable metastases are absent, radical nephrectomy may be performed following early ligation of the renal artery. At surgery, the aim is to gain control of the vena cava as quickly as possible, avoiding dislodgement of the tumor thrombus. It is impossible for the renal vein to be safely occluded until the arterial supply of the kidney is controlled. In this situation, preoperative renal artery occlusion is a helpful adjunct to surgery. After this is accomplished, attention can be turned to the vena cava without added dissection being required to the artery. Vascular control of the vena cava is obtained above and below the tumor thrombus. The renal vein can be opened at its junction with the vena cava, and the tumor thrombus can gently be removed.[16]

Surgical excision is the preferred treatment for renal cell carcinoma, offering the only chance for cure of the disease. Various adjunctive treatments have been employed, without much success, in attempts to cure or control the disease. These include radiation therapy, chemotherapy and hormonal therapy, immunotherapy, and excision of distant solitary metastases.

Radiation therapy is a controversial form of treatment for renal cell carcinoma.[16] Definitive radiation is rarely employed because renal cell carcinoma is a relatively radioresistant tumor. Postoperative irradiation may be employed in instances where there is lymphatic invasion, perinephric spread, incomplete removal of primary tumor, or metastases that cannot be excised[10] Irradiation can be used for palliation to decrease pain, the size of large masses, or hematuria from renal cell carcinoma.

Chemotherapy and hormonal therapy results are disappointing. Renal cell carcinoma remains one of the tumors most refractory to standard chemotherapy. Although progestational treatment has been employed in the past, there remain no single or combination chemotherapy agents, hormonal agents, or combinations of chemotherapy and hormonal agents that have been shown to be effective in patients with Stage IV disease.[4,5,16]

Immunotherapy requires further investigation. The identification of monocolonal antibodies may provide a basis for specific treatment. However, the ability of such antibodies to act on large bodies of solid tumors remains in doubt.[4]

Excision of solitary metastases (especially brain, liver, and bone) along with nephrectomy have resulted in occasional cures.[5]

Approximately 30% of patients have metastatic disease at diagnosis.[4] In patients with metastatic disease, palliative nephrectomy has been employed for relief of local pain, for hemorrhage, or for severe hormonal or paraneoplastic symptoms resulting from the primary tumor.[5,16] This type of surgery is justified in patients who are likely to survive several months.[4,16]

Prognosis. The most important determinant of prognosis in renal cell carcinoma is the pathological stage of the tumor when it is initially diagnosed and treated.[16] Five-year survival following radical nephrectomy for Stage I renal cell carcinoma ranges from 60% to 75%, while patients with Stage II lesions have a survival from 47% to 65%.[17,22,27]

Patients with renal vein or inferior vena caval involvement have five-year survival of 25% to 50%, whereas it is 12% to 25% for patients with regional lymph node involvement or extracapsular extension.[16,21] Patients with effective surgical removal of renal vein or inferior vena caval thrombus have shown 5-year survival rates of 25% to 50%.[19,27] It is hoped that improved survival will result from earlier diagnosis of "incidental" carcinomas found on excretory urograms and tomograms and on abdominal computed tomography scans.[5]

Nursing Management

The nursing care of patients with renal cell carcinoma requires a knowledge of the disease process, the various treatments employed for management of the disease or its accompanying symptoms, and specific goals of therapy. Renal cell carcinoma is a life-threatening disease that may require extensive, radical treatment. Because nurses may be caring for patients at all stages of their disease it is incumbent on them to provide support, instruction, and skilled care at many levels.

Some patients may be candidates for *renal artery occlusion* preceding radical nephrectomy, when there is vena caval tumor involvement. Provision of skilled nursing care is dependent on a knowledge of the procedure and the treatment of the side-effects resulting from it. Teaching is an important component of nursing care for both patients facing this procedure and subsequent radical nephrectomy, and their family members.

Nursing Diagnosis. Possible nursing diagnoses, secondary to the renal artery occlusion procedure, include anxiety, and alterations in comfort related to the procedure and resulting from the postinfarction syndrome. The patient will experience pain, nausea and vomiting, and fever, side-effects that are inherent to the syndrome.

Goals. General patient goals should center around attempts to decrease anxiety through knowledge of the procedure, including the reason why it is being performed, its temporary side-effects, and its expected benefits. Efforts should be made to minimize physical discomfort resulting from the procedure and to assure the patient that the experienced side-effects are only temporary.

Interventions. Patient teaching is an important component of care. Patients facing renal artery occlusion must be taught about the procedure. They should understand that the procedure enhances the ability to control the primary renal tumor. Occlusion of the renal artery prior to radical nephrectomy allows for a reduction of tumor size and vascularity. Patients should understand that the procedure is preliminary to radical nephrectomy. They should be instructed that the postinfarction syndrome associated with the procedure is temporary and should last less than 3 days. Patients and family members must be taught that the postinfarction syndrome encompasses the side-effects of pain, nausea and vomiting, and fever.

In order to maintain patient comfort during the postinfarction period, a number of interventions are indicated. Patients should receive parenteral narcotics for the significant amount of pain that they will almost immediately experience. Antipyretics may be administered to control temperature elevations that may persist for several days. With temperatures above 102.6°F (39°C), blood cultures should be drawn.[10] Antibiotics are indicated only in the presence of proven infection or in patients who are at risk of developing infection within the necrotic tumor mass.[10]

Mild to moderate nausea and vomiting may be treated with antiemetics. Use of such agents may also help to decrease the patient's anxiety. Accurate monitoring of intake and output is essential during this period of fluid loss. Intravenous fluid replacement may be necessary if the patient's oral intake is not adequate.

Evaluation. Patients who have been adequately instructed about renal artery occlusion and the postinfarction syndrome will be less anxious about the procedure. Patient comfort will be evidenced by palliation of pain, control of temperature elevation, and minimization of gastrointestinal complaints with maintenance of adequate fluid and electrolyte balance.

Radical nephrectomy is the treatment of choice for many patients with renal cell carcinoma. The patient facing such an extensive procedure requires specialized teaching preoperatively and astute nursing care and assessment postoperatively. The specific interventions and outcome criteria for the patient with renal cell carcinoma is found in the Nursing Care Plan for the Patient Undergoing Radical Nephrectomy. This is only a guide; each patient has individualized needs and hence individual nursing care plans.

Renal Pelvic and Ureteral Neoplasms

Tumors of the renal pelvis and ureter are relatively rare. Transitional cell and squamous cell carcinoma of the renal pelvis account for approximately 5% of all renal tumors.[10] The incidence of renal pelvic carcinoma is approximately 1 per 183,000 population.[20] Carcinoma of the ureter accounts for less than 1% of all genitourinary neoplasms.[10] Approximately two thirds of these tumors occur in the lower one third of the urether.[16]

Renal pelvic and ureteral tumors usually occur in the sixth to seventh decades of life and are rarely seen in persons less than 30 years old.[16] The tumors are twice as common in males as females.[16]

Etiology

Specific chemicals are associated with the incidence of transitional cell carcinoma of the upper urinary tract. Persons who have worked for long periods of time in the aniline dye, rubber, textile, and plastic industries have shown an increased incidence of transitional cell carcinoma.[16]

Phenacetin-containing analgesics have also been shown to place users at an increased risk for cancer of the renal pelvis. Tobacco, combined with such analgesics, seems to exert a synergistic effect on the renal pelvis. Similarly, tobacco use alone shows a strong correlation with cancer of the ureter and renal pelvis.[11] It is also believed that some renal pelvic tumors might result from chronic irritation and inflammation secondary to calculous disease.[5]

Pathophysiology

Transitional cell carcinoma alone or with squamous or glandular differentiation accounts for 90% of all tumors of the renal pelvis and ureter.[16] The spread of transitional cell carcinoma occurs by direct extension or by metastasis by means of hematogenous of lymphatic routes.[5,16] The regional lymph nodes are most often involved before other sites of metastasis. The most common sites of metastasis include lung, liver, lymph nodes, and bone.[16]

Clinical Manifestations

The most common presenting symptom, occurring in nearly 75% of patients with renal pelvic and ureteral tumors, is hematuria.[16] Hematuria may present early or late in the disease. Most often it is gross and painless.

Approximately one third of patients with ureteral carcinoma will experience flank pain.[10] Pain over the kidney may be caused by acute ureteral colic from the passage of blood clots through the ureter or from ureteral obstruction.[10,16]

Additional presenting symptoms may include urinary frequency, dysuria, fever of unknown origin, back pain, malaise, weight loss, or inanition.[10,13,16] Palpation usually does not detect any abnormality. However, a palpable renal mass secondary to hydronephrosis may be present in a thin patient.

Medical Management

Diagnosis. A variety of radiological and cytological studies are useful in diagnosing carcinomas of the renal pelvis and ureter. The following tests are routinely performed for diagnostic purposes:[5,10,16]

Cystoscopy is important in diagnosing renal pelvis carcinoma. The procedure allows the physician to visualize blood spilling from a ureteral orifice and to localize the bleeding source. It is also an important test in the diagnosis of ureteral carcinoma. Cystoscopic visualization of the ureteral orifice and submucosal tunnel will permit identification of a tumor low in the ureter.

Excretory urography (intravenous pyelogram) will depict a defect of pelvic-filling in patients with carcinoma of the renal pelvis. It should be performed with *retrograde urography* in patients suspected of ureteral carcinoma.

Cytological examination of urine is helpful in diagnosing transitional cell carcinomas of the urinary tract. Retrograde brushings of the ureter and renal pelvis may yield valuable material for diagnosis.

Renal arteriography differentiates tumors of renal parenchymal origin from those arising in the collecting system.

Bulb ureterography, performed under fluoroscopy, is the preferred study for diagnosing ureteral tumors. The ureter that has been dilated below the kidney appears as the classic "goblet sign."

(*Text continues on page 805*)

NURSING CARE PLAN FOR THE PATIENT UNDERGOING RADICAL NEPHRECTOMY

NURSING DIAGNOSIS/PROBLEM 1: Anxiety related to fear of the diagnosis of renal cell carcinoma and the loss of a kidney by radical nephrectomy

Nursing Interventions	Rationale	Outcome Criteria
1. Establish rapport with patient and family and observe their behavior with regard to the diagnosis and impending surgery. a. Promote expressions of anxiety. b. Assist the patient and family to verbalize feelings. c. Provide reassurance and support.	1. Nurse is responsible for meeting the educational needs of patient and family. Patient and family concerns will be identified and level of anxiety will be assessed.	1. Supportive, trusting relationship will be established. The patient and family will seek information about the surgical procedure and postoperative care. Patient and family will verbalize fears regarding diagnosis, will verbalize decrease in level of anxiety.
2. Teach patient and family what radical nephrectomy is, why it is indicated, and what it is hoped to accomplish. (Reinforce physician's instruction through the use of pictures and diagrams.)	2. Radical nephrectomy is accomplished by early ligation of the renal artery and renal vein and en bloc removal of the kidney and adrenal gland with the surrounding Gerota's fascia, followed by regional lymphadenectomy.[16]	2. Patient and family will verbalize understanding of the extent of the surgery and the reason for it. The family is supportive to the patient.
3. Instruct patient that the remaining kidney will assume the work of both kidneys.	3. Many patients are fearful that they will not live normally with only one kidney.	3. Patient's fear about functioning with one remaining kidney will be abated.
4. Provide preoperative teaching to patient and family (including what to expect following surgery).	4. Patient independence is promoted through preparatory educational instruction.	4. Patient will verbalize activities he will perform and how he can participate in his care and contribute to a positive postoperative outcome.
5. Preoperatively, the patient's affected side is cleansed and shaved from the nipple to midthigh.	5. The patient will have an incision made either in his flank or abdomen. The cleansing will help guard against infection.	5. No postoperative infection occurs.

NURSING DIAGNOSIS/PROBLEM 2: Potential postoperative complications (respiratory infection, shock, pain, wound infection, fluid and electrolyte imbalance, and gastrointestinal distention) related to radical nephrectomy surgery

Nursing Interventions	Rationale	Outcome Criteria
1. Check lung sounds, observe for any signs of dyspnea. A regular schedule of turning, coughing, and deep breathing is established (usually every 2 hr). Assist the patient and support the operative site.	1. Prevention of atelectasis and/or pneumonia. Early detection of pneumothrax. Deep breathing is likely to be painful, possibly predisposing to shallow respirations.[28]	1. No evidence of respiratory complications. Absence of fever, dyspnea, or lung congestion.
2. Check vital signs every 2–4 hr; be alert to the signs of shock.	2. Prevention or early detection of hemorrhagic shock. Secondary hemorrhage may develop due to delayed healing and the sloughing of renal tissue.[28]	2. Normal vital signs, normal skin color and temperature
3. Check incisional dressing every 4 hr (especially under the patient's back if he has a flank incision).[9]		3. No evidence of bloody drainage.

(Continued)

NURSING CARE PLAN FOR THE PATIENT UNDERGOING RADICAL NEPHRECTOMY (*Continued*)

Nursing Interventions	Rationale	Outcome Criteria
4. Determine the source and severity of pain. Administer analgesics as ordered. Position with a small pillow placed between the lower costal margin and the iliac crest when the patient is on his side to reduce discomfort by relieving pain on the incision.[28]	4. Some discomfort may result from the hyperextended lateral position the patient was placed in during surgery for maximum exposure and facilitation of the surgical procedure.	4. Patient verbalizes an adequate reduction or absence of pain and resumption of comfort.
5. Observe incisional dressing every 4 hr during the first 24–48 hr.	5. Dressings usually require changing or reinforcement once per shift early in the postoperative period.[9]	5. Absence of fever and any abnormal wound conditions, including purulent exudate, erythema, edema, dehiscence, or hematoma.
6. Observe the incision for presence of edema, erythema, ecchymosis, hematoma, or wound dehiscence.[9]	6. Patients with cancer are often in marginal nutritional status, which increases the danger of wound infection and wound dehiscence.	6. An accurate assessment of wound appearance will be maintained and abnormalities will be noted as they occur so that appropriate interventions may be promptly instituted.
7. Note the presence of purulent wound drainage.[9] Obtain wound culture.	7. This indicates infection. culturing will identify the microbial source of the infection and will define the necessary antibiotic treatment.	
8. Temperature should be taken every 4 hr.	8. Elevation of temperature ($\geq$ 101°F) may indicate the presence of a wound infection.[9]	8. Temperature elevation remains under 101°F. If temperature increases $\geq$ 101°F, the physician is notified.
9. Monitor the patient's fluid and electrolyte status carefully.[9] a. Monitor intravenous infusion volume and rate. Strict record of intake and output b. Be alert to the signs of electrolyte imbalance, including changes in level of consciousness, changes in respiratory status (rate and depth), cardiac abnormalities, and abnormalities in muscle tone. c. Be alert to signs of fluid overload, including pulmonary congestion or central venous pressure elevation.	9. Any abnormalities that arise place the remaining kidney at risk for complications and/or deterioration. Prompt attention to abnormalities may prevent irreversible consequences. Removal of the adrenal gland in conjunction with the diseased kidney may contribute to a possible fluid imbalance.	9. Patient retains appropriate fluid and electrolyte status. • Adequate hydration is maintained. • Remaining kidney is functioning within its normal capacity. • Early detection and reporting of any manifestations of complications
10. Monitor gastrointestinal function.[9]	10. A period of intestinal atony often follows this surgery.	10. Resumption of bowel sounds within 24–48 hr and passage of flatus.
a. Restrict oral intake until bowel sounds are heard and flatus is passed (usually 24–48 hr).	a. Bowel sound resumption and passage of flatus indicate that the intestines are regaining their function.	a. Absence of abdominal distention or nausea and vomiting following resumption of oral intake
b. Be alert to symptoms of distention, nausea, or vomiting following resumption of oral intake.	b. Premature oral intake may cause nausea and vomiting, abdominal distention, and abdominal discomfort.	

(*Continued*)

NURSING CARE PLAN FOR THE PATIENT UNDERGOING RADICAL NEPHRECTOMY (*Continued*)

Nursing Interventions	Rationale
c. Clear liquids are given orally and intake is increased as tolerated based on the physician's orders.	c. Oral intake is resumed when intestinal peristalsis is reestablished.

NURSING DIAGNOSIS/PROBLEM 3: Knowledge deficit of home care and continued medical follow-up

Nursing Interventions	Rationale	Outcome Criteria
1. Provide discharge teaching to patient and family regarding self-care needs. a. Explain indications, side-effects, dosage, and schedule for all discharge medications. b. Explain that the patient may experience incisional pain and continued fatigue as a normal effect of the surgery for several weeks.	1. This instruction will prepare patient to return to an independent position outside hospital and help him to establish realistic goals with regard to recovery.	1. In discussions, patient will evidence understanding of discharge instructions and an understanding of realistic expectations for himself upon discharge.
2. Instruct the patient to notify the physician if any of the following occur:[9] a. Chills, fever, hematuria, flank pain b. Sudden decrease in urinary output in spite of maintenance of normal fluid intake c. Weight loss, bone pain, change in mental status, or numbness or weakness of extremities	2. Renal damage must be prevented by immediate medical intervention.[9] a. May indicate urinary tract infection b. May indicate renal failure c. May indicate metastatic spread of tumor	2. Patient will state the signs of impending renal problems. ▪ He will indicate accurately when to call the physician. ▪ Kidney damage will be avoided and possible spread of tumor will be identified. ▪ Patient will return to the physician for follow-up care.
3. Provide patient with discharge diet instruction	3. Diet following radical nephrectomy will be individualized for each patient depending on the status and function of the remaining kidney.	3. Patient will verbalize the diet and/or fluid restrictions that he must adhere to, and the reasons for such restrictions.
4. Provide patient with information related to follow-up medical care (need for periodic appointments for physical examination and diagnostic examination).	4. It will be necessary for the physician to monitor the patient's kidney function and to check for tumor spread.	4. Patient will have knowledge and a written record of his initial follow-up appointment following discharge. He will verbalize an understanding of why periodic checkups are required and will have a general idea of how often he will need to be seen by the physician.
5. Assess home support to determine: a. Whether a care-giver will be available to assist the patient for the first few postoperative weeks; b. Whether the care-giver is able to properly monitor the patient's status and recognize possible complications.	5. The patient and family often benefit from professional reassurance in the home for the first few weeks following discharge. Professional monitoring of the patient's status may be indicated. The patient and family may need nursing assistance if further treatment is indicated.	5. Patient and family will cope adequately with recovery and possible further therapy.
6. Refer the patient and family to a community nursing agency for continued nursing care in the home.		

Treatment. The treatment of choice for transitional cell carcinoma of the renal pelvis or ureter is radical nephroureterectomy.[5,16] This procedure includes removal of the kidney, ureter, the attached portion of bladder on the involved side and the surrounding lymphatic structures. Ureter removal prevents the tendency for transitional cell pelvic tumors to "seed" down the ureter into the bladder, or to be multifocal.[5] This procedure is indicated for patients with invasive disease whose radiological studies indicate renal pelvic tumor and whose cytologic studies are positive. It is also indicated in patients whose tumor is present at a site other than the distal ureter.[10] Less radical procedures such as distal ureterectomy with ureteral implantation may be performed when noninvasive disease occurs in the lower one third of the ureter.[10]

In the absence of performing the surgeries already mentioned, palliative measures may be taken to prevent obstruction of the ureter by tumor. A urinary diversion may be performed or a flexible silicon ureteral stent may be placed for maintenance of patency.[10]

Chemotherapy is not effective in treating advanced carcinomas of the renal pelvis or ureter. Radiation therapy remains an unproven adjunct in controlling residual tumor, unresectable tumor, or local recurrence. Radiotherapy may be useful in treating inoperable or disseminated tumors.[5,10,16]

Prognosis. Delay in diagnosis, often resulting from lack of significant symptoms, leads to delay in treatment and ultimately a poor prognosis for patients with urothelial tumors.[16] Symptoms may be overlooked for periods up to 2 years.

Depth of tumor invasion seems to be the most accurate indicator of survival. Generally, patients with highly invasive tumors have a worse prognosis than those with superficial low-stage lesions.[13]

Nursing Management

Nursing care of the patient undergoing surgery for transitional cell carcinoma of the renal pelvis or ureter is very similar to that required for the patient undergoing surgery for renal cell carcinoma or carcinoma of the bladder.

As with any grave disorder such as this, the patient and family will experience a great deal of anxiety about the impending surgery and its outcome. Providing as much information about the surgical procedure, what it involves, and what the patient will experience postoperatively will alleviate some of this anxiety and promote a supportive atmosphere for expression of feelings.

In the postoperative period, there are potential complications of respiratory difficulties, shock, pain, wound infection, fluid and electrolyte imbalance, and gastrointestinal discomfort. Carrying out comfort measures and ongoing evaluation are essential in detecting and eliminating these potential problems. Check lung sounds for signs of dyspnea and vital signs every 2 to 4 hours for any evidence of hemorrhagic shock. Determine the source and severity of pain and administer analgesics as ordered. Observe the incisional dressing and check for the presence of edema, erythema, hematoma or wound dehiscence, as well as for any evidence of purulent drainage. Fluid and electrolyte status is determined by monitoring IV volume and rate, maintaining strict intake and output records, and observing the patient for any signs of electrolyte imbalance such as changes in level of consciousness, respiratory rate, or cardiac function.

Once the patient has recovered and is preparing to go home, the nurse should offer discharge planning information related to home care procedures, medication, possible complications, diet instruction, and follow-up medical care. The details for all these interventions, with rationale and expected outcomes, are given in the accompanying Nursing Care Plan for the Patient Undergoing Radical Nephrectomy, and can be extrapolated to fit the needs of the patient undergoing nephroureterectomy.

Bladder Neoplasms

Bladder carcinoma is the most common urinary tract neoplasm. Transitional cell carcinomas represent 90% to 95% of all primary bladder cancers. Epidermoid and squamous cell carcinomas constitute 5% to 7% of primary bladder carcinomas, while only 1% to 2% are adenocarcinomas.[26] Eighty-four percent of all bladder cancers occur on the lateral and posterior walls of the bladder, whereas 40% occur on the trigone.[5] An estimated 30,000 new cases of bladder cancer occur in the United States annually.[5,20] This tumor is responsible for 2.5% of all cancer deaths in the United States.[5]

Bladder cancer is three times more common in men than in women and is seen four times more often in whites than blacks. It is most common in the 50- to 70-year age-group. The average age at diagnosis is 68.[26] The incidence of bladder cancer varies with geographic location. It is more frequently encountered in highly industrial areas.

Etiology

Numerous carcinogens have been implicated in the development of bladder carcinoma. Aromatic amines, used in the rubber, leather, and dye industries, are the best known carcinogens.[26] A latency period of 6 to 20 years exists from the time of the exposure to these carcinogens in humans until tumor transformation.[5]

Cigarette smokers are twice as likely to develop bladder carcinomas as nonsmokers.[3] Similarly, persons who experience chemical cystitis, associated with cyclophosphamide, or who ingest large quantities of phenacetin are at higher risk for the development of bladder carcinoma.[26]

Chronic bladder infections and calculous disease are believed to be associated with the development of squamous cell carcinoma of the bladder.[5] Specifically, infection with *Schistosoma haematobium* causes chronic irritation of the bladder mucosa. As a result, this parasite is suspected as a factor in the development of bladder carcinoma. Artificial sweeteners such as cyclamates and saccharin have been suggested as etiologic agents; however, studies have failed to provide definitive evidence of an increased risk in heavy users of such agents.[14]

Pathophysiology

Transitional cell carcinoma of the bladder is characterized by an ability to develop multiple recurrences in multiple separate areas in the bladder, ureters, renal pelvis, and prostatic ducts. Twenty-five percent of patients with bladder carcinoma will initially present with multiple separate tumors in the bladder.[26] Thirty percent of patients with one bladder carcinoma at diagnosis will develop new or recurrent tumor within 5 years.[12] The risk of tumor recurrence is primarily related to the cytological differentiation of the initial tumor cells and to the number of tumors present at the time of diagnosis.[26]

The natural course of bladder tumors is unpredictable. The extent of disease at diagnosis is important in defining risk of additional bladder tumors and in defining initial management.[26] At initial diagnosis, 82% of patients have a tumor or tumors confined to the bladder, 9% have regional disease, and 6% have distant metastases.[20] A definition of bladder cancer staging follows.

- Stage 0 — Carcinoma *in situ* and superficial tumor limited to the mucosa
- Stage A — Superficial tumor extending into the submucosa
- Stage B_1 — Involvement of superficial muscle layers of bladder
- Stage B_2 — Deep invasion of muscle layers of bladder
- Stage C — Extension through serosal surface of the bladder or perivesical fat
- Stage D_1 — Metastatic invasion of pelvic lymph nodes or adjacent pelvic organs
- Stage D_2 — Metastasis beyond the pelvis

The most common sites of disseminated metastatic disease are lung, bone, and liver. Patients who have not been treated with cystectomy or pelvic radiation also have a high incidence of tumor penetration into the pelvic soft tissues, vagina, and rectum.[26]

Clinical Manifestations

Gross hematuria is the most common initial symptom in 75% of bladder cancer patients.[5] Virtually all patients will present with microscopic hematuria.[5] The next most common symptom is frequent bladder irritability and dysuria, occurring in one third of patients.[5,26] This symptom increases in the later stages of the disease.

It is important to note that the above symptoms often suggest urinary tract infection. Urinary tract infections must be carefully evaluated, especially in older persons, so that an early bladder carcinoma is not overlooked.[26] Advanced cases may present with symptoms of rectal obstruction, pelvic pain from local extension or nerve root involvement, or lower extremity edema secondary to lymphatic or venous occlusion.

Medical Management

Diagnosis

Certain radiological, surgical, and cytological procedures are critical to the diagnosis and staging of bladder carcinoma. Accurate staging based on the following procedures will lead to appropriate treatment planning and a prediction of eventual prognosis.[5,26]

Excretory urography (intravenous pyelogram) is useful in detecting a renal mass, stone, ureteral obstruction, lymph node involvement, or other tumors of the pelvocaliceal system or ureters.

Cystoscopy with biopsy of visualized lesions is the definitive procedure for diagnosing bladder cancer and determining the extent of tumor. Repeat cystoscopies at regular intervals are important to rule out recurrence following successful treatment.

Bimanual examination of the bladder while the patient is under anesthesia is an important staging procedure that provides useful information about local extent of the tumor.

Urine cytology is a useful adjunct in detecting malignant cells following resection of bladder rather than as an initial diagnostic procedure.

Treatment

Treatment of bladder carcinoma may involve a single surgical procedure or a combination of therapies including surgery, radiation, and/or chemotherapy. Medical management is dependent on the extent of the disease (stage), the general health of the patient, previous treatment, and the person's history of tumor recurrence rate.[5] For the purpose of discussing treatment, bladder carcinoma may be divided into three categories: superficial, invasive, and metastatic disease.

Superficial Transitional Cell Carcinoma (Stages 0, A, B_1). *Transurethral resection* or transurethral resection with fulguration will adequately control tumor that is singular, superficial, shows no muscle invasion, and shows a slow recurrence rate.[5,26] Transurethral resection alone is not sufficient for patients with Stage A or B_1 tumors that are multiple or occur in association with carcinoma *in situ*.

There is a risk of recurrence and multiplicity of tumors in patients with superficial bladder tumors. Therefore, cystoscopy should be performed on these patients every 3 months for 2 years, then every 6 months for 3 more years.[26] If suspicious lesions are found, they should be biopsied immediately.

Patients who are treated for superficial tumors but are at a high risk for recurrence may benefit from *intravesical chemotherapy* with agents such as thio-TEPA, doxorubicin, or mitomycin C.[24] Thio-TEPA has been widely used and may be safely administered into the bladder. Results have shown complete eradication of visible superficial carcinomas in 50% to 60% of cases.[26]

Segmental bladder resection (partial cystectomy) may be performed for large, single, superficial transitional cell carcinomas located in the dome of the bladder or the lateral wall. Patients with diffuse or multiple recurrent disease that is resistant to intravesical chemotherapy, may benefit from simple cystectomy with placement of an ileal urinary conduit.[5,26]

The role of *radiation therapy* in the treatment of superficial transitional cell carcinomas has not been clearly defined. Intercavity radium may be indicated following transurethral resection. The use of external beam radiation is still under investigation. Radiation treatment is indicated only after traditional surgical measures such as transurethral resection and fulguration, and applications of topical chemotherapy have failed to control the tumor.[5]

Invasive Transitional Cell Carcinoma (Stages B_2, C). *Total cystectomy* is indicated in bladder tumors that are invasive or anaplastic or that involve the trigone for patients who have a reasonable life expectancy.[5] This radical procedure requires permanent urinary diversion and often includes resection of local pelvic lymph nodes.[5] When performed in the male patient the surgery includes the removal of the bladder, prostate, seminal vesicles, and often the urethra. It invariably results in sexual impotence. In female patients the procedure involves removal of the bladder and the urethra.[5,26]

The surgery may be performed as two procedures (with urinary diversion and staging first, followed by cystectomy) or as one procedure.[5] Forms of *urinary diversion* that are commonly performed include the ileal loop, colon loop, ureterosigmoidostomy, ureteroileosigmoidostomy, cutaneous ureterostomy, and rectosigmoid bladder. Cutaneous vesicostomy, cutaneous urethrostomy, and continent vesicostomy are less commonly performed.[10]

Used prior to surgery, *radiation therapy* has been reported to be a safe adjunct that seems to enhance the control of invasive bladder carcinoma.[5,26] Alternative treatment with radiation therapy may be indicated when medical conditions prevent combinations of preoperative radiation followed by surgery.[5] Clinical investigations continue into the role of radiation therapy in the management of invasive bladder carcinoma.

The role of *systemic chemotherapy* (following radiation and cystectomy) in the possible prevention of systemic metastases is currently under investigation.

Advanced Metastatic Disease. The primary goal of treatment of patients with advanced bladder carcinoma is symptom management and palliative treatment of disease. Painful bone lesions, painful urination, and bleeding are symptoms caused by advanced lesions and may be effectively palliated with radiation therapy. Instillation of 10% formalin is often useful in controlling life-threatening bladder hemorrhaging.[26] In selected cases, simple cystectomy and urinary diversion may be performed when repeated episodes of bladder hemorrhage occur or when ureteral obstruction is severe.[10,26]

Currently, there is no established systemic chemotherapeutic drug protocol for the treatment of metastatic bladder carcinoma.[5] Cisplatin is the single most effective chemotherapeutic agent in bladder carcinoma. In many patients it causes a significant reduction of both symptoms and measurable tumor masses.[26] Cyclophosphamide, methotrexate, vinblastine, doxorubicin, 5-fluorouracil, and mitomycin C are additional chemotherapeutic drugs that have shown some therapeutic value in disseminated bladder cancer.

Patients with advanced bladder carcinoma should be carefully evaluated before vigorous treatments are employed. Careful evaluation of the goals of treatment should always be made. This evaluation is particularly important in elderly or debilitated patients. Treatment goals for such patients should concentrate on improved comfort and enhanced functional capacity.

Prognosis

The depth of tumor invasion into the bladder wall (stage) is the most important factor in predicting the ultimate prognosis of a particular lesion.[5] Patients with prior histories of bladder tumors have poorer outcomes. For patients without a history of bladder carcinoma, prognosis for survival is poorer as the initial tumor size increases.[15]

The overall 5-year survival rate for all patients with disease confined to the bladder is 71% to 76%.[8] For patients with local extension or distant metastases, the 5-year survival rate is only 5% to 23%.[8] To date, the best survival rates for patients with invasive bladder cancer have resulted from the combination of cystectomy and adjuvant radiation therapy.[15]

Nursing Management

Patients with carcinoma of the bladder may undergo a variety of treatments depending on the extent of their disease. Patients with superficial bladder tumors may undergo transurethral resection, transurethral resection with fulguration, or partial cystectomy. Patients with invasive tumors often face the more radical total cystectomy with permanent urinary diversion. Advanced metastatic disease is usually treated symptomatically, the goal of treatment being palliation of the disease. The nurse plays an important role in caring for patients with bladder cancer. Her knowledge of the disease process and her technical expertise in caring for patients undergoing such procedures will influence the patient's understanding of, and ability to undergo, the procedures. It will also influence the patient's ability to cope with the physical and emotional changes the procedures impose.

Transurethral Resection: Nursing Management

Nursing Diagnosis. Nursing diagnoses specifically related to patients undergoing transurethral resection and fulguration include knowledge deficit regarding perioperative events; potential for postoperative complications such as shock, infection, voiding difficulties, and pain; potential for complications arising from inadequate management of the indwelling urethral catheter and continuous bladder irrigation; and patient/family knowledge deficit regarding self-care following discharge.

Goals. Nursing goals relate to education of the patient with regard to the procedure that will be performed, what to expect postoperatively, and how to manage independently on discharge from the hospital. Additional goals relate to the prevention of postoperative complications and maintenance of comfort.

Preoperative Interventions. Patients undergoing transurethral resection and fulguration of bladder tumors require preoperative instruction. The procedure, whereby a resectoscope is inserted through the urethra, a clear solution is infused into the bladder for visibility, and an electric current is used to resect and cauterize the tumors, should be thoroughly explained to the patient. It should also be explained that an indwelling urethral catheter will be placed following the procedure and will remain in place for 1 to 5 days, depending on tumor size and extent of bleeding, and that the urine will be slightly bloody early in the postoperative period.[9] Continuous bladder irrigation (which will require approximately 24 hours of bed rest postoperatively) may also be employed. The patient should be instructed that hospitalization will last anywhere from 2 to 7 days.

Postoperative Interventions. Potential postoperative side-effects should be anticipated. Because severe bleeding may occur following resection of tumors, the patient should be observed for *shock*. Vital signs should be checked every 4 hours and careful attention should be paid to an increased pulse and respiratory rate, a decreased blood pressure, diaphoresis, pallor, and apprehension. Hypovolemic shock may occur if the tumors are highly vascular or if complete hemostasis is not accomplished.[9]

Prevention and treatment of *infection* may be accomplished by closely monitoring the patient's temperature every 4 hours and by investigating further possible sites of infection when the temperature is $\geq$ 101° F (38° C). If manipulation of the urethral catheter is required during irrigation, it is suggested that the temperature be taken every 2 hours. This will help detect any infection resulting from introduction of bacteria into the urinary tract.[9] Following removal of the catheter the patient should be observed closely for signs of inability to resume the preoperative voiding pattern and for dysuria. In evaluation of intake following catheter removal, determine if the inability to void is a problem. For instance, an intake of 500 ml should necessitate voiding within 3 to 4 hours.

Pain is an expected postoperative complication that should be thoroughly assessed with regard to location, intensity, and frequency. The nurse should be alert to the signs of pain that may result from an obstructed catheter, or of irritation of the bladder at the surgical site caused by the catheter.[9] Analgesics should be administered as ordered following assessment of catheter patency, fixation to avoid irritation at the urethral orifice, or pull that may be causing bladder neck irritation.

Proper *care of the indwelling catheter* will help prevent any untoward complications following surgery. Attention should be paid to the color of the urine and the presence of clots. Frank bloody urine is not normally present following this type of surgery.[9] Any cessation of urine output, despite hand irrigation of the catheter, should be promptly reported. The nurse should be familiar with the signs of bladder perforation, which include suprapubic pain, abdominal rigidity, decreasing catheter drainage in spite of good hydration, and fever.[9] If bladder perforation is suspected, the physician should be immediately notified and oral intake should be held.

If continuous *bladder irrigation* is instituted following surgery, the nurse should observe the patient for the presence of any bladder distention or abdominal discomfort that may indicate an obstruction. She should further note how freely the drainage flows and the color of the drainage. The norm is a clear or slightly blood-tinged color.[26]

In the absence of any postoperative complications and in preparation for discharge, the patient should receive thorough *discharge instruction*. The patient should be instructed that occasional hematuria may be expected for several weeks following discharge. The patient should be instructed to notify the physician if any of these signs, which include fever, chills, and flank pain, are present. The physician should also be notified at the sign of any urethral blockage (if the patient is unable to void for 6 hours or more in spite of normal fluid intake), or if frank bloody urine continues in spite of an increased fluid intake (possibly indicating hemorrhage).[9]

Follow-up care for the patient with superficial bladder cancer who has undergone transurethral resection and fulguration will require repeat cystoscopies at regular intervals. Urine samples will also be obtained on a regular basis to check for the presence of any malignant cells. The person will need ongoing support, encouragement, and reassurance.

Evaluation. Following appropriate care and instruction, the patient undergoing transurethral resection and fulguration will be able to explain the procedure that is to be performed. He will further be able to verbalize some of the expected postoperative experiences. Postoperative complications will be readily detected and kept to a minimum as a result of astute nursing intervention. The patient and family will be able to describe possible complications after discharge, their manifestations, and actions to take if they should occur. The patient will keep appointments for the periodic follow-up care that he will routinely receive.

Partial and Total Cystectomy: Nursing Management

Nursing Diagnosis. Nursing diagnoses related to the patient undergoing *partial cystectomy* include knowledge deficit of the patient and family with regard to the extent of the surgery and the expected postoperative outcome and experiences; potential for postoperative complications of shock, abnormal wound conditions, voiding difficulties, and pain; potential problems arising from improper management of the indwelling urethral catheter; patient and family knowledge deficit regarding plans for and continued care following discharge. In addition to the above-mentioned diagnoses, the patient undergoing total cystectomy faces potentially overwhelming emotional complications related to sexual impotence, and adjustment to and care of a permanent urinary diversion.

Goals. Goals for the patient undergoing partial cystectomy are similar to those for the patient undergoing transurethral resection and fulguration. Additional goals for the person facing total cystectomy will center around preparation for resumption of a relatively normal active life, and promotion of expression of feelings related to sexual impotence and placement of a permanent urinary diversion. A final goal will be eventual acceptance of and knowledge about the care of the urinary diversion.

Preoperative Interventions. Preoperative teaching for patients facing cystectomy should include a description of the procedure involved. *Partial cystectomy* patients can expect excision of the bladder tumor and some of the normal tissues surrounding it. Postoperatively, patients will have an indwelling urethral catheter in place for approximately 5 days. A drain will exit from the incision site, and it will be covered with a dressing that will be changed periodically. The patient is instructed that the urine will be sightly bloody for several days following surgery.

Preoperative teaching for the patient who will undergo *total cystectomy* is quite extensive. The patient should be taught that the procedure involves removal of the bladder, prostate, seminal vesicles, and possibly the urethra (the bladder and urethra in females) and that it invariably results in impotence. It further involves ureteral transplantation for permanent urinary diversion (see section Urinary Diversion below).

Postoperative Interventions. Postoperative complications will be minimized through ongoing patient assessment and prompt nursing intervention. Blood loss from partial cystectomy should be minimal. The same signs and symptoms of shock that are observed in the patient who has undergone transurethral resection and fulguration are applicable to patients undergoing partial cystectomy. Symptoms of impending shock should be reported immediately.

The potential for *wound complications* is present following partial cystectomy. The patient's physical status is weakened as a result of surgery and of the malignancy itself. The dressing should be checked every shift. According to the physician's orders, a wet dressing should either be reinforced or changed using aseptic technique. The wound should be observed for signs of infection such as purulent drainage. A wound culture should be taken in the presence of such drainage. Culture results will help identify any infecting organisms and help to define appropriate antibiotic treatment.

The patient's temperature should be taken every 4 hours. With an elevation of temperature to ≥ 101°F (38°C), a *wound infection* is suspected. Any wound dehiscence should be reported to the physician. An ongoing record of the presence of any edema, erythema, or ecchymosis at the wound site should also be maintained.[9]

Voiding difficulties may arise following partial cystectomy. Initially, bladder capacity may be lessened to as little as 75 ml to 100 ml, and the patient may need to void frequently for the first few weeks following surgery. This should be only a temporary condition, since the bladder should eventually stretch to regain its full presurgical capacity.

Pain assessment and intervention in the partial cystectomy patient are indentical to that of the patient having undergone transurethral resection and fulguration. The one difference in the cystectomy patient is that the pain source may be the incisional site.

Detection and prevention of complications with regard to the management of the *indwelling urethral catheter* involves observing the urine for the passage of frank blood. There should be little bleeding into the bladder following partial cystectomy, and the urine should be slightly bloody to clear within 48 hours following surgery.[9] With any catheter irrigation, the nurse should be careful not to overdistend the bladder with irrigant. This may result in disruption of the surgical site.[9] The amount of irrigant that can safely be instilled and that must be returned should be established by the physician.

In addition to the complex physical care that is required postoperatively, patients who undergo total cystectomy require comprehensive *psychological support.* The patient's self-concept and feelings regarding sexuality will be threatened by the loss of potency. The change in body image because of the loss of the normal pattern of function resulting from the diversion procedure may cause feelings of shame, depression, and anger (see Chap. 57).

The patient's reactions require thoughtful attention on the part of the nurse. She should encourage expression of his feelings and those of his family and assure the patient that his feelings are normal. The patient needs time to adjust to the changes. The nurse should try to decrease the patient's despair, and help promote acceptance and motivation. Referring the patient to a stoma club for his continued education and support is particularly appropriate.

Discharge Teaching. Discharge teaching for the patient who has undergone partial cystectomy is an important component of care. The patient should be informed that he may experience continued incisional discomfort and fatigue for several weeks following discharge.[9] The patient should be instructed to notify the physician at any signs of urinary tract infection (*e.g.,* chills, fever, flank pain), wound infection (increasing pain at incision site), or if there is blood in his urine (possibly indicative of urinary tract infection or tumor recurrence). Follow-up medical care is similar to that required for patients following transurethral resection and fulguration.

A visiting nurse referral is a necessary intervention for the patient who has undergone total cystectomy. The visiting nurse may continue with and reinforce the extensive discharge teaching about the urinary diversion that was begun in the hospital. She will be valuable in helping the patient adapt to his body image alteration and in providing ongoing physical care and psychological support. A good nurse-to-nurse communication network will be established as a result of such a referral.

Evaluation. Outcome criteria for the patient who has undergone partial cystectomy will include the patient's ability to accurately describe the procedure and the expected postoperative course. The patient will state the discharge instructions and follow-up care. In addition, postoperative complications will be avoided or detected immediately, and the proper interventions will be instituted.

It is hoped that the patient who undergoes total cystectomy will express his feelings related to the surgery and the tremendous physical changes it will impose. Goal achievement will also be related to the patient's ability to care for the stoma and to resume as normal a lifestyle as possible.

Urinary Diversion: Nursing Management

Alteration in the anatomical pathway of urine flow is related to surgical correction of pathological problems within the renal–excretory system. Various types of diversion of urinary flow are possible; the type selected depends on the nature of the problem.

Ileal Conduit. An ileal conduit is the most common type of urinary diversion. The surgical indications include cancer of the bladder, adult neurogenic bladder, and interstitial cystitis and trauma that is irreparable.

An ileal conduit consists of a section of bowel into which the ureters have been transplanted. A small portion of the ileum (stoma) is brought out onto the abdominal wall resulting in a flow of urine from this intestinal stoma (Fig. 60–1). The surgical procedure consists of excision of the ureters from the bladder and transplantation into the segment of the ileum. The ileum section is resected from the intestinal tract along with its mesentery since the mesentery contains the blood supply necessary to maintain tissue viability. The ends of the ileum from which the segment was taken are anastomosed together to reestablish intestinal continuity. The segment of the ileum into which the ureters are transplanted is sutured closed and the other end is brought out onto the abdominal wall. It is referred to as the stoma.

The ileal segment does not serve as a reservoir. The urine flow from the stoma is continuous. Obviously, this is an abnormal means of urine flow.

Nursing Diagnosis. The abnormality of urinary flow and the need to wear special devices to collect the urine and to care for the devices and the skin often underlie problems of body image and self-esteem as well as specific difficulties in managing the equipment and preventing complications of infection and skin excoriation.

Urinary diversion creates problems similar to those experienced by patients and families when treatment of bowel pathologies necessitates diversion of fecal flow through an intestinal stoma on the abdominal wall (colostomy, ileostomy). The reader is referred to Chapter 80 where the nursing care of patients with bowel diversion is discussed in detail.

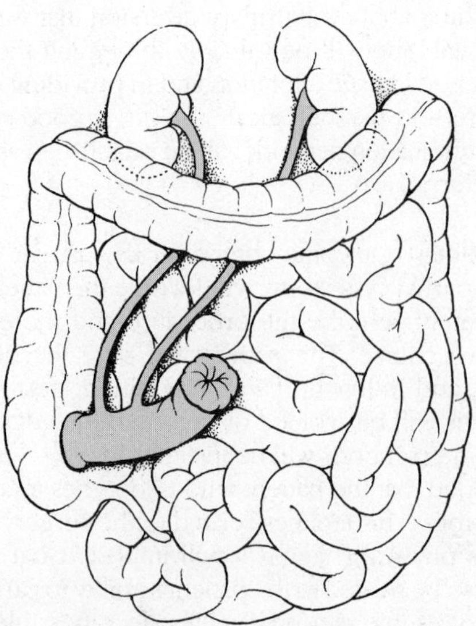

FIGURE 60–1 Ileal conduit.

Goals. The goals of nursing are to support the patient and family throughout the entire experience. Specifically, the goals are to prepare the patient preoperatively; to acquaint the patient with the surgical procedure and what to expect postoperatively; to promote recovery from the surgical procedure; to prevent potential postoperative complications; to teach the patient how to care for the stoma, about the selection and care of equipment; the signs and symptoms of possible complications and actions to take, and sources of support in the community; and to counsel regarding adaptation to this change in body structure. It is essential that nursing care be individualized to the patient and family. Each of these goals and evaluation of its achievement is discussed in the following subsections.

Preoperative and Immediate Postoperative Interventions. Interventions in the preoperative period include teaching and reinforcing the patient's knowledge base and providing emotional support, and an explanation of what can be expected postoperatively. Postoperative interventions consist of assessing the stoma for viability, adequacy of urine drainage, mucous plugging, and pouch fit.

Determining adequate urinary output is imperative. Urine output from the stoma occurs immediately and is continuous, especially while the patient is receiving IV fluids. The urine should become clear yellow after a few days postoperatively. Hematuria is to be expected in the initial postoperative phase, and it should gradually decrease. If it occurs later on, a physician should be notified. Stents (splinting catheters) are used sometimes by surgeons to keep the urine pathways patent. They are removed on the fifth to tenth day postoperatively. The nurse must observe the stents for urine flow and report if there is no flow from either stent. Urine will flow from the stoma as well as the stents. Measurement of the amount of urine output is essential for comparison with the volume of intake. An imbalance between intake and output suggests a problem of renal function, ureter patency, or mucous plugging.

The abdominal drainage pouch needs to be connected to a straight drain collection container when the patient is in bed or during the night. This prevents the pouch from becoming too heavy, which results in leakage. It also prevents stagnant urine in the pouch, which leads to increased bacteria and greater risk of urinary tract infection.

Because the intestine produces mucus it is normal for patients with an ileal or colon conduit to have mucus in the urine. If this is a problem in plugging the spout of the pouch or the tubing of the night drain, there are special solutions available to dissolve the mucus. (Check with stoma equipment suppliers.) Urinary pouches are drainable and can be disposable or temporary. They have a push- , pull- , or twist-type of valve opening that adapts to night drainage. They are available with or without an antireflux valve. The antireflux valve prevents the stoma from being bathed in urine that has collected in the pouch.

Preoperative and Immediate Postoperative Evaluation. Outcome criteria for achievement of goals of preoperative and postoperative care are

1. Patient ability to describe change in urinary drainage that will occur with surgery
2. Patient expression of confidence in regard to outcome of surgery and acceptance of the need for the surgery
3. Stoma appears pink
4. Urine flow is continuous and from both ureters
5. Intake and output balance
6. Mucous plugging does not occur
7. Urine clears to yellow color within 3–5 days postoperatively
8. Drainage pouch is attached to straight drainage container when patient is in bed

Urinary Leakage

Interventions. Nursing interventions to prevent complications or detect their onset early in order that treatment may be instituted promptly are essential. Urinary leakage from anastomosis sites is a potential complication in the immediate postoperative period prior to complete wound healing. Close observation of high-risk patients in the immediate postoperative period for signs and symptoms of urinary leakage is one intervention. The urine leaks into the peritoneal cavity, causing *peritonitis.*

Manifestations of urinary leakage are a sudden decrease in urinary output, presence of abdominal/perineal drainage, abdominal distention and tenderness, prolonged ileus, and fever. These signs and symptoms of peritonitis are detected by taking frequent vital signs, maintaining an accurate intake and output record, assessing the abdomen for distention and tenderness, and assessing wound drainage. Detection of suspicious signs or symptoms should be reported promptly to the physician. It is possible for a leakage site to heal spontaneously; however, it often requires surgical drainage and repair of the anastomosis site.

Patients most prone to urinary leakage are those with potential healing difficulty. Healing may be problematic because of poor nutrition status and/or previous tissue trauma. For instance, persons with diabetes mellitus often have marginal nutritional status that predisposes to impairment of wound healing. Preoperative irradiation as a form of treatment for the pathology does traumatize tissue and impair the healing process.

Preventive interventions include recognition of the high risk in the preoperative period and consultation with the physician and nutritionist regarding improvement of nutritional status. Improvement measures include supplemental protein feedings, increase in vitamin C and B intake, and control of other disease problems such as diabetes mellitus (see Chap. 74). Vitamin supplements should be included in postoperative intravenous therapy. Other measures include assistance with position changes and mobility to avoid undue stress on the suture line.

Evaluation. Outcome criteria for evaluating nursing interventions relative to potential danger of urinary leakage are

1. Absence of signs or symptoms as noted above
2. Wound healing occurs without delay or separation of wound edges
3. If urine leakage occurs, it is recognized promptly and treatment is initiated immediately.

Fluid and Electrolyte Balance

Interventions. The goal of interventions is to prevent fluid and electrolyte imbalance. There is a risk of metabolic acidosis, hypokalemia, and hyperchloremia when ureters are surgically implanted into the ileum, jejunum, or sigmoid colon. These problems result from reabsorption of electrolytes from the intestines when the urine pools in an intestinal pouch for a period of time. The chlorides are reabsorbed, leading to metabolic acidosis if the kidney cannot excrete the excess chlorides. The factors that usually contribute to development of this problem are a long conduit, prolonged time of urine contact with the conduit mucosa, and the presence of impaired renal function. These problems rarely occur with the ileal conduit because the urine remains in the conduit so briefly.

Nursing actions consist of monitoring laboratory reports of pH and serum electrolytes, observing for signs and symptoms of metabolic acidosis and hypokalemia (see Chaps. 13 and 14), and instructing the patient and family about the problem, emphasizing the need to consult with the physician if the symptoms occur. Although fluid and electrolyte imbalance is not common, the patient should be aware of the possibility and the action to take.

Evaluation. The goal of fluid and electrolyte balance will be achieved if.

1. The pH and serum electrolytes remain within normal range.
2. No signs or symptoms of metabolic acidosis or hypokalemia are present.
3. The patient can explain the early signs and symptoms of metabolic acidosis and hypokalemia and the action to take if this occurs.

Potential Infection

Interventions. The goal of nursing is to prevent the occurrence of infection. In the event infection does occur, the goal is early detection and correction of the problem. Residual urine in the conduit, bacterial invasion in the stoma, and ureteroileal reflux are all reasons for a high incidence of urinary tract infections after conduit surgery. Contributing factors include improper hygienic practices when applying the pouch, an alkaline urine, and inadquate fluid intake. Preventive measures include the use of the straight drainage system when the patient is in bed to avoid the presence of stagnant urine in the pouch, a change of pouches every 5 to 7 days, cleaning of the pouch with dishwashing detergent or pouch-cleaning agents followed by white vinegar rinse, and use of clean technique in applying the pouch. The nurse should institute these practices in the hospital and teach them to the patient and family member. Other preventive interventions are to encourage a fluid intake of 2500 ml to

3000 ml every day to promote urine flow, and maintenance of a urine pH at 6.5. An acid urine inhibits bacterial growth. Acid-ash foods include eggs, cheese, whole grains, meat, prunes, cranberries, and plums. The patient should be taught to use chemosticks to determine urine pH, and to adjust nutritional intake accordingly.

Urinary tract infections are likely to occur sometimes, and the patient should be forewarned. Detection of the presence of infection depends on monitoring for fever, flank pain, chills, odoriferous urine, and hematuria. If these manifestations are detected, the physician should be notified. Urine cultures may be desired. In the hospital, the urine speciman should be obtained by using a double- or single- lumen catheter and sterile technique. The patient will need to come to the doctor's office or clinic if the infection occurs after discharge.

Evaluation. Outcome criteria for prevention of potential infection are

1. The patient drinks 2500–3000 ml of fluids each day.
2. Urine pH is maintained in acid range.
3. The patient demonstrates the use of clean technique in applying the urinary pouch.
4. The patient states the pouch is attched to straight drainage when he is in bed.
5. The patient states he changes the pouch every 5–7 days.
6. The patient describes the pouch-cleaning techniques as cleaning with dishwashing detergent followed by a white vinegar rinse.
7. The patient can state the manifestations of infection and that their presence should be reported to the physician.

Obstruction

Interventions. One nursing goal is to prevent the occurrence of factors that predispose to obstruction, namely, edema at the ureteroileal junction, stenosis of the stoma, and peristomal hyperplasia. A second goal is early detection of impending obstruction and prompt reporting to the physician. Postoperatively, the inflammatory process occurs at the site of anastomoses. Edema at the ureteroileal junction or at the fascial level is a possibility. Inflammation accompanying infection of the conduit and ureters may also precipitate obstruction. It is difficult to prevent this occurrence since the usual measures for decreasing edema (*i.e.,* cold applications, elevation, *etc.,* as discussed in Chap. 15) cannot be instituted at the ureteroileal junction.

Detection of obstruction at the ureteroileal junction depends on monitoring of intake and output relationships. Decreased urinary output is one manifestation of obstruction. Undetected obstruction may result in hydronephrosis and renal damage. The physician should be notified of any decrease in urinary output. If stents are in place, it is possible to determine which ureteroileal junction is affected.

Stricture can occur in the stoma at the level of the skin, muscle, fascia, any level of the ileal segment, or at the ureteroileal junction; the result is obstruction, stasis of urine, dilation of the intestinal conduit, and infection. Causes of strictures are inflammation and scarring of the stoma and skin due to prolonged contact with alkaline urine, inflammation accompanying infection, and growth or weight gain of the patient. If a No. 18 French catheter cannot be passed into the stoma of an adult or if there is increased residual urine, stenosis is usually present. An intravenous pyelogram (IVP) or loopogram can be helpful for diagnosis. The patient may be asymptomatic unless urinary stasis is present or there is a urinary tract infection.

Peristomal hyperplasia may present as a wartlike appearance around the stoma. Eventually, the hyperplastic tissue impinges on the stoma, and obstruction may result. A factor contributing to development of peristomal hyperplasia is prolonged contact of alkaline urine on the skin. Such contact occurs when the stomal opening in the pouch or faceplate is too large. The stomal opening in the appliance should be no more than 1/16 inch larger than the stoma.

Nursing interventions include the prevention and management of peristomal skin hyperplasia, acidification of alkaline urine, and avoidance of stomal scarring by using an adequate-sized opening in the faceplate. The patient must be given an accurate-sized stomal pattern and cautioned that the stoma will shrink in size and the pattern will need to be changed in a couple of months. Patients and family members should be taught how to measure stoma size but, as an added precaution, a follow-up appointment should be made for consultation with the nurse regarding the calibration of the stoma. At this time the patient should be provided with a new pouch or faceplate with correct stoma opening.

If irritation of the skin is present, the problem is treated by using a skin barrier until it has resolved (Fig. 60–2). When a new pouch is applied, the stoma area should be pretreated for 10 minutes with a white vinegar soak. A cool air-dryer can be used on the peristomal area for several minutes before applying the pouch.

Evaluation. Criteria for evaluating goal achievement relative to obstruction are.

1. No indications of the existence of peristomal hyperplasia.
2. The patient uses a pouch with an opening no greater than 1/16 inch larger than the stoma.
3. The patient demonstrates accurately how to measure the stoma pattern.
4. Patient uses a skin barrier when skin irritation occurs.
5. The patient uses white vinegar soak to treat skin irritation prior to applying a new pouch.
6. The patient accurately states the manifestations of impending obstruction and the need to notify the physician if these occur (decreased urinary output, inability to pass a No. 18 catheter into the stoma or, if passed, there is residual urine in the conduit).

Ammonia Salt Encrustation

Interventions. The nursing goal is to prevent the occurrence of ammonia salt encrustations on the stoma. Encrustations present as a white substance that cannot be

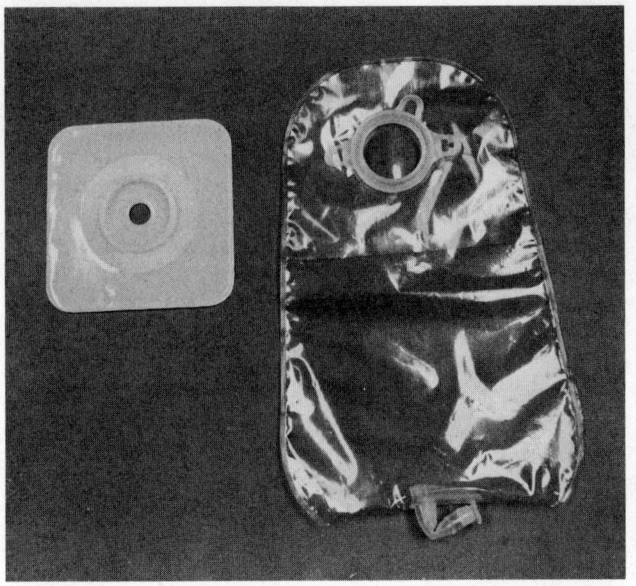

A

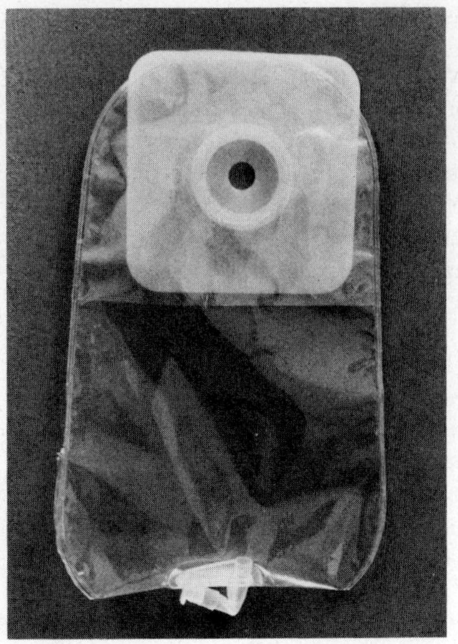

B

FIGURE 60–2 Skin protective barrier used with urostomy pouch. (*A*) Squibb Stomahesive wafer (left) and Sur-Fit urostomy pouch (right). (*B*) Stomahesive wafer with pouch attached.

removed from the stoma or as a sandpaperlike substance that appears around the stoma opening on the faceplate. The appearance of the crystals is usually associated with an alkaline urine, although occasionally the crystals may be acidic. If crystals are present, the urine pH should be determined prior to initiating treatment.

Since the usual situation is for the crystals to be associated with alkaline urine, prevention is by maintenance of an acid urine pH of about 6.5. This can be accomplished by an acid-ash dietary intake (see prevention of infection above) and ascorbic acid (vitamin C) along with avoidance of alkaline-ash foods such as milk, vegetables, citrus fruits, and carbonated beverages. The use of sodium bicarbonate (a home remedy for "upset" stomach) should be avoided. Externally, cleaning of the skin and pouch with full-strength or dilution of 1:2 water and vinegar solution is both a preventive and treatment intervention. If crystals are present the stoma should be bathed with 1 oz of white vinegar daily for 15 to 20 minutes. The use of the night drain to prevent urine from bathing the stoma is essential. It appears that crystals are a more frequent occurrence with rubber as contrasted with plastic pouches. If the crystals should be associated with an acid pH, then the recommended treatment is cleansing with a sodium bicarbonate solution. The patient needs careful instruction about this complication, including how to recognize it and how to determine urine pH. Prevention and treatment consultation with the enterostomy therapist is encouraged.

Evaluation. Goal achievement is attained if.

1. The patient does not experience crystal formation.
2. Crystal formation clears readily with use of the above-described recommended treatment (vinegar for alkaline crystals and sodium bicarbonate for acid crystals).
3. The patient can describe the problem and treatment accurately.

Urinary Calculus

Interventions. The nursing goals are prevention of the complication of urinary calculus and early detection if preventive measures fail (see Chap. 61). Patient adherence to a preventive regimen is a necessary element for goal achievement; therefore, patient and family teaching is an important intervention not only as part of the discharge planning but throughout the long-term follow-up consultation service. The need to involve the patient and family applies to all previously discussed preventive interventions. They are interventions subsumed under the broad nursing responsibility of promoting maximum level of wellness.

Preventive interventions relative to development of urinary calculus depend on a knowledge of predisposing factors. These factors are immobility, inadequate fluid intake, presence of urea-splitting urinary tract organisms that are most apt to be in alkaline urine, occurrence of pyelonephritis, retention of residual urine in the conduit, ureteral dilation, hyperchloremic acidosis, and impaired renal function. The first four of these factors can be influenced by patient adherence to preventive measures. Unfortunately, the structural problems of conduit length, the collection of residual urine in the conduit, and the often resulting reabsorption of chloride ions as well as pathological causes for renal function impairment are not amenable to preventive nursing interventions.

Patient teaching should emphasize the preventive interventions of regular exercise, fluid intake of 2.5 liters to 3 liters/day, maintenance of an acid urine through dietary intake as previously described, adherence to a daily regimen of adequate rest, nutrient intake, and avoidance of crowds and other situations where there is a high risk of exposure to infectious organisms. Since the development of urinary calculus is associated with both urine stasis and the presence of bacteria, prevention focuses on achieving a dilute urine with a low bacterial count. Other nursing interventions that contribute to prevention include treating stomal and skin conditions that lead to stasis and obstruction (see previous sections of this chapter).

Nurses may work with patients undergoing surgical reconstruction of the conduit to shorten it and thereby lessen the danger of residual urine contributing to infection, calculus, and hyperchloremia. Sometimes the physician will prescribe hydrochlorothiazide (HCTz) to decrease urinary excretion of calcium. Persons receiving this medication usually require a potassium supplement since the diuresis promotes potassium excretion.

Patients are taught signs and symptoms of urinary calculus and instructed to notify their physicians if these should occur. The signs and symptoms include flank pain, nausea, chills, fever, and hematuria. The patient is also taught to strain his urine since the stone may be passed and it is desirable to have it analyzed to determine its composition. Stone formation is discussed in Chapter 61.

Evaluation. Criteria for goal achievement are patient reports of

1. A fluid intake of 2.5–3 liters/day
2. Consistent urine pH of 6–6.5
3. Maintenance of a regimen of adequate rest and exercise
4. Freedom from infections
5. Accurate signs and symptoms of urinary calculus and actions to take if they should occur

Stomal Management Problems

Interventions. Other stomal management problems are similar to those experienced by persons with intestinal diversions. These include stoma prolapse and retraction, parastomal hernia, and peristomal skin breakdown. These problems and sexuality problems are discussed in detail in Chapter 80.

Interventions for Continuity of Care. Patients need to be taught the importance of lifetime follow-up care. This will include IVPs, routine renal function studies, urinalysis (UA), urine culture, and determination of conduit residual (normal is 3 ml to 5 ml). The purpose is to detect potential problems early. The problems may be disturbances in renal function, infection, or anatomical changes. Patients also need routine follow-up by an enterostomal therapy nurse to monitor self-care activities to assure prevention of complications.

Community support groups such as ostomy clubs are often very helpful to some people. These organizations are discussed in Chapter 80. Literature written for the person with urinary diversion is available from the local branch of the American Cancer Society, appliance companies such as Hollister, Inc., and from the local branch of the United Ostomy Association.

Adult Polycystic Disease of the Kidneys

Cystic disorders of the kidney represent malformations in which normal cell forms are replaced by abnormal tissue.[25] With the exception of the simple renal cyst, adult polycystic disease is the most common cystic disorder of the kidney.[6] It is often characterized by bilaterally enlarged kidneys with grapelike, fluid-filled clusters.[25] This disease is an inherited disorder with distinct anatomical characteristics, predictable progressive course, and a clinical picture that recurs among affected individuals and families.[6]

Adult polycystic disease typically manifests itself during the fifth decade of life. It affects both sexes equally and follows a similar clinical course in both men and women.[6,28] Presenting symptoms and progressive renal failure manifest at similar chronological ages from generation to generation in each affected family.[6]

Etiology

Adult polycystic disease is often found in more than one family member and in successive generations. A family history of the condition or of less specific renal disease is found in 75% to 80% of cases.[6] It is transmitted as a mendelian dominant trait with complete penetrance among predisposed individuals who survive to the ninth decade.[6]

Pathophysiology

As cysts enlarge within the kidney, pressure on adjacent organs results as does stretching of the renal capsule and tension on suspensory kidney tissues.[6] Renal enlargement occurs as a result of multiple cyst expansion in which functional tissue and blood vessels are compromised. Renal failure eventually results from the ultimate compression of adjacent, previously functioning nephrons.[6] Signs of increasing renal failure are manifested with progression of the disease. The blood pressure rises along with blood nitrogenous waste levels. As electrolyte and fluid imbalances occur, the patient enters a terminal uremic state.[28]

Various clinical conditions are associated with adult polycystic kidney disease. Hepatic cysts occur in approximately 30% of patients.[6] Additional cysts are often found in other organs, including the pancreas, testis, spleen, ovary, lung, thyroid, and uterus.[6] Neoplasia has been identified in the adult polycystic kidney. Cerebral aneurysms also occur in association with this disease.

Clinical Manifestations

Individuals with adult polycystic disease remain asymptomatic during the first 3 to 4 decades of life.[28] When it manifests itself, the disease initially presents as abdominal discomfort followed by bilateral nephromegaly and, ultimately, by renal failure.[6] Depending on the duration and extent of renal involvement, elevated blood pressure and azotemia may be present.[6]

Bilaterally palpable kidneys are evident in two thirds of patients with polycystic kidney disease.[6] Renal colic accompanied by massive hematuria may be present, resulting from hemorrhage into a cyst. Occasionally, patients may present with oliguria resulting from cystic ureteral occlusion. If calcification occurs in the affected kidneys, patients may present with signs of ureteral stone.[6] Because cystic kidneys are prone to infection, patients with adult polycystic disease initially may present with gram-negative sepsis.[6]

Medical Management

Diagnosis. The diagnosis of adult polycystic kidney disease largely results from clinical examination, history, and the outcome of the following radiological tests:[6]

Excretory urography (intravenous pyelogram) will show bilateral but irregular enlargement of the kidneys in patients with adult polycystic disease. Calcification will be evident in approximately 50% of patients, and the calyceal system will be distorted.

Nephrotomography will show mottling and irregular opacification of the renal substance. Large numbers of cysts will give a "Swiss cheese" appearance to the organs involved.

Ultrasonography is a useful diagnostic test that is a noninvasive alternative to urography or arteriography.

Retrograde pyelography is used cautiously because it increases the risk of urinary tract infection. It has been suggested for diagnostic use only when neoplasia or obstruction are suspected in the face of adult polycystic kidney disease.

The clinical diagnosis of adult polycystic disease is further based on the physical examination and patient history. Often, the nodular surface of the polycystic kidney is felt on physical examination. Urinalysis is generally unremarkable but may show 1 to 2 (+) protein, some granular casts, and slight hematuria and pyuria.[6] Finally, a family history positive for adult polycystic kidney disease, early deaths, and renal diseases is highly suggestive of the presence of the disorder.[6]

Treatment. The treatment for adult polycystic kidney disease is nonspecific. Attention is paid to the treatment of clinical conditions and symptoms that result from the disease. Chronic azotemia that occurs during the progression of renal failure should be treated by conventional therapeutic measures. High blood pressure may also be treated conventionally, with special attention to the presence of urinary salt-wasting, which may indicate the need to discontinue antihypertensive treatment.[6] The presence of hypovolemia is treated with salt and water replacement. Urinary tract infections may not respond to periodic or chronic conventional treatment. Ultimately, nephrectomy may be indicated for the control of such infections.[6]

Surgery performed on cysts is indicated only to reestablish urinary flow in the face of ureteropelvic obstruction from expanding cysts. This once routine cyst "deroofing" procedure actually has been shown to accelerate azotemia.[6] Nephrectomy may be indicated to control massive hematuria. As renal failure progresses, the patient is generally maintained on hemodialysis. Eventually the patient may be considered a candidate for renal transplantation.

Prognosis. When the diagnosis of adult polycystic kidney disease has been established, the prognosis is almost always poor. The degree of compression and cystic damage to the parenchymal tissue will determine the patient's length of survival.[28] A 10-year survival is characteristic for individuals who experience the associated renal failure before the age of 50.[6] The course is more rapid in persons who become azotemic after the age of 50.[6] When the blood urea nitrogen concentration reaches 40 mg/dl, the average survival declines to just over 2 years.

Nursing Management

Nursing Diagnosis. Examples of diagnoses for patients with adult polycystic kidney disease include potential for complications arising from the renal dysfunction (*e.g.,* infection, high blood pressure, fluid and electrolyte problems) and pain related to cystic distention of tissues; and anxiety related to fear of death and the realization that one may be perpetuating an inheritable disease.

Goals. Realistic nursing goals include maintenance of patient comfort through palliation of pain, management of the accompanying signs of urinary infection (including fever and urinary discomfort), management of hematuria, and identification and management of progressive renal failure, including high blood pressure, fluid and electrolyte imbalances, and uremia. Teaching the patient and family with regard to the cause and possible prevention of the disease in future generations, as well as what the patient may expect to experience as the disease progresses, are additional goals.

Interventions. Adult polycystic kidney disease patients should be treated symptomatically when clinical manifestations or complications of the disease arise. Patients who experience lumbar and abdominal pain that increases with exertion and/or colicky pain associated with the passage of clots should receive a thorough pain assessment by the nurse. Analgesics should be administered as ordered and periods of bed rest should be encouraged. Patients experiencing urinary tract infections should have their temperatures monitored every 4 hours. Urine culture and sensitivity tests should be monitored closely and appropriate antipyretic and antibiotic therapy should be instituted as ordered. Any changes in micturition should be noted, and oral fluids should be encouraged (unless contraindicated by the compromised renal status).

Hematuria is a common manifestation of adult polycystic kidney disease that merits close monitoring. A continuing record should be kept of urine characteristics. Pulse and blood pressure should be monitored at least every 4 hours, and the patient should be observed for signs of shock. Continued hematuria may contribute to an underlying anemia, requiring transfusion. Because hematuria is also a common manifestation of renal malignancy, the nurse must be especially alert to its presence in adult polycystic disease patients who develop it following renal transplantation without having had prior nephrectomy.

Patients with adult polycystic disease should have their blood pressures monitored every 4 hours. They should be observed and questioned for signs of high blood pressure, including morning occipital headaches, dizziness or lightheadedness, shortness of breath, paroxysmal nocturnal dyspnea, cough, edema, or chest pain. In the presence of high blood pressure, antihypertensive medications should be administered as ordered. The patient's fluid status should be monitored carefully. It should also be remembered that antihypertensive therapy may need to be discontinued in the presence of urinary salt-wasting.

With the continued progression of disease and renal failure the nurse must provide ongoing assessment and intervention. Caring for the patient with progressive renal failure is a challenging and complex task requiring specialized knowledge.

In trying to maintain patient comfort, special attention should be paid to the patient's fluid and electrolyte status and the progessive uremia that will occur. Treatment with salt and water will be necessary if hypovolemia results. As uremia progresses the nurse must intervene when adverse changes in the integument, gastrointestinal system, metabolism, fluid–electrolyte and acid–basic status, pulmonary, neurological, cardiovascular, hematological, endocrine, and skeletal systems arise (see Chap. 57)

The patient with adult polycystic disease faces many emotional upheavals. The initial confirmation of diagnosis, the progressive debilitation of the disease, and the burden of knowing that the patient may be passing it on to successive generations are all psychological issues with which the patient must deal. The nurse can be instrumental in providing the necessary comprehensive instruction about the disease and the disease process. Additionally, the nurse may provide assurance to the patient that clinical symptoms of the disease will be treated as they arise and that the patient's comfort will be maintained.

The nurse may help to prepare the patient for future treatment by introducing him to the concept of and teaching him about renal dialysis and possible renal transplant. Finally, the nurse may help the patient deal with any anger or guilt related to passing the disease on to future generations by arranging for genetic counseling.

Evaluation. As a result of appropriate nursing interventions, patients will report maintenance of comfort. Through comprehensive patient instruction and counseling, patients will discuss the disease with understanding of its nature. Discussion will indicate accurate knowledge of the disease and the risks of passing it on to future generations. The patient will also be able to make decisions about future care such as dialysis and possible renal transplantation.

References

1. Bennington JL, Laubscher FL: Epidemiologic studies on carcinoma of the kidney. Cancer 21(6):1069–1071, 1968
2. Boyland E, Dukes CE, Grover PL, Mitchley BCV: The induction of renal tumours by feeding lead acetate to rats. Br J Cancer 16(2):283–297, June 1962
3. Cole P, Monson RR, Haning H, Friedell GH: Smoking and cancer of the lower urinary tract, New Engl J Med 284(3):129–134, January 1971
4. DeKernion JB: Treatment of advanced renal cell carcinoma—Traditional methods and innovative approaches. J Urol 130(1):2–7, July 1983
5. Frank IN, Keys HM, McCune CS: Urologic and male genital cancers. In Rubin P (ed): Clinical Oncology: A Multidisciplinary Approach, 6th ed. pp 198–220. American Cancer Society, 1983
6. Gardner KD Jr: Cystic disorders of the kidney. In Flamenbaum W, Hamburger RJ (eds): Nephrology: An Approach to the Patient with Renal Disease, pp 424–440. Philadelphia, JB Lippincott, 1982
7. Garnick MB: Advanced renal cell cancer. Kidney Int 20(1):127–136, July 1981
8. Hopkins SC, Ford KS, Soloway MS: Invasive bladder cancer: Support for screening. J Urol 130(1):61–64, July 1983
9. Lerner J, Khan Z: Manual of Urologic Nursing. St. Louis, CV Mosby, 1982
10. McConnell EA, Zimmerman MF: Care of Patients with Urologic Problems. Philadelphia, JB Lippicott, 1983
11. McCredie M, Steward JH, Ford JM, Analgescis and tobacco as risk factors for cancer of the ureter and renal pelvis. J Urol 130(1):28–30, July 1983
12. Melicow MM: Tumors of the urinary bladder: A clinicopathological analysis of over 2500 specimens and biopsies. J Urol 74(4):498–521, October 1955
13. Mills C, Vaughan ED Jr: Carcinoma of the ureter: Natural history, management and 5-year survival. J Urol 129(5):275–277, February 1983
14. Morrison AS, Buring JE: Artificial sweetners and cancer of the lower urinary tract. New Engl J Med 302(10):537–541, March 1980
15. Narayana AS, Loening SA, Sylmen DJ, Culp DA: Bladder cancer: Factors affecting survival. J Urol 130(1):56–60, July 1983
16. Richie JP, Garnick MB: Primary renal and ureteral cancer. In Rieselbach RE, Garnick MB (eds): Cancer and the Kidney, pp 662–706. Philadelphia, Lea & Febiger, 1982
17. Robson CJ, Churchill BM, Anderson W: The results of radical nephrectromy for renal cell carcinoma. American Association of Genito-Urinary Surgeons 60:122–129, 1968
18. Saitoh H: Distant metastasis of renal adenocarcinoma. Cancer 48(6):1487–1491, September 1981
19. Schefft P, Novick AC, Straffon RA, Stewart BH: Surgery for renal cell carcinoma extending into the inferior vena cava. J Urol 120(1):28–31, July 1978
20. Silverberg E, Lubera JA: Cancer statistics, 1983. CA—A Cancer Journal for Clinicians 33(1):3–26, 1983
21. Siminovitch JMP, Montie JE, Straffon RA: Prognostic indicators in renal adenocarcinoma. J Urol 130(1):20–23, July 1983
22. Skinner DG, Colvin RB, Vermillion CD et al: Diagnosis and management of renal cell carcinoma. A clinical and pathologic study of 309 cases. Cancer 28(5):1165–1177, November 1971
23. Smith CT: Disorders of the male reproductive and genitourinary systems. In Hincker EA, Malasanos L: The Little, Brown Manual of Medical-Surgical Nursing, pp 1065–1111. Boston, Little, Brown & Co, 1983
24. Soloway MS: The management of superficial bladder cancer. Cancer 45(7):1856–1865, April 1980
25. Suhayda R: Disorders of the renal system. In Hincker EA, Mal-

asanos L: The Little, Brown Manual of Medical-Surgical Nursing, pp 941–1008. Boston, Little, Brown & Co, 1983

26. Trump DL: Update on dx and management of bladder cancer. Geriatrics 37(7):87–91, 1982
27. Waters WB, Richie JP: Aggressive surgical approach to renal cell carcinoma: Review of 130 cases. J Urol 122(2):306–309, September 1979
28. Watson JE: Medical-Surgical Nursing and Related Physiology. Toronto, WB Saunders, 1979

Bibliography

Broadwell D, Jackson B: Principles of Ostomy Care, Chaps 18 and 22. St. Louis, CV Mosby, 1982

Brubacher L, Beard P: A helpful new handout for your ostomy patients. RN, pp 34–37, 1983

Watt R: Ostomies: Why, How and Where. Nurs Clin North Am 402: 1976

Chapter 61

Urolithiasis

Constance J. Hirnle

The presence of stones in the urinary system is referred to as *urolithiasis*. The stone itself is referred to as a *calculus*. Stone formation can occur anywhere in the urinary tract, but most frequently lithiasis formation begins in the kidney. Stones can vary in size, from sand- or gravel-sized particles that freely pass out of the urinary system to a large staghorn calculus that can encompass the entire renal pelvis and must be surgically removed.

Epidemiological factors of calculi are not fully understood. Heredity plays a role because it influences an individual's anatomy and biochemical makeup. Imposed on our genetically determined physical self are environmental factors, such as geography, diet, and lifestyle, which can contribute positively or negatively to stone formation. Underdeveloped countries of the world, especially Southeast Asia, report high incidences of bladder stones, perhaps related to dietary deficiencies. The incidence of upper tract (kidneys and ureters) urolithiasis is more common in developed countries of the world, including the United States. Within the United States the southeastern states constitute the "stone belt" area where the incidence of urolithiasis is greatly increased. One hypothesis for this is that the "soft" water consumed in the stone belt area is a contributing factor in stone formation.[8] Also, the warm climate of the southeastern states may predispose individuals to dehydration, which can increase the saturation content of the urine and thus increase the likelihood of stone formation. Calculi may occur in any age group, but most commonly occur between the ages of 20 to 55 years. Men are more commonly affected than women.

About 65% of renal stones are calcium based, composed of calcium phosphate, calcium oxalate, or a combination of the two (Fig. 61–1). Of the remaining 35%, 15% are magnesium ammonium phosphate (struvite), 10% are uric acid, and 10% are cystine stones.[6] Each classification of stone has its own unique etiology.

Etiology/Pathophysiology

Calcium Stones

Although the etilogy of calcium stone formation is not fully understood, several significant factors have been researched more fully in the last decade. The role of hypercalciuria and increased absorption of oxalate in the formation of calcium stones is now better understood, as is idiopathic hypercalciuria.

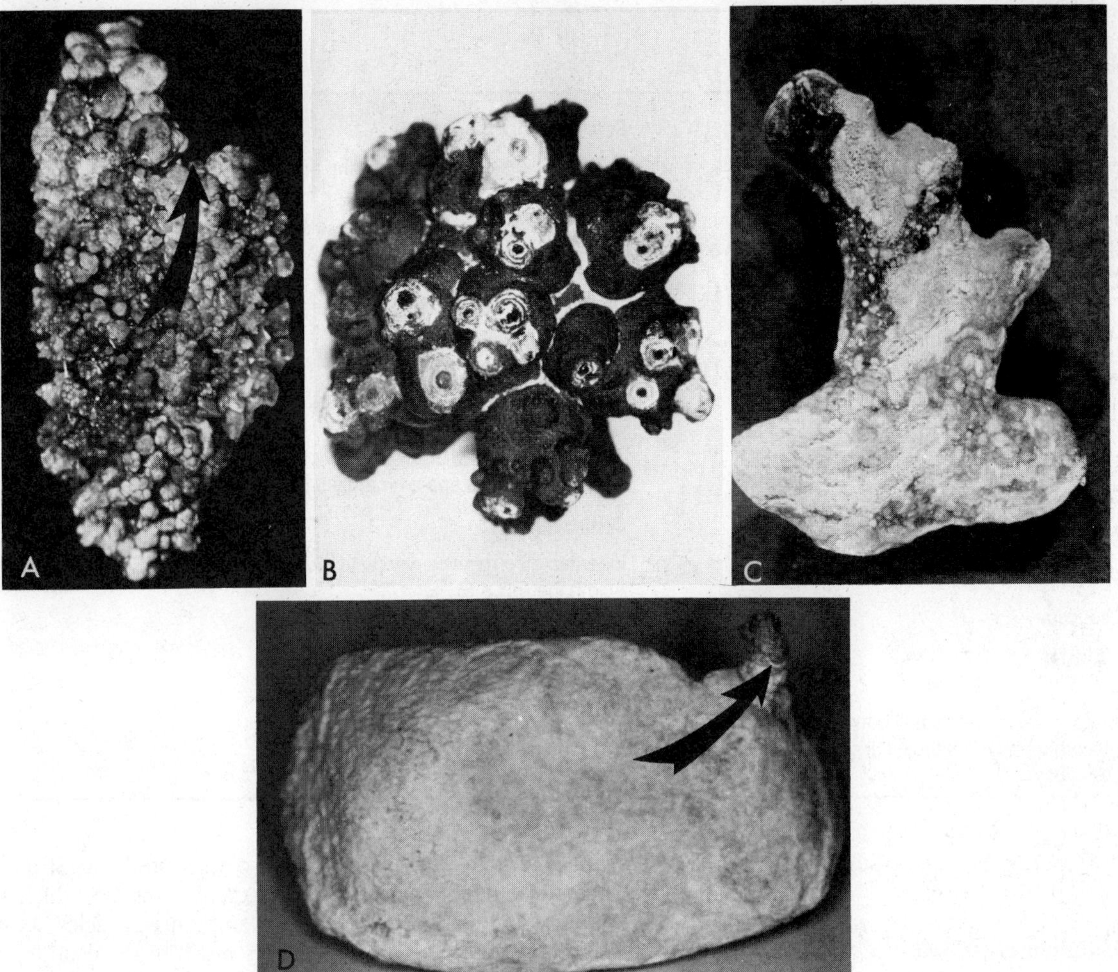

FIGURE 61–1 Examples of urinary calculi. (*A*) Calcium oxalate monohydrate (whewellite). Actual size 5 × 8 cm. Arrow indicates indentation of point of attachment of stone to papilla. This is sometimes called a "mulberry stone." (*B*) Uric acid calculus. Actual size 2.3 cm. Sometimes called a "jack stone." (*C*) Staghorn calculus of magnesium ammonium phosphate (struvite). Actual size 4.5 × 7 cm. (*D*) Bladder calculus of magnesium ammonium phosphate (struvite), which has formed on piece of nonabsorbable suture (*arrow*). Patients who produced stones in *C* and *D* both had chronic urinary infection *Proteus mirabilis.* (Orach GW: Urinary lithiasis. In Harrison JH, Gittes R, Perlmutter A et al [eds]: Campbell's Urology, 4th ed, p 816. Philadelphia, WB Saunders, 1978)

Hypercalciuria. Hypercalciuria can be defined as urinary calcium greater than 4 mg/kg/24 hr.[2] Hyperexcretion of calcium into the urine can be caused by specific metabolic problems, which, when isolated, can often be successfully treated. Increased urinary calcium can be related to increased absorption of calcium from the bone, increased absorption of calcium from the intestine, or impaired renal tubular absorption of calcium in the kidney. Pathologies that can lead to hypercalciuria by extracting calcium from the bone or intestine or leaking it from the kidney are listed in Table 61–1. In addition to these pathologies, certain medications can cause hypercalciuria, namely, exogenous steroids (*e.g.*, ACTH), furosemide, ammonium chloride, acetazolamide, excessive thyroid hormone, and excessive intake of vitamin D.

In approximately 35% of calcium stone formers, serum calcium levels are within normal limits; thus their hypercalciuria is designated as idiopathic. Pak and associates hypothesize that excess calcium excretion is the result of impaired renal tubular reabsorption (renal hypercalcium) or intestinal hyperabsorption of calcium (absorptive hypercalciuria).[6]

Hyperuricosuria. In addition to hypercalciuria, high levels of uric acid in the urine correlate positively with calcium stone formation. Coe hypothesizes that uric crystals can act as a nidus for calcium oxalate stone formation and that high levels of uric acid lower the degree of calcium supersaturation required to initiate crystal formation. Coe also feels that urate crystals and perhaps uric acid crystals can absorb large, molecular-weight polyanions that act to inhibit the growth of calcium oxalate crystals.[3] Hyperuricosuria is

TABLE 61–1
Pathologies Related to Urinary Stone Formation

Calcium Stones (↑ absorption of Ca^{2+} from bone)	***Struvite Stones***
Hyperparathyroidism	Infection caused by urea-splitting organism
Paget's disease	*Proteus mirabilis*
Malignant tumors that cause osteolysis (*e.g.*, breast, prostate, lung)	*Pseudomonas*
Cushing's disease	*Klebsiella*
Immobility	*Staphylococcus*
	Alkaline urinary pH > 7.0
Hypercalciuria (↑ absorption of Ca^{2+} from gut)	***Uric Acid Crystal Stones***
Excessive intake of vitamin D	Saturation of urate in urine
Sarcoidosis	Increased uric acid production (*e.g.*, gout, myeloproliferative disorder)
Milk-alkali syndrome	Administration of uricosuric agents (*e.g.*, probenecid)
Impaired Renal Tubular Absorption of Ca^{2+}	Acidic urine pH of approximately 5.5
Renal tubular necrosis	***Cystine Stones***
Hyperuricosuria (↑ urinary uric acid)	Inherited disorder of amino acid metabolism
Purine-rich diet	Acid urine (pH 5.5)
Uric acid overproduction	
↑ Absorption of Oxalate	
Familial oxaluria	
Postoperatively, ileal resections or small bowel bypass	
Overdosage of ascorbic acid or methoxyflurane anesthetic	
Severe Ca^{2+} restriction	

generally caused by a purine-rich diet or uric acid overproduction.

Increased Absorption of Oxalate. Oxalate is the end product of the metabolism of certain amino acids. Increased urinary levels of oxalate can crystallize into stones. Hyperoxaluria can be the result of familial oxaluria, sever calcium restriction, or the overdosage of ascorbic acid or methoxyflurane anesthetic. Most commonly, increased oxalate absorption is secondary to inflammatory bowel disease or small bowel bypass surgery. It is thought that the malabsorption present in these conditions increases the fat available to bind with calcium, which frees up oxalate, thus increasing the liklihood of oxalate being absorbed in the intestine. Approximately 7% to 10% of patients with malabsorption will develop urolithiasis.[4]

Properties of Calcium Stones. Calcium phosphate stones are yellow or brown in color, varying in hardness, and frequently laminated. They are radiopaque and visualize well on x-ray. Calcium oxalate stones are usually small, hard, and rough. They are dark in color and often covered by sharp spicules. They, too, visualize on x-ray. Staghorn formation can occur in calcium phosphate stones but are rare in calcium oxalate stones.

Struvite Stones

Triple phosphate, or struvite, stones always occur with an infection caused by a urea-splitting organism. Most commonly this organism is *Proteus mirabilis* but *Pseudomonas, Klebsiella,* and *Staphylococcus* are also associated with struvite stones. Such bacteria contain the enzyme urease, which is capable of splitting urea into two ammonia particles. As ammonia is liberated, urine becomes much more alkaline, with a pH greater than 7.0. Alkaline urine facilitates the precipitation of magnesium ammonium phosphate, thus creating a supersaturated solution that fosters stone development. Often bacteria is incorporated into the stone during its formation, making treatment of the infection difficult since reinfection is common.

Properties of Struvite Stones. Struvite stones are yellowish in color and somewhat friable. Often they can form on preexisting calcium stones, and laminations may indicate the presence of calcium oxalate or calcium phosphate. Struvite stones are moderately opaque and will visualize on x-ray.

Uric Acid Stones

Uric acid stones occur when urine becomes supersaturated with urate. Hyperuricuria can be a result of increased uric acid production such as can occur in gout or in myeloproliferative disease in which there is a rapid cell turnover. Most uric stone formers have idiopathic hyperuricuria, which is characterized by normal serum uric acid levels but elevated urinary uric levels. Purine-rich diets or the administration of uricosuric agents such as probenecid can also cause hyperuricosuria, thus contributing to uric stone formation. Regardless of the factors causing the hyperuricosuria, uric stones only precipitate in an acidic urine (pH 5.5).

Properties of Uric Acid Stones. Uric acid stones are usually small and hard, varying in color from yellow to reddish brown. Often these stones occur bilaterally in multiple numbers. Uric acid stones are nonopaque on x-ray and can be visualized as filling defects on an intravenous pyelogram.

Cystine Stones

Cystine stone formation is due to an inherited autosomal recessive disorder of amino acid metabolism, which results in cystinuria. In this metabolic disorder, renal tubular absorption of cystine, as well as lysine, argenine, and homocystine, is impaired, Cystine is relatively insoluble; thus precipitation and stone formation is common. Cystine stones, like uric acid stones, form only in acidic urine. Since this error in metabolism is inherited, cystine stone formation can occur in very young children and follow them through adulthood.

Properties of Cystine Stones. Cystine stones are light yellow or yellow brown in color and tend not to occur singly. Multiple cystine stones can combine together into large staghorn masses. Cystine stones are only slightly opaque and difficult to visualize on x-ray.

Lower Urinary Tract Lithiasis

Urolithiasis most frequently occurs in the upper urinary tract. If a stone migrates all the way to the bladder, it will most often be passed without difficulty. Occasionally, a stone cannot be passed owing to a lower urinary tract obstruction, such as benign prostatic hypertrophy. The stone can continue to grow until it becomes quite large.

Stones can originate in the bladder, where they can form in diverticula or secondary to lower urinary tract obstruction and urinary stasis.[1] Bladder calculi were very common in 18th and 19th century Europe, but today them seem to be generally restricted to young boys in underdeveloped countries of the Middle and Far East. Their occurrence in this population may be related to protein deficiences.

Clinical Manifestations

The signs and symptoms exhibited by the patient with urolithiasis depend on the size, shape, location, and movement of the calculi. Small calculi, less than .5 mm in diameter, frequently pass freely from the urinary system without causing symptoms. Larger stones, as they migrate down the ureter, cause pain. In addition to pain, indications of urinary obstruction or infection often are present.

Pain

Renal colic is a group of symptoms associated with movement of calculus through narrowing anatomical points in the ureter that causes obstruction of urine. Renal colic is abrupt, severe pain that radiates from the kidney. Colic is most commonly observed as the stone leaves the kidney and migrates into the ureter at the ureteropelvic junction. Severe costovertebral angle pain that radiates throughout the flank area to the abdomen and groin is common. As the stone travels down the ureter, other points of narrowing can cause renal colic to reoccur. As this happens, the pain is localized lower in the abdomen, radiating to the bladder, vulva, or scrotum. The severity of renal colic is such that the patient "doubles up," writhing in pain. At times this pain cannot be controlled with narcotics. The pain of renal colic is thought to be caused by muscle spasms induced by the stretching and obstruction of the ureter by the calculus.

Severe pain of this sort often causes an elevation of heart rate and blood pressure. Respiratory rate is also often elevated and can become "grunting" in nature during severe spasm of colicky pain.

In addition to severe pain, nausea and vomiting are commonly associated with renal colic because the autonomic nervous system innervation of the celiac ganglion serves both the kidney and stomach. Abdominal distention can also occur.

In contrast to renal colic, a dull, aching flank or abdominal pain may be associated with urolithiasis. This is usually the result of inflammation or chronic renal impairment secondary to hydronephrosis.

Urinary Symptoms

Urinary output is usually not affected by the presence of a calculus, since often urolithiasis occurs only in one kidney, and complete obstruction of the ureter does not always occur. The presence of renal calculi can cause hydronephrosis if the ureter is obstructed, which will eventually lead to renal damage.

The patient may complain of urgency and frequency, especially if the calculus has lodged near the bladder. Inflammation in the area around the bladder neck can cause pain on urination.

Urinalysis often reveals microscopic or gross hematuria that is the result of trauma to the mucosa of the urinary system. If the stone has completely obstructed the ureter, hematuria may be absent. Pyuria is often present, especially in the presence of an infection. Urinary tract infection is often accompanied by fever, chills, and malaise.

Medical Management

Diagnosis

The patient who presents with renal colic, hematuria, and/or infection is diagnostically worked up to confirm the presence or absence of a stone and to help develop an appropriate therapeutic plan of management. Urinalysis and urine for culture and sensitivity are helpful in determining the presence of urinary tract infection. Blood chemistries are often ordered for calcium, phosphorus, uric acid, potassium, and chloride. Renal function tests (serum creatinine and blood urea nitrogen) are ordered to identify renal damage. A 24-hour urine collection for creatinine clearance, calcium, phosphorus, cystine, oxalate, and uric acid helps to identify supersaturation of these components in the urine that can predispose an individual to stone formation. Since 90% of renal stones are radiopaque, radiographic studies are helpful in confirming stone presence and pinpointing stone location. Intravenous pyelogram, retrograde pyelography, excretory urograms, renal scans, and ultrasound may be ordered in addition to a routine KUP (kidney, ureter, bladder) x-ray.

From information derived from patient examination, history, and diagnostic tests, the physician must decide whether to treat the urolithiasis medically or intervene surgically. Treatment depends on the size and location of the calculus, the presence or absence of infection, the status of the involved kidney and ureter, the renal function of the patient, and the degree of pain the patient is experiencing. Sugery is generally indicated if infection is present and cannot be eradicated with antibiotic therapy, if there is progressive renal damage, if the stone is causing obstruction of urine flow, or if the stone causes severe pain.[5]

Treatment

Information obtained from the diagnostic tests, in addition to the history elicited from the patient, helps the physician to identify the type of calculus that is present. The diagnostic process is greatly enhanced if the patient passes any calculus that can be analyzed to determine the stone's composition. Identification of stone type is important, since medical management varies for each type of renal stone. In fact, methods used to prevent one type of stone may enhance the development of another type of calculus.

Adequate hydration is the most significant method of treatment for any type of stone. Fluids are usually increased to above 4000 ml/24 hours to produce urine that is more dilute than extracellular fluid. Urinary output should be greater than 3000 ml/24 hours. In addition to preventing stone formation, adequate hydration can aid stone passage, since increasing urinary output will elevate hydrostatic pressure behind the stone.

Medical management is aimed at decreasing the concentration of crystals that precipitate out of solution to form stones when concentrations approach saturation levels. Pharmacological agents, as well as dietary management, are helpful in accomplishing this. In addition to decreasing saturation levels of certain urinary components, altering the pH of the urine can be helpful in preventing certain types of calculus formation.

Calcium stones are most effectively treated with hydration, thiazide diuretics, and phosphates. If the stone is calcium phosphate based, acidification of the urine will also be helpful. Struvite stones are most frequently managed with hydration, antibiotic therapy, and acidification of urine. Hydration, alkalinization of urine, and allopurinal therapy are most commonly employed for uric acid stones. Cystine stones respond best to hydration, alkalinization of urine, and the administration of D-penicillamine.

Dietary therapy is sometimes helpful in treating urolithiasis. Uric acid stones are treated with a low-purine diet, whereas oxalate-based stones can be treated with a low-oxalate diet. Foods to avoid in a low-purine diet are meats, spinach, beans, peas, tea, coffee, chocolate, and alcohol. In a low-oxalate diet, the foods to avoid include asparagus, cabbage, celery, chocolate, lamb, rhubarb, spinach, tomatoes, beets, nuts, tea, citrus fruits, and cranberries.

Many physicians recommend a moderate restriction of both calcium and phosphorus (Shorr's regimen) for calcium- or phosphate-based stones. Recent research questions the usefulness of the diet, since urinary calcium levels are only slightly lowered by dietary restriction of calcium. Also, such a diet can decrease the level of pyrophosphates, which have been demonstrated to inhibit the growth of calcium phosphate crystals.[4] In addition to altering the crystalloid composition of the urine, dietary therapies are helpful in altering urinary pH. An acid-ash diet (encourages eggs, meat, poultry, cereals, cranberries, prunes, grapes, asparagus, tomatoes, and corn) increases the acidity of the urine and therefore is recommended for calcium phosphate stones and struvite stones. Alkalinization of urine using an alkaline-ash diet (includes milk, rhubarb, vegetables, tomatoes, and fruit except those included in acid-ash diet) is useful for uric acid or cystine stones. Good compliance with restrictive diets, especially for long periods of time, is difficult to obtain. For this reason, dietary management is often not the most significant preventative factor for the patient with urolithiasis.

Chemolysis, a method of dissolving stones, has been successfully used for struvite, uric acid, and cystine stones. A chemolytic solution (either alkylating or acidifying agents) is instilled by means of a percutaneous nephrostomy tube to the location of the stone and then drained from the area by another nephrostomy tube. This avoids buildup of pressure in the renal pelvis. Chemolysis is contraindicated when infection is present, which is often the case in struvite stones that readily dissolve.[9]

Surgical Treatment

Surgical intervention is generally required for stones that are greater than 1 cm in size. Various surgical procedures used for stone removal are listed in Table 61–2. Incisions made at various points along the urinary tract, depending on the location of the stone. A nephrostomy tube may be inserted into the renal pelvis to ensure adequate drainage of urine and prevent hydronephrosis. A nephrectomy may be necessary if hydronephrosis secondary to obstruction from a calculus has caused renal damage. At times, a partial nephrectomy is indicated if multiple stones have lodged themselves into one area of the kidney and are difficult to remove individually because of their location. Postoperative hemorrhage is more common when the surgery directly involves the kidney, since this area is very vascular. Other postoperative considerations include the following: prevention of infection, prevention of pulmonary complication, prevention of paralytic ileus, adequate fluid and electrolyte balance, and pain control.

Recent developments in less invasive surgical procedures for patients with urolithiasis have greatly decreased the cost and length of hospital stay as well as the trauma and complications that the patient experiences. Percutaneous ultrasonic lithotripsy (PUL) is a procedure in which percutaneous guide wire is inserted through the flank into the kidney. Dilators are placed over the guide wire to permit the insertion of a tube, similar to a small cystoscope, that can be advanced to the location of the stone. Small stones can be removed using forceps. If the stone is too large to be removed in this manner, an instrument capable of dispersing ultrasound waves is inserted. The ultrasound waves fragment the stone into smaller pieces that can then be mechanically removed or flushed out of the system with an irrigating solution and a suction catheter. Extracorporeal shock wave lithotripsy (ESWL) is a totally noninvasive procedure used to crush renal calculi. The patient is placed in a tank of water through which spark-induced shock waves are propagated. These shock waves cause the calculus to be pulverized into many minute particles that can easily be removed during normal urination.[10]

Prognosis

Prognosis of urolithiasis is variable. If the underlying causative factor, such as hyperparathyroidism, can be identified and successfully treated, the prognosis is excellent that renal calculi will not occur. Reoccurrence varies from 8% to 80%, depending on stone type, with an average 25% reoccurrence rate during the 2- to 3-year period following the first stone.[2] Reoccurrence becomes more frequent following each subsequent stone formation. For many individuals with renal calculi, prevention becomes a lifetime process.

TABLE 61–2
Surgical Intervention for Urolithiasis

Surgery	*Indications*
Open Procedures	
Nephrolithotomy	Incision into kidney to remove stone
Nephrectomy (partial or total)	Removal of part of or entire kidney (when severe damage has been done to the kidney from calculus)
Pyelolithotomy	Stone removal from the renal pelvis
Ureterolithotomy	Stone removal from ureter
Cystolithectomy	Stone removal from bladder
Litholapaxy	Crushing of urolithiasis with lithotrite; small stone fragment can then be flushed from urinary tract
Closed Procedures	
Percutaneous ultrasonic lithotripsy (PUL)	Ultrasound used to fragment large calculus so fragments can be mechanically removed or flushed out of the system
Extracorporeal shock wave lithotripsy (ESWL)	Patient is placed in tank of water through which shock waves are sent to pulverize stone that is then passed during urination

Nursing Management

Assessment and Nursing Diagnosis

It is important to elicit any factors from the patient's history that may have contributed to stone formation (Table 61–3). Dietary patterns, fluid intake, and medication history are especially helpful to aid the nurse in planning teaching needs of the patient. In addition to the patient admitted with urolithiasis, assessment of this information should be made for any patient having increased potential for the formation of renal calculi. High-risk groups would include immobilized individuals (*e.g.,* quadraplegics, and individuals on bed rest), patients undergoing cancer chemotherapy, individuals with urinary tract infections, dehydrated individuals, and individuals with the medical problems listed in Table 61–1.

Nursing diagnosis for the individual with renal calculi may include alterations in comfort; potential for infection; knowledge deficit regarding therapeutic management program; anxiety regarding pain, hospitalization, and possibility of surgery; impairment of urinary elimination or function; and change in body image. The patient who has undergone surgery to remove urinary calculi may have the following nursing problems: potential for postoperative hemorrhage, potential for pulmonary complications, alterations in comfort, potential for infection, alterations in urinary elimination and function, alterations in body image, and alterations in bowel elimination. For nursing management of patients with urolithiasis, see the Nursing Care Plan for the Patient with Urolithiasis; the plan would have to be modified to meet the individual needs of patients.

TABLE 61–3
Assessment Factors Specific to Patients with Urinary Calculus Disease

- Present and past medical history
  - Medical treatment and surgical procedures on and outside the genitourinary tract
  - Urinary tract infection
  - Periods of prolonged illness with immobilization or dehydration
  - Gout
  - Malignant neoplasms
  - Endocrinopathies
- Family histories
- Present and past geographic residences
- Age
- Sex
- Occupation
- Dietary habits
- Fluid intake
- Vitamin intake
- Medication history
  - Steroids
  - Alkalizing agents
- Pain
  - Location
  - Intensity
  - Character and quality
  - Chronology
- Pain response
  - Psychological
  - Behavioral
  - Affective

(From McConnell E, Zimmerman M: Care of Patients with Urologic Problems, 76. Philadephia, JB Lippincott, 1983)

NURSING CARE PLAN FOR THE PATIENT WITH UROLITHIASIS

NURSING DIAGNOSIS/PROBLEM 1: Alterations in comfort secondary to renal colic, trauma to renal and urinary tissues, and inflammation.

GOAL 1.1: To relieve pain.

Nursing Interventions	Rationale	Outcome Criteria
1. Administer pain medication (narcotic–antagonist) or antispasmodics.	1. Pharmacological intervention to relieve pain.	1–4. a. Patient claims pain no greater than 4, on a scale of 1 to 10. b. Patient passes stone. c. Pain does not interfere with activities of daily living. d. Pain does not interrupt patient's sleep.
2. Encourage patient to let the nursing staff know when he begins to experience pain.	2. Out-of-control pain requires more medication to obtain relief. Allow patient a degree of control in pain management.	
3. Notify the physician if pain is not relieved with current pain order.	3. Physician may need to alter pain prescription for adequate control.	
4. Positive comments and approach that pain medication will be effective.	4. Lessen patient anxiety and increase placebo effect.	
5. Moist heat or sitz baths.	5. Stimulation of heat receptors rather than pain receptors.	
6. Distraction.	6. Focuses patient's attention away from painful stimuli.	
7. Relaxation techniques.	7. Decrease muscle tension and focus concentration on area other than pain.	

GOAL 1.2: To detect passage of stone.

Nursing Interventions	Rationale	Outcome Criteria
1. Strain all urine.	1. To detect stone when it passes; save so analysis can detect stone composition.	1–2. a. Stone is found in urine. b. Radiographic studies indicate absence of calculi. c. Pain abates.
2. Increase fluids to more than 4000 ml/24 hr. Space evenly over 24 hr (1 glass/hour while awake, 2 glasses once during the middle of the night).	2. Increases hydrostatic pressure behind stone to aid in moving it out of the urinary tract. Prevents supersaturation of urine, which can add to stone mass or help create new calculi.	

NURSING DIAGNOSIS/PROBLEM 2: Potential for urinary infection related to stasis of urine.

GOAL 2: To prevent or control urinary tract infection.

Nursing Interventions	Rationale	Outcome Criteria
1. Monitor vital signs every 4 hr, noting deviations from baseline indicative of infection (↑ temp, ↑ pulse).	1. Elevation of temperature or pulse may be indication of infection.	1–2. a. Urine bacteria count less than 100,000/ml urine b. Temperature 37°C Patient promptly reports symptoms of infection (*e.g.*, flank pain, dysuria, chills, hematuria) to the nurse. c. Can demonstrate how to test urinary pH.
2. Monitor urine culture, urinalysis, and WBC. Report deviations from baseline indicative of infection to physician.	2. Physician needs to be alerted to abnormalities in infection so medical intervention can be instituted to control infection.	

(*Continued*)

NURSING CARE PLAN FOR THE PATIENT WITH UROLITHIASIS (*Continued*)

Nursing Interventions	Rationale	Outcome Criteria
3. Administer antibiotics as ordered.	3. Pharmacological intervention to lower infection.	
4. Increase fluids to 400 ml (given throughout 24-hr period).	4. Encourages frequent urination, which avoids urinary stasis	
5. Encourage ambulation.	5. Prevents urinary stasis	
6. Alter pH of urine (<6) for patient with struvite stones:	6. Struvite stones (those stones commonly associated with infection) develop in an alkaline urine.	
a. Teach about acid-ash diet (encourage foods such as eggs, meat, poultry, fish, cereals; fruits and vegetables such as cranberries, prunes, grapes, tomatoes).	a. Acidification of urine prevents stone growth. Foods on acid-ash diet help acidify urine.	a. Can relate foods included in therapeutic diet
b. Teach specific medications to acidify urine.	b. Medication helps to acidify urine.	
c. Teach patient how to test urine pH with Nitrazine paper.	c. Indicates pH of urine so patient can evaluate how successful he is in acidifying urine.	

Goals

Nursing goals for the patient with urinary calculi center around relief of pain, prevention or adequate treatment of infection, passage or removal of the calculi, maintenance of normal renal function, and adequate knowledge regarding therapeutic regimen.

Nursing Interventions

Adequate Hydration. Adequate hydration is most significant for the patient with urinary lithiasis. The nurse must teach the patient how to incorporate a high fluid intake into his lifestyle. Most physicians prefer that fluid intake is above 4000 ml/24-hour period. It is important to translate this into terms the patient can understand, such as one 8-oz glass of water or juice every hour while awake and two 8-oz glasses when the patient awakens during the night to use the bathroom. It is important to space fluid intake so that transient dehydration will not occur. Patients can be taught to measure specific gravity of their urine to ascertain that urine is sufficiently dilute. It is also important to increase fluid intake during periods of potential dehydration, as in hot weather, fever, vomiting, or diarrhea. Intravenous fluids are sometimes necessary if adequate hydration cannot be maintained.

Urine-Straining for Calculi. Urine must be strained with gauze to detect stone when passage occurs. It is important that the patient be instructed how to do this. Any stones obtained should be saved and sent to the lab for content analysis. Such information is important in developing an appropriate plan for medical management.

The nursing plan should promote as much *mobility* as possible for the patient to prevent urinary stasis. Ambulating in the halls frequently during the day is one way to accomplish this. The patient should be encouraged to empty his bladder at least every 2 hours. If the patient is successful in his hydration program, this is easy to accomplish.

Pain Control. Pain control is an important factor for the patient with renal stones. If the patient is not experiencing renal colic, he may be anxious that the pain will soon return. Adequate doses of narcotics should be administered for the pain relief without fear of narcotic addiction. If pain relief is inadequate, the physician should be notified. Support and reassurance can be helpful to allay the anxiety and help the patient cope with the discomfort he is experiencing.

To help ensure patient compliance, the nurse should institute a teaching plan that helps that patient understand how medications or dietary regimens inhibit his particular calculus development. Dietitians and pharmacists can be helpful in outlining the plan, which then can be reinforced by the nurse. It is essential that such a teaching plan occur far enough prior to discharge that reinforcement of content can be given, as well as questions answered. Teaching the patient how to test urinary pH with nitrogen paper is important so that the patient can evaluate the effectiveness of pharmacological and dietary measures.

Postoperative Management. Following open surgical procedures for calculi removal, the postoperative patient must be assessed frequently to detect postoperative hemorrhage, which is common when surgery involves a highly vascular organ such as the kidney. It is necessary to monitor vital signs, wound drainage, and urinary output. Large amounts of serosanguineous drainage can be expected following some renal surgeries. Dressings should be examined and changed frequently.

Nephrostomy tubes are used postoperatively to drain urine from the renal pelvis. It is important to ensure patency of these tubes to avoid buildup of pressure that would ultimately result in renal damage. Tubes should be checked frequently for kinks or plugs. Positioning the patient with pillows can help to prevent pressure on the tubes and decrease the possibility of occlusion of the tube. Nephrostomy tubes should never be clamped. If a nephrostomy tube appear to be plugged, sterile irrigation is permissible with a physician's order. Care must be taken to avoid causing infection or increasing pressure within the renal pelvis. Irrigations should be limited to 4 ml to 6 ml of sterile saline. Nephrostomy site of insertion should be checked for bleeding.

General postoperative measures should be instituted to prevent respiratory complications. Deep breathing and coughing, use of incentive spirometry, and early ambulation help prevent atelectasis and postoperative respiratory problems (see Chap. 8).

Evaluation

Outcome criteria that specifically denote the successful attainment of the nursing goals are important in the evaluation process for the patient with urolithiasis. Specific outcome criteria are listed in the Sample Care Plan for the Patient with Urolithiasis.

References

1. Banner M, Pollack H: Urolithiasis in the lower urinary tract. Semin Roentgenol 17(2):140, April 1982
2. Coe F: Nephrolithiasis: Pathogenesis and Treatment. Chicago, Year Book Medical Publishers, 1978
3. Coe F, Parks J: Hyperuricosuria and calcium nephrolithiasis. Urol Clin North Am 8(2):227, June 1981
4. Menon M, Krishman CS: Evaluation and medical management of the patient with calcium stone disease. Urol Clin North Am 10 (4):599–605, November 1983
5. Nemoy N: Axioms on renal calculi. Hospital Medicine 15:15, February 1979
6. Pak C: The spectrum of pathogenesis of hypercalciuria. Urol Clin North Am 8(2):247, June 1981
7. Robbins S, Angell M, Kumar V: Basic Pathology. Philadelphia, WB Saunders, 1981
8. Rodgers A, Spector M: Human stones. Endeavors 5(3), 1981
9. Smith A, Lee W: Percutaneous stone removal procedure including irrigation. Urol Clin North Am 10(4):724, November 1983
10. Sound, shock waves shatter kidney stones. JAMA 249(18):2434, May 1983

Bibliography

Brenner B, Rector F: The Kidney, 2nd ed. Philadelphia, WB Saunders, 1981

Chaptman R, Bonica J: Acute pain: Current concepts. Upjohn: A Scope Publication, 1983

Derrick F, Carter W: Kidney stone disease: Evaluation and management. Postgrad Med 66(4), October 1979

Fleisch H et al: Urolithiasis Research. WY Plenum Press, 1976

Gault P: How to break the kidney stone cycle. Nursing 78 8:24–31, December 1978

Gracie WA, Ransohoff DF: The natural history of silent gallstones. New Engl J Med 307(13):798–800, September 1982

Kinney AB, Blount M: Effect of cranberry juice on urinary pH. Nurs Res 28:287, 1979

Lyles K, Drezner M: An overview of calcium homeostasis in humans. Urol Clin North Am 8(2):209–226, June 1981

Maki T: Pathogenesis of calcium bilirubinate gallstones: Role of E coli, B-glucuronidase and coagulation by inorganic ions, polyelectrolytes and agitation. Ann Surg 164:90, 1966

McConnell E, Zimmerman M: Care of the Patient with Urologic Problems. Philadephia, JB Lippincott, 1983

Metheny N: Renal stones and urinary pH. Am J Nurs, pp 1372–1375, September 1982

Nelter F: Ciba Collection of Medical Illustrations, Vol. 3, Digestive System—Part III, Liver Biliary Tract and Pancreas; Vol. 6, Kidneys, Ureters and Urinary Bladder. CIBA Pharmaceutical Co, 1964

Resnick M: Evaluation and management of infection stone. Urol Clin North Am 8(2):265–276, June 1981

Sodeman W, Sodeman T: Pathologic Physiology: Mechanisms of Disease, 6th ed. Philadelphia, WB Saunders, 1979

UNIT VII

Nursing Care of Patients with Alterations in Neurological Function

Chapter 62

Review of Anatomy and Physiology
Nervous System

Barbara R. Landau

The nervous system is commonly divided into the central nervous system (CNS), which is the brain and spinal cord, and the peripheral nervous system, which consists of 12 pairs of cranial nerves that arise from the brain and 31 pairs of spinal nerves from the spinal cord. The nervous system is also divided into the somatic and the autonomic nervous system (ANS). The somatic nervous system supplies skeletal muscle and carries sensory information from many parts of the body. The autonomic nervous system is a motor system that innervates smooth and cardiac muscle and some glands.

The Brain and Related Structures

The Brain

The brain is commonly divided into the brain stem and the greatly enlarged cerebral hemispheres (Fig. 62–1).

The Brain Stem

The brain stem consists of the medulla, pons, and midbrain. It contains fiber tracts connecting the brain and spinal cord, central connections for cranial nerves, several important control centers including those for heart rate, blood pressure, and breathing, and the reticular formation that extends through the posterior portion of the brain stem. The reticular formation is a region of many synapses and small neurons, and it is important for many somatic and autonomic activities. At its superior end the midbrain divides into two cerebral peduncles, one of which enters each cerebral hemisphere.

The cerebellum is not part of the brain stem, but it is part of the hindbrain. It is separated from the brain stem by the fourth ventricle, but it is connected to the brain stem by three paired fiber bundles, the cerebellar peduncles.

The Forebrain

The diencephalon is a continuation of the brain stem on either side of the third ventricle. Its major components are the thalamus and hypothalamus. The thalamus consists of several groups of nuclei with important relay functions. They have been classified according to the type of information they transmit, as sensory relay, motor relay, limbic relay nuclei, association nuclei (to cortical association areas), and nonspecific or diffuse nuclei (to the entire cortex). The hypothalamus contains important centers for control of visceral and other functions, and it controls the pituitary gland.

The cerebral hemispheres consist of the cerebral cortex, which is a thin layer of gray matter on the surface, the basal

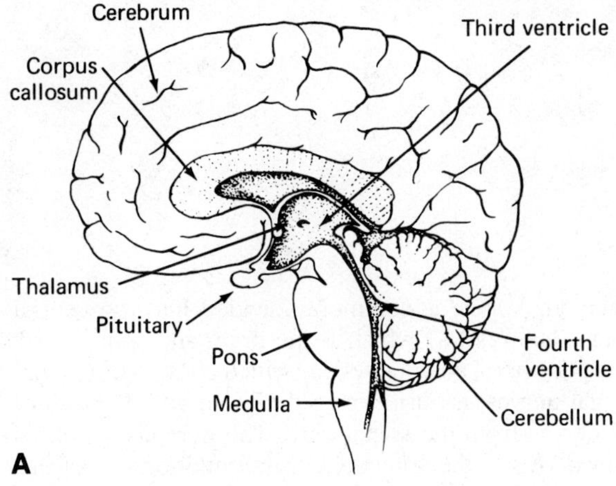

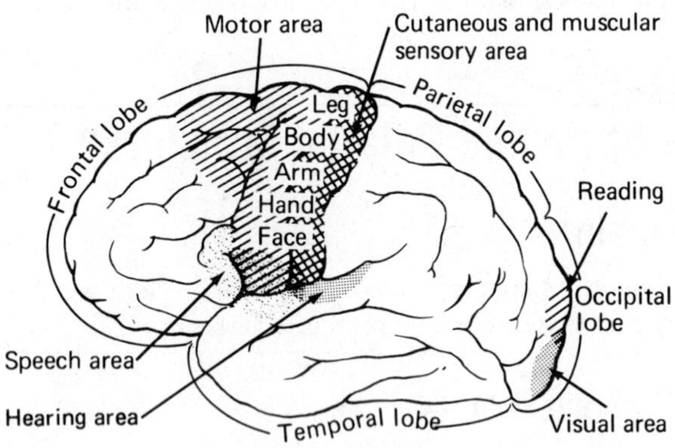

FIGURE 62–1 (*A*) Major structures of the brain. (*B*) Diagrammatic representation of approximate areas of the brain that control various functions.

ganglia (really basal nuclei) deep in the hemispheres, and white fiber tracts. The fiber tracts connect one part of the cortex to another (association fibers), one hemisphere with the other (commissural fibers), or the cortex with other parts of the brain or spinal cord (projection fibers).

The cerebral surface is marked by ridges (gyri) and grooves (sulci) that greatly increase the area and hence the amount of cortical gray matter. The hemispheres are divided into lobes, each named for the bone that covers it. The lobes are separated by prominent fissures or sulci, except for the occipital lobe, whose boundaries are less clearly delineated. The precentral gyrus, which is in the frontal lobe anterior to the central sulcus, contains the primary motor area associated with skeletal muscle activity. The postcentral gyrus, which is the parietal lobe behind the central sulcus, contains the primary receiving area for sensory pathways from the body surface and is known as the somatosensory area. The temporal lobe contains the primary receiving area for audition, and the occipital lobe contains the visual receiving area. Association areas are adjacent to the senory receiving areas.

The rhinecephalon includes olfactory structures on the ventral surface of the forebrain, and tracts that connect with several parts of the brain. In humans the olfactory role is not well developed, but as the limbic system, its connections with the hypothalamus and other centers serve important integrative functions.

Cranial Nerves

The first two cranial nerves arise from outgrowths of the forebrain, but the others arise from the brain stem in a manner rather similar to spinal nerves (Fig. 62–2). Cell bodies of sensory neurons are in ganglia outside the CNS, whereas those of somatic and autonomic motor neurons are in individual nuclei. Most cranial nerves are mixed, but some are entirely sensory and several are entirely motor. The cranial nerves and their components are summarized in Table 62–1.

Related Structures

The Ventricles

The CNS developed embryologically from a tube that remains as the ventricles in the brain and the central canal in the spinal cord. The large paired lateral ventricles are in the cerebral hemispheres and have extensions into each lobe. They communicate through interventricular foramina with the narrow midline third ventricle. The tiny cerebral aqueduct connects the third and fourth ventricles.

The Cranial Meninges and Cerebrospinal Fluid

The brain is enclosed by the same meningeal layers as the spinal cord—dura mater, arachnoid, and pia mater—and these layers are continuous through the foramen magnum. The cranial dura, however, has two layers: the outermost is in close contact with the cranial periosteum and the inner layer forms folds that help to protect the brain and limit its movement. The falx cerebri is in the longitudinal fissure between the hemispheres, and the tentorium cerebelli forms a roof over the cerebellum, separating it from the cerebrum. Large venous sinuses are located in both the free and attached edges of the dural folds.

Cerebrospinal fluid (CSF) fills the ventricles and the subarachnoid space around the brain and spinal cord. It is formed in the ventricles by the choroid plexuses. Cerebrospinal fluid resembles plasma, but it contains virtually no protein and is generally under only a slight pressure (10 to 20 mmHg.) The CSF circulates slowly from the lateral to the third and fourth ventricles, and through openings in the roof of the fourth ventricle out into the subarachnoid space. Tiny arachnoid projections (arachnoid villi) protrude into the large venous sinuses, and the CSF filters through them into the venous sinuses. The CSF must be removed at the same rate that it is formed, and if its flow is blocked, pressure may become very high in the ventricles and they may become enlarged, at the expense of brain tissue. The CSF provides an important protection for the brain, partly by acting as a cushion against blows and partly by lending buoyancy to the very soft brain tissue which, in effect, reduces brain weight.

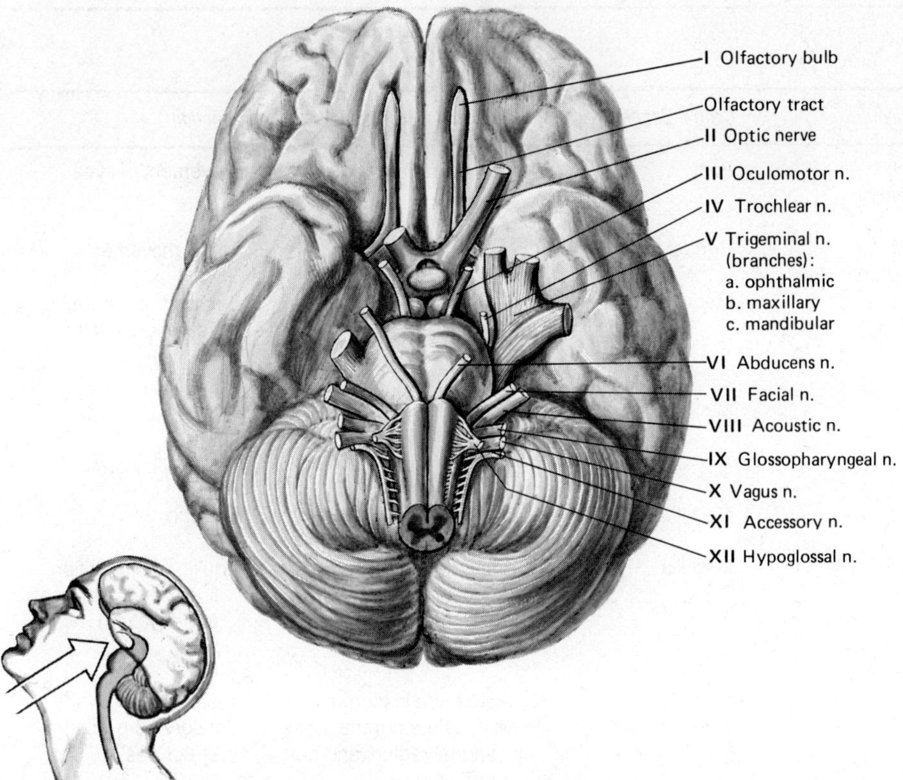

FIGURE 62–2 Base of brain, showing origin of the cranial nerves.

TABLE 62–1
The Cranial Nerves

Nerve	*Components*	*Central Connections*	*Peripheral Connections*	*Function*
I. Olfactory	Afferent	Olfactory tract and bulb	Olfactory epithelium in nasal cavity	Smell
II. Optic	Afferent	Optic chiasm and tract	Photoreceptors in retina	Vision
III. Oculomotor*	Efferent (somatic)	Midbrain	Extraocular muscles (superior, inferior, and medial rectus; inferior oblique)	Movement of eyes
	Efferent (visceral)	Midbrain	Ciliary muscle and pupillary constrictors	Accommodation for near vision, constriction of pupils
IV. Trochlear*	Efferent (somatic)	Midbrain	Extraocular muscles (superior oblique)	Movement of eyes
V. Trigeminal	Afferent	Pons	Skin and mucous membrane	General sensations
Ophthalmic division			Forehead, orbit, nasal cavity	
Maxillary division			Maxillary region, teeth of upper jaw	
Mandibular division			Mandibular region, teeth of lower jaw	
Motor division	Efferent (somatic)	Pons	Muscles of mastication	Mastication
	Afferent	Midbrain	Proprioceptors on muscles of mastication	Muscle sense

(*Continued*)

TABLE 62–1
The Cranial Nerves (Continued)

Nerve	Components	Central Connections	Peripheral Connections	Function
VI. Abducens*	Efferent (somatic)	Pons	Extraocular muscle (lateral rectus)	Movement of eyes
VII. Facial	Efferent (somatic)	Caudal pons	Muscles of facial expression	Facial movements
	Efferent (visceral)	Medulla	Salivary glands (sublingual and submaxillary; lacrimal glands)	Secretion of saliva; secretion of tears
	Afferent	Medulla	Taste buds near tip of tongue	Taste
VIII. Vestibulocochlearis				
Cochlear	Afferent	Medulla	Receptors in spiral organs of inner ear	Hearing
Vestibular	Afferent	Medulla	Receptors in semicircular canals, utricle, and saccule (vestibular apparatus in inner ear)	Equilibrium (position, linear and rotary acceleration)
IX. Glossopharyngeal	Afferent	Medulla	Taste buds in tongue	Taste
	Afferent	Medulla	Mucous membrane, pharyngeal region, and carotid sinus	Sensory from visceral structures†
	Efferent (visceral)	Medulla	Salivary gland (parotid)	Secretion of saliva
	Efferent (somatic)	Medulla	Muscles of pharynx	Swallowing
X. Vagus	Efferent (visceral)	Medulla	Cardiac pacemaker and muscle; smooth muscle and glands of thorax and abdomen	Regulation of visceral structures (parasympathetic)
	Efferent (somatic)	Medulla	Muscles of pharynx and larynx	Swallowing, control of larynx
	Afferent	Medulla	Viscera of thorax and abdomen	Sensory from visceral structures†
XI. Spinal accessory	Efferent (somatic)	Medulla	Muscles of pharynx and larynx (distributed with vagus)	Swallowing, control of larynx
	Efferent (somatic)	Upper cervical segments of spinal cord (enters through foramen magnum)	Sternocleidomastoid and trapezius muscles	Movement of head and shoulder
XII. Hypoglossal*	Efferent (somatic)	Medulla	Extrinsic and intrinsic muscles of tongue	Movement of tongue

* Nerves III, IV, VI, and XII also contain afferent fibers from proprioceptors in extraocular muscles and muscle of tongue. They serve muscle sense.
† Some visceral afferents reach the level of consciousness and cause sensation, but others do not, and hence do not cause a sensation (such as afferents from receptors in blood vessels that detect blood pressure).

Blood Supply to the Brain

The arterial supply to the brain comes from the internal carotid and vertebral arteries. The internal carotid arteries branch into the anterior cerebrals to the medial surface of the hemispheres, and the middle cerebral flow to the lateral surface. The vertebral arteries join on the surface of the medulla to form the basilar artery, which gives off branches to the brain stem and cerebellum before terminating in the posterior cerebral arteries to the posterior and inferior portions of the hemispheres. Tiny communicating arteries connect these arteries and theoretically make it possible to maintain a blood supply if flow in one of the major arteries is blocked.

Venous blood drains into surface veins in the subarachnoid space, which empty into one of the large venous sinuses in the dural folds. The sinuses converge and eventually drain into a sinus that becomes the internal jugular vein as it leaves the skull.

The Spinal Cord, Spinal Nerves, and Spinal Reflexes

Anatomy of the Spinal Cord

The spinal cord extends from the foramen magnum to about the level of the second lumbar vertebra (L2). There are 31 pairs of spinal nerves: 8 cervical, 12 thoracic, 5 lumbar, 5 sacral, and 1 coccygeal. They emerge from the spinal cord at regular intervals, but since the cord is shorter than the vertebral canal, the nerve roots must descend in the canal to exit through an intervertebral foramen at the proper level. Below L2 the vertebral canal contains only spinal nerve roots (the cauda equina), and it is the preferred site for lumbar puncture (Fig. 62–3).

Spinal Nerves and Their Distribution

Upon emerging from the vertebral canal, each spinal nerve divides into a small posterior ramus that supplies intrinsic muscles of the back and the skin over them, and a larger anterior ramus that follows around the body wall to the anterior midline, giving off cutaneous and muscular branches. The distribution of spinal nerves is clearly shown in the trunk as strips of skin known as dermatomes (Fig. 62–4).

Spinal Reflexes

Reflexes are involved in virtually everything a person does, and although most are quite complex, they are all governed by the same principles as the simplest spinal reflexes. As the response to a stimulus, the minimal reflex requires something to detect the stimulus (a sensory receptor), something to respond to it (an effector), and a connection between them (nerve fibers and a synapse). This connection, however, usually involves more than a single synapse, and is commonly called a center.

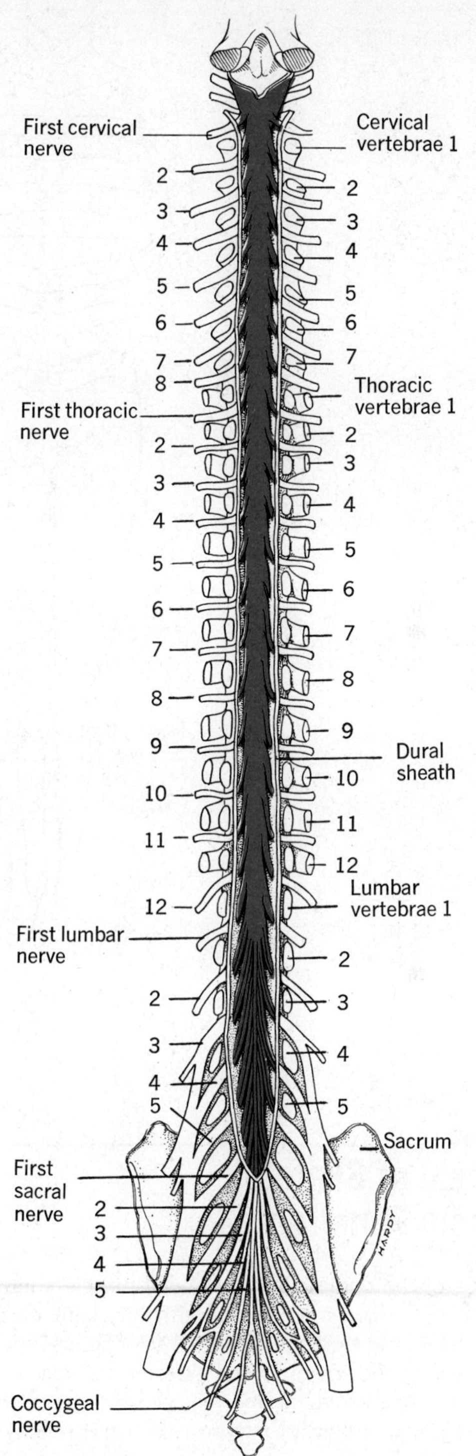

FIGURE 62–3 Spinal cord lying within the vertebral canal. Spinous processes and laminae have been removed; dura and arachnoid have been opened. Spinal nerves are numbered on the left side; vertebrae are numbered on the right side.

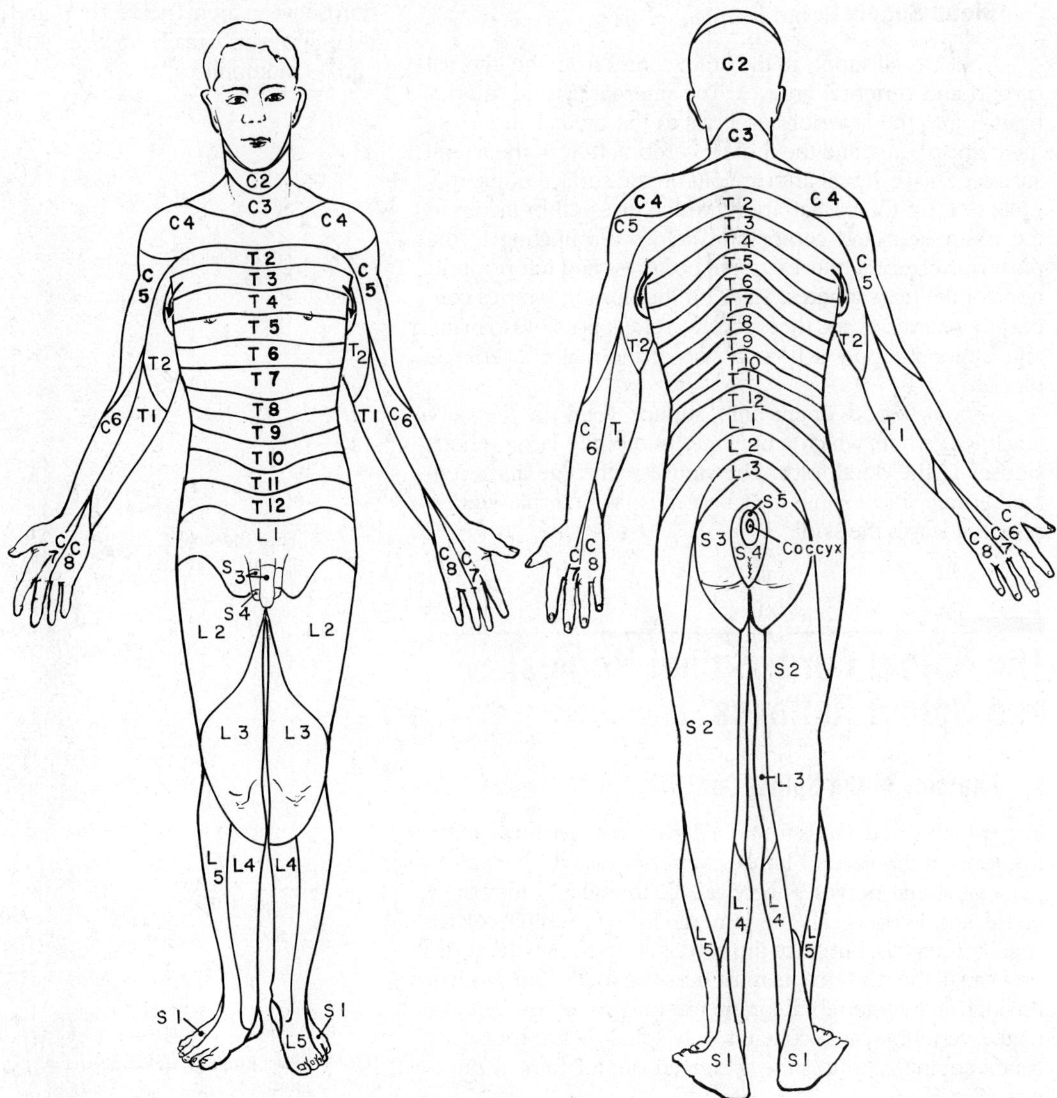

FIGURE 62–4 Cutaneous distribution of spinal nerves (dermatomes). (Barr ML, Kiernan JA: The Human Nervous System: An Anatomical Viewpoint, 4th ed. New York, Harper & Row, 1983)

Control of Skeletal Muscle Function

Because of the complexity of skeletal muscle control, it is convenient to dismantle the smoothly operating mechanism and consider the elements separately. Somatic motor actions can be approached from several different but related aspects: as postural or movement and manipulation; as extensor or flexor; as tonic or phasic; or as nonvoluntary (reflex) or truly voluntary (willed).

Postural control involves mechanisms to resist gravity and provide a stable base of support for other movements. Postural adjustments are carried out mainly by extensor or antigravity muscles, and the responses are generally tonic and nonvoluntary, often below the level of consciousness.

Movement and manipulation activities include skilled precision movements such as those of the fingers and some of the limb movements that move the body. They are more likely to involve flexor muscles, phasic contractions such as the rhythmic movements of walking, and to be truly voluntary.

Both types of activity require integrative mechanisms to coordinate different muscle groups and to direct complex patterns of movement. The centers that control these varied aspects of somatic motor function are located at nearly every level from spinal cord to the cerebral cortex.

Coordination

The cerebellum is the structure primarily concerned with coordination. The three pairs of cerebellar peduncles connect it with the spinal cord, the pons, and the midbrain.

The cerebellum receives input from muscle spindles (unconscious proprioceptors) by way of the spinocerebellar tracts, collateral branches of ascending fibers (conscious proprioceptors), the vestibular apparatus by way of vestibular nuclei in the brainstem, and finally a very important input from the cerebral cortex by way of nuclei in the pons. The output of the cerebellum is to the motor neurons by way of the reticulospinal, vestibulospinal, and rubrospinal tracts, and to the cerebral cortex by way of motor relay nuclei in the thalamus.

The cerebellum may be considered as a comparator. Its input from the cortex provides information about the directions sent to the muscles and what the muscles *should be* doing, and input from the spinal cord reports what the muscles *are* doing. The cerebellum then acts to correct any discrepancies by calling for modifications in the motor output of both the cortex and the other pathways to the motor neurons. Cerebellar lesions cause errors in rate, range, force, and direction of movements (missing or overshoot), performing movements in parts rather than smoothly (dissection of movements), inability to perform rapidly alternating movements (supination–pronation), and intention tremors (which appear only when a movement is attempted).

The Autonomic Nervous System

The autonomic nervous system (ANS) controls visceral effectors: cardiac and smooth muscle, and some glands. As an involuntary system, all of its actions are reflex, and although it is an efferent system, its reflex nature requires an afferent input. The afferent side is often overlooked because its organization is the same as somatic afferents, and, in fact, many afferent fibers influence both somatic and autonomic efferents.

The ANS has two divisions, sympathetic and parasympathetic. Many visceral organs are supplied by both divisions, and in these organs the two divisions usually have opposing actions (Table 62–2).

The parasympathetic nervous system is also known as the craniosacral division because it arises from the brain and sacral cord. The cranial component comes from four cranial nerves: III (oculomotor), VII (facial), IX (glossopharyngeal), and X (vagus). Postganglionic cell bodies are in the wall of the organ. The sacral component is carried in the pelvic nerve, which is formed from spinal nerves S2, S3, and S4, and supplies the pelvic viscera and genitalia.

TABLE 62–2
Some Important Effects of Autonomic Stimulation

Effector	*Sympathetic (adrenegic)*	*Parasympathetic (cholinergic)*
Cardiac muscle and pacemaker	Stimulation Acceleration	Inhibition Deceleration
Smooth muscle		
Skin (piloerectors)*	Contraction	
Digestive system	Inhibition	Contraction, increase tone and motility
Urinary bladder	Inhibition	Contraction (empties)
Bronchioles	Dilation	Constriction
Pupil	Dilation	Constriction
Blood vessels		
Cutaneous*	Constriction	
Skeletal muscle	Some dilation (a few fibers cause constriction, and some are cholinergic)	
Viscera (most)	Constriction	(Dilation in a very few organs)
Glands		
Lacrimal		Secretion
Respiratory passages	Inhibition	Secretion
Digestive system		
Salivary	Scant, viscous secretion	Profuse, watery secretion
Stomach	Inhibition (?)	Secretion
Intestine	Inhibition (?)	Secretion
Pancreas (exocrine)	Decreased secretion	Increased secretion
Liver	Release glucose into bloodstream	
Adrenal medulla	Secretion	
Sweat glands*	Secretion (cholinergic)	

* *Note:* Skin structures have no parasympathetic innervation.

Functions

Autonomic actions tend to be integrative and regulatory. Whereas the somatic nervous system responds to changes in the external environment, the autonomic nervous system responds to changes in the internal environment. The ANS plays a major role in maintaining the constancy of that internal environment (*i.e.,* homeostasis), and is the chief regulator of most of the organ systems that control the internal environment.

The specific actions of the two divisions of the ANS are shown in Table 62–2. Several conclusions can be drawn from the table, as follows:

1. In organs that have a dual innervation, actions are generally opposing, but in glands with a dual innervation, the actions are different but not necessarily opposing.
2. Some glands are innervated by only one division.
3. The skin receives only a sympathetic innervation.
4. Almost all blood vessels receive only a sympathetic innervation.
5. All smooth muscle does not show the same response to one division.
6. The sympathetic division does not always excite or increase responses.

The sympathetic nervous system often discharges as a unit. The effects of such a mass discharge are those associated with the mobilization of resources and the expenditure of energy needed to meet an emergency. The familiar fight–flight response includes cardiac acceleration, vasoconstriction that reduces blood flow to skin and viscera, inhibition of the digestive system, epinephrine secretion by the adrenal medulla, and release of glucose by the liver.

Although it is an endocrine gland, the adrenal medulla is an integral part of the sympathetic nervous system. It is under sympathetic control and the actions of its hormones (chiefly epinephrine, and some norepinephrine) are those of the sympathetic nervous system, and their release as part of the sympathetic mass discharge reinforces the response.

The sympathetic division is not essential to life. Sympathectomized laboratory animals can survive very well, but do not cope well with stresses such as cold. The sympathetic nervous system is quite capable of discrete response in which activity of an individual organ is altered independently.

The parasympathetic nervous system is organized for discrete, localized responses of individual organs; a parasympathetic mass discharge would not be advantageous. Parasympathetic actions, in contrast to sympathetic actions, tend to be of a more restorative and conservational nature.

Some portion of each division is active at all times. In some organs one division is tonically active and exerts major control. For example, the parasympathetic innervation to the heart dominates, while sympathetic action controls blood vessels, most of which receive no parasympathetic innervation.

Bibliography

Chusid JG: Correlative Neuroanatomy and Functional Neurology, 18th ed. Los Altos CA, Lange Medical Publications, 1982

Eyzaguirre C, Fidone SJ: Physiology of the Nervous System, 2nd ed. Chicago, Year Book Medical Publishers, 1975

Ganong WF: Review of Medical Physiology, 11th ed. Los Altos CA, Lange Medical Publications, 1983

Landau BR: Essential Human Anatomy and Physiology, 2nd ed. Glenview, IL, Scott, Foresman and Company, 1980

Noback CR, Demarest RJ: The Human Nervous System, 3rd ed. New York, McGraw-Hill, 1981

Patton HD, Sundsten JW, Crill WE, Swanson PD: Introduction to Basic Neurology. Philadelphia, WB Saunders, 1976

Somjen GG: Neurophysiology—The Essentials. Baltimore, Williams & Wilkins, 1983

Vander AJ, Sherman JS, Luciano DS: Human Physiology—The Mechanisms of Body Function, 3rd ed. New York, McGraw-Hill, 1980

Chapter 63

Assessment of Neurological Function

Karen Booth McCormick

Assessment of nervous system function consists of general observation of the patient, the gathering of data from the patient's history, and a systematic neurological examination. Both nurses and physicians perform neurological assessments, sharing some of the same methods and at times the same goals (*e.g.,* detection of change in baseline neurological status), but for the most part their focus is different. Physicians make neurological assessments for the primary purpose of localizing pathology and making a diagnosis. Nurses make neurological assessments for the primary purpose of determining the types of deficits the patient has and how these impact his life.

General Observation

A directed but general observation of the patient and how he relates to his environment can be extremely useful in the assessment of the nervous system. Observation of the general behavior of the patient may be done at the initial contact, before the formal process of taking the history begins.

Level of Consciousness

If the patient is in bed, is he awake or sleeping? If he is awake, does he appear to be alert and attentive? Does he respond appropriately to his environment or does he appear confused? Is he drowsy? If he is drowsy, will he stay awake as long as interaction is required or will he fall asleep in the middle of a conversation? If he is drowsy or asleep, what kind of stimulus does it take to elicit a response, for example, voice, shaking, noxious stimuli, and what is the nature of his response, for example, opens eyes, attempts to remove the noxious stimulus, abnormal posturing of an extremity, or no response at all, even to deep noxious stimulation?

General Appearance

How old does the patient appear? Is he well groomed with cleanliness of his body and clothes? Are his clothes properly placed on his body? Does he wear glasses or use a hearing aid or other prostheses? Are there any obvious asymmetries of his face or extremities? Is there any eye deviation? Are there any wounds, burns, scrapes, or bruises on his extremities? Are there any obvious birthmarks or skin tumors?

Affect. Is his affect appropriate to the setting and his condition? Does he appear depressed, or glib and unconcerned? Does he appear to be tense? Does he appear to be in pain, for example, does he protect a body part, assume a stilted or rigid posture, and attempt to minimize movement; is his face drawn up or contorted?

Gait. Does the gait appear normal with normal stepping and arm swing? Is the gait slow, with swinging (circumduction) of the leg from the hip in order to clear the ground? Is one leg lifted abnormally high in order to clear the ground? Does the foot drop? Does it clear the ground? Is there scuffing of the toes of the shoes? Is the gait wide-based or unsteady; is there swaying, staggering, or reeling? Is the gait characterized by a "slapping" of the feet against the ground as the heel hits the ground first followed by the toes in an exaggerated or overly hard stamping manner (sensory ataxia)? Is the gait slow and shuffling (*e.g.,* Parkinson's disease, senile gait, or apraxic gait)?

Movement. Do the patient's movements seem to be smooth, coordinated, and natural, and are they carried out at a normal pace? Are the movements slow? Do any body parts assume unnatural positions? Are movements jerky or uncoordinated? Are there any involuntary movements, for example, tremors, facial grimacing, brief jerks of an extremity or body part, writhing movements, or flailing movements?

Any abnormalities should be noted and recorded later as the initial part of the examination; likewise, if the patient appears to be in good health and there are no obvious abnormalites, this should also be recorded.

Ongoing Assessment. General observation of the patient's behavior, of course, is not limited to part of the formal neurological assessment but is an ongoing process that assumes paramount importance in the daily care of the patient with a neurological illness. The nurse is in an ideal position to make pertinent observations of the behavior of the patient and how he interacts with his environment. It is not at all uncommon for the nurse to be the first to note that a patient has a neurological deficit that was not noted on formal examination but becomes apparent as the patient goes about the tasks of daily living. Thus, the nurse must at least be familiar with the behavioral neurological deficits in order to be aware of what to observe when providing care to the patient with a neurological disease.

Medical History

The medical history serves many purposes. Its primary purpose is to provide health care providers with a thorough history of the patient's state of health. In the process of meeting this goal, it also

1. Provides necessary information for making a diagnosis, both medical and nursing (many neurological disorders may be accurately diagnosed on the basis of the history alone)
2. Provides direction to the subsequent physical examination, both medical and nursing; that is, if the patient's problem suggests a difficulty with language, that portion of the examination that tests language functions will be expanded
3. Provides information that introduces us to the patient as an individual
4. Provides information about the patient's strengths and weaknesses and how he generally copes with problems and illnesses
5. Provides information which portrays that patient's health potential and which may also signal that the patient is at risk for incurring other illnesses or injuries
6. Provides a basis for health teaching
7. Provides part of the information from which medical and nursing care may be planned.

For the nurse, the patient's history becomes integral to making a nursing diagnosis and planning subsequent care. Unless the nurse is functioning in a role as the person responsible for the patient's medical history and physical, for example, as a nurse practitioner or a clinical nurse specialist, she can modify the medical history and direct her interview to those aspects that will meeting nursing care goals. Such a format will be presented later in this chapter.

It should be noted that the patient interview, though conducted for the purpose of obtaining a history, also provides an excellent opportunity for establishing rapport with the patient. The interviewer should be an attentive listener with a warm and reassuring demeanor and should conduct herself in a caring and professional manner. The patient is often frightened by the assessment process and worried about the outcome. Some of the information needed for a thorough history may make the patient feel threatened and thus defensive and possibly uncooperative. Every effort should be made to make the patient feel comfortable and safe in sharing information about his personal life.

Neurological History

Some of the data sought in the patient's history assumes particular significance when interviewing a patient with a neurological disorder. The *introductory information* should make special note of the source of the information. Sometimes the patient is unable to give the history because of altered level of consciousness, or a thought or language disorder, and the history must be obtained from a relative, friend, or even past medical records. The ancestral heritage, or nationality, of the patient may be important, in that some neurological disorders are seen more commonly in, but usually not limited to, individuals with a given heritage (such as Mediterranean or Scandinavian). Where the patient has lived and traveled may play a role in his illness. For instance, individuals who have spent their childhood years in northern latitudes (north of 37°) may have an increased risk of developing multiple sclerosis.[1] Also, exposure to some infectious processes are endemic to certain areas, for example, coccidioidomycosis is common in the Southwest and malaria in the tropics. In addition, inquiry regarding the patient's handedness should be made.

The history of the *present illness/problem* should provide a detailed account of each symptom, its nature (*i.e.,* location, quality, and severity), date of onset, precipitating factors, and duration (*i.e.,* constant, intermittent, or worse at any particular time of day). It should also be noted what, if anything, makes the symptom worse or better, and what has been the general pattern of progression (*i.e.,* rapid, static, progressively worse, remitting, and exacerbating).

The *past medical history,* in addition to the established format, should provide information regarding any chronic or recent exposures to toxins or chemicals. A thorough review of the nature of the patient's occupation and hobbies, with a focus on exposure to lead-based paints, insecticides, mercury, and the like, will generally elicit this information. Recent exposure to viruses or recent vaccinations should be noted. Recent insect, spider, tick, snake, or scorpion bites or stings should also be noted. An inquiry for the history of any fairly recent injury should be made. All *childhood illnesses* and *major injuries* should be documented, and particular attention should be given to the *developmental history,* including the perinatal history (*e.g.,* difficult labor or prematurity).

The *family history* is also very important. Many neurological disorders are familial or hereditary. Questioning of the patient should be directed toward the history in any family members of problems with headaches, weakness or paralysis, loss of sensation, involuntary movements or tremors, or retardation or dementia.

The *neurological portion of the review of systems* should be expanded to include any history of problems that may be associated with nervous system dysfunction.

Often when the patient complains of a neurological symptom, it is necessary to determine exactly what he means. For example, it is not uncommon for a patient to state that his arm or leg is weak, when in actuality it is numb. Clarification of what the patient is experiencing is also necessary in determining the nature of the symptom. Many times the nature or characteristics of the symptom suggest one diagnosis over another. A throbbing, severe, unilateral headache lasting about 6 to 24 hours and associated with photophobia, nausea, and vomiting suggests a diagnosis of migraine, whereas a constant, unremitting, generalized headache described as a feeling of a tight band around the head and lasting for days, weeks, or even months is usually characteristic of a tension muscle contraction headache.

Certain common neurological symptoms such as pain, headache, vertigo, numbness, and visual disturbances constitute historical data that should be obtained.

Pain. The exact *location* of the pain should be established. Does the pain involve more than one area? Does it seem to be in these areas simultaneously or does it radiate from one area to another? If it radiates, what is the path of its movement?

The *quality* of the pain should be ascertained. Is it throbbing, aching, burning, boring, dull, or lancinating (*i.e.,* sharp, knifelike, or stabbing)? Is it deep or superficial? Is there any tenderness over the area? One should be careful not to "put words into the patient's mouth." It may be helpful to ask the patient, "If you were going to cause this pain in someone else, what would you use to produce it?"

What is the *severity* of the pain? Is it mild, moderate, or severe? The patient can be asked to grade his pain on a scale of 1 to 5 (with 1 being mild and 5 being intolerably severe). What is the *duration* and *timing* of the pain? Is it intermittent, lasting only a few seconds? Does it last for minutes or hours? Is it always present, day after day? Does it interfere with sleep? Is it worse at any particular time of the day?

Are there any *precipitating factors* such as movement, weather changes, stress, sneezing, or straining? What *alleviates* the pain? Does rest, heat, or cold, or analgesics (type, dosage, frequency) relieve the pain or make it better? Are there any *associated symptoms* such as nausea or vomiting, changes in temperature or color of a part, or any swelling?

Headache. Much of the above section is relevant to the headache history. Special attention should be given to the location of the headache, especially regarding whether it is unilateral or bilateral, throbbing or aching, worse in the morning on awakening (elevated intracranial pressure) or worse as the day progresses (tension), associated with photophobia, nausea, or vomiting, precipiated or made worse by straining, sneezing, stress, or use of alcohol. What relieves the headache—for example, a change in posture or medication? An inquiry regarding the patient's habits can sometimes provide a clue to the etiology; occipital neuralgia, a headache resembling tension headache, can be caused by pressure to the occipital area incurred when reading in bed with the head propped up against a hard surface.

Vertigo. The patient may mean different things when he complains of dizziness or light-headedness. It should be determined what the patient means by the use of these terms. Vertigo is the sensation of movement or spinning of the self or of the environment. Are there any associated symptoms of nausea, vomiting, ataxia, tinnitus, impaired hearing, or alteration of consciousness (*e.g.,* fainting, or feeling of unreality or detachment)? Does anything aggravate or alleviate the dizziness, such as position changes or closing the eyes?

Numbness. Determine if the patient means weakness rather than, or in addition to, numbness. Ask the patient to map out the involved areas. What is the nature of the numbness? Is it associated with tingling as if the part is "going to sleep," or peculiar sensations of creeping or crawling (paresthesias)? Is it also associated with pain? Does a certain position or activity precipitate or worsen the numbness? Has the patient ever injured himself or burned himself without being aware of it? Is the numbness intermittent or consistent? Does it precede headache or loss of consciousness or tonic–clonic movements of an extremity? If a preprinted neurological examination form that illustrates an anterior and posterior view of the body is available, the patient can be asked to shade in the areas that he feels are the ones affected (this does not substitute for a sensory examination).

Visual Disturbances. It is not uncommon for the patient to refer to double vision (diplopia) as blurred vision. In fact, many visual disturbances are often described as other than what they are. Visual disturbances may take the form of a generalized decreased visual acuity, loss of vision in an area of the visual field, a distortion of vision (such as wavy shapes), double vision, or total loss of vision. One should determine if the disturbance is constant or intermittent in nature (*e.g.,* migraine prodrome or transient ischemic attack). Does anything make it better? Closing one eye relieves diplopia; it does not matter which eye is closed since diplopia usually results from dysfunction of the coordination of eye movements. Does anything make it worse, such as eyestrain? Does it first appear or become worse as the day progresses (*e.g.*, diplopia seen in myasthenia gravis)?

In the course of taking the patient's history, the nurse might elicit information that suggests the presence of a seizure disorder. For information regarding what behaviors indicate a seizure disorder and how to obtain a seizure history, the reader is referred to Chapter 65.

Neurological Examination

Examination of the nervous system provides information regarding the functional integrity of neurological systems. A deficit or group of deficits, because of the way in which the nervous system is organized, will often provide the information needed to localize the area of the pathological process. This information, combined with the history, allows determination of the nature of the pathological process, for example, neoplastic, vascular, infectious, and degenerative. Further diagnostic tests such as angiography, myelography, or computerized tomography serve to define even further the precise location and often the nature and extent of the lesion; many diagnostic tests also provide information regarding the integrity of surrounding areas.

The nurse, unless functioning in an expanded role, need not acquire the art and skill of conducting a complete neurological examination. She should, however, have a basic understanding of what functions are being tested, what constitute normal and abnormal responses, and what these responses indicate. This knowledge will enable the nurse to correlate neurological deficits exhibited by the patient with the anatomical area of pathology or dysfunction. This information, along with a basic understanding of neuroanatomy and neurophysiology, provides the theoretical background necessary for the identification as well as the anticipation of possible changes in the patient's neurological status when they occur. A format for a neurological examination that is oriented toward the goals of nursing, and that is especially useful in the hospital or home setting, will be presented later in this chapter.

The neurological examination is a part of the physical examination. For the most part, the entire physical examination is done, even when the focus is neurological. This is especially important if the patient has not had a recent physical examination. Occasionally, however, only the neurological examination is done.

The medical model for the neurological examination is divided into six major areas: mental status, cranial nerves, motor system, reflexes, sensory function, and cerebellar function. The examiner may conduct the examination in any sequence preferred (*e.g.*, testing all sensory functions including cranial nerves at once, and likewise for motor functions), but the examination is documented in an orderly fashion similar to that listed above (Fig. 63–1).[4]

General Observations

A surprising amount of information is obtained in the process of making general observations of the patient and in the process of obtaining the history (*e.g.*, status, language, and articulation of speech). When recording the examination, the general observations should be noted in a concise, descriptive paragraph that precedes the formal examination.

Vital Signs

Following the general observations, the vital signs should be noted. The patient's temperature, right and left radial pulses, respiration, right and left brachial blood pressures, as well as a lying and standing blood pressure (immediate, and after 3 minutes), and the patient's weight and height should be recorded. Many neurological symptoms can be due to cerebral vascular ischemia from a variety of causes. Postural (orthostatic) hypotension can cause dizziness or syncopal attacks. A difference in systolic blood pressures (of at least 20 mmHg), accompanied by differences in the quality and rate of the right and left radial pulses, in the presence of symptoms of vertebrobasilar insufficiency (*i.e.*, dizziness, visual loss, blurring, or diplopia, syncope, ataxia, dysarthria, and sensory and motor loss of the face and extremities) may indicate cerebral ischemia. The ischemia occurs secondary to a "steal" of blood from the vertebrobasilar arteries into the brachial artery. The brachial artery "steals" the blood because it is partially obstructed (lower pressure gradient). This condition is called subclavian steal syndrome.

Mental Status

The mental status examination follows in the recording sequence. Actually, much of it has been done while obtaining the history. An important point to remember in the assessment of mental status is to conduct those portions that need to be tested specifically in such a way that the patient does not feel that his intelligence is being challenged.

The mental status examination is divided into six parts. These include general appearance and behavior, stream of talk, mood and affective responses, content of thought, intellectual capacity, and sensorium.

After making those observations noted above, the examiner can specifically test the patient's short-term memory by giving him three unrelated words to remember. After all three words have been given to the patient, he should be asked to repeat them immediately and also to recall them 5 minutes later. In the 5-minute interval, the patient is distracted with other parts of the examination. Another area that needs to be tested specifically is the patient's ability to perform calculations. Generally, he is asked to do "serial sevens." This task requires the patient to subtract 7 from 100, 7 from the remainder, and so on. One can also request the patient to multiply 33 × 4 or spell "world" backward.[15]

FIGURE 63–1 Neurological exam form. (Prepared by Teresa M. Chmelir, RN, MN)

Neurological Exam

Handedness ____________

Gait ____________

Tandem ____________

Heels, toes ____________

Romberg ____________

Mental Status

Level of consc. OX3 ____________

Naming objects ____________

Memory: Recent ____________

Remote ____________

Retention ____________

Calculations ____________

Speech

Cranial Nerves

I. Smell ____________

II. V. acuity ____________

Fundoscopic ____________

Visual fields ____________

III, IV, VI. EOM ____________

Nystagmus, diplopia ____________

Pupils & converg. ____________

V. Facial sens. LT, PP ____________

Masseters ____________

VII. Facial movements

Smile, look up ____________

Purse lips, close eyes ____________

VIII. Hear whisper ____________

Rinne (air vs. bone) ____________

Weber (forehead) ____________

IX, X. Gag, swallowing ____________

Palatal elevation ____________

XI. Turn head (SCM) ____________

Shrug shoulders (Trap) ____________

XII. Tongue (midline) ____________

Invol. movements ____________

Motor

Strength ____________

Bulk, tone ____________

Pronator drift ____________

Invol. movements ____________

Sensory

Light touch ____________

Pain (sharp/dull) ____________

Vibration ____________

Position sense ____________

Stereognosis ____________

Graphesthesia ____________

Double simult. stim. ____________

Cerebellum

Finger to nose ____________

RAM's ____________

Heel to shin ____________

Reflexes

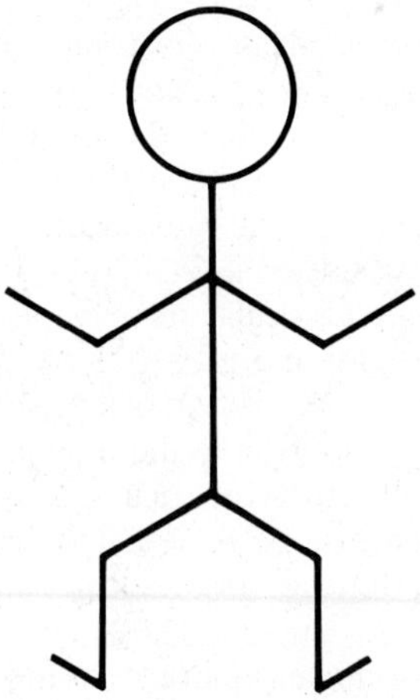

Patient's name ____________

Date ____________

Cranial Nerves

Cranial nerve function is tested next. There are 12 paired cranial nerves (see Chap. 62). Each member of the pair innervates structures on the same side from which it arises (the ipsilateral side).

Ofactory Nerve. The first cranial nerve, the olfactory nerve, serves the sense of smell. Smell is tested by asking the patient to identify or indicate that he is able to smell a non-irritating substance (such as coffee, cloves, oil of cinnamon, or lemon).

Optic Nerve. The second cranial nerve is the optic nerve. The optic nerve may be inspected directly by ophthalmoscopy; its function may be assessed by testing visual acuity and visual fields. Visual acuity can be tested by having the patient read from a visual acuity chart or by reading small print at a distance (*e.g.,* a magazine or newspaper).

The optic nerve is examined by inspecting the optic fundus through an ophthalmoscope. Papilledema (edema of the optic disc) may signify increased intracranial pressure. It is characterized by blurring of the disc margins, venous distention with loss of venous pulsations, obliteration of the physiological cup, and later, disc elevation and hemorrhages.

Oculomotor, Trochlear, and Abducens Nerves. The functions of cranial nerves III, IV, and VI, the oculomotor, trochlear, and abducens are tested together. These nerves supply the muscles that coordinate eye movements. The integrity of these nerves is assessed by testing extraocular movements (EOMs) and pupillary responses. Extraocular movements are tested by requesting the patient to visually track an object in all gaze directions without moving his head. Then, he is also requested to follow an object as it approaches his nose. The eyes should move to their full range and in a coordinated fashion (conjugately). An important point to remember is that a lesion of one of these cranial nerves causes a weakness of one of the ipsilateral extraocular muscles. A weakness of an extraocular muscle will result in the dominance of its opposing muscle; thus the eye will be deviated to the strong side.

While assessing extraocular movements, the examiner should also observe for the presence of nystagmus. *Nystagmus* is an involuntary oscillation of the eyes. Usually there is a fast and a slow component to the oscillation. Nystagmus may be in horizontal, vertical, or rotary planes or directions. Sometimes the form may be mixed. The presence of nystagmus indicates dysfunction of the ocular system, the labyrinth or vestibular nerve, the medial longitudinal fasciculus, brain stem vestibular nuclei and tracts, or the cerebellum.

The pupillary response of the eye is tested by shining a bright light (preferably that of a focused beam of light, such as a flashlight—do not use overhead lamps) into one eye at a time. The patient should be instructed to focus his vision on a far object in order to prevent constriction of the pupil as it accommodates while looking at a near object. The normal pupil will constrict in a brisk fashion in response to the light. When one pupil constricts, the other constricts as well; this is called consensual response, and its presence also reflects the integrity of the oculomotor nerve. The consensual response, tested by observing for constriction of the pupil in one eye when a light is directed into the opposite eye, is also assessed. The examiner should also note the equality of the size of the pupils; pupillary inequality is termed *anisocoria.* The pupils should be round. An irregular or oval-shaped pupil has been associated with increased intracranial pressure.[11] Finally, the ability of the pupil to constrict on accommodation is tested. This can be done at the same time that convergence, an extraocular movement, is tested, by requesting the patient to focus on an object that is brought in toward his nose.

Lesions of the oculomotor, trochlear, and abducens nerves can occur as a result of neuropathies, infectious processes, trauma, or space-occupying lesions such as neoplasms, hematomas, or aneurysms. An oculomotor paralysis occurs with herniation of the uncus (basal, medial temporal lobe) into the transtentorial notch. Its appearance requires emergency action.

Trigeminal Nerve. The fifth cranial nerve, the trigeminal nerve, has sensory and motor components. Sensory modalities include touch, pain and temperature, and proprioception. The sensory component of the nerve is much greater than the motor component. The major function of the trigeminal nerve includes sensations of the face, cornea, and mucous membranes of nasal and oral cavities, and movements of the muscles of mastication. Sensory functions (tactile and pain) of the trigeminal nerve are tested by determining the patient's ability to feel light touch and pinprick over the areas of the face innervated by the ophthalmic, maxillary, and mandibular divisions of the fifth nerve.

Sensation of the cornea is carried over the ophthalmic division of the fifth cranial nerve. It may be tested by lightly touching the cornea with a wisp of cotton. This maneuver should elicit a reflex blink. An absent corneal blink reflex is due either to impaired corneal sensation (afferent component) or impairment of the closure of the eyelid (efferent component), which is innervated by the seventh (facial) cranial nerve.

The motor functions of the trigeminal nerve are tested by assessing the muscle bulk of the temporalis and masseter muscles and symmetry of movement of the masseters and the lateral pterygoids. Observe the temporal muscles for symmetry of bulk; a hollow in the temple can be indicative of atrophy of this muscle. Symmetry of bulk and strength of the masseters is determined by requesting the patient to bite down while the examiner palpates the masseters.

Facial Nerve. The seventh cranial nerve, the facial nerve, primarily is a motor nerve that supplies the muscles for facial expression and the stapedius muscle of the middle ear. A small sensory component serves taste over the ipsilateral anterior two thirds of the tongue.

Motor functions of the facial nerve are tested by asking the patient to wrinkle his forehead, close and hold his eyes tightly shut while the examiner attempts to open them, show his teeth, purse his lips, and frown. Any asymmetry of facial movement should be noted. Likewise, with the patient's face at rest, any asymmetry such as smoothing of the forehead or flattening of the nasolabial fold should also be observed.

Taste is tested by requesting the patient to extend his tongue while the examiner places a sweet, salty, or sour substance on one half of the anterior portion of the tongue. He should be able to determine the nature of the substance while his tongue remains protruded. The patient is instructed to rinse his mouth between testings.

Acoustic Nerve. The eighth cranial nerve, the acoustic nerve, is comprised of two nerves—one, the cochlear; the other, the vestibular. The cochlear nerve transmits impulses from the organ of Corti, and it is involved in hearing. The vestibular nerve transmits proprioceptive impulses from the saccule, utricle, and semicircular canals, and it is involved in the maintenance of equilibrium and orientation in space.[3]

Hearing is grossly tested by asking the patient if he can hear finger rustling (*i.e.,* rubbing the fingers together beside the patient's ear) or the ticking of a watch. An asymmetry in the distance that these sounds can be heard in each ear should be noted. Following this, the ability of the patient to detect sound waves through bone and air is tested using a vibrating tuning fork (512 cps) on the patient's mastoid processes and asking the patient if he can hear the sound and to indicate when he can no longer hear it. Normally, air conduction of sound is better than bone conduction. If bone conduction is better, it implies that a conduction hearing loss is present; that is, that the lesion lies within the mechanisms of the ear itself. This can be due to excessive wax in the ear canal, a damaged eardrum, or otosclerosis. If hearing is decreased for both air and bone conduction, a neurosensory lesion (one in the cochlear nerve) is most likely the cause.

Vestibular nerve function is most commonly assessed by observation of nystagmus. In the screening neurological examination, the presence or absence of nystagmus is generally noted while observing the patient with his eyes at rest and again during extraocular movements (discussed earlier under the examination of cranial nerves III, IV, and VI). Spontaneous nystagmus is always abnormal. Nystagmus that is induced by positional changes of the head and extraocular movements is generally abnormal; however, a few beats of nystagmus on extreme lateral gaze can be normal. Nystagmus may be noted with alcohol intoxication and certain drug toxicants (most notably phenytoin).

Glossopharyngeal and Vagus Nerves. Functions of the ninth (glossopharyngeal) and tenth (vagus) cranial nerves are tested together since they share most of the same functions. They both are mixed sensory and motor nerves. They function together to effect swallowing, and they participate in speech articulation. The tenth cranial nerve alone supplies the larynx. The ninth cranial nerve alone serves taste sensation over the posterior one third of the tongue (not tested).

The patient's speech has already been assessed during the accounting of his history. If any speech deficit is suspected, further testing is done.

The patient who has a palatal weakness will also experience difficulty swallowing (dysphagia). The presence or absence of such a problem should be elicited in the history.

Glossopharyngeal and vagus nerve functioning can be tested by observing for elevation of the soft palate when the patient says "Ah. . . . " A failure of one side to elevate indicates a paralysis on that side. The gag reflex is tested by touching a tongue blade to one side of the palatal arch and then the other. An absence of the gag reflex can be due to either a ninth nerve lesion (afferent component) or to a tenth nerve lesion (efferent component). Failure of the palate to elevate symmetrically on phonation (volitional) in the presence of an intact gag reflex when the affected side is stimulated (reflex) is indicative of an upper motor neuron lesion.[7]

Accessory Nerve. The eleventh cranial nerve, the accessory, is a motor nerve that supplies the sternocleidomastoid (SCM) and trapezius muscles. Its function is tested by observing these muscles for symmetry of bulk and movement. When testing the sternocleidomastoid, request the patient to turn (not tilt) his head to one side at a time and to hold it there against the examiner's resistance. To test both SCMs, ask the patient to forcefully push his head forward against resistance. A weakness in one sternocleidomastoid will result in a weakness of head-turning to the opposite side. The trapezius is tested by instructing the patient to raise his shoulders against the examiner's resistance. Observe for any swinging of the scapula during this maneuver.

Hypoglossal Nerve. The twelth cranial nerve, the hypoglossal, is a motor nerve that supplies the tongue. Its action is to protrude the tongue forward; therefore, a weakness of one side will cause deviation of the tongue to the side of the weakness (*i.e.,* the strong side pushes the tongue forward unopposed) when the tongue is protruded. To assess the integrity of the hypoglossal nerve, instruct the patient to protrude his tongue. Inspect for deviation and the presence of atrophy or fasciculations (muscle twitching).

Motor System

Examination of the motor system comprises assessment of symmetry of muscle bulk, tone, and strength. Decrease in muscle bulk (atrophy) and decrease in muscle tone (hypotonia), when associated with muscle weakness (paresis) or paralysis, are abnormal signs associated with lower motor neuron (LMN) lesions. Hypotonia and a generalized muscular weakness or decrease in energy (asthenia) are also a feature of cerebellar lesions. An increase in muscle tone (hypertonia) when associated with paresis or paralysis is indicative of an upper motor neuron (UMN) lesion. UMN lesions are not generally associated with atrophy, but disuse atrophy is seen with long-standing UMN deficits. Hypertonia is also noted in Parkinson's disease; it is not accompanied by muscle weakness.

Muscle Bulk and Tone. Inspection of muscle bulk is completed by observing and palpating muscle groups to determine the presence or absence of wasting (atrophy). Inspection of muscle bulk provides some information about muscle tone as well. Normally, there is a certain degree of muscular tension in the relaxed muscle. This is known as tonus. Sometimes a "flabby" muscle noted on palpation is a sign of hypotonia. To further assess tonus, the degree of resistance of muscle groups to passive stretch is determined. The patient is instructed to relax totally and to let the examiner move his limbs.

If there is absolutely no resistance in the muscles to movement, the muscles are said to be *flaccid* or *atonic*. If the tone seems to be only decreased, it is noted as *hypotonia*. An increased resistance of the muscles to passive stretch is called *hypertonia*. This exaggerated muscle tone may be described as spasticity or rigidity. The term *spasticity* is usually reserved to describe the hypertonicity present with an upper motor neuron lesion, and it is characterized by an increased resistance to passive stretch, especially noted in flexor muscle groups in the upper extremities. This resistance is felt only on initiation of the movement (a brisk movement), and will "give way" as the examiner continues the movement. This characteristic has prompted the use of the term "clasp-knife" spasticity. The term *rigidity* describes the type of hypertonicity noted in the muscles of patients who have Parkinson's disease (or other extrapyramidal system disorders). Rigidity is characterized by a steady, persistent resistance to passive stretch in both flexor and extensor muscle groups. This phenomenon has led to the descriptive phrases "lead-pipe" rigidity, or "plastic" rigidity. Cogwheel rigidity is seen in patients with Parkinson's disease and is manifested by a ratchetlike jerking noted in the extremity on passive movement. Another type of rigidity, known as paratonia (gegenhalten), is seen in patients who have frontal lobe dysfunction. These patients may be confused, suffer from dementia or "senility," or may even be in "light" coma (stupor). This type of rigidity is also a lead-pipe rigidity; however, it is noted in muscle groups in which weakness or paralysis is absent. The patient has no control over this response, although it will often appear to the caretaker (or examiner) that it is a purposeful resistance.

Muscle Strength. Strength of the major muscle groups is assessed by asking the patient to move his head, trunk, and limbs against the examiner's resistance. The degree of the strength of movement that the patient demonstrates is noted and recorded.

The test for pronator drift is performed by requesting the patient to hold his arms outstretched in front of him, with palms held upward. Observe for any pronation of his hands. Pronation indicates weakness.

The patient's *gait* provides information about the motor system as well as the extrapyramidal, cerebellar, and sensory systems. Ask the patient to walk down a corridor. Observe for any abnormalities previously discussed. Also ask the patient to walk on his heels (L4 and L5) and toes (S1 and S2). While the gait is being tested, it is also convenient to observe the patient walking tandem (*i.e.,* heel-to-toe in a straight line). Note any swaying; abnormalities are suggestive of cerebellar dysfunction.

Reflexes

Reflex testing comprises muscle stretch reflexes (myotatic reflexes), superficial reflexes, and other special reflexes (*i.e.,* auditory, peripheral, palmomental, snout, and so on) that may or may not be tested along with the others.

Muscle Stretch Reflexes. The muscle stretch reflexes (MSRs) tested in the screening neurological examination include the jaw, biceps, triceps, quadriceps, femoralis (patellar), and triceps surae (Achilles). These reflexes are observed for symmetry when tested bilaterally and for the briskness of reflex movement.

Superficial Reflexes. Superficial reflexes are elicited by stimulation of the skin. Generally, the superficial reflexes tested in the screening neurological examination include the abdominal reflexes and the plantar responses of the feet. The response to stimulation is recorded as present, absent, or equivocal (*i.e.,* present or difficult to determine).

The abdominal reflexes are tested by stroking the skin surface of the abdomen in each of the four quadrants; the direction of the stroke should be toward the umbilicus. The broken edge of a tongue blade can be used as a stimulus instrument. A normal response is the movement of the umbilicus toward the quadrant stimulated.

The plantar response is tested by stroking the sole of the foot with a blunt instrument such as the broken edge of a tongue blade, the handle of a reflex hammer, or a key. The stimulus should be applied firmly but gently to the lateral aspect of the sole, beginning at the heel and stopping short of the base of the toes. A normal response is a flexion of the toes (a flexor-plantar response). An abnormal response is one in which the great toe extends upward (an extensor-plantar response, or Babinski reflex).

Cerebellar Function

The major function of the cerebellum is to coordinate the rate, regularity, and force of voluntary muscle contraction. Thus, the cerebellum affects the smooth and accurate functioning of all voluntary muscles including those used for eye movements and speech. Individuals with cerebellar lesions tend to manifest varying degrees of ataxia (dystaxia), hypontonia, nystagmus, and dysarthria.

Dystaxia can be noted in the upper extremities when testing for finger-to-nose coordination. The patient is asked to touch the tip of the examiner's finger with the tip of his forefinger (each hand tested separately) and then to touch his own nose, and to repeat this maneuver several times while the examiner moves the location of her finger each time. A consistent undershooting or overshooting the target is called dysmetria. Heel-to-shin testing is another testing for dystaxia, but in the lower extremities. The patient should be seated or supine; he is asked to take the heel of one foot and to very accurately, without deviation, move it down the shin of his other leg. Deficits in any of these maneuvers indicate an ipsilateral cerebellar lesion.

The patient's ability to perform rapid, alternating move-

TABLE 63–1
Manifestations of Movement Disorders

Chorea—involuntary, rapid, brief, jerky movements occurring at an irregular rate in the extremities and possibly the face (grimacing)

Athetosis—involuntary, slow, sinuous (writhing) movements of the extremities, head, and trunk

Ballismus—involuntary, violent, flinging movements of the extremities, usually limited to one side of the body (hemiballismus). Thought to be a form of chorea

Dystonia—involuntary, sustained athetoid posturing of an extremity, head, or trunk

Resting tremor—also known as Parkinsonian tremor; a coarse, rhythmic tremor noted with the limb in repose; it is suppressed or diminished by voluntary movement. When limb is truly at rest (during sleep), the tremor disappears.

Intention tremor—a jerky, more or less rhythmic tremor noted *during* the performance of a precise, voluntary movement (as in touching examiner's finger); may seriously interfere with performance of skilled acts; absent when limbs are at rest and during the initial part of a movement

Action tremor—also known as a postural tremor; a fine, rhythmic tremor noted when the extremities are actively maintained in a certain position, such as with arms outstretched. Some examples of tremors of this type include benign essential tremor, familial tremor, and tremor noted with hyperthyroidism.

Akinesia—paucity of movement (reduced movement) of an affected part in the absence of weakness or paralysis; habitual movements (such as crossing the legs and turning the head) are reduced or absent.

Bradykinesia—slowness of movement

ments is also evaluated. He is instructed to alternately slap his thigh with first the palm of his hand and then the back of his hand as fast as possible. It is not uncommon for individuals to perform better with the dominant hand, especially when they are tested singly.

The speech observed in cerebellar dysfunction is dysarthric, but it may also exhibit a peculiar quality called "scanning speech." This type of speech is characterized by alternating patterns of slowness and explosiveness as each syllable is spoken.

During the cerebellar examination the patient should also be observed for any manifestations of basal ganglia dysfunction such as involuntary movements (*i.e.*, chorea, athetosis, ballismus, and resting tremor), akinesia, or bradykinesia (see Table 63–1).

Sensory Function

Examination of the sensory system tests the modalities of touch, pain, temperature, proprioception, and vibratory discrimination. Included here also are tests of the higher integrative cortical sensory functions. The sensory examination relies on subjective responses of the patient. The screening sensory examination is a gross testing of somatic sensory sensibilities.

Tactile sensation is tested by lightly touching the patient's hands, arms, trunk, feet, and legs with a wisp of cotton. The patient is first shown what the examiner will be doing and instructed on how he is to respond, for example, "Say yes every time you feel me touch you." The test is then conducted, as are all sensory examinations, with the patient's eyes closed.

Pain and temperature discriminations are tested in the same manner, substituting a pin with a head (sharp/dull) and tubes of warm and cold water. If any deficit to sensation of light touch, pinprick, or temperature is noted, the examiner should map out the involved areas by applying the test stimulus in the area in which the patient reports decreased or absent sensitivity, and move the stimulus progressively outward, noting where the patient reports he feels a change.

Nursing Assessment

The nursing model for neurological assessment makes many of the same observations as the medical model but organizes this data into functional categories. This method is especially relevant to the practice of nursing, which involves making nursing diagnoses and the prescription (nursing orders) and implementation of nursing interventions.

The functional categories for neurological assessment, developed by Mitchell, Cammermeyer, Ozuna, and Woods, around which the patient's neurological examination is based, include consciousness, mentation, movement, sensation, integrated regulatory function, and coping with disability.[12] These authors have outlined their functional approach to the patient's history and examination as it pertains to neurological dysfunction. It is the disorder of movement and how this affects the patient's daily living that is the concern of the nurse.

The serial assessment of neurological function in an individual patient assumes a prominent role in the day-to-day activities of the nurse. An ongoing assessment not only provides information from which current nursing orders (plan of care) are written, but also provides information that alerts the nurse to any possible life-threatening changes in the patient's neurological status.

When orders for "neuro checks" are written, these usually comprise those signs that, if a deterioration were to occur, would signify a critical or potentially life-threatening event in the patient's neurological status. These signs typically include the patient's level of consciousness (Glasgow Coma Scale score), pupillary equality and light responses, motor ability, and when appropriate, sensory appreciation. When intracranial pathology is not present (*e.g.*, postoperative laminectomy), it is sufficient to observe for motor and sensory changes only. When an intracranial space-occupying lesion is present, the threat of expansion and decreased intracranial compliance is always present. Expansion of contents within the intracranial compartments (*e.g.*, hematoma, neoplasm, edema, and obstructive hydrocephalus) may cause portions of the brain to shift (herniation), with eventual compromise of the vascular supply to the brain stem, and subsequent death of the patient (Fig. 63–2).

With central, downward transtentorial herniation, a decreasing level of consciousness is usually the first sign of neurological deterioration. The nurse should be alert to even subtle signs of a change in the patient's level of consciousness. This may be indicated first by the patient's sleeping more than usual and may gradually progress, with the patient becoming more and more drowsy until he is difficult to arouse.

With uncal herniation, a dilating pupil that is at first sluggishly reactive may be the first sign of neurological worsening. As the herniation progresses, which it may do quite rapidly, depressed consciousness, posturing of extremities, and brain stem abnormalities may be noted.

When acute neurological deterioration is a possibility, it is most important to evaluate the patient's neurological signs at appropriate intervals throughout the day and night. Never eliminate a neuro check, assuming that the patient is sleeping and needs his rest. He may be slipping into coma. When making neurological assessments, the nurse must remember that any loss of function or change from baseline represents deterioration, and the physician should be notified. The experienced neuroscience nurse is generally able to determine when a change in status necessitates prompt notification of a physician. For nurses who are not yet comfortable with recognizing critical neurological events, report to the physician any change that has been noted.

Neurodiagnostic Tests

There is a wide variety of diagnostic tests employed to aid in the diagnosis of nervous system diasease. Some of these tests, including skull and spine x-rays, CT scans, electroencephalograms, electromyography and nerve conduction velocity studies, brain scans, cerebral blood flow, angiography, lumbar punctures and myelography, are presented in Table 63–2.[5,9,13] New diagnostic tests, such as nuclear magnetic resonance (NMR) imaging and positron emission tomography (PET) scans, are being developed at a rapid pace. Many of these new procedures promise to revolutionize the diagnosis and treatment of neurological dysfunction. The CT scan has already revolutionized neurodiagnosis.

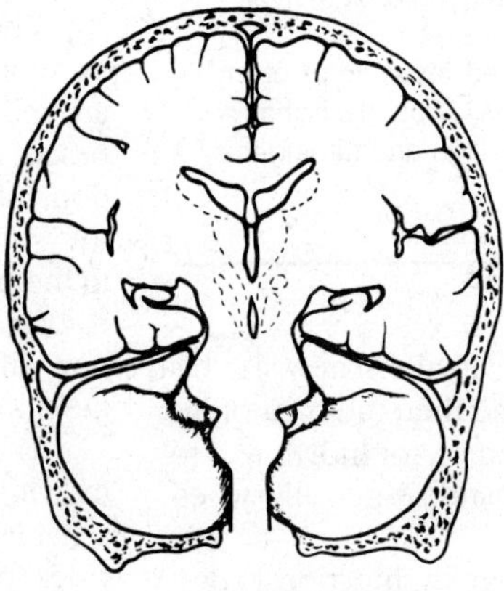

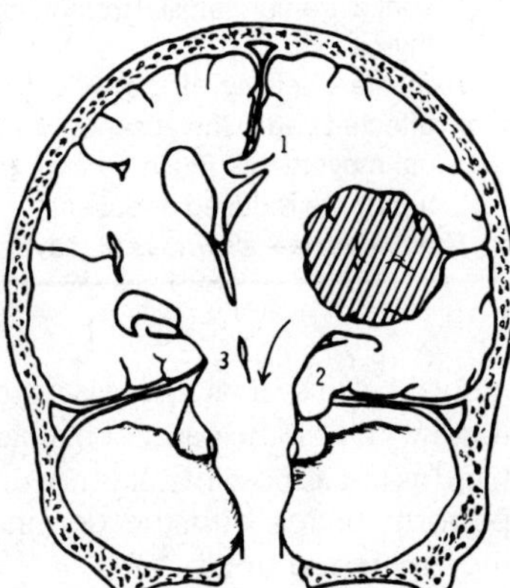

FIGURE 63–2 Intracranial shifts from supratentorial lesions: (*1*) herniation of the cingulate gyrus under the falx; (*2*) herniation of the temporal lobe into the tentorial notch; (*3*) downward displacement of the brain stem through notch. (Plum F, Posner J: Diagnosis of Stupor and Coma, 2nd ed. Contemporary Neurology Series. Philadelphia, FA Davis, 1972)

TABLE 63–2
Neurodiagnostic Tests

Skull Films:

Definition: Radiographs of skull to detect abnormalities of skull and to demonstrate selected intracranial pathology

Purpose

Detect skull fracture
Location of pineal body
Detect erosion of sella turcica
Detect alteration in bone density
Observe for vascular markings
Observe size and shape of skull

Nursing Considerations

Remove metallic items from hair.
Note unusually thick head dressings or heavy braids on requisition.

Spine Films:

Definition: Radiographs of spine to detect bony changes

Purpose

Detect vertebral fracture
Detect bone erosion
Detect degenerative changes
Detect calcification
Detect narrowing of vertebral canal

Nursing Considerations

Remove metallic objects from around neck or body.
When fracture suspected, avoid flexion or rotation of spine; use three-man lift during transfers to and from x-ray table, and use fourth person to support head if cervical fracture suspected.

(*Continued*)

TABLE 63–2
Neurodiagnostic Tests *(Continued)*

Spine Films: Nursing Considerations (cont'd)

May need to assist technician in obtaining clear view of lower cervical vertebrae when fracture suspected: shoulders are pulled down with head and neck maintained in alignment

Computerized Axial Tomography (CT) Scan:

Definition: Computerized reconstruction of body part by passage of multiple x-ray beams through area and measurement of signals based on different density of various tissues

Purpose

Detect intracranial space-occupying lesions
Detect cerebral edema
Detect intracranial hypertension
Detect hydrocephalus
Detect cerebral infarction
Detect cerebral atrophy
Detect subarachnoid hemorrhage

Nursing Considerations

Remove metallic objects from hair.
Patient must remain absolutely still; may require sedation if not contraindicated
Clear liquids only 4 to 6 hr before test if contrast material is used (reduces nausea and vomiting)
Patient should be well hydrated before, during, and after study if contrast material used (observe fluid restriction orders if ordered).
Observe for allergic reaction to iodinated contrast material.

Electroencephalography:

Definition: Recording of spontaneous electrical impulses of the brain from scalp electrodes; when recorded directly from cortical surface during surgery, it is termed electrocorticography

Purpose

Detect abnormal electrical activity
Monitor status of coma on continuing basis
Cerebral mapping during surgery to remove epileptogenic foci (electrocorticography)

Nursing Considerations

Explain procedure to patient; allay any fears or apprehension: no possibility of shock, cannot "read" mind
Hair should be clean, without oils or sprays.
No caffeine at least 24 hr prior to testing
Medication may be ordered for patient if sleep electroencephalogram (EEG) desired
Withhold anticonvulsant medication only when specifically ordered by physician.
Wash hair following procedure to remove EEG paste; may require several washings

Electromyography (EMG) and Nerve Conduction Velocity (NCV) Studies:

Definition: EMG records electrical activity in muscles at rest, during voluntary contraction, and in response to electrical stimulation. NCV records speed of conduction in motor and sensory fibers of peripheral nerves.

Electromyography (EMG) and Nerve Conduction Velocity (NCV) Studies (cont'd):

Purpose

Detect neuromuscular disorders

Nursing Considerations

Explain procedure to patient; small electrode needles will be inserted.
Most patients experience mild discomfort; to some, it is relatively painful.

Brain Scan:

Definition: Administration of small amount of radiopharmaceutical (oral, IV, intra-arterial, or inhalation) to measure tissue uptake

Purpose

Screening and following course of brain tumors and cerebral vascular disease

Nursing Considerations

Reassure patient radiation hazard is negligible.
Instruct patient he will have to remain still for 45 to 60 minutes.

Cerebral Blood Flow (CBF) Study:

Definition: Measurement of total or local (regional) CBF to determine areas of increased or reduced blood supply by inhalation, intra-arterial, or intravenous administration of a radiopharmaceutical

Purpose

Estimate risk of cerebral ischemia prior to surgical procedures
Evaluate CBF during and following surgery
Evaluate CBF in cerebral vascular accident
Determine presence of CBF in significant increase in intracranial pressure
Possible role in diagnosis and treatment of dementias

Nursing Considerations

Reassure patient that radiation hazard is negligible.
Observe arterial puncture site for signs of hematoma: may cause respiratory distress if carotid injection
Observe for change in neurological status
Observe vital signs as ordered; bradycardia may occur with vagal irritation during carotid puncture (atropine will correct problem)
Bed rest for at least 6 hrs

Angiography:

Definition: Intra-arterial injection of contrast material with simultaneous radiographs of head and neck to visualize intracranial and extracranial vessels

Purpose

Detect aneurysm or arteriovenous malformation (AVM)
Detect vasospasm following subarachnoid hemorrhage either spontaneous in origin or secondary to trauma
Detect extracranial or intracranial vascular occlusive disease
Further delineate neoplasms or evaluate their blood supply

(Continued)

TABLE 63–2
Neurodiagnostic Tests *(Continued)*

Angiography (cont'd):

Nursing Considerations

Explain procedure to patient; may experience hot, flushing sensation when dye is injected

Contrast material is injected into femoral, brachial, or carotid arteries.

Remove metallic clips from hair.

Make sure patient is not allegic to iodine.

Clear liquids 4 to 6 hr before testing; patient should be well hydrated to reduce risk of renal damage; IV often ordered to ensure adequate hydration before, during, and after procedure; also provides access for medications if needed

Premedicate per orders.

Postprocedure:

Observe arterial puncture site for bleeding or hematoma; pressure dressing is usually in place; may have ice pack to area ordered

Observe pulse for quality (distal to puncture site): diminished or absent pulse may indicate occlusion of vessel by thrombus or from hematoma; also observe limb for color and temperature

Observe for bradycardia and hypotension; occurs occasionally with vagal irritation in carotid artery; more common with carotid puncture but can be seen with catheterization of vessel as well; condition reverses with administration of atropine

Observe for any change in neurological status; risk of stroke or ischemia following angiography secondary to embolus, thrombus, or vasospasm

Bed rest (may have head elevated) for 12 to 24 hr; if femoral puncture, must keep leg extended and immobile for several hours to prevent dislodgment of clot

Lumbar Puncture

Definition: Introduction of needle into spinal subarachnoid space (usually at L4–5 or L3–4 vertebral interspace)

Purpose

Examination of cerebrospinal fluid

Introduction of contrast material for radiological procedures

Introduction of medication

Serial punctures to remove bloody CSF following subarachnoid hemorrahge

Measure CSF pressure (hazardous if intracranial hypertension suspected)

Spinal anesthesia

Nursing Considerations

Explain procedure to patient; local anesthetic usually used

Assist patient to assume "fetal position": lateral recumbent position with back arched, head and knees flexed on chest (ideal if chin touches knees), so that maximal widening of intervertebral space is achieved.

Remain with patient to encourage maintenance of desired position and to allay apprehension.

Postprocedure

Remain flat in bed 6 to 24 hr (may lie on side).

Encourage fluids if not contraindicated.

Medicate as needed for headache.

Observe for change in neurological status.

May develop fever and nuchal rigidity secondary to aseptic meningitis.

Lumbar Puncture (cont'd):

If pressure significantly elevated, observe patient closely for change in neurological status (may precipitate herniation of uncus or cerebellar tonsils).

Myelography:

Definition: Introduction of a radiopaque solution, oil-soluble or water-soluble, into the spinal subarachnoid space with fluoroscopic and radiographic observation

Purpose

Detect vertebral disc disease

Detect intramedullary or extramedullary spinal cord tumors or syringomyelia

Nursing Considerations

Explain procedure to patient; will require a lumbar puncture (sometimes cisternal puncture performed)

Patient will be restrained to x-ray table while table is tilted to allow movement of dye (may not be necessary for lumbar examination when metrizamide is used).

Premedicate patient as ordered.

Some physicians give loading doses of phenytoin prior to procedure if metrizamide is used (may cause generalized seizures if enters cranial subarachnoid space)

Postprocedure for Pantopaque (oil-soluble):

Flat in bed for 6 to 24 hr; may turn to side

Encourage fluids.

Observe at regular intervals for any change in neurological status (motor/sensory).

Medicate for pain or headache as needed.

Head of bed may be ordered elevated if all of contrast material not removed.

Postprocedure for metrizamide (water-soluble):

Supine with head elevated 30° for at least 8 hr to prevent rapid entry into cranial subarachnoid space (SAS)

Patient should be kept as quiet as possible.

Encourage fluids.

Observe for any change in neurological status.

Observe for generalized seizures.

Avoid administration of phenothiazines (they lower seizure threshold).

Be alert for appearance of confusion, disorientation, and nausea about 6 hr after testing when drug crosses blood–brain barrier.

Isotope Cisternography:

Definition: Introduction of radioactive isotope into lumbar, or occasionally cervical, subarachonid space to determine

CSF flow characteristics

Purpose

Identify presence of communicating hydrocephalus

Identify CSF leak

Evaluate functioning of CSF shunt

Nursing Considerations

Keep patient flat 8 to 24 hr following lumbar puncture.

Encourage fluids, if not contraindicated.

Inform patient of necessity of repeated scans (*e.g.,* 3, 6, 12, 24, 48, and 72 hr after injection).

Summary

The assessment of nervous system function comprises a patient history, general observation of the patient, a detailed neurological examination, and appropriate diagnostic tests. When the patient is hospitalized, this information is supplemented by daily observation of the patient. In the process of obtaining (or reviewing) this information, the nurse is able to identify potential or actual deficits with which the patient may need to cope; she also may anticipate how this dysfunction might affect the patient's ability to engage in daily physical, mental, social, and recreational activities. The consideration of this data along with information about the patient as an individual enables the nurse to more effectively plan and provide his care.

References

1. Adams RD, Victor M: Principles of Neurology. New York, McGraw-Hill, 1977
2. Bakerman S: A, B, C's of Interpretive Laboratory Data. 1983 (Author is publisher)
3. Brodal A: Neurological Anatomy, 3rd ed. New York, Oxford University Press, 1981
4. Chmelir T: Neurological Exam. Unpublished paper, 1984
5. Core Curriculum for Neuroscience Nursing. American Association of Neuroscience Nurses, 1984
6. DeJong RN: Case taking and the neurologic examination. In Baker AB, Baker LH (eds): Clinical Neurology 1:1–83, 1977
7. DeMyer W: Techniques of the Neurologic Examination, 3rd ed. New York, McGraw-Hill, 1980
8. Heilman KM, Valenstein E: Clinical Neuropsychology. New York, Oxford University Press, 1979
9. Hickey J: The Clinical Practice of Neurological and Neurosurgical Nursing. Philadelphia, JB Lippincott, 1981
10. Jennett WB, Plum F: The persistent vegetative state. Lancet 1:734–737, 1972
11. Marshall LF, Barba D, Toole BM, Bowers SA: The oval pupil: Clinical significance and relationship to intracranial hypertension. J Neurosurg 58:566–568, 1983
12. Mitchell PH, Cammermeyer M, Ozuna J, Woods NF: Neurological Assessment for Nursing Practice. Reston, Reston Publishing Company, 1984
13. Nebe DE: Diagnostic studies. In Snyder M (ed): A Guide to Neurological and Neurosurgical Nursing. New York, John Wiley & Sons, 1983
14. Plum F, Posner JB: The Diagnosis of Stupor and Coma, 3rd ed. Philadelphia, FA Davis, 1980
15. Strub RL, Black FW: The Mental Status Examination. Philadelphia, FA Davis, 1977
16. Teasdale G, Jennett B: Assessment of coma and impaired consciousness. Lancet 2:81–83, 1976

Chapter 64

Nursing Strategies for Common Neurological Problems

Nursing Diagnosis Interventions Evaluation

Judy Hill Ozuna

Because the human nervous system influences a broad spectrum of human functioning, disease or injury of the central nervous system (CNS) manifests itself in many ways. The resulting nervous system dysfunction is influenced as much by the location of the lesion as it is by the pathology. The dysfunction may be evident by either excess or deficit phenomena, or both. For instance, dysfunction in movement may be from paralysis (deficit) or from involuntary movements such as tremor (excess).

Because a goal of nursing is to assist patients with deficits in self-care and daily living tasks, common neurological problems are presented from a functional perspective. Once the nurse has identified neurological dysfunction, the next step is to determine how it affects daily living and whether there is actual or potential influence on other aspects of daily living. Once the nursing diagnosis is made, intervention strategies are developed.

Alterations in Consciousness

Consciousness has two components: content and arousal.[16] The content of consciousness includes cognitive and affective functioning and is addressed in the section Alterations in Cognitive Functioning. Arousal is the degree of awareness of self and the environment. It corresponds to a continuum in which wakefulness is on the homeostatic end and coma is on the pathological end of the continuum. A point on this continuum is most often referred to as the level of consciousness. It is obvious that both components of consciousness are prerequisite to any kind of self-care.

Alteration of consciousness outside of psychiatric disease most often implies disruption of the reticular activating system in the brain stem and thalamus. Although clouding of consciousness (*e.g.*, confusion and decreased attention) can occur in conditions affecting one of the cerebral hemispheres (*i.e.*, stroke, tumor), coma itself is the result of damage to the reticular activating system or extensive damage to both cerebral hemispheres.[16] Conditions that create loss of arousal by bilateral hemisphere disturbance include bilateral stroke, rapidly expanding intracerebral mass lesions (*e.g.*, hemorrhage, tumor, or sudden malfunction of an intraventricular shunt), and a variety of metabolic disorders (*e.g.*, liver or renal failure, diabetes, fluid-electrolyte imbalance, vitamin deficiency, and gastrointestinal disease).

Alterations in consciousness may be rapid in onset or gradual and sustained. Implications and nursing care differ somewhat for each. Temporary, intermittent alterations in consciousness such as those seen in some types of seizure and in syncope will not be discussed in great detail here. In general nursing care for these problems should focus on prevention of injury by anticipating the attack and providing physical safety measures such as keeping bedside rails up when patients are in bed and accompanying patients when they are out of bed.

Alterations in Consciousness of Rapid Onset

Conditions commonly causing acute alterations in consciousness include stroke, cerebral hematoma, head trauma, rapidly expanding cerebral tumors, and intracerebral hemorrhage. In this context rapid onset means onset within minutes or hours. A rapid change in level of consciousness has serious implications for any patient with an expanding mass of tissue (*e.g.,* blood, tumor, cerebrospinal fluid) in the cerebral hemispheres. Such a change signifies the beginning of herniation syndrome, which is downward displacement of the supratentorial brain contents into the brain stem. The resulting pressure on the brain stem can disrupt the protective reflexes and even the cardiac and respiratory regulatory centers in the medulla if the condition is not reversed.

Assessment. Nursing care standards for the unconscious patient are outlined in Table 64–1. Assessment is the first priority, which determines the nursing care to be delivered. Remember that assessment of an unconscious patient must be based on his responses to stimuli (*e.g.,* speech, touch, pain, and light) because he cannot communicate or respond to commands. The patient's family needs to be assessed regarding their perception of the patient's condition and their coping mechanisms. They should be encourage to verbalize their feelings and concerns, for they are often frightened and confused, and have feelings of helplessness. Both the family and the health care staff should be aware that although the patient may appear not to know what is going on around him, he may hear what is being said.

Assessing the unconscious patient deserves special attention for the following reasons:

1. The patient who presents with acute onset of unconsciousness requires urgent evaluation in order to determine the cause of the impairment and, when appropriate, to implement prompt intervention.

TABLE 64–1
Nursing Care Standards for the Unconscious Patient

Standard: The patient will attain, maintain, or regain his highest level of consciousness.
The family possesses the knowledge, attitude, and skills to interact with the patient with altered consciousness.

Assessment: The nurse assesses, records, and reports the following:

Patient:
1. Behavioral response to stimuli:
   eye movement, speech, movement, sensation
2. Pupillary size and reactivity:
   direct, consensual
3. Eye movements
4. Brain stem reflexes:
   swallowing, cough, gag, corneal

Family:
1. Perception of consciousness, coma, cognition
2. Preference for teaching–learning strategies
3. Readiness for learning

Nursing Diagnosis	*Outcome*	*Process*
High risk for neurological deterioration related to increased intracranial pressure	Changes in neurological status detected by measurable criteria.	Assess, record, and report consciousness, specifically deterioration. Avoid or minimize increased intracranial pressure by: 1. Controlling environmental stimuli 2. Positioning to avoid restriction of venous outflow 3. Implementing measures to prevent increased intrathoracic pressure 4. Maintaining normothermia 5. When ordered, restricting fluids and free water If consciousness decreases, prepare for any of the following: 1. Administration of medications 2. Hyperventilation 3. Insertion of intracranial monitoring device 4. Withdrawal of cerebrospinal fluid 5. Induction of barbiturate therapy 6. Removal of bone or infarcted brain

(Continued)

TABLE 64–1
Nursing Care Standards for the Unconscious Patient (*Continued*)

Nursing Diagnosis	*Outcome*	*Process*
Inability to control or maintain human responses: related to altered consciousness	Until patient regains control of human responses: 1. Elimination patterns are maintained as measured by daily records of fecal and urinary output. 2. Nutritional requirements are maintained as measured by daily intake/output, calorie counts, and weights. 3. Mobility and skin integrity are maintained as measued by range of movement and absence of decubital ulcers. 4. Hygiene needs are met as measured by appropriate condition of skin, hair and mouth, and absence of odors. 5. Communication and sensory input needs are met as measured by daily auditory, visual, and tactile stimulation. 6. Sleep and rest are maintained as measured by daily periods of uninterrupted rest.	1. Assesses stool consistency and frequency. Begins bowel program if necessary. Monitors urine output, fluid intake. 2. Ensures adequate calorie and fluid intake. 3. Performs range of motion regularly. Positions in correct alignment. Avoids prolonged pressure on bony prominences. 4. Provides daily hygiene, including diligent mouth care. 5. Provides regular verbal communication and appropriate tactile, auditory, and visual stimulation.
	Family verbalizes that patient has been cared for with respect for privacy and individuality.	Controls environment to ensure privacy during patient interventions. Uses patient's preferred name.
Sensory perceptual alteration related to altered consciousness	Patient is involved in program of sensory stimulation.	Coordinates program that includes tactile, gustatory, olfactory, visual, and auditory stimuli.
Potential for ineffective family coping related to patient's death	Family verbalizes that patient experiences a dignified death and was treated with kindness and respect.	Supports family members in verbalizing their feelings. Supports family throughout the grieving process
Knowledge deficit (family) of altered consciousness	Family distinguishes between: 1. Comatose patient (who does not open eyes) 2. Awake patient (who opens eyes) 3. Aware patient (who opens eyes and follows commands)	Teaches meaning of the following behavioral responses: 1. Eye movement 2. Movement 3. Following commands 4. Speech Teaches definition of terms related to behavioral responses
Change in pattern of family interaction with patient related to altered consciousness	Family participates in patient's care.	Identifies verbal and nonverbal cues of desire to interact with and care for patient

(Adapted from Nursing Standards Committee, American Association of Neuroscience Nurses, 1982)

2. The unconscious patient is at risk for developing life-threatening complications secondary to loss of protective reflexes; these deficits may be noted during examination.
3. Special assessment techniques are required, since the patient is not able to cooperate with the examination.

The patient's history is of great importance, and it should be obtained at the earliest opportunity from family members or friends. The general cardiovascular and respiratory status of the patient is evaluated first so that any compromise that may exist can be promptly treated. The patient should be inspected thoroughly for any visible clues, such as trauma, that might be the cause of the loss of consciousness. An alteration in either quantity or quality of awareness diminishes consciousness.

Assessment of consciousness is based on the ability of the individual to respond in a psychologically meaningful way to his environment. This response may be diminished to the point that it compromises only an attempt by the patient to remove a noxious stimulus (*e.g.,* pulling the hand away when pressure is applied). One can see, however, that this behavior though compromised does reflect some degree of a purposeful or meaningful activity. One should remember that the determination of a patient's conscious state is evaluated by his ability to respond. When a patient gives no evidence of wakeful psychological awareness, it is assumed that he is unconscious; in fact, there presently is no way in which one can be absolutely certain that awareness does not exist.

When describing a patient with an altered level of consciousness, it is best to avoid terms such as stuporous, obtunded, and somnolent, since these terms are not standardized and have different meanings to different individuals. Rather, the behavior of the patient in response to stimuli should be described.

Assessment of patients with impaired consciousness has been facilitated by the development of an assessment tool called the Glasgow Coma Scale (Table 64–2). Primarily, it determines the degree of conscious impairment by evaluating behavioral responses in three areas: motor responses, verbal responses, and eye-opening. The examiner lists, in each category, the *best* response given by the patient. Each response is weighted numerically so that the overall response may be quantified.

If a noxious stimulus must be used when stimulating a patient in order to obtain a response, it is proposed that this consist of a standardized stimulus of pressure applied to the nailbed (Fig. 64–1). Family members and friends should be informed of why noxious stimuli are used in the assessment process.

The term *coma,* or *comatose,* is reserved to describe those individuals who make no psychologically meaningful response to stimuli and who do not open their eyes to stimuli. The term *vegetative state* (though it has a distasteful connotation, it denotes autonomic or vegetative integrity) has come to describe those individuals who make no psychologically meaningful response to stimuli, but who exhibit periods of eye-opening.[10]

Once consciousness is impaired, assessment of brain stem functioning provides a measure of brain stem impair-

TABLE 64–2
The Glasgow Coma Scale*

		Score
Eye-opening	*Spontaneous*—eyes open spontaneously, independent of stimuli	4
	To voice—open to any verbal approach, not necessarily to the command to open the eyes	3
	To pain—should be tested by stimulus applied to limbs because grimacing associated with supraorbital pressure may cause eye closure	2
	Nil—eyes remain closed	1
Best motor response	*Obeys commands*—moves limb to command	6
	Localizes to pain—noxious stimulus causes limb to move so as to remove it	5
	Withdraws to pain—semipurposeful response; movement of extremity away from stimulus but no attempt made to remove stimulus	4
	Abnormal flexion—adduction of arm with flexion at elbow and wrist (decorticate posturing)	3
	Extensor response—adduction, internal rotation, and extension of arm (decerebrate posturing)	2
	Nil—no movement of limb	1
Best verbal response	*Oriented*—implies awareness of self and environment (with orientation to person, place, and time)	5
	Confused—responds to questions in a conversational manner, but responses indicate varying degrees of disorientation and confusion	4
	Inappropriate—intelligible articulation, but speech is used only in a random or exclamatory way (*e.g.,* shouting and swearing); no sustained conversation is possible	3
	Incomprehensible—moaning and groaning without recognizable words	2
	Nil—no verbalization	1

* The score from each section is added to obtain the GSC score; the minimum score possible is 3, the maximum is 15. The motor response is determined by testing the upper extremities.

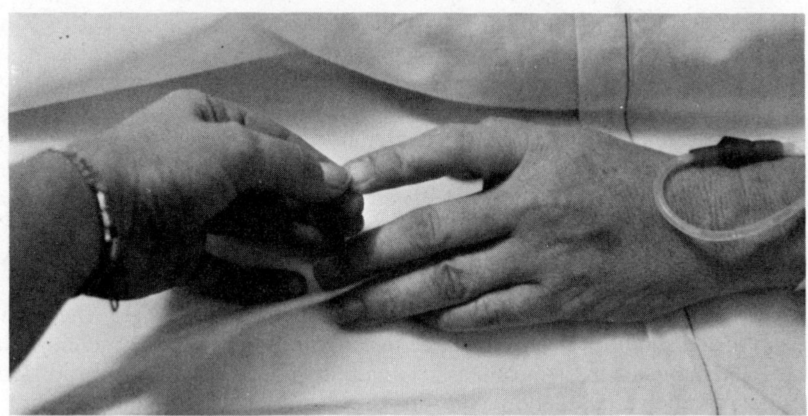

FIGURE 64–1 Applying pressure to the fingernail is one type of stimuli to use in assessing the patient's level of consciousness. (Decision Audiovisual Media. Neurological Care Series. Philadelphia, JB Lippincott)

ment. The optic nerve can be assessed by testing the pupillary light reflexes. The sudden emergence of a *dilated, nonreactive pupil* is of special import, signifying the onset of herniation of the uncus (temporal lobe), which, if allowed to progress, compromises the vascular supply to the brain stem, with death ensuing. Often the first indication of oculomotor compression is a pupil that begins to react sluggishly to light.

In the unconscious patient, extraocular movements may be evaluated by testing *oculocephalic and oculovestibular responses.* An oculocephalic response (doll's head maneuver) is tested by rotating the patient's head from side to side. This maneuver in a patient with a depressed level of consciousness will cause the eyes to roll to the opposite side of the head-turn. Absence of this response indicates brain stem dysfunction at the level of the lower pons or below (a grave prognostic sign). *This maneuver should not be done on a patient with head injury* until cervical spine injury has been ruled out.

Oculovestibular responses are tested by raising the patient's head 30 degrees and instilling 20 ml of ice water into the external auditory canal (cold caloric irrigation). In an unconscious patient, a "normal" response is conjugate deviation of the eyes toward the irrigated side. This maneuver tests the integrity of the vestibular portion of cranial nerve VIII, as well as the function of cranial nerves III and VI. *This test should not be done unless the tympanic membrane has been demonstrated to be intact.*

The classic Cushing's response (increased blood pressure, widening pulse pressure, and decreased pulse) as a sign of increasing intracranial pressure (ICP) is usually a late sign. It should not be relied on for an early indication of neurological deterioration. It results from ischemia of the vasomotor centers in the lower brain stem. Damage to the cardiovascular regulating centers in the lower brain stem can result in cardiac dysfunction, especially arrhythmias.

Certain respiratory patterns may be seen in unconscious patients. One of the most common patterns is Cheyne-Stokes respiration (CSR). CSR is characterized by repeated cycles of waxing and waning of the *depth* of respirations (crescendo–decrescendo), each cycle being followed by a period of apnea.

Apneustic breathing is characterized by an inspiratory pause. It is most often associated with pontine infarction. Ataxic breathing, or Biot's respiration, is characterized by a completely irregular, random pattern of both depth and rate of breathing. Its appearances signifies medullary compromise and impending respiratory failure.

It is also important to assess function of the protective reflexes: eye blink (for protection of the cornea) and cough and gag reflexes (for protection of the airway) as well as cardiac and respiratory function. The cough and gag reflexes are especially important because aspiration of saliva, stomach contents, secretions, and food into the lungs is a real danger in the unconscious patient. Maintenance of an adequate airway is a high priority. If the airway is obstructed, an artificial airway may be required. The patient should positioned on his side with head slightly elevated (unless contraindicated) so that the tongue does not fall back and occlude the airway (Fig. 64–2). If secretions are a problem, frequent suctioning is indicated.

The key element in the assessment of the unconscious patient, or any patient with neurological dysfunction who is at risk for losing additional function, is to detect any deterioration at the earliest possible moment. Early detection allows, when appropriate, prompt intervention and, when possible, a reversal of the progression. Especially peculiar to the central nervous system is the characteristic that a delay in intervention in an acutely evolving process may change a potentially reversible condition to one that is irreversible.

Interventions. The nursing diagnoses that are likely to be made for the unconscious patient include high risk for neurological deterioration related to increased intracranial pressure, alterations in patterns of elimination and nutritional intake, immobility, potential skin breakdown, and sensory perception alterations. For the family, the problems revolve around coping difficulties and knowledge deficit.

The nursing strategies for increased intracranial pressure are covered in Chapter 69, Neurological Trauma. For those nursing diagnoses stemming from the patient's inability to control or maintain body functions, the nurse must determine which body functions are affected and perform activities of daily living that the patient cannot do on his own. The nurse must protect the patient from physical injury re-

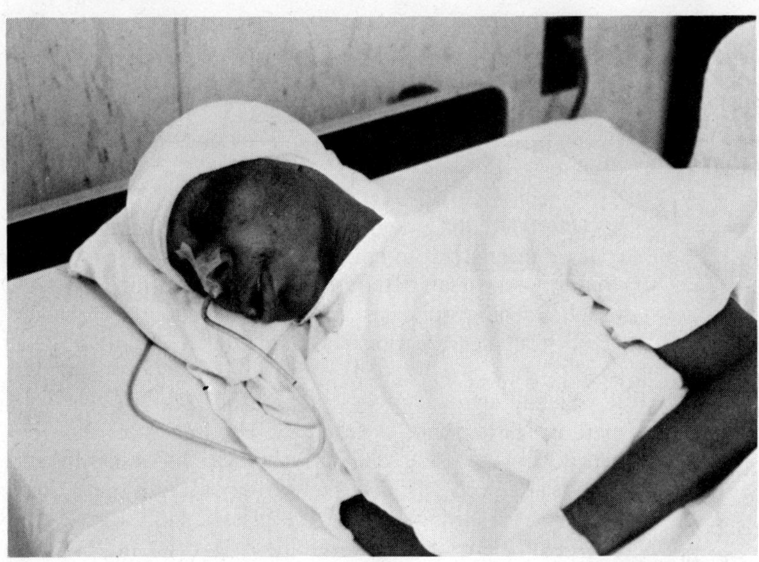

FIGURE 64–2 Proper positioning of the unconscious patient; the head is elevated and turned to the side. (Decision Audiovisual Media. Neurological Care Series. Philadelphia, JB Lippincott)

lated to immobility or related to excessive movement that is seen in some patients emerging from coma. The nurse must make sure the side rails of the bed are up at all times and that restraints on the limbs and trunk are not inhibiting circulation or limiting motion to the extent that contractures are developing.

Sustained Alterations in Consciousness

Although some patients in coma regain consciousness, others do not or they remain in coma for prolonged periods (weeks to months). Patients in the latter two categories suffer from conditions such as extensive stroke or significant head injury. In other situations patient may have gradual onset of alteration in consciousness. This implies a slow neuropathological process. Causes for this include degenerative diseases of the nervous system, metabolic encephalopathies, slow-growing mass lesions (*e.g.,* chronic subdural hematoma, tumor, and hydrocephalus). Some patients may regain consciousness through medical intervention (*e.g.,* evacuation of a subdural hematoma or placement of a ,shunt for hydrocephalus). Others may never regain consciousness.

Interventions. Nursing diagnosis and interventions include those described for rapid-onset alterations in consciousness, although the Glasgow Coma Scale is not useful for assessing patients in long-term coma. The care of patients not likely to regain consciousness is especially difficult from several viewpoints. These patients are at the highest risk for developing complications, and they require the most care. The impact on the family is tremendous. They must face the loss of their family member as an independent, interactive human being. They must grapple with the decision to place him in a nursing care facility or attempt to care for him at home. They as well as the care-givers may face an ethical dilemma: should life support measures be discontinued? The nurse must be cognizant of these issues in working with families of patients in prolonged coma and offer appropriate resources to them. These may involve referral to social work services, chaplain services, community agencies, and national foundations.

Evaluation. The patient will maintain an adequate airway with either type of alteration in consciousness and will be free from physical injury related to the immobility of altered consciousness.

Alterations in Cognitive Functioning

Mental functioning is the sum of congitive and affective mental processes. Cognitive functions include attention, memory, language, perception, planning, judgment, insight, and problem solving. These give one the ability to understand the meaning of symbols (letters and numbers), form, and spatial relationships and to receive, interpret, and integrate incoming stimuli and produce willed motor acts in the form of speech and complex behaviors. Affective mental process forms the basis of one's personality and emotions. Because processes of the human mind are so complex, ones sees a wide variety of deficits in cognitive functioning with neurological disease. They can range from mild memory impairment to major language, memory, and visual–spatial problems.

In contrast to alterations in consciousness, pathology causing alterations in cognitive functioning occurs at a higher level in the cerebrum, specifically in the cerebral cortex limbic system. Causes of disturbances in mental abilities include metabolic disorders (*e.g.,* diabetes, pulmonary disease, hepatic or renal failure, cardiopulmonary insufficiency, and hypothyroidism), drug intoxication, transient ischemic attacks, fluid and electrolyte imbalances, nutritional deficiencies, head trauma, and degenerative diseases.

Psychiatric diseases can also cause problems in mentation. However, these will not be addressed in this chapter, even though conditions such as depression and schizophrenia have been linked to physiological pathology. The most basic mental functions are attentiveness, memory, and language. Without these, more complex functions cannot take place.[20]

Attentiveness Problems

Consider how difficult it would be to assess a person's cognitive abilities if he is constantly being distracted by someone passing by or by noise from a conversation near him. Being able to attend to a specific stimulus without being distracted by extraneous environmental stimuli (*i.e.*, paying attention) is essential for communication and learning to take place. Common causes of decreased attentiveness or distractibility are diffuse brain dysfunction due to metabolic disturbance, drug intoxication, systemic infection, and bilateral cortical damage due to head trauma, encephalopathies, multiple infarctions, and encephalitis.

Assessment. Attentiveness can be checked by simply observing the patient or asking him if he has difficulty concentrating. Formal assessment involves asking the patient to repeat randomly selected groups of numbers. Normal persons of average intelligence can repeat five to seven digits.[20] Another problem of attention involves inattention to stimuli on the side of the body opposite a unilateral brain lesion. This is sometimes called hemi-inattention. It may range from inability to perceive a touch stimulus on the affected side when both sides of the body are touched simultaneously (double simultaneous stimulation) to total lack of awareness of the affected side of the body and of any stimulus coming from that side. This syndrome is presented later under the section Agnosia.

Interventions. It is important that the nurse determines the cause of decreased attention because it may be due to something other than pathological causes. Anxiety causes distractibility, and depression produces disinterest and reduced arousal.[20] Efforts to conduct patient education will be fruitless if the patient is too distractible. Family members may need to be taught the information instead.

Memory Problems

Problems with memory are commonly seen in neurological disease. They can be caused by any disease affecting the temporal lobes (an essential component of the memory circuit) including trauma, tumor infarction, hemorrhage, infection, degenerative disease, and seizure.

Memory difficulties can range from minor inconvenience to devastating incapacity. Minor memory problems are frequently reported in epileptic patients, probably as much a result of antiepileptic therapy as of the seizures themselves. Memory is severely affected in persons who have had herpes simplex encephalitis because this disease selectively damages the temporal lobes. They may not have any short-term memory and consequently have great difficulty managing day-to-day affairs. One woman forgot how to make coffee if she didn't do it every day. She had to keep an indexed notebook to help her keep track of her experiences and her daily plans. People with Alzheimer's disease suffer progressive loss of memory due to the degenerative nature of the disease.

Interventions. For memory problems that tend not to change, the nurse can employ interventions such as repetition and rehearsal, demonstration, cues and memory aids, varied teaching strategies, and positive feedback. These and other strategies are presented with more detail in Table 64–3.

Slater suggests several approaches for patients with memory disturbance.[18] Orientation to reality can be enhanced by use of a calendar, photographs of family and friends and home, a clock, a television or a radio, and familiar objects. Hearing aid and eye glasses should always be worn by patients during wakefulness. The patient's environment should be ordered, structured, and consistent. For instance, furniture and personal items should be arranged in the same way every day. Verbal interaction should include simple, concrete directions and explanations and avoidance of abstractions.

Memory dysfunctions have significant implications for patient education and discharge planning. The nurse should make sure that if a patient cannot remember or understand explanations of procedures, medication schedules, and home care activities, family members or future care-givers must be given the appropriate information about patient care.

Aphasia

Language is a major factor in our ability to interact with others. It is the foundation on which our social interactions occur and is perhaps the most important means by which we learn new things. Clearly, difficulties with understanding or expressing language have far-reaching implications.

Language is the use of symbols to communicate wishes, needs, and ideas. The centers of language for most people are in the left hemisphere of the brain (Fig. 64–3). Wernicke's area, which is in the area of the angular gyrus, is normally thought of as the center for speech comprehension. However, it also has a part in speaking (as evidenced by the speech difficulties of people with lesions in this area) as well as a major role in reading and writing.[6] Broca's area, which is in the posterior inferior frontal lobe, is the center for verbal expression. These areas are connected to each other by fibers composing the arcuate fasciculus. Wernicke's area receives visual input (for reading) from the occipital lobes and auditory input (for speech comprehension) from the temporal lobes. Language dysfunction can occur as a result of damage in the centers themselves or their connecting pathways.

There are many types of aphasia. Two major types are receptive or fluent aphasia (involving Wernicke's area) and expressive or nonfluent aphasia (involving Broca's area). In *receptive aphasia* the patient can hear the sounds of speech but cannot understand what is being said. He also tends to make errors in the use of words. In *expressive aphasia* there is difficulty in expressing thoughts verbally. In reality most

TABLE 64–3
Teaching Approaches for the Patient with Memory Disturbance

Teaching Approach	*Rationale*
Provide for repetition and rehearsal.	Memory is facilitated by repeated practice; forgetting occurs with inactivity. Consistency is a form of repetition.
Make information meaningful. Combine demonstration with explanation. Show how teaching relates to life situations. Relate material to be learned to meaningful situations.	Meaningful information is important in the organization of memory and activates the reticular formation to facilitate attention and arousal. Organization facilitates memory. When an activity is of value to a person, it serves as a reinforcement to performance.
Allow sufficient time for a response.	More time may be needed for the person to process information and produce a response.
Use cues and memory aids.	Recognition is easier than recall; recall requires a memory search, whereas recognition does not.
Proceed from simple to complex.	The more difficult the task, the more deleterious is a given degree of cortical destruction.
Use multiple modalities directed at the same activity.	The more the brain senses an event, the more it remembers it.
Adjust the teaching approach to the patient's strengths and weaknesses.	Persons with left hemisphere lesions have difficulty learning verbal material. Persons with right hemisphere lesions have difficulty retaining visual nonverbal material.
Expect that the patient will learn.	The power of expectation alone can positively influence others. Some learning is possible even with severe memory disturbance.
Provide positive feedback.	Reinforcement facilitates learning. Patients with memory impairment may forget their own success.

(Adapted from Mahoney EK: Alterations in cognitive functioning in the brain damaged patient. Nurs Clin North Am 15(2):288–289, 1980)

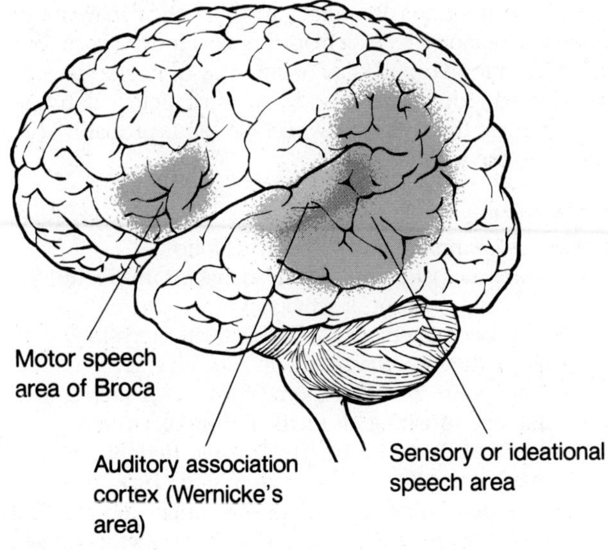

FIGURE 64-3 Sensory and motor language areas. These areas are connected by the superior longitudinal (arcuate) fasciculus.

aphasias are rarely clear-cut in their presentation because many brain lesions involve parts of both language centers or their connecting fibers. Therefore, one usually sees a mixture of comprehension and expressive difficulties. Use of labels for identifying an aphasia is not that useful for nursing care. What is more useful is an accurate description of what language dysfunctions exist and what abilities remain intact so that communication can be built around the remaining abilities.

Loss of language can have devastating and far-reaching effects on a person's life. Patients with expressive language problems become very frustrated with their inability to communicate needs and thoughts. Patients with receptive language difficulties have great difficulty learning new things. Marital relationships may become strained, work may no longer be possible, and the patient may totally withdraw from social situations. Formal speech therapy is the means by which language rehabilitation is achieved both in the hospital and after discharge. The nurse should attempt to support the therapeutic approaches initiated by the speech pathologist.

Interventions. The nurse can use a variety of interventions to support the patient experiencing a language deficit. Verbal communications should be kept short and simple. Much can be communicated nonverbally by both the patient and the nurse through the use of pantomime, gesture, and visual cues. The use of speech should not be avoided, however, because most authorities believe the best therapy is continued hearing of speech.[21] In addition, the nurse should offer only a few choices for the patient's verbal response and allow him plenty of time to respond. The patient should be treated as an adult; avoid talking down to him.

The nurse should be face to face with the patient, looking at him and using attentive but relaxed facial expression and body language to enhance the quality of communication. She should be honest in telling the patient when she cannot understand him and encourage him to let her know when he doesn't understand her. Continuing to offer encouragement and reinforcement when success is achieved is essential. The environment should be free from distractions during verbal interactions, and frequent multisensory and social stimulation should be included in the plan of care.[11]

For the purpose of outlining nursing care, language problems are separated into two categories: comprehension and expression deficits.

COMPREHENSION DEFICIT

- Use pantomime and gestures.
- Use visual cues.
- Speak with short, simple and specific phrases of speech.
- Do not overestimate comprehension.

EXPRESSION DEFICIT

- Ask yes–no questions.
- Anticipate needs.
- Be attentive to key words in the patient's speech for cues.
- Use writing board or alphabet board if reading and writing are intact.
- Use words the patient uses it some speech is present.

Without intact attention, memory, and language function, it is difficult to assess other aspects of cognitive functioning and even the rest of nervous system function. For instance, the nurse cannot determine the patient's general knowledge nor even expect him to be able to learn new things (about his illness or his self-care). She cannot get an accurate assessment of his motor function if he cannot follow commands, or of his sensory function if he cannot express himself. In these situations one must rely on evaluation of responses to stimuli to assess neurological function.

Agnosia

Agnosia is the inability to understand the meaning or significance of a particular sensory stimulus, although the sensory pathways and the sensorium are relatively intact. Lesions causing agnosia usually occur in areas where interpretation of sensory input occurs, most commonly in the parietal lobes but occasionally in the occipitotemporal area as well.[14] There are a variety of agnosias, including verbal, tactile, and visual agnosias (Table 64–4), because there are several types of sensory inputs. *Verbal* agnosia is the inability to understand the spoken word (fluent or receptive agnosia). *Tactile* agnosia is the inability to identify an object by its feel (astereoagnosia). *Visual* agnosia is the inability to name an object when looking at it.

TABLE 64–4
Agnosias

Stimulus type—definition, terminology
Verbal—inability to understand spoken word (fluent or receptive aphasia)
Tactile—inability to identify an object by feeling it (astereoagnosia)
Visual—inability to name or tell use of an object by seeing it
Seeing a human face—inability to recognize a person by seeing only his face (prosopagnosia)

Except for verbal agnosia, the agnosias are typified by the ability of the remaining senses to correctly identify the stimulus. Therefore, nursing care could be directed toward having the patient use the ***uninvolved*** senses to compensate for the deficit. An example is to have the patient with *prosopagnosia* (the inability to recognize a person's face) listen to the voice of someone he knows in order to identify him, or to have the patient with visual agnosia feel an object in order to identify it.

Anosognosia is the inability to recognize one's own disease or defect. The neglect syndrome, of which anosognosia is a part, has a global effect on the patient because the patient's image of himself is distorted. It is usually seen with right parietal lobe lesions, although it can be seen with lesions in the dominant parietal lobe, frontal lobes, or basal ganglia.[19] One can ask a conscious patient with a dense left-sided hemiplegia (resulting from a stroke in the right parietal lobe) what happened to him and he will deny that anything is wrong. One may show him his paralyzed arm and he will deny that it belongs to him.

Hemi-inattention is another aspect of the neglect syndrome.[4] It is characterized by inattention to one half of one's body as well as to one half of the space around him (on one side of the midline). Patients with this deficit may not respond to a person speaking from the unattended space. They may neglect food on one half of their tray or neglect to dress the affected side of their body. A visual field cut usually accompanies the neglect syndrome and probably contributes to the inattention.

Interventions. Nursing care for patients with hemi-inattention is summarized by Booth as follows:[4]

1. Place the patient in a room so that his unaffected side is facing the central activity in the room.
2. Approach the patient from his unaffected side.
3. Place the food toward the unaffected side.
4. Encourage the patient to perform ADLs, such as shaving and brushing his teeth, in front of a mirror.

The last practice may be of questionable benefit since patients may omit the mirror image side. However, with constant feedback from the nurse, the patient can attend to the affected side. In face, this is the focus of nursing intervention in the rehabilitation phase. Also, because the patient's ability to process verbal input (a left hemisphere function in most people) is usually intact, the nurse should use verbal instructions. She should not use demonstration or pantomime because visual–spatial abilities (a right hemisphere function) are probably impaired. She should keep verbal distractions to a minimum, keep the room well lighted and free of clutter, establish clear horizontal and vertical reference points, and place the patient's unaffected side near the wall when working with his affected extremities in order to minimize distraction and assist him in focusing his attention on his affected extremity.

Neglect syndrome has significant implications for both acute nursing care and long-term rehabilitation. Patients with neglect syndrome often attempt to get out of bed, and because they do not recognize their hemiplegia, proceed to fall. It is generally believed that the rehabilitation outcome of these patients is worse than those with left hemisphere lesions. However, some aspects of neglect behavior can be modified. In general, the techniques involve intensive training, focused attention, repetition, feedback regarding performance, and operant conditioning.[4]

Apraxia

The apraxias are disorders in carrying out learned movement and cannot be accounted for either by weakness, uncoordination, or sensory loss, or by incomprehension of or inattention to commands.[7] There are several types of apraxia: constructional (inability to copy geometric drawings), dressings apraxia (inability to dress oneself), ideomotor apraxia (inability to perform symbolic common gestures such as saluting and shaking hands), and ideational apraxia (inability to use objects in an appropriate manner). See Table 64–5 for a summary overview.

The translation of a command into a motor act involves many structures in the cerebral hemispheres. Interpretation of language commands (verbal or written) occurs in Wernicke's area. The order must then travel either to the ipsilateral motor cortex or via the corpus callosum to the contralateral motor cortex where the message is sent down the pyramidal tracts and out the central nervous system to skeletal muscles. Apraxias are generally ascribed to lesions in the cerebral cortex of either hemisphere, specifically in the premotor area of the frontal lobes and parts of the parietal lobes. Constructional and dressing apraxias have most often been seen with right-sided lesions and ideomotor apraxia with left-sided lesions. It has been reported, however, that apraxia can occur with subcortical white matter lesions and even lesions in the basal ganglia and thalamus.[1]

TABLE 64–5
Types of Apraxia

Constructional—inability to copy geometric drawings
Dressing—inability to dress oneself in proper sequence or even dress at all
Ideomotor—inability to perform symbolic, common gestures, *e.g.,* blow out a match, salute, write with an imaginary pen (not clinically important since people may retain ability to perform motor activities)*
Ideational or utilization—inability to appropriately use objects (*e.g.,* hammers, matches, and drinking cup)

*Agostoni E, Coletti A, Orlando G et al: Apraxia in deep cerebral lesions. J Neurol Neurosurg Psychiatry 46:804–808, 1983

Interventions. Apraxias can affect numerous daily living routines, including basic hygiene and grooming, dressing oneself, cooking, and work. Consider how difficult it would be to perform these activities if one could not correctly manipulate common objects (*e.g.,* water faucet, comb and brush, clothing, pots and pans, and knife). Nursing care is directed toward doing for the patient what he cannot do for himself and providing assistance in tasks he can partially complete. The first step, however, is to recognize that the problem is apraxia (or dyspraxia) and not misinterpret it as lack of cooperation, stubbornness, aphasia, or paralysis. In general the patient with apraxia can perform whole tasks more easily than parts or steps of tasks. He may do better if instruction is given outlining the goal but not the method (*e.g.,* "Here's the chair," not "Stand up, lean forward, turn around."). Sometimes no instruction and a gesture will work better. Remember, the problem is that the verbal command cannot reach the motor centers. Automatic activities may be possible when intentional ones are not. For instance, if handed a cup, the patient may be able to drink, but be unable to if told to drink. He will probably do best in a relaxed, nondemanding atmosphere in which little attention is paid to his disabilities.[21]

Another point to remember is that response to command for axial movements ("Look up," "Open your eyes," "Bend your head down," "Stand," "Bend over.") are often preserved in dyspractic patients.[7] The nurse may be able to creatively mesh the patient's ability to respond to these commands with his intact automatic movements in the plan of care. In addition, some patients appear to develop the ability to "self-signal" when given a command to perform a movement with the dyspractic hand. Such patients can do the action first with the unaffected limb that somehow signals the affected limb to initiate it correctly. Others may be able to use nonverbal signaling in which they use precursor motor activities to perform the commanded movement (*e.g.,* pretend to strike a match and bring it to the face in order to complete the command to "Blow out a match.").[7]

Behavior Changes and Impaired Thought Processes

It is not uncommon or surprising to see behavioral changes with diseases of the brain. After all, the brain is what gives humans their personality and emotions, and guides their psychological and physical selves. Behavior changes and impairment of thought processes (*e.g.,* judgment, insight, planning and problem solving) can result from a variety of disorders. Damage to the frontal lobes frequently yields a constellation of behavioral abnormalities known as the frontal lobe syndrome. This can include personality changes, disinhibition, impulsiveness, inattention, mood lability, poor judgment and difficulty with abstraction.[17] Cerebral atrophy, seen in Alzheimer's disease, Pick's disease, Creutzfeldt-Jakob disease, alcoholic dementia, Huntington's disease and neurosyphilis, causes problems with a variety of higher cognitive functions and can lead to regressive, child-like behavior. Psychological and personality changes are frequent sequelae of head injury and constitute the post-traumatic or postconcussion syndrome. Symptoms include headache, irritability, dizziness, diminished concentration, and hypersensitivity to certain stimuli (*e.g.,* noise and crowds).[23] Intellectual function and memory are not usually or are only minimally impaired. The symptoms tend to diminish with time, although they may persist for several months or longer.[17]

Some feel that uncontrolled temporal lobe epilepsy leads to personality and behavior changes (*e.g.,* sober affect, heightened philosophical/religious interests, circumstantiality, aggression, altered sexuality, and rigid personality),[3] although this is still quite controversial.[22] Left temporal epileptic discharges are supposedly associated with depression, hypergraphia, and paranoia, whereas right-sided discharges are associated with emotional lability and denial of unpleasant aspects of behavior.

Interventions. A variety of interventions have been proposed for behavior change and impaired thought processes. Orienting the patient to reality, speaking in short sentences with simple words, communicating face to face with the patient, keeping the environment free from distractions and structuring the patient's surroundings in an orderly consistent way are means of dealing with alterations in thought processes. Inappropriate behavior may be handled by reinforcing appropriate behavior, ignoring inappropriate activity, setting limits, and diverting the patient from destructive behavior. For a more detailed overview of care see the accompanying Nursing Care Plan for Selected Behavior Problems Related to Brain Injury.

Evaluation

Evaluation of the nursing care of patients with alterations in cognitive functioning involves regular, formal assessment of the changes in the individual's cognitive functions.

Alterations in Movement

Movement is the major form of output of the nervous system except for endocrine function. For the purpose of this section, movement refers to voluntary coordinated skeletal muscle movement. Many parts of the nervous system are involved in movement: primary and association motor cortex in the frontal lobes, basal ganglia, cerebellum, descending pathways, and peripheral nerves (including the cranial nerves). Although not part of the nervous system, skeletal muscle must also be intact for normal execution of movement. Any

NURSING CARE PLAN FOR SELECTED BEHAVIOR PROBLEMS RELATED TO BRAIN INJURY

NURSING DIAGNOSIS/PROBLEM 1: Alteration in thought processes related to brain injury
GOAL 1: Patient will demonstrate improved orientation and sense of reality.

Nursing Interventions	Rationale	Outcome Criteria
1. Employ orientation to reality: use orienting objects such as clock, radio, television; photographs of family, friends, staff; use memory board or schedule for activities.	1. Constant reminders help maintain orientation in patients with memory deficits.	1. Demonstrates some awareness of time, place, and person
2. Avoid too many different caregivers.	2. Confused patients become disturbed by a constantly changing staff.	2. Exhibits feeling of ease with staff
3. Use multiple sensory modalities to orient patient.	3. The more ways the brain receives information, the more it remembers it.	3. Demonstrates sense of reality
4. Use short sentences and simple words.	4. Brain injury makes it difficult to process complex sentences.	4. Exhibits understanding of content being communicated
5. Use face-to-face contact; keep environment free from distractions.	5. These measures help to focus patient's attention.	5. Exhibits attentive behavior
6. Keep environment structured, ordered, and consistent.	6. Inconsistency fosters confusion; repetition and structure enhance retention.	6. Demonstrates some awareness of time, place, and person

(*Continued*)

NURSING CARE PLAN FOR SELECTED BEHAVIOR PROBLEMS RELATED TO BRAIN INJURY *(Continued)*

NURSING DIAGNOSIS/PROBLEM 2: Potential for violence related to brain injury as evidenced by aggressive outbursts and insecurity
GOAL 2: Patient will demonstrate socially acceptable behavior.

Nursing Interventions	Rationale	Outcome Criteria
1. Maintain calm, firm attitude	1. This helps communicate a nonthreatening, but authoritative presence.	1. Reduction in or absence of violent, aggressive outbursts
2. Use two or three people for care.	2. When patient becomes physically abusive, several staff can help protect both patient and family from injury.	2. Patient and staff are free from injury.
3. Avoid overstimulation: regulate visitors and visiting hours; avoid excessive TV watching, loud noises, numerous demands, frequent touching; use a private room; place in "time out" room that is away from activity for short intervals if patient becomes agitated.	3. Too much stimulation precipitates aggressive behavior.	3. Appears secure and comfortable

NURSING DIAGNOSIS/PROBLEM 3: Inappropriate behavior related to brain injury
GOAL 3: Patient will demonstrate socially acceptable behavior.

Nursing Interventions	Rationale	Outcome Criteria
1. Reinforce appropriate behavior; ignore inappropriate behavior.	1. Positive reinforcement encourages a behavior; lack of reinforcement extinguishes a behavior.	1. Inappropriate behaviors become less frequent; appropriate ones more frequent.
2. Set limits on patient's behaviors.	2. Established guidelines for behavior help patient monitor himself.	2. Follows guidelines for behavior
3. Use diversion for destructive behavior.	3. Focusing on another activity can redirect patient's behavior.	3. Destructive behavior becomes less frequent.

disease or condition that involves any of these structures can lead to alterations in movement.

Because nurses are concerned with how neurological disease affects function,[12] nursing interventions in this section will focus on common motor dysfunctions—altered motor aspects of seeing, eye closing, facial expression, eating, speaking, and limb movement.

Altered Motor Aspects of Seeing

In order for the eyes to see a unified image, they must move together or conjugately, in a coordinated fashion. When they do not move together, double vision occurs. Dysfunction of eye movements can be caused by paresis/palsy of cranial nerves III, IV, or VI, or by incoordination of extraocular movements. Double vision can be very disturbing to an individual, even to the point of making him nauseous.

Interventions. The simplest intervention for double vision due to cranial nerve palsy is patching one eye, thereby allowing only one image to be seen instead of two. If both eyes have good vision, the patch should be switched to the other eye periodically. Patching one eye may not help double vision resulting from nystagmus because it will not prevent or alleviate the rapid to and fro moving of the eye.

Altered Blink or Eye Closing

Two common causes of altered eye blink are cranial nerve VII damage and Parkinson's disease. Paralysis of the orbicularis oculis muscle innervated by cranial nerve VII results in inability to close the eye and to blink. This can be significant for two reasons. Corneal ulceration can occur due to inadequate lubrication and subsequent drying, and one's appearance can be altered to the degree that the person becomes socially withdrawn.

In Parkinson's disease, automatic movements such as eye blinking, swallowing, and swinging the arms while walking are reduced. In this condition the initiation, pace, and rhythm of movement is altered, not from muscle paralysis but from neurochemical disturbance in the basal ganglia. The normal blink rate of ten or more times per minutes is severely reduced, increasing the risk of corneal damage.

Interventions. Interventions for decreased or absent eye blink are the same, regardless of the cause. Regular application of eyedrops every hour may avoid the need for the most drastic option of patching the eye closed. However, if the patient complains of severe pain in the eye, one should immediately suspect corneal damage. In this situation patching the eye may be the only option.

Altered Facial Expression

Weakness of the facial muscles can be due to lesions in several parts of the nervous system—the cerebrum (motor cortex, internal capsule, brain stem, corticobulbar tract, and cranial nerve VII nuclei), and the peripheral axon of cranial nerve VII. The pattern of hemiparesis depends on the location of the lesion. Lesions rostral to the cranial nerve nucleus (*e.g.,* stroke) will cause paresis/paralysis only of the lower face ("central facial" paresis). This is because the eyes and forehead receive innervation from *both* cerebral hemispheres. In contrast, a lesion involving the cranial nerve nucleus or its peripheral axon will cause total paralysis of one half of the face on the ipsilateral side. For although both hemispheres supply the upper face muscles, the final common pathway for those fibers is via the peripheral axon of the cranial nerve VII on that side of the face. Consequently the cosmetic, and therefore self-image, effect is much more severe with a lower motor neuron (LMN) lesion than with an upper motor neuron (UMN) lesion. Lesions affecting the motor component of cranial nerve V, which helps close the jaw, also affect facial movements and expression. Speaking may be affected if there is inadequate jaw closure or the perioral muscles are weak (sounds using the lips cannot be made). Likewise, eating may be affected because food becomes lodged in the paretic side of the mouth.

Interventions. Most UMN lesions and some LMN lesions (*e.g.,* myasthenia gravis and amyotrophic lateral sclerosis) involving the face usually affect the tongue and throat muscles as well, making eating not only difficult but dangerous because of the potential for aspiration. Interventions for these implications will be addressed in the next section.

Altered Movements in Eating

The movements of eating include opening the mouth, chewing, manipulating the food with the tongue, and swallowing it. These movements involve cranial nerves V, VII, IX, X, and XII. Lesions affecting these nerves can involve the cerebrum, brain stem, peripheral nerve, and neuromuscular junction. In general, upper motor neuron lesions cause less severe problems than lower motor neuron lesions because the throat musculature receives bilateral innervation from the cortex. However, in most cases the disability is severe enough to warrant the special measures described below.

The most important implications of altered movements of eating are danger of aspiration and altered nutrition. If the epiglottis cannot close completely during attempts to swallow, food or secretions may slip into the trachea rather than pass down the esophagus. The airway may become totally occluded, leading to respiratory arrest, or the aspirated contents may pass into the lungs and cause aspiration pneumonitis. Alterations in swallowing are often accompanied by decreased or absent gag reflex. Because of the inability to perceive food or secretions in the pharynx, the stimulus to close the epiglottis is not generated, adding to the potential for aspiration. Chewing and swallowing difficulties may necessitate enteral feedings, by means of nasogastric, cervical esophagostomy, gastrostomy, or jejunostomy routes. Patients who are conscious may lose their appetite because eating is so closely associated with social interactions. These patients may withdraw from social occasions (including family meals) due to an altered self-image, decreased self-esteem, and loss of independence.

Larsen provides a helpful overview of swallowing problems and interventions.[9] Deficits in swallowing, also called dysphagia, can range from mild impairment to total dysfunction. There are two major types of dysphagia in patients with neurological disease: paralytic dysphagia and pseudobulbar dysphagia. *Paralytic dysphagia* is a result of lower motor neuron disease that involves the cranial nerves or their nuclei in the brain stem. It involves muscle weakness and impairment of oral reflexes relative to the extent and site of the lesion. *Pseudobulbar dysphagia* results from upper motor neuron disease, for instance, cerebral stroke or trauma. Patients with this problem will have spastic muscles of the face and oropharynx and hyperactive reflexes due to loss of inhibitory influence from the cortex.

Interventions. In both situations thorough assessment of eating movements should be made prior to feeding the patient. The nurse should test for strength of jaw opening and closing, tongue movement, soft palate elevation, cough and gag reflexes, and for degree of laryngeal elevation with attempts to swallow. The ability to swallow may be tested by giving ice chips, since they provide a cold stimulus and texture, both of which enhance swallowing mechanisms. Besides, if the patient does aspirate some of the ice, it will be unlikely to damage the lungs or lead to pneumonia.

Rehabilitation for partial paralytic dysphagia involves strengthening the muscles that are partially functional. However, one should keep in mind that return of the ability to eat a regular diet may never be achieved because damaged reflexes may never return to normal. Using an oral feeding tube is an excellent means of stimulating muscles and will not endanger the patient if it gets into the larynx, since it can be retrieved readily. In addition, the patient can be encouraged to consciously think about the substance in his mouth, and about swallowing it. Conscious awareness of swallowing

TABLE 64–6
Foods in Dysphagia

Desirable	*Undesirable*
Medium boiled eggs	Uncooked milk (increases phlegm)
Sliced canned peaches	Soft, fresh bread (sticky)
Gelatin cubes	Bananas (sticky)
Custard	Applesauce, purees (break apart, can be aspirated)
Mashed potatoes	
Cooked milk products,* (creamed soups, puddings)	

* Bringing milk to its boiling point breaks down the protein chains.

can enhance the involuntary reflexes. Certain foods and textures are tolerated better than others. Examples are listed in Table 64–6. The best foods are those that have consistency and can be formed into a nonsticky bolus.

Patients with pseudobulbar dysphagia will have more difficulty with liquids than solids because liquids do not stimulate the sensory mechanisms in the mouth as well. They may not tolerate a feeding tube because of hyperactive gag reflexes. Approaches for a patient with left hemisphere damage will differ from those with right hemisphere damage. Because speech may be impaired with left hemisphere damage, the patient can become overwhelmed and confused if eating and conversation are attempted simultaneously. It is best to avoid distracting him with conversation while he is eating, although simple one-word commands may help. He should sit bolt upright in bed when eating with the neck slightly flexed, as should all patients with swallowing problems, unless contraindicated. The patient with a right hemisphere lesion may have a dyspraxia that involves difficulty figuring out how to get the food from the plate to his mouth, how much to chew, and when to swallow. He needs to be talked through each step in eating, with sufficient time allowed for a response. It is best to consult a speech pathologist, if one is available, for thorough assessment and care planning of patients with swallowing problems.

Patients with Parkinson's disease may develop swallowing problems for two reasons: impaired swallowing movements, and buildup of saliva due to lack of spontaneous, automatic swallowing. The rate of swallowing is reduced, and eating becomes slower and more deliberate. Food tends to collect in the mouth and back of the throat, which may lead to choking and coughing episodes. These patients need to be reminded to think about the steps of swallowing. They should take small amounts at a time, chew well using both sides of the mouth, and eat slowly. They should make a conscious effort to swallow saliva often.[2]

Alterations in Speaking

The motor aspects of speaking involve the muscles of the mouth, jaw, tongue, lips, soft palate, and throat. Phonation, the generation of speech sounds, is a result of the controlled passage of air through contracted vocal cords. These are innervated by the vagus nerve (cranial nerve X). The articulation or formation of speech sounds is governed by muscles in the mouth, lips, tongue, and soft palate. These muscles are innervated by cranial nerve VII, IX, X, and XII. Both voluntary control and coordination of these muscles is essential for intelligible speech. Therefore, the cerebellum and the motor cortex respectively, as well as their connecting pathways, must be intact for normal speech.

The inability to phonate, called *aphonia,* is usually the result of a laryngectomy. That is, there is no possible way to make speech sounds, except by expelling air from the esophagus through the mouth. Whispering is possible if the vocal cords are paralyzed, because it is simply the result of expelling air from the lungs through the mouth. Changes in phonation and articulation can have profound effects on daily living because they affect speech, the primary form of human communication. When a person cannot express his needs or wants except by gestures, writing, or use of a mechanical communicating device, the spontaneity of communication is lost, as is the "color" of speech provided by modulating inflection, cadence, and emphasis. The likelihood of withdrawal from human interaction is high.

Dysarthria or slurred speech is the result of the inability to coordinate speech sounds, which can result from cortical, cerebellar, or cranial nerve dysfunction or from drug intoxication (*e.g.,* alcohol, antiepileptic medication). Patients with physical disease may be erroneously perceived as drunk, which could add to preexisting low self-esteem.

Patients with Parkinson's disease have difficulty speaking because of incoordination and decreased movements of muscles that control respiration, phonation, articulation, and prosody (the rate, rhythm, and intonation of speaking).

Interventions. One should encourage the use of writing or sign language by patients who cannot speak. Phrase boards can help communicate common basic needs. It is important to communicate with these patients regularly since they may tend to withdraw from human interaction, and it is important to remember that none of the above methods is an adequate substitute for the spontaneous conversational speech of everyday living. Patients with dysarthria should be advised to speak slowly and deliberately so that they can be understood. Families and coworkers should be informed that the patient's speech is not a result of alcohol intoxication, and they should be encouraged to allow him plenty of time to communicate his needs and ideas. Speech improvement exercises for patients with Parkinson's disease are available in booklets provided by the American Parkinson Disease Foundation.[2]

Alterations in Limb Movement

Alterations in limb movement can range from minor weakness in one muscle group (from mononeuropathy of a peripheral nerve) to total body paralysis (*e.g.,* high cervical spine lesions or amyotrophic lateral sclerosis). They can range from minor incoordination (due to alcohol intoxication) to total inability to keep one's balance (due to cerebellar degeneration). They can be characterized by a lack of spontaneous movement or bradykinesia as seen in Parkinson's disease, or they can involve excessive involuntary movements as seen in Huntington's chorea or stroke involving the basal ganglia. The extent of the alteration in movement correlates directly with the impact on daily living.

For patients with quadriplegia, tasks as simple as feeding oneself and daily hygiene are impossible. Wheelchair-bound individuals have limitations in accessibility to work and recreation. Weakness or paralysis in only one limb can cause some people great distress. It takes longer to do common, everyday activities. The individual must do more planning and allow more time to complete daily grooming and hygiene tasks. Involuntary movements can also affect mobility, as well as body image. Excessive movements can make it just as difficult to perform activities of daily living as does weakness or paralysis. A lot of energy is used and there may be difficulty maintaining adequate nutrition. Further, the person may withdraw from social interaction out of concern over the reactions he receives in public. Any patient who is immobilized in bed is at risk for all the hazards of immobility: pressure sores, venous stasis with thrombophlebitis, urinary stasis and infection, constipation, contractures, and osteoporosis. These problems are addressed in Nursing Care Plan for the Immobile Patient.

Interventions. A major goal of nursing is to keep the patient as independent as possible. If his condition allows it, he should be encouraged to walk. If he is in danger of falling or is confused, he should ambulate with assistance. If this is too dangerous, he should use a wheelchair. Patients with severe incoordination on one side should be encouraged to use the limbs of the other side. Sometimes weighted devices, such as a pen or drinking cup, can facilitate their use. Cups or glasses should be filled only half full to avoid spillage. Only as a last resort should a patient be fed by someone else.

There are a variety of interventions for patients with bradykinesia. Pacing boards can be used for speaking, and tapping a rhythm can help pace walking. Control of involuntary movements other than by medication is very difficult although some patients have developed unique methods. Some sit on the affected limb or limbs, or wedge them between themselves and the couch or chair. Others consciously tense the muscles in the affected limb or do unnoticeable voluntary movements such as grabbing a coin in their pocket to eliminate the resting tremor of parkinsonism. These interventions are not intended to constitute a comprehensive list.

Alterations in Sensation

To review, the special senses include smell, sight, hearing, maintaining equilibrium, and taste. The somatic senses, or ones that the whole body feels, are touch, pressure, pain, heat and cold, vibration, and position sense. Alterations in sensation can affect a single special sense, or a combination thereof. Causes of sensory dysfunctions range from lesions in peripheral nerves and ascending pathways in the spinal cord to brain stem lesions in the thalamus and sensory cortex in the brain. Since each modality is carried by a specific set of nerve fibers, the location of the lesion will determine the type and extent of sensory dysfunction.

Alteration of Smell

Anosmia (lack of ability to smell) often occurs after basilar skull fracture. The olfactory fibers traversing the delicate cribriform plate become easily severed when there is trauma to that area. The lack of smell at first glance appears to be a somewhat benign and insignificant disability. After all, smell is not essential for safety, nor particularly important to maintain life. However, it is easy to recall how disappointing it is not to be able to smell or taste one's food when ill with a cold. Food simply does not have the same appeal as it does when smell is intact. Smell, in fact, is what determines the flavor of one's food. Anosmia or decreased sense of smell, therefore, can lead to serious consequences by affecting one's appetite. This could be one of the reasons that the elderly tend to have poor nutrition, since loss of olfactory neurons often accompanies aging.

Interventions. Nursing care in general is aimed at enhancing the remaining abilities, whether they be motor or sensory, to make up for the dysfunction. In the case of decreased smell, one can increase the appeal of food by creating a nice visual presentation: beautify the setting for the meal, use colorful foods, use a variety of textures and temperatures, and make eating a social occasion in which others are also eating.

Alterations in Seeing

Blindness can take several forms, depending on the cause and the location of the lesion. Pathology within the retina of one eye can lead to monocular blindness. Glaucoma and optic nerve damage can cause blindness of this type. Transient monocular blindness, *amaurosis fugax,* results from a small plaque that dislodges from the carotid artery and travels into the ophthalmic artery and then into the retina. Transient blindness can also occur with some types of migraine headaches, as a result of vascular spasm. Blindness can occur in only part of the visual field if a part of the optic pathways is damaged.

Interventions. Total blindness can have a severe impact on daily living. For most people it means a drastic change in the home and at work. Patients must adjust to using non-visual cues to move about, perform ADLs, and work.

For patients withwiht visual field cuts as a result of stroke, tumor, or brain surgery, a few simple interventions should be used. Initially, the patient may not realize he has a vision field cut. He should be reminded to turn his head to see the part of the environment that is in the field cut, for instance, the food tray or visitors and care-givers. The patient's bed should be placed so that the major activity of the ward is within the intact visual field. Later, during the rehabilitation phase, the position may be reversed so as to force the patient to pay attention to the side of the field cut.

Alterations of Hearing

This disturbance has received a lot of attention in regard to industrial settings and the youth population, for it is

NURSING CARE PLAN FOR THE IMMOBILE PATIENT

NURSING DIAGNOSIS/PROBLEM 1: Potential for impaired gas exchange related to aspiration and atelectasis from physical immobility

GOAL 1: Maintain patent airway, facilitate gas exchange, and prevent aspiration and atelectasis

Nursing Interventions	Rationale	Outcome Criteria
1. Position patient in a side-lying or head-elevated position, with head slightly in extension.	1. The tongue cannot occlude the airway; the movement of diaphragm and chest muscles are facilitated for deep breathing in this position.	1. Airway is patent; chest excursions and diaphragm movements are seen with each respiration.
2. Suction oral and nasal pharynx as needed; suction trachea if endotracheal or tracheosomy tube is in place.	2. Secretions accumulating in the airway inhibit air flow to the lungs.	2. Respirations are free from gurgling sounds; tracheal tubing is free from secretions.
3. Turn patient at least every 2 hours; have patient cough and deep breathe if he is capable.	3. These activities help clear secretions and maintain a patent airway, thereby preventing atelectasis.	3. Breath sounds are normal.
4. Check for residual tube-feeding formula before delivering next feeding, and administer feedings slowly, carefully.	4. Tube feedings may be regurgitated resulting in aspiration.	4. There is no aspiration.

NURSING DIAGNOSIS/PROBLEM 2: Potential alteration in tissue perfusion related to physical immobility

GOAL 2: Stimulate normal circulation, prevent circulatory stasis and clotting, and preserve the integument

Nursing Interventions	Rationale	Outcome Criteria
1. Turn at least every 2 hours.	1. Frequent change of position enhances circulation to the skin, muscles, and joints.	1. Skin is free of reddened areas.
2. Avoid placing bony prominences in positions likely to cause excessive pressure on them.	2. Decubitus ulcers occur most fruqently over bony prominences.	2. Skin is free from pressure sores.
3. Place elastic support hose on legs.	3. External pressure provided by hose prevents pooling of venous blood in legs, thereby preventing thrombophlebitis.	3. Legs are free of focal areas of tenderness, redness, and heat.

NURSING DIAGNOSIS/PROBLEM 3: Potential alteration in bowel and bladder elimination and alteration in nutrition, less than body requirements, due to physical immobility

GOAL 3: Maintain good hydration and nutrition, prevent urinary tract infection, and fecal impaction

Nursing Interventions	Rationale	Outcome Criteria
1. Measure body weight daily.	1. Weight loss is an indicator of poor hydration and/or inadequate caloric intake.	1. Optimal body weight is maintained.
2. Maintain fluid intake of 2000–3000 ml of fluid daily and adequate caloric intake for patient's needs (determined by dietician).	2. Bed rest increases the rate of tissue breakdown, thus adequate nutrition is essential; ample fluid intake is necessary to keep urine dilute and ensures "flushing" of urinary tract, which helps prevent stone formation and infection and prevents stool from becoming hard and impacted.	2. Fluid intake is 2000–3000 ml daily; urine is clear and free of sediment; stool is well formed and passes at least every 3 days.

(Continued)

NURSING CARE PLAN FOR THE IMMOBILE PATIENT *(Continued)*

NURSING DIAGNOSIS/PROBLEM 4: Activity intolerance and potential for injury related to osteoporosis
GOAL 4: Minmize osteoporosis and prevent falls

Nursing Interventions	Rationale	Outcome Criteria
1. Ambulate patient whenever possible; if not, stand with assistance.	1. Pull of gravity and stress on long bones strengthens them.	1. Patient is free from fractures.
2. Attend patient while ambulating; use safety belt around patient's waist if necessary; use proper technique when transferring patient.	2. Increased calcium loss due to prolonged bed rest increases likelihood of fractures.	2. Patient is free from injury and fractures.

NURSING DIAGNOSIS/PROBLEM 5: Potential for impaired physical mobility related to muscle wasting and contractures
GOAL 5: Maintain normal function, prevent contractures, and prevent subluxation and other joint injuries

Nursing Interventions	Rationale	Outcome Criteria
1. For spastic limbs position them opposite to the spastic position:	1. These positions help prevent contactures and enhance normal movement.	1. Patient is free from contractures.
a. Upper extremities: position shoulder forward (protracted), extend elbow, supinate forearm, rest arms on lapboard (not shoulder sling).	a. A lapboard supports the shoulder without contributing to development of contractures.	
b. Lower extremities: position hip forward (protracted), avoid use of footboard.	b. Pressure on the feet by a footboard increases extensor spasticity and leads to plantar flexion (foot drop).	
c. Limit time spent in supine position	c. Supine position increases spasticity.	
2. For flaccid limbs: a. Use a footboard. b. Support arm in a sling.	2. Footboard supports the flaccid foot, preventing foot drop. Sling prevents shoulder subluxation.	2. Absence of foot drop and shoulder subluxation
3. Encourage active range of motion of nonparalyzed limbs; provide passive range of motion in paralyzed limbs.	3. Disuse of muscles leads to muscle wasting; range of motion maintains joint mobility.	3. Absence of muscle wasting in nonparalyzed limbs, absence of contractures.

known that chronic exposure to loud noise, whether it is from machinery or music, destroys the tiny hair cells in the cochlea that transform sounds into nerve impulses. Many other conditions lead to decreased ability to hear. Loss of hair cells also occurs as a function of aging. Otosclerosis, hardening of the tiny bones in the middle ear, prevent them from vibrating and conducting sound waves to the inner ear. In addition, lesions involving the auditory pathways from the inner ear to the auditory cortex in the temporal lobe (*i.e.,* acoustic neuroma and trauma) can cause loss of hearing.

Interventions. Decreased hearing has perhaps more impact on social interaction than any aspect of daily living. Because our social being depends so much on verbal interactions with others, it is reasonable to expect some degree of social withdrawal in persons with decreased hearing. These people do best when only one person talks to them, fairly close and without extraneous noises. Many can read lips to enhance their perception of what is said, and therefore one should directly face the person when speaking to him. Persons who are totally deaf, as well as their families, usually are taught to use sign language. In the initial stage, however, communication can be facilitated by simply writing or using a reader board.

Alterations in Maintaining Equilibrium

Keeping one's balance is the result of an intricate feedback loop between the sensory inputs from the labyrinths of the inner ear and the proprioceptors in the legs, and the motor outputs of the cerebellum and cerebral cortex to the skeletal muscle. Therefore, a disturbance in any of these structures can cause balance problems. Common causes include peripheral neuropathy, acoustic neuroma, and cerebellar insult. The foremost implication of dysfunction in maintaining equilibrium is safety. It is well known that falls are a common cause of iatrogenic injury in hospitals. In most cases they are the results of patient's losing their balance.

Interventions. Patients must be carefully monitored when they ambulate for the first time. Their needs, especially for elimination, must be anticipated so that they are not tempted to get out of bed before they are capable of doing so safely. Wheelchairs or safety belts may be employed to prevent falling.

Some patients adjust to balance problems by using a wide-based gait. Others may complain of dizziness and even nausea. A complaint of dizziness could mean feeling faint or experiencing vertigo. *Vertigo* is the term for the sensation of feeling that either the person is spinning or the world around him is spinning. It is to be distinguished from feeling faint or about to black out. Patients complaining of vertigo should be kept in the position that is most comfortable for them.

Alterations of Taste

One rarely sees alteration of taste alone, because there are two cranial nerves that carry taste fibers (VII and IX) and both of these have other functions. Alteration in taste has implications similar to alteration of smell. Loss of taste is seen in the elderly as a result of physical loss of taste buds.

Because appetite may be decreased, the physical appeal of food should be enhanced as described earlier.

Alterations in Somatic Sensations

Somatic sensory modalities are touch/pressure, pain/temperature, and vibration/position sense. Lesions influencing somatic sensations can occur in the receptors themselves, the peripheral nerves, the ascending nerve tracts, the thalamus, and the sensory cortex. Because each sensory modality is carried by a different set of ascending fibers, one may see only touch, or only pain/temperature sensation affected; or one may see an apparent "dissociation" of sensory deficits—loss of pain and temperature on one side of the body and loss of touch on the other side (Brown-Séquard syndrome). The special and somatic sensations are important, for they give us information about both our internal and our external environments.

Interventions. Deficits in sensation pose problems in personal safety. We are all aware that decreased touch and pain sensation can lead to tissue injury by way of pressure sores, burns, abrasions, and the like. Patients who are alert and responsive to education should be reminded to use their special senses (especially sight) to detect closeness to danger (*e.g.*, a stove) and beginning pressure sores. The guiding principle of management is to capitalize on the patient's remaining abilities and encourage him to use intact senses to monitor his well-being.

Pain is a syndrome of excessive sensation and it has many etiologies. Post-traumatic acute pain from accidents or surgery is usually short-lived and relatively ameliorated by analgesic medication. If that pain cannot be reduced, it can lead to serious consequences. Postoperative pain may inhibit one's ability to cough and deep breathe, which is vital for preventing pneumonia and atelectasis. Chronic pain is a more serious and more debilitating problem that has many psychosocial as well as physical sequelae. The management of chronic pain is very complex, and the reader is referred to Chapter 9 for more information.

Alterations in Integrated Autonomic Regulation

A number of fundamental human functions that have the autonomic nervous system as their major effector are integrated at several levels of the nervous system. These functions include breathing, circulation, temperature control, ingestion/digestion, elimination, sexual function, and emotional experience. A great many primary neurological disorders interfere with such regulation at one or more levels.

Homeostatic regulatory function may take place at several levels—spinal cord and brain stem reflex centers, hypothalamus, and perhaps limbic cortex. All integrated regulatory systems have at least four levels of control: voluntary control at the cerebral cortex, brain stem and spinal cord autonomic reflexes, and peripheral control at the involved organ.[13] Therefore, disruption of nervous system functioning at any of these four levels can potentially disrupt integrated regulation of one or more of the functions listed. Breathing and circulation are covered extensively in Units IV and V of this volume. The remaining functions and implications of their dysfunction and nursing interventions are presented here.

Alterations in Temperature Control

Maintenance of body temperature within a fairly narrow range is critical for normal functioning of all body cells. Behavioral means of body temperature control (*i.e.*, putting on or taking off clothing, moving to an appropriate environment) are governed by the cerebral cortex. An example of someone who does not have this ability is the patient who is unconscious regardless of the cause. He does not perceive that he is too hot or too cold, nor can he manipulate his environment to help regulate his body temperature. In cool environments (less than 21° C) such as the operating room he is at risk for hypothermia.

The centers for autonomic regulation of body temperature are located in the hypothalamus. Patients with subarachnoid hemorrhage and other lesions in the region of the floor of the third ventricle may develop aseptic hyperthermia because of damage to the anterior hypothalamus where the heat loss center is located.

Spinal reflex control of temperature involves the autonomic functions required to dilate and constrict the blood vessels in the skin and cause sweating. Nervous system disease that influences any of these areas, their interconnecting pathways, or innervation of the effector organs can lead to a disturbance of body temperature regulation. The patient with spinal cord lesions in the acute stage of spinal shock becomes poikilothermic (takes on the temperature of the environment).

Interventions. Nursing care for these people and for unconscious patients involves careful monitoring of body core temperature and appropriate measures to bring body temperature into the homeostatic range. For hypothermic patients this would include putting on extra clothing or blankets or raising the room temperature, and perhaps providing warmed humidifed air, which increases body temperature internally through the lungs.[15] Measures for hyperthermic patients would include tepid sponging, cooling blankets, fans, and lowering the room temperature.

Alterations in Ingestion/Digestion

Ingestion includes initiation of eating behavior (cortical and limbic control) and chewing and swallowing (motor functions described earlier). Digestion, the mechanical and chemical alteration of food in the gastrointestinal tract, is predominantly an autonomic nervous system activity, mediated by a balance of sympathetic and parasympathetic impulses. Therefore, disturbance in cortical, brain stem, spinal cord, or peripheral nerves can affect ingestion/digestion. Cerebral hemisphere lesions can impair conscious food seeking and eating behavior. Stroke and other paralyzing lesions can affect the ability to chew and swallow, as can blockage of neuromuscular transmission (as in myasthenia gravis). Interventions for dysphagia (difficulty in swallowing) have been mentioned earlier.

Interventions. A common disturbance in digestion is paralytic ileus, which is frequent after spinal cord injury and abdominal surgery and may be seen in critically ill patients. Patients may complain of feeling full, constipated, or distended. Vomiting may occur and may lead to aspiration if swallowing, coughing, and gag reflexes are dysfunctional. Interventions include monitoring of bowel sounds before food or enteral feedings are offered.

Alterations in Elimination

Alterations in bowel and bladder function occur frequently in persons with a variety of neurological disorders because control of elimination occurs at all levels of the nervous system. The motor cortex acts to inhibit reflex emptying of the bowel and bladder. The sensory cortex is important for appreciation of bladder and rectal distention and enables voluntary initiation of micturition and evacuation. Pathways between the cortex and the sacral segments are important for autonomic control of the micturition reflex and probably of the evacuation reflex. The spinal reflex arcs for elimination are located in the sacral segments. Therefore lesions involving any of these structures can affect elimination. Damage to the frontal lobes of the brain from trauma, hemorrhage, or tumor can lead to incontinence due to lack of inhibition of the voiding and defecation reflexes. When this problem affects micturition it is called *uninhibited neurogenic bladder*. This problem can also occur with lesions in the tracts from the cerebral cortex to the midbrain–pontine micturition centers, or from the pons to the sacral spinal cord. Disorders such as multiple sclerosis, spinal cord injury, transverse myelitis, and tumors can interrupt nerve impulse transmission to and from sacral spinal cord and cortex. If the interruption is complete, the resulting effect on micturition is reflex voiding in which the bladder fills and empties in a reflex fashion. The condition is called *reflex neurogenic bladder*. Damage to the reflex arc for micturition, which is located in the sacral spinal cord, alters the micturition reflex. The problem is called *autonomous neurogenic bladder* and is characterized by distention and bladder filling without contractions.

The implications of altered urinary elimination are significant. Inadequate management of bladder dysfunction can lead to overdistention, formation of calculi, and infection. Complications resulting from an improperly managed neurogenic bladder are a leading cause of death in the paraplegic individual.[8] Urgency, frequency and incontinence in the conscious person forces him to be very careful in planning physical activities and fluid intake so that the need to urinate occurs only at appropriate and convenient places. Embarrassment over accidents and fear of potential ones may alter social activity, work, and recreation. Family members may unconsciously reject the person who requires constant cleaning up. This may eventually lead to placement in a nursing home.

Interventions. Although a majority of bladder dysfunctions can be placed in one of these categories, there are instances in which the dysfunction is a mixture of several types. Accurate diagnosis of the type of bladder dysfunction is best made by a urologist and is dependent on the history, presence of the bulbocavernous reflex, intravenous pyelogram, cystometrogram, and electromyography. Bladder reconditioning programs that match the dysfunction are then established. Table 64–7 summarizes the programs for each type of bladder problem.

Bowel dysfunction may be easier to manage than bladder dysfunction, but it can lead to complications such as fecal impaction with overflow diarrhea, obstipation, and even ileus. Frequent stool incontinence can lead to urinary tract infection and decubitus formation.

The purpose of a bowel program is to establish regular evacuation at a schedule time, to avoid incontinence, constipation and impaction, and to avoid social embarrassment.

TABLE 64–7
Programs for Bladder Reconditioning

Uninhibited Bladder

Many patients with uninhibited bladders have brain damage as a result of stroke, tumor, or trauma. Diminished awareness and understanding may limit the patient's ability to cooperate with a bladder program.

Two goals of a reconditioning program for such patients are (1) increase the length of time between voiding, and (2) eliminate episodes of incontinence.

Steps that may be taken to achieve these goals include the following:

1. Provide stimulation to increase the patient's awareness of surroundings and body functions. For example, take patient to the toilet facilities.
2. A schedule for toileting should be specified at time intervals based on the patient's bladder capacity and voiding pattern. The time interval should be estimated from the most recent voiding.
3. Have the patient assume the optimal position for voiding, if feasible, to allow for relaxation of the external urinary sphincter and perineal muscles. The sitting position is optimal for females; the standing position is best for males.
4. Use methods designed to stimulate voiding and to relax the patient, such as pouring water over the perineum or allowing water to run from the tap.

Reflex Bladder

A goal of a bladder reconditioning program for patients with reflex bladders is a residual urine of less than 50 ml, achieved with the use of trigger mechanisms to initiate reflex voiding. The following steps may be used to achieve this goal:

1. Instruct the patient to empty his or her bladder every 4 hours.
2. Teach the patient to use cutaneous trigger mechanisms to stimulate the voiding reflex. These mechanisms include pulling of the pubic hairs, massage of the abdomen; pinching, slapping, or stroking of the skin; and digital rectal stimulation.
3. Avoid the use of the Credé maneuver with a reflex bladder, for it may cause damage to the urethra and vesicoureteral reflux if the external sphincter is contracted.

Autonomous Bladder

A goal of a bladder reconditioning program for patients with autonomous bladders is a residual urine of less than 75 ml with the use of the Credé and Valsalva maneuvers. Steps that may be taken to achieve this aim include the following:

1. Instruct the patient in the use of the Credé maneuver with or without the Valsala maneuver.
2. Encourage the patient to do strengthening exercises for the abdominal muscles to develop maximal power of abdominal pressure and to ensure satisfactory voidings with the least amount of residual urine possible.
3. Instruct the patient to empty the bladder when its capacity is approximately 350 ml. Determine the time interval by correlating fluid intake with the predicted urinary output based on the voiding pattern.

Motor Paralytic Bladder

A goal of a bladder reconditioning program for patients with motor paralytic bladders is to use Credé and Valsalva maneuvers to empty the bladder, achieving volumes of residual urine of less than 75 ml. To accomplish this goal, one may follow these steps:

1. Implement interventions similar to those used for patients with autonomous bladders.
2. Teach intermittent self-catheterization if the patient is unable to empty the bladder efficiently with Credé or Valsalva maneuvers.

Sensory Paralytic Bladder

A goal of a bladder reconditioning program for patients with sensory paralytic bladders is to empty the bladder according to a preplanned voiding schedule. To accomplish this goal one may follow the steps listed below:

1. Instruct the patient to empty his or her bladder every 3 hours instead of waiting for a sensation of bladder fullness.
2. Initiate intermittent self-catheterization in patients with bladder and atonicity and large volumes of residual urine.

(From Johnson J: Rehabilitative aspects of neurological bladder dysfunction. Nurs Clin North Am 15(2):293–307, 1980

Before initiating a program, the nurse should first assess the person's bowel history, his appetite and diet preferences, the medication he is taking, his mobility, his communication abilities, and his potential for cooperation. The nurse should find out what time of the day the person wants his bowel program, since some patients may prefer times other than the morning.

A common bowel program is one based on providing a stimulus to initiate reflex evacuation of the bowel. In general, the patient begins the program by drinking hot liquid and eating some food. This facilitates the gastrocolic and duodenocolic reflexes generated by distention of the stomach and duodenum and produces peristalsis. Twenty to thirty minutes after the meal, a suppository is inserted high into the rectum, making sure that it is in contact with rectal mucosa. This further stimulates peristalsis of the lower colon and rectum. Care must be taken not to insert the suppository into stool because it will not be effective. The patient should be on the toilet or a commode 15 minutes after the suppository is inserted. The sitting position is important, because gravity and the squatting position assist in expulsion of stool.

If evacuation does not occur, digital stimulation is instituted 30 minutes after the suppository was inserted. Digital stimulation consists of placing a gloved and lubricated forefinger into the rectum and gently pressing against the rectal wall in a circular fashion until the sphincter relaxes. This may need to be repeated. The patient may assist by deep breathing and bearing down. Total time spent on the toilet or commode should be limited to 1 hour. If spontaneous evacuation does not occur, the bowel contents should be removed manually.

The bowel program should be repeated every 2 to 3 days. If the stool is regularly hard, an oral stool softener such as docusate sodium (Colace) may be helpful. Agents that produce bulk in the gastrointestinal tract, such as Metamucil, are also useful in establishing bowel regularity. Caution should be taken to make only one change in the bowel program at a time so that the effectiveness of a given intervention can be evaluated.

Alterations in Sexual Response

Disorders at any level of the nervous system have the potential to influence some or all of the phases of sexual response (desire, excitement, and orgasm). Cerebral lesions may inhibit the desire phase or the reflex responses of the excitement phase. Brain stem and spinal cord lesions may interrupt cognitive-mediated desire and the effector systems necessary to achieve intercourse (*e.g.*, penile erection). Neuropathies and spinal cord lesions that affect sensation in large parts of the body, particularly the erotic zones, may decrease the sensory components of desire. Finally, autonomic neuropathies, lesions in the sacral segments and cauda equina, and peripheral neuropathies may prevent any reflex activity in the excitement and orgasmic phases, while leaving desire intact.[13]

Preservation of reflex activity in the genital area makes intercourse potentially achievable for the male with spinal cord damage. Loss of such reflexes prevents intercourse, but does not prevent sexual expression and is not necessarily damaging to sexual health. Persons with dysfunction of physical sexual response do not lose their sexuality and can achieve intimacy and affection without physical intercourse.

Interventions. Nursing interventions require tactful inquiry and an open, nonjudgmental attitude in teaching and counseling. This is a difficult goal to measure because decisions about sexuality are entwined with the patient's value system.

Alterations in Emotional Response

The limbic system is generally thought to be the seat of emotions, although the cerebral neocortex is thought to participate by "fine tuning" the emotion. Examples of this might include inhibiting expression of an emotion, analyzing an emotional experience, and learning from an emotional experience. Limbic system input to the hypothalamus generates autonomic and skeletal muscle behavior in response to the emotion (*e.g.*, sweating and muscle tension).

Because transmission of these impulses to the effector organs (autonomic system and skeletal muscle) is through the brain stem and spinal cord, lesions at any level can affect some components of the emotional experience. Bilateral frontal lobe lesions often produce a "flat" affect, or lack of emotion. Frontal lobe lesions may also disinhibit emotional outflow, resulting in inappropriate laughing or crying. The influence of seizure activity in regions of the limbic system may cause changes in emotional response as described earlier. Although cognitive appreciation of emotional experience is not affected by lesions in the spinal cord, the "gut" feelings are not present because they are blocked from reaching the cerebrum.

Finally, emotion can influence symptoms associated with neurological disease. Many people with epilepsy have more seizures during periods of emotional stress or even excitement. Those with cataplexy may have attacks during periods of stress or laughter. Because the neural substrates for emotion and regulatory function share the same brain areas, transmitter substances, and pathways, it is not surprising that aggravation of neurological symptoms occurs during times of emotional upheaval.

Interventions. The nurse should evaluate the relationship of a patient's emotional responses to the neurological illness. If certain emotional states precipitate the illness, the nurse should help the patient find ways to avoid them, or help the patient learn to recognize them as precipitating factors so that self-protection measures can be employed. For instance, if emotional excitement routinely precipitates an epileptic seizure, the patient may need to make sure he is accompanied by someone or is sitting or lying down during events that are likely to lead to that emotional state. If emotional lability or flat affect is a physiologically determined outcome of neurological illness, the nurse should communicate this to other care-givers and to the patient's family so that the patient's behavior is not perceived as a negative reaction to their interactions with him. Finally, if certain emotional responses are psychological reactions to neurological illness, the nurse may need to offer guidance and counseling to help the patient cope with his illness. See Chapter 3 for more information on coping with illness.

Evaluation

The patient's remaining abilities in autonomic regulation will be enhanced to promote the remaining functions in the activities of daily living.

Summary

Neurological disease affects a wide range of human functioning. For nursing purposes human functioning governed by the nervous system can be categorized into five major areas: consciousness, cognitive functioning, movement, sensation, and integrated autonomic regulation. The nurse needs to determine which aspects of these functions are affected and how they influence self-care and daily living. From these data she can develop and implement the patient care plan.

References

1. Agostoni E, Coletti A, Orlando G et al: Apraxia in deep cerebral lesions. J Neurol Neurosurg Psychiatry 46:804–808, 1983
2. American Parkinson Disease Association. Speech problems and swallowing problems in Parkinson's disease. February, 1983
3. Bear D: The significance of behavior change in temporal lobe epilepsy. McLean Hospital Journal 6:9–21, 1977
4. Booth K: The neglect syndrome. J Neurosurg Nurs 14(1):38–43, 1982
5. Brigman C, Dickey C, Zegeer LJ: The agitated, aggressive patient. Am J Nurs 83:1409–1412, 1983
6. Geschwind N: Specialization of the human brain. Sci Am 241(3):180–202, 1979
7. Geschwind N: The apraxias: Neural mechanisms of disorders of learned movement. American Scientist 63:181–195, 1975
8. Krane RJ, Siroky MB: Clinical Neurology, p 159. Boston, Little, Brown, Co, 1979
9. Larsen G: Chewing and swallowing. In Martin N, Holt NB, Hicks D (eds): Comprehensive Rehabilitation Nursing, pp 173–185. New York, McGraw-Hill, 1981
10. Mahoney EK: Alterations in cognitive functioning in the brain damaged patient. Nurs Clin North Am 15(2):283–292, 1980
11. Menikheim ML, Loen M: Impairments in verbal communication. In Snyder M (ed): A Guide to Neurological and Neurosurgical Nursing, pp 228–245. New York, John Wiley & Sons, 1983
12. Mitchell PH, Irvin NJ: Neurologic examination: Nursing assessment for nursing purposes. J Neurosurg Nurs 9:23–28, 1977
13. Mitchell PH, Cammermeyer M, Ozuna J, Woods NF: Neurologic Assessment for Nursing Practice. Reston VA, Reston Publishing Company, 1984
14. Nardelli E, Buonnano F, Coccia G et al: Prosopagnosia. Eur Neuro 21:289–297, 1982
15. Pflug AE, Aasheim GM, Foster C, Martin RW: Prevention of post-anesthesia shivering. Can Aanaesth Soc J 25(1):43–49, 1978
16. Plum F, Posner JW: The Diagnosis of Stupor and Coma. Philadelphia, FA Davis, 1980
17. Slater MC: Altered levels of consciousness: Impaired thought processes. In Snyder M (ed): A Guide to Neurological and Neurosurgical Nursing, pp 157–188. New York, John Wiley & Sons, 1983
18. Staas WE, DeNault PM: Bowel control. American Family Practitioner 7(1):90–100, 1973
19. Stein S, Volpe B: Classical "parietal" neglect syndrome after subcortical right frontal lobe infarction. Neurology 33:797–799, 1983
20. Strub RL, Black FW: The Mental Status Examination in Neurology. Philadelphia, FA Davis Company, 1977
21. Taylor S, Ballenger S: Neurologic Dysfunction and Nursing Interventions, pp 358–359. New York, McGraw-Hill, 1980
22. Trimble M: Personality disturbances in epilepsy. Neurology 33:1332–1334, 1983
23. Voris H: Craniocerebral trauma. In Baker AB, Baker LH (eds): Clinical Neurology, vol 2, p 12. Hagerstown, Harper & Row, 1975

Chapter 65

Seizures

Judy Hill Ozuna

A seizure is a physical manifestation of paroxysmal and abnormal electrical firing of neurons in the brain. The term *seizure disorder* may refer to any number of conditions that result in such a paroxysmal electrical discharge. These conditions could be metabolic or structural in nature. Epilepsy, however, is the medical term for the condition of having recurring seizures. The term epilepsy should not be used unless a person has a second seizure that occurs spontaneously and without an immediate preceding metabolic cause. Unfortunately, epilepsy is sometimes euphemistically referred to as a "seizure disorder" because for many people the word epilepsy has negative connotations. The avoidance of the medical term epilepsy is unfortunate because it perpetuates the social stigma against epilepsy and it causes patients great distress when they later learn that what they have is epilepsy.

Epilepsy

Most people with epilepsy are otherwise healthy. That is, between seizures they can function as any healthy person can. They are at risk for physical harm only during a seizure. Therefore, people with epilepsy often suffer less from the seizures themselves than from the psychosocial problems that accompany this "invisible" disorder. Their daily lives are affected a great deal because of still existing, albeit improving, negative attitudes about epilepsy. People who witness seizures in public are frequently frightened and draw away from the person or else they misinterpret the behavior as having a psychiatric origin. This in turn causes the epileptic person to withdraw from society. It can create a loss of self-esteem and an inability to cope. Another common psychosocial problem of people with epilepsy is difficulty in finding and keeping jobs.[24] Much of this is due to misconceptions on the part of the employers. Some of it is due to the individual's own inadequate social skills, which evolved from societal and family reactions to epilepsy. Another significant difficulty in the social arena is the restriction on driving an automobile. This makes it very difficult for epileptic persons to get to work, even if they do get a job. It also has a negative impact on their already restricted social and recreational activities. It is important for nurses to keep these potential problems in mind while caring for persons with epilepsy.

Epilepsy is a chronic disorder that requires antiepileptic drug therapy, usually throughout life. Consequently, compliance with medication therapy can be a problem, as can drug toxicity. Nurses need to be knowledgeable of the goals and principles of antiepileptic therapy, pharmacology, and pharmacokinetics and of strategies to improve compliance in order to assist patients in achieving improved seizure control.

Etiology

A seizure is generally a sign of underlying pathology involving the brain. It may be the first sign of nervous system disease (*e.g.,* brain tumor), or it may be a sign of a systemic or metabolic derangement. In a metabolic disturbance, the normal chemical environment of the brain is altered. This produces progressive irritation of the cerebral cortex, resulting in hyperexcitability of neurons and a lower seizure threshold. The hyperexcitable neurons begin to fire spontaneously in a non-normal fashion and this leads to the clinical seizure. Seizures resulting from systemic and metabolic disturbances are not considered epileptic if the seizures cease when the underlying problem is corrected. For example, a seizure that results from hypoglycemia and is controlled by an infusion of glucose would not be considered epileptic. The more common metabolic and systemic disturbances that can cause seizures are listed in Table 65–1.

In contrast to systemic and metabolic causes of seizures, structural brain damage and inherent "faulty wiring" of the brain circuitry (as seen in generalized absence epilepsy) cause recurring seizures that cannot be controlled except by chronic use of antiepileptic medication. There are many causes of structural brain damage such as head trauma, degenerative diseases (*e.g.,* Alzheimer's disease, Huntington's chorea, and multiple sclerosis), tumors, cerebral vascular disorders, and infection. Some of these disorders along with the percentage of cases that develop epilepsy are presented in Table 65–2.

Trauma. Trauma is one of the primary causes of cortical damage. People who develop recurring seizures from head injury are said to have post-traumatic epilepsy. The risk of developing post-traumatic epilepsy depends on the duration of unconsciousness, whether the dura was penetrated, the degree of direct cortical damage, and genetic predisposition to seizures.[5] Post-traumatic epilepsy usually begins within 2 years of the injury. For this reason antiepileptic therapy is often instituted as soon as possible for prophylaxis. (See Chapter 69, Neurological Trauma for more information on post-traumatic epilepsy.) It is believed that the higher incidence of epilepsy in firstborn children may also be due to trauma. The hypothesis is that as the baby passes through the semi-rigid pelvic cavity during delivery, the temporal lobes of the brain are pressed against the tentorium, resulting in hypoxic brain damage and subsequent scarring.[16] This damage may not be apparent at birth, and seizures resulting from this damage usually do not occur until after the child reaches school age. Specific causes of epilepsy cluster in certain age-groups,[1] as shown in Table 65–3.

Although many causes of epilepsy have been identified, three fourths of all epilepsy cannot be attributed to a specific cause and is termed idiopathic.

Heredity. The role of heredity in the etiology of epilepsy has been difficult to determine owing to the problems of separating genetic from environmental or acquired influence. Most authorities agree, however, that first-degree relatives of a person with epilepsy appear to have 2% to 5%

TABLE 65–1
Metabolic and Systemic Causes of Seizures

A. Electrolyte imbalance
   - Acidosis
   - Heavy metal poisoning
   - Hypocalcemia
   - Hypocapnea
   - Hypoglycemia
   - Hypoxia
   - Sodium–potasium imbalance
   - Systemic diseases (liver, renal failure, *etc.*)
   - Toxemia of pregnancy
   - Water intoxication

B. Infections
   - Meningitis
   - Encephalitis
   - Brain abscess

C. Withdrawal of sedative–hypnotic drugs
   - Alcohol
   - Antiepileptic drugs
   - Barbiturates
   - Benzodiazepines

D. Iatrogenic drug overdose
   - Theopylline
   - Penicillin

(Adapted from Ozuna J, Cammermeyer M: Epilepsy, A Course Syllabus for Independent Study. University of Washington, Seattle, 1983)

TABLE 65–2
Structural Causes of Seizures

	Cases that Develop Epilepsy (%)
Head trauma	7*
Degenerative diseases	
Alzheimer's	25–33
Creutzfeldt-Jakob	60
Huntington's chorea	3–16
Multiple sclerosis	8
Pick's disease	
Tumors	
Genetic diseases	
Cerebral vascular disorders	20
Infections	17–34
Encephalitis	
Meningitis	
Brain abscess	
Febrile seizures	5

* Incidence varies with type of head injury.
(Ozuna J, Cammermeyer M: Epilepsy, A Course Syllabus for Independent Study. University of Washington, Seattle, 1983)

TABLE 65–3
Causes of Recurrent Seizures in Different Age Groups

Age of Onset (Years)	*Probable Cause*
Infancy, 0–2	Congenital maldevelopment, birth injury, metabolic disorders (*e.g.*, hypocalcemia, hypoglycemia), vitamin B_6 deficiency, phenylketonuria, and others
Childhood, 2–10	Perinatal anoxia, injury at birth or later, infections, thrombosis of cerebral arteries or veins, or indeterminate cause (idiopathic epilepsy)
Adolescence, 10–18	Idiopathic epilepsy, trauma, or congenital defects
Early adulthood, 18–25	Idiopathic epilepsy, trauma, neoplasm, or withdrawal from alcohol or other sedative–hyponotic drugs
Middle age, 35–60	Trauma, neoplasm, vascular disease, or alcohol or drug withdrawal.
Late life, over 60	Vascular disease, neoplasm, or degenerative disease

(Adams RA, Victor M: Principles of Neurology. New York, McGraw-Hill, 1981, p. 225)

risk for also having epilepsy. This risk decreases with increasing genetic distance, and increases with increasing number of affected family members.[13] Typical absence or classic petit mal epilepsy tends to have the strongest hereditary component, with the risk to first-degree relatives possibly being as high as 8%.[25] In addition, there are several single genetic disorders that cause epilepsy and there is also evidence that some families carry a predisposition for epilepsy in the form of an inherently low threshold to seizure-producing stimuli such as trauma, disease, or fever.[13]

Febrile seizures, for instance, tend to occur in certain families. They occur in about 5% of children under the age of 5. They are tonic/clonic convulsions that accompany fever, although the fever may not be very high. Febrile seizures do not carry a great risk for the development of epilepsy, since only 2% to 6% of children with febrile convulsions subsequently developed epilepsy.[13] The risk depends on the aspects of the seizure itself and the status of the child prior to the onset of febrile seizures.[11]

Precipitating Factors. There are factors that increase the likelihood of seizures in some people with epilepsy. These are called precipitating factors. It is probable that these factors somehow lower the seizure threshold although the actual mechanism is unknown. In fact, there may be more than one mechanism, because the nature of the factors is so variable. There is no doubt that certain physical and psychological factors provoke seizures in susceptible people. These factors will vary from person to person, but they are consistent within the same person. Common precipitating factors are emotional stress, fatigue, loss of sleep, menstrual periods, fever, and other illness. In some cases specific sensory stimuli (*e.g.*, startling noises, music, light flashes) and specific activities (*e.g.*, eating, reading, mental arithmetic) precipitate seizures. However, the most important common precipitating factor is failure to take medication as prescribed, or noncompliance.[17]

Prevalence. Between 0.5% and 2% of the population, or from 1 million to 4 million people in the United States have epilepsy. The onset of epilepsy occurs before the age of 20 years in 80% of cases. Accurate figures of the prevalence of epilepsy are difficult to obtain for two reasons. The first is variability in making a diagnosis of epilepsy in people who have recurring seizures from febrile illness, recurring electrolyte imbalance, multiple infectious processes, or brain tumors, to name a few. An example of this is the person who at one time had seizures due to a brain tumor but no longer has them since the tumor was removed. Is he considered epileptic because he is still taking epileptic medication prophylactically? The second reason is that for a wide variety of reasons many persons with epilepsy do not report their seizures. They may wish to avoid the social stigma, to maintain their driver's license, to avoid job discrimination, or simply to maintain privacy.

A seizure is only a symptom of a complex physiological event within the brain. Seizures may result from metabolic imbalance, in which case they are reversible and preventable. These seizures are not epileptic. Recurring seizures that result from structural damage or inherent faulty wiring are referred to as epileptic seizures and are treated with antiepileptic medication.

Pathophysiology

Seizures are the result of paroxysmal excessive hypersynchronous discharge of neurons. This means that seizures arise only from gray matter and not from white matter of the brain. Recall that gray matter contains nerve cell bodies and white matter contains fiber tracks or the axons of the nerve cells. Because nerve cells are excitable cells, any disturbance that creates the likelihood for increased firing can lead to a seizure. Epileptic neurons can recruit adjacent neurons to fire abnormally also. The direction of the spread of the epileptic activity is dependent on cellular mechanisms that determine pathways of least resistance. An example of this anatomical spread is the Jacksonian seizure, in which there are clonic movements that may begin in the face and then spread to involve the arm and then the leg of the same side.

At times epileptic neurons may fire abnormally and not recruit adjacent neurons. This may result in what is called ***interictal discharges,*** that is, discharges that occur between the actual seizures. A clinical seizure will not occur until enough neurons are firing abnormally and for a long enough period of time, usually more than 5 seconds. This concept is important in discussing the diagnosis of epilepsy. The electroencephalogram (EEG) is useful in diagnosing epilepsy even though the patient may not have the seizure during the recording. If interictal epileptiform discharges appear, the diagnosis of epilepsy may be made.

There are several experimental models that have been developed to study the mechanisms of epilepsy. They will not be discussed in great detail here, and it is still not clear exactly which mechanisms are present in patients with epilepsy. There is evidence of a disturbance in the excitatory and inhibitory synapses impinging on the epileptic neuron.[25] There is also indication of different degrees of epileptic neurons within the epileptic focus. The most severely epileptic nerve cells can stimulate the next level of epileptic nerve cells and thereby generate a seizure by recruiting the adjacent neurons.[28]

In addition, several chemical and structural alterations have been observed, both within the epileptic focus and outside it, and they have provided evidence of possible mechanisms for epileptic activity.[18] One is the loss of inhibitory neurons (usually from hypoxia) in the cerebellum, neocortex, and certain other structures in the cerebrum. Loss of this inhibitory influence leads to seizures in many experimental situations. Another alteration is the loss of spines on the dendrites of neurons in the epileptic focus, which may be a reason for their hyperexcitability.[14] It is common to see proliferation of fibrous astrocytes (glial scarring) in the epileptic focus, although the exact role this may play in generating seizures is still not clear.[18] Alteration in enzymes and neurotransmitter substances within the brain may also play a part in epileptic activity.[18]

The phenomenon of "kindling" is an important aspect of epilepsy pathogenesis. It appears that repetitive electrical discharges from an epileptic focus can reproduce or "kindle" long-lasting and possibly permanent changes in neuronal excitability, both locally and in distant areas of the brain.[20] This presents an interesting and important implication for human epilepsy: seizures can beget more seizures. Clinical experience indicates that the longer seizures go without control, the less likely they are to be controlled. Therefore, a vigorous attempt must be made to control epilepsy in the early stages.

Classification of Epileptic Seizures

Epileptic seizures are currently classified according to the International Classification of Epileptic Seizures, originally developed in 1970[12] and revised in 1981.[7] This system classifies seizures according to their clinical manifestations and their electroencephalographic correlates. The system permits more specific definition of seizure types, enhances determination of appropriate drug treatment, and increases knowledge of the effectiveness of treatment and the prognosis of each seizure type. In the past, seizures were divided into *grand mal* and *petit mal.* Whereas grand mal was used to describe a generalized tonic-clonic convulsion, petit mal was used to name any seizure that was not a convulsion. As can be seen in Table 65–4, these terms are very inadequate because there are, in fact, many more types of seizures. Use

TABLE 65–4
International Classification of Epileptic Seizures

I. Partial seizures (seizures beginning locally)
  A. Simple partial seizures (consciousness not impaired)
    1. With motor symptoms
    2. With somatosensory or special sensory symptoms
    3. With autonomic symptoms
    4. With psychic symptoms
  B. Complex partial seizures (with impairment of consciousness)
    1. Beginning as simple partial seizures and progressing to impairment of consciousness
      a. With no other features
      b. With features as in A, 1–4
      c. With automatisms
    2. With impairment of consciousness at onset
      a. With no other features
      b. With features as in A, 1–4
      c. With automatisms

II. Generalized seizures (bilaterally symmetrical and without local onset)
  A. Absence seizures
    1. Typical
    2. Atypical
  B. Myoclonic seizures
  C. Clonic seizures
  D. Tonic seizures
  E. Tonic/clonic seizures
  F. Atonic seizures

III. Unclassified epileptic seizures (inadequate or incomplete data)

(Abstracted from Commission on Classification and Terminology of the International League Against Epilepsy. Proposal for Revised Clinical and Electroencephalographic Classification of Epileptic Seizures. Epilepsia 22:489–501, 1981)

of the former labels can cause confusion both for lay and professional people.

The International Classification lists two major categories: (1) partial and (2) generalized seizures. The specific types of seizures under each category are listed in Table 65–4.

Partial Seizures

Partial seizures are the most common form of epilepsy, occurring in about 67% of all adult patients with epilepsy and in about 40% of all children with epilepsy.[9] Partial seizures originate from a specific focus or scar in the cerebral cortex. The location of the focus determines the clinical presentation of the seizure; for instance, if the discharging focus is located in the motor cortex in the right cerebral hemisphere where hand movements originate, twitching of the left hand may occur. Other sensory, motor, cognitive or emotional phenomena may occur if the discharging focus is located in the part of the brain that governs that particular function. The clinical manifestation of a partial seizure can involve any of the functions of the brain, of which there are many. Partial seizures are further divided into simple partial and complex partial seizures, as indicated in Table 65–4. The major distinction between these two types is that consciousness is not impaired in simple partial seizures and it is impaired in complex partial seizures

Clinical Manifestations. Clinical manifestations of *simple partial seizures* include stiffening or jerking of a limb on one side of the face, head turning or eye deviation (motor symptoms), tingling sensations in a body part (somatosensory symptoms), ringing in the ears or visual distortions (special sensory symptoms), "butterflies" in the stomach, or respiratory and cardiac changes (autonomic symptoms), and a feeling of *deja vu* or forced thinking (psychic symptoms).

Complex partial seizures, as their name implies, can involve a variety of behavioral, emotional, affective, and cognitive functions in addition to alteration of consciousness. Although the location of the discharging focus is often in the temporal lobe, hence the term *temporal lobe seizure,* complex partial seizures can also arise from other parts of the brain, often from the frontal lobes. They usually last longer than 1 minute and are frequently followed by a period of postictal confusion.

The most common manifestations of complex partial seizures are lip smacking and automatisms. They are sometimes called psychomotor seizures. A person may continue an activity that was initiated before the seizure began, such as counting out change or picking up items from a grocery shelf, but after the seizure the person does not remember the activity performed during the seizure. Other automatisms are less organized, such as picking at clothing, fumbling with objects (real or imaginary), or simply walking away. Many say that they can hear someone call to them during their seizure, but they cannot respond verbally or physically to commands. If they do speak, it is gibberish or mumbling. If someone tries to restrain them during a seizure, they can become combative or agitated. They are not malicious, nor are they directing their aggression to any person. It is as if their brains are driving them to execute a behavior and if someone tries to prevent them from doing so, they resist to the point of becoming aggressive. Individuals who exhibit this behavior during a seizure are often misunderstood and sometimes erroneously committed to psychiatric or corrective institutions.

Sometimes the sole manifestation of a complex partial seizure may be clouding of consciousness or a confused state without any motor or sensory components. This type of seizure should be distinguished from a generalized absence (petit mal) seizure because the preferred drug treatment for the two disorders differs. A complex partial seizure usually lasts longer (several seconds to 1 or 2 minutes), and full consciousness returns slowly rather than abruptly when the seizure is over. Figure 65–1 shows the EEG of a person having a complex partial seizure.

If the electrical discharge from an epileptic focus remains confined to a limited area, the seizure will remain focal or partial in nature. In some cases, however, the electrical activity spreads to involve the entire brain, culminating in a generalized tonic/clonic seizure. The seizure is then said to be a *secondarily generalized* seizure. Any tonic/clonic seizure that is preceded by an aura or warning (sensory phenomenon) or unilateral motor activity is a partial seizure that becomes secondarily generalized. Many tonic/clonic seizures that appear to be generalized from the onset may actually be secondarily generalized seizures, but the preceding partial component may be so brief that it is undetected by the patient, the observer, or even the EEG. Unlike a primary generalized tonic/clonic seizure, the secondarily generalized seizure may result in temporary paralysis of a body part. This is called Todd's paralysis and it always resolves after varying lengths of time, usually within 24 hours.[6]

Generalized Seizures

The clinical onset of a generalized seizure is immediate. There is no warning that the seizure is beginning. The EEG shows diffuse abnormal electrical discharge involving both cerebral hemispheres without any evidence of focal onset. The clinical manifestations of the seizure will vary with the type of generalized seizure. Almost all primary generalized epilepsies are genetically transmitted and almost all genetically determined epilepsies are expressed as primary generalized seizures. [9] About 20% of adults and children with epilepsy have primary generalized seizures.[9]

Tonic/Clonic (Grand Mal) Seizures. The most common generalized seizure is the tonic/clonic or grand mal seizure. This seizure is characterized by sudden loss of consciousness, often with a cry, followed by stiffening of the body for several seconds (tonic phase) and subsequent jerking of the extremities (clonic phase). The seizure lasts only 1 to 2 minutes. During the tonic phase, the person's jaws clamp shut and respirations cease. This can cause cyanosis suggesting that the person is in acute respiratory distress, but this is short-lived and respirations usually resume within several seconds. The seizure often terminates with a very loud sigh. This is followed usually by a period of very deep sleep, which may last a few minutes to several hours.

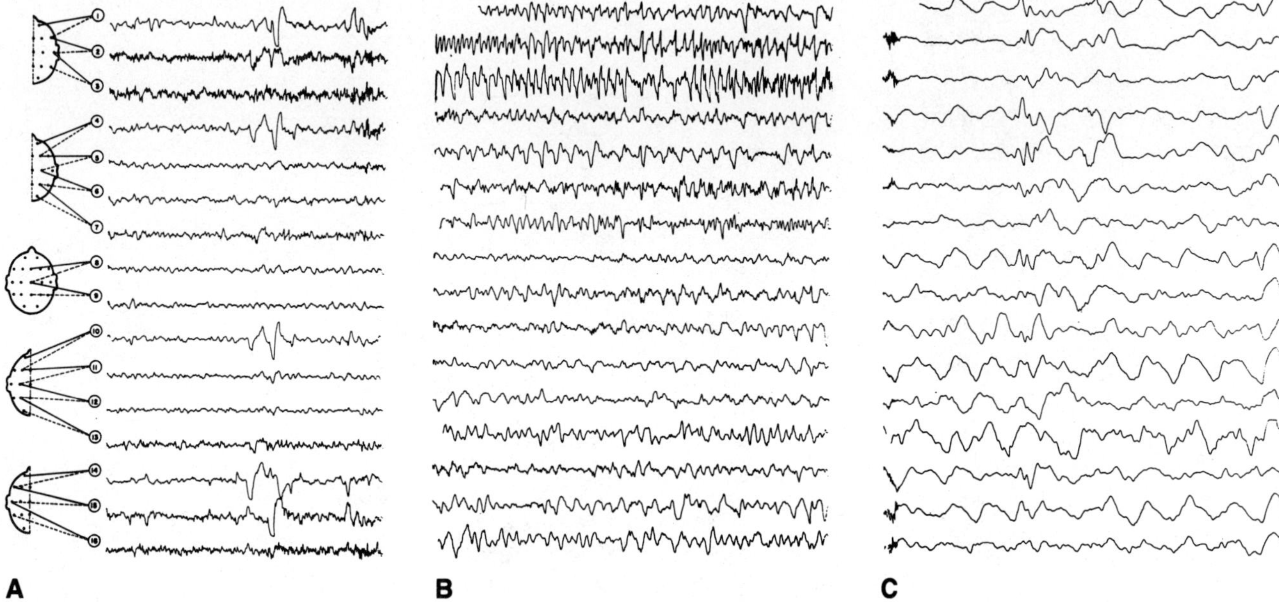

FIGURE 65–1 (*A*) EEG showing preictal sample of essentially normal brain wave activity in a patient with partial complex seizures. (*B*) EEG during partial complex seizure. Rhythmic sharp waves and fast activity are evident in the right frontotemporal area. The patient is exhibiting automatisms. (*C*) EEG showing postictal phase of complex partial seizure. There is generalized slowing of brain wave activity and voltage suppression on the right. (Courtesy of Robert Wilkus, MD, Regional Epilepsy Center, University of Washington, Seattle)

People may not feel "normal" for several hours after that and sometimes for even days. The person may complain of very sore muscles after the seizure. This is often a clue that a tonic/clonic seizure has occurred in a person whose seizure may not have been witnessed. Although tongue biting and incontinence are frequently associated with tonic/clonic seizures, they may not occur and their presence is not a requirement for the seizure to be classified as tonic/clonic.

During the seizure, the EEG shows rhythmic discharges of 10 cps or more, decreasing in frequency and increasing in amplitude during the tonic phase. This pattern is interrupted by slow waves during the clonic phase with a spike and wave pattern followed by postictal depression and slowing.[25] Figure 65–2 shows the EEG of a person having a generalized tonic/clonic seizure.

Absence (Petit Mal) Seizures. Absence seizures are further subdivided into *typical* and *atypical* absence. *Typical absence,* also known as classic or pure petit mal, is a specific seizure type and it should not be confused with other non–tonic/clonic seizures. Typical absences occur in 4% of all patients with epilepsy.[9] Typical absences are manifested by brief loss of contact with the environment and a blank stare lasting only a few seconds, followed by abrupt return to consciousness. There may be blinking of the eyelids, or simple automatisms (*e.g.,* chewing, lip smacking) or mild body movements. In addition, the EEG shows typical, bilaterally synchronous and symmetric 3 cps spike-and-wave activity.

The onset of typical absence or petit mal seizures usually occurs in childhood. In many cases these seizures cease when the person reaches adulthood. However, if typical absences are accompanied by generalized tonic/clonic spells, the prognosis is less favorable. Although the absence spells may decrease or cease, the tonic/clonic spells will often persist. Only 5% to 25% of pure absence (not combined with tonic/clonic) seizures return within 5 years after drug withdrawal, but 65% of absence combined with tonic/clonic seizures return within 5 years after cessation of treatment.[9]

Atypical absence seizures clinically resemble true petit mal seizures. The primary difference between typical and atypical absence seizures is based on the EEG and the age of the person. During the atypical seizure the spike-and-wave activity is present but the frequency varies from 2 cps to 4 cps. Atypical seizures may occur either in children or adults. Figure 65–3 is an EEG showing a generalized interictal epileptiform discharge in an adult male with atypical absence seizures.

Myoclonic and Atonic Seizures. Other generalized seizures include myoclonic and atonic seizures. A myoclonic seizure is characterized by sudden excessive jerk of the body or extremities. These seizures are very brief and may occur in clusters. The EEG shows generalized burst discharges that correlate with muscle activity. Atonic seizures were formerly called drop attacks or falling spells. They were also called akinetic seizures. They involve sudden loss of muscle tone, usually causing the person to fall to the ground. However, the person is conscious by the time he hits the ground and is usually able to assume normal activity immediately. Because

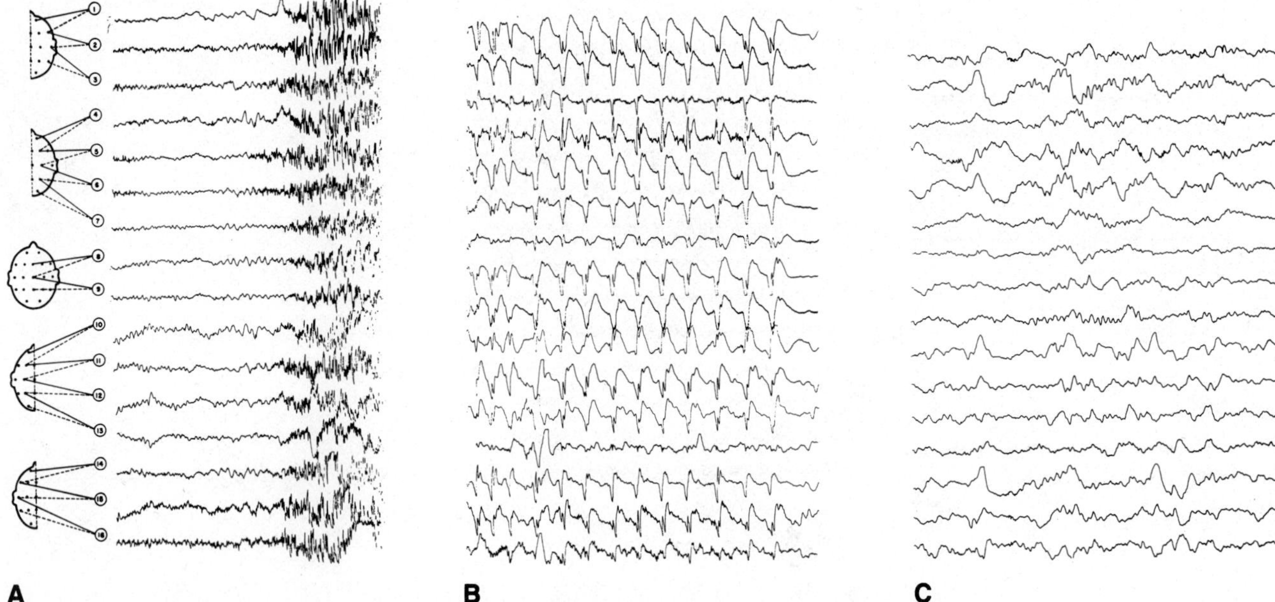

FIGURE 65–2 (*A*) EEG showing onset of generalized tonic–clonic seizures, of the tonic phase. Brain activity becomes obscured by electrical activity from scalp muscles (EMG activity) as the patient stiffens. (*B*) EGG showing clonic phase of tonic–clonic seizure. Abnormal spike and wave discharges are seen in all leads. (*C*) EEG showing postictal phase of tonic–clonic seizure. There is generalized slowing of brain activity. The patient is comatose. (Courtesy of Robert Wilkus, MD, Regional Epilepsy Center, University of Washington, Seattle)

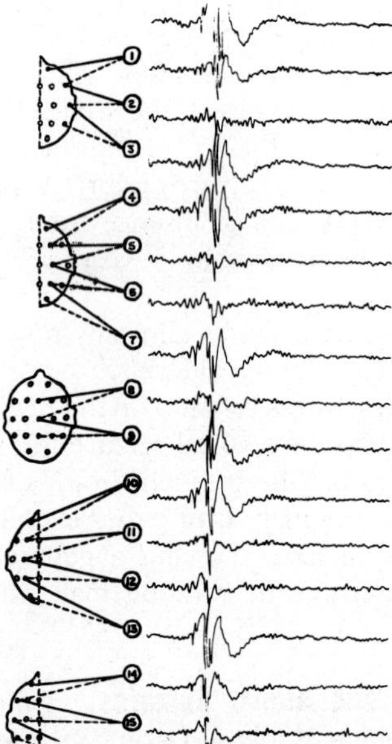

FIGURE 65–3 EEG showing a generalized interictal epileptiform discharge in a man with atypical absence seizures. (Courtesy of Veterans Administration Medical Center, Seattle, Washington)

persons with this type of seizure often hit their faces and heads, they may need to wear protective helmets. The EEG pattern may show polyspikes and waves or flattening or low voltage fast activity.

Status Epilepticus

Status epilepticus (SE) is defined in many ways, but most definitions include a statement that SE involves seizure activity lasting for at least 30 minutes.[15] This term is often interpreted to include persons who do not regain consciousness between successive seizures. There are as many kinds of SE as there are types of seizures.This condition is harmful to the nerve cells of the brain, and it can lead to neuronal death. Generalized tonic/clonic status epilepticus is the most life threatening of the common forms of SE and will be the focus of the following discussion.

Causes and Prognosis. A review by Lovely and Ozuna of some patient series indicated that over half of all cases of SE are due to symptomatic causes.[15] In adults, these included cerebral tumors, cerebral vascular disease, infection, head trauma, metabolic disorders, and drug abuse (alcohol and barbiturates). In studies of children only, cryptogenic causes accounted for over one half of the cases of SE before the age of 15 years. The symptomatic causes of SE that were most common in children were acute brain injury (*e.g.,* meningitis, encephalitis, subdural hematoma, dehydration and electrolyte disorders, anoxic injury, and exogenous toxins) and chronic encephalopathy (*e.g.,* birth injury, progressive and nonprogressive encephalopathy, and congenital brain defects).

The overall mortality rate associated with SE is as high as 20%, with the rate increasing as the duration of SE increases. Death may be due to SE itself or to the underlying pathology.

Patients with underlying pathology often respond poorly to conventional treatment. Tonic/clonic SE, which is present in only 1% to 5% of all patients with a history of epilepsy, accounts for one third of all epilepsy-related deaths.[3] The most common cause of SE in epileptic patients is noncompliance. Morbidity, the incidence of neurological sequelae after SE, is 12% to 37%.[15] The morbidity rate is highest among infants and decreases successively with age. The vulnerability of the immature brain has been substantiated by experimental studies in young rats and by clinical studies of children. Seizures producing brain damage in adults usually exceed 6 hours duration; in infants and small children damage can follow seizures lasting only 1 to 2 hours.[19]

Management. SE, especially of the tonic/clonic type, is a medical emergency. The nurse may be responsible for initiating several actions when a patient is admitted in status epilepticus. First of all, respiratory and ECG monitoring is required. An intravenous line should be started for administration of fluid and drugs. This line can also be used later for obtaining blood samples as needed. Blood is usually taken to screen for possible causes of SE. This includes analysis of glucose, electrolytes, blood urea nitrogen, and toxic substance levels. Blood cultures might also be taken if sepsis is suspected. Complete blood count is often done as well. If SE does not respond readily to treatment, a urinary catheter should be inserted. Urine may be monitored for volume, myoglobulinemia, and sepsis and toxicity screening. A nasogastric tube is inserted to prevent aspiration of vomitus or secretions.

The seizure itself must be carefully observed because it can give valuable clues to the diagnosis of the type and cause of SE. Seizure observation will be discussed later under Nursing Management. General neurological functions should be assessed and monitored throughout the episode of SE. This includes monitoring of the level of consciousness, particularly between attacks, pupil size equality and reactivity, and gross motor and sensory function. The person with SE must also be observed for the presence of head trauma, bruises, and/or fractures of the body and limbs, and for needle marks. The last sign may indicate drug abuse as the cause of SE.

The usual drug treatment for SE is an initial dose of intravenous diazepam (Valium) or lorazepam (Ativan). Because these drugs are short-acting, they need to be followed with a longer acting antiepileptic medication, usually phenytoin (Dilantin) or phenobarbital. The nurse should be aware of the side-effects of these medications and monitor the patient for presence of the side-effects during the course of treatment.

Diagnosis

History

The history is the most valuable component of the workup for a person with possible epilepsy. The nurse can be very helpful in this portion of the diagnostic workup by obtaining a complete description of the seizure activity, either from a family member or someone who has witnessed the seizure. Often the patient cannot describe the seizure because he is not conscious during the spell. Details about the seizure should include any precipitating factors, the presence or absence of a warning and the nature of the warning, the seizure activity, the postictal experience of the patient, and the frequency of the seizures. Other aspects of the patient's history should include the age at onset, the perinatal history including growth and development and the birth history, the presence or absence of febrile seizures, any family history of epilepsy, any prior treatment, and any illnesses or injuries that might be a cause for epilepsy.

Lab Studies/EEG

Laboratory studies are done to rule out various causes for seizures. Routine blood and urine studies are often done for baseline information. Electrolytes and blood chemistries will be evaluated to identify possible metabolic causes for seizures. Other tests will be done to identify intracranial pathology. These include CT scan, cerebral angiography, and lumbar puncture as indicated.

The *EEG* is the major diagnostic test in the workup of a person with seizures. Even though the patient may not have a seizure during the recording of the EEG, the presence of interictal epileptiform discharges will help confirm the diagnosis. However, epileptic patients do not always exhibit interictal discharges during brain wave testing. The EEG takes only a short sample of brain wave activity, since the test lasts only 30 to 90 minutes. Therefore, negative results do not rule out epilepsy. Repeated EEGs increase the likelihood of getting positive results. On the other hand, certain epileptiform discharges may fail to produce changes detectable in the scalp recording.

Routine scalp EEGs record only amplified brain waves from the superficial regions of the brain by means of scalp electrodes, so that discharges occurring deep within the brain may be covered by other activity before they reach the scalp. Sometimes special electrode leads are used to record from structures beneath the surface of the brain. These include nasopharyngeal leads, which are placed up the nose; sphenoidal leads, which are placed percutaneously beneath the sphenoid region of the skull; depth electrodes, which are planted directly into brain tissue; and cortical strip electrodes, which are placed subdurally over the surface of the brain.

Neuropsychological testing may be done in the evaluation of persons presenting with seizures. The purpose of neuropsychological testing is to determine if there is brain dysfunction and to determine if the pattern of change in brain function is indicative of a destructive lesion. Neuropsychological testing involves evaluation of cognitive functions and personality and emotional traits.

Medical Management

Pharmacotherapy

The major medical treatment for epilepsy is antiepileptic medication. Epileptic seizures can be controlled in 50% to 95% of cases with this form of treatment depending on seizure type.[9] The choice of antiepileptic drug depends on the seizure type, the side-effects of the medication, and the preference of the patient. Some patients may choose a drug that is cheaper even though the efficacy may not be as good as one that is more expensive. Others decide that they do not like the secondary side-effects, for instance, gum hypertrophy and excess growth of facial hair associated with phenytoin use.

The principles of antiepileptic therapy are similar to those of other medications that are taken chronically. A single drug is usually tried first. The dose of the drug is usually pushed either to the point of controlling seizures or to the point of producing toxic side-effects. The goal of therapy is to obtain maximum control of seizures with minimal side-effects.

If a single first-line drug is not effective, it will be tapered and stopped while a second first-line drug is added. If a single drug does not appear to work effectively, a combination of drugs may then be tried. Serum drug level determinations are frequently made in order to determine if the dose of drug is enough to achieve a therapeutic level, that is, one that will control seizures. In general, levels below the therapeutic range are likely not to control seizures and levels above the range are likely to cause toxic side-effects. The drug half-life is the major determinant of the dosing interval. Drugs with a long half-life do not need to be taken as frequently as drugs with a short half-life.

Table 65–5 lists each major antiepileptic drug, the seizure types that each is effective in controlling, the drug half-life, the therapeutic serum level range, the common side-effects, and known drug interactions.

Side-Effects. The side-effects of antiepileptic medication can be classified into two categories. Dose related side-effects involve the central nervous system. They usually include disturbances in coordination and in mental functioning. Idiosyncratic allergic and metabolic side-effects are in the second category. They usually affect organs outside the central nervous system. These include liver toxicity, bone marrow suppression, skin rash, gingival hyperplasia, and folic acid deficiency.

Assessment for dose related side-effects of antiepileptic medication can be evaluated by the nurse. The eyes are tested for nystagmus. Although nystagmus is a pathological sign in other disorders, nystagmus without diplopia in the epileptic person is nothing more than evidence of presence

TABLE 65–5
Antiepileptic Drugs

Drug	*Type of Seizure*	*Adult Dose & Half-Life*	*Therapeutic Serum Level*	*Side-Effects Precautions*	*Drug Interactions*
Phenytoin Dilantin 50 mg tabs and 100 mg caps	Generalized—tonic/clonic, not for absence type (will make worse); partial focal	200–600 mg dose in single or split dose 5–8 mg/kg/day Half-life 7–22 hr	10–25 mcg/ml	Ataxia, diplopia, nystagmus, dysarthria, gingival hyperplasia, hirsutism, fetal abnormalities, peripheral neuropathy (yearly folate and B_{12} levels)	With benzodiazepines, bishydroxycoumarin, chloramphenicol, disulfiram, ethosuximide, isoniazid, methylphenidate HCL, phenothiazines, phenylbutazone, salicylic acid, cimetidine—↑ serum level of phenytoin With phenobarbital, carbamazepine, clonazepam, dexamethasone, digoxin, ethanol—↓ serum level of phenytoin With digoxin, bishydroxycoumarin, metyrapone—↓ in digoxin, hydroxycoumarin, and metyrapone levels With folate, can result in ↓ half-life of phenytoin With valproic acid can lead to ↑ free phenytoin level

(Continued)

TABLE 65–5
Antiepileptic Drugs *(Continued)*

Drug	*Type of Seizure*	*Adult Dose & Half-Life*	*Therapeutic Serum Level*	*Side-Effects Precautions*	*Drug Interactions*
Phenobarbital 15, 30, 60, 100 mg tabs	Generalized—tonic/clonic partial focal	60–200 mg/day in single or split dose half-life 96 hr	10–30 mcg/ml	Drowsiness, loss of libido, loss of mental alacrity, depression, irritability in children; may lead to withdrawal seizures if withdrawn too rapidly	With phenothiazine—can cause sedation and ↑ metabolism of phenothiazide leading to CNS depression With diazepam can cause ↓ BP and pulse and ↓ phenobarbital level With phenylbutazone can cause ↑ metabolism of phenylbutazone With phenytoin can lead to ↓ phenytoin level and ↓ phenobarbital level and half-life With bishydroxycoumarin leads to ↑ bleeding time if phenobarbital stopped With clonazepam leads to ↓ phenobarbital level With valproic acid leads to ↑ phenobarbital level
Primidone Mysoline 50 and 250 mg tabs; 100 mg chewable tabs	Generalized—tonic/clonic Partial focal	250–750 mg/day Half-life: primidone 3–12 hr; phenobarbital metabolite 48–144 hr	Primidone, 6–12 mcg/ml Phenobarbital, 10–30 mcg/ml	Ataxia, drowsiness, depression; may lead to withdrawal seizures if withdrawn too rapidly	With isoniazid can cause ↑ serum primidone level With phenytoin, carbamazapine can ↑ conversion to phenobarbital
Carbamazepine (CBZ) Tegretol 200 mg tabs	Generalized—tonic/clonic Partial focal	600–1800 mg/day Half-life: initially, 12–30 hr; chronic, 7–12 hr	6–12 mcg/ml	Nystagmus, nausea and vomiting, rash, edema, dizziness, blood dyscrasias (monthly CBC, platelet count)	With phenytoin can cause ↓ CBZ level With propoxyphene ↑ CBZ level
Valproic acid Depakene 250 mg caps Depakote 250, 500 mg tabs	Generalized—tonic/clonic, typical and atypical absence, atonic, myoclonic Partial focal that are refractory	1500–3000 mg/day Half-life 9–13 hr	50–100 mcg/ml	Ataxia, drowsiness, nausea, tremor, temporary alopecia, decreased liver function (SGOT and periodic follow-up)	With phenobarbital can cause ↑ phenobarbital level With phenytoin can cause ↑ free phenytoin level

(*Continued*)

TABLE 65-5
Antiepileptic Drugs (*Continued*)

Drug	*Type of Seizure*	*Adult Dose & Half-Life*	*Therapeutic Serum Level*	*Side-Effects Precautions*	*Drug Interactions*
Ethosuximide Zarontin 250 mg caps	Generalized—typical and atypical absence	1000–2000 mg/day Half-life 24–72 hr	40–100 mcg/ml	Drowsiness, dizziness, nausea and vomiting, headache, rash	
Clonazepam Clonopin 5, 1, 2 mg tabs	Generalized—typical and atypical absence attacks (when not responsive to ethosuximide), atonic, myoclonic	2–8 mg/day in split dose Half-life 18–50 hr	.013–.072 mcg/ml	Drowsiness, ataxia, behavioral changes, hypersalivation, increased bronchial secretions; may lead to withdrawal seizures if withdrawn too rapidly	With valproic acid may cause absence attacks
Methsuximide Celontin 150, 300 mg caps	Generalized—typical and atyptical absence attacks that are refractory Partial focal that are refractory Partial focal that are refractory	300–1200 mg dose		Drowsiness, dizziness, ataxia, nausea, rash, blood dyscrasias (check CBC)	With phenytoin can cause increase in tonic/clonic seizures With phenytoin ↑ phenytoin level With phenobarbital ↓ phenobarbital level

(Ozuna J, Cammermeyer M: Epilepsy, A Course Syllabus for Independent Study. Department of Physiological Nursing, University of Washington, 1983)

of the antiepileptic medication. If the patient complains of double vision or difficulty in seeing, he may be experiencing some toxicity. Coordination is tested by finger-to-nose movement and tandem walking. Other tests include examination of gait and the Romberg sign (ability to maintain an upright posture with the eyes closed and feet together). Patients experiencing dose-related toxicity often complain of feeling "drunk." One should be aware that complaints of mental dulling are a subjective sign of drug toxicity. A general rule is that drug dosages should not be changed unless the side-effects are interfering with daily living, or unless the seizures are not controlled.

Surgical Treatment

In some patients who have intractable seizures, surgical removal of the epileptic focus may be possible. To be considered a candidate for this type of surgery, very strict criteria must be met. First, there must be evidence that seizures cannot be controlled in spite of trials of several drugs. Second, the epileptic focus must be identifiable and localized. Third, the focus must be in an area of the brain that will not leave an unacceptable neurological deficit such as paralysis or aphasia if it is excised. Complex partial seizures are the most common seizure treated by surgery. The focus of this seizure type is often found in the anterior temporal and/or inferior frontal regions of the cortex. Fortunately, both of these areas can be excised without causing neurological deficit.

The operative risks are less than average. Mortality risk is less than 1%. Morbidity risk is about 2% due to hemorrhage and infection.[21] Most of the centers that perform cortical resection surgery yield the same outcome data; of those who meet the criteria and have the operation, 30% to 40% will become seizure free at least for several years, another 30% to 40% will obtain a significant decrease in their seizure frequency, and about 20% will experience no change in seizure frequency. Therefore, the success of surgery in controlling seizures is quite good. However, the outcome in terms of psychosocial adjustment does not always correlate with seizure control. One study found that reduction of seizures after surgery did not improve employment status in those who were unemployed prior to surgery.[2] This may mean that evaluation of psychosocial status is just as important as evaluation of the seizure focus in the workup for epilepsy surgery.

Other types of surgery are used in severely intractable epilepsy and are performed in only rare cases. Stereotactic surgery may be used to obliterate deep epileptic foci. Section of the corpus callosum may be done as a last resort to prevent intractable multifocal partial seizures from secondarily generalizing into frequent tonic/clonic seizures. Hemispherectomy (complete removal of cortex in one hemisphere) may also be done for intractable multifocal epilepsy, localized to one, usually already severely damaged hemisphere.

Other Treatments

Other innovative therapies for management of intractable seizures have been developed, but their efficacy has not been proven. This includes a form of *operant conditioning* that involves training the person to generate a certain type of brain wave frequency that is known to be resistant to the development of seizures.[26,27] The other is *cerebellar stimulation,* which involves application of electrical current to the cerebellum, thereby stimulating the inhibitory influences of the cerebellum on to the cortical structures in order to prevent seizure activity.[8] This method is still highly controversial.

Nursing Management

This section will be divided into two parts. The first part will address nursing management of patients during a seizure. The second part will focus on the long-term implications of epilepsy and the nursing management that pertains to them.

Care During Seizures

The care of a patient during a seizure should focus primarily on maintaining a safe environment. The seizure that has the greatest risk for causing injury and even fatality is the generalized tonic/clonic seizure, although there is potential for injury with any seizure that involves alteration of consciousness. The two major goals for nursing care during a seizure are protection from injury and prevention of aspiration. In most cases the nurse will not be present at the onset of the seizure, so that it will not be possible to put an oral airway or padded tongue blade between the person's teeth. Once the tonic phase begins, the jaws clamp shut and no amount of human force can open them.

Side rails should be raised at all times for the patients who are in bed and who are at risk for having seizures. If a seizure does happen and the patient is not in bed, the nurse should remove furniture and other hard objects from the area. The person's head should be cradled if he is on the floor so that he does not bang his head. No attempt should be made to restrain the person. The patient should be turned to his side to allow the tongue to fall away from the airway and allow drainage of the excessive saliva that accumulates during the seizure. The nurse should remain with the patient until he regains consciousness. Nursing Care Plan for the Patient with Tonic/Clonic Seizures details the management of this type of seizure patient (see p 885).

Patients having complex partial seizures pose a different risk. Although they may not fall and hurt themselves, they may wander off or move into dangerous areas. Nurses should follow the patient but not try to restrain him. The nurse should calmly try to coax the patient back to his room. She should not forcefully grab him, however, because he may become aggressive.

The nurse should be aware of things to look for during the seizure so that she can document what occurs during the seizure. This includes noting the time of onset and the duration of the seizure. The activity of the patient at the time of onset should also be noted; for instance, was the patient sleeping. Other points to include are whether there is any focal onset to the seizure and the detailed description of the sequence of events. This includes the behavior, motor movements, sensory phenomena, and postural tone as well as incontinence or tongue biting. Autonomic changes such as pupillary dilation, cyanosis, altered respirations, perspiration, and skin paleness should also be noted. It is very important to observe laterality of movement, especially eye deviation, head turning, or extension of a limb during the seizure, since this may indicate a focal origin of the seizure.

Long-Term Management

Nursing management of the long-term effects of epilepsy involve assessment of psychosocial functioning, since this is often the major effect that epilepsy has on a person's life. Fear and anxiety play a major part in a person's adjustment to epilepsy. This has many dimensions. A person may fear death or injury during the seizure. He may fear loss of his job. He may fear the rejection of others if he has a seizure in public or if his condition becomes known to his friends and family. The person may go through a grieving process once the diagnosis of epilepsy has been made. The grieving may be related to the loss of self-control or the loss of independence. Loss of independence may be perceived because of the need to take medication, the inability to drive a car legally, or family concern over leaving the patient alone and unattended.

Persons with epilepsy may develop a role disturbance and an alteration in self-concept. The person may no longer feel well even though he is physically well between seizures. He may feel that his role as a student, parent, breadwinner, or homemaker has changed since the onset of epilepsy. Some persons may develop an ineffective coping mechanism of using seizures for secondary gain. For instance, an epileptic child may threaten to have seizures if parental discipline is carried too far.

Social isolation is another problem that may occur in patients with epilepsy. A person may withdraw from social situations or even from family and work. This is often related to fear of rejection. The nurse should encourage the patient to discuss his feelings and refer him to resources such as those to be described.

Health Education

A major area of concern for nurses is lack of knowledge among persons with epilepsy. Ignorance and misconceptions can be the root of many psychosocial problems and even of compliance problems. It is important that the nurse assess the patient's knowledge of epilepsy and of the medications used to treat it. Table 65–6 outlines a teaching approach for patient education. The Epilepsy Foundation of America, which has local chapters in many major cities in the United States, provides both written and audiovisual materials on a wide variety of topics in epilepsy for both children and adults. Many local chapters provide these materials. They also sponsor service programs such as self-help groups, family support groups, job clubs, and field trips. If there is evidence of noncompliance based on low serum drug levels, the nurse should evaluate the reasons for possible noncompliance. These include denial, forgetfulness, fear of medication, fear of the side-effects of medication, and simple lack of understanding. Once a thorough assessment of the causes of noncompliance are obtained, interventions can be developed and implemented.[22]

TABLE 65–6
Teaching Plan for a Patient with Epilepsy

Outcome Criteria	*Teaching Plan*	*Evaluation*
I. Patient and family state patient is likely to have another seizure (acknowledge susceptibility)	Review with patient and family: 1. Anatomy/physiology of nerve impulse transmission in brain 2. Probable cause of patient's seizures 3. Pathophysiology of epilepsy 4. Body functions governed by specific brain regions and how patient's seizures relate to these functions (Fig. 65–1)	Patient and family regularly indicate knowledge of susceptibility to recurring seizures.
II. Patient and family recognize possible consequences of seizures on patient's life.	Review with patient and family:	Evidence that patient has adjusted to his epilepsy
1. More seizures there are, less likely to be controlled	1. Seizures beget more seizures	1. Demonstrates acceptance of epilepsy
2. Risk of physical injury during seizure	2. Physical danger if patient loses consciousness, falls, or drives during seizure	2. Admits having seizures if they have occurred
3. Difficulty finding employment	3. Benefits and risks of telling employer about having epilepsy	3. Gainfully employed according to abilities
4. Inabiilty to legally drive if not seizure free	4. State law on driving	
III. Patient and family demonstrate positive actions toward controlling patient's seizures	Review with patient and family:	Evidence that patient is taking health action for his epilepsy
1. Identifies names of prescribed medications, dosage, time schedule, side-effects	1. All aspects of medication regimen	1. Obtains maximal seizure control with minimal side effects
2. States understanding of differences in dosage needs for individuals	2. Use of serum level determinations	2. Maintains therapeutic serum drug levels
3. Lists factors that precipitate his seizures	3. How to avoid, better handle precipitating factors	3. Gives no history of activities or situations that precipitate his seizures
4. States understanding of need for follow-up by health provider		4. Returns regularly for follow-up visits
5. States advantages/disadvantages of ID tags	5. Pros and cons of ID tags	5. Has made logical decision about wearing ID tags
6. Demonstrates appropriate first aid procedure for all seizure types	6. First aid procedures	6. Shows minimal, if any, physical injury after a seizure

(Ozuna J, Cammermeyer M: Learning needs of the epilepsy patient. In Van Meter M (Ed): Neurologic Care, A Guide for Patient Education, pp 133–151. New York, Appleton-Century-Crofts, 1982)

NURSING CARE PLAN FOR THE PATIENT WITH TONIC/CLONIC SEIZURES

NURSING DIAGNOSIS/PROBLEM: Potential for injury related to generalized tonic/clonic seizure activity
GOALS: Prevent injury and alleviate anxiety

Nursing Interventions	Rationale	Outcome Criteria
1. Remove objects from patient's surroundings; raise bed side rails (should be padded); if patient is on the floor, place soft padding under his head; do not restrain patient; loosen tight clothing.	1. Seizure activity involves very forceful muscle contractions that may lead to injury if body part hits hard object.	1. Patient is free from injury.
2. If patient gives enough warning before teeth become clenched, place padded tongue blade or oral airway, or soft cloth between teeth; do not force objects between closed jaws.	2. The jaw generates 1000 lb/square inch when tightly clenched. Forcing objects between the teeth may break either the teeth or the object, and fragments may be aspirated. A bitten tongue heals well and does not pose any significant danger to the patient.	2. Patient is free from aspiration, broken teeth.
3. As seizure activity subsides, turn patient's head and body to the side.	3. Gravity helps draw the tongue away from the airway, enhancing ventilation and facilitating drainage of pooled secretions out of the mouth, thereby preventing aspiration.	3. Respirations are adequate and patient is free from aspiration.
4. Remain with the patient until he regains consciousness; assess his neurological status and vital signs postictally.	4. The patient may injure himself, or he may have further seizure activity.	4. Patient is free from injury.
5. Note and record seizure activity as well as preictal and postictal status.	5. Accurate description of the seizure events is the most important information for making any medical diagnosis.	5. Seizure events are documented.
6. Offer comfort and reassurance.	6. Patients are often embarrassed after a seizure.	6. Patient is free from psychological stress.

Evaluation

The criteria for evaluating goal achievement for the person experiencing a seizure are contained in Nursing Care Plan for the Patient with Tonic/Clonic Seizures.

The person will have avoided injury and will demonstrate adequate respirations and a clear airway with no aspiration. He will have gained an understanding of the mechanism of epilepsy and the means of controlling it, and he will adhere to the drug regimen and indicate an ability to cope with this disorder. A large portion of the difficulties people with epilepsy face stems from public ignorance and misconceptions about this disorder and those who have it. Nurses have a responsibility not only to care for patients with epilepsy, but also to increase public knowledge and understanding so that persons with epilepsy can be free from stigma, stereotype, and social isolation.

References

1. Adams RA, Victor M: Principles of Neurology. New York, McGraw-Hill, 1977, p 225
2. Augustine EA, Novelly RA, Mattson RH et al: Occupational adjustment following neurosurgical treatment of epilepsy. Ann Neurol 15(1):68–72, 1984
3. Browne TR: Drug Therapy Reviews: Drug therapy of status epilepticus. Am J Hosp Pharm 35:915–922, 1978
4. Caveness WF, Merritt HH, Gallup GH: A survey of public attitudes toward epilepsy in 1974 with an indication of trends over the past twenty-five years. Epilepsia 15:532–536, 1974
5. Caveness W et al: The nature of posttraumatic epilepsy. J Neurosurg 50:533–545, 1979
6. Chabria S, Shope JT: Medical aspect of epilepsy: An overview. In Black RB, Hermann BP, Shope JT (eds): Nursing Management of Epilepsy, pp 1–23. Rockville: Aspen Publications, 1982

7. Commission on Classification and Terminology of the International League Against Epilepsy: Proposal for revised clinical and electroencephalographic classification of epileptic seizures. Epilepsia 22:489–501, 1981
8. Cooper IS: Cerebellar Stimulation in Man. New York, Raven Press, 1978
9. Delgado-Escueta AV, Treiman DM, Walsh GO: The treatable epilepsies, Part I. New Engl J Med 308(25):1508–1514, 1983
10. Epilepsy Foundation of America. Basic Statistics on the Epilepsies. Philadelphia, FA Davis, 1975
11. Fishman MA: An approach to the management of children with febrile seizures: A child neurologist's point of view. In Nelson KB, Ellenberg JH (eds): Febrile Seizures, pp 87–92. New York, Raven Press, 1981
12. Gastaut H: Clinical and electroencephalographical classification of epileptic seizures. Epilepsia 11:102–113, 1970
13. Jennings M, Bird T: Genetic influences in epilepsy. Am J Dis Child 135:450–457, 1981
14. Loeser JD, Howe JF: Deafferentation and neuronal injury. In: Epilepsy, A Window to Brain Mechanisms. pp 123–133. New York, Raven Press, 1980
15. Lovely MP, Ozuna J: Status epilepticus. In Nikas D (ed): The Critically Ill Neurosurgical Patient, pp 125–139. Edinburgh, Churchill-Livingstone, 1982
16. Matheison G: Pathology and pathophysiology. In: Laidlaw J, Richens A (eds): A Textbook of Epilepsy, pp 437–453. Edinburgh, Churchhill-Livingstone, 1982
17. Mattson R, Lerner E, Dix G: Precipitating and inhibiting factors in epilepsy. Epilepsia 15:271–272, 1974
18. Meldrum B: Pathology and pathophysiology. In Laidlaw J, Richens A (eds): A Textbook of Epilepsy, pp 456–487. Edinburgh, Churchill-Livingstone, 1982
19. Meldrum B: Physiological changes during prolonged seizures and epileptic brain damage. Neuropediatrie 9(3):203–212, 1978
20. Morrell F: Physiology and histochemistry of the mirror focus. In Jasper HH, Ward AA, Pope A (eds): Basic Mechanisms of the Epilepsies, pp 357–370. Boston, Little, Brown Co, 1969
21. Ojemann GA: Basic mechanisms implicated in surgical treatments of epilepsy. In Lockard JS, Ward AA (eds): Epilepsy: A Window to Brain Mechanisms, pp 261–277. New York, Raven Press, 1980
22. Ozuna J: Compliance with therapeutic regimens: Issues, answers, and research questions. J Neurosurg Nurs 13(1):1–6, 1981.
23. Ozuna J, Cammermeyer M: Epilepsy, A Course Syllabus for Independent Study. University of Washington, Seattle, 1983
24. Perlman L: The person with epilepsy: Life style, needs, expectations. In Pietsch S (ed): A Needs Assessment Survey of the Clients of the National Epilepsy League. Chicago, National Epilepsy League, 1977
25. Solomon G, Kutt H, Plum F: Clinical Management of Seizures. Philadelphia, WB Saunders, 1983
26. Sterman B: Biofeedback and epilepsy. Human Nature, pp 50–79, May, 1978
27. Wyler AR, Robbins CA, Dodrill CB: EEG operant conditioning for control of epilepsy Epilepsia 20:279–286, 1979
28. Wyler A, Ward AA: Epileptic neurons. In: Epilepsy, A Window to Brain Mechanisms, pp 51–68. New York, Raven Press, 1980

Chapter 66

Cerebrovascular Disorders

Patricia A. Osborne

Cerebral Ischemia and Infarction

The health problems of cerebral ischemia and infarction may be caused by any condition that affects cerebral blood flow and perfusion of brain tissue. The most common conditions are cerebral vascular disorders causing occlusions or hemorrhages of cerebral arteries. *Cerebral ischemia* refers to a disturbance in brain *function* from diminished cerebral perfusion; neurological deficits may be reversed if the perfusion is restored. *Cerebral infarction* implies that cell death has occurred from continued impairment of perfusion; brain *structure* is affected, leaving permanent neurological deficits.

Cerebral infarctions are also referred to as cerebral vascular accidents (CVA) or strokes. A stroke, however, is not a disease state. It is simply a descriptive term for a group of disorders and is actually an outcome of the underlying cerebral vascular disorder. Strokes are the third most common cause of death in the United States and a major cause of disability. The annual incidence of stroke is 138/100,000 people with an overall mortality of 91/100,000 people per year.[72] Strokes most frequently occur in the elderly with their incidence increasing in proportion to age. Yet, despite the current increasing age of the general population, the incidence of strokes has been declining in recent years.[22] This is presumably due to prevention, early detection, and improved treatment of risk factors. Nevertheless, strokes remain a major health and social problem. In the Framingham Study, which evaluated 5184 persons with stroke an average of 7 years after the stroke occurred, 71% of survivors had an impaired vocational capacity, 31% required assistance in self-care activities, 20% needed assistance with ambulation, and 16% were institutionalized.[25]

The National Survey of Stroke (1980) estimated the economic cost of all strokes to be 7.3 billion dollars per annum. Thus, cerebral infarction can be a severe, disabling condition to society as a whole, as well as to the individual and family.

In this chapter, the health/illness problems of cerebral ischemia and infarction are presented in two sections; those resulting from cerebral vascular occlusions and those from hemorrhages. The definition, etiology, pathophysiology, clinical manifestations, and medical management of each disorder are described. Even though there are similarities among the two groups of disorders, many important differences exist that this approach will clarify.

The nursing management of people who suffer cerebral ischemia or infarctions are presented next, utilizing nursing diagnoses common to these health/illness problems. The focus initially is on the acute and rehabilitative phases of health management. Specific nursing management of the presenting problem (cerebral ischemia or infarction) is described here with reference to the underlying cause (occlusion or hemorrhage) when appropriate. The remaining section describes nursing diagnoses that are derived from the effect of the disorders and resultant neurological dysfunctions on a patient's daily life. For each diagnosis, analysis of assessment data, goals, interventions, and outcome criteria are addressed. The purpose of this approach is to help organize a tremendous amount of information related to the health/illness problem into diagnostic categories that nurses are licensed to treat and held accountable for in current nursing practice.

Cerebrovascular Occlusions: TIA and Stroke

Definition and Classification

The two most common cerebrovascular disorders causing ischemia and infarction are cerebral thrombosis and embolism. Cerebral thrombosis accounts for 53% of infarctions, whereas cerebral embolism is the cause of approximately 31%.[47]

Cerebral thrombosis refers to the formation and development of a blood clot or thrombus in a cerebral vessel, primarily arteries. It is highly associated with atherosclerosis and hypertension. Atherosclerotic plaques may begin forming in childhood and adolescence, yet symptoms are usually not seen until later in life. These plaques cause narrowing and stenosis of arteries as discussed in Chapter 22, Atherosclerosis. An abnormal clot or thrombus may form on the plaque resulting in occlusion of the artery. Blood flow is dangerously diminished or completely stopped to the area of the brain normally supplied by the vessel. The most frequent sites for development of a thrombus are bifurcations of the major cerebral arteries, with a large proportion occurring in extracranial vessels.

In *cerebral embolism,* occlusion of a vessel occurs when substances such as fragments of blood clots, tumor, fat, bacteria, or air are dislodged from the site of formation and carried by the bloodstream to occlude small, distal cerebral arteries. These emboli are most commonly associated with heart disease or atherosclerosis in extracranial or intracranial arteries.

Cerebral ischemia and infarction from these occlusions may further be classified by the temporal nature of progression and regression of the deficits. The occlusion of blood vessels may cause transient ischemic episodes or a complete infarction.

TIA. A transient ischemic attack (TIA) is defined as a temporary episode of focal neurological dysfunction presumed to be of vascular origin. It begins very rapidly and resolves completely, leaving no residual neurological deficits. It is most easily thought of as analogous to angina pectoris. The duration of each attack is only a matter of minutes, usually 2 to 15 minutes, but may last up to 24 hours. TIAs are usually caused by occlusions in either the carotid artery system or the vertebrobasilar system. Multiple TIAs may occur for several years without subequent infarction, or an infarction may follow within hours or days of the first TIA. In the Framingham study, with follow-up of 26 years on 5184 patients, 222 (56.5%) infarctions were preceded by TIAs, which is not a significantly large number, yet 40% of the patients who did have a TIA subsequently experienced a cerebral infarction.[25]

Stroke. A *stroke-in-evolution* refers to progressive or continuous neurological impairment over a period of several hours or days. This is usually related to extension or growth of a thrombus or multiple emboli that causes a gradual stepwise impairment in cerebral blood flow and an increase in neurological deficits. In a stroke or infarction, the maximal neurological deficit is present from the onset. The patient may deteriorate in the first 1 to 5 days from cerebral edema, but once this resolves, the neurological deficits stabilize and may improve somewhat.

Etiology

Atherosclerosis is the major factor underlying occlusions of cerebral arteries. The atherosclerotic process may cause thrombosis of the artery, or be a source of microemboli.

Many other factors are associated with or increase the risk of developing a cerebrovascular occlusion, with the major ones related to the development of atherosclerosis. Hypertension is the most important factor, particularly for cerebral thrombosis. An elevated systemic pressure may drive the atherosclerosis into arterial walls, thus decreasing the resiliency of the artery. Even without atherosclerosis, hypertension may cause structural changes in arterial walls. In both situations, cerebral autoregulation may be impaired and cerebral blood flow (CBF) altered. Many cardiac diseases are also considered risk factors, either by causing hypertension or as a source of emboli to the brain.

Pathophysiology

Cerebral ischemia and infarction occur only when there is a significant decrease in perfusion of brain tissue. There is a wide margin of safety between optimal tissue perfusion and hypoperfusion. The latter does not occur unless the cerebral perfusion pressure (CPP) decreases to two-thirds of the optimal level. At this time, electrical dysfunction of neurons impairs brain function, and clinical signs of ischemia become evident. If blood flow and perfusion are restored, these symptoms will resolve as in a TIA. The margin between hypoperfusion and cellular malfunction is much smaller. Cell metabolism is disturbed with a CPP 20% of optimum, and death occurs soon thereafter.[9] Thus, once signs of ischemia have occurred from hypoperfusion, cell death and cerebral infarction may follow with resultant permanent neurological dysfunction. The area of infarction occurs in brain tissue supplied directly by the occluded artery. A zone of hypoperfusion around the infarcted area is usually seen, the extent of which depends primarily on the integrity of collateral blood flow and development of cerebral edema.

A partial or total arterial occlusion may occur without any or very minimal evidence of neurological dysfunction.

There are many factors involved in the pathogenesis of cerebral ischemia and infarction, such as the location and speed of the occlusion; blood pressure; oxygen, carbon dioxide, and glucose levels; blood volume and viscosity; and presence of other vascular anomalies or occlusions.[9] These factors, known as *modifiers of ischemia,* determine whether or not a cerebral occlusion will cause ischemia or infarction, and if so, to what extent.

Location of Occluded Artery. The location of an occluded artery is important primarily for the extent of collateral circulation available. The blood supply to the brain is derived primarily from cerebral arteries that serve as branches of the circle of Willis (Fig. 66–1). If the occlusion occurs extracranially or in an intracranial artery proximal to the circle of Willis, blood flow from the contralateral internal carotid artery (ICA) or the posterior circulation is diverted through the cirlce of Willis to the cerebral arteries normally supplied by the occluded vessel. If the collateral blood flow is adequate to sustain cerebral perfusion of all brain areas, then ischemia or infarction may not occur. Since the internal carotid artery supplies such a large number of cerebral arteries and thus a large area of brain tissue, failure of the collateral circulation will result in a large area of ischemia or an extensive infarct on the side of the occluded artery.

Collateral flow or the development of anastomotic channels may also be present around an occlusion in intracranial arteries distal to the circle of Willis. The most distal and smallest arteries, however, usually do not have a significant collateral circulation, thus areas of the brain supplied by these arteries are more susceptible to a decrease in blood flow. Since these intracranial arteries supply smaller areas of brain tissue than the carotid system, the resultant damage may be less.

Speed of Occlusion. When an artery becomes gradually occluded, as with atherosclerosis leading to thrombosis, tolerance to the obstruction develops from the sustained pressure gradient. This allows time for the development of collateral flow, thus preventing or lessening the extent of ischemia or infarction. If the occlusion occurs rapidly, as with an embolus, there is little time for collateral flow to develop prior to the insult. Neurological dysfunction will occur more suddenly, and the extent of the infarction may possibly be greater than with a thrombosis. Therefore, the speed of occlusion is an important factor.

Blood Pressure. Both the stability and actual level of blood pressure are major factors in the pathogenesis of ischemia or infarction. After a cerebral insult, cerebral autoregulation is impaired at the site of the insult and in distal arteries. The brain is unable to regulate cerebral blood flow in relation to blood pressure and metabolic demands of the brain; cerebral blood flow and perfusion thus are directly dependent on the systemic blood pressure. A low blood pressure may not be adequate to maintain collateral circulation, and the cerebral perfusion pressure decreases. Hypertension, particularly abrupt fluctuations in systolic pressure, may precipitate a hemorrhage through damaged vessel walls or lead to the development of cerebral edema with resultant intracranial hypertension.

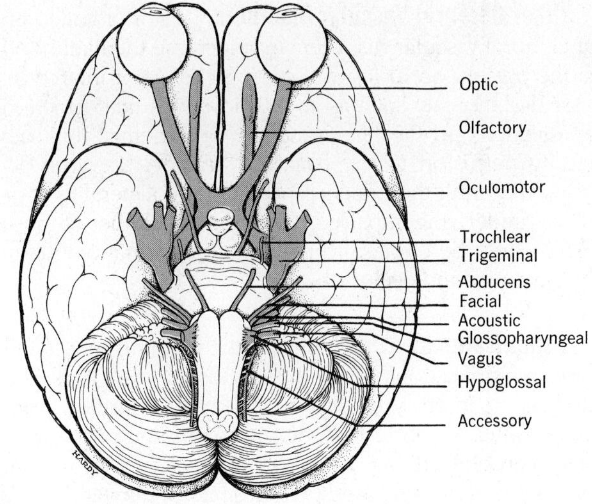

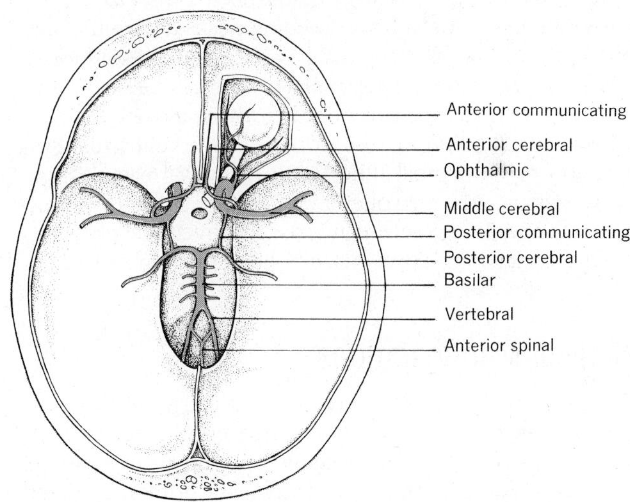

FIGURE 66–1 (*A*) The circle of Willis as seen at the base of a brain that has been removed from the skull. (*B*) Blood supply to the brain (circle of Willis) shown in relation to the base of the skull.

Levels of CO_2 and O_2. Normally autoregulation is influenced by levels of CO_2 and O_2 such that hypercapnea and hypoxemia will cause vasodilation and increase cerebral blood flow. In brain areas with impaired autoregulation, this relationship is altered, and changes in CO_2 and O_2 may aggravate or extend areas of ischemia. The loss of cerebral autoregulation prevents the brain from compensating for the metabolic imbalances.

Increased Blood Viscosity. Increased blood viscosity as seen in polycythemia or *extreme dehydration* may cause sludging of blood and adherence of blood particles to atheromatous plaques. Any of these factors may directly occlude arteries or impede blood flow through smaller collateral vessels. A low plasma volume may worsen ischemia or infarction by reducing cardiac output or increasing blood viscosity.

Other Cerebral Vascular Disorders. Prior or concomitant cerebral vascular disorders may increase the likelihood that the present occlusion will cause ischemia or infarction. A vascular anomaly such as an arteriovenous malformation may divert blood flow from the site of ischemia, thus decreasing perfusion to the damaged brain. A previous occlusion may limit the brain's capability for collateral flow or indicate underlying impaired autoregulation. Either of these factors would be enough to precipitate ischemia or infarction from a second occlusion.

Complications. In addition to the ischemia modifying factors, complications from the occlusion may limit the brain's compensatory mechanisms and cause further brain damage. After an occlusion, the most common problem is that of cerebral edema. In the absence of autoregulation, elevations of systemic blood pressure may precipitate development of edema by increasing cerebral blood flow in the damaged brain area. Plasma proteins leak out of the overdistended capillaries, drawing fluid from the vascular system into brain tissue. Usually the swelling peaks during the second to fourth day after the insult, with gradual resolution.[68] When edema is severe, intracranial pressure increases, blood flow and perfusion are reduced further, and areas of ischemia or infarction may be worsened. The ventricular system and cerebrospinal fluid (CSF) pathways may also become obstructed, or swollen brain tissue may be displaced across the midline. A severe increase in intracranial pressure, if left untreated, may precipitate brain herniation and death.

Clinical Manifestations

The presentation and course of an occlusive disorder is primarily dependent on the type and severity of the disorder, whether it is a transient ischemic episode or a complete infarction. The clinical manifestations are primarily related to the location of the occluded vessel and the development of secondary neurological complications.

TIA Manifestations

Transient ischemic attacks (TIA) begin very suddenly and are of short duration. Signs and symptoms are present only during an attack, and the neurological examination may be completely normal after the episode. If a person experiences recurrent TIAs of similar symptomatology, the underlying cause is most likely thrombosis or emboli arising from a major extracranial or cerebral artery. Blood flow is diminished to the same area of the brain in each attack. If, however, TIAs recur with variable symptomatology, the cause is usually emboli from the heart lodging in different intracranial arteries and affecting more than one brain area.

The symptoms of TIA depend on the arteries involved. Carotid and cerebral artery TIAs manifest symptoms such as blindness in one eye, hemiplegia, hemianesthesia, speech disturbance, and confusion. *Vertebrobasilar artery TIAs* include the following symptoms: dizziness, diplopia, numbness, visual defects in one or both fields, and dysarthria.

Stroke Manifestations

The presentation and course of a *cerebral infarction* varies depending on the etiology of the cerebral occlusion. The evolution of a thrombotic infarct is more variable than an embolic or hemorrhagic one. The gradual or stepwise onset reflects the slow impairment of blood flow as the atherosclerotic plaque enlarges and occludes the artery. Deficits may develop over a period of days to weeks during which prodromal episodes of TIAs may occur with improvement between attacks. The acute infarct often occurs during sleep or within 1 hour after rising. Headache accompanying the onset is rare, yet hypertension and evidence of vascular disease elsewhere in the body is common. Changes occur over the first few days from increased stenosis, occlusion, cerebral edema, or from subsequent emboli.

Occlusions from cerebral emboli evolve very abruptly, usually without warning and are unrelated to activity. As with TIAs, if the symptomatology is similar in each episode the source of emboli is most often an intra-arterial plaque or thrombus, whereas if it is variable reflecting involvement of multiple brain areas, the source is most likely cardiac. An embolus may stay at the initial site of occlusion or it may break up into fragments and travel to other brain areas.

Thrombotic occlusions may occur in either the carotid artery or vertebral and basilar arteries. The majority arise in the internal carotid artery, causing infarction in the anterior two thirds of the ipsilateral cerebral hemisphere. Cerebral emboli usually occlude intracranial arterial branches with the middle cerebral artery (MCA) being the most frequent site followed by the basilar and posterior cerebral arteries. Loss of consciousness at the beginning of an infarct is rare unless the brain stem or both cerebral hemispheres are involved. Changes or deterioration in consciousness along with worsening of other neurological deficits would suggest development of cerebral edema or hemorrhage that would increase intracerebral pressure (ICP). Neurological deficits are numerous, and they vary depending on the occluded artery. The range of symptoms include possible loss of consciousness, hemiplegia, aphasia, visual field defects, and dysarthria.

Diagnosis

The history, physical, and neurological examination often yield the most valuable information in diagnosing the presence of cerebral ischemia and infarction. Laboratory tests and procedures, both invasive and noninvasive, are required to determine the etiology of the insult. An accurate diagnosis is vital since the medical treatment depends on the etiology and presence of concomitant disorders.

Assessment

History. Since many patients do not present to the hospital until symptoms have resolved (as with TIA) or their condition has deteriorated so that consciousness is impaired, the history must be obtained or verified by a family member or significant other. Important details of the history include the temporal nature of the onset; history of TIA and their characteristics; presence of risk factors; prior medication use, particularly anticoagulants, antihypertensive, and cardiac drugs; and initial symptoms and their progression prior to admission.

Physical Examination. Physical examination includes assessment of all systems, with extensive evaluation of neurological and cardiovascular status. The neurological examination assesses the presence and extent of deficits to determine the location of the arterial occlusion. If deficits are worsening over time or if new ones are developing, frequent examinations are necessary to differentiate between an evolving infarction and secondary complications.

The cardiovascular system is evaluated as a possible source of cerebral occlusion and for associated risk factors. Also the ability of the heart to provide adequate cardiac output and cerebral blood flow must be assessed. Blood pressure is monitored for the presence of hypertension, which is commonly a compensatory mechanism after the insult, but may also be a sign of underlying cardiac disease. Hypotension may indicate an inability to support cerebral blood flow. Changes in blood pressure, particularly abrupt fluctuation, are important to note because they may precipitate a hemorrhage through damaged cerebral vessels. Changes in pulse pressures may indicate aortic disease as well as a late sign of brain herniation (shifting of brain tissue as a result of pressure).

Diagnostic Tests. A *CT scan* is the most commonly utilized diagnostic test. It may differentiate an infarction caused by arterial occlusion from that of hemorrhage, but it does not differentiate an embolic from a thrombotic occlusion. The presence of cerebral edema, hydrocephalus, or mass lesions are also visualized. Other types of brain scans utilizing radioisotopes or radionuclides are available but not as common. *Nuclear magnetic resonance* (NMR) is a new procedure that yields more detailed information than a CT scan, but at present it is not widely available. *Positron emission tomography* (PET scan) is capable of evaluating cerebral hemodynamics and metabolism by intravenous injection of radio-labeled metabolic substrates. This may be indicated particularly if neurosurgical treatment of the occlusion is considered.

The *lumbar puncture* (spinal tap) evaluates the cerebrospinal fluid and its pressure. Significant findings include increased protein with a thrombotic infarct, and elevated white blood cells with septic emboli or infection. Presence of blood indicates a hemorrhagic infarct. If intracranial pressure is elevated, the lumbar puncture is usually deferred, since withdrawal of fluid may precipitate brain herniation.

Routine x-rays of skull, cervical spine, and soft tissue of the neck are performed to assess the presence of carotid calcifications that may impair circulation. An *EEG* differentiates TIAs from seizure disorders or may localize the area of infarction from which seizures are arising.

An *arteriogram* (angiogram) is the most invasive procedure performed. It is necessary to definitively diagnose the presence, location, and extent of arterial occlusion and collateral blood flow. It is performed particularly if the diagnosis is questionable or surgical treatment is indicated.

Noninvasive tests of carotid function assess the origin of a bruit, the extent of occlusion, and the circulatory hemodynamics of carotid blood flow. There are two categories of tests, direct and indirect.[2]

Medical Management

After appropriate first aid and stabilization of the patient's condition, treatment of cerebral ischemia and infarction is directed at the cause of the disorder to relieve the pathological process and prevent recurrent episodes. The focus of treatment varies depending on the extent of residual neurological deficits. If the episode was transient, the major treatment is control of risk factors by medical or surgical interventions to prevent further occlusions. Once a fixed neurological deficit has occurred, treatment is aimed at preventing complications and further infarctions and at rehabilitation of the patient.

Treatment of TIAs

By the time the person suspected of having a TIA presents to a hospital, the episode has often resolved. Neurological status is monitored closely, however, for recurrent attacks or progression to an infarction. Ischemic attacks caused by hypertension, hypotension, and arrhythmias of blood disorders are managed by treating the underlying medical problem. TIAs caused by arterial occlusions, such as thrombosis or emboli, are treated with medications or surgery.

Drug Therapy

Two classes of pharmacological agents are currently utilized: anticoagulants and platelet antiaggregant drugs. Much controversy exists on the relative effectiveness of each class. A review of the evidence supporting the use of *anticoagulants* after a TIA is not convincing since most conclusions on the benefits are based on very weak data.[4] If the source of a TIA is an embolus from a myocardial infarction, mitral stenosis, or prosthetic heart valve, anticoagulants may be indicated for a period of weeks to many months. These drugs are usually not utilized for longer than 6 months, however, because the risk of cerebral hemorrhage is great and their long-term benefit controversial. Treatment is usually begun wtih heparin sodium either by continuous or intermittent intravenous infusion every 4 to 6 hours. The dosage is adjusted to maintain the activated partial thromboplastin time (APTT) at two to two and a half times the normal control as measured 3 to 4 hours after the medication is administered. If long-term anticoagulation is indicated, heparin is discontinued and oral preparations such as warfarin sodium (Coumadin) and dicumarol are given. Since these drugs increase the risk of hemorrhages, they must be discontinued prior to angiography or surgery.

Platelet antiaggregant drugs are most often the drug of choice for prevention of recurrent TIAs or subsequent infarction. Even with these, however, evidence on the effectiveness is controversial, since there are few randomized controlled studies. Three drugs are currently available: sulfinpyrazone (Anturane), dipyridamole (Persantine), and aspirin. Literature to date has demonstrated that sulfinpyrazone is of no proven value and dipyridamole is inconclusive, while aspirin in a dosage of 1300 mg per day is effective in decreasing the incidence of subsequent strokes and death by 31% in drug-treated as compared to control groups.[4] The rationale for their usage is based on the fact that many TIAs are related to platelet-induced thrombosis. Low dosages of aspirin act to inhibit platelets that synthesize thrombus-inducing prostaglandins and vasoconstrictive substances. In large doses (2g to 3g/day), the beneficial inhibition of platelet action is counteracted and arterial thrombosis may be precipitated. Persantine, 50 mg four times a day, is often given with low dose aspirin since it potentiates its antiplatelet action.

Surgery

Surgery may be performed to prevent recurrent TIAs and infarctions after a patient's condition has stabilized or in lieu of pharmacological treatment. It is most often done for occlusions in the extracranial portion of the carotid artery, since this is most accessible neurosurgically and has the lowest risk. There are, however, techniques available for intracranial or vertebrobasilar occlusions.

Carotid Endarterectomy. Carotid endarterectomy is the most common procedure for treatment of extracranial carotid stenosis. It is primarily indicated when the stenosis has compromised the anterior cerebral circulation resulting in a TIA. It may also be done when an asymptomatic bruit is present because this is an early sign of underlying stenosis. The procedure removes the atherosclerotic plaque from the arterial wall, thus increasing cerebral blood flow. The combined operative mortality and morbidity is low, less than 2%, yet it rises in patients with major cardiopulmonary disorders.[65] The first 24 hours following surgery are the most critical for the development of cerebral ischemia from embolization during surgery, thrombosis of the endarterectomy site, or intolerance of temporary carotid clamping. Other possible complications include airway obstruction from a hematoma in the neck and cranial nerve damage.[5]

Arterial Bypass. When a carotid artery is totally occluded or the occlusion is caused by intracranial atherosclerotic disease, arterial bypass or anastomotic procedures may be indicated. Various types of procedures include subclavian-to-carotid bypass for occlusion of the inferior cerebral artery, vertebrobasilar revascularization for vertebrobasilar artery occlusion, and superficial temporal artery and middle cerebral artery anastomosis for intracranial occlusion.[39] These procedures restore blood flow to damaged tissue by rerouting blood from an area proximal to the occlusion to a distal point on the artery.

Treatment of Stroke

Initial treatment in cerebral infarction focuses on stabilizing the patient's condition and preventing or relieving complications of the cerebral insult. This involves all health care providers, and is begun immediately with general supportive care of all bodily systems. In addition, treatment is aimed at prevention of further infarction and rehabilitation. Prevention of further infarction involves primarily medical treatment, with a few surgical interventions currently available. It is not possible to restore infarcted tissue, yet neurological deficits may be lessened by increasing cerebral blood flow and perfusion to ischemic areas surrounding the infarction. Measures to restore this circulation and arrest pathological processes can be categorized into three main objectives.

Increase Cerebral Blood Flow and Perfusion

Bed Rest: Strict bed rest is maintained until the patient is medically stable. The head of the bed is usually kept flat or minimally elevated if cerebral edema is present.

Blood Pressure Control: The primary goal is to keep blood pressure stable at a pressure high enough to maintain adequate cerebral perfusion without causing further increases in intracranial pressure or precipitating a hemorrhage. Immediately after an infarction, an elevated blood pressure is a transient compensatory mechanism and is not treated. If the hypertension does not resolve by itself, however, medications to decrease the pressure are utilized. If hypotension develops, these medications are discontinued and if necessary, the pressure is elevated with fluid administration. Vasodilators are rarely used to increase blood flow to the brain.

Maintain Optimal Oxygenation: Insuring a patent airway and adequate ventilation is vital in preventing hypoxia and hypercapnia. Both of these conditions may cause further brain damage by precipitating vasodilation and potentially increasing intracranial pressure. Close attention to respiratory status is particularly important when vertebrobasilar insufficiency is suspected of causing a brain stem or cerebellar infarction. Methods of insuring adequate oxygenation include maintaining a patent airway with positioning and suctioning; monitoring ventilation by arterial blood gases; and preventing atelectasis, aspiration, and pneumonia. If ventilation is inadequate, mechanical-assisted ventilation is indicated, particularly if consciousness is impaired.

Maintain Adequate Cardiac Output: Conditions such as shock, blood loss, fluid and electrolyte imbalances, and pooling of blood in the lower extremities must be treated immediately to maintain cardiac output and adequate blood flow to the brain. Underlying cardiac disorders such as myocardial infarction, coronary artery disease, arrhythmias, or valvular heart disease are managed with appropriate medical treatment for the disorder.

Correct Blood Abnormalities: Disorders such as anemia, polycythemia, or elevated blood viscosity caused by dehydration or other causes must be corrected so that circulation is maintained without precipitating further occlusions of blood vessels.

Decrease Cerebral Edema

Treatment is directed at dehydration of the brain, promoting restitution of the blood-brain barrier, and preventing further cerebral ischemia or hemorrhage from elevated intracranial pressure.[67] Edema occurring after an ischemic episode is more refractory to treatment than edema that occurs after a cerebral trauma or tumor, though fluid restrictions and medications are still utilized. Hyperosmolar agents such as mannitol, glycerol, and low-molecular-weight dextran (Rheomacrodex) have been effective, as well as diuretics such as ethacrynic acid (Edecrin) and Furosemide (Lasix).

Neurological status must be monitored closely, particularly with the use of mannitol, since a rebound elevation of intracranial pressure above pretreatment levels may occur after stopping the drug.

Glycerol, if given early, has been the most beneficial agent. Caution must be used in patients with diabetes mellitus or extreme dehydration, as the drug may precipitate a nonketogenic hyperosmolar hyperglycemia.

The use of steroids such as dexamethasone (Decadron) and prednisone is controversial with little data supporting its benefit, yet these drugs are commonly utilized. When the edema is severe or nonresponsive to the above treatments, controlled hyperventilation may be utilized to decrease intracranial pressure.

Prevent Further Occlusions

Control of risk factors is the major aspect of prevention. Pharmacological agents and surgery to remove the underlying pathological process are utilized, yet their benefit is questionable after an extensive infarction. Anticoagulants are given when the cause is a noninfective embolus or if the patient presents with an evolving stroke. Anticoagulation is usually maintained for 2 weeks and then gradually discontinued.

Surgical Options

Surgical options for cerebral infarctions are limited. Surgery may be performed in stable patients with mild residual deficits if the occlusion is neurosurgically accessible. Surgery is contraindicated in patients with severe deficits from an extensive infarct, an evolving infarct, severe diffuse intracranial disease, or severe systemic disease. Emergency surgery is performed if a hemorrhage occurred after an occlusion or if a massive cerebellar infarction caused acute obstructive hydrocephalus with compression of the brain stem. Both of these conditions are life threatening and are treated by the surgical removal of the infarcted cerebellum.

Prognosis

TIA. Prognosis after a TIA is usually measured in terms of recurrent symptoms and long-term mortality. It is generally thought that one third of patients will experience recurrent TIAs, one third will have subsequent infarctions, and one third will have no further problems. Studies have demonstrated rates of subsequent cerebral infarctions as low as 4.8%[49] to a high of 40%.[31,47,80] A relatively high incidence of myocardial infarction has also been demonstrated after TIAs, with a rate of 21% in 390 patients over a 5-year period.[31]

The presence of risk factors significantly affects the outcome of patients after a TIA. Muuronen and Kaste found that hypertension worsens chances for survival.[49] Patients with normal blood pressures had a 100% chance for survival 1 year after a TIA, 94% after 5 years, and 76% after 10 years. These chances decreased considerably in patients with hypertension: there was a 95% chance of survival after 1 year, 80% after 5 years, and only 49% 10 years after the initial TIA. Further evaluation of risk factors such as heart disease, peripheral vascular disease and diabetes mellitus, in addition to hypertension did not influence the risk of cerebral infarction, but it did increase the risk of subsequent myocardial infarction and thus mortality.[49]

Stroke. The majority of patients survive the initial insult to the brain unless massive infarction of the brain stem occurs. The mortality after a thrombotic infarction (30% to 40%) is slightly higher than that after an embolic one (20% to 30%).[43] Patients who have the poorest prognosis are those with infarctions of the brain stem causing deep coma or cerebellar infarctions. Even small infarcts of the cerebellum may be fatal from resultant brain stem compression or obstructive hydrocephalus. Large infarcts of the cerebral hemispheres, with or without brain stem involvement, also have a poor prognosis since extensive cerebral edema can lead quickly to supratentorial herniation and death. Survival of such patients depends primarily on maintaining bodily systems and preventing or treating complications rapidly.

Age negatively influences a person's chance for recovery and survival because of the normal changes in brain structure and function that occur with aging, and an increased incidence of other health problems. Any complications, such as pneumonia and pulmonary embolus and infections, hinder recovery and potentially cause death in patients severely disabled from the cerebral insult.

If a patient does survive the initial infarct, his condition usually improves. After a small infarction with few residual neurological deficits, recovery may begin in a few hours or days and almost complete recovery may occur. Patients with more severe deficits show less improvement over a longer period of time, particularly for recovery of movement and language functions. Small gains in function may continue for a year or more, but for all practical purposes, residual deficits present 6 months after the infarct most likely are permanent.

Nursing Management

The nursing management for cerebral occlusions is covered later in the section entitled Nursing Management of the Stroke Patient.

Cerebrovascular Hemorrhages

Cerebral ischemia and infarction may occur from ruptures of cerebral arteries either directly into the brain tissue (intracerebral hemorrhage) or into the subarachnoid space (subarachnoid hemorrhage). As a whole, cerebral hemorrhages are the third most frequent cause of stroke syndromes. Only 10% of cerebral infarctions are caused by intracerebral hemorrhages and 6% from subarachnoid hemorrhages,[47] yet the resultant mortality and morbidity is higher than that associated with occlusive disorders. There are many neurological and vascular disorders that cause and precipitate hemorrhages, but the most common are primary or hypertensive intracerebral hemorrhages and subarachoid hemorrhages from intracerebral aneurysms and anteriovenous malformations (AVM).

Intracerebral Hemorrhages

Intracerebral hemorrhages are defined as ruptures of cerebral arteries directly into brain tissue. The vessels most commonly involved are deep penetrating arteries. The hemorrhages vary in size from petechial (dots) or small slit hemorrhages to massive ones several centimeters in diameter. They occur most frequently after the age of 50 with the incidence increasing in respect to age.[69]

Etiology and Pathophysiology

Intracerebral hemorrhages may occur from a variety of causes, but the most common is hypertension, causing a primary or hypertensive intracerebral hemorrhage. The exact nature of the underlying vascular lesion is not fully understood. Structural changes in arterial walls from hypertension may be further aggravated by the presence of atherosclerosis. There is a loss of elasticity and thinning of arterial walls that impairs cerebral autoregulation. The exact cause of the rupture is usually unknown, but it is probably related to sudden severe fluctuations in blood pressure, precipitating a rupture through the damaged arterial walls. The incidence of other risk factors such as diabetes mellitus and cardiac disease has been relatively minor.[47]

When an *intracerebral artery ruptures,* blood may diffuse throughout a large area disrupting nerve cell function and synaptic transmission or it may form a hematoma. As the hematoma increases in volume, tissue is displaced and compressed. Cerebral ischemia occurs from the interruption of blood flow and hypoperfusion, or from compression of brain tissue. With continued compression and impaired perfusion, areas of infarction develop as nerve cells are destroyed. Large hematomas may require surgical removal, although with smaller hemorrhages, phagocytes and macrophages eventually remove the blood. After 2 to 6 months, the blood has resolved so that only an orange-stained area is visible on a CT scan at the initial site of hemorrhage.[10]

Clinical Manifestations

Intracerebral hemorrhages occur without warning and most often when a person is up and active. Although manifestations develop gradually in the majority of patients, the full extent of deficits are present at onset in approximately 34% of patients.[47] A severe headache often occurs and is accompanied by signs of meningeal irritation if bleeding extends into the subarachnoid space. The neurological deficits that develop vary in relation to the size and site of hemorrhage. The symptoms include muscle weakness in the face, arms, or legs, eye deviation, flaccid limbs, aphasia, ataxia, hemiplegia, nausea, vomiting, stiff neck, dysarthria, and possibly loss of consciousness. The patient's condition may deteriorate as a hematoma accumulates or other complications causing intracranial hypertension arise.

The course of a patient's condition after any hemorrhage depends to a large extent on the development and severity of complications. If these conditions do not develop or are reversed quickly with appropriate treatment, many of the neurological deficits will resolve or lessen in severity over time. Recurrent intracerebral hemorrhages from the same site are rare, but they may occur from other areas if severe underlying cerebrovascular disease or hypertension is present. Subsequent development of seizure disorders is not uncommon as a late manifestation.

Treatment

The treatment of a patient after an intracerebral hemorrhage is similar to that of a patient with infarction from a cerebral occlusion. The primary goal is to restore and maintain the cerebral circulation and to prevent further ischemia and infarction. This is accomplished primarily with medical management.

Medical measures are aimed at increasing perfusion and oxygenation of brain tissue. After a severe hemorrhage or in the presence of any complications, intensive monitoring of blood pressure and intracranial pressure are instituted. During the acute phase, strict bed rest is maintained and the head of the bed is elevated a little more than after an occlusion, usually 15 to 30 degrees. This will promote venous drainage and reduce cerebral edema; elevation greater than this may impair cerebral blood flow to the brain.

Control of blood pressure is vital to ensure cerebral perfusion and prevent further hemorrhages. Initially, hypertension may be left untreated and monitored closely. If it remains elevated, medications are given to maintain a stable blood pressure without abrupt fluctuations. Actual blood pressure limits vary with each individual according to their baseline pressures and the presence of intracranial hypertension.

Measures to maintain *optimal oxygenation* and adequate cardiac output are similar to those described for occlusive disorders. Assisted or controlled ventilation may be utilized if consciousness is impaired or controlled hyperventilation is required to control intracranial pressure. Cardiac function is monitored with a continuous ECG and invasive catheters as needed. Cardiac disorders are treated with appropirate medications. Fluid administration is regulated to maintain cerebral blood flow, but restrictions may be required to decrease cerebral edema.

The *treatment of cerebral edema,* in addition to the general measures outlined earlier in the chapter, includes pharmacological agents such as steroids, hyperosmolar agents, or diuretics. When intracranial pressure is high and unable to be controlled with standard measures, barbiturate therapy may be utilized. High dosages of barbiturates are given to purposely put the patient in a coma in an effort to decrease cerebral metabolism and control edema. The treatment is still considered experimental and carries a high risk of complications, and thus is utilized only as a last resort in many institutions.[70]

Surgery is indicated if a large hematoma is causing severe intracranial hypertension, or if a cerebellar hemorrhage is causing brain stem compression. If hydrocephalus develops, initially a ventricular catheter is placed for drainage of cerebrospinal fluid. The hydrocephalus usually resolves as obstructing blood dissolves or is surgically removed. After a severe hemorrhage, however, a permanent shunt may be required for treatment of chronic hydrocephalus. Two types of shunts are utilized: a ventriculo-atrial (VA) shunt or a ventriculo-peritoneal (VP) shunt. In both types, infection as well as blockage of the shunt are major complications often requiring shunt removal or revision.

Prognosis. Intracerebral hemorrhages have a graver prognosis than cerebral occlusions or subarachnoid hemorrhages. Fifty to 70% of people die within the first 1 to 3 days after an intracerebral hemorrhage, usually from brain herniation.[35] If patients do survive this initial period, full recovery is often very good. Since the advent of the CT scan, a higher incidence of intracerebral hemorrhages has been found, yet survival rates have improved dramatically.[17] These changes may be attributed to better detection of small hemorrhages and quicker treatment.

Subarachnoid Hemorrhages

Intracranial Aneurysms

The most common cause of subarachnoid hemorrhage (SAH) is an intracranial aneurysm, which accounts for approximately 50% of all spontaneous SAHs.[40, 57] They are rare in children, with the highest incidence occurring between the ages of 35 and 65. There are three types of aneurysms: mycotic, fusiform, and saccular, with the latter being the most predominant. Saccular, or berry, aneurysms are saclike dilatations in the walls of arteries (Fig. 66–2). They generally arise from bifurcations of the major proximal intracranial arteries around the circle of Willis, with 85% found in the anterior cerebral circulation and 15% in the posterior circulation.[13] Aneurysms may occur singly or multiple ones may be found in various locations in the cerebral circulation (Fig. 66–3). Data from both clinical and postmortem studies indicate that if a person has one aneurysm there is a 20% to 25% chance that more are present.[76]

How and why aneurysms occur is still a matter of considerable controversy. The main hypotheses attribute the defect either to congenital origins, postnatal changes in arterial walls from degenerative or inflammatory processes, or a combination of the two.[63] The role of preexisting hypertension and atheromatous plaques in relation to aneurysm formation is still being questioned.

Pathophysiology

The growth of an aneurysm is most easily explained by a biophysical hypothesis which states that the initiating factor is a mechanically induced degeneration of the internal elastic membrane from hemodynamic forces within the vessel.[19] The site of maximum stress is at the apex of a bifurcation to which high velocity blood flow transmits pulsatile forces. This energy of moving blood is transformed to pressure energy that eventually causes destruction of the internal elastic membrane. The turbulence and vibrations from the pulsatile blood flow act on the weakened wall to increase the size of the aneurysm and further decrease wall thickness.

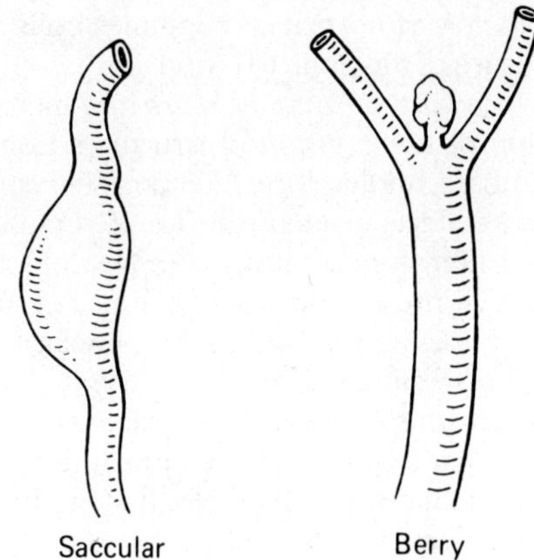

FIGURE 66–2 Saccular and berry aneurysms.

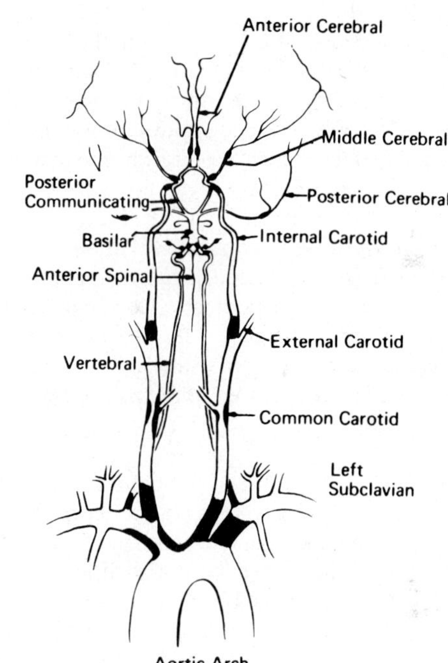

FIGURE 66–3 Major locations for cerebral aneurysms. (Beeson PB, McDermott W: Textbook of Medicine. Philadelphia, WB Saunders)

A rupture of an intracranial aneurysm occurs when the combination of intra-aneurysmal pressure, aneurysm size, and thinning of the vessel wall overpowers the structural components of the artery.[19]

If a person survives the initial rupture, bleeding into the subarachnoid space is stopped by local tissue pressure and the formation of a fibrin plug at the site of the rupture. There is also an initial elevation in intracranial pressure after the rupture, which is thought to be a protective mechanism preventing disruption of the fibrin clot.[53] The subarachnoid hemorrhage causes generalized and focal disturbances of brain function; some may be ischemic in nature and others may develop into infarctions. The disturbances of brain function occur primarily in three ways:

1. *Disruption* of normal cerebral metabolism by direct exposure of the brain to blood.
2. *Increased intracranial pressure and* mechanical distortion or *compression* of structures from blood in the subarachnoid space: After an aneurysm ruptures, blood collects around the site of rupture and may form a hematoma, causing compression of tissue. Intracranial pressure may rise because of the mass effect of the hematoma, further impairing cerebral blood flow and perfusion.
3. *Arterial vasospasm,* which is characterized by an abnormal narrowing of the cerebral arteries. The vasospasm reduces cerebral blood flow, but causes a marked increase in cerebral blood volume.[26] Vasospasm usually does not occur until after the third day postrupture, reaches a peak on day 6 to 8, and may persist for 2 to 4 weeks.[20,30,74] The etiology of vasospasm is unclear, but it is generally accepted that the collection of blood around the ruptured aneurysm is a significant factor.[64] Many researchers have attempted to identify spasmogenic chemicals (*e.g.,* serotonin, catecholamines, prostaglandins, and histamine) that are released from the clotted blood, causing vasoconstriction of the surrounding vessels.[11,30,82] The release and breakdown of erythrocytes has also been implicated.[55] Autonomic nervous system dysfunction, specifically sympathetic hyperactivity, has been hypothesized to occur secondary to hypothalamic damage.[16,75] It is most likely that a combination of spasmogenic substances and autonomic dysfunction are involved in the pathogenesis of vasospasm.

Rebleeding. Extension of ischemic areas or development of infarctions may also be a consequence of complications. The most dangerous and fatal is that of recurrent hemorrhage or rebleeding. After the initial rupture, ideally the fibrin plug remains in place until the damaged wall repairs itself. Fibrinolysis of the clot begins a few days after the rupture, reaches a peak by the end of the first week, and often persists up to 3 weeks.[48] This period coincides with the time of the greatest danger for rebleeding, which is generally considered to be 7 to 14 days after a subarachnoid hemorrhage. If a rebleed does occur, the ischemia and infarction is more extensive and the prognosis for survival is greatly reduced. The risk of rebleeding is enhanced by the loss of cerebral autoregulation because the aneurysm is then subjected to any alterations in blood pressure and volume. Other complications such as cerebral edema, hydrocephalus, systemic hypotension, cardiac arrhythmias, or cardiac failure may worsen the ischemia or infarction by decreasing cerebral perfusion. Early ischemic deficits are usually caused by primary pathological factors such as the presence of blood or a mass, while delayed ischemic deficits are most commonly related to rebleeding and vasospasm.

Clinical Manifestations

The majority of patients with intracranial aneurysms are not diagnosed as such until the aneurysm has ruptured and caused a subarachnoid hemorrhage. Certain warning signs prior to a rupture, ranging from persistent headaches or focal neurological signs to loss of consciousness have been noted in at least 10% to 59% of patients.[40,73] These symptoms are attributed to either expansion of the aneurysm, minor bleeding, or ischemia from spasm or occlusion of the vessel. Usually the first sign of rupture is a sudden, excruciating headache that may or may not be followed by a loss of consciousness. Manifestations of meningeal irritation may be present, such as nausea, vomiting, neck and back pain, nuchal rigidity, and photophobia. Hypertension is present prior to the onset in the majority of patients and is always present immediately after the rupture.

Transient or persistent neurological deficits may develop from the onset, again depending on the location of the aneurysm and size of the rupture. After a minor bleed into the subarachnoid space, few if any focal deficits occur; if present, they are related to cranial nerve dysfunction. Bitemporal hemianopsia (tunnel vision) is a sign of an aneurysm compressing the second cranial nerve at the optic chiasm. A third nerve palsy (oculomotor nerve) is manifested by ptosis, diplopia, pupillary dilatation, and divergent strabismus. Lower cranial nerve palsies are infrequent unless brain herniation develops. With larger bleeds, major hemispheric deficits may be present causing disturbances of brain function in relation to the affected artery. Disturbances such as changes in appetite, sleep, or behavior, and fever or cardiac abnormalities may be attributed to hypothalamic damage.

Arteriovenous Malformations

Arteriovenous malformations (AVMs) are developmental abnormalities in which the normal separation between the arterial and venous systems is absent; there is no vascular bed from which perfusion of brain tissue and exchange of metabolites occurs. The anomaly consists of hypertrophic dilated arteries that feed into thin-walled vessels and connect directly into dilated draining veins (Fig. 66–4). AVMs are present from birth, but the onset of symptoms is usually not until the ages of 10 to 30. They are a significant cause of infarctions in young people.[35] They vary in size from a few millimeters to a large mass of tortuous vessels. The most common locations for an AVM are the posterior portions of the cerebral hemispheres; however, they may be found in any area of the brain, brain stem, or spinal cord. Often they arise from major intracranial arteries lying in the subarachnoid space, but they may extend deep into the brain parenchyma.

The AVMs may change in size over time with the smaller ones enlarging, those of moderate size usually remaining the same, while the largest may actually decrease in size.[76] Arteries adjacent to an AVM are essentially normal vessels, yet over time they too may become dilated and tortuous as they are forced to carry an increased blood supply. The dilated, draining veins often develop into a huge aneurysmal sac from the pressure of the large artificial blood flow on the vessel walls.

The common risk factors associated with occlusive disorders are generally not implicated in the development of AVMs. Hypertension may be seen as a compensatory mechanism at the time of AVM rupture, but often the blood pres-

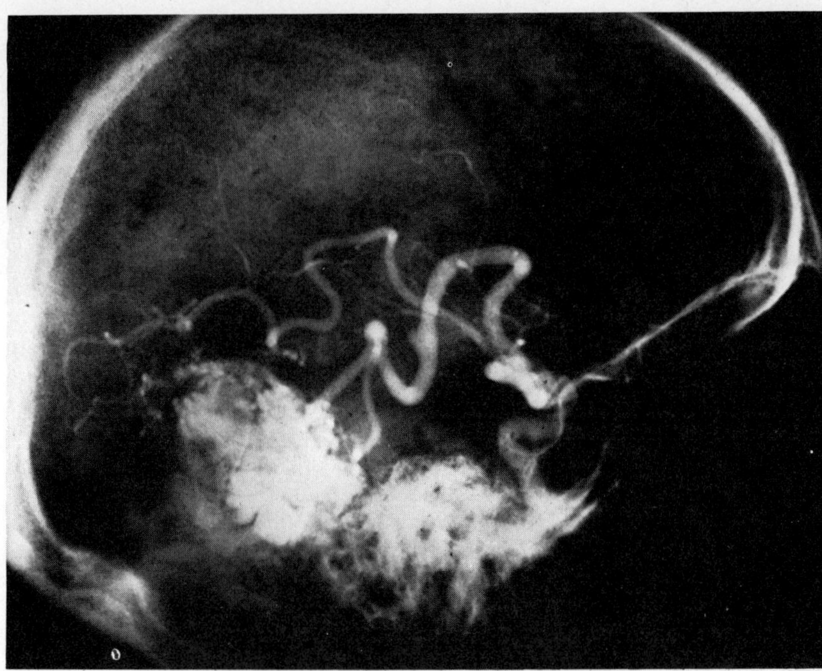

FIGURE 66–4 AV malformations consist of dilated arterial and venous channels with the apex pointing toward the lateral ventricle. They cause headaches, seizures, subarachnoid hemorrhage, increased ICP, and strokelike syndromes. (Smith RR: Essentials of Neurosurgery. Philadelphia, JB Lippincott, 1980)

sure is entirely normal preceding the event. Underlying cardiac disease may be present, particularly in the presence of large AVMs that increase cardiac output, but it is not a common factor. The effect of lifestyle, habits, and emotional stress on the rupture of an AVM as well as on the rupture of an aneurysm is an area of controversy that needs further clarification. These factors, as they contribute to general stress and the development of other disorders, must not be minimized because they influence the outcome and prognosis of the subarachnoid hemorrhages.

Pathophysiology

Arteriovenous malformations (AVMs) do not have to rupture to cause cerebral ischemia or infarction. Because the normal communication between the arterial and venous system is absent, arterial blood is shunted directly from the arterial feeders to the draining veins without perfusion of underlying brain tissue. If adequate collateral flow is present, brain tissue underneath and around the AVM may remain normal. If an AVM enlarges in size, however, it may draw a disproportionate share of the cerebral blood flow away from surrounding areas so that collateral vessels are unable to maintain cerebral perfusion. The brain tissue underlying and surrounding the AVM becomes ischemic or infarcted. Cerebral autoregulation, which normally controls cerebral blood flow, is impaired in the dilated hypertrophic vessels; thus, as is the case with aneurysms, systemic hypotension, hypoxia, metabolic imbalances, or cardiac disturbances may all worsen the ischemic or infarcted areas.

Cerebral ischemia and infarction are most severe when an AVM ruptures. What actually causes or precipitates this hemorrhage is often unknown. Interestingly, it is the smaller AVMs that rupture most frequently.[76] AVMs located on the cerebral hemispheres or brain stem primarily rupture into the subarachnoid space, whereas those on deeper penetrating arteries bleed predominantly into brain tissue. In either case, ischemia and infarction develop from disruption of metabolism caused by the presence of blood, mechanical displacement and compression from a hematoma, or elevated intracranial pressure. Delayed ischemic deficits or infarctions occur, again as with aneuryms, primarily from cerebral edema, hydrocephalus, vasospasm, and rebleeding episodes.

Treatment

After a subarachnoid hemorrhage (SAH) the immediate goal is to restore and maintain cerebral blood flow and perfusion of brain tissue. Then the pathological process causing the subarachnoid hemorrhage, either an aneurysm or arteriovenous malformation, can often be arrested and removed. Both medical and surgical interventions are utilized, although controversy exists regarding the benefits and timing of each. Management is directed primarily at prevention of rebleeding and arterial vasospasm. Unfortunately, this is difficult because the time of greatest risk for both complications is similar and treatment of one may aggravate or precipitate the development of the other complication.

Medical Management

Aneurysm precautions are routinely utilized and include general medical and nursing measures that decrease stimuli and stress while promoting rest and relaxation. Medications for sedation are usually given if the patient is alert, agitated, or confused. Phenobarbital is usually the drug of choice since it may also act as an anticonvulsant to protect against seizures. The general guideline is to titrate the dosage so that the patient sleeps undisturbed but is easily aroused for monitoring of neurological status.

Control of blood pressure is the major aspect of treatment and the most difficult. Controlled hypotension used to be the treatment of choice to prevent rebleeding, but precipitation of vasospasm often outweighed this benefit. Currently, the goal of treatment is to maintain a normotensive blood pressure. Avoiding sudden fluctuations, particularly of the systolic pressure, is the most important factor, since a sudden change will precipitate a rebleed more often than a high steady pressure. If blood pressure is elevated, antihypertensive agents or diuretics are carefully titrated against fluid or plasma administration to obtain a smooth and gradual decrease in blood pressure while maintaining cerebral blood flow. Measures to maintain adequate oxygenation and cardiac output as noted in the previous sections are instituted.

Control of intracranial pressure after the initial rupture is important to prevent permanent neurological deficits. A ventricular catheter is frequently used for monitoring intracranial pressure as well as to treat hydrocephalus. Medications to decrease cerebral edema are given along with mild fluid restrictions if vasospasm is not present.

To *prevent rebleeding* until surgery can be safely performed, antifibrinolytic agents are commonly given to prevent lysis of the clot at the site of the rupture. Aminocaproic acid (Amicar) is the most common agent utilized, and is usually given by continuous intravenous infusion. It retards normal fibrinolysis of the clot by inhibiting the formation of plasmin from plasminogen.[21] Treatment is continued until surgery, or for at least 2 weeks when the acute risk of rebleeding diminishes.

For *management of arterial vasospasm,* there is no accepted universal treatment since the pathophysiology of the problem is still unclear. The goals of current treatment, however, are to increase perfusion pressure and cerebral blood flow and to decrease cerebral vascular resistance and improve intravascular rheology.[18,21,58] Fluid administration with low-molecular-weight dextram (Rheomacrodex) or albumin improves the rheology of the microcirculation by keeping blood vessels open so that tissue may be perfused. Medications to dilate cerebral arteries are also utilized. They increase cerebral blood flow and perfusion by improving cardiac output and altering peripheral vascular resistance, as well as directly dilating the cerebral arteries. The latter effect may be accomplished by blocking calcium flow across cell membranes. Examples of medication regimens include isoproterenol hydrochloride (Isuprel) and aminophylline; nitroprusside (Nitropress); and nifedipine (Procardia) and verapamil hydrochloride (Calan). These drugs, particularly Isuprel, may cause arrhythmias, thus lidocaine hydrochloride is often given prophylactically. Administration of reserpine and kanamycin sulfate is thought to prevent vasospasm by depleting serotonin, a vasoconstrictive substance.[82] Induced hypertension by fluid administration and medications will increase perfusion pressure and volume, but it is usually not utilized unless the aneurysm or arteriovenous malformation has been surgically obliterated, or all other attempts to decrease vasospasm have failed.

Surgical Management

Emergency surgery is performed only for removal of life-threatening hematomas. If hydrocephalus is present, causing intracranial hypertension, ventricular catheters are inserted immediately, but permanent shunt procedures are delayed until a later date. The only definitive way to prevent rebleeding from an aneurysm or arteriovenous malformation is surgical removal of the vascular anomaly.

For intracranial aneurysms, the size, shape, location, and number of aneurysms determine the feasibility and type of surgical procedure. Clipping of the aneurysm is the only method of fully obliterating the anomaly. It can only be done on accessible aneurysms with a "neck" upon which a metal clip is placed (Fig. 66–5). If the aneurysm is very large or does not have a neck, trapping or gluing procedures are performed to stabilize the aneurysmal wall and prevent rebleeding. When multiple aneurysms are present, surgery becomes more difficult. If the aneurysm that ruptured can be identified, that one is clipped. Other accessible aneurysms may be clipped at the same time or in a subsequent operation. If multiple aneurysms are present on the same side of the brain, carotid ligation may be chosen to decrease the risk of rebleeding as long as adequate collateral circulation is present.[76]

The timing of surgery is critical and controversial. If the patient is in good neurological condition (Grades I and II), many surgeons recommend early surgery prior to the third day after the hemorrhage. Aside from decreasing the risk of rebleeding, early surgery may decrease the incidence of vasospasm because the clot around the aneurysm and blood in the subarachnoid space is removed. If vasospasm does occur, vigorous treatment may be instituted postoperatively to decrease late ischemic deficits. If the patient is in poor neurological condition (Grade III–V), either from the initial hemorrhage or secondary complications, surgery is usually delayed at least 2 weeks or until he is medically stable. Patients in Grade VI condition are usually not surgical candidates and rarely survive the initial rupture.

Nonsurgical procedures to occlude intracranial aneurysms have recently been developed. During arteriograms, detachable balloons may be inserted into the aneurysmal sac to occlude the anomaly. The procedure is still considered experimental because serious complications, such as occlusion of the entire artery, precipitation of an embolus, or rupture or refilling of the aneurysm, may occur.[14]

Desired surgical treatment for an arteriovenous malformation (AVM) is complete removal by resection; however, this procedure can be performed only in approximately 50% of the cases.[76] If the AVM is not easily accessible or if it is too large, ligation of the feeding arteries may decrease the size of the anomaly. This will diminish the risk of rebleeding, minimize ischemia, and allow easier dissection at a later date. More recently, laser treatment has been utilized preoperatively to coagulate and contract blood vessels to decrease the size of the lesion.

Neuroradiological procedures are available for AVMs that are not amenable to surgery, or are done to decrease blood supply to an AVM prior to surgery. Artificial embolization of the AVM, by introduction of artificial Silastic spheres, metallic pellets, or liquid glue into the feeding arteries, clots the AVM and decreases its size. Detachable balloon procedures are also being developed to obtain the same effect. Both procedures carry a high risk of extending ischemia and infarctions, or precipitating hemorrhages. The proton beam

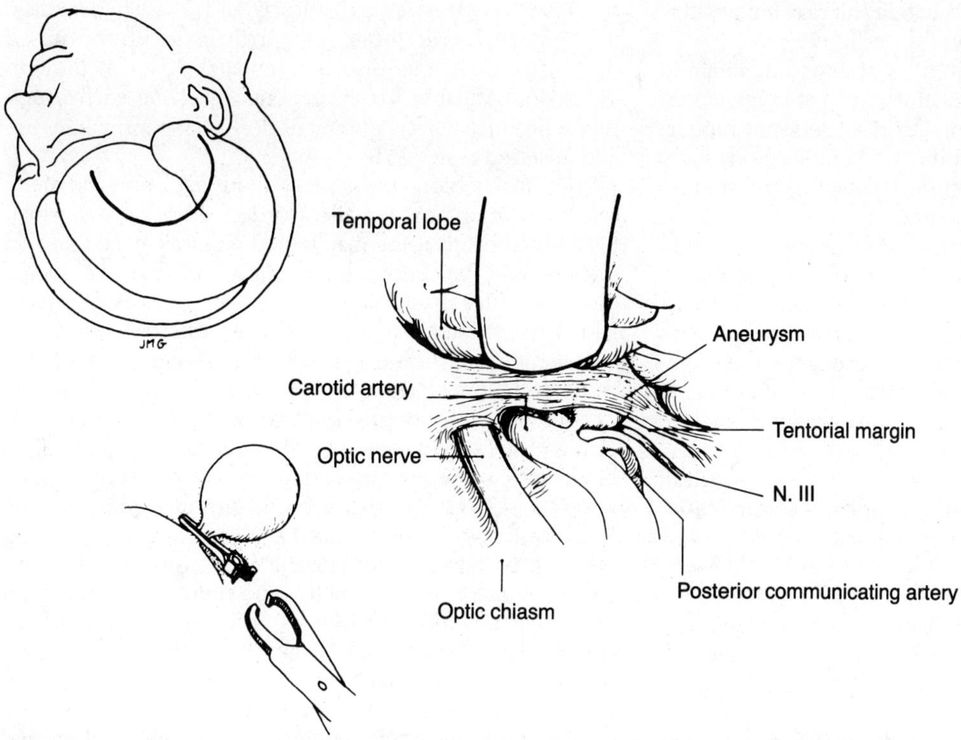

FIGURE 66–5 Clipping or a ligation of the aneurysmal neck provides the best protection against rebleeding, although the initial risk may be slightly higher. (Smith RR: Essentials of Neurosurgery. Philadelphia, JB Lippincott, 1980)

procedure utilizes radiation energy to decrease the size of the AVM. It is used most often for deep AVMs and those in critical brain areas.

Nursing Management of the Stroke Patient

The previous sections have described basic information on cerebral ischemia and infarction and the medical management of these problems. Many neurological dysfunctions may occur as a result of these disorders, including disturbances of consciousness, mentation, movement, sensation, integrated regulation, and coping abilities. Nursing management is directed at treatment of the dysfunctions and its effect on daily living. Nursing strategies to treat common neurological dysfunctions are presented in Chapter 64, which the reader is referred to as needed. The following sections will address these dysfunctions as etiologies of common nursing diagnoses. Specific nursing strategies pertaining to the treatment of the patient with cerebral ischemia or infarction are presented.

Health management refers to all interventions evolving from a physician's or nurse's orders that are directed at or influence the primary health problem, cerebral ischemia or infarction. In the acute phase, the nurse is responsible for this management because the patient is usually incapable of doing so himself. The health management deficit or core problem may arise from neurological dysfunction in any area (*e.g.,* consciousness, mentation, movement, sensation, coping, or integrated functions), or enforced dependency from therapeutic treatment regimens (*e.g.,* bed rest and aneurysm precautions). The effects of aging on normal bodily functions and the presence of any cardiovascular or respiratory disturbances contribute to a patient's health as well as his ability to manage it.

Acute Phase

Nursing Assessment

Initial and ongoing assessment of neurological status is vital to detect life-threatening situations and evaluate the type and severity of deficits for their effect on daily life. The nurse must first evaluate the patient's level of consciousness, both arousal and content (cognitive mentation), and the presence or absence of protective reflexes to determine priorities of care. The type and timing of all nursing care activities must also be evaluated carefully for their influence on the patient's condition since many of them may alter blood pressure and intracranial pressure.

All bodily systems must be monitored in the acute phase; however, cardiovascular and respiratory systems as well as fluid and electrolyte status have the most direct effect on brain function. The cardiovascular system is assessed for its ability to maintain an adequate cardiac output and cerebral perfusion. Disorders such as myocardial ischemia, arrhythmias, and blood pressure instability all may impair cardiac output, cerebral blood flow, and perfusion.

Respiratory status is evaluated for ability to maintain a patent airway and adequate ventilation and thus oxygenation of brain tissue. Preexisting pulmonary disorders may hinder ventilatory efforts as will development of complications such as congestive heart failure, pneumonia, aspiration, pulmonary embolism, and the effects of immobility.

Assessment of fluid and electrolyte status involves evaluation of the renal as well as cardiovascular and respiratory systems. Fluid overload may occur from impaired cardiac function or rapid fluid administration, and may precipitate a hemorrhage or cerebral edema with a resultant increase in intracranial pressure. Fluid deficits may develop after use of diuretics, hyperosmolar agents, or fluid restrictions and extend ischemia or infarction by causing hypotension or vasospasm. Electrolyte imbalances may worsen neurological status either directly (*i.e.,* acidosis precipitates cerebrovasodilation) or indirectly (*i.e.,* hyperkalemia impairs cardiac function).

Goal. The goal of nursing care for a patient with an acute health management deficit is to maintain or attain the integrity and optimal functioning of the nervous system by preventing or minimizing cerebral ischemia or infarction. Medically this is obtained by cerebral blood flow and perfusion, and arresting and removing the pathological process when possible. Nursing management focuses on implementation of prescribed medical treatments and prevention and early detection of complications.

Interventions. General nursing interventions that pertain to both occlusive and hemorrhagic causes of cerebral ischemia or infarction are presented first, followed by specific management issues for the different disorders. TIAs are not addressed separately. Patients who experience these usually do not require as much intensive monitoring as a patient with a cerebral infarction; the extent and type of nursing management will depend on the patient's condition and how recently the event occurred. For care of an unconscious patient, the reader is referred to Table 64–2 in Chapter 64 for nursing standards.

General Nursing Measures

Neurological Status. Continuously assess and monitor neurological status. Hourly checks of consciousness, movement, pupillary responses, protective reflexes, and vital signs are required initially after the insult and then can be done every 2 to 4 hours as the patient stabilizes. In noncomatose patients, a more thorough neurological examination should be performed to detect subtle changes as well as to identify deficits that may impair a patient's functional ability.

Cardiovascular Status. Assess and monitor cardiovascular status. An ECG is done on admission, and continuous monitoring is utilized if the patient's condition is unstable or if cardiac disease is suspected as a cause. Heart rate and rhythm are assessed for arrhythmias, and prescribed medications given to correct these. Since arrhythmias may be caused by drugs to treat other disorders, antiarrhythmic medication should be available for all patients receiving such drugs. Blood products to correct any underlying abnormalities are administered as needed.

Control of blood pressure by fluid regulation and medications is important for all disorders. The level at which blood pressure is to be maintained will vary depending on the etiology, presence of complications, and preexisting disorders. After an occlusion, blood pressure is usually maintained at normotensive levels or higher, whereas after a hemorrhage, hypotension may be desired. Blood pressure control in patients with aneurysms is difficult. To prevent or treat vasospasm, mild hypertension may be desired to keep cerebral arteries patent, however this increases the risk of rebleeding. To prevent rebleeding, blood pressure is often lowered to decrease pressure and turbulence against the weakened wall of the aneurysm. When lowering of blood pressure is required, the nurse is responsible for administering the medications, usually mild diuretics or antihypertensive agents, monitoring the effectiveness of the agents, and observing for adverse effects. If blood pressure elevation is required, intravenous fluids or plasma volume expanders are administered. The reader is referred to Grand[24] and O'Brien and Pallett[54] for commonly used medications and nursing considerations.

Respiratory Status. Maintain patent airway and adequate ventilation to minimize hypoxia and hypercapnea. Routine pulmonary care with coughing and deep breathing (avoid strenuous coughing with increased intracranial pressure and incentive spirometers are utilized in alert patients. Postural drainage is usually contraindicated in the acute phase since changes in position may increase intracranial pressure, and chest physical therapy (percussion and vibration) should be performed carefully and only as ordered. Suctioning may be necessary to maintain a patent airway, but care must be taken to hyperoxygenate the patient pre- and post-suctioning, and proper technique utilized to minimize intracranial pressure elevations.[46,67]

Oxygen is administered to prevent hypoxemia and hypoxia with the method of administration (*e.g.,* prongs, masks, tracheostomy) dependent on the patient's ventilatory capabilities and neurological status. If the patient's consciousness is impaired or protective reflexes are lost, assisted or controlled mechanical ventilation may be instituted. If controlled hyperventilation is prescribed to decrease intracranial pressure, blood gases are monitored closely. Patients are weaned slowly off a ventilator to prevent rebound acidosis, which may cause cerebral vasodilation. A respiratory therapist should be consulted for proper assessment and assistance with all respiratory treatment.

Infection. Prevent infections and maintain normal body temperature to decrease metabolic demands. Measures to prevent infections are basic to all nursing care and include excellent hygiene, care of equipment (*e.g.,* respiratory and ventriculostomy equipment, urinary catheters, and intravenous lines), and prevention of aspiration. Body temperature may also be elevated in the absence of infection from hypothalamic dysfunction after a subarachnoid hemorrhage. Acetaminophen (Tylenol), fans, and cooling blankets are utilized as prescribed, but care must be taken to prevent shivering since this may increase blood pressure.

Cerebral Edema. Prevent or treat cerebral edema. Steroids, diuretics, and hyperosmolar agents are administered as prescribed. When steroids are utilized, antacids are routinely given with each dose or every 2 hours to minimize gastric irritation. When fluid restrictions are used, fluids should be given in small amounts and spaced throughout the day. Blood and urine tests are monitored as well as mental status changes, vital signs, skin turgor, daily weights, and intake and output for signs of excessive dehydration.

Hydrocephalus. When ventriculostomies are utilized, the amount of drainage must be recorded and the site of insertion kept clean to prevent infections. Symptoms of hydrocephalus that indicate shunt malfunction or obstruction include mental status changes, gait disturbance, and urinary incontinence. If the patient is confused, safety precautions to prevent injury must be instituted. If chronic hydrocephalus develops, a permanent shunt may be placed surgically, requiring routine preoperative and postoperative care of neurosurgical patients. Major complications to observe for after a shunt procedure include shunt obstruction, subdural hematoma, infection, and seizures.

Blood Pressure and Intracranial Pressure. It is important to prevent sudden fluctuations in blood pressure or elevations in intracranial pressure. Patients are maintained on bed rest with the head of the bed flat or minimally elevated after an occlusion, and elevated 15 to 30 degrees after a hemorrhage. Before bed rest is discontinued, particularly after an occlusion, postural vital signs must be monitored. Autonomic disturbances, brain stem damage, fluid imbalances, or impaired cardiac function may all cause a precipitous drop in blood pressure with a change in posture. Neck flexion and rotation must be avoided with careful positioning, sandbags to stabilize the head, and placement of objects in front of the patient to minimize head turning.[46,66]

The number and duration of Valsalva maneuvers should be limited since this causes an increase in intrathoracic pressure, a decrease in venous return, and a rebound elevation in blood pressure. This is particularly important after a subarachnoid hemorrhage because changes in the cerebrovascular system and cerebrospinal fluid during a Valsalva maneuver have also been documented.[6,28] These sudden changes may precipitate rupture of an aneurysm or arteriovenous malformation, especially if they occur repeatedly. If the patient is alert, he should be encouraged to breathe out during any activity that involves a Valsalva maneuver, for example, micturition, straining at stool, use of bedpan, or bending.[37] Valsalva maneuvers also occur with activities such as coughing, sneezing, vomiting, and suctioning; although one cannot always avoid these activities, measures to prevent or minimize their frequency are important. Isometric or static exercises should be avoided since these increase blood pressure, particularly in conjunction with a Valsalva maneuver. Patients should be instructed not to push against a footboard or mattress or to lift or carry objects since these are all forms of static exercise.

Nursing interventions should be spaced out so that only one activity is performed per hour whenever possible. For example, a patient should not be suctioned, turned, put on the bedpan, and have range-of-motion exercises at the same time. Change in intracranial pressure have been demonstrated with some basic nursing interventions, with a cumulative elevation noted when these activities are grouped together.[46]

Nursing Measures for Occlusive Disorders

Anticoagulation Therapy. Administer anticoagulants or platelet antiaggregants as prescribed. Prothrombin time must be monitored daily at a consistent time as well as electrolytes because of the diuretic effect of heparin. Protamine sulfate and vitamin K (antidotes for anticoagulants) should be available for emergency usage. With all drugs, one must observe for bleeding; hematuria is usually the first sign, but bleeding may occur in the gums, stools, stomach (check vomitus or nasogastric aspirate) and skin (petechiae, ecchymosis).

Anticonvulsant Therapy. Administer anticonvulsants as prescribed while monitoring drug levels and observing for adverse effects. The nurse should be aware of all possible drug interactions. Dilantin may potentiate the effects of anticoagulants, and therefore the dosage of the latter often needs to be adjusted and the patient observed closely for bleeding. The nurse should record all characteristics of seizures since these often help localize the area of brain damage. Safety precautions should be instituted when a patient is at risk for injury from the seizures.

Postoperative Care. Postoperative care of a patient after surgery for an occlusive disorder involves close monitoring of neurological and cardiovascular status. After a carotid endarterectomy care includes maintaining the head of the bed flat until vital signs are stable; monitoring neurological signs hourly, observing specifically for contralateral hemiparesis and cranial nerve dysfunction; checking gag and swallow ability prior to resuming oral intake; monitoring blood pressure; and keeping intubation equipment at the beside because of neck hematoma, which may cause tracheal obstruction and laryngeal nerve damage.[5] Development of a neck hematoma may be assessed by checking neck size, location of cricoid cartilage, hoarseness, and respiratory distress.

Nursing Measures for Subarachnoid Hemorrhage

Aneurysm Precautions. Maintain aneurysm precautions, but individualize these measures to each patient's condition, previous lifestyle, and tolerance to the restrictions. If any of the restrictions increase rather than decrease anxiety, they may be modified accordingly with the physician's approval. Common measures include the following:

1. A private, quiet room kept darkened because of photophobia.
2. Minimization of all sudden noises: disconnect or lower volume on the phone and paging system in the room, and place monitors outside the room.
3. Strict bed rest with the head of the bed elevated approximately 20°. Assist patient with turning and positioning to minimize static muscle contractions, neck flexion, and rotation.
4. Passive range of motion only—no isometrics or active exercises.
5. Limitation of the number and duration of Valsalva maneuvers as noted previously. Encourage the patient to take a deep breath during any activity involving a Valsalva effort. Stool softeners are usually given to decrease straining at stool, but these may potentially increase the Valsalva effort if the patient is unable to expel soft stool with weakened abdominal muscles. The use of a bedpan may also increase a Valsalva effort and potentiate constipation. Halpern has demonstrated that the frequency, intensity, and duration of Valsalva maneuvers increases with constipation and bedpan use.[27,28] Thus, if a patient is in good neurological condition (Grades I and II), a commode should be considered to minimize these complications.
6. Avoidance of enemas, since distention of the lower colon may causes an adverse vagal effect. Rectal thermometers will not cause a vagal effect, but may precipitate a Valsalva maneuver.
7. Administration of prescribed sedatives, usually phenobarbital, so that the patient sleeps undisturbed, yet is easily aroused. Avoid restraining patients because this may increase agitation.
8. Administration of analgesics prior to onset of pain to maintain comfort.
9. Maintenance of fluid restrictions for controlled hypotension or treatment of cerebral edema. Extreme hot and cold fluids, as well as caffeine, may be limited because of their stimulant effects.
10. Avoidance of unnecessary interruptions and stimuli. Limit the number and length of visits. TV and radio may be allowed to prevent sensory deprivation in a stable patient.

Rebleeding. Administer antifibrinolytic therapy to prevent rebleeding as prescribed. This is usually given by continuous IV infusion with a controlled device. The nurse must observe for adverse effects of this treatment, which include nausea, anorexia, abdominal cramps, diarrhea with oral preparation, dizziness, headaches, and thrombosis. For the latter effect, the infusion site must be checked routinely for phlebitis or infiltration. Antiembolic compression boots are utilized to decrease venous stasis and prevent clotting in the lower extremities. Calf and thigh circumference should be measured; skin should be observed for redness, warmth, and tenderness; and peripheral pulses should be palpated for presence and symmetry.[33]

Vasospasms. Administer medications and fluids to prevent or treat vasospasm as prescribed. Many of the medications require IV infusion with a controlled device and close monitoring in an intensive care unit since their dosages are titrated according to cardiovascular as well as neurological status.

Fluid Volume. Monitor intake and output, daily weights, serum and urine osmolalities, and electrolytes, and maintain fluid restrictions for syndrome of inappropriate secretion of antidiuretic hormone (SIADH).

Preoperative and Postoperative Care. Preoperative preparation of a patient with an aneurysm or arteriovenous malformation may require additional sedation to prevent rebleeding. Teaching must be done very carefully, informing the patient of risks and procedures in a manner that will minimize anxiety. Having a family member present during teaching and the morning before surgery is often helpful. Postoperative care includes all routine measures and monitoring after a craniotomy with careful regulation of blood pressure. It is important to remember that the patient may be hypovolemic with decreased nutritional reserves from preoperative and operative medications. This may cause postoperative hypotension and vasospasm, both of which may potentiate cerebral ischemia; thus, fluid replacement is vital.[32] Bed rest is maintained until the patient is neurologically stable, but other aneurysm precautions may be discontinued if the aneurysm or arteriovenous malformation was surgically occluded.

Evaluation

The outcome of a patient's acute health management status is globally evaluated by the severity and extent of neurological dysfunctions. Ideally for a patient with a TIA no further attacks or progression to an infarction occurs, and the patient is able to resume prior functional abilities. If an infarction did occur, improvement or neurological functions would indicate achievement of the goal. Further rehabilitation may be required to attain an optimal level of functioning in daily life. As the patient moves from the acute to the rehabilitative phase, he will become a more active participant in his health management.

Outcome may also be evaluated specifically by the development of problems arising in other bodily systems that have direct effects on cerebral blood flow and perfusion.

Potential for alteration in cardiac output and tissue perfusion is assessed by maintenance of blood pressure and heart rate within prescribed limits and maintenance of cerebral perfusion pressure by prevention and treatment of intracranial hypertension.

Potential for ineffective breathing patterns or airway clearance is evaluated by presence of a clear airway and lungs on auscultation, maintenance of blood gases within normal or prescribed limits, and maintenance of ventilatory capacity within normal limits.

Potential for fluid volume alterations, either overload or deficit, may be complications of or desired outcomes of treatments. A fluid volume deficit may be the desired state for the treatment of cerebral edema and intracranial hypertension, whereas a fluid volume overload may be a desired outcome for treatment of vasospasm. Criteria for evaluation of these problems then depends on the effect of the abnormality on body systems. The goal is to maintain vascular volume at an appropriate level to treat the pathophysiological disorder, yet to not adversely affect other bodily systems.

Potential for alteration in temperature regulation is evaluated by body temperature, the occurrence of shivering, and development of infectious processes.

Rehabilitation Phase

Nursing Assessment

After a patient's condition has stabilized, the focus of health management is prevention of recurrent episodes. For patients with TIAs, this is particularly important since TIAs are considered warning signs for both cerebral and myocardial infarctions. In this rehabilitative phase, the nurse may continue to manage many aspects of the patient's health, but emphasis should be directed at teaching the patient and family to assume a more active role.

The etiology of a health management deficit is primarily related to the patient's functional capabilities, level of knowledge, and presence of risk factors that predispose a patient to recurrent episodes.

The patient's functional capabilities to manage his own health are best determined by the amount of enforced dependency present, that is, whether the patient is dependent on another person or object for management of his health. All human functions must be assessed, with the categories of consciousness, mentation, and movement being particularly important. If a patient's consciousness is impaired, then he may be totally dependent on another person for all care. Disturbances in mentation (*e.g.,* poor memory, receptive aphasia, and decreased insight or judgement) may enhance a patient's dependency on others and hinder compliance with instructions or medications. Problems with movement, such as hemiplegia or paresis, have obvious implications; the patient physically may not be able to perform ADLs or prepare special meals.

The patient's and family members' level of knowledge and beliefs regarding the health problem, the benefits and risks of prescribed treatment, and the effect of all of these factors on the patient's life must be assessed. Knowledge deficits and misbeliefs may hinder compliance with health management and adaptation to the neurological disorder.

Finally, the presence of any risk factors for recurrent episodes must be evaluated as well as the benefits and risks of prescribed treatment regimens. These will influence the extent of the health management deficit and serve as a basis for planning intervention.

Goal. The goal is that the patient and family will possess the knowledge, beliefs, and capabilities to maintain or attain health management for prevention of further cerebral ischemia or infarction. Further medical or surgical interventions may be indicated. The focus of this section is teaching the patient and family to control common risk factors by the appropriate use of medications and lifestyle adjustments.

Interventions

Initial nursing management, interventions, and teaching about the control of risk factors is begun in the acute care setting. Ideally all patients should then be referred to a stroke prevention program. If a cardiac disorder precipitated or developed as a consequence of the cerebral episode, cardiac rehabilitation may also be indicated.

General Nursing Measures. General nursing measures in the rehabilitation phase include several foci. Patients and families should be instructed on signs and symptoms of recurrent ischemic episodes or infarction and on appropriate first-aid measures. They should be aware of late complications such as seizure disorders or exacerbation of cerebral edema and hydrocephalus. If patients are maintained on steriods, they should be instructed to prevent infections and observe for bleeding.

Blood pressure and maintenance of adequate cardiac output remain the most vital issues for both occlusive and hemorrhagic disorders. Medications may be prescribed for treatment of hypertension, arrhythmias or other cardiac disorders, diabetes, and hyperlipidemia. Teaching about medications should be done in conjunction with methods of monitoring their effectiveness and adverse effects.

Lifestyle adjustments are recommended to minimize risk factors for cerebral and myocardial infarctions. Dietary restrictions or changes may be prescribed for control of hypertension, diabetes, hyperlipidemia, or weight reduction. A nutritional consultation should be obtained for necessary teaching and monitoring effectiveness. Activity and exercise restrictions are primarily dependent on mobility impairments and activity tolerance. If cardiac disease is present, a stress test should be performed and activity monitored closely in conjunction with cardiovascular status. If the patient's previous lifestyle was sedentary, attempts to increase exercise, particularly if weight reduction is desired, are indicated. This is done slowly with the avoidance of strenuous exercises that may cause sudden changes in blood pressure. Habits such as cigarette smoking, recreational drugs, and excessive ETOH use are discouraged. The type and amount of emotional stress and past and present coping strategies must be evaluated for their effect on the patient's health as well as adaptation. Referral to a support group or individual therapist is strongly suggested to cope with emotional stress and life changes from the neurological disorder. Pamphlets for patient and family teaching are listed under suggested readings at the end of this chapter.

Specific Nursing Measures. The specific nursing measures focus on the problem of bleeding. If a patient is maintained on anticoagulants or platelet antiaggregants after a cerebral occlusion, teaching should include basics of the medication regimen, necessary blood monitoring, and observation of adverse effects, especially bleeding. Drug interactions must be explained and patients cautioned against taking *any* medications unless prescribed by their physician.

After a subarachnoid hemorrhage, antifibrinolytics and drugs for vasospasm are not used for an extended period of time; prevention of a recurrent episode is primarily dependent on control of blood pressure by medications and lifestyle modifications. Certain activities may be restricted, such as heavy lifting, bending, and strenuous exercise. Sexual intercourse is usually not contraindicated but modification of positioning may be suggested.

Evaluation

After teaching and referral to appropriate resources, the patient and family should be capable of and feel comfortable in managing the patient's health. Methods of evaluating their knowledge and capabilities to measure outcome criteria may include ability to explains signs and symptoms of recurrent episodes and demonstrate appropriate first aid treatment, to identify risk factors and explain the plan for treatment for each, to describe their medication regimens and methods of monitoring for adverse effects, to demonstrate how to check blood pressure and heart rate and other tests as prescribed, and to explain or plan changes in lifestyle in relation to the patient's mobility impairments and activity tolerance. The established plans and interventions must be coordinated with a rehabilitation program, ambulatory care professionals, or a home health agency to ensure follow-up in these areas.

General Nursing Diagnoses

Impaired Thought Processes

Nursing Assessment

The two cerebral hemispheres are thought to be dominant or responsible for different cognitive processes; thus manifestations of impaired thought processes will vary depending on the location and extent of the cerebral ischemic episode or infarction. The left hemisphere is important for reasoning in a logical, successive manner, and for the ability of abstraction, language, calculations, analyzing details, marking time, and verbal memory. The right hemisphere is often described as more intuitive and relates things as they really are. It is imaginative, subjective (relates in feelings), and simultaneous (perceives the whole picture or concept rather than focusing on details). The right brain often communicates in pictures and is extremely important for spatial perceptual relationships and nonverbal (performance) memory.[61] A patient's behavioral style also varies: patients with left hemispheric damage are often slow and cautious, whereas those with right-sided damage are described as quick and impulsive. The reader is referred to Chapter 64 for an in-depth discussion of these impairments.

To accurately assess the presence and extent of cognitive impairment, arousal must be intact and some form of communication must be available. Formal mental status examinations and neuropsychological testing will detect deficits, but close observation and interaction with the patient is necessary to assess the influence of this dysfunction on self-care and daily life.

Goal. The first priority for management is for the patient to maintain or attain thought processes and capabilities that will enable him to relate and interact safely with his environment. This is necessary for learning new coping strategies to adapt to the changes in lifestyle brought on by the neurological disorder.

Interventions

Neuropsychological testing should be obtained as soon as possible to diagnose and verify the type and extent of deficits. A plan for managing the problems can then be devised, utilizing the patient's intact cognitive abilities and avoiding stimuli or situations beyond the patient's ability that may increase anxiety or frustration. The family should be involved with establishing this plan since they can contribute important information about the patient's prior personality, behavior, and intellect that influences the current situation. When cognitive deficits are severely impairing functional abilities, cognitive retraining programs should be investigated for a more thorough and formal approach.

Impaired Concentration. For impaired concentration and attention span, short time periods for teaching should be utilized in a structured environment to minimize distractions. Topics should be summarized frequently, and the patient should be refocused and oriented on the task or subject being addressed. If the patient has limited ability to shift from one task to another, present only one activity or topic at a time to minimize frustration. Reasoning and problem solving will be impaired when a patient has very concrete thought processes. Information needs to be explained very simply and concretely, breaking things up into small logical steps. Often problem-solving simulated sessions are helpful; however, if the patient is not able to carry over learned information to other situations, the sessions need to be done repetitively, using familiar situations.

Impaired Memory. Impaired memory will interfere with almost all functional abilities. Patients with impaired verbal memory (usually left hemisphere damage) will retain information best when demonstrations or pantomime are utilized. For patients with impaired performance or nonverbal memory, verbal and written information is usually retained best. With any memory and learning difficulties, repetition of instructions and tasks is vital. Perseveration or inappropriate repetition of a word or activity may also be encountered and is a frustrating problem that hinders learning and completion of tasks. When this occurs, the patient is not able to stop it himself. The cycle has to be broken by intervention from another person and is best accomplished by changing the topic or task. Scolding the patient or asking him to stop will only increase the patient's frustration and anxiety.

Behavioral Problems. Behavioral problems often interfere with appropriate thought processes and learning. Confusion and aggressive and inappropriate behavior may occur after a cerebral infarction that involves frontal and temporal lobes and other limbic system structures. A patient is often unable to interpret his feelings and thus responds inappropriately, or he lacks the ability to control responses. The patient may feel angry or frustrated, yet not know why. He may become overwhelmed by these feelings if he remains in the presence of the stimulus or situation that evoked the feeling. Behavior then becomes disorganized, with exaggerated or inappropriate responses.

To counteract this, techniques to minimize frustration and anxiety should be employed. Conversations, as well as activities and the environment, need to be structured since the patient does not have the internal ability to structure or organize his feelings and responses. If a patient is expressing frustration, anger, or sadness, acknowledge his feelings and interpret their meanings for him. Asking open-ended questions at this time (*e.g.,* How do your feel?, Why are you acting like this?) will only aggravate the situation. Stimuli or situations that precipitate the disorganized or uninhibited behavior should be identified and avoided.

If a patient does lose control of his behavior and becomes confused, agitated, or angry, it is necessary to remove the patient from the stimulus as quickly as possible. Reasoning or explanations at this time will not stop the escalation, and the use of restraints often escalates the situation and should be avoided unless the patient or another person is in danger. When these behavioral problems are present, it is vital to share the management techniques with all staff, family members, and visitors so that a consistent approach is utilized (See section Ineffective Coping Strategies later in this chapter.)

Evaluation

Nursing management of impaired thought processes is evaluated in terms of the patient's ability to learn and adapt to the changes in his health and daily life. This can initially be assessed by observing the patient's ability to attend to a stimulus, retain information, interpret its meaning, recall and apply this information to other situations, and communicate needs and desires appropriately and safely. These abilities should be evaluated with nonfamiliar as well as familiar people or situations. The patient may do well in the latter situation, but be totally nonfunctional when faced with a new situation. The patient and family should be aware of the specific cognitive limitations and demonstrate methods of compensating for them. If behavior is a problem, the family and patient should be able to identify precipitants of inappropriate behavior and demonstrate methods of preventing and controlling them in a calm manner.

Impaired Communication

Nursing Assessment

There are many forms of communication, both verbal and nonverbal, that may be impaired directly from the cerebral insult or indirectly by medications that alter awareness, cognition, behavior, or sensory perception. The first priority of assessment is to determine the type and extent of communication deficit as well as intact functions that may be utilized to compensate for the impairment.

Aphasia usually occurs after damage to the dominant hemisphere. There are many forms of aphasia, which include difficulty with comprehension (receptive), speaking (expressive), naming (anomia), reading (alexia), or writing (agraphia). Discrete focal lesions may cause only one form of aphasia, but mixed types are usually manifested. The presence of a language disturbance may be grossly evaluated by listening to fluency of speech and to grammar or abnormal word usage and by assessing the patient's understanding of instructions and his ability to name objects, read, and write.

Other disorders that interfere with verbal communication include *dysarthria,* verbal *dyspraxia* (difficulty approximating speech sounds despite intact facial muscles), and *aphonia.* The first two disorders often occur after cortical damage, while dysarthria may also be due to cerebellar or brain stem infarctions. Aphonia is not a usual consequence of cerebral ischemia or infarction, but disturbances in phonation may occur from laryngeal nerve damage after a carotid endarterectomy or tracheal intubation.

The *emotional component* of communication may be impaired after damage to the right or nondominant cerebral hemisphere. These patients exhibit no difficulties in speaking or understanding words, but their ability to express emotions by tone or melody of speech may be lost. They may also have difficulty discriminating and identifying emotions in someone else's voice, and they respond inappropriately to humorous situations.[71]

Nonverbal communication or "body language" may be altered from problems in moving or seeing. Weakness of the facial muscles, lips, or tongue may cause an inability to smile, frown, or kiss, whereas decreased visual acuity, field cuts, or ocular gaze disturbances may hinder eye contact with others. The person with a hemiplegia or paresis may have difficulty emphasizing speech with gestures or expressing feelings by touching or hugging another person. A patient's ability to communicate nonverbally can be assessed easily during a routine neurological examination and by observation of their interactions with other people.

The importance and significance of a communication deficit varies for individual patients and is dependent on a person's personality, education, cultural and social background, and lifestyle. Educational level, as well as the patient's native language, is extremely important to assess prior to planning interventions so that appropriate words are utilized.

Goal. Regardless of the type and etiology of communication problem, the goal for all patients is to maintain or attain some form of communication to enable interaction with other people and the environment. Failure to establish some form of communication may cause other problems such as potential for injury, social isolation, impaired self-concept or esteem, and self-care deficits. It is important to recognize the psychological impact of communication problems because a resultant depression or anxiety may hinder management and adaptation.

Interventions

After the type and extent of communication deficit has been identified, an alternative method of communication should be established. Both the impaired and the compensatory communication methods should be clearly written on the patient's medical record and care plan, and shared with the family. Putting a sign over the patient's bed is not desirable or appropriate since it may be perceived as degrading and increase feelings of helplessness and frustration. A speech consultant should be obtained for assistance in planning communication methods and initiating therapy as soon as the patient's neurological status stabilizes.

In addition to the practical strategies for management of aphasia (see Chap. 64), anticipating a patient's needs by observing nonverbal behavior and structuring activities so that the patient can anticipate routines help decrease anxiety and compensate for the communication deficit. When nonverbal communication or the emotional component of speech is impaired, the nurse must listen to and observe the patient carefully to determine the emphasis and meaning of words. By overlooking these facets of communication, messages may be lost or misinterpreted quite easily.

The use of flash cards with pictures of words, an alphabet board, or writing may be utilized for a patient with expressive aphasia or impaired auditory comprehension. If he cannot point to the correct responses, head or eye movements in the direction of the correct word, letter, or picture are substituted. Once neurological deficits have stabilized, alternative communication methods for long-term use may be investigated, such as a small electronic communicator that types out messages or a computer that is activated by hand, eye, head, or breathing movements.

Evaluation

The desired outcome for all patients with a communication deficit is that basic needs and desires are satisfied. The patient should be free from injury while self-care needs are met by the nurse, patient, or family member. The patient's and family's knowledge and understanding of teaching may be evaluated by observing the patient and his interaction with others. Effects of medications, sensory perceptual disturbances, and psychological reactions often cannot be avoided. Strategies to minimize or counteract their influence may be evaluated by observing the extent to which these hinder communication and self-care. If any of these factors are causing significant problems, they should be identified as separate nursing diagnoses, and specific interventions should be instituted.

Sensory–Perceptual Alterations

Nursing Assessment

Sensory–perceptual disturbances may involve primary senses or higher cortical sensory functions. The primary senses most often affected are seeing and feeling (somatic sensation). Visual disturbances may include temporary diminished acuity or blindness from a TIA (amaurosis fugax), cortical blindness from an occipital lobe infarct, visual field cuts such as homonymous or bitemporal hemianopsias, diplopia, and nystagmus or ocular gaze disturbances. Impaired somatic sensation may be manifested by a partial loss of feeling in the face or an extremity from a cortical or brain stem infarction. Abnormal sensations may also occur, such as disabling pain from a thalamic infarct. It is important to remember that aging diminishes the acuity of sensory modalities so that deficits may be more pronounced in the elderly; the elderly patient may also have limited intact modalities to compensate for impaired functions.

Higher cortical sensory and perceptual abilities are disturbed or lost usually with damage to the right parietal lobe. Examples of such dysfunctions include hemi-inattention, anosognosia, impaired spatial orientation (*i.e.,* difficulty distinguishing right from left, localizing body parts or objects, and route finding), and visual, tactile, or auditory agnosias.

Treatment regimens may also aggravate or cause sensory–perceptual alterations. These disturbances are enhanced in the presence of actual sensory deficits; when one modality is diminished, the others become more sensitive and thus more susceptible to sensory perceptual changes in the environment. Sensory deprivation (restriction of sensory stimuli) or perceptual deprivation (absence or lack of meaningful stimuli) may result from prolonged bed rest or aneurysm precautions. Sensory–perceptual overload may develop in an intensive care unit with a large amount of nonmeaningful stimuli. The concomitant use of CNS depressants may contribute to these problems by altering awareness of surroundings, whereas CNS stimulants cause distorted perceptions. Patients with these sensory–perceptual alterations may exhibit acute anxiety, hallucinations, delusions, and confusion and disorientation, as well as worsening of cognitive abilities.[45]

Goal. The goals of management for sensory–perceptual alterations include maintaining or attaining the patient's maximum sensory function, self-care ability, and comfort and preventing sensory–perceptual alterations caused by changes in environmental stimuli.

Interventions

Identifying intact abilities is a priority so that they may be utilized to accommodate for impaired sensory functions. Identifying sensory–perceptual deficits from parietal lobe damage is often difficult, but it is extremely important since these deficits usually impair a patient's functional recovery more so than language deficits. Since these patients often retain verbal skills, their abilities are overestimated by themselves and by others, and subtle problem areas are often overlooked. The manner in which any deficits influence basic ADLs and safety should be clear documented. O'Brien and Pallett offer specific strategies for many common perceptual problems,[59] examples of which are presented in Table 66–1.

Safety precautions to prevent injury should be instituted and they include arranging a clutter-free environment within the field of vision, using an eye patch alternating on each eye if diplopia is present, teaching the patient with an ocular gaze palsy or field cut to scan the environment, and regulating water temperature to prevent burns for a patient with altered somatic sensation.

TABLE 66–1
Nursing Strategies for Sensory-Perceptual Alterations

Perceptual Problem	*Example*	*Nursing Interventions*
A. *Disorders related to perception of self and illness*		
1. Inattention to one side of the body that can involve motor, tactile, and visual modalities	1. The patient will be unable to perceive touch on the affected side when both sides of the body are touched simultaneously, but will be able to feel a single touch on the affected side only.	1. Remind the patient of any motor, tactile, or visual inattention that might interfere with functional activities.
2. Lack of concern for hemiplegia or other motor or sensory deficits	2. Tendency to leave extremities in awkward or dangerous positions. The patient may allow arm to dangle over side of bed or may run over foot with wheelchair.	2. Teach patient to position the affected extremities carefully, using his unaffected hand to do so. Use sling for an affected arm that has little or no muscle tone.
3. Lack of awareness of hemiplegia or other motor or sensory deficits	3. Attribution of the problem to some minor somatic complaint. The patient may insist upon getting out of bed unassisted.	3. Observe the patient closely and anticipate his needs. In spite of repeated explanations, he will have difficulty retaining information about deficits.
4. Denial of hemiplegia or other motor and sensory deficits	4. Attempt at walking on the paralyzed leg. The patient may insist that his affected extremities have adequate strength.	4. Encourage handling the affected limb to reinforce awareness of the affected side. Teach methods of performing activities that will ensure safety.
B. *Disorders related to perception of space and body image*		
1. Unilateral spatial neglect. Lack of awareness of one side of the body that can involve motor, tactile, and visual modalities	1. Failure to recognize people approaching from affected side. On the neglected side, the patient may bump into objects, fail to use his limbs, and ignore visual and tactile stimuli. He may walk to one side and turn only to the right.	1. Increase stimulation to affected side and encourage interaction of staff and visitors with neglected side. Have the patient handle his limbs and teach him to bathe, dress, and position them. Place TV on that side.
a. Hemianopsia	a. Neglect of visual input from the affected side, for example, visitors, staff members, food, or objects on a tray located on the affected side	a. Place objects on his unaffected side. Instruct him to visually scan his physical environment.
2. Defects in localizing objects in space, estimating size, and judging distance	2. Difficulty in abstracting one object from others surrounding it, *e.g.*, in distinguishing food on a tray from the rest of background	2. When working with the patient, close the curtain or door. Eliminate objects except those that the patient is using, *e.g.*, soap and washcloth. Do not have flowers, *etc.* on the table for these will distract him.
3. Defects in route-finding	3. The patient will have difficulty learning new routes. He may even get lost finding his way on once familiar routes because he has no sense of direction or awareness of the relationship of turns to the point he is trying to reach.	3. The patient should never be sent alone on a new route or be allowed to leave familiar, safe surroundings unattended. In familiar territory, he should always have clearly written instructions with identification of landmarks that will help him identify the direction to a given destination.
a. Defective topographical memory	a. Difficulty in recalling and describing routes or spatial characteristics of familiar surroundings. For example, arrangement of furniture in a room, location or doorway to room	a. Provide a clue to routes or objects, for example, a piece of colored tape on the patient's bed to distinguish it from other beds.
4. Reading and counting disabilities. Inability to align columns and rows of digits	4. When counting, the patient gets lost in proceeding from one unit to another and may forget items that have already been counted.	4. Provide the patient with exercises in copying figures and placing them in columns for computation.

(*Continued*)

TABLE 66–1
Nursing Strategies for Sensory-Perceptual Alterations *(Continued)*

Perceptual Problem	*Example*	*Nursing Interventions*
a. Inability to tell time	a. Inability to read the time or set the hands of a clock or watch	a. When establishing schedules, orient the patient to time frequently by associating passage of time with the arrival of visitors, serving of meals, or appointments for scheduled therapy.
b. Reading and counting	b. Loss of directional orientations with respect to printed material. Patient may begin reading anywhere on the line.	b. Assist in directional orientation. Have patient use finger or ruler to follow the printed line.
5. Right–left disorientation. Inability to discriminate	5. The patient will be unable to distinguish right and left sides of himself or others. Patient is unable to follow directions or instructions that rely on comprehension of the concepts "right" and "left."	5. Use descriptive adjectives such as the "weak" arm or "good" leg to refer to the body, and descriptive phrases such as "blue," the door "next to the bed" in directions.
C. Apraxia		
1. Inability to perform a learned movement voluntarily	1. Difficulty in using the hand as in eating, threading a needle, or writing. The patient may demonstrate extraordinary delays and be clumsy. Difficulty with movements of the mouth; this may interfere with speech, chewing, and swallowing. Difficulty in initiating purposeful actions, such as walking, sitting, and rising	1. Encourage the patient to feed himself independently. If necessary, guide his hand to his mouth but have him complete the action. With repetition, some patients improve in performance. Speech, occupation, and physical therapy can provide some exercise to improve or compensate for some of the deficits. Teach individual components of an activity separately. Then proceed to integrate components into a completed activity.
2. Constructional apraxia	2. Difficulty in assembling apparatus requiring interpretations of directions, as in "do-it-yourself" kits	2. Instruct the patient to reply more on touch than on vision when arranging objects. This is also a safety measure, for example, in handling sharp objects.
a. Inability to put together 2-dimensional units to form 3-dimensional figures and patterns.	a. Difficulty in arranging objects according to clear spatial awareness, for example, setting a table with dishes and silverware	
b. Inability to analyze visually, piece by piece, in order to construct a whole	b. Inability to place the hands of a clock appropriately	
c. Inability to reproduce simple patterns through arrangement of separate parts or through drawings		
3. Dressing apraxia	3. Inability to put on clothes properly. The relationships of parts of garments is disturbed. The patient may put clothes on backwards or have difficulty finding a sleeve or he may neglect to clothe one half of the body.	3. Instruct patient in dressing himself. For some patients, repetition of an activity results in improved performance. Sometimes visual clues are helpful, *e.g.*, colored labels sewn on the neck or sleeve of a garment.

(Adapted from O'Brien MT, Pallett PJ: Total Care of The Stroke Patient, pp 146–150. Boston, Little, Brown & Co, 1978)

When hemi-inattention is present, usually one would approach the patient from his unaffected side. During the rehabilitative phase, however, the patient is encouraged to use his affected body parts; the room is arranged so that the patient is forced to look to the affected side.[8] When agnosias are present, sensory stimuli should be identified and interpreted simply each time the stimulus is introduced, and the patient should be instructed to use his unaffected senses to identify objects. For example, a patient with a visual agnosia should feel objects to identify them and determine how to use them correctly.

For relief of pain from sensory disturbances, analgesics

are prescribed. These must be monitored carefully because sensory–perceptual deprivation may be accentuated if a patient's awareness is altered by the drugs. Comfort measures such as positioning, cool or warm cloths, distraction, diversion, and deep breathing exercises may be helpful. Relaxation techniques involving progressive muscle relaxation should not be utilized in patients with increased intracranial pressure since isometric exercise is contraindicated. Other techniques, such as meditation or visual imagery, may precipitate seizures in susceptible patients. Only stable patients should attempt these with supervised instruction.

To prevent sensory–perceptual deprivation, ideally the patient should be placed in a room with an alert patient. When a patient is on bed rest, particularly with aneurysm precautions, the amount and type of stimuli is monitored in relation to the patient's responses. If stimuli increase anxiety, the amount of stimuli should be minimized, and meaningful stimuli that require interactions with others or the environment should be introduced. If photophobia is not severe, maintaining normal light–dark cycles in the room will help decrease perceptual distortions. Occupational and recreational therapists may help provide varied and meaningful stimuli to the patient.

Evaluation

First and foremost, the patient should be free from injury when sensory or perceptual impairments are present. The patient should receive adequate sensory and perceptual stimulation at a level that does not hinder psychological and physiological condition. This can be evaluated easily by documenting changes in psychological and physiological status that cannot be explained solely on the basis of any other problem. Specifically after a subarachnoid hemorrhage, the desired outcome would be that no recurrent hemorrhage occurred from sensory and perceptual stimulation.

The outcome of management for sensory–perceptual alterations can be further evaluated by a patient's ability to perform ADLs utilizing appropriate aids and intact sensory modalities. He should also be in control of his pain, as evidenced by verbal and nonverbal behavior. When these outcomes are not met, additional problems (*i.e.,* self-care deficit, alteration in comfort) are identified and treated accordingly.

Impaired Physical Mobility and Self-Care Deficit

Nursing Assessment

Problems with mobility and self-care are addressed together since their development and outcome are highly interdependent. Manifestations of mobility impairments may range from an inability to turn oneself in bed, sit, stand, transfer, ambulate, or use one's arms and hands. Impaired mobility may interfere with self-care abilities such as toileting, bathing, dressing, grooming, or feeding.

Neurological deficits from ischemia or infarction of brain areas necessary for movement are the major causes of both problems. Deficits and their causes include weakness or paralysis of one or more extremities (motor cortex or brain stem), abnormal movements or difficulty initiating movement (basal ganglia), impaired coordination (cerebellum), apraxia (parietal lobes), or total loss of voluntary movement and abnormal posturing (brain stem damage). A change in muscle tone and reflexes also hinders mobility and functional use of extremities. After a typical hemispheric infarction, muscle spasticity with hyperreflexia develops from the loss of cortical inhibition on lower motor nerves. If untreated, contractures potentially may occur that further limit movement and self-care.

Ischemia or infarctions of other brain areas also influence the presence and extent of these problems. Alterations in consciousness and mentation will hinder a patient's ability to learn voluntary movement or the use of adaptive aids. Movement and ADLs may also be impaired from difficulties in feeling, seeing, or localizing body parts in relation to the environment. The patient will be predisposed to injury, and will be unsafe, hesitant, or unable to perform ADLs or to walk.

Concomitant health problems, such as cardiac or respiratory disorders, may limit a patient's tolerance for activity. Sedative drugs or toxicity from anticonvulsants may decrease a patient's alertness and coordination. Therepeutic treatments (*i.e.,* bed rest, aneurysm precautions, or attached monitors and IV lines) may cause an enforced immobility and dependency for self-care; the immobility may increase weakness and may promote disuse atrophy and contractures. Finally, ineffective coping may hinder a patient's motivation and ability to participate in a rehabilitation program.

In addition to assessing the etiology of the problems, the degree of independence a patient exhibits when performing these activities at their optimal level of functioning must be evaluated. Independence is determined by the need for adaptive aids or assistance from one or more persons, whether it is for supervision or complete care. A patient in the latter situation is actually in the most dependent role and will require the greatest amount of external resources and support.

Thus all human functions, therapeutic regimens, and needs for assistance must be assessed and treated. The following interventions focus on management of neurological dysfunctions, primarily motor, as they relate to the presenting problems.

Goal. The long-term goal of both mobility and self-care deficits is for the patient to maintain or attain an optimum degree of functioning and independence in daily life. After an infarction, it may take weeks to several months before this goal can be adequately assessed because of slow gains in functions. There are many short-term goals in the acute and early rehabilitative phases that are essential for restoration of functional abilities and independence. A full range of motion (active and passive) of all extremities and joints is maintained or attained, as well as maintenance or improvement of muscle strength and coordination. Pain or discomfort may arise from complications of immobility (*e.g.,* contractures or bedsores). Preventing these and assisting the patient to maintain or attain control of his pain contributes to independence in mobility and self-care.

Interventions

When a patient is on strict bed rest, proper positioning, body alignment, and passive range-of-motion (ROM) exercises are necessary to prevent contractures and disuse atrophy and preserve residual function. Active ROM and isometric exercises are contraindicated because of their effects on blood pressure and intracranial pressure. Flaccid extremities are supported by pillows, trochanter rolls, or sandbags to maintain the extremities in functional positions. If spasticity is present, extremities should not be kept in flexed positions since this favors development of flexion contractures. Sustained pressure against a hard surface, such as a footboard or hand splints, may increase spasticity; soft rolls or pillows are used to keep hands and feet in functional positions. Turning and repositioning every 2 hours, or as indicated by skin integrity, helps prevent contractures and skin breakdown and maintain comfort.

Once the patient is medically stable, physical and occupational therapy consultants should be obtained to begin a more active rehabilitation program emphasizing functional independence in mobility and ADL. It is important to consider all cognitive, communication, sensory, spatial, and perceptual deficits in this phase when structuring teaching sessions and environment.

To increase mobility, training in bed mobility is initiated first. An upright position is resumed gradually to prevent sudden blood pressure alterations, beginning with bed-sitting techniques and pivot transfer to chairs. To increase strength and coordination of extremities, more active exercises and teaching are required. When some lower extremity function is intact, the patient first practices standing and maintaining balance, then progresses to ambulation training. Instruction on usage of aids, such as a cane or walker, are usually required. Use of a wheelchair may be necessary with severe lower extremity weakness, paralysis, or a lower activity tolerance.

Techniques to increase upper extremity strength and function and improve self-care abilities are begun while the patient is on bed rest. A sling prevents subluxation of the shoulder joint, while splints or soft rolls maintain functional positions of the hands. Specific aids such as built-up utensils, plate guards, or high-rimmed bowls make it easier for a patient to feed himself. Trays are arranged simply within the patient's field of vision, and dishes are presented one at a time to minimize confusion. If the nondominant hand is used, there may naturally be less coordination; beginning with finger foods will help improve coordination. Initially containers should be opened for the patient, and foods should be prepared to decrease frustration. Gradually the patient should be encouraged to perform these activities for himself.

Many aids are available to assist with other self-care activities, such as long-handled brushes, built-up toothbrushes, mitted washcloths, and Velcro straps on clothing. A tub seat, rails and raised toilet seat in the bathroom will ensure safety and make bathing and toileting tasks much easier.

For all self-care activities, the process should be broken down into simple steps, with feedback and encouragement given at successful completion of each step. If errors are made, tell the patient what was wrong, but do not perform the task for him unless it is obvious that he cannot do so himself. Assisting a patient at this time, while acknowledging and praising him for his efforts and accomplishments, is vital if the patient is to attempt the task again. Bardach presents two types of remedial techniques for patients with visual–perceptual or cognitive deficits that can be utilized by nurses to enhance a patient's self-care abilities.[3]

SYSTEMATIC SIMPLIFICATION OF DEMANDS

1. Break down a specific task into small steps (*e.g.,* dressing).
2. Give patient cues at each step until he is able to complete it (*i.e.,* dress self).
3. Each time the patient gets dressed, systematically decrease the number of cues until he performs it without help or with a minimal number of cues.

COMPENSATION FOR DEFICITS

1. Determine the deficit and its effect on self-care.
2. Devise method so that the patient understands and is aware of the deficit (*e.g.,* if hemi-inattention, show the patient the affected limb).
3. Teach the patient methods to compensate for the deficit (*i.e.,* hold onto his affected arm to increase awareness and prevent injury or use a sling).

Differences between functions of the right and left sides of the brain are important to remember. A patient with right hemisphere damage will do better if verbal instructions are given. Encouraging a patient to talk himself through the task and putting a list of necessary steps on a mirror are extremely helpful. When hemi-inattention is present, the patient needs to be reminded to bathe and dress the neglected side of his body; performing these activities in front of a mirror may provide visual input to counteract the neglect.[8] Structure and supervision of these activities minimizes the patient's impulsiveness and overestimation of his capabilities. A patient with left hemisphere damage will learn self-care abilities better when pantomime and demonstrations are utilized. The patient may be slow and cautious; thus constant feedback is necessary.

For all patients, environmental distractions should be minimized, and sufficient time allowed for completion of the task. This is time consuming for the nurse, yet a hurried approach with frequent interruptions will interfere with the patient's learning and performance, as well as impair his self-esteem by making him feel inadequate or a bother to the nurses.

Evaluation

The outcome of mobility and self-care deficits is measured in three ways: the extent of functional abilities, the degree of independence in performing these functions, and prevention of complications from immobility. Functional abilities can be assessed by observing the patient's mobility in turning, sitting, transferring, standing, and walking. Performance of self-care activities is evaluated by observing the patient bathing, dressing, toileting, and eating. The degree of independence is measured by the manner in which the patient is able to perform these activities, either with the assistance of adaptive devices, supervision, or actual assistance from one or more persons. Complications of immobility, such as frozen shoulder, disuse atrophy, or contractures are evaluated for their direct effect on movement and self-care with interventions modified accordingly.

Immobility may also lead to the development of other problems, such as potential for injury, sensory–perceptual deprivation, discomfort, ineffective gas exchange, impaired skin integrity, or altered urinary or bowel elimination. When these occur, they are evaluated and treated as separated patient problems, yet their influence on mobility and self-care must not be overlooked.

Alteration in Nutritional Status

Nursing Assessment

Nutritional disturbances in the acute phase are usually characterized by an intake less then body requirements. The opposite may have been present preinfarction (*i.e.,* obesity or hyperlipidemia). Inadequate nutrition may be assessed generally by monitoring dietary intake, elimination, body weight, skin integrity and turgor, mucous membranes, laboratory values, vital signs and neurological status; the latter two are particularly important for detecting fluid and electrolyte disturbances.

There are often many possible causes of inadequate nutrition. The disturbance is often an effect of treatments such as intravenous fluids without adequate electrolyte supplementation, prolonged or inadequate tube feedings without hydration, hyperosmolar agents or diuretics, or dietary and fluid restrictions. Specific neurological deficits may impair one's ability to ingest food. The primary problem is dysphagia caused by cortical or brain stem infarctions. Poor intake may also be related to visual and perceptual disturbances (*e.g.,* the patient is unable to see or neglects the food on his plate), motor or sensory deficits (*e.g.,* difficulty preparing food and getting it into one's mouth), depression (*e.g.,* decreased appetite), or cognitive and communicative deficits (*e.g.,* inability to express food preferences and learn adaptive techniques). Anorexia, and nausea and vomiting, which may be manifestations of meningeal irritation after a subarachnoid hemorrhage or gastric irritation from adverse effects of medications, further limit nutritional intake.

Goal. The immediate goal during the acute phase is for the patient to maintain or attain adequate nutrition and hydration to ensure functioning of all bodily systems. When dysphagia is present, the patient (and family) must also maintain or attain the knowledge and skills necessary to chew and swallow safely, or use alternative methods to ensure adequate nutrition and hydration.

Interventions

Initially patients are maintained on intravenous fluids until consciousness and protective reflexes are fully assessed, or if surgery is being considered. When a patient is alert and has an intact gag reflex, oral alimentation is preferred. Tube feedings are utilized, usually beginning with a nasogastric tube, if consciousness is impaired or the gag reflex is ineffective. If tube feedings are required long-term, alternative types are considered.

When dysphagia is present, a speech pathologist should be consulted for evaluation and appropriate therapy.[36] After a cerebral infarction, pseudobulbar dysphagia may be seen with spastic muscles and a hyperactive gag reflex. The reader is referred to Chapter 64 for specific techniques to treat this dysphagia. Meals should be small and given frequently, four or five times per day. Solids are much easier to swallow than liquids, especially thin, clear liquids. Water should be avoided or, if given, ice water is tolerated best. Foods should be high in texture, taste, temperature, and smell to stimulate the senses and improve muscle function. A nutritional consultation should be obtained for all patients to determine caloric and nutritional requirements. When eating, it is vital that the patient is sitting upright or positioned at 45 degrees to prevent aspiration and to allow gravity to assist with swallowing.

To minimize or prevent nausea, antacids 1 hour before and after meals or every 2 to 4 hours are given. If vomiting or gastrointestinal bleeding occurs, oral foods are withheld while the problem is treated.

Evaluation

The adequacy of a patient's nutritional and hydration status may be evaluated objectively by monitoring skin integrity and turgor, mucous membranes, daily weights, intake and output records, and laboratory tests. The occurrence of infections, rate of wound healing, and overall recovery are general measures of outcome. If these do not progress as expected, inadequate nutrition should be suspected, and an immediate consultation with the physician and dietician is necessary.

Chewing and swallowing abilities are evaluated by examination and observation. The patient should be able to demonstrate appropriate techniques to facilitate swallowing, prevent aspiration, and compensate for hand, visual, and perceptual impairments. If tube feedings are utilized on a long-term basis, the patient's and family's knowledge and skills in administering these are evaluated by return demonstration of feeding techniques, care of the tube, and formula preparation.

Alteration in Bowel Elimination

Nursing Assessment

Impaired bowel elimination may be manifested by fecal incontinence, diarrhea, or constipation. Incontinence may occur after an infarction from loss of cortical inhibitory mechanisms resulting in uninhibited contractions of the bowel. Incontinence may also be a problem in patients with an impaired consciousness, a decreased awareness or perception of the need to defecate, and inability to communicate the need to defecate, or an inability to physically get to the bathroom resulting from mobility, visual, or spatial–perceptual problems. Diarrhea and constipation are usually iatrogenic, but underlying bowel disorders, laxative use, and poor dietary habits may be contributing factors. Iatrogenic diarrhea is often related to the adverse effects of medications, such as kanamycin, oral Amicar, certain antacids, and to tube feedings. Constipation, however, is the most frequently encountered disturbance.

Immobility from neurological deficits and enforced bed rest are the major factors favoring development of constipation, as does the unnatural position required in using a bedpan. Dehydration from fluid restrictions and medications, poor dietary intake, the use of constipating medications (*e.g.,* narcotics, sedatives, anticonvulsants, and some antacids), the inability to communicate the need to defecate, or irregular bowel routines are additional causes of constipation.

In addition to the above factors, previous bowel habits and the use of aids are important factors to assess. Bowel records should be kept to record the frequency, consistency, color, and odor of stool, the presence of blood (guiac test), and time of defecation to accurately diagnose the problem and establish a plan of care.

Goal. Management of altered bowel elimination is directed at maintaining or attaining regular elimination patterns of soft formed stool with a minimum of Valsalva effort. This latter part is extremely important in patients after a subarachnoid hemorrhage to prevent rebleeding episodes. If bowel elimination is a chronic problem (*i.e.,* fecal constipation, incontinence), the patient and family should possess the knowledge and skills to continue a bowel program at home and prevent secondary complications such as skin breakdown and fecal impactions.

Interventions

Medications that alter a patient's awareness and perceptions and cause constipation or diarrhea should be avoided whenever possible. If antacids are routinely given, alternating between magnesium-based (diarrhea producing) antacids and aluminum-based (constipating) antacids will help regulate bowel patterns.

Constipation. Establishing a consistent routine for bowel elimination and anticipating a patient's need to defecate are necessary to prevent constipation and decrease fecal incontinence. Patients should be given a bedpan or preferably be taken to the bathroom or commode at a specific time each day. Suppositories given prior to this on a daily basis stimulate defecation; after a while, digital rectal stimulation by itself may be adequate to stimulate elimination. For patients who are unable to perceive or interpret the need to defecate or who are confused or agitated, these measures may not be adequate to prevent incontinence. It may be necessary to take the patient to the bathroom a half hour after each meal and observe nonverbal behavior between meals to anticipate needs.

Specific treatment of constipation requires removing or minimizing all contributing or predisposing factors. As soon as possible, the patient should be allowed to use the commode rather than a bedpan, and general activity should be gradually increased. For patients on anuerysm precautions or those with severe vertebrobasilar occlusions, the benefits of a commode have to be weighed against the detrimental effects of a change in posture on blood pressure and intracranial pressure. Fluids should be liberalized to a least 2000 ml/day once the danger of cerebral edema has lessened. Reliance on laxatives should be avoided since their frequent usage may worsen bowel patterns. If the patient is able to swallow, Metamucil one to three times daily with prune juice at bedtime is recommended in addition to regulation of dietary habits to include foods high in fiber and roughage. Stool softeners alone, particularly in patients on fluid restrictions, are usually ineffective. Agents that stimulate peristalsis, suppositories, or oral preparations should be given with the stool softeners if a patient is unable to defecate for two days. Enemas should be avoided, particularly in patients with a subarachnoid hemorrhage, since they may cause an adverse vagal reaction and interfere with bowel retraining efforts.

Diarrhea. When diarrhea occurs, the patient must first be checked for the presence of a fecal impaction or any systemic disorder that may be causing the diarrhea. If an impaction has been ruled out, agents to counteract the diarrhea, such as Kaopectate or Lomotil, may be prescribed. Medications that contribute to diarrhea should be discontinued if possible, and dietary and fluid intake regulated accordingly.

Whatever regimen is effective to prevent or treat bowel elimination disturbances should be taught to the patient and family. Since this is often a topic of embarrassment for many people, it should be discussed in privacy and with discretion. Inability to control one's bowels often impairs one's self-esteem and image. Patients should be told that these are common yet treatable problems and should be allowed to verbalize their concerns.

Evaluation

The easiest way to evaluate the outcome of bowel elimination disturbances is to keep a stool chart for monitoring frequency, timing, and consistency of stool, as well as effectiveness of intervention. The passage of hard stools, or less than 3 days of stools per week, indicate constipation, whereas greater than three stools per day are considered abnormally frequent.[12,41] The effect of Valsalva maneuvers on a patient's neurological and cardiovascular status should also be monitored by observing the patient while defecating.

Other problems may develop as a consequence of impaired bowel elimination. Fluid deficits or electrolyte disturbances may result from diarrhea or fecal incontinence. If these develop, other measures for their management are necessary in addition to treatment of the elimination problem.

Alteration in Urinary Elimination

Nursing Assessment

Urinary incontinence is the predominant manifestation of impaired urinary elimination. As with bowel incontinence, it usually results from a loss of cortical inhibition causing uninhibited bladder contraction, but it may also be related to a urinary tract infection or overflow from bladder distention. As with bowel elimination, other neurological dysfunctions may contribute to urinary problems. Urinary tract infections are usually iatrogenic problems caused by incomplete emptying of the bladder caused by immobility or indwelling urinary catheters.

Urinary function is assessed by monitoring voiding patterns (*i.e.,* timing, frequency, and amount), presence of incontinence, residual urine volumes by straight catheterization, and the patient's perception of bladder fullness and voiding sensation. When a urinary infection is suspected, urinary cultures should be obtained. If incontinence is a problem, the type of incontinence must be determined, whether a continual leakage, stress incontinence, or sudden vomiting of large amounts. Tests to evaluate bladder capacity and integrity of sphincter tone are useful for diagnosing the cause and planning appropriate treatment.

Goal. Nursing management is directed at maintaining or attaining normal voiding patterns (with minimal Valsalva efforts in the acute phase). To decrease urinary incontinence, measures to prevent infections, avoid overdistention, and encourage adequate storage of urine are necessary.

Interventions

As with the treatment of bowel elimination problems, medications that alter a patient's awareness or perception of the need to urinate should be avoided. Environmental stimulation may increase the patient's awareness of bodily functions and surroundings. The patient should be taught how to palpate his lower abdomen to check bladder distention and use Credé techniques to enhance emptying of the bladder. Examples of bladder reconditioning programs are presented in Chapter 64.

Indwelling catheters should be avoided unless a patient is comatose or urinary output needs to be monitored closely. Toileting every 2 hours is recommended, with the length of time between voids gradually increased. If the patient is unaware of urinary incontinence, it is difficult to retrain the patient in this manner. Keeping the patient clean and dry is often the most that can be done. As soon as possible, the patient should utilize the commode or bathroom, so that gravity will enhance emptying. If nocturnal incontinence occurs, fluids and any diuretic medications should be restricted after dinner so that the patient does not have to urinate at night.

If these strategies fail to control incontinence, intermittent catheterization at regular intervals may be indicated. External catheters for males may be helpful if a patient is unable to get out of bed or is confused. Medications to decrease uninhibited bladder contractions may be prescribed with or without catheterization.

To prevent urinary tract infections, the above methods to avoid urinary retention are necessary. If indwelling catheters are utilized, frequent perineal and catheter care is required, and constant urinary irrigations may be prescribed. Medications may be given to acidify the urine, but the patient must be monitored closely for development of lithiasis.

Evaluation

Outcomes of nursing management for these problems are the ability of the patient to completely empty his bladder, remain clean and dry between voids, and be free of infection. These can be objectively evaluated by monitoring the length of time between voidings, the presence of incontinence, residual volumes after urination, and urinary cultures. Effectiveness of medications to lower the pH of the urine can be evaluated by testing urine acidity.

The patient and family should possess the knowledge, skills, and capability to maintain normal urinary patterns and prevent infections. This may require extensive teaching and practice if indwelling catheters or intermittent catheterization are utilized.

Sleep Pattern Disturbance

Nursing Assessment

Humans normally progress through four stages of sleep (non-REM stages) followed by a period of REM (rapid eye movement) sleep. The latter begins 90 minutes after sleep onset and then may recur at 90-minute intervals throughout the night.[7] Disturbances in these normal sleep-cycles may be characterized by insomnia (*i.e.,* difficulty falling asleep, frequent awakenings, or arising too early), total sleep deprivation, or selective deprivation of certain sleep stages. The manifestations of these problems are varied; they include fatigue, confusion, cognitive or perceptual impairments, or inappropriate behavior. Without REM sleep, for instance, people may exhibit greater excitability and hallucinatory behavior with prominent aggression and defensiveness.[7] These problems may negatively affect a person's daily functioning, as well as ability to cope with the neurological disorder.

When assessing the cause of the sleep disturbance, first consider the location of the cerebral insult. Brain areas important in the genesis and maintenance of sleep include the brain stem reticular formation, the hypothalamus, and their interconnections. Infarctions in these areas will disrupt sleep–wake cycles. For example, infarction of the posterior hypothalamus may cause somnolence, destruction of the mid-pons may result in persistent wakefulness, and damage of the lower brain stem may cause insomnia.[7] Other neurological dysfunctions may cause sleep disturbances. Mobility impairments, pain, or discomfort may hinder sleep from an inability to move and get comfortable. Nocturnal seizures, urinary or fecal incontinence, and respiratory or cardiac disturbances are frequent causes of nocturnal awakenings. Fear, anxiety, or depression may cause insomnia or sleep deprivation.

Medications must also be considered for their influence on sleep. CNS-stimulating agents (reserpine or caffeine) may contribute to insomnia. Many antihypertensive and cardiac drugs inhibit REM sleep, whereas benzodiazepines, barbiturates, anticholinergics, and catecholamines affect the deep sleep stages.

The frequency and timing of nursing care activities and other hospital routines may be contributing factors of sleep disturbances. Awakening a patient for hourly vital signs or turning interrupts sleep cycles or causes total sleep deprivation. The detrimental effect of these nursing activities may be enhanced in the presence of environmental deprivation or excessive stimulation.

The severity of sleep disturbance is evaluated in terms of its influence on daily functioning. Knowledge of prior sleep habits and the patient's prior responses to disturbed or inadequate sleep helps to evaluate current problems and plan interventions. To objectively assess sleep patterns, a patient should be observed during sleep for quality and duration. During the day, the amount of naps required and presence of cognitive or behavioral disturbances that are not solely related to brain damage should be noted. Often sleep recordings with EEG monitoring are helpful to identify sleep disturbances and their etiology.

Goal. The goal of nursing management is for the patient to maintain or attain a normal sleep–wake cycle according to prior habits and present needs. Unfortunately, in the acute phase normal cycles are often impossible to achieve because of the need for constant monitoring and treatment. The goal then becomes attainment of adequate sleep and rest to prevent untoward physiological disturbances. When a sleep disturbance is a manifestation of the cerebral infarction, interventions may be limited; management focuses on supportive care and removal of other factors that may contribute to the sleep problem.

Interventions

To prevent sleep disturbances, the environment should be modified to decrease extraneous, nonmeaningful stimuli at night, and to provide stimuli that decrease anxiety and aid orientation. Physiological conditions such as dyspnea, incontinence, or pain should be treated with appropriate measures. Medications that interrupt sleep cycles should be avoided. Nursing care activities should be scheduled to limit the number of awakenings at night. If this results in performing many things at once, the detrimental effect of sustained stimulation and activity on intracranial pressure and blood pressure needs to be considered first. Procedures that increase anxiety should be avoided prior to sleep. Encouraging verbalization of concerns, along with soothing back rubs, often promotes sleep better than any medications.

Specifically for the management of patients who become confused or agitated in the evening (sundown syndrome), the environment should be made as familiar as possible, and daily routines and bedtime rituals should be established.[38] It is helpful to have consistent personnel assigned to the patient to decrease confusion. Simple explanations should be given to the patient prior to changes in routines and personnel because sudden alterations may precipitate or exacerbate behavioral and sleep disturbances.

Evaluation

The presence of sleep disturbances and effectiveness of nursing intervention can be evaluated subjectively by the patient's perception of the quality of his sleep and by how rested he feels on awakening and throughout the day. Observation of the patient at night is helpful to determine whether or not the patient is actually sleeping and to evaluate stages of sleep. During sleep, one should observe a lack of purposeful movement, closed eyelids, heavy slow breathing, and diminished responses to external stimuli. During REM sleep, movement of the eyes under closed lids may be observed. Evaluation also includes the patient's ability to perform self-care, participate in health management, and cope effectively with the disorder. When the basic need of sleep and rest is not met, disturbances will arise in these areas.

Sexual Dysfunction

Nursing Assessment

Assessment of sexual dysfunction involves evaluating three components of sexuality: ability and method of sexual expression and behavior, libido, and sexual roles and identity. Any or all of these may be impaired after a cerebral infarction.

Methods of sexual expression and behavior are commonly altered owing to residual mobility impairments. Problems may range from difficulty expressing intimacy of affection by kissing, hugging, or holding hands, to performing or enjoying sexual intercourse. Adverse effects of medications, depressions, lack of privacy within a hospital, or lack of knowledge regarding limitations and alternative methods may all add to these difficulties.

A change in sexual libido or interest is another potential cause of sexual dysfunction. Changes, either an increase or decrease, may be related to adverse effects of medication, psychological reactions to the health problem, or infarction or limbic system structures. Since the temporal lobe is often affected by occlusive disorders and the hypothalamus is damaged after rupture of an aneurysm around the circle of Willis, dysfunction of these limbic areas may be a more common cause of sexual problems than is usually suspected.

Changes in a person's sexual roles and identity almost always occur after a cerebral insult. The ability to perform one's role as a spouse, partner, or parent may be impaired as well as one's perception of oneself as a male or female. These roles and identities may be altered by neurological deficits affecting the patient's competence in self-care, mobility, and social activities. Actual changes in a person's appearance from the neurological deficits or medications (*e.g.,* steroids and Dilantin may have masculinizing effects) may hinder one's sexual identify as will the attitudes of other people. After a stroke, people are often perceived and treated as a child or victim with their sexual needs and capabilities overlooked.

Assessment of sexual function also includes baseline data regarding a patient's previous sexuality, sociocultural norms, developmental levels, and age. Age is important to consider since cerebral ischemia or infarction may affect any age-group, but the resultant sexual concerns and norms will vary among the different ages.

If a potential or actual sexual dysfunction has been identified, the effect of this on a person's daily life must then be evaluated. This is often difficult in the acute care setting, with subjective information primarily being obtained from the patient or family. The information, however, may serve as a guide for planning interventions and referring the patient to appropriate professionals and community resources.

Goal. The goal and extent of nursing management of sexual dysfunction will vary more so than other patient problems depending on the etiology of the infarction, the acuity of the patient's condition, and the type of facility. Basic goals that should be addressed for all patients and families include allowing the patient or family to express sexual concerns and promoting sexual health and a positive self-concept.[81] If specific sexual concerns or problems are identified, a nurse knowledgeable and comfortable talking about sexuality may address these or refer the patient to a therapist or psychologist. The goal of management is then directed at assisting the patient to maintain or attain satisfactory and enjoyable sexual expression and behavior.

Interventions

A helpful and important nursing intervention is to "give permission" to the patient and family to talk about sexual concerns.[81] It is important not to project one's own values or concerns at this time. Promoting general sexual health may involve teaching about the effect of the patient's health problem on sexuality, as well as his need for sexual expression to maintain health. Specific teaching may be needed about appropriate contraception in young females (*e.g.,* avoiding the birth control pill after a subarachnoid hemorrhage) and prevention of infections to which they may be more susceptible, especially if they are on steroids. A positive self-concept may be fostered by acknowledging the person's maleness or femaleness in a respectful manner, utilizing the person's appropriate name, treating the person in an adult manner, and providing privacy. Anticipatory guidance regarding possible problem areas and available resources helps decrease anxiety and promote positive coping strategies.

For specific disturbances in sexual expression and behavior, many alternatives are feasible. Often suggestions on different positions for sexual intercourse, which will decrease interference from a catheter, ease mobility, or enhance pleasure, are all that is needed. Before any specific suggestions are made, however, the physician should first be consulted about the effect of the activity on the patient's health and suggested limitations. If a patient has an unclipped aneurysm or arteriovenous malformation, he will probably be advised against resuming sexual intercourse for a while, or different positions or methods of sexual expression will be suggested. The exact length of time and type of restrictions depend primarily on the severity of the cerebral insult, the integrity of the cerebral circulation, and cardiovascular status. If adverse effects of medications are interfering with functioning, the physician should be consulted regarding a change in drugs. If depression or complex sexual concerns are present, counseling should be encouraged. The reader as well as patients are referred to the book *Toward Intimacy* (see Suggested Readings at the end of this chapter), which focuses on family planning and sexual concerns of disabled women.

Evaluation

The most important outcome criteria is that the patient and family have the opportunity to express and feel comfortable about expressing sexual concerns and their influence on daily life. Effectiveness of teaching and anticipatory guidance may be evaluated by the patient's and family's ability to relate potential and actual problem areas, limitations or restrictions imposed by the health problem, and available resources for counseling or assistance. Evaluating a person's sexual self-concept is difficult in the hospital setting. One often has to depend on subjective statements from the patient as to how he perceives himself or herself; however, observation of a patient's interactions with family, friends, or staff may elicit subtle discrepancies. It is important to remember that the development of a positive sexual self-concept after a severe cerebral injury will take time, and the nurse should not expect attainment of this during the acute hospitalization.

Ineffective Coping Strategies

Nursing Assessment

The term *coping* refers to the strategies a person utilizes to adapt to a physiological or psychological problem or change.[44] From previous sections of this Chapter, it is obvious that there are many potential problem areas and changes that occur after a cerebral ischemic episode or infarction. Patients have to cope with the acute change in their health status and the possibility of death and to learn new strategies to cope with residual neurological dysfunctions. A person's coping strategies are effective as long as the person perceives that the strategies bring him relief. When the strategies do not do this, and the resultant problem or change is impairing the person's ability to function in daily life, the coping strategies are considered inadequate.

Manifestations of ineffective coping are varied and may include physiological changes (*e.g.,* tachycardia, hypertension, sweating, anorexia, or insomnia); inappropriate or exaggerated behavioral responses (*e.g.,* agitation or uncontrolled anger); or emotional reactions of anxiety, fear, or depression.

Assessment of a patient's coping abilities involves evaluation of current stressors (*i.e.,* problems or changes) and resources, both internal and external, that the patient utilizes to cope with the stressors. Knowledge of a patient's previous methods of coping, sociocultural influences and values, and age and developmental level are necessary, since these factors will influence the patient's perceptions and reactions to current situations.

Problems or changes arising after a cerebral insult may be assessed in relation to how they affect a patient's basic needs. Utilizing Maslow's hierarchy of needs one can easily see how all basic needs may be altered or unmet.[42] Basic physiological needs (*e.g.,* need for oxygen, circulation, nutrition, elimination, and so on) may be altered directly from the cerebral ischemic episode or infarction, its complications, or preexisting risk factors. Safety may be impaired with any mobility problem, seizures, sensory deficits, or spatial–

perceptual problems. The need for love or belonging may be unmet because of sexual dysfunction, social isolation, or discrimination. Self-esteem may be impaired from any loss or change in one's body image, roles and relationships, and level of independence and from the attitudes of others.

If any of the above needs are unmet, a patient's ability to pursue self-fulfillment or self-actualization will be hindered; this latter need is also affected by cognitive deficits. If basic needs are altered or unmet, demands on a patient's daily life are increased, requiring more resources and coping strategies.

External resources must be assessed for their availability and capability of providing assistance to the patient. The most important resource is support and assistance from family, friends, and community agencies. Overs and Healy emphasize the need to view the patient in relation to the family unit and resultant changes in roles after a cerebral infarction.[56] Values and beliefs concerning one's role within a family and society, however, are very difficult to change, particularly in elderly patients whose values are determined by traditions (*i.e.,* the male as provider and the female as caretaker of the family). The authors stressed the need to supplement family supports to aid adaptation rather than try to change such values or beliefs.

DeJong in a study of 84 patients with strokes also recognized the need for family and additional supports.[15] He found that the most important predictor of a patient's ability to live independently was marital status; that is, married patients had a greater chance of living in a less restricted environment. Financial resources, the availability of barrier-free housing and transportation, and adaptive aids or equipment are also considered external supports that assist patients to cope with neurological dysfunctions. DeJong also found that the most important predictor of a patient's ability to have a productive lifestyle was the ability to get into a motor vehicle.[15] Thus, this should be included in mobility training, and alternative means of transportation should be examined.

When assessing a patient's internal resources and abilities to cope with change, emotional responses and behavior are most easily evaluated. Behavioral strategies may be categorized as methods of avoiding, circumventing, or confronting a situation or change.[44] It is important to remember, however, that any emotional or behavioral response is dependent on brain function. The manner in which the body responds to a change of stress is dependent on integration of incoming sensory stimuli, arousal mechanisms in the brain stem, cortical areas for perception and interpretation of stimuli, the limbic system for emotional reactions, the hypothalamic–pituitary axis for autonomic and endocrine responses, and the motor system for reflex and voluntary reactions to the stimuli. Ischemia or infarction of any of these brain areas may affect a patient's ability to adapt to a change or stress. Stimuli may not be perceived, arousal may not be activated, interpretations of stimuli may be distorted or lost, or responses may be exaggerated or inappropriate to the situation.

Impairments of consciousness, sensation, and movement are most readily identified as factors hindering a patient's internal coping mechanisms. However cognitive, behavioral, or emotional impairments are just as important. If a patient has difficulty interpreting incoming stimuli or controlling his responses, he may become easily confused or agitated when faced with a sudden change or stress. If the patient is left in the presence of the stimulus, behavior may deteriorate with inappropriate or exaggerated responses.

Chronic adaptation to changes or problems may also be severely impaired with cognitive, behavioral, or emotional disabilities. Learning new techniques to compensate for impaired functional abilities will be difficult in the presence of memory deficits, decreased attention and concentration, impaired judgment, insight, and problem-solving abilities. Denial, which may be identified as a behavioral coping strategy to avoid a stressful situation, may also be a manifestation of right parietal lobe damage. The occurrence of depression, which may be a response to a change or loss, may also be related to brain damage or medications. Clinical depressions have occurred more frequently in patients with left hemispheric infarctions, suggesting a structural rather than situational cause of the depression in these patients.[62] Any of these deficits may limit or prevent a patient from utilizing past coping strategies or learning new ones to adapt to the neurological disorder.

Goal. The goal of nursing management for the patient with actual or potential ineffective coping strategies is to assist the patient and family to maintain or attain a balance between demands on daily life and available resources. Effective coping is attained when the patient perceives that his coping strategies bring him relief. When this does not occur, nursing management is directed at helping the patient attain more effective coping strategies and strengthen external resources. When the cerebral insult has altered a patient's internal coping abilities, nursing management should also be directed at teaching the patient and family methods of compensating for the impaired functions.

Interventions

Factors that influence demands on daily life should be removed, corrected, or minimized whenever possible. The first priorities in the acute phase are to address basic physiological needs and maintain safety. Long-term safety and security needs should be identified as early as possible because they will influence a patient's ability for self-care, his level of independence, and his predisposition after hospitalization. Management of any problems affecting love, belonging, and self-esteem are more difficult; they require a multidisciplinary approach and close family involvement. Referral to a social worker or psychologist is usually helpful for counseling to address specific problem areas.

When external resources, particularly family supports, are lacking, it is necessary to mobilize additional support from friends, neighbors, or community agencies (*e.g.,* stroke clubs). The spouse or care-giver in the home should be involved in all care in order to learn how to assist the patient to live in a less restricted home environment. Referral to vocational and financial assistance programs should be made when a patient's job capabilities or income is affected. Rehabilitation programs and home health care agencies may provide additional supports so that a patient may live independently. If these supports are inadequate, alternative care facilities, such as chronic care hospitals or nursing homes, may be needed.

If the patient's internal resources to cope with change or stress are impaired from the cerebral insult, the nurse has to provide assistance, structure, or take over for the impaired functions. For patients with impaired consciousness or sensation, this is done by sensing changes or threats to his safety, taking action to protect the patient from injury, or correcting the problem for him. If the patient has cognitive, emotional, or behavioral disturbances, management is more difficult. The nurse must provide external structure and control to compensate for the patient's lack of internal control. This can be done by structuring a patient's environment and daily routines to minimize sudden changes or confusion. Conversation is also structured, particularly with a patient who has difficulty interpreting stimuli or feelings. In this case, changes or stimuli should be acknowledged and interpreted for the patient, and open-ended questions should be avoided. Stimuli that precipitate inappropriate or exaggerated behavior should be identified and avoided whenever possible. When a patient is unable to control his behavior or feelings, he must be removed or distracted from the stimulus or situation. Once the patient has calmed down, the inappropriate responses may be discussed and more effective coping strategies promoted. (See previous section Impaired Thought Processes.)

Most patients will benefit from counseling to help adapt to the many changes and stresses. The effectiveness and type of counseling, however, depends on the nature of the cognitive, emotional, or behavioral impairments. It is best if counseling is practical in orientation, rather than insight-oriented, when a patient does not have the cognitive abilities necessary for analysis. Behavioral modification programs may help promote effective coping strategies and discourage inappropriate responses. Teaching the family how to provide structure for the patient and control his behavior is vital to maintain consistency and ensure effectiveness of the techniques. It is important to recognize the strain this places on family members. They have to adapt to and accept the changes in the patient, as well as subsequent changes in family dynamics and roles. Family counseling should be stressed as an integral part of any rehabilitation program.

Evaluation

The desired outcome is that the patient and family will maintain or attain adequate resources, both internal and external, to cope with the demands of daily life. This can be evaluated by observing the way that the patient responds to a change or problem. Effective coping strategies should bring subjective and objective relief to the patient and not impair his safety. The patient and family should be able to identify factors that increase demands on daily life and know how to remove or minimize them. They should be aware of limitations in external resources and know how to supplement these with community support. If the patient's internal coping abilities are impaired, both the patient and family should be able to identify factors that hinder coping and demonstrate methods of avoiding these or compensating for impaired functions. To evaluate the effectiveness of teaching, patient–family interactions should be observed in the hospital and at home if possible.

Effectiveness of nursing management is further evaluated by the patient's objective and subjective abilities to manage in a home environment as demonstrated by the degree of compentence in self-care abilities, mobility, and social functions. The patient may be dependent on adaptive aids or another person, yet the accomplishment of these activities in as independent a setting as possible is the desired goal of any rehabilitative process.

Summary

Cerebral ischemia and infarctions may potentially alter all human functions, and they have a significant risk of morbidity and death. Advances in medical treatment have decreased mortality rates, but residual neurological dysfunctions still interfere with all aspects of daily life. The overall outcome is often an enforced dependency on objects or other people. Adaptation to such an outcome is extremely difficult for many people; it requires extensive teaching and support beginning immediately after the insult.

Many potential problem areas have been presented in this chapter. All of these problems will not occur for every patient, but some may experience additional problems to those reviewed here. Nursing care of these people is complex, requiring integration of acute care and rehabilitative knowledge and skills, patience, and understanding. With this care, many people can adapt to their disorder and attain a functional and rewarding life.

References

1. Adams HP Jr, Nibbelink DW, Torner JC, Sahs AL: Antifibrinolytic therapy in patients with aneurysmal subarachnoid hemorrhage. In Sahs AL, Nibbelink DW, Torner JC (eds): Aneurysmal Subarachnoid Hemorrhage—Report of the Cooperative Study, p 331. Baltimore, Urban and Schwarzenberg, 1981
2. Ball PM: Preventing stroke through noninvasive carotid artery assessment. J Neurosurg Nurs 14(4):182, 1982
3. Bardach JL: Psychological considerations in hemiplegia. In Cobb AB (ed): Medical and Psychological Aspects of Disability, p 71. Springfield IL, Charles C Thomas, 1973
4. Barnett HJM: Medical management of cerebral transient ischemic attacks. In Meyer JS, Shaw TS (eds): Diagnosis and Management of Stroke and TIAS, p 123. Reading MA, Addison-Wesley Publishing Co, 1982
5. Baum PL: Carotid endarterectomy—one strike against stroke. Nursing 83 13(3):50, 1983
6. Berman JA, Halpern A, Shaftel N et al: The cerebrovascular dynamics of bowel function. Angiology 11:437, 1960
7. Boddy J: Brain Systems and Psychological Concepts, p 211. New York, John Wiley & Sons, 1978
8. Booth K: The neglect syndrome. J Neurosurg Nurs 14(1):38, 1982
9. Carney AL, Anderson EM: The system approach to brain blood flow. In Carney AL, Anderson EM (eds): Diagnosis and Treat-

ment of Brain Ischemia, Advances in Neurology, vol. 30. New York, Raven Press, 1981

10. Chusid JG: Correlative Neuroanatomy and Functional Neurology, 17th ed, p 305. Los Altos CA, Lange Medical Publications, 1979
11. Cohen RJ, Allen GS: Effects of subarachnoid blood and spasmodic agents on cerebral vasculature. In Wilkins R (ed): Cerebral Arterial Spasm, p 287. Baltimore, Williams & Wilkins, 1980
12. Connel AM, Hilton C, Irvine G et al: Variation of bowel habit in two population samples. Br Med J 2:1095, 1965
13. Crowell RM, Zervas NT: Management of intracranial aneurysms. Med Clin North Am 63(4):695, 1979
14. Debrun G, Fox AJ: Interventional neuroradiology in the treatment of cerebral aneurysms. In Hopkins LN, Long DM (eds): Clinical Management of Intracranial Aneurysms, p 273. New York, Raven Press, 1982
15. DeJong G, Branch LG: Predicting the stroke patient's ability to live independently. Stroke 13(5):648, 1982
16. Doshi R, Neil-Dwyer G: A clinicopathological study of patients following a subarachnoid hemorrhage. J Neurosurg 52:295, 1980
17. Drury I, Whisnant JP, Garraway WM: Primary intracerebral hemorrhage: Impact of CT on incidence. Neurology 34(5):653, 1984
18. Fein JM: Preoperative vasospasm: Diagnosis and treatment. In Hopkins LN, Long DM (eds): Clinical Management of Intracranial Aneurysms, p 111. New York, Raven Press, 1982
19. Ferguson GG: Physical factors in the initiation, growth, and rupture of human intracranial saccular aneurysms. J Neurosurg 37:666, 1972
20. Fisher CM, Robertson GH, Ojemann RG: Cerebral vasospasm with ruptured saccular aneurysm—the clinical manifestations. Neurosurgery 1(3):245, 1977
21. Flamm, ES: Antifibrinolysis and the preoperative management of subarachnoid hemorrhage. In Hopkins LN, Long DM (eds): Clinical Management of Intracranial Aneurysms, p 49. New York, Raven Press, 1982
22. Garraway W, Whisnant JP, Furkin AJ et al: The declining incidence of stroke. New Engl J Med 300:449, 1979
23. Graf CJ, Torner JC, Perret GE, Nibbelink DW: Cooperative aneurysm study. Long-term follow-up evaluation of randomized study. In Sahs AL, Nibbelink DW, Torner JC (eds): Aneurysmal Subarachnoid Hemorrhage—Report of the Cooperative Study, p 203. Baltimore, Urban and Schwarzenberg, 1981
24. Grand W: Preoperative blood pressure in the aneurysm patient. In Hopkins LN, Long DM (eds): Clinical Management of Intracranial Aneurysms, p 29. New York, Raven Press, 1982
25. Gresham GE, Phillips TF, Wolf PA et al: Epidemiologic profile of long-term stroke disability: Framingham study. Arch Phys Med Rehabil 60(11):487, 1979
26. Grubb RL Jr: Cerebral hemodynamics and metabolism in subarachnoid hemorrhage. In Hopkins LN, Long DM (eds): Clinical Management of Intracranial Aneurysms, p 163. New York, Raven Press, 1982
27. Halpern A, Shaftel N, Selman D, Birch HG: The cardiovascular dynamics of bowel function. Angiology 11:99, 1960
28. Halpern A, Shaftel N, Selman D et al: The straining forces of bowel function. Angiology 11:426, 1960
29. Heros RC: Cerebellar hemorrhage and infarction. Stroke 13(1):106, 1982
30. Heros RC, Zervas NT, Negoro M: Cerebral vasospasm. Surg Neurol 5:354, 1976
31. Heyman A, Wilkinson WE, Hurwitz BJ et al: Risk of ischemic heart disease in patients with TIA. Neurology 34(5):626, 1984
32. Hopkins LN: Postoperative management of the aneurysm patient. In Hopkins LN, Long DM (eds): Clinical Management of Intracranial Aneurysms, p 295. New York, Raven Press, 1982
33. Hunter, C: Nursing problems of patients undergoing aminocaproic acid treatment for subarachnoid hemorrhage due to aneurysm. J Neurosurg Nurs 11(3):160, 1979
34. Jane JA, Winn HR, Richardson AE: The natural history of intracranial aneurysms: Rebleeding rates during the acute and long-term period and implication for surgical management. Clin Neurosurg 24:176, 1977
35. Jankovic J: Differential diagnosis of stroke. In Meyer JS, Shaw TS (eds): Diagnosis and Management of Stroke and TIAS, p 77. Reading MA, Addison-Wesley Publishing Co, 1982
36. Larsen, GL: Chewing and swallowing. In Martin N, Hoh NB, Hicks D (eds): Comprehensive Rehabilitation Nursing, p 173. New York, McGraw-Hill, 1981
37. Lee K: Aneurysm precautions: A physiologic basis for minimizing rebleeding. Heart Lung 9(2):336, 1980
38. Lee K: Rest and comfort status. In Mitchell PM, Loustau A (eds): Concepts Basic to Nursing, 3rd ed, p 603. New York, McGraw-Hill, 1981
39. Levinthal R: Neurosurgical management of cerebral transient ischemic attacks and subarachnoid hemorrhage. In Meyer JS, Shaw TS (eds): Diagnosis and Management of Stroke and TIA, p 208. Reading MA, Addison-Wesley Publishing Co, 1982
40. Locksley HB: Natural history of subarachnoid hemorrhage, intracranial aneurysms, and arteriovenous malformations. In Sahs AL, Perret GE, Locksley HB, Nishioka H (eds): Intracranial Aneurysms and Subarachnoid Hemorrhage, p 37. Philadelphia, JB Lippincott, 1969
41. Martelli H, Deveroede G, Arhan P et al: Alimentary tract: Some parameters of large bowel motility in normal men. Gastroenterology 75:612, 1978
42. Maslow A: A theory of human motivation. Psychol Rev 50:370, 1943
43. Meyer JS: Course, prognosis, and medical management of patients with acute stroke. In Meyer JS, Shaw TS (eds): Diagnosis and Management of Stroke and TIA, p 156. Reading MA, Addison-Wesley Publishing Co, 1982
44. Mitchell PH: Psychosocial and mental-emotional status. In Mitchell PM, Loustau A (eds): Concepts Basic to Nursing, 3rd ed, p 223. New York, McGraw-Hill, 1981
45. Mitchell PH: Sensory status. In Mitchell PM, Loustau A (eds): Concepts Basic to Nursing, 3rd ed, p 309. New York, McGraw-Hill, 1981
46. Mitchell PH, Mauss NK: Relationship of patient-nurse activity to intracranial pressure variations: A pilot study. Nurs Res 27(1):4, 1978
47. Mohr JP, Caplan LR, Melski JW et al: Harvard cooperative stroke registry: A prospective registry of patients hospitalized with stroke. Neurology 28:754, 1978
48. Mullan S: Conservative treatment of the recently ruptured aneurysm. Surg Neurol 3:27, 1975
49. Muuronen A, Kaste M: Outcome of 314 patients with transient ischemic attacks. Stroke 13:24, 1982
50. Nibbelink DW: Antihypertensive and antifibrinolytic therapy following subarachnoid hemorrhage from ruptured intracranial aneurysm. In Sahs AD, Nibbelink DW, Torner JC (eds): Aneurysmal Subarachnoid Hemorrhage—Report of the Cooperative Study, p 287. Baltimore, Urban and Schwarzenberg, 1981
51. Nibbelink DW, Torner JC, Henderson WG: Antifibrinolytic therapy in recent onset subarachnoid hemorrhage. In Sahs AL, Nibbelink DW, Torner JC (eds): Aneurysmal Subarachnoid Hemorrhage—Report of the Cooperative Study, p 297. Baltimore, Urban and Schwarzenberg, 1981
52. Nibbelink DW, Torner JC, Henderson WG: Randomized treatment study—Regulated bedrest. In Sahs AL, Nibbelink DW, Torner JC (eds): Aneurysmal Subarachnoid Hemorrhage—Report of the Cooperative Study, p 27. Baltimore, Urban and Schwarzenberg, 1981

53. Nornes H, Magnaes B: Intracranial pressure in patients with ruptured saccular aneurysms. J Neurosurg 36:537, 1972
54. O'Brien MT, Pallett PJ: Total Care of the Stroke Patient. Boston MA, Little, Brown & Co, 1978
55. Osaka K, Handa H, Okamoto S: Subarachnoid erythrocytes and their contribution to cerebral vasospasm. In Wilkins R (ed): Cerebral Arterial Spasm, p 313. Baltimore, Williams & Wilkins, 1980
56. Overs RP, Healy JR: Stroke patients: Their spouses, families and the community. In Cobb AB (ed): Medical and Psychological Aspects of Disability, p 87. Springfield IL, Charles C Thomas, 1973
57. Parkarinen S: Incidence, etiology, and prognosis of primary subarachnoid hemorrhage: A study based on 584 cases diagnosed in a defined urban population during a defined period. Acta Neurol Scand 43 (Suppl 29):1, 1967
58. Peck, S: Calcium blocking agents for treatment of cerebral vasospasm. J Neurosurg Nurs 15(3):123, 1983
59. Post KD, Flamm ES, Goodgold A, Ransohoff J: Ruptured intracranial aneurysms—case morbidity and mortality. J Neurosurg 46:290, 1977
60. Ransohoff J, Goodgold A, Benjamin MV: Preoperative management of patients with ruptured intracranial aneurysms. J Neurosurg 36:525, 1972
61. Richardson K: Right brain–left brain: The nurse consultant and behavior change following stroke. JPNMHS 20(5):37, 1982
62. Robinson RG, Price TR: Post-stroke depressive disorders: A follow-up study of 103 patients. Stroke 13(5):635, 1982
63. Sahs AL: Observations on the pathology of saccular aneurysms. In Sahs AL, Perret GE, Locksley HB, Nishioka H (eds): Intracranial Aneurysms and Subarachnoid Hemorrhage, p 24. Philadelphia, JB Lippincott, 1969
64. Saito I, Sano K: Vasospasm following rupture of cerebral aneurysms. Neurol Med Chir (Tokyo) 19:103, 1979
65. Seiden MR: Practical Management of Chronic Neurologic Problems, p 197. New York, Appleton-Century Crofts, 1981
66. Shalit MN, Umansky F: Effect of routine bedside procedures on intracranial pressure. Isr J Med Sci 13(9):881, 1977
67. Shapiro HM: Intracranial hypertension: Therapeutic and anesthetic considerations. Anesthesiology 43(4):445, 1975
68. Shaw CM, Alvord EC Jr, Berry RG: Swelling of the brain following ischemic infarction with arterial occlusion. Arch Neurol 1:161, 1959
69. Shaw T, Meyer J: Aging and cerebrovascular disease. In Meyer JS, Shaw T (eds): Diagnosis and Management of Stroke and TIA, p 1 Reading MA, Addison-Wesley Publishing Co, 1982
70. Spetzler RF, Selman WR: Barbiturate-induced coma for the treatment of subarachnoid hemorrhage. In Hopkins LN, Long DM (eds): Clinical Management of Intracranial Aneurysms, p 155. New York, Raven Press, 1982
71. Strub RL, Black FW: Organic Brain Syndromes, p 213. Philadelphia, FA Davis, 1981
72. US Department of Health Education and Welfare: National Survey of Stroke, NIH Publication No. 80-2069. Washington DC, US Government Printing Office, 1980
73. Waga S, Ohtsubo K, Handa H: Warning signs in intracranial aneurysms. Surg Neurol 3:15, 1975
74. Weir B, Grace M, Hansen J, Rothberg C: Time course of vasospasm in man. J Neurosurg 48:173, 1978
75. Wilkins RH: Hypothalamic dysfunction and intracranial arterial spasms. Surg Neurol 4:472, 1975
76. Wilkins RH: Multiple aneurysms and associated arteriovenous malformations: Operative considerations. In Hopkins LN, Long DM (eds): Clinical Management of Intracranial Aneurysms, p 193. New York, Raven Press, 1982
77. Wilkins RH: The pathogenesis and pathophysiology of intracranial arterial spasm and its role in the timing of operations for aneurysm. In Hopkins LN, Long DM (eds): Clinical Management of Intracranial Aneurysms, p 101. New York, Raven Press, 1982
78. Winn HR, Richardson AE, Jane JA: The assessment of the natural history of single cerebral aneurysms that have ruptured. In Hopkins LN, Long DM (eds): Clinical Management of Intracranial Aneurysms, p 1. New York, Raven Press, 1982
79. Winn HR, Richardson AE, O'Brien W, Jane JA: The long-term prognosis in untreated cerebral aneurysms. II. Late morbidity and mortality. Ann Neurol 4(5):418, 1978
80. Wolf P, Kannel W: Controllable risk factors for stroke: Preventive implications of trends in stroke mortality. In Meyer JS, Shaw TS (eds): Diagnosis and Management of Stroke and TIA, p 25. Reading MA, Addison-Wesley Publishing Co, 1982
81. Woods NF: Sexuality status. In Mitchell PM, Loustau A (eds): Concepts Basic to Nursing, 3rd ed, p 265. New York, McGraw-Hill 1981
82. Zervas NT, Kistler J, Ploetz J: Effect of reserpine and kanamycin on postoperative delayed ischemic deficits in patients with subarachnoid hemorrhage after aneurysm rupture. In Wilkins R (ed): Cerebral Artery Spasm, p 514. Baltimore, Williams & Wilkins, 1980

Bibliography

Benoliel JQ, McCorkle R, Young K: Development of a social dependency scale. Research in Nursing and Health 3:3, 1980

Boss BJ: Dysphasia, dyspraxia and dysarthria: Distinguishing features, Part I. J Neurosurg Nurs 16(3):151, 1984

Dix PE, Ridder ME: The adolescent with a stroke. J Neurosurg Nurs 15(2):80, 1983

Finch K: Vasospasm secondary to subarachnoid hemorrhage: The current controversy, research, and nursing dilemmas. J Neurosurg Nurs 12(4):199, 1980

Fode NC, Laws ER, Sundt MT Jr: Communicating hydrocephalus after subarachnoid hemorrhage: Results of shunt procedures. J Neurosurg Nurs 11(4):253, 1979

Fordyce WE, Jones RH: The efficacy of oral and pantomime instructions for hemiplegic patients. Arch Phys Med Rehabil 47:676, 1966

Franco LM: Syndrome of inappropriate secretion of antidiuretic hormone. J Neurosurg Nurs 14(5):276, 1982

Galbraith SL: Management of patients with subarachnoid hemorrhage. Nursing Times, October 25:1852, 1979

Gerk MK, Kassell NF: Cerebral vasospasm: Update and implications. J Neurosurg Nurs 12(2):66, 1980

Geschwind N: Specializations of the human brain. Sci Am 241(3):180, 1979

Grabois M: Rehabilitation of patients with completed stroke. In Meyer JS, Shaw TS (eds): Diagnosis and Management of Stroke and TIAs, p 267. Reading MA, Addison-Wesley Publishing Co, 1982

Katzman R, Terry R: Normal aging of the nervous system. In Katzman R, Terry RD (eds): The Neurology of Aging. Philadelphia, FA Davis, 1983

Leonberg SC, Elliott FH: Prevention of recurrent stroke. Stroke 12(6):731, 1981

Malone PE, Whitehead JM: Speech and language rehabilitation following stroke. In Meyer JS, Shaw TS (eds): Diagnosis and Management of Stroke and TIA, p 292. Reading MA, Addison-Wesley Publishing Co, 1982

Norman S: Diagnostic categories for the patient with a right hemisphere lesion. Am J Nurs 79(12):2126, 1979

Raizner AE: Cardiologic considerations in managing patients with stroke. In Meyer JS, Shaw TS (eds): Diagnosis and Management of Stroke and TIA, p 237. Reading MA, Addison-Wesley Publishing Co, 1982

Sawitzke S, Teter A: Arteriovenous malformations of the brain. General review including role of embolization. J Neurosurg Nurs 8(2):132, 1976

Taylor S, Ballenger S: Neurologic Dysfunctions and Nursing Interventions. New York, McGraw-Hill, 1980

Zegeer LJ: Nursing care of the patient with brain edema. J Neurosurg Nurs 14(5):268–275, 1982

Suggested Readings for Patient and Family

Books

Task Force on Concerns of Physically Disabled Women. Toward Intimacy. Snohomish County, Washington, Planned Parenthood, 1977

Pamphlets

American Heart Association National Center, 7320 Greenville Avenue, Dallas, Texas 75231

- Aphasia and the Family
- Body Language
- Do It Yourself Again—Self-Help Devices for the Stroke Patient
- Fact Sheet on Heart Attack, Stroke, and Risk Factors
- Low Sodium Cookbook (Massachusetts Affiliate of American Heart Assoc)
- Recipes for Fat-Controlled Low Cholesterol Meats
- Stand Up to Stroke
- Strike Back at Stroke
- Strokes—A Guide for the Family
- Stroke—Why Do They Behave That Way?
- Up and Around—A Booklet to Aid the Stroke Patient in Activities of Daily Living

Chapter 67

Intracranial and Spinal Cord Tumors

Marci-Lee Catanzaro

The word *neoplasm* implies an abnormal growth of cells. The proliferation of cells may be benign or malignant and may infiltrate nervous system tissue, causing widespread destruction of neurons and supportive structures. Because nerve cells in the central nervous system do not normally regenerate, destruction of cells by tumor infiltration or compromise of their normal function has permanent sequelae.

Tumors in the nervous system may be classified in a variety of ways. Some of the more common classification systems include

- The type of cells from which the tumor arises
- The level of the nervous system involved
- The relationship of the tumor to the dura
- Whether the tumor is primary or secondary

The location of the tumor within the nervous system is the most important determinant of the functional deficit that the patient will experience.

Etiology

The etiology of symptoms attributed to nervous system dysfunction result from compression or destruction of normal neural tissue and from chemical alterations in these cells. For example, symptoms of central nervous system neoplasia result when tumors destroy the tissues in which they are situated, displace and compress tissues around them, or alter metabolism of the cells. The space-occupying properties of tumors may cause an increase in intracranial pressure by obstructing vascular flow, by obstructing the reabsorption of the cerebrospinal fluid, and by increasing the intracranial contents by their very presence.

Neurological disturbances of movement, sensation, consciousness, mentation, and integrated regulation are determined by the size, location, and the invasive qualities of the abnormal cell growth. The ability of the patient to cope with the resulting disruptions to daily living will depend on the extent of the loss and the remaining resources available to adjust to changes. Treatment of tumors may further compromise the functional ability of the individual as chemotherapy, radiation, or surgery affects normal cells.

Tumors of the central nervous system account for greater than 2% of annual cancer deaths. It is estimated that there are 13,700 new cases of primary central nervous system tumors annually. These tumors account for about 10,000 deaths each year.[3] Secondary or metastatic brain tumors contribute significantly to mortality and morbidity from neoplasia. Of all persons who die of cancer, 22% have intracranial metastases at the time of autopsy; however, Adams and Victor pointed out that autopsy is not always done and often does not include the brain, resulting in artificially low estimates.[1]

It is estimated that there are 4,000 new spinal cord tumors diagnosed annually. Most of these tumors are benign;

however, significant morbidity and residual disability often result.

Intracranial Tumors

Pathophysiology

The symptoms that result from an intracranial tumor are a function of certain principles of physics and physiology. The cranial vault has a restricted volume that is occupied by brain tissue, blood, and cerebrospinal fluid. The Monro-Kellie hypothesis states that the bulk of these elements must be constant, and that any increase in one element must be at the expense of one or more of the others. A tumor growing in one part of the brain must displace blood, cerebrospinal fluid, or both. The first response to tumor growth is for cerebrospinal fluid to be displaced to the spinal and the perioptic subarachnoid space. Increased fluid in the perioptic subarachnoid space compromises venous drainage and is manifest by papilledema or "choked disks." Papilledema appears through an ophthalmoscope as a blurred or elevated optic disc. This appearance is caused by edema at the point where the optic nerve enters the eyeball. As brain tissue adjacent to the tumor is compressed by the expanding lesion, capillary pressure and permeability are increased and the blood–brain barrier is weakened. Plasma enters the extracellular space to produce a vasogenic type of cerebral edema that is confined to cerebral white matter. This type of edema develops rapidly and further increases the intracranial contents. As compensatory mechanisms fail, intracranial pressure increases and may progress to brain herniation.

Classification and Etiology

Statistics on the types of intracranial tumor are difficult to obtain. *Glioblastoma multiforme,* which includes malignant glioma and astrocytoma grades III and IV, are the most common central nervous system tumors in adults and account for 50% of all primary brain tumors. Glioblastoma multiforme are rapidly growing and uniformly fatal with a median survival of 8 to 9 months. They occur most commonly in the cerebrum in people between the ages of 40 and 60 years. Gliomas account for about one quarter of spinal cord tumors and occur in a host who is an average of 38 years of age.[3]

Meningiomas are the second most common type of intracranial tumor. Persons in the fifth decade of life are most likely to develop this type of brain tumor. The prognosis for the person with a meningioma is generally more favorable and is dependent on its location and the extent of excision. Approximately 60% of meningiomas can be cured with complete tumor removal. Meningiomas and schwannomas account for 56% of spinal cord tumors and occur most often in the thoracic segment.[3]

Pituitary adenomas account for 12% to 18% of intracranial tumors. They are almost never malignant and often asymptomatic. Manifestations of these tumors are frequently endocrine disorders secondary to abnormal hormone secretion.

There are no known causes of human gliomas. Most childhood tumors are considered to be developmental in origin. Meningiomas are associated with chromosome 22 abnormalities, and retinoblastomas have a significant hereditary component. It is estimated that as high as 40% of brain tumors are metastatic. The primary tumor is most often in the lung, breast, or kidney. Metastatic lesions to the spinal cord are from the breast and lung. The incidence of metastatic disease is steadily increasing. Reasons for this include increasing incidence of lung cancer, increasing age of the population, and increased survival of persons with cancer.

Evidence of metastatic lesions in the brain are an ominous sign in neoplastic disease. Posner has reported that the median survival for nontreated brain metastasis is approximately 1 month.[8] Treatment with adrenocorticosteroids alleviate symptoms but prolong survival by only 2 months. Total brain irradiation and surgical resection of the tumor increase median survival to a maximum of 6 months.

The age of the individual is an important factor in the biology of brain tumors. The incidence of central nervous system tumors is significantly greater in children than adults. The most common tumors in children are the medulloblastoma and brain stem gliomas.[7] Oligodendrogliomas occur most often in the cerebral hemisphere of young adults. Meningiomas and glioblastomas have the highest incidence around age 50. Heredity plays a significant role in the development of retinoblastomas, neurofibromas, and hemangioblastomas.[1]

The type of tumor cell determines certain characteristics of the disease. A glioblastoma is an invasive and highly malignant tumor that progresses rapidly, whereas a meningioma is a benign tumor that is slowly progressive and produces its symptoms by compression.

Clinical Manifestations

The clinical manifestations of neoplastic changes in the nervous system are largely related to the portion of the nervous system from which the disorder arises (Fig. 67–1). Major

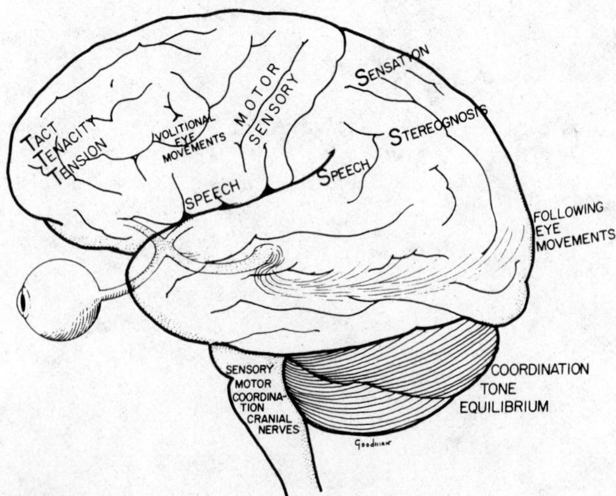

FIGURE 67–1 Functional significance of intracranial tumors of the cerebral cortex, cerebellum, and brain stem. (Hardy JD: Rhoads Textbook of Surgery, 5th ed. Philadelphia, JB Lippincott, 1977)

centers for the integration of motor activity are located in the frontal lobe of the cerebrum. A tumor in this area of the brain produces spastic weakness of the legs, disturbances of the bowel and bladder sphincters, and difficulty speaking secondary to motor involvement of the muscles of articulation. The parietal lobe controls sensation of light touch, two-point discrimination, stereognosis, and joint position. The occipital lobe controls visual reception. The temporal lobe plays a major role in the sensations of hearing, smell, taste, and vestibular functioning. A lesion in the temporal lobe may cause difficulty in interpreting sensations, olfactory or gustatory hallucinations, psychomotor seizures, or aphasia and dyslexia with right–left disorientation. The nuclei of cranial nerves III through XII are located in the brain stem. Neoplastic lesions in the brain stem will compromise the motor or sensory functions controlled by those nerves. For an overview of the signs and symptoms of cerebral neoplasia, see Table 67–1.

The cerebellum plays a major role in the coordination of muscular movement. The patient with a cerebellar tumor will exhibit misdirected or jerky movements, a tendency to fall or drift toward the affected side, and diminished tendon reflexes on the side of the tumor.

Medical Management

The most common type of brain tumor is the glioblastoma. The multicentricity and diffuse nature of this tumor makes complete surgical excision impossible. Radiotherapy and chemotherapy have been shown to increase survival rates; however, even with treatment, survival beyond 2 years is exceptional. Recently, combined treatment with surgery, chemotherapy, and radiation have resulted in increased mean survival time.

Nitrosoureas have been demonstrated to be the most effective drugs in the treatment of malignant gliomas. They increase the mean survival time from 35 to 45 weeks. Lomustine (CCNU) and carmustine (BCNU, BiCNU) are the nitrosoureas most commonly used in the treatment of gliomas.[5,9]

Surgical excision of astrocytomas and oligodendrogliomas have increased survival times. A significant number of patients have a recurrent oligodendroglioma within a few months of operation. Reticulum cell sarcoma and lymphoma are highly sensitive to radiotherapy, which extends survival for several years.

A meningioma that occurs on an accessible surface of the central nervous system can be cured by complete surgical excision. Carefully planned radiation is used when surgical excision is impossible or incomplete. Regardless of the treatment, meningioma tends to recur. The systemic and intra-arterial administration of chemotherapy combined with radiotherapy has been encouraging in the treatment of medulloblastoma. Approximately two thirds of the cases survive for 5 years.

Surgical excision followed by radiotherapy is used for a single site of metastatic carcinoma. Multiple metastases are treated with radiotherapy and steroids such as dexamethasone (Decadron), which are used to decrease cerebral edema associated with tumor growth. Treatment extends survival for an average of 6 months. Only 5% to 10% of people with central nervous system metastasis survive for 2 years.[1]

Nursing Interventions

One way in which the nurse can be instrumental in preventing further deterioration is by being alert to early signs and symptoms of intracranial lesions and encouraging medical evaluation. Headache in adults is an early sign of many tumors. This headache may be described as dull or sharp and as mild or severe. Headache is most prominent during sleep or on awakening, and it is believed to be caused by vasodilation secondary to decreased gravity drainage associated with the recumbent position and with a buildup of CO_2.[2] The patient may experience vomiting with or without

TABLE 67–1
Signs and Symptoms of Cerebral Neoplasia

Location	*Function*	*Signs and Symptoms*
Frontal lobes	Integrated regulation Mentation Movement	Muscle weakness Bowel/bladder disturbances Impaired memory and judgment Emotional lability Non-fluent aphasia Tactile, position, and vibratory sensation
Parietal lobes	Sensation	Paresthesias
Occipital lobes	Visual sensation	Agnosia Homonymous hemianopsia Visual illusions and hallucinations
Temporal lobes	Special senses	↓ Hearing Tinnitus Olfactory or gustatory hallucinations Vertigo Fluent aphasia

nausea. The vomiting may be projectile and is not associated with food intake. Personality changes, notably irritability, indifference, apathy, and lack of spontaneity are common. These behavioral signs are most often reported by family members. Seizures may precede other symptoms by months. The aura and pattern of the seizure may be helpful in localizing the tumor; therefore, an accurate description of these events is essential. The location of the tumor will determine other signs and symptoms. For example, a tumor in the cerebellum will cause ataxia and nystagmus, whereas one in the lower frontal lobe or posterior fossa will cause papilledema. Some symptoms may arise from lesions in different parts of the brain. Alterations in movement may arise from a tumor in the motor cortex, motor tracts, or cerebellum.

Seizures may occur in the patient with a primary or metastatic brain tumor. They may be an early or late sign of an intracranial mass or they may be a late sequelae of a supratentorial craniotomy. Nursing care involves taking seizure precautions by keeping the side rail up and protecting the patient from injury.

Craniotomy. The patient undergoing craniotomy for histological diagnosis or resection of an intracranial neoplasm must be supported toward maximum physiological and psychological function. For details of nursing management, see the Nursing Care Plan for the Patient Undergoing Craniotomy for a Neoplasm. The reason for and the extent of the surgery, and the surgical approach will determine the nursing care the patient requires. A tumor located in the cerebellum or at the cerebellar–pontine angle is usually approached through the posterior fossa. This area is in close proximity to the respiratory centers in the brain stem; therefore, the patient must be closely monitored for at least 24 hours for sudden apnea. Blood gas determinations are required if respiratory rate or volume changes, or if the patient develops lethargy, restlessness, or other signs of respiratory embarrassment.

The patient with frontal or temporal lobe surgery is likely to have periorbital edema. Tight head dressings may contribute to the edema. Edema makes it difficult to check pupils. Elevating the head of the bed 20 to 30 degrees, applying cold compresses to the eyes, and loosening the head dressing may decrease the edema.

Intracranial Hypertension. A situation that increases blood pressure, causes cerebral vasodilation, obstructs venous outflow, or obstructs the flow of cerebrospinal fluid may create a substantial increase in intracranial pressure. The patient with an intracranial neoplasm is at risk for the development of inadequate cerebral profusion secondary to intracranial hypertension (increased intracranial pressure). Intracranial hypertension may result from an increase in the volume of brain tissue secondary to tumor growth. Trauma to brain tissue caused by surgical intervention, radiation, or chemotherapeutic agents may cause cerebral edema. Tumor growth may increase intracranial pressure (ICP) by altering cerebral blood flow or impairing circulation of cerebrospinal fluid.

Goals for the patient with a potential for intracranial hypertension secondary to tumor growth or surgical trauma include

1. Early detection of increasing intracranial pressure
2. Prevention of transient and sustained increases of intracranial pressure in the presence of existing intracranial hypertension
3. Reduction of intracranial pressure to levels that permit adequate brain perfusion.

Early detection of intracranial hypertension requires direct measurement of intracranial pressure. Clinical signs are neither a reliable nor a valid measure of intracranial pressure. They are, however, essential in detecting deteriorating neurological status. Documentation of neurological status at regular intervals is essential in any patient at risk for intracranial hypertension. Prevention of transient and sustained increases of ICP and the reduction of ICP levels are presented in Chapter 69, Neurological Trauma.

Reliable and valid measures of intracranial pressure can be achieved only by direct measurement of intracranial pressure. Signs and symptoms such as headache, vomiting, and papilledema may be indicators of intracranial hypertension. Changes in level of consciousness, changes in pupil equality and reactivity, widening pulse pressure, and bradycardia, which are classically associated with increased ICP, are actually signs of brain stem dysfunction. When they result from intracranial hypertension, they are a late sign indicating that the brain stem is impaired and that transtentorial brain herniation is occurring. Measurement of intracranial pressure may be done through the use of an intraventricular cannula or by subdural, epidural, or subarachnoid devices.

Evaluation

Early identification and prevention of further deterioration of neurological function may be evaluated by frequent and consistent nursing assessment of the patient's functional status in the areas of movement, sensation, consciousness, mentation, and integrated regulation. The findings of the nursing assessments must be documented and communicated to other members of the health care team. Secondary disability resulting from immobility, sensory overload or deprivation associated with hospitalization, tissue hypoxia, and iatrogenic disorders are prevented or at least minimized.

The patient's ability to achieve optimum levels of functioning, considering the capabilities and limitations that remain may be assessed by the person's ability to perform self-care activities. The patient's age, sex, role in the family and society, previous level of wellness, and the extent of disease are important considerations in determining when optimum functioning has been achieved.

Spinal Cord Tumors

Pathophysiology

Tumors of the spinal cord vary considerably from those of the brain. They are considerably less frequent, are more often benign, and produce their effects mainly by compression of the spinal cord rather than by invasion. Spinal cord tumors are classified as intramedullary or extramedullary. Intramedullary tumors arise within the substance of the spi-

NURSING CARE PLAN FOR THE PATIENT UNDERGOING CRANIOTOMY FOR A NEOPLASM

NURSING DIAGNOSIS/PROBLEM 1: Anxiety related to uncertainty about effects of surgery
GOAL: Reduce anxiety

Nursing Interventions	Rationale	Outcome Criteria
1. Assess current level of consciousness and ability to understand.	1. Pathological changes secondary to tumor may alter consciousness and mentation.	1. Patient asks appropriate questions concerning risks and aftereffects of surgery.
2. Provide opportunity to discuss concerns about the effects of surgery.	2. Brain surgery is often viewed as causing gross alterations in personality.	2. Patient/family verbalize concerns about the future.
3. Explain events and procedures to patient and family concerning: a. Head shaved b. Lengthy procedure c. Location and intensity of immediate postoperative care	3. Feelings of dismay often accompany loss of hair.	3. Accepts loss of hair; family not alarmed at length of procedure or intensive monitoring.
4. Involve family and significant others in preoperative preparation.	4. Family can recognize subtle changes in patient and can offer psychological support.	4. Family reports positive and negative changes in patient. Family acts in supportive and reassuring manner.
5. Prepare for postop appearance: a. Dressing b. Severe swelling and discoloration around face and eyes (greater 2–3 days postop)	5. Unexpected size of dressing and progressive increase in swelling and discoloration increase fear and anxiety.	5. Patient and family convey understanding of postoperative appearance.

NURSING DIAGNOSIS/PROBLEM 2: Alteration in neurological function related to impairment or destruction of brain cells secondary to neoplastic cell changes
GOAL 1: Early identification and prevention of further deterioration of neurological function

Nursing Interventions	Rationale	Outcome Criteria
1. Assess, document, and report the functional status in the areas of movement, sensation, consciousness, mentation, integrated regulation, and coping.	1. Monitoring the stability or instability of nervous system disease. Detect life-threatening nervous system dysfunction.	1. Ideally, further deterioration in neurological function is prevented. Physiological and psychological function are maintained to the extent possible or supplemented when necessary.
2. Frequency of assessment ranges from every 15 minutes to daily, depending on the stability of the patient.	2. Detect abnormal nervous system function in order to determine alterations in self-care activities.	2. All life-threatening alterations are detected as they occur and do not progress to brain herniation.

GOAL 2: Prevent further damage to brain cells secondary to tissue hypoxia

Nursing Interventions

1. Prevent transient and sustained increases in intracranial pressure.
2. Using ICP monitor, continuously assess pressure, noting changes with environmental stimuli and nursing care.

(Continued)

NURSING CARE PLAN FOR THE PATIENT UNDERGOING CRANIOTOMY FOR A NEOPLASM *(Continued)*

Nursing Interventions	Rationale	Outcome Criteria
3. Reduce ICP to levels that permit adequate brain perfusion by administering medications and other therapeutic measures as ordered. 4. Prevent or manage seizures. 5. Prevent complications of immobility.		
6. Observe for evidence of: a. Increased drowsiness b. Focal weakness c. Change in pupils d. Variations in blood pressure or pulse	6. Intracranial hemorrhage or hematoma could be fatal if not immediately corrected.	6. Early signs of increasing intracranial pathology are detected.
7. Administer mild analgesics or codeine for pain.	7. Sedatives are contraindicated since they mask signs of neurological deterioration. Headache and meningeal irritation following craniotomy tend to be mild. Narcotics mask signs of neurological deterioration and depress respirations.	7. Medications do not complicate accurate assessment.

GOAL 3: Achieve optimum level of functioning, considering capabilities and limitations

Nursing Interventions	Rationale	Outcome Criteria
1. Reassess, document, and report functional status. a. Identify strengths that can be used to increase self-care. b. Anticipate additional deficits based on knowledge of pathophysiology.	1. Detect alterations in self-care activities.	1. Patient performs self-care activities at a maximum level based on capabilities and limitations.

NURSING DIAGNOSIS/PROBLEM 3: Body image disturbance related to altered body function and appearance
GOAL: Optimize body functioning and appearance

Nursing Interventions	Rationale	Outcome Criteria
1. Gradually increase independence. 2. Provide skull cap, scarf, or wig.	1. Promoting maximum independence encourages integration of losses and increased focus on remaining abilities.	1–2. Patient integrates change in appearance into body image.
3. Praise patient for things well done. 4. Encourage participation in ADLs.		3–5. Patient strives to utilize remaining abilities.
5. Provide necessary PT, OT, and speech therapy.	5. Relearning abilities lost through neuronal damage requires significant retraining.	
6. Realistically discuss expected improvement in appearance/function.		

nal cord, invading and destroying tracts and central gray structures. Extramedullary tumors arise in the vertebral bodies or extradural tissues.

Tumors that cause compression of the spinal cord produce symptoms gradually over a period of weeks and months. Initially motor symptoms predominate and begin on the ipsilateral (same) side. Sensory symptoms often begin with a tingling paresthesia and progress to loss of pain and temperature, and finally loss of vibration, touch, and position sense (see Table 67–2).

Lesions within the spinal canal may interrupt nerve roots or spinal nerves and result in symptoms at one level of the body. Lesions of the dorsal root or spinal nerve produce radicular pain (limited to one or more dermatomes) and areas of paresthesia, hyperesthesia, or loss of cutaneous sensation in a dermatome distribution. Lesions of the anterior root produce weakness, atrophy, loss of reflexes, and loss of muscle tone.

Spinal cord lesions may also interrupt major ascending sensory and motor pathways and may affect all sensory modalities and motor function below the level of injury. Lesions of one half of the spinal cord result in Brown-Séquard syndrome in which there is loss of pain and temperature perception contralateral to the lesion and ipsilateral loss of position, vibratory, and fine or discriminatory touch, with ipsilateral motor deficit.

Damage to the posterior column is commonly caused by tumors. Symptoms include loss or decrease in position and vibratory sense, possibly paresthesia, and loss of discrete localization. Touch, temperature, and pain sensations remain intact.

A tumor that involves the nerve roots will produce pain in the distribution of a sensory nerve root. This pain may be knifelike, a dull ache, or a combination of both. Other sensory changes include paresthesias, impaired touch, and perception of pinprick. Motor disturbances include muscle cramps, atrophy, fasciculations, and loss of tendon reflex. A knowledge of the neuroanatomy of the spinal cord will allow the nurse to anticipate the expected deficits in patients with tumors at varying locations throughout the spinal cord.

Medical Management

The medical management of spinal cord tumors varies with the nature of the lesion and the clinical condition of the patient. Intradural–extramedullary tumors are best managed with early excision. Intramedullary gliomas require microscopic excision and radiotherapy. A combination of radiotherapy, endocrine therapy, and chemotherapy is used to treat epidural carcinoma and lymphoma. Laminectomy is often performed to allow access to the tumor for diagnostic purposes and to prevent irreversible compressive effects with infarction of the spinal cord.[1]

Nursing Interventions

The nursing management of the patient with a spinal cord tumor does not differ from that of the patient with a spinal cord injury. The deficits that the patient experiences will be related to the level of the tumor. Pain, sensory and motor deficits, and sphincter disturbances are likely to require nursing intervention.

TABLE 67–2
Signs and Symptoms of Spinal Cord Tumors

Classification	*Common Types*	*Signs and Symptoms*
Intramedullary	Glioma Ependymoma Astrocytoma	Progressive spastic paraparesis ↑ Deep tendon reflex (DTR) below level of tumor Babinski sign Wasting, fasciculations of segmental muscles Dissociated sensory loss
Extramedullary	Meningioma Neurofibroma Sarcoma	*Nerve root:* Sensory loss Paresthesias Wasting along distribution of root(s) *Posterior:* Proprioceptive deficits Paresthesias Ataxia *Anterior:* Progressive motor weakness Spasticity ↑ DTR Babinski sign *Lateral:* Brown-Séquard syndrome

Nursing Management Overview

Nursing management of the patient with tumors of the central nervous system encompasses every phase and facet of nursing. This group of patients presents an opportunity to exercise diligence and skill unequaled by any other group of patients. The ultimate success of therapeutic intervention is highly dependent on the quality of nursing care that the patient receives during the diagnostic, treatment, and long-term management phases of the disease.

Roles of the nurse in the management of patients with neoplasia include direct care-provider, coordinator, counselor, and educator. To fulfill these roles, the nurse must understand the following:

- Location and type of the tumor
- Pathophysiology of the tumor
- Effect the tumor will have on movement, sensation, consciousness, mentation, integrated regulation, and the ability to cope with the disease
- Diagnostic procedures to be performed
- Treatment protocol

Since most brain tumors progress to death in a relatively short period of time, it is important for the nurse to understand the psychosocial responses of the patient and significant others to a life-threatening illness.

Cell changes in the central nervous system that result from disease or its treatment have widespread effects on human response. The resulting nursing diagnoses include altered patterns of nutrition–metabolism, activity–exercise, and cognition–perception. Other nursing diagnoses include altered elimination, sexual function, sleep–rest cycles, and role relationships. Fear of the diagnosis and treatment are common when tumors are involved. Body image disturbances result from altered body function and appearance and result in negative feelings or perceptions about the body, repeated focusing on past function or appearance, and shame or guilt.

The nursing goal for the patient includes the early identification and prevention of further deterioration of neurological function, compensation for the effects of the disease on daily life, and optimization of body functioning and appearance.

References

1. Adams RD, Victor M: Principles of Neurology, 3rd ed. New York, McGraw-Hill, 1981
2. American Association of Neurosurgical Nurses: Core Curriculum for Neurosurgical Nursing. Chicago, Author, 1977
3. American Cancer Society: Cancer Facts and Figures. New York, American Cancer Society, 1985
4. Blass JP, Plum F: Metabolic encephalopathies in older adults. In Katzman R, Terry R (eds): The Neurology of Aging. Philadelphia, FA Davis, 1983
5. Bloom HJG: Intracranial tumors: Response and resistance to therapeutic endeavors. Int J Radiat Oncol Biol Phys 8:1083, 1982
6. Ganong WF: Review of Medical Physiology, 11th ed. Los Altos, CA Lange Medical Publications, 1983
7. Koos WT, Miller MT: Intracranial Tumors of Infants and Children. St Louis. CV Mosby, 1971
8. Posner JB: Clinical manifestations of brain metastasis. In Weiss L, Gilber HA, Posner JB (eds): Brain Metastasis. Boston, GK Hall, 1980
9. Rosenblum ML, Gerosa MA, Dougherty DV, Wilson CB: Improved treatment of a brain-tumor model: Advantages of single over multiple dose BCNU schedules. J Neurosurg 58:177, 1983

Bibliography

Aring CD: Metabolic encephalopathy: Neurologic and psychiatric considerations. Heart Lung 11:516, 1982

Burgess KE: Neurological disturbance in the patient with an intracranial neoplasm: Sources and implications for nursing care. J Neurosurg Nurs 15:237, 1983

Fode NC, Laws ER, Northcutt RC: Pituitary tumors and hypertension: Implications for neurosurgical nurses. J Neurosurg Nurs 15:33, 1983

Gargan R: Nursing management of the patient with meningeal carcinomatosis. J Neurosurg Nurs 12:184, 1980

Hill SA, Neuwelt EA: Intra-arterial chemotherapy following blood-brain barrier disruption in a patient with malignant glioma. J Neurosurg Nurs 14:94, 1982

Jones CC, Cayard CH: Care of ICP monitoring devices: A nursing responsibility. J Neurosurg Nurs 14:255, 1982

Lamb S: Interstitial radiation for the treatment of brain tumors using the stereotactic method. J Neurosurg Nurs 12:138, 1980

Mitchell PH: Intracranial hypertension: Implications of research for nursing care. J Neurosurg Nurs 12:145, 1980

Rhodes M, Grosser B: Complications of posterior fossa craniotomy. J Neurosurg Nurs 15:9, 1983

Segal G: A primer of Brain Tumors, 3rd ed. Chicago, Association for Brain Tumor Research, 1985

Segal G: Treatment of Brain Tumors. Chicago, Association for Brain Tumor Research, 1983

Stewart C: Current concepts of chemotherapy for brain tumors. J Neurosurg Nurs 12:97, 1980

Taylor JW, Ballenger S: Neurological Dysfunction and Nursing Intervention. New York, McGraw-Hill, 1980

Wujcik D: Meningeal carcinomatosis: Diagnosis, treatment, and nursing care. Oncology Nursing Forum 10(2):35, 1983

Zegeer LJ: Nursing care of the patient with brain edema. J Neurosurg Nurs 14:268, 1982

Chapter 68

Infectious and Degenerative Neurological Disorders

Marci-Lee Catanzaro

Infections of the Nervous System

The vast majority of human diseases are of known etiology. They are produced by microorganisms, notably bacteria, viruses, rickettsiae, fungi, mycoplasma, protozoa, or nematodes. Sulfonamide drugs and antibiotics have markedly decreased the incidence of infections, including those of the central nervous system (CNS). Infections of the CNS, however, are not rare and present grave danger for their victim.

Microorganisms are responsible for causing infectious diseases of the nervous system. These infectious diseases may be classified according to the causative organism such as bacteria, virus, or rickettsia. Infectious diseases may also be viewed as acute or chronic. Some infective organisms give rise to disorders of the nervous system by causing granulomatous infiltration of the cells or by producing toxins that interfere with normal cell function.

Much has been learned about the means by which microorganisms initiate infections and produce tissue injury, the influence of host resistance, and the mechanism of recovery. Much of this knowledge has not yet found direct application to human disease in a way that allows us to predictably alter the course of uncomplicated infectious disease. Infections of the central nervous system produce symptoms by causing the neurons to cease normal functioning or to take on new characteristics.

Pathophysiology

The spinal and cranial bones and the dura mater make the suprasegmental structures associated with sensation, movement, and cognition notably invulnerable to infective agents. Protective mechanisms may fail when

- Suppuration occurs in the middle ear, mastoid cells, or frontal, ethmoid, and sphenoid sinuses.
- An osteomyelitic focus erodes the inner table of bone and invades the dura, subdural space, pia, arachnoid, or the brain substance.
- Infective emboli from the lungs and heart are carried to the brain.
- A contaminant is introduced through a penetrating injury, a congenital sinus tract, or an invasive procedure such as a lumbar puncture.[24]

The spinal epidural space is considerably more vulnerable to infection than the intracranial space. Once infection is established, it spreads rapidly to the other cerebrospinal structures. Bacteremia or septicemia rarely involves the central nervous system. However, bacteremia associated with pneumonia is a frequent forerunner of bacterial meningitis.

Bacterial Infections

Bacterial Meningitis

Among the bacterial infections, blood-borne (hematogenous) bacterial meningitis is usually caused by a single microorganism. In the adult these organisms are most often *Diplococcus pneumoniae, Hemophilus influenzae,* and *Neisseria meningitidis.* The most common infecting organisms in the neonate are *Escherichia coli* and group B streptococcus. Infants and children most commonly develop bacterial meningitis from *Hemophilus influenza.* Infections of the suprasegmental structures that result from emboli carried from the lungs and heart and those that extend from other structures, notably the ears, are commonly mixed infections.

Bacteria in the subarachnoid space cause an inflammatory reaction in the pia mater and arachnoid, the cerebrospinal fluid, and the ventricles. Initially, there is congestion of meningeal vessels and migration of neutrophils into the subarachnoid space. As exudate increases, it extends into the sheaths of cranial and spinal nerves and for a very short distance into perivascular spaces of the cortex. By the second week of the inflammatory process the cellular exudates are deposited in two layers. Just beneath the arachnoid membrane is a layer of polymorphonuclear leukocytes and fibrin. Plasma cells and macrophages form the layer next to the pia mater. The exudates result in fibrosis of the arachnoid and a walling off of pockets of exudates.[2]

Resolution of the inflammatory process is largely dependent on the stage at which the process is arrested. With early intervention, no residual changes in the arachnoid occur. Infection that is allowed to persist for several weeks results in permanent fibrous overgrowth of meninges and in adhesions between pia mater and arachnoid and the arachnoid and dura mater. An infrequent and late sequela is chronic adhesive arachnoiditis or chronic meningomyelitis. These conditions result in pain, weakness, and atrophy and may progress to spastic ataxia with sphincter disturbances.

Clinical Manifestations

The clinical manifestations of bacterial meningitis differ between infants and adults. Infants cannot complain of headache, the most common complaint of older individuals. Fever, generalized convulsions, and disorders of consciousness, such as drowsiness, are usual manifestations common to all age-groups. A bulging fontanel occurs in infants. Older children and adults frequently experience stiffness of the neck on forward bending (nuchal rigidity).

Cerebrospinal fluid (CSF) demonstrates pleocytosis with leukocyte counts ranging from 1,000 to 100,000/cubic millimeter (normal 0–5/cu mm). Neutrophils comprise 85% to 90% of the total leukocytes. CSF pressure is consistently elevated above 180 mm H_2O and may be over 400 mm H_2O, suggesting brain swelling and the potential for transtentorial herniation. Protein levels are almost always above 45 mg/100 ml and may exceed 500 mg/100 ml. Glucose levels are usually lower than 40 mg/100 ml. The causative agent is often identified through Gram stain.

The mortality rate for bacterial meningitis is related to the infective organism and to the age of the host. The mortality rate for meningococcal meningitis ranges from 5% to 15%, whereas it is 15% to 30% in pneumococcal meningitis. A disproportionate number of deaths occur in the neonate and in the elderly. Approximately half of the infants who survive pneumococcal meningitis show serious neurological sequelae. The majority of adults recover and show no residual neurological deficits.[2]

Treatment

Bacterial meningitis is a medical emergency. It is treated with intravenous antibiotics for a period of 10 to 14 days. Penicillin G is the drug of choice for pneumococcal or meningococcal meningitis. Infections caused by Enterobacteriaceae and *Pseudomonas* are treated with gentamicin. Brain swelling associated with infection is treated with adrenocortical steroids and with osmotic diuretics.[2]

Nursing Interventions

The patient with meningococcal meningitis is at risk for development of adrenal insufficiency and must be observed for hypotension, respiratory collapse, and petechiae. The nursing diagnoses include alterations in cardiac output, impaired gas exchange, and alteration in both cerebral and peripheral perfusion. Prompt intervention is essential.

It is not uncommon for the patient with bacterial meningitis to have a high fever with increased pulse and respiratory rates. Levels of consciousness may decrease as the infection compromises cerebral function. A reliable method of assessing levels of consciousness and reporting this information is essential. The Glasgow Coma Scale is one such instrument for serial assessment of consciousness in the acutely ill patient. This scale incorporates eye opening, motor response, and verbal response to stimuli. It is often combined with charts on which to record pupil size and reaction to light and motor strength,[11,22]

Prescribed treatment protocols will include antibiotic administration, usually by the intravenous route. It is important that the antibiotic be administered on time and continued for the prescribed period even when clinical improvement is evident. Measures to reduce fever may include antipyretic medications, hypothermia blankets, or iced saline or alcohol baths. Anticonvulsants may be used to prevent seizures.

In the acute phase of central nervous system infection, such as meningitis and encephalitis, the patient is hyperirritable and experiences hyperalgesia. It is important to reduce environmental stimuli by keeping the room darkened and as quiet as possible. Avoid unnecessary moving of the patient. The patient may be unable to perform self-care activities and will need assistance with these in order to remain clean and comfortable. The prevention of complications will depend, to a large extent, on the nature and duration of the infection. The patient with bacterial meningitis will be debilitated much longer than the one with viral meningitis. Immobility is a major cause of complications in any seriously ill patient. Nursing care to prevent these complications is included in Chapter 64, Nursing Strategies for Common Neurological Problems.

Bacterial Toxins

Some diseases of the nervous system are caused by toxin-producing bacteria. The most common of these diseases are diphtheria, tetanus, and botulism.

Tetanus. Tetanus is caused by the toxin produced by *Clostridium tetani.* The way in which this endotoxin acts is not fully understood but it appears to interfere with the motor neuron reflex arc in the spinal cord and brain stem in much the same way as strychnine. The tetanus toxin may also disrupt normal neural function at the cerebral cortical level and in the sympathetic nervous system.

Prevention of tetanus through immunization is the first line of defense. Immunization should be renewed through a booster dose of tetanus toxoid administered every 10 years. The person with an injury that carries a threat of tetanus is treated with toxoid. Persons who have never been immunized or who have never received a booster dose of toxoid receive both toxoid and human antitoxin. Tetanus is treated at the onset with a single dose of antitoxin and a course of penicillin. Surgical débridement of the wound is imperative, and the tissue around the wound is infiltrated with antitoxin. Short-acting barbiturates and chlorpromazine are used to sedate the patient and to suppress the muscle spasms.[2]

Diphtheria. The toxin of *Corynebacterium diphtheriae* is produced in the inflammatory exudate in the throat and trachea. Eighty percent of cases of diphtheria do not progress to the central nervous system. Those cases that do progress predictably affect the trigeminal, facial, vagus, and hypoglossal cranial nerves and may produce sensorimotor polyneuropathy.

There is no specific treatment for the neurological complications of diphtheria. Immediate treatment with antitoxin tends to lessen the incidence and severity of complications.

Botulism. The presynaptic endings at the neuromuscular junction are affected by the toxin produced by *Clostridium botulinum.* This exotoxin interferes in some poorly understood way with the release of acetylcholine quanta. Adams and Victor noted that more than half of the reported cases of botulism occur in the states of California, Washington, Colorado, New Mexico, and Oregon.[2]

Trivalent antiserum is available for the treatment of botulism. Recovery, however, is most dependent on the effectiveness of supportive care, such as maintenance of respiratory function and fluid and electrolyte balance.

Viral Infections

With the possible exception of rabies, viral infections of the central nervous system occur as a complication of systemic infection. Unlike bacteria that rapidly affect all types of cells, viruses tend to be confined to a particular type of cell. For example, viral infections of the meningeal cells result in benign *aseptic meningitis. Encephalitis* is caused by a viral infection of the parenchymal cells of the brain. The motor neurons of the cranial and spinal nerves are particularly vulnerable to the viruses that cause *poliomyelitis.*

In spite of the widespread prevalence of viruses in the environment, viral infections of the nervous system are an uncommon occurrence. Normally the reticuloendothelial system clears viral particles from the blood before they have an opportunity to invade the nervous system. Even though viral meningitis is more common than its bacterial counterpart, little is known about its pathogenesis because recovery is almost always inevitable and sequelae are uncommon.[1,8]

Chronic viral infections are increasingly implicated in many diseases of the central nervous system formerly thought to be pure degenerative diseases. Viruses enter the body and rather than producing an acute illness remain clinically silent for long periods of time. They may or may not produce cytopathic changes during the silent period. The role of the immune system in the development of chronic viral infections is unknown. It has been hypothesized that the virus is kept in check by normal immunologic mechanisms during the long incubation period and that disease occurs when these defenses fail. *Kuru, progressive multifocal leukoencephalopathy*, and *subacute sclerosing panencephalitis* have been identified as slow virus infections. Changes in the nervous system in these diseases simulate degenerative processes to such as extent that other major degenerative disease of the central nervous system, such as Parkinson's disease, multiple sclerosis, and amyotrophic lateral sclerosis, are being reexamined for possible connections to chronic viral infections.

Herpes Zoster (Shingles)

Reactivation of a previous viral infection can occur with a virus. An example of this is herpes zoster which is caused by the same virus as chickenpox. Although the pathogenesis is not fully understood, it is generally agreed that herpes zoster or shingles is a spontaneous reactivation of a varicella infection that was latent in the sensory ganglia following the primary infection. The virus moves along sensory nerves from cutaneous vesicles to the sensory ganglion. It remains latent until activated, perhaps by waning immunity. At that time it moves down the axon to the skin. The virus has been demonstrated in skin lesions. Inflammatory reactions in the segmental nerve, its sensory ganglion, and the posterior horn of the spinal column have been a consistent finding.[2]

The disease occurs at a rate of 3 to 5 cases/1000 persons per year. Unlike chickenpox, herpes zoster is not communicable except to persons with no immunity to chickenpox. It has no seasonal variation and does not occur in epidemics. Chickenpox is associated with childhood, whereas the incidence of herpes zoster increases with age. The sexes are equally affected. One side of the body is as likely to be affected as the other.[19]

Herpes zoster is characterized by radicular pain and vesicular cutaneous eruptions. Itching, tingling, or burning sensations involving the affected dermatome usually precede the vesicular cutaneous eruptions by several days. The tense clear vesicles on an erythematous base appear within 3 to 4 days. The vesicles become cloudy after a few days and dry, crusted, and scaly after 5 to 10 days. The pain usually persists for 1 to 4 weeks but may last months or years. In some cases there is a segmental sensory loss and motor palsy.

Viral diseases of the nervous system are usually self-limiting. There is no specific treatment. Medical management is directed toward alleviating the symptoms. For example, analgesics and lotions or powders applied to the skin lesions are prescribed for herpes zoster.

Landry-Guillain-Barré Syndrome

Landry-Guillain-Barré syndrome is an example of another mechanism by which viruses cause disease by mediating an immunologic reaction directed at CNS tissue. The exact cause of the syndrome is unknown, although there is evidence that after a virus infection, there is a cell-mediated immunologic reaction directed at peripheral myelin. There is frequently a history of antecedent viral infection, followed by cross-reactivity of the viral-coat protein with a protein in peripheral myelin and subsequent demyelination. The disease affects mainly the Schwann cells that synthesize and maintain peripheral nerve myelin. Initially there is a severe inflammatory reaction with accumulation of cells around veins in peripheral nerves and lymphocytic infiltration into peripheral nerve fibers near points where motor and ventral roots fuse. Later there is edema of the myelin sheath and subsequent fragmentation of myelin. In response to changes in the peripheral axon, the anterior horn cell and lower motor neuron undergo a process known as chromatolysis, in which the cell body becomes enlarged and cell function is impaired. This sequence of events is potentially reversible if the distal disease process is resolved.

The syndrome is nonseasonal and nonepidemic. It affects males and females equally and occurs between the ages of 8 months and 81 years of age. There are 1.7 cases/100,000 population.[18] Weakness is the major clinical manifestation. It is more or less symmetrical and evolves over a period of several days. Paralysis tends to progress from distal to proximal; from lower extremities to upper extremities; then to trunk, intercostal, and neck muscles; and finally to cranial nerves. Sensory aberrations such as pain, paresthesias, and anesthesia vary widely from patient to patient or may be absent. Signs of generalized infection, such as fever and lymphadenopathy, are notably absent. Spinal fluid is initially normal but protein levels begin to rise after several days, reaching a peak in 4 to 6 weeks. Nerve conduction velocities become slowed early in the disease process, and denervation potentials tend to appear later if at all.

Nursing Interventions

Because the progression of paralysis eventually affects all body systems, the patient requires support for basic physiological needs. The most pressing need is to maintain respiratory exchange. As the weakness and paralysis progress, eventually the intercostal muscles become paralyzed, affecting respiration. Respiratory failure is predictable, and ventilatory support by means of a respirator will be needed for weeks.

Nursing interventions call for continual assessment of vital signs and indications of progressive weakness and paralysis. The parameters assessed include mentation, consciousness, dyspnea, skin color, chest movement, and lung sounds. Blood gases, tidal volume, and vital capacity are checked frequently as a measurement of pulmonary function. A tracheostomy set and respirator should be at hand for emergency use in view of the fact that ventilatory support will be required.

To avoid atelectasis and pneumonia, the patient should be encouraged to cough and breathe deeply as long as muscle strength allows. Chest physiotherapy, frequent turning, and suctioning should be instituted as needed to clear the bronchi and facilitate breathing. The patient needs constant reassurance that the condition is temporary and will eventually abate.

There is also a potential for circulatory collapse owing to the paralysis affecting the autonomic mechanisms that control circulation. Sinus tachycardia or bradycardia, fluctuations in blood pressure, and either profuse diaphoresis or lack of sweating can result. To prevent circulatory collapse the nurse should frequently assess cardiac rate and rhythm and blood pressure, minimize positive pressure during mechanical ventilation, and avoid sudden position changes that could tax the body's compensatory mechanism and result in cardiac collapse.

Progressive paralysis eventually affects the patient's ability to chew and swallow, thereby interfering with nutritional intake. Nursing interventions include assessing how well the patient can chew and swallow during mealtime. When the ability to chew and swallow becomes compromised as a result of paralysis, gavage feedings or hyperalimentation may be instituted as needed. Throughout the course of the disease, the nurse assesses the patient's hydration status, urinary output, vital signs, and daily weight.

The psychosocial needs of the patient with Landry-Guillain-Barré syndrome often outweigh the needs for intensive physical care. When adequate ventilatory status is maintained, these patients are fully alert and conscious of their environment. A person who before the onset of disease was healthy and independent in all activities of daily living progressively becomes totally dependent on other persons and on machines for survival. A nurse who developed this disease reported that her experience was a continual nightmare as paralysis progressed and the diagnosis was uncertain.[3] Constant support, reassurance, and explanations are essential. The patient must understand the normal course of progressive paralysis and subsequent remission of the paralysis. It is reassuring to know that the disease is temporary and that the staff providing for care anticipates the next level of disability and is prepared to deal with it in a timely fashion.

The Nursing Care Plan for the Patient with Landry-Guillain-Barré Syndrome includes criteria for the goals of maintaining adequate ventilation, preventing circulatory collapse, and maintaining positive nitrogen balance.

Spirochetal Infection: Neurosyphilis

Syphilis is a well-known spirochetal venereal disease. Within 3 to 18 months of untreated infection, the causative organism, *Treponema pallidum,* invades the central nervous system, causing an asymptomatic meningitis. This state may persist for many years before the chronic, progressive changes become evident. The cell changes that occur are thought to be the result of an exaggerated or hypersensitivity response. Meningeal thickening, brain atrophy, ventricular enlargement, and granular ependymitis are evident. The perivascular spaces are filled with lymphocytes and mononuclear and plasma cells. Nerve cells disappear, and rod-shaped microgliocytes and abnormal astrocytes are present. Meningeal fibrosis with obstructive hydrocephalus is present in many cases.[2]

The incidence of neurosyphilis has declined dramatically in the second half of this century. However, the incidence of primary syphilis has actually increased in recent years so that we may expect to see an increase in neurosyphilis in the future. As noted earlier, there is a lengthy period during which the treponeme lives in the central nervous system, and it causes a chronic, progressive inflammation of the parenchymal cells. During this stage of the disease, diagnosis can be made by analysis of CSF. Spinal fluid abnormalities include (1) an increase in gamma globulin, (2) positive serological tests, (3) an increase in lymphocytes, and (4) elevation of the globulin fraction of protein. The patient with fully developed neurosyphilis exhibits progressive mental and physical degeneration, including dementia, dysarthria, myoclonic jerks, intention tremor, seizures, hyperreflexia, and pathological reflexes.

Nursing Management

Assessment and Nursing Diagnosis

The specific treatment for infections of the central nervous system will depend on the infecting organism and the

NURSING CARE PLAN FOR THE PATIENT WITH LANDRY-GUILLAIN-BARRÉ SYNDROME

NURSING DIAGNOSIS/PROBLEM 1: Inadequate pulmonary ventilation related to progressive muscle weakness
GOAL: Maintain adequate ventilation

Nursing Interventions	Rationale	Outcome Criteria
1. Assess, document, and report ▪ Progression of weakness ▪ Mentation ▪ Consciousness ▪ Dyspnea ▪ Skin color ▪ Chest movements ▪ Lung sounds ▪ Subjective complaints	1. Weakness progresses and finally affects respiration, paralyzing intercostal muscles. ▪ Reduced O_2 to the brain results in decreased cerebral metabolism and function.	1. Signs of progressive muscle weakness are identified early. ▪ Respiratory problems are anticipated. ▪ Appropriate ventilatory support is initiated.
2. Obtain blood gases, tidal volume, and vital capacity, as ordered.	2. Laboratory determinations of pulmonary function provide objective data on which to plan care.	2. Laboratory values are consistent with observed condition of patient and are used in planning care.
3. Obtain tracheostomy set and respirator for emergency use.	3. Respiratory failure is a predictable and manageable complication. ▪ Ventilatory support will be needed for weeks; tracheostomy is the method of choice to prevent damage to oral and tracheal mucosa from endotracheal or nasogastric tubes. ▪ Ventilation, not perfusion, is the problem. O_2 is seldom required.	3. Unnecessary delay is avoided when ventilatory support is needed. ▪ Respiratory failure is recognized early and appropriate support is initiated.
4. Encourage patient to cough and deep breathe, as paralysis allows. a. Institute IPPB, chest physiotherapy, frequent turning, and suction as necessary.	4. Paralysis of preganglionic fibers of the vagus nerve result in an inability of the bronchi to constrict and dilate alternately.	4. Atelectasis and pneumonia are prevented. ▪ Respiratory therapy does not fatigue patient, resulting in exacerbation of symptoms.

(Continued)

NURSING CARE PLAN FOR THE PATIENT WITH LANDRY-GUILLAIN-BARRÉ SYNDROME (*Continued*)

NURSING DIAGNOSIS/PROBLEM 2: Alteration in cardiac output (potential circulatory collapse) related to autonomic dysfunction
GOAL: Prevent circulatory collapse

Nursing Interventions	Rationale	Outcome Criteria
1. Assess, document, and record cardiac rate and rhythm, blood pressure, and sweating.	1. Helps in determining the effect of disease on autonomic function and provides a baseline to compare progression of disease.	1. Altered autonomic function is detected early.
2. Minimize positive pressure during mechanical ventilation. 3. Avoid sudden position change.	2–3. Stimuli to the autonomic nervous system may exceed compensatory mechanism, resulting in circulatory collapse.	2–3. Factors that contribute to autonomic dysfunction are minimized.

NURSING DIAGNOSIS/PROBLEM 3: Alterations in nutrition related to inability to chew and swallow food
GOAL: Maintain positive nitrogen balance.

Nursing Interventions	Rationale	Outcome Criteria
1. Assess function of cranial nerves associated with chewing and swallowing prior to each feeding.	1. Muscle weakness secondary to paralysis of cranial nerves results in an inability to meet caloric requirements.	1. Cranial nerve dysfunction is detected early and self-care deficits are anticipated.
2. Institute gavage feedings or hyperalimentation, as necessary.	2. The critically ill have increased needs for calories, carbohydrates, fats, and fluids.	2. The patient does not aspirate food.
3. Assess hydration state, urinary output, vital signs, and daily weight. Obtain blood for electrolyte determinations.	3. Patients on supplemental feedings are at risk for fluid and electrolyte imbalance.	3. Parameters used to assess nutritional state remain within normal limits.

site of infection. Nursing management of patients with CNS infections is directed toward the following:[9]

1. Assessing the patient's condition
2. Carrying out the prescribed treatment protocol
3. Providing supportive care
4. Preventing complications
5. Enhancing rehabilitation

The clinical manifestations of infections are similar to infections in other body systems. Fever, general malaise, and serological evidence of the body's immune response are evident. Infections of the central nervous system may affect a particular structure throughout the nervous system. For example, meningitis affects the meninges and poliomyelitis attacks the motor neurons of the cranial and spinal nerves.

Assessment of the patient with CNS infection includes

- Vital signs
- Level of consciousness
- Cranial nerve functions (*e.g.,* pupil size and reaction to light, eye movements, visual fields)
- Motor function
- Sensory function
- Mentation

Sequelae of CNS infections may range from minor disabilities that will resolve over time to serious disability requiring an aggressive rehabilitation plan. The nurse is the one who is with the patient most and is in a position to provide valuable information about the patient's self-care abilities.

Goals. Overall goals for the nursing management of patients with infections of the central nervous system include supporting normal function during the period of acute illness, preventing complications, and enhancing the full recovery of the patient.

Intervention

Patients with infections of the central nervous system exhibit self-care deficits in the areas of movement, sensation, consciousness, and mentation. Nursing care for these deficits is included in Chapter 64, Nursing Strategies for Common Neurological Problems.

Patients with pathological conditions of the central nervous system are at risk for developing a variety of complications secondary to immobility and sensory deprivation or overload associated with altered neurological functioning. An important goal in the nursing management of these patients is to prevent these problems. This goal will be achieved when early signs and symptoms of problems are recognized and intervention is initiated to prevent sequelae of immobility and sensory alterations.

Many patients with infections of the central nervous system are in severely compromised states and their condition will change rapidly. The close observation provided by the nurse must be documented in such a way that others on the health care team can compare the patient's progress over time. Deteriorating neurological function must be identified promptly and communicated to the physician in a timely fashion. It is reassuring to the patient, also, to know that those providing care anticipate changes and are prepared to manage them appropriately. Specific goals in the care of the patient with Landry-Guillian-Barré syndrome include maintaining adequate ventilation, preventing circulatory collapse, and assuring positive nitrogen balance (see Nursing Care Plan).

Degenerative Diseases of the Nervous System

As life expectancy continues to increase, degenerative diseases of the central nervous system assume a position of increasing importance. These degenerative diseases include Alzheimer's disease and Parkinson's disease, which are sufficiently common as to have become household words. Muscular dystrophy and myasthenia gravis, although not degenerative diseases of the nervous system, result in clinical manifestations that are similiar to many of the degenerative diseases.

Definition and Classification

Degenerative diseases are a group of disorders in which there is a gradual, generally symmetric, relentlessly progressive wasting of structural elements of the nervous system. Many diseases formerly classified as degenerative are now known to be caused by metabolic disorders, immunologic disorders, toxins, nutritional deficiencies, or chronic viral infections. Within our lifetime, the list of degenerative disease will continue to shrink as scientists discover the causes of these disorders.

Classification of diseases according to their etiology is common. Degenerative diseases, however, cannot be classified in this way because the etiology is unknown. These diseases are grouped as follows:

1. Disorders of mentation with or without other neurological abnormalities. Senile dementia of the Alzheimer's type is an example of a dementing disease without other neurological manifestations. An example of a dementia with concomitant movement disorder is Huntington's disease.
2. Disorders of movement including abnormalities of posture and movement, ataxia, and muscular weakness. Parkinson's disease, spasmodic torticollis, and familial tremor are examples of progressive abnormalities of posture and movement. Diseases exemplifying muscle weakness include amyotropic lateral sclerosis, muscular dystrophy, and myasthenia gravis.
3. Disorders that result in abnormalities of movement, sensation, and mentation. This group of disorders is exemplified by multiple sclerosis.

Etiology

Degenerative diseases are characterized by loss of cells in the nervous system. Much has been learned about the anatomical changes that occur in these diseases. Still a mystery is the mechanism by which these degenerative changes begin and progress relentlessly. These diseases begin insidiously and run a gradually progressive course that may extend over many years. In the early stages of disease, changes in function may be so slight that the patient may be unaware of them.

The structural changes that occur in some disease states resemble those changes associated with aging. As aging occurs, there is a thinning of gray and white matter, especially in the superior temporal and frontal gyri and the frontal cortex. There is a decrease in the extracellular compartment volume that is associated with a decrease in cellular efficiency. Within the cell, there is an accumulation of lipofuscin and neurofibrillary tangles. Biochemical changes, including decreased oxygen consumption by brain tissue and an overall decrease in neurochemical transmission efficiency, are believed to play a significant role in the overall decrease in neuronal metabolism.[23] These changes have led some researchers to speculate that degenerative diseases are just an acceleration of normal aging. There is little scientific evidence to support this theory.

The role of chronic viral infections in degenerative diseases is a current topic of extensive research. It is known that viruses can remain latent in the body, later to become active and cause structural damage to cells. The exact mechanism by which this occurs eludes scientists.

The immune system has also been implicated in degenerative diseases. Diseases formerly thought to be degenerative are now known to be autoimmune disorders. For example, there is considerable evidence that myasthenia gravis is a defect in neuromuscular transmission that results when an antibody to the acetylcholine receptors prevents depolarization of the motor end plate.[9]

Senile (Alzheimer's) Dementia

Progressive dementia can occur with or without other neurological abnormalities. Senile dementia of the Alzheimer type (SDAT), Pick's disease, and postencephalitic and post-traumatic dementias are examples of progressive dementia without other neurological abnormalities. Examples of dementias accompanied by other neurological abnormalities are Huntington's disease, Jakob-Creutzfeldt disease, and cerebrocerebellar degeneration.

Pathophysiology

Dementia is a broad diagnostic category that includes disorders characterized by deterioration in intellectual functioning. In recent years it has become evident that dementia is the result of pathological changes in the brain and is not inevitable with aging. Genetic and unknown environmental factors are thought to predispose a person to senile dementia of the Alzheimer type. Within the brain there is a loss of nerve cells in the substantia nigra, basal ganglia, and cortex with excessive formation of senile plaques in the neocortex and hippocampus. Neurofibrillary tangles appear in the neocortex and there is a loss of neurotransmitters in the cortex and hippocampus, particularly choline acetyltransferase and somatostatin. It is believed that symptoms do not appear until after a certain number of tissue alterations occur and that the threshold for symptoms is individualized and associated with the extent of redundancy in the neural circuitry.[25]

Senile dementia of the Alzheimer type affects more than a half million people in the United States. It accounts for about half of the nursing home admissions and is implicated in more than 100,000 deaths per year.[25] Dementias are frequently subdivided according to their severity. For example, a person with severe dementia has lost the ability to live independently. Over 50 diseases have been noted to cause dementia. Alzheimer's disease accounts for more than half of all causes of dementia, and nearly one quarter of cases are caused by vascular disease of the brain. Other diseases, such as Huntington's, Pick's, and Parkinson's disease and metabolic, toxic, and inflammatory or infectious processes account for the remaining causes.

Clinical Manifestations

Clinical manifestations of Alzheimer-type dementia include loss of memory, difficulty in speaking and writing secondary to memory loss, loss of conceptualization and arithmetic ability, and forgetfulness in common activities. The person with advanced senile dementia of the Alzheimer type may be expected to have difficulty performing daily activities such as dressing, eating, and washing. There are difficulties relating to others and alterations in personality that are often expressed as paranoia. The person experiences an overall deterioration of health and usually dies from aspiration pneumonia.[5]

Medical science has yet to discover a way to prevent the structural and degenerative changes that occur with aging. Neurological changes as a result of normal aging are seldom the cause of clinically significant loss of function. When neurological dysfunction becomes evident in the elderly, it is important to differentiate the normal changes in neurological functioning that occur with aging from those changes suggesting a disease process. Stewart pointed out that cerebral vascular disease is evident in 84% of the population over the age of 65 years.[23] In many cases, treatment of the vascular disease improves the neurological function of the person. The incidence of some neurological diseases, such as Parkinson's disease and trigeminal neuralgia, increases with age. Concurrent disease states and nutritional deficiencies may further compromise neurological function already impaired by normal aging.

Various drugs have been tried and proven to have no effect on the progression of dementia. These treatments have included vasodilators and stimulants, L-dopa, and massive doses of vitamins. Aberrant behavior often responds to chlorpromazine and related drugs.

Nursing Interventions

Senile dementia of the Alzheimer type is a progressive disorder. Nursing management must be formulated according to the degree of dementia demonstrated by the patient at the present time. A cognitive function scale was developed by Reisberg and colleagues[21] and later adapted.[20] This scale ranges from level 1 (normal), with no functional impairment to level 7 (late dementia), with loss of intelligible vocabulary and all motor abilities, stupor, and finally coma. Table 68–1 presents a guide for assessing the functional capacity of the patient at each level of the disease. A concise overview of the care involved is presented in the Nursing Care Plan for the Hospitalized Patient with Senile Dementia of the Alzheimer Type (SDAT).

Nursing management of the hospitalized patient with

TABLE 68–1
Functional Assessment of Patients with Senile Dementia (Alzheimer's)

1. Does the person have subjective complaints of memory loss or memory deficit?
2. Does the person complain of slight memory loss, forget where familiar objects are placed, or forget familiar names?
3. Is the person appropriately concerned about memory loss?
4. Are others, such as family members and employers, aware of clear-cut deficits?
5. Can the person recall the content of a story, either read or told?
6. Does the person try to hide signs of impaired mentation?
7. Is there objective evidence on neuropsychiatric examination of memory and concentration deficits?
8. Can the person manage complex tasks?
9. Has there been a change in affect?
10. Does the person remember such things as telephone numbers, dates of important events, and names of close members of the family?
11. Is the person oriented to time, person, and place?
12. Has there been a change in sleep/wake cycles?
13. Can the person utter any meaningful sounds, perform psychomotor skills, and maintain urinary and fecal continence?

NURSING CARE PLAN FOR THE HOSPITALIZED PATIENT WITH SENILE DEMENTIA OF THE ALZHEIMER TYPE (SDAT)

NURSING DIAGNOSIS/PROBLEM: Altered cognitive and perceptual abilities related to loss of nerve cells

GOAL 1: Establish effective communication

Nursing Interventions	Rationale	Outcome Criteria
1. Assess current level of cognitive function. 2. Contact family about current functional and coping behaviors. 3. Initiate and maintain face-to-face contact. 4. Reorient person with each contact.	1–2. Knowledge of current deficits and coping behaviors will provide guidance for establishing plan of care. Knowledge of abilities will permit maximum use of strengths.	1–9. Patient will be able to communicate at some level and follow directions.
5. Communicate information in a distraction-free environment. 6. Explain exactly what is to be done. Give simple, specific directions and information.	5. Distraction will inhibit memory storage.	
7. Post information the patient must remember, if reading ability is intact. 8. Label bathroom, bed, *etc.,* if necessary. 9. Focus interaction on what is familiar and meaningful.	7. Memory aids facilitate establishing new memory store.	

GOAL 2: Provide safe, structured environment

Nursing Interventions	Rationale	Outcome Criteria
1. Place patient in location where observation is easy (near nurses' station, with reliable roommate, or where family can stay).	1. The patient with dementia is easily confused by new surroundings.	1. Patient will remain safe and relatively stable.
2. Establish and maintain consistent environment, including staff personnel. 3. Remove all potentially dangerous objects (*e.g.,* razor, scissors, matches).	2. The ability to adjust to a new environment and learn new material is severely limited.	
4. Approach patient in calm, unhurried, firm but tolerant manner.	4. The behavior of others is mirrored in the patient's behavior.	

GOAL 3: Maintain optimum function

Nursing Interventions	Rationale	Outcome Criteria
1. Initiate physical and occupational therapy.	1. Abnormal reflexes produce severe motor impairment and flexion contractures.	1. Normal mobility is retained as long as possible.
2. Encourage self-care within ability.	2. Enhances sense of competency.	2. Performs self-care activities within ability when reminded.
3. Administer antianxiety and antipsychotic agents as ordered.	3. Controls anxious and agitated behavior.	3. Patient remains in control of behavior.
4. Keep patient awake during the day.		4. Patient sleeps during the night.
5. Provide finger foods if ability to use utensils is limited.	5. As dementia progresses the patient may have no appetite or interest in food.	5. Adequate nutrition is maintained.
6. Encourage high-fiber diet with adequate fluids.		

dementia must take into consideration the fact that most demented individuals tend to decompensate in unfamiliar surroundings. The ability to learn new material is impaired before remote memory is lost. Therefore, the patient may be able to function independently while at home but be unable to learn ways of carrying out activities of daily living with even subtle differences in the hospital environment.[4]

The establishment of effective communication and provision of a safe, structured environment will be of concern when working with the hospitalized patient with dementia. To assess safety, place the patient in a room near the nurse's station where he can be easily observed and remove any dangerous objects from his immediate environment. Establish and maintain a consistent environment by reorienting the patient to room and personnel, returning items to the same location, assigning the same nursing personnel, following routines, and including familiar objects from home whenever possible.

It is equally important to promote as much effective communication as possible. Maintaining face-to-face contact, conveying information in an environment that is free from distractions, and explaining what is to be done in simple specific sentences are means of achieving this goal. It may also be helpful to provide memory aids such as labeling items in the room, assuming that the patient's reading ability is still intact.

To maintain optimum functioning, the patient should be encouraged to carry out self-care activities as much as possible and should be assured proper nutritional intake. The patient should be engaged in some kind of physical therapy during the day to keep him awake during daylight hours and to allow for sleep during the night. Anxious and agitated behavior may be controlled through the administration of antianxiety or antipsychotic agents as prescribed.

Family Teaching

As dementia progresses, more and more care is required outside the hospital and the burden of the family increases. Family members must understand the nature of the disease and the fact that altered cognitive and perceptual abilities are the result of a disease process over which the person has no control. Family members will need instructions on

- Establishing effective communication with the patient
- Maintaining mobility and cognitive activity appropriate to the patient's level of fitness
- Maintaining usual patterns of elimination and sleep/wake patterns
- Maintaining optimum nutritional status

As the person with Alzheimer's disease becomes progressively more disabled, the family will need assistance in preparing for increased care. They will need support as they experience grief over the gradual loss of the personality they knew. Various community organizations and self-help groups such as ADREA, have been formed to support family members through the long and agonizing process of coping with Alzheimer's-type dementia. A variety of books have been published for the lay public that are helpful to some family members attempting to manage a severely disabled person.[14]

Huntington's Disease

Huntington's disease is an inherited disease that affects both sexes equally. Pathologically, there is degeneration and severe loss of small neurons in the caudate and posterior two thirds of the putamen and marked atrophy of the frontal lobes of the cortex. Clinical manifestations occur between 25 and 45 years of age and progress without remission to death in about 15 years. The disease often manifests itself by slight alterations in character. The patient becomes suspicious and irritable, and behavior progresses to impulsive and eccentric and finally to virtual psychosis. Abnormalities of movement begin as a slight restlessness and progress to constant choreiform movements that involve the entire musculature.

In the early stages of the disease, phenothiazines and butyrophenones may suppress abnormal movements and alleviate eccentric behavior or emotional lability. As the disease progresses, the effectiveness of these drugs decreases.

Parkinson's Disease

It has been reported that 1% of the population over the age of 50 years is affected by Parkinson's disease. The disease occurs in all ethnic groups, countries, and socioeconomic classes. It typically has its onset between the ages of 40 and 70 years with a peak age of onset in the sixth decade of life.[14] A parkinsonian syndrome is also seen after manganese, lead, carbon monoxide, and carbon disulfide poisoning. Certain drugs, notably the phenothiazines and reserpine, can induce similar symptoms. It is important that the degenerative disease be differentiated from the treatable parkinsonian syndrome arising from toxicity.

Parkinson's disease involves a progressive dopamine deficiency state resulting from loss or damage to cells in the substantia nigra and other pigmented nuclei. In the absence of sufficient dopamine, excitatory mechanisms go unopposed. The classic triad of symptoms in Parkinson's disease include tremor, rigidity of limbs, and poverty of movement. Poverty of movement is manifested by masked faces, diminished arm swing, tiny handwriting, an inability to perform two stereotyped patterns of motor activity simultaneously, and difficulty initiating movement. Rigidity is evidenced in resistance to movement producing cogwheeling, which is a rhythmical fluctuation in the intensity of resistance. Tremor is slow and rhythmic and occurs when voluntary muscles are relaxed.

Pharmacological agents commonly used to manage the symptoms of Parkinson's disease include levodopa and dopa decarboxylase inhibitors, dopamine agonists, antiviral agents, anticholinergics, and antihistamines (see Table 68–2). Levodopa (Larodopa, Dopar) alone or with a dopa decarboxylase inhibitor (Sinemet) are used to decrease tremor, increase speed and flexibility of movement, and decrease

TABLE 68–2
Drugs Used to Manage Symptoms of Parkinson's Disease

Classification	*Chemical*	*Trade Name*	*Effects*
Dopamine precursor Decarboxylase inhibitor	Levadopa Levodopa and carbidopa	Dopar Larodopa Senimet	*Therapeutic:* Decreased tremor and rigidity; increased speed and flexibility of movement *Adverse:* Nausea, vomiting, pink or red urine that turns dark on standing, postural hypotension, dyskinesias, hallucinations, aberrant behavior, increased heart rate, and palpitations
Dopamine agonist	Bromocriptine Pergolide Lisuride	Parlodel	*Therapeutic:* Same as L-dopa; may alleviate "on-off" effect *Adverse:* Same as L-dopa; hallucinations may be more prominent.
Anti-cholinergic	Biperiden Cycrimine HCl Procyclidine HCl Trihexypenidyl HCl Benztropine mesylate	Akineton Pagitane Kemadrin Artane Tremin Cogentin	*Therapeutic:* Decreased tremor and rigidity; no change in bradykinesia *Adverse:* Constipation, urinary retention, intestinal obstruction
Antiviral	Amantadine HCl	Symmetrel	*Therapeutic:* Same as L-dopa; less helpful for tremor *Adverse:* Same as anticholinergics; potentiates anti-cholinergics
Anti-histamines	Chlorphenoxamine HCl Diphenhydramine HCl Orphenadrine HCl	Phenoxene Benadryl hydrochloride Dissipal	*Therapeutic:* Less effective than L-dopa; may increase tremor *Adverse:* Drowsiness, dizziness, hypotension, headache, weakness

Evaluation Criteria:

1. Can the patient describe changes in symptoms due to the drug?
2. Does the examiner notice changes in tremor, rigidity, and duration of sustained finger tapping?
3. Does the patient and family recognize the difference between increased tremor and the onset of dyskinesia and choreiform movements?
4. Is evaluation by care-providers sought when new side-effects of symptoms appear?
5. Does the patient acknowledge that side-effects such as dry mouth are a trade-off for decreased symptoms?
6. Does the patient have all prescriptions filled at the same pharmacy to decrease the possibility of additive effects of drugs?
7. Can the patient articulate the name and dose of the drug(s) taken?

rigidity. After treatment with levodopa for several years, some patients develop an "on–off" effect in which the therapeutic benefits of the drug alternate with no improvement in symptoms. This effect can sometimes be alleviated with a dopamine agonist such as bromocriptine (Parlodel), pergolide, or lisuride. Amantadine HCl (Symmetrel), an antiviral agent, has been found helpful in decreasing the symptoms of Parkinson's disease. Anticholinergic and antihistamine drugs with anticholinergic effects have been used to decrease tremor and rigidity, but they have no effect on bradykinesia.[16]

Exercise programs are often prescribed for the patient with Parkinson's disease. These exercises can improve mobility, balance, and coordination and can increase independence in activities of daily living. The American Parkinson Disease Association publishes a home exercise manual that can assist the patient to carry out the regular exercise program at home.[11] These exercises are designed to incorporate mobility and general exercise for major body parts, to build up tolerance to exercise, and to further improve finer coordination skills and balance. In some areas, group exercises programs are available to the person with Parkinson's disease. These programs provide supervision in exercise and the social support of group interaction.

Friedreich's Ataxia

There are at least 60 different diseases and syndromes causing progressive ataxia. In many of these no attempt has been made to scientifically study the neuroanatomical changes that occur in the central nervous system. Friedreich's ataxia, an inherited disorder, has been considered a prototype of progressive ataxia. Pathologically, the spinal cord is small and the posterior columns and the corticospinal and spinocerebellar tracts are depleted of medullated fibers. A reduction in the nerve cell population occurs in numerous other areas of the CNS.

The disease is most commonly inherited as an autosomal recessive trait and has an onset of ataxic gait at about age 12. By age 30, nearly all patients are wheelchair-bound or bedridden. The upper extremities become ataxtic. Speech becomes progressively slow, slurred, explosive, and finally incomprehensible. Mentation remains intact. Myocardial muscle fibers are also affected by the disease. It is believed that the conducting system in the heart degenerates. Many patients die as a result of cardiac arrhythmias or congestive heart failure. There is no medical intervention to halt the progression of the disease or to ameliorate the symptoms.

Amyotrophic Lateral Sclerosis

Amyotrophic lateral sclerosis (ALS) or Lou Gehrig's disease is the most common of the motor system diseases that result in progressive muscular weakness. Other diseases in this category include progressive spinal muscular atrophy, progressive bulbar palsy, and primary lateral sclerosis. These diseases are progressive degenerative disorders of the motor neurons in the spinal cord, brain stem, and motor cortex. The exact etiology of these diseases is unknown. A genetic component has been implicated in some forms of muscular atrophy. It is estimated that between 5% and 10% of patients with ALS have a family history of the disease that is generally inherited as an autosomal dominant pattern. ALS occurs sporadically in the population with an incidence (number of new cases per year) of 1.4 cases/100,000 population. The prevalence (number of cases existing in the population) of ALS ranges from 2.5 to 7 cases/100,000 population. The male/female ratio is 1.4 : 1 in those under 65 years of age and equal beyond that age.[26]

Most typically, the first indications of the disease are awkwardness in tasks requiring fine finger movements, a subjective feeling of stiffness of the fingers, and slight weakness or wasting of the hand muscles. Cramping and twitching of arm and shoulder muscles may be present. Within a short period of time, spasticity of the legs and generalized hyperreflexia develop. Eventually the muscle weakness spreads to the neck, tongue, pharyngeal and laryngeal muscles, and trunk. Sensory and sphincter function are preserved. Death commonly occurs within 5 years of onset from respiratory paralysis.

Like the other degenerative diseases, no treatment has been found to alter the course of ALS. Experimental treatment with thyroid-stimulating hormone (TSH) has produced transient improvement in muscle function in some patients.

Myasthenia Gravis

Myasthenia gravis is not a degenerative disease as such, but it is believed to be caused by an autoimmune reaction. The action potential in muscle is generated by nerve impulses in motor nerve fibers at specialized sites known as motor end plates or the neuromuscular junction. The synapse between the nerve and muscle fiber membrane requires the presence of a chemical neurotransmitter called acetylcholine (ACh). In myasthenia gravis, there is a reduction in the number of acetylcholine receptors. The disease affects 1 in 25,000 people. It has an unusual age and sex distribution in that women typically develop the disease between the ages of 20 and 30 years, whereas men do not develop myasthenia gravis until ages 60 or 70. Women are affected twice as often as men.[7]

The disease is characterized by generalized weakness and fatigability of voluntary muscles. Classification is based on the severity of the symptoms and ranges from ocular myasthenia that involves the ocular muscles only, causing ptosis and diplopia, through fulminating myasthenia in which there is bulbar involvement. The course of the disease is unpredictable. Some patients have a mild and slowly progressive course, whereas others have a rapid, stormy course, with exacerbations accompanied by respiratory failure. Respiratory failure and intercurrent respiratory infections are the most common causes of death.

Follicular hyperplasia of the thymus gland occurs in nearly all persons with myasthenia gravis, and thymectomy is carried out in practically all patients. Prednisone and anticholinesterase drugs, neostigmine (Prostigmin) and pyridostigmine (Mestinon), are used to counteract myasthenic weakness. Immunosuppressive drugs including steroids and cytotoxic drugs, such as azathioprine (Imuran) and cyclophosphamide (Cytoxan) have been used alone or combined with other therapies.[12]

The peak effect of drugs varies with the individual. Knowing when the maximum strength of muscles occurs following drug administration makes it possible to schedule activities to coincide with this peak. Patients who have difficulty chewing and swallowing may be able to eat a meal at the peak of drug action. Semi-solid foods may be easier to swallow than liquids or solids. Hot foods tend to increase muscle weakness.

Organization is a key to efficient use of the myasthenic person's energy. Learning to pace activities, set realistic goals, and conserve energy by such things as using a stool in the kitchen will greatly improve functional abilities. Resources are available through the Myasthenia Gravis Foundation and the Muscular Dystrophy Association.

Myasthenic Crisis. Anticholinesterase drugs, which are used to alleviate the symptoms of muscle weakness in the person with myasthenia gravis, can cause a cholinergic crisis that occurs when excessive medication blocks acetylcholine receptor sites and results in increased muscle weakness and respiratory paralysis. Myasthenic crisis, on the other hand, can lead to profound weakness and respiratory paralysis because of too low a dose of the drug. The demand for anticholinesterase is increased by infection, trauma, stress, changes in endocrine balance, temperature extremes, hypokalemia, or stress. Administration of medication on time is critical, since a delay of 15 to 20 minutes may result in increased symptoms.[12]

Cholinergic or myasthenic crises may occur suddenly and without warning. Initially the typical signs of respiratory difficulty (increased respiratory rate, nasal flaring, and intercostal or suprasternal retractions) may not be apparent. Subtle changes such as apprehension and insomnia are common. Chest expansion decreases, and the patient experiences dysphagia, dysarthria, and dysphonia. Respiratory paralysis occurs followed by changes in blood gases, blood pressure, and pulse rate.

Changes in vital signs are a late sign of crisis. Observe the patient for changes in speech, posture, facial expression, degree of ptosis, and extent of extraocular movements.[12] The patient often knows when a crisis is approaching before overt signs are apparent. Early assessment of impending crisis includes the careful examination of muscle strength in the upper extremities, neck, and face.

Tensilon and Prostigmin for treatment of myasthenic crisis and atropine for cholinergic crisis should be easily accessible. Also needed is respiratory support equipment such as suction catheters, ventilator bag, oxygen, and an intubation tray.

Crises in myasthenia do not always occur in the controlled hospital setting. Persons with this disease must know how to contact emergency assistance. They should wear identification that includes their diagnosis, drugs and dosages, contraindicated medications, and the physician's name and phone number.

Muscular Dystrophy

The muscular dystrophies are diseases of skeletal muscles. They are included here because the clinical presentation of progressive muscle weakness closely parallels diseases of neurological origin. There are at least nine classes of progressive, hereditary diseases of muscle in which there is degeneration and loss of muscle fibers.[2] These diseases are usually familial in origin, often carried by the female and affecting the male. Pathologically, there is atrophy with wide variation in muscle fiber size. Eventually muscle is replaced by fat and connective tissue.

Severe generalized muscular dystrophy of children begins in early childhood, usually before the sixth year of life. The incidence is estimated at 3 cases/100,000 population. The disease occurs predominantly in males and has a strong familial liability. The most common forms are Duchenne's and Erb's dystrophy. Weakness and hypertrophy begin in the shoulder and hip girdles and eventually affect the arms and hands, as well as the abdomen. Hypertrophy of cardiac muscle is often the cause of death.

Some forms of muscular dystrophy appear later in life and affect only selected muscle groups. Fascioscapulohumeral dystrophy presents during the second or third decade of life as weakness of the face and shoulders. Pelvic muscles may become involved later. Scapulohumeral (limb-girdle) dystrophy affects the shoulder or shoulder and pelvic muscles, while progressive external ophthalmoplegia affects only the extraocular muscles.

There is no specific treatment for any of the muscular dystrophies. Quinine may temporarily relieve myotonia but has no effect on muscle atrophy. Complications of bone fractures, pulmonary infections, and cardiac decompensation are treated symptomatically.

Multiple Sclerosis

The cause of the pathological changes that occur in multiple sclerosis is unknown; however, much evidence has been accumulated to suggest that an immunologic disorder plays a significant role in the pathogenesis of demyelination. Pathologically, the macrophage destroys myelin throughout the brain and spinal cord. The oligodendrocytes that would ordinarily produce new myelin fail to do so. Astrocytes form a scar that interrupts the normal flow of impulses across the nerve fiber. A genetic predisposition to the disease may be one determinant of risk for the development of this disease.

As myelin is destroyed it is replaced by sclerotic plaques that interfere with normal nerve conduction. The classic triad of symptoms includes nystagmus, scanning speech, and tremor. However, disorders of sensation, bowel and bladder disorders, and movement disorders are common. Mentation disorders are apparent in some persons with multiple sclerosis.

The disease has some unique epidemiological characteristics. It occurs most often in parts of Europe and North America that lie between 40 and 60 degrees north latitude and in the southern portion of New Zealand and Australia. Where a person is born and raised is more critical to the development of multiple sclerosis than where the person lives at the time of onset. The disease more commonly affects women and has a greater prevalence in higher socioeconomic groups.

Hundreds of therapeutic interventions have been proposed for multiple sclerosis, none of which has halted the progression of demyelinization. ACTH and corticotropin are used to decrease the symptoms resulting from acute inflammation associated with demyelination. The usual duration of therapy with these drugs is 10 to 14 days. Many of the clinical trials now are aimed at altering the immune system. Meanwhile, therapy is centered on minimizing the effect of symptoms on daily living.

Care of the person with multiple sclerosis is directed toward maintaining general well-being. Toward this end, the person must learn to

1. Avoid excessive fatigue
2. Avoid extremes of temperature
3. Prevent exposure to infection
4. Undertake early and vigorous treatment when infection occurs
5. Balance rest and exercise within their capacity
6. Eat a nutritious and well-balanced diet

Pharmacological agents may play an important role in the managment of multiple sclerosis. Acute exacerbations of the disease may be treated with ACTH or corticosteroids. Spasticity may be managed with diazepam (Valium), dantrolene sodium (Dantrium), or baclofen (Lioresal). Neurogenic bladder may be treated with cholinergic drugs (*e.g.*, bethanechol chloride) or anticholinergic drugs (*e.g.*, propantheline bromide, oxybutynin chloride). The patient should know the name, dose, and expected effects of each drug. A journal is helpful in developing an ability to recognize positive and negative effects of medication.[16]

The person with multiple sclerosis may have multiple and varied problems, including impaired vision, sensory changes, altered mobility, tremor, altered elimination, and impaired communication. These problems are addressed in the Nursing Care Plan for the Patient with Multiple Sclerosis. Additionally, the person has information needs in the areas of disease process, treatment, drug therapy, and follow-up care. Other problems exist in the areas of sexuality, emotional adjustment (*e.g.,* denial, depression, and euphoria), and social and vocational adjustment.[15]

NURSING CARE PLAN FOR THE PATIENT WITH MULTIPLE SCLEROSIS

NURSING DIAGNOSIS/PROBLEM: Impaired mobility, altered sensation, tremor, visual and speech impairment, and bowel and bladder dysfunction related to myelin loss

GOAL 1: Maximize visual function and safety

Nursing Interventions	Rationale	Outcome Criteria
1. Check visual acuity on hospital admission or outpatient visit.	1. Vision may change gradually or suddenly as a result of demyelinization of optic nerve.	1. Visual changes are assessed early and needed action is taken.
2. Advise primary care-provider of changes in vision.	2. Acute optic neuritis may require drug therapy.	2. Further damage to optic nerve from swelling is prevented.
3. Instruct patient with diplopia to use eye patch and to alternate the patch between eyes at least daily.	3. Eye patch relieves diplopia but will cause blindness if used on the same eye continually.	3. Patient uses eye patch when diplopia is present; alternates patch as directed.
4. Reassure patient that blindness from MS is unusual.	4. Knowing that symptoms are transient will decrease anxiety.	4. Patient verbalizes that visual impairment is unlikely to lead to blindness.

GOAL 2: Prevent injury and maximize level of functioning

Nursing Interventions	Rationale	Outcome Criteria
1. Assess and record sensory impairment and mobility level at hospital admission, weekly while on inpatient unit, and at each outpatient visit.	1. Accurate knowledge of current functional level is essential for care planning.	1. Care plan is individualized and based on current functional level of patient.
2. Instruct patient in safety measures such as: a. Testing bath water temperature with unaffected extremity or with thermometer b. Using a pot holder when cooking c. Avoiding the use of electric heating pads d. Wearing gloves in cold weather	2. MS may decrease temperature perception.	2. Thermal and cold injury is prevented.
3. Teach patient to use visual clues to overcome deficits in touch and position sense.	3. Visual feedback may help the person compensate for loss of touch and position sense.	3. Patient is able to maintain maximal level of function.
4. Discuss need for mobility aids, as needed.	4. The use of canes, crutches walkers, and wheelchairs may prevent falls.	4. Patient recognizes appropriate assistive devices for ambulation inside and outside the home.

(*Continued*)

NURSING CARE PLAN FOR THE PATIENT WITH MULTIPLE SCLEROSIS (*Continued*)

GOAL 3: Establish effective communication

Nursing Interventions	Rationale	Outcome Criteria
1. Observe communiation patterns to determine if they are effective.	1. Dysarthria and scanning speech interfere with communication.	1–4. Patient is able to communicate effectively.
2. Encourage patient to speak slowly.	2. Slowing the rate of speech improves understandability.	
3. Refer to speech pathologist, if needed.	3–4. Learning new ways of communicating requires specialized assistance.	
4. Encourage patient to learn the use of assistive devices.		

GOAL 4: Maintains bowel and bladder function

Nursing Interventions	Rationale	Outcome Criteria
1. Assess and report patient's dietary and elimination patterns.	1–2. Abdominal muscle weakness and inactivity contribute to constipation and fecal incontinence.	1–2. Patient has bowel movement every 2–3 days, abdomen is soft, and there is no fecal impaction.
2. Initiate bowel training program, if needed.		
3. Instruct patient on need for high-fiber diet and adequate fluid intake.		3. Patient demonstrates satisfactory intake.
4. Assess and report urinary function: a. Frequency b. Urgency c. Incontinence d. Recurrent infection	4. Demyelination of neuroanatomic pathways serving the bladder will result in failure to empty or failure to store urine.	4. Accurate records of function allow for individualized care planning.
5. Teach the patient to follow the regimen established to manage urinary dysfunction.	5. Drugs, mechanical assistance, or intermittent catheterization may be necessary to minimize the effects of neurogenic bladder.	5. Patient reports decreased symptoms, maintains continence, and avoids urinary tract infection.

Nursing Management

Assessment and Nursing Diagnosis

The group of degenerative diseases considered in this chapter are diverse in the type and extent of symptoms they produce. The nurse who is hospital-based may see these patients at the time of diagnosis, during a period of reevaluation as the disease progresses, or when they are hospitalized for other disorders. Nursing assessment focuses on the functional deficits experienced by these patients. These deficits fall into the categories of movement, sensation, and mentation. In addition, the patient will be taking medications to control symptoms. These patients will need careful assessment in terms of the therapeutic and nontherapeutic effects of the drugs.

Self-care deficits are common in persons with disorders of movement and severe deficits in mentation. Patterns of elimination may be altered because of muscle weakness or the person's ability to provide self-care in these areas. The person who is unable to eat independently may experience nutritional and metabolic alterations, and the person who maintains the same caloric intake while becoming progressively less active has the potential for obesity. Progressive inability to care for oneself and to perform accustomed role responsibilities result in altered self-concept and the potential for ineffective coping. In sum, the person with a degenerative disease has the potential for developing problems in all areas of function.

Goals. The goals for patients with degenerative diseases of the nervous system include

1. Maintaining normal function under as many circumstances and for as long as possible

2. Preventing immobility and sensory deprivation or overload associated with altered neurological function
3. Providing information so that the patient and family can manage the disease independently outside the hospital

Interventions

The challenge in working with patients with degenerative diseases is to keep them as independent as possible for as long as possible. This requires the cooperation of all members of the health care team, including the patient. An integrated program of physical, psychological, educational, vocational, and recreational therapies is essential.

Patients with pathological conditions of the central nervous system are at risk for developing a variety of complications secondary to immobility and sensory deprivation or overload associated with altered neurological functioning. An important goal in the nursing management of these patients is to prevent these problems. This goal will be achieved when early signs and symptoms of problems are recognized, and intervention is initiated to prevent sequelae of immobility and sensory alterations.

Patients with degenerative diseases will spend the majority of their life with their disease outside the hospital and the direct supervision of health care professionals. These patients and their family members must learn the daily management of the disease, including the therapeutic regimen.

References

1. Adams RD, Petersdorf RG: Pyrogenic infections of the central nervous system. In Petersdorf RG, Adams RD, Braunwal E et al (eds): Harrison's Principles of Internal Medicine, 10th ed. New York, McGraw-Hill, 1983
2. Adams RD, Victor M: Principles of Neurology, 2nd ed. New York, McGraw-Hill, 1981
3. Blanco K, Cuomo N: From the other side of the bedrail: A personal experience with Guillain-Barré syndrome. J Neurosurg Nurs 15:355, 1983
4. Boss BJ: The dementias. J Neurosurg Nurs, 15:87, 1983
5. Brody H: Neuroanatomy and neuropathology of aging. In Buzze EW, Blazer DG (eds): Handbook of Geriatric Psychiatry. New York, Van Nostrand Reinhold, 1980
6. Catanzaro M: Nursing care of the person with MS. Am J Nurs 80:286, 1980
7. Drachman D: Myasthenia gravis. New Engl J Med 298:136,186, 1978
8. Harter DH, Petersdorf RG, Adams RD: Viral diseases of the central nervous system: Aseptic meningitis and encephalitis. In Petersdorf RG, Adams RD, Braunwal E et al (eds): Harrison's Principles of Internal Medicine, 10th ed. New York, McGraw-Hill, 1983
9. Hickey J: The Clinical Practice of Neurological and Neurosurgical Nursing. Philadelphia, JB Lippincott, 1981
10. Hrovath M: Myasthenia gravis: A nursing approach. J Neurosurg Nurs 14:7, 1982
11. Jones C: Glasgow coma scale. Am J Nurs 79:1551, 1979
12. Kess R: Suddenly in crisis: Unpredictable myasthenia. Am J Nurs 84:994, 1984
13. Lavigne J: Home exercises for patients with Parkinson's disease. The American Parkinson Disease Association.
14. Mace NL, Rabins PV: The 36-hour day. Baltimore, John Hopkins University, 1981
15. McDonnell M, Hentgen J, Holland N, Levison PW: Problem oriented nursing care plans. Am J Nurs 80:292, 1980
16. Mithcell PH, Catanzaro M: Learning needs in chronic neurologic disease. In MJ VanMeter (ed): Neurologic Care: A Guide for Patient Education. New York, Appleton-Century-Crofts, 1982
17. National Institute of Neurological and Communicative Disorders and Stroke. Special Report: Parkinson's disease. Washington DC, Author, 1981
18. Prydun M: Guillain-Barré syndrome: Disease process. J Neurosurg Nurs 15:27, 1983
19. Ray CG: Chickenpox (varicella) and herpes zoster. In Petersdorf RG, Adams RD, Braunwal E et al (eds): Harrison's Principles of Internal Medicine, 10th ed. New York, McGraw-Hill, 1983
20. Reisburg B: Stages of cognitive decline. Am J Nurs 84:225, 1984
21. Reisberg B et al: The global deterioration scale for assessment of primary degenerative dementia. Am J Psychiatry, 139:1136, 1982
22. Rimel RW, Tyson GW: The neurologic examination in patients with central nervous system trauma. J Neurosurg Nurs 11:148, 1979
23. Stewart CM: Age-related changes in the nervous system. J Neurosurg Nurs 14:69, 1982
24. Taylor JW, Ballenger S: Neurological Dysfunctions and Nursing Intervention. New York, McGraw-Hill, 1980
25. Terry R, Katzman R: Senile dementia of the Alzheimer type: Defining a disease. In Katzman R, Terry R: The neurology of aging. Philadelphia, FA Davis, 1983
26. Varon MI: The current status of amyotrophic lateral sclerosis (memorandum). Amyotrophic Lateral Sclerosis Society of America, February 19, 1981

Bibliography

American Association of Neurosurgical Nurses: Core Curriculum for Neuroscience Nursing. Chicago, Author, 1983

Barry L: The patient with myasthenia gravis really needs you. Nursing 82 12(7):50, 1982

Bolton RM: Creutzfeldt-Jakob disease. J Neurosurg Nurs 14:1, 1982

Boss BJ: Acute mood and behavior disturbances of neurological origin: Acute confusional states. J Neurosurg Nurs 14:61, 1982

Douvoisin R: Parkinson's Disease: A Guide for Patients and Family. New York, Raven Press, 1978

Garrett E: Parkinsonism: Forgotten consideration in medical treatment and nursing care. J Neurosurg Nurs 14:13, 1982

Jemison-Smith P, Hubbel H: Guillian-Barré syndrome. Critical Care Update 10(6):12, 1983

Pajk M: Alzheimer's disease inpatient care. Am J Nurs 84:216, 1984

Power PW: Family intervention in rehabilitation of patient with Huntington disease. Arch Phys Med Rehabil 63:441, 1982

Scheinberg L: Multiple Sclerosis: A Guide for Patients and Families. New York: Raven Press, 1983

Stern G, Lees A: Parkinson's Disease: The Facts. New York, Oxford University Press, 1982

Tikkanen PL: Landry-Guillian-Barré-Strohl syndrome. Am J Neurosurg Nurs 14:74, 1982

Trockman G: Working with the confused or delirious patient: Caring for the confused or delirious patient. Am J Nurs 78:1495, 1978

Wolanin MO, Phillips LRF: Confusion: Prevention and Care. St Louis, CV Mosby, 1983

Chapter 69

Neurological Trauma

Karen Booth McCormick

Head Trauma

Incidence and Epidemiology

Head trauma has become a major health problem with serious medical and socioeconomic consequences.

Statistics compiled in recent years have consistently demonstrated the rate of occurrence for head injury in males to be twice that for females. Motor vehicle accidents account for nearly half of all head injuries and are most common in the 15- to 24-year-old age-group.[22] Further, 70% of patients who were comatose following head injury sustained their head injuries in motor vehicle accidents.[28]

Substance abuse, primarily alcohol, is known to increase the risk of an accident. The risk of an alcohol-related accident is ten times that of chance when the blood alcohol level is >150 mg/100 ml.[21] Health education of society, especially youth, regarding the significant increased risk of accidents while under the influence of alcohol and other central nervous system depressants or hallucinogens must continue to be foremost. Reduction of the speed limit and use of seat belts reduced fatal and severe injuries four times over that encountered in motor vehicle accidents in which seat belts were not used.[38] Use of helmets has been shown to decrease severity of injury in motorcycle, bicycle, and work-related accidents.[21]

Etiology and Classification

Head injuries may be classified in a variety of ways. They may be classified as closed injuries (blunt or nonmissile injuries) and open injuries (missile or penetrating). Basically, *closed injuries* are those in which there has been no break in continuity of the skull with regard to intracranial contents and the environment. *Open injuries* are those in which communication between intracranial structures and the environment has occured.

Skull fractures are classified as nondepressed, linear, or depressed. Most basal skull fractures are linear and single, but they may be compound–depressed (*e.g.,* sinus cavity bone fragmented and pushed into the brain). A depressed fracture may consist of an area of indentation pressing on the brain or it may be compound, with comminuted fragments pushed into the brain.

Pathophysiology

In order to understand the mechanics of brain injury one must consider the properties of the brain, the structures that encase it, and what happens when kinetic energy is applied or transferred to the head. The brain possesses gellike properties and is contained in a rigid structure, the skull.

Acceleration and deceleration are the two types of forces that may be applied to the head during blunt impact. Acceleration occurs when a moving object strikes the stationary head. Deceleration occurs when the moving head strikes a stationary object. These forces may cause both linear and rotational movements of the brain within the skull. For example, when an individual's head strikes the windshield of a car, the brain, having gained momentum from the movement, is thrown against the then stationary skull. The brain, in the process of this forward and/or lateral movement, sustains injuries to its surface (contact phenomena) as well as to the brain parenchyma (shear, tensile, and compressive strains). Cortical surface injuries are caused by the impact of the cerebral hemispheres against the skull and dural partitions. The ventral portions of the cerebral hemispheres are "scraped" across the bony projections, and ridges of the basal skull and the brain stem may strike the edge of the tentorium. Structures within the brain may be disrupted by the sliding of one tissue over another (shear strain), by tissue being pulled apart, or by tissue being subjected to compression. Cortical vessels may be torn by both the displacement of the brain as well as by pressure gradients.[25,27,35,36]

In addition to acceleration–deceleration forces (blunt injuries), the brain may also be damaged by penetrating forces (missile and stab wounds) and by compressive forces (crush injuries). Indirect injuries to the brain may also occur with whiplash types of injuries and by a fall on the buttocks.

Primary and Secondary Brain Damage

Head injury results in both primary and secondary damage to the brain. Primary damage occurs as a direct result of the injury itself, whereas secondary damage occurs as a result of the effects of the primary damage.

Primary damage, resulting from direct or indirect impact damage to the head, can cause focal structural damage such as skull fracture, cortical contusion, and cerebral cavitation.

Cerebral lacerations may result from depressed bone fragments as well as from penetrating wounds such as those produced by missile or stab wounds.

Blunt injuries, penetrating injuries, and crush injuries to the head may all produce extensive local brain damage without an associated loss of consciousness; loss of consciousness is a result of diffuse phenomena.

Concussion is a result of diffuse injury to the brain. Cerebral concussion has traditionally been defined as a brief loss of consciousness associated with a period of amnesia that occurs as a result of direct or indirect impact to the head. Experimental studies and clinical evidence suggest that concussion may be a graded phenomenon ranging from Stage I, consisting of a very brief period of mild confusion only (alteration of consciousness) without an associated total loss of consciousness, to Stage IV, which is associated with posttraumatic amnesia (PTA) and retrograde amnesia (RGA)—amnesia for events preceding the concussion.[35]

The primary focus of both medicine and nursing is to prevent, or at least minimize, the effects of secondary brain damage. Secondary brain damage arises from intracranial expanding lesions and brain swelling, which may produce increased intracranial pressure (ICP) as well as brain shifts and herniation syndromes, leading to permanent neurological deficit or death if not promptly treated (or if the condition does not respond to treatment).

Hematomas

Expanding mass lesions within the cranium may take the form of epidural or subdural hematomas or intracerebral hematomas. An *epidural hematoma* (Fig. 69–1) is a solid clot of blood that occurs as a result of arterial and/or venous bleeding above the dura (between the periosteal dura and the skull). It is often associated with a linear fracture of the temporal bone that traverses, and lacerates, the middle meningeal artery. The bleeding proceeds rapidly, and because of the volume and the rapidity with which the mass expands (less time for the brain to compensate), prompt action to evacuate the hematoma is neccesary to avert catastrophe. Epidural hematomas are most frequently seen in the temporoparietal areas, but they also occur in frontal, occipital, and posterior fossa areas. There may be little or no underlying brain damage. Loss of consciousness may be delayed, immediate and prolonged, or brief at the onset of impact followed by a lucid interval, followed by delayed loss of consciousness (this was previously considered to be the classic presentation

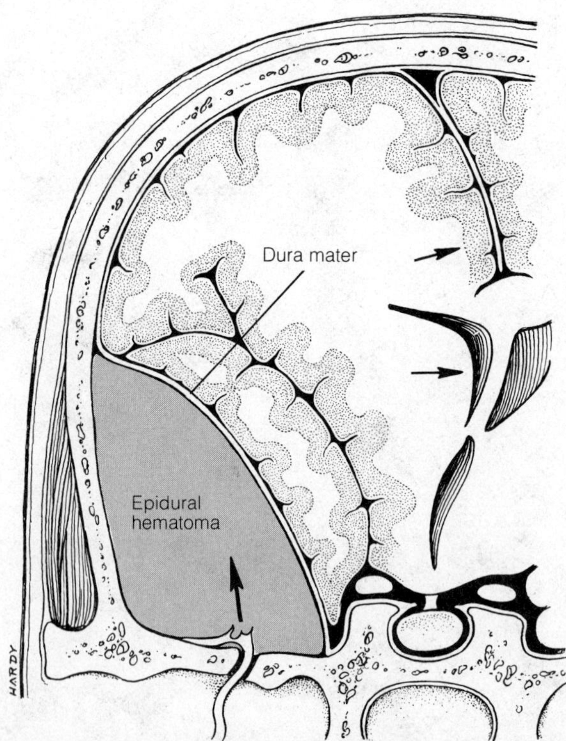

FIGURE 69–1 Epidural hematoma. The dark area in the lower left of the drawing represents the hematoma. Note the broken blood vessel and the shift of midline structures.

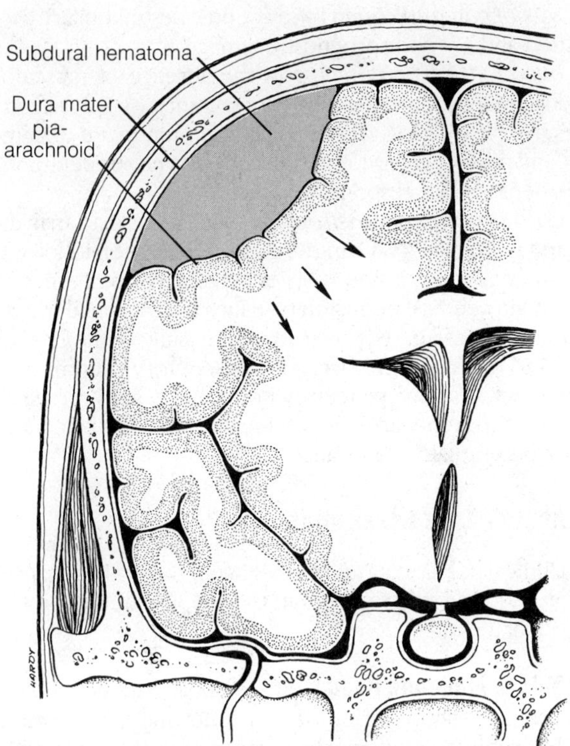

FIGURE 69–2 Subdural hematoma. The dark area in the upper left of the drawing represents the hematoma. Note the shift of midline structures.

of an epidural hematoma. When these hematomas are diagnosed and evacuated promptly, the prognosis for full recovery is usually excellent.

A *subdural hematoma* is a collection of blood (clotted in the acute state) located between the dura and the arachnoid (Fig. 69–2). Its formation may arise from a variety of sources. Pressure gradients occurring with impact injury may cause disruption of bridging cortical veins; there may be generalized subdural bleeding (not uncommon in head injuries) which, combined with severe injuries, may be sufficient to create a mass effect; and lacerations of the brain itself may cause subdural collections of blood. Acute subdural hematomas are often associated with a poorer prognosis because they are generally seen in more severe head injuries. A subdural hematoma may be categorized as acute, with symptomatology occuring within 1 to 3 days of injuries; subacute, with symptomatology occurring within 4 days to 2 weeks after injury; and chronic, which gives rise to symptoms after 2 weeks of injury.[27] Subdural hematomas may be associated with underlying contusions, intracerebral hematomas, and necrotic brain.

Intracerebral hematoma usually develops from extravasation of blood from the small intracerebral vessels. They tend to be more common in the frontal lobe but are also seen in the temporal lobe. They are often associated with contusions and subdural hematomas and may also arise from direct laceration of the brain.

Brain Swelling

Focal brain swelling often accompanies contusions and intracerebral hematomas and, as such, acts as an expanding mass lesion, serving to complicate these lesions further. This type of swelling is due to vasogenic edema. Edema fluid formation develops in areas where there has been a breakdown in the integrity of the blood–brain barrier.

Diffuse brain swelling may be due to cerebral vascular engorgement occurring in response to the immediate effects of impact to the head; however, the etiology of this type of brain swelling remains under investigation.[25]

In summary, intracranial expanding lesions add to the morbidity and mortality of head injury by causing brain shifts and herniation of brain structures. In addition, intracerebral space-occupying lesions cause brain swelling. An increase in intracranial pressure, observed with expanding mass lesions, may cause brain herniation as well. It may also compromise perfusion of the brain. A review of intracranial pressure dynamics is essential in understanding the pathophysiology and treatment of head trauma.

Intracranial Pressure

The dynamics of intracranial pressure (ICP) can be defined as the pressure exerted by the brain constituents, namely blood, cerebrospinal fluid, and brain tissue, within the rigid skull. Normal ICP is 0–10 mmHg (torr), which corresponds to 0–136 mmH_2O. The very upper limit of normal is 15 mmHg or 204 mmH_2O.[26]

An increase in intracranial pressure results from an addition to the volume of any of the intracranial constituents. For example, an obstruction of the cerebrospinal fluid pathways, preventing the circulation and absorption of CSF into the venous sinuses, an intracranial space-occupying lesion, or an increase in blood volume, all add to the overall intracranial volume.

The ability for compensation within the intracranial compartments is termed *compliance* (or elastance). When addition to intracranial volume is tolerated without an increase in ICP, compliance is said to be high; Elastance, because it is the inverse of compliance, is said to be low. As volume is added to the intracranial compartments, a critical point is eventually reached wherein compensation is no longer possible. At this point, an addition of even a small volume will cause a large and precipitous rise in intracranial pressure, so that compliance is low (or elastance is high) and ICP increases.[26] Generally, a large but slowly expanding mass is more easily compensated than a small, rapidly expanding one.

Intracranial pressure may influence as well as be influenced by cerebral blood flow (CBF). Normally, CBF is maintained at a constant level, regardless of the blood pressure, through a mechanism inherent in the blood vessels called *autoregulation.* Autoregulation of the diameter of the cerebral vessels normally functions at levels of mean systemic arterial pressures between 60–145 mmHg. Autoregulation, however, is frequently lost, either focally or generally, early in the process of brain compression. It is frequently nonexistent in patients who are comatose or who have intracranial hypertension. Cerebral vessels may continue to be sensitive to changes in Pa_{CO_2} after head injury, though this effect may be somewhat reduced. Normal Pa_{CO_2} is 35–45 mmHg. An increase in Pa_{CO_2} levels, or hypercarbia (such as that which may occur secondary to inadequate pulmonary ventilation) produces cerebral vasodilatation, while hypocarbia produces cerebral vasoconstriction. Arterial oxygen levels will influence the cerebral blood flow if it falls below 50–60 mmHg, at which point it causes cerebral vasodilatation.

Any condition that interferes with venous outflow, the venous return of blood from the brain, increases cerebral blood volume (CBV), and may cause a significant rise in intracranial pressure. Any increase in intra-abdominal or intrathoracic pressure, such as occurs with Valsalva maneuvers, will cause a concomitant rise in juglar venous pressure, and further increase ICP.

Clinical Manifestations

Physicians and nurses are often dependent on the individuals who witnessed the trauma and those who first arrived at the accident scene (police, fire department, emergency medical technicians) for valuable information regarding the condition of the patient at that time. Such information includes any signs of apnea, loss of consciousness, pupillary response, eye deviation, or seizures.

Emergency Room Assessment

Once the patient arrives in the emergency room, a full examination is conducted to determine the extent of all injuries that might have been incurred as a result of the trauma.

External evidence of head injury includes scalp contusions, lacerations, and hematomas. The presence of periorbital ecchymosis (racoon's eyes) and blood behind the tympanic membrane (hemotympanum) suggest a basal skull fracture. Bleeding from the external auditory canal may signify a basal skull fracture or it also may signify laceration to the canal itself. Occasionally cerebrospinal fluid otorrhea may be observed, which, of course, is pathognomonic of basal skull fracture. Battle's sign, ecchymosis of the mastoid area, is not demonstrated until 2 to 3 days after trauma, and also indicates basal skull fracture.

Depressed skull fractures may be palpated by noting a "step-off" ridge. Sometimes a depressed skull fracture is obvious on visible inspection.

Alteration in either mental status or consciousness points to cerebral dysfunction either from the head injury alone, or in combination with a postictal state (following a seizure), alcohol intoxication, drug abuse, hypoxia, or hypovolemia. If the patient is awake and oriented, history of loss of consciousness at the scene and the presence of amnesia should be noted. The Glasgow Coma Scale score should of course be documented. If the patient is unresponsive, information regarding whether or not a lucid interval was present prior to his arrival in the emergency room should be sought.

Loss of gag and cough reflexes indicates medullary dysfunction and is a poor prognostic sign.

Impaired motor function in the absence of musculoskeletal trauma indicates focal brain injury or spinal cord injury. *Sensory deficits* due to focal brain injury are uncommon and when they are noted usually are not evident until the patient is more responsive.

Cardiopulmonary dysfunction, such as cardiac arrhythmia and ischemic ECG changes, is commonly seen following head injury. Hypertension is observed and may be necessary to maintain cerebral perfusion pressure if intracranial hypertension is present. Hypotension is usually indicative of trauma to other systems. Irregular respiratory patterns may be present. Usually patients who present with irregular respiratory patterns are unconscious and are intubated and placed on ventilatory assistance.

Acute Phase Assessment

Clinical manifestations of head injury during hospitalization in the acute phase may vary widely depending on the severity of the injury.

Mild to Moderate Head Injury. Those patients who are admitted for a short period of time following a concussion, which is a mild to moderate head injury, are admitted so that they may be observed for delayed signs of complication. Signs and symptoms that may be observed in a patient who has sustained a mild to moderate head injury during this phase may include mild disorientation, post-traumatic amnesia, short-term memory deficits, headache, nausea and vomiting, light-headedness, positional vertigo, hearing impairment, facial weakness, and other focal symptoms (usually indicative of cortical contusion) such as dysphasia or weakness of an extremity.

Abnormal signs and symptoms must be evaluated in terms of the baseline examination. Evidence of potentially serious complication includes decreasing level of consciousness, abnormal pupillary light response, anisocoria, and any other focal neurological deficits that were not previously present. Focal neurological signs include cranial nerve dysfunction, motor weakness, receptive or expressive dysphasia, or focal seizure. Appearance of a CSF leak is indicative of a basal skull fracture, and is of concern because it is a potential source for meningitis.

Moderate to Severe Head Injury. Patients with moderate to severe head injury will manifest clinical signs of prolonged unconsciousness (greater than 24 hours) associated with or without brain stem dysfunction signs. Abnormal flexor or extensor posturing of the extremities, either spontaneous or on stimulation, may be evident. Brain swelling and increased intracranial pressure may be present, and the patient may show clinical signs of brain herniation, which is either in the process of being treated or has not responded to treatment (refer to Chap. 63 for brain herniation syndromes). These patients may also have focal neurological deficits such as hemiparesis and cranial nerve dysfunction. Generalized or focal motor seizures may occur.

Recovery Phase Symptoms

Postconcussion Syndrome. Following mild head trauma, many patients will note a variety of problems, which have come to be known as postconcussion syndrome. This syndrome comprises headache, dizziness–vertigo, poor concentration, memory impairment, fatigue, irritability, depression, insomnia, and alcohol intolerance. Many investigators have contended that these problems are mainly a result of psychological factors; however, there is increasing evidence that these problems do have an organic basis. It is not uncommon for patients to continue to have these problems for months following the head injury.

Prolonged Disabilities. Once the patient begins improving from a moderate to severe head injury, other neurological deficits, which were not noted earlier because of impaired consciousness, become apparent. Physical disabilities, if present, certainly add to the difficulties of the recovery process, but it is the cognitive–psychosocial impairments that by far create the most significant problems in the reintegration of the patient into society. Cognitive deficits can impede the patient's return to school or work, his interaction with his family, friends and coworkers, and even his ability to participate in rehabilitation. Some patients with severe head injury never return to their former selves. Many of the physical disabilities that persist after head injury are due to focal and multifocal brain damage; the cognitive–psychosocial impairments, however, seem to be related to diffuse brain damage. Neurological deficits and disabilities that may be noted in the recovery phase, some of which may be permanent, include anosmia, visual impairment, hearing impairment, language impairment, motor impairment, sensory impairment, pain problems, impairment of higher cortical integrative functions, cognitive impairment, and psychosocial behavioral deficits.

Post-traumatic Epilepsy. The risk of developing late post-traumatic epilepsy following blunt head trauma in general is about 5% overall.[21] Of those patients who develop late post-traumatic epilepsy, most will have their first seizure within a year of injury, though onset of epilepsy up to 4 years later is not uncommon. Generally, with each advancing year that the patient does not develop post-traumatic epilepsy his chance of doing so decreases.

Seizures may be generalized with a focal onset or primarily generalized. Complex partial seizures are also seen. For a review of seizure disorders, see Chapter 65.

Following Post-traumatic Coma. As patients begin to recover from post-traumatic coma they continue to have impairment of consciousness and mental status. They may sleep a lot, appear totally disinterested in their environment, and take no initiative to feed or groom themselves. They are usually incontinent. They verbalize little, if at all.

As they improve they may spend more time awake (often at night) and will manifest confused behavior. They will attempt to get out of their bed or chair when they are unsafe to do so. They may be combative. They may verbalize in answer to questions (and often give confused and disoriented responses), but they will seldom carry on a conversation. They usually continue to be incontinent. They may feed themselves but not uncommonly will have an apraxia for eating. They will not know how to use utensils, they may eat with their hands, drink from bowls, eat butter, or pour salad dressing on their meat or dessert, and so on. They may even attempt to eat their napkin or the menu on their tray.

Following this phase, they gradually will begin to be more appropriate. They may verbalize more, but they still rarely carry on a conversation. They often have a very flat affect. They may or may not continue to be disoriented. They may still manifest confused behavior at night.

Patients who have had significant head trauma in which there was a moderate degree of subarachnoid hemorrhage are at risk of developing a communicating hydrocephalus. Serial CT scans, especially in patients who begin to deteriorate, may show progressively enlarging ventricles. These patients may eventually require a shunting procedure in order to provide a means whereby cerebrospinal fluid may be continually drained from the cerebral ventricles.

The improvement made during this phase may take place over weeks to months. It is not uncommon that, once a patient reaches a certain level wherein he spends more time awake and demonstrates more appropriate behavior, he will improve rapidly with noticeable daily gains. This improvement, however, is just the beginning; it signifies that the patient is ready to benefit from a formal rehabilitation program.

Medical Management

Diagnosis

The diagnosis of craniocerebral trauma is dependent on the history of trauma and presence of impaired consciousness, associated with or without abnormal findings on the neurological examination. External evidence of head injury may or may not be present. The goals of the diagnosis of intracranial damage, as outlined by Becker and coworkers, include[3]

1. To define as quickly as possible the presence of major mass lesions that require surgical removal, preferably and ideally before herniation syndromes are evident
2. To determine abnormal intracranial function in order to guide and direct appropriate operative and non-operative therapy
3. To localize the number, size, and nature of all brain injuries to classify obstacles to ongoing management and to provide accuracy in predicting outcome
4. To identify all scalp and skull injuries, which may be a source of both immediate and delayed brain insults

The diagnosis of *skull fracture* can occasionally be made on inspection and palpation. Skull films and CT scans are the diagnostic tests used. Basal skull fractures are most often diagnosed indirectly by clinical evidence; this type of fracture often does not appear on skull films.

Cortical contusions are often diagnosed by the presence

of focal neurological deficits. CT scans are sometimes negative, especially immediately after trauma. Serial scans are recommended to monitor the development or expansions of contusions (contusion plus edema), or their possible evolution into intracerebral hematomas.

Intracranial hematomas are either epidural, subdural, or intracerebral. They are most frequently diagnosed by CT scanning. Development of focal neurological signs that were not previously present or deterioration of the patient's level of consciousness should alert everyone to the possibility of an expanding mass lesion.

Intracerebral hematomas are high density lesions and are often surrounded by areas of low density (edema). All of these lesions may produce a shift in midline structures.

Brain edema often produces a "mass effect" that causes displacement, distortion, and compression of the ventricles. If edema is great and intracranial pressure is elevated, the ventricles may appear only as slits and the basal cisterns may be obliterated.

Subarachnoid hemorrhage is very common in head injury. The CT scan will demonstrate this as high density areas in the basal cisterns, sylvian fissure, and interhemisphere fissure.

Intracranial pressure (ICP) may be measured by a variety of techniques. Proponents of ICP monitoring maintain that it allows for early diagnosis and rational therapeutic intervention. In addition, monitoring can assist in the evaluation of therapy such as positioning, suctioning, osmotherapy, hyperventilation and CSF drainage. Basically there are three methods of monitoring ICP (intraventricular, subarachnoid, and epidural); these methods measure the ICP by means of different routes.

Emergency and Acute Care

The greatest priority in the treatment of craniocerebral trauma at the scene is the establishment of an *airway.* After the patient's airway is cleared and an airway is established, 100% oxygen is delivered. Hypoxemia is common in the head-injury patient and, if not corrected, can further damage the brain. Special technique in establishing an airway is required because of the possibility of an associated cervical spine injury.

Second in importance is the maintenance of *circulation.* An intravenous line is inserted whether or not it appears to be needed at the scene. This provides a prompt access should volume replacement or medications be required enroute to the hosptial. A preferred solution is 5% dextrose in Ringer's lactate.

Treatment in the acute phase allows for a more thorough assessment. *Scalp lacerations* are carefully inspected for underlying depressed fracture, cleaned, irrigated, and sutured. Scalp lacerations, if associated with skull fracture, can provide avenues for intracranial infection.

Depressed skull fractures require operation to irrigate, débride, and elevate the depressed bone fragments. Patients who have persistent CSF leaks following basal skull fractures usually require dural repairs.

Cortical contusions do not require surgical evacuation, but serial scans should be obtained, should they evolve into intracerebral hematomas.

Intracranial hematomas, unless they are very small, require prompt surgical evacuation. Intracerebral hematomas may also be associated with contused and necrotic brain. This tissue is excised, since it may act as an expanding mass with surrounding edema.

A major portion of the initial care of the patient with head trauma is directed toward the reduction of secondary insults to the brain. These result in brain shifts and herniation with increased ICP and brain swelling.

Measures to Reduce Intracranial Pressure

Some of the methods used to reduce *intracranial hypertension* include (1) CSF drainage, (2) osmotherapy, (3) diuretics, (4) steroids, (5) hyperventilation, (6) hypothermia, and (7) barbiturates. Management regimens may differ among neurosurgeons.

CSF drainage may be accomplished by removing small amounts of cerebrospinal fluid on an intermittent basis or through continuous drainage and is usually followed by a prompt reduction in ICP.

Osmotherapy is directed at dehydrating the brain. Osmotic diuretics shrink the size of normal brain but have little effect on diseased brain. The goal is to achieve the most effective level of serum osmolality; that is, the level which promotes dehydration of the brain and minimizes water and electrolyte disturbances. The most commonly employed osmotic diuretic is mannitol. An intravenous (IV) bolus of 1 g/kg is usually given rapidly. Mannitol has a peak effect in 25 minutes. When giving mannitol on an emergency basis on the general nursing unit, one should make certain that the patient has an indwelling urinary bladder catheter. Osmotherapy may be combined with fluid restriction. Dehydration, however, should not cause hypovolemia. It is recommended that IV intake equal urine output. All IV medication should be included in the daily allotment of IV fluid administration. Free-water overload is to be avoided. Nurses must be alert to electrolyte imbalances and undesired levels of serum osmolality. Deviations should be reported to the physician.

The use of *steroids* in head injury remains controversial. When used, high doses may be administered.

Hyperventilation with a ventilator is very effective in decreasing intracranial pressure. It lowers Pa_{CO_2}, which in turn causes vasoconstriction and thereby reduces cerebral blood volume (CBV). However, hypercarbia and hypoxemia must be avoided because they can result in an enormous increase in ICP.

Hypothermia reduces cerebral metabolism and cerebral blood flow. It has been used in the treatment of head-injured patients. However, because of associated systemic complications occurring with its use, it has fallen into disfavor. Even when patients are not placed on a hypothermia regimen, fever always should be aggressively treated since hyperthermia to any degree is detrimental. Neurogenic fevers often respond better to external cooling than to medications, but both methods should be used. Sponges with tepid water and alcohol are still effective, and should be instituted promptly if a cooling blanket is not available. Fans are also effective.

Barbiturate therapy is generally reserved for management of the patient with uncontrolled intracranial hypertension. Barbiturates are thought to reduce intracranial pressure by causing arteriolar constriction and subsequent reduction of cerebral blood flow and cerebral blood volume. Barbiturates also decrease the cerebral metabolic rate, stabilize cell membranes (decrease cerebral edema formation), and act as free radical scavengers to reduce damage of metabolites from ischemia.[40] The patient's response to noxious stimuli is also reduced, averting the increases in ICP that are attendant to the daily care of the patient.

Other Treatment Concerns

Hyponatremia. Hyponatremia is not an uncommon occurrence in patients with head injury or other intracranial pathology. One of the most common causes of hyponatremia in the neurosurgical patient is the syndome of inappropriate secretion of antidiuretic hormone (SIADH). Another common cause, hopefully not seen in the neurosurgical patient, is fluid overload. Hyponatremia can also be seen as a complication of mechanical ventilation.[21] SIADH is characterized by water retention in the presence of hypo-osmolar serum. Hyponatremia is significant when the serum sodium is less than 130 mEq/liter (normal is 135–145 mEq/liter). It can be a serious complication, especially if levels fall to as low as 115–127 mEq/liter, because it results in cerebral edema. It should always suspected with decreasing levels of consciousness. Hyponatremia can also precipitate generalized seizures. Treatment consists of fluid restriction to 800 ml or less per day.[21] If the hyponatremia is severe and does not respond to fluid restriction, occasionally a 3% intravenous solution of sodium chloride (300 ml) is administered.

Hypernatremia. Hypernatremia may result from diabetes insipidus, excessive administration of osmotic diuretics, excessive protein intake from formula tube feedings (not enough free water is, or can be, given with the formula), or from insufficient fluid intake (especially at risk are patients who are confused and are not receiving IV fluids—they generally will not drink enough fluids on their own). Diabetes insipidus results from dysfunction of the posterior pituitary gland (decreased release of antidiuretic hormone), and it may occur with neoplasms, operative procedures, and trauma in the region of the hypothalamus and pituitary. It is characterized by polyuria with low specific gravity (1.000 to 1.006). A patient who is awake will also have polydipsia and may be able to replace the large volume of urine output in that manner; a patient who has a depressed level of consciousness, however, will have an impaired thirst mechanism. The urine output may be massive, leading to life-threatening hypovolemia.

Treatment consists of the administration of vasopressin, either water-soluble or in oil. Vasopressin tannate in oil has a longer duration of action (48 to 72 hours); however, if the vial in which it is dispensed is not warmed and thoroughly shaken for a period of minutes, the vasopressin is not adequately dispensed in the solution, and it is ineffective. Vasopressin in oil should effect a change in urine excretion to 20 to 30 minutes; if urine excretion is not reduced in this length of time there is a high probability that the medication was not properly administered. Aqueous vasopressin is easy to administer and acts within a few minutes; however, its duration of action is 3 to 4 hours.

Pulmonary Insufficiency. Aspiration pneumonia (aspiration immediately after head trauma), chest trauma, atelectasis, pulmonary edema, pulmonary embolism, fat embolism, and adult respiratory distress syndrome (ARDS) are all possible pulmonary insufficiency complications of head injury. Hypoxemia can be catastrophic to an already compromised brain.

Neurogenic pulmonary edema is thought to occur as a result of a massive sympathetic discharge from the hypothalamus. This causes a brief systemic vasoconstriction that redistributes a large volume of blood to the pulmonary vasculature with resulting pulmonary edema. Refer to Chapters 30 and 31 for a review of the management of pulmonary insufficiency.

Coagulopathies. Coagulopathies of all types may be seen in the head-injured patient. Both hypercoagulability and hypocoagulability are observed.[21] Disseminated intravascular coagulation (DIC) has also been observed in head-injured patients. The brain has a rich supply of thromboplastin and it is postulated that following trauma to the brain, thromboplastin is released. This causes the cycle of events that lead to DIC. DIC is usually treated with heparin; however, the use of heparin in a head-injured patient is ill-advised. For further information about DIC and its management, refer to Chapter 54.

Hypermetabolic States. Severely head-injured patients have been shown to develop hypermetabolic states at a level similar to that seen in burn patients.[16] It is now recognized that enteral feedings of high protein and high calories are not sufficient to maintain positive protein and caloric balance. Although parenteral feedings have been advocated, this method is not without drawbacks, especially since fluid overload and administration of high glucose solutions are contraindicated in head-injured patients. Studies are presently being conducted to determine the efficacy and safety of parenteral feedings to head trauma patients.

Early Post-traumatic Seizures. Early post-traumatic seizures (those occurring within the first week of injury) occur in about 5% of patients with blunt head trauma (penetrating head injuries have a higher incidence). These seizures may be generalized or focal. Standard therapy is to treat the seizure with phenytoin. An IV loading dose of phenytoin is administered followed by maintenance doses of phenytoin. Generally, patients are asked to continue taking phenytoin for 1 year after head trauma. The efficacy of phenytoin as a prophylaxis for post-traumatic epilepsy, however, is in dispute and is currently being studied.

Postconcussion Syndrome. Patients who have symptoms of postconcussion syndrome (see previous section in this chapter) should be reassured that these symptoms are a part of the recovery process and that they are temporary. The length of time a person experiences these symptoms is variable, and this should also be related to the patient. Headache may be treated with mild analgesics. If positional vertigo is a problem, the patient should be instructed to avoid those positions which precipitate it. An ears, nose, and throat consult is appropriate. Generally the patient should be encouraged to resume his usual activities as tolerated. The patient should not be made to feel that he is an invalid; however, neither should he be made to feel that his problems are unfounded.

Recovery Phase Treatment

Treatment of patients with moderate to severe head injury in the recovery phase is directed toward assisting the patient to advance along the continuum of coma, wakeful unresponsiveness, and confusion, agitation, or social withdrawal, to personal and interpersonal awareness. Physical and cognitive–perceptual deficits may be present in varying degrees and may not be fully recovered. Treatment is generally directed toward improving motor control and perceptual dysfunction, reality orientation, treatment of communication disorders, remediation of cognitive deficits, and treatment of behavioral deficits.[37] The overall emphasis is that of reintegration of the patient to being a functioning member of his family and community. Both the patient and his family will require assistance in the reintegration process.[37]

Nursing Management: Acute Phase

Assessment and Nursing Diagnosis

Nursing and medicine share many of the same treatment goals in the care of the patient with acute head injury. Nursing diagnosis and care are directed toward the early recognition and treatment of potentially life-threatening events. In addition, the nurse functions as a patient/family advocate and as a support to the patient's family (significant others) as well. Among the appropriate nursing diagnoses are potential ineffective airway clearance, potential cognitive impairment, potential alterations in fluid volume, and potential sensory–perceptual alterations related to the head injury.

Goals. The nursing goals of patients who are in the acute phase of a head injury are directed toward maintaining physiological function and early treatment of potentially life-threatening events.

Nursing Interventions

It is imperative that the nurse be able to detect subtle changes in the patient's neurological status at the earliest possible moment. Appropriate intervention is based on the recognition of these changes as well as the understanding of the pathophysiological mechanisms involved in head trauma.

Intracranial Pressure Considerations. One way in which the nurse can ensure that her practice in the care of the patient with head injury can make a difference is to use nursing measures that may minimize rises in intracranial pressure. These include properly positioning the patient to enhance cerebral venous drainage, giving diligent pulmonary care, avoiding fluid overload, maintaining normal body temperature, recognizing abnormal laboratory values (including arterial blood gases and electrolytes), administering medication on time to prevent agitation, and recognizing seizure activity.

In cases where the patient's intracranial pressure is being monitored, the nurse should make note of what patient care activities cause an increase in intracranial pressure, and, where possible, modify the patient's care accordingly. Theoretically, it may be better to space nursing care activities that have been shown to increase intracranial pressure (*e.g.,* suctioning, turning) so that the duration of the elevation in ICP is kept to a minimum.

Changes in intracranial pressure when turning patients has been observed, though the effects have not been consistent. Mitchell recommends that the nurse be alert to increases in ICP when turning patients.[29] If increased ICP repeatedly occurs in a given position, that position should be avoided for that patient. Head rotation in such a manner that it potentially obstructs the jugular vein should also be avoided.[24] Pillows that cause flexion at the neck should also be avoided.

In one study conducted by Mitchell and Mauss, conversation about the patient at the bedside caused a consistent rise in ICP.[30] If the patient is undergoing intracranial pressure monitoring, the nurse can watch for this effect and, if it is noted, curtail conversation at the bedside during this acute phase. One should always be mindful of conversations at the bedside of any unconcious patient. These patients may be unresponsive, but this does not mean that one can infer with certainty that they do not hear. Table 69–1 lists some of the nursing measures that may be effective in minimizing elevations in intracranial pressure.

Respiratory Considerations. To minimize hypoxia while suctioning, the duration of suctioning should be only 15 seconds. Limiting the duration of suctioning has been noted to be more effective than hyperinflating the lungs prior to suctioning.[29]

Respiratory insufficiency caused by atelectasis or pneumonia must not be allowed to develop. Turning the patient side to side when feasible, suctioning, and PEEP (positive end expiratory pressure) during assisted ventilation are measures that help prevent respiratory complications. Every one of these measures, however, may also have a deleterious effect by raising intracranial pressure, so that caution must be used in carrying out these procedures.

Assisted ventilation with PEEP has been shown to increase ICP in some patients, probably due to the concomitant increase in intrathoracic pressure. Mitchell notes that head elevation may reduce the risk of increased intracranial pres-

TABLE 69–1
Measures That May Minimize Rise in Intracranial Pressure

- Maintain proper positioning
  1. Keep head of bed elevated.
  2. Maintain patient's head in neutral position.
     a. No pillows
     b. Prevent head from tilting to the side
  3. Turn patient all in one piece.
  4. Avoid severe hip flexion.
- Minimize patient's agitation.
  1. Limit suctioning to 15 seconds or less.
  2. Space nursing care activities to minimize duration of increases in intracranial pressure.
  3. Avoid conversations at the bedside.
  4. Medicate appropriately.
- Decrease chance of Valsalva maneuvers.
  1. Monitor frequency and consistency of patient's stools.
     a. Administer stool softeners as necessary.
  2. If patient is awake, do not allow him to assist with position changes.
     a. Instruct him to exhale during changes in position.
- Maintain normothermia.
  1. Administer antipyretic medication and provide external cooling promptly.
- Recognize and treat seizures promptly.
- Provide excellent pulmonary care.
  1. Prevent hypoxemia and hypercarbia.
- Avoid fluid overload.
  1. Be alert to hyponatremia.

sure associated with PEEP.[29] All patients with intracranial hypertension, whenever possible, should have their head elevated 30 degrees. This has been shown to promote venous outflow and thereby reduce intracranial pressure.

Family Support. Families (including significant others) of the acutely head-injured patient are in need of support in many ways. They need to be prepared for what to expect before they first see their loved one. The nurse can minimize the psychological trauma if she takes the time to tell the family how the patient appears and about the various equipment that may be placed in the room. The family needs answers to its questions. Information provided to them should be truthful as well as sensitive. They need to be allowed access to the patient. One should not forget that a person requiring hospitalization does not cease to exist as a member of his family and, as such, both he and they continue to have rights to be together as much as possible without compromising patient care. Families need to feel that they can obtain information about the patient at any time, and receive explanations about procedures and patient care activities. They need "permission" to "take time off" from attendance at the bedside so that they can meet their own personal needs. They need to be prepared for possible outcomes at appropriate times. For instance, when it appears that the patient will survive the initial acute phase, it is not the time to make predictions to the family about the physical and mental disabilities that the patient may be left with. It is sufficient to let them know that recovery may be a long process, lasting weeks to months (even years). When it appears that the patient's recovery may be an extended one, the patient's family may benefit from attending meetings sponsored by the National Head Injury Foundation, which sponsors support groups in many states.

Evaluation

When the patient has survived the acute phase with minimal physiological complications, the goals for that phase will have been achieved. The patient then moves into a recovery phase, requiring nursing care with a different focus.

Nursing Management: Recovery Phase

Assessment and Nursing Diagnosis

Analysis of assessment data from the acute phase is incorporated into the recovery phase. The diagnoses include the potential for growth in family coping and the potential for impaired functioning related to the head injury.

Goals. The nursing care of patients who are recovering from head injury is directed toward preventing complications and maximizing the patient's steadily, albeit sometimes slowly, improving abilities. Second, the nurse should be able to provide care to the patient that is appropriate for each deficit as well as for him as an individual.

Nursing Interventions

The nurse must first be able to identify the deficits that the patient may have. For example, in addition to noting that the patient is confused and disoriented and has a hemiparesis, the nurse should also be able to recognize if the patient has a visual field defect, expressive or receptive aphasia, apraxia, hemi-inattention, or cognitive dysfunction. The nurse who provides care to the patient with a neurological disorder must have more than an acquaintance with rehabilitation principles and techniques. Rehabilitation does not begin when the patient is transferred to a rehabilitation unit. It is started as soon as possible after injury.

The nurse should consult with the patient's therapists so that consistency in the care of the patient may be provided. The family should also be included in this process. The patient's potential for maximal recovery is enhanced when nurse, family, and therapists are all working together with a common goal and consistent plan for the care of the patient. Once the patient is able, he too becomes an active participant in his care.

Outside of the family, it is the nurse who best knows the patient. It is she who attends the patient 24 hours a day. The nurse is in an ideal position to note the patient's abilities, disabilities, his response to various therapies, and his needs. The nurse can obtain valuable information from the patient's family about him as an individual and as a family member. And it is the nurse who provides feedback about the patient's progress to other members of the health care team. The patient who has suffered brain damage, perhaps more than any other patient, needs an individualized and consistent plan of care. It is the nurse who both provides and coordinates this endeavor.

Evaluation

The person recovering from head injury will not have preventable complications and will maximize his improving abilities. The patient will have his care provided on an individualized basis.

Spinal Cord Injury

Epidemiology

Recent studies have estimated the annual occurrence of spinal cord injury in the United States to number 10,000 per years.[22] This estimate does not include persons who died at the scene of the accident or who were dead on arrival at the hospital. Young adults and adolescents incur the highest percentage of spinal cord injuries, with 30% to 50% of injuries occurring in persons between the ages of 15 and 24, and about another 30% occurring in the 25- to 44-year age-group.[5,22,32] Efforts need to be directed at reducing the number of accidents due to motor vehicle accidents (MVAs), falls, and sports activities (*e.g.,* diving, trampoline, football) in general. Use of seat belts has reduced overall incidence of injury sustained in MVAs by 70% in one report.[6] However, neither lap belts, shoulder harnesses, nor the three-point lap-sash seat belts has been shown to be effective in reducing spinal cord injuries in posterior crashes, and they have been found to be only minimally effective in lateral crashes.[23] Many injuries sustained in car accidents could be avoided if the degree of extension and flexion permitted the head were reduced.[13]

Mechanism of Spinal Injury

Fractures of the spine may or may not cause injury to the spinal cord, and the spinal cord may be injured without evidence of injury to the vertebrae. When spinal cord injury does occur, it poses a serious threat to the life and health of the individual.

The forces that produce injury to the spinal cord are the same as those that act to produce injury to the head. These forces include acceleration, deceleration, and deformation. They cause injury to tissue by compression (pushing materials together), tension (tearing materials apart), shearing (sliding of portions of material on other portions),[13] and penetration (gunshot wound, stab wounds).

The types of injuries sustained by the *cervical spine* are mainly due to flexion (most common), rotation, and extension movements of the neck and to axial forces applied to the spinal column. The cervical spine is particularly vulnerable to injury because of its mobility and because it supports a heavy and mobile head at one end while being attached to a rigid thorax at the other.

The *thoracic spine* has considerable structural stability. For a closed injury to occur at this level, a great deal of force has to have been applied. Most injuries occur when the force is applied in an axial direction, such as that which occurs in a fall on the buttocks, or one in which a seated airline passenger is involved in a crash landing. Flexion injuries can occur when either the lower part of the body is fixed and the upper part of the body flexes sharply over a fulcrum or vice versa.[11] The thoracic spine also is more subject to penetrating injuries (*e.g.,* gunshot wounds, stab wounds).

The *lumbar spine,* though flexible, is less often injured than the cervical spine because the lumbar spine has more muscle and ligamentous support. Closed injuries of the lumbar spine occur during flexion, extension, or rotation movements as well as when an axial force is applied to the spine, with the most common causes being motor vehicle accidents and falls. The lumbar spine also is more likely to be involved in penetrating wounds.[10]

Injuries to the *sacral spine* alone are rare. When they do occur, they are usually a result of an axial force applied during a fall in which the person lands on his buttocks.

Classification of Spinal Injuries

Injuries to the spine are classified according both to type and mechanics of injury. Injuries are also regarded to be stable or unstable. Stability is determined by the integrity of the major supporting ligaments, that is, the interspinous ligament, the anterior and posterior ligaments, and the articular facets. Generally, if any two of these ligaments are torn or if the articulating facets are broken or dislocated, the injury is considered to be unstable.

Spinal cord injury is classified as complete or incomplete depending on the presence or absence of neurological function remaining. A *complete* lesion is defined as one in which all voluntary motor, sensory, and vasomotor functions are absent below the level of the injury. An *incomplete* lesion is one in which some degree of either voluntary motor or sensory function, or both, remains below the level of the lesion. Complete and incomplete lesions in cervical cord injuries are differentiated on the basis of whether sacral sensation is absent and whether there is voluntary control of sacral innervated muscles and sphincter tone. When all these are absent, the lesion may be considered to be complete. If sacral sensation is present or if sphincter control is intact, the lesion is incomplete.[39] Some of the incomplete cord lesions follow patterns that are permitted by cord anatomy and type of injury to the spinal cord (Table 69–2).

Pathophysiology

Pathophysiological mechanisms of spinal cord injury include concussion, contusion, ischemia, edema, stretching (distraction) of cord tissue, laceration, hematomyelia, and transection (anatomical or functional).

Animal studies have shown that immediately after spinal cord injury there exists within the cord a brief moment in which only the electron microscope can detect a minimal tissue change. This moment is, however, associated with complete motor and sensory loss below the level of the lesion. Why this occurs with only minute tissue change is not known. It has been postulated that the basis for loss of function could be physiochemical.

TABLE 69–2
Incomplete Spinal Cord Lesions

Syndrome	*Mechanism*	*Clinical Manifestations*
Anterior spinal cord syndrome	Usually results from a hyperextension injury that may cause compression of anterior portion of spinal cord or the anterior spinal artery	Complete paralysis, decreased pain and temperature sensation, and intact touch, position, and vibratory sensation below the level of injury
Central spinal cord syndrome	Usually results from a hyperextension injury but also can result from a hyperflexion injury; individuals with narrowing of cervical spinal canal are especially at risk, *e.g.*, elderly	Motor loss in arms (LMN type) is greater than loss in legs (UMN type); variable sensory deficits; sometimes bladder and bowel function preserved (these fibers are in peripheral area of spinal cord). LMN weakness in arms occurs either because of associated injury to cervical spinal roots or to anterior horn cells only; also innervation to the arms from the corticospinal tract lies medial in the spinal cord, accounting for arm weakness greater than legs, but not for LMN weakness
Brown-Séquard syndrome	An anatomical or functional transection of the spinal cord; usually results from penetrating wounds	Paralysis and absent vibratory and position sense below level of lesion on same side as lesion; loss of pain and temperature below level of lesion on side opposite the lesion

Following this very brief period (several minutes), small petechiae appear in the injured cord segment along with some bleeding into the subarachnoid space. This is followed by edema and hemorrhage, appearing first in the gray matter of the contused segment, and then spreading both to segments above and below, as well as to the peripheral white matter.

The initial hemorrhage, which consisted of a small extravasation of blood, may progress to the point of occupying most of the injured tissue and this, in turn, leads to tissue necrosis. Two days after injury there appears to be an inflammatory response in the tissue. One week after the injury fibroblasts are present and formation of scar tissue begins.[8]

Research presently is being conducted to determine ways in which the series of events leading to tissue necrosis and eventual fibrosis can be interrupted, thus possibly preventing complete and irreversible spinal cord damage.

Clinical Manifestations

The clinical manifestations of spinal cord injury is dependent on the level of the injury as well as whether it is a complete or incomplete lesion. Loss of motor function and sensation differ according to the spinal cord levels affected (see Tables 69–3 and 69–4).

Spinal Shock

Spinal shock is a condition in which there is immediate, complete loss of all reflex, motor, sensory, and autonomic activity below the level of cord injury. This state may last several days to several weeks. When it resolves, if the lesion has not been a complete one, return of sensory and motor function in the areas that were spared will be noted; if the lesion was complete, reflex activity, often excessive, will return with the cord segments operating on a simple reflex arc basis.[41] Often, return of the bulbocavernosus reflex is the first sign that spinal shock is resolving. The bulbocavernosus reflex is elicited by applying direct pressure over the bulbocavernous muscle behind the scrotum and pinching the glans penis, causing the muscle to contract.

Clinical signs of spinal shock, which appear below the level of the lesion, include flaccid paralysis, areflexia, loss of function of all sensory modalities, respiratory insufficiency with cervical and thoracic injuries, hypotension, bradycardia, hypothermia, paralytic ileus, oliguria (sometimes less than 2 ml/minute), urinary retention with overflow, and fecal retention.

Once spinal shock resolves, if the lesion is complete many of the problems listed above remain, although respiratory function may improve with patient teaching. In an incomplete lesion gastric motility improves; bladder emptying will become either upper motor neuron or lower motor neuron in type; and hypotension, including postural hypotension, may improve. Other problems that may arise in the first couple of weeks after injury include pulmonary edema, cardiac arrest, venous thrombosis, pulmonary embolism, and gastric ulcers. The patient also will probably experience normal feelings of denial, anger, and depression during the acute phase following his injury.

Problems that may be encountered later and may continue to be problems for the rest of the patient's life include urinary tract infections, renal failure, osteoporosis, severe flexor spasms, pressure sores, and autonomic dysreflexia. Problems associated with spinal cord injury will be more fully discussed later in the chapter under the section Nursing Management.

TABLE 69–3
Segmental Spinal Cord Level and Function

Level	*Function*
C1–C6	Neck flexors
C1–T1	Neck extensors
C3, C4, C5	Supply diaphragm
C5, C6	Shoulder movement, raise arm (deltoid); flexion of elbow (biceps); C6 externally rotates the arm (supinates)
C6, C7, C8	Extends elbow and wrist (triceps and wrist extensors); pronates wrist
C7, C8, T1	Flexes wrist
C8, T1	Supply small muscles of the hand
T1–T6	Intercostals and trunk above the waist
T7–L1	Abdominal muscles
L1, L2, L3, L4	Thigh flexion
L2, L3, L4	Thigh adduction
L4, L5, S1	Thigh abduction
L5, S1, S2	Extension of leg at the hip (gluteus maximus)
L2, L3, L4	Extension of leg at the knee (quadriceps femoris)
L4, L5, S1, S2	Flexion of leg at the knee (hamstrings)
L4, L5, S1	Dorsiflexion of foot (tibialis anterior)
L4, L5, S1	Extension of toes
L5, S1, S2	Plantar flexion of foot
L5, S1, S2	Flexion of toes

(Adapted from DeMyer W: Techniques of the Neurologic Examination, 3rd ed. New York, McGraw-Hill Book, 1980)

TABLE 69–4
Segmenal Spinal Cord Level and Sensation

Level	*Area of Sensation*
C5	Deltoid
C6	Thumb
C7	Middle finger
C8	Little finger
T4	Nipple line
T10	Umbilicus
L5	Big toe
S1	Little toe
S2–S5	Perineal sensation

Paralysis

Upper motor neuron (UMN) paralysis occurs with spinal cord injury when the long descending motor tracts in the white matter are interrupted. This results in a spastic paralysis (once spinal shock resolves) below the level of the lesion. Because of the excessive tone, the affected muscles do not atrophy, although once the spasticity diminishes disuse atrophy may occur. A UMN paralysis has particular implications for the patient. Spasticity may become a problem, especially for the individual with paraplegia, if painful flexor spasms develop. If the cord lesion is above T12 the patient will develop a reflex neurogenic bladder (one that fills and evacuates by automatic reflex). In males, the ability to have a reflex erection is usually possible, but there is no orgasmic sensation. Ejaculation, though, is sometimes possible.

Lower motor neuron (LMN) paralysis occurs with spinal cord injury when there is damage to the spinal cord at the S2–S4 segments (conus medullaris) or their spinal roots (cauda equina). An LMN lesion results in a flaccid paralysis. Because the muscles lack tone, atrophy of the affected muscles develops. An LMN paralysis also connotes specific types of dysfunction. If the lesion is at T12 or below, the patient will usually have an atonic, areflexic neurogenic bladder, which will distend to accomodate large volumes of urine before overflow incontinence occurs. With cauda equina lesions and incomplete spinal cord injury the bladder may have patchy sensory/motor innervation and will require urologic evaluation to determine what types of problems may be encountered. Evacuation of the bowel will require volitional increases of abdominal pressure as well as manual evacuating. Volitional and reflex erection in males is abolished if S2–S5 cord segments are damaged or their roots are damaged. Patients with incomplete lesions may manifest a variety of experiences, for example, a voluntary (psychic) erection but no sensory feedback.

Medical Management

The goals in the management of any person who is suspected of having sustained a spinal cord injury include preventing additional damage to either the bony, ligamentous, or neural elements; treating the neurological injury; and realigning the spine to ensure stability and reduce pain.[9]

Emergency Treatment

At the scene of the accident, anyone who has sustained a head injury should be suspected of having sustained a spinal injury. Anyone who complains of severe, localized neck pain may have suffered a spinal injury. Anyone who is unable to move one or more limbs is treated as having had a spinal injury. Anyone who reports decreased sensation in the trunk or extremities is treated as having had a spinal injury. In addition, anyone who has been involved in an accident and is unconscious is likewise suspected of having a spinal injury.

It has been reported that 10% of patients with quadriplegia developed quadriplegia after their initial injury.[9,33] In the initial management of patients with a suspected injury to the spine, the patient should not be moved until proper assistance and equipment is available, unless massive bleeding or respiratory distress is present. In addition, the patient's head and neck position should not be changed. The person should be covered to maintain body warmth. A spine board should be used to transport the patient. The patient will remain on this spine board during all transports outside and in the hospital, until the spinal injury has either been ruled out or it has been reduced or stabilized. Good head-neck-body alignment is maintained at all times. Maintenance of an adequate airway always takes precedence and any respiratory distress must first be attended.

Acute Care

Once the patient is in the emergency department and respiratory and cardiovascular adequacy has been established, *assessment of neurological function* follows. A history that details how the accident happened is important and often provides clues for the mechanism and type of injury that may have been sustained. A careful, detailed neurological examination is imperative to determine a reliable, accurate baseline documenting the presence or absence and precise localization of remaining neurological function. This is especially important in determining the best treatment modalities. In the patient with apparent cervical cord transection, every effort should be made to determine the presence of sacral sensation and function.

Radiographs of the spine, often with special views, is then undertaken. A physician or an experienced neurological nurse should be present when the films are taken. Once the nature and extent of the injury are determined, the appropriate treatment is instituted. Occasionally, myelography is needed to further delineate the extent of injury. This procedure is undertaken cautiously and only when it is felt that the knowledge gained from it will favorably affect the patient's outcome.

Neck Pain. When there is no neurological deficit and the x-ray studies are negative for bony vertebral injury but the patient complains of neck pain, he probably has sustained a hyperextension or hyperflexion injury of the neck. Generally, the more severe injuries have immediate onset of pain, but usually severe pain is delayed for 24 to 48 hours after injury. The sternocleidomastoid muscles may be swollen and tender, and pain may radiate into one or both shoulders. The pain may also radiate to the occiput and retro-orbital areas. Weeks after the accident the patient may experience headache, tinnitus, vertigo, pain in the ears, transitory obscuration of vision, and vasomotor disturbances of the face.[14] Persistence of these problems is more commonly seen following hyperextension acceleration injuries. The whiplash injury is a *real* injury and should not be dismissed as neuroticism. Degenerative changes in the spine 7 years after acceleration injuries at a rate of six times what would be expected for the age-groups has been reported by Hohl.[14]

Treatment of neck pain, if it is severe, includes neck splinting with a cervical collar. One week of bed rest, in order to remove the weight of the head from the neck, may be necessary. Traction is used to reduce muscle spasm, but it should only be used if it reduces pain. The patient should be encouraged to return to work in about a week, but he should avoid any extension of the neck. Emotional or muscular tension should be avoided. Application of moist heat and deep heat to the neck may also help relieve pain. Muscle relaxants and narcotic analgesics may be helpful initially, but the patient's reliance on these medications should be discouraged. Recently, the anti-inflammatory agent ibuprofen has successfully reduced the pain associated with these injuries. Dunsker provides the following axiom: If the patient's injury was severe enough to require 1 week of bed rest, he will probably have daily discomfort for at least 6 weeks; if at the end of 6 weeks daily pain is still present, he may continue to have intermittent discomfort for an additional 6 to 12 months.[14]

Bony and Ligamentous Injury. Treatment of this type of spine injury is based on the extent of the injury and its stability. If minor fractures of the cervical spine only (*e.g.,* chip fractures of the body, unilateral fracture of a facet, lateral or spinous process fracture) are demonstrated on x-ray film, immobilization with a hard cervical collar or brace for 6 to 8 weeks is all that is required. The hospital stay should be short. Major vertebral injury, if it is stable, requires a period of immobilization with skeletal head traction, followed by the wearing of a brace, followed by a soft cervical collar. An unstable cervical injury will require reduction (realignment of vertebrae) with skeletal head traction followed by application of a Halo brace, which will be worn for the next 3 to 4 months. Flexion and extension spine films to check for recurrent dislocation should be done immediately after removal of the brace and again in 3 months and 1 year. Hyperextension cervical injuries require immobilization with skeletal head traction for 6 weeks, followed by a brace in *flexion* for 6 to 8 weeks. Extension of the neck should be avoided in cervical extension injuries since this will cause progression of the neurological deficit.

Simple Thoracic Injuries. Simple thoracic injuries require immobilization in bed with hyperextension of the spine for 4 to 6 weeks. Following this a form-fitting plaster jacket is worn for an additional 3 months, followed by an extension brace for 3 to 4 months.

Lumbar Fractures. Lumbar fractures usually require treatment with bed rest with the spine in extension for 6 to 8 weeks followed by a plaster jacket for 3 months, and an extension brace for an additional 3 months. A lumbar sprain should be treated with a week to 10 days of bed rest and pelvic traction, 25 lb (with knees flexed) to reduce muscle spasm. Muscle relaxants, analgesics, and anti-inflammatory

TABLE 69–5
Williams Flexion Exercises for Back Pain

Pelvic tilt: Lie flat on your back with knees bent. Tilt your pelvis back toward the floor and tighten your abdominal muscles. Hold for 10 seconds and relax. This exercise may also be done while standing with your back against a wall.

Knee-to-chest: Lie flat on your back with knees bent. Grasp your knees with your hands. Bring one knee up to your chest, flattening your low back against the floor; hold for 10 seconds. Then repeat with the other knee. Continue alternating knees, to tolerance. Then grasp both knees and bring them both to your chest while flattening your low back against the floor. Hold to tolerance.

Partial sit-up: Lie on your back with one to two pillows under your head and shoulders. Flex your knees. While tightening your abdominal muscles and pushing your low back toward the floor (pelvic tilt), raise your head and shoulders slightly off the floor with your arms outstretched in front of you. Do not attempt to sit all the way up.

agents may also be given. The patient should be taught Williams exercises, as described in Table 69–5. Sacral fractures are usually treated with 6 to 8 weeks of bed rest with the patient flat in bed.

Surgery. Occasionally surgery is indicated for vertebral injury. It is generally undertaken only when there is progression of neurological deficit despite adequate reduction and stabilization of the spine and when there is a good chance that a neurological deficit may be improved with the removal of compressive elements (*e.g.*, anterior cord syndrome in which bony fragments are visualized extruding into the spinal canal, and cauda equina injuries in which there is injury to nerve roots). Surgery may also be indicated for a lesion that is felt to be incomplete, but in which severe dislocation is present. Severe dislocation in the thoracic spine may eventually cause disfigurement that may hamper the patient's ability to care for himself.

Investigational Treatment. Several treatment regimens under investigation may be encountered. Use of systemic steroids is generally advocated in the treatment of spinal cord injury even though its effectiveness in preventing or improving neurological dysfunction has not been established. Studies investigating the effectiveness of steroids and their effectiveness at different doses are presently being undertaken. It has been postulated that steroids stabilize cell membranes and they preserve lysosome integrity, thereby preventing the release of proteolytic enzymes and subsequent edema. Many neurosurgeons feel that steroids do benefit the clinical status of the patient, and on that basis advocate their early administration (within the first 4 to 6 hours after injury or sooner) until the results of studies are available.[33,42] Studies are also currently being conducted to evaluate the efficacy of naloxone and of local hypothermia in the treatment of humans with spinal cord injury.

Nursing Management

Assessment and Nursing Diagnosis

Problems that the patient may develop during the acute and rehabilitation phases of recovery cover a wide range depending on the degree of disability.

Potential nursing diagnoses relate to several body system dysfunctions and to psychological reactions and may include the following:

1. Alteration in respiratory function related to paralysis, ineffective cough, atelectasis, pneumonia, hypoventilation, and ventilator dependency
2. Alteration in cardiovascular status related to loss of sympathetic innervation, vasodilation, and immobility
3. Alteration in nutrition and fluid volume balance
4. Alteration in bowel elimination and function related to spinal shock, loss of volitional motor control, paralytic ileus, constipation, and impaction
5. Alteration in urinary elimination and function related to spinal shock urinary stasis, urinary retention, and infection
6. Alteration in skin integrity
7. Potential for pain, contracture, physical injury, perceptual disturbances, anxiety, coping difficulty, sexual dysfunction, and self-concept disturbances

Table 69–6 provides a list of nursing diagnoses commonly seen in patients with spinal cord injury.

Goals. The nursing care of patients with spinal cord injury is directed toward the goals of ensuring that the patient will experience no additional damage to the spinal cord. The nurse should provide appropriate, individualized intervention for the dysfunction that results from the spinal cord injury, and the patient should receive the coordinated efforts of all health care professionals to assure maximum recovery. The patient and his family should receive education regarding his injury, care, and potential.

Interventions

Respiratory Insufficiency. If the lesion is cervical or high thoracic, the patient will experience varying degrees of respiratory insufficiency. The muscles of respiration include the intercostals, abdominals, and the diaphragm. The intercostal and abdominal muscles are innervated by thoracic cord segments; the diaphragm is supplied by C3, C4, and C5 cord segments. High cervical cord lesions are associated with a high mortality, but increasing numbers of these patients are surviving and are being maintained on artificial respirators and, eventually, portable lung respirators. Some patients are candidates for electrophrenic nerve stimulators. Patients with midcervical and high thoracic cord lesions breathe diaphragmatically. The vital capacity is often less than 1 liter. Other problems that compromise pulmonary function include the inability to cough and the development of atelectasis and pneumonia. Improper positioning of the patient and gastric dilatation can also produce respiratory

TABLE 69–6
Nursing Diagnoses Common in Spinal Cord-Injured Patients

Neurological

At risk for further neurological deficits and further spinal cord damage secondary to unstable fracture, bony compression, spinal cord edema, circulatory impairment

Potential for pain at level of injury due to nerve root involvement

Respiratory

At risk for hypoventilation due to paresis/paralysis of diaphragm, intercostal musculature, fatigue

Alterations in respiratory function secondary to ineffective cough due to paresis/paralysis of diaphragm, intercostal and/or abdominal muscles

Potential for atelectasis and pneumonia secondary to inability to handle secretions and immobility

At risk for pulmonary embolism secondary to vasodilation, deep vein thrombosis, and immobilization

At risk for respirator dependency due to muscle paresis/paralysis, long-term ventilatory support, and fear of inability to breathe

Cardiovascular

Alterations in cardiovascular status secondary to loss of sympathetic innervation

At risk for deep vein thrombosis due to vasodilatation and immobilization

Potential for orthostatic hypotension due to loss of sympathetic innervation, vasodilatation and prolonged immobilization

Nutritional

Potential for stress ulcers secondary to the stress response and steroid therapy

Alteration in nutrition: less than body requirements

At risk for fluid volume deficit (or iatrogenic fluid volume overload)

Genitourinary

Alteration in bowel function due to spinal shock and loss of volitional motor control

Potential for paralytic ileus due to loss of sympathetic innevation

At risk for constipation and impaction due to paralytic ileus and immobilization

Alterations in bladder function secondary to spinal shock or damage to reflex arc (atonic bladder)

At risk for urinary stasis, urinary infection, and urinary retention due to involuntary voiding reflex (or absence of voiding reflex)

Potential for autonomic dysreflexia due to bladder or bowel distention or skin stimulation

Miscellaneous

Alterations in temperature regulation due to loss of sympathetic innervation

Alterations in skin integrity due to circulatory impairment, immobilization, and catabolic state

Potential for contractures due to paralysis, spasticity, and immobilization

At risk for physical injury

Psychological

At risk for perceptual disturbances due to environment, sensory deprivation, and immobilization

At risk for anxiety

Potential for altered coping mechanisms

Potential for alterations in self-concept

Potential for lack of acceptance of disability

Potential for altered sexual response

(Giubilato RT: Acute care of the high-level quadriplegic patient. J Neurosurg Nurs 14:128–132, 1982)

insufficiency by compromising diaphragmatic functioning. For these patients vital capacities should be measured at least every 8 hours. Arterial blood gases should be monitored frequently, and any hypoxia should be treated immediately. Intermittent positive pressure breathing (IPPB) is administered at least four times per day, and each treatment should be followed by suction and assistive coughing. As vital capacity improves, and if chest films are negative, the frequency of IPPB treatments may be decreased. In most patients, with the use of these methods maximum vital capacity is usually achieved in 8 to 10 weeks.[7]

The patient may be assisted to cough with the use of an abdominal binder and intermittent manual pressure on the chest wall. Regular turning is imperative, but the prone position should be avoided since this position promotes hypoventilation. Patients with quadriplegia breathe more effectively when supine and in positions with their heads slightly downward. The sitting position has been reported to reduce inspiratory capacity.[7]

Pulmonary Edema. Pulmonary edema can also be a problem in the acute spinal cord–injured patient, especially if the lesion is high. The exact mechanism by which this occurs is not understood; it may be induced by autonomic dysfunction, but it most certainly can be seen with the overzealous administration of intravenous fluids. All reports warn against attempts at correcting low urine output with large volumes of fluid replacement. The oliguria encountered immediately after injury is seen with spinal shock. Measurement of pulmonary artery pressure, or the central venous pressure, is helpful in monitoring the patient to see if fluid replacement is necessary.

Cardiovascular Problems. Patients with high cervical cord lesions often have cardiovascular problems, specifically bradycardia, secondary to the loss of autonomic activity. Occasionally a patient may develop marked bradycardia and cardiac arrest during suctioning secondary to a vasovagal reflex. Vagal sensory receptors present in the trachea and bronchi and mechanical irritation of these may result in reflex bradycardia. Patients who are at highest risk of developing profound bradycardia and cardiac arrest are those who are hypoxic. It is essential to ensure that the patient is well-ventilated before carrying out suctioning procedures.

Venous Thrombosis and Pulmonary Embolism. These problems are a particular threat in the first 2 to 3 weeks following injury, and the patient with a cervical or high thoracic injury remains at risk for developing these problems for the first 3 months after injury. Immobilization, paralysis, and vasomotor paralysis associated with decreased pulmonary ventilation and decreased venous return are all factors that contribute to venous stasis. Factors that influence blood coagulability include age, obesity, anemia, infection, hypoproteinemia, hyperglobulinemia, and metabolic changes of potassium and calcium. Many of these may exist in any one patient.

The most frequent site of thrombosis is in the legs. The lower extremities should be inspected regularly for swelling, and the patient should be observed for a low-grade fever. These signs can be obscured by postural edema and a urinary tract infection. Frequent turning of the patient, prevention of pressure on the calves, raising the foot of the bed, and antiembolic stockings reduce the risk of thrombus formation.

Pulmonary embolism occurs more frequently in complete lesions than incomplete lesions, with the highest incidence in cervical and thoracic cord lesions.

Paralytic Ileus. Paralysis of peristalsis occurs immediately following cervical and thoracic spinal cord transections. Paralytic ileus can develop rapidly and its presence can seriously compromise respiratory function because it interferes with the function of the diaphragm. Every patient with spinal shock should have a nasogastric tube placed, and suctioning of gastric contents should be done as necessary. The patient should not take any nourishment by mouth until bowel sounds return. Once peristalsis resumes, clear liquids, which are advanced to a regular diet as tolerated, can be initiated.

Body Temperature. The patient with cervical and high thoracic cord lesions is unable to regulate his body temperature in response to ambient temperatures. This occurs because the normal sympathetic connection between the midbrain and sympathetic plexuses is interrupted. Usually patients are hypothermic but if the ambient temperature is hot, they may become hyperthermic. They are unable to sweat in response to increased temperatures. This situation is aggravated by decreased heat loss through the lungs. Immediate measures should be taken to externally cool the patient (*e.g.*, tepid sponges, fans, ice).

Postural Hypotension. Spinal cord injury above the level of T5 results in postural hypotension when changing from the horizontal to the vertical position. Premonitory symptoms may include blurring followed by loss of vision, giddiness, and tinnitus.

Regular and frequent turning from the supine to lateral positions in the acute stage is an important stimulus to restore vasomotor control.[17] Thigh-high elastic stockings and an abdominal binder should be applied before the patient is raised. Once the patient reaches the stage where he can be upright, the upright position should be assumed in slowly progressing increments, advancing them as is tolerated. The patient can also be encouraged to drink fluids before he is scheduled to be up.

Bladder Dysfunction. Guttman lists the primary goals in the management of any type of neurogenic bladder, whether UMN or LMN, to be:

1. Prevention of infection
2. Prevention of overdistention of the bladder
3. Prevention of local damage to the urethra and bladder
4. Maintenance or restoration of satisfactory bladder capacity
5. Making the patient catheter-free as soon as possible

Intermittent catheterization has been shown to be the most effective method of bladder drainage in the acute phase of spinal cord injury. It reduces the incidence of urinary tract infection and predisposes to early recovery of bladder function.[17,42] O'Donnel and Taylor state that the goal of therapy is to achieve a balanced bladder. They describe the balanced bladder as one that has low voiding pressures, no outlet obstruction, and a sterile, low residual volume (< 100 ml) of urine. They further state that most patients, 80% to 90%, will achieve balanced bladder function with intermittent catheterization or a suprapubic cystocath.[34]

Factors that influence the patient's ability to perform his own intermittent catheterization, if he continues this type of bladder management once he is home, include his ability to use his hands, his motivation and reliability, his educability, and his psychosocial environment.

Long-term bladder management begins with the initiation of bladder training. Prevention of urinary tract infection is very important (the most common cause of death in patients with spinal cord injury is renal failure). Attempts to keep the bladder flushed with large volumes of fluid (except at night), and the attempt to maintain urine acidity with, for example, ascorbic acid or cranberry juice is made.

Bowel Dysfunction. Absence of peristalsis during spinal shock will result in a bowel dysfunction evidenced by the retention of feces. Initially this is managed by giving a cleansing enema after the return of bowel sounds (usually 2 to 3 days after the injury). Once the bowel has been cleansed and the patient is eating, bowel training begins. The goal of bowel training is to achieve bowel evacuation at the same time every day. This will save the patient much anxiety. Stool softeners should be administered on a daily basis as needed. A Bisacodyl or glycerine suppository is given every day at the same time, preferably after a meal, until regular evacuation is obtained. The patient with an LMN lesion may also require manual evacuation of stool.

Spasms. Painful flexor spasms may seriously interfere with the patient's ability to participate in rehabilitation and self-care. Many different medications are prescribed for the treatment of spasticity. The more common medications are diazepam, dantrolene, and baclofen. The presence of pressure sores and urinary tract infection has been reported to increase the tendency to develop flexor spasms.

Mobility. Prolonged bed rest, especially when combined with immobility, causes changes in mineral metabolism; osteoporosis may result. Frequent changes in the patient's position along with passive exercises may reduce osteoporosis. A high-protein diet is also advocated.

Autonomic Dysreflexia. Autonomic dysreflexia consists of a massive, uncompensated sympathetic discharge that may occur in patients with lesions about T7 in response to a noxious stimulus (often a visceral stimulus). It is manifested by paroxysmal hypertension, pounding headache, facial flushing, sweating above the lesion, nausea, and bradycardia. It usually develops later in the course of the recovery process and is most frequently seen with the presence of a distended bladder. Sometimes fecal impaction or sexual activity will also precipitate it. It may constitute a medical emergency, and the patient's head should be raised to promote a reduction in blood pressure. The offending stimulus should be removed at once though the trigger mechanism is not always apparent. A fast-acting antihypertensive medication may need to be given, such as Apresoline. Removal of a fecal impaction should not be attempted until the patient's blood pressure is under control.

Skin Breakdown. The spinal cord-injured patient is especially at risk for developing pressure sores. In the acute stage he is on bed rest, he cannot move himself, and he has decreased circulation to the skin. He may also be in a state of catabolism, with increased caloric and protein needs. Still, there is never an excuse for a patient who is dependent on the nursing staff for care to develop pressure sores.

The patient should be turned from side to side and it is imperative that this is done at least every 2 hours. The patient's skin must be kept meticulously clean to avoid skin irritation. Care should be taken to avoid scraping the patient's skin on the bed sheet since an abrasion could provide a site for further tissue breakdown. The skin should be inspected at every turn for the presence of any reddened areas and, if present, they should be massaged to stimulate circulation to the area. There are many special beds and padding now available that make the skin care of the patient with spinal cord injury much easier to manage.

Contractures. Passive range of motion of the patient's limbs should be done at least twice a day. Development of muscle contractures will greatly reduce the patient's rehabilition potential. Occasionally spasticity may be so pronounced that range of motion is difficult to perform and does not prevent the development of contractures. Diligent range of motion of the patient's limbs during spinal shock may reduce the chance for development of severe spasticity.[17]

Sexual Dysfunction. Sexual dysfunction may have a tremendous impact on the patient's self-esteem, body image, and role and gender identity. Patients should be made aware that sexual counseling is available to them. This is usually undertaken by a trained therapist. The emphasis in counseling is usually placed on alternative methods of providing sexual satisfaction for the patient and his partner. Upper motor and lower motor neuron lesions will present with different types of sexual dysfunction (See previous section, Paralysis).

Psychosocial Reactions. The sudden onset of loss of function is a devastating psychosocial experience. Initially, when the patient is acutely ill, he may not fully realize the implication of what has happened to him. The experience of being unable to move and unable to feel a large part of the body, coupled with spending 24 hours a day looking at a wall or ceiling (in the intensive care unit) and disruption of normal sleep can create a great deal of anxiety in itself. Occasionally patients who are on turning frames begin to hallucinate during this stage.

Once the full impact of what has happened begins to register, the patient may respond in a variety of ways, and this may, in large part, depend on how he has coped with problems before. Not every patient will experience denial, anger, depression, and acceptance. The nurse must allow for the patient to express (or not express) his feelings as he desires. The patient should be made to feel that the nursing staff will support him. The nurse should be respectful of the patient's integrity, considerate of his feelings, and truthful and sensitive in answering his questions. The nurse needs to be aware that the patient needs to feel that he has control over what is happening to him and when. Consultation with the patient in developing a mutually agreeable plan of care is important. Give the patient as much control as is possible.

Primary nursing is an excellent way for the nurse to truly get to know the patient as an individual; likewise the patient has an opportunity to feel comfortable with one special nurse. Continuity of care is very important in the care of the spinal cord-injured patient. This should be provided be a detailed and explicit nursing care plan, so that when the primary nurse is not on duty, another nurse will know what should be done for the patient and how it should be done.

The family often shares as many of the anxieties and fears for the future as the patient. They should be made to feel that they can express these feelings to the nurse. They should be included in the patient's care whenever possible, but this should be gradual so they do not become overwhelmed. The nurse should provide periods of privacy for husbands and wives if this is possible.

Rehabilitation. Rehabilitation begins as soon as the patient is stable. All members of the health care team should be involved in the rehabilitation process. The goal of the rehabilitation process is to assist the patient in achieving his maximum potential. Emphasis is placed on the abilities of the patient rather than his disabilities. The patient and his family are integral members of the rehabilitation team.

Evaluation

The patient will experience no additional damage to the spinal cord, and he will receive individualized intervention for the dysfunction. The patient will demonstrate maximal recovery of function relative to his injury, and he will show evidence of learning regarding his injury, care, and recovery potential.

Intervertebral Disc Disease

Etiology

It is estimated that approximately 80% of the population will experience back pain during the course of their lives. One third of those afflicted will be incapacitated for varying lengths of time. In addition, back pain accounts for one quarter of all sick-leave days, and the average industrial disability claim related to back pain amounts to 123 days. Most cases of back pain diagnosed as "lumbar–sacral strain/sprain" are the result of disc disease.[12]

Incidence of cervical and lumbar disc disease, contrary to previous thought, is not correlated to gender, type of work or body build.[12] Factors that do appear to play a significant role in the development of disc disease include age and trauma. Frequently, patients with lumbar disc disease report an injury prior to the onset of symptoms, though many may not recall such an event.[1, 12, 19, 31] About 90% of patients with cervical disc disease do not recall a prior injury.[15]

Disc disease is thought to occur as a result of degenerative changes in the intervertebral disc, mechanical stress incurred secondary to the degenerative changes, and additional mechanical stress to the vertebral discs, especially lumbar discs, caused by poor posture, weak muscles, and lifting objects while the back is in a flexed or rotated position.[12]

Pathophysiology

The spine is composed of 33 vertebrae: 7 cervical, 12 thoracic, 5 lumbar, 5 sacral, and 4 coccygeal vertebrae. Each vertebral body, from the second cervical through the fifth lumbar, is separated from the underlying vertebral body by a disc. The intervertebral disc provides a cushion or shock absorber between the vertebrae, acts to equalize pressures over the vertebral surface, and serves as an articulation between the vertebral bodies.[12, 31] There is a variety of stresses that the intervertebral disc is subjected to during normal movement of the spine. Compression, flexion, hypertension, and rotational forces all produce stress in the disc. The lumbar vertebrae, in particular, are subjected to more stress than other vertebrae.

Intervertebral discs undergo gradual degeneration with age. By the fourth decade there are retrogressive changes in the cartilaginous plate, degenerative changes in the annulus (the outer layer), and decreased fluid volume in the nucleus pulposus (the inner core). Progression of these changes with advancing age results in erosion of the vertebral body by the bulging discs, tears in the posterior annulus, calcification of the disc, and replacement of the nucleus pulposus and fibrocartilage.

It has been postulated that the degenerative changes in the nucleus pulposus that cause a decrease in the protein content may initially act as an oncotic agent resulting in an uptake of fluid by the nucleus.[12, 15] This high intradiscal pressure may then cause a rupture in the annulus with relatively minor stress.

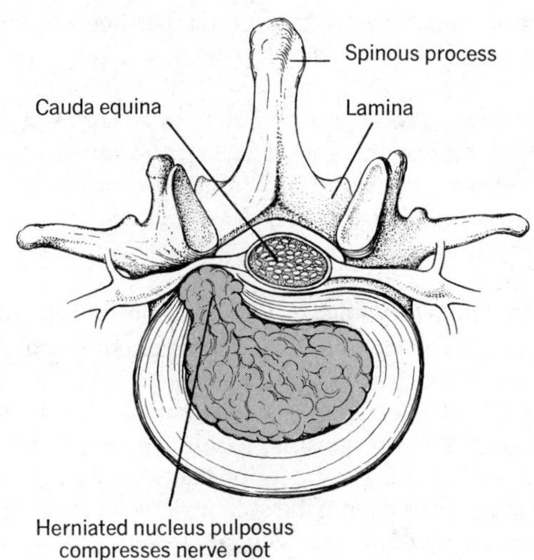

FIGURE 69–3 Ruptured vertebral disc.

With degenerative changes in the disc, it has been established that additional stress is placed on the vertebral facets, and ligaments. The constant stress on the ligaments and articular surfaces of the vertebrae, produced by the increased mobility of vertebral bodies, stimulates the formation of new bone. The stretching of the posterior ligament by the bulging disc also stimulates new bone growth, and this ligament may become thickened and calcified. This overgrowth of bone (osteophytic formation) further serves to impinge on neural structures.

It is the protrusion of disc substance, either the bulging annulus fibrosus itself or the herniated nucleus pulposus (HNP), through the weak posterior longitudinal ligament that has been termed *protruded intervertebral disc* (Fig. 69–3).

The most common site for disc herniation to occur is in the lumbar region at L4-5 and L5–S1 disc interspaces. The next most common site is at L3-4. Disc herniation in the cervical area is less common. The most common cervical site is at the C5-6 and C6-7 intervertebral spaces. Thoracic disc herniation is rare, occurring in approximately 1% of all herniated discs.[2, 19] When thoracic disc herniation does occur, it usually occurs between T9 and T12. The most common site is at the T11-12 interspace, and the disc tends to herniate centrally rather than laterally.

Clinical Manifestations

Protruded Lumbar Disc. The patient who has symptoms of lumbar disc disease usually presents with back pain. The pain is thought to be due to irritation of pain fibers that result from the stretching of the posterior annulus and posterior longitudinal ligaments.[12] The pain may be gradual in onset, with a dull aching quality or it may be sudden and severe, with accompanying muscle spasm. The pain in both cases is aggravated by activity (any motion whatsoever precipitates severe pain when muscle spasm is present) and is relieved by rest.

Within a few days or weeks the back pain gradually subsides. If the episode has not resulted in impingement of the spinal nerve root by disc protrusion, the patient will be asymptomatic until the next episode, usually precipitated by a minor trauma, such as an awkward movement. If the herniation has compressed a spinal nerve root, the subsiding back pain is replaced by a boring, aching pain in the buttock and posterior or posterolateral aspect of the thigh and calf; this pain is termed *sciatica*. It may be accompanied by numbness and tingling radiating into the foot. Leg pain is often relieved by lying on the unaffected side, with the painful leg in a flexed position. Physical exertion, sneezing, coughing, or straining may aggravate both back and leg pain.

The patient with symptomatic lumbar disc disease will usually assume a characteristic stance in an attempt to minimize back and leg pain. The posture, assumed because of paravertebral muscle spasm and an attempt to flatten (or straighten) the curvature of the lumbar spine, is a slight forward tilting of the trunk (Fig. 69–4). Position is changed in a careful, slow manner with a great deal of guarding of the back, and the patient will prefer to stand rather than sit. The gait will be slow and deliberate. The patient may also hold the affected leg in slight flexion at the hip and knee to reduce stretching of the sciatic nerve. When observing the patient's back, some scoliosis may be noted and there may be evidence of increased paravertebral muscle tension. Local tenderness over the involved vertebra and paravertebral muscles may also be present.

On examination, combinations of pain and paresthesia with diminished sensory, motor, and reflex function may be noted in the distribution of the affected spinal nerve. Symptoms of spinal nerve root involvement, usually due to nerve root compression, are called radiculopathy. Pain and other sensory changes may be precipitated or aggravated by various maneuvers that place tension on the sciatic nerve.

Rarely, a central herniation of disc material into the lumbar vertebral canal in the presence of a narrow canal will cause compression of the cauda equina. The cauda equina is composed of lumbar–sacral spinal nerve roots. Compression at this level may cause a flaccid paraparesis, loss of sphincter tone, depressed or absent lower extremity muscle stretch reflexes, and sensory disturbances.

Protruded Cervical Disc. A protruded cervical disc, because the herniation usually occurs in a posterocentral or posterolateral direction, may compress the cervical spinal cord, the cervical spinal roots, or both. Cervical cord symptoms may also be caused by compromise of the cervical vascular supply by impinging structures.

Symptoms usually begin with posterior neck pain that may be concomitant with paravertebral muscle spasm (Fig. 69–5). With the passing of a variable length of time the pain may begin to radiate into the arm and is accompanied by tingling and numbness in the distribution of the affected cervical nerve root (Fig. 69–6). Symptoms may be aggravated by sneezing, coughing, or straining.

Protruded Thoracic Disc. The rare event of thoracic disc protrusion usually causes cord compression because the lower thoracic vertebral canal is narrower and because herniations are usually in a posterior and central direction. Again, cord involvement at this level may also be a result of compromise of the vascular supply.

Most patients do not give a preceding history of trauma, and often the symptoms are chronic (a 2 to 4 year history is common) and progressive.[2, 19] The patient usually complains of generalized back pain that is mild to moderate in severity. Limitation of movement of the back, scoliosis, and paravertebral muscle spasm may be present.

Numbness in the lower extremities, which may gradually ascend, is a common complaint; it may be unilateral or bilateral. Diminished appreciation for pain and temperature sensation and the presence of paresthesias are also common.

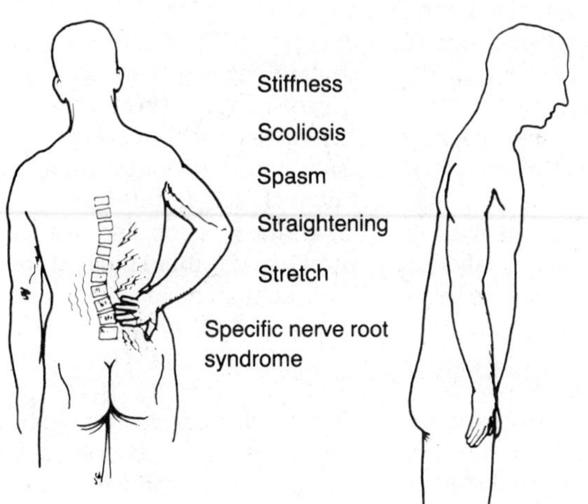

FIGURE 69–4 The spinal signs of lumbar disc herniation (Smith RR: Essentials of Neurosurgery. Philadelphia, JB Lippincott, 1980)

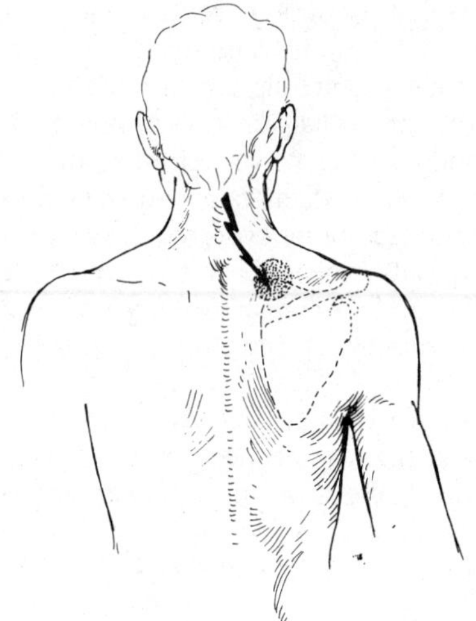

FIGURE 69–5 Pattern of pain radiation with a lateral protrusion of a cervical disc. (Hoppenfeld S; Orthopaedic Neurology. Philadelphia, JB Lippincott, 1977)

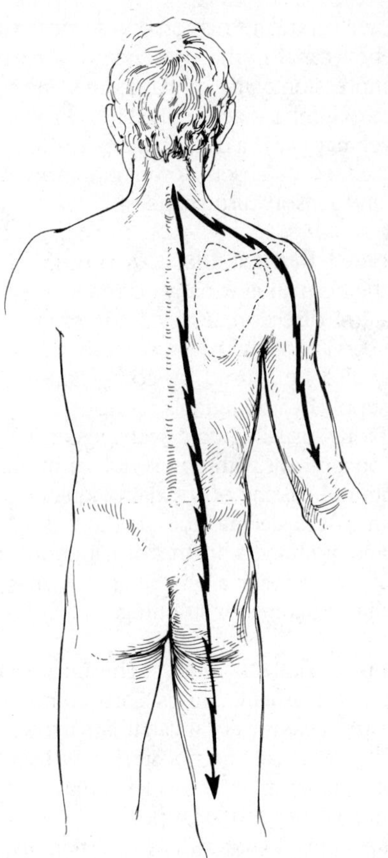

FIGURE 69–6 Pattern of pain radiation with a midline herniated cervical disc. (Hoppenfeld S: Orthopaedic Neurology. Philadelphia, JB Lippincott, 1977)

In addition, the patient may note an unsteady gait, bladder and bowel disturbances, and sexual dysfunction.

Spondylosis. The term spondylosis generally refers to the degenerative osteophytic changes in the discs, vertebrae, and ligaments that occur at more than one level. There usually is no history of trauma, although as already noted, if the degenerative changes are already present a very minor traumatic event may precipitate onset of symptoms. Symptomatic cervical spondylosis is more common than symptomatic lumbar spondylosis. Degenerative changes cause osteophytic overgrowth. This bony overgrowth results in encroachment of the spinal nerve roots and the spinal cord.

Cervical spondylosis may result in both nerve root and spinal cord compression (myelopathy), giving rise to both lower motor neuron and upper motor neuron dysfunction signs. Lower motor neuron signs will be noted in the distribution of the affected spinal nerve roots (sensory, motor, or both) that supply the arm, and upper motor neuron signs will be noted in the arms (depending on the level of spinal cord compression) and legs. Spondylotic changes are common with aging and, depending on the severity, may or may not give rise to symptoms. The task then becomes one of correlating the patient's signs and symptoms to the exact level(s) of spondylotic changes.

Posterior neck pain is also a common complaint in cervical spondylosis. Differentiating spondylosis from an acutely hernitated disc is made possible with spine films and CT scanning.

Spondylolysis and Spondylolisthesis. Spondylolysis is thought to be a congenital anomaly that affects the lumbar vertebrae (most commonly at L5). The defect consists of a loss of bony continuity in the neural arch.[1] This defect allows the forward displacement of one vertebral body on the vertebral body below it; this subluxation is called spondylolisthesis. Spondylolisthesis may also occur without a bony, structural defect.

Approximately 5% of the population may have spondylolysis. It is not always symptomatic and, when it is, symptoms usually do not appear until around the age of 35. Symptoms include low back pain that is aggravated by weight bearing, lifting, and moving, especially extension movements. Leg pain may be present and is the result of compression of spinal nerve roots.[12]

On examination, a steplike deformity sometimes may be palpated over the spinous processes at the lumbosacral area. The pelvis may be rotated forward.

Medical Management

Diagnosis

Diagnosis is, of course, dependent on an accurate history and physical examination. In addition, a few diagnostic tests have proven beneficial in the diagnosis of degenerative intervertebral disc disease.

Plain radiographs (x-rays) of the spine may show disease other than a herniated disc that is responsible for the patient's symptoms. These may include rheumatoid arthritis and osteoarthritis, vertebral fracture, neoplasm, congenital anomalies, infectious processes, and significant differences in leg length.[12,19] Plain x-ray studies usually do not show a herniated disc; what may be demonstrated are degenerative changes indicative of disc disease such as narrowing of disc interspaces or the presence of osteophytes.

Computerized tomography (CT) of the spine is especially useful in demonstrating changes associated with degenerative disc disease. CT scanning has proven most helpful in showing a narrow spinal canal (spinal stenosis).

Myelography is usually employed only when surgical intervention is the treatment choice. In this instance, a myelogram is used to delineate the level of disc protrusion as well as to rule out the presence of other spinal lesions that may not have been demonstrated on plain spine films.

Treatment

Prevention of symptomatic disc disease should be advocated through health education. Many schools and workplaces provide instruction on the prevention of back injury. Preventive measures include maintenance of proper posture while standing, sitting, or walking, good muscle tone, and the employment of good body mechanics when lifting. In addition, properly constructed chairs and car seats, firm mattresses for sleeping, and chairs and worktables that are maintained at the proper height to reduce strain on the neck and back have proven to be helpful.

Conservative Treatment. Most patients with symptomatic degenerative disc disease respond to conservative treatment. The principle of conservative treatment is to protect the affected disc from additional strain and to provide rest of the affected spinal area to promote healing by fibrosis.[12] Conservative treatment for patients who have disc disease at any vertebral level is generally based on rest, avoidance of activities or postures that aggravate the condition, and external support of the affected body area. Pelvic traction has not been found to be beneficial in the treatment of lumbar disc disease. Cervical traction has been found to be effective in some people with pain from cervical disc disease. Table 69–7 lists specific measures employed in the conservative management of disc disease.

Surgical Treatment. Surgical treatment of disc disease is advocated when the patient's symptoms fail to subside with conservative treatment, recurrent attacks of severe pain and radiculopathy prevent the patient from leading a normal life, nerve root compression has resulted in weakness in an extremity part, or symptoms of spinal cord or cauda equina compression are present (urgent surgery is necessary when this occurs).

Surgical treatment for *lumbar disc herniation* is undertaken to remove the entire nuclear disc (discectomy) and cartilaginous plate, leaving only a "horseshoe" of annulus on the anterior and lateral sides.[12] Sometimes it is not possible to remove the entire disc. In order to gain access to the protruded disc, a portion of a lamina (laminotomy) or sometimes the entire lamina (laminectomy) is usually removed. If the disc protrusion is found to be entirely lateral, only the lamina on the affected side needs to be opened (hemilaminotomy or hemilaminectomy). Occasionally, narrowing of the intervertebral foramen and entrapment of the nerve root by osteophytic processes may require enlargement of the foramen (foraminotomy). Fusion of lumbar vertebrae is indicated only when there is instability of the neural arch created by disc disease or surgical procedures undertaken to achieve adequate decompression of the nerve root.

Approximately two thirds of patients who have had surgery for lumbar disc removal have good to excellent results. Of the remaining one third of patients, one half experience improvement of their symptoms and one half do not improve. Generally, patients who primarily have back pain fare worse than those whose symptoms are primarily due to root compression.[12]

Complications that may attend lumbar discectomy include injury to the nerve root; injury to the dural sac causing a tear and a cerebrospinal fluid leak; injury to abdominal vessels or organs; inflammation or infection of the disc space; mechanical instability of the spine; chronic adhesive arachnoiditis; and severe pain from improved sensation following nerve root decompression, muscle spasm, or inadequate disc removal.[12,20] Delayed epidural hematoma that causes cord compression is also a possible complication. Its presence requires emergent reoperation for evacuation of the clot and hemostasis.

Surgical treatment for *cervical disc disease* may include hemilaminotomy or hemilaminectomy, posterior discectomy, foraminotomy, posterior fusion, or anterior discectomy with or without fusion. The surgical procedure selected is one that affords the maximum exposure needed for adequate decompression of the cervical spinal canal or intervertebral foramina and that carries the least risk. If a herniated disc is present and a posterior discectomy is performed, the surgeon usually will remove only the extruded disc fragments (of which there are usually several), and will not enter the annulus to remove all of the nuclear disc material. Complete nuclear disc removal in the cervical region is not neces-

TABLE 69–7
Conservative Treatment for Symptomatic Disc Disease

I. Lumbar Disc Problems
   A. *Mild to moderate symptoms:*
      1. Decrease activity in general; includes resting in bed when pain increases.
      2. Avoid lifting, bending, or standing.
      3. Sleep on a firm mattress.
      4. Application of heat to low back if this seems to improve comfort.
      5. Wear lumbar corset.
      6. Take pain medication as needed.
      7. Continue above treatments until symptoms subside; if symptoms do not subside or if they increase at end of 1 week, contact physician.
      8. Once pain subsides, perform Williams flexion exercises or isometric exercises to strengthen abdominal and back muscles.
   B. *Severe symptoms:*
      1. Strict bed rest on a firm mattress, in position of comfort
      2. Take pain medication at prescribed intervals.
      3. When symptoms subside, follow instructions for mild to moderate symptoms.
      4. Strict bed rest may be enforced for up to 3–4 weeks before the treatment can be considered to have failed to improve symptoms.

II. Cervical Disc Problems
   A. *Mild to moderate symptoms:*
      1. Wear soft cervical collar.
      2. Avoid any activity that increases pain.
      3. Take pain medication as needed.
      4. Continue above treatments until symptoms subside; if symptoms do not subside or if they increase at the end of 1 week, contact physician.
   B. *Severe symptoms:*
      1. Bed rest with very flat pillow
      2. Intermittent cervical traction with 5–8 lb of weight; if pain is not relieved, or made worse, at the end of 24 hours, discontinue traction.
      3. Apply heat if it improves symptoms.
      4. Take pain medication at prescribed intervals.
      5. When symptoms subside, follow instructions for mild to moderate symptoms.
      6. If symptoms do not subside within the time frame given you by physician, recontact physician.

sary because the incidence of recurrent cervical disc protrusion at the same site is less than 1%.[15]

The anterior cervical approach is most often indicated for the patient who has signs of spinal cord compression from a herniated disc or from spondylotic processes at only one or two levels. The anterior approach is favored when cervical myelopathy is present because it provides more direct access to the area of pathology, allows restoration of the anterior contour of the spinal canal, and does not interfere with neck stability.[8] Anterior discectomy may be performed with or without fusion of the vertebral bodies. Most often total removal of the disc is done and a bone graft, usually taken from the anterior, superior part of the iliac crest, is wedged into the disc interspace.

Complications of posterior cervical operations include wound infection, soft tissue hematoma, injury to the spinal cord or nerve roots, spinal cord compression due to epidural hematoma, air embolism (more likely if the sitting position is used), subcutaneous wound dishiscence, and vertebral instability.[8]

Complications of anterior cervical operations include wound infection, intraoperative or delayed postoperative hemorrhage with compromise of the airway, injury to the soft tissue of the neck (*e.g.,* esophagus, trachea, and carotid artery), laryngeal nerve damage, damage to nerve roots, and pneumothorax (rare). Injury to the spinal cord is, by report, exceedingly rare.[8]

Nursing Management

Assessment and Nursing Diagnosis

Analysis of assessment data determines the course of treatment and the appropriate nursing management plan. The appropriate nursing diagnoses may include potential activity intolerance related to the dysfunction, impaired physical mobility related to disc disease, and alteration in comfort related to pain from the disc disease.

Goals. The goals for the patient with degenerative disc disease include his knowing how to minimize the stress to his back or neck, maintaining good posture, and practicing proper body mechanics. For the patient who requires surgical intervention, the goals also include the patient's being free from anxiety related to the procedures of the surgery and of the postoperative care; absence of perioperative complications, and resumption of normal activities of daily living.

Nursing Interventions: Conservative Treatment

Exercise Teaching. The patient who has degenerative disc disease especially needs to know how to minimize the stress to his back or neck so that he can reduce the number of repeated injuries and possibly avoid the necessity of having surgery. Maintenance of good posture and the practice of proper body mechanics is essential. The patient with exaggerated lumbar lordosis (swayback) and weak abdominal muscles will place additional stress on his lumbar vertebrae and discs. Strengthening of abdominal muscles will reduce the degree of lumbar curvature and improve posture. The nurse can teach the patient how to perform the Williams flexion exercises, a popular prescription for patients who need to strengthen the abdominal and erector spinae muscles of the back (see Table 69–5). Some physicians believe that flexion exercises are potentially harmful to the person with disc disease and instead advocate simple isometric exercises designed to strengthen abdominal and erector spinae muscles.[12] Exercises undertaken to strengthen abdominal and back musculature should be performed during asymptomatic periods; the individual with moderate to acute low back pain should totally rest his back.

Posture. Maintenance of good posture while sitting and sleeping is also important. Avoidance of slouching while sitting and avoidance of prolonged periods of sitting will reduce lumbar stress. Extended periods of driving a car can be quite stressful to the back. No individual with episodes of back or neck pain should ever sleep on his stomach (prone position). This position increases the lordotic lumbar curve. For patients with cervical disc disease, the prone position will require them to maintain their head in a rotated, lateral position for an extended period of time. These patients should also be cautioned against sleeping with thick pillows under the head (exaggerated flexion of the neck) and falling asleep in an awkward posture (*e.g.,* while sitting or semi-reclining on the sofa). Again, some physicians favor exercises of the head and neck to maintain normal range of motion and others believe that once significant cervical disease is present, even normal movements of the neck will serve to hasten and increase osteophyte formation.[15]

Body Mechanics. The patient with evidence of disc disease should be taught proper body mechanics with emphasis placed on avoiding lifting while in a flexed or rotated position and making certain that all objects that are lifted are held close to the chest. It has been proposed that the single most important factor in producing stress to the lumbar spine is the distance between the weight lifted and the back.[12] A lumbar corset should be worn during times when it is known beforehand that a planned activity will place increased stress on the spine. Lifting heavy objects may also stress the cervical spine by pulling the arms. Reaching for objects, as well as lifting them, while in an awkward posture can increase stress to the neck.

Activity Level. Patients who are experiencing mild to moderate back or neck pain should reduce their activity (see Table 69–7). The patient with mild low back pain should pay particular attention to his posture and body mechanics. Actually when the patient is having pain, he almost always will automatically move his body in the correct manner because the least deviation from good body mechanics will produce an immediate increase in pain. In general, the spine should always be kept straight or slightly flexed with the entire trunk moving in one piece (or as one unit); all rotation and extension movements should be avoided. A lumbar corset worn during acute episodes of mild to moderate back pain offers support to the back and abdominal muscles and decreases stress to the lumbar vertebrae. Similarly, a soft cervical collar will provide the same benefits to the cervical vertebrae.

Sitting. The patient who has mild to moderate back pain should be advised to avoid long periods of sitting; when he must sit, he should sit in a straight-back chair with his back held straight against the back (a pillow behind the back may be necessary), with his legs flexed at the hips and knees, and with his feet resting on a footstool. Elevating the knees above the hips reduces strain on the back. When only mild back pain is present, the patient may find that lying on the floor and performing the knee–chest exercise (see Table 69–5) may reduce his discomfort.

Bed Rest. Bed rest during periods of increased back discomfort is essential in reducing stress to the vertebrae and back musculature caused by normal activities such as standing, walking, and sitting. The patient may be more comfortable lying flat on his back (or with his head elevated only slightly) with his legs elevated on pillows. This position decreases lumbar strain by flattening the lumbar curve. Care should be taken to avoid applying direct pressure at the back of the knees. Intermittent flexion and extension of the feet will act as a deterrent to thrombus formation in the legs. If the patient has leg pain, he may be more comfortable when lying on his unaffected side and flexing his painful leg to reduce tension on the sciatic nerve. A pillow placed between his legs will maintain proper alignment of his hip and reduce tension on back musculature. Bed rest is also beneficial for relief of cervical pain by eliminating the weight of the head and minimizing neck motion. Mild non-narcotic analgesics and nonsteroid anti-inflammatory agents may be prescribed for patients during recurrent episodes of mild to moderate back and neck pain.

Of special note is the occurrence of muscle spasm in the back or neck. The patient who has muscle spasm is usually in severe pain. These patients should be given enough analgesic medication to significantly reduce or stop the pain. Onset of muscle spasm results in a cycle of muscle spasm–pain–increased muscle spasm. Codeine (or sometimes stronger medication) along with a muscle relaxant may provide enough analgesia and sedation to break this cycle.

Most importantly, patients with disc disease should be taught to take particular care of their backs or necks at the first sign of pain. Increasing activity *does not* "work it out." By reducing activity, the patient may very well avert a more severe injury that will then incapacitate him for a week or two, or more. This approach does not apply to the patient with chronic pain. This patient is not able to obtain relief from pain by either conservative or surgical measures; therefore, he is taught to live with his pain and proceed as much as is possible with normal daily activities.

The patient with severe pain is placed on strict bed rest, either at home or in the hospital; he is usually allowed bathroom privileges. The nurse must emphasize the importance of adhering to bed rest. Every time the patient gets out of bed, stress is placed on the spine. In order to maximize the benefits of conservative treatment the patient must remain in bed as much as possible.

Patients with severe neck or back pain, especially when it is accompanied by radiculopathy, are often hospitalized so that an accurate evaluation of the efficacy of conservative treatment may be made, and early detection of any increase in neurological deficit may be made. Nursing measures indicated for the person who has had an episode of severe back or neck pain and who has been hospitalized for conservative management are listed in Table 69–8.

Preoperative and Postoperative Nursing Interventions

The patient whose pain and radicular symptoms do not subside with conservative treatment will need surgery. The nurse should help to allay any of the patient's fears by explaining all diagnostic procedures throughly, the type of surgery planned, and what he might expect after surgery. Routine preoperative teaching including deep-breathing exercises should be done. Most surgical spine procedures for disc disease do not require an extended period of bed rest. In most instances, the patient will be able to stand to void on the night of surgery.

Postoperatively, the patient's vital signs and neurological signs should be monitored at least 1 to 2 hours following his return from the recovery room. This interval may be increased the following day to every 4 hours through postoperative day 3, and then possibly to once a shift, if the patient's condition permits. The frequency of monitoring vital or neurological signs is automatically increased whenever an abnormality is detected. Any onset of a new neurological deficit (sensory or motor) or any worsening of a previously existing neurological deficit should be reported to the physician at once. It may indicate development of a spinal epidural hematoma, the presence of which may cause irreversible neurological deficit from spinal cord compression. The presence of a spinal epidural hematoma is a surgical emergency.

Following a Lumbar Discectomy. Following a lumbar discectomy, the patient will usually have orders to remain flat on his back for 1 to 2 hours in order to promote hemostasis. He is then log-rolled side to side every 2 hours. In most instances, he may stand to void the night of surgery; he will probably require the assistance of two people, even if he has learned the technique of getting in and out of bed preoperatively, as described in Table 69–8. The patient should be watched carefully for urinary retention. If he is unable to void 8 to 12 hours after surgery (depending on fluid intake) he may require a one-time catheterization. All measures to assist the patient to void should first be tried. Persistent urinary retention should be reported to the physician.

The patient's dressing should be monitored every 2 hours for evidence of bleeding or cerebrospinal fluid leak. Usually, if the surgeon has had to repair a dural tear, he will increase the length of time that the patient must remain flat in bed in order to reduce tension placed on the dural sutures and minimize the risk of cerebrospinal fluid leak.

Pain medication should be administered to the patient around the clock (rather than prn) for at least the first 24 hours. Narcotic analgesics are usually ordered for the first 3 postoperative days.

TABLE 69–8
Nursing Care of the Patient with Severe Back and Neck Pain

Activity

1. Enforce bed rest and explain to patient why it is important.
2. Place bed boards under mattress.
3. Facilitate patient's compliance with bed rest.
   a. Assist patient with hygiene. Patient should not strain to reach any body part; he should remain flat in bed. Nurse should assist with most of bath.
   b. Provide opportunity for patient to brush his teeth in AM and after meals.
   c. Provide easy access to nurses' call light.
4. If bathroom privileges are allowed, instruct patient with low back pain on how to get out of bed without placing undue stress on the back.
   a. Patient should turn to his side with his knees flexed and carefully slide to the edge of the bed while keeping the spine straight (nurse may need to assist by pulling the patient to the side of the bed by pulling draw sheet).
   b. The patient then pushes himself to a sitting position from a side-lying position by keeping his spine straight while pushing on the bed with his upper hand placed in front of his chest.
   c. Then he uses his lower arm to assist with weight bearing.
   d. Sitting should be kept to a minimum.
   e. The patient should be sitting on the edge of the bed before attempting to stand and should keep his spine as straight as possible while coming to a standing position.
   f. The reverse procedure is followed for getting back into bed.
5. Encourage patient to wear lumbar corset or cervical collar when upright.
6. Patient should wear antiembolic stockings (nurse will need to assist patient with their application); he should be taught to flex and extend his feet at intervals.

Positioning

1. Patient should assume position of comfort.
   a. If there is lumbar pain, patient may be more comfortable lying flat on back (or with head slightly elevated) with his legs elevated and flexed at the hips and knees; elevation of both the knees and footgatch will minimize pressure placed at back of knees.
   b. If leg pain is present, patient may be more comfortable lying on his unaffected side, with painful leg flexed.
   c. If cervical pain is present, the head of the patient's bed should be flat, or elevated slightly for cervical traction; a flat pillow is permitted to prevent neck extension; flexion of the neck is also to be avoided.
2. Prone position is prohibited for back and neck pain.

Immobility

1. Nurse should be aware of the problems associated with immobility and plan nursing care accordingly.

Medications

1. Common medications used include analgesics, nonsteroid anti-inflammatory agents, muscle relaxants, and stool softeners.
2. Pain medication should be given around the clock rather than prn if patient is in acute phase.
3. Antacids may need to be administered if anti-inflammatory medications are given.

Diet

1. High-fiber diet reduces straining with bowel elimination.
2. Weight reduction may be indicated in order to reduce stress on spine.

Heat Treatments

1. Deep ultrasonic heat treatment may be most beneficial.
2. Moist heat is better than dry heat.
3. Nurse should be aware of safety precautions when applying heat and using heat appliances.

Neurological Signs

1. Patient's baseline values should be established.
   a. If cervical disc disease is present, sensory and motor testing of all extremities should be done.
   b. If lumbar disc disease is present, sensory and motor testing of lower extremities should be done.
2. Observe patient for any onset of, or increase in, neurological deficit; a patient with sudden onset of symptoms of spinal cord compression or cauda equina compression requires immediate surgery.

Psychosocial Support

1. Provide patient opportunity to express concerns or fears and, when appropriate, provide teaching.
2. Patient may be worried about
   a. Extended period of time away from home or work
   b. Finances: he may have reduced income when not working and may worry about how to pay for hospital bill
   c. Losing his job because of extended or repeated absences; losing his job because of activity restrictions
   d. Whether he can continue his type of work if it requires frequent lifting, straining, or prolonged periods of sitting or driving
   e. Having support of spouse, children, or coworkers for reduced activity level
   f. Sexual activity precipitating recurrent episodes of pain
   g. Not getting enough pain medication to relieve pain
   h. Addiction to analgesics or muscle relaxants
   i. Increasing disability and alteration of lifestyle
   j. Surgery or anesthesia
3. Patient education should be given regarding posture, body mechanics, exercises, and activity level during recurrent episodes.

The patient may be ambulated on the first postoperative day, depending on his tolerance. Administration of pain medication 20 to 30 minutes before the patient is assisted out of bed or ambulated is helpful in reducing the patient's pain and anxiety. It is wise to have two people available to assist with ambulation until the nurse feels the patient's safety is not at risk. Some analgesics and muscle relaxants may produce orthostatic hypotension or dizziness. Antiembolic stockings may reduce the risk of orthostatic hypotension.

The patient may be able to care for himself by the second postoperative day, except for bathing his back and legs. Sutures are usually removed about 7 days after surgery, and the patient may begin to shower 1 to 2 days after the sutures are removed.

On occasion the patient's pain may increase about 3 days after surgery. This may be due to improved sensation in the nerve root or it may be due to muscle spasm. The pain may be relieved by returning the patient to bed rest, especially if it is due to muscle spasm, and administering around-the-clock narcotic analgesics, muscle relaxants, or both for another 48 hours. The patient should be reassured that it is temporary.

If the patient's condition permits, his ambulation is progressively increased. Sitting is kept to an absolute minimum. Most patients can be discharged about 1 week after surgery with activity restrictions for the next 2 weeks, including minimal sitting. Gradual increase in activity is then allowed, with return to light work in 1 to 2 months. A follow-up appointment with the physician is scheduled for 6 weeks after surgery. Discharge teaching should include reinforcement of good posture and proper body mechanics. An exercise regimen, to begin very gradually and only when the patient can tolerate it, is given to the patient. Other commonly given discharge instructions are presented in Table 69–9.

Following Cervical Discectomy. The patient who has posterior cervical discectomy will require much of the same postoperative care as the patient with a lumbar discectomy with regard to observation of vital and neurological signs, observation of the dressing, and frequency of turning. The head should be kept flat with only a flat pad (a folded blanket or sheet) under the head to prevent lateral flexion while side-lying and hyperextension while lying on the back (Fig. 69–7). A soft cervical collar will also provide support and limit neck motion while the patient is in bed. The patient may be allowed out of bed with a collar the day after surgery. He may be up as much as is tolerated. The length of time the cervical collar must be worn depends on the patient's condition and the surgeon's preference.

The patient generally is able to care for himself 1 to 2 days following surgery, but he should be cautioned not to strain or pull with his arms in doing his care. A shower is permitted when sutures are removed and this often coincides with the day of discharge from the hospital.

Discharge instructions include instructions to avoid straining the neck in any way. The patient should avoid driv-

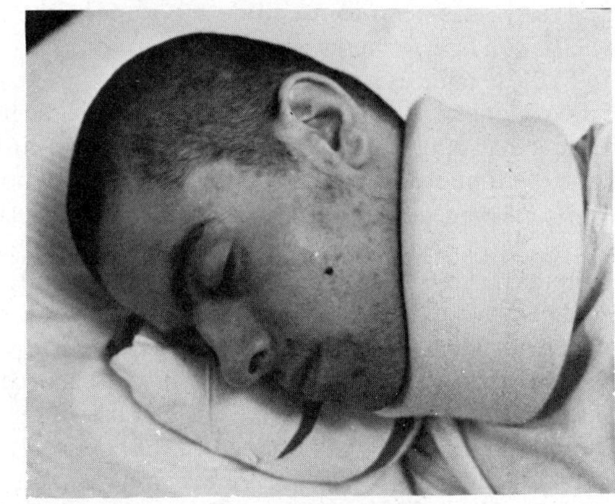

FIGURE 69–7 Head position following a cervical laminectomy. (Decision Audiovisual Media. Neurological Care Series. Philadelphia, JB Lippincott)

TABLE 69–9
Commonly Prescribed Postoperative Discharge Instructions

1. *Operative site:* Observe for signs of infection, *e.g.*, fever, increased pain, inflammation, or drainage. Notify the physician at once.
2. *Bathing:* May shower if sutures are out. Avoid tub baths for at least 3 weeks due to risk of slipping and difficulty in maintaining erect spine.
3. *Pain:* Take pain medication as needed; increase in pain should be reported to physician.
4. *Activity:* Guided by level of discomfort. For the first 2 weeks, minimal exertion, avoid standing or sitting for long periods, and rest lying down as much as possible.
5. *Lumbar corset:* Follow physician's instructions. May need to wear for 6 months. Some physicians may not advocate a lumbar corset.
6. *Diet:* If overweight, weight reduction is essential in reducing chances of disc reherniation or herniation at another level. High-fiber diet will reduce straining with bowel elimination.
7. *Sports:* Strenuous activity prohibited until physician instructs you otherwise.
8. *Sex:* You may resume sexual activity when you feel comfortable to do so.
9. *Driving:* Avoid for at least 3 weeks; when driving is resumed, position your seat closer to the steering wheel to prevent stress to the back. ALWAYS WEAR A SEAT BELT, both as a passenger and a driver.
10. *Work:* Light work may be resumed within 1 to 2 months; heavier work should be avoided until physician approves—to be determined at 6-week follow-up appointment.
11. Practice good posture and body mechanics.
    a. *Standing:* Avoid for long periods; keep spine erect, abdomen pulled in; bending one knee can reduce stress to low back.
    b. *Sitting:* Avoid soft chairs and deep couches; straight-back chairs are best; a small footstool reduces stress to the back if you keep your knees flexed (do not extend legs straight out on a footstool while sitting).
    c. *Lifting:* Avoid whenever possible. If necessary, turn and face the object. Bend at the knees and hips—NEVER AT THE WAIST. Hold the object close to your chest and stand up. NEVER turn and lift simultaneously.
    d. *Shoes:* Wear low-heeled shoes; high heels increase the curve of your low back and place stress on your back.

(Adapted from Sutcliffe S: Comprehensive nursing care: The patient with a ruptured lumbar disc. J Neurosurg Nurs 10:86–91, 1978)

ing a car, reaching, lifting, and sports activities until his physician has advised him it is acceptable to do so.

The patient who has had an *anterior cervical discectomy* will be placed on bed rest for 12 to 24 hours. During this time, in addition to frequent monitoring of the patient's vital and neurological signs, the nurse should carefully observe the operative site for evidence of undue swelling. Postoperative bleeding or hemorrhage can compromise the patient's airway. Often a postoperative drain is present; this is usually removed the day after surgery. Most patients have throat discomfort and difficulty swallowing for a few days after surgery. Humidified air, throat lozenges, and viscous Xylocaine will add to the patient's comfort. A soft diet until he can comfortably swallow solid food will be necessary. If the laryngeal nerve has been damaged during surgery, the patient will have a hoarse, husky voice that does not improve. Generally, these injuries never recover.

If the patient has had a fusion, a postoperative x-ray film is taken the day after surgery before he is allowed to be upright. If the film confirms the proper position of the bone graft, he is allowed to be up as tolerated. Some physicians advocate a hard cervical collar while the patient is up and others prefer no collar. Often the use of a collar depends on the number of vertebral levels operated and vertebral stability. These patients usually only require codeine for pain management; they often indicate that their greatest source of discomfort is the hip from which the bone graft was taken.

The physician should be notified of the sudden recurrence of radicular pain. Its occurrence may indicate that the bone graft has slipped. A lateral cervical spine film will need to be taken and another operation will have to be performed if the bone graft has slipped.

Most patients can be discharged 4 to 8 days after surgery. They may resume light activity but should avoid riding in or driving a car (other than the trip home). They should immediately report any signs of infection or increased pain to their physicians. The physician will want to evaluate the patient between the eighth and ninth postoperative weeks. Cervical spine films will be made at this time to determine the status of the bone graft. If full fusion has occurred, the patient may resume full activity. If fusion has not taken place, he will be placed in a cervical collar for the next 8 weeks. Repeat x-ray films will be taken at intervals until fusion is demonstrated.

Evaluation

The patient with intervertebral disc disease will utilize appropriate body mechanics, will maintain good posture, and will experience minimal to no stress to the back and neck. The patient who has experienced surgery for disc disease will demonstrate minimal to no anxiety related to the operative procedure and postoperative nursing care, will experience no postoperative complications, and will resume normal activities of daily living in a reasonably prompt period of time.

References

1. Adams RD, Victor M: Principles of Neurology. New York, McGraw-Hill, 1977
2. Arbit E, Patterson RH Jr: Extradural spinal cord and nerve root compression from benign lesions of the dorsal area. In Youmans JR (ed): Neurological Surgery, 3rd ed, vol 3, pp 2562–2573. Philadelphia, WB Saunders, 1982
3. Becker DP, Miller JD, Young HF et al: Diagnosis and treatment of head injury in adults. In Youmans JR (ed): Neurological Surgery, 2nd ed, vol 4, pp 2251–2259. Philadelphia, WB Saunders, 1982
4. Boles R: Facial, auditory, and vestibular nerve injuries associated with basilar skull fractures. In Youmans JR (ed): Neurological Surgery, 2nd ed, vol 4, pp 2251–2259. Philadelphia, WB Saunders, 1982
5. Bracken MB, Freeman DH, Hellenbrand K: Incidence of acute traumatic hospitalized spinal cord injury in the United States, 1970–1971. Am J Epidemiol 113:615–622, 1981
6. Carter ER: Traumatic spinal cord injuries due to automobile accidents. South Med J 70:709–710, 1977
7. Carter RE: Medical management of pulmonary complications of spinal cord injury. In Thompson RA, Green JR (eds): Adv Neurol 22:269, 1979
8. Clark K: Anterior operative approach for benign extradural cervical lesions. In Youmans JR (ed): Neurological Surgery, 3rd ed, vol 3, pp 2613–2628. Philadelphia, WB Saunders, 1982
9. Clark K: Injuries to the cervical spine and spinal cord. In Youmans JR (ed): Neurological Surgery, 2nd ed, vol 3, pp 2318–2337. Philadelphia, WB Saunders, 1982
10. Clark K: Injuries to the lumbar spine. In Youmans JR (ed): Neurological Surgery, 2nd ed, vol 3, pp 2356–2361. Philadelphia, WB Saunders, 1982
11. Clark K: Management of thoracic spinal column injuries. In Youmans JR (ed): Neurological Surgery, 2nd ed, vol 3, pp 2344–2355. Philadelphia, WB Saunders, 1982
12. Davis CH Jr: Extradural spinal cord and nerve root compression from benign lesions of the lumbar area. In Youmans JR (ed): Neurological Surgery, 3rd ed, vol 3, pp 2535–2561. Philadephia, WB Saunders, 1982
13. Dohn DF: Hyperextension-hyperflexion injuries of the cervical spine. In Youmans JR (ed): Neurological Surgery, vol 2, pp 1075–1083. Philadelphia, WB Saunders, 1973
14. Dunsker SB: Hyperextension and hyperflexion injuries of the cervical spine. In Youmans JR (ed): Neurological Surgery, 2nd ed, vol 3, pp 2338–2343. Philadelphia, WB Saunders, 1982
15. Ehni G: Extradural spinal cord and nerve root compression from benign lesions of the cervical area. In Youmans JR (ed): Neurological Surgery, 3rd ed, vol 3, pp 2574–2612. Philadelphia, WB Saunders, 1982
16. Gadisseux P, Ward JD, Young HF, Becker DP: Nutrition and the neurosurgical patient. J Neurosurg 60:219–232, 1984
17. Guttman L: Spinal Cord Injuries. Comprehensive Management and Research, 2nd ed. London, Blackwell Scientific Publications, 1976
18. Healy GB: Current concepts in otolaryngology: Hearing loss and vertigo secondary to head injury. New Engl J Med 306:1029–1031, 1982
19. Hinton RC: Backache. In Samuels MA (ed): Manual of Nerologic Therapeutics, 2nd ed, pp 71–82. Boston, Little, Brown & Co, 1982
20. Howe JR: Manual of Patient Care in Neurosurgery, 2nd ed. Boston, Little, Brown & Co, 1983
21. Jennett B, Teasdale G: Management of Head Injuries. Philadelphia, FA Davis, 1981
22. Kalsbeek WD, McLaurin RL, Harris BSH, Miller JD: The national head and spinal cord injury survey: Major findings. J Neurosurg (Suppl) 53:S19–S31, 1980
23. Kilberg JK, Robinson S: Automotive crash injury report (No. 6), 1823–1830, 1967. In: Early Management of Acute Spinal Cord Injury, pp 59–66. New York, Raven Press, 1982
24. Lipe HP, Mitchell PH: Positioning the patient with intracranial hypertension: How turning and head rotation affect the internal jugular vein. Paper presented at Annual Meeting, American Association of Neurosurgical Nurses, Los Angeles CA, 1979

25. Miller JD: Physiology of trauma. Clin Neurosurg 29:103–130, 1982
26. Miller JD: Volume and pressure in the craniospinal axis. Clin Neurosurg 22:76–105, 1975
27. Miller JD, Becker DP: General principles and pathophysiology of head injury. In Youmans JR (ed): Neurological Surgery, 2nd ed, vol 4, pp 1896–2083. Philadelphia, WB Saunders, 1982
28. Miller JD, Butterworth JF, Gudeman SK et al: Further experiences in the management of severe head injury. J Neurosurg 54:389–299, 1981
29. Mitchell PD: Intracranial hypertension: Implications of research for nursing care. J Neurosurg Nurs 12:145–154, 1980
30. Mitchell PD, Mauss NK: Relationship of patient-nurse activity to intracranial pressure variations: A pilot study. Nurs Res 27:4–10, 1978
31. Mulder DW, Dale AJD: Spinal cord tumors and disks. In Baker AB, Baker LH (eds): Clinical Neurology, vol 3, pp 1–28. New York, Harper & Row, 1977
32. National Spinal Cord Injury Model Systems Conference: Proceedings. Phoenix AZ, National Spinal Cord Injury Data Research Center, 1978
33. Norell H: The early management of spinal injuries. Clin Neurosurg 27:385–400, 1979
34. O'Donnel WF, Taylor R: Genitourinary problems of spinal cord trauma. Curr Probl Surg 17:216–228, 1980
35. Ommaya AK: Mechanisms of cerebral concussion, contusions, and other effects of head injury. In Youmans JR (ed): Neurological Surgery, 2nd ed, vol 4, pp 1877–1895. Philadelphia, WB Saunders, 1982
36. Pitts LH: Neurological evaluation of the head injury patient. Clin Neurosurg 29:203–224, 1982
37. Rosenthal M, Griffith ER, Bond MR, Miller JD: Rehabilitation of the Head-Injured Adult. Phildelphia, WB Saunders, 1983
38. Seat belts: The overwhelming evidence. Br Med J 1:593–594, 1977
39. Thompson GB: Acute cervical spinal cord injury: Clinical assessment and classification of neurological deficit. In Tator CH (ed): Early Management of Acute Spinal Cord Injury, pp 1–24. New York, Raven Press, 1982
40. Turner M: Intracranial hypertension. Crit Care Q 2:67–76, 1979
41. White RF, Yashon D: General care of cervical spine injuries. In Youmans JR (ed): Neurological Surgery, vol 2, pp 1049–1066. Philadelphia, WB Saunders, 1973
42. White RJ: Advances in the treatment of cervical cord injuries. Clin Neurosurg 26:556–569, 1979

Bibliography

Albin MS, Hung T, Babinski MJ: Epidemiology, emergency and acute care: Advances in physiopathology and treatment. Curr Prob Surg 17:190–240, 1980

Caveness WF: Incidence of craniocerebral trauma in the United States in 1976 with trend from 1970–1975. Adv Neurol 22:1–3, 1979

Eidelberg E: The pathophysiology of spinal cord injury. Radiol Clin North Am 15:241–246, 1977

From "regeneration" to prostheses: Research on spinal cord injury. JAMA 245:1293–1297, 1981

Gertzbein SD: Traffic-related cervical spinal injuries and seat belts. In Tator CH (ed): Early Management of Acute Spinal Cord Injury, pp 59–66. New York, Raven Press, 1982

Griffith ER: Types of disability. In Rosenthal M, Griffith ER, Bond MR, Miller JD (eds): Rehabilitation of the Head-Injured Adult, pp 23–32. Philadelphia, FA Davis, 1983

Hansebout RR: A comprehensive review of methods of improving cord recovery after acute spinal cord injury. In Tator CH (ed): Early Management of Acute Spinal Cord Injury, pp 181–195. New York, Raven Press, 1982

Hardy AG, Rossier AB: Spinal Cord Injuries: Orthopedic and Neurological Aspects. Stuttgart, Georg Thieme, 1975

Jennett B: Scale and scope of the problem. In Rosenthal M, Griffith ER, Bond MR, Miller JD (eds): Rehabilitation of the Head-Injured Adult, pp 1–8. Philadelphia, FA Davis, 1983

Kraus JF: Epidemiologic features of head and spinal cord injury. In Schoenberg BS (ed): Advances in Neurology, vol 19, pp 261–278. New York, Raven Press, 1978

Kraus JF, Franti CE, Riggins RS et al: Incidence of traumatic spinal cord lesions. J Chronic Dis 28:471–492, 1975

Langfitt TW: Clinical methods for monitoring intracranial pressure and measuring cerebral blood flow. Clin Neurosurg 22:302–320, 1975

Levine JE, Becker DP: Reversal of incipient brain death from head-injured apnea at the scene of accidents. New Engl J Med 301:109, 1979

Lundberg N: Continuous recording and control of ventricular fluid pressure in neurosurgical practice. Acta Psychiatr Neurol Scandia 149 (Suppl 36):1–93, 1960

Michaelis LE: Epidemiology of spinal cord injury. In Vinkin PJ, Bruyn GW (eds): Handbook of Neurology, vol 25, part 1, pp 141–143. New York, American Elsevier Publishing Company, 1976

Miller JD: Early evaluation and management. In Rosenthal M, Griffith ER, Bond MR, Miller JD (eds): Rehabilitation of the Head-Injured Adult, pp 37–58. Philadelphia, FA Davis, 1983

Miller JD, Becker DP, Ward JD et al: Significance of intracranial hypertension in severe head injury. J Neurosurg 47:503–516, 1977

Mitchell DE, Adams JH: Primary focal impact damage to the brainstem in blunt head injuries: Does it exist? Lancet 2:215–218, 1973

Ommaya AK, Gennarelli TA: Cerebral concussion and traumatic unconciousness: Correlations of experimental and clinical observations on blunt head injuries. Brain 97:633–654, 1974

Ricci MM: Intracranial hypertension: Barbiturate therapy and the role of the nurse. J Neurosurg Nurs 11:247–252, 1979

Chapter 70

Alterations in Special Senses

Vision and Hearing Problems

Gretchen B. Stengel

Throughout her career, the nurse will encounter patients with sensory–perceptual problems. Whether caring for a patient with a specific problem of the sensory system itself or caring for a patient with other concurrent health problems, the nurse needs to know the major causes of sensory loss and be aware of how sensory loss affects lifestyle.

Our senses allow us to perceive and thereby interact with our environment. When a person is unable to perceive his environment meaningfully, sensory deprivation results, as has been discussed in Chapter 10.

Milder forms of visual and auditory impairment inhibit our ability to enjoy and interact with our environment, resulting in boredom and isolation. This is particularly true for persons with hearing deficits, since social communication is almost entirely dependent on the ability to hear. People with sensory impairments may become increasingly restricted in the ability to read, use the telephone, enjoy television or radio, attend lectures, plays and musical offerings, or partake in social gatherings. Especially for deaf people, the world can become a very monotonous and lonely place, and acute or chronic psychological problems, particularly paranoia and dementia, can become secondary manifestations of their sensory loss.

Sensory loss can also affect an individual's ability to comply with medical treatment. Visual deficits make it difficult to read directions on medications, packaging labels, or pamphlets pertaining to health care. Auditory deficits encumber communication with health professionals and make health teaching time consuming, awkward, and often ineffective. Changes in taste caused by aging predispose the elderly to increase their use of salt and sugar, two condiments frequently contraindicated in this age-group. Proprioceptive and visual problems may curtail prescribed exercise programs. Each of these losses may become a barrier to quality health care.

Nursing Management of Persons with Sensory Loss

Assessment and Nursing Diagnosis

Prior to devising a plan of care for any patient suffering sensory loss, the nurse needs a thorough understanding of the extent of the loss and its impact on the patient's preferred lifestyle. A complete history, inclusive of social activities, hobbies, living arrangements, and recreational activities, and a general examination of the involved system should be made.

Potential nursing diagnoses include sensory–perceptual alteration, ineffective coping, grieving, social isolation, disturbance in self-concept, and injury related to trauma.

Goals. The goals for care of the patient with visual impairment or hearing loss are that the patient will be able to effectively carry out the activities of daily living within the limitations of the loss.

Interventions for the Visually Impaired

To be classified as *legally blind,* one must have a visual field limitation of 20 degrees or less, or best corrected central distance vision of 20/200 in the better eye. The problems and limitations that being blind imposes on lifestyle are immense and difficult for a sighted person to imagine. Most people who become blind lose their sight after age 20. Usually the loss occurs gradually, allowing a period of time for adjustment, but it may occur suddenly if due to an accident. In either case, the patient has to learn new patterns of eating, dressing, grooming, and navigating his environment. He may also need to learn a new job, a different way of continuing his education, or different hobbies and pastimes. As with any loss, the newly blinded person will need to go through a process of grieving and a period of adjusting to an altered body image.

A blind person relies on his senses of touch and hearing, as well as memory, to provide information previously acquired visually. Although to some extent almost all blind persons must depend on others to meet some of their needs, for some elderly, who may also have deficits of hearing and short-term memory, the loss of sight may force them to become totally dependent. In our Western culture, where independence is valued so highly, this is often the most difficult adjustment of all to make, not only for the afflicted individual but also for those with whom he lives.

Numerous aids and devices are available specifically designed to assist the visually impaired. A list of these may be obtained by contacting the appropriate agencies. Additionally, many libraries provide books in braille, as well as tapes and records on various subjects, that are available to the legally blind. White canes and guide dogs help many blind people increase their independence outside the home. Guidelines to observe when interacting with a visually impaired person are listed in Table 70–1. These strategies can be modified for persons with less severe disability.

Interventions for the Hearing Impaired

The loss of hearing severely limits the ability to engage in social interaction, and people who have a disabling hearing loss must learn alternate methods of communicating. Although the loss of hearing is usually gradual, adjusting to it is never easy. If vision is good, these people can learn to lip read and use other visual cues such as facial expressions, body language, and gestures to participate in conversation. Sign language is also available for those motivated to learn it. However, since many hearing-impaired persons are elderly and also have poor vision, these options frequently are not usable alternatives.

Some hearing-impaired persons, primarily those with a conductive type of hearing loss, may benefit from using a hearing aid to increase the intensity of sound. Most of these devices are small and can be worn unobtrusively behind or within the ear. The purchase of a hearing aid should only be made following a complete evaluation by a qualified audiologist and otologist.

Because hearing aids are expensive, particular care should be used when handling them, and when not in use they should be stored away from heat and sunlight, preferably with the batteries removed. The ear mold should be kept clean of cerumen and washed with soap and water, taking care not to get the hearing aid itself wet. The ear mold may also need to be reshaped as the person grows older, since the length of the auditory canal increases with age. Learning to use a hearing aid takes time and can be difficult, especially for persons with a sensorineural type of loss for whom the benefits may not be as great as those with a conductive type of loss.

Loss of hearing is not only a burden for those afflicted, but it can also be a burden for those who live with and care for these people. Guidelines to facilitate communicating with the hearing impaired are found in Table 70–2.

Evaluation

The patient has made effective adjustment to life within the limitations of his sensory–perceptual impairment.

Vision Problems

Cataracts

Etiology and Clinical Manifestations

A cataract is an opacity or clouding of the normally clear, crystalline lens of the eye. It can be a congenital abnormality, the result of trauma, or caused by drugs or metabolic disease. However, the most common cause of cataracts is aging. For reasons not well understood, some people develop cataracts at a younger age than others. Fortunately for these people, the opaque lens can be surgically removed and, barring problems of the remaining eye structures, vision can be restored using an artificial lens.

Generally cataracts occur bilaterally in person over 60 years of age and are manifested by a gradual blurring vision (Fig. 70–1). This usually affects distance vision first and generally can be compensated in the early stages by prescription changes. Patients with cataracts may also complain of problems with glare, headaches, and irritability. The diagnosis is confirmed by direct visualization of the lens opacity.

Medical Management

Considering that almost all people over the age of 70 manifest some degree of opacity,[10] few cataracts advance to the stage where surgery is required. The indications for cataract surgery have broadened markedly in the last several decades, and it is no longer necessary to wait until the cata-

TABLE 70–1
Guidelines for Interaction with the Visually-Impaired Person

- Always identify yourself before touching the person.
- Always indicate the presence of others in the environment.
- Explain all strange noises and any procedures to be done fully prior to starting them.
- When orienting the patient to his environment, walk with him, having him identify the location of the call bell, bedside stand, bathroom facilities, sink, chairs, closet, nurses station, and so on.
- Be sure doors are not left partially ajar and that items and pieces of furniture are not rearranged without telling the patient about the change. Memorizing where things are located is the primary way a blind person functions independently.
- When walking with a blind person, always have him rest his hand on your forearm or grasp the back of your upper arm. This allows him to sense your direction and better maintain his balance. Provide him verbal notice of any changes in terrain or direction.
- As you would with any person, ask if you can assist him rather than assume he needs or wants your help. An overprotective attitude toward a blind person tends to foster dependence and insecurity rather than independence and security.

TABLE 70–2
Guidelines for Interaction with the Hearing-Impaired Person

- Always obtain the person's attention before attempting to talk with him.
- Position yourself in the person's direct line of vision with adequate light on your face.
- Use alternative words and gestures if what you initially said was not heard.
- Use a low tone of voice, and keep it low, despite any increase in volume.
- Do not shout.
- Do not cover or distort mouth movements.
- Use short phrases.
- Speak slowly toward the deaf person's better ear.
- Reduce or eliminate background noise as much as possible.
- Write out any words that seem to be difficult to understand.
- Never touch a deaf person without first alerting him.

ract is fully mature before it can be removed. The decision to have cataract surgery should be based on several factors. Among these are the degree of visual limitation and rate of cataract growth; the degree to which ADLs, job performance, and pastime activities being compromised; the condition of the retina and cornea; and future plans and potential lifestyle changes.

Usually cataract surgery is performed on only one eye at a time. Preoperative medications are given to relax the patient so that, once the anesthetic is injected, patients often fall asleep during surgery. The use of local anesthesia minimizes the common postoperative side-effects of nausea, vomiting, coughing, and disorientation, and it is especially advantageous when the patient is elderly or has a compromised respiratory system.

An intracapsular extraction is the procedure commonly used to remove a cataract. This type of operation removes the entire lens and its capsule (Fig. 70–2). An alternate procedure is an extracapsular extraction that leaves the posterior capsule of the lens intact. Either surgery entails making a 140–160 degree incision, instilling a fibrinolytic and proteolytic enzyme to break down the zonules holding the lens, removing the lens with or without its capsule, and closing the wound with silk, nylon, or vicril sutures. An iridectomy is routinely done to prevent a secondary glaucoma from occurring if the vitreous moves forward and blocks the flow of aqueous humor from the eye. Unless an intraocular lens is implanted during surgery, vision following surgery is restored by using either cataract glasses or a contact lens.

Another method of removing cataracts is by phacoemulsification. This procedure uses ultrasound to break up the lens, and an irrigation–aspiration system to remove the lens fragment from the anterior chamber. The advantage of removing the lens by phacoemulsification is that recovery time is shortened owing to the smaller incision required. This procedure is generally restricted to young persons whose lenses are soft and who are not having an intraocular lens implanted.

In recent years the use of microscopes, allowing finer suture material and instrumentation, and the perfection of the intraocular lens have combined not only to increase the number of cataract surgeries performed but also to improve their visual outcome. Although controversy still exists concerning the lower age limit for implantation surgery, an intraocular lens implant is now being considered for any older cataract patient with an otherwise healthy eye.[9] Also, an increasing number of patients are now undergoing a "secondary" intraocular lens implant several years following their primary cataract surgery.

Nursing Management Plan

Assessment and Nursing Diagnosis

The analysis of data for the patient who has had cataract surgery is similar to that presented earlier for sensory loss. The appropriate nursing diagnoses include sensory–perceptual alteration: visual, potential for injury: trauma, and impaired home maintenance management.

Goals. Following cataract surgery, patients need to be protected from and cautioned against participating in any activity that would increase intraocular pressure or place strain on the suture line, such as lifting, pushing or pulling heavy objects, and bending over instead of squatting.

Interventions

Complications that can occur as a result of inappropriate activities include iris prolapse, hemorrhage, and vitreous loss, which can precipitate retinal detachment. Patients are usually allowed out of bed the day of surgery and discharged

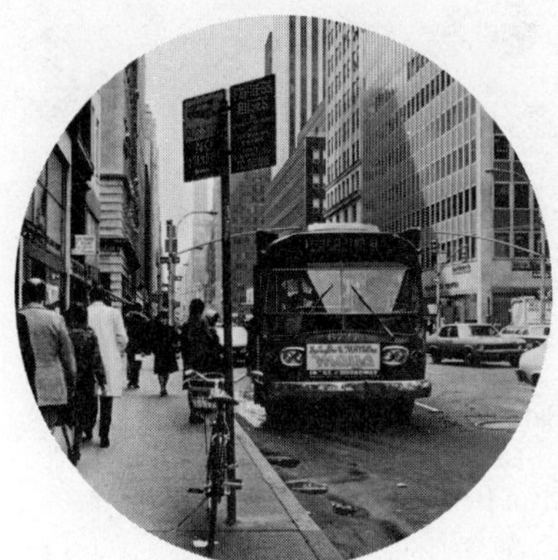

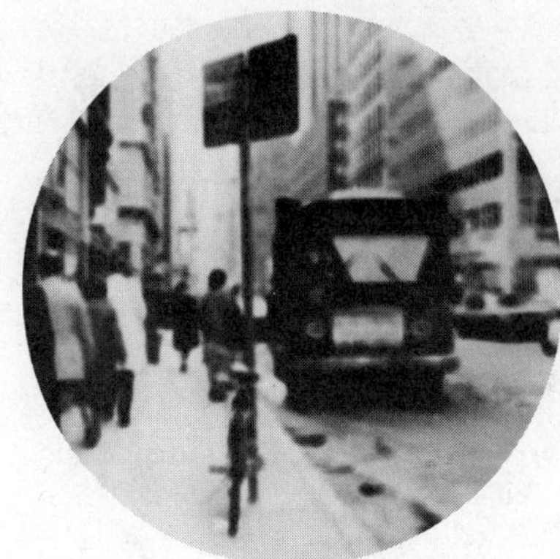

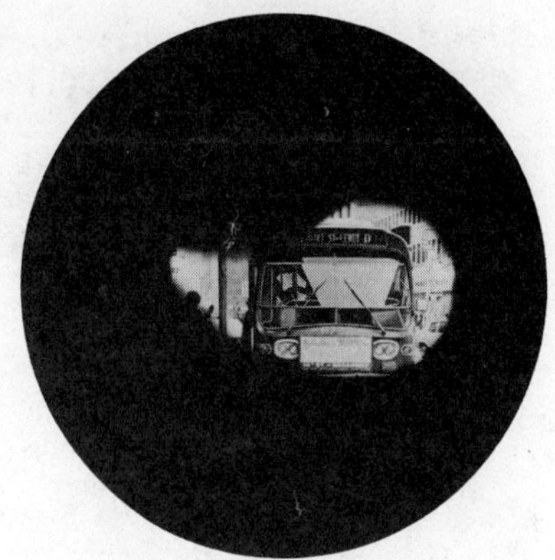

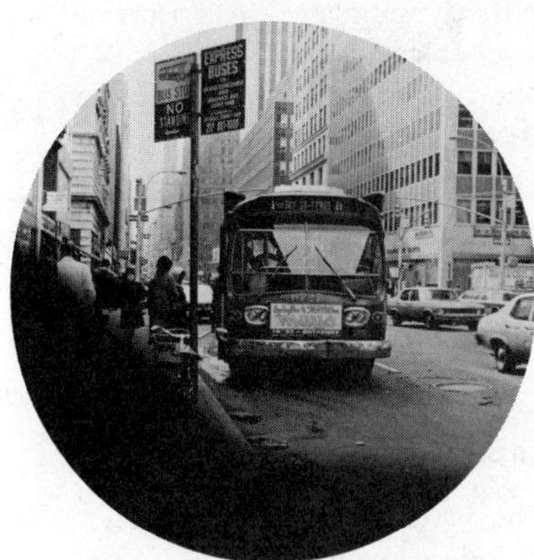

FIGURE 70–1 Vision of persons with various eye conditions. (Courtesy of The Light-house, The New York Association for the Blind)

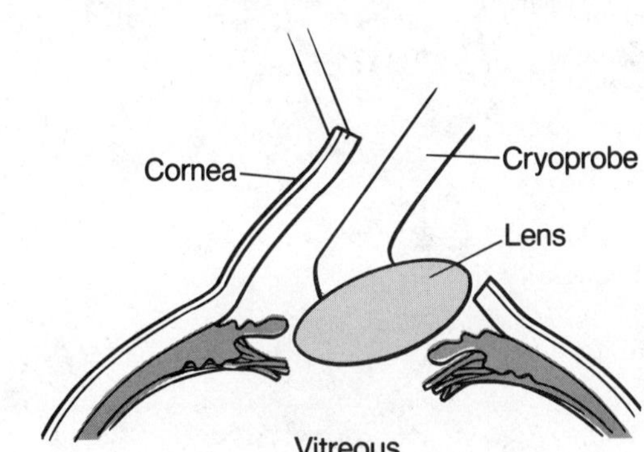

FIGURE 70–2 Intracapsular cataract extraction using a cryoprobe.

in 1 to 3 days. Some patients are operated on in a day surgery center and are discharged the day of surgery. Pain is mild and limited to a scratchy feeling or dull ache. The patient is advised to wear an eye shield at night and protect the eye during the day with either an eye shield, patch, or glasses. Drops and ointments are prescribed to counteract postoperative iritis, dilate the eye, and guard against infection.

Restoration of vision following surgery will vary, depending on the type of surgery performed and the abilities and preferences of the patient. If an intraocular lens has been implanted, postoperative vision will approximate the quality of vision prior to cataract formation. Reading glasses will be required for near vision or conventional glasses may be prescribed to correct astigmatism or any remaining refractive error.

If an intraocular lens has not been implanted, the patient must use either cataract glasses or a contact lens to restore vision. Cataract glasses provide good central vision, but they have several drawbacks that can make adjusting to them difficult. Because they are positioned 14 to 15 mm in front of the natural lens position, cataract glasses restrict peripheral vision and magnify the visual field 33%. This causes objects to appear closer than they are and makes straight lines look curved and distorted and, unless both lenses have been removed, double vision occurs because the brain cannot fuse two images of such differing size. Learning to wear cataract glasses takes time and perseverance. Initially the patient should be cautioned against trying to walk with the glasses on, and particular care should be exercised when pouring hot liquids or cooking. With continued practice, the time required to adjust to cataract glasses is 1 to 2 months.

A contact lens more closely approximates the natural position of the lens and magnifies the visual field about 6%. The lower magnification allows fusion to occur so that double vision is not a problem if only one lens has been removed. Handicapped persons or those who lack the man-

NURSING CARE PLAN FOR THE POSTOPERATIVE CATARACT PATIENT

NURSING DIAGNOSIS/PROBLEM 1: Potential for injury: trauma, related to visual loss
GOAL 1: To prevent injury related to visual loss

Nursing Interventions	Rationale	Outcome Criteria
1. Orient patient to environment; ensure patient knows location of bathroom and call bell.	1. Knowledge of environment increases patient's independence and ability to request help when needed.	1. Patient is oriented to surroundings and knows location of vital items.
2. Ambulate with assistance.	2. Reliance on a sighted person reduces risk of falls and injury.	2. Patient requests assistance when getting out of bed and ambulating.
3. Keep area unobstructed and free of hazards.	3. Obstacles, spills, doors partly ajar, *etc.,* increase likelihood of injury.	3. Patient ambulates in area free from obstacles.
4. Maintain continuity of environment and objects in it.	4. The patient relies on memory to assist him with his activities of daily living.	4. The patient will not sustain an injury related to ambulating with a visual loss.

NURSING DIAGNOSIS/PROBLEM 2: Potential for postoperative injury or trauma related to increased intraocular pressure
GOAL: To prevent injury to the eye related to increased intraocular pressure

Nursing Interventions	Rationale	Outcome Criteria
1. Position patient on unoperative side with pillows.	1. Side-lying position eliminates perssure on the suture line.	1–7. The patient will not experience vision changes or loss as a result of vitreous prolapse, vitreous loss, or hemorrhage from activities that increase intraocular pressure or place strain on the suture line.
2. Patch operative eye. Use protective shield if ordered by physician.	2. Patch and shield protect eye from accidental injury.	
3. Use restraints only as last resort.	3. Restraints may cause patient to become more agitated and restless.	
4. Administer prophylactic medications as ordered by physician to prevent nausea and constipation.	4. Vomiting and straining to defecate increase intraocular pressure.	
5. Instruct patient not to lift, pull, or push heavy objects.	5. Intraocular pressure is increased by these maneuvers.	
6. Teach patient to squat rather than bend over.	6. Maintaining the head in an upright position decreases intraocular pressure.	
7. Teach patient techniques to safely administer drops and ointment.	7. Injury can result from poor technique of administration.	

NURSING DIAGNOSIS/PROBLEM 3: Potential sensory–perceptual alterations: visual, related to removal of the lens
GOAL: To prevent confusion, restlessness, and anxiety related to sensory–perceptual alterations of visual origin

Nursing Interventions	Rationale	Outcome Criteria
1. Stimulate alternate senses of touch and hearing. a. Provide verbal contact frequently. b. Touch patient as a means of communication rather than solely for care-giving activities.	1. Patient relies on the senses of touch and hearing to maintain orientation to his environment.	1–4. The patient will not experience confusion, restlessness, or anxiety related to visual sensory–perceptual alteration.

(Continued)

NURSING CARE PLAN FOR THE POSTOPERATIVE CATARACT PATIENT *(Continued)*

Nursing Interventions	Rationale
2. Ambulate patient early in post-operative period.	2. Resuming normal activities increases sense or orientation.
3. Refrain from using bilateral patches, restraints, and side rails.	3. Patches and restraints limit meaningful contact and increase perceptual distortion.
4. Use discretion when administering sedating medications.	4. Most cataract patients are elderly, and confusion is a frequent drug side-effect.

NURSING DIAGNOSIS/PROBLEM 4: Potential for impaired home maintenance management related to postoperative precautions limiting all activities that potenitally could increase intraocular pressure
GOAL: To prevent potenital injury secondary to increased intraocular pressure

Nursing Interventions	Rationale	Outcome Criteria
1. Instruct patient to arrange cooking utensils to eliminate lifting and bending.	1–2. Lifting and bending increase intraocular pressure.	1–3. Patient will be free from injury due to the complications of vitreous loss, vitreous prolapse, or hemorrhage secondary to increased intraocular pressure.
2. Help patient plan home management activities, *i.e.,* food purchases, cleaning.		
3. Ensure adequate availability of persons to provide help as needed.	3. Situations can occur that are unplanned or that require assistance from others.	

ual dexterity required to manipulate a contact lens may have extended-wear soft contacts prescribed. These soft lenses can be left in place for several weeks to months and changed in the doctor's office or by a family member.

Evaluation

The patient will not experience the adverse consequences of participating in activities that increase intraocular pressure or place strain on the suture line. For a more complete discussion see the accompanying Nursing Care Plan for the Postoperative Cataract Patient.

Glaucoma

Definition and Etiology. Glaucoma is the third major cause of blindness in the United States, affecting approximately 2% of the population over 40 years of age.[4] It occurs when the flow of aqueous humor from the eye is blocked, causing the intraocular pressure to increase and reflexively damage the optic nerve, creating a permanent loss of vision.

Pathology and Clinical Manifestations. Glaucoma can be classified as congenital, primary, or secondary, as a complication of injury, infection, surgery, or prolonged use of topical steroids. There are two forms of primary glaucoma, open-angle (also called wide-angle, chronic, or simple glaucoma) and narrow-angle (also called acute or angle-closure glaucoma). Of these, the most common form is open-angle.

Open-Angle Glaucoma

Open-angle glaucoma occurs bilaterally and is caused by degenerative changes of the trabecular meshwork that block the flow of aqueous humor from the eye. As the flow of aqueous humor diminishes relative to its production, intraocular pressure increases and damage to the ocular nerve occurs, giving it a cuplike appearance. Because the condition develops gradually and asymptomatically, rarely is the patient aware that anything is wrong with his eyes. Initially vision is lost peripherally and therefore goes unnoticed. Occasionally patients complain of a dull, morning headache that disappears on awakening. Although most cases of open-angle glaucoma are diagnosed during a routine eye examination, if the condition persists undetected or untreated, the glaucoma patient will become permanently blind.

The diagnosis of open-angle glaucoma is based on direct examination of the optic disc for cupping, evaluation of the visual fields, and measurements of the intraocular pressure. Serial pressure readings above 20–24 mmHg are generally considered suspect, and provocative tests may be used to confirm the diagnosis. The simplest of these tests involves drinking a quart of fluid, having the patient sit in a dark room for half an hour, and then remeasuring the intraocular pressure. An elevation of more than 7 mmHg is considered diagnostic.

Treatment. The confirmed diagnosis of glaucoma requires the patient to accept that he has a chronic condition requiring treatment for the rest of his life. Medications and dosage regimens to control introcular pressure will vary based on individual response. However, the goal of therapy is always the same, which is to maintain intraocular pressure within the normal range and prevent damage to the optic nerve.

The treatment of glaucoma usually involves taking drops one to five times a day. Cholinergic solutions (*e.g.,* pilocarpine hydrochloride, carbachol, echothiophate iodide) are frequently used to constrict the pupil and contract the ciliary muscle, thereby enhancing the flow of aqueous humor from the eye. Because these drugs cause headaches and make it difficult to see, compliance with therapy, especially for younger patients and people with central cataracts, can be a problem.

Since 1978, the drug timolol maleate (Timoptic) has been available, and it is increasingly being used as the drug of choice for glaucoma therapy. Timolol is a β-adrenergic blocking agent that lowers intraocular pressure by decreasing the production of aqueous humor. Because it has few visual or systemic side-effects and only needs to be used one or twice a day, compliance with therapy is improved. Similar to other β-adrenergic blocking agents, this drug is contraindicated in patients with a history of bronchial asthma, severe chronic destructive pulmonary disease, and cardiac failure.

Oral medications to control intraocular pressure are carbonic anhydrase inhibitors such as acetazolamide. These drugs also inhibit the production of aqueous humor, and in difficult-to-control cases may be prescribed up to four times a day in addition to the drop regimen. Side-effects of carbonic anhydrase inhibitors include fatigue, nausea, anorexia, and mild paresthesias of the face and extremities. Hypokalemia can also occur if the patient is on other diuretics, and long-term therapy with acetazolamide has been correlated with an increased incidence of renal calculi. A list of the common drugs used to treat glaucoma and their side-effects may be found in Table 70–3.

Because open-angle glaucoma is a chronic disease devoid of symptoms, it can be difficult to convince patients that they must remain on treatment, particularly if they are experiencing adverse side-effects of the medication. Glaucoma patients should have their intraocular pressure checked every 2 to 3 months, and undergo periodic field examinations to ensure proper control of their condition. If the intraocular pressure remains elevated despite treatment or if peripheral vision continues to be lost, surgery is indicated.

Narrow-Angle Glaucoma

In narrow-angle glaucoma the flow of aqueous humor from the eye is completely blocked, causing a sudden rise in intraocular pressure. Unlike people with open-angle glaucoma, these patients have a normal trabecular meshwork and normal intraocular pressure but an abnormal, anatomically narrowed anterior chamber. Attacks of narrow-angle glaucoma may be triggered by trauma, pupil dilation, stress, or any ocular change that pushes the iris forward, such as hemorrhage or a swollen lens. Unlike open-angle glaucoma, attacks of narrow-angle glaucoma occur suddenly, and permanent loss of vision can occur within 48 to 72 hours. For this reason, medical attention must be sought immediately.

Symptoms of narrow-angle glaucoma are a sudden onset of blurred vision, a rainbow-colored halo around lights, and excruciating eye pain, often severe enough to cause nausea, vomiting, and abdominal discomfort. The affected eye will have an inflamed, watery appearance, a cloudy cornea, a fixed and dilated pupil, and markedly elevated intraocular pressure.

Treatment. Treatment of narrow-angle glaucoma consists of administering miotic drops (*e.g.,* pilocarpine, 4%) every 5 minutes to constrict the pupil and pull it away from the trabeculum. Carbonic anhydrase inhibitors (*e.g.,* acetazolamide) and an osmotic diuresis agent (*e.g.,* glycerin) may also be used. An analgesic (*e.g.,* meperidine, 75–100 mg IM) should be given to relieve pain and associated nausea. If the measures are successful, intravenous mannitol may be given. Once the intraocular pressure has been lowered, surgery is generally scheduled on an emergency basis. Because the conditions that predispose a patient to narrow-angle glaucoma occur in both eyes, prophylactic surgery is almost always performed on the other eye at the same time.

Surgical Management of Glaucoma

In addition to the medications previously discussed, surgical treatment is utilized. Surgery for glaucoma consists of establishing an alternate pathway for the aqueous humor to drain away from the eye. Any one of several different types of surgery may be done. For patients with narrow-angle glaucoma, bilateral peripheral iridectomies are generally the surgery of choice. This procedure permits the aqueous to flow from the posterior chamber to the anterior chamber, and it keeps the iris from bulging forward and obscuring the angle. In open-angle glaucoma or in narrow-angle glaucoma if a large portion of the trabecular meshwork is nonfunctional owing to synechiae (adhesions of the iris to the cornea), a trephination or trabeculetomy is usually recommended.

A trephination removes a piece of the sclera, allowing the aqueous to flow from the anterior chamber under a conjunctival flap and be absorbed into the conjunctival blood vessels. A trabeculectomy places an opening into the anterior chamber under a partial thickness scleral flap. In this procedure an iridectomy is also done to prevent the iris from prolapsing into the opening and obstructing the flow of fluid.

Since the late 1970s, the argon laser beam has been used as an alternative to surgical treatment of both open-angle and narrow-angle glaucoma. The advantage of laser therapy is that, since a surgical incision is not required, it can be done on an outpatient basis, eliminating the need for hospitalization, anesthesia, and a prolonged postoperative recovery period. Although the long-range effect of argon laser therapy is still being evaluated, initial follow-up studies indicate that

TABLE 70-3
Drugs Commonly Used in the Treatment of Glaucoma

Drug	Form	Dose	Action	Adverse Effects
Cholinergic Agents (Parasympathomimetics)				
Pilocarpine	.25–10% solution	gtt 1–2, q 4–6 hr	These drugs act by simulating the effect of acetylcholine on the smooth muscle cells of the eye, resulting in accommodation and pupillary constriction (miosis). Constriction of the ciliary muscle stretches the trabecular meshwork, enlarging the drainage channels and lowering intraocular pressure.	Spasm of accommodation, blurred vision, brow ache, headache, miosis *Systemic:* Nausea, vomiting, sweating, abdominal cramps, diarrhea, salivation, general fatigue, weakness, and depression
Carbachol	.75–3% solution	gtt 1–2, q 8–12 hr		
Anticholinesterase Agents				
Physostigmine	.25–1% solution	gtt 1–2, q 4–6 hr	These drugs act by inhibiting the action of cholinesterase, thereby increasing the concentration of acetylcholine. The net result is an increase in parasympathetic activity similar to cholinergic agents.	Potential for severe, if not fatal, side-effects if not administered in carefully controlled doses. Discontinue 2 weeks prior to surgery since interaction with succinylcholine can cause profound respiratory depression. Headache, blurred vision, eye pain, iris cysts, cataracts, posterior synechiae, and dilated vessels of the conjunctiva *Systemic:* Bradycardia, nausea, vomiting, diarrhea, sweating, abdominal cramps, general fatigue and weakness, depression
Demecarium bromide	.125–.25% solution	gtt 1–2, bid		
Echothiophate iodide	.06–.125% solution	gtt 1–2, bid		
Isoflurophate	.01–.1% solution	gtt 1–2, bid		
Adrenergic Agents (Sympathomimetics)				
Epinephrine borate	1% solution	gtt 1–2, bid	These drugs reduce aqueous production by constricting the conjunctival blood vessels. They also increase aqueous outflow by stimulating adrenergic receptors in the angle structures of the eye. Because of their mydriatic effect, these drugs cannot be used for patients with anatomically narrow angles.	Headache, brow ache, eye ache, lid and conjunctival hypersensitivity, maculopathy, and conjunctival hyperemia *Systemic:* Tachycardia, faintness, anxiety, nosebleeds, hypertension, trembling
Epinephrine hydrochloride	2% solution	gtt 1–2, bid		
Epinephrine bitartrate	2% solution	gtt 1–2, bid		
β-Adrenergic Blocking Agents (Sympatholytics)				
Timolol maleate	.25–.5% solution	gtt 1–2, bid	A derivative of propranolol, this drug acts by blocking adrenergic nerve cell effector sites, thereby decreasing aqueous production. Pupil size is unaffected.	Few ocular side-effects; occasional superficial punctate keratitis *Systemic:* Same as for propranolol, bradycardia, exacerbation of PVD, bronchoconstriction, depression, weakness, fatigue, disorientation, and memory loss Contraindicated in patients with congestive heart failure and asthma
Carbonic Anhydrase Inhibitors				
Acetazolamide	125–250 mg tablets	tabs 1, q 6–12 hr	These drugs inhibit the enzyme carbonic anhydrase, resulting in inhibition of aqueous humor production and diuresis.	Numbness and tingling of fingers and toes, anorexia, nausea, vomiting, diarrhea, fatigue, depression, hypokalemia, and renal calculi Monitor serum potassium in patients receiving concurrent therapy with thiazide diuretics or digoxin.
Methazolamide	50 mg tablet	tabs 1, q 6–8 hr		
Dichlorphenamide	50 mg tablet	tabs 1, q 6–8 hr		
Ethoxzolamide	125 mg tablet	tab 1, q 6–8 hr		

argon laser iridotomies are often preferable to surgical iridectomies for the narrow-angle glaucoma patient, and they are a valuable adjunct to the clinical management of the patient with open-angle glaucoma.[12]

In some difficult to control cases of glaucoma, an attempt may be made to partially destroy the cells of the ciliary body to reduce aqueous production. These procedures involve the use of diathermy, cryothermy, or laser, and are generally measures of last resort.

Nursing Management

Assessment and Nursing Diagnosis

The appropriate nursing diagnoses for the patient with glaucoma include sensory–perceptual alteration: visual, potential fear and anxiety related to glaucoma, and disturbance in self-concept.

Goals. The goals for the patient with glaucoma include understanding the nature of glaucoma and demonstrating acceptance of the treatment regimen.

Interventions

Postoperative care of the glaucoma patient will vary with the specific type of surgery performed and the preferences of the surgeon. Since the incision required is smaller and since intraocular structures are not disturbed, postoperative restrictions are less prohibitive than are those for patients having cataract surgery. Drops and ointments are prescribed based on the need to either dilate or constrict the pupil, and they vary with the nature of the surgery, the depth of the anterior chamber, the intraocular pressure, and the amount of inflammation present.

Compliance with medication regimens and periodic evaluations of both introcular pressure and peripheral vision are imperative. The patient must realize that, although treatment does not restore vision, it does prevent further loss. Fully understanding the nature of glaucoma and its untreated consequences will enhance patient acceptance. The nurse, through teaching skills and an ability to discern patient fears and concerns, is a key person toward gaining this acceptance. Suggested guidelines for teaching the glaucoma patient are presented in Table 70–4.

TABLE 70–4
Teaching Guidelines for Glaucoma Patients

- Wear a Medic Alert bracelet or carry a card indicating that you have glaucoma and what medications you are taking.
- Have a backup supply of medication at home, work, or when traveling.
- Read labels of over-the-counter medications carefully to ensure that they are not contraindicated for persons with glaucoma.
- Inform any physician or other person prescribing medications that you have glaucoma.
- Refrain from ingesting large quantities of liquids, especially those containing caffeine.
- Try to avoid stressful or physically exhaustive situations. If this is not possible, check with your opthalmologist; a temporary increase in medication may be indicated.
- Comply with prescribed therapy and scheduled checkups.

Evaluation

The patient will demonstrate understanding of glaucoma, will not suffer any further loss of vision, and his intraocular pressure will remain within the normal range.

Retinal Disorders

Macular Degeneration

Definition and Etiology. Macular degeneration, or loss of central vision, is a common, frustrating condition afflicting a significant number of elderly people. It is the leading cause of new cases of legal blindness in the United States in persons over 65, and is thought to be present in mild form in about 11% of the elderly.[7]

Pathology and Clinical Manifestations. Macular degeneration occurs bilaterally, and is characterized by the growth of new blood vessels into the macular area that totally obscure central vision. Its cause is thought to be vascular in origin, since the macula, which is normally devoid of blood vessels and receives its nourishment from the underlying choroid, is particularly vulnerable to arteriosclerotic changes that accompany aging. Various forms of the disease exist and are termed disciform degeneration, exudative or hemorrhagic maculopathy, and involutional or atrophic maculopathy.

Early symptoms of macular degeneration may include distortion of straight lines, a scotoma, or an intermittent blurring of central vision that gradually worsens over time. Fortunately, peripheral vision remains unaffected, and is adequate for getting about in familiar places and performing the routine tasks of daily living.

By using their peripheral vision, persons with macular degeneration can generally maintain their independence; however they are limited in their ability to do any task requiring fine central vision, that is, reading, writing, sewing, or participating in crafts and hobbies. These patients are appropriately fearful and frustrated over their loss. Nurses need to reassure these people that, barring any other retinal problem, they will not become totally blind, and will always be able to care for themselves.

Medical Management. About 10% of patients with macular degeneration have a form of the disease that can be treated in its early stages by argon laser photocoagulation. This treatment seals the abnormal new blood vessels, preventing bleeding, fluid leakage, and attendant scar tissue formation. Early recognition of this particular form of macular degeneration is particularly important, since the disease remains in its treatable stage for a very limited period of time. Various other therapies, including steroids, vitamins, and circulatory agents, have been tried for other forms of macular degeneration but, unfortunately, none has ever been found effective in altering the progressive nature of the disease.

Retinal Detachment

Definition, Etiology, and Pathology. As the name implies, a retinal detachment occurs when fluid collects between the sensory lining of the eye, containing the rods and cones and the pigment epithelium beneath it, causing the two layers to separate. The fluid may be an exudate from an underlying blood vessel, in which case the condition is termed a *serous* detachment or, more commonly, it comes from the vitreous passing through a hole in the retina, in which case the condition is termed a *rhegmatogenous* detachment.

Predisposing factors include age, vitreous traction, myopia, aphakia, diabetic retinopthy, inflammatory conditions of the vitreous, and trauma. Persons diagnosed as having a retinal detachment in one eye should have the other eye carefully examined also, since there is a 15% chance of it developing a retinal detachment as well.[6]

Clinical Manifestations. Symptoms of an impending detachment include intermittent momentary flashes of light resembling sun glinting off metal. Often these are associated with the appearance of multiple black floating spots, called floaters, in the field of vision. Central vision may be normal or poor depending on macular involvement. Commonly the patient complains of a black shadow cutting across his peripheral field of vision. There is no pain or sensation associated with retinal detachment.

Medical Management. If detected early before the retina has actually detached, treatment consists of cryotherapy or laser photocoagulation to create a scar and seal the retinal hole. Often this can be done on an outpatient basis. However, if the retina has become separated from its underlying layer, more extensive surgery will be necessary, since without treatment the entire retina will gradually detach, causing the eye to become completely blind.

Retinal detachment patients are usually admitted directly to the hospital from their opthalmologist's office. Because of this, they tend to be scared and anxious and need appropriate realistic reassurance. These patients are usually placed on strict bed rest, with the head of the bed flat or elevated depending on the location of the detachment. Head movement generally is restricted, and bilateral patches may be ordered to minimize eye movement. These restrictions help limit extension of the detachment and allow realignment of the retina against the pigmented epithelium, reducing the need to drain subretinal fluid. To gain their full cooperation, retinal detachment patients need to fully understand the rationale for these restrictions. Additionally, the nursing care plan should include interventions to enhance patient comfort while on bed rest and reduce the risks of immobility.

Surgery. The two types of surgery done to repair a detached retina are scleral implantation and scleral buckling. In both procedures the area around the retinal tear is first scarred by applying either diathermy or cryothermy to the exterior surface of the globe. If the detachment is relatively small, a silicone sponge implant is placed over the detached area to exert external pressure and bring the choroid into contact with the retina. Indenting the globe in this manner reduces the pull of the vitreous on the weakened retina. If a large portion of the retina has detached, a circling band of silicone is usually placed around the entire globe either in addition to or in place of the silicone sponge, as shown in Figure 70–3. If subretinal fluid prohibits the retina from coming in contact with the pigmented epithelium, the fluid is drained from the eye through an opening made in the sclera and choroid layers. Retinal detachment surgery can be long and tedious, taxing the skills and patience of the best surgical team. Its outcome will depend on the size of the detachment, whether or not the macular area is involved, and the amount of time elapsed prior to surgery.

Following surgery, the postoperative patient generally is allowed out of bed within 24 to 48 hours and is discharged from the hospital within a week. Head and eye movements remain restricted for several weeks, sometimes by having the

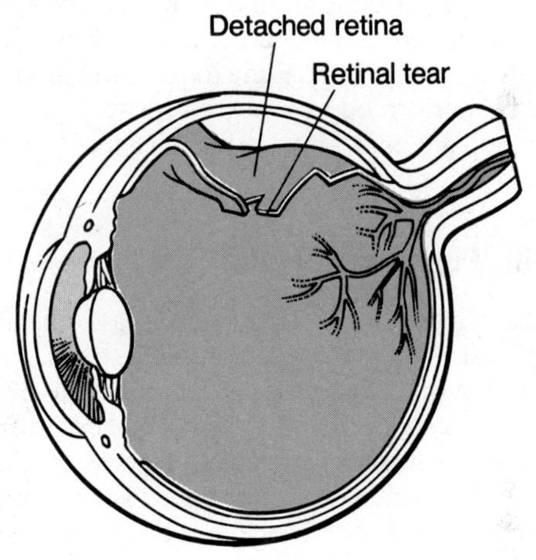

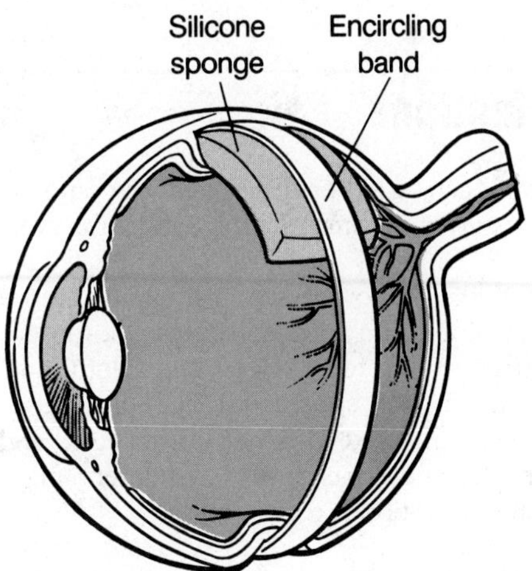

FIGURE 70–3 Surgical repair of detached retina: silicone sponge implant with encircling band. When the buckle is tightened, the implant indents the sclera holding the choroid and retina together.

patient wear pinhole glasses. Jarring activities are prohibited, and the patient is cautioned against reading, lifting heavy objects, bending over, moving his head quickly, and driving. Athletic activities, such as playing tennis and golf, should not be resumed for several months until approved by the physician. Because surgery may alter the shape of the eye, the patient's glass prescription may need to be changed following recovery.

Diabetic Retinopathy

The incidence of diabetic retinopathy as a complication of diabetes increases with the duration and severity of the diabetic condition, and it can be classified as either nonproliferative or proliferative. The nonproliferative form is characterized by dilation of the blood vessels, microaneurysms, blot hemorrhages, and retinal edema. The proliferative form is more severe, and is characterized by the growth of new blood vessels onto the surface and into the vitreous. These vessels can hemorrhage, causing partial or complete loss of vision. Treatment by laser photocoagulation can frequently be used to seal off new vessels and prevent hemorrhage, but it does not stop progression of the disease. Other complications of diabetic retinopathy include vitreous scarring and retinal detachment. If vitreous hemorrhage or scarring has occurred, a vitrectomy to remove blood or scar tissue may be performed. A more extensive discussion of diabetic retinopathy may be found in Chapter 74, Diabetes Mellitus.

Retinitis Pigmentosa

Retinitis pigmentosa is a genetic disease that initially destroys the rod cells of the eye. Because these cells perceive black and white vision, the earliest symptom of this disorder, usually first noticed during childhood or adolescence, is night blindness. Symptoms gradually progress over a number of years to a total loss of peripheral vision. Eventually, macular vision may also be lost. Presently no treatment has been found to halt or slow the progression of the disease. Genetic counseling is advised.

Eye Infections

Eye infections can be either acute or chronic, and can involve either the external or internal structures of the eye.

Hordeolum. A hordeolum, commonly referred to as a sty, is an infection of a sebaceous gland of the eyelid. The affected area becomes red, swollen, and painful, and without treatment usually will spontaneously rupture and resolve. Hot packs may be used to hasten the process and relieve discomfort. An antibiotic drop or ointment may be prescribed if the condition is recurrent.

Chalazion. A chalazion is similar to a hordeolum but occurs in a deeper gland of the lid. These tend to be more chronic, alternately becoming reddened and inflamed and then quieting to a cystlike swelling. The best treatment for a chalazion is excision using local anesthesia. Following the procedure, antibiotic drops should be used to prevent recurrence.

Blepharitis. Blepharitis is a chronic infection of the eyelids and lash follicles characterized by red, itchy, granulated lid margins. It is particularly common among elderly nursing home patients who may be chronically anemic, and is frequently associated with seborrheic dermatitis of the scalp and eyebrows. Persons with blepharitis often complain of general eye irritation, photophobia, and a feeling that their eyes are tired all the time. Daily treatment consists of removing the scales, using an antibiotic ointment, and practicing good hygiene.

Conjunctivitis. The cause of conjunctivitis may be either a bacterial or viral infection, or an allergic reaction of the conjunctiva. It is characterized by redness, tearing, itching, photophobia, and a scratchy feeling. Discharge is always present, but will vary in nature and amount depending on the causative organism. An acute bacterial form of conjunctivitis is common among schoolchildren and is highly contagious. These infections respond well to treatment with topical sulfur or antibiotic preparations. Care should be taken not to infect the other eye or other persons with whom the patient comes in contact.

Trachoma. Trachoma is a highly contagious, chronic infectious disease of the conjunctiva and cornea caused by a microorganism. Although rare in the Western world, it is the major cause of blindness in the Eastern world. Trachoma responds well to treatment with topical and systemic antibiotics.

Keratitis. Keratitis can be caused by any one of several factors, and refers to an inflammation of the cornea that may be either superficial, deep, or ulcerative. Its symptoms include pain, irritation, photophobia, tearing, and blepharospasm. Although the treatment of keratitis depends on the cause, it usually includes patching the eye unless infection is involved, prescribing topical or systemic antibiotics, applying warm compresses, and using mydriatics to dilate the pupil. Corticosteroids may also be prescribed unless the cause is herpes simplex virus, in which case they are contraindicated. Systemic but not topical anesthetics may be ordered for pain. Keratitis should always be treated promptly; otherwise corneal ulceration with permanent scarring and loss of vision may result.

Corneal Transplant. If extensive corneal scarring and loss of vision has occurred, a corneal transplant or keratoplasty may be indicated. This procedure, which is also done for keratoconus and for trauma or pain secondary to bullous keratopathy, uses a donated cadaver cornea to replace the diseased cornea. The graft may be either full-thickness (penetrating keratoplasty) or partial-thickness (lamellar keratoplasty), depending on the depth of the scar formation. In the last 20 years the development of microsurgery and monofilament suture material has greatly improved the outcome of keratoplasty.

Following surgery, keratoplasty patients should adhere to the same restrictions that are ordered for other ophthalmology patients who have had intraocular surgery. Major complications to guard against are infection and displacement, which can cause the graft to become opaque.[8]

Uveitis. Uveitis is an inflammation of the uveal tract, which includes the iris, ciliary body, and choroid. The iris is the most common structure afflicted and, in this form, the term acute anteroir uveitis or iritis is used to describe the condition. Symptoms of uveitis include pain and irritation, photophobia, and blurred vision. Prompt treatment with topical or systemic corticosteroids to reduce inflammation, and with mydriatics to prevent formation of synechiae (adhesions) is imperative. Complications of uveitis include secondary glaucoma, cataracts, retinal detachment, and macular degeneration.[11]

Sympathetic Ophthalmia. Sympathetic ophthalmia is a rare but severe form of uveitis. It occurs following severe injury or infection involving the uveal track of one eye (the exciting eye). Ten days to several years later, the opposite eye (sympathizing eye) can also develop a severe uveitis which, if untreated, results in complete blindness. For this reasons, it is recommended that a severely injured eye always be removed within 10 days.

Enucleation. In addition to the concern about sympathetic ophthalmia, enucleation (surgical removal of an eye) is also recommended for a blind, painful eye or when an intraocular malignancy exists. When an enucleation is done, the globe is removed and the muscles are attached to a magnetic implant that allows movement of a magnetized prosthetic eye shield postoperatively. Hemorrhage is the major concern following surgery, and is guarded by using a large pressure dressing. The eye shield, painted to match the remaining eye, can be fitted approximately 2 weeks postoperatively. Teaching includes daily care of the socket and prosthesis, and techniques for inserting and removing the shield.

Trauma to the Eye

Mild forms of eye trauma include abrasions, foreign bodies, and chemical burns. Abrasions of the corneal epithelium are characterized by pain, photophobia, and tearing. An antibiotic drop and an eye patch for 24 hours to eliminate irritation from the upper lid are usually prescribed. Foreign bodies not embedded in the cornea can frequently be irrigated from the eye or, if they are visible on the sclera, they can be removed with a cotton applicator. Foreign material embedded in the cornea should always be removed by an opthalmologist. Chemical burns are treated by immediately irrigating the eye with copious amounts of water or saline, if available. The eye should be patched, and the patient referred to an ophthalmologist for further evaluation and treatment.

Severe trauma to an eye must be evaluated by an ophthalmologist immediately. Both eyes should be lightly patched to eliminate eye movement, the patient placed in a recumbent position, and all exertion avoided. The patient should refrain from rubbing the injured eye or squeezing the lids, since any additional pressure can cause further injury.

Nursing Management of the Ophthalmology Patient

Assessment and Nursing Diagnosis

The eyes should be thoroughly examined by an ophthalmologist or optometrist periodically throughout life. In young adulthood, this should be done every 5 years, or as indicated by symptoms. After age 40, examinations should be done every 2 to 5 years, and more frequently in a family with a positive ophthalmic history for detached retina or glaucoma.

A routine eye examination consists of a refraction; an external inspection of the brows, lids, conjunctiva, sclera, iris, and cornea; a rough approximation of visual fields; an evaluation of the extraocular muscle movements and pupillary response to light; an assessment of the internal structures of the eye; and a measurement of the intraocular pressure. A detailed description of eye assessment may be found in textbooks on physical assessment.

The term *refraction* refers to the procedure used to determine the degree of visual focusing error that may or may not be present. In the *emmetropic* (normal) eye, light rays are bent as they pass through the cornea and lens and come to focus directly on the macula. In the *hyperopic* (farsighted) eye, the eye is smaller than normal and the light rays come to focus behind the macula. A convex lens is used to correct this problem. In the *myopic* (nearsighted) eye, the eye is larger than normal and the light rays come to focus in front of the macula. A concave lens is used to correct this problem.

Other terms with which the nurse should be familiar are *astigmatism,* referring to an irregular curvature of the cornea, *presbyopia,* referring to the loss of accommodation with age, and *strabismus*, referring to a condition in which the optical axis of both eyes cannot be directed toward the same object.

The cause of strabismus may be either paralytic, resulting from paralysis of the eye muscle or nonparalytic, resulting from an inherited abnormality; in either case, diplopia (double vision) results. In a young child, the conflicting second image will be disregarded and result in poor visual development of the unused eye, a condition called amblyopia ex anopsia. Treatment of strabismus is aimed at realigning the optical axis of the eyes to establish binocular vision, and may include patching the unused eye, wearing corrective glasses, visual training, or surgery.

The nursing diagnoses for patients with ophthalmic disorders include sensory–perceptual alterations: visual, potential for injury related to vision impairment, potential anxiety or fear related to visual deficit, alteration in comfort: pain related to the ophthalmic disorder, social isolation, and potential disturbance in self-concept.

Goals. The goals for the patient with ophthalmic disorders include orientation to time and place, freedom from injury potentially resulting from vision impairment, effective coping with fear and anxiety, absence of pain and discomfort, and the ability to carry out activities of daily living.

Interventions

The eyes are naturally bathed by their own protective lubricating tears. Therefore, it only is necessary to wash around the eyes and remove any dried material from the inner canthus. Occasionally the nurse may be required to irrigate an eye to remove debris, chemicals, or crusted material from the lid margins. This is done by directing a stream of warm, isotonic solution across the eyeball and along the conjunctiva, while holding the lids open and having the patient look first up and then down. The fluid should flow temporally and never be directed forcefully onto the cornea.

To protect the eyes from trauma, shatterproof glasses should be worn whenever working near machinery or with tools that could throw off potentially penetrating material. Similarly, protective eyewear should be worn during some sports activities and whenever there is excessive exposure to very bright light, as in skiing, sailing, and certain industrial occupations. Eyestrain (prolonged exertion of the ciliary muscles of accommodation) can be avoided by using adequate lighting, correct lens prescriptions, and by periodically resting the eyes by looking into the distance whenever engaged in prolonged near distance work. The eyes should never be rubbed excessively or habitually, since this increases the liklihood of introducing bacteria into the eyes, causing a low grade infection.

Whenever ophthalmic medications are administered, the patient should be approached out of his direct line of vision, and the nurse should rest the heel of her hand on the patient's cheekbone, to guard against accidentally poking the eye. Then, with the patient's head tipped back, the eyes rolled upward, and the lower lid held away from the eyeball, one or two drops of medication can be instilled into the pocket formed by the everted lower lid. If an ointment is to be applied, the same technique should be followed, and a small, ribbonlike quantity of ointment placed along the entire surface of the everted lower lid (Fig. 70–4).

In both cases, the medication is fully dispensed across the surface of the eye when the patient blinks. When applying medications, the tip of the applicator should never touch the eyelids or lashes, and preparations should never be placed or dropped directly onto the eyeball itself.

Whenever an eye is patched, the primary precaution to observe is to be certain that the cornea is fully protected by the eyelids. This can be done by using at least three pieces of tape, and placing them diagonally across the patch from the cheekbone to the forehead. This technique allows facial movements to occur without loosening the tape or causing it to pull against the patient's skin.

Preoperative Nursing Management

As with any patient, the nurse will want to thoroughly orient the patient to his new surroundings and the people in it. Since the patient's vision may be more impaired following surgery and he will likely be medicated, the location of the

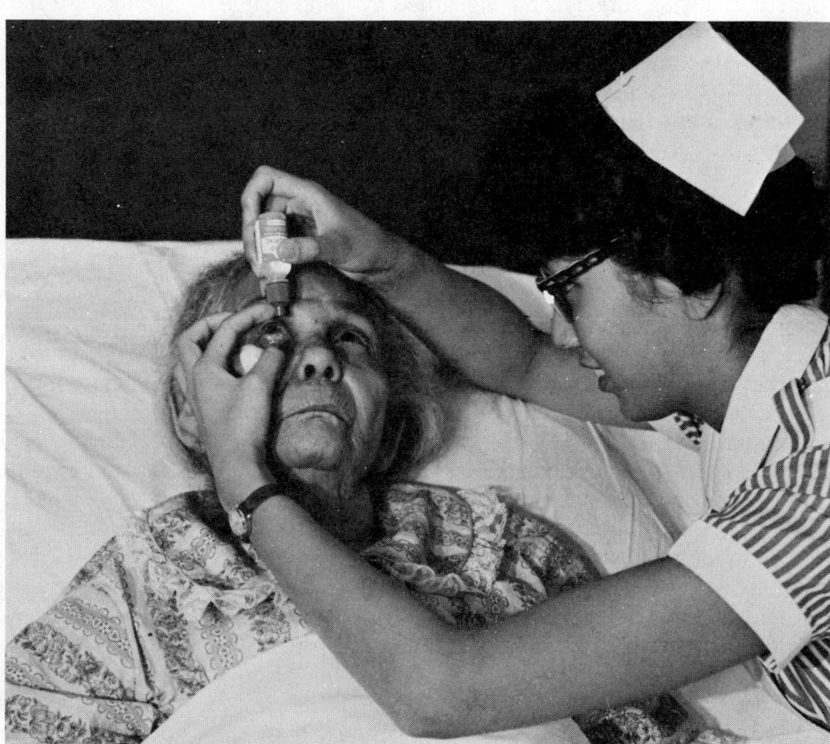

FIGURE 70–4 Technique for instilling ophthalmic drops and ointment. When instilling eye drops, instruct the patient to look upward, then lightly pull down the lower lid to form a receptacle for the dropped medication.

bathroom and call light are particularly important. This is especially significant for elderly patients who frequently have nocturia, secondary to normal age-related changes of the renal system and possible diuretic therapy.

The nurse must be clearly informed as to the patient's diagnosis, and what operative procedure is being performed on which eye. She must not assume that the patient can provide this information, since he either may be medicated or may not have absorbed what he has been told, owing to anxiety or concern about asking foolish questions. By evaluating the patient's level of understanding at this time, the nurse can begin to formulate a teaching plan of care.

Preoperative orders will specify how each eye is to be prepared and what drop routine will be required. These orders must be followed exactly. A preoperative enema or laxative may be ordered the night before surgery, as well as a shower and shampoo, if these activities are to be restricted postoperatively. If the eye lashes are to be cut, this is generally done by the ophthalmologist in the operating room prior to surgery. Each surgeon has his own routine, with which the nurse will become familiar.

Preoperative teaching should include warnings against any postoperative activity that would increase intraocular pressure. These activities include placing the head in a dependent position, straining on defecation, the Valsalva maneuver, coughing, sneezing, and vomiting. Because ophthalmic patients are often elderly and may have some degree of hearing loss, the nurse needs to be certain that the patient has heard and understood the information she is giving.

Patient fears often focus on concerns of pain and how long the eyes will be bandaged. The answers to these questions are variable with the nature of the surgery and the practices of the surgeon. However, pain is generally confined to a dull ache and is well controlled postoperatively, and improved closure techniques have made bilateral patches no longer mandatory.

Postoperative Nursing Management

Goals following ophthalmic surgery are to protect the operative eye from pressure, prevent increases in intraocular pressure, prevent intraocular infection, prevent sensory deprivation and disorientation, and prevent complications of immobility. Generally patients are allowed out of bed within 24 hours of surgery. However, while in bed patients should have the side rails up and the call bell within reach at all times. They should be instructed to lie on their unoperated side or back, with the bed flat or slightly elevated, depending on the postoperative orders.

The operative eye should be securely patched, and may have a protective metal shield over it. Initially the unoperative eye may also be patched to minimize eye movements. However, if the patient becomes restless, confused, or disoriented, the patch should be removed to help counteract the effects of sensory deprivation. Restraints are almost always contraindicated, since they tend to increase restlessness, and straining against them can dangerously elevate intraocular pressure. Personal items should be arranged within reach and assistance given, as for anyone with limited vision.

As previously mentioned, all activities that increase intraocular pressure should be avoided, and the patient should be cautioned against putting any external pressure on the eye by rubbing, squinting, or squeezing his eyelids. As with any postoperative patient, aseptic techniques must be observed whenever dressings are changed. During the initial postoperative period, this is usually done by the surgeon himself. Signs and symptoms of postoperative complications of which the surgeon should be notified include sudden, sharp, or excessive pain; bloody, purulent, or clear, viscous discharge; and temperature elevation.

Sensory deprivation and immobility are nursing concepts and diagnoses that every ophthalmology nurse should be familiar with. Because the majority of ophthalmology patients are elderly and may have chronic problems of sensory loss and bone and joint disease, the management of these problems frequently needs to be addressed on the care plan of patients undergoing ophthalmic surgery. Chapters 10 and 87 provide a full discussion of nursing interventions for patients suffering sensory deprivation and immobility, keeping in mind the restrictions mentioned above.

Evaluation

The patient will be oriented to time and place, will not have injuries related to his visual deficit, will cope effectively with fear and anxiety related to his disorder, will not evidence pain or discomfort related to his ophthalmic disorder, and will be able to carry out activities of daily living.

Hearing Problems

Ear Infections

Ear infections can be either acute or chronic, can involve either the internal or external structures of the ear, and may be either bacterial, viral, or fungal in nature.

External Otitis

External otitis of the ear refers to an infection or inflammation of the external ear. It can range from mild to severe, and is usually caused by chronic irritation. Incorrect or excessive cleaning of the ears, contact dermatitis from soap, shampoo, or metal, and swimming are often predisposing factors. These infections are generally bacterial in nature, but they may be fungal. Signs and symptoms of external otitis include redness, swelling, itching, crusting and scaling of the inflamed tissues. In its more acute form, pain, adenopathy, fever, and discharge may be present.

Treatment is generally with topical antibiotics (*e.g.,* neomycin sulfate, bacitracin) unless acute symptoms indicate that systemic antibiotics are warranted. Analgesics are given for pain. The auricle and ear canal should be kept clean and dry. Topical corticosteroids may be prescribed to reduce inflammation, and antiseptic compresses may be used to help control weeping of the affected tissue. Often external otitis is refractory to treatment, and the patient experiences recurrence whenever the predisposing factors prevail. Using earplugs when swimming or bathing may help to reduce recurrence.

Otitis Media

The term otitis media basically refers to three types of infections or inflammations that can occur in the middle ear. Acute otitis media commonly occurs in children, whose short, straight eustachian tubes, enlarged pharyngeal lymphoid tissue, and frequent upper respiratory infections predispose them to middle ear infections. Chronic otitis media is the most common middle ear infection of the adult, and is associated with previous episodes of acute otitis media. The third type of otitis media, serous otitis media, frequently occurs in children, but it can occur at any age. In this condition the eustachian tube fails to function properly, resulting in sterile fluid collecting in the middle ear. Due to the proximity of neighboring structure, complications of otitis media can be severe and life threatening. They include mastoiditis, labyrinthitis, meningitis, brain abscess, facial paralysis, and conductive hearing loss.

Acute Otitis Media. Acute otitis media is also referred to as suppurative otitis media. It usually follows or accompanies an upper respiratory tract disease when the normally sterile middle ear becomes infected by nasopharyngeal bacteria. Symptoms include severe ear pain, a feeling of fullness and pressure, hearing loss, fever, and chills. On inspection the tympanic membrane appears dull and red, with dilated blood vessels. At first it may retract, but later bulges, as secretions accumulate in the middle ear. Unless antibiotic treatment is initiated, rupture of the membrane with purulent otorrhea may occur.

For severe bulging or if symptoms continue despite treatment, a myringotomy (surgical incision of the tympanic membrane) is recommended. Additional treatment consists of bed rest, analgesics, antipyretics, and broad-spectrum systemic antibiotics. Cold compresses may help relieve pain, or warm compresses may be ordered to hasten resolution. Acute otitis media almost always responds well to treatment, and the once common complication of mastoiditis (infection of the mastoid bone) is rarely seen today, except in cases of inadequate therapy. If mastoiditis does occur with abscess formation, surgical drainage is required.

Chronic Otitis Media. Chronic otitis media occurs when the middle ear and mastoid cells become chronically infected. There is usually a history of of recurrent or inadequately treated acute otitis media, and the eardrum is almost always perforated. Symptoms include a continuous or intermittent discharge from the ear (which may be foul-smelling) and conductive hearing loss. The condition is usually painless. If the posterior margin of the tympanic membranes is ruptured, epithelial tissue from the external canal can grow into the middle ear, forming a cholesteatoma (cystlike mass). This in turn can cause erosion of adjacent bones and tissue, resulting in ossicle or neurological damage.

Treatment of chronic otitis media consists of using local and systemic antibiotics along with ear irrigations to remove debris and promote drainage. Resolution of chronic otitis media may include a mastoidectomy to remove infected material, and a tympanoplasty to restructure the sound-conducting mechanism of the middle ear.

A *mastoidectomy,* although rare since the advent of antibiotics, may be required if the mastoid process becomes infected as a complication of otitis media. During this surgery, all diseased tissue is excised, including the ossicles of the middle ear if they are involved. Complications of mastoid surgery include facial nerve paralysis, meningitis, and deafness, if the ossicles must be removed.

Serous Otitis Media. Serous otitis media, also referred to as otitis media with effusion, "glue ear," secretory otitis media, and nonsupportive otitis media, occurs when there is an effusion of fluid into the middle ear owing to negative middle ear pressure. It may be caused by either the eustachian tube failing to equalize middle ear pressure or an allergic reaction of the mucous membrane. Symptoms include a feeling of fullness, conductive hearing loss, and mild pain. It can be differentiated from acute otitis media by lack of severe pain and fever. Initially the tympanic membrane is retracted, and then gradually becomes less mobile as fluid accumulates in the middle ear. Tympanometry, an objective means for determining middle ear pressure, may be performed to aid in diagnosis.

Treatment of serous otitis media is aimed at equalizing the pressure on either side of the tympanic membrane, and may include decongestants and antihistamines to unblock the eustachian tube, fluid aspiration by needle or through a myringotomy incision, or ventilation tubes placed in the tympanic membrane. When tympanotomy tubes are inserted, they may be left in place for weeks to months, and the patient should be cautioned against getting water into his ears when swimming or bathing.

Labyrinthitis

Labyrinthitis is an infection of the vestibular and cochlear labyrinth. It may occur following an upper respiratory infection, an episode of acute otitis media, an exacerbation of chronic otitis media, or mastoiditis. Symptoms of labyrinthitis are severe vertigo, with nausea and vomiting, tinnitus, and nystagmus; its treatment includes bed rest, sedation, and antibiotics if infection is present. Although attacks of labyrinthitis may last several days, recovery is usually complete with minimal hearing loss. An acute purulent form of labyrinthitis can result in total destruction of the affected structures and total loss of hearing. In these cases, surgery, usually a mastoidectomy to remove all infected material, is often necessary.

Trauma to the Ear

Trauma to the ear may be in the form of objects inserted into the external ear canal or a severe blow to the side of the head. Other than vegetable matter, most objects can be removed by irrigation or with forceps. Vegetable matter (*e.g.,* beans, peas) should always be removed by instrumentation, since water will cause them to swell and become impacted. Insects that penetrate the ear canal can be suffocated by instilling a drop of oil into the ear prior to removing them by irrigation.

If the eardrum has been perforated by trauma, symptoms will include pain, deafness, and occasional bleeding. Fortunately, most traumatic perforations heal spontaneously with minimal loss of hearing. Antibiotics may be prescribed to guard against middle ear infection, and the patient should avoid getting water into the ear. A myringoplasty may be done if spontaneous healing does not occur.

A severe blow to the head can dislocate the ossicles of the middle ear and cause a conductive loss of hearing. Treatment consists of surgical reconstruction of the ossicular chain.

Conductive Hearing Loss

A conductive hearing loss is caused by any disorder or disease that interrupts the conduction of sound from the external ear to the sensory receptors in the cochlea. It may be caused by impacted cerumen, damage to the tympanic membrane, middle ear infection, or failure of the ossicles to transmit sound, as in otosclerosis.

Cerumen Impaction. Cerumen, a substance secreted by glands lining the external ear canal, functions to protect the ear by trapping bacteria and dust. In some persons, and as a normal consequence of aging, an increased accumulation of cerumen occurs that can dry, become impacted, and occlude the auditory canal, causing a conductive hearing loss. The condition is usually asymptomatic, although some persons may notice a loss of hearing and feeling of fullness, particularly if the wax absorbs moisture and swells.

Treatment of impacted cerumen is first to soften it with a solution of mineral oil or hydrogen peroxide and then irrigate the ear canal with a syringe or water pick set on low speed. Irrigating solutions should always be warmed to body temperature, and the fluid should be injected along the upper wall of the ear canal, never forcefully toward the eardrum. An ear irrigation should never be done if there is a history of a perforated eardrum or if inflammation is present. Cerumen can also be removed under direct visualization with a curette. Cotton-tipped applicators should not be used, since they tend to further impact the cerumen.

Tympanic Membrane Damage. The tympanic membrane may be perforated as the result of injury or infection, or it may be perforated surgically (myringotomy) if it appears that spontaneous rupture is imminent. In either case, healing usually occurs within 24 hours, and until then, no water should enter the ear. Because scarring of the tympanic membrane following a myringotomy is minimal, there usually is no loss of hearing. However, more extensive scarring of the membrane can occur with repeated perforations and can cause a conductive hearing loss. Chronic perforation of the tympanic membrane is a complication of otitis media and requires surgical correction.

Middle Ear Infections. Middle ear infections cause loss of hearing either by destroying the ossicles or by fluid accumulation interfering with ossicle function. Ear infections and their treatment were discussed earlier in this chapter.

Otosclerosis. Otosclerosis is a relatively common, usually bilateral hearing disorder that occurs predominately in females, beginning in young adulthood. It is characterized by an abnormal growth of spongy bone in the middle ear that eventually immobilizes the stapes, resulting in conductive hearing loss. The primary symptom of the disease, usually first noticed in the late teens, is a gradual loss of hearing associated with tinnitus. In about 50% of the cases there is a family history of deafness. Although patients with otosclerosis hear well with a hearing aid, because of their young age they generally seek surgery in the form of stapedectomy. Surgery improves hearing in more than 80% of the cases operated.

Ear Surgery

Most surgery on the ear consists of procedures to reconstruct the delicate structures of the middle ear in an attempt to restore hearing to persons who have a conductive hearing loss. It may also be done to remove benign or malignant growths or to excise infection.

Surgery on the *tympanic membrane* consists of either a *myringotomy,* the surgical incision of the membrane to relieve pressure in the middle ear, or a *Type I tympanoplasty,* the surgical repair of a perforated eardrum by use of a graft. In cases of recurrent otitis media, a ventilating tube may be placed in the membrane to relieve pressure and allow drainage. These tubes are not uncomfortable, and they can be left in place for weeks, during which time the ear must be protected from water.

Surgery on the *middle ear* is referred to by the general term *tympanoplasty.* The extent of surgery is indicated by the use of Roman numerals. As mentioned above, Type I tympanoplasty involves surgical reconstruction of the tympanic membrane. Type II tympanoplasty involves reconstruction of the malleus; Type III tympanoplasty is the reconstruction of the malleus and incus; Type IV tympanoplasty is the reconstruction of the malleus, incus, and most of the stapes; and Type V tympanoplasty includes the mobilization of the stapes as well.

A *stapedectomy* is the procedure of choice for persons who have otosclerosis. This procedure involves removing either a portion or all of the immobilized stapes. If only a portion of the stapes is removed and the footplate is left, an opening is made in it through which a prosthesis is placed and attached to the incus. If the entire stapes is removed, a graft is placed over the oval window, and a prosthesis is attached from it to the incus.

Still in the experimental stage is a procedure known as the *cochlear implant.* In this surgery, electrodes are placed in or just outside the internal ear in the hope of stimulating any surviving nerve fibers. In the future as technology improves, this procedures offers the greatest hope to patients suffering profound sensory deafness.

Sensorineural Hearing Loss

Etiology

A sensorineural hearing loss is caused by any disorder or disease that affects the cochlea or auditory nerve, interrupting the sensory reception of sound or its transmission to the interpretive areas of the brain. Causes of sensorineural hearing loss include noise-induced hearing loss, Meniere's disease, viral infection, acoustic tumors, ototoxic drugs, trauma, and degenerative changes of aging, commonly referred to as presbycusis. With the exception of ototoxicity, which is usually reversible, sensorineural hearing loss is almost always permanent. Hearing aids, which amplify but do not clarify sounds, are of little benefit, since people with this type of hearing loss lose the ability to discriminate sounds.

Pathology and Clinical Manifestations

Noise-Induced Hearing Loss. Prolonged exposure to high noise levels or brief exposure to excessively loud noise can temporarily or permanently damage the delicate structures of the organ of Corti. If the hearing loss is the result of a blast of noise, as occurs from an explosion or shotgun, it will be most pronounced immediately following the insult, with spontaneous improvement occurring in days to weeks. If the hearing loss is the result of exposure to noise over a continuous length of time, as occurs in many occupations and to devotees of amplified rock music, the damage will be permanent and irreversible. In either case, the hearing loss occurs first in the high-frequency sounds and, with continued exposure, extends to affect the lower-frequency sounds, making speech discrimination increasingly difficult. The best treatment of noise-induced hearing loss is prevention. As indicated above, hearing aids are of little help, and rarely are worn if prescribed. Although damage to the organ of Corti is irreversible once it has occurred, additional hearing loss can be prevented by eliminating further noise exposure. Provisions of the Occupational Safety and Health Act (OSHA) presently require workers in noisy industries to wear protective ear covering, limit their exposure to high noise levels, and have their hearing periodically monitored.

Viral Infection. Hearing loss may be a complication of viral infection. Among the diseases known to cause deafness are mumps, measles, chickenpox, and poliomyelitis. Fortunately, this complication is rare since the advent of immunization.

Ototoxic Drugs. Many drugs are potentially ototoxic, causing temporary or permanent loss of hearing. Among these are the aminoglycoside antibiotics (primarly streptomycin sulfate, gentamicin sulfate, and viomycin sulfate), diuretics (primarily ethacrynic acid and furosemide), antimalarial agents (primarily quinine sulfate), and salicylates. In addition to auditory disturbance, these drugs also cause vestibular disturbance, vertigo, and light-headedness. Individual response varies, and all patients on these drugs should have their blood levels and hearing monitored closely. This is especially important in cases of impaired renal function and when these drugs are prescribed in combination with one another or in high dosages.

Presbycusis. Presbycusis is a general term used to refer to the sensorineural hearing loss commonly associated with aging. Various factors are thought to contribute to the etiology of presbycusis; among these are heredity, environment, metabolism, and circulation. Exposure to noise, as previously described under noise-induced hearing loss, is felt to be a major contributing factor in the development of presbycusis. A strong correlation has also been found between the incidence of atherosclerosis and presbycusis,[3] indicating that impaired circulation may be a factor.

The degree of hearing loss with presbycusis may be so slight that it is imperceptible except by audiometric studies, or so severe that it is profoundly disabling. Similar to noise-induced hearing loss, impairment is first noticed in the high-frequency sounds and later progresses to involve the lower frequencies. Persons with presbycusis also complain that they hear, but cannot discriminate, what is being said to them. This occurs because the soft sounds of *f, s, th, ch,* and *sh* are among the first sounds lost, later followed by loss of the hard consonant sounds such as *p, t, b,* and *d.* The lower-frequency vowel sounds are generally well-preserved.[5]

Hearing aids may be of some help to patients who have a coexisting conductive hearing loss, but for most people they are of little value, since they amplify all frequencies without improving the clarity of what is being said.

Disorders of Equilibrium

Problems of equilibrium arise from disorders of the vestibular labyrinth. They include labyrinthitis, previously discussed under infections of the inner ear, and Meniere's disease.

Meniere's Disease. Meniere's disease is a chronic disease of unknown etiology characterized by severe, recurrent attacks of vertigo associated with nausea and vomiting, tinnitus, and hearing loss. These attacks occur suddenly, usually several times a year, and can last for hours or days, totally incapacitating the patient. Initially the associated hearing loss fluctuates, but gradually it becomes permanent, and worsens over years.

The exact cause of Meniere's disease is unknown, but it appears to relate to an abnormality of either the formation or absorption of endolymph.[2] Structurally, the cochlear duct dilates, which is thought to account for the gradual loss of hearing.

Medical Management. Treatment of Meniere's disease is directed toward reducing the amount of endolymph by diuresis, restricting salt and fluid, and by using antihistamines and nicotine acid to provide local vasodilation. Sedatives and antianxiety agents are frequently used to relieve associated psychiatric symptoms. An especially acute attack may be relieved by giving atropine sulfate to block autonomic nervous system function. In rare cases not relieved by conservative treatment, surgery may be necessary.

Nursing Management of the Otology Patient

Assessment and Nursing Diagnosis

Symptoms indicating problems with the auditory system include loss of hearing, pain, discharge, tinnitus, dizziness, and a feeling of fullness. The nursing diagnoses include sensory–perceptual alteration: auditory, alterations in comfort related to pain, potential for injury related to trauma, social isolation related to impaired communication, and disturbance in self-concept.

A routine ear examination includes an assessment of hearing and balance, inspection of the auricle and ear canal, and otoscopic evaluation of the tympanic membrane. More extensive evaluation may include audiometric evaluation, caloric stimulation, neurological testing, and x-ray examination.

Goals. General goals of nursing care of the otology patient include protection from preventable hearing loss and maintenance of preferred amount of social interaction. Specific goals of surgical care are to prevent infection and the dislocation of any prosthetic devices or grafts inserted during surgery.

Interventions

Care of the ears primarily involves keeping them clean and protecting them from trauma and infection. Objects should never be inserted into the ear past the point of vision, and the ears should be cleaned with nothing smaller than a small finger or by irrigation, as previously described for the removal of cerumen. If there is a history of infection or tympanic membrane perforation, the ear should be protected from water to guard against infection. During an upper respiratory infection, the nose should never be blown forcefully, nor should so much pressure be created in the upper nasal passages that infected secretions are forced into the middle ear by way of the eustachian tube. For the same reason, persons with a history of ear infections and small children should be advised against flying in nonpressurized aircraft, especially if they have an upper respiratory infection.

Protecting the ears from trauma due to prolonged exposure to noise is of particular concern in Western industrialized societies, where people are exposed daily to noise levels that can damage the sensitive organ of Corti. Persons who in their daily work or enjoyment of hobbies and recreational opportunities subject themselves to the trauma of loud noise should always wear ear plugs or ear protectors. Federal regulations now make this mandatory in certain occupations. Health educators need to increase public awareness of those situations that currently are not regulated and yet pose a threat of hearing loss, for example, hunting, working with power tools, and exposure to amplified music.

Preoperative Nursing Considerations. As with any surgical patient, the nurse will want to thoroughly orient the patient to his environment. It is important that the patient understands the nature of his impending surgery and the potential complications from it. The patient's hair should be washed the night before surgery and the area around the auricle shaved. Ear drops, ointments, irrigations, and hot or cold compresses may be ordered to decreased any inflammation or relieve discomfort. A twisted piece of sterile gauze or a commercially prepared ear wick may be used to help remove drainage by capillary action. These should be changed frequently and should never be compressed but, rather, inserted loosely into the external meatus. If the patient is experiencing vertigo, care should be taken to avoid accidents, for example, with side rails or call bell. These patients may rest more comfortably in a quiet, darkened room. Accompanying nausea and vomiting can be treated with antiemetics and parenteral fluids.

Postoperative Nursing Considerations. Aseptic technique should be used whenever the ear dressing or drainage is handled, and the patient should refrain as much as possible from coughing, sneezing, or blowing his nose immediatley following surgery. These actions potentially could force material up the eustachian tube or by pressure dislodge middle ear prostheses and grafts. The nurse should ensure that the ear is kept dry, and monitor her patient for symptoms of facial nerve paralysis, meningitis, and infection. Vertigo, which may accompany some forms of surgery, can best be treated by keeping the patient flat and providing appropriate safety measures. Postoperative medications for the otology patient may include all or any of the following: antibiotics, antiemetics, analgesics, sedatives, and antihistamines. It is important to remind patients that the true outcome of their surgery cannot be fully assessed until dressings are removed and all postoperative swelling subsides.

Evaluation

The patient will maintain social contacts, will not have preventable loss of hearing, will not have infection, and will not have complications related to surgery.

References

1. Beales PH: Acquired deafness: Causes and Treatment. The Practitioner, Vol 277:915–925, June 1982
2. Birrell JF: Logan Turner's Diseases of the Nose, Throat, and Ear. London, John Wright and Sons, 1982
3. Gilad O, Glorig A: Presbycusis: The aging ear, Part I. Journal of American Auditory Society Vol 4, No 5:195–206, 1979
4. Kilroy JL: Care and teaching of patients with glaucoma. Nurs Clin North Am (3):393–404, 1981
5. Larsen G: Ear problems. In Carnevali D, Patrick M: Nursing Management of the Elderly. Phildelphia, JB Lippincott, 1979

6. Moore CR: Scleral buckling for retinal detachment. AORN (3):495, 1982
7. National Eye Institute: Laser treatment found effective in preventing blindness from senile macular degeneration. J Am Geriatr Soc 31(4):238–239, 1983
8. Romanes G: Transplantation and the eye. Practitioner, Vol 226, May 1982
9. Stark WJ, Leske MC, Worthen DM, Murray GC: Trends in cataract surgery and intraocular lenses in the United States. Am J Ophthalmol 96:304–310, 1983
10. Taisch E, Taisch DP, Metz HS: Problems of the eyes. In O'Hara, Deverezux, Andrus, Scott (eds): Eldercare, a Guide to Clinical Geriatrics, p 266. New York, Grune and Stratton, 1981
11. Vaughan D, Asbury T: General Ophthalmology, 10th ed. Los Altos CA, Lange Medical Publications, 1983
12. Wilkinson EL, Christensen RE: Laser treatment for glaucoma. West J Med 140(2):271–272, 1984

Bibliography

Andreason MD: Color vision defects in the elderly. Journal of Gerontology and Nursing (7):383–384, 1980

Bain DJG: Acute otitis media in general practice. Practitioner 225(1361):1568–1575, 1981

Bluestone CD: Otitis media: New aspects of etiology, pathogenesis, diagnosis and treatment. Consultant (12):66–79, 1979

Boyd-Monk H: Cataract surgery: New techniques you'll be involved with. Nursing 77, pp 56–61, June 1977

Boyd-Monk H: Retinal detachment and vitrectomy: Nursing care. Nurs Clin North Am 16(3):433-451, 1981

Cataract surgery: Providing total patient care. Helping Geriatric Patients, A Nursing Photobook. Nursing 83, pp 65–69, April 1983

Chignell AH: Advances in the treatment of retinal disorders. Practitioner 226:1691–1697, October 1982

Cooling RJ: The injured eye. Practitioner 226:849–858, May 1982

Dangel M, Havener W: Drugs and the aging eye. Geriatrics, pp 133–140, March 1981

DeWeese DD, Saunder WH: Textbook of Otolaryngology, 6th ed. St Louis, CV Mosby, 1982

Ellis RA: Advances in cataract surgery. Occupational Health Nursing 29(7):34–38, 1981

Engelstein JM: Cataract Surgery, Current Options and Problems. Orlando FL, Grune and Stratton, 1984

Freese AS: Cataracts and their Treatment. New York, Public Affairs Pamphlets, 1980

Freese AS: Glaucoma—Diagnosis, Treatment, Prevention. New York, Public Affairs Pamphlets, 1979

Gallagher MA: Organ transplantation series: Corneal transplantation. Am J Nurs 81(10):1845, 1981

Gilad O, Glorig A: Presbycusis: The aging ear, Part II. Journal of American Auditory Society 4(6):207–217, 1979

Harker LA: Effusions and infections. Emergency Medicine 12(20):24–27, November 30, 1980

Harrison CJ: Managing ears that won't get better. Consultant 22(4):283–299, 1982

Havener WH: Ocular Pharmacology, 4th ed. St Louis, CV Mosby, 1978

Hayes PL: Treatment and nursing care of corneal disease. Nurs Clin North Am 16(3):383–392, 1982

Hodes BL, Choromokos EA: Glaucoma. Postgrad Med pp 111–120, July 1978

Irvine PW: The hearing-impaired elderly patient. Postgrad Med 72(4):115–118, 1982

Jakobiec FA, Siegelman J: Advanced Techniques in Ocular Surgery. Philadelphia, WB Saunders, 1984

Jeglum EL: Ocular therapeutics. Nurs Clin North Am 16(3):453–477, 1981

Kolder HE: The latest in cateract therapy. Consultant 21(4):147–153, 1981

Luntz MH, Harrison R, Schenker HI: Glaucoma Surgery. Baltimore, Williams & Wilkins, 1984

MacFadyen JS: Caring for the patient with a primary retinal detachment. Am J Nurs 80, No. (5):920–921, May 1980

McCoy K: Cataracts and intraocular lenses: From cloudy to clear. Nurs Clin North Am 16(3):405–414, 1981

McLoy K: The ear (Section III) in Birrell JF (ed): Logan Turner's Diseases of the Nose, Throat and Ear, 9th ed. Boston, Wright, 1982

Mathalone MBR: Ophthalmic emergencies. Practitioner 225:1151–1155, August 1981

More on macular degeneration and lasers. Massachusetts General Hospital Newsletter 2(1), July 1983

Ohta R, Carlin M, Harmon B: Auditory acuity and performance on the mental status questionnaire in the elderly. J Am Geriatr Soc 29(10):476–478, 1981

Pollack IP: Laser iridotomy in the treatment of angle-closure glaucoma. Ann Ophthalmol 13(5):549–550, 1981

Sensory changes in the elder (programmed instruction). Am J Nurs 81(10):1851–1880, 1981

Resler MM, Tumulty G: Glaucoma update. Am J Nurs 83(5):752–756, 1983

Sataloff RT, Colton CM: Otitis media: A common childhood infection. Am J Nurs 81(8):1480–1483, 1981

Sataloff RT, Vassallo LA: Choosing the right hearing aid. Hosp Pract 16(5):32A–32S, 1981

Smith J: Focusing your care for the patient with an intraocular lens implant. RN, pp 46–50, March 1978

Smith JF, Nachazel DP: Ophthalmologic Nursing. Boston, Little Brown & Co, 1980

Thomas PD, Hunt WC, Garry PJ et al: Hearing acuity in a healthy elderly population: Effects on emotional, cognitive and social status. J Gerontol 38(3):321–325, 1983

Todd B: Using eye drops and ointments safetey. Geriatric Nursing, pp 53–57, January–February 1983

Tripathi RC, Tripathi BJ: Lens morphology, aging and cataract. J Gerontol 38(3):258–270, 1983

Weinstock FJ: What your aging patient may want to know about cataracts. Geriatrics, 57–60, December 1978

Wertz R: Alternatives to standard cataract surgery. Postgrad Med pp 96–105, July 1978

Wong EK, Wang S, Leopold IH: How ophthalmic drugs can fool you. RN, March 1980

Wong DL, Dornan LR: Nursing care in childhood cancer: Retinoblastomia. AJN, p 425, March 1982

Yang HK, Kline OR Jr: Posterior Chamber Lens Implant Surgery. New York, Raven Press, 1983

UNIT VIII

Nursing Care of Patients with Alterations in Endocrine Function

Chapter 71

Review of Anatomy and Physiology
Endocrine System

Barbara R. Landau

The endocrine system is one of the body's two control systems, the other being the nervous system. The relationship between the two systems is described in Chapter 12. The nervous system controls action of such effectors as skeletal, smooth, and cardiac muscle, and some glands, whereas target cells for the endocrine system include virtually every cell in the body. Glands of the endocrine system are distributed throughout the body, some as separate organs and others as cell clusters or isolated cells in an organ with other functions (Fig. 71–1). Endocrine glands are those glands that produce a specific substance, a hormone, which is transported in the bloodstream to a distant target organ to exert a specific action.

Hormones generally affect the rates of ongoing processes, particularly processes that are important to the overall body economy. Hormones help to

- Regulate the energy supply by actions on processes for digestion of foods, and for storage, conversion, release, and utilization of energy.
- Control composition of the extracellular fluid, specifically water and electrolytes (Na^+, K^+, Ca^{2+}, PO_4^{2-}).
- Activate mechanisms for coping with a wide variety of stressful conditions, *e.g.,* trauma, cold, and dehydration.
- Regulate such basic mechanisms as growth, development, and reproduction.

Mechanisms of Hormone Action

In spite of the great number of hormones and variety of actions, there are remarkable similarities in their mechanisms of action. First, a hormone must "recognize" its target organ, and then activate the proper response mechanism in the target cell. The receptor is the key to both processes.

Hormone Receptors

Receptors are proteins which contain binding sites that have an affinity for a particular molecule, that is, the hormone. The specificity of the receptor is the means by which a hormone recognizes its target organ. A hormone cannot act upon a cell that does not have receptors for it. Formation of a hormone–receptor complex initiates the specific target cell response.

Receptor protein is subject to control by cellular processes. Additional receptors can be synthesized and inserted into the plasma membrane, or they can be removed and degraded. Thus the "sensitivity" to a hormone can be altered by changing the number of available receptor sites. Hormone effectiveness can also be altered by extracellular factors that destroy, inactivate, or perhaps occupy, receptor binding sites.

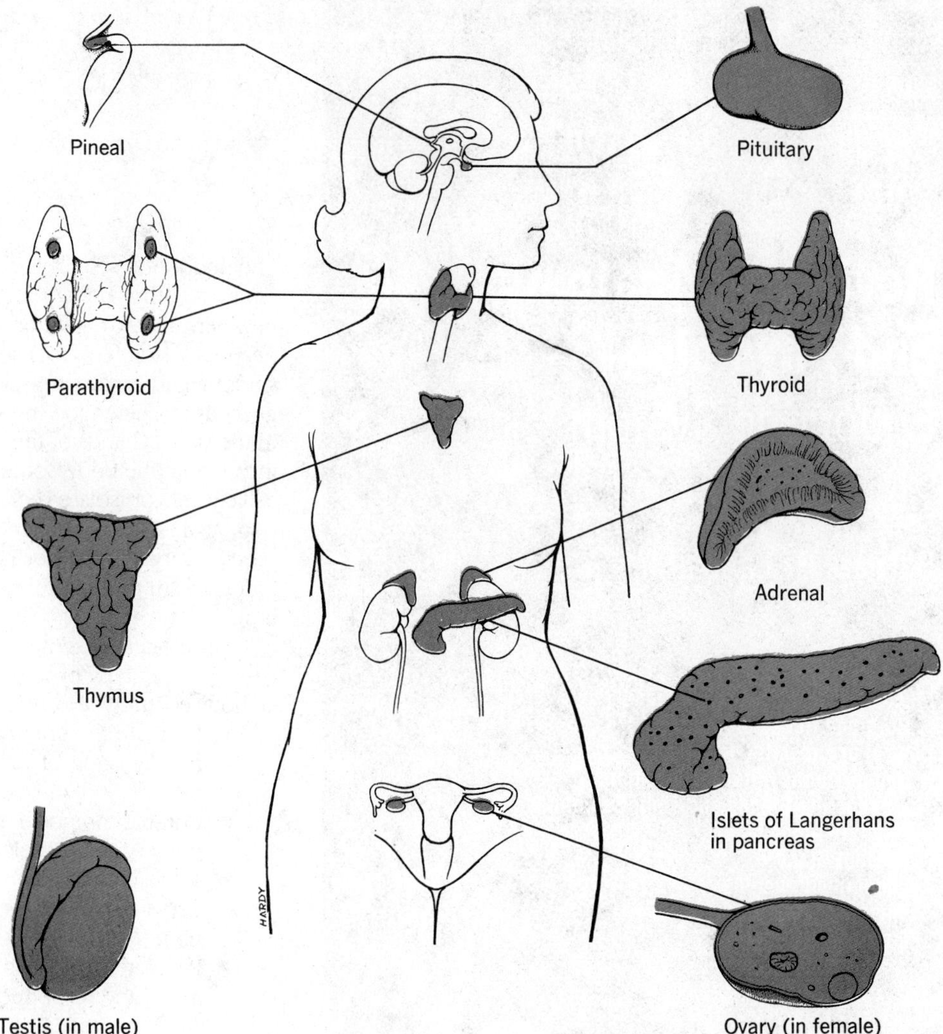

FIGURE 71–1 General location of the major endocrine glands.

Control of Endocrine Function

Endocrine functions and hormone actions are determined by factors that regulate hormone levels and those that determine hormone effectiveness. Plasma hormone levels depend on the balance between the rates of hormone secretion and hormone removal or inactivation. Hormone effectiveness is determined peripherally at the target cell, and it is affected by such factors as the availability and affinity of hormone receptors and by the availability of substrate (*i.e.,* enzymes to activate) and energy sources (*e.g.,* ATP). The best understood controls are those of hormone secretion rates.

Negative feedback systems, in which hormone secretion is regulated by the substance the hormone regulates, are among the simplest and most important regulatory mechanisms. For example, blood glucose level is the major determinant of insulin secretion, and calcium is the main regulator of parathormone secretion. A longer feedback loop operates for hormones whose secretion is controlled by anterior pituitary hormones, since the hormone secreted by the target organ inhibits the pituitary rather than the target organ.

Some endocrine glands respond to direct neural (autonomic) action. The adrenal medulla is entirely under autonomic control. In most glands, neural regulation is secondary to other controls.

The brain, however, exerts control over most endocrine action by way of the hypothalamus, which receives input from many parts of the brain and exerts neural influence over many autonomic functions. The hypothalamus also controls the posterior pituitary and regulates the anterior pituitary and all the endocrine glands controlled by it. Brain control of endocrine functions should be no suprise because endocrine responses must be coordinated with the needs of the entire body, not merely the level of some substance or process. The endocrine system lacks both a sensory system to monitor conditions widely and mechanisms to integrate and coordinate its responses. The nervous system, therefore, does the sensory monitoring and integrating and directs much of the overall action of the endocrines. The hypothalamus, with its close ties to the limbic system and other parts of the brain, provides the connections by which emotions may affect hormone secretion.

Hypothalamic–Pituitary Relations

Brain control of hormone secretion depends on the unique anatomical and functional relationship between the hypothalamus and pituitary gland (Fig. 71–2).

The *posterior lobe* maintains its connection with the brain, and it is innervated by neurons from the hypothalamus. These are neuroendocrine cells with cell bodies in the hypothalamic nuclei, and axons that pass through the pituitary stalk to end in close proximity to capillaries in the posterior pituitary gland. The blood supply to the posterior lobe comes directly from hypophyseal arteries, and is separate from that to the anterior lobe. The substances released by the hypothalamic nerve endings enter capillaries in the posterior lobe to be distributed throughout the body as hormones of the posterior lobe. They are antidiuretic hormone (ADH, vasopressin) and oxytocin. The posterior pituitary gland is not a true endocrine gland because it does not produce any hormones.

Cells of the *anterior lobe* produce several hormones, and since most of them act on other endocrine glands, the anterior pituitary was once thought to be the "master gland." The only significant innervation to the anterior lobe is to its blood vessels; there is none to the secretory cells. The anterior lobe receives its blood supply directly by way of the

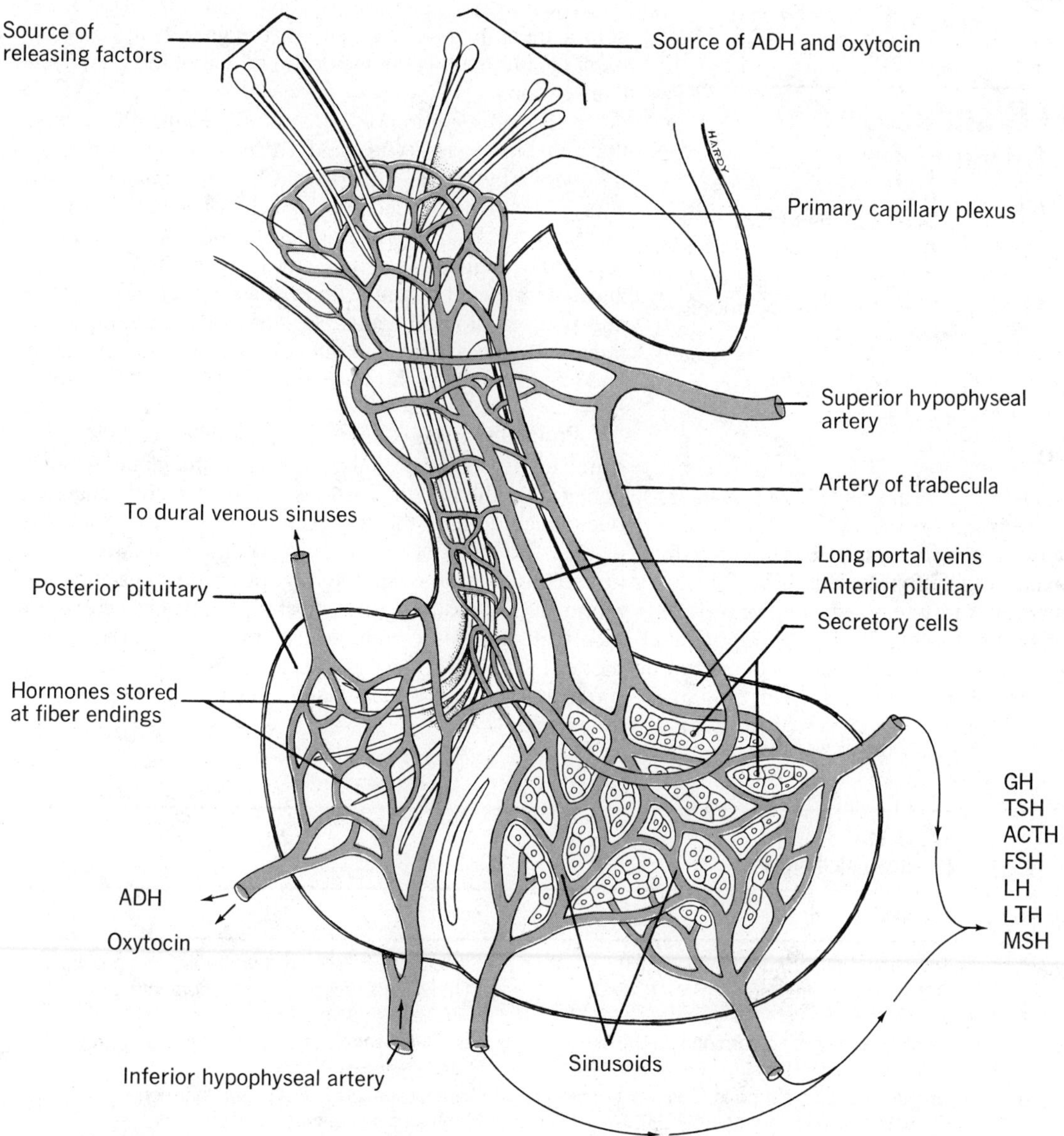

FIGURE 71–2 Diagram of the hypothalamus and the anterior and posterior pituitary. Hypothalamus releasing or inhibiting hormones are transported to the anterior pituitary by way of the portal vessels. ADH and oxytocin are produced by nerve cells in the supraoptic and paraventricular nuclei of the hypothalamus and then transported through the nerve axon to the posterior pituitary where they are released into the circulation.

hypothalamus. Arteries that supply the anterior lobe first break into capillaries in the hypothalamus near the origin of the pituitary stalk, then drain into sinusoidal veins that pass to the anterior lobe, and break into a second capillary bed. This vascular arrangement is the hypophyseal portal system. Neurosecretions are taken up by the capillaries and transported by the hypophyseal portal vessels to the anterior lobe where they diffuse from the bloodstream and act upon the secretory cells. The hypothalamic neurosecretions are *releasing hormones* because they stimulate secretion of anterior lobe hormones. There are releasing hormones for all of the anterior pituitary hormones, and inhibitory hormones for growth hormone and prolactin whose target organs are not endocrine glands and thus would not be inhibited by negative feedback (Table 71–1).

The Endocrine Glands and Their Secretions

The endocrine glands and the major actions of their hormones are summarized in Table 71–2. The following discussion supplements the table by focusing on certain pertinent and significant aspects of some of the glands and hormones.

Pituitary Gland

Anterior Pituitary

Growth hormone (GH) and prolactin (PRL) exert their actions on nonendocrine target organs, but the other anterior lobe hormones act on endocrine glands to cause growth and development as well as secretion. Two of these, follicle stimulating hormone (FSH) and luteinizing hormone (LH) (which are produced by the same cells), serve important functions, namely, stimulation of the development of ovarian follicles and formation of corpora lutea in females, and increased spermatogenesis in males. Adrenocorticotropic hormone (ACTH) is formed from a prohormone that is also the precursor of several other substances, including β-lipotropin (β-LPH) and β-endorphins, which are secreted in small amounts by the ACTH-producing cells.

Growth Hormone. Growth hormone stimulates growth in the epiphyseal plates of growing long bones by stimulating mitosis in chondroblasts and consequently their formation of cartilage matrix. Cartilage growth delays closure of the epiphyses and prolongs linear growth of long bones. In the absence of GH the epiphyses close before the bones reach normal length, and too much GH leads to accelerated and continued growth, which may lead to gigantism. Excess GH after growth is completed leads to thickening of certain bones, known as acromegaly.

The metabolic effects of GH on protein are anabolic and complement their skeletal actions. The growth and development of soft tissue is in proportion to that of the framework that supports it.

Although secretion of GH is controlled mainly by hypothalamic hormones (GRH and GIH/somatostatin) that are influenced by neural input to the hypothalamus, it is also affected by metabolic factors. Growth hormone secretion is increased by high amino acid levels and hypoglycemia, is reduced by high levels of free fatty acids and hyperglycemia, and is influenced by the actions of a number of hormones and pharmacological agents. Because of the interaction of these substances, it is often difficult to assign specific causes and effects with any assurance.

Prolactin. The primary action of prolactin (PRL) is to stimulate secretion of milk in postpartum females, but it depends on the previous actions of estrogen and progesterone, which develop the secretory capacity of the mammary glands. The effect of PRL in males is unknown. Most of the time PRL secretion is inhibited by prolactin inhibitory hormone (PIH, dopamine), but during pregnancy secretion is increased under the influence of prolactin-releasing hormone (PRH), and it reaches a peak at parturition. Continued prolactin secretion is maintained in response to suckling by the infant.

TABLE 71–1
Hypothalamic Hormones

Hormone	*Action*
Thyrotropin-releasing hormone (TRH)	Stimulates secretion of thyrotropin, also prolactin
Corticotropin-releasing hormone (CRH)	Stimulates secretion of adrenocorticotropic hormone, also β-lipotropin
Luteinizing-releasing hormone (LRH), or gonadotropin-releasing hormone (GnRH)	Stimulates secretion of follicle-stimulating hormone and luteinizing hormone
Growth-releasing hormone (GRH)	Stimulates secretion of growth hormone
Prolactin-releasing hormone (PRH)	Stimulates secretion of prolactin
Growth hormone inhibitory hormone (GIH), or somatostatin	Inhibits growth hormone secretion, also thyrotropin
Prolactin inhibitory hormone (PIH), or dopamine	Inhibits prolactin secretion
Antidiuretic hormone (ADH) or vasopressin, released from posterior pituitary	See Table 71–2
Oxytocin, released from posterior pituitary	See Table 71–2

TABLE 71–2
The Endocrine Glands and Their Hormones

Hormone	*Major Control of Secretion**	*Major Actions*
Anterior Pituitary (Adenohypophysis)		
Growth Hormone (GH, somatotropin) *peptide*	Growth hormone releasing hormone (GRH); growth hormone inhibitory hormone (GIH, somatostatin)	Stimulates body growth; stimulates growth of epiphyseal cartilage in long bones; metabolic actions include effects on carbohydrate and lipid; some actions via somatomedins
Thyroid-stimulating hormone (TSH, thyrotropin) *glycoprotein*	Thyrotropin-releasing hormone (TRH)	Stimulates growth and secretion by thyroid gland
Adrenocorticotropic hormone (ACTH) *peptide*	Corticotropin-releasing hormone (CRH)	Stimulates growth and secretion by adrenal cortex
Follicle-stimulating hormone (FSH) *glycoprotein*	Luteinizing hormone releasing hormone (LRH), gonadotropin-releasing hormone (GnRH)	Stimulates growth and development of ovarian follicles in female; stimulate spermatogenesis in male
Luteinizing hormone (LH), or interstitial cell stimulating hormone (ICSH) *glycoprotein*	Luteinizing hormone releasing hormone (LRH), gonadotropin-releasing hormone (GnRH)	Stimulates ovulation, formation of corpus luteum, secretion of estrogen by follicle, and estrogen and progesterone by corpus luteum in female Stimulates secretion of testosterone by interstitial cells in male
Prolactin (PRL) *peptide*	Prolactin-releasing hormone (PRH); prolactin inhibitory hormone (PIH, dopamine)	Stimulates secretion by mammary glands
Posterior Pituitary (Neurohypophysis)		
Antidiuretic hormone (ADH, vasopressin) *peptide*	Osmotic pressure of plasma via hypothalamic osmoreceptors (increased OP reduces hormone release)	Increases water reabsorption in collecting ducts of kidney; decreases urine volume
Oxytocin *peptide*	Neuroendocrine reflexes initiated by stimulation of receptors in uterus and mammary glands	Contraction of uterine smooth muscle; ejection of milk from mammary glands (contraction of myoepithelial cells)
Adrenal Medulla		
Epinephrine and norepinephrine *amines*	Sympathetic nervous system	Sympathomimetic; metabolic actions include increased blood level of glucose and release of fatty acids into bloodstream
Adrenal Cortex		
Mineralocorticoids (aldosterone, corticosterone) *steroids*	Angiotensin II, also ACTH, ↓ plasma levels of Na^+ ↑ plasma levels of K^+	Increases sodium reabsorption in distal tubules of kidney, decreases excretion; decreases potassium reabsorption, increases excretion
Glucocorticoids (cortisol, hydrocortisone, deoxycorticosterone) *steroids*	Adrenocorticotropic hormone (ACTH)	Metabolic actions, including protein catabolism, increased levels of glucose and fatty acids in blood; aids in withstanding stress; in large doses suppresses inflammatory reaction
Androgens (dehydroepiandrosterone, DHEA) *steroids*	ACTH	No significant effects at normal levels
Thyroid Gland		
Thyroxin (T_4) and Triiodothyronine (T_3) *amines*	Thyroid-stimulating hormone (thyrotropin, TSH)	Increases oxygen consumption and metabolic rates of almost all cells
Calcitonin (CT) *peptide*	Calcium level in blood (increase stimulates)	Lowers calcium in blood, mainly by increasing mineral deposit in bone
Parathyroid Gland		
Parathormone (PTH) *peptide*	Calcium level in blood (decrease stimulates)	Raises calcium level in blood, by increasing withdrawal from bone, increasing reabsorption in kidney; decreases phosphate reabsorption; increases absorption from digestive tract by action on vitamin D

(*Continued*)

TABLE 71–2
The Endocrine Glands and Their Hormones (Continued)

Hormone	*Major Control of Secretion**	*Major Actions*
Pancreatic Islands		
Insulin *polypeptide*	Blood glucose level (increase stimulates, decrease inhibits); also metabolic stimuli	Lowers blood glucose level, increases entry of glucose into cells; metabolic actions include storage of glycogen, fat, and synthesis of protein
Glucagon *peptide*	Decreased blood glucose level; other metabolic stimuli	Raises blood glucose level, causes glycogenolysis, gluconeogenesis, and lipolysis with release of glucose and fatty acids into bloodstream
Somatostatin (GIH) *peptide*	Increased glucose, amino acids; also various metabolic stimuli	Inhibits release of insulin, glucagon, and several gastrointestinal hormones
Testis		
Testosterone *steroid*	Interstitial cell stimulating hormone (ICSH, LH)	Stimulates growth and development of male sex organs and sex characteristics; aids spermatogenesis
Ovary		
Estrogens (estradiol, estriol, estrone) *steroids*	Luteinizing hormone (LH)	Stimulates growth and development of female sex organs and sex characteristics
Progesterone *steroid*	Luteinizing hormone (LH)	Stimulates further development and differentiation of sex organs
Relaxin *polypeptide*		Loosening (relaxation) or pubic symphysis and pelvic ligaments; aids in dilatation of cervix of uterus at end of pregnancy
Placenta		
Human chorionic gonadotropin (HCG) *glycoprotein*		Maintains corpus luteum beyond usual life span, stimulates it to secrete estrogen and progesterone in early pregnancy
Human chorionic somatomammotropin (HCS, chorionic growth hormone–prolactin, human placental lactogen) *protein*		Growth hormone-like actions during pregnancy (maternal, not fetal)
Estrogen *steroid* Progesterone *steroid*		Together estrogen and progesterone stimulate continued growth and development of sex organs, especially endometrium during pregnancy; also mammary glands
Stomach		
Gastrin *peptide*	Vagal stimulation, presence of certain substances in stomach	Secretion by gastric mucosa, especially of hydrochloric acid
Small Intestine (Duodenum)		
Cholecystokinin-pancreozymin (CCK) *peptide*	Fat, protein digestion products in duodenum	Secretion of digestive enzymes by exocrine pancreas; contraction of gall bladder
Secretin *peptide*	Acid (low pH) in duodenum	Secretion of high-bicarbonate fluids by exocrine pancreas
Kidney		
Erythropoietin *glycoprotein*	Hypoxia (in kidney)	Increases rate of erythropoiesis in bone marrow (may also be formed by action of renal erythropoietic factor on a protein from liver)
Renin *protein* (enzyme)	Fall in renal blood flow and pressure; decreased sodium transport in renal tubule	Activates angiotensin I to angiotensin II (peptide), which is a powerful vasoconstrictor; increases secretion of aldosterone
1,25-dihydroxycholecalciferol (Vitamin D) *steroid*	Formation enhanced by parathormone	Increases blood calcium by increased intestinal absorption; causes bone resorption

* In addition to negative feedback

Posterior Pituitary

The posterior pituitary lobe hormones, antidiuretic hormone (ADH, vasopressin) and oxytocin, are really hypothalamic hormones. They are synthesized in neurons in the hypothalamus and travel down their axons to the posterior lobe. They are released from the nerve endings on the arrival of action potentials and enter nearby capillaries.

ADH. The chief action of ADH is to increase the permeability to water in cells of collecting ducts of the kidney, which allows more water to be reabsorbed from the tubular lumen. The volume of urine is reduced, but its tonicity is increased.

Secretion of ADH is controlled mainly by the effect of plasma osmotic pressure on osmoreceptors in the hypothalamus. The osmoreceptors increase ADH release when the osmotic pressure rises, and inhibit it when osmotic pressure falls. Secretion is also caused by stimulation of low pressure baroreceptors in the atria and great veins. These baroreceptors respond to lowered central venous pressure, such as might be caused by hemorrhage. Antidiuretic hormone plays a very important homeostatic role. By adjusting fluid loss to maintain tonicity of the plasma, it maintains tonicity of the extracellular fluid. It has a half-life of about 18 minutes and must be secreted continually; a lack of ADH results in excessive loss of fluid (diabetes insipidus).

Oxytocin. Oxytocin causes contraction of cells in the mammary gland and of smooth muscle cells of the pregnant uterus. Their contraction forces milk from the alveoli into the secretory ducts. Oxytocin release is part of a neuroendocrine reflex. Tactile stimulation of receptors in the nipple causes action potentials in typical afferent neurons, which reach the hypothalamus and cause release of oxytocin into the bloodstream.

Uterine smooth muscle becomes increasingly sensitive to oxytocin during the course of pregnancy, and in late pregnancy the number of oxytocin receptors also increases. Although oxytocin is not believed to initiate labor, its secretion rises after labor has begun. Tactile receptors in the cervix are stimulated by increasing pressure from the head of the fetus as labor begins. Afferent neurons from these receptors cause release of oxytocin, which increases the intensity of labor contractions.

Adrenal Gland

The encapsulated adrenal glands are situated in the perirenal fat atop the kidneys. They consist of two different glands that have come to be associated anatomically. The adrenal medulla is of neural origin and is, in effect, a sympathetic ganglion whose postganglionic neurons lack axons. It is innervated by sympathetic preganglionic (cholinergic) neurons. It secretes epinephrine and norepinephrine, and the actions of its hormones are essentially those of the sympathetic nervous system.

The adrenal cortex accounts for about 90% of the weight of the gland. Although it completely encloses the medulla, its secretory cells are apparently not innervated.

The gland has a very rich blood supply. The arteries form a plexus under the capsule that provides arteries to the cortex and sinusoids that pass between the cords of cortical cells to reach the medulla. The adrenal medulla therefore receives blood that contains cortical secretions. The adrenal veins empty into the renal veins, which drain directly into the inferior vena cava rather than the portal system.

Adrenal Medulla

Catecholamines secreted by the adrenal medulla include epinephrine (80%), norepinephrine (20%), and a small amount of dopamine. The overall actions of epinephrine and norepinephrine are similar but there are differences due largely to the distribution of receptors. There are α and β receptors in the plasma membranes of target cells, and they have been subdivided into α_1 and α_2 and β_1 and β_2 receptors. Norepinephrine and epinephrine have roughly equal affinity for the receptors, except that norepinephrine binds β_2 receptors very weakly.

Alpha$_1$ receptors are widely distributed in smooth muscle, including blood vessels, where they cause contraction (constriction). Alpha$_2$ receptors are not as widely distributed, being found mainly in presynaptic nerve endings where they modulate (mostly inhibit) the release of norepinephrine by these neurons.

Beta$_1$ receptors are found mainly in the heart where they increase all aspects of cardiac function. Beta$_2$ receptors are more widely distributed, especially in smooth muscle, where the action is inhibitory (relaxation). Thus, these catecholamines cause smooth muscle contraction by binding α receptors, and inhibit smooth muscle by binding β_2 receptors. Most of their metabolic actions involve binding of β receptors, actions in which epinephrine is much more potent than norepinephrine.

Differences between the cardiovascular actions of epinephrine and norepinephrine are significant. Both increase cardiac action (rate and force of contraction) by means of β_1 receptors, and both stimulate vascular smooth muscle (vasoconstriction) by means of α_1 receptors, which raise total peripheral resistance and mean arterial pressure. Epinephrine relaxes vascular smooth muscle (vasodilatation) by means of β_2 receptors, which are present particularly in skeletal muscle vessels. Since epinephrine causes constriction in some vascular beds and dilatation in others, it has much less effect on total peripheral resistance and arterial pressure. When epinephrine is injected (experimentally), the peripheral resistance falls slightly and mean arterial pressure changes very little (a slight rise in systolic pressure, a slight fall in diastolic pressure, and a rise in pulse pressure). Because norepinephrine lacks the dilator action, its injection causes a marked increase in peripheral resistance and raises arterial pressure. The result of this is a reflex slowing of the heart and consequent reduction in cardiac output.

Adrenal Cortex

Adrenal cortical hormones are synthesized from cholesterol, much of which is obtained from circulating low-density lipoproteins (LDLs). Adrenal cortical hormones fall into three groups: mineralocorticoids, glucocorticoids, and androgens. Mineralocorticoids, which are produced by cells in the outermost layer of the adrenal cortex, regulate Na^+ and K^+ in the extracellular fluid. The hormones secreted are aldosterone and deoxycorticosterone. They are produced in approximately equal amounts, but aldosterone is more potent and is the only one of physiological significance. Glucocorticoids are produced by cells of the middle and inner layers. The hormones secreted are cortisol (hydrocortisone) and smaller amounts of corticosterone. Large doses have a powerful anti-inflammatory action. Androgens are produced by cells of the same two layers. Dehydroepiandrosterone (DHEA) is the major androgen, although small amounts of testosterone and also progesterone and estrogen may be released. Approximately equal amounts of androgens are secreted in male and female, but DHEA is not very potent and has no significant effect when secreted in normal amounts.

Adrenocorticotropic hormone stimulates the adrenal cortex, especially the middle and inner layers. Hypophysectomy leads to atrophy of these layers but not of the outermost layer. Adrenocorticotropic hormone secretion is caused by corticotropin-releasing hormone (CRH) from the hypothalamus, and is inhibited by negative feedback of glucocorticoids (cortisol). A variety of "stressful" stimuli increase the release of CRH and cause marked increases in secretion of ACTH and glucocorticoids. Andrenocorticotropic hormone also increases the secretion of aldosterone, and its secretion is not dependent on ACTH. Angiotensin II, increased K^+, and decreased Na^+ act directly on the outermost layer of the adrenal cortex.

Mineralocorticoids. Mineralocorticoids include aldosterone and deoxycorticosterone. Aldosterone acts in the kidney, on cells of the distal tubules and proximal collecting ducts to increase reabsorption of Na^+ from the tubules. Sodium ions diffuse into tubular cells from the lumen and are actively transported out the other side into the interstitium from which they enter capillaries. Aldosterone also reduces the sodium loss in saliva, sweat, and gastric juice. Although aldosterone controls reabsorption of only about 2% of the sodium reabsorbed, this fraction is essential. The balance of sodium intake and excretion is very carefully regulated, and a 2-% decrease in reabsorption would be enough to upset that balance. It is because of the sodium-retaining action of the mineralocorticoids that the adrenal cortex is essential to life.

Aldosterone also increases the excretion of K^+, (or perhaps of H^+) in exchange for Na^+. Increased reabsorption of sodium is thus accompanied by greater excretion of K^+ or H^+ in proportions that are determined by pH and acid–base mechanisms. More potassium is excreted when the pH is relatively high (an alkaline load).

Glucocorticoids. Metabolic actions of the glucocorticoids are many, varied, interrelated, and not completely understood, but in general they maintain the energy supply and the blood glucose level during fasting for tissues that depend on them. This energy is supplied by an increased breakdown of protein and release of amino acids into the bloodstream, by breakdown of fat that increases circulating free fatty acids and by glycogenolysis in the liver and muscle, which subsequently release glucose from the liver and lactate from muscle. The glucose released from the liver is obtained both from glycogenolysis and gluconeogenesis from amino acids released by protein catabolism.

Glucocorticoids exert important "permissive" actions in which their presence is necessary for certain other actions to occur, including the actions of catecholamines and glucagon. In the absence of glucocorticoids, for example, vascular smooth muscle does not respond well to epinephrine, and there is dilatation of blood vessels with accompanying fall in blood pressure and loss of fluid from capillaries.

In pharmacological doses glucocorticoids exert a marked anti-inflammatory action. They suppress the inflammatory response at several levels and remove most of the symptoms. Glucocorticoids act by

1. Blocking the release of histamine that normally accompanies the combination of certain types of antibodies and antigens (but they do not block the antigen–antibody binding)
2. Reducing the migration of neutrophils, monocytes, and lymphocytes to the site of injury (chemotaxis)
3. Stabilizing lysosomal membranes, thereby reducing the release of lysosomal enzymes and their phagocytic actions
4. Inhibiting the action of fibroblasts that form connective tissue fibers, thus slowing repair

Such high levels of glucocorticoids, by blocking the symptoms of inflammation, mask the presence of bacterial infection, which may then spread undetected and unchecked. Since large doses inhibit the release of ACTH, cessation of such therapy may be followed by marked adrenal insufficiency.

Endocrine Pancreas

The endocrine portion of the pancreas consists of clusters of endocrine cells called the pancreatic islets or islands of Langerhans, which are scattered throughout the exocrine pancreas. Several types of secretory cells have been identified: A cells, which secrete glucagon; B cells, which produce insulin; D cells, which produce somatostatin (GIH); and F cells, which produce a pancreatic polypeptide. The hormones are released into the portal vein and pass through the liver before reaching the general circulation, and about half of the insulin and more than half of the glucagon are inactivated in the liver.

Insulin. Insulin receptors are found on the membranes of almost all cells. Some actions are exerted at the membrane and some inside the cell. The receptor-insulin complexes tend to aggregate, and then are taken into the cell. They eventually reach lysosomes and are inactivated.

The best known action of insulin is lowering the blood glucose level, but it also has important effects on fat and protein metabolism, all of which are anabolic. Insulin favors the storage of fuel sources, which is particularly important because most other metabolic hormones are catabolic in one or more actions. Insulin increases the entry of glucose into cells that transport glucose by facilitated diffusion. It activates several enzymes, including some that increase glycogenesis in the liver and skeletal muscle and including several glycolytic enzymes, and it inhibits some of the enzymes for gluconeogenesis.

Insulin inhibits breakdown and release of fatty acids from adipose tissue and favors lipogenesis from glucose owing to the increased entry of glucose into fat cells. Insulin increases the entry of amino acids into cells and their incorporation into protein. These anabolic actions reduce protein breakdown and release of amino acids, which indirectly reduces gluconeogenesis in the liver.

Together these actions lower the plasma levels of glucose, lipid, and amino acids by causing their entry into cells and conversion to glycogen, fat, or body protein. Because insulin favors the use of glucose for fuel and the storage of any excess energy source, it is of particular importance after a meal (absorptive state) when plasma levels of these substances are elevated. When insulin levels are low (postabsorptive state), as in fasting or diabetes mellitus, the blood glucose levels rise because glucose does not readily enter cells to be used or stored as glycogen or fat, and the glycogenolysis and gluconeogenesis in the liver lead to release of more glucose from the liver. The catabolic actions of other hormones on protein and lipid are not counteracted, and the increased levels of amino acids contribute to gluconeogenesis. The elevated fatty acid levels provide an energy source, but may lead to ketosis because of a limited ability to metabolize the ketone bodies formed when fatty acids are oxidized.

Insulin causes K^+ to enter cells, which lowers the extracellular K^+ levels. Insulin secretion is reduced in K^+ depletion. Exercise increases glucose entry into skeletal muscle cells and therefore reduces insulin requirements.

Insulin secretion is controlled largely by the blood glucose level in a direct feedback mechanism, but a variety of other factors also affect it. In addition to high plasma glucose levels, insulin secretion is increased by elevated blood levels of amino acids, gastrointestinal hormones (secretin, gastrin, and CCK), and glucagon and by vagal stimulation and β-adrenergic stimulators. Its secretion is inhibited by somatostatin, α-adrenergic stimulators, and low blood glucose.

Glucagon. Glucagon is chemically similar to the intestinal hormone secretin, and they share some actions. Glucagon is also secreted in small amounts by cells of the stomach and duodenum. Its secretion is increased by such factors as increased plasma levels of amino acids and cortisol, sympathetic stimulation, exercise, and various "stressful" stimuli, and it is inhibited by insulin, glucose, and somatostatin.

The actions of glucagon are similar to those of epinephrine. Glucagon acts primarily in the liver, and it is generally antagonistic to insulin. The role of glucagon has been described as prevention of hypoglycemia and making energy sources available between meals; it mobilizes energy sources. The actions are generally hyperglycemic, owing to glycogenolysis and gluconeogenesis in the liver, and the release of glucose from the liver. It also increases the breakdown of fat and release of fatty acids and glycerol into the circulation, and thus is ketogenic.

The insulin/glucagon ratio is an important consideration. The ratio is high when glucose is available and is being stored, but low when glucose supply is low. A number of enzymes involved in metabolic regulation (*i.e.*, glycolysis, glycogenolysis, Krebs cycle, fatty acid metabolism) are either activated or inactivated, depending on the relative amounts of insulin and glucagon.

Thyroid Gland

The thyroid gland consists of numerous spherical follicles. The thyroid hormones, thyroxine (T_4) and triiodothyronine (T_3), are synthesized and stored in the follicles. Clusters of interstitial cells between the follicles produce calcitonin.

Thyroid hormones are unique in their iodine content. The follicle cells have a great ability to trap iodine, as iodide (I^-). They actively pump it into the cells, where its concentration is 10 to 100 times greater than in the plasma.

In the circulation, the hormones are almost entirely bound to one of several plasma proteins (T_4, 99.98% and T_3, 99.8%). Unbound molecules diffuse into target cells and bind receptors in the nucleus. T_3 is three to four times more potent than T_4, and it binds more readily. T_4 is converted to T_3 in many cells, and some believe the conversion is necessary for it to act.

The major effect of thyroid hormones is increased oxygen consumption of almost all tissues (exceptions include the brain, anterior pituitary, and spleen). Most of the other effects are secondary to the increased metabolic rate. Thyroid hormones are closely associated with the catecholamines. Several thyroid hormone actions resemble β-adrenergic effects. They increase the number of β-adrenergic receptors in the heart. Thyroid hormones are essential for normal brain development, and also speed mental action in adults. The latter is dependent on actions on specific processes rather than increased metabolic rate, since thyroid hormones do not increase brain oxygen consumption.

Secretion of thyroid hormones is increased by thyroid-stimulating hormone (TSH) from the anterior pituitary, and inhibited by negative feedback of T_3 and T_4. Thyroid-stimulating hormone is secreted in response to thyrotropin-releasing hormone (TRH) from the hypothalamus, which is also inhibited by negative feedback of thyroid hormones.

Parathyroid Glands

The parathyroid glands consist of several tiny bits of gland embedded in the posterior surface of the thyroid gland. They secrete parathormone (PTH), which raises the plasma calcium level. PTH secretion is controlled directly by plasma calcium, so that a fall in calcium causes secretion and a rise inhibits it. Parathormone is the major factor in the regulation of calcium and phosphorus in the extracellular fluid, with the assistance of calcitonin (CT) from the thyroid gland and vitamin D. Together they help to control the movement of calcium and phosphate in and out of the extracellular fluid by actions on bone, kidney, and digestive tract (Fig. 71–3).

About 99% of the body's calcium is in bone. The remainder is primarily in the extracellular fluid, since calcium is essentially an extracellular ion. Of the 10 mg/dl (4.5–5 mEq/liter) of calcium in the plasma, nearly half is protein bound. Small amounts of calcium are necessary for a variety of vital

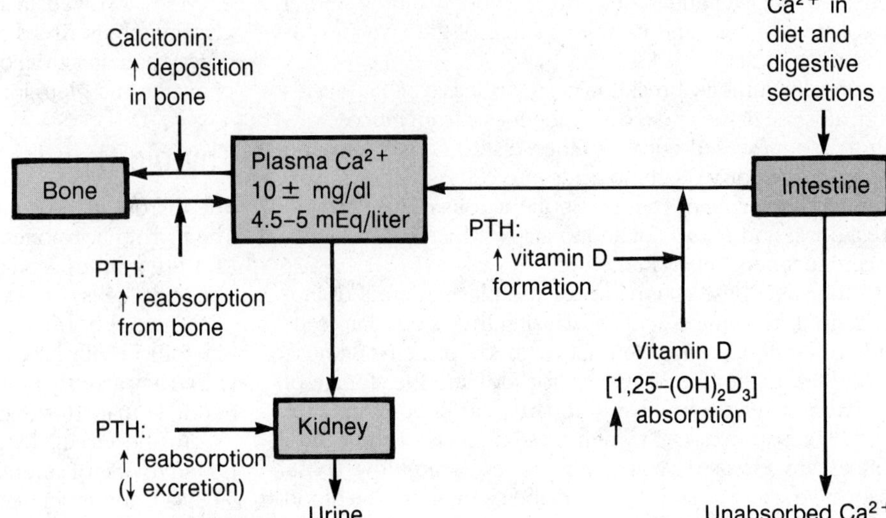

FIGURE 71–3 Hormonal regulation of calcium metabolism.

processes: blood clotting, normal contraction of cardiac and skeletal muscle, release of neurotransmitters and other secretions, and normal excitability of nerve and muscle cells. The latter is the most critical, however, for this action is responsible for the hypocalcemic tetany associated with lack of PTH. Calcium lowers the excitability (raises the threshold) of these cells by increasing the amount of depolarization needed to produce an action potential. When extracellular calcium is low, the excitability is increased (threshold is lowered), leading to unwanted action potentials that cause muscle contractions and tetany. The condition can be fatal if the muscles of respiration are affected.

Parathormone. Parathormone (PTH) prevents a fall in plasma calcium levels in several ways. It causes withdrawal (resorption) of calcium from bone, by stimulating osteocytes and osteoclasts. They take up Ca^{2+} from adjacent bone matrix and then actively transport it out the other side of the cell where it enters capillaries. It reduces renal excretion of Ca^{2+} by increasing active transport of Ca^{2+} from the lumen of distal tubules in the kidney. Since bone mineral is a calcium-phosphate complex, withdrawal of mineral increases plasma levels as well as phosphate calcium. Parathormone increases excretion of inorganic phosphate, thereby preventing phosphatemia when bone mineral is resorbed. Normally phosphorus is actively reabsorbed from the proximal tubules. PTH inhibits this process, so more phosphorus is excreted. Parathormone also increases absorption of calcium from the gut.

Calcitonin. Calcitonin (CT) from the thyroid gland acts as a PTH antagonist. It tends to lower calcium levels, and its secretion is increased when the plasma calcium level rises, and inhibited when the plasma calcium level falls. Calcitonin reduces bone resorption, probably by lowering Ca^{2+} permeability of the bone cells. It also increases phosphate excretion by the kindey. The physiological role of CT is questionable, because there is no known "deficiency" condition. Its role may be to serve as a check or restraint on PTH activity in bone.

Vitamin D. Although a precursor of 1,25-dihydroxycholecalciferol is obtained in the diet, the active form is produced in the body, so that it qualifies as a hormone. Sunlight (ultraviolet light) activates certain prohormones in the skin, which are transported to the liver for modification and then to the kidney for final activation, a step that is enhanced by PTH. The main action of Vitamin D is on the wall of the digestive tract where it increases active transport (absorption) of calcium and phosphate, and therefore helps to assure adequate levels of the ions needed for mineralization of bone.

Bibliography

Ganong WF: Review of Medical Physiology, 11th ed, Chaps 17–24. Los Altos CA, Lange Medical Publications, 1983

Greenspan FS, Forsham PH: Basic and Clinical Endocrinology, 1st ed. Los Altos CA, Lange Medical Publications, 1983

Leeson TS, Leeson CR: Histology, 4th ed. Philadelphia, WB Saunders, 1981

Sawin CT: Endocrine Physiology, Part X. In Ross G: Essentials of Human Physiology, 2nd ed, Chaps 37–42. Chicago, Year Book Medical Publishers, 1982

Chapter 72

Assessment of Endocrine Function

Christine A. Larson

The regulatory effects of the endocrine system are diverse and affect most of the bodily functions. Endocrine disorders are the result of overproduction or underproduction of one or more hormones. The many signs and symptoms of endocrine dysfunction are expressions of the accentuation or absence of the hormone's physiological actions. Because of the widespread effects of hormones on the body, endocrine syndromes can produce a confusing clinical picture, sometimes mimicking disorders of vastly different etiologies.

The subtleties of early endocrine manifestations are easily illustrated. Most hormones affect energy metabolism and muscle function, so that their deficit may lead to weight changes, fatigue, and apathy, vague symptoms that can be attributed to many physiological and psychological causes. Indeed, many patients are labeled as depressed, malingering, or simply psychoneurotic, while the true cause of endocrinologic dysfunction goes undiagnosed and untreated. In late stages of endocrine dysfunction, however, obvious changes in the patient's physical habitus make recognition easier.[3]

The health practitioner must be thorough and alert to all pertinent information, both subjective and objective, obtained during the course of history taking and physical examination, and should be suspicious of any reported or observed changes in mental acuity, emotional stability, energy levels, weight, appetite, skin, and libido. (See Table 72–1.) Some of the more general signs of endocrine dysfunction are the easiest to overlook and as different as blood pressure changes, menstrual irregularities, and psychiatric illness. Although careful history taking and physical examination can provide presumptive evidence of an endocrine abnormality, the definitive diagnosis invariably depends on the laboratory data.

History

Direct examination of the endocrine system is difficult because of the anatomical positioning of most endocrine organs. However, information from the patient can supply important clues to their functioning. A thorough history should be obtained from the patient or the person acting on the patient's behalf. Questioning of this person is important because mental acuity is often compromised in many pathological endocrine states, making the patient a vague and inaccurate historian. The following information is more endocrine-specific and should be included in data gathering. (See Chapters 101 and 102 for gonadotropic disorders.)

Present State of Health

Patients with endocrine disease often present with nonspecific complaints. The chief complaint may not relate to just one but a group of symptoms. The most common presenting problems include fatigue, weakness, menstrual changes, weight changes, and bone pains. It is important to determine if the appearance of these symptoms has been gradual or sudden and what the patient has done about them. It is also essential to know what medication, prescribed or nonprescribed, the patient has been taking. Medication history is significant because some drugs can mimic or cause endocrine disease and interfere with diagnostic laboratory tests, and others are used to control or treat endocrine disorders.

Health History

In addition to usual questions about past medical, surgical, obstetrical, or traumatic events, details about birth weight, growth rate, weight patterns, and stages of physical and emotional development should be sought. To obtain information related to growth or development in the child or adolescent, family doctors and school records may be invaluable sources.

Specific information required may vary depending on the presenting condition. For instance, data regarding past radiation therapy to the head and neck are especially important when thyroid nodules are suspected.

Family History

Along with routine questioning, information about thyroid disease and diabetes mellitus should be included since these conditions have a familial tendency. Questions about a family history of growth, weight, and developmental problems and hirsutism are also important in distinguishing an abnormality from a normal family tendency.

Social and Personal History

Since some endocrine conditions are exacerbated by stress, the patient should be asked about recent emotional upheaval in the workplace or at home and to identify any current physical or emotional stressors. Many endocrine disorders require lifelong management and medication (*e.g.,* Addison's disease, diabetes mellitus, and hypothyroidism). Information about the patient's usual coping patterns is essential for proper counseling. Perhaps of greatest importance is the patient's perception of the impact his condition and prescribed treatment has on his lifestyle.

Review of Systems

When recording the review of systems, information about the following should be included.

GENERAL

Has the patient experienced increased fatigue, weakness, or lethargy?
What is the level of activity tolerance, *i.e.,* Can the patient climb a flight of stairs without feeling short of breath? At what times of day is he most fatigued?
Have there been changes in sleep patterns? What are these changes?
Has there been a gradual or sudden weight gain or loss? How much weight over how long a time?
Has linear growth been accelerated or delayed (especially in the child)?
Has the number of infections experienced increased?
Has there been any noticeable increase in heat or cold temperature intolerance?

HEAD AND NECK

Has the patient experienced headaches? How often and what kind?
Have there been any noticeable changes in vision (*e.g.,* diplopia)?
Has his voice changed, becoming more hoarse or gruff?
Has the patient experienced any neck pain?
If so, does it radiate to the ear?

SKIN

Have there been any noticeable changes in skin such as:
- Increased or decreased pigmentation?
- Excessive or decreased perspiration?
- Increased oiliness or dryness?
- Delayed wound healing?
- Increased bruising?
- Edema or puffiness?
- Decreased, excessive, or abnormal distribution of body hair?

CARDIORESPIRATORY

Has the patient experienced any episodes of palpitations?
Does he experience vertigo on arising from a reclining position?
Has there been any noticeable breathing difficulty or exertional dyspnea?

GASTROINTESTINAL

Has there been increase or decrease in appetite?
What is the amount and type of food intake on an average daily basis?
What is the average alcohol consumption per day or week?
Have there been problems with nausea, vomiting, diarrhea, or constipation?

URINARY

Has there been a sudden increase or decrease in the frequency of urination? What is the approximate volume of urine passed?
Must the patient awaken at night to urinate?
Has there been a noticeable increase in thirst? Is it insatiable?
What is the average fluid intake per day? What kinds of fluids?

REPRODUCTIVE

What was the age of onset and speed of advancement through pubertal stages?
At what age was the start of menarche? Date of last menstrual period?

Have there been changes in the menstrual cycle?
Has there been a decline in libido?
Are there concerns about impotency?
Have the breasts (man or woman) been secreting a discharge or milk (galactorrhea)?

NEUROLOGICAL

Have there been any reported mental changes such as depression, inappropriate euphoria, frequent crying spells, or increased irritability?
Are there complaints of increased anxiety, nervousness, or memory impairment?
Has the patient noticed tremors of his extremities during periods of sustained posture?
Has the patient experienced numbness or tingling of his face or extremities?
Are feelings of weakness generalized or localized?

MUSCULOSKELETAL

Has the patient experienced bone pains, arthralgia, or muscle cramps?
Have the changes in size or proportion of the head, hands, feet, or tongue been noticed (*e.g.*, increases in hat, glove, or ring size)?
Has there been a series of fractures over the past few years?

Physical Assessment

The clinical approach to physical assessment will differ according to the presenting problem. Thus if the patient is of shorter than normal stature, the signs and symptoms of pituitary or thyroid deficiency should be sought with particular vigor because the pituitary and the thyroid are important glands associated with growth. Table 72–1 lists clues that may alert the nurse to the presence of endocrine dysfunction. Physical assessment of the endocrine system focuses primarily on obtaining data by means of inspection and palpation. Except for determining the extent of secondary disorders, the use of auscultation and percussion is limited.

Inspection

When collecting objective data, the nurse should pay particular attention to the patient's growth and developmental status and keep in mind the patient's age, race, and familial or genetic predisposition when deciding whether variations noted in growth, pubertal development, and hair distribution are within normal limits. Endocrine dysfunction can mildly or markedly alter the maturation of the body. To determine whether or not the abnormal physical characteristics observed in the patient are indeed pathological or are simply inherited traits, family members should be examined for similar traits (*e.g.*, abnormal stature or unusual fat distribution). The patient's mental acuity, behavior, and pattern of speech can also be assessed during history taking.

GENERAL APPEARANCE

Level of consciousness and alertness
Appearance neat or disheveled, dress appropriate or inappropriate
Facial expression and posture (any evidence of distress, discomfort, fatigue, apathy, or anxiety)
Shape of face (note roundness or puffiness)
Apparent dyspnea

PHYSICAL CHARACTERISTICS

Height
Body frame (small, medium, or large)
Limb growth (span)*
Upper/lower body ratio†
Weight, appropriateness to height and body frame
Body alignment and symmetry of paired structures
Abnormal appearance or absence of *secondary* sex characteristics, *i.e.,* development of breasts and external genitalia
Abnormal milk discharge from breasts
Shape and proportion of head, facial features, hands and feet

INTEGUMENT

Color and areas of increased or absent pigmentation (skin and mucous membranes)
Skin temperature and turgor
Dryness, scaliness, oiliness, increased perspiration
Atrophic or leathery appearance
Bruises or rashes
Lesions and unhealed cuts
Edema, dependent or periorbital
Purplish striae on abdomen, breasts, and upper thighs

BODY HAIR

Appropriate distribution
Excess (hirsutism) or absence of body hair
Texture (brittle, coarse, or fine)
Head hair easily pulled out or resistant to pulling

EYES

Visual acuity
Fields of vision (particularly note peripheral vision loss)
Eyelids normal or drooping (lid lag)
Extraocular movements present
Shape and size (check for exophthalmos)
Clarity of cornea (check for cataracts)
Nystagmus
Retinal fields for diabetic retinopathy or optic atrophy

MUSCULOSKELETON

Presence of tremors or paresthesias (include tongue)
Strength and tone (ability to lift legs, arms, or head against moderate counterpressure by examiner)

* The distance between the upper extremities, from the tip of one middle finger to the other, with the arms outstretched. In the adult, the span should approximately equal the height.

† Normally the ground-to-pubis distance is slightly shorter than that between the pubis and crown.

TABLE 72–1
Clinical Manifestations and Their Common Endocrine Causes*

Clinical Manifestation	*Endocrine Disorder*
Neurological	
Fatigue	Adrenal insufficiency, hypothyroidism, hypoglycemia, acromegaly, hyperparathyroidism
Nervousness	Hypoglycemia, pheochromocytoma, thyrotoxicosis
Confusion, somnolence, coma	Diabetic ketoacidosis, severe hypoglycemia, syndrome of inappropriate antidiuretic hormone (SIADH), hypothyroidism
Paresthesias	Hypothyroidism, hypoparathyroidism, acromegaly, diabetes mellitus
Headache	Pituitary tumors, pheochromocytoma, hyperaldosteronism, hypoglycemia
Psychosis	Hypoglycemia, hypothyroidism, hyperthyroidism, Cushing's syndrome, syndrome of inappropriate antidiuretic hormone (SIADH), hyperparathyroidism, adrenal insufficiency
Cardiovascular	
Hypertension	Hyperaldosteronism, Cushing's syndrome, hypothyroidism, hyperparathyroidism, pheochromocytoma
Orthostatic hypotension	Adrenal insufficiency, hyperaldosteronism, diabetes mellitus, pheochromocytoma
Bradycardia	Hypothyroidism
Tachycardia or tachyarrhythmia	Hyperthyroidism, pheochromocytoma, adrenal insufficiency
Congestive heart failure	Hyperthyroidism, hypothyroidism, Cushing's syndrome
Gastrointestinal	
Anorexia	Adrenal insufficiency, hypothyroidism, hyperparathyroidism
Peptic ulcer	Cushing's syndrome, multiple endocrine adenomatosis (MEN) Type I
Diarrhea	Hyperthyroidism, adrenal insufficiency, thyroid carcinoma
Constipation	Hyperparathyroidism, hypothyroidism, pheochromocytoma
Weight loss	Adrenal insufficiency, hyperthyroidism, diabetes mellitus, pheochromocytoma, diabetes insipidus
Abdominal pain	Adrenal insufficiency, hyperparathyroidism, hyperthyroidism, diabetes mellitus
Musculoskeletal	
Weakness	Hyperthyroidism, hypothyroidism, Cushing's syndrome, adrenal insufficiency, hyperparathyroidism, hypoparathyroidism, hyperaldosteronism
Pathological fractures	Cushing's syndrome, hyperparathyroidism
Joint pain	Hypothyroidism, acromegaly
Bone pain	Hyperparathyroidism, Cushing's syndrome
Bone thickening	Acromegaly
Reproductive	
Amenorrhea	Hyperthyroidism, hypogonadism, Cushing's syndrome, acromegaly, pituitary tumor, Sheehan's syndrome
Loss of libido of impotency	Hypogonadism, hypothyroidism, adrenal insufficiency, acromegaly, diabetes mellitus
Gynecomastia	Hypogonadism, thyroid dysfunction, pituitary tumor
Urologic	
Polyuria	Hyperparathyroidism, hyperaldosteronism, diabetes insipidus, diabetes mellitus
Kidney stones	Cushing's syndrome, hyperparathyroidism, acromegaly
Integumentary	
Hirsutism	Adrenal hyperfunction, congenital adrenal hyperplasia, acromegaly
Hair loss	Hypoparathyroidism, hypothyroidism, Cushing's syndrome, various autoimmune disorders
Sparse body hair	Pituitary insufficiency, adrenal insufficiency, hypogonadism

(*Continued*)

TABLE 72–1
Clinical Manifestations and Their Common Endocrine Causes* *(Continued)*

Clinical Manifestation	*Endocrine Disorder*
Integumentary	
Hyperpigmentation	Addison's disease, hyperthyroidism, ectopic ACTH production
Vitiligo	Many autoimmune endocrine diseases
Profuse diaphoresis	Acromegaly, hyperthyroidism, hypoglycemia, pheochromocytoma
Atrophic, fine skin	Cushing's syndrome, hypothyroidism
Thick, leathery skin	Acromegaly
Ecchymosis	Cushing's syndrome
Edema	Cushing's syndrome, hypothyroidism
Ocular/Visual	
Diplopia	Graves' disease, hypoglycemia, pituitary tumor
Visual field deficit	Pituitary tumor
Periorbital swelling	Hypothyroidism, Graves' disease
Exophthalmos	Graves' disease, Hashimoto's thyroiditis
Body Habitus	
Round face	Cushing's syndrome, pseudohypoparathyroidism
Short stature	Prepubertal growth hormone deficiency, childhood hypothyroidism, childhood Cushing's syndrome, pseudohypoparathyroidism
Abnormally tall stature	Prepubertal growth hormone excess
Laboratory Findings	
Anemia	Adrenal insufficiency, pituitary insufficiency, thyroid dysfunction, hyperparathyroidism
Hyponatremia	Syndrome of inappropriate antidiuretic hormone (SIADH), adrenal insufficiency, pituitary insufficiency, hypothyroidism
Hypokalemia	Cushing's syndrome, hyperaldosteronism
Hyperkalemia	Adrenal insufficiency
Hypocalcemia	Hypoparathyroidism
Hypercalcemia	Hyperparathyroidism, adrenal insufficiency, hyperthyroidism

* Based on information found in Harvey AM: Practice of Medicine, 12th ed. New York, Appleton-Century-Crofts, 1980

Degree of muscle atrophy (note symmetry)
Shape of spine (look for evidence of kyphosis and lordosis)
Deep tendon reflexes*

VOICE

Appropriateness of speech patterns
Quality (hoarseness and volume)

VITAL SIGNS

Elevated or decreased body temperature
Hypertension (paroxysmal?)
Orthostatic hypotension
Tachycardia or bradycardia

Palpation of Thyroid Gland

The thyroid gland is one of the few endocrine organs (the other being the gonads) that are routinely examined by palpation. Palpation provides information about its size, shape, symmetry, and tenderness. The examiner must be familiar with the anatomical position of the midline neck structures. The hyoid bone, thyroid cartilage, cricoid cartilage, and tracheal rings should be identified before palpating.

*A complete neurological examination is advisable.

The neck is first inspected for obvious thyroid tissue. Usually the position of the thyroid gland is not visible. A feature that distinguishes the thyroid from other masses in the neck is its upward movement on swallowing. This movement occurs because of the intimate connection between the gland and larynx. Palpation of the thyroid gland can be done using a posterior or anterior approach. With either approach, the examiner must use care to avoid exerting too much pressure upon the delicate structures.

Posterior Approach. The patient should be seated with the examiner standing directly behind him. With fingers curved and both thumbs resting on the back of the patient's neck, the index and middle fingers of both hands should gently feel for the thyroid isthmus and anterior surfaces of

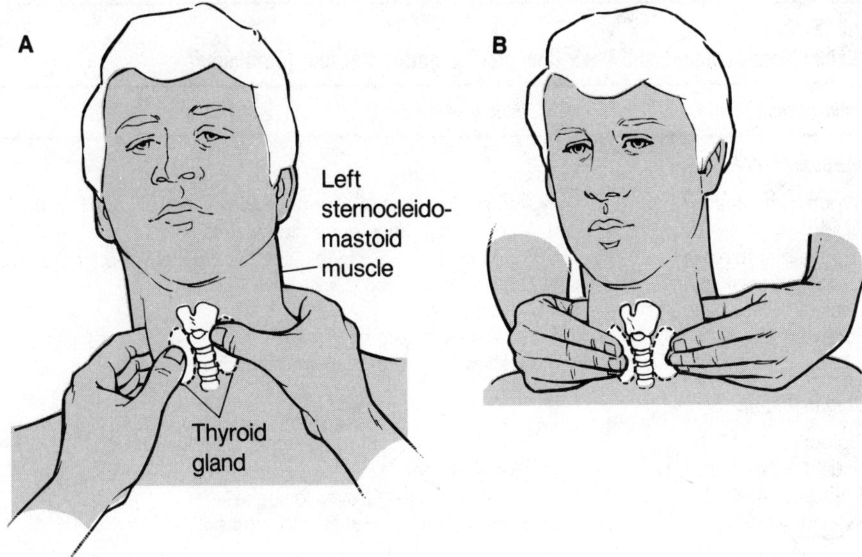

FIGURE 72–1 Palpation of the thyroid gland. (*A*) Anterior approach. (*B*) Posterior approach.

the lateral lobes. The isthmus may be more readily located by asking the patient to swallow.

To palpate the right lobe, the patient is asked to flex his neck slightly forward and to the right. This relaxes the neck muscles and facilitates examination. With the fingers on the left hand, the examiner then displaces the thyroid gland to the right. The right thumb is placed behind the sternocleidomastoid muscle, and the index and middle fingers are used to palpate the right lateral lobe of the thyroid. To facilitate palpation, the patient again is asked to swallow. The procedure for palpating the left lobe is simply the reverse, displacing the gland with the right hand and palpating with the left.[10] (Fig. 72–1, *A*). In most patients the gland itself cannot be felt, but the isthmus is distinguishable. If palpable, the thyroid gland should feel smooth. An enlarged thyroid usually feels finely lobulated, like a well-defined organ. Thyroid nodules feel like firm protuberances or swellings. A firm, fixed nodule may indicate the presence of a tumor. Pain or tenderness is an indication of acute inflammation and acute thyroiditis.[5]

Anterior Approach. The examiner stands in front of the patient. The isthmus is palpated just below the cricoid cartilage with the plamar aspects of the second and third fingers. Again, palpation is enhanced by having the patient swallow. The isthmus should move upward. To feel the right lobe, the patient's neck should be slightly flexed and tilted to the right. In this approach, the examiner displaces the thyroid to the left with the right hand. The left middle and index fingers are hooked behind the sternocleidomastoid muscle and the right lobe is palpated with the left thumb. The palpating fingers should be below or at the lower level of the thyroid cartilage. The procedure is reversed to palpate the left lobe.[1] (Fig. 72–1, *B*).

Although the examiner may prefer one approach, both approaches may be required to detect subtle abnormalities of the thyroid gland. The examiner should palpate as much of the gland as possible, carefully recording the size, consistency, configuration, and number of abnormal nodules present. If the thyroid gland is believed to be enlarged, it should be auscultated. Hypertrophy of the gland increases blood flow through thyroid arteries and produces vibrations that can be heard with a stethoscope as a bruit.

Laboratory Studies

Hormones in body fluids are found in extremely small concentrations, requiring measurement techniques that are very sensitive and precise. The three methods of measurement are bioassays, chemical assays, and displacement assays.

Bioassays are generally used only for research purposes, since they tend to be cumbersome and lack sufficient sensitivity. *Chemical assays* are more useful clinically for measuring hormones and their metabolites in either serum or urine. *Displacement assays,* also termed *radioimmunoassays* (RIA), are the most commonly used and precise method of measurement. This kind of assay depends on the use of radionuclide labeling and specific binding reagents, such as antibodies, specific binding proteins, cellular receptors, and enzymes. This technique accurately detects very small concentrations of many hormones (as well as some peptides, vitamins, and drugs) and demonstrates good sensitivity and specificity.[8]

Laboratory evaluation of patients with endocrine problems is directed toward two goals. Initially, baseline studies are done to measure circulating levels of hormones suspected to be in excessive or deficient amounts. If a hormone is found in abnormal quantity, more definitive studies are done to determine the exact location of the disorder. Toward achieving the latter goal, it is helpful to use stimulation and suppression tests. *Stimulation tests* are done to determine whether a low circulating level of a particular hormone is a problem of function or of control. For example, an adrenocorticotropin hormone (ACTH) stimulation test can be performed if a patient is suspected of having adrenal hypofunction. This test may help in determining if the hypofunction is a primary problem in the adrenal cortex itself or if it is secondary to a pituitary lesion.[6] Thus, if the adrenal cortex does not secrete more cortisol in response to administered ACTH, a diagnosis of primary hypofunction of the adrenal cortex can be made.

Suppression tests are more useful in evaluating abnormal hyperfunction of specific organs. For example, glucose normally suppresses growth hormone (GH) levels. If GH is not suppressed after ingestion of a glucose load, an abnormality in GH secretion, such as occurs in acromegaly, is suspected.[6]

It should be noted that measurement of a hormone in the blood is limited to the hormone level within the body at the time the specimen is drawn. A single determination of a specific hormone can reflect neither the diurnal fluctuations nor the temporary changes in circulating levels that normally occur with many hormones. Therefore repeated measurements, with consideration given to diurnal hormone variations, give more reliable results.[8] More accurate than random blood sampling is the 24-hour urine analysis that measures levels of specific hormones and their metabolites. This method reflects normal hormone fluctuations within the body.

Stress, poor nutritional status, and drug therapy all may influence hormonal secretion. Many of the tests are invasive, causing the patient some discomfort and anxiety, which in turn may affect the levels of stress hormones and alter test accuracy. It is important for the nurse to prepare the patient for diagnostic testing in the best way to reduce stress. Acknowledging a patient's anxiety is a good way to begin. Clear instructions should be given as to the purpose and method of testing, and what to expect before and after the test. Physical preparation may vary from one institution to another. Scheduling of the test is often a nursing responsibility, and consideration should be given to the effects of diurnal fluctuations of some circulating hormones. For example, cortisol levels usually peak in the early morning hours and ebb in the evening. Therefore, peak and baseline blood levels of cortisol should be drawn at 8 AM and 8 PM (or 4 PM), respectively. In addition to laboratory studies, radiography, computerized axial tomography (CAT scan) and pneumoencephalography (for pituitary tumors) may be done.

Diagnostic tests of endocrine function are outlined in Table 72–2. They are grouped according to specific glandular etiology. The purpose, procedure, and interpretation of each test is briefly described. In addition, considerations relevant to the nursing care of the patient before and after each test are discussed.

TABLE 72–2
Outline of Endocrine Diagnostic Studies[2,4,5,7,9–15]

Study	*Purpose and Procedure*	*Interpretation*	*Nursing Considerations*
Pituitary Function Tests			
Blood Studies			
Basal growth hormone levels	To screen for hypopituitary states and acromegaly. A radioimmunoassay of blood is taken after an overnight fast.	Normal values: Males, <5 ng/ml Females, <8 ng/ml Increased levels are diagnostic of acromegaly. Values <1 ng/ml may indicate hypopituitarism.	NPO after midnight if blood drawn between 7 and 8 AM. Patient should be at rest for at least 1.5 hr before test because activity increases GH levels. No smoking before and during test. The following drugs may elevate GH levels: β-adrenergic drugs, alcohol, and oral contraceptives.
Growth hormone stimulation test	To screen for hypopituitarism. After overnight fast and before ambulation, arginine HCl 0.5 g/kg is infused IV over 30 min. Regular insulin, 0.1–1.5 U/kg, may be infused instead. Blood samples for GH are drawn 30, 60, and 90 min after infusion. Exercise may also be used as stimulation. The patient exercises on a bicycle ergometer against known resistance for 10 min. Blood samples of GH are drawn 25 min following start of exercise.	A threefold rise over baseline GH should be seen. Subnormal response should be reconfirmed by repeating test after a 24-hr wait. Low values are indicative of hypopituitarism.	NPO after midnight if blood drawn in early AM. Bedrest for at least 1.5 hr before test. When insulin is used, observe carefully for severe hypoglycemic reaction. Dextrose 50% should be readily available. This test is contraindicated for patients with Addison's disease, myocardial infarction, and epilepsy. No stimulation of GH is seen in many overweight individuals.

(*Continued*)

TABLE 72–2
Outline of Endocrine Diagnostic Studies[2,4,5,7,9–15] *(Continued)*

Study	*Purpose and Procedure*	*Interpretation*	*Nursing Considerations*
Pituitary Function Tests			
Glucose suppression test	To screen for acromegaly. After an overnight fast and during bed rest, GH is measured before and 1 hr after oral 100-g glucose administration.	Normal values: <1 ng/ml Persistant elevation is diagnostic of acromegaly.	Patient should be rested 1.5 hr before and during testing.
Basal prolactin levels	Done when pituitary tumors suspected. An early morning blood sample is drawn.	Normal values: Males, 1–20 ng/ml Females, 1–25 ng/ml Values >300 ng/ml is highly indicative of pituitary tumors. Values of 100–300 ng/ml seen in 50% of patients with pituitary tumors	Npo after midnight. Instruct patient to avoid exercise and breast stimulation prior to test. The following drugs may cause elevations in prolactin levels: phenothiazines, reserpine, estrogen, and tricyclic antidepressants.
Water deprivation test	To evaluate antidiuretic hormone secretion. Water is withheld and hourly serum and urine osmolality samples are obtained. This test is done until 3 consecutive urine samples have about equal osmolarity (a plateau); may take 6–8 hr	Normal values: Serum = 285–295 mOsm/liter Urine = 300–800 mOsm/liter Diabetes insipidus is suspected with the following values at plateau: Serum = >300 mOsm/liter Urine = <300 mOsm/liter	Describe test to patient. Obtain hourly urine specimens. Monitor specific gravity of urine. Assess for dehydration. Use measures to abate thirst. Test is contraindicated in hypercalcemic states.
Other Studies			
Skull x-ray films Computerized axial tomography (CT scans)	To screen for a variety of pituitary diseases. A sagittal and frontal views are obtained. The sella turcica is assessed for size, volume, and erosion. Measurements should be compared with those of the normal sella turcica.	Abnormalities may be indicative of diseases of the hypothalamic pituitary axis. Focal bulging and anterior wall thinning of the sella turcica may be early signs of microadenoma.	No special preparation required except describe study to patient.
Thyroid Function Tests			
Blood Studies			
Thyroxine concentration [T_4(RIA)]	To evaluate thyroid function. Simple blood sample is drawn to measure serum thyroxine level, using radioimmunoassay technique.	Normal values: 5–12 μg/dl Elevation indicates hyperthyroidism. Decreased values indicate hypothyroidism. *Note:* 5 out of 100 normal individuals have abnormal levels. If T_4 levels are abnormal, thyroid-binding globulin (TBG) should be measured.	No special preparation required. Lowered plasma-binding proteins, as seen in malnutrition and liver disease, may give low values. Low values are also seen after administration of salicylates, glucocorticoids, and phenytoin. High values may be seen in pregnancy and with oral contraceptive use.
Triiodothyronine concentration [T_3(RIA)]	Useful in conjunction with T_4 in screening for thyroid hyperfunction in the presence of a normal T_4. Only a routine blood sample is required. Radioimmunoassay technique is used.	Normal values: 75–225 ng/dl Elevated values indicate hyperthyroidism. Not a useful test in hypothyroidism	Same as for T_4 except it is not affected by salicylates or phenytoin
Resin triiodothyronine uptake (RT_3U)	Indirectly measures thyroid-binding globulin in (TBG) capacity. Radioactive T_3 is added to blood sample to bind with unoccupied sites on TBG. The amounts of bound T_3 are measured.	Normal values: 25–30% of radioactive T_3 will bind High values seen in hyperthyroidism Low values seen in hypothyroidism	No special preparation required. False-positive readings seen in pregnancy and with estrogen use. False-negative values seen with drugs such as phenytoin and salicylates.

(Continued)

TABLE 72–2
Outline of Endocrine Diagnostic Studies[2,4,5,7,9–15] *(Continued)*

Study	*Purpose and Procedure*	*Interpretation*	*Nursing Considerations*
Thyroid Function Tests			
Free T_4 index (FT_4I)	A good measurement of T_4 levels despite variable levels of plasma thyroid-binding proteins It multiplies values of RT_3U and T_4.	Normal values: 3.8–14.9 units Low values may be seen in hypothyroidism. High values seen in hyperthyroidism	No special preparation required.
Radioactive iodine (^{131}I) uptake (RAIU)	A common measurement of thyroid activity. A tracer dose of ^{131}I is given IV or PO. Serum uptake measurements are taken 4, 6, 8, 24 and, perhaps, 48 hr after dosing. A 24-hr urine sample is also obtained. Radioactive iodine is often combined with a thyroid scan.	Normal values: *Serum:* 15–35% uptake of ^{131}I in 24 hr. Early uptake indicates hyperthyroidism. Delayed uptake indicates hypothyroidism. *Urine:* Excretion of 40–60% ^{131}I in 24 hr. Low values indicate hyperthyroidism. High values indicate hypothyroidism.	Many iodine preparations can interfere with ^{131}I studies and should be discontinued before testing, such as iodine-rich foods (seafood), some cough medicines, and radiopaque dyes. Nephrotic syndrome can increase ^{131}I uptake. Glucocorticoids and sulfonylureas decrease ^{131}I uptake. The patient should by reassured about the minimal risk from the radioactive preparation. Nursing responsibility includes accurate 24-hr urine collection.
Thyroid stimulation hormone (TSH) stimulation test	To evaluate thyroid function and differentiate between primary and secondary hypothyroidism. TSH, 10 U, is given IM daily for 3 days. Baseline ^{131}I uptake and protein bound iodine (PBI) tests are done on day before test. They are repeated on day 3.	^{131}I uptake of >10% and PBI of 7–11 μg/dl support the diagnosis of secondary hypothyroidism or euthyroidism.	Patient may continue to take thyroid medications throughout test. Avoid intake of iodinated preparations that may alter ^{131}I uptake test.
Thyronine releasing hormone (TRH) stimulation test	To evaluate pituitary–thyroid axis, TSH reserve, and borderline hypothyroidism or hyperthyroidism. Blood is drawn to measure baseline TSH (normal values: 1.9–5.4 μU/ml). TRH, 200–500 μg, is then given IV. TSH measurements are made at 0, 30, and 60 min after infusion (drawing at 45 min is optional).	Normal value shows doubling of baseline values, with peak in 30 min. Primary hypothyroidism shows high baseline values and exaggerated rise. Secondary hypothyroidism produces normal rise with delayed peak. Hyperthyroidism produces no marked rise.	Test should be done after an overnight fast and the patient in a well-rested state. Patient should be forewarned of multiple blood draws. Pregnancy and postmenopausal states create high baseline TSH values.
Other Studies			
Thyroid scan	To evaluate location, size, shape, uniformity, and anatomical function of the thyroid gland. Commonly used to evaluate thyroid nodules. A tracer dose of ^{131}I or $^{99m}TcO_4$ is given IV. At 2, 6, and 24 hr a scintillation scanner is moved over the thyroid, producing an electromagnetic map (a scintogram), which records distribution of radioactive uptake by the gland.	Adenomas may appear as "cold" or "hot" spots. Graves' disease gives a diffuse appearance and Hashimoto's thyroiditis gives a mottled picture.	The patient should be given instruction and reassurance about the nature of the test.

(Continued)

TABLE 72–2
Outline of Endocrine Diagnostic Studies[2,4,5,7,9–15] *(Continued)*

Study	*Purpose and Procedure*	*Interpretation*	*Nursing Considerations*
Thyroid Function Tests			
Basal metabolic rate (MBR)	To evaluate metabolic actions of the thyroid hormone indirectly by measurement of oxygen consumption under specific conditions. O_2 uptake is measured using an oxygen-filled spirometer with coupled kymograph through which the relaxed patient breathes. The patient's oxygen uptake is compared with standards for sex, age, and body surface area. Results are expressed in percentage above and below normal. This test is not as conclusive as those listed above.	Normal values: −10%–+10% Values above 10% may indicate hyperthyroidism.	To obtain a true baseline value, the patient must be well-rested, warm, comfortable, emotionally at ease, and have fasted for at least 12 hr. Anxiety can give falsely high readings, so the patient should be calmed by thorough reassurances. Many other things can alter the values, such as environmental noises, psychosis, Paget's disease, smoking, Addison's disease, emphysema, and pheochromocytoma.
Achilles tendon reflex recording	To evaluate the speed of the Achilles tendon reflex. A magnet electrode is strapped to the heel and generates an electric current as the foot and magnet move in response to tapping of the Achilles tendon. It is of little diagnostic value in hyperthyroidism.	A visible delay in reflex time is seen in 90% of persons with hypothyroidism.	The patient must receive explanations of the unusual test procedure.
Parathyroid Function Tests			
Blood Studies			
Parathyroid hormone (PTH)	To evaluate PTH levels in the serum by a radioimmunoassay method. Normally measured in conjunction with serum calcium. A routine blood sample is required.	Normal values vary but have an inverse relationship to calcium. If elevated PTH levels are seen along with elevated serum calcium levels, primary hyperparathyroidism is suspected.	No special preparations are required
Total serum calcium	An important test in screening for parathyroid disease. A routine blood draw is done. The calcium value should be corrected for decreases in serum albumin: Ca^{2+} mg/dl = measured Ca^{2+} mg/dl minus 0.8(4.5 g/dl, patient's serum albumin)	Normal values: 9–11 mg/dl or 4.5–5.5 mEq/liter High values may indicate primary hyperparathyroidism. Low values may indicate hypoparathyroidism. Low values are also seen in vitamin D deficiency and malabsorption syndrome.	Measurements are best obtained in the fasting state. Otherwise, no special preparation is required.
Serum phosphate	To evaluate the level of inorganic phosphorus in the blood. A routine blood sample is required.	Normal values: 1.3–1.75 mEq/liter or 2.5–4.5 mg/dl Elevations seen in hypoparathyroidism, renal failure, and laxative abuse. Low values seen in hyperparathyroidism, osteomalacia, rickets, and malabsorption syndrome.	No special preparation required

(Continued)

TABLE 72–2
Outline of Endocrine Diagnostic Studies[2,4,5,7,9–15] *(Continued)*

Study	*Purpose and Procedure*	*Interpretation*	*Nursing Considerations*
Parathyroid Function Tests			
Urine Studies			
Nephrogenous cyclic adenosine phosphatase (cAMP)	To screen for possible hyperparathyroid disorders. With patient recumbent, 0.9% saline is infused at 150 ml/hr, starting 2 hr before test. A bladder catheter is inserted for precise 2-hr urine collection. The urine is measured for creatinine clearance, cAMP, and volume. Midway through urine collection a serum sample of cAMP and creatinine are measured. Total nephrogenous cAMP = cAMP excreted minus cAMP filtered	Normal values: 1.0–3.5 nMol/dl Elevations are indicative of hyperparathyroidism.	Careful preprocedure instruction, aseptic catheter insertion, and precisely timed urine collection are essential.
Calcium excretion test	To evaluate parathyroid activity. Calcium is measured in urine collected for 24 hr. It usually has a linear relationship to serum calcium.	Normal values: Males, <4 mg/kg ideal body weight Females, <3 mg/kg ideal body weight High values may indicate hyperparathyroidism. Hypercalciuria is seen in nearly all hypercalcemic states.	Pretest explanation to the patient and accurate 24 hr-urine collection are required. Increased intake of protein, magnesium, and vitamin D elevate the values.
Phosphorus excretion test	To evaluate parathyroid (PTH) activity. Phosphorus is measured from urine collected for 24 hr. A PTH test is often done concurrently. It normally has an inverse relationship to PTH.	Normal values: 1000 mg excreted in 24 hr Increased phosphorus excretion is seen in hyperparathyroidism.	Pretest explanations to the patient and an accurate 24-hr urine collection are required.
Other Studies			
Skeletal radiography Bone scans	May be used in conjunction to evaluate bone density changes and deformity that may have resulted from abnormally high calcium resorption from excessive PTH secretion	Bone density can be assessed, but a loss of 25% may be needed before a report of decreased bone density can be made.	No special preparation is required except for explanation of the procedure
Adrenal Cortex Function Tests			
Blood Studies			
Plasma cortisol	To evaluate serum cortisol levels to assess adrenocortical function. Routine blood sample is drawn. Usually repeated sampling is made for conclusive results.	Normal values: 8 AM = 10–30 μg/dl 8 PM = 10 μg/dl (Note that 8 PM levels are normally <50% of 8 AM levels Elevations may be seen in adrenocortical hyperfunction, such as occurs with Cushing's syndrome. Normal to low values are seen in adrenocortical insufficiency, such as Addison's disease.	Blood specimens must be drawn to coincide with circadian rhythm, usually at 8 AM and 4 or 8 PM. Draw time should be marked on the laboratory slip. The patient's stress, which may elevate values, must be minimized. A fasting sample is preferred.

(Continued)

TABLE 72–2
Outline of Endocrine Diagnostic Studies[2,4,5,7,9–15] *(Continued)*

Study	*Purpose and Procedure*	*Interpretation*	*Nursing Considerations*
Adrenal Cortex Function Tests			
Dexamethasone suppression test	To evaluate adrenocortical activity when hyperfunction is suspected. Has some degree of usefulness in distinguishing adrenocortical hyperplasia from adrenal tumors. Dexamethasone 1 mg PO is given at midnight and plasma cortisol is drawn at 8 AM the following day. Often is done in conjunction with urinary 17-hydroxycorticoids (17-OHCS) test	Normal values: <6 mg/dl; values >13 mg/dl may indicate Cushing's syndrome.	A sedative may be given at hour of sleep to ensure a good night's rest. False-positive results may be recorded in acutely ill or very anxious patients or in those taking interfering drugs (*e.g.*, phenytoin and estrogens). A fasting sample is preferred.
ACTH stimulation test	Useful in screening for adrenocortical insufficiency. Two methods may be used: 1. ACTH, 250 μg, is given IM and plasma cortisol levels are measured before and 30 and 60 min after injection. 2. ACTH (or its analog) infused IV, 25–50 U/500 ml normal saline, over 8 hr for 3 days. Routine plasma cortisol levels are obtained, along with three 24-hr urine collections, for 17-OHCS. Baseline plasma cortisol and urinary 17-OHCS should be measured.	Normal values: *Serum:* Cortisol should double from baseline. *Urine:* 17-OHCS should increase 4 to 5 times baseline levels. Little or no response to ACTH is seen in primary adrenocortical insufficiency. A normal response is seen in secondary adrenocortical insufficiency or chronic iatrogenic adrenal suppression.	Explanation of procedure to patient Collection of specimens on time is important. Urine is best collected from 8 AM to 8 AM
Urine Studies			
17-Hydroxycorticoids (17-OHCS)	To evaluate urinary levels of glucocorticoid metabolites. Normal adrenals secrete cortisol at a rate of 20 mg/day of which <50% is excreted in urine as hydroxysteroids.	Normal values: Males = 3–12 mg/24 hr Females = 3–10 mg/24 hr High values are seen with hyperfunction of the adrenal cortex.	Explain procedure to patient. Refrigerate urine specimen or use laboratory-supplied preservative.
17-Ketosteroids (17-KS)	To evaluate adrenocortical activity. 17-KS are weak anabolic androgens and are measured from a 24-hr urine collection. It is often done in conjunction with adrenal stimulation and depression tests.	Normal values: Males, 5–23 mg/24 hr Females, 3–15 mg/24 hr High levels are seen with adrenocortical hyperfunction. Low levels are seen with adrenocortical hyperfunction of the adrenal and pituitary glands.	Same as for 17-OHCS. Low levels may also be seen with myxedema, exogenous steroids, and starvation.
Metyrapone test (metapyrone)	Differentiates adrenocortical hyperplasia from adrenal tumors by testing intactness of pituitary–adrenal feedback mechanism. Before test, baseline 24-hr urine for 17-OHCS is collected. Metyrapone, 750 mg PO (which blocks cortisol synthesis) is given every 4 hr for 24 hr. A 24-hr urine collection is obtained concurrently and again on the following day. An ACTH stimulation test should precede the test to assess adrenal responsiveness to ACTH.	Normal values: A 2-fold to 4-fold rise in 17-OHCS An even greater response is seen with pituitary-dependent Cushing's syndrome and no response is seen in the presence of an adrenal tumor.	Same as for urinary 17-OHCS test. Nurse must be alert for signs of adrenal insufficiency, which may be induced by metyrapone. This drug should be given with food to allay the common side-effects of nausea and vertigo.

(*Continued*)

TABLE 72–2
Outline of Endocrine Diagnostic Studies[2,4,5,7,9–15] *(Continued)*

Study	*Purpose and Procedure*	*Interpretation*	*Nursing Considerations*
Adrenal Cortex Function Tests			
Fludrocortisone suppression test	To screen for primary aldosteronism. Fludrocortisone, 0.1 mg PO, is given every 6 hr for 3 days. A 24-hr urine specimen is collected the day before testing and on day 3 to measure the level of excreted aldosterone. This test is usually done along with plasma renin activity tests.	Normal values: <20 μg/24 hr High values, along with low plasma renin activity, is indicative of primary aldosteronism.	To explain the procedure to the patient. An accurate 24-hr urine collection is needed. A low salt diet (<2 g/day), stress, and diuretics will all increase aldosterone.
Adrenal Medulla Function Tests			
Blood Studies			
Plasma catecholamines	Screening test for pheochromocytoma. An intravenous catheter is inserted and blood sampling done 15 to 20 min after venipuncture. This technique is used to minimize the patient's response to pain.	Normal values: 150–325 pg/ml A 3-fold to 4-fold increase over normal levels would be indicative of pheochromocytoma. This test is not as diagnostic as the urinary test.	The patient should be supine in a quiet, comfortable environment for 30–40 min before the test. The patient's anxiety, which can elevate values, should be minimized.
Urinary Studies			
Vanillylmandelic acid (VMA)	A 24-hr urine specimen is used to screen for pheochromocytoma. Measures urinary excretion of catecholamine metabolites	Normal values: <7 mg/24 hr This value may vary, depending on laboratory procedure. High values are seen with pheochromocytoma.	A 24-hr urine collection should be kept at a pH of 3 or less, by adding HCl (preservative). Drugs such as methyldopa, reserpine, and bronchodilators will elevate values. The physician should be consulted about stopping these drugs 3 days before the test if possible. The following foods also cause spurious elevations in VMA and should be avoided: coffee, tea, chocolate, vanilla extract, and bananas.
Metanephrines	A 24-hr urine test used to screen for pheochromocytoma. The procedure is similar to that of the VMA test.	Normal values: <1.3 mg/24 hr	Same as for VMA test
Pancreas (Endocrine) Function Test			
Blood Studies			
Fasting blood sugar (FBS)	To evaluate circulating amounts of glucose. It helps assess the presence or control of diabetes mellitus. A routine blood draw follows an overnight fast.	Normal values: 70–120 mg/dl Elevated levels suggest further studies are required to rule out diabetes mellitus.	The study requires a 12-hr fast. Patient started on NPO at hour of sleep for a morning blood specimen.
Two hour postprandial test	To evaluate glucose metabolism. Blood glucose levels are drawn 2 hr after a high carbohydrate meal or a glucose load of 100 g.	Normal values: 70–120 mg/dl Blood glucose should return to fasting levels. If levels remain high, diabetes mellitus may be indicated.	Responsible for notifying laboratory of exact time for specimen draw to ensure accuracy of test

(Continued)

TABLE 72–2
Outline of Endocrine Diagnostic Studies[2,4,5,7,9–15] *(Continued)*

Study	*Purpose and Procedure*	*Interpretation*	*Nursing Considerations*
Pancreas (Endocrine) Function Test			
Glucose tolerance test (GTT)	To evaluate insulin response to glucose loading. A fasting blood sugar value is obtained. The patient is then given 50–200 g (1.75 g/kg body weight) of glucose orally (or IV if oral intake is not possible). Blood samples are drawn at $\frac{1}{2}$, 1, 2, and 3 hr. Sometimes a 4- or 5-hr sample is collected.	Normal values: Fasting = 70–120 mg/dl $\frac{1}{2}$ hr = 100–180 mg/dl 1 hr = 90–170 mg/dl 2 hr = 75–135 mg/dl 3 hr = normal levels Elevations are seen with diabetes mellitus or adrenal hyperfunction. Low values may indicate screening for hypoglycemia.	NPO after midnight. The patient is given a glucose load along with an explanation of the frequent blood draws. Oral contraceptives, smoking, steroids, salicylates, diuretics, and phenytoin can impair glucose-tolerance results.
Urine Studies			
Glucose (Clinitest, Diastix, Multistix, Labstix, Tes-Tape)	To evaluate urinary glucose concentration by a copper reduction or an enzyme method. Usually correlates urine glucose with serum glucose levels and may be used to guide insulin therapy.	The test evaluation varies according to the method used. Instructions on package should be followed carefully.	A fresh, second urine specimen is preferred. Because of the different tests available, package directions should be followed. Some drugs affect accuracy of test, such as large doses of ascorbic acid, chloral hydrate, levodopa, salicylates, isoniazid, tetracyclines, and cephalosporins. These can give false-positive readings.
Ketones (Acetest, Ketostix, Labstix, Multistix)	To measure amounts of ketone bodies excreted in the urine. Evaluates alterations in fat metabolism	No ketone bodies should be found in the urine; however, readings vary Package instructions should be followed. Ketones are found in the presence of ketoacidosis due to diabetes mellitus or starvation.	A freshly voided specimen is used. Follow package directions.

Summary

Most endocrine disorders begin insidiously and progress slowly. Early in the course of a disease the clinical manifestations may be subtle, making detection difficult. Recognition of the disorder in its late stages, however, is easier as the physical signs of endocrine dysfunction become obvious. Unfortunately, by the time the diagnosis is made, many of the gross physical changes are irreversible. A carefully taken history and a thorough physical examination greatly aid early detection. Once an abnormality within the endocrine system is suspected, the next step is to identify its specific signs and symptoms. Laboratory data are then obtained to support or negate the suspicion and to guide management.

Although laboratory measurements of hormonal concentrations in body fluids are theoretically the best clues to hormonal status, it should be remembered that many factors (such as drugs or low plasma albumen) can influence the accuracy of the laboratory findings. The nurse is responsible for the preparation and support of the patient before, during, and after testing. Appropriate scheduling of tests and proper collection of specimens are also nursing responsibilities. Finally, many of these tests are uncomfortable and costly. The nurse, therefore, plays an important role in promoting the accuracy and minimizing unnecessary repetitions of the laboratory studies.

References

1. Bates B, Hoekelman R: A Guide to Physical Examination. Philadelphia, JB Lippincott, 1983
2. Burman KD: Interpretation of thyroid function tests in systemically ill patients. Critical Care Quarterly 6(3):1–11, 1983
3. Conn HF: Current Diagnosis 6. Philadelphia, WB Saunders, 1980
4. Cryer PE: Diagnostic endocrinology, 2nd ed. New York, Oxford University Press, 1979

5. DeGroot LJ, Cahill GF, Odell WD et al (eds): Endocrinology, vol. 1. New York, Grune & Stratton, 1979
6. Harvey AM: Practice of Medicine, 12th ed. New York, Appleton-Century-Crofts, 1980
7. Hershman JM: Management of Endocrine Disorders. Philadelphia, Lea & Febiger, 1980
8. Howanitz PJ, Howanitz JH: Evaluation of endocrine function. In Henry JB (ed): Clinical Diagnosis and Management by Laboratory Methods. Philadelphia, WB Saunders, 1979
9. Kinderlehrer DA: Thyroid function tests. Am Fam Physician 21(5):116–120, 1980
10. Malasanos L, Barkauskas V, Moss M et al: Health Assessment, 2nd ed. St Louis, CV Mosby, 1981
11. Morrow LB: Clinical evaluation of pituitary adenomas. Postgrad Med 68:155–164, 1980
12. Reeves ML, Forhan SE, Skyler JS et al: Comparison of methods for blood glucose monitoring. Diabetes Care 4:404–406, 1981
13. Wats NJ, Keffer N: Practical endocrine diagnosis. Philadelphia, Lea & Febiger, 1982
14. Widman FK: Clinical Interpretation of Laboratory Tests, 9th ed. Philadelphia, FA Davis, 1983
15. Williams RH (ed): Textbook of Endocrinology. Philadelphia, WB Saunders, 1981

Bibliography

Bains J, Walfish PG: The assessment of thyroid function and structure. Otolaryngol Clin North Am 11:419–443, 1978

Bouchnier IAD, Morris JS (eds): Clinical Skills: A system of clinical examination. London, WB Saunders, 1976

Burnside JW (ed): Physical Diagnosis, 16th ed. Baltimore, Williams & Wilkins, 1981

DeFronzo R: Glucose intolerance and aging. Diabetes Care 4:493–501, 1981

Dillon RG: Handbook of Endocrinology, 2nd ed. Philadelphia, Lea & Febiger, 1980

Ezrin C, Godden JO, Volpe R (eds): Systematic endocrinology. Hagerstown, Harper & Row, 1982

Fairchild RS: Diabetes insipidus: A review. Critical Care Quarterly 3:111–118, 1980

Felig P, Baxter JD, Broadus AE et al (eds): Endocrinology and Metabolism. New York, McGraw-Hill, 1981

Gold EM: Cushing's syndrome: A tripartite entity. Hosp Pract 14:67–75, 1979

Hall R: Fundamentals of Clinical Endocrinology, 3rd ed. New York, Year Book Medical Publishers, 1981

Hart IR, Newton RW: Endocrinology, vol 2. Baltimore, University Park Press, 1983

Hellman R: The evaluation and management of hyperthyroid crisis. Critical Care Quarterly 2:77–92, 1980

Humes H, Warins R, Brenner B: Disorders of water balance. Hosp Pract 14:133–145, 1979

Isselbacher K, Adams RD, Braunwald E et al (eds): Harrison's Principles of Internal Medicine, 9th ed. New York, McGraw-Hill, 1980

Jubiz W: Endocrinology: A Logical Approach for Clinicians. New York, McGraw-Hill, 1979

Katz FH: Adrenocortical diseases: Identification and management. Postgrad Med 66:52–65, 1979

Keeson CM, Young RE, Talwar D et al: Glycosylated hemoglobin in the diagnosis of non-insulin-dependent diabetes mellitus. Diabetes Care 5:395–398, 1982

Kozak G: Clinical Diabetes Mellitus. Philadelphia, WB Saunders, 1982

Miller JM, Hamburger JI, Kine S: Diagnosis of thyroid nodules. JAMA 241:481–484, 1979

Prior JA, Silberstein J, Stang J: Physical Diagnosis: The History and Examination of the Patient. St Louis, CV Mosby, 1981

Surr CW: New blood-glucose monitoring products (part 1). Nursing 13:42–45, 1983

Surr CW: New blood-glucose monitoring products (part 2). Nursing 13:58–62, 1983

Vaitukaitis JL: Current endocrinology. Basic and Clinical Aspects. New York, Elsevier, 1982

Chapter 73

Nursing Strategies for Common Endocrine Problems

Nursing Diagnosis Interventions Evaluation

Christine A. Larson

The endocrine system, in conjunction with the nervous system, has the complex task of maintaining physiological and psychological integrity. It is involved in a variety of continuous adaptive processes. In the pursuit of maintaining homeostasis, the endocrine system has a profound influence on the regulation of energy metabolism, stress response, growth and development, personality development, and fluid and electrolyte balance.

Individuals with endocrine disorders present with widely diverse clinical manifestations. No body system is unaffected by hormonal influence. Yet, despite this diversity and regardless of their specific etiologies, the problems that patients must cope with are similar. Once the diagnosis of altered endocrine function has been made, the nurse should anticipate the general needs of the patient. Many endocrine syndromes are chronic and may have a marked impact on the patient's lifestyle, sometimes causing dramatic changes in the patient's physical appearance that can injure his self-esteem. The nurse is then challenged to assist the patient in coping with, and controlling, the underlying endocrine dysfunction. Occasionally, impaired endocrine function brings about severe metabolic disruption, requiring the nurse to make astute, ongoing assessments and to implement acute lifesaving measures.

In this chapter, common nursing diagnoses/problems associated with disruption of the endocrine systems are discussed. For each problem identified, nursing strategies are outlined along with general criteria for evaluating the effectiveness of nursing interventions. The management of patients with specific endocrine disorders is discussed in their respective chapters.

Alterations in Fluid Volume

Extracellular Volume Deficit

Nursing Diagnosis/Problem. Extracellular volume (ECV) deficit can occur as a result of hypofunction of the adrenal cortex or from severe osmotic diuresis related to hyperglycemia found in diabetic ketoacidosis and hyperosmolar hyperglycemic nonketotic coma (HHNK). Volume depletion is due to an increase in renal excretion of sodium and water. The fluid loss from the extracellular spaces (intravascular and interstitial) can leave the patient with mild to severe hypovolemia. Chronic ECV depletion is the most common disorder, and the patient can often be managed at home by simply increasing oral fluid intake. However, the condition may exacerbate into an acute crisis, resulting in profound shock, requiring acute interventions with rapid parenteral volume replacement. The defining characteristics of the diagnosis of extracellular volume deficit include decreased urine output, weight loss, hemoconcentration, decreased blood pressure, elevated pulse, decreased skin turgor, thirst, dry mucous membranes, and concentrated urine.

Interventions. In general, nursing responsibilities should focus on assessing the patient's hypovolemic status. Observations by the nurse are important in guiding therapy and are useful in monitoring the patient's response to treatment. Close scrutiny of the patient's blood pressure is essential and should frequently include evaluations for orthostatic hypotension. To do this, the blood pressure and pulse are first obtained with the patient in a supine, flat position. Then the blood pressure and pulse are obtained with the patient in sitting and standing positions. A drop in systolic pressure of 10 mmHg to 20 mmHg and in diastolic pressure of 10 mmHg, together with an increase in pulse rate, is indicative of orthostatic hypotension. Orthostatic hypotension is a hallmark sign of extracellular volume depletion. Persons demonstrating orthostatic hypotension should be cautioned against quickly changing from a recumbent to an upright position because vertigo or syncope may occur.

Poor skin turgor and dry mucous membranes are other nursing observations that support the diagnosis of extracellular volume depletion. These should be watched for and recorded. The determination of poor skin turgor is made by pinching the skin which, rather than quickly resuming shape when released, remains wrinkled for up to 20 seconds.[3] Accurate intake and output records must also be kept, and abnormal routes of fluid loss, such as perspiration, vomiting, and diarrhea, monitored. Obtaining urinary specific gravities can help assess the degree of dehydration. In addition, daily weights, taken at the same time and on the same measuring scale, should be obtained. Volume depletion is often accompanied by a drop in weight but may not be if the patient has an intracellular volume excess as well. Specific nursing assessment of fluid status is discussed in Chapter 13.

If the patient is able to tolerate an oral intake, fluids should be offered frequently. Keeping fluids readily available is particularly important to the confused, bedfast, or immobilized patient. Body fluid losses are best replaced with tomato juice, milk, or bouillon rather than plain water, which may predispose the person to an added problem of water (intracellular volume) excess.[5]

Evaluation. The expected outcome of treatment is a return to normal volume status. The patient should demonstrate vital signs within his normal limits, no orthostatic hypotension, relief of symptoms of dehydration, and an adequate urine output of at least 25 to 30 ml/hour with urine specific gravity within 1.005–1.020.

Extracellular Volume Excess

Nursing Diagnosis/Problem. Extracellular volume excess occurs in individuals with hyperfunction of the adrenal cortex, such as occurs with Cushing's syndrome and aldosteronism and may be present with hypothyroidism. The increase in volume results from excessive renal retention of sodium and water. Defining characteristics may include high blood pressure, tachycardia, edema, and distended jugular veins.

Interventions. The nurse is responsible for determining the presence of, and patient's tolerance to, volume overload. Of greatest concern is the individual with a compromised cardiovascular system. An increase in circulating volume may greatly tax an ailing heart and lead to cardiac decompensation. Signs of volume overload include elevations in blood pressure, increase in pulse rate, jugular vein distention, pulmonary crackles, and dependent edema. Extreme dyspnea or angina are serious symptoms requiring prompt referral and medical intervention. Daily weighing can provide extremely useful information to guide therapy. Weight gains coincide with fluid retention; a 1-lb weight gain is approximately equivalent to 500 ml of retained fluid.

Often patients are restricted to 1200 ml to 1500 ml of fluid per day. The restriction can cause distressing thirst and is not always well tolerated. Explaining the purpose of this therapy and working closely with the patient in implementing it will greatly aid in its success. The amounts of liquids allowed per shift should be entered in the patient's care plan and posted by his bedside. The nurse can help allay his thirst by providing hard candy to suck or gum to chew. Either one can stimulate salivation and reduce the craving for liquids. When possible, the patient should be allowed to choose the types of liquids to be included in his diet. Serving well-chilled liquids in a glass with a false bottom and having the patient swish the fluid around in his mouth before swallowing may increase satisfaction. Good oral care moistens mucous membranes and is also important in alleviating thirst. In the alert patient, sham drinking may be tried. This technique consists of taking a mouthful of liquid, swishing it around the mouth, and expectorating it. Sham drinking relieves thirst by moistening mucous membranes without increasing fluid intake.[5]

Restricting sodium intake to less than 4 g/day may also be required. Discussing with the patient the use of salt substitutes and the avoidance of high sodium foods (such as canned vegetables and dairy products) is extremely helpful. Low sodium foods include cereal, fruits, fresh vegetables, potatoes, and honey. Because of salt restrictions, food may seem bland and unappetizing. Use of other seasonings (such as lemon, basil, herbs, and mint) will improve the taste. To replace salt in soups and stews, vinegar may be used, 2 to 3 teaspoons of vinegar : 4 to 6 quarts of liquid.[3]

Evaluation. The expected outcome of adopting these measures is the return of the patient to a normal volemic state, detectable in a proportionate drop in body weight and the absence of dependent edema, pulmonary crackles, and jugular vein distention. The patient will be able to relate causative factors to ECV excess and comply with fluid and sodium intake restrictions.

Alterations in Tissue Perfusion Related to High Blood Pressure

Nursing Diagnosis/Problem. Severe high blood pressure and tachycardia result from an exaggerated catecholamine response in pheochromocytoma and hyperfunction of the thyroid gland. Hyperaldosteronism may also elevate blood pressure. High blood pressure can produce dramatic manifestations in the patient, creating discomfort, and sometimes it has dire consequences. Cerebral ischemia due to decreased cerebral blood flow and myocardial ischemia resulting from increased afterload on the heart are of particular concern.

Interventions. Nursing considerations are aimed at preventing precipitous increases in blood pressure. Of equal importance is watching for the potential complications known to occur with extreme increases in blood pressure or from the side-effects of administered antihypertensives. The patient's blood pressure should be carefully monitored at regular times, as dictated by the acuteness of the patient's condition. Blood pressure may increase continuously or have paroxysmal increases. Many factors are known to precipitate paroxysmal attacks of severe high blood pressure. These factors should be discussed with the patient so that they can be avoided. Among them are stress, exercise, postural position changes, straining, and sudden extreme environmental temperature changes. During episodes of extreme high blood pressure, the patient's neurological status should be evaluated for deleterious effects of increased blood pressure. The patient may demonstrate pupillary changes or manifestations of stroke, such as changes in level of consciousness, hemiphagia, or aphasia. Early detection of any of these changes prompts early treatment and perhaps can minimize damage.

Some patients, particularly those with pheochromocytoma, may require the intravenous infusion of potent antihypertensive drugs. Many of these drugs are titrated to response of the patient's blood pressure. Because most potent antihypertensives also have important side-effects, their administration must be closely monitored by the nurse.

Evaluation. The expected outcome for the patient is an abolition of paroxysmal episodes of high blood pressure with a reasonable decrease in blood pressure. The patient will be able to relate causes and preventive measures for high blood pressure. Also desired is early detection and treatment of complications.

Alterations in Electrolyte Balance

Hypokalemia

Nursing Diagnosis/Problem. Alterations in various hormonal concentrations can severely disrupt potassium balance with life-threatening consequences. Hypokalemia occurs with Cushing's syndrome and hyperaldosteronism and is caused by increased renal excretion of potassium.

Interventions. The nurse's primary role in this problem is in watching for and preventing potassium depletion. Patients likely to have potassium depletion must be identified, and their serum potassium levels must be closely monitored. Some signs of hypokalemia include neuromuscular weakness, cardiac arrhythmias, and paralytic ileus. These and other manifestations of hypokalemia are discussed in Chapter 76. Some patients may be receiving digitalis and diuretic therapy to treat the problem of fluid volume excess. These individuals need to be aware of the symptoms of digitalis toxicity, which is potentiated by hypokalemia (*i.e.,* anorexia, nausea, vomiting, and irregular pulse).[7]

To prevent hypokalemia, a sufficient dietary intake of potassium is essential. The patient and his family can be taught the importance of including potassium-rich foods in the diet. A dietician may be able to assist. Foods with high potassium content include citrus fruits, melons, bananas, baked white potatoes, avocados, beans, squash, prunes, dates, and maple syrup.[8]

Evaluation. With appropriate nursing interventions, the expected outcome for this patient is a serum potassium level within the normal range. The patient and his family should be able to name at least seven foods rich in potassium and be able to discuss the importance of including such foods in the diet.

Hyperkalemia

Nursing Diagnosis/Problem. Hyperkalemia is an important problem encountered in patients with hypofunction of the adrenal cortex (Addison's disease). Potassium is retained in excessive amounts by the kidney.

Interventions. The management of severe hyperkalemia is primarily pharmacological. The nurse's responsibility is the proper administration of the appropriate drugs prescribed by the physician. Hyperkalemia, like hypokalemia, can produce an array of physical manifestations for which the nurse must watch. Among them are nausea, diarrhea, cramps, and muscular weakness. Since the myocardium is markedly depressed when potassium levels are high, an electrocardiogram should be obtained. Potassium elevations produce tall peaked T waves and, at toxic levels, widened QRS complexes.[7] Arrhythmias may also be seen and require immediate intervention. The nurse can also focus on preventing exacerbation of the endocrine disorder because it can potentiate hyperkalemia. The major intervention in the latter goal is education of the patient, to be discussed later in this chapter. Included in the teaching program is instruction about a low potassium diet.

Evaluation. The expected outcome for the patient is a normal serum potassium level and an absence of the physical signs of hyperkalemia. In addition, the person will avoid food high in potassium content and discuss the rationale for this.

Hypercalcemia

Nursing Diagnosis/Problem. Hypercalcemia occurs in patients with hyperparathyroidism and, occasionally, with hyperfunction of the thyroid gland. The most prominent cause is a hormonally induced increase in calcium resorption from bones, leading to excessive serum calcium levels. Some endocrine disorders can result in varying degrees of immobility by depressing physical and emotional function.

Immobility itself robs the bones of calcium, and may result in high serum calcium levels.

Interventions. The nurse needs to be alert to patients in danger of hypercalcemia. High calcium levels can predispose a patient to serious, yet preventable, consequences. Serum calcium should be monitored along with serum phosphorus. Serum calcium and serum phosphorus are inversely related. Physical manifestations to watch for include thirst, polyuria, Chvostek and Trosseau signs, and gastrointestinal symptoms such as anorexia, nausea, and constipation.[3] The therapy is determined by the severity and etiology of the problem. As urinary calcium levels increase, so too does the risk of developing renal calculi. Signs of renal calculi include flank pain, dysuria, and hematuria. Screening for calculi may be done by straining all urine through gauze for stone analysis. The procedure for urine straining should be taught to the patient along with the need to restrict calcium in the diet. Renal stones composed of calcium oxalate or calcium phosphate are formed in alkaline urine; therefore, foods and drugs which promote an acid urine are administered. Acidifying foods include cranberries, prunes, asparagus, grapes, tomatoes, corn, meat, poultry, fish, cereal, and eggs.[3]

The affected patient often has "brittle bones," due to increased calcium resorption, and is prone to pathological fractures. Therefore, ambulatory assistance should be readily available to prevent serious falls. A program of activities that is designed to diminish calcium resorption and that will provide mild to moderate bone stress could be implemented. Such a program should be adjusted to the patient's tolerance to physical activity.

An increased intake of fluids (especially isotonic fluids) is important, since patients with hypercalcemia tend to have excessive polyuria and are prone to extracellular volume deficit. Augmenting fluid intake also decreases the threat of renal calculi. Careful recording of intake and output, along with administration of parenteral fluids, are required. To help encourage oral fluid intake, incentives such as preferred beverage can be implemented.

Evaluation. The expected outcome for the patient is a serum calcium level within normal limits. Also desired is the absence of preventable complications, such as an extracellular volume deficit, renal calculi, and pathological fractures due to personal injury.

Alterations in Activity Tolerance Related to Fatigue

Nursing Diagnosis/Problem. Fatigue is a symptom found in nearly all endocrine disorders. It is most often due to altered glucose and energy metabolism. Some endocrine problems can cause protein catabolism leading to muscle wasting. Muscle wasting can cause marked weakness and inability to manage routine daily activities. The patient's activity tolerance may be further compromised by backaches and joint pain if osteoporosis is present. Debility can range in severity from mild exertional dyspnea to near total dependency.

Interventions. The nurse must first assess the extent of the patient's disability. Can the patient walk unassisted with sufficient coordination? What personal hygienic care is the patient capable of managing? What is the patient's perception of his activity limitations? The latter is important. How the patient perceives decompensation of his physical abilities and its impact on his lifestyle profoundly influences his coping abilities. Consideration of this should be incorporated into short- and long-term nursing strategies.

A major nursing goal is to prevent or minimize fatigue. The nurse should provide assistance with whatever essential tasks the patient is unable to handle. Careful planning and scheduling of the patient's activities is necessary to ensure adequate rest and to reduce energy expenditure. Consultation between health care team members and the patient about the spacing of activities, such as meals, hygienic care, visitors, and diagnostic studies, is extremely helpful. Such scheduling can be incorporated into the patient's care plan to provide continuity of care. A sincere positive attitude on behalf of the nurse can encourage improvement in the patient's mobility status.[6]

Assessing the patient's stamina and response to exercise can help gauge the degree of gradual activity progression. Vital signs (blood pressure, pulse, and respirations) are taken before and immediately after exercise. After 3 to 5 minutes of rest, the vital signs are repeated. Activity should be decreased, or discontinued, if the patient experiences dyspnea, vertigo, chest pain, confusion, an increase in diastolic blood pressure of 15 mmHg, a drop in systolic blood pressure, or a greatly decreased or irregular pulse rate.[4]

In long-term management, the physical structure of the patient's home environment should be appraised. Are there stairs to be negotiated? Where is the bathroom situated? Are there others around to assist the patient with particularly fatiguing activities? Rearranging furniture or sleeping quarters may be necessary. Together the nurse, patient, and family members can evaluate the patient's normal daily routine, determining which activities the patient can do, must do, and enjoys doing. This joint evaluation is important in planning a flexible daily schedule that allows a maximum amount of rest, yet enough tolerated activity to provide the patient with some sense of independence and well-being.

Evaluation. With prudent measures to conserve and restore his energy, it is expected that the patient will progress to the optimum level of mobility and demonstrate a reasonable ability to manage daily activities. With increased stamina the patient's self-esteem will, it is hoped, increase.

Alterations in Carbohydrate Metabolism

Hyperglycemia

Nursing Diagnosis/Problem. Hyperglycemia is seen in diabetes mellitus, hyperfunction of the adrenal cortex, pheochromocytoma, and conditions causing elevations in growth hormone secretion. Defining characteristics may include elevated fasting blood glucose levels (> 120 mg/dl), thirst, polyuria, and hunger.

Interventions. When the diagnosis has been made, the nurse is responsible for frequent monitoring of the patient's blood and urine glucose levels, using whatever means of data collection is available (see Chap. 74). The patient can be taught these monitoring methods for home use. Because hyperglycemia can cause osmotic diuresis, the intake and output of patients must be accurately recorded. In addition, the patient's hydration status should be assessed by observing skin turgor and mucous membranes. If his urinary output is far in excess of his fluid intake, and if signs of dehydration exist, provision of appropriate oral and parenteral fluids is indicated.

Depending on the etiology and severity of the patient's underlying problem, an adjustment in caloric intake may be required. If such a reduction is ordered, the nurse needs to carefully explain this to the patient and his family. It is important to identify the person responsible for the buying and preparation of the patient's food. This person must have a clear understanding of the prescribed diet. It is also helpful to involve a dietician, who will discuss specifics of the diet prescription and how to measure foods and use food exchanges. Written information on the specifics of the diabetic diet can help the patient in managing the prescribed diet at home. In diet planning, the patient's food preferences, cultural differences, and economic status must be taken into account.

Sometimes insulin is required to lower blood sugar. When insulin is administered, the type of insulin used, dose, route, and site of injection must be accurately documented. In addition, the patient should be observed for insulin effects. Long-term dietary restrictions and insulin injections may be necessary. Effective teaching is essential for the patient's compliance and for control of his disease. (see Chap. 74).

Physical and emotional stress can cause catecholamine-induced gluconeogenesis and glycogenolysis, exaggerating hyperglycemia. Nursing measures aimed at stress reduction are important. The patient should be encouraged to obtain prompt treatment for even mild illnesses and to increase the activities he finds most restful and relaxing. The nurse can help him identify and cope with potential stressors.

Evaluation. The expected patient outcome of treatment is maintenance of a normal blood sugar concentration. The patient should be able to discuss dietary management, measurements of blood and urine glucose, and the importance of reducing stress.

Hypoglycemia

Nursing Diagnosis/Problem. Hypoglycemia can result from hypofunction of the adrenal cortex, from pancreatic insulinomas, or as a response to therapy in insulin-dependent diabetes mellitus and can be a serious finding. As blood sugar falls, the glucose-dependent brain cells starve and eventually die.

Interventions. Prevention of hypoglycemia is the primary nursing concern. Interventions are usually directed toward educating the patient. The importance of routine meal scheduling, which includes bedtime snacks, is emphasized. Skipped meals or irregular eating patterns are to be avoided because meal omission can cause deleterious drops in blood glucose. A high carbohydrate snack close at hand is essential and should be taken at the first signs of hypoglycemia.

The physical manifestations of hypoglycemia are central nervous system related and can vary among individuals. Symptoms include nervousness, tremors, diaphoresis, hunger, slurred speech, and confusion. Ingestion of a high carbohydrate substance can quickly alleviate symptoms. If swallowing is difficult, placing the high glucose substance beneath the tongue allows for rapid absorption and relief of symptoms. However, if hypoglycemia is severe, the patient may require hospitalization and an intravenous dose of 50%-dextrose solution. Nursing management of hypoglycemia is discussed in detail in Chapter 74.

Evaluation. With preventive measures and early interventions, the expected treatment outcome is a blood glucose level within normal limits. The patient and his family should be able to describe the symptoms of hypoglycemia, and its prevention and treatment.

Impaired Nutritional Intake Related to Gastrointestinal Distress

Nursing Diagnosis/Problem. Most endocrine disorders cause some degree of gastrointestinal disturbance. Anorexia, nausea, and vomiting are frequently seen. Contributing to the problem can be the treatment regimen itself, the prescribed medications, and diet. Such symptoms can impair the patient's nutritional intake. As nutritional intake falls, the body is forced into a catabolic state, with protein wasting, which increases the patient's fatigue, and weight loss. The patient with endocrine dysfunction is already subject to infection and delayed wound healing. Malnutrition greatly augments the problem as it decreases serum albumin, iron-binding capacity, and lymphocyte count.

Interventions. Nursing interventions play an important role in promoting adequate nutrition. Before developing a plan of care, the nurse must consider the patient's underlying health problem, nutritional status, ideal body weight, age, and activity level. His daily weight should be obtained and can serve as an important indication of nutritional status and the effectiveness of the nursing interventions. A 10% weight loss in the past month is considered significant.[4]

As mentioned earlier, many hormonal drugs can affect the patient's nutritional intake. Unfortunately, most of these patients are required to take these medications for life. If the drug cannot be changed, the pharmacist can be consulted for suggestions for modifying their administration. Sometimes taking them with food, or changing the times at which they are taken, can diminish their gastrointestinal side-effects.

When planning dietary modifications, it is important to consider the patient's culture and food preferences. The clinical dietician, if available, can provide invaluable assistance in ascertaining the dietary needs of the patient, and can perform a baseline nutritional assessment and determine the patient's daily caloric requirements. Small, frequent, and attractively served meals can increase the patient's enthusiasm for eating. Varying the foods to allow for different textures and tastes can increase meal appeal. Good oral hygiene, before and after meals, along with encouragement of some independence at mealtimes may help. The physician can be consulted about the use of vitamins and mineral supplements because these substances often have a stimulating effect on the patient's appetite. Encourage the individual to choose food items as close to actual eating times as possible and to avoid overly rich, sweet, greasy, or fried foods.[4]

Ileus, obstruction of the intestines, may result from an electrolyte imbalance due to an underlying endocrine disorder. Therefore, absence of bowel tones and distention of the abdomen should be watched for in patients at risk.

For many patients, a modified diet is a major part of the total treatment program. Before he is discharged, the patient and those responsible for his meal preparation must receive dietary instructions, in which both the nurse and the dietician can participate, giving consideration to the individual's social and economic status. Certain food supplements and special diet foods can be expensive. Persons on a special diet can avoid high costs by learning how to select from food purchased for the whole family. Some diets may require the elimination, substitution, or measurement of particular foods. Whatever the dietary modification, a well-balanced diet can be obtained through selection of the proper foods.

Irregular eating habits or skipped meals may have serious consequences in some endocrine disorders, most notably diabetes mellitus and Addison's disease, where hypoglycemia is of great concern. Instruction on how to adjust the diet and purchase and prepare food should be given to patients and their families. In addition, the purpose of the prescribed diet should be carefully explained. Compliance is increased when perceived benefits outweigh the perceived hardships of dietary restrictions.

Evaluation. The expected outcome of treatment is a sufficient nutritional intake to promote anabolism and maintain the desired body weight. If a modified diet is prescribed, the patient or whoever prepares his food should be able to explain its purpose, the types of foods to be limited, how to measure and prepare foods, and how food substitutes are used.

Increased Potential for Infection and Delayed Wound Healing

Nursing Diagnosis/Problem. This problem is of concern in many endocrine disorders, particularly diabetes mellitus, adrenal disorders, and hypothyroidism, and results largely from depression of the immune response and poor nutrition.

Interventions. The nurse's concern, then, is in preventing infection and promoting wound healing. Keeping this in mind, the nurse must be especially scrupulous in the aseptic techniques used during invasive procedures, such as bladder catheterization, care of the intravenous site, dressing changes, and the like. The patient's temperature is monitored closely and white blood cell counts are made routinely to detect early signs of infection. Such patients require diligent skin, oral, and respiratory hygiene to prevent nosocomial infection. Wound healing is delayed in these patients and risk of postoperative evisceration is abnormally high. The incision should be supported when the patient coughs or moves about in bed, to minimize stress on the wound. Frequent monitoring and documentation of the incision's appearance are extremely important. Furthermore, a good nutritional intake, especially a diet rich in protein and vitamins A and C, is essential in promoting wound healing.[3]

In some patients, such as those with Cushing's syndrome, the inflammatory response may be diminished or absent. Typical signs of infection are often masked, making early detection difficult. Therefore the nurse must be particularly observant, noting, along with purulent wound drainage, any localized pain and loss of function.

In assigning hospital beds, the nurse should isolate the patient at risk from patients with contagious diseases. At home, the patient is instructed to avoid large crowds or contact with people who are suffering from upper respiratory tract infections, influenza, or other communicable diseases. The physician should be notified if the patient develops cold symptoms or early signs of other infections.

The patient also needs to be aware that even minor cuts and trauma will take longer than normal to heal and are more subject to infection. The patient should be taught not to wear ill-fitting shoes and to avoid walking barefoot outdoors. The feet are located quite a distance from the heart and blood flow is less, thus the feet are particularly subject to delayed wound healing. The safety of the activities normally engaged in by the individual should be evaluated and may need to be adjusted according to the degree of immunosuppression and impact on his self-esteem. Sometimes what the patient "wants to do," and "should do," are not in agreement. The patient's decision to engage in activities that may be harmful is his own to make but he must be made aware of the risks involved.

Evaluation. The expected outcome is that the patient will remain infection-free and that wound healing will be complete. In the event that infection does occur, early detection is desired. There should be no elevations in body temperature, signs of infection (respiratory or urinary), or purulent wound drainage. The patient should be able to name at least five ways to minimize the risk of infection.

Potential for Injury

Nursing Diagnosis/Problem. All endocrine disorders will subject the patient to increased risk of personal injury, either because of muscle weakness, sensorial changes, protein catabolism, or osteoporosis (pathological fractures).

Falls are especially common and can seriously injure or incapacitate the patient.

Interventions. Nursing strategies are aimed at preventing injury to the patient. The individual's strength and coordination should be assessed. Is he able to walk unassisted? If not, what degree of assistance does he require—a cane, a walker, an assistant? Is the patient's sensorium intact? Is he oriented to person, place, and time? In the hospital, the patient can be instructed to be out of bed only with someone in attendance. His cane or walker and call light should always be kept close at hand. For the confused patient, soft restraints may be required. When restraints are used, concerns for the patient's safety should be explained to the family. Frequent reorientation can be given to such patients. Utilization of night-lights is recommended. Personal pictures, a wall clock, and a large daily calendar are sometimes helpful. Nursing care should be consistent and conscientious.

The patient's immediate environment can be rearranged to minimize safety hazards. For example, the bed should be left in the down position with side rails up. Chairs, stools, and trash cans should be moved aside, allowing a clear path to the bathroom. A well-lit room can also prevent him from stumbling over unseen objects. At home, family pets, such as small dogs and cats, should be restrained to avoid being underfoot. Small throw rugs are potential hazards since they are common causes of slips and falls. Providing nonskid surfaces in the bathtub and shower, and on the patient's shoes and slippers can also prevent mishaps. Sunglasses may be worn outside to reduce glare.[4] The nurse, patient, and family members can evaluate the home environment and plan appropriate changes to facilitate the patient's mobility and safety.

Evaluation. The expected outcome of instituting these interventions is a decreased risk or incidence of accidental injury. The person will identify factors that increase the potential for injury and utilize preventive measures. Ideally, the safety of the patient can be accomplished at the same time that his mobility is maximized.

Altered Body Image

Nursing Diagnosis/Problem. Many endocrine disorders have profound effects on physical characteristics, causing changes in soft-tissue distribution, stature, and skin pigmentation. Abnormalities in the pituitary secretion of growth hormone can lead to structural changes such as dwarfism, gigantism, or acromegaly. Abnormalities of the adrenal cortex can result in hyperpigmentation, altered fat distribution and, perhaps, abnormal secondary sex characteristics. Disorders in these and other endocrine glands may also cause sexual impotency. Altered self-concept may affect role performance and interpersonal relationships. Patient reactions may include social withdrawal, increased dependence, or self-destructive behavior.

Interventions. Whatever the etiology, the problems for the affected patient are obvious. Self-esteem is greatly challenged. Fortunately, many body changes disappear as the underlying problem is corrected. However, some aberrant physical characteristics do not. While the problem exists, the nurse needs to be sensitive to the patient's need for acceptance. The patient's feelings must be acknowledged and allowed expression. The nurse can explore personal strength and coping resources with the patient and make referrals for psychological counseling as necessary. Individual, group, or family counseling may be indicated to further assess and strengthen the person's coping resources.

To promote better self-esteem, the patient should be out of bed and dressed every day, as physical tolerance allows. Good grooming enhances physical appearance and should be encouraged. An accepting and nonthreatening environment is essential toward reconstruction of an altered body image. By providing accurate information, the nurse can clarify any misconceptions the patient has about himself, his care, or his care-givers.[4] Establishment of realistic, attainable short-term goals may increase the patient's sense of accomplishment. The nurse should offer positive reinforcements for actual achievements but avoid false praise. Support for the patient need not only center on the nurse–patient relationship but may also involve family members. The coping abilities of the patient's companions must be strengthened if they are to provide sufficient, long-term support for the patient at home. Activities the patient especially enjoys and is physically able to tolerate, such as painting or fishing, can be encouraged. Resumption of as normal a lifestyle as possible may help the patient to cope with any physical changes in his appearance.

Evaluation. The expected outcome is an improvement in the patient's self-image, as demonstrated by verbalizing positive feelings about himself, resuming role-related activities, and showing an increased involvement in outside interests.

Ineffective Coping

Nursing Diagnosis/Problem. Severe coping intolerance to physical and emotional stress is seen in the patient with hypofunction of the adrenal cortex due to a marked decrease in energy reserves. Stress intolerance is also seen as a result of exaggerated catecholamine response in patients with hyperfunction of the thyroid gland. The defining characteristics may include severe anxiety, insomnia, somatic complaints, inability to problem-solve, and deterioration of interpersonal relationships.

Interventions. Providing an environment that is free of emotional or physical stressors is an immense challenge for the nurse. It is advisable to remove excessive environmental stimulation and develop an atmosphere of empathic understanding. The nurse should speak slowly and calmly and focus on the present situation, giving feedback about current reality and avoid making excess demands on the patient.[4] This individual may react inappropriately, with extreme agitation or tears. Family members and close friends should be made aware that this behavior is a result of the disease and not to be taken personally. Voiced anger or retaliatory remarks may only aggravate the patient's condition.

Present and potential life stressors could be identified through careful interviewing. Listening carefully as the patient speaks, observing facial expressions, gestures, body position, eye contact, and voice intensity is valuable. The nurse, with the patient and his family and close associates, can develop a care plan for the hospital and home, to minimize anxiety and provide consistency of care. Sparing the patient unexpected bad news or personal and environmental change is desired whenever possible. Relaxation techniques can also be effective in some cases, such as guided imagery or progressive relaxation technique. (Table 73–1 provides effective steps in relaxation techniques). Quiet activities, such as needlepoint or puzzles, can provide soothing diversion and decrease stress levels. The actual stress response, however, is difficult to control consciously. Indoor temperatures should be kept fairly constant. Ambient temperature swings are often not well tolerated. The nurse can be very helpful by assigning the hospitalized patient to a quiet room, away from disturbing lights and sounds. Delivery of patient care should be calm, caring, and consistent. The scheduling of care can be adjusted to allow for uninterrupted sleep periods. In addition, the patient must be instructed to notify the physician of any illnesses or minor surgeries. This instruction is particularly important for the patient with adrenal insufficiency because the daily steroid dose may need to be increased. Even a seemingly minor upper respiratory infection may result in acute adrenal crisis and extreme physical prostration.

TABLE 73–1
Progressive Relaxation Technique

Progressive relaxation involves systematic constriction and relaxation of muscle groups, beginning with the face and finishing with the feet. Combined with rhythmic breathing, this exercise helps the individual to focus on quiet inner body processes and provides one way to constructively manage stress. It takes approximately 15 to 30 minutes to complete.

1. Remove glasses and shoes; wear loose clothing.
2. Assume comfortable sitting or reclining postiion; avoid lying completely flat (this is to decrease the risk of falling asleep).
3. Begin with slow, rhythmic breathing.
   a. Close your eyes or stare at a spot and take a slow deep breath.
   b. Exhale the breath slowly.
4. Continue rhythmic breathing at a slow steady pace, feeling the tension leave your body with each breath; feel the heaviness of all extremities.
5. Begin progressive relaxation of muscle groups:
   a. During inhalation, tighten your muscles
   b. During exhalation, relax your muscles
   c. Suggested order for tension–relaxation cycle (tension technique in parentheses)
      Face, jaw, mouth (squint eyes, wrinkle brow)
      Neck (pull chin to neck)
      Right hand (make a fist)
      Right arm (bend elbow in tightly)
      Left hand (make a fist)
      Left arm (bend elbow in tightly)
      Back, shoulders, chest (shrug shoulders up tightly)
      Abdomen (pull stomach in and bear down on chair)
      Right upper leg (push leg down)
      Right lower leg and foot (point toes toward body)
      Left upper leg (push leg down)
      Left lower leg and foot (point toes toward body)
6. Practice technique slowly.
7. End relaxation session when you are ready by counting to three, inhaling deeply, and saying, "I'm relaxed."

(Adapted from Carpenito LJ: Nursing Diagnosis: Application to Clinical Practice. Philadelphia, JB Lippincott, 1983)

Evaluation. With the implementation of nursing interventions, the expected outcome is a decrease in controllable emotional and physical stressors. The patient will verbalize feelings related to his emotional state, manifest decreased muscle tension, and express satisfaction with sleep patterns. It is also hoped that family members will demonstrate their increased tolerance of the patient's behavior by considerate dialogue and regular visits.

Alterations in Bowel Elimination

Nursing Diagnosis/Problem. Many endocrine disorders can cause either constipation or diarrhea because of altered electrolyte balance and prolonged immobility, which can affect peristalsis.

Interventions. The nurse can prevent constipation from occurring by first reviewing the patient's normal defecation pattern. A balanced diet is essential in promoting normal bowel elimination. Dietary considerations can be discussed with the patient, taking into account food preferences and allowances. For a normal daily bowel movement, approximately 800 g of raw fruits (with skins) and vegetables (*e.g.,* lettuce, cabbage, turnips, brussels sprouts, broccoli, cauliflower) should be included in daily intake. Whole grain breads, cereals, nuts, and seeds are also encouraged. Bran intake should be increased gradually since it may irritate the gastrointestinal tract, causing flatulence and diarrhea. A liberal fluid intake of at least 2 liters/day (8 to 10 glasses) is also advised unless contraindicated.[4] Bowel tones are assessed to determine the presence of an ileus. A daily routine can be established and a stimulus for defecation provided, such as coffee or prune juice. Assisting the patient to attain a normal semi-squatting position allows optimum usage of abdominal muscles and the effect of gravity.[1] Physical activity, in accordance with the patient's level of fatigue and activity tolerance, may be encouraged to promote peristalsis.

Diarrhea, on the other hand, may be found in patients with hyperfunction of the thyroid gland. In this case the nurse should discuss with the patient the avoidance of foods that increase peristalsis, such as highly seasoned and bulky foods. If diarrhea is severe, the patient should be assessed for fluid and electrolyte losses as discussed earlier in this chapter. These losses must be replaced. Fluids such as apple juice, bouillon, and diluted cola and ginger ale are encouraged.

Milk products are to be avoided until normal stool consistency has returned.

Evaluation. The expected outcome for the patient is a return to normal bowel function. The patient will be able to accurately discuss methods to reduce problems with bowel elimination.

Knowledge Deficit

Nursing Diagnosis/Problem. Most endocrine problems are chornic and require long-term management. Patient teaching is essential to control the underlying disease, minimize exacerbations of the disorder, and facilitate compliance to the prescribed therapy.

Interventions. When the acute symptoms subside and the patient's emotional and physical condition allows, education about the disease and its treatment begins. Family members should be included to offer support and assistance at home. Including the family is particularly important for patients with emotional and mental instability. Information included in the teaching program will vary, depending on the specific disorder, the individual patient needs, and institutional policy. The patient's stage of acceptance of his disease, level of cognitive ability, ethnic background, and sensory intactness must be assessed before formal dissemination of information begins.[2]

Consistency in patient teaching is important. Therefore, the information given to the patient and how the patient responds to the instruction should be accurately documented. It is preferable to give nonthreatening information before more anxiety-producing information. Both informal and formal teaching methods can be incorporated. Written handouts can facilitate the learning experiences and are especially useful for reference when the patient has left the hospital. Solicitation of expressed feelings, concerns, and questions by the patient are encouraged in order to clarify any misconceptions that may exist.

Effective patient teaching not only minimizes the patient's stress and increases his coping abilities, but also dramatically affects the course and management of most endocrine problems. Its importance cannot be overemphasized. Use of resource persons within the hospital (such as the pharmacist and the dietician) to help develop the teaching program and provide individualized patient instruction makes a more effective program. Topics to include in the teaching program are general information about the endocrine disorder, the prescribed medications, dietary modifications, methods for minimizing the risk of infection and personal injury, and the role of stress in relation to the disease. Table 73–2 provides specific points to emphasize under each of the categories.

Evaluation. The effectiveness of the teaching program can be determined by the attainment of the teaching goals. It is hoped that, with sensitive instruction, not only will the patient's compliance to therapeutic regimens improve, but the underlying disease process will eventually stabilize. The patient or family members will actively participate in the desired health behaviors, appropriately discuss information related to the specific endocrine disorder, and experience a general decrease in anxiety.

TABLE 73–2
Patient Education in Endocrine Disorders

1. The endocrine disorder
   a. Its general pathophysiology
   b. The general aims of therapy
   c. What conditions can exacerbate the illness
2. Prescribed medications
   a. Name, dose, route, frequency
   b. General actions of drug
   c. Side-effects to watch for
   d. When to discontinue drug or change dosage
   e. What to do when unable to take drug
3. Dietary modifications
   a. Purpose of diet
   b. Types and amounts of foods to be added to diet
   c. What foods to avoid
   d. How foods are measured
   e. What food substitutes may be used
4. How to minimize risk of infection and personal injury
   a. Avoid crowds and contagious people
   b. Clear the home of potential safety hazards
   c. Avoid walking barefoot and wear well-fitting shoes
   d. Notify physician of early cold, or influenza, symptoms and wounds that are slow to heal
5. Stress as related to the disease
   a. Identify physical and emotional stessor
   b. How can stress, or its effects, be diminished
   c. Discuss relaxation techniques
   d. Identify coping strategies and support persons
6. The importance of regular health evaluations
7. The importance of wearing a Medic-Alert identification bracelet or necklace
8. The avoidance of taking over-the-counter medications without first consulting the physician or primary health care provider

Summary

The effects of endocrine dysfunction on the body can manifest chronically or acutely and often with astounding variability and complexity. The patient's physical, mental, and emotional integrity are often severely affected. Nursing evaluations play a major role in determining the patient's level of dysfunction and response to therapy. The focus of nursing interventions will vary according to the type and degree of the endocrine dysfunction. Goals may range from restoration of fluid and electrolyte balance to restoration of the patient to a reasonable ability to manage activities of daily living; from promotion of improved patient self-esteem to promotion of long-term compliance to the therapeutic regimen.

Perhaps the greatest challenge for nurses lies in helping patients with endocrine disorders to cope with their diseases. Armed with a basic understanding of the underlying endocrine pathophysiology and using a calm, consistent, conscientious approach, the nurse can assist the patient by seeking out and strengthening his coping resources. Vital to the long-term disease management in nearly all endocrine disorders is education of the patient. The effective teaching program covers all pertinent aspects regarding the specific disease and treatment. The patient's family should be included to facilitate support and continuity of management when the patient returns home.

References

1. Aman RA: Treating the patient, not the constipation. Am J Nurs 80:1634–1635, 1980
2. Bille D (ed): Practical Approaches to Patient Teaching. Boston, Little, Brown & Co, 1981
3. Brunner LS, Suddarth DS (eds): The Lippincott Manual of Nursing Practice, 3rd ed. Philadelphia, JB Lippincott, 1983
4. Carpenito LJ: Nursing Diagnosis: Application to Clinical Practice. Philadelphia, JB Lippincott, 1983
5. Felver L: Understanding the electrolyte maze. Am J Nurs 80:1591–1595, 1980
6. Meissner DS: Evaluate your patient's level of independence. Nursing 10:72–73, 1980
7. Tucker SM, Breeding MA, Canobbio MM et al: Patient Care Standards. St Louis, CV Mosby, 1980

Bibliography

Allen S: Step by Step: Renew a patient's initiative. Nursing 81, 11:56–57, 1981

Billings C: Emotional first aid. Am J Nurs 80(11):2005–2009, 1980

Blevins D (ed): The Diabetic and Nursing Care. New York, McGraw-Hill, 1979

David AJ: Disability, home care and the caretaking role in family life. J Adv Nurs 5:474–484, 1980

Goldstein V: Caretaker role fatigue. Nurs Outlook 29:23–30, 1981

Hebert P, Breeding P: Self-care after hypophysectomy. J Neurosurg Nurs 11(2):118–120, 1979

Jenkins EH: Living with thyrotoxicosis. Am J Nurs 80(5):956–958, 1980

Martin D: Enjoyable activity for everyone. Geriatric Nursing 2:210–213, 1981

Muthe NC: Endocrinology: A Nursing Approach. Boston, Little, Brown & Co, 1981

Redman B: The Process of Patient Teaching in Nursing. St Louis, CV Mosby, 1981

Riffle K: Falls: Kinds, causes and prevention. Geriatric Nursing 3:165–169, 1982

Sanford SJ: Dysfunction of the adrenal gland: Physiologic considerations and nursing problems. Nurs Clin North Am: 15:481–488, 1980

Sneid DS: Hyperosmolar hyperglycemic nonketotic coma. Critical Care Quarterly 3(2):29–41, 1980

Urrows ST: Physiology of body fluids. Nurs Clin North Am 15:603–615, 1980

Wake MM, Brensinger JF: The nurse's role in hypothyroidism. Nurs Clin North Am 15:453–467, 1980

White V, Kumagi L: Preoperative endocrine and metabolic considerations. Med Clin North Am 63:1321–1334, 1979

Ziegler J: Physical reconditioning. Nursing 80, 10:67–69, 1980

Chapter 74

Diabetes Mellitus

Carol A. Blainey

It is critically important for the professional nurse to understand diabetes,* related physiology, pathophysiology, the multifaceted components of management, and the psychosocial impacts of this chronic condition that affects people of all ages. It is the nurse who interprets the concepts and teaches people to live with and control their diabetes. The vast majority of patients are not hospitalized and, indeed, for those who are hospitalized, a major goal is early discharge; hence day-to-day and minute-to-minute management of diabetes is under the control of the patient, his family members, and friends.

It has been established that effective teaching of people who have diabetes is a continuous process for the duration of the individual's life. Updating and reinforcement of learning helps the patient to attain maximum quality of self-management.[1,22] As more and more is learned about diabetes through research, changes in its care and management are continually being made. It is the professional nurse's challenge to understand, integrate, and explain to people who have diabetes the reasons for changes in management as they occur. The state of knowledge and treatment of diabetes is in evolution, giving rise to differences in opinions among health professionals. These differences in opinions can confuse and cause patients anxiety, and it is the nurse who assists them in understanding the origins of the different opinions and in coming to some resolution of the differences as they ultimately determine their own treatment regimens in conjunction with a multidisciplinary team approach (RN, MD, RD, *etc.*). Therefore, the nature of the condition and the need for continuous education mandate education for self-care as the primary contribution nurses make in the health care of people who have diabetes.

Basis for Nursing Management

Definition

The definition of diabetes remains elusive. In the strict sense, diabetes is a syndrome rather than a disease because there are no clear-cut etiologic factors or pathogenesis, no consistent clinical findings, and no specific laboratory tests. Abnormalities of the endocrine secretion of the pancreas (either an absolute or relative insufficiency of insulin, an insufficient number of insulin receptor sites on cells, or a combination of the two abnormalities) results in alterations in the metabolism of the food that is eaten (carbohydrates, fats, and proteins). Eventually structural abnormalities develop in a num-

*Wherever the term diabetes appears in this chapter it is meant to refer to diabetes mellitus.

ber of different body tissues. Four general components of the syndrome are:

- Hyperglycemia
- Large vessel (macrovascular) disease
- Small vessel (microvascular) disease
- Neuropathy

A useful working definition of diabetes is as follows: a symptomatic or asymptomatic state of altered carbohydrate metabolism, characterized by fasting blood glucose levels in excess of 140 mg/dl and by blood glucose values in excess of 200 mg/dl if a glucose tolerance test is done.[10]

Epidemiology

In the United States diabetes is one of the common chronic diseases. There are now over 6 million cases of diagnosed diabetes and an estimated 5 million undiagnosed cases. The prevalence of diabetes in the United States has shown a steady increase and this trend is expected to continue. Several factors are thought to contribute to the increase:

- Decreased death rate among people who have diabetes
- Over-all increased life expectancy
- Increased prevalence of obesity
- Increased number of diabetics having children
- Growing public awareness from community education.

It has been estimated that 60% of Americans with diabetes are over 55 years of age or older. Clearly, diabetes represents a major health problem in the United States. Discovering the undiagnosed cases and teaching sound self-management to all those with a diagnosis of diabetes is a major task for health professionals.

Classification

Diabetes is a condition that presents in many different forms. Seven different classifications of diabetes have been identified by the National Diabetes Data Group and National Institutes of Health and endorsed by the American Diabetes Association and the World Health Organization (Table 74–1). Two of the seven classifications, Insulin-Dependent Diabetes Mellitus (IDDM) and Non-Insulin-Dependent Diabetes Mellitus (NIDDM), constitute the great majority of all cases.

Insulin-Dependent Diabetes Mellitus. IDDM accounts for about 10% of the total cases of diabetes and usually presents in people of normal weight and 25 years of age and younger; however, IDDM has occurred in individuals of all ages. The clinical manifestations are abrupt onset of the classic symptoms: polyuria, polydipsia, polyphasia, weight loss, and malaise. These symptoms rapidly, in a matter of hours, progress to ketoacidosis. Since people with IDDM produce essentially no endogenous insulin, they will always require exogenous sources of insulin to prevent ketoacidosis and hence to sustain life. In general, the more serious complications of large vessel and small vessel changes and neuropathies are associated with IDDM than with NIDDM.

Non-Insulin-Dependent Diabetes Mellitus. The second major classification of diabetes is NIDDM, which accounts for about 80% of the total cases of diabetes in the United States. There is often no discernible onset of the symptoms and frequently the condition is noted through routine physical examinations and laboratory testing. Usually, people with NIDDM are over 40 years of age and obese. They may have the classic symptoms of polyuria, polydipsia, and polyphasia or less specific indications, such as infections of the skin, urinary tract, or vagina.

The advent of the radioimmunoassay for insulin in the 1960s revealed that people with NIDDM usually have the same levels of circulating endogenous insulin as do lean normal people. Although they may be symptomatic without additional insulin, they will not become ketoacidotic. The primary treatment for them is weight loss. The incidence of hypertension, angina, myocardial infarction, changes in renal and retinal blood vessels, and neuropathies is higher than in the general population and less than in people with IDDM.

Etiology

Charles Best and Fredrick Banting (1921) are credited with isolating insulin as one of the internal secretions of the pancreas. More than 60 years later, however, the cause of diabetes and hence a cure is still unknown. Rosaline Yallow's development of the radioimmunoassay for insulin in 1960 revealed that the circulating insulin levels of people with NIDDM are the same as those of lean normal people. This finding began the differentiation of IDDM and NIDDM as separate syndromes.

Insulin-Dependent Diabetes Mellitus (IDDM). What is known of the etiology of IDDM points to multifactorial elements involving genetics and the environment. The histocompatibility locus antigens (HLA), located on chromosome 6 in humans, are genetic markers that determine immune responses. In white populations in which IDDM is the predominate form, there is a striking relationship between IDDM and the presence of certain antigens. Islet cell antibodies were found at the time that the diagnosis of IDDM was made. This finding suggested abnormal immune responses and autoimmunity as causative factors. Onset of IDDM after viral infections and a seasonal cycle of onset suggested that IDDM may be a manifestation of a viral infection.[33]

Non-Insulin-Dependent Diabetes Mellitus (NIDDM). In NIDDM, the genetic factors of etiology include a high prevalence of relatives with NIDDM. The incidence of NIDDM markedly increases when a community moves from a traditional to a modernized lifestyle, changing its diet from low-calorie, high-fiber foods to high-calorie, refined foods, and its lifestyle from an active (physical) to a more sedentary form. Current data suggest that people with NIDDM have (1) insulin resistance, that is, insufficient numbers of insulin receptor sites, which are located on membranes of almost all cells, and (2) an impaired ability to secrete insulin.[28] This combination of factors of impaired secretory ability and unresponsiveness works to multiply effects. The reverse would

TABLE 74–1
Classification of Diabetes Mellitus and Other Categories of Glucose Intolerance

Current Names	*Previous Names*	*Clinical Characteristics*
Insulin-dependent diabetes mellitus (IDDM), Type I	Juvenile diabetes (JD), juvenile-onset diabetes (JOD), ketosis-prone diabetes, brittle diabetes	Little or no endogenous insulin: requires exogenous insulin for survival. Onset at any age, usually at young age (<25). Causes believed to be genetic, environmental or acquired, probably involving abnormal immune responses
Non-insulin-dependent diabetes mellitus (NIDDM), Type II	Adult-onset diabetes (AOD), maturity-onset diabetes (MOD), ketosis-resistant diabetes, stable diabetes, maturity-onset diabetes of the young (MODY)	Rarely develop ketosis except during infections or severe stress. Produce varying amounts of endogenous insulin, occasionally require exogenous insulin. Most are obese and over 40 years of age at onset. Cause thought to be genetic coupled with environmental factors
Diabetes mellitus associated with other conditions or syndromes	Secondary diabetes	Accompanied by conditions known or thought to cause diabetes mellitus: pancreatic or hormonal disease, drugs or chemical toxicity, abnormal insulin receptors, or certain genetic syndromes
Impaired glucose tolerance (IGT) a. Nonobese b. Obese	Asymptomatic diabetes, chemical diabetes, subclinical diabetes, borderline diabetes, latent diabetes	Glucose levels are between normal and diabetic levels. Increased susceptibility to atherosclerotic disease
Gestational diabetes (GDM)	Gestational diabetes	Women whose diabetes begins or is noted during pregnancy
Previous abnormality of glucose intolerance (PrevAGT)	Latent diabetes, prediabetes	Past history of elevated blood glucose, now have normal levels
Potential abnormality of glucose intolerance (PotAGT)	Potential diabetes, prediabetes	Never had glucose intolerance but considered at high risk due to several reasons, including relatives with diabetes, mothers of babies who weigh more than 9 lb at birth, obesity

(Adapted from Medical World News, October 29, 1979, pp 52–53)

also be true, for example, if after weight loss and regular physical exercise there was an increase in the number of receptor sites and a continuing deficit in secretory ability, the net result would be less severe NIDDM.

Pathology and Pathophysiology

The basis of the pathology of diabetes is poorly understood. Results of a 10-year prospective study of diabetic individuals (The Diabetes Control and Complication Trial [DCCT]) begun in 1983 are expected to provide data that will help to explain the development of the structural and hence functional changes in blood vessels and nerves. Several theories have been advanced to explain the changes. One theory is that in the presence of high glucose levels, basement membrane is thickened in every capillary bed in the body.[15] How the thickening of the basement membrane occurs and what relationship this change has to aging in general, and to renal and retinal disease specifically, is not clear. There are data to support a trend toward basement membrane thinning when blood glucose levels in diabetic individuals are normalized.[21]

The DCCT will assess the effects of control strict enough to maintain blood glucose levels within normal ranges (80 to 120 mg/dl). The study is designed to determine whether strict control of blood glucose level will prevent or delay the onset of changes in large and small blood vessels and in neurological functioning.

Mechanisms for Maintaining Plasma Glucose Homeostasis

Throughout the life of a normal healthy individual, blood glucose concentration is confined within narrow limits, between 60 and 120 mg/dl of blood. The immediate goal of maintenance of adequate glucose levels is to provide a constant supply of glucose to the brain, because of the very small energy stores in the brain itself and because the brain normally uses only glucose for energy. Nerve tissues, erythrocytes, and cells of the intestines, liver, and kidney tubules do not require insulin for transfer of glucose. Insulin is required to facilitate the transport of glucose into skeletal and cardiac muscle and into adipose tissue.

Glucose, as a product of digestion, flows to the liver through the portal vein. Once in the liver, the glucose is either used or stored, depending on the current blood glucose level. The ability to maintain glucose concentrations within the very narrow limits is mainly through the biological opposition of two pancreatic hormones, glucagon and insulin. The insulin–glucagon mechanism is primarily responsible for the steady, even supply of plasma glucose despite periods of no nutrient intake, exercise, or stress, or despite a high carbohydrate meal.

The beta cells of the islets of Langerhans in the pancreas continously monitor blood glucose and then secrete insulin (which lowers blood glucose) in appropriate amounts to maintain a normal level. Simultaneously, if glucose levels drop, for instance, after large energy expenditures or long periods of fasting, the alpha cells of the islets of Langerhans secrete glucagon (which raises blood glucose by stimulating the release of glycogen from the liver) to restore blood glucose levels. Normally, some insulin is secreted all the time; glucagon is secreted only during periods of high energy expenditure or fasting.[29]

The Role of Insulin

Understanding the role of insulin is important in the management of people with diabetes because insulin affects the metabolism of carbohydrates, protein, and fats. The most obvious and easily demonstrated effect of insulin lack is on carbohydrate metabolism, that is, hyperglycemia and glucosuria. However, the effects of insulin on the metabolism and storage of fats and protein are important.

Insulin Effects on Carbohydrate Metabolism. Insulin is primarily an anabolic hormone and works by means of a feedback system in response to carbohydrate intake, causing the liver to suppress glycogen release (glycogenolysis) and suppressing the formation of new glucose from noncarbohydrate stores (gluconeogenesis). Hence, a major function of insulin is the storage of any glucose in excess of that needed to maintain blood glucose levels betweeen 60 and 120 mg/dl. A second fundamental effect of insulin on carbohydrate metabolism is to accelerate the use of glucose by heart muscle, the diaphragm, skeletal muscles, and adipose tissue. Under normal conditions the rate of glucose use is determined largely by the rate at which glucose enters the cell. Glucose entry is not a process of simple diffusion but is a process of active transport. Transport is stimulated by insulin and leads directly to accelerated glucose utilization.

Insulin Effects on Fat Metabolism. Insulin has widespread effects on fat formation and fat mobilization. The fact that insulin increases the formation of fat has been clear since the first emaciated diabetic patient demonstrated a pad of adipose tissue after treatment with insulin. Insulin prevents the accumulation of fatty deposits in the liver by forming fatty acids from excess glucose after glycogen concentration in the liver reaches 5% to 6% of liver mass. The fatty acids so formed are then transported to adipose cells for storage. Another important effect of insulin in fat metabolism is to regulate the balance between fatty acid storage and fatty acid utilization in adipose cells. Insulin favors net fatty acid storage in adipose tissue by inhibiting the activity of hormone-sensitive lipase, an enzyme that catalyzes the breakdown of stored triglycerides, which in turn inhibits the release of fatty acids into the plasma.

Insulin suppresses ketosis by inhibiting the formation of ketone bodies in the following way. During insulin lack and in the presence of excess fatty acids in the liver, excess amounts of acetoacetic acid are formed by the liver cells and released from the liver into the circulation. Some of the acetoacetic acid is converted into beta-hydroxybutyric acid and acetone. These two substances and acetoacetic acid are called *ketone bodies*. When large amounts of ketone bodies are in body fluids the condition is called ketosis. Evidence of the effects of insufficient insulin on fat metabolism is demonstrated by elevated plasma cholesterol and elevated triglyceride levels.

Insulin Effects on Protein Metabolism. Insulin favors the conservation of protein and restrains the use of amino acids for the synthesis of glucose. The mechanisms through which insulin enhances protein storage are not as well understood as are the mechanisms of storage of carbohydrates and fats. However, in the absence of insulin all protein synthesis and storage stops and the catabolism of protein increases. Large amounts of amino acids are put into plasma and reused directly for energy or converted to glucose through gluconeogenesis. This process results in protein wasting, weight loss, and weakness, which are classic signs and symptoms of diabetes.

Glucagon

The action of glucagon is opposite that of insulin. Glucagon serves as a catabolic hormone for mobilizing fuel from newly formed glucose entering the liver, from cell stores of glycogen (glycogenolysis), and from free fatty acids and glycerol emerging from fat tissue (gluconeogenesis). These actions, glycogenolysis and gluconeogenesis, work to prevent

TABLE 74–2
Summary of the Actions of Insulin and Glucagon

Insulin Actions (Anabolic)

1. Activates transport of glucose into cells
2. Stores food materials in muscle, liver, and adipose tissue
3. Prevents loss of depot fat
4. Prevents accumulation of fatty deposits in liver
5. Suppresses ketosis by inhibiting formation of ketone bodies
6. Favors fatty acid storage in adipose tissue by activating enzymes that catalize breakdown of stored triglycerides
7. Restrains use of amino acids for synthesis of glucose
8. Favors conservation of protein
9. Stimulates protein synthesis within tissues

Glucagon Actions (Catabolic)

1. Releases newly formed glucose from liver
2. Breaks down glycogen from cell stores (glycogenolysis)
3. Breaks down fat cells, releasing free fatty acids and glycerol (gluconeogenesis)

hypoglycemia in fasting states or between meals. The actions of glucagon are clearly illustrated by the example of some diabetic individuals who have difficulty controlling their blood glucose levels because hypoglycemia is not quickly relieved by the oral intake of concentrated carbohydrates. These individuals should keep a supply of glucagon for injection intramuscularly to promote rapid mobilization of glucose and resolution of the hypoglycemia.

Constantly maintaining normal blood glucose levels in a variety of situations, that is, eating and fasting and maintaining effective metabolism of carbohydrates, proteins, and fats, requires complex integration of many physiological mechanisms. Insulin and glucagon are two important agents responsible for maintaining glucose homeostasis. Table 74–2 provides a summary of the actions of insulin and glucagon.

Anterior Pituitary

Anterior pituitary (adenohypophysis) controls in a major way the metabolic functions that affect blood glucose. The anterior portion of the pituitary gland, which lies in the sella turcica at the base of the brain and is connected with the hypothalamus by the hypophyseal stalk, plays a major role in the control of metabolic functions that affect blood glucose. The specific hormones coming from the pituitary that have a direct influence on blood glucose levels are:

1. Growth hormone (GH)
2. Adrenocorticotropic hormone (ACTH), which controls the secretion of some of the adrenocortical hormones, *i.e.*, glucocorticoids (cortisone from the adrenals), which in turn affect the metabolism of glucose, proteins, and fats through a catabolic action
3. Thyrotropin, which controls the rate of secretion of thyroxine by the thyroid gland. Thyroxine in turn controls the rates of most of the chemical reactions in the entire body.

Actions of these hormones tend to increase blood glucose; insulin alone lowers blood glucose. For a complete review of metabolic processes the reader is referred to a current textbook of physiology. Several references are listed in the Bibliography at the end of this chapter.

Summary

Briefly, the onset of diabetes (from insufficient production of insulin in the case of insulin-dependent diabetes mellitus, and impaired insulin secretion, utilization, and insulin resistance in the case of non-insulin-dependent diabetes mellitus) leads to the accumulation of plasma glucose because of the inability of the liver to store glucose as glycogen or to move glucose into the body cells. In an attempt to provide adequate energy to the body cells, first body stores of glycogen are broken down into glucose (glycogenolysis). Next, large amounts of stored fats are broken down (gluconeogenesis), resulting in ketosis. At the same time, stored proteins and amino acids are broken down and appear in the plasma, and are used directly for energy or converted to glucose through gluconeogenesis. However, in the face of insufficient or ineffective insulin, the blood glucose continues to increase as no glucose is moved into cells and used for energy. The buildup of blood glucose results in an increase of plasma osmolarity, and an osmotic diuresis ensues. Glucosuria generally occurs when the plasma glucose rises above 180 mg/dl. The renal threshold for glucose varies and changes with time, usually increasing. As these processes continue, the cardinal symptoms and signs of diabetes occur: polyuria, polydipsia, polyphasia, weight loss, and malaise. In IDDM the onset of signs and symptoms is abrupt and pronounced. In NIDDM some individuals may have such an insidious or mild onset of the signs and symptoms that they may have adapted and recognized the changes only on hindsight. Some individuals with NIDDM are asymptomatic.

Clinical Manifestations

Manifestations of diabetes vary widely among different people. In individuals with IDDM (10% of all diabetics), the presenting clinical manifestations are the classic signs and symptoms often sufficiently advanced as to include ketoacidosis. In persons with NIDDM (80% to 90% of all diabetic individuals), the presenting clinical manifestations always include hyperglycemia and usually polyuria and polydipsia, but not ketoacidosis. In persons with NIDDM, hyperglycemia is not infrequently a serendipitous finding made when a chronic urinary tract, vaginal, or skin infection is investigated. Hypertension and slow-to-heal skin wounds are frequently associated with diabetes.

Acute Manifestations

Ketoacidosis

Ketoacidosis is the most acute manifestation of IDDM, is the most frequent reason for which diabetic patients under age 20 are admitted to the hospital, and accounts for about 14% of all hospital admissions.[16] The worldwide mortality rate from an episode of ketoacidosis since 1950 has been reported as 10% (range from 1% to 19%).[3,31] Ketoacidosis can become the presenting event of IDDM if a person is unaware of having diabetes. In an individual with known IDDM, ketoacidosis can occur whenever an intercurrent illness, infection, or emotional stress upsets the usual balance of food intake, exercise, and insulin. Usually, the cause is a failure to increase exogenous insulin dosages to levels sufficiently high enough to control the blood glucose. Occasionally, ketoacidosis results from an inappropriate decrease or even omission of insulin. Ketoacidosis does not occur suddenly but develops over a period of several hours or days. Pathophysiological events leading to hyperglycemia and ketosis are described in the preceding section and are summarized in Figure 74–1. If this situation remains uncorrected, dehydration and acidosis overwhelm the body's buffering system, and respiratory compensation is inadequate for the keto acid load. Coma and death can ensue. (See Chap. 13 and 14 on fluid and electrolytes and acid–base balance.) A summary of history, clinical findings, and laboratory findings in diabetic ketoacidosis found in Table 74–3.

Treatment of ketoacidosis includes insulin administration and restoration of fluids and electrolytes. The generally accepted method of insulin administration is low-dose, continuous intravenous infusion of regular insulin. Dosage depends on the severity of ketoacidosis and the physician's preference. Insulin immediately restores the movement of glucose into the body cells and halts gluconeogenesis. Intravenous fluids are used to correct the volume depletion. Initially, normal saline or lactated Ringer's solution is used, with subsequent fluid choices depending on ongoing hourly

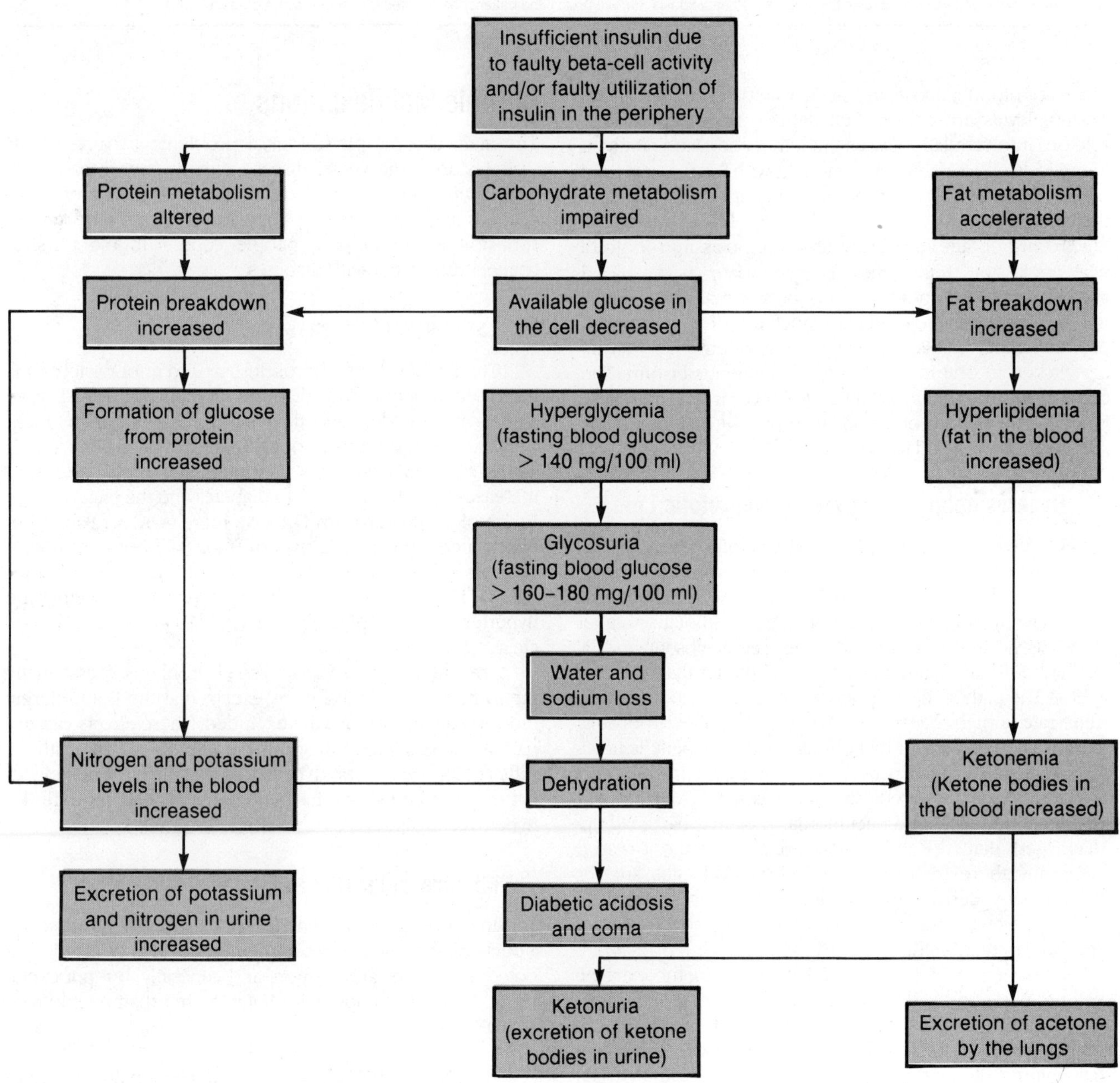

FIGURE 74–1 Pathogenesis of diabetic ketoacidosis.

TABLE 74–3
Summary of Diagnostic Findings in Diabetic Ketoacidosis

History	Clinical Findings	Laboratory Findings
Undiagnosed IDDM Intercurrent illness Emotional stress Omission of insulin In person with IDDM	Stupor, drowsiness Flushed facies Soft or sunken eyeballs Hypothermia Acetone breath Thirst Signs of dehydration Kussmaul's respirations (deep sighing) Hypotension Tachycardia Volume Depletion	Serum ketones Hyperglycemia (300 mg/dl) Acidosis Bicarbonate, 10 mEq/liter Glycosuria Ketonuria Also check levels of potasium, chloride, creatinine, sodium

Note: Variations occur according to cause of the ketoacidosis, for example, if the patient has an infection fever may be present.

results of blood glucose and electrolyte determinations. Potassium levels are critical. Cell damage from ketoacidosis releases intracellular potassium into the blood with resultant high levels of potassium. As treatment with insulin and fluid proceeds, cell walls repair and potassium is moved back into the body cells with resultant depletion of blood potassium. Electrocardiogram and serum levels of potassium indicate when potassium replacement is appropriate. As the blood glucose returns to normal levels over a matter of hours, intravenous fluids are changed to include some dextrose to prevent hypoglycemia. Gradually, as the patient improves, he is switched to oral feedings and subcutaneous insulin. The cause of the ketoacidosis (infection, myocardial infarction, lack of information, or compliance difficulties) should by now be identified and treated.

Hyperosmolar Hyperglycemic Nonketotic Coma

Hyperosmolar hyperglycemic nonketotic coma (HHNC) is a metabolic disturbance that usually occurs in people 60 years and older who have NIDDM, in whom the glucose levels are higher than 500 mg/dl, serum osmolality higher than 330 mOsm/kg, serum and urine acetone absent, arterial pH higher than 7.3, and plasma HCO_3^- higher than 20 mEq/liter.[24] The pathogenesis is poorly understood and the mortality rate is high, between 40% and 60%.[25] The prodromal period is usually much longer than that of diabetic ketoacidosis, and a majority of patients have had a concurrent illness or stressor, such as cerebrovascular accident (CVA), myocardial infarction (MI), and pneumonia. They may have had undiagnosed diabetes that is exacerbated by the stressor. Generally, there are a variety of neurological signs, such as hemisensory deficits and hemiparesis and focal seizures, which can evoke the most common misdiagnosis—that of cerebrovascular accident.

Treatment of HHNC is aimed at correcting the extreme volume depletion and the hyperosmolar state, and then detecting and treating the underlying illness. Maintaining a high degree of suspicion to keep alert to all sources of potential volume depletion in the elderly person with NIDDM works toward early detection and hence toward more successful treatment of HHNC.

Chronic Manifestations

The main chronic physiological problems associated with diabetes are large vessel disease, small vessel disease, and neuropathy. Since little is known of the causes of these changes and care is mainly supportive, nurses have key responsibilities in helping people cope with the physical changes associated with diabetes.

Large Vessel Disease

The incidence of atherosclerosis and arteriosclerosis is increased in people with diabetes. Diabetic individuals have angina at an earlier age than do nondiabetic individuals. Coronary heart disease accounts for half of the deaths among adults with NIDDM, and the incidence of hypertension increases with the duration of diabetes and the patient's age. In the older person with NIDDM, there is a correlation between increased systolic hypertension and both peripheral vascular disease and cerebral vascular disease. Whether NIDDM is a cause of the systolic hypertension or whether the hypertension is simply reflecting changes in the vessels is not clear.[7]

Treatment of these large vessel problems is essentially the same as for nondiabetics, except that the β-adrenergic blocking agents are usually excluded. These agents can impair counterregulatory responses and blunt the sympathetic reflex response to hypoglycemia, so that the diabetic individual may not be aware of a hypoglycemia reaction until the hypoglycemia is severe or prolonged.

Microvascular Disease

In diabetes, the first change in the small blood vessels is a thickening of the basement membrane. This change is first noted in the eyes and kidneys and generally, but not exclusively, occurs in people with IDDM rather than people with NIDDM.

Diabetic Retinopathy. Diabetic retinopathy is one of the leading causes of new blindness in adults in the United States. Annually there are 5000 new cases of blindness due to diabetes.[31] Diabetic changes in eyes can be divided into two major groups, nonproliferative and proliferative retinopathy.

In *nonproliferative retinopathy* three basic pathological processes occur: (1) increased retinal vascular permeability, (2) structural alteration of the retinal capillaries, and (3) vaso-obliteration. Nonproliferative retinopathy may progress very slowly with little interference to the vision (Fig. 74–2).

Proliferative retinopathy is a growth of fibrovascular tissue on the inner surface of the retina and is thought to be caused by retinal ischemia (Fig. 74–3). Newly formed vessels develop in the area between the retinal and vitreous gel. Fibrous tissue is associated with the new vessels and this tends to cause tension on the retina, resulting in hemorrhage into the vitreous and in retinal distortion and detachment (Fig. 74–4). Early detection of proliferative retinopathy allows treatment with laser photocoagulation to stop the proliferation of new blood vessels. Vitrectomy is done to remove blood when a hemorrhage occurs. The nursing section later in this chapter includes a section on the special needs of the blind diabetic individual.

Nephropathy. Nephropathy is another manifestation of microvascular changes associated with diabetes. Structural and functional changes become evident within months of the onset of IDDM. Glomeruli enlarge and the glomerular filtration rate increases. Diffuse and nodular glomerulosclerosis can be demonstrated histologically, although these changes generally do not cause clinical renal problems in the first 10

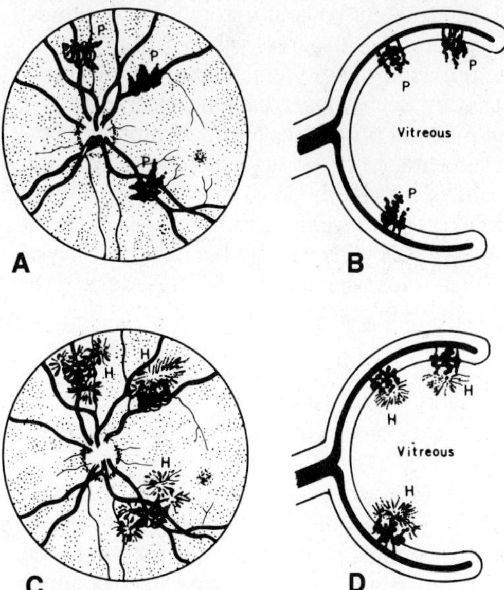

FIGURE 74–3 Proliferative retinopathy is the more severe form of the disease. (*A*) Vessels (*P*) have sprouted from the existing ones, proliferating into the vitreous. (*B*) Cross section of the eye shows the same new vessels growing into the vitreous. (*C*) Hemorrhages which commonly develop surround the new or proliferating vessels. (*D*) Cross section shows hemorrhages (*H*) leaking into the vitreous from proliferating vessels. (Reprinted with permission from Association for Education and Rehabilitation of the Blind and Visually Impaired, successor organization to American Association of Workers for the Blind which published Blindness Annual, 1969. Cf. page 28.)

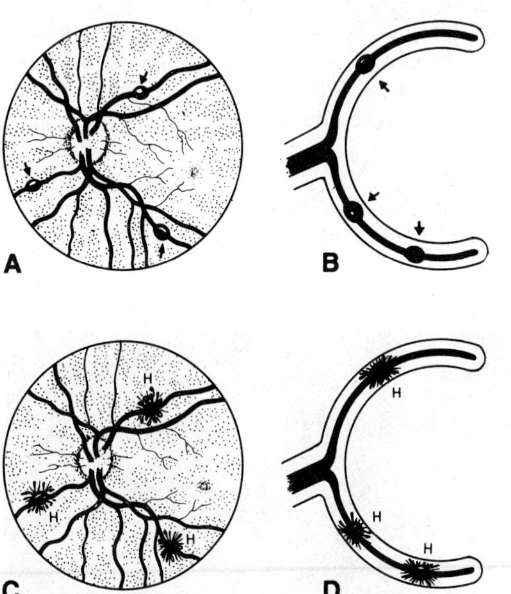

FIGURE 74–2 In the milder or nonproliferative form of diabetic retinopathy, the blood vessel damage is contained within the retina. (*A*) Damage first occurs in the walls of the retinal capillaries. Arrows point to areas in the capillary wall which balloon out, forming aneurysms. (*B*) Cross section of the eye also shows aneurysms. (*C*) The walls of the aneurysms are weak, and blood can easily flow through them. (*D*) The cross section shows these hemorrhages contained within the retina. (Reprinted with permission from Association for Education and Rehabilitation of the Blind and Visually Impaired, successor organization to American Association of Workers for the Blind, which published Blindness Annual, 1969. Cf. page 27.)

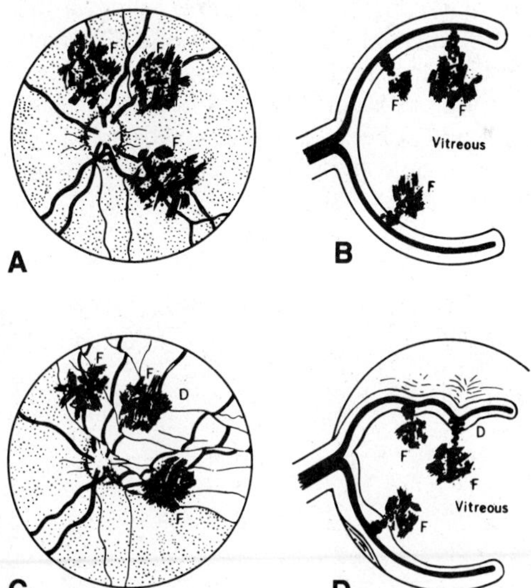

FIGURE 74–4 Hemorrhages into the vitreous which accompany proliferative diabetic retinopathy are often replaced by fibrous or scar tissue that forms in the vitreous. (*A*) Ophthalmoscopic view shows this fibrous tissue (*F*). (*B*) Cross section depicts the same process with fibrous tissue forming in the vitreous. (*C*) Traction from the fibrous tissue has pulled on the retina and caused a detachment (*D*). (*D*) Cross-sectional sketch of the retinal detachment shows the fibrous tissue pulling the retina into the vitreous. (Reprinted with permission from Association for Education and Rehabilitation of the Blind and Visually Impaired, successor organization to American Association of Workers for the Blind which published Blindness Annual, 1969. Cf. page 29.)

years of IDDM. Intermittent proteinuria is the first clinical renal complication and may progress within 1 to 3 years to persistent proteinuria and subsequent decline in renal function, as measured by decreasing creatinine clearance. The decline in renal function progresses to renal failure about 5 years after the appearance of persistent proteinuria. Early treatment of nephropathy has been to strive to keep blood glucose and blood pressure within normal ranges. Approximately 20% to 25% of all patients who begin renal dialysis have diabetes. Renal transplantation has been performed in the case of renal failure in people with IDDM.

Neuropathies

Neuropathies associated with diabetes have been reported as having an incidence of from 50% to 60% in all diabetic individuals. The variation in percentage is a function of the problem of defining diabetic neuropathy. This complication of diabetes generally, but not exclusively, occurs in persons in older age-groups who may have neuropathies from other causes as well as having typical age-related changes. As mentioned in the section on blood vessel complications, diabetes is a leading risk factor of cerebrovascular accidents. In general, diabetic neuropathies cause a slowing of nerve conduction and loss of tendon reflexes. The diabetic peripheral neuropathies can be described as being symmetrical, of slow, progressive onset, and of a stocking-glove distribution on the feet and hands. The sensory changes can cause dysfunction through weakness and atrophy of distal muscles of the hands and feet.

Autonomic nervous system involvement is manifested in a wide variety of dysfunctions. Absence of sweating of the feet, atrophy of the skin, and malformations of the toenails are common. Postural hypotension and nocturnal diarrhea are frequent. Gastric atony is not common but creates major problems of management because of uneven absorption of meals. Sexual impotence in all diabetic males over 30 years of age has been estimated at 50%.[8,23]

Combined Neurological and Vascular Problems

Sexual impotence in diabetic men is believed to have a vascular and neurological basis. Psychogenic factors are well established as causes of sexual dysfunction, and drug and alcohol abuse are also associated with impotence. Generally, the investigation of impotence begins by ruling out any other endocrine cause. Efforts are made to get the blood glucose and blood pressure under the best control possible. Additional treatment modalities include psychological counseling to determine causes, relieve anxiety, and examine alternative methods of sexual expression. Surgical implantations to simulate penile erection are available.

Sexual dysfunction in women has been reported as a vague complaint of decreasing enjoyment of coitus and the specific complaint of decreased lubrication. Discerning causes of sexual dysfunction in women are complicated by the frequent occurrence of urinary tract infections and vaginal infections.

Foot Problems. The feet of diabetic individuals merit special emphasis because of the frequency of the need for amputation to remove infected areas that do not heal. The incidence of amputations of the lower extremities of diabetic individuals is 20,000 per year.[31] The problems have a basis in vascular and neurological changes resulting from diabetes.[17] The angiopathies lead to atrophic skin changes and decreased circulation, so that an injury on the feet occurs more easily, is more readily infected, is more difficult to reach with systemic antibiotics, and thus is slow to heal (Fig. 74–5). Concomitantly, the neuropathies result in decreased sensation and muscle atrophy, with changes in pressure points on the feet. Without pain to alert the person to injury and to remind him or her to protect the injured area, injuries occur, and healing is slowed.

In young people with IDDM, neuropathies can be present without the angiopathy. Hence, injury to the feet may occur because of decreased sensation, but with adequate

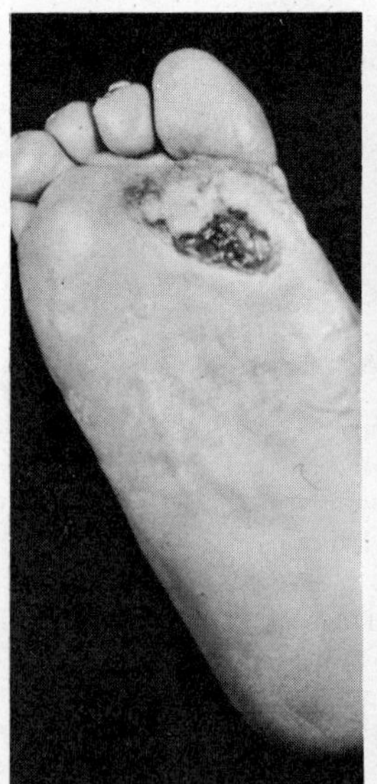

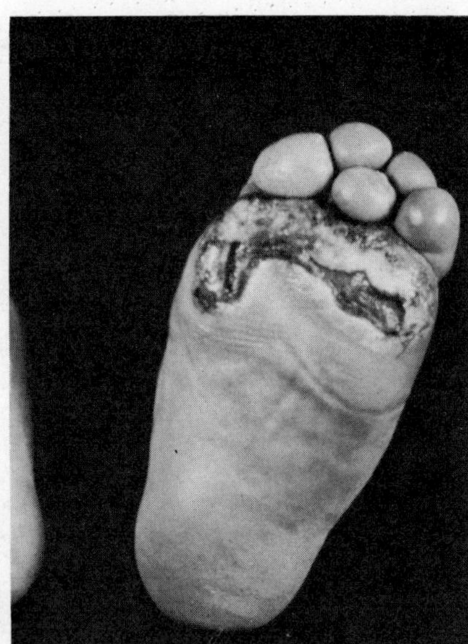

FIGURE 74–5 Severe ulceration of feet secondary to diabetic neuropathy. (Ezrin C, Godden JO, Volpe R [eds]: Systematic Endocrinology, 2nd ed, p 424. New York, Harper & Row, 1979)

circulation healing occurs quickly if stress is taken off the injured area. Details of preventive measures in regard to care of the feet are discussed later in the nursing section of this chapter.

Emotional Manifestations

Psychosocial reactions and adaptations to receiving a diagnosis of diabetes generally parallel the reactions to any chronic condition: disbelief, developing awareness, reorganization, and resolution. Diabetes is somewhat more complex in that there are continual changes because of development of the disease as well as in the treatment of symptoms. In addition, body image alteration and adaptation are complicated by no visible physical change in the body with the diagnosis of diabetes. Hence, adaptation may be slowed as the phase of denial is prolonged.

There is substantial evidence that diabetic control is altered by emotional stress. Internal motivation to maintain adherence to treatment plans is clearly affected by emotional states. High anxiety states and depression are frequently associated with diabetes and its concomitant requirement of permanently changed lifestyles, threats to previous life plans, and the endlessness of treatment.[12]

Medical Management

Diagnosis

Diagnosis of Diabetes in Adults. Diagnosis of diabetes in adults requires one or more of the following criteria:

1. Obvious elevation of plasma glucose, coupled with the classic signs and symptoms: polyuria, polydipsia, polyphasia, glucosuria, and malaise, or
2. A fasting blood glucose concentration of 140 mg/dl or higher, or
3. A plasma glucose concentration of 200 mg/dl or higher at 1 and 2 hours after a 75-g oral glucose challenge. The person must have had a 3-day preparatory diet that includes at least 150 g of carbohydrate.

Aging is associated with progressive glucose intolerance. This process begins in the third and fourth decade of life and continues. The basis of the glucose intolerance of aging appears to be tissue unresponsiveness to insulin.[5] It is unclear whether it is a normal part of aging or a disease process. In the past, upward adjustment of random blood glucose levels were made for the elderly, although fasting blood glucose levels are minimally affected by age. Currently, the diagnostic criteria for fasting glucose remain the same for all adults, a fasting blood glucose above 140 mg/dl is considered to be the critical criterion for a diagnosis of diabetes. Random blood glucose levels may be elevated in the elderly; however, if the fasting blood glucose level is below 140 mg/dl that person does not have diabetes.

Diagnosis of Diabetes in Children. The diagnosis of diabetes in children requires the following criteria:

1. Classic signs and symptoms of diabetes: polyuria, polydipsia, glycosuria, polyphagia, rapid weight loss, and fatigue
2. Elevated random plasma glucose levels of 200 mg/dl or higher[24]

Oral Glucose Tolerance Tests. Oral glucose tolerance test (OGTT) are not done as frequently as in the past because of the previous diagnostic criteria, the rationale being that if the fasting blood glucose is elevated, then the blood glucose will surely be elevated after a glucose challenge. Occasionally, however, the OGTT is done when stress or gestational diabetes is suspected. The procedure for an OGTT is as follows:

1. An unrestricted diet that includes at least 150 g of carbohydrate is eaten for 3 days prior to the test.
2. A fast of at least 10 hours, but no more than 16 hours, immediately before the test. Water is allowed.
3. Collection of a fasting blood glucose sample, with the person seated. Smoking is not allowed at any time during the test.
4. Receipt by adults of 75 g of glucose and children of 1.75 g/kg of bodyweight, up to a maximum of 75 g of glucose. Zero time is the beginning of taking the oral glucose over a period not exceeding 5 minutes.
5. Blood glucose levels are drawn at 30-minute intervals for 2 hours.

Treatment

The management of this chronic condition that is inextricably linked to food intake is in reality under the control of the person who has the condition. Hence, the primary treatment modality is education for self-management. A general overview of the medical management of diabetes is included here. Details of the content of the education for the various components of management are included in the nursing section later in this chapter, because the professional nurse is the health professional most qualified to coordinate the educational process of patients.

Diet. Since management of diabetes is so closely involved with eating, *meal plans* have always been the central focus of care. Before 1923 and the advent of insulin therapy, diet was the only treatment and a great variety of approaches were tried, from starvation to taking nearly spoiled food. Since insulin has been available, varying combinations of foods have been suggested, with controversy about how much carbohydrate should be included. Many health professionals believed that carbohydrates should be severely restricted, which necessitated the increase of protein and fat in the meal plan.

Currently, most health professionals believe that the high fat diet is more detrimental to diabetic individuals than is a high carbohydrate diet, especially when there is an increase in more complex carbohydrates. The usual composition of diet for a diabetic is 50% carbohydrate, 30% to 40% protein, and 10% to 20% fat. Research studies are now in progress to evaluate the effects on blood glucose exerted by simple vs. complex carbohydrates. In addition to the composition of the meal plan, the main diet therapy for obese individuals with NIDDM is a low-calorie diet for weight loss.

Exercise. Exercise has always been a component of treatment in diabetes, but currently focus on this modality of treatment has increased as exercise for everyone has received renewed attention. Exercise as a means to weight control by increasing the nonfat body weight portion of body weight has been added to the beneficial effects of exercise for improved cardiovascular and emotional status.[2]

Insulin. Insulin and oral hypoglycemic agents are the pharmacological components of management in diabetes. Current data on types of insulin and oral agents are discussed in the nursing management section later in this chapter. The choices for insulin therapy are considerably increased, and physicians make choices that are then altered as time reveals the individual's response to the specific drug. Opinions about the usefulness of oral agents remain controversial and are again up to the physician's discretion in regard to how much information and freedom of choice to give to his patients. People with IDDM take only insulin and people with NIDDM are treated initially with diet therapy and exercise and then with oral agents or insulin according to the physician's decision.

Coping with Chronic Disease. Coping with diabetes and managing the activities of daily living are complex and demanding and are certainly a part of the management of any chronic disease. Integrating the necessary changes into the lifestyle and maintaining the motivation to continue the activities unaffected by diabetes are important details of care that determine the degree to which a person will be able to follow therapeutic regimens. A large component of treatment is providing information and giving support to diabetic individuals as they deal with the emotional reaction to integrating the event of a serious chronic disease with the fact that it has some genetic basis. Clearly, helping people cope with changes of health status are within the realm of professional nursing and are discussed later in the nursing section of this chapter.

Measurements of the Effects of Treatment

Short-term effects of the treatment of diabetes can be measured by the abatement of symptoms and of blood glucose levels. Long-term effects of treatment can be measured by lowered plasma cholesterol and lowered triglycerides and perhaps by the prevention or delay of the onset of the complications of diabetes. For the latter we must wait for the results of the 10-year prospective study now in progress. Blood glucose levels can be measured by glucose monitoring strips, conventional laboratory methods, and hemoglobin A_{1c} testing.

Self Blood-Glucose Monitoring. Self blood-glucose monitoring (SBGM) is based on using chemically impregnated strips that react with the glucose in blood. Color reagents are impregnated into the strips, and a color change occurs as a result of the oxygen released when glucose reacts with the glucose oxidase enzyme in the strip. The individual pricks the skin on the side of a finger with an automatic spring-loaded instrument (Autolet or Autoclix are examples) or a lancet. Next, a hanging drop of blood is placed on the pad of the strip using care of avoid touching the pad. After a period of time that may be different in different brands of strips, but is usually 60 seconds, the pad is wiped or washed with water and then another time period elapses, usually 15 seconds. Then the strip is compared to a color chart to determine the blood glucose. Various meters have been developed to read the strips, using a needle or digital readout (Fig. 74–6). The frequency of self blood glucose testing is very individual and determined by the patient, nurse, and physician. Usually people with IDDM test two to four times daily: before meals, at bedtime, and any other time they wish to confirm the level of glucose in their blood. A pregnant diabetic individual may be testing up to seven times a day. Self blood-glucose testing has provided patients with a means to measure their own blood glucose levels that is more precise than urine test results. Patients can then make judgments about daily or hourly adjustment of food intake, exercise, and insulin and have direct feedback on how these variables influence their glucose control. On clinic visits conventional laboratory procedures are useful for validating the accuracy of self blood-glucose testing, and provide data about the level of glucose in the blood at a particular time rather than control of the blood glucose over time. SBGM is invaluable in assisting the diabetic and his physician and nurse to recognize and treat early diabetic ketoacidosis at home, possibly preventing hospitalization.

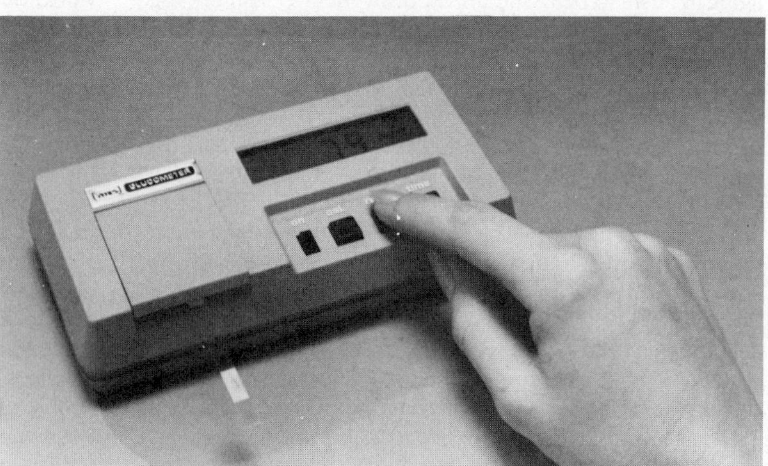

FIGURE 74–6 An example of a commercially available glucometer which measures electronically the amount of glucose in the blood. (Courtesy of Ames Division, Miles Laboratory, Inc.)

Glycosolated Hemoglobin A_{1c}. Glycosolated hemoglobin A_{1c} is a naturally occurring nonenzymatic, postsynthesis modification of hemoglobin that results in the attachment of glucose to the red blood cell (protein hemoglobin). The modification is irreversible and is produced slowly and continuously throughout the 120-day life span of erythrocytes. The blood level of hemoglobin A_{1c} has been shown to be an indicator of the average blood glucose concentration over the preceding 1 to 3 months. Normal levels of hemogblobin A_{1c} vary with the particular laboratory test, and levels in diabetic individuals may be two to three times normal. This test removes the problem of spurious results reported by patients or the more common event of patients rigorously controlling food intake for a few days preceding clinic visits, so that their blood glucose levels are not reflective of their more typical food intake patterns. Hemoglobin A (HbA) now serves as a marker for glucose control. Goals to maintain the glucose level as near to normal as possible can now be followed on a continuum with the advent of HbA.

Urine Testing. Before the advent of self blood-glucose testing, the only means patients had to monitor their self-management was urine testing. Urine testing was never considered a precise measure of blood glucose for many reasons. Circulatory and renal function changes related to diabetes or aging clouded the accuracy of the testing. The state of bladder function affected results in that the patient may have had residual urine in the bladder that influenced subsequent urine tests. Many drugs affect the results of urine testing. Considering all of these factors, urine testing still offers useful data. On a day-to-day basis that evolves into a week-to-week pattern, control over time can be estimated. Marked changes in blood glucose levels are also reflected in the patterns of urine tests. When cost and discomfort are considered, urine testing is still appropriate, particularly for elderly individuals with NIDDM who are not going to be making major changes in their treatment.

Whether patients should test first-voided urine specimens or random urine specimens is tied to what information is sought. If an estimate of current blood glucose levels is desired, a second or third voided specimen is needed and self blood-glucose monitoring would be best. If information is sought about weekly control of blood glucose, urine specimens that represent aliquots of urine since the last voiding provide more useful data.

Urine testing for glucose can be done at home by using Clinitest tablets or various dipstick methods. All forms of urine testing use a method that compares colors with color charts. Methods, directions, and timing are given on the packages, and it is imperative that the timing be precise. Care must be taken to avoid touching either the tablets or the portions of the dipstick that will come into contact with the urine being tested.

Testing for ketones is conducted in the same way as for glucose. Every person with diabetes needs to have the means and knowledge to test for ketones in the urine and blood when illness occurs. Ketone testing provides a critical piece of data when diabetic individuals make decisions regarding the need to call a health care professional. Normally, no ketones are present in the urine. How to manage glucose levels during intercurrent illness is discussed later in the nursing management section of this chapter.

To obtain a 24-hour urine specimen, a person voids and discards a specimen, notes the time, and then collects all urine produced during the next 24 hours. Analysis of the 24-hour specimen gives data about blood glucose control for that 24-hour period. Normally, individuals lose no glucose in their urine. In addition to glucose, the 24-hour urine specimen can be examined for protein and creatinine, and creatinine clearance can be calculated as a means of monitoring renal status.

Prognosis

The advent of insulin prolonged the life expectancy of diabetic individuals to a considerable degree. Currently, with sound management of diabetic ketoacidosis, the prognosis of diabetes is dependent on the amount of end-stage disease that develops. Actual death rates from diabetes are difficult to obtain, since mortality statistics generally do not specify contributing causes of death. Data that are available indicate that diabetes is the fifth leading cause of death from disease. The report from the National Commission on Diabetes in 1975 suggested that diabetes and its complications are responsible for more than 300,000 deaths annually in the United States. The most frequent cause of death for people with diabetes is myocardial infarction. Estimates of life expectancy in people with diabetes vary greatly, but all agree that life expectancy is decreased.

Nursing Management Plan

Self-Care Education

The prime nursing management responsibility of diabetic individuals is education for self-management. Education for self-care is cost-effective because it decreases hospital admissions. Communication is the mechanism through which nurses assist people to manage their activities of daily living (ADL) in the face of alterations in health. Empirical data have indicated that the type of communication is a factor in the effectiveness of health professional intervention. Studies to verify the empirical data have begun. For example, people have been found to have higher comprehension of their therapeutic regimens when clinicians used in combination of statements that (1) demonstrated respect for the patient, (2) shared current clinical data, and (3) acknowledged patient statements.[18] It follows that if people understand their regimens they will be more likely to adhere to the plan.

Because nurses have a broad objective of assisting people to manage their ADL in the face of change, time spent establishing a relationship of mutual respect is cost-effective. Giving people information about diabetes without assessment or establishing a relationship will not result in the individual's understanding and hence adhering to the suggested treatment.

Major ways education can be implemented is through nurses acting as role models when care is given to hospitalized patients and by emphasizing important areas during outpatient visits. For example, during hospitalization and at outpatient and home visits, nurses can give attention to the care of the patient's feet. Direct instruction, either in individualized programs or through more formal group classes, are other methods of teaching self-management.

Assessment

Assessment of the individual with diabetes is threefold: physical, psychosocial, and educational.

Physical Assessment

Assessment is designed first to establish a baseline from which changes can be measured, second to detect any evidence of complications related to diabetes, and third to discover any other conditions that might be complicated by diabetes. High risk clinical manifestations of diabetes are related to: (1) circulation, (2) nutrition, (3) the integument, (4) the senses, (5) elimination, (6) sexuality, (7) rest, and (8) comfort. After establishing the presence of any deficit or alteration, the nurse can then document and the effects of these manifestations on the chosen lifestyle and ADLs of that individual.

Psychosocial Assessment

A major element of psychosocial assessment in people who have diabetes is to consider the individual's ability to cope with having a chronic, constantly changing condition that is intimately involved with eating. Coping with the body image alteration that occurs when people learn they have diabetes is compounded by no visible change in their bodies. Having no physical change to view complicates the grieving process and tends to prolong the denial stage. In addition, no concessions by others are made to the diabetic individual as is often the case in more visible chronic diseases, such as arthritis. Diabetes requires that people deal endlessly with the condition and they are constantly reminded that they have diabetes by their awareness of what they can or cannot eat. Many culturally designated occasions involve eating, so that people with diabetes are required to focus on their condition at these important times.

Another element to consider is that the need to inform other people of the potential need for help during hypoglycemia invades privacy. Personal priorities may require reordering or change.

Some people attach stigma to any condition that involves genetic transmission. This genetically transmissible component of diabetes causes many people to have recollections of relatives with diabetes. Time and childhood perceptions may have distorted reality, leaving frightening and often incorrect expectations of what the future holds. Also, having diabetes causes a reexamination of plans made for the future, such as vocational choice, marriage, and reproduction. Finally, individuals may focus concern on the fact that people with diabetes die at an earlier age as compared with nondiabetic individuals.

Educational Assessment

Diabetes mandates self-care because continuous control of blood glucose is needed. Complex new information about the management of diabetes is being added all the time and must be learned. Lifestyles may need to be changed and several times daily self-inflicted needle pricks may be required for blood testing and insulin injections. Educational prerequisites of sound self-management are as follows:

- *Psychomotor skills* should be sufficient to test blood or urine, to give insulin injections, and to take care of the feet. Physical disabilities, such as blindness or mobility deficits, may necessitate some adaptations of the usual methods of testing and injection. Visual acuity may be temporarily altered by uncontrolled diabetes, but this condition will improve with treatment, so that some learning modalities may need revision as vision improves.
- *Cognitive skills* needed include the ability to take in, understand, and apply new information. Degree of visual acuity, literacy level, and any learning disability are of considerable importance. Diabetic individuals describe a feeling of being in a dream or being unable to focus their thoughts when their blood glucose is highly elevated.
- *Affective strengths* prerequisite to learning self-care are emotional stability and coping abilities. Consideration of the diabetic person's social support systems or lack of support is a major component of educational assessment in determining whether the individual's personal priorities will allow sufficient attention to self-care.

A person's health beliefs regarding the seriousness of diabetes and the usefulness of treatment influence the success of treatment. Also, the individual's attitudes toward health care providers are crucial to effective intervention. Locus of control, attitudes toward adherence to treatment regimens, and interest in learning about diabetes all provide information that will guide educational interventions.

The following are pivotal questions to pose relative to determining a person's level of understanding and to detecting difficulties in coping with ADL in relation to diabetes:

- How has diabetes affected your body?
- How do you feel diabetes will affect your body over time?
- What do you believe caused your diabetes?
- How do you feel diabetes has or will affect your life?
- What do you believe you can do to minimize the effects of diabetes?
- Where does treating your diabetes rank in your current personal priority list?

Nursing Diagnoses

The nature of this metabolic disease encompasses every functional area of the body and has the potential to have an impact on all ADLs. The main concern of nursing is teaching self-care, and this provides a way of approaching nursing diagnosis. Deficits in knowledge of self-care can have a psychosocial basis or can be caused by knowledge deficits, skill deficits, or sensory-perceptual alterations that prevent self-care. Examples of some nursing diagnoses for people with a recent clinical diagnosis of diabetes are

- Disturbance of self-concept related to a recent diagnosis of diabetes, leading to inability to learn
- Knowledge deficit related to management of recurrent insulin reactions
- Skill deficits, *e.g.,* insulin injection techniques, and home blood glucose monitoring methods, leading to inability to do self-care
- Fear of the consequences of recent diagnosis of diabetes, leading to an inability to learn

As the individual adjusts to the initial impact of the medical diagnosis, the nursing diagnoses change. Some examples of this phase are

- Denial of diabetes leading to neglect of self-care, *i.e.,* does not take insulin, test blood glucose, or follow meal plan
- Inability to decrease body weight, leading to control of NIDDM
- Nonadherence to self-care related to varied eating patterns imposed by family needs or social events

When people have a known, long-standing diagnosis of diabetes, nursing diagnoses might be

- Alteration in home management of diabetes related to inability to follow suggested meal plans, leading to high glycosolated hemoglobin A_{1c}
- Potential for impairment of skin integrity related to angiopathy and neuropathy, leading to lack of sensation in feet
- Sexual dysfunction related to neurological and vascular changes from diabetes, leading to depression about impotence

Clearly, careful individualized deliberate assessment and continuing updating and refining of nursing diagnoses are prerequisite to effective interventions.

Goals

Given the current state of knowledge about diabetes, general goals for people who have diabetes are

- Maintenance of blood glucose in as near a normal range as possible, 60 to 120 mg/dl, with no episodes of hypoglycemia/hyperglycemia
- Achievement and maintenance of ideal body weight
- Understanding, acceptance, and implementation of the prescribed treatment regimen
- Movement toward adaptation to this chronic condition
- Confidence in being capable of coping with diabetes

These goals are obviously intertwined and mediated by that interdependency. Interpretation and adaptation are necessary in making these general goals applicable to specific individuals.

Nursing Interventions

As mentioned above, the prime intervention in management of diabetic individuals is education for self-care. When the person receives the medical diagnosis of diabetes, he is most often overwhelmed, confused, and frightened. For many individuals with NIDDM, the diagnosis is not unexpected because other family members have had the same diagnosis. These people are often initially less overwhelmed but more depressed. Diabetic individuals report having been upset to a degree to which they could not effectively cope, for a period of 6 months to a year. Some report that everything said and given them to read during that time was as if the information was spoken or written in a language they could not comprehend. In the face of this response of the patient, his family and friends of necessity must manage the diabetes.

If health professionals fail to evaluate the impact and the person's response to the impact of a diagnosis of diabetes, their efforts at best will be ineffective and at worst will work to undermine the confidence patients have in the usefulness of maintaining contact with health professionals. This situation can be approached by first dealing only with the requisites of survival, waiting until some adaptation has occurred and then moving to more comprehensive teaching. For example, if the person has IDDM, insulin is needed at least once daily and constitutes the number one priority. Closely tied to insulin administration are blood glucose determination, measurement of dose, maintenance of a sterile syringe and needle, site rotation, and injection technique. Helping the person and his family achieve proficiency in these areas and then adding to them works toward managing the problem of information overload and coping disabilities.

For people with NIDDM, the priority is weight loss. One approach to weight loss has been to hospitalize overweight people with NIDDM so that they can be monitored closely while a treatment of total dietary fast is instituted to bring the blood glucose under control and to begin behavioral modification of caloric intake. Outpatient intensive diet therapy, with weekly or daily meetings with health professionals, is sometimes the initial treatment protocol for people with NIDDM.

As the person shows some adaptation to the medical diagnosis, more breadth and depth of material presented can be added. Patients become able to profit from independent reading and group classes. Strong support and care to avoid overloading them with information and responsibility during the initial stages of self-management are crucial when developing long-term attitudes toward self-care abilities. Positive attitudes toward health care professionals and sustained contact with health care professionals are important for optimum health over time.

Education of the individual with diabetes encompasses a working knowledge of nutrition, exercise, the hypoglycemic agents they will need, and the hygiene and psychosocial adaptations expected of them.

Nutrition

Meal plans are the basis of treatment of all types of diabetes. They are designed to primarily control and systematize the intake of carbohydrates so as to minimize the stress on the impaired blood glucose regulating mechanism. In general, the goals of nutritional therapy are similar in all types of diabetes, except for a reduction in the calorie intake of obese persons with NIDDM. Goals of nutritional therapy in diabetes are the following

1. A caloric intake appropriate for attaining and maintaining ideal body weight. Amounts of calories are determined by age, sex, height, weight, usual activity level, and growth and developmental needs.
2. An adequate intake of all essential nutrients
3. Modifications in volume and kinds of nutrients as required in the management of complications of diabetes or other existing or potential conditions
4. A spacing of food intake to (a) match absorption with adequate levels of insulin in the liver and the peripheral circulation, and (b) protect the individual from hypoglycemia during sleeping
5. Integration of meal plans with exercise and medications

Calorie Allocation. The most efficacious meal plan for people who have diabetes has been a subject of continuing debate. Before the availability of insulin, restriction of carbohydrates and calories was the only course of treatment. Currently, the trend is toward liberalization of carbohydrate intake (50% to 60% of total calories) with emphasis on increasing the proportions of complex carbohydrates and fiber while avoiding concentrated refined sugar, mainly to control calories. In general, fat intake should be no more than 35% of total calories and an emphasis placed on unsaturated fats as suggested by the American Heart Association. This leaves about 25% of total calories for protein. Controlling fat intake necessitates an easing of the restrictions on carbohydrates, since many sources of protein also contain fat. Achieving metabolic control of diabetes mainly through nutrition, especially weight control, has the desired effect of lowering insulin requirements and hence the potential for wide variations in blood glucose.

Management of sodium intake can be considered at the same time as eating habits are evaluated. The usual daily requirement of 1100 mg to 3300 mg of sodium is frequently exceeded, which aggravates the problem of high blood pressure, a common symptom in people with diabetes.

It is often the physician who determines the appropriate caloric intake and the proportions of carbohydrate, protein, and fat. Then the dietition or nurse, or both meet with the patient to transcribe the diet prescription into a meal plan.

Consideration is given to the following: (1) religious and cultural influences on diet, (2) national origins, (3) social status, (4) economic status, (5) who prepares the meals, and (6) who eats with the patient. Meal plans for people who have diabetes are appropriate for everyone and can serve as a focus for sound nutrition in the entire family group. Using former patterns of eating as guides to minimize the amount of change works to aid in adherence to the therapeutic diet.

Exchange Lists. Diabetic exchange lists are the usual method of teaching people sound nutrition and weight control. Foods appropriate for people with diabetes are classified into six groups, determined by the composition of the food (Table 74–4). Each group contains similar kinds and amounts of food according to the nutritional value of carbohydrates, proteins, and fats. Foods within each group can be exchanged for any other food within that same group. When the correct proportions of the individual's dietary requirements have been established, the dietitian determines what exchanges are appropriate from each exchange list. Learning the sizes of portions of servings is an important part of gaining control of dietary intake. Whether people weigh or measure portions is a matter of choice, but it is necessary to gain a correct concept of amount. This technique together with an understanding of diabetic exchanges will allow the person to eat anywhere.

Special foods are rarely necessary for people who have diabetes. Reading labels of canned, frozen, or processed foods will alert them to the sugar and salt contents. When the desire is to decrease sugar and salt content, general guidelines for fruits, vegetables, and meats are as follows: fresh is better than frozen, and frozen is better than canned. Rinsing canned or frozen items in water before use can decrease the amount of sugar and sodium.

TABLE 74–4
Exchange Lists for Meal Planning*,†

Foods are grouped together on the basis of the carbohydrate, protein, fat content for a designated serving size.

List 1	Milk exchanges Includes nonfat, low fat, and whole milk. One exchange of milk contains 12 g of carbohydrates, 8 g of protein, a trace of fat, and 80 Cal.
List 2	Vegetable exchanges One exchange of vegetables contains about 5 g of carbohydrate, 2 g of protein, and 25 Cal.
List 3	Fruit exchanges One exchange of fruit contains 10 g of carbohydrates and 40 Cal.
List 4	Bread exchanges Includes bread, cereal, and starchy vegetables. One exchange of bread contains 15 g of carbohydrates, 2 g of protein, and 70 Cal.
List 5	Lean meat One exchange (1 oz) contains 7 g of protein, 3 g of fat, and 55 Cal. Medium-fat meat As for lean meat and omit one half of fat exchange from the meal plan. High-fat meat As for lean meat and omit one fat exchange from the meal plan.
List 6	Fat One exchange of fat contains 5 g of fat and 45 Cal.

* Exchange list with actual food items and portions and meal plans of specific calorie amounts can be obtained from dietitions or the local chapter of the American Diabetic Association.

† The exchange lists are based on material in the exchange lists for Meal Planning prepared by Committees of the American Diabetes Association, Inc. and the American Diabetic Association in cooperation with the National Institute of Arthritis, Metabolism, and Digestive Diseases, and the National Heart and Lung Institute, National Institutes of Health, and the Public Health Service, US Department of Health, Education and Welfare.

Eating Patterns. Changing patterns of food intake, whether to decrease weight or decrease concentrated carbohydrates, has had a low sustained success rate. People who have diabetes must learn that their meal plan is the main treatment of their condition. A slender figure may be an esthetic goal for everyone but in the diabetic individual it is a necessity for health. Having diabetic individuals keep records of everything they eat, when, and what they were doing at the time will provide data for initiating behavior modification plans. Rewarding oneself in ways that do not involve eating is a creative practice. Fasting under the guidance of health professionals has been used to gain control of blood glucose and to initiate a change in eating habits for people with NIDDM; however, crash dieting does not as a rule result in a sustained weight loss. Making up one's mind that oral intake will require control for the rest of one's life is necessary; some groups that have the common goal of lifetime weight control have had sustained success.

Although management of meal plans are the primary responsibility of registered dietitians, nurses with their opportunity for frequent and ongoing contact with patients are in a pivitol position to help them gain control of their meal plans. Primary means are personal role modeling, interest in and frequent discussion about meal plans, and methods of sustained changes in nonproductive eating habits.

Dietary Modifications During Intercurrent Illness. When diabetic individuals (with IDDM or NIDDM) have brief illnesses, such as upper respiratory infections or gastrointestinal disturbances, their blood glucose levels usually rise. This rise occurs in the face of decreased intake and elevated body temperature. Infections cause insulin resistance, but it is not known how. An important part of self-care is learning a general protocol to follow when an illness intervenes. This protocol is of course in addition to the usual regimen of rest, warmth, and control of fever. Of utmost importance is regularly, every 4 hours, determining blood glucose level, either through self blood-glucose monitoring or by estimating blood glucose from the results of urine tests. All diabetic individuals, when they are ill, need to have the equipment and ability to check every 4 hours for the presence of ketones in the urine.

The individual taking insulin should continue the usual dosage schedule. Minimum 24-hour liquid carbohydrate intake is 150 g, that is, 7 ½ cups of *sugar-containing* liquid, such as ginger ale, apple juice, gelatin, or milk. This amount of carbohydrate will provide sufficient glucose to minimize the breakdown of stored glucose. In addition to the liquid, the usual foods are helpful during illness: water, broth, crackers, bread, and eggs.

During illness an important decision for patients is when to notify a health professional. There are 4 criteria:

1. Inability to take at least 7½ cups of carbohydrate-containing liquid every 24 hours
2. Vomiting for 4 or more hours without relief
3. Detection of ketones in the urine
4. Either blood glucose or urine tests show higher than usual levels for several days

If any one of these conditions is met then the person's health care provider should be notified.

SUMMARY OF CARE DURING INTERCURRENT ILLNESS

1. Test blood for glucose or test urine for glucose every 4 hours.
2. Test urine for ketones every 4 hours.
3. Take usual dose of insulin.
4. Take at least 7½ cups of carbohydrate-containing liquid every 24 hours.
5. Call health care professional if urine shows ketones, if unable to take adequate liquid, or if blood or urine tests show higher than usual glucose levels for several days.

Exercise

The American Diabetic Association's (ADA) logo is a triangle shape to represent the three current aims of the ADA: research, detection, and education. In the past, ADA's logo was a triangular balance scale to represent the three modes of treatment of diabetes: diet, exercise, and hypoglycemic agents. During recent years there has been a surge of interest in the exercise component of care, reflecting an increased interest in exercise among the general population. How exercise lowers blood glucose is not clear; however, it has been suggested that insulin receptors become more sensitive to insulin, which in turn facilitates the movement of insulin and glucose into the body cells.[30] In addition to the well-known benefits of physical exercise, that is, improved circulation, increased sense of well-being, increased strength and endurance, for diabetic individuals the effect of exercise may be to lower the doses of insulin required to keep blood glucose under control. Exercise programs can be instituted by beginning gradually, incorporating preexercise stretching, regularly checking heart rates to prevent going over maximum heart rates as determined by age, and then ending the exercise session with a gradual cool-down by slowing down the exercise for the last 5 minutes.

Striving for daily regularity in amounts and types of exercise allows preplanning of what to eat and of insulin dosages. When individuals are not able to maintain even, daily exercise programs, they can work with their health professional to determine different eating and insulin schedules for active and sedentary days. For example, university students may be physically inactive during weekly classes and then physically very active during weekends.

When exercise is spontaneous, eating 5 g to 10 g of glucose (*i.e.,* one fruit exchange) before the exercise and repeating the intake if the exercise is prolonged will prevent hypoglycemic episodes. After illness or hospitalization when exercise may be curtailed, diabetic individuals may note hypoglycemia on resuming more activity and need to lower insulin doses. Posthospitalization hypoglycemia is the main reason why people are no longer hospitalized to begin conventional insulin therapy.

Certainly every diabetic individual needs an evaluation by a health professional before beginning any exercise and to have the professional modify the exercise programs according to the patient's physical state. The use of exercise as treatment can make a considerable improvement in the overall well-being of diabetic individuals. People with NIDDM can augment their efforts at weight control by using gradually increasing exercise to tone their muscles and increase the percentage of their lean body mass. People with IDDM need not believe they must curtail their physical activity, unless they have some existing contraindication, such as compromised circulation to vital organs. There are data to support the use of exercise postprandially by people with IDDM, to prevent rapid rises in blood glucose after meals.[4]

Smoking and Diabetes

Of course smoking is detrimental to health (see Unit IV). In the case of diabetes, the typical patterns of the detrimental effects of smoking are exaggerated, particularly those in the vascular system. Hence cessation of smoking is imperative if the highest level of wellness is to be achieved by the diabetic individual.

Insulin

Insulin therapy was instituted in 1923, following its discovery. From that time until the development of biosynthetic human insulin in 1979, all insulin was derived from the pancreas of pork and beef, with pork being the most nearly like human insulin. The process of removing contaminants from beef and pork insulin steadily improved, resulting in very pure forms of pork insulin. Currently, there are many forms of beef and pork insulin available, and biosynthetic insulin (BSI) became available to the general public in the fall of 1983. It is important to keep in mind that insulin is a hormone that can control diabetes but is not a cure for diabetes. The use of insulin pumps works toward meeting the objective of mimicking the physiological function of a normal pancreas; however, the pump cannot detect glucose levels and is not economically feasible nor appropriate for all diabetic individuals.

In nondiabetic individuals the beta cells of the islets of Langerhans secrete insulin in the range of 40 units a day in response to food intake and elevated blood glucose. In addition the beta cells have about 200 units of insulin in reserve. The individual with IDDM has no or an insufficient ability to provide adequate endogenous insulin, so that exogenous insulin is required. The usefulness for people with NIDDM of taking insulin is a debatable issue. Generally the problem in the individual with NIDDM is not insufficient insulin but tissue unresponsiveness to insulin, and therefore taking more insulin seems to have little value. However, some individuals who have NIDDM and who have been unable to reduce their body weights take insulin in an effort to bring the blood glucose levels nearer to normal ranges. Individuals with gestational or other stress-related diabetes may require insulin for short periods. Taking insulin intermittently carries the risk of developing antibodies to insulin; then when the need for exogenous insulin again arises larger amounts of insulin will be required.

Types of Insulin. The several forms of insulin are given in Table 74–5. They can be divided into three main categories, based on the onset, peak, and duration of action. They are (1) rapid action with a short duration, (2) intermediate onset, action, and duration, and (3) a delayed onset with a prolonged action. The rapid-action, short-duration insulin was developed first. The modified or intermediate forms of insulin were developed later to minimize the number of daily injections, by adding preparations that make regular insulin less soluble and thereby delay the absorption and hence action of the insulin. The first prolonged-action insulin was protamine zinc insulin (PZI). This insulin was developed by Hagedorn of Denmark. He added protamine, a basic protein obtained from the sperm of a fish, but it had no rapid action. Next came neutral protamine Hagedorn (NPH), globin zinc, and lente insulin. NPH, globin zinc, and lente insulins are mixtures of regular and protamine insulins and so have a relatively rapid onset and yet have prolonged action.

Biosynthetic insulin (BSI), or human insulin, either is made by enzymatically removing a protein in pork insulin and replacing it with a human protein made by a bacterium or is produced entirely by bacteria. The actions of BSI and

TABLE 74–5
Summary of Action of the Various Insulin Preparations

Type	*Preparation*	*Onset* (hr)*	*Peak* (hr)*	*Duration* (hr)*
Rapid-acting	Crystalline	½–1	2–4	8
	Zinc insulin (regular)	½–1	2–4	14
	Semilente	½–1	5–7	12–16
Intermediate-acting	Isophane insulin injection (NPH)	2	6–12	20–30
	Lente	2	6–12	24–28
Long-acting	Protamine zinc injection (PZI)	6–8	14–24	36 +
	Ultralente	7	18–24	36 +

** Actual times of onset, peak, and duration vary greatly in individuals according to their present activity and circulatory status.*

pure pork insulin are very similar in action and elicit about the same antibody response.

Human insulin is available as regular, NPH, and lente insulin. Insulin is prescribed in units of insulin per milliliter. U 40 is available for administering very low doses to children, and U 500 is available for the rare instance of insulin resistance. Before U 100 was available only U 40 and U 80 could be obtained. These strengths were replaced with U 100 to avoid errors related to using U 40 insulin with a U 80 syringe and vice versa.

Regular Insulin. Regular insulin is crystal clear, whereas longer-acting forms of insulin are cloudy. Regular insulin is used when a rapid and short action is desired, such as when treating ketoacidosis and in using insulin pumps when a continuous action is desired. Regular insulin is the only form that can be administered intravenously. Regular insulin is used by a diabetic person to control blood glucose to offset the need to eat to meet the action of long-acting insulin taken several hours previously. This technique requires three to four doses of regular insulin daily, just as was required before the delayed action insulins were available. The multiple-dose schedule can be followed in the usual manner or through a small needle (25 to 27 gauge) left in the subcutaneous tissue. The abdomen is the favored site when using this technique, and the needle is changed every 1 to 3 days. Regular insulin can be mixed with a longer-acting form to control the blood glucose in relation to the first meal taken after a period of sleep.

Modified Forms of Regular Insulin. Modified forms of regular insulin with additives that delay absorption and hence prolong duration of action are appropriately used by diabetic individuals whose blood glucose is relatively easily controlled. Individuals within the classification of IDDM seem to produce quite variable amounts of endogenous insulin. This range provides an explanation for the wide variations in ease of control of IDDM. Some of these individuals retain some ability to produce endogenous insulin, which provides a continuous background of insulin. They need to augment their own insulin secretion with one or two daily injections of modified or a mix of regular and modified insulin, but they retain the ability to produce some endogenous insulin.

Mixed Insulins. If regular and modified insulin are to be mixed for injection using one syringe, the following procedure should be used to avoid contamination of regular insulin with modified insulin. First a sterile needle should be placed in the vial containing the modified insulin to release any negative pressure in the vial. Next the regular insulin is drawn up in the usual sterile manner. Finally the modified insulin is drawn into the syringe containing the regular insulin, taking care to prevent any regular insulin from entering the vial containing modified insulin. The syringe should be gently rotated to mix the two insulins.

Determining the correct type, dose, and timing of insulin is a continuous process. The diabetic individual's constantly changing physical and emotional status mandates frequent reevaluation of the appropriateness of the current insulin therapy schedule. Nurses can assist patients to deal with the lack of a stable regimen through continual assessment, education efforts, and development of support systems among health professionals, friends, and family.

Injection Technique

Teaching individuals to administer insulin to themselves is a particularly important challenge for nurses. Aversion to injection stems from fear of pain and the admission of a chronic illness adding up to a seemingly overwhelming task. People in the throes of striving to cope with a new diagnosis of IDDM or facing a failure at achieving weight loss in NIDDM are those most often affected. Depending on their physical state at the time, they may have additional difficulties with attention span, vision impairment, and slowed manual dexterity all resulting from elevated blood glucose. In the face of these interferences the individual must learn self-administration of insulin. First of all the skin must be penetrated with a needle. Only when that has been accomplished can any focus on what else needs to be learned be expected, such as how to minimize the trauma of injection, and sterile technique. After one successful experience at self-injection using sterile saline, more detail can be given regarding injection. If the nurse can recall her own first experience at inserting a needle in someone else, some of the feelings of injection of oneself can be captured. Ending the session with a second injection of sterile saline works to leave the person with a sense of achievement and confidence. Providing detailed written instructions of exactly what was said or a tape recording of the session for the person to review later is helpful.

The objective in administering insulin subcutaneously is to place the insulin in the potential space between fat and muscle tissue. No studies have been done to establish a correct method of injecting insulin. Pinching up some skin and inserting the needle at a 90° angle to the pinch and a 45° angle to the extremity or abdomen has been generally believed to achieve the objective (Fig. 74–7). It was thought

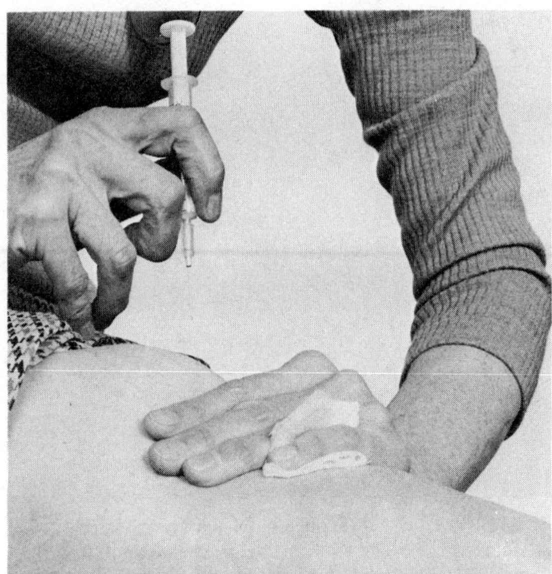

FIGURE 74–7 Technique for self-injection of insulin.

desirable to maintain the pinch throughout the injection with one hand while aspirating with the little finger of the other hand that is holding the syringe. Some people may lack the manual dexterity needed for this technique. Some health professionals are currently advocating the pinch method only for use in abdominal sites by people of normal weight. For other injection sites, for example, arms and legs, they suggest stretching the skin and injecting at a 90° angle to the skin. The rationale for this technique is that it gives, theoretically, more consistent placement of the insulin using a ½-inch needle and it is simpler. The benefit of massaging the site of injection is of current research interest. Studies have demonstrated improved control of postprandial blood glucose when injection sites are massaged before eating each meal throughout the day.[6]

Injection Sites. Any area of subcutaneous tissue can be used for insulin injection. It is generally agreed that rotation of sites avoids scarring. In the past there were problems with lipodystrophies. Lipodystrophies are areas of swelling or areas of atrophy related to insulin injections (Fig. 74–8). Advent of the more pure forms of insulin seems to have minimized the number of lipodystrophies. Rotating the injection sites programs each injection 1 inch in every direction from other injection sites, and no injection site is used more frequently than once every 6 weeks. A method of rotation is illustrated in Figure 74–9.

Selection of the site requires consideration of several factors. (1) Hard physical activity involving the injected area has been associated with more rapid absorption and subsequent hypoglycemia. So if the person is going to be physically active, use of abdominal sites would be the most appropriate. (2) Absorption is more comparable from sites in the same general area. For example, injections into the arms and legs are absorbed at different rates. Use of sites on the same extremity and rotating within that site should result in more similar absorption rates on a day-to-day basis.

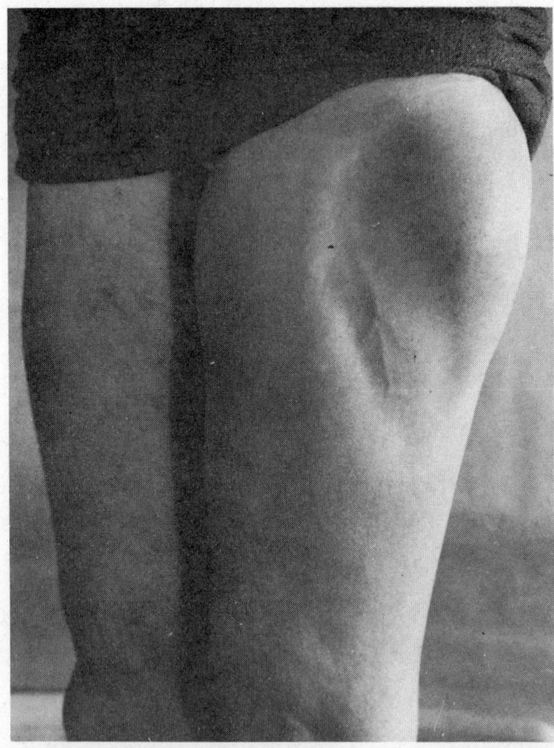

FIGURE 74–8 Severe insulin-induced fat atrophy. Atrophy has caused disfigurement at site of daily insulin injections in left thigh. (Ezrin C, Godden JO, Volpe R [eds]: Systematic Endocrinology, 2nd ed. New York, Harper & Row, 1979)

Local reactions to the injected insulin may occur, usually during the initial treatment. The reactions are manifested by redness, swelling, and itching at the site of injection. The first signs and symptoms usually appear 2 to 12 hours after injection, reaching a peak in 18 to 24 hours, and after 3 to 4 weeks of insulin therapy the reactions slowly subside. Changing the insulin from all beef to all pork, or vice versa or from NPH to lente occasionally prevents the reactions. It is hoped that BSI will not cause local reactions. On rare occasions a person will require desensitization.

Syringes. Most people prefer ½-inch disposable syringes with very small bore needles (27 to 28 gauge). Some still prefer glass syringes for reasons of lower cost and ease of use. Sterility of glass syringes can be achieved by boiling in water and storage in a sterile container with the syringe and plunger separated. Another method of storing a glass syringe is to separate the syringe and plunger and place them in a container of 70% isopropyl alcohol. When ready to use, the two parts are reassembled and the plunger is pushed in and out several times to remove any alcohol. A needle is attached and the insulin is drawn up and injected.

There is evidence that outpatients can safely reuse disposable syringes for up to 2 months.[13, 26] After each injection the syringe and attached needle can be replaced in the packet and kept in refrigeration. When the needle becomes dull it is replaced with a new sterile needle.[9] In a study of 30 patients no clinical or bacteriological evidence of infection was found. One syringe out of 60 showed bacterial growth.[9] Cleaning injection sites with soap and water or alcohol is easily done. However, infections resulting from no cleansing of skin prior to injections have not been demonstrated.

Tips on insulin injection are listed in Table 74–6.

Pump Therapy

A small but growing number of people with IDDM are using insulin pumps to attempt to maintain their blood glucose within normal ranges. Regular insulin is delivered continuously through a small 26 to 27 gauge needle in the subcutaneous tissue, usually of the abdomen. Tubing connects the needle to a syringe containing regular insulin. The syringe is powered by batteries that are wired to a mechanism that very slowly depresses the plunger of the syringe. In addition to the slowly and continuously administered regular insulin, a bolus of regular insulin is given before meals. This bolus is administered from the same syringe, usually by depressing a button on the pump. The needle site and tubing are changed every 2 to 3 days. The entire pump, batteries, and syringe, are housed in a container measuring approximately 4½ inches × 3 inches × 1 inch. It is worn strapped to the chest under clothing or attached to the belt (Fig. 74–10).

Potential hazards associated with the use of insulin pumps are related to (1) mechanical hazards of too much

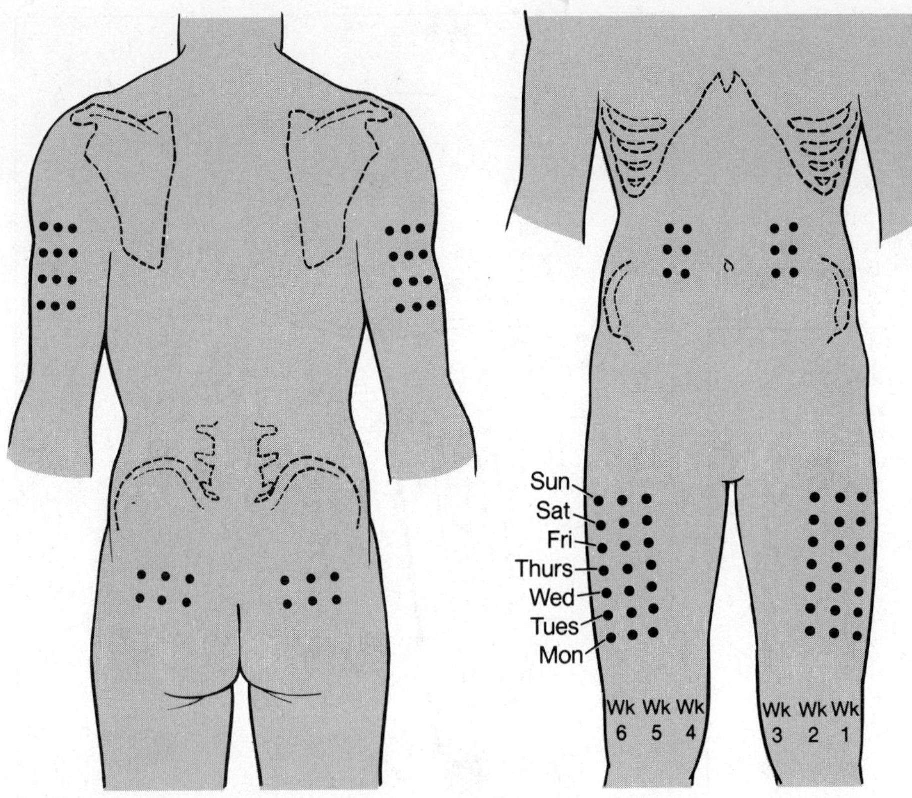

FIGURE 74–9 Insulin injection sites and rotation schedule.

TABLE 74–6
Tips on Insulin Injection

1. Keep the insulin vial in current use in a place where the temperature will not exceed 70°F or go below 32°F. Refrigerate extra vials.
2. Roll the insulin vial between hands to mix it, do not shake it.
3. If mixing regular insulin with a modified insulin, always draw regular insulin first to avoid contamination of rapid-acting insulin with prolonged-action insulin and to keep the dosage proportions the same.
4. To minimize bubbles within the bore of the syringe, wet the syringe bore with insulin up to the dosage level, inject it back into the vial, then draw the desired dosage.
5. Check the dosage carefully in a good light.
6. Select the site and clean it with alcohol. Let the alcohol dry before inserting the needle.
7. Insert the needle bevel up.
8. If using an insulin with a prolonged action, inject over no more than a 2- to 4-second time span to avoid insulin clogging in the tip of the needle.

insulin being delivered with subsequent hypoglycemia or too little insulin being delivered with resultant hyperglycemia and (2) inflammation or infection at the needle sites. Most individuals using insulin pumps report feeling better physically, having more energy, and preferring the more spontaneous lifestyle the pump allows. They are no longer required to eat at times dictated by the action of prolonged-action insulin taken several hours earlier.

Insulin pump therapy is still too new for the long-term effects on the typical patterns of complications from IDDM to have been evaluated. However, the short-term effects are showing that the glycosolated hemoglobins are more normal in people on pump therapy. Individuals must be willing to undergo intensive education, often hospitalization, to learn self-management of IDDM with insulin pump therapy. Learning requires considerable motivation and willingness to devote time to doing frequent blood glucose monitoring. In addition, insulin pump therapy mandates the continuous availability of nurses knowledgeable and skillful at teaching self-management of diabetes.

Oral Hypoglycemic Agents

Oral hypoglycemic agents, sulfonylureas, are used to treat NIDDM when diet and exercise therapy have failed to bring blood glucose toward normal ranges. In rare instances, oral agents are used in conjunction with insulin for patients with IDDM whose blood glucose has proved difficult to control. The mode of action of the sulfonylureas is not completely known, but it is believed that they enhance synthesis and release of insulin from beta cells. These drugs are not effective in the absence of functioning beta cells. There is some evidence that the sulfonylureas act to increase insulin sensitivity of extrapancreatic tissues, perhaps by increasing the number of insulin binding sites on these cells. Sulfonylureas available in the United States are listed in Table 74–7. Mechanisms by which the second-generation sulfonylureas improve glucose tolerance parallel those of the first generation of these drugs. Before 1977 phenformin hydrochloride, a biguanide, was available in the United States

FIGURE 74–10 Infusion insulin pump. (*A*) Schematic drawing of infusion pump. (B) Insulin pump in place. (View *A* courtesy of Cardiac Pacemakers, Inc., St. Paul, Minnesota)

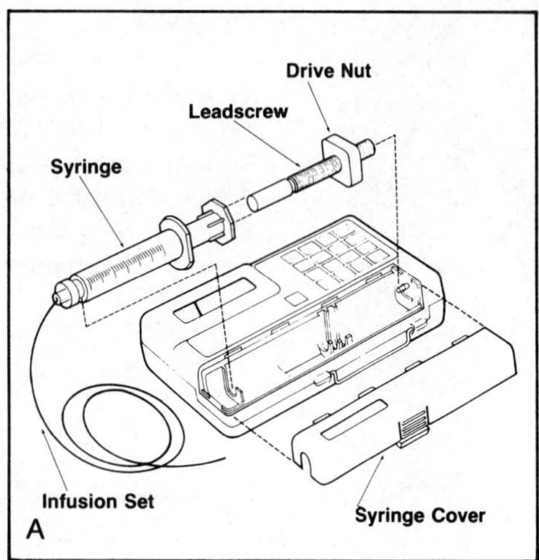

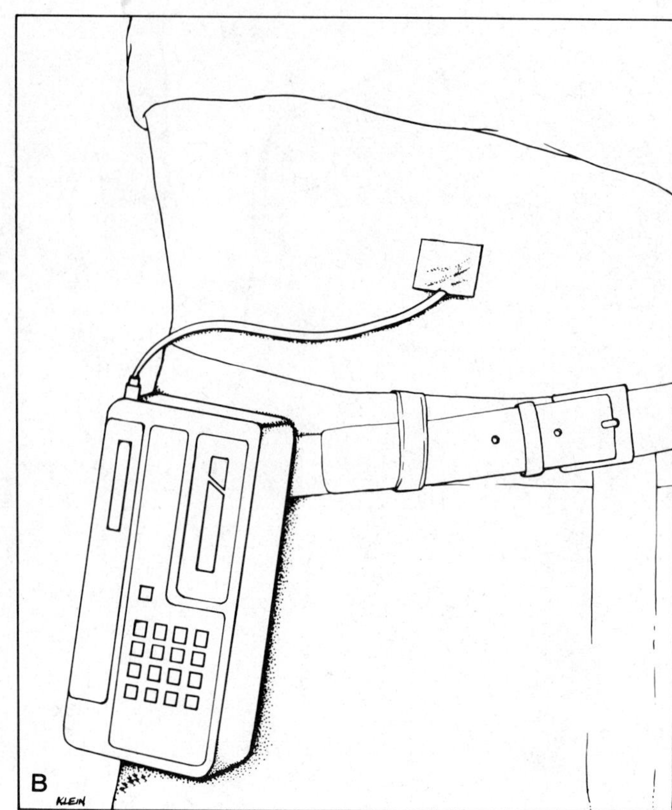

as an oral hypoglycemic drug. The mechanism of action was unknown but was believed to be extrapancreatic, acting in some way on peripheral tissues to increase glucose uptake. Because of its dangerous side-effect, lactic acidosis, phenformin hydrochloride was removed from the market by the US Food and Drug Administration. Currently (1983), buformin hydrochloride, another biguanide with action similar to phenformin, is under investigation and is not yet on the market.

People who are beginning therapeutic trials of sulfonylureas require close monitoring for the first 7 days to establish the effectiveness of the drugs. Individuals may be responsive to one sulfonylurea and not to another. They need to know why, how, and when to do self blood-glucose monitoring or urine testing to ensure early detection of high or low blood glucose levels. Cognitive understanding and psychomotor skill with blood or urine testing can be documented through return demonstrations by the patient. Telephone calls between clinic visits are a simple method of follow-up until an effective regimen is established. As with insulin therapy, it is imperative that people understand and value that the sulfonylureas are treatment and not cure for their diabetes and that following their meal plan and regular exercise are required for optimum management of their diabetes.

TABLE 74–7
Oral Hypoglycemic Agents Available in the United States

	Half-life (hr)	*Duration (hr)*	*Dosage Range*
First-Generation Sulfonylureas			
Acetohexamide (Dymelor)	5–8	12–24	0.25–1.5 g*
Chlorpropamide (Diabinese)	30–36	60	0.1–0.5 g†
Tolazamide (Tolinase)	7	10–14	0.1–1.0 g§
Tolbutamide (Orinase)	4–6	6–12	0.5–3 g§
Second-Generation Sulfonylureas			
Glyburide (Micronase, Diabeta)	5–16	16	2.5–30 mg*
Glipizide‡ (Glibenase)	3–7	6	2.5–30 mg*

* Divided or single dose
† Single dose
‡ Currently not available in the USA
§ Divided doses

Hypoglycemia

A main hazard of the treatment of diabetes with insulin and oral hypoglycemic agents is hypoglycemia. Hypoglycemia can cause damage to the neurons of the cerebral cortex. Results of lack of adequate glucose to the cerebral cortex can cause injury, for example, the person loses consciousness and falls down. Brain cells in general do not require insulin to utilize glucose; however, they have very little ability to store glucose. When the blood glucose level drops below

50 mg/dl in spite of the body's counterregulatory mechanisms, hypoglycemia is the result.

Hypoglycemia can occur whenever the three-way balance of diet, exercise, and hypoglycemic agents is disrupted, for example, decreased food intake, delayed food intake, additional exercise, or an erroneously large dose of insulin or sulfonylurea. Everyone taking hypoglycemic agents, sulfonylureas, or insulin must be able to recognize the signs and symptoms of hypoglycemia to know the correct action to take. Hypoglycemia is potentially a very serious complication because of the effects it has on the cerebral cortex, resulting in slowed thinking at a time when rapid, correct action is crucial to reversing the hypoglycemia. In addition, complications from diabetes may result in damage to the autonomic nervous system, which in turn may prevent the individual from quickly becoming aware of the signs and symptoms of hypoglycemia. The rapidity with which a hypoglycemic reaction occurs of course depends on many factors, but it is primarily related to the rapidity of action of the specific hypoglycemic agent.

Regular insulin usually causes rapid onset of hypoglycemia, whereas the prolonged-action insulins cause slower onset of signs and symptoms. When the cause of the hypoglycemic reaction is a sulfonylurea, the onset of signs and symptoms is slow and easily mistaken for some other cause of change in level of consciousness. Hypoglycemia can be divided into four phases, in which two components are apparent: autonomic nervous system responses and central nervous system depression.

Phase I Parasympathetic phase, with hunger, nausea, bradycardia, and hypotension

Phase II Beginning of diminishing cerebral function, with lethargy, apathy, and difficulty in talking and concentration

Phase III Sympathetic phase with diaphoresis, tachycardia, tremor, and increased blood pressure

Phase IV Further cerebral dysfunction, with coma and convulsions[24]

When hypoglycemia occurs during sleep, patients may experience nightmares, damp bedclothes, and more than usual disarrangement of their bedclothes.

Treatment of Hypoglycemia. Clearly the objective of treating hypoglycemia is to rapidly restore blood glucose to normal ranges, without overshooting and causing hyperglycemia. With the availability of blood glucose testing with a fingerstick blood sample and immediate reading of results there are likely to be fewer times when actual blood glucose levels are unknown. Treatment of hypgolycemia in conscious individuals includes ingestion of 10 g of rapidly absorbed carbohydrate: 2 sugar cubes, 2 to 3 small pieces of hard candy, 5 lifesavers, or 4 oz of juice or sugared soda. If there is no diminution of signs and symptoms in 5 minutes, the same dose of carbohydrate is repeated. When the symptoms abate, the individual needs to have the next scheduled meal or snack early to prevent a return of the hypoglycemia.

If the person is unconscious and is near health professionals, 10 g to 50 g of 50% glucose is administered intravenously. If the person is unconscious but is not near health professionals, syrup, honey, or one of the commercially available glucose preparations can be placed in the buccal cavity of the mouth after the person is placed in a side-lying position. Glucagon can be administered intramuscularly to the unconscious person, although raising the blood glucose by this method is slower than by the oral or intravenous routes. When the cause of the hypoglycemia is a sulfonylurea, the patient usually requires admission to the hospital for 2 to 3 days for close monitoring and continuous intravenous glucose *because of the long duration of action of the oral agents.*

After the hypoglycemic episode has been treated, it is important for the individual to retrace the events that led up to the incident, to detect anything that could have caused the hypoglycemia. Obviously, prevention of hypoglycemia is preferable to treating it, and this can be accomplished through careful education of patients regarding the balance of food intake, exercise, and hypoglycemic agents, early detection of hypoglycemia, and even spacing of food intake and exercise. Diabetic individuals who are taking insulin should have as part of their daily meal plan, a midmorning, midafternoon, and bedtime snack. All diabetic individuals should wear a bracelet or necklace that identifies their diabetic state. They should also carry a source of rapidly absorbed carbohydrate to ensure that they receive immediate treatment in the event of hypoglycemia. Diabetic individuals need to inform family, friends, and co-workers of their condition and to explain signs and symptoms of hypoglycemia and the appropriate treatment in the event that they are not able to help themselves.

If there is any doubt as to the cause of hypoglycemic-like signs and symptoms, treatment for hypoglycemia should be administered without delay. If the signs and symptoms are of hypoglycemia, the symptoms will quickly abate and if they are caused by something else, the small amount of carbohydrate will have done no harm.

Loss of Vision

As mentioned in an earlier section of this chapter, diabetes is the leading systemic cause of loss of vision. In addition to the retinopathies associated with diabetes, cataracts are commonly found in people who have diabetes. The changes in the lens are identical to cataracts associated with aging; however, the incidence is increased and the changes occur at an earlier age in diabetic individuals.

When vision loss is partial, there are a number of devices that allow the individual to remain independent, such as insulin needle guides that fit over the vial of insulin, and small magnifying lenses that can be attached to the insulin syringe. Urine test strips that are four times regular size are available. Self blood-glucose monitoring systems that have a brightly colored, large print, digital readout can be used. Instructions can be prepared with bold, large-sized print.

When vision loss is complete, the diabetic individual requires daily contact with someone who can examine his feet, read blood or urine test results, and draw up insulin. Though not the most desirable procedure, insulin can be drawn up before it is needed and kept under refrigeration. The diabetic person can remove the syringe from the refrigerator a few minutes before doing the injection to bring the insulin to room temperature, and can then gently rotate the syringe to distribute any suspension that has precipitated out. So long as the amount of regular insulin is in a 1 : 1 or larger ratio to modified insulin no change occurs in the insulin. The Bibliography at the end of this chapter lists articles that give specific details regarding devices for the visually impaired diabetic individual.

Hygiene

Hygiene for diabetic individuals differs little from that for people who do not have diabetes. In the main there is simply a need to be more deliberate, particularly with oral hygiene and care of the feet. Dental work may temporarily disrupt control of diabetes; therefore, sound preventive care works to eliminate this disruption. There is some evidence that movement of white cells, leukotaxis, is slowed in individuals who have diabetes, which implies that diabetic individuals may incur infectious processes more easily. Once an infectious process is established, control of diabetes may be disrupted and healing of the infection may be delayed.

The Feet. The feet of diabetic individuals merit special, deliberate care because of the possible presence of neuropathy and angiopathy and the potentially serious complications of injury and infection. The potential foot problems have causes that may be combinations of impaired circulation, decreased sensation, and possible atrophy of muscles of the feet due to neuropathy. Problems of the feet usually occur in the older individual, but young individuals with IDDM may have neuropathy to the extent that they are not aware of injuries to their feet. A complicating factor is that people assign importance to pain and if injuries do not hurt they believe the injury is not serious, and hence they will pay little attention to measures of prevention and care.

The objectives of education for care of the feet are to have people (1) value the importance of looking at or having someone else look at their feet on a daily basis and (2) maintain an intact uncalloused integument over their feet. Table 74–8 presents an overview for care of the feet.

TABLE 74–8
Foot Care for a Patient with Diabetes Mellitus

1. Assess feet daily (or have someone else do it) for red areas or broken skin and sensation. Ask physician to examine feet at clinic visits.
2. Wash and dry feet daily with attention to areas between toes.
3. If skin is dry, soak feet for 5–20 minutes in warm soapy water, rinse, and dry. Apply a bland cream to feet and heels but not between toes. Check temperature of water with elbow.
4. If skin is moist, bathe feet in daily shower or bath, dry carefully between toes.
5. If callous formation is present, rub area with a pumice stone while feet are wet, then rub with a towel. Do not use chemical agents to remove corns or callous formation.
6. Immediately after bathing, while toenails are softened, cut nails straight across, and smooth with an emery board. (If unable to see or reach feet, have someone else cut toenails.)
7. Inspect inside of shoes for foreign objects, nail points, or wrinkled padding.
8. Wear shoes and stockings that are not tight and give room for movement of toes. Wear shoes with moderately high heels.
9. Break in new shoes gradually.
10. Tie shoes loosely but firmly.
11. If feet perspire, change shoes and stockings during the day.
12. Do not smoke tobacco.
13. Avoid any one position for long periods of time.
14. Do not sit with legs crossed.
15. Avoid more than a right angle bend when sitting.
16. Prevent pressure on back of knees from the use of a chair that is too high.
17. Walk as much as can be tolerated daily.
18. Do not place feet near source of heat: fireplace, heater, heating pads, or hot water bottle. If feet are cold at night, wear socks.
19. Protect feet from injury by wearing shoes or stockings at all times.
20. Use a light at night.

Podiatrists and sometimes physical therapists can assist people if muscle atrophy from a neurological cause or if any malalignment of bones has occurred. Shoes with extra depth and padding, custom-made to evenly distribute body weight, can relieve and prevent problems. During clinic visits, home visits, or hospitalizations deliberate attention from nurses to the condition of the feet serves to emphasize the importance of daily visual inspection and care. See Table 74–9 for a summary of assessment of the feet.

Psychosocial Adaptations

Individuals adapting to the chronic condition of diabetes go through the same process of grieving and adaptation as is involved in adjusting to a diagnosis of any chronic deterioration. With diabetes the situation is complicated by the lack of any visible physical change to initiate movement through the grieving sequence of denial, developing awareness, reorganization, and resolution. Because treatment of diabetes centers on food intake, its presence is constantly in the mind and there is no escape from it. Fear of completely losing control of oneself through hypoglycemia or ketoacidotic coma constitutes a serious threat. Real and potential changes in lifestyle and life plans contribute to the major adaptations required in diabetes. The magnitude of the changes and threats are greater in IDDM but still exist in NIDDM.

Education for self-management works to give the diabetic person a sense of control through an understanding of the pathophysiology of diabetes and its treatment, and provides up-to-date information from which to make informed judgments about important life choices. Specific psychosocial intervention involves the deliberate teaching of strategies to develop coping abilities that may be needed in the predictable crises of diabetes.[11] Crisis are likely to occur during initial diagnosis and onset of the disease as well as during sudden changes in blood glucose control, and there

TABLE 74–9
Assessment of the Feet

1. Compare color of feet one with the other and with that of the rest of the body.
2. Compare color of feet when elevated and when even with, and below the level of the heart.
3. Compare temperature of toes with that of the ankles of both feet.
4. Assess the quality of sensation, using cotton-tipped applicator. Do not prick skin.
5. Assess the quality of dorsalis pedis and posterior tibial pulses.
6. Check for thickened or incorrectly cut toenails.
7. Examine toes for fungal infections of the toenails (onychomycosis) and between the toes (tinea pedis).
8. Examine for beaks in the skin.
9. Examine for callous formation.
10. Find out if person smokes tobacco.
11. Determine whether the person uses restrictive clothing on feet or legs (stockings, garters, undergarments, or shoes).
12. Determine whether the person routinely sits with legs crossed.
13. Determine whether the patient or other person examines the feet daily.
14. Determine the person's usual amount and kind of daily exercise.

are the normal developmental crisis associated with childhood, adolescence, marriage, parenting, and aging. In addition, there is the ongoing burden of living with diabetes for the rest of one's life, which can include crisis related to disease-specific symptoms, hospitalizations, managing complicated therapeutic regimens, failure to achieve therapeutic responses, and the threat of imminent or early death. Although crisis is a time of distress and demand, it can be a time of growth. People are alert and focused on their health and this can facilitate learning.

Use of anticipatory coping, which teaches preparedness and adaptive strategies before a crisis occurs, can diminish the disruption caused by the crisis and help keep events in realistic perspective. Specific strategies include developing or fostering emotional support systems of families, friends, or groups; developing sound patterns for acquiring the new knowledge and skills necessary for tackling developing medical problems; and setting up systems for child care, transportation, and emergency aid before it is needed.

Having the ability to preplan and learn in anticipation of needs indicates that an individual has worked through at least a portion of the grieving process. For those people who have not made any move toward adaptation, anticipatory coping strategies may help them along toward adaptation by helping them decrease some of their anxiety.

Evaluation of Goal Achievement

When nurses come in contact with diabetic individuals in any setting, outcome criteria for nursing interventions are the objectives of programs for teaching self-management of diabetes. Problem-oriented record systems are a method of documenting achievement of the objectives and long-term desired changes in self-care. When diabetic individuals are hospitalized, current understanding of self-management can be documented and further teaching–learning sessions can be planned. Clearly, specific nursing outcomes related to the need for the diabetic person's hospitalization will be required. The goals of educational programs have been reached when a diabetic person is

- Able to describe the alterations in his or her body that resulted in diabetes
- Able to describe how interactions of food intake, exercise, and hypoglycemic agents affect blood glucose
- Able to state his or her ideal body weight
- Able to correctly test urine or do self blood-glucose and urine ketone monitoring
- Able to describe onset, peak, and duration of action of the prescribed hypoglycemia agent
- Able to describe signs and symptoms of hypoglycemia, how to avoid hypoglycemia, and how to treat hypoglycemia
- Able to inject the correct dose of insulin using sterile technique
- Able to describe rotation of sites of injections of insulin
- Able to describe correct action during an intercurrent illness, including how to determine correct dosages of insulin, fluid needs, and when to call a health care provider
- Able to describe correct care for feet
- At all times carrying a source of sugar and identification regarding diabetes
- Able to express how having diabetes has affected his or her life

Summary

Assisting people of all ages and their families and friends to correctly manage their diabetes and still have lifestyles that are fulfilling is a challenge for a professional nurse. As indicated in the preceding pages, meeting this challenge requires the nurse to draw on all elements of her professional education and experience.

References

1. Anderson R: Defining and evaluating diabetes patient education. Diabetes Care 6:619–620, 1983
2. Barnard RJ, Lattimore L, Holly R et al: Response of non-insulin dependent diabetic patients to an intensive program of diet and exercise. Diabetes Care 5:370–375, 1982
3. Beigelman PM: Severe diabetes ketoacidosis, 482 episodes in 257 patients: Experience of three years. Diabetes 20:490–500, 1971
4. Caron D: The effect of postprandial exercise on meal-related glucose intolerance in insulin-dependent diabetic individuals. Diabetes Care 5:364–370, 1982
5. deFronzo R: Glucose intolerance and aging. Diabetes Care 4:493–501, 1981
6. Dillon R: Improved serum insulin profiles in diabetic individuals

who massage their insulin injection site. Diabetes Care 6:399–401, 1983

7. Drury PL: Diabetes and hypertension. Diabetologia 24:1–9, 1983
8. Ellenberg M: Impotence in diabetes: The neurological factor. Ann Intern Med 75:213–219, 1971
9. Grennough A, Cockcroft PM, Bloom A: Disposable syringes for insulin injection. Br Med J 1:1467–1468, 1979
10. Guthrie DW, Guthrie RA: Nursing Management of Diabetes Mellitus. St Louis, CV Mosby, 1982
11. Hamburg B, Inoff GE: Coping with predictable crisis of diabetes. Diabetes Care 6:409–416, 1983
12. Hansen S, Pollets D: Psychological aspects of diabetes mellitus—a critical review. Diabetes Care 2:227, 1979
13. Hodge RH, Krongaard M, Sande MA, Kaiser DL: Multiple use of disposable insulin syringe needle units. JAMA 244:266–267, 1980
14. Keen H, Jarrett J: Complications of diabetes, 2nd ed. London, Edward Arnold, 1982
15. Kilo C, Vogler N, Williamson J: Muscle capillary basement membrane changes related to aging and to diabetes mellitus. Diabetes 21:881–898, 1972
16. Kyner J: Diabetic ketoacidosis. Critical Care Quarterly 3:65–75, 1980
17. Levin, Marvin, Lawrence: The Diabetic Foot, 3rd ed. St Louis, CV Mosby, 1983
18. Mazzuca S, Weinberger M, Kurpius D et al: Clinical communication associated with diabetic patients' comprehension of their therapeutic regimen. Diabetes Care 6:347–350, 1983
19. Mitchell P, Loustau A: Concepts Basic to Nursing, 3rd ed. New York, McGraw-Hill, 1981
20. National Diabetes Data Group 1979. Diabetes 28:1039–1057, 1979
21. Peterson C, Jones R, Esterly J et al: Changes in basement membrane thickening and pulse volume concomitant with improved glucose control and exercise in patients with insulin-dependent diabetes mellitus. Diabetes Care 3:586–589, 1980
22. Pichert J: Not all medicines (or patient education programs) are the same. Diabetes Care 6:618–619, 1983
23. Schiavi RC, Hogan B: Psychological aspects of sexual problems. Diabetes Care 2:9–17, 1979
24. Schnatz JD: Diabetes Mellitus: Problems in Management, p 240. Menlo Park, California, Addison-Wesley, 1982
25. Sneid DS: Hyperosmolar hyperglycemic nonketotic coma. Critical Care Quarterly 3:29–43, 1980
26. Stepanas TV, Turley H, Tuohy EA: Reuse of disposable insulin syringes. Med J Aust 1:311–312, 1982
27. Tucker S, Breeding M, Canobbio M et al: Patient Care Standards, 3rd ed. St Louis, CV Mosby, 1984
28. Turner RC, Holman RR, Mathew DR, Peto J: Relative contributions of insulin deficiency and insulin resistance in maturity-onset diabetes. The Lancet 1:596–597, 1982
29. Unger R: Diabetes and the alpha cell. Diabetes 25:136–151, 1976
30. Vranic M, Kawamori R: Essential roles of insulin and glucagon in regulating glucose fluxes during exercise in dogs. Diabetes (Suppl) 28:45–52, 1979
31. White C: Diabetes Mellitus: The Continuing Challenge. Report of the National Diabetes Advisory Board. NIH Publication No. 83-2624. Washington DC, US Department of Health and Human Services, Public Health Service, National Institutes of Health, 1983
32. White C: Keeping up. Facts and Comparisons 777, St Louis, Facts and Comparisons Inc, 1983
33. Yoon JW, Austin M, Onodera T, Notkins AL: Virus-induced diabetes mellitus: Isolation of a virus from the pancreas of a child with diabetic ketoacidosis. N Engl J Med 300:1173–1179, 1979

Bibliography

Abrams AC: Clinical Drug Therapy: Rationales for Nursing Practice. Philadelphia, JB Lippincott, 1983

Beland I, Passos JY: Clinical Nursing: Pathophysiology and Psychosocial Approaches, 4th ed. New York, Macmillan, 1981

Bierman J, Toohey B: The Diabetic's Sports and Exercise Book. Philadelphia, JB Lippincott, 1977

Bleicher SJ: Symposium on home glucose monitoring. Diabetes Care 3:57, 1980

Bliss M: The Discovery of Insulin. Chicago, University of Chicago Press, 1982

Bratusca-Marrain PR: Insulin counteracting hormones: Their impact on glucose metabolism. Diabetologia 24:74–79, 1983

Clark AP: Diabetic ketoacidosis. In Kenner CV et al (eds): Critical Care Nursing, pp 515–535. Boston, Little, Brown Co, 1981

Davis W: Factors affecting the educational diagnosis of diabetic patients. Diabetes Care 4:275–278, 1981

Dudley J: The diabetes educator's role in teaching the diabetic patient. Diabetes Care 3:127, 1980

Dye B, Blainey C, Brye P, Palmer J: Starting the person with diabetes on insulin in the outpatient setting: Teaching guide for physicians and nurses. J Fam Pract 53:341–348, 1977

Fredholm N: The insulin pump: New method of insulin delivery. Am J Nurs 81:2024, 1981

Guyton AC: Textbook of Medical Physiology, 6th ed. Philadelphia, WB Saunders, 1981

Metzger MJ: A new test for blood sugar. Am J Nurs 83:763–764, 1983

Miller B, White NE: Diabetes assessment guide. Am J Nurs 80:1314–1316, 1980

Peterson CM: Symposium on optimal insulin delivery. Diabetes Care Suppl 5:1–103, 1982

Porter A: Symposium on diabetes: Patient education and care. Nurs Clin North Am, 1977

Rifkin H (ed): The Physician's Guide to Type II Diabetes (NIDDM): Diagnosis and Treatment. American Diabetes Association, 1984

Schade D, Eaton P, Carlson G et al: Future therapy of the insulin dependent diabetic patient: The implantable insulin delivery system. Diabetes Care 4:319, 1981

Skyler JS: Symposium on human insulin of recombinant DNA origin. Diabetes Care 5 (Suppl 2):1–186, 1982

Strauss AL, Glaser BG: Chronic Illness and the Quality of Life. St Louis, CV Mosby, 1975

Suitor CW, Hunter MF: Nutrition: Principles and Application in Health Promotion. Philadelphia, JB Lippincott, 1980

Tyler G, Steel JM, Ewing DJ et al: Sexual responsiveness in diabetic women. Diabetologia 24:166–171, 1983

Watkins PJ, Edmonds ME: Sympathetic nerve failure in diabetics. Diabetologia 25:73–77, 1983

Williams RH: Textbook of Endocrinology, 6th ed. Philadelphia, WB Saunders, 1981

Chapter 75

Disorders of the Thyroid and Parathyroid Glands

Christine A. Larson

Thyroid Gland

Disorders of the thyroid gland are relatively common occurrences and, if diabetes mellitus is excluded, they account for as much as four fifths of all endocrine problems. Diseases of the thyroid gland are characterized by enlargement of the gland, alterations in hormonal secretion, or both. Clinical manifestations arise as a result of local compression on neck structures from increased glandular size and the generalized effects of hormonal excess or deficit. The latter can produce a wide variety of physiological and metabolic effects. In this chapter disorders of both hyperfunction and hypofunction of the thyroid and parathyroid glands are discussed.

Hyperfunction of the Thyroid Gland: Hyperthyroidism

Hyperthyroidism (thyrotoxicosis) is a clinical syndrome characterized by increased circulating levels of thyroid hormones, that is, thyroxine, triiodothyronine, or both. The most common variety of hyperthyroidism is Graves' disease, an autoimmune disorder also known as diffuse toxic goiter. Less commonly, hyperthyroidism may result from a toxic nodular goiter.[27] Causes of hyperthyroidism are listed in Table 75–1.

Graves' Disease

Etiology and Pathology

Graves' disease, also termed Parry's or Basedow's disease, is a common disorder that can occur at any age. It is, however, most frequently seen in women between the third and fourth decades of life. In nongoiterous areas of the world, the ratio of predominance in women may be as high as 7 : 1. An increased incidence in monozygotic twins points toward an inherited factor, probably an autosomal recessive gene.[17]

The underlying problem in Graves' disease is a derangement of the intrinsic mechanism that normally adjusts thyroid hormone secretion to meet the metabolic needs of the body tissues. Its pathogenesis is not known. It was once thought to be a result of oversecretion of thyroid-stimulating hormone (TSH) from the anterior pituitary. At present, it is believed to be due to an autoimmune process in which the body reacts inappropriately to its own thyroid tissue. The thyroid tissue is perceived by the body as antigenic or foreign. It is theorized that a substance known as long-acting thyroid stimulator (LATS), now called thyroid-stimulating antibody (TSA_b), is produced by the lymphocytes in response to the perceived thyroid antigens. It is believed that TSA_b competes for TSH receptor sites on the thyroid membrane. The action of this antibody is to stimulate increased release of thyroid hormones (thyroxine and triiodothyronine). In addition, TSA_b is capable of increasing thyroidal iodine uptake and inducing thyroidal hyperplasia. Thyroid-stimulating antibodies are found in only 40% to 80% of patients with Graves' disease, and their presence or absence does not consistently relate to thyroid hyperactivity. Recent data suggest there may be other thyrotropic-antibody processes involved.[2,7]

Despite the etiology, the thyroid gland becomes diffusely enlarged, soft, vascular, and nodule free. Graves' disease is often marked by periods of remission or exacerbations. Its onset typically follows a period of acute emotional or physical stress.

Clinical Manifestations

Signs and symptoms of Graves' disease are variable and are related to the metabolic effects of the thyroid hormones on the body tissues. Manifestations also arise from increased sympathetic nervous system activity associated with the disease. The severity of the disease relates not only to the degree of hormone excess but to its rapidity of onset, its duration, and the patient's age. The most serious consequence of any form of hyperthyroidism is the exacerbation of the disease into a thyroid storm.

Hair and Skin Changes. Hair and skin changes occur owing to excessive thyroid hormone. The increased metabolic effects of thyroid hormone cause hair to become fine and sparse and to lose pigment prematurely. Women may demonstrate some recession of the temporal hairline. In addition, nails become thin and brittle, and the distal portion of the nail tends to separate from the bed (onycholysis). This finding is particularly noticeable on the fourth digit bilaterally. Increased sympathetic activity is demonstrated by warm, moist skin. The patient often complains of increased perspiration and a marked intolerance to heat. The elbows, palms, and soles may appear reddened. This redness may be accompanied by vitiligo (white patches on the skin) in 7% of the cases.[11] Occasionally pretibial myxedema (dermopathy) occurs over the dorsum of the legs and feet (Fig. 75–1). It appears as raised, circumscribed, thickened, hyperpigmented, orange peellike patches of skin that are often itchy and painful. This unique manifestation is probably the result of localized mucopolysaccharide deposition, the cause of which is unknown.

Behavior and Mentation Changes. Behavior and metabolic changes occur owing to excessive thyroid hormone. Increased circulating levels of thyroxine (T_4) accelerate cerebral functioning. The patient may have difficulty in concentrating and may manifest emotional instability by wide swings of mood and, occasionally, episodes of overt psychosis. Increased muscle tone often creates fine tremors, making the patient appear clumsy. His handwriting becomes shaky,

TABLE 75–1
Causes of Hyperthyroidism

Graves' disease (diffuse toxic goiter), the most common variety, is an autoimmune disorder.

Toxic nodular goiter, a less common variety, is not an autoimmune disorder.

Toxic thyroid adenoma is a small, benign nodule on the thyroid gland that autonomously secretes thyroid hormone.

Metastatic thyroid carcinoma (usually follicular) results in hypersecretion of thyroid hormones.

Thyroiditis causes a transient increase in the secretion of thyroid hormones and is due to inflammation or lymphocytic infiltration of the thyroid gland.

Factitious thyrotoxicosis is the result of excessive, or chronic, ingestion of exogenous thyroid hormone by emotionally unstable patients in an attemtp to lose weight.

Malignancies with circulating thyroid stimulators results in excessive thyroid stimulation and increased thyroid hormone production. Human chorionic gonadotropin (HCG) has TSH-like effects and is secreted in choriocarcinomas of the placenta, hydatiform moles, and embryonal cell carcinomas of the testes.

TSH-secreting tumor of the pituitary gland causes overstimulation of the thyroid gland.

Jodbasedow effect is occasionally seen in older individuals with nontoxic multinodular goiter who are exposed to large amounts of exogenous iodine.

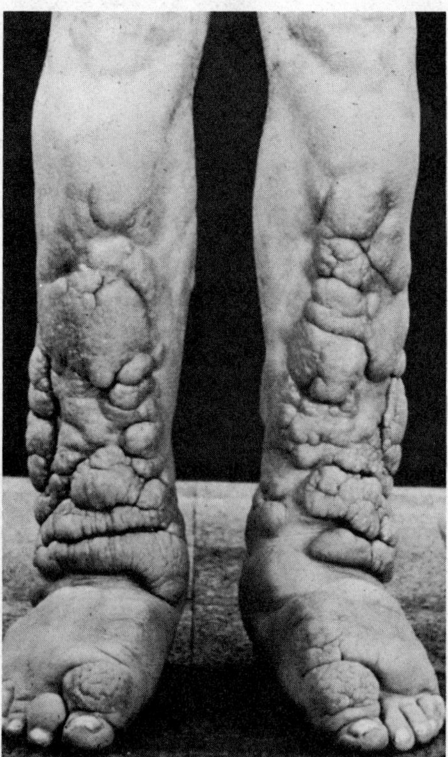

FIGURE 75–1 Severe pretibial myxedema. (Ezrin C, Godden JO, Volpe R [eds]: Systematic Endocrinology, 2nd ed, p 107. New York, Harper & Row, 1979)

he frequently drops things, and he suffers frequent insomnia. His overall behavior is one of nervousness and irritability.

Cardiovascular Changes. The whole cardiovascular system is accelerated because of the increase in catecholamine levels and elevated metabolic rate.[27] Tachycardia, with a full bounding pulse, increases cardiac output and blood pressure and widens the pulse pressure. The elderly are particularly subject to arrhythmias, especially paroxysmal atrial tachycardia and atrial fibrillation. Angina pectoris can occur as heart rate increases. Heart sounds become intensified and, occasionally, a systolic murmur is heard at the mid to lower left sternal border. This murmur may disappear after the hyperthyroidism is controlled. The point of maximum intensity (PMI) is usually readily visible in the precordial region. The signs and symptoms of congestive heart failure may be seen in chronic, untreated hyperthyroidism. Extreme vascularity of the gland with increased blood flow through the thyroid arteries usually results in a bruit that can be heard or palpated over the enlarged gland.[13]

Neuromuscular Changes. Loss of muscular strength and fatigue from muscle wasting and proximal myopathy are prominent symptoms. The patient usually complains of inability to climb stairs or rise from a chair. Exertional dyspnea, without evidence of cardiac failure, is common. These changes are manifestations of increased protein catabolism. Localized or generalized paralysis may be seen in association with hypokalemia. Paralysis, however, is not common. More often, osteoporosis and acropachy (thickening of fingers or toes) are experienced.[1]

Gastrointestinal Changes. The patient usually experiences an increase in appetite, yet has a sustained weight loss. The hypermetabolic effects of the disease cause gastrointestinal hypermotility, with nausea, vomiting, increased bowel tones, diarrhea, and occasionally, abdominal pain and cramping. Diarrhea is not always present, especially in the elderly patient. Concomitant liver disease with jaundice and pruritis may also occur.[2]

Ocular Changes. It is not certain what causes the *ophthalmopathy,* yet it is a characteristic finding in individuals with Graves' disease. Occasionally, a patient with Hashimoto's thyroiditis has exophthalmos but this is rare.[2] This type of thyroiditis will be discussed later in the chapter. The eyes appear prominent, with the sclera visible completely around the iris. Exophthalmus is thought to be due to a combined effect of upper lid retraction and mucopolysaccharide and fluid accumulation in the retro-orbital tissues, and it can be somewhat asymmetrical, even unilateral. The forward displacement of the eyeballs in their orbits (proptosis) gives the patient a startled or "frog-eyed" appearance (Fig. 75–2). If exophthalmus is severe, the lids may not be able to close completely, and periorbital edema may give them a puffy appearance. Extraocular muscle function may be diminished, causing varying degrees of strabismus. Occasionally, conjunctivitis, diplopia, decreased visual acuity, "burning" in the eyes, and increased tearing (or dryness) will occur. It should be noted that severe exophthalmus is not a common finding and that these ocular changes can occur in the absence of hyperthyroidism.[12]

Gynecological Changes. Some women with hyperthyroidism experience oligomenorrhea or amenorrhea, decreased fertility, and a tendency toward spontaneous abortion. Impotency and decreased libido are common complaints in men.

Thyroid Enlargement. The thyroid gland typically increases to 3 to 4 times its normal size. On rare occasions, no

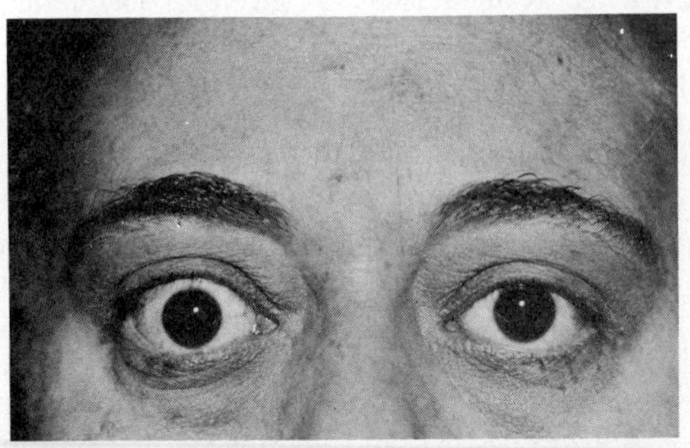
A

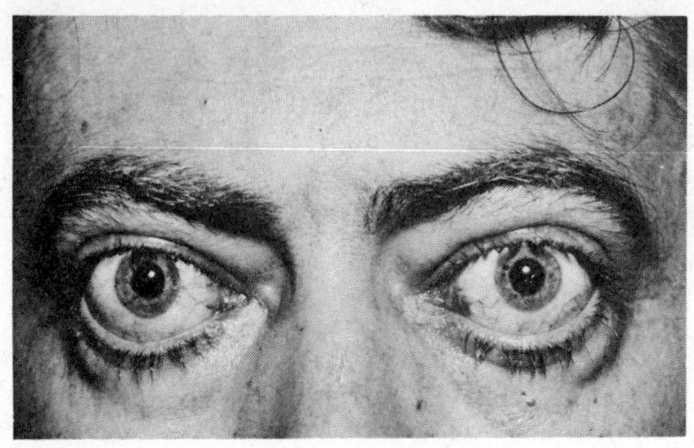
B

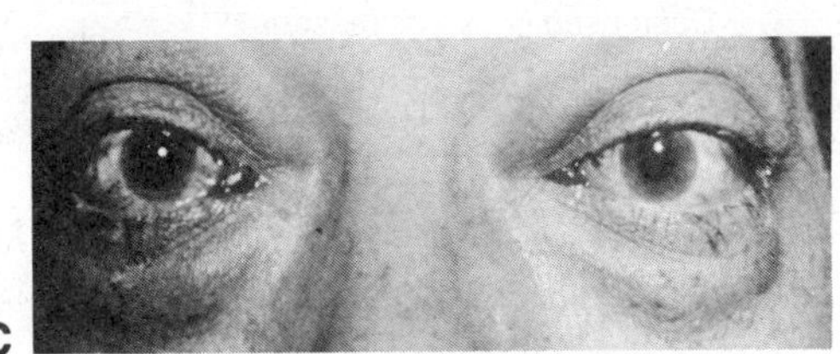
C

FIGURE 75–2 Examples of different degrees of ophthalmopathy due to Graves' disease. (*A*) Upper lid retraction. (*B*) Lower lid retraction. (*C*) Lid fullness. (Werner SC, Ingbar SH: The Thyroid, 4th ed, pp 664–666. New York, Harper & Row, 1978)

enlargement is noted. The gland increases symmetrically and may be lobulated, and it characteristically feels rather firm and beefy. A hyperplastic pyramidal lobe is often palpable.[13]

Radioimmunoassay shows increases in serum thyroxine (T_4) or triiodothyronine (T_3), or both. In some hyperthyroid states, T_3 is elevated by as much as 3% and exceeds the amount of T_4. A thyroid suppression test evaluates whether there is pituitary control of the gland. If, after administration of T_3, ^{131}I uptake is less than 50% of the pretest measurement, hyperthyroidism is not the diagnosis. Using another test, hyperthyroidism is present if thyroid-stimulating hormone (TSH) fails to rise within 30 minutes after administration of thyroid-releasing hormone (TRH). Other laboratory findings include increased serum protein bound iodine (PBI) and decreased serum cholesterol and total lipids.[4] (Table 75–2 summarizes the laboratory tests conducted to detect thyroid dysfunction.) Specific diagnostic studies of thyroid function are discussed in Chapter 72.

Toxic Nodular Goiter. Toxic nodular goiter is typically observed in middle-aged or elderly men and women with a preexisting goiter. Unlike the onset of symptoms in Graves' disease, which may extend over a few months to a year, the clinical manifestations of toxic nodular goiter take much longer to appear. Several years may pass before the diagnosis is made. This condition appears to arise as a pathological evolution of single or multinodular goiter; it is not an autoimmune disorder. Quite simply, the gland becomes unsuppressible by normal feedback mechanisms and overproduces the thyroid hormones. Because of its slow onset and the age of the patient when it appears, toxic nodular goiter is often accompanied by cardiovascular manifestations such as angina and congestive heart failure, proximal muscular weakness and other signs of myopathy. The disorder is also, but less commonly, associated with exophthalmos.[13]

TABLE 75–2
Summary of Laboratory Tests for Thyroid Dysfunction

Test	*Hyperthyroidism (Graves' disease)*	*Hypothyroidism (primary)*
Serum T_4	Increased*	Decreased
Serum T_3	Increased	Normal or decreased
T_3 resin uptake (RT_3U)	Increased	Decreased†
Radioactive iodine uptake (^{131}I uptake)	Increased	Decreased
Protein binding iodine (PBI)	Increased	Decreased
Thyroid-stimulating hormone (TSH)	Decreased	Increased‡
Serum cholesterol	Decreased	Increased
Achilles tendon reflex	Rapid	Slow
Basal metabolic rate (BMR)	Increased	Decreased

* T_4 may be normal in patient with T_3 thyrotoxicosis.
† RT_3U may be increased in patients with goiterous hypothyroidism.
‡ TSH is decreased in secondary hypothyroidism.

Medical Management

The diagnosis of hyperthyroidism is usually based on clinical manifestations, laboratory data, and radionuclide scanning of the thyroid gland. When the diagnosis of Graves' disease has been made, there are three main ways of treating it: drugs, radioactive iodine, and surgery. The appropriate choice is influenced by the patient's age, parity, and size of the goiter. The patient should be told about the three kinds of treatment, the procedures involved, their advantages and disadvantages, and potential complications, and should participate in the choice.[1] Treatment is usually designed to interfere with thyroid hormone synthesis by drugs or ablation of thyroid tissue, using surgery or radioiodide therapy.

Antithyroid Drugs. In essentially all cases, antithyroid drugs control excessive production of thyroid hormone. It takes approximately 4 to 8 weeks to achieve a clinically euthyroid (normal thyroid) state, although physical improvement may be seen sooner. In the United States only two drugs are available, propylthiouracil (PTU) and methimazole (Tapazole). Carbimazole is used extensively in Great Britain. Antithyroid drugs are most often used in children, young adults, pregnant women, and as preoperative preparations to ensure euthyroid status in patients who are to be treated surgically. These drugs are also used in patients who cannot for some reason be treated surgically.

Of the two available drugs, PTU has the advantage of speed of action, and can cause hypermetabolic symptoms to subside relatively quickly. This drug acts by blocking peripheral conversion of T_4 to T_3 in the liver. On the other hand, methimazole has a longer half-life and can be given in much smaller amounts. Although symptoms may disappear, these antithyroid drugs must be continued for 6 months to 2 years. For most adults, initial doses of PTU, 100 mg to 150 mg every 8 hours, or of methimazole, 20 mg to 30 mg every 12 hours, will usually be required.[13] Higher doses may be needed for some individuals. Smaller doses are given for maintenance therapy. Sometimes, exogenous thyroxine is given when the patient's plasma T_4 levels fall into the hypothyroid range. Exogenous thyroxine obviates the need to determine the dosage by titration and prevents the risk of sudden drug-induced hypothyroidism.

When giving antithyroid drugs the nurse should be alert to their side-effects, of which skin rashes and transient fever are the most common. These manifestations usually disappear after treatment has been discontinued. Less common but more serious are leukopenia, thrombocytopenia, elevated levels of liver enzymes, and agranulocytosis. Agranulocytosis is potentially lethal and is manifested by high fever, sore throat, and mouth lesions.[1] The patient should be alerted to these side-effects and urged to report their appearance promptly. The patient should be cautioned against purchasing over-the-counter cough remedies because they may contain significant amounts of iodine, which can potentiate the actions of antithyroid drugs.

Adjunctive Drug Therapy. Adjunctive drug therapy can also be used. *Iodide* is one of the best agents available for inhibiting hormone release, yet its effects are transient and incomplete; therefore, iodide is not satisfactory for chronic use. It is, however, useful in patients who require rapid correction of their hyperthyroid state. Iodide must only be given several hours after initiation of an antithyroid drug that blocks hormone synthesis; if not, it may actually exacerbate hyperthyroidism. *Iodine* is also used before surgery to reduce the size and vascularity of the thyroid gland. There are various types of iodide preparations available for use, most notably saturated solution of potassium iodide (SSKI) and Lugol's solution. The latter is a preparation containing both iodine and iodide, but it has no advantage over SSKI.[7] Iodide solutions have an unpleasant salty taste, so they should be diluted in a full glass of water, juice, or milk and be administered after meals. Iodide solutions are best taken through a straw, since they may stain the teeth. Patients on iodine therapy should be observed for signs of iodine toxicity. Toxic signs include swelling of the buccal mucosa, coryza, rashes, and excessive salivation. The physician should be notified of these symptoms because the drug may need to be discontinued or the dose adjusted. (See Table 75–3 for usual drug doses.)

Adrenergic Antagonists. Adrenergic antagonists can also be used to alleviate symptoms due to increased stimulation of the sympathetic nervous system. The current choice is propranolol (Inderal), but others may be as effective. Indications for use of propranolol include tachycardia, agitation, diaphoresis, and tremor. Beta blocking agents are particularly suited for use in thyroid storm without evidence of acute congestive heart failure. Doses of at least 160 mg daily are usually required. Propranolol or other β-blocker should be discontinued as soon as the patient's state has become euthyroid.[27]

Radioactive Iodide. Radioactive idodide is a relatively simple, effective, and inexpensive form of therapy, and it is the best treatment available for toxic nodular goiters. Administration is usually by mouth in the form of a radionuclide, most frequently ^{131}I. For Graves' disease, a single dose of 2 mCi to 10 mCi is typical. Much higher doses are used for toxic nodular goiter. Radioactive iodine is taken up by the thyroid, which is, in part, destroyed in the process. The higher the dose, the more thyroid tissue will be destroyed. Symptomatic improvement begins after 2 to 4 weeks, but a euthyroid state is usually not achieved until approximately 3 months after administration of the single dose.[13]

The need to be concerned about radioactive destruction of the gonads as a consequence of this mode of therapy has not been substantiated by research. Still, patients of child-

TABLE 75–3
Common Iodide/Iodine Compounds

Drug	*Preparations*	*Usual Dosage Range*	*Remarks*
Potassium iodide (various manufacturers)	Liquid—325 mg/5 ml, 500 mg/15 ml Tablets—650 mg Enteric-coated tablets—300 mg	Adults—300 mg to 650 mg every 4 hr to 6 hr Children—250 mg to 1000 mg daily in divided doses	Useful for hyperthyroidism, thyrotoxic crisis (with antithyroid drugs), preoperatively for thyroidectomy, and to facilitate bronchial drainage and cough in chronic pulmonary diseases. Discontinue if skin rash appears.
Saturated solution potassium iodide (SSKI)	Solution—1 gm/ml	0.3 ml to 0.6 ml 4 to 12 times/day diluted in water, juice, or milk	Commonly used presurgically for reducing size and fragility of thyroid gland. Do not allow to stand uncovered for prolonged periods of time because solution may evaporate. Slight discoloration of solution does not affect potency.
Potassium iodide—Niacinamide hydroiodide (Iodo-Niacin)	Tablets—135 mg potassium iodide and 25 mg niacinamide hydroiodide	Adults—2 tablets 3 times/day Children—1 tablet 3 times/day	Indicated to facilitate cough and bronchial drainage, for prophylaxis of goiter, and management of hyperthyroidism.
Sodium iodide (various manufacturers)	Injection—10%, 20%	*Thyroid crisis*—1 g to 2 g by IV infusion every 2 to 6 days	Primarily used for acute treatment of thyroid crisis. Be alert for development of acute iodism (*e.g.,* metallic taste, stomatitis, sneezing, vomiting, swollen salivary glands) and pulmonary edema.
Strong iodine solution (Lugol's solution)	Solution—5% iodine and 10% potassium iodide	0.1 ml to 0.3 ml 3 times/day (usually for 10 days to 14 days before thyroidectomy)	Principally used to prepare thyroid gland for surgery; also used with an antithyroid drug for treating thyrotoxic crisis. Discontinue if signs of iodism appear (see above). Administer solution diluted in juice, milk, or water, preferably after meals.

(Malseed R: Quick Reference to Drug Therapy and Nursing Considerations, p 420. Philadelphia, JB Lippincott, 1983. With permission)

bearing age should sign a consent form before starting treatment. The fear that use of ^{131}I will lead to thyroid cancer has not been statistically supported either.[2] Perhaps of greater concern is the sudden appearance of hypothyroidism that occurs in 10% of patients treated with radioactive iodine. Secondary hypothyroidism can usually be treated by the exogenous administration of thyroxine. Patients treated with smaller doses (<30 mCi) of ^{131}I can be allowed to go home. Higher doses require hospitalization of the patient. Nursing considerations for patients on radioactive iodide therapy are outlined in Table 75–4.

Sodium ipodate (Oragraphin) has been shown to lower serum T_3 levels by as much as 50% within 24 hours of administration. It is more rapid acting than antithyroid drugs, but its potential usefulness is still under investigation. Other pharmacological agents used on occasion are lithium carbonate, glucocorticoids, and immunosuppressive agents such as 6-mercaptopurine. None of these drugs has demonstrated long-term effectiveness in disease control.

TABLE 75–4
Nursing Considerations for the Patient on Radioactive Iodide (^{131}I) Therapy

1. Before ^{131}I administration, an overnight fast is required because the presence of food delays absorption.
2. Antithyroid drugs should be discontinued 3 to 4 days before administration of ^{131}I.
3. Liquid ^{131}I dose is given in a glass or plastic cup because wax and paper cups may absorb the material.
4. In childbearing women, ^{131}I should only be given during or 10 days after menstruation.
5. Solid food should not be eaten for 2 hours after ^{131}I administration, to reduce the risk of vomiting and loss of the isotope.
6. Intake of liquids should be encouraged and the patient must be urged to urinate frequently because ^{131}I will concentrate in the urine.
7. Because the urine and feces will remain slightly radioactive for 24 to 48 hours, the toilet should be flushed two or three times after each use by the patient.
8. The patient should be urged to avoid coughing or expectorating for 24 hours, if possible.
9. The patient who immediately goes home should restrict contact with small children and sleep alone for two nights.
10. For the patient receiving more than 30 mCi of ^{131}I, hospitalization is required. Only nurses who are not pregnant should be assigned to care for the patient. Contact by nurses should be limited to 30 minutes per shift, per person, during the first day. The time of contact may be increased to 1 hour per shift the second day.
11. The perspiration of the patient on high doses of ^{131}I is radioactive, and the linen should be considered contaminated.
12. Gloves should be worn when handling the patient's urine, contaminated linen, and soiled Kleenex. Care of radioactive waste should be handled according to hospital policy.
13. Visiting is usually restricted the first day.
14. The patient must be warned that he may experience marked thyroid tenderness immediately after ^{131}I administration.
15. The patient should be instructed to watch for and report signs of hypothyroidism (fatigue, vertigo, muscle cramps, puffy eyelids, cold and pale skin, and decreased gastrointestinal motility).

Surgical Treatment. Before the common use of antithyroid drugs and radioactive iodine therapy, *subtotal thyroidectomy* (partial removal of the thyroid gland) was the usual treatment for hyperthyroidism and is still used for persons, young adults and children especially, who cannot be treated successfully with drugs. Preoperatively, the patient must be made euthyroid with drugs. An iodine preparation (potassium iodide or Lugol's solution) is given for 10 consecutive days. Antithyroid drugs are given in conjunction with this, but are discontinued 2 days before the operation. Up to 90% of the thyroid may have to be removed to effectively alleviate hyperthyroid symptoms. A complete thyroidectomy is usually performed in the case of a malignancy. Complications of surgical interventions are relatively uncommon but quite severe. The risks include anesthesia mishaps, death during surgery, laryngeal nerve damage (with vocal cord paralysis), hypoparathyroidism with tetany and, most frequently, hypothyroidism. The last two complications are difficult to avoid because of the nature of the operation.[18]

After ablative treatment, by either radioactive iodine or surgery, patients will require lifelong medical supervision and thyroid hormone replacement. If a subtotal thyroidectomy is performed, the remaining tissue may be sufficient to provide the necessary amount of thyroid hormones. However, the residual tissue may undergo hyperplasia, resulting in recurrent hyperthyroidism.[13]

Medical Management of Hyperthyroid Ophthalmopathy. Medical management includes instillation of 0.5% to 1% methylcellulose eye drops to provide soothing comfort. Diuresis, obtained using chlorothiazide, may be attempted to decrease retro-orbital edema. If exophthalmos progresses, with deterioration of the ocular muscle, large doses of glucocorticoids (*e.g.*, prednisone) may be used. In cases of severe exophthalmos, which causes pressure on the optic nerve, surgical decompression is necessary to prevent blindness and usually removal of part of the bony orbit is also performed, to relieve intraorbital pressure.[2] Tarsorrhaphy (suturing the eyelids together) may be required to extend the eyelids over the bulging eyeballs if they cannot be closed during sleep. The intervention prevents corneal ulceration. Unfortunately, successful treatment of hyperthyroidism does not necessarily result in reduction of the ophthalmopathy.[12]

Nursing Management Plan

Nursing care of the hyperthyroid patient is directed toward controlling many of the manifestations resulting from elevated levels of circulating thyroid hormone and accelerated metabolism.

In general, nursing interventions are directed at

1. Assisting the patient to cope with the anxiety and irritability brought on by the condition

2. Promoting nutritional intake to counter the increase in protein catabolism resulting in weight loss and muscle weakness
3. Initiating measures to deal with elevated body temperature and with gastrointestinal discomfort brought on by diarrhea, abdominal cramps, and possible dehydration
4. Protecting the patient's eyes from possible injury as a result of exophthalmos
5. Monitoring for elevated blood pressure, signs of arrhythmias, and emotional stress.

The specific nursing diagnoses and nursing interventions for each of these measures are given in detail in Nursing Care Plan for the Patient with Hyperthyroidism. It addresses several major problem areas and is intended to be general in its scope. Individualizations are necessary to apply this care plan effectively in meeting specific patient needs.

(*Text continues on page 1063*)

NURSING CARE PLAN FOR THE PATIENT WITH HYPERTHYROIDISM

NURSING DIAGNOSIS/PROBLEM 1: Ineffective coping (individual) related to excessive anxiety manifested by irritability, insomnia, and decompensation of interpersonal relationships

GOAL 1.1: To reduce anxiety and promote adaptive coping mechanisms

Nursing Interventions	Rationale	Outcome Criteria
1. Promote a restful environment a. Maintain a calm, relaxing atmosphere away from disturbing sounds. b. Carefully select potential roommates. c. Schedule activities and nursing procedure to allow sufficient rest periods. d. Restrict visitors as necessary. e. Administer sedatives as ordered when indicated. f. Give consistent, calm nursing care. g. Encourage quiet diversional activities, such as puzzles and needlepoint; provide soothing back rubs.	1. a–g. Anxiety aggravated by increased serum thyroxine (T_4) tends to create a sense of danger and loss of control. Increased motor activity and unpredictable responses can occur to even minor external stimuli. Eliminating unnecessary external stimuli and providing a restful environment can increase the patient's sense of control and security, and promote sleep.[5]	1–6. The patient will: a. Voice feelings related to his emotional state. b. Identify his coping patterns and personal strengths. c. Make time for relaxing activities. d. Demonstrate an optimal balance of rest and activity, reporting improved sleep patterns. e. Maintain healthy relationship with family or friends.
2. Encourage expressions of feelings.	2. Discussion of feelings allows consensual validation and the foundation of trust.[3] Behavior and physical changes often create feelings of frustration and altered self-concept.	
3. Watch for tremor and assist with activities that are difficult for the patient to manage.	3. Tremor, due to increased circulating T_4, can greatly interfere with the patient's ability to manipulate objects, often leading to greater frustration and anxiety.	
4. Reassure the patient and family that any irritable behavior is largely disease-related and may be controlled with appropriate treatment.	4. Disturbed coping mechanisms can cause alienation between the patient and those significant to him.	
5. Instruct the family to avoid sharing disturbing news with the patient; carefully explain all nursing and medical procedures.	5. Clear explanations and instructions help to allay stress.	
6. Avoid stimulus such as tea, coffee, and cocoa.	6. Such stimulants may aggravate irritability and tremor.	

(*Continued*)

NURSING CARE PLAN FOR THE PATIENT WITH HYPERTHYROIDISM (*Continued*)

NURSING DIAGNOSIS/PROBLEM 2: Altered nutritional status related to increased protein catabolism, leading to weight loss, muscular weakness, and integumentary changes

GOAL 2.1: To promote sufficient nutritional intake to maintain a positive nitrogen balance and anabolism

Nursing Interventions	Rationale	Outcome Criteria
1. Weigh daily at same time, using same scale.	1. Inability to meet metabolic requirements results in weight loss.	1–5. The patient will: a. Achieve and maintain ideal body weight. b. Demonstrate no skin breakdown. c. Demonstrate increased physical stamina. d. Discuss rationale for the prescribed diet.
2. Provide a well-balanced diet, high in carbohydrates and proteins with up to 4000 Cal a day. Give between-meal snacks and vitamin supplements.	2. To obtain a 1-lb weight gain requires approximately 3000 Cal above metabolic requirements.[3]	
3. Examine skin for breakdown.	3. Poor nutritional status results in the skin's decreased ability to regenerate and repair itself.	
4. Monitor serum albumin, hemoglobin, and lymphocyte levels.	4. A nutritional deficit can result in decreased serum albumin, hemoglobin, and lymphocyte levels. Assessment of these parameters provides valuable information about the patient's nutritional status.	
5. Progress activity gradually and alternate with rest periods.	5. The patient's activity endurance increases when energy expenditure is balanced with energy restoration periods.	

NURSING DIAGNOSIS/PROBLEM 3: Heat intolerance related to increased metabolic rate, resulting in elevated body temperature, diaphoresis, and general discomfort

GOAL 3.1: To promote comfort and increased tolerance to ambient temperature

Nursing Interventions	Rationale	Outcome Criteria
1. Provide a cool, well-ventilated environment and loose, cool clothing.	1. A response to circulating catecholamines in hyperthyroidism results in an exaggerated increase in metabolic rate with vasodilatation and heat intolerance.	1–4. The patient will: a. Voice decreased discomfort related to heat and diaphoresis. b. Carry out activities aimed at "heat relief." c. Take in sufficient fluid to counter fluid loss from diaphoresis. d. Maintain normal body temperature.
2. Monitor patient's temperature and relieve fever with nonaspirin antipyretics.	2. The abnormal increase in basal metabolic rate may produce elevations in body temperature.	
3. Change damp clothing and linen frequently. Encourage good hygiene with cool, tepid bath.	3. The hyperthyroid patient is often subject to diaphoretic episodes caused by heat intolerance. Good hygiene and dry clothing promotes comfort and skin intactness.	
4. Monitor fluid intake and output. Encourage patient to make up perspiration losses by increasing fluid intake (up to 3000–4000 ml/day).	4. Severe diaphoresis can cause a loss of up to 2500 ml/day. Continued loss without replacement will result in dehydration.	

(*Continued*)

NURSING CARE PLAN FOR THE PATIENT WITH HYPERTHYROIDISM (Continued)

NURSING DIAGNOSIS/PROBLEM 4: Potential for accidental injury related to tremor, fatigue, and osteoporosis, which may result in preventable accidents

GOAL 4.1: To prevent the incidence of accidental injury and encourage safe mobility

Nursing Interventions	Rationale	Outcome Criteria
1. Assist the patient with ambulation as necessary. Keep call-bell well within the patient's reach.	1. Hyperthyroidism can cause proximal myopathy and fatigue. Weakness may result in loss of balance and falls. Hyperthyroidism also promotes osteoporosis, which increases susceptibility to bone fracture.	1–4. The patient will be able to identify factors that increase the potential for injury and use safety measures to prevent injury. No incidence of accidental injury related to tremor or falls. The patient will experience increased, safe mobility.
2. Clear environment of potential hazards and obstacles to mobility. Provide nonskid slippers or shoes for ambulation.	2. Accidents occur frequently from stumbling over obstacles, such as wastebaskets, toys, small animals and from slipping on small throw rugs and wet floors.	
3. Supervise and caution against smoking.	3. Tremor of the hands and upper extremities potentiate dropping of objects. A dropped cigarette is an extreme fire hazard.	
4. Provide adequate lighting, with soft light at night. Keep light switch easily accessible.	4. Poor lighting may obscure potential obstacles to mobility.	

NURSING DIAGNOSIS/PROBLEM 5: Potential alterations in bowel elimination related to diarrhea, which may result in abdominal cramping and dehydration

GOAL 5.1: To return to normal bowel functioning

Nursing Interventions	Rationale	Outcome Criteria
1. Monitor frequency and type of bowel movements. Ausculate bowel tones.	1. Hyperperistalsis with diarrhea and abdominal cramping is a response to increased circulating thyroid hormones.	1–3. Fewer complaints of abdominal cramping. Stools will be firmer and less frequent.
2. Give no foods that are highly seasoned, bulky, or have high roughage content (*i.e.,* raw fruits and vegetables).	2. Intestinal irritants, such as highly seasoned foods and roughage, promote hyperperistalsis.	
3. Monitor for signs and symptoms of dehydration if diarrhea persists. Replace fluid losses through stools with increased fluid intake.	3. Rapid transit of feces through large intestine results in less water absorption and a liquid stool, which increases the risk of dehydration.	

(Continued)

NURSING CARE PLAN FOR THE PATIENT WITH HYPERTHYROIDISM (*Continued*)

NURSING DIAGNOSIS/PROBLEM 6: Potential injury to eyes related to exophthalmus, manifested by discomfort and loss of visual acuity

GOAL 6.1: To prevent eye injury and promote retention of optimum vision

Nursing Interventions	Rationale	Outcome Criteria
1. Protect the patient's eyes from irritants and injury:[12] a. Shield the patient's eyes from excessive light, dust, *etc.* with eyepatches or eyeglasses. b. Moisten cornea and conjunctiva with isotonic eye drops. c. Cover or tape eyelids shut, especially at night, if eyelids do not close completely. d. Cool, moist, compresses can help soothe irritated eyes.	1. a–d. The combination of retroorbital edema and upper lid retraction may cause eyes to appear "bulging" and prevent complete lid closure. The cornea is in jeopardy of damage because of drying and irritants. Measures are taken to prevent corneal drying and contact with irritants.	1–2. No evidence of corneal damage will occur and vision will remain unimpaired.
2. Frequently examine corneas for clarity and intactness.	2. The irritation and drying effects on the cornea can cause conjunctivitis and progress to visual deterioration.	
3. Instruct patient to report any changes in visual acuity.	3. Prompt reporting of visual changes is essential for successful treatment and preservation of visual acuity.	3. The patient will: a. Actively participate in measures to protect eyes from injury. b. Promptly notify physician of changes in visual acuity.

NURSING DIAGNOSIS/PROBLEM 7: Alterations in cardiac output related to hypermetabolic responses that may result in high blood pressure, heart failure, and arrhythmia

GOAL 7.1: To promote stable cardiovascular functioning

Nursing Interventions	Rationale	Outcome Criteria
1. Monitor frequently the patient's cardiovascular status. a. Monitor blood pressure and pulse; report persistent elevations in either. b. Look for potentially dangerous arrhythmias. Monitor rate and regularity of pulse. Have patient report episodes of palpitations, vertigo, or angina. c. Look for signs of heart failure: jugular vein distention, edema, pulmonary congestion, dyspnea.	1. a–c. The hypermetabolic effects of increased thyroid functioning results in vasoconstriction and stimulation of myocardial functioning, causing elevations in pulse, blood pressure, and the potential for arrhythmias (tachycardia and ventricular irritability). Decompensation of the heart can occur, resulting in overt signs of congestive heart failure.	1–3. Blood pressure and pulse will be maintained with or near normal limits. There will be no evidence of heart failure of arrhythmias. The patient will identify factors that increase cardiac workload and minimize these as much as possible.
2. Minimize emotional and physical stress. Balance activity and rest periods.	2. Stress increases circulating catecholamines, which further increase the workload on the heart.	
3. Administer antihypertensives, cardiotonics, and antiarrhythmics as ordered.	3. Appropriate administration of prescribed cardiovascular drugs is essential in preventing serious cardiopulmonary complications related to hyperthyroidism.	

Nursing Care of the Patient with a Thyroidectomy

Preoperative Care. Preoperatively, the nurse should provide the patient with a restful and calm environment. Assigning the patient to a room away from disturbing sights and sounds, such as the nursing station or elevator, is helpful. A pleasant window view and relaxing radio music can provide soothing diversion. Visitors should be cautioned against distressing conversation and boisterous activity. Consistent nursing care, frequent back rubs, and scheduled rest periods can be extremely beneficial.

The hyperthyroid patient is often catabolic, with muscle wasting and a poor nutritional intake. To restore a positive nitrogen balance, a diet high in carbohydrates, protein, and supplementary vitamins is encouraged. In addition, the nurse is responsible for administering antithyroid drugs to render the patient euthyroid. Reasons for prescribed medications should be carefully explained to the patient. The medicines are best tolerated if taken with meals. Side-effects of antithyroid drugs need to be watched for and reported.

Immediate presurgical preparation includes the usual preoperative explanations of what the patient can expect postoperatively, such as deep breathing, coughing, turning, the taking of frequent vital signs, and the administration of intravenous infusions and oxygen. Special considerations, such as how to move the head and neck to minimize incisional stress, should be explained. A special effort must be made to ensure the patient a good night's sleep before the surgery.

Postoperative Care. Postoperatively, aside from the recording of routine vital signs and the measurement of intake and output to assess volume status, there are three precautions that require nursing attention: the prevention of airway obstruction, laryngeal nerve damage, and tetany.

Tracheal Compression. Tracheal compression can be caused by postoperative hemorrhage or tissue swelling, and most often occurs 12 to 14 hours after surgery.[1] Choking and either irregular or stridulous breathing may indicate pressure upon the trachea. A tracheostomy set should remain in the patient's room, along with oxygen and suction, for at least 48 hours for use in the event of acute airway obstruction. Assessments also include observation of incisional swelling or hemorrhage. The latter is sometimes best assessed at the sides of the dressing or at the back of the patient's neck, where blood tends to accumulate. The patient's head must be adequately supported when he is moving about or turning in bed, to ease tension on the neck incision. Sandbags or pillows can be used to immobilize the head. A semi-Fowler's position is best, if the patient can tolerate it, since this position minimizes swelling.

Laryngeal Nerve Damage. Damage to the laryngeal nerve is best investigated after the patient recovers from anesthesia. Signs and symptoms include hoarseness or a weak whispery voice. These voice changes may be due to temporary postoperative swelling and may be transient, but hoarseness should not persist longer than 4 days. The patient is cautioned to avoid talking unless absolutely necessary. Writing on a pad or "magic slate" may ease communication. It should be remembered that bilateral laryngeal nerve damage can cause paralysis of the glottis and precipitate suffocation.[21]

Tetany. The likelihood of tetany developing depends on the number of parathyroid glands removed during surgery. Early signs include tingling of the toes and fingers and around the mouth. Later signs include positive Chvostek's and Trousseau's signs and grand mal seizures. In Chvostek's sign, the facial muscles go into a spasm when they are gently tapped. In Trousseau's sign, carpopedal spasms of the arm result when the upper arm is compressed. Calcium chloride must be readily available for emergency intravenous infusion.

Acute Thyroid Storm. An acute thyroid storm may develop postoperatively because of inadequate preoperative preparation and increased thyroid hormone release during surgical manipulation of the gland. The nurse must observe and report early signs of this emergency. When discharged from the hospital the patient needs to be aware of the importance of continued medical follow-up. Not only are signs of hypothyroidism to be watched for, but signs of hyperthyroidism as well. The thyroid tissue remaining after subtotal thyroidectomy may eventually regenerate, causing recurrent episodes of hyperthyroidism. This too must be watched for.

Thyrotoxic Crisis (Thyroid Storm)

Thyrotoxic crisis represents an extreme exaggeration of the clinical manifestations of hyperthyroidism and is a true medical emergency. It is a complication usually associated with Grave's disease (75%), although it can occur in patients with toxic nodular goiter. The precipitating causes are infections, surgery, and other trauma. Less common causes include severe stress (such as fear or extreme heat), radioactive iodine therapy, excessive palpation of the thyroid gland, and diabetic ketoacidosis.[10] Thyroid storm is characterized by fever (sometimes hyperpyrexia with temperature as high as 106° F [40.7° C]), marked tachycardia with arrhythmias, diarrhea, profuse diaphoresis, and hypotension. If untreated, it can progress rapidly to delirium, coma, cardiovascular collapse, and death.[20]

The diagnosis of thyrotoxic crisis must be made early and appropriate treatment given, because the mortality from thyroid storm is approximately 20%. Therapeutic interventions include temperature control with a hypothermia blanket, replacement of fluid volume, administration of glucocorticoids (steroids acutely lower T_4 and T_3 in the plasma), and high doses of antithyroid drugs. Propranolol can be administered to achieve β-adrenergic blockade and inhibit the peripheral manifestations of thyroid hormone excess. Should congestive heart failure develop in thyroid storm, propranolol is contraindicated.[15] Other supportive measures can be initiated to improve clinical status and prevent death (Table 75–5).

TABLE 75-5
Treatment of Thyroid Storm

1. Propylthiouracil or methimazole: 900–1200 mg/day by mouth or by nasogastric tube, in 3 or 4 divided doses
2. Iodine: 30 drops of potassium iodide daily by mouth or 1–2 g/day of sodium iodide by slow IV infusion
3. Propranolol: 160 mg/day by mouth in 4 divided doses or 1–2 mg by slow IV every 4 hours
4. IV glucose solutions
5. Reversal of dehydration and restoration of electrolyte balance
6. Cooling blanket for hyperpyrexia
7. Digitalis preparation, if indicated
8. Treatment of underlying precipitating cause (*i.e.*, infection, pulmonary embolism, or diabetic ketoacidosis)
9. Definitive control of the crisis: ablation of the thyroid gland with ^{131}I or by surgical removal (subtotal thyroidectomy)

(Adapted from Klein IL, Levey GS: Thyroid emergencies: Thyroid storm and myxedema coma. Topics in Emergency Medicine 5(4):33–39, 1984)

Hypofunction of the Thyroid Gland: Hypothyroidism

Hypothyroidism (Gull's disease) is a relatively common metabolic state caused by a deficiency in circulating thyroid hormones. Adult onset of severe hypothyroidism is sometimes known as *myxedema;* hypothyroidism occurring in infancy and childhood is termed *congenital hypothyriodism.*

Etiology and Pathophysiology

In adults, the cause of hypothyroidism is most often iatrogenic, following ablative treatment for hyperthyroidism, either surgery (thyroidectomy) or radioactive iodine therapy.[1] Drug therapy with antithyroid and iodide preparations are not infrequent causes. Spontaneous hypothyroidism can also be secondary to chronic immune thyroiditis (Hashimoto's disease) and other inflammatory conditions, such as amyloidosis and sarcoidosis. Less commonly, hypothyroidism results from decreased TSH secretion by the pituitary, failure of the hypothalamus to produce thyrotropin-releasing hormone (TRH), and inability of the thyroid to synthesize hormones because of dietary iodine deficiency. Myxedema is most prevelant in women of middle age or older.[27]

In infants, hypothyroidism results from a congenital absence or underdevelopment of the thyroid gland, or it may be caused by a severe iodine deficiency suffered by the mother during pregnancy. Less frequently, an enzymatic defect in thyroxine synthesis is inherited as an autosomal recessive trait. Over the age of 2, congenital hypothyroidism is usually secondary to chronic, autoimmune thyroiditis. Hypothyroidism occurs three times more often in girls than in boys and often produces profound abnormalities in growth and development.[1,22] In both adults and children, hypothyroidism results in a slowing of nearly all metabolic processes within the body.

Clinical Manifestations

The signs and symptoms of hypothyrodism are related not only to the degree of thyroid hormone deficit present but to the age of onset. The manifestations of hypothyroidism are somewhat different in adults and children.

Typically, the early clinical features of adult hypothyroidism are varied and vague. The onset of symptoms is usually insidious, and may progress over years before detection occurs.

As metabolic processes slow, the patient experiences easy *fatigability.* Motivation declines and physical inertia sets in. Increased somnolence, with the patient falling asleep at inopportune times, is a common occurrence. The voice often becomes low-pitched, slow, and rough.[8]

The *skin* becomes cool to the touch and dry and scaley—so scaly in fact that large flakes are shed from knees and elbows.[13] Mucopolysaccharide infiltration of the subcutaneous tissue, along with overgrowth of the horny layer of the epidermis, make the skin appear thickened or "doughy." A yellow orange discoloration of the skin may also become apparent, especially on the palms. This discoloration is due to *hypercarotinemia,* which is secondary to failure of the liver to convert carotene to vitamin A and is a result of thyroid hormone deficiency. Hair loss is common. Eyebrows become sparse (with the outer third missing) and nails become brittle. A puffy face along with periorbital edema is particularly noticeable, along with upper eyelid drooping. The tongue is sometimes enlarged and protrudes from the mouth.[2]

Ordinarily, the patient appears unusually placid with slowed intellectual functioning. However, agitation and frank psychosis may occur and are accompanied by paranoid ideation, suicidal tendencies, and hallucinations.[2] Paresthesias of the hands and diminished hearing are common. These annoying signs are probably the result of mucoprotein deposits on the median and eighth cranial nerves, respectively. Cerebellar dysfunction may appear in the form of ataxia, intention tremor, and nystagmus. The patient's movements often appear slow and clumsy. Reflexes also demonstrate delayed relaxation time, especially in the Achilles tendon. The drop in metabolic rate often makes the patient hypothermic and intolerant of cold.

A slowed pulse rate, decreased cardiac output, and poor peripheral circulation are sometimes seen. Occasionally, the heart may appear enlarged either because of ventricular dilatation or because of pericardial effusion. Pleural effusions and ascites due to liver impairment and hypoproteinemia may also be present. Hypothyroid individuals are often predisposed to atherosclerosis, because depressed liver functioning elevates blood cholesterol levels.[27]

Aching muscle and stiffness of joint are frequent early complaints in hypothyroidism. Thickening of the joint capsule, arthritis, and bursitis are common. Discomfort also derives from abnormal sensitivity to cold. As the metabolic rate falls, heat production diminishes.

Constipation is a frequent complaint because of the decreased motility of the bowel. More serious occurrences are intestinal ileus and megacolon. Weight gain, due probably in large part to fluid retention, is characteristic.

Irregular menstrual periods and severe menorrhagia are common in young women. Decreased libido is the rule for both sexes. Fertility is usually diminished but pregnancy is possible. Unless the mother's hypothyroidism is drug-related, the newborn is often euthyroid.[22]

If the enlargement is primary, it may be caused by a diffuse goiter. Its presence, however, virtually excludes the possibility of pituitary, or hypothalamic, insufficiency as a cause of hypothyroidism.

With the failure of the metabolic processes, along with hepatic and renal impairment, *coma* ensues. It usually develops gradually, with progressive stupor, hypoventilation, hypotension, water excess, hypoglycemia, and severe hypothermia. Positive, bilateral Babinski signs are usually present. Rapid development of myxedema coma may occur with severe stress (such as sepsis and exposure to cold) or with trauma and administration of central nervous system (CNS) depressants.[13] Coma is particularly common in the elderly with concurrent medical problems. Chronic hypothyroidism mortality may be as high as 60% to 70%.

Diagnostic Tests. Radioimmunoassay reveals low T_4 and T_3 levels. In hypothyroidism due to primary thyroid insufficiency, TSH levels will be high. Decreased TSH levels are found in hypothyroidism due to hypothalamic or pituitary insufficiency and are occasionally found in euthyroid states. Other findings include elevations in serum cholesterol, alkaline phosphatase, triglycerides, prolactin, carotene, and liver enzymes. In addition, normocytic, normochromic anemia is observed. Laboratory data in myxedema coma show low serum sodium and low albumin, along with a decreased pH and increased Pa_{CO_2} (due to respiratory hypoventilation). Electrocardiographic abnormalities include flattened or inverted T waves, minor ST-segment depressions, and low-amplitude QRS complexes. A thyroid scan (^{131}I uptake test) demonstrates impaired uptake.[27]

Clinical Manifestations in Infants and Children

Characteristic signs of hypothyroidism in infancy develop at 3 to 6 months of age and may be delayed in the breast-fed infant, since some thyroid hormone is contained in breast milk. Usually the infant is described as "a good baby" sleeping excessively with only an occasional hoarse cry.[1] Its development, both mental and physical, is delayed. Its deep tendon reflexes are diminished and it makes slow awkward movements. Its abdomen is often protuberant, and it has an umbilical hernia because its abdominal muscles are hypotonic. The infant also has feeding problems and constipation. Liver impairment interferes with conjugation of bilirubin, and the child may become jaundiced. The tongue is enlarged, making breathing noisy and sometimes causing airway obstruction. The classic physical features include a short forehead, wide-set puffy eyes, wrinkled eyelids, broad flat nose, dull sparse hair, and cold dry skin. Mental retardation is typically profound but may be limited, depending on how soon thyroid hormone replacement therapy begins.[22]

A child who develops hypothyroidism after the age of 2 is less likely to develop severe mental retardation. The reason is probably that CNS maturation is complete at this age. The detection of hypothyroidism is usually based on statural growth retardation (due to delayed epiphyseal maturation), obesity, and a head that appears abnormally large in relation to the stunted extremities. Radiographic examination reveals immature bone age, epiphyseal dysgenesis, and retarded dental development. Sexual maturation is also delayed.[1] The laboratory data found with cretinism are the same as those observed with adult hypothyroidism.

Medical Management

The first therapeutic goal is to identify the underlying cause and correct it, if possible. For instance, a patient with chronic obstructive lung disease who has been taking medications with high iodine content can be improved by decreasing or discontinuing the offending drug.[13] In congenital hypothyroidism, an early diagnosis and appropriate treatment is essential to minimize mental retardation. Hormone deficiency is corrected by gradually replacing thyroid hormone. The drug of choice is levothyroxine (T_4). Other medications used with success include liothyronine (T_3), liotrix (synthetic mixture of T_3 and T_4), and USP desiccated thyroid. Drug doses are gradually increased to prevent the sudden onset of thyroid storm. Doses are proportionately higher for children than for adults, because thyroid hormone is more quickly metabolized in children. (See Table 75–6 for usual doses of various thyroid hormone preparations.) Lifelong replacement is usually indicated.[27]

Myxedema coma is corrected by immediate intravenous administration of levothyroxine or liothyronine, with maintenance doses every 8 to 12 hours. Hypoventilation necessitates oxygenation and, perhaps, mechanical ventilation. Correction of hypothermia is done judiciously. The application of external heat may dramatically shunt blood to the periphery, further decreasing blood pressure and compromising vital organs, such as the brain and kidneys. Blankets should suffice.[13] Hypoglycemia can be promptly treated with an intravenous bolus of 50% dextrose. A water restriction to less than 1 liter/day can help correct hyponatremia, if present. Secondary problems such as infection, myocardial infarction, and gastrointestinal hemorrhage require appropriate and specific management.[19]

Nursing Management Plan

Nursing interventions for the patient with hypothyroidism are aimed at restoring a normal metabolic state, preventing complications of the disease, and stengthening long-term coping resources to better handle the chronic nature of the disease. For the patient with congenital hypothyroidism, a nursing aim is to provide sufficient psychological support to the parents, who must now deal with a child who may be mentally retarded. The nurse should help these parents focus on their child's strengths rather than on his weaknesses, adopting a positive yet realistic attitude. Controlled, stimulating activities may help the child to reach maximum potential.[1] Referrals to a variety of supportive community agencies can be made.

TABLE 75–6
Common Thyroid Hormone Replacement Drugs*

Drug	*Dosage*	*Nursing Considerations*
Levothyroxine sodium—T_4 (L-Thyroxone, Levothroid, Levoid, Noroxine, Synthroid)	*Oral:* 0.1 mg/day initially; increase by 0.05–0.1 mg increments every 1–3 weeks until desired response achieved Use lower dose in the elderly. *Parenteral:* IV dose: 0.2–0.5 mg initially for myxedema coma Maintenance dose: 0.1–0.3 mg daily	Levothyroxine sodium is a synthetic form of the natural T_4. Give oral doses in morning, before breakfast. Discontinue levothyroxine before transferring to liothyronine. Mix parenteral dose in normal saline. Levothyroxine may exacerbate underlying diseases, such as Addison's disease, diabetes insipidus, and diabetes mellitus.
Liothyronine sodium—T_3 (Cytomel)	*Oral:* For hypothyroidism: initially 25 g daily, with maintenance 25–75 g daily For myxedema coma: initially 5 g daily. Maintenance dose: Increase all doses by 12.5–25 g every 1–2 weeks, until desired effects are achieved.	Liothyronine is a synthetic form of the natural T_3. Has a more rapid onset and shorter duration than L-thyroxine. When transferring to levothyroxine, start levothyroxine, then discontinue liothyronine after several days. Liothyronine sodium is used in the T_3 suppression test.
Liotrix (Euthroid, Thyrolar)	*Oral:* Initially give 15–30 mg daily, gradually increasing dose every 1–2 weeks.	This drug is a mixture of synthetic T_4 and T_3 in a fixed ratio of 4 : 1. Report headache in the Euthroid patient, since dosage adjustment or change to another thyroid preparation may be necessary.
Thyroid, dessicated (Armour thyroid, S-P-T, Thermoloid, Thyrar, Thyroteric, Proloid)	*Oral:* *In myxedema:* Give 16 mg daily for 2 weeks, then 32 mg/day for 2 weeks; then 65 mg/day. Thereafter dosage increased as needed: maintenance dose is 65–130 mg/day *Hypothyroidism without myxedema:* Initially 65 mg/day increased by 65 mg every month until desired effects achieved	Is a preparation of dessicated animal thyroid gland Administer as single dose before breakfast. Observe patient closely for adverse effects, such as palpitations, angina pectoris, and hypertension. Teach patient to monitor own pulse and consult physician if it remains over 100. Drug may potentiate anticoagulants, requiring decreased doses. Avoid ingestion of foods high in iodine (*i.e.*, turnips, cabbage, soybeans, kelp, and some breads)

* Replacement therapy for thyroid products is based on the following equivalency: 60 mg liotrix = 65 mg dessicated thyroid = 0.1 mg levothyroxine (T_4) = 25 g liothyronine (T_3).

For the adult patient, one of the major nursing challenges is to help the patient deal with the psychosocial and cognitive effects that result from the slowed metabolic processes characteristic of the disease. The altered thought processes reflected in confusion, lethargy, and intellectual impairment must be dealt with by implementing measures to promote optimum levels of cognitive functioning. The same is true for the fatigue and lethargy that compromises the patient's ability to carry out activities of daily living. Interventions to increase the patient's level of functioning are part of the effort to overcome these self-care deficits. Changes in physical appearance and stamina that result in an altered body image and a lack of self-esteem and respect require careful attention to enhance the patient's coping abilities. In the realm of physical problems that arise for the patient with hypothyroidism, the nurse would not only administer the pharmacotherapy prescribed but would also be alert for gastrointestinal problems such as constipation, nausea, and cramps resulting from the slowdown in peristalsis and for potential lowering of cardiac output that could lead to congestive heart failure. The specific interventions for each of these problems are discussed in detail in Nursing Care Plan for the Patient with Hypothyrodism. As with the other care plans presented, the interventions should be individualized to meet the specific needs of each patient.

Simple Goiter

Simple goiter (nontoxic goiter) is enlargement of the thyroid gland that is not the result of inflammation or neoplasia and does not become exacerbated into hyperthyroidism or hypothyroidism. It has also been described in terms of *endemic* or *sporadic* goiter.[2] Endemic goiter usually refers to thyroid enlargement that results from etiologic factors common to a particular region. Sporadic goiters connote goiters arising in nonendemic areas from a stimulus that is not shared by the general population. Because these terms can lead to some confusion, simple, or nontoxic, goiter is the preferred term.[13]

(*Text continues on page 1071*)

NURSING CARE PLAN FOR THE PATIENT WITH HYPOTHYROIDISM

NURSING DIAGNOSIS/PROBLEM 1: Alterations in thought processes related to slowed metabolic processes that result in confusion, lethargy, and impaired intellect

GOAL 1.1: To promote optimum level of cognitive functioning

Nursing Interventions	Rationale	Outcome Criteria
1. Evaluate the patient's level of consciousness and frequently reorient the patient to persons, places, and time. Put a calendar and clock in the room. 2. Maintain a nonstressful environment. Provide consistent, patient, and sensitive nursing care. 3. Provide sufficient sensory stimulation by giving regular back rubs and displaying colorful wall hangings (preferably items from home).	1. Receiving and accurately interpreting incoming stimuli from the environment is essential for optimum emotional and physical functioning. 2. Stress can decrease the efficiency at which the patient can adequately receive and process information. 3. Sensory deprivation can result in perceptual distortions, altered time sense, anxiety, and hallucinations. Familiar environments promote orientation and a sense of well-being.	1–3, 5–6. The patient will: a. Demonstrate optimum contact with reality: oriented to person, place, and time. Make reality-based statements. b. Demonstrate increased motivation. c. Approximately communicate his needs.
4. Discuss the nature of the patient's behavioral changes with the patient's family and close friends.	4. Inappropriate behavior may cause anxiety and alienation in family members and friends.	4. The family will discuss rationale for cognitive changes in patient and continue to demonstrate support.
5. Allow adequate time for patient to express himself. Also speak slowly and clearly to patient.	5. Reduced metabolic functioning and mental acuity often produces a slowing of speech. More time is required for the patient to process and react to information. In addition, hearing is sometimes diminished.	
6. Avoid use of sedatives and hypnotics (*i.e.,* narcotics, barbiturates, anesthetics). If administration of these drugs are necessary, lowered dosage is imperative.	6. Hypothyroid patients demonstrate increased sensitivity to sedatives and hypnotics.	

NURSING DIAGNOSIS/PROBLEM 2: Cold intolerance related to slowed metabolic processes may result in mild hypothermia and discomfort

GOAL 2.1: To promote comfort and increased tolerance to ambient temperatures

Nursing Interventions	Rationale	Outcome Criteria
1. Maintain a warm environment. Provide cotton blankets, warm robe, socks, *etc.,* as required for warmth. Avoid exposing patient to sudden drafts. 2. Monitor the patient's temperature routinely. 3. Provide warm beverages to drink.	1. Hypothyroidism results in reduced metabolic processes that impair the patient's ability to adapt to cooler temperatures. 2. As metabolic functions slow, body temperature falls. 3. Cold foods and beverages may potentiate chilling in the patient.	1–3. Body temperature will remain within normal limits. The patient will: a. Express satisfaction with an increase in comfort. b. Use measures to promote warmth.

(Continued)

NURSING CARE PLAN FOR THE PATIENT WITH HYPOTHYROIDISM (*Continued*)

NURSING DIAGNOSIS/PROBLEM 3: Alterations in skin integrity related to edema and excessive dryness that may result in skin breakdown

GOAL 3.1: To prevent disruption in skin integrity

Nursing Interventions	Rationale	Outcome Criteria
1. Monitor skin for edema, increasing hair loss, and lesions.	1. Hypothyroidism results in thickening and drying of skin, along with generalized hair loss. This along with edema creates an increased risk of skin breakdown.	1–3. There will be no evidence of skin breakdown. The patient will discuss and participate in measures aimed at preventing skin breakdown.
2. Prevent skin breakdown: a. Use oils or lotion during and after baths. b. Administer skin care to pressure points at least four times a day and apply sheepskin or foam to patient's heels and elbows. c. Avoid harsh soaps and rough towels. Blot skin dry; do not rub. d. Provide a diet high in protein, carbohydrates, and vitamins. e. Promote optimum sleep.	2. Dry skin and edema impair the skin's function as a protective barrier and promote skin breakdowns. a. Oils and lotions may temporarily relieve the skin's extreme dryness. b. Areas of greatest risk of breakdown (pressure points) require extra protection. c. Harsh soaps and vigorous towel drying may simply increase dryness of the skin. d. An inadequate intake of protein, carbohydrates, and vitamins can impair tissue regeneration. e. Inadequate sleep causes high levels of chalone (a hormone that depresses epidermic regeneration).[5]	
3. Teach patient and family members how to identify and prevent skin breakdown.	3. The patient and family assume primary responsibility in the long-term prevention of integumentary impairment.	

NURSING DIAGNOSIS/PROBLEM 4: Alterations in bowel elimination related to constipation may result in nausea and cramping

GOAL 4.1: To resume normal bowel functioning

Nursing Interventions	Rationale	Outcome Criteria
1. Monitor bowel tones, abdominal size, and frequency of stools.	1. Peristalsis slows because of hypofunction of the thyroid gland, resulting in constipation. An enlarged abdomen may suggest a megacolon or ascites, both of which are sometimes seen in hypothyroidism.	1–3. A return to normal bowel elimination patterns with soft formed stool. The patient will practice health behaviors aimed at reducing constipation.

(*Continued*)

NURSING CARE PLAN FOR THE PATIENT WITH HYPOTHYROIDISM (*Continued*)

Nursing Interventions	Rationale
2. Promote the frequency and softening of stools. a. Encourage intake of a diet with foods high in fiber, such as raw vegetables and bran. Fluids are encouraged only if signs of heart failure are absent. b. Encourage adequate exercise to the level of the patient's tolerance.	2. a. Foods high in fiber act as bowel irritants to stimulate peristalsis. An increased fluid intake will increase the water content of the stools. b. Activity also promotes peristalsis, which produces softer stools.
3. Caution patient against straining at stool. Assist the patient in assuming a more natural position (semi-squatting) during defecation.	3. Straining at stool increases intra-abdominal pressure and creates stress on an already compromised heart. A semi-squatting position allows optimal use of abdominal muscles and the effects of gravity.

NURSING DIAGNOSIS/PROBLEM 5: Self-care deficit related to fatigue, confusion, and generalized discomfort, resulting in impaired ability to perform activities of daily living

GOAL 5.1: To preserve and promote optimal level of functioning in managing self-care activities

Nursing Interventions	Rationale	Outcome Criteria
1. Evaluate the patient's ability and endurance in performing self-care activities, such as feeding self, bathing, toileting, grooming, *etc.* Discontinue activity if the patient experiences dyspnea, vertigo, or extreme tachycardia.	1. Self-care deficit often results from decreased stamina, confusion, or mobility impairment due to discomfort. Some activities may cause excessive energy expenditure, resulting in dyspnea and elevations in pulse rate.	1–4. The patient will: a. Perform self-care activities at an optimal level. b. Express satisfaction with accomplishments despite limitations. c. Demonstrate improved physical endurance and motivation.
2. Gradually increase activity levels. Plan rest periods according to the patient's daily activities.	2. Endurance is improved when energy expenditure is well matched by energy conservation.	
3. Allow patient to participate in activity schedules and goals. Explore with patient and his family possible incentives (*e.g.,* performing a task such as a handicraft). Give encouragement for attained activity goals. Promote a sincere, positive "can do" attitude.	3. Patient participation incentives and encouragement can increase motivation toward achieving self-care goals.	
4. Provide soothing back rubs, diversional activities, and mild analgesics. Place warm pads over areas of discomfort.	4. Pain may result from effusion and thickening of joint capsules, and result in limited mobility. Back rubs and distraction techniques can effectively minimize discomfort.	

(*Continued*)

NURSING CARE PLAN FOR THE PATIENT WITH HYPOTHYROIDISM (Continued)

NURSING DIAGNOSIS/PROBLEM 6: Alterations in cardiac output related to impaired metabolic functions, resulting in potential for heart failure

GOAL 6.1: To prevent and detect early congestive heart failure

Nursing Interventions	Rationale	Outcome Criteria
1. Monitor cardiovascular performance; evaluate blood pressure and pulse; watch for signs of congestive heart failure, pulmonary crackles, dependent edema, heart gallop sounds, and jugular vein distention; monitor weight daily.	1. Hypothyroidism causes reduction in cardiac rate, force of contraction, and cardiac output. Myocardial functioning is further compromised by pericardial effusion, cardiac hypertrophy, and coronary artery disease. Evidence of right and lef ventricular dysfunction often results.	1–4. The patient will: a. Demonstrate cardiac tolerance to activity (*i.e.,* stable blood pressure, pulse, and respirations). b. Manifest no signs of congestive heart failure. c. Identify factors that increase cardiac workload. d. Promptly report signs of cardiac intolerance to exercise.
2. Provide diet low in cholesterol and sodium. Monitor serum cholesterol levels.	2. Altered lipid metabolism results in elevated cholesterol levels, which potentiates coronary heart disease. An increase in sodium intake can increase fluid retention and create greater circulating volume, causing further stress on the heart.	
3. Minimize physical and emotional stressors.	3. Stress increases circulating catecholamines, which can adversely tax an already compromised heart.	
4. Plan nursing strategies to promote rest; scheduling sufficient rest periods between activities. Ask patient to report dyspnea, chest pain, vertigo, palpitations, or irregular pulse with or without exercise.	4. Physical activity can place great demand on the cardiac workload and should be well balanced with rest. Warning signs that the heart is not coping with the demands placed on it include chest pain, dyspnea, pulse alterations, and vertigo.	

NURSING DIAGNOSIS/PROBLEM 7: Altered body image related to changes in physical appearance and stamina, resulting in a decreased self-esteem, depression, frustration, anger, or social withdrawal

GOAL 7.1: To promote self-confidence and assist with reconstruction of body image

Nursing Interventions	Rationale	Outcome Criteria
1. Provide an environment conducive to expression of feelings. Be understanding and consistent in care delivery. a. Respect patient's wishes for privacy. b. Maintain an open, positive, and accepting attitude toward the patient.	1. The marked changes in physical appearance and stamina can be distressing. a. Discussion of feelings allows consensual validation and may help clarify misconceptions the patient may have regarding his disease, care, and the care-givers. b. Acceptance of the patient's abilities and limitations facilitates trust in, and success of, the therapeutic program.	1–4. The patient will: a. Express feelings related to his emotional state. b. Identify personal strengths and abilities. c. Make positive statements about his appearance. d. Actively maintain interpersonal relationships with those he cares about.
2. Encourage good personal hygiene and grooming.	2. Good personal hygiene enhances physical appearance and may aid self-esteem.	

(*Continued*)

NURSING CARE PLAN FOR THE PATIENT WITH HYPOTHYROIDISM (*Continued*)

Nursing Interventions	Rationale
3. Work with patient to identify realistic and easily attained goals. Plan care to allow sufficient time for the patient to accomplish tasks.	3. Unrealistic goals beyond the patient's capabilities can lead to further frustration and hamper movement toward growth of self-confidence. Daily goals, such as writing a letter, may be appropriate.
4. Assist family members in understanding and helping patient's physical and mental changes.	4. The family must be able to support the patient who may have a long-term coping deficit. Family members may go through a grieving period related to the patient's physical and behavioral changes. These feelings must be explored and allowed expression.

Etiology and Pathophysiology

Simple goiters arise when, for some reason, the thyroid gland cannot secrete enough thyroid hormone to meet metabolic requirements. As a compensatory mechanism, the thyroid gland undergoes hyperplasia to increase thyroid hormone synthesis. Normal levels of TSH are usually seen. The problem lies within the thyroid tissue itself. Depletion of glandular organic iodine and impaired intrathyroid hormone synthesis make the thyroid tissue more sensitive to circulating TSH. This increased sensitivity is probably responsible for the goitrogenesis and results in increased hormone synthesis. Therefore, despite an underlying impairment of hormone production, the patient remains metabolically normal.[7]

One cause of nontoxic goiter is insufficient iodine intake, which occurs where there is iodide-deficient soil and water or where malnutrition includes iodine deficiency. Such areas include central Africa and the highlands of New Guinea. There are also so-called goitrous belts in the United States, in the Midwest, Northwest, and Great Lakes regions.[1] Another cause is the ingestion of excessive amounts of goitrogenic foods or the use of goitrogenic drugs. Goitrogenic foods contain substances that inhibit T_4 production. Examples of such foods are rutabagas, cabbage, turnips, peanuts, soybeans, peas, leafy green vegetables, peaches, strawberries, carrots, and radishes. Goitrogenic drugs include thyroid inhibitors, phenylbutazone, sulfonylurea, para-aminosalicylic acid, cobalt, and lithium.[2]

Simple goiters are found most frequently in women, particularly during adolescence, pregnancy, and menopause. In highly endemic areas, practically all adults may have some degree of thyroid enlargement.[27]

Clinical Manifestations

The degree of thyroid enlargement may vary from a small, single nodule to a massive, multinodular goiter the size of a large melon (Fig. 75–3). Since the patient's metabolism has essentially not altered, the clinical manifestations are primarily those of the mechanical sequelae of increased gland size, such as respiratory difficulty and dysphagia caused by compression and displacement of the trachea or esophagus. Hoarseness due to compression of the recurrent laryngeal nerve may occur, but is rare, however, in simple goiter and is often more suggestive of a thyroid neoplasm. Very large goiters may cause superior mediastinal obstruction and impede venous return. Such obstruction can cause vertigo or syncope when the patient raises his arms above his head (Pemberton effect).[1]

Medical Management

For the diagnosis to be made, other disorders with similar clinical effects must be ruled out. Such disorders include Graves' disease, Hashimoto's thyroiditis, and thyroid carcinoma. Laboratory findings for nontoxic goiter include high or normal TSH or T_3 serum concentrations, low normal to normal serum concentrations of T_4 and PBI, and normal or elevated ^{131}I uptake.

The goal of treatment is to diminish the size of the thyroid gland. Exogenous thyroid hormone replacement (with levothyroxine or liothyronine) is usually given to inhibit TSH secretion and allow the gland to rest. If the goiter is a result of iodine deficiency, small doses of iodide (Lugol's solution or potassium iodide solution) are given. If ingested goitrogenic agents are the suspected cause, treatment is often accomplished by withdrawing and avoiding these substances. For a large goiter that is unresponsive to therapy and is accompanied by symptoms related to compression, a subtotal thyroidectomy may be required.

Nursing Management Plan

Nursing considerations in the care of individuals with simple goiter is focused on preventive and supportive care.

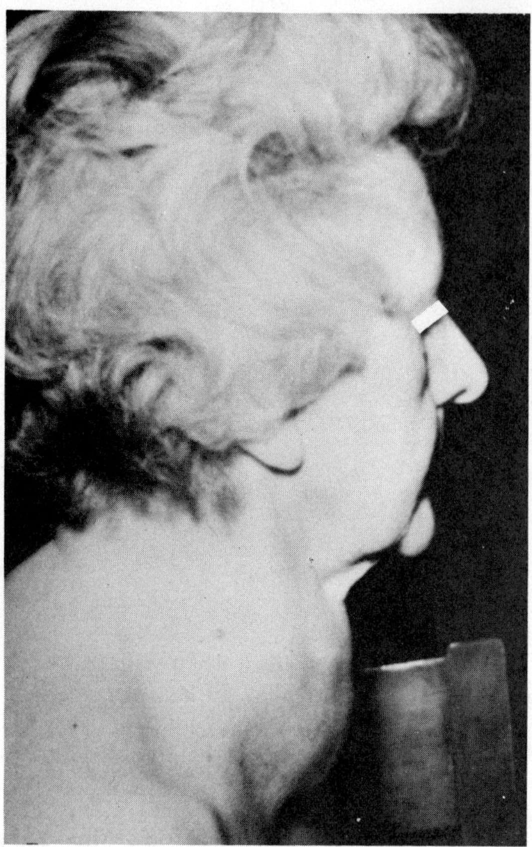

FIGURE 75–3 Large nontoxic multinodular goiter. (Werner SC, Ingbar SH: The Thyroid, 4th ed, p 519. New York, Harper & Row, 1978)

Assessment and Nursing Diagnosis. A knowledge deficit by the general population about the cause and treatment of simple goiter is the prevailing problem nurses must deal with. This problem can be of great concern in areas where endemic goiter is particularly prevalent. In addition, nurses must help the patient cope with altered body image that may occur in response to the disfiguring nature of the disease.

Goals. Primary nursing goals are aimed at public education, particularly in endemic areas, about the prevention of goiter. Additional goals include facilitating proper use and understanding of prescribed antithyroid medications and promoting a positive self-image despite the presence of a disfiguring goiter.

Interventions. Individuals at risk for developing simple goiter should be advised to avoid goitrogenic foods that were discussed previously under Etiology. Instructions need to be given about the most economical way to supply the minimum daily iodine requirements (150 mcg to 300 mcg) to prevent goiter.[3] Foods high in iodine include shellfish, seaweed, and iodized salt. The nurse should provide sensitive emotional support because the patient's self-concept may be disturbed. Maintaining a positive, open environment conducive to expression of feelings is desired. The nurse can explore realistic strengths and resources with the patient to divert intense focusing on the unattractive goiter. If surgical intervention is not appropriate or if the goiter is unresponsive to therapy, the patient may be shown creative ways to camouflage or direct attention away from the goiter, such as the use of scarfs, high collars, long pendants, and attractive facial makeup.

Evaluation of Goal Achievement. Ideally, a decline in the incidence of simple goiter will be seen. Yet, this goal may be a long time in attaining. Although preventive medicine in this country has accelerated over the past decade, major gaps in public health education still exist. The incidence of endemic goiter has declined, yet preventable cases continue to persist. It is also hoped that the patient will maintain a healthy body image as demonstrated by active participation in role-related activities and positive self-esteem.

Thyroiditis

Thyroiditis is primarily characterized by inflammation, enlargement, and dysfunction of the thyroid gland. Etiology can be quite varied, yet two important types are generally recognized: chronic and subacute thyroiditis.

Chronic Thyroiditis. Chronic thyroiditis is most commonly associated with an autoimmune process in which the body produces antibodies in defensive response to perceived thyroid tissue antigens. There is marked lymphocytic infiltration of thyroid tissue (*Hashimoto's thyroiditis*). Goiter is an important feature of the disease, involving the entire gland. Typically the thyroid feels soft and "rubbery" on palpation, and the enlargement may not always be symmetrical. Despite this enlargement, no thyroid bruit can be auscultated. As the disease progresses and the thyroid parenchyma is replaced more and more by lymphocytes and fibrous tissue, symptoms of hypothyroidism become more apparent.[2,4] Hashimoto's thyroiditis is frequently found in conjunction with other autoimmune disorders, pernicious anemia, lupus erythematosus, rheumatoid arthritis, Addison's disease, and even Graves' disease itself. It is usually found in women between the ages 30 and 50, but it may also occur in young children. Except for the sensation of localized compression on neck structures, the disorder itself is usually asymptomatic. As the thyroid tissue becomes progressively nonfunctional, idiopathic myxedema can occur. Treatment focuses primarily on replacing thyroid hormone, as required, and is usually sufficient to reduce thyroid size and relieve symptoms of hypothyroidism.[23]

Subacute Thyroiditis. Subacute thyroiditis (de Quervain's thyroiditis, granulomatous thyroiditis) is an inflammatory condition that causes painful enlargement of the thyroid gland. It frequently occurs several weeks after a viral infection, such as an upper respiratory infection, mumps, and coxsackievirus or adenovirus infection. However, the viral connection has not been proven. The patient typically presents with thyroid gland enlargement and tenderness. Pain may radiate to the ears. Fever, malaise, and signs of hyperthyroidism are commonly observed. Leukocytosis, elevated sedimentation rate, and high serum T_4 levels are usually seen early in the course of the thyroiditis. After 2 to 4 weeks, transient periods of hypothyroidism with decreased serum T_4 and ^{131}I uptake levels occur. Recovery takes approximately 2 to 4 months or more.[13]

Subacute thyroiditis is a rather benign disorder and is usually treated symptomatically with success. Aspirin or acetaminophen, for fever and discomfort, usually suffices. In severe cases, glucocorticoids (such as prednisone) may be used for their steroidal anti-inflammatory effects. Acute pyogenic thyroditis, a rare disorder caused by a bacterial infection, should be suspected if there is little response to steroid therapy. In this case, antibiotics should be administered.[2]

Nursing Management Plan

Nursing care is usually directed toward support of medical management and focuses on the general needs of the patient with an infectious process.

Assessment and Nursing Diagnosis. Patient problems related to thyroiditis include alterations in comfort due to the painful inflammatory process and elevated temperature and a potential diversional activity deficit related to the monotony of confinement during the recovery period.

Goals. Selected nursing interventions will provide appropriate external stimuli to prevent boredom and promote the general comfort of the patient.

Interventions. The patient should be instructed on the proper use of mild analgesics and antipyretics to relieve fever and discomfort. Providing appropriate diversional activity not only allays boredom but may help promote patient comfort. With the patient's assistance the nurse can create a cheerful, pleasant environment (*e.g.,* well-lighted and flowers) with plenty of reading materials and conversational pieces. The patient should be encouraged to wear street clothes during the day if feasible and participate in appropriate quiet activities (*e.g.,* drawing, knitting, reading, and writing). The television should not be the only source of diversional activity. Clearly informing the patient about the nature of his illness and its treatment may aid the patient in tolerating his activity restrictions.

Evaluation of Goal Achievement. It is hoped, with successful interventions, that the patient will relate improvement in level of comfort and successfully engage in diversional activity.

Thyroid Neoplasm

Perhaps one of the commonest abnormalities of the thyroid gland is the development of a nodule, a localized area of enlargement. Approximately 90% of these nodules are either benign adenomas or cysts. The remaining nodules are carcinomatous lesions of varying malignancy. True adenomas are single, encapsulated nodules, most of which are hypofunctional, but some may function autonomously to produce thyroid hormone.[2] When radioisotope scanning is done, using either pertechnetate or ^{131}I, accumulation of the isotope within the nodule can make the nodule appear as "hot" or "cold" (Figure 75–4). The hot nodule accumulates greater amounts of isotope than the surrounding tissue. Thyroid hormone may or may not be produced in excess by the adenoma. Nevertheless, these nodules are almost always benign. Several may, however, go through degenerative changes and become "cold" nodules. Less radioactive isotope is taken up by the cold nodule on a thyroid scan. Although cold nodules have a higher tendency toward malig-

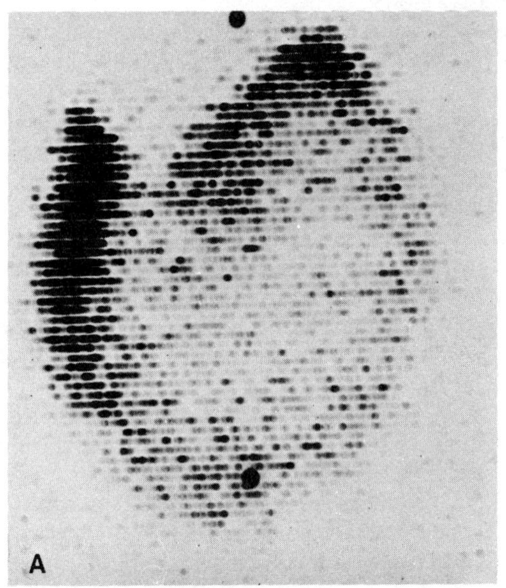

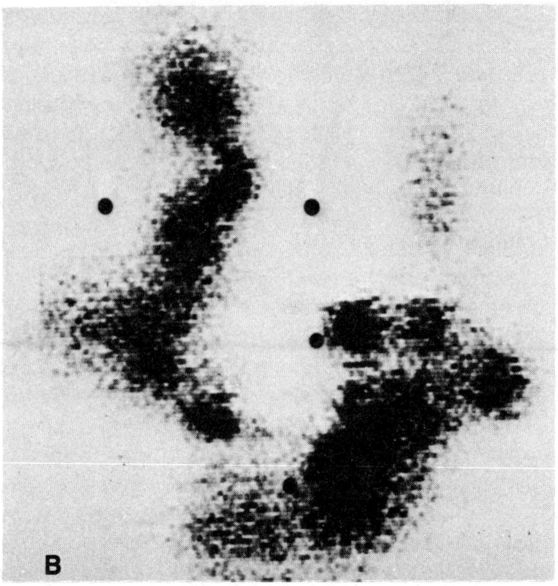

FIGURE 75–4 Thyroid scans showing "cold" nonfunctioning nodule (*A*) and a "hot spot" functioning nodule (*B*). (Werner SC, Ingbar SH: The Thyroid, 4th ed, pp 307, 314. New York, Harper & Row, 1978)

nancy, it should be remembered that 90% of such lesions are still benign. Often needle biopsy of the nodule along with ultrasound (sonography) are done to determine if a malignancy does exist.[13] If the nodules are benign, conservative treatment, if any, is preferred. If the patient shows signs of hyperthyroidism, radioactive iodide therapy is prescribed. Surgery is indicated only when other therapeutic measures fail.

Etiology. Carcinoma of the thyroid gland is exceedingly rare, usually affecting middle-aged women. It often is the result of prolonged radiation to the head and neck. The carcinomas encompass a wide spectrum ranging from a rather benign tumor (papillary carcinoma) to a highly malignant, invasive tumor (anaplastic carcinoma); the forms in between include follicular and medullary tumors. They are defined as follows:

1. *Papillary carcinoma,* is a nonencapsulated, slow-growing neoplasm with peak incidence in the third or fourth decade. It accounts for 50% to 80% of all thyroid carcinomas and has the best prognosis of a 90%, 10-year survival rate.
2. *Follicular carcinoma,* is a slow-growing, encapsulated tumor with a tendency toward vascular invasion and metastasis. It accounts for 10% to 15% of thyroid malignancies and has a peak incidence in the fourth and fifth decades of age. Survival rates are similar to those of papillary carcinoma if no metastasis has occurred. Otherwise, there is a 35%, 10-year survival rate.
3. *Medullary carcinoma* reaches peak incidence in the fourth to sixth decades but occurs at any age. It represents 7% of all thyroid carcinomas and may occasionally be associated with a genetic (autosomal dominant trait) predisposition. Ten-year survival rate is 60%, although this drops markedly with metastasis.
4. *Anaplastic thyroid carcinomas* account for 15% of thyroid malignancies in the United States and 50% in Europe. They rarely occur in patients under 35 years of age. This carcinoma is highly invasive and has a very poor prognosis, with death occuring within 6 to 12 months.

Fortunately papillary carcinomas are the most common, constituting 80% to 90% of all thyroid carcinomas.[13]

Clinical Manifestations and Therapy. The clinical manifestations of thyroid malignancies depend on the type of carcinoma, degree of metastases, and the age of the patient, and these factors also determine the mode of therapy to be used. Since papillary tumors often carry an excellent prognosis (80% survival, often 10 years), aggressive treatment need not be necessary.[13] For most thyroid carcinomas, a partial or total thyroidectomy is required together with excision of affected lymph nodes. Should residual tissue remain or a threat of distant metastases exist, ablative therapy using radioactive iodine can be used. These treatment modalities are least effective against anaplastic carcinoma. In these more malignant tumors, irradiation and chemotherapy can be attempted, but success has been only moderate. Anaplastic carcinoma usually kills 75% of its victims within 1 year.

Nursing Management. Nursing care of these patients is the same as that of the patient with a thyroidectomy, as discussed previously. General nursing interventions for patients with cancer can be found in Chapters 11 and 19.

Parathyroid Glands

The parathyroid glands are four, small bean-shaped structures located immediately posterior to the thyroid gland. Parathyroid hormone, sometimes called parathormone, is essential for calcium and phosphate homeostasis. Two major disorders of the parathyroids can occur, resulting from hyperfunction or hypofunction of these glands.

Hyperfunction of the Parathyroid Glands: Hyperparathyroidism

Etiology and Pathophysiology

Hypoparathyroidism is a syndrome caused by chronic hypersecretion of parathyroid hormone (PTH) by one or more of the four glands. The disorder can occur as *primary* or *secondary* hyperparathyroidism.

Primary hyperparathyroidism is a common disorder that arises within the gland itself. It is accompanied by parathyroid gland enlargement and increased secretion of PTH. Solitary adenomas account for 90% of primary hyperparathyroidism.[13] Other causes include multiple adenomas, carcinoma, and hyperplasia of all four parathyroid glands. It may also occur in the syndrome of multiple endocrine neoplasms (MEN) Type I (Werner's syndrome) or MEN Type II (Sipple's syndrome) (see Chap. 77). Occasionally this disorder can be attributed to neck and thyroid irradiation therapy given several decades previously. Primary hyperparathyroidism is more commonly found in the third to fifth decade of life, but it can be found in children. It is also two to three times more common in women than men.[1]

Hyperfunction of the parathyroid glands stimulates the mobilization of ionized calcium within the body. The kidney increases the rate of calcium resorption from the glomerular filtrate, with resulting augmentation of renal clearance of phosphate. Despite the decreasd calcim clearance, there is hypercalciuria because of the presence of marked hypercalcemia.[9] Also calcium is resorbed from the bone at an accelerated rate. In the presence of normal vitamin D levels, additional calcium is transferred from the intestinal lumen (in the duodenum and proximal jejunum) to the intestinal wall cell and into the plasma. The end result is a marked elevation in serum calcium[25] (see Fig. 75–5).

Secondary hyperparathyroidism is precipitated by low serum levels of ionized calcium in individuals with normal functioning parathyroid glands. To compensate for low circulating calcium levels, PTH production and secretion are increased. Parathyroid hyperplasia develops. There also appears to be some underlying resistance to the metabolic

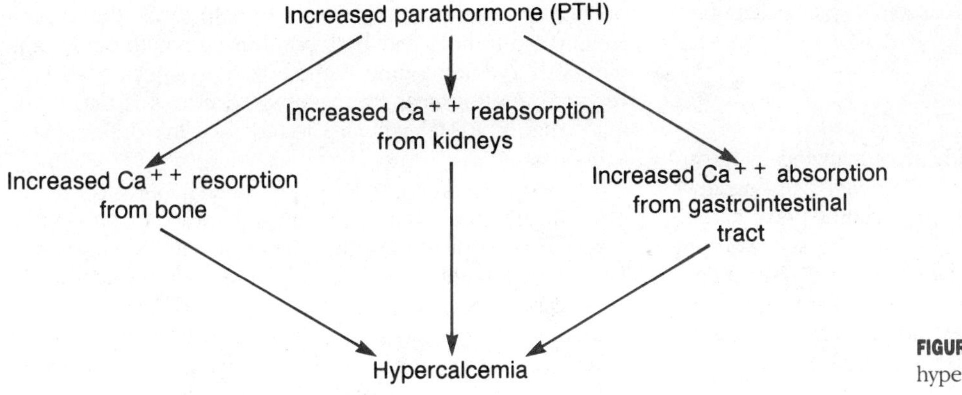

FIGURE 75–5 Primary hyperparathyroidism.

actions of PTH. Although the exact mechanism is not known, conditions that produce mild hypocalcemia (thus precipitating hyperparathyroidism) include rickets, certain forms of osteomalacia, vitamin D deficiency, calcium deprivation, chronic renal failure, steatorrhea, and pseudohyperparathyroidism.[13] Secondary hyperparathyroidism usually does not result in hypercalcemia because normal feedback control mechanisms remain intact and regulate hormone secretions. No serious clinical consequences occur except in chronic renal failure.

Clinical Manifestations

The clinical effects of primary hyperparathyroidism result from high circulating levels of ionized calcium and low serum phosphate levels. It presents several different faces and is often difficult to diagnose. About one third of the patients are asymptomatic. In patients who are symptomatic, clinical manifestations are usually vague and found in various body systems, most importantly the neuromuscular, skeletal, and renal systems.[14]

Renal Signs. Recurring kidney stones (*nephrolithiasis*), which may lead to renal insufficiency, are the most consistent finding of primary hyperparathyroidism. The formation of renal calculi is precipitated by the high calcium and phosphate content of the urine. Along with kidney stones, the patient experiences renal colic (pain), recurrent urinary tract infections, and polyuria. The polyuria is secondary to the kidney's decreased ability to concentrate urine.

Musculoskeletal Signs. Chronic *low back pain, bone tenderness, bone deformities* and *pathological fractures* due to generalized bone demineralization and osteoporosis may occur as calcium is reabsorbed in excessive amounts from the skeletal system. The areas of resorption are replaced by characteristic cysts, tumors, and areas of osteitis fibrosa. Other findings may include pseudogout, synovitis, spinal kyphosis, osteoclastic bone tumors, and loss of the laminal dura that surrounds the teeth.[11] Superperiosteal resorption found in the phalanges, long bones, pelvis, and the lateral ends of clavicles, along with the "salt and pepper" appearance of the skull, are the most specific radiographic bone changes observed.[13]

Marked *proximal muscle weakness and atrophy* are clinical features of the disease, and are due to a decrease in muscle contractility. High serum calcium levels greatly elevate the resting membrane potential of muscle cells, thereby decreasing excitability of nerve and muscle cell membranes. There is general muscle atony, reflexes are depressed or absent, and there is a lack of coordination. The patient complains of easy fatigability and experiences difficulty in negotiating stairs. In some individuals, abnormal fasciculations are noted on the tongue.

Neurological Effects. *Mild to severe psychomotor* or *behavioral disturbances* may be observed. Disorientation, confusion, memory loss, even frank psychosis with paranoia and hallucinations may occur. More often general malaise, lethargy, and drowsiness are experienced, but they can progress into stupor and coma in cases of severe hypercalcemia.[14]

Gastrointestinal Symptoms. Hyperparathyroidism is often associated with mild *gastrointestinal symptoms.* Nausea, vomiting, and anorexia are often seen with accompanying weight loss. Peptic ulcers may form because of the stimulatory effects of PTH on gastric secretion. There also seems to be a strong association with acute pancreatitis since both diseases appear together with some frequency.[13] The reasons for this are not entirely known. If the pancreatitis is severe enough it can induce hypoglycemia and epigastric pain. Unrelated problems, such as constipation and vague abdominal discomfort, may also be experienced.

Cardiovascular Manifestations. Occasional electrocardiographic changes include flattened or inverted P waves, alcoved S-T segments, widened T waves, and shortened Q-T intervals. Bradycardia with bursts of tachycardia and atrioventricular block may also ensue. Calcification of arteries can infrequently lead to high blood pressure and heart disease. Patients become extremely sensitive to the effects of digitalis.[16]

Other Signs. Calcification of the cornea of the eye (band keratopathy), a severe occipital headache, decreased auditory acuity, and pruritus of the skin are less common features of this disorder. Their presence is related to high serum calcium and low serum phosphate levels.[2] Metabolic acidosis due to impaired renal reabsorption of sodium bicarbonate, which often parallels increased phosphate clearance, may also be present.

Diagnostic Evaluation

High serum PTH levels, with accompanying hypercalcemia, are characteristic findings in primary hyperparathyroidism. Elevations in serum chloride, alkaline phosphatase, uric acid, and creatinine levels may also be seen. Serum phosphorus levels are typically decreased. In secondary hyperparathyroidism serum calcium levels are normal or slightly decreased and serum phosphorus levels are variable.

It should be noted that hyperparathyroidism is difficult to diagnose because symptoms are often vague or absent. There are also many causes for hypercalcemia (see Table 75–7). The diagnosis, therefore, is one of exclusion, ruling out other potential problems. Positive findings on physical examination in addition to hypercalcemia and elevated serum PTH levels usually confirm the diagnosis.[16]

Medical Management

Treatment is aimed at the underlying cause and at alleviating symptoms. It is often dictated by the nature of the disorder and the severity of hypercalcemia. Surgical removal of the parathyroid tumor, in the case of adenomas or carcinomas, is often required. Hyperplasia of the parathyroid glands may necessitate removal of all but one half of one gland. A portion of parathyroid gland must be left to supply sufficient amounts of PTH. Many symptoms of the disease disappear within days after surgery. Serum calcium usually returns to normal within 24 hours. The surgical procedure itself can be a difficult one. Sometimes ectopic tumors lie within the mediastinum, thymus, pericardial sac, or carotid artery, requiring thoracotomy and sternal splitting.[13] Several preoperative measures can be taken to help locate the tumor. Parathyroid tumors may be located using parathyroid scanning with ^{75}Semethionine. Catheterization of neck veins with venous sampling near the parathyroid glands is also helpful.[27] Higher PTH levels are found in veins draining the adenoma.

If surgery is contraindicated and hypercalcemia is marked, the patient can be managed with oral phosphate supplements (phosphosoda, Hyperphos-K, Neutra-Phos). These supplements can effectively lower serum calcium levels and prevent formation of kidney stone.[13] Symptomatic treatment of hypercalcemia may also be necessary. In these instances, rapid volume replacement with normal saline is often indicated to reexpand circulating blood volume that may have been reduced by polyuria. This intervention also promotes excretion of urinary calcium and discourages the formation of kidney stones. Diuretics, such as furosemide (Lasix) and ethacrynic acid, are prescribed to minimize renal tubular reabsorption of calcium. Thiazides, however, *should not* be used because they promote calcium retention within the kidney and can severely worsen the problem. Mithramycin, an antibiotic, inhibits bone resorption by decreasing osteoclastic activity and is often used successfully to lower serum calcium levels. Calcitonin, a hormone produced by the parafollicular cells of the thyroid, also inhibits bone resorption and promotes renal excretion of calcium. Its short half-life and tendency toward refractoriness make it more suitable for adjunct rather than frontline therapy.[9] See Table 75–8 for a summary of the medical management of hyperparathyroidism.

Appropriate therapy is directed to other, poorly tolerated manifestations of this disease, such as behavioral abnormalities, gastrointestinal disturbances, and musculoskeletal discomfort. Untreated, hyperparathyroidism with severe hypercalcemia can progress to renal failure and ultimately death.

TABLE 75–7
Causes of Hypercalcemia

Increased calcium resorption from bone:
Primary hyperparathyroidism
Malignancy with or without bone metastases
Ectopic PTH secretion
Production of vitamin D-like substance
Leukemia, lymphomas, and multiple myeloma
Prolonged immobility
Vitamin A intoxication
Hyperthyroidism
Increased calcium resorption by renal tubules:
Thiazide diuretics
Renal disease
Polyuric phase of acute renal failure
Increased gastrointestinal calcium absorption:
Vitamin D intoxication
Sarcoidosis
Tuberculosis
Other:
Adrenal insufficiency
Milk-alkali syndrome
Chronic renal dialysis

Nursing Management Plan

When surgery is not performed, nursing interventions are aimed at decreasing serum calcium levels and minimizing potential complications of the disease. Common problems in the patient with hyperparathyroidism include potential alteration in urinary elimination related to renal stones; potential gastrointestinal disturbances related to peptic ulcer formation; activity intolerance related to weakness and fatigue; potential alteration in cardiac output and function related to arrhythmias and hemodynamic changes; potential injury related to falls and pathological fractures; and ineffective coping related to an altered body image. The nursing goals, interventions, and outcome criteria for each of these nursing diagnoses are presented in Nursing Care Plan for the Patient with Hyperparathyroidism.

Nursing Care of the Patient Following Surgical Removal of the Parathyroids

When surgery is performed, postoperative care is similar to that for the patient with a thyroidectomy. Close monitoring of the patient's vital signs and volume status is required; the patient may be in danger of overhydration during

TABLE 75–8
Medical Management of Hyperparathyroidism with Hypercalcemic Crisis

Drug	*Dose*
Acute Stage (24 hr or less)	
Normal saline	2 liters over 3 hr (if dehydration severe), followed by infusion of 150–300 ml/hr
Furosemide (Lasix)	Up to 3.2 g over 48 hr
Phosphate (In-Phos or Hyper-Phos)	1.5 g IV over 6–8 hr
Renal dialysis	Use calcium-free dialysate.
Ethylenediaminotetracetate (EDTA)	Infuse in normal saline, not more than 3 g in 24 hr
Intermediate Stage (1–7 days)	
Mithramycin	15–25 μg/kg IV, push or infusion. Repeat dose in 72 hr
Calcitonin (Calcimar)	4 U/kg IM every 12 hr
Prednisone	40–60 mg/day

(Adapted from Lukert BP: Hypercalcemia. Critical Care Quarterly 3:11–18, 1980)

the first few days. A tracheostomy set is kept at the patient's bedside for use should incisional hemorrhage or edema cause obstruction of the airway. As with the patient with a thyroidectomy, a semi-Fowler's position is recommended along with cautious head and neck movement and sandbag support. This will help decrease the edema and thus minimize risk of tracheal pressure. Assessing the degree of respiratory distress and watching for swelling at the operative site and alterations in mentation are important nursing interventions.

Transient, but sometimes profound, hypocalcemia may follow surgery as calcium is presumably sucked up into "hungry bones," causing a marked lowering of serum calcium levels.[13] Monitoring laboratory data for low serum calcium and low serum magnesium can alert the nurse to these potential postoperative problems. Ongoing monitoring of serum potassium and sodium values is also indicated, since treatment may adversely affect their levels. Early signs of resulting tetany include complaints of tingling in the hands and around the mouth. These symptoms may subside or progress to severe neuromuscular irritability with convulsions. Early manifestations should be reported immediately and calcium chloride IV should be made available for emergency administration.

Early in the postoperative course, ambulation is encouraged. The patient may find the exertion uncomfortable but it provides sufficient bone stress to speed up bone recalcification.[9]

Hypofunction of the Parathyroid Glands: Hypoparathyroidism

Etiology and Pathophysiology

Hypoparathyroidism is a syndrome characterized by a deficiency of PTH secretion and a subsequent lowering of serum calcium. Probably the most common cause of this disorder is surgical removal of or trauma to the parathyroid glands or their vascular supply (*acquired hypoparathyroidism*).[1] Acquired hypoparathyroidism can also result, although more rarely, from thyroid irradiation or infiltrative diseases of the parathyroid glands, such as neoplasms, sarcoidosis, hemochromocytosis, amyloidosis, and tuberculosis. *Idiopathic hypoparathyroidism* is generally attributed to an autoimmune process similar to Hashimoto's thyroiditis. This particular disease entity is usually detected in childhood. Less commonly, a congenital absence of the parathyroids and thymus can occur (DiGeorge syndrome).[13] There is a transient and reversible form of hypoparathyroidism induced by low serum levels of magnesium. In all these forms, PTH secretion is decreased. As a result there is a disruption of calcium and phosphorus metabolism. More calcium is lost through the gastrointestinal and renal systems, and bone resorption decreases. Because there is an inverse relationship between calcium and phosphorus, the circulating levels of the latter increase.[2]

Pseudohypoparathyroidism. There is a rare, genetic disorder known as pseudohypoparathyroidism. Although it demonstrates the clinical manifestations of hypoparathyroidism, it is characterized by an *increase* in PTH secretion with hyperplasia of the parathyroid glands. The problem in this disorder is not with PTH secretion but with end-organ response. The kidney and bone somehow become resistant to the normal effects of PTH. Thus the high circulating levels of PTH have little impact and low serum calcium levels are the result. The pathophysiology of this disorder remains unknown.[13]

Clinical Manifestations

Mild hypoparathyroidism is usually asymptomatic, but when present, the symptoms most often reflect altered neuromuscular irritability due to lowered serum calcium levels.

(Text continues on page 1083)

NURSING CARE PLAN FOR THE PATIENT WITH HYPERPARATHYROIDISM

NURSING DIAGNOSIS/PROBLEM 1: Potential for alterations in urinary elimination related to renal stones, which may result in hematuria and pain

GOAL 1.1: To prevent and detect early renal stone formation

Nursing Interventions	Rationale	Outcome Criteria
1. Administer a fluid intake of at least 3000 ml/day as tolerated. (Parenteral fluids may be necessary if the patient is unable to ingest more than 2500 ml of fluid orally a day.)	1. Approximately 90% of renal stones contain calcium or magnesium in combination with phosphate or oxalate. Hyperparathyroidism causes high urinary calcium levels, which promote the formation of stones. A dilute urine reduces the concentration of urinary crystalloids and minimizes the risk of stone formation.[1] Therefore, a large fluid intake is encouraged.	1–4, 6–7. Absence of renal stone as evidenced by no complaints (renal colic), hematuria, nausea, chills, and fever. Patient will adopt behaviors aimed at reducing risk of renal stone formation, such as increased fluid intake and ingestion of a diet high in acid ash content and low in calcium content. Patient will demonstrate appropriate skill in straining own urines.
2. Strain all urine through gauze mesh and instruct the patient in this procedure.	2. The majority of stones are small enough to be passed by the patient. These stones should be analyzed for composition, which helps in determining appropriate therapy. The procedure for urine straining is discussed in Chapter 61.	
3. Administer drugs for acidifying urine and increase patient's dietary intake of foods and liquids high in acid ash.	3. Renal stones composed of calcium oxalate or calcium phosphate are formed in alkaline urine. Food high in acid ash content and drugs such as ascorbic acid (vitamin C) and methenamine mandelate (Mandelamine) create an acidic urine, thus decreasing the likelihood of stone formation.[1] (See Chapter 73 for specifics of dietary management.)	
4. Decrease ingestion of foods and substances high in calcium content and avoid excessive intake of Vitamin D.	4. A high calcium ingestion may further aggravate the problem, increasing the formation of renal stones. Foods high in calcium content include dairy products. Some antacid preparations, particularly Tums, contain large amounts of calcium and should be avoided. Vitamin D increases the stimulation of parathyroid hormone.	
5. Monitor for signs of renal stones (flank pain, hematuria, nausea, vomiting and chills).	5. Stones may occlude the opening to a ureter, resulting in an increase in the force of ureteral peristaltic contractions, which can produce flank pain with possible radiation into the groin and genitalia with accompanying signs of hematuria, nausea, chills, and fever.	5. Signs of renal stones detected at onset.

(Continued)

NURSING CARE PLAN FOR THE PATIENT WITH HYPERPARATHYROIDISM (*Continued*)

Nursing Interventions	Rationale
6. Monitor urinary output.	6. Hypercalcemia and resulting hypercalciuria interferes with the concentrating ability of the kidneys and can result in polyuria with eventual risk of dehydration.
7. Monitor urine pH.	7. Renal stones resulting from hypercalciuria are more likely to develop in alkaline urine. A urinary pH of 5 or less is desired to decrease the risk of renal stone formation.[1]

NURSING DIAGNOSIS/PROBLEM 2: Potential gastrointestinal disturbances secondary to hyperparathyroidism, resulting in peptic ulcer formation and anorexia

GOAL 2.1: To prevent or detect early peptic ulcer formation

Nursing Interventions	Rationale	Outcome Criteria
1. Monitor patient for complaints of heartburn or epigastric pain.	1. Parathyroid hormone has a stimulatory effect on gastric secretions that can greatly potentiate the risk of peptic ulcer formation. As erosion of the gastric mucosa occurs, discomfort is felt. It may be sharply localized pain in the epigastric region or be perceived as heartburn.[1]	1–2. Signs of peptic ulcer formation detected at onset
2. Guaiac emesis and stools for blood.	2. A bleeding ulcer may manifest itself as hematemesis (bloody or coffee ground) and black stools. Guaiac materials are often required to determine occult quantities of blood.	
3. Consult physician about prescribed diet and antacids. Instruct patient to avoid caffeine-containing beverages and aspirin-containing drugs, and to eat meals at appropriate times.	3. The patient's symptoms may be relieved with the ingestion of frequent small feedings to neutralize stomach acids. Antacids (low in calcium) may be administered 1 hour after meals and at bedtime. Ingestion of irritating substances should be avoided, such as caffeine beverages and aspirin-containing drugs.	3. The patient will: a. Be free of peptic ulcer symptoms: have no epigastric pain, have no hematemesis, and have guaiac-negative stools. b. Adopt behaviors to minimize peptic ulcer formation or pain. Eat meals at appropriate times; avoid foods and substances that cause pain; use antacids.

GOAL 2.2: To stimulate appetite to promote sufficient nutritional intake to meet metabolic needs

Nursing Interventions	Rationale	Outcome Criteria
1. Monitor daily weight. Refer patient for nutritional assessment if indicated.	1. Weight loss usually accompanies a deficit in protein and caloric intake and is a valuable gauge of nutritional status. Comparisons should be made between the patient's premorbid and ideal body weights. Assessing baseline caloric requirements for the patient may be helpful.	1–2. The patient will: a. Report improved appetite. b. Attain and maintain nutritional balances: attain or maintain desired body weight.

(Continued)

NURSING CARE PLAN FOR THE PATIENT WITH HYPERPARATHYROIDISM (*Continued*)

Nursing Interventions	Rationale
2. Improve psychological desire for food: a. Determine the patient's eating habits, cultural preferences, and allow independence at mealtimes. b. Promote good oral hygiene. c. Provide frequent, appropriately sized meals that are attractively served at the proper temperature.	2. Numerous psychological elements join physiological factors in promoting anorexia: a. Allowing the patient as much input into his food preferences and as much independence at mealtimes as possible may improve his sense of control, minimize frustration, and improve appetite. b. Poor oral hygiene can adversely alter the taste of food. c. Smaller food portions, served attractively, can appear less overwhelming to the patient who lacks the desire yet knows the importance of eating.

NURSING DIAGNOSIS/PROBLEM 3: Decreased activity tolerance related to weakness and fatigue, which may result in apathy and discouragement

GOAL 3.1: To promote improved activity endurance and maintenance of optimal level of physical functioning

Nursing Interventions	Rationale	Outcome Criteria
1. Progress activity gradually: a. Gradually increase activity according to the patient's tolerance (note heart rate and respirations). b. Space activities to allow sufficient rest periods. c. Assist patient with strenuous but necessary activities. d. Encourage ambulation with assistance as necessary.	1. a–d. Muscular weakness results from altered cell membrane potentials, which decrease the excitability of nerve and muscle cells. There is marked proximal muscle weakness and atrophy. Exercise is poorly tolerated (increased heart rate and dyspnea) and must be spaced with sufficient rest periods. Gradual active muscle use can improve muscle tone and stamina.	1–2. An observable increase in physical strength and stamina
2. Provide incentive for patient involvement in activity. a. Allow patient to set functional activity goals. b. Promote a sincere "can do" attitude regarding the patient's mobility status.	2. Fatigue often brings discouragement and apathy. a. Encouraging the patient to actively participate in goal-setting promotes a sense of control and potentiates goal attainment. b. Providing a positive environment conveys to the patient the belief that he can improve his level of functioning, thereby promoting achievement.	

(*Continued*)

NURSING CARE PLAN FOR THE PATIENT WITH HYPERPARATHYROIDISM (*Continued*)

NURSING DIAGNOSIS/PROBLEM 4: Potential for altered cardiovascular performance secondary to hypercalcemia, which may result in cardiac arrhythmais and hemodynamic changes

GOAL 4.1: To prevent or detect early cardiovascular changes related to hypercalcemia

Nursing Interventions	Rationale	Outcome Criteria
1. Monitor blood pressure and pulse routinely. Instruct patient to promptly report episodes of palpitations or vertigo.	1. A normal calcium balance is essential for proper electrical and mechanical functioning of the heart. Hypercalcemia can predispose the patient to bradycardia with bursts of tachycardia. During these episodes, blood pressure may fall creating symptoms of vertigo and syncope. Infrequently, calcification of arteries may result in chronic hypertension.	1–2. Blood pressure and pulse will remain within the patient's normal limits. The patient will promptly report to the nurse or physician any episodes of palpitations or vertigo.
2. Administer digitalis preparations with extreme caution.	2. Hypercalcemia increases the sensitivity of the myocardium to digitalis, thus potentiating digitalis toxicity.	

NURSING DIAGNOSIS/PROBLEM 5: Potential for accidental injury related to generalized bone demineralization and weakness, which may result in pathological fractures and falls

GOAL 5.1: To prevent incidence of accidental injury related to falls and pathological fractures

Nursing Interventions	Rationale	Outcome Criteria
1. Provide a safe environment a. Position furniture as necessary and remove unnecessary equipment and small throw rugs. b. Patient should wear nonskid slippers. c. Assist with ambulation as necessary.	1. a–c. Individuals who are unsteady because of weakness are more likely to trip over obstacles. Parathyroid hormone stimulates the release of calcium from bones, which leads to demineralized and osteoporotic bones. Such bones are prone to pathological fractures with resultant falls. Assisting the patient as necessary and clearing the environment of potential hazards can minimize the risk of falls.	1–4. No incidence of accidental injury related to falls. The patient will: a. Identify factors that increase the potential for injury. b. Use safety measures to prevent injury.
2. Confer with patient and family about the home environment, identifying potential hazards and safety precautions.	2. Early problem solving about potential home environmental hazards can help prevent injury and facilitate the patient's mobility after discharge.	
3. Encourage gradual activity as tolerated to include isometric exercises and moderate weight bearing.	3. Active exercise can improve muscle tone and endurance while some degree of bone stress is necessary to encourage calcium resorption into bones.	

(*Continued*)

NURSING CARE PLAN FOR THE PATIENT WITH HYPERPARATHYROIDISM (*Continued*)

Nursing Interventions	Rationale
4. Instruct patient to avoid lifting and carrying heavy objects or from frequent bending.	4. Strenuous lifting and bending may potentiate compression fractures of the spine because of generalized demineralization of the vertebral bodies.[3]

NURSING DIAGNOSIS/PROBLEM 6: Altered body image related to various physical changes, which may result in feelings of lowered self-esteem, depression, anger, and social withdrawal

GOAL 6.1: To promote self-confidence and to assist with reconstruction of altered body image

Nursing Interventions	Rationale	Outcome Criteria
1. Provide an environment conducive for self-expression.	1. Body image is a mental concept a person has about himself, and it is intimately linked with his subjective judgment of his physical and social competence.[5] The numerous physical changes caused by hyperparathyroidism can be emotionally devastating. The nurse can provide important support during times of extreme intrapersonal vulnerability.	1–4. The patient will demonstrate improved self-concept as evidenced by his: a. Ability to make positive statements about his appearance or abilities. b. Resumption of role-related responsibilities.
a. Respect the patient's wishes for privacy.	a. Intrusive procedures and behaviors can threaten an individual's sense of wholeness.	
b. Maintain an open, positive, and accepting attitude toward the patient.	b. A closed, negative attitude can threaten the patient's adaptation to physical changes and jeopardize trust in, and success of, therapeutic interventions.	
c. Refer patient for psychological counseling as necessary.	c. To promote successful adaptive behaviors, long-term therapy may be necessary to explore with the patient his attitudes, values, and usual coping styles.	
2. Assist the patient in identifying personal strengths, coping resources, and supper persons.	2. In helping the patient to identify sources of support, he is more likely to utilize them. Identifying realistic strengths may help minimize exaggeration of perceived failures.	
3. Clarify any misconceptions the patient may have about himself, his care, or his care-givers.	3. A maladaptive response by a patient to altered body image may include an inaccurate perception of his own abilities and the benefits of treatment.	
4. Include family members or close friends in planning emotional support.	4. Family members also may go through a grieving process related to changes in the patient's physical and emotional changes. These feelings should be explored and allowed expression. The family must be able to provide sound support for the patient who may have a long-term coping deficit.	

Acute Hypocalcemic Tetany. Acute hypocalcemic tetany starts with numbness and tingling of the fingers, toes, and around the lips. Laryngospasm, causing respiratory distress with stridor (a crowing sound), may follow and is a serious finding because it can progress to cyanosis and respiratory arrest.[1] A feeling of constriction in the throat with painful spasms of the smooth and skeletal muscles and dysphagia are typical in tetany. Cramps in individual muscle groups in the legs and feet may cause acute pain and difficulty in walking. *Trousseau's sign* is carpopedal spasm caused by ischemia of the arm when compression is applied to the upper arm. *Chvostek's sign* is facial muscle spasm elicited by tapping on the facial muscles or branches of the facial nerve. Chronic tetany is typically unilateral. All forms of tetany can lead to partial or grand mal seizures. These signs of tetany usually accompany a lowering of ionized calcium levels in the serum to approximately 30% below normal. The neuromuscular irritability relates to a decrease in resting membrane potential and to increased excitability of muscle and nerve cells.[9]

Mental Abnormalities. Sometimes mental abnormalities will occur. Irritability, confusion, depression, anxiety, memory impairment, emotional lability, and frank psychosis have been observed. These signs may be related to calcification of various parts of the nervous system. Complaints of headaches and general fatigue are not uncommon. Papillary edema from intracranial pressure may develop, because fluid retention may occur.[13]

Cardiovascular Effects. Low serum calcium levels can markedly alter the mechanical and electrophysiological behavior of the heart. Decreased myocardial contractility often accompanies a decrease in cardiac output. Electrocardiographic changes include longer QRS and Q-T intervals.[9] Patients with hypoparathyroid neuromuscular irritability become very insensitive to the effects of digitalis.

Integumentary Changes. Integumentary changes occur chiefly in young patients with idiopathic hypoparathyroidism and include dry, lackluster, and pluckable hair and patchy alopecia. The skin appears dry and scaly. Fingernails become brittle, malformed, and have transverse grooves. Skin infections, usually moniliasis, are frequent.

Teeth and Eye Changes. A characteristic feature of hypoparathyroidism in early life is weakening of the tooth enamel and blunting of the tooth roots, which causes the teeth to stain, crack, and decay easily. Eyes often develop cataracts.[2]

Pseudohypoparathyroidism. Signs and symptoms of pseudohypoparathyroidism are the same as those described for hypoparathyroidism, but it additionally has some unique characteristics. The patient demonstrates some degree of mental retardation, along with a short, stocky and obese stature and a round face. The hands and feet are also disproportionately small because of the shortening of one or more metacarpal or metatarsal bones. This shortening is readily recognized by having the patient clench his fist. A dimple will appear over the head of the affected bone.[7]

All patients with hypoparathyroidism exhibit decreased serum PTH levels along with hypocalcemia, and 70% have increased urinary calcium levels. Serum phosphorus levels are usually greatly elevated. Pseudohypoparathyroidism differs only in that PTH levels are elevated.

Medical Management

The aims of treatment are (1) to prevent hypocalcemic tetany and (2) to minimize the side-effects and complications of the disorder. *Acute tetany* requires intravenous administration of calcium gluconate, calcium gluceptate, or calcium chloride to raise serum calcium levels. Calcium chloride is particuarly irritating and may cause tissue necrosis if infiltrated into the surrounding tissue. All intravenous calcium preparations are best diluted in 100 ml of 5% dextrose in water and infused for 10 to 15 minutes. Airway management is of immediate concern should convulsions occur. Muscle relaxants (*e.g.,* diazepam) can also be given to decrease neuromuscular irritability. Tetany can be prevented by oral calcium replacement. A daily intake of 1 g to 2 g of calcium by diet or supplementation is necessary. In addition, vitamin D supplements are given to enhance calcium absorption within the gastrointestinal tract. The doses of calcium and vitamin D should be gradually reduced as serum calcium levels return to normal. Lifelong calcium replacement is usually required in all irreversible forms of hypoparathyroidism. The patient is also instructed to eat a diet low in phosphate and high in bulk. Aluminum hydroxide (Amphojel, Basaljel) can be taken initially to lower serum phosphate levels.[9]

Nursing Management Plan

Nursing care of the hypoparathyroid patient is essentially the same as that given to the individual following surgical removal of the parathyroid glands, which was discussed earlier in this chapter.

Assessment and Nursing Diagnosis. The major problem the patient must face and the nurse must consider are those related to low serum calcium. Most important are the potential alteration in effective airway and potential self-injury related to tetanic seizures. Another nursing diagnosis is knowledge deficit of both patient and family regarding long-term management of hypoparathyroidism that is essential in promoting disease control.

Goals. The goals of nursing interventions are aimed at promoting an adequate airway and minimizing both the risk of tetanic seizures and the risk of bodily injury should seizures occur. A more long-term goal involves facilitating patient understanding of prescribed therapy and promoting control of the disease process.

Interventions. The patient with hypoparathyroidism requires close observation for manifestations of hypocalcemia and tetany. Signs of low serum calcium have already been discussed in this chapter. The patient should be instructed to watch for any paresthesias, such as numbness and tingling of the extremities or minor muscle twitching, and report these symptoms at once. In acutely hypocalcemic patients, seizure precautions should be maintained. Precautions against seizure include padded side rails, an artificial airway (or padded tongue blade), and a warning to the patient not to smoke unattended.

Calcium gluconate should be kept close at hand in the event of acute tetany. All calcium preparations are best given slowly to minimize sudden high levels of serum calcium. High serum calcium levels precipitate potentially lethal cardiac arrhythmias. Digitalized patients are particularly vulnerable. Constant measurements of electrocardiographic and vital signs are recommended. Should calcium chloride be administered, watch for signs of infiltration. Calcium chloride is particularly irritating to tissues and tissue necrosis may ensue. The infiltrated tissues should be diluted with saline infiltration.

In the presence of mild tetany, symptoms can be improved if the patient rebreathes his own exhaled air. To do this the patient is asked to breathe in and out of a paper bag or plastic glove. This maneuver decreases exhaled carbon dioxide, increases blood levels of carbonic acid, and subsequently lowers serum pH. The resulting acidotic environment enhances the solubility and degree of available ionized calcium in the blood.[25] Thus, the physiologically active form of calcium is increased, temporarily minimizing tetany. If the patient cannot cooperate sufficiently in this therapy, the nurse can help by firmly placing a rebreather mask, or glove, over the patient's mouth and pinching close the patient's nose. Several "free" breaths should be allowed intermittently to provide sufficient oxygen intake.

Care of the patient with chronic hypoparathyroidism focuses primarily on his education. The patient and his family should be taught how to plan a diet high in calcium and vitamin D and low in phosphate. Foods rich in calcium include milk and milk products, molasses, and turnip greens. Antacids such as Amphojel, Riopan, and Maalox can be taken before meals to reduce phosphate absorption and raise serum calcium levels.[5] Tums, an over-the-counter antacid, can also increase calcium absorption. Supplementary oral preparations of calcium gluconate or calcium chloride are usually prescribed by the physician.

Intake of vitamin D supplements, in doses ranging from 50,000 to 250,000 units per day, or dihydrotachysterol (a vitamin D compound) may also be encouraged to promote gastrointestinal calcium absorption and calcium to mobilize from the bone. It is also thought to promote phosphate excretion. Dietary sources of vitamin D include fortified milk, fish liver oils, sardines, and egg yolks. Because of the high serum phosphate levels, the patient should be instructed to avoid taking laxatives or enemas high in phosphate. Dry, scaly skin, common in hypoparathyroidism, can be softened with frequent applications of oil-based creams. Harsh soaps should be avoided.[3]

Evaluation of Goal Achievement. Several observations can indicate goal achievement. First there will be maintenance of a patent oral airway and the absence of injury related to seizure activity. Serum calcium will remain within normal limits. The patient will be able to accurately discuss the nature of his illness and the rationale for prescribed therapy. In addition, the patient will increase his dietary intake with foods rich in calcium and vitamin D.

Summary

The role of the nurse in caring for patients with disorders of the thyroid and parathyroid glands is an important one. Concepts of pathophysiology, altered metabolism, and electrolyte imbalances generate a set of specific patient problems and form the basis for related nursing interventions. The nurse must remain ever vigilant for exacerbations of these underlying diseases, whose dramatic presentations include such medical emergencies as acute thyrotoxicosis, myxedema coma, and hypocalcemic tetany. Accurate and ongoing assessment of the patient's physical and emotional status is essential in providing effective acute care and in assisting the patient to cope with long-term management of his disease.

References

1. Arcangelo VP: Disorders of the thyroid and parathyroid. In Diseases: Nurses Reference Library, Nursing 83. Springhouse: Intermed Communications, 1983
2. Beeson PB, McDermott W: Textbook of Medicine. Philadelphia, WB Saunders, 1981
3. Brunner LS, Suddarth DS (eds): The Lippincott Manual of Nursing Practice, 3rd ed. Philadelphia, JB Lippincott, 1982
4. Brown J, Solomon DH, Beall GN et al: Autoimmune thyroid diseases—Graves' and Hashimoto's. Ann Intern Med 88:378–381, 1978
5. Carpenito LJ: Nursing Diagnosis: Application to Clinical Practice. Philadelphia, JB Lippincott, 1983
6. Chernow B (ed): Pharmacologic Approach to the Critically Ill Patient. Baltimore, Williams & Wilkins, 1983
7. DeGroot L et al: Endocrinology, Vol 3. New York, Grune & Stratton, 1979
8. Dillon RG: Handbook of Endocrinology, 2nd ed. Philadelphia, Lea & Febiger, 1980
9. DuRubertis FR: Hypercalcemia and hypocalcemia. Topics in Emergency Medicine 5:64–73, 1984
10. Evangelisti JT, Thorpe CJ: Thyroid storm—a nursing crisis. Heart Lung 12:184–193, 1978
11. Giraud FT: Hypoparathyroidism. In Conn HF et al (eds): Current Diagnosis Six. Philadelphia, WB Saunders, 1980
12. Gorman CA: The presentation and management of endocrine ophthalmopathy. Clin Endocrinol Metabol 7:67–96, 1978
13. Harvey AM, Johns RJ, Owens AH et al (eds): Practice of Medicine, 20th ed. New York, Appleton-Century-Crofts, 1980
14. Heath H, Hodgson SF, Kennedy MA: Primary hyperparathyroidism. N Engl J Med 302(4):189–193, 1980
15. Hellman R: The evaluation and management of hyperthyroid crises. Critical Care Quarterly, 3:77–92, 1980
16. Hoffman JT, Newby TB: Hypercalcemia in primary hyperparathyroidism. Nurs Clin North Am 15:469–480, 1980
17. Jenkins EH: Living with thyrotoxicosis. Am J Nurs 80:956–958, 1980

18. Katz AD, Bronson D: Total thyroidectomy. Am J Surg 136:450–454, 1978
19. Klein IL, Levey GS: Thyroid emergencies: Thyroid storm and myxedema. Topics in Emergency Medicine 5:33–39, 1984
20. Klein IL, Levey GS: Thyroid storm. Hospital Medicine 19:34a–34p, 1982
21. Krueger J, Ray J: Endocrine Problems in Nursing. St Louis, CV Mosby, 1976
22. La Franchi S: Hypothyroidism. Pediatr Clin North Am 26:33–51, 1979
23. Lee WN: Thyroiditis, hyperthyroidism and tumors. Pediatr Clin North Am 26:53–64, 1979
24. Lukert BP: Hypercalcemia. Critical Care Quarterly 3:11–18, 1980
25. McFadden EA, Zaloga GP: Calcium regulation. Critical Care Quarterly 6:12-21, 1983
26. Wake MM, Brensinger JF: The nurse's role in hypothyroidism. Nurs Clin North Am 15:453–467, 1980
27. Williams RH: Textbook of Endocrinology, 6th ed. Philadelphia, WB Saunders, 1980

Bibliography

Ashcraft MW, Van Herle AJ: Management of thyroid nodules, II: Scanning techniques, thyroid suppression and fine needle aspiration. Head Neck Surg 3:216–230, 1981

Beahrs OH: Operative management of hyperparathyroidism. Milit Med 146:98–99, 1981

Coe FL, Fairis MJ: Does mild asymptomatic hyperparathyroidism require surgery? N Engl J Med 302:224–225, 1980

Coulombe P, Dussault J, Walker P: Catecholamine metabolism in thyroid disease. J Clin Endocrinol Metab 44:1185, 1977

Cryer PE: Diagnostic Endocrinology, 2nd ed. New York, Oxford University Press, 1979

Dillion RG: Handbook of Endocrinology, 2nd ed. Philadelphia, Lea & Febiger, 1980

Doresio T: Hypercalcemic crisis. Heart Lung 7:425–434, 1978

Esselstyn CB: Parathyroid surgery. Surg Clin North Am 59:77–81, 1979

Feek CM, Sawers JS, Irvine WJ et al: Combination of postassium iodide and propranolol in preparation of patients with Graves' disease for thyroid surgery. N Engl J Med 302(16):883–885, 1980

Fuller E: Intervening promptly in myxedema coma. Patient Care 18:67–76, 1984

Geola F, Chopra L: Hyperthyroidism and hypothyroidism. Medical Times 108:64–68, 73–74, 1980

Gurmond JH, Wilson SG: Post-irradiation thyroid disorders. Am J Nurs 80:1256–1258, 1980

Hall R: Fundamentals of Clinical Endocrinology, 3rd ed. New York, Year Book Medical Publishers, 1981

Hart IR, Newton RW: Endocrinology, Vol 2. Baltimore, University Park Press, 1983

Hellman R, Kelly K, Mason W: Propranolol for thyroid storm. N Engl J Med 297:671–672, 1977

Hershman JM: Management of Endocrine Disorders. Philadelphia, Lea & Febiger, 1980

Honigman RE: Thyroid function tests. Nursing '82 12:68–71, 1982

Jubiz W: Endocrinology: A Logical Approach for Clinicians. New York, McGraw-Hill, 1979

Mannix H, Pyrtek LJ, Crombie HD et al: Hyperparathyroidism in the elderly. Am J Surg 139:581–585, 1980

Meek JC: Myxedema coma. Critical Care Quarterly 3:131–137, 1980

Muthe NC: Endocrinology: A Nursing Approach. Boston: Little, Brown & Co, 1981

O'Riordan JH: Calcium and the endocrine system. Practitioner 226:237–241, 1982

Roberts JW: Symptomatic hyperparathyroidism. Surg Clin North Am 62:225–228, 1982

Ryan WG: Endocrine Disorders: A Pathologic Approach. Chicago, Year Book Medical Publishers, 1980

Solitary nodule? Is surgery indicated? Patient Care 17:119–153, 1983

Urbanic RC, Mazzaferri EL: Thyrotoxic crisis and myxedema coma. Heart Lung 7:435–447, 1978

Vaitukaitis JL: Current Endocrinology: Basic and Clinical Aspects. New York, Elsevier, 1982

Werner SC, Ingbar SI (eds): The Thyroid. New York, Harper & Row, 1978

White V, Kumagi L: Preoperative endocrine and metabolic considerations. Med Clin North Am 63:1321–1334, 1979

Chapter 76

Disorders of the Adrenal Glands

Christine A. Larson

Each of the paired adrenal glands consists of two unrelated organs, the cortex and the medulla, which, except for their location upon the upper poles of the kidneys, have little in common. Together the cortex and medulla contribute to the body's successful physical and emotional adaptation to changes in the internal and external environment. Only the cortex, however, is essential for life.

This chapter presents separately the dysfunctions of the cortex and medulla. A discussion of their etiology, pathophysiology, clinical manifestations, and disease management is presented for specific disorders.

The adrenal cortex is the body's only source of glucocorticoids and mineralocorticoids, and is a supplementary source of androgens and estrogens. The bodily impact of most of the cortical hormones is essential for survival. Glucocorticoids, of which cortisol is the most important, exert widespread effects on body metabolism and play a major role in the body's coping defenses against internal and external stressors. Mineralocorticoids, particularly aldosterone, are important regulators of fluid and electrolyte imbalance. The androgens have the least physiological impact of all adrenocortical hormones, but they do contribute to the development of secondary sex characteristics.[21] Dysfunction of the adrenal cortex will result in either the elimination or the exaggeration of some or all of the adrenocortical hormone effects.

Hyperfunction of the Adrenal Cortex

Glucocorticoid Excess: Cushing's Syndrome

Etiology and Pathophysiology

The excessive circulation of cortisol, with its resulting characteristic manifestations, is known as Cushing's syndrome. Although it is usually associated with elevated glucocorticoid levels, it may be accompanied by excessive androgen secretion. The etiology of this disorder can fall into one of the following categories:

1. *Primary Cushing's syndrome:* Excessive cortisol secretion due to an intra-adrenal neoplasm (adenoma or carcinoma)
2. *Secondary Cushing's syndrome:* Excessive cortisol secretion resulting from an extra-adrenal abnormality.
   a. *Pituitary-dependent Cushing's syndrome* (Cushing's disease): Adrenal hyperplasia with increased

cortisol secretion, resulting from increased release of adrenocorticotropic hormone (ACTH) secondary to a pituitary or hypothalamic lesion
   b. *Ectopic Cushing's syndrome:* Excessive autonomous secretion of ACTH or cortisol by a non-pituitary, nonadrenal neoplasm
3. *Iatrogenically-induced Cushing's syndrome:* Elevated cortisol levels due to overzealous or chronic administration of exogenous glucocorticoids

Adrenal neoplasms account for 25% of all cases of Cushing's syndrome. This percentage is higher in children. Benign adrenal adenomas are the most common and tend to encapsulate within the adrenal tissue. Carcinomas tend to infiltrate the adrenal vasculature and to metastasize.[11,13,18] Neoplasms usually occur unilaterally. Increased adrenal production of cortisol suppresses endogenous secretion of ACTH by the anterior pituitary gland by means of a negative feedback mechanism. As ACTH levels fall, the unaffected adrenal cortex lacks sufficient stimulation and atrophies (Fig. 76–1, *A* and *B*).

Pituitary-dependent Cushing's syndrome is most often a disorder of hypothalamic origin in which there is increased release of corticotropin releasing factor (CRF) from the hypothalamus. The resulting excessive secretion of ACTH by the pituitary causes bilateral adrenal hyperplasia and cortisol overproduction (Fig. 76–2, *A*). ACTH secretion continues despite the high circulating cortisol levels, indicating an abnormality in the feedback mechanism.[7,21]

Ectopic ACTH-producing tumors remain a rare cause of the clinical manifestations of cortisol excess (Fig. 76–2, *B*). The most common tumors associated with non-endocrine ACTH production include carcinomas of the lung, pancreas, gallbladder, and thymus.[13] The rapid growth of these tumors often brings about the patient's demise before the clinical signs of Cushing's syndrome become apparent. A far more common cause of Cushing's syndrome is supraphysiological doses of glucocorticoids. Synthetic steroids with glucocorticoid activity, such as cortisone acetate and prednisone, enjoy widespread use because of their effective anti-inflammatory and anti-immunologic effects. Table 76–1 lists common clinical uses for exogenous steroid administration. The resulting elevation in circulating cortisol suppresses ACTH output and causes bilateral adrenal atrophy. Although the patient demonstrates the clinical manifestations of Cushing's syndrome, acute adrenal insufficiency can suddenly occur if the steroid is discontinued abruptly.

Clinical Manifestations

The signs and symptoms of Cushing's syndrome represent an exaggeration of the physiological actions of cortisol, and in some instances, of androgens.

Moderate Central Obesity. A common finding is common central obesity, which is due to alterations in fat deposition. The exact mechanism responsible is not known. Atypical fat distribution usually involves the trunk, especially the cervicodorsal region ("buffalo hump"), supraclavicular areas, and abdomen. The abdomen appears large and pendulous. Fat also distributes about the face, in the cheeks and under the chin, imparting a round and plethoric (moon face) appearance (Fig. 76–3). Although the patient appears obese, the extremities are quite scrawny in comparison with the rest of the body. The extremities are thin due to protein wasting, which occurs in cortisol excess. If the patient is massively obese (300 lb or more) and has obese extremities, the diagnosis of Cushing's syndrome is unlikely. Patients with non-endocrine, ACTH-producing tumors may not always show signs of obesity because of the wasting and debilitating nature of the neoplastic process.[22]

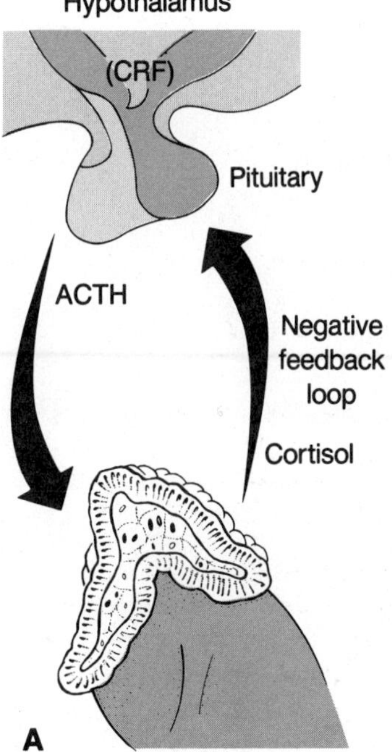

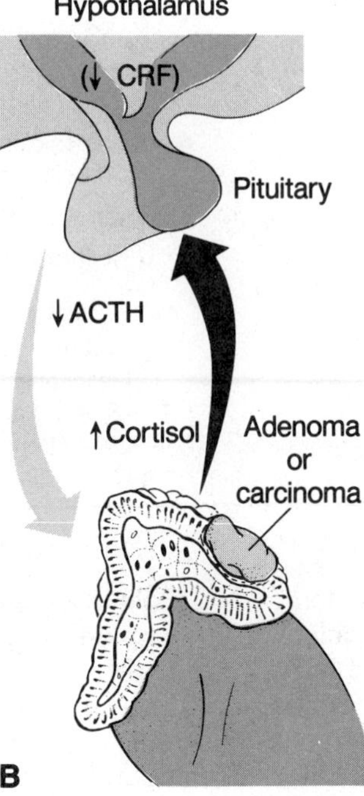

FIGURE 76–1 Pathophysiology of Cushing's syndrome: schematic showing normal hypothalamic–pituitary axis (*A*) and primary Cushing's syndrome (*B*).

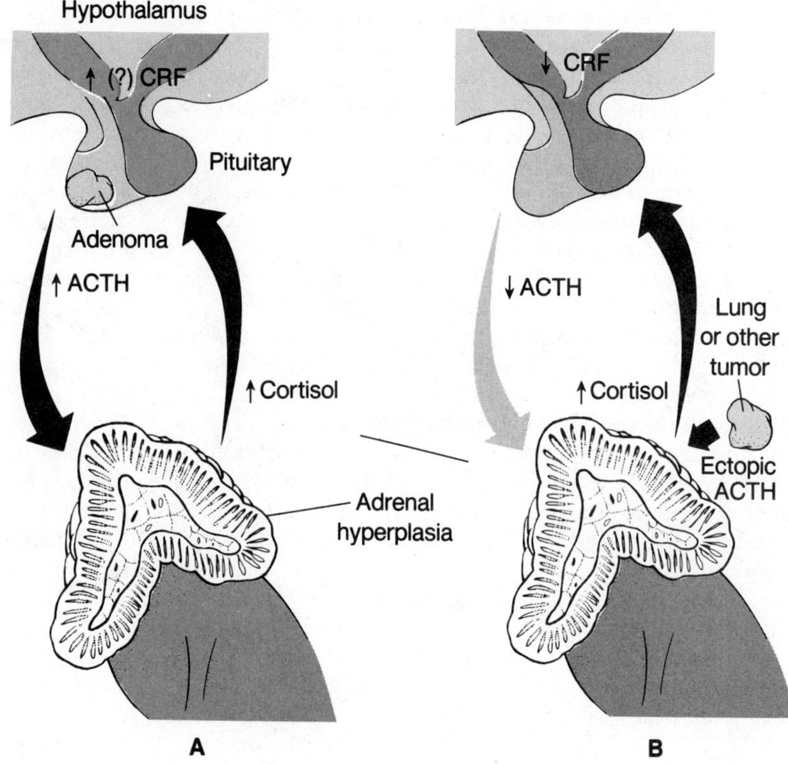

FIGURE 76–2 Secondary Cushing's syndrome. (*A*) Pituitary-dependent Cushing's disease. (*B*) Ectopic Cushing's syndrome.

TABLE 76–1
Clinical Use of Glucocorticoids

Endocrinology
- Acute and chronic adrenal insufficiency
- Congenital adrenal hyperplasia

Rheumatology
- Rheumatology
- Systemic lupus erythematosus
- Polymyalgia rehumatica
- Polyarteritis nodosa
- Polymyositis

Hematology
- Hemolytic anemia
- Idiopathic thrombocytopenic purpura
- Leukemia

Allergy
- Anaphylaxis
- Angioneurotic edema
- Drug reactions
- Contact dermatitis
- Stevens-Johnson syndrome
- Urticaria

Gastroenterology
- Ulcerative colitis
- Chronic active hepatitis
- Regional enteritis
- Celiac sprue

Dermatology
- Used topically in many skin diseases

Pulmonary
- Bronchial asthma
- Bronchiolitis
- Chronic obstructive pulmonary disease

Nephrology
- Nephrotic syndrome

Miscellaneous
- Cerebral edema and increased intracranial pressure
- Malignancies
- Myocarditis
- Organ transplantation
- Ocular diseases

Muscular Weakness. Muscular weakness, predominately in the muscles of the pelvic girdle and extremities, secondary to loss of muscle mass may be experienced and is a result of increased protein catabolism. The patient may complain of difficulty in climbing stairs or getting up from a low sitting position.

Skin Changes. Another expression of protein catabolism is skin change. The skin becomes thin, fragile, paperlike and liable to injury. Striae, which are pink and purplish and wider than 1 cm, are usually present on the abdomen, breast, buttocks and axillae.[21] These skin changes are due to weakening of the collagenous fibers in and under the skin. Protein

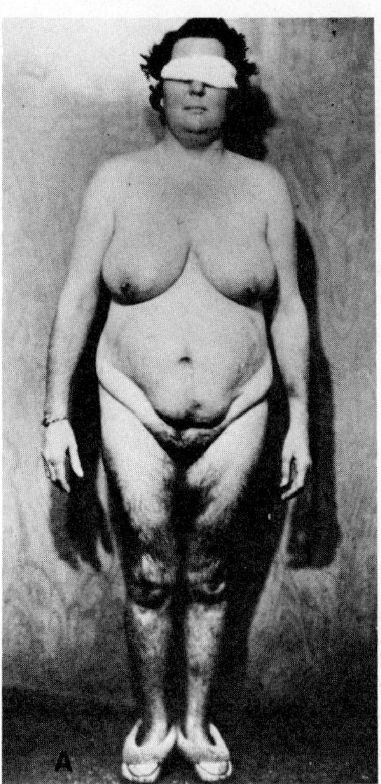

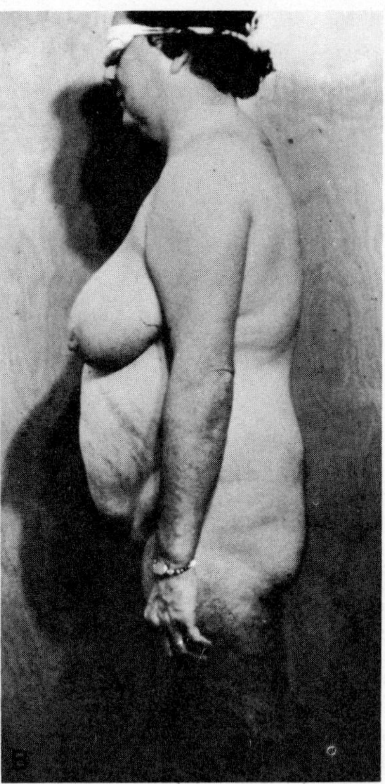

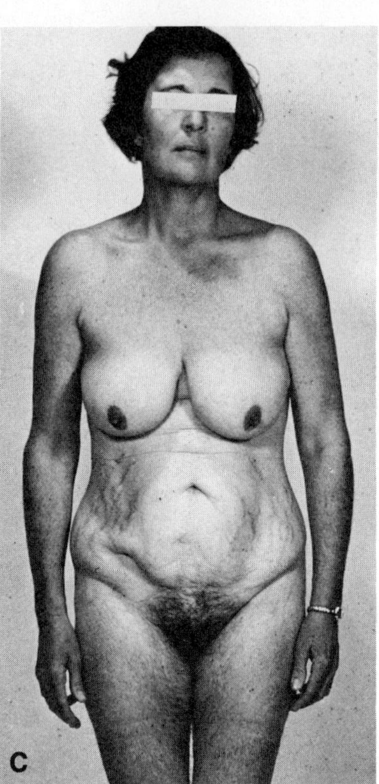

FIGURE 76–3 Cushing's syndrome. (*A*) Truncal obesity, striae, moon face, and hirsutism. (*B*) Lateral view of same patient shows obvious buffalo hump, and lateral abdominal striae are more clearly seen than in front view. (*C*) Same patient is shown following cure of Cushing's syndrome by removal of both adrenals, which were hyperplastic. Note regression of obesity and moon face, and increase in pigmentation, particularly of the areolae. This pigmentation is probably caused by a pituitary oversecretion of ACTH. (Ezrin C, Godden JO, Volpe R [eds]: Systemic Endocrinology, 2nd ed, p 208. New York, Harper & Row, 1979)

wasting also takes toll of blood vessels. Capillary fragility leads to an increased tendency toward bruising and hematoma formation.

Hyperpigmentation of the skin is found in about one third of patients with Cushing's syndrome.[13] It is usually the result of increased circulating ACTH, either ectopic or pituitary dependent. It is almost exclusively found in secondary Cushing's syndrome and is a useful diagnostic sign in ruling out the presence of an adrenal tumor.

Impaired Glucose Tolerance. Hyperglycemia and impaired glucose tolerance are present in about one half of patients with Cushing's syndrome. Elevated cortisol levels promote exaggerated hepatic gluconeogenesis and decrease glucose uptake by adipose and muscle cells. Despite the presence of hyperglycemia, serum insulin levels are also elevated, indicating marked insulin resistance. Glucosuria may be seen, but ketoacidosis is an uncommon finding. Individuals with underlying, or latent, diabetes mellitus are not able to tolerate this increased glucose load. Exacerbations of their disease may occur, requiring careful management.[9,13]

Peptic Ulcers. Peptic ulcers may form because cortisol excess promotes acidic gastric secretions and pepsin production. Because cortisol also inhibits gastric mucus production susceptibility to ulcer formation is increased.

High Blood Pressure. Mild to moderate high blood pressure is found in most individuals with Cushing's syndrome. The mineralocorticoid activity of cortisol excess promotes renal retention of sodium and water. This expansion of extracellular volume is one of the causes of observed high blood pressure. Another probable cause is the cortisol-induced hypersensitivity of blood vessels to circulating catecholamines, resulting in widespread vasoconstriction.[6] Whatever the cause, high blood pressure predisposes the patient to the development of coronory heart disease and stroke.

Osteoporosis. A particularly unwelcome feature of Cushing's syndrome is osteoporosis, which can result in compression fractures of the spine, pathological fractures of the long bones, and persistent backaches. Cortisol is thought to increase calcium resorption from the bone and inhibit collagen synthesis, thus interfering with bone formation and replenishment.[13] Children with Cushing's syndrome usually experience arrest in linear growth.

Increased Risk of Infection. The anti-inflammatory properties of cortisol can greatly retard the body's healing mechanisms and increase risk of infection. Early signs of infection, such as fever and inflammation, may not appear, thus delaying early identification and treatment of infection.[17] Suprainfections by opportunistic microbes are frequently seen.

Virilization. Virilization may be seen in women as a result of increased androgen secretion. Among the signs are hirsutism, thinning scalp hair, acne, decreased libido, an enlarged clitoris, and menstrual changes ranging from irregularity to total cessation. Except for precocious sexual development in young boys, the abnormal masculinizing effects of excess adrenal androgens on males are few.

Psychological Manifestations. Insomnia, depression, anxiety, mood swings, and frank psychosis may be observed.[13] Sometimes patients are admitted first to the psychiatric unit during exacerbations of their disease. The cause of the exacerbations is unknown but appears to relate to increased circulating levels of cortisol and ACTH. Some emotional instability may be the patient's response to altered body image and decreased self-esteem.

Hematologic Changes. Red blood cell and granulocyte counts may be elevated. Lymphopenia and a decrease in eosinophils may also be observed. Hypokalemia occurs in 20% of cases, because cortisol promotes potassium excretion in the renal tubules. Increased plasma cortisol levels, with loss of normal diurnal variations, along with elevated urinary levels of steroid metabolites (17-hydroxycorticoids and ketogenic steroids) are always seen. However, elevations in plasma ACTH are only found in secondary Cushing's syndrome. Low ACTH values are seen in primary and iatrogenically-induced Cushing's syndrome.[5, 21]

Many of the clinical manifestations of Cushing's syndrome can be reversed with the correction of the underlying cause (see Fig. 76–3).

Medical Management

The diagnosis of Cushing's syndrome is not difficult to make because of the striking physical manifestations of this disorder. Useful clinical clues to the diagnosis of Cushing's syndrome include (1) muscle weakness; (2) thinning of the skin, with ecchymoses; (3) osteoporosis; and (4) hypokalemic alkalosis. Once suspicion arises, laboratory confirmation must be made.

Treatment of Cushing's syndrome is directed toward alleviating the underlying cause. The etiology of the disorder should first be identified through a series of serum and urine diagnostic tests (see Chap. 72). The presence of adrenal, pituitary, or nonendocrine tumors can be determined using ultrasound, angiography, radiographic studies, and computerized axial tomography (CAT scan). If a pituitary tumor has been identified, there is a choice of therapies to consider. Each has met with varying degrees of success. More often the treatment of choice for the adult patient is surgical removal of the pituitary tumor or of the entire gland (hypophysectomy). Emerging techniques allow the removal of pituitary microadenomas, using a transphenoidal approach, without removing the normal pituitary tissue. (Transphenoidal hypophysectomy is discussed in Chapter 77.)

The gland may also be destroyed using local needle implants of ^{90}Y (a radioactive isotope), radioactive gold, or cryosurgery. Still another treatment modality employs pituitary irradiation in dosages of 4000 or 5000 rads over a 30-day period. Complete remission can be achieved, but it often requires several months. This treatment is most effective in minor cases of pituitary-dependent Cushing's syndrome in children.[22]

For tumors of the adrenal cortex, surgical resection of the tumor by adrenalectomy is necessary. Typically, tumors are unilateral and only the affected adrenal gland is removed. Because the adrenal tumor promotes excessive cortisol secretion from the affected gland, ACTH is often suppressed. The fall in ACTH levels then results in atrophy of the unaffected gland. These consequences require that the patient receive steroid replacement therapy following unilateral adrenalectomy until the atrophied gland can resume normal functioning. However, lifelong steroid replacement is mandatory for bilateral adrenalectomy.[3]

Ectopic Cushing's syndrome requires excision of the ectopic tumor. Often the neoplasm cannot be removed either because of its location or because it has metastasized. The prognosis is usually poor and treatment usually incorporates palliative measures.

Pharmaceutical therapy may be indicated for patients for whom surgical interventions are unsuitable. Three agents are most commonly used to inhibit cortisol synthesis and thus decrease manifestations of hypercortisolism: aminoglutethimide, metyrapone and, o,p′DDD (mitotane). Aminoglutethimide (Elipten) inhibits cholesterol conversion to pregnenolone, thus effectively blocking cortisol production. It is fairly rapid-acting and its side-effects range from gastrointestinal disturbances to somnolence and skin rashes. Metyrapone only partly blocks cortisol synthesis somewhere along the biochemical pathway. It is best used in conjunction with aminoglutethimide. The drug o,p′DDD is a particularly potent adrenal inhibitor. Its mechanism of action is unknown and it can lead to acute adrenal insufficiency. Its more common side-effects resemble those of aminoglutethimide.[21]

Other pharmaceutical agents occasionally used are those that act on the central nervous system. Cyproheptadine, a serotonin antagonist, inhibits ACTH secretion, making it most suitable for treating pituitary-dependent Cushing's syndrome. This drug is relatively new and results have not been consistent. The most common side-effects include lethargy and weight gain.

If Cushing's syndrome is a result of chronic use or high doses of exogenous glucocorticoids, signs and symptoms can be reduced with gradual dose reduction or discontinuation of steroid therapy. In some cases alternative therapy can be attempted.

Symptomatic relief of hypertension, hypokalemia, and metabolic alkalosis can be treated with the mineralocorticoid antagonist spironolactone (Aldactone).[13]

Nursing Management Plan

Manifestations of Cushing's syndrome are varied and must be approached with astuteness, patience, and creativity. The majority of nursing interventions are aimed at alleviating as many as possible of the distressing signs and symptoms of the disorder, most notably fluid and electrolyte imbalance.

Additional goals include

- Preventing accidental injury from falls or pathological fractures that may result from osteoporosis and muscle weakness
- Guarding against or detecting infection that may result from an impaired immune response brought on by an increase in circulating glucocorticoids
- Encouraging increased activity to overcome the immobility imposed by weakness and fatigue
- Promoting coping strategies to deal with the change in body image.

A sample care plan describing the details of nursing interventions and expected outcomes for the related nursing diagnoses is presented in the Nursing Care Plan for the Patient with Cushing's Syndrome. Individualization, of course, is necessary to meet each patient's needs.

(*Text continues on page 1096*)

NURSING CARE PLAN FOR THE PATIENT WITH CUSHING'S SYNDROME

NURSING DIAGNOSIS/PROBLEM 1: Potential alterations in fluid volume related to extracellular volume (ECV) excess, which may result in dependent edema, jugular vein distention, hypertension, and pulmonary congestion.

GOAL 1.1: To prevent and detect early extracellular volume excess

Nursing Interventions	Rationale	Outcome Criteria
1. Assess for ECV excess daily or as necessary.	1. Hyperfunction of the adrenal cortex results in increased glucocorticoid and mineralocorticoid release. Both types of hormones promote renal reabsorption of sodium and water, thus expanding the extracellular compartment (interstitium and intravascular).	1. Detection of ECV at its onset.
a. Monitor blood pressure and pulse.	a. Blood pressure and pulses may be elevated.	
b. Measure and record intake and output.	b. Urine output may fall well below fluid intake.	
c. Record weight daily.	c. One liter of fluid retention corresponds to approximately 2 lb of weight gain.[3]	
d. Watch for and record edema, jugular vein distention, and pulmonary crackles.	d. As the extracellular compartment expands, dependent edema, increased jugular vein distention, and pulmonary crackles are observed.	
2. Restrict fluid intake to 2000 ml or less per day as ordered. a. Dilute parenteral (IV) medications with sterile water vs. saline when possible.	2. Fluid restriction can help minimize the risk and degree of fluid retention. Isotonic solutions expand the ECV compartment more rapidly than do hypotonic solutions, thus pharmacy may be asked to mix IV medications in sterile water instead of saline. All types of fluids, however, should be limited as much as possible.	2–3. Absence of the signs and symptoms of ECV excess: blood pressure and pulse will remain within the patient's premorbid range and no sudden weight gains, edema, jugular vein distention, and pulmonary crackles.

(*Continued*)

NURSING CARE PLAN FOR THE PATIENT WITH CUSHING'S SYNDROME *(Continued)*

Nursing Interventions	Rationale
3. Limit sodium intake to less than 2 g/day (5 g salt) or as ordered. Review Chapter 70 for sodium restricted diet.	3. Limiting sodium intake decreases the sodium "load" presented to the kidneys, eventually resulting in an overall decrease in retained sodium and water. It is important to remember that table salt does not entirely consist of sodium. There is approximately 393 mg of sodium in 1 g of salt. Foods with high sodium content to be avoided include dairy products, canned foods, and foods with added preservatives. Some medications may also be high sodium sources, such as various antacids, pain remedies, cough syrups, and sedatives.

NURSING DIAGNOSIS/PROBLEM 2: Potential electrolyte imbalance related to hypokalemia (potassium deficit), which may result in cardiac arrhythmias, muscular weakness, and paresthesias.

GOAL 2.1: To prevent and to detect early hypokalemia

Nursing Interventions	Rationale	Outcome Criteria
1. Assess periodically serum potassium.	1. Increased secretion of mineralocorticoid (aldosterone) decreases renal tubule reabsorption of potassium, resulting in increased urinary potassium loss and hypokalemia.	1. Hypokalemia detected at its onset.
2. Assess and instruct patient to monitor and report signs of hypokalemia, such as weakness, hypoactive reflexes, disorientation, paralytic ileus, and polyuria.	2. Potassium is important in maintaining cell membrane stability in the cardiovascular, neuromuscular, and renal systems. The result of hypokalemia is prolonged myocardial repolarization, decreased neuromuscular function, and an inability of the kidneys to concentrate urine.	2–3. Absence of hypokalemia evidenced by normal serum potassium levels and no physical signs and symptoms of hypokalemia.
3. Replace potassium. a. Increase dietary intake of foods with high potassium content. b. Dispense potassium supplements as ordered. c. Discuss purposes of potassium replacement with patient and family.	3. a–b. To prevent hypokalemia, urinary potassium losses must be replaced with the high potassium diets discussed in Chap. 73. c. Understanding the rationale for potassium replacement therapy will increase patient compliance.	

(Continued)

NURSING CARE PLAN FOR THE PATIENT WITH CUSHING'S SYNDROME (*Continued*)

NURSING DIAGNOSIS/PROBLEM 3: Potential for accidental injury related to osteoporosis and muscle weakness, which may result in falls and pathological fractures.

GOAL 3.1: To prevent accidental injury related to falls and pathological fractures

Nursing Interventions	Rationale	Outcome Criteria
1. Provide a safe environment: rearrange furniture to enhance mobility, use a night-light, remove unnecessary equipment from room, patient should wear nonskid slippers. Confer with patient and family about necessary rearrangement of home environment prior to discharge, and assist patient with ambulation.	1. Osteoporosis can result in bone fragility and increases the risk of vertebral collapse and pathological hip fractures, which may precipitate falls. Individuals unsteady because of weakness are even more likely to trip over unseen obstacles. A well-lighted environment clear of potential obstacles and ambulatory assistance can minimize the risk of falls.	1–3. No incident of accidental injury related to falls.
2. Encourage active isometric exercises as tolerated.	2. Active exercise may help increase muscle tone and also provide sufficient bone stress to prevent further bone demineralization.	
3. Instruct patient to avoid heavy lifting, carrying heavy weights, or bending over a great deal.	3. Cushing's syndrome potentiates osteoporosis. Heavy lifting and similar strenuous activity can promote compression fractures of the vertebral bodies.[3]	

NURSING DIAGNOSIS/PROBLEM 4: Potential for infection and prolonged wound healing related to impaired immune response from increased circulating glucocorticoids

GOAL 4.1: To prevent and to detect early infection

Nursing Interventions	Rationale	Outcome Criteria
1. Place patient in a noninfectious environment. a. Instruct patient to avoid crowds and persons with upper respiratory infections or other contagious ailments.	1. The anti-inflammatory properties of cortisol greatly increases the risk of infection. One of the body's first lines of defense against invading pathogens is lost; therefore, potential sources of infection must be avoided.	1–3. No evidence of preventable infections. Infection detected at its onset.
2. Monitor the patient's white blood cell count and complaints of discomfort.	2. Normal inflammatory response is lost and the typical early manifestations of infection (*i.e.,* fever, inflammation) may not be seen. Complaints of increased malaise may be the first sign of infection.	
3. Use very strict aseptic technique when caring for skin lesions or performing invasive procedures.	3. Invasive hospital procedures penetrate the skin barrier, thus exposing the patient to potential sources of infection.	

(*Continued*)

NURSING CARE PLAN FOR THE PATIENT WITH CUSHING'S SYNDROME (*Continued*)

GOAL 4.2: To promote complete wound healing

Nursing Interventions	Rationale	Outcome Criteria
1. Monitor wounds for persistent drainage and localized pain.	1. The anti-inflammatory and protein wasting properties of cortisol can interfere with the body's healing mechanism. Wound closure will be delayed and prone to infection.	1–3. All wounds will heal within a reasonable time frame. Operative wounds will not be subject to infection or evisceration.
2. Instruct patient to avoid cuts, bruises, and trauma; injections should be given only as necessary.	2. Weakening of the collagen matrix of the skin and subcutaneous tissues increases the susceptibility to trauma and delays wound healing.	
3. Encourage the patient to increase dietary intake of protein and vitamins A and C.	3. An intake of protein and vitamins A and C are important in the formation of collagen, a protein that helps support and reconstruct body tissues.	

NURSING DIAGNOSIS/PROBLEM 5: Decreased activity tolerance related to weakness and fatigue, which may result in impaired performance of self-care activities and frustration

GOAL 5.1: To promote improved activity tolerance

Nursing Interventions	Rationale	Outcome Criteria
1. Conserve energy expenditures when possible.	1. Muscular weakness results from protein catabolism and loss of muscle mass, especially in the pelvic girdle and extremities.	1–2. The patient will: progress to the optimal activity level possible, identify factors and carry out behavior that promotes activity tolerance, and report satisfaction with level of physical abilities.
a. Assist patient with activities when necessary (especially with arising from a bed or chair).	a. Because of muscle wasting in the lower extremities, arising from a reclining position may be particularly difficult.	
b. Progress activity gradually, spacing activities to allow sufficient rest periods.	b. Sufficient rest periods are essential in restoring energy and alleviating fatigue. Progressive grading of activity improves physical endurance and prevents overwhelming the patient. It also allows the patient to "see" progress being made.	
2. Provide incentive for involvement in activity.	2. Activity intolerance often breeds discourgement and apathy.	
a. Assist the patient in setting realistic achievable activity goals.	a. Allowing the patient to participate in setting activity goals promotes incentive, success, and progress.	
b. Promote a sincere "can do" attitude regarding the patient's mobility status.	b. Providing a positive environment conveys to the patient the belief that he can improve his level of functioning, thus encouraging goal achievement.	

(*Continued*)

NURSING CARE PLAN FOR THE PATIENT WITH CUSHING'S SYNDROME (*Continued*)

NURSING DIAGNOSIS/PROBLEM 6: Alterations in body image related to physical and behavioral changes, which may result in feelings of lowered self-esteem, frustration, depression, and withdrawal.

GOAL 6.1: To promote self-confidence and to assist with reconstruction of altered body image

Nursing Interventions	Rationale	Outcome Criteria
1. Provide an environment conducive to self-expression.	1. Body image is a mental idea a person has about himself and is intimately linked with his subjective judgments about his physical and social competence. In Cushing's syndrome the muscle wasting, altered fat distribution, and androgenic symptoms are particularly distressing.	1–4. The patient will demonstrate improved self-esteem as evidenced by: ability to make positive statements about his appearance and abilities, resumption of role-related responsibilities, and ability to discuss the causes of observed physical changes and rationale of treatment.
a. Respect the patient's wish for privacy.	a. Intrusive procedures and behaviors can threaten an individual's sense of integrity.	
b. Provide consistent nursing care and maintain an open, accepting attitude toward the patient.	b. An empathetic, open, and honest attitude by the nurse can facilitate a patient's trust and self-expression.	
c. Refer patient for psychological counseling as needed.	c. Long-term therapy may be required to more thoroughly explore the patient's attitudes, emotional status, and coping abilities.	
2. Assist the patient in identifying coping resources and support persons.	2. In helping the patient identify sources of support, he is more likely to use such resources to facilitate his coping abilities.	
3. Clarify any misconceptions the patient may have about himself, his care, or his care-givers.	3. A maladaptive response to changes in body image may include inaccurate perceptions of one's abilities and the benefits of therapy. Many cushingoid features disappear after treatment and this must be made clear to the patient. Mental changes may also create misconceptions and feelings of paranoia.	
4. Include the patient's family in planning emotional support. Assess the family's coping status.	4. Family members also may go through a grieving process related to the patient's overt physical and mental changes. These feelings should be explored and allowed expression. The family must be able to provide a sound support base for the patient who may have long-term coping needs.	

Mineralocorticoid Excess: Aldosteronism

Etiology and Pathophysiology

Aldosteronism develops from excessive secretion of aldosterone, the most potent mineralocorticoid, from the adrenal cortex. It is not usually accompanied by alterations in the other adrenocortical hormones. The two types of aldosteronism are based on etiology:[17]

- *Primary aldosteronism* (Conn's syndrome) is caused by oversecretion of aldosterone either by an adrenal adenoma (80% of cases) or by bilateral adrenal hyperplasia (20%).
- *Secondary aldosteronism* is the term applied when aldosterone secretion from both adrenal cortices is stimulated by sources extraneous to the adrenals. The common finding in all cases is an elevated renin level. The causes include
  - Pregnancy
  - Hypovolemia
  - Congestive heart failure
  - Cirrhosis of the liver
  - Chronic renal failure
  - Bartter's syndrome
  - Use of oral contraceptive
  - Therapy with diuretics
  - Malignant hypertension
  - Idiopathic cyclic edema
  - Renin-secreting tumors

Primary aldosteronism was once thought to be a common cause of high blood pressure. It is now believed that it accounts for less than 1% of the hypertensive population. It is found twice as frequently in women as in men, and the majority of its victims are between 30 and 50 years of age. In primary aldosteronism, the normal feedback control for regulating aldosterone secretion is lacking. Aldosterone is produced and secreted regardless of body needs and in defiance of normal suppressive stimuli (Fig. 76–4). Although multiple adrenal tumors may be found, a single, small, benign adrenal adenoma is more likely. Carcinomas very rarely cause primary aldosteronism.[15]

Secondary aldosteronism is usually the result of a decrease in the effective plasma volume or perfusion pressure detected by the renal stretch receptors in the juxtaglomerular apparatus in the kidney. The resulting release of renin and subsequent activation of angiotensin II stimulate aldosterone release. Aldosterone stimulates the exchange of sodium for potassium in the distal tubule of the kidney, leading to sodium retention, potassium excretion, volume expansion, and an increase in blood pressure.

Clinical Manifestations

The signs and symptoms of aldosteronism result from an exaggeration of aldosterone's effects on the kidney. The hallmark signs of primary aldosteronism are high blood pressure and hypokalemia.

Chronic licorice ingestion gives rise to a similar condition that is called pseudoaldosteronism. Black licorice contains glycyrrhizic acid, a substance that evokes similar aldosterone effects in the distal tubules, and it can produce symptoms that are easily confused with those of primary aldosteronism.[13]

Hypertension. Increased sodium and water retention by the kidney, with subsequent volume expansion, can cause dramatic elevations in blood pressure. Patients may complain of severe headaches and visual disturbances. The risk of

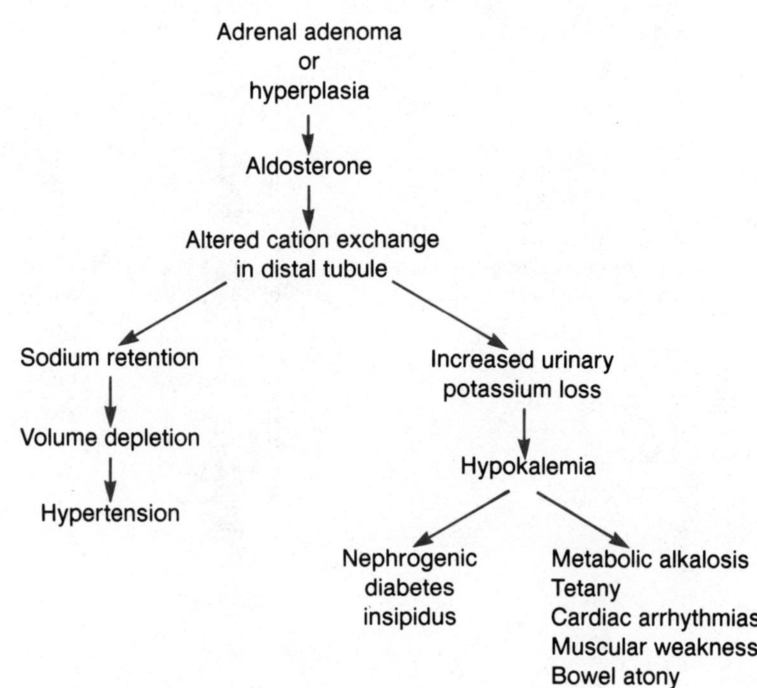

FIGURE 76–4 Pathophysiology of primary aldosteronism.

cerebrovascular accidents in heightened. Left ventricular enlargement may be noted in some patients as a cardiac adaptation to high blood pressure. In individuals with heart disease, the threat of congestive heart failure causes great concern. The hemodilution from the increased blood volume results in a lowered hematocrit. Surprisingly, edema is rarely seen in primary aldosteronism. The reason is that increased glomerular filtration rate and renal tubular damage evoke polyuria. Edema, however, is a common occurrence in secondary aldosteronism.[15]

Hypokalemia. Spontaneous hypokalemia in the presence of high blood pressure should raise suspicions of primary aldosteronism. Excessive renal excretion of potassium is a direct effect of aldosterone excess. Urinary potassium excretion of more than 30 mEq/day is usually seen.[13] Potassium wasting often leads to muscular weakness and cardiac arrhythmias because of alterations in neuromuscular activity. Nephrogenic diabetes insipidus that results from chronic hypokalemia is another cause of polyuria. Something renders the cells of the renal tubules incapable of responding to antidiuretic hormone and free water is increasingly excreted, but the exact cause is not understood. This excessive excretion of water can be reversed with potassium replacement.

When potassium levels fall, hydrogen ions move into the cells to replace potassium losses and maintain electroneutrality and into the urine in the tubules in exchange for sodium ions. The result of this hydrogen-ion shifting is metabolic alkalosis. Signs of tetany may be seen, because metabolic alkalosis reduces the amounts of free ionized calcium in the plasma.

Elevations in both urinary potassium and plasma aldosterone levels (>30 mEq/day) will be seen. Despite a high sodium intake of at least 300 mEq/day, urine and plasma aldosterone levels remain inappropriately elevated. Plasma renin levels will be lowered in primary aldosteronism and elevated in secondary aldosteronism.

Medical Management

For patients with primary aldosteronism the differential diagnosis of adrenal adenoma or bilateral adrenal hyperplasia must be made. Radionuclide adrenal scans may help visualize the underlying pathological changes. Preferred treatment for adrenal tumors is partial or total adrenalectomy, to which response is often good. It may take up to 1 month or more after surgery for blood pressure and suppressed renin levels to return to normal.[21]

Before the surgery, the high blood pressure and hypokalemia can be treated with an aldosterone antagonist, spironolactone (100 mg to 400 mg/day), which inhibits aldosterone synthesis and its effects on the distal tubules. Other diuretics should be avoided because they may further reduce potassium levels and precipitate serious cardiac arrhythmias. Potassium supplements are, of course, very important and are given according to the amount of potassium deficit. Sodium intake should also be restricted. As less sodium is presented to the distal tubules, less potassium is excreted in exchange for sodium.

Patients with bilateral adrenal hyperplasia are less responsive to surgical interventions and are usually treated medically. Secondary aldosteronism is treated symptomatically, with management focused on alleviating the underlying cause. Aldosteronism can have lethal consequences but, with early diagnosis, it can be easily managed and even cured.

Nursing Management Plan

Nursing considerations are aimed at evaluating the degree of high blood pressure and hypokalemia, their sequelae, and the response to therapy. Patient teaching also plays an integral part in successful management of these patients.

Assessment and Nursing Diagnosis. Possible nursing diagnoses related to high blood pressure include potential alterations in tissue perfusion (stroke), alterations in comfort (headache), and ineffective individual or family coping. Alterations in electrolytes related to hypokalemia can be evidenced by neuromuscular weaknesses, paresthesias, and cardiac arrhythmias. Another possible nursing diagnosis is knowledge deficit related to proper management of aldosteronism that can result in noncompliance and loss of control of the disease process.

Goals. Patient goals are related to the identified nursing diagnosis. General patient goals include early detection and prevention of stroke, promotion of comfort, maintenance of normal serum potassium levels, and increased knowledge about the nature of the disease and its treatment and compliance with the therapeutic interventions.

Interventions. High blood pressure is related to increased renal retention of sodium and water. Blood pressure should be closely and routinely monitored along with lung auscultations, daily weights, and an accurate recording of intake and output. The degree of edema, although it is not common in primary aldosteronism, is assessed in all dependent areas of the body. Attempts to minimize elevations in blood pressure should be made. The patient must be cautioned to avoid overexertion and straining at stool. Laxatives may be ordered and increasing bulk in the diet is encouraged. The nurse must watch for the potential side-effects of prescribed antihypertensive medications.[1]

One of the dangers of high blood pressure is stroke; therefore, neurological assessments should be ongoing. Headaches are common and should be treated with mild analgesics, relaxation techniques, and cold packs. Patients treated medically should learn how to monitor their own blood pressure. In addition, instruction about prescribed medications and their purpose and side-effects should be included in patient education.

Serum potassium levels must be closely observed and physical manifestations of hypokalemia watched for. The signs include muscular weakness, metabolic alkalosis, tetanus, paresthesias, a positive Chvostek's sign (see Chap. 72), and arrhythmias. A diet low in sodium and high in potassium is encouraged. If adrenalectomy is recommended, preoperative preparation is given. (See section Nursing Care of the Adrenalectomy Patient at the end of this chapter.)

Evaluation of Goal Achievement. Goal achievement can be assessed by the stabilization of blood pressure and the absence of, or early detection of, altered cerebral perfusion. The patient is able to accurately discuss the nature of his illness and the appropriate use of antihypertensive medication. The patient will also discuss and participate in behaviors aimed at reducing blood pressure. Finally, serum potassium levels will remain at normal levels with the patient adhering to the prescribed high potassium diet.

Androgen Excess: Adrenogenital Syndrome

Etiology and Pathology

The adrenogenital syndrome is a virilization syndrome that results from excessive production of adrenal androgens. These androgens are eventually converted to testosterone, which accounts for the observed virilism. The syndrome may be inherited (congenital adrenal hyperplasia [CAH]) or acquired (adrenal virilism). Acquired adrenal virilism is relatively rare, and is usually secondary to a virilizing tumor (adenoma or carcinoma) of the adrenal cortex. It can be found at any age and in men and women but is twice as likely to occur in women.[1,11]

Congenital adrenal hyperplasia is the most common adrenal disorder in infancy and childhood. It has a genetic predisposition, and is transmitted as an autosomal recessive trait. Any one of the six enzymes required for cortisol and possibly aldosterone production may be deficient. The cortisol deficit stimulates increased production of ACTH, which in turn stimulates the adrenal cortex, resulting in excessive androgen release. In some forms of CAH, excessive ACTH secretion stimulates the production of certain cortisol precursors that promote salt wasting.[1] As these compounds increase and aldosterone levels fall, an acute adrenal crisis may be precipitated.

Clinical Manifestations

The external genitalia of the newborn female with *congenital adrenal hyperplasia* (CAH) are usually ambiguous (female pseudohermaphroditism). The clitoris is enlarged and has a urethral opening at its base. There is also some degree of labial fusion. Virilism persists as she grows older. Newborn males with the syndrome demonstrate no obvious abnormality. They do, however, experience precocious sexual development, with accentuated masculine characteristics prior to puberty. Both males and females have rapid bone growth and at first appear tall for their ages, but early epiphyseal closure results in short adult stature. Salt-wasting CAH, with acute adrenal crisis, results in death during the newborn's first week of life, which is due to vomiting, dehydration, hyponatremia, and hyperkalemia.[1,14]

Clinical manifestations of *acquired adrenal virilism* vary with the patient's age at onset. Prepubescent girls develop pubic hair and clitoral enlargement, with no breast enlargement at puberty and delayed menses. Prepubescent boys demonstrate hirsutism with penis and prostate development equal in size to those of the adult male. The testes, however, fail to mature.

Adult females are extremely hirsute, with dense hair distribution on the extremities and trunk, and pubic hair extending to the navel. In addition, they have acne, deep voices, temporal baldness, increased muscle mass, decreased breast size, enlarged clitoris, uterine atrophy, amenorrhea, and a general development of male habits. Virilizing syndromes are less obvious in adult males. Characteristic laboratory findings include greatly elevated serum testosterone levels and increased urinary 17-ketosteroids.[1,14]

Medical Management

Treatment depends on the type of lesion suspected. In CAH, there is a defect in cortisol production with a resultant increase in ACTH secretion. Increased circulating levels of ACTH produce the characteristic adrenal hyperplasia and excessive androgen release. The therapy, then, consists of administering glucocorticoids to shut off the negative feedback loop and suppress pituitary ACTH secretion.[1]

Early diagnosis of adrenogenital syndrome in the newborn with ambiguous genitalia is essential to avoid errors in sex assignment. Surgery can be used to correct the labial fusion and other defects. Children usually respond well to steroid therapy and most remain on it throughout life.

In adults with virilizing adrenal tumors, prompt surgical excision is required. When metastasis has occurred, antitumor drugs, such as o,p′-DDD, are used with or without local irradiation.

Nursing Management Plan

Nursing care for these patients is essentially the same as that for adrenalectomy patients. The nurse must also be sensitive to the patient's and the family's difficulties in coping with the sexual ambiguity.

Assessment and Nursing Diagnosis. Care of patients with adrenocortical hyperfunction and those undergoing adrenalectomy surgery is discussed elsewhere in this chapter. Problems specific to individuals with adrenogenital syndromes are related to the ambiguous sexual characteristics. Nursing diagnoses include alterations in body image and ineffective coping by the patient and family members. Defining characteristics for such diagnoses might manifest as signs of grieving, withdrawal from social contacts, self-destructive behavior, neglect or overprotectiveness by family members, and distortion of reality concerning the client's health problem.

Goals. Through selective interventions the nurse will try to assist the patient with reconstruction of body image; to assess the competency of coping abilities of both the patient and his family and to restore coping resources and mutually supportive problem-solving abilities among family members.

Interventions. The nurse should facilitate a trusting nurse/patient (or family) relationship by promoting an environment conducive to expression of feelings. Clarify misconceptions related to the disorder and its treatment and provide reliable information about the nature of the disorder and realities of therapy. Family members are encouraged to participate in the patient's care. Usual coping patterns should be assessed, along with family strengths and weaknesses, and constructive alternative behaviors discussed. Avoid negative criticism, yet give only realistic praise. The patient should be related to as either male or female according to the genetic predisposition or the individual's preference. Chapter 73 discusses in greater detail the care of patients with coping and self-esteem problems.

Evaluation of Goal Achievement. Goal attainment will be reflected by the ability of both patient and family to verbalize true feelings related to the disorder, its treatment and prognosis, and their use of healthy coping behaviors. The patient will also demonstrate reconstruction of an altered body image with a strong, positive gender identification.

Hypofunction of the Adrenal Cortex: Adrenocortical Insufficiency

Etiology and Pathology

Adrenocortical insufficiency includes all conditions in which suppression of the adrenal is accompanied by a marked decreased in production and secretion of adrenocortical hormones. The various types of adrenal insufficiency fall into two general categories based on etiology.[17]

1. *Primary adrenal insufficiency* (Addison's disease) results from intrinsic pathological changes in both adrenal glands
2. *Secondary adrenal insufficiency* is caused by a deficit in ACTH, due either to pathological changes in the anterior pituitary gland or to adrenal suppression by exogenously administered steroids

The most common cause of Addison's disease is idiopathic atrophy of the adrenal glands, probably the result of some autoimmune process in which circulating adrenal antibodies slowly destroy the glands. Patients often have a family history of adrenal insufficiency. They may also have concurrent autoimmune disorders involving the thyroid gland and gonads. Tuberculosis, one the most common cause of primary adrenal insufficiency, is now rarely encountered. Accounting for even fewer cases are infiltrative diseases such as bilateral metastases, amyloidosis, leukemia, and sarcoidosis. Destruction of 90% of the glands usually occurs before clinical signs of adrenal insufficiency appear.[13] Causes of adrenocortical insufficiency are listed in Table 76–2.

TABLE 76–2
Causes of Adrenocortical Insufficiency

- I. Primary adrenal insufficiency
  - A. Intrinsic destruction of adrenal gland
    1. Idiopathic atrophy, autoimmune
    2. Tuberculosis
    3. Histoplasmosis
    4. Infiltrative diseases; sarcoidosis, hemochromatosis, leukemia, malignancies
    5. Septicemia (menigococcal or staphylococcal)
    6. Surgical removal of adrenal glands
    7. Hemorrhage from anticoagulants
  - B. Metabolic failure of hormone production
    1. Inhibitive and cytotoxic drugs (metyrapone and o, p′-DDD)
- II. Secondary adrenal insufficiency
  - A. Pituitary disease
    1. Postpartum necrosis (Sheehan's syndrome)
    2. Pituitary tumors (chromophobe adenoma, craniopharyngioma)
    3. Idiopathic destruction
    4. Granulomas (leukemia, hemochromatosis)
    5. Metastatic diseases
    6. Trauma, surgery
  - B. Suppression of hypothalamic–pituitary axis
    1. Abrupt cessation of chronic exogenous steroid administration

Primary adrenal insufficiency (Addison's disease) can occur at any age and is found equally in men and women (Fig. 76–5, *A*). It is a relatively uncommon, chronic disorder, found in 1 case per 100,000 population. As the level of adrenocortical hormones falls, ACTH secretion is increased by the anterior pituitary by means of the intrinsic feedback mechanism.

Because of the widespread use of exogenous steroids, iatrogenic secondary adrenal insufficiency is encountered much more often. In females, endogenous secondary adrenal insufficiency is caused by postpartum pituitary infarction (Sheehan's syndrome), by a pituitary tumor, or it is idiopathic. In males, approximately half have a pituitary tumor, while in the remaining half no discernible cause can be found. In secondary adrenal insufficiency, a decrease in circulating ACTH with a resulting decrease in adrenocortical hormones is found[13] (Figure 76–5, *B*). Aldosterone may not be markedly decreased because other factors besides ACTH are responsible for regulating aldosterone secretion.

Clinical Manifestations

Whatever the etiology, hypofunction of the adrenal cortex interferes with the body's ability to handle internal and external stress. The signs and symptoms observed in adrenal insufficiency are related to deficiencies in both aldosterone and cortisol.

Fluid and Electrolyte Imbalances. Aldosterone deficiency renders the distal tubules of the nephron incapable of conserving sodium. As a result, sodium is lost through the

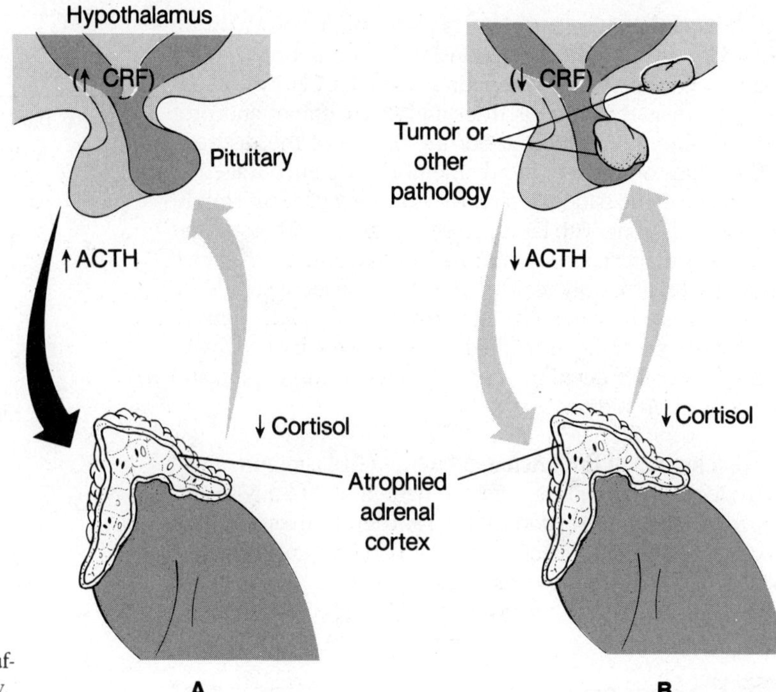

FIGURE 76–5 Pathophysiology of adrenocortical insufficiency. (*A*) Primary Addison's disease. (*B*) Secondary.

kidneys. The volume of the extracellular fluid is depleted; blood volume decreases and blood pressure falls. *Postural hypotension* (standing blood pressure rarely rising above 110 systolic) and *syncope* is a common occurrence, and in severe cases profound hypovolemic shock occurs. The heart size becomes smaller in response to the chronic decrease in cardiac output.

An impaired ability to conserve sodium in the nephron and appropriately excrete the water load leads to *hyponatremia*. As serum sodium levels reach 120 mEq/liter or less, dizziness, confusion, and neuromuscular irritability result. Potassium levels rise (*hyperkalemia*) as the cation exchange in the distal tubule can no longer take place at a normal rate. Cardiac electrophysiological changes can occur as a result and are manifested by sharp peaking T waves, broadened QRS complexes and, in severe cases, mechanical cardiac standstill. Markedly elevated potassium levels may also result in ascending paralysis with flaccid quadriplegia and mixed sensory defects.[11]

Hypoglycemia. A lowering of the blood sugar level (*hypoglycemia*) is seen in approximately half the patients with adrenal insufficiency. The absence of cortisol results in a fall in hepatic gluconeogenesis and a rise in tissue glucose uptake. Hypoglycemia is the result. This problem is even more common in patients with secondary adrenal insufficiency because there is suppression of other pituitary hormones that play a role in glucose metabolism. One example is growth hormone. Periods of fasting are not well tolerated by individuals with hypofunction of the adrenal cortex and can seriously affect them.

Fatigue. Perhaps the most consistent finding in adrenal insufficiency is that of fatigue and weakness, which early in the disease may appear sporadically and only in times of stress. Weakness may progress to the point that fatigue is continuous, and the patient is bedridden. Often the voice becomes weak and indistinct, usually because of cortisol deficit with altered carbohydrate metabolism and potassium wasting.

Hyperpigmentation. Hyperpigmentation is a striking although inconsistent feature of adrenal insufficiency, commonly appearing as a diffuse brown, bronze, or tan darkening over exposed and unexposed areas of the body. It is particularly prevalent over elbows, knees, and other pressure areas. Common sites include the areolae, the creases of the hand, scars, and the anogenital area. Sometimes small, black freckles appear over the forehead, neck, and face. Bluish black splotches in the mucous membranes, such as the gums and vaginal surfaces, are also seen.[13] *Vitiligo,* a condition of patchy depigmentation surrounded by areas of increased pigmentation, is also common, and is usually encountered in primary adrenal insufficiency (Fig. 76–6).

Gastrointestinal Signs. Anorexia, nausea, vomiting, diarrhea, and ill-defined abdominal pain are frequent findings in adrenal insufficiency. They primarily result from a cortisol deficit. The symptoms tend to cause weight loss and augment the problem of dehydration, which in turn contributes to hypotension.

Stress. Irritability, restlessness, and confusion are frequently observed in patients with adrenal insufficiency. These signs, along with the loss of vigor, often make the individual appear apathetic and may invoke accusations of malingering. Patients may become increasingly anxious, lethargic, and incapable of leading productive lives.[21] Extreme

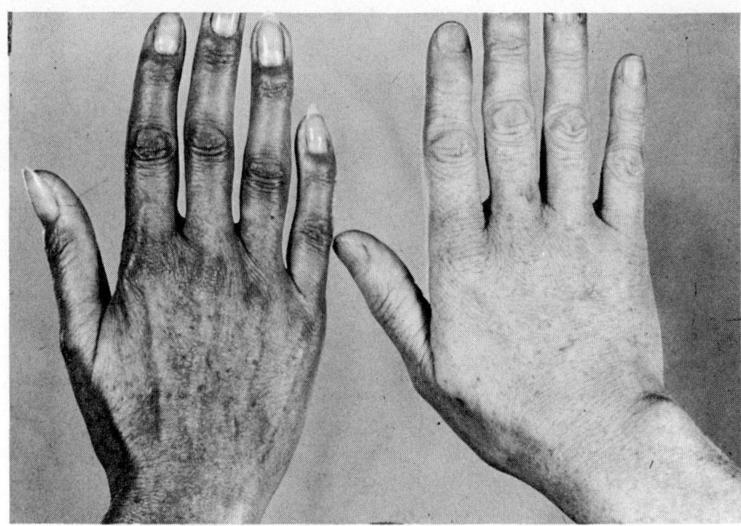

FIGURE 76–6 Pigmentation of hand on left is due to Addison's disease. Normal hand shown on right. (Ezrin C, Godden JO, Volpe R [eds]: Systematic Endocrinology, 2nd ed, p 214. New York, Harper & Row, 1979)

incapacitating prostration can occur in the presence of even mild emotional or physical stress (*e.g.,* a cold).

Sexual Effects. Adrenal androgen deficiency is usually of little consequence in the male because testicular androgen production is sufficient. In the female, however, axillary and pubic hair become scanty. Amenorrhea and decreased libido may also be experienced.

Laboratory Values. Hypofunction of the adrenal cortex is accompanied by a fall in circulating plasma cortisol and low values for urinary 17-hydroxycorticoids (17-OHCS) and 17-ketosteroids (17-KS). In primary adrenal insufficiency, plasma ACTH values are elevated, whereas the opposite is true in secondary adrenal insufficiency. An ACTH stimulation test will cause cortisol levels to rise if a pituitary deficiency exists. Failure of cortisol to rise is seen in primary adrenal disorders. In addition, abnormal findings include hyperkalemia, hyponatremia, hypochloremia, hypoglycemia, and an increased blood urea nitrogen.[5]

Diagnosis. Recognition of the disease in the early stages is often difficult. The clinical manifestations are shared by many debilitating disorders. Suspicions should always arise if any patient has a syndrome of hypotension, weakness, anorexia, and weight loss. Hypofunction of the adrenal cortex, if undiagnosed and untreated, carries a poor and frequently fatal prognosis.

Acute Adrenal Crisis

The manifestations of primary adrenal insufficiency are usually insidious and chronic in their development. However, Addison's disease can become exacerbated into a lethal crisis, so that prompt interventions are necessary to avoid death. Acute adrenal crisis usually occurs because the Addison's disease has not been properly controlled with hormone replacement therapy or the patient has suffered from marked physical or emotional stress. Individuals chronically receiving pharmacological doses of corticosteriods for a variety of reasons may also be subject to acute adrenal crisis if corticosteroid therapy is abruptly terminated. The crisis results because ACTH secretion is suppressed and subsequent disuse atrophy of the adrenal glands has taken place. Bilateral adrenal hemorrhage secondary to heparin therapy is another common cause of acute adrenal crisis.

Acute adrenal crisis can also occur in an individual who was previously well, and is seen most frequently as a consequence of severe fulminating infections, such as meningococcal or staphylococcal septicemia (Waterhouse-Friderichsen syndrome).[1] Other causes include bilateral adrenalectomy and sudden pituitary destruction.

The signs and symptoms of acute adrenal crisis are an exaggeration of those of chronic adrenal insufficiency. In addition, petechial hemorrhages may be observed on the skin. Most important and most lethal are profound hypovolemic shock, hyperkalemia, and hypoglycemia.[17]

Acute Medical Management. In acute adrenal crisis, therapy is directed toward rapidly increasing circulating levels of cortisol and replacing the extracellular volume deficit, which may be as much as 20%. A rapid intravenous infusion of 5% dextrose in normal saline is given. Cortisol (hydrocortisone phosphate, Solu-Cortef) is administered intravenously and repeated every 6 hours until acute symptoms subside.[16] It may also be added to the normal saline infusion. Hydrocortisone does not totally replace mineralocorticoid stores, but as long as enough saline is administered this is of little concern initially. Hyperkalemia usually responds dramatically to cortisol–saline administration and generally requires no other therapy in the acute stage.[18]

Ongoing hemodynamic monitoring of central venous pressures or pulmonary artery wedge pressures is usually helpful to accurately assess volume status. Frequent electrocardiograms and serum electrolytes may also be ordered.

Acute Nursing Management Plan. Nursing care of the patient with acute adrenal crisis is directed toward lifesaving measures. Assessing and maintaining circulating volume is paramount. Frequent evaluation of vital signs, urine output, and hemodynamic parameters, along with monitoring heart rhythm for the presence of serious arrhythmias, is necessary. Signs of saline excess from overaggressive fluid restoration must be guarded against, watching out for pulmonary rales, edema, jugular vein distention, and heart gallops.[20]

Volume status is not the only thing requiring close scrutiny. The patient's somnolent state may compromise the airway. Therefore, airway patency must be closely monitored, and suction and oxygen must be kept close at hand. A calm approach, with careful explanations of the procedures, can help alleviate excessive stress and put less demand on an already compromised cardiovascular system.

Chronic Adrenal Insufficiency

Chronic Medical Management. Addison's disease is a relentless, usually incurable disorder requiring hormone replacement for life. Glucocorticoid replacement is satisfactorily achieved with administration of oral cortisone acetate, 20 mg to 25 mg in the morning and 10 mg to 12.5 mg in the afternoon.[19] The larger morning dose is given to mimic the normal diurnal pattern of cortisol secretion (circadian rhythm) within the body. Equivalent doses of other glucocorticoids, such as prednisone and prednisolone, may also be used. (See Table 76–3 for the guide to proper steroid administration.) Doses are usually increased twofold or fourfold during times of stress, such as during minor surgery, dental work, or infections. Side-effects vary and can affect numerous body systems (see Table 76–4).

Some individuals with primary adrenal insufficiency may require aldosterone replacement. Fludrocortisone acetate (Florinef), a mineralocorticoid, is given 0.1 mg every day or three times a week. Patients with secondary adrenal insufficiency usually have sufficient aldosterone secretion and may not require mineralocorticoid replacement. The patient may be told to increase salt intake in the diet, particularly during episodes of profuse sweating. Up to 8 g of salt may need to be added to the everyday diet.[21]

It is wise for the patient to keep an injectable steroid readily available at all times in the event of his being found unconscious or because of vomiting or an intercurrent illness that prevents him from taking oral steroid supplements. Often suggested is a small, well-labeled kit containing 100 mg of hydrocortisone phosphate solution in a sterile syringe ready for injection. An identification bracelet stating the patient's name, the name and phone number of the nearest kin, and the physician's name and phone number should also be worn. If the patient is found injured or unconscious, the Medic-Alert bracelet should instruct the person in attendance to inject the hydrocortisone found in the patient's possession. (General guidelines for the patient taking steroids are listed in Table 76–5).

Chronic Nursing Management Plan. Long-term nursing considerations are aimed at control of the disease. Patient teaching is essential for ensuring compliance to the therapeutic regimens. Proper self-administration of steroids, re-

TABLE 76–3
Characteristics of Pharmacological Adrenocorticosteroids

Trade Names	*USP Name*	*Relative Potency of Anti-inflammatory Drugs (cortisol = 1)*	*Relative Potency of Mineralocorticoids (aldosterone = 1)*
Glucocorticoids			
Decadron, Deronil, Dexameth, Hexadrol	Dexamethasone*	30	0
Celestone	Betamethasone	30	0
Medrol	Methylprednisolone*	6	0.4
Aristocort, Kenacort	Triamcinolone†	5	0
Deltasone, Deltra, Meticorten, Paracort	Prednisone	4	0.8
Delta-Cortef	Prednisolone	4	0.8
Cortef, Cortifan, Cortril, Hydrocortone	hydrocortisone* (cortisol)	1	0.6
Cortogen, Cortone	Cortisone	0.8	0.6
Mineralocorticoids			
Cortef-f, Florinef	Fludrocortisone (9-fludrocortisol)	10	80.8
Cortate, Decortin, Doca	Desoxycorticosterone (DOC)	0	20.0

* May come in intravenous preparations
† A topical agent

TABLE 76–4
Side-Effects of Glucocorticoid Therapy

Fluid and Electrolyte Imbalances
- Hypokalemia (hypokalemic alkalosis)
- Hypocalcemia
- Edema

Cardiovascular Effects
- Hypertension
- Congestive heart failure
- Atherosclerosis

Neurological Manifestations
- Psychotic reactions
- Nervousness
- Seizures
- Neuritis
- Headache

Dermatological Signs
- Skin atrophy
- Ecchymosis
- Acne
- Striae
- Impaired wound healing

Musculoskeletal Deficiencies
- Osteoporosis
- Muscle wasting
- Pathological fractures
- Stunted growth

Ophthalmic Abnormalities
- Glaucoma
- Corneal lesions

Gastrointestinal Disturbances
- Nausea
- Peptic ulcer
- Abdominal distention
- Pancreatitis

Body Habitus Changes
- Moon face
- Obese trunk
- Thin extremities

Other Anomalies
- Glucosuria
- Hyperglycemia
- Menstrual irregularities

TABLE 76–5
Advice to Patients Taking Steroids

1. The drug should be taken as prescribed. *DO NOT ALTER DOSE OR STOP MEDICATION WITHOUT CONSULTING YOUR PHYSICIAN*! Sudden cessation of drug may precipitate an adrenal crisis. Gradual drug withdrawal is essential.
2. Take oral drug at mealtimes or with snack to reduce gastric irritation.
3. With alternate-day therapy (often used for patients on long-term therapy): take twice the usual daily dose of glucocorticoid every other morning, preferably before 9 AM.
4. With daily administration of glucocorticoid: mimic the normal physiological diurnal rhythm in the body. Take the higher doses of glucocorticoid around 8 AM, with lesser dose being taken during the afternoon or evening.
5. Establish your baseline data regarding blood pressure, weight, and sleep pattern, and continually assess them throughout the period of steroid administration.
6. If ordered, eat a diet high in potassium and low in sodium. Potassium-rich foods include: leafy vegetables, avocado, citrus fruit, bananas, and whole grains. Sodium-rich food to be avoided include snack foods, bouillon, sauces, luncheon meats, canned vegetables, and cheeses.
7. Notify your physician if you experience disease exacerbations or are subjected to severe stress, such as infection or injury. Dose readjustment may be necessary.
8. If you have substantial or borderline diabetes mellitus your blood and urine glucose levels will be closely monitored.
9. Report the appearance of undesirable side-effects, such as excessive weight gain, edema, marked muscle weakness, bone pain, hypertension, depression, headache, polyuria, and the development of an infection.
10. Use of a firm mattress and bed board (patients with persistent backache).
11. Avoid infectious people and immediately report an infection if one is suspected. Report delays in wound healing and vague feelings of being "sick." (Because your immune system is suppressed, infections may be masked.)
12. Obtain a Medic-Alert identification bracelet, describing your condition, drug, and dose.
13. See your physician on a regular basis.

duction of stress, correct diet, and the importance of medical follow-up are included in the teaching.

Aside from the teaching program, the nursing care of a patient with Addison's disease includes

1. Maintaining normal fluid and electrolyte balance to offset potential extracellular volume deficit and hyperkalemia
2. Minimizing physical and emotional stress and encouraging coping measures to deal with the patient's emotional lability
3. Promoting optimium physical activity in self-care to overcome muscle weakness and fatigue
4. Providing good nutrition to prevent hypoglycemia
5. Encouraging adherence to the treatment plan in the face of long-term management.

Specific nursing diagnoses, goals, interventions and expected outcomes are presented in the Nursing Care Plan for the Patient with Addison's Disease. It is important for the nurse to emphasize that normal life patterns can be reestablished with supplemental adrenocorticoid therapy. Indeed, prognosis is generally good for patients with proper control of the disease. Like diabetes mellitus, the control of Addison's disease is a lifelong responsibility.

(*Text continues on page 1109*)

NURSING CARE PLAN FOR THE PATIENT WITH ADDISON'S DISEASE

NURSING DIAGNOSIS/PROBLEM 1: Alterations in fluid volume related to extracellular volume (ECV) deficit, which may result in dehydration and hypovolemic shock.

GOAL 1.1: To detect early ECV deficit and to maintain a normovolemic state

Nursing Interventions	Rationale	Outcome Criteria
1. Watch for extracellular volume deficit daily or necessary.	1. Adrenocortical insufficiency results in a decreased release of mineralocorticoid (aldosterone), which promotes renal losses of water and sodium. An ECV deficit may ensue.	1. ECV deficit detected at its onset.
a. Monitor blood pressure and pulse (note orthostatic hypotension).	a. Excessive losses from the extracellular compartment may lead to dehydration and shock, which is manifested by orthostatic hypotension and tachycardia.	
b. Measure and record intake and output.	b. A 1-liter loss from the extracellular fluid compartment approximately reflects a 2 lb weight loss.	
c. Record daily weights.	c. Excessive urinary output relative to fluid intake can herald the risk of dehydration. Other routes of fluid loss (*i.e.,* diarrhea, perspiration, and respirations) should also be included in the assessment.	
d. Watch for and record skin turgor and condition of mucous membranes.	d. Dehydration is typically manifested by dry mucous membranes and poor skin turgor.	
2. Encourage fluid intake of at least 3000 ml/day.	2. The patient with Addison's disease can experience tremendous urinary fluid losses that can create marked extracellular volume depletion. These fluid losses must be replaced.	2–5. The patient will demonstrate a normovolemic status as evidence by: no orthostatic hypotension, moist mucous membranes, and urine output of 30 ml/hour.
3. Increase salt by at least 5 g/day.	3. An increased dietary intake of sodium is encouraged to offset large renal losses of sodium. Five grams of salt equals 2 g of sodium. Normal sodium intake is 5–10 g daily. This amount should be increased in the Addison's patient.	
4. Administer parenteral fluids as ordered.	4. Excessive fluid losses may result in severe dehydration and hypovolemic shock necessitating rapid parenteral replacement of isotonic solutions. Normal saline is used because of its physiological sodium content.	
5. Caution patient to avoid arising quickly from a sitting or reclining position.	5. Extracellular fluid deficit is usually accompanied by orthostatic hypotension and can cause extreme vertigo or syncope when arising from a sitting or recumbent position.	

(Continued)

NURSING CARE PLAN FOR THE PATIENT WITH ADDISON'S DISEASE *(Continued)*

NURSING DIAGNOSIS/PROBLEM 2: Potential alterations in electrolyte balance related to hyperkalemia, which may result in electrocardiographic changes and muscle weakness or paralysis.

GOAL 2.1: To prevent or to detect early hyperkalemia

Nursing Interventions	Rationale	Outcome Criteria
1. Monitor serum potassium values.	1. As aldosterone levels fall because of adrenocortical insufficiency, renal-tubule excretion of potassium is decreased, resulting in higher circulating potassium levels.	1–3. Absence of hyperkalemia as evidenced by: normal serum potassium levels and no neuromuscular or cardiovascular signs of hyperkalemia.
2. Watch for signs of hyperkalemia, such as muscle weakness, paresthesias, paralysis, cardiac arrhythmias, and gastrointestinal upset.	2. Potassium is a major intracellular cation essential for normal neuromuscular activity. High serum potassium levels can cause disturbances in muscle function of the heart (widened QRS complexes, prolonged Q-T interval, ventricular fibrillation), the skeletal muscles (muscle weakness, paraesthesia, or paralysis), and the gastrointestinal system (nausea, diarrhea).	1–2. Elevated serum potassium and signs and symptoms of hyperkalemia detected at its onset.
3. Encourage an intake of a low potassium diet. Instruct the patient of the importance of such a diet.	3. To prevent further potassium loading, a restriction on potassium intake should be instituted. Foods high in potassium and thus to be avoided include bananas, melons, prunes, dates, citrus fruits, avocadoes, molasses, and some salt substitutes. Understanding the rationale of such a diet will increase the patient's compliance.	

NURSING DIAGNOSIS/PROBLEM 3: Coping deficit related to decreased cortisol levels, which may result in extreme emotional liability and stress intolerance

GOAL 3.1: To minimize physical and emotional stressors

Nursing Interventions	Rationale	Outcome Criteria
1. Control environmental stressors.	1. The patient with Addison's disease often experiences mental changes such as depression, irritability, anxiety, and apprehension. Normal stress responses are lacking. Extreme prostration may occur after even mild environmental stress.	1–4. The patient will: not be emotionally labile and not exhibit intolerance to stress.
a. Reduce noise from loud talking, radios, or clamor of nurse's station.	a. A noisy environment can be distressing to individuals, particularly in unfamiliar surroundings.	
b. Keep room temperature constant. Bed socks and a warm robe may be used.	b. Temperature extremes can produce physical stress as cardiovascular changes occur to maintain stable body core temperature.	

(Continued)

NURSING CARE PLAN FOR THE PATIENT WITH ADDISON'S DISEASE (*Continued*)

Nursing Interventions	Rationale
c. Encourage arrangement of familiar items (*e.g.,* photographs) around bedside.	c. Unfamiliar surroundings, especially the alien confines of a hospital, can be particularly stressful. Personal articles, family photos, *etc.,* can reduce patient's unease.
2. Deliver consistent nursing care by means of the use of primary caregiver and specific care planning.	2. A nurse who is known and trusted by the patient, and care given with continuity can be reassuring to the patient.
3. Encourage family members to avoid conveying disturbing news to the patient, especially during more stressful periods.	3. Bad news and family squabbles are emotionally stressful and can further compromise the patient who lacks coping stability.
4. Explain all procedures carefully.	4. Careful explanations can help minimize anxiety induced by the unknown.

GOAL 3.2: To facilitate the use of coping strategies and stress relaxation techniques

Nursing Interventions	Rationale	Outcome Criteria
1. Provide an environment conducive of self-expression.	1. Encouraging the patient to verbalize feelings aids in the assessment of his sense of situational control and personal coping strategies. It allows for validation of feelings.	1–2. The patient will: voice feelings related to his emotional state and suggest and carry out alternative coping strategies. Decreased manifestations of emotional ability.
2. Instruct patient on stress-relaxing techniques and assist in practice of them. The following is an example: a. Assume a comfortable lying or sitting position with eyes closed; b. Keep environmental noise low or use soft music; c. Concentrate on slow, deep breathing and feel the heaviness of all extremities; d. If muscles are tense, tighten and relax each muscle group from feet to head; and e. Allow a minimum of 15–20 min for this.	2. Stress relaxation technique is an "emotion-focused" coping strategy to aid in reducing stress-related physiological and emotional manifestations (see Chap. 73 for more discussion).	

(*Continued*)

NURSING CARE PLAN FOR THE PATIENT WITH ADDISON'S DISEASE (*Continued*)

NURSING DIAGNOSIS/PROBLEM 4: Activity intolerance related to muscle weakness and fatigue, which can result in frustration, apathy, and impaired performance of self-care activities.

GOAL 4.1: To promote optimal level of physical functioning

Nursing Interventions	Rationale	Outcome Criteria
1. Reduce energy expenditure when possible.	1. Muscle weakness and fatigue is brought on by altered carbohydrate metabolism and potassium wasting. Reducing energy demands can increase physical endurance.	1–2. The patient will: progress to highest activity level possible, identify factors and carry out behaviors that promote activity tolerance, and report satisfaction with level of physical abilities.
a. Plan rest periods according to the patient's daily schedule (between activities).	a. Sufficient rest periods helps restore rapidly depleted energy stores.	
b. Activities should be increased gradually.	b. Progressive buildup of activities promotes tolerance and physical endurance, and the patient's endurance directly affects the rehabilitation process.	
2. Provide incentive for involvement in and progress of activity.	2. Activity intolerance often breeds frustration, discouragement, and apathy.	
a. Help patient set appropriate activity schedule and goals.	a. Achievable goals can bring about even small successes to inspire the patient.	
b. Convey a positive attitude to the patient regarding his mobility status.	b. A positive attitude conveys to the patient a belief that he can improve his level of functioning, thus encouraging goal attainment.	

NURSING DIAGNOSIS/PROBLEM 5: Alterations in nutritional status related to nausea and anorexia, which may result in a greater risk of hypoglycemia.

GOAL 5.1: To prevent hypoglycemic episodes through promotion of sufficient nutrional intake to meet caloric requirements

Nursing Interventions	Rationale	Outcome Criteria
1. Encourage the desire to eat.	1. Anorexia and nausea are vague manifestations of cortisol deficit, having both physiological and psychological foundations.	1–4. The patient will: take in sufficient protein, carbohydrate, and calories to meet body requirements; report increased desire to eat; maintain normal blood glucose levels with no signs and symptoms of hypoglycemia; avoid meal omissions; and discuss rationale for the importance of maintaining a sufficient nutritional intake.
a. Maintain good oral hygiene.	a. Good oral hygiene improves the taste of food and can increase the desire to eat.	
b. Provide frequent, appropriately sized meals that are attractively served at proper temperature.	b. Smaller, attractively served meals appear less overwhelming to the patient who lacks the desire to eat.	
c. Determine the patient's eating habits and cultural preference and allow independence at mealtimes.	c. Allowing the patient as much input into his food preferences and as much independence as possible may improve his sense of control, minimize frustration, and improve appetite.	

(*Continued*)

NURSING CARE PLAN FOR THE PATIENT WITH ADDISON'S DISEASE (*Continued*)

Nursing Interventions	Rationale
2. Monitor serum glucose levels.	2. A deficit in cortisol results in reduced hepatic gluconeogenesis, thus decreasing circulating blood glucose levels.
3. Provide a diet high in protein and carbohydrates and encourage between-meals and bedtime snacks.	3. Adults require a 1600–3000 Cal intake (based on age, body size, emotional state, activity level, and metabolism) to meet the average daily metabolic requirements. Intermittent snacks decrease the risk of episodic hypoglycemia.
4. Caution patient to avoid periods of fasting or meal omission.	4. Fasting is not well tolerated by individuals with Addison's disease because compensatory hepatic gluconeogenesis is impaired.

NURSING DIAGNOSIS/PROBLEM 6: Potential noncompliance to long-term disease management related to the chronic nature of the disease, resulting in exacerbation of the disorder

GOAL 6.1: To promote patient compliance and disease control

Nursing Interventions	Rationale	Outcome Criteria
1. Assess patient's perception of his illness and its treatment.	1. Inaccurate perceptions held by the patient about his disease and its treatment must be identified and corrected. Misunderstandings of the nature and seriousness of the illness and susceptibility to complications can greatly affect compliance.	1–3. The patient will: verbalize fears, frustrations, and anxiety related to the disease or its treatment. The patient will have accurate perceptions about the nature of the disease and its treatment. The patient will accurately discuss the nature of the illness, the importance of lifelong management, and the prescribed treatment as listed. The patient will actively participate in the health behaviors prescribed or desired for disease control.
2. Encourage the patient to express any fears or frustrations he has related to his health needs.	2. Fears and frustrations about prescribed treatment (whether valid or not) can interfere with compliance and must be discussed openly for effective problem solving to take place.	
3. Teach patient and his family about the nature of the disease, the importance of lifelong management, and the following prescribed treatment plan: intake of high sodium, high protein, high carbohydrate, low potassium diet; avoid omitting meals; proper self-administration of steroids (see Table 76–5); increased fluid intake; wearing Medic-Alert identification bracelet naming the disease and emergency procedures; carrying at all times an emergency kit with hydrocortisone or dexamethasone for parenteral use; and the importance of lifelong regular medical checkups.	3. Teaching is important for longterm control of Addison's disease. It requires active participation of the patient and family to enhance learning retention. Information should be conveyed clearly and in a relaxed environment with repetition and written handouts. A thorough understanding of the illness and its treatment can aid in the patient's acceptance and successful participation in disease management.	

Hyperfunction of the Adrenal Medulla: Pheochromocytoma

The adrenal medulla is, in reality, an extension of the sympathetic nervous system. The medullary production of catecholamines, epinephrine, and norepinephrine is important in protecting the individual from hypoglycemia and in mobilizing energy stores for use in times of preconceived danger. The principal disorder of the adrenal medulla is pheochromocytoma.

Etiology and Pathology

Pheochromocytoma is a rare, often benign tumor that originates from the chromaffin cells and secretes catecholamines in excess. These tumors can be malignant but are difficult to differentiate histologically. Some tumors may be found in extra-adrenal structures, especially in paraganglionic tissue within the sympathetic nervous system. However, the majority (85%) reside within the medulla of one or both adrenal glands. The right gland is affected more often than the left.[13] Overproduction of epinephrine only occurs in adrenal pheochromocytomas, whereas excessive norepinephrine production can be found in both adrenal and extra-adrenal tumors.

The incidence of pheochromocytoma is small, occuring in about 36,000 Americans and accounting for fewer than 1000 deaths annually. It commonly occurs between the fourth and sixth decades in less than 1% of patients with high blood pressure but can be found at any age in men and women.[1]

Clinical Manifestations

All symptoms of pheochromocytoma are related to the increased circulation of catecholamines and their effects on body tissues. The hallmark manifestation of these tumors is high blood pressure. In the classic presentation, high blood pressure is paroxysmal with blood pressure elevations of 200 to 300 mmHg systolic and 150 to 175 mmHg diastolic, in response to spontaneous and paroxysmal release of catecholamines. In many individuals, sustained high blood pressure makes it difficult to distinguish pheochromocytoma from essential hypertension. They will, however, have paroxysmal attacks at some point in their disease.[4] Curiously, two thirds of all patients with pheochromocytoma will demonstrate postural hypotension.

Other symptoms associated with catecholamine excess are palpitations, profuse diaphoresis, vertigo, pounding headaches, nervousness, flushing, and pallor. Still others are nausea and vomiting, constipation, abdominal pain, penile pain, and dysuria. These symptoms are probably provoked by spincter spasm and decreased peristalsis.[6] The insulin-inhibitive and hepatic glycogenolytic effects of catecholamines often produces hyperglycemia with glucosuria, polyuria, and polydipsia. In 14% of patients with pheochromocytoma, signs are atypical or absent.

Paroxysmal attacks can occur spontaneously or be induced by a variety of stimuli such as physical exertion, strong emotions, cold, smoking, eating, alcohol, some anesthetic agents, intercourse, position change, bladder distention, or straining at stool.[6] Paroxysmal attacks may also be precipitated by tyramine-containing foods (such as cheese) and monoamine oxidase (MAO) inhibiting drugs, usually taken in conjunction. Sometimes the effects of combined ingestion of MAO inhibitors and tyramine-rich foods may mimic pheochromocytoma, and a differential diagnosis must be made.

The conditions most likely to be confused with pheochromocytoma are intracranial lesions, transient ischemic attacks, hyperthyroidism, anxiety reactions, menopause, essential hypertension, and angina pectoris. Pheochromocytoma can also occur in conjunction with medullary carcinoma of the thyroid gland and hyperparathyroidism. The combined disease entity is known as multiple endocrine neoplasia type II (MEN type II, Sipple's syndrome.)[9]

Medical Management

The diagnosis of pheochromocytoma can be made in about 90% of patients on the basis of laboratory data. Screening 24-hour urine collections for catecholamines and their metabolites is the most common diagnostic tool. Urinary metanephrine, a catecholamine derivative, gives the most reliable measurement. Urinary vanillylmandelic acid (VMA), a metabolite of epinephrine, can also be measured, but it is more difficult to measure accurately.[4] Elevation in either metanephrine or VMA levels is indicative of pheochromocytoma. (See Chapter 72 for specific laboratory studies.)

Surgical removal of the tumor is the treatment of choice and is successful in 90% of cases. The tumor is usually located by angiography, intravenous pyelograms, and CAT scans. To prevent intraoperative and postoperative complications, patients often undergo pharmacological control of their symptoms during the week before surgery. Adrenergic blocking agents, such as phenoxybenzamine (Dibenzyline) and propranolol (Inderal), drugs which inhibit the systemic effects of catecholamines, may be administered. An intravenous infusion of phentolamine (Regitine), an α-adrenergic blocking agent, may be administered during surgery to prevent extremely high blood pressure that often occurs with induction of anesthesia and tumor manipulation. Intravenous nitroprusside (a potent vasodilator) may also be used for intraoperative control or for management of paroxysmal hypertensive crises. An alternative class of drugs is being used with increasing frequency to stabilize patients preoperatively or to control symptoms in patients with pheochromocytoma who are not candidates for surgery. This class of drugs works to inhibit synthesis of catecholamines. One such drug is metyrosine (Demser), which inhibits hydroxylase, an important enzyme in the synthesis of norepinephrine.[5]

For patients for whom surgery is not possible or for those who are not improved by surgery, long-term control with adrenergic blocking agents is prescribed. From preliminary reports a new drug, alpha-methyl-para-tyrosine, appears quite promising for these individuals.

Postoperatively, shock is of greatest concern, and it is usually combated with volume expanders and vasopressor agents. It should be noted, however, that this shock may be unresponsive to norepinephrine infusion.[6] If the tumor has originated in the adrenal gland, then postoperative care is the same as that following an adrenalectomy.

Nursing Management Plan

A major nursing consideration is the identification of the hypertensive patients with accompanying signs of excessive catecholamine discharge, and their referral for definitive evaluation.

Assessment and Nursing Diagnosis. Once the diagnosis of pheochromocytoma has been made the greatest nursing concern is related to severe episodic high blood pressure. Nursing diagnoses might include alterations in comfort due to headaches,. and potential for alteration in tissue perfusion (stroke) resulting in neurological deficits. Another problem may be anxiety related to headache discomfort and increased circulating catecholamines due to the nature of the illness.

Goals. With effective nursing interventions, it is hoped that there will be stabilization of blood pressure, early detection or prevention of neurological impairment, and promotion of comfort and relaxation.

Interventions. Throughout the hospital stay, careful assessment of vital signs and emotional support is an essential part of the nursing care plan. The patient should be on bed rest with the head of the bed elevated at least 45 degrees to take advantage of the orthostatic drop in blood pressure known to occur in many patients with pheochromocytoma.[5] Potential triggers for hypertensive attacks might include controlling room temperature, administering stool softeners to prevent constipation, and providing a calm environment for the patient. While awaiting surgical intervention, the patient may be receiving sympathetic blocking agents. The side-effects of these drugs include nasal congestion, tachycardia, arrhythmias, gastrointestinal disturbance, and flushing. These adverse effects should be discussed with the patient and closely monitored. During times of exaggerated elevations in blood pressure, the associated headache may be quite severe yet unresponsive to prescribed analgesics. Relaxation techniques (see Chap. 73) and cutaneous stimulation, such as cold packs and back rubs, may be tried. Throughout the hypertensive episode, neurological assessments should be made and changes reported.

Evaluation of Goal Achievement. Expected outcomes of nursing interventions include the return of blood pressure within normal limits. The patient will manifest no signs of neurological deterioration and report improvement in level of comfort. Finally the patient will discuss the purpose and side-effects of prescribed drugs and utilize behaviors aimed at reducing the risk of paroxysmal hypertensive attacks.

Nursing Care of the Adrenalectomy Patient

Surgical removal of part of the adrenal glands or one or both adrenal glands (adrenalectomy) is performed as treatment for a variety of disorders of the adrenal cortex and medulla. Surgery of this type has greater risks for the patient than most other surgical procedures. Manipulation of the glands can cause an excessive release of adrenal hormones into the circulation.

Preoperative Care. Nutritional support is important in promoting optimum physical stamina to withstand the rigors of surgery and improve wound healing postoperatively. A diet high in protein and vitamins is helpful, especially since glucocorticoid excess produces a state of catabolism. Electrolyte imbalances should also be corrected, for example, potassium supplements and foods rich in potassium are given to patients with hyperfunction of the adrenal cortex.

Emotional preparation for the adrenalectomy is similar to that for other operations. The surgical procedure is explained and also what postoperative activities can be expected. The patient should be informed about intravenous infusions, hemodynamic monitoring techniques, nasogastric suctioning, and the like. Instructions about postoperative coughing, deep breathing, and turning in bed give the patient confidence and ensure compliance. This compliance is particularly important because these patients are prone to infection.

Postoperative Care. After a bilateral adrenalectomy, the patient becomes suddenly depleted of adrenocortical hormones and adrenal medullary catecholamines. The patient behaves as any individual with adrenal insufficiency and is likely to suffer an acute adrenal crisis.

Blood pressure, along with fluid and electrolyte levels, can fluctuate widely postoperatively, especially in the first 48 hours. Electrocardiographic monitoring and arterial, central venous and, at times, pulmonary artery wedge pressure monitoring are done during and after surgery. Replacement glucocorticoids are given intravenously until oral doses are tolerated. Cortisol may be given on the day of surgery to help the patient withstand the stress of surgery. Hypovolemic shock is combated with appropriate fluid replacement and vasopressors. Nursing assessments are important in evaluating the patient's response to therapy. Intake and output must be accurately measured, and vital signs must be measured frequently. The nurse must also be alert for signs of adrenal insufficiency, such as lethargy, apathy, nausea and vomiting, hypoglycemia, and hypokalemia. These signs should be reported immediately.

Immediately after surgery, the patient is maintained by taking nothing by mouth. Diet is gradually introduced according to tolerance. When oral intake is possible, a diet relatively high in protein and carbohydrates is prescribed. Periods of prolonged fasting may not be well tolerated by these patients and should be avoided because fasting can precipitate hypoglycemic episodes. The nurse should anticipate stressful situations for the patient and prevent them. Sufficient rest periods along with comfort measures are also given.

Because wound healing may be impaired, wound drainage and temperature should be monitored. Only strict aseptic techniques are used in dressing changes. Splinting the wound during coughing and turning helps alleviate wound stress. In preparing for discharge, comprehensive teaching is carried out to help the patient cope with lifelong management of adrenal insufficiency. The teaching plan would be similar to that for the patient with Addison's disease.

Summary

Disorders of the adrenal gland are varied and demonstrate a staggering array of clinical manifestations. The problems encountered by patients with adrenal dysfunction result from either an excess or a deficit of adrenal hormones. Caring for individuals with adrenal disorders requires a basic understanding of normal adrenal physiology and the actions of adrenal hormones. Early identification and referral of patients with adrenal abnormality are common nursing goals. The physical manifestations of these abnormalities can be both frightening and discouraging to the sufferer. Psychological support is as important as physiological support in helping these patients cope with their illness and in alleviating the stress that they are poorly able to tolerate. Because of the chronic nature of many adrenal disorders, educating the patient to comply with the necessary therapeutic regimens is especially important in establishing control of the disease process.

References

1. Arcangelo VP: Adrenal disorders. Diseases: Nurses Reference Library. Nursing 83 Books. Springhouse, Intermed Communications, 1983
2. Brunner LS, Suddarth DS (eds): The Lippincott Manual of Nursing Practice, 3rd ed. Philadelphia, JB Lippincott, 1982
3. Byyny RL: Preventing adrenal insufficiency during surgery. Postgrad Med 67:219–225, 1980
4. Camunas C: Pheochromocytoma. Am J Nurs 83: 887–891, 1983
5. Cryer PE et al: Diagnostic Endocrinology, 2nd ed. New York, Oxford University Press, 1979
6. Engleman K: The adrenal medulla and the sympathetic nervous system. In Wyngaarden JB, Smith LH (eds): Cecil's Textbook of Medicine, 16th ed. Philadelphia, WB Saunders, 1982
7. Gold EM: Cushing's syndrome: A tripartite entity. Hosp Pract 14:67–75, 1979
8. Gotch PM: Teaching patients about adrenal corticosteroids. Am J Nurs 81:78–81, 1981
9. Harvey AM, Johns RJ, Owens AH et al (eds): The Principles and Practice of Medicine, 20th ed. New York, Appleton-Century-Crofts, 1980
10. Hurwitz, LS: Nursing implication of selected pediatric endocrine problems. Nurs Clin North Am 15:525–534, 1980
11. Isselbacher KJ, Adams RD, Braunwald E et al (eds): Harrison's Principles of Internal Medicine, 9th ed. New York, McGraw-Hill, 1980
12. James VH (ed): The Adrenal Gland. New York, Raven Press, 1979
13. Jubiz W: Endocrinology: A Logical Approach for Clinicians. New York, McGraw-Hill, 1979
14. Kaplan S: Disorders of the adrenal gland, I. Pediatr Clin North Am 26:77–89, 1979
15. Nicholls MG, Espiner EA, Highes H et al: Primary aldosteronism. Am J Med 59:334–342, 1978
16. Rush DR, Hamburger SC: Drugs used in endocrine metabolic emergencies. Critical Care Quarterly 3:1–8, 1980
17. Sanford SJ: Dysfunction of the adrenal gland: Physiological considerations and nursing problems. Nurs Clin North Am 15:481–498, 1980
18. Schimke RN: Adrenal insufficiency. Critical Care Quarterly 3:19–27, 1980
19. Schteingart DE: Cushing's disease: An update. Drug Ther 8:125–135, 1978
20. Tzagournis M: Acute adrenal insufficiency. Heart Lung, 7:603–609, 1978
21. Williams RH (ed): Textbook of Endocrinology. Philadelphia, WB Saunders, 1981
22. Wilson CB, Tyrrell JB, Fitzgerald P: Cushing's disease revisited. Am J Surg 138:77–79, 1979

Bibliography

Atuk NO: Pheochromocytoma: Diagnosis, localization and treatment. Hosp Pract 18:186–202, 1983

Bissada NK: Surgical diseases of the adrenal gland. Am Fam Physician 15:130–135, 1977

Dillon RG: Handbook of Endocrinolgoy, 2nd ed. Philadelphia, Lea & Febiger, 1980

Gever LN: Reducing the side-effects of steroid therapy. Nursing 80 10:59, 1980

Gold EM: The Cushing's syndromes: Changing views of diagnosis and treatment. Ann Intern Med 90:829–844, 1979

Hall R: Fundamentals of Clinical Endocrinology, 3rd ed. Chicago, Year Book Medical Publishers, 1981

Hart IR, Newton RW: Endocrinology, Vol 2. Baltimore, University Park Press, 1983

Hershman JM: Management of Endocrine Disorders. Philadelphia, Lea & Febiger, 1980

Javadpour N, Woltering EA, Brennan MF et al: Adrenal neoplasms. Curr Probl Surg 17:1–52, 1980

Jones SG: Adrenal patient—proceed with caution. RN 45:66–72, 1982

Jones SG: Bilateral adrenalectomy: Post-op dangers to watch for. RN 45(2):66–69, 1982

Katz FH: Adrenocortical diseases: Identification and management. Postgrad Med 66:52–65, 1979

Koppers LE: Pheochromocytoma—critical care. Critical Care Quarterly 3:93–97, 1980

Krueger J, Ray J: Endocrine Problems in Nursing. St Louis, CV Mosby, 1976

Prinz RA, Brooks MH, Lawrence AM et al: Cushing's disease: The role of adrenalectomy and autotransplantation. Surg Clin North Am 59(1):159–165, 1979

Rincon J, Greenblatt RB, Schwartz RP et al: Not Cushing's syndrome. Am Fam Physician 19(5):77–86, 1979

Robinson AG: Acute adrenal insufficiency: Addisonian crisis. Topics in Emergency Medicine 5:40–44, 1984

Ryan WG: Endocrine Disorders: A Pathologic Approach. Chicago, Year Book Medical Publishers, 1980

Tepley JF, Lawrence GH: Pheochromocytoma. Am J Surg 140:107–111, 1980

Toward safer use of topical steroids. Emergency Medicine 30:12, 1980

Voorhess M: Disorders of the adrenal medulla and multiple endocrine adenomatosis. Pediatr Clin North Am 26:209–222, 1979

White DJ, Williamson K: What to watch for with synthetic adrenocortical steroids. RN 43:37–39, 1980

White V, Kumagi L: Preoperative endocrine and metabolic considerations. Med Clin North Am 63:1321–1334, 1979

Chapter 77

Disorders of the Pituitary Gland and Hypothalamus

Christine A. Larson

The pituitary–hypothalamic axis exerts prime control over the body's hormonal functions. The intimate relationship between the hypothalamus and the pituitary gland and their effects on other endocrine structures are discussed in Chapter 71. A disorder arising in the hypothalamus or in the pituitary gland can produce a variety of abnormalities within the target organs, such as the thyroid, adrenals and gonads. Alterations in the secretion of pituitary hormones can be selective, involving an increase in one or more hormones and a concomitant suppression of others. In consequence, it is extremely difficult to classify and describe all possible pituitary syndromes.[9] The diversity creates a challenge for nurses to meet the complex needs of patients with pituitary disorders.

Dysfunctions of the anterior and posterior pituitary lobes will be discussed separately in this chapter. To gain a better understanding of the complexity of pituitary syndromes, the reader is encouraged first to review Chapter 71 on the anatomy and physiology of the endocrine system.

The anterior pituitary (adenohypophysis) is sometimes referred to as the master gland because it produces and secretes six major trophic hormones that affect not only target glands but have widespread effects on body tissues. Together these hormones greatly influence the body's metabolism, stature, sexual maturation, and intellectual development.[6] Release or inhibition of these trophic hormones occurs in response to the secretion of releasing or inhibiting hormones from the hypothalamus. The hypothalamus, in turn, is responsible for continuous surveillance of the body's internal and external environment. Through a dynamic adaptive process, it assists the body in meeting its changing needs. Certain pathological conditions can give rise to excessive release of one or more pituitary hormones. The target gland or tissue of that hormone will respond with overactivity, unless the gland itself is diseased and unable to respond. For instance, increased release of adrenocorticotropic hormone (ACTH) will cause excessive stimulation of the adrenal cortex, resulting in Cushing's syndrome. The opposite is also true. Decreased secretion of a trophic hormone can cause hypofunction of the target gland. Disorders will be discussed as consequences of either hyperfunction or hypofunction of the anterior pituitary gland.

Hyperfunction of the Anterior Pituitary Gland: Hyperpituitarism

Hyperpituitarism is the excessive production and secretion of one or more trophic hormones from the anterior pituitary gland. Hypersecretion is most often the result of a secreting pituitary adenoma. The incidence of pituitary adenomas is less than 1/100,000 population per year.[10] Pituitary adenomas are found primarily in the 30- to 50-year age-group, but may occur in much younger individuals. The manifestations of these adenomas vary according to the type of tumor involved (acidophil, chromotrope, or basophil), the nature of the trophic hormone secreted, and the age of the individual. Aberrations of growth hormone and prolactin secretion are the most common disturbances associated with hyperfunction of the anterior pituitary gland. The consequences of excessive prolactin secretion (galactorrhea) are discussed in Chapter 102. Since excesses of other trophic hormones are discussed in chapters pertaining to disorders of their target glands, only disturbances of growth hormone secretion will be examined here.

Growth Hormone Excess: Acromegaly and Gigantism

Etiology and Pathophysiology

Acromegaly is the result of sustained hypersecretion of growth hormone (GH) by benign acidophilic (or mixed acidophilic and chromophobe) tumors of the pituitary. Malignancies are less common causes. It is a relatively rare, chronic disease of middle age affecting men and women equally. Acromegaly is characterized by continued growth of bone and connective tissue in the acral (distal) parts of the body, that is, the hands, feet, and face.[9] The disease most frequently becomes conspicuous during the third and fourth decades of life, although a few patients can trace the onset of disease to adolescence or, even more rarely, to childhood.

When there is hypersecretion of GH prior to the onset of puberty (closure of the epiphyseal plates), longitudinal growth accelerates and the result is *gigantism*. An arbitrary definition of gigantism is attainment of height that is three standard deviations above the normal mean height for the age.[13] True gigantism is an extremely rare disease which, like acromegaly, usually results from a pituitary adenoma. Fifty percent of individuals with gigantism have acromegalic features (Fig. 77–1). It is not uncommon to see these giants attain heights of 8 ft or more, have disproportionately long limbs, and weigh over 300 lb. These statural abnormalities (without the acromegalic features) may be due to inherited traits or may be part of a hypogonadal (eunuchoid) syndrome. Such causes must be ruled out.

Both acromegaly and gigantism may be accompanied by signs of hypersecretion of other trophic hormones. However, as the disease progresses and the tumor enlarges, pressure from the expanding tumor mass may actually cause hyposecretion of the trophic hormones. The patient with gigantism usually dies before the age of 21, often succumbing to infection and various hormonal imbalances.[6]

Clinical Manifestations

The clinical features of acromegaly fall into three major groups:

1. Symptoms caused by pressure from the increasing tumor mass

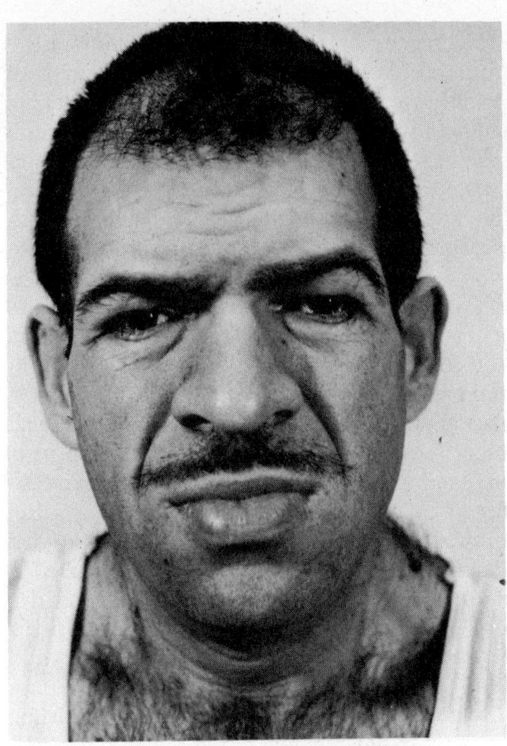

FIGURE 77–1 One of the characteristics of acromegaly is coarsening of the facial features. (Ezrin C, Godden JO, Volpe R [eds]: Systemic Endocrinology, 2nd ed, p 67. New York, Harper & Row, 1979)

2. Metabolic changes produced by excessive GH secretion and altered secretion of other trophic hormones
3. Symptoms due to enlargement of bones, soft tissues, and viscera

The onset of acromegaly is often so insidious and subtle that it escapes early detection.

Tumor Pressure. The pituitary gland rests within a cranial vault, known as the sella turcica. Headaches are the most common local manifestation of pituitary tumors, with or without marked pituitary enlargement. The headache is usually variable in intensity and location. Visual defects, characteristically bitemporal hemianopia, occur as pressure increases on the inferior aspect of the optic chiasm.[10] Another sign of increasing pressure is optic pallor detected on retinal examination. If this pressure is not relieved, eventual blindness with optic atrophy results. Rarely do signs of confusion and memory impairment occur. Equally uncommon yet potential symptoms are related to suprasellar extension of the tumor. These symptoms might include dysfunction of the third, fourth, or sixth cranial nerves, along with alterations in appetite, sleep, and temperature regulation.

Growth Hormone Excess. Growth hormone directly inhibits peripheral glucose uptake and antagonizes the effects of insulin, thus hypersecretion of GH predisposes the patient to hyperglycemia. Glucose intolerance is present in 50% of affected patients but overt diabetes mellitus occurs in only 10% to 15%. The usual symptoms accompany hyperglycemia, such as polyuria and polydipsia. However, ketoacidosis and vascular complications are exceedingly rare.[13] Growth hormone increases renal tubular reabsorption of phosphate while promoting excretion of urinary calcium. The latter results in high urinary concentration of calcium and increases the incidence of renal stones, often found in acromegalics. Excessive levels of GH also increase the basal metabolic rate and cause hypertrophy of sweat glands with hyperhidrosis (profuse diaphoresis). Most patients find the latter symptom particularly distressing. Hypertension is found in 30% of acromegalics, but the reason for this is unclear.[10] It may be related to adrenocortical stimulation with increased cortisol secretion.

Increased production of other trophic hormones, most notably prolactin, ACTH, and gonadotropins may be evident, but with no consistency in their manifestations. Hyperprolactinemia more commonly accompanies growth hormone excess, manifested by complaints of amenorrhea and galactorrhea (inappropriate, excessive breast milk secretion) in women or impotency in males. Libido may be increased at the onset of acromegaly but is lost as the course of the disease progresses.[13] Hirsutism, with unwanted facial hair, is occasionally present in female acromegalics.

Musculoskeletal Hypertrophy. Increased circulating levels of GH result in enlargement of the skeleton, muscle, soft tissue, and viscera and in thickening of the skin. These changes are so slow in evolving that they often go unrecognized for years, until the disease has become exceedingly advanced. There is often a history of progressive increases in shoe, hat, and glove size. The patient may notice that old rings are becoming increasingly tight. Although the patient is often overweight and appears large, he is typically not obese.

In acromegaly, bone overgrowth is the most striking feature. The brow ridges are prominent, giving the forehead a jutting or "neanderthal" appearance. As the maxilla lengthens, the teeth are spread apart. The ribs and clavicles widen and lengthen considerably. Anterior–posterior thickening of the vertebral bodies may produce thoracic kyphosis, making forward flexion of the spine difficult. The long bones are broadened. The legs become bowed and produce a characteristic rolling gait.[9] Soft-tissue mass is greatly increased, giving the hands a thick, fleshy spadelike appearance and causing enlargement of the tongue, lips, ears, and nose. Facial wrinkles become exaggerated. Vocal cords thicken, causing deepening of the voice in 50% of patients.[13] The skin appears oily, thick, and has a rubbery texture.

Continued growth of cartilage, bones, and soft tissues of the hands and wrist results in carpal tunnel syndrome, caused by compression of the median nerve with acroparesthesias in 30% of acromegalics.[10] Other peripheral nerves may also be involved. In addition, synovial and capsular changes in the joints, along with cartilage hypertrophy, frequently cause arthralgias and deforming arthritis.

Hypertrophy of skeletal muscles and easy fatigability are common in acromegaly. Atrophy of large muscle groups may be found in the later stages of the disease. The viscera are generally enlarged. The brain, lungs, thyroid, kidneys, salivary glands, and heart are enlarged twofold to fivefold. Hepatomegaly and splenomegaly can occur but, if they are seen, the presence of a secondary disease must be ruled out. Hypertrophy of the heart, along with altered fat metabolism, predisposes the patient to the development of atherosclerosis and cardiac decompensation. Ventricular ectopic beats and intraventricular conduction defects are common. Death is often due to cardiovascular disease or pituitary apoplexy (expansion or hemorrhage of the pituitary tumor).[7]

Medical Management

The key to treatment is early diagnosis. Initial suspicion of the disease arises with the appearance of the classic acromegalic features. Comparing the patient's current appearance with old photographs is often helpful. Radioimmunoassay demonstrates increased plasma GH levels. However, random sampling can be misleading, since GH is not secreted at a steady rate.[9] Stimuli such as food ingestion, stress, sleep, exercise, and diurnal variation markedly affect GH concentration. It is known that glucose normally suppresses GH secretion. Therefore, the diagnosis of acromegaly can be confirmed when a glucose infusion fails to lower serum GH levels. (See diagnostic studies in Chapter 72.) Radiographic studies of the skull reveal an enlarged and distorted sella turcica. Assessment of visual fields and acuity can help determine the extent of pressure on the optic chiasm. Computerized axial tomography (CT scan), arteriography, and pneumoencephalography can evaluate the presence and extent of the pituitary lesion.

Treatment is aimed at normalizing serum GH levels without affecting normal pituitary functioning. Therapeutic approaches using irradiation or surgery are enjoying widespread use at present.

Surgery. When the tumor has extended beyond the sella turcica, surgical intervention is recommended. Removal of the pituitary gland (hypophysectomy) can be done by means of a transfrontal craniotomy when the tumor is found to involve the optic chiasm. However, transphenoidal hypophysectomy is the procedure of choice.[4] Selective removal of the adenoma or, in rare cases, total removal of the pituitary gland can be done using this simple, relatively safe surgical procedure. An incision is made in the inner aspect of the upper lip at the gum line. The pituitary gland is reached by entering through the nasal septum and the sphenoid sinus; visualization is aided by use of a microscope (Fig. 77–2). In nearly 90% of patients, improvement of acromegaly has been reported following transphenoidal hypophysectomy.[9] Complications are relatively few, especially if the posterior pituitary gland remains intact. Cryosurgery has also frequently been done to debulk pituitary tumors. The incidence of hypopituitarism is high postoperatively with all surgical procedures and requires attention.

Irradiation. Several means of irradiation can be employed with varying degrees of success. External irradiation can alleviate some symptoms temporarily, but often requires extremely high doses (5500 rads), which can damage adjacent brain tissue. Irradiation with accelerated proton beams can focus directly upon the pituitary gland and is able to deliver over 9000 rads while sparing surrounding tissue. Proton irradiation has a very high degree of success. Unfortunately, the maximal benefits may not become apparent for 3 to 5 years.[10] Radioactive implantation of the pituitary with

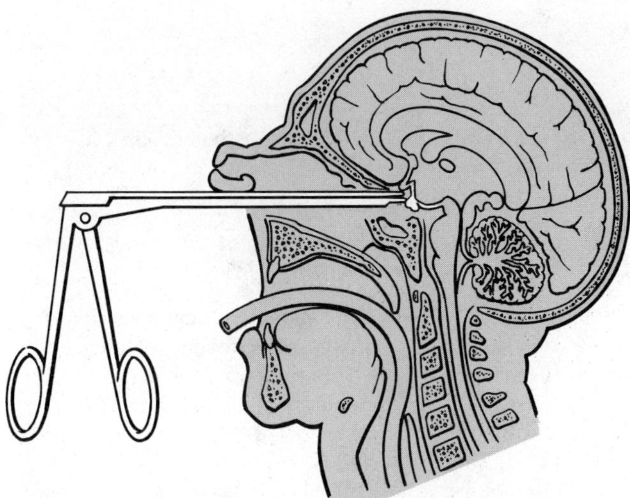

FIGURE 77–2 Transsphenoidal hypophysectomy for surgical approach to the pituitary gland.

yttrium (^{90}Y) and other radionuclides is performed more frequently in Europe than in the United States. While reported to be effective, troublesome complications such as persistent rhinorrhea and meningitis are common.

Pharmacotherapy. Pharmaceutical interventions have not proved successful for long-term use. Bromocryptine (a dopamine antagonist) is probably the most promising among pharmaceutical agents for management of acromegaly. This drug paradoxically inhibits GH secretion in patients with acromegaly, but its effects are only transitory. Side-effects of bromocryptine (Parlodel), such as gastrointestinal disturbances and postural hypotension, can be avoided by gradually increasing the dose to desired levels over several days. Other drugs, used with less success, include estrogens, chlorpromazine, and medroxyprogesterone.[10] Pharmaceutical intervention is not recommended as first-line management of acromegaly. It is more often prescribed as adjunctive therapy for patients for whom surgery and irradiation are inappropriate.

Ablative pituitary therapy results in permanent deficiency of the trophic hormones supplied by the anterior pituitary. Pituitary hormones are essential for life. Instead of replacing the trophic hormones, which is difficult to do on a long-term basis, the essential hormones produced by the target organs are supplied, such as glucocorticoids, thyroid hormones, and sex hormones. The prognosis is variable and depends on both the underlying cause and the age of onset of altered GH secretion. Often, medical help is not sought until late in the disease when neurological symptoms appear. It should be realized that treatment does not reverse many of the physical manifestations of acromega'.[13]

Nursing Management Plan

With careful and consistent assessment, the nurse can identify an individual with probable GH excess. Identification is easier perhaps for nurses working in outpatient clinics or home health agencies because they often have the opportunity to see a patient repeatedly for an extended period of time. These nurses are more likely to observe the chronic physical changes consistent with acromegaly and gigantism. The growth and developmental patterns in children should be carefully monitored. Sudden accelerations of growth, incongruent with familial traits, justify referral for further evaluation. Questioning adults about continual increases in ring, hat, glove, or shoe size can provide valuable information. If coarse features consistent with acromegaly are noted, the patient should be asked to bring in serial photographs depicting himself over time.[7]

When the diagnosis is made, nursing care should focus on helping the patient cope with undesirable changes in his appearance. Preventing or alleviating complications of the disease is also an important consideration. A sample nursing care plan is outlined in Nursing Care Plan for the Patient with Acromegaly.

Preoperative Care

Before surgery, an attempt to alleviate the patient's fear should be made with an honest, understandable explanation of the scheduled operation and the expected postoperative procedures. Hydrocortisone therapy often begins the night before surgery, because glucocorticoid levels will drop dramatically immediately after surgery.[2] The possibility of postoperative sterility due to hyposecretion of gonadotropin should also be discussed. An environment conducive to ventilation of personal feelings and discussing the patient's concerns must be maintained.

Postoperative Care Following Transphenoidal Hypophysectomy

If a craniotomy is done to correct the pituitary lesion, the postoperative care is that which is routinely indicated for the patient with a craniotomy (see Chap. 67). More often, transphenoidal hypophysectomy is the procedure chosen. Postoperative measures specific for this approach will be described here. Neurological assessments should be made to detect increased intracranial pressure. Vital signs, level of consciousness, pupil equality and responsiveness to light, and motor and sensory function are evaluated. The head of the bed should remain elevated at a 30° angle to promote venous return, thus minimizing intracranial swelling and headache. Headache is a common postoperative complaint. Several other measures can be useful in decreasing intracranial pressure and limiting stress on the operative site within the sella turcica. The patient should be discouraged from coughing, sneezing, or bending at the waist. Stool softeners can be administered to prevent constipation and straining at stool.

Nasal Drainage. The nose is usually packed with gauze for 48 to 72 hours after surgery. It is important for the nurse to carefully assess the amount and type of nasal drainage. Leakage of cerebrospinal fluid from the operative site is a major complication of this surgical procedure. Clear nasal drainage or constant swallowing should alert the nurse to a possible cerebrospinal leak. Normal nasal drainage is devoid

(*Text continues on page 1120*)

NURSING CARE PLAN FOR THE PATIENT WITH ACROMEGALY

NURSING DIAGNOSIS/PROBLEM 1: Altered body image related to the acquired features of acromegaly, which may result in frustration, decreased self-esteem, depression, anger, or social withdrawal.

GOAL 1.1: To promote self-confidence and to assist with reconstruction of altered body image

Nursing Interventions	Rationale	Outcome Criteria
1. Provide an environment conducive to self-expression.	1. The marked changes in body features and libido often associated with acromegaly can be distressing. The patient may hold negative (valid or invalid) subjective judgments about his physical and social competence. Feelings of isolation may ensue. Rebuilding of self-esteem requires a foundation of trust.	1–6. The patient will demonstrate improved self-esteem as evidenced by: ability to make positive statements about his abilities and reassumption of role-related responsibilities.
a. Respect the patient's wishes for privacy.	a. Intrusive procedures and behaviors can threaten the patient's already altered sense of wholeness.	
b. Maintain an open, positive, and accepting attitude toward the patient.	b. Acceptance of the patient's abilities and limitations along with an open, positive attitude enhances the patient's trust in, and success of, the therapeutic program.	
c. Refer to psychological counseling as needed.	c. To promote successful adaptive behaviors, a more in-depth exploration of the patient's attitudes, values, and coping styles may be necessary.	
2. Set reasonable tasks and realistic goals for patient to attain.	2. Unrealistic goals beyond the patient's capabilities can lead to further frustration and hamper growth of self-esteem.	
3. Assist patient in identifying personal strengths and coping resources.	3. Helping the patient identify personal strengths may help minimize his exaggeration of perceived failures. Recognition of sources of support may promote use of such resources.	
4. Clarify any misconceptions the patient may have about himself, his care, and his care-givers.	4. A maladaptive response by a patient to altered body image may include an inaccurate perception of his own abilities and the benefits of treatment.	
5. Encourage maintenance of the patient's role-related responsibilities as he is able.	5. Depression may cause withdrawal by the patient from others and role-related responsibilities that can further damage his self-esteem. Having the patient do as much for himself as he is able can bring a sense of self-worth.	

(Continued)

NURSING CARE PLAN FOR THE PATIENT WITH ACROMEGALY (*Continued*)

Nursing Interventions	Rationale
6. Include family members in planning strategies for emotional support.	6. The family must be able to provide sound support for the patient who may have a long-term coping deficit. Family members may also go through a grieving period related to the patient's physical changes. These feelings must be explored and allowed ventilation.

NURSING DIAGNOSIS/PROBLEM 2: Potential alterations in sensory input related to an enlarging pituitary tumor, which can result in diminished visual acuity and peripheral vision.

GOAL 2.1: To detect early and treat visual impairment

Nursing Interventions	Rationale	Outcome Criteria
1. Routinely assess and document visual acuity, peripheral vision, and extraocular movement.	1. As the pituitary gland tumor enlarges, pressure increases on the inferior aspect of the optic chiasm, which typically results in bitemporal hemianopia. Unrelieved pressure will lead to eventual blindness. Dysfunction of the third, fourth, and sixth cranial nerves may also occur, resulting in abnormal extraocular movement.[9]	1–2. There will be no further deterioration in visual acuity. The patient will promptly notify the nurse or physician of any perceived change in vision.
2. Refer patient for appropriate follow-up if visual changes occur.	2. Early interventions are essential if visual changes occur because increasing pressure in the optic chiasm can result in optic nerve atrophy and irreversible blindness.	

GOAL 2.2: To prevent accidental injury related to visual impairment

Nursing Interventions	Rationale	Outcome Criteria
1. Provide a safe environment.	1. Sensoriperceptual problems greatly increase the risk of accidental injury.	1. There will be no incidence of accidental injury related to visual impairment.
a. Orient patient to placement of furniture, personal items, and toilet facilities in the room.	a. Stumbling over unseen obstacles in unfamiliar surroundings is a serious concern in the visually impaired.	
b. When addressing the patient assume a position within the patient's central field of vision.	b. Bitemporal blindness is the most common visual disturbance found in patients with acromegaly.	

(*Continued*)

NURSING CARE PLAN FOR THE PATIENT WITH ACROMEGALY (*Continued*)

NURSING DIAGNOSIS/PROBLEM 3: Alterations in verbal communication related to slowed, disarticulate speech, which may result in unmet needs and frustration.

GOAL 3.1: To promote optional communications that will facilitate the patient's self-expression and meet the patient's needs

Nursing Interventions	Rationale	Outcome Criteria
1. Allow the patient adequate time to express his problems.	1. Acromegaly results in enlargement of the tongue and thickening of the vocal cords, which may result in garbled and delayed speech. Patience and time are necessary to allow for optimal articulation of the patient's needs.	1–3. The patient will: a. Demonstrate improved ability to express himself; b. Relate decreased frustration with communication; and c. Use alternative methods to enhance communication.
2. Anticipate the patient's needs whenever possible.	2. Speech is a fundamental way of expressing desires and feelings. Poor communication can cause feelings of frustration, anger, confusion, and depression. Accurate anticipation of the patient's needs may decrease such feelings.	
3. Provide alternative methods of communication, such as pad and pencil.	3. Although speech may be affected, the acromegalic is usually able to comprehend the spoken and written word (unless blind). Having the opportunity to clarify his desires using alternative communication methods (*e.g.,* writing) may work to reduce frustration and facilitate fulfillment of the patient's needs.	

NURSING DIAGNOSIS/PROBLEM 4: Alterations in personal hygiene related to profuse diaphoresis and skin oiliness, which may result in general discomfort and affect body image.

GOAL 4.1: To promote optimal personal hygiene and prevent discomfort related to profuse diaphoresis

Nursing Interventions	Rationale	Outcome Criteria
1. Encourage good hygiene with at least daily baths using soap and water.	1. Growth hormone excess often results in hypertrophy of various dermal glands, including sweat glands, which results in profuse diaphoresis and skin oiliness. Because body odor is enhanced by such secretions, frequent baths are important.	1–5. The patient will: a. Appear well groomed; b. Not have offensive odor; c. Carry out behaviors necessary to promote good personal hygiene; d. Appear well hydrated; e. Relate sincere feelings of comfort; f. Demonstrate improved self-esteem (see Problem #1).
2. Change clothing and bedding as needed because of perspiration.	2. Profuse diaphoresis can quickly dampen bedding and clothing, creating discomfort for the patient.	
3. Avoid oil-based lotions on the skin.	3. Skin of an acromegalic is thick and oily, often causing clogged pores and pimples. Oil-based creams and lotions can aggravate the problem.	

(*Continued*)

NURSING CARE PLAN FOR THE PATIENT WITH ACROMEGALY (*Continued*)

Nursing Interventions	Rationale
4. Frequently examine the skin for breakdown.	4. Excessive moisture can cause skin excoriation, particularly at the body folds.
5. Encourage a sufficient fluid intake.	5. Extreme diaphoresis can result in fluid loss of greater than 1 liter in 24 hr. An adequate fluid intake is necessary to prevent possible dehydration.

NURSING DIAGNOSIS/PROBLEM 5: Potential discomfort related to acroparesthesias and arthralgias, which may result in impaired mobility, safety risks, and discouragement.

GOAL 5.1: To reduce discomfort and facilitate safe mobility

Nursing Interventions	Rationale	Outcome Criteria
1. Assess the degree and location of paresthesis and pain. a. Have patient rate pain on scale of 10 (0 = absence of pain; 10 = worst pain).	1. Growth hormone excess can cause an overgrowth of cartilage, bone, and soft tissues, resulting in compression of nerves in the wrist and ankles, thus creating acroparesthesias. In addition, synovial and capsular changes in the joints can frequently cause arthralgia pain. a. Scaling the pain helps the patient effectively describe the pain intensity and response to treatment.	1–4. The patient will: a. Receive validation that the pain exists; b. Relate a reduction in pain and discomfort; c. Demonstrate improved mobility; and d. Behave in such a way that ensures personal safety while he is active.
2. Assist patient with activities as necessary.	2. Ambulation may be compromised because of joint pain or paresthesias of the feet. Such impairments can result in limited activity tolerance or increased risk of falls. Manual dexterity may be decreased becaue of arthralgia, leading to inability to carry out even simple tasks.	
3. Caution patient about handling objects that are potentially hot.	3. Paresthesias of the hands can decrease the patient's ability to accurately gauge temperatures, thus increasing the risk of burns.	
4. Promote a sincere "can do" attitude regarding the patient's pain relief and mobility status.	4. A positive attitude conveys to the patient the belief that he can adjust to activity limitations and improve level of comfort. An optimistic outlook potentiates success of interventions.	

(*Continued*)

NURSING CARE PLAN FOR THE PATIENT WITH ACROMEGALY (*Continued*)

NURSING DIAGNOSIS/PROBLEM 6: Potential glucose intolerance related to excessive hormone, resulting in hyperglycemia and glucosuria

GOAL 6.1: To maintain normal serum and urine glucose levels

Nursing Interventions	Rationale	Outcome Criteria
1. Routinely monitor blood and urine glucose levels.	1. Growth hormone antagonizes the effects of insulin and inhibits peripheral-tissue glucose uptake. Glucose intolerance is found in 50% of acromegalics.	1–4. The patient will: a. Maintain fasting blood glucose of 130–140 mg and glucose-free urine; b. Identify current life stressors and carry out interventions aimed at stress reduction; and c. Adhere to the therapeutic regimen (diet, drugs, and glucose testing).
2. With the patient identify and plan ways to minimize physical, emotional, or environmental stressors.	2. Sress increases the release of cortisol from the adrenal cortex, which stimulates glucose production by means of gluconeogenesis and glycogenolysis.	
3. Place patient on calorie-controlled diet as ordered.	3. A calorie and carbohydrate restriction may be ordered to minimize the glucose load on the system, which already has impaired glucose metabolism.	
4. Administer hypoglycemic agents as ordered.	4. Less than 30% of acromegalics develop overt diabetes mellitus and even fewer require insulin administrations routinely. If diet control alone cannot be achieved, oral hypoglycemic agents may be used.[7]	

of glucose; therefore, the drainage can be tested with a glucose-sensitive strip, such as those used to test glucosuria. A positive result confirms that cerebrospinal fluid is leaking.[2] Such leakage is often accompanied by a persistent and severe supraorbital headache, usually caused when cerebrospinal fluid enters the sinuses. Typically, cerebrospinal fluid leaks resolve in 72 hours with bed rest and head elevation. Antibiotics can be given prophylactically to prevent meningitis.

Possible Adrenal Crisis. Because ACTH can no longer be secreted by the pituitary gland, the patient is in danger of developing acute adrenal insufficiency. Careful surveillance for signs of acute adrenal crisis should be initiated. (See the section Acute Adrenal Crisis in Chapter 76.) Cortisone replacement must be administered regularly and will be required on a lifelong basis. Postoperatively, release of other trophic hormones from target organs may be suppressed due to lack of pituitary releasing hormones. The degree and long-term nature of replacement therapy of specific hormones may not be known with any certainty for several weeks. Hypofunction of all target organs should be evaluated on an acute and long-term basis.

ADH Deficiency. The hypophysectomy may interfere with the hypothalamic stalk and posterior lobe of the pituitary gland, resulting in a deficiency of antidiuretic hormone (ADH). This deficiency is usually temporary, resolving in 2 to 3 weeks. However, its effects are quite dramatic and can prove fatal if specific interventions are not immediately undertaken. Careful monitoring of urine output and specific gravity is essential. A deficiency in ADH will lead to an excessive output of dilute urine, a condition known as diabetes insipidus. Aggressive fluid replacement is usually necessary. Fluid replacement is often guided by urinary output; therefore, a very accurate assessment of output must be made. Pitressin can be administered, as needed, if urine output continues to exceed 300 to 400 ml/hour or if the urine remains dilute with specific gravity below 1.004.[9]

Other Measures. Other immediate postoperative nursing considerations include administration of mild analgesics and cool compresses to the forehead to relieve persistent headaches. If no cerebrospinal fluid leaks are observed, the patient can be up and walking within 24 hours. Since the patient is forced to mouth-breathe because his nose is packed, good oral care is important.

Health Teaching. Long-term care following hypophysectomy is primarily aimed at educating the patient. The importance of continuing hormonal replacement should be emphasized. It is important that the patient and his family understand the nature of the drugs and their doses, routes, time of administration, and side-effects. They should be cautioned against abruptly discontinuing these hormone replacements. They should also be instructed on how to watch for signs of the various hormonal deficiencies. Wearing an identification bracelet and keeping a list of prescribed medications can aid the patient in obtaining appropriate medical care should an emergency arise. Careful lifelong medical follow-up is crucial for the successful management of these patients.

Following surgery, testosterone can be given to men experiencing impotency or alterations in libido. For women, atrophy of the vaginal mucosa is often a problem.[10] Younger women can be treated with estrogens. These changes in sexual and reproductive functioning are often of considerable concern to the patient. Encouraging patients to express their feelings about this matter can prove beneficial. Sometimes referral for appropriate psychological counseling can be made.

Hypofunction of the Anterior Pituitary: Hypopituitarism

Etiology and Pathophysiology

Hypopituitarism is a complex syndrome marked by hyposecretion of trophic hormones from the anterior pituitary gland, with secondary atrophy of the target organs. Pituitary insufficiency may result from destruction of the gland by trauma, irradiation (therapy for head and neck tumors), surgical removal, infections, infiltrative diseases, vascular lesions, and pituitary tumors. Genetic predisposition and hypothalamic lesions can also cause pituitary insufficiency. Other causes are listed in Table 77–1. The terms *panhypopituitarism* and *Simmond's disease* are used synonymously to denote a total absence of pituitary trophic hormones. Nonsecreting pituitary tumors, particularly chromophobe adenoma, are the most common cause of hypopituitarism in the adult male.[4] In children hypopituitarism is usually secondary to a congenital anomaly or to pituitary adenomas (craniophayrngioma). Postpartum necrosis of the pituitary gland due to ischemia (Sheehan's syndrome) is the most common cause of hypopituitarism in females.[9] Sheehan's syndrome usually follows postpartum uterine hemorrhagic shock, although it can be associated with other causes. Typically this syndrome develops insidiously over a decade or more. Failure to lactate, involution of the breasts, and persistent amenorrhea, followed by loss of axillary and pubic hair are early manifestations.[13] Occasionally, anterior pituitary hormone deficiencies will occur acutely during the puerperium, resulting in diabetes insipidus, hypoglycemia, and sudden death.

Clinical Manifestations

The clinical features of hypopituitarism depend on the age of the patient, the type of hormonal deficiency, and the speed at which the disease progresses. Usually, symptoms of this disease develop slowly and demonstrate a great deal of variability. Sometimes, however, symptoms will suddenly appear, as in severe postpartum pituitary necrosis. Regardless of the etiology of the pituitary failure, selective deficiencies of trophic hormones, with failure of their target organs, can occur. The clinical picture can be dominated by either adrenocortical insufficiency, hypothyroidism, or hypogonadism, but if panhypopituitarism is present all three may be present.

TABLE 77–1
Causes of Pituitary Insufficiency

Tumors
Chromophobe adenoma
Craniopharyngioma
Trauma
Surgery
Irradiation
Infectious processes
Infiltrative diseases
Postpartum uterine hemorrhagic shock (Sheehan's syndrome)
Diabetes mellitus
Sickle cell disease
Collagen vascular disease

As ACTH secretion falls, the adrenal glands fail and glucocorticoid production decreases. Hypoglycemia is often the prevailing manifestation of cortisol deficiency. Vertigo, weakness, headaches, gastrointestinal disturbances, abdominal cramps, alopecia, and weight loss may also be discovered on physical examination. As in patients with Addison's disease, the individual with hypopituitarism is often intolerant of physical and emotional stress. Minor surgery or an acute infection can predispose the patient to an adrenal crisis, manifested by extreme prostration, hyponatremia, and hypotension. The severity of adenocortical insufficiency is reduced somewhat as mineralocorticoid secretion is relatively undisturbed by ACTH deficiencies.

A lack of thyroid-stimulating hormone (TSH) results in hypofunction of the thyroid gland. As thyroid hormone levels fall, the patient may experience easy fatigability, intolerance to cold, and paresthesias of the extremities. Slowed deep tendon reflexes, orthostatic hypotension, and bradycardia can be observed. The skin often appears thin, cool, and dry and scaly, and there are fine wrinkles about the eyes. The hair becomes dry, brittle, and is readily lost. Pallor also occurs but is usually the result of decreased secretion of melanocyte-stimulating hormone (MSH).[9] Sometimes mental aberrations can appear, earning the patient a diagnosis of some psychiatric disorder.

Amenorrhea, failure to lactate, impotence, decreased libido, infertility, atrophic external genitalia, and loss of pubic hair commonly follow testosterone and estrogen deficiency. In males, loss of total body hair is sometimes a very striking feature of the disease.[10]

The effects of GH deficiency are most evident in childhood before the epiphyses close. Growth becomes stunted resulting in *sexual ateliotic dwarfism.* Maximum stature is usually at least 40% below normal while body proportions remain unaffected (Fig. 77–3). These normal body proportions distinguish the pituitary dwarf from other forms of

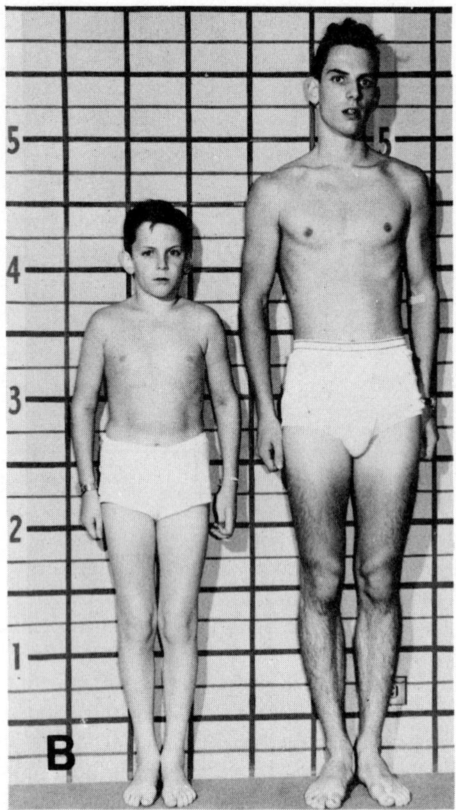

FIGURE 77–3 Anterior pituitary deficiency and growth failure. These twins are 17 years old. The affected twin on the left has a height of a 9½ year old. (Ezrin C, Godden JO, Volpe R [eds]: Systemic Endocrinology, 2nd ed, p 533. New York, Harper & Row, 1979)

dwarfism.[7] Puberty is delayed but full sexual maturity is usually attained with fertility intact.

When a tumor is the underlying cause of pituitary failure, signs of increasing intracellular or extracellular tumor expansion may be seen. Like expanding secreting tumors, enlarged nonsecreting pituitary tumors may produce pressure on the optic chiasm, creating visual field defects and alterations in visual acuity.

Diagnostic evaluation must confirm pathosis of the anterior pituitary or hypothalamus and rule out primary disease of the target organs (adrenals, gonads, and thyroid). The GH reserve test is the most sensitive index of pituitary insufficiency. In affected individuals GH serum levels fail to rise in response to insulin-induced hypoglycemia or to administration of L-dopa. More definitive testing is discussed in Chapter 72. Radiographic examinations of the skull, CT scanning, pneumoencephalography, or cerebral angiography may be done to confirm the presence of intracellular or extracellular tumors.

Treatment of hypopituitarism and panhypopituitarism is usually aimed at replacing target gland hormones found to be in deficient supply. Hormone replacement may include cortisol, thyroxine, and androgens (or cyclic estrogen). Prolactin is usually not replaced because few troubling symptoms occur with its deficiency. For patients of childbearing age, follicle-stimulating hormone (FSH) and human chorionic gonadotropin (HCG) may be given to improve fertility. Dwarfism can be treated with some success if the diagnosis is made before puberty. Administration of human growth hormone (HGH) stimulates growth by as much as 4 inches to 6 inches the first year. Recombinant DNA technology has made HGH more readily available than was previously possible using only cadaver-derived HGH. Pituitary trophic hormones are usually not prescribed because of the extreme expense involved and the need for daily injections.[6]

If a pituitary tumor is present, ablative therapy using surgery or irradiation may be performed. These modes of treatment are discussed in earlier sections of this chapter.

As with other endocrine disorders, the nurse plays a major role in identifying and referring patients with suspected hypofunction of the pituitary gland. An understanding of the hormonal effects on the body is essential in properly screening and managing the patient with hypopituitarism. Individuals suspected of likely pituitary failure should be followed closely. Such persons include the woman who experiences a hemorrhagic or hypotensive episode during childbirth and fails to lactate after the delivery. The nursing care of the patient with hypopituitarism is quite complex and may vary according to the specific hormone deficiencies of the target organs. Care of the patient with adrenal or thyroid hypofunction is dealt with in Chapters 75 and 76.

Assessment and Nursing Diagnosis. Although the problems encountered by the patient with hypopituitarism may vary greatly depending on the extent of involvement of the target glands, one problem occurs with some constancy. The patient is at great risk of decreased self-esteem as a result of the abnormalities in physical appearance and sexual functioning. This alteration in self-concept may greatly impair the patient's coping abilities and his ability to relate meaningfully with others.

Goals. Nursing efforts are aimed at reconstruction of the altered body image, to promote self-confidence and facilitate the use of adaptive coping behaviors.

Interventions. Strong emotional support is essential for the patient who is trying to cope with changes in body habitus and functioning. In establishing a trusting nurse–patient relationship, the nurse creates an environment conducive to the expression of feelings. A positive, realistic attitude by the nurse can assist in the individual's adaptation to the altered self-concept. In addition one may find ways in which to foster feelings of personal achievement, such as setting achievable daily goals or involvement in hobbies such as exercising, sewing, woodworking, and painting.[3] It is also useful to assess the patient's support systems and to problem-solve in ways to correct deficiencies. Finally the nurse can be of great help by providing reliable information about the nature of the disease and its treatment to the patient and his family. This allows for clarification of any misconceptions the person has about himself, his care, or his care-providers. It also provides a foundation on which the individual and his family can form realistic and acceptable personal expectations.

Evaluation of Goal Achievement. Through appropriate interventions it is hoped that the patient will develop an improved self-concept as demonstrated by making positive and realistic statements of his abilities. Goal achievement can also be observed by the patient's ability to verbalize feelings related to his emotional state, to assume role-related responsibilities with some confidence, and to develop mutual support between self and family.

Hypopituitary Crisis (Pituitary Apoplexy)

Pituitary apoplexy is a clinical syndrome manifested by profound weakness and altered mentation, ranging from complaints of extreme fatigue, syncope, and confusion to irreversible coma.[9] A sudden, severe headache along with nuchal rigidity, hypotension, bradycardia, hypothermia, and various visual defects such as diplopia, extraocular palsies, and photosensitivity may also be part of the constellation of clinical symptoms.

Pituitary apoplexy is found in 5% to 10% of patients with pituitary adenomas. It is thought to be associated with rapid enlargement of the tumor and hemorrhagic necrosis within the pituitary mass. the syndrome can be precipitated by stress induced by an emotional crisis, infection, surgery, trauma, exposure to cold, or prolonged fasting.[10] Other conditions predisposing the patient to a hypopituitary crisis include mechanical ventilation, anticoagulation therapy, and administration of CNS depressants (*e.g.*, morphine sulfate and barbiturates) to which the hypopituitary patient is extremely sensitive. The variability in the clinical manifestations of the disorder is probably related to the extent and direction of tumor expansion.

Management of pituitary apoplexy is a matter of some controversy. Usually corticosteroids are given to reduce cerebral edema and correct secondary adrenal insufficiency. Symptomatic treatment is given to correct underlying fluid and electrolyte derangements, ventilatory problems, and other treatable manifestations of the disorder. If necessary, prompt surgical pituitary decompression by means of a transphenoidal approach is done.[17]

Nursing care of the patient experiencing a transphenoidal hypophysectomy is discussed earlier in this chapter.

Disorders of the Posterior Pituitary

The posterior pituitary (neurohypophysis) is part of the neurosecretory system together with the hypothalamus. Vasopressin (antidiuretic hormone, ADH) and oxytocin are produced within the supraoptic nuclei of the hypothalamus. These hormones travel along the supraoptic hypophysial tract to the posterior pituitary where they are stored and then released into the circulation in response to physiological stimuli. Only disorders producing excessive or deficient levels of ADH will be discussed here.

ADH Excess: Syndrome of Inappropriate ADH

Etiology and Pathophysiology

Antidiuretic hormone is normally secreted in response to serum osmolality as monitored by osmoreceptors in the hypothalamus. Hyperosmolality results in increased ADH secretion, which promotes renal water reabsorption. Conversely, hypo-osmolality causes suppression of ADH and thus increases renal water excretion. The syndrome of inappropriate ADH (SIADH) is characterized by persistent ADH secretion despite serum hypo-osmolality, and predisposes the patient to water intoxication and hyponatremia. As the blood volume expands, aldosterone is suppressed and an increase in renal sodium excretion results. The urine becomes concentrated and urinary sodium values increase. The progressive loss of sodium through the kidneys further exaggerates hyponatremia, sometimes to lethal levels.

The syndrome of inappropriate ADH is associated with numerous conditions in response to stress, many drugs, pulmonary and CNS diseases, and in association with malignant tumors (Table 77–2). Tumor association has been implicated in as many as 80% of all cases of SIADH.[11] Tumors, particularly oat cell carcinomas, known to produce ADH ectopically, are independent of hypothalamic control. Bronchogenic malignancies probably account for most of the ectopic ADH production, although tumors involving virtually all body systems have been implicated.[8]

Drugs induce SIADH in various ways, either by increasing hypothalamic ADH production or by potentiating ADH's effects on the renal tubules. Central nervous system diseases probably reduce the sensitivity of the osmoreceptors, resulting in inappropriate secretion of ADH. The mechanism for this resetting of osmolality "sensors" is not entirely understood. Nor is it clear how limbic stimulation by extreme stress stimulates increased ADH production, although this phenomenon has been observed.[10]

Clinical Manifestations

The symptoms observed in SIADH are related to the underlying etiology and the degree of hyponatremia. The manifestations are generally neurological and nonspecific. Patients are usually asymptomatic until serum sodium values fall below 120 mEq/liter. As water intoxication develops and brain cells swell, clinical signs will include headaches, confusion, increasing stupor, muscle twitching, seizures, or coma. Gastrointestinal disturbances with anorexia, nausea, and vomiting may also occur. Edema is usually absent, except in severe hyponatremia, because water is distributed between the intracellular and extracellular compartment.[10]

TABLE 77–2
Causes of the Syndrome of Inappropriate ADH (SIADH)

Ectopic ADH	
Malignancies	
Lung carcinoma (oat cell, most common)	
Pancreatic carcinoma	
Gastrointestinal carcinoma	
Lymphoma	
Tuberculosis	
Endogenous ADH	
Stress	
Trauma	
Surgery	
Pulmonary diseases (most kinds)	
Central nervous system diseases	
Brain abscess	
Meningitis	
Subarachnoid hemorrhage	
Viral infections	
Psychosis	
Head injury	
Drugs	
Vasopressin	Tricyclic antidepressants
Oxytocin	Chlorpropamide
Vincristine	Thiazides
Barbiturates	Cyclophosphamide
Nicotine	Clofibrate
Tegretol	Morphine

Medical Management

Once the presence of hyponatremia has been established by at least two separate serum sodium determinations, other causes should be ruled out. Recognition of such causes as Addison's disease, cirrhosis, cardiac failure, and overaggressive water intake is usually not too difficult. The diagnosis of SIADH can often be made by obtaining simultaneous urine and serum samples to test for osmolality. The serum osmolality will be abnormally low with inappropriate hyperosmolality of the urine. Any patient with a normal serum sodium value does *not* have SIADH.[8] Corroborative laboratory data include increased urine sodium values, low blood urea nitrogen (BUN), low creatinine, hypocalcemia, hypokalemia, and hypouricemia.

Treatment of SIADH can focus either on treating the underlying cause or on alleviating water excess. Many patients can be managed by fluid restriction alone. Fluids (especially water) can be limited to 1000 ml/24 hours. Demeclocycline, 600 mg to 1200 mg/day, given orally can often restore serum sodium levels within 2 weeks. The drug works by making the renal tubule insensitive to ADH, and producing nephrogenic diabetes insipidus. Lithium carbonate can be used to obtain this same effect, but has rather serious side-effects.[8]

If hyponatremia persists or becomes life-threatening, and it is associated with profound neurological consequences, rapid infusion of 300 ml to 500 ml of hypertonic (3% to 5%) saline can be given to quickly alleviate symptoms. This procedure is usually followed by water restriction and administration of diuretics such as furosemide (Lasix). Furosemide helps minimize the risk of cardiac failure, which is potentiated by the underlying excess volume load and the bolus of hypertonic solution. Potassium replacement is given if serum levels fall.[16] The syndrome of inappropriate ADH is often transient. The prognosis is usually determined by the severity of the underlying disease.

Nursing Management Plan

Nursing care of the patient with SIADH is primarily directed toward prevention and early detection of the disorder, and support of medical treatment.

Assessment and Nursing Diagnosis. Owing to the nature of the illness, the major problem the nurse must deal with is alteration in fluid volume related to water (intracellular volume) excess. This nursing diagnosis has many implications for nursing management, requiring astute observations and creative interventions.

Goals. The goals of nursing interventions are the identification of persons at risk for and the prevention of SIADH. Once the diagnosis of SIADH has been established, nursing actions are aimed at reestablishing and maintaining a normal volume status.

Interventions. Initially, those individuals at greater risk of developing SIADH should be identified. (Review causes of SIADH in Table 77–2). Interventions are then focused on preventing abnormal ADH secretion. Minimizing stress and pain in the postoperative and post-trauma patient often helps in decreasing ADH secretion. Adapting a calm, unhurried approach in caring for the patient and administering adequate analgesics to ensure the patient's comfort are important. Drugs that provoke increased ADH secretion, such as morphine, should be avoided. Serum sodium values must also be routinely monitored with suspicions of SIADH increasing when serum sodium levels fall below 130 mEq/liter.

Fluid balance can be assessed by accurately monitoring fluctuations in daily weight, along with intake and output. The nurse should be alert to decreases in urinary output with concurrent increases in its specific gravity. Although these signs often signify dehydration, they may represent SIADH when accompanied by signs of hyponatremia and overhydration. Neurological assessment contributes to the evaluation of water balance. Increasing lethargy is one of the earliest signs of marked hyponatremia.

Once the diagnosis of SIADH has been made, promoting a fluid restriction of 1000 ml to 1200 ml/day is necessary. The amount of fluid allowed per shift should be marked clearly on the patient's care plan, placed at the patient's bedside, and discussed with the dietary department. The patient should also be informed of the purpose of this therapy. To promote patient comfort and allay thirst, liquids are served well chilled and in a thick-bottomed glass to give the illusion of greater volume. Good oral care may help prevent annoying mouth dryness and thirst. Fortunately, great thirst is not a serious problem in SIADH.

Keeping the head of the patient's bed elevated at least

15° to 30° enhances blood return to the heart, increases left atrial filling pressure eliciting, it is hoped, a drop in ADH secretion. Before being discharged, the patient with chronic SIADH must be taught the signs and symptoms of hyponatremia and hypokalemia so that he can monitor his own response to therapy. Dietary supplementation of sodium and potassium is also discussed. Hypokalemia is usually a problem when diuretics have been administered. Electrolyte replacement preparations are varied and often cause some degree of gastric distress. These preparations should be well diluted and given at meal times to improve drug tolerance and patient compliance. The patient should also be assisted in planning liquid intake, making the most of restricted allowances.

Evaluation of Goal Achievement. Goal achievement can be assessed in the patient by the maintenance of normal serum sodium levels and the absence of the signs and symptoms of hyponatremia. In addition the patient will demonstrate compliance to fluid intake restrictions, as ordered, and be able to appropriately discuss the rationale for such restrictions.

TABLE 77–3
Causes of Neurogenic Diabetes Insipidus (DI)

Primary Causes
Idiopathic (most common)
Familial

Secondary (Acquired) Causes
Head trauma
Neurosurgery
Tumors
  Primary pituitary tumors
  Craniopharyngioma
  Metastatic carcinoma
  Acute leukemia
Granulomatous diseases
  Tuberculosis
  Sarcoidosis
  Histiocytosis
  Syphilis
Infections
  Meningitis
  Encephalitis
Vascular (aneurysms)
Drugs
  Diphenylhydantoin
  Alcohol

ADH Deficit: Diabetes Insipidus

Etiology and Pathophysiology

Diabetes insipidus (DI) is a disorder characterized by the kidney's inability to conserve water. It results from (1) a hypothalamic pituitary defect in ADH synthesis or release (neurogenic DI) or (2) renal tubular resistance to ADH (nephrogenic DI).[16] The numerous causes of DI are listed in Table 77–3.

Neurogenic DI is a relatively rare disturbance, occurring equally in both men and women, usually between the ages of 10 and 20.[10] An idiopathic cause is determined in 45% to 50% of these patients. A genetic reduction in ADH neurosecretory cells within the hypothalamus (familial DI) is far less common. Increasingly, neurogenic DI is a consequence of therapeutic ablative interventions within the region of the pituitary and hypothalamus. Such procedures include hypophysectomy, cryosurgery, and irradiation.

Nephrogenic DI also has many causes that render the renal tubules insensitive to ADH. A familial disorder resulting in this type of DI is caused by a genetic defect within the renal tubules and, unlike neurogenic DI, is inherited primarily by males. Nephrogenic DI rarely results in the massive polyuria characteristic of neurogenic DI. Regardless of the underlying etiology, the patient with DI is unable to concentrate his urine and thus excretes large amounts of diluted urine.[5]

Clinical Manifestations

In severe neurogenic DI with a near-total shutdown of ADH release, urine output may reach or exceed 10 to 16 liters/day with urinary specific gravity readings remaining below 1.005.[10] Not surprisingly, extreme thirst and polydipsia accompany the polyuria. If able to respond to this thirst by taking in sufficient quantities of water, the patient can usually manage quite well. However, frequent voidings and excessive thirst can markedly affect his sleeping patterns, causing fatigue and irritability. Less severe forms of neurogenic DI, with suboptimal levels of ADH, result in urine outputs of a little over 4 liters/day. Nephrogenic DI produces less dramatic polyuria, with a urine output of 2 to 3 liters/day.[18]

Concern arises when a patient is not able to respond adequately to thirst because his level of consciousness is altered or he is hindered by physical immobility. Should this happen, signs of dehydration and hypernatremia can develop rapidly. Such signs include poor tissue turgor, dry mucous membranes, postural hypotension, tachycardia, muscular weakness, and increasing somnolence. Despite marked dehydration and increased serum osmolality (>280 mOsm/liter), the urine typically remains dilute. Diabetes insipidus sometimes appears transiently within 1 or 2 days after cerebrovascular trauma.[5] Relief of intracranial pressure may cause these symptoms to disappear as quickly as they developed.

Medical Management

Diabetes insipidus must be distinguished from other causes of polyuria, most notably psychogenic polydipsia. The latter is due to an emotional disturbance and is associated with overhydration rather than dehydration. A good history and physical examination are required to determine the probable cause of the polyuria and evaluate the state of hydration. An extremely useful procedure is to obtain simultaneous urine and blood samples to test the osmolality. In the patient with DI, urine osmolality will be low whereas serum osmolality is high, in contrast to the individual with psychogenic polydipsia in whom both urine and blood samples will demonstrate low osmolality. A water deprivation test can be done to evaluate the concentrating ability of the kidneys and must be done with great caution because dangerous hypovolemic levels may result (see Chap. 72). A safer, more rapid test in diagnosing DI is the administration of ADH by nasal spray or injection. Prompt relief of symptoms, with decreased urine output and increased specific gravity, is conclusive of neurogenic DI.[10] Nephrogenic DI will not respond to exogenous ADH.

Treatment of DI is dependent on the cause and clinical manifestation. In the alert patient fluid replacement is usually sufficiently controlled by quenching the thirst with a large amount of fluids. Intravenous water replacement is required when urine output exceeds 250 ml/hour for 2 consecutive hours (6 to 7 liters/day) and when the patient who is unable for some reason to respond to thirst.[16] In addition, various forms of vasopressin are available for treating neurogenic DI. After head trauma or neurosurgery, aqueous vasopressin, 5 units to 10 units subcutaneously, is the drug of choice. A longer acting preparation is used for persistent, severe DI. Vasopressin tannate, an oil suspension, is given intramuscularly in doses of 2.5 units to 5 units and is effective for 48 to 96 hours. Lysine vasopressin, a nasal spray, will effectively control polyuria for only a few hours, requiring 4 doses a day. A preferred drug, desmopressin, is given intranasally, and its effects last for 8 to 20 hours.[18]

Sometimes pharmaceutical agents are used in place of hormonal therapy to increase the release of ADH or enhance its actions on the kidney, but only when the posterior pituitary has some residual capacity to secrete ADH. Chlorpropamide (Diabinese), an oral hypoglycemic agent, may be used in doses of 250 mg to 500 mg/day. Hypoglycemia may accompany the use of this drug. Therefore, the patient should be instructed to eat regular meals and avoid meal omissions.[9]

Nephrogenic DI will not respond to any of the pharmacological agents referred to above. Thiazide diuretics have a paradoxical effect on patients with nephrogenic DI by reducing urine output, presumably by causing sodium depletion. Thiazide diuretics, along with dietary salt restriction, can effectively decrease urine output by as much as one third to one half in individuals with nephrogenic DI.[10]

Nursing Management Plan

Assessment and Nursing Diagnosis. The primary nursing diagnosis in relation to DI is alterations in fluid volume related to water deficit, which can, if not corrected, progress into profound hypovolemia. In the case of chronic DI, problems related to ineffective coping and knowledge deficit may also be seen. The latter may be of particular concern if the patient is to safely and effectively self-administer the unusual pharmaceutical agents used in the treatment of DI.

Goals. The major goals in the care of the individual with DI is the restoration and maintenance of a normal volume status. In addition the nurse would strive to facilitate an increase in the patient's knowledge of his illness and its successful management, and to promote patient compliance to prescribed therapy.

Interventions. Daily weights and careful monitoring of intake and output are essential. The nurse is responsible for ensuring that lost fluids are replaced either orally or parenterally. Urine specific gravity should be measured, but it cannot be used as a guide to fluid replacement. If the patient is able to tolerate oral intake, liquids need to be readily available in sufficient supply, and his state of hydration should be frequently monitored. Signs of hypovolemia are hypotension, tachycardia, loss of tissue turgor, and weight loss. Serum sodium values must be closely monitored; as water depletion increases so will the serum sodium levels (>145 mEq/liter). Conversely, water intoxication from overzealous rehydration may greatly lower the sodium values (<135 mEq/liter).

Before he is discharged the patient is advised to obtain a medical identification bracelet and to carry the prescribed medication at all times. The patient needs to know not only how to monitor intake and output but also how to appropriately administer his drugs. He must be taught the proper injection or intranasal administration techniques. Vasopressin tannate in oil, for instance, must be warmed because of its viscosity.[14] How to roll the vial in the hands to ensure uniform dispersion of the drug should be demonstrated. In using the vasopressin nasal spray, the patient is instructed that nasal congestion due to allergy or colds can impair the drug's effectiveness, so that the dose has to be changed. In addition, these nasal spray preparations must not be inhaled because they may cause coughing, chest tightness, and dyspnea. Even when given properly, these nasal sprays can cause irritation of the nasal mucosa, conjunctivitis, and bronchopulmonary allergic reactions. Overmedication with all forms of ADH preparations can precipitate hypervolemia. The patient should immediately report to his physician any signs of volume excess, such as weight gain, dyspnea, or angina.

Evaluation of Goal Achievement. The success of nursing management would be evidenced by the return of the patient's serum sodium values to normal levels and the absence of symptoms related to hypovolemia. The patient will describe the disease process, causes and procedures for disease control, and actively participate in the prescribed health behaviors, such as properly administering medications and wearing a medical identification bracelet.

Multiple Endocrine Neoplasia

Multiple endocrine neoplasia (MEN) is a syndrome in which two or more endocrine glands develop hyperplasia, adenoma, or carcinoma, concurrently or consecutively.[7] This concomitant failure of multiple endocrine organs is usually inherited as an autosomal dominant trait. Men and women are equally affected and the disorder can occur at any age. At present two types of MEN are recognized: MEN Type I (Werner's syndrome) and MEN Type II (Sipple's syndrome).

Multiple endocrine neoplasia, Type I is associated with adenomas of the parathyroid glands, pancreatic islet cells, and the pituitary gland. Parathyroid adenomas are usually multiple. Nearly 90% of the patients with MEN Type I have hyperparathyroidism, although hypercalcemic crises are rare. Hyperplasia of the pancreatic islet cells may be present. Nonbeta islet cells commonly secrete gastrin and, with excess secretion, produce Zollenger-Ellison syndrome, which is characterized by malabsorption, diarrhea, and peptic ulcer formation. In addition, hypoglycemia may result from increased insulin production from the beta islet cells of the pancreas. Most pituitary adenomas found in MEN Type I are nonfunctional chromophobe tumors. However, 30% of these tumors may be hyperfunctioning and lead to acromegaly, Cushing's syndrome, or hyperprolactinemia.[9]

Multiple endocrine neoplasia, Type II is associated with medullary carcinoma of the thyroid, pheochromocytoma, and occasionally hyperparathyroidism. The thyroid carcinoma may be metastatic and often secretes high levels of calcitonin. Pheochromocytoma occurs bilaterally in over 50% of cases and extra-adrenal tumors are rare.[13] Patients with familial pheochromocytoma have clinically indistinguishable clinical manifestations from sporadically occurring pheochromocytoma. Symptoms include headache, hypertension, and palpitation.[10]

Treatment of MEN depends on which organs are involved. Eradication of the tumors and management of residual symptoms are required. In MEN Type I, peptic ulceration associated with Zollinger-Ellison syndrome is of primary concern. Such ulcers do not respond well to conventional therapy. Besides tumor resection, a radical gastric resection may be necessary. Hypoglycemia is managed with administration of oral or intravenous glucose to maintain blood sugar within a normal range. In MEN Type II pheochromocytoma is managed with antihypertensive drugs and resection of the adrenal medullary tumor.[9] Specific treatment procedures for hyperparathyroidism, pheochromocytoma, pituitary adenomas, and pancreatic insulinomas can be found in their respective chapters.

References

1. Brunner LS, Suddarth DS (eds): Lippincott Manual of Nursing Practice, 3rd ed. Philadelphia, JB Lippincott, 1982
2. Camunas CE: Transphenoidal hypophysectomy. Am J Nurs 80:1820–1823, 1980
3. Carpenito LJ: Nursing Diagnosis: Application to Clinical Practice. Philadelphia, JB Lippincott, 1983
4. Clancy J, Abruzzi L: Pituitary tumors, growth disease: Nurses' intervention of patients with pituitary tumor. J Neurosurg Nurs 10:24–28, 1978
5. Fairchild RS: Diabetes insipidus: A review. Critical Care Quarterly 3:111–118, 1980
6. Frazier SD: Growth disorders in children. Pediatr Clin North Am 26:1–14, 1979
7. Garfano CD: Pituitary disorders. In Diseases: Nurses Reference Library, Nursing 83. Springhouse, Intermed Communications, 1983
8. Hamburger S, Rush D: Syndrome of inappropriate secretion of antidiuretic hormone. Critical Care Quarterly 3:119–129, 1980
9. Harvey AM, Johns RJ, Owens AH et al (eds): The Principles and Practice of Medicine, 20th ed. New York, Appleton-Century-Crofts, 1980
10. Jubix W: Endocrinology: A Logical Approach for Clinicians. New York, McGraw-Hill, 1979
11. Kubo W, Grant M: The syndrome of inappropriate antidiuretic hormone. Heart Lung 7:469–475, 1978
12. Mathes-Albuire B, Alguire P: Autoimmune polyglandular syndromes. Am Fam Prac 29:149–152, 1984
13. Nelson DH: Disease of the adenohypophysis. In Isselbacher K et al (eds): Harrison's Principles of Internal Medicine, 9th ed. New York, McGraw-Hill, 1980
14. Rush DR, Hamburger JC: Drugs used in endocrine metabolic emergencies. Critical Care Quarterly 2:1–9, 1980
15. Solomon BL: The hypothalamus and the pituitary gland: An overview. Nurs Clin North Am 15:435–451, 1980
16. Streeten DH, Moses AM, Miller M: Disorders of the neurohypophysis. In Isselbacher KJ et al (eds): Harrison's Principles of Internal Medicine, 9th ed. New York, McGraw-Hill, 1980
17. Verbalis JG, Robinson AG: Hypopituitarism. Topics in Emergency Medicine 5:74–78, 1984
18. Zucker AR, Chernow B: Diabetes insipidus and the syndrome of inappropriate antidiuretic hormone release. Critical Care Quarterly 6:63–74, 1983

Bibliography

Balestrieri F, Chernow B, Rainey T: Post-craniotomy diabetes insipidus: Who's at risk: Crit Care Med 18:108–110, 1982

Cooperman D, Malarkey W: Pituitary apoplexy. Heart Lung 7:450–454, 1978

Costen G: Endocrine disorders associated with tumors of the pituitary and hypothalamus. Pediatr Clin North Am 26:15–31, 1979

DeGroot LJ, Cahill GF, Odell WD et al (eds): Endocrinology. New York, Grune & Stratton, 1979

DeTroyer A: Demeclocycline: Treatment for syndrome of inappropriate antidiuretic hormone secretion. JAMA 237:2723–2726, 1977

Franco LM: Syndrome of inappropriate secretion of antidiuretic hormone. J Neurosurg Nurs 14:276–279, 1982

Hall R: Fundamentals of Clinical Endocrinology, 3rd ed. Chicago, Year Book Medical Publishers, 1981

Hart IR, Newton RW: Endocrinology, Vol 2. Baltimore, University Park Press, 1983

Hau TH: Current management of diabetes insipidus. Compr Ther 6:22–25, 1980

Herbert D, Breeding P: Self-care after hypophysectomy. J Neurosurg Nurs 11:118–120, 1979

Hershman JM: Management of Endocrine Disorders. Philadelphia, Lea & Febiger, 1980

Krueger J, Ray J: Endocrine Problems in Nursing. St Louis, CV Mosby, 1976

Markowitz S, Sherman L, Kolodny HD et al: Acute pituitary vascular accident (pituitary apoplexy). Med Clin North Am 65(1):105–116, 1981

McGregor AM, Scanlon MF, Hall K et al: Reduction in size of a pituitary tumor by bromocriptine therapy. N Engl J Med 300:291–293, 1979

McInerney M: Prolactin producing pituitary adenomas. J Neurosurg Nurs 13:15–17, 1981

Moens J: Coping with diabetes insipidus. Convalescent Nursing 75:18–20, 1979

Morrow LB: Clinical evaluation of pituitary adenomas. Postgrad Med 68:155–164, 1980

Moses AM: Diabetes insipidus and ADH regulation. Hosp Pract 12:37–44, 1977

Moses AM, Notman D: Diabetes insipidus and syndrome of inappropriate antidiuretic hormone secretion (SIADH). Adv Intern Med 27:73–100, 1982

Neufeld M, Mclaren N, Blizzard R: Autoimmune polyglandular syndromes. Pediatr Ann 9:154–162, 1980

Oliver RE, Jamison RL: Diabetes insipidus: A physiologic approach to diagnosis. Postgrad Med 68:120–131, 1980

Ross JL, Shenkman L: Diabetes insipidus. Compr Ther 5:30–35, 1979

Shiner G: Human growth hormone: Potentials for treatment are broadened. Resources Reporter 12:1–5, 1980

Sowers DK, Sowers JR: Pituitary emergencies. Critical Care Quarterly 3:45–54, 1980

Stillman MJ: Transphenoidal hypophysectomy for pituitary tumors. J Neurosurg Nurs 13:117–122, 1981

Verbalis JG: Hypernatremia and hyponatremia. Topics in Emergency Medicine 5:79–89, 1984

Williams RH (ed): Textbook of Endocrinology. Philadelphia, WB Saunders, 1981

Wilson CB, Dempsey LC: Transphenoidal micro-surgical removal of 250 pituitary adenomas. J Neurosurg 48:13, 1978

UNIT IX

Nursing Care of Patients with Alterations in Gastrointestinal Function

Chapter 78

Review of Anatomy and Physiology

Gastrointestinal System

Barbara R. Landau

The function of the gastrointestinal (GI) system is to prepare ingested material for entry into the body (the bloodstream). The preparation involves digestion, transport, absorption, and elimination of unabsorbed material. These processes are carried out in a tube that extends through the body from mouth to anus. As food put into it is carried along by muscle action, large quantities of secretions are poured in from glands in the wall of the tube or outside of it. Fluid, electrolytes, and digested materials are absorbed, and the remainder is excreted.

Structure of the Gastrointestinal Tract

The digestive system consists of the organs of this continuous tube, plus several accessory organs, namely the salivary glands, pancreas, liver, and gallbladder, as shown in Figure 78–1.

The digestive tract is interrupted by several sphincters which help to regulate the passage of material. They are the upper and lower esophageal sphincters, the pyloric sphincter, the ileocecal valve, and the internal and external anal sphincters.

Blood Supply. Organs in the abdominal cavity are supplied by branches of the celiac axis: the splenic, left gastric, and hepatic arteries, which supply the stomach, liver, pancreas, and duodenum; the superior mesenteric artery to the small intestine and first part of the colon; and the inferior mesenteric to the rest of the colon and most of the rectum. Branches from the anterior division of the internal iliac supply the lower rectum and perineum.

Veins that drain the abdominal organs converge to form the hepatic portal vein, which carries the nutrient-rich blood from the digestive tract to the liver. The hepatic veins carry it to the inferior vena cava.

Peritoneum. The peritoneum forms a continuous serosal sheet which lines the abdominal cavity and covers the organs in it, forming the peritoneal sac or cavity (Fig. 78–2). Organs outside of this sac, such as the pancreas, are retroperitoneal, as are the kidneys and pelvic organs. Many organs of the abdominal cavity are suspended and supported by folds of peritoneum.

Digestive Muscle Function. Digestive tract smooth muscle demonstrates a certain level of tone that varies with the membrane potential; it increases with hypopolarization and decreases with hyperpolarization. The muscle cells also respond directly to stretch without neural participation, for

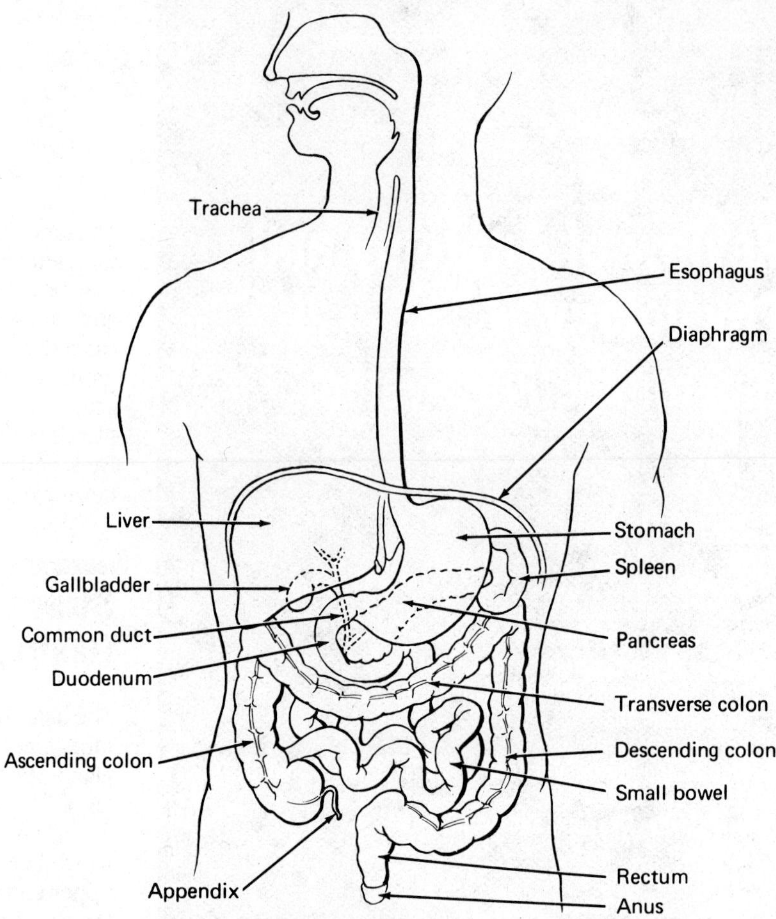

FIGURE 78–1 Diagram of the gastroinestinal tract.

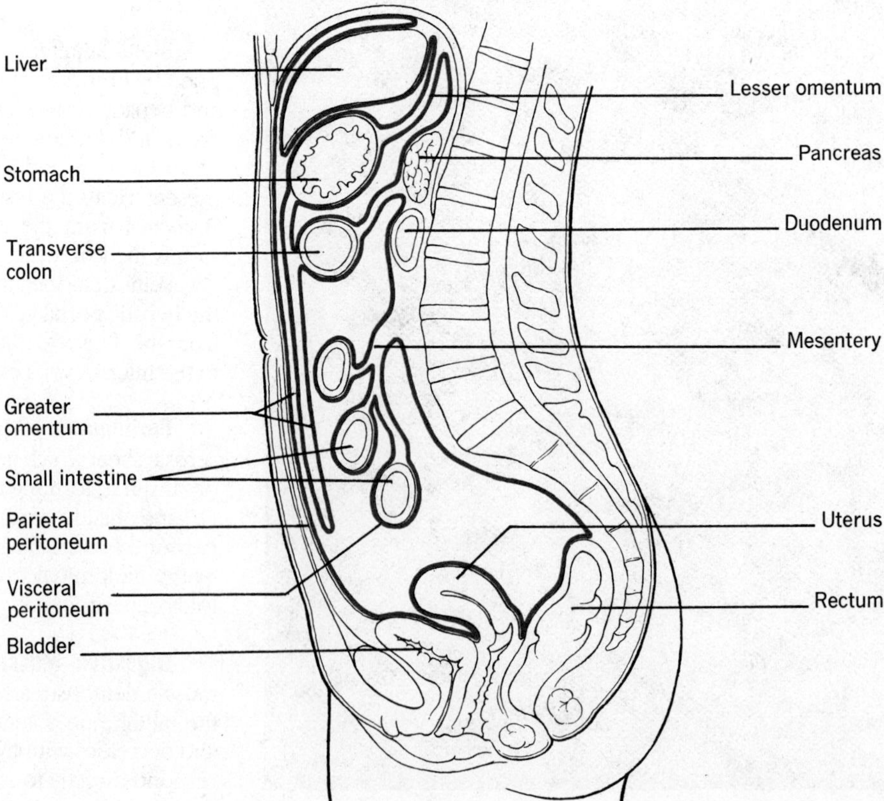

FIGURE 78–2 Reflections of the peritoneum as seen in sagittal section.

stretch itself hypopolarizes the membrane and raises excitability, an important mechanism of local control.

These properties combine to produce several types of motor activity in the GI tract. Peristalsis is a wave of contraction that moves caudally at a velocity and frequency determined by the velocity and frequency of the slow wave. With food in the stomach, distention and other stimuli raise the excitability of muscle cells, so that when the slow wave reaches them, there is sufficient depolarization during the hypopolarization phase to produce a contraction which moves toward the pylorus. Although peristalsis also occurs in the small intestine, rhythmic segmentation is more characteristic. Intestinal pacemaker cells develop slow waves, but as local conditions in the small intestine vary more, a given site undergoes alternate contraction and relaxation while segments on either side are relaxing and contracting. This action pushes the contents back and forth, mixing them with secretions. Because the frequency is higher in the upper part of the intestine, there is a general tendency of the material to slowly progress in a caudal direction.

Control of Gastrointestinal Function

Both the automaticity of GI smooth muscle and the action of secretory cells that produce the digestive juices are externally controlled. These controls are primarily neural and hormonal.

Neural Controls

Smooth muscle of the GI tract receives innervation from both divisions of the autonomic nervous system (Fig. 78–3). The sympathetic supply to abdominal structures arises from the cord between T6 and L3 and passes, by way of the splanchnic nerves, to synapse in a collateral ganglion. Sympathetic stimulation and epinephrine inhibits GI smooth muscle (except sphincters), but is excitatory to vascular smooth muscle.

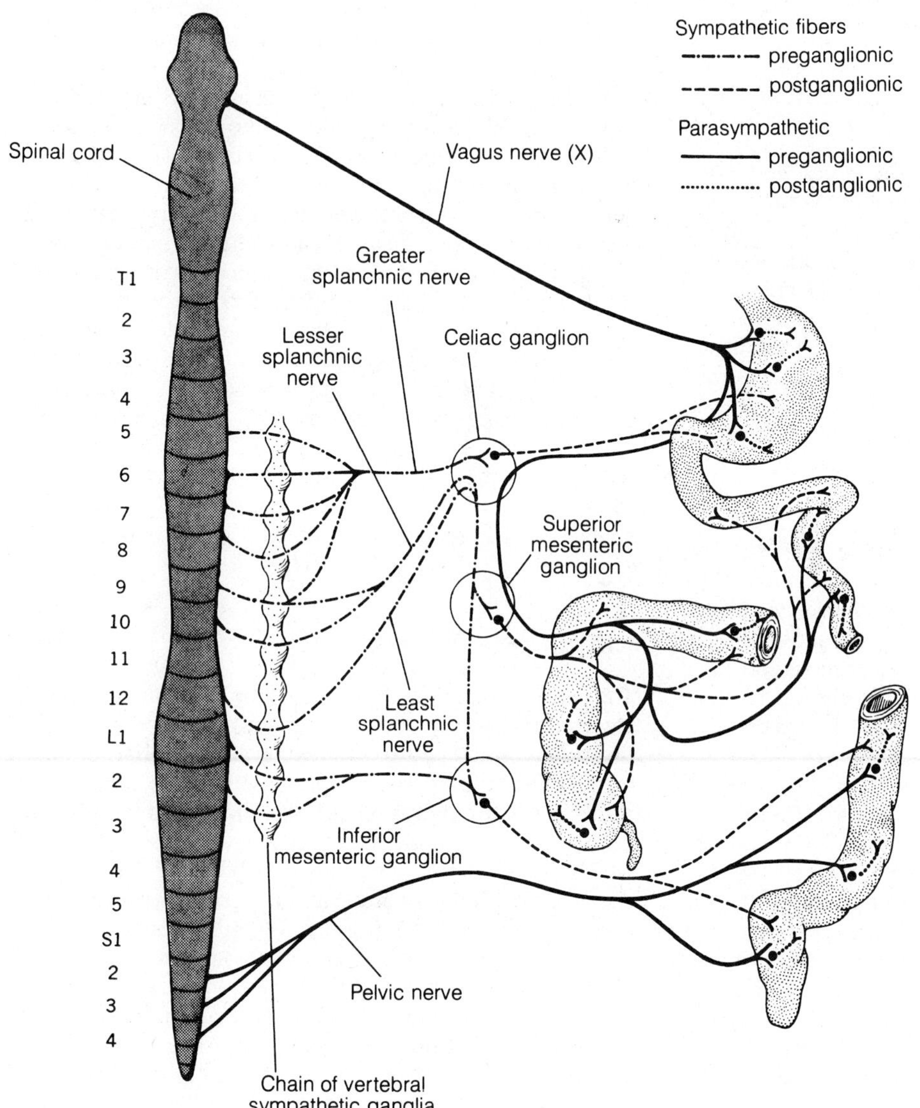

FIGURE 78–3 The autonomic innervation of the gastrointestinal tract. (Drawing by Edith Tagrin in Beck WS: Human Design. New York, Harcourt Brace Jovanovich, 1971. Copyright 1971 by Harcourt Brace Jovanovich, Inc. Used by permission of the publisher.)

The parasympathetic innervation is supplied mainly by the vagus nerve except for the lower part of the colon and rectum which are innervated by the pelvic nerve (S2–4). Parasympathetic stimulation generally increases motor activity (except in sphincters) and causes secretion of some glands. There is little parasympathetic innervation to blood vessels, but in glands the acetylcholine from secretory fibers is a vasodilator and increases blood flow during secretion, as do some metabolites. Sympathetic stimulation causes vasodilation in glands with β-adrenergic receptors.

The myenteric and submucous plexuses present a situation that is unique to the GI tract, and constitute what is known as the intrinsic innervation of the intestines. Many of these neurons are parasympathetic postganglionic fibers that terminate on effector cells, but some arise from sensory receptors and function as sensory neurons, while others are interneurons which connect them. The plexuses can function independent of the extrinsic innervation (connections with the central nervous system) to provide a means by which a small part of the intestine can respond to local conditions in that segment, as a "local reflex." Because it is particularly well-developed in the lower part of the digestive tract, denervation has little effect on much of the intestinal function. Some sympathetic neurons end on motor neurons of the intrinsic system.

Humoral Controls

The GI tract has been said to be the largest endocrine gland in the body, secreting more hormones than any other. The endocrine cells are widely distributed throughout the epithelium. Of the rather large number of substances known to be produced in the GI tract, only four meet the criteria of a true hormone. Others have been identified, but as there is a question as to whether they are produced in sufficient amounts under physiological conditions, they are termed "candidate hormones" (Table 78–1). Many of them also act as neurotransmitters, or as paracrine agents by diffusing to nearby target cells, and many of them are produced in other parts of the body, especially the brain.

The true GI hormones are gastrin, cholecystokinin (CCK), secretin, and gastroinhibitory peptide (GIP). All affect a number of GI functions in large doses, but their physiological actions are few. Gastrin is produced by cells in gastric glands in the antrum of the stomach and returns to find its target cells in the stomach. Its main actions are secretion of hydrochloric acid (HCl) by parietal cells and a trophic (growth-stimulating) action on mucosa of the gastrointestinal tract.

Cholecystokinin (CCK), which was once thought to be two different hormones, has two types of action. As its name suggests, one action is to cause the gallbladder to contract, and the other, which reflects its other identity (as pancreozymin), is to stimulate secretion of enzyme-rich pancreatic juice. Secretin, the first hormone to be discovered, causes release of pancreatic juice that has a high bicarbonate content. Gastroinhibitory peptide (GIP) inhibits both motor and secretory activity of the stomach, and thus slows gastric emptying. CCK, secretin, and GIP are all secreted by the duodenal mucosa in response to stimulation by the intestinal contents.

Histamine is not a hormone, but a large amount is present in the stomach and it is a potent stimulus to acid secretion. Prostaglandins, a ubiquitous class of compounds, exert a protective action for gastric mucosa against acids, and some prostaglandins alter intestinal motility.

Secretory and Motor Functions of the Gastrointestinal Tract

Oral Cavity, Pharynx, and Esophagus

The oral cavity receives saliva produced by the parotid, submandibular, and sublingual glands. It contains fluid, electrolytes, mucus, and salivary amylase (ptyalin), which initiates the hydrolysis of starch (Table 78–2). Saliva is needed for taste because taste buds respond only to substances in solution, and as a lubricant to aid in forming a bolus for swallowing. Salivary secretion is under reflex control, and is increased by stimulation of receptors in the oral cavity (dryness, touch) and by input from other parts of the brain.

Motor activity in the oral cavity consists of masticatory movements, which break down the ingested material and mix it with the salivary secretion. Although swallowing is a reflex act, it is initiated voluntarily. In the initial or oral phase, the tongue moves the bolus toward the pharynx, which triggers a complex sequence of events. In the pharyngeal phase, muscles of the soft palate, uvula, and pharynx contract to block off the nasal cavity, and the larynx moves up and forward, tipping the epiglottis to deflect food from the larynx. Sequential contraction of pharyngeal muscles moves the bolus into the esophagus, and the upper esophageal sphincter is temporarily relaxed. The contraction continues as a peristaltic wave down the skeletal and smooth muscle of the esophagus (as the esophageal phase). A vagally mediated reflex causes the lower esophageal sphincter to relax and to allow passage of food into the stomach. The sphincter normally prevents regurgitation of gastric contents into the esophagus.

Stomach

The gastric secretion is produced by cells in the gastric glands. Parietal cells secrete HCl at a pH of about 1.0. The hydrogen ions (H^+) are obtained by the hydrolysis of water in the cells and are actively pumped into the lumen. The remaining hydroxide ions (OH^-) are formed into the bicarbonate radical, HCO_3^- (catalyzed by carbonic anhydrase) which diffuses into the bloodstream (causing the "alkaline tide"). Chloride ions diffuse into the parietal cells and are actively pumped into the lumen. Pepsin, produced by the chief cells, is a proteolytic enzyme formed as the inactive pepsinogen and activated in the lumen by HCl. Mucus, which is formed by surface epithelial cells and mucous neck cells in the glands, helps protect the mucosa from frictional and chemical abuse.

The parietal cells also produce the "intrinsic factor,"

TABLE 78–1
Gastrointestinal Hormones and Some "Candidate" Hormones

Hormone	*Source*	*Probable Stimulus*	*Physiologic Actions*
Gastrin	Gastric antrum, duodenum	Acid (pH above 2.0), protein, vagal stimulation	Increases gastric secretion, especially of acid Increases antral motility Trophic action on gastric mucosa
Cholecystokinin (CCK)	Duodenum, jejunum	Peptides, amino acids, long-chain fatty acids	Increases pancreatic secretion of enzyme Causes contraction of gallbladder Inhibits gastrin-mediated acid secretion Potentiates actions of secretin
Secretin	Duodenum, jejunum	Acid in duodenum, (pH below 4.5)	Increases secretion of HCO_3^- by epithelium of pancreatic and biliary ducts Inhibits gastric motility and secretion Potentiates action of CCK
Gastric inhibitory peptide (GIP)	Duodenum, jejunum	Glucose and fatty acid in duodenum	Inhibits gastric motility and secretion Slows gastric emptying Enhances insulin secretion in response to glucose
Vasoactive peptide (VIP)	Neurons of intrinsic plexuses, stomach through colon	Unknown	Inhibits smooth muscle of gastrointestinal tract and blood vessels, thus decreases motility and increases blood flow Increases gastric secretion of acid and pepsin Increases pancreatic secretion of water and HCO_3^-
Motilin	Duodenum, jejunum	Released in cyclic fashion in fasting animals	Initiates intestinal motility during interdigestive periods
Chymodenin	Duodenum	Fat??	Increases pancreatic secretion of chymotrypsinogen
Bulbogastrone	Duodenal bulb	Acid in duodenum	Inhibits gastric secretion of acid (gastrin antagonist)
Bombesin	Stomach through colon, also nerve endings		Increases release of gastrin and CCK
Villikinin	Duodenum	Chyme in duodenum??	Increases contraction of intestinal villi
Pancreatic polypeptide	Pancreatic islets	Secreted after eating, especially protein, also vagal stimulation	Inhibits pancreatic secretion (organic and inorganic components)
Somatostatin	Nerve and endocrine cells in intestinal mucosa, pancreas, and brain	Mixed meal, acid?	Multiple inhibitory actions (Inhibits secretion of gastrin, secretin, GIP, VIP, and motilin)

TABLE 78–2
The Principle Digestive Enzymes

Source	*Enzyme*	*Substrate*	*Products*	*Comment*
Salivary glands	Salivary amylase	Starch	Disaccharides, mainly maltose	Inactivated when mixed with acid in stomach
Stomach	Pepsin (*pepsinogen*)	Proteins, polypeptides	Polypeptides	Pepsinogen activated by HCl (low pH)
Exocrine pancreas	Trypsin (*Trypsinogen*)	Proteins, polypeptides	Polypeptides	Trypsinogen activated by enterokinase
	Chymotrypsin (*Chymotrypsinogen*)	Proteins, polypeptides	Polypeptides	Chymotrypsinogen activated by trypsin
	Carboxypeptidase (*Procarboxypeptidase*)	Polypeptides	Smaller polypeptides, amino acids*	Procarboxypeptidase activated by trypsin; acts at carboxyl end of chain
	Pancreatic amylase	Starch	Disaccharides, mainly glucose	
	Pancreatic lipase	Triacylglycerides	Monoacylglycerides*, fatty acids*, glycerol*	Effectiveness increased by emulsifying action of bile salts
	Pancreatic enterase	Cholesterol esters	Cholesterol*	
	Deoxyribonuclease	DNA	Nucleotides	
	Ribonucleases	RNA	Nucleotides	
Intestinal mucosa	Aminopeptidase	Polypeptides	Small polypeptides, amino acids*	Acts at amino (N-terminal) end of chain
	Dipeptidases	Dipeptides	Amino acids*	
	Disaccharidases	Disaccharides	Monosaccharides*	
	Maltase	Maltose	Glucose*	
	Sucrase	Sucrose	Glucose*, fructose*	
	Lactase	Lactose	Glucose*, galactose*	
	Nucleases and related enzymes	Nucleic acids	Pentoses*, purine*, and pyrimidine* bases, phosphate*	
	Enterokinase	Trypsinogen	Trypsin	No digestive action *per se*

* Absorbable form

which binds vitamin B_{12} and enables the vitamin to be absorbed from the intestine in the ileum. A lack of intrinsic factor results in pernicious anemia.

Gastric secretion is related to the presence of food. The first or cephalic phase occurs before food enters the stomach. It is a preparatory secretion, mediated by vagal action initiated by stimuli similar to those that cause salivary secretion. The second or gastric phase is a response to signals from the stomach, including an increase in pH due to food in the stomach that causes gastrin release, and distention which acts through the intrinsic network and vagal reflexes to increase acid and enzyme secretion. The third or intestinal phase occurs after food has left the stomach and is apparently due to the presence of some gastrin-secreting cells in the intestinal mucosa; it causes but scant volume.

The stomach normally has enough tone that it is quite small, but it relaxes as food enters (receptive relaxation). Motility increases as the stomach fills owing to stimulation of intrinsic and extrinsic nerves, which raises the excitability of muscle cells. Weak peristaltic contractions begin to appear in the body of the stomach. Successive contractions become stronger, especially in the antral region. This churning in the antral region is where most of the gastric mixing and digestion occur.

The stomach emptying rate depends upon the pressure gradient across the pyloric sphincter. In general, signals from the stomach tend to increase motility and hasten emptying, while signals from the duodenum tend to inhibit motility and slow emptying. The duodenum exerts major control over gastric emptying, and if it is removed, emptying occurs very rapidly (dumping). On the average, the stomach is usually empty some 2 to 4 hours after a meal.

Small Intestine

Chyme entering the duodenum is acid and contains fats, partially digested starches and proteins, and gastric and salivary secretions. Pancreatic juice and bile are added, entering the duodenum a few centimeters below the pylorus, and there is a sizable intestinal secretion. The small intestine is the major site of digestion and absorption.

Food in the intestine increases motor activity resulting in peristaltic waves.

Exocrine Pancreas

The pancreas is a rather diffuse organ with its head located in the curve of the duodenum and its tail trailing off toward the spleen. It is both an exocrine and endocrine organ, but it is the exocrine portion that has important digestive functions. Secretory cells of the exocrine pancreas are arranged as acini around a tiny lumen from which a duct arises. The pancreatic duct empties into the duodenum with the bile duct. Pancreatic juice contains several proteolytic enzymes, including trypsin and chymotrypsin, which are released in inactive form; an amylase which, like that in saliva, yields disaccharides; and pancreatic lipase, which is the only significant lipase.

The secretion of pancreatic juice is controlled primarily by hormones produced by the duodenal mucosa. CCK release occurs when fat and partially digested protein are present, and causes acinar cells to secrete a small volume of pancreatic juice with high enzyme content. Secretin, released when acid is present, stimulates pancreatic duct cells to put out a large volume of secretion with a high bicarbonate content. Vagal stimulation also increases the production of pancreatic juice.

Liver

The liver has a number of varied roles, many of them concerned with metabolism. Its chief role in digestion is the production of bile, which is actually an excretory product.

Structure of the Liver. The liver is the largest organ in the body (after the skin). It receives blood from the hepatic artery and the portal vein (from the digestive tract), and sends blood by the hepatic vein to the inferior vena cava. The hepatic artery and portal vein and the common bile duct reach the liver in the lesser omentum.

The liver is organized into lobules (Fig. 78–4). Each lobule has a central vein (a tributary of the hepatic vein) with plates or sheets of liver cells radiating out from it. The spaces between the sheets of liver cells contain the liver sinusoids, whose endothelial cells form discontinuous capillaries. They are very porous. There are macrophages in the sinusoids. Around the periphery of the lobules are branches of the hepatic artery, portal vein, and bile ducts (the "hepatic triad"). The sinusoids receive blood from both the hepatic artery and the portal vein which flows toward the central vein. As blood flows through the sinusoids, nutrients and other substances are taken up by liver cells, and substances that were stored, produced, or metabolized by the liver enter the sinusoids.

Bile Formation and Release. Bile contains cholesterol; bile salts, which are steroids derived from cholesterol; bile pigments, which are derived from the metabolism of hemoglobin and give bile its characteristic color; and electrolytes. Bile aids digestion because the bile salts are good emulsifying agents; by reducing the surface tension, large fat globules form many smaller ones, which improves the effectiveness of pancreatic lipase.

Bile released from the liver cells enters tiny bile canaliculi that lie between liver cells, and is carried to the bile ducts at the edges of the lobule which converge to the hepatic duct. The cystic duct from the gallbladder joins the hepatic duct to form the common bile duct which enters the duodenum. Since the duodenal opening is usually closed, bile tends to back up into the cystic duct and gallbladder.

Intestinal Secretion

The intestinal mucosa produces several enzymes to complete the digestion of disaccharides and peptides. These enzymes are not truly secreted, however, for they are located on the microvilli of epithelial cells. With the high rate of turnover of intestinal epithelium, the displaced cells soon disintegrate and release their enzymes into the lumen.

Large Intestine and Rectum

The large intestine is shorter in length but greater in diameter than the small intestine. The colon (the portion of the large intestine which extends from the cecum to the rectum) is characterized by a sizable bacterial population which causes fermentation of some sugars, degradation of some remaining proteins, and some breakdown of indigestible materials such as cellulose.

The colon shows considerably less motor and secretory activity than the small intestine. Movements are generally rather sluggish and consist mostly of weak segmentation and peristalsis. These movements are mediated through both the intrinsic and extrinsic innervation. Once or twice a day, strong peristaltic waves, known as mass peristalsis or peristaltic rush, sweep for some distance and move colonic contents into the normally empty rectum. They may be triggered by food in the stomach (the gastrocolic reflex), probably by gastrin release. Movement of material into the rectum causes distention and the sensation of fullness, and is the stimulus for the defecation reflex, which requires, in addition to contractions in the lower colon and rectum, relaxation of the internal and external sphincters, and contraction of abdominal, diaphragm, and expiratory muscles. The skeletal muscle of the external sphincter provides the means to override the involuntary portion of the reflex act.

Digestion and Absorption

The gastric mucous membrane is a tight, relatively impermeable membrane that helps protect underlying tissue from hydrogen ions. It permits very little absorption, except for some weak acids (salicylates, including aspirin) and ethyl

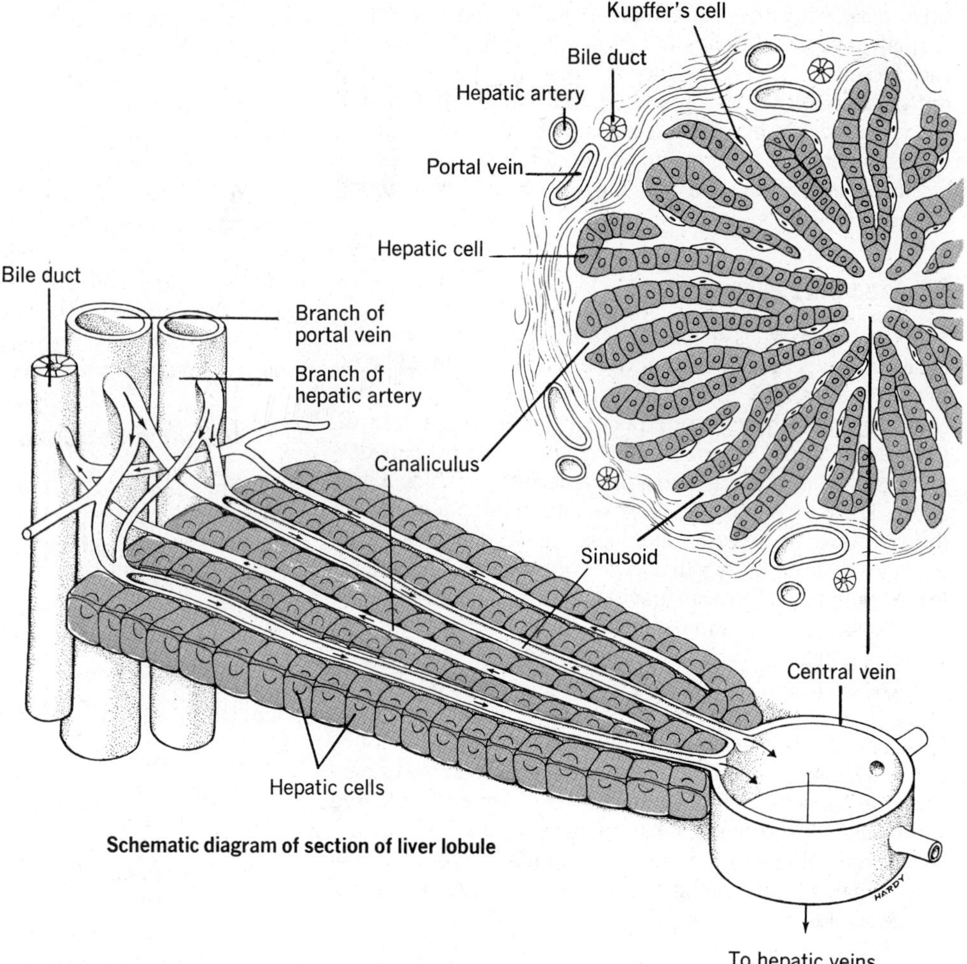

FIGURE 78–4 Diagram of liver lobule showing blood vessels and bile ducts.

alcohol. Digestion occurs primarily in the duodenum and early jejunum, and absorption begins as soon as materials are reduced to absorbable molecules. Absorption involves not only ingested material, but also several liters of secretions produced by the digestive organs. Most of the nutrients and much of the fluid have been removed by the end of the jejunum, and most of the remaining fluid and electrolytes are absorbed from the ileum.

Carbohydrates

Carbohydrates are absorbed as monosaccharides, mainly glucose. Salivary and pancreatic amylases yield disaccharides, with the final breakdown carried out by membrane-bound disaccharidases in the intestinal mucosa. Glucose is actively transported by co-transport with sodium (as it is in renal tubules). The carrier molecule also binds sodium, and the glucose is carried into the cell only when sodium moves into the cell down its electrochemical gradient (Fig. 78–5). Glucose then diffuses from the basal side of the cell into the extracellular fluid and enters the bloodstream. Galactose is actively transported by the same carrier. Fructose is absorbed by facilitated diffusion, and pentoses by simple diffusion.

Protein

About half the protein to be digested comes from ingested foods, the other half from enzymes secreted into the intestine and from desquamated mucosal cells. Large protein molecules are broken by enzymes that are released in inactive forms (pepsin, trypsin, chymotrypsin). They have similar actions, but attack different amino acid linkages. Gastric and pancreatic digestion leave mostly di- and tripeptides, some of which are absorbed, but most of which are broken down by intestinal peptidases and absorbed as amino acids. Absorption of amino acids is an active process mediated by several carrier molecules (for basic, acidic, neutral, and amino acids). All involve co-transport with sodium in the same manner as glucose.

Fat

Pancreatic lipase is the only significant lipolytic enzyme; with the assistance of the bile salts, it readily removes fatty

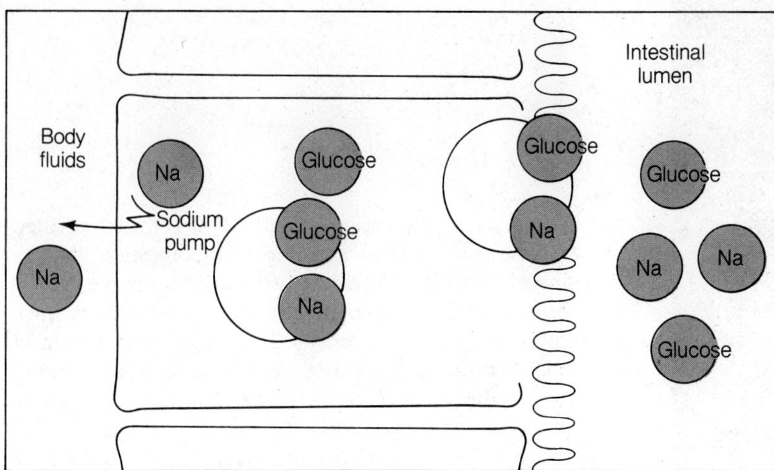

FIGURE 78–5 Diagram of the hypothetical sodium-dependent transport system for glucose. The concentration of glucose builds up within the intestinal cell until a diffusion gradient develops, causing glucose to move into the body fluids. Sodium is transported out of the cell by the energy-dependent (ATP) sodium pump. This creates the gradient needed to operate the transport system.

acids from the 1- and 3-bonds of neutral fats (triacylglycerides); the final fatty acid is removed only very slowly.

Short-chain fatty acids and glycerol diffuse through the mucosal cells and enter the portal circulation, but long-chain fatty acids (and monoacylglycerides) are re-esterified in the mucosal cells. Cholesterol and phospholipids are added to form chylomicrons, which leave the cell by exocytosis and enter lymphatic capillaries (lacteals) in the villi. Most fats therefore bypass the portal circulation and enter the general circulation.

Water and Electrolytes

A large volume of fluid is absorbed with electrolytes, mostly from the small intestine. For the most part the absorption is controlled by local conditions rather than neural or hormonal factors. Rapid breakdown of large molecules may increase the osmotic pressure in the intestine and cause fluid to enter, while active transport of ions and molecules creates an osmotic gradient for fluid absorption. The active sodium ion (Na^+) is particularly important, for its removal is coupled with absorption of many other substances, by co-transport or by electrochemical gradients. In the ileum and colon chlorine ions (Cl^-) are actively absorbed in exchange for HCO_3^-, and in the colon active Na^+ absorption creates an electrical gradient that causes potassium ions (K^+) to be excreted.

The absorption of calcium and iron are externally regulated. Calcium absorption is increased by vitamin D, whose final activation is brought about by parathormone. Iron absorption is controlled in part by the amount of iron stored (as ferritin) in the intestinal mucosa.

Material that is excreted in the stools is about 75% water. The solid portion contains indigestible material (fiber, cellulose), bacteria, and the debris of desquamated mucosal cells.

Several days are normally required for material to pass through the digestive tract. This includes 2 to 4 hours in the stomach, about 6 to 8 hours in the small intestine, and some 2 to 3 days in the colon, an average of 3 to 4 days. Alterations in the rate of passage change the amount of time available for transport processes to occur. More rapid passage reduces fluid absorption and creates electrolyte problems, particularly with K^+ loss. These problems are more critical in infants and children, who have less fluid reserve.

Bibliography

Crouch JE: Functional Human Anatomy, ed 3, chap 21, pp 470–515. Philadelphia, Lea & Febiger, 1978

Davenport HW: Physiology of the Digestive Tract, ed 4. Chicago, Year Book Medical Publishers, 1977

Davenport HW: A Digest of Digestion, ed 2. Chicago, Year Book Medical Publishers, 1978

Ganong WF: Review of Medical Physiology, ed 11, chap 25, 26, pp 377–413. Los Altos, CA, Lange Medical Publications, 1983

Johnson LR: Gastrointestinal Physiology. St. Louis, CV Mosby, 1977

Landau BR: Essential Human Anatomy and Physiology, ed 2, chap 22, 23, pp 541–588. Glenview, IL, Scott, Foresman, 1980

Sernka TJ, Jacobson ED: Gastrointestinal Physiology—The Essentials, ed 2. Baltimore, Williams & Wilkins, 1983

Chapter 79

Assessment of Gastrointestinal Function

Linda M. Simmons

The functions of the gastrointestinal (GI) system, as indicated in the previous chapter, include ingestion, digestion, absorption, and elimination. Nutrients and medications are usually introduced into the body by the mouth and alimentary tract. Nutrients must then be processed or changed to a form of substrate that the body can use for energy and tissue building. This is the process of digestion. Following digestion, nutrients must be absorbed by the bloodstream and delivered to organs and tissues for the metabolism required for cellular repair, tissue building, or the production of energy. The final process in the utilization of ingested nutrients is the elimination of metabolic waste products. The structures and organs involved in GI function include the mouth, esophagus, stomach, small intestine, colon, and rectum. Because of their role in digestion and metabolism, the liver, gallbladder, and pancreas are also considered part of the GI system. Alterations in any of these functions can result in health problems ranging from minor discomforts (*e.g.,* transient nausea) to life-threatening conditions (*e.g.,* massive hemorrhage, carcinoma).

The GI system is intimately associated with many other somatic functions. Dysfunction of almost any body system may give rise to GI signs and symptoms, or symptoms may reflect primary GI disease. For instance, one of the manifestations of inadequate heart function is nausea and vomiting. This is probably related to impaired central nervous system function. Also, GI side-effects are common for an uncountable number of both prescription and over-the-counter drugs. Therefore, GI dysfunction may occur in patients being treated for a wide variety of health problems (*e.g.,* orthopedic, endocrine, and so forth). Precise assessment may be challenging for the health practitioner because symptoms are often numerous and vague. However, nursing assessment is crucial for identifying problems amenable to both direct nursing interventions and indirect interventions such as notification and consultation with the physician and teaching of patients, families, and other care-givers. Assessment is the first step of the nursing process.

Direct examination of some structures in the GI system is possible using invasive techniques and state-of-the-art technology. However, indirect evidence of dysfunction or pathology gained by careful history and physical examination is invaluable for precise and complete patient evaluation.

The nurse's role in data collection regarding the patient's GI status includes obtaining an accurate history and performing physical assessment as well as assisting the patient before, during, and after any necessary diagnostic tests. The nursing diagnosis is based on information obtained by the above activities. Although the nurse should assess all patients in a systematic way, each patient requires an individualized approach to questioning and physical examination. All assessment measures should be performed with consideration to the patient's age, stage of development, chief complaint, present physical condition, and previously obtained baseline data, if available.

Gastrointestinal History

Much of the information required for assessment of GI function is available from a complete general health history which supplies helpful subjective information. Whether the patient is hospitalized or seen in a clinic setting when undergoing evaluation for GI symptoms, it is the physician who usually completes the medical history and physical examination. The nurse should review these data in order to avoid repeating the entire health history. Additional data are then collected based on the patient's present symptoms of GI dysfunction. If the patient is in acute pain or other distress, the nurse should focus questioning on the presenting signs and symptoms and defer questioning about related areas until the patient is more comfortable.

History is extremely important because GI complaints are often numerous, varied, and vague. Sometimes, with the patient's consent, it is helpful to have a family member or significant other present during the history-taking interview to clarify and supplement information. Other sources of information include the patient's medical record, when available, and interviews with other professional staff.

Because "normal" GI function may vary widely from person to person, it is important to identify those symptoms that reflect change from the patient's norm. The health practitioner should appreciate that some persons may find discussing GI functions embarrassing and should use a matter-of-fact tone during questioning.

Dietary Practices

Assessment would not be complete without evaluation of the patient's nutritional status and dietary practices, often factors in GI dysfunction. Much of the nutritional assessment is based on the diet history. The most accurate method for evaluating dietary adequacy is the "food diary." The patient or staff records all foods and fluids taken for a typical 24 to 48 hours. When a diary is impractical, the nurse should question the patient regarding food intake during the preceding 24 hours. The nurse, often with the assistance of a clinical dietician, evaluates quality and quantity of nutrients ingested and identifies ideal body weight (IBW) range. If need for change is indicated, consideration must be given to the patient's preferences, daily work, personal schedule, and financial resources. The relationship between the occurrence of GI symptoms and food intake can provide important clues in the overall assessment of GI function.

Some GI symptoms (*e.g.,* nausea, anorexia), although not of a serious nature by themselves, can lead to serious problems if a reduced intake of calories and protein results. Certain groups of individuals, because of increased needs or decreased resources are at a particularly high risk for nutritional deficiencies. These groups include infants and children, adolescents, pregnant and lactating women, economically disadvantaged persons, persons who have had GI surgery resulting in absorption problems, and elderly persons. Older persons, in general, constitute a particularly high-risk group for malnutrition for several reasons (see Table 79–1).

TABLE 79–1
Risk Factors for Nutritional Inadequacy in Elderly Persons

Reduced income
Decreased mobility resulting in difficulty shopping
Changes in tastes sensations
Loneliness
Increase in sedentary habits
Physical debilitation
Lack of knowledge of what constitutes sound nutrition
Cognitive impairment (forgetting to eat)

Approach to Data Collection

The following are *examples* of questions meant to elicit general as well as symptom-specific data regarding the status of the GI system. The extent of questioning depends on the patient's symptoms as well as previously documented information. The data obtained should augment information obtained by the physician during the general health history.

General Changes or Problems

Has there been a recent change in energy level?
Was there a major crisis in the patient's life (*e.g.,* death of a family member, loss of a job)?
Is the patient more easily fatigued lately?
Have there been recent appetite changes?

Patient and Family Medical History

Does the patient have a history of GI-related illness?
Has the patient had previous surgery for GI problems (*e.g.,* gastrectomy, cholecystectomy)?
Are there any concurrent diseases or health problems?
Is the patient taking any prescription or over-the-counter medicines?
Is there a family history of GI disorders, including carcinoma of the GI tract?

Nutritional Data

Has there been a recent weight loss or gain?
Was the weight change intentional or inadvertent?
Was the weight change sudden or gradual?
Are there disturbances following ingestion of food?
Has there been a recent change in usual meal times, environment, or meal companions?
What constitutes a typical day's diet intake? Obtain recent hour diet diary or 24- to 48-hour food recall.
Have there been recent changes in eating habits?
What is the usual alcohol intake, daily or weekly?
Is there a new or recurrent food intolerance? Specify.
Is there pain or discomfort before or after meals?
Is there tooth sensitivity to hot or cold?

Oral and Esophageal Changes or Problems

Have there been recent changes in the surface texture of the lips, tongue, gums, or mouth lining?
Has the patient noticed any sores or lumps in the mouth area?
Is there any pain in the mouth area?
Is there any difficulty moving the tongue?
Have there been recent changes in the amount or character of saliva? Disagreeable taste?
Is there any difficulty speaking?
Have there been any recent gum problems (*i.e.*, bleeding or recession)?
Have there been recent dental problems?
Is the patient edentulous?
Does the patient have any dental prostheses?
Is there any difficulty chewing or swallowing?
Is there pain on swallowing (odynophagia)?
Are there complaints of eructation or heartburn?

Stomach and Digestion

Does the patient report recent indigestion episodes?
Does the patient experience fullness after eating?
Is there a history of abdominal trauma or surgery?
Does the patient experience abdominal cramps?
Has the patient experienced nausea and/or vomiting?
Has the patient vomited blood or coffee-ground-like material?
Are there any complaints of abdominal pain? If so, obtain symptom-specific data including the following:
 Factors which initiate the symptom (*e.g.*, situation or specific food).
 Symptom onset relative to causative factor.
 Symptom character and location.
 Symptom duration.
 Factors which improve or worsen the symptom.
 Extent to which the symptom(s) interfere with usual daily activities.

Bowel Function

Has there been a recent change in bowel habits?
Has there been a change in the frequency, color, or character of stools?
What does the patient do to stimulate defacation?
How often does the patient use laxatives or antidiarrheal agents?
Has any bleeding with stool been noticed? If so, symptom-specific data to obtain include the following:
 Color of blood, bright red or dark, tarry.
 Estimation of blood loss. (*Note:* This is difficult because a few drops of blood in the toilet may appear to be a few cups.)
 Frequency of blood appearing with a stool.
Is there any pain with defecation?
Does the patient strain at stool?
Is there a history of hemorrhoids?
Does the patient complain of flatulence?
Is there a history of bowel surgery?
Does the patient have an ostomy? What does the routine care involve?

General Symptoms

Is there a history of yellow discoloration of the skin or sclera of the eyes?
Has there been any noticeable edema of the extremities?

Physical Assessment

A physical examination is often performed by the physician when a patient is admitted to the hospital or seen in an outpatient clinic, but there are occasions when the nurse must perform a part or all ot the physical assessment. During the care of patients, specific problems may evolve, manifested by new or different symptomatology. For GI-related symptoms, subjective data can be expanded by history-taking. Further evaluation of GI status requires systematic physical assessment. Both types of data are necessary as a basis for the nurse's clinical judgment.

Objective data about the patient's GI status are collected using physical examination including the techniques of inspection, auscultation, percussion, and palpation. General guidelines for physical examination include the following:

- Wash hands.
- Warm hands and stethoscope.
- Have necessary equipment assembled ready to use.
- Drape the patient for maximum privacy, minimum exposure.
- Explain all procedures, have the patient relax.
- Conduct examination based on history data.

The validity of the data obtained from physical assessment depends on the examiner's knowledge of GI anatomy. When documenting findings, include a simple illustrative diagram whenever possible. The actual approach to physical assessment will be governed by the patient's symptoms revealed during the history. For example, if the patient's chief complaint is mouth soreness, a thorough investigation of the lower intestinal tract may not be warranted.

General Observations

A common approach to the assessment of GI function begins with the inspection of the patient's overall appearance. The lighting in the examination room should provide even illumination. Areas to observe include body build type, stature, evidence of malnutrition (over or underweight), skin color and tone, and evidence of being in acute distress (*e.g.*, facial grimace, hands guarding abdomen). Measure vital signs, including lying and sittling pulse and blood pressure. Orthostatic hypotension may be an indication of bleeding. Measure and record anthropometric data including weight, height, and triceps skinfold thickness. Height and weight data are compared to ideal body weight range (Table 79–2). Proceed with the exam using a cephalocaudal approach. The nurse should be particularly alert to signs of malignancy, especially when seeing patients in the home environment or clinic setting, in order to suggest physician consultation. These signs occur with increasing frequency in elderly persons.

TABLE 79–2
Metropolitan Height and Weight Tables, 1983

Men					Women				
Height					Height				
Feet	*Inches*	*Small Frame*	*Medium Frame*	*Large Frame*	*Feet*	*Inches*	*Small Frame*	*Medium Frame*	*Large Frame*
5	2	128–134	131–141	138–150	4	10	102–111	109–121	118–131
5	3	130–136	133–143	140–153	4	11	103–113	111–123	120–134
5	4	132–138	135–145	142–156	5	0	104–115	113–126	122–137
5	5	134–140	137–148	144–160	5	1	106–118	115–129	125–140
5	6	136–142	139–151	146–164	5	2	108–121	118–132	128–143
5	7	138–145	142–154	149–168	5	3	111–124	121–135	131–147
5	8	140–148	145–157	152–172	5	4	114–127	124–138	134–151
5	9	142–151	148–160	155–176	5	5	117–130	127–141	137–155
5	10	144–154	151–163	158–180	5	6	120–133	130–144	140–159
5	11	146–157	154–166	161–184	5	7	123–136	133–147	143–163
6	0	149–160	157–170	164–188	5	8	126–139	136–150	146–167
6	1	152–164	160–174	168–192	5	9	129–142	139–153	149–170
6	2	155–168	164–178	172–197	5	10	132–145	142–156	152–173
6	3	158–172	167–182	176–202	5	11	135–148	145–159	155–176
6	4	162–176	171–187	181–207	6	0	138–151	148–162	158–179

Weights at ages 25–59 based on lowest mortality. Weight in pounds according to frame (in indoor clothing weighing 5 lb, shoes with 1-inch heels).

Weights at ages 25–59 based on lowest mortality. Weight in pounds according to frame (in indoor clothing weighing 3 lb, shoes with 1-inch heels).

(Courtesy of the Metropolitan Life Insurance Co, New York, 1983)

Mouth and Pharynx

Equipment needed: flashlight, tongue depressor. Ask patient to remove lipstick.

Inspection: Observe for symmetry of lips and surface texture. Note cracks, lesions, presence or absence of drainage. Note scars and malformations. Inspect oral mucosa for smoothness and pink color. Note any white spots, patches, discoloration, roughened texture, inflammation, ulceration. Shiny buccal mucosa is a normal variation in the elderly. Note number of teeth and condition. Note loose teeth. Gingiva should be smooth and pink. If edentulous, inspect for reddened (dark) spots from ill-fitting dentures. Observe dentures for fit. Have patient remove dentures to observe ridge for evidence of pressure areas. Inspect uvula for midling position. Observe tongue mobility for symmetry and limited motion.

Palpation: Examine lips, buccal mucosa, and tongue for presence of lumps. Note whether lumps are fixed or movable.

Esophagus

Cannot directly examine without instrumentation. Most data about esophageal dysfunction are obtained by history and diagnostic tests.

Stomach

Not usually palpable. Assessed during examination of the abdomen, and by instrumentation when indicated.

Abdomen

Equipment needed: stethoscope with diaphragm and bell. It is recommended that inspection, auscultation, and percussion be performed prior to palpation of the abdomen because palpation may disrupt intestinal peristaltic activity and alter bowel sounds (*i.e.,* stimulate or subdue sounds). The diaphragm of the stethoscope is used to auscultate bowel sounds while the bell detects vascular sounds.

Inspection: Observe for symmetry and visible peristalsis. Note visible masses and hernias. Note any distention; measure abdominal girth. Note presence of ostomies, scars, and striae. Inspect for distended blood vessels and jaundice. Umbilicus should be inverted. Observe skin color. Note jaundice, petechiae.

Auscultation: Auscultation of the abdomen should be performed in a quiet setting to aviod interference with and misinterpretation of abdominal sounds. As always, explain to the patient what you are going to do. Warm the stethoscope between your hands. Determine the presence or absence of bowel sounds in all four quadrants. Note high-pitched sounds which may occur proximal to obstruction. Note presence or absence of abnormal vascular sounds (*e.g.,* aortic or renal bruits).

Percussion: Abdominal percussion is performed to estimate the location and size of abdominal organs and structures. The usual technique involves placing the middle finger of one hand flat on the abdomen. Percussion sounds are elicited by striking or thumping the distal joint of the flat middle finger with the tip of the flexed middle finger of the other hand (Fig. 79–1). Percuss from quadrant to quadrant.

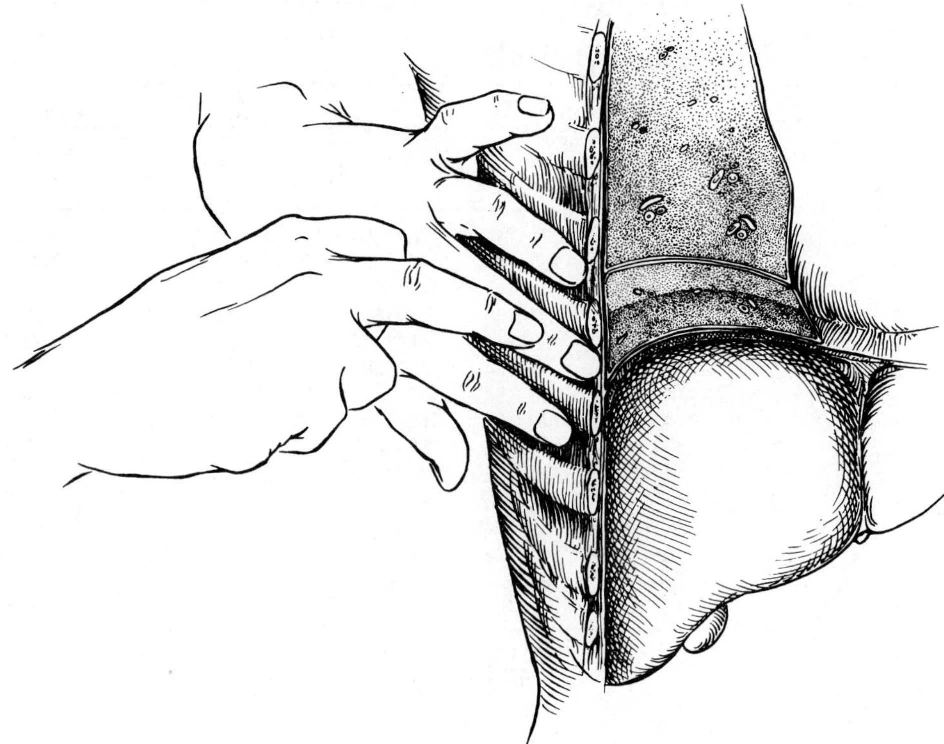

FIGURE 79–1 Detection of upper border of liver dullness. Absolute dullness is compared to relative dullness and to resonance on percussion. This technique may be practiced on any normal chest.

Tympanic sounds are heard over an air-filled bowel. Dullness is present over stool-filled colon or ascitic fluid. Normally, the lower liver border is at or above the costal margin and may not be palpable. The upper border of the liver is determined because it indicates the size of the right lobe. Dullness in the left upper quadrant may indicate splenic enlargement.

Findings are documented by noting in which quadrant of the abdomen they are located (Fig. 79–2).

Palpation: The fourth step in physical assessment of the abdomen is palpation, for which there are several acceptable techniques. The most common method consists of light palpation followed by deep palpation. During light palpation, using the pads of the fingertips, the examiner can identify muscle tenderness and resistance. Ordinarily, quadrants should be examined in the same order used for auscultation and percussion. However, if the patient complains of localized abdominal pain, examine that quadrant last. Findings are expressed as they compare to the other quadrants. With fingers together, press smoothly and gently in all quadrants. If muscular resistance or rigidity is noted, have the patient take a deep breath and exhale. Persistent involuntary rigidity may be a sign of acute peritonitis which requires prompt notification of the physician because immediate medical intervention is necessary. Also feel for masses and assess skin temperature at this time.

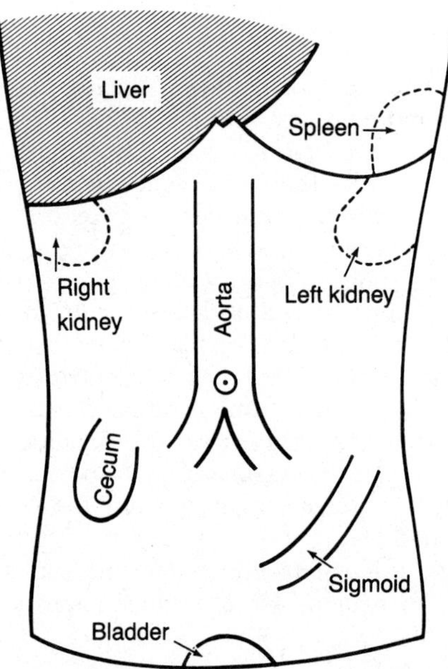

FIGURE 79–2 Internal anatomy. Placement of abdominal organs. Those organs drawn with solid lines are palpable in normals, whereas those drawn with dotted lines are usually palpable in disease.

The abdominal assessment is completed using the technique of deep palpation, which is performed to identify organ position, tenderness, or masses. This advanced technique should be used only after it has been demonstrated and performed under supervision. Bimanual palpation is best, pressing the fingers about 3 inches into the abdomen toward the back (Fig. 79–3). Systematically palpate one quadrant at a time. Be gentle in areas of tenderness. Note rebound pain when fingertips are quickly withdrawn, which indicates inflammation. If a mass is palpated, note its location, size, mobility, and consistency. In some circumstances this technique is contraindicated. One such situation is when bruits

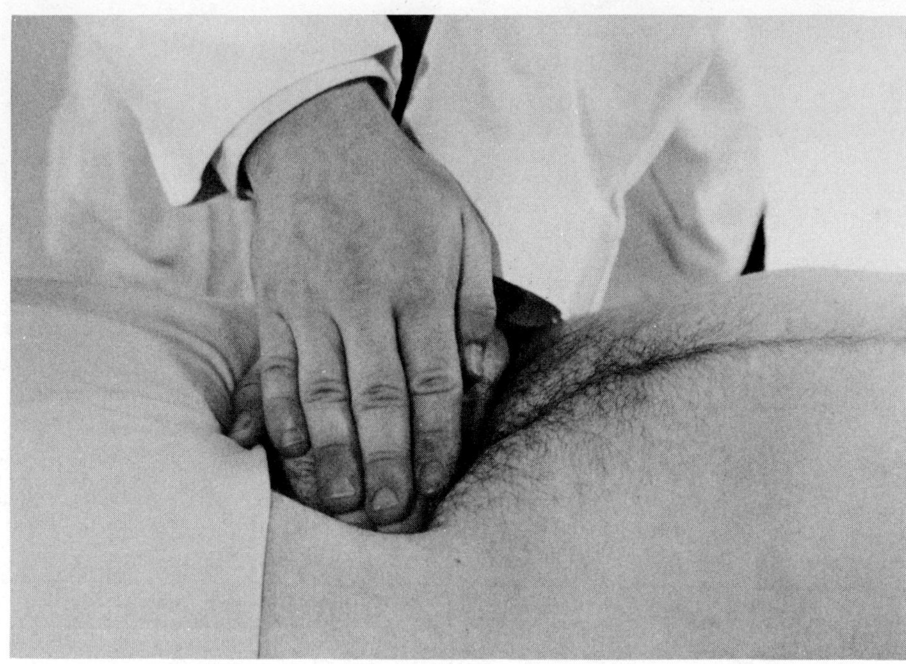

FIGURE 79–3 Technique for bimanual palpation.

are auscultated and arterial perfusion to the lower extremities is reduced. These are manifestations of a dissecting aortic aneurysm, which is an uncommon but very serious condition which requires immediate medical intervention.

Liver

The lower edge of the liver may be palpated by placing the fingertips of one hand on the right side of the abdomen under the *costal* margin at the midclavicular line. Have the patient breathe in deeply, exhale, and inhale a second time. During the second inspiration, press the fingertips gently inward and upward. The lower liver border should tap the examiner's fingertips as it is pushed downward by the diaphragm. The upper liver border is identified by percussion (discussed above), and the normal span from dome (top) to bottom is 10 to 15 cm. The normal liver may not be palpable in some patients. Note hepatic enlargement or tenderness to palpation.

Spleen

The spleen is normally not palpable owing to its position under the ribs. However, the examiner can palpate for splenic enlargement by performing maneuvers similar to liver palpation under the left *costal* margin (Fig. 79–4). Begin with light palpation and follow with deep palpation. A tender spleen should not be deeply palpated, and this finding should be reported to the physician.

Gallbladder

The gallbladder is not directly examined using the above techniques. However, tenderness of this organ may be manifested during light and deep palpation. Inflammation of the gallbladder may be signaled if the patient has splinting respirations or "catches" his or her breath when asked to breathe deeply. Physical examination provides some indirect evidence of hepatic, splenic, gallbladder, and pancreatic function. More definitive data of dysfunction are revealed from laboratory tests and other diagnostic studies.

Perianal Region

The terminus of the GI tract is assessed using the techniaues of inspection and palpation. The examiner should visualize the perianal area and note unusual coloration, lesions, external hemorrhoids, or prolapsed rectal tissue. Document unusual odor or drainage as well. Prepare the patient for palpation or digital examination by explaining what will be done and enlisting his or her cooperation. This technique may be used to check for suspected fecal impaction. Reassure the patient that he or she may feel some discomfort but not pain. Never use force when inserting the lubricated gloved finger through the rectal sphincter. Gently palpate for nodules. Note tenderness, mucous, or blood, as well as the presence of stool. If stool is present on the glove after examination it is tested for occult blood. Offer the patient tissue or a towelette for cleansing after the examination.

Diagnostic Tests

Gastrointestinal symptomatology, as discussed previously, may be vague, making it difficult to identify specific causes of dysfunction by history taking and physical examination alone. Assessment is usually augmented with diagnostic tests including laboratory analysis of serum, urine, stool, and

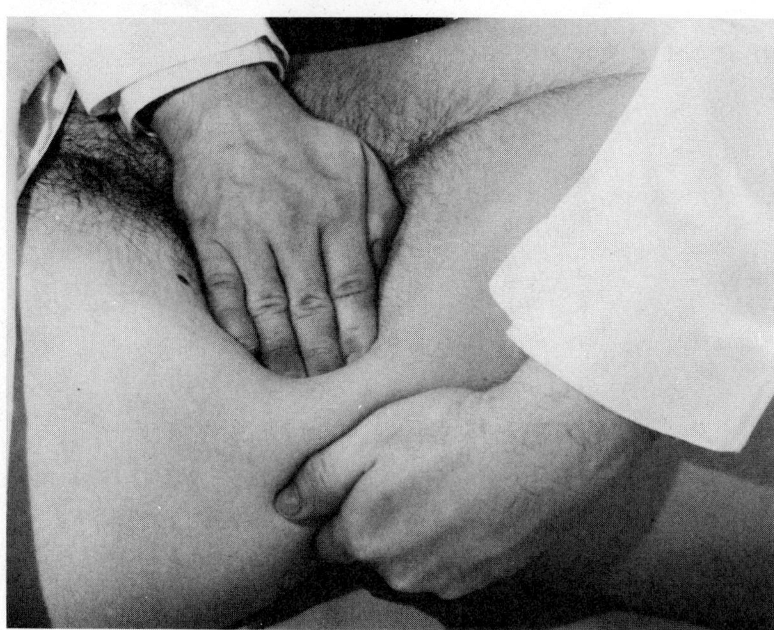

FIGURE 79–4 Bimanual palpation: one hand anteriorly and the other posteriorly, patient supine. The fingers of the posterior left hand press the posterior abdominal wall forward.

gastric secretions, contrast radiography, and endoscopic examination. It is not uncommon for patients with GI dysfunction to undergo several tests for diagnosis and monitoring of specific disorders. The nurse must keep in mind the time-consuming, costly, and sometimes unpleasant aspects of these tests.

Pretest Preparation

Although many of the tests are considered routine by nurses, they are not routine for the patient. Even a simple venipuncture requires patient preparation. Pretest preparation includes careful explanation about the test the patient is to undergo. When the nurse is unfamiliar with the facility's procedure or the range of normal values for a particular test, he or she should consult the laboratory personnel. The nurse uses this information in two ways: to instruct the patient before the test and to plan aftercare. Except in emergencies this teaching should be scheduled so as to allow the patient time to ask questions and voice any concerns. A spouse, family member, or significant other should be included in the preparation, unless the patient objects. The patient should be given written explanations. Some diagnostic studies (*e.g.,* endoscopy and biopsy) require signed consent. It is the nurse's responsibility to see that this is accomplished according to the facility policy. The patient should not be given any premedications (*i.e.,* sedatives or narcotics) until signed consent is obtained.

Premedication may be ordered before tests of an invasive nature (*e.g.,* gastroscopy) in order to decrease test-related anxiety and discomfort as well as minimize secretions. As with any drug, the nurse must check for any known drug allergies. Side-effects of the premedication must be noted promptly and emergency care given as necessary. Emergency resuscitative equipment should be readily available and its use familiar to all personnel. Narcan, a narcotic antagonist, should be available in the event of narcotic-induced respiratory depression. Because many diagnostic tests for GI dysfunction are performed on an outpatient basis, the patient should be told to plan for a ride home if sedative medications will be used before or during the procedure. Vital signs should be taken and recorded before and during procedures involving medications or invasive techniques.

When test procedures require the patient to assume a position he or she may find embarrassing, care must be taken to drape in order to minimize exposure. Throughout any procedure, the nurse should question and observe the patient to determine level of discomfort and tolerance of the procedure.

Elderly Patients. Special consideration must be given to the needs and potential problems of elderly patients undergoing diagnostic studies. If sensory deficits are evident, pretest instructions should be given slowly, loudly enough, and be accompanied by written instructions. A family member or significant other should accompany the patient.

Two common problems for many older patients undergoing GI tests are fatigue and dehydration. Because some examinations (*e.g.,* barium enema or colonoscopy) often leave the patient feeling weak and fatigued, the planning should include rest when the patient returns to the nursing unit or home, in the case of an outpatient. Fluid loss can result from multiple enemas, laxatives, and other cleansing procedures required before certain examinations (*e.g.,* barium enema, sigmoidoscopy). Oral fluid replacement must be encouraged in these patients unless contraindicated.

Post-Test Considerations

The patient must be given clear verbal and written instructions following the test. Include when the diet may be resumed, activity restrictions if any, medication resumption, and symptoms to report. Include the telephone number of the physician, nurse, or department to call should problems or questions arise.

The nurse should be aware of the normal range of values for diagnostic tests. Normal values may differ depending on the laboratory or center making the determinations. Knowledge of the test is important in order to instruct the patient prior to the test as well as to plan aftercare.

Several of these studies involve direct visualization of a part of the gastrointestinal tract. Included in this category are esophagoscopy (direct visualization of the esophageal mucosa), gastroscopy (direct visualization of the gastric mucosa), proctoscopy and sigmoidoscopy (direct visualization of the mucosa of the distal segment of the colon and rectum).

Radiological procedures include barium enemas and barium swallows, small bowel radiography, cholecystography, and cholangiography. Other studies depend on specimen examination, such as gastric analysis and stool analysis.

Table 79–3 contains information about the purpose and procedure of common GI diagnostic studies, the normal values and clinical significance of findings as well as nursing considerations for each test.

TABLE 79–3
Common GI Diagnostic Studies

Study	*Purpose and Procedures*	*Clinical Significance*	*Nursing Considerations*
Esophagoscopy	Direct visualization of the esophageal mucosa for inspection, biopsy, or removal of foreign body. A flexible fiberoptic endoscope is passed orally into the esophagus (~ 30 cm)	Site of bleeding or abnormality may be precisely located. Nodules or lesions may be biopsied. Causes for swallowing discomfort or difficulty may be identified.	*Pretest (Esophagoscopy and gastroscopy)* Explain test to patient, including use of premedication. Describe sensations patient may experience. Explain approximate length of procedure. Determine if written consent is signed. NPO 6 hr–8 hr before test. Remove dentures and eyeglasses. Have patient void. Enlist cooperation and support throughout procedure. Patient is unable to talk and has no gag reflex during test. An IV may be started and maintained for possible emergency medications. Have suction available. *Post test:* No food or fluids until gag reflex returns (~ 2 hr–4 hr). Rest at least 1 hr after test. Check vital signs q 30 min for 2 hr. Assess for complications (*e.g.*, perforation). Instruct patient to report swallowing difficulty, bloody or tarry stools, or pain 24 or more hr after test.
Gastroscopy	Direct visualization of gastric mucosa. To identify location of ulcer or upper GI bleeding. Biopsy may be included to differentiate between benign and malignant lesions. A flexible fiberoptic endoscope is passed orally into the stomach.	Normal mucosa shows no bleeding or ulcers. Newer scopes permit direct treatment of small gastric bleeding sites by cauterization or laser treatment.	
Esophagastroduodenoscopy (EGD)	In addition to above, the pylorus and duodenum are visualized. May be extended to explore pancreas and gallbladder (ERCP, see below).	Same as above	Same as for esophagoscopy. Patient may need to belch to expel air insufflated during test.

(*Continued*)

TABLE 79–3
Common GI Diagnostic Studies *(Continued)*

Study	*Purpose and Procedures*	*Clinical Significance*	*Nursing Considerations*
Endoscopic retrograde cholangiopancreatography (ERCP)	An extension of EGD (above) to explore pancreatic and common bile duct fluoroscopically for gallstones or obstruction. A cannula is threaded through the fiberoptic scope into the common bile and pancreatic ducts. Contrast media is instilled and several x-rays are taken.	Normal findings are negative for gallstones, and no obstruction is seen in pancreatic and common bile ducts, gallbladder and duodenal papilla. Abnormal results may include stones, stenosis, or malignancy.	Same as above. In addition, an IV is started before the procedure. Glucagon IV may be given to inhibit duodenal activity. NPO for 12 hr before test. Check vital signs q 30 min after test for 4 hr. Observe for complications including urinary retention, cholangitis, and pancreatitis (fever, abdominal tenderness, pain).
Proctoscopy and sigmoidoscopy	Direct visualization of mucosa of distal segment of the colon and rectum. Rigid instrument allows visualization of up to 20 cm of colon. A flexible fiberoptic sigmoidoscope may be inserted up to 65 cm. This is a routine screening procedure for colon cancer for males over 40 yr, with family history. Biopsy may be performed during the procedure.	Up to 75% of colon neoplasms are within the range of visualization of the flexible instrument. Normal findings include temporary hyperemia and excess mucus secondary to the enema. Abnormal findings: decreased mucus, bleeding, edema, polyps, ulcers, and carcinoma.	*Pretest:* Light supper and light breakfast. Can be performed on an outpatient basis, without special preparation. If there is stool in the rectum, a suppository or enema may be required for evacuation. Knee–chest of Sims' position. *Post test:* After exam, allow for rest. Offer fluids and food before patient returns home. Instruct patient to report pain, bleeding, or fever following the procedure.
Colonscopy	Direct visualization of colonic mucosa up to ileocecal valve (~ 130 cm–180 cm) using a flexible fiberoptic colonscope. Purposes: locate site of bleeding, identify polyps, tumors, diverticuli, remove foreign bodies. Brush border cytology and/or biopsy may be performed during the procedure.	Normal: no evidence of polyps, tumors, or bleeding. Abnormal findings may include polyps, malignancy, inflammatory bowel, disease, ischemia, vascular anomaly. Contraindicated in presence of massive acute bleeding, recent colonic surgery, active inflammatory disease, acute abdomen, or suspected recent bowel perforation.	*Pretest:* Written informed consent. Clear liquids for 72 hr prior to test. NPO for 8 hr prior to test. Laxatives 1 day–3 days before, as ordered. Enemas morning before, as ordered. VS before test. *During test:* Running IV for analgesia/light anethesia. Explanation and support throughout test. Patient may experience gas pain. Drugs used include narcotics, sedatives, and possibly anticholinergics, to relieve bowel spasm. Have narcotic antagonist available (*e.g.*, Narcan). *Post test:* VS q 30 min till stable. Encourage fluids. Observe for bleeding and signs of perforation. If polypectomy performed, low-fiber diet for 2 wk. Patient should not drive home. Elderly patients should be observed for cardiovascular problems. This test is fatiguing, extra rest required.

(Continued)

TABLE 79–3
Common GI Diagnostic Studies *(Continued)*

Study	*Purpose and Procedures*	*Clinical Significance*	*Nursing Considerations*
Radiologic Procedures			
	Visualization of areas of GI tract using contrast media and x-rays		
Barium enema (lower GI series)	To visualize the position, movement and filling of the segments of the colon. Liquid barium is introduced by enema, and x-rays are taken with and without fluoroscopy. For more definitive visualization, air may also be injected into the colon as a second contrast medium. If abdominal scans, ultrasound, or proctoscopy is also indicated, these procedures must be done prior to barium enema.	Abnormal findings include tumors, fistulae, diverticuli, obstruction, stenosis, inflammation, ulcerative colitis, polyps, megacolon, active bleeding.	*Pretest:* Written informed consent. Explain procedure. It may be lengthy Bowel preparation must be through, or colon won't visualize well. Provide written instruction to outpatients. Clear liquids evening before test, NPO after midnight. Laxatives and enemas as orderd. On morning of test hold oral medications or check with physician about different route of administration (*e.g.*, parenteral). Procedure is uncomfortable and tiring, especially for elderly patients. *Post test:* Increase fluid intake. Observe for electrolyte imbalance. Provide/encourage rest. Provide written instructions for outpatients. Laxatives, as ordered, to expel barium and prevent constipation, especially if the patient is pre-op. Stools are light colored until barium is eliminated. Instruct to report pain, bloating, bleeding, or absence of stool. Stress importance of elimination of barium (it can harden in the bowel and cause obstruction or perforation).
Upper GI (gastric radiography) (barium swallow)	To visualize the position, shape, and activity of the esophagus, stomach, duodenum, and jejunum. A liquid barium suspension is swallowed during fluoroscopy after a preliminary x-ray.	Abnormal findings may indicate congenital anomalies, hiatus hernia, esophageal and gastric diverticulitis, pyloric stenosis, peptic ulcer, tumor, polyps, gastritis, or foreign bodies.	*Pretest:* NPO after midnight. Laxatives and enemas not necessary unless this test will follow a barium enema. *Post test:* Offer food and fluids. Laxative, if necessary, to expel barium. Stool color is light until barium is evacuated. Observe for rectal bleeding. A follow-up x-ray 24 hr later may be scheduled. Stress importance of elimination of barium.

(Continued)

TABLE 79–3
Common GI Diagnostic Studies *(Continued)*

Study	*Purpose and Procedures*	*Clinical Significance*	*Nursing Considerations*
Radiologic Procedures			
Small bowel radiography (small bowel follow-through)	To visualize the contours and motility of the small bowel by the use of barium or other contrast material. Contrast material is swallowed during fluoroscopy and x-ray films are taken. This test is often done immediately after upper GI.	Abnormal results may reveal ulcerative colitis, tumors, obstruction, Meckel's diverticulum, regional enteritis (Crohn's disease), intussusception, atresia, intra-abdominal hernias, filling defects.	*Pretest:* If done with UGI, total time for test is increased and more fatigue is likely. Explain what to expect to the patient. NPO after midnight. Written instructions to outpatients. Identify drugs patient may be taking which affect motility (*e.g.*, narcotics, anticholinergics, metaclopramide and anti-ulcer drugs) and alert physician. *Post test:* Offer food and fluids. Allow for extra rest. Laxatives as directed to prevent constipation. Observe color of stool for completeness of barium evacuation.
Cholecystogram	To visualize the gallbladder by the use of contrast material taken orally. X-rays films are taken first of the dye-filled gallbladder. Following a fatty meal, x-rays are taken of the stimulated gallbladder.	Normal findings include the absence of stones (cholelithiasis) and normal emptying of the gallbladder following a fatty meal. Abnormal results include the presence of stones, obstruction, nonvisualization.	*Pretest:* Explain test to patient. Contrast tablets given after low-fat evening meal. Usually six tablets are taken, one every 5 min. Enema and laxatives, as directed. NPO after midnight. *Post test:* Unless other diagnostic tests are planned, usual diet is resumed. Extra fluids needed to restore hydration.
Cholangiogram	To visualize the hepatic, cystic, and common ducts for patency. May be performed in three ways: 1) IV method consists of injection of dye intravenously and x-rays are taken of dye excretion by the liver; 2) After gallbladder surgery, dye is injected directly into the biliary tract by a drainage tube left in place; 3) Intraoperatively, dye is directly injected into the ducts and visualized as well as x-rayed.	Normal findings include patency of hepatic, cystic, and common ducts. Abnormal results include stones in any area of the biliary tree, obstruction, tumors, or nonvisualization.	*Pretest:* 1) IV cholangiogram. NPO after midnight, laxatives and enemas as directed. Explain procedure including approximate length of procedure (about 4 hr). Inquire about dye allergies. 2) Postoperative and 3) Intraoperative techniques, prepare as surgical patient. *Post test:* 1) IV technique. Encourage fluid intake. Provide or promote rest. Resume diet as directed. 2) Postoperative, and 3) intraoperative technique, provide postoperative nursing care.

(Continued)

TABLE 79–3
Common GI Diagnostic Studies *(Continued)*

Study	*Purpose and Procedures*	*Clinical Significance*	*Nursing Considerations*
Radiologic Procedures			
Exfoliative (brush border) cytology	To examine cells lining the GI tract to distinguish between benign and malignant disease. Includes cells of the esophagus, stomach, pancreatic and gallbladder drainage, small intestine, and colon. Cells are obtained by either of two methods: 1) Saline lavage through nasogastric tube or proctoscope or 2) during endoscopy.	Normal findings are negative for benign and malignant cellular changes. Abnormal esophageal cells may indicate malignancy, folic acid or vitamin B_{12} deficiency, esophagitis. Abnormal gastric cells may indicate malignancy, gastritis, pernicious anemia, granulomatous inflammation. Abnormal duodenal, pancreatic and/or gallbladder cells may indicate malignancy. Abnormal colon cells may indicate malignancy, ulcerative colitis, or ileitis.	Explain procedure to patient. Obtain written consent. Assist to pass nasogastric tube or swallow endoscopic tube. (See endoscopy.) This can be an uncomfortable procedure. *Pretest:* Liquid diet. For colon studies, laxatives and cleansing enemas are given. *Post test:* Provide fluids, food, and extra rest. Anticipate anxiety concerning results of examination.
Gastric analysis with histamine or histalog	To obtain and analyze gastric contents for amount of hydrochloric acid (HCl) secreted in response to betazole hydrochloride or histamine injection. A nasogastric tube is inserted, and multiple specimens of gastric contents are aspirated before and after subcutaneous injection.	Increased hydrochloric acid secretion after histamine injection may indicate duodenal ulcer. Decreased or absent secretion of HCl may indicate gastric malignancy. Absence of HCl may also indicate pernicious anemia. Increased HCl and presence of food in stomach after fasting suggests obstruction. There may be increased or decreased HCl secretion in the presence of a gastric ulcer.	*Pretest:* Explain test to patient, including drugs used. Obtain careful drug and allergy history. If histamine is used, a skin test should be performed first to rule out allergic response. Have epinephrine on hand to counteract problems from histamine. Histalog causes fewer systemic side-effects. NOP for 12 hr. Avoid drugs affecting gastric secretion 1 day–2 days before test. Other considerations as for all patients with NG tube. *Post test:* Observe vital signs for effects of drug used. Remove tube quickly. May eat if no nausea is present.
Gastric analysis with insulin (insulin tolerance test, Hollander test)	To obtain and analyze gastric contents for the amount of hydrochloric acid secreted in response to a subcutaneous injection of insulin. This is a test for comleteness of vagotomy (see surgical management of patient with peptic ulcer, Chapter 83).	Normally, reduced blood sugar level stimulates the vagus to increase secretion of hydrochloric acid. Normal finding without vagotomy is increased HCl secretion after insulin injection. Post vagotomy, there should be no HCl secreted in response to insulin.	*Pretest:* See above. Be prepared for hypoglycemic response to the regular insulin injection. Have sweetened fruit juice on hand, as well as dextrose 50% for intravenous injection readily available. *Post test:* Same as for gastric analysis with histamine or histalog.
Stool for occult blood	To detect presence of blood in stool. Specimen is obtained during rectal examination or from results of bowel movement. Stool is tested with a reagent.	Normal: Negative. Blood in stool may indicate GI tract bleeding, related to colitis, peptic ulcer, carcinoma, gastritis, or diverticulitis.	*Pretest:* If orthotoluidine is used (Hematest, Occultest) patient must have meat-free diet for 4 days. Other tests for occult blood do not require dietary restrictions. *Post test:* No specific follow-up.

Bibliography

Caly JC: Assessing adults' nutrition. Am J Nurs 77(10):1605, 1977

Carr-Locke D: Colonscopy and sigmoidoscopy. Nursing Times 79(24):72–75, 1983

Carr-Locke D: Update on gastrointestinal endoscopy. 2. Endoscopic retrograde cholangiopancreatography. Nursing Times 79(23):50–52, 1983

Curtis C: Colonoscopy: The nurse's role. Am J Nurs 75(3):430–432, 1975

Dansky KH: Assessing children's nutrition. Am J Nurs 77(10):1610, 1977

Fishbach R: A Manual of Laboratory Diagnostic Tests, ed 2. Philadelphia, JB Lippincott, 1984

French RM: The Nurse's Guide to Diagnostic Procedures, ed 5. New York, McGraw-Hill, 1980

Holt RW, Wherry DC: Why flexible fiberoptic sigmoidoscopy is important in the geriatric patient. Geriatrics 34(5):85, 1979

Hoppe MC, Descalso J, Kapp SR: Gastrointestinal disease: Nutritional implications. Nurs Clin North Am 18(1):47, 1983

Jirovec MM: The gastrointestinal system. In Armstrong ME, Dickason EJ, Howe J, Jones DA, Snider MJ (eds): Handbook of Clinical Nursing. New York, John Wiley, 1984

King CE, Toskes RP: Breath analysis. When and how to use it in GI and liver disease. Consultant 23(11):117, 1983

Klein AE: Medical Tests and You. New York, Grosset & Dunlap, 1977

Liebermann TR, Baines M: Gastrointestinal fiberoptic endoscopy. Diagnostic and therapeutic aspects. Surg Clin North Am 59(5):787, 1979

Margen S, Allen LH: What to look for in the nutritional examination. Consultant 16(3):43, 1976

Spiro HM: Clinical Gastroenterology, ed 3. New York, Macmillan, 1983

Steinheber FU: Bleeding from the lower gastrointestinal tract: Diagnostic approach. Hosp Med 19(5):121–129, 1983

Talbot TM, MacKeigan JM: Colonic endoscopy in perspective. Surg Clin North Am 58(3):459, 1978

Chapter 80

Nursing Strategies for Common Gastrointestinal Problems

Nursing Diagnosis Interventions Evaluation

Margaret Heitkemper
Lynda Brubacher

Gastrointestinal (GI) tract problems are often manifested in the form of alterations in dietary intake, elimination, and absorption. Specific therapies used in the treatment of disease may also promote alterations in dietary intake and elimination.

Alterations in Nutrition

Nausea and Vomiting

Nursing Diagnosis

Inadequate nutritional intake may be related to inability of the gastrointestinal tract to tolerate food or liquids and manifested in nausea and vomiting. Nausea and vomiting are two of the most common symptoms experienced by patients. The underlying causative factors may be GI pathology or disturbance in function of other body systems. Nausea and vomiting are problems which are frequently discussed together because they often occur together.

Nausea. Nausea is a subjective sensation described as the inclination or desire to vomit. This subjective feeling is often accompanied by physiological changes including hypotension, tachycardia, tachypnea, and increased salivary secretion. Nausea is often described in relation to GI symptoms including abdominal heaviness, queasiness, or a sinking feeling. Nausea results in variable degrees of anorexia. Patients with nausea often experience a worsening or intensifying of the symptom with the thought, sight, or smell of food.

The neurological connections and central processing center for the sensation of nausea remains to be determined. Peripheral receptors for nausea are probably located in visceral organs. Abdominal injuries as well as increases in visceral organ pressure (*e.g.,* obstruction) frequently result in complaints of nausea. Nausea and vomiting are common complaints of postoperative patients. Cerebral input can also produce the sensation of nausea. The sight of something offensive, as well as emotional upset, can produce the sensation of nausea. Nausea can be chemically induced. It is a frequent side-effect of a variety of medications including antibiotics and chemotherapeutic agents used in the treatment of cancer.

Vomiting. Vomiting, the forceful expulsion of gastric and/or intestinal contents through the mouth, is a reflex phenomenon. Vomiting frequently follows or occurs with nausea; however, vomiting can occur with or without nausea. More is known about the physiological pathways for vomiting than for nausea. A vomiting center located in the medulla of the brain stem has been identified. This vomiting center receives input from both peripheral and central afferents. Peripheral afferents originate in the visceral organs (*e.g.,* myocardium, GI tract, uterus, bladders, kidneys) and travel by way of the spinal cord to the brain stem. Central input from the cerebral cortex to the vomiting center includes information from the senses (*e.g.,* sight, sound, smell) as well as psychological input. Furthermore, the vomiting center receives information from the chemoreceptor trigger zone. The chemoreceptor trigger zone is a small, diffuse area located in the hypothalamus at the floor of the fourth ventricle, and as such is exposed to both cerebral spinal fluid and cerebral blood supply. Emetic substances in the blood activate the vomiting center by this route.

Once the vomiting center has been activated through stimulation of peripheral receptors, chemoreceptor trigger zone, or cerebral cortex, vomiting is initiated. The act of vomiting is a complex reflex. The esophagus and upper stomach relax, while abdominal muscles begin to contract. This results in an increase in intra-abdominal pressure which exerts pressure on the passive stomach.

Interventions

In some situations, the stimulus to nausea/vomiting can be eliminated or reduced. The nausea/vomiting resulting from viral infection, dietary indiscretion, and/or emotional stimuli is generally self-limiting. The patient is on nothing per mouth until the symptoms subside, and then is started on clear liquids at room temperature.

The goals of nursing care for the patient with nausea/vomiting include (1) assessing and recording the intensity of the symptoms and characteristics of the emesis; (2) removing the stimulus when possible, providing pharmacologic relief as ordered, and monitoring the efficacy as well as side-effects; (3) optimizing nutritional status; (4) preventing complications such as fluid and electrolyte imbalances and aspiration; and (5) maximizing patient comfort.

The monitoring of the patient's emesis may include noting the color, pH, volume, and the presence of bile and blood. The presence of bright red blood may be indicative of an esophageal tear which can occur with vigorous vomiting. In patients with suspected or known diagnosis of ulcer disease, the emesis is guaiaced for occult blood. Greenish-colored emesis is indicative of bile. Extremely foul-smelling emesis may be a sign of pyloric obstruction, while foul-smelling emesis with fecal material may occur in the patient with an intestinal obstruction.

The second goal of nursing care is to remove the stimulus when possible. This may include evaluating medication side-effects, examining dietary indiscretions or ingestion of contaminated food, and attempting to eliminate or reduce emotional stimuli which are producing the symptom. Pharmacological agents are frequently prescribed for patients with severe and/or prolonged nausea/vomiting. These drugs are listed in Table 80–1 as well as common side-effects associated with these drugs. Patients on antiemetic agents are monitored for both the effectiveness of the medication in relieving symptoms and for central nervous system side-effects.

The third goal of nursing therapy is to optimize the patient's nutritional status. Both nausea and vomiting can result in significant reductions in dietary intake. Patients who are vomiting will be NPO until the symptom subsides. The lack of dietary intake for 24 to 48 hours is not critical in persons with normal body weight and no other pathologies. However, for those patients with chronic recurring nausea related to drug therapy or pathology, reductions in oral intake may put the individual at risk for malnutrition. Elderly persons may also experience significant problems (*e.g.,* hypoglycemia, dehydration, orthostatic hypotension) when fluids and food are withheld, which is compounded by the loss of fluids with vomiting.

Ongoing assessment of the patient's report of nausea is important in planning nutritional interventions. The nurse must determine whether nausea occurs at certain times during the day or if it is related to drug therapy or food types. If prescribed, antiemetic medications are administered prior to meals. Meals or nutritional supplements are planned for times that the patient is less likely to be nauseated. Frequently nauseated patients fare better with dry foods such as dry toast and crackers, while foods with a high-fat content are poorly tolerated. The patient's nutritional intake is mon-

TABLE 80–1
Commonly Used Drugs for Nausea/Vomiting

Drug	*Examples*	*Action*	*Side-effects*
Antihistamines	Dramamine (dimenhydrinate) Gravol Bonine (meclizine)	Central depressant effect on chemoreceptor trigger zone and vestibular system	Drowsiness Dry mouth Lassitude
Phenothiazine	Thorazine (chlorpromazine) Stelazine (trifluoperazine) Compazine (prochlorperazine)	Chemoreceptor and vomiting center inhibition	CNS: sedation Parkinsonian symptoms
Metoclopramide	Maxeran Reglan	Increase gastric emptying Sedative effect on chemoreceptor trigger zone	Drowsiness Confusion Parkinsonian symptoms

itored by recording the caloric intake, while nutritional status may be monitored by anthropometric measurements and blood chemistry determinations.

A fourth goal of nursing interventions for the patient with nausea/vomiting is to maintain fluid and electrolyte balance. The lack of oral intake as well as loss of fluids with vomiting can result in dehydration and electrolyte imbalances, in particular of sodium, potassium, and hydrogen. The elderly patient is at risk for developing fluid and electrolyte imbalances even with vomiting of short duration.

The patient with prolonged or severe vomiting will be given intravenous fluid replacement to reduce the risk of electrolyte imbalances. Serum electrolyte levels need to be monitored. An accurate intake and output record is kept by the nurse. Physical assessment of the patient's hydration status is done at regular intervals.

Another goal is prevention of aspiration of the emesis, which is a serious complication of vomiting. The elderly patient with a reduced gag reflex and the unconscious patient are particularly at risk for aspiration. Aspiration of emesis into the pulmonary system can result in pneumonia and seriously jeopardize the recovery of the patient. Patients who are vomiting and unconscious patients should be kept with their head lowered and on their side to reduce the risk of aspiration.

The fifth goal of nursing care is to provide patient comfort. Nausea and vomiting are distressing symptoms which impact on the patient's comfort. As such, the patient's outlook and sense of psychological well-being are affected. Patient compliance to the therapeutic regimens may also be influenced by nausea/vomiting.

Patients who are experiencing nausea and vomiting should be encouraged to take slow, deep breaths. Relaxation techniques have proven helpful in cancer patients with nausea induced by chemotherapy.[4] Soiled gowns and linens should be changed immediately to facilitate patient comfort. The patient needs to have ready access to a clean emesis basin and tissues. Good oral care will reduce patient discomfort.

Evaluation

Outcome criteria of therapeutic interventions for the patient with nausea and vomiting include a reduction in nausea/vomiting, patient report of increased comfort, maintenance of weight, absence of aspiration, balanced intake and output, normal serum electrolyte and bicarbonate levels.

Anorexia

Nursing Diagnosis

Nutritional intake less than body requirements is related to interference with normal ingestion of nutrients and manifested by anorexia (loss of appetite), emotional disturbances, and problems in ingesting foods. The lack of appetite may be the result of the disease itself (*e.g.,* cancer) or therapy such as surgery, radiation, chemotherapy. Anorexia is also a common symptom of depression. Anorexia in general creates a challenge to both nurses and dietitians to increase the patient's oral intake. Drug therapy can purposely or inadvertently produce anorexia. Lack of appetite can result in significant reductions in oral intake and loss of body weight.

Interventions

The goals of nursing care are to prevent complications associated with decreased food intake and to increase dietary intake by appetite stimulation. The first goal is met by careful and continuous monitoring of the patient's dietary intake by calorie counts or with 24-hour dietary recall. The patient's nutritional and hydration states are monitored. Protein-calorie malnutrition may be treated by the institution of enteral/parenteral feeding. Vitamin supplements need to be provided. The anorexia may be relieved spontaneously by the removal of the causative agent such as chemotherapeutic agents or radiation.

The second goal of improving diet intake may be promoted by consulting with the dietitian in determining dietary intake and patient likes and dislikes, and planning meals which include foods that the patient likes and can tolerate. Dietary plans for patients with anorexia frequently incorporate the use of small, frequent meals. For the patient with depression, appetite may be improved as the condition improves with the use of antidepressants.

Anorexia Nervosa

Nursing Diagnosis

Alteration in nutritional intake may be related to an emotional disturbance relative to food intake and manifested in severe weight loss (anorexia nervosa). Anorexia nervosa is a problem which affects primarily young women and girls, and can result in significant alterations in body weight. The name anorexia nervosa is actually a misnomer in that these patients have a normal appetite. In fact, patients with anorexia nervosa may consume a normal or greater than normal diet, but self-induced vomiting and diarrhea result in nutritional deficits. While the cause of anorexia nervosa is unknown, it is most frequently considered a psychiatric disorder. Numerous etiologic factors and mechanisms have been suggested. A current theory is that anorexia nervosa develops in a young girl as a response to abnormal family dynamics. Food is rejected as an act of defiance.[14] There is also evidence that anorexia nervosa may be the result of hypothalamic dysfunction.[17] The disease does affect young men; however females affected outnumber males 20 to 1.

Characteristics of anorexia nervosa include self-induced weight loss which is significant, various psychological disturbances, and marked physiological changes. Characteristics of the individual with anorexia nervosa include self-critical personality; an early puberty; a recent family crisis such as divorce or a death; or perceptual problem, in that body size is overestimated. Anorexia nervosa patients frequently come from upper socioeconomic families. A common initiating event is a weigh-loss program in which a limit is not set and the individual continues to diet to beyond 25% loss of normal body weight. Physical manifestations of anorexia include weight loss, protein–calorie malnutrition, hypothermia, anemia, bradycardia, hypokalemia and a variety of other problems related to nutritional deficiencies, and extensive use of cathartics or self-induced emesis. Repeated self-induced vomiting will result in destruction of teeth due to exposure to hydrochloric acid. The female patient with anorexia nervosa also becomes amenorrheic. The physical symptoms often look like thyroid dysfunction, so thyroid dysfunction must be ruled out by thyroid hormone (T_4, T_3) measurements. Unlike the patient with either malnutrition or hypothyroidism, lethargy is not a problem. In fact, some patients may exercise strenuously (jogging, biking, swimming).

Interventions

Interventions when the patient has anorexia nervosa center around the prevention of life-threatening complications. Anorexia nervosa is a chronic problem and, as a result, long-term plans are warranted. Patients with anorexia nervosa are admitted to the hospital when there are fluid and electrolyte problems and when weight loss has occurred to an extreme (greater than 40% loss of normal weight) or in a short period of time (25%–30% in less than 3 months). Causes of death for the patient with anorexia nervosa are infection and/or cardiac arrhythmia which may be related to hypokalemia. Hypokalemia alkalosis develops as a result of diuretic and laxative use. The serum level may drop as low as 1.5 mEq. Intravenous administration of fluids and electrolytes is initiated to correct imbalances.

An interdisciplinary team including physician, psychologist/psychiatrist, nurse, and dietitian collaborate to plan weight-gain strategies. An optimal weight gain is 2.5 lb to 4 lb/wk. The use of force feedings such as tube feeding and TPN are contraindicated unless the situation is life-threatening. The patient frequently resists these therapies and will attempt to pull out tubes and intravenous lines. A diet is planned which includes foods that the patient likes. A low-lactose and low-fat diet is recommended during the early repletion period because enzymes for the digestion of these substances are decreased with starvation. Patients are weighed at regular intervals.

Nurses can play a critical role by developing a trusting relationship, providing reassurance, allowing the patient to verbalize feelings and fears regarding weight, and carefully supervising at mealtimes. This latter involves preventing the patient from vomiting or disposing of food. At present, pharmacological therapy for anorexia nervosa has not proved universally successful.

Families of patients with anorexia nervosa frequently need support and reassurance. They usually need to be involved in psychotherapy. Because of the exposure anorexia nervosa has received in the popular press, parents may blame themselves for the problem. The nurse should be open to family members expressing their concerns as well as maintaining an optimistic viewpoint on the situation.

Evaluation

Outcome criteria for the patient with anorexia include improved appetite as evidenced by subjective report and recorded dietary intake, increased caloric intake, and increase or maintenance of body weight. The success of interventions for the person with anorexia nervosa is evidenced by an increase in body weight, a decrease in the use of laxatives or emetic agents, and the patient's ability to openly discuss the problem and give recognition to its emotional basis.

Oral Trauma

Nursing Diagnosis

Interference with normal nutritional intake is also associated with traumatic conditions and malformations requiring reconstructive surgery. These conditions include fractures of the jaw, mandibular deformities, and temporomandibular joint dysfunction syndrome (disharmony in a component of the occlusal system such as abnormal bite). Immobilization of the fractured sections of the jaw inhibits normal chewing as do some of the surgical procedures to correct jaw deformities.

The aims of interventions for the person with restricted mobility of the jaw are prevention of aspiration if nausea and vomiting should occur, prevention of oral infection, maintenance of oral hygiene and of adequate nutritional intake. Fractured jaws and soft tissue injury often occur together. The break in tissue continuity necessitates prophylactic injections of tetanus and antibiotics. Cleansing of the oral cavity, suturing, and wiring of the jaw are accomplished in surgery. The procedure may be done on an outpatient basis. The patient must be observed closely for nausea and vomiting. The *patient/family must be instructed to cut the elastic bands or wires if vomiting should occur.* Scissors or wirecutters should be available *at all times.* Suction should also be available in the immediate postoperative period. Usually the tip of the suction catheter can be inserted through a tooth gap in the mouth or through the nares to the nasopharynx.

Edema of the mouth occurs after trauma or corrective surgery. The patient needs to be watched closely to be certain the swelling is not sufficiently extensive to interfere with respirations. Maintenance of a semi-Fowler's position for 24 to 48 hours after treatment will help to prevent excessive edema. If it does occur, the outpatient should return for immediate attention in the emergency room. If the patient is hospitalized, the physician is notified immediately. The treatment is a tracheostomy.

Patients need to be taught how to clean the oral cavity. The procedure will vary depending on the extent of trauma and of restricted mobility of the jaw. Patients/families must be taught about the necessary dietary modifications. A liquid diet taken through a straw or with the use of an aseptosyringe with catheter attached is necessary if the jaw is wired. The liquids should be high-calorie and reinforced with protein, vitamins, and minerals. Large quantities of high-calorie formula should not be taken at one time because it may precipitate nausea and vomiting. Written instructions about dietary modifications should be provided to the patient and family.

Evaluation

The patient with restricted jaw mobility and/or soft tissue trauma and his or her family should be able to accurately describe how to release the rubber bands or wires if vomiting occurs and actions to take if edema causes respiratory distress or signs of infection occur (increased pain, temperature); patient should demonstrate ability to do oral hygiene; patient or family should report adherence to dietary modifications and patient should maintain pre-trauma body weight.

Interference with Digestion

Nursing Diagnosis

Alteration in digestion may be related to a decrease or absence of hydrochloric HCl acid secretion in the stomach and manifested as fatigue and weight loss. A relative lack of HCl acid is referred to as hypochlorhydria. The lack of acid is most commonly the result of a loss of the acid-secreting gastric mucosa cells due to pernicious anemia, gastritis, gastric cancer, or gastric resection. In these patients the intragastric pH is often 6 or higher. Hypochlorhydria is frequently observed in elderly patients, which may be the result of chronic atrophic gastritis or normal cell loss with age. Achlorhydria or hypochlorhydria is also associated with alcoholism, tuberculosis, sprue, parasitic infections, and hyperthyroidism. Diagnosis is by measurement of intragastric or gastric aspirant pH during both basal conditions and following maximal stimulation of HCl acid secretion with histamine or pentagastrin. Anemia is usually present because of malabsorption of iron.

Interventions

The goals of nursing interventions are to teach the patient about medication administration, the need for routine follow-up to monitor anemia, and, if possible, reassurance that hyposecretion of acid is not indicative of major pathology.

The replacement of hydrochloric acid is initiated in the patient with achlorhydria or hypochlorhydria. The patient is instructed to take the dilute hydrochloric acid solution at mealtimes and to sip the solution slowly through a straw to prevent corrosion of teeth enamel. Because of the relationship of hypochlorhydria and pernicious anemia, it is desirable to reassess the patient periodically for signs of pernicious anemia, including routine blood work. Pernicious anemia is a condition in which there is a lack of the intrinsic factor normally present in the gastric juices. The factor is essential for the absorption of vitamin B_{12} and/or folic acid which in turn are necessary for maturation of erythrocytes. The latter is treated with parenteral injections of vitamin B_{12}.

It is important to teach the patient about the problem and to provide reassurance, when possible, that the problem is not life-threatening. This reassurance is not possible if the underlying problem is cancer. The explanations and reassurance should reduce stress and unnecessary concern.

In situations of reduced acid secretion, a thorough work-up including endoscopy is initiated to rule out the existence of gastric carcinoma. Periodic follow-up exams may also be necessary to monitor changes in the gastric lining. The nurse must reassure the patient when the results of physical examination are negative but must also discuss the importance of adhering to periodic follow-up examinations.

Evaluation

Criteria for goal evaluation are (1) the patient adheres to the instructions; (2) patient reports decreased discomfort with meals and improved nutritional intake; (3) hemoglobin level is within normal limits and patient expresses a decrease in anxiety; (4) when indicated, the patient adheres to a schedule of periodic reexamination.

Malabsorption

Nursing Diagnosis

Alteration in nutrition may be related to inability to absorb one or more of the dietary constituents (carbohydrate, protein, and fat) and is manifested in weight loss, fatigue, diarrhea, and abdominal cramping. Malabsorption occurs in a number of patients who have GI pathology or have had GI resections. Malabsorption syndromes can also develop in patients who have genetic deficiencies in digestive enzymes.

Some patients will have problems with absorption of all three dietary constituents. For example, patients who develop short-bowel syndrome following resection of a portion of the small bowel have problems with absorption due to decreased functional surface area. However, within 3 to 6 months after the surgery, there is sufficient hypertrophy of the remaining mucosa to provide adequate nutrition if the person has six to eight feedings a day. The diet given is high in protein and carbohydrates and low in fat (approximately 60 g) because problems with fat absorption frequently last up to 1 year.

Patients may have problems with absorption of only one of the three nutrients. The most common problems are lactose intolerance and protein malabsorption. ***Lactose intolerance*** (malabsorption) occurs when there is insufficient or no enzyme to deal with the amount of lactose (a disaccharide) delivered to the small intestine. Estimates of the incidence of lactose intolerance range from 15% to 50 % in the North American adult population. The most frequent cases, primary lactase deficiency, is genetically determined. Secondary causes of lactose intolerance include disorders of the small intestine (*e.g.,* inflammatory bowel disease or regional enteritis), celiac, sprue, acute gastrointestinal infections, and massive bowel resection. Patients who have had gastric surgery often develop lactose intolerance due to dumping or rapid gastric emptying.

When lactose is ingested by a patient with inadequate lactase enzyme, the disaccharide remains in the intestinal lumen. As a result of its osmotic nature, water is retained in the lumen or pulled from the intestinal mucosa. In the colon, the sugar is then acted on by the normal bacteria that reside there. The patient complains of abdominal cramping, discomfort, and nausea, and may experience diarrhea. There is no known cure for primary lactase deficiency.

Protein malabsorption is often caused by celiac disease. In celiac disease, the patient has a permanent intolerance to gluten, the protein found in wheat, rye, barley, and buckwheat. Celiac disease is known by a variety of names including gluten-sensitive enteropathy, nontropical sprue, idiopathic steatorrhea, and celiac sprue. Celiac disease is most common in western and southern European Caucasians and their descendants. In adults, the disease is more prevalent in women than men.

The exact cause of celiac disease is not known, but there is a strong genetic component. Specifically, in celiac disease there is a lack of the enzyme that degrades N-pyrrolidone peptide. As a result, when gluten-containing foods are ingested, there is an increase in the amount of this peptide, which then interferes with the normal function of intestinal mucosal cells. If prolonged, histological changes in the intestinal epithelial cells occur. These changes, however, can be reversed if the offending agent is removed from the diet.

Interventions: Lactose Malabsorption

The goals of nursing care are to reduce lactose intake in the lactose-intolerant patient and thereby promote patient comfort, and to prevent inadequate calcium intake. The first goal is accomplished through nutritional counseling. The amount of lactose tolerated by an individual is frequently variable and depends upon the source of the lactose and other foods with which it is eaten. The patient is encouraged to remove lactose-containing foods from the diet. The patient should avoid milk and ice cream. Cheese is often well tolerated. However, the majority of recommended lactose-restricted diets are too strict for most adults. Although they contain similar lactose content as plain milk, foods such as buttermilk and yogurt are frequently tolerated because of their increased osmolarity, which results in decreased gastric emptying and decreased entry time into the small intestine. Products such as Lact-aid, a preparation containing lactase, can be added to milk products to break down lactose. The Lact-aid is incubated with the milk in the refrigerator 24 hours prior to its use, and often has a sweeter taste than plain milk. For some patients with severe lactase deficiency, symptoms may remain after the exclusion of dairy products from the diet. The intake of other sources of lactose need to be investigated including caramel candies, chocolate, cordial liqueurs, and some instant foods.

The second goal of nursing management is to prevent calcium imbalance. Long-term reduction in dairy product intake may seriously reduce the amount of calcium intake. This may aggravate osteoporosis, particularly in postmenopausal women. A dietary history is important to determine additional sources of calcium in the diet. The addition of calcium supplements may be necessary. Tums is an over-the-counter, inexpensive source of calcium.

Evaluation. The success of nursing therapeutics is determined by patient reports of a decrease in lactose intake, decrease in GI symptoms such as cramping and diarrhea, the intake of calcium supplements adequate to achieve recommended levels, and maintenance of body weight.

Interventions: Protein Malabsorption

The goals for nursing interventions are (1) prevention of complications by dietary counseling; (2) patient acceptance of dietary restrictions; (3) a regain and maintenance of body weight.

Nutritional counseling is the primary therapy for the patient with gluten intolerance. Patients often fare better when sample meal plans along with a list of substitutions are provided rather than merely a list of foods to be avoided.

Nutritional assessment, including anthropometric measurements and biochemical determinations, is done at regular intervals in those patients with complications including diarrhea and malabsorption.

The second goal is patient acceptance of dietary restrictions or patient adherence to the treatment plan. This may be difficult for the patient in whom the gluten-free diet varies markedly from lifelong dietary habits or the patient whose family members continue to eat prohibited foods such as breads and cereals. The patient is instructed on the risks of dietary indiscretions. Patient teaching regarding diet is focused on those foods that can be tolerated. Teenagers who have been gluten-intolerant since childhood may have particular problems in adherence to the diet, due to peer pressure.

Evaluation. Outcome criteria for the patient with gluten intolerance include patient reports of absence of acute episodes of diarrhea, dietary intake that adheres to prescribed foods, and maintenance of normal body weight.

Enteral Replacement Therapy

Tube Feeding

Alteration in nutrition related to inability to ingest food may require enteral nutrition. Situations in which this may occur are obstructions, decreased level of consciousness, and reconstructive surgical procedures. When the GI tract is functional and nutritional support is necessary, tube feedings may be initiated. Tube feeding is an artificial means of supplying calories by a tube. Enteral feedings are not suitable for patients who have an inadequate amount of functioning bowel (*e.g.*, inflammatory bowel disease), severe GI disturbances which result in intractable vomiting, obstruction, or upper GI bleeding. In general, tube feedings are used for the maintenance of body weight rather than to promote significant weight gains. Tube feedings can be delivered by a tube passed through the nose to the stomach (nasogastric) or to the intestine (nasointestinal) (Fig. 80–1). Placement of the feeding tube into the small intestine is thought to reduce the likelihood of aspiration because the pyloric sphincter inhibits backflow of intestinal contents into the stomach and hence regurgitation. The nasoenteric feeding tube placement is estimated by measuring from the tip of the nose to the earlobe, then to the xiphoid process, and increasing the length by 5 cm.[13] (See Fig. 80–2.)

Tube Insertion

Tube insertion may be performed by a nurse. For the patient, the passage of the tube is likely to produce anxiety. Careful explanation of the procedure as well as the benefits to the patient and time for questions and answers, when possible, may help to alleviate this anxiety.

For tube insertion, the patient should be in an upright position. If the patient is unconscious or on bedrest, the head of the bed is elevated. Most NG and NI tubes are marked at regular intervals to denote distance into the GI tract. The first 2 to 4 inches of the tube are well-lubricated with a water-soluble lubricant to facilitate passage of the tube through the naris. The patient is questioned regarding any nasal abnormality (*e.g.,* deviated septum, broken nose). Such information may also be present on the patient's chart. Once the naris has been selected, the tube is inserted through the naris and to the pharynx. At this point, the patient is instructed to swallow to facilitate passage of the tube to the stomach. If allowable, small sips of water are also helpful in passage of the tube down the esophagus.

In an alert, conscious patient, the inadvertent passage of the tube into the respiratory tract will produce coughing and choking. Other measures to determine gastric placement of the tube include gastric aspiration of gastric juice with a 60-ml syringe or the infusion of air through the tube while the abdomen is auscultated with a stethoscope. The escape of air is heard through the stethoscope.

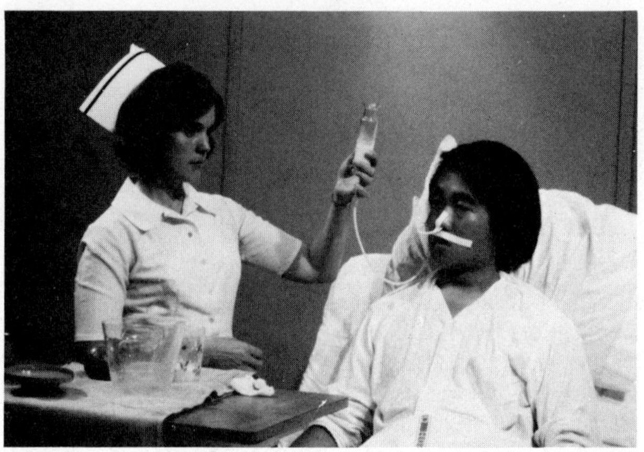

FIGURE 80–1 Tube feeding.

The end of the NG tube is secured by taping it to the patient's nose. To avoid trauma to the naris, the tube should extend straight out from the naris for a short distance and then be brought up over the nose and taped to the forehead so as not to obstruct vision. The tube may also be attached to the patient's gown to prevent accidental displacement of the tube.

The end of an NI tube may or may not be secured. If the tube is to travel through the intestine, it should not be attached until the tube reaches the desired area in the intestine. The weighted end of the tube, as well as peristaltic waves of the stomach and duodenum, facilitate this movement. The right side-lying position or ambulation will further promote passage of the tube. Once the tube tip is in its preferred location, it is secured.

Surgical placement of the feeding tube directly into the esophagus, stomach, or intestine may be done. A *cervical esophagostomy* may be used for feeding in the patient who has had head and neck surgery. A *gastrostomy* tube may be placed in the patient on long-term tube feeding to reduce nasal and pharyngeal irritation produced by nasogastric and nasointestinal tube and to decrease the risk of aspiration. A *jejunostomy* tube may be placed in the patient with upper gastrointestinal tract pathology.

Types of Tube Diets

Tube placement may determine the type of diet utilized. Tube feedings may be classified as blenderized, chemically defined, oral supplements and elemental diets. The diets currently used are presented in Table 80–2. A regular diet may be blenderized for use by the patient on home tube feedings because its base is the normal diet eaten by the rest of the family. However, these blenderized diets are often milk-based and thus may be a problem for the patient who has relative lactose intolerance.

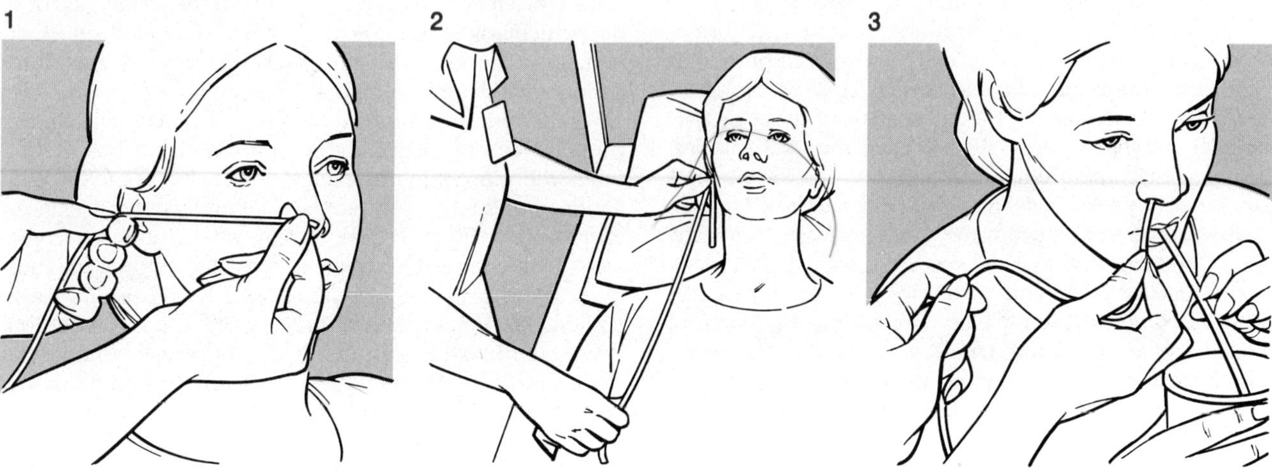

FIGURE 80–2 Inserting a nasogastric tube.

TABLE 80–2
Common Types of Tube-Feeding Diets

Type	*Constituents*	*Uses*
Blenderized	Milk-based, high-protein content	Elderly persons whose digestive and absorptive functions are intact Given by NG tube
Chemically defined diets (*e.g.*, Ensure, Isocal, Sustacal, Ensure Plus)	Lactose-free, nutritionally complete when adequate calories are given	Specifically designed for tube feeding; well-tolerated by majority of tube-fed elderly patients Given by small-diameter transpyloric feeding tubes or NG
Oral supplements (*e.g.*, Ensure, Sustacal)	Lactose-free, nutritionally complete when adequate calories are given	Given by mouth as a supplement to increase nutrient or calorie intake
Elemental diets (*e.g.*, Vivonex)	Lactose-free, clear liquid, amino acids in peptide protein composition	Elderly persons with impaired digestion; cause minimal stimulation of pancreatic biliary, intestinal secretion Given by small-bore feeding tube or NG

Chemically defined (polymeric) diets contain high-molecular-weight sources of protein, carbohydrate, and fat. Because these diets contain whole protein as well as a greater percentage of fat, they are often more palatable than elemental diets and thus many of them can be used as oral supplements for patients who need additional calories. The palatability of these diets can be enhanced by the use of flavored additives. These diets are complete in that they contain all the recommended daily allowances for vitamins and minerals. The osmolality is variable for the commercially prepared formulas which deliver approximately 1 kcal/ml. Those formulas which deliver 1.5 kcal/ml are hyperosmolar and thus need to be delivered at a constant, slow rate to avoid symptoms of tube-feeding intolerance. Most, but not all, of the commercially prepared formulas are lactose-free.

Elemental diets, also referred to as monomeric formulas, are composed of amino acids or hydrolyzed protein as the protein source and oligosaccharides or disaccharides as the carbohydrate source. The fat content of these diets is variable, anywhere from 1% to 30% of the total calories. Elemental diets require minimal digestion and for the most part are readily absorbed. This type of diet may be preferable for the patient with inflammatory bowel disease, pancreatic insufficiency, or short-bowel syndrome, in which the digestive function of the intestinal tract is compromised. Elemental diets are frequently bitter to taste and are therefore designed to be administered by a tube. Because of the hyperosmolar nature of the solution, these diets are generally given at a specified rate by an infusion pump. Most pumps are battery-operated which facilitates patient ambulation.

Commercially prepared formulas which can be adjusted to meet individual patient needs are also available (*e.g.*, products that contain amino acids and are low in electrolytes K, Mg, and PO4 for patients with chronic renal disease).

Complications

Complications of tube feeding are divided into mechanical, metabolic, and gastrointestinal (Table 80–3). Mechanical complications include problems related to the tube such as obstruction and dislocation. With the use of smaller-sized feeding tubes, the risk for these complications increases. For the patient on intermittent feedings, the feeding tube is flushed with water after each feeding. The tube is also irrigated after the administration of medications by the tube. Clogging of the tube will require tube removal and the insertion of a new tube. This is stressful for the patient and may be particularly so for the patient who has nasal mucosal irritation. The use of blenderized diets may be limited to patients who have larger lumen tubes (*e.g.*, Fr 12).

Dislocation of the feeding tube may occur due to improper anchoring of the tube at its proximal end. Nasogastric tubes will move into the small intestine due to the forceful contractions of the antral stomach. Gastrostomy and jejunostomy tubes may also travel distally when sutures become loose. The gastrostomy tube may block the pylorus and thus prevent the emptying of gastric contents and produce distention and regurgitation. Tube position following insertion is checked by x-ray and then the point of entry should be marked with permanent ink so that tube position can be checked prior to each feeding.

Aspiration. Aspiration of the tube-feeding formula into the pulmonary system is a serious complication of tube feed-

TABLE 80–3
Complications of Tube Feeding

Classification	*Preventive Nursing Interventions*
Mechanical	
Tube-clogging	Flush tube with water after medications and diet administration
Nasal/pharyngeal irritation	Use of small lumen, pliable tubes Nose and mouth care every day Monitor nose and throat for signs of bleeding and infection Moisten tissues with normal saline applicators and swabs
Aspiration	Maintain patient at greater than 45-degree angle during feeding and for 1 hr postfeeding Insert air into tube and listen over stomach to determine proper tube placement Monitor for symptoms of gastric reflux—patient complains of heartburn, epigastric distress Check for abdominal distention, residual volumes prior to feeding Stop formula infusion in patient who is vomiting Check tube placement in patient with a gastrostomy tube
Dislocation of feeding tube	Ascertain tube placement prior to each feeding; clearly mark feeding tube at insertion site
Metabolic	
Hyperglycemia	Monitor urinary glucose levels every shift for the first week, then 3–4 days/week
Hyperglycemic nonketotic coma	Monitor urinary glucose levels at regular intervals; observe for alterations in mentation
Hypernatremia, dehydration	Assess fluid balance; note increase in fluid loss (*e.g.*, vomiting, diarrhea, daily body weights) Increase water content administered with or between feedings
Tube-feeding syndrome	Monitor the patient's serum electrolytes, Na, Cl, BUN Increase water intake
Gastrointestinal	
Diarrhea	Evaluate appropriateness of diet and method of administration including: ▪ Lactose content ▪ Osmolality ▪ Temperature ▪ Rate of administration ▪ Volume delivered/hour ▪ Mixing with medications; check medication instruction for timing in relation to feeding Initiate tube feeding at ¼ to ½ concentration and increase over 24–48 hr
Bacterial contamination	Change feeding bag and tubing each 24 hr; rinse bag after ech feeding; careful handwashing prior to handling tube Use unit dose formula Feeding to hang no longer than 12 hr
Constipation	Evaluate diet; may indicate need to change from elemental to chemically defined diet

ing. Aspiration may occur as a result of improper positioning of the patient ($< 30°$), position of the feeding tube, and the lack of a gag reflex because of the disease process. Nasogastric tubes by their very presence may result in an incompetence of the lower esophageal sphincter thus limiting the natural barrier between the stomach and esophagus. Gastrostomy tubes are thought to decrease the likelihood of aspiration because of the lack of interference with the lower esophageal sphincter. Nasointestinal tubes are also recommended for patients with problems of aspiration. Aspiration is a certain risk in patients who vomit in response to tube feeding. However, aspiration can occur without overt signs of vomiting, particularly in patients with a diminished gag reflex or an endotracheal tube in place.

Manifestations of aspiration include respiratory distress or failure, sputum production, increased respiratory rate, heart rate, and infiltrate observed on chest x-ray. The results of aspirating gastric contents into the pulmonary system will depend upon the amount and pH of the gastric contents.

Nursing interventions for the patient to prevent aspiration include (1) determining tube position following insertion by injection of air through the tube and listening for the sound over the upper abdomen with a stethoscope; (2) aspirating gastric contents prior to each feeding; (3) checking amount of gastric residual prior to each intermittent feeding or every 2 to 4 hours in the patient on continuous feeding and, if greater than 150 ml is present, the feeding is withheld until the residual volume is rechecked 30 minutes later; (4) maintaining head elevation at a minimum of 30° to 45° during and for 1 hour following feedings; (5) monitoring for abdominal distention; (6) discontinuing the tube-feeding infusion if the patient vomits or complains of nausea.

Nasopharyngeal Irritation. Nasopharyngeal irritation may occur due to the insertion and constant presence of a nasogastric tube. The use of small lumen pliable tubes has reduced the degree of irritation, however, many institutions continue to use large (Fr 14–18) tubes made of less pliable material. The patient whose general health status is marginal is at a high risk for tissue breakdown. The nasal mucosa should be moistened with normal saline applicators or swabs. Manipulation or movement of the tube within the nose is at the least uncomfortable and can be quite painful. The patient with a nasogastric tube may also have oral mucosa problems due to mouth breathing and decreased stimulation of saliva. Good oral care is critical in these patients as well as routine monitoring of the mucosal tissue for bleeding or infection. When possible, patients should be allowed to suck on hard candy or ice chips.

Metabolic Complications. Metabolic complications may be precipitated by a change in physiological status of the patient and the constituents of the diet. These complications include hyperglycemia, hyperglycemic nonketotic coma, hypernatremia, and tube-feeding syndrome. Hyperglycemia, as evidenced by increases in fasting blood glucose levels and the presence of glucose in urine, may result from the carbohydrate content of the diet or relative insulin insensitivity due to sepsis, age, or undiagnosed diabetes mellitus. The patient may have sufficient insulin secretion to prevent ketosis but not enough to handle the hyperglycemia. The patient is monitored at regular intervals during the first week for manifestations of hyperglycemia. If elevations in blood glucose and urinary glucose occur, the rate of diet administration is reduced and/or rapid-acting insulin may be administered. For the patient with undetected hyperglycemia and glucosuria, dehydration may occur due to the osmotic pull of glucose in the urine. The end result would be hyperglycemic nonketotic coma. The early manifestations of this syndrome are mental changes (*e.g.,* confusion) which go undetected in the tube-fed patient who has neurological impairment or may be ascribed to behavioral problems in the older patient. The treatment of hyperglycemic nonketosis is the administration of insulin and an increase in hydration.

Fluid Problems. Inadequate fluid administration and/or increased fluid losses due to diarrhea, perspiration, and vomiting can result in dehydration of the tube-fed patient. Dehydration is a common problem in patients on tube feeding. Additional fluids (water, saline) are added to the total volume of tube feedings to reduce the likelihood of this complication. Most commercial formulas contain approximately 850 ml water/liter and, therefore, additional fluid is required depending upon the patient's tube-feeding intake and metabolic status. These fluid needs will also be increased in the patient who is experiencing vomiting or diarrhea and increased insensible water loss.

The tube-fed patient who is comatose is particularly vulnerable to dehydration because of an inability to respond to thirst. The patient receiving radiation or chemotherapy may think the manifestations such as dry tongue are expected outcomes of the therapy. Again, elderly patients are particularly at risk for developing complications related to dehydration. The intake and output record must be monitored. When intake is not greater than output by 500 to 1000 ml or greater if the patient is febrile, additional free water should be added.[1] When indices point to dehydration additional water may be administered with the feeding or between feedings. For the patient with manifestations of saline depletion, sodium chloride may be added to the feeding.

For the patients with fluid overload problems (*e.g.,* congestive heart failure) more concentrated formulas which contain 1.5 kcal/ml may be preferred. Because these formulas have a greater osmolarity they must be delivered at a constant slow rate to decrease the likelihood of osmotic diarrhea. Overhydration may occur in the patient with renal or hepatic diseases. When significant overload occurs diuretics may be warranted. The patient's hydration level is assessed by monitoring serum sodium levels, skin turgor, and mentation levels.

Tube-Feeding Syndrome. Tube-feeding syndrome is a complex of electrolyte imbalances which may develop in the tube-fed patient.[6] Possible contributing factors include renal tubular dysfunction; primary water deficit; adrenal corticosteroid secretion producing sodium retention; and advanced age and renal arteriosclerosis.[18] Manifestations include elevated serum sodium and chloride levels and urea-nitrogen. The syndrome is treated by increasing the amount of free water which is administered. Tube-fed patients may develop problems of potassium balance. Hyperkalemia is most likely to develop in the patient who is in metabolic acidosis or is on an enteral diet with a high potassium content. Hypokalemia may result from insulin administration.

Gastrointestinal Complications.. When the patient is receiving enteral therapy gastrointestinal complications including nausea/vomiting, diarrhea, and constipation, can occur. Diarrhea is perhaps the most common complication associated with enteral nutrition. Diarrhea may result from the method of administration (*e.g.,* rate, volume, temperature) as well as the diet composition (*e.g.,* osmolarity, lactose content). It is recommended that tube feedings be initiated gradually at ¼ concentration and increased to ½ strength and finally to full strength during the first week of tube feeding.[8] The rate of administration will vary with the physician's order for continuous or intermittent bolus feedings. Continuous feedings are administered at a range of 75 to 150 ml/hour and the rate is controlled by a pump. The pump is movable to permit patient mobility. Patients with a nasointestinal or a jejunostomy tube are most commonly fed by continuous feeding. Intermittent feedings are given in boluses of 200 to 400 ml, four to six times a day. Feedings are delivered over a 1 to 2 hour period by gravity drip and may be the method of choice for the patient with a nasogastric or gastrostomy tube.

The advent of unit dose commercial diets negates the need for warming up tube feeding prior to administration. There is probably little difference in patient tolerance of warm (body temperature) versus room temperature feedings. However, blenderized diets which are kept refrigerated should be warmed to room temperature prior to infusion.

Patients who have problems related to osmolality of the tube feedings are treated by adding water to the feeding, thereby reducing the osmolality. However, the replacement of formula with water will reduce the overall caloric intake of the patient.

Bacterial Contamination. Bacterial contamination of the formula may also result in GI problems including diarrhea. Hospital policies dictate the regularity of changing the disposable feeding equipment. Bags and tubing are generally changed every 24 hours. Formula should not hang for longer than 12 hours. The most important preventive measure for bacterial contamination is careful handwashing prior to setting up the feeding apparatus and handling the formula. Can tops and openers need to be wiped clean prior to opening. Formula which has been stored in the refrigerator for 48 hours or greater should not be used. After each feeding the tube is clamped off to prevent leakage or contamination.

Constipation. For patients on long-term tube-feeding, constipation may become a problem due to the lack of fiber in the diet. A careful bowel record must be maintained. Patients on elemental diets may have a bowel movement only once a week. Patients on polymeric diets may pass a stool every 2 to 3 days, which may differ markedly from the patient's normal bowel pattern. Constipation can result in abdominal discomfort in the patient. Treatment of the constipation is discussed later in this chapter.

Psychosocial Concerns. The psychological impact of receiving calories by a tube needs to be considered. Mealtime for most individuals is a social time which may also have religious or cultural implications for the patient. The lack of control over the type, amount, and time of diet delivery may be distressing to some patients. Patients need assurance that the tube feeding is temporary, if this is the situation. The patient's right to privacy needs to be considered. For many patients the constant presence of an NG tube may be distressing because it is a visible sign of disease or an eating problem. For the patient receiving tube feedings, comfort can be enhanced by the changing of bed linens and clothes which are soiled by spillage or leakage of the formula.

With the advent of smaller tubes and commercially prepared diets, tube feedings can be managed by patients and their families at home. For home tube feedings, patients are instructed on tube insertion, care and maintenance of equipment, as well as the manifestation of complications.

Evaluation

Successful administration of enteral feeding is determined by the absence of adverse responses, maintenance of body weight, and patient understanding of the process, when possible.

Parenteral Replacement Therapy

Total Parenteral Nutrition

Alteration in nutrition related to inability to digest or absorb food may require *total parenteral nutrition* (TPN). *In parenteral alimentation,* calories are provided in the form of carbohydrates, fats, and amino acids. The percentage of dietary constituents is dependent upon the patient's problem and caloric needs. Unlike tube feeding, total parenteral nutrition can increase body weight with administration of sufficient calories. To avoid protein malnutrition a certain percentage of the calories will be provided by protein. Calories can be delivered by two parenteral routes: peripheral and central.

Peripheral Vein Alimentation. Solutions which can be delivered through the peripheral veins are limited to lipids and isotonic amino acid solutions. Hypertonic glucose and amino acid solutions can be administered through a peripheral vein but necessitate frequent changes of the insertion site due to irritation of the vein produced by these solutions. These solutions increase the risk for thrombophlebitis and, therefore, the insertion site must be changed every 24 to 48 hours.[12] Peripheral parenteral nutrition can be used to maintain a positive nitrogen balance but cannot reverse a negative nitrogen balance. It may be the route of choice for the patient who cannot tolerate central vein catheterization or who has had an infected central insertion site. Lipid solutions can be delivered through a peripheral vein with generally no greater than 500 to 1000 ml administered per day. The amino acid content should not exceed 4% and the dextrose content should be greater than 7%.

Central Vein Alimentation. For long-term administration of a hypertonic solution, total parenteral nutrition (TPN), a central vein is selected. The most frequently used vein is the superior vena cava (Fig. 80–3) The vein is catheterized under sterile conditions in an operating room. The catheter is inserted by percutaneous puncture or by a cutdown. This site is not used in the patient who has a burn in this area, has had a mastectomy, or the patient who has had radical neck surgery. The superior vena cava is accessed via the external jugular, internal jugular, or subclavian vein.

TPN Solutions

TPN solutions are composed of dextrose and amino acids. Generally, 25% of the solution is dextrose which contributes to the high osmolality of the solution. Amino acids (5%–10%) are present in variable concentrations depending upon the degree of physiological stress the patient is under. Only essential amino acids are administered to those patients with kidney or liver failure who have problems with urea excretion. Electrolytes and minerals are included or added to solutions dependent upon the patient's electrolyte status.

The number of calories prescribed by the physician is constantly evaluated. Undernutrition will result in muscle metabolism while overnutrition can result in fatty infiltration of the liver. Frequently the infusion of the TPN solution is controlled by use of an infusion pump. Two types of pumps are available, those that control the drip rate and those which control the volume. In-line filters are present in the system to remove air bubbles, particles, and, possibly, microorganisms. Solutions should be examined prior to administration, and the expiration date must be noted. Clouding of the solution indicates deterioration, and the solution should be discarded.

For the first day of TPN, only a fraction of the total caloric requirements is given. The caloric content of the infusate is increased over the first several days of TPN to allow for adaptation of the patient to the diet. During the first week of TPN, blood electrolyte, glucose, urea nitrogen, and protein are determined at regular intervals. Complications of TPN are most apt to occur when administration of the solution is initiated because of the concentration of nutrients. Adjustments are usually necessary during the first week. Stabilization on TPN generally requires 7 to 10 days. Caloric intake is greater than 2000 cal/day and consists of carbohydrate and crystalline amino acids or protein hydrolysate.

Interventions

Nursing interventions are directed toward (1) preparing the patient for insertion of the central line; (2) preventing complications associated with parenteral alimentation or minimizing complications by early detection and prompt treatment; (3) administering the prescribed solution at the specified rate; (4) teaching the patient about the treatment; (5) supporting the patient and family; and (6) monitoring the effect of the treatment.

Patient Preparation. The upper chest is washed, shaved, and cleaned with an antiseptic solution prior to the insertion of a central vein catheter. A local anesthetic is used. A small skin incision is made, and the catheter is tunneled a short distance through the subcataneous tissue prior to its insertion into the vein. This separates the point of entry of the catheter into the vein from its entry into the skin. The

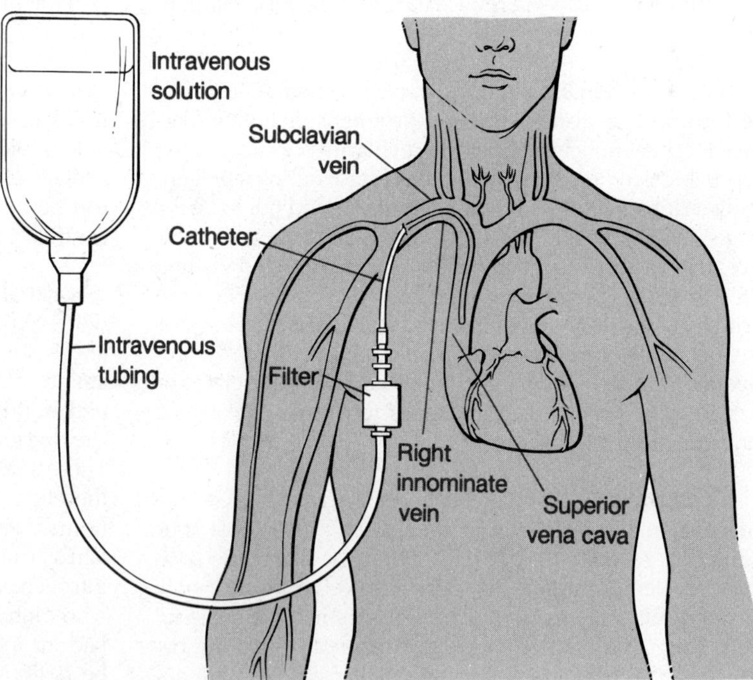

FIGURE 80–3 Hyperalimentation showing catheter placed directly into subclavian vein and threaded into innominate vein and superior vena cava.

position of the radiopaque catheter is checked by x-ray. Serious complications such as hydrothorax and pneumothorax accompanying catheter insertion rarely occur and are more likely to occur in the patient who is malnourished or frail. The catheter is locked with a Luer lock cap when TPN solutions are not being administered. A heparin lock flush is injected into the cap to minimize the possibility of clotting.

Infection. A major concern with both central and peripheral alimentation is to decrease the potential for infection. The nurse involved in assessing for manifestations of wound infection and sepsis (see Chap. 15). The entry site of the catheter is covered with an occlusive dressing which is changed (usually every 48 hours) under strict aseptic conditions. Some commercial dressings permit observation of the wound without requiring removal of the dressing. The wound is monitored for drainage as well as leakage of the TPN solution. Manifestations of catheter-related sepsis include chills, fever, increased white blood count. When catheter infection is suspected the catheter is removed, the tip and blood are sent for cultures, and antibiotics are initiated.

Other catheter-related complications are venous thrombosis and septic thrombophlebitis which may be related to infection, dehydration, or tissue irritation by the catheter tip. These complications also necessitate removal of the catheter. Patient problems with parenteral nutrition include mechanical and metabolic complications. Table 80–4 lists the common complications associated with parenteral nutrition.

Hyperglycemia. Hyperglycemia is a common problem, especially in patients who are hypermetabolic. The hyperglycemia may be the result of insulin resistance, too high a glucose load, or unsuspected diabetes mellitus. Increased renal clearance of glucose will produce an osmotic drag within the renal tubules and increased urine output which may result in dehydration and the potential for hyperosmolar coma. Excess glucose is converted to fat, producing large amounts of carbon dioxide and water. Furthermore, glucose-induced lipogenesis can cause hepatic lipid deposition which may compromise liver function. Insulin may be administered to facilitate glucose uptake by cells. If electrolyte imbalance occurs, the composition of electrolytes in the infusate can be altered. The BUN is monitored to detect a build-up of urea or nitrogenous waste products which may be toxic to a variety of systems including the central nervous system. This is particularly important in the patient with inadequate renal function (*e.g.,* chronic renal failure). Serum albumin levels may be measured as a rough estimate of nutritional adequacy.

Overhydration is another potential problem due to the volume of fluid infused. Accurate intake and output records are important. The patient is weighed daily, and manifestations of overhydration such as edema and mentation changes (*e.g.,* confusion) are monitored. At high risk are patients with renal or cardiac disease and those who have sepsis. Patients who resume oral intake while on TPN are also at risk for overhydration, therefore the volume of oral intake needs to be recorded. Electrolyte problems include hypophosphatemia, hypokalemia, and hypomagnesemia which occur as a result of rapid cellular uptake of glucose.

Evaluation of nutritional adequacy includes anthropometric measurements such as midarm circumference and skinfold thickness, as well as daily weights. Biochemical measurements (*e.g.,* serum albumin) are indicative of nutritional adequacy.

Biochemical changes are also dependent upon the primary pathophysiology as well as the nutritional therapy. For patients on long-term alimentation liver function tests may also be done. In some patients, long-term TPN has resulted in fatty infiltrations in the liver and alteration in liver function as manifested by increases in liver enzymes. Numerous medications are incompatible with the protein solution of TPN solutions. Therefore all medications are checked for their compatibility with the TPN solution prior to administration by the TPN catheter.

Patient/Family Teaching. Instruction of the patient and his or her family regarding solution administration and monitoring for manifestations of infection usually takes about a week. Patients who are candidates for home TPN therapy are evaluated in relation to ability to handle the equipment, to understand the information, and to solve problems. For many patients, home TPN has economical and psychological advantages over hospitalization for TPN. Patients and their families usually need a visiting nurse to assist with dressing changes during the first several weeks after discharge. Some patients prefer to infuse solutions from 10 PM to 10 AM to facilitate activity during the daytime. Whenever possible, oral intake (400–600 ml/day) should be encouraged. For the patient with limited or no oral intake, mouth care is critical.

Evaluation

The success of TPN is determined by the maintenance of positive nitrogen balance, maintenance of or gain in body weight, and the absence of metabolic or mechanical complications. For the patients on long-term home TPN, patient teaching is evaluated by body weight, lack of infection at the insertion site, patient/family ability to state and demonstrate appropriate care of the insertion site and administration and storage of the nutritional solution, and patient/family expressions of acceptance of the required modifications of lifestyle.

Excess Food Intake

Nursing Diagnosis

Alteration in nutrition related to excess food intake may be manifested by obesity. Nutritional intake in excess of body requirements is related to many factors. Although the normal control of feeding behavior appears to reside primarily in the central nervous system, peripheral receptors from the throat, GI tract, and liver contribute to regulation of diet intake.[10] In the CNS, two hypothalamic nuclei, the lateral and ventral medial, appear to be important in eating behavior. Although not firmly established, a genetic predisposition to body size may be present. Feeding behavior is also influenced by social and psychological factors.

In the United States and other industrialized countries,

TABLE 80–4
Complications of Total Parenteral Nutrition

Problems	Causes	Nursing Measures
Metabolic		
Hyperglycemia Glucosuria Osmotic dehydration Hyperosmolar coma	Glucose intolerance Increased infusion rate Undetected diabetes mellitus Excessive glucose load	Monitor urine and serum glucose levels Observe for changes in mentation, confusion Increased urine output Administer insulin per order If decreased level of consciousness, stop the infusion
Overhydration	Excessive fluid infusion Increased oral intake Particularly at risk: ▪ Renal patients ▪ Cardiac disease ▪ Sepsis	Monitor urine output, body weights Observe for manifestations including changes in mentation, edema Stop infusion/notify physician regarding change in fluid volume Administer diuretics per order
Hypophosphatemia	Rapid uptake due to glucose transport into cell	Monitor for lethargy, peripheral paraesthesia, ECG changes, serum phosphate levels Administer phosphate supplement per order
Hypokalemia	Rapid uptake due to glucose transport into cell	Monitor serum potassium, muscle weakness, paralysis, respiratory insufficiency Administer potassium supplement per order
Hypomagnesemia	Rapid uptake due to glucose transport into cell	Monitor serum magnesium levels; monitor for tingling sensations around the mouth, paresthesia in fingers, change in mentation Administer magnesium supplement per order
Liver dysfunction (elevation in liver enzymes, bilirubin)	Fat infiltration of liver	
Vitamin deficiency	Manifestations of individual vitamin deficiencies	Administration of vitamin supplements
Mechanical		
Tube clogging	Insufficient heparin when infusion stopped	Catheter is irrigated with a heparin-containing solution after use
Wound infection	Contamination	Dressing changes are done at regular intervals by qualified staff members. Use of Op-Site dressing which allows for observation.
Leakage	Cracking of the tubing Improper connection	Replacement of tubing Check patient's gown or bedding for leakage

obesity is a common problem. It is estimated that between 32% and 40% of Americans are overweight. The definition of obesity is variable but is generally defined as 20% over ideal body weight. Ideal body weight is based upon the height and sex of the individual. The Metropolitan Life Insurance Company height and weight tables provide the ideal body weights. Morbid obesity is defined as 100 lb or 100% or more over ideal body weight.

Obesity can result in significant health problems as well as produce psychological and social problems for the person. Health-related problems associated with obesity include diabetes mellitus, cholecystitis, and cardiovascular disease. The principal cause of death in morbidly obese persons is cardiovascular disease. Obesity is associated with increased morbidity and decreased life expectancy. Obesity, or overweight, is also associated with negative social consequences (*i.e.,* prejudices).

Obesity can be described as a psychophysiological disorder. The cause of obesity are multiple and overlapping. In general, caloric intake exceeds caloric need. This may be due to excesses in caloric intake or decreases in energy expenditure. Both phenomena may result from an alteration in the hypothalamic setpoint. The setpoint is the body weight around which the body will defend (*i.e.,* overeat to regain weight when body weight falls below the setpoint). In obese individuals the setpoint may be higher than that for a normal weight person.

Evidence for the setpoint theory is based on animal studies as well as the observation that most obese individuals return to their obese weight following a variety of weight-reduction programs.[16] The setpoint may be genetically determined because there is a familial tendency to obesity. However, it is difficult to separate genetically determined tendencies from learned eating or energy expenditure habits.

Obese individuals may be more responsive to food-related external cues than to internal cues of satiety.[7] Obese individuals also have an increase in the number of fat cells, which may be genetically determined or the result of early dietary patterns. However, the link between adipocytes and the central control of eating behavior remains to be determined.

Interventions

Nursing goals for the obese patient include (1) weight loss and (2) maintenance of weight loss once it has been attained. Interventions focus on patient education regarding treatment strategies, dietary counseling, and the avoidance of fad diets or weight-loss programs which promise easy and rapid weight loss, and encouraging the patient during the weight-reduction program. The most effective treatment of obesity is that which provides for long-term control, because the positive effects of weight loss on morbidity are dependent upon long-term weight reduction. Therapies for obesity include behavioral modification, pharmacological agents, and surgery. None of these therapies correct the underlying problem but they do facilitate the reduction of body weight and, hence, reduce the morbidity and mortality associated with obesity. However, pharmacological and surgical therapies do have risks for the patient.

Behavioral Modification. Behavioral modification programs are directed at altering and changing the stimuli associated with eating, and modifying eating habits to reduce caloric intake. Lifelong eating habits are difficult to modify, particularly on a long-term basis. Behavioral modification programs, which may be with a therapist or in a group setting, operate under the theory that overeating is a learned behavior. Therefore, weight reduction can be accomplished by modifying eating behavior. These types of programs focus on the behavior of eating rather than the diet *per se.* Strategies include taking smaller bites, eating at specified times during the day, and identifying eating cues (*e.g.,* emotional upsets, depression) for eating. However, many of the self-help groups such as TOPS (take off pounds sensibly) and Weight Watchers also provide diet education which includes a reduction in total daily calories, an exercise plan, and may include social support mechanism.

Pharmacological Therapy. Pharmacological treatment of obesity is used cautiously in select patients due to the side-effects and addictive nature of drugs such as the amphetamines which may be used to control appetite. These drugs act by suppressing the appetite center, however, they have a variety of other central nervous system effects as well.

Exercise. With restricted dietary intake, there is generally a loss of body weight during the first 2 to 3 weeks. However, with further restriction in caloric intake, the basal metabolic rate also decreases. Therefore, restriction in calories must be accompanied by an increase in physical activity or exercise to further decrease body weight. For the person who is overweight and has had limited exercise, the exercises should be introduced gradually and increased over time to meet the patient's tolerance.

Maintenance Diet. Once the ideal body weight has been achieved the individual must continue on a maintenance diet because the tendency to gain weight is a lifelong problem.

Due to the increased risk of morbidity associated with obesity, patients are frequently counseled by physicians and nurses to reduce body weight. A reduction in caloric intake below energy requirements will result in weight reduction. Such counseling needs to be preceded by an evaluation of the patient's dietary history and habits. The role of food in the person's life, both from a social and cultural viewpoint, is often difficult to determine. Evaluation of the patient may reveal a pattern of dieting, weight loss, and regaining weight. Patient education needs include the avoidance of drastic and fad diets which can, if prolonged, result in significant nutritional deficiencies. The patient needs to be wary of diets that offer rapid losses in body weight. Most diets which restrict calories will result in a rapid loss of body weight initially. However, this loss is due to loss of water.

Motivation. Motivation is an important factor in any weight-reduction program. The patient must see the need to reduce his or her weight. Frequently, conditions such as cardiovascular impairments (*e.g.,* hypertension) motivate the patient to seek help in weight reduction. Nurses can facilitate this motivation by encouraging the patient in weight-reduction efforts. Patients need to set a realistic goal for weight reduction. This is often determined by body build and the degree of obesity. The patient is instructed to weigh himself at regular intervals at the same time of day and with the same amount of clothing on.

Evaluation

The success of any weight-reduction program is evidenced by a decrease in body weight which is maintained. The patient will report adherence to dietary habits that facilitate weight loss or maintenance of weight loss. Patients who do not alter their dietary habits or who consume high-calorie foods and liquids at frequent intervals may fail to lose weight.

Surgical Intervention for Obesity

Patients who are candidates for weight-reducing surgeries have undergone other forms of therapy with minimal success. The patient has also had a thorough work-up to rule out potential endocrine imbalances which may have produced the obesity. For some patients, however, surgical therapy may be the last option to decrease the morbidity associated with long-term obesity. Part of the routine surgical work-up will frequently include a psychiatric evaluation. The purpose of this evaluation is to determine which patients may have problems during the postoperative period.

Jejunoileal Bypass. Surgical interventions include jejunoileal bypass in which a segment of the small intestine is bypassed, thus decreasing the surface area of the intestine available for dietary absorption. Thus, weight loss is produced by a process of malabsorption. This type of surgery was more commonly performed in the early and mid 1970's. It is not used as frequently today because of the incidence of late complications following surgery. These complications include liver failure, arthritis, myositis, tenosynovitis, and dermatitis, and are thought to result from colonic bacteria overgrowth in the excluded intestine.[9] Other problems include megacolon (dilatation of the colon), bypass enteritis, intussusception, and obstruction. A variety of other problems develop due to the malabsorption produced by the surgery. These include electrolyte and acid–base imbalances, vitamin deficiencies, and protein malnutrition.

Gastric-Reduction Operations. The basic principle of gastric-reduction surgeries is to decrease the size of the stomach and thus limit the amount of food that can be consumed. The volume that the resected stomach will hold will vary between surgical techniques, but will be between 30 and 50 ml. The outlet between the stomach and intestine is narrowed to prevent gastric dumping syndrome.

One type of gastric reduction is the gastric bypass, in which the proximal portion of the stomach is anastomosed to the small intestine. Weight reduction is produced due to decreased dietary intake. Similar to this is gastroplasty, or gastric stapling, in which the stomach is partitioned into two segments, leaving a small canal to connect the two segments. As a result, the amount of food that the stomach can hold is drastically reduced. Gastroplasty is used more frequently than gastric bypass because it is technically easier to perform and it has been associated with fewer long-term complications. However, it has been associated with a less permanent weight loss. With gastric partitioning there is an estimated overall mortality rate of about 4% and morbidity from 10% to 20%.[6]

Interventions. Goals of nursing after surgical intervention for gastric bypass include teaching appropriate eating habits, which are important to prevent disruption of the staple line and to prevent obstruction of the channel, which is 1 cm or less. These habits are:

1. Three meals a day.
2. Solid foods only at mealtime.
3. Eat slowly, mealtime should be at least 40 minutes long.
4. Chew foods completely.
5. Avoid foods that cannot be chewed completely; spit out foods that cannot be chewed.
6. Drink 1500 to 2000 ml water daily; between meals, avoid high-calorie soft drink. Fluids should be taken in small sips to avoid stretching of the pouch.
7. Select foods from the basic food groups.
8. Stop eating when the sensation of fullness is present; overeating can result in vomiting.[2,9]

These practices will instill good eating habits and facilitate weight loss. Weight loss is also facilitated by the avoidance of high-calorie drinks such as milkshakes, sodas, beer. Tolerance to individual foods will vary between patients. Certain foods which are particularly intolerable for many patients include tough meats such as hamburger, membranes from oranges and grapefruit, fibrous vegetables, highly spiced foods, fried foods, concentrated sweets, and milk.[9] The elimination of such foods from the diet may result in inadequate protein intake. Following gastric surgery patients are at risk for developing vitamin deficiencies including thiamine, folate, B_{12}, and iron. Manifestations of these deficiencies include lethargy, weakness, paresthesias, ataxia, confusion. Patients are taught the importance of daily iron and vitamin supplements. Blood levels are measured at routine follow-up appointments.

Alterations in Bowel Elimination

Diarrhea

Nursing Diagnosis

Alteration in bowel elimination is related to disorders of the bowel and is manifested in frequent, nonformed stools. Diarrhea can produce an interruption in the activities of normal living as well as discomfort. Most cases of diarrhea are self-limiting, and require no intervention, however, some patients with more severe forms of diarrhea may require hospitalization for replacement of fluid and electrolytes. In older adults diarrhea can result in serious complications due to drastic reductions in fluid and electrolytes. Recurrent diarrhea may be an indication of underlying GI pathology. Generally, diarrhea is referred to as an increase in stool number per day and a decrease in consistency from solid to liquid. In most cases of diarrhea, these two characteristics occur together.

An average of 9 liters of fluid travel through the GI tract daily, with only 1% to 2% of this fluid excreted in the stool. In diarrhea, the water content of the stool increases with the severity of diarrhea. The additional water in the stool may be the result of inadequate intestinal absorption of fluid or from increased fluid secretion by mucosal cells.

Interventions

The goals of nursing management for the patient with diarrhea are to (1) maintain optimal fluid and electrolyte status; (2) promote optimal nutrition; (3) optimize patient comfort and safety; and (4) promote activities of daily living.

Fluid and Electrolyte Status. Potential disturbances in fluid and electrolyte balance result from loss of fluid and, if prolonged, dehydration will occur. Dehydration, loss of 10% body weight, may necessitate the need for parenteral repletion of fluids. Fecal losses which exceed 3 to 4 liters/day necessitate parenteral fluids. Along with water loss, there are losses of electrolytes, including sodium and potassium. The sodium loss, along with water loss, will produce manifestations of saline deficiency. Thus, the patient will complain of thirst, fatigue, and weight loss. Signs of dehydration include loss of skin turgor, orthostatic hypotension, and, if prolonged, changes in mentation. Signs and symptoms of hypokalemia include fatigue, ECG changes, and lethargy.

In mild, self-limiting cases of diarrhea, the patient takes only clear liquids to promote bowel rest during the first 12 to 24 hours. If nausea or vomiting are not present, sodium and potassium can be replenished by glucose–electrolyte solutions. Oral glucose–electrolyte solutions such as Pedialyte or Gatorade, containing glucose, sodium, and potassium, are frequently recommended, as are products such as cola, ginger ale, and root beer. The diet is then resumed gradually starting with dry toast and crackers. In older adults even a relatively minor bout of diarrhea can result in a drastic reduction in circulating volume, and thus these patients are at risk for dehydration and subsequent cardiovascular changes.

For the patient with moderate to severe diarrhea, fluid and electrolyte replacement is critical. Because orthostatic hypotension may be present, the patient needs ready access to a bedpan or bedside commode. The patient may be placed on bedrest and bowel rest with solid food withheld for 12 to 24 hours or longer depending upon duration of the diarrhea. Intravenous fluid replacement is instituted when manifestations of dehydration or nausea and vomiting are present.

The patient's hydration status is evaluated by monitoring intake and output records, skin turgor, serum electrolyte levels, and mentation status. The patient with diarrhea, regardless of the underlying pathology, needs to be monitored for the frequency and consistency of bowel movements.

Nutritional Status. The second nursing goal is to support body needs for adequate nutrition. The patient may not have sufficient nutrient intake or man not absorb sufficient foodstuffs, resulting in loss of body weight. Most episodes of diarrhea due to viral agents are self-limiting, and thus, limited nutritional intake for 24 hours will not result in serious complications. In situations where the diarrhea persists (prolonged gastroenteritis, dumping syndrome), short-bowel syndrome, malabsorption will result due to hypermotility of the intestine, which reduces the digestive and absorptive time of the gut.

Interventions include careful records of the patient's weight as well as intake and output records in order to facilitate the assessment of the patient's nutritional status and planning of nutritional interventions. Other measurements which are used include white blood count, serum albumin levels, and skinfold thickness. None of these indicators is sufficient as the sole determinant of nutritional status. Patients who exhibit signs of malnutrition or who are placed on bowel rest due to diarrhea or bleeding may require parenteral alimentation to maintain body weight or elemental diets which can be absorbed readily from the intestine.

Comfort. A third goal is to prevent skin breakdown and to promote patient comfort secondary to diarrhea. Patients with prolonged or recurrent diarrhea may experience problems with skin excoriation, particularly if incontinence is a problem. The diarrhea stool can be irritating to the anal tissue. The perineum needs to be checked at regular intervals for redness, excoriation, and tissue breakdown. Patients are taught to wipe the anal area after each bowel movement. Older patients with problems of mobility may need assistance to accomplish this. Appropriate skin care for the patient with excoriated perianal tissue may include heat lamp exposure for 15 minutes each 8 hours and/or the application of antiseptic solution. Sitz baths using an antiseptic agent may be used to prevent infection and promote comfort.

Activity Level. The fourth goal is to promote maximum activities of daily living. Patients with chronic diarrhea due to a functional disorder or due to known pathology of the intestine often experience alterations in ability to carry out daily activities. Patients in whom fecal incontinence occurs concomitantly with diarrhea must deal with a potential socially embarrassing situation. There is the inconvenience of constantly searching out restrooms in public places or the work environment. As such, the patient may reduce social contacts as well as decrease mobility, which may ultimately result in social isolation. The patient requires support from staff as well as family members to deal with the problem of fecal incontinence. Some patients may opt for protective underpads which may provide increased social mobility.

Patients with recurrent episodes of prolonged diarrhea may be treated with antidiarrheal agents. These drugs are listed in Table 80–5. Patients are instructed on the use of such medications, how to avoid overusage, and potential side-effects. Overuse of all antidiarrheal agents can produce constipation or obstruction. Symptoms of fecal incontinence which is secondary to constipation may be misinterpreted as diarrhea. Other drugs such as corticosteroids, antibiotics,

TABLE 80-5
Antidiarrheal Agents

Type	*Action*	*Side-Effects*
Opiates Paregoric Codiene (60 mg q8 hr)	↓ Small and large intestine motility ↑ Intestinal water and electrolyte absorption	CNS depression Sedation Addiction
Synthetic Opiates Loperamide hydrochloride (Imodium) (2 mg bid, total of 16 mg/day) Diphenoxylate hydrochloride (Lomotil)		Abdominal cramps Constipation Nausea/vomiting Dry mouth Drowsiness
Absorbants Kaopectate	Absorbs excess fluid	
Antispasmodics Atropine Tincture of belladonna	↓ Intestinal motility	
Bulk-forming agents: Metamucil, Effersyllium	Absorb excess fluid	

and replacement enzymes are used for specific patients who have underlying GI pathology as discussed in following chapters.

Evaluation

The success of management is evident by a decrease in diarrhea and the passage of formed stool. The adequacy of fluid and electrolyte replacement is determined by the absence of orthostatic hypotension and manifestations of electrolyte imbalance, serum electrolyte levels within normal limits, and the presence of a clear sensorium. The effectiveness of nutritional therapies for patients with chronic problems of diarrhea is determined by decreased incidence of diarrhea and the maintenance of body weight. Other determinants of goal achievement are the patient reports a decrease in discomfort, maintains an intact skin, and increases self-care activities.

Constipation

Nursing Diagnosis

Constipation is related to prolonged retention of stool or feces in the intestine or rectum and manifested in infrequent bowel movements. The determination of constipation is dependent upon normal bowel habits. A bowel movement each day is not normal for every person. Some patients' normal bowel patterns include a bowel movement every 3 to 4 days, while in others, two to three bowel movements each day is the norm. Constipation is also described as the passage of dry, hard stool which occurs as a result of water absorption of the colon. Therefore, constipation is defined as an increase in the interval between bowel movements (generally 3 or more days) and/or the passage of a dry, hard stool with straining.

Constipation can result from a multitude of factors, including gastrointestinal and extragastrointestinal. Common causes of constipation include change in diet (*e.g.,* reduced fiber content), decreased fluid intake, immobility, decreased appetite, and pharmacological agents which decrease intestinal transit (*e.g.,* opiates) or increase fluid absorption in the colon. Constipation is a problem whose prevalence increase with age. Prolonged and indiscriminate use of cathartics can result in decreased motility of the colon as well.

Functional alterations in bowel motility are also thought to account for constipation in a portion of patients. Hypotonic colon is relatively common in older adults. It is associated with fecal incontinence due to overflow. Constipation can also occur as a result of gastrointestinal pathophysiology such as obstruction in the intestine and colon which decreases the amount of feces delivered to the rectum. Hemorrhoids and anal fissures, which make passage of the stool painful, may cause constipation because the afflicted person ignores the urge to defecate in order to avoid the discomfort. Ischemic bowel disease may result in delayed intestinal transit.

Interventions

The goals of nursing management are to (1) relieve constipation, (2) prevent recurrence, and (3) promote comfort. Relief from constipation may be accomplished through the use of laxatives, enemas, and suppositories. The ideal laxative is not yet available. Laxatives are categorized as wetting agents, lubricants, bulk-forming agents, and stimulants (Table 80–6). The type of laxative prescribed is based on the degree of constipation, medical history, and other medications that the patient is taking.

A second goal of nursing care is to prevent recurrence of constipation. Patient education is an important component of the therapy for constipation. Patients need to be taught normal bowel function and actions to achieve normalcy. The actions are to heed the urge to defecate, eat a diet that includes roughage, drink 1½ quarts to 2 quarts of fluid a day, and include some physical activity in the daily regimen. Laxatives should not be used on a long-term basis to manage constipation. Indiscriminate and long-term use of laxatives is often a cause of diarrhea. When laxatives are used, they should be used at the lowest dose and withdrawn gradually. Patients need to be instructed on the harmful side-effects of laxatives.

Constipation produces abdominal discomfort (*e.g.*, sensation of fullness, cramping, pain), as well as straining at passage of the stool. One method of preventing constipation is by the addition of bran to soft or liquid foods which are in the individual's normal diet. A total of 30 to 60 g daily is recommended. The patient needs to take a glass of liquid at each meal. Other foods such as raw fruits and vegetables may not be as effective as bran because the fiber content is less than that of bran. Bran does not require refrigeration and can be stored easily, therefore, people can pack it easily when traveling. The inclusion of dietary fiber may be difficult for some patients. The introduction of bran into the diet will produce an increase in flatus and possibly abdominal discomfort. The patient should be told that the flatus will decrease with time. Some patients find the use of psyllium

TABLE 80–6
Pharmacological Therapies for Constipation

Type	*Brand Name*	*Action*	*Precautions*
Wetting agents (surfactants)	Colace Doxinate Surfak	Promote softening and emulsification of the stool; 50–200 mg	Not given with mineral oil
Lubricants	Mineral oil, 15/45 ml/1–3x daily	Softens stools	Taken between meals to prevent interference with absorption of fat-soluble vitamins
Bulk-forming agents	Metamucil, 2–4 g/3x daily, ½ to 1 glass H_2O Effersyllium	Nonabsorbable hydrophilic→swell and thus softens stool	Before or after other drugs
Stimulants			
Small intestine	Castor oil (rapid onset)	Stimulates secretion of small bowel	Small bowel malabsorption Prolonged use results in damage to Auerbach's plexus
Colon	ExLax Bisacodyl (Dulcolax) senna, cascara, aloes		
Osmotic stimulants	Mg sulfate, hypertonic phosphate Milk of Magnesia Lactulose (slow onset), 1–2 Tb (10–20 g) daily		Increased gas, bloating
Suppositories			Cramps
Rapid onset	Glycerin	↑ Water secretion in distal colon	
	Dulcolax Senokot	Ganglion cells of Auerbach's plexus direct irritants	
Enemas			
Rapid onset			
Oil retention		Remove fecal impactions by softening the stool	

(Metamucil) compounds more palatable than bran cereal. In elderly patients with dentition problems, this form may be more easily taken. Patients who have constipation which involves the expulsion of a dry, hard stool may benefit from the use of stool softeners.

The third goal is to promote comfort and prevent alterations in lifestyle. Good bowel habits imply defecating as soon as the urge to defecate is felt. In persons who do not, the feces remains, and greater water absorption occurs. The neural stimulation produced by the distending bowel adapts with time, and the urge is no longer felt, while the bowel continues to distend. The patient should be in an upright position to facilitate defecation. Therefore, the patient on bedrest should be placed on the bedpan and the head of the bed elevated. The use of the commode or bathroom is the best and should be encouraged whenever the person's health permits.

Exercise may also be beneficial to the patient with constipation, in particular those patients in whom inactivity is also present. Patients who are inactive as a result of neuromuscular disease such as Parkinson's disease, strokes, multiple sclerosis, and spinal cord injury frequently have problems with constipation which may be improved by the addition of regular exercise.

Evaluation

Goals are achieved if the frequency and regularity of bowel movements increase and the patient reports a decrease in abdominal discomfort and an increase in ease of defecation.

Diarrhea Alternating with Constipation

Nursing Diagnosis

Diarrhea alternating with constipation is related to irritable bowel syndrome (IBS) and is manifested by alteration in bowel habits accompanied by abdominal discomfort which lasts for greater than 3 months.[14] Irritable bowel syndrome is not a specific disease, and there is no specific pathology associated with the symptoms. A wide range of symptoms has been associated with this syndrome including diarrhea, constipation, and abdominal discomfort. Constipation and abdominal discomfort are thought to arise from intestinal spasm or other alterations in intestinal motility. Irritable bowel syndrome has been noted to occur frequently in patients who suffer from psychiatric problems such as depression, hypochondria, and hysteria.

Diagnosis is made after other diseases have been ruled out. For the patient with GI symptoms, the diagnosis of irritable bowel syndrome may provide reassurance that there is no intestinal or colon cancer. Patients with this disorder do not appear to be at increased risk for other GI diseases.

Interventions

The goals of nursing management are to (1) promote optimal elimination patterns; (2) educate the patient regarding treatment measures, especially dietary changes and medication; and (3) promote comfort. An irritable bowel is most frequently managed by the addition of fiber (20 g of bran) to the diet. Fiber slows down the movement of the fecal mass in patients with diarrhea or loose stools and increases the fecal movement in patients with constipation. Fiber also draws water into the lumen and results in a softer stool which is easier to pass. Fats, which decrease intestinal transit, may produce symptoms of bloating and constipation in patients with an irritable bowel and should be avoided. Similarly, known gas-producing foods should also be avoided. Bulk-forming agents such as hydrophilic colloids may be of benefit in patients when constipation predominates and may be met with greater acceptance by the patient than bran. Similar to bran, these products are associated with increased flatus and bloating when they are initially started. These preparations do not work immediately, but rather it may be several days before the patient notices the effect.

For patients who are more prone to diarrhea, antidiarrheal agents may be used intermittently to control diarrhea. Although anticholinergics have long been used in the management of GI symptoms, these drugs have many side-effects which may be particularly hazardous to the elderly client, and thus are not commonly used in patients with irritable bowel syndrome. However, when the patient is treated with anticholinergics or antispasmodics, these drugs are given 30 to 45 minutes prior to eating. Patients need to be instructed on the use of these medications and to monitor for side-effects.

Evaluation

Goal achievement is attained when the patient reports a decrease in abdominal discomfort, in the incidence of diarrhea or constipation, and adherence to prescribed therapy including medications.

Paralytic Ileus

Nursing Diagnosis

Absence of segmental intestinal motility is related to a disruption in the normal peristalsis of the bowel and manifested by abdominal discomfort, distention, vomiting, and absence of bowel tones. Abdominal distention may not be present in patients who have nasointestinal tubes in place for bowel decompression. X-ray visualization of the abdomen reveals a bowel filled with air. Paralytic ileus is a problem frequently encountered by patients who have undergone a major physiological stress (*e.g.,* trauma, burns) or who have had abdominal surgery which required manipulation of the bowel. The etiology is unknown, but it is thought to be due to the release of catecholamines, which inhibit intestinal motility and thus result in decreased movement of intestinal contents through the segment affected. Paralytic ileus may also occur as a result of inflammation or infection of the bowel or the abdominal organs (*e.g.,* pancreatitis, peritonitis, inflammatory bowel disease).

If undetected, paralytic ileus can result in significant problems for the patient. These problems include obstruction to the movement of intestinal contents proximal to the segment of bowel which is "paralytic," pooling of secretions in the affected portion, and fluid and electrolyte imbalance.

Interventions

The goals of nursing interventions for patients with paralytic ileus are (1) early recognition of the problem, (2) promotion of comfort; and (3) maintenance of fluid balance. The condition is suspected in the postoperative patient who does not have bowel sounds. Surgical patients at high risk for paralytic ileus receive no fluid or food per mouth and will have a nasogastric (NG) or nasointestinal (NI) tube in place and connected to a suction apparatus. The NG or NI tube is left in place until the return of bowel sounds or the passage of stool or flatus. During this time the patient's hydration is maintained by intravenous fluid administration. Paralytic ileus is frequently self-limiting and subsides within 2 to 3 days.

Nasogastric Intubation

Nasogastric (NG) or *nasointestinal (NI) tubes* are placed in patients for a variety of reasons, including decreased or absent intestinal motility. Other reasons are for diagnostic purposes such as the determination of gastric juice pH under basal or stimulated conditions, to aspirate gastric contents prior to surgery or following drug overdose. An NG tube may be used to decompress the stomach in patients experiencing GI hemorrhage or surgery. In these situations the proximal end of the tube is attached to a suction apparatus. The amount of fluid and blood loss can be ascertained by measuring the aspirant content. The presence of the NG tube in the patient with an upper GI bleed allows for the instillation of irrigation solutions (*e.g.,* iced normal saline) or medications such as antacids. Aspiration of gastric or intestinal contents is critical for the patient who will undergo surgery for an intestinal or pyloric obstruction. Intestinal decompression is frequently accomplished by long tubes which are weighted to facilitate the movement of the tube from the stomach to intestine. Examples of such tubes include the Miller-Abbot and Cantor tubes. During the postoperative period NG or NI tubes are used to decompress the intestine to reduce pressure on the suture line as well as to decrease the possibility of obstruction due to paralytic ileus. As discussed earlier in this chapter, NG or NI tubes may be used for tube feeding.

Suction may be used to empty gastric or intestinal contents. This is accomplished by mechanical aspiration either by gravity or, more commonly, by a device such as the Gomco suction machine. The amount of pressure exerted by these devices will be dependent upon the size of the tube. For example, a greater amount of pressure is required to aspirate through a small lumen tube than a large lumen tube. A maximum of 25 mmHg pressure is used because beyond this point, mucosal injury is likely to occur. The *Salem Sump* tube has a vent which prevents the suction tube tip from attaching to tissue in contrast to the *Levin* tube which does not have a vent.

Suction may be continuous or intermittent. Intermittent suction helps to maintain tube patency. The amount of pressure as well as the intermittency of the suction is prescribed by the physician. Multiple lumen tubes are frequently used for decompression.

Irrigation of the nasogastric tube may be required to prevent clogging of the tube. The amount and timing of NG irrigation are prescribed by the physician. For the postgastric surgery patient, irrigation is a sterile procedure. The irrigation solution is infused manually, and the tube is reattached to suction. The return of the irrigation solution is monitored. If there is no return, the patient is observed for manifestations of obstruction, and the physician is consulted.

Nursing Care

The presence of an NG or NI tube can produce nasal irritation and potential for *mucosal breakdown.* Elderly patients are at risk due to increased fragility of mucosal tissue and decreased wound-healing response. Patients on chemotherapy may also be at greater risk for complications of mucosal breakdown. The patient's naris needs to be checked for bleeding. A water-soluble lubricant can be applied to the tube at the point of insertion into the nose. For prolonged tube placement, the tube will be replaced every 2 to 3 weeks, alternating nares if possible.

Oral care is also paramount in the patient with an NG or NI tube. If possible, the patient is encouraged to brush his teeth and to rinse his mouth. For the patient unable to do this, and who also has diminished gag reflex, normal saline swabs and hydrogen peroxide swabs are used to clean the oral cavity. Patients may benefit from chewing gum or sucking on hard candy, if permissible. The lips are moistened with a water-soluble lubricant. This is important because most patients with a tube in place will mouth-breathe. The nursing interventions to prevent problems of nasal mucosal irritation were discussed in the section on tube feeding.

Proper placement of the tube is important. Once an NG placement has been verified by x-ray visualization, the point of entry into the nose is marked with a permanent ink pen. Then, after the tube is manipulated or temporarily dislodged, it can be returned to its original location.

Patients with an NG or NI tube which is attached to suction are at risk for problems with fluid and electrolyte imbalance. Careful monitoring of intake including irrigating solutions and output is critical. The color and characteristics of the aspirant are important to record. The patient is frequently on intravenous fluid replacement to reduce the risk of dehydration and electrolyte imbalance. The patient's hydration status is monitored by body weight, skin turgor, edema, mental status, and serum electrolyte levels.

Bowel Resections: Colostomy and Ileostomy

Intestinal Stomas

Alteration in bowel elimination is related to surgical creation of an intestinal stoma. Pathologies requiring bowel reconstruction and abdominal intestinal stomas include cancer, diverticulitis, and ulcerative colitis. A stoma, an opening into a body cavity or organ, can be temporary or permanent. The specific type refers to the portion of the gastrointestinal or urinary tract that is brought to the skin surface. A temporary stoma is used when surgical closure is anticipated in the future. Conditions that may require a temporary stoma include perforating diverticulitis, obstructed colon, traumatic intestinal perforation, volvulus and rectovaginal fistula. Closure depends on several factors. Some stomas are done with the intent of closure but become permanent because of the patient's age, the disease process, general condition, or because of poor surgical risk. If a person with a temporary stoma is discharged from the hospital before closure, it is important that he learn as much about his care as the person with a permanent stoma.

A permanent stoma may be required in cancer of the rectum, sigmoid colon, or bladder or because of trauma. A permanent stoma is surgically created when the distal portion of the bowel (or urinary tract) has been removed or if the pathology distal to the stoma makes closure and normal function impossible.

An end stoma consists of one or two stomas such as is created in a double-barrel colostomy. In the double-barrel colostomy, the proximal stoma is the functioning stoma; the distal stoma is nonfunctioning (Fig. 80–4).

A loop stoma consists of an intact segment of bowel looped through the abdomen, rather than severed (Fig. 80–5). This loop of bowel is stabilized with a plastic rod for 7 to 10 days postoperatively. There is one stoma that has two openings. Effluent drains from the proximal opening. Because of the close proximity of the two openings, effluent may spill over into the distal segment. This can be a colostomy, ileostomy, or urostomy but is most commonly done as a transverse colostomy.

Bowel diversion leading to the construction of a stoma may take the form of an ileostomy or a colostomy. In an ileostomy, the opening is made into the ileum. In a colostomy, an opening is made anywhere along the ascending, transverse, descending, or sigmoid colon. The colostomy may be double barrel or result in an end or loop stoma, with the site of the disease determining its location.

Stoma Equipment

The appropriate use of stoma equipment can be an area of confusion for nurses as well as patients unless they have guidance and knowledge of the equipment and its potential problems. Basic terminology can be misleading. While people refer to a collecting device as a pouch, appliance, or bag, the important thing to remember is to describe the collecting device in a positive manner. Identifying it as a pouch usually conveys a positive image. There are two general types of disposable pouches available: drainable and nondrainable. Other pouch variables include with or without skin barriers, starter openings or standard openings, urinary or fecal, clear or opaque, snap-on pouches with skin barriers, as well as various shapes and sizes (Fig. 80–6). Some pouches are lightweight and disposable after using them 1 to 7 days.

There are two types of reusable pouches, one-piece and two-piece. The faceplate is a round or oval disk made of plastic or rubber with the stoma opening in the center. The faceplate adheres around the stoma with the use of adhesives, cements, or a skin barrier. The faceplate is permanently attached to the pouch with the one-piece system. On two-piece equipment the faceplate and pouch are attached separately. Reusable equipment can be worn for several days before being removed. Durability depends on several things: the material used in construction, the care the equipment receives, and the effluent's chemical reaction to the material. The pouches need to be discarded and replaced if odor is present after thorough cleansing or if they become brittle.

The choice of faceplates depends on the anatomical configuration around the stoma and the type of stoma. Faceplates may be flat, flexible, rigid, or have varying degrees of convexity. Patients need recommendations and assistance in addition to follow-up instructions from an enterostomal ther-

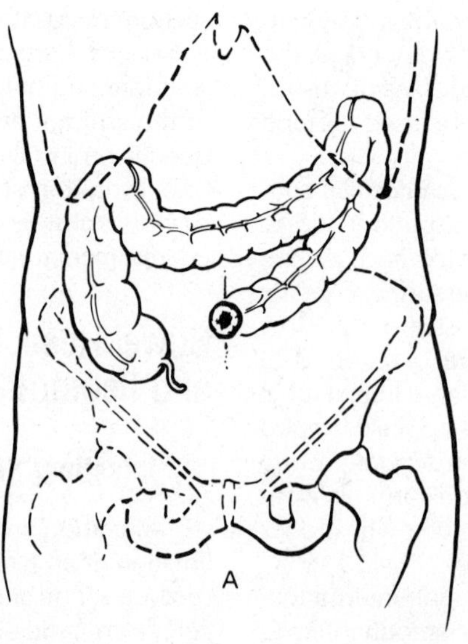

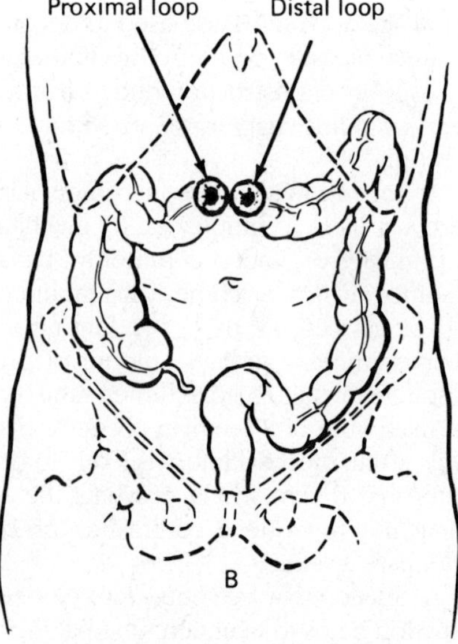

FIGURE 80–4 (*A*) One type of single-barreled colostomy. The distal portion of the bowel has been removed, and the colostomy is permanent. (*B*) One type of double-barreled colostomy, showing proximal and distal loops. This type of colostomy may or may not be permanent.

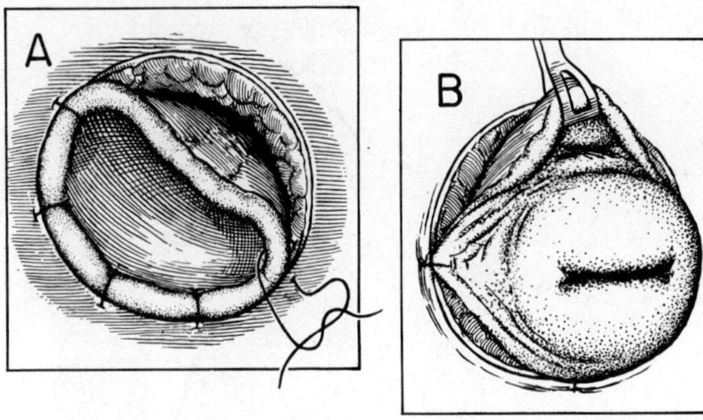

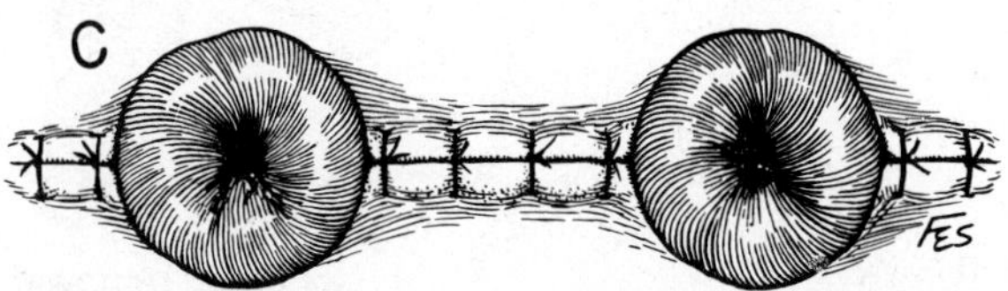

FIGURE 80–5 (*A*) Permanent end colostomy. Bowel is being sutured to the skin with several interrupted absorbable sutures. (*B*) Loop colostomy. The proximal afferent functional limb is placed inferior to the nonfunctioning distal limb, the orifice of which is in relation to the Babcock clamp. (*C*) Divided colostomy with a bridge of skin between the afferent and efferent limbs. (Veidenheimer MC: Carcinoma of the rectum. In Hardy JD [ed]: Rhoads Textbook of Surgery, 5th ed. Philadelphia, JB Lippincott, 1977)

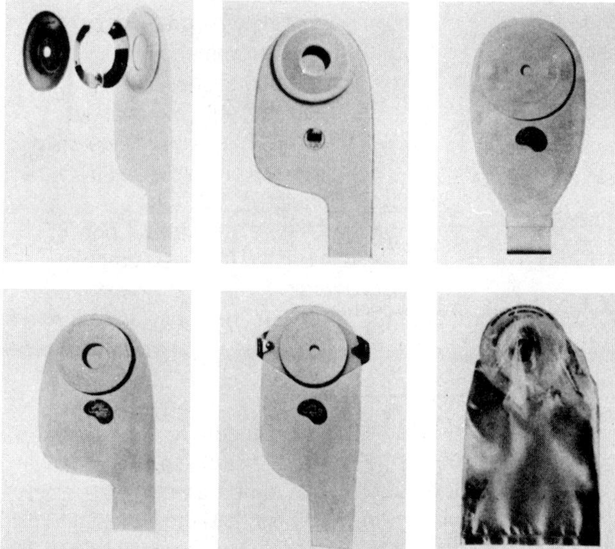

FIGURE 80–6 The permanent stoma appliance. A variety of permanent ileostomy appliances are available from the manufacturer. The features of these appliances vary as to pouch size, pouch length, pouch shape, and faceplate (disk) design. (United Surgical Corp.)

apy (ET) nurse if they use this equipment. The reusable pouch is usually applied only after the postoperative stomal edema subsides, approximately several weeks postoperatively. Periodic stoma calibration is necessary. Reusable equipment is most frequently used on patients with urinary diversions and ileostomies. Modifications have to be made over a period of time due to weight change, change in the contour of the abdomen, and the stoma size.

There are many types of pouches available, and one type is not appropriate for each patient. An ideal system protects the skin, contains the odor and effluent, and is not noticeable under clothing. An adequate seal provides optimal skin protection. Drainage should not collect between the stoma and the outer edge of the pouch. Close observation is necessary to detect drainage collecting around the stoma as it will result in skin breakdown. Other considerations which determine the selection of equipment include the size and contour of the abdomen, the size of the stoma, and the type and frequency of the effluent that is emitted (Fig. 80–7). In addition, the patient's disabilities, mental and physical status, manual dexterity, physical activities, financial situation, personal preference, and comfort must be considered in equipment selection. Other pertinent factors in pouch selection are patient sensitivities, noise created by the pouch, whether it has a starter or standard stoma opening, and the availability of the equipment.

There are three methods of adhering a pouch to the body: use of a skin barrier, double-faced adhesive disk or adhesive on a disposable pouch, and surgical cement or adhesive spray. Combinations of all three are sometimes effective. The choice is based on the following:

1. *Stoma effluent.* Effluent that has potential for being irritating needs a protective barrier (*i.e.,* small bowel effluent).
2. *Anatomical characteristics.* A smooth surface around the stoma can be achieved through the use of skin barriers or pastes.
3. *Sensitivities.* If a patient's skin is sensitive to adhesives or skin barriers, it would be a contraindication in using that particular product.
4. *Patient preference.* This contributes to adaptation.
5. *Disabilities.* This may necessitate a simple method of application
6. *Current skin problems.* The short-term use of a skin barrier may be needed until skin irritation has been resolved.

Texture and temperature of the skin also influence the selection of the skin barrier. Patient activities, cost, and climate are other factors to consider.

Adhesives are available as double-faced adhesive disks, silicone spray, or liquid skin cement. They will provide adhesion to reusable faceplates, increase the adhesive surfaces of the pouch if the adhesive area is too small, or increase adherence of the adhesive on a pouch. In certain instances, adhesives make it possible to reuse disposable equipment. If adhesive is on the patient for several days, it is usually easy to remove. If it is well-adhered, there are solvents specially made to assist in removing pouches. The skin needs to be washed well after using solvents. Caution needs to be exercised when using skin cement. If the cement is not allowed to dry before the pouch is sealed to the skin, severe chemical burns may occur. Allergic reactions sometimes occur because cements contain rubber derivatives.

Belts support the weight of the pouch but are not intended to hold it on. They are beneficial when a convex faceplate is used. Caution needs to be exercised, as they can

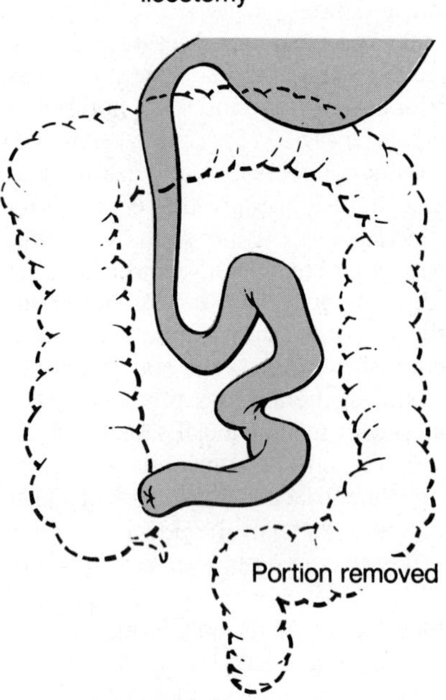

Effluent Characteristics
- Liquid to pasty
- Slightly odorous
- Damaging to peristomal skin
- Frequency of drainage: often (approx. 800 ml/24 hr)

Equipment Recommended
- Drainable
- Disposable or reusable
- Skin barrier

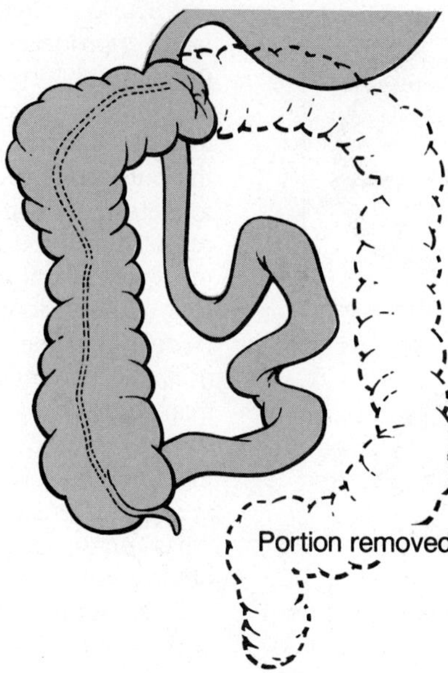

Effluent Characteristics
- Semiliquid to soft
- Malodorous
- Damaging to peristomal skin
- Frequency of drainage: several times in 24 hr

Equipment Recommended
- Drainable, disposable, or reusable
- Skin barrier

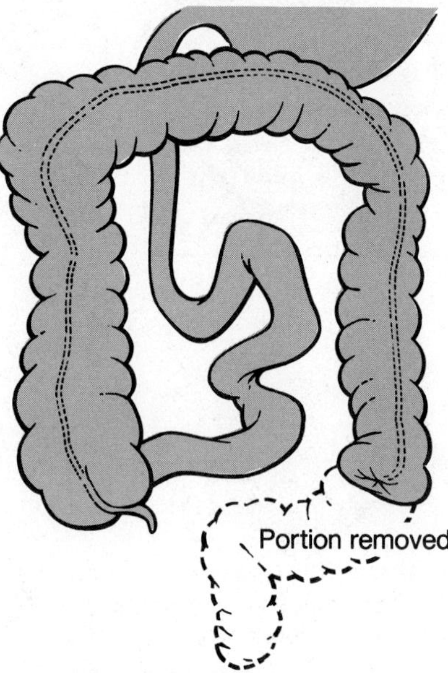

Effluent Characteristics
- Semiformed to formed
- Malodorous
- May irrigate
- Frequency of drainage: once or twice every 24 hr may be predictable

Equipment Recommended
- Closed end; disposable if regulated with removal not more than once or twice daily
- Stoma cap or gauze pad if regulated
- Disposable; drainable if not regulated (required emptying when 1/3 full)

FIGURE 80–7 Stoma equipment needed on the basis type of procedure and the characteristics of the effluent (output).

gravitate to the waistline, pulling the faceplate to the stoma, harming tissue, and perhaps lacerating the stoma. They can cause skin irritation if they are too tight. Paraplegics and quadraplegics need special attention to this potential problem. "Picture framing," applying one strip of tape to all four edges of the pouch where it attaches to the body, is a method of support which distributes the weight of the pouch and enhances the seal.

Nursing Management

Preoperative Interventions

Preoperative preparation is ideally given to the patient several days before surgery except when an accident or other emergency necessitates immediate treatment. In an emergency situation, preoperative teaching is kept to a minimum in order not to overload the patient and increase anxiety. The teaching would be part of the postoperative management.

When the procedure is scheduled as elective surgery, preoperative teaching can be of benefit to the patient and the family. The enterostomal therapy (ET) nurse needs to be consulted. Enterostomal therapy is a nursing specialty devoted to the rehabilitation of people with stomas. Preoperative preparation includes assessing the patient's knowledge base. The nurse determines the patient and family expectations from surgery, and understanding of the diagnosis. The nurse can clarify misconceptions and terms by asking such questions as: "What does this mean to you?" "What is your understanding of this?" "Have you known anyone with a stoma?" The information that must be clearly explained is gastrointestinal (or urinary) tract function and how a stoma alters the structure. It is best to use basic pamphlets and diagrams to demonstrate points. The explanation includes the appropriate size, color, location of the stoma, and the type of drainage to expect after surgery. The patient may be shown the pouches used to contain the effluent, and the routine care is described. However, it is important to remember that it is common for people to hear only information that is acceptable and to blank out the part that is unacceptable. A limited understanding of medical terminology, a reluctance to ask questions, anxiety, and trying to assimilate too much information at one time interferes with the learning process.

It is desirable to determine current stressors in the patient's life and to discuss the patient's lifestyle before illness and during this illness. This information will be used in helping the patient to learn self-care after surgery and to plan a daily routine. The nurse needs to be aware of the patient's limitations, level of maturity, mental status, learning ability, manual dexterity, and visual acuity. The patient should be encouraged to express fears and anxieties as well as how he or she perceives the surgery affecting lifestyle. In order to plan a teaching approach, the nurse determines if the patient has an easier time learning new information by reading, observing a demonstration, doing a specific task, or one-to-one interaction. Talking to another person with a stoma can be beneficial to some patients, and the United Ostomy Association provides this service with the consent of the patient and physician. Discuss with the patient and family their perceptions of each other's roles in self-care or supportive care. Patients need assistance in developing realistic goals and expectations of their care.

Preoperative physical preparation will include all that is discussed in Chapter 8. In addition, antibiotics are given to decrease the bacterial flora of the bowel and thus minimize the danger of infection because the bowel will be excised. Any other special drains as may be anticipated should be explained.

Marking of the stoma site is necessary because an improperly placed stoma can result in skin irritation, frequent leakage of drainage around the pouch, and frustration to the patient. An enterostomal therapy nurse needs to be consulted preoperatively for marking of the stoma site. Various anatomical factors influence proper stoma placement. The stoma should be placed away from the bony prominences, the umbilicus, waistline, costal margins, creases, folds, incisions, or scars. The stoma should not be proximal to prosthetic equipment, pendulous breasts, existing abdominal hernias, or to other stomas or fistulae. The stoma needs to be visually accessible. On a protuberant abdomen, higher stoma placement is recommended.

Postoperative Care

Following surgery, the stoma is assessed at regular intervals to determine if there is adequate blood supply or if edema is excessive. The color of the stoma is an indication of blood supply. A stoma that is rosé to brick red reflects a viable stoma mucosa. A pale color may indicate anemia. A blanching, dark red to purple color indicates inadequate blood supply to the stoma or bowel. Causative factors may include adhesions, a low flow of blood or excessive tension on the bowel at the time the stoma was constructed. Sustained color changes must be reported to the surgeon.

Mild to moderate edema is considered normal in the initial postoperative period. Moderate to severe edema may be due to a variety of causes, including possible trauma to the stoma, obstruction, food allergy, or gastroenteritis. Bleeding from the stoma must also be assessed. A small amount of oozing from the stoma is normal. However, moderate to extensive bleeding could indicate a coagulation problem and internal gastrointestinal bleeding. Signs of moderate to excessive bleeding must be reported to the physician.

Skin Care. The skin around the stoma is vulnerable to irritation by adhesives or other agents used to secure the pouch to the skin. To avoid skin trauma, remove the pouch by gently pushing down on the skin while pulling up on the pouch. Warm water or a mild solvent made to be used on peristomal skin will allow for easy removal. If a solvent is used, it must be washed from the skin because it can be irritating. The skin needs to be cleansed gently. Rubbing vigorously or using a harsh cleanser is discouraged. A mild, nongreasy soap is preferred. The skin must be rinsed well and patted dry.

Pouch Application. The principles of pouch application include:

1. Measure the stoma. Prepare the skin barrier to fit accurately. The stoma opening in the pouch should be slightly larger than the stoma.
2. The skin should be clean and dry.
3. Change the pouch on a routine basis, before leakage occurs. Approximately every 3 days is appropriate in the immediate postoperative period. Every 5 to 7 days is usually appropriate later one.
4. Try to change the pouch when minimal output is expected (*i.e.,* don't plan a pouch change right after a meal). Change it if burning or itching is present under the pouch.
5. Assess stoma viability, suture and skin integrity.
6. Assess amount of output, color, and consistency.

Intake and Output. Accurate intake and output measurement is important in all types of stoma patients. It is particularly important in ileostomy patients because they are vulnerable to electrolyte imbalance. The collection device needs to be checked frequently for the type and amount of output. Emptying the pouch when it is ⅓ full or if it is inflated with gas is an important step to prevent leakage from a heavy pouch.

Care of the Perineal Wound. When a person has an abdominal perineal resection, the anus, rectum, and the lower colon are removed through the perineal wound. This wound will heal by primary or secondary intention. If there is extensive infection it will be left open to heal by secondary intention. The nursing care will involve dressing changes, wound irrigations, and sitz baths. If the perineum is partially closed with the insertion of Penrose drains, there will be drainage. Dressings are changed frequently to prevent odor and discomfort, and to maintain asepsis. If the perineum is completely closed, catheters are placed in the pelvic cavity and brought out to the skin through stab wounds on each side of the closed perineal wound. These catheters are removed several days postoperatively. The perineal wound is frequently a source of discomfort. The patient may feel like he wants to evacuate and he finds sitting uncomfortable. Providing a soft cushion will add to his comfort.[3]

Patient Teaching. Teaching a patient self-care is a gradual process that needs to start with brief explanations of routine care. Involvement of the patient is dependent on physical and emotional readiness. It is important that the nurse have an accepting attitude and not show disgust or be repulsed by the stoma or drainage. If the patient senses rejection it affects adjustment to the situation. Proper use of the stoma equipment is important to the physical and emotional well-being of the patient. In order for the patient to learn, adequate time must be provided free from interruptions and with assurance of privacy. Teaching and discharge planning need to include:

1. A knowledge of anatomical and physiological alterations and how this relates to daily living
2. Management of drainage and the appliance
3. Care of the stoma and peristomal skin
4. Care of the incision and perineal wound
5. Medication precautions required because of absorption and elimination change
6. Nutritional requirements
7. Odor control
8. Sexual implications
9. Clothing
10. Activities including travel
11. Signs and symptoms requiring medical attention[3]

See Table 80–7 as a guideline for teaching the stoma patient.

Colostomy Irrigation

There is some controversy regarding colostomy irrigation. Some enterostomal therapy nurses and physicians feel it contributes to a person's adjustment, while others feel it is unnecessary and unnatural. If the patient will be managing his colostomy with irrigation, he needs to be instructed and to be able to do return demonstrations before discharge or be followed closely as an outpatient if he learns irrigation after discharge.

Use of a stoma cone or soft catheter with a dam minimizes the danger of perforation by the catheter (Fig. 80–8). Safety precautions that patients need to know are to never force a catheter into a stoma or insert it more than 2 to 3 inches, and to never use a hard plastic catheter or lubricate a catheter with Vaseline, as this hardens plastic (water-soluble lubricant is recommended). The amount of solution recommended is 500 ml to 1000 ml of tepid water instilled over 5 to 10 minutes. Using more than 1000 ml of water is discouraged unless the patient's bowel is being prepared for colostomy closure. Instruct the patient to irrigate approximately the same time every day or every other day if he is trying to gain control with irrigation. Have the patient sit on a padded chair in front of the toilet if there is a tender perineal wound or if the patient is unable to tolerate sitting on the toilet for several minutes.

Loss of control or spillage between irrigations can occur if the patient becomes emotionally upset or has a change in dietary habit. Other contributing factors are improper irrigation technique or a parastomal hernia. If loss of control or diarrhea occurs, a drainable pouch needs to be applied. Irrigating needs to be temporarily discontinued if diarrhea occurs. Constipation can become a problem if the patient is on frequent doses of medication that contribute to this problem (*e.g.*, codeine, iron, or antidepresssants). Increasing dietary roughage, fluid intake, and exercise can be helpful in preventing constipation. A mild laxative and stool softener combination can be a short-term solution.

Patients become alarmed if no fluid returns after irrigating. This can happen occasionally if they are dehydrated. If fluid backs up in the tubing during irrigation, it could mean one of several things. The abdominal muscles may be tense; have the patient relax and take slow, deep breaths. Impaction is a possibility, or maybe the regulator controlling the flow of irrigation fluid needs to be opened more. If elimination of stool occurs several times throughout the day on a regular basis, it is probably a waste of time to irrigate. However, irrigation techniques need to be evaluated by an enterostomal therapy nurse before discontinuing this procedure.

Psychological Support

Psychological support of the patient with a stoma is essential. Many patients feel mutilated and are emotionally traumatized by facing a change in elimination. They need a safe, nonjudgmental environment to express feelings and emotions openly. The reason for surgery influences people's reactions and adjustment. If the stoma is temporary, the person was probably not well prepared because of the emergent nature. The patient will frequently focus on the fact that the stoma is temporary when faced with learning self-care. If the person was ill for a number of years with colitis, it is frequently a relief to be free of the discomfort associated with the disease. If the patient is faced with the diagnosis of cancer, the initial concern of a threat of life frequently overshadows concerns of having a stoma. It is not uncommon for the patient to experience feelings of depression, anger, grief, fear, resentment, or rejection. If these feelings aren't resolved after a period of time, professional help may be necessary.

Defense mechanisms can be used as an adjustment technique. Those frequently seen in stoma patients are repression, regression, and displacement. Repression is demonstrated by the patient forgetting things that make him uncomfortable. Repetition regarding the details of self-care is required. In regression, a patient frequently returns to earlier behavior patterns, may become dependent, and either refuses or is unable to appropriately assume self-care within a reasonable time. Displacement occurs when the patient vents anger towards others rather than on the actual problem.[11]

A large percentage of patients react negatively when they initially see their stoma. They need an explanation and reassurance regarding the appearance. Patients should not be forced to look at their stoma. When they are emotionally ready, they will become involved with their care and be able to look at their stoma.

The response of close family members to the stoma is an important factor in a patient's adjustment. Family members need to be informed and to receive special attention in order to be supportive. The first year is a period of extensive adjust-

TABLE 80–7
Health Care Maintenance of the Stoma Patient

Potential Problems	*Contributing Factors*	*Prevention*	*Management*
Care Common to the Patient with an Ileostomy or Colostomy			
Gas	Air swallowing, omission of meals, ingested food or beverage that produces gas (*e.g.*, food from the cabbage family, dried beans, dairy products, carbonated beverages, beer, apple juice, and onions).	Avoid or reduce consumption of foods that cause gas. Avoid skipping meals.	Release gas from the pouch opening.
Odor	Poor hygiene. Food that produces odor (*e.g.*, onions, fish, cabbage, and spices).	Change pouch regularly. Clean the end of the pouch after emptying. Use of pouch or oral deodorants. Use of an odor-proof pouch.	Dispose of reusable equipment if odor is present after thorough cleansing. Ventilate area well during pouch change or when emptying. Use a room deodorant.
Care Specific to a Patient with a Sigmoid or Descending Colostomy			
Constipation	Certain medications (*e.g.*, narcotics, iron). Eating habits (*e.g.*, not enough roughage in diet or inadequate fluid intake). Inadequate physical activity.	Ingest food with bulk-forming properties (*e.g.*, fruit, vegetables, bran). Take at least 8 glasses of fluids per day. Increase activity level.	Determine contributing factors. Take prescribed medication.
Care Specific to a Patient with an Ileostomy or Ascending Colostomy or Right Transverse Colostomy			
Obstruction *Note:* Symptoms could be any of the following: ▪ Thin liquid discharge ▪ Constant output ▪ Foul odor ▪ Cramping ▪ Distended abdomen ▪ Vomiting ▪ No ileostomy output ▪ Stoma edema	Inability of the skin around the stoma to stretch. Small aperture through the abdominal wall. Inability to chew food well (*e.g.*, edentulous). Ingestion of high-roughage foods without adequate chopping or without adequate fluid intake.	Eat the following with discretion in terms of amounts per meal and chew thoroughly: coconut, nuts, popcorn, celery, dried fruit, seeds, and other high-roughage food.	Contact a physician. Take prescribed pain medication (parenteral recommended). Nasogastric suction. Use of stoma lavage by a trained person. (30–50 ml of normal saline is instilled with a catheter and syringe with fluid returning before adding more.) Remove faceplate (stoma edema could result in a lacerated stoma if the faceplate isn't removed). Lie down or get into a knee–chest position. *Note:* Some obstructions resolve spontaneously.
▪ Fluid and electrolyte depletion (K, Na) *Note:* Because the colon has been removed, absorption of fluids and electrolytes may be reduced	High output without adequate replacement of fluids and electrolytes.	Take adequate fluids, especially during increased fluid loss (*e.g.*, diarrhea and diaphoresis). Take fluids that replace electrolyte loss (*e.g.*, Orange Crush, bouillon, and tea). Know signs of fluid depletion: marked thirst, decreased urinary output, fatigue, dry skin and mucous membranes.	Contract a physician if high output doesn't resolve within a few hours. Intravenous fluids.

(*Continued*)

TABLE 80–7
Health Care Maintenance of the Stoma Patient *(Continued)*

Potential Problems	*Contributing Factors*	*Prevention*	*Management*
Care Specific to a Patient with an Ileostomy or Ascending Colostomy or Right Transverse Colostomy			
Medication problems (patient with ileostomy)		Avoid sustained-release medications. They are unreliable for the person with an ileostomy. Never take laxatives or irrigate the stoma. Use only potassium-retaining types of diuretics. Return to clinic for vitamin B_{12} injections about every 3 months if terminal ileum has been removed. Check with the physician. Do not use stool softeners; they are unnecessary.	
Diarrhea *Note:* Know proper definition of diarrhea in relationship to anatomical location of the stoma.	Ingestion of contaminated food or beverage. Ingestion of antacids or other medicine. Impaction (sigmoid or descending colostomy). Irradiated bowel. Emotional upset. Ingestion of food with laxative properties. Chemotherapy.	Be aware of medications, foods, or beverages that have laxative properties. Prevent impaction by preventing constipation. (See prevention of constipation.)	Take prescribed drugs. Eat applesauce, bananas, boiled milk, or rice to thicken stool. Increase fluid intake with sodium and potassium (*e.g.*, broth, Orange Crush, tea).[17]

(Brubacher L, Beard P: A helpful new handout for your ostomy patients. RN, p 36–37, August 1983)

ment to physical concerns such as fear of sounds, odor, leakage, and fears regarding close relationships and society. They need encouragement to return to normal function and expand their lives as they recover.

Sexuality

Some people are concerned that their sexual function may be altered after stoma surgery. Health-care professionals need guidelines and appropriate methods of counseling patients regarding sexual concerns. The nurse needs to know what sexual problems may be present because of the surgery and what can be suggested to the couple to help them to cope with these problems. It is important to keep up to date on this knowledge through reading current literature and attendance at workshops and seminars. The nurse needs to be aware of her feelings, values, and predjudices relative to sex. It is sometimes helpful to arrange for a meeting between a sexually active person who has had stoma surgery and the patient who is to have stomal surgery so they can talk. The United Ostomy Association has booklets available on the topics of "Sex, Courtship and the Single Ostomate," "Sex and the Male Ostomate," and "Sex and the Female Ostomate." Sexual problems may be attributable to preexisting conditions. Patients should be advised to regain physical strength before expecting optimal sexual function. Medications such as certain types of antidepressants, antihypertensives, tranquilizers, and antihistamines contribute to sexual problems in some people. Antispasmodics sometimes interfere with orgasm in female patients. Excessive alcohol consumption can interfere with sexual function as well.

Pregnancy

During pregnancy the stoma may become larger at the base because of the increased size of the abdomen. The increased size of the stoma and configuration of the abdomen usually requires a change in the type of equipment from a reusable pouch to a disposable pouch. The stoma may elongate and have an increased tendency to bleed because of the increased pressure from the fetus, resulting in decreased venous return.

Complications

Obstruction can be caused by adhesions or food blockage. Food blockage is more common in the ileostomy

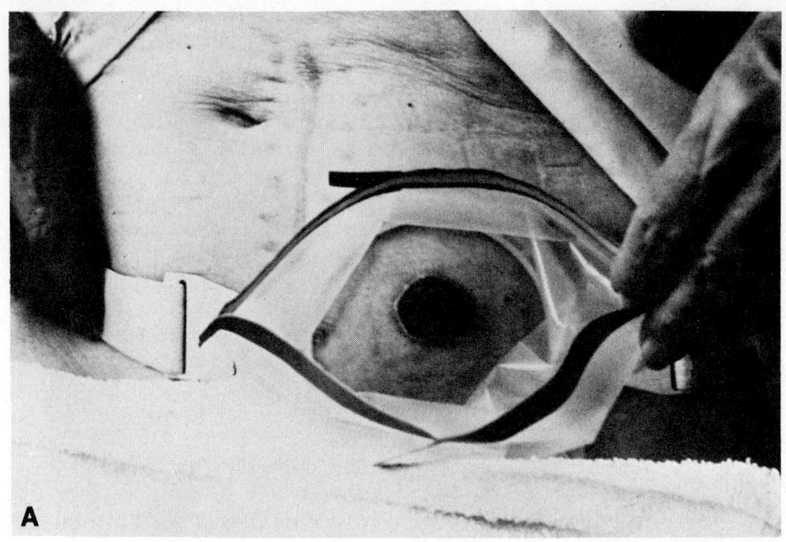

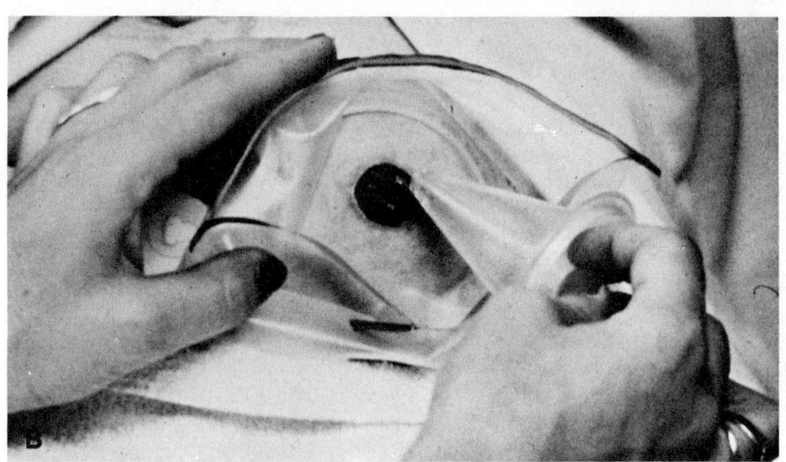

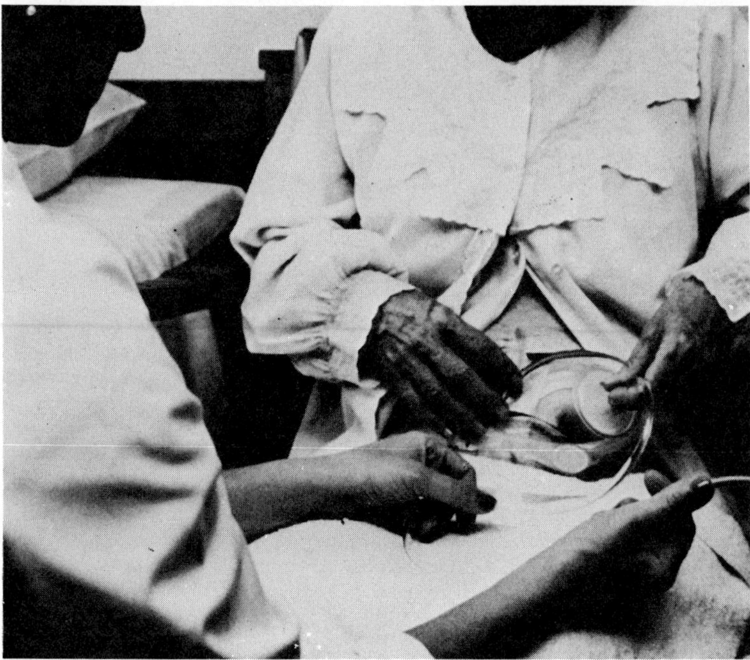

FIGURE 80–8 (*A*) The patient has a plastic irrigating sleeve secured with a belt around the exposed colostomy stoma. (*B*) The lubricated cone is gently introduced into the stoma at an angle so that it follows the natural path of the colon. (*C*) The patient holds the cone firmly as the nurse opens the flow-control clamp, which allows the irrigating solution to enter the colon.

patient. Symptoms of blockage include a change in discharge from semi-solid to thin liquid, foul odor, cramping, abdominal distention, and vomiting. Always check the stoma for edema if obstruction is present. Application of a disposable pouch with the proper stoma opening can prevent constriction from the pouch.

Wound infection is a common complication of colon surgery. Adequate preoperative preparation, meticulous surgical technique, and adequate drainage contribute to infection-free wounds. It is also important to have a well-secured pouch so that the incision is not contaminated with leakage of drainage. Wound infection may be treated by incision and drainage, parenteral antibiotics, local moist heat, and wet-to-dry dressings.[3]

Retraction of the stoma can create a problem in obtaining an adequate seal from the pouch. Retraction can occur from "scar tissue formation around the stoma with shrinkage of the fascial supportive structures that pulls the stoma inward."[3]

Prolapse (protrusion) of the stoma through the abdominal wall occurs in the presence of weak abdominal muscles or if there is inadequate surgical securing of the supportive structures of the stoma. A prolapsed stoma must be carefully reduced by a physician. Following reduction, the patient should lie flat and replace reusable stoma equipment with a temporary disposable pouch. The color of the stoma must be observed closely because there is a risk of impaired circulation.

Stenosis is a narrowing of the stoma lumen. This can result from scar tissue at the junction of the stoma mucosa and the skin. If stenosis causes symptoms of obstruction, surgical correction is indicated.

Parastomal hernias occur more frequently in patients with sudden weight gain, wound infection, or if the stoma is surgically created outside the rectus muscle. When parastomal hernias occur there can be a problem with the pouch fitting properly. The patient needs to be evaluated by a surgeon for possible repair.

Peristomal skin breakdown can be associated with one or more of the following factors:

1. Injury from the effluent because of excessive amount, loose consistency, and irritant composition
2. Medications
3. Underlying disease and treatment
4. Surgical construction and location of the stoma
5. Inadequate skill of those caring for the patient
6. Lack of interest of the patient in self-care
7. Nonavailability of proper supplies.[3]

Products used to prevent or treat skin breakdown include skin barriers, stomahesive and karaya powder, and skin sealants.

References

1. Bernard M, Forlaw L: Complications and their prevention. In Rombeau JL, Caldwell M (eds): Clinical Nutrition, vol 1, Enteral and Tube Feeding, Chap 29, p 542–569. Philadelphia, WB Saunders, 1984
2. Brazeau P: Dietary management of morbidly obese patients who undergo gastroplasty. Can J Surg 27:132, 1984
3. Broadwell D, Jackson B: Principles of Ostomy Care, chap 20, 25. St. Louis, CV Mosby, 1982
4. Colanch PH: Relaxation training for control of nausea and vomiting in patients receiving chemotherapy. Cancer Nursing 6:277–283, 1983
5. Feighner JP, Robins E, Guze SB, Woodruff RA Jr, Winokeer G, Munoz R: Diagnostic criteria for use in psychiatric research. Arch Gen Psychiatry 26:57–63, 1972
6. Freeman JB, Burchett H: Failure rate with gastric partitioning for morbid obesity. Am J Surg 145:113–118, 1983
7. Grinker J, et al: Taste sensitivity and susceptibility to external influence in obese and normal weight subjects. J Pers Soc Psychol 22:320, 1972
8. Konstantinides N, Shronts E: Tube feeding: Managing the basics. Am J Nurs 9:1312–1318, 1983
9. Linner JH: Surgery for Morbid Obesity, New York, Springer-Verlag, 1984
10. Lytle LD: Contorl of eating behavior. In Wurtman RJ, Wurtman JJ (eds): Nutrition and the Brain, vol 2. New York, Raven Press, 1977
11. Mahoney J: A Guide to Ostomy Nursing Care, p 91. Boston, Little, Brown & Co, 1976
12. Moghissi K, Boore JRP: Parenteral and Enteral Nutrition for Nurses. Rockville MD, ASPEN, 1983
13. Rombeau JL, Jacobs DO: Nasoenteric tube feeding. In Rombeau JL, Caldwell M (eds): Clinical Nutrition, vol 1, Enteral and Tube Feeding, chap 16, p 261–274. Philadelphia, WB Saunders, 1984
14. Rosman BL, Minuchin S, Baker L, Liebman R: A family approach to anorexia nervosa: Study, treatment, and outcome. In Vigersky RA (ed): Anorexia Nervosa, p 341–348. New York, Raven Press, 1977
15. Shipes E, Lehr S: Sexual Counseling for Ostomates, p 86. Springfield, Charles C Thomas, 1980
16. Stunkard AF: Behavioral treatments of obesity: Failure to maintain weight loss. In Stuart RB (ed): Behavioral Self-Management, Strategies, Techniques, and Outcomes. New York, Brunner/Mazel, 1977
17. Szmukler GI: Drug treatment of anorexic states. In Silverstone T (ed): Drugs and Appetite. New York, Academic Press, 1982
18. Walike BC, Walike JC, Hanson RL: Nasogastric tube feeding: Clinical complications and current progress of reserach. Health Team 2:33–35, 1975

Bibliography

Broadwell D: Sorrells Summary of Your Ileostomy Care, p 18–19. Bard Consumer Products Div, 1976

Brubacher L, Beard P: A helpful new handout for your ostomy patientes. RN 34–37, August 1983

Del Rio D, Williams K, Esvelt B: Handbook of Enteral Nutrition: A Practical Guide to Tube Feeding. El Segundo, CA, Medical Specifics Publishing, 1982

Freeman JB: First Canadian symposium on the surgical treatment of morbid obesity: Part I: Overview. Can J Surg 27:119–120, 1984

Lenneberg E, Mendelssohn A: Colostomies, A Guide, p 23. United Ostomy Association, Inc., 1974

Michener WM: Special problems of the adolescent: Abdominal pain, growth, anorexia. In Farmer RG, Achkar E, Fleshler B (eds): Clinical Gastroenterology. New York, Raven Press, 1983

Schuster MM: Constipation. In Bayless T (ed): Current Therapy in Gastroenterology and Liver Disease: 1984–1985. St. Louis, CV Mosby, 1984

Chapter 81

Neoplastic and Degenerative Gastrointestinal Disorders

Christine E. Reheis

For most people a diagnosis of cancer carries with it the connotation of a slow, painful, gradually debilitating progression to death. Unfortunately, in some situations this is an accurate interpretation. However, in other situations it is an erroneous impression. The prognosis, course, and treatment of malignancies that occur in different parts of the gastrointestinal tract are discussed in this chapter. The nurse will need this information in working as a member of the health care team and in developing individualized plans for the nursing management of patients.

Cancer at various sites along the gastrointestinal trace has some commonalities. Common nursing problems relate to the perceived significance of the diagnosis; the pain associated with increasing tumor size and pressure on surrounding tissues; nutritional deficits accompanying problems of ingestion, digestion, absorption, or metabolism of nutrients; weakness and physiological changes associated with surgical intervention; and education about the disease, its treatment, and its long-term management.

Potential nursing diagnoses are fear and anxiety related to the life-threatening nature of the disease, and the unknowns about the treatment; discomfort related to the disease process and treatment; alteration in nutritional intake related to disease process; and knowledge deficits about the disease and its management. Many of these diagnoses are discussed extensively in preceding sections of the text (Chapters 8, 9, 19, and 80). Therefore, these nursing diagnoses are acknowledged in this chapter but not discussed in detail except for the distinctive features pertinent to nursing management of patients with specific types of disorders.

Cancer of the Mouth

Cancer of the Lip

Definition and Etiology

The lip is the most common site of cancer of the oral cavity. Ninety to ninety-five percent of lip malignancies are located on the lower lip.[40] The most common type of lip cancer is squamous cell carcinoma. The highest incidence occurs between the ages of 55 and 65. It occurs more frequently in men than in women. Carcinoma of the lip is most often seen in white male smokers with fair or ruddy complexions, light hair, and gray or blue eyes. It is rare in blacks, being up to 10 times more common in whites.[41] In the United States, it is more common in the southern states than the northern.

Prolonged exposure to solar radiation has been implicated as a major factor in the development of carcinoma of the lip. This disease is commonly seen in persons with outdoor occupations who have heavy exposure to the sun.

Cigarette and pipe smoking is associated with a high incidence of lip cancer. It is believed that the direct inhalation of tobacco smoke and the chronic lip irritation generated within the cigarette or pipe from the high temperatures of the smoke may be causative factors.

Lip irritation may also occur from dentures that do not fit, sharp, jagged teeth, and chronically infected gingiva. Lack or absence of dental hygiene is frequently seen in patients with carcinoma of the lip.[40]

Generally, squamous cell carcinomas of the lower lip are well-differentiated and the incidence of metastases is low (less than 10%). When metastases occur, the disease progresses in an orderly fashion. Local and regional metastases of lip cancer occur in the submental and submaxillary lymph nodes. With more advanced cases, metastases can occur in the jugular, carotid, and supraclavicular areas. With further tumor enlargement, mandibular involvement may occur, and bone erosion becomes apparent on x-ray.[4]

Clinical Manifestations

Early symptoms of cancer of the lip include the presence of a blister or induration that arises in an area of leukoplakia. History of a recurrent, nonhealing lip sore that repeatedly forms a dry crust and bleeds on removal is characteristic of lip carcinoma. The crusting may exist for many years before infiltration develops. Most lip carcinomas remain localized as papillary or ulcerative lesions for long periods of time. Gradually, these tumors increase in size.

As carcinoma of the lip advances and extension of tumor into the skin of the lip is seen, secondary infection and necrosis develop. The tumor becomes ulcerated, tender, and swollen. It is surrounded by erythema, and purulent exudate forms in the center. In the presence of infection, pain and tenderness are common.

Medical Management

Diagnosis. Clinical examination of the primary lesion includes palpation of the tumor with two fingers to determine its infiltration and extension. Punch biopsy of the lesion with subsequent histologic examination will help to differentiate benign lip lesions from malignant carcinomas.

Palpation of the submental, submaxillary, and cervical lymph nodes is carried out to determine the presence of metastases. Normal cervical lymph nodes are generally soft, flat, mobile, and less than 1 cm in size. Metastatic cervical lymph nodes are readily detected once they grow beyond 1 cm in diameter. They are hard, and either oval or round.[44]

Treatment. Two treatment modalities for cancer of the lip currently exist: surgery and interstitial or transcutaneous radiation therapy. The specific treatment that is chosen is tailored to cell grade, tumor location, and the presence or absence of metastatic lymph nodes.

Small carcinomas of the lip may be treated with either surgery or external beam radiotherapy, with equally acceptable prognostic, cosmetic, and functional results.[11] Surgery is the preferred treatment for extensive cancer involving the mandible, or for cancer associated with significant soft tissue loss which will necessitate major reconstruction after the tumor is controlled by radiation therapy. Surgery is also indicated when radiation treatment fails. For any lip tumor with metastases to lymph nodes, the treatment of choice is surgery combined with radiotherapy. A radical neck dissection (including possible removal of the periosteum or a cortical margin of the mandible) combined with adjuvant radiation therapy is performed in the presence of palpable cervical lymph node metastases. Prophylactic or elective neck dissection or radiation in the absence of clinically palpable lymph nodes is not indicated for patients with lip cancer[16] because there is a low frequency rate of regional metastases.

Prognosis. Cancer of the lip has one of the highest cure rates of all head and neck cancers. The prominent location of the tumor allows the individual to detect it and presumably seek treatment at an early stage. The 5-year survival rates for patients treated for lower lip cancer are greater than 90% when no cervical metastases are present. When cervical metastases are present, the prognosis is reduced, with a 5-year survival rate of 45% to 50%.

Cancer of the Tongue

Definition and Etiology

With regard to cancer biology and behavior, the tongue may be divided into two distinct parts: the oral anterior (mobile) two thirds, and the posterior one third or base. Cancers of the anterior tongue are considered to be oral cavity malignancies. Cancers of the posterior tongue are considered malignancies of the oropharynx.

In the United States, cancers of the tongue represent approximately 1% to 1.6% of all malignancies. By contrast, in India cancers of the tongue are responsible for 30% to 47% of all malignancies.[21] Of all head and neck diseases, cancers of the tongue cause the greatest number of deaths among Americans.[38] With the exception of carcinoma of the lip, carcinoma of the tongue is the most common oral malignancy.

More than 95% of the malignancies developing in the tongue are squamous cell carcinomas. The remaining 5% consist of tumors of minor salivary glands, undifferentiated carcinomas, or sarcomas. Most cancers of the tongue (75%) arise in the anterior two thirds.

Carcinoma of the tongue occurs most commonly in the middle to the later decades of life. The highest incidence occurs in the sixth decade. The disease is predominantly one of men; however, the incidence is steadily increasing among women.[29]

The use of tobacco in one form or another is probably the most important single etiologic factor for cancer of the tongue. Other factors include irritation of the tongue from jagged teeth, use of spices and hot foods, avitaminosis, alcoholism, cirrhosis of the liver, syphilis, and chemical poisoning. Betel-nut chewing is believed to be directly related to the high incidence of carcinoma of the tongue in India and Asia.[21]

Pathophysiology

Carcinoma of the tongue may be papillary (exophytic) or infiltrative. These two types of tumors differ both in behavior and histology. The exophytic tumors are usually more differentiated, not infiltrative, and less likely to immediately metastasize to cervical lymph nodes. The infiltrative tumors are usually more anaplastic and undifferentiated; they spread rapidly through the musculature of the tongue, and metastasize early to the cervical lymph nodes or to distant sites. Infiltrative tumors also recur frequently.[29]

Because the tongue is endowed with a rich supply of lymphatics, squamous cell carcinoma is often found to have metastasized to lymph nodes by the time diagnosis is made. Tumors originating from the anterior portion of the oral tongue usually metastasize to the submandibular and midjugular lymph nodes. Tumors arising from the posterior portion of the oral tongue often metastasize to the subdigastric and upper jugular lymph nodes.[41] Carcinomas of both the oral tongue and the base of the tongue can spread to the floor of the mouth, producing total fixation of the tongue.

Clinical Manifestations

During the early stages, symptoms of carcinoma of the tongue may be negligible. Lesions present on the oral tongue may be indurated, nontender ulcers. Patients may complain of irritation or a canker sore, and they rarely seek medical attention. As the tumor enlarges, pain develops. Pain is referred through the lingual and auriculotemporal nerves directly to the external auditory meatus and to the temporomandibular joint. Lumps in the neck, bleeding, dysphagia, odynophagia, otalgia, and fixation of the tongue with resultant slurring of speech are late signs and symptoms indicating advanced carcinoma of the oral tongue.

Carcinoma arising in the base of the tongue is often asymptomatic. As a result, early diagnosis of tumors at this site is rare. Moderately advanced tumors of the base of the tongue may be accompanied by pain and unilateral sore throat. Odynophagia, dysphagia, otalgia, hemorrhage, and "hot potato" voice may be associated with large tumors in this area. Often, the only presenting symptom of this disease is a neck mass.[41]

Medical Management

Diagnosis. Clinical inspection of the tongue may uncover the presence of any suspicious lesions. The base of the tongue cannot be easily seen or examine with a tongue depressor. Therefore, a laryngoscopic examination is important in diagnosing carcinomas of the base of the tongue. This examination is also useful for tumor mapping and biopsy to establish the extent and nature of the tumor before treatment is instituted.

Careful palpation of the base of the tongue may uncover the presence of tumor that may not be apparent visually. It may also help to evaluate the extent of the disease. Because of the high frequency of cervical lymph node metastases at diagnosis, careful palpation of lymph nodes is essential.

Biopsy of any suspicious lesions found on the tongue is important in establishing a definitive diagnosis of cancer. Lateral xerograms of the base of the tongue and hypopharynx may be useful in revealing the fissure-like formation of an infiltrative tumor.[41]

Treatment. Radiation therapy and surgery are treatments of choice for the management of carcinoma of the tongue. Treatment choices are currently based on tumor size, location, histologic grading, and the presence or absence of cervical lymph node metastases.

Small cancers of the oral tongue can be effectively controlled by either surgery or radiotherapy. Moderately advanced, medium-sized tumors involving the adjacent floor of the mouth may be treated surgically with partial glossectomy, partial mandibulectomy, and radical neck dissection. Treatment of advanced (greater than 4 cm) oral tongue cancers with deep muscular invasion is combined surgery and radiation therapy.

When radiation therapy is employed for treatment of carcinoma of the oral tongue, it is accomplished by means of comprehensive external beam therapy to the primary site and first echelon lymph nodes. The primary tumor then receives boost radiation either by interstitial implant or intraoral cone electron beam therapy. For advanced disease, interstitial implantation or intraoral cone therapy is ineffective. As a result, external beam therapy is employed exclusively in combination with surgery. With the exception of small, exophytic, mucosal lesions, treatment of carcinoma of the oral tongue must include treatment of regional lymph nodes because of the high incidence of metastases.[41]

The necessary surgical treatment for carcinoma of the base of the tongue usually includes excision of the entire tongue (total glossectomy) and laryngectomy. In addition to the mutilation and functional deformity caused by such primary surgery, marginal disease recurrent at the primary site and nodal neck disease may often occur following surgery. As a result, radiotherapy may be favored as the primary treatment of choice. Radiotherapy may also be used in combination with surgery, or with surgery and chemotherapy.[13]

Prognosis. Prognosis of *carcinoma of the oral tongue* varies depending upon tumor size and the presence of regional metastases. For small (less than 2 cm), well-differentiated oral tongue tumors without evidence of metastases, the 5-year survival rate has been reported as high as 85%. For larger tumors (greater than 4 cm) with cervical lymph node metastases, the survival rate decreases to approximately 25%.[10]

Patients with *carcinoma of the base of the tongue* have very poor survival rates. Small, early tumors of the base of the tongue are uncommon. Often, by the time diagnosis is made, occult disease has spread beyond the palpable limits of the tumor, neck lymph node metastasis has occurred (often bilaterally), and a relatively high incidence of distant metastases is also present.

Nursing Management

Nursing Diagnosis

Nursing diagnoses for patients with cancer of the lip or tongue facing surgery, radiation therapy, or both, are as follows: debilitated nutritional state related to the local or systemic effects of the cancer or the side-effects imposed by surgery or radiation therapy; potential for oral infection; alteration in comfort (pain); potential for inadequate healing related to nutritional deficits and alterations in oral mucosa; potential for complications arising from treatments or the presence of tumor (*e.g.*, xerostomia or excessive salivation and difficulty in maintenance of a patent oral airway); impairment communication; patient fears and concerns about the diagnosis and treatment; and knowledge deficit regarding the disease process, treatment options, and discharge instructions.

Nursing care may be very complex depending on the location of the lesion, the extent of the disease, the type of treatment employed, and the patient/family response to the problem. The nurse must consider the educational needs of the patient and family, psychological support of both patient and family, preparation of the patient for the treatment(s), and care of the patient during the following treatment, including management of treatment side-effects or any complications that arise following treatment. Nursing care will also include an evaluation of the patient's rehabilitative needs and referral to appropriate nursing and other rehabilitative community resources. All nursing care plans must be individualized to the particular patient/family.

Goals. The goals of nursing management are to promote adequate nutritional intake to maintain body needs and achieve wound healing; to prevent oral infection; to alleviate discomfort; to prevent interference with oral airway; to maintain communication; to alleviate fear; to teach the patient and family self care to prevent infection and promote healing; and to assist the patient to cope with a new body image if necessary.

Interventions

Nutritional Support. Careful attention must be directed toward the nutritional needs of the patient before, during, and following therapy. The location, size, or discomfort caused by the tumor may interfere with the patient's ability to ingest a nutritionally balanced diet, as may the side-effects imposed by surgery or radiation therapy. This may be reflected in weight loss, poor wound healing, and a generally debilitated condition.

It is important to assess the patient's limitations in eating and swallowing (local and systemic). For the patient whose oral intake is limited by the physical presence of the tumor, the use of plastic straws or children's feeding utensils may be helpful. Foods should be soft or liquid to facilitate eating.

Small, frequent, attractive meals of favorite foods may be less likely to overwhelm the patient and promote intake. The smell of foods is important, as is the temperature and extent of seasoning. Providing oral care prior to meals to remove any oral odors, debris, or bad tastes that exist may also encourage the patient to eat. The patient who is unable to eat by mouth may need to be fed by nasogastric tube or parenteral nutrition (Chapter 80).

Oral Care. In addition to facilitating eating, meticulous oral care is important preceding and following surgery and radiation therapy. The mouth must be kept clean to reduce the chance of infection, promote healing, and increase the patient's self-confidence by helping to reduce or eliminate mouth odor.

The nurse should perform routine oral assessments prior to, during, and following treatment. Such examinations should focus on the condition of the mouth; the condition and color of the oral tissues, including the presence of any swelling, erythema, dryness, or oral lesions; and the condition of the teeth. Any changes that occur during or following treatment should be recorded and reported.

Assuming that there are no contraindications, the patient is encouraged to brush his teeth often with a soft toothbrush. Any dentures that are present should receive frequent care and cleaning. Any irritations caused by dentures should be investigated and corrected; this is especially important if the patient is receiving radiation therapy of the mouth. The combination of tissue changes caused by radiation and friction caused by the dentures may result in painful oral ulcerations that may become infected. Analgesics or topical anesthetics may be prescribed in the presence of oral ulceration resulting from treatment.

Oral irrigations, with solutions such as normal saline that are directed to all parts of the mouth, are encouraged. Irrigations will aid healing, minimize the chance of infections, promote comfort, and help maintain oral cleanliness by loosening and eliminating mucus and necrotic material.

Xerostomia (dryness of the mouth) is an uncomfortable side-effect that often develops when the salivary glands lie within the field of radiation therapy or are affected by surgical treatment. This problem may be counteracted by encouraging the patient to increase his oral fluid intake. He should be cautioned to avoid tobacco, foods, and liquids such as alcohol that will cause further dryness or be irritating to the oral mucosa. The use of lemon glycerin swabs and commercial mouthwashes is discouraged because these products promote further dryness. Salivary flow may be stimulated with chewing gum or lemon drops. The patient may also fine one of the commercially available artificial saliva preparations beneficial. Humidification of a dry environment may also be helpful.

In contrast to those patients experiencing xerostomia, some patients may experience excessive salivation both pre- and postoperatively. Drooling is a problem that some patients must constantly deal with and one that often proves to be very embarrassing. If the condition is a temporary one following surgical treatment and one that is fairly severe, mechanical suction may be used initially by the nurse and later by the patient to routinely remove the secretions. Mild drooling may be aided through administration of anticholinergic drugs and also by teaching the patient to swallow more frequently and carry a supply of mouth wipes at all times. Oral reconstructive surgery may be indicated in cases where drooling is severe.[9]

Maintaining a patent airway is of utmost importance in patients who experience excess salivation, in those who are recovering from surgery in the immediate postoperative period, and in patients with possible obstructive tumors, especially prior to treatment. Immediately following surgery the patient is placed in a supine position with head turned to the side, or in the lateral position, to allow drainage from the mouth. Suctioning is performed with care in the postoperative period, so that suture lines and sensitive oral tissues are not disturbed. If the size and location of the tumor threatens to obstruct the airway, treatment should be initiated as soon as possible, and the patient should be observed closely for any breathing difficulties.

Communication Concerns. Patients who undergo surgery for cancer of the tongue maybe faced with a speech impairment following surgery. The nursing care of such persons requires patience and understanding of the patient's fear and frustration. To facilitate communication, the patient should be provided with paper and a pencil. A referral to speech pathology should be made so that the patient is thoroughly evaluated and appropriate speech training is begun. Finding a person who has undergone similar surgery and rehabilitation to meet with the patient may help provide encouragement and needed incentive. The American Cancer Society may be of service in helping to locate former patients for this purpose.

Emotional Support. In addition to the physical care that is required, patients with cancers of the oral cavity and oropharynx require extensive psychological support and understanding. The patient is likely to be frightened about the diagnosis of cancer and the treatment he faces. He will be concerned with his appearance and the changes that treatment will impose. Other common areas of immediate concern include drooling, fear of pain, and difficulty in communicating, eating, and swallowing.

The nurse must work toward establishing open communication with the patient. A caring and trusting relationship will encourage the patient to express his fears and concerns. In return, the nurse will be able to provide continued guidance, encouragement, and education. She will also work with family members and friends in eliciting their ongoing thoughtful support of the patient.

Health Teaching and Discharge Planning. The patient's need for knowledge will be great. Information that should be discussed with patient and family are the disease and its natural history, options for treatment, and the patient's and family's understanding of the physician's explanation of treatments. These explanations may need to be reinforced or clarified. The patient will have concerns about preparations for therapeutic treatment and will want to know how treatment will physically affect him (including temporary and permanent side-effects). The patient will need to be instructed as to how he may participate in his own care to promote recovery.

The nurse will facilitate patient and family learning by establishing a teaching plan that will be implemented at the time of diagnosis and carried through discharge. Discharge planning and teaching must be thorough and complete for patients who have been treated for cancer of the lip or tongue. An individualized plan for home care should be formulated among the members of the health care team, the patient, and his family. Each member of the team will be responsible for providing detailed information to the patient and family. Such information will include dietary instruction, information about speech therapy and rehabilitation (when appropriate), and instructions on dressing changes and management of excess oral secretion by suctioning (when appropriate).

The nurse is ultimately responsible for reviewing discharge instructions and reinforcing teaching. She should instruct the patient and home care givers about certain potential problems. They should be aware of the signs of hemorage, infection, and airway obstruction, and when to notify the physician. She should provide the patient with information pertaining to his first follow-up medical visit outside the hospital and explain that periodic follow-up examinations are necessary to monitor his progress.

Finally, an assessment should be made of the patient's physical and psychological condition at discharge, the care that is required at home and its complexity, and the ability of the care givers to provide care. Based on this assessment and in conjunction with patient and family wishes, a home health referral may be made. Additionally, referrals to any rehabilitative services that are indicated should be made at this time. Referrals to community agencies will facilitate recovery and readjustment back into the community.

Evaluation

Outcome criteria for goal achievements are as follows:

1. The patient maintains or regains weight to pretreatment level.
2. The oral mucosa is maintained free of infection.
3. The patient reports minimal oral discomfort.
4. A clear oral airway is maintained.
5. The patient expresses a decrease in anxiety.
6. The patient and family discuss feelings and concerns about the diagnosis and outcome of treatment.
7. The patient and family accurately describe and perform oral self-care procedures.
8. The patient and family discuss openly and accurately the disease, treatment, expected outcomes, and potential problems.

Esophageal and Gastrointestinal Cancers

Cancer of the Esophagus

Definition and Etiology

Esophageal cancer has one of the widest geographic variations in incidence of any human cancer. In the United States it represents only 5% of all gastrointestinal cancer, and accounts for 2% of all cancer deaths. In some parts of the world cancer of the esophagus is the leading cause of death. The incidence is highest in the Far East, with a rate of 46.3 per 100,000 men over age 35 in Japan, as compared with 10 per 100,000 in the United States.[33]

From Iran through central Asia to northern China, there is an area of strikingly increased incidence that has been called "the esophageal cancer belt."[36] There has also been an increasing incidence of esophageal cancer in Africa since World War II. Other areas exhibiting high incidences of esophageal cancer include Scotland, the Soviet Union, the Scandinavian countries, Curacao, and coastal South Carolina (primarily among black males).[33]

Pathophysiology

Squamous cell carcinoma accounts for 98% of all esophageal cancers. THe occurrence of squamous cell carcinoma of the esophagus is equally divided between the upper and lower half.

The rich network of lymphatics in submucosal and mucosal layers of the esophagus make early dissemination of esophageal cancers common. Submucosal spread 4 to 5 cm on either side of the primary lesion is not unusual. Involvement of the trachea, left main stem bronchus, recurrent nerves, carotids, and aorta are often observed at the time of diagnosis.[34] Esophgeal tumors may produce severe local symptoms due to mediastinal involvement, pericardial involvement, or the production of tracheoesophageal fistulae.[24]

Spread of disease by way of the bloodstream is common in esophageal malignancies. Liver, lung, and bone are commonly affected. Cervical esophageal tumors often spread through lymphatic channels to anterior jugular and supraclavicular nodes.

Clinical Manifestations

The primary symptom of esophageal cancer is dysphagia. It is present in 90% of patients with the disease. Dysphagia is usually painless, insidious, and slowly progressive. It is initially noted with the ingestion of solid foods. As the esophagus narrows with tumor progression, dysphagia eventually progresses to difficulty in swallowing liquids, including saliva. Weight loss is a related, common clinical finding in most patients. Additional symptoms include malaise and anorexia.[33]

Signs and symptoms of advanced disease are often the initial indicators of esophageal cancer. Complete obstruction of the esophagus by tumor may cause nausea and vomiting either with or without aspiration. Persistent cough may be present secondary to tracheal involvement or presence of tracheoesophageal fistula. Persistent hoarseness may result from extensive mediastinal involvement, resulting in recurrent laryngeal nerve compression. The presence of aortoesophageal fistulae will result in hemoptysis from rapid exsanguinating hemorrhage.

Medical Management

Diagnosis. A useful diagnostic test for detection of cancer of the esophagus is the barium esophagogram. This test will show an abrupt narrowing of the barium column at the tumor site. This visualization is distinctly different from the concentric tapers narrowing seen with benign stricture of the esophagus.

Esophagoscopy and biopsy are used to establish a pathologic diagnosis of esophageal cancer. With the combination of esophageal brushings and multiple biopsies, the diagnosis of squamous cell carcinoma of the esophagus can be made with greater than 90% accuracy.[36]

Treatment. Patients with tumors of the middle and distal one third of the esophagus who do not have metastatic disease or locally advanced tumor into the mediastinum are treated surgically. Patients with carcinoma of the cervical esophagus are not considered candidates for resection because these tumors have commonly already invaded the larynx, trachea, carotid arteries, or spinal column.[24]

The preferred "curative" surgical approach for appropriate surgical candidates is radical esophagectomy with esophagogastrostomy. The surgical technique employs a thoracoabdominal approach, with laparotomy and right-sided thoracotomy. After the diseased portion of the esophagus is removed, esophagogastrostomy involves bringing the stomach into the chest and implanting the proximal end of the esophagus into it. Esophageal resection may be complicated by a number of problems including anastomotic leaks, strictures, wound infection, and complications such as pulmonary insufficiency, pulmonary embolism, and congestive heart failure. Such problems increase morbidity, and may lead to a high incidence of postoperative mortality.[24]

In patients who have advanced disease, extensive local unresectable tumor with obstruction, or complications such as tracheoesophageal fistula, a palliative bypass without resection may be indicated.[34] Palliative treatment of esophageal cancer and its debilitating symptoms such as dysphagia may also be achieved through radiation therapy. Radiation therapy is the treatment of choice for carcinoma of the cervical esophagus since resection of these tumors is rare.

Prognosis. The diagnosis of cancer of the esophagus inherently carries with it a poor prognosis. Considering all patients, the 5-year survival rate varies between 2% and 6% regardless of the treatment modality employed.[15] The delay in diagnosis resulting from a lack of early signs and symptoms of the disease is the single most important reason for the poor survival rates.[34]

Cancer of the Stomach

Definition and Etiology

Adenocarcinoma accounts for more than 97% of all gastric malignancies. More than 50% of gastric adenocarcinomas are located in the pyloric and antral regions. The incidence of gastric carcinoma is highest in Japan, Chile, and Iceland, and has been steadily growing in these countries since 1950. In contrast, the incidence of gastric cancer in the United States has declined by approximately 50% between 1930 and 1975.

A number of environmental factors have been associated with the development of gastric carcinoma, including eating pickled and highly salted or smoked foods, and working in occupations such as coal mining, farming (nitrate fertilizer exposure), nickel refining, lumber, and rubber processing.[34]

Preexisting diseases may influence the development of gastric carcinoma. There is a high incidence of gastric adenocarcinoma (5% to 10%) in patients with pernicious anemia. Although controversy exists about gastric ulcers, they do not appear to be directly associated with gastric carcinoma.[24] However, the occurrence of gastric carcinoma in the gastric remnant many years (15 to 20) following surgery for histologically proven benign peptic ulcer is not uncommon. Bile reflux may play a part in the progressive development of these gastric stump cancers.

Pathophysiology and Clinical Manifestations

Gastric carcinoma can spread along mucusal surfaces and infiltrate the gastric wall, resulting in widespread inflammation, or it can extend outside the stomach to organs such as the omentum, liver, pancreas, and colon. Spread also occurs to nearby lymph nodes and by the blood to the liver.

The early diagnosis of gastric carcinoma is difficult owing to the lack of specific presenting signs and symptoms. Mild upper abdominal discomfort (with or without anorexia and weight loss) which does not respond to typical medical management may represent a possible gastric carcinoma. Similarly, gastric carcinoma should be suspected in persons presenting with ulcer symptoms that do not respond to routine medical treatment, and in the presence of iron deficiency anemia which lacks an obvious cause.[33]

Unfortunately, many gastric cancers do not produce symptoms until the disease has metastasized. Advanced disease may manifest itself with complaints such as early satiety, dysphagia, significant weight loss, ascites, and hepatomegaly.[24]

Medical Management

Diagnosis. Gastroscopy allows the stomach mucosa to be visualized and gastric secretions to be removed and analyzed for malignant cells. Carcinoma must be ruled out if achlorhydria is present. A typical gastric ulcer which does not heal completely as shown by x-ray film in 4 to 6 weeks must be suspected as possibly being malignant.

The upper gastrointestinal (GI) roentgenographic study is the study most commonly used to detect gastric cancer. Upper GI, double-contrast barium studies can determine abnormalities in almost 90% of patients with symptomatic gastric carcinoma. A double-contrast study allows for careful examination of the proximal stomach where malignant lesions might be missed by conventional barium studies.[24]

Treatment. The type of gastric surgery performed depends on the location of the neoplasm in the stomach and the extent of the disease. The procedures consist of wide excision of the cancer site and may include adjacent tissues. The excision may be subtotal or total gastrectomy and may include a portion of the esophagus for cancer of the proximal stomach and a portion of the duodenum for cancer of the distal stomach (see Fig. 81–1). A splenectomy may be required if the gastric lesion directly invades the spleen, and node-bearing tissues may also be excised. The surgical procedure for total gastrectomy is esophagojejunostomy; for partial gastrectomy it is either gastroduodenostomy or gastrojejunostomy. In the presence of high-grade obstruction resulting from gastric tumor, some palliation and re-establishment of enteral feeding may be achieved with a feeding jejunostomy. Palliative bypass procedures do not seem to be of any benefit to patients whose tumors cannot be curatively or palliatively resected.

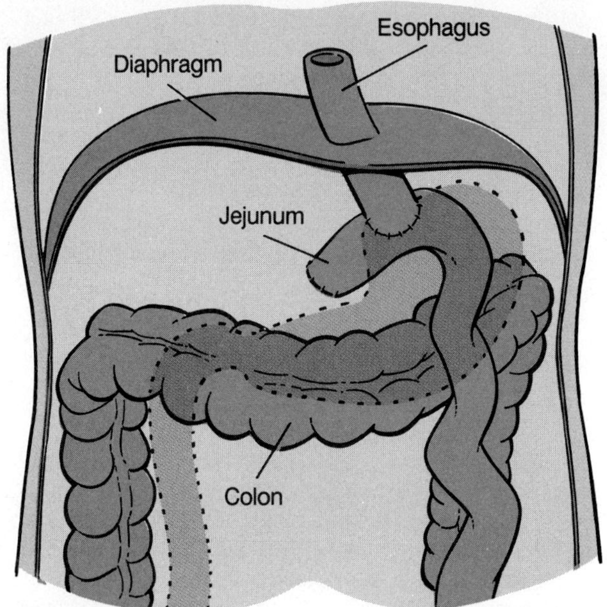

FIGURE 81–1 Total gastrectomy with esophagojejunostomy.

Radiation therapy and chemotherapy have been employed in the treatment of gastric carcinoma with varying results. Radiation therapy does not appear to improve survival in patients with locally residual or recurrent gastric carcinoma. Radiation therapy is, however, useful in the palliation of pain, particularly from bony metastases. Radiation combined with chemotherapy, particularly 5-fluorouracil, appears to be beneficial in patients with locally advanced or recurrent gastric carcinoma.[24]

Prognosis. The overall outlook for patients with gastric cancer is generally poor. The results following gastric resection vary with the amount of gastric involvement and the type of surgery performed. The overall 10-year survival rate for patients who are candidates for "curative" gastric surgery varies between 5% and 25%.[24]

Cancer of the Small Intestine

Definition and Etiology

Tumors of the small intestine comprise approximately 1.5% of all benign and malignant gastrointestinal neoplasms. The most common type is a carcinoma tumor most frequently located in the terminal ileum.[31]

Malignant tumors of the small intestine occur about as frequently in men as in women. These tumors present most commonly in the fifth to sixth decades of life.[31]

The etiology of small bowel tumors is not known. Presumably the large mucosal surface of the small bowel frequently comes in contact with many enteric carcinogenic substances, yet the incidence of primary cancers of the small intestine is very small. The transit time is relatively short as contrasted with the large intestine, where the incidence of cancer is much higher.

Pathophysiology and Clinical Manifestations

Tumors of the small intestine are usually small lesions less than 1.5 cm in diameter. These tumors have slow rates of local spread and metastases. However, because of their small size and deep mucosal site of origin, the primary tumors often do not disturb the physiology of the host enough to cause clinical symptoms. Symptoms often do not occur until invasion and metastases have taken place. Spread beyond the primary tumor site results in invasion of the muscular layer, then spread to the peritoneum and mesentery.

Obstruction is the most common symptom signaling the presence of a small bowel neoplasm. Vague, intermittent abdominal pain which may be described as "cramps" usually results from partial bowel obstruction caused by these tumors. Bleeding is present in over half of symptomatic patients. An abdominal mass may be present with or without other symptoms.

Other clinical signs and symptoms of small bowel lesions include anorexia, nausea, vomiting, diarrhea, anemia, fever, and weight loss. Regional enteritis may also be present in association with small bowel carcinoma.[33]

Medical Management

Diagnosis. Radiographic studies including abdominal x-rays and barium contrast studies of the small bowel will identify tumors. Evaluation of gastrointestinal bleeding may be accomplished by passing a small bowel tube. To determine the level of bleeding, the tube is aspirated frequently and examined for occult blood. Superior mesenteric arteriography, when used during the period of active bleeding, will help to identify the site of the bleeding.

Treatment. Most lesions of the small intestine are treated surgically. Segmental resection is performed for removal of benign tumors. Extended resection and anastomosis are performed for malignant lesions.[33] A right colectomy and an ileotransverse colostomy are usually performed for malignancies of the terminal ileum. Carcinomas of the small bowel metastasize to mesenteric lymph nodes. As a result, wide surgical resection of the neoplasm and regional lymph nodes is the necessary treatment of choice. Carcinomas of the duodenum may require radical pancreaticoduodenectomy. Even when disease has spread beyond the scope of total surgical excision in cancers of the small intestine, palliative surgery is performed to help relieve pain and lessen the change of obstruction, perforation, and hemorrhage.[34]

Prognosis. Malignant tumors of the small intestine generally have a poor prognosis.

Cancer of the Colon and Rectum

Definition and Etiology

The incidence of colorectal cancer and the resulting death rates are high in countries such as the United States, Great Britain, Canada, and northern Western Europe, where colorectal malignancies account for about two-thirds of all alimentary tract cancers. (These same countries show low incidences of esophageal and gastric cancers. The reverse is true for countries such as Japan and Finland, where the incidence of lower alimentary tract cancer is very low compared with the high incidence and death rates resulting from esophageal and gastric cancers.[24]) Nearly 130,000 new cases of colorectal cancer are diagnosed annually in the United States. More than 59,000 Americans will die annually as a result of colorectal cancer. Only lung cancer causes more annual deaths than colorectal cancer in men, and only breast cancer kills more women each year than large bowel cancer.[38]

Ninety-five percent of colorectal cancers are adenocarcinomas. Carcinoid tumors, leiomyosarcomas, and lymphomas are presented in lesser degrees. Fifty percent occur in the rectum.[33]

Dietary fiber, which leads to an increase in stool bulk, has been correlated with a lowered incidence of large bowel cancer. It has been proposed that diets low in fiber result in prolonged transit time of stool. It is hypothesized that if there is a carcinogen in the feces that can induce and promote colon cancer, then slow transit time will allow longer exposure of the colon mucosa to carcinogens, thus increasing the risk of developing colon cancer.[24] Rural Africans, who eat diets high in natural fiber, have relatively rapid fecal transit time through the colon and correspondingly low incidences of colonic cancer. Individuals from Western nations whose diets characteristically lack fiber and contain large amounts of refined carbohydrates have slower fecal transit times. These nations report high incidences of colon cancer.[24]

Dietary fat may also play a significant part in the development of colon cancer. Metabolism of fats within the intestines results in production of acid and neutral steroids and their metabolites that structurally resemble some carcinogens. Additionally, diets high in fat cause increased secretion of bile acids into the gut, which may be associated with colon cancer.[33]

Ulcerative colitis has a definite risk of colon cancer. The increased colorectal cancer risk only involves patients with colitis involving the entire bowel (pancolitis). Granulomatous colitis (Crohn's disease) is also associated with with an increased risk of colon cancer. Patients diagnosed with Crohn's disease of the colon before the age of 21 have a higher likelihood of developing colon cancer than the normal population. These persons will also develop these cancers at earlier ages.[24] Familial polyposis of the colon is an autosomal-dominant, hereditary condition which affects both sexes. Polyps usually increase in number until a typical patient has polyps involving the entire colon. Large bowel cancer may be anticipated in 100% of patients with multiple polyposis. Most of these patients develop cancer by the ages of 35 to 40 years.[24]

Other factors that have been mentioned as possible contributors to colorectal carcinoma include viruses, agricultural chemicals, and excessive beer drinking. Patients who have had partial resection of the colon for cancer are at increased risk for developing a new primary tumor in the remaining portion of the colon. Patients with histories of previous breast, endometrial, or bladder cancer also seem to be at increased risk for developing colon cancer.[7]

Pathophysiology

On gross examination, large bowel cancer may be growing from the bowel wall into the lumen, producing a papillary mass which threatens obstruction.

Colorectal cancer generally grows slowly. It may remain localized for long periods of time. Spread of the tumor may occur by direct extension into the bowel wall, direct infiltration of adjacent tissues, invasion of lymphatic vessels and nodes, invasion of the bloodstream, transperitoneal implantation, or intraluminal transplantation.[39] Distant metastasis most commonly involves the liver and then lung.[12]

Clinical Manifestations

Clinical features associated with colorectal carcinomas relate to tumor size and location. Tumors of the right colon usually present with vague symptoms of abdominal pain and mild anemia. Gross bleeding is uncommon with tumors of the right colon; however, slow blood loss from fungating tumors is not uncommon, and stools are frequently positive for occult blood. In addition, almost 40% of patients with cecal carcinomas will have a palpable right lower quadrant mass on physical examination.[24] Obstruction resulting from right colon tumors is uncommon.

Tumors of the left colon usually present with symptoms of obstruction. Patients with left colon lesions often present with intermittent crampy lower abdominal pain and fullness. The pain, related to gradual progressive obstruction, is often relieved with defecation or the passage of flatus. Change in the caliber of stools is also common in patients with left-sided colon carcinomas. Overt bleeding is associated with carcinoma of the colon in 50% of patients with left-sided lesions.[7]

If the symptoms of intermittent bowel obstruction are not recognized and acted on, complete bowel obstruction will eventually occur. Patients exhibiting complete bowel obstruction will experience severe abdominal pain, increasing abdominal distention, vomiting, and constipation. Such patients present with surgical emergencies requiring decompressive procedures.[23]

Obstructive symptoms are uncommon in patients with rectal carcinoma, owing to the large caliber of the rectum. Rectal bleeding is the most common complaint of patients with rectal cancer. Eighty percent of patients with rectal carcinoma have symptomatic bleeding. Bleeding may be evidenced as gross blood mixed with feces, blood on the outside of feces, or rectal bleeding after straining at stool.[32]

Changes in bowel habits are reported by greater than 70% of patients with rectal carcinoma. These symptoms include alternating constipation and diarrhea, decrease stool caliber, and tenesmus accompanied by a feeling of incomplete rectal evacuation. In patients with rectal cancer, pain is reported as a symptom in less than 25% of cases. Dull, boring pelvic pain may be present late in the disease when it has spread beyond local lymph nodes and invaded perirectal structures.[7]

Rectal carcinoma is often accessible to direct palpation on physical examination. Sixty-five to eighty percent of rectal carcinomas can be palpated on a careful rectal examination.

Patients who are suspected of having colorectal cancer may exhibit physical signs of metastatic disease. Such signs include the following: supraclavicular adenopathy, an enlarged nodular liver, ascites, palpably enlarged and firm ovaries, and nodules in the region of the umbilicus.[23]

Medical Management

Diagnosis. The patient should be questioned about a history of previous diagnosis and treatment for polyps and ulcerative or granulomatous colitis. Information should be elicited as to whether other family members have been diagnosed with colorectal carcinoma or other cancers. The patient should further be questioned about the presence of any rectal bleeding, changes in bowel habits, presence of any abdominal pain, recent weight loss, or whether the patient has been told he is anemic.

A rectal examination is necessary. In women, the examination should be rectal–vaginal so that lesions as high as 13 cm may be detected. Half of all rectal carcinomas may be detected by digital examination.[33] Patients should further be examined for any signs of metastatic disease.

Patients who are suspected of colon cancer should undergo proctosigmoidoscopy. This procedure allows for visualization of 25 cm of colonic mucosa past the rectosigmoid junction. Any lesions present should be biopsied and examined for mobility (to help predict the extent of tumor involvement). Two out of three cancers of the colon and rectum can be seen and biopsied through the sigmoidoscope.[35]

Barium enema is an important diagnostic tool in the evaluation of unexplained abdominal mass, in the presence of iron-deficient anemia (especially when occult blood is present in the stools), and in the face of overt rectal bleeding when there is no obvious active bleeding site in the anus or rectum. If the sigmoidoscopy is positive, the barium enema is helpful in delineating the extent of the pathology and in ruling out other colonic lesions. The use of air-contrast barium enema improves diagnostic accuracy greatly. The air-contrast technique allows small polyps of tumors that might otherwise be missed to be easily identified.[24]

Colonoscopy allows direct visualization of the entire colonic mucoa. It should be performed to the cecum in all patients with unexplained gastrointestinal blood loss and in patients with positive or equivocal barium enemas. Even in patients who have colon cancer diagnosed by barium enema, additional polyps may be found by colonoscopy.

Carcinoembryonic antigen (CEA) levels, once believed to be specific immunologic markers for the diagnosis of colon cancer, have been found to be elevated with other cancers and inflammatory bowel diseases. CEA levels should be measured, however, because of their important prognostic value. It has been shown that in patients with primary colorectal cancer, the likelihood of recurrent disease within 2 years approximates 80% in the face of an elevated CEA (>2.5 ng/ml). If the preoperative CEA is <2.5 ng/ml, the recurrent rate approximates 30%.[3]

Mass screening may lead to early detection of colorectal cancer. The American Cancer Society recommends a routine annual digital rectal examination for all persons 40 years of age and older. A stool guaiac (Hemocult slide) test should be added at age 50 on an annual basis. At age 50 and over, the American Cancer Society further recommends that sigmoidoscopy be performed every 3 to 5 years after two initial negative sigmoidoscopies 1 year apart.[14]

Treatment. The particular surgical approach chosen for treatment of colorectal carcinoma depends upon the tumor site. Colorectal carcinomas are removed by wide segmental resection of the colon and the mesentery with intestinal anastomosis or abdominoperineal (A–P) resection and permanent colostomy depending upon the level of the cancer. The surgical procedure of choice for patients with right colon lesions is a right hemicolectomy. Patients with left colon lesions above the peritoneal reflection will undergo left hemicolectomy.

Low-lying colorectal cancers may be treated by a number of surgical procedures. The two major procedures include the combined A–P resection in which the rectum and anus are completely removed and the patient receives a permanent colostomy, and the low anterior resection in which the rectal tumor is removed and the continuity of the bowel retained. The position of the tumor usually dictates whether a low anterior or an A–P resection is performed. Persons who have had previous colon carcinoma should have total abdominal colectomy. Patients with familial polyposis syndrome require total colectomy to prevent the occurrence of malignant transformation.[7]

Chemotherapy has been used in an attempt to treat advanced colorectal cancer. However, in spite of the large numbers of patients who have been treated with single agents and combination regimens, there is no convincing evidence that any systemic treatment results in improved survival.[24] Regional chemotherapy involves the delivery of chemotherapeutic drugs directly to organs containing metastatic tumor (such as the liver) by way of a catheter placed in an artery which directly supplies the organ. Hepatic artery infusion studies have been carried out with the delivery of drugs such as 5-fluorouracil and floxuridine (FUDR). It is hoped that long-term hepatic arterial infusion in patients with metastatic colon cancer will provide maximum exposure of the tumor to chemotherapeutic drugs and minimal exposure of normal tissues (such as bone marrow and gastrointestinal tract) to the toxic effects of the drugs.[24] Clinical studies are similarly being carried out with fully implanted devices such as the Infusaid pump and subsequent hepatic arterial infusion of FUDR. Patients who have received combined postoperative adjuvant radiation therapy and chemotherapy following surgery for rectal carcinoma show significantly fewer recurrences and significantly better survival rates than patients receiving chemotherapy alone, radiation therapy alone, or no therapy at all.[34]

Prognosis. The 5-year survival rate for all patients with primary colorectal cancer ranges from 40% to 50%.[38] The location of the tumor may be significant, as it is generally recognized that tumors of the ascending (right) colon have a somewhat more favorable prognosis than those of the descending (left) colon, or rectum.

Nursing Management

Nursing Diagnosis

As in the previous section, the problems of patients with cancer along the gastrointestinal tract relate to the perceived significance of the disease, the discomfort associated with tumor compression of surrounding tissues, the alteration in nutritional status, and the care requirements associated with the particular treatment. The diagnoses are fear related to the life-threatening nature of the diagnosis; alteration in comfort; alteration in nutritional intake; potential for complications associated with surgery, radiation, or chemotherapy; self-care deficits; and knowledge deficits relative to the diagnosis, treatment, and follow-up care.

The nursing care required by patients undergoing resection of a portion of the gastrointestinal tract with anastomosis to re-establish continuity will vary somewhat depending upon the location and extent of the procedure. The potential postoperative complications include atelectasis or pneumonia, pain, fluid and electrolyte imbalance, abnormal wound conditions, leakage from the anastomotic site, abdominal distention, inadequate dietary intake, and weight loss. Patients having surgery of the esophagus will have chest tubes in place postoperatively because the procedure requires entry into the chest cavity. Potential complications include bleeding and clot obstruction of the drainage tubes. Patients having stomach surgery (*e.g.,* gastrojejunostomy) will have a duodenal stump which is sutured close. A potential complication is rupture of the duodenal suture line.

Patients having small bowel resection and anastomosis could develop duodenal fistulas, paralytic ileus, and malabsorption syndrome. The potential postoperative complications following colon surgery, especially an A–P resection, include urinary retention or incontinence in men, discomfort, and potential infection of the perineal wound.

Goals. The goals of nursing management are to reduce anxiety; assist the patient and family to cope with the stress of an operative procedure; promote comfort; promote improved nutritional status; prevent postoperative complications; promote recovery from surgery; and educate the patient and family about the disease, treatment, and self care following discharge.

Preoperative Interventions

Patients who are diagnosed as having a malignancy of the gastrointestinal tract are usually also told that they need surgery. The patient should be given an explanation of his disease and the treatment (potentially curative or palliative).

The nurse provides reinforcement of the physician's information and often clarification. This knowledge should aid the patient in making decisions about his care. Knowledge of the disease and its treatment should help to allay anxiety. Opportunity should be provided the patient and family to discuss their feelings and concerns about the diagnosis, treatment, and treatment outcome.

The patient must also be informed about the physical preparation for surgery and the postoperative experiences. Likewise, the patient who is to receive adjuvant or palliative radiation therapy must receive information about how such treatment will affect him and its possible side-effects. The patient who is to have disfiguring surgery, such as an A–P resection with colostomy, must understand the procedure and the fact that it is permanent.

Preoperative preparation of the patient will include correction of existing nutritional problems by means of elemental diet feeding or total parenteral nutrition. In many cases, a weight gain will be necessary before surgery is attempted, as will corrections of any hemoglobin, protein, fluid or electrolyte deficits that may exist. The patient should be informed that an intravenous line will be in place for the administration of intravenous fluids, blood, and medications.

The presence of malnutrition may lead to decreased blood volume, hemoconcentration, alterations in fluid and electrolyte balance, and decreased resistance to infection. As a result, the patient may require preoperative blood transfusions to restore blood volume, and intravenous administration of fluids and electrolytes to correct any imbalances that may exist. Meticulous maintenance of a complete intake and output record beginning preoperatively and continuing throughout the postoperative period will help to ensure that adequate fluid balance is maintained and will alert the nurse to any possibility of fluid imbalance.

Preparation of the bowel for surgery requires mechanical cleansing and reduction of intestinal bacterial flora in addition to decreasing fecal bulk by dietary means several days prior to surgery. The bowel may be cleansed by the administration of laxatives, enemas, or colonic irrigations. To prevent the risk of peritoneal cavity contamination at the time of surgery and to suppress the bacterial flora in the intestine, oral antibiotics such as kanamycin, neomycin, and erythromycin are administered. Patients with intestinal obstruction should not undergo mechanical cleansing or antibiotic treatment.

Further preoperative preparation includes the insertion of a nasogastric tube to remove accumulated air or fluid, help facilitate surgery, and minimize abdominal distention postoperatively. A Foley catheter is inserted prior to surgery to ensure that the bladder is empty during surgery and thus reduce the possibility of bladder trauma. Placement of the Foley catheter will help with the hourly evaluation of output postoperatively. The indwelling catheter is also useful since many patients experience considerable problems with voiding postoperatively.

The patient whose surgery includes placement of a colostomy should be referred to the enterostomal therapist preoperatively. Comprehensive teaching, assistance, and ongoing psychological support is provided by this specialist. Ongoing collaboration with the enterostomal therapist will afford the nurse the opportunity to reinforce teaching and evaluate patient performance according to a coordinated plan of care. (For detailed information about nursing care of the patient with a colostomy, see Chapter 80).

If the problem is esophageal obstruction, excess saliva and increased drooling are often present. In order to minimize the possibility of aspiration of secretions, the nurse must assist the patient with the removal of secretions. At all times during the pre- and postoperative period, maintenance of a patent airway is essential. Constant attention to optimal oral hygiene is also essential both pre- and postoperatively. Frequent mouth care, including elimination of secretions, tooth brushing, and oral rinses, is encouraged (especially before meals) to ensure that any odor, foul breath, or bad taste is eliminated. The patient should also be informed that closed chest drainage tubes will be placed during surgery because the thoracic cavity will be entered. In addition to preparing the patient for the surgical experience, preoperative teaching may also help to minimize or prevent postoperative complications.

Postoperative Interventions

Pulmonary Considerations. Pulmonary complications may arise early in the postoperative period following gastrointestinal surgery. The nurse must continually assess the patient's pulmonary status. Routine lung assessment includes checking the patient's lung sounds for congestion and establishing a routine schedule (every 1–2 hr) of turning, coughing, and deep-breathing. Analgesics may be administered prior to these coughing and deep-breathing procedures in order to minimize incisional pain and increase patient compliance. Early ambulation is also encouraged. As a result of this routine, it is anticipated that postoperative complications of pneumonia and atelectasis will be prevented.

Immediate postoperative care of the patient who undergoes esophageal resection is similar to that required for patients undergoing thoracic surgery. Because the surgical incision is near the diaphragm, the patient may be reluctant to cough and breathe deeply. In an effort to prevent pulmonary complications, expectorants and bronchodilators may be prescribed. Maintenance of vigorous pulmonary care will help to remove an accumulation of secretions which might cause respiratory complications such as aspiration pneumonia. Following surgery, the patient should be placed first in a semi-Fowler's and later in a Fowler's position. Such positioning will help prevent a reflux of gastric secretions.

Wound Care. The wounds of all patients must be observed frequently for any signs of infection including purulent drainage, erythema, or edema. If wound infection is suspected a culture should be obtained, and antibiotic therapy should be instituted on the basis of culture results. Dressing changes should be carried out under aseptic technique. The patient's incision is suspected as a site of infection whenever a temperature elevation ($\geq 101°F$) is present.

Anastomotic Leakage. A temperature elevation may also signal the presence of anastomotic leakage. An anastomosis involving the esophagus has a greater tendency to leak than any other anastomotic site in the gastrointestinal tract. This complication must be recognized and dealt with immediately because a leaking gastroesophageal anastomosis may lead to death. Leakage may be caused by tension of the suture line, the patient's inability to heal, or an impaired blood supply of the organ to which the esophagus is attached.[19]

Leakage is usually apparent within the first postoperative week. The nurse should be alerted to this complication upon noting inflammation, a low-grade fever, and fluid accumulation in the pleural space.[19] An anastomotic leak should also be suspected in the presence of increased pulse and respiration rates and signs of shock. Early recognition of this problem will lead to prompt treatment involving drainage of the thoracic cavity or reoperation to repair the anastomosis.

Following radical subtotal gastrectomy and reconstruction, there is a danger of leakage from the duodenal stump.[19] Observe the patient closely for any signs of duodenal "blowout," including sudden pain, temperature elevation, tachycardia, and abdominal rigidity. Report appearance of any of these signs immediately so that treatment may be initiated. Treatment will include fluid and electrolyte replacement and duodenal stump drainage.

Abdominal Distention. The patient's nasogastric drainage system should be continually assessed to assure patency and thus avert associated gastrointestinal problems. The patient's abdominal girth should be measured and recorded every shift, and the presence of any abdominal distention should be immediately reported. The patient should not be given anything by mouth until peristalsis returns and the nasogastric tube is discontinued.

When distention of the small bowel occurs, as with paralytic ileus, the capacity of the intestine to absorb fluid is altered. As distention progresses, intestinal secretions increase as absorption decreases; consequently, an imbalance of fluid and electrolytes results. Arterial and venous blood flow obstruction occurs as pressure within the distended small intestine builds. Edema and transudation of plasma into the peritoneal cavity then occurs. Ultimately, there is a decrease in the extracellular fluid volume. Oliguria and postural hypotension result from the extracellular fluid volume deficit. Hypokalemia occurs secondary to increased renal excretion of potassium and its isolation in the small intestine.

Fluid Balance. A precise intake and output record should be maintained which includes a measurement of all oral and parenteral fluids administered, and all output including urine, emesis, and nasogastric or intestinal tube drainage (color, odor, and consistency should be noted in addition to volume). Urine output and specific gravity should be measured every hour. A decrease in urine output to < 40 ml/hr or any change in specific gravity should be reported (high specific gravity may indicate inadequate fluid replacement).

A replacement of fluid and electrolyte losses will include the administration of intravenous fluids with sodium chloride, sodium bicarbonate, and potassium added. Blood levels of sodium, potassium, and bicarbonate, and pH of the blood should be checked routinely. Vital signs including blood pressure, pulse, respirations, and temperature should be monitored frequently to detect any signs of circulatory collapse.[19]

A Foley catheter will usually remain in place for 3 to 5 days following surgery to assist in evaluation of fluid balance status. It is also helpful for the male patient following an abdominal perineal resection since urinary retention and incontinence can occur. It will also help keep the perineal dressing dry. Men should understand from the onset that resection of the presacral nerves and sympathetic fibers may result in sexual impotence postoperatively. The patient should receive pre- and postoperative counseling about this problem.

Pain Control. Analgesics should be administered as ordered following a thorough assessment to determine the location, nature, and duration of the patient's pain. Positioning the patient in a modified Fowler's position may further contribute to his postoperative comfort by decreasing pull on the suture line and promoting ease of respiration. However, the patient who has had an A–P resection may experience considerable discomfort from the perineal wound. Comfortable positioning may be difficult, and a sensation of wanting to evacuate the rectum may result from the presence of packing, perineal drainage, pressure, and pain in the wound. It is unlikely that the patient will be able to sit or lie in a recumbent position following surgery, owing to the pressure that this position will exert on the perineal wound. Perineal wound separation may occur as a result of pressure that is placed on the area when the patient assumes a recumbent position. To guard against this, the patient is taught to assume a lateral position and to change position every 2 hours.

Nutritional Support. When oral fluids are reinstituted, they are begun sparingly. Initially, the patient is given small amounts of water. The amount is then increased based on the patient's tolerance. The patient's total parenteral nutrition is maintained to provide necessary nutrients and prevent further dietary deficiencies. Oral dietary intake will complement parenteral intake. The patient's diet is advanced as tolerated. For the patient having esophageal or stomach surgery, bland foods are offered until the patient is able to eat six small meals per day and drink 120 ml of fluid between meals. Regurgitation may result from the patient eating too fast or too much. Regurgitation may also signify the presence of edema along the suture line which is preventing fluids and solids from moving into the intestinal tract. As a result, nasogastric suction may need to be reinstituted until the edema has subsided.[9]

When oral feedings are reinstituted, the postgastric surgery patient should be observed for signs and symptoms of the dumping syndrome. The patient should be taught the manifestations of the syndrome and how to avert it through proper dietary intake and habits. This problem is discussed in Chapter 83.

Discharge Planning. Preparation for discharge include comprehensive instructions related to the patient's care outside of the hospital. These instructions and plans for home care and follow-up medical care will be provided by members of the hospital health care team including the nurse, dietitian, enterostomal therapist, physician, and social worker. The patient and family will be active participants in planning for discharge. Comprehensive dietary instruction should be provided by the dietitian and reinforced by the nurse. The patient should be taught to weigh himself daily and should be taught what he should and should not eat, how much, and how often. Eating should be encouraged because weight loss is a common and continuing problem following surgery. Problems that might arise following small bowel surgery are diarrhea and malabsorption syndrome (see Chapter 80).

Adequate discharge preparation will include a written list of the patient's medications and why they are being given, when they are to be taken, and the possible side-effects of each. Treatments such as sitz baths and dressing changes for patients after A–P surgery should be taught both family and patient prior to discharge (see Chapter 80). The patient should also receive instructions about conditions or circumstances that warrant physician notification. He should be provided with information related to his first follow-up visit to the physician following hospitalization. He should also understand why periodic medical visits are necessary to assess his progress and monitor his medical status.

In addition to complications that might arise following surgical treatment, complications and side-effects may also occur in conjunction with radiation therapy. Radiation therapy is usually received following discharge from the hospital. It is important for the patient to understand that the problems associated with therapy are only temporary and will subside following the cessation of treatment. Possible side-effects related to radiation therapy include anorexia, diarrhea, and crampy abdominal pain. These generally result from hypermotility of the gastrointestinal tract.[19] The clinic nurse should continue assessment of the patient throughout therapy, and side-effects should be treated symptomatically as they arise. By providing information, understanding, and support throughout treatment, the nurse will encourage the patient and contribute positively to the therapeutic regime.

Cancer of the colon and rectum is a major health problem in the United States. Because it is such a common disease among Americans, it is important for nurses to support the early detection and treatment of colorectal cancer through public education and promotion of participation in screening programs. Particular attention should be focused on persons who are at high risk for development of the disease, which would include family of patients being treated for the disease.

A visiting nurse referral will provide ongoing assessment, assistance, and encouragement to the patient and family at home. She will help the patient and family with any physical care procedures that need to be carried on in the home, as well as provide valuable psychological support. She will be an ongoing resource and source of information. Provision of skilled nursing care at home and comprehensive teaching prior to discharge should minimize anxieties on the part of the patient and family. As a result, the patient and family will be adequately prepared for home care and complications will be avoided.

Outcome criteria for goal achievement are as follows:

1. The patient and family accurately describe the operative procedure and postoperative treatment.
2. The patient and family discuss feelings and concerns about the diagnosis and treatment.
3. The patient expresses a decrease in anxiety.
4. The patient states that pain is controlled with treatment measures.
5. Evidence of adequate nutrition status is achieved preoperatively and maintained postoperatively.
6. Complications are prevented (*e.g.,* vital signs are stable, weight is stable, nasogastric drainage is maintained, intake and output are balanced, lungs are clear, abdominal girth is stable, serum electrolytes are within normal limits).
7. The patient accurately describes potential side-effects of radiation treatment and how to manage these effects.

Cancer of the Pancreas

Definition and Etiology

The majority of neoplasms of the exocrine pancreas are adenocarcinomas. Most arise from ductal epithelium (>80% of tumors), the remainder primarily from acinar tissue. Two thirds of pancreatic tumors arise in the head of the pancreas; the remainder are found in the body and tail.[1,34]

Although these tumors are relatively rare, comprising only 2% to 3% of all forms of cancer, the incidence of pancreatic carcinoma has increased almost 300% over the last 40 years. Approximately 25,000 new cases are diagnosed annually. In the United States, pancreatic carcinoma is currently the fourth most common cancer in men and the fifth most common in women.[12] It is the fifth most frequent cause of cancer death in the United States.[20]

Three major factors are believed to be associated with an increased risk of pancreatic carcinoma; they include diabetes mellitus, tobacco use, and diet. There is some evidence to suggest that in women with diabetes mellitus, pancreatic cancer is two to six times more common than in nondiabetic women. This association does not exist for men.[24]

Cigarette smokers have at least a twofold increased risk for developing pancreatic cancer. No increased incidence has been demonstrated for pipe or cigar smokers, thereby suggesting that the carcinogenic effect is dependent upon inhalation of tobacco smoke containing nitrosamines and other metabolites. Pancreatic cancer occurs 10 years earlier in cigarette smokers than in nonsmokers.

Diets high in meat and fat are correlated with an increased risk of pancreatic cancer in humans. Coffee consumption has also been correlated with pancreatic cancer. Exposure to chemicals such as benzidine, betanaphthylamine, and alkylating chemotherapeutic drugs may be related to the higher incidence of pancreatic cancer in chemical workers.[5,28]

Carcinoma of the pancreas produces a hard, nodular, poorly defined enlargement of the portion of the gland where it originates. When first seen, the majority of cases are advanced, with early nerve sheath and vascular invasion. Tumors in the head of the pancreas may invade adjacent structures, and lead to obstruction of the portal vein, duodenum, and inferior vena cava.[1] Carcinomas of the body and tail of the pancreas may remain asymptomatic for long periods. They may later become apparent as large, palpable tumor masses, frequently invading surrounding structures such as splenic arteries, splenic veins, and the stomach.[34]

The most frequent sites of metastases are the nearby lymph nodes. In the end stages of the disease, liver metastases are almost always present.

Clinical Manifestations

Most patients with carcinoma of the pancreas present with the insidious onset of asthenia, anorexia, weight loss, gaseousness, and nausea. Weight loss is the most common symptom and may be rapid and marked. It results from an associated diabetes mellitus, from a coexisting maldigestive syndrome, or from anorexia from the disease or from chronic pain. Blockage of the common bile duct by carcinoma at the head of the pancreas results in jaundice. Blockage of the pancreative duct by tumor may cause acute pancreatitis. Portal hypertension with the development of esophageal varices may result from tumor invasion or compression of the portal venous system. Pancreatic tumor invasion of the stomach may result in gastrointestinal bleeding.[20] A dull, boring pain confined to the epigastrium or back is present in most patients. Emotional disturbances, characterized by depression, agitation, and anxiety, have also been reported in a majority of patients.[20,34]

The above symptoms precede the slow and progressive jaundice associated with carcinoma of the head of the pancreas. The jaundice is persistent and is accompanied by pruritus. Elevated levels of serum bilirubin and alkaline phosphatase are present in patients with obstructive jaundice as a manifestion of carcinoma of the head of the pancreas.

With carcinoma of the body of the pancreas, as the tumor enlarges, infringement of the nerve plexus around the celiac ganglia results in severe back pain. The pain is often persistent and is heightened by eating or lying down. Pain may be relieved by sitting up or bending forward.[1,20,34] Jaundice occurs late in the course of patients with carcinoma of the body and tail of the pancreas.[20] It usually results from advanced disease causing bile duct obstruction or liver metastases.[20]

Severe weight loss and weakness associated with metastases to other organs are symptoms initially seen with carcinoma of the tail of the pancreas. Additionally, a palpable abdominal tumor is often the most common finding.[1] Late in the disease maldigestion.[20]

Medical Management

Diagnosis. An upper gastrointestinal (GI) series identifies gastric outlet obstruction or invasion and compression or obstruction of the duodenum by tumor in the head of the pancreas. Unfortunately, these findings signify relatively advanced tumors, rendering the upper GI series useless for early diagnosis. Other tests that make possible an early diagnosis of pancreatic cancer are ultrasonograph, computed tomography (CT) scans, endoscopic retrograde cholangiopancreatogram (ERCP), and arteriography.

Treatment. The only chance of cure for pancreatic carcinoma is by surgery.[25] The only patients who are cured by surgery are those with cancer of the head of the pancreas who do not show evidence of metastases. Patients with body and tail carcinoma present with locally advanced disease and are not curable. Surgical resection for cure is possible in less than 25% of pancreatic cancer diseases who are explored.

One surgical procedure is the radical pancreaticoduodenectomy (Whipple procedure), which involves resection of the pancreatic head, the duodenum, the distal stomach, and the distal part of the common bile duct. The entire duodenum is resected; the pancreatic duct is implanted into the jejunum, which is anastomosed to the common hepatic duct; and a gastrojejunostomy is performed. The other surgical procedure that may be performed is the total pancreatectomy, in which the entire pancreas is removed with the distal stomach and duodenum.[1]

In patients who are not resectable for cure, palliative bypass procedures are often performed. Gastroenterostomy and biliary bypass may prevent subsequent duodenal or biliary obstruction, and may be beneficial in patients who are to receive postoperative radiation or chemotherapy.[34] Such bypass procedures decrease the risk of serious obstructive complications that could limit the success of additional treatment with radiation or chemotherapy.

Radiation therapy has been employed with limited success in the treatment of pancreatic carcinoma. Radiation appears to be most effective in patients with localized or regional disease.

Chemotherapy for pancreatic cancer has provided some tumor regression and palliation of symptoms. Although complete responses and long-term disease-free survivals have not yet been achieved, the advantages of tumor regression, control of symptoms, and some prolongation of survival in patients responding to chemotherapy make the approach worthwhile.

Prognosis. Carcinoma of the pancreas is a rapidly progressive disease which has usually metastasized by the time diagnosis has been made. Ninety percent of patients with untreated pancreatic carcinomas will die within 1 year of diagnosis.

Nursing Management

Nursing Diagnosis

Problems of patients undergoing pancreatic surgery are related to perceived significance of the diagnosis, alteration in comfort and nutrition, and potential for complications following surgery. The nursing diagnoses are fear related to the life-threatening nature of the disease and treatment; alteration in comfort related to the disease process; alteration in nutritional status and in fluid and electrolyte balance related to inadequate pancreatic function; potential for postoperative complications; and knowledge deficits about the disease, treatment, and follow-up care. Potential postoperative complications include pneumonia, hemorrhage, wound infection, and disturbances in digestion and absorption of nutrients.

Goals. The goals of nursing management are to alleviate fears, promote comfort, maintain nutritional status and fluid and electrolyte balance, prevent complications of surgery or detect them promptly, assist the patient in recovery from surgery, and educate the patient and family about the disease, treatment, and follow-up care.

Interventions

Nursing interventions of patients having pancreative surgery are similar to those discussed for patients having surgery for cancer of the gastrointestinal tract. Only specific additions or differences are discussed in this section.

Nursing interventions preoperatively center around establishing rapport with the patient and family, gaining their confidence in the skill of the nursing staff, and educating them about the operative procedure and the postoperative care.

Postoperatively, close observations of patient status are necessary to detect impending complications. Interventions to promote airway clearance, maintain fluid and electrolyte balance, promote adequate drainage from the nasogastric and other drainage tubes, keep wounds clean and dry, maintain urine output, and control pain will contribute to prevention of complications. Particular interventions include careful monitoring of blood pressure and comparison with preoperative baseline. Hypotension often occurs following pancreatic surgery because of the division of the sympathetic fibers to the mesentery following radical resection. In the presence of hypotension, vasopressor drugs may be necessary for 24 to 48 hours.[29]

The nurse must maintain the patency and adequate drainage of the gastrointestinal tubes and drains. These tubes and drains are placed to maintain decompression of the pancreas, jejunum, biliary tract, and stomach. Patency of the system is necessary to minimize distention and ischemic pressure. Kinking of tubes and drains must be prevented. The type as well as amount of drainage must be determined and recorded.

Hemorrhage may occur from leakage of activated pancreatic juice and digestion of neighboring arteries.[12] The nurse must check stools for blood and be alert for changes in vital signs. Prothrombin levels are also determined frequently, and Vitamin K may need to be administered. (Vitamin K production is impaired because of the disease process.)

Intraperitoneal infection is the single greatest threat to the patient. The infection is likely to be located beneath the diaphragm, beneath the liver, or adjacent to a leaking anastomosis of the biliary or pancreatic jejunostomies.[12] The nurse must be alert to signs of infection, such as increasing temperature and pulse and patient expression of an increase in pain intensity.

Diabetes mellitus is a possible consequence of a Whipple procedure and a definite consequence of a total pancreatectomy. The nurse must be alert to signs of hyperglycemia such as blurred vision, irritability, puritus, glycosuria and manifestations of metabolic acidosis. The patient will need insulin replacement for the remainder of his life.

Usually, total parenteral nutrition is continued for 2 to 3 days following surgery since it takes time for the anastomotic sites to heal sufficiently to start oral intake. The combination of pancreatic insufficiency, maldigestion, malabsorption, and possible diabetes mellitus predisposes the patient to severe nutritional deficiencies. The nurse should monitor the patient's nutritional status. She should also be alert to frothy, light-colored stools that may contain undigested fat. Pancreatic enzyme insufficiency may result in nondigestion of ingested fat and protein. Replacement with pancreatic enzyme tablets will need to be continued throughout life.

Education of the patient and family for home care will ease the transition to assumption of responsibility for self-care or family care. Referrals must be made to community home health nurses and other community resources as indicated by individual patient needs.

Evaluation

Outcome criteria are as follows:

1. The patient and family accurately describe treatment and prescribed follow-up care.
2. The patient and family discuss concerns and fears about the disease and treatment.
3. The patient and family express a decrease in anxiety.
4. The patient states the pain is controlled by measures used.
5. The patient does not manifest signs of complications.
6. The patient and family accurately describe manifestations that warrant discussion with the physician.

Cancer of the Liver

Definition and Etiology

The majority of primary malignant tumors of the liver are adenocarcinomas. There are two major cell types: those arising from the parenchymal liver cell (hepatoma or hepatocellular carcinoma) and those arising from the bile duct cell (cholangioma or cholangiocarcinoma).[1] Ninety percent of all primary liver tumors are hepatocellular carcinomas.[2]

Primary hepatic carcinoma is rare in the United States, representing about 2% of all cancers.[1] This incidence contrasts sharply with the incidence in areas such as sub-Saharan Africa and the Far East, where this disease may represent 20% to 40% of all cancers. Hepatocellular cancer is the second most common cancer found in Southeast Asia. In the East African Bantu, four out of every five autopsies show hepatocellular carcinoma.

A strong association exists between cirrhosis of the liver and primary liver carcinoma. Cirrhosis is present in approxiamtely 70% to 75% of patients with carcinoma of the liver. It is believed that approximately 4% of patients with cirrhosis will eventually develop hepatoma. Similarly, there is a strong correlation between hepatitis B virus and the development of primary hepatocellular carcinoma.[34]

Pathophysiology

Hepatic cancer may present as a large, single nodule or as multiple satellite tumor nodules around a large primary lesion. Death ensues from liver failure, often with no evidence that the cancer has spread beyond the liver. However, primary liver carcinoma may spread by centrifugal growth within the liver, by parasinoidal extension to the other parts of the liver, by retrograde venous extension into the portal vein, and by invasion of the lymphatics.[1]

Clinical Manifestations

Several years of illness may precede the onset of symptoms in patients with primary hepatic carcinoma. The symptoms are seldom characteristic and, in some cases, hepatocellular carcinoma may remain completely asymptomatic. Initial symptoms of hepatic cancer may include nonspecific complaints of upper abdominal pain, weakness, weight loss, lassitude, sensations of fullness or bloating, and anorexia.[33] As the tumor grows, pain may become constant and more severe, and may radiate into the back. Almost 70% of patients have pain and weight loss.[1]

Hepatocellular carcinoma should be suspected in patients with cirrhosis who manifest unexplained clinical deterioration such as increasing abdominal girth, impaired mental status, and weakness. Sudden hypotension or abdominal pain may be observed in patients with rapid hemorrhage into the tumor mass or the peritoneal cavity.[34]

Physical findings noted in patients with hepatoma are those of chronic liver disease (see following section). Hepatomegaly is present in almost all patients. The liver is hard, nodular, and tender. A hard, irregular lump may be felt in the right upper quadrant, continuous with the liver. If the left lobe is involved, the mass is epigastric. Hepatic bruits may be heard in nearly 25% of patients.

Medical Management

Diagnosis. Primary carcinoma of the liver must be differentiated from metastatic carcinoma, which is the most frequent type of tumor found in the liver. Cancer should always be suspected in patients with cirrhosis who exhibit a rapid increase in liver size and who display the signs and symptoms mentioned above. Diagnostic and laboratory tests include the following:

- *Radioisotope scans* of the liver with substances such as radioactive technetium-99m colloid are especially useful in diagnosing lesions larger than 2 cm in diameter.
- *Laboratory studies* include serum alkaline phosphatase, which is almost always elevated even if jaundice has not yet appeared. Elevation of particular isoenzymes of alkaline phosphatase are characteristic of specific primary liver carcinomas.
- *Needle biopsy* of the liver is especially useful if a definite palpable nodule can be biopsied.
- *Computed tomography (CT) scans* will help to identify and localize mass tumor lesions. They are also useful in helping to determine biopsy sites.
- *Selective hepatic arteriography* is valuable for tumor diagnosis, for localization, to determine operability, and to follow the effects of therapy.

Treatment. Surgical excision is the only definitive treatment for primary carcinoma of the liver. Up to 90% of the liver may be removed with eventual survival in the treatment of hepatic carcinomas. Total hepatectomy and liver replacement (liver transplantation) have been carried out in selected patients with variable results. If the patient survives the surgery, the immunosuppression necessary to prevent rejection favors recurrence and metastases.

Radiation therapy is of little value in the treatment of primary liver cancers. The tumors are essentially radioresistant, and liver tolerance lies in a subcancercidal dose range of 3000 rad.[1]

Palliative treatment may be accomplished by systemic chemotherapy, hepatic arterial infusion of chemotherapy, hepatic arterial ligation, hepatic arterial embolization, or a combination of methods. Chemotherapeutic drugs administered systemically or by way of the cannulated hepatic artery have been shown to bring about temporary hepatic tumor regression. Intravenous treatment with single agents such as adriamycin and 5-fluorouracil has yielded limited response rates.

Prognosis. The resectability rate for all hepatic tumors is very low. Usually the tumor has involved both lobes of the liver or has metastasized distally when the diagnosis is first made. Resection is possible in less than 1% of tumors. The course of the disease is rapid if the tumor is nonresectable.[1]

Nursing Management

Nursing Diagnosis

Problems of patients undergoing hepatic lobectomy are anxiety and fear related to the diagnosis, alteration in comfort and nutrition, and potential for complications following surgery. The nursing diagnoses are fear related to the life-threatening nature of the disease; alteration in comfort; potential alteration in nutritional status and fluid and electrolyte balance related to interference with liver function; potential for postoperative complications; and knowledge deficit about the disease, treatment, and follow-up care. Potential postoperative complications include pneumonia, atelectasis, hemorrhage, wound infection, and disturbances in liver function (hypoglycemia, alteration in protein synthesis and lipid metabolism, and alteration in synthesis of vitamin K).

Goals. The goals of nursing management are to alleviate fears, promote comfort, maintain nutritional status and fluid and electrolyte balance, prevent complications of surgery or detect them promptly, assist the patient in recovery from surgery, and educate the patient and family about the disease, treatment, and follow-up care.

Interventions

Patients who are to undergo hepatic lobectomy for primary carcinoma of the liver require preoperative teaching. The patient may express fear related to the loss of part of his liver. The patient should be taught that removal of up to 90% of the liver is compatible with life. Furthermore, he should understand that the blood supply will augment rapid regeneration and that normal liver mass and function will return within 6 months following surgery.[19]

Preoperatively, the patient is taught why various procedures are performed and why certain medications are administered. Daily colonic irrigations and administration of antibiotics prior to surgery will help to minimize any postoperative infection in the face of further abdominal exploration and surgery that is needed at the time of resection. Administration of vitamins such as vitamin K (to help restore blood clotting mechanisms) and vitamins A, D, C, and B complex (when jaundice is present) should be explained to the patient. Postoperative administration of steroids may serve to increase liver regeneration and help prevent fibrosis.

The patient requires constant attention for the first 2 to 3 days. Vital signs should be monitored every 15 minutes until they are stable, and then every hour for 24 to 48 hours. The risk of hemorrhage is very great in the patient who has undergone hepatic lobectomy. Dressings should be checked frequently for oozing or bleeding. Even when the patient is allowed to dangle his feet (approximately 3 days following surgery) and progress to ambulation, his vital signs must be watched closely. The pulse, blood pressure, and respiration rate should be monitored closely before and after any form of exertion.

Because surgery involves opening the thoracic cavity, the patient will have in place underwater chest drainage tubes connected to underwater-seal drainage bottles when he returns from surgery. Appropriate nursing assessment and care of this system is essential to maintain proper functioning and avoid complications.

Careful monitoring of the patient's intake and output will alert the nurse to any fluid and electrolyte problems that may occur. Hypovolemia may result from extensive blood loss. A precise record of the patient's intake (including intravenous infusions, blood infusions, and oral intake when the Levin tube is discontinued and an oral diet is reinstituted) and output (including chest tube drainage, suction drainage from the Levin tube, and urine output) should be maintained postoperatively. The patient should be observed for any signs of electrolyte imbalance, including changes in the level of consciousness, changes in respiratory rate or depth, the presence of cardiac abnormalities, or any muscle tone abnormalities.

Lung sounds should be checked frequently and, in an attempt to prevent postoperative respiratory complications such as pneumonia or atelectasis, a schedule of turning, coughing, and deep breathing is maintained every 2 hours. This is especially important because atelectasis often results from the splinting of the upper abdominal muscle that is done as a result of the location of the incision.

Turning and coughing may be painful for the patient who has undergone hepatic lobectomy. The nurse can be of assistance in helping the patient cough by placing both hands over the incision site as a splint. Comfort may further be afforded and lung expansion promoted by placing the patient in a semi-Fowler's position. Assessment of the patient's discomfort should be an ongoing process postoperatively. Appropriate analgesics should be administered as ordered following a definition of the level and source of the pain.

The patient's dressing should be observed closely during the postoperative period. Because the possibility of hemorrhage exists, dressings should be checked frequently for oozing or bleeding. Care of the wound site will depend upon the surgeon's orders. The dressing may need to be routinely reinforced, or aseptic dressing changes may be ordered.

Observation of the patient for any signs of infection postoperatively will include taking the patient's temperature every 4 hours (temperature $\geq$ 101°F may indicate the presence of a wound infection); observing the wound for the presence of any purulent drainage; and, when appropriate, observing the wound site for the presence of abnormalities such as edema or erythema. Identification of any of the above may be indicative of a wound infection requiring prompt medical attention. Wound culturing when infection is suspected will help to define appropriate antibiotic treatment.

The potential for serious metabolic abnormalities exists following hepatic lobectomy. The patient should be observed for hypoglycemia. Decreased glyconeogenesis may cause a precipitous fall in blood sugar. To prevent this, a constant infusion of 10% glucose may be required for the first 48 hours.[9] Protein synthesis and lipid metabolism are altered following resection, necessitating albumin infusions. The serum albumin level falls sharply for 10 days after extensive liver resection. Albumin replacement may be necessary for 3 to 4 days or until a normal level is achieved.[19]

Discharge Planning. Throughout the patient's hospital course, discharge planning should be occurring between patient, family, and nurse. The patient should receive appropriate dietary instruction following removal of the Levin tube. Approximately 5 days postoperatively, when the Levin tube is removed, the patient may ingest up to 60 g/day of protein.[19] Diet will progress gradually from clear liquids to semisoft, soft, and regular as tolerated. A dietary consultation will provide the patient and family with the knowledge necessary for the maintenance of an appropriate nutritionally balanced diet at home.

Another important component of discharge planning is self-care. Early in the postoperative period the patient is allowed to dangle his feet. Early ambulation is encouraged as the patient increases participation in his care. An assessment should be made of the patient's home situation to ascertain whether he will have access to home care should he need it.

In preparation for discharge the patient should receive written instructions about any special procedures he is to follow and under what circumstances he should call the physician. He should understand why he is taking specific medications, the side-effects of the medications, and any special precautions related to their administration. Prior to discharge, return follow-up care should be planned with the patient and family. A home-care nursing referral will help to reinforce teaching begun in the hospital and to monitor the patient's progress at home.

Evaluation

Outcome criteria for goal achievement are as follows:

1. The patient and family discuss openly their concerns about the diagnosis, treatment and outcome.
2. The patient expresses a decrease in anxiety.
3. The patient states the pain is controlled by measures used.
4. The patient does not manifest signs of complications, *e.g.,*
   Vital signs remain stable.
   Lungs are clear.
   Chest drainage is maintained until discontinued.
   Nasogastric drainage is maintained until discontinued.
   No abdominal distention exists.
   Serum electrolytes are within normal limits.
   No signs of wound infection (edema, redness) are apparent.
   Blood sugar and serum proteins are maintained with replacement.
   Weight is maintained.
5. Abnormalities in any of the above-listed manifestations are detected promptly and the physician consulted.
6. The patient and family accurately describe treatment and prescribed follow-up care.

Cirrhosis of the Liver

Definition and Etiology

Cirrhosis of the liver is one of the oldest diseases known to man. The disease represents chronic degenerative tissue changes that occur in the liver.

The three main types of cirrhosis are *alcoholic* (Laennec's, portal, or fatty), *postnecrotic* (toxic, nodular, or posthepatic), and *biliary* (cholangitic, or obstructive).

Alcoholic cirrhosis is the most common type seen in the North America, many parts of Western Europe, and South America. The incidence of alcoholic cirrhosis is higher in men. Typically, the average onset of symptoms occur at about 50 years of age.[22] Postnecrotic cirrhosis is the most common type of cirrhosis found throughout the world. Viral hepatitis is believed to be associated with the development of postnecrotic cirrhosis. Women are affected with postnecrotic cirrhosis as often as men.[22] Biliary cirrhosis is defined by clinical and chemical signs of chronic impairment of bile excretion and evidence of progressive liver destruction around the intrahepatic bile ducts. The development of biliary cirrhosis may be associated with atypical (cholestatic) hepatitis, and chronic bile duct obstruction by postoperative strictures or by gallstones, usually with superimposed cholangitis infections. Most patients with primary biliary cirrhosis are middle-aged women.[22] Because alcoholic cirrhosis is the type of cirrhosis most frequently encountered in the United States, further discussion is primarily center on this particular condition.

Chronic alcoholism is believed to be responsible for 90% of cirrhosis in men and 70% in women. Ten to twenty percent of chronic alcoholic patients have clinical or morphologic evidence of cirrhosis. It is apparent that the amount and duration of alcohol ingestion are determining factors in the development of alcoholic cirrhosis, rather than the type of alcohol consumed. Characteristically, the patient with alcoholic cirrhosis has consumed one or more pints of whiskey, several quarts of wine, or an equivalent amount of beer daily for at least 10 years.[22]

Malnutrition is recognized as another factor that contributes to the development of alcoholic cirrhosis. Alcoholic patients' diets are typically protein and vitamin deficient. They often develop additional clinical problems such as Wernicke-Korsakoff disease and folate deficiency, which are characteristic of debilitated nutritional states.

Pathophysiology

Hepatic cirrhosis results in massive disturbance and disruption of liver function. Destruction of parenchymal cells occurs with subsequent formation of, and replacement with, dense fibrosis scar tissue. Disruption of the normal liver lobular architecture occurs, along with formation of nodules of liver parenchyma surrounded by fibrous tissue.

As the disease advances, three major complications threaten patients with any type of cirrhosis: portal hypertension, fluid retention, and hepatic encephalopathy. *Portal hypertension* is directly associated with fibrosis and resulting structural changes in the liver. Regenerative nodules that form in the presence of severe fibrosis act as obstructions to the flow of portal blood through the liver. A rise in portal venous pressure (portal hypertension) results from the impaired portal blood flow. The consequence of increased portal pressure in cirrhosis is increased blood flow around the liver. The major sites of collateral flow include dilated veins around the rectum (hemorrhoids), cardioesophageal junction (esophagogastric varices), and retroperitoneal space and falciform ligament of the liver (periumbilical or abdominal wall collaterals). The major complication of portal hypertension is massive hemorrhage from the thin-walled, fragile varices in the upper stomach and lower esophagus. Such variceal bleeding often occurs as a painless, massive hematemesis or melena that cannot be correlated with any precipitating factor.[22]

Fluid retention in the form of ascites and edema is a common complication associated with the progression of cirrhosis. Ascites represents the accumulation of large quantities of fluid within the perintoneal cavity. In the cirrhotic patient, ascites may result from the disturbance of both local and systemic mechanisms that regulate the movement of fluids and electrolytes. Local factors that favor the development of ascites include portal hypertension and increased hepatic lymph flow. Systemic factors that contribute to the development of ascites in the cirrhotic patient include the presence of decreased plasma colloid oncotic pressure, hyperaldosteronism, and impaired water excretion.[22]

Hepatic encephalopathy (hepatic coma) is a metabolic disorder of the nervous system that may occur as cirrhosis progresses. This condition is believed to result from the accumulation of various toxic substances (such as ammonia) within the brain. This occurs when these substances, after having been absorbed from the intestine, are unable to be metabolized by the cirrhotic liver.

Hepatic encephalopathy may be seen in patients with stable, inactive cirrhosis following predisposing events such as gastrointestinal bleeding, an increase in dietary protein intake, electrolyte disturbances, and acute infections.[22] Hepatic encephalopathy is characterized by disturbances in consciousness, changing neurologic signs (rigidity, hyperreflexia), distinctive electroencephalographic changes, and "flapping tremor."[22] If not treated promptly, this condition rapidly results in death.

Clinical Manifestations

The onset of alcoholic cirrhosis may be subtle and the disease may go unrecognized for several years. After 10 years or more of chronic alcoholism, however, symptoms of progressive liver dysfunction, fluid retention, and portal hypertension may manifest themselves.[18] The patient may experience increasing weakness and fatigability, anorexia, slight weight loss, jaundice, intermittent ankle edema, and increasing abdominal girth due to ascites. The physical examination usually reveals a firm and enlarged liver, muscle wasting, a palpable spleen, palmar erythema, ascites, spider angiomas, jaundice, male gynecomastia and testicular atrophy, and female menstrual irregularity or amenorrhea.

As the disease progresses, the patient with alcoholic cirrhosis becomes increasingly weak and emaciated, and chronically jaundiced. Ascites increases, as do signs of portal hypertension such as the development of extensive portal–systemic venous collaterals around the rectum (hemorrhoids), cardioesophageal junction and retroperitoneal space, and falciform ligament of the liver (periumbilical or abdominal wall collaterals). Hepatic encephalopathy may eventually ensue.

The results of laboratory tests indicate the loss of liver function. Anemia may be present, resulting from gastrointestinal blood loss, folic acid deficiency, hypersplenism (portal hypertension produces venus congestion of the spleen), and the direct toxic effect of alcohol on the bone marrow. Hypersplenism and the toxic effect of alcohol on the bone marrow may also cause leukopenia and thrombocytopenia. Hyperbilirubinemia and variable elevations of serum alkaline phosphatase will be reflected in liver function tests results.

Additionally, the serum albumin is often decreased, while globulins are increased. When the disease is severe, clotting mechanisms are disturbed. As a result, there is a prolongation of the prothrombin and partial thromboplastin times. An elevated level of blood ammonia is representative of impaired liver function and shunting of portal blood around the liver and into the systemic circulation in the cirrhotic patient.

Further possible indications of the presence of alcoholic cirrhosis may include evidence of a diabetic type of glucose intolerance and the presence of respiratory alkalosis. Hypomagnesemia is also commonly seen. The presence of dilutional hyponatremia and hypokalemia reflective of secondary hyperaldosteronism are often seen in cirrhotic patients with ascites and edema.

Medical Management

Diagnosis

Alcoholic cirrhosis is strongly suspected in patients who have a history of chronic, excessive alcohol consumption that has continued over a long period of time. Additionally, the presence of various signs and symptoms of chronic liver disease, laboratory data that indicate abnormal liver function, and hepatomegaly may provide additional evidence that is suggestive of this disease.[18]

The definite diagnosis of cirrhosis is established by gross or microscopic examination of the liver. A percutaneous liver biopsy should be performed to confirm the diagnosis and define the stage of the disease. The presence of esophageal varices evidenced by barium-contrast x-ray studies or upper gastrointestinal endoscopy is also suggestive of cirrhosis.[17]

Treatment

Nutritional Measures. Complete abstinence from alcohol is the essential component of treatment for the patient with alcoholic cirrhosis. Additionally, attempts are made to improve the patient's nutritional status and promote healing of the damaged liver. The patient is placed on a diet containing at least 1 g protein per kilogram of body weight and 2000 to 3000 calories per day (provided there is no evidence of impending hepatic coma).[22] Daily administration of multivitamin capsules provides additional nutritive supplementation. Folic acid deficiency is treated with replacement therapy. Large parenteral doses of thiamine are also administered to these patients in the presence of Wernicke-Korsakoff disease.

Management of Variceal Hemorrhage. Primary treatment of alcoholic cirrhosis further includes management of any major complications that may arise. Generally, *portal hypertension* that results from established cirrhosis is not reversible. *Hemorrhage of established varices,* therefore, may pose a life-threatening situation for the patient.

In the face of massive hematemesis or melena resulting from ruptured varices, quantitative replacement of blood loss is essential to prevent further deterioration of liver function. Additionally, endoscopic or radiographic studies are employed to provide definitive demonstration of esophageal varices, location of the actual bleeding site, and exclusion of other causes of gastrointestinal hemorrhage. Variceal hemorrhage may be temporarily controlled by infusion of vasopressin, balloon tamponade, left gastric vein occlusion, or endoscopic sclerosis of varices.[22]

A continuous infusion of vasopressin (initially approximately 0.4 units/min) can reduce or stop variceal hemorrhage. This action is accomplished by the drug's lowering of splanchnic blood flow and portal pressure. Vasopressin is administered with caution either intravenously or directly in the superior mesenteric artery. Its use may prove harmful to patients with ischemic heart disease.[17]

The Sengstaken-Blakemore tube or a modified single balloon tube may be employed as a mechanical means to stop variceal bleeding. The Sengstaken-Blakemore gastric and esophageal balloon tubes are designed to compress the submucosal veins and thereby tamponade the bleeding sites. (Fig. 81–2). Use of the balloon tamponade or vasopressin infusion therapy should be regarded as temporary measures to control hemorrhage; these measures have significant incidences of relapse. If both methods fail to control the bleeding, transhepatic catheterization and occlusion of the left gastric vein may cause variceal hemorrhage to cease. An additional method aimed at controlling acute bleeding may be provided by directly injecting sclerosing solutions such as anolamine oleate into the varices by way of the endoscope.[17,22]

Emergency surgical shunting procedures may be employed to control acute hemorrhage and prevent exsanguination. Although such procedures carry a high risk of mortality (25%–50%), they are usually effective in preventing future variceal bleeding, and permitting significant recovery of liver function. Nonemergent, elective surgical shunt procedures (portacaval, splenorenal) may be performed in order to prevent initial or recurrent variceal hemorrhage. The portacaval shunt diverts the blood into the low pressure caval vein to reduce portal pressure (Fig. 81–3). This procedure involves anastomosis of the portal vein to the inferior vena cava. As a result, portal pressure decreases, and hepatic arterial flow increases; splanchnic venous pressure decreases, and collateral circulation disappears. The splen-

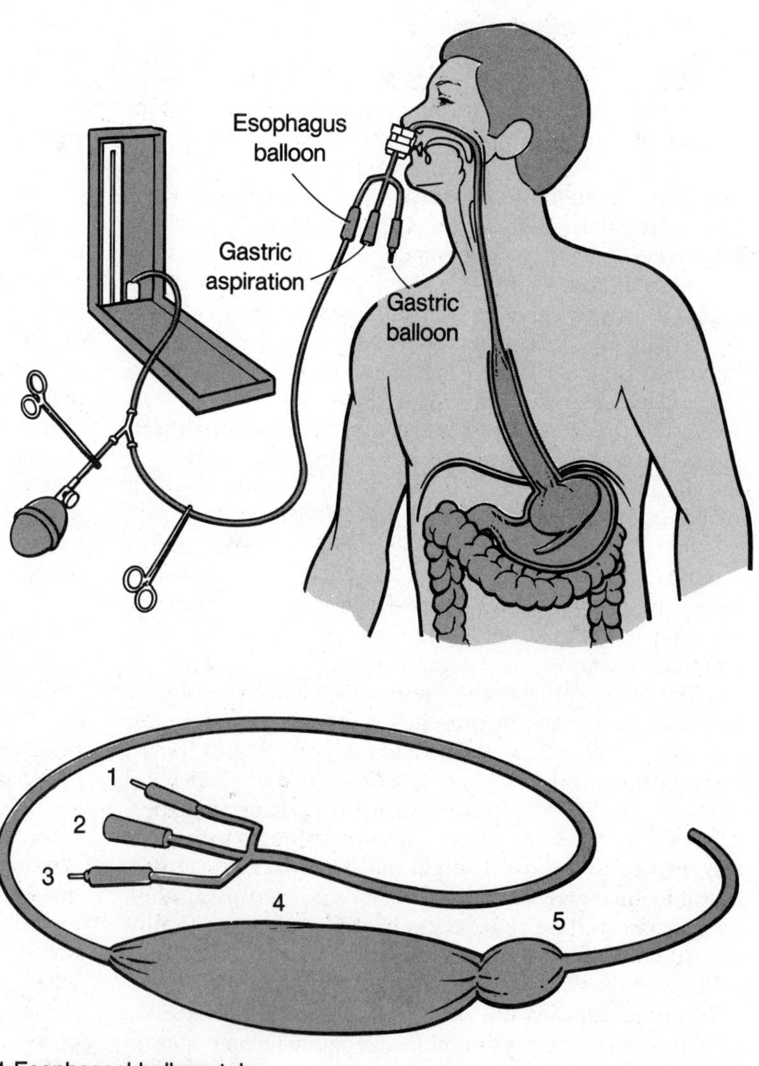

FIGURE 81–2 Use of Sengstaken-Blakemore tube to treat bleeding esophageal varices.

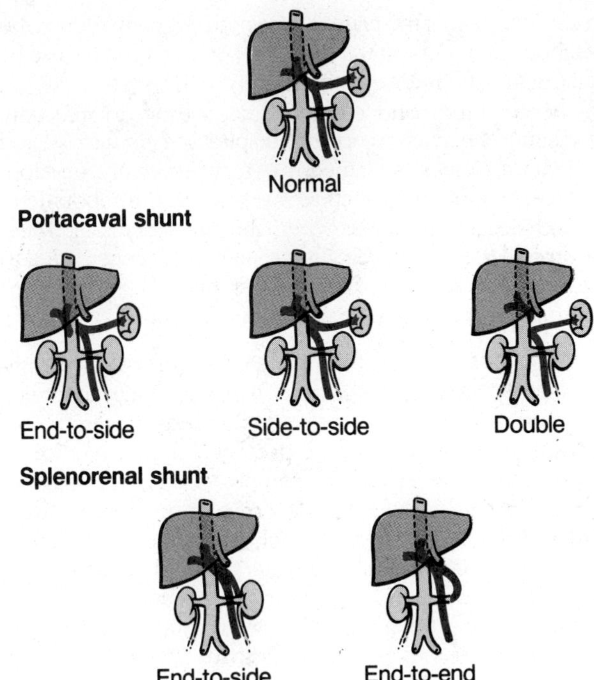

FIGURE 81-3 Schematic presentation of portacaval and splenorenal shunt procedures.

orenal shunt involves removal of the spleen with the anastomosis of the splenic vein to the left renal vein.[19]

Management of Fluid Retention and Ascites. In addition to prompt detection and correction of any variceal hemorrhage, patients suffering from alcoholic cirrhosis must often receive treatment for the complication of fluid retention. The cirrhotic patient with ascites should be placed on bedrest, and strict fluid and sodium restrictions should be instituted. Sodium intake is restricted to 30 mEq per day and fluid intake is limited to 1500 ml per day if hyponatremia is marked.[22] (At the same time, it is necessary to ensure that adequate amounts of protein and calories are ingested to promote healing of the damaged liver.) Loss of ascites should occur gradually in order to avoid serious consequences that may result from acute changes in plasma volume. The goal of therapy is aimed at a loss of not more than 1 kg/day of body weight in the presence of ascites and peripheral edema, and not more than 0.5 kg/day in patients with ascites only.[22] Daily weights monitor the amount of fluid lost.

If no change in weight is observed following 1 week of bed rest, and fluid and sodium restrictions, then spironolactone is administered. Small doses of furosemide may be administered with caution to patients whose ascites fails to respond to treatment. Aggressive diuretic therapy should be avoided because it may be complicated by depletion of plasma volume and reduction of renal function. It is necessary to continously monitor the patient's fluid and electrolyte status. Administration of albumin infusions may be necessary to restore plasma volume if significiant intravascular volume depletion occurs. Rapid diuresis of the patient may result in hypokalemic alkalosis, which enhances hepatic encephalopathy.[22]

Short-term control of intractable ascites may also be afforded through the surgical implantation of a plastic shunt between the peritoneal cavity and the superior vena cava (LaVeen shunt). As a result of this procedure, ascitic fluid is continuously reinfused into the venous system. This procedure may be accompanied by complications such as infection and disseminated intravascular coagulation.[22] It is contraindicated in patients with coma, varices infection, coagulopathy, or congestive failure.

Therapeutic paracentesis is performed when the cirrhotic patient with ascites is experiencing acute respiratory distress, or is in danger of rupturing an umbilical hernia. Up to 3 liters of ascites may be removed over a 4-hour period. Acites fluid removed in this way tends to reaccumulated within several days. The paracentesis may therefore need to be repeated until a diuresis is established. The paracentesis procedure should not be performed repeatedly in patients with cirrhosis because it may lead to protein and volume depletion, hemorrhage, infection of the ascitic fluid, and chronic ascites leak.[22]

Management of Hepatic Encephalopathy. An additional possible complication of alcoholic cirrhosis that requires prompt recognition and management is hepatic encephalopathy. All patients with alcoholic cirrhosis should be observed for personality changes, mood disturbances, confusion, inability to perform self-care activities, a deterioration in handwriting, unusual somnolence, and asterixis, which may signal the onset of hepatic encephalopathy. The treatment of this conditon centers around decreasing ammonia production in the colon and eliminating or treating factors that precipitate the encephalopathy,[6] such as upper gastrointestinal tract bleeding. Further, all protein should temporarily be removed from the diet until patient improvement is evidenced and protein can again be tolerated. (Chronic hepatic encephalopathy is treated with protein restriction of 30 or 40 g/day.) Fluid and electrolyte abnormalities such as hypokalemic alkalosis should be immediately corrected. Sedatives, analgesics, and tranquilizers previously prescribed should be discontinued since they cannot be metabolized by the liver.[22]

Prognosis

Patients with alcoholic cirrhosis who abstain from alcohol and maintain nutritionally well-balanced intakes have a 5-year survival rate of approximately 60%. Patients who continue to drink have a 40% 5-year survival rate. Death rates are higher in patients who experience complications of alcoholic cirrhosis such as variceal hemorrhage, ascites, or hepatic encephalopathy.

Nursing Management

Nursing Diagnosis

Nursing diagnoses for patients with cirrhosis of the liver are alterations in nutritional intake related to excessive ingestion of alcohol and decreased metabolic function of the liver; ineffective coping related to alcohol addiction; self-care deficit related to physiological changes from liver dysfunction and resulting physical debilitation; alterations in comfort related to pruritus and pain; potential hemorrhage related to altered clotting mechanisms and portal hypertension; alteration in fluid and electrolyte balance related to ascites; alteration in mental function related to increased level of serum ammonia; and knowledge deficit about treatment of the disease and follow-up care.

The extent of nursing care relative to each diagnosis will vary with the phase of illness, and the severity and duration of the disease. For example, nursing management when working with the newly diagnosed patient may emphasize assisting the patient to cope with the diagnosis and change behavior relative to alcoholic intake, whereas the emphasis may be on assisting in the physical treatment when the patient is hemorrhaging from esophageal varices.

Goals. Goals for the patient with alcoholic cirrhosis include an improved nutritional intake; increased tolerance of activity and the ability to perform activities of daily living; maintenance of skin integrity with an absence of skin breakdown; maintenance of comfort by diminishing pruritis and alleviating or minimizing pain; decreased risk of bleeding; decreased evidence of ascites and pedal edema; improved mental status; compliance with a program of abstinence from alcohol; and knowledge of discharge instructions and follow-up medical care.

Interventions

The patient with alcoholic cirrhosis is generally physically debilitated. Attempts are made to reverse this condition and correct the patient's nutritionally deficient status. Daily weights are maintained in addition to strict records of intake and output.

Nutritional Intake. Because of the importance of nutrition, the patient must be encouraged to eat. He should be offered three to four small meals supplemented with foods such as eggnog or ice cream, and low-sodium snacks. Encouragement to eat may be enhanced by provided palatable meals that are planned according to the patient's preferences as much as possible and that are served in an environment that is conducive to appetite stimulation.

Frequent oral hygiene may also make food more appealing to the patient. In the presence of nausea, antiemetics should be administered 30 to 45 minutes prior to the meal. (Compazine and Vistaril should be avoided as these drugs depend on the liver for detoxification.) Patients who have severe anorexia, those who are vomiting, or those who are just unable to eat may require feeding by nasogastric tube or parenteral hyperalimentation.

When hepatic encephalopathy is present, protein is temporarily eliminated from the diet. Foods or fluids high in carbohydrates are administered to the patient instead. As the patient improves, protein intake is restored to a level that is tolerable and safe. (For example, protein may be added in increments of 20 g up to a total of 60 g.)[19]

Managing Fatigue. An impaired nutritional status may contribute to the patient's easy fatigability and decreased activity level. The patient must be protected against excessive fatigue. Bed rest is recommended, and nursing care focuses on conservation of the patient's strength. Rest will reduce the metabolic demands on the liver, conserve oxygen for use by vital organs, and increases the liver's blood supply.

Because the patient is more susceptible to infection, efforts must be taken to prevent respiratory, circulatory, and vascular difficulties. Such measures may prevent the development of complications such as pneumonia, thrombophlebitis, and decubitus ulcers. When the nutritional status improves and the patient regains strength, he is encouraged to gradually increase his activity. Rest periods are planned along with increasing activity and mild exercise.[9,42]

Skin Care. Care of the patient's skin is of utmost importance in view of the increased susceptibility to breakdown and infection. Such susceptibility results from the patient's decreased mobility, the presence of any jaundice or subcutaneous edema, and the compromised nutritional and immune status. The use of an alternating pressure mattress or foam egg-crate mattress will help guard against decubitus development. In addition, the patient should be turned and his position changed every 2 hours if he is unable to do this for himself. Skin trauma may be prevented by avoiding the use of adhesive tapes and irritating soaps. The application of lotion may be soothing to the skin. Because the skin over the abdomen is generally quite taut, gentle applications of lotion to this particular area may provide comfort.[19]

The presence of pruritus may be quite uncomfortable for the patient. Attempts should be made to prevent dry skin by avoiding soaps and applying oil-based lotions. Administration of antihistamines and cholestyramine (Cuemid) may also provide relief. Generally, 6 to 10 mg of Cuemid is administered daily, and relief is obtained in 4 to 7 days.[19]

Pain Management. Patient comfort may also be adversely affected by the presence of pain (especially cramping of the small bowel and aching in the region of the liver). The status of the patient's pain should be assessed and appropriate measures should be instituted to alleviate it. Techniques such as distraction, relaxation, cutaneous stimulation, and positioning may prove to be useful adjuncts or replacements to analgesic therapy. Caution must be taken when administering analgesics to the patient with alcoholic cirrhosis. Analgesics such as morphine, acetaminophen, codeine, and Darvon are metabolized by the liver and should be restricted when liver disease is severe.[19]

Bleeding Precaution. Any evidence of bleeding should be immediately reported. The nurse should institute appropriate preventive measures to protect the patient from trauma and bruising. Side rails can be padded for protection. Any patient ambulation should be done with assistance. When injections are given, the smallest-gauge needle possible should be used. Following the injection, pressure should be applied to the site until all evidence of bleeding has stopped. Soft-bristled toothbrushes are recommended to guard against any gingival trauma. A soft diet will guard against mechanical trauma to weakened varices. The patient should further be instructed against straining at stool, vigorous nose-blowing, and coughing. The patient's urine, stools, and emesis should be observed for bleeding.[42] Salicylates and any drugs that erode esophageal mucosa should be avoided.

Hemorrhaging esophageal varices is an emergency required immediate intervention to prevent shock and death. Maintenance of a patent airway is the immediate priority; the patient should be positioned on his side to facilitiate this. The patient's vital signs should be monitored frequently (every 15 min) during the acute bleeding episode. The nurse should be alert to the signs of hypovolemia (cold, clammy skin; blood pressure drop; tachycardia; restlessness; and increased or shallow peripheral pulse). Arterial or central venous pressure (CVP) readings will also be taken frequently to monitor the patient's blood volume status. The patient often requires oxygen to prevent hypoxia. The patient will require intravenous fluids to maintain fluid and electrolyte balance. He will also require a Foley catheter to facilitate hourly urine output measurements. (Urinary output should be maintained between 30 and 50 ml/hr.) Replacement of lost blood by transfusions of fresh blood is also important.

Sengstaken-Blakemore Tube Management. The Sengstaken-Blakemore tube has three openings: one for gastric aspiration, one for inflating the esophageal balloon, and one for inflating the gastric balloon (see Fig. 81–2). The function of each lumen should be clearly marked. The esophageal balloon, which applies direct pressure to the esophageal veins, is inflated usually to a pressure of 20 to 40 mmHg, and the gastric balloon, which applies pressure at the cardiac orifice of the stomach, is inflated to keep the tube in place. Traction may be applied to the tube to prevent the gastric balloon from falling back into the stomach. The third lumen is used to suction blood and gastric secretions from the stomach. Iced saline lavage may be used in the stomach balloon in order to decrease blood flow and cause vasoconstriction.

The nurse must know how much pressure should exist in both balloons and how much traction should be applied. Ulceration may develop in the stomach or esophagus if the tube is left in place too long or at too high a pressure. To guard against this the balloon may be deflated for 5 minutes at periodic intervals. There is a chance that the tube might rupture causing airway obstruction and aspiration of gastric contents. Asphyxiation may result from the traction pulling the tube into the oropharynx. Because of the possibility of complications, the patient must be observed very closely.[9]

To prevent gastric acid reflux and to facilitate ventilation, the patient with an esophageal tube is placed in a low or semi-Fowler's position. The nurse should listen to the patient's lung sounds frequently to assess for any signs of aspiration of secretions. Airway obstruction may occur because secretions cannot easily pass around the tube. Oropharyngeal suction may be indicated.[19]

Vasopressin may be administered to the patient also in an attempt to temporarily control bleeding. The effectiveness of this treatment is evidenced by the appearance of the gastric draining. Bleeding should be controlled by this method in 4 to 6 hours.[42]

Respiratory Care. Postoperative nursing care of the patient having a shunt procedure is similar to that required for general abdominal surgery. A vigorous program to maintain a clear airway should be strictly followed postoperatively. The patient is at high risk for pulmonary complications because of the close proximity of the surgical area to the diaphragm and the possible presence of ascites. The nurse should be aware of the possible complications that may arise postoperatively including hemodynamic shock, hepatic encephalopathy, electrolyte imbalance, metabolic and respiratory alkalosis, delirium tremens, and seizures.[9]

The patient with cirrhosis and ascites may experience dyspnea, which may be indicative of either ascites accumulation or hydrothorax. Ventilation is facilitated by placing the patient in a low or semi-Fowler's position and providing pillows for support, especially under the abdomen.

Neurological Concerns. Nursing care requires comprehensive, ongoing assessment and documentation of the patient's mental and neurological status. When patients have jaundice, ascites, and portal hypertension, signs of coma should be expected. Most drugs in the sedative, antiemetic, analgesic, and tranquilizer categories are metabolized by the liver; therefore, they should be avoided.

Treatment of hepatic coma may require administration of magnesium sulfate and normal saline enemas to inhibit further ammonia formation and remove blood from the intestine. Neomycin is given orally to inhibit the formation of ammonia. In addition, oral administration of lactulose or enemas of lactulose decrease ammonia absorption.

Psychosocial Support. It is evident that the patient suffering from alcoholic cirrhosis is one who faces numerous serious disease complications and requires comprehensive physical care. Because the patient faces such rigorous therapy and in addition is required to permanently abstain from alcohol, he requires patient and thoughtful psychological guidance and support. The patient's unwillingness or inability to comply is understandable. He must, however, understand the detrimental implications of his continued drinking as they relate to his own health and the lives of others. Support and guidance in this difficult effort may be provided to patients and family members through affiliation with organizations such as Alcoholics Anonymous, Al-Anon, and Ala-Teen.

Discharge Planning. In preparation for discharge, members of the health care team provide comprehensive discharge teaching to the patient and family members. Written instructions should specifically outline the patient's dietary recommendations and restrictions. The patient should also be provided with detailed information outlining the types of medications he is receiving. He should have an understanding of his physical limitations and under what circumstances the physician should be notified. He should have knowledge of his follow-up medical appointment following discharge, and understand the importance of periodic medical examinations. A visiting nurse may provide additional care and support in the home that is needed and desired by the patient and family.

Evaluation

Outcome criteria for goal achievement are as follows:

1. The patient reports a food intake which is consistent with a nutritionally balanced diet.

2. Weight gain without increased edema or ascites is evident.
3. The patient reports a decrease or an absence of anorexia and gastrointestinal disturbances.
4. The patient demonstrates an increase in performance of activities of daily living.
5. Skin integrity is maintained.
6. The patient reports a decrease or an absence of pruritus and pain.
7. There is an absence of signs of bleeding (stool negative for occult blood, no emesis, vital signs stable).
8. There is a decrease in or an absence of pedal edema.
9. The patient is oriented and converses appropriately.
10. The patient accurately describes treatment to be followed.
11. The patient and family report abstinence from alcohol.

References

1. Adams JT, Poulter CA, Pandya KJ: Cancer of the major digestive glands: Pancreas, liver bile ducts, gallbladder. In Rubin P (ed): Clinical Oncology, A Multidisciplinary Approach, 6th ed, pp 178–189. American Cancer Society, 1983
2. Adson MA: Diagnosis and surgical treatment of primary and secondary solid hepatic tumors in the adult. Surg Clin North Am 61(1):181–196, 1981
3. Band PR, Beck IT, Dinner PJ, Miller AB: Two-year follow-up study of patients with known serum concentrations of carcinoembryonic antigen. Can Med Assoc J 117(6):657–659, 1977
4. Baker SR, Krause CJ: Cancer of the lip. In Suen JY, Myers EN (eds): Cancer of the Head and Neck, pp 280–300. New York, Churchill Livingstone, 1981
5. Bates RR: Chemical carcinogenesis and the pancreas. J Surg Oncol 7(2):143–149, 1975
6. Borowsky SA: Cirrhosis. In Gitnick G (ed): Gastroenterology, pp 213–232. New York, John Wiley & Sons, 1983
7. Brooks WS, Moore MR: Carcinoma of the colon. In Galambos JT, Hersh T (eds): Digestive Disease, pp 522–529. Boston, Butterworth Publishers, 1983
8. Brunner L: Medical and nursing postoperative management for Whipple procedure. Nursing '73 3(12):48–49, 1973
9. Brunner LS, Suddarth DS: Textbook of Medical Surgical Nursing, 5th ed. Philadelphia, JB Lippincott, 1984
10. Calcaterra TC, Juillard G: Head and neck neoplasms; Cancer of the oral cavity and oropharynx. In Haskell CM (ed): Cancer Treatment, pp 522–568. Philadelphia, WB Saunders, 1980
11. Deer DA: The role of radiotherapy in combined treatment of malignant neoplasms of the head and neck. In Donald PJ (ed): Head and Neck Cancer: Management of the Difficult Case, pp 340–358. Philadelphia, WB Saunders, 1984
12. del Regato JA, Spjut HJ: Cancer of the digestive tract. In Ackerman and del Regato's Cancer: Diagnosis, Treatment, and Prognosis, 5th ed. pp 572–611. St Louis, CV Mosby, 1977
13. Donald PJ: Oropharynx and tongue base. In Donald PJ (ed): Head and Neck Cancer: Management of the DIfficult Case, pp 40–61. Philadelphia, WB Saunders, 1984
14 Eddy DM: Guidelines for the cancer-related checkup: Recommendations and rationale. CA 30(4):208–215, 1980
15. Errington RD: The role of conventional and fast neutron radiotherapy. In Hodgson HJF, Bloom SR (eds): Gastrointestinal and Hepatobiliary Cancer, pp 355–375. Boston, Butterworth Publishers, 1983
16. Fitzpatrick PJ: Cancer of the lip. Otolaryngology 13(1):32–36, 1984
17. Galambos JT: Bleeding varices. In Galambos JT, Hersh T (eds): Digestive Disease, pp 433–441. Boston, Butterworth Publishers, 1983
18. Galambos JT: Cirrhosis. In Galambos JT, Hersh T (eds): Digestive Diseases, pp 408–432. Boston, Butterworth Publishers, 1983
19. Given BA, Simmons SJ: Gastroenterology in Clinical Nursing, 4th ed. St Louis, CV Mosby, 1984
20. Hersh T: Carcinoma of the pancreas. In Galambos JT, Hersh T (eds): Digestive Diseases, pp 344–348. Boston, Butterworth Publishers, 1983
21. Higginson J, Muir CS: Epidemiology of cancer. In Holland JF, Frei E III (eds): Cancer Medicine, pp 257–327. Philadelphia, Lea & Febiger, 1982
22. LaMont JT, Koff RS, Isselbacher KJ: Cirrhosis. In Petersdorf RG, Adams RD, Braunwald E, Isselbacher KJ, Martin JB, Wilson JD (eds): Harrison's Principles of Internal Medicine, 10th ed. 10, pp 1804–1978. New York, McGraw-Hill, 1984
23. Leffall LD, Stearns MW: Early diagnosis of colorectal cancer. CA 24(2 & 3):152–159, 1974
24. Macdonald JS: Gastrointestinal Cancer: Update 1984. Chicago, Sieber & McIntyre, 1984
25. Macdonald JS, Gunderson LL, Cohn I Jr: Cancer of the pancreas. In DeVita VT, Hellman S, Rosenberg SA (eds): Principles and Practice of Oncology, pp 563–589. Philadelphia, JB Lippincott, 1981
26. Macdonald JS, Gunderson LL, Cohn I Jr: Cancer of the stomach. In DeVita VT, Hellman S, Rosenberg SA (eds): Principles and Practice of Oncology, pp 534–562. Philadelphia, JB Lippincott, 1981
27. MacMahon B: Risk factors for cancer of the pancreas. Cancer 50(11):2676–2680, 1982
28. Mancuso TF, El-Attaw AA: Cohort study of workers exposed to betanaphthylamine and benzidine. J Occup Med 9(6):277–285, 1967
29. Martis CS: Carcinoma of the tongue: Evaluation of surgical treatment of 123 cases. J Oral Maxillofac Surg 40(6):277–347, 1982
30. Moertel CG: The esophagus. In Holland JF, Frei E III (eds): Cancer Medicine, pp 1739–1753. Philadelphia, Lea & Febiger, 1982
31. Moertel CG: Small intestine. In Holland JF, Frei E III (eds): Cancer Medicine, pp 1808–1818. Philadelphia, Lea & Febiger, 1982
32. Moertel CG. Thynne GS: Large bowel. In Holland JF, Frei E III (eds): Cancer Medicine, pp 1830–1859. Philadelphia, Lea & Febiger, 1982
33. Morton JM, Poulter CA, Pandya KJ: Alimentary tract cancer. In Rubin P (ed): Clinical Oncology, A Multidisciplinary Approach, 6th ed, pp 154–176. American Cancer Society, 1983
34. Ramming KP: Management of malignancies of the gastrointestinal tract. In Gitnick G (ed): Gastroenterology, pp 323–368. New York, John Wiley & Sons, 1983
35. Recht KA, Belis JA, Kandzari SJ et al: Ureterosigmoidostomy followed by carcinoma of the colon. Cancer 44(4): 1538–1542, 1979
36. Roseberg JC, Schwade JG, Vaitkevicius VK: Cancer of the esophagus. In DeVita VT, Hellman S. Rosenberg SA (eds): Principles and Practice of Oncology, pp 499–533. Philadelphia, JB Lippincott, 1981
37. Shedd DP: Cancer of the head and neck. In Holland JF, Frei E III (eds): Cancer Medicine, pp 1671–1685. Philadelphia, Lea & Febiger, 1982
38. Silverberg E, Lubera JA: Cancer statistics, 1983. CA 33(1):9–25, 1983

39. Speese-Owens N, Rutkowski J: Nursing care of the patient with cancer of the gastrointestinal system. In Bouchard-Kurtz R, Speese-Owens N: Nursing Care of the Cancer Patient, 4th ed, pp 358–387. St Louis, CV Mosby, 1981
40. Trias AA, Fresneda AC, Semeraro C: Surgical treatment of carcinoma of the lip. J Dermatol Surg Oncol 8(5):367–376, 1982
41. Wang CC: Radiation Therapy for Head and Neck Neoplasms. Boston, John Wright—PSG, 1983
42. Watson JE: Medical-Surgical Nursing and Related Physiology, 2nd ed. Toronto, WB Saunders, 1979
43. Wynder EL, Bross IJ: A study of etiological factors in cancer of the esophagus. Cancer 14(2):389–413, 1961
44. Zagars G, Norante JD: Head and neck tumors. In Rubin P (ed): Clinical Oncology, A Multidisciplinary Approach, 6th ed, pp 230–261. American Cancer Society, 1983

Chapter 82

Infectious and Inflammatory Gastrointestinal Disorders

Margaret Heitkemper
Deborah Martin

Infection and inflammation of the gastrointestinal (GI) tract occur in patients as a result of a variety of factors including environmental, genetic, and autoimmune. Regardless of the precipitating factor, the problems produced by both inflammation and infection will depend upon the area or organ involved, the severity of the disease, and the degree of malabsorption or malnutrition. Infectious agents affect primarily the stomach, intestine, and liver, while inflammation, which occurs in response to infection, injury, or autoimmune disease, may occur in any organ of the GI tract including the liver, pancreas, or gallbladder.

Common problems associated with infection or inflammatory diseases are those related to the inflammatory process, malabsorption, and fluid and electrolyte imbalances. This chapter will consider common infections and inflammatory diseases in the same order that food and fluid enter and leave the body; therefore it will start with infectious disorders affecting the oral cavity.

Herpes Simplex

A relatively common infectious disorder affecting the lips in adults is herpes simplex. Herpes simplex viruses (HSV) belong to a large family of DNA (deoxyribonucleic acid) viruses called the herpes viruses. The initial infection with each virus is called a *primary infection.* Each of the herpes viruses, including HSV, has the capability of persisting in the host after the primary infection has resolved. HSV resides in neural cells and is capable of reactivation at a later time. A recurrent infection is said to occur at the time of reactivation.

Herpes simplex viruses are commonly identified as two serotypes (HSV-1, HSV-2). In the majority of cases, HSV-1 is involved in infections of the mouth, with HSV-2 involved in genital tract infections. The incubation period of HSV infections ranges from 2 to 20 days. The source of HSV which infects man *is* man alone: there is no animal reservoir. Close contact is required for the spread of herpetic infections. Primary infection occurs when the virus (in contaminated secretions) is introduced into the body by a mucous membrane or through a cut on the skin surface. The person spreading the virus may or may not have a clinically apparent lesion. For approximately 3 to 4 weeks after the primary infection, virus particles continue to be shed. The length of viral shedding is shorter (3–5 days) after recurrent infections. Nosocomial transmission of herpes virus I has occurred in an intensive care unit.

Etiology and Pathophysiology

Once the HSV enters a cell, it begins to replicate and produces mature virions which take over the cell machinery.

The vesicle, which forms on the skin as a result of HSV infection, contains leukocytes, multinucleated giant cells, and swollen epidermal cells.[13] Necrosis occurs only in deep tissue infections. After the active infection resolves, the viral particles travel up the peripheral nerves and maintain themselves in sensory nerve ganglia. Reactivation occurs when some stimulus (*e.g.,* cold, fever, menses, stress, trauma) releases the viral particles, and they retrace their journey down the nerve to the skin. There they multiply, and new lesions occur. Recurrent infections tend to occur at the same site as the initial infection. Individuals with impaired immunity, especially cell-mediated immunity, have the most severe infections.

Clinical Manifestations

Primary infections of herpes simplex can occur at the mucocutaneous junction on the skin, in the mouth, tonsils, and genital areas. Lesions appear as numerous, small vesicles which turn into shallow, gray, painful ulcers. Infections of the lips and mouth, the most common site of infection, can range from nonapparent to severe gingivostomatitis. In addition to the blisters, symptoms often include fever, constitutional signs, and local adenopathy. Primary infections are more severe than recurrent infections. Primary infections may persist for 2 to 3 weeks, whereas recurrent infections usually resolve within a week.

More severe infections are associated with severe health problems such as burned patients and immunocompromised cancer patients. Patients with cancer involving the lymphatic and hematopoietic systems, or transplant patients, often experience recurring herpes infections due to alterations in their immune systems from their therapy or disease processes. Manifestations of more severe infection can include not only local signs of herpes, but esophageal involvement, encephalitis, meningitis, or disseminated infections as well.

Medical Management

Patients with herpes simplex (HSV-1) do not normally require medical intervention, though they may develop these infections while hospitalized for other reasons. Immunocompromised patients may experience disseminated herpes and will require medical care.

Nursing Management

Nursing Diagnosis

The nurse should determine the patient's understanding of herpes simplex I and how to prevent its spread. The hospital nurse should assess for its presence in immunocompromised patients with a history of herpes infections.

Goals. The major nursing goals are to prevent the spread of herpes within the hospital and educate the patient to understand the disease and prevent its spread.

Interventions

The nurse must take precautions to prevent transfer of the herpes viruses of an infected patient to him- herself or to another patient. When coming into direct contact with herpetic lesions or secretions, contact isolation protocols should be followed. For this type of isolation, gloves and gowns are used if infective material will be touched, and masks are used if the nurse will have close contact with the patient. Handwashing is essential after caring for these persons.

Herpes simplex can be transmitted even though active lesions are not obvious. Therefore, the routine use of gloves during oral and tracheal suctioning is a good prophylactic measure.

Patients with localized infections should be taught the length of the infectious period and how to avoid infecting others. For example, persons with herpes simplex I should not kiss others until the lesions have healed.

Evaluation

Outcome criteria are: (1) absence of spread of infection, (2) patient accurately describes the disease and how to prevent its spread, and (3) patient reports behavior compatible with prevention of spread.

Dental Caries and Periodontal Disease

The two most common infectious/inflammatory conditions affecting the teeth are dental caries and periodontal disease. Dental caries are cavities in the enamel of the teeth. Periodontal disease is an inflammatory degenerative condition of the supporting structures of the teeth. Both of these diseases are chronic in nature and have alternating periods of tissue damage and repair. The diseases affect children and adults of all ages.

Etiology and Pathophysiology

The causative factor for both dental caries and periodontal disease is the thin film of saliva, bacteria, and bacterial end products that covers the teeth (dental plaque) and a diet that contains refined carbohydrates. Refined carbohydrates provide the nutrients for bacteria to metabolize and produce acid. The bacterial acid in the dental plaque removes the tooth mineral (demineralization) by a process of microscopic penetrations of the enamel surface (pores) and eventual penetration of bacteria. When a cavity finally occurs, it becomes a site for producing a bacterial population which is then available to seed other areas in the mouth. Dental caries are a potential problem as long as natural teeth are retained.

Periodontal disease results from the action of the metabolic end products of the bacteria on the gingiva. The initial lesion is inflamed gums. As the disease progresses, the space between the gingiva and the tooth (sulcus) deepens and the extent of inflammation increases. Eventually, the inflammatory process damages the epithelial attachment to the tooth (at the bottom of the sulcus) and the danger of chronic infection increases. The disease may progress over many years to involve loss of connective tissue and bone. The loss of supporting tissue causes the teeth to become mobile, and the teeth are lost if the disease is not treated.

Clinical Manifestations

Examination of the oral cavity of a person with dental caries would reveal plaque buildup on the teeth. The patient might complain of tooth pain. If the patient has periodontal disease, the gums would be inflamed, hypertrophied, painful, and may bleed. The teeth may be loose.

Medical Management

The physician notes the condition of the teeth as part of the physical examination, and if necessary the patient is referred to a dentist for treatment of dental caries and periodontal disease. If treated early, both conditions can be prevented from requiring extraction. If infection is present in a patient who is hospitalized for another problem, the physician may treat the condition with antibiotics to prevent the spread of infection and refer the patient to the dentist after discharge.

Nursing Management

Nursing Diagnosis

The nursing diagnoses related to dental condition are alteration in comfort, impairment of oral hygiene, potential for oral infection, potential for inadequate nutritional intake, and knowledge deficit. A nursing assessment should include examination of the oral cavity. Teeth with heavy dental plaque can be a source of infection especially in the patient having a surgical procedure or the patient who is critically ill.

Goals. The goals of nursing care are to assist the patient in achieving a clean oral cavity and to teach the patient how to prevent development of dental caries and periodontal disease.

Interventions

If the gums are painful and swollen, warm saline mouth rinses will cleanse and soothe the tissues. Water should be used because it has a neutral pH of 7.0. As a cleansing agent, hydrogen peroxide will oxidize protein and thereby remove organisms from inaccessible areas, especially deep sulci. Brushing and flossing will help to remove plaque.

An important nursing function is to teach hospitalized patients and the public how to prevent caries and periodontal disease. The three approaches are to reduce bacterial contact with the teeth, reduce the intake of sugar, and increase the resistance of teeth with appropriate use of fluorides. Teeth should be brushed after eating using a fluoride toothpaste. The brushing should be thorough (3–5 minutes), should include all available surfaces, and the bristles should be angled toward the gums to assure that they enter crevices. Flossing should follow brushing to reduce the extent of plaque between the teeth.

The development of dental caries is related to the intake of sugar. When sugar and bacteria are present, acid production occurs. Frequent intake of sugar is more harmful than eating a large amount at one time because in the former situation the teeth are continuously exposed to the sugar. If the sugar is eaten, the teeth should be brushed thoroughly after ingestion or at least the mouth rinsed with water. Another means of modifying the effect of sugar is to eat a piece of cheese or some nuts after the sweets as these foods will decrease the amount of acid production.

Fluoridation of water supply in the community results in a reduction in the incidence of dental caries. Topical fluoride application and fluoride rinses increase resistance to caries. They are also recommended for prevention of periodontal disease. Daily use of fluoride solutions disrupts bacterial metabolism and the production of acid end products.

Evaluation

The criteria for goal achievement are: (1) the teeth are clean and the gingiva are not inflamed, (2) the patient can accurately describe oral hygiene measures that will prevent dental caries and periodontal disease, and (3) the patient reports adhering to the measures taught. In the community, a follow-up survey of the group taught (*e.g.,* school children, adult groups) would indicate adherence to the preventive measures.

Infections of the Oral Cavity

The most common infections of the oral cavity and salivary glands are necrotizing gingivitis (Vincent's stomatitis), parotitis, and Ludwig's angina. Necrotizing gingivitis is an ulceromembranous infectious disease affecting the gingiva, tonsils, pharynx, and mucous membrane of the oral cavity. Parotitis is an inflammation of the parotid gland. Ludwig's angina is an infection of the sublingual and submandibular spaces.

Etiology and Pathophysiology

The initiating factors in oral infections are poor oral hygiene, dental caries, and abscesses, and a high bacterial population in the oral cavity. Contributing factors are low tissue resistance because of nutritional deficiency and marginal general health status. The organisms are usually a combination of an anaerobic spirochete and fusiform bacillus. Parotitis can also result from dehydration and increased salivation.

Clinical Manifestations

The oral cavity of the patient with an infection is inflamed, painful, and the gums usually are bleeding. The breath is malodorous. The gums may be ulcerated and covered with a gray exudate. The systemic signs of infection (fever, leukocytosis) are present as is lymphadenopathy. If the tonsils and pharynx are affected, the patient may complain of a sore throat and difficulty in swallowing. Severe edema could precipitate respiratory distress. The onset of parotitis is usually sudden. The gland becomes swollen, tender, warm to touch, and reddened. It is accompanied by chills, fever, and leukocytosis. Postoperative patients are at risk especially if they become dehydrated or do not receive adequate oral hygiene.

Medical Management

Diagnosis. A scraping of the affected tissue will produce secretions for a culture. Microscopic examination of the culture identifies the causative organisms.

Treatment. The treatment consists of oral hygiene to clean the mouth, debridement of the exudate, and antimicrobial therapy. Antibiotics prescribed are usually penicillin G or chloramphenicol. If the airway becomes obstructed, a tracheostomy would be performed.

Prognosis. Prompt treatment with an appropriate antibiotic will usually control the infection. Prevention of reinfection is dependent on oral hygiene and dental treatment.

Nursing Management

Nursing Diagnosis

The common nursing diagnoses for patients with oral cavity infections are alteration in comfort, alteration in nutritional intake, potential for spread of infection, and knowledge deficit regarding oral hygiene. The discomfort and inadequate nutritional intake are related to the inflamed, painful, and bleeding condition of the gums, the fetid odor, and loss of appetite. The systemic signs of infection, fever and malaise, contribute to the discomfort.

Goals. The goals of nursing care are to prevent parotitis postoperatively, promote adequate fluid intake, relieve discomfort, improve oral hygiene status, teach the patient measures to prevent recurrence of the problem, and assist in controlling the infection.

Interventions

Identification of patients at high risk for parotitis is essential. These patients should be taught how to do thorough oral hygiene preoperatively. Postoperatively, the nurse should maintain good oral hygiene if the patient is unable to do this care. Adequate fluid intake should be encouraged or, if the patient is not permitted oral fluids, frequent saline mouth rinses are necessary.

Discomfort may be relieved with warm saline mouth rinses, and the use of hydrogen peroxide rinses will clear the oral cavity. Administration of analgesics is important for pain relief.

Adequate nutritional intake of vitamin C for wound healing is encouraged through offering bland fruit juices such as cranberry juice. Fluids will be less irritating than a diet of solid foods. Milk shakes, ice cream, custards, and other bland foods may be tolerated if the infection is not severe.

Administration of prescribed antibiotics is essential for control of the infection. The patient must be monitored for signs of respiratory distress. To prevent recurrence of the infection, the patient and family are taught the oral hygiene measures described for the prevention of dental caries.

Evaluation

The criteria for goal achievement are:

1. No evidence of parotitis in postoperative patients.
2. Patient reports a decrease or absence of discomfort following analgesic administration and oral hygiene.
3. Temperature and leukocyte count returns to normal range.
4. Patient describes oral hygiene measures that will prevent recurrence.
5. Patient reports using preventive measures.
6. Patient reports no difficulty with respiration, or if patient's respirations become difficult and the swelling increases, the physician is consulted immediately. A tracheostomy tray is kept in the patient's room.

Gastritis

As the name implies, gastritis is an inflammation of the gastric mucosa. Gastritis is generally classified as either acute superficial gastritis or chronic gastritis. These types are markedly different both in terms of etiology and course of the disease. Acute gastritis is frequently the result of ingestion of an irritating or contaminated substance and is self-limiting, while chronic gastritis is an ongoing problem which will result in the loss of normal gastric mucosa.

Acute Gastritis

Acute gastritis is a benign and self-limiting inflammation of the gastric mucosa which is usually due to an exogenous substance, that is, the ingestion of an irritating substance. Endoscopic exam of the stomach of a person with acute gastritis reveals a reddened and edematous gastric mucosa and possibly the presence of superficial erosions in the mucosa layer. Abstinence from the causative agent will facilitate the healing of the injured mucosa.

Etiology and Pathophysiology

Causative factors include chemicals (*e.g.*, alcohol, salicylates, caffeine, spicy foods), mechanical or thermal injury, or ingestion of bacteria in contaminated food. Reflux of duodenal contents containing bile acids (as a result of vigorous vomiting) into the stomach will also produce acute gastritis and, if repeated or prolonged, can result in chronic gastritis or predispose to gastric ulcer formation.

Regardless of the etiologic factor, in acute gastritis the irritation of, or injury to, the gastric mucosa evokes a local inflammatory response. The mucosa becomes edematous with inflammatory cells moving into the affected area, and vascular congestion results. Small areas of erosion of the gastric mucosa may also be present in one spot or throughout the stomach.

Clinical Manifestations

A few hours after the ingestion of an irritating substance the patient complains of epigastric pressure or pain, and malaise. Depending upon the severity of inflammation and extent of area involved, the patient may experience nausea and/or vomiting. Diarrhea may occur if the small and large intestines are involved as well.

Medical Management

Diagnosis is generally by the patient's history. Upon abdominal exam the patient may have some epigastric tenderness. Patients with acute gastritis are often treated on an outpatient basis. The focus of treatment is on symptomatic relief as well as prevention of recurrence. Symptomatic relief may mean restricting food intake until the inflammation and nausea and vomiting have subsided. Antacids may be beneficial to patients who experience epigastric discomfort. Due to the regenerative ability of the gastric epithelium, acute gastritis is self-limiting, and the chances for complete recovery are excellent

Nursing Management

Nursing Diagnosis and Goal. Because the patient with acute gastritis is treated primarily on an outpatient basis, the office nurse or emergency room nurse will determine the patient's awareness of etiologic factors and need for education relative to prevention and carrying out of prescribed therapy. The patient may also need to be evaluated relative to knowledge of medications or foods which are known irritants to the gastric mucosa. The goal is to assist the patient in taking appropriate action to prevent recurrence.

Interventions. Patients may require information regarding use of antacids (*e.g.,* timing dosages, side-effects) and other medications which may be prescribed for symptomatic treatment. Nutrition should be discussed with the patient and counseling given regarding the use of spicy foods and fluids containing caffeine. When acute gastritis is the result of chronic alcohol abuse, the patient should be counseled to seek assistance for alcohol abuse.

Evaluation. Outcome criteria are a decrease in the incidence of acute gastritis and a report by the patient of a change in nutrition and use of medications as prescribed. Patients with alcohol as a problem would report seeking assistance to overcome alcohol dependence.

Chronic Gastritis

Chronic gastritis or chronic inflammation of the gastric mucosa is a relatively common disorder which develops over a period of months to years. The incidence of chronic gastritis, which is characterized by a thinning of the gastric mucosa and decreased hydrochloric acid (HCl) secretion, increases with age. A variety of exogenous and endogenous factors has been associated with the etiology of gastritis. There now appear to be multiple types of gastritis which differ relative to etiology, location, progression, and treatment.

Etiology and Pathophysiology

Several etiologic mechanisms may be involved in the production of chronic gastritis. It may be the result of an autoimmune disorder. Antibodies directed against the parietal cells have been isolated from patients with chronic gastritis. Concomitantly, these patients frequently have pernicious anemia due to decreased secretion of intrinsic factor and thus decreased absorption of vitamin B_{12} in the ileum. In this type of gastritis, there is a loss of gastric mucosa and a hyposecretion of hydrochloric acid. The fundus and corpus of the stomach are primarily involved. This type of gastritis is frequently referred to as *Type A gastritis.*

Hypersecretory chronic gastritis is frequently seen in patients with peptic ulcer disease. Hypersecretion of hydrochloric acid may result in chronic gastritis, ulcer formation, or both.

Chronic gastritis may also be produced by reflux of duodenal contents containing bile acids into the stomach. The bile acids are destructive to the gastric mucosa and thus result in inflammation. The presence of bile acids in the stomach has also been associated with gastric ulcer formation. Chronic gastritis can occur as a result of prolonged use of gastric irritants such as alcohol and heavy cigarette smoking. This type of gastritis is more diffuse, that is, it is located throughout the stomach rather than one specific anatomical location and it also results in atrophy of the gastric mucosa.

Clinical Manifestations

The symptoms of chronic gastritis will depend upon the etiologic factors and the extent of inflammation. Patients with chronic gastritis may be asymptomatic until sufficient damage is done to result in a decreased gastric-emptying rate which makes the patient experience abdominal discomfort after meals. With the loss of intrinsic factor, patients will develop anemia and, as a result, experience fatigue and neurological problems due to decreased vitamin B_{12} absorption. Patients with gastritis as a result of hypersecretion of acid will experience symptoms similar to peptic ulcer disease, (*e.g.,* epigastric distress). With reflux of duodenal contents, patients frequently experience epigastric distress as well as nausea and possibly vomiting. With advanced gastritis patients may complain of postprandial epigastric heaviness, pyrosis, sour taste, nausea, and vomitus.

Medical Management

Diagnosis Definitive diagnosis of chronic gastritis is by endoscopic visualization and gastric biopsy. Gastric biopsy is also performed to rule out other pathologic changes such as cellular dysplasia. Due to the superficial nature of gastritis, radioscopic visualization is not always beneficial. Gastric secretory studies may be performed to establish the presence of hyperchlorhydria, hypochlorhydria, or even achlorhydria.

Treatment. Treatment of gastritis is dictated by the etiologic factors. Autoimmune or Type A gastritis is treated symptomatically by the parenteral administration of vitamin B_{12}. There is no known treatment for the underlying autoimmune problem. The treatment of hypersecretion of acid is similar to the management of peptic ulcer disease (*e.g.,* antacids, antisecretory agents). Bile reflux is treated by inhibiting the action of bile acids in the stomach. Cholestyramine, a resin, or aluminum hydroxide antacids bind bile acids thus rendering them ineffective in the stomach.

Prognosis. The prognosis of patients with chronic gastritis is dependent upon the etiological factors involved in the disease. Patients with gastritis which results from hypersecretion of HCl or reflux of bile acids may develop gastric ulceration and hemorrhage.

The incidence of gastric carcinoma is higher in people with chronic gastritis than in the general population. However, not all types of gastritis appears to be percursors to cancer. Hypersecretion of acid (which overwhelms the normal gastric mucosal resistance of the stomach) does not result in metaplasia of mucosal cells or atrophy of the mucosa and as such does not appear to be a precursor of gastric cancer. Gastritis which arises as a result of changes within the mucosa itself, such as autoimmune gastritis, may be a precursor to gastric cancer.

Nursing Management

Nursing Diagnosis. Chronic gastritis is a long-term problem which may have an impact on both the patient's comfort and nutritional status. The nurse should assess the patient's knowledge of the problem and make sure he or she understands the need to conform to the medical treatment. Patient problems include discomfort, pain, fatigue, decreased appetite, and the potential for complications including ulceration and hemorrhage.

Goals. The goals of nursing interventions are patient education, prevention of disease progression and complications, maintenance of nutritional status, and control of discomfort.

Interventions. The patient should be given reassurance and support in relation to the disease as a potential precursor to gastric cancer, but nonetheless should be counseled to have an annual medical checkup. The extent of need for emotional support will vary with each individual. The nursing care is directed toward patient education regarding drugs, nutrition, and the importance of routine follow-up care. Drugs (*e.g.,* aspirin, nonsteroidal anti-inflammatory agents) or foods which are known to cause gastric irritation should be avoided. Highly spiced foods as well as coffee and tea should be avoided. The patient may find that small, frequent feedings reduce gastric discomfort. Specific dietary (*e.g.,* bland) regimens have not been shown to be beneficial in the treatment of chronic gastritis. patients need to be instructed on the importance of routine follow-up care and advised to report changes in symptoms or their severity. Over-the-counter preparations, unless recommended, should be avoided for symptomatic relief.

Evaluation. Outcome criteria are patient reports of behavior that includes:

1. Dietary intake in agreement with the prescribed regimen.
2. Avoidance of specific drugs known to cause gastric irritation.
3. Adherence to prescribed drug therapy.
4. Decrease or elimination of pain.
5. Denial of any symptoms or signs of impending complications.
6. Stable weight.
7. Activity level maintained without fatigue.

Enteritis

Enteritis, acute inflammation and infection of the intestine, can be caused by viruses, bacteria, and toxins produced by certain bacteria and parasites. Common causes of viral gastroenteritis are the Norwalk agents, rotavirus (the most common cause of diarrhea in children under age 2), and enteroviruses (coxsackievirus, echoviruses). The most common cause of bacterial gastroenteritis are *Salmonella, Shigella,* and *Campylobacter.* Toxin-associated gastroenteritis is usually caused by *Staphylococcus aureus* or *Clostridium perfringens.* Parasite-caused enteritis is discussed in the following section.

Viruses are by far the most common pathogens, but they are difficult to culture. Of the pathogens described above, only *Salmonella* and *Shigella* isolates are reportable to the Centers for Disease Control (CDC). The numbers of reported isolates of *Salmonella* have been increasing since 1977. Most cases of gastroenteritis occur in the warm summer months, usually between July and November. The warm temperatures during these months are favorable for growth of bacteria.

Bacterial and viral gastrointestinal illnesses are spread by the fecal–oral route. Most cases are acquired by person-to-person contact, although the potential for food- and water-borne outbreaks is ever-present. Many factors, such as numbers of organisms ingested, source of exposure, and host defense mechanisms, determine whether a person will become ill. The large number of organisms necessary to cause *Salmonella* infections makes person-to-person outbreaks unusual. *Salmonella* infections are more likely to be spread in food where, under proper circumstances, organisms can rapidly multiply. In contrast, only 200 organisms of *Shigella* are necessary to cause infection. Therefore, person-to-person outbreaks of shigellosis occur frequently in certain places, particularly under crowded conditions (day-care centers, institutions, jails). *Shigella* can also be spread by water or food. Large outbreaks of both *Salmonella* and *Shigella* have been the result of contaminated food at banquets and restaurants. Nosocomial outbreaks of *Salmonella* have been known to occur when contaminated equipment (*e.g.,* a fiberoptic endoscope) is used on a number of patients.

Etiology

The number of gastrointestinal pathogens is very large (Table 82–1 lists a few of them). Some organisms (*e.g., Shigella* and viruses) are carried only by the human host. Other pathogens (*Salmonella, Campylobacter*) have animal hosts as well. Poultry, beef, and dairy products often become contaminated with *Salmonella* during processing. If the meats are not cooked to the proper temperature, or are mishandled somewhere along the cooking process, the organisms can multiply to numbers sufficient to cause gastrointestinal illness.

Toxins which cause gastrointestinal illness are produced by enterotoxin-producing organisms. The most common type of "food poisoning" in the United States is that due to the toxin of certain *Staphylococcus aureus*. Toxins produced by *S. aureus* is of human origin (*e.g.,* purulent discharges of an infected finger, eye, abscess). When food is contaminated with these organisms and held at or cooked to improper temperatures, toxins are produced. Once these bacterial toxins are ingested, the resulting gastrointestinal illness is usually mild (though uncomfortable) and self-limited, but dehydration can occur. Patients who ingest the preformed bacterial toxins and subsequently become ill are not infectious.

For most bacterial and viral enteric illnesses, persons can be considered infectious while the organisms are incubating and when the person is having overt symptoms or convalescing from a disease. The patient is most infectious while having diarrhea (when large numbers of organisms are being excreted). If hands are not washed with soap and water, particularly after defecating, the organisms can be spread directly to others by hands, by uncooked foods touched by the person, or indirectly through contaminated fomites.

Water supplies, especially in countries with inadequate sanitation, can become polluted with contaminated sewage. Inadvertent cross-connections between sewage and water lines have also occurred. In both instances, widespread bacterial and viral enteritis occurs in persons who consume the contaminated water.

Pathophysiology

The body has a number of natural barriers to pathogens. Initially, gastric acid is effective in killing many bacteria. Conditions under which gastric acidity is reduced (*e.g.,* antacid use, achlorhydria, and gastrectomy) make a person more susceptible to certain bacterial pathogens. Surviving organisms then move into the small intestine where normal microbial flora have some antimicrobial activity against these foreign organisms. If the patient was taking antibiotics such as ampicillin and tetracyclines at the time of exposure, the normal microbial flora may be reduced and predispose the person to infection. The immunosuppressed patient is also at increased risk. Persons at either end of the age spectrum are at risk for more serious disease and complications.

Organisms can produce diarrhea by a number of mechanisms. They can (1) provoke the small and large intestines to secrete large quantities or fluid (often by raising levels of cyclic AMP), (2) cause malabsorption (by deconjugating bile salts), (3) invade and damage intestinal cells directly (as *Shigella* invades the colonic mucosa to produce dysentery).[17]

Vomiting caused by *S. aureus* enterotoxins is probably due to toxin interaction with abdominal viscera. The vagus and sympathetic nerves then carry this sensory stimulus to the vomiting center of the brain.[9]

Clinical Manifestations

Incubation periods of the pathogens which cause gastroenteritis vary from a few hours to a week (Table 82–1). Although symptoms also vary according to the etiologic agent, there are several symptoms of gastroenteritis which are common to all of them. The patient with gastroenteritis will probably experience an acute onset of nausea, vomiting, and/or

TABLE 82–1
Type of Pathogen, Incubation Period, and Symptoms of Common Infections of the Gastrointestinal Tract

			Symptoms			
Pathogen	*Causative Agent*	*Usual Incubation Period*	*Vomiting*	*Diarrhea*	*Abdominal Cramps*	*Fever*
Staphylococcus aureus	toxin	2–6 hr	+	+	+	
Bacillus cereus	toxin	2–12 hr	+	±	±	
Clostridium perfringens	toxin	10–12 hr		+	+	
Vibrio cholerae	bacteria	2–3 days	±	+	±	
Salmonella	bacteria	1–2 days	±	+	+	+
Shigella	bacteria	1–3 days	±	+	±	+
Campylobacter	bacteria	3–5 days	+	+	+	+
Norwalk agent	virus	1–2 days	+	+	+	+
Rotavirus	virus	1–2 days	+	+		+

diarrhea. If the pathogen is bacterial, these symptoms are often accompanied by fever, headache, and blood in the stools. Myalgias and abdominal cramps are frequently present. Illness caused by toxins usually occurs within 2 to 12 hours of eating the contaminated food and rarely includes fever or bloody diarrhea. Once again, the exact set of symptoms is dependent upon the etiologic agent (Table 82–1). No matter what the cause of the diarrhea or vomiting, dehydration is always a possibility. Therefore, the patient will need to be assessed carefully for symptoms of dehydration. Young children and elderly persons are especially susceptible to rapid dehydration.

Medical Management

Diagnosis. A food and travel history are obtained from the patient. If this information and the symptoms seem to indicate the presence of pathogenic bacteria, a stool specimen is sent to the laboratory to be tested for pathogenic bacteria. Few hospital laboratories have the capability of identifying viral pathogens or bacterial toxins. Viral illnesses are routinely diagnosed on the basis of symptoms and negative culture results for bacteria.

Treatment. The use of antibiotics in the treatment of gastroenteritis depends upon the etiologic agent, but most of these illnesses are self-limiting. Antibiotic use is avoided with mild infections caused by some bacteria (*e.g., Salmonella*) as the antibiotics may prolong the carrier state or lead to resistant organisms. Antibiotics are used in the cases of enteric fever, bacteremia, localized infections, and in cases of severe or prolonged diarrhea. Antibiotics are not effective against viral- or toxin-induced illnesses.

Nursing Management

Nursing Diagnosis

Any time a patient presents with acute gastroenteritis, a complete food and travel history should be obtained for the previous 7 days (unless the incubation period is known to be shorter). The patient's understanding of preventive measures (*i.e.,* handwashing and prevention of fecal–oral spread) should be assessed.

Stools should be observed for frequency, consistency, and color. Patients who are hospitalized with gastroenteritis should have their fluid, electrolyte, and acid–base states assessed. Patients should also be assessed for an increase in temperature, headache, relative bradycardia, splenomegaly, and leukopenia—manifestations of enteric fever or bacteremia.

Goals. The goals of the nurse are to prevent spread of the infectious organism in the hospital, maintain the patient's hydration and nutritional status, and to teach the patient about preventing the spread of the infectious organisms.

Interventions

Care of the patient with gastrointestinal illness of infectious origin is similar to care of a patient with hepatitis A discussed in a following section of this chapter. All patients with diarrhea of unknown etiology should be placed on Enteric Precautions until a communicable cause of illness is ruled out.[6] A continent adult with diarrhea can share a room with another adult patient. Patients who are fecally incontinent or who have poor hygiene should have a private room. Persons caring for patients with gastroenteritis should wear gloves and gowns if they are to come into contact with fecally-soiled items (*e.g.,* bedpans). Handwashing after caring for these patients is essential.

If the patient's physician orders a stool specimen, the stool should be delivered to the laboratory immediately after collection. At this time, it will be plated onto the proper culture media for identification of pathogenic organisms. The laboratory should be informed of specific pathogens which are suspected so that the proper media can be used. If there will be a delay between collection and delivery of the stool specimen to the laboratory, correct instructions on preserving the specimen should be obtained from the laboratory ahead of time.

Fluid and electrolyte replacement therapy will need to be carefully monitored and interventions for diarrhea or vomiting instituted. Prior to ambulation, the patient's level of strength and hemodynamic stability should be assessed. Possibly, the patient will need assistance with activities of daily living.

Patients are most infectious while having diarrhea, when millions of organisms are being excreted. As diarrhea resolves, fewer organisms are excreted until they are eventually cleared from the body, usually within a few weeks. (A very small percentage of persons infected with *Salmonella,* however, do become chronic carriers.) Patients who have bacterial or viral gastroenteritis and are food handlers, patient-care providers, or work in or attend day-care centers should be excluded from these activities during their phase of diarrheal illness. It is preferable that a foodhandler no longer be excreting the organism (determined by three consecutive negative stool specimens 24 hours apart, in the case of a bacterial infection) before returning to actual food handling. A public-health nurse may oversee the collection of these specimens once the patient has been discharged from the hospital.

The importance of handwashing should be taught to the patient. Family members should understand the signs and symptoms of illness, the method of transmission of the illness, and methods of preventing spread of the organism.

Evaluation

Criteria for evaluation of goal achievement are:

1. The disease is not spread within the hospital.
2. The patient can accurately describe actions to prevent spread of the infectious agent and reports use of these actions.
3. Intake of fluid equates with fluid output.
4. Blood pressure remains stable.
5. Pulse remains within normal limits.
6. Mucous membrane is moist.
7. Weight remains stable.
8. Stool specimens are negative for organisms three consecutive times.

Parasites

The two organisms that are responsible for the majority of parasite-induced diarrheal illness in the United States are *Giardia lamblia* and *Entamoeba histolytica.* Giardia is more common, but because it is not officially reportable in all states, national counts are not available. Amebiasis (caused by *E. histolytica*) occurs less frequently but can cause a more serious illness.

As are more other infectious forms of gastrointestinal illness, parasitic disease is spread by the fecal–oral route. The primary reservoir of *E. histolytica* and *G. lamblia* is man. In addition, *G. lamblia* can be transmitted by dogs, cats, and wild animals including the beaver. Cysts of both parasites are fairly resistant to destruction and can survive chlorinated water (*e.g.,* in swimming pools) and gastric acidity. Asymptomatic carriers of both illnesses can spread the disease because they pass the infective cysts. The incubation period for both illnesses ranges from 1 to 4 weeks after exposure.

Most *G. lamblia* infections resolve without treatment in 4 to 6 weeks. All persons with *E. histolytica* infections (both asymptomatic and symptomatic) should be treated because they are at risk for later complications.

Endemic levels of both of these diseases are maintained by person-to-person transmission, especially in conditions where overcrowding and poor sanitation occur. Intestinal protozoa can also be transmitted sexually, particularly among male homosexuals. Epidemics have occurred when improperly treated water supplies have become contaminated with the cysts. Nosocomial outbreaks of amebiasis have occurred in mental hospitals, children's homes, and prisons.[15] Severity of illness appears to be higher in immunosuppressed persons.

Etiology

There are two stages in the life cycle of *G. lamblia* and *E. histolytica*—the dormant infective cyst stage and motile trophozoite stage. Infection occurs when a person ingests at least ten cysts. The cysts, unlike the fragile trophozoites, survive the high acidic contents of the stomach. They travel then into the small intestine where the cyst wall disintegrates, and trophozoites are released.

In chronic or asymptomatic infection, the trophozoites detach from the mucosa, round up, and form cyst walls as they pass down the bowel. The cysts, excreted in the feces, are the infectious agent. Under moist conditions, cysts can survive for months outside the host.

Pathophysiology

Giardia lamblia. When ingested by the host, the cysts pass unharmed through the gastric contents and undergo excystation in the duodenum. Attachment of the trophozoites to the intestinal mucosa causes inflammation and edema of the microvilli. These changes in the intestinal mucosa cause diarrhea and sometimes malabsorption syndrome with steatorrhea. A symbiotic relationship between *G. lamblia* and bacteria may account for some cases of symptomatic giardiasis.[4] Patients with severe malabsorption often have other pathogens or coexisting disease.

Entamoeba histolytica. Amebiasis may be a mild illness like giardiasis, or it may be more severe if the parasite invades deeper tissues. Initially, the ameba will cause a tiny area of necrosis. If the ulceration is deep enough, bleeding may occur due to the destruction of small blood vessels. Often extensive ulceration is accompanied by secondary bacterial infections.[2]

Mucosal invasion by trophozoites can result in amebic dysentery or other clinical presentations. Invasion of the submucosa by trophozoites may be followed by their entry into the portal vein system and metastasis of the infection to the liver or other organs. Amebic abscess of the liver, usually the right lobe, is the most common extraintestinal manifestation of *E. histolytica* infections, but hematogenous or direct spread may involve any organ. A certain percentage of infected individuals become chronic cyst-passers.

Clinical Manifestations

Giardia lamblia. The majority of *G. lamblia* infections are asymptomatic. When symptoms occur, patients most often complain of diarrhea, flatulence with distention, abdominal cramps, anorexia, constipation, or diarrhea alternating with constipation. In the most severe forms of the illness, malabsorption syndrome occurs with the passage of foul-smelling, bulky stools and gradual weight loss.

Entamoeba histolytica. The chronic cyst-passer may be asymptomatic or experience nonspecific intestinal complaints, such as alternating periods of loose stools and constipation with flatulence. These patients constitute an important source of infection because they are excreting infective cysts but may not feel ill enough to seek medical attention. In addition, chronic carriers may themselves later develop acute and invasive disease without warning.

Symptoms of amebic dysentery include chills, fever, abdominal cramps, and bloody diarrhea which may progress to intestinal perforation, severe hemorrhage, and death. Individuals with liver abscesses often complain of right upper quadrant pain which, because 85% of liver abscesses occur on the right lobe of the liver, may radiate to the right shoulder. Additional symptoms of abscess formation include malaise, fever, and leukocytosis.

Medical Management

Diagnosis. If a patient presents with signs and symptoms of amebiasis, a history of living/working conditions and foreign travel should be obtained. If giardiasis or amebiasis is suspected, other causes of diarrheal illness (*e.g.,* bacterial) should be ruled out.

Diagnosis of *G. lamblia* or *E. histolytica* is dependent upon identification of trophozoites or cysts by microscopic examination of stool specimens. Diagnosis of amebiasis can be aided by sigmoidoscope and biopsy specimens. The indirect hemagglutination (IHA) serology test is most effective in diagnosing extraintestinal amebiasis as many of these patients are no longer excreting cysts or trophozoites in their stools. Ninety-five percent of patients with extraintestinal amebiasis will demonstrate a positive IHA test (titer ≥ 1 : 128). Family members of patients with amebiasis should submit stool specimens for examination.

Treatment. Individuals with amebiasis or giardiasis are usually treated with antiparasitic drugs on an outpatient basis.

A commonly used drug is metronidazole (Flagyl). The drug dosage is usually 750 mg orally three times a day. Effective therapy requires treatment for 5 to 10 days. This drug is used for both intestinal infections and in the event of liver infection. Tetracycline is also used for treatment. The dose is usually 2 g a day for 7 days. Tetracycline may be used in conjunction with diiodohydroxyquin (Diodoquin).

Prognosis. Patients with amebiasis or giardiasis usually respond favorably to the above-described treatment. However, when the organism travels to the liver, abscesses may form and the person may become severely ill and require hospitalization. Some infected persons may continue to have periods of exacerbations and remissions for months or years.

Nursing Management

Nursing Diagnosis and Goals

The nursing management of patients with parasitic gastrointestinal tract infection is as described for patients with enteritis in the preceding section with the following exceptions.

Interventions

Patients hospitalized with diarrheal illnesses caused by amebiasis or giardiasis should be placed in Enteric Precautions.[6] Patients hospitalized with liver abscesses caused by *E. histolytica* do not have to be placed in Isolation.

The nurse will be responsible for collecting the patient's stool specimens. Because cysts are excreted only intermittently, a series of at least three stool specimens collected on alternate days is often required to detect the infection. Stools examined should be fresh (within 15 minutes of passage) because the trophozoites rapidly lose their motility and identifying characteristics outside the host. If rapid examination is not possible, stools should be preserved in 10% formalin (for cysts) *and* polyvinyl alcohol (PVA) fixative (for trophozoites) for later examination. The nurse should remember that different methods of preserving stool are used if bacterial or viral testing is also to be done by the laboratory.

Methods of preventing parasitic infections should be reviewed with the patient. Campers and backpackers should consider surface water (*e.g.,* rivers, creeks, lakes) to be contaminated. Although iodine-based purification methods are advocated by hiking clubs, the only reliable measure for killing cysts in surface water is to boil the water for at least 10 minutes. Travelers to endemic areas should drink boiled water, bottled or canned carbonated beverages, and eat only cooked foods.[4] Homosexuals should be aware that parasites are transmitted by fecal–oral contact.

Evaluation

Evaluation of goal achievement for patients with parasitic gastrointestinal tract infections is as described for evaluation for patients with viral and bacterial infections in the preceding section.

Chronic Inflammatory Disorders

Chronic inflammatory bowel disease is a term used to encompass several disorders including regional enteritis, ulcerative colitis, and Crohn's colitis. The term inflammatory bowel disease is used frequently to denote these disorders because of the overlap in symptoms, treatment, and nursing management. Furthermore, these disorders are not easy to distinguish diagnostically due to the commonality in presenting symptoms and anatomical location. All chronic inflammatory bowel diseases are associated with multiple gastrointestinal and extragastrointestinal complications. However, the histological appearance of the GI tract differs markedly between these inflammatory diseases. The two most common inflammatory bowel diseases, ulcerative colitis and Crohn's disease (regional enteritis) are contrasted in Table 82–2.

Ulcerative Colitis

Ulcerative colitis is a chronic disease which affects the colon and rectum. Generally, it does not involve the small intestine, although there is a small percentage of patients whose distal small intestine is involved. The ulcerations are most frequently found in the rectum and left colon. The lesions associated with ulcerative colitis are continuous in the sense that the affected tissue is not intermittently distributed throughout the intestine. In ulcerative colitis the inflammation is limited to the mucosal and submucosal layers of the intestinal wall.

The incidence of ulcerative colitis is approximately 5 to 7/100,000. There are two peak-age groups, early twenties and fifties. However, the highest incidence of ulcerative colitis is between 15 and 30 years of age. Although generally considered a disease of young adults, ulcerative colitis can occur in any age group and occurs in both sexes equally. The symptoms, however, may be dismissed in the elderly patient as "normal" age-related changes in GI function. Due to the high incidence of colorectal cancer in this age group, any change in bowel habits needs to be evaluated.

Etiology

The cause or causes of ulcerative colitis are at this time unknown. Individuals with a family member with ulcerative colitis appear to be at greater risk for developing this disease than the general population. The incidence of ulcerative colitis is higher in people of Jewish descent and relatively low in blacks. In some patients ulcerative colitis appears to develop following a bowel infection. However, due to the insidious nature of the onset of the disease, this may not be a cause–effect relationship. Ulcerative colitis may also be an

TABLE 82–2
Comparison of Ulcerative Colitis and Crohn's Disease

	Ulcerative Colitis	*Crohn's Disease*
Location:	Colon	Small intestine, colon
Depth of lesions:	Mucosal, submucosal layers; continuous lesion	All layers of gut wall
Incidence:	More common than Crohn's	
Complications:	Hemorrhage	Hemorrhage, fistula formation, perforation
Manifestations:	Rectal bleeding, bloody stools	Abdominal pain, fever, anal and perianal fistulas, rectal bleeding less common
Etiology:	Unknown, autoimmune Familial tendency Personality factors	Familial tendency Autoimmune?

autoimmune disorder. In some patients with ulcerative colitis, antibodies against the colon epithelial cells in the mucosa have been found. This in turn results in tissue hypersensitivity and increased vulnerability of the colon tissue to the bacteria which normally reside in the colon.

Histological evidence indicates that the initial process in ulcerative colitis is mucosal vasculature congestion which, when prolonged, results in ischemia and necrosis of the mucosal layers. Repeated inflammation will result in loss of normal epithelial cells, and pathologic changes. In persons over 60 years of age, vasculature changes (*i.e.,* ischemia) may be the initiating factor in the etiology of ulcerative colitis.

For many years, the link between psychological factors such as personality and stress and the etiology of ulcerative colitis has been sought. The psychosomatic nature of both ulcerative colitis and Crohn's disease has not been demonstrated by clinical research. However, exacerbation of the diseases is sometimes associated with major physiological and/or psychological stress.

Pathophysiology

The early lesion associated with ulcerative colitis is a granulated mucosa which is red and has diffuse areas of bleeding. With inflammation there is swelling of epithelial cells, necrosis, and eventually loss of cells and the formation of crypts in the mucosa. As lymphocytes, polymorphonuclear leukocytes, and cellular debris collect, these crypts become the site of abscess formation. These abscesses then drain into the intestinal lumen. Eventually the mucosa ulcerates and is vulnerable to bleeding. Inflammatory polyps are frequently observed in the colon of patients with ulcerative colitis.

Clinical Manifestations

Ulcerative colitis has a variable course from its very initiation. For most patients it starts insidiously with symptoms the patient may ascribe to the flu, while in some patients the disease begins abruptly with an acute fulminating episode. The patient may experience recurrent bouts of the disease or acute fulminating episodes. The most common pattern of ulcerative colitis is mild exacerbations of the disease followed by periods in which the patient is asymptomatic. Both ulcerative colitis and Crohn's disease produce multiple extragastrointestinal symptoms which bring the patient to seek help.

The most common symptom of ulcerative colitis is bloody diarrhea. Other common symptoms include pus in the stool, lower abdominal pain, and abdominal tenderness. Generalized manifestations include fever, anorexia, weight loss, nausea, and vomiting. Hematologic evaluation during active disease periods reveals elevated white blood cell count (WBC) and anemia. The signs and symptoms of ulcerative colitis will depend upon the severity of the disease. The classification of severity of ulcerative colitis is discussed below with Crohn's disease.

Crohn's Disease (Regional Enteritis)

Crohn's disease is a chronic, inflammatory, ulcerating disease that may affect any segment of the gastrointestinal tract. It is a chronic disorder marked by exacerbations and remissions. Crohn's disease may develop at any age, including childhood. However, the highest incidence is in the third decade. There are approximately 10,000 new cases diagnosed each year. While the death rates attributed to Crohn's disease and ulcerative colitis are not high, the morbidity and the degree of incapacity are.

Etiology/Pathophysiology

The cause or causes of Crohn's disease are not known at this time. Because there is a familial tendency it may be that this disease is genetically determined. The disease most commonly affects the distal ileum where the intestinal flow is slow and there is therefore increased exposure of the intestinal epithelium to potential irritants, which suggests that as yet undiscovered environmental or dietary factors may be involved. That immunologic factors may also be involved in the etiology is evidenced by inflammatory response observed in the bowel. However, at this time, there is little supportive evidence for any of these as the sole cause of Crohn's disease.

Unlike ulcerative colitis, all layers of the intestinal wall are involved in Crohn's disease. This is why fistula and submucosal abscess formation are more common in patients with Crohn's disease as compared to ulcerative colitis. The disease affects patches of intestinal tissue, affected areas being separated by normal tissue. Crohn's disease can affect any segment of the GI tract from the mouth to the anus. Most patients have involvement of the distal small intestine (50%), perianal (30%), and colon (20%). The rectum, which is typically involved in ulcerative colitis, is usually spared in Crohn's disease; however, there are exceptions. Crohn's disease and ulcerative colitis are classified as acute-severe, moderate, mild, or quiescent active disease.

Clinical Manifestations

The signs and symptoms of Crohn's colitis are similar to that of ulcerative colitis. Regardless of anatomical location, Crohn's disease generally has an insidious onset. Rectal bleeding is not as common in patients with Crohn's as in ulcerative colitis. Depending upon the segments of the intestine involved by Crohn's disease, the stool may contain occult blood. However, the other symptoms of Crohn's colitis are similar to that of ulcerative colitis which makes diagnosis based solely on symptoms impossible.

Patients with Crohn's disease who have involvement of the upper gastrointestinal tract (*i.e.,* stomach, duodenum) experience symptoms which are similar to those experienced with peptic ulcer disease. When the distal small intestine is involved, problems with malnutrition due to inadequate absorption are more pronounced.

Acute-severe disease. During acute-severe colitis the patient manifests symptoms of full-blown inflammatory process. Grossly bloody diarrhea (greater than six stools per 24 hours), fever, anemia, nausea, vomiting, and abdominal pain are associated with acute-severe colitis. Dehydration occurs due to loss of fluids from diarrhea, fever, and vomiting. As a result, the patient will have cardiovascular changes indicative of reduced blood volume (*e.g.,* tachycardia, orthostatic hypotension). The patient is acutely ill and requires hospitalization. If the symptoms of acute-severe colitis are unrelieved by medical management, surgical therapy may be necessary. The mortality rate of patients with acute-severe inflammatory bowel disease is approximately 20%.

Acute-moderate disease. Patients with acute-moderate colitis may also have grossly bloody diarrhea, abdominal pain, fever, and nausea. However, the severity of the symptoms is not as great as in the patient with acute-severe disease. The patient can sometimes be managed at home if family or friends are available to assist with care.

Mild active disease. Patients with mild active disease do not have fever or other systemic symptoms. Gastrointestinal symptoms include abdominal tenderness, cramping pain, and/or change in bowel patterns (*i.e.,* constipation or diarrhea). These patients are generally treated symptomatically. However, it is important to keep in mind that both Crohn's disease and ulcerative colitis can rapidly progress from mild to acute-severe active disease.

Because of the similarities in complications, medical management, and nursing management, Crohn's disease and ulcerative colitis are discussed together. Specific differences between the diseases in relation to these categories are presented.

Complications

Intractability. The most common complication accompanying inflammatory bowel disease is intractability of symptoms. Recurrent bouts of active disease and limited remissions occur in a number of patients with ulcerative colitis and Crohn's disease. This is one of the reasons that patients elect to have surgical therapy.

Perforation. With chronic inflammation and loss of cells there is thinning of the intestinal wall, which predisposes to intestinal perforation. The risk of perforation is greater for patients with Crohn's disease because it affects all layers of the wall. This is a serious complication, due to the spilling of intestinal contents into the peritoneal cavity and the resultant peritonitis. Perforation generally produces a sudden onset of pain in the lower abdomen. However, the manifestations of perforation and peritonitis may be masked if the patient is receiving steroids.

Fistula formation. With inflammation of intestinal tissue there is swelling of the mucosal tissue and fistula formation. Fistula formation is a frequent complication of Crohn's disease, due to the increased intraluminal pressure required to propel contents through an affected segment of the intestine. These fistulas can extend into bowel loops or surrounding tissues such as the bladder. Generally fistula development in the bladder, manifested by pyuria or fecaluria, is a sign of advanced Crohn's disease.

Hemorrhage. The severity of the bleeding will depend upon the length of the colon involved. Large segments of colon tissue that bleed will result in substantial blood loss. Massive bleeding is a primary indication for surgical intervention.

Toxic megacolon. Toxic megacolon occurs as a result of paralysis of the motor neurons in the colon. Feces are unable to move through this segment, resulting in a dilatation of the colon and obstruction above the level of paralysis. Toxic megacolon greatly increases the risk of perforation and may necessitate an emergency colectomy.

Obstruction. As a result of inflammation and edema of the intestinal tissue, the lumen of the intestine may become markedly narrow and result in obstruction (Fig. 82–1). This obstruction can generally be alleviated by the use of anti-inflammatory agents.

Malabsorption. This complication is most likely to develop in patients with Crohn's disease which involves the small intestine. There is decreased absorption of vitamin B_{12}, folate, and iron, resulting in anemia. If the jejunum is involved, the patient experiences lactose intolerance due to inadequate lactase enzyme. The larger the area of small intes-

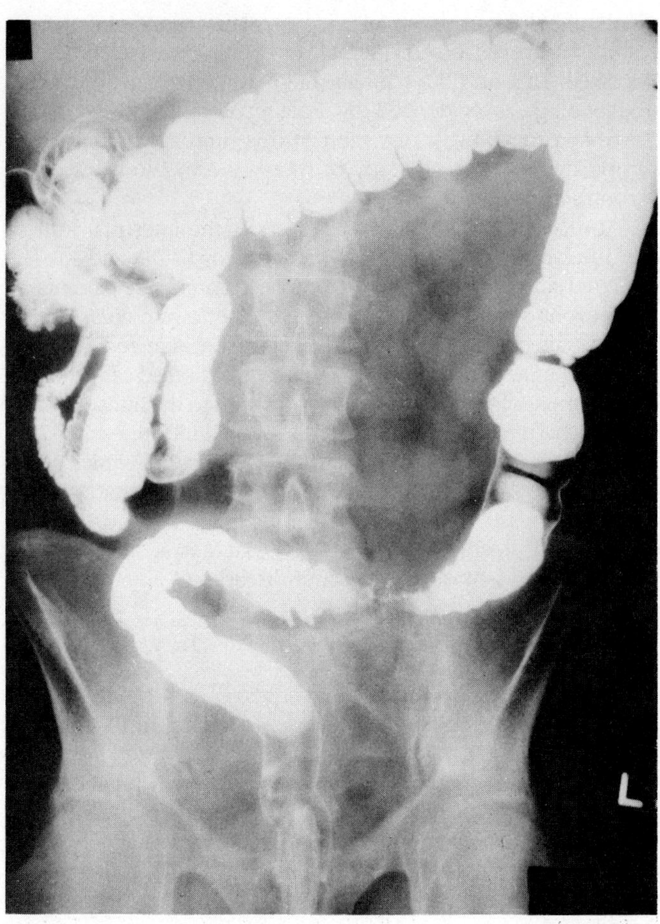

FIGURE 82–1 Barium enema x-ray examination showing a stricture in the sigmoid colon caused by Crohn's disease. The patient had already undergone resection of the terminal ileum and right colon for Crohn's disease. (Eastwood GL: Core Textbook of Gastroenterology, p 143. Philadelphia, JB Lippincott, 1984)

tine affected by Crohn's disease, the greater the likelihood and severity of malabsorption.

Extraintestinal complications. Ulcerative colitis and Crohn's disease have been linked to over 100 complications, many of which are extraintestinal. Extraintestinal complications of inflammatory bowel disease include hepatic and biliary disease; skin, ocular, and oral lesions; and musculoskeletal problems (*e.g.,* arthritis).

Susceptibility to neoplasia. The link of inflammatory bowel disease to colorectal cancer is associated with the duration of the bowel disease. Patients who have had ulcerative colitis for longer than 7 years are at high risk for colorectal cancer. The cancer occurs in this group of patients at a younger age than with the general population. Right-sided colon cancer is the most common location of cancer in this group. The risk for intestinal cancer is also high for patients with Crohn's disease. Patients who have had Crohn's disease for 15 to 20 years are at risk for either small intestine or colon cancer. The presence of intestinal or colon cancer is often missed because the symptoms are similar to the disease itself. The American Gastroenterological Association recommends annual sigmoidoscopy with rectal biopsy and barium enema staggered at 6-month intervals, and colonoscopy every 2 years as a means of detecting cell changes of a malignant nature.

Medical Management

Diagnosis

A diagnostic differentiation between Crohn's disease and ulcerative colitis is difficult because of the similarities in etiology and manifestations. When Crohn's disease affects the colon, the primary site of ulcerative colitis, it is even more difficult to distinguish between the two diseases. Diagnostic tests include sigmoidoscopy, flat plate of abdomen, barium enema (once perforation has been ruled out), as well as blood counts, and stool examinations.

Treatment

The treatment for Crohn's disease and ulcerative colitis is similar. However Crohn's disease, which generally persists longer due to the depth of the lesions, will probably be treated for a longer period of time. The goals of patient management are to promote and maintain remission of the disease. This is accomplished through pharmacologic therapies to reduce inflammation and infection and to alleviate symptoms. If this goal is not achieved, then surgical therapy is indicated.

Pharmacologic Therapy. *Sulfasalazine* is the most commonly prescribed medication for inflammatory bowel disease. Despite the fact that this drug is commonly used, its mechanism of action is not yet completely understood. Its modes of action appear to be both anti-inflammatory and antimicrobial. Sulfasalazine seems to be most effective for patients with moderate-to-mild inflammatory bowel disease, and may be used as adjunctive therapy in patients with acute-severe disease. Patients are started on sulfasalazine gradually, with the dosage increased in a stepwise fashion. Many of the side-effects of this drug are dose-dependent. These side-effects include nausea and vomiting. Enteric-coated sulfasalazine (En-Azulfidine) has proved helpful in reducing these upper GI side-effects. Sensitization to the drug is manifested by a fever and/or rash. Patients can be successfully desensitized to the drug. Severe side-effects of the drug include bone marrow depression and hepatic toxicity. Other potential side-effects include temporary oligospermia and decreased sperm motility, which, considering the young age group involved, may be an important factor in limiting the drug therapy. Patients on long-term sulfasalazine therapy exhibit folate deficiency which can be corrected by folic acid replacement.

Because of their anti-inflammatory and immunosuppressive actions, *steroids* are used in patients with inflammatory bowel disease. However, the degree to which steroids are used in the management of inflammatory bowel disease depends on the severity of the disease. Parenteral steroids are used for acute-severe active inflammation. Steroids at this time are the most effective drug for treating acute-severe inflammatory bowel disease. Oral steroids are frequently used for moderate and mild disease. Steroid therapy may or may not be used for the patient in remission. Steroid therapy is also beneficial in reducing the severity of extragastrointestinal complication such as iritis, uveitis, and arthritis. To reduce the long-term side-effects of cortisol prednisone is given on an alternate-day schedule. Adrenocorticotropin hormone (ACTH) may be given parenterally to stimulate adrenal production of endogenous cortisol and has been shown to be beneficial in treatment of inflammatory bowel disease. Other medications may be used as adjunct therapy to reduce the amount of steroid taken. For the patient who is nutritionally depleted, steroids, which are catabolic hormones, may add to the potential for complications.

Hydrocortisone enemas may be used for patients with ulcerative colitis who have distal colon involvement. Generally, the enema is composed of 100 mg hydrocortisone in 60 ml of saline which is given as a retention enema at bedtime. This administration route may be used for 1 to 3 weeks and has been shown to be effective in decreasing rectal bleeding, tenesmus (intense rectal urgency), and diarrhea. Steroid foam preparations may also be effective when applied to the distal colon. Similarly, rectal suppositories of 10 to 15 mg hydrocortisone or 5 to 10 mg prednisone may also be beneficial.

Although steroids appear to be helpful in most patients with inflammatory bowel disease, they do not cure either ulcerative colitis or Crohn's disease. Furthermore, steroids do not guarantee complete remission of the disease. Due to the depth of the intestinal lesions with Crohn's disease, patients will be on steroid therapy for a prolonged period of time.

Azathioprine and *mercaptopurine* are *immunosuppressive agents* which are used for the treatment of Crohn's disease and ulcerative colitis. These drugs decrease lymphocyte cytotoxicity and suppress cell-mediated immunity. However, their specific mechanism of action in relation to inflammatory bowel disease is not known. Azathioprine has some steroid-sparing action, in that less steroid can be used when combined with azathioprine. Due to the uncertainty of long-term side-effects of these drugs, they usually are not used in patients under 50 years of age.

A commonly used *antibacterial agent* is *metronidazole (Flagyl).* This drug is generally used in combination with sulfasalazine or prednisone. The side-effects of this drug, including taste alterations, Antabuse-like effects, and neuropathy, as well as its unknown long-term effects on intestinal microflora, are important considerations, especially in the treatment of young patients.

Pharmacologic therapy also includes drugs to provide *symptomatic* relief. These include antidiarrheal agents such as *loperamide* and *diphenoxylate.* Anticholinergics may be prescribed. However, gastrointestinal (*e.g.,* bowel obstruction) and extragastrointestinal side-effects associated with these drugs make them of limited value. Antispasmodic drugs (*e.g.,* Pro-Banthine) may be prescribed for abdominal cramping and diarrhea. Other drugs that decrease GI motility, such as codeine, may also be used.

Surgical Treatment. For approximately 10% of patients with inflammatory bowel disease, medical management will not be sufficient for symptom control. For these patients surgical resection of the bowel is performed to remove the site of the symptoms. Other reasons for surgical intervention include the presence of complications including perforation, hemorrhage, obstruction, toxic megacolon, abscesses, or fistula formation. Surgical treatment for ulcerative colitis generally involves removal of the colon and rectum (proctolectomy). The patient is left with a permanent ileostomy. This procedure in the patient with ulcerative colitis is curative. The higher-than-normal risk of colon cancer in this group of patients is eliminated with surgery.

Surgical therapy for Crohn's disease will depend upon the site and extent of the disease. The surgery consists of removal of the diseased portion with anastomosis of the proximal and distal portions of the intestine. Removal of the affected tissue is not always curative for Crohn's disease. Approximately 50% of patients experience return of the disease in another segment of bowel within 10 years of the surgery.

Prognosis

The patient who is treated and controlled with drugs will often experience periods of exacerbation over the years. This is a chronic disease, however, if the acute episodes can be controlled with drugs, this is usually preferred to surgical treatment. As indicated earlier, the risk of malignancy is present. As indicated above, surgical treatment is curative for patients with ulcerative colitis. Patients with Crohn's disease will likely have a recurrence of the disease in a remaining section of the bowel.

Nursing Management

Nursing Diagnosis

Nursing diagnoses commonly occurring in patients with Crohn's disease or ulcerative colitis relate to the long-term nature of the disease and the effect of the disease on the intestine and resulting manifestations. These diagnoses often include ineffective coping skills on the part of both the patient and family, fluid volume deficits, alteration in nutritional status, self-care deficits, and alteration in bowel patterns. The degree of alteration is influenced by the severity of the disease and by the inner resources of the person.

Goals. The goals of therapy are to assist the patient in coping physiologically and psychologically with the acute episode or with surgical treatment. This includes maintenance of fluid and electrolyte balance and adequate nutritional status, alleviation of discomfort, prevention of complications, patient ability to discuss concerns and feelings about the disease, and patient ability to assume self-care.

Interventions

During acute-severe colitis, patients are admitted to the hospital. The patient may be on bowel rest, which consists of no food or fluids by mouth and a nasogastric or nasointestinal tube to suction gastric or intestinal contents. Parenteral fluids are administered to compensate for loss of fluids by exudative diarrhea, fever, suctioning, and possibly vomiting. Patients need to be monitored for abnormalities in electrolyte levels. In particular, hypokalemia is a problem of patients with acute-severe colitis. Orthostatic hypotension as a result of fluid loss may necessitate the use of a bedpan rather than the bathroom or bedside commode. Vital signs should be checked at regular intervals (every hour) during the acute phase. Accurate intake and output records including the number, consistency, color, and odor of stools should be recorded.

Depending upon the nutritional status of the patient. TPN (total parenteral nutrition) or enteral liquid diets may be initiated to replace protein which is lost during exudative diarrhea. However, TPN is frequently reserved for those patients with malnutrition who will be undergoing surgery. Nutritional status is monitored by daily weights and by serum levels of nonprotein nitrogen.

Stools need to be assessed for frequency and the presence of blood, pus, or mucus. The patient is monitored for abdominal distention and abdominal pain which may be indicative of obstruction.

In caring for the patient with acute-severe colitis, the nurse will also administer appropriate medications to decrease inflammation, provide symptomatic relief, and promote comfort. Pharmacological therapy for acute colitis includes parenteral steroids (*e.g.*, hydrocortisone 300–400 mg) and sulfasalazine. Sulfasalazine (Azulfidine) is not as beneficial as steroids in the patient with acute-severe colitis because it must be taken orally and may be detrimental to bowel rest. Antidiarrheal agents may be used for severe diarrhea; however, these drugs have been associated with the occurrence of toxic megacolon and for this reason may be avoided. The nurse needs to monitor the effects of all drugs administered in relation to symptomatic relief and side-effects.

Patients with moderate active colitis may be treated on an outpatient basis. These patients usually require medication and nutritional information which need to be planned on an individual basis. Teaching is the primary nursing intervention for the patient with moderate or mild active disease. Bowel rest may not be required in these patients. Oral sulfasalazine (0.5 to 1 mg q.i.d.) and prednisone (40 mg po daily) are frequently used. A high-calorie, high-protein, low-roughage diet is recommended during the active phase of the disease. Milk and milk products as well as irritating foods need to be avoided. Agents that precipitate diarrhea, including coffee, alcohol, fruit and vegetable skins, seeds, corn, and nuts, should be avoided. Frequently patients with ulcerative colitis and Crohn's disease exhibit symptoms of lactose intolerance. Because milk products are a major source of calcium for many persons, and because steroids predispose to calcium loss, an additional source of calcium should be recommended. Vitamin and mineral replacements will need to be made particularly in those patients who have small intestine involvement.

Like patients with moderate active disease, patients with mild active inflammatory bowel disease are managed on an outpatient basis, except during acute exacerbation when fluid and electrolyte replacement is required, or during periods of rectal bleeding. Patients need to be encouraged to report flulike symptoms including diarrhea, nausea, abdominal cramping. The use of over-the-counter preparations for GI symptoms must be strongly discouraged.

Patients with inflammatory bowel disease may experience chronic fatigue. Many patients are 10 to 20% below ideal body weight. Furthermore, specific nutritional deficits may be present. Protein loss as a result of diarrhea is the most common cause of nutritional deficit. Diet therapy needs to be planned individually according to the stage of the disease. During an acute-severe episode the patient may be on complete bowel rest or a liquid diet. Total parenteral nutrition may be used in some patients with acute-severe colitis. However, it is primarily used preoperatively to improve the nutritional status of the patient requiring surgery and postoperatively. Elemental or chemically defined diets may be used during acute-severe colitis or enteritis. The emphasis in nutritional therapy during remission is on a normal diet.

Malnutrition, undernutrition, and chronic diarrhea indicate the importance of optimal skin care. The patient's skin needs to be examined at regular intervals for redness and excoriation. Patients who experience urgency and incontinency at times should have ready access to the bedpan.

Patients with inflammatory bowel disease require emotional support from members of the health team. Much has been written about the personality type of the patient with ulcerative colitis. These patients are described as insecure and sensitive, with a tendency to be dependent. Such characteristics may be attributed to the chronic nature and uncertainty of the disease as well as the severity of the symptoms.

Patients need time, encouragement, and opportunity to verbalize their feelings. The nurse should be patient and accepting of the person's emotional needs. Kindly but frank discussions of the disease and the person's perspective on the disease should assist the person in working through emotional responses to the problem. All procedures need to be carefully explained to the patient with time allowed for questions and discussion. Psychiatric therapy may be recommended, and the patient needs support and encouragement to follow through on this recommendation.

Evaluation

Outcome criteria for the patient being treated conservatively for Crohn's disease or ulcerative colitis are:

1. The frequency of stools decreases, the stool is formed and brown in color.
2. Patient reports relief of abdominal discomfort.
3. Fluid intake and output balance.
4. Blood pressure and pulse are within normal range.
5. Oral nutritional intake increases.
6. Patient accurately describes action of medications, possible side-effects, and prescribed schedule for taking them.
7. Patient and family openly talk about the disease, their emotional responses to it, and plans for coping with the problem on a long-term basis.
8. Patient gradually assumes responsibility for activities of daily living without experiencing fatigue.

Nursing Management in Surgical Resection

Preoperative Nursing Interventions

During the preoperative period for the patient undergoing elective, nonemergent bowel resection with anastomosis, the medical and nursing care focuses on correction of malnutrition, fluid and electrolyte imbalances, decreased blood volume, and intestinal distention. Patients with acute-severe disease are poor surgical candidates due to bowel inflammation and systemic symptoms. The bowel is prepared for surgery with sulfasalizine or neomycin. The purpose is to minimize the bacterial level and hence the danger of infection of the abdominal cavity. Special precautions and methods are used during the resection of the bowel to assure that fecal contents are not spilled into the abdominal cavity.

Patients need to be taught about the surgical procedure. Information about the length of the normal bowel will reassure them that the bowel can be resutured without tension. In contrast to the patient having an ileostomy, the person having a resection with anastomosis will not have a major, obvious change in body image. The patient may be fearful of the surgery but also usually may welcome it as a means of symptom relief.

Because the disease is continuous along the bowel, the usual surgical procedure for ulcerative colitis is an ileostomy. Tne procedure consists of removal of the entire bowel. This is known as an abdominal perineal resection. The bowel is severed at the ileum which is then brought out onto the abdomen. The stoma is the slightly everted mucous membrane lining of the ileum. The abdominal wall incision for stoma placement is small and located away from the main incision through which the surgery is performed. The underlying tissues constrict around the ileal stoma thereby preventing contamination from skin organisms. After the bowel is free from blood vessels and fibrous attachments, the patient is repositioned in a side-lying or jackknife position to facilitate removal of the entire bowel including the rectum. The surgical procedure was diagrammed and the nursing care of these patients was discussed in Chapter 80.

Patients with Crohn's disease may have a segmental bowel resection with anastomosis of the nondiseased portions of the bowel. The segmental nature of the disease permits this type of surgery. The following discussion focuses on care of patients with resection and anastomosis.

Postoperative Nursing Interventions

After resection with anastomosis the patient will have a nasointestinal tube in place to remove gas and intestinal secretions which may put pressure on the suture line. Drainage from the tube needs to be monitored for color, consistency, volume, and presence of blood. The volume of output should decrease over the initial 24 to 48 hours after surgery. Potential early postoperative complications include hemorrhage and hypoxia. Patient vital signs should be assessed every 4 hours, or more often if indicated.

Patients are maintained on intravenous fluid replacement and possibly TPN for several days after surgery. During this period fluid and electrolytes are monitored for imbalances due to losses from suctioning. Once bowel function has returned (as evidenced by presence of bowel tones and passing of flatus) and initial healing of the anastomotic site has occurred, the nasogastric tube is removed. Oral intake will be resumed gradually beginning around day 4 or 5 if bowel function has returned.

Adaptation to oral feeding will depend upon the location and length of intestine removed. Resection of the small intestine involving the jejunum will produce problems in absorption of fluid and electrolytes, fat, and vitamins A, D, E, and K. Removal of the distal small intestine (ileum) will result in vitamin B_{12} malabsorption and fat malabsorption due to loss of bile salts. Resection of the ileocecal valve may produce increases in intestinal motility as well as movement of colonic bacteria into the small intestine. Weight loss generally occurs during the postoperative period after bowel surgery. Regain of weight and strength is a gradual process. Nutritional supplements may be necessary for a period of many months. However, symptomatic relief usually is followed by an improvement in both mental and physical status.

Evaluation

Preoperatively, goal achievement would be evidenced in the patient and family ability to explain the operative procedure, the treatments to expect postoperatively, and the actions the patient will take to cooperate with these treatments, thereby preventing potential complications. Other evidence of goal achievement is a balance in fluid intake and output, weight stability, normal serum protein levels, normal blood pressure, and completion of a course of antibiotic therapy.

Postoperatively, criteria for goal achievement are:

1. Patient report of minimal abdominal discomfort which decreases throughout the postoperative period.
2. Increase in self-care ability throughout postoperative period, with patient reporting decrease in fatigue and weakness.
3. Patient openly discusses feelings about surgery and the disease.
4. Patient reports plans for future activities which are realistic and in agreement with teaching about postoperative activities.
5. No evidence of postoperative complications: wound clean and dry; lungs clear to auscultation and percussion; abdomen soft; bowel tones heard by 4th to 5th postoperative day, flatus passed, has bowel movement; fluid intake and output balance; vital signs remain stable; serum electrolytes within normal range; nasogastric drainage gradually decreases in volume, fluid is clear.

Diverticulosis and Diverticulitis

A diverticulum is a blind outpouching or protrusion of the intestinal mucosa through the muscle coat (Fig. 82–2). Diverticulosis refers to the presence of these outpouchings while diverticulitis indicates an acute inflammation of these pouches. When the outpouching becomes impacted with fecal contents this results in inflammation and/or perforation. Diverticula vary markedly both in size and number, but are most commonly found in the sigmoid colon.

Because manifestations and diagnostic tools do not clearly distinguish between diverticulosis and diverticulitis, the two are often referred to collectively as diverticular disease. Diverticular disease is a relatively common problem with 30% of people over 60 years of age and as many as 50% over 80 years of age afflicted. It is extremely uncommon in persons under 30 years of age.

Etiology and Pathophysiology

The formation of these pouches may be related to several factors. The incidence of diverticular disease increases with age. With aging there is weakening of musculature and as a result the increase in intraluminal pressure pushes out

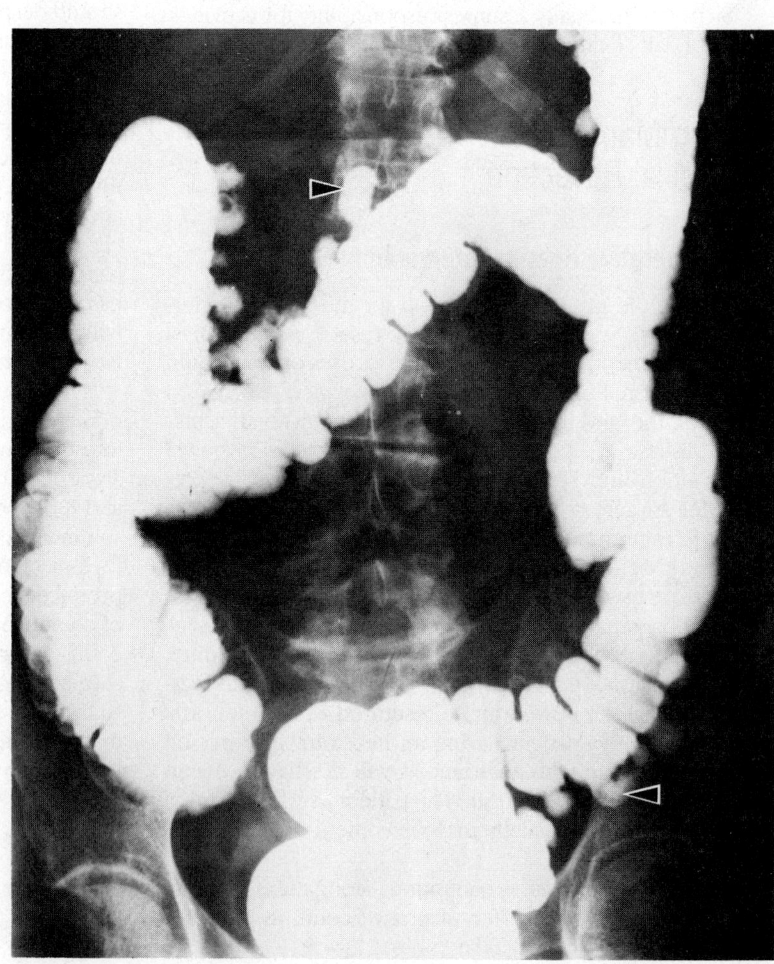

FIGURE 82–2 Barium enema x-ray examination showing numerous diverticula throughout the colon. The arrows indicate two of the many diverticula. (Eastwood GL: Core Textbook of Gastroenterology, p 181. Philadelphia, JB Lippincott, 1984)

part of the intestinal wall. However, not all elderly persons exhibit diverticulosis and thus it is probably not a normal aging change. Diverticular disease that appears in middle age is associated with a thickening of the intestinal wall. Diverticular disease has also been found in patients with a history of ulcerative colitis and Crohn's disease. The incidence is higher in affluent countries, indicating perhaps that environment or nutrition may contribute to the etiology. Low-fiber diets which utilize refined sugar are common in affluent countries. These diets result in increased intraluminal pressure and, as a consequence, precipitate diverticulosis. Chronic constipation and obesity are also risk factors for diverticulosis. In some patients, diverticular disease may occur as a result of vascular changes in the intestinal circulation. Ischemic bowel changes (*e.g.,* decreased blood flow due to congestive heart failure) may put the person at greater risk for developing diverticulosis. In some patients, muscular abnormalities with spasm of the sigmoid colon probably precede diverticular disease.

Clinical Manifestations

The patient with diverticulosis is frequently asymptomatic until the pouch becomes inflamed. The most common symptom associated with diverticular disease is abdominal discomfort or pain in the lower left quadrant. For some patients the discomfort is modified by diet or bowel movements. Intermittent rectal bleeding which is not associated with stool consistency is another common manifestation of diverticular disease. Diverticular disease is one of the common causes of blood in the stool of elderly patients. If the diverticulum impinges on a ureter or the bladder, urinary tract problems may be present.

With diverticulitis the patient feels a steady pain in the lower left quadrant along the path of the colon. Pain in the lower back may be present as a result of referred pain. Constipation is the usual symptom. However, diarrhea sometimes occurs. The abdomen is tender to touch and the patient may demonstrate some guarding on the left side. Other symptoms of generalized inflammation are also present including fever, elevated white blood cell count, and nausea.

Medical Management

Diagnosis. Diverticular disease is diagnosed by patient's history, physical findings, and barium enema exam. X-ray examination is delayed until inflammation has subsided. Because of similarities in manifestations, colorectal cancer should be ruled out as part of the diagnostic work-up.

Treatment. Once diverticular disease has been diagnosed, the focus of medical management is on preventing infection or inflammation of the diverticula. Uncomplicated diverticular disease is treated by dietary changes including a low-roughage, high-fiber diet. Bulk-forming agents such as psyllium hydrophilic mucilloid (Metamucil) and stool softeners are often prescribed. There is no known cure for diverticulosis.

Medical therapy for acute diverticulitis is the administration of broad-spectrum antibiotics because the causative factor is usually bacteria present in the diverticula. Depending upon the severity of the disease, changes in diet may be necessary including a low-fiber diet until signs and symptoms of infection subside. Symptomatic treatment of abdominal discomfort includes the use of pain medications and antispasmodic drugs.

Complications. Diverticulitis is generally self-limiting; however, complications may arise. The complications of diverticular disease include the following: (1) perforation of the diverticulum resulting in peritonitis, (2) perforation into an adjoining tissue such as the urinary bladder, (3) abscess formation at the site of the diverticulum, (4) hemorrhage, and (5) obstruction. These complications may or may not result in the need for surgical resection of the affected tissue. When a diverticulum perforates, emergency surgical intervention is usually indicated. A temporary colostomy is performed to divert the fecal flow and prevent further peritoneal contamination. Later, the affected portion of the bowel may be resected. However, in some cases, the perforation will resolve without surgical intervention. Obstruction and bleeding from the diverticula are common and in many situations will subside without surgical intervention.

Surgical intervention consists of a temporary double-barreled colostomy. A segment of the bowel proximal to the diseased portion is brought out onto the abdomen. Openings are made in the bowel wall to divert the fecal flow out of the stoma (colostomy). This is a temporary measure to divert fecal flow away from the inflamed and perhaps perforated area. Once the inflammation has subsided (2–3 months), the surgeon will close the temporary colostomy and may do a resection of the diseased portion. The nondiseased portions of the bowel are sutured together (see Chapter 80).

Nursing Management

Nursing Diagnosis

Patient problems with diverticular disease include abdominal discomfort, alteration in bowel patterns, self-care deficits, anxiety, and potential for systemic toxicity related to perforation and peritonitis. These problems relate to the interference with intestinal motility as a result of the outpouchings of the intestinal mucosa and weakness of the muscle coat. Data obtained from the patient are a history of bowel function; usually the patient indicates that constipation is a problem. The history of dietary habits may reveal a low-fiber diet, which decreases the bulk of the stool. Patients may express anxiety about the nature of the problem and its prognosis. If abdominal discomfort is severe, this may interfere with self-care ability. It is not uncommon to admit older patients in acute abdominal distress from a perforated diverticulum. Data to collect include vital signs, hydration status, and discussion of pain intensity. The physician should be notified because emergency surgery may be necessary.

Goals. The goals of nursing interventions are to prevent the development of diverticula, to prevent infection and inflammation in patients with the disease, and to assist patients who need surgical treatment to recover from this treatment.

Interventions

Because diverticula cannot be eliminated other than by surgical resection, the emphasis of therapy is on prevention of diverticular disease. Health teaching of patients and the public aims at decreasing the presence of risk factors such as chronic constipation, low-fiber diet, and obesity. Increased fiber or bran in the diet increases the bulk of the stool and thereby promotes intestinal motility and decreases straining at stool. Decreased intraluminal pressure may prove beneficial both in reducing the formation of diverticula as well as decreasing the likelihood of impaction of an existing diverticulum.

In uncomplicated diverticular disease, the focus is on patient teaching. The goal is to prevent inflammation. Necessary alterations in diet may not be readily accepted by the patient when they vary from lifelong dietary habits. During asymptomatic periods a high-fiber diet should be eaten, excluding indigestible fiber such as apple skins. The introduction of foods high in fiber may need to be done gradually; for example, substituting whole grain breads for white bread; the introduction of root vegetables, fruits, and nuts. Foods which contain high levels of fiber also increase intestinal gas and therefore, for some patients for whom gas is a problem, these foods definitely need to be incorporated into the diet gradually.

The patient with chronic constipation may need to be placed on a bowel program. The addition of bran 50 to 90 g per day will facilitate fecal movement and avoid marked increases in intraluminal pressure. However, harsh laxatives should be avoided. Patients need to be taught to observe for symptoms of diverticulitis (*i.e.,* changes in bowel patterns, and mucus and blood in the stool). Health teaching should include advising persons who experience changes in bowel habits and/or rectal bleeding to seek medical treatment. These symptoms should be investigated due to the possibility of colorectal cancer which is especially high in the elderly population.

Patients requiring a temporary colostomy need assistance in coping physically and mentally with this sudden change in health status and body image. Depression is common despite reassurances that the colostomy is temporary. Nurses can help the person to cope with the problem through interpersonal interactions that include listening and encouragement as well as discussions of the person's feelings. The care of the patient with colostomy is discussed in Chapter 80.

Patients with temporary colostomy as a result of a perforated diverticulum are often in the older age group. Elderly people often have more difficulty coping emotionally with unexpected changes in health status than do younger people, and their physical stamina is often marginal. Therefore, the recovery period after surgical intervention may be prolonged in the elderly and may necessitate transfer to a long-term care facility for convalescence, particularly if family resources are minimal. The patient may stay in this institution until inflammation of the bowel has subsided sufficiently to permit closure of the colostomy. During this convalescence at home or in the long-term care institution the patient should be taught self-care.

Following surgery to close the colostomy, the patient usually improves quickly. During the postoperative period, the patient should be taught the actions to take to prevent a recurrence of the acute inflammation process. These actions were presented in the above section on prevention of inflammation.

Evaluation

Goal achievement relative to education of the public to prevent occurrence of the disease could be determined by a follow-up contact with the group or person taught. The persons would describe, through written or verbal communication, changes in behavior that included an increase in dietary fiber, regularity in bowel elimination, avoidance of straining at stool, and avoidance of a diet high in refined sugars.

Goal achievement with patients who have diverticula is measured by patient reports of the above-cited actions. In addition, the patient would report not using harsh laxatives, absence of mucous and blood in the stool, and no changes in bowel patterns.

Criteria for the patient having surgery for perforated diverticulum are:

1. Patient expresses emotional responses to the colostomy.
2. Patient accurately describes the surgical procedure and the future treatment.
3. Patient demonstrates increasing ability to care for self including colostomy care.
4. Patient demonstrates increasing strength by increasing participation in activities of daily living.
5. No postoperative complications occur.

Pancreatitis

Pancreatitis is a serious inflammation of the pancreas which results in obstruction of the outflow of pancreatic secretions. Etiologic factors are associated with age and sex. Those patients in which gallbladder disease is the precipitating cause are more likely to be female and in their fifth or sixth decade of life, whereas patients with pancreatitis associated with alcohol abuse are usually younger and are predominantly male.

Pancreatitis is classified according to pathological processes. *Acute interstitial pancreatitis* is characterized by edema and inflammation of the interstitium. It is secondary to other diseases (*e.g.,* gallbladder disease), and the pancreas should return to normal function after the inflammation subsides. *Acute hemorrhagic pancreatitis* is characterized by diffuse areas of inflammation and hemorrhage. In this type of acute pancreatitis portions of the pancreas become necrotic; this results in fibrosis of the pancreas and loss of function. This type of pancreatitis is most frequently associated with prolonged alcohol use. Chronic pancreatitis is a progressive, destructive disease in which normal tissue is replaced by connective tissue. The end result is pancreatic insufficiency.

Etiology and Pathophysiology

Acute pancreatitis has been associated with several factors including (1) preexisting disorders such as biliary disease, (2) postoperative trauma, (3) drugs, (4) pregnancy, (5) hypercalcemia (*e.g.,* hyperparathyroidism), (6) infections, and (7) alcohol ingestion. Chronic pancreatitis develops after repeated episodes of acute pancreatitis due to chronic alcohol abuse (chronic calcifying pancreatitis) or chronic obstruction of the bile duct (chronic obstructive pancreatitis). Sometimes chronic pancreatitis develops with a negative history of acute events.

Regardless of the initiating event, the inflammation of the pancreas appears to be produced by activation or release of pancreatic enzymes (*e.g.,* lipase, trypsin) within the pancreas itself. Why this autodigestion of the pancreas occurs is not known at this time. Obstruction of the pancreatic duct as a result of gallbladder disease, lithiasis, spasm or stenosis of the sphincter of Oddi, or a direct blow to the pancreas will result in a backup of pancreatic secretions. As the pressure increases due to continued production of pancreatic enzymes, the duct will rupture, spilling these enzymes into the parenchymal tissues of the pancreas.

Alcohol appears to have a direct metabolic effect on pancreatic tissue resulting in protein precipitation which causes the ducts to dilate and the acinar cells to atrophy. Eventually, necrosis of the pancreas occurs.

Clinical Manifestations

The signs and symptoms of acute pancreatitis will depend upon the severity of the attack. Patients with mild pancreatitis may be asymptomatic, but most do experience abdominal discomfort or steady epigastric pain which may radiate to the back. Eating generally intensifies the pain. Patients complain of nausea and sometimes of vomiting, which does not relieve the discomfort. Nausea and vomiting are most likely to occur after a period of overeating or overdrinking.

In patients with a severe attack of acute pancreatitis the signs and symptoms are more dramatic. The patient complains of severe pain, the vomiting is more persistent, and there is increased abdominal rigidity and decreased bowel activity. On physical exam, the patient has a rigid abdomen with tenderness to touch. Generalized manifestations include fever, elevated white blood cell count, and hypotension. Hypotension may be the result of both the loss of fluid and enzymes into the peritoneal cavity and the release of bradykinin and kallikrein. Laboratory studies show an elevation in serum and urine amylase, serum lipase, hypocalcemia, hypoalbuminemia, and, in some patients, hyperglycemia due to increased glucagon release.

Chronic pancreatitis is characterized by periods of exacerbations and remission. Manifestations during acute recurrent attacks are as described above. As the disease progresses, pancreatic insufficiency results in decreased production of the enzyme lipase which results in fat malabsorption and steatorrhea. Protein malabsorption may also occur and result in a decrease in muscle mass and loss of body weight.

Medical Management

Diagnosis. Pancreatitis is suspected in the patient with a history of associated factors as indicated above and with steady, epigastric abdominal pain and tenderness. Laboratory analysis for pancreatic enzymes serum or urine amylase, and serum lipase provides evidence about the existence of pancreatic disease but does not give information of the severity of the disease.

X-ray visualization of the abdomen is done to determine if fluid is present in the peritoneal cavity. Upper-gastrointestinal x-ray may be performed to rule out the possibility of duodenal ulcer. Ultrasonography is done to exclude the possibility of gallstones.

Other diagnostic measures especially when chronic pancreatitis is suspected are endoscopic visualization (endoscopic retrograde cholangiopancreatography of the bile duct), pancreatic biopsy, and the secretion-stimulation test in which secretion is administered intravenously and gastric-duodenal secretion is collected by a double lumen tube. Due to loss of normal tissue from the acinar pancreas, there is a reduction in the secretion of both enzymes and bicarbonate fluid.

Treatment. The goals of medical therapy are to eliminate the precipitating events (whether they be cholelithiasis, hypercalcemia, infection, hyperlipidemia, alcoholism, or pancreatic duct damage) to decrease further pancreatic damage and to provide systemic support for the patient during repair of the damaged tissue. Patients with acute pancreatitis secondary to biliary disease respond well to surgical correction of gallbladder disease. Hypercalcemia secondary to hyperparathyroidism will be corrected by surgical resection of the parathyroid gland. Patients with chronic alcohol abuse will require appropriate counseling to abstain from alcohol. Chronic pancreatitis is an irreversible process, hence, treatment focuses on prevention of acute acerbations, symptomatic relief, and treatment of pancreatic insufficiency.

Pancreatic stimulation is reduced by decreasing the release of secretin, the intestinal hormone which normally stimulates the release of enzymes and bicarbonate from the pancreas. Secretin is released by the presence of acidic chyme in the duodenum. Therefore, interventions directed toward reducing the acidic content of the intestinal lumen include antacids via a nasogastric tube, histamine receptor blockers (*e.g.,* cimetidine, ranitidine), and nothing per mouth. Nasogastric suction of gastric contents to reduce pancreatic stimulation has long been used in the treatment of acute pancreatitis. The suction tube is clamped for 20 to 30 minutes after installation of the antacid. In patients with mild or moderate pancreatitis, the use of nasogastric suction may not be necessary.[5]

Pain relief is important in the patient with acute pancreatitis. The usual drug is meperidine (50–100 mg) every 4 to 6 hours. Morphine is contraindicated because it causes spasm of the sphincter of Oddi, which will further decrease pancreatic outflow. Intravenous therapy is initiated to replace fluids and electrolytes lost by escape into the peritoneal cavity, through nasogastric suctioning, and lack of oral intake. Often subclavian lines are used for nutritional therapy because the need for parenteral fluids is of relatively long duration.

In chronic pancreatitis, pancreatic insufficiency is treated with pancreatic enzyme supplements. Enzymes given at the beginning and in the middle of the meal help to improve digestion and absorption. An H_2-blocker or antacid may be used in conjunction with the pancreatic enzymes to reduce HCl acid breakdown of the enzymes in the stomach. A low-fat diet is prescribed to reduce discomfort and steatorrhea.

Prognosis. Uncomplicated pancreatitis is generally self-limiting. In mild pancreatitis the symptoms will subside in 3 to 4 days. Patients with severe acute pancreatitis without complications will generally have pain and abdominal tenderness for 1 to 2 weeks. Biliary tract obstruction, most commonly due to cholelithiasis, is the usual cause of recurrent acute pancreatitis. These recurrent bouts rarely result in significant damage and pancreatic insufficiency. When the underlying problem is alcoholism, the prognosis is guarded because of the long-term damage to the pancreas and because the outcome depends on abstinence from alcohol. Prognosis for chronic pancreatitis is poor because there is no known curative treatment.

Complications. Pancreatic secretions which leak from the inflamed pancreas can produce extrapancreatic problems including (1) pancreatic ascites; (2) necrosis of the large and small bowels, resulting in spasm and possibly obstruction; (3) GI bleeding from gastritis; (4) jaundice, due to gallstone or compression of the common bile duct.

Pseudocysts are a distinctive complication of pancreatitis (Fig. 82–3). A pseudocyst is a cyst that is lined only by inflammatory fibrous tissue. About 10% of the patients with pancreatitis related to chronic alcohol abuse will develop a pseudocyst. Such cysts are rare following pancreatitis due to obstruction. Pseudocysts result from autodigestion of the pancreas and the replacement of tissue with liquefied necrotic material. The size of the cyst is variable and will depend to some degree on the amount of the pancreas which is blocked. These cysts contain pancreatic enzymes. The pseudocyst may disappear spontaneously as a result of draining. Pseudocysts are manifested clinically by a palpable mass in the epigastrium, abdominal pain, fever, and tenderness. Pseudocysts can be diagnosed by ultrasonography. Treatment of the pseudocyst will depend on the patient's symptoms and condition. In the asymptomatic patient with active pancreatitis, the cyst may be left to drain on its own. In other patients, who exhibit persistent fever, pain, and laboratory evidence of acute pancreatitis, percutaneous drainage may be required.

Nursing Management

Nursing Diagnosis

In general, nursing diagnoses are related to the effect of pancreatitis on the energy level of the patient and hence the ability to perform activities of daily living; on the toxic systemic effects of the disease; the patient's need for assistance in repairing tissue damage; and on the therapy required to

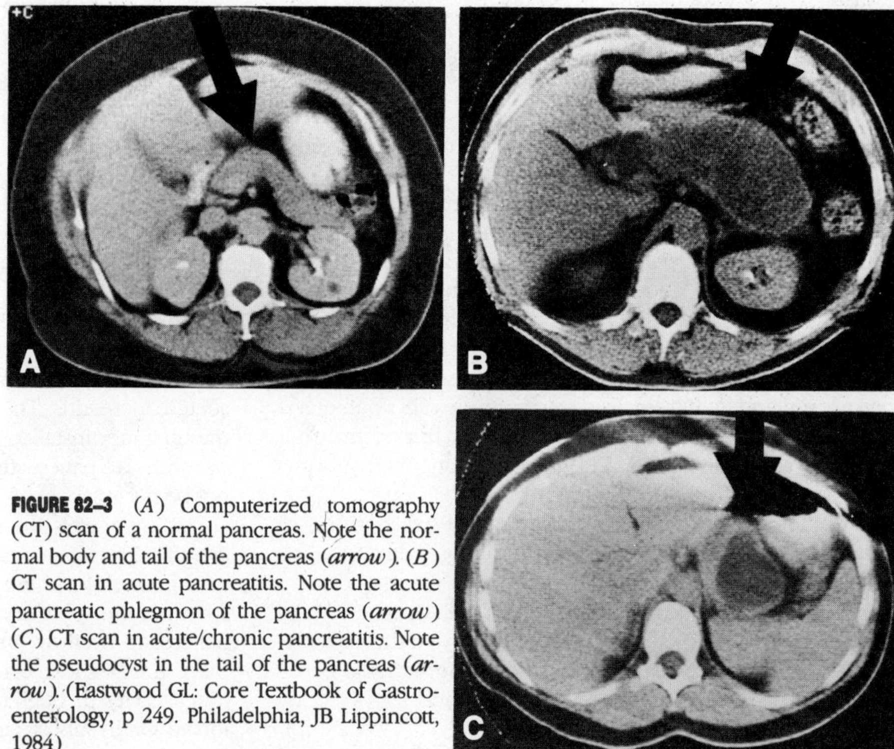

FIGURE 82–3 (*A*) Computerized tomography (CT) scan of a normal pancreas. Note the normal body and tail of the pancreas (*arrow*). (*B*) CT scan in acute pancreatitis. Note the acute pancreatic phlegmon of the pancreas (*arrow*) (*C*) CT scan in acute/chronic pancreatitis. Note the pseudocyst in the tail of the pancreas (*arrow*). (Eastwood GL: Core Textbook of Gastroenterology, p 249. Philadelphia, JB Lippincott, 1984)

manage the etiologic factor. Diagnoses commonly made are self-care deficits, anxiety, alteration in comfort, alteration in bowel elimination, fluid volume deficits, knowledge deficits, alteration in nutrition (decreased absorption of fat and protein), and disturbance in self-concept. For patients with chronic pancreatitis additional diagnoses may include potential for anticipatory grieving, spiritual distress, and fear. These latter problems are individual and relate to the person's ability to cope with the inevitability of death. All diagnoses must be individualized for the particular patient. Many of these diagnoses and related interventions are discussed in Chapter 80.

Goals. The goals of nursing care are to reduce pain and discomfort, prevent shock, provide fluid and electrolyte replacement, promote adequate nutrition, prevent or reduce secondary symptoms, and work with the patient to teach and promote acceptance of changes in lifestyle necessary to prevent recurrence and to support the patient/family in the terminal stages of a chronic disease.

Interventions

Patients with acute pancreatitis (either an initial occurrence or an acute exacerbation of a chronic disease) are frequently hospitalized. The stimulation of the pancreas is reduced in hopes of decreasing autodigestion. The patient receives no food or fluids by mouth, and parenteral fluid replacement is initiated. Because parenteral fluids are given over a relatively long period of time, particular attention must be directed toward prevention and early detection of inflammation at the insertion site. A nasogastric or nasointestinal tube will be inserted to remove further stimulation.

During an acute attack of pancreatitis the patient's cardiovascular status needs to be assessed frequently for signs of shock. Vital signs, skin color, temperature and moisture, and mental acuity are monitored at frequent intervals to detect impending shock. Shock is the leading cause of death in the patient with acute pancreatitis. The movement of fluid into the abdominal cavity may produce a significant drop in circulating blood volume and hence in cardiac output. Renal function is assessed by monitoring urine output. Other problems associated with acute pancreatitis include fluid and electrolyte (*e.g.,* sodium, potassium, chloride, calcium) imbalances, severe abdominal pain, and malnutrition. Assessment of fluid intake and output and attention to laboratory reports of electrolyte levels as well as signs of electrolyte disturbance are necessary assessment measures. Pain is increased with hypokalemia and the patient complains of extreme fatigue. Muscle strength is decreased.

Pain medications are administered at periodic intervals to provide a stable level for pain relief. Other methods of pain relief are lowering anxiety level through explanations, reassurance, encouraging and listening to expressions of emotional responses, and use of diversional therapy. The patient's pain level is assessed, and the effectiveness of pharmacological therapy is evaluated. Overmedication as well as alcohol withdrawal may result in behavioral changes ranging from lethargy to agitation. Counseling sessions with family and the patient are necessary to promote understanding and to develop approaches for coping with behavioral changes. In preparation for home care, referral to visiting nurse services is often a source of assistance to patients and families.

The patient is closely monitored for the presence of complications. Gastritis or superficial erosions of the gastric mucosa can be assessed by guaiacing stools for occult blood. The administration of H_2-blockers and antacids will reduce the likelihood of GI bleeding. Ascites or collection of fluid in the abdominal cavity may occur as a result of inflammation and increased capillary permeability. The ascites may further increase abdominal pain and contribute to respiratory impairment due to incomplete chest expansion. The patient requires instruction and assistance in coughing and deep breathing to reduce the risk of pneumonia.

Malabsorption and malnutrition may be problems if the duration of the inflammatory process is prolonged. Restricted oral intake and anorexia as well as increased metabolic rate may leave the patient at risk for protein–calorie malnutrition. Temporary insufficient pancreatic enzymes may produce problems with fat absorption and steatorrhea. The patient's nutritional status needs to be evaluated continuously. This includes recording all oral intake, both solid and liquid, daily weights, records of stools including color and consistency, and blood analysis for proteins and electrolytes.

After the acute phase, oral nutrition will be resumed. However, paralytic ileus is a complication associated with acute pancreatitis and therefore bowel function should be assessed prior to resumption of oral intake. A low-fat, high-calorie diet is ordered. Patient tolerance of the diet is assessed by patient complaints, the absence of diarrhea and steatorrhea. If enzyme replacement therapy is ordered, the patient and family are taught its purpose and the guidelines for taking the preparations with meals.

Long-term problems are related to malabsorption. Malabsorption of fat-soluble vitamins K and D may result in bleeding tendencies, and musculoskeletal changes. The patient will probably be on vitamin supplement therapy. High-protein oral supplements may also be beneficial.

During the recovery phase, the patient's knowledge of the disease and causative or precipitating factors is evaluated. The patient with chronic pancreatitis needs support and encouragement to comply with medical regimens. If necessary, the patient should be referred to alcohol treatment programs; family cooperation and assistance are essential.

Evaluation

Outcome criteria for goal achievement in the nursing management of patients with pancreatitis are:

1. Vital signs stable.
2. Fluid intake and output balance.
3. Mucous membranes moist.
4. Weight stable.
5. Serum protein and electrolytes within normal limits.
6. Nasogastric drainage clear, and amount within normal limits.
7. Patient reports minimal discomfort from pain.
8. Patient and family discuss emotional responses to the disease and concerns about the prognosis.

9. Patient and family accurately describe necessary actions to prevent recurrence.
10. Family provide verbal reassurance and support to the patient.
11. Patient reports carrying out self-care activities to extent possible as determined by disease progression.
12. Patient and family work with support groups (*e.g.*, religious advisor, visiting nurses, hospice) as the circumstances indicate (individualized).

Chronic Pancreatitis

Chronic pancreatitis refers to the presence of histological alterations of the pancreas. It is a progressive, destructive disease of the pancreas in which normal tissue is replaced by connective tissue. The end result of chronic pancreatitis is pancreatic insufficiency. Chronic pancreatitis may develop in patients after repeated episodes of acute pancreatitis due to chronic alcohol abuse or chronic obstruction of the common bile duct. However, there are patients with chronic pancreatitis who give a negative history for acute pancreatitis.

Chronic pancreatitis can be separated into two types: chronic calcifying pancreatitis and chronic obstructive pancreatitis. Chronic calcifying pancreatitis is the more common type. Chronic pancreatitis most frequently occurs in people between the ages of 40 and 60. Chronic calcifying pancreatitis is more frequent in men with a history of alcohol abuse, while that associated with chronic obstruction is more frequent in women.

Etiology and Pathophysiology

Chronic calcifying pancreatitis is related to chronic alcohol ingestion. The mechanism of alcohol's action is not completely understood, but there appears to be a direct metabolic effect of alcohol on pancreatic tissue, resulting in protein precipitation. As a result the ducts must dilate and acinar cells atrophy. Eventually necrosis of the pancreas will occur. Chronic obstructive pancreatitis may also be the result of blockage or spasm at the sphincter of Oddi, which results in a backup of pancreatic secretions and dilatation of the ducts.

Clinical Manifestations

Chronic pancreatitis is characterized by acute bouts of abdominal pain interspersed by pain-free periods. On physical exam the patient may complain of abdominal tenderness. As the disease progresses the periods of pain become more frequent. The pain experienced by the patient is similar to acute pancreatitis in that it is severe and is unrelieved by food.

Malabsorption is a problem caused by pancreatic insufficiency. Decreased lipase enzyme from the pancreas results in fat malabsorption and steatorrhea. Protein malabsorption may also occur and results in a decrease in muscle mass and loss of body weight. Similar to acute pancreatitis, chronic pancreatitis produces elevations in serum and urinary amylase as well as elevations in bilirubin.

Medical Management

Diagnosis. Chronic pancreatitis is diagnosed from laboratory findings, endoscopic visualization (endoscopic retrograde cholangiopancreatography of the bile duct), or pancreatic biopsy. The secretin-stimulation test in which secretin is administered intravenously and gastric-duodenal secretion is collected by a double lumen tube may also be used. Due to loss of normal tissue from the acinar pancreas, there is a reduction in the secretion of both enzymes and bicarbonate fluid. Ultrasound may be used to determine the presence of gallstones as well as the presence of pseudocysts.

Treatment. Chronic pancreatitis is an irreversible process and as such there is no curative treatment at this time. Hence treatment is focused on preventing acute exacerbations of the disease, on symptomatic relief, and on treating pancreatic insufficiency.

Pancreatic insufficiency is treated by the use of pancreatic enzyme supplements. Enzymes given at the beginning and in the middle of a meal help to improve digestion and absorption. An H_2-blocker or antacids may be used in conjunction with the pancreatic enzymes to reduce HCl breakdown of the enzymes in the stomach.

Pharmacological agents are prescribed to provide pain relief and reduce nausea and vomiting. A low-fat diet is encouraged to reduce discomfort and steatorrhea.

Nursing Management

Nursing Diagnosis

Patient problems during an acute attack of chronic pancreatitis are similar to those experienced in acute pancreatitis. In addition, because the disease is progressive, common diagnoses are alteration in absorption of fat and proteins; alteration in bowel function as a result of malabsorption of fat; self-care deficits, increasing pain, weakness, and fatigue; potential for anticipatory grieving, spiritual distress, anxiety, and fear. These latter problems are individual and relate to the person's ability to cope with the inevitability of death (see Chapter 11).

Because the disease is progressive the patient experiences intermittent problems with pain, anorexia, nausea, vomiting, hyperglycemia (if the endocrine portion of the pancreas is involved), jaundice, and abnormal serum levels of pancreatic enzymes. When a major part of the pancreas no longer functions, malabsorption becomes a primary problem as a result of pancreatic insufficiency. Malabsorption produces diarrhea, steatorrhea, weight loss, and symptoms of fat-soluble vitamin deficiency (see Chapter 80). Central nervous system changes may occur as a result of malnutrition, and dependency on pain relievers may result from persistent and often severe pain.

Interventions

A patient with chronic pancreatitis needs support and encouragement to comply with medical regimens. In the periods between acute exacerbations, the focus is on monitoring for and preventing aggravation of the disease. Substances which are known to aggravate pancreatitis, such as alcohol, need to be avoided. if necessary, the patient should be referred to alcohol treatment programs; family cooperation and assistance are essential.

Nutritional status is assessed at regular intervals. Signs and symptoms of fat malabsorption include steatorrhea and weight loss. The patient is instructed to adhere to the low-fat diet. Because fat makes up a significant percentage of the average diet, adherence to the diet may be difficult. The nurse works with the dietitian to provide practical suggestions and sample meal plans so that caloric and protein requirements can be met. The patient and family are taught the importance of enzyme replacement therapy and the guidelines for taking enzyme preparations with meals.

Long-term problems of chronic pancreatitis and pancreatic insufficiency are related to malabsorption. The patient may manifest problems related to fat-soluble vitamin malabsorption including bleeding tendencies (vitamin K) and musculoskeletal changes (vitamin D). The patient will probably be on vitamin supplement therapy to correct nutritional imbalances. High-protein oral supplements may also be beneficial.

The patient's pain level is assessed and the effectiveness of pharmacological therapy evaluated. Overmedication as well as alcohol withdrawal may result in behavioral changes ranging from lethargy to agitation. Counseling sessions with family as well as the patient are necessary to promote understanding and to develop approaches for coping with behavioral changes. Referral to visiting nurse services is often a source of assistance to patients and families.

Ascites or collection of fluid in the abdominal cavity may occur as a result of inflammation and increased capillary permeability. The ascites may further increase abdominal pain as well as contribute to respiratory impairment due to incomplete chest expansion. The patient requires instruction and assistance in coughing and deep breathing to reduce the risk of pneumonia.

Nursing interventions during acute phases of chronic pancreatitis are similar to those discussed for patients with primary acute pancreatitis. The patient is often admitted to the hospital for intravenous fluid therapy, or total parenteral nutrition may be instituted in the case of the malnourished patient.

Malnutrition results in weakness, and often the patient needs assistance with personal hygiene, although maximum level of self-care should be encouraged to prevent further wasting from inactivity. Control of pain is a major problem; the pain is severe, and analgesic levels must be maintained. If the patient is maintained at home in the terminal phases, visiting nurses and hospice can assist with pain control including measures to relieve anxiety and fear. Spiritual assistance may be desirable depending on the patient's religious beliefs (see Chapter 11).

Evaluation

The success of therapeutic intervention is determined by evaluation of patient's nutritional status, pain level, and ability to cope with the inevitable outcome of the disease.

Outcome criteria are:

1. Patient and family report a nutritional intake compatible with that prescribed and taught.
2. Patient reports minimal discomfort from pain.
3. Few or no acute, severe flare-ups of the disease occur.
4. Patient reports carrying out self-care activities to extent possible as determined by disease progression.
5. Patient and family discuss disease outcome openly.
6. Patient and family work with support groups (*e.g.*, religious advisor, visiting nurses, hospice) as the circumstances indicate (individualized).

Cholecystitis

Cholecystitis is an acute inflammation of the gallbladder, which is the storage site for bile produced by the liver. In over 90% of the patients the cause of the inflammation is bile stasis secondary to gallstone impaction of the cystic duct. Because gallstone formation occurs in approximately 10% of the general population, there is a potential for acute cholecystitis occurring in a significant number of people.

Etiology and Pathophysiology

The most common cause of cholecystitis is cholelithiasis or gallstone formation (Fig. 82–4). Gallstones are composed of the substances which are normally found in the bile (*i.e.*, cholesterol, bilirubin). Stones may be pure cholesterol or bilirubin but more frequently are mixed in composition. Approximately 10% of the total United States population and 30% of patients over 65 years of age have cholesterol gallstones. Cholelithiasis affects women four times as frequently as males. Persons at risk for gallstones include those with a positive family history, obesity, diabetes mellitus, Crohn's disease, and those who have had jejunoileal bypass surgery for morbid obesity. Other predisposing factors include sedentary lifestyle, multiparity in women, and high cholesterol intake.

The exact cause of gallstone formation is not known, however, it appears to be a problem in metabolism which results in a change in the composition of bile. Excess in the cholesterol content of bile produced by the liver results in precipitation of cholesterol in the gallbladder. The precipitation of bile constituents is facilitated by gallbladder stasis which occurs as a result of delayed gallbladder emptying.

Cholecystitis can also be produced by surgical trauma or injury to the gallbladder. However, this is a relatively rare cause of cholecystitis.

Clinical Manifestations

Patients with cholecystitis may have a history of biliary colic produced by obstruction of the cystic duct. The pain is usually sudden in onset, located in the epigastrium or right upper quadrant with radiation to right shoulder or scapula. The marked increase in pain may produce restlessness and nausea/vomiting. The pain may be intense as it results from spasms of the obstructed duct. The pain usually subsides

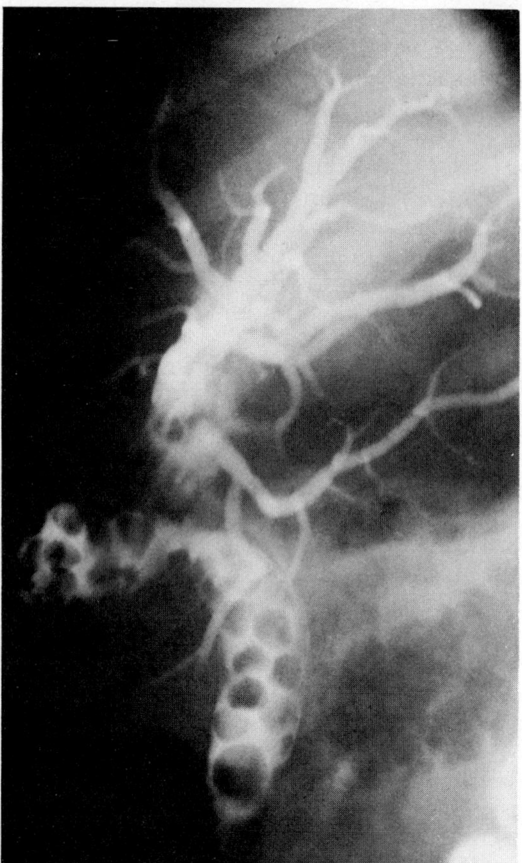

FIGURE 82–4 Percutaneous transhepatic cholangiogram demonstrating radiolucent stones within the gallbladder and a dilated common bile duct. (Eastwood GL: Core Textbook of Gastroenterology. Philadelphia, JB Lippincott, 1984)

with time, generally within a few hours. A low-grade fever may be present.

Patients with acute cholecystitis frequently exhibit gastrointestinal disturbances (*e.g.,* pain nausea, vomiting) after a high-fat meal. Other complaints may include flatulence, indigestion, and abdominal distention. The patient with inadequate bile secretion will exhibit problems related to lack of fat-soluble vitamin absorption, because these vitamins are absorbed in the GI tract similar to the way dietary fats are absorbed. Vitamin K, which is essential for clotting, is a fat-soluble vitamin, therefore, patients may manifest problems with bleeding. Malabsorption of fat-soluble vitamins A, D, and E may result in musculoskeletal changes.

In acute cholecystitis the gallbladder is generally palpable and the patient experiences tenderness on the right side. In approximately 20% of the patients, jaundice due to obstruction will be present. The blockage of bile flow causes increased bile pressure in the hepatic and liver ducts. The liver is unable to clear the blood of bilirubin, and its increase in the blood gives a yellow tone to the patient's conjunctiva and eventually the skin. If present, the stool may contain fat (steatorrhea) and may be clay-colored because fat is not absorbed and bile is not present in the intestine to give it the brown color. The urine may be bile-colored because the kidney will attempt to compensate by secreting bilirubin.

Medical Management

Diagnosis. Calcified gallstones can be seen by x-ray examination. An intravenous cholangiogram may be performed to determine cystic duct obstruction. Ultrasonography may also be performed to determine the presence of gallstones. Another diagnostic tool for acute cholecystitis is the HIDA scan. Laboratory tests include liver function tests (*e.g.,* direct and indirect bilirubin and enzymes SGOT and LDG). These test results may be elevated because of the inability of the liver to clear the blood. If pancreatic function is compromised by the gallstone, serum amylase levels will be elevated.

Treatment. Medical therapy is directed at eliminating the cause of the inflammation, reducing inflammation, controlling infection, reducing pain, and preventing recurrence.

During the acute phase of cholecystitis, therapy is directed at resting the gallbladder. When the patient is experiencing nausea and vomiting, gastric suction may be instituted and the patient restricted to nothing per mouth. Fluid and electrolyte replacement is initiated. Pharmacological agents are administered to reduce discomfort (*e.g.,* narcotics) and to reduce gallbladder contractions or spasms (*e.g.,* antispasmodics, anticholinergics). Antibiotics are given if an infection is present. Dissolution of the gallstone may be accomplished through ultrasound treatment or once the inflammation has subsided, the gallbladder may be surgically removed. In patients without nausea and vomiting and following resolution of the acute phase, a low-cholesterol, low-fat diet is frequently recommended to decrease gallbladder stimulation.

Prognosis. In some patients with acute cholecystitis and cholelithiasis the disease may become chronic. Chronic cholecystitis is similar to acute cholecystitis except the symptoms are less abrupt in onset. The patient may have a history of longstanding fat intolerance, or steatorrhea, and dyspepsia. The usual treatment for both acute and chronic cholecystitis which results from gallstones is surgical removal of the gallbladder (cholecystectomy). At the same time stones trapped in the cystic duct or common bile duct are removed (choledocholithotomy). The gallbladder is not necessary for life, and patients function normally without the gallbladder.

Nursing Management

Nursing Diagnosis

Problems commonly identified in patients with acute cholecystitis are discomfort related to distention of tissues from the inflammatory process and to nausea and vomiting; fluid volume deficit related to vomiting and absence of intake; self-care deficit because of discomfort and weakness; potential for complications related to obstruction of bile flow, resulting in inadequate absorption of vitamins and fat; and knowledge deficit concerning actions to prevent recurrence of an acute attack.

Patients with acute cholecystitis frequently exhibit gastrointestinal disturbances, flatulence, indigestion, and abdominal distention. The patient with inadequate bile secretion will exhibit problems related to lack of the fat-soluble vitamin absorption resulting in problems with bleeding and musculoskeletal changes. Skin color and color of the sclera need to be assessed to determine the presence of jaundice. Jaundice occurs if the obstruction to bile flow causes a distention of bile ducts in the liver and hence inability of the liver to clear the blood of bilirubin. If present, the urine and stool color must be noted. The stool may contain fat (steatorrhea) and may be clay-colored. The urine may be bile-colored.

Assessment of the patient's knowledge level about the disease, precipitators of an acute incidence, and how to prevent this occurrence is important. Knowledge of diagnostic measures and surgical procedure, if this is recommended, are other assessment factors.

If surgical treatment is done the patient will need the usual pre- and postoperative assessments as discussed in Chapter 8. Postoperative assessment must include observations of drainage amount and color if a wound drain or common bile duct drainage tube (T-tube) is used. The surgical incision may be a horizontal one located just below the rib cage. Muscles are severed in making this incision, and wound pain can be intense when the patient changes position, coughs, and deep breathes.

Goals. The goals of nursing are to relieve discomfort, assist in the control of fluid volume, promote self-care to the maximum extent possible, to detect early manifestations of impending complications, to promote behavior changes which will prevent recurrence of the problem, and, in the event surgery is indicated, the goal is to promote uneventful recovery from surgery.

Interventions

During the acute phase of cholecystitis, the nursing goals are to provide symptomatic relief. Pain medications are given to relieve abdominal pain. Patients in severe pain who manifest autonomic symptoms, including diaphoresis and hypotension, need to have vital signs monitored at regular intervals. The nurse needs to record time, severity, and frequency of symptoms as well as the response of the patient to pharmacological interventions. Antiemetic drugs are given to reduce nausea and vomiting. Fluid and electrolyte balance needs to be monitored in those patients with vomiting and NG suction. Dehydration may be a problem unless the patient is receiving intravenous therapy. If jaundice (yellowish color of sclera and skin) is present, symptomatic relief from pruritus is warranted. High blood levels of bilirubin result in seepage of it from the blood into the tissues, causing tissue irritation. Calamine lotion, antihistamines, and soft linen help to decrease pruritus.

After the acute phase, the nurse needs to help identify risk factors for recurrence. it is known that certain population groups are at risk for developing gallstones and gallbladder disease. The reduction in cholesterol intake in such patients and the reduction of weight in obese subjects are appropriate interventions to reduce the risk of active gallbladder disease. The patient should know that dietary factors are important in reducing recurrence of the disease. The patient on long-term, conservative medical management should be on a low-fat diet. In particular, dairy products, fried foods, rich pastries, and nuts need to be avoided. The number of calories will depend on the nutritional status of the patient.

Preoperative Nursing Interventions. In the patient who is undergoing cholecystectomy, preoperative nursing care is focused on patient teaching. Cholecystectomy is frequently done on an elective basis. Therefore, weight reduction for the obese patient can be instituted prior to surgery. For patients with malnutrition, a high-calorie, high-protein, and high-carbohydrate diet is recommended. During the preoperative period bleeding problems are determined and treated. The operative procedures needs to be explained to the patient, in particular the fact that the loss of the gallbladder will not significantly hinder lifestyle. Patients are taught to cough and deep breathe while splinting the incision area because it is painful for patients postoperatively.

Postoperative Nursing Interventions. The patient who has a cholecystectomy will usually have a Penrose drain positioned in the gallbladder bed and exiting onto the abdominal surface through a stab wound located within close proximity to the surgical incision. If the presence of a stone necessitated an exploration of the common bile duct, the patient will also have a T-tube emerging from another stab wound. The Penrose drain, used to prevent accumulation of fluid in the gallbladder bed, will be covered with a dry, sterile dressing. In general, the drainage is serosanguineous with a small amount of bile during the first 24 hours. The dressing will require frequent changes during the first 24 hours postoperatively because bile can be irritating to the skin.

The T-tube is attached to a closed drainage system to reduce the risk of impaired bile flow through the biliary system after surgery. Trauma to the common bile duct with surgery stimulates the inflammatory process. Inflammation of the duct could cause obstruction to bile flow. The T-tube also prevents contracture and stenosis of the duct during healing. Patients with a T-tube in place need to be in a semi- or low-Fowler's position. The amount and color of drainage needs to be measured at regular intervals. The patency of the T-tube should be checked. If the tubing is kinked or the drainage bag is above the level of the incision, backup of bile and bile reflux will occur.

Skin care around the Penrose drain or T-tube drain is critical because bile salts can be corrosive to the skin. The T-tube should be checked around the site of entry for drainage which would indicate a leak in the system. The skin should be cleaned each time the dressing is changed; Betadine ointment may be applied at the insertion site as a precaution against infection. The patient must be taught how to clean around the T-tube, empty the drainage bag, and prevent pull on the tube. The patient may be discharged with the T-tube in place. It would be removed in the doctor's office at a follow-up visit. A visiting-nurse referral may be indicated to provide support and at-home teaching.

Evaluation

Outcome criteria for the patient with acute cholecystitis are:

1. Patient reports a decrease and eventual absence of abdominal pain.
2. Fluid intake and output balance.
3. Nasogastric drainage is maintained during the acute phase.
4. Patient reports an increase in energy level and participates in self-care to extent possible.
5. No manifestations of jaundice, clay-colored stools, or steatorrhea are present or, if present, the physician is consulted.
6. The patient accurately describes foods that should be avoided, such as fried foods, gravies, nuts, dairy products, and rich pastries.

If the patient has surgery to remove the gallbladder, the outcome criteria in addition to those described in Chapter 8 are:

1. Drainage from the T-tube is maintained (if one present).
2. Absence of signs of skin irritation and infection around the T-tube or Penrose drain.
3. Patient reports relief of discomfort following administration of analgesics.
4. Patient increases participation in self-care each postoperative day.
5. Fluid intake and output balance.
6. Patient cooperates in postoperative measures to prevent complications (*e.g.,* respiratory—coughing and deep breathing).
7. Patient accurately describes measures to take during early convalescence including care of T-tube, caution in lifting, increasing physical activity, and return visit to the surgeon.

Hepatitis

Acute hepatitis is a common yet serious disease of the liver. Inflammation of the liver (the literal meaning of the word hepatitis) can result from a wide variety of pathologic conditions. Not all types of hepatitis are communicable. There are, for example, instances where liver injury is due to adverse reactions to certain drugs such as analgesics (*e.g.,* aspirin, acetaminophen), antibiotics (*e.g.,* tetracycline), and antineoplastic agents (*e.g.,* 6-mercaptopurine). However, most of the hepatitis seen in any given community is caused by infectious agents. Although a number of bacteria and viruses (*e.g.,* Epstein-Barr virus, cytomegalovirus) can cause hepatitis, the overwhelming majority of infectious hepatitis cases are due to infection with either hepatitis A virus (HAV) or hepatitis B virus (HBV).

At this time, there are three classifications of viral hepatitis: hepatitis A, hepatitis B, and non-A, non-B (Table 82–3). The causative agents of hepatitis A (HAV) and hepatitis B (HBV) have been identified. Hepatitis non-A, non-B is an

TABLE 82–3
Comparison of the Various Forms of Viral Hepatitis

	Hepatitis A	*Hepatitis B*	*Non-A, Non B Hepatitis*
Previous name:	Infectious hepatitis	Serum hepatitis	
Transmission:	Fecal–oral, person-to-person, food-borne	Direct inoculation, person-to-person	Direct inoculation, transfusions
Diagnosis of acute case:	Anti-HAV IgM	HBsAg and/or Anti-HBc	Rule out Hepatitis A and hepatitis B
Acquired immunity:	Lifetime	Lifetime	Lifetime
Incubation period:	15–50 days	50–180 days	40–160 days
Onset:	Abrupt	Insidious	Insidious(?)
Course of illness:	Short, acute	Prolonged, acute, and chronic	Intermediate, acute, and chronic
Complications and carrier state:	Unusual	5–10% of acute cases have complications; carrier state +	Carrier state possible
Prophylaxis with immune globulin:	ISG	HBIG/ISG	
Vaccine available:	No	Yes	No

exclusionary category into which all other cases of viral hepatitis fall. Non-A, non-B is probably caused by one of at least three viruses which will be given names as they are identified.

Viral hepatitis is a reportable disease in all 50 states. Cases are reported by local health authorities through the state health departments to the Centers for Disease Control (CDC) in Atlanta, Georgia. In 1982, 56,773 cases of viral hepatitis were reported to the CDC.[3] This figure underrepresents the actual number of cases of viral hepatitis, as many cases are asymptomatic and never diagnosed. Hepatitis A shows seasonal variation which tends to peak in late summer and early fall. Over half of the cases of all types of hepatitis are reported in the 20- to 39-year-old age group, though it occurs in people of all ages. More than twice as many males as females are reported to have hepatitis B.

Hepatitis A

Hepatitis A, sometimes referred to as "infectious hepatitis" or "short incubation hepatitis," is spread predominantly by the fecal–oral route. The HAV virus is excreted in large quantities in the feces for 2 weeks before and 1 week after onset of symptoms. It is during the time of HAV excretion that the person is considered communicable. The presence of HAV in the bloodstream or in other body fluids is transient and does not contribute significantly to the transmission of disease.

Conditions that facilitate the spread of hepatitis A include crowding and poor hygiene. Foodborne outbreaks have occurred in restaurants (due to an infectious foodhandler who unknowingly contaminates food or by the ingestion of raw shellfish harvested from waters contaminated by HAV). Person-to-person outbreaks have occurred in daycare centers, especially those caring for children in diapers (where the disease is not easily diagnosed, as most young children are anicteric, and the virus can be easily spread among children and staff).

Nosocomial transmission of HAV in hospitals is unusual because most cases of hepatitis A do not require hospitalization and the use of the proper enteric isolation precautions, primarily good handwashing, will prevent spread of the disease. Thus, nosocomial spread of hepatitis A has been reported only rarely.[11,14] In these outbreaks, staff members did not realize a patient was excreting HAV because the patient was admitted with an unrelated diagnosis while incubating hepatitis A, or the patient acquired the disease during an extended stay in the hospital. In either case, the patient subsequently developed diarrhea while excreting HAV, was not placed in isolation, and exposed the unsuspecting employees to the virus. Any patient with diarrhea should be considered potentially infectious, and appropriate Enteric Isolation precautions should be taken.

Hepatitis B

Hepatitis B, also known as "serum hepatitis," is primarily spread through infectious blood and/or blood products. Other body secretions such as saliva, semen, and urine can contain the HBV but are less frequently associated with transmission of the disease. Introduction of infectious material into mucous membranes (*e.g.,* eyes, mouth) and into cuts has led to infection, as has intimate sexual contact. Accidental needle puncture with HBV-contaminated needles or parenteral inoculation with contaminated blood, plasma, or serum are common routes of entry into the host. HBV can also be transmitted by shared needles of illicit drug users. A form of vertical transmission, that is, spread of the organism between an infected mother and her neonate, can occur, primarily through exposure to infectious blood during the perinatal period.

Populations at risk for developing hepatitis B include health-care professionals who are frequently exposed to blood, laboratory personnel, dialysis unit staff members and patients, clients and staff of institutions for the mentally retarded, dentists and dental practitioners, close contacts of patients with a current HBV infection, illicit parenteral drug users, male homosexuals, and immigrants and refugees from areas of high-HBV endemicity (*e.g.,* Southeast Asia or Sub-Saharan Africa). Nosocomial transmission of HBV occurs most frequently after accidental needle puncture with an HBV-contaminated needle or when an HBV-contaminated blood or blood product comes in contact with a mucous membrane or minute cut, abrasion, or burn.[7]

Etiology

The first causative agent of viral hepatitis, the HBV or Dane particle, was identified in 1970. The inner core of the spherical HBV particle contains hepatitis B core antigen (HBcAg) and hepatitis B "e" antigen (HBeAg). Hepatitis B surface antigen (HBsAg) surrounds both the HBcAg and HBeAg. In addition, HBsAg can be found free within the bloodstream and has been used in the diagnosis of hepatitis B for many years.

The HAV was identified in 1973 and contains the hepatitis A antigen (HAAg). As the stool becomes negative for virus, the serum antibody (anti-HAV IgM) quickly reaches its peak levels in the bloodstream. Anti-HAV IgM is a useful diagnostic serological marker because of its early presence (2 weeks, 3 months after infection). Although IgM antibody quickly disappears, another antibody (anti-HAV IgG) is produced which remains detectable for life.

The causative agent(s) for non-A, non-B have not been identified, though an antigen can be detected 7 to 10 days after infection.[16] Apparently, only a weak antibody response occurs, making diagnosis difficult. Thus, 90% of post-transfusion hepatitis is caused by non-A, non-B viruses.

Pathophysiology

The basic pathophysiology of hepatitis A, B, and non-A, non-B is identical. During an acute case of viral hepatitis, inflammation of the liver is generalized, and small focal areas of cellular necrosis occur. The necrosis is associated with both a leukocytic and histocytic response and infiltration.[16] The surviving cells retain glycogen. Fatty changes do not occur. The changes which occur in the liver interfere with normal functions (*i.e.,* breakdown of bilirubin, metabolism of drugs, and synthesis of protein).

Viral hepatitis can be a multisystem infection although the liver is the principal organ affected. Regional lymph nodes are enlarged. Splenomegaly, acute pancreatitis, and myocarditis can occur.

During the acute stage of illness, the levels of liver enzymes, AST (SGOT) and ALT (SGPT) are dramatically elevated. By the time jaundice occurs, these enzymes may be more than eight times their normal values.[8] The AST and ALT levels reach their peak in the icteric phase of illness. Once recovery occurs, these levels fall rapidly, but remain slightly abnormal for several weeks afterwards. Only mild elevations (one to three times normal) occur in alkaline phosphatase and LDH levels. CPK levels are normal in viral hepatitis. Bilirubin levels are usually elevated in viral hepatitis. Jaundice can be detected when the bilirubin level is ≥2.5 mg/dl. Urine may turn dark before icterus is visible.[8]

Recovery, accompanied by regeneration of liver cells, is aided by the scavenger activity of the reticuloendothelial system and occurs in the vast majority of hepatitis patients. In fact, 99.5% of hepatitis A and 90% to 95% of hepatitis B patients have complete recovery with resulting lifetime immunity.[8]

Clinical Manifestations

Incubation periods for the three classifications of viral hepatitis vary: hepatitis A is 15 to 50 days; hepatitis B is 50 to 180 days; non-A, non-B is 40 to 160 days (Table 82–3). Symptoms of hepatitis range from asymptomatic to severe, sometimes fatal, cases. As many as 50% of hepatitis cases, especially hepatitis B, may be asymptomatic or anicteric depending on factors such as age and general health of the patient prior to infection. Anicteric cases may have mild flu-like symptoms and are usually not recognized as having hepatitis.

When symptoms occur, their onset is abrupt for hepatitis A and insidious for hepatitis B and non-A, non-B. The clinical course is similar for all three forms though both hepatitis B and non-A, non-B tend to be more severe, have a longer clinical course, and can be associated with a serum-sickness-like syndrome. Symptoms usually occur in two phases: preicteric and icteric. Prior to the onset of jaundice the patient may complain of malaise, anorexia, intermittent nausea and vomiting, fever, headache, and a dull pain in the right upper quadrant which is not affected by meals, antacids, or position. Loss of desire for cigarette smoking often occurs. Diarrhea or constipation can occur, but these symptoms are not characteristic of hepatitis in all cases. In 70% of cases, the liver is palpable with a smooth, tender edge. Jaundice usually occurs 3 to 10 days after onset of symptoms. Often the patient begins to feel better once jaundice is present though malaise and jaundice may continue for weeks. Weight loss of 10 or more pounds is not unusual. Approximately 5% to 10% of all hepatitis B infections lead to the HBV carrier state or chronic liver disease. As many as 10% to 40% of non-A, non-B hepatitis cases will eventually develop some form of chronic liver disease, and a carrier state probably exists.

Complications

A very rare and serious complication, *fulminant hepatitis,* occurs in less than 5% of hepatitis cases and is defined by the appearance of hepatic failure or encephalopathy. Fulminant hepatitis usually occurs within 7 to 14 days after onset of hepatitis and is caused by severe necrosis of the liver. Supportive care in an ICU is essential to allow the liver time to heal. Initial symptoms include increasing lethargy, somnolence, and personality changes. If hepatic failure continues, the patient may become stuporous and fall into a coma. Mortality rates are 65% to 80%.[12] Death is frequently due to uncontrolled bleeding.

Chronic persistent hepatitis, the most common chronic sequela of hepatitis B, is marked by chronic inflammatory cells in the liver but necrosis and fibrosis are absent. Patients are generally healthy, but have intermittent or continuous elevation of liver enzymes. Jaundice is usually absent. Most cases eventually have resolution of infection, but some cases develop chronic active hepatitis.

Chronic active hepatitis is a more serious complication of hepatitis. Patients often present with symptoms of fatigue, anorexia, and weight loss, with recurrent episodes of jaundice. This disease can also be present in a clinically asymptomatic person. Liver enzymes are variably elevated. Piecemeal necrosis and occasional scarring of the liver are present. Patients with extensive liver damage (*i.e.,* portal-to-central bridging hepatic necrosis) have a tendency to develop *cirrhosis* (refer to Chapter 81). An extremely rare but serious long-term complication of HBV infection is *hepatocellular carcinoma.*

Medical Management

Diagnosis. Diagnosis of an acute case of hepatitis A is based on clinical symptoms, exposure history, elevated AST and ALT enzymes, and the presence of either anti-HAV IgM in the serum (when this test is available) or the presence of HBsAg in the serum.

Previous infections with hepatitis A are identified by a serum anti-HAV IgG result. For hepatitis B, resolving infections are usually indicated by anti-HBe, anti-HBc, and anti-HBs.

Treatment. Hepatitis is usually a self-limiting disease. Treatment for hepatitis cases is supportive, and the degree of intervention depends on the initial health of the patient. Young, healthy patients can usually recover on modified bedrest in their homes. Once symptoms abate, these persons can slowly return to their usual activities. If a relapse occurs, the patient should return to bedrest.

Persons who have severe nausea and vomiting, underlying pathology, high bilirubin levels (>10 mg/dl), ALT (SGPT) levels >50 times normal, or prolonged protimes may require hospitalization. Once symptoms abate, the patient may be discharged for convalescence at home.

Medications have not been found to be useful in arresting or altering the course of hepatitis. Only the most essential medications should be given in the acute phase of illness. Drugs which are detoxified in or excreted by the liver should be avoided. Sedatives should be avoided, if possible. Acetaminophen in low doses may be preferable to aspirin as an analgesic due to its lack of effect on the gastric mucosa and on platelet function. Corticosteroids are not recommended for treatment of uncomplicated viral hepatitis. They may actually prolong the course of the illness and increase the risk of sequelae.[8] Corticosteroids have sometimes been prescribed for patients who have biopsy and clinical evidence of progressive disease, although the role of such medication is uncertain at this time.

Exposure histories of family members and close contacts of hepatitis A or B patients should be done to determine who needs prophylaxis.

Prevention. Hepatitis B vaccine is now available for high-risk personnel (*e.g.,* ER staff, OR staff, laboratory technicians, dialysis staff) for prevention of hepatitis B. Three injections are required over a 6-month time period to provide immunity. Many hospitals are now providing vaccine for high-risk personnel. An initial screening may be conducted to determine employees who are already immune to hepatitis B (*i.e.,* those with anti-HBs). Of course, these immune individuals would not need to be vaccinated. Hepatitis B vaccine can also be given to family members at risk and persons with high-risk lifestyles.

Postexposure prophylaxis. Immune globulin (IG) is effective in ameliorating symptoms of hepatitis A in those who have had direct, fecal–oral contact (*e.g.,* household contact, day-care center case contact) with a hepatitis A case during time of infectiousness (2 weeks before and 1 week after onset of symptoms).

Hepatitis B immune globulin (HBIG) is recommended as prophylaxis against hepatitis B for susceptible personnel who have a single parenteral, oral, or mucosal exposure to HBV-infected blood, secretions, or excretions *known* to be positive for hepatitis B surface antigen (HBsAG—formerly known as HAA, AA).

Nursing Management

Nursing Diagnosis

Nursing diagnoses for the patient with hepatitis are related to the communicability of all three types of hepatitis and to the disturbance in liver function that is disrupted by the disease. The common diagnoses are self-care deficits related to the fatigue and weakness that accompanies the change in liver function, alteration in comfort related to the inflammation of the liver, alteration in nutritional intake related to nausea and vomiting, and potential for transmission of the disease to other people. The diagnoses need to be individualized to the particular patient. The nurse should assess the patient's level of infectiousness and resultant needs for isolation and/or prevention of spread of the disease. Assessment should also include observations of nutritional status, skin care needs, weight, level of fatigue, vital signs, recognition of pending complications, and the patient's knowledge of the disease.

Goals. The goals of nursing interventions are to prevent the spread of the disease in the hospital, maintain the patient's nutritional status, alleviate discomfort, recognize and report signs and symptoms of complications, and teach the patient about the disease and prevention of its spread.

Interventions

Control and containment of hepatitis A within a hospital is easy if basic hygienic techniques are followed. Hepatitis A is spread primarily by the fecal–oral route. The patient is most infectious prior to the onset of jaundice and for a week thereafter. During the time of infectiousness, the patient should be placed on Enteric Precautions.[6]

A patient with acute hepatitis A who is fecally continent is not likely to spread the disease and does not necessarily need a private room. The patient should be reminded to wash his or her hands with soap and water after using the rest room. The nurse should wear gloves and a gown when handling a bedpan or a fecally contaminated item; handwashing with soap and water is always important after contact with the patient and potentially infectious, contaminated articles. Of course, it is not always known that patients have an enteric infection while they are in the hospital. Therefore, it is always important to wash hands well and to treat feces or fecally contaminated items as though they may be infectious. See the accompanying Nursing Care Plan for the Patient with Hepatitis A.

A patient who is positive for HBsAg or who has non-A, non-B hepatitis should be placed on Blood/Body Fluid Precautions.[6] Any time an employee is to handle blood or body fluids from an HBsAg-positive or a non-A, non-B patient, gloves and gowns should be worn. Care should be taken to avoid splashing blood or serum onto the employee's mucous membranes or getting these secretions into cuts. In fact, if the employee has cuts on his or her hands, gloves should be worn while caring for these patients, Feces from these patients are not infectious unless the patient is experiencing gastrointestinal bleeding. Care should be taken in the disposal of needles used for these patients. Needles should not be recapped or bent; they should be placed in an impervious, prominently labeled container which is kept inside the room. For any patient in isolation, disposable articles contaminated with infectious material should be discarded. Reusable articles should be double-bagged and labeled before being sent for decontamination and reprocessing.

The patient's level of strength should be assessed and considered before activities are undertaken. While symptomatic, the patient should be on modified bedrest. Once symptoms abate, the patient should slowly return to routine activities. Alcoholic intake should be avoided until late in the convalescent period because the liver metabolizes alcohol. A low-fat, high-carbohydrate diet may be more palatable to the anorexic patient.

The nurse should explain to the patient precautions to take to avoid transmission of the disease to others and medications which should be avoided. Patients who are HBsAg-positive or who have been diagnosed with non-A, non-B should not donate blood or blood products.

Evaluation

The disease does not spread within the hospital. The patient's nutritional status will be maintained and discomfort will be minimized. The patient will understand the disease and how to prevent its spread.

(*Text continues on page 1240*)

NURSING CARE PLAN FOR THE PATIENT WITH HEPATITIS A

NURSING DIAGNOSIS/PROBLEM 1: Alteration in activity tolerance due to decreased ability of liver to synthesize proteins and metabolize nutrients and medications.

GOAL 1.1: To prevent further stress on liver function.

Nursing Interventions	Rationale	Outcome Criteria
1. Promote rest.	1. The liver requires time to heal. Increased levels of activity place greater demands on the liver.	1. Patient expresses diminishing feelings of weakness and fatigue. Gradual increase in self-care.
2. Avoid giving medications which must be detoxified in or excreted by the liver, including sedatives.	2. When medications cannot be detoxified by the liver, toxic levels could develop in the body. Many sedatives are detoxified or excreted by the liver. Also, sedatives mask signs and symptoms of impending hepatic coma.	2. Toxic levels of medications will not occur in the patient's bloodstream.
3. Teach the patient to avoid alcoholic beverages during the recovery period.	3. Alcohol is detoxified by the liver.	3. The patient will avoid alcohol during the acute phase of illness.

GOAL 1.2: Monitor the patient's liver function.

Nursing Interventions	Rationale	Outcome Criteria
1. Assess for signs and symptoms of fulminant hepatitis including lethargy, somnolence, and personality changes. Document changes. Consult with physician regarding any changes.	1. These are signs of liver failure. Toxic substances accumulate in the blood because the liver is unable to metabolize them.	1. Detect and report these signs and symptoms before coma occurs.
2. Monitor the patient's ALT, AST, bilirubin levels, and prothrombin.	2. Elevated liver enzymes and bilirubin levels indicate the degree of liver involvement. The prothrombin time may be elevated if the liver is unable to synthesize prothrombin. Also, there may be a decreased amount of vitamin K absorbed by the gut.	2. Consult with the physician regarding laboratory values that are elevated.
3. If prothrombin times are elevated, watch for signs and symptoms of bleeding.	3. Prolonged prothrombin times indicate the blood is taking longer to clot.	3. Early detection of abnormal bleeding.
4. Assess and document the color of the: • Skin • Stools • Sclera • Urine	4. Increased levels of bilirubin in the bloodstream cause the skin, urine, and sclera to be jaundiced. Stools will be pale and light gray.	4. Early detection of abnormalities indicative of decreasing liver function.

GOAL 1.3: Alleviate the patient's pruritus.

Nursing Interventions	Rationale	Outcome Criteria
1. Assess the patient's level of discomfort.	1. The buildup of bilirubin in the patient's skin may cause pruritus.	1. The patient will have minimal pruritus.

(Continued)

NURSING CARE PLAN FOR THE PATIENT WITH HEPATITIS A (*Continued*)

Nursing Interventions	Rationale
2. Keep the patient's skin from becoming dry by using emollient creams; teach patient to avoid frequent baths and irritating clothes.	2. Dry skin can cause pruritus.
3. Encourage the use of loose clothing, preferable made of cotton.	3. Perspiration can augment pruritus. Cotton allows perspiration to evaporate quickly.

NURSING DIAGNOSIS/PROBLEM 2: Potential for unintentional spread of hepatitis A due to inadequate knowledge.
GOAL 2: To prevent spread of infection by the fecal–oral route.

Nursing Interventions	Rationale	Outcome Criteria
1. The patient will be placed on Enteric Precautions until 1 week after the onset of jaundice.	1. The patient's feces are infectious 2 weeks before and 1 week after the onset of symptoms.	1. No patients in or employees of the hospital will develop hepatitis A.
2. The nurse entering the patient's room will follow Enteric Isolation precautions: • Wearing gloves for touching infective material. • Wearing a gown if soiling is likely. • Washing hands with soap and water before leaving the room. Articles contaminated with infective material should be discarded or bagged and labeled before being sent for decontamination and reprocessing.	2. Hepatitis A virus is spread by the fecal–oral route. The nurse wants to prevent spread of the virus from the patient to self or to other patients.	2. Nosocomial transmission of the virus will not occur.
3. The nurse will teach the patient how to prevent spread of the virus: • Handwashing with soap and running water is essenital after defecation. • Handwashing is essential prior to preparing food for others.	3. Hands which may be contaminated by the virus, especially after defecation, can spread the virus to others, directly or by food. Soap, running water, and scrubbing of the hands should remove the virus particles.	3. The patient and family will accuately decribe how to prevent spread of the virus and will follow procedures taught.

NURSING DIAGNOSIS/PROBLEM 3: Alteration in nutritional intake (less than body requirements) to assist the regeneration of hepatic cells.
GOAL 3: To assist the patient in developing an acceptable dietary plan.

Nursing Interventions	Rationale	Outcome Criteria
1. Assess the patient's level of appetite and nausea.	1. Patients with hepatitis often are anorexic and nauseated.	1. The patient will assist in developing an appealing diet.
2. Determine and offer types of foods which appeal to the patient.	2. Often the patient with hepatitis finds high-carbohydrate, low-fat diets more appetizing.	2. Dietary intake will be adequate to meet wound-healing needs.
3. Offer high-caloric foods in small amounts at frequent intervals.	3. Small amounts of foods may be more tolerable than large amounts.	
4. Prohibit cigarette smoking in the patient's room.	4. Cigarette smoke can create nausea in patients with hepatitis.	
5. Consult with dietitian as needed.		

One measure of goal achievement is the absence of spread of the disease within the hospital or, if the patient is at home, absence of the disease in other members of the family. Other outcome criteria are: the patient accurately explains the disease, its treatment, and actions to prevent spread; the patient is observed to carry out proper handwashing procedures; the patient reports increasing ability to perform activities of daily living without fatigue; nutritional intake of a low-fat, high-carbohydrate diet is adequate; weight is maintained; patient reports a decrease or absence of abdominal discomfort.

Peritonitis/Peritoneal Abscess

Peritonitis is an inflammation of the peritoneum which occurs as a result of bacterial or chemical contamination. Peritonitis may result in the formation of a peritoneal abscess, which is a collection of purulent material surrounded by inflamed tissue.

Etiology and Pathophysiology

Peritonitis can occur from entry of GI contents into the peritoneal cavity following perforation anywhere along the GI tract or in any of the abdominal organs including ovaries and fallopian tubes. Organisms commonly associated with peritonitis include *Escherichia coli* (most common), streptococci, staphylococci, pneumococci, and *Pseudomonas*. Spillage of pancreatic enzymes can also cause destruction of tissue and peritonitis. Other causes are abdominal trauma and postoperative complication (*e.g.*, leakage from an anastomosis). Peritonitis is the most common cause of death following abdominal surgery. With the introduction of bacteria into the sterile abdominal cavity, there is a localized, intense inflammatory response. The extent of the inflammation will depend upon the cause or the amount of bacterial contamination. Peritonitis may stay localized in one area and become walled off by fibrous inflammatory tissue resulting in an abscess, or it may become generalized throughout the peritoneal cavity.

Clinical Manifestations

The patient with peritonitis has abdominal discomfort as well as systemic manifestations of an inflammatory response. The patient is febrile, and may be nauseous and vomiting. Perforation of the intestine produces pain, and the patient may be in shock (*e.g.*, tachycardia, tachypnea, hypotension) as a result of fluid loss into the abdominal cavity and pain. Intestinal motility is decreased, and paralytic ileus, which occurs as a result of local inflammation and irritation, is a common complication of peritonitis. The abdomen on physical exam is tender to touch and very rigid. Pain is intensified with movement. The patient may have abdominal distention due to movement of fluid into the abdominal cavity and decreased gastrointestinal motility. Peritonitis, if undetected and untreated, has a high mortality rate. Therefore, the focus is on prevention and aggressive treatment.

Medical Management

Diagnosis. Peritonitis and peritoneal abscess are diagnosed from patient history, physical examination, and x-ray visualization of the abdomen. Laboratory values, such as elevated white blood cell count, are indicative of an infection. Fluid and electrolyte imbalances are due to loss of fluids and protein into the abdominal cavity.

Treatment. Medical treatment is directed at correcting fluid and electrolyte imbalances, arresting the infection, relieving abdominal pain, and supporting the patient in the toxic period. Parenteral antibiotics are utilized to control infection. Analgesics are given to reduce discomfort and anxiety. Morphine is not frequently used because it decreases GI motility. Fluid and electrolyte replacement is initiated to correct imbalances. Nasogastric drainage may be instituted, especially if paralytic ileus is present. This will decrease the distention of the GI tract resulting from absence of motility. If the peritonitis or peritoneal abscess is the result of perforation, surgical intervention may be necessary to close the intestinal wall and to remove fluid and exudative material from the peritoneum. Surgery may be performed after fluid replacement is sufficient to correct symptoms of shock.

Nursing Management

Nursing Diagnosis

The problems usually present in the patient with peritonitis are related to fluid loss into the peritoneal cavity, the presence of infection, and the systemic toxic state. The diagnoses are fluid volume deficit, alteration in comfort, alteration in self-care ability, potential for complication of shock, anxiety, alteration in bowel function, and potential for alteration in mental acuity.

Patients at risk for peritonitis or with this diagnosis should be assessed every 15 to 30 minutes for signs of shock (see Chapter 24). Observations of abdominal girth must be made to determine progression of abdominal distention. Recording of quantity and consistency of vomitus is necessary. Pain, and the response to control measures, needs to be determined. Assessment must include record of intake and output. Monitoring of intravenous therapy and nasogastric drainage is essential. Assessment for potential complications of bed rest, such as respiratory infection and skin trauma, will be carried out daily as will assessment of the patient's ability for self-care. The severity of the illness usually results in signs of high anxiety and fear in both the patient and family.

Goals. The goals of nursing interventions for the patient with peritonitis are: to relieve discomfort, to detect early manifestations of further complications, to promote recovery from infection, and to alleviate anxiety and fear.

Interventions

The patient with peritonitis or peritoneal abscess is acutely ill. Intravenous fluids are initiated and the nurse needs to monitor the patient's fluid balance. Vital signs are checked frequently to observe for changes in blood pressure and heart rate. A nasogastric or nasointestinal tube may be inserted, particularly in the patient with a perforation. The purpose of the nasointestinal tube is to reduce the movement of gastrointestinal contents into the abdominal cavity. The patient who does not have a perforation may have a nasogastric tube inserted if a paralytic ileus exists. The patients without nasogastric or nasointestinal drainage are usually not given food or fluid orally until the motility of the gastrointestinal tract has been determined. The patient with such a drainage tube is also not given any nourishment by mouth. Antibiotics are administered intravenously.

Pain control includes administering prescribed analgesics and providing comfort measures, both physical and emotional. It may include assisting the person to cope with the life-threatening nature of the situation. Families will also need help in understanding the illness and its treatment. The seriousness of the situation may place considerable stress on the family, and nursing support will be essential. The patient and family may desire counseling from a spiritual advisor (see Chapter 11).

Monitoring of the patient's progress is a major interdependent nursing function. Early detection of a change in physical status may make it possible for the physician to apply medical interventions promptly.

Evaluation

The patient should be prevented from going into irreversible shock. Recovery may be slow but the process will be with minimal discomfort. Fluid and electrolyte imbalances will be avoided. Personal hygiene needs will be met, and the complications of bed rest, such as respiratory infections and skin trauma, will be avoided.

The criteria for goal achievement are:

1. Patient reports decrease in discomfort following administration of analgesics.
2. Fluid intake and output balance.
3. Blood pressure and heart rate remain within normal limits and, if not, the physician is consulted.
4. Fever gradually declines over the period of antibiotic administration.
5. The patient and family openly discuss their concerns and fears.
6. The patient and family express a decrease in anxiety.

References

1. Balart LA: The sequelae of hepatitis B infection. Current Concepts in Gastroenterology 8:12–16, 1983
2. Brown HW, Neva FA: Basic Clinical Parasitology. Norwalk CT, Appleton-Century-Crofts, 1983
3. Centers for Disease Control. Annual summary 1982: Reported morbidity and mortality in the United States. Morbidity Mortality Weekly Rep 31(54), 1983
4. Craft JC: Giardia and giardiasis in childhood. Ped Infec Dis 1:196–211, 1982
5. Field B, Hepner G, Shabot M, Schwartz A, State D, Worthern N, Wilson R: Nasogastric suction in alcoholic pancreatitis. Science 24:339–344, 1979
6. Garner JS, Simmons BP: Guideline for isolation precautions in hospitals. Infection Control 4(suppl):245–325, 1983
7. Gurevich I: Viral hepatitis. Am J Nurs 83:571–586, 1983
8. Hoofnagle JH: Acute hepatitis. In Mandell GL, Douglas RG, Bennett JE (ed): Principles and Pratice of Infectious Diseases, pp 1043–1062. New York, Wiley, 1979
9. Hughes JM: Food poisoning. In Mandell GL, Douglas RG, Bennett JE (eds): Principles and Practices of Infectious Diseases, pp 907–923. New York, Wiley, 1979
10. Krogstad DJ, Spencer HC, Healy GR: Amebiasis. N Engl J Med 298:262–265, 1978
11. Orenstein WA, Wu E, Wilkins J, Robinson K, Francis DP, Timko N, Wayne R: Hospitacquired hepatitis A: Report of an outbreak. Pediatrics 67:494–497, 1981
12. Perrillo RP, Aach RD: The clinical course and chronic sequelae of hepatitis B virus infection. Seminars in Liver Disease 1:15–25, 1981
13. Rawls WE: Herpes simplex virus type 1 and 2 and herpes virus simiae. In Lennette EH, Schmidt NJ (eds): Diagnostic Procedure for Viral, Rickettsial and Chlamydial Infections, pp 309–315. Washington DC, American Public Health Association, Inc., 1979
14. Seeberg S, Brandberg A, Hermodsson S, Larsson P, Lundgren S: Hospital outbreak of hepatitis A secondary to blood exchange in a baby. Lancet 1:1155–1156, 1981
15. Sexton DJ: Amebiasis in a mental institution: Serologic and epidemiologic studies. Am J Epidemiol 100:414–423, 1974
16. Sherlock S: Virus hepatitis. In: Diseases of the Liver and Biliary System, pp 244–265. Oxford, Blackwell, 1981
17. Spiro HM: Clinical Gastroenterology. New York, Macmillan, 1977

Bibliography

Almy TP, Howell DA: Diverticular disease of the colon. N Engl J Med 302:324–330, 1980

Anderson SJ et al: Enteral nutrition for hospitalized patients. Plast Surg Nurs, 3(4):93–94, 1983

Block JE: Surgical management of Crohn's colitis. N Engl J Med 302:1068–1070, 1980

Buchman TG, Roizman B, Adams G, Stover GH: Restriction endonuclease fingerprinting of herpes simplex virus DNA: A novel epidemiological tool applied to a nosocomial outbreak. J Infect Dis 138:488–498, 1978

Castro AF, Tuxien P: Inflammatory bowel disease. Surg Clin North Am 58:573–582, 1978

Dietzen DC: Surgery of the pancreas. SGAJ 5(4):5–6, 1983

DiMagno EP: Answers to questions on acute pancreatitis. Hosp Med 19(10):91, 95–101, 104–105, 1983

Diverticulosis (pictorial). Nurs Mirror Nov 9:157, 1983

Editorial: Guidelines for using gastrointestinal tubes. Nursing 13(12):57–59, 1983

Hammerberg O, Watts J, Chernesky M, Luchsinger I, Rawls W: An outbreak of herpes simplex virus type 1 in an intensive care nursery. Ped Infect Dis 2:290–294, 1983

Harris N: Controlling dental diseases: State of the art. Health Values: Achieving High Level Wellness 8(1):31–37, 1984

Kirsner JB: Observation on the medical treatment of inflammatory bowel disease. JAMA 243:557–563, 1980

Managing the patient with concurrent life-threatening conditions. Nursing 14(6):60–64, 1984

Morran CG et al: Randomized controlled trial of physiotherapy for postoperative pulmonary complications. Br J Anaesth 55(11):1113–1117, 1983

Painter N: Diverticular disease of the colon: A bane of the elderly. Geriatrics 31:89–94, 1976

Petersdorf R et al: Harrison's Principles of Internal Medicine. New York, McGraw Hill, 1983

Plumley PF, Francis B: Dietary management of diverticular disease. J Am Diet Assoc 63:527–530, 1973

Rodman MJ: An update on the new drugs you are dispending (cholelithiasis). RN, 47(4):67–70, 1984

Sabiston D (ed): Davis-Christopher Textbook of Surgery. Philadelphia, WB Saunders, 1981

Siram K et al: Home enteral hyperalimentation catheter: Surgical technique and problem solving. Nutr Support Ser 4(3):32, 36, 1984

Smith J et al: An inside view: Endoscopic retrograde cholangiopancreatophy. Nurs Mirror, Nov 3, 157(22):30–33, 1983

Smith L, Thier S: Pathophysiology. Philadelphia, WB Saunders, 1981

Speedie G: Nursology of mouth care: Preventing, comforting and seeking activities related to mouth care. J of Advanced Nursing 8:33–40, 1983

Ulrich RS: View through a window may influence recovery from surgery (psychosocial factors). Science April 27, 224:420–421, 1984

VanLandingham SB et al: Pancreatic pseudocyst. Hosp Med, 20(1):71–72, 77–78, 81–83, 1984

Chapter 83

Ulcers of the Gastrointestinal Tract

Margaret Heitkemper
Linda M. Simmons

Gastrointestinal ulceration represents one of the most common pathophysiological problems of the GI tract as well as one of the most serious. The treatment of ulcer disease as well as ulcerlike symptoms accounts for a significant portion of over-the-counter pharmaceutical agents purchased by consumers. Ulceration, in general, implies a break in the normal continuity of the mucosal lining, the depth of which may vary from superficial lesion (erosion) to a full thickness lesion which results in perforation.

Classification

Gastrointestinal ulcers are frequently classified according to etiology (*e.g.,* peptic or stress). Peptic ulcers refer to those ulcerations produced by an imbalance in hydrochloric (HCl) acid and proteolytic enzyme secretion and the natural protective barrier of the stomach and intestine. Generally, peptic ulcer disease is a chronic disease marked by exacerbations and remissions. Stress ulcers or acute focal necrosis are generally considered to be acute lesions of the GI tract which occur in response to a major physiological stressor such as trauma, hemorrhage, cardiovascular insult, or burns. Because of inherent differences in the etiology and pathophysiology of peptic ulcer disease and stress ulcers, these types of GI ulcerations are discussed separately.

Peptic Ulcers

Peptic ulcers are also classified according to anatomical location (esophageal, gastric, duodenal, or jejunal) and depth of the ulceration. Superficial ulcerations which penetrate into the mucosal layer of the stomach or duodenum are referred to as *erosions.* These superficial lesions are not readily detectable by x-ray visualization. Deeper lesions penetrate the mucosal layer and perhaps extend into the muscular layers of the intestinal wall. Perforation, a life-threatening condition, occurs when the ulcer penetrates through all layers of the intestinal wall, allowing gastric or intestinal contents to spill into the abdominal cavity of into an adjoining organ.

Because of the intense inflammatory response accompanying Crohn's disease and ulcerative colitis, they are discussed in the preceding chapter.

Definition and Incidence

Peptic ulcer disease, in general, is a chronic and recurring disorder of the GI tract. It is projected that one out of ten persons will experience peptic ulcer disease at some point in life. Patients with peptic ulcer disease (PUD) frequently have a long history of exacerbation and remission.

However, with the advent of new pharmacological agents (*e.g.,* histamine receptor blockers), which promote ulcer healing, the number of patients admitted to the hospital with a primary diagnosis of peptic ulcer disease is decreasing.

Peptic ulcers occur in those areas of the GI tract exposed to hydrochloric (HCl) acid and the proteolytic enzyme, pepsin. Regardless of the location of the benign ulcer, the common denominator for peptic ulcers is the presence of HCl acid. Although peptic ulcers occur in the stomach and duodenum, the most common site for peptic ulcer formation is the duodenum which is "downstream" from the site of acid secretion. Some patients may have ulcers in both the stomach and the duodenum. Ulcerations in the jejunum due to inadequate buffering of HCl acid in the duodenum are infrequent. However, patients who have had a gastric resection and gastroenterostomy, in which gastric contents bypass the duodenum, jejunal tissue may be exposed to acidic contents. Peptic ulcer disease encompasses a variety of disorders which result in destruction or ulceration of the GI mucosa.

Ulcers, in general, occur more frequently in men than women. However there appears to be an increasing incidence among women, particularly employed women who have family responsibilities as well. In the United States, duodenal ulcer disease appears to be more common in urban areas than in rural environments. The peak incidence of duodenal ulcers is in the fourth to fifth decade while gastric ulcers are most commonly observed in people in their sixth decade. A small percentage of patients will have multiple ulcers with both the stomach and duodenum affected.

Etiology and Pathophysiology

The presence of food in the stomach results in the release of HCl from the parietal cells of the stomach. The mechanisms for HCl release are multiple and, for the most part, interrelated. Stimulators of acid secretion include the vagus nerve which releases acetylcholine which then stimulates the parietal cells to secrete HCl. Central nervous system control over acid secretion is mediated by the vagus nerve. The antral hormone gastrin, which is released in response to food in the stomach, stimulates the release of HCl acid. The release of HCl acid is also stimulated by histamine which is present in the gastric mucosa. Histamine stimulates acid secretion by specific histamine receptors on parietal cells.

When acid is secreted and the gastric pH drops to 2 or 3, the conversion of pepsinogens (inactive forms of the enzymes secreted by the gastric chief cells) to pepsin is facilitated. Although not essential for protein digestion, pepsin does initiate protein digestion in the stomach.

Under normal circumstances, the gastric mucosa is protected from autodigestion by pepsin because of the presence of the gastric mucosal barrier. While the exact anatomical components of this barrier are not known, it is hypothesized that it is composed of the following protective elements: (1) the mucus secreted by cells lining the stomach, (2) tight junctions between the epithelial cells which prevent the back diffusion of HCl acid. The regenerative ability of the epithelial cells which permits rapid recovery from mucosal injury is a contributing factor to the barrier. The pathogenesis of ulcer disease seems to be related to either an excess of acid-peptic activity or a disruption of one of the components of the gastric mucosal barrier. For example, the ingestion of aspirin, steroids, nonsteroidal anti-inflammatory drugs (*e.g.,* indomethacin), alcohol, or bile salts can result in increased permeability of the epithelial cell barrier allowing the back diffusion of HCl acid.

There appears to be a hereditary predisposition to peptic ulcer disease, in that a person with a family member with ulcer disease has an increased risk of developing an ulcer as compared to the general population. However, it is not known whether this is related to increase in basal (nonstimulated) or stimulated acid secretion, or a decrease in protective mechanisms. In general, the amount of acid secretion varies from person to person, and the pattern of acid secretion within each person varies depending upon the time of day, diet, gastric contents, hunger, stress (both psychological and physical), and the presence of other pathophysiological problems. Genetic, environmental, and experiential factors all influence acid secretions.

By itself, hypersecretion of HCl acid from the parietal cells can produce gastric and more commonly, duodenal ulcers. Patients who have Zollinger-Ellison syndrome, in which high levels of gastrin are secreted from a tumor in the pancreas, exhibit multiple ulcers in both the duodenum and stomach. Ulcers occur when acid secretion exceeds the mucosal protective mechanisms or the ability of the stomach to buffer the acid. They can result from the ingestion of substances which are destructive to the gastric and duodenal epithelium, as well as hypersecretion of HCl acid. Cytoprotection of the gastric epithelium may be compromised in the patient receiving alkylating drugs such as those used in chemotherapy. These drugs decrease RNA synthesis and hence, reduce the mitosis of epithelial cells. Due to the decreased ability of the epithelial cells to replace themselves, such drugs leave the gastric mucosa particularly vulnerable to erosion formation. In the stomach when the normal defense of the gastric mucosal barrier is overwhelmed, HCl acid can then diffuse back from the gastric lumen into the mucosal layer. The acid along with pepsin is destructive to the epithelial cells and capillaries.

Peptic ulcer disease has been associated with diet, in that foods which stimulate acid secretion are though to be ulcerogenic. Certain constituents of foods such as caffeine or theophylline may be aggravating to the person with ulcer disease, but there is no evidence that these constituents by themselves are ulcerogenic.

While peptic ulcer disease is the result of an imbalance of corrosive versus protective forces, there appear to be anatomical differences that influence the importance of these factors. Manifestations of the disease and medical management are related to anatomical location of the ulcers along the GI tract, as discussed below.

Esophageal Peptic Ulcers

Pathophysiology

Erosions or ulceration of esophageal mucosa may occur in the patient with reflux esophagitis. The presence of an incompetent lower esophageal sphincter or hiatal hernia will predispose to reflux of aciditic gastric contents into the lower portion of the esophagus. Gastric acid along with proteolytic pepsin in gastric juice can be destructive to the esophageal mucosa. The outcome will be inflammation (*i.e.*, esophagitis) and, if prolonged, ulcer development.

Clinical Manifestations

Patients with reflux esophagitis complain of "heartburn" or epigastric distress which may radiate to the back or lower abdomen. Recurrent esophagitis and the replacement of mucosa with scar tissue can result in esophageal stricture. Patients with Zollinger-Ellison syndrome who have hypersecretion of gastric acid also have a high incidence of esophageal disease. Likewise patients with diabetic neuropathy who exhibit delayed gastric emptying are also at risk for reflux esophagitis, as well as patients with a nasogastric tube in place which keeps the lower esophageal sphincter between the stomach and the esophagus open.

Gastric Peptic Ulcers

Description and Incidence

Gastric ulcers can develop in any portion of the stomach but are most frequently found in the antrum of the stomach, which is located proximal to the pylorus, and the lesser curvature of the stomach. Typically, a gastric ulcer is round or oval shaped and has the appearance of a punched out cavity with an inflammatory base. Patients with gastric ulcers are generally older than patients with duodenal ulcers. The increased use of nonsteroidal anti-inflammatory drugs for chronic diseases such as arthritis may be a precipitating factor. Family history also appears to be an important factor in determining patients at risk for developing a gastric ulcer.

Etiology

As discussed earlier, peptic ulcers occur as a result of an imbalance in the secretion of HCl acid and the mucosal resistance factors. However, in some patients hypersecretion of HCl does not appear to be a causative factor in the etiology of the gastric ulcer, because gastric ulcers may be associated with reduced or normal basal acid output. The patient with a gastric ulcer who also has duodenal peptic ulcer disease frequently exhibits an acid secretion pattern similar to that of duodenal ulcer patients. In patients who do not demonstrate acid hypersecretion, the etiology appears to be an impairment of the normal protective mechanisms of the stomach. Agents which have been shown to be destructive to the gastric mucosal barrier with chronic ingestion include aspirin, corticosteroids, nonsteroidal anti-inflammatory drugs, and reserpine. It has been suggested that aspirin may be responsible for up to 15% of all gastric ulcers. However, the link between pharmacological agents and ulcer development is not clearcut, because patients taking these drugs are likely to have a systemic disorder which in itself may be a factor in the development of the ulcer. The reflux of intestinal contents containing bile salts as well as the reflux of pancreatic and intestinal alkaline contents into the stomach have been shown to be destructive to the gastric mucosa. Gastric ulcers may develop in patients with a history of gastritis due to hypersecretion of HCl acid.

Clinical Manifestations

Signs and symptoms of gastric ulcers are unpredictable and in some cases asymptomatic. As many as one-third of the patients with gastric ulcers who are 65 or older may be asymptomatic with a gastric ulcer.[2] The decrease in ulcer-type pain in older patients may be due to decreased visceral pain sensitivity. This observation coupled with the increased incidence of gastric ulcers in older patients, indicates the need for careful nursing assessment of the patient with unexplained anemia, loss of appetite, or decreased body weight. Although some patients may complain of nausea and vomiting these are not common symptoms of a gastric ulcer. The signs and symptoms produced by the complications of gastric ulcer disease are more discernible than the symptoms of gastric ulcer disease itself.

Therefore, it can be seen that there are no clearcut signs of gastric peptic ulcer disease. Patients may have some epigastric tenderness as well as loss of weight and dull, aching epigastric pain, which frequently radiates to the back, sternum, or lower abdomen. The patient may also complain of nocturnal epigastric pain occuring 1 to 2 hours after going to bed. The cause of pain is less predictable for the patient with gastric ulcers than for the patient with duodenal ulcers. While for many gastric ulcer patients pain is relieved by food or antacids, the pain-food-relief cycle is not always present and in some patients the ingestion of food may produce or increase epigastric discomfort. When the pain is aggravated by food, the patient has a decrease in appetitite and a resulting weight loss. Laboratory determinations may reveal mild to moderate anemia. Long-standing gastric ulcer disease will produce loss of gastric epithelial cells and thus reduced acid secretion or acholorhydria which may also produce anemia due to decreased intrinsic factor and decreased absorption of vitamin B_{12} in the small intestine.

Gastric ulcers are a serious problem both in relation to the primary complications including hemorrhage, perforation, obstruction, and the increased incidence of gastric cancer in patients with a history of gastric ulcers (see Chapter 81). Similarities and differences between gastric and duodenal peptic ulcers are shown in Table 83–1.

Duodenal Peptic Ulcers

Description and Incidence

Peptic ulcer disease involving the duodenum is more common than are gastric ulcers. Approximately 200,000 new cases are diagnosed annually. Unlike gastric ulcers, peptic ulcers are rarely associated with malignancies. Duodenal ulcers are characteristically deep, penetrating through the submucosal layers of the intestinal wall. These ulcers are generally located in the proximal duodenum within close proximity of the (pylorus junction, duodenal bulb). As noted

TABLE 83–1
Comparison of Gastric and Duodenal Ulcers

	Gastric	*Duodenal*
Location:	Distal stomach, antrum, lesser curvature	Proximal duodenum, duodenal bulb
Incidence:	5th–6th decade; men greater than women; most common ulcer in over 65 age group	4th–5th decade; men greter than women; most common ulcer in under 65 age group
Symptoms:	Epigastric pain, relieved or aggravated by food anorexia	Epigastric pain, pain-food-relief cycle
Etiological factors:	Disruption of gastric mucosal barrier Ulcerogenic drugs: Aspirin Nonsteroidal anti-inflammatory Steroids Bile reflux History of chronic gastritis High, normal, or low acid secretion	Hypersecretion of HCl acid Ulcerogenic drugs Psychosocial stress Seasonal variations Blood group O
Hereditary predisposition:	Yes	Yes
Malignancy:	7%–8%	Rare

earlier, the anatomical location of the duodenum makes it "downstream" from the site of acid secretion.

Etiology

Duodenal ulcers may result from increased gastric acid secretion, defective duodenal alkalinization or decreased resistance of the duodenal mucosa to acid. Most persons with duodenal ulcers have higher than normal HCl acid secretion rates under both basal conditions and under conditions of maximal stimulation with histamine or pentagastrin (a synthetic form of the antral hormone gastrin which is a potent stimulator of HCl acid secretion). The excess hydrochloric acid reaching the duodenum may be the result of an increase in the number of parietal cells, an increased acid secretion in response to a meal, or a defect in the ability to shut off acid secretion once it has been initiated.

A genetic factor may be present in etiology because a person with a family member with a duodenal ulcer is at three times the risk for developing an ulcer than are persons without a family history. Persons with Type O blood appear to have tendency toward duodenal ulcer development. It has long been thought that peptic ulcer disease is associated with psychosocial stress or an inability to deal with stress. While the relationship between stress and peptic ulcer disease remains to be determined, case reports of persons with ulcer disease indicate that some patients with ulcer disease do experience a larger number of psychosocial stressful events, or that they are more sensitive to this type of stress.[7]

In a certain percentage of patients with both acute and chronic ulcer disease, stressful events often precede symptoms, as well as complications. Personality characteristics may be a factor in transient or chronic elevations in gastric acid secretion. Stress with its activation of the autonomic nervous system and increase in acid secretion may aggravate ulcer disease or potentiate ulcer development. Seasonal variations in the recurrence or exacerbation of symptoms have been observed, with spring and fall having the highest incidence of reported ulcer symptoms. Other factors associated with duodenal ulcer disease include cigarette smoking, as well as cirrhosis and chronic renal failure.

Clinical Manifestations

The most common complaint of patients who have duodenal ulcers is "heartburn" or pain in the epigastric area. Patients may describe this pain as burning, aching, or hungerlike. Similar to the pain of gastric ulcers, it may radiate to the lower abdomen, sternum, or back. This pain generally follows a pain-food-relief cycle in that food relieves the pain by buffering HCl acid during exacerbation of the ulcer disease. Although patients may complain of pain at bedtime, pain in the morning is not a frequent complaint. This is probably related to decreased HCl acid secretion during the night. Characteristically, this pain occurs 1 to 3 hours after a meal and is often relieved by food or antacids. Some patients with duodenal ulcer disease actually gain weight due to the frequency of meals rather than experiencing weight loss. Patients with recurring ulcer disease frequently experience a clustering of symptoms lasting days to weeks, followed by pain-free periods. This ulcer-type pain, however, may also occur in persons who do not have any histological evidence of duodenal or gastric ulcer disease. It is important to note that not all patients with duodenal ulcer disease will experience or complain of epigastric pain.

In many patients symptoms do not always correlate with the presence or absence of active disease. Some patients with symptoms of heartburn or epigastric distress may not have active disease, while an asymptomatic patient may hemorrhage. Manifestations of an acute hemorrhage may include hematemesis, melena, and orthostatic hypotension. Patients who experience a slow bleed from the ulcer may complain of weakness, fatigue, and symptoms of cardiac failure. Nausea and vomiting are uncommon complaints with duodenal ulcer disease. However, with gastric outlet obstruction because of scarring and stenosis, the patient may have vomiting several hours after eating, as well as anorexia and weight loss. Laboratory evaluation may reveal a mild to moderate anemia.

The nurse needs to evaluate the patient's complaint of epigastric pain and determine if a change in location or duration of the pain has occurred. Often a change in the nature of pain denotes the existence of complications.

Complications

Intractability. When ulcer symptoms are not resolved with medication, diet, and environmental modification, the symptoms are termed intractable. Intractability is the most common complication of peptic ulcer disease. The unrelenting discomfort associated with this condition has a significant impact on a person's lifestyle. It is the most common reason for gastric surgery.

Hemorrhage. Bleeding is a common complication of peptic ulcers. Ulceration leading to erosion of blood vessels occurs in 25% of patients. The most common site for the hemorrhage is the posterior aspect of the duodenal bulb. Symptoms may be mild or severe.

Among the presenting signs of GI hemorrhage are anemia, stool which is positive for occult blood, or black tarry stools. Tarry stools may indicate either ongoing bleeding or bleeding that occurred within the past few days. Signs and symptoms are related to the amount and rate of blood loss and include tachycardia, hypotensions, and fatigue.

Because a large number of patients will experience hemorrhage without pain or discomfort, the nurse needs to carefully assess changes in vital signs. For example, the patient with a history of high blood pressure may exhibit a drop in blood pressure as a result of hemorrhage but this decrease may result in a blood pressure reading with normal limits. Therefore, the patient's blood pressure and heart rate are evaluated with respect to their normal baseline level as well as determination of orthostatic hypotension.

Symptoms which indicate a need for prompt intervention include hematemesis and, ultimately, shock due to blood loss. Depending on the extent of bleeding, the patient may require a NG (nasogastric) or naso-intestinal tube, saline lavage, blood transfusions, and possibly surgery. The mortality rate associated with hemorrhage is 3% to 10%. The mortality rate increases significantly in the over 60 age group due to the impact of blood loss on coexisting conditions (*e.g.*, cardiovascular and renal disease).

While the presence of acute GI bleeding may be indicative of ulcer disease, upper GI bleeding may be the result of other processes such as bleeding esophageal varices, esophagitis, gastritis, or blood dyscracia.

Perforation. A small percentage (about 5%) of ulcers will perforate. This is a very serious, potentially life-threatening occurrence. Accounting for 65% of all ulcer deaths, perforation occurs when the ulcer erodes the entire thickness of the gastric or duodenal mucosal and muscular wall. Perforation can occur in chronic ulcer disease or be the first symptom of an acute problem. Depending on ulcer location, perforation may extend into adjoining structures and become sealed off (*e.g.*, perforation of posterior wall of the duodenum into the pancreas). Pancreatitis, a very serious potentially lethal infection, may result. Perforation may also extend into the peritoneum. Consequently partially digested food, acid, digestive enzymes, and bacteria freely invade the sterile abdominal area. The resulting infection is termed *peritonitis*. The patient with a perforated ulcer is at high risk for peritonitis and prompt surgical intervention is necessary. Surgical repair of the perforation may involve closure of the immediate area or more extensive resection of the ulcer.

With perforation, the patient experiences sudden onset of severe abdominal pain. As a result of both the pain and the leakage of gastric and intestinal contents, the patient will exhibit signs and symptoms of shock. The abdomen is rigid to palpation and silent to auscultation. X-ray films are taken to diagnose perforation as the escape of air from the stomach shows up as free air in the abdominal cavity.

Stenosis/Obstruction. About 5% of chronic peptic ulcers result in gastric outlet obstruction. Stensosis is due to inflammation, edema, scarring, and pylorospasm. Depending upon the degree of inflammation or scar tissue, complete obstruction of the pylorus or intestine may occur. Both stenosis and obstruction are more common in duodenal ulcer disease than in esophageal or gastric ulcer disease. Symptoms of stenosis/obstruction include anorexia, bloating, and nausea after eating. When this is a chronic problem, loss of body weight will result. Severe obstruction results in vomiting which may be projectile and foul-smelling due to prolonged stasis of stomach contents.

The patient with gastric or intestinal obstruction requires hospitalization for the treatment of this complication. A nasogastric or naso-intestinal tube is inserted and intermittent suction is initiated to empty the stomach or intestine and allow inflammation and edema to subside. Intravenous (IV) therapy is initiated to replace fluids and electrolytes which are lost as a result of vomiting or suctioning. Surgical intervention may be necessary to relieve the obstruction.

Medical Management

Diagnosis

The presence of peptic ulcer may first be suspected from the patient's history and physical examination. About one-third of the patients with peptic ulcers are asymptomatic until a complication such as hemorrhage or perforation occurs. The presence of occult blood in the stool may be the first sign in an asymptomatic patient. Because both patients with gastric and duodenal ulcers experience ulcer pain, it is not possible to distinguish between the two based on symptoms. Patients with symptoms of GI dysfunction often undergo a number of diagnostic tests to pinpoint the cause of symptoms. The nurse's role in patient preparation for diagnostic procedures as well as after care are discussed in Chapter 79.

To determine or evaluate the ulcer size and depth, the patient may be scheduled for GI endoscopy in which a flexible fiberoptic endoscopic instrument is passed into the esophagus, stomach, or duodenum for visualization of the lumen wall. Because endoscopic visualization permits direct view of the ulcer, it can be determined if the ulcer is currently bleeding. New scopes allow for cauterization of vessels to decrease bleeding or laser therapy to increase healing. Manometric and pH monitoring will provide information on the pressure of the lower esophageal sphincter as well as the pH of the lower esophagus.

For the patient with a gastric ulcer, tissue biopsies from multiple sites in the stomach, as well as brush cytology or wash saline cytology may also be performed at the time of endoscopic exam to rule out the possibility of gastric cancer. Although not as accurate as endoscopic examination to diagnose superficial ulcers or erosions, upper GI x-ray series using barium as the contrast material may also be employed in the diagnosis of ulcer disease.

Analysis of gastric contents may be performed to identify gastric pathology as well as to determine the effectiveness of antisecretory drug therapy. Both basal and maximally stimulated HCl acid secretion are measured to determine if hypersecretion of HCl acid is an etiologic factor in patients with gastric or duodenal ulcers. A serum gastrin level determination may also be performed. Patients who have a history of chronic gastritis and gastric ulcers may have high levels of serum gastrin, because gastrin is released from the antrum in response to a low intragastric pH. A fasting gastrin level may also be determined to rule out Zollinger-Ellison syndrome, because these patients have high levels of the hormone secreted by the pancreas.

Treatment

The aims of medical therapies for peptic ulcer disease include the following:

1. To alleviate symptoms.
2. To minimize the offensive factors responsible for the ulceration.
3. To optimize the conditions that promote healing.
4. To prevent recurrence and complications.

Medical management includes pharmacologic, dietary, and environmental interventions.

Medications for peptic ulcers generally fall into three categories; acid-neutralizers (*e.g.,* antacids), antisecretory agents (*e.g.,* histamine (H_2) receptor antagonists and anticholinergics), and cytoprotective agents (*e.g.,* sucralfate). These drugs may be used individually or in combination to promote ulcer healing or to prevent recurrence of ulcers.

Antacids

Antacids have long been the cornerstone for symptomatic relief and promotion of healing in patients with peptic ulcer disease. The primary purpose of antacid administration is to neutralize gastric (hydrochloric) acid, which will then secondarily promote healing and prevent tissue breakdown. Antacids are usually given to keep the gastric pH about 5.0 which then inhibits the conversion of pepsinogen to its active form, pepsin.[3] Most antacids consist of aluminum, magnesium, calcium, or bicarbonate, either as single agents or in various combinations (Table 83–2). The numerous antacid preparations vary in their capability to neutralize acid. Antacids also vary in their sodium content. Because of the frequency of antacid administration in ulcer disease, the sodium content may be an important consideration, especially for patients with congestive heart failure and high blood pressure. Some preparations have the advantage of being sugar-free which may also be an important consideration in some patients (Table 83–2).

SIDE-EFFECTS. The most common side-effects of antacid therapy are changes in bowel function. Magnesium-containing agents tend to cause diarrhea while aluminum and calcium antacids cause constipation. These side-effects are counterbalanced in products that contain both magnesium and aluminum. Magnesium-containing antacids are contraindicated for patients with renal failure. Aluminum-containing antacids also place the patient at risk for phosphorus depletion due to the binding of aluminum with dietary phosphorus to form an insoluble compound which is then excreted in feces. The latter type is preferred for patients with renal failure, in order to reduce hyperphosphatemia and urinary phosphatic calculi formation. Calcium-containing antacids have a distinct disadvantage in that they may cause acid rebound, or hypersecretion of acid. Unbound or free calcium has been shown to stimulate the release of the hormone gastrin from the antral mucosa which then stimulates the release of HCl acid. Sodium bicarbonate, although an effective neutralizing agent, is usually avoided because it is systemically absorbed, may produce metabolic alkalosis, acid rebound, and has a high sodium content.

Because patients on antacid therapy for ulcer disease are on these medications for a prolonged period and patient compliance to the regimen is critical, the selection of the antacid is often made on the basis of taste and the effect on bowel activity. To alleviate the occurrence of side-effects, alternate or combination (*e.g.,* aluminum–magnesium preparations) therapy is often prescribed.

THERAPEUTIC ACTION. The therapeutic action of antacids is prolonged when they are administered between meals (*i.e.,* 1–2 hours after meals and at bedtime). The usual dose and frequency is 30 to 60 ml of liquid antacids or 1 to 2 tablets, after meals and at bedtime. For severe pain, antacids may be taken as often as hourly. Tablets should be chewed well and followed by a glass of water. Liquid suspensions must be shaken well and should be followed by a sip of water to ensure passage into the stomach. Of the two forms of antacids the liquid form as been shown to be more effective in neutralizing HCl acid and less expensive for long-term use.

Administration of antacids with other medications (*e.g.,* tetracyclines, cimetidine) may interfere with drug absorption. Therefore, administration times of other oral drugs should be staggered. Elderly patients as well as patients with concomitant cardiovascular and renal problems, need to be

TABLE 83–2
Antacids

Generic Name	*Trade Name*	*Dose*	*ANC* (mEq)*	*Sodium (mg)*
Aluminum hydroxide gel	Ampogel	Between meals, h.s.		
	tabs	2 tabs, 3–6 times/day	9.0	0.3/tab
	susp	10 ml, 3–6 times/day	6.5	0.3/5 ml
	Alternagel	5 ml, 3–6 times/day	12.0	2.0/5 ml
Aluminum phosphate gel	Phosphagel	q2h, between meals, h.s. 15–30 ml	1.5	12.5
Dihydroxyaluminum amino-acetate	Robalate	1–2s, between meals, h.s.	7	
Dihydroxyaluminum sodium carbonate	Rolaids	1–2 tabs prn	7.5–8	53
Aluminum carbonate gel, basic	Basalgel			
	caps	1–2 q2h	13	2.8
	tabs	1–2 q2h	14	2.1
	susp, res	5–10 ml, q2h	14	2.4
	susp, extra strength	5 ml, q2h	11	23.0
Magnesium hydroxide	Milk of Magnesia	1–2 tabs, 4 times/day 5–10 ml, 4 times/day	13.5	
Magaldrate	Riopan	Between meals, h.s.		
	tabs	1–2	13.5	0.3
	susp	5–10 ml	13.5	0.3
Calcium carbonate	Alka-2	1–4 tabs prn	10	
	Tums	1–4 tabs prn	10	2.7
	Trialka	2–6 tabs prn		salt-free
Aluminum hydroxide, magnesium hydroxide	Maalox Susp†	30–30 ml, 1 and 3 hrs pc, h.s.	13.5	1.35
Aluminum hydroxide, magnesium hydroxide, simethicone	Gelucil Liq†	30–60 ml, 1 and 3 hrs pc, h.s.	12	0.7
Calcium carbonate, glycine	Titralac†	30–60 ml, 1 and 3 hrs pc, h.s.	19	11
Aluminum hydroxide, magnesium hydroxide, calcium carbonate	Camalox†	30–60 ml, 1 and 3 hrs pc, h.s.	18	2.5
Aluminum hydroxide, magnesium hydroxide, simethicone	Mylanta†	30–60 ml, 1 and 3 hr pc, h.s.	12.7	0.68

Note: Aluminum hyroxide may decrease the absorption of digoxin, isoniazid, phenytoin, corticosteroids, quinidine, warfarin, and oral iron.
*Acid neutralizing capacity in mEq, per capsule, tablet or 5 ml.
† Sugar-free.

assessed and carefully monitored for bowel changes, edema from sodium retention, and alterations in renal function while taking antacids.

Antisecretory Agents

H_2 BLOCKERS. Antisecretory agents inhibit the secretion of HCl acid from the parietal or oxyntic (acid-secreting) cells in the stomach by blocking the histamine H_2-receptors (histamine H_2-receptor antagonists). These drugs are commonly referred to as *H_2-blockers.* H_2-blockers are prescribed for prevention as well as healing of peptic ulcers. Relief of pain associated with peptic ulcer disease is often managed with H_2-blockers alone or in combination with anatacids. The major drugs in this category are cimetidine (Tagamet) and ranitidine (Zantac) (Table 83–3).

Therapy with cimetidine is indicated for patients with an

TABLE 83–3
H_2-Blockers

Generic Name	*Trade Name*	*Purpose*	*Dose*	*Route*	*Side-effects*
Cimetidine	Tagamet	Antiulcer	300 mg, qid, with meals and h.s.	po, IM, IV in 100 ml NS or D5W over 15–20 minutes	Confusion, impotence, vitamin B_{12} malabsorption, diarrhea
		Prophylaxis	400 mg h.s.		
Ranitidine	Zantac	Decreases gastric acid secretion	300 mg every 8–12 hrs 150 mg, bid	po	Dizziness, rash, muscle pain, gynecomastia, constipation

active ulcer or for the patient who has suffered a major insult (*e.g.*, trauma, burn) in which stress ulcer may occur. For the hospitalized patient the usual dose of cimetidine is 300 mg PO or IV, four times a day. Oral cimetidine is most effective when given 30 to 60 minutes before meals. Intravenous doses must be diluted with a compatible solution (*e.g.*, sodium chloride) and directly injected over no less than 2 minutes or intermittently infused over 15 to 20 minutes.

Because cimetidine is metabolized in the liver and eliminated primarily by the kidneys, the dosage should be reduced to 300 mg twice a day if renal or hepatic function is impaired. Cimetidine should be avoided for 24 hours prior to gastric analysis or serum gastrin level determination because it interferes with obtaining baseline data. It may potentiate the action of oral anticoagulants, chlordiazepoxide, diazepam, and theophylline and decrease the absorption of tetracyclines. Cimetidine may also cause a false postive Hemoccult test for the presence of gastric bleeding if the test is performed within 15 minutes or oral cimetidine administration.

Outpatient therapy with cimetidine usually consists of 300 mg orally with each meal and at bedtime. For ulcer prophylaxis, the daily dose is 400 mg at bedtime. Antacids, if needed, should not be administered within 1 hour of cimetidine dose. Cimetidine should be tapered or discontinued gradually to reduce the possibility of ulcer recurrence.

The elderly must be observed closely for side-effects of cimetidine especially symptoms of central nervous system (CNS) dysfunction (*i.e.*, confusion, focal twitching, dizziness, and seizures). The nurse and patient should also be alert for signs and symptoms of impaired renal or hepatic function.

Ranitidine is similar in action to cimetidine but only available in the oral dosage form. The usual dose is 150 mg orally twice a day. The advantage of ranitidine over cimetidine is that it can be therapeutic in smaller doses which are given less frequently and, subsequently, result in fewer side-effects. The cautions for elderly patients receiving cimetidine also apply to ranitidine.

Nursing Responsibilities for patients receiving H_2-blockers include observations for the desired effect (*i.e.*, pain relief, as well as adverse effects, predominantly headache, dizziness, rash, fatigue, constipation, and diarrhea, in addition to the CNS symtpoms previously listed. Patients receiving H_2-blockers need to understand the importance of adhering to prescribed dose and timing of medication in relation to meals. Patients are generally maintained on the H_2-blockers until healing is established. At that time, the patient's medication may be either gradually reduced or continued to prevent ulcer recurrence. Patients who develop pain upon discontinuation of H_2-blocker drugs should promptly report their symptoms to the physician as there is a possibility of ulcer recurrence or development of complications (*e.g.*, perforation).

ANTICHOLINERGICS. Another group of antisecretory agents is the anticholinergics. Anticholinergic drugs have been used for many years to reduce gastric acid secretion and hypermotility. The agents are muscarinic cholinergic receptor blocking agents. These drugs act by decreasing acetylcholine-stimulated HCl acid secretion and reducing contractile activity of the stomach. Atropine, belladonna, and banthine-containing preparations are in this group (Table 83–4).

The major disadvantages of anticholinergics, when given in doses high enough to relieve ulcer symptoms, are the side-effects, including urinary retention, dry mouth, blurred vision, and tacycardia. Elderly patients, in particular, must be monitored for cardiovascular, urinary, and CNS disturbances. In the stomach, anticholinergics reduce gastric emptying by a decrease in gastric motility which increases exposure of the gastric mucosa to irritating substances, and may increase gastric pain and discomfort. Furthermore, it is not known what role gastric stasis plays in the etiology of gastric cancer. Due to these side-effects and the advent of H_2-blockers, anticholinergics are of limited use for long-term gastric and duodenal ulcer therapy. However, anticholinergics may be used in combination with antacids or H_2-blockers for duodenal ulcer pain relief.

Cytoprotective Agents

Cytoprotective agents are a nonabsorbable aluminum salt of sulfated disaccharide such as sucralfate (Carafate). This agent exerts a protective effect by forming a complex which coats ulcerated mucosal tissue, and also inhibits pepsin activity. Because it is nonabsorbable it is used for the treatment of

TABLE 83–4
Anticholinergics

Generic Name	*Trade Name*	*Usual Dose Range*
Atropine	Atropine	0.3–0.6 mg p.o., a.c. and h.s.
Belladonna		0.3–1.0 ml p.o.
Atropine, scopolamine, hyoscyamine HBr, phenobarbital	Donnatal	3–8 tabs/day
Belladonna extract, phenobarbital	Belap	15 mg, 3–4 times/day, a.c. and h.s.
Dicyclomine	Bentyl	20–40 mg, p.o., IM 3 or 4 times/day, a.c. and h.s.
Propantheline bromide	Pro-Banthine	15 mg TID a.c., 30 mg h.s. Elderly 7.5 mg TID Adult maximum, 120–240 mg/day

Side-effects of Anticholinergic Drugs in General:

Dry mouth, blurred vision, voiding difficulty, constipation, tachycardia, confusion, disorientation, mydriasis, central nervous system stimulation.

Contraindications for the Use of Anticholinergics:

Hypersensitivity to belladonna alkaloids, narrow-angle glaucoma, cardiac disease, GI tract obstruction, myasthenia gravis, prostatic hypertrophy, paralytic ileum.

duodenal ulcers in patients in which drug metabolism is a problem. Furthermore, because sucralfate is nonabsorbable, it has few known side-effects. However, some patients do experience nausea after taking the drug. The usual dose is 1 g four times a day, given 1 to 2 hours before meals and at bed time. Other medications should be given at different times, if possible, because sucralfate interferes with drug absorption, especially tetracyclines. Anatacids, if prescribed, should be taken ½ to 1 hour before or after sucralfate. At this time, it is recommended that sucralfate therapy should not be continued for more than 8 weeks.

Endogenous prostaglandins are thought to play a role in cytoprotection of GI mucosa, therefore, synthetic analogues are presently being evaluated for their efficacy and safety in preventing and treating duodenal ulcers. Side-effects of synthetic protaglandins are pronounced and include diarrhea, nausea, vomiting, abdominal cramps, and cardiovascular alterations. However, synthetic protaglandins, in particular the E-type, require very small doses and consequently side-effects are minimized. Although these drugs are used in other countries, at this writing the Federal Drug Administration (FDA) has not approved the use of synthetic prostaglandins in the US for the treatment of peptic ulcer disease.

Pharmacological therapy using antacids and H_2-blockers (*e.g.*, cimetidine) either separately or in combination, results in healing 85% to 95% of peptic ulcers within 6 weeks.[4] Sucralfate appears to compare favorably with cimetidine in healing duodenal ulcers. Anticholinergics are often prescribed as adjunctive therapy in combination with antacids and H_2-blockers.

Dietary Modification

The role of diet in the management of peptic ulcers is controversial. The rationale for dietary restrictions and inclusion of bland foods has not been scientifically supported.[1] Essentially all foods and beverages cause gastric acid secretion. Although milk and other dietary products neutralize acid, it has been shown that milk actually stimulates relatively more HCl acid secretion than either carbonated beverages or coffee.[5] In fact, high quantities of dairy products may induce "acid rebound."

When dietary modification is indicated, the aim is prevention of gastric irritation and relief of the distressing symptoms of pain and burning before and after meals. The most important factor in diet adaptation for the patient with a peptic ulcer is the person's tolerance. Certain substances such as spicy foods cause dyspepsia in some persons. It may be wise to reduce or eliminate caffeine and alcohol consumption. Smoking should be avoided as it has been shown to delay ulcer healing, regardless of the therapy. Persons with hyperlipidemia and those at risk for cardiovascular problems should reduce their intake of fats (which are present in high amounts in dairy products).

Surgical Management

In spite of medical management, many persons with peptic ulcers experience complications which require surgical interventions. The aims of surgery are removal of ulcerated tissue and reduction of the secretion of HCl acid.

Indications for surgical intervention are:

1. When medical management does not result in symptom relief (*i.e.*, intractability).
2. When serious life-threatening complications occur (*e.g.*, hemorrhage, perforation, and obstruction).
3. When there is possible malignancy.

The most common types of surgical interventions are *gastrectomy, vagotomy,* and *pyloroplasty.* Usually some combination of these procedures is performed.

Gastrectomy involves removal of a portion of the stomach, most commonly the distal one-half or two-thirds of the stomach is resected. This type of surgery is performed to remove the ulcerated tissue itself as well as a large portion of the acid-secreting cells. Gastrectomy is generally performed for recurrent gastric ulcers, nonhealing ulcers, or hemorrhage. A type of gastrectomy, antrectomy involves removal of that portion of the stomach containing gastrin-secreting cells. The remaining portion of the stomach is anastomosed either to the duodenum (Billroth I) or jejunum (Billroth II); see Fig. 83–1.

Vagotomy involves sectioning or severing the vagus nerve in the region of its innervation to the stomach (Fig. 83–1c). The purpose of vagotomy is to reduce the source of vagally stimulated HCl acid. Vagotomy may be performed alone. However, the procedure is often combined with gastrectomy in an effort to enhance healing and to reduce the possibility of ulcer recurrence. The types of vagotomy are truncal, selective, and highly selective.

Truncal vagotomy consists of severing both the posterior and anterior trunks of the vagus nerve just prior to its juncture in the stomach. The loss of vagal input to the stomach results in reduced HCl acid secretion as well as decreased gastric motility and emptying. Selective vagotomy involves sectioning the vagus and interrupting only those branches innervating the stomach, but sparing celiac, hepatic, pancreatic, and other branches. Highly selective vagotomy (also called parietal cell vagotomy or proximal gastric vagotomy) involves sectioning only that portion of the vagus nerve which innervates the acid-secreting cells of the stomach and spares innervation to the antrum and other structures. The possible side-effects of vagotomy, delayed gastric emptying, diarrhea, and gallstones, are less severe after selective vagotomy than after a truncal vagotomy. However, the 10-year recurrence rate associated with selective vagotomy is higher than with truncal.

Pyloroplasty is the surgical repair or reopening of the pylorus, and it is performed to enhance gastric emptying. Pyloroplaysty, or an alternate type of drainage procedure (*e.g.*, gastrojejunostomy), must accompany surgical procedures that interfere with gastric emptying (*i.e.*, antrectomy, truncal, and selective vagotomy). The vagus nerve modulates gastric emptying, therefore, lack of vagal innervation results in the potential for gastric stasis. Vagotomy with pyloroplasty is the procedure of choice for elderly patients and individuals considered poor surgical risks. The stomach and duodenum remain intact, therefore there are fewer postsurgical complications.

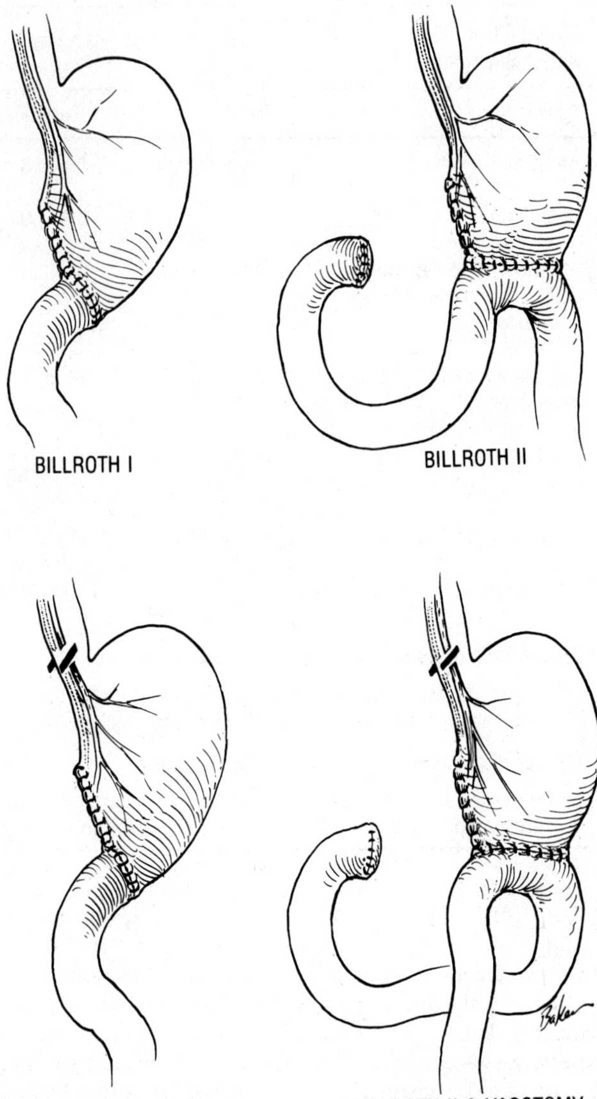

FIGURE 83–1 Diagrammatic representation of distal partial gastrectomy, with gastrointestinal continuity being restored by gastroduodenostomy (Billroth I) and gastrojejunostomy (Billroth II), with and without truncal vagotomy. (Sleisenger MH, Fordtran JS [eds]: Gastrointestinal Disease, 2nd ed. Philadelphia, WB Saunders, 1978)

Photocoagulation

Endoscopic laser photocoagulation is a new nonsurgical approach to control bleeding from gastric erosions. Laser is an acronym for *l*ight *a*mplification by the *s*timulated *e*mission of *r*adar. The fiber which delivers the laser beam is threaded through one of the channels of a fiberoptic endoscope. Following local anesthesia, the endoscope is passed orally to the ulcer site. The physician can visualize the bleeding area and direct the laser to specific areas. After treatment the nurse should caution the patient to avoid food and fluids by mouth until the local anesthesia is no longer effective and normal swallowing has returned. This usually takes about 2 hours. The procedure may be indicated for elderly patients and persons who are considered poor surgical risks. If laser treatment is unsuccessful in controlling bleeding, gastric surgery may be required.

Nursing Management

The problems of persons with peptic ulcers are related to pain control, adequate nutrition, potential for complications, patient understanding and adherence to a treatment regimen, and recovery from surgery when this treatment is necessary. Nursing care focuses on assisting the patient in coping with these problems.

Assessment and Nursing Diagnosis

Alteration in patient comfort is related to the pain accompanying the tissue damage or even perforation at the lesion site and the manifestations of nausea and vomiting which also result from tissue damage or complications of the disease such as bleeding or obstruction. During the acute or active phase, the patient is assessed for the frequency and severity of abdominal pain, nausea, and vomiting. The patient with an active bleeding ulcer needs to be monitored for bleeding by testing stools and emesis for occult blood. Vital signs are taken at frequent intervals for signs of reduced blood volume (*e.g.*, hypotension, tachycardia). A nasogastric tube may be placed with intermittent suction to reduce gastric stimulation as well as to monitor gastric secretion for bleeding. The amount and color of gastric output needs to be noted. The patient is assessed for possible complications including obstruction, perforation, and gastric stasis. Abdominal distention, abdominal rigidity, presence or absence of bowel tones and bowel function are data relevant to possible obstruction, perforation, or bleeding.

Alteration in nutritional status may accompany the discomfort and sensations of nausea. Determinations of relationships of pain and food intake are important. Data that give evidence of nutritional status include blood protein levels, weight loss, and lowered hematocrit and hemoglobin.

Assessment of anxiety level provides data regarding possible factors contributing to the development of the disease and interference with healing. Conversations with the patient should be structured to help identify situations that are stressful and methods the person uses to cope with these situations. Assessment should determine if the patient accepts the fact that anxiety may be a contributing factor and is willing to discuss mental health practices.

Nurses need to determine patients' knowledge regarding medications that are prescribed and the intent to carry out this therapy. Conversations regarding medications should be initiated early in the course of hospitalization to allow sufficient time for patient education.

Goals. The goals of nursing management are to (1) relieve abdominal discomfort, (2) maintain or restore adequate nutrition, (3) prevent or detect recurrence and complications, (4) assist the patient to cope with stressful situations, (5) educate the patient about the illness and treatment regimen and (6) assist the patient to cope with a surgical intervention when this is indicated.

Interventions

Promotion of physical and emotional rest is crucial. Antacids may be required hourly, possibly in combination with other antisecretory agents. If hospitalization is necessary, a nasogastric tube may be inserted and food and fluids withheld. Gastric decompression using intermittent suction relieves discomfort and nausea. The patient is maintained on IV therapy during this time. Frequent mouth care and lubrication of the nares are important comfort measures. Patency of the nasogastric or naso-intestinal tube must be maintained (Fig. 83–2). Reassurance and the rationale for treatment measures should be offered. The accompanying nursing care plan elucidates more specific nursing intervention for pain control, potential bleeding, and nutrition (p 1255).

The chronic features of peptic ulcer disease require the patient to adhere to a medication schedule and, usually, some activity and dietary adaptations as well. Medication compliance, in particular antacid therapy, is generally good during symptomatic periods, but decreases with the subsiding of symptoms. Compliance with recommendations about diet, smoking, and stress reduction is often poor when the patient is asymptomatic. Having an understanding of the disease and the rationale for treatment may enhance patient compliance with medication schedule and lifestyle adaptations.

Diet Management. Nursing management includes shared responsibility for dietary counseling with the clinical dietician. Frequent small meals (*i.e.*, six meals per day), are usually helpful. Patients need to be informed about label reading in order to determine constituents of prepared and processed foods. Mealtimes should be as stress-free as possible. Nutritional guidance is based on the patient's current eating habits. Patients who are anemic may need dietary counseling to increase dietary intake of iron because use of iron supplements frequently results in dyspepsia. Patient acceptance of dietary modification may depend on whether or not pain relief is obtained with smaller meals and avoidance of foods and substances that are particularly irritating.

Patient Teaching. Patients with peptic ulcer disease need knowledge concerning the recommended treatment regimen and long-term follow up care in order to avoid recurrence or complications. Knowing the cause or contributing factors of the disease may be the single most important factor in determining compliance with recommended adaptations. The patient needs to know the desired effects of the prescribed medications as well as the side-effects which may occur. It is especially important to discourage the use of over-the-counter medications which could interfere with healing (*e.g.*, aspirin).

Another nursing responsibility includes the evaluation of drug therapy the patient may be on for other health problems. It is important to identify those drugs which are known to produce ulceration (*i.e.*, aspirin, steroids, and nonsteroidal anti-inflammatory agents). The physician must be consulted about the continued use of these drugs. Patients with

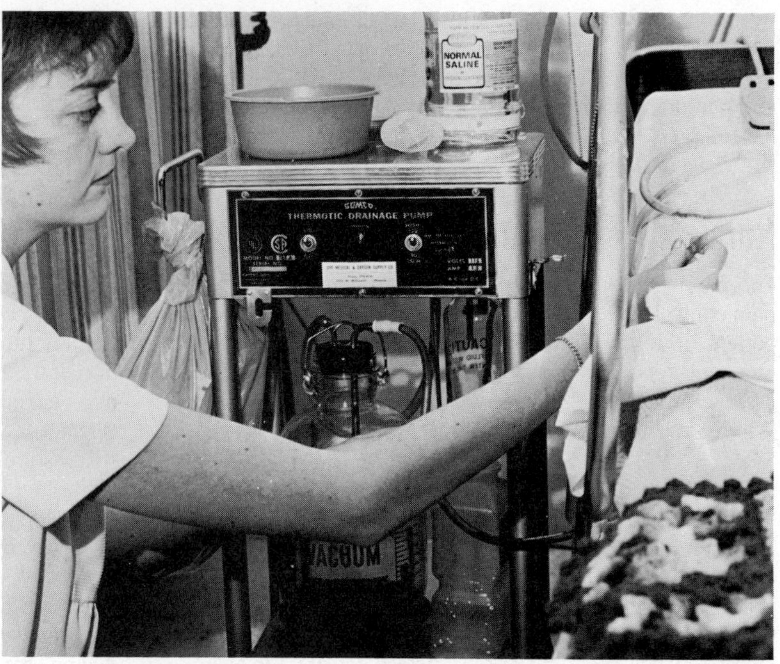

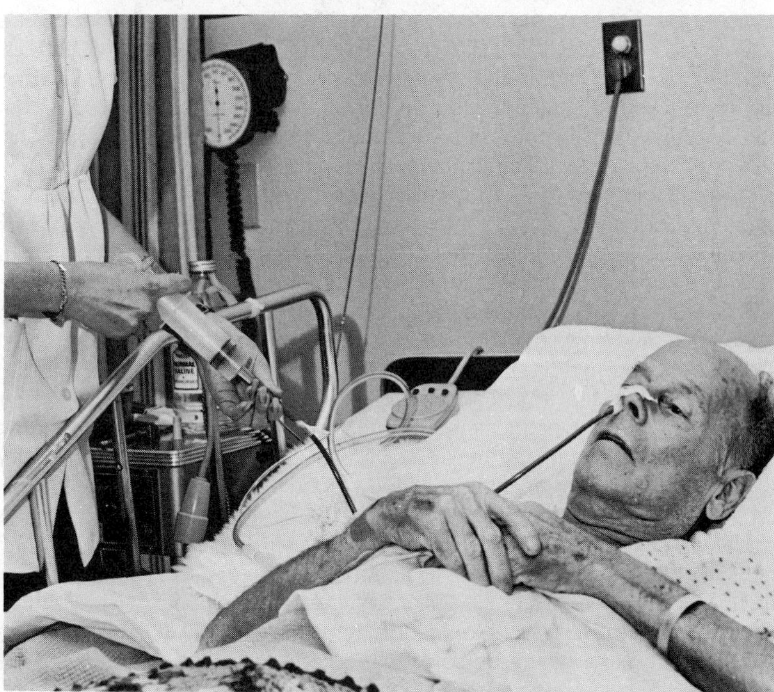

FIGURE 83–2 Patients with peptic ulcers frequently require nasogastric suctioning. The nurse is responsible for irrigating the tube and assessing drainage return.

cardiovascular and renal problems need to be monitored for edema from sodium retention.

Psychosocial Support. Patients with duodenal ulcer disease need supportive therapy as well. The patient needs to be reassured that duodenal ulcers are primarily benign in nature. Although new pharmacological treatments have greatly improved the healing rate of duodenal ulcers and decreased recurrence, a high percentage of patients diagnosed with a duodenal ulcer will have a recurrence of the disease within 1 year of diagnosis. Because of the increased incidence of gastric cancer in people with a history of gastric ulcer, patients with gastric ulcer disease may need additional emotional support; they may also need to be reevaluated at regular intervals.

Emotional Factors. Patient education includes fostering an understanding of the impact of environmental factors such as stress upon the aggravation of ulcer disease. While researchers debate the link between "stress" and peptic ulcer disease, cognizant or subconcious stress have been associated with exacerbation or recurrence of the disease in some patients.

Clearly emotions, via neural and hormonal activity, have a pronounced effect on the functions of the GI tract, in particular, motility and secretion. It has long been known that prolonged elevations in adrenal cortisol secretion, such as accompanies physical and psychological stress, lead to ulceration. It is within the nurse's role to assist the patient to identify stressful aspects of his or her life and to promote stress-reduction activities (*e.g.*, relaxation or biofeedback techniques, physical exercise, and psychotherapy). Physical and emotional rest is also an effective means to decrease the quantity or intensity of stressors.

Despite pharmacologic and dietary therapy and lifestyle adaptations, there are a number of patients (about 15%) whose ulcers will not heal. One factor which is associated with delayed ulcer healing is cigarette smoking. While the

NURSING CARE PLAN FOR THE PATIENT WITH PEPTIC ULCER DISEASE

NURSING DIAGNOSIS: Alteration in comfort related to irritation of ulcerated mucosal tissue
GOAL 1: To reduce or eliminate mucosal irritation

Nursing Interventions	Rationale	Outcome Criteria
Acute episode Promote physical and emotional rest. Offer sedatives as prescribed. Explain therapeutic regimen. Provide opportunity for patient to express feelings and concerns. Administer prescribed medications on time. If an NG tube is used: Maintain patency. Provide for frequent mouth care.	Anxiety may stimulate the vagus nerve which results in acid secretion. Medications may neutralize acid, block acid secretion, or inhibit pepsin activity. Drainage of gastric secretions relieves pressure on ulcerated tissue.	No subjective complaints of abdominal pain. No nausea or vomiting. Absence of sensation of bloating. Talks about feelings and concerns. Has relaxed facial expression and body posture.
Chronic phase 1. Instruct patient about medication schedule. a. Stress importance of continuing medications for specified period of time. b. Inform about side-effects of medications. c. Assist to set up staggered drug schedule if taking other medications. d. Discourage use of over-the-counter drugs without physician consultation. e. Provide rationale for pharmacologic regimen.	Medications are important in decreasing irritation of ulcerated mucosa. To accomplish this purpose, they must be taken at specified time period.	Patient adheres to prescribed medication schedule. No complaints of discomfort associated with meals. Verbalizes understanding of medication program. • Dosage, timing • Staggering other medications • Continuation of therapy even when asymptomatic
2. Provide guidelines for dietary modification. a. Discuss possible irritating effects of caffeine, alcohol, spicy foods, and carbonated beverages. b. Encourage several small meals. c. Keep meal times as stress-free as possible. d. Rest for 30 to 60 minutes after meals.	Spicy foods may cause dyspepsia; caffeine and alcohol may stimulate acid secretion. Anxiety increases acid secretion through vagal stimulation. Small meals may prevent distension and bloating.	Patient identifies and avoids those foods which cause discomfort. Absence of symptoms related to food intolerance.

(Continued)

NURSING CARE PLAN FOR THE PATIENT WITH PEPTIC ULCER DISEASE (*Continued*)

NURSING DIAGNOSIS 2: Potential/actual inadequacy of circulating blood volume related to bleeding in the GI tract.
GOAL 1: To prevent bleeding and subsequent loss of circulating blood volume.

Nursing Interventions	Rationale	Outcome Criteria
1. Administer antacids, if prescribed, to keep gastric pH above 5.0. 2. Administer antisecretory drugs, if precribed at appropriate intervals. 3. Monitor stool for presence of occult blood. 4. Instruct patient to avoid irritating foods and beverages.	An acid pH increases ulcerated tissue trauma and may result in erosions of blood vessel wall. A loss of blood volume decreases cardiac output and oxygen supply to tissues.	No GI bleeding as evidenced by the following: a. Stool specimen is negative for occult blood. b. NG aspirate or emesis has a pH over 5.0 and is negative for occult blood. c. Hct and Hgb within normal limits. d. Vital signs within normal limits for patient. e. Absence of signs and symptoms listed above.

GOAL 2: Early detection and treatment of bleeding from ulcer site.

Nursing Interventions	Rationale	Outcome Criteria
1. Check stool regularly for presence of occult blood. 2. Test emesis, if any, for blood content. 3. Monitor vital signs, skin color, and temperature. 4. Assess blood pressure and pulse, lying and sitting for orthostatic changes. 5. Monitor hematocrit and hemoglobin levels on a regular basis. 6. Monitor for expressions of weakness, fatigue. 7. Provide rationale for necessary diagnostic tests (*e.g.,* endoscopy). 8. Assess for hyperperistalsis characterized by increased bowel sounds. 9. Document amount, color, and consistency of gastric output.	Bleeding from an ulcerated site results in blood in the stool and emesis. A loss of blood volume decreases cardiac output and oxygen supply to tissues. Bleeding results in a decrease in number of red blood cells. Blood in the stool is irritating to intestinal mucosa and stimulates peristalsis. Blood in gastric output has the appearance of coffee grounds. Calculation of fluid and blood replacement depends on accurate record of loss.	Signs and symptoms of GI bleeding are detected before profound cardiovascular alterations ensue. Bleeding is terminated following prompt intervention. If possible, patient expresses confidence in decisions of health-care team.

NURSING DIAGNOSIS 3: Potential alteration in nutrition, related to discomfort associated with eating.
GOAL: Maintain/restore adequate nutrition.

Nursing Interventions	Rationale	Outcome Criteria
1. Implement diet program: nonirritating food, small meals, and rest.		1. No complaints of discomfort associated with meals. Patient verbalizes understanding of relationship of dietary management to ulcer disease. Patient gives report indicating adequate nutritional intake.

(*Continued*)

NURSING CARE PLAN FOR THE PATIENT WITH PEPTIC ULCER DISEASE (*Continued*)

Nursing Interventions	Rationale	Outcome Criteria
2. Promote absorption of nutrients by the following measures: a. Avoid antacids that induce diarrhea. b. Reduce carbohydrate intake to minimize the occurrence of rapid gastric empyting (dumping syndrome). c. Reduce or eliminate fluid intake during meals.	Absorption of nutrients is required to meet energy needs, maintain body weight, and promote healing.	2. Weight within range of ideal body weight. Absence of sensation of bloating.

relationship between smoking and ulcer healing is not understood, patients with ulcer disease who smoke should be encouraged to quit or reduce the number of cigarettes.

Because recurrence and complications are not uncommon, patients should be instructed to seek medical intervention if ulcer symptoms recur. The sample care plan highlights some of the common problems of patients with peptic ulcers. The key to successful nursing management is the individualization of approaches to every patient.

Evaluation

Outcome criteria for the patient with peptic ulcer are:

1. Patient states the pain is decreased or relieved.
2. NG tube, if present, is patent.
3. Absence of abdominal distention.
4. Oral cavity is moist, teeth clean.
5. Patient reports adherence to prescribed antacid therapy. Accurately states action of antacid.
6. Patient reports adherence to dietary therapy
7. Patient reports actions taken to relieve stressful situations.

Perioperative Nursing Management

Preoperative Interventions

Preoperative nursing management includes preparing the patient for surgery by informing the patient and family of what to expect during hospitalization. Often, most preliminary diagnostic tests are completed on an outpatient basis prior to admission. While the physician is responsible for informing the patient about the proposed surgical procedure(s), risks, and possible alternatives for treatment, the nurse should determine the patient's understanding of this information. Any misunderstandings about the surgical procedure should be clarified. Pictures or diagrams may promote understanding. The nurse's discussion should include information about routine pre- and postoperative measures (*e.g.,* no fluid/food by mouth (NPO) from the evening before surgery, analgesia, IV therapy, use of the nasogastric tube, and gradual diet resumption when intestinal function returns and incision lines have healed). The patient requires support and reassurance, during the preoperative period, as well as an opportunity to have questions answered. (Refer to Chapter 8 for care of the patient undergoing surgery.)

Postoperative Intervention

After gastric surgery the patient's primary needs cluster around comfort, gastric decompression, pain relief, and nutrition. Immediately after surgery, the nurse's responsibilities include assessment of the patient's vital signs and other parameters indicative of the patient's hemodynamic and fluid balance status. Along with the routine postoperative measures, including pulmonary toilet and wound care, the nurse will monitor gastric output through the nasogastric tube. Gastric output will be bloody for about 12 hours but should lighten considerably by the first operative day. The nasogastric tube must be observed closely for patency. Without a physician's order, the NG tube should not be repositioned or irrigated by the nurse, as this may disrupt the anastomosis suture line. When irrigation is performed per physician's order, it is a sterile procedure. The patient is monitored for complications including bleeding and obstruction. Bleeding, increased abdominal pain, cessation of drainage, and vomiting around the nasogastric tube necessitate contacting the physician.

The nurse should be particularly alert for evidence of new or continued bleeding as well as fluid and electrolyte imbalance. Signs and symptoms of problems include bright red returns from the NG tube more than 24 hours after surgery, decreased blood pressure, increased pulse rate, diminished level of consciousness, cardiac irritability, pallor, poor skin turgor, and muscle twitching.

Incisional discomfort is to be expected as with any abdominal surgery. Parenteral narcotics are usually given as needed for analgesia. Nausea may be a serious problem, not only because of discomfort, but, if followed by vomiting, the retching will put strain on the suture line. Antiemetics may be prescribed as needed. The patient remains NPO until bowel sounds are auscultated or passage of flatus or stool occurs. With the resumption of bowel activity, the physician may order small amounts of water or other clear liquids by mouth, while the NG tube is clamped but remains in place. If this is not tolerated (*e.g.,* the patient becomes nauseated), the NG tube may be unclamped and reconnected to suction. Liquids may be tried again in several hours or according to the physician's order. If fluids are tolerated, the NG tube is generally removed and diet is slowly and carefully resumed. The removal of the NG tube is a positive sign of progression of convalescence and should be used to encourage the patient about satisfactory progress.

Long-Term Complications

The nurse has a key role in the education of the patient who has undergone ulcer surgery. The goals are prevention and early detection of long-term complications and successful adaptations for resumption of a healthy lifestyle.

Dumping Syndrome. Following gastrectomy, the most common complication is "dumping syndrome." Dumping is probably caused by rapid gastric emptying of hyperosmolar fluid and substances into the duodenum. As a result, the hyperosmolar chyme pulls water from the mucosal tissue into the intestinal lumen. This produces both an increase in intestinal volume and a decrease in circulating blood volume. Rapid gastric emptying and inadequate mixing of food with gastric and intestinal enzymes will eventually produce malabsorption.

Symptoms of dumping syndrome can be very uncomfortable and include cramps, nausea, palpitations, sweating, diarrhea, and weakness. Onset of symptoms generally occurs 30 to 60 minutes after eating. The syndrome is more pronounced after a high-carbohydrate meal because this stimulates the release of insulin. However, the insulin is in excess of need because of the inadequate absorption of the meal.

The following approaches may be suggested to minimize symptoms of dumping syndrome:

1. Eat small, frequent meals, 4 to 6 times a day.
2. Avoid high-carbohydrate foods, especially those with large amounts of refined sugar.
3. Include in diet more protein and fat, which empty more slowly from the stomach than carbohydrates.
4. Drink fluids between meals, not with meals.
5. Plan to rest for about 30 minutes after meals.

Dumping syndrome is usually self-limiting and often resolves in 6 to 12 months after surgery; however, for a small percentage of patients, this may be a life-long problem.

Pernicious Anemia. Pernicious anemia is a possible long-term complication because removal of acid-producing cells also eliminates production of intrinsic factor required for absorption of vitamin B_{12}, which is needed for formation of red blood cells. For signs, symptoms, and treatment, refer to Chapter 53. Symptoms of pernicious anemia may not appear until several months following surgery. Treatment involves the parenteral administration of vitamin B_{12}.

Weight Loss and Inadequate Nutrition. After surgery, weight loss and inadequate nutrition may result from inability to eat large meals or from problems with distention and dumping. There can also be undernutrition because of poor absorption of nutrients. Follow-up care should include careful nutritional and hematological assessment by the nurse. Problems may require consultation with the clinical dietician.

Carcinoma. Cancer of the gastric stump may be a long-range complication of gastrectomy for benign ulcer disease. Malignant lesions are often discovered in the seventh decade.[6] Therefore, follow-up care should include investigation of new or recurrent symptoms for possible malignancy. Early detection of malignancy and prompt intervention are the goals for a successful outcome.

Evaluation

Outcome criteria for the person who has surgical treatment for peptic ulcer are:

1. Patient and family accurately describe proposed surgery, treatment expected after surgery, and cooperative actions expected of patient.
2. Patient reports relief of pain with use of analgesic after surgery.
3. Nasogastric tube remains patent, abdomen is soft, bowel tones present.
4. Patient is free of manifestations of complications.
5. Patient cooperative in postoperative care (*i.e.,* coughing and deep breathing).
6. Lungs are clear to auscultation.
7. Wound is clean, free of evidence of infection.
8. Patient reports use of specific measures to prevent dumping syndrome; measures apparently successful.
9. Patient sleeps well.
10. Patient reports adherence to recommended dietary modifications.

Stress Ulcers

Description/Evidence

Stress ulcers are acute focal necrosis of the gastric and duodenal mucosa. Acute stress ulcers of the stomach or small intestine have been observed in patients following major trauma, cardiovascular insult, burns, and surgery. These ulcers are generally superficial in that they are limited to the mucosal and submucosal layers of the stomach and intestine. However, they are generally multiple, and hemorrhage from the sites is an emergency situation. Once bleeding is initiated it is difficult to control, so the focus is on prevention of ulcers in those patients who are at risk. Prevention is critical because these patients due to their primary diagnosis are poor surgical risks.

Etiology/Pathophysiology

While the precise pathophysiological mechanism of acute stress ulcer formation remains to be elucidated, marked reduction in gastrointestinal, in particular mucosal, blood flow appears to play a critical role in the subsequent ischemia and necrosis of the mucosa tissue. Major physiological insults, such as hemorrhage, shock, or burns, reduce cardiac output. To compensate for the reduction in circulating volume, vasoconstriction of the splanchnic circulation occurs. If prolonged, the reduction in splanchnic blood flow will result in ischemia which ultimately destroys the gastric mucosal barrier. Disruption of the barrier permits the back diffusion of HCl acid which is destructive to capillaries and mucosal cells. While the cardiovascular changes accompanying a major physiological insult appear to be the critical etiologic factor, hypersecretion of HCl acid may also be a causative factor. Physiological stressors activate the central nervous system which results in vagal activation as well as adrenal glucocorticoid secretion. Both of these factors may facilitate the demise of the gastric mucosal barrier.

Clinical Manifestations

Patients with acute stress ulcers are generally asymptomatic. Frequently the earliest sign is hemorrhage. Hemorrhage generally occurs 2 to 10 days following the initial insult.

Medical Management

Diagnosis. Diagnosis is by endoscopic visualization because ulcers are superficial and not readily visualized by x-ray.

Treatment. Treatment of stress ulcers focuses on prevention of both ulcers and complications in those who are at risk: major trauma patients, surgery patients, patients who have undergone burns, cardiovascular insult, or septicemia. For example, patients admitted to the coronary care unit for myocardial infarction are frequently started on H_2-receptor blocker for prophylaxis. Other preventive measures include the placement of a nasogastric tube for aspiration of gastric contents. The gastric pH is monitored at regular intervals (every 1–2 hours), and antacids are administered to maintain the intragastric pH greater than 5.0 or 5.5.

Prognosis. Acute stress ulcers carry a mortality rate of about 50% because of the condition of the patient and the multiple ulcer sites which hemorrhage.

Nursing Management

Assessment and Nursing Diagnosis

Patients with high risk for stress ulcers as described above need to be monitored carefully. Expressions of abdominal pain or discomfort need careful attention. Testing of emesis and stools for blood is necessary.

Goals of nursing management of the critically ill patient at risk for stress ulcer development are to: (1) monitor for manifestations of stress ulcers, (2) maintain the intragastric pH greater than 5 to decrease the likelihood of tissue erosion and hemorrhage, and (3) maintain optimal cardiovascular status by administration of fluid and electrolytes as prescribed.

Interventions

Patients at risk for stress ulcer formation need to be identified. Sometimes the nurse may have to take the initiative in bringing this to the attention of the physician. If a nasogastric tube is in place as a preventive or treatment measure the intragastric contents can be monitored by a pH probe or by gastric aspiration. Generally, antacids are ordered (30–60 ml) every 1 to 2 hours to maintain the intragastric pH above 5 or 5.5. Bowel sounds are monitored. A marked increase or decrease in bowel sounds may be indicative of hemorrhage. Because hemorrhage from stress ulcer may be the first overt manifestation, vital signs are monitored at frequent intervals, and stools and emesis guiaiced for occult blood. The patient who is at risk for stress ulcers is usually critically ill. The nursing care will include nursing interventions to achieve goals related to the primary medical and nursing diagnoses. The nursing interventions in the evident ulcerations occur as described under peptic ulcers.

Evaluation

Absence of manifestations of peptic ulcers in the critically ill person or early detection and prompt treatment, maintenance of a gastric pH greater than 5, and stable vital signs indicative of adequate cardiovascular status are the desired outcomes.

Ulcers of the small and large intestine are addressed in the preceding chapter.

References

1. American Dietetic Association position paper on bland diet in the treatment of chronic duodenal ulcer disease. J Am Diet Assoc 59:244, 1971
2. Clinch O, Banerjce Ak, Ostrick G: Absence of abdominal pain in elderly patients with peptic ulcers. Age Ageing 13:120–123, 1984
3. Craig CR, Stitzel RE (eds): Modern Pharmacology. Boston, Little, Brown & Co, 1982
4. Ippoliti AF: Evolution in the medical treatment of peptic ulcer disease. Drug Therapy July: 97–112, 1983
5. McArthur K, Hogan D, Isenberg JI: Relative stimulatory effects of commonly ingested beverages on gastric acid secretion in humans. Gastroenterology 83:199–203, 1982
6. Neimark S, Rogers AI: Carcinoma of gastric remnant after surgery for benign peptic ulcer. Postgraduate Med Dec 72(6):245–247, 1982
7. Peters MN, Richardson CT: Stressful life events, acid hypersecretion and ulcer disease. Gastroenterology 84:114–119, 1983

Bibliography

Brunner L: What to do (and what to teach your patients) about peptic ulcer. Nursing 76 6:27, 1976

Dwyer RM, Yellin AE, Craig J, Cherlow J, Bass M: Gastric hemostasis by laser phototherapy in man. JAMA 236(12): 1976

Eisenhouer LA, Gerald MC: The Nurse's 1984–85 Guide to Drug

Therapy, Drug Profiles for Patient Care. Englewood Cliffs, NJ, Prentice Hall, 1984

Facts and Comparisons. Loose Leaf Drug Information Service. St. Louis, JB Lippincott, 1983

Fall DJ: Gastrointestinal disorders. In Price SA, Wilson LM (eds): Pathophysiology: Clinical Concepts of Disease Processes, 2nd ed. New York, McGraw-Hill, 1982

Frank-Stromborg M, Stromborg P: Test your knowledge of caring for the patient with peptic ulcer. Nursing 82 11:66–69, 1982

Givens BA, Simmon SJ: Gastroenterology in Clinical Nursing, 4th ed. St. Louis, CV Mosby, 1984

Govoni LE, Hayes JE: Drugs and Nursing Implications, 4th ed. Norwalk, CT, Appleton-Century-Crofts, 1982

Isenberg JI: Therapy of peptic ulcer. JAMA 233:540–542, 1975

Kiefhaber P: European experience in laser photocoagulation in GI tract. In Endoscopic Control of GI Bleeding. Boca Raton, FL, CRC Press, 1981

Peters MN, Richardson CT: Stressful life events, acid hypersecretion and ulcer disease. Gastroenterology 84:114–119, 1983

Piper DW: Antacids and anticholinergic therapy. Clinical Gastroenterology 2:361, 1973

Spiro HM: Clinical Gastroenterology, 3rd ed. New York, Macmillan, 1983

Waddy M: Light surgery. Nursing Mirror 155(19): 1982

Welsh JD: Diet therapy of peptic ulcer disease. Gastroenterology 72:740–745, 1977

Chapter 84

Gastrointestinal Structural Disorders

Denise Davignon

Herniations

A hernia (rupture) is the abnormal protrusion of a viscus outside its normal cavity. The hernia ring is the ring of muscular tissue (opening) through which the viscus protrudes. The opening in the cavity wall through which the viscus protrudes may vary in size and may be congenital or acquired. The protrusion of the viscus may be intermittent or continuous, depending on the type and severity of the hernia. While the term may apply to any body part (e.g. herniated disc, cerebral hernia), it more commonly refers to a protrusion of an abdominal viscus from the abdominal cavity.

Etiology and Pathophysiology

Hernias are caused by a combination of a weakening or defect in the muscle wall and increased intra-abdominal pressure. The muscular wall defects may arise from congenital variants, including impairments of collagen tissue and musculature integrity, or from previous surgical intervention. Acquired muscle wall weakness may develop as a result of trauma or with the aging process.

Intra-abdominal pressure is increased under a number of circumstances and with certain pathological states. These include pregnancy, obesity, bearing down (Valsalva's maneuver) as with chronic constipation, straining associated with use of incorrect technique when lifting weights or other heavy objects, pushing or pulling, ascites, chronic cough, or an enlarging tumor or lesion. Increased abdominal pressure will not likely cause a hernia unless a muscle wall weakness coexists.

Classification

Abdominal hernias may be classified according to (1) the anatomical location and (2) the severity of protrusion. The more commonly occurring locations are hiatal (diaphragmatic), incisional (ventral), umbilical, inguinal (direct or indirect), or femoral.

The severity may be described with one of four terms: reducible, irreducible, incarcerated, or strangulated. When a hernia is *reducible* the protruding viscus recedes into the abdomen mechanically when the client is supine, or can be manually replaced by gently pushing the mass back into the cavity. An *irreducible* hernia cannot be replaced in the abdominal cavity by any method. An *incarcerated* hernia is one in which the protruding viscus is both irreducible and obstructed. This condition eventually leads to obstructed blood flow to or from the viscus and the hernia is referred to as *strangulated.* The last two situations are serious and differentiation between the two is difficult.

Incarcerated and strangulated hernias are considered to be surgical emergencies because the viscus will become acutely obstructed, and with its vascular supply compromised it will rapidly become necrotic and gangrenous. The intestines or the bladder, as in the case of the femoral hernia, are the organs likely to be contained in the herniated sac and therefore affected by this process. Indirect inguinal hernias, umbilical, and femoral hernias are more likely to strangulate than others because these sacs have smaller necks and tend to be surrounded by rigid rings of tissue as contrasted with direct inguinal hernias which tend to have broader necks. Also, over time, adhesions may develop between a hernial sac and its contents and result in an irreducible or incarcerated hernia. The types of hernias are listed and described in Table 84–1.

Hiatal (Esophageal) Hernia

In a hiatal hernia, a portion of the stomach protrudes through a defect in the diaphragm wall at the point where the esophagus passes through the diaphragm (Fig. 84–1).

Clinical Manifestations

Hiatal hernias may be asymptomatic or may have mild to severe symptomatology. The size of the hernia and amount of stomach compression contribute to this range of clinical symptoms. The most common clinical manifestation is the patient complaint of "heartburn" (pyrosis, dyspepsia) caused by the reflux of gastric juices into the esophagus and the subsequent irritation of the esophageal mucosa (reflux esophagitis). This symptom is described as a burning or tight feeling substernally or in the throat, neck, or back. The pa-

TABLE 84–1
Types of Hernias

Type and Incidence	*Description*
1. Hiatal: 1% (diaphragmatic)	
a. Sliding	*Junction* of esophagus and stomach moves above level of diaphragm. Over 75% of hiatal hernias are sliding.
b. Rolling	*Fundus and greater curvature of* stomach roll through diaphragmatic opening for the esophagus; gastroesophageal junction remains in normal position below diaphragm. Hiatal hernias become increasingly frequent after age 50 and reported in 67% of those over 60. (Schuster)
2. Inguinal: 75%	
a. Indirect	Protrusion of viscus through the inguinal ring; hernial sac follows the spermatic cord (male) or round (Poupart's) ligament (female) through the inguinal canal and often on into scrotum or labia
b. Direct	Sac passes directly through posterior inguinal wall and into inguinal canal in an area of weakness (vs through inguinal ring as with indirect). May occur in older persons secondary to decrease of collagen fibers in area.
3. Femoral: 6%; (male > female)	Protrusion of viscus through femoral ring into femoral canal appears below the inguinal (Poupart's) ligament.
4. Incisional: 10% (ventral)	Protrusion occurs through weakness in abdominal wall at site of previous surgery. Occurs most often when impaired healing (infection, poor nutriton, multiple surgeries in same location) and in obese persons.
5. Umbilical: 3%	Protrusion of viscus through umbilical opening. Common in obese persons and those with ascites and cirrhosis or when intrathoracic pressure is increased as with chronic bronchitis and asthma.
Some Rarer Types: 2%	
6. Epigastric	Fatty hernia of linea albea
7. Obdurator	Mass in femoral triangle
8. Spigelian	Occurs above inguinal ligament

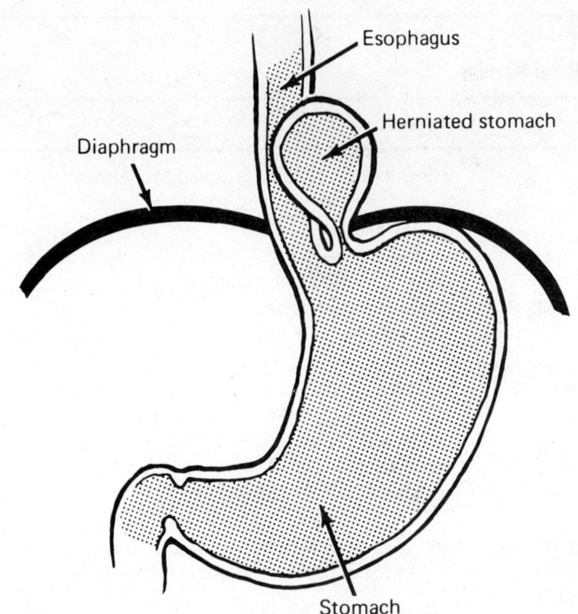

FIGURE 84–1 Esophageal hiatus hernia, paraesophageal type. The herniated portion of the stomach protrudes through the diaphragm into the chest cavity.

tient may also complain of liquid in the throat or mouth described variously as bitter, acid, burning hot, or sour tasting. This regurgitation of gastric contents and the heartburn are aggravated by recumbent, stooping, or bending positions, especially if following meals. Smoking, alcohol, tea, coffee, and stress may also precipitate pain. Other symptoms include the following: dysphagia (difficulty swallowing) due to muscle spasm, edema, or stricture of the esophagus; painful swallowing; or bleeding due to the esophageal inflammation. Such symptoms may represent complications of hiatal hernia, severe esophagitis, strangulation of the herniated stomach, and gastrointestinal hemorrhage. Anemia may occur due to occult bleeding from the esophageal mucosa.

Medical Management

Diagnosis. In many persons hiatal hernia is symptomless. When there is pain it may closely resemble angina pectoris (deep, steady pain, or occasional burning pain in the xiphoid region) or that of gallbladder or peptic ulcer disease.

Barium swallow studies (x-ray) and rigid esophagoscopy can be performed to help define the location of the esophogastric junction relative to the diaphmragmatic hiatus. Often these measures are not precise and flexible endoscopy may be performed, both to facilitate a more accurate measurement of the level of the esophogastric junction and to observe for diaphragmatic defects separate from the esophageal hiatus. Esophageal biopsy and cytology specimens may be obtained to assess the extent of esophagitis and to rule out the diagnosis of carcinoma or polyps. Motility studies, esophageal pH recordings, and lower esophageal pressure (LES) recordings can be done to provide additional diagnostic information, but these are not routinely used in clinical practice.

Treatment. The purpose of treatment is to alleviate the problem of gastric reflux by minimizing or preventing reflux and to protect the esophageal mucosa from refluxed gastric contents. Alleviating gastric reflux will thereby control symptoms and reduce the risk of esophagitis, hemorrhage due to erosion, stenosis, and stricture formation. For sliding hiatal hernias, generally conservative measures are prescribed such as eating smaller, more frequent meals, avoiding highly seasoned food or carbonated beverages, caffeine and alcohol, remaining in an upright position after meals, elevating the head and shoulders when supine and taking drugs such as antacids to relieve symptoms. Surgical intervention is recommended only when conservative measures fail to relieve symptoms or when complications occur as in the case of massive hiatal hernia. Paraesophageal hernias require surgical treatment. Conservative treatment is outlined in Table 84–2.

Surgical Treatment. For a sliding hiatal hernia, surgery is aimed at restoring normal anatomy by replacing the gastroesophageal junction below the level of the diaphragm. Often a fundoplication (anti-reflux procedure) and vagotomy (to decrease acid production) are also performed. The Nissen fundoplication is one of several types of surgical procedures and consists of a transabdominal approach in restoring the esophageal junction to its normal position, strengthening the esophageal hiatus, and then wrapping the fundus of the stomach around the lower esophagus which helps to reinforce the sphincter. Other procedures that may be selected are the Hill repair (posterior gastroplexy) and the Belsey Mark IV (transthoracic approach). Surgery may be performed through the abdomen or the thoracic cavity depending upon the surgeon and the patient's condition.

Operative treatment of a paraesophageal hernia is indicated in most cases due to a high risk for complications. With surgical repair the herniated stomach is restored in the abdominal cavity and fixed by sutures (anterior gastroplexy). The enlarged diaphragmatic hiatus is then sutured tightly around the gastroesophageal junction.

Prognosis. It has been estimated that roughly 90% of persons having surgical repair for *sliding hiatal hernia* have good results with the remaining 10% experiencing recurrent or persistent reflux. Recurrent symptoms of reflux are apparently more common than actual anatomical recurrence of the hernia.[10] Causes of anatomic recurrence may include inadequate surgical repair, excessive tension on the point of fixation due to a shortening of the esophagus, weakening of muscle or fascial structures with aging, obesity, or atrophy.

There is usually good management with surgical repair for *paraesophageal hernias*. Weakened muscles of the diaphragm can contribute to poor surgical results.

Inguinal Hernias

Diagnosis of inguinal hernia is made based on history and physical examination findings. Hernias are rarely symptomatic and therefore they are often detected during the

TABLE 84–2
Conservative Treatment for Sliding Hiatal Hernias

Treatment Measure	*Rationale*
Smaller more frequent meals.	Prevent gastric bloating caused by overdistention of the stomach with increased dietary intake.
Reduce or avoid highly seasoned foods, carbonated beverages, certain fruit juices, chocolate.	Prevent heartburn sometimes associated with intake of these foods.
Reduce or avoid the use of caffeine, nicotine, alcohol, fatty foods.	Maintain tone of lower esophageal sphincter (LES), a 3–6 cm zone of increased pressure just above gastroesophageal junction, which may become relaxed with the intake of certain substances (food, beverages, drugs).
Avoid bending or a recumbent position especially after a meal; use pillows to elevate head and shoulders when supine; sleep in a slightly inclined position with the head of the bed 4–6 inches higher (approximately 30°) than the foot.	Use of gravity to maintain the stomach and its contents below the level of the diaphragm.
Weight reduction if obese; treat chronic cough; wear loosely fitting garments.	Decrease intra-abdominal and intrathoracic pressures that might otherwise interfere with swallowing and gastric emptying and favor the backward flow of gastric contents.
Use of drugs for symptomatic treatment	
Antacids	Antacids neutralize gastric acid.
Silicone	Silicone coats the esophaeal mucosa.
Alginate	Alginate (alginic acid) and antacids (gaviscon) will create a surface solution on gastric contents that adheres to and protects esophageal mucosa if reflux occurs.
Surface anesthetics	Surface anesthetics and antacids relieves pain associated with reflux.
Urecholine/histamine	Urecholine/histamine thought to affect LES tone.
Metaclopramide	Metaclopramide affects LES tone, stimulates esophageal peristalsis, and improves gastric emptying.

course of a routine physical exam, or the patient may notice a visible swelling or bulging in the groin (Fig. 84–2). When there are symptoms they often occur as the hernia becomes enlarged and are generally more pronounced with indirect rather than direct hernias. The patient will complain of a "pulling" sensation or discomfort which may be relieved when the hernia is reduced.

Physical Examination. The differentiation between direct and indirect inguinal hernia is made by a thorough examination. On inspection with the patient standing and straining, the hernia appears as a round, symmetrical bulge at the level of the external ring. An indirect hernia appears more elliptical over the inguinal canal and may descend into the scrotum. If there is a direct hernia, the posterior wall of the inguinal canal is relaxed or non-palpable with the patient supine (versus normally firm) and the hernia will protrude against the examining finger when the patient coughs or strains. An indirect inguinal hernia will come down the inguinal canal against the side of the upward and laterally directed index finger. Finally, the direct hernia usually disappears when the patient is supine whereas the indirect hernia may or may not be reducible.

Indirect inguinal hernias must be differentiated from a number of other conditions that can occur in the groin. These include lymphadenopathy, abscesses of the groin, hydrocele, varicocele, undescended testes, and hemorrhage in the patient taking anticoagulants.

Treatment. Conservative treatment consists of having the patient wear a truss to hold the viscus in place. Large uncomfortable protruding hernias can be maintained in a

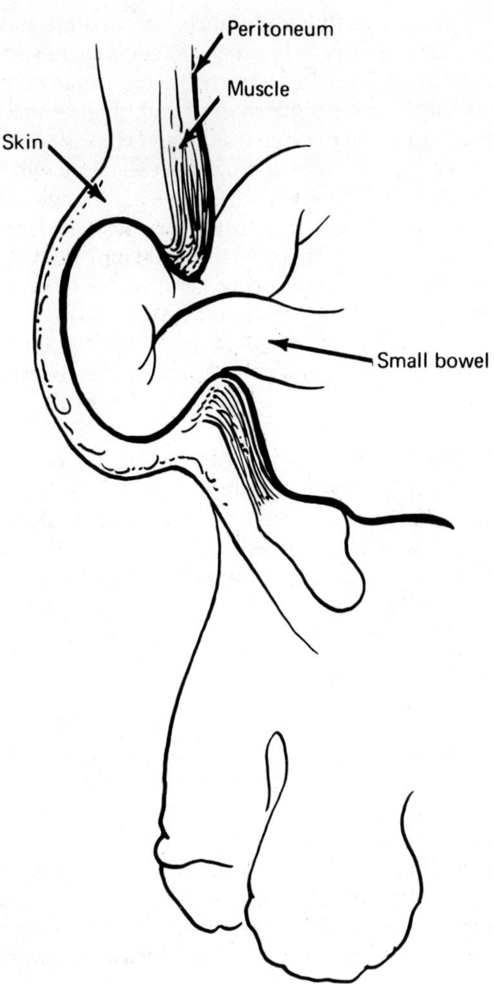

FIGURE 84–2 Inguinal hernia, demonstrating how the small bowel can become caught in the herniated sac.

reduced state to decrease discomfort and minimize the risk of strangulation.

Surgical Treatment. Indirect hernias should be surgically repaired, regardless of the patient's age, because of their tendency to incarcerate, obstruct, and strangulate. Unless there are specific contraindications these risks outweigh those associated with an operation.

A herniorrhaphy (surgical repair of hernia) is somewhat different for young adults than for older adults. For both groups surgery consists of ligation and removal of the hernial sac with a reduction in size of the inguinal ring. Additionally, it is necessary with the older patient to perform a hernioplasty to strengthen any weakened area with the patients' own fascia or with a synthetic mesh material. When an incarcerated hernia has spontaneously reduced, surgery may also include exploration of the abdomen to determine the viability of the small intestines. This may be performed within the same incision or by a separate vertical incision. There are variations in the techniques of surgical repair depending on the location, size, and amount of tissue weakness. Common names of repair techniques include Bassini, Halsted, and Shouldice. The latter two are variations of the basic Bassini repair.

The recurrence rate for indirect hernias is between 2% and 30% and between 4% and 33% for direct inguinal hernias. A number of conditions are known to predispose the patient to recurrence of the hernia. These include chronic cough, constipation, poor tissue turgor, postoperative wound infection, prostatism, and operative errors.

Nursing Interventions. The patient should be cautioned not to use force to reduce the hernia because such pressure could rupture a strangulated mass. Other precautions include instructing the patient to apply firm pressure over the hernia before coughing or straining, to avoid lifting heavy objects, and to lose weight if excessively overweight. The patient should also be taught to be on the alert for signs of hernia strangulation including abdominal pain or pain in the region of the hernia, swelling, tenderness, an inability to reduce the hernia or discoloration of tissues over the swelling.

In the postoperative period, nursing care includes administering the prescribed medication for pain and assessing how effectively it relieves the patient's postoperative discomfort. An additional pain relief measure is the application of ice bags to the groin area to reduce swelling and discomfort from the surgical trauma. To prevent wound dehiscence the patient should be instructed to avoid heavy coughing and to splint the incision if coughing is unavoidable. The tension caused by sneezing can be offset by advising the patient to sneeze with the mouth open. Stool softeners and fluids should be encouraged to help establish a regular bowel pattern and to avoid straining which could also result in wound dehiscence. Until the wound has healed, the patient should be advised not to lift anything heavier than a large book and should not drive a car until a follow-up visit to the surgeon.

Intestinal Obstructions

Intestinal obstruction is the interference with the normal progression of bowel contents. An obstruction may be partial, allowing some passage of contents, or complete and can occur at any point along the bowel. Adhesions, strangulated inguinal hernias, and neoplasms are the three most common causes of intestinal obstructions. Other causes are volvulus, intussusception, diverticulum, and polyps.

Obstructions may be classified as mechanical or strangulated. Mechanical refers to obstructions in which the blood supply to the bowel is adequate in contrast with strangulated obstructions in which the blood supply to the bowel is compromised.

Pathophysiology

There are differences in pathophysiology between mechanical obstruction and strangulation obstruction. The major physiologic disorder with *mechanical* obstruction is the accumulation of gas and fluid proximal to the section of the obstructed bowel which in turn leads to bowel distention and edema and increased, intense peristalsis. Fluid and electrolyte imbalance occurs as the intestines increase secretions and decrease absorption in response to the initial distention; fluids and electrolytes are then lost to the lumen, the edematous bowel wall, the free peritoneal fluid, and by vomiting or nasogastric suction. Intense peristalsis occurs as the bowel attempts to overcome the obstruction; this may traumatize the bowel, causing further edema and swelling. With fluid and electrolyte loss, the extracellular space becomes depleted resulting in hemoconcentration, hypovolemia, renal insufficiency, shock, and death.

A *strangulated* obstruction includes an occlusion of the blood supply to a portion of the bowel and an obstruction of the bowel lumen. Venous return from the strangulated bowel segment is blocked and results in extravasation of bloody fluid into the bowl lumen and bowel wall. At the same time the gangrenous bowel leaks toxic breakdown products into the peritoneal cavity causing peritonitis.

Clinical Manifestations

Initial symptoms of complete mechanical obstruction are abdominal pain, inability to pass gas and stool by the rectum, followed by abdominal distention. With a partial obstruction, diarrhea is common and there may be some elimination of gas and feces distal to a high obstruction. With progression of the obstruction severe continuous abdominal cramps are felt in conjunction with hyperperistalsis. As the regular waves of peristalsis become intermittent, the patient's colicky cramps are interspersed with inactive periods of 3 to 5 minutes if the obstruction is high in the intestine and 6 to 10 minutes with lower obstruction. The pain is diffuse across the upper abdomen with a high obstruction, midabdominal with lower ileal obstruction, lower abdominal with colon obstruction, and in the lower abdomen and perineum with rectosigmoid obstruction. If the obstruction is not relieved the cramps abate and a generalized abdominal discomfort is described. With a high obstruction a reflex vomiting occurs soon after the bowel obstructs and is followed by attacks of vomiting. With a low obstruction, vomiting does not occur until a day or two following obstruction. The vomitus may be copious, malodorous, and dark and may effectively decompress the bowel when there is a high obstruction.

Medical Management

Diagnosis. Because the pathologic processes that result in dehydration and distention occur gradually, the physical exam may be normal within the first 24 hours of mechanical obstruction. However, strangulation obstruction produces more marked symptoms early. In both types there is guarding and tenderness of the abdomen during palpation however if a mass is felt the obstructed bowel may be strangulated. On auscultation there will be high-pitched, metallic sounds when pain is felt and an absence of bowel sounds in between attacks of pain. Within 48 to 72 hours vital signs and physical exam findings become increasingly abnormal as the body progressively responds to the obstruction with distention, fluid imbalance, dehydration, and hypovolemia. Early laboratory findings include a slight rise in Hct (in response to fluid loss) and BUN (as urine output decreases). Later, with progression of pathological responses, there will be a fall in plasma sodium and chloride. Metabolic acidosis is common. The white blood cell count will be elevated (15,000–25,000/mm^3) if the bowel is strangulated. Primary mesenteric vascular occlusion may be considered if the white blood cell count is 40,000 to 60,000/mm^3. Radiographic study is a valuable diagnostic tool and will demonstrate gas fluid levels suggestive of intestinal obstruction. Further radiographic studies may be done, including barium enema, intravenous urography, or contrast dye studies by mouth or nasogastric tube.

Treatment. Treatment measures consist of fluid and electrolyte replacement, decompression of the bowel, and an operative procedure to correct the cause of obstruction. The type of surgical treatment will vary depending on the etiology of the obstruction. The procedure may be a resection of an obstructed or strangulated segment and subsequent anastomosis, anastomosis around an obstruction, or formation of a stoma proximal to the obstructed segment. If a gallstone is causing the obstruction, an enterotomy is performed to remove it. If the obstruction if caused by adhesions, intussusception, or an incarcerated hernia, surgery consists of lysis (surgical removal), manipulation-reduction, and reduction respectively and the bowel is not opened.

Adhesions are tight bands of scar tissue that occur around and between body organs, and are the result of scar tissue shrinkage over time. In the abdomen, these often occur months or years after surgery, or radiation. They can be symptomatic and cause an intestinal obstruction when they form around a portion of a bowel and partially or completely obstruct the lumen. Treatment consists of lysis of the scar tissue.

Volvulus is a twisting or rotation of the bowel around itself producing a partial or complete obstruction (Fig. 84–3). It occurs more frequently in the sigmoid colon (85%) than the cecum (15%). Volvulus is associated with severe chronic constipation seen primarily in those with severe psychiatric or neurologic disorders and the inactive elderly with advanced cardiovascular and pulmonary disease. Initial treatment for volvulus of the sigmoid is nonoperative and consists of insertion of a rectal tube by a sigmoid scope to deflate the distended bowel distal to the obstruction. The tube is left in place for 2 to 3 days until normal bowel function resumes. This is followed by surgical resection of the area of volvulus and anastomosis.

Intussusception is the invagination or telescoping of a proximal section of bowel into the lumen of the distal section. It most frequently occurs spontaneously in infants, but can occur in adults, and then is usually the result of a polyp which causes the intussusception. Large nodes in the mesentary may be an etiological factor. Most intussusceptions begin in the ileocecal valve and extend through a variable length of the colon and occasionally prolapse through the anus. The bowel may become obstructed with the invagination or as a result of secondary edema. Treatment consists of reduction that may occur during barium enema administered for diag-

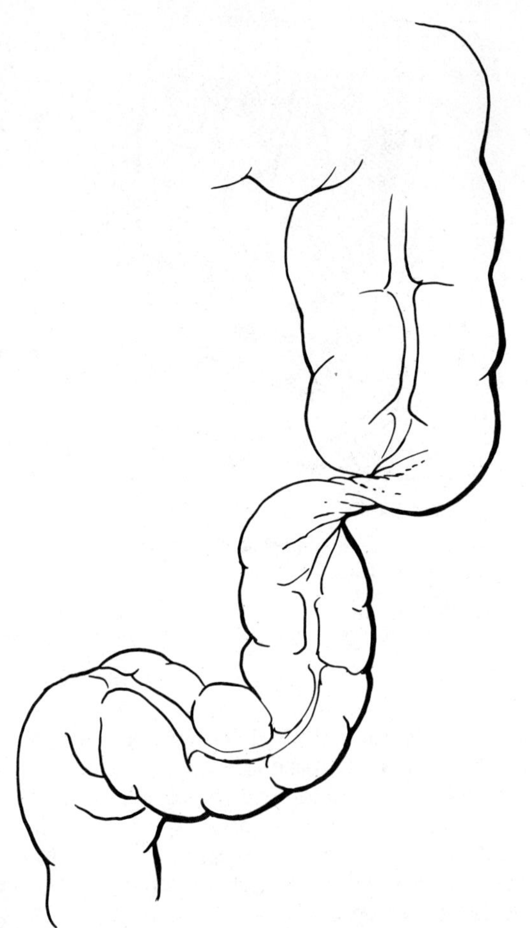

FIGURE 84–3 Volvulus of the colon. The twisting can cause complete obstruction.

nostic purposes or a surgical reduction consisting of manual progressive compression of the bowel.

Diverticulum is a herniation of intestinal mucosa through a weakened area in the muscle wall of the intestine. Multiple herniated sacs, or outpouchings are referred to as *diverticulosis,* and if inflammation and irritation is present the condition is referred to as *diverticulitis.* Diverticulitis may cause secondary problems including bowel obstruction, perforation with abscess and fistula formation, or perforation with peritonitis and hemorrhage. Initial treatment consists of fluid replacement, antibiotics, and nasogastric suction. If symptoms are not relieved, surgical treatment is performed. Surgery may include a colostomy if there is a perforation or a resection of the portion of bowel that contains the diverticuli.

A *polyp* is a mass of tissue that arises from mucosa and protrudes into the lumen of the gastrointestinal tract. Polyps commonly arise in the sigmoid colon and rectum and though they are frequently asymptomatic, they may bleed. They may occur singly or in groups. There are several types. Juvenile polyps occur mainly in children but occasionally develop in young adults, and have no malignant potential. *Adenomatous polyps* are the most commonly occurring neoplasm of the colon and rectum. They are usually pedunculated, firm tumors, less than 1 cm in size and occur with increasing frequency after age 21. A *villous adenoma* (papillary adenoma) is a polypoid lesion with frondlike projections. They are poorly demarcated and because of their smooth, soft surface, difficult to detect by palpation. They have a small but definitely malignant potential. *Familial polyposis* is a rare hereditary disease characterized by the appearance of many adenomas in the colon and rectum in adolescence and the progression to carcinoma of the colon if left untreated. All polyps should be removed because of the uncertainty of their evolution to carcinomas. They can be removed by colonscopy or sigmoidoscopy when the polyps are small. When there is invasive malignancy a resection is performed and when the diagnosis is familial polyposis an abdominal colectomy is indicated with resection of rectum and anus terminal ileostomy.

Fecal incontinence is the major postsurgical complication when the polyps are in the rectum, and is reported as high as 60%. Adequate reconstruction of the rectum and the presence of normal neurological function within the pelvic region reduce the risk for incontinence. Stenosis of the anal mucocutaneous suture line is another complication, and treatment consists of dilation or anoplasty.

Nursing Management

Assessment

A careful evaluation of symptoms and gastrointestinal function will help differentiate between small and large bowel obstruction and will aid in determining if there are any problems requiring immediate therapeutic attention, such as fluid replacement. Acute obstruction of the small intestines usually manifests itself in a triad of symptoms and signs—vomiting, abdominal distention, and cramping (colicky abdominal pain). A grossly enlarged abdomen may be a result of gastrointestinal distension that occurs when fluid and gas accumulate in the bowel or if there is peritonitis. A visible churning in a distended abdomen is usually diagnostic of a small bowel obstruction. Tenderness and rigidity or signs of abdominal bulge should be reported to the physician immediately.

Peristaltic sounds are evaluated by auscultating the abdomen. Hyperperistalsis or borborygmus (loud, high-pitched rushing sound occurring simultaneously with colicky pain) may indicate obstruction of the small intestines. A lack of bowel sound would indicate an absence of bowel motility that may be associated with inflammation or gangrene late in the course of a severe complete obstruction or strangulation. The physician is contacted immediately if hyperperistalsis or absence of bowel tones are detected or not detected.

Other signs to note include temperature, pulse, respirations, and laboratory data—CBC, serum electrolytes, and BUN. Elevations in temperature, pulse respirations, and white blood count may indicate infection and peritonitis that may be associated with an acute or late stage of chronic obstruction. Potassium, sodium, and chloride values will be decreased due to the retention of electrolyte-rich fluids in the bowel and their subsequent loss in the peritoneal cavity or by vomiting. BUN will increase initially as the body responds to decreased fluids and electrolyte concentrations by decreasing output.

Interventions

While the patient is awaiting surgery, there is a need to administer IV fluids and electrolyte therapy and possibly administer nutrients through parenteral hyperalimentation. Blood levels of sodium, potassium, bicarbonate, and blood pH are monitored to evaluate the effectiveness of IV therapy. Careful observations and recording are made of intake and output including IV solutions, oral food and fluid (if the patient is not NPO), emesis, drainage from intestinal tubes, and urinary output. Nasoenteric suctioning may be ordered to decompress the bowel above the site of the obstruction by removing fluid and gas and relieving vomiting and bowel distention.

The emotional reactions of patients with intestinal obstruction are frequently intense and reflect deep felt distress and pain. Providing emotional support and encouraging discussion regarding concerns and fears are ways by which the nurse can help release this pent-up anxiety. Efforts should be made to enlist the support of others (pastor, family) when appropriate. The care of patients having intestinal surgery is discussed in Chapters 81 and 82.

Hemorrhoids

Definition

Hemorrhoids (piles) are varicose (enlarged) veins in the hemorrhoidal plexus of the mucous membranes of the anal canal. Because the veins are normally very large and dilated and the mucosal tissues in which they lie are bulky and engorged with blood during defecation, hemorrhoidal disease is described as an exaggeration of normal anatomy. Many people have them and they often appear, become symptomatic and then resolve spontaneously, frequently leaving an external skin tag (fibrous connective tissue covered with skin). Hemorrhoids may be internal and external, or if occurring in both locations they are referred to as mixed hemorrhoids. Internal hemorrhoids occur in the vascular cushions of the mucous membrane of the upper portion of the anal canal. External hemorrhoids occur in the venules of the smooth skin in the lower portion of the canal (see Fig. 84–4). Prolapsed hemorrhoids are internal hemorrhoids that have protruded outside the anal canal. A thrombosed hemorrhoid is one in which the blood has clotted; it may become infected or result in a skin tag.

Etiology/Pathophysiology

In many cases there is no identifiable cause of this increased dilation and pressure; however, several factors have been implicated in the causation. Straining during defecation, resisting the urge to defecate, the absence of venous valves, standing for prolonged periods, pregnancy, and portal hypertension associated with cirrhosis are thought to result in the excess engorgement of anal cushions and obstruction of venous return. Hereditary weakness of vessels may also contribute to this process.

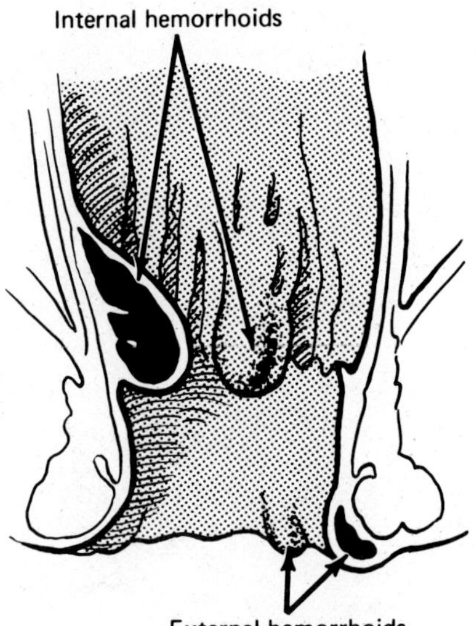

FIGURE 84–4 Internal and external hemorrhoids.

Hemorrhoids develop with repeated episodes of tense engorgement of the anal musocsal cushions. Injury may result, causing bleeding from the capillaries and damage to the normal supports of the anal cushions, eventually resulting in a tendency to prolapse.

Clinical Manifestations

External hemorrhoids are often asymptomatic. When one becomes thrombosed the patient will experience acute pain. The mass may be palpable and visible outside the anus. Internal hemorrhoids are intermittently symptomatic. Symptoms may include pruritis ani (itching in the anal region), discomfort, and bleeding with bowel movements. Large internal hemorrhoids may prolapse with straining on bowel movements.

Medical Management

Diagnosis. The diagnosis is made based on the history (relative to associated causative factors), symptoms, and physical examination.

Treatment. Initial treatment of a painful prolapsed hemorrhoid may include reducing the hemorrhoid if possible, bedrest in a prone, Trendelenburg's position, and cold witch hazel compresses. Further treatment can be performed on an outpatient basis. The thrombosed area is injected with topical anesthestic and the hemorrhoid excised, with electrocoagulation of the bleeding points. Initial treatment for nonpainful thrombosed hemorrhoids or bleeding internal hemorrhoids should be nonsurgical, and directed at restoring regular, nonconstipated bowel patterns through rigorous attention to dietary factors that contribute to constipation and those that promote soft formed stool.

Uncomplicated bleeding internal hemorrhoids can also be treated nonsurgically on an outpatient basis with a procedure called rubber band ligation. Rubber band ligation is performed without anesthesia and consists of placing a rubber band on the rectal mucosa above the internal hemorrhoid, via an instrument inserted into the rectum. In roughly a week's time, the resulting tissue constriction causes a sloughing of the tissue distal to the rubber band and leaves an area of inflammation that eventually fibroses. Repeated procedures can be performed every 6 to 8 weeks and up to two to three areas can be ligated each time. Another procedure that may be used instead of the rubber band treatment is injection of the tissue with a sclerosing substance.

Cryotherapy is a technique used to freeze hemorrhoid tissues with liquid nitrogen. However, cryosurgery can cause severe pain, prolonged wound healing, and profuse discharge. It also can result in anal strictures and incontinence.

Hemorrhoidectomy is indicated when there are large hemorrhoids, bleeding, pain, and prolapse. Surgery may also be required in the immediate postpartum period for women who have had severe hemorrhoids during pregnancy with prolapse or thrombosis occurring at the time of delivery. Surgery consists of removal of all the hemorrhoidal tissue through ligation and excision. The many variations in surgical technique are commonly aimed at minimizing scarring in the anal canal, preserving anal sphincter function, and retaining an anal orifice large enough to allow nonpainful elimination of a normal bowel movement.

Nursing Management

Nursing Diagnosis and Interventions

Following a hemorrhoidectomy, the major nursing diagnoses are alteration in comfort, pain, and alteration in elimination related to the surgical procedure. Interventions include administering pain medication regularly for the first 24 to 48 hours after surgery to control pain, encouraging sitz baths to relieve discomfort and promote healing by increasing circulation to the perianal area, and providing a sponge or foam ring or donut for the patient to sit on to alleviate pressure on the perianal area. It is important to avoid constipation which may result if the patient resists the urge to have a bowel movement because of rectal pain. Administer stool softeners and encourage fluid intake to facilitate defecation. Instruct the patient to avoid straining during bowel movements and to use ointments, suppositories, creams, or other preparations to help shrink or anesthetize swollen mucous membranes.

Because internal hemorrhoids may reoccur, a patient teaching program should be instituted that stresses dietary intake of fluids (approximately 2 qt daily), and fibers (fruits and vegetables), the use of stool softeners as needed and the importance of avoiding straining during defecation. Instruct the patient to observe for rectal bleeding and to have regular rectal examinations.

Prognosis

There is a more permanent result with ligation technique than with the injection technique because loss of hemorrhoidal tissue is more precise with ligation. Multiple applications of the rubber band may be required to achieve complete relief of symptoms. Hemorrhoidectomy is very good for achieving symptom relief. Complications for this procedure, however, include infection and abscess formation with resulting pain and stenosis of involved tissue; the reported incidence of infection is 0.2%.

References

1. Abdu R: Repair of paracolostomy hernias with marlex mesh. Dis Colon Rectum 25(6):529, 1982
2. Block M: Managing the silent, atypical acute abdomen. Geriatrics 38(9):50, 1983
3. Delp M, Manning RT: Major's Physical Diagnosis: An introduction to the Clinical Process. Philadelphia, WB Saunders, 1981
4. Lewis SM, Collier IC: Medical Surgical Nursing: Assessment and Management of Clinical Problems. New York, McGraw-Hill, 1983
5. Loebl S, Sprato G, Heckheimer E: The Nurses Drug Handbook, 3rd ed. New York, John Wiley and Sons, 1983
6. Pearson FG, et al: Massive hiatal hernia with incarceration: A report of 53 cases. Ann Thorac Surg 35(1):45, 1983
7. Roussel JG, Prins JG: Hernia abdominalis permagna: A staged repair with the temporary use of prostatic material. Surgery 92(5):906, 1982
8. Sabiston DC (ed): Textbook of Surgery, 11th ed. Philadelphia: WB Saunders, 1977
9. Schwartz SI, Shires GT, Spencer FC, Storer EH (eds): Principles of Surgery. New York, McGraw-Hill, 1984
10. Way L: Current Surgical Diagnosis and Treatment, 6th ed. Los Altos, Lange Medical Publications, 1983

UNIT X

Nursing Care of Patients with Alterations in Musculoskeletal Function

Chapter 85

Review of Anatomy and Physiology

Musculoskeletal System

Barbara R. Landau

The musculoskeletal system provides a supporting framework for the body and its parts, permits and causes movements of the parts, and is responsible for the form and shape of the body. It consists of the bones of the skeleton, the joints that connect them, and the muscles that move them. The bones are rigid to provide the necessary support, but movement is possible because they are flexibly connected. The bones are levers and the joints are the fulcrums about which the levers rotate. Muscles are attached to the bony scaffold in a manner that allows them to exert force on the levers and move them.

The Skeleton and Bones

The most obvious function of the skeleton is as a supporting framework for the body; all body parts are attached to it directly or indirectly. Some bones serve important protective functions; those of the cranium and vertebral column encase the fragile tissue of the brain and spinal cord, and bones of the rib cage shield the thoracic viscera. Because of the high mineral content of the intercellular material, bone is an important storage site of calcium and phosphorus, and a reservoir from which they may be withdrawn. It is also the site of blood cell formation, for the hematopoietic tissue is located in the interstices of the red bone marrow of certain bones.

In addition to bone, the skeleton contains cartilage as well as fibrous connective tissue. They are all characterized by an abundance of intercellular material, and it is the specific properties of the intercellular material that distinguishes bone and cartilage from other tissues.

The intercellular material or matrix of bone consists of fibers and ground substance. The fibers are almost entirely collagenous and more abundant than one might expect. The minerals give bone its rigidity and hardness and make up about two thirds of its weight. The organic component of bone (*i.e.,* the cells, fibers, and nonmineral part of the ground substance) give bone a certain strength, toughness, and flexibility.

Bone Structure

Bones may be classified by their shape as long, short, flat, or irregular bones. Long bones are found only in the extremities; short bones include such bones as the tarsal and carpals; flat bones are in the cranium; and irregular bones are those of the vertebrae.

A typical long bone consists of a shaft or diaphysis and two ends or epiphyses (Fig. 85–1). It is covered by periosteum except for the articular surfaces, which are covered by a thin layer of hyaline cartilage, the articular cartilage. The periosteum, which is continuous with the deep fascia of surrounding muscles, contains blood vessels and cells that

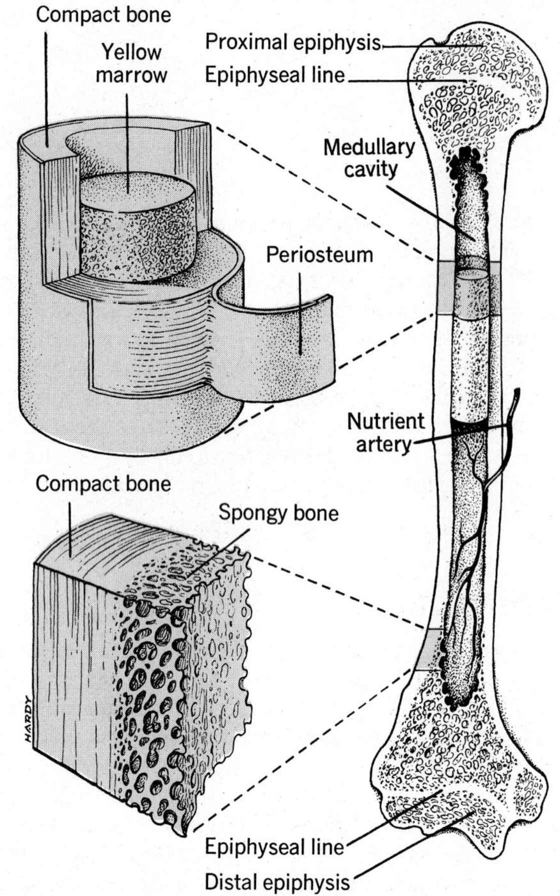

FIGURE 85–1 Diagram of a long bone shown in longitudinal section.

have the potential to become bone-forming cells under certain conditions.

The outer portion of long bones is composed of dense compact bone, which is quite thick in the diaphysis and thin at the epiphyses (see Fig. 85–1). In the center of the shaft is the marrow cavity, which is occupied largely by fat cells and hence is called yellow marrow. It is lined with a thin film of connective tissue, the endosteum. The epiphyses contain a delicate latticework of cancellous or spongy bone. Hematopoietic cells occupy the spaces between trabeculae of cancellous bone, and this area is the red bone marrow. In early life red marrow occupies most of the interior portion of the bone, but it is largely replaced by yellow marrow later. In the adult, most of the hematopoietic activity is restricted to a few bones (*i.e.,* sternum, iliac crest), but others retain the potential to become active once more. Bones other than long bones consist of a thin layer of compact bone on the surface and cancellous bone in the interior, but with no marrow cavity.

Microscopically, compact bone is organized in units known as osteons or haversian systems (Fig. 85–2). The closely packed osteons consist of concentric rings or lamellae surrounding a tiny central or haversian canal that contains blood vessels and some connective tissue. There are lacunae, each of which contains a bone cell or osteocyte, along the junctions between lamellae. The isolated osteocytes communicate with other bone cells and indirectly with the blood vessel in the canal by way of slender processes that lie in tiny canaliculi in the lamellae. Since the bone matrix will not support diffusion, the metabolic needs of the osteocytes are met by these cell processes.

The blood supply for bones comes mainly from the nutrient arteries that enter the compact bone through nutrient foramina. In long bones most vessels enter in the region of the diaphysis and break into branches. Some branches enter the marrow cavity and others enter cancellous bone of the epiphyses. Arteries to osteons pass through channels that penetrate the compact bone and communicate with central canals. Venous blood from bone returns in veins that course through the same channels, but in the opposite direction.

Bone is a living dynamic tissue. Bone development is a continuous process, with osteoclasts constantly eroding bone to reshape it, while osteoblasts are forming new bone elsewhere. Since one of the actions of osteoclasts is withdrawal of calcium from bone, they also participate in regulating calcium levels in the blood.

Bone Metabolism

The regulation of bone metabolism is inseparable from the regulation of calcium metabolism, and both are under the same hormonal controls. Bone mineral is a complex crystallized salt, primarily calcium phosphate. Bone accounts for about 99% of the body calcium and about 90% of body phosphate. Some of the bone calcium is in readily available form, but most is in a relatively stable, slowly exchangeable form.

The serum calcium level must be kept within a fairly narrow range (around 10 mg/dl, 5 mEq/liter), and bone is the bank where calcium may be deposited or withdrawn to maintain that level. A slight change in bone calcium content will cause a major change in calcium level in the blood and other soft tissues. Over a period of time, however, the rate of bone formation and mineralization must equal the rate of bone resorption or the total bone mass will change.

If one assumes a dietary intake of calcium that is sufficient to meet the needs (which may not be a valid assumption), then the balance of calcium and phosphate is controlled largely by three hormones: parathormone (PTH) from the parathyroid glands, calcitonin (CT) from the thyroid, and vitamin D (1,25-dihydroxycholecalciferol, 1,25-$[OH]_2D_3$). Formation of the latter involves the action of the skin, liver, and kidney, with the final active form being released from the kidney. A low serum calcium level increases PTH release, and high serum calcium inhibits it. PTH raises serum calcium levels by withdrawing calcium from the bone (resorption), by reducing renal excretion of calcium (by increased reabsorption), and by facilitating absorption of calcium from the intestine (indirectly by stimulating vitamin D production). It also increases renal excretion of phosphate. PTH increases the number of osteoclasts as well as their activity (it increases their permeability to calcium), and it also increases the permeability of osteocytes to calcium.

The small fraction of the calcium that is in the soft tissues

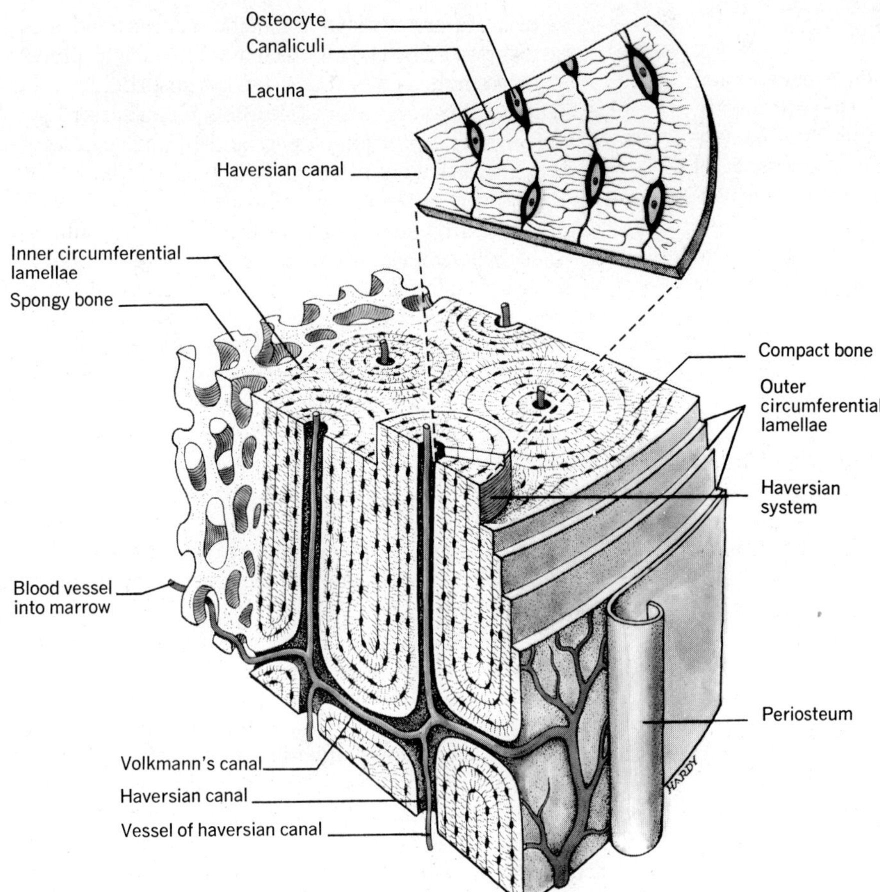

FIGURE 85–2 Diagram of haversian systems as seen in a wedge of compact bone tissue. The periosteum has been peeled back to show a blood vessel entering one of Volkmann's canals. *Upper right:* sketch showing osteocytes lying within lacunae; canaliculi permit interstitial fluid to reach each lacuna.

has many functions, but the one most sensitive to low serum calcium is the stability of nerve and muscle cell membranes. Low calcium causes an increase in excitability (lower threshold), which leads to inappropriate muscle contractions and perhaps tetany.

Calcitonin, on the other hand, acts to lower serum calcium, and its secretion is elicited when serum calcium levels are high. The primary action of calcitonin is to inhibit bone resorption by decreasing the permeability of the membranes of osteoclasts and osteocytes to calcium. It also increases renal excretion of calcium and phosphate. The homeostatic role of calcitonin is not yet established, since its absence has no significant effect on bone metabolism as long as PTH is available.

The primary action of vitamin D (which can be considered a hormone because it is produced in the body and transported in the bloodstream to distant target cells) is to increase the absorption of calcium and phosphorus from the intestine. The resultant increase in serum calcium and phosphate levels facilitates the mineralization of bone. Vitamin D also exerts a permissive effect on many of the actions of PTH, including the withdrawal of mineral from bone.

A number of other hormones affect bone metabolism and mineralization. The adrenal glucocorticoids, through their catabolic actions on protein, reduce the organic component of bone. They also reduce calcium and phosphate absorption from the intestine and increase their excretion. Thyroid hormones raise levels of calcium in blood and urine. Estrogens tend to inhibit the action of PTH, an important consideration in the development of osteoporosis in postmenopausal women.

During the growth years the metabolic balance is shifted in favor of bone formation, which involves additional hormones. Chief among them is growth hormone from the anterior lobe of the pituitary, whose general action is to promote uptake of amino acids and synthesis of protein by cells. The hormone promotes growth of the soft tissues, especially muscle but also the organic component of bone. The actions of growth hormone on the skeleton are indirect, however, for the hormone stimulates production of somatomedins by the liver, and they carry out its actions. The specific action on the skeleton is stimulation of mitotic activity of chondroblasts in the cartilage model, especially in long bones. Their proliferation and growth thickens the epiphyseal disk, which delays its disappearance and prolongs linear growth of the bone.

Androgens, which have a powerful anabolic effect on protein, also stimulate the growth of the cartilage of the epiphyseal disk that leads to the growth spurt that occurs in boys at puberty. Androgens, however, cause an abrupt end to linear bone growth by bringing about the disappearance of the cartilage and final fusion of the bone.

Articulations

The articulations hold the bones of the skeleton together and are necessary for movement. They differ in structure according to the roles they serve. Joints differ in the type of connecting material between the bones, in the type and range of movement permitted (if any), and in the shapes of the articulating surfaces of the bones. Articulations have been classified and subdivided on the basis of all these criteria. One system, based on movement, classifies joints as synarthroses (no movement), amphiarthroses (minimal movement or "give") and diarthroses (freely movable).

Classification of Joints

A useful classification is based first on the type of connecting material, with subdivisions according to movements and articular surfaces.

1. Fibrous joints—Bones are joined by fibrous connective tissue.
   a. *Sutures*—between cranial bones. Immovable due to interlocking junctions between the bones and short numerous connecting fibers.
   b. *Syndesmoses*—forms an interosseous membrane or ligament. Fibers are somewhat longer, and permit a slight "give." An example is the distal tibiofibular joint.
2. Cartilaginous joints—Bones are joined by cartilage, supported by ligaments, and permit only slight movement.
   a. *Synchondroses*—hyaline cartilage between the bones. The best example is between the diaphysis and epiphyses of growing long bones; another example is the costochondral joints.
   b. *Symphyses*—fibrocartilage between the bones, and a thin layer of hyaline cartilage covering articular surfaces. Examples are the pubic symphysis and the joints between bodies of the vertebrae. The fibers in the fibrocartilage of the intervertebral disk are arranged in a specific manner, and the disk has a fibrogelatinous material (nucleus pulposus) in the center that is a shock absorber.
3. *Synovial joints*—the movable joints, characterized by the presence of a joint cavity and hyaline cartilage over the articular surfaces of the bones (Fig. 85–3). The joint is enclosed by a fibrous joint capsule and reinforced by supporting ligaments. The capsule is lined by a synovial membrane whose cells produce the synovial fluid, which reduces friction between the moving bones. Since articular cartilage is avascular, the synovial fluid is important to it, and changes in the fluid's composition may lead to degenerative changes in the articular cartilage. In adults, cartilage cells rarely undergo mitosis.

Movements at Joints

The amount and type of movement possible at a particular joint depends on the structure of the articulating portions of the bones involved.

Joint Axes. Virtually all movement is a form of rotation. One end of the bone is relatively fixed and the other end rotates about it. The bone is a lever whose fulcrum is at the fixed end. A line through the fulcrum and perpendicular to the plane of movement is the axis of that movement. For the elbow joint, the axis is a transverse line through the joint (the plane of rotation is a sagittal plane). The elbow is said to be a uniaxial joint because the only movements possible (flexion and extension) occur about a transverse axis. Flexor muscles cross the joint anterior to the axis, and extensor muscles cross the joint posterior to it. Movements in other planes are prevented by the shape of the bones and the supporting ligaments.

Uniaxial joints may be ***hinge joints*** such as the elbow, or *pivot joints* such as the radioulnar joint. The latter is a special joint with a roughly longitudinal axis. The movements are pronation and supination.

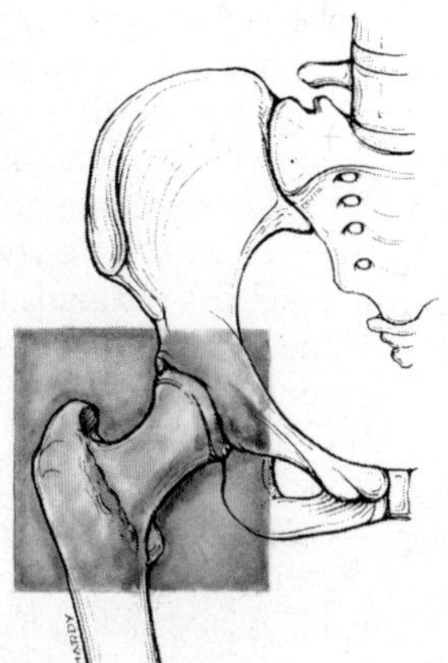

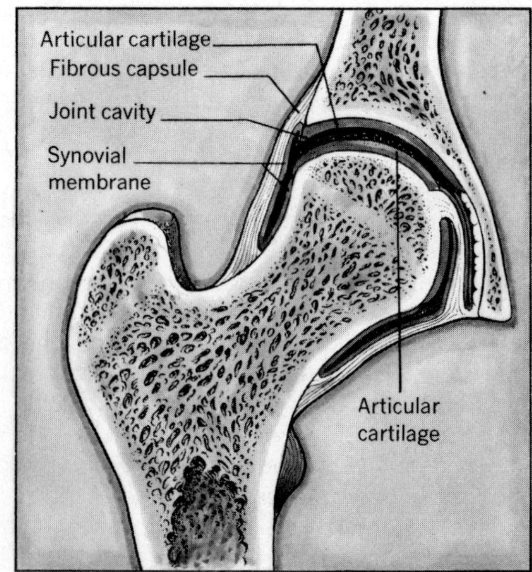

FIGURE 85–3 Hip joint, showing structure of synovial joints. Joint cavities have been enlarged.

Biaxial joints permit movements about either of two axes, and in two planes. They may be *condyloid joints* such as the atlanto-occipital, radiocarpal (wrist), or metacarpophalangeal joints, or *saddle joints* such as the carpometacarpal joint of the thumb. The axes are transverse (flexion and extension) and anteroposterior for abduction and adduction. Muscles that cause abduction cross the joint lateral to the axis, and adductors cross medial to it. The axes of the saddle joint are similar, except that they are slightly angled.

Multiaxial joints, which have more than two axes, include *ball-and-sockets joints* and *gliding joints.* Ball-and-socket joints such as the hip and shoulder have a third axis, a vertical or longitudinal axis about which medial and lateral rotation of the femur or humerus may occur. In movements at gliding joints, such as those between carpal and tarsal bones, the bones slide over one another rather than rotate. The movements are slight, and axes usually are not described for them.

Skeletal Muscle

Skeletal muscles generate the force to move the body parts. They make up about 40% of the total body weight and therefore have considerable impact on the body's energy requirements. Connective tissue surrounds each muscle fiber (endomysium), each bundle of fibers (epimysium), and each muscle (perimysium). The latter is part of the deep fascia. Blood vessels and nerves run in the connective tissue septa. Muscle attachments are either fleshy or fibrous. Fleshy attachments are those in which muscle fibers arise directly from the bone. Fibrous attachments are tendons or aponeuroses and are much stronger.

At rest skeletal muscles have a relatively low metabolic rate, and they obtain most of their energy by oxidizing fatty acids brought by the blood stream. During exercise the metabolic rate may increase 100-fold or even 1000-fold for short periods. Muscle cells must provide the energy to sustain such bursts, since cardiovascular adjustments cannot increase blood flow enough, either in time or quantity, to meet such requirements.

Bibliography

Crouch JE: Functional Human Anatomy, 3rd ed, Chaps 8–11. Philadelphia, Lea & Febiger, 1978

Ganong WF: Review of Medical Physiology, 11th ed, Chap 3. Los Altos CA, Lange Medical Publications, 1983

Landau BR: Essential Human Anatomy and Physiology, 2nd ed, Chaps 4–7. Glenview IL, Scott, Foresman and Company, 1980

Patton HD, Sundsten JW, Crill WE, Swanson PD: Introduction to Basic Neurology, Chap 6. Philadelphia, WB Saunders, 1976

Ross G: Essentials of Human Physiology, 2nd ed, Chap 3. Chicago, Year Book Medical Publishers, 1982

Rosse C, Clawson DK: The Musculoskeletal System in Health and Disease. Hagerstown MD, Harper & Row, 1980

Vander AJ, Sherman JH, Luciano DS: Human Physiology: The Mechanisms of Body Function, 3rd ed. New York, McGraw Hill, 1980

Chapter 86

Assessment of Musculoskeletal Function

Martha J. Lentz

History

In an effort to accurately assess the musculoskeletal system, many different technologies such as radiograph, bone scan, and arthroscopic examination have been developed. However, in spite of all the advances in technology, the most important part of a complete assessment of the musculoskeletal system remains the history. The underlying nature of the problem can often be inferred from the mechanism of injury or from the pattern of onset. A stress fracture may not be visible on radiograph, but could be identifiable using a bone scan at greater risk and cost to the patient. Obtaining a careful history of the patient's pattern of exercise, and any recent changes in this pattern, can aid in identifying the presence of a stress fracture before it is visualized by radiograph. This is particularly true when the history is coupled with the findings from the physical examination.

Onset and Course

The detailed history begins with a complete description of the onset and course of the problem. The patient should be asked to give a complete description of what happened or what precipitated the current episode, and when it happened or how long the current problem has existed. This includes knowing if the onset was sudden, as in a traumatic injury, or if it was a gradually developing condition. Has this problem occurred before or is this the first time? If it has occurred before, how long has it been since the last episode? If the problem had a traumatic onset, the patient should describe as completely as possible the mechanism of injury. Did he experience a blow or a fall? If a twisting motion occurred, in what direction was it? Was there the sound of a pop or a crack heard or felt at the time of the accident?

Changes Experienced

When the problem has had an acute onset, the changes that were present at the time of injury frequently are very different from what the nurse observes on initial examination of the patient. The patient should be asked to describe as completely as possible what changes he observed after the accident. Was there immediate pain, discoloration, or swelling? If there were no immediate changes, did they develop later and over what length of time? What type of treatment, if any, did the patient use? Application of heat can turn the appearance of a relatively minor sprain into the swollen and red look of a more severe injury. Conversely, prompt application of cold can limit swelling and bleeding of a severely injured joint. A thorough history of what happened can help sort out the correct interpretation of the observed signs.

When the condition has had a gradual onset, the questions asked should elicit information as to when the problem was first noticed. Attention should be directed to what area was first affected and whether that remained the same or has changed. Is the problem restricted to a single area, such as a single limb or joint, vs. involving widespread areas of the body? Again, how the affected area appears in terms of swelling and redness should be described.

Information as to what makes the condition better or worse can be appropriately considered for problems having either a gradual or an acute onset. What patient actions or conditions help to reduce pain, swelling, or inflammation? For example, does the patient take anti-inflammatory medication or use heat to successfully reduce pain and stiffness? Are there activities or conditions that result in increased pain or swelling? The timing of reported pain and stiffness or swelling may also provide information about the underlying problem. For example, morning pain and stiffness involving multiple joints is a frequent sign of rheumatoid arthritis, and pain that only occurs in the front of the knee when walking up stairs is often a sign of chondromalacia of the patella. Information about joint instability or locking of the joint will provide additional insight into the underlying nature of the problem.

Impact on Daily Activities

General information about any effect the problem has on the patient's ability to carry out activities of daily living should also be obtained. Is the patient able to work and maintain a home? Can the patient comb his hair, bathe, get dressed and undressed? Does the patient require any assistive devices or use other compensating techniques? When evaluating the impact of these alterations, it is important to consider them in the context of the patient's usual activity patterns. Recurrent twisting of the ankle may not appear to have a very serious impact on a person whose job does not require walking; however, the recurrent ankle problem could represent a significant disruption in lifestyle by preventing the person's usual recreational activity of jogging. Information obtained should include alterations in all activities of daily living—recreational, social, and work.

Physical Examination

The basic techniques used in the physical examination of the musculoskeletal system are inspection and palpation. The symmetry between both sides of the body in contour and mass is observed. Evidence of wasting, the presence of masses or deformities, and changes in skin color are noted. Observation of range of motion and of the ability to make smooth and coordinated movements involving multiple joints is essential. Palpation is used to detect joint instability and bone continuity, to evaluate deformities and swelling, and to localize pain by eliciting tenderness. Tenderness is pain produced by pressure exerted on the affected area during palpation. Inspection and palpation are done both in the general overview and in evaluating the status of specific areas of the musculoskeletal system.

General Overview

The physical examination begins with observing the patient's posture from the front, back, and sides. Curvature of the spine or other deformity, evidence of muscle wasting or masses, and variation in skin color should be noted. Any conspicuous changes in joint appearance, such as swelling or deformity, are recorded for further examination.

The patient's gait should be evaluated for smoothness, length of stride, and general balance. When walking, weight should be distributed evenly, with knees and toes pointed forward. An adult usually walks with 2 inches to 4 inches between the heels and with steps about 15 inches in length. A widened stance or shorter step is often seen with aging, fatigue, pain, muscle weakness, or decreased sense of balance. Slapping, scraping, and dragging sounds should be noted. For example, the patient with peroneal nerve palsy will raise the knees to avoid dragging the toes of the affected side, and then the foot will slap down with an easily heard sound after the heel strike.

When observing the patient's gait, any use of assistive devices should be noted. If possible the evaluation should be made with and without the use of assistive devices, such as crutches or walkers. The type of footwear usually worn by the patient should be evaluated. The shoes worn by many women contribute to poor posture, poor foot balance, and pain that can disrupt their gait. The wear pattern on the heels and soles indicates the pattern of foot strike and follow-through of the stride and helps to identify abnormalities.

Observations of simple tasks, such as the patient's ability to remove clothes, can provide information about specific musculoskeletal functions requiring further examination. For example, limitations in shoulder-joint range of motion may be indicated by difficulty in removing a shirt or sweater; difficulty in bending over to remove shoes and stockings suggests the need for careful evaluation of the lower back and hip joint; and problems with the joints of the hands may be evidenced by difficulty in using buttons. In addition to noting any such problems, the patient's adaptation should be noted. Can the patient perform the needed tasks by using assistive devices or flexion of associated joints to overcome restricted range of the primary joints, such as flexing the neck forward to reduce the shoulder joint range needed to remove clothes?

Muscle Mass

Changes in joints or injuries to parts of the skeletal system are often associated with changes in the muscles that move the affected part. For example, knee injuries such as a torn meniscus are often associated with a rapid decrease in the size of the quadriceps femoris muscles. Equivalence of muscle mass can be estimated by measuring the circumference of the affected extremity and comparing it to the unaffected extremity (Fig. 86–1). Muscles do not have good landmarks; therefore, all measurements are made by a measured distance from a bony landmark. In the example of

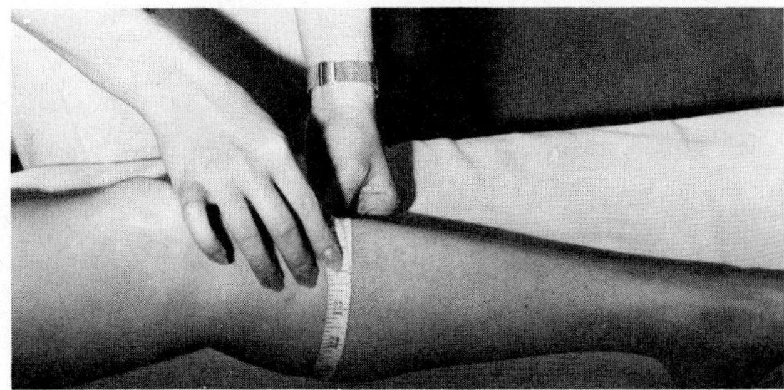

FIGURE 86–1 Muscle mass can be determined by measuring the circumference of the affected extremity with a tape measure and comparing it to the unaffected extremity.

changes in the quadriceps muscles, the level for measuring the circumference is made by measuring up the same distance from the joint margin of the femoral condyles on each leg to determine if the muscles are equal in size.

Power

Power is assessed on a graduated scale consisting of six functional levels:[1]

0 = No contraction
1 = Flicker or trace of contraction
2 = Active movement with gravity eliminated
3 = Active movement against gravity
4 = Active movement against gravity and resistance
5 = Normal power

Resistance can be applied by the examiner holding the limb and exerting several pounds of pressure that the patient is then asked to overcome. Power should be evaluated repeatedly in cases of acute trauma. Progressive changes in the ability to contract muscle groups are indicative of alterations occurring in the neuromuscular function.

Range of Motion

When evaluating range of motion, both active and passive range should be assessed. Great intraindividual difference in range of motion occurs; thus the affected joint should be compared with the unaffected side. Passive range of motion will be greater only in those cases in which innervation to the muscles or the attachment of the muscle involved in moving the joint has been disrupted. Evaluation of range of motion should be done for most patients; even those patients without obvious deformity or complaints should be evaluated to ensure that impairment in joint range does not impact on the ability to perform other functions. For example, a woman having a mastectomy may experience reduction in shoulder range of motion that can frustrate rehabilitative efforts.

The particular types of movement that need to be evaluated depend on the type of joint involved, as shown in Table 86–1. Hinge joints, such as the knee, require only the evaluation of the ability to flex and extend. Ball and socket joints (hip joint) and complex joints (wrist) that can move in multiple directions need each direction of movement evaluated. The movements include internal and external rotation, adduction (movement toward midline), abduction (movement away from midline), eversion, and inversion. The basic elements of range of motion assessment is the same for the different joint type whether it is a large joint like the knee or a small joint in a finger.

All muscle groups involved in supporting and moving a joint are used when the joint is put through full range of motion. Destruction of joint surfaces, as with rheumatoid arthritis, can limit the range and smoothness of joint motion. Changes in surrounding tissues, such as with decreased elasticity of fibrous connective tissue or shortening of attached muscle groups, will also limit joint range of motion. Evaluation of range of motion requires that in extension and flexion the joint be moved beyond neutral anatomical position. Full active extension must be observed when evaluating movement of the fingers and toes. Inherent tissue elasticity, coupled with simple relaxation after flexion, can result in the fingers and toes returning to the position of anatomical rest without active contraction of the muscles responsible for joint extension.

Where there is alteration in range of motion, observation and palpation of the joints are done. The shape, size, and alignment of the joint should be noted. The joint should be palpated for warmth, tenderness, and crepitus (a grinding or grating sensation felt as two rough surfaces rub against each other). Comparison is made between the two sides of the body.

Neurovascular Assessment

Whenever the integrity of the skeleton is disrupted, there is potential for harm to the surrounding soft tissue, especially to the neurovascular system. The mechanism of injury or bone fragments at a fracture site may cause immediate damage to the nerves and blood vessels. Subsequent swelling or pressure from casts or excessive tension from traction can also result in damage to the neurovascular system. Adequacy of function and changes in the neurovascular system should be evaluated at regular intervals and the findings recorded. The length of the intervals between checks depends on the severity of the initial injury and on the observed status of the neurovascular system. As a general guideline, neurovascular assessment is done hourly for the first 24 hours after the initial injury, surgery, application of traction, or the application of a cast. If after that time no evidence of neurovascular compromise is apparent, assessment is then done every 2 to 4 hours. Evaluation consists of checking circulation, motion, and sensation.

Circulation. Evaluation of circulatory status of an extremity involves checking for pulses, capillary refill, color, and temperature. The radial pulse is most commonly palpated. In the leg the dorsalis pedis, which can be palpated between the first and second metatarsals on the dorsum of the foot, is the most commonly evaluated pulse (Fig. 86–2). The posteriortibial pulse, which can be felt posterior to the medial malleolus, should also be checked. Because these pulses are difficult to locate, especially if there is swelling, the sites at which they could initially be palpated should be marked on the skin with an ink marker.

TABLE 86–1
Primary Types of Joint Motions

Joint	Motion	Comments
Spine		
Cervical, lumbar and thoracic	Extension Flexion Lateral flexion Rotation	Lumbar and thoracic tested together
Upper extremities		
Shoulder	Flexion Extension Hyperextension Abduction Adduction Rotation	Rotation tested with elbow flexed
Elbow	Extension Flexion Rotation	Rotation is called *supination* (to turn palms up) and *pronation* (to turn palms down).
Wrist	Flexion Extension Ulnar deviation Radial deviation	
Hand	Flexion Extension Abduction Adduction Opposition	Abduction is done with fingers and thumb. Opposition is done with thumb and fingers.
Lower extremities		
Hip	Flexion Extension Hyperextension Abduction Adduction Internal and external rotation	Flexion and rotation are done with knee flexed.
Knee	Flexion Extension	
Ankle and foot	Flexion Extension Eversion Inversion	Ankle and toe flexion is called *dorsiflexion;* extension is called *plantar flexion.*

Capillary refill is assessed by applying pressure to the nailbed until it turns white, then releasing the pressure (Fig. 86–3). There should be a rapid return of color to the site. The rate of capillary return is compared with the unaffected side. Slow or sluggish capillary return indicates reduced arterial flow. However, if there is both reduced arterial flow and obstructed venous outflow, capillary refill may appear to be normal.

When the circulation is intact the normal skin color of fingers and toes has an underlying reddish tone. Interference with arterial circulation can be indicated by a pale or ashen color in lightly pigmented skin and by a dull ashen color in heavily pigmented skin. A bluish tone or cyanotic color, which may indicate decreased venous return, can be best observed in the nailbeds. Again the affected extremity should be compared with the unaffected side, since great individual differences exist in normal skin color. Normal vascular changes in response to environmental cooling may also affect the observed skin color.

When blood supply is reduced to an extremity, its temperature will be lower than one with intact circulation. Temperature is evaluated by feeling the skin with the dorsal surface of the examiner's fingers. The skin on the back of the hand is more sensitive to temperature than the skin on the palmar surface. The temperature of the affected extremity is compared to the unaffected extremity. As with skin color,

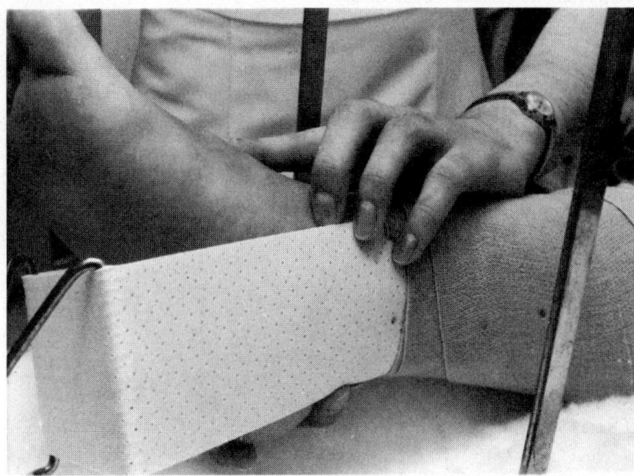

FIGURE 86–2 Palpating the pedal pulse in an affected extremity is one way of evaluation circulation.

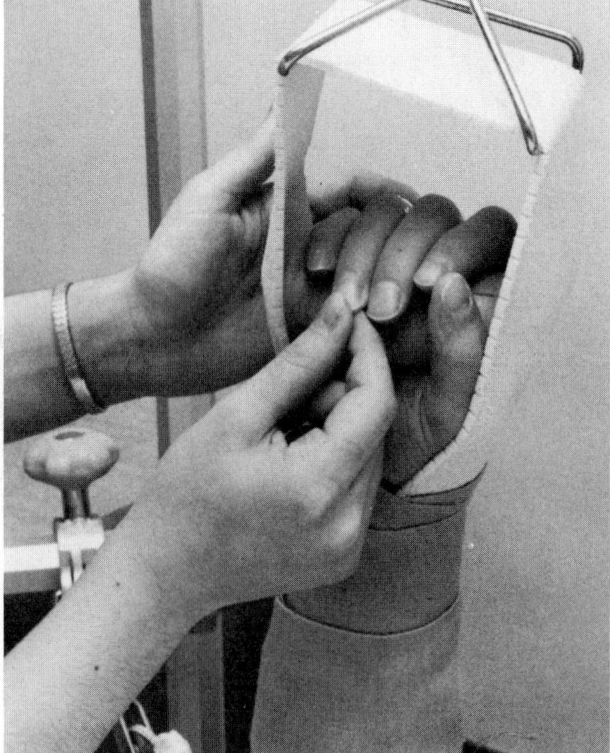

FIGURE 86–3 Capillary refill time is evaluated by applying pressure to the nailbed and determining how long it takes for color to return to the nailbed after the pressure is released.

skin temperature may be influenced by environmental cooling especially if ice bags or a wet cast are being applied to the extremity. Assessment of circulatory status does not rest on any one of these signs but is evaluated on the basis of information obtained from each of these four parameters.

Motion. Evaluation of motion requires that muscle groups below the level of injury be actively contracted. Changes in the ability to actively contract muscles reflect a compromised ability of the nervous system to initiate movement or of muscle to carry out the movement. As was indicated in the section on range of motion, it is important to note whether the movement is the result of active muscle contraction or simply the result of the inherent tissue elasticity. The power of the movement should also be evaluated using the scale listed in the section on power. The power of the muscle groups on the affected side are compared with the same muscle groups on the unaffected side. When assessing the client's ability to contract the involved muscle groups, it is important to evaluate whether reduced movement or power is due to impaired function or to active restriction of movement secondary to pain or fear of causing pain.

Sensation. Changes in sensation can vary from minor reduction to complete loss of sensation. The pattern of sensation loss provides information on the site at which impairment is occurring. Changes in nerve function can result from the initial injury or may occur progressively secondary to anoxia, decreased circulation, or as the result of pressure. Paresthesias, such as numbness, tingling, and burning, result from a nerve's decreased ability to accurately transmit impulses. The focal area of assessment below the level of injury depends on the nerve distribution that is most likely to have been damaged by the specific injury or treatment (Table 86–2). When assessing sensory changes, care must be taken to distinguish between adjacent nerve distributions. For example, in the lower leg the peroneal nerve splits into two branches. The superficial peroneal nerve can be evaluated over the greater portion of the dorsal surface of the foot. The deep peroneal nerve is evaluated in the restricted area of the dorsal surface of the first web space (Fig. 86–4). Baseline information should be obtained so that later observations can be compared and progressive dysfunction can be distinguished from that occurring at the initial injury. Sensory function is tested by pricking the surface of the skin with a sharp object, like a pin. Care should be taken to avoid breaking the skin.

Summary

The primary modes of obtaining information about alterations in the musculoskeletal system are from a careful history and systematic examination using observation and palpation. Careful assessment of the history should be made and ongoing patient information obtained.

Special Diagnostic Procedures

The primary methods of identifying and characterizing an alteration in the musculoskeletal system are by the history and physical examination. The use of special diagnostic procedures can further facilitate the precise characterization of the alteration. These diagnostic procedures include the use of radiographs, sampling of fluids in a joint, electromyographic measurement, and direct visualization of the joint by arthroscope.

TABLE 86–2
Signs and Symptoms of Neurovascular Impairment for Lower Leg and Forearm

Compartment	*Structure*	*Signs and Symptoms*
Lower leg		
Anterior	Tibialis anterior Extensor hallucis longus Extensor digitorum longus Deep peroneal nerve	Inability to dorsiflex toes and foot Pain on passive plantar flexion of toes and foot Hypoesthesia of dorsal forst web space
Deep posterior	Tibialis posterior Flexor hallucis longus Flexor digitorum longus Posterior tibial nerve	Weak plantar flexion of toes and foot inversion Pain on passive toe extension and foot eversion Hypoesthesia of plantar surface of the foot
Forearm		
Volar	Flexor muscles of wrist and fingers Median nerve Ulnar nerve	Weak wrist and finger flexion Pain on passive wrist and finger extension Hypoesthesia of volar aspect of the fingers

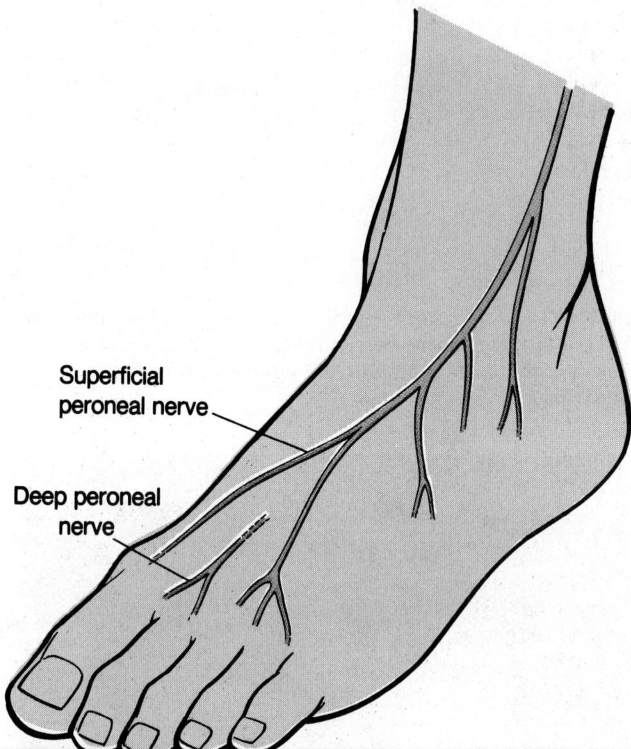

FIGURE 86–4 Cutaneous distribution of common peroneal nerve on the dorsum of the foot. Only at the small area of the first web space can the deep peroneal nerve be evaluated.

Among the earliest of the specialized diagnostic procedures developed was the radiograph. Bones are radiopaque (not readily allowing the passage of radiation), having high density as a result of high mineral content. Changes in bone density and shape can indicate the presence of a fracture, thinning of the bone as in osteoporosis, or the presence of abnormal growth as with a bone spur.

Often an injured bone will appear normal when only a single view is taken, but when the bone is observed from another angle the deformity can be visualized. Preparation prior to the patient going for radiographs should include the number and type of films that are planned, and the reason for taking views from different angles. If the patient is aware that radiographs will be taken from several angles and of the importance of the different positions, the level of anxiety and pain experienced may be reduced or at least better tolerated.

Tomography or *laminography* are specialized methods of taking multiple radiographic films. These procedures involve taking many films showing different layers or slices of the tissue of interest. Computed tomography, which uses computer control of the radiation, provides imaging that differentiates the radiographic densities of different tissue types, allowing the visualization of lesions not possible with conventional tomography. Patients may be concerned with both the amount of equipment involved and the amount of exposure to radiation. The patient should be reassured that more equipment does not mean more discomfort and that the amount of radiation is kept to a minimum by the precise computer control.

The previous radiographic procedures have relied on the natural differences in tissue density to differentiate structures within the film. Such procedures work well with identifying changes in the bony structures but do not allow adequate visualization of changes in cartilage and other soft tissue structures. To help in identifying problems with nonbone structures, radiopaque dyes may be injected into the area to be examined and then radiographic films taken. The pattern of dye distribution is then evaluated for abnormal restriction or extension. This type of procedure is referred to as an *arthrogram* and is frequently done to examine for tears in the cartilage of joints such as the knee. Similar procedures involving the use of radiopaque dyes to examine structures associated with the spine have been given specific labels. A *myelogram,* which involves injecting a radiopaque dye into the subarachnoid space, allows the detection of a protruding nucleus pulposus or soft tissue tumor in the vertebral canal. A *diskogram* is used to detect an abnormal disk by the extension of an injected radiopaque dye beyond the normal range for an intact disk.

Another method of identifying changes that cannot be detected by standard radiographic techniques is through the use of radionuclides. A radionuclide that has a high affinity for bone is injected. Areas of high blood flow and high metabolic activity pick up greater concentrations of the radionuclide and thus can be visualized. This procedure is commonly referred to as a *bone scan.* Among the conditions that can be detected and localized by a bone scan are primary and metastatic bone tumors, osteomyelitis, and stress fractures. Areas of decreased metabolic activity may also be identified by their low level of radionuclide uptake, as in avascular necrosis.

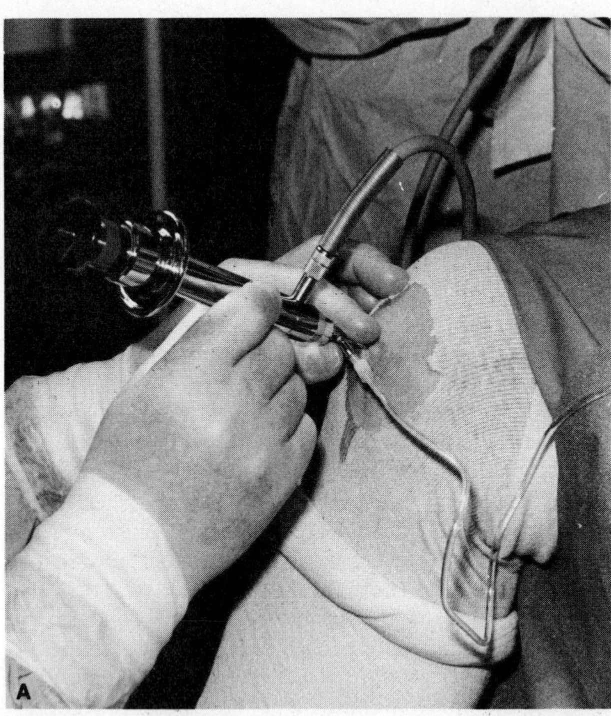

FIGURE 86–5 Arthroscopic examination of the knee. The fiberoptic scope is inserted into the knee (*A*) to allow visualization of the joint. *B* shows the normal field of the arthroscope; *C* shows a torn meniscus.

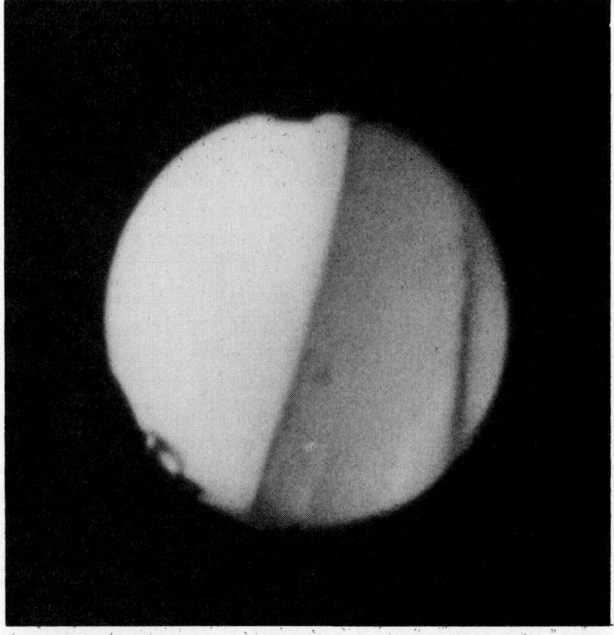

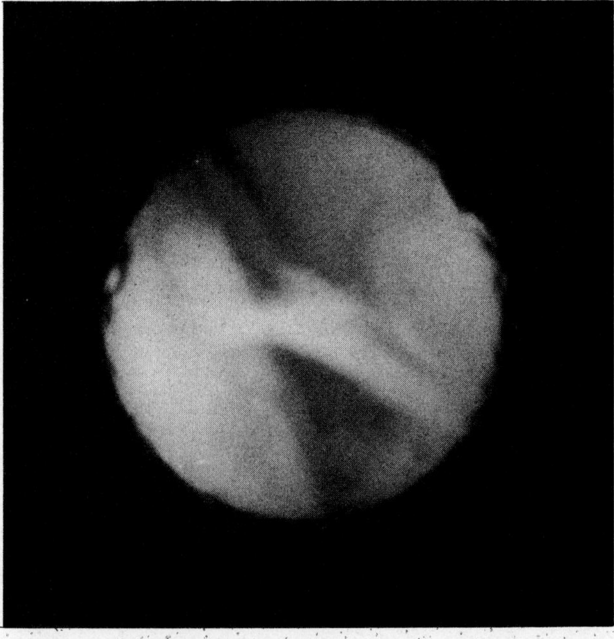

Joint Aspiration

If there is effusion in the joint it may be necessary to determine if the fluid is synovial in origin or the result of infection or bleeding. An *arthrocentesis* in which a needle is inserted into the joint and fluid removed for future examination may be done. This procedure is done under local sterile conditions to avoid introducing any infectious organism into the joint space. The arthrocentesis can at the same time be used as treatment in draining off the fluid to relieve pressure within the joint space.

Electromyograph

Measurement of electrical activity in a muscle or muscle group is made by means of surface electrodes. The procedure is analogous to that used in obtaining an electrocardiograph. By the type of alteration in electrical activity it is possible to distinguish between disorders of nerve and nerve conduction and between muscle diseases.

Arthroscopic Examination

Arthroscopic examination allows for direct or indirect (with a video camera) visualization of structures in a joint. A fiberoptic scope is inserted into a joint through a small skin incision. The joint is perfused with normal saline to provide space between tissue for easier visualization. The structures of the joint, including soft tissue and joint lining, can then be evaluated for change (Fig. 86–5). Originally the arthroscope was used only as a diagnostic procedure, and almost exclusively in the knee. Today both diagnosis and treatment procedures are performed by means of the arthroscope and have involved nearly every joint.

Treatment procedures have included the removal of torn cartilage and the repair of torn ligaments. Additional incisions are made to introduce instruments needed to remove or repair damaged structures. Because there is much less disruption of the adjacent muscles and ligaments, rehabilitation time is markedly reduced. Injuries in the past that could have resulted in an athlete missing an entire season result in only a few missed games or races. Arthroscopic examination and treatment, because it can be done under local anesthesia and with such minimal restriction of post-treatment activity, can allow for the examination and treatment of joint conditions of elderly patients with much less risk than was previously possible.

Arthroscopic examination is usually done using local anesthesia supplemented by sedatives. However, general anesthesia may be used especially if there is the possibility of needing an open procedure following the initial diagnostic examination. Following the arthroscopic examination there will typically be one to several small incisions covered with bandages. The joint area may be wrapped in an elastic wrap to minimize swelling and provide some stability of the joint. The degree of activity allowed will depend more on the type of the initial injury than on the arthroscopic procedure that was done.

Reference

1. Medical Research Council: Aids to the Examination of the Peripheral Nervous System (Memorandum No. 45). London, Her Majesty's Stationery Office, 1976

Bibliography

Adams JC: Outline of Orthopedics, 9th ed. Edinburgh, Churchill Livingstone, 1981

Bates B: A Guide to Physical Examination. Philadelphia, JB Lippincott, 1983

Birnbaum JS: The Musculoskeletal Manual. New York, Academic Press, 1982

Drucker MM: Arthroscopic surgery of the knee joint. AORN J 36:585–593, 1982

Farrell J: Orthopedic pain: What does it Mean? Am J Nurs 84:466–469, 1984

Garrick JG: The sports medicine patient. NCNA 16:759–766, 1981

Lenman JAR, Ritchie AE: Clinical Electromyography, 3rd ed. London, Pitman, 1983

McRae R: Clinical Orthopaedic Examination, 2nd ed. Edinburgh, Churchill Livingstone, 1983

Rosse C, Clawson DK: Introduction to the Musculoskeletal System. New York, Harper & Row, 1970

Salter RB: Textbook of Disorders and Injuries of the Musculoskeletal System, 2nd ed. Baltimore, Williams & Wilkins, 1983

Wassel A: Nursing assessment of injuries to the lower extremity. NCNA 16:739–748, 1981

Wassel AC: Sport medicine: Acute and overuse injuries. Orthopedic Nursing 3:29–33, 1984

Chapter 87

Nursing Strategies for Common Musculoskeletal Problems

Nursing Diagnosis
Interventions
Evaluation

Karen A. Waxdahl

The scope of orthopedic nursing practice has been defined as encompassing "those nursing activities which assist the individual to modify his lifestyle and environment so that he can attain optimum neuro-musculo-skeletal function compatible with his life goals."[41]

This chapter considers the principles used to implement the nursing process for the patient experiencing alterations in musculoskeletal structure or function. The nursing strategies apply to patients with traumatic, infectious, inflammatory, or neoplastic disorders. The assessment phase, as described in the previous chapter, consists of both a thorough general assessment as well as a specialty assessment to arrive at nursing diagnoses pertinent to the orthopedic patient. The nurse applies the knowledge of the healing process and of specific treatment modalities to develop the nursing care plan.

Potential for Injury Related to Neurological and Vascular Damage

Nursing Diagnoses

Patients with problems affecting the musculoskeletal system are at risk for neurological and vascular damage for a number of reasons. Nerves and blood vessels may be affected by an injury, a surgical procedure, the swelling associated with trauma, or a therapeutic modality employed to immobilize the extremity. Casts, traction, or even the position of the extremity have the potential for placing enough pressure on neurovascular structures to produce ischemia and affect their function. Neurovascular assessment of the extremities is one of the most important observations made by nurses caring for orthopedic patients because the potential for impairment is extremely common.

Analysis of Assessment Data. Neurovascular assessment consists of evaluating the distal portion of the extremity; most frequently the toes and fingers are observed. The three components of a neurovascular examination are circulation, sensation, and motion. Circulation and sensation may be tested by applying pressure to the finger or toes. When the fingernail (or toenail) is compressed and then immedi-

Note: The views expressed in this chapter are those of the author and do not reflect official policy of the United States Army or the Department of Defense.

ately released, the color should return to a normal pink hue. This indicates normal capillary refill time. The patient should also be able to move or extend the fingers on request (Fig. 87–1).

The frequency of assessment depends on the patient's specific diagnosis and status; the location of the problem within the musculoskeletal system; the physician's orders; and the length of time since injury, surgery, or cast or traction application. It is the responsibility of the professional nurse to ensure the existence of orders specifying assessment frequency and to increase the frequency if a problem is suspected.

Interventions

Elevation of the extremity and application of ice to the trauma site are methods effective for minimizing swelling and thus maintaining the circulation to muscles and nerves. Continuous assessment of their effects is essential.

Elevation. Elevating an extremity uses principles of gravity flow as well as decreasing hydrostatic pressure in blood vessels to reduce edema.[5] With immobilization of an injured extremity, the skeletal muscle pump is compromised. The muscles are not contracting normally and are not milking the venous blood toward the heart as effectively as in the erect and moving person. Actively moving the fingers or toes will also help to reduce edema by using the muscle pump. The presence of arterial disease may make elevation contraindicated in some instances.

For elevation to be effective in reducing swelling, the extremity must be elevated above the level of the heart. This means that if the leg is to be elevated, the patient cannot raise the head of his bed to an upright position because his leg would no longer be above the level of his heart. Lower extremities may be elevated by raising the foot of the bed and by using pillows under the leg. Unless the person is in a flexed-knee cast, the bed should be elevated so that the leg is extended. This means elevating the knee gatch along with the foot of the bed. Failure to raise the knee gatch will result in hyperextension of the knee and much discomfort for the patient. Upper extremities can be elevated on pillows or they can be suspended from an intravenous pole by using stockinette or commercially available slings. Whatever method of elevation is used, the entire extremity must be supported, and the distal joints must always be higher than those proximal. For example, the wrist is higher than the elbow, and the elbow is above the shoulder.

Ice. Ice has long been used for minimizing swelling in acute trauma. Swelling reaches its peak in approximately 24 to 48 hours and should subside thereafter. Ice is most frequently used for the initial 48 to 72 hours after injury or surgical intervention. Most physicians order continuous ice application, although it is occasionally ordered as intermittent.

The reduction of swelling with ice results from the vasoconstriction caused by the cooling. The vasoconstriction produces a decreased blood flow, a decrease in the amount of hemorrhage, and a reduced inflammatory response. The histamine release is blocked and therefore the usual vasodilatation and subsequent accumulation of exudates do not occur to as great an extent.

In a study done to evaluate types of cooling devices, it was found that ice chips in a plastic bag produced the greatest lowering of tissue temperatures.[32] Other devices evaluated were the frozen gel packs and the packs that use an endothermic chemical reaction to produce the cold temperatures.

Ice-filled hot water bottles are an effective way to apply ice. The water bottles are safer to use than ordinary plastic bags since there is less chance of leaking and tearing. Ice bags should be wrapped to reduce moisture and be placed along both sides of the extremity as opposed to on top of a cast. The weight of an ice bag can cause patient discomfort as well as cause depressions in the cast if the cast is wet.

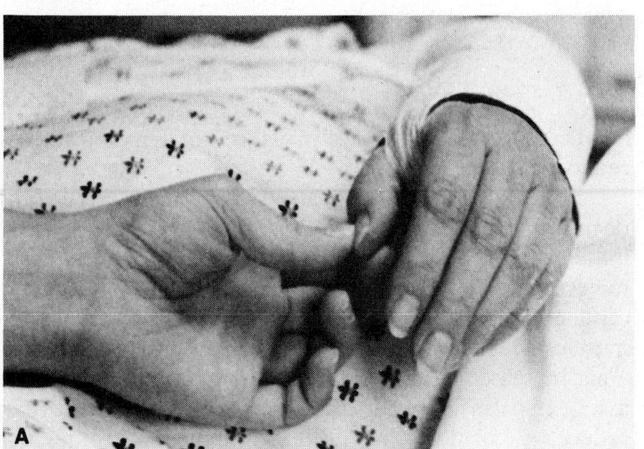

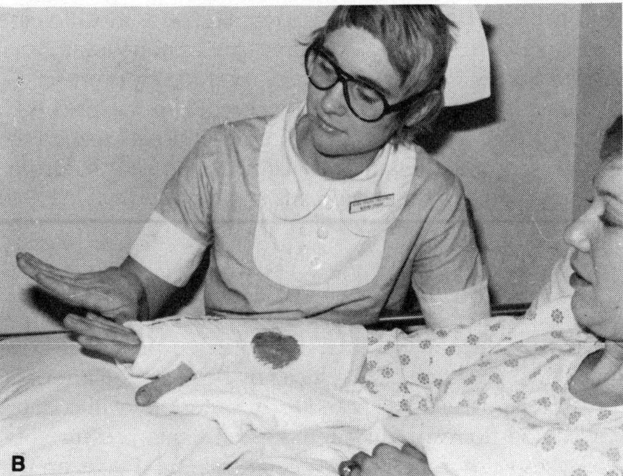

FIGURE 87–1 Neurovascular assessment is essential in patients with musculoskeletal disorders being treated by constrictive devices such as casts. (*A*) Circulation and sensation are being evaluated. (*B*) Motion is being assessed.

Evaluation of Neurovascular Status

The distal portion of the involved extremity will be

- Pink in color
- Warm to the touch
- With capillary refill time less than 3 seconds
- Without swelling or with only mild swelling
- With strong pulse
- Without numbness and tingling
- With sensation present to light touch
- Demonstrating full active range of motion

Potential for Impaired Function Related to Neurovascular Complications

Compartment Syndrome

A condition in which increased tissue pressure within a closed space compromises the circulation to local neuromuscular structures is known as compartment syndrome. Sheaths of inelastic fascia surround skeletal muscles and blood vessels; the closed space formed by this fascia is called a compartment. The leg has three compartments and the forearm has three (Fig. 87–2). A sustained pressure increase within a compartment is not tolerated because the fascia does not stretch with the swelling. Because the swelling is not dispersed, the outcome of the pressure buildup is compression of the blood vessels, a reduction in capillary blood perfusion, and tissue ischemia. If allowed to persist, an extremity with contractures and severe functional disabilities may result. Therefore, early recognition and treatment are essential.

Etiology. Increased pressure in a muscle compartment is caused by either a reduction in size of the compartment or an increase in the volume of the compartment contents. Casts, tight dressings, or the eschar from burns can restrict the size of the compartment. Problems that increase the contents are edema, bleeding, intravenous infiltration, crush injuries, and muscle hypertrophy from overuse.[25,34] The edema and hemorrhage associated with fractures both contribute to a larger volume inside a closed space. The fractures most often associated with compartment syndrome are those of the proximal tibia and supracondylar fractures of the humerus.[34]

Pathophysiology. Elevated intracompartmental pressure results in a cycle of ischemia and edema. The etiologic factors produce an increase in the tissue pressure. If the interstitial pressure rises sufficiently between the arteriolar pressure and the tissue pressure, the arterioles will collapse and blood flow is reduced. Increased tissue pressure also collapses veins if it exceeds venous pressure. However, if in response to an accumulation of metabolites, the capillary flow increases, the return to the venules will increase venous pressure and open the veins. The increased venous pressure decreases the arteriovenous pressure gradient and further reduces blood flow.

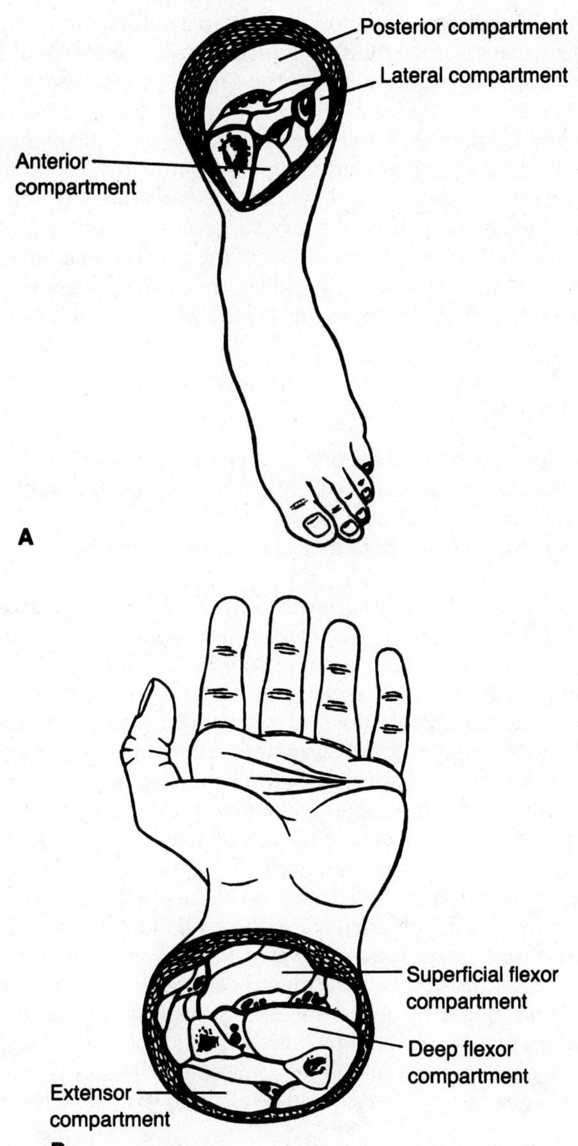

FIGURE 87–2 (*A*) Cross section of leg showing compartments outlined by heavy lines. (*B*) Cross section of forearm showing compartments outlined by heavy lines.

Both of these mechanisms, the arteriolar closing and the decrease in the arteriovenous pressure gradient, result in ischemia. Ischemic muscle releases histamine, and histamine causes capillary dilatation. The resultant increase in capillary permeability allows transudation of plasma into the muscle, which produces more swelling and further ischemia. Increased intracompartmental pressure may also cause a reflex spasm of larger arteries in the muscle to further reduce circulation.[11,12,25] Compartment syndrome that progresses for longer than 12 hours is likely to produce irreversible damage to muscles and nerves.[25] A classic example is Volkmann's contracture of the hand (Fig. 87–3).

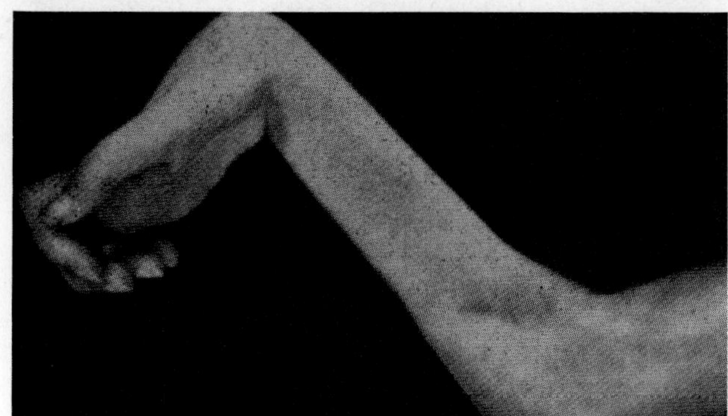

FIGURE 87–3 Volkmann's contractures. (Boyes JH: Bunnell's Surgery of the Hand, 5th ed. Philadelphia, JB Lippincott, 1970)

Clinical Manifestations. The onset of this syndrome varies from 2 hours to 6 days following trauma.[26] Early recognition of the signs and symptoms is a shared responsibility between physicians and nurses. Assessment of a patient at high risk for compartment syndrome may be necessary as frequently as every 30 minutes. Accurate reporting and documentation of observations and actions taken is critical.

Pain is the most important symptom of compartment syndrome. The pain is out of proportion to that expected from the primary problem, and it is progressive and unremitting. It is frequently described as deep and throbbing. Analgesics in the usual doses do not relieve the pain as expected. Actually, physicians may not order analgesics for patients at high risk for this syndrome so as not to mask the symptoms. Pain from fractures should decrease gradually after immobilization of the fracture and when it does not, this provides an important clue to a developing vascular problem.

A second symptom is pain resulting from the passive stretch of the ischemic muscle when passive flexion or extension of the fingers or toes is attempted. Other symptoms that may occur are a decrease in active motion of the digits (paralysis) and paresthesia and hypoesthesia in the nerve distribution. The pulse cannot be relied on as a clue to the presence or absence of compartmental syndrome. Because the tissue pressure is rarely high enough to occlude major arteries, the pulse and capillary refill remain intact. There are also various methods available allowing physicians to measure intracompartmental pressure as a more objective means of diagnosing the syndrome.

Management. Immediately on noting the symptoms of compartment syndrome, the nurse must notify the physician and place the extremity at the level of the heart. Elevation of the extremity in the presence of increased tissue pressure in a closed space diminishes local blood pressure and is, therefore, contraindicated.[27] Any constricting casts or dressings are removed immediately.

If the symptoms do not resolve within 30 to 60 minutes after the removal of dressings, a surgical decompression by fasciotomy is necessary. The surgeon makes an incision through the fascia along the length of the compartment. This procedure permits the muscle to swell more freely without circulatory compression. Once the swelling has subsided (probably 3 to 5 days), the patient may be returned to the operating room for a delayed primary closure of the wound, or a skin graft may be done to cover the wound.

Peroneal Nerve Palsy

Definition and Pathophysiology. This condition is one in which there is a partial or complete paralysis of the peroneal nerve. The patient with an ischemic peroneal nerve develops weakness in the dorsiflexors of the foot and a foot drop deformity. This nerve is very vulnerable to pressure since it lies between the skin and the head and neck of the fibula with very little subcutaneous tissue to protect it. The nerve can become ischemic from casts, dressings, thromboembolic hose that are too tightly applied over the fibular head, or from lying with the leg externally rotated so that there is pressure from the bed over the fibular head. The elderly patient is especially susceptible to peroneal compression because of reduced subcutaneous tissue between the nerve and the bone. Furthermore, reduced muscle tone leads the lower extremities into external rotation when the patient is lying supine.

Clinical Manifestations and Management. Initially, the patient may complain of numbness and paresthesias over the peroneal nerve distribution. Simply relieving the pressure at this point will prevent loss of function. Interventions such as repositioning the leg, rewrapping constricting dressings, or trimming a cast or bending the edge of a cast outward will be effective. If the pressure continues and the patient loses his ability to actively dorsiflex the foot, more vigorous nursing intervention will be required. Strategies useful in recovering and maintaining peroneal function are passive dorsiflexion exercises to the foot and support of the foot with a padded footboard. The patient may need to use a dorsiflexion orthosis for walking.

Potential for Neurological and Vascular Damage or Injury Related to Restrictive Immobilizing Devices

The previous discussion alluded frequently to the cast as a contributing factor in the potential for neurological and vascular damage or injury. The challenge to the nurse caring for the patient in a cast is not only in preventing neurovascular compromise, but also in safeguarding the efficiency of the cast, promoting the patient's comfort in the cast, and preventing other complications. Most patients in casts spend very little time in the hospital, and thus teaching the patient to care for himself and his cast at home is an extremely important aspect of nursing care.

Casts

The rigid immobilizing device known as a cast is made up of layers of plaster of paris bandages or of layers of synthetic materials. Plaster of paris is still the most frequently used material. However, synthetic materials are becoming increasingly popular and must be understood.

Casts are primarily used for temporary immobilization such as

- Immobilization of bone fragments during fracture healing
- Postoperative immobilization during the healing process
- Prevention or correction of deformities (*e.g.*, with scoliosis or arthritis)
- Promoting rest during disease processes
- Permitting early weight bearing

Some of the more common types of casts and examples of conditions for which they may be used follows. The list is by no means complete. A wide variety of casts are in use today and there are just as many variations on a given cast to accomplish a given treatment goal.

Types of Casts

- A *long arm cast* extends from the axillary fold to the proximal palmar crease and is used for fractures of the forearm, elbow, and distal humerus and for postoperative immobilization of the same (Fig. 87–4, *A*).
- A *short arm cast* extends from below the elbow to the proximal crease of the hand and is used to treat hand and wrist fractures and for postoperative immobilization of the hand and wrist (Fig. 87–4, *B*).
- A *hanging arm cast* is a modified long arm cast with a sling around the neck and is applied so that the weight of the cast exerts traction on the humerus. The patient must remain in the upright, sitting position so that the cast "hangs." This cast is used for distal humeral fractures (Fig. 87–4, *C*).
- A *long leg cast* is one that extends from the upper thigh to the toes and is indicated for fractures of the tibia and fibula, unstable ankle fractures, and injuries to the distal femur and knee (Fig. 87–4, *D*).
- A *short leg cast* extends from below the knees to the toes and is used in the treatment of ankle fractures, ligament injuries in the ankle, and fractures of the tarsals (Fig. 87–4, *E*).
- A *long leg cylinder cast* extends from the proximal thigh to just above the medial and lateral malleoli. It is used for stable injuries and postoperative immobilization of the knee joint, distal femur, and proximal tibia (Fig. 87–4, *F*).
- A *hip spica cast* incorporates the trunk and one or both lower extremities to immobilize the hip joint(s). The cast is used to treat fractures of the pelvis, hip, and femur and is also used for postoperative immobilization of these structures (Fig. 87–4, *G*).
- A *cast-brace* consists of a thigh cuff and a patellar tendon weight-bearing cast connected with knee hinges. It is used to treat femoral shaft fractures and fractures of the tibial plateau. The advantages of this cast are maintaining knee joint motion and permitting early ambulation, which stimulates osteogenesis. The thigh cuff is molded to allow the soft tissue hydrostatic pressure to dynamically immobilize fracture fragments; in other words, the soft tissues exert a compression force to maintain alignment of the bone.

Cast Materials

The gypsum powder in a *plaster of paris* cast is bound to gauze bandages and is supplied in rolls or strips of various widths. When the roll or strip is placed in tepid water, an

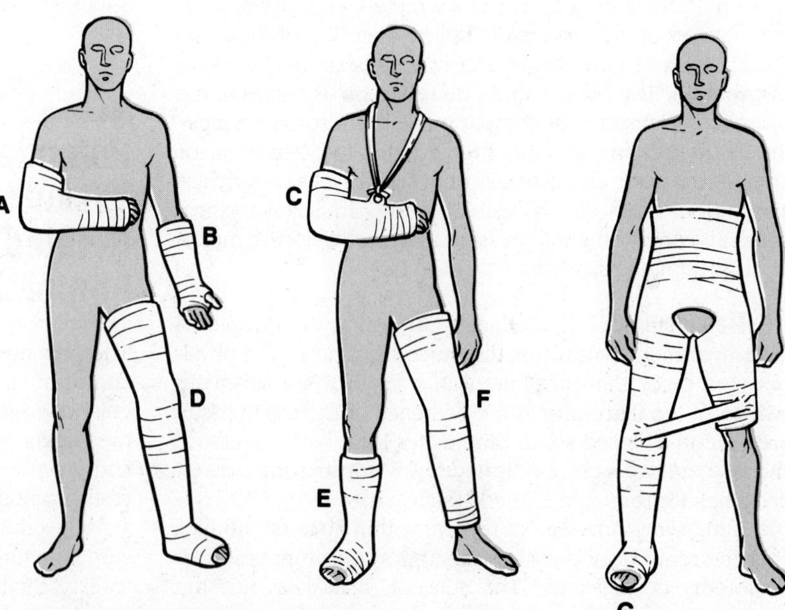

FIGURE 87–4 (*A*) Long arm cast. (*B*) Short arm cast. (*C*) Hanging arm cast. (*D*) Long leg cast. (*E*) Short leg cast. (*F*) Long leg cylinder cast. (*G*) A one and one-half hip spica cast.

exothermic chemical reaction occurs during which the gypsum and water form crystals that lock with each other through the gauze. The plaster then "sets," forming a rigid dressing. Setting time varies from 2 to 8 minutes depending on the type of plaster and the water temperature.

Setting time should not be confused with drying time. Complete drying of the cast may take from 24 to 48 hours depending on the thickness of the cast. Casts dry as the water evaporates. Once the water evaporates, little air-filled pockets remain, leaving the cast porous. A cast is much lighter in weight once the water has evaporated.

The advantages of plaster of paris materials include their being relatively inexpensive, their ease in molding, and their requiring no special equipment to apply. A major disadvantage is that plaster casts cannot be immersed in water. When wet, casts become soft and break. Soiled areas can only be cleansed with a slightly damp cloth. Another disadvantage of plaster casts is that it takes 24 to 48 hours to dry, thus delaying weight-bearing ambulation.

Synthetic Materials. Three types of synthetic cast materials are available: fiberglass, thermoplastic, and polyester/cotton knit. They consist of a fabric impregnated with a water-activated substance. However, there is one type of fiberglass material that is impregnated with a photosensitive resin and requires a special ultraviolet light to harden it.

There are several advantages to synthetic casts. Weight bearing can occur approximately 30 minutes after application since no drying time is needed. Immediate weight bearing is a convenience for all patients with casts, but it becomes most beneficial in caring for the elderly with the risks inherent to immobility. Synthetic casts are also very lightweight and, again, this feature is especially useful for elderly persons in whom a heavy plaster cast would stress those joints proximal to the cast. These casts can be fully immersed in water without interrupting the integrity of the cast. Therefore the patient may shower or swim if allowed by the physician.[20] Techniques for drying the cast are discussed later in the chapter.

Disadvantages of synthetic casts are the extra skills needed in application and their expense. Depending on the material used, synthetics are three to eight times more expensive than plaster.[20] Thus plaster will probably continue to be the material of choice for initial casting and for those situations where the cast is changed frequently. For a very thorough discussion of synthetic casts, see the article by Lane and Lee.[20]

Cast Application

The cast must be applied to closely conform to the contours of the extremity in order to provide adequate immobilization and decrease the risk of skin irritation. Another principle followed is immobilizing the joints above and below a fracture, the rationale being that both ends of the bone need to be immobilized to prevent motion at the fracture site. Motion at the site interferes with healing and has the potential of increasing soft tissue damage.

The steps in cast application are listed in Table 87–1 and are essentially the same whether plaster or synthetic materials are used. Cast technicians and physicians most frequently apply casts, although nurses who have been trained also apply them.

TABLE 87–1
Steps in Application of Casts

1. Skin is inspected for the condition of skin and wounds.
2. Extremity is placed in desired position.
3. Stockinette may be applied over the extremity.
4. Cast padding is applied around the extremity.
5. Felt or foam is placed to pad bony prominences.
6. Plaster bandage is dipped into water.
7. Plaster is rolled onto the extremity and is molded to the contours during the process.
8. Plaster splints (strips) may be placed in areas where extra strength is needed.
9. Edges are trimmed to the desired margin, and the stockinette or padding are rolled back on the cast and held in place with more plaster.
10. Excess plaster is cleaned off the patient.

Nursing Diagnoses and Interventions

The nursing care is organized here under specific nursing diagnoses. The same diagnoses will not apply to all patients; they must be individualized based on the assessment data collected.

Knowledge Deficit and Potential Anxiety

Assessment focuses on what the patient verbalizes about previous exposure to casts, including knowledge of his present condition and understanding of what the physician has told him, the amount of his pain, and his emotional response to his current situation. The amount of information given to the patient prior to casting will depend on the evaluation of this assessment data and also the time available for preparation. Instructions that may be included are what will be done to make him more comfortable during the procedure, the type of cast and reason for use, and how the cast is applied. The patient should be told about the heat he will feel from the exothermic reaction, that the cast will become lighter as the water evaporates (if plaster is used), and whether or not he will be allowed to walk on the cast. Patients having a body cast applied over their chest should be informed of the feeling of shortness of breath that may occur.

Knowledge of what to expect during and after the procedure helps to alleviate the patient's anxiety. Other measures effective for relief of apprehension include answering his questions honestly, handling the affected extremity very carefully, providing support and reassurance throughout the procedure, and providing privacy.

Potential for Injury

Potential for physical injury is related to heat production by cast materials. Heat is normally felt by the patient during cast application owing to the chemical reaction occurring between the cast material and water. The patient should not feel that he is being burned, and care must be taken not to burn him. Ensuring that the dipping water is not too hot is one safety measure.

The cast should be placed on fabric-covered pillows or a bath blanket rather than on plastic pillows and should not be covered with sheets or anything else. Plastic pillows or coverings interfere with heat dissipation and have the potential to cause burns under the cast. If the cast is handled properly, the heat dissipates in 10 to 15 minutes and the cast then feels cold and clammy. The cast still should not be covered, though, because exposure to air promotes drying.

Potential for Neurovascular Compromise

The patient with a cast is at risk for neurocirculatory problems because of the circumferential and rigid nature of the cast. The cast does not allow for expansion when swelling occurs and, therefore, increases the pressure on blood vessels and nerves. In addition, improper handling of the cast or poorly placed padding and improper positioning of the extremity may cause neurovascular compromise.

Neurovascular assessment has been discussed earlier in this chapter. It should be accomplished every hour for the first 24 hours and then every 4 hours if the status is normal for the patient. It is very important to have a precast assessment documented to use as a baseline.

Elevating the extremity above heart level and applying ice to the traumatized area are strategies to prevent neurovascular impairment. If compromise is observed, the extremity may be elevated higher and repositioned. If there is not a rapid return to the previous state, the physician should be notified.

A constricting cast may need to be split or bivalved. Splitting the cast, which involves using a cast cutter to cut a strip down the anterior aspect of the cast, allows for more swelling without tissue constriction. If necessary, the cast can be spread open further by using a device called a cast spreader (Fig. 87–5).

When a cast is split into two sections, it has been bivalved. It is cut down the medial and lateral aspects to leave an anterior and a posterior piece. The sections can be spread as necessary and the two parts can be wrapped with an elastic bandage to maintain the position of the extremity. Whether a cast is split or bivalved, the padding underneath must be cut with a scissors. Cutting the plaster will do no good if the padding is still circumferentially constricting. Either splitting or bivalving is often done immediately after cast application as a prophylactic measure when moderate to severe swelling is anticipated.

Potential for Impairment of Skin Integrity

Persons with casts are at risk for pressure areas over bony prominences and at cast edges. The most valuable assessment technique for pressure areas is listening to the patients. Their complaints should never be ignored. Patients usually report burning pain in the areas of pressure. If this pain should suddenly cease, it does not mean all is well, but indicates that ulceration with destruction of the superficial nerve endings has occurred. A patient may also complain of the cast rubbing or irritating his skin. This is especially common around cast edges. Skin under the edges can be observed using a flashlight.

In addition to patient complaints, another indication of a problem is that the cast feels warm to the touch over a developing pressure sore, or an area of drainage appears. Assessment should occur at least every 8 hours and more frequently if the patient is at high risk for skin breakdown. High risk patients include the elderly with less subcutaneous tissue "padding," those persons with sensory deficits in the casted area, and those with a history of skin breakdown.

Handling and Drying the Cast. Prevention of skin problems related to the cast begins with proper handling of the cast. A wet plaster cast is prone to indentations from fingers and firm surfaces, and the dents in turn place excessive pressure on the skin under the cast. During drying, casts must be handled with the palms of the hand rather than with the fingers since fingertips cause indentations (Fig. 87–6). The cast should be placed on pillows for cushioning; the mattresses used in orthopedic areas are quite firm and could

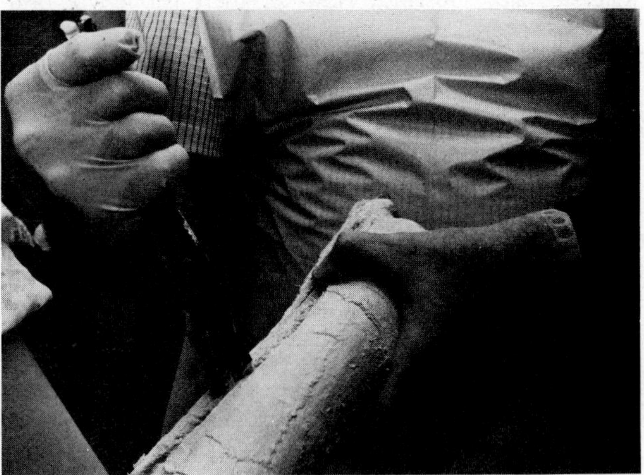

A

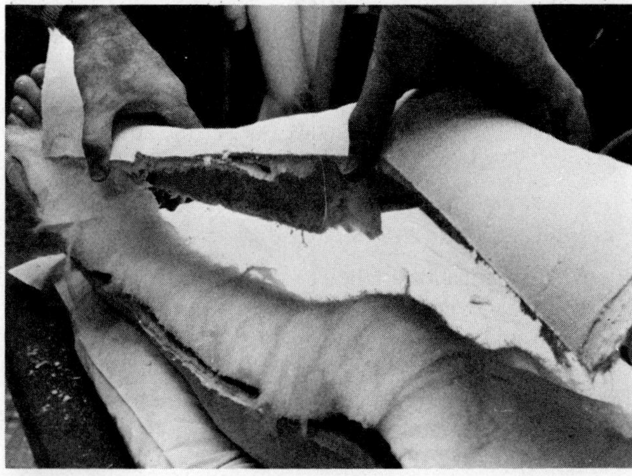

B

FIGURE 87–5 (*A* and *B*) Bivalving and splitting a cast is one way to relieve undue pressure threatening neurovascular function.

flatten the cast. Patients should be cautioned against placing their wet casts on flat surfaces or sharp edges.

Since a wet cast increases the risk of pressure areas, attention is given to facilitating the evaporation of water from the plaster. The cast should be left open to the air and not covered with blankets. Unless contraindicated, the patient should be turned every 2 to 3 hours for exposure of all surfaces to air. Turning a patient in a body cast or hip spica cast may be delayed a few hours to prevent the cast from changing position. The use of fans, hair dryers, or heat lamps is not recommended for drying casts because they may cause burns or dry the outer layers and leave wet the inner layers next to the skin. A cast should dry from the inside out, and it is best accomplished by natural evaporation.

Petaling the Cast Edges. Once the cast dries, attention should be given to the cast edges. If the edges have been finished by rolling the stockinette or cast padding back over the cast, there is less chance of skin irritation. Edges that are not finished can be petaled. Petals are made from adhesive tape or moleskin cut into 2- to 3-inch strips with the corners of one end rounded (Fig. 87–7). The rounded end is placed just inside the cast edge, and the strip is pulled over the edge and taped to the cast.

If a patient reports continual irritation at the edges, the edge can be bent back slightly with a duckbill cast bender. The rough edges of some synthetic casts can be smoothed with a nail file or emery board. Lotion may be applied to areas surrounding the cast, but never underneath. When applied under the edges, lotion may accumulate and macerate the skin.

Protecting the Perineal Area. Patients in hip spica and body casts also require special attention to skin around the perineal area. Plaster and padding wet with urine not only macerates the skin, but the odor causes discomfort and embarrassment for the patient. Once the plaster becomes soiled there is really no effective way to clean it; thus the key is to protect the cast. First, waterproof material can be tucked under the edges in the groin and buttocks area or the material can be "petaled" onto the edges. Second, proper placement on the bedpan helps avoid wet plaster. The patient may turn to his side with help, and the nurse places the bedpan parallel to the cast and the patient rolls onto his back and the bedpan. Once the patient is off the bedpan, the waterproof material can be removed and the perineal area washed and dried thoroughly.

Pain. Never ignore complaints is a cardinal rule in caring for patients in casts. If they report burning pain, pressure, or irritation, and the discomfort is not resolved by the previously mentioned strategies or repositioning, then the problem should be reported immediately. The physician may elect to remove the cast, bivalve it, or window it. It is much easier to prevent pressure sores than to treat them.

Windowing consists of cutting a square or rectangular area from the cast over an area to relieve pressure or inspect a wound (Fig. 87–8). The skin underneath can be inspected or wound care can be done through the window. The piece of plaster removed must be saved because it will be replaced and held in place with an elastic wrap. If the windows were left open, the tissue in the uncovered area would swell and bulge through the window. There would then be pressure and skin breakdown at the window margins.

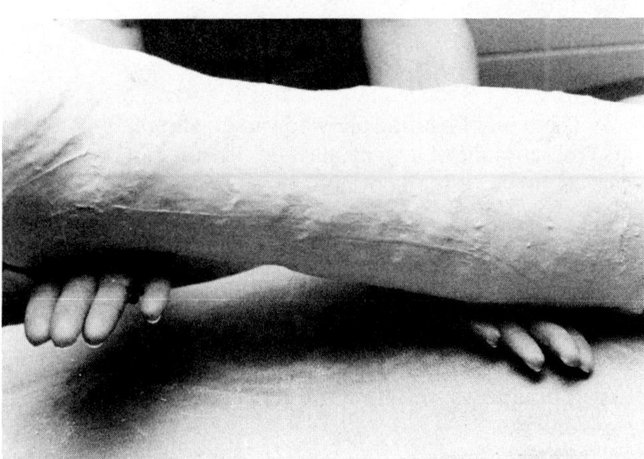

FIGURE 87–6 The correct way to handle a wet cast is to use the palms of the hands, not the fingertips.

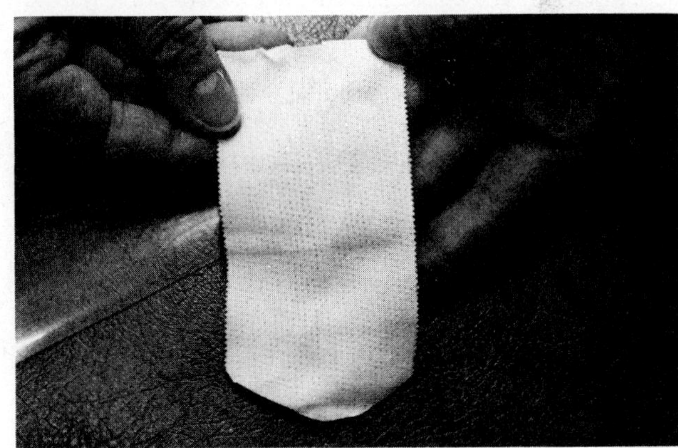

A

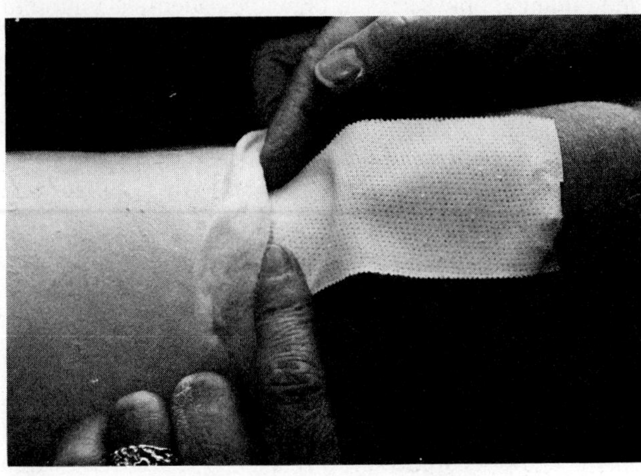

B

FIGURE 87–7 (*A* and *B*) The edges of a cast can be protected by using "petals" of adhesive tape.

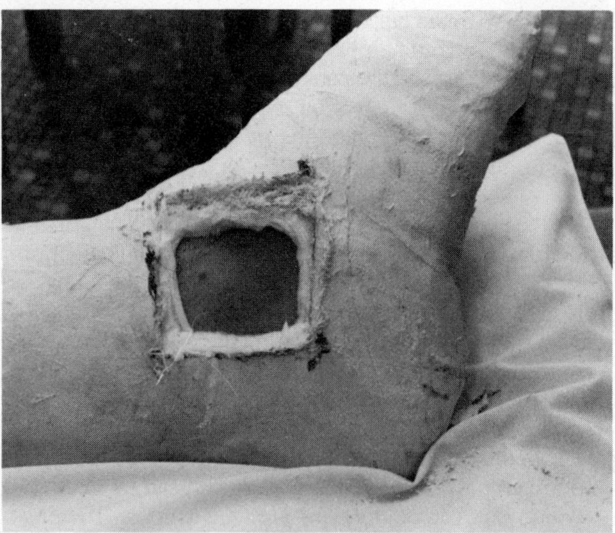

FIGURE 87–8 Windowing a cast relieves pressure and provides access to skin area.

Potential for Infection

The signs and symptoms of an infection include noticeable drainage on the cast; a musty, unpleasant odor; warmth over the area; localized pain; and a fever. Assessing for infection can be done along with skin assessment. To note odor, smell the cast at the edges from about 1 inch away. A sour smell is normal, but a musty odor may signify an infection. Running the hands along the cast can detect a "hot spot."

If drainage appears, it may be green or yellow in color and should be differentiated from expected drainage. Red or reddish brown drainage is normal over a surgical wound. The bloody drainage may not appear for several days and may appear as a larger area as the days go by. This is only the result of the porous plaster gradually absorbing the bloody drainage from the wound. And because the plaster is so porous, the bleeding may look like a larger volume than it really is.[14] Some authorities state that there is no need to outline the drainage on the cast since drainage is expected, and outlining only serves to draw the patient's attention to the bleeding.[14,31]

Impaired Physical Mobility

The amount of mobility may range from complete bed rest to full weight-bearing ambulation. The physician will order the activity level for patients with lower extremity casts, body casts, or hip spica casts. Patients with only an upper extremity cast are usually ambulatory and can use a sling to support the cast. Assistive devices such as crutches, canes, or walkers, which may be necessary for patients with lower extremity involvement, are discussed in a later section.

If weight bearing is allowed in the cast, either a walking heel or a cast boot is needed. A walking heel is made of hard rubber and is secured to the plantar surface of the cast with a plaster wrap. The patient usually will need to have his shoe built up for the uninvolved side because a walking heel adds height. Cast boots are worn over the cast and can be removed at will. They do not significantly elevate the foot, so that no shoe buildup is necessary.

Range-of-motion exercises should be done several times daily for all unaffected joints to prevent joint stiffness and muscle atrophy. When prescribed by the physician, isometric exercises are started for those muscles involved in the injury. The nurse or physical therapist also teaches a program of exercises designed to improve strength in those muscles that will be needed for transfers or crutch walking.

Alteration in Comfort: Itching

Itching under casts is a common and annoying problem since the area is not accessible to scratching or any of the usual methods of relieving an itch. Sources of irritation and itching under a cast include the padding, plaster crumbs, dry skin, and perspiration. A normal desquamation process occurs in the skin and a yellow-grayish sebaceous exudate with flakes of dead skin accumulates under the cast and becomes very itchy. Some persons are sensitive to the cast materials and develop a contact dermatitis.

Helping the patient to relieve the itching can be quite a challenge. Patients should be instructed to *never* put coat hangers, knitting needles, pencils, or other objects into their casts to scratch. In addition to the possibility of these objects becoming caught in the cast and causing pressure areas, they may break the skin and result in an infection. The padding may also be wrinkled with these objects, and pressure and ultimately tissue necrosis may occur. Persons should also be instructed not to pour talcum powder or cornstarch into the cast because these substances cake and irritate the skin and thus produce itching. Antihistamines, such as diphenhydramine hydrochloride, may reduce itching but their sedative effect poses a safety problem, and many patients find the sedation unacceptable.

Blowing cool air from a hair dryer into the cast reduces itching, but it is of no value if the cast is snug. Another strategy that can be used to relieve itching is to apply ice to a contralateral site corresponding to the itching site.[47] Ice is inexpensive and readily available. The rationale for this approach is similar to that for using contralateral pain relief measures.

Self-Care Deficit: Bathing

The type of bathing allowed varies with the type of cast and the amount of activity allowed. Plaster casts cannot get wet, as previously mentioned. However, this does not preclude bathing or showering with proper precautions. Patients with upper extremity casts or short leg casts may take tub baths if they are careful in holding the extremity out of the water. Cast protectors for use in showering are commercially available for both arm and leg casts. They consist of a plastic covering and a method to secure the plastic above the cast. A double plastic bag secured with tape at the top works the same way.

Whichever method is used, it must be very secure to prevent leaks. It is also necessary to ensure that the physician has approved showering for the person. All patients, and especially those on crutches, should be cautioned about the wet, slippery floors in the shower room. For unsteady or elderly patients, a shower in the wheelchair is the safest strategy. Most orthopedic units have a shower that will accommodate a wheelchair. At home, tub chairs can be installed to provide this security.

Synthetic casts are immersible in water if the stockinette and padding are also synthetic. If so, and the physician approves, these patients can shower or swim. The person who plans to do so must be instructed very carefully in procedures for drying the cast and in the dangers of skin maceration if it is improperly dried. To dry the cast, it is first blotted with a towel. Then a hair dryer is used to dry all surfaces. The hair dryer should be on a cool or warm setting except when drying a Hexcelite cast, when a cool setting must be used since heating this material causes it to soften.[19] Drying the cast thoroughly may take up to 3 hours and the patient should be thoroughly apprised of this. He may forego the pleasures of a swim or use shower protectors because of the time commitment. The advantage of immersible synthetic casts is probably most beneficial to the person who is in a body cast for several months.

Knowledge Deficit of Cast Care at Home

The extent to which a person with a cast can care for himself at home depends on the type of cast and the resources available in the home. Assessment of each patient's situation must be accomplished early in the hospitalization for discharge planning to be effective.

Home care instructions for the person in a cast should include

- Neurovascular assessment and symptoms that warrant notifying the doctor
- Correct elevation and ice application
- Skin care and danger signs of pressure and infection
- Techniques for showering and bathing
- Correct use of crutches, walkers, or slings
- Types of modification of clothing
- Activity allowed
- Exercises to be performed and their frequency
- Measures to relieve itching
- Positioning techniques to enhance comfort

Removing the Cast. When it is time for the cast to be removed, teaching is needed to prepare the patient. The nurse explains the procedure for cutting the cast and discusses the appearance of the extremity. There is a sour-smelling, yellow-gray exudate caked on the skin. The patient should gently cleanse the area with soap and water and then apply lotion to restore moisture. Vigorous scrubbing in an attempt to remove all the exudate in one washing causes breaks in the skin. The extremity that has been casted will appear smaller than the opposite one owing to muscle atrophy. The structures are weakened; therefore, the arm or leg should be handled gently. Discomfort may also be present in muscles and joints that have not been used, but this should gradually subside with rehabilitation.

This complication, associated with body or hip spica casts that cover the abdomen, warrants immediate intervention. The syndrome is an acute obstruction of the duodenum, probably caused by mechanical compression of a portion of the duodenum by the superior mesenteric artery. Gastric and duodenal dilatation result.[40]

Symptoms include persistent nausea and vomiting, resulting in life-threatening electrolyte imbalances. Abdominal distention and pain are also seen. Treatment consists of decompression using a nasogastric tube, fluid and electrolyte replacement with IV therapy, maintenance of npo status, and removal of the cast.

The syndrome may be suspected in individuals who become quite anxious and claustrophobic in their casts. They may have difficulty breathing and experience gastric fullness after eating. The nausea and vomiting may be present, but it is not so severe as in cast syndrome. Cutting a window over the abdomen and developing a supportive relationship with the patient may relieve the symptoms. Occasionally, the cast needs to be bivalved and the anterior half removed.

Evaluation

Expected outcomes for the patient in a cast include

- Neurovascular status of affected extremity intact
- Patient describes signs of neurovascular impairment and demonstrates correct elevation and ice application.
- No skin breakdown observed or complaints of pressure voiced
- Person demonstrates activities of daily living, including bathing techniques.
- Patient demonstrates safe use of assistive devices.
- Person describes measures to enhance comfort.
- Person demonstrates exercises.
- Person lists/describes when to call the physician.

Impaired Physical Mobility Related to Musculoskeletal Disorders

Confronted with the word immobility, the health care professional immediately associates it with another: complications. Preventing or minimizing the complications of immobility is one of the greatest challenges for the nurse caring for orthopedic patients.

Prior to considering the problems associated with immobility, it is important to consider the positive aspects. Resting the body or a part of it is one of the most common therapeutic methods used for musculoskeletal disease and injury. The most commonly used measure, the cast, has been thoroughly discussed. Traction, another common method, will be considered later in this section. But first, a look at the reasons for immobilization is in order.

Immobility and Healing

Immobilization is necessary for the healing of most injuries to the musculoskeletal structures. Painful joints and muscles resulting from disease of musculoskeletal structures are frequently rested in splints or casts or simply not used to enhance comfort.

Bone. Bone heals by creating new bone. The process of osteogenesis is necessary to reestablish the continuity of bone. This is different from soft tissues, which heal with a fibrous tissue scar. A fibrous tissue bridge would not be strong enough to support skeletal functions. Bones take longer to heal than other structures, and if they are inadequately aligned when immobilized, then healing may be delayed or faulty alignment and deformity may result.

The process of fracture healing can be divided into the following stages:

1. *Hematoma formation.* A blood clot is formed between the bone fragments as a result of the bleeding from torn blood vessels in the area. The hematoma provides a structure upon which the fibrin network can build. Because of the disrupted blood supply, the cells on both edges of the fracture line die.
2. *Cellular proliferation.* The cells at the torn ends proliferate and differentiate into granulation tissue that forms a soft tissue bridge across the bone ends. Meanwhile, the process of phagocytosis is occurring, removing red blood cells and dead tissue.
3. *Callus formation.* The granulation tissue differentiates into a loosely woven cartilage and bone matrix through the actions of chondroblasts and osteoblasts. This process takes place between 6 and 21 days after the injury, but the bone is not yet strong enough to bear weight.
4. *Ossification.* Calcium salts are deposited in the callus, and the bone becomes rigid and healing is complete. The process takes place in 3 to 10 weeks after injury.
5. *Remodeling.* The bone is returned to its normal shape and contour by the action of osteoclasts resorbing excess bone and osteoblasts forming new bone where additional strength is needed. Muscle contraction and weight-bearing stresses placed on bone determine the shape and strength of the bone. Therefore, the remodeling stage may take several years.

Tendons. When ruptured, tendons do not really heal themselves. The ends need to be sutured surgically. They then heal when connective tissue from the surrounding tissues penetrates between the sutured ends and deposits collagen. Ultimately tendon fibers are formed. Tendons are immobilized during healing because mobilization during this time seems to produce hypertrophy of the tendon.[8]

Ligaments. Ligaments also need to be sutured when a complete tear occurs. If not sutured, they heal with a gap of fibrous tissue between the ends and a weak ligament results, leading to joint instability. Ligaments heal by collagen formed by fibroblastic activity of both the ligament itself and of the surrounding tissues. Immobilization of ligaments is necessary to prevent stress on the suture line.[8]

Muscles. Partial tears of muscle heal by regeneration of the fibers, while more complete tears may require surgical intervention. Rest ranging from temporary cessation of the activity that precipitated the injury to splinting is the treatment of choice.

Nursing Diagnoses and Interventions

Complications Related to Immobility

The human body was designed for motion and when inactivity results from orthopedic disease, injury, or treatment, there are predictable adverse physiological effects on many body systems. Nursing attention to preventing or minimizing these effects, as well as detecting problems early, has a significant effect on the ultimate rehabilitation of the patient. Because the potential for complication secondary to immobility is a very significant aspect of orthopedic patient care, a concise review follows. Greater detail can be found in the sections discussing nursing diagnoses related to specific body systems.

Potential Impairment of Skin Integrity

Skin disruption can take many forms, including pressure sores, abrasions, and maceration. It is one of the most problematic complications. Prolonged pressure over bony prominences; friction from wrinkled sheets; the shearing force applied to the skin when sliding a patient up and down in bed; and moisture from urine, feces, and perspiration all lead to skin breakdown. Factors that contribute to the potential for loss of skin integrity include advancing age, malnutrition, sensory losses, inability to alter position, obesity, and sedating medication.[2,39]

Skin, especially that over bony prominences, should be assessed at least every 8 hours, and more frequently in persons at greater risk. Skin becoming ischemic from pressure is reddened, warmer, and may be edematous. A reddened area that does not return to normal coloration 30 to 60 minutes after the pressure is relieved is a danger sign and requires very vigorous nursing attention.

The most significant nursing strategy in preventing skin breakdown is removing pressure or preventing concentrations of pressure. Turning the patient every 2 hours is the standard effective measure. The turning frequency must be individualized to the patient's condition.

Other important nursing strategies are aimed at maintaining or improving the health of the skin tissues. Gentle massage over bony prominences increases the circulation to the area. Careful cleansing and thorough drying of the perineal area of the incontinent patient are vital to preventing excoriation. Prevention of dehydration and provision of adequate nutrients are also very important.

Many devices are available to assist in skin care for those persons at risk. Egg crate mattresses, sheepskins, elbow and heel protectors, air mattresses, and flotation pads all distribute pressure over a larger area. Alternating pressure mattresses function to change the pressure points every few minutes. An alternating pressure mattress that also has an airflow system where air flows through the sheets and onto the patient is quite effective in preventing skin maceration in those patients who are incontinent or who perspire excessively.

The patient who cannot be turned, such as one in traction, can be taught to shift his weight or lift his hips off the bed by lifting up on the trapeze on an hourly basis (Fig. 87–9). Patients who cannot lift themselves should be lifted when being repositioned or moved up in bed to prevent shearing forces on the skin. Lifting patients when placing them on the bedpan, as opposed to sliding it under them, also avoids the shearing force. Pillows placed under the legs elevate the heels off the bed when the patient is supine.

Alteration in Peripheral Tissue Perfusion

Not only is thromboembolic disease a complication of immobility, it is also recognized as the most common complication of lower extremity surgery or trauma.[1] Etiology of deep vein thrombosis is a combination of venous stasis, local trauma to the vein, and hypercoagulability. Refer to Chapter 21 for further discussion.

Symptoms of deep vein thrombosis include calf or thigh tenderness, warmth over the site, edema of the extremity, and a positive Homans' sign (pain in the calf muscle upon passive dorsiflexion of the foot). All of these symptoms need not be present and, indeed, a patient can have a thrombosis without any symptoms. Detection of symptoms involves observing for erythema and edema, palpating for tenderness and temperature, and passively dorsiflexing the patient's feet. Calf circumference may be measured and recorded on a daily basis for those persons at high risk.

Nursing actions to prevent the problem are aimed at increasing venous flow. The most effective measure is calf pumping. This exercise, which must be done several times per hour, consists of having the patient dorsiflex and plantarflex his feet. If his leg is casted and he cannot move his ankle, he can move his toes. Calf pumping increases the action of the muscle pump and therefore, the venous flow. Antiembolic hose increase venous flow as well.

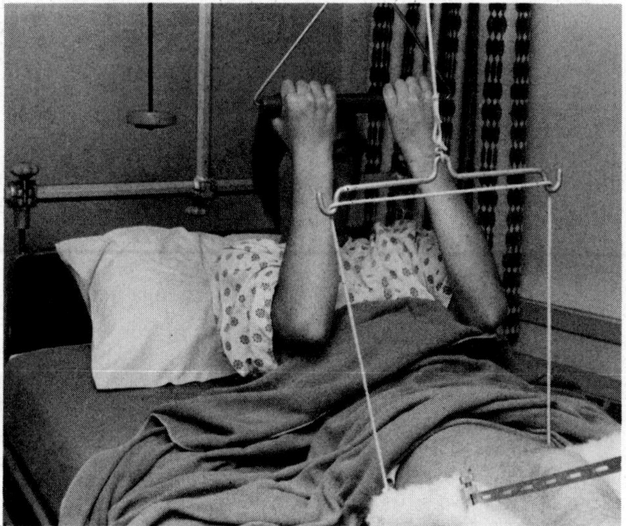

FIGURE 87–9 The patient can use the trapeze to pull himself up in bed and relieve pressure.

Alteration in Balance Related to Orthostatic Hypotension

This complication results from an excessive volume of blood pooling in the lower extremities and abdominal viscera. Bed rest compromises the ability of the peripheral vessels to constrict when assuming the upright posture. Upon rising, the blood pressure falls and the patient is dizzy and may faint.

Preventive strategies involve putting the patient in as much of an upright posture, during bed rest, as his condition will allow. Use of elastic stockings or bandages that externally compress the vessels may also help.

It is important to remember this effect of bed rest when getting patients out of bed the first few times. They need to change positions slowly and gradually. Give them time to adjust to the sitting position prior to moving them to a standing position. A tilt table is frequently used for persons who have been on bed rest for long periods. They are brought into a standing posture very gradually as their blood pressure is monitored and their responses observed (Fig. 87–10).

Alteration in Bowel Elimination: Constipation

Lack of activity, changes in diet and fluid intake, lack of privacy, having to use a bedpan, and narcotic analgesics all contribute to constipation. Weakened abdominal and perineal muscles as a result of immobility interfere with the ability to pass this hard, dry stool.

Measures to prevent constipation must be individualized for the patient and the extent of his immobilization. Increasing fluid intake, adding more fruit and vegetables to the diet, a glass of prune juice daily, exercising the abdominal muscles, stool softeners, and laxatives can be used. The upright position is the natural one for defecation and should be used if possible. However, the orthopedic patient often cannot be in the upright position because of traction, casts, or pain. It is important that these patients establish a routine and be provided with complete privacy. Elderly persons frequently already use some method to ensure their daily bowel movement, such as coffee, prune juice, or laxatives. These methods should be determined and continued. Patients with hard, dry stool, no bowel movement for 3 to 4 days, or watery stools, are constipated and at risk for developing fecal impaction and require more intensive efforts aimed at prevention.

Ineffective Airway Clearance

Hypostatic pneumonia results from stasis of secretions. It is not necessarily a problem for the young, healthy person once he is off narcotic analgesics. But it must be actively prevented in the very weak, ill, or elderly patient. The respiratory muscles are weakened by bed rest, and there is a

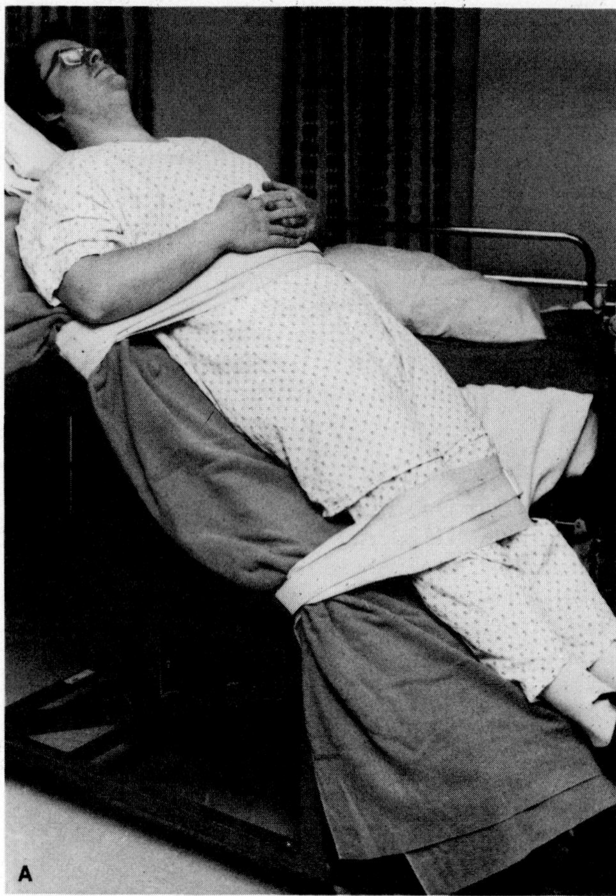

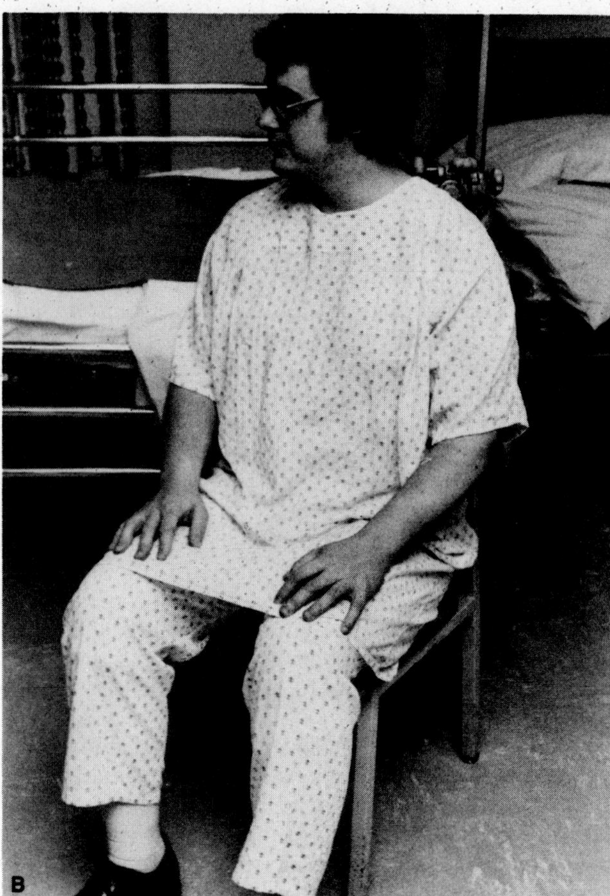

FIGURE 87–10 (*A* and *B*) A tilt table can be used to slowly bring a patient from a lying position to an upright position after an extended period of bedrest.

decrease in the stimulus to breathing. The patient may be too weak to cough out the secretions accumulating in the bronchioles. Signs and symptoms of hypostatic pneumonia include rapid pulse, greenish yellow mucus, cough, fever, pain with respirations, and labored respirations.

Preventing the pooling of respiratory secretions involves turning the patient every 2 hours if possible and having him cough and breathe deeply every 2 hours. Use of an incentive spirometer may be necessary. Encouraging any type of activity will stimulate deeper breathing.

Impaired Physical Mobility Related to Muscle Atrophy

Muscle mass and strength is retained through active contraction of the fibers. With inactivity, there is a decrease in size and strength of muscle. Muscle atrophy leads to even less endurance and more fatigue and, thus, to even less activity. The loss of muscle tone that results affects the body's ability to maintain an upright posture against gravity, and a longer period of rehabilitation is necessary.

Muscle atrophy is prevented by active range of motion to all joints not immobilized and by isometric muscle-setting exercises. The exercises should be done at least every 3 to 4 hours. Often, a physical therapist will prescribe an exercise program for the patient directed toward minimizing disuse atrophy and strengthening muscles that will be needed for use of crutches or walkers and transferring into chairs.

Muscles that lose tone can become permanently stretched or shortened from incorrect positioning, and joint contractures then occur. Prevention of contractures is discussed in a later section.

Potential for Disuse Osteoporosis

Disuse osteoporosis refers to bone mass reduction as a result of loss of muscle tone and mass and decreases in the physical stresses that impact bone remodeling and formation.[13] It can be generalized or located in a specific body part. Since more bone is resorbed than is formed, a negative calcium balance accompanies the bone loss. Therefore, in addition to the potential for weakened, fragile bones there is the problem of hypercalciuria. This type of osteoporosis is considered reversible if the individual is mobilized within a certain period of time, but becomes irreversible if immobility is prolonged.[17] The duration of immobility before irreversible loss occurs is not known.

The most widely accepted theory as to the cause of disuse osteoporosis is loss of the compressive, weight-bearing stress on the bone.[10,44,45] It follows from this that active weight-bearing activities alone are effective in retarding bone loss. Various isotonic and isometric exercises and devices have been tried in the space program, but none have met with success in reducing bone loss.[49,50]

It appears that the inclusion in care plans of isometric or isotonic exercises or plantar flexion against a footboard specifically to slow bone loss is unnecessary. These activities are, however, important in preventing disuse muscle atrophy and contractures and should not be excluded from a plan of care.

For some orthopedic patients, active weight bearing is impossible. For others, active weight bearing with a tilt table or circo-electric bed may be possible. It does appear from the literature that approximately 3 hours of weight-bearing stress is necessary daily.[15]

There is no way of assessing the amount of bone loss in the clinical setting. Therefore, an important consideration is preventing injury to these patients. Gentle handling of an extremity after its removal from a cast can prevent refracture. Lifting and moving immobilized patients very carefully is important since their fracture threshold may be very low.

Alteration in Elimination

Alteration in elimination in this instance is related to urinary stasis and renal calculi. In the supine position, urine pools in the renal calices and pelvis and also in the bladder. Compounding the problem, the patient may have difficulty relaxing the external urethral sphincter to void when he is required to use the bedpan. One outcome of urine retention is a urinary tract infection.

All patients on bed rest should be assessed for bladder distention, bladder discomfort, and frequency and amount of voiding. A patient voiding small amounts on a frequent basis may be overflowing; that is, he has a full bladder, but is eliminating only enough to relieve the pressure. Incontinence is another indication of overflow retention. Strategies to prevent urine retention are similar to those for preventing constipation. Placing the patient in an upright position, or as near to it as his condition allows, and providing privacy are most helpful. Running water in the room and pouring warm water over the perineum may stimulate micturition. If the patient is still unable to void, the physician must be notified and a catheterization may be ordered.

As mentioned earlier, the hypercalciuria that accompanies osteoporosis predisposes to the formation of renal calculi. In their classic study on the effects of bed rest, Dietrick, Whedon, and Shorr[9] found that although urinary calcium doubled, the factors that influence the solubility of urinary calcium reflected no change. Urine volume increased only slightly. The urine pH increased (became more alkaline), and there was no change in citric acid secretion. These findings, combined with urinary stasis and the presence of bacteria, favor the formation of calcium phosphate urinary tract stones. The most common sites for stones are the renal pelvis and urinary bladder.

Careful assessment of immobilized individuals for a history of stones, the presence of a urinary tract infection, or urine retention is essential for identifying patients at high risk. Renal colic, urethral colic, diarrhea, and abdominal discomfort are signs and symptoms of renal calculi. Maintaining an adequate fluid intake will help to prevent urinary stasis and decrease urine concentration to slow stone formation.

Evaluation

Expected outcomes for the patient with impaired physical mobility include

- No skin breakdown observed or complaints of pressure voiced
- Demonstrates effective exercises for increasing peripheral venous return
- No evidence of dizziness or loss of balance related to a drop in blood pressure with position change
- No evidence of constipation
- Demonstrates deep breathing exercises and has no evidence of pooling of secretions
- Demonstrates adequate muscle strength and bone density through activities of daily living
- Demonstrates no evidence of urinary stasis or calculi formation

Traction: A Method of Immobilization

Caring for the patient in traction is a challenge for any nurse. Knowledge of the principles of traction not only ensures delivery of effective nursing care, but also makes the process more interesting. These patients may be immobilized for long periods and require ingenuity in providing the emotional as well as the physical aspects of care.

Principles of Traction

Traction is a pulling force applied in a specific direction to a body part by manual or mechanical means. The pulling force usually is applied with a system of weights, ropes, and pulleys. It is used to align and maintain the alignment of the fragments of a fracture, to overcome muscle spasm, to stretch muscles and tendons, or to hold the extremity in position and thus prevent more injury.

To be effective in aligning fractures and maintaining that alignment, traction must overcome the deforming effect of the mechanical force that caused the fracture, the effect of the muscle pull, and the effect of gravity. The force that caused the fracture often leaves the bone fragments displaced. A pulling force (traction) not only pulls on the bone fragments to align them, but also on the surrounding soft tissues that help to hold the fragments in place. The muscle spasms that accompany fractures pull on both ends of the bone and cause bowing deformity or overriding of the bone fragments.[22] The traction force has to be slightly greater than the muscle force to overcome deformity from muscle spasm. It follows that the amount of weight needed to apply the pulling force to a bone surrounded by large muscles is greater than that needed for areas of smaller muscle mass. Gravity pulling on a fracture site also results in deformity, and traction correctly applied overcomes the bowing effect of gravity on the fracture fragments.

Skin Traction and Skeletal Traction

Traction may exert the pulling force on the bones in two ways. It may be applied to the skin with the force then transmitted indirectly to the skeleton. This type is known as skin traction. The second type is skeletal traction, in which the traction is applied directly to skeletal structures.

Skin traction is accomplished using weight that pulls on tapes, foam straps, or plastic materials applied to the skin. The skin does not tolerate large amounts of weight for long periods of time. Five to ten lb is the amount of pull the skin will tolerate without breaking down. It also may be released temporarily to provide skin care. Different types of skin traction include Bucks traction, pelvic traction with a pelvic belt, and cervical traction with a cervical halter (Table 87–2).

Skeletal traction is applied directly to bone with wires, pins, or tongs placed into or through bones. Skeletal traction is used when the force must be continuous and when heavier weights are required to overcome muscle spasm. The usual amount of weight seen is 25 to 40 lb. Types of skeletal traction include balanced skeletal traction, overhead arm traction, and cervical traction with tongs (Table 87–3).

Countertraction. Countertraction is a force equal to that of traction that pulls in the opposite direction. Without it, the patient would not be balanced against the traction. The

TABLE 87–2
Types of Skin Traction

Bucks Traction

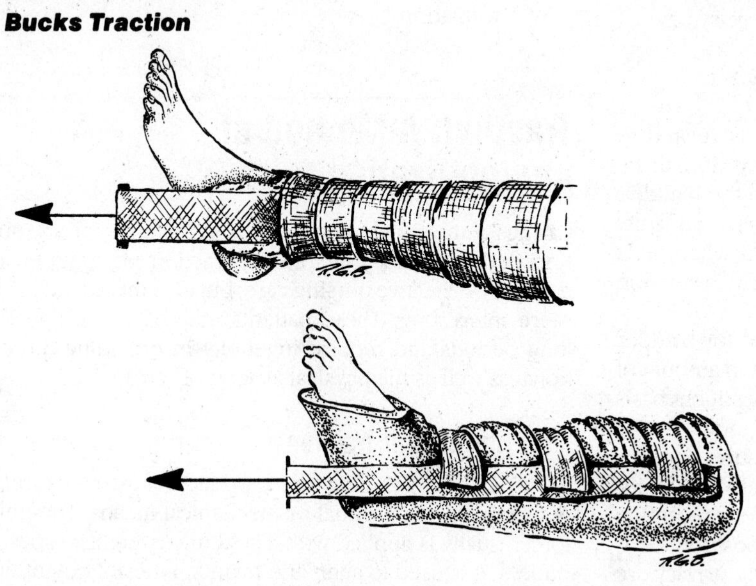

Application: Either applied with straps and an elastic wrap or with a traction boot
Indications: Temporary immobilization of a fractured hip, low back pain, locked knees
Note: May be continuous or may be temporarily released. Skin and neurovascular status must be observed closely.

Pelvic Traction with Pelvic Belt

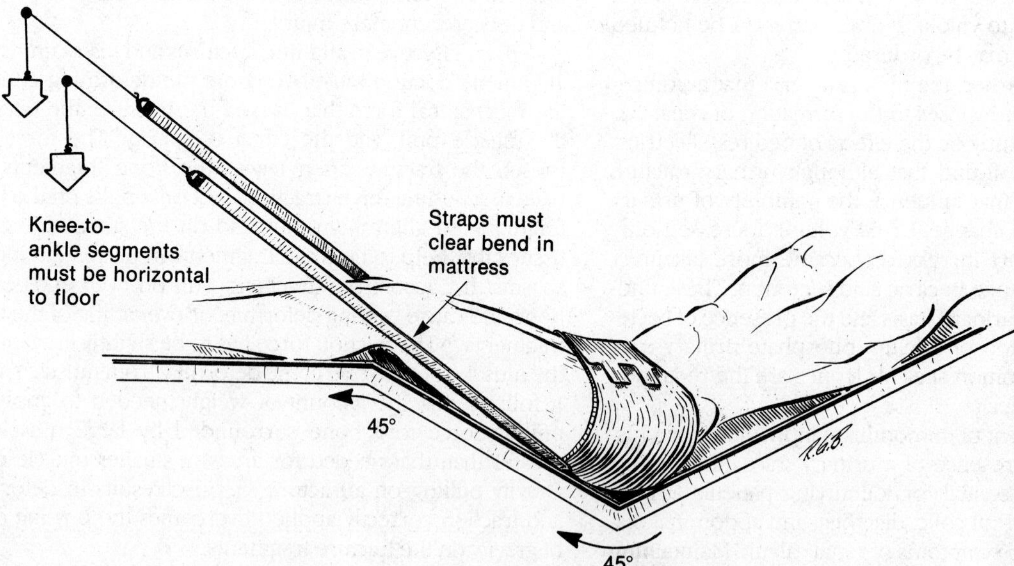

Application: Applied with a pelvic belt that has straps on lateral aspects that extend to pulleys. Pull is on the lumbar spine.
Indications: Low back pain
Note: Patient should have hips and knees flexed at about 45 degrees. Usually is intermittent

(Continued)

traction force would pull the patient toward it, and the patient could end up pressed against the foot or the side of the bed, thereby decreasing the effectiveness of the traction. The weight of the patient's body provides some countertraction. The body weight can be enhanced by use of trochanter rolls or positioning devices, by using shock blocks to elevate the bed itself, or elevating the head of the bed. With balanced-suspension traction, a counter-pulling system of weights and pulleys provides much of the countertraction.

The principles of caring for patients in traction are listed in Table 87–4. Nursing care of the patient in skin traction is illustrated in a discussion of Bucks traction and that of skeletal traction through discussion of balanced suspension skeletal traction applied to the femur.

Bucks Traction

Bucks traction is longitudinal traction applied to one or both lower extremities. Most frequently it is used on one leg to promote comfort and reduce muscle spasm in patients with fractured hips while they are awaiting surgical fixation. Five to eight lb of weight is sufficient to adequately immobilize the extremity. Other uses include correcting or preventing lower extremity contractures, locked knees, or low back pain.

Bucks traction is frequently applied by nurses. One method of application involves applying adhesive, moleskin, or foam straps along the medial and lateral aspects of the leg, followed by wrapping an elastic bandage around the leg (Fig. 87–11, *A*). Adhesive or moleskin straps adhere to the skin and thus have the potential to cause blistering and skin breakdown. Foam straps are not adherent and must be wrapped securely enough to prevent their slipping, but not so tight as to constrict circulation. The elastic bandage is wrapped from the ankle to the knee, using a modified figure-eight wrap to provide even compression. Excessive pressure must be avoided over the Achilles tendon, the malleoli, and the proximal fibula (where the peroneal nerve lies close to the skin). Once the straps and wrap are in place, a spreader bar or footplate is attached. These devices must be wide enough to spread the tapes enough to keep pressure off the malleoli and sides of the foot. A rope is attached to the spreader bar, put through a pulley at the foot of the bed, and the weight is attached. The physician orders the amount of weight to be used.

The newer method of applying Bucks traction uses a foam rubber boot (Fig. 87–11, *B*). The boot fastens around the extremity with Velcro closures. It has straps down the medial and lateral aspects and a device at the foot end for attachment of the rope and weights. Thromboembolic hose may be worn on the extremity underneath the boot.

Bucks traction is usually temporary. Nonetheless, the

TABLE 87–2
Types of Skin Traction *(Continued)*

Cervical Traction with Cervical Halter

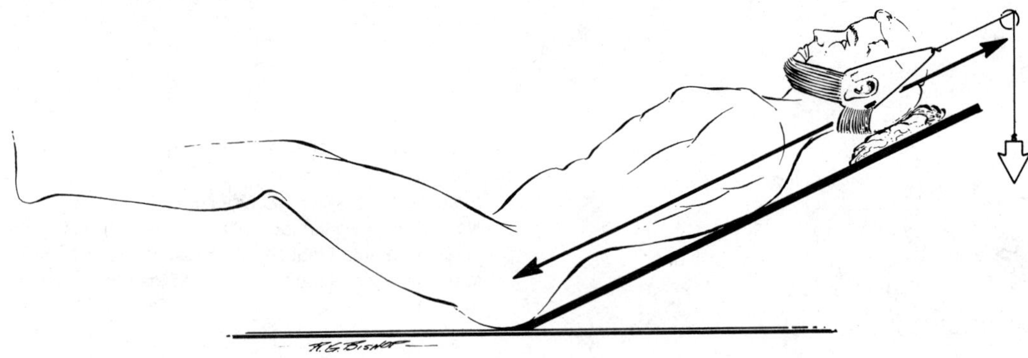

Application: Uses a head halter and a spreader bar to apply pull to occiput and thus the neck and shoulder muscles
Indicators: "Whiplash," neck pain or strain
Note: Usually is intermittent. Pressure areas are the chin, occiput, and ears. Males without beards should shave daily for added comfort.

(Drawings from Lewis RC Jr: Handbook of Traction, Casting and Splinting Techniques. Philadelphia, JB Lippincott, 1977)

TABLE 87–3
Types of Skeletal Traction

Balanced Skeletal Traction

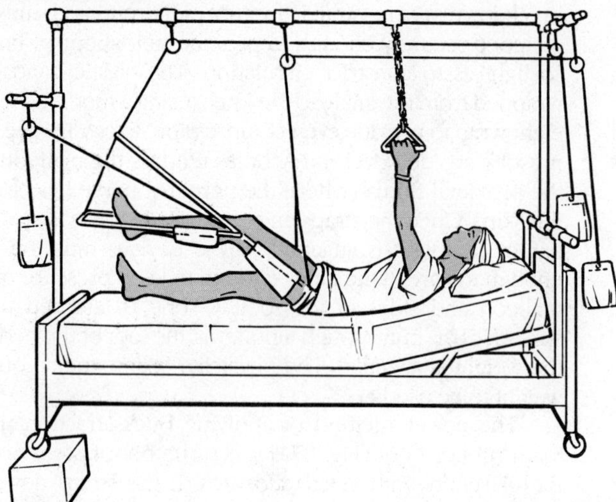

Application: Pin is inserted through the proximal tibia or distal femur, and leg is suspended off the bed in balanced system.
Indications: Fractures of the femur
Note: Always continuous. Never lift up on the traction weights.

Overhead Arm Traction

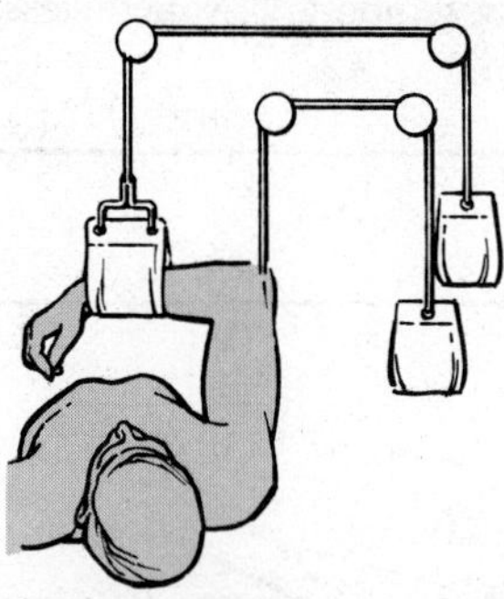

Application: Pin is inserted through the olecranon, and the forearm is suspended in a sling.
Indications: Fractures of the humerus
Note: Always continuous

Cervical Traction with Tongs

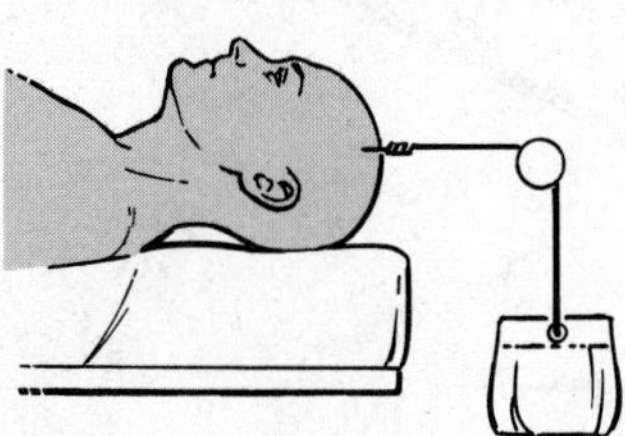

Application: Crutchfield or Vinke tongs are inserted into the skull.
Indications: Cervical fractures or dislocations
Note: Always continuous. Patient may be on a turning frame. It is recommended that sandbags be kept at the bedside for immobilization of the head if the tongs should come out.

patient is on bed rest and at risk for disuse complications. A trapeze on the bed is essential for helping the person move about in bed and for getting on and off the bedpan. Back care is best accomplished by having the patient use the trapeze to lift his upper body. The bed can be changed from top to bottom. If the patient must be turned for back care or linen changes, he can be turned 45 degrees to either side. A pillow is placed between his legs for maintaining body alignment during turning. Specific care related to nursing diagnoses for the patient in Bucks traction is discussed below.

Nursing Diagnoses and Interventions

Potential for Neurovascular Compromise. The injury or disease plus the Bucks traction place the patient at risk. Neurovascular assessment is done every hour for 24 hours and then every 4 hours if the status is normal. If edema occurs in the foot, the elastic wrap or the boot straps may be too tight. It is often necessary to include the foot when wrapping the elastic bandage to prevent or control the edema.

The nursing staff also needs to be on the alert for pero-

TABLE 87–4
Principles of Caring for the Patient in Traction

- The established line of pull must be maintained. The patient's body alignment may need adjustment. Pulleys and extension bars should not be moved.
- Traction is usually continuous. Some types of skin traction are intermittent. Weights must never be removed from skeletal traction.
- The traction setup must be free from friction that could interfere with the amount of pull. Heavy linens should not be draped over ropes.
- Weights should hang freely and not touch the floor or drag on the bed.
- There must be countertraction. Without the opposite pull the patient is pulled toward the traction force.
- Footplates against the foot of the bed or a knot in contact with the pulley interferes with the pull. These areas must be observed frequently. Ropes must also be in the center of the pulley.
- The bed should be equipped with a trapeze. The pàtient can move up in bed by holding onto the trapeze and bending the unaffected leg. With his unaffected foot flat on the bed, he can push into the mattress and move himself.
- Patients in traction should be placed on a firm mattress to prevent contractures and the friction and back strain created by a sagging mattress.
- Active motion of all unaffected joints must be maintained by range-of-motion exercises every 3 to 4 hours during waking hours.

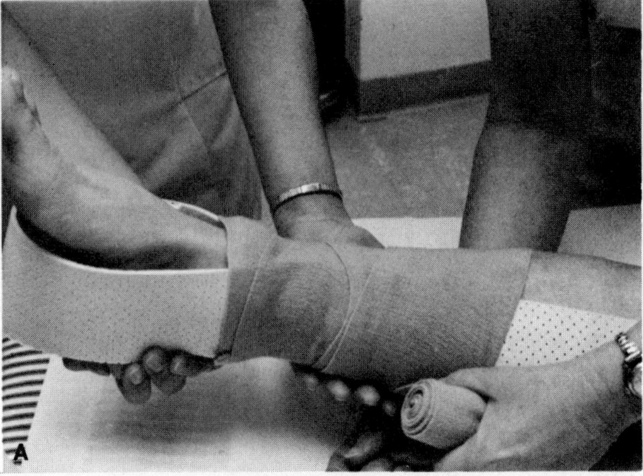

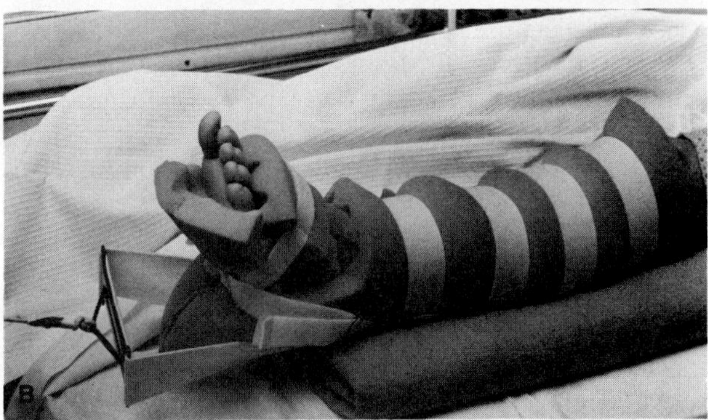

FIGURE 87–11 Buck's traction, using mole skin and tape (*A*) or a foam rubber boot (*B*).

neal nerve palsy when using this traction. Pressure from the elastic wrap or the boot over the fibular head can leave the peroneal nerve ischemic. Also, if the patient's leg is externally rotated, pressure may be exerted over this nerve. A good habit to develop is having the patient dorsiflex his affected foot each time the nurse enters the room. If weakness or sensory loss are noted, loosening the straps of the boot or rewrapping the elastic bandage will probably relieve it. Physician's preferences or local policies should be checked prior to removing the traction. However, Bucks traction usually should be released and rewrapped every 8 hours. This prevents long-term pressure on nerves and circulatory constriction. It also provides an opportunity to assess and care for the skin.

Potential Impairment of Skin Integrity Related to Immobility. The skin within the traction device and the heels are especially at risk. The skin over the fibular head, the tibia, and the malleoli are in danger from pressure created by the wrap, the straps, and the pulling force. Frequent rewrapping and observation of the skin are necessary to avoid skin breakdown. It may be necessary to pad these areas.

Heels are a problem. If left alone, they dig into the mattress, a situation that creates a great deal of pressure, and they will break down within hours. They can be kept off the bed by placing a small pillow or a bath blanket underneath the calf. There are also foam devices on the market designed for keeping heels off the bed (Fig. 87–12). In using these devices, the nurse needs to carefully observe the Achilles tendon for pressure. Heel protectors may also be used. The heels should be gently massaged every 4 hours to increase circulation. Heel protectors or other devices are not a substi-

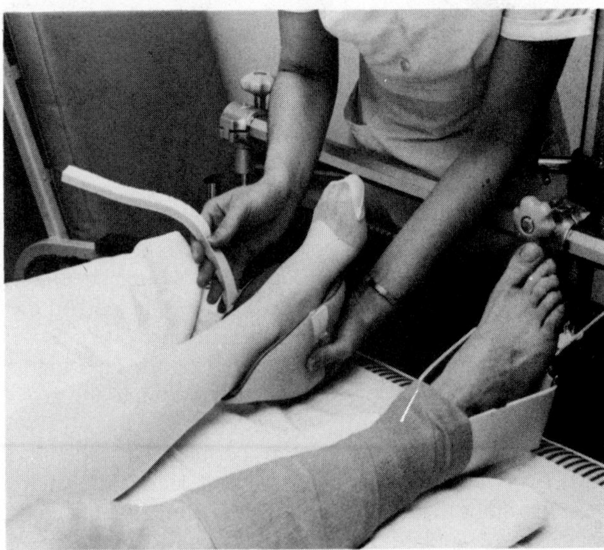

FIGURE 87–12 Protecting the heel from pressure in a patient in Buck's traction.

tute for massage and close observation. Redness and blistering are signs of a developing pressure sore.

The foam traction boot must also be removed at least every 8 hours. The foam is convoluted on the inner aspect and can produce a significant amount of pressure. Simply loosening the straps is not sufficient. The boot should be removed so that the entire leg and the heels can be inspected.

Evaluation

Expected outcomes for the patient in traction include

- Neurovascular status of the affected extremity intact
- Integrity of the skin intact

Skeletal Traction

Balanced skeletal traction is used most frequently to treat fractures of the femur. It consists of traction applied through a pin placed in the distal femur or the proximal tibia and of a balanced-suspension system where the leg is supported off the bed by a system of ropes, pulleys, and weights. Skeletal traction is continuous; once applied it is not removed. As previously stated, 25 to 40 lb of weight may be used, and it can be left in place 3 to 4 months if necessary.

Pin placement is done by the physician either in the operating room, the emergency area, or the patient's room. A local anesthetic can be used if the patient does not require a general or regional anesthetic for other reasons. If the procedure is done under local anesthesia, the patient is given a parenteral analgesic. Small skin incisions are made over the site, and the pin is threaded through the bone. A traction bow is applied to the pin, and the rope and weights are attached to this bow. The pin used may be either a Steinmann pin or a Kirchner wire. Some physicians also apply casts around the pin for added pin stability and to protect against infection at the sites.

Once the traction is on, the balanced-suspension system is applied. Most frequently, a Thomas splint and Pearson attachment are used. Sheepskin slings or towels are attached to the rods to support the extremity in the splints. The Thomas half-ring splint supports the thigh, and the Pearson attachment supports the lower leg and allows for knee flexion. Once suspended, the hip and knee are flexed and the lower leg is lying parallel to the mattress (Fig. 87–13).

The half-ring can be applied either on the anterior or posterior thigh. Either way, the ring will press into the groin and some extra padding may be needed.

A balanced-suspension setup permits the patient to move easily and comfortably in bed. It allows the entire lower extremity to function and move as a unit. If the skeletal traction were applied without the suspension, movement would occur at the fracture site rather than at the hip joint each time the patient moved. The patient can be moved up and down in bed and lift himself up off the bed for skin care and bedpan use without discomfort and without motion at the fracture site.

The amount of weight and the position of the leg are determined by the physician. Although the patient is able to move around in bed, he may experience discomfort and need assistance to get into the correct position. An accurate method of communicating the correct position of each patient in balanced skeletal traction is to take a photograph of the patient and attach it at the head of his bed or to his nursing care plan.

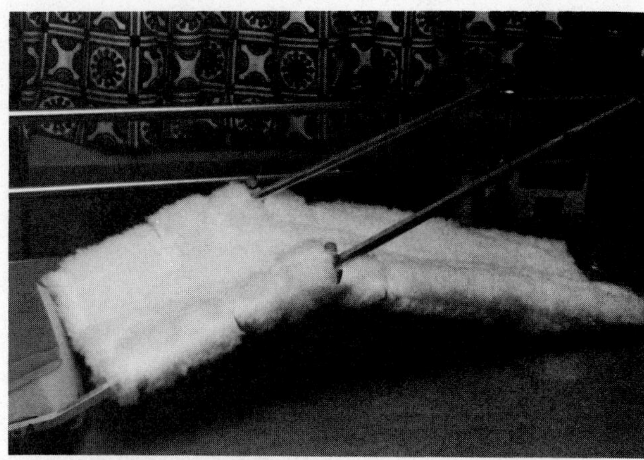

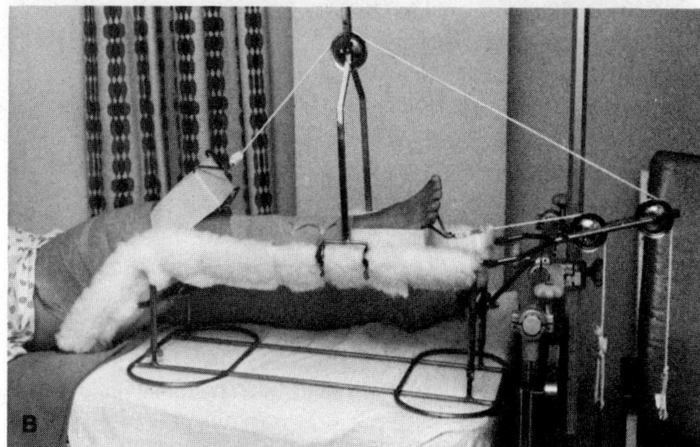

FIGURE 87–13 (*A* and *B*) Thomas splint and Pearson attachment with sheepskin covering.

The nursing staff is responsible for maintaining the effectiveness of the traction as well as preventing the complications associated with immobility and the traction equipment. This patient, usually the active adolescent or young adult male, requires a very understanding yet firm nursing staff to help him tolerate this forced inactivity.

Nursing Diagnoses and Interventions

Potential for Neurovascular Compromise. Hourly assessment of the neurovascular status is required for at least the first 24 hours. The physician should be notified of any compromise. If the pin was placed in the proximal tibia, it may be close to the peroneal nerve. The splints may also be placing pressure on this nerve as well as the femoral, popliteal, and sural nerves. For neurovascular changes thought to be a result of pressure from splints, the nurse can shift the splints enough to relieve pressure without disrupting the traction.

Inflammation (neuritis) of the ulnar nerve may occur when the patient uses his elbows to push himself up in bed.

The ulnar nerve is quite superficial as it passes over the medial epicondyle of the humerus and as such is quite susceptible to pressure. the patient reports numbness and tingling in the ulnar distribution of his hands. The problem is usually resolved by teaching the patient to use his overhead trapeze to move himself in bed. Elbow protectors or padding may also be used.

Potential for Impairment of Skin Integrity Related to Immobility. The heels, sacrum, and elbows are the bony prominences particularly susceptible to pressure in the average traction patient. Protectors may be applied to heels and elbows. They do not relieve pressure, but instead distribute it over a wider area. Therefore, heels and elbows should be assessed and massaged every 3 to 4 hours.

Heels require vigorous attention, and the heel of the leg in traction requires special care. If it is resting on the slings, it should be well padded with sheepskin or foam. The slings should be removed or pushed back several times daily to remove pressure from the heel totally. This measure places additional pressure over the Achilles tendon so that area must be padded well also.

If a footplate is in use, it must be removed at regular intervals to prevent pressure sores on the plantar surface of the foot. All pressure sores heal slowly, but due to the nature of the skin on the foot's sole, these take even longer. Skin breakdown on the foot could delay ambulation when fracture healing is sufficient to permit it.

The most effective way to protect the sacrum is to have the patient use his trapeze and lift his buttocks off the bed hourly or during every television commercial. Egg crate mattresses, sheepskins, or alternating pressure mattresses are also helpful.

The traction equipment itself creates some hazards for the skin. Corks, rubber stoppers, or adhesive tape placed on the pin protect the opposite leg from the sharp ends. Wrinkles in the slings supporting the leg in the Thomas splint and Pearson attachment add unnecessary pressure. The slings should be checked and repositioned frequently. The metal parts of the splint and the ropes suspending it may place pressure anywhere along the limb, especially if the patient is obese.

Particularly problematic is the half-ring at the proximal end of the Thomas splint. If countertraction is insufficient, the ring presses into the groin. In this case, the physician may need to add more weight to the balance system. If the ring is posterior so that the patient is sitting on it, the skin needs to be observed very closely. When pressure from the ring exists, the tendency is to pad it. However, this padding should be removed frequently to prevent its becoming a pressure source.

Potential for Infection. The pin sites should be assessed every shift for redness, drainage, edema, warmth, or increased tenderness. The physician is notified if any of these signs appear. Normally, there is slight serous drainage due to the foreign body reaction of the bone to the pin. This drainage should not be purulent.

Physicians vary greatly in their preferences as to how much care is given to the pin sites. The nursing staff should be aware of these preferences and have either a written physician's order or unit policies for pin care. Some physicians prefer that nothing be done to the sites. The rationale here is that when the site is left undisturbed there is less chance of contaminating the pin tract. This does not relieve the nurse of responsibility to observe the site frequently.

Other physicians prefer that the sites be cleansed one or two times daily with peroxide or iodine-containing solutions and then have iodine ointments applied at the insertion sites. The rationale for cleansing around the pins is to keep the pin sites open to allow for free drainage of serous fluid so that it does not become a medium for bacteria. Whatever type of pin care is ordered, it must be performed using aseptic technique. Osteomyelitis, as the end result of a pin tract infection, is a chronic disabling condition that could have been prevented.

Diversional Activity Deficit. A nursing diagnosis of diversional activity deficit applies to the patient who complains of boredom, becomes inattentive, or is restless.[7] It is the result of a monotonous environment with little interesting activity. It may be discovered, upon further assessment, that the patient is experiencing social isolation or sensory deprivation or overload rather than diversional activity deficit.

Varying the environment and the daily routine can help to alleviate these feelings. Allow the patient to make decisions about when routines, such as bathing, will be done. If the bed can be moved, rolling the patient into the hall, the lounge areas, or outdoor patios does wonders for his spirits. Find out what sedentary activities the person is interested in and ask occupational therapy or recreation departments to provide activities to occupy his time. Allow the patient time to ventilate. It is also important to drop into the patient's room just to talk when there are no tasks to be done for him. Find out his interests and discuss them. This activity can communicate that the nursing staff respects him as an individual and not just a patient.

Powerlessness Related to Hospitalization. Although a diagnosis of powerlessness related to hospitalization will not apply to every patient in traction, it occurs frequently enough for consideration. Many factors contribute to the perception of loss of control. Lack of privacy, lack of knowledge, social isolation, violation of personal space, and dependence on others for activities of daily living are causes. Patients experiencing a feeling of powerlessness respond in various ways. They may express their frustration over inability to control events. They may respond to their situation with depression, apathy, anger, or aggressive behavior, and they may be hesitant to make decisions.

To plan nursing interventions, the causative factors must be identified and the patient can be assisted to determine what in his current environment he can control. Allow the patient to make decisions about when routine activities are carried out, when he prefers visitors, and how his room is arranged. Keep the patient informed about his condition and plan for care. If it is not possible to provide all necessary information, the nurse can arrange for the patient to meet with the health care provider who can.

Respecting the patient's right to privacy is one of the most beneficial interventions. Provide the patient with planned periods of time when he will not be interrupted. Knock on the door before entering his room. Respect his possessions and ask his permission to get items from his bedside stand when necessary. Ensure that the patient's body is not left exposed during bathing or treatments. Providing the patient uninterrupted privacy for sexual expression, either by himself or with a significant other, is also important.

Keeping his belongings, call bell, and television control within his reach will contribute to the patient's sense of control in his environment. It is also helpful if he has access to calendars and newspapers and that he be able to continue with those daily habits that can be arranged in the hospital. For example, the patient who always watches the evening news should have his schedule arranged so that he may continue to do so.

Evaluation

Expected outcomes for the patient include

- Neurovascular status of extremity intact
- Absence of the signs and symptoms of immobility complications
- Skin intact
- No evidence of infection at the pin site
- Participates in diversional activities
- Identifies situational factors that he can control
- Participates in decisions about care and discharge planning

Gait and Mobility Problems Due to Musculoskeletal Disorders

Gait is the pattern of walking requiring the coordinated actions of muscles and joints. When joint range of motion is decreased, muscle weakness is present, or central nervous system balance is affected, a limp or exaggerated gait motion compensates. The assessment of gait is discussed in Chapter 86. The nursing diagnosis/problem is impaired physical mobility. The intervention is providing assistance.

Many aids are available to increase a person's mobility. Braces, crutches, walkers, and canes—when used appropriately—make it possible for patients with deformities or disabilities, joint pains, or fractures to move around in their environment.

Braces

Braces and splints are used to immobilize painful joints for comfort or to prevent fatigue during ambulation. They may also be used to prevent motion in a portion of the leg to permit ambulation. Examples are knee braces that support unstable knees or a short leg brace that is designed to prevent or correct foot drop.

Crutches

Crutches are the ambulatory aid used most frequently. There are various types available for use with different injuries, disabilities, or muscle strengths. Crutches are used during healing of sprains or fractures, after surgery for protection of repairs, and after amputations. Permanent use of crutches may be anticipated for some musculoskeletal and neuromuscular disorders. Physical therapy departments usually fit the patient for crutches and provide the instructions. However nurses need to know the basics so they are able to assess whether the patient is using the crutches correctly on a continuing basis as well as to instruct patients in the absence of a physical therapist.

Preparing for Crutch Walking. Walking with crutches requires strong upper extremities. While the patient is in bed or in the wheelchair, there are exercises he can do to strengthen the muscles he will be using. He can do push-ups from the prone position. Sitting push-ups can be done either in bed or in a wheelchair by pushing down with the hands, extending the elbows, and lifting the buttocks off the bed or chair.

Isometric exercises such as gluteal setting and quadriceps setting on the unaffected leg are necessary to maintain the strength of those muscles for ambulation. For gluteal setting, instruct the patient to squeeze his buttocks together and hold for a count of ten. To teach the individual to tighten his quadriceps muscle, instruct him to tighten the muscle by pushing the back of his knee into the bed.

Fitting the Crutches. Though there are several types of crutches available, axillary crutches are the most common and will be the ones considered here. When a patient is measured for crutches, the overall height of the crutch should be 2 to 3 finger widths below the anterior axillary fold when the crutch tips are 6 inches to 9 inches diagonally in front of the toes. The handpiece should be positioned so that the elbow is flexed 25 degrees to 30 degrees when the handpiece is grasped.

The Three-Point Crutch Gait. The most common gait used for orthopedic patients is the three-point nonweight-bearing gait. It is used when one leg cannot bear weight. To walk, both of the crutches and the involved extremity are advanced, the body weight is then supported on the crutches through the hands and on the unaffected extremity (3 points). Weight should not be placed on the axillae, but on the hands. Then with full weight supported on the hands, the unaffected leg swings to the crutches to again yield three points of contact.

Protecting the Crutch-Walking Person from Physical Injury. Patients should wear well-fitting, low-heeled or flat shoes. It is a good idea to place a belt securely around the patient's waist and to hold on to it from behind until his gait is steady. A belt gives the assistant some control if the patient should lose his balance. The rubber tips on the ends of the crutches must be intact.

Persons should walk erect with the head up. Crutch-walking patients must be instructed not to lean on their crutches because they could develop a "crutch palsy." Pressure on axillary nerves and blood vessels causes numbness and tingling in the hands. If allowed to persist, permanent disability may occur.

The patient on crutches must be taught to look for hazards in his environment. Crutches may slip on wet floors, ice, throw rugs on floors, or almost any obstacle on the floor, so the patient should observe the areas in front of him. He also needs to be warned that it is more difficult to walk on carpeting.

Canes

Canes are used for balance and to reduce weight-bearing stress on a knee or hip, and to reduce weakness or instability in one leg. A cane is held in the hand opposite the affected extremity. The cane height should allow 15 degrees to 30 degrees of elbow flexion. For walking, the cane is advanced at the same time as the involved leg, thus shifting the weight onto the unaffected leg.

Walkers

Walkers provide a wide base of support and thus the most security for ambulation. They are often used by elderly persons. To walk, the patient lifts the walker and advances it a short distance and then steps forward. Many patients can progress from the walker to crutches as they gain strength.

Evaluation

Expected outcomes for the patient using ambulatory aids are

- Demonstrates the correct gait with the aid
- Demonstrates safe ambulation
- Describes hazards in the environment that could cause accidents

Problems of Joint Motion, Rest, and Activity

Situations interfering with joint range of motion are of many types. Stiffness and contractures result from pain, immobility, inflammatory processes, fractures, and dislocations. Nurses must take a very active role in preventing limitation of motion and in teaching patients to maintain their maximal range of motion.

Loss of mobility due to disuse often begins with joint pain. Individuals tend not to move joints that are painful to protect themselves from the pain. Joint stiffness can also follow a fracture near or through a joint surface by formation of periarticular adhesions. Inflammatory processes interfere with joint motion as fibrous tissue forms around and between the joint surfaces to restrict motion.

Contractures are the end result of immobility. This deformity occurs when muscles are held in a shortened or contracted position for a prolonged period. Although it is much less common, a contracture may also occur when muscles are held in the stretched position.

Nursing Diagnoses and Interventions

Alteration in Comfort Related to Joint Stiffness

Joint stiffness can be defined as a feeling of discomfort or restriction when the patient attempts to move a joint after an inactive period.[42] The inactive period may be as short as an hour. The stiffness may occur after rest, with activity relieving it or it may occur after activity, in which case it is relieved by rest.

Heat is often effective in relieving joint stiffness. It softens the fibrous tissue around the joint for easier motion as well as produces an analgesic effect. Heat can be in the form of tub baths, showers, hot packs, or heating pads. Range-of-motion exercises are more comfortable and effective when done immediately after heat application. Patients with joint problems, however, should be cautioned about avoiding excessive exercise. It is better to exercise for short periods and increase the number of exercise periods in a day. A good rule of thumb is that if joint pain lasts for longer than ½ hour after exercise, the exercise was too vigorous.

There are many assistive devices available for persons with pain or impairment of joint motion. Crutches, canes, or walkers can be used to reduce weight-bearing stresses on lower extremities. Elevated toilet seats make it easier to get on and off toilets. There are aids to help open door knobs and jar lids, long-handled reachers for obtaining items from the floor, long-handled shoe horns, eating utensils with builtup handles, and meat cutters. Devices that help in dressing such as zipper pulls, devices to help button clothing, and devices to put on stockings are available. Velcro closures on clothing and shoes are very helpful. Patients in need of these aids can be referred to occupational and physical therapists for determination of the best aids for the individual and for instructions in their use.

Persons with joint involvement need instructions for protecting their joints from further injury. Alternating rest with activity and alternating sitting and standing tasks varies joint use. Frequently used objects can be placed in easily accessible areas to decrease the need to reach and bend. Sliding an object along a countertop requires less energy and joint motion than picking it up. Clothing that is worn together, for example a skirt and blouse, can be hung together in closets. The occupational therapist again is an excellent resource person for assisting the patient to modify his daily activities to protect his joints.

The most effective measure to prevent joint stiffness is movement through the full range of motion of the joints. Active range of motion is preferable. However, if the muscles are paralyzed, passive range of motion is necessary. When doing passive range of motion, do not force the joint beyond its point of resistance. Doing so could have the opposite effect, causing more damage and further loss of motion.

Impaired Physical Mobility Related to Contractures

If joint motion is reduced by contractures, much more energy is required for a person to move and he will fatigue more easily. His rehabilitation may be greatly prolonged. Contractures as a result of immobility are preventable. Attention must be given to correct positioning of the patient and to frequent changing of the position. No position is a good position if it is continuous.

Some common contractures, their definitions, and prophylactic nursing measures are listed in Table 87–5. Flexion contractures are most common because flexor muscles are stronger than extensors. Patients also tend to lie in positions of flexion and adduction in attempts to relieve back and joint discomfort, to keep warm, and to feel secure. Comfort measures such as back rubs, warm drinks, extra blankets, and psychological support may alleviate these needs. The patient should spend frequent periods in the position of extension as well as doing active or passive range of motion.

TABLE 87–5
Nursing Strategies to Prevent Specific Joint Contractures

1. *Foot drop:* Deformity of the foot in plantar flexion as a result of shortening of the Achilles tendon and stretching of the anterior leg muscles
   a. Use a padded footboard or pillows to maintain the functional position of the foot. Remove the footboard several times daily for range of motion to the foot.
   b. Keep the bedclothes from putting pressure on the toes and foot.
2. *Knee flexion contracture:* Caused by contraction of the hamstring muscles with prolonged knee flexion
   a. Use pillows under knees judiciously.
   b. Allow for frequent full extension of the legs.
   c. Avoid prolonged sitting.
3. *Hip flexion contracture:* Contracture of muscles that flex the hip, resulting from prolonged sitting or a soft, sagging mattress
   a. Use a firm mattress or bedboards.
   b. Place the patient in a flat position for periods.
   c. Unless contraindicated, place the patient in the prone position daily.
4. *External rotation contractures of lower extremities:* Outward rotation at the hip joints due to relaxation of muscles
   a. A sandbag or pillow can be placed at the thigh or lower leg. Avoid placing sandbags at the fibular head, which would place pressure on the peroneal nerve.
   b. Use a trochanter roll. It is made by rolling a towel or bath blanket into a roll and placing it under the greater trochanter of the femur.
5. *Adduction contracture of the lower extremities:* Contracture of the hip adductor muscles most often related to lying on the side without support between the legs
   a. Place pillows between the legs when the patient is side-lying.
   b. Use an abduction pillow between the legs when the patient is supine.
6. *Adduction contracture of the upper extremities:* Results from contracture of pectoral muscles from lying or sitting with arms adducted
   a. Place supports between the arms and torso.
   b. Encourage hair combing, fastening the gown in the back, and lying the arms abducted.

Evaluation

Expected outcomes for the patient experiencing problems with joint range of motion include

- Individual demonstrates active or passive range-of-motion exercises or significant other demonstrates passive range of motion.
- Individual describes/demonstrates correct use of assistive devices and ambulation aids.
- Individual describes/demonstrates joint protection activities.
- Absences of joint contractures after a period of immobility

Pain Due to Musculoskeletal Problems

The discomfort associated with his condition is probably the patient's most immediate concern. Without relief from it, he cannot mobilize his resources toward coping with his disease or injury. If his pain is not alleviated it is very difficult for him to concentrate on an exercise program or any instructions he is receiving.

Nursing Diagnoses and Interventions

Alteration in Comfort: Muscle Spasms

Muscle spasms often occur after a sprain or a fracture, after surgery, or with a joint inflammation. They are involuntary contractions that start as a response to local pain and to the products of injury. These contractions are sustained and use a large amount of the available nutrients. In addition, some of the blood vessels are compressed. The resulting ischemia causes tissue damage, and substances are released that cause more pain. The additional pain produces more spasms.[46]

Patients experiencing muscle spasm will usually report it. They state that their muscles are jumping or they feel the ends of their bones grating. Occasionally, the nurse will actually observe the muscle activity. When the muscle tires, patients may report a poorly localized aching.

Muscle spasms are expected to gradually subside after immobilization with splints, casts, or traction. Application of ice is also an effective strategy for reducing spasms. The cold acts by decreasing the excitability of the muscle afferents.[46]

When chronic muscle spasms are the problem, both heat and cold have been recommended. Examples of conditions associated with chronic spasms are back and neck pain and arthritic joints. Heat may relax the muscle and reduce the tone; cold usually provides greater pain relief.

Alteration in Comfort: Pain

Pain is associated with almost all musculoskeletal disorders and can be quite severe and difficult to manage. The pain may be the acute pain associated with traumatic injuries or surgical procedures or it may be chronic in nature. Low back pain is the most common chronic pain syndrome associated with the musculoskeletal system.

Assessment of pain (see Chap. 9) is an ongoing process. It is necessary to determine the current cause of the pain so that the most appropriate strategy can be chosen. It is also important to continually assess the effects of each strategy or combination of strategies.

Pain in a musculoskeletal structure not only interferes with the patient's comfort, but can produce significant disability. A person with joint pain who does not move the joint as a protective mechanism may end up with a contracture. A patient with a fracture who does not exercise because of pain or fear of pain develops muscle atrophy and joint stiffness. In the instance of low back pain the socioeconomic impact must be considered when an individual is not able to work.

Nurses caring for orthopedic patients will use a variety of measures to provide pain relief. Knowledge of the patient's problem, a thorough assessment of the patient's pain and his response to it, and knowledgeable use of pain relief measures will contribute to achievement of goals relative to pain relief.

Drug Therapy for Pain

Many patients with traumatic injuries or surgical procedures involving musculoskeletal structures require narcotic *analgesics* for a period of time. How much and how long will depend on the patient and the nature of the insult. It is important for nurses to gain as much knowledge as they can about pain and the pharmacology of analgesic drugs to enable them to use drugs most effectively.

There has been a recent trend to undertreat patients in severe pain with narcotics. Studies have demonstrated that significant numbers of patients (41% and 73%) treated with narcotic analgesics still experienced moderate to severe pain.[24,48] The fear of causing addiction was identified as a major reason why physicians order insufficient doses of narcotics in insufficient frequencies and why nurses may withhold narcotics from patients in pain. Actually, there is little chance of addiction when the patient is experiencing pain.[24,28] Patients usually stop taking the drug when their pain is gone.

The patient's response to the drug is the best indication of how much he needs and how frequently he may need it. The recommended doses in the pharmacology references are just that—recommended doses. When the first prescribed dose is administered, observe the effects. Document the amount of pain relief, the length of time it took for the patient to feel relief, and the duration of action. If the pain returns before the patient can have another dose, the dose may be too low or the time between doses is too long. If he still has pain an hour after administration when most drugs should be reaching their peak effect, the dose may be too low. Conversely, if the patient is very sedated or respiratory depression develops, the dose may be too high.[29] Remember, however, that patients can be quite sedated and still experience pain. In that case, he may need a different drug.

It is the nurse's responsibility to report the patient's response to analgesics to the physician and ask for changes if the patient's pain is not relieved. The drug orders can be changed. Musculoskeletal pain can be quite severe and can last several days. Inadequate pain relief can impair the patient's ability to cope with his entire situation and prolong his reports of pain.

The best approach to pain relief is a preventive one.[29] This means giving analgesics before the pain becomes severe. Some patients may choose to delay taking medication until the pain becomes unbearable. It is much more difficult to control and may require larger drug doses when pain is that severe. Getting control of the pain may require around-the-clock administration rather than a prn basis for a period of time. This approach is especially useful when switching from injectable to oral drugs.

Besides narcotics, drugs useful for relieving musculoskeletal pain are aspirin, acetaminophen, and the other nonsteroidal anti-inflammatory drugs. Tricyclic antidepressants are being used successfully in some chronic pain situations.[28]

Distraction

The strategy of *distraction* can be defined as directing the attention away from the painful sensation and toward other stimuli.[28] It does not take the pain away, but it reduces the perception of the discomfort and increases the person's tolerance. Distraction is only effective as long as the person is directing his attention elsewhere. When distraction ends, the person again becomes aware of the pain.[30]

The most effective distraction methods are those that use a combination of auditory, visual, or tactile–kinesthetic stimuli.[28] Auditory input may be music or being read to by another person. Examples of visual methods are slide-viewing or staring at a stationary object. Touch–movement stimuli may result from rhythmic breathing, being held, or rocking. There is no solid empirical evidence yet as to exactly how distraction interferes with pain impulse transmission, but it does work and should be encouraged.

There is a need for more widespread recognition by health professionals that patients do use distraction. Physicians, nurses, and technicians use distraction regularly to divert patients' attention from uncomfortable procedures. Yet, as Wiener identified in studying low back pain patients on an orthopedic unit, many nurses are quick to judge the amount of pain patients are having by their behavior at a particular moment without looking at whether or not the patients are using distraction techniques.[52] Nurses need to obtain a careful history of methods patients are using to relieve pain and then support that use.

Because of the short-term effects of distraction, patients could be medicated (or treated in another manner) while they are engaged in distraction so that their medication will be taking effect when distraction ends. The nurse and the patient could plan together how they will use distraction and other pain relief measures to achieve maximal results.

One research finding is that only slowly rising pain is amenable to distraction.[33] It is difficult for a patient to gain control over pain that rapidly increases in intensity. Therefore, if a painful procedure is anticipated, it is helpful to begin distraction methods beforehand.

Cold and Heat Applications

Cold relieves pain as well as muscle spasm. Cold slows nerve conduction velocity in sensory and motor nerves and thus slows the conduction of pain impulses to the brain. Cold is being used more frequently now than ever before since patients find that it acts quickly and the effects last longer than those of heat.

Cold can be applied in several ways, including ice bags and commercially available cold packs. Cold damp towels may also be used. If using ice packs, a towel or pad of some type should be placed between the patient's skin and the pack to avoid damaging the skin. Ice massage to the lower back is effective in producing temporary local anesthesia in chronic back pain.

Heat probably is not as effective in relieving pain as is cold, but some patients find it preferable. Heat increases the pain threshold by depressing the excitability of free nerve endings and peripheral nerve fibers, which is similar to what cold does.[21]

Heat can be applied with electric heating pads, warm moist packs, heat lamps, or warm tub baths and showers. Physical therapists use paraffin baths, diathermy, whirlpool baths, and hydrocollator packs to apply heat. In hospitals, the use of heat usually requires a physician's order.

Heat is not used immediately after trauma because it may cause an increase in bleeding and edema. It should be used with caution in patients with sensory deficits and in patients who are sedated or unable to communicate.

Other nursing strategies useful for patients with musculoskeletal pain include relaxation techniques, positioning, and other cutaneous stimulation techniques. Cutaneous stimulation may include massage and application of menthol ointments. A combination of techniques is often most effective in relieving pain.

Evaluation

Expected outcomes for the person experiencing pain are as follows. The patient

- Verbalizes comfort
- Demonstrates or discusses use of appropriate noninvasive pain relief measures
- Discusses appropriate use of analgesics for his situation
- Demonstrates improved mobility as comfort increases
- Identifies activities that increase discomfort and avoids or modifies those activities

Low Back Pain

The problem of low back pain is a very common one and deserves consideration. Studies done in several countries demonstrate that 80% of the population will experience some degree of back pain during a lifetime.[36] In the 30- to 60-year age-group, investigations have reported it to be the most expensive health problem.[35] The number of workdays lost due to low back pain is probably second only to the days lost from upper respiratory infections.[19,35] Back pain, therefore, is a significant socioeconomic problem.

Attacks of acute back pain may begin around the age of 25.[37] Pain in 90% of the persons will subside within 2 months.[37] But it does have a tendency to recur, although subsequent attacks may not be as severe.

The exact cause of most back pain remains unknown. Epidemiological studies have found that bank clerks, farmers, heavy industrial workers, and nurses were likely to have low back pain at a younger age.[51] Truck drivers have a very high incidence of back pain.[18,43] Prolonged sitting plus the transmission of vibratory forces to the spine may be the mechanism for this pain.[51] More sedentary workers also develop low back pain, but they do not lose as much time from work as the person whose occupation involves heavier manual labor.

Nursing Interventions

With a problem as prevalent as this one, it is inevitable that professional nurses will encounter patients with recurrent low back pain for which no cause is found. Nurses can assist the patient to improve his comfort, mobility, and ability to perform activities of daily living. The activities outlined here that reduce stress on the lower back and increase muscular support to the spine may also help prevent further episodes of low back pain. It should be remembered, however, that each patient's pain, disability, psychosocial outlook, and general health is individual. Therefore, an instructional program must be planned in collaboration with other health-care team members after a thorough patient assessment.

Positioning

A very comfortable position for the patient to assume is the psoas position. In this position, the person lies on the back with a small pillow under the head and with the hips and knees flexed nearly 90 degrees, the legs resting on a chair. This can also be accomplished in bed by supporting the legs with pillows. With the hips and knees bent, the psoas muscle relaxes to decrease the load on the lumbar spine.[23] Because of the psoas relaxation, this position is recommended for 20-minute periods three times a day.

Persons with back pain often are most comfortable sleeping on a very firm mattress. They should be encouraged to try various positions in bed until they find those most comfortable for them.

A variety of studies on sitting in various types of chairs have been done. During unrelaxed, unsupported sitting, the load on the lumbar spine is greater than during standing.[38] This is probably due to the pelvis tilting backward with a flattening of the lumbar lordosis.[23] During supported sitting the loads are less because part of the weight of the body is supported by the backrest. The lowest intradiskal pressure and electromyelogram activity of the paraspinal muscles were found with the subject sitting in a chair with a backrest angle of 120 degrees and a 5-cm lumbar support. The highest intradiskal pressure was found when sitting in a straight-back chair with no lumbar support. In all types of chairs, the use of arm rests decreased the intradiskal pressure.[35] The implications are to assist the patient to identify chairs that may be more comfortable for him. If there is no lumbar support, a rolled towel or very small pillow placed in the lower back area will suffice. A patient's feet should always reach the floor when sitting; if they do not, stools or pillows should be used to support them. Studies done on car drivers' seats recommended the same backrest angle and lumbar support as for a chair.[4] In addition, these investigators recommended the use of automatic transmissions, since both pushing in the clutch and shifting gears increased intradiskal pressure.

The thoughts on standing posture are somewhat conflicting. It has often been suggested that one foot be placed on a stool or a lower shelf while standing for long periods, such as during ironing or doing dishes. This position relaxes the psoas muscle, but it also flattens the lordotic curve and there is evidence that flattening the curve increases pressure in the intervertebral disk. Until there is more definitive data, it is suggested that nurses assist the patient in determining which position might be comfortable for him. It may be that the subjective information which suggests lifting one leg as the most comfortable is correct, but it is not yet documented.[51]

Lifting

Numerous studies on lifting have been done since patients with back pain all experience increases in pain with increased loads. Nachemson reported that the most significant factor is the distance of the load from the body.[35] The crucial point is to keep the load close to the body from the time it is picked up until it is put down again. Another important item to teach patients is to always face the object they will be lifting. It has been demonstrated that both disk pressure and intra-abdominal pressure increase when the trunk is loaded in lateral flexion and in rotation.[3]

Persons should also be aware that whenever there is a choice between pushing or pulling a load, the pushing should be chosen. There is a smaller increase in disk load with pushing.[51]

Exercising

Traditionally, sit-up exercises have been used to strengthen abdominal muscles with the goal of increasing intra-abdominal pressure. An increase in intra-abdominal pressure produces an air or fluid cushion that creates turgor in the soft tissues to support the spine.[51] However, it has not been demonstrated empirically that abdominal strength determines the ability to increase intra-abdominal pressure.[16]

If sit-ups are to be done, a curl or half sit-up is recommended. The patient begins supine with the knees flexed and lifts the head and shoulders just until the shoulder blades clear the surface. The patient should wait for acute pain to subside before beginning sit-up exercises.

Cady and co-workers studied 1652 firefighters for 3 years to determine the effects of strength and fitness on subsequent back injuries. On the basis of objective measurements of fitness, the firefighters were placed in one of three categories: Least Fit, Middle Fit, and Most Fit. The results revealed that physical fitness and conditioning are preventive measures for back injuries and that further investigation is warranted in other occupational groups. The Least Fit had 7.1% injured, the Middle Fit 3.2%, and the Most Fit 0.8% injured.[6]

The benefits of exercise are well known to nurses. In addition to conditioning body structures and improving their endurance, exercise increases mental alertness and provides for a sense of accomplishment. Also with vigorous exercise, there may be an increase in the endorphin levels, which decreases pain and in general makes a person feel better. Recommended exercises are walking, running, swimming, and bicycling. Whichever is chosen by the patient, it should be done at least three times a week for 20 minutes. As with any aerobics program, the patient should start slowly and work up to the 20-minute period.

Activities to Avoid

There are several activities that should be avoided. Bilateral straight-leg raising has often been recommended for abdominal strengthening but it has not been shown to activate the abdominal muscles. Instead, the psoas muscle pulls the lumbar area into lordosis.[23]

Leaning forward, whether from the standing or sitting position, increases intradiskal pressures and should be avoided. If it is necessary to bend over to accomplish a task, sit down next to it or move it to a higher surface. When sitting at a desk or table, move the body in as close as possible to avoid forward bending.

Obesity, of course, should be avoided. It not only increases the compressive forces on the spine but also increases the anterior load just as if the individual were carrying a heavy box.

Nurses do have an important role in assisting patients to improve their comfort and to prevent further episodes of low back pain. Assessing patients, evaluating new research reports, and conducting investigations are all part of nursing's responsibility in determining how best to affect the quality of life for the person with low back pain.

References

1. Aaron RK, Ciombor D: Venous thromboembolis in the orthopedic patient. Surg Clin North Am 63:529, 1983
2. Ahmed MC: Choosing the best method to manage pressure ulcers. Nurses' Drug Alert (special report) 4:113, 1980
3. Andersson GBJ, Orentgren R, Nachemson A: Intradiskal pressure, intra-abdominal pressure, and myoelectric back muscle activity related to posture and loading. Clin Orthop 129:156, 1977
4. Andersson GBJ, Orentgren R, Nachemson A, Elfstrom G: Lumbar disc pressure and myoelectric back muscle activity during sitting, IV. Studies on a car driver's seat. Scand J Rehabil Med 6:128, 1974
5. Ashton H: The effect of increased tissue pressure on blood flow. Clin Orthop 113:15, 1975
6. Cady LD, Bischoff DP, O'Connell ER et al: Strength and fitness

and subsequent back injuries in fire fighters. J Occup Med 21:269, 1979

7. Carpenito LJ: Nursing Diagnosis Application to Clinical Practice. Philadelphia, JB Lippincott, 1983
8. Cruess RL, Dumont J: Healing of bone, tendon, and ligament. In Rockwood CA, Green DP (eds): Fractures, vol. 1. Philadelphia, JB Lippincott, 1975
9. Dietrick JE, Whedon GD, Shorr E: Effects of immobilization upon various metabolic and physiologic functions of normal men. Am J Med 4:3, 1948
10. Donaldson CL, Hulley SB, Vogel JM et al: Effect of prolonged bed rest on bone mineral. Metabolism 19:1071, 1970
11. Evarts CM: Complications. In Rockwood CA, Green DP (eds): Fractures, vol. 1. Philadelphia, JB Lippincott, 1975
12. Glancy GL: Compartmental syndromes. ONA Journal 2:148, 1975
13. Goldring SR, Krane SM: Metabolic bone disease. DM 27:1, 1981
14. Hankin FM, Gragg AS, Kaufer H: Bleeding beneath postoperative plaster casts. Orthopaedic Nursing 2:27, 1983
15. Issekutz B, Blizzard JJ, Birkhead NC, Rodahl K: Effect of prolonged bedrest on urinary calcium output. J Appl Physiol 21:1013, 1966
16. Jackson CP, Brown MD: Analysis of current approaches and a practical guide to prescription of exercise. Clin Orthop 179:46, 1983
17. Jaworski ZFG: Physiology and pathology of bone remodeling. Orthop Clin North Am 12:485, 1981
18. Kelsey J: An epidemiological study of acute herniated lumbar intervertebral discs. Rheumatol Rehabil 14:144, 1975
19. Kelsey JL: Idiopathic low back pain: Magnitude of the problem. In White AA, Gordon SL (eds): American Academy of Orthopaedic Surgeons Symposium on Idiopathic Low Back Pain. St Louis, CV Mosby, 1982
20. Lane PL, Lee MM: New synthetic casts: What nurses need to know. Orthopedic Nursing 1:13, November–December, 1982
21. Lehmann JF, Warren CG, Scham SM: Therapeutic heat and cold. Clin Orthop 99:207, 1974
22. Lewis RC Jr: Handbook of Traction, Casting and Splinting Techniques. Philadelphia, JB Lippincott, 1977
23. Lindh M: Biomechanics of the lumbar spine. In Frankel VH, Nordin M (eds): Basic Biomechanics of the Skeletal System. Philadelphia, Lea & Febiger, 1980
24. Marks RM, Sachar EJ: Undertreatment of medical inpatients with narcotic analgesics. Ann Intern Med 78:173, 1973
25. Matsen FA: Compartmental syndrome: An unified concept. Clin Orthop 113:8, 1975
26. Matsen FA, Clawson DK: The deep posterior compartmental syndrome of the leg. J Bone Joint Surg 57A:34, 1975
27. Matsen FA, Winquist RA, Krugmire RB: Diagnosis and management of compartmental syndromes. J Bone Joint Surg 62A:286, 1980
28. McCaffery M: Nursing Management of the Patient with Pain, 2nd ed, pp 92, 99, 206, 222. Philadelphia, JB Lippincott, 1979
29. McCaffery M: Patients shouldn't have to suffer: How to relieve pain with injectable narcotics. Nursing 10:34, October, 1980
30. McCaffery M: Relieving pain with noninvasive techniques. Nursing 10:54, December, 1980
31. McFarland MB: Encircling cast drainage: Is it valuable? Orthopaedic Nursing 3:41, 1984
32. McMaster WC, Liddle S, Waugh TR: Laboratory evaluation of various cold therapy modalities. Am J Sports Med 6:291, 1978
33. Melzack R, Weisz AZ, Sprague LT: Stratagems for controlling pain: Contributions of auditory stimulation and suggestion. Exp Neurol 8:239, 1963
34. Mubarak SJ, Hargens AR: Acute compartment syndromes. Surg Clin North Am 63:539, 1983
35. Nachemson AL: The lumbar spine: An orthopaedic challenge. Spine 1:59, 1976
36. Nachemson AL: A critical look at the treatment for low back pain. Scand J Rehabil Med 11:143, 1979
37. Nachemson AL: The natural course of low back pain. In White AA, Gordon SL (eds): American Academy of Orthopaedic Surgeons Symposium on Idiopathic Low Back Pain. St Louis, CV Mosby, 1982
38. Nachemson AL, Morris JM: In vivo measurements of intradiscal pressure: Discometry, a method for the determination of pressure in the lower lumbar discs. J Bone Joint Surg 46A:1077, 1964
39. Natow AB: Nutrition in prevention and treatment of decubitus ulcers. Topics in Clinical Nursing 5:39, 1983
40. Nelson JP, Ferris DO, Ivins JC: The cast syndrome. Postgrad Med 42:457, 1967
41. Orthopedic Nurses' Association, American Nurses' Association Division on Medical–Surgical Nursing Practice: Standards of Orthopedic Nursing Practice. Kansas City, American Nurses' Association, 1975
42. Polley HF, Hunder GG: Rheumatologic Interviewing and Physical Examination of the Joints, 2nd ed. Philadelphia, WB Saunders, 1978
43. Snook SH: Low back pain in industry. In White AA, Gordon SL (eds): American Academy of Orthopaedic Surgeons Symposium on Idiopathic Low Back Pain. St Louis, CV Mosby, 1982
44. Steinberg ME, Trueta J: Effects of activity on bone growth and development in the rat. Clin Orthop 156:52, 1981
45. Vaughn J: The Physiology of Bone, 3rd ed. New York, Oxford, 1981
46. Warren CG: The use of heat and cold in the treatment of common musculoskeletal disorders. In Kessler RM, Hertling D (eds): Management of Common Musculoskeletal Disorders. Philadelphia, Harper & Row, 1983
47. Waxdahl KA: Effects of Application of Ice on Itching. Unpublished master's thesis, University of Washington, 1982
48. Weis OF, Sriwatanakul K, Alloza JL et al: Attitudes of patients, housestaff, and nurses toward postoperative analgesic care. Anesth Analg 62:70, 1983
49. Whedon GD, Lutwak L, Rambaut PC et al: Mineral and nitrogen balance study observations: The second manned Skylab mission. Aviat Space Environ Med 47:391, 1976
50. Whedon GD, Lutwak L, Reid J et al: Mineral and nitrogen metabolic studies on Skylab orbital space flights. Trans Assoc Am Physicians 87:95, 1974
51. White AA, Panjabi MM: Clinical Biomechanics of the Spine, pp 279, 281, 308, 329, 332–333. Philadelphia, JB Lippincott, 1978
52. Wiener CL: Pain assessment on an orthopedic ward. Nurs Outlook 23:508, 1975

Chapter 88

Musculoskeletal Trauma

Dee Malchow

Musculoskeletal trauma is defined as an injury from external force to the skeleton and therefore to all tissues surrounding it. As nurses we are concerned not only with the impact on the skeleton and the tissues adjacent to it but also with structures enclosed or supported by it. When the bones break, the muscles cannot move; blood vessels are ruptured and circulation is impaired; and nerve supply is interrupted so further movement and sensation is blocked. Thus, we are concerned with more than the skeletal injury; we have an awareness of probable assault to adjacent structures as well.

There are many ways of causing or predisposing an individual to musculoskeletal trauma. Accidents are probably the most obvious cause and may occur at home (*e.g.,* falls in bathtub, downstairs, or over phone cord), at work (*e.g.,* lifting, using machinery, dropping things), or from motor driven vehicles (*e.g.,* impact within or outside a car, boat, motorcycle, or train) to give a few examples. Motor vehicles often cause severe injury to several other systems in addition to musculoskeletal trauma because of the intense impact involved. Most sport and recreational activities involve risk of injury from persistent vigorous action. The degree of injury may range, for example, from tennis elbow (inflammation of the elbow joint) to a compound fracture of the femur from ski racing.

Occasionally, unexpected injury may result from rather innocent activities. For example, the ankle may twist slightly and be fractured or sprained just from getting up from a chair; or a jaw may dislocate from an extra-wide yawn.

Pathological fractures are common when the individual has a predisposing condition such as cancer or osteoporosis. Aging itself can also predispose a person to injury because of a natural increase in the brittleness of the bones and a loss of balance and coordination. Often aging is accompanied by diminishing vision, hearing, and touch that would otherwise warn the individual of a dangerous situation. Other conditions that the elderly may face are cerebral ischemia (decreased blood supply to the brain), dizziness, arthritis, and muscular weakness, all of which predispose the sufferer to injury.[10]

In treating this type of injury the goal is to immobilize the affected area until healing occurs. Support and immobilization are commonly achieved through casts, splints, and slings. Internally, pins, screws, rods, or wires may be used. In achieving and maintaining proper alignment of the broken ends, traction may be applied.

Although immobilization is the goal, it can often result in stiffness of the muscles and joints. To counteract this, active and passive motion of the extremity is promoted. Some forms of treatment (*i.e.,* rods and pins) allow movement from the early stage. Other supports (*i.e.,* casts and splints) are more restrictive and allow only limited motion. Physical therapy can be invaluable in these cases by permitting normal healing and maintaining optimum function.

Soft Tissue Injuries

Contusions. A blow or blunt force (*e.g.*, a kick or fall) applied to the soft tissues is usually the cause of a contusion. The resulting injury to the blood vessels will cause localized bleeding and therefore the bruised effect, or ecchymosis, common to this injury. The skin becomes discolored, first turning red and purple from the small vessel hemorrhage. As it heals and the fluids are resorbed, it will become brown and then yellow before regaining its normal color. Besides the discoloration, symptoms include localized tenderness and swelling.

Occasionally a sac of blood may develop, called a hematoma. Like the contusion, hematomas are usually absorbed by the system but require more time. The physician may elect to aspirate this collection of fluid and clotted blood or remove it surgically to enhance healing.

Strains. Strains are small, incomplete muscle tears that have caused some bleeding into the tissues. They are caused by overstretching or overexertion of a local group of muscles. They often occur during sports activities, with muscle fatigue or a sudden twisting action. A strain involves the muscle–tendon unit and not the ligaments.

Symptoms include sudden severe local pain, which may be incapacitating. Passive stretching of the affected area may provide some relief, but tenderness continues and swelling rapidly follows. Ecchymosis may appear. A radiograph to rule out possible fracture is needed.

Sprain. When the ligaments are torn or detached in a muscular injury, it is called a sprain. Usually the cause is similar to that of a strain—a wrenching or twisting action, often during sports activities. Along with the ligament tear, there is also ecchymosis from ruptured blood vessels. Avulsion fractures (*i.e.*, the pull of a ligament or tendon dislodges a bone fragment) are not uncommon in this kind of injury, and therefore a radiograph is needed.

Loss of function is obvious, and protection of the injured site is vital. Providing stability for a joint while at the same time providing for its mobility is the key function of a ligament. A torn ligament obviously lacks this stability. Other symptoms include swelling and severe pain. Occasionally the disability is not quickly apparent but becomes so 2 to 3 hours after the injury has occurred.

Nursing Management

Assessment and Nursing Diagnosis

Based on the assessment data, nursing history, and clinical symptoms, the major nursing diagnoses are alteration in comfort due to pain from soft tissue injuries and impaired physical mobility secondary to pain and loss of function of affected areas.

Goals and Interventions

Immediate application of cold for about the first 24 to 48 hours will minimize bleeding, swelling, and pain in soft tissue injuries. After this initial period, intermittent heat will promote circulation and healing. Usually a series of 15- to 30-minute applications four times daily is desirable. This intervention will promote the healing goals of vasodilation, absorption, and repair.

Strains and sprains are also best managed with immediate elevation and immobilization. An elastic pressure bandage is commonly used to achieve immobilization. Since the patient or a member of his family will need to reapply this bandage at intervals (every 8 hours for skin integrity), they should be carefully taught the principles of its application. Special care should be taken to demonstrate a snug supportive wrap that does not impede circulation. For more severe cases, immobilization can be ensured by applying either a cast or a splint. In some sprains where the ligament is completely ruptured, surgical repair may be necessary. Weight bearing can be allowed as tolerated, or the use of a cane or crutches may be required. A sprain of the ligaments in the cervical spine (as from a "whiplash" injury) will require a cervical collar to effect immobilization and relieve pressure.

Activity during the recovery phase varies with the extent of injury. A contusion responds most effectively to passive and active motion, within the limits of pain. Sprains, however, require more guarded activity during rehabilitation. The key principle that the patient must understand is that too much activity will disrupt healing and may cause further injury.[1] Exercise should progress slowly. Any swelling or pain at the injured site should signal immediate termination of the activity. With proper care a strain should heal completely in 3 to 6 weeks.

Evaluation

Healing time for a sprain is generally a month. When totally healed as evidenced by decreased pain and increased mobility, exercise and activity in moderation can begin. Patient education should stress that incomplete healing or repeated injury will cause the joint to be unstable. Careful management of its healing will minimize the joint's future susceptibility to injury.

Dislocations

Definition and Etiology

A dislocation occurs when the articulating surfaces of a joint are out of normal anatomical contact. They are essentially "out of joint" A partial separation of a joint is called a *subluxation.* The force required to produce this type of injury is usually greater than that causing a sprain or strain. Sometimes, however, this occurrence may be spontaneous; underlying pathological conditions such as arthritis, congenital weakness, or previous trauma in the same area may be responsible.

Pathophysiology

Dislocation creates severe distortion and stress on the associated joint structures, blood vessels, and nerves. If not relieved, nerve palsy or avascular necrosis (tissue death due to insufficient blood supply) may result. Also, the synovial nourishment to the cartilage is often disrupted. Without this the cartilage quickly deteriorates, resulting in a chronic painful joint with limited motion. A dislocation, therefore, because of its potential for permanent impairment must be regarded as a serious injury with a worse potential.

Clinical Manifestations

Clinical manifestations can include (1) pain, (2) limited motion, (3) shortening of the extremity, (4) a change in the joint's contour, (5) muscle spasm, and (6) a change in the joint's axis. Radiographs will confirm the diagnosis, discover whether the joint surface is fractured, and aid in its *reduction* (i.e., bringing the displaced parts into normal position).

Medical Management

Some dislocations will reduce themselves, leaving only a sprain. Usually reduction is done by a physician. Anesthesia is generally required for this most painful procedure in which the head of the bone is manipulated slowly and carefully back into the joint cavity. If soft tissue damage and edema are excessive, the dislocation may require open reduction (surgery). For example, the ruptured ligaments associated with severe knee injuries would require surgical intervention.

Nursing Management

Assessment and Nursing Diagnosis

Based on the nursing assessment, history, and clinical manifestations, the nursing diagnoses are alteration in comfort due to pain from the dislocation and impaired physical mobility related to the dislocated joint.

Goals and Interventions

Immediate care is aimed at limiting further trauma to the area by immobilizing the limb and applying cold to minimize edema. When reduction is achieved, it is important to keep the joint immobilized with a cast or by splinting and bandaging until healing is complete. Cold may be applied. Nursing management includes careful observation for pain, cyanosis, tingling or numbness, and limited motion of the distal joints. Observation for vascular or neurological compromise is common to all orthopedic injuries that require snug, supportive dressings. Regular assessment of skin color, temperature, and sensation must be made, and the bandage checked for inside or outside constriction. Muscle spasms may occur and may require management with prescribed analgesic or antispasmodic agents.

Immobilization should continue for 3 to 6 weeks, and during this time the adjacent joints should be actively exercised. When healing is complete, moderate, active movement of the joint is encouraged. Patient education should include the potential harm of passive stretch (not active extension of joint) at this stage. To prevent future injury and instability of the dislocated joint, it is helpful to tape or otherwise support it during athletics. Some degree of traumatic arthritis is likely to occur after any dislocation.[7]

Fractures

Fractures, quite simply, are breaks in the normal continuity of a bone. Every fracture results in soft tissue injury to some extent. Usually, however, a broken bone is not critical or dangerous unless it is accompanied by hemorrhage or shock, or both.

Bones have a high degree of hardness and strength, which is combined with a high level of resilience. Generally a significant impact is required to break them.

Etiology

Typical causes of fractures are[9]

- *Direct force* (the most frequent cause) breaking the bone at the point of contact
- A *shear force,* producing a torsion or twisting of the bone with a resultant fracture distant from the point of contact (*e.g.,* forceful twisting of the hand could result in a forearm fracture)
- *Strong, sudden muscle contraction* (*e.g.,* a rib may fracture with a severe coughing spell)
- *Muscle fatigue,* depriving the bones of the necessary support required for exertion and causing an uneven pull on them (*e.g.,* a skier often will sustain a break during a fall late in the day when muscles are fatigued)
- *Pathological conditions,* demineralizing the bone mass to a point at which it may break spontaneously. Examples of these conditions are osteoporosis (increased porosity of the bone), bone tumors (tumors decalcify bone), malnutrition, disuse, and metabolic disorders (*e.g.,* poor mineral absorption and hormonal changes)

Bones become weakened when they are not used. Osteogenesis, or the development of bones, is stimulated with weight bearing and activity. Conversely, with disuse the natural process of resorption of old bone cells is not balanced with osteogenesis. The bones become porous and therefore highly susceptible to fracture.

This risk of fracture is compounded in the hospital setting with prolonged bed rest and generalized weakness and ambulation in a strange environment, particularly if the patient is elderly, has other physical disabilities, or has undergone diagnostic tests or treatments. Awareness that all hospitalized patients are more susceptible to fractures than when healthy is a key to their prevention.

Types of Fractures

The types of fractures are many and varied. Only a few of the more than 150 will be discussed here (Fig. 88–1). Fractures can be described in many ways. The following are among the most common:

- *Simple or closed fracture:* The skin is intact over the site of fracture.
- *Compound or open fracture:* An external wound makes contact with the underlying fracture. Either an external object penetrates the skin and soft tissue and then breaks the bone (*e.g.,* when a car fender strikes the leg of a pedestrian) or the bone ends rupture the tissue and skin from the inside on fracture.
- *Incomplete:* Only one side of the bone breaks through the periosteum (*i.e.,* the fracture line only extends part way through the bone. This is often called a greenstick or willow fracture.
- *Complete:* The break or fracture line goes completely through the bone, and the periosteum is disrupted on both sides.
- *Impacted or telescoped:* One part of the fractured bone is driven into the other part.
- *Displaced:* The bone ends at the fracture site are pulled apart or separated from each other.
- *Complicated:* A body organ or other tissues sustain injury from the fracture (*e.g.,* a fractured rib may puncture a lung or disrupt nerves or blood vessels).
- *Comminuted:* The bone is broken in several pieces, often from a crush injury.
- *Hairline:* A thin break line occurs with no displacement of the bone.
- *Avulsion:* A bone fragment is pulled away at the attachment of a tendon or ligament.

The direction of the fracture line is used to further describe the break. Examples are

- *Transverse:* The fracture line is straight across or at right angles to the bone.
- *Linear:* The break goes up and down or parallel to the bone. It is sometimes called a longitudinal fracture.
- *Oblique:* The break line is at an angle to the bone shaft, usually about 45 degrees.
- *Spiral:* The break line twists around the bone. Sometimes this is called a torsion fracture and is caused by a twisting force.

The description of a fracture may include its cause.

- *Stress:* Too much activity to which the bone is not accustomed causes the break.
- *Pathological:* The bone has a preexisting disease that predisposes it to a fracture.

The location of a fracture on the bone may further be used to describe it. Such terms as epiphyseal, epicondylar (above a condyle), and articular (fracture at the joint), extracapsular (outside the joint) or intracapsular (inside the joint) fall into this category.

To be descriptive, most fractures can be and are described by several of the above terms. For example, in high-impact trauma it is possible to have a compound, comminuted, midshaft fracture of the tibia or a closed, nondisplaced stress fracture of a metatarsal head. These terms provide a quick description of the fracture, its location, its severity, whether it involves other tissues, and often its cause.

Clinical Manifestations

The symptoms or effects of a fracture are, in most circumstances, obvious. They include pain, deformity, swelling, discoloration, loss of function, crepitation, and abnormal motion. In the case of a compound fracture, the actual bone ends may still be protruding through the skin. Symptoms may be combined or inapparent. Routine radiographs of suspected injuries will aid in the diagnosis of asymptomatic fractures. The common fracture symptoms can be described as follows:

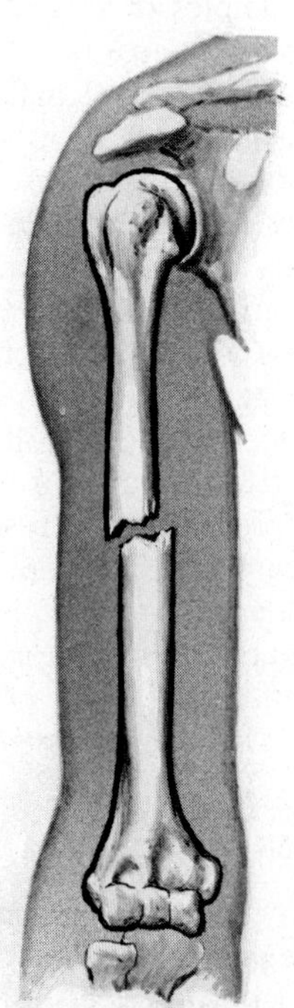
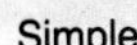

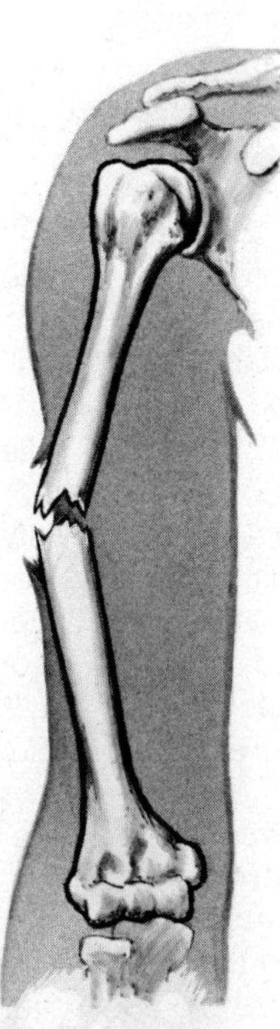

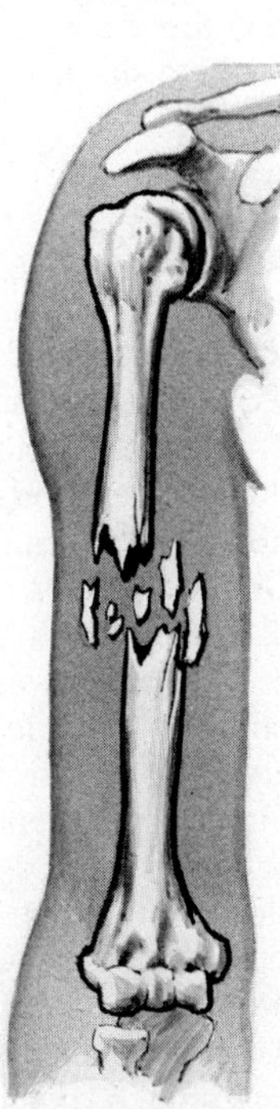

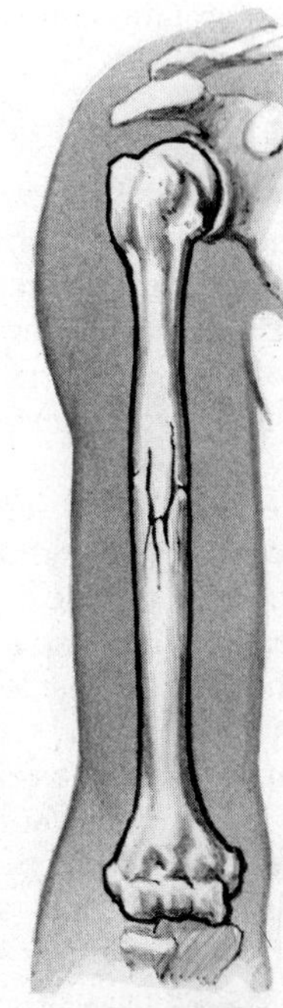

FIGURE 88–1 Types of fractures.

- *Pain* is nearly always present and usually severe, especially until the bone ends have been immobilized. The pain is intensified by injury to adjacent structures, swelling, muscle spasm, and any movement of the bone fragments. In some cases injury to sensory nerves may reduce the pain.
- *Ecchymosis* (bruising) and swelling result from the injury and bleeding, but may not be obvious for several days. These phenomena always occur to some degree, even if they are not noticeable, because a bone cannot break without damaging adjacent soft tissues.
- The *abnormal appearance* of the area around the fracture may be quite obvious, since changes occur according to the type of fracture and degree of angulation and depression of the bone.
- *Shortening of the bone* is common, especially when long bones are involved, and the strong muscles cause the edges of the bone to overlap.
- *Loss of normal function* and abnormal mobility are other typical symptoms. Often these symptoms are obvious, but if the injuries are subtle, a comparison with the unaffected extremity will help to confirm the diagnosis. Loss of function is due to the functional dependence of muscles on the stability of the bone to which they are attached.
- *Muscle spasms* may intensify the pain and the degree of deformity. Muscle rigidity, however, often causes a natural splinting effect, which keeps the bone ends immobile initially.

A grating noise (crepitus) can often be heard with movement of the injured part. It is caused by the edges of the broken bone rubbing together, and although it confirms the fracture it also causes soft tissue damage, and therefore should be avoided.[10]

Confirmation of the presence and degree of fracture are determined by a radiograph. The radiological examination is always necessary to identify the exact location and direction of the fracture line.

In summary, the determination of a fracture most often is associated with a specific trauma. The identification of the break is derived from a combination of the patient's history, a physical examination, and radiographic findings. Since occasionally the above described signs and symptoms may be minimal or lacking (as with a hairline or impacted fracture) it is vital to include the radiographic findings.

Unlike some other specialized tissues in the body, bone heals by restoring itself. This is not merely scar formation around the broken ends but regeneration of the bone tissue, a process that occurs in several distinct stages. Bone healing is discussed in Chapter 87.

Medical Management

The principles to consider when treating fractures are reduction, immobilization, and rehabilitation.

- *Reduction* is the attempt to restore the bone's normal alignment, position, and length.
- *Immobilization* is needed to keep the fragmented ends still and in place until time allows healing to occur.
- *Rehabilitation,* returning the affected part to normal strength and function, is the goal of fracture management.

There are three main approaches to fracture treatment and reduction. They are traction, closed reduction, and open reduction. Many variations of these approaches are possible. Reduction is not always necessary. In some cases, such as a nondisplaced fracture, the bone ends are already together and will only require a splint or sling to maintain their position. In other cases, normal positioning or realignment of multiple fragments (as with a comminuted fracture) is not possible, so that some shortening or angulation cannot be avoided. Some fractures are best treated by combining several approaches. A femur fracture, for example, may initially require balanced traction and then having an intramedullary rod inserted (open reduction). These techniques will be discussed in greater detail later.

Before bone reduction (or "setting") is begun, the patient should be prepared. A thorough explanation of the procedure and its expected outcome is vital to the patient, who will also need medication for pain in time for it to be effective. The affected area should be cleaned gently, kept elevated, and handled carefully.

Although not vital, it is desirable to reduce a fracture as soon as possible. For one thing, accumulation of blood and fluids will make the tissues less elastic, and for obvious reasons, the bone will be easier to reduce before it starts healing.

A fracture is not an isolated injury. When considering its reduction, one must also consider the repair or allow the healing of adjacent tissues. Surgical repair of major nerves, blood vessels, tendons, skin, and so on may be required. Soft tissue edema is relieved with elevation, cold application, and muscle activity (when possible). Under the direction of the physical therapist, muscle activity will also minimize joint stiffness and promote healing.

The three basic reduction methods are traction, closed reduction, and open reduction.

Traction. Traction is the application of a mechanical pull to the body that permits fracture reduction. When the pulling force is applied in one direction, there must be an equal pull in the opposite direction (countertraction). Usually the opposite pull is the patient's own body weight on an inclined bed frame, but it can also take the form of weights hung at the opposite end of the bed.

The purpose of the traction is to overcome the effect of muscle spasm while the bone ends align normally. Sustained traction will also minimize pain, maintain alignment, and permit some joint exercises. A full discussion of traction is presented in Chapter 87.

Closed Reduction. Closed reduction is obtained with manual traction and manipulation of those fractures that can be reduced without surgery. It is a painful procedure and requires some degree of anesthesia. If local anesthesia is used, the patient will usually not be hospitalized. Instead, the bone will be reduced, radiographs will be taken to ensure proper alignment, and the patient will be sent home wearing a cast.

Once accurate reduction is achieved, it is very often

maintained with the help of a *cast*. The purpose of the cast is to provide protection and support during healing. A cast is essentially a temporary external skeleton. A full discussion of casts is presented in Chapter 87.

Open Reduction. Many fractures are best treated in surgery by open reduction. These types of fractures include open contaminated wounds, those with bone ends displaced, those with tissue or material caught between the fragments, and those that cannot be reduced with the closed approach. Reduction of femur fractures and those at or near joints are typically treated by open reduction. Sometimes the prolonged bed rest required with traction reduction is too great a risk (*e.g.,* for an elderly person), and therefore the surgical approach is chosen.

During the operation, a variety of *internal fixation devices* can be used to hold the bone fragments in place until proper healing has occurred. These devices include metallic wires, screws, pins, plates, nails, or rods (Fig. 88–2). They are attached to the cortical bone on either side of the break or (with rods) through the bone's medullary canal. The chief advantages of these forms of stabilization are that secure, accurate, long-term alignment is achieved, and early patient mobility can be allowed.

Metal devices are not a substitute for actual bone healing. Over a period of time they will bend and break if good bone healing does not occur. A few disadvantages of internal fixation are that (1) contamination may be introduced into the fracture sites, (2) circulation may be significantly disrupted by the devices, and (3) the devices may further damage adjacent bone, nerves, or other nearby tissue.

Other problems that may develop include actual mechanical failure (from inadequate insertion and stabilization), material failure (faulty or damaged devices), localized inflammation or allergic response, and disuse osteoporosis (*i.e.,* the bone stress is taken up by the metal so the bone does not regenerate adequately). In spite of these potential problems, internal fixation is often the most desirable and effective course of treatment.

The choice of when to use open reduction depends on several factors. If the injury is already an open fracture, internal fixation will be done immediately to minimize risk of infection. A closed fracture allows more time flexibility. Usually it is best done in 24 to 48 hours, but it may be delayed a week or two, especially if, meanwhile, stable traction can be maintained.

Small bone plates have also been utilized more recently in the treatment of facial fractures. Immediate stability and enhanced cosmesis are advantages of this approach.

Nursing Management

Assessment and Nursing Diagnosis

Initial first aid intervention and related principles will be discussed here very briefly. Details of first aid medical management of fractures should be sought in appropriate specialized texts.

At the scene of injury, the primary concern is for airway patency, cardiopulmonary function, hemorrhage, and shock. Once these are determined to be under control, fracture management can be pursued. The nursing diagnoses include the potential for ineffective airway clearance, alteration in cardiac output, alteration in comfort due to pain, and fluid volume deficit related to the injuries.

Preoperatively the patient needs to be thoroughly informed of the procedure and its postoperative expectations. The nursing diagnosis of anxiety related to the surgical procedure requires that emotional support and the opportunity

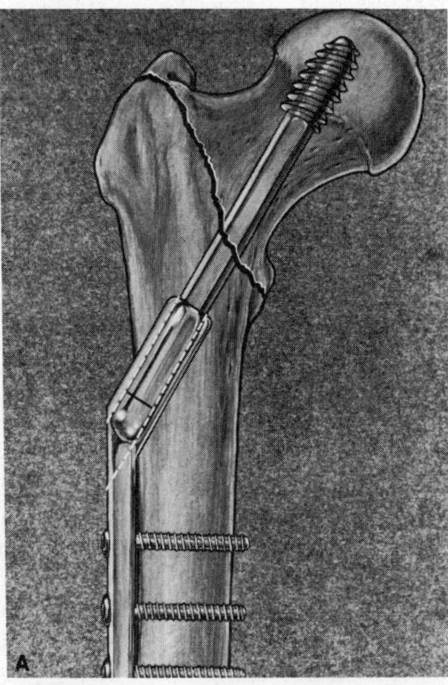

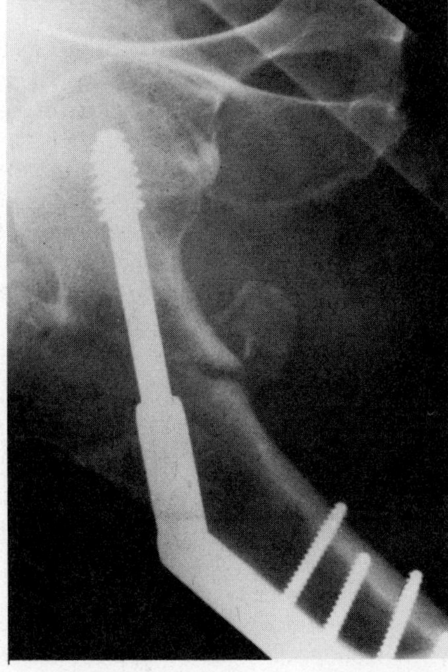

FIGURE 88–2 (*A* and *B*) Sliding hip screw, used in internal fixation for trochanteric fractures. (Courtesy of Department of Orthopaedics, Harborview Medical Center, Seattle)

for both patient and family to ask questions should be provided, when possible. Since surgery will result in actual skin impairment, the skin must be thoroughly cleansed to minimize the risk of infection.

Fixators appear rather ominous or as one nurse described it, "formidable."[12] The nursing diagnosis is fear of pain related to traction. For this reason psychological preparation of the patient is important. Reassurance should persuade the patient that pain is not a problem once the traction is in place. Encouragement is provided with early mobility and the patient's involvement in care of the device.

The limb with a new external fixator is initially elevated to limit pain and edema. Careful observation for signs of neuromuscular problems and infection is needed. As with skeletal traction, routine pin care is required. (See the section on traction in Chapter 87.) The clamps on the fixator frame must not be adjusted.[1]

Goals

The most important goal with a suspected fracture is to keep the site of injury immobile. Do not move the patient unless there is danger. While preparing for transportation to a health care facility, the fracture must be splinted securely. If the fracture is in the leg, stabilize the fracture by bandaging the two legs together. The arm can be put in a sling or bandaged to the chest. A well-padded splint secured over clothing is ideal. The purpose of "splinting them where they lie" is to prevent further tissue damage, pain, and hemorrhage. If movement is absolutely essential before splinting the fracture, someone should apply traction by maintaining a slow steady pull along the long axis of the injured bone. If this is done properly, both rotation and angulation of the fragments will be prevented.

Even though the nurse has evaluated the patient initially, she must be consistently aware of his overall condition. Changes in his condition may occur, for example, shock may set in; therefore, focus on the fracture should not limit the nurse's total awareness.

Assessment of the nerve and vascular impairment that often accompanies fractures is important. Sensation may be diminished distal to the injury. Consider that a spinal cord injury may also be present or may occur if the patient is moved, and treat the patient accordingly (see Chap. 69). Circulatory status is determined by the presence and strength of distal pulses as well as by the color and warmth of the extremity beyond the injury. (See evaluation of circulation under the section Cast Application in Chapter 87.)

The nursing goals for the patient in traction are that the patient is comfortable and accepting the fixator as well as being involved in its care. The limb shows signs of good circulation, has mobility within its limits, and has normal sensations distal to the injury. When the bone has healed, the patient eventually achieves his previous level of activity without residual effects.

Interventions

Pain is nearly always severe with a fracture but less if the fracture site is kept immobile. Administration of a narcotic on arrival to the hospital is desirable if no head injury is present. Soothing conversation and a controlled and reassuring manner will aid in calming the patient and minimizing his pain.

Physical evaluation will necessitate the removal of clothing at the site of the injury, and they should be gently removed or cut away. Before swelling occurs, constricting items such as watches, rings, and bracelets should be removed.

If the fracture is *open (compound),* the wound should be covered with a sterile or clean dressing. No effort should be made to push back the exposed bone. Even if the bone is not exposed, a compound fracture may be present where the skin has been broken. Bleeding can be controlled by local pressure over the wound. A tourniquet should be avoided unless the extent of bleeding is threatening the patient's life. If a tourniquet is used, it must be loosened at frequent intervals (every 5 minutes) to keep from totally impeding the circulation to the area.

Care should be taken to splint the open fracture as it is. Any attempt to apply traction or straighten the extremity may pull the exposed bone back inside the skin and cause further damage to nerve, blood vessels, and other tissues. It could also introduce gross contamination in the form of dirt, hair, and foreign matter into the wound.

Splinting. The approach to splinting varies. As mentioned above, the padded splint is best, but an extremity can be bandaged to and supported by another part of the body. Commercial splints are made of aluminum, wood, cardboard, and inflatable plastic (air splints). Some types of air splints are shown in Fig. 88–3. When commercial splints are not available a splint can be fashioned from such items as rolled newspaper, padded boards, sticks, rolled blankets, or even golf clubs and baseball bats.

Proper splinting will immobilize the fractured bone ends and simultaneously minimize further damage, pain, deformity, muscle spasm, shock, and hemorrhage. It will also promote healing by permitting clot formation at the fracture site, which is an important step in bone healing.

Principles of normal body alignment, keeping the joints above and below the fracture immobile, and protection of soft tissues by adequate padding must be considered when splinting. A well-applied, rigid splint will stabilize the entire bone by being secured firmly above and below the fracture site. Once immobilized the injured extremity can be elevated to minimize edema.

Care should be taken to ensure that circulation is not impaired by the splint. The integrity of the soft tissues and the skin will be maintained if the splint is carefully padded. If splinting is done properly, the joints at either end of the fracture will be completely immobilized.

Postoperative Care

Postoperatively the nursing care is similar to that for any other major operative procedure (see Chap. 8). Further immobilization with casting or traction may be applied in the operating room. In any case an overhead trapeze will be useful for optimal postoperative care. The affected arm or leg

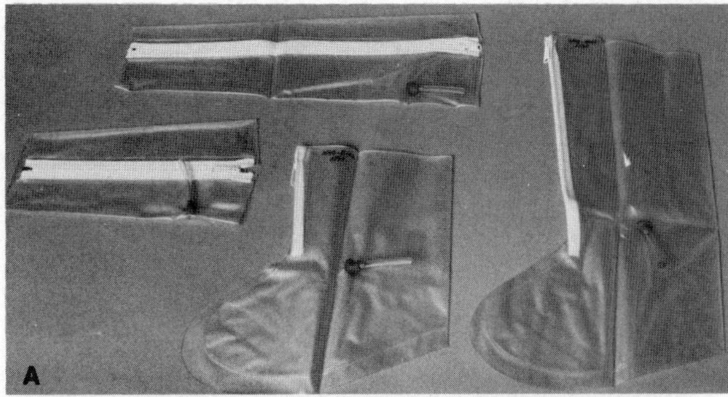

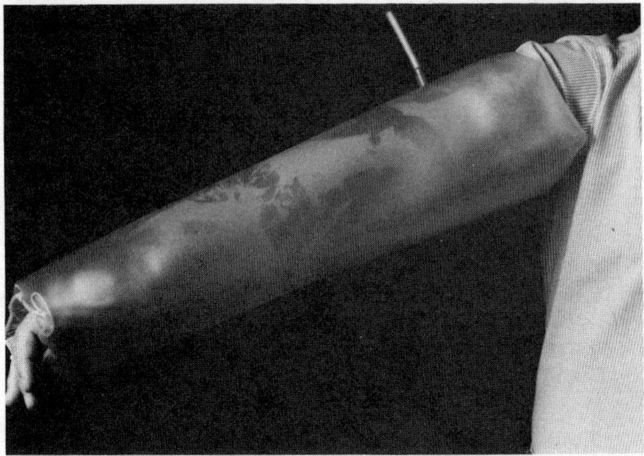

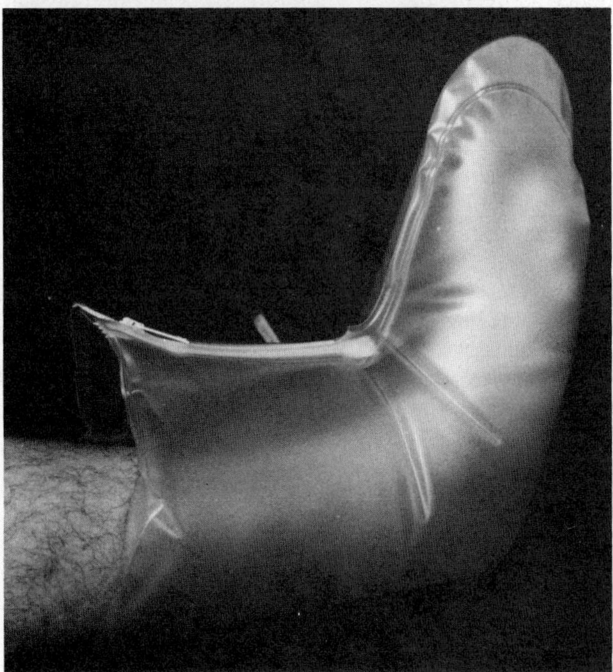

FIGURE 88–3 Air splints. (*A*) Various sizes of air splints. (*B*) An air splint in place on an arm; note that the fingers are exposed for assessment. (*C*) Air splint for foot or ankle.

is elevated to promote venous return. The surgical wound is inspected and managed as any postoperative wound would be. Because of the need to dissect the deep muscles, there is often a greater amount of wound drainage from an orthopedic procedure. Expectation of some excess drainage must be considered when monitoring the wound, dressing, and Hemovac (low-suction drainage device).

Pain is an individual problem, but generally it is quite intense after orthopedic surgery. Usually liberal doses of narcotics are given for the first 24 to 72 hours. Commonly a dramatic decrease in pain will occur during this period. The administration of analgesics should then diminish accordingly. Again, pain is individual and must be evaluated as such. Most orthopedic procedures give rise to prolonged musculoskeletal complaints. The risk of drug dependency arises when the severe postoperative pain subsides and the long-term discomforts of bone healing are managed with stronger drugs than necessary. Often diversion or nursing measures such as positioning, massage, and reassurance can be most effective during this period.

When a fracture is accompanied by an open wound with extensive soft tissue damage it has become common to apply an *external fixator.*[11] This device is also useful when the fracture is severely comminuted, fails to heal, or becomes infected.

The bone is stabilized with skeletal pins or wires, which are inserted in the bone fragments and then attached to an external stainless steel framework (Fig. 88–4). These devices immobilize the bone, provide easy access to the wound, and permit early patient mobility.

Evaluation

The nursing interventions of emergency fracture management can be evaluated by achievement of several observable criteria.

- The airway is kept patent and respiratory distress is eliminated.
- Blood loss is controlled by minimizing direct bleeding, thereby stabilizing vital signs.
- Contamination of the open wound is kept minimal.
- Pain is minimized by immobilizing and elevating the injured part.

The goals of both medical and nursing management are to regain correct alignment, regain function, and return the patient to his previous activities as soon as possible.

Once the patient has had surgery or traction placement, evaluation of the circulation must be done regularly. The nurse is in a key position to monitor this and needs to report any significant changes immediately to prevent irreversible damage. As with the casted patient, one thorough method of observation comprises the five Ps: pain, pallor, pulselessness, paresthesia, and paralysis. Also, skin temperature and color along with degree of swelling are important symptoms.

Complications of Fractures

Fracture complications that can seriously threaten life and limb are shock, fat embolism, and compartment syndrome. Delayed complications include avascular necrosis, delayed union, and nonunion.

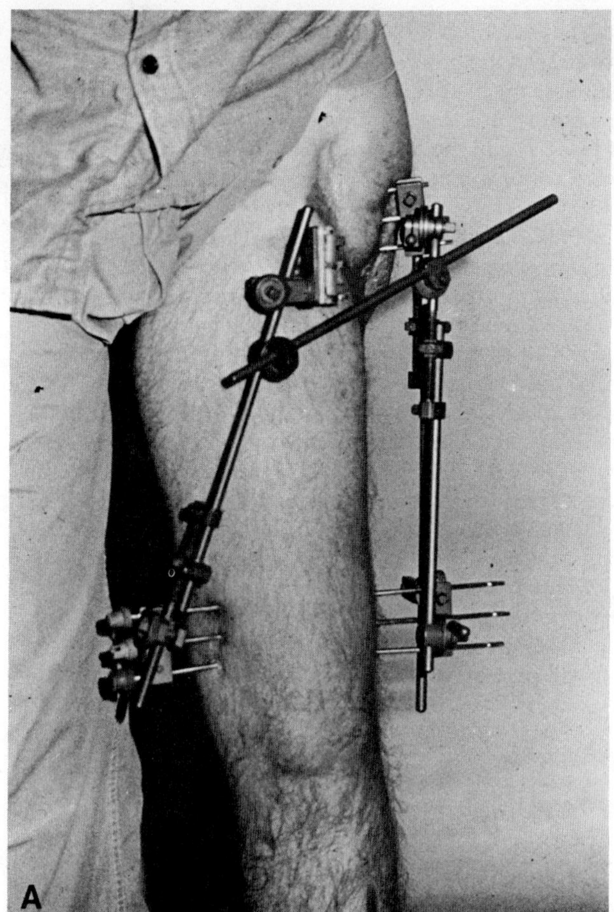

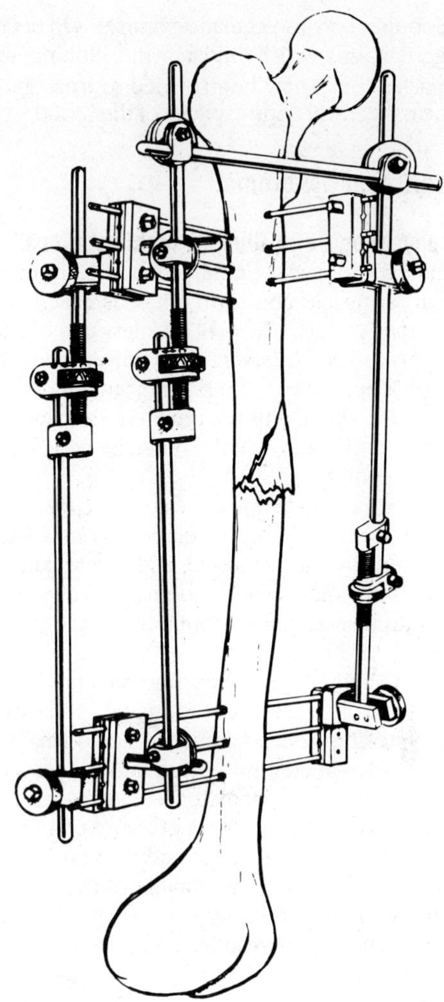

FIGURE 88–4 (*A* and *B*) External fixators. (Gossling HR, Pillsbury SL [eds]: Complications of Fracture Management, pp 131, 431. Philadelphia, JB Lippincott, 1984)

Hypovolemic Shock and Fat Embolism

Hypovolemic shock due to excessive loss of blood both externally and internally can be a real threat with some fractures. Open fractures are particularly at risk, but bones such as the femur, pelvis, and ribs and vertebrae can cause extensive bleeding into the tissues. The very vascular nature of these bones adds to this risk.

When the first aid management has stopped further blood loss, the body's depleted fluid volume needs to be replaced intravenously. Adequate fracture splinting and pain-killing drugs are then provided. (See further discussion of shock management in Chapter 24.)

A syndrome unique to the patient with lower extremity or multiple fractures is a *fat embolism.* This syndrome results in 20% of the fatalities from fractures.[15] It is believed that in the period following severe fractures of the long bones, fat globules are released from the bone marrow into the bloodstream. Another theory (metabolic) suggests that "catecholamines elevated by the patient's stress reaction cause mobilization of fatty acids and the development of fat globules in the blood stream."[3] In either circumstance, these globules combine with platelets to form emboli. Severe problems are caused when these emboli lodge in the brain, lungs, heart, and kidneys.

Clinical Manifestations. Appearance of the symptoms of shock or embolism is rapid and usually occurs within the first 48 hours following the injury. Mentally a person will show agitation, restlessness, and delirium symptoms similar to those of alcohol withdrawal symptoms. Involvement of the heart and lungs will result in tachypnea, tachycardia, dyspnea, wheezing, and copious amounts of thick white sputum. Hypoxia is evident with arterial blood gases below 60 mmHg. A chest radiograph shows a scattered infiltration. Petechiae will often appear in areas such as the buccal membranes, conjunctival sacs, axillae, and across the chest.

Medical Management. Treatment focuses on giving the patient respiratory support until the crisis has passed. Oxygen is immediately administered in high concentrations. If needed, other respiratory interventions will be initiated, such as intermittent positive pressure breathing (IPPB), suctioning, intubation, and a respirator. Steroids may be given to decrease the lung inflammation and cerebral edema.

Heparin is often given to improve blood flow and break

down fat globules. Low-molecular dextran aids in decreasing platelet aggregation, which initiates the clotting cascade. Blood or packed cells may be provided to treat shock and increase the oxygen-carrying capacity of the blood.

Compartment Syndrome

Pathophysiology and Clinical Manifestations. When edema in an extremity associated with a fracture minimizes circulation to a muscle compartment, it is called compartment syndrome (see also Chap. 87). Unless this condition is quickly recognized and intervention is started, compartment syndrome can jeopardize the limb. If not attended to in 6 to 8 hours, the muscle tissue will not receive blood and will die. Therefore, it is imperative that the nurse be consistently observant for the condition.

Commonly this syndrome can be suspected in a closed fracture of the forearm or lower leg. Symptoms include excessive pain, tense swollen muscle, and severe pain on passive stretch. There may also be edema, pulselessness, erythema, and diminished neurovascular function.

Medical Management. In some facilities it may be possible to actually measure the tissue pressure by a pressure-monitoring device (similar to hemodynamic pressure monitoring). A needle is inserted into the suspect compartment. The mercury manometer will give a reading (the normal range is 10 to 20 mmHg). A pressure of 45 mmHg or above signals the need for surgical intervention.

Surgical decompression is obtained through a fasciotomy. Failure to make this intervention, when necessary, within the first 6 hours will result in some tissue necrosis and will jeopardize the limb.

Avascular Necrosis

Pathophysiology and Clinical Manifestations. Avascular necrosis of bone means bone death due to a lack of blood supply. It can occur to any bone from a number of causes. Our focus here is its etiology in relation to fractures and dislocations. The area most often affected by this condition is the neck of the femur. Its effects are delayed from the time of the bone fracture. As the patient begins to move, he experiences pain and limitation of function. A radiograph will show that the devitalized bone is collapsing structurally. Occasionally the bone may collapse, but it will be resorbed and replaced by new bone. In most cases, however, surgical intervention is necessary. This may call for bone grafts to revitalize the area, replacement of the lost bone by a prosthesis, or joint fusion.

Delayed Union and Nonunion

Delayed union and nonunion are terms given to the failure of bone to form a union (heal) in the normal time frame after fracture. Delayed union may not require further treatment. With nonunion, however, the healing has stopped and some intervention is necessary.

Predisposing conditions to delayed union or nonunion are infection, poor circulation, ineffective immobilization (callus formation is disrupted), inadequate reduction of the fracture, and the poor general condition of the patient. The location of the injury may also increase the risk of nonunion. For example, fractures of the neck of the femur (usually in the elderly) and the lower third of the tibia (usually in the adolescent or young adult) are often sites of nonunion.

Medical Management. Treatment is aimed at speeding up healing and restoring bone integrity. Surgical intervention can include débridement and internal fixation with or without bone grafting. Electrotherapy has also been used successfully in some cases. Electrodes are implanted at the site of fracture or else external electromagnetic coils are placed in the dressing above the nonunion. The electrical stimulation enhances deposition of minerals and bone formation.[4] For 10 to 12 hours a day pulsing electromagnetic currents are delivered to the area (Fig. 88–5). The success rate using electrotherapy is comparable to that for bone grafting (about 75%).

When healing does not occur, the patient may need to wear a protective, supportive brace and remain on crutches indefinitely. In some cases it may be obvious that an artificial limb will provide the patient with more function, freedom, and comfort. The patient should be aware that this is an option.

Nursing Management

Assessment and Nursing Diagnosis

The health-care team should be aware of the extensive long-term stress that nonunion places on the patient. The patient requires much sympathetic support and occasional intervention as he faces and deals with multiple hospitalizations, an altered body image, inactivity, decreased independence, chronic pain, impatience, irritability, and decreasing support from family and friends.[2] The nurse is in a strategic position to recognize the early indications of complications of fractures, administer promptly the treatment plan as ordered, and allay the patient's apprehension. The appropriate nursing diagnoses include disturbance in self-concept, impaired physical mobility, alteration in comfort due to pain, and disabled or ineffective family coping related to the complications of fractures.

Goals

The nursing goals for the patient with complications of fractures are that the patient will have the indications of complications recognized early; demonstrate an understanding of the treatment plan; and express less apprehension and anxiety regarding the complications.

Interventions

Providing opportunities for verbal interaction, encouragement, realistic goal-setting, and maximum use of support systems is helpful. Keeping long bone fractures immobilized and avoiding massage of the area and any sudden movement can be effective in preventing fat embolism.

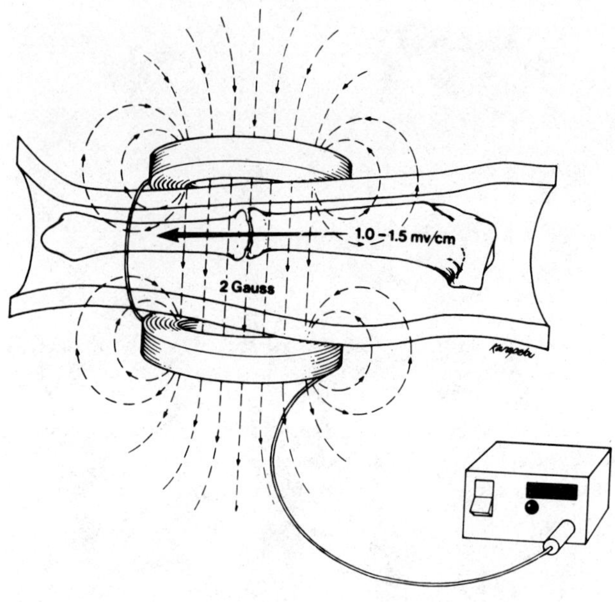

A

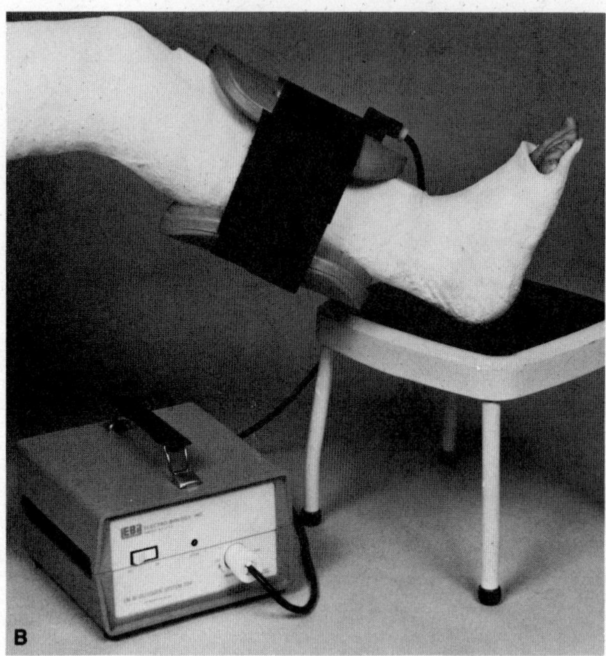

B

FIGURE 88–5 (*A*) Principles of application in the treatment of nonunion in electromagnetic fields. The pair of coils is mounted anteriorly and posteriorly on the surface of the cast and is plugged into the pulse generator. The generator, which is attached to the 110-volt line, "drives" the coils with 10 to 18 volts, depending in part on the distance between the coils. As current flows in the coils, a pulsing electromagnetic field is established between the pair, penetrating the cast and the soft tissues. The field is weak (average, 2 gauss) and the magnetic flux lines (B field), which are at right angles to the bone in this configuration, induce a voltage drop (E field, at a right cycle to the B field) along the long axis of the tibia of 1 mv/cm to 1.5 mv/cm. (*B*) Noninvasive method of inducing osteogenesis. Electromagnetic fields are created about the nonunion site between the pads. For nonunion of the tibia, a thigh-length cast is necessary. Note that the knee is fixed in 30° flexion to eliminate tensile forces. (View *A* from Bassett CAL, Mitchell SN, Gaston SR: Treatment of ununited tibial diaphyseal fractures with pulsing electromagnetic fields. J Bone Joint Surg 63A:511, 1981. View *B* courtesy of Electro-Biology, Inc., Fairfield, New Jersey. In Turek SL: Orthopaedics: Principles and Their Application, 4th ed, Vol 1, p 67. Philadelphia, JB Lippincott, 1984)

When a compartment syndrome is suspected, all restrictive dressings should be loosened (*e.g.,* bivalve casts) and the limb should be kept flat. Elevation will further restrict blood supply to the area.

Monitoring of symptoms and pressure readings should be done regularly (usually hourly). When possible, the patient should be well informed of the problem and instructed to report any significant changes in symptoms immediately. Again the skilled, informed nurse is extremely important in identifying and reporting the condition immediately. Although the syndrome itself cannot be prevented, its complications can.

Discussion of typical fracture treatment has covered the usual approach of casts, traction, and surgery. Because of the prevalence of hip fractures in the elderly and their need for in-hospital care, nursing management is detailed in the Nursing Care Plan for the Patient with a Hip Fracture.

Evaluation

As a result of general fracture management, the patient will understand the type and degree of fracture, the therapeutic management and overall aim of treatment. The patient will be comfortable with his progress and with his ability to cope with it. An understanding of care needed throughout convalescence is also imperative. Essentially, the aim is to return the patient to his previous active role in society as soon as possible. The specific aim is to restore the injured part and its adjacent joints to their normal function, mobility, and strength.

Amputation

When a limb is damaged or diseased beyond repair, its surgical removal is called amputation. Although to most this word has a very negative implication, it is in fact a positive step. Amputation is actually constructive surgery. The destruction, from whatever cause, has already happened to the limb. The condition of the limb has deteriorated to a point at which it threatens life or, most certainly, the quality of life. To then remove that destroyed or nonfunctional portion is the first step in returning the individual to a normal place in society.

Surgical amputation, if done properly, is a meticulous,

(*Text continues on page 1326*)

NURSING CARE PLAN FOR THE PATIENT WITH A HIP FRACTURE

PREOPERATIVE CARE

GOAL 1: Relief of hip discomfort by immobilizing and stabilizing the fracture

Nursing Interventions	Rationale	Outcome Criteria
1. Initially, promote patient comfort by:		
a. Comfortably positioning him in bed.	a. Immobility and proper positioning prevent further injury from the fracture and lessen pain.	a. Patient able to say he experiences less pain.
b. Applying Bucks traction or sandbags, or both as ordered.	b. Traction aids in reducing fracture and keeping it immobile.	b. Traction is in proper alignment.
c. Administering analgesics as ordered and needed.	c. Pain relief will minimize restlessness and agitation and promote cooperation with therapeutic regimen.	c–d. Patient appears restful.
d. Giving individualized basic nursing care for rest and comfort.		

GOAL 2: Minimize stress, fear, and potential disorientation resulting from injury and anticipated surgery

Nursing Interventions	Rationale	Outcome Criteria
1. Explain extent of injury, planned treatment, and expected hospital course. a. Assure patient that discomfort will be minimized with surgical reduction.	1. Stress and fear are reduced with knowledge, understanding, and familiarity.	1. Patient appears less anxious; asks appropriate questions; relates understanding of injury and plan of care.
2. Encourage independence and choices where possible (*e.g.*, food, clothing, hygiene, daily schedule).	2. More control creates less helplessness and more involvement in plan of care and its outcome.	2. Patient participates in development of health care plan.
3. Encourage support of family, spiritual beliefs, and friends.	3. Sharing anxieties and grief lessens them.	3. Patient is able to use available resources and support systems.
4. Promote use of familiar objects (*e.g.*, clothing, lap robe, pictures, and aids such as glasses, dentures, hearing aid).	4. Familiar items and aids will minimize fears and mental confusion.	4. Patient is mentally alert.
5. Determine preinjury orientation of limb.	5. Potential for development of mental confusion from injury and unfamiliar surroundings	
6. Use aids to orientation (*e.g.*, clocks, calendars, TV). Minimize number of staff working with patient.		6. Patient can demonstrate orientation to time, place, and person.

GOAL 3: Prevent problems of inactivity and secondary medical problems

Nursing Interventions	Rationale	Outcome Criteria
1. Encourage breathing exercises.	1. They help keep lungs clear and free from congestion.	1. Lungs are clear.
2. Regularly inspect legs and promptly report any circulatory impairment.	2. Early diagnosis and treatment will minimize thromboembolic complications.	2. Circulation is improved.

(Continued)

NURSING CARE PLAN FOR THE PATIENT WITH A HIP FRACTURE (*Continued*)

Nursing Interventions	Rationale	Outcome Criteria
a. Administer prescribed low-dose anticoagulant.	a. Effective prophylaxis for emboli formation	
b. Promote calf-pumping exercises.	b. Promotes good circulation and venous return in the leg	
c. Provide and promote wear of antiembolic stockings.		
3. Inspect and massage bony prominences (*e.g.*, heels, sacrum, elbows) at least three times a day.	3. Aid in maintaining skin integrity	3. No evidence of skin breakdown or excessive pressure or moisture
a. Change position of patient every 1–2 hr, as traction allows.	a. Relieves areas of pressure	
b. Use special mattresses (*e.g.*, air, water, convoluted) and sheepskin.	b. Minimizes the areas of skin subjected to pressure and shear	
c. Keep patient's skin clean and dry.		
4. Monitor stool and urine output.	4. Urinary stasis and constipation are common problems for the bedridden, especially among the elderly.	4. Stool and urine output are normal. No signs of constipation.
a. Encourage fluid intake.		
b. Administer stool softeners as ordered.		
c. Avoid use of catheters, if possible.	c. Catheters will often introduce infection into bladder and decrease patient's ability to control bladder function.	c. No signs of urinary tract infection. Adequate urine volume.

POSTOPERATIVE CARE FOLLOWING HIP-FRACTURE REDUCTION

GOAL 1: Promote relief of pain due to postoperative state

Nursing Interventions	Rationale	Outcome Criteria
1. Administer prescribed pain medication as needed.	1. "Normal" pain related to surgery usually requires strong analgesics for 24–48 hr.	1. Pain is lessened.
a. Assess degree of relief.	a. Ensures that medication is adequate	a. Patient is alert.
b. Keeps legs abducted with pillows or splint.	b. Supports legs and keeps site of surgical reduction in neutral position	b. Fracture correctly positioned and supported
c. Reposition frequently.		

GOAL 2: Patient involved in therapeutic regimen and prevention of inadequate healing of fracture and wound

Nursing Interventions	Rationale	Outcome Criteria
1. Convey plan of care to patient, and modify and individualize it to his needs.	1. Over-dependency on others can be related to need for assistance in performing basic self-care.	1. Cooperating to meet basic self-care needs
2. Encourage nutritional and fluid intake that is high in protein and vitamins.	2. Promotes wound healing and maintains overall health status	2. Well-balanced diet eaten with extra fluids

(*Continued*)

NURSING CARE PLAN FOR THE PATIENT WITH A HIP FRACTURE (*Continued*)

Nursing Interventions	Rationale	Outcome Criteria
3. Encourage activities and exercises: a. Deep breathing and coughing b. Calf pumping c. Range-of-motion exercises d. Quad sets and gluteal sets	3. They keep lungs uncongested and stimulate circulation around the fracture.	
4. Promote safe mobility with direction and coordination of a physical therapist. a. Assist patient into wheelchair several times a day. b. Supervise use of ambulatory aid.	4. Fracture and reduction cause significant temporary restriction of mobility.	4. Patient is able to move independently in bed. a. To participate in transfer to wheelchair b. To walk with the aid of crutches, cane, or walker
5. Make discharge plans to allow for temporary lessened mobility.		5. Eventually preoperative activity level resumed

PREVENTING COMPLICATIONS FROM FRACTURE DAMAGE OR SURGICAL INTERVENTION

GOAL: Avoidance of potentially long-term problems related to fracture and surgery

Nursing Interventions	Rationale	Outcome Criteria
1. Watch for symptoms such as fever, odor, amount, and consistency of wound discharge and for failure of wound edges to heal.	1. Infection is a risk with any deep open wound (surgery).	1. No sign of deep infection
2. Assess degree of discomfort and any limited or decreased range of motion, or deformity.	2. Nonunion, avascular necrosis, and failure of an internal fixation device are potential risks.	
a. Refer for radiologic evaluation.	a. Radiography will confirm or rule out above complications.	a. No radiologic evidence of these postoperative complications.

highly skilled, plastic (builds up and molds tissues) and reconstructive procedure. It must be planned and performed with great care. The *residual limb* (remaining portion of an amputated limb) will be facing great demands for which it was not made. It will be expected to maneuver a sophisticated, bulky artificial limb. If the amputation is of part of the leg, the residual limb will be required to tolerate the entire weight of the body.

Etiology

The cause of amputation in the majority of cases is peripheral vascular disease (disease of the smaller, outlying blood vessels). This condition develops most often in mid or later life and is often a complication of diabetes mellitus. A second factor that is consistently prevalent in a dysvascular (*i.e.,* poor-circulation) limb requiring amputation is a history of heavy smoking. In Sweden, studies to determine the causes of amputation have been going on over a 30-year period. Some of those investigated had a family history of vascular disease, some were elderly, and some had diabetes, but *all* were smokers![14] (Peripheral vascular disease and its implications are discussed in Chapters 47 and 48 in more detail.)

External force or traumatic injury is the third factor, and it is the cause of about 20% of all amputations.[8] This category includes such assaults as motor-vehicle accidents (*e.g.,* motorcycles, cars, trains, boats), falls, burns (*e.g.,* electrical, thermal, chemical), war injuries, gunshot wounds, frostbite, and explosions. Nearly all amputations of the arm are due to traumatic injury. The fourth factor, tumors and congenital disorders, both cause about 5% of all amputations and usually affect the child population.

These four factors are the main causes of limb removal. Other conditions associated with amputation such as osteomyelitis (bone infection), gangrene, crushing injuries, nonhealing trophic ulcers, and septic wounds can usually be included in one of the four categories. Osteomyelitis, for example, is usually the outcome of an old trauma, and nonhealing ulcers are often a symptom of peripheral vascular disease. This section will focus on care of the traumatic amputee.

Medical Management

The traumatic injury that is evaluated for an amputation is often a large open extremity wound sustained in grossly contaminated circumstances (*e.g.,* in a motorcycle accident). A large loss of blood is not uncommon and efforts to stop the flow and replace the blood are vital. Physiological shock can be expected with this loss of fluid (see Chap. 24). Careful effort should be made to check for accompanying injuries. The obvious major wound may distract the health care team from other significant but less obvious injuries.

Partial or complete amputation requires intense evaluation by the trauma team. Pursuing salvage of the limb will require assessment of the circulation, nerve supply, and degree of bone and soft tissue destruction. Medical management will first involve consideration of reimplantation. In most cases reimplantation is not feasible. If it is considered, the following factors are necessary for this option to be feasible:

- The severed limb should have been handled carefully, by wrapping it in a sterile (or clean) drape, and kept cool.
- The patient must be in good general health and be capable of following a careful and disciplined management program.
- A properly equipped operating room and a skilled team to perform microvascular surgery must be available.
- The injury will be best dealt with if it has been incurred as a result of a clean, continued incision with minimal contamination rather than as a result of the extensive destruction of a crushing, twisting, or tearing injury.

The highest success rate is attained with finger reimplants and with the upper extremity in general. Besides the need for large nerves to regenerate in a leg reimplant, the demand of weight bearing is usually too severe to reattach the distal portion. Above all, the risk of introducing massive infection into the system is considerable with reimplantation, and the bigger the extremity, the greater is that risk. Furthermore, the almost inevitable lack of function and sensation accompanied by the presence of pain, edema, and cellulitis nearly always makes amputation the preferred course with a severed leg. However, the potential for success with implants is greater in children, whose capacity for renewed growth and cellular activity is greater. Children's nerves, in particular, have a better chance of reestablishing themselves.

Surgical Procedure. When the option of salvaging a limb has been ruled out, the following surgical procedure is pursued. In most cases, the damaged extremity is removed, the bone is beveled, and vascular flaps of muscle and soft tissue that have been left attached are used to cover the bone. Surgeons try to preserve as much length as possible while removing the limb at a level that will heal. Healing is dependent on the circulation to the area and its freedom from disease and infection.

Selection of the appropriate level at which to amputate for both upper and lower extremities is shown in Figure 88–6. Proximity of the joint is always considered when making the selection. Efforts are made to preserve the joints whenever possible, but there must be a minimal distance from the joints if a prosthesis is to be used with success. For example, a residual limb preserved to below the knee must have at least 3 inches of tibia remaining to permit adequate function of the artificial limb.

In most cases the final determination of preserved length will be made in the operating room. Here the skin bleeding and tissue infection or destruction are evaluated directly. Scant bleeding will indicate the need for raising the level, to ensure healing. A common procedure used by many

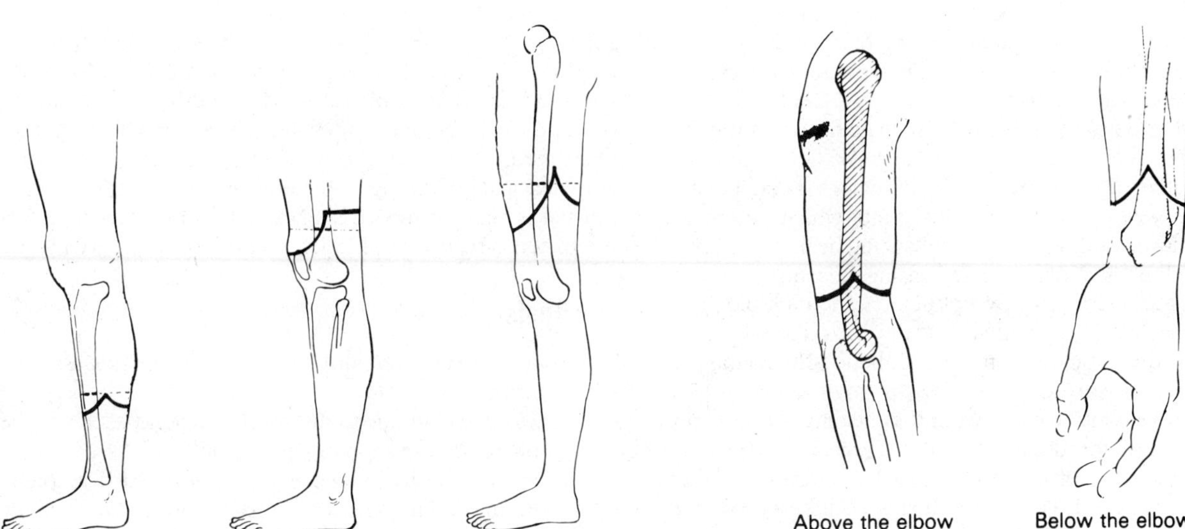

FIGURE 88–6 Appropriate levels at which to amputate in upper and lower extremities. (Turek SL: Orthopedics: Principles and Their Application, 4th ed, Vol 2. Philadelphia, JB Lippincott, 1984)

surgeons is the injection of a fluorescein dye, which will permeate the healthy vascularized tissue and make it visible.

In amputation surgery, the procedure is often done in two stages. The initial surgery is the primary or open procedure, leaving the wound open for a few days to drain purulent or infectious material. This approach is especially advisable for a contaminated traumatic amputation.

The second stage of final closure and any necessary revision is done after 5 to 7 days. Usually an incision tube will be left in place to drain off blood and serous fluid. Should the tube ever become dislodged, it should never be reinserted because that would expose the wound to infection. Instead it must be removed and the physician must be informed. Normally this tube is removed after the first 24 to 72 hours.

Soft vs. Rigid Dressings. Two types of *postoperative dressings* are commonly used with an amputation. One is the soft dressing, which is similar to most postoperative dressings. It is applied when the residual limb is wrapped with soft compressive dressings. Many physicians prefer to use this dressing because it allows easier wound observation, with only a simple dressing change. The other is the rigid dressing or immediate-fit postoperative cast, use of which is the preferred approach in many medical centers for several reasons that will be discussed later. The cast is fabricated around the residual limb in the operating room directly over the postoperative dressings. A sterile stump sock is applied over the cast and then felt pads are placed to relieve pressure points. A cushioned end-pad is put over the end of the stump, and elastic plaster is wrapped over it all. An adjustable metal unit called a pylon is attached to the distal end of the cast. To this a length of pipe, precisely measured for the patient, is connected and a foot ankle assembly is attached on the end of that (Fig. 88–7). This cast will be changed 3 or 4 times before the definitive prosthetic fitting is begun.

The immediate-fit postsurgical cast has several advantages for the patient. The first advantage is psychological. Although the unit is not cosmetically attractive, it affords a degree of encouragement to the patient by providing a substitute foot in place of the one that has been removed. Weight bearing for the traumatic amputee will begin in 2 or 3 days. Resuming ambulation even to a limited degree provides another psychological bonus.

Another advantage of the immediate-fit cast is the fact that it protects the stump. In so doing it also helps minimize postoperative pain. One of its key advantages is that it exerts rigid compression on the residual limb, which minimizes postoperative swelling, thereby enhancing healing and shaping of the limb in addition to decreasing the pain.

With the option of early ambulation, the multiple problems of inactivity are avoided. Initially, the patient has only toe-touch weight bearing on the prosthetic side. By the second cast change in 7 to 10 days, he will begin applying 15 lb to 20 lb, providing that the wound is healing satisfactorily. Healing is monitored closely by the physical therapist. The patient should never commit his total weight on this cast, even if the wound is completely healed. Unlike a final prosthesis, the fit, durability, and transfer of weight on the limb is not as precise. Usually a maximum of 40 lb to 50 lb is advised while walking with crutch support.

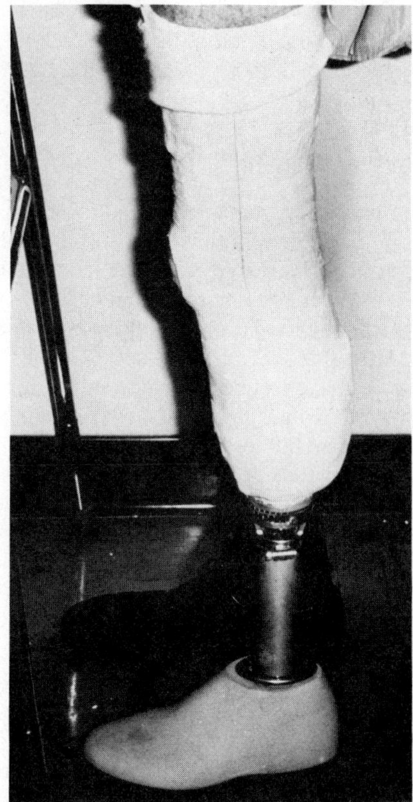

FIGURE 88–7 Immediate-fit cast with pylon. (Courtesy of Prosthetics Research Study, Seattle)

Nursing Management

Assessment and Nursing Diagnosis

Much of the nursing management is unique to the amputee. All possible support and intervention will be needed to restore function to the arm amputee and to help the leg amputee walk again. A significant loss has occurred. The appropriate nursing diagnoses include disturbance in self-concept, impaired physical mobility, and potential for grieving and ineffective coping related to the loss of the amputated limb. The stigma of the altered body image is a part of this loss. Dealing with the grief reaction that accompanies amputation and having a general awareness that grief is normal is vital for the nurse. Nonjudgmental acceptance of the patient's reaction to his loss will expedite his grief work.

Goals

Specific goals that could be established include assisting the amputee to

1. Manage pain due to the surgical wound itself and the phantom sensation phenomenon.
2. Prevent postoperative complications such as pneumonia and thrombophlebitis, as well as other conditions associated with inactivity.
3. Promote wound healing and monitor for barriers to wound healing.

4. Promote optimal mobility and independent living. This goal will be realized in different ways and to different degrees according to the individual. For example, a young person with an amputation below the knee can be expected to enjoy nearly the same activities as before. An elderly person with an amputation above the knee, on the other hand, will have significant difficulty in attempting to function and navigate as before. The young person would walk with a prosthesis and no other aid. The elderly person might choose to forego a prosthesis and use a wheelchair, especially if the limitations of cardiovascular function are a consideration.
5. Cope with the grief reaction due to the considerable loss faced by the amputee. Expressions of grief at this time are not only typical but very desirable. It is through this difficult process that they will be able to reestablish themselves psychologically and become remotivated and resume satisfactory lifestyles, while accepting the changes that have occurred.

Preoperative Interventions

The assault of amputation is severe both physically and psychologically. Preoperative management should be directed at helping the individual attain the highest physical and emotional level possible. This will be his initial step in preparation for wearing a prosthesis. An optimum physical condition and an accepting mind will promote his adjustment to this loss.

Physically, in leg amputations, which are the more prevalent kind, the focus should be on strengthening the patient's upper body and remaining leg in preparation for walking with the aid of crutches. Physical therapy can be an adjunct in teaching how to transfer from wheelchair to bed and vice versa and teaching the three-point gait, for example. Other normal preoperative teaching for promoting such things as lung function and overall circulation is, of course, necessary.

Because of the intense emotion that usually accompanies amputation, it is well for the nurse to assist in interpreting and reinforcing the surgeon's explanation to the patient. If the patient and his family can learn to accept their reaction of shock and grief, this acceptance will help them feel more at ease and more able to talk about it with less embarrassment. When their concerns are voiced, which of them are unfounded and which may warrant more support and information at a later date can then be determined. Common fears are being less acceptable to others, lifelong invalidism, less locomotion, change in homemaking practices, and loss or change of job. Rather than attempt problem solving at this point, one should listen compassionately and avoid being judgmental. Too much factual information at this time may be beyond the comprehension of the distraught patient.

Postoperative Interventions

The common occurrence of phantom sensation (the feeling of the missing extremity still being there) should be mentioned before surgery, so that the patient is not unduly disturbed by this postoperative sensation. This phenomenon is very normal and is discussed in more detail later. The nurse will use routine cast care as well as routine postoperative care. The cast must be kept away from hard surfaces to avoid uneven pressure and indentations until the cast has dried (about 24 hours). A cast dryer is not usually recommended since it may promote bleeding. The skin near the edges of the cast must be checked regularly for too much pressure or irritation.

A waist belt will be attached to the cast to keep it from slipping down, especially during transfers and while walking. The waist belt should be kept on and fitting snugly, although it can be loosened for comfort while the patient is in bed. If the cast should become too loose or slip off, the physician should be notified, and the residual limb should be wrapped immediately with an elastic compression bandage. No attempt should be made to put the cast back on should it come off, since it may cause uneven pressure on the tissues. For further details on cast management see Nursing Care Plan for Amputee Cast Management.

Pain

The first goal of pain management involves several issues. Postoperatively it is typical for the new amputee to experience severe pain for a day or two. Usually this diminishes significantly by the third or fourth day. During this time the nurse should conscientiously provide the pain medication ordered. The physician should be notified if the patient does not seem to obtain adequate relief from the medication. Although the pain is quite significant in the early stages, like other orthopedic pain it normally will diminish dramatically within the first week. Very often a very mild analgesic is the only requirement for comfort after that. It is noteworthy here that dependence on strong medication for pain relief is a great risk for amputees. This is especially so if, before the amputation, the patient has undergone prolonged unsuccessful treatment on his injured limb. Unfortunately, the new amputee may become accustomed to the effect of the medication and not be aware that the actual level of pain has diminished. The habit of asking for the drug on a routine basis, along with the need to want to escape from the reality of what has happened, will often cause the amputee to request the drug in excess of need. The medical staff too often will respond by providing long-term medication because the injury is so conspicuous and severe. Being firm and informative on this point will be to the advantage of the patient. Consider that the amputee will have enough to deal with without the added assault of drug dependency.

Conservative efforts to manage pain postoperatively could include elevation of the affected limb. Some relief is often provided by this measure, but it should not be utilized after the first 24 to 48 hours because it may lead to joint contracture. This complication will be discussed later. No ice should be applied to the wound area, especially in the presence of any circulatory problems.

Phantom Sensation

The phantom sensation is unique to the amputee. It is best referred to by the health care providers as a sensation rather than phantom "pain," because of the suggestibility of

NURSING CARE PLAN FOR AMPUTEE CAST MANAGEMENT

GOAL: Prevent uneven pressure on cast and promote full range of motion of residual limb

Nursing Interventions	Rationale	Outcome Criteria
1. Rest casted limb while damp on soft flexible surface (*e.g.,* pillow, bed).	1. To maintain cast integrity and prevent pressure areas	1. Cast is smooth and hard with no cracks or breaks.
2. Elevate casted limb on pillows, about 45° or whatever is comfortable.	2. To decrease swelling and pain immediately after surgery	2. Cast is snug but not tight or uncomfortable.
3. Ensure that residual limb maintains full ROM (range of motion): Keep residual limb flat after first 48 hr; turn the patient face down 2 or 3 times/day for 1 hr; instruct patient in ROM exercises; observe and document frequency of ROM exercises actually performed.	3. To prevent contractures of residual limb	3. Patient is able to demonstrate with no difficulty full ROM of residual limb. Later, is able to demonstrate use of prosthesis with no hindrance from joints.
4. Check that waist belt and cast strap are secure.	4. To maintain proper cast positioning	4. Cast is firmly in place; patella felt in center position through opening in below-knee cast.
5. Contact physical therapist for coordination of weight bearing and ambulation.	5. To begin early mobility and weight bearing	5. Patient is able to transfer and walk or propel himself safely within therapeutic guidelines.
6. If cast comes off, wrap limb immediately in ace bandages, elevate it, and notify physician.	6. To prevent edema in the residual limb and to protect it.	6. Limb has retained size and shape provided by initial cast.

the term. This is not to imply that the sensation is not real. In fact it is a very common, strong sensation experienced by most amputees.[5] Usually it is described as being a tingly, uncomfortable, odd sensation similar to that of bumping your "funny bone," but with the definite feeling that all or part of the missing extremity is still there. At times it can be intense and may be described as cramping, burning, or piercing, but it usually is not ongoing or totally unmanageable. Medical explanation for this phenomena is varied and scant, yet it does recognize that most amputees feel it to a degree. The sensation is usually strongest immediately postoperatively and tends to diminish as the wound heals and as the limb itself matures. Occasionally the patient may have preoperative numbness in the extremity (as with certain injuries) so there typically will be no experience of the phantom sensation at all. The feeling can probably best be described as similar to what a person feels after removing his watch or hat and it still seems to be there.

Efforts to relieve this uncomfortable sensation include activity and diversion, since as with any discomfort, getting the mind off of it will help. Other conservative measures include massage or pressure to the residual limb. If a cast is in place, pressure from a pillow or towel pulled against the end of it will generally help give relief. After the wound has healed the patient will often become quite adept at locating the exact nerve area on the residual limb that will respond to massage, pressure, or change of position.

Significant, continuous phantom pain, as such, in the missing limb is actually quite unusual. Even those who do experience it usually report that it is very sporadic. For these people, temporary management with certain neurological drugs (*e.g.,* Tegretol and Dilantin) and certain tricyclic antidepressants (*e.g.,* Sinequan) may be effective.

Postoperative Complications

Preventing postoperative complications requires careful routine inspection of the wound (when possible) and monitoring of other signs and symptoms. One consideration would be to look for hemorrhage, but in reality hemorrhage is extremely rare and is merely something the nurse should be aware of.

Wound Healing. Wound healing is enhanced by good nutrition and adequate rest. A short course of oral antibiotics (48 to 72 hours) is advisable in avoiding infections. Early awareness of potential signs of infection will aid in initiating immediate treatment and preventing further involvement. If the wound is covered with a rigid dressing then other symptoms to monitor for are increasing or persistent pain, foul smelling or increased drainage (on the cast), fever, and edema.

Contractures. Contractures are a devastating barrier to successful prosthetic rehabilitation and are essentially preventable. The nurse needs to give the patient full understanding and involvement. Such efforts as range-of-motion exercises to the affected extremity and lying in a prone position (lying on the abdomen) two or three times a day are a part of this prevention. A written reminder of these for the patient to take home is advisable, especially if there is a delay in the fit or use of the prosthesis.

Self-Care. Self care should be encouraged as much and as soon as possible. Ambulation on crutches or parallel bars is often begun the second day. The physical therapist will be responsible for managing this as well as for the extent of weight bearing on the pylon cast. For the arm amputee, occupational therapy will provide optimum prosthetic and single-arm independence.

Cultural background can be a help or hindrance to realization of these goals. For example, one elderly Chinese lady with whom the author once worked had undergone foot binding as a young girl (an old Chinese custom used to keep girls' feet small and dainty). The resulting deformity of her remaining foot was a barrier to learning to walk again after her above-knee amputation. However, her culture also promoted respect and care for the elderly by their families. Her daughter's family took her back home, working consistently and patiently with her as she learned to walk safely with her prosthesis and a walker.

Grief Reaction. The nurse needs to be aware that losing an extremity at any level is similar to experiencing the death of a loved one.[13] A *grief reaction* to some extent will be an important step in the patient's adjustment to his condition. As with a death, the usual steps in grief reaction are denial, anger, depression, anxiety, and adaptation. Remember that all patients are individuals and may go through these steps in their own pattern and time frame. Some may not get past denial until they have left the hospital.

A compassionate, listening ear is appreciated by the patient. Sharing grief lessens it. Give permission for him to cry (crying is a normal reaction to this kind of situation). All of the patient's support systems should be fully utilized (*e.g.*, family, spiritual beliefs, and friends).

When the patient seems receptive, arrange a visit with a successful amputee. This is usually very motivating and encouraging to the new amputee.

Adjusting to Amputation. Adjusting to an amputation is often approached differently, depending on one's age. The young often have not had time to build their mental defenses, but their physical being is strong. The elderly, on the other hand, have usually lived through severe losses in their past and know that good living may still be ahead. However, they often face the physical barriers of an aging body and debilitating disease conditions. Some may see this loss as a sign that the rest of their body also is approaching death.[6]

Evaluation

If the goals of nursing management have been adhered to, the patient will be essentially free of pain. The patient will say that he is free of pain and appears to be comfortable; his need for drugs is minimal with only an occasional non-narcotic analgesic needed; and the phantom sensation is not distressing or unmanageable. He will have no complications associated with amputation. The residual limb has healed well in 3 to 5 weeks; there are no signs of hemorrhage, infection, or skin breakdown; the patient can demonstrate full range of motion at all joints. He has resumed his previous level of independence and optimum mobility. He performs activities of daily living; he walks unaided with a prosthesis, crutches, cane, or he uses a wheelchair without assistance (as appropriate). His grief reaction is expressed appropriately in the direction of adaptation and adjustment. He makes use of the support systems available to him; he has begun to set appropriate goals and is working towards them (*e.g.*, job, recreation, and social activities); he participates in his health-care regimen; he maximizes his abilities and accepts his limitations; he accepts changes of body image; and he projects self-confidence.

Summary

In summary, musculoskeletal trauma can include a wide range of injury from contusions to amputations. Severe trauma may result in a combination of injuries to the soft tissues, bones, joints, and often to other systems as well. Satisfactory recovery and rehabilitation will depend on several factors that can all be positively affected by high quality nursing intervention. Understanding of prevention, first aid, medical management, the healing process, and the psychological impact will help the nurse in assisting the patient achieve optimum function and adjustment following his injury.

References

1. Brunner L, Suddarth D: Medical-Surgical Nursing, 5th ed. Philadelphia, JB Lippincott, 1984
2. Clark J, Malchow D: How to avoid errors in limb salvage decisions. Orthopaedic Review 13:48, 1984
3. Del Bueno DJ: Recognizing fat embolism in patients. RN 36:48, 1973
4. Elliott J: Electrical stimulation of bone growth wins clinical acceptance. Medical News 243:1402, 1980
5. Haber WB: Reactions to loss of limb: Physiological and psychological aspects. Ann NY Acad Sci 74:18, 1985
6. Huslin H: On psychologic amputation. Orthopaedic Review 6(3):37, 1977
7. Jones D et al: Medical-Surgical Nursing, 2nd ed. New York, McGraw-Hill, 1982
8. Kay HW, Newman JD: Relative incidences of new amputations. Orthotics and Prosthetics 29:6, 1975
9. Kerr A: Orthopedic Nursing Procedures, 3rd ed. New York, Springer, 1980
10. Luckmann J, Sorenson K: Medical-Surgical Nursing. Philadelphia, WB Saunders, 1980
11. Mears DC: Materials and Orthopaedic Surgery. Baltimore, Williams & Wilkins, 1979
12. Meredith S: Formidable: That's the only word for the external fixation device—and for the care it demands. RN 42:19, 1979

13. Parkes CM, Napier MM: Psychiatric sequelae of amputation. Br J Psychol 9:440, 1975
14. Persson BM: Amputation surgery in review. Speech presented at the ISPO Conference, Bologna, Italy, 1980
15. Spickler L: Fat embolism. ONA Journal 2:146, 1975

Bibliography

Allgower M, Spieger PG: Internal fixation of fractures. Clin Orthop 138:26, 1979

Alves R, Martin RA: An overview of orthotics and prosthetics. ONA Journal 4:231, 1977

An alternative to amputation. Emergency Medicine 11:42, 1979

Atlas of Limb Prosthetics. St Louis, CV Mosby, 1981

Baker JL: Nursing care study: Traumatic sub-total amputation of the right hand. Nursing Times 74:323, 1978

Baker WH et al: The healing of below knee amputations; a comparison of soft and plaster dressing. Am J Surg 133:716, 1977

Beasley R: Symposium on management of upper limb amputations. Orthop Clin North Am 12:4, 1981

Bentley G: Operative Surgery: Orthopaedics, part 1. London, Butterworths, 1979

Bonamo JJ: More than just a sprained ankle. Emergency Medicine 9:97, 1977

Brooker A, Edwards C: External Fixation: The Current State of the Art. Baltimore, Williams & Wilkins, 1979

Brown S: Avoiding postop pitfalls with hip fracture patients. RN 45(5):49–53, 1982

Brunner L, Suddarth D: Medical-Surgical Nursing, 5th ed. Philadelphia, JB Lippincott, 1984

Buck B, Lee AD: Amputation: Two views. Nurs Clin North Am 11:641, 1976

Buckwalter K et al: Pain assessment and management in the patient with a fracture. J Nurs Care 14(7):17, 1981

Burgess EM: Disarticulation of the knee. Arch Surg 112:1250, 1977

Burgess EM: Immediate postsurgical prosthetic fitting: A system of amputee management. Phys Ther 51:139, 1971

Burgess EM, Matsen FA: Determining amputation levels in peripheral vascular disease. Journal Bone Joint Surgery, 1483, 1981

Burkhalter WE et al: The upper extremity amputee: Early and immediate postsurgical prosthetic fitting. Journal Bone Joint Surgery (Am) 58:46, 1976

Calderone MS: Doctor, will it leave a scar? Front Radiat Ther Onc 14:130, 1980

Campbell D, Kempson G: Which external fixation device? Injury 12(4):291, 1981

Cheney R: Immediate postsurgical prosthetics in the management of below-knee amputees. ONA Journal 4:260, 1977

Clark J, Malchow D: How to avoid errors in limb salvage decisions. Orthopaedic Review 13(4):47, 1984

Clark M, Shapiro D: Life and limb. Newsweek, January 15, 1979

Coleman A: Rehabilitation of the elderly amputee: A review of the literature. ONA Journal 6(7): 281, 1979

Compere C: Electromagnetic field and bones. JAMA 247(5):669, 1982

Connolly J: DePalma's The Management of Fractures and Dislocations: An Atlas, 3rd ed. Philadelphia, WB Saunders, 1981

Copley IJ: No matter what you call it, it's still pain to the patient. RN 41:64, 1978

Crossland S, Deyerle W: Compartmental syndrome. Nursing 10(11): 51, 1980

Curry K: Construction of a customized pylon: Simple, quick, and functional . . . allowing trial weight bearing. Phys Ther 61(7):71, 1981

Davis R: The classic: The aims of internal fixation. Clin Orthop 138:23, 1979

Day HJB: The assessment and description of amputee activity. Prosthet Orthot Int 5:23, 1981

Dealing with emergency amputations. Nursing 10(4):82, 1980

Deyerle WM, Crossland SA: Broken legs are to be walked on. Am J Nurs 77:1927, 1977

Donahoo CA, Dimon JH III: Orthopedic Nursing. Boston, Little, Brown & Co, 1977

Donahoo C, Spickler L: Core Curriculum of Orthopedic Nursing. Atlanta, Orthopedic Nurses Association, 1980

Dorr L: Treatment of hip fractures in elderly and senile patients. Orthop Clin North Am 12(1):153, 1981

Duerksen J: Hip fractures: Special considerations for the elderly patient. Orthop Nurs 1(1):11–19, 1982

Dunhery E: Fractured hip: How to position and mobilize patient—without undoing their surgery. RN 42(6):44, 1979

Edmonson A, Crenshaw H: Campbell's Operative Orthopaedics, 6th ed. St Louis, CV Mosby, 1980

Edwards C et al: Management of compound tibial fractures using external fixation. Am Surg 45(3):190, 1979

Effeney DJ et al: Transmetatarsal amputation. Arch Surg 112:1366, 1977

Eversmann WW Jr: Ankle fracture in adults. Hospital Medicine 14:84, 1978

Farrell J: Casts, your patients, and you—Part I: A review of basic procedures. Nursing 8(10):65, 1978

Farrell J: Casts, your patients, and you—Part II: A review of arm and leg cast procedures. Nursing 8(11):57, 1978

Farrell J: Casts,your patients, and you—Part III: A review of hip spica procedures. Nursing 8(12):53, 1978

Farrell J: Illustrated Guide to Orthopedic Nursing, 2nd ed. Philadelphia, JB Lippincott, 1982

Farrell J: Nursing care of the patient in a cast brace. Nurs Clin North Am 11(4):717, 1976

Finch RA, MacDougal M, Tibbs DJ, Morris PJ: Amputation for vascular disease: The experience of a peripheral vascular unit. Br J Surg 67:233, 1980

Fighting fat after fracture. Emergency Medicine 10:221, 1978

Foort J: How amputees feel about amputation. Orthotics and Prosthetics 28:21, 1974

Gale PS: The musculoskeletal system. McGraw-Hill Handbook of Clinical Nursing. New York, McGraw-Hill, 1979

Gartland JJ: Fundamentals of Orthopedics, 4th ed. Philadelphia, WB Saunders, 1978

Gong H Jr: Fat embolism syndrome: A puzzling phenomenon. Postgrad Med 62:40, 1977

Green DP: The sprained wrist. Am Fam Physician 19:114, 1979

Grossling H, Donohue T: The fat embolism syndrome. JAMA 241(25):2740, 1979

Haber WB: Reactions to loss of limb: Physiological and psychological aspects. Ann NY Acad Sci 74(1):14, 1958

Hartman JT: Fracture Management: A Practical Approach. London, Henry Kimpton Publishers, 1978

Harvey-Smith W: Stress fractures. Nurse Pract 3:46, 1979

Hay B et al: External fixation: Option for fractures. AORN J 34(3):417, 1981

Heilem F: Epidemilogy of hip fracture. A review with implications for the physical therapist. Phys Ther 59(10):1221, 1979

Heppenstall R: Fracture Treatment and Healing. Philadelphia, WB Saunders, 1980

Hierholzer G et al: External fixation: Classification and indications. Arch Orthop Trauma Surg 92:175, 1978

Hilt N, Cogburn S: Manual of Orthopedics. St Louis, CV Mosby, 1981

Hittenberger D: Extra-ambulatory activities and the amputee. Clinical Prosthetics and Orthotics 6(4), 1982

Huffer JM: Traumatic injuries: Office treatment of fractures. Postgrad Med 62:199, 1977

Jacobs R et al: Internal fixation of intertrochanteric hip fractures: A clinical and biomechanical study. Clin Orthop 146:62, 1980

Jones DA et al: Medical-Surgical Nursing, 2nd ed. New York, McGraw-Hill, 1982

Kalman R: Altered appearance, altered relationships. Am J Psychiatry 138(3):391, 1981

Kay HW, Newman JD: Relative incidences of new amputations. Orthopedics and Prosthetics 29(2):3, 1975

Kegel B et al: Functional capabilities of lower extremity amputees. Arch Phys Med Rehabil 59:109, 1978

Kegel B et al: Recreational activities of lower extremity amputees: A survey. Arch Phys Med Rehabil 61, 1980

Keller C, Laros G: Indications for open reduction of femoral neck fractures. Clin Orthop 152:131, 1980

Kerr A: Orthopedic Nursing Procedures, 3rd ed. New York, Springer, 1980

Kryschyshen P, Fisher K: External fixation for complicated fractures. Am J Nurs 80(2):256, 1980

Kuska B: Acute onset of compartment syndrome. JEN 8(2):75, 1982

Lamb K: Effects of positioning of postoperative fractured-hip patients as related to comfort. Nurs Res 28(5):291–294, 1979

Larson CB, Gould M: Orthopedic Nursing, 9th ed. St Louis, CV Mosby, 1978

Lentz M: Selected aspects of reconditioning secondary to immobilization. Nurs Clin North Am 16(4):729, 1981

Luckmann J, Sorenson K: Medical-Surgical Nursing, 2nd ed. Philadelphia, WB Saunders, 1980

Lupien A: Head off compartment syndrome before it's too late. RN 43(12):38, 1980

Malone J: Rehabilitation for lower extremity amputation. Arch Surg 116(1):93, 1981

Meador R: Learning to live with a new leg. Am J Nurs 79:1339, 1979

Mears D, Fu F: Modern concepts of external skeletal fixation of the pelvis. Clin Orthop 151:65, 1980

Mender J et al: Open fractures of the tibia. Clin Orthop 156:98–104, 1981

Meredith S: Formidable: That's the only word for the external fixation device—and for the care it demands. RN 42(12):19, 1979

Miller L: Orthopedic patients in an ambulatory facility. Nurs Clin North Am 16(4):749, 1981

Mourad L: Nursing Care of Adults with Orthopedic Conditions. New York, John Wiley & Sons, 1980

Muller ME et al: Manual of Internal Fixation, 2nd ed. New York, Springer-Verlag, 1979

Muslin H et al: On psychologic amputation. Orthopaedic Review 6(3):37, 1977

Parkes CM: Reaction to the loss of a limb. Nursing Mirror 148(1):36, 1975

Passo SS: The musculoskeletal system. McGraw-Hill Handbook of Clinical Nursing. New York, McGraw-Hill, 1979

Pfefferbaum B, Pasnau R: Post amputation grief. Nurs Clin North Am 2(4):687, 1976

Powell M: Orthopaedic Nursing and Rehabilitation, 8th ed. New York, John Wiley & Sons, 1980

Roaf R, Hodkinson L: Textbook of Orthopaedic Nursing, 3rd ed. Oxford, Blackwell Scientific, 1980

Roon AJ et al: Below-knee amputation: A modern approach. Am J Surg 134:153, 1977

Ross N: Volkmann's ischaemic contracture: A complication following elbow injuries. ONA Journal 6(5):211, 1979

Rubin G, Fliess D: Devices to enable persons with amputation to participate in sports. Arch Phys Med Rehabil 64:37, 1983

Salter RB: Textbook of Disorders and Injuries of the Musculoskeletal System. Baltimore, Williams & Wilkins, 1970

Schontag H et al: External fixation as an alternative when treating 2nd and 3rd degree open lower leg fractures. Arch Orthop Trauma Surg 97(1):13, 1980

Smith A: Common problems of lower extremity amputees. Orthop Clin North Am 13(3):569, 1982

Stillman MJ: Experiences in clinical problem solving—Mike J.: A young man with a fractured femur. RN 41(7):63, 1978

Taggart M: Body image: Looking beyond the mirror. Journal of Practical Nursing 27:25, 1977

Taylor A: External fixation of fractures: A simple method. Injury 12(3):213, 1980

Troup I, Wood M: Total Care of the Lower Limb Amputee. London, Pittman, 1982

Unthoff H: Current concepts of internal fixation of fractures. Can J Surg 23(3):213, 1980

Wagner FW Jr: The diabetic foot and amputation of the foot. In Mann RA: Duvries Surgery of the Foot, 4th ed. St Louis, CV Mosby, 1979

Walters J: Coping with a leg amputation. Am J Nurs 81(7):1349, 1981

Wassel A: Nursing assessment of injuries to the lower extremity. Nurs Clin North Am 16(4):739, 1981

Waters RL et al: Energy cost of walking of amputees: The influence of level amputation. Nursing Times 74:1490, 1978

Webb JK: The orthopedic management and rehabilitation of patients with multiple skeletal injuries. Orthop Clin North Am 9:569, 1978

Wu Y et al: An innovative removable rigid dressing technique for below-the-knee amputation. J Bone Joint Surg (Am) 61A(5):724, 1979

Chapter 89

Musculoskeletal Inflammation and Connective Tissue Disorders

Terry F. Cicero

Inflammatory disorders of the musculoskeletal system include a wide variety of conditions of varying etiologies. Bacterial invasion of the bone and joints can directly initiate the inflammatory process. Osteomyelitis and tuberculosis of the spine are examples in this category.

The connective tissue diseases (rheumatic) are a group of disorders with diffuse involvement of skeletal muscles, bones, and joints. Although many of the diseases have systemic manifestations, the most prevalent symptoms are musculoskeletal in origin. The inflammatory process in this group of disorders may be the result of immunologic aberrations (*e.g.,* rheumatoid arthritis, systemic lupus erythematosus, and systemic sclerosis), postbacterial infections in other areas of the body (*e.g.,* Reiter's syndrome), metabolic processes (*e.g.,* gout), or a combination of these.

The purpose of this chapter is to discuss the epidemiology, pathology, and medical and nursing management of the more common inflammatory disorders of the musculoskeletal system.

Common themes occur throughout the chapter. Most of the disorders are, or have the potential to be, chronic and debilitating. Patient management is uniformly concerned with the problems of pain, varying degrees of immobility or functional impairment, and alterations in body image.

Osteomyelitis

Osteomyelitis is a bacterial infection of the bone. Pathogenic organisms can enter the bone through trauma or surgery, or during skeletal traction in which pins or tongs are used (external source). Bacteria may also enter the bloodstream from infections in other areas of the body and spread to the bone (internal foci). Examples of such infections are pharyngitis, otitis media, infected skin lesions, sinus infections, dental abscess, or phlebitis associated with heroin users.[20,22] Factors that enhance the development of bone infections as a complication of closed fractures are diabetes, debilitation, and alcoholism.[5] Osteomyelitis is most frequently seen in children, and it can be acute or chronic.

Etiology and Pathophysiology

The organisms frequently associated with osteomyelitis are *Staphylococcus aureus* and *Streptococcus pyogenes*. Occasionally pneumococcus may be responsible, since it predominates in the oral cavity and in the paracranial sinuses.

Osteomyelitis most frequently occurs in the metaphyseal area of long bones. This area is vascular but the circulation is sluggish. The vessel walls contain few polymorphonuclear leukocytes, and the metaphyseal area is the weakest point in growing bone.[8] Once the bacteria become established in the bone, the infection spreads through the medullary canal to the subperiosteal region of the bone. The infection can push through the epiphyseal plate and into the joint capsule, resulting in septic arthritis. The formation of a subperiosteal abscess elevates the periosteum and separates a segment of bone from its blood and nutrient supply. The ischemic area of bone becomes necrotic and is referred to as *sequestrum* (Fig. 89–1). As the disease progresses, the elevated periosteum stimulates osteoblastic activity, and new immature bone, or involucrum, is laid down over the sequestrum. Frequently the new bone contains perforations called cloacae that allow sequestrum to yield draining sinuses.

Clinical Manifestations

In the acute phase there is malaise, general weakness, vague aching, and swelling over the affected bone. In children, the mother may notice the child's reluctance to use the extremity. As the disease progresses, chills, high fever, and severe tenderness over the bone are pronounced. Muscle spasms are common, because the joint is held in a flexed, protective position.

In the chronic phase as the bacteria continue to thrive in the scar tissue, the patient complains of attacks of pain, with swelling and inflammation over the affected bone. Temperature, white cell count, and erthrocyte sedimentation rate (ESR) are elevated, but the toxemia is not as severe. Draining sinuses are a common problem. Radiographs reveal large irregular cavities and dense areas where sequestrum is forming.

Medical Management

In the acute phase early identification and eradication of the infective organism is the primary aim of treatment. Laboratory tests show leukocytosis, an elevated ESR, and positive blood cultures (prior to institution of antibiotic therapy). Radiographs initially show no changes, but within 2 weeks of the onset reveal an elevated periosteum and mottling in the metaphysis. Intravenous antibiotic therapy is instituted after blood specimens and needle aspiration of abscesses are sent for culture and sensitivity. A combination of two broad-spectrum antibiotics such as nafcillin (Nafcil), cefazolin (Kefzol), cephalothin (Keflin), or methicillin (Staphcillin) are used until sensitivities are known. Antibiotics frequently do not penetrate well into the infected area, and therefore high serum levels of the drugs are necessary. Probenecid (Benemid) is given to decrease the rate of antibiotic excretion from the kidney, thus prolonging the serum levels of the drug.[20] Antibiotic therapy can last for 6 weeks to 1 year.

Surgical exploration, débridement, and drainage of sequestra or abscesses are indicated if the patient does not respond to antibiotic therapy within 24 to 48 hours.

The limb is usually immobilized in a cast or splint to decrease spread of infection and reduce pain. Narcotic or non-narcotic analgesics may be ordered to control pain. Transfusions may be necessary if anemia is present.

Long-term combination surgery and antibiotic therapy is required to manage *chronic osteomyelitis.* All necrotic and infected bone and tissue must be removed through sequestrectomy or saucerization before healing can occur. The extremity is placed in a cast with a window for access to care for the wound. The wound may be surgically closed over an irrigation catheter for local antibiotics, or it may be packed with dressing to facilitate drainage. Management of chronic osteomyelitis frequently entails skin grafting after the infection heals.

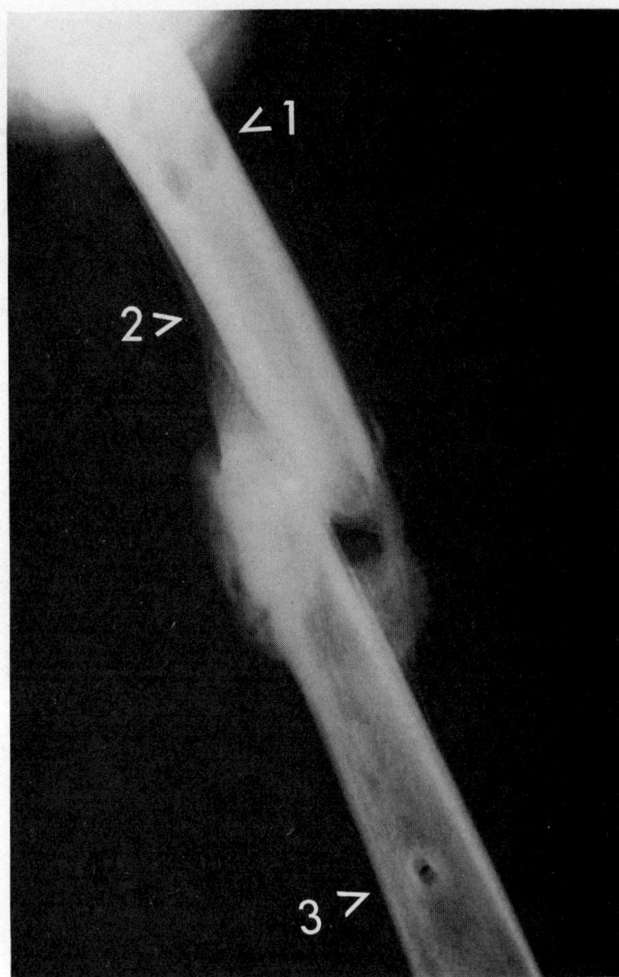

FIGURE 89–1 X-ray film of developing osteomyelitis in a femur with a healing fracture: (*1*) sequestra; (*2*) elevated periosteum; (*3*) skeletal pin site (not to be confused with sequestra).

Nursing Management

Assessment and Nursing Diagnosis

Information derived from the nursing history and physical assessment identify problems for nursing management. The major nursing problems include pain secondary to inflammation and debris in the bone, potential inadequate wound healing, and anxiety secondary to inadequate knowledge about treatment. Problems related to the hazards of

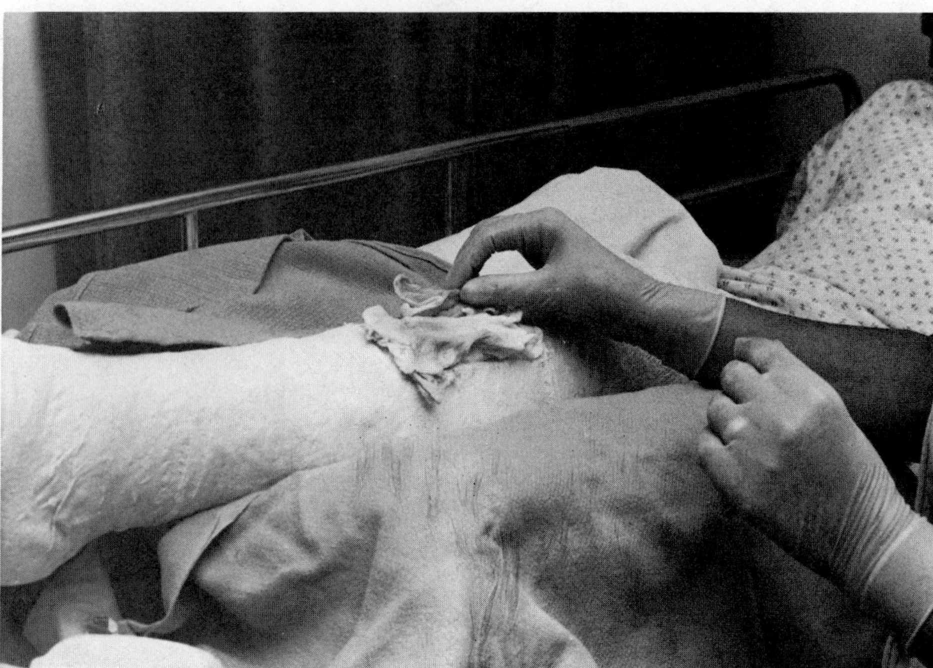

FIGURE 89–2 Dressing and cast care in osteomyelitis. Any dressing changes must be done using strict sterile technique and extreme gentleness in handling the affected part.

immobility and cast care are also a consideration and are discussed in Chapter 87.

In addition to the nursing problems already stated, emotional manifestation from frequent, lengthy hospitalizations and alterations in body image secondary to draining wounds and skin grafts are problems confronted in caring for patients with chronic osteomyelitis. The nursing problems associated with care of skin grafts are discussed in Chapter 97.

Goals. The major goals for patients with osteomyelitis are to relieve the pain and prevent bone and wound infection. It is also important to provide adequate nutritional support and to reduce anxiety about the treatment as well as negative feelings about body image.

Interventions

Osteomyelitis is very painful, and the affected extremity must always be handled carefully. When turning or repositioning the patient, arrange for sufficient help so that one nurse can support and prevent the extremity from twisting while the other nurse repositions the trunk. A firm mattress and good body alignment are essential. Adequate support with firm pillows or splints on affected joints reduces pain and muscle spasm. Stool softeners, laxatives, and enemas may be required if narcotic analgesics are given for pain.

Development of additional painful areas or spikes in temperature while on treatment warrant investigation, since they may indicate a secondary infection or extension of the existing infection.

Aseptic technique is imperative if there is a draining sinus or wound. Wounds or irrigation systems may need to be managed through the window of a cast (Fig. 89–2). Keeping the cast dry is a major challenge. Sterile plastic and abundant fluff dressings around the window edge provide temporary protection.

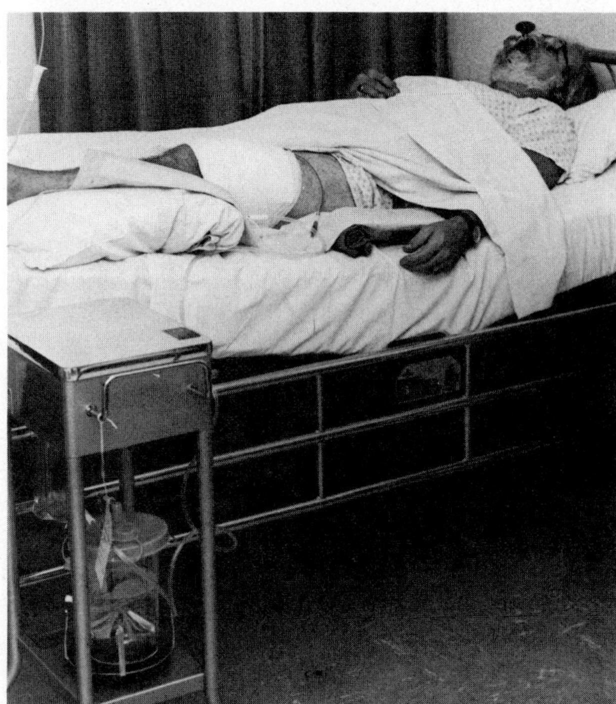

FIGURE 89–3 Irrigation systems in the management of osteomyelitis frequently involve a Hemovac or suction unit.

Irrigation of antibiotics into the wound are a sterile procedure and often involve a Hemovac, Jackson Pratt, or other suction unit (Fig. 89–3). Input and outflow measurements of the irrigant are monitored on an hourly basis. Explicit instructions from the surgeon are needed regarding what action to take if the unit becomes clogged.

Periodically, samples of the drainage may be obtained for culture and sensitivity. Wound and skin precautions must be strictly adhered to when handling contaminated dressings, linen, and equipment. Careful hand washing is essential to prevent cross-infection to other patients.

Infections greatly increase the metabolic demands of the body. High-protein, high-calorie meals promote healing and ensure positive nitrogen balance. A multivitamin supplement may be ordered. Fluids are encouraged to 3000 ml/day for hydration and to prevent renal complications from heavy antibiotic use.

Patients need to be aware of the serious nature and therapy of the disease. They should be given time and opportunities to express their questions and concerns regarding surgical procedures and long-term antibiotic therapy. As their condition merits, providing passes to leave the hospital between treatments helps alleviate the depression and boredom that accompany long-term hospitalization.

The patient's self-image may be impaired as a result of the wound irrigation system, draining sinuses, or an unsightly fresh skin graft. The wounds, casts, and drainage also become odorous. Supportive measures to provide comfort, honest answers to questions about the condition, and allowing the patient to verbalize his feelings demonstrate respect for the patient and his needs.

Evaluation

The patient will

1. Obtain relief of pain:
   a. Expresses no complaint of pain with exercise
   b. Is able to sleep without pain
   c. Has no physiological or nonverbal indicators of pain *e.g.,* increased pulse and grimacing
2. Demonstrate no sign of bone and wound infection:
   a. Expresses no complaint of pain
   b. Exhibits no purulent drainage from sinuses or dressings
   c. Remains afebrile
   d. Serum leukocyte and sedimentation rates are normal
3. Demonstrate optimal nutritional status:
   a. Consumes 3 high-calorie/high-protein meals/day
   b. Intake of 3000 ml fluids/day, unless contraindicated
   c. Exhibits normal serum protein levels
   d. Has increasing energy level
4. Demonstrate a decrease in anxiety about treatment:
   a. Expresses feelings regarding care
   b. Verbalizes an accurate description of treatment procedure
   c. Participates in self-care
5. Have realistic concept of altered body image:
   a. Free of depression
   b. Demonstrates interest and participates in self-care
   c. Verbalizes feelings/frustrations concerning condition

Tuberculosis of the Spine

The most common and most debilitating type of chronic bone infection is due to tuberculosis. The incidence of skeletal tuberculosis has greatly decreased in the past 20 years because of better diagnostic techniques, tuberculin testing of cattle, pasteurization of milk, and discovery of antituberculosis drugs. Skeletal involvement, however, still accounts for 3% of all diagnosed tuberculosis.[3]

Etiology and Pathophysiology

The tubercle bacillus *Mycobacterium tuberculosis* is the causative organism. The bacteria can affect any bone or joint in the body, but the spine is the most commonly involved site, constituting 50% of reported skeletal cases.[28] Invasion of the vertebrae is secondary to circulatory transport from the primary foci, usually the lungs.

Following bacterial invasion of the vertebral body, inflammation occurs resulting in areas of ischemia and necrosis. The bone softens and collapses, causing deformities of the spine. Displacement of the intervertebral disk causes spinal cord compression, pain, and paralysis.

Abscesses, composed of serum, leukocytes, bone debris, and bacteria, form and migrate onto either side of the spine. They can result in draining sinuses.

Clinical Manifestations

Symptoms of tuberculosis of the spine are usually insidious. Anorexia, weight loss, fatigue, and general malaise occur, with night sweats and intermittent evening temperature rise. The spine is stiff, with painful, limited motion from ankylosis. There is often a hunchback deformity that is tender to palpation. The vertebral muscles have frequent spasms.

The most serious complications of spinal tuberculosis are neurological, and they occur in 20% of the patients.[28] Pressure and stretching of the spinal cord from inflammatory edema, compression deformities, thrombosis, or abscess formation result in motor weakness or paralysis. Meningitis occurs if abscesses rupture through the dura membrane.

Medical Management

Diagnosis is confirmed through radiograph and laboratory studies. Radiographs show collapse of vertebral bodies, loss of intervertebral disk space, and paraspinal abscesses. Sputum cultures and tissue biopsies reveal tubercle bacilli. Tuberculin skin tests are generally positive, and there is usually an elevated leukocyte count.

Treatment of tuberculosis of the spine includes immobilization, chemotherapy, and possible débridement–decompression surgery. Traditionally the patient was immobilized on a plaster bed for long periods. This method is still in use, but the efficacy of complete bed rest is unproven. Contemporary treatment immobilizes the spine in a cast or brace while allowing the patient to resume his normal daily activities.[19] The period of immobilization is lengthy, lasting from 6 to 18 months.

Chemotherapy utilizes a combination of the antituberculosis drugs: streptomycin sulfate, *p*-aminosalicylic acid (PAS), isonicotinic acid hydrazide (INAH), rifampin, ethambutol, and ethionamide. These drugs are taken for a 1- to 2-year period and are associated with significant side-effects: eighth cranial nerve damage from streptomycin and liver toxicity and bone marrow depression from rifampin. Drug therapy is discussed in detail in Chapter 28. The use of corticosteroids is controversial, but they may be given to reduce neurological complications. Therapeutic response is gauged by radiography and a reduced erythrocyte sedimentation rate, which are performed at 3- to 6-month intervals.

Orthopedic surgery is indicated for progressive bone destruction or increase in abscess size after 3 months of conservative treatment. Débridement and decompression procedures are performed when neurological complications develop or do not recede after a 4-week trial of medications and rest. Chemotherapy is always given with surgery.

Nursing Management

The nursing assessment, diagnosis, goals, and interventions for the patient with tuberculosis of the spine are similar to care of the patient with chronic osteomyelitis. The common nursing problems are pain, immobilization, draining sinuses, and impaired nutritional status. Additional nursing management problems relate to education of the patient and family with tuberculosis (Chap. 28), spinal cord injury (Chap. 69), and meningitis (Chap. 68).

Rheumatoid Arthritis

Rheumatoid arthritis (RA) is a chronic progressive systemic disease characterized by inflammation of diarthrodial joints. Rheumatoid arthritis is associated with multiple extra-articular manifestations such as anemia, osteoporosis, and skin, cardiac, ocular, vascular, pulmonary, and cardiac dysfunction. The disease affects 2% to 6% of the adult US population and includes all races.[12] The onset most commonly occurs in the 20- to 40-year age-group, with a 3:1 female preponderance.[16]

Etiology

The cause of rheumatoid arthritis remains unknown, but it is thought to be an autoimmune mechanism (see Chap. 16). There is a higher incidence of positive rheumatoid factor (RF) in the serum of RA patients than the general population. Rheumatoid factor is a laboratory measure of immunoglobulin IgG or IgM that reacts with the IgG antibodies produced by lymphocytes in synovial fluid. Rheumatoid factor also occurs in other diseases, such as subacute bacterial endocarditis, syphilis, hepatitis, viral infections, and chronic fibrosing lung disease, so that its presence is not diagnostic for rheumatoid arthritis.

A genetic predisposition to developing rheumatoid arthritis has recently been demonstrated.[4] An antigen found on human leukocyte antigen (HLA, the histocompatability antigen) has been found in 50% of diagnosed RA patients.[16] Other possible etiologic factors are infective agents and endocrine abnormalities. It is likely that rheumatoid arthritis results from a combination of several factors.

Pathophysiology

Although rheumatoid arthritis is a systemic disease, the primary target organ is the synovial joints. The initiating event in the pathological process is inflammation of the synovial membrane as lymphocytes and plasma cells infiltrate the joint, causing hyperemia, congestion, and pain. Antigen–antibody complexing occurs as inflammatory cells produce IgG, IgA, and IgM (rheumatoid factors). These complexes are engulfed by phagocytic cells that eventually rupture and release lysosomal enzymes that further attack the synovial lining.[4] The synovial lining thickens and forms a mass called *pannus* (granulation tissue), which adheres to and erodes the articular cartilage. As the process continues, bone is exposed, joint space is lost, and adhesions and bony fibrosis ultimately lead to ankylosis. Subluxation (partial dislocation) may occur from cartilage loss, ligament weakening, and disuse muscle atrophy.

Clinical Manifestations

The clinical course of rheumatoid arthritis is extremely variable and characterized by periods of remission and exacerbations. The onset is usually insidious, with joint inflammation preceding the systemic symptoms of fatigue, malaise, anorexia, weight loss, low grade fever, myalgias, and parasthesias.

The onset can also be explosive, with high fever and profound disability. The explosive form is associated with a good prognosis and often permanent remission, whereas an insidious onset with extra-articular involvement has the poorest prognosis.[13]

Joint involvement is usually symmetrical and accompanied by complaints of morning stiffness. Symptoms often begin in the hands, especially the proximal interphalangeal (PIP) and metacarpophalangeal (MCP) joints (Fig. 89–4). As the disease progresses, the metatarsophalangeal, wrist, knee, elbow, ankle, and shoulder joints are affected. Any diarthrodial (freely moveable) joint may be involved, including the temporomandibular, intervertebral facet, or the cricoarytenoid joint of the larynx.

Synovitis is present with soft tissue edema, warmth, tenderness, and pain with motion. Joint movement is limited owing to synovial effusions, splinting, and muscle spasms. Characteristic flexion contractures and fixed deformities of the hands and feet are due to fibrosis of the tendons and ligaments of the joint capsule (Fig. 89–5).

Extra-articular manifestations are numerous and may be life threatening (Fig. 89–6). They occur in one out of every five RA patients.[16] The most common extra-articular symptoms are subcutaneous nodules, occurring in 20% of patients.[4] They are spongy, freely moveable, and are usually found over bony prominences such as the olecranon, occiput, or fingers. They can also be located on the sclera, pleura, or heart valves. The nodules have a necrotic center sur-

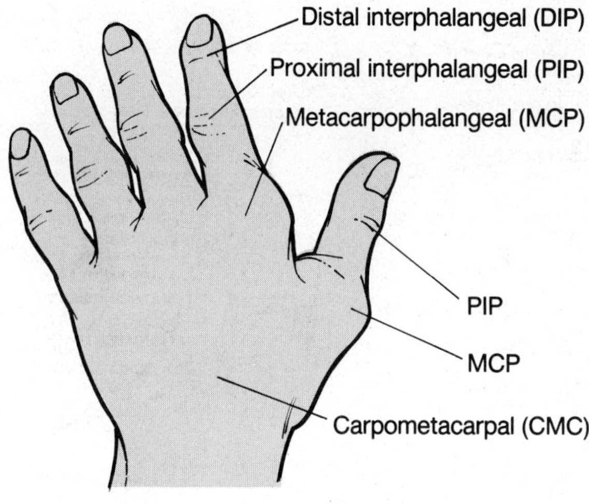

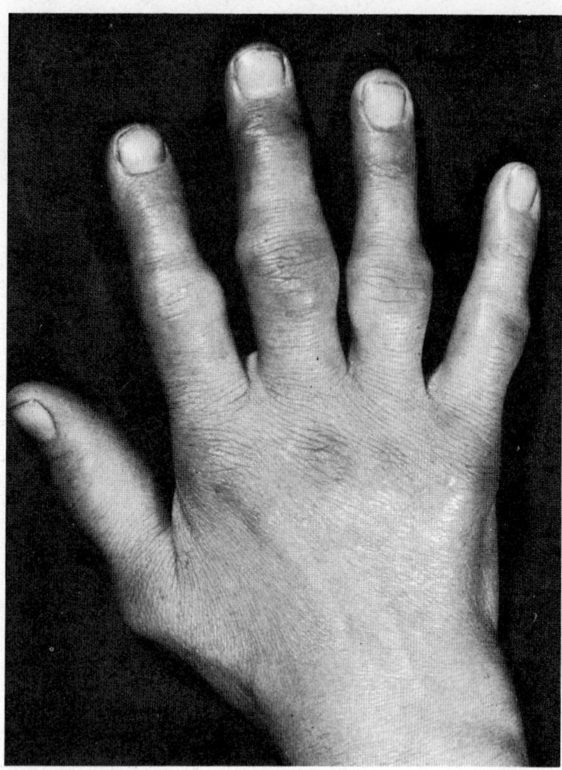

FIGURE 89–4 Joint involvement in the hands in rheumatoid arthritis. (View *B* from Utsinger PD, Zvaifler NJ, Ehrlich GE [eds]: Rheumatoid Arthritis: Etiology, Diagnosis, Management, p 288. Philadelphia, JB Lippincott, 1985)

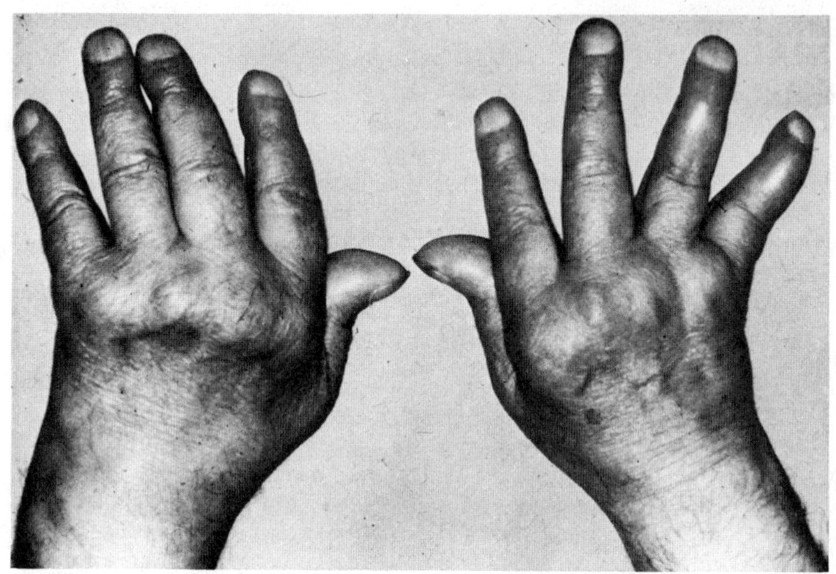

FIGURE 89–5 Synovitis of the mcp joints, ulnar deviation, and "swan-neck" deformity of the right fourth and fifth digits. (Utsinger PD, Zvaifler NJ, Ehrlich GE [eds]: Rheumatoid Arthritis: Etiology, Diagnosis, Management, p 289. Philadelphia, JB Lippincott, 1985)

rounded by tissue, producing large amounts of collagenase, an enzyme that destroys connective tissue. Rheumatic nodules can become infected, ulcerate, or limit the function of a joint.

Sjögren's syndrome occurs in 10% to 25% of patients and is characterized by decreased saliva (xerostomia) and lacrimal secretions (keratoconjunctivitis sicca). Women with Sjögren's syndrome may have decreased vaginal secretions and complain of painful sexual intercourse (dyspareunia).

Cardiac, pulmonary, and renal involvement are the most serious consequences of rheumatoid arthritis. Systemic symptoms are either drug induced or the result of vasculitis and antigen–antibody tissue invasion.

Medical Management

The primary clinical goal in treating rheumatoid arthritis is to achieve remission. Treatment, however, is dependent on the severity and extent of the disease process and on the degree of functional limitation, disability, or deformity.

Diagnosis. Laboratory evaluations have a limited role in the diagnosis and management of patients with rheuma-

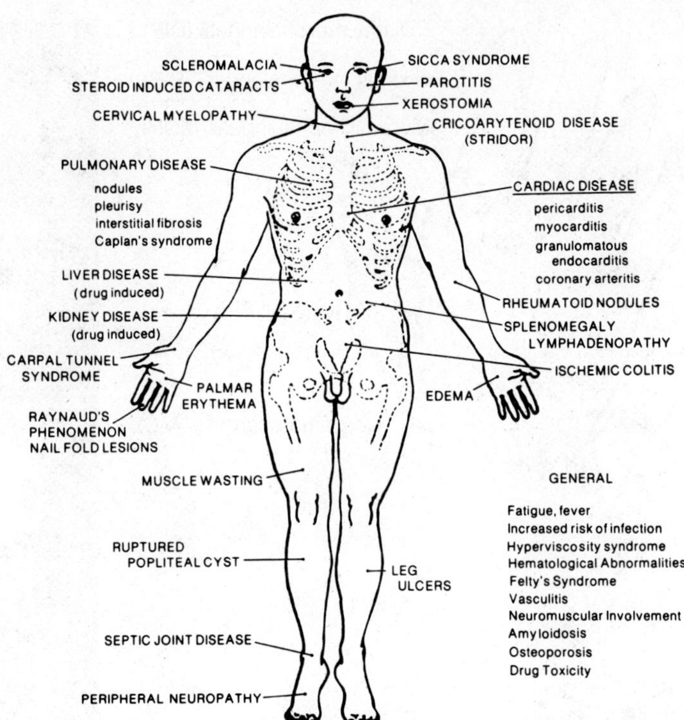

FIGURE 89–6 Signs and symptoms of systemic disease in rheumatoid arthritis. (Calin A: Differential Diagnosis in Rheumatology: An Atlas for the Physician, p 119. Philadelphia, JB Lippincott, 1984)

toid arthritis. The erthrocyte sedimentation rate (ESR) is usually elevated during periods of exacerbation, and it is the single most important test of inflammatory activity. C-reactive protein, a glycoprotein that appears during any inflammation, is elevated in 70% to 80% of patients.[16] Rheumatoid factor, positive in 75% to 90% of RA patients, and antinuclear antibodies (ANA), positive in 25%, denote abnormal immune activity.

Other common laboratory results are normocytic anemia, leukocytosis, and increased platelets. Synovial fluid samples reveal increased white blood cell count. Radiograph of the involved joints depicts effusions, osteopenia, marginal erosions, and joint narrowing or misalignment.

When rheumatoid arthritis is newly diagnosed, conservative measures such as rest periods, physical therapy, splints, and salicylates are employed. Patient education about the disease, principles of joint protection, and the importance of compliance with a treatment regimen is standard.

Pharmacotherapy. Aspirin is the mainstay of anti-inflammatory therapy owing to its potent anti-inflammatory, analgesic, and antipyretic actions. Aspirin is available in a variety of forms aimed at reducing its most significant side-effect, gastrointestinal toxicity. It must be taken in high doses throughout the day to achieve and maintain adequate blood levels.

A large variety of nonsteroidal anti-inflammatory agents (NSAIs) are available for patients who fail to respond to salicylate therapy. These medications include indomethacin (Indocin), phenylbutazone (Butazolidin), and the newer agents ibuprofen (Motrin), naproxen (Naprosyn), tolmetin (Tolectin), fenoprofen (Nalfon), piroxicam (Feldene), and sulindac (Clinoril). The newer compounds were developed in an effort to reduce gastrointestinal intolerance.

For patients with persistent articular inflammation, one of several remission-inducing agents can be tried. They include hydroxychloroquine sulfate (Plaquenil), gold, and D-penicillamine (Depen, Cuprimine). Gold is presently available only in intramuscular preparations, and therapy must be administered weekly for 3 to 6 months before progress is seen. Once remission occurs, the interval between injections is gradually lengthened. Triethylphosphine (Auranofin), an orally administered gold preparation, is currently under investigation.[6,11,15]

Intra-articular and systemic corticosteroids often dramatically alleviate pain and inflammation, but they are associated with numerous side-effects, and their use is controversial.

Cytotoxic agents such as cyclophosphamide (Cytoxan), azathioprine (Imuran), methotrexate, and others, although not approved by the FDA for treatment of rheumatoid arthritis, have afforded some relief to patients with particularly severe and resistant forms of the disease. Therapy aims at suppressing the immune mechanisms that are thought to be responsible for the inflammation. The goal of therapy is to administer long-term, low-dose therapy without causing significant bone marrow depression. Table 89–1 summarizes the drugs most frequently used in treating rheumatoid arthritis and identifies the major nursing considerations related to their administration.

Surgery. *Operative procedures* are also available to improve joint function and decrease pain. Synovectomies are considered in patients who have inflammatory activity in

TABLE 89–1
Medications Used in Rheumatoid Arthritis

Drug	*Action*	*Nursing Considerations*
Anti-inflammatory Agents		
Salicylates (aspirin)	Thought to inhibit prostaglandin synthesis Anti-inflammatory, analgesic, antipyretic Available in many forms: buffered, enteric-coated, prolonged action, caffeine Therapeutic serum salicylate levels of 18–25 mg/100 ml	Minimize gastrointestinal intolerance by administering with meals or antacids. Potential for gastric ulcers is increased if taken when drinking alcohol. Advise patients not to buy in large quantities and to smell tablets prior to ingestion for vinegar odor (acetic acid). If present, discard all tablets. Instruct patients to report petechiae, bleeding gums, bloody or black stools, tinnitus or dizziness.
Nonsteroidal Anti-inflammatory Agents (NSAIDs)		
Indomethacin (Indocin)	Similar to aspirin Palliative use only in active stages of moderate to severe RA	*For all the nonsteroidal anti-inflammatory agents:* Administer with meals or antacids to minimize gastrointestinal side-effects.
Phenylbutazone (Butazolidin)	Mode of action not known Anti-inflammatory, antipyretic, analgesic, uricosuric	Gastrointestinal ulceration and hemorrhage are the most common symptoms. Can cause dizziness and light-headedness Need to monitor hepatic and renal function
Oxyphenbutazone (Tandearil)	Same as Butazolidin Has less ulcerogenic activity than phenylbutazone	Report signs of abnormal bleeding due to drug-induced prolonged bleeding time
Fenoprofen calcium (Nalfon)	Mode of action of all the following NSAIDs are unknown but possibly related to inhibition of prostaglandin synthesis. Have the same actions as the above Decreases serum uric acid	Inhibits platelet aggregation and prolongs bleeding time Cross-sensitivity to other NSAID has been reported Has lower incidence of gastrointestinal symptoms
Ibuprofen (Motrin, Rufen)	Same as Nalfon, but no effect on uric acid	Associated with Stevens-Johnson syndrome (an acute inflammatory skin reaction) and fluid retention and edema
Naproxen (Naprosyn)	Longer half-life than some other NSAIDs, thus requires less frequent administration	
Piroxicam (Feldene)	The longest acting of the NSAIDs; requires only 1 dose/24 hr	
Sulindac (Clinoril)		Associated with Stevens-Johnson syndrome, peripheral edema, and congestive heart failure
Tolmetin sodium (Tolectin, Tolectin DS)		Na^+, water retention, hypertension, and some blood dyscrasias
Remission-Inducing Agents		
Hydroxychloroquine sulfate (Plaquenil)	An antimalarial compound with anti-inflammatory actions Stabilizes lysosomal membranes Used in conjunction with salicylates Prescribed for treatment of RA and systemic lupus erythematosus Maximum benefit may not occur until 6 months of therapy	Minimize gastrointestinal effects by administering with meals Irreversible retinopathy can progress even after therapy is discontinued. Advise patients to have ophthalmology exams every 4 to 6 months

(*Continued*)

TABLE 89–1
Medications Used in Rheumatoid Arthritis *(Continued)*

Drug	*Action*	*Nursing Considerations*
Remission-Inducing Agents		
Gold sodium thiomalate (Myochrysine)	*Water-soluble:* rapid absorption Anti-inflammatory joint action of both gold preparations is unknown, but may be related to gold uptake by macrophages and inhibition of phagocytosis.	Patient to remain recumbent for 15 to 30 minutes past injection to overcome nitrotoid reaction—flushing, fainting, dizziness Adverse effects: stomatitis, rash, reversible nephrotic syndrome with proteinuria, and rare blood dyscrasias
Aurothioglucose (Solganal) (An oral form is under investigation)	*Oil-suspension:* slower acting, to reduce the side-effects Both preparations are given by IM injections weekly for an indefinite period. Can be taken in conjunction with salicylates Maximum benefit may not occur until 3 to 6 months of therapy	Prior to each injection: urinalysis for protein and blood, CBC with differential, platelet count Increased need for salicylates while on gold therapy indicates a decreased response to the gold.
Glucocorticosteroids		
Prednisone (Deltasone) Prednisolone	Synthetic hydrocortisone Inhibits phagocytosis and interferes with tissue granulation Immunosuppressive: decreased number of circulating lymphocytes and reduction in antibody titers Used for short-term, acute flare-ups	Administer with meals or antacids to reduce gastrointestinal irritation. Has a cumulative effect on bone metabolism, which can be reversed with vitamin D administration Follow BP, weight, serum K, and glucose closely. Adverse reactions: diabetes, sodium and water retention, hypertension, hypokalemia, osteoporosis, muscle wasting, gastric ulcers, perforation, hemorrhage, glaucoma, cushingoid features
Intra-articular Corticosteroids		
Aristospan, Hydeltra, Kenalog, Decadron LA, Celestone	Predominantly localized, with mild systemic effects Injections lower intra-articular temperature, which decreases collagen and cartilage breakdown	Be alert to potential systemic effects. Relieves pain so that patients can undergo physical therapy. Given in 3 to 4 intermittent injections (one every 3 months)
D-Penicillamine (Cuprimine, Depen)	Mechanism of action not known, but appears related to inhibition of collage formation and dissociation of macrophages Potentiation of hematological and renal toxicity if taken with antimalarials, cytotoxins, gold, Tandearil, or Butazolidin	Cross-sensitivity between penicillin and penicillamine May interfere with absorption of vitamin B_6 Monitor CBC, platelets, and urinalysis every 2 weeks. Special attention to skin pressure areas, since drug increases skin friability Adverse reactions: unusual skin wrinkling and rashes, dysgeusia (loss of taste) reversible, thrombocytopenia, anemia, nephrotoxicity, and hepatotoxicity
Immunosuppressive Drugs		
Cyclophosphamide (Cytoxan)	Mechanism of action is not known, but it modifies the body's autoimmune response.	Monitor CBC, platelets, liver and kidney function weekly.
Azathioprine (Imuran)	Given in low dose to prevent bone marrow depression May be given with steroids Given only if patient has severe RA and is not responsive to other therapy	Carcinogenic—advise patients concerning contraception Adverse reactions: highly toxic, bone marrow depression (especially leukopenia), stomatitis, gastrointestinal ulcerations, alopecia, renal toxicity, hepatotoxicity, and reduced resistance to infection Watch for overgrowth of opportunistic organisms (*e.g.*, yeast, fungus).

only one to five joints. The procedure, accomplished through an arthroscope, removes the adherent pannus before the joint degenerates. Joint replacements are considered for patients with severe deformities, significant functional disabilities, or poorly controlled pain.

Experimental treatments with strong potential include thoracic duct drainage, plasmapheresis, and lymphoid irradiation.[26]

Nursing Management

Assessment and Nursing Diagnosis

Based on the assessment data, nursing history, and severity of disease involvement, unlimited nursing challenges are possible. The nursing problems most frequently encountered are joint pain and stiffness; impaired mobility secondary to joint pain and deformity; inability to perform ADLs; altered self-image secondary to loss of independence, deformity, and chronic illness; and inadequate nutrient intake related to malaise and gastrointestinal disturbances from medications. Additionally there is an increased potential for pressure sores secondary to decreased mobility and medication side-effects, and noncompliance with therapeutic regimen secondary to the grieving process and societal lure to try unproven remedies.

Goals. The major goals are interrelated with many of the nursing problems. The initial goal is to decrease pain and reduce inflammation. Measures are also directed at increasing joint mobility and muscle strength in order to prevent deformities and promote independence in carrying out ADLs. All of these factors will assist the patient to maintain a positive body image. Adhering to the treatment protocol, engaging in daily activities, and maintaining adequate nutritional support constitute the major goals of a patient and family educational program.

Interventions

Full treatment of the patient requires an interdisciplinary approach to include nurses, physicians, social workers, dieticians, and occupational and physical therapists. Much of the nurse's responsibility lies in patient and family teaching. Nursing interventions are described in detail in Nursing Care Plan for the Patient with Rheumatoid Arthritis.

Pain is controlled with medications combined with heat or cold applications and frequent rest periods. Both heat and cold decrease muscle spasm, increase joint range of motion, and improve exercise performance. Cold therapy is more effective for acutely inflamed joints, and heat for chronic pain. Superficial heat, through moist hot packs, hydrotherapy, and paraffin dips, provides shallow penetration. Deep heat (diathermy, ultrasound) actually penetrates the joint with heat. The benefits of deep vs. superficial heat have not been established.

Rest and relaxation are essential to minimize the fatigue associated with systemic disease and relieve the stress of weight bearing on the joints. Rest periods are correlated with disease activity; as inflammation increases, more rest is required.

A regular exercise program is the heart of treatment to keep joints mobile. Pain and inflammation cause the patient to immobilize the joint. Motion is further limited by muscle spasms. Range-of-motion and muscle-strengthening (isometrics) exercises are used in conjunction with heat/cold and analgesics.[24] Adjustments in the program are made when systemic or joint symptoms increase or decrease. Excessive strain on joints should be avoided at all costs. Guidelines for joint protection are outlined in Table 89–2.

Patient independence is encouraged within individual limits. Many aspects of self-care can be accomplished if the patient is given additional time for task completion.[21]

There are numerous self-help devices available to help the patient to dress, bathe, eat, and groom. Canes, walkers, and custom-made shoes provide support and prevent falls. Increased independence in self-care fosters a positive self-image.

Patient education is an integral part of therapy. The patient must be knowledgeable about the disease, his symptoms, his treatment program, and available community resources.

Patient education should also address quackery. Unfortunately, there are many unproven remedies that advertise a cure for arthritis. Over 1 billion dollars per year is spent on dietary gimmicks (*e.g.,* cod liver oil and vitamins), herbal medicines, dimethyl sulfoxide (DMSO), and copper bracelets. Illegal medications are available from China and Mexico that often contain unknown quantities of corticosteroids, indeomethacin, or phenylbutazone. Communication between patients, nurses, and physicians is imperative concerning any change in the therapeutic regimen.

Evaluation

Evaluation of nursing interventions, specified as outcome criteria, is as follows.

(*Text continues on page 1347*)

TABLE 89–2
Patient Guidelines for Joint Protection in Rheumatoid Arthritis

1. Learn to respond to pain by decreasing activity.
2. Always use your biggest muscles and strongest joints.
3. Alternate light and heavy tasks.
4. Take frequent rest periods.
5. Participate in jobs or activities that can be easily interrupted if pain develops.
6. Don't remain in one position for long periods.
7. Use lightweight equipment and self-help devices.
8. Eliminate unnecessary tasks.
9. Maintain good posture while at work or rest.
10. Warm, swollen joints should be used as little as possible (only range-of-motion exercises).

(Adapted from Simpson CF, Dickinson GR: Exercise. AJN 83(2):275, 1983)

NURSING CARE PLAN FOR THE PATIENT WITH RHEUMATOID ARTHRITIS

NURSING DIAGNOSIS/PROBLEM 1: Alterations in comfort and pain related to joint pain and stiffness
GOAL 1: Control pain and reduce inflammation

Nursing Interventions	Rationale	Outcome Criteria
1. Administer pain medications and remissive agents as ordered.	1. Salicylates and NSAIDs are used to relieve inflammation and pain. Remissive agents are used to arrest the progress of the disease.	1. Absense of nonverbal clues of pain (*e.g.*, limping, grimace, rubbing an affected joint)
a. Be alert to the side-effects (Table 89-1).		
b. Instruct patient not to omit his doses of anti-inflammatory agents.	b. Anti-inflammatory agents require high blood levels, which fall with missed doses.	b. No signs of inflammation (*e.g.*, redness, warmth, swelling)
2. Apply hot or cold therapy to affected stiff joints.	2. Provides temporary pain relief by raising the pain threshold.[23]	
a. Contraindications: Do not use deep heat for acutely inflamed joints.	a. Increased temperature possibly accelerates cartilage destruction[23]	
b. Do not use hydrotherapy in elderly with cardiovascular or respiratory problems.	b. Leads to increased body temperature, pulse, and oxygen consumption, and to decreased blood pressure (vasodilation)	
c. Do not use for patients with vasculitis or Raynaud's phenomenon.	c. Cold temperatures result in vasoconstriction and initiate vasospasm.	
3. Advise patient to take a hot tub bath or shower on arising.	3. Shortens the period of morning stiffness	
4. Provide regular rest periods at scheduled intervals.	4. A *balance* of rest with exercise is important: too much rest causes joint stiffening; not enough causes damage and decreased stamina.	4. a–b. The patient will: — Increase rest and sleep during inflammatory peirods of the disease.
a. During excerbations, provide more rest with joints in functional positions.	a. Systemic rest helps control fatigue and joint inflammation.	— Take rest periods before and after exercise.
b. Splint actively affected joints whenever not being used.	b. Joint rest decreases the inflammation and pain associated with daily activities.	
5. Teach patients relaxation techniques (stress reduction).	5. Emotional stress aggravates systemic and articula activity.	5. The patient practices relaxation techniques.

NURSING DIAGNOSIS/PROBLEM 2: Impaired physical mobility and function related to splinting from pain, resulting in muscle atrophy
GOAL 2.1: Increase joint mobility and muscle strength through regular exercise program
GOAL 2.2: Prevent formation of deformities

Nursing Interventions	Rationale	Outcome Criteria
1. Engage in a regular therapeutic exercise program. a. Do full range-of-motion exercises several times daily. b. Perform smooth and slow.	1. Pain and swelling often limit joint use, and resulting inactivity causes decreased joint range, decreased muscle strength, and loss of function. Flexion deformities occur readily in rheumatoid joints.	1. The patient: — Actively participates in a regular exercise program. — Experiences no pain 15 minutes past completion of exercise.

(*Continued*)

NURSING CARE PLAN FOR THE PATIENT WITH RHEUMATOID ARTHRITIS (*Continued*)

Nursing Interventions	Rationale	Outcome Criteria
c. Stop exercising if there is much pain or if the existing pain intensifies. d. Coordinate exercise periods when anti-inflammatory medications are at their peak. e. Perform exercises after hot or cold therapy.		— Exhibits no signs of muscle atrophy from nonuse, or shows improvement in atrophy that was initially present.
2. Maintain good body alignment and correct posture when walking, sitting, or in bed.	2. Correct joint alignment reduces strain on muscles, ligaments, tendons, and joints.	2. Exhibits no disuse muscle atrophy or increase in pretreatment deformity

NURSING DIAGNOSIS/PROBLEM 3: Self-care deficits related to decreased energy level and deformities
GOAL 3: Independent performance of ADLs

Nursing Interventions	Rationale	Outcome Criteria
1. Regular exercise periods	1. Exercise helps to maintain physical and mental health.	
2. With help from physical therapy, teach patient self-care activities. a. Use lightweight self-help devices (PT or OT can provide): *i.e.*, long-handled combs, toothbrushes, shoehorn; velcro and snaps instead of ties, buttons, or hooks.	2. Fine, delicate movements increase joint stress, increase pain, and contribute to deformity.	2. The patient will: — Feed self without assistance — Bathe/groom self without assistance — Dress self without assistance — Ambulate inside and outside home — Cook, clean, shop for self
3. Be alert to limitations, but allow sufficient time for patient to complete tasks.	3. Pain, stiffness, deformities, and relearning ways of performing tasks require additional time.	

NURSING DIAGNOSIS/PROBLEM 4: Disturbance in self-concept related to loss of independence, deformity, and chronic illness
GOAL 4.1: Attainment of a positive self-image

Nursing Interventions	Rationale	Outcome Criteria
1. Encourage self-care activities within range of ability.	1. Independent daily functioning decreases the fear, anxiety, and anger that accompanies debilitating illness and helps to improve self-concept.	
2. Encourage patients and families to express their feelings of anxiety, fear, or hostility. 3. Identify methods of positively dealing with tension (*e.g.*, swimming, hot tub, and music).	2. Suppressed feelings increase the interfamily stress and often accentuate the patient's negative feelings about himself.	2–3. The patient: — Identifies his feelings — Expresses feelings to health care workers — Expresses feelings to family members — Participates in activities that decrease tension — Participates in social activities

(*Continued*)

NURSING CARE PLAN FOR THE PATIENT WITH RHEUMATOID ARTHRITIS (*Continued*)

GOAL 4.2: Patient and family participation in an ongoing educational program

Nursing Interventions	Rationale	Outcome Criteria
1. Assess patient/family knowledge regarding disease and individual treatment plan.	1. To identify knowledge deficits so teaching can begin at the right level	1. Patient and family can: — Briefly describe RA and pathology — Describe individual treatment plan — Identify side-effects of their medications
2. Discuss and clarify misconceptions about RA and its treatment (*e.g.*, folklore—copper bracelets, chestnut seeds in pockets, cod liver oil, *etc.*).	2. Patients waste money and delay necessary treatment when trying unproven remedies. (THERE IS NO CURE FOR RA!)	2. Ask health team questions prior to participating in "new cures."
3. Provide information for discharge planning: — Medications — Exercise/rest — Joint protection		
4. Provide social service consultation to help arrange financial assistance if necessary.	4. Specialized self-help devices, rehabilitation services, and frequent hospitalizations are a financial drain.	

NURSING DIAGNOSIS/PROBLEM 5: Alteration in nutrition (less than body requirements) related to malaise from systemic disease and side-effects from medication therapy

GOAL 5: Maintain adequate nutritional support, and reduce incidence of gastrointestinal disturbances from medications

Nursing Interventions	Rationale	Outcome Criteria
1. Provide diet high in protein, iron, vitamins, with snacks in between meals and at HS. a. Administer vitamin and mineral supplements as ordered. b. Follow a program of calorie reduction with high-protein if the patient is overweight.	1. RA is a systemic disease often associated with anorexia, anemia, and weight loss. a–b. Adequate calories, protein, and nutrients are necessary for tissue repair. Inflammation and stress of the disease increase daily calorie requirements.	1. The patient will: — Consume at least three well-balanced, high-protein meals/day — Follow a calorie-reduced diet if prescribed — Maintain weight within 10% of ideal
2. Correct patient misconceptions about dietary fads that claim to "cure arthritis."	2. There is no scientific evidence to support claims that any particular foods, vitamins, or minerals positively affect the prognosis of RA.	2. Does not participate in food fads without first consulting health team members

The patient will:

- Have decreased pain and reduced inflammation
- Have increased joint mobility and muscle strength
- Avoid deformities
- Perform independent ADLs
- Maintain adequate nutritional support
- Sustain a positive self-image
- Participate in an educational program

Osteoarthritis (Degenerative Joint Disease)

Osteoarthritis (OA) is the most common form of connective tissue disease. Over 16 million Americans seek medical attention for the condition each year, and between 50% to 70% of the US adult population show some radiological evidence of degenerative joint disease.[16,18] Unlike rheumatoid arthritis, osteoarthritis is not a systemic disorder. Although it is generally noninflammatory, there is an inflammatory component.

Etiology and Pathophysiology

The cause of osteoarthritis is unknown, but it is frequently referred to as a "wear and tear" disease. Certain factors such as congenital abnormalities, trauma, obesity, genetic predisposition, and metabolic or endocrine abnormalities are thought to influence the degenerative process.[16]

Osteoarthritis is characterized by the breakdown of cartilage in the diarthrodial joints. As the cartilage thins, the joint space narrows. Bone grates against bone with subsequent ulceration in the subchondral bone plates. As the disease progresses, the capsule and synovial membranes thicken, the proximal bone hypertrophies, and bone cysts develop. The net effect is pain and loss of stability of the joint.

Clinical Manifestations

The most prominent patient complaint is joint pain that gradually worsens with activity and is relieved by rest. Stiffness may occur after periods of inactivity or upon arising. Usually stiffness lasts less than 30 minutes and improves with exercise. Crepitus, a crunching or grating sound, often occurs during joint movement, and is due to eroded articular surfaces rubbing each other. Muscle spasms frequently occur, and joint mobility may be restricted. Effusions accumulate, giving the joints a swollen appearance, but warmth is present only when osteoarthritis is inflammatory. Unlike rheumatoid arthritis, joint involvement is usually asymmetric, and affects one or more of the following joints: distal interphalangeal (DIP), proximal interphalangeal (PIP), carpometacarpal (CMC), and first metatarsophalangeal (see Fig. 89–4). Herberden's nodes often are present on the end joints of the fingers, as shown in Figure 89–7.

Cervical and lumbosacral spine involvement with spur formation (bony growth) is a frequent occurrence but rarely causes major problems.

Degeneration of the large, weight-bearing joints is the most severe and debilitating form of the disease. It develops slowly and involves the hip and knee joints.

Medical Management

Osteoarthritis is frequently diagnosed by x-ray before the patient has physical complaints. Radiographs may reveal soft tissue swelling, joint space narrowing, bony erosions, cysts, osteophytes (bony outgrowths), and deformity. Medi-

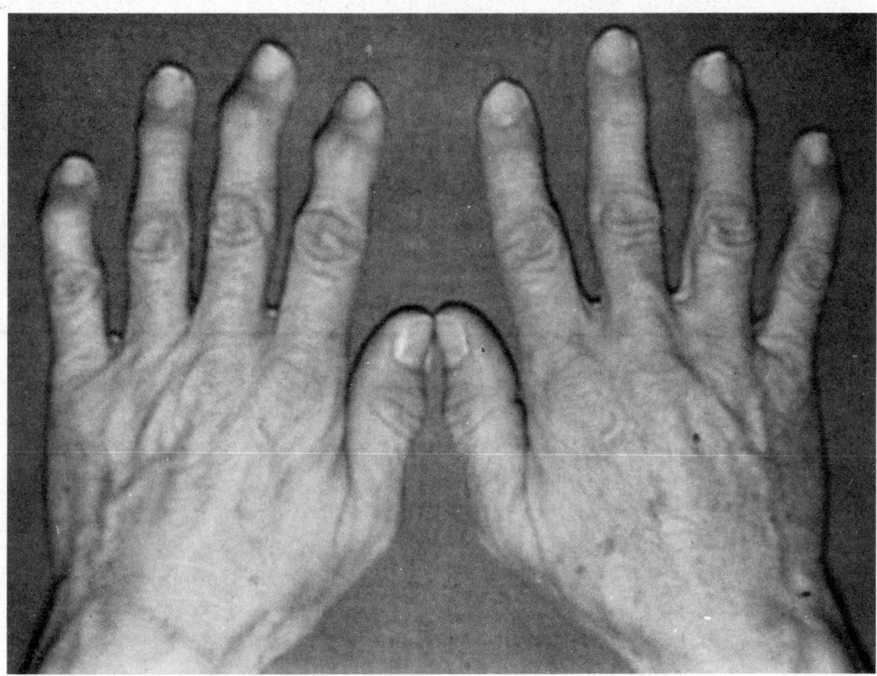

FIGURE 89–7 Heberden's nodes on end joints of fingers in rheumatoid arthritis and osteoarthritis. (Calin A: Differential Diagnosis in Rheumatology: An Atlas for the Physician, p 116. Philadelphia, JB Lippincott, 1984)

cal management of osteoarthritis is mainly aimed at pain relief. Moderate doses of aspirin or acetominophen (Tylenol) are sufficient, as opposed to the high doses needed to provide anti-inflammatory action in rheumatoid arthritis. The large, weight-bearing joints are occasionally inflamed, and the nonsteroidal, anti-inflammatory agents may be helpful (see Table 89–1). Corticosteroids are rarely needed and can cause further bone deterioration. Patients with extensive joint destruction may need total knee or hip replacements to relieve pain and restore joint function.[17]

Joint Replacement. Replacement of joints because of degenerative conditions (*e.g.*, rheumatoid arthritis, osteoarthritis) or trauma has become widely accepted and successful. The new joints are mechanical implants that replace the injured or degenerated joint, providing surfaces that permit smooth articulation. Joint replacement results in improved function and relief of pain. They are used predominantly in the finger, knee, and hip joints, the hip joint being the most common.

The material used for joint replacements varies with the joint, but metal, high density polyethelene, and silastic are the typical components. Methyl methacrylate is the bone-bonding agent used to cement the prostheses in place.

The primary medical goals for all joint replacements are to relieve pain, improve function, and prevent infection. The surgical procedure and postoperative care varies with the particular joint being replaced and its usual anatomical and physiological characteristics. Because total hip joint replacement is the surgery most frequently done, it is the only one discussed here. The care of patients undergoing replacement from other joints can be abstracted from these concepts and principles.

Total hip replacement consists of replacing the acetabular socket with a plastic cup socket and the femoral head and neck with a metal femoral prosthesis (Fig. 89–8). Both of these components are cemented in place with methyl methacrylate. These new surfaces provide for smooth articulation for improved function, relief of pain, increased ambulation, and stability.

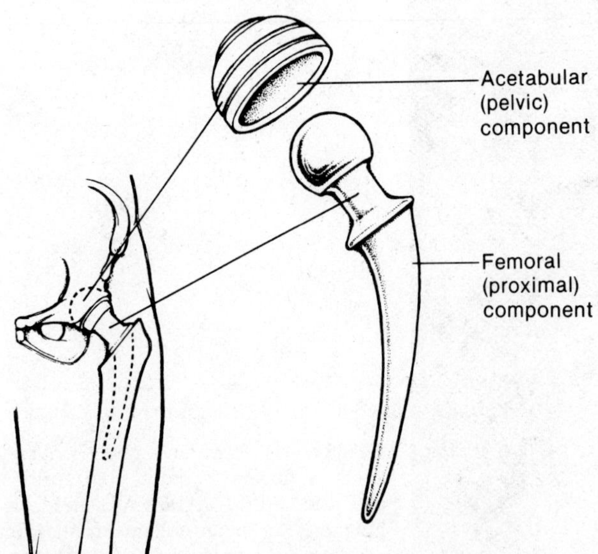

FIGURE 89–8 Total hip joint prosthesis.

The only contraindications for joint replacement are the presence of active infection or inadequate bone for cementing the prostheses. The primary potential complications are dislocation of the femoral head from the acetabular socket during the immediate postoperative phase, or the possibility of infection which could lead to prosthesis failure.

Nursing Management

Assessment and Nursing Diagnosis. Based on the assessment data, nursing history, and clinical symptoms, the major nursing problems encountered are pain and stiffness secondary to joint degeneration, impaired mobility secondary to joint pain and deformity, and inability to perform activities of daily living. For the patient undergoing joint replacement, the nursing problems also include the potential for infection related to the surgical procedure and the potential for impaired mobility related to possible dislocation of the prosthetic joint.

Goals. The major nursing goals for the patient with osteoarthritis are to relieve pain, promote increased joint mobility and strength, prevent formation of deformities, and encourage independent performance of ADLs.

The additional goals for the patient undergoing total joint replacement are to prevent infection and dislocation and to improve joint mobility and function.

Interventions. The major role of nursing in the treatment of patients with osteoarthritis is helping the patient to manage the disease by himself. Although gross deformities are not prevalent in osteoarthritis, joint pain and stiffness are debilitating and disabling. The basic principles—exercise, rest/relaxation, joint protection, and nutrition—are generally the same as for patients with rheumatoid arthritis. The nursing interventions and evaluation criteria for these principles are detailed in Nursing Care Plan for the Patient with Rheumatoid Arthritis.

For the patient who needs a total joint replacement procedure, the nurse needs to be actively involved from the time the decision is made. Preoperative teaching includes muscle exercises, coughing and deep breathing, positioning, and transfer techniques that will be expected in the postoperative period. Because many of the patients having total hip replacements are older, the potential for pulmonary complications is greater owing to the general anesthesia, limited activity, and age-related respiratory changes. For that reason, many elderly patients receive spinal anesthesia rather than general anesthesia.

In order to prevent hip joint dislocation and to promote optimal healing, the patient is taught muscle exercises to strengthen the upper extremities as well as the muscles of the affected lower extremity. Upper extremity strength is needed to use an overhead trapeze for in-bed positioning, and crutches and walker for ambulation. The strength of the muscles surrounding the affected joint contributes to prevention of dislocation. Consequently, isometric exercises of the quadriceps and gluteal muscles are an important preoperative consideration.

Postoperatively, the main considerations for nursing care include positioning, pain control, prevention of infection and thrombus formation, and exercise and ambulation.

Positioning of the patient is an important aspect of preventing dislocation. The affected leg must be in an abduction position to allow the prosthetic femoral head to be securely located in the plastic acetabular cup. This position of abduction is promoted through the use of abduction splints and a wedge-shaped pillow, or several pillows.

Positioning is also important to promote limited hip flexion (45°–60°). The patient is taught to avoid positions with 60° to up to 90° or more of flexion, such as sitting upright in a chair or on a commode. Having semireclining chairs and elevated toilet seats available is essential in the early postoperative period.

Positioning the patient to prevent adduction and flexion is essential in the early postoperative period when the patient is particularly susceptible to dislocation. In order to change positions periodically, the patient is turned about 45° with the aid of a trapeze, splint, and pillows. The head of the bed should not be elevated more than 30° to 45°, nor should the operated leg approach or cross the midline of the body, in order to prevent dislocation.

Preventing infection of the surgical site as well as preventing pneumonia are also goals following joint replacement. Encouraging deep-breathing through coughing, and use of an incentive spirometer or other positive-pressure breathing equipment is the best prevention for pulmonary problems such as atelectasis and pneumonia. Preventing infection of the surgical site is primarily the responsibility of the surgical team. Early detection of symptoms of infection is vital in the postoperative period. The nurse should observe for classic signs of infection (see Chap 17).

Preventing thromboembolism is a nursing consideration in the immediate postoperative period. Flexing the feet and ankles stimulates blood flow and venous return in the lower leg, and prevents venous stasis. Anti-embolic stockings are used to avoid venous stasis, and observing for pressure sites under the stockings is essential. Observation and testing for classic signs of thrombophlebitis is part of the nurse's daily assessment. Low-dose anticoagulants or aspirin may be employed in some patients.

The amount of medication needed for pain control varies with each patient. Many patients report that the amount of pain they experience postoperatively is less than what they experienced before surgery. Parenteral analgesics/narcotics may be used in the first 24 to 48 hours, with lesser amounts of oral medication needed after that time. Muscle spasms, periods of exercise and ambulation, and discomfort due to pressure from edema at the surgical site may contribute to periodic needs for pain medication. Giving an analgesic about 20 to 30 minutes before physical therapy or ambulation exercise may be useful in encouraging involvement in these activities. However, in order to prevent falls, the nurse should be alert to any dizziness or balance problems that may accompany the medication.

Increased pain on the operative side accompanied by muscle spasm may be the first indication of dislocation. The nurse will assess for other indicators of dislocation such as abnormal rotation of the leg, shortening of the leg as shown by comparing alignment of both feet and knees, and increased discomfort of the operated limb with any motion. Dislocation is a complication that must be recognized and reduced quickly because circulatory and nerve damage may result. As the operative site heals and the muscles increase in strength, the danger of dislocation diminishes.

In preparing the patient for discharge, the importance of continued exercise, steadily increasing ambulation, and continued avoidance of adduction and flexion beyond prescribed limits become the focus of patient education. Walking tends to be the best activity to provide exercise and ambulation in the recovery period. If permitted and the patient enjoys it, swimming is also a helpful activity.

In order to prevent dislocation during the early months, planning should be done with the family to ensure the availability of apparatuses (walker, crutches, elevated toilet seat) and adaptations (higher chairs, a recliner, or other items) that the patient will need. In avoiding positions of flexion and adduction, the patient should never dress himself, cross his legs, or bend over from a sitting position to reach for something. For many activities the patient will need assistance from others for several months.

Evaluation. The patient will

1. Obtain relief of pain with activities of daily living and at rest.
2. Demonstrate improved joint mobility and stability in walking gait and in standing balance.
3. Demonstrate no indications of infection at the surgical site or in the respiratory system.
4. Experience no dislocation of the joint prosthesis following the replacement procedure.
5. Experience no thrombophlebitis or venous stasis problems.

Gout

Gout is an inflammatory disorder resulting from deposition of uric acid crystals in the joints and tissues. It is one of the oldest arthritic diseases, and was originally described by Hippocrates in 400 BC. The disease is characterized by recurrent acute, painful arthritic attacks, usually in the great toe joint.

Etiology

Uric acid is the end product of purine metabolism. Purines are derived from the diet (exogenous) or are synthesized within the body (endogenous). Uric acid is eliminated by the kidney. Persistent hyperuricemia is the hallmark of gout and is caused by overproduction or undersecretion of uric acid.

Primary gout is caused by an inherited defect of purine biosynthesis leading to an overproduction of uric acid, or a genetic dysfunction of renal excretion of uric acid. Primary gout accounts for 80% of all cases, of which 95% are males.[27]

The initial arthritic attack usually occurs in the fourth or fifth decade of life.

Secondary gout is an acquired disease, secondary to hematopoietic, renal, or nutritional disorders.[9] Polycythemia vera, multiple myeloma, and the leukemias are associated with rapid cell turnover and increased uric acid production. Irradiation of tumors and administration of cytotoxic chemotherapy also cause massive cellular destruction and acute increases in urate production.

Chronic renal failure or drug effects on the kidneys may impair uric acid excretion. Aspirin, thiazide diuretics, and some antituberculosis medications (pyrazinamide) are associated with hyperuricemia.

Development of gout has been reported with myxedema, hyperparathyroidism, postmyocardial infarction, hypertension, toxemia of pregnancy, and respiratory acidosis—symptoms possibly related to the renal complications of these diseases.[9]

Pathophysiology

Acute attacks of gout occur when the serum becomes hypersaturated with uric acid, and crystals precipitate into the joints and soft tissues, forming nodules called *tophi.*

Pain and inflammation are due to uric crystals, within the joints, being engulfed by leukocytes and forming phagosome. Lysosomal digestive enzymes are released into the phagosome to break down the crystals. The negative charge of the crystals rupture the phagosomal membrane, releasing digestive enzymes into the joint cavity. Self-digestion ensues, attracting more leukocytes, and the inflammatory cycle repeats.

Clinical Manifestations

The onset of gout is usually an abrupt, acutely painful arthritic attack, developing overnight. In 75% of patients, the big toe is the first joint affected.[7] The affected toe is swollen, reddened, warm, and extremely tender. The pressure of bedcovers on the joint may be intolerable. A fever may be present during the acute phase. The episode resolves within a week if left untreated; however, reoccurrence is common, and the intervals between attacks is variable.

Chronic gout is uncommon, but it develops if hyperuricemia is untreated for many years. Patient history reveals recurrent attacks, increasing in frequency and number of involved joints over the years. Arthritic symptoms become persistent with pain and swelling of many joints. Morning stiffness may be a complaint as multiple tophi result in deformity and restricted movement (Fig. 89–9).

Kidney stones develop in 10% to 20% of patients with gout. Chronic renal failure may be due to hypertension of tubular damage induced by uric acid crystals. Less than 10% of gout patients die from renal insufficiency.[27]

Medical Management

Diagnosis is based on the development of an acute attack, in the presence of persistent hyperuricemia. The presence of uric acid crystals in an aspirated sample of synovial fluid confirms the diagnosis. A 24-hour urine specimen for uric acid, and laboratory studies of renal function guide treatment.

The treatment of gout has two components: treatment of the acute attack and long-term management of hyperuricemia after the attack subsides.

Management of the acute attack involves relieving pain and inflammation. NSAIDs are the mainstay of treatment (see Table 89–1). Indomethacin is generally the most rapid agent in reducing gout pain.

Colchicine has been used for acute attacks for 200 years and is thought to act by stabilizing lysosomal membranes. A positive response to colchicine is regarded as a diagnostic indicator of gout. The therapeutic dose, however, is close to the toxic dose, resulting in nausea, vomiting, and diarrhea. The aim is to build up the blood level (1 mg/2 hours) until the gouty attack ends or toxicity occurs. Joint pain and inflammation may not subside for 8 to 24 hours. Corticosteroids are effective in reducing the joint inflammation in acute attacks, but there is a high frequency of recurrence after treatment is withdrawn.

There are two main groups of pharmacological agents

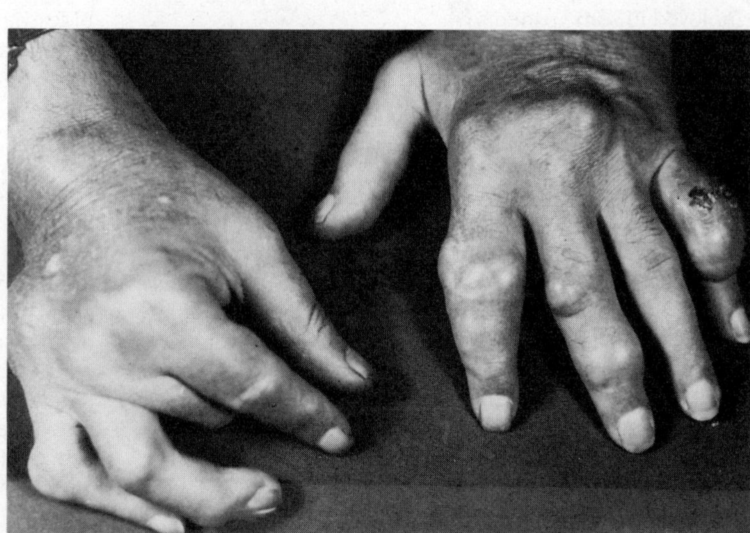

FIGURE 89–9 Severe gouty arthritis of the hands. (Turek SL: Orthopaedics: Principles and Their Application, Vol 1, p 248. Philadelphia, JB Lippincott, 1984)

that lower the serum uric acid after the acute attack has resolved. The agents either block the formation of uric acid (*e.g.*, allopurinol) or promote resorption of tissue deposits and excretion of uric acid (*e.g.*, probenecid and sulfinpyrazone). Nonsalicylate anti-inflammatory agents or colchicine should be administered concomitantly in the early months of treatment since these drugs can precipitate acute gouty attacks as tissue deposits are mobilized. Long-term therapy is required in patients who have more than two acute attacks in a year, have secondary gout, tophi, or a high persistent serum uric acid level.

Nursing Management

Nursing Diagnosis

Based on the clinical manifestations, nursing history, and assessment data, the major nursing problem for the patient with an acute gouty attack is intense pain secondary to joint inflammation. Nursing problems for the patient with chronic gout include potential reoccurrence of severe joint pain, potential renal failure secondary to uric acid stone formation, and potential draining sinuses due to tophi eruptions.

Goals. The major goals for the patient with gout are to relieve joint pain and prevent renal stone formation and draining skin lesions. To achieve these goals, an added goal is to encourage the patient to adhere to the therapeutic regimen.

Interventions

During an acute gouty attack, pain relief is the chief goal for both patient and nurse. Anti-inflammatory agents and colchicine are the mainstay of treatment, but pain relief may take from 2 to 24 hours. Narcotic analgesics may be necessary until the definitive treatment is effective. Other nursing measures to relieve pain include bed rest, with the affected extremity splinted and elevated. A bed cradle is utilized to prevent sheets from causing pressure on tender joints. Cold packs applied to the joints may reduce the inflammation. Early ambulation is not only intolerable because of severe pain, but it may precipitate an acute reoccurrence.

After the acute attack has subsided, long-term therapy is started to control serum uric acid levels. Usually the memory of severe pain is vivid enough to ensure full cooperation. The patient will take the medication for his lifetime and will need education concerning self-administration and side-effects. Allopurinol, Benemid, and Anturane have very few side-effects; gastrointestinal disturbances are the most common. The patient should be instructed not to take aspirin or other salicylate-containing medications if taking Benemid or Anturane, due to antagonistic actions.

Patient education of dietary restrictions is usually not required. A normal protein intake has a relatively small effect on blood uric acid levels; however, glandular meats, sardines, and shellfish are particularly rich in purine and should be avoided. Other dietary measures may include instruction to eat alkaline foods such as potatoes and milk, which increase the urine pH and inhibit the precipitation of uric acid crystals in the kidney.

Formation of kidney stones is a constant threat. Unless contraindicated, patients should drink at least 3000 ml of fluid per day to promote excretion of uric acid. Large fluid intake is especially important in the early stages of Benemid or Anturane therapy, since resorption and mobilization of tissue uric acid deposits result in excessively high urine and serum urate concentrations. Additionally, hospitalized patients need careful monitoring of their intake and output and laboratory studies of kidney function.

Soft tissue tophi formation in chronic gout patients needs special attention. Clothing, shoes, and linen rub and irritate superficial tophi, causing ulcerations and draining sinuses. The drainage is chalky white, consisting of large numbers of uric acid crystals. Meticulous skin care and a light, sterile dressing will prevent lesions from becoming infected. Soft slippers, gloves, and protective clothing over superficial tophi may prevent their rupture.

Evaluation

The patient will

1. Experience relief of joint pain:
   a. Is free of current pain and inflammation
   b. Experiences no future acute gouty attacks
2. Adhere to long-term therapy:
   a. Self-administers medications in the absence of acute gouty attacks
   b. Experiences no further tophi formation
3. Be free of renal stone formation:
   a. Serum uric acid levels in normal range
   b. Drinks 3000 ml/day of fluids
   c. Maintains a urine pH of 7 or higher
4. Show no signs of draining tophi:
   a. Experiences a decrease in number of tophi
   b. Exhibits no inflammation or purulent drainage from tophi

Systemic Lupus Erythematosus

Systemic lupus erythematosus (SLE) is a chronic, multisystem, autoimmune disease. It was named after the characteristic butterfly rash across the nose and cheeks that is likened to the damage from the bite of a hungry wolf. The disease was once thought to be relatively rare and always fatal. Better diagnostic techniques have hastened confirmation of the disease, and have shown SLE to be common, occurring in 1 out of every 700 people. Early diagnosis and treatment have also improved the prognosis. The 10-year survival rate is currently 50%.[10]

Etiology

The cause of SLE is unknown, but it is believed to involve immunologic and environmental factors. There is a genetic predisposition, and it is possible that a viral infection may be responsible. Environmental factors that are associated with acute exacerbations are physical stresses of infections, surgery, or pregnancy; emotional tension; and ultraviolet light, either artificial or natural. A variety of drugs may precipitate the clinical features of SLE, including procainamide (Pronestyl), hydralazine (Apresoline), isoniazid (INH), chlorpromazine (Phenergan), diphenylhydantoin (Dilantin), and quinidine. The symptoms resolve when the offending drug is discontinued.

The disease occurs five times more frequently in female adolescents and adult women of childbearing age than in men. Approximately 12% of lupus patients develop their disease after age 50.

Pathophysiology

There is considerable evidence implicating immunologic abnormalities in the pathogenesis of SLE. Tissue injury is mediated by the disposition of circulating immune complexes along the basement membranes in many organs and vessels. Although many organs may be involved, the kidney is particularly susceptible to injury, and lupus-induced nephritis is the most frequent cause of death. In 1979 Maddison and Reicklin found lupus glomerulonephritis to occur from anti-DNA (antinuclear antibody) complexed with DNA being deposited in the glomerulus. Complement, a series of proteins in the serum, become fixed to the antigen–antibody complex and trigger the inflammatory process.

The pathogenesis of drug-induced lupus is unclear, but a few hypotheses are being investigated. Several of the medications, procainamide, hydralazine, and isoniazid, have similar chemical properties, and are associated with the development of anti-DNA. Results of several studies indicate that the drugs alter DNA and increase the immune system's reactivity.[10] Another explanation is that the drugs alter the immune mechanism and decrease the body's tolerance to self-antigen.

Clinical Manifestations

The onset of SLE can be insidious or acute. Usually the onset is insidious in the elderly, with symptoms of weakness, anorexia, malaise, fatigue, and arthritis. Younger patients frequently have an acute onset with fever and severe multisystem involvement. The course of the disease is characterized by periods of remission and exacerbations. When the disease is active, there may be a reoccurrence of previous symptoms, or totally new symptoms.

Polyarthritis and polymyositis, particularly of the hip and shoulder, are present in 90% of patients, and frequently are the initial symptoms.

Skin involvement is prominent, occurring in 80% of patients. Typically there is a raised, scaly, reddened "butterfly" rash on the face. Rashes also occur on the neck, extremities, or trunk, along with ulcerations of the oral and nasal mucosa. Exposure to ultraviolet light often aggravates skin involvement. Alopecia (hair loss) is a frequent finding.

Kidney disease is present in 50% of patients, manifested by hematuria, proteinuria, and tubular acidosis. Neurological complications, due to microinfarcts, occur in 50% of patients. These include peripheral neuropathies, seizures, psychoses, or other signs of mental deterioration.

Inflammation of the vessels (vasculitis) decreases blood supply, and accounts for injury and dysfunction to other organs. Pleuritis, interstitial fibrosis, pericarditis, peritonitis, hepatitis, and gastrointestinal irritation are typical findings. Peripheral vascular disease and renal involvement cause hypertension in many SLE patients.

Medical Management

In 1971, the American Rheumatism Association developed criteria for the diagnosis of SLE. Diagnosis is confirmed if the patient has any of the criteria listed below:

Facial erythema
Discoid lupus (involves only the skin)
Alopecia
Raynaud's phenomenon
Oral or nasal ulceration
Photosensitivity
Pleuritis/pericarditis
Arthritis without deformity
Psychosis/convulsions
Lupus erythematosus (LE) cells
Chronic false-positive test for syphilis
Profuse proteinuria
Cellular casts
Anemia, leukopenia, and thrombocytopenia

Mild to moderate anemia, leukopenia, and thrombocytopenia is common, and often mirrors disease activity. The erthrocyte sedimentation rate is usually elevated when the disease is active. Other laboratory findings will be specific to the organs that are involved. Antinuclear antibodies (ANA) are the most sensitive screening test for SLE, and are present in 95% of patients. Anti-DNA are specific to SLE, and are positive in 70% of patients. The lupus erythematosus factor (LE) is usually positive during the course of the disease.

Treatment of SLE involves prevention of complications and symptomatic treatment during the active phase of the disease. During remission, patients may require no therapy.

Prophylactic use of antibiotics should be avoided because lupus patients have a high incidence of hypersensitivity. Other known lupus-inducing medications should be closely monitored and discontinued if symptoms arise.

Joint and muscle symptoms are treated with salicylates. Plaquenil is especially useful for treating arthritis and skin rashes. Corticosteroids are the mainstay of therapy for severely ill patients with nephritis and neurological complications. There are significant side-effects associated with the use of steroids. Table 89–1 discusses the medications used in rheumatoid arthritis and the actions and implications of drug therapy that would be similar for SLE.

Immunosuppressive therapy with cyclophosphamide or azathioprine is still controversial. Their use has been limited to severe, life-threatening complications that are not responding to steroids.

Nursing Management

Assessment and Nursing Diagnosis

Patients are frequently hospitalized during acute exacerbations with a wide array of symptoms. They may also be hospitalized when in remission, for reasons unrelated to SLE. Based on the clinical manifestations and nursing assessment, the major nursing problems include pain and discomfort secondary to joint and muscle inflammation; disruptions in skin integrity secondary to rashes and lesions; major infections secondary to neutropenia and steroid therapy; self-care deficit secondary to fatigue, weakness, and pain; and emotional swings due to neurological involvement or ineffectual coping mechanisms.

Goals. The major goals for the lupus patient with the above nursing problems are to relieve pain and discomfort, maintain skin integrity, minimize risk of infection, decrease fatigue and weakness, maintain optimal nutrition, increase independence in ADLs, and decrease emotional swings.

Interventions

In addition to drug therapy, joint and muscle pain is managed with bed rest. Supporting the joints with pillows may reduce the discomfort and enable the patient to sleep. Active or passive ROM exercises, after the acute inflammation has subsided, prevent stiffness and muscle atrophy.

Skin rashes and lesions are often tender and irritating. Meticulous hygiene will prevent breakdown, decrease itching, and minimize the risk of local infections. Topical corticosteroids may be used to decrease inflammation. Avoidance of ultraviolet light through sun-blocking creams, long-sleeved clothing, hats, and sunglasses decrease skin involvement from photosensitivity.

Patients are particularly susceptible to infection and should be instructed to avoid people with known infections, especially upper respiratory or urinary tract infections. Hospitalized patients have vital signs taken every 4 hours. Total body cultures (blood, urine, sputum) are taken for increased temperatures. If the patient is severely neutropenic, protective (reverse) isolation is indicated.

Fatigue and weakness are the most frequently occurring problems. Patients are encouraged to space their daily activities and plan frequent rest periods throughout the day.

Anorexia from gastrointestinal irritations, side-effects of medications, and generalized malaise may lead to weight loss. Six small, high-protein meals per day encourage adequate calorie and protein intake. Soft, pureed foods may be ordered if the patient is dysphagic. Supplemental, high-protein-calorie drinks (Ensure) help assure adequate nutrition.

Fatigue, weakness, and arthralgias may decrease the patient's ability or willingness to provide independent self-care. Spacing of daily activities and frequent rest periods may enhance the ability to dress, feed, and groom. Other measures to help the patient increase his independence are discussed under Nursing Care Plan for the Patient with Rheumatoid Arthritis.

Emotional aberrations, hopelessness, depression, and fear are common with any chronic illness. The nurse can encourage verbalization of fears to health care professionals or to a close friend or family member. Social workers may direct the patient to community resources for homemaking or financial assistance if this is the source of concern.

Evaluation

Evaluation of the nursing interventions for the major goals are listed below as outcome criteria. The patient will:

1. Have absence of pain and discomfort:
   a. Expresses no subjective complaints of pain
   b. Actively participates in activities of daily living
   c. Has no restricted joint motion
2. Maintain skin integrity:
   a. Has no skin ulcerations
   b. Demonstrates no itching of rashes and lesions
   c. Existing rashes have decreased erythema
   d. Wears sun protection and limits exposure to ultraviolet light
3. Experience no major infection:
   a. Remains afebrile
   b. Is free of urinary tract or respiratory infections
   c. Avoids exposure to adults and children with infections
4. Have decreased fatigue and weakness:
   a. Spaces activities during the day
   b. Takes 2 to 3 rest periods (½ hour) during the day
   c. Sleeps 8 to 12 hours at night
5. Maintain optimal nutrition:
   a. Eats at least 3 balanced meals/day
   b. Takes vitamin/mineral supplement, if ordered
   c. Maintains within 10% of ideal body weight
6. Be able to dress, feed, and groom self without assistance
7. Experience decreased emotional swings:
   a. Verbalizes fears and concerns to health care professionals or significant others
   b. Contacts community sources for financial assistance
   c. Socializes with friends and family
   d. Actively participates in social activities and hobbies

Progressive Systemic Sclerosis (Scleroderma)

Progressive systemic sclerosis (PSS) is a progressive connective tissue disease. It is characterized by hardening and thickening of cutaneous and visceral connective tissues.

Etiology and Pathophysiology

The etiology is unknown, although it is theorized that a dysfunction of the immune system is involved.

The disease occurs in women two to three times as often as men. Onset usually occurs in the 25- to 50-year age-group, and it rarely affects children.

The disease begins with microvasculitis, usually of the dermis. Edema and inflammation of the involved tissues lead to ischemia, fibrosis, and excessive collagen disposition. The tissues lose their elasticity and become smooth, thick, tight, and shiny. The skin is frequently involved, but other tissues, including blood vessels, lungs, esophagus, gastrointestinal tract, heart, and kidneys, can be affected.

Progressive systemic sclerosis, like lupus erythematosus, has remissions and exacerbations. Patients may live a long time with a mild, slowly progressing case. If vital organs become involved, the disease may rapidly progress to death. The leading cause of death is renal failure.

Clinical Manifestations

The term scleroderma means "hard skin," and describes the initial skin involvement. The fingers are often the first affected, and resemble sausages from the accompanying edema and thickening. Raynaud's phenomenon is a frequent symptom, with pain and discoloration of the fingers from vasospasm that is aggravated by cold. Progression occurs as the arms, face, and chest become affected. Facial skin becomes tight and masklike, without expression. Normal skin folds around the eyes and forehead disappear. The mouth becomes rigid, with restricted movement of the lips. Swallowing can be difficult. Respiration may be impaired as the chest skin firms and limits chest expansion. Pain and stiffness of the fingers and extremities often render them immobile and useless. Contractures and disuse atrophy result in deformity.

Tissues of other organs are affected as the disease progresses. Proteinuria, hematuria, and hypertension accompany renal involvement.

Medical Management

Laboratory studies are not helpful in making the diagnosis. Skin biopsies are the most specific. Elevated ESR, rheumatoid factor, and positive antinuclear antibodies (ANA) may be demonstrated. Other organ-specific tests may be useful in defining the extent of the disease. There is no therapy available that prevents or retards the progression of sclerosis in PSS. Para-aminobenzoic acid (PABA) has been used with variable results. Colchicine and penicillamine are currently under investigation because of their inhibitory effects on collagen disposition. Steroids are commonly used, but their efficacy is unproved. Captopril (Capoten), an angiotension II enzyme inhibitor, has recently shown promise in treating renal involvement.

Treatment of progressive systemic sclerosis is symptomatic and is directed at the organ system involved. Pain and arthritic symptoms respond to aspirin and NSAIDs. Physical therapy and exercise retard formation of contractures and muscle atrophy.

Vasospasm of the hands from Raynaud's phenomenon can be decreased by limiting exposure to cold temperatures. Smoking is discouraged because of its vasoconstrictive effects. Vasodilators (*e.g.,* Aldomet) may also be of benefit.

Nursing Management

Assessment and Nursing Diagnosis. Nursing assessment, diagnosis, goals, and interventions for the patient with scleroderma is similar to the care of the patient with systemic lupus erythematosus. Two additional nursing problems may be encountered: pressure sores secondary to immobility and vascular changes, and dysphagia secondary to oroesophageal involvement. Nursing care of patients with pressure sores and dysphagia are discussed in Chapters 93 and 64.

Avascular Necrosis

Avascular necrosis of bone involves the death or infarction of bone as a result of a lack of oxygen and nutrient delivery to the bone cells. Although avascular necrosis is not very common because of the well-developed vascular system of bone by means of the haversian canal, it is a potential complication of rheumatoid arthritis, systemic lupus erythematosus, and prolonged corticosteroid therapy. Pain, restricted joint movement, and gait disturbances are the most common associated problems. Avascular necrosis is most often a late complication of a fracture of the femoral neck. Further discussion on assessment and management of avascular necrosis is in Chapter 88.

Seronegative Arthropathies

The seronegative arthropathies are a group of rheumatic diseases with similar pathological, radiological, and clinical features. They are seronegative for rheumatoid factor and are generally positive for HLA-B27, the histocompatibility antigen. They tend to be milder and less progressive than seropositive rheumatoid arthritis. Ankylosing spondylitis and Reiter's syndrome will be discussed, although the seronegative arthropathies also include postinfectious reactive arthropathies, psoriatic arthritis, and enteric spondylitis.

The nursing problems, goals, and interventions are similar to those for patients with rheumatoid arthritis and osteoarthritis, and they can be extracted from discussions on those disorders.

Ankylosing Spondylitis (Marie-Strümpell Disease)

Ankylosing spondylitis is a chronic, progressive, inflammatory disease of the spine and sacroiliac joint. It affects 1% of the population and occurs in men four times as often as in females.[4] It usually occurs in adolescence or early adulthood between 10 and 30 years of age, and it has a familial predominance.

Etiology. The cause of the disease is unknown; however, recent tissue-typing research has found that over 70% of diagnosed patients belong to the same tissue group, HLA-B27.[1,19]

Pathophysiology. The disease begins in the sacroiliac joints and advances up the spine. Inflammation of the joints is followed by fibrosis and then ankylosis, as the joints and disk spaces are replaced by bone. The final result is a completely rigid "bamboo spine," as evidenced by radiograph.

Clinical Manifestations. The early symptoms are low backache and morning stiffness. As the dorsal and lumbar spine become involved, motion of the back and chest expansion are restricted. Eventually the entire spine becomes fixed and immobile. Systemic symptoms include fatigue, fever, and loss of weight. Irisitis, cardiac conduction disturbances (first-degree AV block) and pulmonary fibrosis may develop.[2]

Medical Management. There is no treatment to prevent or retard progression of ankylosing spondylitis. Since stiffening of the spine is inevitable, the goals of therapy are to relieve pain, maintain an optimal posture, and prevent respiratory complications.

Laboratory studies reveal a normal ESR and mild anemia. The rheumatoid factor is usually not present, but HLA-B27 is present in 90% of cases.

Pain is treated with salicylates, NSAIDs, and heat. X-ray therapy has been used for severe pain, but it is usually contraindicated because of the dangerous side-effects of myelitis and malignant degeneration.

The patient is instructed to maintain an erect posture when sitting or standing, to prevent flexion deformities. The mattress should be very firm, and the head should never be elevated with a pillow. Splints or a back brace may provide support. Frequent rest periods through the day are encouraged.

Surgical procedures such as corrective osteotomy for marked deformities of the spine or total hip replacement are occasionally indicated. Initially the patient's symptoms are improved, but stiffness invariably reoccurs.

Nursing Management

The nursing problems most frequently encountered are joint pain and stiffness, impaired physical mobility secondary to joint pain and deformity, and inability to perform activities of daily living. These problems are similar to those for patients with rheumatoid arthritis and osteoarthritis. The goals, interventions, and evaluation outcome criteria can be extracted from discussions on those disorders.

Reiter's Syndrome (Brodie's Disease)

Reiter's syndrome is a connective tissue disorder that has been classically defined as a triad of arthritis, urethritis, and conjunctivitis. It is most common in 20- to 40-year-old men. Recent evidence suggests women may be victims more frequently than previously recognized.[12, 25]

Etiology. The disease is thought to be triggered by infection of the genitourinary or gastrointestinal systems. No causative organisms have been identified, but it frequently occurs 14 days after exposure to venereal disease or dysentery.[14]

HLA-B27 is present in 75% to 95% of patients, and it may indicate an immunologic association with the disease.[12]

Clinical Manifestations. Symptoms of Reiter's syndrome include prostatitis, penile or vaginal lesions, and a urethral discharge. A mild, burning conjunctivitis and lesions on the hands and feet are common. The joints most commonly involved are the feet, ankles, and knees. The spine may become involved with ankylosing spondylitis.

Other complications rarely associated with Reiter's syndrome are aortic insufficiency, cardiac conduction disturbances, and pancarditis.

Medical Management. The main goal of treatment is to minimize pain and inflammation in the involved joints. Salicylates generally provide adequate pain relief, but Indocin, Butazolidin, and Feldene may be used for severe inflammation. Corticosteroids may be helpful for patients unresponsive to the previous drugs. Antibiotics are not helpful because no organism can be positively cultured.

Nursing Management

The major problems for patients with Reiter's syndrome are musculoskeletal in origin. These problems include pain and stiffness secondary to joint degeneration, impaired mobility secondary to joint pain and deformity, and inability to perform activities of daily living. Additionally, there is a potential for altered self-image secondary to loss of independence, deformity, and lesions on the hands and feet. These problems are similar to those for patients with rheumatoid arthritis and osteoarthritis. The goals, interventions, and evaluation criteria can be extracted from discussions on those disorders.

References

1. Brewerton DA, James DC: The histocompatibility antigen (HL-A27) and disease. Semin Arthritis Rheum 4:191, 1975
2. Brown HE: Ankylosing spondylitis. In Talbott JH (ed): Clinical Rheumatology, 2nd ed. New York, Elsevier Science Publishers, 1981
3. Brunner LS, Suddarth DS: Textbook of Medical Surgical Nursing, 5th ed. Philadelphia, JB Lippincott, 1984
4. Calin A: Diagnosis and Management of Rheumatoid Arthritis. Menlo Park CA, Addison-Wesley, 1983
5. Canale ST, Phil J, Watson FM et al: Acute osteomyelitis complicating closed fractures. J Bone Joint Surg (Am) 57:415, 1975
6. Clark SR: Drugs and remedies. Am J Nurs 83(2):266, 1983
7. Doyle D: Gout. Nursing Mirror Nov 11:xvi, 1981
8. Drummond-Webb JJ, Schnaid E: Acute osteomyelitis complicating a simple fracture. S Am Med J 64:915, 26 Nov 1983
9. Emmerson BT: Hyperuricaemia and Gout in Clinical Practice. Australia, ADIS Health Science Press, 1983
10. Giansiracusa DF, Kantrowitz FG: Rheumatic and Metabolic Bone Diseases in the Elderly. Lexington MA, The Collamore Press, 1982
11. Govoni LE, Hayes JE: Drugs and Nursing Implications, 4th ed. Norwalk CT, Appleton-Century-Crofts, 1982
12. Gottlieb NL: Reiter's syndrome. In Talbott JH (ed): Clinical Rheumatology, 2nd ed. New York, Elsevier Science Publishers, 1981
13. Harris ED: Evaluation of pathophysiology and drug effects on rheumatoid arthritis. Am J Med Oct 31:56, 1983

14. Hart FD: Seronegative arthropathies. Nursing Mirror Nov 11:vi, 1981
15. Haslock I: Arthritis in old age: Drug treatment. In Wright V (ed): Bone and Joint Disease in the Elderly. New York, Churchill Livingston, 1983
16. Koerner ME, Dickenson GR: Adult arthritis, a look at some of its forms. Am J Nurs 83(2):254, 1983
17. Lance EM: The effect of joint replacement on rheumatoid synovitis and its significance. Arthritis Rheum (Suppl) 25:59, 1982
18. MacLauren J, Lorig K: Osteoarthritis, management requires sound patient teaching. J Prac Nurs 31(7):17, 1981
19. Monk GJE: Orthopaedics for Undergraduates, 2nd ed. Oxford, Oxford University Press, 1981
20. Phillips K: Osteomyelitis of the skull. J Neurosurg Nurs 14(5): 280, 1982
21. Pinals RS, Masi AT, Larsen RA et al: Preliminary criteria for clinical remission in rheumatoid arthritis. Arthritis Rheum 24:1308, 1981
22. Rocca RF et al: Preliminary skeletal infection in heroin users: A clinical characterization, diagnosis and therapy. Clin Orthop 144:238, 1979
23. Simpson EF: Heat, cold or both. Am J Nurs 83(2):271, 1983
24. Simpson EF, Dickenson GR: Exercise. Am J Nurs 83(2):273, 1983
25. Smith DL, Rennet DM, Regan MG: Reiter's disease in women. Arthritis Rheum 23:335, 1980
26. Strand CV, Clark SR: Adult arthritis, drugs and remedies. Am J Nurs 83(2):266, 1983
27. Talbott JH: Gout and hyperuricemia. In Talbott JH (ed): Clinical Rheumatology, 2nd ed. New York, Elsevier Science Publishers, 1981
28. Tuli SM: Tuberculosis of the Spine. New Delhi, Amerind Publishing, 1975

Bibliography

Altman RD: Systemic lupus erythematosus. In Talbot JH (ed): Clinical Rheumatology, 2nd ed. New York, Elsevier Science Publishers, 1981

Altman RD: Scleroderma. In Talbot JH (ed): Clinical Rheumatology, 2nd ed. New York, Elsevier Science Publishers, 1981

Arthritis Foundation: Primer on the Rheumatic Diseases, 7th ed. New York, The Foundation, 1973. Reprinted from JAMA (Suppl), 224 April 30, 1973

Bunch TW, O'Duffy JD: Disease modifying drugs for progressive rheumatoid arthritis. Mayo Clin Proc 55:161, 1980

Calin A: Editorial: HLA-B27 in 1982: Reappraisal of a clinical test. Ann Intern Med 96:114, 1982

Cohen AS et al: Preliminary criteria for the classification of SLE. Bull Rheum Dis 21:643, 1971

deToledo CH et al: The patient with scoliosis. Am J Nurs 79:1587, 1979

Elliott J: Vertebral osteomyelitis goes undiagnosed. JAMA 243(14): 1410, 1980

Farrell J: Illustrated Guide to Orthopedic Nursing, 2nd ed. Philadelphia, JB Lippincott, 1982

Gault SJ, Spyker JM: Beneficial effect of immobilization of joints in rheumatoid and related arthritides: A splint study using sequential analysis. Arthritis Rheum 12:34, 1969

Gerber LH: Aids and appliances. In Wright V (ed): Bone and Joint Diseases in the Elderly. New York, Churchill Livingston, 1983

Griffiths DLI: The operative treatment of tuberculosis of the spine. J Bone Joint Surg 57B:111, 1975

Hart FD: Osteoarthritis and rheumatoid arthritis. Nursing Mirror Nov 11:ii, 1981

Hart FD: Disseminated connective tissue diseases. Nursing Mirror Nov 11:xiii, 1981

Horvath S, Hollander J: Intra-articular temperature as a measure of joint reaction. J Clin Invest 28:469, 1949

Howell DS: Osteoarthritis. In Talbott JH (ed): Clinical Rheumatology, 2nd ed. New York, Elsevier Science Publishers, 1981

Kahn MA, Khan MK: Diagnostic value of HLA-B27 testing and ankylosing spondylitis and Reiter's syndrome. Ann Intern Med 96:70, 1982

Lopez-Overjero JA, Saal SD, DAngelo WA et al: Reversal of vascular and renal crises of scleroderma by oral angiotensin-converting enzyme blockade. N Engl J Med 300:1417, 1979

Machover S, Spaecky AJ: Effect of isometric exercise on the quadriceps muscle in patients with rheumatoid arthritis. Arch Phys Med 47:737, Nov 1966

Maddison RF, Martin MFR, Scott DGI: Other connective tissue disorders. In Wright V (ed): Bone and Joint Disease in the Elderly. New York, Churchill Livingston, 1983

Nickolson RA: Twenty years of bone and joint surgery in Bradford. J Bone Joint Surg 56B:760, 1974

Nysather JO, Katz AE, Lenth JL: The immune system: Its development and functions. Am J Nurs 76:1614, 1978

Price SA, Wilson LM: Pathophysiology, Clinical Concepts of Disease Processes, 2nd ed. New York, McGraw-Hill, 1982

Shiokawa Y, Abe T, Yamauchi Y: New Horizons in Rheumatoid Arthritis. Amsterdam, Excerpta Medica, 1981

Smith RR: Essentials of Neurosurgery. Philadelphia, WB Saunders, 1980

Stahl NI, Klippel JH: Recognizing drug induced lupus syndromes. Drug Therapy (Hospital) Sept:80, 1978

Stevens MB: Rheumatoid arthritis. In Wright V (ed): Bone and Joint Disease of the Elderly. New York, Churchill Livingston, 1983

Testa NN: Surgery for arthritis: What can and cannot be done. Consultant 18:142, 1978

Tilkian SM, Conover MB, Tilkian AG: Clinical Implications of Laboratory Tests, 3rd ed. St Louis, CV Mosby, 1983

Torbett MP, Ervin JC: The patient with systemic lupus erythematosus. Am J Nurs 77:1299, 1977

Tucker SM, Breeding MA, Canobbio MA et al: Patient Care Standards, 2nd ed. St Louis, CV Mosby, 1982

White J: Teaching patients to manage systemic lupus erythematosus. Nurs 78 8(9):26, 1978

White JF et al: Rheumatology Nursing. Nursing 79 10:108, 1979

Williams SR: Nutrition and diet therapy, 4th ed. St Louis, CV Mosby, 1982

Chapter 90

Metabolic, Structural, and Neoplastic Conditions of Musculoskeletal Origin

Terry F. Cicero

Bone is a dynamic organ that is constantly being remodeled. The rates of bone formation and resorption can be altered by external factors (*e.g.,* diet, sunlight, and trauma) or internal factors (*e.g.,* digestion and endocrine function).

The purpose of this chapter is to discuss the epidemiology, pathology, and medical and nursing management of specific musculoskeletal disorders that alter the cellular structure and function of bone.

Common metabolic disorders that result in abnormal formation of bone matrix, and their complications will be discussed. These disorders are treatable and frequently preventable. The problems of pain management and potential pathological fractures are common to all the disorders discussed.

There is a variety of different tumors of the musculoskeletal system. They are classified according to their cells of origin and occur either as benign tumors, primary malignant sarcomas, or secondary carcinomas from tumors in other parts of the body. Occasionally benign tumors develop into malignancies. It is beyond the scope of this chapter to consider all the tumors involving the skeletal system, but the most frequently occurring tumor will be discussed, tumor of the bone cells, or osteosarcoma.

Scoliosis, although usually a congenital spinal deformity, will be discussed because it is a potential complication of many of the other disorders.

Osteoporosis

Osteoporosis refers to a group of diseases characterized by a reduction of total skeletal mass and density, without changes in the mineral composition. The imbalance of bone homeostasis occurs because the rate of bone formation is less than rates of bone resorption. The calcium/protein ratio of the existing bone remains normal. The most significant aspect of osteoporosis is that the reduced skeletal volume is not strong enough to provide adequate mechanical support, resulting in increased risk of fracture under conditions of normal skeletal stress. The most vulnerable sites for fracture are the distal radius (Colles' fracture), the proximal femur, and the thoracic and lumbar vertebrae.

Etiology

Osteoporosis can result from aging, low-bone-mineral density at maturity, changes in estrogen status, immobility, nutritional deficiencies, excessive catabolic agents (*e.g.,* corticosteroids, thyroid dysfunction), or any combination of these. Rarer types are related to hepatic or biliary cirrhosis, radiation osteonecrosis, or prolonged heparin therapy.[14]

It is characteristically a disease of white women who are 65 years or older. Bone density parallels skin pigmentation, whites having the least bone mass and blacks having the most.

Pathophysiology

The major types of osteoporosis can be differentiated biochemically and by radiograph. However 30% of the bone mass can be lost before osteopenia can be identified by x-ray. Fig. 90–1 shows an example of a normal spine and one with osteoporosis.

In women the rates of bone formation and resorption remain equal until about age 40, when formation remains the same but resorption increases. Reduction in estrogen is the principal factor in postmenopausal and oophorectomized patients, since estrogen replacement is known to decrease the rate of bone loss. Estrogen-related bone loss is estimated to be 8% every 10 years.

Although age-related bone loss does occur in men, it generally starts 15 to 20 years later, and it proceeds at a slower rate (4% every 10 years). Other age-related events are impaired hepatic hydroxylation of vitamin D, a decreased ability of the intestine to absorb dietary calcium, and reduced renal production of 1-,2-,4-dihydroxyvitamin D.

Excessive catabolic agents, as seen with long-term corticosteroid therapy, Cushing's syndrome, or hyperthyroidism, initially increase bone resorption with compensatory rapid bone formation. However this early homeostatic action fails, and bone formation decreases while resorption continues. Profound bone loss results. In contrast to postmenopausal osteoporosis with low urinary calcium excretion, steroid-related osteoporosis is characterized by hypercalcemia and decreased serum alkaline phosphate due to a renal tubule phosphate leak. The degree of bone loss is directly proportional to the length of steroid therapy. The progression of bone loss halts when therapy is discontinued, but the bone mass deficit is usually not replaced.

Immobilization from prolonged bed rest, paralysis, or casts reduces the skeletal stress of weight bearing and muscle contraction needed to stimulate bone formation. This type of osteoporosis is associated with elevated alkaline phosphate levels.

Reduced calcium and vitamin D intake over a long pe-

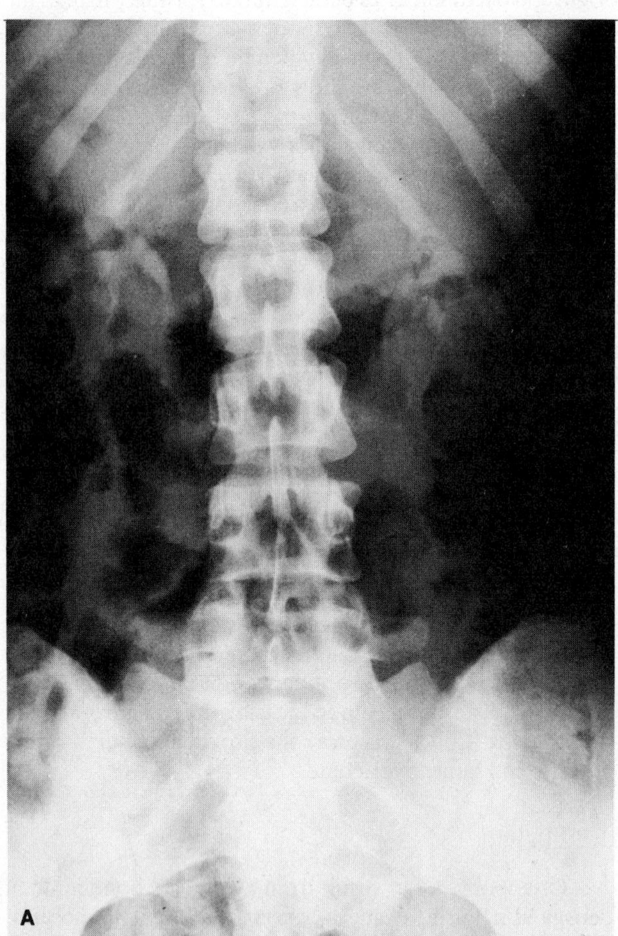

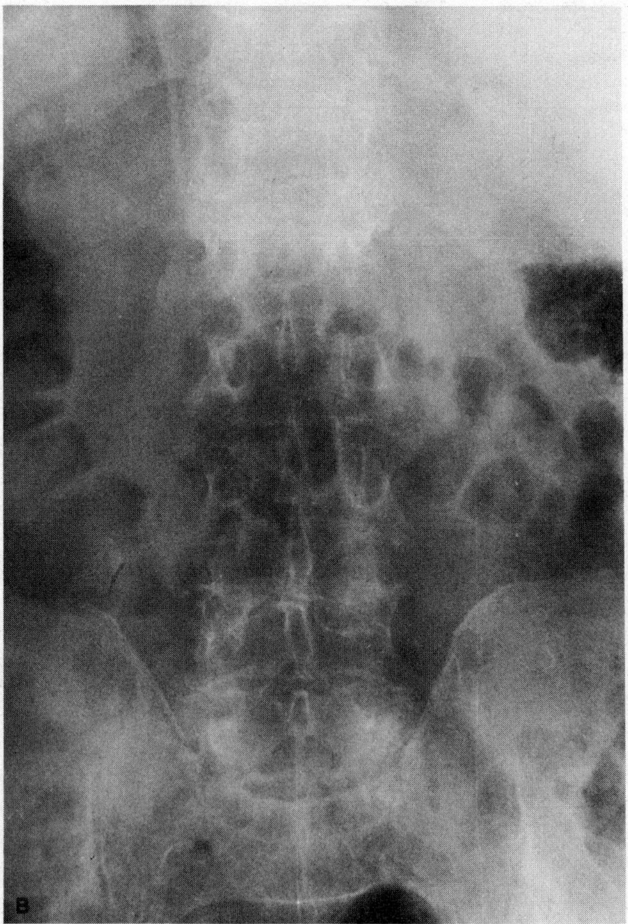

FIGURE 90–1 (*A*) Normal spine. Vertebral bodies are well defined and "white" because of an adequate amount of calcium. (*B*) Osteoporosis of the spine. The bones have a "washed out" appearance because of mineral loss. Vertebral bodies are somewhat compressed.

riod play a key role in the initiation of osteoporosis. Dairy products and leafy green vegetables are the main sources of calcium in the diet. Adults require 800 mg of calcium per day, yet the estimated average consumption is 300 mg to 500 mg/24 hours. The effects of aging boost the daily requirements for a postmenopausal woman to 1500 mg/day to prevent bone loss. Metabolites of vitamin D stimulate bone synthesis and augment absorption of calcium from the intestines. Patients who have had a gastrectomy or those with intestinal malabsorption illnesses are at further risk for nutritional calcium deficits.

Clinical Manifestations

The most common presenting symptom is back pain of varying degrees and increasing curvature of the spine (kyphosis). Both are due to compression fracture of one or more of the lower thoracic or lumbar vertebrae. These fractures are generally not related to significant trauma. The back pain worsens with movement and is associated with spasms of the paravertebral muscles. There is localized tenderness at the site of fracture. If multiple compression fractures have occurred over time, scoliosis (lateral curvature of the spine) and kyphosis (dowager's hump) result in loss of height from 1 inch to 6 inches. As kyphosis becomes more pronounced, the ribs angle downward and the thoracic cage telescopes into the pelvis.[6] This shortens the trunk and causes the stomach to pouch outward as the stomach muscles relax (Fig. 90–2). The height loss can be estimated by measuring the patient's arm span from longest fingertip to fingertip, which usually is equal to his earlier normal adult height. Corticosteroids may exaggerate the kyphosis as the "buffalo hump" fat distribution is superimposed over the dowager's hump of osteoporosis. The patient may also complain of weakness, fatigue, shortness of breath, and poor appetite, all of which could be related to posture changes.

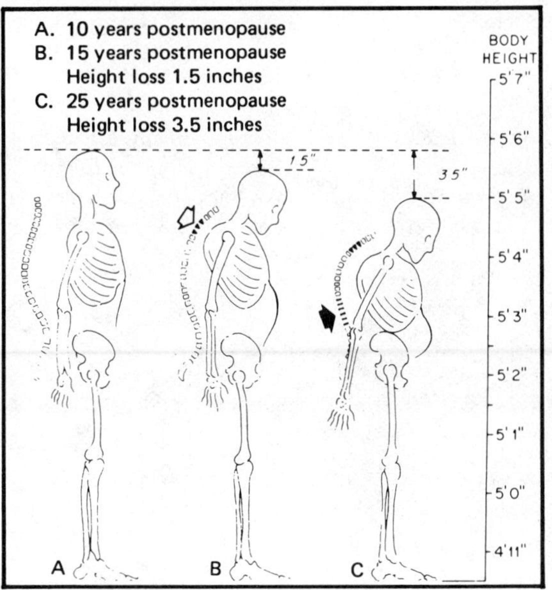

FIGURE 90–2 Posture changes associated with osteoporosis and aging. (Courtesy of the Wilson Research Foundation)

Osteoporosis may be discovered as a result of a Colles' fracture or a hip fracture. More than 75% of all hip fractures are related to osteoporosis.

Medical Management

Prophylaxis is the best approach, since the treatment of established osteoporosis does not replenish the lost bone mass but rather halts the progression. Preventative measures include identification of individuals at risk, diet, and early ambulation or range-of-motion exercises for surgical, casted, or bedridden patients.

Conventional therapies for clinical osteoporosis include dietary replacement of protein, calcium, and vitamins with additional supplements. Low-dose oral estrogen therapy (Premarin) has proved effective in reducing negative calcium balance. Its use, though, has been associated with stroke, hypertension, thrombosis, myocardial infarction, and a ninefold increase in risk of uterine cancer. It is imperative that patients receiving estrogen report irregular vaginal bleeding, have Pap smears every 6 months, and perform monthly breast self-examinations. Women who have had a hysterectomy can be given estrogen without fear of endometrial cancer.

Other measures include administration of oral fluoride salts, which act to stimulate new bone formation and inhibit resorption.[28] The main adverse effect is gastrointestinal upset. Calcitonin, a thyroid hormone that decreases bone loss, parathyroid hormone, and anabolic steroids (stanozolol) are also being used.[19] The efficacy of these agents is unproven and considered experimental.

Pain management includes local heat, analgesics, avoiding straining from constipation, and early ambulation. Compression fractures generally heal by themselves, however Colles' and hip fractures may require casts, traction, or hip-pinning as discussed in Chapters 87 and 88.

Nursing Management

Assessment and Nursing Diagnosis

Patients are generally not admitted to the hospital with a primary diagnosis of osteoporosis. It may be a secondary diagnosis related to a bone fracture, or totally unrelated to the admitting diagnosis. The major nursing problems for patients with osteoporosis, regardless of etiology, include acute or chronic pain secondary to pathological fractures and muscle spasm; stress fractures secondary to decreased skeletal strength; potential for falls related to decreased muscle strength; and inadequate nutritional intake, especially protein, calcium, and vitamin D.

Goals. The goals for patients with varying degrees of osteoporosis are that the patient will be free of pain from fractures and muscle spasms; not suffer additional fractures during the hospital stay and through increased home safety; increase his level of physical activity; and increase his dietary intake of protein, calcium, and vitamin D.

(*Text continues on page 1362*)

NURSING CARE PLAN FOR THE PATIENT WITH OSTEOPOROSIS

NURSING DIAGNOSIS/PROBLEM 1: Alterations in comfort and pain related to vertebral compression fractures and paravertebral muscle spasm
GOAL 1: Relief of pain

Nursing Interventions	Rationale	Outcome Criteria for Goal Achievement
1. Thorough assessment of any new or acute complaints of pain 2. Bed for several days during episodes of acute pain 3. Administer pain medication and muscle relaxants as prescribed.	1. Spontaneous fractures may occur without significant trauma. 2. Compression fractures heal by themselves and new fractures are aggravated by motion. a. Bed rest for extended periods promotes demineralization and should be avoided. b. Intermittent rest periods relieve stress from abnormal posture.	1–3. The patient: —Experiences relief of pain ▪ At rest ▪ During activity —Appears comfortable ▪ No expressions of anxiety on face ▪ Has periods of uninterrupted sleep

NURSING DIAGNOSIS/PROBLEM 2: Potential for injury related to decreased skeletal strength from porous and fragile bone
GOAL 2: Preventing injury and additional fractures

Nursing Interventions	Rationale	Outcome Criteria for Goal Achievement
1. Use care when turning or transferring the patient a. Logroll when turning from side to side. 2. Raise commode seat in the bathroom. 3. Provide walker or cane if unsteady when ambulating. 4. Patient to wear nonskid slippers or shoes when ambulating	1. Spontaneous fractures may result from simple movement. a. Logrolling keeps spine straight. 2. Will reduce stress on spine from sitting at low position 3. Provides support and can prevent unsteadiness	1–4. The patient: a. Shows no signs of additional fractures b. Is free of episodes of acute pain, especially following activity c. Ambulates safely and with reduced risk of falling
5. Discharge instructions: a. Avoid sudden bending and lifting of heavy objects. b Avoid walking on snow and ice. c. Remove scatter rugs. d. Don't wax floors. e. Be sure lamp cords aren't draped across walking areas. f. Leave night light on. g. Install handrails and nonskid surface in bathtub.	5. The elderly often have decreased stability on their feet, poor eyesight, and the need to use the bathroom during the night. These present a safety hazard that results in falls and fractures.	5. The patient will: a. Identify verbally 4 to 5 methods for making the home safer b. Will not experience new fractures as the result of slipping or falling

(Continued)

NURSING CARE PLAN FOR THE PATIENT WITH OSTEOPOROSIS *(Continued)*

GOAL 3: Adequate dietary intake to prevent bone resorption

Nursing Interventions	Rationale	Outcome Criteria for Goal Achievement
1. Provide high-protein diet with snacks in between meals and at H.S. a. Calcium, 1500 mg/day for post-menopausal women (800 mg/day for other adults) b. Vitamin D, 375 IU/day c. Dark leafy vegetables d. Dairy products and milk fortified with vitamin D	1. The rate of bone resorption is slowed by increased protein and calcium. Vitamin D is necessary for calcium to be absorbed by the intestines.	1–2. The patient will: a. Eat 3 balanced meals/day. b. Consume 1500 mg or 800 mg calcium, as required.
2. Administer calcium and vitamin D supplements as ordered.		
3. Administer estrogen, fluoride, calcitonin, or anabolic agents, if ordered.	3. Estrogen therapy retards bone loss and reduces the body's negative calcium balance.	3. The patient will demonstrate the correct method of self-breast-check.

NURSING DIAGNOSIS/PROBLEM 3: Activity intolerance and impaired physical mobility related to compression fractures and reduced musculoskeletal stamina

GOAL 1: Increased participation in activity program

Nursing Interventions	Rationale	Outcome Criteria for Goal Achievement
1. In hospital:		1–2. The patient:
a. Evaluate ability and motivation to exercise independently.	a. Age, pain, poor health, and orthopedic problems often impose physical and mental limitations.	a. Actively participates in the exercise program
b. Schedule active or passive range-of-motion exercises.	b. Demineralization of bone and disuse muscle atrophy is decreased through regular exercise.	b. Uses assistance devices (if necessary)
c. Arrange for any needed assistance devices.	c. Elderly are frequently unsteady on their feet.	c. Joins and regularly attends a group with a compatible and approved program
2. Discharge planning:		
a. Encourage patient to join an exercise group through YWCA or Senior Citizens.	a. Organized programs increase motivation and stimulate continued participation from the positive psychological benefits.	
b. Instruct patient in a *daily* exercise program within his individual limitations *e.g.,* walking, swimming, bicycle riding		

Interventions

Pain can often be managed by bed rest for several days with a firm mattress and pillows to provide adequate support. Williams' position (head of bed raised and knees bent) may be the most comfortable if the patient has significant back pain. Extreme care and gentleness must be used in moving and turning the patient. Logrolling with a pillow between the knees is the best method for positioning the patient from side to side. Analgesics are often required, and if they are of the narcotic group, the nurse must be alert to the possibility of constipation, which would be compounded by bed rest. (A more detailed overview of nursing interventions is presented in Nursing Care Plan for the Patient with Osteoporosis on pp 1360–1361.)

Exercise through passive or active range of motion is a priority to decrease the demineralization of the bones. Physical therapy may be consulted to assess the patient's capabilities and assist in the exercise program. Safety measures such as nonskid slippers and walkers or canes may be provided if the patient is ambulatory.

The patient's eating habits need to be evaluated to ensure an adequate intake of protein, calcium, and vitamin D. If the patient has a poor appetite, smaller meals with between-meal nourishment may be indicated.

Patient education for discharge should address home pain management, exercise, safety, and nutrition. There may be specific instructions concerning home medications or discharge diagnosis, such as hip-pinning.

Evaluation

Evaluation criteria for the problems and related nursing interventions are

- Absence of pain from spontaneous fractures
- No additional fractures
- Increased level of physical activity
- Increased intake of protein, calcium, and vitamin D

Osteomalacia

Osteomalacia is a metabolic bone disease characterized by softening and deformity of mature bone due to deficient mineralization. It is an adult form of rickets, a childhood bone-softening disease caused by inadequate intake and synthesis of vitamin D. Nutritional rickets in children is uncommon in the United States because of vitamin D fortification of milk and food products.

Etiology

Osteomalacia results from lack of minerals for normal osteoblastic–osteoclastic activity. The deficiencies may be due to poor dietary intakes, postgastrectomy syndromes (*e.g.,* Crohn's disease and ulcerative colitis), hepatitis, excessive kidney loss of serum phosphorus, and exhaustion of skeletal minerals from repeated pregnancies and long-term lactation. Prolonged use of drugs such as phenytoin (Dilantin) or phenobarbital, which disrupts vitamin D metabolism in the liver; antacids (*i.e.,* aluminum hydroxide), which bind phosphates; and corticosteroids, which decrease intestinal calcium absorption, all increase the risk of osteomalacia.[12]

Pathophysiology

In contrast to osteoporosis, where there is a decreased rate of but normal mineralization of the newly formed bone, osteomalacia has a marked increase in abnormal nonmineralized bone. The result is decreased skeletal strength, softening and bowing of the bones, accompanied with pain and tenderness. Generalized weakness may be due to impaired oxygen delivery to the muscles from decreased red blood cell adenosine triphosphate (ATP), secondary to hypophosphatemia. More than one pathophysiological factor may be at work in any given patient.

The aging process itself is responsible for some degree of malabsorption, but if it is compounded by gastrointestinal disorders, vitamin D and calcium absorption is further compromised. Gastrectomy, small bowel resections, and biliary obstructions decrease fat absorption. Vitamin D is fat-soluble, and along with calcium, is simply excreted. Crohn's disease and ulcerative colitis are associated with diarrhea and lack of food and mineral absorption from lack of time of food's being in the bowel. Hepatic disorders decrease the conversion of vitamin D into its active metabolites, 25-hydroxyvitamin D.

Adequate renal function is also necessary for conversion of vitamin D into active metabolites. Furthermore, the acidosis that accompanies kidney failure leads to increased parathormone release and increased skeletal calcium loss.

Clinical Manifestations

The presenting symptoms include bone pain, muscle weakness, skeletal deformities, and fractures.[10] At first, the skeletal pains are vague and poorly localized. As the disease progresses, the pain is nagging to severe. The patient may develop a waddle or limp, since lifting the feet and climbing stairs becomes difficult and painful. The softening of the bones may result in lateral bowing of the legs, bending of the femoral neck, and angulation of the sternum. The trunk shortens from deformity of the spine, usually kyphosis and occasionally scoliosis. As with osteoporosis, compression fractures may occur with minimal trauma, and they often go unnoticed by the patient.

Medical Management

Typical laboratory findings are a low or normal serum calcium and low serum phosphorus. These values may fluctuate according to the immediate state of vitamin D correction. Serum alkaline phosphatase is usually elevated.

A characteristic radiographic finding that helps differentiate osteomalacia from osteoporosis are Looser's zones, or pseudofractures. These are bands of decalcification that run perpendicular or oblique to the surface of the bone and are particularly common in the ribs, scapula, pubic rami, and femoral neck.[10] Since these occur most frequently where major arteries cross bone, it is believed that the mechanical stresses of the pulsating arteries may be responsible.

The treatment of osteomalacia includes correction of the predisposing disorder, exposure to sun (the skin manufactures vitamin D when exposed to ultraviolet light), phosphate repletion, and calcium/vitamin D supplementation.[16] If a diagnosis of osteomalacia cannot be established, a positive response to a therapeutic trial of vitamin D will confirm its presence.

Nursing Management

Assessment and Nursing Diagnosis

The clinical symptoms of pain, weakness, and fractures, along with a positive diagnosis of osteomalacia, guide specific areas for the nursing history and assessment. These include an assessment of pain, motor function, diet, and bowel function.

The major nursing problems encountered are bone pain and tenderness, pathological stress fractures secondary to decreased skeletal strength, and potential for falls secondary to bone deformities and decreased muscle strength.

Goals. Analysis of information obtained from the medical and nursing assessment identify specific goals for individual patients. The goals usually identified are to relieve the bone pain and enhance remineralization of the bone and to prevent the disease from recurring.

Interventions

Pain management should be individualized based on the severity of the pain and any limitations of the patient's activities as a result. Generally pain will decrease with the same interventions that are used for pain management in the osteoporotic patient.

The skeletal problems of softening, fractures, and Looser's zones generally resolve when the underlying disease or dietary deficiency is treated. While the bone is remineralizing, safety precautions as for the osteoporotic patient will decrease the risk of further fractures.

Calcium and vitamin D supplements are the most widely accepted method for remineralizing the bone. A diet high in vitamin D or supplements is recommended if the demineralization was from nutritional deficiencies. If the patient has a malabsorption condition, ultraviolet irradiation from natural or mechanical sources is recommended in addition to vitamin D and calcium supplements.

Once the bone is remineralized and the fractures healed, prevention of recurrence is facilitated by patient education and continued treatment of any ongoing, predisposing conditions. Patient education is directed at dietary management, home administration of supplements, increasing the exposure to sunlight, and the importance of maintaining follow-up appointments with the physician.

Evaluation

Evaluation of the nursing interventions for the major goals includes the following outcome criteria.

The patient

1. Is free of bone pain
   a. Has no complaints of pain
   b. Has periods of uninterrupted sleep
   c. Is able to participate in activities of daily living
2. Demonstrates remineralization of the bone
   a. Progression of skeleton deformities ceases
   b. No further stress fractures occur
   c. X-ray and biochemical findings confirm improvement
3. Prevents disease recurrence
   a. Adheres to increased dietary intake of calcium and vitamin D
   b. Self-administers mineral/vitamin supplements
   c. Maintains checkup appointments
   d. Increases exposure to sunlight

Scoliosis

Scoliosis is a lateral curvature of the spine that can occur in the thoracic, lumbar, or thoracolumbar section of the spine. In addition to the lateral curve, the vertebral bodies are often rotated.

Etiology and Pathophysiology

Scoliosis occurs in two forms: postural and structural. Postural scoliosis is due to poor posture from muscular weakness or from a discrepancy in leg length that results in compensatory changes in the spine as the individual stands erect. Structural scoliosis can result from *congenital anomalies* of the vertebral body, muscle imbalance from *neurological lesions* (*e.g.*, poliomyelitis and cerebral palsy), or *idiopathic causes* in which the pathology is unknown. Idiopathic scoliosis is the most common form and is classified according to age of onset. Adolescent iodiopathic scoliosis occurs predominantly in girls, and the curve rapidly progresses from age 10 to maturity.[9]

Clinical Manifestations

Scoliosis rarely presents subjective symptoms until the deformity is well established. This often delays diagnosing and treating the condition unless it is noticed during a routine medical examination. The adolescent may notice that "one hip sticks out" or there is a "rib hump" that is accentuated by bending over (Fig. 90–3). Parents may observe that the child's pants legs are different lengths or that dresses hang poorly. The patient may complain of fatigue or backache. A severe curve will reduce the patient's height and can cause dyspnea from interference with lung function and efficiency. Patients with grossly deformed chests are prone to recurrent pulmonary infections and possible paresthesias and paralysis from excessive traction on the spinal cord.[25] During examination, a plumb line is dropped from the patient's occiput, and lateral deviation of the spine is noted (Fig. 90–4). The patient's back is also examined for discrepancies in shoulder, elbow, or iliac crest height. The mobility of the spine is also noted and helps to determine the method of treatment.

Diagnosis of scoliosis is confirmed by anteroposterior radiograph, which aids in measuring the degree of the curve.

Medical Management

The treatment goal for the patient with scoliosis is to end up with the smallest deformity possible when the child has stopped growing. The course of treatment can be conservative or operative. Variables that determine the treatment method include the age of onset, the angle, and the mobility of the curve, as well as the child's emotional status and attitude of the parent.

Conservative Treatment. Conservative treatment involves the use of exercises and braces to strengthen the torso muscles and keep the curve from progressing. Exercise alone is prescribed for curves less than 20 degrees. The program includes pelvic tilts, sit-ups, push-ups, hyperextension, and deep-breathing exercise. The spine is reevaluated every 3 months.

The Milwaukee brace is used in addition to exercises if the scoliosis curve is greater than 20 degrees, or if the curve increases 3 degrees to 4 degrees while the patient is on an exercise program. The brace is adjustable and is periodically refitted by the orthopedic surgeon. It is worn 23 hours/day until bone growth is complete (Fig. 90–5).

Operative Treatment. Operative treatment is considered for patients not responding to a conservative approach, or with a curve of 45 degrees. Surgical procedures involve decorticating and excising the spinous processes and facet joints, using bone chips as grafts to line up the fusion, and immobilizing the spine internally by Harrington rods, Dwyer screws, or Lugue rods. Postoperatively, patients wear a Risser body cast for 6 months (Fig. 90–6), followed by a Milwaukee brace for another 3 to 6 months. Patients who have had Lugue instrumentation do not need a postoperative brace or cast because of the increased spinal stability with this procedure.[1,2,3]

Nursing Management

Spinal fusions for scoliosis are a major surgical procedure associated with significant complications, which include sur-

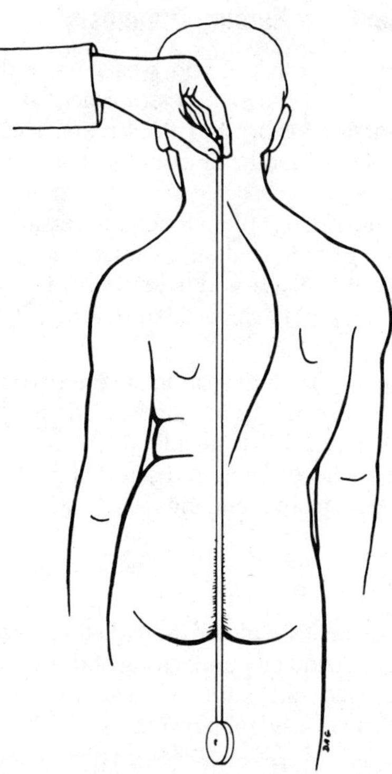

FIGURE 90–4 Scoliosis can be detected by use of the plumb line.

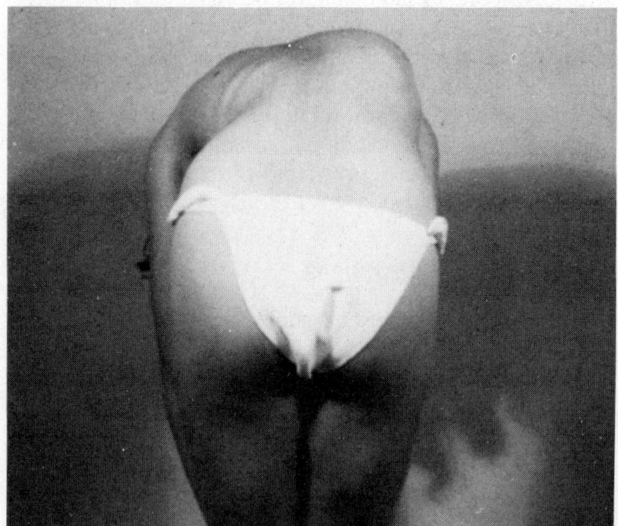

FIGURE 90–3 Scoliosis becomes apparent when the patient bends over. (O'Connor BJ: Scoliosis: Classification and diagnosis in pediatric orthopedics. ONA J 3:84, 1976)

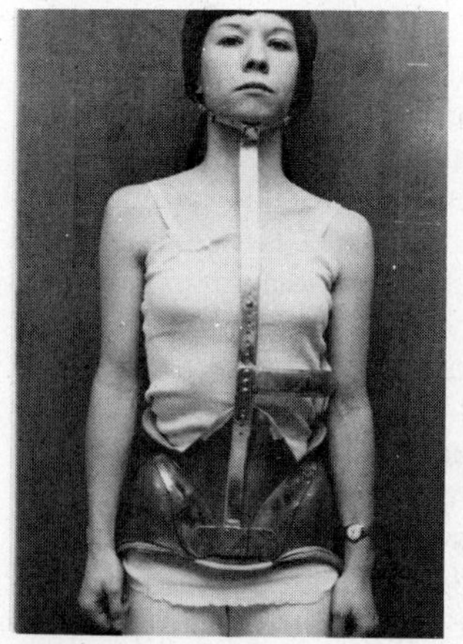

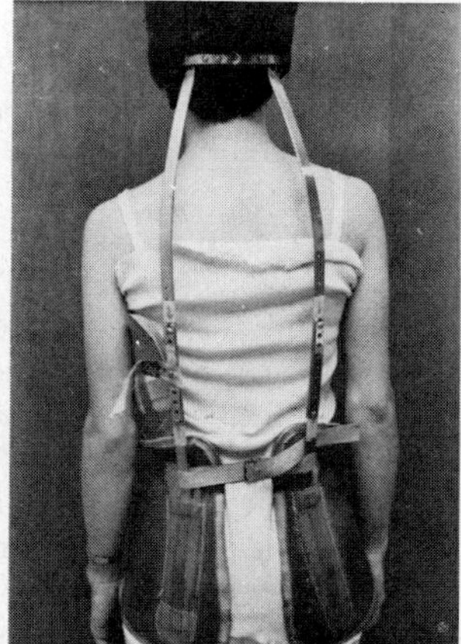

FIGURE 90–5 Milwaukee brace used in treatment of scoliosis.

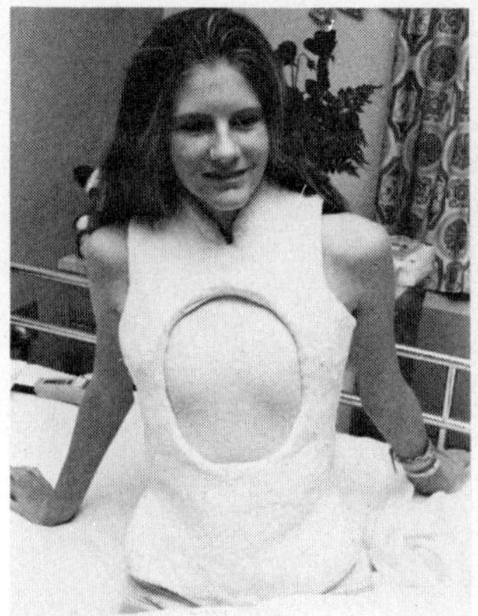
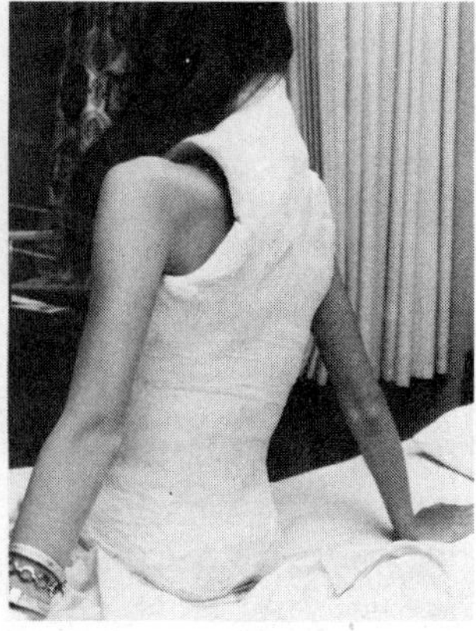

FIGURE 90–6 Risser cast is applied following spinal surgery in scoliosis.

gical wound infection, pneumonia, and neurological deficits. The typical types of nursing problems and interventions required for a patient undergoing surgery can be found in Chapter 8. Cast care and care of a patient undergoing a laminectomy or spinal fusion are discussed in Chapters 87 and 69 respectively.

Paget's Disease (Osteitis Deformans)

Paget's disease is a chronic bone disease of geriatric patients, affecting 2% to 4 percent of people 60 years old. It is characterized by excessive bone resorption and deposition. It results in softening, enlargement, and severe deformity of the skeleton. The disease usually affects multiple areas of the skeleton (polyostotic). The spine, femur, skull, pelvis, and tibia are the most commonly involved bones. Monostotic, or single bone involvement, occurs in 10% of patients with Paget's disease. The disease occurs more commonly in Anglo-Saxon people, and there is often a family history of the disease.

Etiology and Pathophysiology

At present, the etiology of Paget's disease is unknown. Several of the possible causes being exposed include a slow viral infection, a biochemical collagen defect, and a benign neoplastic condition that precedes sarcomatous degeneration.[11,24,26]

The progression of bone involvement in Paget's disease is divided into two stages. In the initial stage there is increased osteoclastic activity, resulting in excessive bone resorption. The characteristic bowing occurs at this stage while the bones are soft. In the second stage there is a compensatory increase in bone formation. This osteoblastic activity causes thickening of the bone in an irregular mosaic pattern. Enlargement of the bone is accompanied by increased vascularity.

Clinical Manifestations

Patients with Paget's disease have a wide spectrum of clinical findings. Many patients are asymptomatic, and the disease may be detected inadvertently from an elevated alkaline phosphatase level or from radiographic studies performed for other reasons. The more severe form of the disease can render gross deformity, pain, and a variety of metabolic, rheumatological, and neurological complications.

The disease rarely causes pain in the early stages; however, when it does occur it is typically a chronic, deep ache, which is more noticeable at night. An abrupt increase in the intensity of pain suggests that a stress fracture has occurred or the development of malignant degeneration (osteosarcoma).[7] The patient usually seeks advice because of the associated deformities. The most obvious changes are the anterior bowing of the tibia, femur, and humerus. The affected bones develop multiple arteriovenous fistulas that have been associated with high-output cardiac failure.

Fractures of the neck of the femur are a common complication. Involvement of the spine most frequently involves the lumbosacral region. As the disease progresses, the spine becomes thicker and compressed. The patient's height shortens and kyphosis develops. Bone enlargement in this area can result in severe back pain from pressure on the nerve root. Paraplegia from spinal cord compression also occurs. The cranium also thickens, especially in the frontal area. The patient may say his hat size increases every year. Occasionally the skull invaginates. Deafness, hydrocephalus, and other neurological symptoms can result. Figure 90–7 demonstrates the classic posture of the patient with Paget's disease.

The serum alkaline phosphatase level is usually elevated from the increased osteoblastic activity. Urinary hydroxyproline excretion is also elevated and indicates increased collagen turnover. The serum calcium levels are normal but may be increased if the patient is immobilized. Hyperuricemia is seen in about 50% of the male patients; 25% of these men have clinical evidence of gout.[7]

Medical Management

Asymptomatic patients with Paget's disease require no medical treatment. Those with minimal pain can often be helped with analgesics. Nonsteroidal, anti-inflammatory agents such as indomethacin (Indocin) or piroxicam (Feldene) may be used to relieve rheumatological symptoms.

Specific antipagetic medications, for example, calcitonin, disodium etidronate (EHDP), and mithramycin (Mithracin) all suppress bone resorption and are used only on patients with serious forms of the disease. Clinical indicators for suppressive therapy are severe bone pain, high-output cardiac failure, recurrent renal calculi secondary to hypercalciuria, multiple fractures, neurological complications, and bone involvement that may result in disabling deformity.

Calcitonin, a polypeptide hormone, has been used since 1963, and it reduces bone pain in 60% of patients.[12] Salmon, porcine, and human calcitonin are available, but only salmon calcitonin is used in this country.[27] Calcitonin decreases bone resorption by reducing the number of osteoclasts and

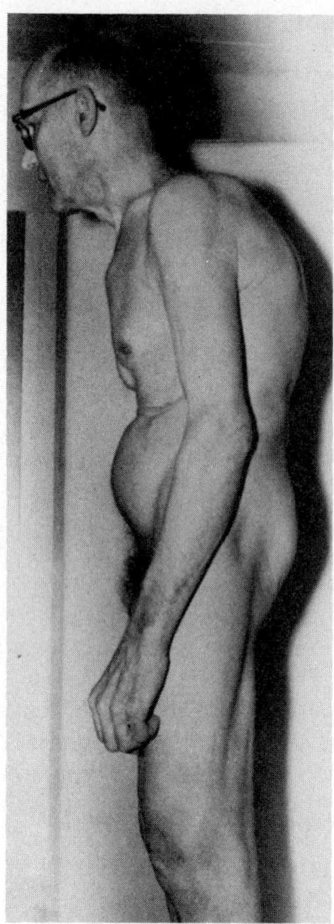

FIGURE 90–7 Paget's disease, affecting mainly the spine, the pelvis, and left femur. (Turek SL: Orthopaedics: Principles and Their Application, Vol 1, p 737. Philadelphia, JB Lippincott, 1984)

altering their ability to resorb bone. Bone formed after calcitonin therapy has normal structure. Along with pain relief, the hormone reduces complications during and following orthopedic surgery of pagetic bone. A fall in skin temperature over involved bone and a decrease in cardiac output can occur. Generally, hearing deficits and other neurological symptoms do not improve with calcitonin therapy. The drug is given as a daily subcutaneous injection for approximately 3 months. Nausea occurs in 10% of patients. Facial flushing, paresthesias, fever, urticaria, and local skin reaction are other possible side-effects.

Disodium etidronate, a diphosphate, is administered orally for no longer than 6 months. If symptoms reoccur, another 6-month regimen may be given. The drug decreases both bone resorption and formation and is very effective in alleviating bone pain. The main side-effect is mild diarrhea.

Mithramycin, a cytotoxic antibiotic, is not a first choice treatment because of hepatic, renal, and platelet toxicity.[12] The drug has been shown to suppress bone turnover and substantially reduce pain. Mithramycin is given intravenously in subturmoricidal doses for 7 days. Minor side-effects include nausea, vomiting, and persistent malaise. Frequent laboratory testing of BUN, creatinine, SGOT, SGPT, platelets, and clotting factors monitor the toxic effects of the drug.

Improvements in bone can be monitored by decreasing levels of serum alkaline phosphatase and decreased hydroxyproline excretion.

Surgery may be required to repair fractures or improve neurological symptoms. The most frequently performed procedures are total hip replacement, internal fracture fixation, and decompressive procedures of the cranium or spine. Occasionally ventriculojugular shunts may be performed to improve associated hydrocephalus.[4]

Nursing Management

Assessment and Nursing Diagnosis

Based on the clinical manifestations, the nurse must assess to what extent that patient's symptoms interfere with his daily routine and how they can be improved. The major nursing problems for the patient with Paget's disease include bone pain secondary to altered skeletal metabolism, stress fractures secondary to abnormal bone metabolism, decreased physical activity secondary to bone pain and deformity, and hearing deficits related to abnormal skull growth.

Goals. Information obtained from the nursing assessment identify individual goals for the patient's care. The goals usually identified are to relieve the bone pain, arrest further deformity or fracture, maintain skeletal function, and manage any hearing deficit.

Interventions

The pain of Paget's disease can usually be managed with analgesics and anti-inflammatory agents such as aspirin, ibuprofen (Motrin), or indomethacin (Indocin). Splinting, immobilization, or bed rest generally are not helpful. Sudden onset of severe pain usually indicates a fracture, nerve compression, or malignant degeneration, and requires further medical evaluation.

Management of fractures is determined by their location. Healing is usually rapid, but it can be unpredictable. Spinal compression fractures heal spontaneously with bed rest. Tibial, humeral and femoral fractures are treated with traction or with external or internal fixation. Nonunion femoral neck fractures are the most troublesome to treat and usually necessitate a total hip replacement or bone grafting.

The progression of bone deformities is treated by the administration of bone suppressor medications. Nurses need to be cognizant of the side-effects as previously discussed. Nurses are often involved in educating the patients concerning home drug administration and the importance of follow-up appointments.

Although the bone suppressors can arrest further deformities, they cannot reverse those that exist and that are limiting the patient's skeletal function. If the limited function is the result of painful, involved joints, joint replacements may be beneficial. Pain and muscle weakness associated with nerve impingement from spinal cord compression can also limit the patient's mobility. Laminectomies and decompression procedures often give symptomatic relief. Calcitonin therapy may be instituted 1 to 2 weeks before surgery to decrease the vascularity of the involved bone and to limit bleeding.

If the patient's gait is impaired, he may be unsteady on his feet and at risk for falling. Mobility may be improved through use of assistance devices such as walkers and canes. The nurse might suggest installation of bathtub rails to prevent bathroom accidents.

Deafness from compression of the eighth cranial nerve can be managed by hearing aids and by alternative communication techniques such as lip reading or sign language. A speech therapist may be consulted to help plan and implement a means of communication. If the patient is hospitalized, his hearing impairment must be documented on the Kardex, along with specific information concerning his communication pattern, whether he wears a hearing aid, and which ear is involved.

Evaluation

The patient

1. Is free of bone pain:
   a. Has no complaints of pain
   b. Has periods of uninterrupted sleep
   c. Is able to participate in activities of daily living
2. Has arrest of further deformity or fracture:
   a. Visible progression of skeletal deformities ceases
   b. X-ray and serum alkaline phosphatase levels confirm bone improvement
   c. No further stress fractures occur
3. Maintains skeletal function:
   a. Is able to move joints freely without pain
   b. Uses walker or cane for stability and assistance
   c. Is able to participate in activities of daily living
4. Manages any hearing deficit:
   a. Wears hearing aid
   b. Uses lip reading or sign language to augment communication
   c. Is able to understand and respond in conversations

Osteosarcoma

Primary osteogenic sarcoma (osteosarcoma) is a highly malignant tumor associated with a 5-year survival rate of approximately 20% after a curative amputation. The poor prognosis is due to rapid metastasis of the tumor to the lung.

Etiology and Pathophysiology

Osteosarcoma occurs in the metaphyses of the long bones, usually in the distal femur, the proximal tibia, and the proximal humerus. It is a disease of adolescents and young adults between the ages of 12 and 20 years. It may occur in adults over 50 years of age who have Paget's disease. There is a slight male predominance.

The histological appearance is either osteolytic, in which the tumor erodes the bone cortex and erupts into the soft tissues, or osteoblastic, in which new bone is formed. The hallmark of the tumor is the malignant spindle cells that produce osteoid.[18] The periosteum is lifted from the bone as the tumor expands, and new bone is laid down in spindles radiating away from the center of the tumor. This creates a "sunburst" effect on the roentgenogram.[25] Metastasis is usually to the lungs, carried by the bloodstream.

Clinical Manifestations

The patient often seeks medical attention because of a swelling over a bone. The bone is often tender to palpation. A dull ache is common, but severe pain is rare in the early stages of the tumor. The skin over the mass is often warm from increased circulation in the area. There may be limited range of motion from joint involvement. Cachexia, severe pain, and malaise are later and more ominous symptoms.

Medical Management

The major medical goals for treating patients with primary osteosarcoma are gross removal of the tumor, destruction of all micrometastases, and rehabilitation of the patient as soon as possible. This requires a multidisciplinary health team, to include nurses, surgeons, radiologist, oncologist, physical and occupational therapists, and social workers.

Diagnostic indicators include an elevated serum alkaline phosphatase level, bone marrow aspiration, bone scans, gallium scans, and CT scan (computerized tomography), which help differentiate and determine the extent of the disease. Chest x-rays and lung tomography identify patients who have metastatic disease.

Amputation of the limb above the tumor or involved joint needs to be performed following a biopsy to confirm the neoplastic diagnosis. Many centers advocate immediate rehabilitation through early fitting of prostheses and early weight bearing to provide psychological benefits. This facilitates healing of the stump through decreased edema and pain. Immediate fitting is risky if the patient is reluctant, debilitated, diabetic, or on prolonged corticosteroids.

Some research cancer centers are investigating limb-preservation surgery as an alternative to amputation. The tumor is resected and the bone defect is replaced with a custom-fitted prosthetic implant.[13] Study patients are highly selected for small tumor size. The procedure includes preoperative and postoperative chemotherapy.

Before the 1970s, the major limiting factor in the management of osteosarcoma was the early development of pulmonary metastasis. Since that time and the advent of chemotherapy in combination with surgery the 5-year survival rate has improved from 20% to 40% to 60%.[8] The choice of chemotherapeutic agents is not clear. However, the antimitotic drugs being used in different combinations are high-dose methotrexate, citrovorum, Adriamycin, and vincristine. The treatments may be started before or after surgery, and repeated at intervals for as long as 2 years. Progress is monitored through lung tomography and laboratory tests. A decrease in a previously elevated serum alkaline phosphatase level indicates a positive response to treatment.

The efficacy of prophylactic lung irradiation, immunotherapy, and surgical resection of pulmonary macrometastases in improving survival rates is still unclear, but under investigation.[5, 20, 22]

Nursing Management

Assessment and Nursing Diagnosis

Based on the clinical manifestations and on what avenue of medical management is chosen for the patient, the nurse will be an integral member of the health care team. Preoperatively, nursing function includes assessing the patient's learning needs, coping strategies, nutritional status, and rehabilitative potential. Postoperative assessment is directed at evaluating pain, wound healing, and early rehabilitation. During chemotherapy, nursing assessment will be concerned with the complications associated with the drugs and with continued rehabilitation.

The major nursing problems for caring for the patient with osteosarcoma include pain secondary to neoplastic growth or operative procedure, altered body image and coping difficulties secondary to loss of limb and decreased independence, all the potential problems related to complications of a major operative procedure (*e.g.*, pulmonary emboli, thrombophlebitis, wound infection, and pneumonia), and all nursing problems related to the patient undergoing chemotherapy (see Chap. 19).

Goals. The goals for the patient with osteosarcoma will change depending on his phase of treatment. The major goals are to relieve pain; minimize postoperative complications; promote early rehabilitation and independence; and minimize complications from chemotherapeutic regimen.

Interventions

Bone pain is managed preoperatively and postoperatively by narcotic or non-narcotic analgesics. Immobilization of the involved area through bed rest, splints, sandbags, or pillows may be helpful. Emotional support is provided by encouraging verbalization of fears and explaining all procedures.

The postoperative complications of stump infection, pulmonary emboli, thrombophlebitis, pneumonia, muscle wasting, and contractures are minimized by coughing and deep breathing routines, incentive spirometry, frequent vital signs, and early ambulation. Adequate calories and protein and fluids to 3000 ml/day are provided. (See Chapter 88 for nursing care of the amputee patient.)

A rehabilitation program begins at the first preoperative encounter and continues throughout the patient's care. The patient is encouraged to actively participate in his care. Active or passive range-of-motion exercises are provided. Early ambulation with the prosthesis and crutch training promote resumption of independent functioning.

Surgery, rehabilitation, prostheses, and maintenance can be a financial burden. To help with these concerns the social worker can be a liaison between the family and potential community resources.

The patient undergoing irradiation or chemotherapy has many physical and emotional needs because the side-effects of osteosarcoma can be devastating. Specific nursing concerns and interventions for the patient undergoing these treatments are described in Chapter 19.

Evaluation

The patient

1. Is free of pain
   a. Has no complaints of pain
   b. Has periods of uninterrupted sleep
   c. Actively participates in exercise program
   d. Ambulates with crutches and/or prosthesis
2. Has minimal postoperative complications
   a. Remains afebrile
   b. Has clear breath sounds
   c. Shows no evidence of thrombophlebitis or pulmonary emboli
   d. Has a healing stump incision
   e. Maintains optimal state of nutrition
3. Demonstrates rehabilitation and indnependence
   a. Actively participates in exercise program
   b. Ambulates with crutches and/or prosthesis
   c. Participates in activities of daily living
4. Adheres to and his minimal complications from chemotherapy
   a. Takes prescribed medications
   b. Keeps appointments with physician
   c. Anticipates side-effects of chemotherapy
   d. Copes with alterations in physical appearance and energy level

References

1. Adjemiar L: Scoliosis surgery. ONAJ 5:9, 1978
2. Allard JL, Dibble SL: Scoliosis surgery. A look at lugue rods. Am J Nurs 5:609, 1984
3. Anderson: Treat with bracing. Am J Nurs 9:1592, 1979
4. Barry HC: Orthopedic aspects of Paget's disease of bone. Arthritis Rheum 32(10):1128, 1980
5. Breur K et al: Prophylactic irradiation of the lungs to prevent development of pulmonary metastases in patients with osteosarcoma of the limbs. In: Sarcomas of Soft Tissue and Bone in Childhood. National Cancer Institute Monograph 56, 1981
6. Brunner LS, Suddarth DS: Textbook of Medical Surgical Nursing, 5th ed. Philadelphia, JB Lippincott, 1984
7. Cawley MI: Complications of Paget's disease of the bone. Gerontology 29(4):276, 1983
8. Cortes EP, Holland JF: Adjuvant chemotherapy for primary osteogenic sarcoma. Surg Clin North Am 6:1391, 1981
9. Farrel J: Illustrated Guide to Orthopedic Nursing, 2nd ed. Philadelphia, JB Lippincott, 1982
10. Frame B, Pargitt AM: Osteomalacia, current concepts. Ann Intern Med 89:966, 1978
11. Francis MJD, Smith R: Evidence of a generalized connective tissue defect in Paget's disease of the bone. Lancet 1:841, 1974
12. Giansiracusa DL, Kantrowitz FG: Rheumatic and Metabolic Bone Diseases in the Elderly. Lexington, The Collamore Press, 1982
13. Goorin AM et al: Adjuvant chemotherapy for osteosarcoma, a decade of experience. Surg Clin North Am 61(6):1379, 1981

14. Gordon G, Vaugh C: Osteoporosis: Early detection, prevention, and treatment. Consultant 21(1):64, 1980
15. Hardman M: Multiple myeloma, suppressing the problem. Nursing Mirror 154(10):47, 1982
16. Haussler MR, McCain TA: Basic and clinical concepts related to Vitamin D metabolism and actions. N Engl J Med 297:974, 1977
17. Hays K, Rafferty DC: Care of the patient with malignant lymphoma. Nurs Clin North Am 17(4):689, 1982
18. Kissane JM et al: Sarcomas of bone in childhood: Pathologic aspects. In: Sarcomas of Soft Tissue and Bone in Childhood. National Cancer Institute Monograph 56, 1981
19. Lane JM, Vigorita VJ: Current concepts, osteoporosis. J Bone Joint Surg 65A(2):274, 1983
20. Leventhal BG: Immunotherapy of sarcomas. In: Sarcomas of Soft Tissue and Bone in Childhood. National Cancer Institute Monograph 56, 1981
21. Levitt DZ: Multiple myeloma. Am J Nurs 81(7):1345, 1981
22. Marcove RC, Rosen G: En bloc resections for osteogenic sarcoma. In: Sarcomas of Soft Tissue and Bone in Childhood. National Cancer Institute Monograph 56, 1981
23. McIntyre OR: Current concepts in cancer, multiple myeloma. N Engl J Med 301(4):193, 1979
24. Mills BG, Singer FR: Nuclear inclusions in Paget's disease of bone. Science 194:201, 1976
25. Monk GJE: Orthopaedics for Undergraduates, 2nd ed. Oxford, Oxford University Press, 1981
26. Rassmussen H, Bordier P: The Physiological and Cellular Basis of Metabolic Disease. Baltimore, Williams Wilkins, 1974
27. Singer FR: Paget's Disease of Bone. New York, Plenum Medical, 1977
28. Skillman TG: Can osteoporosis be prevented? Geriatrics 35(2):95, 1980

Bibliography

Altman RD: Paget's disease. In Talbott JH (ed): Clinical Rheumatology, 2nd ed. New York, Elsevier Science, 1981

Barry HC: Orthopedic aspects of Paget's disease of bone. Arthritis Rheum 23(10):1128, 1980

Breur K, Schweisguth O, Cohen P et al: Prophylactic irradiation of the lungs to prevent development of pulmonary metastases in patients with osteosarcoma of the limbs. Surg Clin North Am 61(6):1371, 1981

Buckness E: Scoliosis, the curve that made Teri taller. Nursing Mirror 1219:34, 1979

Burnside IM: Nursing and the Aged. New York, McGraw-Hill, 1976

Eiber F: Adjuvant treatment of osteosarcoma. Surg Clin North Am 61(6):1371, 1981

Exton-Smith NA: Metabolic bone disease. In Wright V (ed): Bone and Joint Disease in the Elderly. New York, Churchill Livingston, 1983

Gilchristi GS, Pritchard DJ, Dahlin DC et al: Management of osteogenic sarcoma: A perspective based on the Mayo Clinic experience. Surg Clin North Am 61(6):1371, 1981

Kissane JM, Askin FB, Nesbit ME et al: Sarcomas of Bone in Childhood: Pathologic aspects. In: Sarcomas of Soft Tissue and Bone in Childhood. National Cancer Institute Monograph 56, 1981

Kudelka M: Breaking news on osteoporosis. AJN 84(6):708, 1984

Lane JM, Vigorita UJ: Osteoporosis. Current Concepts Review 65A(2):274, 1983

McFadden EA, Zaloga GP: Calcium regulation. Critical Care Quarterly 6(3):12, 1983

Nordin: Osteoporosis. In Wright V: Bone and Joint Disease in the Elderly. New York, Churchill Livingston, 1983

Price SA, Wilson LM: Pathophysiology: Clinical Concepts of Disease Processes, 2nd ed. New York, McGraw-Hill, 1982

Richards M: Osteoporosis. Geriatric Nursing 3(2):98, 1982

Rosen G, Niren A, Caparros B et al: Osteogenic sarcoma: Eighty-percent, three-year, disease-free survival with combination chemotherapy. In: Sarcomas of Soft Tissue and Bone in Childhood. National Cancer Institute Monograph 56, 1981

Taylor HC, Teitelbaum SL, Langert PW: Symptomatic osteomalacia after jejunoileal bypass surgery in a patient with primary hyperparathyroidism. Gastroenterology 85(3):735, 1983

Tilkian SM, Conover MB, Tilkian AG: Clinical Implications of Laboratory Tests, 3rd ed. St Louis, CV Mosby, 1983

Tucker SM, Breeding MA, Canobbio MA et al: Patient Care Standards, 2nd ed. St Louis, CV Mosby, 1980

UNIT XI

Nursing Care of Patients with Alterations in Integument Function

Chapter 91

Review of Anatomy and Physiology

Integument System

Barbara R. Landau

Function of the Skin

The integument is made up of skin and the structures derived from it. Skin covers the external surface of the body and is continuous with the mucous membranes that line the internal surfaces of the digestive, respiratory, and urogenital systems. Skin is similar to mucous membranes in many respects; both consist of a surface epithelial layer and an undelying connective tissue layer. The chief difference is the layer of keratinized material on the skin surface, but skin structure is also adapted in many other ways to serve its special functions.

The most obvious function of the skin is to protect the cells and their internal environment from hazards of the external environment. Skin is able to withstand mechanical forces such as pressure and frictional abrasion, it limits loss of fluid to the external environment, and it provides a barrier to the invasion of microorganisms. It also protects against, or at least minimizes, the effects of chemical, osmotic, and thermal stresses, and of ultraviolet radiation from the sun. Skin is also important in the formation of vitamin D; it contains a precursor which the ultraviolet rays convert to a more active form. Skin makes several important contributions to the regulation of body temperature. Cutaneous vessels control heat loss by regulating the volume of warm blood, and hence the amount of heat, brought to the surface. Secretion by the sweat glands may increase heat loss. Fat in the skin and subcutaneous tissue provides insulation. Finally, skin is one of the most important sense organs we have. Numerous sensory receptors provide information about the environment at the body surface. Pain receptors are the first to come to mind, but all of the sensory receptors contribute to the protective function of skin. Temperature receptors provide information about environmental temperature needed by the temperature-regulating centers. Touch and pressure receptors provide proprioceptive input as well as general sensory information to the central nervous system.

Skin Structure

The skin consists of the epidermis and the dermis or corium (Fig. 91–1). Epidermis is the surface epithelium and is of ectodermal origin. It rests upon the dermis, a rather dense connective tissue layer of mesodermal origin. Beneath the skin is a layer of loose connective tissue, the subcutaneous tissue, or hypodermis. It is not actually part of the skin, but is intimately associated with it functionally.

Blood vessels and lymphatics are totally absent from the epidermis; they are located in the dermis and underlying

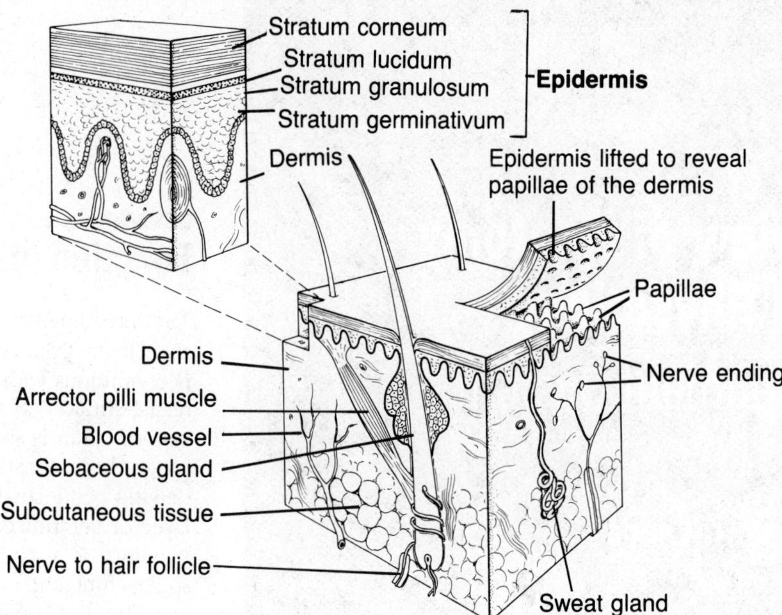

FIGURE 91–1 Structure of the skin.

subcutaneous tissue. Nerve endings, however, are found in both dermis and epidermis. Those in the epidermis are mainly bare nerve endings. The dermis contains both bare nerve endings and more specialized encapsulated endings, as well as motor fibers to blood vessels, the arrector pili muscles, and sweat glands.

There are several important derivatives or appendages of skin—the nails, hair and hair follicles, sebaceous glands, and sweat glands. They are all of epidermal origin, but are located mainly in the dermis or even the subcutaneous tissue.

Epidermis

The external surface of the epidermis is marked by various types of ridges. There are tension lines which seemingly run at random and mark the skin surface into small polygonal areas. The lines are usually quite faint and are most apparent in hairy skin, as on the dorsum of the hand or forearm. Flexure lines are found in the skin over joints, such as the interphalangeal joints and the palm of the hand. Perhaps the most distinctive makings are the parallel ridges and grooves on the palmar surface of the hand and fingers and the soles of the feet. They are sometimes called *friction ridges* because their presence on the gripping surface improves the ability to grasp and manipulate objects with the hands, or to get a good "footing" for locomotion. The patterns of loops, whorls, and arches formed by the ridges begin to appear about the thirteenth week of intrauterine life and maintain the same pattern throughout life. Because they are unique to each individual, fingerprints, palmprints, and footprints can be used for indentification.

Skin is sometimes described as thin or thick, the difference being largely due to characteristics of the epidermis rather than the whole skin. Thin or hairy skin covers most of the body surface. In addition to hairs and hair follicles, it has sebaceous glands and sweat glands. Thick skin is found on the soles of the feet and palms of the hand and flexor surfaces of the digits. It lacks hairs and hair follicles and sebaceous glands, but has sweat glands.

Structure of Epidermis

Epithelial cells of the epidermis have a high regenerative capacity; the entire layer is replaced about every 15 to 30 days, depending upon its location. Mitosis occurs in the deepest layers, and the cells are gradually displaced toward the surface as a result of subsequent mitoses. The cells undergo marked changes as they are pushed upward and farther from the blood vessels which bring needed sustenance. On the basis of these changes, five layers have been identifid in the epidermis. They are usually described in thick skin where they are more apparent.

1. *Stratum germinativum* or basal layer is the deepest layer. Mitoses occur most frequently in this layer, but are not limited to it. The basal cells are cuboidal or columnar in shape and are separated from the dermis by a rather thick basal lamina which provides for cohesion between epithelial cells and underlying tissues.
2. *Stratum spinosum* is sometimes called the "prickle cell" layer because of the appearance of its cells. As the cells are displaced toward the surface, they become somewhat flattened and elongated, with their long axis parallel to the skin surface. Numerous cytoplasmic extensions, or "spines," protrude from the cell surfaces to meet those from adjacent cells, and are firmly bound to them by desmosomes.

3. *Stratum granulosum* or granular layer consists of several layers of cells characterized by the presence of cytoplasmic granules which contain keratohyaline, a precursor to keratin. The cells become more flattened in this layer, and the cytoplasmic extensions disappear, although the desmosomes and fibrils remain. Sensory nerve endings of the epidermis do not reach beyond this layer.
4. *Stratum lucidum* or clear layer, which is named for the clear or translucent appearance of its cells, can be identified readily only in thick skin. The cells are very flat, and the cell boundaries are less distinct.
5. *Stratum corneum* or horny layer, which is the surface layer, consists of dead cells—the scalelike remnants of cells from which all internal structures have disappeared (except keratin filaments). In deeper portions of the stratum corneum, the cell layers are packed rather densely and adhere to one another tightly, but near the surface they are more loosely packed and less firmly bound. They make up the material that is continually being shed from the skin surface. In thick skin, especially of the sole of the foot, the stratum corneum may be as thick as all the other layers combined, but in the thin skin of more protected areas it is only a few layers thick.

Skin Color and Melanin

Skin color depends upon the presence of three pigments, melanin, carotene, and hemoglobin. The effect of the hemoglobin depends upon the volume of blood flowing through the cutaneous vessels, the hemoglobin content of the blood, and whether it is in the oxy- or deoxy- form. Because the epidermis is avascular, the hemoglobin is in the dermis. A yellow pigment, carotene, is present in the stratum corneum and also in adipose cells of the subcutaneous tissue.

Melanin, the most important pigment of the skin, exists as dark brown granules produced by melanocytes. These cells are located between the basal cells in the deepest layer of the epidermis, and also around the base of hair follicles. Newly synthesized melanin accumulates as granules which migrate along the melanocyte processes and are eventually transferred to the epithelial cells ("injected" into them) where they remain. Melanin, therefore, is produced in melanocytes but stored in the epithelial cells.

Ultraviolet light from the sun initially increases the migration and distribution of melanin granules, and later increases the production of melanin leading to tanning of the skin. In humans, melanocyte-stimulating hormone (MSH) from the intermediate lobe of the pituitary gland is not secreted as a separate hormone, but its amino acid sequence is part of the adrenocorticotropic hormone (ACTH) molecule, and ACTH increases melanin production. In adrenal insufficiency there is typically increased ACTH production (due to reduced negative feedback of corticoids) and increased skin pigmentation.

Members of dark-skinned races have about the same number of melanocytes as those with light skin, but their melanocytes have more and larger melanin granules. Albinism is the result of an absence of melanin. It may occur in any race and is usually due to a genetic disorder in which one or more of the enzymes needed for melanin synthesis is missing.

Dermis

Beneath the epidermis is the dermis or corium, a layer of dense connective tissue with its numerous collagenous, elastic, and reticular fibers (Fig. 91–2). It is thickest (about 3 mm) in the palms and soles, and thinnest on the eyelid and penis where it may be only 0.5 mm thick.

The superficial or papillary layer of dermis lies in the valleys between the epidermal ridges and forms the dermal papillae. The thicker reticular layer is beneath it. Capillary loops extend up into the papillae to supply the metabolically active cells of the epidermis (primarily the basal cells). There are numerous sensory nerve endings in the dermal papillae, primarily encapsulated endings believed to be associated with touch and temperature, and also some bare nerve endings (pain).

The reticular layer is a denser connective tissue (in spite of the name). Numerous bundles of collagen fibers tend to be oriented longitudinally in the extremities and transversely in the trunk, forming what are sometimes known as *cleavage lines.* Stretching the skin by rapid growth, as by a tumor or pregnancy, may partially rupture some collagen fibers and result in scar formation.

As a person ages, collagenous fibers develop more cross-linkages and become more stable and less flexible. Elastic fibers also develop cross-linkages and may fray with continued stress, while reticular fibers tend to be replaced by collagenous fibers. The density of the ground substance increases as its fluid content falls. As a result, aging skin loses its elasticity and resiliency, and wrinkles begin to form.

Sweat glands and sebaceous glands lie in the reticular layer, and the base of most hair follicles is in its deeper part. The arrector pili muscles are small bundles of smooth muscle fibers that arise in the papillary layer of the dermis and insert on the shaft of hair follicles. In some locations, skeletal muscle fibers, such as the muscles of facial expression, insert in the dermis.

Subcutaneous Tissue

The skin is attached to underlying structures by a layer of loose connective tissue known as subcutaneous tissue. Its fibers are continuous superficially with those of the dermis (Fig. 91–2) and below with those of the deep fascia surrounding skeletal muscle, or the periosteum or perichondrium of skeletal elements. There are fewer fibers in regions where the skin is loosely attached (more freely movable), but fibers are more abundant and heavier in regions such as the palms and soles. Subcutaneous tissue contains numerous fat cells and fat deposits, which in some areas of the body may reach a thickness of 3 cm or more. The eyelids, penis, and scrotum, however, are devoid of adipose cells and fat deposits. In infants and young people this layer, the panniculus adiposus,

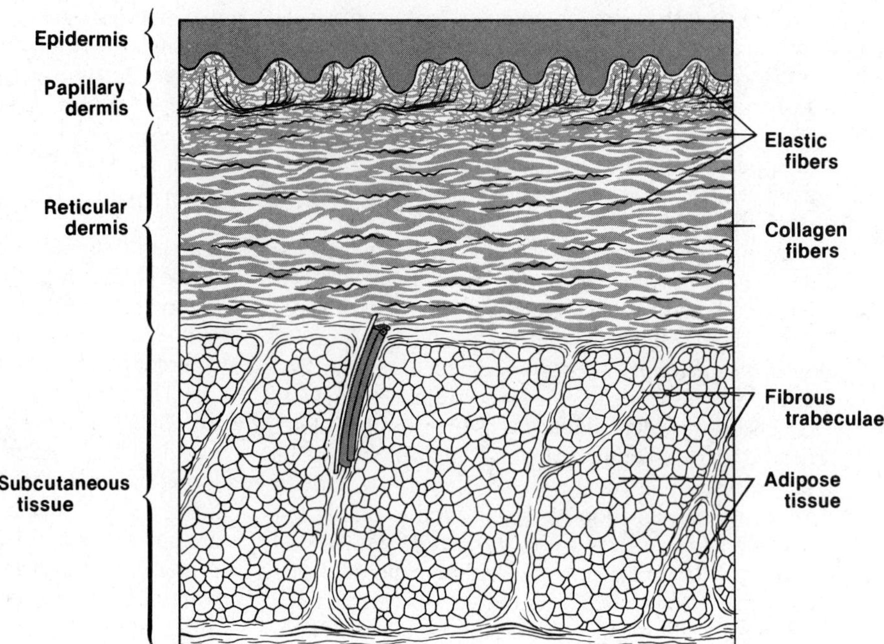

FIGURE 91–2 The dermis. (Dobson RL, Abele DC: The Practice of Dematology, p 8. Philadelphia, JB Lippincott, 1985)

is rather uniform over the entire body surface, but in adults it becomes thinner in some areas and thicker in others. Its thickness and distribution vary with the sex of the person and other factors.

Blood Vessels and Nerves

Arteries enter the subcutaneous tissue from deeper regions and form a plexus along the junction with the dermis. Deep branches from this plexus supply subcutaneous tissues including fat cells, and superficial branches supply sweat glands and the base of deeper hair follicles. The more superficial branches also form a plexus along the junction of the papillary and reticular layers of the dermis. The capillary loops found in each dermal papilla arise from this plexus, as do branches to more superficial parts of hair follicles, and sebaceous glands. The capillaries drain into venules which lead into venous plexuses at several levels and then into veins in the subcutaneous tissue. There are also numerous arteriovenous anastomoses, which can be opened to greatly increase cutaneous blood flow—an important aspect of temperature regulation. Atrophy of the capillary loops and superficial capillary networks occurs with aging, which not only reduces the blood supply for epithelial cells but also reduces the effectiveness of the cutaneous blood flow in regulating heat loss from the skin.

The skin and related structures serve an important sensory role; the many and varied sense organs monitor conditions in the external environment. The cutaneous nerves run with larger blood vessels in the subcutaneous tissue and send branches to nerve plexuses at several layers in the dermis. Nerve fibers from these plexuses supply the dermis and epidermis, as well as the subcutaneous tissue. There are numerous sensory receptors that respond to pain, touch, hot, cold, and pressure. Bare nerve endings, usually associated with pain, penetrate the deeper layers of the epidermis.

There are also a number of motor fibers; they are autonomic sympathetic fibers that innervate smooth muscle of the blood vessels and arrector pili muscles, and secretory cells of the sweat glands. (*Note:* there are no parasympathetic fibers in skin.)

Appendages of the Skin

Nails

The dorsal surface of distal phalanges of the fingers and toes has a tough horny cover, the nail plate. Keratin in the nail plate has a high sulfur content, which may explain its toughness and resistance to chemicals. The nail plate rests on the epithelium of the nail bed, which consists of only the deeper layers of the epidermis (germinativum and spinosum).

The nail plate is translucent and its pink coloring is due to the numerous blood vessels in the nail bed underneath. Slight pressure on the free edge of the nail causes the area to blanch as blood is forced from these vessels. A delayed return of color after the release of pressure may indicate low blood pressure or cutaneous vasoconstriction. The whitened crescent at the proximal end of the nail is the lunula. Its significance is unknown, but it may result from reduced vascularity of the underlying portion of the nail bed (which contains the actively proliferating epithelium).

Hair

Hairs grow from hair follicles which are found in all skin except the thick skin of the soles and palms and a few other sites such as the lips and areas of urogenital openings. The abundance and characteristics of the hair vary with the age, sex, race, and genetic makeup of the individual, as well as the part of the body. Most hair is quite fine, but that of eyelashes and eyebrows is coarse, and at puberty coarse hairs appear in the pubic and axillary areas. In postpubertal males the beard becomes quite coarse, and body hair in other areas also becomes somewhat coarser. Hairs do not grow continuously; growth periods of variable length are followed by shorter periods of inactivity. On the scalp periods of growth last several years and inactive periods last for 2 or 3 months. Growth cycles are not synchronized, but occur in a mosaic pattern in different parts of the body.

Hair color is determined by the pigment produced by melanocytes which are present among the epidermal cells of the matrix. They are larger than melanocytes of the surface epithelium, but like them, produce melanin granules which are transferred to the newly formed cells in the bulb of the hair. Melanin granules are especially abundant in the cells that will become the cortex of the hair. Slight differences in the chemical composition of the melanin cause subtle variations in hair color. Absence of pigment leaves silvery white hair, and gray hair is a mixture of white and pigmented hair.

Hair follicles usually lie at an angle to the skin surface. An arrector pili muscle lies on the side toward which the hair slopes (Fig. 91–1). Each is a small bundle of smooth muscle fibers which arise in the papillary region of the dermis and attach to the sheath of the hair follicle. Their contraction, which is caused by sympathetic stimulation, pulls the hair into a more perpendicular position. In furred animals, piloerection improves the insulating qualities of the fur because more air is trapped between the hairs, and it is also part of the generalized sympathetic discharge associated with the response to anger or fear. In humans, a similar response occurs, but the result is not improved insulation, only the characteristic pimpling of the skin known as "gooseflesh" caused by movement of the hair. Sensory nerve endings that surround hair follicles are stimulated by movement of the hair. They are very sensitive; the movement of a single hair on the back of the hand can be detected.

Sebaceous Glands

Sebaceous glands are found over the entire skin surface, except the thick skin of the palms and soles. In hairy skin they are associated with hair follicles and secrete into them. In some areas (lips) the ducts may open directly on the skin surface. Sebaceous glands are more numerous and larger on the face and scalp.

The oily secretion of sebaceous glands known as sebum is made up of lipid material plus the debris of disrupted cells. It is released from the short ducts into hair follicles alongside the hairs, and slowly works its way to the skin surface. Lipolysis, with the formation of fatty acids, may occur in hair follicles. Sebaceous glands, which secrete more or less continuously, are not under neural control but are stimulated by hormones. The larger glands of the face and scalp are particularly sensitive to androgens from the testis in males and from the adrenal cortex and ovary in females. Disturbances in the secretion and flow of sebum are major factors in development of acne. Comedones (blackheads) result if the material hardens in the ducts. In elderly persons the sebaceous glands may atrophy. Sebum does, however, have some weak bacteriocidal and fungicidal actions.

Sweat Glands

Sweat glands are distributed over almost the entire skin surface, except the glans penis and margins of the lips. Two types of sweat glands are identified; eccrine glands are the typical sweat glands and are widely distributed, especially on the palms and soles; apocrine glands are larger and found in limited areas, chiefly the axillary region.

The product of the eccrine secretory cells resembles an untrafiltrate of plasma. It contains sodium, potassium, urea, lactate, and ammonia, among other things. The fluid that reaches the skin surface, however, is a hypotonic solution. This is possible because there is an active transport mechanism, a sodium pump, in the cells of the secretory duct. These cells actively remove sodium from the lumen of the duct, resulting in the hypotonic fluid.

The sweat glands are stimulated by sympathetic fibers, but they are cholinergic. Sweat glands are important in temperature regulation; evaporation of sweat from the skin surface has a powerful cooling effect, so it is not surprising that there is neural input from the heat loss centers in the hypothalamus. Persons with congenital absence of sweat glands (or malfunction due to disease) have difficulty in dissipating heat and are prone to heat stroke. Sweat secretion may also be elicited by nonthermal stimuli of sympathetic origin. Fear and anxiety result in sweating which appears initially in the palms and soles, and then in other areas—the so-called cold sweat.

The apocrine sweat glands are found mainly in the axilla. They are much larger than eccrine sweat glands and in most cases their secretory ducts open into the canal of a hair follicle rather than on the skin surface, and their secretion is more viscous and contains more protein. They receive an adrenergic sympathetic innervation; secretion is increased by stressful stimuli such as fright or pain, but not by heat. Apocrine sweat glands are more dependent upon sex hormones; they appear and begin to function at the time of puberty, and in females secretion varies with the menstrual cycle. When secreted, apocrine sweat is odorless, but upon exposure to the ever-present cutaneous bacteria, it acquires a characteristic odor. This is considered undesirable in our society and much effort and expense goes into preventing (or masking) it. For many animals, however, the secretions of these glands provide important means of recognition, sexual attraction, or territorial marking.

Bibliography

Bloom W, Fawcett DW: A Textbook of Histology, 10th ed. chap 23, pp 563–597. Philadelphia, WB Saunders, 1975

Crouch JE: Functional Human Anatomy, 3rd ed. chap 6, pp 72–82. Philadelphia, Lea & Febiger, 1978

Junqueira LC, Carneiro J: Basic Histology, 4th ed. chap 19. Los Altos, CA, Lange Medical Publications, 1984

Landau BR: Essential Human Anatomy and Physiology, 2nd ed. pp 66–74. Glenview, IL, Scott, Foresman and Company, 1980

Leeson TS, Leeson CR: Histology, 4th ed. chap 10, pp 308–327. Philadelphia, WB Saunders, 1981

Warwick R, Williams PL: Gray's Anatomy, 35th British ed. pp 1159–1169. Philadelphia, WB Saunders, 1973

Chapter 92

Assessment of Integument Function

Susan Pfister
Pauline M. Bruno

The two main components of assessing the skin are the same as those for assessing other organ systems: a comprehensive history for background information, followed by hands-on physical examination. A third component, psychosocial assessment, is included for this particular system because of the impact alterations in physical appearance can have on a person in modern society.

History

Integumentary assessment begins with the patient's family history. Information should be elicited concerning skin disorder tendencies and the occurrence of systemic metabolic diseases because such disorders may be manifested by skin eruptions or color changes (*e.g.,* the frequent skin infections and the dry, itchy, atrophic skin seen in diabetes mellitus). The family's cultural beliefs, religious and ethnic practices that could affect health behaviors and influence the condition of the skin should be included.

An overall picture of the patient's past and current health provides a basis from which specific needs and problems can be identified. Those factors influencing the patient's general health include occupation, lifestyle behaviors and social habits, dietary considerations, usual patterns of skin care, use of pharmacologic agents, and the presence of acute or chronic disease, especially collagen, renal, or hepatic disease. The occurrence of any past skin abnormalities should be discussed plus any known allergic reactions—food, drug, contact. Exposure to chemicals, solvents, or radiation should be explored, and any major physical trauma or surgery should be documented. Recent changes in any of the aforementioned areas are important to note.

The patient's description of his or her current state of health may give clues to the presence of a dermatologic condition. For example, the patient with a skin disorder may present only with symptoms of pain or pruritus.[5] The patient should then be questioned regarding any change in the texture or color of the skin including the genital region, appearance of any rash (even if transient), any change in hair, nails, or oral mucous membranes. If a rash, lesion, or other skin change is present, information concerning the pattern of onset, appearance, location, duration, and presence of any exudate should be obtained.

Physical Assessment

Two main tools are used in physical assessment of the integumentary system; inspection and palpation. Both tools are used in two phases. The first phase involves looking at the skin for its overall condition—color, texture, moisture, turgor, and temperature. The second phase consists of more detailed examination of specific skin abnormalities (*e.g.,* lesions, rashes, hematomas). Both of these phases will be discussed in more detail. It is important to include examination of the hair, nails, mucous membranes of the mouth, intertriginous areas (skin folds), and the skin surrounding the genital and anal regions.

General Condition of the Integument

The overall skin color should be observed prior to further assessment. Possible variations in color tone are bronze, brown, yellow, red or ruddy hues, pallor, and cyanosis. A blue, cyanotic color results from decreased oxygenation of tissues and may be seen in cardiopulmonary disorders such as congestive heart failure. A yellow cast localized in the sclera or generalized in the skin may indicate liver disease such as hepatitis. The decreased color or pallor seen in anemia and shock results from an altered amount or distribution of oxyhemoglobin. For an overview of skin color variations and their causative factors see Table 92–1.

Patients with skin of natural pigmentation other than the shades commonly labeled as white may be more difficult to assess in this area. The tongue, lips, nail beds, and buccal mucosa are less pigmented areas and as such may be the best indicators of potential pallor or cyanosis. Keep in mind that the ambient temperature and the patient's emotional status may mask color changes or create temporary but misleading changes.

The status of the blood supply to the skin should be assessed with notation of any bleeding or ecchymosis. The presence of multiple ecchymotic areas could be indicative of blood-clotting deficiencies. The moisture content of the skin as evidenced by external dryness, clamminess (sweat), or oiliness is important to note, as is the presence of edema. Edema results in taut, smooth, shiny skin over the affected area. It is most evident over bony prominences and in dependent areas (*i.e.,* the sacral area, pedal area, and lower extremities).

Skin turgor (elasticity) is one indicator of the patient's degree of total body hydration. The mobility and turgor of the skin can be measured by lightly pinching a fold of skin and observing the time it takes to return to its original position (Fig. 92–1). Loss of turgor is indicated by persistence of the skin fold for a time after pinching and may be present in dehydration, senile cutaneous atrophy, or rapid loss of body tissue in weight reduction. The best location for testing skin turgor is over the sternum where subcutaneous tissue is minimal.

The temperature of the skin (cool, warm, hot) should be noted. This can be addressed more accurately if the skin is touched by the back of the examiner's fingers. Additional factors to assess include texture and thickness of the skin which reflect age, environmental exposure, and trauma. The presence of any skin lesions or other abnormalities should be noted. Skin lesions are described in the following section.

Fingernails and toenails should be inspected and palpated for their color, shape, consistency (brittle), and the presence of any lesions. The hair should also be examined for its appearance (dull or shiny), quantity, texture, and distribution. Integumentary changes that occur in conjunction with specific disease states are covered in those chapters which focus on the major system involved (*i.e.,* clubbing of the fingers, in the respiratory and cardiovascular assessment chapters, 26 and 34).

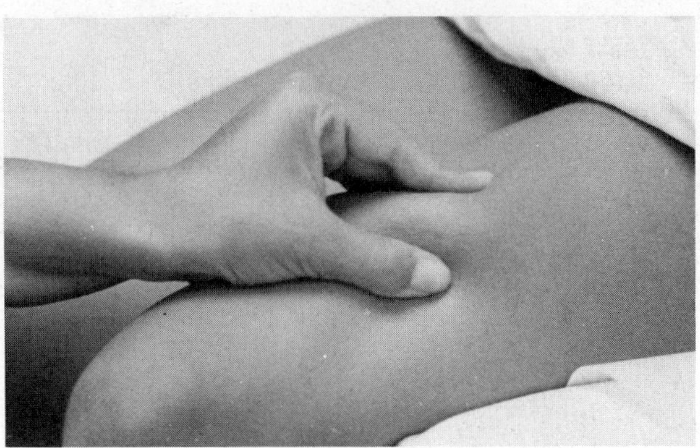

FIGURE 92–1 Testing skin turgor.

Specific Alterations of the Integument

There are four major observations to be made when assessing any type of skin lesion or disorder:

1. Color of the lesion or affected area
2. Anatomic distribution of the lesion or rash
3. Configuration of groups of lesions
4. Morphology of individual lesions.

When inspecting a lesion, it is important to describe the brightness of a lesion's color as well as the color itself. The distribution of a skin disorder could be localized, bandlike, generalized, involving intertriginous areas, or involving exposed surfaces. Groups of lesions may be clustered, annular, linear, or irregular with no distinct pattern. The size of the individual lesion or the skin area covered by a disorder should be recorded using metric measurements.

Skin Lesions and Altered Skin Integrity

Individual lesions may be generally categorized as primary or secondary. Primary lesions are those disorders arising from previously normal skin and include maculae, papules, nodules, tumors, polyps, wheals, blisters, cysts, pustules, and abscesses. Secondary lesions are changes that appear following a primary lesion (*e.g.,* formation of scar tissue or crusts from dried burn vesicles).[1] Primary lesions may be further described as nonelevated, elevated-solid, or fluid-filled elevations. A basic description and illustration of the major primary and secondary lesions can be found in Table 92–2.

Urticaria, an inflammatory skin condition, is characterized by the eruption of pale papules or wheals which are associated with severe itching. This disorder usually results from contact with external irritants such as foods, insect bites, pollens, or drugs. Drug reactions may also manifest as

(*Text continues on page 1382*)

TABLE 92–1
Skin Color Variations and Causative Factors

Color	*Process*	*Causative Factors*	*Typical Localization*
Brown	Deposition of melanin	Genetic	Generalized
		Sunlight	Exposed area
		Pregnancy	Face, nipples, areolae, linea nigra, vulva
		Addison's disease	Exposed area, points of pressure and friction, nipples, genitalia, palmar creases, recent scars; often generalized
Grayish tan, bronze, or grayish blue	Deposition of melanin and hemosiderin	Hemochromatosis	Exposed areas, genitalia, and scars; often generalized
Blue (cyanosis)	Increased amount of reduced hemoglobin secondary to hypoxia		
	▪ Peripheral	Anxiety or cold environment	Nails; sometimes lips
	▪ Central (arterial)	Heart or lung disease	Lips, mouth, and nails
Reddish blue	Combination of increase in total amount of hemoglobin, increase in reduced hemoglobin and capillary stasis	Polycythemia	Face, conjunctiva, mouth, hands, feet
Red (Erythema)	Increased visibility of normal oxyhemoglobin:		
	▪ Dilatation or increased numbers of superficial blood vessels or increased blood flow	Fever, blushing, alcohol intake, local inflammation	Face and upper chest or local area of inflammation
	▪ Decreased oxygen utilization in the skin	Cold exposure	The cold area (*e.g.*, ears)
Yellow			
Jaundice	Increased bilirubin levels	Liver disease, red blood cell hemolysis	First in sclera, then mucous membranes and generalized
Chronic uremia	Retention of urinary chromogens, superimposed on the pallor of anemia	Chronic renal disease	Most evident in exposed areas, may be generalized; does not involve sclera or mucous membranes
Decreased color			
Depigmentation	Decreased melanin	Albinism	Generalized lack of pigment in skin, hair, eyes
		Vitiligo	Patchy, symmetrical, often involving the exposed areas
Pallor	Decreased visibility of oxyhemoglobin:		
	▪ Decreased blood flow in superficial vessels	Syncope, shock, some normal variations	Most evident in face, conjunctiva, mouth, nails
	▪ Decreased amount of oxyhemoglobin	Anemia	Most evident in face, conjunctiva, mouth, nails

(Modified from Bates B: A Guide to Physical Examination, 3rd ed. Philadelphia, JB Lippincott, 1983)

TABLE 92–2
Basic Types of Skin Lesions

Primary Lesions (May Arise from Previously Normal Skin)

Circumscribed, Flat, Nonpalpable Changes in Skin Color

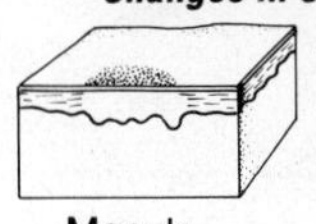
Macule

Macule—Small, up to 1 cm.*
Example: freckle, petechia

Patch—Larger than 1 cm.
Example: vitiligo

Palpable Elevated Solid Masses

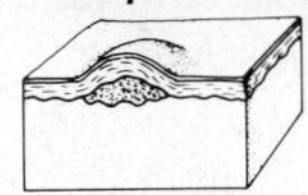
Papule

Papule—Up to 0.5 cm.
Example: an elevated nevus

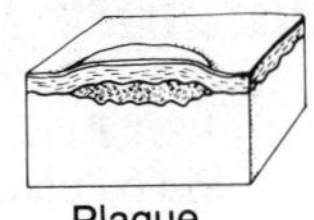
Plaque

Plaque—A flat, elevated surface larger than 0.5 cm, often formed by the coalescence of papules

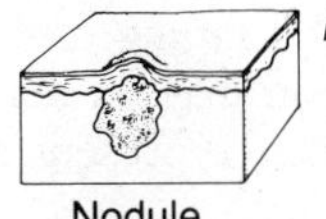
Nodule

Nodule—0.5 cm to 2 cm; often deeper and firmer than a papule

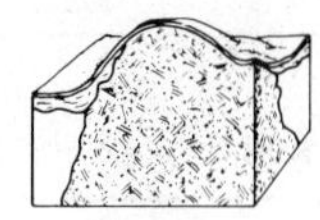
Tumor

Tumor—Larger than 1–2 cm.

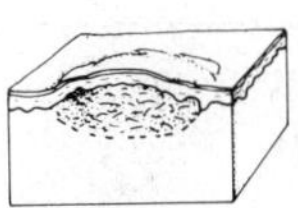
Wheal

Wheal—A slightly irregular, relatively transient, superficial area of localized skin edema.
Example: mosquito bite, hive

Circumscribed Superficial Elevations of the Skin Formed by Free Fluid in a Cavity within the Skin Layers

Vesicle

Vesicle—Up to 0.5 cm; filled with serous fluid.
Example: herpes simplex

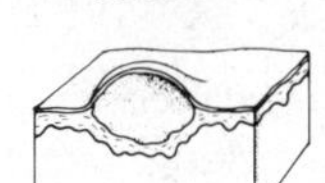
Bulla

Bulla—Greater than 0.5 cm; filled with serous fluid.
Example: 2nd degree burn

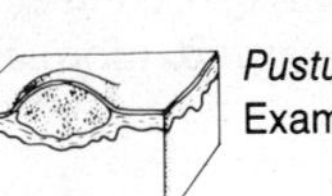
Pustule

Pustule—Filled with pus.
Example: acne, impetigo

Secondary Lesions (Result from Changes in Primary Lesions)

Loss of Skin Surface

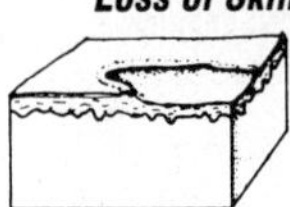
Erosions

Erosion—Loss of the superficial epidermis; surface is moist but does not bleed.
Example: moist area after the rupture of a vesicle, as in chickenpox

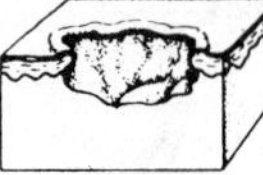
Ulcers

Ulcer—A deeper loss of skin surface; may bleed and scar.
Examples: stasis ulcer of venous insufficiency, syphilitic chancre

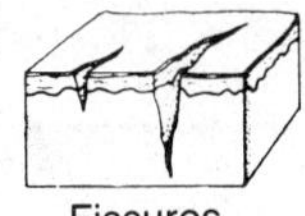
Fissures

Fissure—A linear crack in the skin.
Example: athlete's foot

Material on the Skin Surface

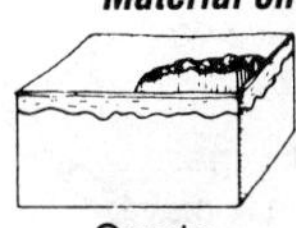
Crusts

Crust—The dried residue of serum, pus, or blood.
Example: impetigo

Scales

Scale—A thin flake of exfoliated epidermis.
Examples: dandruff, dry skin, psoriasis

Miscellaneous

Lichenification—Thickening and roughening of the skin with increased visibility of the normal skin furrows.
Example: atopic dermatitis

Scar—Replacement of destroyed tissue by fibrous tissue

Atrophy—Thinning of the skin with loss of the normal skin furrows; the skin looks shinier and more translucent than normal.
Example: arterial insufficiency

Excoriation—A scratch mark

Keloid—Hypertrophied scar tissue

* Authorities vary somewhat in their definitions of skin lesions by size. Dimensions given in this table should be considered approximate, not rigid.

macular lesions over the shoulders, back, chest, or entire body. Nodules are commonly seen with gout, rheumatoid arthritis, and Hodgkin's disease, and may present as growths in various glands. Basal cell carcinoma is the most common type of skin cancer and presents with papules progressing to ulcers usually located on the face between the hairline and the upper lip. Nevi (moles, birthmarks) are congenital dislocations of a circumscribed area of the skin due to pigmentation and are quite common in occurrence. Certain infectious conditions such as herpes zoster may present with fluid-filled lesions on the skin. Paronychia, an inflammation of the structures in the distal phalanx of the finger, may also occur with some infections.

Other disorders result in breaks of the continuity of the skin described as fissures, cracking, excoriation, and decubitus. Trauma is the major contributing factor to the occurrence of ecchymosis, abrasions, contusions, and hematomas. These conditions are covered more thoroughly in other chapters. Documentation of the above observations related to integumentary assessment is crucial. The use of accurate and precise terminology in describing skin disorders is essential for communication among health-team members. This communication paves the way for accurate medical diagnosis and initiation of appropriate treatment to relieve the disorder.

Laboratory Tests

Once a dermatological problem has been identified, inspected, and palpated, one of several laboratory tests may be indicated to determine the most effective treatment. A superficial scraping of the skin disorder for microscopic examination may be helpful in identifying the type of lesion. If exudate is present, a culture and sensitivity test may be done

TABLE 92–3
Changes of the Integument Caused by Aging

Structure	*Process Involved*	*Observable Change*
Skin*	Loss of sweat and sebaceous glands	Dry, flaky skin
	Altered melanocyte activity	Pallor; mottling and roughness of exposed area; pigment, accumulations on backs of hands, face, genitoanal region.
	Connective tissue/collagen changes	Thin, translucent skin; decreased tissue turgor (resiliency)
	Loss of elasticity	Skin folds and wrinkles—most obvious in exposed surfaces (*e.g.*, face; furrowing)
	Loss of subcutaneous adipose tissue	Furrowing
	Fragility of dermal blood vessels	Purpura, especially on back of hands and on forearms
	Diminished vascular supply	Decrease in rosy appearance of skin and mucous membrane
Nails	General changes	Slowed growth Disappearance of lunula Development of longitudinal ridges
	Overgrowth of horny, keratinized layers	Thickened, brittle nails; toenails may become curved or hooked.
	Deposition of calcium	Dull, yellow nails
Hair	General changes	Loss of hair from scalp, axillary, and pubic areas (loss progresses from periphery inward)
	Facial hair:	
	▪ Decreased estrogen production to oppose androgens	Increased facial hair in women
	▪ General	Increased growth of hair on eyebrows, nostrils, and borders of ears in men
	Decreased melanocyte activity Decreased density of hair follicles	Gray axillary hair: the degree of axillary graying correlates most precisely with age.
	Hereditary factors	Gray scalp hair

* Decreased effectiveness of skin as a thermal insulator, a barrier to microorganism access, and a protector from injury and water loss

to reveal specific organisms which may be susceptible to certain medications. For suspected fungal infections, the diagnosis may be confirmed with either a culture or a microscopic examination utilizing a preparation of potassium hydroxide (KOH).[4] The Wood's light test is helpful in diagnosing scalp infections caused by a particular group of spore-producing microorganisms. The spores, located on hair strands, fluoresce an apple-green under the Wood's light.[6]

Biopsy of skin tissue is indicated for those disorders that manifest changes in color, size, or shape. Nonhealing lesions, abnormal growths, or tumors are also biopsied. Nursing responsibilities include preprocedure discussion with the patient regarding the reason for the biopsy, the procedure involved, and the time required for test results.

Psychosocial Assessment

In addition to history taking and physical assessment, the psychosocial dimension should be explored as a third component of integumentary assessment. A person's appearance, much of which is reflected through the skin, is a major factor in interpersonal relationships, especially when making the initial contact or first impression. Body language and particularly facial expressions are nonverbal means of communication. The skin also serves as a major organ of communication through the act of touching. Touching serves as a psychological tool of acceptance.[3] Depending on the type and extent of skin problem, the person with a skin disorder may be ignored, shunned, or the victim of open stares, looks of disgust, or ridicule. This is due, in part, to America's advertised love affair with youth and beauty. As a result, the person who lives with a dermatological problem may not suffer physical pain but may suffer immeasurable psychological pain.

Emotional reactions which may be experienced by the person with a skin disorder include embarrassment, anxiety, frustration, anger, depression, and rejection. The patient may have feelings of lowered self-esteem plus those of guilt and disgust in relation to his or her own physical appearance. Nursing implications for helping someone deal with these reactions include listening to the patient vent thoughts and feelings. The nurse can show acceptance of the patient through facial expressions, tone of voice, and, perhaps most, through touch. With regard to touch, discussing the fears of family and friends plus the needs of the patient will often clear the way for increased closeness and support among those involved. Touch during the process of physical assessment can set the tone for acceptance by health professionals at the initial patient contact whether in a clinic, physician's office, hospital, or home.

Changes of the Integument Caused by Aging

Throughout the process of assessment of the skin it is important to consider universal changes that take place with age. Although these changes occur in all aging people, the quality and time of onset of the changes are variable among individuals. Environmental exposure, heredity, and degree of skin pigmentation may affect or contribute to the types of changes that occur in the skin, nails, and hair (see Table 92–3). The loss of elasticity and subcutaneous adipose tissue combined with collagen changes results in the common wrinkling and furrowing of aged skin. The weathered appearance and leathery feel of older skin is directly related to years of sun exposure. Nails of the fingers and toes become thickened and brittle due to keratosis. Reduced melanin activity plus hereditary factors contribute to the graying of scalp hair. Increased growth of facial hair may occur in women due to an alteration in the hormonal balance of estrogen and androgen.[2]

In addition to these normal aging changes, certain skin disorders are fairly common in the aged population. The occurrence of these disorders may be related to factors such as lifestyle and physiological aging changes (see Table 92–4). Aging decreases the skin's effectiveness as a barrier to infection. Consequently, the older patient is more susceptible to bacterial, viral, and fungal infections. Once they have achieved access, these organisms are harder to combat due

TABLE 92–4
Alterations in Skin of Elderly Persons

Contributing Factors

1. Decrease in peripheral vascular circulation influencing the response to physical trauma and temperature variation
2. Atrophy of the reticular endothelial system leading to depression of the immune response
3. Malnutrition
4. Life-long exposure to sunlight
5. Exposure to radiation therapy and drugs (chemicals)
6. Genetic predisposition to aging changes
7. Emotional responses to stresses of life
8. Changes in responsiveness of nerve endings to sensory stimuli

Common Alterations

- Alterations in cell growth
  - Thickening of keratinizing cells
  - Benign epidermal tumors
  - Premalignant tumors
  - Malignant tumors
- Infections
  - Bacterial
  - Viral
  - Fungal
- Vascular disturbance
  - Benign vascular tumors
  - Inadequate blood flow—atrophy, stasis dermatitis, ulcerations
- Hypersensitive responses
  - Contact dermatitis

(Modified from Bruno P: Skin problems. In Carnevali DL, Patrick M [eds]: Nursing Management for the Elderly. Philadelphia, JB Lippincott, 1985)

to depression of the aged person's immune system. The depressed immune response plus years of exposure to sun, radiation, drugs, or other chemicals, contribute to those disorders resulting from altered cell growth. Many older people live in a state of chronic malnutrition due to financial constraints or other problems. This poor nutritional status leads to a general debilitated condition which predisposes the older person to disorders of many kinds, including those of the integumentary system.

References

1. Bates B: A Guide to Physical Examination, 3rd ed. Philadelphia, JB Lippincott, 1983
2. Bruno P: Skin problems. In Carnevali DL, Patrick M (eds): Nursing Management for the Elderly, Philadelphia, JB Lipincott, 1985
3. Delaney VL, North C: Skin assessment. Topics in Clinical Nursing 5(2):5–10, 1983
4. Fitzpatrick TB, Polano MK, Suurmond D: Color Atlas and Synopsis of Clinical Dermatology. New York, McGraw-Hill, 1983
5. Hillman RS, Goodell BW, Grundy SM, McArthur JR, Moller JH: Clinical Skills: Interviewing, History Taking, and Physical Diagnosis, New York, McGraw-Hill, 1981
6. Rudolph AH: Surefire ways to treat fungal infections of the skin, scalp, and nails. Modern Medicine, pp 122–141, January 1985

Bibliography

Carnevali DL, Patrick M (eds): Nursing Management for the Elderly, 2nd ed. Philadelphia, JB Lippincott, 1986

DeGowin EL, DeGowin RL: Bedside Diagnostic Examination, 4th ed. New York, Macmillan, 1981

Dossey L: The skin: What is it? Topics in Clinical Nursing 5(2):1–4, 1983

Kenney RA: Physiology of Aging. Chicago, Year Book Medical Publishers, 1982

Porth C, Kapke K: Aging and the skin. Geriatric Nursing 4(3):158–162, 1983

Chapter 93

Nursing Strategies for Common Integument Problems

Nursing Diagnosis Interventions Evaluation

Linda M. Dunn

Nursing care for patients with alterations in the skin focuses on the physiological and psychological responses to the disorder. The skin serves critical physiological functions by supporting and protecting the internal organs and participating in temperature regulation, as well as psychological functions by contributing to outward appearance and formation of self-concept. Nursing identifies individual patient responses and creates strategies to assist the patient in coping and adapting to the impairment.

Potential Impairment of Skin Integrity Related to Positional Trauma (Pressure Sores)

Assessment and Nursing Diagnosis

Positional trauma is a descriptive phrase for excoriations and ulcerations of tissue overlying weight-bearing bony prominences. The terms *pressure sore, bedsore,* and *decubitus ulcer* are also used interchangeably to describe the same phenomenon. Elderly people or those with mobility restrictions are highly susceptible to this condition. Necrosis will result from pressure of sufficient extent and duration to interfere with adequate blood flow, tissue nutrition, and oxygen. There is little consistency from one person to another in the extent and duration of pressure necessary to result in tissue damage.

Whether or not a person will develop positional trauma is influenced by many variables. Individual susceptibility depends on the developmental dynamics explained in the following principles.[1]

Duration and extent of pressure on weight-bearing bony prominences varies with position. The longer the sustained pressure, the greater the danger is of interference with circulation, nutrition, and oxygenation of tissue. Because mean capillary pressure is 25 mmHg, positional pressure readily occludes the microcirculation.

The extent of pressure on ischial tuberosities is greater when a person is sitting in a chair with the feet supported than with the feet hanging free. Distributing the weight along the posterior thighs by allowing the feet to hang free does not focus pressure on one site. The pressure on the sacral area also varies directly with the extent of the elevation of the head of the bed.[4] Persons in semi- or high Fowler's position for cardiovascular/respiratory problems are at increased risk for postural pressure lesions of the sacrum and buttocks.

Shearing forces on sacral tissues vary directly with increasing elevation of the head of the bed.[3] Gravity pull displaces the underlying subcutaneous tissue downward while the outer skin tissues adhere to the bed linen. This uneven tissue shift distorts the anatomy of those blood vessels, causing angulation and interference with circulation.

Extent of pressure varies with body build.[4] The tissues of an obese person disburse the weight over a large surface, whereas weight-bearing pressure is concentrated over the bony prominences of thin persons. However, the blood supply to the subcutaneous tissue of an obese person is not proportionately increased, and overall tissue nutrition and oxygenation may be marginal because the interstitial area for transport of nutrients is greater.[1]

Perception of and response to painful stimuli are decreased in depressed persons and absent in areas of the body that are paralyzed. The stimuli may not be perceived or generate a response. A person capable of self-movement must change position in response to painful stimuli to protect tissues from trauma. Persons such as the comatose, the debilitated, and those who are partially paralyzed, who are incapable of self-movement are prone to postural trauma.

Other factors influence susceptibility to tissue trauma. The presence of systemic disorders, such as infections which increase body temperature, increases the metabolic rate of cells and heat and body fluid losses. Tissues in this situation are less resistant to trauma. Additionally, rough, wrinkled, damp bed linen may contribute to skin maceration and irritation. Dampness may result from the heat of plastic draw sheets or from incontinence.

Interventions

The goals for nursing management of the patient with positional tissue trauma are to prevent the formation or extension of pressure-damaged tissue, to maintain adequate nutrition and fluid intake, and to relieve discomfort associated with the tissue damage.

Detection of increased susceptibility to positional tissue trauma is a nursing responsibility. Daily assessment for changes in mobility, emotional status, nutritional intake, general health, and condition of bed linen should provide data necessary for making judgments about susceptibility.[1]

Preventive measures should be initiated promptly for those who are at risk for positional tissue trauma. The type of measure selected will vary with the situation and potential for trauma. Sheepskin, an alternating pressure mattress, or perhaps a gel pad under the buttocks area and an hourly turn schedule are examples of nursing interventions which may be employed. The turn schedule should use all positions possible before returning to the initial position, thus avoiding the cumulative effects from sustained pressure.[1]

The incidence of trauma to tissues over weight-bearing bony prominences remains high.[2] At the present time, no one method appears to promote healing of superficial lesions to an extent greater than other methods, even though the literature is replete with suggestions for therapy. Keeping the area clean, exposing it to the drying effects of air, and avoiding additional pressure trauma usually result in healing if nutrition is maintained and the person does not become more debilitated. Because superficial lesions do not penetrate the full thickness of the skin, they tend to be painful but usually heal quickly if kept clean and free of pressure interference with circulation.

Wound healing is by secondary intention. Granulation tissue fills the center crater and the epithelial cells gradually migrate over the area, meet and seal the wound with scar tissue. Adequate calories, proteins, and vitamins are essential for wound healing. Vitamin C functions in collagen formation, and the B vitamins are needed for a normal blood supply.

Large ulcerations include full skin thickness and deeper muscle layers. The trauma may include necrosis of the deeper areas within a large crater. The rim is often undermined extensively. If cleansing with hydrogen peroxide, irrigating the undermined area, exposure to air, and elimination of weight bearing on the site do not permit healing by granulation and scar tissue, the ulcer may need surgical debridement and skin grafting.[1]

Evaluation

The outcome criteria for the prevention of the formation or extension of pressure damaged tissue are:

- The skin is without persistent redness or dusky redness over areas of potential trauma.
- The skin is free of blisters or breaks in the continuity.

The outcome criteria for maintaining adequate nutrition and fluid intake are:

- The person has adequate food and fluid intake relative to the daily requirements of the person's situation.
- The skin will have normal turgor.

The outcome criteria for relief of discomfort related to tissue damage are:

- The patient recognizes the need to change positions regularly.
- The patient relates verbally the diminishment of relief of pain.

Alteration in Comfort: Pruritus

Assessment and Nursing Diagnosis

Pruritus (itching) is an unpleasant, irritating cutaneous sensation for which scratching is the most common self-treatment. Scratching is a protective mechanism for removing noxious stimuli; however it may damage the skin, impair its function as a barrier, and ultimately lead to secondary infection.

One of the most frequent causes of pruritus is dry skin. Dry skin is rough, has fine flakes, is less flexible, and feels dry to the touch. As the skin becomes drier, it cracks, or fissures may occur. Elderly persons often experience dry skin due to an age-related loss of moisture in the tissues and changes in the ability of the epidermis to retain water. With aging, there is a decrease in secretion of skin lipids which help hold water in and retard evaporation from the skin. Decreased environmental humidity promotes dehydration and dryness of the skin which triggers pruritus. Paradoxically, extremely high humidity can cause sweat retention leading to itching.

Pruritus may occur from local irritations, such as foreign bodies, plant products, wool, and insects, or it may be a manifestation of a systemic disease. Generalized pruritus is frequently seen in diabetes mellitus, chronic renal insufficiency, liver disease (especially with biliary obstruction), leukemias, internal malignancies, and lymphomas (especially Hodgkin's disease). Drug hypersensitivities may itch, with or without an obvious rash. Several infectious diseases such as chickenpox and measles cause pruritus; however, many infectious diseases manifested by a rash do not.

Anxiety and excessive motion are demonstrated by persons with severe pruritus. Energy is expended by constant rubbing, scratching, and twisting in an effort to relieve the discomfort. Scratching increases blood flow to the area and worsens the sensation, easily creating an itch–scratch–itch cycle.

Pruritus may disrupt or prevent initiation of sleep, and is frequently worse at night due to a decrease in diversional activities and the warmth of bed covers which promotes further vasodilatation.

Interventions

The goals for nursing management of the patient with pruritus are to relieve the discomfort of itching, to prevent or relieve situations which cause pruritus, and to prevent damage to the skin.

Several techniques may be employed to relieve the misery of the pruritic patient. Cold or cool applications will promote vasoconstriction and provide soothing relief and comfort. These may be given as full baths, or as soaks or compresses to the involved area. They will also help rehydrate the skin. Tranquilizers may be employed in severe acute pruritus to control agitation, hyperactivity, and anxiety. Sedatives may be used judiciously particularly when pruritus interferes with sleep. Topical steroid applications are useful in decreasing inflammation and vasodilatation. Diversional activities that the nurse can create with the help of the patient and family may be beneficial in focusing the patient's attention away from the irritation. The use of techniques such as relaxation and visual imagery may temper the patient's anxiety and contribute to the efficacy of the other treatment modalities.

The nurse and patient should jointly identify factors that stimulate or aggravate pruritus and remove them, when possible, from the patient's activities or environment. The treatment for dry skin is simply directed towards rehydration and avoidance of drying factors. Chemicals such as domestic cleaners and solvents that remove skin lipids should be avoided. Soap should only be used in bathing the axilla and genitals as it also removes protective skin oils. Where used, it should be thoroughly rinsed off the skin. Using tepid bath water and patting rather than rubbing the skin dry avoids the vasodilatation caused by heat and friction. Oils, added to the bath water, form a thin film over the skin which may reduce dryness; however, extreme caution must be taught to the patient because bath oils create a very slippery bathtub surface. Applying lubricating creams and ointments immediately after bathing is probably more effective, however, in retaining water and treating dry skin. Nonperfumed lotions containing lanolin are preferable. Rehydration of the skin may be enhanced by increasing the relative humidity in the environment. Cool mist room humidifiers may be helpful during dry winter months.

Breaking the itch–scratch–itch cycle is essential for preventing skin damage triggered by pruritus. All measures to remove the stimulant and provide symptomatic relief should be considered even to the extent of sedation if it is the only remaining method of offering respite to damaged skin. Fingernails may need to be cut short or covered with gauze mittens to prevent further tissue trauma.

Evaluation

The outcome criteria related to relief of the discomfort of pruritus are:

- Patient reports reduction or relief in the sensation of pruritus.
- Skin is without the marks caused by scratching, such as excoriations or long linear parallel fingernail lines.
- Skin color over the affected area is normal for patient.

The outcome criteria related to prevention or relief from situations which cause pruritus are:

- Skin appears smooth and flexible without flaking or dryness.
- Patient is able to articulate factors that stimulate or worsen pruritus.
- Patient incorporates measures to prevent excessive dryness in daily hygiene practices (if dry skin is a causative factor).

The outcome criterion related to prevention of damage to the skin is:

- Patient reduces or ceases all motor activity in response to pruritus, such as scratching and rubbing the area.

Disturbance in Self-Concept Related to Changes in Skin Appearance

Assessment and Nursing Diagnosis

The way in which a person views, feels, or thinks about himself or herself comprises self-concept. An important component of self-concept is an individual's mental image of his or her body. Appearance of the skin contributes a significant aspect to formation of body image. We make immediate judgments based on the small area of skin covering a person's face. Characteristics of the skin (color, texture, wrinkles, blemishes, and scars) provide a major aspect of physical attraction. Changes in the appearance of the skin, whether from disease, surgery, trauma, or normal aging, may create a disturbance in self-concept if the person fails to accept and adapt to the change in body image.

The skin is also a sensitive means of communication. A simple touch can convey a variety of emotions such as love, empathy, and concern. Touch also plays an important part in sexual expression. Skin disorders are obvious and aesthetically unappealing and may lead to self- or other-imposed social isolation.

The impact of skin changes on self-identity and self-concept greatly depends on an individual's perception of the change or alteration. People vary widely in how focused and concerned they are with physical appearance and to what extent they perceive an alteration threatens their attractiveness. Surgical scars are proudly displayed by some, while to others they evoke feelings of shame and failure. The facial lines and changes in contour that accompany normal aging may be gradually incorporated into the self-concept of some, while others experience depression and seek extensive measures to battle the process. Additionally, the nurse's perception of the significance of the alteration may blind him or her to the patient's need for support. Therefore, a patient's concern with an altered skin appearance should not be casually dismissed as merely being of cosmetic importance or because it will eventually go away.

Patients may communicate disturbances in self-concept by indirectly conveying negative feelings about the way they view themselves. The alert nurse will learn to recognize such signals as refusal to look in the mirror or at the body part; withdrawal from social contacts; unwillingness to discuss the disfigurement; self-neglect; and grieving behaviors, such as weeping, anger, or depression.

Interventions

The goals for nursing care are that the patient will be encouraged to express feelings, to acquire or retain a positive self-concept, and to accept and adapt to the changes in body image.

Open expression of feelings is the first step toward acceptance of an alteration in the appearance of the skin, and consequently a change in body image. The nurse can encourage this expression by conveying acceptance and sensitivity to the patient's concern. Asking open-ended questions is less anxiety-producing and invites the patient to select priority areas. The nurse who has established a trusting, therapeutic relationship can help the patient articulate perceptions of the problem and feelings of self-worth by listening attentively and accepting the patient's feelings without judging or advising. Verbal expression helps clarify thoughts and will aid the patient in decision making and adaptation. The nurse should avoid socializing or joking with the patient in an effort to divert attention as this encourages the patient to avoid critical issues and assume a cooperative patient role.

Strategies to foster a positive self-image and self-concept should be thoughtfully incorporated into nurse–patient interactions. It will be easier for the patient to accept a change in appearance if acceptance is demonstrated by the caregivers. Nonverbal communication can transmit powerful judgments. It is important for the nurse to establish eye contact and maintain a controlled facial expression particularly when the patient has obvious facial skin abnormalities such as scars, burns, severe rashes, or birthmarks. Self-esteem is affected when it is apparent that others avoid social contact, looking, or touching.

The message nursing hopes to convey to the patient is that he or she has value and worth despite changes in body appearance. Encourage autonomy by respecting any routines or rituals the patient demonstrates in personal hygiene and allowing self-care whenever possible. Offer praise and support when the patient takes pride and interest in his or her appearance. By demonstrating respect for the patient, you will encourage feelings of self-respect and acceptance.

Patients undergoing changes in body image are in crisis. The nurse needs to observe for excessive stress and behaviors that may be interpreted as a request for emotional support. Answering questions and clarifying misconceptions provide the patient with accurate, objective information. A discussion of past experiences in coping with illness and stress builds confidence for facing the present challenge. The nurse needs to accept each person's unique pattern of adjustment, to be available when support is needed, and to avoid forcing the patient into rapid adaptation to any change in body image.

Evaluation

Outcome criteria for evaluating goal achievement are that the patient:

- Discusses feelings about the changes in body appearance
- Interacts socially with family, friends, staff
- Participates in own care and hygiene; and relates acceptance or contentment with his or her body.

Altered Skin Function in Temperature Regulation

Assessment and Nursing Diagnosis

Alteration in body temperature regulation may be manifested by impairment in heat conservation, secondary to changes in the skin, or by impairment in heat loss, secondary to changes in the skin.

The skin, under the influence of the hypothalamus and the sympathetic nervous system, is a critical factor in the regulation of body temperature. Body temperature is a measure of the balance between heat production and heat loss. Heat is generated in the body as a result of metabolic activity. Heat production can be accelerated by such conditions as exercise, shivering, hyperthyroidism, infections, trauma, and emotions.

The skin functions as an organ in temperature regulation by three mechanisms. Blood vessels called papillary capillaries are contained near the body surface in the dermal layer of the skin. When the body temperature is judged by the hypothalamus to be elevated, blood (carrying heat) is increased to the papillary capillaries which facilitates the transfer of heat from the body to the environment. Heat can be lost from the body surface as a result of peripheral vasodilatation by radiation (heat transfer to an object without physical contact), conduction (heat transfer to an object by direct physical contact), or convection (heat loss by means of a current of air). Similarly, when the body or environmental temperature is too low, vasoconstriction of papillary capillaries occurs which conserves heat by decreasing skin blood flow which discourages body surface heat loss.

The second mechanism by which the skin participates in the control of body temperature is through the evaporation of water released from the sweat glands. Vaporization of water from the body surface cools the blood as it circulates through the skin. The sweat glands are contained in the dermal layer of the skin.

The third function in temperature regulation served by the skin is contributed by the innermost layer, the subcutaneous tissue. Subcutaneous tissue (fat) insulates the underlying tissues and organs from environmental extremes in temperature, particularly cold.

Dysfunction or destruction of the layers of the skin may alter the body's ability to maintain a stable body temperature. Heat conservation is impaired in elderly persons due to an age-related degeneration of the papillary capillaries, resulting in compromised oxygenation and nutrition to the skin. Subcutaneous tissue diminishes with age, reducing the insulating capability of the skin. This progressive impairment of vascular circulation and tissue nutrition and loss of subcutaneous tissue predisposes elderly persons to a feeling of being cold, especially in cool environments. When the environmental temperature is low, the protective response is peripheral vasoconstriction to conserve body heat, but this response in the elderly diminishes blood flow in the skin because of the fewer papillary capillaries.

Any debilitating disease or chronic illness that leads to a nutritionally deficient state can eliminate or reduce the subcutaneous layer of the skin, subsequently jeopardizing heat conservation. Clinical examples of this process include cardiac disease, intestinal dysfunction or malabsorption syndromes, anorexia nervosa, cognitive disorders that interfere with nutritional intake, or cancer particularly when associated with chemotherapy.

Regulation of body temperature is altered by accelerated heat loss through impairments of the skin's integrity. Not only is the protective mechanism of the skin against foreign invasion lost, but also rapid heat dissipation is facilitated by direct communication between the external environment and the internal body tissues. Examples of heat loss by this mechanism include: full thickness, extensive area burns; exposure of internal organs to the cool operating room environment; large, open wounds, especially those frequently exposed during dressing changes and fluid irrigations; and large, full thickness decubitus ulcers.

Dysfunction of the skin may, in addition to impairing heat conservation, interfere with heat dissipation. The sweat glands are controlled by the hypothalamus which responds to an increase in skin or blood temperature. There is a decrease in the size, number, and function of the sweat glands with aging which impairs adaptation to increases in internal or environmental temperatures. Therefore, elderly persons are more suseptible to heat exhaustion.

Interventions

The goals of nursing management for the patient with impaired heat conservation are to reduce or control heat loss, to maintain a physiologic body temperature, and to promote patient comfort.

The goals of nursing management for the patient with impaired mechanisms for heat loss are to facilitate heat dissipation and to maintain a physiologic body temperature.

The maintenance of body temperature within a normal range is essential for proper functioning of the central nervous system and chemical reactions throughout the body. Nursing has a primary role in monitoring the body temperature of patients. Accurate determination of body temperature requires an accurate instrument, proper placement for the appropriate length of time, and accurate reading of the instrument. Knowledgeable evaluation of the results of therapy to regulate body temperature relies upon consistently accurate measurements.

Maintenance of a constant room temperature of approximately 72°F (22.5°C) is recommended for patients with impaired heat conservation. Patient education for self-care for the elderly, particularly during the cold winter months, should recommend wearing hat and gloves outside (much heat loss occurs from the head and hands); wearing close-knit undergarments; selecting wool clothing because it provides better insulation; wearing socks on cold feet at night; staying indoors on windy days to avoid the windchill effect; using sheet blankets; adding extra clothing in the morning when metabolic activity is lowest; and using small frequent meals and warm liquids to provide heat to the body. Community resources may be explored for elderly persons on limited, fixed incomes who may be unable to pay winter heating bills and are at risk for life-threatening hypothermia.

Efforts should be made, during delivery of nursing care to patients with open wounds and exposed tissues and organs, to curb the amount of heat lost to the environment. Unless contraindicated, open wounds should be covered. Irrigating solutions should be warmed to room temperature before using. Wound care should be performed quickly and efficiently to limit the time of exposure. Raising the ambient temperature during this time may be beneficial.

Nurses may incorporate several considerations into nursing management of patients sensitive to cold. Care must be taken during bed baths to expose only small areas at a time, keeping the rest of the body covered, warm, and dry. The nurse caring for the postoperative patient should closely monitor body temperature until it returns to normal. This may be facilitated by the use of heated blankets or commercially prepared heating pads. The placement of patient beds away from cold windows or outside walls will reduce the amount of heat lost through radiation.

Nursing interventions for patients with impairment of mechanisms to dissipate heat are directed toward patient education. Wearing loose, light clothing in hot weather is recommended. Outdoor activity is best scheduled during early morning or evening hours. Working in the shade, alternating between work and rest, and wearing a hat to protect the head from intense heat will reduce the adverse effects of hot weather.

Evaluation

The outcome criteria used for the evaluation of nursing interventions reflect the stated goals:

- Body temperature between 96.8°F (36°C) and 99.5°F (37.5°C)
- No visible shaking, shivering, or patient complaints of feeling cold
- Patient report feeling comfortable
- Skin feels warm and dry (not cold or hot to touch).

Summary

Nursing has the unique role within the health-care team of developing and implementing strategies that will facilitate successful adaptation or complete elimination of the human responses that accompany health problems. Dysfunction or discomfort of the skin can be a manifestation of many altered health states. Skin manifestations that occur in response to other disorders or conditions have been included in other sections of this book. A continuation of this discussion of the maintenance of skin integrity and functioning can be found in Chapter 15 dealing with wound healing, Chapter 43 dealing with peripheral vascular disease, and Chapter 95 dealing with burns and pressure lesions.

References

1. Bruno P: Skin problems. In Carnevali DL, Patrick M (eds): Nursing Management for the Elderly, pp 460–462. Philadelphia, JB Lippincott, 1985
2. Bruno P: Variables associated with the development of postural tissue trauma. Unpublished doctoral dissertation, University of California, San Francisco, 1971
3. Goth KE: Clinical observations and experimental studies of pathogenesis of decubitus ulcers. Acta Chira Scandia 87(Suppl 76):198–200, 1942
4. Lindan O, et al: Pressure distribution in the surface of the human body. Arch Phys Med Rehabil 46:378–385, 1965

Bibliography

Bruya M: Body temperature status. In Mitchell P, Loustau A (eds): Concepts Basic to Nursing, 3rd ed. New York, McGraw-Hill, 1981

Campbell C: Nursing Diagnosis and Intervention in Nursing Practice, 2nd ed. New York, Wiley Medical Publication, 1976

Carnevali D, Patrick M: Nursing Management for the Elderly. Philadelphia, JB Lippincott, 1979

Carpenito LJ: Handbook of Nursing Diagnosis. Philadelphia, JB Lippincott, 1984

Finch C, Hayflick L: Handbook of the Biology of Aging. New York, Van Nostrand Reinhold, 1977

Murray R: Principles of nursing intervention for the adult patient with body image changes. Nurs Clin. North Am 7:697, 1972

Parrish J: Dermatology and Skin Care. New York: McGraw-Hill, 1975

Chapter 94

Infectious and Inflammatory Skin Disorders

Barbara S. Innes

Infections

The skin is constantly exposed to both pathogenic and nonpathogenic organisms. While many of these organisms are easily removed by washing, many others remain on the skin and become resident flora. Normally, the skin acts as a protective mechanism against the invasion of these pathogens into the underlying tissues of the body. An intact integument does this very effectively. However, when the skin loses its integrity or otherwise does not function properly, these opportunistic organisms become foci for the development of infectious processes.

Skin infections may be either primary or secondary. Primary infections usually occur on otherwise intact skin, while secondary infections develop in skin areas which have already been damaged by trauma or other skin lesions, such as ulcers and psoriasis. The categories of skin infections discussed in this chapter include bacterial, fungal, and viral.

Bacterial Infections

Because of the normal protective properties of the skin, bacterial infections are usually secondary in nature. The causative organisms require entry through the skin, but they are readily available when the opportunity occurs.

Impetigo

Etiology and Pathophysiology. Impetigo is a common superficial infection often thought of as a children's disease. However, it is highly contagious and adults also develop the infecion, especially those who have frequent contact with children such as parents and teachers. It is an endemic disease with an apparent increased incidence in the summer and early fall and evidence of higher incidence rates in tropical climates. Poor hygiene has traditionally been considered a predisposing factor; however, recent studies can find no definite relationship.[1] Transmission of the disease is by direct skin-to-skin contact, especially with infected skin lesions.

There are two main forms of impetigo: vesicular and bullous. The main distinction is the causative organism. Each form can also be recognized by the initial and continuing lesion development.

The more common form of the disease is vesicular impetigo which is caused by group A beta-hemolytic streptococci. The lesions, which usually appear on the extremities, begin as small papules which quickly become fluid-filled vesicles; these lesions then rapidly develop into pustules which rupture, usually within 24 hours. The fluid in the pustules forms a characteristic thick golden-yellow (honey-colored), crumbly, crust (Fig. 94–1). This crust can be removed, but new crusts form to take its place. The surrounding skin, as well as that under the crusts, is usually erythemic and weeping. The lesions increase in both size and number by extension. The crusted areas frequently become colonized by staphylococci from the adjacent skin.

Bullous impetigo is generally found on the face, buttocks, trunk, and perineum. The causative organism is coagulase-positive staphylococci. These lesions begin as small vesicles which rapidly develop into flaccid bullae (Fig. 94–2). The bullae generally erupt in 1 to 2 days leaving a superficial eroded area which is covered by a thin, light brown, lacquerlike crust. The surrounding skin is usually asymptomatic.

Clinical Manifestations. The main clinical manifestation is the development of skin lesions as described above. Pruritis is often present with both forms of the disease. Generally, neither type of impetigo causes systemic symptoms, although regional lymphadenitis may be present with vesicular impetigo.

Medical Management. Diagnosis is usually established by the appearance and course of the skin lesions. Gram stain culture of the vesicular fluid may be done if necessary to definitely establish the causative organism.

In very mild cases of impetigo, topical therapy with antibiotics may be sufficient. However, especially because of the streptococcal organisms, systemic antibiotics are often used. The primary agent is penicillin with penicillinase-resistant penicillin being used in resistant cases. Erythromycin may be used in penicillin-allergic patients. It is important to inspect other members of the patient's family and treat them as necessary.

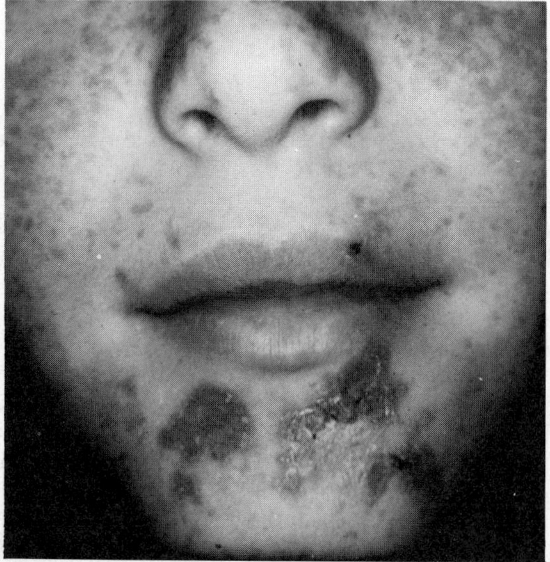

FIGURE 94–1 The crusted lesions of impetigo. (Dobson RL, Abele DC: The Practice of Dermatology, p 17. Phildelphia, JB Lippincott, 1985)

Full recovery from impetigo is the norm, although there is the potential of developing post-streptococcal glomerulonephritis. This complication is the reason that penicillin is usually used early in the medical management regimen. Recurrence of the disease is rare if treatment is continued for 5 to 10 days after the lesions dry up.

Nursing Management

Assessment and Nursing Diagnosis. The nursing diagnoses are related to the impaired integrity of the skin, the patient's need to properly follow the medical treatment regimen, and prevention of further infection.

The specific diagnoses are:

- Psychological discomfort due to contagious skin disease
- Impaired skin integrity
- Potential development of secondary infection
- Knowledge deficits related to self-care of the involved area and prevention of recurrence and spread of the disease.

It is important for the nurse to carefully inspect any suspicious skin lesions and to question the patient about contacts with infected persons, origin and course of lesions, and the presence of itching. Lymph nodes may be palpated for swelling or tenderness.

Interventions. The goals of nursing management are that the patient will not experience embarrassment, will avoid secondary infection and extension of the lesions, and learn necessary self-care of the infected area and preventive precautions.

Because impetigo is often associated with poor personal hygiene, the development of this disease is usually accompanied by embarrassment. The nurse needs to reassure the patient that lack of cleanliness is not necessarily associated with incidence of the disease. The nurse also needs to make sure that embarrassment does not prevent the patient from seeking appropriate medical care.

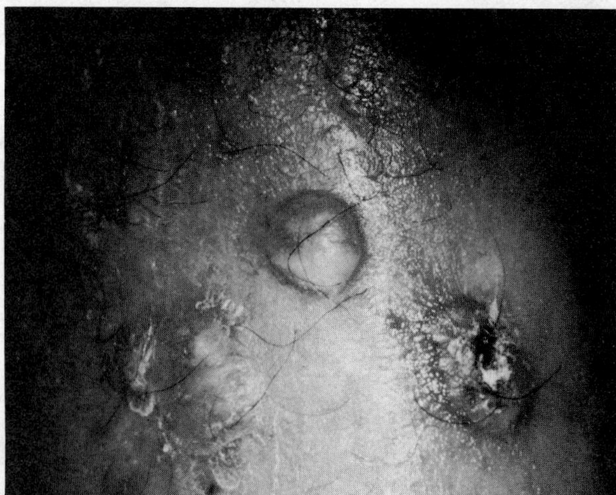

FIGURE 94–2 Bullous impetigo. (Dobson RL, Abele DC: The Practice of Dermatology, p 206. Philadelphia, JB Lippincott, 1985)

Topical care of the infected area and surrounding skin both prevents the development of secondary infection and facilitates healing of the lesions. The crusts must be removed to prevent harboring of the causative organisms. These crusts may be soaked off with cool, wet compresses; if necessary, the area may be scrubbed to effectively remove all crusts. If topical antibiotic agents are being used, the patient needs to be instructed in their proper application. The patient must be encouraged to continue taking prescribed systemic antibiotics for the full course of treatment. The whole family should be inspected for the presence of impetigo lesions.

Evaluation. Outcome criteria for goal achievement are:

1. Patient will seek follow-up medical care appropriately for self and family members as necessary.
2. There will be no secondary infections of the lesions.
3. Patient accurately demonstrates self-care of the infected area.
4. Patient accurately describes self-administration of prescribed medications.
5. Patient describes appropriate measures to prevent spreading and recurrence of the disease.

Furuncles and Carbuncles

Etiology and Pathophysiology. A *furuncle* or boil is a staphylococcal infection of a hair follicle or sebaceous gland, often representing an extension of a superficial folliculitis. These infections often occur in hairy areas of the body, especially where there is perspiration and friction; this includes the neck, face, axillae, and buttocks. The lesion develops into a hard, red, tender nodule which often erupts, discharging purulent drainage.

A *carbuncle* is a deeper infection involving several follicles, often representing a collection of furuncles. As with furuncles, the causative organism is generally a coagulase-positive staphylococcus. These infectious foci usually occur in the thick, inelastic, fibrous skin such as on the posterior neck and back. The involved area of the skin is usually red, indurated, and painful with multiple pustules and several draining points with purulent drainage. Carbuncles may extend to become significant abscesses.

Clinical Manifestations. The presence of a hard, red, tender nodule with or without purulent drainage is the primary manifestation of this disease process. Furuncles are rarely accompanied by systemic symptoms. Carbuncles, however, are frequently associated with fever, pain, and malaise. Leukocytosis is often present with carbuncles.

Medical Management. The extensiveness of the involved area and the presence of systemic symptoms help differentiate carbuncles from furuncles. Gram stains and cultures of the drainage may be used to definitively establish the causative organism.

Systemic antibiotics to eradicate the causative organisms are frequently the primary medical treatment. Hot packs may be recommended to help the body localize and mobilize its normal phagocytic response. Surgical incision and drainage of the lesion may be necessary. After the surgical drainage of the lesion, topical antibiotics may be used to prevent secondary infection.

If the medical treatment regimen is effective, recovery is complete as soon as the lesion area is organism-free and healed. There are complications, however, that may prolong the disease process and cause other deficits. Bacteremia is a potential complication of carbuncles.

Nursing Management

Assessment and Nursing Diagnoses. Nursing diagnoses for patients with furuncles or carbuncles are related to the impaired integrity of the skin, the patient's needs to properly follow the medical treatment regimen, and prevention of spread of the infecting organisms.

The specific diagnoses are:

- Impaired skin integrity
- Potential development of secondary infection
- Knowledge deficits related to self-care of the infected area and prevention of the spread of the infecting organisms.

The nurse's assessment will involve monitoring both the affected local area and the development of systemic progression. The infected area and surrounding tissue are inspected for redness, hardness, and the type and amount of drainage. The patient is questioned about the degree of pain and malaise. Frequent measurement of vital signs helps to monitor the body's systemic response.

Interventions. The goals of nursing management are that the patient will have healing of the skin lesions, avoid secondary infection and extension of the lesions, and learn necessary self-care of the infected and surrounding area and measures to prevent spread of the organisms.

Appropriate wound care is necessary both to facilitate healing and to prevent extension of the current process as well as a secondary infection. The infected area and surrounding skin should be washed with a mild soap and water at least twice a day or as necessary to keep the drainage from prolonged contact with the skin. Because of the danger of breaking down the protective wall surrounding the infection, the lesion should not be squeezed or "popped." In the presence of drainage, the wound should be covered with a dressing, which should be changed twice daily or as necessary to keep the wound dry. Because the infecting organism is a pathogen, it is important that the dressings be handled with care to prevent spread of the organisms to others.

Moist, warm compresses may be used to help the body localize the infectious process and to mobilize the body's defense mechanisms through increased vascularization in the affected area. These may be applied four times daily or more often. The patient needs to be taught to avoid burns from compresses that are too hot.

Supportive measures may be needed if the patient is experiencing systemic symptoms. Nursing interventions may be necessary to control pain and fever. Adequate fluids, nutrition, and rest will support the body's healing mechanisms.

Evaluation. Outcome criteria for goal achievement are as follows:

1. A clean wound with no signs of infection
2. Patient accurately demonstrates appropriate self-care of the affected area.
3. Patient describes appropriate measures to prevent spread of the infecting organisms to self or others.

Cellulitis and Erysipelas

Etiology and Pathophysiology. *Cellulitis* is an infection, usually caused by streptococcal and staphylococcal organisms, that involves the upper layers of the dermis and the subcutaneous tissue. It is nonsuppurative and diffuse, and it spreads along the connective tissue planes. The origin of the infection is generally by invasion of the infecting organisms through a break in the integument or by spread through the lymphatics from another infected area. The classic signs of an inflammatory process—redness, swelling, pain—are present. The lesion may progress to central necrosis and suppuration.

Erysipelas is a rare type of cellulitis. Its distinctive characteristic is the presence of well-demarcated borders rather than the diffuse character of cellulitis. It is more superficial with the development of a red plaque which spreads rapidly with distinct, raised borders (Fig. 94–3). It has a sudden, acute onset, and the patient feels quite ill.

Clinical Manifestations. The primary manifestation is the lesion which is reddened, swollen, painful, and warm. The demarcation of the borders is as described above. There may be red streaks leading from the affected area along the adjacent lymphatics and lymphadenopathy may be present. Systemic symptoms, such as fever, chills, and malaise will likely be present. Leukocytosis will be present.

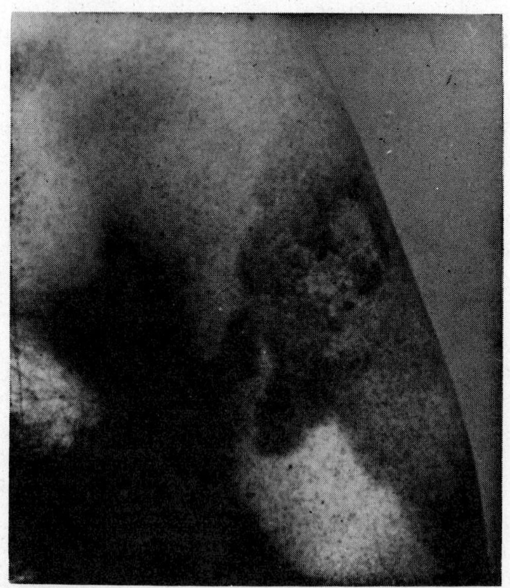

FIGURE 94–3 Erysipedas. (Dobson RL, Abele DC: The Practice of Dermatology, p 210. Philadelphia, JB Lippincott, 1985)

Medical Management. A culture and sensitivity test may be done of the affected area or drainage to definitively identify the causative organism and to help in the selection of the appropriate antibiotic.

Systemic treatment with the appropriate antibiotic is the mainstay of the medical regimen. Rest and elevation of the affected part is recommended. Hot packs may be used to help wall off the infectious process and to mobilize the body's defense mechanisms. Treatment with the appropriate antibiotic will be continued for several days to several weeks after clearing of the lesion; the longer treatment times are used especially with erysipelas. Adequate medical treatment should effect a complete recovery from the disease, although bacteremia is not an unusual complication.

Nursing Management

Assessment and Nursing Diagnoses. The nursing diagnoses for patients with cellulitis or erysipelas are related to impairment of skin integrity, pain management, and the patient's need to follow the prescribed medical regimen. The specific nursing diagnoses are:

- Impaired skin integrity
- Potential for secondary infection
- Alteration in comfort related to the infectious process
- Knowledge deficits related to self-care.

Nursing assessment is primarily aimed at evaluating the progression or regression of the disease process. The involved area and surrounding tissues should be inspected for redness, warmth, swelling, and the presence of drainage. Local lymphatic paths should be observed for red streaks. The patient should be questioned about pain and malaise. Frequent measurement of vital signs is important to the systemic response to the disease.

Interventions. The goals of nursing management are that the patient will experience healing of the skin, avoid secondary infection, have relief from pain, and learn self-care measures.

The nursing interventions are generally those described above for the management of furuncles and carbuncles. Because the involved area is usually larger with cellulitis and erysipelas and the disease is more acute, the interventions need to be intensified. Bedrest is essential and, if the affected part is an extremity, it must be immobilized and elevated. Drainage will be present only if the affected area has been opened surgically; in this case, all precautions must be taken to prevent spread of the infecting organisms.

Evaluation. The outcome criteria for evaluation of the nursing management of patients with cellulitis and erysipelas are the same as for furuncles and carbuncles.

Fungal Infections

Fungi are plant organisms which are found everywhere in nature and become opportunistic when exposed to the skin of an appropriate host. Host susceptibility seems to be increased when the immune system is compromised or overcome with other factors. The two main forms of cutaneous fungal infection are those caused by dermophytes as discussed here and candidiasis, as discussed in Chapter 101.

Dermatophyte Infection (Ringworm: Tinea Infections)

Etiology and Pathology. The most common form of fungal infection is that caused by dermatophytes (also called ringworm). This infection is classified by its location: tinea pedis (athlete's foot), tinea cruris (groin area), tinea corporis (body), and tinea capitis (scalp). The fungi may enter through breaks in the skin or through the respiratory or gastrointestinal tracts. A typical cutaneous lesion is annular in shape with inflammatory activity in the border zone while the center of the lesion is either normal or has minimal scaling (Fig. 94–4). It is thought that the fungus needs noninflamed tissue for its support and so proliferates outward into healthy tissue, leaving the center portion to heal. Darkness, moisture, and maceration support growth of the invading fungi.

Clinical Manifestations. The manifestations of the disease process somewhat differ according to the anatomical location.

Tinea pedis is seen most frequently in the toe web spaces (Fig. 94–5) and is manifested by intense pruritis, scaling, cracking, vesicles, maceration, and a foul odor; there may also be chronic scaling of the soles of the feet.

Tinea cruris typically begins as a hyperpigmented, dry eruption with minimal scaling and well-demarcated borders which may involve the groin, perineum, and perianal area.

Tinea corporis often begins as a small papule or plaque which grows slowly and peripherally as described above.

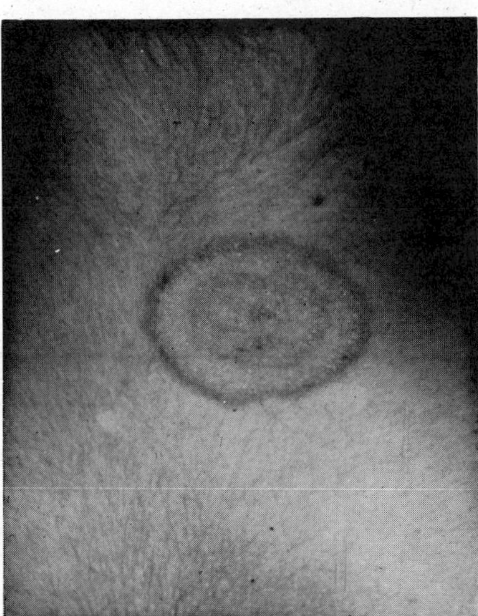

FIGURE 94–4 Tinea corporis in an annular configuration. (Dobson RL, Abele DC: The Practice of Dermatology, p 12. Philadelphia, JB Lippincott, 1985)

Tinea capitis, primarily a disease of children, forms annular patches with hairs broken off a few millimeters above the scalp. Pruritis is usually present with all forms.

Medical Management. The medical treatment for dermatophytes involves avoidance of a suitable environment for growth and the use of antifungal medications. The involved areas must be exposed to the air and allowed to dry in order to facilitate healing and prevent further growth. Topical antifungal agents, such as miconazole and clotrimazole, may be used for minor lesions. Systemic treatment with an antifungal, antibiotic agent, such as griseofulvin or ketoconazole, is often necessary. Acute episodes of tinea pedis may be treated with potassium permanganate or Burow's solution soaks to remove the crusts and scales. Secondary infections must be treated appropriately. A change in lifestyle to prevent a suitable environment for fungal growth is paramount in the prevention of reinfection.

Nursing Management

Assessment and Nursing Diagnoses. The nursing diagnoses for patients with dermatophyte infection are related to impaired integrity of the skin, the patient's need to follow the prescribed medical treatment regimen, and prevention of recurrence of the disease. Specific diagnoses are:

- Impaired skin integrity
- Potential secondary infection
- Knowledge deficits related to self-care of the infected area and prevention of recurrence.

The nursing assessment involves inspection of the involved area. Observations should be made of the location and distribution of lesions, amount of scaling, and degree of moistness of the area. The patient should be questioned about the degree of pruritis present.

Interventions. The goals of nursing management are that the patient will experience skin healing, prevent secondary infection, and learn to prevent recurrence of the infection.

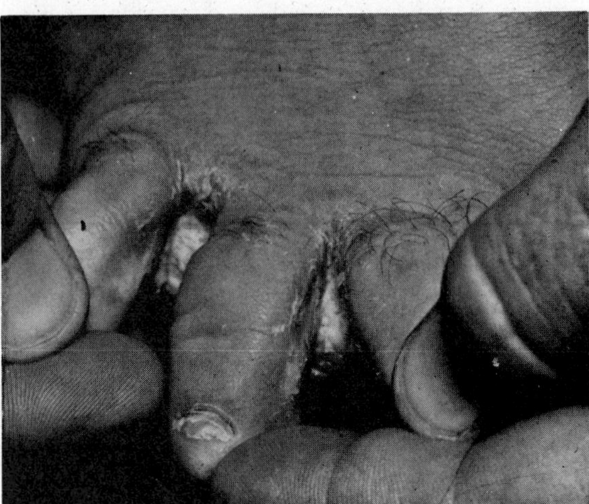

FIGURE 94–5 Tinea pedis. (Dobson RL, Abele DC: The Practice of Dermatology, p 183. Philadelphia, JB Lippincott, 1985)

Except for periods when the infected area may be soaked to remove crusts and scales, it should be kept dry and free from friction. If possible, it should be exposed to the air for long periods. Topical agents should be applied as prescribed, and this treatment should be continued for several weeks after disappearance of the lesions to avoid recurrence.

Prevention of infection is very important, especially with tinea pedis. The main preventive measure is to keep the feet dry and clean. The feet should be washed with soap and water at least daily, usually at the end of the day. Clean, cotton socks or hosiery with cotton feet should be worn. Cotton wadding may be used between the toes at night to prevent maceration. Shoes should be of "breathable" material, and the same pair should not be worn 2 days in a row. Dusting the feet, including between the toes, with talcum or an antifungal powder may help keep the feet dry. When possible, the person should go barefoot to facilitate air-drying.

Persons with tinea cruris shold avoid synthetic underwear and tight-fitting clothes; talcum or antifungal powder in this area may also help to prevent accumulated moisture.

Evaluation. The outcome criteria for nursing management are:

1. Patient demonstrates appropriate self-care of the affected area.
2. Clear skin with no signs of scaling, maceration, annular patches, crusts, or secondary infection
3. Patient accurately describes measures to avoid reinfection.

Viral Infection: Herpes Zoster (Shingles)

Etiology and Pathology. Herpes zoster is caused by the varicella-zoster virus (VZV). Primary infection in a person without resistance to the organism will develop into chickenpox; a person who has had chickenpox previously will develop zoster. Herpes zoster is a disease occurring especially in elderly persons whose immune systems have become less competent, and in immunosuppressed patients.

The disease is limited locally to the sensory nerve ganglia, the sensory nerve fibers, and the skin. The development of herpes zoster may represent a reactivation of the organisms which have remained dormant in the spinal ganglia or cranial nerve ganglia since the original varicella infection; this reactivation process may be stress-related. There is also evidence that the disease may be transmitted through direct contact with cutaneous zoster lesions on another person and that VZV in the nasopharynx may be spread through aerolization. The virus can be found in the vesicles as long as 7 days after their appearance.[3]

The primary characteristic of herpes zoster is the distribution of the lesions in a bandlike pattern along a dermatome, most frequently found unilaterally on the thorax or face. The typical rash begins with a patch of erythema which evolves into grouped papules; these lesions progress into vesicles with clear fluid to pustules with purulent fluid. Some lesions grow in size until they become bullae (Fig. 94–6). Lesions generally continue to erupt for several days to 2 weeks, last for about a week, and then crust.

Clinical Manifestations. As with other skin infections, the primary clinical manifestation is the lesion pattern described above. Another hallmark of the disease is pain. Itching and paresthesia usually precede the onset of the rash by up to 48 hours. The patient may experience systemic prodromal signs, such as malaise and low-grade fever. Neuralgia along the affected dermatome can be severe and debilitating and may persist after the rash disappears, in which case, it is called postherpetic neuralgia. Postherpetic neuralgia occurs in 11% to 70% of the patients and is more common in elderly persons.[4] Patients may not be able to tolerate clothing touching the area and the pain sometimes mimics myocardial infarction or pleurisy.

Medical Management. Appearance and especially distribution of the lesions is usually enough to establish the diagnosis.

Because herpes zoster is self-limiting and of relatively short duration, treatment may be only for symptomatic relief. Corticosteroids, cold compresses, and analgesics may be used to relieve the pain. Burow's solution soaks or aqueous or alcoholic shake lotions may be used to dry the lesions. Some medications may be used to shorten the course of the disease and to reduce symptoms, although their actual end results continue to be investigated. These include vidarabine, which must be started early in the course of the disease if it is to be effective, and acyclovir. The use of interferon is also being investigated.

Probably the most frustrating problem to treat is the postherpetic neuralgia. This symptom may last for a period of 2 to 6 months after the rash disappears and has been reported to last indefinitely in some individuals. The medications mentioned above may reduce the incidence of this complication. Systemic corticosteroids started early in the disease seem to decrease the occurrence. Analgesic therapy may need to be continued for a long time. Tricyclic antidepressants have been effective with some. Work is being done with sympathetic nerve blocks, transcutaneous electric nerve stimulators, and behavioral therapies in attempts to control this pain.

Nursing Management

Assessment and Nursing Diagnoses. The nursing diagnoses for patients with herpes zoster are related to impaired integrity of the skin, pain, the patient's need to properly care for the affected area, and the patient's need to know how to avoid spreading the organisms. Specific diagnoses are:

- Impaired skin integrity
- Altered comfort level related to the painful lesions
- Knowledge deficits related to self-care of the affected area and to measures to prevent transmission of the organisms.

The nursing assessment involves monitoring the progress of the disease process and identification of complica-

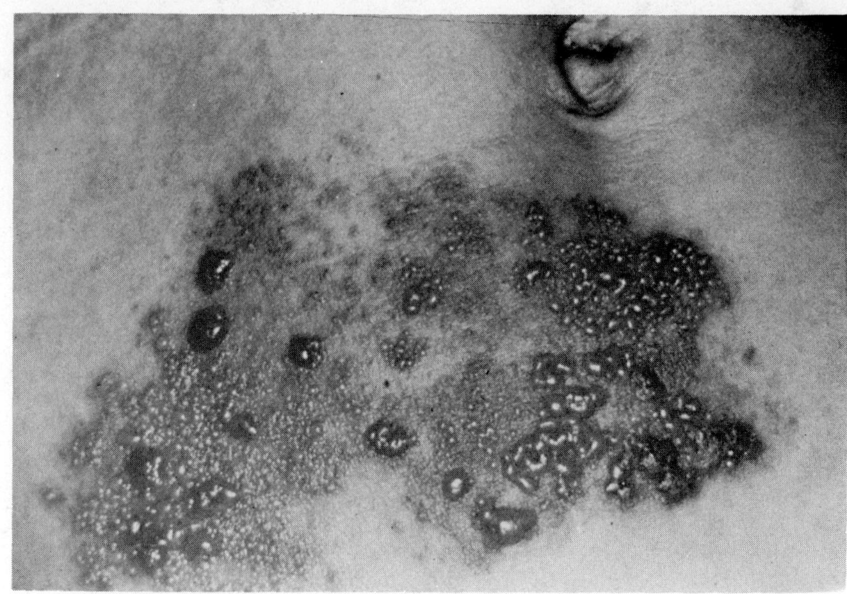

FIGURE 94–6 Grouped vesicles of herpes zoster. (Dobson RL, Abele DC: The Practice of Dermatology, p 16. Philadelphia, JB Lippincott, 1985)

tions. The affected skin area should be inspected for progression of the lesions and signs of secondary infection, although the development of the latter is very rare. It is important to assess the patient's pain: severity, location, duration, and effectiveness of previous interventions.

Interventions. The goals of nursing management are that the patient will experience healing, participate in pain management, and learn self-care of the affected area and measures to prevent transmission of the organisms.

Care of the affected skin area is primarily a matter of keeping the skin clean and free of moisture and the application of medications as indicated by the medical regimen. The area should also be protected from friction and other trauma.

The primary need for nursing intervention is in the area of pain management. Analgesics may be used, although they are often not very effective. Cool compresses or showers may be used. Many times the patient cannot tolerate restrictive clothing, so the nurse needs to be creative in helping the patient find clothing that will not be restrictive or cause friction on the affected area and yet will be acceptable for the person to wear in public. The patient will also frequently experience depression because of the severity or duration of the pain. The patient and significant others need to be supported and reassured.

Because herpes zoster is considered to be contagious through direct contact with lesions and their drainage, precautions must be taken to prevent spread of the disease. The patient needs to be careful not to autoinfect himself, especially in the eye. Dressings, clothing, and linens must be handled with care. In the hospital, wound and skin precautions are usually used as long as there is any drainage from the lesions. Meticulous handwashing is essential.

Evaluation. The outcome criteria for goal achievement are:

1. The involved area of the skin will heal with no sequelae.
2. Patient describes adequate pain management.
3. Patient describes appropriate care of the affected area.
4. Patient accurately describes measures to prevent spread of the disease.

Hypersensitivities

Hypersensitivity reactions account for about half of the skin diseases. Skin sequelae, such as hives and itching, are often the first sign of an allergic reaction. The variety of causative agents is almost infinite. Drugs, food, clothing, footwear, cosmetics, hair dye, and metal jewelry are only a few. The resin of certain plants, such as poison oak, poison ivy, and poison sumac, causes allergic dermatitis reactions when it comes in contact with the skin. This section will discuss two types of hypersensitivity reactions of the skin: contact dermatitis and pemphigus.

Contact Dermatitis

Etiology and Pathology. Contact dermatitis indicates an inflammatory response of the skin to various chemical or physical factors. There are two subdivisions: irritant contact dermatitis and allergic contact dermatitis. Although the basic approach to both is the same, they have different pathophysiological mechanisms.

In irritant contact dermatitis, the degree of response is directly related to the chemical or physical properties of the substance as well as the time of exposure. The skin reaction ranges from mild erythema to vesicles and papules to erosions and ulceration (Fig. 94–7).

Allergic contact dermatitis is a manifestation of delayed

hypersensitivity resulting from contact with an allergen. It represents a T-lymph–antigen reaction. The visible results are an eczematous reaction: erythema, edema, vesiculation, stinging, and itching (Fig. 94–8).

Clinical Manifestations. The skin lesions described above are the most common manifestation. The patient will also experience itching and/or burning. Secondary infections may be present because of persistent scratching.

Medical Management. The key to specific diagnosis is finding the exact causative agent. Tracking this down may require very careful and creative interviewing. Patch testing of the skin for specific allergens may be done.

Removal of and avoidance of the irritant or allergen is the mainstay of treatment. A drying alcohol shake lotion or calamine lotion may be used. Topical or systemic corticosteroids may be needed to reduce the inflammatory response. Antihistamines may be necessary to relieve pruritis.

If the irritant or allergen can be identified and avoided, the prognosis is excellent. Continued contact with these agents can lead to a more systemic histamine reaction and/or chronic eczematous dermatitis, showing dry, scaly, thickened, inelastic, and fissured skin.

Nursing Management

Assessment and Nursing Diagnoses. The nursing diagnoses for patients with contact dermatitis relate to the impaired integrity of the skin, the need to relieve the itching and burning, and the patient's need to follow the medical treatment.

Specific nursing diagnoses are:

- Potential development of secondary infection
- Altered comfort due to itching or burning
- Knowledge deficits related to self-care of the affected area and to measures needed to prevent recurrences.

Nursing assessment is primarily related to monitoring progression of the skin lesions. The affected area is inspected for signs of infection (redness and purulent drainage) and extension of the lesions. The patient is questioned about itching or burning. The nurse may also play an important role in identifying the causative agent through careful interviewing of the patient.

Interventions. The goals of nursing management are that the patient will experience healing of the affected area, prevent secondary infection, relieve itching and burning, and learn about self-care of the affected area and how to avoid recurrences.

Care of the affected area involves keeping it clean. Soaks with cool Burow's solution or Epsom salt solution may help relieve the itching. If the skin is not broken, soaking in colloidal oatmeal or cornstarch baths may be soothing. Alcohol shake lotions may also be used to dry the area. Antihistamines may be necessary.

A crucial part of the long-term care for this patient is the identification and then avoidance of the causative agent(s). The nurse may help the patient develop creative ways of

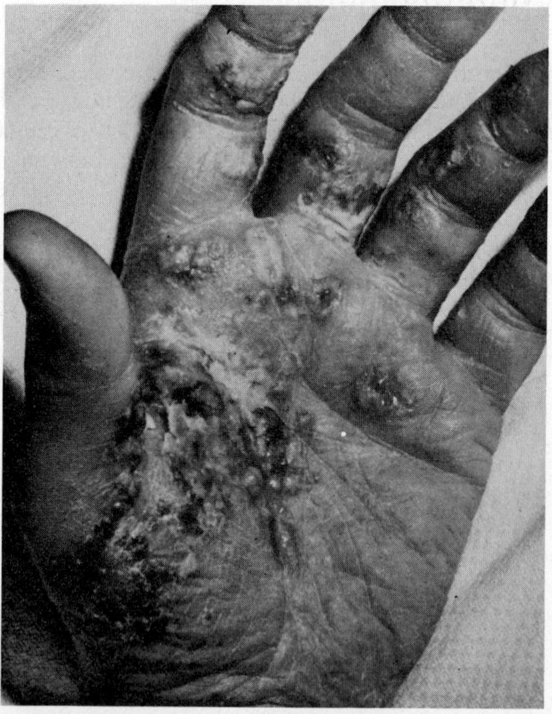

FIGURE 94–7 Severe primary irritant contact dermatitis. (Dobson RL, Abele DC: The Practice of Dermatology, p 38. Philadelphia, JB Lippincott, 1985)

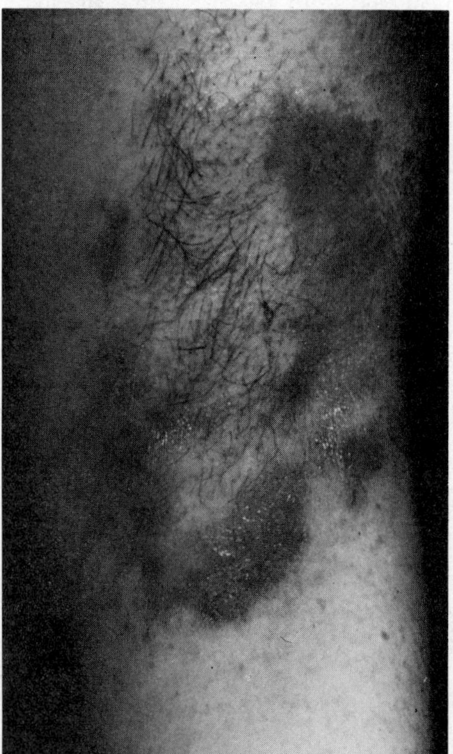

FIGURE 94–8 Allergic contact dermatitis due to clothing. (Dobson RL, Abele DC: The Practice of Dermatology, p 39. Philadelphia, JB Lippincott, 1985)

avoiding skin contact with irritants or allergens when exposure to them is possible, such as may occur in the home or work place. An example of this is the use of cotton-lined rubber gloves when working with certain agents.

Evaluation. Outcome criteria for goal achievement are:

1. Clear skin with no lesions or signs of secondary infection
2. Patient describes appropriate self-care of the affected area.
3. Patient accurately describes measures to prevent recurrence.

Pemphigus

Etiology and Pathology. Pemphigus is a chronic bullous disease that is not too common, but the incidence may be rising. It seems to be a disease especially of elderly persons. The basic mechanism is an antigen–antibody reaction localized in the intracellular cement substance of the epidermis. The result is the formation of bullae (blisters) which range from 1 to 10 cm in size. The blisters are found on otherwise normal-appearing skin and mucous membrances. These bullae enlarge and progress to painful erosions with crusting and oozing. The epidermis can usually be separated from the dermis with gentle trauma, such as rubbing across both the affected and unaffected skin. Because the eroded areas heal slowly, the patient often has large denuded areas of skin. In untreated patients, the disease progresses with the development of more extensive large thin-walled bullae filled with clear or yellow fluid (Fig. 94–9).

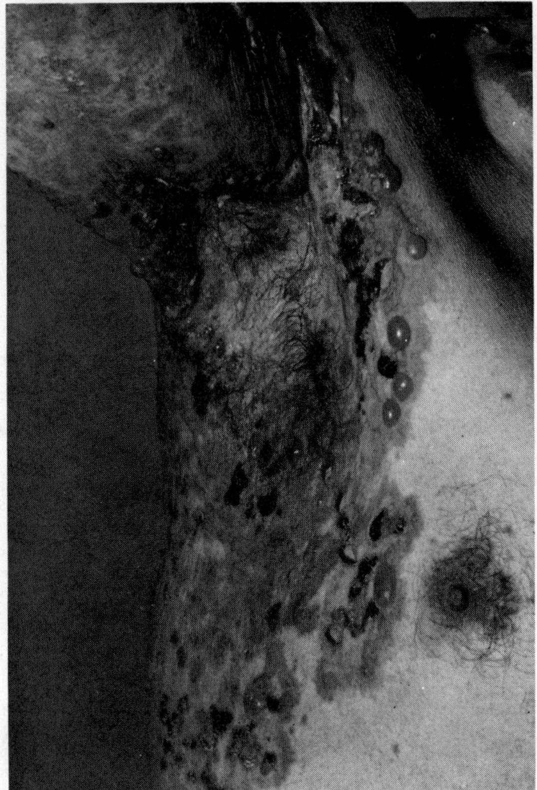

FIGURE 94–9 Bullous pemphigoid. (Dobson RL, Abele DC: The Practice of Dermatology, p 103. Philadelphia, JB Lippincott, 1985)

Clinical Manifestations. The appearance of lesions as described above are the primary manifestation. The affected areas are painful, and there may be a foul odor. Secondary infections are common. If the patient has large denuded areas of skin, fluid and electrolyte imbalances may be present.

Medical Management. The primary medical intervention is high-dose steroids which must be started early in the disease process. This therapy is continued until the patient is in definite remission. Immunosuppressives have been used to supplement the steroids. Secondary infections and fluid and electrolyte imbalances must be treated as indicated.

A few years ago, the prognosis for a patient with pemphigus was very poor. The institution of steroid therapy has changed this picture, although there is still a high mortality rate for patients with extensive disease. The concern is for patients with large denuded areas because of the high risk of infection and the incidence of complications due to fluid and electrolyte loss and stress-related body system failures.

Nursing Management

Assessment and Nursing Diagnoses. The nursing diagnoses for patients with pemphigus relate to the impaired skin integrity and the patient's need to follow proper medical treatment.

Specific nursing diagnoses are:

- Impaired skin integrity
- Potential development of secondary infection
- Altered fluid and electrolyte balance
- Altered comfort due to pain
- Altered nutritional needs
- Altered temperature regulation
- Knowledge deficits about self-care of the affected area.

Nursing assessment involves monitoring of the affected area as well as monitoring the patient for systemic reactions. The skin should be inspected for erythema, bullae formation and rupture, and drainage. The patient should be questioned about the degree of pain. The nurse needs to monitor vital signs, intake and output, nutritional intake, and urine glucose frequently.

Interventions. The goals of nursing management of the patient with pemphigus are that he or she will have healing of the affected skin, adequately manage pain, not experience complications due to denuded skin areas, and learn self-care of the affected area.

In milder forms of the disease, skin cleanliness and care are important. Cool wet dressings may both protect the blistered areas and be soothing. Potassium permanganate baths help prevent infection and may help to control the characteristic odor emanating from these lesions. Friction and pressure to these areas must be avoided. More advanced disease, in which there are large denuded skin areas, requires nursing interventions similar to that for burn patients.

Evaluation. Outcome criteria for goal achievement are:

1. Clean, well-healed skin in the affected area
2. Adequate relief of pain
3. Adequate fluid and electrolyte balance
4. Patient describes appropriate self-care of the affected area.

Vascular Change: Stasis Dermatitis

Etiology and Pathology. Stasis dermatitis is a common disorder and is the result of peripheral vascular disease of the lower legs. It may or may not be accompanied by skin ulceration.

It usually begins with edema in the ankle near the internal malleolus, especially at the end of the day. The onset may be spontaneous or may be secondary to trauma in the region; there is often a history of varicose veins or deep venous thrombosis. As the process continues, erythema of the skin may develop and the area may become either very dry or weeping and moist. This poorly nourished tissue then becomes a prime environment for ulcer formation (Fig. 94–10). These ulcers are very hard to heal and the resulting scar tissue increases the chances of even more ulceration.

Clinical Manifestation. The main clinical manifestation of stasis dermatitis is the appearance of the skin which was described above. The patient may also complain of either pruritis or of pain caused by the poor circulation to the area. The symptoms may be relieved by rest and elevation of the extremity, especially in its earlier stages.

Medical Management. The main goal of medical treatment is to reduce the high venous pressure in the affected limb. This may be done in a variety of ways, including bedrest with the leg elevated. If the patient cannot maintain bedrest, a compromise is sought. The patient is taught to keep the leg elevated as much as possible and to avoid long periods of standing. Compression of the vessels may be accomplished through the use of elastic bandages or elastic compression stockings.

Nursing Management

Assessment and Nursing Diagnoses. The nursing diagnoses for the patient with stasis dermatitis relates to potential skin infection, pain management, and prevention of skin ulceration and extension of the venous insufficiency. The diagnoses are:

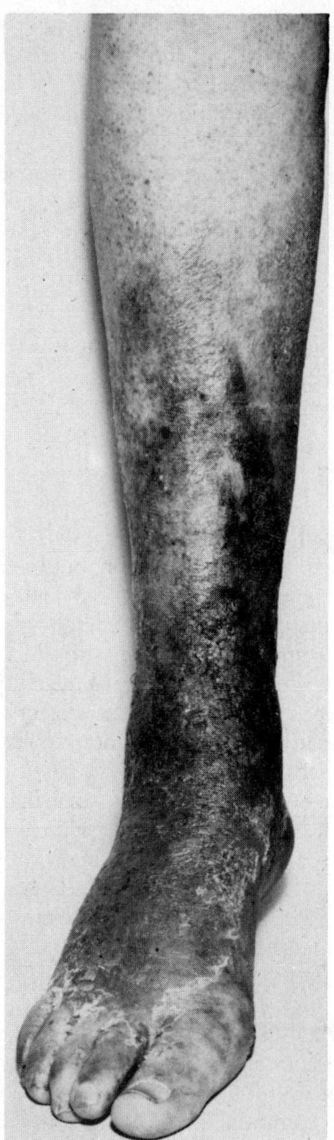

FIGURE 94–10 Stasis dermatitis. (Dobson RL, Abele DC: The Practice of Dermatology, p 50. Philadelphia, JB Lippincott, 1985)

- Potential skin infection
- Alteration in comfort due to pain
- Potential impairment of skin integrity due to ulceration
- Knowledge deficits regarding preventive measures.

Frequent assessment of the skin condition is essential. This involves physical inspection as well as questioning the patient about progression of the discoloration or ulceration. The nurse may ask about situations that make the poor circulation or pain better or worse. The nurse also needs to question the patient about treatments used at home.

Interventions. The goals of nursing management are that the patient will prevent secondary skin infection and prevent ulcer formation, experience effective pain management, and learn necessary self-care in the prevention of ulceration and progression of the disease.

If the skin is weeping and broken, it must be kept clean and dry. Burow's solution compresses may be applied three to four times a day followed by air drying. Steroid ointments may be ordered to reduce the inflammation.

As mentioned above, pain may be effectively managed with rest and elevation of the limb. If this is not sufficient, mild analgesics may be used.

Prevention of ulceration and disease progression are paramount parts of nursing management. It is important that the patient have the necessary knowledge for self-care in this area. The patient must be taught to avoid long periods of standing and to elevate the affected limb as much as possible, at least for 15 to 20-minute periods several times a day. The nurse may need to help the patient devise means for doing this that will have the least interference with daily activities. If the patient is to wear elastic bandages or elastic stockings, he or she must be taught the correct way to apply them as well as the necessity for consistent use of these devices. The patient needs to clean and inspect the affected limb at least once daily so that ulcerations can be detected early. It is also important to avoid trauma to the affected area because the area is so vulnerable. Any signs of infection or ulceration should be reported to a health-care professional immediately.

Proper nutrition and weight control need to be maintained during this time. Follow-up support resources should be identified for the patient to facilitate continued loss of weight as necessary.

Evaluation. Outcome criteria for goal achievement are:

1. No signs of infection or ulceration in the affected area
2. Patient will describe adequate pain management.
3. Patient will describe appropriate measures to prevent ulcer formation and progression of the disease process.

References

1. Becker L, Tschen E: Common bacterial infections of the skin. Primary Care 10:397, 1983
2. Fuller E: Herpes zoster: What can you do to help? Pt Care 17:165, 1983
3. Truesdell M: The scourge of the aged: Herpes zoster. J Gerontol Nurs 9:220, 1983
4. Yardley D, et al: Herpes zoster. Am Fam Physician 28:138, 1983

Bibliography

Ackerman A, Niven J, Grant-Kels J: Differential Diagnosis in Dermatopathology. Philadelphia, Lea & Febiger, 1982

Bannick S: Skin Diseases: Diagnosis and Management in Clinical Practice. Menlo Park, CA, Addison-Wesley, 1982

Caserio R: Bites, rashes, and itches. How to identify and treat them. Postgrad Med 73:267, 1983

Dahl M: Common Office Dermatology. New York, Grune & Stratton, 1983

Ecker R: Contact dermatitis. Hosp Med 20:41, 1984

Flaxman B: Pruritis: Identifying and treating the causes. Postgrad Med 69:177, 1981

Galen W: Dermatitis. Primary Care 10:355, 1983

Griffin D: Shingles: Dealing with the recurrent virus. Consultant 23:231, 1983

Hess F, Graff J: Skin and soft tissue infections. Top Emerg Med 4:72, 1982

Jorizzo J: The itchy patient. Primary Care 10:339, 1983

Kirkis E: Herpes zoster: What precautions are enough? RN 45:137, 1982

Labson L: "Doctor, I can't stand this itching!" Patient Care 18:89, 1984

Lamb C: Dermatologic problem? Which therapy? Patient Care 17:37, 1983

Lever W, Schaumburg-Lever G: Treatment of pemphigus vulgaris. Arch Dermatol 120:44, 1984

Lucey J, et al: Herpes Whitlow. Am J Nurs 84:60, 1984

Maddin S: Current Dermatologic Therapy. Philadelphia, WB Saunders, 1982

McKay M: Topical dermatologic therapy. Primary Care 10:513, 1983

Patel H, et al: Bullous pemphigoid and pemphigus vulgaris. Ann Allergy 50:144, 1983

Roenigk H: Office Dermatology. Baltimore, Williams & Wilkins, 1981

Schachner L, et al: A therapeutic update of superficial skin infections. Ped Clin North Am 30:397, 1983

Tunnessen W: Cutaneous infections. Ped Clin North Am 30:515, 1983

Vasarinsh P: Clinical Dermatology: Diagnosis and Therapy of Common Skin Diseases. Boston, Butterworths, 1982

Chapter 95

Neoplastic Skin Disorders and Related Dermatologic Conditions

Barbara S. Innes

Malignant Neoplasms

Skin cancers are the most frequently occurring of all neoplasms. It is estimated that 500,000 new cases of basal cell and squamous cell carcinomas and 14,000 cases of malignant melanoma are diagnosed each year. The rate for basal cell and squamous cell carcinomas represents 20% of all cancer in men and 10% to 15% in women.[21,23] At the same time, however, skin cancer is generally the easiest of all the cancers to treat. The cure rate for nonmelanomas is over 95% and for stage I melanomas, 80%.[21] While skin cancers do metastasize, this usually does not occur until quite late in the disease process and because most lesions are very visible, treatment is ordinarily instituted before the invasion occurs.

Risk Factors

The etiology of each specific type of skin cancer will be discussed below. However, the risk factors for the whole category are so similar that a general discussion will be used as an introduction to further consideration of the pathology and management of skin cancer.

Although hereditary factors and chemical exposure are definite contributors in the development of skin cancer, the most important is exposure to the sun. In most instances, it is the cumulative effects of long-term exposure to the sun, particularly the ultraviolet-B rays, that cause the development of premalignant and malignant skin lesions. Those parts of the skin that are most exposed are the prime targets for sun damage; these include the face, neck, ears, and hands. Normally, the melanin system located in the lower parts of the epidermis is activated by the sun's rays and acts as an ultraviolet filter. Over the years, the skin loses its normal elasticity, becomes wrinkled and leathery, and lesions begin to appear. At first, these lesions are nonmalignant and may only be discolorations; however, over time, these skin changes may become malignant. The results of sun exposure are accentuated by ultraviolet-A rays, heat, and wind.

Certain hereditary factors are considered indicative of high risk for skin malignancies. These include light-skinned, blue- or gray-eyed people with red or blond hair. People with darker skin and higher levels of protective melanin are much less likely to develop skin neoplasms resulting from sun exposure. Freckling and easy-burning are also considered warning signs for future malignancy. The following classification scale can be used to determine the skin cancer risk of an individual:

Rank	*Skin Response*
I	Always burns, never tans
II	Usually burns, tans only with difficulty
III	Sometimes burns mildly, tans fairly easily
IV	Rarely burns, tans very easily

Chemical exposures are also thought to contribute to the development of skin malignancies. Arsenic ingestion is a prime suspect with certain insecticides identified as a common source. Chronic exposure to polycyclic aromatic hydrocarbons, such as may be found with coal products manufacturers, roofers, creosote coaters, and cotton spinners, is a common finding among people with skin neoplasmas.[4] Nitrosoureas and nitrogen mustard are carcinogenic with chronic exposure.[12]

Finally, there are some personal predisposing factors that increase the person's risk of developing skin cancer. People with a history of previous skin diseases or allergies have a higher incidence of skin malignancy. Areas of radiation dermatitis and healed burn scars are at especially high risk.

This chapter presents the three major types of skin cancer: basal cell carcinoma, squamous carcinoma, and malignant melanoma. Also included is a discussion of cutaneous T-cell lymphoma and Kaposi's sarcoma, diseases that are occurring with increasing frequency.

Basal Cell Carcinoma

Etiology and Pathology

Basal cell carcinoma is the most frequent form of skin cancer. Although it may appear at any age, it most often develops in the fourth or fifth decade of life. Men are affected more than women, and the lesions usually develop in skin areas having long-term sun exposure; these include the head and neck, back, forearms, and hands.

There are five different types of basal cell carcinomas: noduloulcerative, pigmented, superficial, sclerosing, and recurrent. The noduloulcerative lesions are the most common type, In the beginning stages, the appear as waxy, translucent, pearly papules. Telangiectatic (dilated) blood vessels are usually present within and around the lesion. The center of the lesion may form an ulcer crater (Fig. 95–1), and it frequently bleeds with minor trauma. Pigmented lesions resemble noduloulcerative lesions except that they are speckled with a blue or black color. Superficial basal cell carcinomas are often harder to recognize because they are not as visible as the previous two types. They usually present as an erythematous patch or scale with an irregular border and resemble dermatitis (Fig. 95–2). Sclerosing lesions do not ulcerate until their very late stages and appear early as an indistinct area with a yellowish white color. Recurrent carcinomas typically appear as a small papule within a previously treated area.[7]

Clinical Manifestations

The main manifestation of basal cell carcinomas is the appearance of skin lesions as described above. Sometimes, the person will describe burning or itching in the site. Frequently, there is a history of frequent bleeding in the involved area.

Medical Management

Treatment of these lesions is designed to completely remove the malignant cells and prevent recurrence while, at the same time, sacrificing the least amount of normal tissue. This is done by one or more of several modalities: curettage and electrodesiccation, cryosurgery, surgical excision, radia-

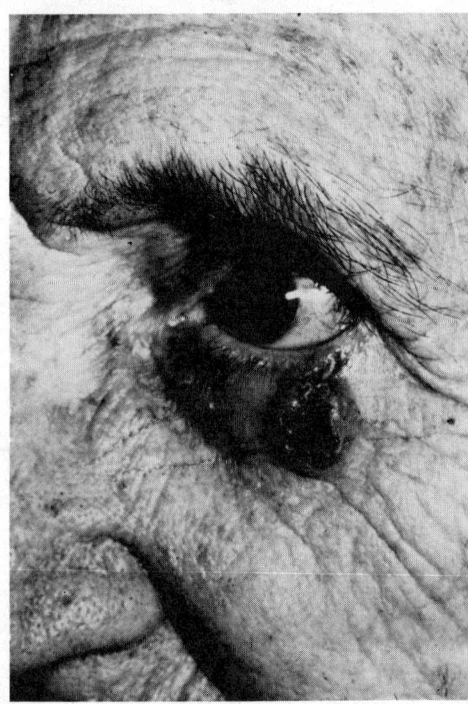

FIGURE 95–1 Nodular basal cell carcinoma with central ulceration. (Dobson RL, Abele DC: The Practice of Dermatology, p 278. Philadelphia, JB Lippincott, 1985)

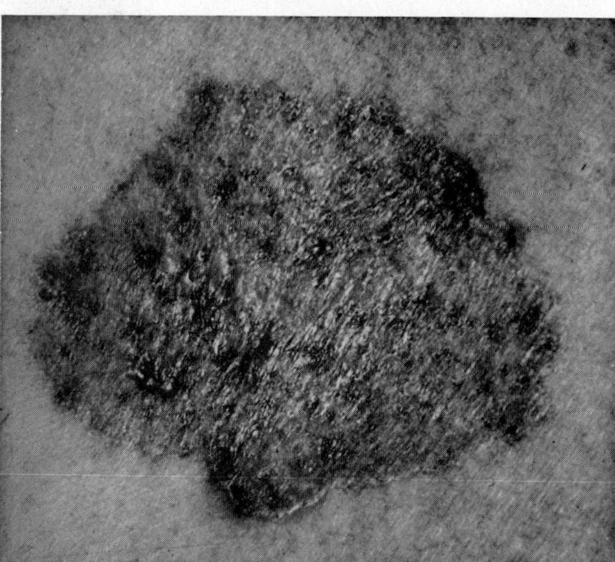

FIGURE 95–2 Superficial spreading basal cell carcinoma. Note threadlike border on lower portion of tumor. (Dobson RL, Abele DC: The Practice of Dermatology, p 280. Philadelphia, JB Lippincott, 1985)

tion, and topical chemotherapy. The decision about the appropriate treatment mode is made after considering several variables, including size and depth of the lesion, the specific anatomical location, duration of the lesion, condition of the surrounding skin, the age and general health status of the person, whether the lesion is a primary or recurrent one, and whether there is a single lesion or multiple ones.[1]

Curettage and electrodesiccation is the easiest and most commonly used treatment for basal cell carcinoma, especially for lesions in their early stages when they are less than 2 cm in diameter. It consists of scraping the surface of the lesion with a currette and then applying a mild electrical current to achieve homeostasis and destroy any malignant cells remaining within the scraped area. An open wound remains which must granulate and heals by secondary intention.

Cryosurgery involves freezing the tissue, killing the cells exposed to the cold source. Thermocouple needles are usually placed into the tissue at the base of the lesion so the freezing process can be monitored. Liquid nitrogen is the primary freezing agent used. The tissue is frozen to a temperature of −25 to −30° C; it is often allowed to thaw and then is refrozen. The frozen area is obvious during the treatment because it becomes white and icy-looking. There is usually edema in the treated site for several days with a period of serous exudate and weeping occurring for 2 to 3 weeks. An eschar forms about 4 weeks after the treatment, and the wound heals by secondary intention. It is important to note that cryosurgery done on black skin may leave a permanently depigmented area.

Surgical excision, which is generally done for lesions over 2 cm in size, is usually done under local anesthesia, although extensively involved areas may necessitate general anesthesia for better relaxation. The surgical area must extend beyond all borders of the malignant lesion and, if the area is large, skin grafting may be done to facilitate healing and to provide for a good cosmetic result.

A special type of surgery, called Moh's "microscopically

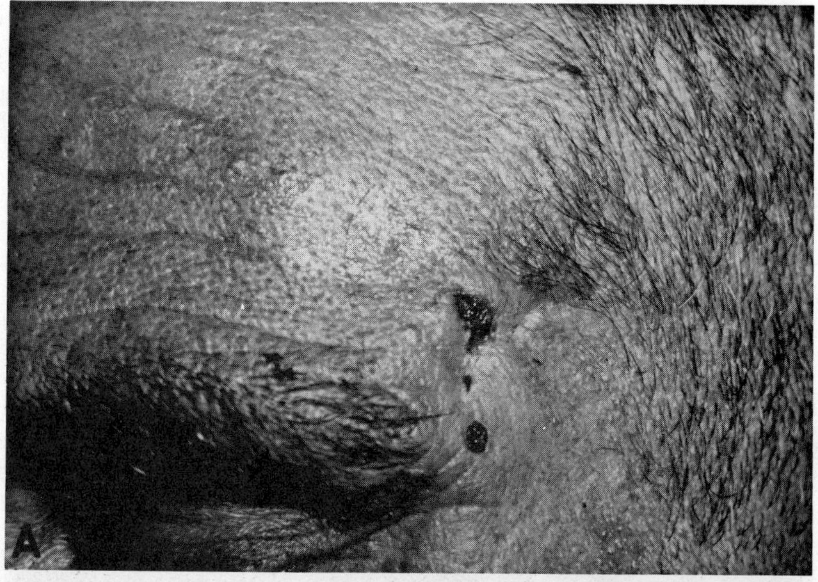

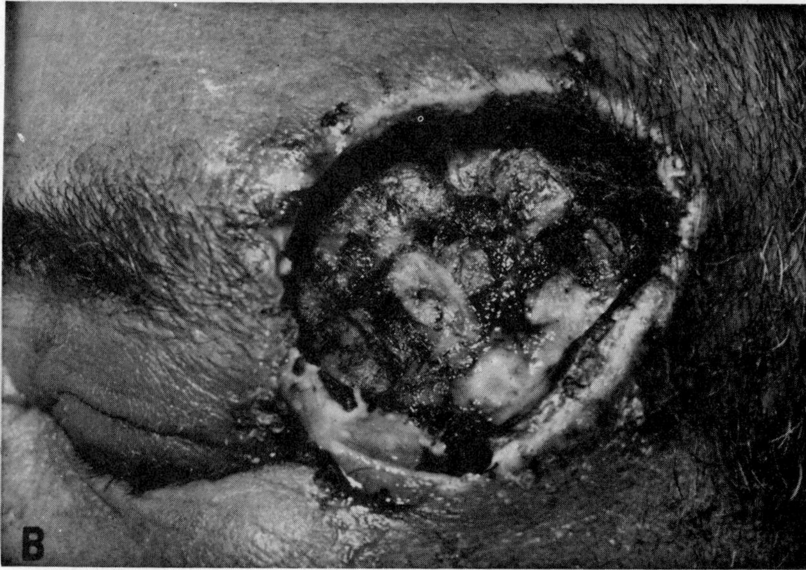

FIGURE 95–3 (*A*) A recurrent basal cell carcinoma adjacent to left eyebrow. (*B*) The extent of the tumor as revealed by microscopically controlled surgery. (Dobson RL, Abele DC: The Practice of Dermatology, p 281. Philadelphia, JB Lippincott, 1985)

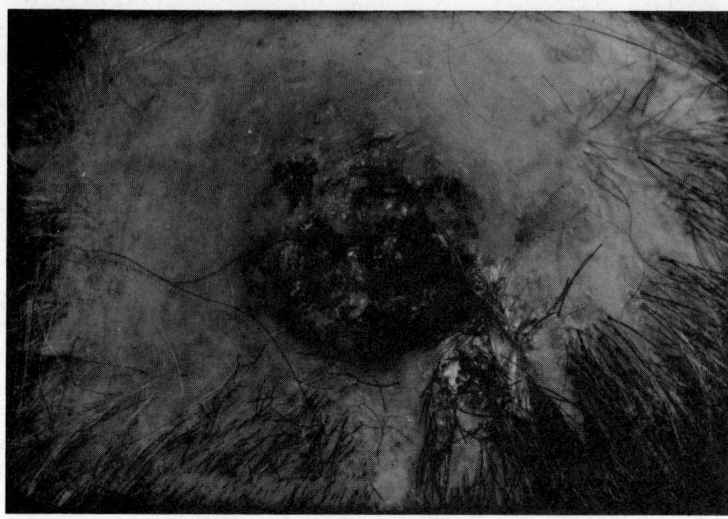

FIGURE 95–4 Squamous cell carcnoma arising in an old burn scar. (Dobson RL, Abele DC: The Practice of Dermatology, p 282. Philadelphia, JB Lippincott, 1985)

controlled excision" or "Moh's surgery, fresh tissue technique" may be used to excise the malignant tissue (Fig. 95–3). It is recommended for recurrent tumors; large lesions, especially those located around the nose, eye, and ear; and lesions arising in areas of radiation dermatitis. In this technique, which requires special training for the surgeon, tissue is excised from the lesion area and the speciman is carefully marked with dyes so that its corresponding points in the wound crater can be located exactly. The tissue speciman is then examined cell by cell under the microscope. If malignant cells are found on the surface of the speciman, more tissue is removed from the exact corresponding area of the wound. This process is repeated until no further cells are found on the surface of the frozen section indicating that all the malignant cells have been removed from the skin. In this procedure, chemical fixatives used to be applied to the surface of the lesion which allowed a bloodless field during the excision; however, with the newer surgical instruments, this is no longer necessary.[18]

Radiation therapy is often used in areas around the eyes, the tip of the nose, and where damage to vital structures is a significant risk of the other methods. Because of the danger of additional malignancy occurring later in the irradiated areas, this treatment mode is usually confined to older persons. The treated area may become reddened and blistered for several weeks.

Topical chemotherapy, the application of a topical antineoplastic solution, (*e.g.,* flourouracil, trichloroacetic acid), may be used to destroy the malignant cells. This treatment usually involves at least daily application of the medication for several weeks. Its use for overt cancers is controversial.[1,17]

With the possible exception of topical chemotherapy, the treatment modes have a well-documented success rate. All are above 90% successful. As mentioned above, lesions caught early in their development have an excellent prognosis. However, if metastasis has occurred, the cure rate is severely affected.

There is an additional treatment mode being studied. It involves the application of heat to the lesion, bringing it to approximately 42° C. The mechanism of action is not fully understood, but it may involve accumulation of nuclear protein in the cells, damage to the plasma membranes, or an enzymatic reaction which kills the cell. The sources used for this hyperthermic treatment include ultrasound, radiofrequency, and microwave. More controlled studies are necessary before the treatment gains wide acceptance.[8]

Prognosis. Basal cell carcinomas are very slow growing and rarely metastasize. The time interval between onset of the disease and the development of metastasis ranges from 4 to 25 years with a mean of 11 years.[16] However, the diagnosis of metastasis indicates a poor prognosis for the person. The usual sites for metastases are the lymph nodes, bone, lung, and liver.

Squamous Cell Carcinoma

Squamous cell carcinomas occur less frequently than do basal cell tumors. Their etiology, medical management, and nursing management have many similarities to those of basal cell carcinomas although there are a few differences. Bowen's disease is a name sometimes used for the *in situ* phase of squamous cell carcinoma.

Etiology and Pathophysiology

Squamous cell tumors arise in the keratinizing cells of the epidermis. They are usually prefaced by premalignant tumors such as actinic keratosis which is discussed later in the chapter.

The most common sites for squamous cell tumors are the sun-exposed areas of the skin, especially the malar region, lips, and dorsum of the hands. They are frequently found in old burn scars or sinus tracts, areas of radiation dermatitis, and skin spaces having a history of chronic inflammatory processes (Fig. 95–4). Squamous cell lesions also develop on mucous membranes exposed to chronic irritation, such as from pipe smoking and dentures.

Clinical Manifestations

The typical squamous cell lesion presents as a flesh-colored, firm, slowly enlarging nodule or a punched-out ulceration. It may, however, be seen as a scaly, reddish brown plaque with an underlying induration and irregular borders. Sometimes, the lesion is not clinically visible and will not be identified until it has metastasized.

Medical Management

Diagnosis and Treatment. The diagnosis and treatment of squamous cell carcinoma are very similar to those of basal cell carcinoma. The primary difference lies in the slight variation in treatment modalities. Surgical excision may be a bit more extensive with wider margins being taken to ensure complete removal of the malignant cells. Systemic antineoplastic chemotherapy may be used earlier in the disease process than with basal cell carcinoma. Immunotherapy may also be added to the treatment protocol.

Prognosis. As with basal cell carcinomas, these lesions are slow-growing and rarely metastasize, although *de novo* tumors are more aggressive and demonstrate a 10% metastasis rate.[5] The 5-year cure rate following microscopically controlled excision is estimated to be over 93%.[9]

Nursing Management

Assessment and Nursing Diagnoses

Nursing diagnoses for patients with basal or squamous cell carcinoma relate to the perceived significance of the diagnosis, care of the wound following treatment, and the need for prevention and follow-up treatment.

The nursing diagnoses are:

- Fear related to the life-threatening associations with the diagnosis
- Potential for wound infection
- Knowledge deficits related to prevention of recurrence and self-care of the wound after treatment.

Nursing assessment is especially important in the initial diagnostic phase. It is important for the nurse to include careful inspection of the skin in any assessment. Any suspicious area should be closely examined, and the person should be questioned about its history. Special attention should be given to the lesion's duration and recent changes in its character. Bleeding or ulcerating tendencies of the area should be determined. Pertinent information should be communicated to the appropriate person.

Interventions

The goals of nursing management are to alleviate fear and anxiety, to prevent infection, and to teach the patient necessary self-care of the wound and preventive precautions.

Many people have a high anxiety about a diagnosis of cancer, even though skin cancer has such a high cure rate. Therefore, the nurse may need to help the person work through this fear. In addition, sometimes the treatment leaves a cosmetic change in the person, and adaptation to this new body image may be necessary. Listening and helping the person talk to significant others about feelings and needs facilitate adjustment to the diagnosis of skin cancer and to the lifestyle changes that may be necessary to prevent recurrences.

Appropriate wound care is necessary after most treatments to facilitate healing with the least amount of disfigurement. It is important to avoid infection and to allow wounds to heal without disruption. This care ranges from simply keeping the wound clean to changing dressings using appropriate technique. Any dressings used should be of the nonadhesive type to avoid interference with the granulation process within the wound. Because treatments are generally done on an ambulatory basis, careful instructions must be provided so that good wound care can be provided at home.

Education is probably the most important nursing intervention. As with any other disease process, prevention is the best treatment. Because cumulative sun radiation is the prime causative factor in the development of both basal and squamous cell carcinoma, people must be taught to avoid prolonged exposure to ultraviolet-B rays. Protective clothing should be worn, and sunscreen lotions with para-aminobenzoic acid (PABA) should be applied liberally and frequently. Times in the sun should avoid those hours (10 AM to 3 PM) when radiation is most intense. People who are at high risk for development of skin cancer should be taught to inspect their skin frequently and to seek medical advice whenever something suspicious is noticed. People who have been treated for skin cancer should receive professional follow-up for the rest of their lives.

Evaluation

Outcome criteria for goal achievement are:

1. Patient discusses feelings and concerns about the diagnosis and outcome of treatment.
2. Patient expresses a decrease in anxiety and a positive feeling about a successful outcome.
3. Patient accurately describes self-care of the wound.
4. A clean wound with no signs of infection (absence of redness, swelling, purulent discharge)
5. Patient accurately describes measures to prevent recurrence of the carcinoma.

Malignant Melanoma

Maligant melanoma is the least common form of primary skin cancer, accounting for less than 2% of all cancers. However, it is the most dangerous because of its high propensity to metastasis and resistance to treatment. In addition, the incidence of this type of neoplasm is growing significantly. In 1930, the rate in the population was 1 : 1500; by 1980, it had risen to 1 : 250; and by the year 2000, it is predicted that the rate of melanoma will be 1 : 150.[24] Approximately 9000 cases of newly diagnosed malignant melanoma are reported annually in the United States, and this type of cancer accounts for almost 5000 deaths each year.[7]

Etiology and Pathophysiology

Malignant melanoma occurs more frequently in males than in females and is mainly a disease of Caucasians, although it does occasionally occur in blacks. The most common site for appearance of the lesions is the lower extremity, although other frequent sites include head and neck, back, chest, abdomen, and upper extremities. Although cutaneous malignant melanoma is the most common form of the disease, primary lesions do appear on other parts of the body. These include the eye, mucous membranes, central nervous system, and autonomic nervous system. These latter melanomas will not be discussed here.

As with the other forms of skin cancer, exposure to the sun appears to be the primary cause of melanoma development. It is hypothesized, however, that rather than accumulation of ultraviolet radiation, intermittent, intense sunburn may be a more important factor. Environmental exposure to carcinogenic compounds, like polychlorinated biphenyls, appears to increase a person's risk. Although the reason is unclear, times of increased hormonal influence, such as in puberty and pregnancy, seem to be correlated with increased melanoma activity. There is some evidence of hereditary tendencies. Finally, the higher incidence of melanoma among immunosuppressed people suggests an immunologic factor.

Malignant melanoma is a neoplasm of the melanin-producing cells, arising primarily in the basal cells of the epidermis. There are four major classifications based on their clinical and histological characteristics: lentigo maligna, superficial spreading malignant, acral-lentiginous, and nodular.

Lentigo maligna melanomas usually first appear in the malar region of the face in elderly persons, although they can occur at any age in any site. They arise from a long-standing patch of brown, tan, or black pigmentation called a lentigo maligna or Hutchinson's freckle. The patch begins as a round, pigmented, smooth macule, but over time, as the lesion enlarges, the borders become irregular. For years, the lesion grows horizontally across the skin surface, then it enters its vertical growth phase, invading the dermis. It is at this time that it becomes a lentigo maligna melanoma.

Superficial spreading melanoma is the most commonly occurring melanoma and appears most frequently on the upper back and lower extremities. It is usually easily visible and presents as a pigmented papule or macule that is typically raised above the surface of the skin (Fig. 95–5). It has irregular borders and varied topography. A bluish color is most ominous, but the lesion may also contain shades of black, brown, tan, red, white, and gray. Variegated color within the lesion is its most striking characteristic. As the lesion grows, it may become nodular and signs of skipped or regressed areas may appear; there is also often a loss of normal skin markings.

Acral-lentiginous melanoma is manifested by lesions that arise around the nails and on the soles and palms. Generally, these lesions are darkly pigmented macules with irregular borders and areas of regression. A range of variegated colors may be seen as with the other types of melanoma. In addition to producing an unusual pigmentation, lesions located near and under the nail often distort the nail itself. This type of melanoma tends to spread across the skin surface for a long time before beginning to invade the dermis.

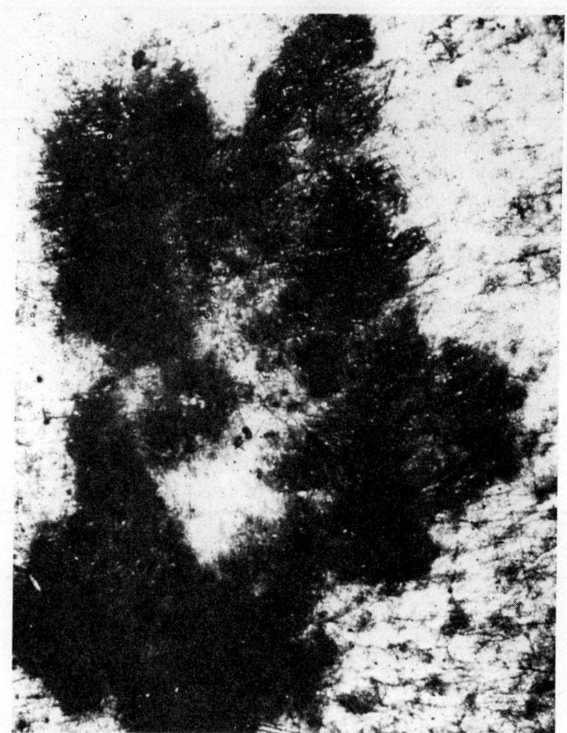

FIGURE 95–5 Superficial spreading melanoma. Note areas of regression. (Dobson RL, Abele DC: The Practice of Dermatology, p 290. Philadelphia, JB Lippincott, 1985)

Nodular melanoma is considered the most dangerous of all the types because it does not have a radial growth stage. From its start, it begins to invade the dermal layer, growing faster, invading more deeply and metastasizing more quickly than any of the three types described above. The lesions appear as either elevated, pedunculated, or convex hard areas that are usually dark brown, blue, or black. They have been described as simulating a blueberry. However, there have also been lesions that were pink or not pigmented at all. This type of melanoma seems not to be correlated to sun exposure and therefore it often appears on parts of the body that are usually covered.

Melanomas generally metastasize by way of the lymphatic system through the lymph nodes and through the vascular system after invading the vein walls. Metastatic lesions may be found locally as satellites located beside or under the main lesion or may be found in distant areas, particularly the bowel, lung, liver, brain, and bone.

Clinical Manifestations

The primary manifestation of malignant melanomas is the appearance of lesions as described above. Assessment of the lesion should include shape, color, consistency, topography, and the presence of satellite lesions. Table 95–1 lists suspicious signs for developing skin lesions.

TABLE 95–1
Suspicious Signs of Malignant Transformation of Nevi (Skin Moles)

Change in size, particularly sudden, rapid growth
Change in color, particularly appearance of red, blue, or white pigmentation, variegated coloration, sudden darkening, leaching of pigmentation onto surrounding skin
Change in shape, particularly rapid elevation or development of irregular borders
Change in consistency, particularly softening or development of friability
Change in topography, particularly development of scaliness, oozing, crusting, erosion, ulceration, or mushroomlike appearance.
Development of pruritis, tenderness, or pain
Development of inflammation with redness or swelling in surrounding skin or development of satellite pigmented areas

(Adapted from Dahl M: Common Office Dermatology, p 140. New York, Grune & Stratton, 1983.

Medical Management

Diagnosis. Diagnosis of malignant melanoma is done primarily through biopsy. As with other neoplastic diseases, the first phase of deciding on a treatment protocol is to determine its classification or stage. A standard staging system has not yet been accepted worldwide and there are several classification systems used for malignant melanoma. One system developed by the New York University Melanoma Cooperative Group divides melanomas into three major categories:

- Stage I—local disease
- Stage II—nodal disease with metastasis to regional lymph nodes
- Stage III—disseminated disease with widespread metastasis

Each stage is then broken in subdivisions.[19] Other systems used include a tumor-node-metastasis (TNM) classification and one that is gaining popularity which looks at level of invasion and thickness of the lesion.

Treatment. The primary treatment for malignant melanoma is surgical excision. Other treatment protocols include chemotherapy, immunotherapy, and radiation.

Surgical Excision. The breadth of the surgical excision used to remove malignant melanomas depends on the size and depth of the lesion. Small, primary melanomas may be removed by simple excision with primary closure of the skin edges while larger, deeper lesions may require extensive excision with split-thickness grafting. Moh's "microscopically controlled excision," described above, may be used. Care must be taken during the surgical procedure to avoid "breakaway" of melanoma cells to the surrounding tissues because these cells are only loosely connected; these liberated cells may be the main cause of recurrent melanomas.

When working with a primary cutaneous lesion with no signs of metastasis, the surgeon also faces the controversial decision about whether or not to do lymph node dissection in the involved region. While this may be helpful in the staging process, there is much debate about the effectiveness of the procedure in terms of treatment. There are data to support both sides of the issue. One recommendation is that elective node dissection should not be performed on the following persons: (1) those with primary lesions that are *in situ* or less than 1 mm thick because the incidence of regional node involvement is so low; (2) those with primary lesions located in the midline of the head and neck or on the trunk; (3) elderly patients whose lesion does not overlie its nodal group; and (4) persons with systemic metastasis because the dissection will not be therapeutic.[19] Patients having regional node dissection in addition to excision of the lesion will require more extensive postoperative wound care.

Chemotherapy. Chemotherapy, most frequently used for palliative treatment of metastatic tumors or for recurrent lesions, may be administered through two main routes: systemic and regional arterial perfusion. There are a variety of chemotherapeutic agents currently used, including DTIC (imidazole carboxamide), vincristine, nitrosoureas, and *cis*-platinum. New agents are being developed continuously.

Systemic chemotherapy is usually achieved intravenously. As with other chemotherapeutic protocols, the administration schedule is designed to attack the malignant cells during their vulnerable stage in the growth process.

Regional arterial perfusion allows the chemotherapeutic agent to be delivered directly into the affected area. The medication is introduced into the artery supplying the region and is pumped by a pump oxygenator into the area for a period of a few hours. During this procedure, the inflow and outflow of blood in the region are controlled so that the agent stays in contact with the surrounding tissues for the intended period of time. Hypothermia is sometimes used to increase the effectiveness of this procedure. This technique is generally used as adjuvant therapy to surgical excision and is considered to be useful in the eradication of melanoma deposits left after the surgical procedure, thereby preventing regional metastasis.

Immunotherapy. Immunotherapy is used to stimulate the body's own immune system to attack the invading cells. This therapy mode has had some success in treating malignant melanomas, especially when used in combination with other treatment modes. It is most frequently used to treat recurrent lesions, although it may be used to limit the growth of a primary tumor. Tumor regression has occurred on occasion, allowing more successful surgical excision. Bacille Calmette Guérin (BCG) is often administered as the challenge agent, although several other substances may be used, such as melanoma cell vaccines, a transfer factor or lymphocyte transfusion.

Radiation. Radiation therapy is the least commonly used treatment because melanomas are considered to be radioresistant. Currently, it is most frequently used for palliation, especially for some of the distant metastatic sites, such as the bone. Internal radiotherapy with radioactive isotopes, such as ^{198}Au may be used to destroy microscopic metastases in stage I lesions and to treat unremovable lymph nodes in stage II melanoma.[3]

Prognosis. As with other forms of cancer, the earlier the disease process can be identified and treated, the greater the change of success for any of the treatment modes described above. The prognosis of people with malignant melanoma depends on several factors, including the size, shape, and location of the lesion and the depth of invasion. When the lesion is under 2 cm, the prognosis is favorable. The main factor involved with depth of invasion is the increasing chance of metastasis which lowers the prognosis. Pedunculation and ulceration are poor prognostic signs. Lesions found on the extremities often have a fairly good outlook, possibly because they are more visible and therefore more likely to be discovered early in their development and possibly because they are located farther from sites of lymphatic drainage. On the other hand, lesions growing on the scalp or trunk have a very poor prognosis.

Nursing Management

Assessment and Nursing Diagnosis

As in other neoplastic diseases, the nursing diagnoses for patients with malignant melanoma relate to the perceived significance of the diagnosis, pain and wound management, and the need for education regarding prevention of lesion recurrence.

The diagnoses are:

- Fear related to the life-threatening associations with the diagnosis
- Alteration in body image
- Alteration in comfort level
- Potential for wound infection
- Knowledge deficits related to prevention of recurrence of the melanoma lesions and self-care of the wound after treatment.

It is often the nurse who first observes suspicious skin tumors either through careful assessment of the skin or in the process of providing routine nursing care. Therefore, it is important for the nurse to be familiar with the lesion characteristics indicating a possible melanoma lesion. These characteristics are described in Table 95–1 and in the preceding lesion descriptions. As with other skin lesions, recent changes are important; however, melanomas often begin with characteristic features which raise suspicions early.

Interventions

The goals of nursing management are to reduce fear and anxiety, to assist the patient to cope with a new body image if necessary, to relieve pain, to prevent wound infection, and to teach the patient necessary self-care of the wound and preventive precautions.

As with any kind of cancer, the diagnosis of malignant melanoma also causes definite fear for both the patient and significant others. Because of the high rate of metastasis with this type of malignancy, the fear of death is even more prevalent than might be expected with the other types of skin cancer. In addition, especially because of the surgical procedure that may be required in the treatment of the lesion, there is frequently a threat to the person's body image. The nurse is usually the resource person who can help these people work through their fears. Creating an environment where the topic and its consequences can be discussed openly is an important step in achieving this goal. This involves application of active listening and counseling skills as well as helping people to be open with each other about their feelings and concerns. It is also important for the nurse to be aware of personal fears and concerns that might block effective intervention in this area.

Because medical management of malignant melanoma almost always involves surgical intervention, pain and wound management are necessary in the postoperative period. The surgical procedure may involve a moderately small incisional area or, if wide excision and skin grafting were necessary, the surgical region may be extensive. The factor will influence the type of nursing intervention necessary to alleviate pain and keep the wound free from infection.

Patient education is an important role for nursing. A person who has had medical treatment for malignant melanoma may need to know about pain and wound management, especially if there is early discharge from the hospital. Nurses can be involved in preventive teaching as they contact people in a variety of settings. Preventive behavior includes avoiding excessive sun exposure, knowing signs and symptoms of suspicious skin lesions, and knowing when and how to seek appropriate medical assistance. Patients who have had melanoma must know the importance of life-long, regular follow-up care. This involves regular inspection of their own skin to check for cutaneous recurrences and examinations by their health-care professional to assess the outcome of the treatment protocol and also to look for recurrences.

Evaluation

Outcome criteria for goal achievement are:

1. Patient and significant others discusses feelings and concerns about the diagnosis and outcome of treatment.
2. Patient expresses a decrease in anxiety and positive feeling about a successful outcome.
3. Patient expresses adequate pain control.
4. A clean wound with no signs of infection (absence of redness, swelling, purulent discharge)
5. Patient accurately describes self-care of the wound.
6. Patient accurately describes measures to prevent recurrence of the melanoma.

Cutaneous T-Cell Lymphoma (Mycosis Fungoides)

Cutaneous T-cell lymphoma, commonly called mycosis fungoides and Sézary syndrome, is a malignancy on the rise in the United States. It is estimated that 400 to 1000 new cases are found each year. This disease occurs most frequently in white and black males with an average age at diagnosis of 52 years.[11]

Etiology and Pathophysiology

The malignant cells in cutaneous T-cell lymphoma are lymphocytes which seem to be attracted to the skin by an unknown factor. It has been theorized that heredity and environment may be contributing factors to the development of the disease. Specific suspicious factors may be the manufacturing of such things as petrochemicals, textiles, and machinery, and a long personal history of skin disease or allergy.

The skin lesions of this disease generally begin superficially as with other types of skin cancer. Initially, they take several forms ranging from eczema to parapsoriasis. As they progress, they extend to the lymph nodes and finally to the visceral organs. The Alibert-Bazin system of classification identifies three developmental phases: premycotic, plaque, and tumor. In the premycotic phase, the lesions appear as nonspecific skin eruptions that may appear and recede in cycles, change in character, or even disappear and then return in the same or a different place on the skin. The plaque phase is signalled by development of an irregular thickening of the skin with elevated plaques (Fig. 95–6). By this time, the lesions are permanent. Then, in the tumor phase, nodular growths occur. These nodules, which may appear on new areas of the skin, may ulcerate, and these ulcerations may occur concurrently with plaques.[10]

Clinical Manifestations

In addition to the skin lesions described above, a common clinical manifestation of the disease is pruritis which may precede or accompany the initial lesions. Severe exfoliation may occur during the premycotic phase. As the disease progresses, advancing skin involvement becomes obvious. The palms and soles may develop hyperkeratosis to the point of painful fissuring. Lesions on the scalp may result in loss of hair. A leonine facies and eversion of the eyelid may be seen in the late stages of the plaque phase. Lymphadenopathy may occur. Because of the open lesions, skin infections may be common.

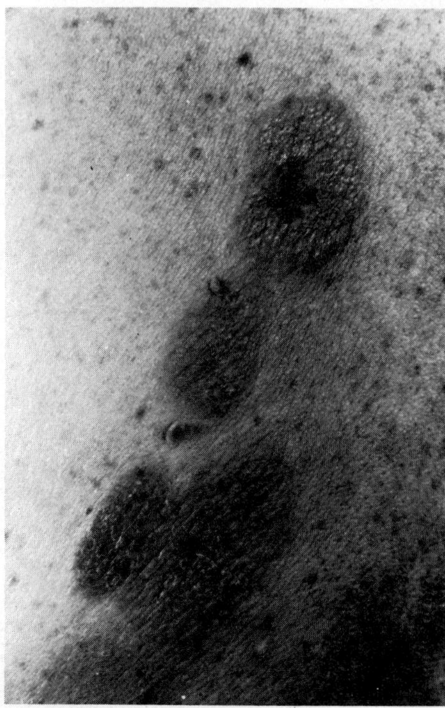

FIGURE 95–6 The plaque stage of mycosis fungoides. (Dobson RL, Abele DC: The Practice of Dermatology, p 299. Philadelphia, JB Lippincott, 1985)

Medical Management

Diagnosis. The diagnosis of cutaneous T-cell lymphoma is established through biopsy. As with any malignancy, staging of the disease is important in planning the medical management needed.

Treatment. There are several treatment modalities for cutanous T-cell lymphoma. These include topical medication, electron beam radiation, psoralen and ultraviolet-A (PUVA) treatment. Systemic chemotherapy is usually used only for advanced cases.

The *topical chemotherapy* usually used is nitrogen mustard applied every day to the entire body except the scalp, unless necessary, and the mucous membranes. Some patients exhibit an allergic reaction in the initial stages of this treatment. If this occurs, the solution should be diluted; the strength of the solution is then increased slowly, thus desensitizing the patient. It is important that the skin be oil-free and that the solution be kept out of the eyes.

Electron beam radiation provides radiation treatment with only superficial penetration. Treatments may be given several times a week. There are a number of side-effects with this method, including radiodermatitis, desquamation, atrophy of the skin and sweat glands, edema, watering eyes and nasal discharge, loss of hair and nails, and joint pain. It is especially important for these patients to avoid strenuous exercise as long as the sweat glands are not functioning properly.

PUVA or psoralen (methoxsalen) and ultraviolet-A light is a common treatment mode for psoriasislike skin diseases. The methoxsalen, which is taken orally about 2 hours before the light treatment, sensitizes the skin to the effects of the light rays. This makes it important for the person to take protective measures against exposure in natural sunlight. Side-effects of this treatment include nausea and vomiting, drying, atrophy, and darkening of the skin, erythema, and an increased incidence of basal cell carcinoma.[10]

Prognosis. The disease is very slow-growing with each stage lasting between months and years. The prognosis is related to the depth of invasion of the disease. Patients with lesions confined to the skin are estimated to have a life span of 9 years, while visceral dissemination shortens this to less than 4 years. The usual sites of distant metastasis include the lymph nodes, liver, spleen, and lungs.

Nursing Management

Assessment and Nursing Diagnosis

Nursing diagnoses for patients with cutaneous T-cell lymphoma relate to the fear of death and altered body image associated with the disease as well as the acute and chronic problems that accompany it.

Specific nursing diagnoses are:

- Fear related to the life-threatening status of the disease
- Alteration in body image due to exfoliative skin
- Altered skin integrity
- Potential for infection
- Impaired maintenance of body heat
- Altered mobility due to contractures
- Impaired nutrition due to anorexia.

In the early stages of the disease, the nurse monitors the condition of the skin. As the disease progresses, continued assessment must be made of the skin, especially in regard to the degree of flaking and presence of open, weeping lesions. The nurse also monitors the patient's level of mobility, body temperature, and nutritional status in order to identify associated problems early in their development.

Interventions

The goals of nursing management are to reduce fear and anxiety, to assist the patient to cope with a changing body image, to maintain skin integrity and prevent infection, to maintain normal body temperature, to maintain appropriate joint mobility, and to provide for adequate nutrition.

Cutaneous T-cell lymphoma is a cancer and, like the others described above, involves fears and concerns about death, body image, and acceptance by others. The concerns about acceptance are accentuated by the severe skin exfoliation that often accompanies this disease. Another factor that makes the psychosocial needs so important is the long-term aspect of the disease; initial interest may wane after awhile. The nurse must usually work with both the patient and family to facilitate working through these psychosocial concerns and to maintain their continued supportive behavior. Self-help groups may provide needed support.

Good skin care is essential. The patient has a continual problem with dry and scaling skin. Because of the open lesions, there is a high danger of skin infection. Personal hygiene must be emphasized, using mild, superfatted soap and medicated bath oils. Creams and ointments may be used to moisturize the skin. Hydrophilic petrolatum with diisopropyl sebacate and isopropyl myristate bath oil and hydrocortisone are especially effective. Ureas increase lubrication of the skin, and methols may be effective in decreasing pruritus. Oral antihistamines may be necessary in the instance of severe itching.

As the disease progresses and the lesions become open, weeping sores, problems of drainage and infection become paramount. Extra blankets may be necessary to counteract the chilling caused by evaporation of the drainage from large parts of the body. There is also a problem when the drainage dries, sticking the patient's clothing or bedclothes to the skin. Sheets of nonadherent dressing material may be used to line the bed or the clothing. Room deodorizers may be necessary to combat the foul odor that often accompanies the drainage. Whirlpool baths and skin debridement may be used in conjunction with antibacterial soaps to fight the infection. Careful hand washing by the nurse is very important.

During acute stages of the disease, the patient becomes seriously ill with erythematous and exfoliating skin, severe pruritis, fever, and a general feeling of being ill. There is much difficulty keeping warm, and a cycle often starts in which dilation and fixation of the blood vessels leads to lack of body heat conservation causing even more chilling. Heat-conserving measures will be needed, but care must be taken not to burn the skin which is very vulnerable.

Contractures are a rather common complication of this disease. In an attempt to get warm and as a response to pain, the patient often huddles into a fetal position and stays there for long periods of time. It is important to do range-of-motion exercises on a regular basis during this phase of the disease. Slow, planned actions with frequent rest periods help accomplish this goal.

Finally, with the significant loss of drainage through the skin and the patient's usual lack of appetite, it is vital for the nurse to be creative in meeting the patient's nutritional needs. It is especially important to provide increased fluid intake and foods high in protein.

The care of patients with cutaneous T-cell lymphoma ranges from minimal supervision of ambulatory care when the disease is in a remissive phase to intensive care during the acute phase. The patient's problems make nursing care a challenge.

Evaluation

Outcome criteria for goal achievement are:

1. Patient and significant others discuss feelings and concerns about the diagnosis and its probable outcome.
2. Patient describes an appropriate psychological support system.
3. Skin will be moist with minimal scaling.
4. There will be no signs of skin infection.
5. The patient will maintain a normal body temperature.
6. The patient will maintain normal joint mobility.
7. The patient's nutritional intake will be adequate to meet needs.

Kaposi's Sarcoma

Kaposi's sarcoma was first described in 1869 and has always been considered a disease primarily affecting men of Mediterranean or Jewish descent, usually in their fifties and sixties. It has also been known that African blacks, young homosexual men, and immunosuppressed people also developed the disease, but these latter groups have been considered insignificant in size. However, with the recent identification and increasing incidence of autoimmune deficiency syndrome (AIDS; see Chap 17), there has been a renewed interest in Kaposi's sarcoma. The progression of Kaposi's sarcoma is often seen as a harbinger of AIDS and is much more aggressive in the AIDS' host than when it occurs as an isolated disease.

Etiology and Pathophysiology

The etiology of this disease is not totally known, although genetics has always been considered a prime factor.

Its link with people having a compromised immune system strongly indicates that it may develop because of an "exhausted" immune system, possibly as a result of multiple infections. There is also continued work to discover a transmissible agent, especially a virus.

The lesions of Kaposi's sarcoma usually begin in the mid-dermis and extend upward into the dermis. They may appear anywhere, including the mucous membranes, and are frequently found on the lower extremities (Fig. 95–7). The lesions may arise as either a patch, plaque, or nodule, although they frequently first appear as a dark blue or purple macule. The lower extremities are the most common initial site with the dorsum of the foot and the area between the toes becoming frequent extension sites. There are four clinical classifications:

1. Nodular—slow growing, found on the extremities
2. Florid "vegetating" or "fungating"—rapid growth, often ulcerated
3. Infiltrate—found in the dermis and deeper structure, often including the bone
4. Lymphadenopathic—aggressive and disseminated, usually affecting children and young adults and not found very often.[23]

Clinical Manifestations

The lesions are the first manifestation of the disease. Then, as the disease progresses, the number of lesions increases and they coalesce into large plaques which often become ulcerated or eroded. Frequently, there is edema of the lower extremities which indicates that invasion into the lymphatics has occurred. Patients often complain of pain and tenderness. Continued progression brings involvement to the gastrointestinal system, spleen, liver, bone, lung, and pleura.

Medical Management

Diagnosis. Diagnosis is generally established through recognition of the lesions. Radiologic and radioisotope studies may be done to establish the extent of disease progression.

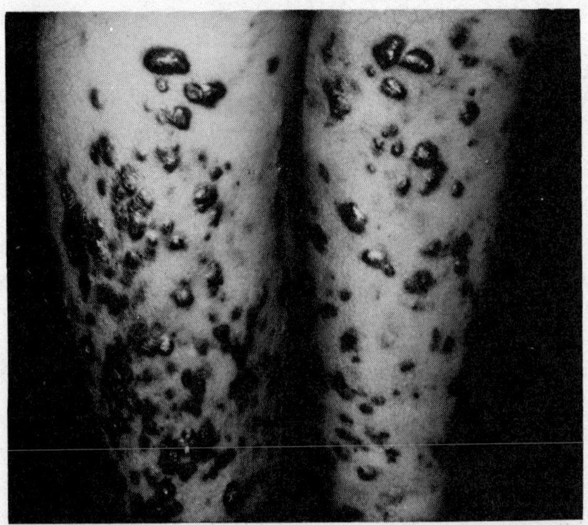

FIGURE 95–7 Kaposi's sarcoma. (Dobson RL, Abele DC: The Practice of Dermatology, p 296. Philadelphia, JB Lippincott, 1985)

Treatment. Radiation has been the classical treatment for Kaposi's sarcoma, especially when the disease is localized. Combination chemotherapy is now being used in more aggressive treatment of the disease. Antineoplastic agents, such as vinblastine, doxorubicin, bleomycin, nitrogen mustard, and actinomycin may be administered intralesionally, intra-arterially, or intravenously. Immunotherapy is also used in an attempt to stabilize the patient's immune system. Bovine-thymic extracts, thymopoietin, monoclonal antibodies, and interferon have been used.

Prognosis. The prognosis for people having Kaposi's sarcoma has become more dim in recent years. Previously, the mean survival rate was 8 to 13 years, but more recently, this survival time has decreased to 3 to 20 *months.*[20]

Nursing Management

Assessment and Nursing Diagnosis

Nursing diagnoses for patients exhibiting signs of Kaposi's sarcoma are related to the fear of death, potential for skin infection, and the need for education regarding sexual activity.

The nursing diagnoses are

- Fear related to the life-threatening implications of the disease
- Potential for skin infection
- Knowledge deficits related to restriction of sexual contacts.

The nurse may identify the lesions of Kaposi's sarcoma during specific skin assessment or routine nursing care. It is important to follow through on the identification of any suspicious skin lesions.

Interventions

The goals of nursing management are to reduce the accompanying fear and anxiety for both the patient and significant others, to prevent skin infection, and to teach the patient about measures to prevent further complications.

As mentioned above, the survival rate with this disease is significantly declining. In addition, its correlation with AIDS has been well-publized in recent years. Therefore, a tentative or positive diagnosis of Kaposi's sarcoma will likely cause high anxiety in the patient as well as in significant others. The nurse needs to be sensitive to this need. The patient may also experience isolation from others. Individual and group counseling may be needed to help the people involved cope with the chronicity and probable outcome of the disease and to help the patient and significant others maintain a supportive relationship.

The kind of skin care needed to prevent infection depends on the status of the lesions. When there are no breaks in the skin, nursing interventions are directed toward maintaining skin integrity. When lesions are open and draining, more intensive measures are needed to prevent secondary infection. Advanced lesions also bleed easily and must be protected from trauma.

Unlike other cutaneous cancers, there does not seem to be a sun-exposure factor in the development of this disease. However, because of the the hypothesized link to sexual activity and because of the accompanying compromised immune system, it must be recommended to the patient that sexual contacts be decreased to reduce the chances of acquiring herpes or cytomegalorvirus.[6, 20]

Evaluation

Outcome criteria for goal achievement are:

1. Patient and significant others discuss feelings and concerns about the disease and its probable outcome.
2. Patient describes an appropriate psychological support system.
3. There are no signs of skin infection.
4. The patient describes appropriate measures to prevent complications through limiting sexual contact.

Nonmalignant Neoplasias

Keratoses

Keratoses are generally benign tumors of the skin, although some varieties are considered to be premalignant. There are two main varieties of this kind of cellular growth: seborrheic keratosis and actinic keratosis.

Etiology and Pathophysiology

Seborrheic Keratosis. Seborrheic keratoses are the most common benign skin tumors that appear in older persons as part of the aging process. The most common sites for these tumors are the trunk, face, scalp, and extremities. The lesions vary from flesh-colored to almost black with tan and brown being the most frequent colors (Fig. 95–8). They may be flat, but are usually verrucous (wartlike). In some areas, like the groin and eyelid, they can develop a pedunculated appearance. They have a "stuck-on" appearance and can usually be partially lifted off the skin, demonstrating some friability. Because of this characteristic tendency, they are easily irritated and may undergo histologic changes so that they resemble malignant growths.

These growths appear suddenly and grow rapidly, increasing both in number and in size of existing lesions. Although they may sometimes be a sign of internal malignancy, these lesions themselves rarely, if ever, become malignant. The main problem associated with them is their cosmetic effect.

Actinic Keratosis. Actinic keratoses are considered to be premalignant lesions, precursors to development of squamous cell carcinoma, although only about 25% progress to this stage.[3] They represent accumulated actinic damage as a direct result of chronic sun exposure and so appear in areas of the skin generally open to sunlight. The lesions appear as scaly papules with an irregular surface and sharp, distinct borders (Fig. 95–9). Colors include yellow, tan, brown, and black. They are frequently covered by a coarse, adherent scale that can be easily peeled off, but which grows back quickly.

Clinical Manifestations

The lesions themselves are the primary clinical manifestation. There may be some pruritis and sometimes

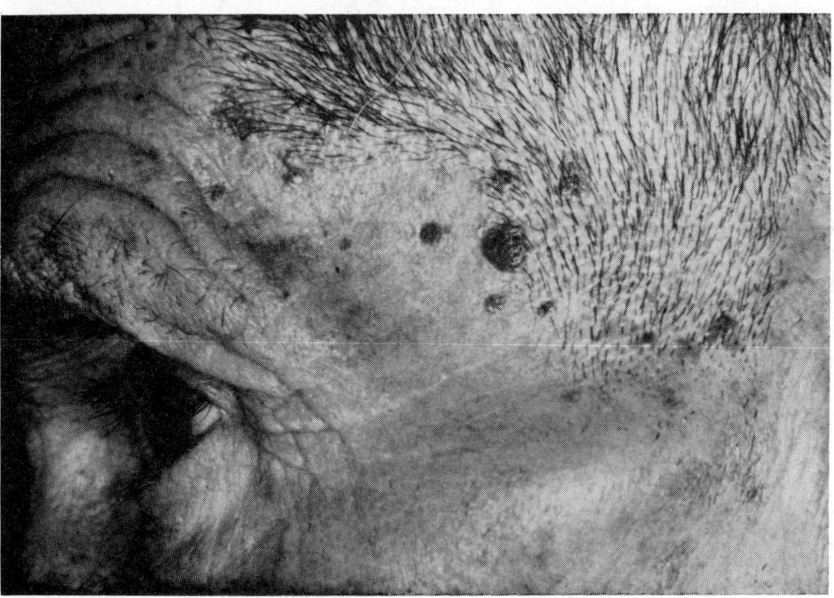

FIGURE 95–8 Early seborrheic keratosis. (Dobson RL, Abele DC: The Practice of Dermatology, p 275. Philadelphia, JB Lippincott, 1985)

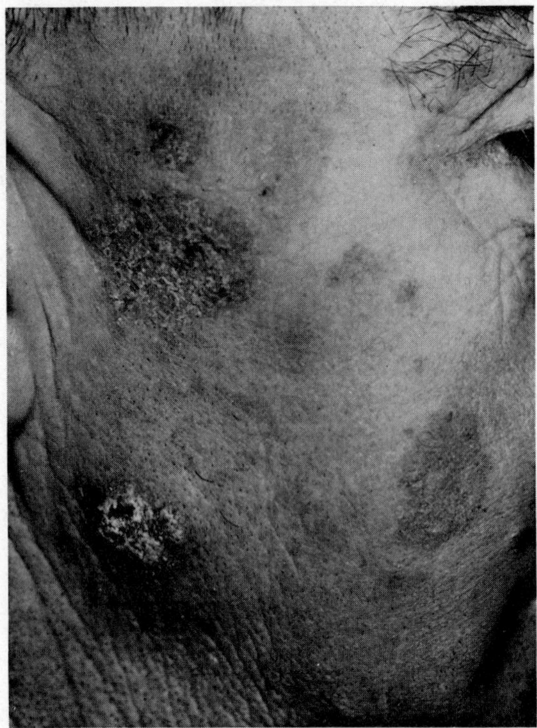

FIGURE 95–9 Actinic keratoses. (Dobson RL, Abele DC: The Practice of Dermatology, p 277. Philadelphia, JB Lippincott, 1985)

some tenderness if the lesion has been irritated. With actinic keratosis, the surrounding skin may show signs of chronic actinic damage, such as mottled pigmentation, telangiectases, and furrowing.

Medical Management

Treatment. Once the diagnosis has been determined, the lesion is removed by cryosurgery, curettage and dessication, scalpel incision, or topical chemotherapy. The topical agent 5-flourouracil is applied to the area for several weeks. The immediate reaction to the chemotherapy treatment is inflammation within 48 to 72 hours following by erosion, then disappearance of the lesion with no significant residual skin effect; it may take several weeks for the healing process to be completed.

Prognosis. Because these lesions are generally nonmalignant, the prognosis is excellent. Once in a while, though, a lesion will become malignant, so medical assessment is suggested for all lesions.

Nursing Management

Assessment and Nursing Diagnosis

Nursing diagnoses for patients with keratoses are related to the prevention of infection after medical treatment and the need for prevention.

The nursing diagnoses are:

- Potential for wound infection
- Knowledge deficits related to prevention of further keratotic lesions.

The primary role of nursing assessment is to identify skin lesions that need medical follow-up. As mentioned above, it is important for the nurse to be aware of suspicious skin lesions.

Interventions

The goals of nursing management are to prevent wound infection and to teach the patient necessary self-care of the wound and preventive measures.

Because the lesion is usually small, the treatment site is simple and requires little care. The area should be kept clean and, if it is easily irritated by clothing, a nonadherent dressing may be placed over it. If topical chemotherapy is being used, the patient should be reminded to follow the prescribed schedule for application for the entire time suggested. Because the healing time is sometimes so long, the person may also need to be encouraged to be patient.

Especially with actinic keratosis, it is important to teach the patient about avoiding sun exposure. Sunscreens with high PABA ratings should be used and protective clothing worn as much as possible.

Evaluation

Outcome criteria for goal achievement are:

1. A clean wound with no signs of infection (absence of redness, swelling, purulent discharge)
2. Patient accurately describes measures to prevent recurrence of keratoses.

Psoriasis

Etiology and Pathophysiology

Psoriasis has been characterized by the advertising media as "the heartbreak of psoriasis." It is a chronic skin disease affected 1% to 2% of the population in the United States. It is a disorder characterized by unpredictable remissions and exacerbations. It affects males and females in equal frequency and, although it can first appear at any age, it usually presents before the age of 30 years. It is rarely found in blacks and American Indians. There is evidence of genetic predisposition, although environmental factors and stress are also considered as significant contributing components.

The basic defect causing this disease is uncontrolled growth of epidermal cells. The exact cause of this process is unknown. However, it appears that three things occur. First, there is an increased mitotic rate of the epidermal cells and a shortened transit time from the basal layer to the corneum stratum. The turnover time of viable epidermal cells goes from its normal rate of 28 days to a new rate of 3 to 4 days. Secondly, there is abnormal keratinization so that the horny layer of the psoriatic lesion sloughs off readily removing protection of the underlying skin. Thirdly, there is dilatation of the upper dermal vessels and periodic discharge of polymorphonuclear leukocytes into the dermal layer.

There are several forms of psoriasis. *Psoriasis vulgaris* is the most common type. It is identified by its well-defined, coinlike, red or salmon-colored scales covered with an adherent silvery scale (Fig. 95–10). The scales are generally quite thick and the edges are well-delineated from the normal surrounding skin. A very typical feature of this form is its symmetry.

Psoriasis guttata involves red or salmon-colored plaques dotting the body in droplike forms. These lesions are distributed like drops of water after a shower. Frequently the patient gives a recent history of an upper respiratory infection.

Psoriasis invernus is identified by its bright red patches. These lesions are usually found in flexural areas, such as the groin, gluteal fold, axillae, and under the breasts. Because these areas are usually moist, scaling is not generally seen. As above, symmetry is a typical finding.

Pustular psoriasis can occur in a generalized form or be restricted to the palms or soles. It is not as common as the above forms of psoriasis, but its presence may indicate significant systemic disease. This form is characterized by the appearance of multiple pinhead-sized, sterile pustules that tend to arise in crops and spread centrifugally. After 1 to 2 days, the skin over the pustules desquamates and new pustules form around the scaling area. This type of psoriasis is often accompanied by fever, malaise, leukocytosis, and the patient may also demonstrate arthralgia and arthritis.

Clinical Manifestations

The most characteristic finding of psoriasis is the appearance of lesions as described above. These lesions may appear anywhere on the body. They are, however, most commonly found on the elbows, knees, scalp, and lower trunk. Nail edges are also often affected with accompanying pitting of the nail itself. The patient also characteristically complains of pruritis in the affected areas, although this finding may be absent.

Two definitive clinical findings in psoriasis are Koebner's isomorphic phenomenon and Auspitz's sign. In *Koebner's isomorphic phenomenon,* there is characteristic reaction that usually occurs 7 to 18 days after trauma to the skin, such as a scratch, acute sunburn, or contact dermatitis. Typical new psoriatic lesions appear along the line of the original injury. *Auspitz's sign* refers to the punctate bleeding points that appear under the scale when it is manually removed. The presence of the latter finding, however, is not very helpful in the diagnostic process, because it usually occurs only in patients whose lesions are obvious from their clinical appearance.

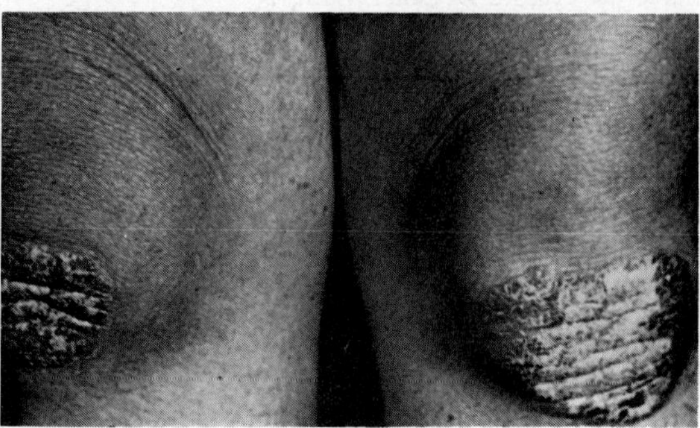

FIGURE 95–10 A typical plaque of psoriasis on the knee. (Dobson RL, Abele DC: The Practice of Dermatology, p 56. Philadelphia, JB Lippincott, 1985)

In *pustular psoriasis,* laboratory studies may show leukocytosis and an elevated sedimentation rate. Otherwise, there are no consistent findings.

Medical Management

Treatment. Besides symptomatic relief, medical treatment is aimed at two main goals: slow down cell proliferation and normalize the keratinization process. This is accomplished primarily through the application of topical agents and the use of phototherapy. Systemic chemotherapy may also be used.

Topical Steroids. The mainstay of treatment of psoriasis is the use of topical steroids. They are used for their anti-inflammatory effects, and they also help lubricate the lesions. Although ointment forms are more effective, they are often not cosmetically acceptable to the patient and creams may be needed in order to gain patient compliance. The medication should be applied two to three times a day, and an occlusive dressing may be used to enhance the effectiveness of the steroid. The underdesirable side-effects of steroids can occur with prolonged use of topical applications.

Topical steroids are expensive and therefore are not generally used when very large body areas are affected. There are also significant side-effects when they are used for long periods. These include adrenal suppression, thinning of the skin and cutaneous atrophy, telangiectasia, development of striae and superimposed fungal and bacterial infections. There may also be rebound effects when the medication is discontinued, and there have been instances when stable disease has been converted to an unstable state.

In severe episodes, corticosteroids may need to be given systemically for a short period of time. They may also be injected intralesionally.

Tar Compounds. Tar compounds may be used alone or in conjunction with ultraviolet light therapy. There is some thought that these compounds depress DNA synthesis; however, their exact therapeutic action is unknown. Their effectiveness in the treatment of psoriasis has been accepted for many decades. Tar compounds are the cheapest treatment available and have the fewest side-effects. However, the crude forms have a bad smell, are very messy, and stain clothing readily. Therefore, patient compliance is a problem in their use. Manufacturers continue to develop new forms which will be more acceptable to patients while at the same time retaining their therapeutic effectiveness. They also cause photosensitization so that patients using them must avoid excessive sun exposure. Use on hairy parts of the body may result in folliculitis.

Tar compounds may be put in bath water, used as shampoos, and applied in ointment and cream forms. Patient compliance is improved if the latter forms can be used only at night.

Anthralin (dithranol) is a coal-tar distillate which inhibits cell growth and is used for this effect in psoriasis. As with the coal tars, it may be used alone or in conjunction with ultraviolet therapy. Its major side-effect is the irritation it causes on the surrounding skin. This can result in redness and blistering. Therefore, it is important that it be applied only to the plaques themselves. Another important problem regards its staining property; all forms stain clothing and the paste form of this medication crumbles and falls off, staining bedding and carpets.

Kerolytic Agents. The thick scales covering psoriatic lesions often interfere with therapeutic penetration of topical medications applied to them. Therefore, kerolytic agents, such as salicylic acid and urea, may be used to remove these scales. These agents may be applied twice a day and the patient then bathes daily in tepid water, removing the scales with nonvigorous friction.

Emollients. Because dry skin is such a major problem in psoriasis, emollients are frequently used to moisturize the skin and to decrease pruritus. White petrolatum is inexpensive and very effective, although its greasiness requires some care with clothing and bedding. There are a number of water-miscible based compounds available over the counter which moisturize the skin without staining clothing. These emollients may be applied in the form of bath oils.

Phototherapy or Photochemotherapy. Visible or ultraviolet radiation may be used alone (phototherapy) or in conjunction with topical agents, such as tar compounds or dithranol, or with systemic psoralens, such as methoxypsoralen, which sensitize the epidermis to the ultraviolet rays (photochemotherapy). This therapy is very effective in the development of remissions, probably through inhibition of DNA synthesis and resultant slowing of cell division. There are, however, significant side-effects (erythema and blistering, pruritus, nausea and vomiting, headache, and dizziness; the latter effects may be caused by the oral psoralens rather than the radiation itself). These symptoms are transient and will disappear when therapy is discontinued. However, there is some concern about long-term effects which include hyperpigmentation and premature skin aging, carcinogenesis, cataract development, impaired cell-mediated immunity, and exacerbation of other photosensitive diseases. These reactions do not become obvious until after 10 to 15 years of therapy, but their possibility must be considered when making the decision about instituting phototherapy.[13]

Sunlight is the cheapest and usually the most convenient form of ultraviolet-B (UVB) phototherapy. In climates where the sun is dependable, the patient may be advised to sunbathe daily. In fact, it has been generally known that psoriatic patients improve during the summer. Care must be taken by these patients, as well as by patients using articifical light sources, to avoid overexposure to the sun. Sunscreens and protective clothing must be used freely during sun exposure times not intended for therapy. Artificial sunlight sources may deliver a more dependable dose of radiation and may be more convenient in many climates.

Other Systemic Agents. Methotrexate and other antimetabolic agents may be used in recalcitrant cases of psoriasis to inhibit cell DNA synthesis and thereby slow cell division. These agents are accepted as therapeutic alternatives and are effective. However, because of their potential toxic effects, they must be used very judiciously. Patients receiving these agents commonly complain of nausea, vomiting, and oral ulceration. Leukopenia, thrombycytopenia, and liver abnormalities are frequently found side-effects.

Retinoids are being investigated for use in the treatment of severe psoriasis. While the specific mechanism of action is not clear, they have been found to be effective in causing remissions of the disease. However, there are several side-effects that must be monitored. Patients frequently report symptoms of dry mucous membranes, alopecia, fragile skin, peeling of soles and palms, and pruritus. There is also evidence of elevated serum triglycerides.[14,15] These agents may also be used in conjunction with PUVA therapy.

Prognosis. Psoriasis is not a curable disease, but one that demonstrates cycles of remission and exacerbation. The course of the disease is very individualized with some patients never being totally free of the disease, while others have only periodic flare-ups with very long clear periods. The disease is primarily a nuisance disease with definite psychological implications because of the reaction of others to the uncosmetic skin appearance. It does not have life-threatening implications, although the high incidence of arthritis in patients having psoriasis means significant pain and immobility problems.

Nursing Management

Assessment and Nursing Diagnosis

Nursing diagnoses for patients with psoriasis relate to the psychological discomfort caused by the disease and its treatment; reduction of dry, scaly skin; and the need for education about how to follow through with medical treatments, the prevention of complications during treatment, and how to reduce the chance of exacerbations.

The nursing diagnoses are:

- Alteration in psychological comfort due to chronicity of the disease and altered body image
- Altered skin integrity due to dryness and erythemic reaction
- Knowledge deficits related to safe maintenance of treatment regimen and measures to reduce exacerbations.

Nursing assessment is primarily of the affected parts of the skin. Careful observation of the lesions for improvement or lack thereof help to guide the treatment regimen. Other parts of the body also need to be observed for development of new lesions. Especially in the beginning of the treatment phase, the nurse also needs to observe the patient's technique in applying the prescribed topical agents to make sure this is being done properly.

Interventions

The goals of nursing management are to help the patient and significant others adjust to the chronicity and altered body image that accompany psoriasis, to promote maximum skin integrity, and to teach the patient the necessary self-care of the skin and preventive precautions.

The diagnosis of psoriasis is very disturbing to the psychological comfort of both the patient and significant others. It is a chronic disease with no cure. The treatments are messy, expensive, and time-consuming. In addition, during active periods of disease, the patient experiences flaking skin and unpleasant lesions which are often repulsive to both the patient and others in the environment. This may cause physical, social, and emotional rejection of the patient. Active listening skills and helping the people involved talk to each other facilitates adjustment to this disease. Support groups may provide needed assistance in this area. There is a growing number of day centers where patients can receive therapy and also meet with other psoriatic patients. The National Psoriasis Foundation can be a helpful resource in the community. The on-going nature of the disease means an on-going need for support, and the nurse often needs to remind especially the significant others of this necessity.

Helping to make the treatment regimen as acceptable as possible facilitates compliance by the patient. Because so many of the topical agents used in the treatment of psoriasis are messy and stain the clothing, the nurse needs to work with the physician and patient to find the most acceptable agent. Alcohol-based tars, which are nongreasy and do not stain the clothing, may be used during the day; water-miscible and oil-miscible vehicles may be saved for night-time use when they do not interfere as much with social interaction. The patient may be encouraged to use emollients either as topical agents or in the bath to help maintain moisturization of the skin.

Prevention of complications of treatment concern two main areas: prevention of further skin irritation and eye protection. Because the patient is responsible for his ongoing care, he needs to be taught how to prevent these complications. While sunlight in the appropriate dosage is therapeutic to patients with psoriasis, too much sun can be harmful. The patient needs to be careful to receive enough sun exposure to produce a therapeutic result, but not enough to burn the skin which will aggravate the psoriasis. What is wanted is a slight skin redness. Patients need to be careful about time of the day, overcast days, and duration of skin exposure. When in the sun during nontreatment times, the patient must be careful to use protective clothing or sunscreens frequently. Patients using coal tar agents or psoralens are particularly photosensitive and must take meticulous precautions against prolonged sun exposure.

Patients using dithranol must be cautioned periodically against getting any of the medication on the skin surrounding the psoriatic lesions. This medication is very irritating to normal skin and may cause extension of the disease as well as severe erythema and blistering.

The eyes must be protected against ultraviolet radiation. Protective goggles must be worn during actual phototherapy and the patient must be sure that this eyewear adequately protects the eyes. Patients who are using photosensitization agents must be careful to wear appropriate sunglasses whenever they are in the sun. Especially when taking psoralens, it is recommended that sunglasses be worn for up to 2 days after taking the medication.

The patient needs to be taught how to stay in remission. This generally means keeping the possible causative factors to a minimum. A generally healthy lifestyle with good nutrition, rest, and exercise help the body maintain its resistance. Emotional stress should be avoided. Illnesses such as colds and the flu should be treated early. Skin trauma, such as cuts and scratches, should be avoided as much as possible. When recurrence of psoriatic lesions occurs, treatment should begin as early as possible in an attempt to avoid a severe episode.

Evaluation

Outcome criteria for goal achievement are:

1. Patient and significant others discuss feelings and concerns about the disease and its treatmen.
2. Patient describes an effective support system.
3. Patient does not experience physical, social, or emotional isolation.
4. The patient consistently follows the prescribed treatment regimen.
5. The patient has minimal dry, flaky skin.
6. The patient describes appropriate protective measures to avoid the complications of therapy.
7. The patient describes appropriate measures to maximize remissions of the disease.

References

1. Albright S: Treatment of skin cancer using multiple modalities. J Am Acad Dermatol 7:143, 1982
2. Anders J, Leach E: Sun versus skin. Am J Nurs 83:1015, 1983
3. Ariel I: Malignant Melanoma. New York, Appleton-Century-Crofts, 1981
4. Bickers D: Skin cancer: Occupational causes. Consult 22:392, 1982
5. Binnick S: Skin Diseases: Diagnosis and Management in Clinical Practice. Menlo Park, Addison-Wesly, 1982
6. Borkovic S, et al: Kaposi's sarcoma. Am Fam Physician 26:133, 1982
7. Dahl M: Common Office Dermatology. New York, Grune & Stratton, 1983
8. Draelos Z, et al: Hyperthermic treatment of cutaneous malignancies. J Am Acad Dermatol 9:623, 1983
9. Dzrebow L, et al: Risk factors for local recurrence of primary cutaneous squamous cell carcinomas. Arch Dermatol 118:900, 1982
10. Eddy J, Selgas-Cordes R, Curran M: Cutaneous T-cell lymphoma. Am J Nurs 84:202, 1984
11. Eddy J, Selgas-Cordes R, Curran M: Sam was dying. . .we had to help him live again. . .mycosis fungoides—An often fatal form of cutaneous T-cell lymphoma. Nursing '81 11:42, 1981

12. Epstein J: Photocarcinogenetic skin cancer and aging. J Am Acad Dermatol 9:487, 1983
13. Farber E, et al: Long-term risks of psoralen and UV-A therapy for psoriasis. Arch Dermatol 119:426, 1983
14. Farber E, et al: Recent advances in the treatment of psoriasis. J Am Acad Dermatol 8:311, 1983
15. Lowe N: Psoriasis therapy: A current perspective. West J Med 139:184, 1983
16. Pollack S: The biology of basal cell carcinoma: A review. J Am Acad Dermatol 7:569, 1982
17. Resnik S: Alternatives to surgery for facial lesions. Consult 19:98, 1979
18. Robinson J: Moh's surgery for skin cancer. Am J Nurs 82:282, 1982
19. Roses D, Harris M, Ackerman A: Diagnosis and Management of Cutaneous Malignant Melanoma. Philadelphia, WB Saunders, 1983
20. Sears H, et al: Kaposi's sarcoma: A deadly new syndrome. Nurs Pract 8:25, 1983
21. Sober A: Diagnosis and management of skin cancer. Cancer 51:2448, 1983
22. Stern R, et al: Skin typing for assessment of skin cancer risk and acute response to UV-B and oral methoxsalen. Arch Dermatol 120:869, 1984
23. Swanson N: Basal cell carcinoma. Treatment modalities and recommendations. Primary Care 10:443, 1983
24. Warshauer D, et al: Sunlight and protection of the skin. Am Fam Physician 27:109, 1983

Bibliography

Ackerman A, Niven J, Grant-Kels: Differential Diagnosis in Dermatopathology. Philadelphia, Lea & Febiger, 1982

Arnold V, et al: Photochemotherapy for psoriasis. Am J Nurs 79:466, 1979

Boer J, et al: Comparison of phototherapy (UV-B) and photochemotherapy (PUVA) for clearing and maintenance therapy of psoriasis. Arch Dermatol 120:52, 1984

Cangialosi C: Plantar keratosis. Why treatment often fails and what to do about it. Postgrad Med 75:128, 1984

Cassileth B, et al: A psychological comparison of patients with malignant melanoma and other dermatologic disorders. J Am Acad Dermatol 7:742, 1982

Coker D, et al: Chemotherapy for metastatic basal cell carcinoma. Arch Dermatol 119:14, 1983

Dubin N, et al: Multivariate risk score for recurrence of cutaneous basal cell carcinomas. Arch Dermatol 119:373, 1983

Fraser M, McGuire D: Skin cancer's early warning system. Am J Nurs 84:1232, 1984

Heckel P: Teaching patients to cope with psoriasis: The unshared disease. Nursing '81 11:49, 1981

Immerman S, et al: Recurrent squamous cell carcinoma of the skin. Cancer 51:1537, 1983

Jelinek J: Aspects of heredity, syndromic associations, and course of conditions in which cutaneous lesions occur solitarily or in multiplicity. J Acad Dermatol 7:526, 1982

Lamberg S, et al: Clinical staging for cutaneous T-cell lymphoma. Ann Intern Med 100:187, 1984

Libbus K: Psoriasis and body image. Nurs Pract 7:15, 1982

Lubritz R, et al: Cryosurgery care rate of actinic keratosis. J Acad Dermatol 7:631, 1982

Menter A: Psoriasis. Hosp Med 20:43, 1984

Petroyzi J, et al: Ultraviolet phototherapy in psoriasis with hydrophilic ointment alone or with crude coal tar. Arch Dermatol Res 272:257, 1982

Ragay A: Skin growths: Differentiating the benign from the malignant. Consult 24:128, 1984

Subrt P, et al: Spreading pigmented actinic keratosis. J Am Acad Dermatol 8:63, 1983

Wolska H, et al: Etretinate in severe psoriasis: Results of a double-blind study and maintenance therapy in pustular psoriasis. J Am Acad Dermatol 9:883, 1983

Zacarian S: Cryosurgery of cutaneous carcinomas. J Am Acad Dermatol 9:947, 1983

Chapter 96

Burn Injuries and Skin Trauma

Janet Marvin

Skin Trauma

Trauma to the integumentary system occurs in numerous ways and ranges from simple lacerations and bruises to major abrasion or degloving injuries and burn injuries. Complications from such injuries range from none or simple linear scars to major tissue loss and systemic complications. Simple injuries to the skin—bruises, lacerations, blisters, ulcerations, hematomas—require minimal care other than cleansing and protection from infections or additional trauma. Major skin trauma, such as large abraded surfaces, burn injuries, crush injuries or degloving injuries, may damage not only the surface of the skin but may involve underlying subcutaneous tissues and may cause major systemic problems such as fluid loss and potential infection or sepsis. Additionally, these injuries may result in major functional loss, pain, and significant psychological sequelae. Because the problems of patients with these major skin injuries are similar to those of patients with major burn injuries, this chapter focuses on the care of the burned patient.

Burn Injuries

Estimating Burn Injuries

The burn injury is defined in two ways: the *extent* or *percent* of body surface area involved, and the *depth* or *amount* of anatomical tissue destroyed.

Percentage Formulas. The *percent* of the total body surface area (TBSA) may be estimated by using a simple formula such as the Rule of Nines devised by Pulaski and Tennison (Fig. 96–1) or a more specific formula such as the Berkow or Lund and Browder (Fig. 96–2).[9,36] Although the Rule of Nines is an easy formula to remember and allows for a quick estimate of burn size, the more specific or detailed formulas allow for a more accurate estimate. Because formulas for fluid resuscitation and caloric intake are based on these estimates, it is necessary for such estimates to be as accurate as possible. When using one of the more detailed formulas for estimations of extent one should not only estimate the extent of the burn but the areas which are not burned. Comparison of the estimates of burned and unburned areas allows for a more accurate estimation of burn size. When estimating the size of small burns, a simple rule to remember is that the palm of the patient's hand represents 1% of body surface area.

Burn Depth. The *depth* of burn is much more difficult to define and may be related to degree of burn (lst, 2nd, 3rd) or to skin thickness (superficial or moderate partial thickness, deep partial thickness, or full thickness). There are currently no tests which accurately define the depth of injury, and even an expert practitioner is often wrong. Knowing how the injury occurred may be somewhat helpful. For example, a steam injury is usually very superficial whereas a flame injury is almost always full thickness. Textbooks abound with clinical descriptions, as seen in Table 96–1, yet in clinical practice one might ask why this is important. Until recently, it really was not important because all burn wounds were managed expectantly with partial thickness wounds allowed to heal over several weeks and full thickness wounds grafted when granulation tissue formed. With the improvements in intensive care, blood banking, and surgical and anesthetic management of patients, burn care has changed, making early excision of deeper wounds feasible. With early excision the morbidity from many of these injuries has been reduced and the functional and cosmetic outcomes have improved.[24] Therefore accurate early diagnosis of wound depth has become much more important.

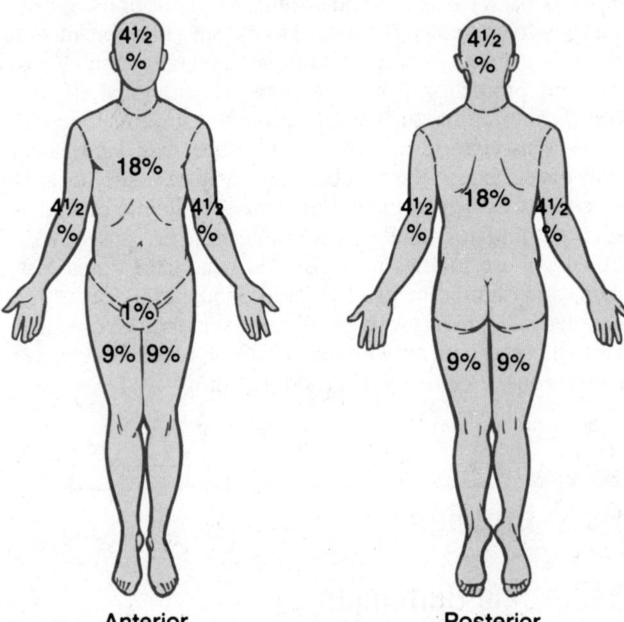

FIGURE 96–1 Rule of nines, a rapid method of estimating percentage of body surface involved.

Currently many techniques to determine wound depth such as light reflection of red, green, and infrared rays, ultrasound, and fluorescent dyes are being investigated.[28,49,58] Although there is a paucity of data to confirm the current clinical impressions, it seems that partial thickness wounds which heal in 3 weeks or less leave minimal residual scars and that full thickness or deeper partial thickness wounds that require more than 3 weeks to heal give rise to thick hypertrophic scars which may limit mobility and present major cosmetic concerns.

Although the depth of the wound is usually judged within a few hours after the injury, the actual depth of the wound may not be accurately judged for 2 to 3 days, especially in the patient with extensive burns. As described by Jackson, the wound initially may have areas of complete necrosis surrounded by areas of stasis and these areas may have adjacent areas of hyperemia.[31] Depending on the adequacy of central and peripheral circulation, the areas of stasis and hyperemia may progress to areas of coagulation necrosis or may have normal vascularity restored. Therefore, until resuscitation is complete and the patient is hemodynamically stable, the evaluation of depth cannot be completed. Likewise as the wounds begin the healing process, if infection or local or systemic hypotension occurs, areas of the wound may become progressively deeper.

Etiology and Epidemiology

Although a review of fire catastrophes (fires causing 25 or more deaths) has shown a decrease thus far in the twentieth century, burn injuries continue to be a major health-care

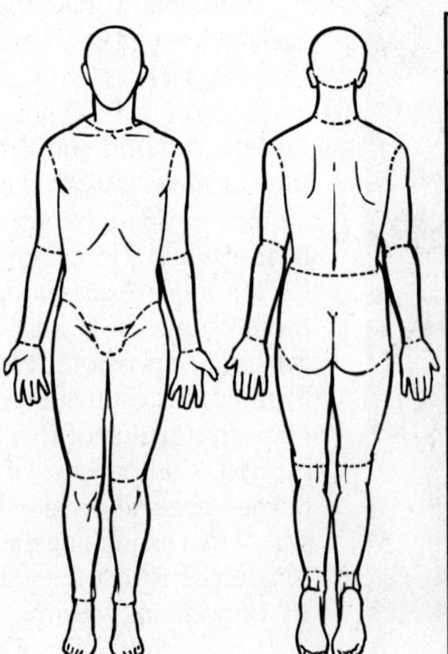

Area	1 yr	1–4 yrs	5–9 yrs	10–14 yrs	15 yrs	Adult	2°	3°
Head	19	17	13	11	9	7		
Neck	2	2	2	2	2	2		
Ant. Trunk	13	13	13	13	13	13		
Post. Trunk	13	13	13	13	13	13		
R. Buttock	2½	2½	2½	2½	2½	2½		
L. Buttock	2½	2½	2½	2½	2½	2½		
Genitalia	1	1	1	1	1	1		
R.U. Arm	4	4	4	4	4	4		
L.U. Arm	4	4	4	4	4	4		
R.L. Arm	3	3	3	3	3	3		
L.L. Arm	3	3	3	3	3	3		
R. Hand	2½	2½	2½	2½	2½	2½		
L. Hand	2½	2½	2½	2½	2½	2½		
R. Thigh	5½	6½	8	8½	9	9½		
L. Thigh	5½	6½	8	8½	9	9½		
R. Leg	5	5	5½	6	6½	7		
L. Leg	5	5	5½	6	6½	7		
R. Foot	3½	3½	3½	3½	3½	3½		
L. Foot	3½	3½	3½	3½	3½	3½		
Total								

FIGURE 96-2 Lund and Browder method of calculating burn size.

TABLE 96–1
Classification of Burn Injury

Depth	*Skin Thickness*	*Anatomical*	*Clinical Appearance*	*Time to Heal*	*Cause*	*Pain*
1st degree	Superficial partial thickness	Epidermal	Pink to red No blisters Slight edema	3–5 days	Sunburn, flash	Discomfort to touch
	Moderate partial thickness	Superficial dermal	Red to pink Moist, weeping Blisters or bullae Edematous	Less than 3 weeks	Brief contact with hot liquids, steam, or hot objects; flash	Very painful
2nd degree	Deep partial thickness	Deep dermal	Pink to pale ivory reticulated pattern Dry appearance	Greater than 3 weeks	Longer contact with hot liquids or objects, chemicals, flames	Pain response variable
3rd degree	Full thickness	Subdermal (fat, muscle, bone)	White, cherry red, brown, or black Thrombosed veins May or may not blister Dry, hard, leathery	Requires grafting for definitive closure	Prolonged contact with hot liquids or objects, flames, chemicals, electrical	Painless to pinprick

problem.[35] Estimates of the number of burn-related injuries vary widely because there is no national reporting system for burn injuries from all sources. Fire service statistics record only those injuries due to fires in which a fire service vehicle response was involved. In most burn case facilities thermal injuries due to flames comprise less than 50% of admission. Scalds, contact injuries, chemical and electrical injuries are much more common than flame burns. In addition, although these injuries combined comprise more than 50% of injuries requiring hospital care, they comprise a much larger percentage of minor burns treated as outpatients.

Scald injuries are far more common in young children, accounting for 50% to 80% of accidents in children under 3.[21,60] The incidence of flame-related injuries increases with age, and they account for 50% or more of injuries in persons older than 18 years of age. Our modern society has been described as the "burn prone society."[40] Our homes are a virtual gold mine of accidents waiting to happen; hot water, electricity, open flames, and flammable liquids are the most frequent causes of home accidents. Carelessness is the cause of 90% of home accidents. Other predisposing factors include alcoholism or alcohol consumption, carelessness, psychiatric illnesses, neurological disorders, associated injuries, and obesity.[37]

The true incidence of either hospitalized or nonhospitalized burn injuries is unknown. In many studies, the overall male-to-female ratio was 2:1. When considered by age groups the male-to-female incidence varies with a 3 : 1 ratio or greater in ages 10 to 49. Children under 4 and adults over 70 approximate a 1 : 1 male-to-female incidence rate. Most studies also indicate a high ratio of nonwhites to whites. For example, in Wallace's study nonwhites accounted for 68% of admissions.[60]

What are the costs of such injuries? In 1982, some 8 million Americans sustained traumatic injuries at an estimated cost to the nation of $61.025 billion.[5] It has been estimated that there are over 2 million burn injuries annually and the cost to the nation is $15 billion to $20 billion. These costs include only the cost of hospitalization, medical care, both acute and rehabilitation, as well as lost wages. This in no way accounts for the emotional cost to patients and families either during the acute injury or over the years that follow.

Pathophysiology and Clinical Manifestations

Burn injuries of greater than 15% to 20% of the body surface area cause significant systemic derangements affecting almost all major body systems. Those most directly affected include the cardiovascular, renal, respiratory, metabolic, immunologic, and the integumentary systems. Although the response is an integrated response; for discussion, the impact on each system will be discussed separately.

Impact of the Burn Injury on the Cardiovascular/Renal System

Injury of any kind to the integument sets in motion a number of processes intended to prevent infection and promote wound healing. These same protective processes are responsible for the many systemic responses seen after the injury. Essentially what is a local phenomenon becomes a systemic process leading to hemodynamic instability and death if the person is not treated.

The local response to tissue injury begins with the release of vasoactive substances from injured tissue which in turn causes vasodilatation and localization of leukocytes and plasma proteins in the area. With burn injuries of greater than 15% to 20% TBSA (total body surface area), this local-

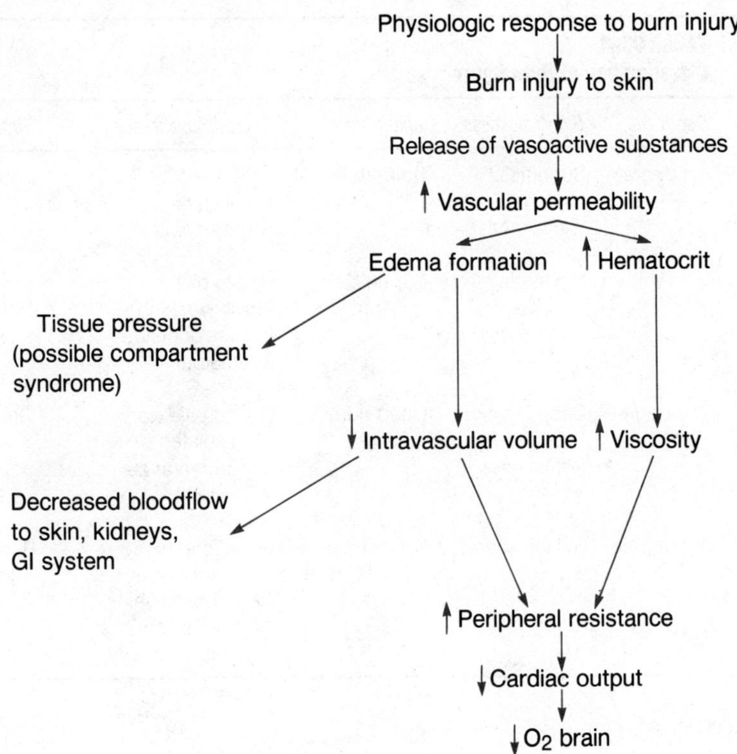

FIGURE 96–3 Physiologic response to burn injury.

ized process becomes systemic with vasodilatation and fluid loss into the interstitial tissues throughout the body. This fluid loss causes massive edema formation, decreased intravascular volume, concentration of red cells and increased blood viscosity (Fig. 96–3).

Within minutes to hours hypovolemia and decreased cardiac output may occur. Blood flow in the peripheral circulation, kidneys, and gastrointestinal tract is decreased. The patient's normal skin becomes cold, pale, and clammy, as blood is shunted to the central circulation. Blood flow to the burn wound is likewise decreased, and if this is not corrected promptly, further tissue destruction occurs. Urine output decreases as the kidneys are stimulated to conserve sodium in an attempt to compensate for the hypovolemia. Gastrointestinal motility is decreased and the lining of the stomach becomes ischemic, thus predisposing the patient to gastric irritation from gastric acid and possible ulceration. Rapid fluid resuscitation to restore the circulatory volume is imperative to prevent the progression of the injury, renal failure, and gastric ulceration.

Renal damage may also occur as a result of rhabdomyolysis (breakdown of striated muscle) caused by myoglobin released as a result of muscle damage. Muscle damage routinely occurs with electrical injuries and often with deep full thickness burn injury. The injury to the kidney in this case may be a combination of low renal perfusion and plugging of the tubules with these proteins.[29] Myoglobinuria is often accompanied by a profound acidosis, and alkalinization of the urine and massive fluid replacement are necessary to prevent permanent renal damage.

Decreased intravascular volume may eventually lead to decreased perfusion of the brain and myocardium. Decreased perfusion of the brain and decreased oxygenation lead to symptoms of confusion and agitation initially, but if the process continues the patient may become comatose. Decreased myocardial function may be the result of diminished flow or may in larger burns result from a circulating myocardial depressant factor.[6]

Impact of the Burn Injury on the Respiratory System: Smoke Inhalation

Smoke inhalation is by far the most common respiratory complication associated with burn injuries, although atelectasis, pneumonia, pulmonary edema (from fluid overload) and adult respiratory distress syndrome from sepsis may also occur.

Smoke inhalation, often spoken of as one condition is actually three:

- Carbon monoxide (CO) intoxication
- Chemical pneumonitis or "smoke poisoning"
- Direct thermal injury.

Each of these injuries may occur concomitantly or independently.

Carbon Monoxide Intoxication. Carbon monoxide intoxication as been reported to cause about 50% of the 12,000 deaths annually that result from fires.[27] The majority of these victims die in the fire and are never seen in a hospital. Carbon monoxide is a gas given off as a by-product of combustion, which has 200 times the affinity for hemoglobin as does oxygen. Carbon monoxide is reversibly bound to the heme pigment and enzymes. Yet despite their great affinity for these proteins, they readily dissociate according to the laws of mass action. The half-life of CO on room air is 4 to 5 hours; on 100% oxygen it is 1 hour, and at 3 atmospheres of hyperbaric oxygen it is 20 to 25 minutes. Although the gas enters the body through the lungs, its major site of injury is the brain and the muscle.

Studies have shown that CO not only causes hypoxemia by combining with the heme pigment in the blood, but also combines with myoglobin in muscle and heme-containing enzymes such as cytochrome oxidase. When CO combines with myoglobin it interferes with normal muscle contraction and has been implicated in decreased myocardial function and cardiac arrhythmias and poor muscle coordination elsewhere. This poor muscle coordination has been said to be one of the factors in limiting the victim's ability to actually get out of a fire.

The brain initially suffers from hypoxemia due to inadequate delivery of oxygen to the brain. Additionally, though, the combination of CO with cytochrome oxidase has been implicated in the delayed or continued coma seen in patients after carboxyhemoglobin (COHgb) levels have returned to normal. In a follow-up study of as long as 3 years, Smith and Brandon reported an overall incidence of 13% of neuropsychiatric disorders, with 40% of these patients having measurable memory impairment.[57] Clinical observations suggest that many of these patients initially have cognitive impairments with difficulty in mathematical and reasoning skills which improve over time.

Clinically the symptoms of CO intoxication vary with the levels of carboxyhemoglobin. Patients with levels of less than 10% usually do not exhibit symptoms, although patients with exercise-induced angina may show a decreased exercise tolerance. At levels above 20%, normal healthy people complain of headache, nausea, vomiting and loss of manual dexterity. At 30%, patients exhibit confusion, lethargy, and ST-segment depression on the electrocardiogram. At levels between 40% and 60%, the patients lapse into coma. Levels about 60% are almost universally fatal.

Chemical Pneumonitis. Chemical pneumonitis, or "smoke poisoning," is a chemical irritation or an injury to the lung resulting from hundreds of by-products of burning materials. Although the mechanism of injury may differ with different by-products, the resulting pathophysiology is similar. Initially there is loss of bronchial epithelial and cilia as well as decreased alveolar surfactant. Within hours tracheal and bronchial epithelium begin to slough, producing a hemorrhagic tracheobronchitis. As the disease progresses, atelectasis occurs and interstitial edema develops, giving a clinical picture of adult respiratory distress syndrome (ARDS). Pulmonary macrophages are poisoned and pulmonary infections occur with great frequency.

Initially the patient with smoke poisoning may exhibit few if any signs or symptoms. Initial arterial blood gas determinations are normal with the presence or absence of a high level of COHgb. The only significant clinical finding may be grossly carbonaceous sputum. As the disease progresses over hours other respiratory signs are seen, including decreases in lung volumes (functional residual capacity (FRC) and vital capacity (VC)), evidence of obstructive airway disease with reduced airflow, increased dead space, and a rather rapid decline in lung compliance.

Interestingly, most of the variability in the pulmonary response seems to be more related to the amount of concomitant burn injury than to the degree of smoke inhalation. Most patients with smoke poisoning alone usually survive if adequate respiratory support is provided; when smoke poisoning which results in ARDS is combined with a burn injury the mortality is about double the mortality of a similar size burn alone, and is far greater than with smoke poisoning alone.

Thermal Injury. Thermal injury to the upper airway is quite common in smoke inhalation, but actual thermal damage below the vocal cords is rare. Only when superheated, moist air (steam) or explosive gases are inhaled have injuries to the lower airways been reported. These injuries are uniformly fatal. On the other hand, thermal injury to the upper airway is quite common. This injury results in blisters and edema formation of the posterior pharynx, larynx, and vocal cords. Edema from this injury may develop rapidly (*i.e.,* minutes to hours) and occlude the airway. Early intubation and waiting for the edema to subside in 48 to 72 hours is the primary treatment. Early clinical signs are variable. Arterial blood gases will usually remain normal until the airway is virtually occluded. Usually the only way to recognize the problem is with a high index of suspicion (*e.g.,* burned in a closed space) and observing for symptoms of increasing hoarseness, difficulty swallowing, and rapid shallow breathing.

Combined Respiratory Injuries. Although any of these three injuries may occur singularly they often occur together, especially smoke poisoning and thermal injury to the upper airway. The diagnosis of each of the problems is based on a high index of suspicion. Patients burned in closed spaces, patients with severe face burns, and patients who present with significant carbonaceous sputum should all be suspect. Careful inspection of oral and pharyngeal mucosa for red, dry, or blistered mucosa is the initial step in diagnosing potential upper airway management problems. Arterial blood gases and COHgb levels should be drawn as baseline and to assist with the diagnosis as the disease process progresses. Continual assessment of respiratory parameters, especially increasing hoarseness and increasing work to breathe, will lead to early diagnosis and intervention.

Impact of the Burn Injury on the Metabolic System

Thermal injury produces one of the most significant metabolic demands seen in humans. Hypermetabolism, negative nitrogen balance, and altered glucose kinetics have all been described.

Hypermetabolism. For the burn patient the degree of hypermetabolism is a linear correlation with the extent of injury up to a burn injury of 40% to 50% of total body surface area (TBSA) at which point the maximal or near maximal level of heat production is attained.[67] Studies have shown that this hypermetabolic response is related to an endogenous reset of metabolic activity and not to evaporative water loss, although environmental conditions have been shown to influence the patient's basic metabolic rate (BMR).[68] Thus patients treated in cooler environments (25°C) may have higher BMR than those treated at 33°C. Studies have also shown that increased production of catecholamines is the major calorigenic mediator responsible for the hypermetabolic response.[67] Likewise, other hormones such as growth hormone, cortisol, and glucagon are known to be elevated at various times after a burn and may contribute to this hypermetabolism.

Why catecholamines are released from the sympathetic nervous system and the adrenal medulla is not well understood, but the only thing that has been shown to decrease BMR and to reset core temperature to a more normal state is central nervous system narcosis. Therefore pain, fear, and anxiety, which are known to increase catecholamines, may play a major role in the whole process.

Alterations in Protein Metabolism. Alterations in protein metabolism also accompany a burn injury. Urinary nitrogen excretion increases markedly. Exudative protein losses through the wound account for 20% to 25% of the total body protein losses initially, but decrease over time as the wound heals. The cause of the majority of protein loss from the body, though, is considered to be the result of breakdown of body stores of protein to produce new glucose in the liver (gluconeogenesis) which as a by-product produces large quantities of urea which is excreted in large quantities (ureagenesis).

The major source of this body protein comes from skeletal muscle as evidenced by the magnitude of nitrogen loss, muscle wasting and decreased muscle strength, serial body composition measurements, muscle biopsies, and studies of 3-methylhistidine excretion.[23] Skeletal muscle breakdown is influenced by hormones, passive and active contractions, and availability of nutrients. Insulin plays a major role peripherally in amino acid uptake or release by muscle tissue. Glucagon does not appear to act peripherally but acts centrally on the liver to favor gluconeogenesis. Catecholamines stimulate the release of lactic acid from muscle tissue. This is followed by the release of three-carbon amino acid fragments which are utilized in the liver to make new glucose. Thus the change in protein catabolism seems to be influenced by changes in levels of catecholamines and changes in the insulin-to-glucagon ratio which both favor gluconeogenesis.

Glucose Kinetics. Glucose kinetics are also altered following burn injury. Initially, during the resuscitation phase, blood glucose is elevated but the mass flow of glucose through the expanded glucose space is only slightly elevated. As the integrity of the extracellular fluid compartment is reestablished, the rate of glucose disappearance is enhanced in spite of a persistent hyperglycemia.[69] This suggests that glucose flow is greater in burn patients. Thus the hyperglycemia in burn patients seems to be the result of increased hepatic glucose production, not altered peripheral disappearance. Therefore a characteristic effect of this phase of metabolism is the increased movement of a large mass of glucose from liver to peripheral tissues. Yet unanswered is the question of why the peripheral tissue of critically ill and injured patients requires the large mass flow of glucose associated with its increased energy cost.

Impact of the Burn Injury on the Immune System

MacMillan reports that of all patients who have burns greater than 30%, nearly three quarters die as a result of sepsis.[38] Although great strides have been made in the prevention and treatment of infection with modern topical and systemic antibiotics, a better understanding of the effect of the burn injury on the immune system is necessary if further improvements in survival are to be achieved. In answer to the question, Why do infections occur in burn patients? Alexander states that infections occur "because environmental and therapeutic factors increase or fail to control the bacterial load or because altered host resistance makes these patients more susceptible."[1]

A major alteration in the host defense response to bacterial invasion of the burn wound is inherent in the wound itself. The loss of the normal integument, the body's first line of defense; the creation of an eschar, the coagulated mass of denatured protein kept warm and moist by the body; and the alteration in vascularity in and near the wound all contribute to the patient's increased susceptibility to infection.

Other less apparent yet equally important alterations that predispose the patient to infection have been described. Many investigators have suggested that a burn-generated toxin may play a role in immune deficiency.[2,52,55] Toxins from the burn eschar and endotoxins from the intestine during episodes of shock have been shown to stimulate the production of prostaglandins which play a role in the regulation of the immune system.[34] Prostaglandin E_2 activates T cells which cause a suppression of the immune response.[63] Prostaglandin E_2 also mediates monocyte suppression activity which is required for the activation of T-suppressor lymphocytes. Prostaglandin E_2-mediated monocyte suppressor activity seems to be under the control of a short lived T-suppressor lymphoctye, which suggests a feedback mechanisms. In addition, several investigators have demonstrated that depressed leukocyte chemotaxis as well as depressed leukocyte phagocytosis exist after burn injury.[20,62] Other investigators have demonstrated depressed intracellular killing capacity of neutrophils following major burn injury.[15,25]

The various components of the immune system including cell-mediated and humoral immunity as well as the complement system have been shown to have a direct effect on opsonization. Opsonin is an antibody that enhances the phagocytosis of bacteria. Decreased antibody production, activation of the complement system, and consumption of opsonins result in decreased phagocytosis. As Saba has demonstrated, opsonins are major determinants of reticuloendothelial function, and thus a decrease in opsonic proteins as seen after major burns or trauma contributes to depression of the phagocytic activity of the reticuloendothelial system.[53] Many of these protein-dependent functions of the immune system may be further aggravated by malnutrition, especially protein malnutrition post burn.

Impact of the Burn Injury on the Integument and the Musculoskeletal System

The integument is obviously most directly involved in the burn injury. Healing of the skin is the primary mechanism by which many of the aforementioned complications may be prevented or attenuated. Also it is the healing process that drives many of the metabolic or immunologic functions. Although the wound receives preferential treatment from the body in the localization of nutrients necessary for repair, if metabolism or host defense mechanisms are impaired, wound healing will not occur normally.

Wound Healing. Initially, injury sets in motion the host defense response to localize white blood cells and plasma proteins to help fight infection. It is from this process that fibroblasts enter the wound and several processes begin: epithelial cells, around epidermal appendages and at the edges of the wound, are stimulated to grow and divide; new vascular buds appear and as new vessels form, protein and other nutrients are delivered to the wound; granulation tissue develops; collagen is formed; some fibroblasts become myofibroblasts and wounds begin to contract. The wound matures over time; although surface healing may occur in a matter of weeks, the scar tissue continues to mature over months to years.

Scar Formation. What causes some wounds to develop hypertrophic scars and others not to is still unknown. Wounds that remain open for longer periods of time (*i.e.,* more than 3 weeks) seem to be more likely to develop hypertrophy. Studies of scar tissue have shown that as the myofibroblasts contract, the collagen fibrils are laid down in a wavy pattern.[3] Eventually as wound contraction continues, the collagen bundles take on a supercoiled appearance and form collagen nodules. As the contracture progresses, the collagen forms a fused mass. Later still, elastic fibers develop in the scar. Final maturity may take a year or more. The scar is said to be mature when it is flat, moderately soft, and has lost the red color.

The red coloration of the scar is caused by the increased vascularity of the scar. As the vascularity decreases, the scar loses the red color and begins to take on the normal pigmentation. The skin overlying the scar becomes pigmented by the migration of pigmented cells from surrounding tissue, and the scar achieves its permanent color. The color of the pigmented scar, though, is often somewhat darker than the surrounding skin. In some cases, migration of cells back into the scar does not occur and the scar may remain white or slightly pink.

Muscle Function. Scar formation and contracture often cause changes in the musculoskeletal system. Loss of muscle function may be a combination of muscle atrophy due to disuse or severe protein malnutrition. Disuse may occur early in the course of therapy because the patient is too ill to actively exercise. Pain and discomfort on movement often inhibit movement even in the not so sick, highly motivated patient. As scar contractures develop during wound maturation, muscle activity may also be limited by the decreased mobility of the overlying skin. This, in turn, leads to muscle shortening and atrophy. Vigorous active exercise, later, as wounds are healed, may be limited by increased oxygen consumption and decreased exercise efficiency. Decreased energy levels, pain, and lack of motivation often make maintenance of an active exercise program impossible. This becomes a vicious circle because as patients lose muscle strength and function they cannot actively stretch the scar tissue, thus preventing contracture of the scar tissue.

Obviously malnutrition, especially protein malnutrition early in the burn course, may also lead to decreased muscle mass, as the body converts protein stores to glucose to meet the necessary energy demands. Adequate nutrition is therefore also necessary if the patient is to regain normal muscle mass and have the energy necessary for exercise.

Muscles and skeletal tissue injury may also be the result of the initial event. Severe flame and electrical burns commonly cause injury to underlying muscles and bone. Significant muscle injury, as is often the case in electrical injury, may necessitate amputation of an extremity.

Bone Injury. Injury to the bone may or may not require removal. For example, injury to the tibia or the calvarium may not require removal, but does require early definitive closure with vascularized flaps to prevent drying of the avascular tissue and osteomyelitis.

Bones, especially in young children, may also be distorted, causing disfigurement and disability. Severe scar contracture can cause subluxation and actual dislocation of joints. This is often seen in hand burns where the skin on the dorsum of the hand contracts and causes subluxation of the metacarpophalangeal joint. This same deformity may occur with burns of the dorsum of the foot as well.

Another complication occasionally seen in burn patients is the development of heterotopic bone formation. These calcium deposits occur most frequently at the elbow joint but have been seen at the shoulder and hip joint. The cause of this abnormal calcium deposit is not known but has been attributed to a number of causes including long-term immobility, aggressive passive range-of-motion exercise, and diets high in protein which may lead to changes in calcium metabolism.[38,39]

Medical Management of the Burned Patient

The diagnosis is by history of the traumatic event and physical appearance. The initial section of this chapter discussed the classification of burns by extent and depth. Estimates of depth are based on appearance, history of type of injury, and newer techniques such as ultrasound and light reflection. The extent and depth of injury control the physiological response and the type of treatment required.

Categories of medical treatment are:

- Fluid resuscitation
- Management of smoke inhalation and pulmonary complications
- Management of metabolic complications
- Prevention and control of sepsis
- Surgical treatment of the wound.

Each of these areas is discussed in the following section. The management of pain is considered in a special section because this is an exceptional and essential area of nurse–physician collaboration. For an overview of the management of the burn patient in the first 24 hours following the burn injury see Table 96–2.

TABLE 96–2
Major Areas of Nursing Management of Patient in First 24 Hours

Respiratory

- Assess adequacy of ventilation.
  - Respiratory rate 16–24
  - Tidal volume normal
  - Absence of hoarseness
  - P_{O_2} less than 120 on F_iO_2 of 40%
- Administer O_2 as indicated.
- Ventilate patient as indicated.

Cardiovascular

- Monitor stabilization parameters.
  - Heart rate 80–120/min
  - BP diastolic greater than 60 torr
  - BP systolic greater than 90 torr
  - CVP 3–12 cm H_2O
  - Urine output 30–70 ml/hr average
  - Urine glucose less than 2+
  - Mentally alert
  - Absence of ileus
- Administer IV fluids to maintain desired parameters.
- For electrical burns, may need to administer $NaHCO_3$ as well as fluids.

Infection Prevention

- Aseptic technique
- Adequate debridement of wounds
- Topical antibacterial therapy
- Tetanus immunization
- Parenteral antibiotics if indicated

Pain Management

- Assess level of discomfort.
- Administer IV narcotics in small frequent doses for maximal relief with minimal side-effects.
- Educate patient and family concerning the burn injury and therapy to allay fears.
- Prevent further tissue injury.
  - Do not allow denuded areas to become dessicated.
  - Keep swelling at a minimum by slight evaluation.
  - Monitor areas of circumferential full thickness burns for signs of circulatory compromise.
- Maintain patient in anticontracture position to prevent long-term physical dysfunction.
- Provide emotional support to allay fears and anxiety.
  - Provide frequent brief explanations about burn injury and therapy.
  - Allow patient to ask questions.
  - If patient is intubated, provide a mechanism of communication.
  - If patient's eyes are swollen shut, treat patient as one would a blind patient when attending the patient's needs.

Fluid Replacement and Resuscitation

Fluid replacement is the cornerstone to the successful treatment and early survival of the burn patient. As described previously under cardiovascular-renal changes after burns, massive fluid shifts and loss of intravascular volume occur rapidly and result in hemodynamic instability and shock. Organ perfusion is diminished and a multitude of complications result, perhaps the most significant of which are renal and cardiac failure and decreased oxygenation of the brain and other tissues.

In general, adults with burns greater than 15% TBSA (total body surface area), children with burns greater than 10% TBSA, and all major electrical burns need immediate intravenous fluid replacement. In most instances patients with smaller burns can be easily resuscitated orally with sodium-containing solutions. For small children a standard pediatric formula containing electrolytes may be used. In older children and adults a solution containing 1/3 teaspoon table salt, 1/3 teaspoon baking soda, and 1000 ml of water may be used. This mixture contains 70 mEq of sodium per liter. This is usually best tolerated when chilled and flavored with lemon juice and sugar.[39]

Formulas for Fluid Replacement

For patients who require intravenous fluid resuscitation, fluid replacement should be prompt and vigorous, but should avoid overreplacement and additional complications. There is great debate in the literature concerning the "best" formula for fluid replacement. Because the portion of the blood that is being lost from the vascular tree is water, electrolytes, and plasma proteins, most of the standard formulas suggest a combination of these components. Some formulas such as the Evans or Brooke formulas recommend giving a combined solution of these components from the beginning.[51] More recently derived formulas, such as the Baxter formula and the Modified Brooke formula or hypertonic saline formulas, begin by giving a combination of sodium and water and give plasma proteins only after 24 hours.[5,50] (See Table 96–3.)

Sodium Replacement. Why the differences in currently used resuscitation formulas? Do they all work equally well? There is no question that the critical component of all formulas is the replacement of the sodium ion, and most formulas recommend the replacement of sodium at a rate of 0.5 to 0.6 mEq/k of body weight/% of total body surface area burned. Therefore, the real controversy is what quantity of free water should be replaced. The Modified Brooke and the Baxter formula both recommend the use of a slightly hypotonic solution (lactated Ringer's) whereas the proponents of hypertonic sodium solutions recommend solutions containing 250 to 300 mEq of sodium per liter. With the hypertonic saline solution there is said to be less edema, decreased occurrence of ileus, and less pulmonary complication which are said to be related to less free water intake. Interestingly, though, because there is a decreased occurrence of ileus, patients are encouraged to continue oral intake of free water. When patients are too ill to continue oral free water intake, their serum sodium tends to increase rapidly, often necessi-

TABLE 96–3
Fluid Resuscitation Formulas (Adults)

Formulas	*1st 24 Hours*	*2nd 24 Hours*	*Total Volume**	*Total Sodium**
Evans formula	Saline 1.0 ml/kg/% Colloid 1.0 ml/kg/% O5W† 2000 ml	Saline 0.5 ml/kg/% Colloid 0.5 ml/kg/% O5W† 1000 ml	7600 ml	880 mEq
Brooke formula	LR‡ 1.5 ml/kg/% Colloid .5 ml/kg/% O5W† 2000 ml	LR‡ 0.75 ml/kg/% Colloid 0.25 ml/kg/% O5W† 1000 ml	7600 ml	770 mEq
Modified Brooke formula	LR‡ ml/kg/%	O5W† and colloid§	5600 ml	728 mEq
Baxter formula	LA‡ 4 ml/kg/%	O5W† and colloid§ +postassium	12000 ml	1456 mEq
Hypertonic saline (New Mexico)	HS‖ 2.5 ml/kg/% (189 mEq Na^+)	O5W† and fresh frozen plasma§ + potassium	7000 ml + oral free	1323 mEq

*First 24 hours for a 70-kg man with a 40% burn
†Dextrose 5% in water
‡Ringer's lactate or other physiological saline solution
§Quantity sufficient to maintain serum sodium < 145 mEq/liter
‖Hypertonic saline

tating the intravenous administration of free water. In studies comparing the hypotonic and hypertonic formulas, the total quantity of sodium and free water are comparatively the same if one counts the oral intake of the hypertonic saline group.[43]

Also of interest, the proponents of hypertonic saline suggest that there are fewer pulmonary complications; this is a claim similar to that of proponents of hypotonic saline solutions. The fact that neither of these formulas recommends the use of plasma proteins within the first 12 to 24 hours may actually be the reason for a decrease in pulmonary complications when using both formulas when compared to those which recommend plasma protein replacement early.

Protein Replacement. In burns greater than 30% TBSA the lungs participate in the initial leak of protein from the capillary bed, and there is some evidence that administration of plasma proteins early (0–12 hours) may contribute to a more significant protein leak.[46] With increased amounts of protein in the interstitial space of the lung, the colloid osmotic pressure is increased and, in turn, leads to increased fluid flux into the lung tissue. This increased interstitial edema may lead to decreased oxygenation and the development of the adult respiratory distress syndrome. Because research has shown that it is possible to restore cardiovascular stability with an electrolyte solution alone it may be wise to reserve the replacement of plasma proteins until capillary integrity returns at 12 to 24 hours.

Fluid Quantity. The exact quantity of fluid to be administered by each of these formulas varies on a 24-hour basis with the weight and burn percentage. The Evans, Brooke, and Modified Brooke formulas recommend 2 to 3 ml/k of body weight/% burn whereas the Parkland formula recommends 4 ml/k of body weight/% burn. Although this again seems like a controversy, the important thing to remember is that each of these formulas is only intended to be a guideline to initiate fluid resuscitation, not a hard and fast rule regarding the total quantity to be given.

Rate of Fluid Replacement. Although the exact quantity as well as the components may vary, the rate at which these formulas are administered remains the same. In each of the formulas, including the hypertonic formulas, it is recommended that one half of the recommended quantity be given in the first 8 hours after injury (not after admission) and that one-fourth of the total solution be given in each of the two remaining 8-hour periods during the first 24 hours. The second 24-hour resuscitation seems to be much less of a controversy. Each of the formulas suggests mostly glucose and water with potassium and plasma or plasma expanders as necessary for maintaining stable cardiovascular parameters.

Monitoring of Fluid Replacement

Because none of the formulas is an absolute predictor of the quantity of fluids any single patient requires for resuscitation, careful monitoring of a combination of clinical and laboratory parameters must be considered. Vital signs, central venous pressure, pulmonary artery pressure, urine output, urine sodium, specific gravity, urine glucose, pigment load, sensorium, signs of adequate peripheral blood flow, gastrointestinal function, and laboratory studies of hematocrit, serum sodium, and blood gases must all be monitored and evaluated in relation to each other.

For example, a pulse rate of 140 in the face of a normal blood pressure, normal central venous pressure, and normal mentation means little, yet an increased pulse rate coupled with decreased mentation and a low blood pressure signifies a problem.

Urine output, although heralded as one of the most useful parameters, has its pitfalls as well. In the adult (70 kg), a normal urine output is usually 0.5 to 1.0 ml/min. Urine outputs, though, may be falsely elevated as a result of the stress response so that if a patient has a high pulse rate, low blood pressure, and a high urine output, the urine should be assessed for the quantity of glucose. Because the stress response may cause an obligatory loss of urine due to glycosuria, additional fluid may be needed to prevent hypovolemia. Urine output also varies from hour to hour, especially at night, because it is partially regulated by cortisol excretion. Therefore, before changes in fluid therapy are made on the basis of an hourly urine volume, the preceding 1 to 2 hours should be evaluated and a judgment made on the mean output over 2 to 3 hours. Specific normal variations for each of the parameters to be evaluated are found in the Nursing Care Section, presented later in this chapter.

Management of Smoke Inhalation

Medical management of smoke inhalation and other pulmonary complications depends on the specific nature of the problem.

Smoke inhalation as described previously is basically three problems—carbon monoxide intoxication, chemical pneumonitis (smoke poisoning), and direct thermal injury. The treatment of each is somewhat different.

Carbon Monoxide Intoxication. Carbon monoxide intoxication is initially treated with 100% oxygen. Frequently the patient who is overcome by carbon monoxide may also require intubation and mechanical ventilation. Occasionally, if the patient remains in a coma after being treated with high levels of oxygen (over 1–2 hours), they may be treated with hyperbaric oxygen. In these cases, if the smoke inhalation is accompanied by a large surface area burn, the risk may outweigh the benefits because it is not unusual for these patients to go into hypovolemic shock while in the hyperbaric chamber. Whether this is caused by physiologic changes related to the hyperbaric treatment or whether it results because it is more difficult to monitor the patient and adjust fluid flow rates is unknown. Unfortunately, the results of hyperbaric oxygen and other modalities of treating the neurologic complications (*i.e.,* dialysis with ultraviolet light or exchange transfusions) have met with little success. The patient with carbon monoxide intoxication who remains comatose after 2 hours of breathing 100% oxygen has little chance for recovery.

Thermal Respiratory Injuries. Treatment of the patient with thermal injury to the posterior pharynx and vocal cords is easily managed with early intubation and waiting 72 hours or so for the edema to subside. The most important aspects of treatment is to recognize early the patient whose airway may become rapidly occluded. A high index of suspicion of any patient burned in a closed space may be the first clue. Increasing hoarseness and difficulty in swallowing are often the first symptoms. Changes in blood gases occur late when the airway is almost totally occluded. Early nasal–tracheal or oral–tracheal intubation is preferred to a tracheostomy because often the external neck is also swollen and it is difficult to palpate the structures of the neck to perform a tracheostomy.

Smoke Poisoning. Treatment of the pulmonary complications caused by the noxious products of smoke is by far the most difficult. Mild cases are treated with humidified oxygen or air, vigorous pulmonary hygiene measures and bronchodilators. If adequate oxygenation cannot be maintained, then intubation, controlled ventilation, and "prophylactic" positive end expiratory pressure (PEEP) may be used. Patients with severe smoke poisoning being treated with PEEP should be monitored by means of a Swan-Ganz catheter to determine pulmonary artery pressure changes and changes in cardiac output. Ventilators are set with the tidal volume near the top of the compliance curve (12–15 ml/kg), and changes in compliance are carefully monitored.

Causes of poor ventilation must be thoroughly investigated. These may include restricted chest wall motion from a constricting eschar, pneumothorax from the high pressure required for ventilation, or mechanical difficulties with the endotracheal tube.

Prophylactic antibiotics are not recommended because they frequently lead to preselection of colonization with more resistant organisms. Frequent monitoring of changes in the amount, color, and consistency of sputum should be accompanied by frequent sputum cultures and Gram's stains to identify early changes in the pulmonary flora. Portable chest x-rays are usually obtained daily and followed as part of the patient's clinical picture. Steriods, although they have been used successfully in severe asthma, are contraindicated in the patient with burns and smoke inhalation. Steroids have been shown by Moylan to increase infection problems and mortality in burn patients by as much as 50% when given to treat smoke inhalation.[42]

With supportive treatment the majority of patients begin to improve on the fifth to seventh day, and can be slowly weaned from ventilatory support.

Long-Term Pulmonary Sequelae

Unfortunately, some patients either do not improve or develop other complications in the second and third week. A common complication at this time is a resistant necrotizing bacterial pneumonia. Most patients who recover do so without long-term sequelae but a few patients develop a restrictive deficit seen on pulmonary function testing. Many in this group have permanently reduced exercise tolerance. As these patients recover it is important that they have repeated pulmonary function testing and in some cases they may need to change occupations during their rehabilitation because of these permanent pulmonary changes.

Management of Metabolic Complications: Nutritional Support

Management of metabolic complications focuses on adequate nutrition as the key factor to recovery in the burn patient. Adequate nutrition will prevent muscle wasting, thus improving functional results; prevent or at least limit many of the immunologic sequelae; and prevent sepsis.

The current questions in managing the nutrition of the burn patient are:

- How many calories?
- How much protein, fat, and carbohydrates?
- What are the best parameters for assessment?

Calorie Intake

Initially calorie intake depends on the patient's prior nutritional status, age, body size, and percentage of body surface area injured. As seen in Table 96–4, the recommended quantities of total calories and the quantities of protein vary widely among nutritional formulas. As with fluid resuscitation formulas, the important thing to remember is that these are only guidelines from which to evaluate how well the patient is doing with such prescribed formulas. Unlike fluid resuscitation formulas, though, patient compliance and tolerances are more of a factor.

Tube Feedings. Unless it is absolutely necessary, the intravenous route of alimentation is not used. Therefore one must administer tube feedings or depend on the patient to eat the required amount. Tube feeding is usually the most reliable enteral route when administered on a continuous basis. Oral feedings although certainly the preferred route when the patient can manage are frequently not appropriate for the patient with a serious burn. Most patients who do not feel well and are in pain do not eat well. To ask a patient to consume 3,000 to 4,000 calories per day is often an impossible request. Patients who try and fail may become less cooperative and refuse all food intake. At this point, if tube feedings are begun, they are viewed as punitive and the patient may become even less cooperative. Beginning tube feedings early and allowing patients to begin to eat as they desire seems to reduce uncooperative behavior and achieve the desired caloric goal more expediently.

Complications of Tube Feedings. Tube feedings are not without complications. The most common complications are:

- Fluid and electrolyte imbalance
- Diarrhea
- Aspiration

Fluid and electrolyte imbalances can usually be prevented by knowing the composition of the tube feeding formulas, carefully monitoring electrolyte status and fluid intake, and administering supplemental electrolytes and free water. Diarrhea is usually a problem of feeding high osmolarity solution too rapidly, although if a milk-based product is used in an adult the diarrhea may be the result of an enzyme deficiency. These problems are best controlled by using a lactose-free solution and starting the feeding with a half-strength solution administered slowly (50 ml/hr). The strength and flow rate can be increased alternately over 3 to 4 days until the desired strength and quantity are achieved.

The danger of *aspiration,* by far the most lethal complication of tube feeding, can be diminished if the head of the bed is kept elevated at 30°, the gastric residuals are measured frequently, and tube placement is carefully monitored. In the burn patient, with the every-present potential that an ileus may develop due to sepsis or fluid and electrolyte imbalances, measuring gastric residuals every 1 to 2 hours is one of the best ways to assess gastric motility and prevent vomiting and aspiration. If the gastric residual is more than twice the amount fed each hour, then the feedings are either stopped temporarily or the flow rate is reduced and the patient is further evaluated.

TABLE 96–4
Comparison of Formulas to Predict the Nutritional Needs of Adult Burn Patients

		Nutritional Requirements		*Nutritional Requirements for 70-kg man with 50% TBSA*	
Formula	*TBSA**	*Calories*	*Protein*	*Calories*	*Protein*
Davis and Liljedahl[17]	1–100%	20 Kcal/kg/day + 70 Kcal/%TBSA/day	1 g/kg/day + 3 g/%TBSA/day	4900 Kcal	220 g
Curreri[16]	0–100%	25 Kcal/kg/day + 70 Kcal/%TBSA/day		3750 Kcal	
Wilmore[65]	>40%	2,000–2,200/m²/day	94/g/m²/day	2640 Kcal	113 g
Muir and Barclay[44]	<20%	35 Kcal/kg/day	1.5 g/kg/day		
	20–30%	40 Kcal/kg/day	2 g/kg/day		
	30–40%	50 Kcal/kg/day	3 g/kg/day		
	40–50%	60 Kcal/kg/day	5 g/kg/day	4200 Kcal	350 g

*Total body surface area

Intravenous Alimentation. When the patient cannot tolerate tube feedings or is unable to meet the required nutritional goals, intravenous alimentation may be necessary. The administration of high-glucose, high-protein formulas may be the only acceptable method of alimentation in the patient with severe injury and multiple complications.

The use of intravenous alimentation can lead to many complications including electrolyte and trace metal imbalances, pneumothorax, hydrothorax, air embolism, and sepsis. Sepsis is the most common complication in burn patients because each time the wound is debrided there are bacteremias which increase the potential for catheter sepsis. For this reason, it is suggested that all intravenous catheters (especially hyperalimentation catheters) be changed at least every 72 hours in the burn patient. As noted in the Nursing Management Section, the hallmark of care of burn patients receiving intravenous nutrition is thorough monitoring for expected results and complications.

Protein, Fat, and Carbohydrate Intake

Protein, fat and carbohydrate intake needs are less well established than total calories required. Protein needs have been stated to be from 1.3 to 5 g/kg of body weight/day depending on the size of burn and age of patient. Wilmore in 1974 recommended 95 g of protein/m^2/day (about 1.3–1.5 g/kg/day).[66] Muir and Barclay recommended 1.5 g/kg/day for burns of less than 20% TBSA in adults and as much as 5 g/kg/day in burns greater than 40% TBSA.[44] Bell et al recommend 3 g/kg/day for children and 1 g/kg/day for adults.[8] Obviously there is little consensus in the literature about the exact quantity of protein needed by the burn patient. There is agreement however that protein needs are increased and that prior protein malnutrition may require additional protein intake.

Until recently, most of the nonprotein caloric intake has been supplied as carbohydrates, especially if the patient was being fed intravenously. Bell et al have suggested that less of the caloric intake should be made up of carbohydrates and more of the intake should be provided by fat.[8] In the case of both intravenous and tube feedings, usually less total volume can be given when fats are substituted for carbohydrates in the solutions. In addition many patients who require caloric levels in excess of 3,000 calories may not tolerate the necessary carbohydrate load. These patients often have difficulty getting rid of the excessive quantity of carbon dioxide and may exhibit increased respiratory rates and acid–base imbalances.

Nutritional Assessment Parameters

Recent literature abounds with a number of different nutritional assessment parameters. A number of these parameters are listed below. Those noted with an asterick (*) are the most reasonable ones for assessing the burn patient.

Test of anergy
Anthropometric measurements
Creatinine height index
Total lymphocyte count
Serum albumin
*Pre-albumin
*Serum transferrin
*Indirect calorimetry
*Nitrogen balance

Anthropometric measures are difficult in the burn patients because of the edema formation or the inability to measure certain body areas because of the wounds. Many parameters such as albumin do not change rapidly enough to be of value. Therefore, those with asterisks provide the best assessment tools with the least variability. Using these parameters and adjusting the caloric requirements by re-estimation as the burn wound heals allow for the best estimates of nutritional needs without overfeeding the patient.

Post-Burn Infection Management

Prevention and management of wound infection is perhaps the single most important aspect of burn care. This includes providing an aseptic environment for care as well as meticulous cleansing and debridement of the wound on a daily basis. In addition, the judicous use of topical and systemic antimicrobial therapy is necessary. Prevention and control of infection must involve a multi-prong approach.

Aseptic Measures. Aseptic environments have long been a part of burn care. Simple or complex systems have been used successfully to aid in the control of the spread of nosocomial infections. Because burn wounds provide an excellent medium in which to grow bacteria, the burn unit is an area of frequent cross-contamination. Organisms of the variety that cause major infectious problems in burn patients, such as *Staphlococcus aureus* or gram-negative infections (*P. Aeruginosa, S. Marcescens,* and *Klebsiella* species) are primarily transmitted by contact spread either on the hands or apron area of personnel or by contact with commonly used equipment.

Attempts to limit the spread of nosocomial infections must therefore limit the possibility of contact spread. This can be accomplished by laminar air flow isolators, meticulous hand washing, wearing aprons when in contact with patients, and eliminating the need for shared equipment or at least thorough disinfecting of shared equipment between uses.

Even with the best of systems to prevent cross-contamination, infection remains a threat to the burn patient. Endogenous bacteria from the patient's skin or the gastrointestinal tract are potential sources of wound infections.

Topical Antimicrobial Agents. Topical antimicrobial agents and daily cleansing and debridement are important in controlling these infections. Currently, there are a number of antimicrobial agents on the market including silver nitrate solution, mafenide acetate cream, and silver sulfadiazine cream. The advantages and side-effects of each are outlined in Table 96–5. There is no one universally best agent. Likewise, without meticulous daily cleansing and debridement of wounds these agents offer minimal infection control.

Systemic Antibiotics. Systemic antibiotics and tetanus toxoid are also a part of prevention and control of infection

TABLE 96-5
Comparison of Advantages and Side-effects of Currently Used Antimicrobial Agents in Burned Patients

Antimicrobial Agent	*Advantages*	*Side-effects*
Silver nitrate solution	Effective against most gram-positive and some gram-negative organisms.	Hyponatremia, hypokalemia, and hypochoridemia Decreased penetration of eschar—not effective against established infection Requires large bulky dressings which limit mobility
Mafenide acetate cream	Effective against wide range of gram-positive and gram-negative organisms Rapidly diffuses through eschar (improved effectiveness in established infections) Permits open treatment of wound, thus increasing mobility	Painful on application May cause hypersensitivity reaction in 5%–7% of all patients Associated with acid–base derangements
Silver sulfadiazine cream	Effective against a wide range of gram-positive and gram-negative organisms Soothing on application Softens the eschar and increases joint mobility Absorbed slowly reducing the chance of nephrotoxcity	May cause a hypersensivitity reaction in 5%–7% of all patients Associated with an initial decrease in WBCs

in these patients. Tetanus toxoid is indicated in all burn wounds no matter how large or small. Although most people in this country have been immunized to tetanus, the burn patient should receive a tetanus booster if it has been more than 5 years since their last booster injection. For the patient who has never been immunized to tetanus, the patient should receive the immunization series as well as tetanus hyperimmune globulin.

Systemic antibiotics are usually reserved to treat specific infections. In the past, prophylactic systemic antibiotics were frequently used to prevent streptococcal or staphylococcal infections but with newer topical therapy this is not usually indicated. In a small number of patients with a propensity to develop infections, such as the diabetic, alcoholic, or patient on steroid therapy, the use of prophylactic antibiotics such as penicillin or other drugs to prevent gram-positive infections may be indicated.

When systemic antibiotics are indicated in the treatment of a specific infection, it is important that an appropriate antibiotic is chosen. Multiple broad-spectrum antibiotics are rarely used. When burn wounds are monitored routinely (two to three times per week with biopsy cultures), the choice of an appropriate antibiotic can usually be made when the patient begins to exhibit signs of sepsis. When aminoglycoside antibiotics are used in burn patients, it is imperative that drug levels be followed carefully. It has been shown that burn patients may require two to three times the normal amount of these antibiotics to achieve therapeutic levels.[70] Unfortunately, this cannot just be assumed but must be measured frequently to eliminate complications from these highly toxic drugs.

Other Antimicrobial Therapies. In addition to standard antimicrobial therapy, current research in the potential use of immunomodulators and techniques such as plasma exchange transfusion to prevent or treat infections in burn patients is being investigated.[30,61] As these therapies are refined and target groups of patients are identified who may benefit from such therapies, the infection problems of these patients may be more easily controlled. As mentioned previously, adequate nutritional support is necessary to support the immune system and prevent sepsis. Equally important to the treatment of infection in the burn patient is the removal of dead tissue. Recent work with early wound excision and grafting has shown a decrease in infectious wound complications.[42]

Debridement of Burn Wounds

Surgical debridement of the burn wound and grafting are the ultimate in debridement and tidy wound care. Improvements in critical care monitoring, blood banking, skin banking, and surgical and anesthetic techniques has led to reinvestigation of surgical debridement of the wound. Janzekovic pioneered the techniques of early excision and grafting in the late 1960s and early 1970s.[32] Today, these techniques have become commonplace in many burn centers and are said to improve the functional and cosmetic outcome for burn patients. Burke has shown, with these techniques and the use of allografts or artificial skin, that improved survival is also possible.[13,14]

Types of Debridement and Grafting

Excision of the burn wound may be accomplilshed in one of two ways: removal of sequential layers of dead tissue until normal tissue is apparent (tangential excision) or removal of all injured tissue and underlying fat to fascia (fascial excision). The advantages to excision and grafting are the early closure of the wound with less risk of infection, decreased scar formation, shortened hospital stay, and early return to work or school. The disadvantages to excision are potentially creating a larger wound if grafts are lost; inducing sepsis if the wound is grossly infected at the time of excision; massive blood loss, especially with tangential excision; and the risks inherent in an operative procedure under anesthesia.

For excision to be successfully completed in the patient with burns of greater than 15% to 20% TBSA, several procedures may be needed. This requires that the first procedure be performed on the third to fifth post-burn day. Usually no more than 15% of the body surface area is excised in one procedure because of the massive blood loss and the need to keep the anesthesia time to a minimum in the critically ill patient. After the first procedure, subsequent procedures may be performed every 2 to 3 days depending on the patient's condition.

The choice of whether a wound will be excised tangentially or fascially will depend on the depth and extent of the wound. Tangential excision lends itself well to the deep dermal or superficial full thickness burn where the graft will survive on the blood supply of the deep dermis or superficial fat. Grafts placed on the deeper fatty layers may not survive due to the minimal blood supply. Deeper full thickness burns may be tangentially excised, if in the opinion of the surgeon the loss of graft is not a risk to the patient's survival. In this case, the risk may be worth the benefit of maintaining as close to normal body contours as possible. When the full thickness areas are extensive and the supply of autograft minimal, the surgeon will usually perform a fascial excision. By removing all of the fat layer and grafting on fascia, the graft is almost certain to survive because the fascia has a good blood supply. The problem with removing the layer of fat is that the fat does not regenerate and the patient is left with loss of normal body contours. For example when the extremities are fascially excised, the patient is left with skinny, spindlelike extremities.

Adequate amounts of autograft may be a problem with any patient with more than a 40% to 50% TBSA burn, and this is always a problem with burns in excess of 70% TBSA. A 40% TBSA burn may present a problem because if the face, hands, feet, perineum, and other difficult-to-harvest areas are spared, there may be less than 20% of the body surface area to cover a 40% TBSA burn. This is always true for the larger burns where the donor areas are always inadequate and may require repeated harvest of healed donor sites to cover the wound. When time for donor skin to regrow (10–15 days) is needed, the excised wound will need to be covered by homograft or other skin substitute. Burke and others are currently developing techniques to use artificial skin or laboratory-grown skin to aid the individual with inadequate donor sites.[7,14]

Burns to the face and anterior neck present an especially difficult problem in terms of grafting. These wounds in the blush area of the body (area above the clavicles) require graft skin from blush areas if a good cosmetic result is to be achieved. Skin from other parts of the body has a yellow cast and gives a terrible color match when applied to the face and anterior neck. When the scalp is not involved, it makes an excellent donor site for face and neck grafts. It can be taken by shaving the head and removing thin split thickness skin leaving the deeply imbedded hair folicles of the scalp in place to regrow. Once the hair regrows, the donor site is completely hidden.

The two major problems in excising and grafting the wound early are the lack of a suitable skin substitute and the ability to define the actual depth of the wound and to judge the best method of excision for the different wound depth. Currently, research is being done in the area of light reflectance techniques, laser doppler, and fluorescent dyes to better define wound depth. This, coupled with the latest development in artificially grown skin or artificial skin substitutes, should eventually lead to even further improvement in survival and cosmetic and functional results.

Prognosis

The prognosis for burned patients depends on many interrelated factors, such as extent and depth of burn, type of burn, type of respiratory tract trauma, age of the patient, and pre-burn health status. In general, the more extensive the burn, the greater the threat to survival even with prompt treatment.

Medical and Nursing Management of Pain

All of the previously discussed treatments of the burned patient require close collaboration between physicians and nurses. Much of the success of therapy depends on the interdependent or collaborative nursing role described in Chapter 2.

Pain management in the burned patient is a joint medical and nursing issue. Even though it is the physician's responsibility to write orders for pain management, it is the nurse's responsibility to assess their effectiveness or lack of effectiveness, and to use non-medication methods of pain control. Physician–nurse joint planning and evaluation of all modalities is essential. Pain management in any patient and especially in the burn patient seems to be a subject prone to confusion, bias, misunderstanding, and frustration.

A recent study on burn patients showed that nurses never gave more than 50% of the daily allowable dose of pain medication and in 30% of the cases gave less than was prescribed.[48] This was during a time that nurses complained that the physicians would not prescribe pain medications appropriately. Heidrick found that although nurses correctly identified when burn patients needed medication for pain, they often withheld medication because of their fear of addiction.[26] Likewise, physicians often underprescribe pain medications based on a similar fear of addiction. These and other biases frequently prevent adequate control of pain in these patients. What, if anything, can be done about this? A better understanding of pharmacological and nonpharmacological approaches by all health-care personnel is a beginning.

Pharmacological Approaches. The mainstay of pain control for centuries has been the use of various pharmacological agents. Narcotics lead the list of potent therapies. Nonnarcotic medications may also be of benefit for smaller burns or as the wound heals. Because pain is more than the sensation of a physical stimulus and is modulated by anxiety, fear, and depression, tranquilizers and antidepressant medications are often helpful. Anesthetic agents in analgesic doses may be used judiciously for severe pain such as that accompanying debridement. These agents include 50% nitrous oxide, ketamine, and short-acting Fentynl-like drugs.[4, 18, 22, 56]

Nonpharmacological Approaches. Nonpharmacological therapies are also useful in certain situations with some burn patients. Hypnosis, biofeedback, and behavior approaches including distraction therapy, imagery, and breathing techniques have been reported to be helpful in some patients.[10, 33, 54, 64] The variable results attributed to many of these techniques may be caused by not choosing the appropriate therapy for the appropriate person or not defining confounding variables (*e.g.,* concomitant use of pain medications or sedatives).

Individualized Plan for Pain Management. Nursing management must begin by evaluating the patient as an individual, including consideration of the patient's past history and response to current therapy. An individualized pain management program is developed in consultation with the patient's physicians, psychologist, and psychiatrist. The key to managing the patient's pain is to develop an individualized program, to continually evaluate and change the program as needed, and to recognize certain universal truths about pain and management. These truths are: pain is an individual experience; pain experiences change from time to time in the same patient; anxiety increases the patient's pain; and pain is easier to manage before the patient reaches his or her level of tolerance. Using these principles and combining pharmacologic and nonpharmacologic techniques will allow for optimal pain management.

Nursing Management of the Burned Patient

Nursing Diagnoses

The nursing diagnoses for a patient with major burns are multiple and complex. The diagnoses vary with the phase of burn injury and the extent of the soft tissue injury (Table 96–6). Problem areas are:

1. Fluid and electrolyte disturbances related to systemic vasodilatation and fluid loss into intestinal spaces, hemolysis, and tissue necrosis
2. Impairment of gas exchange related to carbon monoxide intoxication, upper airway obstruction, or inadequate chest expansion
3. Potential for infection related to burn destruction of tissue, wound contamination, and decreased patient resistance to pathogens
4. Alteration in tissue perfusion related to compartment syndrome
5. Alteration in nutrition (deficit) related to hypermetabolic response to the burn injury
6. Alteration in comfort related to tissue trauma, anxiety, and fear
7. Alteration in mobility and potential for joint contractions related to care requirements and pain
8. Alteration in sensory perception related to toxic state and subsequent reduced auditory, visual, reality-orienting, and time-orienting input, or excess input from the technical care environment
9. Alteration in self-care ability related to cognitive impairment secondary to burn therapy and physical limitations
10. Anxiety related to potential loss of life, body image changes, and loss of ability to work
11. Potential sexual dysfunction related to physical changes or emotional problems
12. Potential impairment of skin integrity related to infection, dryness, and scarring.

Each of these problem areas is discussed in the following sections. See also the accompanying Nursing Care Plan for Preventing Infection in the Burned Patient.

In general, the goals of nursing interventions are to prevent potential complications; monitor patient's response to therapy; collaborate in administration of therapy; promote patient/family knowledge of the treatment, expected outcomes, and cooperation in therapy; and promote patient/family ability to cope effectively with the situation.

Potential Alterations in Fluid and Electrolyte Balance

The potential for disturbances in fluid and electrolyte balance is present in both the immediate postburn phase and the acute phase. The goals of nursing intervention are to prevent imbalances through collaboration with the physician in administration of therapeutic measures and through monitoring the patient's response to therapy. Early detection of impending imbalances is essential.

TABLE 96–6
Nursing Diagnoses Appropriate for an Adult Patient with a Major Burn and Major Soft Tissue Injuries

	Phases of Care for Burn Injuries			
Nursing Diagnosis	*Resuscitation (0–48 hr)*	*Acute (48 hr–discharge)*	*Rehabilitation (post-discharge)*	*Major Soft Tissue Injuries*
Actual field volume deficit	++	+		+
Potential fluid volume excess	+	+		
Potential fluid and electrolyte imbalances	+	+		
Potential impaired as exchange	+	+		
Potential for infection	++	++	+	++
Potential alteration in tissue perfusion	++			+
Deficit in nutrition	++	++	+	+
Alterations in comfort (pain)	++	++	+	++
Decreased mobility and potential joint contracture	+	++	++	++
Actual or potential alterations in sensory perception or disturbances in sleep patterns	++	++	+	
Potential self-care deficit related to cognitive impairment, lack of motivation, or physical impairment	+	++		
Fear, anticipatory anxiety, and spiritual distress	++	++		+
Anticipatory grieving, depression, and social isolation		+	++	+
Activity tolerance decreased		+	++	+
Potential impaired skin integrity (post-healing)			++	
Potential noncompliance secondary to pain, cognitive impairment, lack of motivation, or depression			++	
Potential sexual dysfunction			++	

++ (most likely to occur during this phase)
\+ (may be a problem during this phase)

Assessment and Interventions

Nursing responsibilities include monitoring the effects of the burn injury and the patient's response to therapy. Assessment parameters are many; no one parameter will give an accurate reflection of changes in volume (deficit or excess) or in electrolyte balance.

Fluid Volume Deficits. Parameters that provide data about fluid volume deficits are tachycardia, a central venous pressure (CVP) less than 3 cm H_2O, cardiac output less than 4 liters/min, hypotension, oliguria, increased urine specific gravity, glycosuria, diminished mentation, ileus, hematocrit above 50% and a diminished capillary refill rate. All monitoring equipment (*e.g.*, central venous pressure lines) must be carefully maintained to assure accuracy in measurement. If assessment indicates some of these changes are occurring, the flow rate of fluid administration should be increased. If flow rates must be adjusted more than 20% of the prescribed rate in order to reverse the signs of volume deficit, the physician should be notified so that the patient can be reassessed for complications or additional diagnostic tests.

Fluid Volume Excess. Potential for fluid volume excess is related to difficulty in regulating fluid replacement. Hyponatremia may accompany fluid volume excess. Parameters indicative of fluid excess including increasing CVP (over 12 cm H_2O), pulmonary capillary wedge pressure (PCWP) over 18 torr, confusion, dyspnea, rales, inadequate oxygenation, low cardiac output, normal or increased urine output, decreased urine specific gravity, normal or decreased heart rate, normal or decreased blood pressure, peripheral edema unrelated to burn site, serum sodium less than 130 mEq/liter, decreased serum and urine osmolality. The physician should be notified when these changes are first detected so that therapy may be instituted early to prevent cardiovascular-respiratory compromise. If the patient presents with dyspnea, oxygen may be administered by mask or nasal cannulae.

Fluid replacement should be carefully administered to maintain fluid balance. Calculation and maintenance of appropriate flow rates are essential. Rapid administration of fluid can cause fluid excess and pulmonary edema especially in children and elderly persons. Fluid shifts may necessitate the use of diuretics. These should be administered promptly. Accurate intake and output records must be maintained.

Hypernatremia. Potential for hypernatremia is related to unreplaced evaporative water loss or to osmotic diuresis associated with uncontrolled hyperalimentation or sepsis.

NURSING CARE PLAN FOR PREVENTING INFECTION IN THE BURNED PATIENT

NURSING DIAGNOSIS: Potential wound sepsis related to decreased patient resistance to organisms and wound contamination from body flora and the environment.

GOAL: Colonization of burn wounds will be minimized and systemic sepsis will be prevented.

Nursing Interventions	Rationale	Outcome Criteria
1. Recognize risk factors and early wound changes that may herald sepsis: ▪ Changes in color or character of partial and/or full thickness burns to the body ▪ Potential presence of bacteria, viruses, and fungi in the environment ▪ Multiple invasive procedures and tubes required for optimal management ▪ Decreased or inadequate central and peripheral circulation	1. The burn patient is prone to infection and sepsis from a variety of causes. It is important to recognize these risk factors to plan appropriate preventive therapies.	1–11. Aseptic management of the patient's wounds and environment will be carried out. Colonization of wounds will be prevented or minimized. Systemic sepsis will be prevented or recognized promptly to allow for early treatment. Topical and systemic antibiotic will be administered in a timely, safe manner to prevent infection. Complications and adverse effects of topical and systemic antibiotics will be recognized promptly.
2. Aseptically cleanse and debride burn wounds initially and daily or as prescribed by the physician.	2. Debridement of loose tissue and debris from the wound on a routine basis will lessen the threat of wound infection.	
3. Apply specified topical antibacterial agent immediately after cleansing procedure to prevent contamination and dessication of wound.	3. Topical antibacterial agents are used to control the growth of microorganisms on the wound and to limit their invasion of the wound.	
4. Ensure meticulous total body hygiene (*i.e.,* daily cleansing of noninjured body, hair, nail beds; oral care at least three times/day or more frequently as indicated; prevention or minimization of stool contamination of burn wound).	4. Reservoirs of microorganisms should be eliminated by careful total body hygiene.	
5. Provide total aseptic environment in which to treat the patient.	5. Prevention of cross-contamination requires the maintenance of an aseptic enviornment to prevent the spread of organisms by contact with personnel or inanimate objects within the environment.	
6. Assess frequently (at least every 8 hours) for signs of wound infection. a. Changes in color or character of eschar b. Redness, tenderness, increased heat or pain around the borders of the wound Obtain surveillance cultures under sterile conditions as prescribed.	6. Wounds should be inspected frequently for signs of infection.	

(Continued)

NURSING CARE PLAN FOR PREVENTING INFECTION IN THE BURNED PATIENT (*Continued*)

Nursing Interventions	Rationale
7. Assess frequently (at least every 8 hours) for early and late signs of sepsis. *Early signs* 1. Disorienation 2. Hypo- or hyperthermia 3. Tachypnea 4. Tachycardia 5. Ileus 6. Glycosuria 7. Unexplained acidosis *Late signs* 1. Hypotension 2. WBC < 5000 cells/cubic mm 3. Decreased platelet count 4. Anuria	7. Patients should also be assessed for systemic signs of infection. The presence of three or more of the early or late signs of infection are considered to be diagnostic for sepsis until proven otherwise.
8. Perform aseptic management of all invasive lines and procedures	8. Invasive lines and procedures are additional sources of sepsis in these already immunologically compromised patients.
9. Avoid intravenous lines in leg veins to avoid risk of thrombophlebitis	9. Intravenous cannulae in leg veins are associated with a high risk of thrombophlebitis in the adult burn patient and should be avoided.
10. Administer antibiotic as prescribed. (Careful attention should be paid to timely administration, observation for side-effects, and, when appropriate, the timely drawing of peak and trough levels to maintain safe drug levels.)	10. Burn patients may handle antibiotics differently from most patients; therefore, for safe, effective administration, peak and trough levels should be drawn and the dose adjusted accordingly.
11. Administer tetanus toxoid or tetanus immune globulin as prescribed.	11. All burn wounds are considered tetanus-prone wounds. If the patient has been previously immunized, the immunization should be updated with the administration of tetanus toxoid. If the patient has never been immunized to tetanus, the patient should receive both tetanus toxoid and tetanus hyperimmune globulin.

NURSING DIAGNOSIS: Potential wound sepsis throughout recovery phases related to patient's and family's inadequate knowledge of preventive measures.

GOAL: To prevent recurrence of infection throughout all recovery phases.

Nursing Interventions	Rationale
1. Assess skin integrity and potential for problems with skin integrity Dry scaly skin Rash or pustules Blisters, ulcers Complaints of itching Complaints of lack of normal sensation Complaints of pain, stiffness Complaints of severe pain with cold exposure Inability to direct Decreased elasticity	1. The nearly healed skin of the burn wound is prone to breakdown and infection. Careful inspection of the skin should be a part of the overall assessment process in the rehabilitation phase.

(*Continued*)

NURSING CARE PLAN FOR PREVENTING INFECTION IN THE BURNED PATIENT (*Continued*)

Nursing Interventions	Rationale
2. Instruct patient in home care of wounds. Encourage use of pain medications as needed for wound care.	2. Patient should be provided with oral and written instruction for home care to include: Wound care Pain management Moisturizing lotion Bathing procedures Exposure to sun Pressure garment Splints
3. Prescribe moisturizing lotions to be applied several times/day.	3. Because the newly formed skin is lacking in oil-producing glands, moisturizing lotion should be applied frequently.
4. Instruct patient to bathe with a bland soap and to thoroughly rinse skin after bathing.	
5. Limit exposure to sun for 1 year.	5. Newly formed skin is very sensitive to ultraviolet rays and quickly develops sunburn.
6. Encourage patient to wear pressure garments 23 hr/day (usually for 8–12 months). Encourage use of splints to maximize efforts of exercise.	6. Pressure applied to scar tissue will reduce the thickness of the hypertrophic scar. Splints are often used over joints to maintain the stretching of the scar and maximize the efforts of exercise therapy.
7. Teach patient to inspect skin for pressure areas or blisters and to treat these areas early to prevent infection and ulceration.	7. Any break in the skin has the potential of becoming infected; therefore, the patient should be taught how to deal with these problems when they arise.
8. Explain to patient about pain, stiffness, exerise, and pain associated with cold exposure. (Although most of this lessens over time, pain on cold exposure may persist for years.)	8. Many burn patients have pain and stiffness after periods of inactivity. This is best treated with slow stretching exercise. Also, some patients experience pain in their scars on exposure to cold temperatures. This may be lessened by wearing protective clothing and avoiding prolonged cold exposure.
9. Patients need to be cautioned about their decreased capacity to sweat when exposed to a warm environment and the potential for heat exhaustion.	9. Patients, especially those who have had large areas of their burn wound grafted, may find that they are more prone to intolerance to warm climates because they lack the capacity to sweat.
10. Administer or encourage patient to use medications or topical agents to relieve itching. (This can be an extremely incapacitating problem. It is sometimes relieved by proper use of pressure garments.) If itching interferes with sleep, ask physician to prescribe sedative to lessen sleep disturbances.	10. Itching in the healing wound is a particularly difficult problem to treat. Topical and systemic anti-inflammatory agents may be of some benefit, although for some patients, nothing seems to alleviate this frustrating problem.
11. Caution patient concerning lack of normal sensation in some areas and the potential for injury.	11. As the wound heals, there may be some areas of the wound that lack normal sensation and these areas are more prone to injury or pressure necrosis.

Parameters indicative of hypernatremia are serum sodium above 150 mEq/liter, increase in serum and urine osmolalities, elevation of blood urea nitrogen (BUN), and reduction in urinary sodium. Cardiovascular and central nervous system changes that accompany blood chemistry changes and indicate hypernatremia include rapid pulse, decreased blood pressure, increased urine output, decreased weight, and confusion. Accurate intake and output records and body weights are important. They provide data on which to base judgment of needs for type and amount of fluid replacement.

Hyperkalemia. Burn patients should be assessed frequently, especially in the initial 48 hours after injury, for elevation of serum potassium ($K+$) and for electrocardiographic changes indicative of hyperkalemia. Warning signs include serum potassium above 5 mEq/liter and ECG strips showing peaked T waves, widened QRS, and diminished P waves. Hyperkalemia may progress to ventricular fibrillation or asystole. The physician should be notified of these changes so appropriate therapies can be institute prior to occurrence of fibrillation.

Hyperkalemia can occur in the initial post-burn phase as a result of hemolysis, tissue necrosis, and metabolic acidosis. Fluids should be administered initially at a sufficiently rapid rate to prevent hypoperfusion of the kidney which is the most frequent reason for acidosis. In severe cases of hyperkalemia the nurse may administer calcium gluconate, sodium bicarbonate, glucose and insulin and Kayexalate as prescribed by the physician.

Hypokalemia. Hypokalemia is a potential problem after the initial post-injury phase. Parameters indicative of this state are serum potassium levels below 3.5 mEq/liter and an increased urine potassium level. Hypokalemia may be related to inadequate intravenous fluid administration after the initial 48 hours post-injury. Potassium supplements should be administered as prescribed. Caution must be used because too rapid intravenous administration may induce hyperkalemia.

Mechanical Considerations in IV Therapy. All intervenous lines must be secured to prevent dislodgement; those that must penetrate a burn wound should be sutured in place. Intravenous lines are often difficult to maintain in the burn patient. Stabilization of the line can be a problem if the loss of skin or the greasy ointment used on the burn wound prevents adherence of tape. Aseptic technique must be applied when handling and maintaining invasive lines to reduce the chance of infection.

Evaluation

The goals of nursing will be achieved if the assessment parameters are maintained within normal limits. These parameters would be heart rate or 80–120/min; diastolic blood pressure above 60 torr and systolic above 90 torr; CVP 3–12 cm H_2O; C.O. above 4 liters/min; PCWP less than 18 torr; urine output 30–70 ml/hr; urine free of pigment and glucose; urine specific gravity of 1.010–1.015; normal capillary refilling; hematocrit 40%–50%; absence of ileus; serum Na 136–145 mEq/liter; serum K 3.5–5 mEq/liter; weight will stabilize and patient will be mentally alert.

Other outcome criteria are: monitoring equipment functions properly, patient receives needed volume of fluid over appropriate time period, intravenous lines are maintained safely, and indications of imbalance in fluid or electrolytes are recognized promptly and treated.

Potential for Impaired Gas Exchange

The potential for impaired gas exchange is present in both the immediate post-burn phase and the acute phase of recovery. This potential problem is related to possible carbon monoxide intoxication, upper airway obstruction, inhalation of noxious by-products of smoke, inadequate excursion of the chest wall due to circumferential full thickness burns of the wall or inadequate fluid resuscitation and postoperative respiratory depression. The goals of nursing are to recognize impending gas exchange problems and to successfully treat the condition in collaboration with the physician.

Assessment and Interventions

Clinical judgments about potential gas exchange problems are dependent on knowledge of the burn injury and data from monitoring of specific parameters. The nurse must be aware of the existence of risk factors for smoke inhalation because there is no test specific to the early diagnosis of this occurrence. A history of being in a smoke-filled enclosure, presence of burns of the face, or cicumferential full thickness burns of the chest wall are warning signs. A carboxyhemoglobin of more than 20% and carbonacious sputum are other danger signs.

Respiratory parameters that must be assessed are rate and character of breathing, increasing hoarseness, difficulty in handling secretions and decreased chest wall expansion. Impending airway obstruction may also be diagnosed by changes in mentation (confusion, restlessness, irritability, somnolence, and coma). If the patient shows signs of impending obstruction, then blood gases should be drawn. A P_{CO_2} less than 120 mmHg and an F_IO_2 of 40% indicate hypoxia and a P_{CO_2} greater than 45 mmHg indicates hypercapnea. Changes in P_{O_2} and P_{CO_2} are usually late events which develop when the patient is no longer able to compensate. The pH would be on the low side of the normal range (7.38–7.42) or below normal indicating respiratory acidosis.

If the risk for impairment of gas exchange is high, the patient is intubated. Burn patients who are intubated often have facial burns which make securing the tube very difficult. The creams and ointments used on the burn may make the tube slippery and difficult to secure. When securing the tube, care should be taken not to put pressure on the lateral wall of the nares, the injured areas of the face, ears, or scalp. Excessive pressure will cause tissue necrosis.

Careful attention should be given to maintaining the appropriate settings on the ventilator for the desired respiratory excursion. This is especially important if the ventilator settings are adjusted during suctioning procedures.

Cooperation of the patient is essential to gain the maximum benefit from ventilatory equipment. The procedure and the equipment must be explained carefully in order to allay patient fears. The patient's anxiety is usually increased if he perceives that he has no way to communicate his needs. The patient should be provided with a method to communicate (*e.g.,* word cards). Sedatives or pain medication should be administered as appropriate to allay anxiety and assist the patient to cooperate with the ventilator.

Suctioning frequency should be dependent on the amount of secretion present instead of a preset time interval. Unnecessary suctioning damages the airway and may increase the risk of infection. In any intubated patient, aseptic maintenance of all suction and ventilation equipment is important to reduce the incidence of infection. In the immunologically comprised burn patient, this is even more important because pulmonary macrophages and other immune functions are impaired.

Evaluation

Goal achievement is attained is respiratory problems are promptly diagnosed and referred for treatment before severe impairment occurs. The assessment parameters as noted above will be maintained or returned to normal limits. Patients requiring intubation and ventilation will not develop severe anxiety and will cooperate with ventilator function. Infection will be avoided.

Potential Wound Sepsis

The potential for wound sepsis is present until skin integrity is reestablished in all burned areas and reconstructive surgery is completed. The potential for wound sepsis is related to decreased patient resistance to organisms and wound contamination from body flora and the environment. The goal is to minimize the colonization of burn wounds and prevent systemic sepsis.

Nursing responsibilities focus on four areas:

- Recognition of the signs of impending wound and skin infections
- Maintenance of external and personal hygiene environments which have minimal reservoirs of microorganisms
- Use of aseptic technique in wound care
- Administration of antibiotics.

The specific interventions in each of these areas are presented in the accompanying nursing care plan. The interventions will have to be tailored to the individual needs of each patient.

Potential Alteration in Tissue Perfusion

The potential for alteration in tissue perfusion is usually confined to the initial 48 hours after injury. This problem is apt to occur when the patient has a circumferential full thickness burn, compartment syndrome, or general low flow state (fluid volume deficit). The goal is prevention or early recognition of impending alterations in tissue perfusion.

Assessment and Interventions

The nurse must recognize when risk factors for potential alteration in tissue perfusion are present. Patients at high risk are those with full thickness circumferential burns, electrical injuries or other muscle trauma, or low blood flow states. Extremities of these patients should be carefully monitored for signs and symptoms of inadequate tissue perfusion. Manifestations include a capillary refill of less than 5 seconds; absence of pulses in distal parts of the extremities (hands: radial, palmar arch; feet: posterior tibial artery); pain or paresthesias distal to the burn; decreased nerve and muscle function; cyanosis of unburned areas; and pallor of compartment syndrome area. Clinical judgments are based on the initiation of any of these described signs. The physician should be consulted promptly. Normal fluid volume status is imperative to adequate tissue perfusion. If low blood flow is present this will need to be restored to adequate volume as prescribed.

Slight elevation of the affected extremity may improve venous return but elevation of more than 30 degrees may lead to increased arterial compromise. Elevation should be done to reduce edema but only if compartment syndrome is *not* suspected. With compartment syndrome, even slight elevation may cause further compromise of arterial flow to the inadequately perfused muscle. If the syndrome is suspected, the extremities should be kept level, neither dependent or elevated.

The treatment for compartment syndrome is eschar removal. This procedure is usually done as a ward procedure. The area of full thickness eschar is incised. Patient discomfort is moderate even with the use of sedatives or narcotics. The patient should be instructed about the procedure and assured that the medication will lower the discomfort. The procedure is carried out under aseptic technique.

If a fasciotomy is necessary, this is performed in the operating room under general anesthesia. The patient has to prepared physically and emtoionally for the surgical procedure which may include an amputation. An amputation in necessary if the fasciotomy reveals gross muscle destruction.

Care should be take with all injured extremities to avoid pressure from constricting bed clothing, restraints, or dressings. The extremities of patients with decreased circulation and impaired neurologic functions should be protected from further injury.

Evaluation

Criteria for goal achievement are early detection of signs of decreased tissue perfusion and prevention of major tissue injury. Other criteria are absence of infection if eschar removal or fasciotomies are performed and patient reports of no severe discomfort.

Alteration in Nutrition (Deficit)

The potential for nutritional intake of less than body requirements is present in all phases of care of the burned patient. This potential problem is related to the hypermetabolic response to the burn injury and may be complicated by an ileus, depressed appetite, or ineffective patient coping which is manifested as uncooperative patient behavior. The goal is for the patient to receive the levels of calories and protein that are estimated to be consistent with the burn size and the patient's general condition.

Assessment and Interventions

Calorie and protein intake are monitored to ensure that the patient maintains adequate nutrition. To determine if the recommended intake meets the needs of the patient, serum proteins and nitrogen balance studies are assessed. The nurse must keep intake and output records and daily weights. Danger signals are serum albumin less than 3.5 g/dl; negative nitrogen balance; pre-albumin levels less than 19 mg/dl and transferin levels less than 200 mg/100 ml. The prescribed food and nutritional supplements may have to be administered by tube feedings. Sometimes intravenous alimentation is necessary.

Tube Feeding. For the safe administration of tube feedings the flow rates and concentration must be adjusted to prevent an osmotic diarrhea. The head of the bed should be maintained at 30 degrees or more to lessen the risk of aspiration. The patient should be observed closely to reduce the risk of complications such as aspiration, fluid and electrolyte imbalances, hyperglycemia, glycosuria, diarrhea, and osmotic diuresis. Ileus related to fluid and electrolyte imbalance or sepsis is a common complication in the burn patient.

Gastric residuals are checked regularly (every 2 hours) in the tube-fed patient to detect early ileus and to prevent vomiting and possible aspiration. If the residual is greater than the amount administered over the previous 2 hours, the tube feeding should be discontinued and the physician notified.

Intravenous Alimentation. Intravenous alimentation requires the use of aseptic technique for administration to prevent sepsis. A control device should be used to maintain flow rates in order to prevent iatrogenic hypo- or hyperglycemia. A central venous line should be used unless specifically ordered otherwise. Dressing changes over the insertion site will be according to hospital-established protocol and are ususally done every 48 hours. A transparent dressing will enable the nurse to visualize the insertion site and assess it for signs of infection. If the insertion site is through a burned area, it should be cleansed two to three times per day using the same procedures as for wound care, including the topical antibiotics.

Common complications of intravenous alimentation may be prevented through careful observations for signs of hyper- or hypoglycemia, osmotic diuresis, sepsis and pneumothorax or hydrothorax at the time the catheter is placed or replaced. Blood and urine glucose levels are monitored frequently (every 4–6 hours) to diagnose problems with glucose metabolism. These data become the basis for adjusting the quantity and concentration of the solution administered and to guide insulin therapy. Serum electrolytes and trace metals are determined at least twice weekly. Adjustments are made to prevent excess or deficits of these elements.

Oral Feedings. When the patient is expected to eat a high-calorie, high-protein diet, the food must be presented in the most appealing manner possible and in a timely fashion so that the patient is as comfortable as possible. Painful procedures and the administration of pain medication must be planned so that the patient is maximally comfortable but not sleepy at meal times. Pain is a powerful appetite depressant. The patient must be assisted with eating if self-feeding is not possible or is excessively stressful due to pain. Otherwise self-feeding is encouraged to achieve maximum independence.

To obtain adequate calorie and protein intake between meals, it is necessary to provide supplements. The intake of fluids low in calories or protein (*e.g.,* coffee, tea, diet soda) should be discouraged because these may replace the needed supplements. The nurse should be certain the patient receives foods he or she likes and food should be presented in the most appetizing way possible. Often, presenting only small amounts of food at one time will keep the patient from being overwhelmed, especially if the patient has a depressed appetite.

Evaluation

Goal achievement is attained if weight loss does not exceed 10% of admission weight; serum protein levels return to and are maintained within normal limits; nitrogen balance becomes positive, and calorie and protein intake records indicate estimated needs are met.

Alteration in Comfort

Pain is a problem in all phases of care for the burned patient. It is related to tissue trauma, anxiety, and fear. The goal is to maintain the maximum level of comfort possible given the nature of the injury and the necessary treatments.

Assessment and Interventions

Careful observation of objective and subjective data over time is helpful in adjusting the dose, frequency, and type of medications to be used or to assess the patient's response to nonpharmacologic therapies. Observations indicative of pain include increased pulse rate, diaphoresis, increased agitation, grimacing, and rhythmical movement or no movement of body parts. These observations are especially important for the patient who is intubated and cannot communicate verbally. The nonintubated patient will verbalize the presence of pain and request medications for relief of discomfort. Medications should be given as prescribed and adjustments made according to the patient's response. Data should be obtained and recorded about the relief obtained from various methods that are used. The effectiveness of therapy should be evaluated periodically and recorded so that adjustments can be made based on specific data.

The patient and family should be taught about various pharmacologic and nonpharmacologic therapies that may help to relieve pain. Understanding what to expect should help to relieve the patient's and the family's anxiety. Instruction should include appropriate timing of medications so that pain is kept below levels of intolerance. Other pain relieving actions to be discussed with the patient are the use on non-pain-contingent scheduling of long-acting narcotics such as methadone; use of self-administered medication and the use of adjunctive measures for procedure-related pain (*e.g.,* 50% nitrous oxide, Penthrane, or ketamine).

Nonpharmacologic therapies can be helpful to the patient either with or without accompanying pain medication. The goal of these therapies is to allay anxiety and allow the patient to control the perception of pain. Therapies include assisting the patient to master relaxation techniques, biofeedback, and hypnosis. Anxiety or depression are common emotional responses of burn patients as they attempt to cope with their injury and treatment. Excessive anxiety or depression may accentuate the patient's response to pain and reduce the effectivenss of various therapies. The patient should be assessed for manifestions of anxiety and depression. Pharmacologic treatment of anxiety or depression requires consistent administration of medications over an extended period of time in order to achieve the desired effects. Sedatives may assist in pain management when administered at bedtime to ensure a restful sleep.

Evaluation

Goal achievement relative to pain management is obtained if the patient reports that the pain is controlled at a tolerable level and that he or she has control over pain management. Other criteria are patient cooperation in nonpharmacologic therapies and patient expression of reduced anxiety regarding pain control.

Impaired Mobility

The danger of complications from impaired mobility persists through all phases of care of the burned patient. The enforced immobility is related to care requirements and to precipitation of pain in burned areas with joint movement. The goal is to maintain normal range of motion (ROM) in all joints.

Assessment and Interventions

Early recognition of potential problems with mobility should allow patient care to be planned to lessen the danger and provide necessary alternative therapy. The patient should be assessed for conditions that interfere with mobility, such as intravenous lines, ventilation requirements, and monitoring equipment. Other limiting factors are injuries other than the burn (*e.g.,* fracture), inability of the patient to cooperate with positioning and exercise requirements because of pain and immobilization after grafting to ensure take of the graft.

Burned skin has a great propensity to contract; therefore, joint function must be evaluated frequently. The monitoring of joint function and recording of limitations are usually done by the physical therapist. When the patient cannot maintain mobility of all joints, alternative therapies such as range of motion exercise, positioning and splinting in anticontracture position are imperative. The ROM should be done three to four times each day. Position should be changed every 2 hours to prevent pressure lesions and atelectasis. The use of special beds such as the airfluidized, the ROTO, and the medicus beds or turning frames will help to prevent pressure lesions.

Patients should be assisted to ambulate and exercise as soon as possible. Early ambulation prevents loss of joint function and calcium resorption of bone. Independent activity should be encouraged as early as possible. Exercise and self-care are going to be avoided by the patient if there is inadequate pain control. All nursing measures are interrelated; success in one problem area often depends on success in managing other problems.

Evaluation

Goal achievement is attained if the patient regains mobility as soon as possible after injury and is free of joint contractures and pressure lesions.

Alteration in Sensory Perception

Alterations in sensory perception may be present throughout all post-burn treatment phases. Reduced sensory input may be secondary to diminished or absent auditory, visual, proprioceptive, reality-orienting or time-orienting stimuli, inability to converse with staff (intubation), mental confusion related to physiological disturbances, and social isolation (protective isolation). Sensory overload and sleep deprivation may be secondary to unchanging, persistent stimuli (monitors, ventilators, lights, voices), anxiety, pain, or depression. The goal is prevention of alterations in sensory perception or sleep pattern or, if present, the manifestations will be recognized promptly and the problem corrected.

Assessment and Interventions

Early diagnosis of problems with sensory perception or sleep deprivation is dependent on careful observation and documentation of specific indicants of its existence. These manifestations are:

1. Decreased visual acuity due to facial swelling, eye injury, pre-existing deficits, inability to wear visual aids
2. Decreased auditory acuity due to previous deficit, inability to wear hearing aids, loss of acuity due to toxic effects of drug therapy
3. Irritability, agitation
4. Disorientation
5. Anxiety
6. Depression
7. Wakefulness at night
8. Stressful environment

Many sensory changes may be temporary and the patient and family fears may be allayed by careful explanation and reassurance. Deficits related to inability to wear visual or hearing aids or to edema are of a temporary nature. Frequent reality orientation may lessen the psychological sequelae of alteration in sensory input. Reality orientation includes time of day, day of the month, and identification of personnel. The family should be encouraged to participate in this therapy by making frequent phone calls and visits and by providing audiotapes from family members who may not be able to visit.

Assessment of pain and response to medication given to alleviate it will help to prevent excessive pain stimuli and the accompanying anxiety and depression. Pain assessment may be difficult if the patient cannot communicate verbally. It is necessary to observe for the nonverbal signs and symptoms described earlier.

At times, it may be necessary to restrain the patient for safety reasons. Restraints may increase anxiety and agitation. The patient should be given frequent explanations of the reason for this action. It is important that restraints be used judiciously.

Mental confusion may result from a number of physiological problems, discussed earlier in this section. The reason for mental confusion must be determined, and corrective therapies must be instituted. Patients are often fearful of these periods of disorientation and when lucid may worry about their psychological well-being. These intermittent periods of disorientation should be explained frequently. Intubated patients may become disoriented or agitated from the frustration of being unable to communicate. Methods of communication should be established (*e.g.,* word cards, letter boards, communication computers). Patient disorientation may be increased by the unfamiliar sounds of the care environment. All sounds and unfamiliar equipment should be explained frequently.

Safe care mandates that patients have some mechanism by which they can activate an emergency call or an attendant must be present at all times. Patients must be reassured that they are monitored constantly and assistance is always available.

The patient should be allowed to sleep for as long as possible without interruption from care activities. A minimum of 90 minutes should be provided between care activities to allow for REM sleep. All activities and therapies should be reduced at night, if possible.

Inclusion in the environment of familiar visual and auditory stimuli may help the patient to remain oriented or to reorient himself. This stimuli could be favorite pictures, music, and TV programs.

Evaluation

Indications of goal achievement are:

1. Return to pre-injury levels of visual and auditory acuity
2. Decrease in or absence of periods of disorientation, irritability, agitation, anxiety, and depression
3. Return of sleep patterns to pre-injury status.

Self-Care Deficits

Deficits in self-care are apt to be present in both the immediate post-injury and the acute phases of care. This problem is related to cognitive impairment secondary to burn therapy or anoxia, lack of motivation, or physical limitations. The goal is for the patient to assume self-care as rapidly as his or her condition permits.

Assessment and Interventions

Cooperation of the patient in self-care activities requires physical, emotional, and cognitive ability to perform the required tasks. The patient should be assessed for self-care deficits. These deficits may be difficulty or inability to perform personal hygiene activities, wound care, and exercise therapy. The patient may not be physically capable of completing the required task. Activity tolerance may be low due to general physical condition. Refusal to cooperate with self-care activities when physically possible to do so may indicate problems in coping with the situation or the patient may have a cognitive deficit which limits attention span and memory. A lack of interest or cooperation in self-care may require psychological testing to identify the underlying problem.

Once the patient is judged capable of accomplishing his care, a plan should be made with the patient. The plan should involve the patient in the care, and should be structured to provide for success. The tasks can be divided into small increments to ensure completion and enable the nurse to provide positive reinforcement. The patient should be encouraged to regain independence.

Cognitive deficits may be temporary but are often permanent and may require considerable adjustment for the patient and family. The patient and family will need assistance in accepting and coping with a permanent deficit. Psychological problems which prevent the patient from doing self-care must be treated and until the patient begins to respond to treatment, the family may have to continue to assist with care.

Evaluation

Outcome criteria for goal achievement are:

1. Patient will perform activities of daily living to the best of his physical abilities.
2. Patient will perform wound care accurately and will carry out the prescribed exercise therapy.
3. Cognitive deficits and emotional problems will be accepted or resolved to allow the patient to function independently.

Decreased Activity Tolerance

Decreased activity tolerance will be present in all phases of care of the burned patient but will have its greatest impact in the rehabilitation phase when relearning independence in daily living activities is stressed. This problem is related to prolonged metabolic consequences of the burn injury and to decreased range of joint motion. The goal is for the patient to gradually increase activity tolerance as range of motion improves and physical stamina increases.

Assessment and Interventions

Indicants of level of activity tolerance are the patient's lack of energy to do activities of daily living or to participate in other desired activities, shortness of breath with exercise, an expressed need for frequent rest periods and for more sleep at night, and expressions of having excessive fatigue. It is difficult to make the clinical judgment as to whether the problem is decreased activity tolerance or one of depression. Determination of the patient's pre-morbid exercise tolerance will provide data for assisting the patient in setting goals and developing a planned exercise program. The patient should be instructed to increase activity slowly but on a regular basis and to return to work on a part-time basis for a few weeks before returning to full-time employment. The normal decrease in activity tolerance after an injury should be explained.

Frequent, brief rest periods may help the patient but this should not include sleep in the daytime because this often increases sleep disturbance at night. Sleep problems usually resolve in 3 to 6 months. The patient who continues to have sleep problems should be encouraged to have a complete physical examination. The patient should be reassured that this is usually only a temporary problem. However, if fatigue or shortness of breath continues after several months, the patient should have a physical examination which includes pulmonary function tests. Patients who have had smoke inhalation often have residual constrictive problems.

Evaluation

Indications of goal achievement are:

1. Patient expresses a gradual decrease in fatigue with activity.
2. Normal sleep pattern is regained in 8 to 12 months postinjury.
3. Patient regains pre-morbid exercise tolerance state.

Anxiety and Coping Difficulties

Anxiety may occur in all phases of care of the burned patient. In the initial and acute phases it may be related to potential loss of life and include fear and spiritual distress. Later in the course of treatment it may be related to loss of function and body image changes and may include depression and social isolation. The goals are to assist the patient to work through the grief process without excessive fear, anxiety, depression, or social isolation.

Assessment and Interventions

The emotional adjustment of the burn patient is another joint management problem and includes all health-care professionals who work with this patient. Nursing management of the patient's emotional problems will include the careful assessment, documentation, intervention, and referral of certain problems to other professionals. The degree to which the physician and nurse work together to meet the emotional needs of the patient and involve other health-care providers will not only make a difference in how the patient copes with the acute injury and hospitalization, but also in how he or she will cope with rehabilitation.

The psychological adjustment of the burn patient can usually be classified into three stages: the initial stage of shock or disbelief; the second stage of uncomplicated grief or awareness; and the third stage of rehabilitation or stage of acceptance.[59] During each of these stages, the patient may display frequent behavior changes. He may be happy and cooperative one minute and withdrawn or angry the next. These mood swings are to be expected, and the patient must be helped to understand these changes.

Paramount to optimal emotional support of the patient is the degree of cohesiveness in explanations concerning the patient's care, procedures and therapy, and potential outcome by all members of the staff. Discrepancies or perceived discrepancies in explanations will lead to distrust and feelings of aloneness and depression in the patient. Giving the patient accurate timely information and allowing the patient time to discuss the information will prevent communication problems. Encouraging the patient to express negative as well as positive feelings about his or her injury, care, and progress will alleviate much anxiety and instill a sense of trust. Treating the patient as a part of a family in a social system and assisting the patient in involving family and friends in his care will assist the patient to develop a forward-looking approach, a feeling that he will get better and will be able to once again take his place in society no matter what his disability.[11]

Emotional support of the family or friends is also important. Without adequate knowledge of what to expect, family and friends are of little support. Again, accurate, consistent information given to these individuals will build trust. For patients to trust the staff, they must know that the people significant to them also trust the staff. These individuals must also understand the mood swings that normally accompany the burn injury so that they will know when to be supportive, when to set limits, and how to react to the patient.

Nursing interventions consist of assisting the patient to express fears and anxieties and to develop a hopeful outlook. Regardless of patient behavior as he or she attempts to cope with the problems of loss of life, body image changes, and perhaps loss of ability to work, the nurse needs to convey an acceptance and interest and concern for the patient's well-being. The nurse is a key person in helping the patient to learn to effectively cope with multiple emotional problems.

Evaluation

Outcome criteria are that the patient will talk freely about fears and anxieties, will develop positive feelings about himself, and will reestablish relationships with family and friends.

Potential Noncompliance with Treatment Measures

Noncompliance with treatment may occur in the rehabilitation phase of care when the patient is learning to do wound care. Noncompliance may be secondary to pain, cognitive impairment, lack of motivation, or depression. The goal is for the patient to carry out wound care, exercise therapy, splinting, and wearing of pressure garments.

Assessment and Interventions

Burn patients often must continue their wound care, exercise, and splinting programs for many months postinjury. The rate of noncompliance is variable but important to diagnose early.

Symptoms of noncompliance are:

1. Wound breakdown or increased ulceration
2. Decrease in ROM
3. Increase in contracture formation
4. Splints not being worn or no longer fitting properly due to increased contracture
5. Self-report of increased pain
6. Beginning signs of depression (apathy, weight loss, poor personal hygiene)
7. Inability to describe or carry out previously learned wound care, exercise therapy, and splinting procedures.

The differential diagnosis of the underlying reason for the noncompliance is complex. It may be related to lack of understanding, pain, emotional problems, or cognitive deficits. A psychologist or psychiatrist may need to be consulted for diagnostic purposes. Once the reason for noncompliance is determined, an approach can be developed that will assist the patient to adhere to prescribed therapy. If the problem is cognitive, the teaching techniques can be modified to achieve patient compliance. Referral to community agencies such as Visiting Nurse Service may be appropriate. If the problem has an emotional basis, the patient is encouraged to obtain necessary counseling or medical treatment. Pain is frequently one of the issues in noncompliance and usually can be alleviated by teaching the patient to appropriately use pharmacologic and nonpharmacologic pain-relief therapies.

Evaluation

The goals of care are achieved if the wound begins to heal; ROM improves; splinting and wearing of pressure garments is carried out accurately; manifestations of depression are no longer present; and patient reports a decrease in pain level.

Potential Impairment in Skin Integrity

Impairment of skin integrity may occur in the rehabilitative care of the burned patient. It is related to dry, nonpliable skin, trauma, infection, exposure to sun, temperature extremes, pressure garments, and splinting devices. The goal is healing of burned tissue without injury.

The dangers of skin integrity are infection, dryness, itching, and scarring. The burned areas need to be inspected frequently to detect early signs of these problems. This inspection becomes a patient activity after discharge, therefore, careful instruction and return demonstrations are an essential part of rehabilitative care. The specific measures to be taught are outlined in the nursing care plan for skin care following burns at the end of this chapter. Goal achievement is attained if the burn wounds continue to heal without excessive scarring and without infection.

Potential Sexual Dysfunction

Problems of sexual dysfunction usually do not become evident until the rehabilitative phase of care. The problem is often related to physical changes due to the burn or emotional problems. The goal is for the patient to return to satisfactory sexual function as soon as possible given the particular physical limitations. This problems as well as other problems will vary with each individual patient.

Assessment and Interventions

Situations that predispose the patient to sexual problems are:

1. Loss of or injury to the penis (scar contraction)
2. Injury to the meatus or vaginal opening with scar contracture
3. Painful scars on thighs or in pelvic area
4. Alteration in self-concept
5. Alteration in relationship with significant other
6. Depression.

Whether or not the patient has a physical problem which might interfere with normal sexual function, the nurse should encourage the patient to discuss any perceived or actual problems with sexual function. If a physical limitation is present, this should be discussed prior to discharge. The discussion should be with both the patient and significant other. A frank, open discussion of the problem should help to allay anxiety and frustration.

Changes in patient self-image, lack of understanding on the part of the significant other, or even fear or aversion on the part of sexual partners may contribute to patient concerns. The patient and significant other need assistance in discussing feelings about sexual conduct and in working through alterations in body image. Methods of sexual performance which may increase satisfaction may be suggested. At a later date, some physical problems may be correctable with reconstructive surgery. The patient should be advised of what can be accomplished and encouraged to have the problem corrected.

Summary

Burn patients are perhaps some of the most complex patients for whom a nurse may care. They often test knowledge base, emotional capabilities, and physical endurance. From a knowledge point of view, the nurse must have a broad knowledge of medical–surgical nursing, physiology, pathology, growth and development throughout the life span, psychology, and human relations. The emotional stress of the patient and family as well as those of other staff may become an emotional stress for the nurse. This may push the nurse beyond the ability to cope. Even with the use of the best pain management strategies, the nurse is often the inflictor of pain. This in itself may also push the nurse beyond the ability to cope. Nurses working with burn patients must continually evaluate their own coping strategies and seek help when these strategies no longer work. In addition to the emotional stress, the physical work is demanding. Dressing changes and debridement may require 2 to 3 hours of intensive labor twice a day, this alone may stress the nurse's physical endurance. Taking care of oneself emotionally and physically is the nurse's first responsibility in providing optimal care to the burn patient.

References

1. Alexander JW. The body's response to infection. In Artz CP, Moncrief JA, Pruitt BA, Jr (eds) Burns: A Team Approach, p 114. Philadelphia, WB Saunders, 1979
2. Allgower M, Muller W, Schoenenberger GA: The pathogenetic effect of a specific cutaneous human burn toxin in late mortality and infection after severe burns. In Proceedings of the Second International Symposium on Pharmacological Treatment in Burns. Padua, Piccin Medical Books, 1975
3. Baur PS, Burratt C, Linares HA, et al: Wound contractions, scar contractures, and myofibroblasts: A classical case study. J Trauma 18:8–22, 1978
4. Baskett PJF: Analgesia for the dressing of burns in children: A method using neuroleptanalgesia and Entonox. Postgraduate Med J 48:138–142, 1972
5. Baxter CR, Shrires T: Physiologic response to crystalloid resuscitation of severe burns. Ann NY Acad Sci 150:874–894, 1968
6. Baxter CR, Moncrief JA, Prager MD, Cohen LS: A circulatory myocardial depressant factor in burn shock. In Mather T, Barclay TL, Konickowa Z (eds): Research in Burns, pp 499–502. Bern, Stuttgart, Vienna, Hans Huber Publication, 1971
7. Bell E, Ehrlich HP, Buttle DJ, Nakatsuji T: Living tissue formed in vitro and accepted as a skin-equivalent tissue of full thickness. Science 211:1052–1054, 1981

8. Bell SJ, Molnar JA, Mangino JE, Burke JF: Manual of Nutritional Support of Adult and Pediatric Burn Patients. Boston, Massachusetts General Hospital and Shriners Burns Institute, 1982
9. Berkow SG: A method for estimating the extensiveness of lesions (burns and scalds), based on surface area proportions. AMA Arch Surg 8:138, 1924
10. Bernstein NR: Observations on the use of hypnosis with burned children on a pediatric ward. Int J Clin Exp Hypn 12:1–10, 1965
11. Bernstein NR: Psychosocial results of burns: The damaged self-image. Clin Plast Surg 9:337–346, 1982
12. Burke JF, Quinby WC, Bondoc CC: Primary excision and prompt grafting as routine therapy for the treatment of thermal burns in children. Surg Clin North Am 56:477–494, 1976
13. Burke JF, Wolfe RR, Mullany CS, Mathews DE, Bier DM: Glucose requirements following burn injury. Ann Surg 190:274–285, 1979
14. Burke JF, Yannas IV, Quinby WC, Bondoc CC, Jung WK: Successful use of a physiologically acceptable artificial skin in the treatment of extensive burn injury. Ann Surg 194:413–428, 1981
15. Curreri PW, Heck EI, Browne L, Baxter C: Stimulated neutrophil antibacterial function and prediction of wound sepsis in burned patients. Surgery 74:6–13, 1973
16. Curreri PW, Richmond D, Marvin JA, Baxter CR: Dietary requirements of patients with major burns. J Am Diet Assoc 65:415–417, 1974
17. Davies JWL, Liljedahl SL: Metabolic consequences of an extensive burn. In Polk HC, Stone HH (eds): Contemporary Burn Management, pp 151–169. Boston, Little, Brown and Co., 1971
18. Demling RH, Elerbee S, Jarrett F: Ketamine anesthesia for tangential excision of burn eschar: A Burn unit procedure. J Trauma 18:269–270, 1978
19. Dias DA: Heterotopic para-articular ossification of the elbow with soft tissue contracture in burns. Burns 9:128–134, 1982
20. Edgar MA, Heck E, Okita R, Masters BS, Baxter CR; Defective superoxide production in PMN leukocytes from burned patients. Proc Am Burn Assoc, New Orleans, 1979
21. Feller J, James MH, Jones CA: Burn epidemiology: Focus on youngsters and the aged. J Burn Care Rehab 3(5):284–288, 1982
22. Filkins SA, Cosgrav P, Marvin JA, Engrav LH, Heimbach DM: Self-administered anesthesia: A method of pain control. J Burn Care Rehab 2:33–34, 1981
23. Fitzpatrick GF, Maguid MM, O'Connor NE, Brennan MF: Effects of glucagon on 3 methylhistidine excretion: Muscle proteolysis or ureagenesis? Surg Forum 26:46, 1975
24. Gray DT, Pine RW, Harner TJ, Marvin JA, Engrav LH, Heimbach DM: Early surgical excision versus conventional therapy in patients with 20 to 40 percent burns. A comparative study. Am J Surg 144:76–80, 1982
25. Heck E, Edgar MA, Master BS, Baxter CR: The role of NADH-NADPH oxidase activity in leukocyte function of burned patients. J Trauma 19:49–51, 1979
26. Heidrick G, Perry S, Amand R: Nursing staff attitudes about burn pain. J Burn Care Rehab 2:259-261, 1981
27. Heimbach DM: Smoke inhalation: Current concepts. In Wachtel TL, Kahn V, Frank HA (eds): Current Topics in Burn Care, p 31. Rockville, MD, Aspen Publication, 1983
28. Heimbach DM, Afromowitz MA, Engrav LH, Marvin JA and Perry B: Burn depth estimation—man or machine. J Trauma 24:373–378, 1984
29. Hunt JL, Sato RM, Baxter CR: Acute electric burns. Arch Surg 115:434–438, 1980
30. Ishizawa S, Sakai H, Sartes HE, Larson DL, Daniels JC: Effect of thymosin on T lymphocyte function in patients with acute thermal burns. J Trauma 18:48–52, 1978
31. Jackson DM: The diagnosis of depth of burning, Br J Surg 40:588–596, 1953
32. Janzekovic A: A new concept in the early excision and immediate grafting of burns. J Trauma 10:1103–1108, 1970
33. Knudson-Cooper MS: Relaxation and biofeedback training in the treatment of severely burned children. J Burn Care Rehab 2:102-109, 1981
34. Kremer B, Allgower M, Scholmerich J, Schoenenberger GA: Burn toxin. In Ninnemann JL (ed): The Immune Consequences of Thermal Injury, p 90. Baltimore, Williams & Wilkins, 1981
35. Layton TR, Elhauge ER: U.S. Fire Catastrophes of the 20th Century. J Burn Care Rehab 3:21-28, 1982
36. Lund CC, Browder NC: Estimation of area of burns. Surg Gynecol Obstet 79:352–358, 1944
37. MacArthur JD, Moore. FD: Epidemiology of burn: The burn-prone patient. JAMA 231:259–263, 1975
38. MacMillan BG: The problem of infection in burns. In Hummel RP (ed): Chemical Burn Therapy: A Management and Prevention Guide, pp 335–372. Boston, John Wright. PSG, Inc., 1982
39. Moncrief JA: Replacement therapy. In Artz CP, Moncrief JA, Pruitt BA (eds): Burns: A Team Approach, pp 168–192. Philadelphia, WB Saunders, 1979
40. Moore FD: The burn prone society (editorial). JAMA 231:281–282, 1975
41. Moylan JA: First aid and transportation of burn patients. In Artz CP, Moncrief JA, Pruitt BA, Jr (eds): Burns: A Team Approach, p 153. Philadelphia, WB Saunders, 1979
42. Moylan JA, Chan CK: Inhalation injury: An increasing problem. Ann Surg 188:34–37, 1978
43. Moylan JA, Mason AD, Rogers PW, et al: Postburn shock: A critical evaluation of resuscitation. J Trauma 13:354–358, 1973
44. Muir IFK, Barclay TL: Burns and Their Treatment, 2nd ed. Chicago, Year Book Medical Publishers, 1974
45. Munoz, E: Economic costs of trauma, United States, 1982. J Trauma 24:237–244, 1984
46. Munster AM, Bruck HM, Johns LA, et al: Heterotopic calcification following burns: A prospective study. J Trauma 12:1071–1074, 1973
47. November-Dusansky A, Moylan JA, Linkswiler H, Elson C: Calciuretic response to protein loading in burn patients. Burns 6:198–201, 1980
48. Orgain C, Marvin J, Heimbach DM: Exploring Pain Management Practices. Presented to American Burn Association, New Orleans, LA, March 15–17, 1979
49. Patey H, Scarff RW: The diagnosis of the depth of skin destruction in burns and its bearing on treatment. Br J Surg 32:32–49, 1944
50. Pruitt BA Jr: Fluid and electrolyte replacement in the burn patient. Surg Clin North Am 58:1291–1312, 1978
51. Reiss L, Stirman JA, Artz CP, Davis JH, Amspacher WH: Fluid and electrolyte balance in burns. JAMA 152:1309–1313, 1953
52. Rosenthal, SR: Purified burn toxin and its competition. Surgery 71:527–536, 1972
53. Saba TM, Blumenstock FA, Scoville WA, Bernard H: Cryoprecipitate reversal of opsonic alpha 2-surface binding glycoprotein deficiency in septic surgical and trauma patients. Science 201:622–624, 1978
54. Schafer DW: Hypnosis use on a burn unit. Int J Clin Exp Hypn 21:1–14, 1975
55. Schoenenberger GA: Immunological evidence of the occurrence of a specific antitoxic IgG-fraction in serum of severely burned patients. In Koslowski L, Schmidt K, Hettich R (eds): Burn Injuries: Local Treatment, Toxic Factors, and Infusion Therapy, p 101. Stuttgart, FK Schattauer Verlag, 1979
56. Slogoff S, Allen GW, Wessel JV, Cheney DH: Clinical experience with subanesthetic Ketamine. Anesth Anal Curr Res 53:354–358, 1974

57. Smith JS, Brandon S: Morbidity from acute carbon monoxide poisoning at a three-year follow-up. Br Med J pp 319–321, 1973
58. Steinberg S: Ultrasound gives burns the third degree. Science News 124(15):230, 1983
59. Steiner H, Clark WR: Psychiatric complications of burned adults: A classfication. J Trauma 17:134–143, 1977
60. Wallace BH, Caldwell FT, Meadors FA, Stewart CL: An epidemiologic survey of burn injuries in Arkansas: A focus for prevention. J Burn Care Rehab 5:225-230, 1984
61. Warden GD: The use of plasma exchange in the management of thermally injured patients. In Ninnemann JL (ed): Traumatic Injury: Infection and Other Immunologic Sequelae, p. 219. Baltimore, University Park Press, 1983
62. Warden GD, Mason AD, Pruitt BA Jr: Suppression of leukocyte chemotaxis in vitro by chemotherapeutic agents used in the management of thermal injuries. Ann Surg 181:363–369, 1975
63. Webb DR, Rogerts TJ, Nowowiejski I: Endogenous prostaglandin synthesis and the control of lymphocyte function. Ann NY Acad Sci 332:262–270, 1979
64. Wernick RL, Jaremko ME, Taylor PW: Pain management in severely burned adults: A test of stress innoculation. J Behav Med 4:103-109, 1981
65. Wilmore DW: Energy requirements of seriously burned patients and the influence of caloric intake on the their metabolic rate. In Cowan G Jr, Scheeta W (eds): Intravenous Hyperalimentation, pp 96–108. Philadelphia, Lea & Febiger, 1972
66. Wilmore DW: Nutrition and metabolism following thermal injury. Clin Plast Surg 1:603–619, 1974
67. Wilmore DW, Long JM, Mason AD Jr, Skreen RW, Pruitt BA Jr: Catecholamines: Mediator of the hypermetabolic response to thermal injury. Ann Surg 180:653–669, 1974
68. Wilmore DW, Mason AD Jr, Johnson DW, Pruitt BH Jr: Effect of ambient temperature on heat production and heat loss in burn patients. J Appl Physiology 38:593–597, 1975
69. Wilmore DW, Mason AD Jr, Pruitt BA Jr: Alterations in glucose kinetics following thermal injury. J Trauma 15:697–703, 1975
70. Zaske DE, Sawchuk RJ, Gerding DN, Strate RG: Increased dosage requirements of gentamycin in burn patients. J Trauma 16:824–828, 1976

Chapter 97

Reconstructive Problems

Janet Marvin

Reconstructive (plastic) surgery is the reforming, reshaping, and grafting of tissues for the purpose of improving function and appearance. The person needing reconstructive surgery may have experienced severe trauma from an accident, previous neoplastic surgery, congential defect, or problems associated with change in body contours. Many health professionals, including physicians in various specialties, are often involved in the patient's care over a relatively long period of time. Most of the problems necessitating reconstructive surgery are discussed in other sections including the chapters dealing with burn trauma, massive trauma, and disfiguring neoplastic surgery.

The discussion of reconstructive problems in this chapter relates to the situations in which plastic procedures are helpful, the type of reconstructive procedures, and postoperative considerations. Nursing management of patients having plastic surgery concludes the chapter. Although there are many ways of classifying reconstructive surgical procedures, for the purpose of this discussion, the classification system is as follows:

1. Reconstructive surgery after traumatic injuries
2. Reconstructive surgery for congential defects
3. Reconstructive surgery after ablative cancer surgery
4. Reconstructive procedures for problems of changes in appearance.

Types of Reconstructive Surgery

Reconstructive Surgery After Traumatic Injuries

Initial Treatment

Reconstructive surgery after trauma may be a part of the initial surgical repair of the wound or may be accomplished months or years after the initial repair. In the patient with complex facial lacerations but no other major injury, the surgeon may elect to spend hours carefully repairing the injury thus eliminating the need for later major reconstruction. On the other hand, in the patient with multiple injuries, facial lacerations may be quickly closed after other life-saving procedures are completed, with the intention to revise the scars at a later date. With digit or limb amputation, even in the face of other serious injuries, the decision to replant or to repair and reconstruct later will require the consultation of surgeons from many subspecialties. These decisions will be based on the age, occupation, extremity or digit amputated, and the severity of other injuries.

Degloving injuries may present different problems as to whether to reconstruct initially or to plan on later reconstruction. These injuries frequently leave large open wounds that are best closed initially if wound infection is to be avoided. In some cases, initial reconstruction with flaps and grafts will limit the later reconstructive procedures. Unfortunately, these patients often have sustained other life-threatening injuries, and the open wound must be closed expeditiously. In this case, autografts or biologic dressings such as homografts (cadaver skin) or heterografts (pig skin) may be used to close the wound either permanently or temporarily.

Principles of Wound Care

During the initial care and surgical repair, care must be taken to ensure that as much tissue as possible is preserved and infection is prevented. This care must begin in the prehospital setting and continue through the emergency procedures and into the operating room. The principles of wound care during this phase are outlined as follows:

1. Obtain hemostasis with care not to cause additional injury to tissue.
2. Irrigate wounds thoroughly with saline or water.
3. Remove all visible debris.
4. Cover wound with saline-soaked sponges.
5. Protect wound from contamination.
6. Optimize circulation to the wound.

First, hemostasis must be obtained. This is best accomplished initially by applying direct pressure above the wound, or, if necessary, directly on the wound. When pressure is applied, care must be taken to apply only enough to stop the bleeding and not to deprive the tissues of all circulation. If pressure must be applied for more than 15 to 20 minutes, the pressure should be periodically released, thus allowing circulation in these compromised tissues. If bleeding cannot be stopped with pressure, sutures or electrocautery may be used. Hemostats are rarely used because bleeding vessels usually retract from the wound edges and are most difficult to isolate. Well-placed sutures deep in the wound are usually more effective and less time-consuming than hemostats. They are also less likely to damage the vessels, thereby facilitating reanastomosis.

Thorough irrigation of the wound and removal of debris is extremely important to the prevention of infection. Wound research has shown that irrigation under pressure with either saline or water is preferred to scrubbing and excessive wound manipulation.[11] When pressure irrigations are used, the methods that will prevent further injury to the patient are a syringe with small catheter, blunt needles, or a surgical lavage machine. The use of various soaps, detergents, or antiseptic solutions has been questioned frequently.[1] There is no question that many solutions such as hydrogen peroxide and hexachlorophene may cause further tissue injury especially if they are not thoroughly rinsed from the wound. If an antiseptic agent is used, the preferred choice is Betadine.[8] When used, it should be thoroughly rinsed from the interstices of the wound. Once the wound is thoroughly irrigated, it should be carefully inspected for particles of dirt or debris. Foreign bodies left in the wound are frequently associated with infection. Once the wound is cleansed, sterile dressing soaked in saline should be applied to the wound to prevent additional tissue injury due to drying.

Throughout the cleansing procedures and until the wound is surgically closed, the wound should be protected from contamination. Nosocomial (hospital-acquired) infections account for 5% of all wound infections.[5] To prevent the spread of infection, all personnel must adhere to strict aseptic technique when dealing with open wounds. This requires caps, mask, and gloves to be worn during all direct contact with open wounds. In addition, all equipment and supplies used in wound care should be sterile and handled with aseptic technique. In addition to preventing contamination, the prevention of infection may involve the systemic administration of antibiotics. The use of systemic antibiotics is not recommended for a simple laceration, but may be especially important in the severely injured or compromised patient in whom sepsis is a major threat.[12] If systemic antibiotics are to be effective, they should be administered as soon as possible after the injury.[6] Usually they are administered in the emergency room and then in the operating room if an appropriate period of time has elapsed.

Tetanus immunization should also be checked carefully and if the patient has not had a booster immunization within 5 years, this should be administered.[4] If the patient has never been immunized for tetanus, the first injection of the series and tetanus hyperimmune globulin should be given to the patient. The patient should also receive instruction about how and when to complete the series of immunization.

Postoperative Conditions

Care must be taken to optimize circulation to the wound if infection and additional tissue necrosis are to be prevented. To accomplish this, one must optimize general circulation first. The patient with large open wounds is at high risk of sepsis if allowed to remain in a low-flow state for an extended period of time. Once general circulation is optimal, then circulation to the wound must also be optimized.

Pressure on or about the wound may decrease circulation. To prevent pressure, the nurse should ensure that bandages are not applied too tightly and that the patient is positioned to prevent pressure. Most wounds are best treated with slight elevation. This means that wounds of extremities are positioned just above the level of the heart. In this way, edema may be reduced by improving venous and lymphatic drainage. Care must be taken not to elevate the extremity too high. With elevation of an extremity much above 20 to 30 degrees, arterial flow may be reduced and circulation further compromised. The nurse must also take care that, when elevating the extremities, undue pressure is not placed at the elbow, shoulder, knees, and hip joints. Pressure in these areas may not only impair blood flow but may put increased pressure on nerves and cause neurologic injury.

Optimal management of wounds may make the difference in whether the wound can be closed initially with minimal scar formation or not. If the traumatic wound is grossly contaminated or improperly managed initially, the surgeon may choose a delayed closure procedure. This will surely result in a poor cosmetic result and may require several reconstructive procedures to correct the disfigurement. Delayed closure or improperly closed wounds may cause the patient both physical and emotional disability and must be avoided whenever possible.

Reconstructive Surgery for Congential Defects

Any number of congenital defects are amenable to reconstructive surgery. Such conditions include: cleft lip and palate, hypertelorism syndrome (too much distance between two organs or body parts), polydactyly, hemangiomas, nevi, ear deformities, especially protruding ears, and nasal deformities. Some of these are best repaired during childhood, but others are usually performed after the child matures into adolescence and adulthood. In some cases, the adult has suffered the emotional consequences of such deformities throughout childhood and only as adults avail themselves of corrective surgery. Some of these involve relatively simple procedures while others such as the correction of hypertelorism are very complex and may not be correctable once the patient has reached maturity.

The conditions usually corrected during childhood are cleft lip and palate, hypertelorism, hemangiomas, nevi, and polydactyly. Congential deformities which are usually not corrected until adolescence or adulthood include ear and nasal deformities. Although some people think of the correction of ear deformities as a cosmetic procedure, it is in fact a reconstructive procedure. The deformity occurs because the antihelical fold has not developed. Many young people with protruding ears develop personality problems as they try to overcompensate or draw attention away from the deformity.

Ear and Nose Deformities

Correction of *ear deformities* is best accomplished when the patient recognizes the deformity himself and wishes to have it corrected. In this way, the patient will be able to cooperate with the procedure which is usually done under local anesthesia. The operation remolds the ear cartilage and takes approximately 1 hour. The bandages must remain in place for 1 week to allow the ears to heal in their new position. Usually after the procedure, personality problems resolve as the patient adjusts to a new self-image.

Nasal deformities may be congenital or may result from traumatic injuries. Like ear deformities, nasal deformities may affect the person's self-image and personality. These, too, are best corrected when the patient recognizes the deformity and wishes to have it corrected. This is frequently a procedure done in late adolescence or early adulthood. The procedure is done under local anesthesia and requires the cooperation of the patient. Rhinoplasty reshapes the nose by fracturing the nasal bones, removing excess tissue, and repositioning the nasal bones. The nose is then immobilized with nasal packing and a splint. The immobilization must be maintained for several days. The excessive swelling which accompanies the operation may take 3 to 4 weeks to resolve, but the final results may not be obvious for several months. If bleeding, infection, or displacement of facial bones occur, a second procedure may be required.

Correction of these congenital deformities whether in childhood, adolescence, or adulthood requires cooperation of the patient and health-care personnel. The patient must understand what the procedure may or may not accomplish. Psychologically, the patient must have realistic expectations for how such surgery may affect their lives. The patient who seems to have unrealistic expectations of how the procedure will change their lives should be referred for counseling before the procedure is planned. In this way many unpleasant interactions between the patient and health-care personnel may be avoided, and the patient will get the most benefit from such corrective procedures.

Reconstructive Procedures After Ablative Cancer Surgery

General Considerations

Cancer surgery undertaken for either curative or palliative treatment often results in great tissue loss and excessive deformities. As cancer therapy has improved, with newer techniques of chemotherapy and radiation therapy, more patients are surviving longer and the deformities left by the surgical procedure may be a major issue in whether the patient returns to a normal productive life. The decision of whether to attempt immediate reconstruction at the time of tumor removal or delayed reconstruction depends on whether the surgeon feels that the local tumor is under control.

The advantages of primary reconstruction are improved functional results, especially with head and neck tumors; decreased patient anxiety about appearance; reduction in the number of hospitalizations; fewer postoperative problems related to self-care; and primary reconstruction is usually easier because delayed reconstruction requires operating through a scar. When possible, reconstructive procedures should replace lost tissue with tissue in kind. Often bone, muscle, and soft tissues must be replaced to correct the deformity and restore function. In some cases prosthetic devices may be used as well. The major goal is to restore function and appearance that will be acceptable to the patient.

Surgical Procedures for Breast Cancer

Surgical procedures for the eradication of breast cancer depend on the stage of the cancer. Simple mastectomy, modified radical mastectomy with preservation of the pectoral muscles and removal of axillary lymph nodes, or radical mastectomies and chest wall resection may be performed depending on the stage of the cancer.[7] Surgery for the eradication of the cancer is the prime concern, and reconstructive surgery is a secondary concern. Yet with earlier detection, radical mastectomy is used less and less. The modified radical mastectomy is preferred if reconstructive procedures are to be performed because the pectoral muscles are spared and this makes the reconstructive procedure easier.

In the case of the subcutaneous mastectomy, the skin with the nipple and areola tissues is left intact. Some surgeons prefer to perform a primary reconstruction by placing an implant either in the subcutaneous space or beneath the pectoral muscles. Other surgeons feel that the skin flap created by the initial tissue dissection is traumatized to the extent that blood supply to the skin flap is compromised and a delayed reconstructive procedure may give the best results. In the case of the delayed procedure, the implant is inserted through the old scar and may be placed either subpectorally or subcutaneously. These procedures are fraught with complications such as hematoma, seroma, wound dehiscence, necrosis of the skin, infection, scarring, pain, capsule formation with hardening of the breast, and irregular healing which may result in the improper position of the breast. Because these procedures do not give uniformly good results and because cancer may develop in the remaining breast tissue, the risks and benefits should be thoroughly discussed with the patient several times prior to the procedure.

After modified radical or radical mastectomy, breast reconstruction may be considered. In the younger woman with low-grade malignancy, this may be considered as part of the primary procedure, but reconstruction is usually delayed in these cases for a period of 3 to 12 months. Not all patients who have had mastectomies are candidates for reconstruction and careful medical and psychological examinations of the patient should be included in the preoperative preparation. Usually the reconstructive procedure consists of two stages. The first is the placement of the implant in the subcutaneous or subpectoral space. Once the wound is healed and the area has been stabilized then the nipple and areola can be reconstructed.

In some cases where the original surgery was extensive and required grafting, reconstruction may require chest wall flaps, myocutaneous flaps, or other transposition flaps before an implant can be placed. Chest wall reconstruction may be necessary in the patient with recurrent carcinoma secondary to breast cancer, sarcoma secondary to irradiation, or radiation necrosis of the ribs. In these wounds, prosthetic mesh materials and large pedicle flaps may be necessary to close the chest wall defect. The wounds carry with them high risk and high morbidity because they often involve irradiated tissue.

Head and Neck Cancer

The causes of head and neck cancer can often be attributed to chewing of snuff or betel nuts, smoking of cigarettes or pipes, and continuous exposure to sun and wind.[3] Cancers of the head and neck can usually be diagnosed through a thorough physical examination. Many patients with head and neck cancer have underlying cardiovascular or pulmonary disease which must be diagnosed and treated prior to any surgical procedures. Excessive alcohol ingestion is also associated with head and neck cancer so that liver function tests should be a part of the initial examination. Lumps found in the neck may be primary or metastatic. Usually lumps above the middle of the neck arise from a primary lesion in the cavity of the head or neck. Lumps in the lower neck may represent either a primary lesion above the clavicle or a metastatic lesion below the clavicle. In the case of lesions in the lower neck, gastrointestinal studies, mammograms and intravenous pyelograms should be done to rule out other lesions.

Tumors of the head and neck may include benign lesions such as: granulomas, giant cell tumors, papillomas of the tongue, hemangiomas, lymphangiomas, dermoid cysts, neurofibromas, lymphadenopathies, thyroglossal duct cysts, brachial cleft cysts, tuberculous adenitis, Malherbe's epitheliomas, cystic hygromas, and pigmented nevi. Head and neck tumors which are malignant include: liposarcomas, fibrosarcomas, neurosarcomas, carcinomas of the thyroid, rhabdomyosarcomas, salivary gland tumors, mucoepidermoid carcinomas, malignant granular cell myoblastomas of the tongue, tumors associated with Hodgkin's disease, and malignant melanomas. Most of these malignant tumors can be cured if detected early so that the surgical procedure removes the tumor.

Treatment. Treatment of head and neck tumors include surgery, radiotherapy, chemotherapy, or a combination of the three methods (see Chapters 30 and 81). Evaluation of these patients and decisions about treatment are usually the responsibility of a multidisciplinary team. Head and neck surgeons, radiation oncologists, dentists, medical oncologists, pathologists, anesthesiologists, social workers, and nurse specialists in oncology are usually a part of the primary team. Thoracic surgeons, neurosurgeons, and other medical specialists such as speech therapists and prosthodontists may be used as consultants for the individual patient. Decisions about pre- or postoperative radiation or chemotherapy will be made by consultation with the team. Preoperative radiation or chemotherapy may arrest the spread of the tumor or reduce the size of the lesion. Unfortunately, preoperative radiation may delay wound healing, increase the risk of fistula formation, and cause damage to the carotid artery which may result in sudden hemorrhage. All of these problems must be considered as the plan of treatment is developed.

Postoperative Problems. After surgery for head and neck cancer, the patient may develop upper airway obstruction; hemorrhage, especially of the carotid artery if the patient has had radiation therapy; hematomas under skin flaps; infections; fistula formations; dental caries and mandibular necrosis in patients who have had radiation therapy; and neurological problems related to the resection of one or more of such cranial nerves as the seventh, ninth, tenth, or twelfth. In addition, transection of the vagus nerve may change the voice due to laryngeal damage. Initially, the most disastrous complication may be airway obstruction. Often a tracheostomy is placed at the time of surgery as a precautionary procedure in the high-risk patient. Although some patients may be able to eat soon after the procedure, many patients may require long-term tube feedings for nutritional support.

Reconstructive Surgery for Problems with Appearance

Psychosocial Considerations

Many people have body contours which they feel in some way detracts from their physical attractiveness. These perceived deficits may be the result of normal genetic characteristics such as a large or crooked nose, protruding or receding chin, minimal breast tissue or very large breasts.

Other changes such as sagging facial tissue, drooping eyelids, and sagging breasts, abdomen, or buttocks may be caused by the aging process. Although these changes may not seem important to some people, to others they may actually interfere with self-confidence and interpersonal relationships. If the patient perceives the need for a reconstructive procedure to improve function, appearance, or self-image, the surgery should not be considered unnecessary. However, concerns about seemingly minor body contour changes may be a symptom of a major psychological problem. Patients with such a problem may present the greatest challenges to the health-care team. It is often difficult to differentiate the "normal" patient who wants a simple facelift or augmentation mammoplasty from the patient who sees such a procedure as the answer to everything that is wrong with life. For this reason, although the surgical procedure may be simple, the preoperative evaluation may be very complex. The surgeon who has concerns about the emotional stability of the patient must insist on a preoperative psychological evaluation by a competent psychologist or psychiatrist.[3] This evaluation is not only for the protection of the surgeon, but is often helpful to assist the patients through the postoperative period and later as they deal with their changed appearance and changes in their self-concept and interpersonal relations. Even the person who seems emotionally stable may have some difficulty coping with a changed appearance, self-concept, or interpersonal relationship. An experienced psychologist can often help patients having reconstructive surgery for disfigurement.

Surgical Procedures

Common surgical procedures for disfigurement include otoplasy (correction of protruding ears) and rhinoplasty, which were discussed under congenital deformities; rhytidectomy (face lift); blepharophasty; body contour problems and breast reconstruction.

Rhytidectomy (Face Lift)

Rhytidectomy is usually done in the middle years of life to decrease changes in appearance caused by age. Facial skin ages from exposure to sun and wind, poor nutrition, smoking, excessive alcohol use, and obesity. As the skin of the face ages, it loses its elasticity and firmness, fine wrinkles appear around the eyes, and a general sagging occurs. This process may become quite pronounced as early as the late twenties or early thirties and may be most upsetting to the patient. In the past this has been a problem for which mostly women have sought correction. In the 1980s more and more men are considering facelift surgery for correction of such problems. The emphasis in our society on youth and physical fitness and an increased awareness of the possible enhancement of physical appearance by plastic surgery has led to increased demand for such procedures.

The facelift is usually done under local anesthesia and sedation. The procedure involves making an incision along the temporal hairline, in front of the ear, and proceeds posteriorly into the hairline near the mastoid region (Fig. 97–1). The skin and topmost portion of the subcutaneous layer are

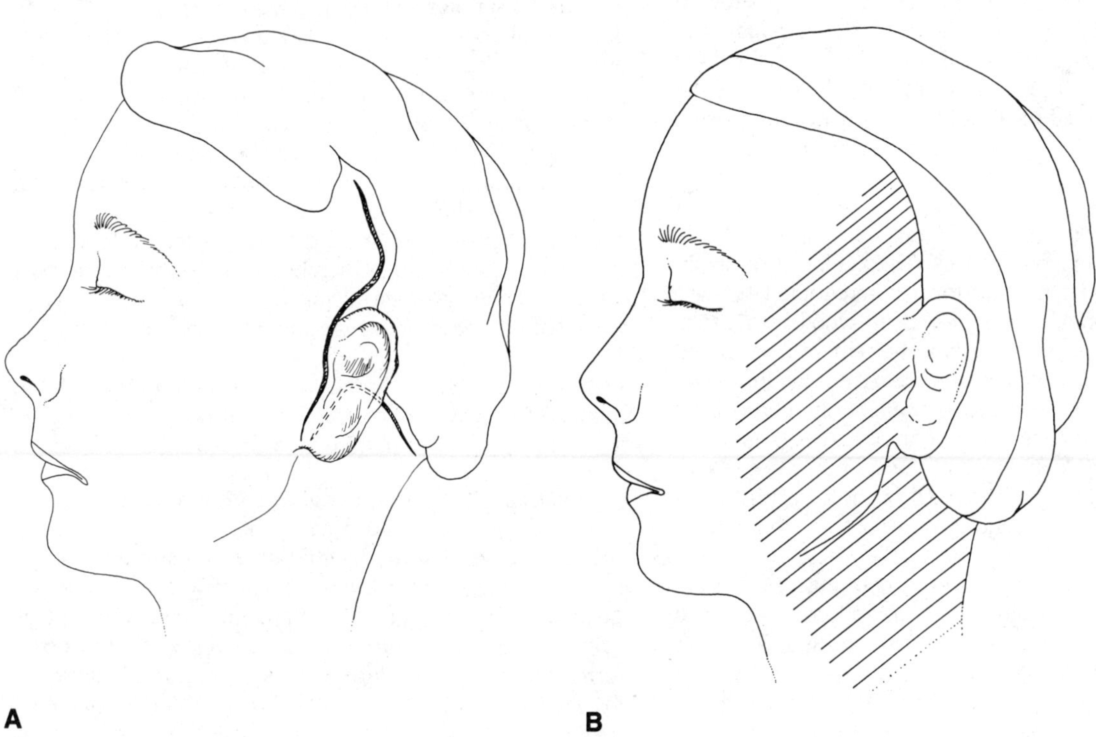

FIGURE 97–1 (*A*) Facelift incision and (*B*) area of undermining of facelift. (Grossman JA: Minor Injuries and Disorders: Surgical and Medical Care, p 278. Philadelphia, JB Lippincott, 1983)

elevated and undermined from the lateral corner of the eye to the lateral corner of the mouth and on the neck to near the midline. The tissue is then pulled posteriorly and superiorly, and the extra tissue is excised. This may involve the removal of ½ to 1½ inches of skin at the edge. Suspension sutures are placed in the hairline in the temporal and mastoid area and remain in place 7 to 10 days. Facial sutures are placed loosely in front of the ear and removed in 5 days. Hematomas under the skin are the most frequent complication and require careful watching for the first 24 to 48 hours.

Because time and gravity continue to pull on the skin of the face, these procedures often have to be repeated. They may be repeated three to four times but eventually the skin becomes thin, shiny, and atrophic. The facelift does not remove the fine wrinkles of aging. This is usually done with a phenol compound creating a superficial chemical burn or by dermabrasion. Both of these procedures create a superficial wound which, when it heals, reduces the wrinkles and tightens the skin. These procedures may be used alone or in combination with a facelift.

Blepharoplasty

Blepharoplasty is performed to remove excessive folds of skin and excessive fat pads around the eyes. The procedure is also done under local anesthesia and is done through incisions in the crease of the upper lid and just below the lash line on the lower lid. The superficial subcutaneous tissue is elevated, the fatty tissue is expressed, and cautery is used to stop any bleeding. The excess tissue is then removed, and tissue is sutured in place. These sutures are usually removed in 48 to 72 hours to reduce the scarring around the needle puncture sites.

Other facial procedures may include lipectomy to remove the fat pad from under the chin or augmentation of the receding chin. The submental lipectomy is usually done as a part of the facelift procedure. The augmentation of the receding chin is often done in conjunction with a rhinoplasty and is augmented with either an alloplastic material or bone graft.

Body Contouring

Body contouring procedures (panniculectomy or abdominal lipectomy) may be performed on people who have lost excessive amounts of weight. Patients who have had stapling procedures of the stomach to help them lose weight often have aprons of fat that must be removed or it interferes with walking. Others who have lost weight often have sacks of empty skin which hang from the upper arms, thighs, and gluteal region. Many women are prone to "riding breeches," a fat deposit on the lateral hips. All of these recontouring procedures are major operations requiring general or spinal anesthesia.

These procedures may result in scar formation especially on the upper arms and thighs. The abdominal scars are more easily hidden in the groin crease and gluteal scar is hidden in the gluteal fold. At least with the abdominal and gluteal procedures if the scars are unsightly they are covered easily by a bathing suit or undergarment. Unfortunately, the scars on the arms, legs, and thighs have a tendency to spread, are often unsightly, and are more difficult to cover by clothing.

Reconstructive Breast Surgery

Reconstructive breast surgery has gained in popularity since the early 1960s when the silicone implant was developed. Abnormalities of the breast may be congenital or acquired. Congential abnormalities may include absence of the nipple (athelia), lack of breast development (amastia), more than two breasts (polymastia), more than two nipples (polythelia), or ectopic breast tissue (usually in the axilla). Acquired abnormalities of the breast may occur as a result of injury caused by burns, trauma, surgical procedures or irradiation. Virginal hypertrophy may occur in girls ages 10 to 15 and result in large ptotic breast. Males, ages 12 to 17, may develop gynecomastia, a benign hypertrophy of the breast which usually resolves over time. This problem in males is sometimes seen in relation to liver disease and endocrine disturbances. Once these other problems are ruled out, if the condition persists, a simple mastectomy may be performed.

In addition to congenital or acquired conditions of the breast, many women are concerned about the size or shape of their normal breasts. Breast development is dependent on a woman's hereditary genes, nutrition, and hormones. Some women have very little breast tissue while other women have an overabundance of breast tissue. One breast may be smaller than the other. Breasts may become ptotic with aging. Many women today seek procedures to correct either congenital, acquired, or inherited abnormalities.

The procedures for correction of these conditions include augmentation mammoplasty, mastopexy, or reduction mammoplasty.

Augmentation Mammoplasty. Augmentation mammoplasty is the simplest of these procedures and is usually done under local anesthesia and sedation (Fig. 97–2). The procedure is safe and relatively trouble free. The most common complication is the formation of a fibrous capsule around the implant. This complication is less of a problem with the newer inflatable implants which can be underinflated to help maintain softness. The most important consideration for the patient who wishes to have augmentation procedure is not the surgical procedure but the psychological well-being of the patient. One must remember that the breast is a sex organ, and many women seeking augmentation procedures are unhappy with their sex life and have low self-esteem. It is wise for any patient requesting this procedure to be evaluated by a psychologist. Some women even find it helpful to continue to see a psychologist for a period of time after the surgical procedure to help them adjust to a new self-image.

Mastopexy. Mastopexy is a procedure used to correct ptosis or sagging of the breast. This is a major operative procedure and requires that the surgeon refashion, reshape, and resuspend the breast tissue. Some women will have adequate breast tissue and others may require silicone implants as well. The patient requiring a mastopexy should be informed that the procedure will require an incision around the areola and will leave more scars than a simple augmentation mammoplasty. When these procedures are done in women of childbearing age who wish to breast feed, care must be taken not to detach the areola and nipple from the ductal system.

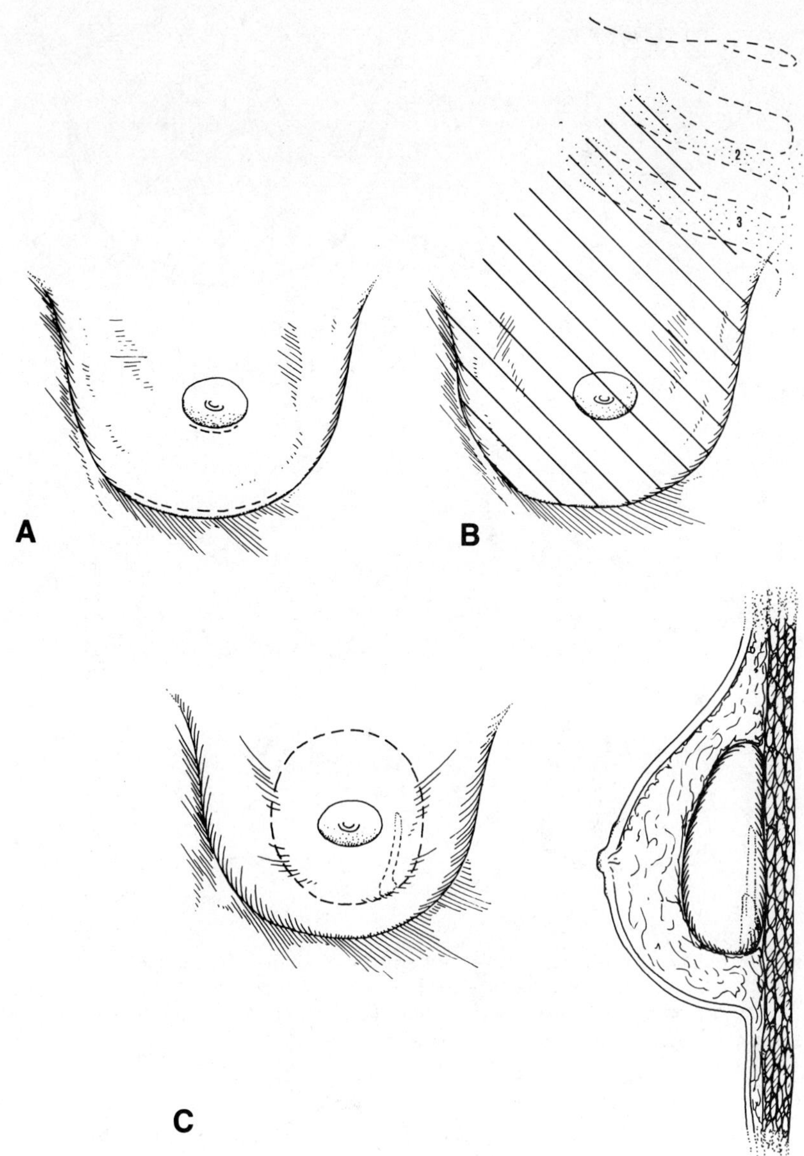

FIGURE 97–2 Augmentation mammoplasty technique. (*A*) Locations of possible incisions. (*B*) Extent of retromammary pocket. (*C*) Implant in pocket. (Grossman JA: Minor Injuries and Disorders: Surgical and Medical Care, p 281. Philadelphia, JB Lippincott, 1984)

Reduction Mammoplasty. Reduction mammoplasty may be performed in the woman with extremely large breasts. This procedure is often performed to reduce back and neck pain caused by the weight of the breast. Some women even have restriction of tidal volume because of their large breasts. Other women may develop brachial plexus impingement and neurologic deficits from the weight of the breast and the brassiere strap. Carcinoma of the breast must be considered in the woman with breast hypertrophy and a thorough history and examination should be completed prior to undertaking the procedure. The procedure is a major operative procedure which usually requires 2 to 4 hours. The tissue removed is always weighed and sent separately for pathologic studies. This procedure not only requires the removal of tissue but also the repositioning of the nipple-areola complex and reshaping and resuspension of the remaining breast tissue (Fig. 97–3).

Complications from this procedure may include hematoma formation, sloughing of the nipple-areola complex, necrosis of skin flaps, and excess scar formation. Because this procedure is usually undertaken to relieve medical problems, such as neck and back pain, most patients are quite satisfied with the results.

Techniques of Plastic Surgery

Although there are a few "standard procedures" in plastic and reconstructive surgery, there are few "standard cases." The techniques available to the plastic surgeon are many, and their applications to a specific patient or problem are varied and require a degree of creativity as well as skill. Although it is beyond the scope of this chapter to describe all the techniques of plastic surgery, a few of the more standard procedures and related postoperative care and potential complications will be discussed.

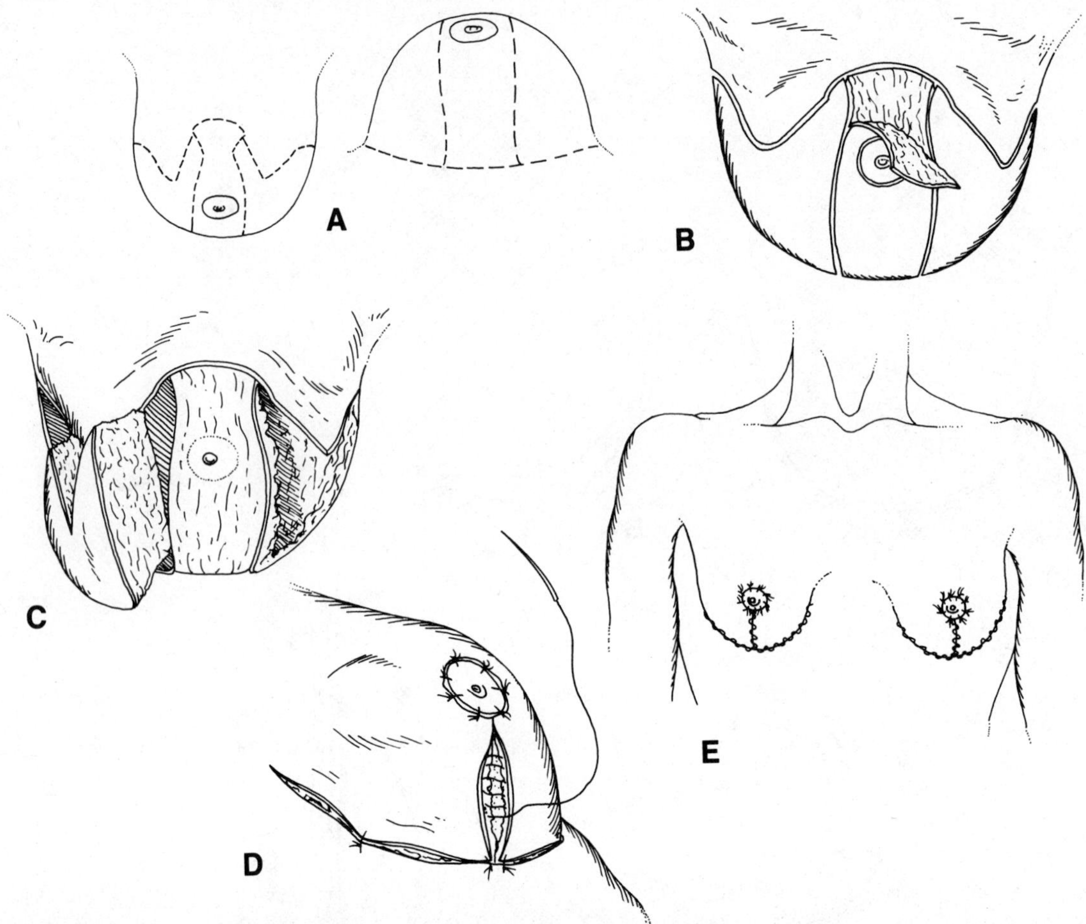

FIGURE 97–3 Method and pattern of reduction mammoplasty. (*A*) Patterns of de-epithelialization and resection marked out. (*B*) De-epithelialization of vertical pedicle for movement of nipple/areola. (*C*) Resection of breast tissue. (*D*) Closure of wounds. (*E*) Final closed wounds. (Grossman JA: Minor Injuries and Disorders: Surgical and Medical Care, p 283. Philadelphia, JB Lippincott, 1984)

Autografts

The free graft or autograft is the removal of tissue from one part of the body (donor site) and application of it to another area of the body (recipient site). The free graft is dependent on the ingrowth of new vessels into the grafted tissue for its blood supply. *Free grafts* may be either *partial-thickness grafts* or *full-thickness grafts* (Fig. 97–4). The partial-thickness or split-thickness graft is usually used to cover large surface defects and can be taken from almost any area of the body. These grafts are frequently used to cover burn wounds, degloving injuries, and large abrasions. The donor site from which the split thickness grafts is taken usually heals by reepithelialization in 10 to 12 days. If necessary, the donor site can be used more than once if it is needed for coverage of large surface areas as in a large burn injury. When split thickness grafts are used to cover facial wounds, it is preferable to use skin from above the clavicle or the inframammary area because this provides the best color match. Skin from other body areas have a yellow tone and do not match the normal blush tone of skin on the face and neck. Sometimes the skin of the scalp is used as a donor site for the face or neck. This not only provides an excellent color match but also leaves a hidden donor site when the hair regrows.

Postoperative Considerations. The partial-thickness or split-thickness graft is applied either as a sheet or as a mesh graft when larger areas are to be covered. The sheet of split-thickness skin gives the best cosmetic results but is the most tenuous during the first 24 to 48 hours postoperatively. When possible, the sheet graft is treated without dressing and inspected frequently for collection of blood, fluid, or pus beneath the graft. If any type of fluid collects under the graft, the blebs must be incised and the fluid expressed to prevent undermining of the graft. The new free graft must be in direct contact with underlying tissue to receive oxygen and other nutrients to support it until new vessels grow into the graft at about 3 to 5 days. The meshed split-thickness graft must be treated with moist dressings to prevent the many cut edges of the graft from drying out.

Because the meshed graft has multiple small holes in it, it is not as prone to being dislodged by the collection of fluid, blood, or pus. Therefore, the meshed graft is often used to close an older granulating wound which may be prone to

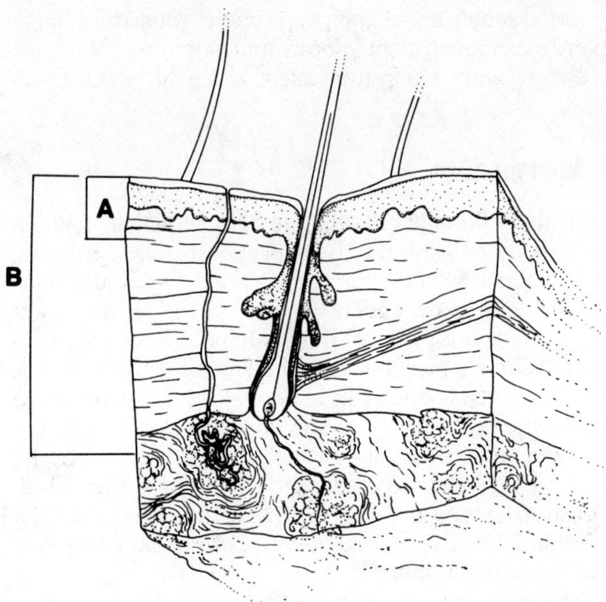

FIGURE 97-4 Microscopic cross section of skin showing (*A*) thickness taken in split-thickness skin graft, and (*B*) thickness taken in full-thickness skin graft. (Grossman JA: Minor Injuries and Disorders: Surgical and Medical Care, p 71. Philadelphia, JB Lippincott, 1984)

infection. The mesh graft does not give as good a cosmetic effect as does the sheet graft because as the interstices of the mesh heal in, there is a pebbly effect created. Over time this pebbly effect may lessen but not always. For this reason, mesh grafts are rarely used on the hand or the face and anterior neck.

One of the most common complications of the split-thickness graft is the scarring of the donor site. Although most donor sites heal with only minimal discoloration of the skin, some may heal with scar hypertrophy. The scar hypertrophy may be related to the depth at which the graft is taken or to infection in the donor site as the wound heals.

Full-thickness grafts require removal of the dermis as well as the epidermis and must be either closed primarily or with a split-thickness skin graft. The full-thickness graft is used in some facial reconstructive procedures and in areas where extreme wearing occurs such as over the heel and Achilles tendon. Although these grafts give a better cosmetic result because they tend to contract less, they are also more tenuous at first because it takes longer for the new vessels to revascularize the graft and it is also more difficult to recognize and treat hematomas or infection under the graft early. The most frequent sites for taking small full-thickness grafts are behind the ear, above the clavicle, in the antecubital fossa, or in the groin or gluteal crease. Primary closure of the graft site is possible if only a small amount of skin is needed.

Other *autogenous tissue* that may be harvested for reconstructive surgery include the dermis, tendons, cartilage, bone, periosteum, mucus membranes, muscles, nerves and composite grafts. The *composite graft* is when two or more tissue types are moved as one such as skin and muscle, skin and cartilage, or muscle, or bone. With the advent of microvascular techniques, large blocks of tissue to include skin, muscle, or bone can be moved and the blood supply restored by microvascular reanastomoses of vessels from the donor site to vessels in the recipient site. The recipient and donor vessels must remain patent to prevent necrosis and sloughing of the tissue. These techniques are frequently used to reconstruct large disfiguring wounds after trauma or ablative cancer surgery. The most common complication of these procedures is avascular necrosis. For example, if a bone graft is performed, the graft must be immobilized next to normal bone to ensure that the graft will be viable. If the graft is not immobilized next to normal bone, the grafted bone will be absorbed.

Skin Flaps

The skin flap is a more conventional way to move tissue from one area to another. In these procedures the vascular pedicle from the donor area is preserved and provides the blood supply to the flap until collateral blood supply develops from the recipient bed. At this time, the vascular pedicle can be cut and the flap reshaped if necessary. There are many different types of pedicle flaps, including the bipedicle, transpositional, rotational or tubed pedicle, and the bilobed pedicle. Flaps may only contain skin and subcutaneous tissue or may be compound flaps which contain muscle, cartilage, or bone. The flap must be carefully designed in relation to the blood supply of both the donor and recipient area. In the donor area, the flap must be designed so that blood supply will not be impaired by stretching or rotation of the donor vessels. The recipient site must also contain an adequate blood supply. Irradiated areas, old scars, or areas of poor vascularity as in venous stasis disease make poor recipient areas and care must be taken to provide margins of normal tissue when possible in the recipient bed.

Z-plasty

In addition to grafts and flaps the Z-plasty is another technique frequently used by the plastic surgeon. The Z-plasty is a procedure that interposes two interdigitating flaps. These procedures are frequently used to correct long linear scars or bands of scar tissue. By changing the direction of a linear scar or placing it in a normal crease line, often an ugly scar can be converted to one that is barely noticeable. By lengthening a scar or band of tissue, often contractures can be corrected and normal movement of a joint can be restored. This procedure and variations of the procedure (*i.e.,* double Z-plasty and W-plasty procedures) are very useful for many reconstructive procedures.

Postoperative Considerations

Postoperative care of grafts, flaps, and Z-plasty procedures requires careful attention to the vascular supply. The transferred tissue should be inspected frequently for signs of vascular compromise. Skin graft may require removal of fluids and clots that accumulate under the graft. The microvascular graft and the flap graft undergo changes in appearance with vascular problems. If the microvascular graft or flap becomes hyperemic it may be a sign of venous congestion or clotting; if it becomes cyanotic or white, it may be indicative of problems with the arterial supply. The Z-plasty must also be observed for the adequacy of circulation. Particular attention should be directed toward the most distal part of the graft because these areas are the most tenuous.

Erythema and swelling around the grafts may signify infection. The graft or flap should be inspected for color, the development of edema, excessive drainage, or changes in temperature. Dressings in and around the graft or flap should be inspected to ensure that they do not become constrictive as edema forms in the wound. Suture lines should also be carefully inspected. Sutures often become too tight as edema forms and may need to be cut to prevent necrosis.

Nursing Management

Nursing Diagnosis

Care of the patient with reconstructive problems requires that the nurse have an in-depth knowledge of wound healing. The nurse must know the expected time course of healing and scar maturation and be able to recognize complications in the wound early so that problems can be corrected and the proliferation of scar tissue decreased. In addition to a knowledge of wound healing, the nurse must be cognizant of the potential psychological problems of the patient having these procedures. Therefore, the nursing diagnoses pertinent to these patients deal with these two major areas of patient care.[10]

The major nursing diagnoses common to this group of patients can be identified, although some of these diagnoses relate specifically to patients having reconstructive surgery for particular problems. However, the nursing management of patients having reconstructive surgery must be individualized.

The major nursing diagnoses include

- Acute alteration in skin perfusion
- Chronic alteration in skin perfusion
- Potential for wound infection
- Potential for skin breakdown or loss of graft or flap
- Potential for nutritional deficits
- Potential ineffective airway clearance
- Potential deficit in diversional activities
- Potential for joint contractures
- Potential for the development of scar tissue
- Impairment of mobility (temporary)
- Self-care deficits
- Bathing and hygiene deficits
- Self-dressing and grooming deficits
- Self-toileting deficits
- Alteration in comfort: pain
- Body image disturbance
- Reactive depression (situational)
- Potential social isolation
- Sexual dysfunction
- Ineffective coping

The goals of nursing are to prevent infection, to maintain blood supply to the graft, to promote wound healing, to achieve maximum patient self-care and mobility, to minimize discomfort, and to help the patient achieve a positive self-image.

Interventions

Acute or Chronic Alteration in Skin Perfusion. Alteration in skin perfusion may be a local or systemic problem. For the trauma patient suffering from acute fluid volume loss, skin perfusion is dependent initially on the restoration of fluid volume. Once normal fluid volume has been reestablished, the nurse must be concerned about local tissue perfusion. To assess adequate local perfusion, the nurse should observe the color, temperature, and capillary refill of the area surrounding the injury, along suture lines, or of the tissue flaps created to cover the defect. This is true for all reconstructive procedures. The cause of decreased local perfusion may be increased edema, poor positioning, tight dressings, or tight sutures.

The nurse may prevent excessive edema formation by positioning the injured part so that it is just above the level of the heart. Because most patients undergoing these types of procedures are alert, the patient needs to be instructed in the appropriate position to relieve edema and prevent stress on the wound. Dressings should be applied firmly but should be checked routinely to be sure that as edema forms they do not impair adequate circulation to the wound. If as edema develops the nurse notes that the skin around the suture line has become tense and develops a red or blue discoloration, the physician should be consulted immediately.

Often clipping a few sutures will mean the difference between tissue necrosis and survival. In some cases chronic alteration in skin perfusion, resulting from venous stasis disease or radiation therapy, may endanger the results of the reconstructive procedure. In these cases increased awareness on the part of the nurse may allow for earlier intervention.

Potential for Wound Infection. With any wound there is always the potential for infection. This potential is greatest in the severely traumatized wound, which may be grossly contaminated, or in wounds created through irradiated tissue. The nurse should observe all wounds for signs of infection which may include: increased heat, redness, swelling, pain, and drainage of purulent material. If wound infection is suspected, the physician should be consulted immediately.

In most cases, the treatment for a wound infection involves removing dead or devitalized tissue, providing adequate drainage, and treatment with antibiotics. Although the removal of tissue is primarily the responsibility of the surgeon, frequent dressing changes and observation of the character and amount of drainage is usually a nursing responsibility. Additionally it is the nurse's responsibility to correctly administer the appropriate antibiotic. To achieve this, the nurse should know the correct dose and possible side-effects of the prescribed antibiotics.

Potential for Skin Breakdown or Loss of Graft or Flap. Injured tissue, skin grafts, or flaps have a potential for breakdown and pressure necrosis. The wound and surrounding tissue should be carefully inspected for signs of breakdown, such as rash, blisters, excoriation, and signs of pressure necrosis, such as red, purple, or blue discoloration. The most common reason for wound breakdown is a reaction to secretions draining from the wound or to the antiseptic solution used to cleanse the wound. In most cases every effort should be made to keep skin surrounding the wound dry and free of drainage. If antiseptic solutions are used to cleanse the wound, they should be rinsed from the wound and surrounding tissues before a dressing is applied. Ointments or drying agents should only be used if prescribed by the physician.

The most common reason for pressure necrosis is either a dressing applied too tightly or the patient lying or sitting on the affected part. To prevent pressure necrosis, the nurse should frequently check the tightness of all dressings and position the patient to prevent pressure on the wound. In some cases foam mattress or flotation or antipressure devices may be used if it is difficult to maintain the patient in the appropriate position.

Potential for Nutritional Deficits. Reconstructive procedures to the face and neck may complicate normal alimentation and thereby create the potential for nutritional deficits. For most patients who are well nourished and require stabilization of the wound for only 2 to 3 weeks, this is rarely a problem. For the severely traumatized person with increased metabolic demands or the cancer patient with prior nutritional deficits, this may be a major concern. Either tube feeding or intravenous nutrition may be necessary. Intravenous nutrition carries with it major consequences such as sepsis, air embolism, or pneumo- or hydrothorax. Tube feedings are usually preferred in these patients unless there are major abdominal problems. Tube feedings are not without risk, especially if the patient is comatose, drowsy from pain medication, or must have the jaws wired as part of the procedure. All patients receiving tube feedings should have the head of the bed elevated at least 30 degrees. For the patient who has his or her jaws wired, wire cutters should be kept at the bedside and the nurse should know which wires to cut to prevent aspiration if the patient vomits.

Potential Ineffective Airway Clearance. Patients with traumatic injuries or who have reconstructive surgery to the face, neck, and chest frequently have airway problems. The most common airway problems include obstruction related to edema or aspiration and atelectasis especially after a lengthy operative procedure. Nursing measures to prevent atelectasis should include coughing and deep breathing exercises, incentive spirometry, and frequent changes in position. (See Chapter 8.) The patient should be observed for changes in patterns of respiration, respiratory rate, or breath sounds. To reduce the change of airway obstruction from edema, the patient's head should be elevated. If the patient has a nasogastric tube, it should be kept patent and the patient should be checked frequently for increased residual gastric secretions. Total airway obstruction is often insiduous or happens acutely and there are few warning signs and symptoms to alert the nurse to an impending problem. With edema formation the only clue present may be increasing hoarseness. Measurements of blood gases and other respiratory parameters will rarely show change until the airway is almost totally obstructed.

Potential Deficit in Diversional Activities. Many patients who undergo reconstructive procedures are generally healthy people. When these patients find themselves confined to bed or unable to carry on their normal life, they frequently become bored, and the potential exists for a deficit in diversional activities. Caring for patients who are bored can be a real challenge. They frequently become the "problem patient" because they have many complaints about their care. Nurses may treat these patients as if they are not really sick and tend to shun them. This often leads to increased behavioral problems. A prehospitalization or preoperative conference with these patients and their families may help the patient understand the confinement of the postoperative period better and help the patient and family plan certain diversional activities. Encouraging the patient to bring hobbies with them to the hospital or even to take up new hobbies while in the hospital may help to alleviate the boredom and make for a more pleasant hospitalization for the patient and staff.

Potential for Joint Contracture. Depending on the procedure performed or the position required to be maintained postoperatively, potential joint contractures either from scar contracture or tendon shortening may be a problem. In some cases, this may be alleviated by proper exercise or splinting. In other cases, for example in someone with a crossleg pedicle flap, a shortened Achilles tendon may be an unfortunate result and may require prolonged rehabilitation once the pedicle is severed. When possible, the nurse should encourage active or passive range of motion in all joints to reduce the potential for this problem.

Potential for Development of Scar Tissue. Most patients presenting themselves for reconstructive procedrues expect to look better postoperatively; however, the potential exists for the development of scar tissue. Unfortunately, although the final result may be an improvement, the initial result may be worse than anticipated. For this reason the nurse and patient must have a thorough understanding of scar maturation. Scar tissue usually matures over a period of 6 to 12 months so that the final results may not be seen for at least a year. This prolonged time frame may be very disturbing to the patient and will require continuous explanation and support from the health-care professionals. Frequent discussions with the patient concerning how they feel about the results may elicit unexpressed fears or anxiety. Patients need to know that it is normal for people to be somewhat disappointed in their results initially. The patient who feels supported during the long scar maturation process is usually happier with the long-term results even if the results are not absolutely perfect.

Impairment of Mobility and Self-Care Deficits. Mobility and self-care deficits may occur postoperatively depending on the type of procedure and area of body involved. The important thing to remember is that often these procedures are performed in otherwise healthy people who may have considerable problems adjusting to their feelings of helplessness. Helping the patient to be as active in self-care as possible will allay some of these feelings. Allowing patients to make decisions about when and what is to be done for them will also help. Since these people are otherwise healthy, it is important to help maintain good grooming habits. If patients feel good about the way they look they will feel more like having company and interacting with others. Preventing self-imposed isolation may be very important to the patient's overall recovery.

Alteration in Comfort. Pain is associated with various reconstructive procedures and may range from mild to severe. Assessing the individual patient's response to pain and providing both pharmacologic and nonpharmacologic therapies to deal with the pain is a major nursing responsibility. Recognizing the interaction between physiologic pain, fear, and anxiety and providing relief for all three is important. While narcotics and anti-anxiety drugs may be helpful in relieving pain, psychological support and teaching the patient methods to reduce anxiety and stress are invaluable.

Body Image Disturbances. Patients who avail themselves of reconstructive procedures are prone to disturbances of body image. These may be mild or severe. As noted previously, part of the preoperative evaluation of these patients should be a psychological consult. Although correcting the deformity may improve the patient's physical appearance without extensive counseling, many of these patients are not happy with the differences they had anticipated in their lives. Often the patient will require extensive counseling pre- and postoperatively to attain the desired changes in their lives.

Reactive Depression (Situational). Even with preoperative counseling many patients develop a reactive depression postoperatively. This may be related to disappointment in the results of the procedure, the postoperative confinement or helplessness imposed by the procedures, the adjustment of the traumatized individual to a new lifestyle or the grief reaction frequently seen in the cancer patient. Assessment should include noting feelings of despair, changes in attention span, sleep disturbances, lower self-esteem, withdrawal or imposed isolation, misdirected anger, irritability, and increased dependency. Patients with these manifestations may require continued psychological counseling postoperatively.

Potential Social Isolation. Many patients who have reconstructive procedures, especially if the procedures involve the face, tend to shun social contacts, therefore there is a potential for social isolation. This has been especially true in the past when women had facelifts and wanted to be completely back to normal before being seen. This trend has somewhat lessened because more and more people, both men and women, are having such procedures. As people become more accepting of the procedures, this trend should lessen. Although there is nothing particularly wrong with some self-imposed isolation, patients should be encouraged to continue to have social contact with family and close friends. If the self-imposed isolation is prolonged or if the patient shuns all social contact, this may be a symptom of severe psychological problems and warrants further assessment.

Sexual Dysfunction. For some patients having reconstructive procedures, sexual dysfunction may be present preoperatively and others may develop the problem postoperatively. In most cases the sexual dysfunction is not a physiologic result of the surgical procedure but may be caused by how the patient feels about himself or herself. Especially when reconstructive procedures involve the female breast, a thorough assessment of the patient's feelings about herself and her perception of sexual adequacy should be part of the preoperative preparation. Counseling should be encouraged if the patient experiences sexual dysfunction either pre- or postoperatively.

Ineffective Coping. Most patients having reconstructive or cosmetic procedures will have some difficulty coping with the enforced changes in lifestyle even though they may be temporary. Usually with the support of family and health-care professionals, these problems will quickly disappear. There will be a few patients who will have prolonged difficulties in coping. They may exhibit the following characteristics: anxiety, fear, anger, inability to solve problems effectively or to meet basic needs, alterations in socialization and role expectations, noncompliance in self-care, high rates of accidents, and verbal manipulation. They may or may not be able to verbalize their inability to cope and may show changes in their normal communication patterns. They may feel that no one is able to understand their problems. These patients need continued psychological counseling and may benefit from self-help groups.

Nursing management of these patients is often difficult and frustrating. Helping the patient to deal with both the physical and psychological problems created by this type of surgery can be a challenge. The gratification for the patient and the staff is often delayed. Having the same nurses involved in all phases of the patient's care from the preoperative evaluation to the final rehabilitation is a goal worth accomplishing to benefit both the patient and the nurse.

Evaluation

Outcome criteria for patients having reconstructive surgery are:

1. Absence of manifestations of infection: redness, pain, swelling, discharge of pus at graft site, and systemic signs of fever, leukocytosis, fatigue, chills
2. Immediate consultation with physician if above signs occur
3. Absence of signs of compromised blood supply to graft: discoloration, necrosis, separation of wound edges
4. Immediate consultation with physician if above signs occur
5. Patient consumes adequate fluids, calories, protein, and carbohydrates to support wound healing (individually determined).
6. Patient participates in activities of interest to him or her and expresses satisfaction of these activities.

7. Skin intact, no signs of excessive pressure, or positional pressure sites
8. Patient exercises to extent possible. Joints are freely movable.
9. Patient performs self-care (hygienic measures) to maximum extent compatible with deficits in mobility.
10. Patient reports minimal discomfort and expresses control over pain management.
11. Patient discusses problems, feelings, and coping techniques. Seeks professional assistance and expresses feelings of increased control and competence in coping with the situation.

References

1. Branemark PI, Ekholm, R: Tissue injury caused by wound disinfectants. J Bone Joint Surg 49-A:48–62, 1967
2. Cancer Facts & Figures 1983, American Cancer Society, 1983
3. Cocke WM, McShane RH, Silverton JS: Essentials of Plastic Surgery, pp 118–135. Boston, Little, Brown and Co., 1979
4. Editorial: The Fifth International Conference on Tetanus, Ronneby, Sweden, 1978. J Trauma 20:191–105, 1980
5. Eickhoff TC: Symposium Keynote Address: Perspectives in Hospital Infection. In Cundy KR, Ball W (eds). Infection Control in Health Care Facilities, p 4. Baltimore, University Park Press, 1977
6. Fuller WD, Hunt J, Altemeier WA: Prophylactic antibiotics in penetrating wounds of the abdomen. J Trauma 12:282–289, 1972
7. Georgiade NG: Reconstructive Breast Surgery, pp 254–317. St. Louis, CV Mosby
8. Georgiade NG, Eiring A., Georgiade R, et al: The effects of various skin sterilization techniques on the viability of skin. Plast Reconstr Surg 21:479–482, 1958
9. Goin MK: Psychological reaction to surgery of the breast. Clinics in Plastic Surg 9(3):347–354, 1982
10. Gordon M: Manual of Nursing Diagnosis. New York, McGraw-Hill, 1982.
11. Stevenson TR, Thacker JG, Rodeheaver GT, Bacchetta C, Edgerton MT, Edlich RF: Cleansing the traumatic wound by high pressure syringe infection. JACEP 5:17–21, 1976
12. Thirlby RC, Blair AJ, Thal ER: The value of prophylactic antibiotics for simple lacerations. Surg Gynecol Obstet 156:212–216, 1983.

UNIT XII

Nursing Care of Patients with Alterations in Reproduction Function

Chapter 98

Review of Anatomy and Physiology

Reproductive System

Barbara R. Landau

The reproductive system is composed of those organs associated with the formation of gametes (germ cells), and their care and transport while in the body (including fertilized ova in females). There are three categories of structures associated with reproduction.

1. Essential or *primary sex organs* are the gonads—the testis and ovary. Gonads produce gametes and sex hormones. The testes produce spermatozoa (sperm) and secrete several androgens, the most important of which is testosterone. Ovaries produce eggs and several estrogens, as well as progesterone. The testes also produce some estrogens and the ovaries produce some androgens.
2. Accessory or *secondary sex organs* play a direct role in reproductive function. They store and transport the gametes (in the epididymis and uterine tubes), and nourish and protect them (in the seminal vesicles and uterus).
3. *Secondary sex characteristics* are not truly reproductive organs because they are not directly involved in the reproductive process, but they are sex-linked hormone-dependent characteristics. Included are growth of the larynx and vocal cords that lower the voice in men, development of the breasts in women, patterns of growth of body hair, differences in body configurations due to the skeletal development (broad shoulders and narrow hips in men and the opposite in women), muscular development, and distribution of subcutaneous adipose tissue.

The Male Reproductive System

The Testes and Scrotum

The testes are suspended outside the body cavity in the scrotum (Fig. 98–1), although they develop inside the abdominal cavity near the kidney. They are connected to the floor of the developing scrotum by a fibrous band, the gubernaculum, and as growth continues, the testes are drawn through the inguinal canal (in the inguinal ligament) into the scrotum, dragging their connections with them. These include the ductus (vas) deferens, spermatic arteries, veins, lymphatics, nerves, some smooth muscle fibers, and several layers of fascia, which together make up the spermatic cord.

The abdominal cavity and peritoneum evaginates into the scrotal sac (vaginal process) anterior to the testes, and eventually becomes sealed off as a closed sac, the tunica vaginalis. The obliterated pathways of the tunica vaginalis and of the testes through the abdominal wall present potential sites of hernia if closure is incomplete.

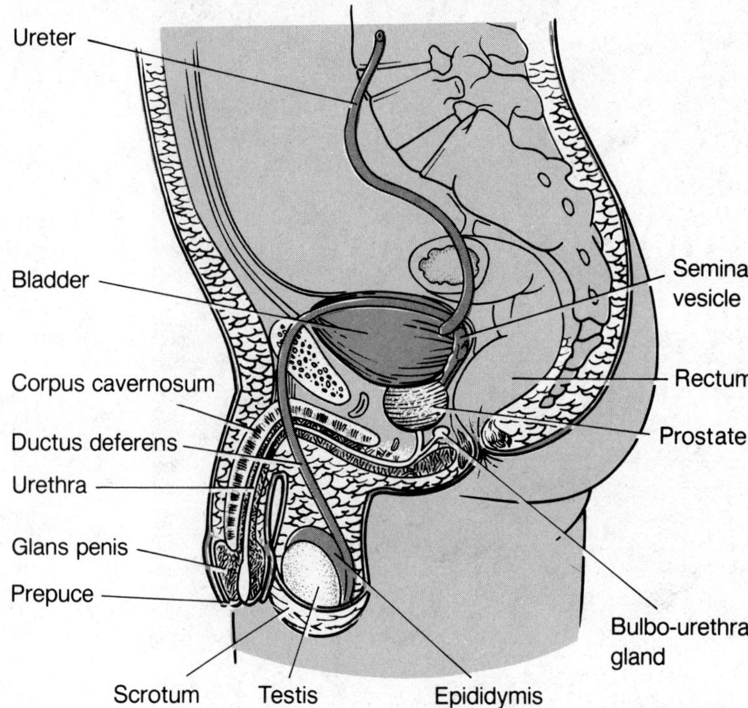

FIGURE 98–1 Organs of the male reproductive system.

Spermatogenesis (the development of sperm) requires a temperature slightly below body temperature. If the testes fail to descend into the scrotum they will not produce viable sperm, a condition known as cryptorchidism. A measure of temperature regulation is provided by muscle fibers in the scrotum whose contraction may raise (or lower) the testes, by dilation or constriction of blood vessels, and by a countercurrent heat exchanger operating between spermatic arteries and veins.

Structure of the Testes

The testes is partitioned into segments that are tightly packed with tortuously coiled seminiferous tubules (Fig. 98–2). Between the seminiferous tubules are clusters of interstitial cells, which are the source of testosterone. The scant interstitial space also contains blood vessels, nerves, and lymphatics. Seminiferous tubules converge to tiny efferent ductules that lead to the epididymis.

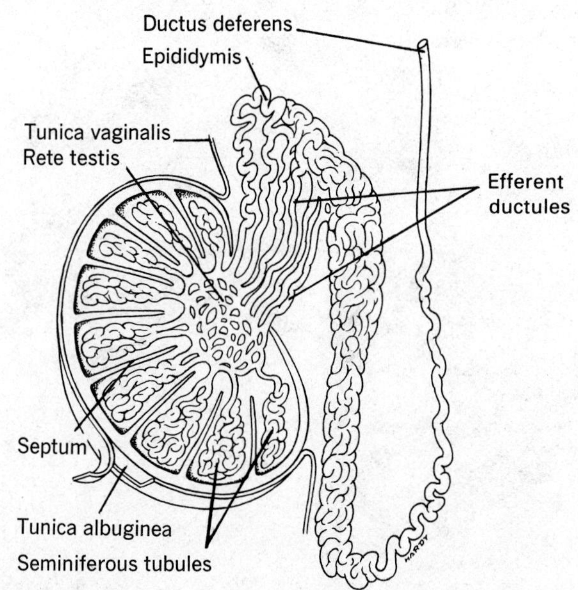

FIGURE 98–2 Structural features of the testis and epididymis.

Transport and Delivery of Sperm

Accessory Organs

The epididymis is a highly coiled tube, with smooth muscle in its walls and very long microvilli on its epithelium. It produces a small amount of fluid that becomes part of the seminal fluid (semen). During the 12 or so days it takes to traverse the epididymis, the sperm undergo the maturational changes necessary for them to become motile and capable of fertilizing an egg.

Upon appropriate stimulation, peristaltic contractions of the epididymal muscle propels the sperm into the ductus (vas) deferens, whose wall contains smooth muscle and ciliated epithelium. The ductus deferens arises from the epididymis near the bottom of the testes and ascends as part of the spermatic cord, retracing the course of the descending testes through the inguinal ligament and into the abdominal cavity. It circles around behind the urinary bladder and ureters, where it is joined by the duct from the seminal vesicle (see Fig. 98–1).

The seminal vesicles produce about 60% of the seminal fluid which, among other things, contains fructose (energy for motile sperm, which have a high energy requirement) and prostaglandins. The ducts converge to form the ejaculatory ducts, which open into the prostatic urethra.

The prostate gland is a doughnut-shaped organ inferior to the urinary bladder through which the urethra passes. Although it is a gland, it contains smooth muscle and a fair amount of connective tissue. Any swelling or enlargement of the prostate can interfere with the passage of urine. It may hypertrophy in later life. The prostatic ducts open into the prostatic urethra and deliver a small amount of fluid that contains a number of substances, among them cholesterol and phospholipids.

The uretha is divided into three parts, the prostatic, membranous, and cavernous (or penile) urethra. The prostatic urethra is the portion in the prostate gland, and the membranous urethra is the short segment that passes through the urogenital diaphragm (between the inferior rami of the pubic bones) as it leaves the body cavity. The cavernous urethra is so named because it is enclosed by highly vascular cavernous tissue of the penis. Tiny bulbourethral glands empty a small amount of mucous secretion into the urethra as it enters the cavernous tissue.

The penis, the male copulatory organ, consists mainly of erectile tissue, called the cavernous bodies: the paired corpora cavernosa and the smaller midline corpus spongiosum that contains the urethra. The cavernous bodies are attached to the urogenital diaphragm at the base of the penis and extend to its tip. The corpus spongiosum ends distally in the glans penis, which is abundantly supplied with tactile receptors. The whole organ is enclosed by a fibrous sheath with limited elasticity.

Erection and Ejaculation

Erection can be initiated as a spinal reflex by stimulation of tactile receptors, particularly those in the glans penis, or by psychogenic stimuli via the limbic system in the brain and pathways descending to the spinal reflex centers. The mechanism involves an increased blood flow into the cavernous tissue. Some of the penile arteries follow a spiraling course en route to the cavernous sinuses, and their thick walls have longitudinal folds in the intima. They are among the few vessels in which dilation is an active process (not just inhibition of constriction). Upon stimulation the vessels straighten and their lumens dilate, which increases the volume of blood in the cavernous tissue. The fibrous sheath around the penis limits expansion, and as the organ becomes engorged with blood the rising pressure in the cavernous sinuses tends to compress the veins, impeding the outflow of venous blood, and the penis becomes quite rigid.

The same stimuli initiate contraction of the smooth muscle in the accessory organs. Peristaltic contractions in the epididymis and ductus deferens move sperm, and contraction of muscle cells in the seminal vesicles and prostate move their secretions into the urethra. Rhythmic contractions of skeletal muscles at the base of the penis lead to the ejaculation of about 2 ml to 4 ml of semen, containing 200 to 300 million sperm (80 to 100 million/ml).

Endocrine Functions of the Testes

Testicular Hormones

The interstitial cells secrete androgens, mainly testosterone. Small amounts of estrogen and progesterone are produced by interstitial cells and by Sertoli cells. The adrenal cortex also produces androgens, mostly dehydroepiandrosterone (DHEA). Testosterone is synthesized from cholesterol and most of it enters the bloodstream. As with all steroids, testosterone is fat-soluble and can diffuse through cell membranes. It binds to a receptor in the target cell cytoplasm and acts in the nucleus to cause formation of mRNA, which leads to snythesis of the protein (enzyme) that carries out a specific action. Testosterone is metabolized in the liver to 15-ketosteroids and excreted in the urine, although some two thirds of the excreted 17-ketosteroids are derived from adrenal cortical steroids.

Testosterone secretion by the fetal testes is necessary for the normal differentiation of male internal and external genitalia (without it, female genitalia develop). It also has an effect on the brain, setting the male pattern of sexual behavior and gonadotropin secretion. After early fetal secretion, minimal amounts are produced until puberty, after which testosterone is secreted continously throughout life, though at a reduced rate in later years.

Control of Testicular Function

Spermatogenesis and hormone secretion are under the control of hormones from the anterior pituitary, and these are under the control of hypothalamic hormones, which gives the brain ultimate control of testicular function. The hypothalamus releases a peptide, gonadotropin releasing hormone (GnRH), into the hypothalamo-hypophyseal portal vessels, which carry it to the anterior pituitary gland to stimulate release of gonadotropins. Luteinizing hormone (LH), also known as interstitial cell-stimulating hormone (ICSH), causes the interstitial cells to produce testosterone. Follicle-stimulating hormone (FSH) initiates spermatogenesis. Some FSH diffuses into Sertoli cells of the seminiferous tubule, causing them to produce an androgen-binding protein, which binds testosterone. Testosterone is needed for the full maturation of sperm, and the binding protein ensures that enough of the testosterone that diffuses into the seminiferous tubules will remain there rather than enter the bloodstream.

The secretion of LH is inhibited by negative feedback of androgens, acting at the level of both the hypothalamus and pituitary. There is evidence that Sertoli cells produce a nonsteroid substance, inhibin, that inhibits pituitary release of FSH.

The Female Reproductive System

In spite of a number of similarities, there are several basic functional differences between male and female reproductive systems. In men from puberty onward, reproductive organ activity and hormone secretion maintain a reasonably constant level, declining only in later years. Sperm are produced continuously—about 30 million each day. In women after puberty, reproductive organ activity and hormone secretion undergo cyclic changes for a period of some 35 years (menarche to menopause). A single egg (usually) develops approximately once each month during that time, for a lifetime total of about 400. All potential ova are formed before birth but remain inactive until appropriately stimulated. Thus, female germ cells are anywhere from about 13 to 50 years old when they finally mature, and they are fertilized by germ cells that have been in existence about 2 to 3 months.

The Ovary and Follicle Development

The ovaries are roughly the size and shape of an almond and are suspended from the posterior surface of the broad ligament (see accessory organs below) by a short fold, the mesovarium. They are covered by a thin layer of connective tissue (tunica albuginea) and a layer of epithelial cells known as the germinal epithelium—because it was once thought to be the source of the germ cells, but is actually part of a modified peritoneal covering.

The substance of the ovary consists mainly of germ cells in various stages of development or degeneration. Over a million germ cells are formed before birth but they begin to degenerate (atresia) almost immediately, and at the time of puberty there are about 400,000 in the two ovaries. In prenatal life the germ cells are oogonia, and at the time of birth they become primary oocytes and begin the first meiotic division. Meiosis is arrested in prophase, however, and is not completed until the time of ovulation so that most never mature.

Oocytes develop in follicles (Fig. 98–3). Each inactive oocyte is surrounded by a single layer of flattened cells enclosed by a basement membrane, known as a primordial follicle. When the follicle is stimulated the oocyte grows, and the surrounding cells increase in size and number and develop into several layers which are called granulosa or follicular cells. A homogeneous noncellular layer, the zona pellucida, appears around the oocyte, and cells from the surrounding stroma become oriented around the follicle as the theca layer. The proliferating granulosa cells soon begin to secrete a fluid (follicular fluid) that creates a space, the antrum, that enlarges as more fluid is produced. The egg with its surrounding cluster of granulosa cells (the cumulus) remains attached to one side of the follicle.

The mature follicle (Graafian follicle) is 1 or 2 cm in diameter and bulges from the surface of the ovary. As ovulation nears, fluid formation increases, and the follicle wall thins and a slight nipple or stigma appears on the exposed surface. Ovulation occurs when the follicle ruptures and follicular fluid flows out into the abdominal cavity. The egg and cumulus are soon flushed out but usually stick to the surface of the ovary. Shortly before ovulation the first meiotic division is completed, forming one secondary oocyte and the first polar body (which is expelled). The second meiotic

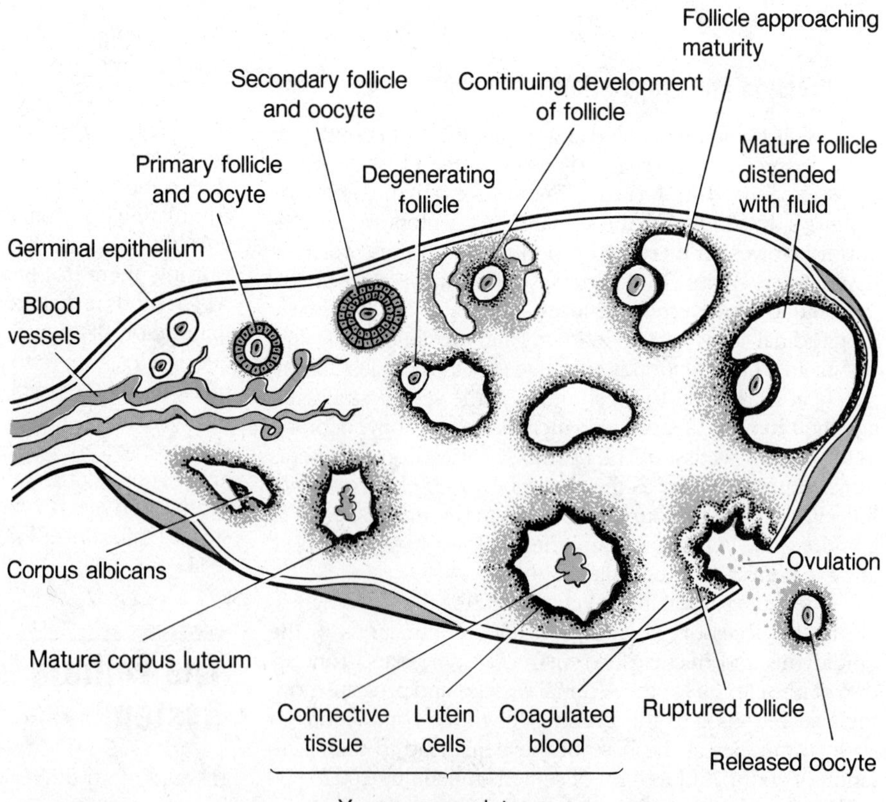

FIGURE 98–3 Schematic diagram of an ovary, showing the sequence of events in the origin, growth, and rupture of an ovarian (graafian) follicle and the formation and the retrogression of corpus luteum. For proper sequence, follow clockwise around ovary, starting at the germinal epithelium (*upper left*).

division begins but is arrested in metaphase and is not completed until, or unless, the egg is fertilized.

After ovulation, the remaining follicle wall collapses and folds in on itself to become the corpus luteum. Granulosa cells hypertrophy and differentiate but do not divide, and a pigmented lipid substance appears in the cytoplasm (hence the name corpus luteum). Theca cells cluster especially between the folds of granulosa cells, and capillaries and fibroblasts invade the cellular mass. The corpus luteum becomes quite large and functions briefly as an endocrine gland, but after a period of 10 to 14 days it begins to slowly regress and is eventually replaced by scar tissue (corpus albicans). If the egg is fertilized, however, the life of the corpus luteum is extended and it becomes even larger. The hormones that it secretes are essential for maintenance of pregnancy during the first 2 to 3 months.

Accessory Organs

Uterine Tubes

The uterine or fallopian tubes extend laterally from either side of the uterus (Fig. 98–4). Their walls contain smooth muscle and the epithelial lining is ciliated, and both are active at the time of ovulation. The fimbriated (fringed) lateral ends of the funnel-shaped uterine tubes are draped over the ovary. As the fimbria moves back and forth over the surface of the ovary, the cumulus containing the egg adheres to it and is drawn into the open end by the ciliary action. The actions of cilia, smooth muscle, and fluid currents move the egg along and in about 3 days it comes to rest midway down the tube, which is the usual site of fertilization. If the oocyte is fertilized it continues toward the uterus, but if it is not fertilized, the oocyte degenerates and is probably phagocytized in the tube.

Uterus

The uterus is a somewhat pear-shaped organ with a thick muscular wall, the myometrium, and a rather small, somewhat triangular lumen. The uterine tubes enter at the upper angles, and the inferior portion tapers to a narrow neck, the cervix, which protrudes into the vagina. The endometrial lining undergoes marked cyclic changes as a result of its sensitivity to ovarian hormones. The deep basal layer adjacent to the myometrium changes very little, but the surface functional layer proliferates and develops glands and increased vascularity with each cycle. It is this layer that is sloughed off in the menstrual flow. The endometrium in the cervical region, however, does not show such marked changes, but does produce mucus whose quantity and properties vary during the cycle.

Vagina

The vagina or birth canal is located between the uretha and rectum. Its upper end surrounds the cervix, and the narrower distal end opens to the exterior. Its wall is a thin fibromuscular coat and the mucosa lacks glands, but its epithelial cells (stratified squamous) undergo characteristic changes during the menstrual cycle.

Ligaments and Peritoneal Folds

The organs of the reproductive system are retroperitoneal and are covered by peritoneum or supported by peritoneal folds. The broad ligament of the uterus forms a fold over the uterine tubes and anterior and posterior surfaces of the uterus, and extends laterally to the body wall. The attachments to the body wall, the suspensory ligaments, provide support for the uterine tubes and ovaries, and passage for the ovarian vessels and nerves. The ovaries are suspended from

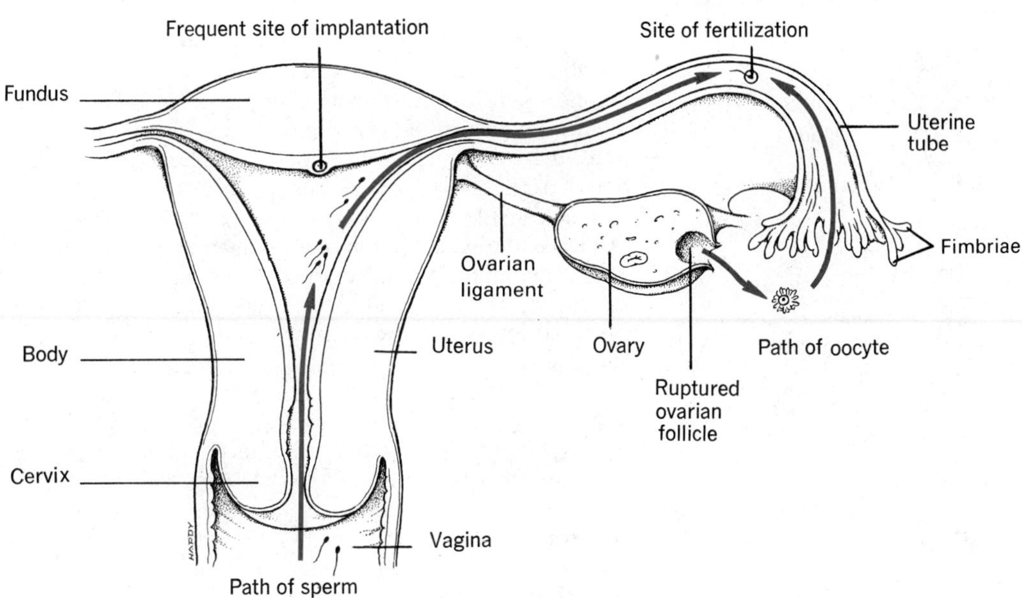

FIGURE 98–4 Schematic drawing of female reproductive organs, showing path of oocyte from ovary into uterine tube. Path of sperm is also shown, as is the usual site of fertilization.

the posterior surface of the broad ligament by a small fold, the mesovarium. The broad ligament encloses the ovarian ligaments, which extend from the uterus to the ovary, and the round ligaments of the uterus, which are embryological remnants that are homologous to the gubernaculum. The round ligaments extend anteriorly from the uterus and pass through the inguinal canal, ending in the labia majora.

External Genitalia

The external genitalia are collectively known as the vulva or pudendum. The perineum is the region of the pelvic outlet and includes the soft tissues between the pubic symphysis and coccyx (Fig. 98–5).

The vestibule is the space that contains the urethral orifice and the vaginal orifice (posteriorly). The latter may be partially covered by a highly vascular mucous membrane, the hymen, which may be absent or may close the opening entirely and may persist after intercourse. The lateral walls of the vestibule are formed by two folds of mucous membrane, the labia minora. Vestibular glands on either side of the vestibule produce a mucous secretion that facilitates movement of the penis during intercourse. At the anterior junction of the labia minora is the clitoris, which contains erectile (cavernous) tissue and is structurally similar to its counterpart, the penis. The labia majora, which lie on either side of the labia minora, are homologous to the scrotum in the male, and are the terminus of the round ligaments of the uterus. Deep to the labia majora on either side of the vagina there is some erectile tissue, the bulb of the vestibule, which corresponds to the bulb and corpus spongiosum of the penis and is also attached to the urogenital diaphragm.

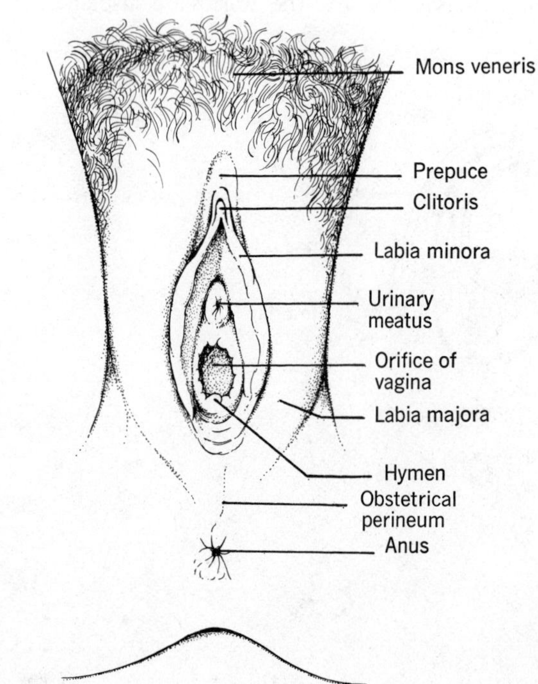

FIGURE 98–5 External genitalia of female.

Endocrine Functions of the Ovary

Ovarian Hormones

The ovary produces several steroid hormones, namely estrogen, progesterone, androgens, and their precursors, as well as relaxin and prostaglandins. The steroid hormones are synthesized from cholesterol, along pathways that are similar to those in the testes and adrenal cortex. Progesterone is an intermediary in all the pathways, and androgens are intermediaries in estrogen synthesis. The ovary is the main source of estrogen and progesterone, but the testes and adrenal cortex produce small amounts, and interconversions are possible in a variety of tissues. Estradiol is the chief estrogen; others are estrone and estriol.

Estrogens are released by both theca and granulosa cells of the developing follicle and the corpus luteum. Theca cells synthesize androgen, some of which is released into the circulation, some is converted to estrogen, but most of the androgen diffuses into the follicle, where granulosa cells convert it to estrogen. Most of the estrogen then diffuses out and enters the bloodstream but some remains in the follicular fluid.

Estrogens are responsible for growth and development of the accessory sex organs and secondary sex characteristics at puberty and for their maintenance thereafter. Estrogens also affect the gonads directly by their stimulatory action on granulosa cell proliferation, and indirectly by their control of gonadotropin secretion.

Many actions of estrogen involve some form of epithelial cell proliferation, including cyclic changes of the epithelial lining of the uterine tubes and vagina, and the endometrium of the uterus. They cause the cervical mucosa to secrete a high volume of watery mucus. Estrogens stimulate growth and development of the myometrium and uterine tubes, and increase excitability of their smooth muscle. The effects on secondary sex characteristics include enlargement of the breasts and growth of a duct system, closure of the epiphyses of long bones, development of the female habitus, including distribution of subcutaneous fat.

Estrogens have a number of metabolic actions, among them maintenance of normal blood vessels and skin conditions, reduced resorption of bone (by antagonizing the action of parathormone), increased tendency to edema by loss of fluid from blood vessels (causing decreased blood volume that leads to renal retention of sodium and water), increased levels of several clotting factors in the blood, and increased circulating levels of high-density lipoproteins (HDL) and reduced levels of low-density lipoproteins (LDL) and cholesterol.

Progesterone is present in only very small amounts until after ovulation, and then remains at a fairly high level until shortly before menstruation. Its effects are much greater on tissues that have been previously exposed to estrogen. Whereas estrogens promote proliferation and growth, progesterone stimulates differentiation of that newly formed tissue. Glands in the endometrium and breasts differentiate and acquire secretory capacity. Progesterone decreases the volume and increases the viscosity of cervical mucus. It also causes the slight rise in body temperature that occurs about the time of ovulation. Progesterone increases the respiratory response to carbon dioxide, resulting in a reduced alveolar P_{CO_2}; it competes with aldosterone in the kidney reducing sodium reabsorption and may lead to increased aldosterone levels. The latter two effects are more pronounced during pregnancy because the progesterone level is quite high.

Control of Ovarian Function

The ovary is controlled by the pituitary gonadotropins, follicle-stimulating hormone (FSH) and luteinizing hormone (LH), and the gonadotropins are controlled by the ovarian hormones and gonadotropin releasing hormone (GnRH) from the hypothalamus. There were formerly thought to be separate releasing hormones for FSH and LH, but it is now quite clear that a single peptide causes secretion of both. GnRH is released in small pulses at 1 to 3 hour intervals, and it seems that the proportion of FSH and LH released may be altered by changing the GnRH pulse interval. Perhaps the major control is exerted by the ovary itself, as feedback from the ovarian hormones. Ordinarily estrogen inhibits both gonadotropin production by the pituitary and GnRH release by the hypothalamus. Under certain conditions, however, estrogen exerts a positive feedback, in which estrogen increases gonadotropin release.

FSH acts on granulosa cells of early follicles, causing production of enzymes needed to convert androgens to estrogen. It also increases the number of LH receptors on granulosa cells (thereby increasing their sensitivity to LH). Synthesis of significant amounts of estrogens requires LH, however, for it stimulates theca cells to produce the androgens by increases in synthesis of the necessary enzymes. LH also stimulates the production of progesterone. Thus although LH is generally considered to be the cause of ovarian hormone secretion, it is clear that the participation of both FSH and LH is required. Estrogen from the follicle and estrogen and progesterone from the corpus luteum inhibit the release of both FSH and LH. The negative feedback seems to be most effective when estrogen levels are in a low to moderate range, for shortly before ovulation estrogen levels become very high and exert a positive feedback effect at both the pituitary and hypothalamus (probably by changing the size and frequency of GnRH pulses). The result is a sharp increase in gonadotropin release, primarily of LH, the so-called LH surge that triggers ovulation.

The Menstrual Cycle

The complex interactions between ovarian and pituitary hormones that cause the cyclic changes in the ovary and other reproductive organs can best be illustrated by noting the events that occur in the course of a single cycle. Figure 98–6 is an attempt to summarize some of these changes and relate them chronologically.

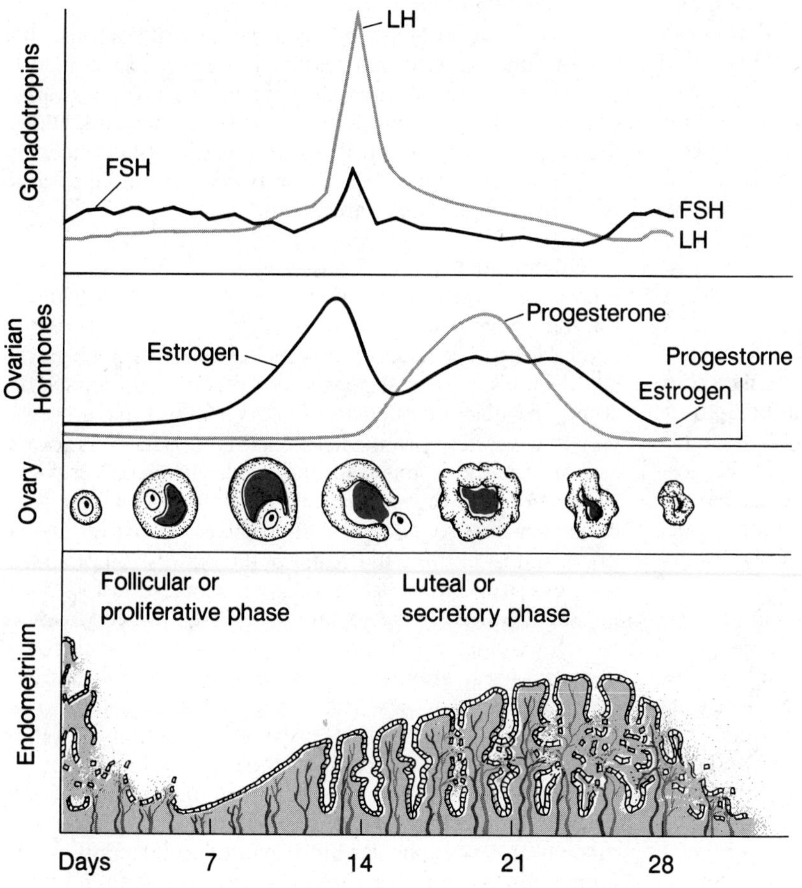

FIGURE 98–6 Summary of events in the menstrual cycle.

In young girls before puberty, FSH and LH are not detectable in the blood. Some follicles occasionally show slight signs of stimulation but do not advance beyond the primary follicle stage, and then undergo atresia. Cycles begin with the secretion of pituitary gonadotropins. A typical 28-day cycle is usually described, but there is considerable variation, especially in young women.

Week 1. The beginning of a cycle is taken as the beginning of menstrual flow, since it is the most readily identified event of the cycle. The menstruum contains cells, connective tissue, glands, and blood vessels of the functional layer of endothelium, and an average of about 30 ml to 50 ml of blood. At the end of 4 to 5 days only the basal layer of endothelium remains, with stubs of remaining blood vessels protruding from the surface.

Secretion of gonadotropin begins to increase before menstruation, and the FSH causes several primordial follicles to show signs of stimulation. The mechanism for "choosing" which follicles will respond is not clear, but several begin to develop and all but one (usually) will become atretic. Estrogen and progesterone levels are initially low, and some of that present may come from adrenal sources. In response to the FSH-induced follicle growth and the increasing number of granulosa cells coupled with LH stimulation of theca cells, the estrogen level begins to rise, and by the end of the first week there are signs of stimulation. The endometrium begins to grow, glands begin to appear, and blood vessels sprout into the thickening endometrium. Signs of stimulation occur in the uterine tube (including increased motility) and other accessory organs.

Week 2. During the second week the endometrium continues to grow, the follicle grows, and estrogen secretion increases. This part of the cycle is often called the proliferative phase in recognition of the endometrial changes, or the follicular phase in recognition of ovarian activity. Estrogen production rises sharply toward the end of the week, increasing by about 300% within about 36 hours. The rapid increase to such a high level elicits the positive feedback causing a great increase in LH secretion (accompanied by a smaller rise in FSH). This is the LH surge that causes ovulation to occur some 24 to 36 hours later, usually about the 14th or 15th day of a 28-day cycle. The follicle ruptures, the ovum is released, and the corpus luteum begins to form. Progesterone levels are very low until the LH surge is underway, which is fortunate, because there is evidence that high levels of progesterone block the positive feedback and LH surge.

Week 3. There is a brief decline in estrogen production as the corpus luteum forms but soon the levels of estrogen and progesterone rise. The corpus luteum becomes quite large, chiefly due to hypertrophy of the granulosa cells (now called granulosa lutein cells). Theca lutein cells undergo less conspicuous changes. Together estrogen and progesterone exert a negative feedback, and the concentrations of FSH and LH decline.

Estrogen continues to stimulate growth and proliferation of the endometrium and other tissues, but the presence of progesterone causes differentiation of those tissues. The growing endometrial glands begin to branch and coil, and soon acquire the capacity to secrete mucus and glycogen. The endometrial arteries grow and become increasingly coiled and are now called spiral arteries. The postovulatory part of the cycle is often known as the secretory phase in recognition of the changes in the endometrium, or as the luteal phase in recognition of ovarian events.

Week 4. In the fourth week the endometrium reaches its maximal development. The corpus luteum begins to lose its effectiveness and secretes less estrogen and progesterone. The cause of this is not known, but several possibilities have been suggested. Perhaps the low levels of gonadotropins (due to high levels of ovarian hormones) provide insufficient stimulus to maintain the corpus luteum. Perhaps prostaglandins, whose secretion is increased by LH, are responsible, or perhaps the corpus luteum is simply "programmed" to function for a limited period of time. Whatever the cause, secretion of estrogen and progesterone declines and all the hormone-dependent tissues show signs of deprivation.

The functional layer of the endometrium begins to shrink and the coiled arteries begin to undergo brief spasms, causing ischemia and damage to the distal tissues. When the vessels relax, there is some blood loss and further destruction of tissue, and with repeated vascular assaults, endometrial deterioration accelerates. By the end of the week (beginning of the next cycle) menstruation begins as the endometrial buildup is lost from the body.

Menstruation is essentially a withdrawal response, for without enough estrogen and progesterone to maintain it, the endometrium disintegrates. The falling levels of ovarian hormones remove inhibition of the pituitary gland, and in the latter part of the fourth week gonadotropin concentration rises, particularly FSH, and with it comes the stimulation of ovarian follicles that starts another cycle.

Menopause. Menopause, which is the cessation of menses, generally occurs in the age range of the early fifties, but the events that lead up to it take place over a period of several years. The ovarian response to gonadotropins gradually declines, and as estrogen secretion falls the cycles become irregular and often anovulatory. By this time, however, very few oocytes (primordial follicles) remain in the ovary.

Most of the changes are the result of reduced estrogen production (menopause has been described as an "estrogen deficiency disease"). There is still some estrogen production, but is almost entirely the result of the conversion of androgens to estrone in peripheral tissues. The levels of FSH and LH are elevated owing to loss of the negative feedback of estrogen. Other effects are due to the absence of estrogen stimulation on granulosa cells and on endometrium and other accessory tissues. There is a gradual atrophy and reduced mucus secretion by cervical, vaginal, and also urethral epithelium, as well as atrophy of the myometrium.

One very common problem is the occurrence of "hot flashes." An increase in core temperature elicits reflex vasodilation and sweating lasting some 10 to 20 minutes and commonly occurring at night. The episodes seem to be related to the decline in estrogen level rather than a low level *per se,* and are probably caused by a central nervous system link with hypothalamic centers affecting temperature regulation and hormone release. Episodes are known to occur in synchrony with pulses of LH release (which are greater in the absence of estrogen inhibition).

Other changes include a gradual decline in bone mass due to increased resorption and decreased formation of bone. There is increased withdrawal of Ca^{2+} from bone, and plasma Ca^{2+} levels are often slightly elevated. There is also a decrease in Ca^{2+} uptake, partly due to a reduced dietary calcium intake and to reduced intestinal absorption. Vitamin D ($1,25(OH)_2D_3$), which increases Ca^{2+} absorption, is also reduced.

Chapter 99

Assessment of Reproductive Function

Joan Shaver

Assessment of reproductive function in both women and men is generally based on determining whether any physical structural or functional alterations in organs or tissues of the reproductive tract exist or whether any cognitive–emotional responses are creating behavioral problems with sexual function. Cultural influences, biases, and taboos produce a block to open communication about this domain of functioning and render the patient susceptible to discomfort at having health-care workers probe the behavioral, physical, or emotional aspects of human responses related to reproductive function. Therefore, a sensitive, caring attitude when assessing this system is imperative in the therapeutic process. Provision of privacy and a nonthreatening questioning style with careful wording and phrasing of questions will enhance patient comfort in disclosing information. A style that conveys nonjudgment of replies but a genuine interest in the described experiences is helpful.

Nursing actions related to assessment of reproductive function involve performing or assisting with physical assessment of the patient. A professional approach to such an examination must be taken, with obvious concern for the dignity of the patient, particularly the privacy that is afforded in the situation. It is usually an excellent opportunity for health teaching about reproductive function. Collection of specimens for assessment is a nursing action that requires knowing proper preparation and processing of various samples and making the patient aware of the goals of the tests and of his or her participation in specimen collection. Although laboratory and diagnostic tests often require special preparation, the important common nursing action is explaining to the patient what to expect and the reason the tests are being performed. Obtaining data from patients requires interviewing skills and knowledge of the relevant information important to the diagnosis of human responses and health problems related to reproduction. Efforts to establish an information-sharing rapport between the patient and the nurse can do much to improve the collection of that data base.

Assessment of reproductive function consists of observing the structural as well as functional status of the patient. Structural examinations include inspection of the tissues and organs of the external genitalia, vagina, and cervix in women, and the penis and scrotum in men (other structures can be palpated); cytological examination of specimen collected from tissues or secretions of the reproductive tract; and visualization techniques. Functional data can be obtained from a gynecological history, including menstrual, sexual, contraceptive, and pregnancy information in women, and a sexual/reproduction history in men; and physiological function tests, including menstrual cycle hormone assays, endometrial, vaginal and cervical changes, body temperature, and tests for pregnancy in women, and hormone and ejaculate assays in men.

Assessment of Reproductive Function in Women

Structural Assessment

Physical Examination

Inspection of the visible tissues of the female external genitalia is a common starting place for determining the normalcy of the reproductive system. This begins with inspection of the mons pubis, labia majora and minora, and perineum and anal region for normal shape, skin integrity, and hair distribution. The clitoris, urethral meatus, and vaginal opening (introitus) can be seen by separating the labia. Tissues should be examined for any swelling, lesions, growths, cell changes, and abnormal coloration, and any abnormal discharge should be noted.

The vagina and cervix of the uterus as internal genitalia can be inspected by inserting a bivalve-blade metal instrument, the speculum, into the vagina. With the blades closed and lubricated with only warm water, the speculum is gently inserted downward and backward fully into the vagina, then opened to observe the cervix (Fig. 99–1). The cervix is about 2 to 3 cm in diameter in nulliparous women (women who have never given birth) and 3 to 5 cm in women who have delivered vaginally. It normally protrudes about 1 to 3 cm into the vagina. The normal cervix is pink and free of lacerations, ulcerations, growths, and inflammation. The uterus opening (the os) is generally small and closed in a woman who has never been pregnant but larger in the adult female who has been pregnant. Discharge or the presence of polyps is abnormal. It is during this phase of the examination that a spatula or cotton-tipped applicator is used to collect a smear from the cervical os, endocervical canal, or posterior fornix of the vagina. The smear may be put on a slide and a fixative applied (a Papanicolaou smear). The cells present are then inspected microscopically for abnormal cellular changes. A specimen obtained from the endocervical canal with a sterile cotton-tipped applicator may be rolled onto a culture medium (Thayer-Martin) plate and incubated for gonorrhea, a sexually transmitted disease.

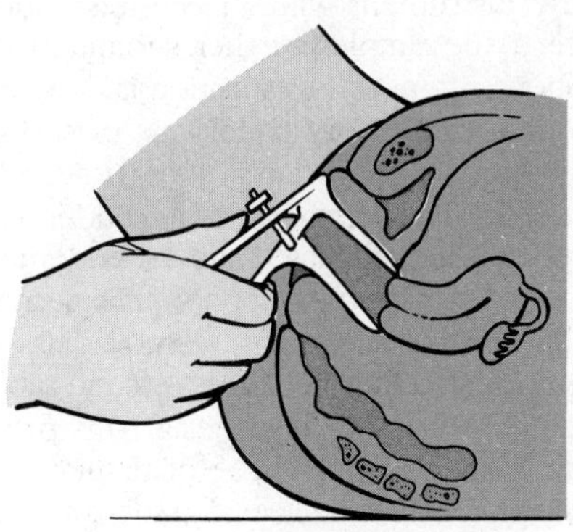

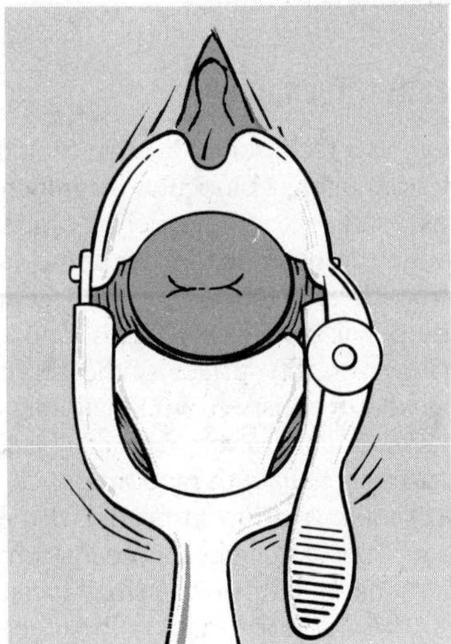

FIGURE 99–1 Vaginal speculum examination.

Normally the vaginal walls should be pink and folded without any discharge. However, the vagina is often a hospitable environment for fungi (*Candida* organisms) and bacterial infection (*Trichomonas, Pseudomonas,* gonorrhea) to flourish, in which case discharge may be noted. A bearing-down maneuver after the speculum has been partly withdrawn should show no protrusion of the cervix or bulging of the anterior or posterior vaginal walls. When there is relaxation of the vaginal walls, the bladder or the rectum can bulge into the vagina, respectively called a cystocele or rectocele. This is a more frequent occurrence as women age.

Following the internal examination with a speculum, a bimanual examination to palpate other structures is usually done by placing two examining fingers in the vagina and a hand on the abdomen (Fig. 99–2). This allows the uterus and adnexa to be palpated. The size, shape, position, mobility, regularity, and consistency of the cervix should be noted. Generally the cervix points posteriorly from the top of the anterior vaginal wall and the fundus of the cervix points anteriorly. Normally the cervix can be freely moved 2 to 3 cm in any direction without causing significant discomfort. Additionally, the uterus should be palpated for position, size, shape, consistency, and mobility with any tenderness or masses noted. The hand that is placed on the abdomen is used to apply pressure in order to palpate the fallopian tubes and ovaries between it and the fingers placed in the vagina. Any enlargement of the organs and tenderness or masses are again noted.

Completion of the internal genitalia examination occurs with rectovaginal abdominal palpation. The middle finger is lubricated and gently inserted into the rectum; the index finger is placed in the vagina. (Fig. 99–3). This method allows the examiner to explore the rectovaginal septum, posterior wall of the uterus, posterior fornix, and cul-de-sac to rule out nodules, scarring, or indurations.[3]

Nursing responsibilities in the physical examination may include performing the physical examination in a practitioner role or assisting a physician during the examination. For obvious reasons, such examinations are potentially embarrassing and anxiety-provoking. Supportive preparation,

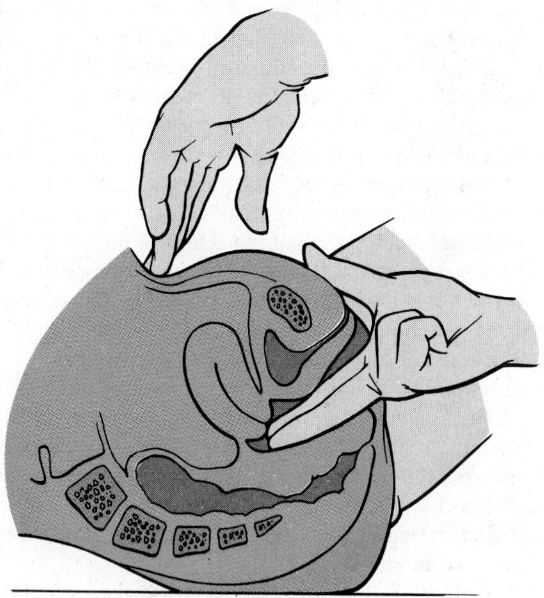

FIGURE 99–2 Assessing and manipulating the uterine cervix.

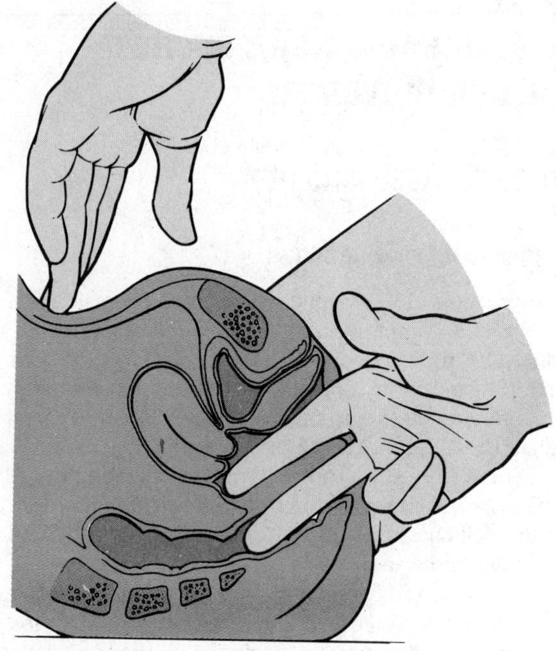

FIGURE 99–3 Retrovaginal–abdominal palpation of internal reproductive organs.

respect for privacy, and ongoing explanations of the procedures are needed. Currently, there is reported success at alleviating some of the anxiety by promoting a much more participative approach with patients. Mirrors are used to have women view the cervix and genital tissues while they are taught to recognize normal aspects and assess any possible abnormalities on an ongoing basis.[4,6]

Cytological Examination

Cytological testing is a screening procedure used to determine if there is any evidence of abnormal cell growth in reproductive tissue. Any such findings would suggest that further investigations be done. As mentioned, specimen may be collected during the vaginal examination using the speculum. Prior to speciman collection, a Schiller's test may be done to detect any signs of abnormal epithelium. Normal cervical squamous epithelial cells contain glycogen and stain dark brown when coated with Lugol's iodine solution. Abnormal epithelial and columnar cells are devoid of glycogen and therefore do not stain. This test is not diagnostic for cancer but indicates areas of abnormal epithelium from which tissue for microscopy should be obtained.

Cytological material should be collected from the cervical canal (endometrial and endocervical secretions) by rotating a saline-moistened, cotton-tipped swab within the cervical canal or by aspirating the secretion with a pipette. Material from the junction of the squamous and columnar epithelium should be collected by scraping and abrading the area with a special spatula. In either case, the material is put on a clean glass slide. Whenever abnormal cells are evident, further tests are needed with samples obtained through culdoscopy or cervical or endometrial biopsy.

Cervical biopsy tissue permits more precise diagnosis of cellular changes than gross inspection or other cytological examination. Small bits of tissue can be removed with a punch biopsy instrument without causing undue pain or bleeding. The tissue samples are then submitted to histological examination and more investigation is done if abnormal cell growth or inflammatory conditions exist. Endometrial biopsy can be done in a clinician's office. However, it is most efficiently done by dilation and curettage under anesthesia in which the cervix is gently dilated and the endometrial lining of the uterus is scraped with a spoon-like, serrated instrument. Histology is then done on the removed tissue to determine any abnormal cellular changes. A cone biopsy can be done in the hospital under anesthesia. This procedure involves taking a cone-shaped piece of tissue including the lesion and most of the cervical canal tissue. Multiple sections can then be cut from the removed tissue and checked for abnormal cells.

Visualization Techniques

Culdoscopy is a technique for inspecting the cervix and vaginal epithelium using a binocular magnifying instrument. Culdoscopy is used to examine pelvic organs. A trocar is inserted through the posterior fornix of the vagina with the woman in knee–chest position. The culdoscope is then inserted into the pelvic cavity. This makes it possible to detect epithelial changes on the surface of the cervix that are not visible with naked eye inspection. Small areas of dysplasia, carcinoma *in situ,* and invasive cancer can be seen and biopsied more accurately than with random punch biopsy.

Laparoscopy allows direct inspection of the pelvic cavity. A high-intensity, fiberoptic light source instrument known as a laparoscope is inserted through a small incision just below the umbilicus. The anterior surface of the uterus, the adnexa, and the posterior cul-de-sac can be viewed in this manner. This procedure may be used to evaluate pelvic pain of unknown origin, and to inspect for small uterine or ovarian masses, infertility problems, congenital anomalies, and ascites.

X-ray tests of the pelvic region may be helpful in the evaluation of various pathologies including pelvic masses or areas of calcification in fibroid tumors or ovarian neoplasms. An important use involves hysterosalpingography in which visualization of the uterine cavity and the fallopian tube lumen is possible after a radiopaque material is injected into the upper reproductive tract. Small intracavity uterine lesions as well as abnormalities in the fallopian tubes can be detected. However, care is taken not to expose pregnant women to x-rays, particularly during the first trimester of pregancy.

Visualization can also be done with *ultrasonic techniques* in some situations. High-frequency sound waves return echoes whenever there is a change in the density of the tissues through which they are passing. Ultrasound can be used to assess normal or abnormal pregnancies including identifying multiple pregnancies and fetal anomalies and assessing fetal growth and placental localization. It can also be used for differential medical diagnosis of various uterine and ovarian enlargements as well as to assess the process of follicle growth and ovulation in infertility studies.[1]

Functional Assessment

Gynecological History

Pertinent information in assessing reproductive function can be obtained by asking the patient about current and past events including menstrual and contraceptive information, pregnancy, and sexual behavior. Many aspects of these histories are considered sensitive areas and patients may be reluctant to share information about them. However, a professional, nonjudgmental approach helps facilitate obtaining relevant information about reproductive health status.

General reproductive information should be ascertained regarding any vaginal discharge and pruritus, breast pain, discharge or lumps, abnormal Pap smears, pelvic pain or abnormal vaginal bleeding, past venereal disease, and pain with intercourse (dyspareunia). A strong family history of gynecological malignancy such as ovarian, uterine, or breast cancer is pertinent information.

One obvious indicator of normal reproductive function in women is the regularity, consistency, and normalcy of the menstrual cycle. A *menstrual history* should include: age at which menstrual periods began (menarche), preparation and reaction to menarche, frequency, duration, and interval of periods, date of last menstrual period, amount of bleeding, any associated pain (type, when it began, duration, interference with daily living, self-management for relief), intermenstrual bleeding, and postcoital or any other symptoms associated with the menstrual cycle.

Usually, first menstruation begins between the ages of 9 and 18 years, within 2 to 4 years after the beginning development of secondary sex characteristics. Monthly cycles then continue usually until the forties or early fifties when last menstruation (menopause) occurs. Alterations in the usually cyclic pattern of menstruation are abnormal and are cause for problem assessment. Periodic bleeding normally occurs every 21 to 45 days (mean = 28.4 days) with flow lasting about 2 to 7 days (mean = 5 days). Average blood loss per menstrual period is only 50 ml to 150 ml. Individual regularity is the general rule but there is considerable variation in cycle length from one woman to another. The preovulation, follicular phase of ovum development has known variability in length from one woman to another. However the postovulation, luteal phase is thought to be normally rather constant at 14 ± 2 days. Abnormal bleeding may take many forms including prolonged or excessive menstrual bleeding (menorrhagia), or spotting or usual amounts of bleeding at irregular intervals (metrorrhagia).

A *contraceptive history* should document the current method being used (if any), duration of use, and problems encountered. Use of oral hormonal preparations and the experience of any side-effects such as thrombosis, migraine, or mood changes or the use of intrauterine devices with any accompanying symptoms such as pain, discharge, other signs of pelvic infection, or late pregnancy loss should be noted.

A detailed *obstetrical history* includes data on the total number of pregnancies, spontaneous and induced abortions, ectopic pregnancies, and premature and term births. Gestational length and pregnancy termination methods (dilatation and curettage, saline abortion, spontaneous vaginal delivery, forceps or cesarean section deliveries) should be ascertained along with any experiences with postpartum complications of lactation, infection, depression, or other complications. In cases where pregnancy has not occurred, the desire for pregnancy and attempts to get pregnant are important information to guide possible referral for infertility assessment.

Sexual History. A complete assessment of reproductive function includes a sexual history of homosexual activity, difficulty with intercourse, or infertility. A brief review of major sexual dysfunction problems and the general etiology of health problems in this area follows. Assessment involves tactful interview of the patient.

Fogel says that women's concerns about sexual functioning tend to cluster around the themes of lack of interest in or feelings for sexual activities, orgasmic difficulties, and pain associated with coitus.[4] The complex etiology of these problems often warrants referral to specialists in the treatment of sexual dysfunction.

General sexual dysfunction in women is manifest as a lack of erotic feeling and responses with no sexual pleasure derived from sexual stimulation. Physiologically there is no significant vaginal lubrication or vasocongestion signs suggestive of the first phase of sexual arousal. Sexually unresponsive women vary in their cognitive/emotional and behavioral reactions to this situation. Some choose to avoid sexual intercourse and find the idea unappealing, others may endure it to preserve a partnership, and still others reportedly enjoy the physical closeness of the act even though they do not receive sexual gratification. Therefore, the coping response will dictate whether or not the experience of general sexual dysfunction is perceived to interfere with daily life and create a health/wellness problem.

Another category of sexual dysfunction is referred to as orgasmic dysfunction in which a woman is sexually responsive, perhaps seeks sexual contact, and demonstrates arousal but is unable to proceed beyond the plateau stage to orgasm. Again the coping response may be such that this condition does not create a health problem for the woman, or it may create negative psychological consequences.

A third category of sexual behavior difficulty is called *vaginismus,* which is relatively rare. Although the tissue and organs of the genitalia appear normal, intense vaginal muscle contraction is present when intercourse is attempted. Many women exhibiting vaginismus are sexually responsive and orgasmic. Theory has it that it may arise as a conditioned response to adverse stimuli associated with actual experiences or fantasies about intercourse or vaginal entry.[4] In the event that this condition or the previously mentioned ones cause distress for a woman, referral to health care specialists in the field of sexual therapy is appropriate. Specific therapies involve extensive education on the physiological and psychological components of sexual behavior, sensate-focusing exercises, communication improvement, and other techniques depending on the nature of the difficulty.

Eliciting a sexual history is frequently difficult for nurses to initiate owing to their own cultural conditioning. However, it is a necessary part of the data base from which diagnoses regarding reproductive function can be made. Although there is no routine way to obtain such information, obvious prerequisites to getting valid information are to have privacy for the interview, move from less sensitive to more sensitive issues, phrase questions in a manner which implies that the specific behavior is not too unusual, and avoid questions that will elicit stereotypic response.[4] For example, a nurse might say "When did you begin to have sexual intercourse?" rather than "Have your ever had sexual intercourse?" Additionally she can say: "There are many forms of sexual expression in people, including having sexual communication with members of the opposite sex or with members of the same sex. How would you describe your own sexual preference?" A further example might to be ask questions in an open-ended manner such as: "People often have questions about their own sexual behavior. Do you have any particular concerns about the sexual aspects of your life?"

Health Education. An opportunity is available for nurses to provide health education during the time that a health history of reproductive function is being taken. Information about normal function can be given, terminology clarified, and assurance expressed. Depending on the life stage of the woman, various aspects of reproductive function are more appropriately emphasized. In adolescents, the emphasis might be on menstrual function and prevention of pregnancy. In young adults, these same issues are important along with preparation for pregnancy. In middle-aged women, more emphasis in health education is placed on the menopause and functioning beyond the reproductive years.

Physiological Function Tests of the Menstrual Cycle

Besides the data obtained from the patient about reproductive function, several objective tests are available to determine whether physiological function is normal or not. Reproductive function depends in large measure on the gonadal, steroid sex hormones, the estrogens and progestins (from the ovaries in females) and the gonadotropins from the hypothalamic/pituitary axis (*i.e.,* follicle-stimulating hormone and luteinizing hormone). Since female reproductive function is cyclic, tests pertinent to the phases of the menstrual cycle are done; for example, the levels of estrogen in the follicular phase and the levels of both estrogen and progesterone in the luteal phase.

Hormone Assays. Hormone assays of ovarian steroid hormones (estrogens and progesterones), or pituitary protein hormones (follicle-stimulating hormone [FSH] or luteinizing hormone [LH]) can be done on plasma or urine using chemical methods or by radioimmunoassay. Radioimmunoassays are capable of quantifying very small concentrations (picograms or one one-millionth of a milligram) of estrone, estradiol, or estriol present in the blood plasma. Careful attention must be paid to documenting where a woman is in her menstrual cycle when samples are taken since levels fluctuate throughout the cycle. Estrogen concentrations are low in the early follicular phase (25 to 75 pg/ml), rise rapidly in the late follicular phase and ovulatory phase (200 to 600 pg/ml), remain elevated during the luteal phase (100 to 300 pg/ml) and decline again at the time of menstruation.

Sometime prior to but especially following ovulation, the normal corpus luteum secretes progesterone. Assessment of progesterone is therefore indicative of successful ovulation and provides initial assessment of absent ovulation (anovulation) as a reason for infertility. Hormonal assays for progesterone are available as they are for estrogen. Progesterone is low in the follicular phase (0.4 to 1 ng/ml) but rises to significant levels in the luteal phase (5 to 15 ng/ml).

Since the function of the ovaries in producing estrogens and progesterone is dependent on FSH and LH (gonadotropins from the hypothalamus/pituitary axis), reproductive function may be changed by alterations in the synthesis, release, action, or degradation of these hormones. Radioimmunoassay of FSH and LH can also be done to determine levels. Highest concentrations of these hormones in plasma occur at midcycle when a surge occurs immediately prior to ovulation.

Tissue and Mucous Smears. Gonadal hormone effects on vaginal, cervical, and endometrial tissues of the reproductive tract can be used as indirect indicators of cyclic hormonal levels. As target tissues for the steroid ovarian hormones, some of their characteristics change with exposure to hormones.

Vaginal smears can be used as an indicator of hormonal function. Under the influence of estrogen, cells of the vagina undergo growth. Basal and parabasal cells proliferate and the epithelium becomes thicker as the cells grow and cornify. When a stained smear of cellular material collected from the upper vagina reveals cornified or precornified cells, the presence of adequate estrogen is surmised. When such cell changes are absent, the influence of estrogen is presumed deficient.

The canal of the cervix contains multiple crypts or glandular structures that secrete mucus into the endocervical canal. The physical characteristics of the mucus vary under the influence of the dominant hormones of the menstrual phases. Just following menstruation the mucus is sparse in amount, viscid, and sticky. Under the influences of increasing estrogens, the quantity of mucus increases until the time of ovulation although viscosity progressively decreases. At the time of ovulation, the mucus is a thin hydrogel, containing mostly water. The mucus at this point is clear and stretchy. The ability of mucus to stretch or spin in a thread is a characteristic called spinnbarkheit. It is quantified by measuring how far mucus can be stretched without breaking. A clear, elastic mucus is believed to facilitate the entry of sperm into the cervical canal for ascension through the uterus to the fallopian tube, which is the site of ovum fertilization. Therefore, the ability of the mucus to stretch is sometimes used as an indicator of the ability of the mucus to support sperm transport and is assessed in infertility considerations. Adequate estrogen production in the follicular phase of ovary follicle development is prerequisite to this change. After ovulation the mucus becomes thicker, cloudy, white or yellow, and tacky. It becomes scant in amount and may disappear in terms of vaginal discharge. Functionally, the thicker mucus seals the cavity of the uterus in case a fertilized ovum has been implanted postovulation.

Cervical mucus can also be assessed by spreading it on a clean glass slide and observing for a pattern of arborization or "ferning" as it dries. The degree of ferning is also influenced by the level of estrogen support. When estrogen levels are low, ferning is absent (occurs after menstruation). This sign progressively increases to a maximum at ovulation when estrogen peaks. Ferning is also inhibited in the second half of the cycle owing to progesterone. This test, if done in the luteal phase of the cycle, can then be used to speculate about the presence of ovulation and the secretion of progesterone. The presence of ferning is believed to be related to the concentration of electrolytes (especially NaCl) in the mucus. Estrogen augments the secretion of salt in the mucous outflow from the glands. Mucus is obtained by inserting an unlubricated speculum into the vagina and visualizing the cervix. A cotton-tipped applicator is inserted into the cervical canal and rotated. The mucus that adheres is placed on the clean glass slide and allowed to dry at room temperature.

Since an outcome of estrogenic activity is proliferation of the endometrial lining of the uterus, a biopsy of the endometrium can be taken and the cells studied histologically for appropriate changes. Under the influence of estrogen, the endometrium increases in thickness and the surface cells appear more columnar. The endometrial glands become tortuous and mitotic (cell division) activity is evident in the epithelial cells. Alternately the influence of progesterone produces a secretory epithelium with attendant cellular changes in the endometrium.

Basal Body Temperature. An indirect but noninvasive method of determining whether postovulation secretion of progesterone is occurring is to measure the basal body temperature over the menstrual cycle. Progesterone is believed to have a thermogenic effect that in many women causes the body temperature to go up roughly 1° F in the last half of the cycle. Women are carefully instructed to take their oral temperature before arising in the morning using a thermometer that has an elongated scale around the range of usual body temperature of 96° to 100° F. In the majority of healthy adult women a biphasic curve is evident when the daily body temperature is graphed over a menstrual cycle. Following menstruation body temperature is reasonably constant until ovulation when a distinct rise of about 1° F is evident and persists until the next menstrual flow.

Test of Physiological Function in Pregnancy

In women of childbearing age, pregnancy is usually suspected when there is a break in menstrual cyclicity. Bodily changes including enlarged, tender breasts, and alterations in appetite or experiences of nausea often may occur concomitantly. As a confirmation of pregnancy, tests to detect human chorionic gonadotropin (HCG) are done. After fertilization of the ovum, and as the trophoblast prepares to implant, HCG is secreted by placental cells and is detectable in the urine or plasma. Common pregnancy tests presently used are immunologic tests based on the reaction of urinary HCG with added serum-containing antibodies (antiserum) to HCG. Most pregnancy tests use agglutination inhibition as an indicator. The urine of pregnant women containing HCG is combined with serum-containing antibodies (antiserum) so that the HCG and antibodies will complex. When this mixture is added to latex particles (on a slide) or sheep red blood cells coated with HCG (in a test tube), agglutination is inhibited since antibody is already complexed, thus serving as a positive test for pregnancy. If the urine does not have HCG in it, the antiserum will complex with HCG-coated sheep red blood cells or the latex particles, causing agglutination or a negative test for pregnancy. The hemagglutination test is a 2-hour test but is more sensitive than the slide test, which takes 2 minutes. Both tests will show false-negative rates if they are performed too early, and false-positives are possible. The hemagglutination test is usually positive by 6 weeks and the slide test by about 7 weeks or more past the last menstrual period.

Assessment of Reproductive Function in Men

Structural Assessment

Physical Examination

In male patients, only the external genitalia of the penis and scrotum are visible for inspection. Sexual maturation is assessed by noting the size and shape of the penis and testes, the color and texture of the scrotal skin, and the type and distribution of the pubic hair. Sexual maturity ratings are often done using Tanner's five stages (Table 99–1). The diagrams accompanying these stages can also be used to educate adolescent patients. If no testicular increase is evident by 13.5 years of age and if pubic hair shows no signs of growth, puberty may be considered delayed although it may not nec-

TABLE 99–1
Sex Maturity Ratings in Boys

	Pubic Hair	Genital: Penis	Genital: Testes and Scrotum
Stage 1	Preadolescent—no pubic hair except for the fine body hair (vellus hair) similar to that on the abdomen	Preadolescent—same size and proportions as in childhood	Preadolescent—same size and proportions as in childhood
Stage 2 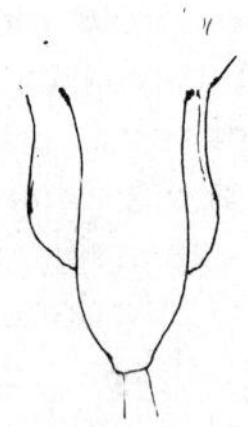	Sparse growth of long, slightly pigmented, downy hair, straight or only slightly curled, chiefly at the base of the penis	Slight or no enlargement	Testes larger; scrotum larger, somewhat reddened, and altered in texture
Stage 3 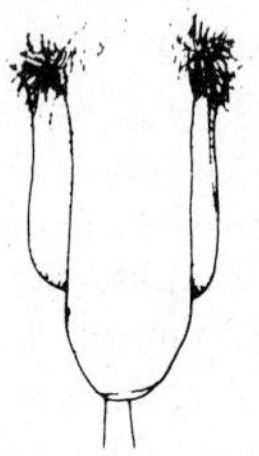	Darker, coarser, curlier hair spreading sparsely over the pubic symphysis	Larger, especially in length	Further enlarged
Stage 4 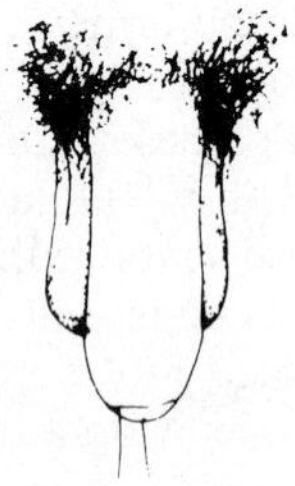	Coarse and curly hair, as in the adult; area covered greater than in stage 3 but not as great as in the adult and not yet including the thighs	Further enlarged in length and breadth, with development of the glans	Further enlarged; scrotal skin darkened
Stage 5 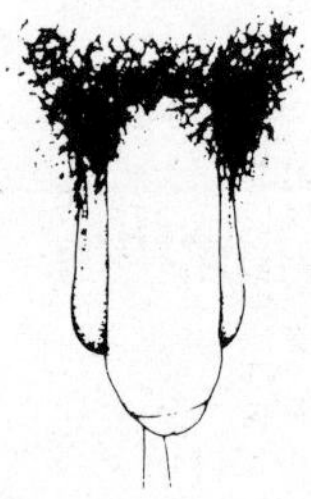	Hair adult in quantity and quality, spread to the medial surfaces of the thighs but not up over the abdomen	Adult in size and shape	Adult in size and shape

(Bates B: A Guide to Physical Examination, 3rd ed. Philadelphia, JB Lippincott,1983)

essarily be of concern. Delay is also suggested if a boy has not reached stage 3 within 4 years of reaching stage 2. If genital development begins before the age of 9 to 9.5 years, it is considered precocious.

Physical examination continues with inspection of the penis including the skin. The prepuce or foreskin if present should be retracted so that the glans tissue can be inspected for lesions, including ulcers, scars, nodules, or signs of inflammation. Retraction of the foreskin should take place easily. Phimosis is adhesion of the prepuce to the glans, making it difficult or impossible to retract. Paraphimosis is a tight prepuce that forms a tight ring around the penis when retracted, leading to painful swelling of the glans. A white, cheesy material known as smegma may normally accumulate under the foreskin. The location of the urethral meatus should be noted at the tip of the penis. By compressing the glans gently between the forefinger and thumb, the meatus should open slightly and the area observed for discharge. Normally there is none. Any discharge should be placed on a glass slide or cultured. The skin around the base of the penis is inspected for excoriations or inflammation. Pubic hair is observed for nits or lice. Palpation of the penis is done to note any tenderness or indurations along the length of the shaft, which could indicate urethal stricture or possible growths.

As with the penis, the scrotum is inspected for contour, symmetry, size, and lesions. Between the thumb and first two fingers, each testis and epididymis is palpated for size, shape, consistency, nodules, and tenderness. The normal size of the testes is variable but the largest should be about 5 cm × 3 cm × 2 cm and of firm consistency. Each spermatic cord with its vas deferens can be palpated along its course from the epididymis to the superficial inguinal canal. If a mass of unknown nature is seen in the scrotum, the area is often transilluminated for further observation.

The inguinal and femoral areas should be inspected carefully for bulges with or without patient straining. A bulge that occurs at rest or appears upon straining suggests a hernia. With the man standing, the index or little finger is directed upward from the distal scrotum, invaginating the scrotal skin until the inguinal canal is felt (Fig. 99–4). If the person is asked to strain, the increased intra-abdominal pressure accentuates any weakness of the internal ring and any herniating mass can be felt.[2] The inguinal canal begins with the internal ring, which is a natural opening in the abdominal wall and extends into the scrotum. The external inguinal ring is the opening between the scrotum and the inguinal canal and is the point where the spermatic cord and vessels enter the inguinal canal. Herniation of abdominal contents through the inguinal canal into the scrotum has potential dire consequences, including injury to abdominal tissues in the event of strangulation (impaired blood flow to the abdominal contents) as well as interference with reproductive function.

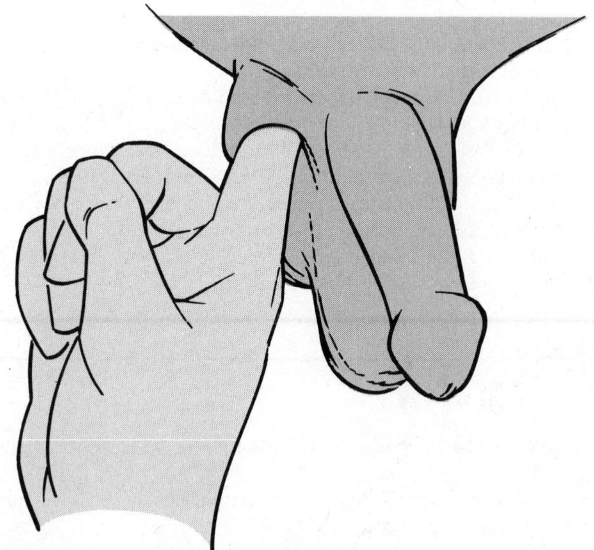

FIGURE 99–4 Examination of the inguinal canal. Note the change in angle from the scrotum to the inguinal canal. The examining finger can palpate easily the entire canal from the external to the internal ring.

The prostate gland, which contributes to the seminal plasma of the ejaculate, can be assessed on rectal examination. It is located anterior to the anterior rectal wall. The posterior aspect of the gland protrudes into the rectal ampulla, which allows this portion to be checked for size, consistency nodules, and tenderness. The size of the normal prostate is variable in individuals but averages about 4 cm in diameter.[7] The seminal vesicles are not normally felt on rectal examination but may be if they are enlarged.

Cytological Examination

In the evaluation of male reproductive function, semen can be collected as a specimen for microscopic evalution of morphology of sperm cells. The seminal fluid is collected by interrupting coitus or inducing ejaculation. Human semen is ejaculated as a fairly viscous, gray-yellowish fluid that forms a solid gel-like substance almost immediately *in vivo* and *in vitro*. The coagulum will usually liquefy spontaneously within 5 to 20 minutes.[5] The spermatozoa are trapped within the coagulated mesh of the seminal plasma. As soon as liquefaction is complete, the spermatozoa begin to move freely and demonstrate motility. This delay in motility has been considered as an opportunity for rest of the sperm cells, perhaps allowing recovery of energy stores for continued motility, therefore protecting viability of the cells. The sample is usually collected after 3 to 5 days of sexual abstinence. The normal volume of ejaculate ranges from 1 ml to 5 ml. The specimen should be collected in a special plastic container and examined preferably in about 1 to 2 hours (see functional assessment section later in the chapter).

Biopsy of testicular tissue is a means by which a specimen for cytology can be obtained. A general anesthetic is required and a needle or excisional biopsy can be done but an open biopsy provides a better specimen.[5] Seminiferous tubules are thus obtained for examination.

Visualization Techniques

In males the structures of the reproductive system are more intricately linked with those of the urinary system than in females. Assessment for conditions of the epididymis or prostate, for example, can involve urinary system visualization tests such as an intravenous pyelogram (contrast medium appears in the bladder by way of excretion by the kidneys), cytoscopy, or urethroscopy.

There are radiological techniques available for assessment of the vas derens, ampulla, seminal vesicles, and ejaculatory duct. The seminal ducts can be filled with contrast media by puncturing the vas deferens at the scrotal level and filling them toward the distal end. Such visualization can show obstruction of the vas deferens, calcification of the vas deferens and seminal vesicles, and problems with the ejaculatory ducts and seminal vesicles.

Functional Assessment

Reproductive Function History

Pertinent self-report data regarding male reproductive function, much like in the female, should focus on evaluation of the sexual history including sexual partnership activity, difficulty with intercourse, and infertility. The interview should explore topics such as sexual development, exposure to drugs, alcohol, or nicotine, and general life-stress factors as well as past diseases. Any complaints of past or current urogenital infections should be noted along with any surgeries that could interfere with the testes or vas deferens.

Sexual dysfunction can take several forms in men.[5] As in women, there can be a lack of erotic feelings (libido). Impotence refers to a reduced or total lack of ability to achieve an erection. This may occur from the onset of sexual activity (called *primary*) or appear after the onset of normal sexual response (called *secondary*). Impotence may be partial (inability to attain or maintain full erection although some erection occurs) or complete (no erection can be initiated). Impotence may also be termed *absolute,* when it is present in every sexual situation or *relative,* when it occurs only in certain situations. A condition known as priapism refers to sustained erection of the penis that is not usually the result of sexual stimulation and gives no pleasurable sensation. It may be very painful and lead to thrombotic changes in the penis. Ejaculation may be premature or retarded. Premature ejaculation usually means that it occurs before penile intromission into the vagina or in less than 2 minutes after intromission. Retarded ejaculation means difficulty even after strong sexual stimulation. As with impotence, ejaculation problems can be primary, secondary, absolute, or relative. Another problem is retrograde ejaculation of the semen backward into the bladder. Orgasm can be absent in men as in women.

As mentioned previously, any sexual behaviors will only be a problem if so evaluated by the patient. However, if they are perceived as interfering with the quality of life, thought should be given to referral to experts in sexual behavior therapy. Disturbances of sexual function can be associated with marital or partnership problems, anxieties over contraception, past negative sexual experiences, lack of knowledge of behavioral function, or various personal factors.

A reproductive function history in men of necessity gets linked to urinary function. Present or past symptoms of scrotal or suprapubic urethral or perineal pain, urethral secretions, sexually transmitted diseases, altered urinary stream, nocturnal or premature ejaculation, either incomplete or reduced, and painful orgasms should be reported.

Physiological Function Tests

Hormone assays are done particularly to assess for infertility in men. Major tests include radioimmunoassays of FSH, LH, prolactin, and testosterone. Plasma levels of testosterone are normally about 0.52 μg/100 ml plasma in young men (18 to 37 years) and 0.38 μg/100 ml in older men (60 to 80 years). Plasma levels of FSH average about 180 ng/ml and LH levels average 64 ng/ml in normal men.[5]

Seminal fluid assays also provide information on aspects of spermatogenesis and auxiliary processes. Analysis should include description of volume, viscosity, and presence of nonliquefied material (determined after 60 minutes), presence of white blood cells (leukocytes) and other cells, aggregation of spermatozoa, sperm density, percent of motile spermatozoa, mean progressive sperm mobility score, percentage of sperm with normal morphology, and percentage of sperm with amorphous heads to those with coiled tails.[5]

The prostrate gland contributes about 13% to 32% of the ejaculate volume, whereas the seminal vesicles contribute 46% to 80%.[8] The components of the semen include water, electrolytes, nitrogenous bases, prostaglandins, citric acid, acid and alkaline phosphatases, zinc, coagulase, and fibrinolysin as well as lipids, proteins, fructose, and other carbohydrate sources. A normal sperm count is about 60 to 200,000 million/ml. At 1 hour after ejaculation, at least 60% of the sperm should be motile as observed under a microscope and at 2 hours, 50% should remain motile.[8] Fructose is contributed mainly by the seminal vesicles, so that deficiency of this sugar implies deficiencies in these structures.

References

1. American College of Obstetrics and Gynecologists Technical Bulletin. Diagnostic Ultrasound in Obstetrics and Gynecology, Women and Health, 7(3/4):55–63, 1982
2. Bates B: A Guide to Physical Examination, 3rd ed. Philadelphia, JB Lippincott, 1983
3. Bellack JP, Bamford PA: Nursing Assessment: A Multidimensional Approach. Monterey CA, Wadsworth Health Sciences Division, 1984
4. Fogel CI, Woods NF: Health Care of Women: A Nursing Perspective. St Louis, CV Mosby, 1981
5. Hafez ES (ed): Human Semen and Fertility Regulation in Men. St Louis, CV Mosby, 1976
6. Latta W, Weismeier E: Effects of an educational gynecological exam on women's attitudes. JOGN 11(2):242–245, 1982
7. Sana JM, Judge RD (eds): Physical Assessment Skills for Nursing Practice, 2nd ed. Boston, Little, Brown & Co, 1982
8. Scott R, Deane RF, Callander R: Urology Illustrated, 2nd ed. New York, Churchill Livingstone, 1982

Bibliography

Glass RH: Office Gynecology, 2nd ed. Baltimore, Williams & Wilkins, 1981

Peckham BM, Shapiro SS: Signs and Symptoms in Gynecology. Philadelphia, JB Lippincott, 1983

Chapter 100

Nursing Strategies for Common Reproductive Problems

Nursing Diagnosis
Interventions
Evaluation

Joan Shaver

This chapter focuses on common health problems and issues affecting the reproductive tract or reproductive behaviors, including alterations in comfort (pain), menstrual bleeding problems, contraception, sterilization, rape-trauma syndrome and perimenopausal transition.

Abnormal Bleeding Patterns

Abnormal vaginal bleeding is the most common gynecological complaint for women and can occur at any age. Abnormal bleeding can occur following pregnancy or its complications, may be due to malignant organic pelvic lesions, or may be due to problems outside the reproductive tract.[10] It can also occur as an abnormal pattern of menstrual bleeding, described by the following terms:

Hypermenorrhea/Hypomenorrhea—Excessive/scant quantity of flow during a menstrual period of normal duration

Menorrhagia—Prolonged flow at regular intervals often with increased amount of blood

Metrorrhagia—Intermenstrual bleeding or bleeding that occurs irregularly between cycles

Menometrorrhagia—A combination of prolonged flow during, and intermittent bleeding between, menstrual periods

Polymenorrhea—Increased frequency of menstrual periods (less than 22 days apart)

Oligomenorrhea—Decreased frequency of menstrual periods that may be associated with some decrease in the duration and quantity of flow (greater than 35 days apart)

Amenorrhea—The failure of menses to start by age 16 years or the absence of menstrual blood flow for more than 3 months in a woman who has established menstruation

Postcoital Bleeding—Vaginal bleeding occurring with or following sexual intercourse

Postmenopausal bleeding—Vaginal bleeding after menopause.

Unusual Menstrual Bleeding. Generally, menstrual cycles regularly associated with hypermenorrhea, menorrhagia, or metrorrhagia (excessive uterine bleeding) suggest organic disease such as a growth. This is reported to occur in 5% to 10 percent of women.[11] Vaginal and cervical lesions such as vaginitis, trauma, cervicitis, cervical polyps, syphilis, and malignancies can cause abnormal bleeding. Bleeding can be associated with endometrial polyps, leiomyoma (benign tumor of the smooth muscle), endometriosis, or uterine malignancies. Tubal lesions such as salpingitis and tubal cancer and ovarian lesions such as cysts and malignancies are also sources of abnormal vaginal bleeding. As well, the presence of an intrauterine device (IUD) for contraception and erratic or prolonged production of progesterone during the luteal phase of the menstrual cycle can induce abnormal bleeding. Polymenorrhea, oligomenorrhea, or amenorrhea tend to suggest disturbances in endocrine control of menstruation. Bleeding associated with pregnancy can accompany threatened abortion, complete or incomplete abortion, missed or habitual abortion, or ectopic pregnancy.

Postmenopausal Bleeding. Bleeding after the time of menopause is typically uterine in origin. The appearance of bleeding in women more than 6 months beyond their last menstrual period requires appropriate medical diagnostic evaluation for malignancy.

Amenorrhea. Menstruation that has never been established or cessation of a previously established pattern of menstrual bleeding constitutes amenorrhea, referred to as either primary or secondary. Primary amenorrhea is usually due to genetic causes or anatomical maldevelopment. If secondary sexual development has been evident for 3 or more years, it is a clue that the uterus is absent, a vaginal septum is causing blockage, or androgen sensitivity or excess is present. Absence of secondary characteristics implies the absence of the ovaries or a disorder of the hypothalamic–pituitary–ovarian axis.

Secondary amenorrhea is believed to have a psychogenic component. It often accompanies major life changes such as moving to a new environment. However it also may accompany rapid weight loss or strenuous exercise.

Amenorrhea can occur in conjunction with normal, hypergonadotropic, or hypogonadotropic function. Normal levels of follicle-stimulating hormone (FSH) and luteinizing hormone (LH) will often accompany developmental abnormalities of the reproductive tract. High gonadotropic levels lead to ovarian failure, and failure of the usual menstrual changes in the uterus, thus preventing menstruation. Low or undetectable gonadotropic levels, genetic or acquired, will also prevent follicular development. Amenorrhea can occur secondary to pituitary tumors, with drug intake, or as a response to stressful environmental conditions. Various drugs such as phenothiazine derivatives, reserpine, ganglionic-blocking agents, alcohol, digitalis, and certain antibiotics can induce amenorrhea by affecting the hypothalamus or inducing anorexia.[13] Intense dieting or development of anorexia nervosa is often associated with low levels of FSH and LH in serum and amenorrhea.[11] Patients who have an overproduction of adrenal or ovarian androgens also will exhibit amenorrhea in conjunction with excessive hair growth on the upper lip, chin, between the breasts, and on the extremities (called hirsutism).[13]

Assessment of Abnormal Bleeding

Unusual Vaginal Bleeding. When women present with abnormal menstrual or intermenstrual bleeding patterns, initial nursing action involves taking a careful history to document the onset, amount, duration, character, and associated symptoms of the bleeding so that a baseline profile can be established. Bleeding is considered abnormal when a regular menstrual bleeding pattern has never been established, when a pattern changes, and when bleeding between periods occurs.[4] Therefore, questions about usual menstrual patterns, the possibility of pregnancy, and contraceptive modes used are asked (Table 100–1).

In terms of excessive menstrual bleeding, it is abnormal if the menstrual cycle is less than 21 days, the duration of menstrual blood loss is more than 7 days, or the volume is such that menstrual pads of adequate absorbency have to be changed very frequently (more than every 1 to 2 hours). Some women are prone to normally heavy menstrual bleeding, and it is of importance whether the current pattern is different from the usual one. An excessive loss is usually considered one in which more than 80 ml is lost in a cycle.[11] Information about the duration of blood loss, time of maximal loss, and whether blood clots are passed is important. In young women, occasional heavy or prolonged bleeding is not cause for great alarm unless there is reason to suspect associated pregnancy complications. A single episode of heavy bleeding may indicate spontaneous abortion or ectopic pregnancy. Sometimes a woman with an IUD or taking oral contraceptives will experience heavy bleeding. Intermenstrual bleeding is of concern at any time, although regular intermenstrual bleeding at midcycle is less worrisome. Spotting, as it is often called, can signal spontaneous abortion, ectopic pregnancy, various gynecological infections, or malignancy.[4] In older women all marked changes in the menstrual bleeding pattern warrant investigation, and bleeding past the time of menopause can be indicative of endometrial cancer.

Other lifestyle factors and associated symptoms should be noted in women complaining of abnormal vaginal bleeding. Moderate to heavy alcohol consumption is associated with scantier menstrual bleeding. Cigarette smokers are five times more likely to have abnormal bleeding although the biochemical reason is not known.[11] Abnormal bleeding is often associated with menstrual cramping and migraine headache. There is an increased prevalence of anxiety and depression, but it is unclear if this is a response to the abnormal bleeding or a predisposing factor. Other symptoms such as pain, lethargy, dyspareunia, and nausea should also be assessed.

A careful pelvic examination will usually follow the history, with observations for reproductive tract lesions. Depending on the reported circumstances of the bleeding, further functional assessment may be done, for example, a pregnancy test or hormone levels.

Amenorrhea. Primary amenorrhea is medically diagnosed by a careful history, physical examination for structural abnormalities, buccal smears to detect chromosomal abnormalities, and progesterone and estrogen–progesterone withdrawal tests. Progesterone is given intramuscularly and the appearance of withdrawal bleeding implies the presence of adequate estrogen and probably a normal pituitary gland, ovaries, and uterus. A combined estrogen–progesterone challenge involves giving the two hormones cyclically as they would normally occur. Failure to induce bleeding suggests endometrial failure. If bleeding occurs, then a 24-hour urinary excretion of pituitary gonad-

TABLE 100–1
Assessment of Abnormal Vaginal (Menstrual, Uterine) Bleeding Patterns

Factor	*Characteristics*	*Concerns*
Bleeding description	Onset	
	Duration	
	Amount	1–2 soaked pads per hour
	Character, color	Extensive clots
	Associated symptoms	Cramps, pain, faintness, weakness
Usual mentrual pattern	Cycle length	<21 days
	Menstrual duration	>7 days
	Regularity	
	Flow severity and type	Heavy or very heavy, clots
	Intermenstrual bleeding	Other than midcycle
	Associated symptoms	Cramps, nausea, mood changes, sleep/eating disorders
Contraception use	Oral contraceptive	Hormone imbalance
	IUD	Bleeding, cramps
Sexual activities	Potential pregnancy	Spontaneous abortion, ectopic pregnancy
Lifestyle factors	Alcohol consumption	Hypomenorrhea
	Cigarette smoking	Abnormal bleeding
	Rapid weight loss, heavy exercise, stress	Amenorrhea
Illnesses and drug intake		Amenorrhea

otropins may be done. High levels suggest primary ovary failure, low levels imply pituitary failure, and normal levels suggest hypothalamic dysfunction.

The most common cause of amenorrhea in women of reproductive age is pregnancy. A careful menstrual and sexual history is warranted. Any associated symptoms of breast tenderness, nausea, vomiting, or fatigue should be noted and a pregnancy test done. When pregnancy is ruled out, disorders of the hypothalamus–pituitary–ovary axis are suspected. Since oral contraceptives can cause amenorrhea, information on birth control methods should be obtained. Some women experience "post-pill" amenorrhea. A history of rapid weight loss, other systemic illnesses, strenuous exercise habits, or drug intake should bé noted because these have all been related to the development of amenorrhea. The history of amenorrhea and oligomenorrhea in which a psychogenic component is surmised should also include questions about major life events and changes such as moving one's home, starting or stopping employment, or difficulties in interpersonal relationships, as well as mood states, fears, and anxieties.

Management of Bleeding Abnormalities

When excessive bleeding is secondary to psychological, endocrine, or genital dysfunction, the primary disorder must be treated. In a large number of patients, the abnormal bleeding is temporary, often due to failure of normal follicular maturation and inadequate progesterone levels in the luteal phase of the menstrual cycle. If this is so, medical treatment involves administering progesterone as a single treatment orally, or over three to six cycles with the drug being given on the 16th to 21st day of the cycle and continued for 5 to 10 days. If estrogen deficiency is suspected, it may be added and given through the first 25 days of the cycle with progesterone being given in the later cycle phases. Since there is evidence that prostaglandins are elevated in menorrhagia, antiprostaglandin compounds (see dysmenorrhea section) have been found to reduce menstrual blood loss. Some patients may be given clomiphene which is an antiestrogen çompound that stimulates LH/FSH release, thereby facilitating ovulation.[11]

Curettage may be therapeutic for excessive bleeding, especially if there is an organic lesion like a polyp, retained placental tissue, or excessive endometrial tissue proliferation. This involves scraping the interior of the uterine cavity with a serrated instrument. Hysterectomy may be done in a few patients in whom none of the above treatments control the bleeding.[11]

Nursing Interventions. Nursing interventions in acute excessive bleeding involve continual monitoring of blood loss and fluid balance including documentation of the number of pads soaked per hour. Blood pressure measurement and the usual observations for shock and evidence of an inadequate circulating volume are necessary. Fluid and blood replacement may be administered as ordered by the physician. Information regarding the existing hemoglobin level, hematocrit, bleeding and clotting time, capillary fragility, platelet count, and clotting factors can guide nursing plans for increased rest and tissue protection if anemia is present or other bleeding tendencies exist.

For the patient, bleeding outside of usual menstrual bleeding is generally viewed as life-threatening and generates fear or anxiety. Reassurance and explanations of the probable reasons for bleeding can be helpful. If ongoing monitoring is required outside of a health care setting, careful explanations of what observations to make are needed. A monthly health diary to systematically record bleeding episodes relative to the menstrual cycle can be helpful in determining whether there is a cyclic pattern of bleeding.

Evaluation. Maintenance of an adequate circulating volume and red blood cell concentration is an obvious goal of therapy for unusual bleeding. Absence of abnormal menstrual or intermenstrual bleeding is indicative of adequate intervention. The ability of the patient to accurately document the bleeding pattern and seek help appropriately helps evaluate nursing interventions.

Alterations in Comfort: Pain

Pain is second to vaginal bleeding as the most common presenting gynecological complaint.[10] Common conditions associated with pelvic pain include painful menstruation (dysmenorrhea), painful sexual intercourse (dyspareunia), ovulatory pain, complications of pregnancy, endometriosis (functional endometrial tissue outside the uterine cavity), pelvic inflammatory disease, and other organic diseases of the uterus, ovaries, and fallopian tubes. Lower abdominal pain can be due to problems outside the reproductive tract and include appendicitis, gastroenteritis, diverticulitis, and urinary tract infections.

Sources of Pain

Deep pain in the body is often imprecise as to segmental location, and pain can be referred to areas removed from the injured or reactive tissue. Therefore pelvic pain can appear to involve diffuse areas of the pelvic cavity. Often pain is generated by inflammatory conditions or abnormal growth conditions of the organs and tissues in the pelvic region (see Chapters 101 and 102), but the following functional situations also give rise to pain.

Ovulatory Pain. Lower abdominal pain occurs in some women with ovulation, a condition called *mittelschmerz*. There is believed to be increased pressure inside the follicle of the ovary prior to rupture. The pressure alone may cause pain, or perhaps the release of some follicular fluid or blood into the peritoneal cavity at ovulation causes a localized peritonitis. The discomfort occurs about the middle of the menstrual cycle, lasts a few hours to a few days, and affects one quadrant of the abdomen or the other, although frequently the right lower quadrant. Slight vaginal bleeding may be associated with the pain.

Dysmenorrhea. Pain associated with the menstrual period is called dysmenorrhea. Although this condition may arise secondarily to pelvic pathology, most often dysmenorrhea has no detectable organic basis and is called primary dysmenorrhea. The true prevalence of primary dysmenorrhea has not been determined but estimates are that upwards of 50% of women have some manifestations of dysmenorrhea[2] and about 20% of women experience severe or disabling dysmenorrhea.[23]

Dysmenorrheic women generally report an unremarkable menarche but begin to have discomfort an average of 3 years later.[10] The incidence of dysmenorrhea peaks in the mid-twenties and decreases after that. The experience of pain and associated symptoms is variable in type and severity among women but can be quite debilitating. It includes lower abdominal spasmodic pain, usually 1 to 3 days prior to and with the onset of menstrual flow, sometimes with radiation to the back and upper thighs. Associated complaints include nausea, vomiting, diarrhea, fatigue, anxiety, depression, and headaches.

Functionally, dysmenorrhea has been associated with hyperactive muscle contractions of the uterus and perhaps reduced blood flow to the endometrium. Of recent interest is information that prostaglandins are high in endometrial tissue with dysmenorrhea. Prostaglandins are known to increase uterine muscle activity and modulate blood flow to the uterus, as well as sensitize nerve endings to the pain-producing effects of other chemical mediators of tissue injury such as bradykinin.

Dyspareunia. Pain with sexual intercourse can occur both with and without observable organic lesions. Anatomical reasons for dyspareunia include congenital defects, inflammatory lesions, and atrophy of the vagina secondary to estrogen deficiency.[10] Pain upon attempts at vaginal penetration suggests vaginismus or involuntary contraction of certain pelvic muscles, an unusually thick hymen, or an inflammatory condition of the vagina. Scarring due to episiotomy or perineal surgery may create painful intercourse. Discomfort felt only with deep penetration of the penis into the vagina may be due to pelvic congestion prior to menstruation, pelvic inflammatory conditions, displacement of the uterus, or endometriosis in portions of the peritoneum. However in many women with this complaint, normal anatomy is evident and pain is assumed to have a psychogenic component, for example, dyspareunia can be related to previous traumatic sexual experiences.

Pelvic Congestion Syndrome. Pelvic congestion syndrome is thought to be due to blood engorgement in the broad ligament and uterus.[12] It is characterized by consistent dull aching pelvic and lower abdominal pain accentuated near the time of menses, dyspareunia, and discomfort with prolonged sitting or standing. The symptoms often tend to merge with those of premenstrual syndrome, such as constipation, diarrhea, gas, cramping, headache, irritability, and depression. Failure to reach orgasm during sexual intercourse, which relieves vascular congestion, has been cited as creating or aggravating this condition and a psychosomatic element has been inferred. No obvious pelvic pathology is usually detectable and this condition remains ill-defined.

Psychogenic Pain. The experience of pain in the lower abdomen or pelvis is often purported to involve conversion of psychic function into a physical manifestation. For women the pelvis could logically be the focus of emotionally triggered pain. It is associated with sexual and reproductive acts that are related intricately to social interrelationships of an intimate and emotionally charged nature. However careful exploration for organic causes is imperative, and psychogenic pain as a diagnosis can be made only after excluding all possible organic reasons. Regardless of whether an organic reason can be found for the pain, the pain is real for the woman experiencing it and it must be treated as a response to a health problem.

Assessment of Pelvic Pain

In general, a diagnosis of alteration in comfort due to pain is made when a patient verbalizes that she is experiencing pain. However, remaining diagnostic processes involve a more complete and helpful description of the pain. This should include information about the experience of pain, its temporal course, and the circumstances surrounding it so that appropriate intervention becomes evident. Often the patient presents with complaints of pain of undetermined type, and the source of the pain can be implied through a careful history.

Several features of the pain should be ascertained, but particularly the location of the pain. The exact site of visceral and deep somatic pain is difficult to ascertain from description but certain typical sites are known. For example, appendicitis begins as pain around the umbilicus but then becomes localized to the right lower quadrant of the abdomen. Unilateral lower quadrant pain accompanies ectopic pregnancy, tumors, or ovarian cysts. Pelvic inflammatory disease tends to be bilateral and involve the entire lower abdomen. It is also important to note pain severity, duration, and whether onset was acute (suggesting rupture or embolus) or gradual (implying a worsening inflammatory or growth process).

Pain may be described using various adjectives, and the patient should be encouraged to describe the experience as fully as possible. Some descriptors of pain include cramping, sharp, burning, aching, throbbing, or fullness. If the character or quality of the pain is described as colicky or intermittent, muscle contraction (or spasm) of a hollow organ is suggested, whereas a dull, throbbing pain occurs more often with chronic inflammatory diseases or tumor growths.

The severity and duration of the pain should be assessed. The relationship with the menstrual cycle is critical. As mentioned, cyclical pain can be functional in nature. Pain after missed periods may indicate complications with pregnancy. Whether or not pain is associated with sexual intercourse should be ascertained. Pain unrelated to the menses involves problems with the nonreproductive organs. A full history of urinary and intestinal tract symptoms is important to elicit. Factors that worsen or improve the pain should be noted. For example, low abdominal pain that follows eating, and perhaps certain foods, suggests a bowel condition. Pain that is increased by a cough, sneeze, or strain can arise from ligament irritation, pelvic inflammation, or peritonitis.

Management of Pelvic Pain

Specific information about the location, duration, severity, onset, character, consistency, cyclicity, and associated circumstances related to pain can help to suggest possible reasons for the pain. When obvious organic reasons for the pain are evident, medical treatment often will involve surgery (for growths or dysfunctional structure) or drugs (for infection or physiological dysfunction). Nursing therapies can involve other nonpharmacological pain management strategies and health teaching.

Dysmenorrhea. The pain associated with ovulation is usually not incapacitating and can spontaneously resolve. It is usually not treated specifically. However, dysmenorrhea can be severe and interfere with a women's daily activities. The treatment of dysmenorrhea can be multifaceted depending on the severity of the problem.

Many women deal with menstrual cramps by taking aspirin. At least part of aspirin's effect is due to its ability to reduce prostaglandin concentrations in tissue, but several newer prostaglandin inhibitors are more potent and effective than aspirin and may be given when dysmenorrhea is severe. These nonsteroidal anti-inflammatory agents, for example, Naprosyn (naproxen), Motrin (ibuprofen), and Ponstel (mefenamic acid), have been found to offer substantial relief to large numbers of women complaining of dysmenorrhea, although not all women. Generally, treatment prior to menstruation is not recommended but rather is prescribed for the first 48 hours of menstruation.[2,3] Contraindications include the presence of gastrointestinal ulcers and hypersensitivity to these drugs. Side-effects are usually mild but gastrointestinal, central nervous system, and other symptoms can occur including indigestion, abdominal pain, vomiting, diarrhea, headache, dizziness, visual or hearing disturbances, depression, or skin rashes.

Oral contraceptives are said to relieve menstrual pain. They prevent ovulation and endometrial development and thereby may also prevent excess prostaglandin activity. This is not a desirable form of therapy for every woman with dysmenorrhea owing to the risks of taking gonadal hormones, but it may help in women for whom this is also a preferred method of contraception.

Other nonpharmacological therapies have been reported to reduce menstrual pain. Symptoms may be affected overall by nutrition. Vitamin B has been suggested for relief of those symptoms associated with menstrual cycle disorder.[4] However, megadoses of this vitamin are not recommended, and toxic reactions to large doses have been experienced. Eating foods high in the B vitamins (such as complex carbohydrates, especially grain products) is a safer alternative. Exercise is reported to have a variable effect on dysmenorrhea. Apparently more athletes report reduced pain upon exercising than increased pain, but the majority of women deny any significant change at all.[14] Acutely, exercise is reported to abate dysmenorrheic pain, perhaps due to the exercise-induced endorphin release or release of prostaglandins that vasodilate endometrial vessels.

Mild heat is helpful to some people since it is believed to relieve high muscle tonus. It probably promotes vasodilation and increases blood flow to the endometrium, believed perhaps to be ischemic. A heating pad, tub bath, or hot shower can be of help.

Cognitive strategies such as biofeedback, general relaxation response, and hypnosis have been used with variable efficacy in treating dysmenorrhea and deserve much more study as a nursing intervention.

Dyspareunia. When an organic cause is known for dyspareunia, treatment involves alleviating the condition, such as treating infections or endometriosis. If lack of vaginal lubrication (a problem for some postmenopausal women) creates dyspareunia, lubricating jellies or creams can be prescribed. Vaginal scarring is amenable to surgical revision as is a thick or imperforate hymen. In cases where there does not appear to be an organic reason for pain, sexual education, counseling, or therapy may be warranted.

Evaluation. Reduced pain experience is the obvious goal of pelvic pain interventions, mainly assessed by patient report. Health teaching will improve knowledge of reproductive function, perhaps give a rationale for the pain, and provide the means to alleviate it. Self-management techniques for pain facilitate developing a sense of control over the situation and expanded ways to cope with pain.

Infertility Problems

A seemingly expanding problem in American culture is the inability to conceive a child when parenthood is desired. Infertility is often defined as an inability to produce a pregnancy after a year or more of sexual relations during which no contraception is used. Primary infertility means that no pregnancy has ever occurred. Secondary or relative infertility refers to infertility after one or more successful pregnancies. Sterility usually denotes the incapacity to conceive due to an absolute, known factor preventing procreation.

The incidence of infertility in the United States has been estimated at between 10% and 15% of all couples of childbearing age, and this number appears to be growing. This, in part, may be due to a rise in sexually transmitted diseases, an increasing incidence of endometriosis, the rising practice of postponing childbearing until a later age, and speculatively on the use of oral contraceptives and intrauterine devices. Both male and female disorders tend to be equally implicated. It is estimated that male factors account for about 40% of infertility, failure to ovulate for about 10% to 15%, tubal problems for another 10% to 30%, and a cervical factor for 5%. In 10% to 20% of couples, there will be no known cause for infertility.[17,22]

Several factors influence the fertility of any couple, but age is certainly one factor. In females, at very young ages, fertility is low but peaks at about 24 years, thereby declining rapidly after age 30. It is rare for pregnancy to occur after age 50. In men, fertility reaches its peak at age 25 and does decline rapidly after age 40 but has been documented in the eighth and ninth decades.[13]

Infertility in women can be attributed to developmental anomalies, metabolic/endocrine disturbances, structural problems secondary to pathophysiology, genetic, or perhaps psychogenic factors. Infections appear as a leading cause of infertility in women owing to the sequelae of scar tissue and adhesions of the uterus, tubes, ovaries, and peritoneal cavity. Pelvic inflammatory disease, endometriosis, ectopic pregnancy, or previous surgical procedures can cause scarring. In general, causes for infertility will be discussed as female factors (ovulatory disorders, cervical, tubal, uterine), male factors, and couple factors (see also Table 100–2).

Female Factors Affecting Fertility

Ovulatory Failure. Failure of ovulation generally occurs because of inadequate follicle maturation, failure of hypothalamus–pituitary–ovary interaction, or interference by excess prolactin secretion. Ovulation failure can occur in spite of normal estrogen production and seemingly normal menstrual periods, with low estrogen amenorrhea, and with amenorrhea in the presence of either high or low FSH/LH or associated with an inadequate corpus luteum. Ovulatory failure can occur secondary to thyroid dysfunction (particularly hypothyroid conditions), excess prolactin secretion, or androgen excess rather than any specific problem within the ovaries. Anovulation with normal levels of ovarian steroid hormones is believed to be precipitated by cognitive/emotional factors. Low estrogen and low FSH/LH amenorrhea can result from failure of FSH and LH synthesis or release from the pituitary or damage to the pituitary or hypothalamus. Low estrogen and high FSH/LH partially describe the insensitive ovary syndrome in which very high levels of estrogen are needed to facilitate ovulation. The inadequate luteal situation is characterized by a menstrual luteal phase shortened by at least 3 days, believed to be due to either inadequate FSH production during ovular ripening or an inadequate LH surge at ovulation.[13]

Fertilization Factors. Infertility can result from the production of cervical mucus that is hostile to sperm penetration and motility. Cervical mucus is most hospitable about 12 to 36 hours before ovulation when it is thin, watery, and clear from adequate pre-ovulatory estrogen. Mucus that is infected or has a high level of antibodies to sperm can cause high sperm mortality.

Fertilization of the ovum by the sperm takes place in the fallopian tube. Muscle contractions of the fimbriated ends of the fallopian tubes are critical to capture of the ovum when released from the ovaries. Movement of the ovum through the fallopian tube depends on muscle contraction, the movements of cilia on the epithelial cells lining the tubes, and the flow of the tubular fluid. Hindrance to ovum availability and a nonconducive fertilization environment can occur owing to structural blockage of the fallopian tubes, failure to capture the ovum, inadequate tube motility, immobile cilia, or inabil-

TABLE 100–2
Major Factors Affecting Infertility

Functional Problem	*Major Disorders*	*Assessment*
Ovulatory failure	Inadequate follicle maturation Disorders Brain–ovary interaction Excess prolactin	Plasma P_4 Basal body temperature Cervical mucus FSH, LH, prolactin, E_2 and P_4 levels in plasma
Implantation failure	Malformed uterus Underdeveloped endometrium Uterine growths	Physical examination Endometrial cell cytology
Testicular failure	Inadequate spermatogenesis Disordered brain–testicular interaction Excess prolactin Traumatic injury to testes Varicocele of testes	Postcoital sperm count Seminal fluid analysis FSH, LH, prolactin, and T_4 levels in plasma; physical examination
Fertilization failure		
Female	Hostile cervical mucus Fimbrial failure to capture ovum Blocked fallopian tube Defective tube motility Inadequate tubular fluid	Ultrasound Laparoscopy Hysterosalpingography Rubin test
Male	Blocked vas or epididymis Inadequate sperm plasma	Microsurgery
Behavioral factors	Major life changes Sexual dysfunction	Health history

ity of the tubular fluid to provide nutritional support for the ovum or sperm.

Implantation Factors. Uterine malformations or scarring after curettage (scraping) of the uterus lining, underdevelopment of the endometrium during the menstrual cycle, and growths in the uterus such as polyps, fibroids, and tumors will prevent implantation of a fertilized ovum.

Male Factors Affecting Fertility

Testicular and Ejaculation Failure. Comparable to ovarian failure, testicular failure can occur. The production of sperm and testosterone by the testes depends on the influence of FSH and LH from the hypothalamus–pituitary–gonad axis, and deficiencies in any part of the axis can create fertility problems. As in the female, elevated prolactin levels will cause gonadal dysfunction.

Spermatozoa are formed from developmental cells in the seminiferous tubules. Maturation takes about 70 days. The sperm are stored in the epididymis and seminal vesicles until ejaculation. Inherited disorders of spermatogenesis can affect male fertility; infection with the mumps virus can impair function; and trauma and pathophysiological processes can affect the testes as can other systemic diseases such as liver disease or diabetes. Chemotherapy for cancer usually has a deleterious effect on sperm production.

Varicosities of the veins that drain the testes (varicocele) can create a higher than normal temperature within the testes, depressing sperm production. The sperm exist and are ejaculated in a plasma that is important to the survival of the sperm. Deficient volumes, infected fluid, or abnormal components can reduce the viability of the sperm. Blockage of the conducting tubes of the vas deferens or epididymis can occur congenitally or be acquired due to infection, trauma, or surgery and will hinder ejaculation of sperm.

Psychogenic and Behavioral Factors Affecting Fertility

The synchrony of the hypothalamus–pituitary–gonad axis in males and females is believed to be prone to emotional and thought influences. Therefore, individuals who are exposed to stressful life situations show evidence of reproductive dysfunction including menstrual irregularity, anovulation, and uterine or tubal infertility in women and testicular failure in males, although the role of stress in infertility is not definitive. Even if psychological factors do not initiate infertility, they may develop in response to it and perhaps compound it or hinder the effectiveness of treatment.

Oftentimes infertility cannot be explained by the evidence of a specific biological disorder in the man or woman. In the couple, sexual problems may be interfering with fertility. Behaviors such as infrequent intercourse, unconsummated relationships, or nonoptimal sexual techniques can influence the process. For example, intercourse may have never taken place because of vaginismus or impotence, or premature ejaculation may prevent impregnation. Position during intercourse or the use of certain lubricants can create problems with facilitating the delivery of sperm to the fallopian tube where fertilization of the ovum takes place.

Assessment of Infertility

Initially, joint consultation with the couple is advisable. This will promote a mutual problem-solving attitude. Although it is frequently the woman who seeks assessment, the man can provide information of importance, be encouraged to ask questions, and participate in the assessment and therapy. Additionally, the partnership can be assessed and serious marital problems exposed. The contact is bound to be stressful and a trusting rapport must be developed between the couple and the health-care provider to obtain diagnostic information regarding fertility.

History. Assessment begins with a history of the problem. A description in the patient's own words including onset and duration of the problem, past attempts at self-treatment or professionally prescribed treatment, the precipitating events to seeking treatment, and the current expectations of treatment should be noted.[22] Additionally, a gynecological, contraceptive, and obstetrical history should be obtained from the woman along with a history of infectious diseases involving the pelvic region or any other gynecological pathologies, such as endometriosis. In the man a urogential history should be taken.

Further information should be sought about lifestyle and environmental factors that can affect fertility, such as alcohol consumption and nicotine and drug use. Factors such as excessive exercise, poor nutrition, abnormal body weight, and stressful life circumstances are important.

Information should be sought regarding sexual practices and knowledge including frequency of intercourse, duration of sexual activity, use of lubricants, positions used, postcoital behaviors (*e.g.,* douching), and satisfaction and areas of concern about the sexual relationship. Additionally, the influence of religious, social and cultural beliefs, the attitudes on sexual practices, and the meaning of and response to infertility should be assessed in order to plan for educational and supportive aspects of therapy.

Ovulation Confirmation. If anovulation is suspected as a reason for infertility a *plasma progesterone* count is a reliable indicator of ovulation if measured in the midluteal phase of the cycle and on serial measures through several cycles. A level of greater than 5 ng/ml is usually accepted as indicating ovulation, although levels twice that are reported to be associated with more frequent conception.[11]

A less reliable but often used method to indicate ovulation is the basal temperature chart. In the first half of the menstrual cycle (follicular phase), the body temperature is low compared to the second half (luteal phase) when the body temperature rises by about 0.5°F to 1.0°F. Classically the temperature drops the day before ovulation and then rises over the next 2 to 4 days. Women are instructed to use a basal body thermometer (which has an elongated range around usual body temperature for easier reading) to record their body temperature before arising in the morning. By keeping a chart all through the menstrual cycle, couples can often tell if the cycles are ovulatory and when they occur, although in retrospect. When observed in conjunction with the *cervical mucus characteristics,* it can indicate which are the most fertile days of the cycle. The presence of an increased volume of clear, watery mucus at the time of ovulation and "ferning" when the mucus is allowed to dry on a slide suggests the presence of ovulation.

Ultrasound can indicate when ovulation is about to occur. Bulging follicles can be seen and ovulation usually occurs within hours of seeing a follicle that is at least 18 cm to 20 cm across.

Tubal Patency. Tubal patency can be tested in several ways. A *laparoscopy* can be used to assess tubal patency and to visualize the uterus, tubes, and ovaries in some detail. Tubal patency is shown by injecting a mixture of normal saline and dye into the cervix and observing it as it passes out of the fimbriated ends of the tubes.

Hysterosalpingography can also be used whereby a radiopaque substance is injected into the uterine cervix by means of a cannula. The uterus and tubes are examined by fluoroscopy as the dye passes through the tubes. This is usually done in a clinic. Occasionally women will complain of shoulder pain presumably due to subphrenic irritation from the dye. This should subside within 12 to 24 hours.[22]

A *Rubin test* involves insufflating carbon dioxide into the cervical canal. With patent tubes, the gas enters the peritoneal cavity, which can be detected by a stethoscope placed on the iliac fossa. Although a relatively safe test, the Rubin test is less preferable than some of the above options because of the discomfort associated with it and because of frequent false-positive readings.[22]

Uterine Development. Samples of endometrial tissue can be taken with curettage under general anesthesia or with a minicurettage in a physician's office or clinic. The cells are tests for genital tuberculosis and examined for cellular changes indicative of progesterone exposure.

Couple Factors. A *postcoital sperm count test* involves assessment of cervical mucus by a health-care provider preferably within 8 hours of sexual intercourse. The couple is asked to abstain from intercourse for 48 hours before the test and to have intercourse within 8 hours of the test. The test is done as close as possible to the peak mucus-production time. Cervical mucus is extracted with a syringe and the number of sperm within the mucus is counted. There should be at least 5 motile sperm per high-power field in mucus taken from the internal os 2 to 3 hours after intercourse.

Male Factors. A basic test of male factors is *analysis of seminal fluid.* Seminal plasma is checked for volume (normally 1 ml to 5 ml), spontaneous liquefaction within 20 minutes of collection, presence of nonliquefied material after 60 minutes, a sperm count of greater than 20 to 40 million/ml, more than 80% normal cell forms, any aggregation of sperm, the percentage of motile sperm (50% to 70%), and biochemical characteristics (pH, fructose).

Tests of hypothalamic dysfunction include assays of plasma FSH, LH, prolactin, and testosterone. In the male, FSH is believed to be needed for proper Leydig cell function, which produces the sperm. High FSH may signify faulty inhibin function and often major damage to germ cells. Deficiency of releasing hormone from the hypothalamus can lead to low levels of both FSH and LH with failure by the testes to produce testosterone. High levels of prolactin will cause testicular dysfunction.

Other tests include chromosome testing, adrenal function tests, testicular biopsy, microsurgery for vas deferens or epididymis blocks, surgery for varicocele, sexually transmitted disease tests, and tests for antibodies produced against testicular cells.

Management of Infertility

Ovulatory Stimulation. Attempts to stimulate ovulation include use of the *synthetic steroid,* clomiphene citrate (Clomide). It acts on the hypothalamic–pituitary axis to enhance secretion of FSH and LH, which stimulate follicle maturation in the ovary. It is given for 5 days in the early follicular phase of the menstrual cycle and used with evidence of adequate follicular function, but not when primary ovarian failure with high FSH and prolactemia is present. The initial trial is with the lowest dose of the drug (50 mg/day) with monitoring of ovulation using methods mentioned previously. Side-effects include hot flushes, palpitations, visual blurring, abdominal distention, bloating, pain or soreness, abnormal ovarian enlargement, multiple ovulations, and increased risk of spontaneous abortions. The risk of multiple pregnancies is high (15% to 20%).[11] Basal body temperature charts are kept to evaluate the response to this drug. If pregnancy does not result but ovulation does, other factors must be assessed. If ovulation is not stimulated, incremental doses of clomiphene can be given to a maximum of 200 mg/day. This may be pursued for three to four cycles, and other treatments may be added such as vitamin C and injections of estradiol or human chorionic gonadotropin (HCG). The HCG is administered intramuscularly 7 to 10 days after clomiphene therapy. Another therapy is pulsed LH-releasing hormone given every 60 to 65 minutes[11] about the time of ovulation to mimic the normal physiological functioning of the hypothalamus and pituitary.

A therapeutic course of *human menopausal gonadotropins* (HMG) or human chorionic gonadotropin (HCG) can be used if clomiphene therapy fails. HMG, a purified preparation of gonadotropins extracted from the urine of postmenopausal women, is given intramuscularly for 7 to 14 days. The response is determined by 24-hour urinary total estrogen excretion or plasma levels of estrogens. When the cervical os is opened and cervical mucus implies a normal pattern of hormone support, HCG is given to stimulate ovulation. The couple is then advised to have intercourse the day of the HCG injection and for 2 days following.[22]

Estrogen measurements are needed to obviate hyperstimulation of the ovaries. This can be a serious consequence of HMG–HCG therapy. In mild cases there is ovarian enlargement, abdominal distention, and weight gain. With severe hyperstimulation, a critical situation can develop including ascites, pleural effusion, electrolyte imbalance, and hypovolemia with oliguria and hypotension.[22]

Ovarian wedge resection, which induces a sustained reduction in circulating testosterone, can be done to remove steroid-producing tissue if interference is found to be due to high levels of testosterone. *Ergot alkaloids* such as clonidine inhibit pituitary secretion of prolactin. They can induce ovulatory function in women with high circulating levels of prolactin as well as in some women with seemingly normal levels.[22]

Structural Correction. Surgical correction of structural anomalies may be done. In women, congenital uterine abnormalities such as bicornuate or septate uterus can be corrected, and the tubes can be reconstructed (tuboplasty) for structural problems, although adhesions secondary to the tissue trauma of surgery are a problem. In men, surgical correction of undescended testicles, hypoepispadias or epispadias blockage of vas deferens or epididymis, varicocele, and other deformities can be done.

Other pathologies such as endometriosis in women need to be treated as do systemic conditions such as diabetes or thyroid conditions in either partner.

Semen Quality. Therapies to improve the quality of semen can be prescribed. These include giving testosterone, which depresses sperm production during treatment, but may produce a rebound of higher levels of gonadotropins when withdrawn. It also has the effect of improving libido. Other gonadal stimulators such as clomiphene can be used in men but often with disappointing results. Gonadotropin-releasing hormone, HMG, or HCG may be administered to elevate the sperm concentration in seminal fluid.

In situations where autoimmune antibodies or antisperm antibodies are formed, *immunosuppressive therapy* (corticosteroids) may be tried. In the antisperm antibody situation, the use of a condom for a 3 to 12 month period to prevent any contact of the female tissue with male sperm may allow the antibody titer to fall. Abstinence from any orogenital sex and sometimes all sexual intercourse for a period of time is usually tried to reduce the antibody level.

Coital Technique Education. Couples need to be counseled on the optimal time in the menstrual cycle to have intercourse, optimal frequency of intercourse, and the most appropriate positions for intercourse as adjunctive therapy to the other therapies. In general, the optimum time is midcycle around the time of presumed ovulation. Education regarding measurement technique and careful self-observation of basal body temperature, cervical mucus, and the cervical os is imperative to determine the optimal time for intercourse. Optimal frequency is about four times or more per week.[22] The couple should aim to have intercourse at least on alternate days in the fertile period. The effect of very frequent intercourse on depleting the sperm count in the ejaculate is suspected but not well documented. In a woman with a normally positioned uterus, an effective position is the male superior position. The woman's thighs are flexed and the hips may be elevated on a pillow. A woman who has a tilted uterus may need to use other positions such as entry from behind. The woman should be counseled to lie in bed, not to urinate for at least 30 to 60 minutes after intercourse, and not to douche. The use of lubricants, jellies, or creams should be avoided since they may have slight spermicidal effects. Saliva is a natural lubricant that can be used if extra lubrication is needed.

Artificial Insemination. Artificial insemination can be done using the partner's sperm, a donor's sperm, or both. Semen is collected by masturbation into a sterile container and used either fresh or quick frozen and thawed at the time of use. The recipient keeps track of basal body temperature to predict the time of ovulation. A clinic visit 2 to 3 days before this is helpful to check on cervical mucus, to measure LH or estrogen levels, and perhaps to measure the growth of a follicle by ultrasound. Two or three inseminations may be done per cycle and the procedure is not usually done longer than 12 months. Usually about three cycles are required for a conception, and pregnancy is purported to be achieved in about 60% of cases.[11]

In general, diligent education of the infertile couple about the reasons for various treatments is an important component of overall therapy. Anxiety and worry over the success of the treatments may in fact introduce psychogenic interference with natural and therapeutically induced function. Reassurance and support are needed although false hopes of creating pregnancy must not be generated.

***In Vitro* Fertilization and Embryo Transplant.** Recently, *in vitro* fertilization and embryo transplant have been developed as therapies for refractory infertility. This may be applied in situations of irreparable tubal damage, infertility of long-standing duration, and where cervical hostility and immunologic problems exist. The process involves aspiration of one or more mature ova from an ovary by laparoscopic or ultrasonic guidance of the harvesting instrument, fertilization of the ova by exposure to the sperm of the partner or donor, culture of the conceptus, and implantation in the uterus.[11] The procedure is expensive and success rates are reported to vary between 0% to 15% although steady improvement is bound to occur as more and more centers have experience with the techniques. Legal and moral problems arise as procedures move to using donor ova as well as sperm or when surrogate mothers are used when the uterus is absent or defective.

Evaluation

Much of nursing intervention related to infertility involves emotional support and health teaching. Evaluation involves the extent to which patients are knowledgeable about medical assessment and treatment goals, preparation for tests, test results and their implications, and appropriate health habits to facilitate pregnancy. Motivation to perform assessments and therapy and comfort in discussing emotional responses can be monitored. Anxiety indicators can be used to gauge the success of supportive care. Acceptance of failure to conceive and consideration of alternative parenting opportunities in cases of refractory infertility may represent evaluative indicators.

Contraception

Common methods of fertility control include steroidal drugs (oral or injectable), intrauterine devices (IUDs), barrier methods, coitus-inhibiting methods (abstinence, withdrawal, and rhythm), sterilization, and planned abortion.

Ovarian Steroid Contraceptives

Oral Contraceptives. Oral contraceptives have been a popular method of birth control since its introduction in the 1960s. The preparations now used are combined estrogen and progesterone pills or progestin only. Estrogen alone does not seem to suppress ovulation as well as the combination of estrogen and progestin. Of the combined forms, the combination is usually ethinyl estradiol or mestranol 30 to 50 μg, plus a progestin (commonly levonorgestrel or norethisterone) 50 to 200 μg. A sequential combination pill allows for the dose of estrogen to remain constant throughout the ovulatory cycle but with a lower dose of progestin in the first half of the cycle than in the last half. This provides an estrogen to progestin ratio that mimics the natural cycle. A preparation is also available which increases both estrogen and progestin in three phases. This lowers the total progestin dose. Progestin-only pills (minipills), usually norethisterone (350 μg) or levonorgestrel (30 μg), are given continuously rather than cyclically.[11]

Exogenous estrogen acts to inhibit FSH release from the pituitary so that follicular development is suppressed and ovulation fails. Progesteronelike drugs inhibit LH release by acting on the pituitary, but do not regularly inhibit ovulation. Progestins act mainly on the cervix and mucus production, making the mucus thick and impermeable to sperm. They can lead to irregular cycles and are often used for patients in whom estrogen is contraindicated, for example, women who are breast-feeding.

Several side-effects have been attributed to oral contraceptives. Estrogen or progesterone excess is suggested when nausea, vomiting, dizziness, migraine headaches, edema, breast enlargement, heavy menstrual bleeding, acne, increased facial hair growth, or loss of sexual desire occur.[8] Users of minipills suffer significantly more menstrual irregularities with spotting, breakthrough bleeding, and short cycles than combination pill users.

More severe outcomes also have been associated with oral contraceptive use including high blood pressure, urinary tract infections, gallbladder disease, superficial and deep-vein leg thrombosis, and cerebral vascular disease.

Implants and Injectables. These types of contraceptive agents are emerging as new methods. These methods aim to prolong the action of a one-time hormone administration. Two long-acting progestin steroids, depomedroxyprogesterone acetate (Depo-Provera) and norethisterone enanthate, when injected, can act for about 2 or 3 months. Implantable steroids in polymer forms including microcapsules, spheres, or pellets for continuous slow drug release are being studied. However, some polymers are nonbiodegradable necessitating removal of the device when exhausted and, therefore, testing of biodegradable polymers for drug delivery is continuing. The implants are inserted under the skin, usually on the inside of the forearm using a trocar, a potentially uncomfortable procedure.

Another method of contraceptive steroid delivery is the *vaginal ring,* a device made of a biocompatible substance (*e.g.,* Silastic) impregnated with a drug (*e.g.,* medroxyprogesterone acetate). Such rings can be inserted and removed by the woman. Protocols include wearing the ring 3 weeks out of the cycle or continuously. Side-effects are similar to those found with other methods of steroidal administration.

Intrauterine Devices (IUDs)

The availability of antibiotics effective against uterine infections and the use of polyethylene as an inert plastic allowed the development of devices that could be inserted and retained in the uterus. The likely mode of action of an IUD is to prevent implantation of a blastocyst, perhaps by a nonspecific foreign body reaction. The failure rate is between 1 to 6 per 100 users for the first year. Side-effects are a significant problem with this form of contraception including pain, bleeding, and expulsion. Even more seriously, any pregnancy has a higher risk of being ectopic, or, if intrauterine, of being spontaneously aborted. A greater risk of sepsis is associated with this method as compared to other means of birth control.[8] Newer IUDs releasing substances such as copper or steroidal hormones, for example, progesterone, have been shown to be highly effective as a contraceptive and relatively safe. Some research is being done to impregnant IUDs with substances to reduce bleeding or pain including progestins, antifibrinolytic agents, certain enzyme inhibitors (*e.g.,* protease), and prostaglandin inhibitors.

Barrier and Spermicidal Methods

These contraceptive methods include preventing sperm from entering the vagina (condoms) or the uterus (diaphragms and cervical caps), or chemically killing the sperm in the vagina (foams, creams, and jellies). Use of barrier methods has increased in recent years, partly due to evidence of unwanted risks with oral contraceptive use.

Condoms. Condoms can be obtained either dry or prelubricated in individual packages. Application must occur during the coital act when penis erection is present. The sensitivity of the penis is reportedly reduced somewhat, making this method objectionable to some men. One major advantage is that it has the potential to interfere with the spread of sexually transmitted disease.

Spermicides. The barrier methods used by women involve spermicidal agents alone or with mechanical devices such as diaphragms or cervical caps. Spermicides are effective if used properly and come in the form of creams, jellies, pressurized foam, foaming tablets, or suppositories for deposit directly into the vagina. These products are safe, available, convenient, and offer some protection against sexually transmitted disease. Disadvantages are that they tend to be messy to use, should be used within a short time of coitus, and can cause burning or allergic-type reactions in some women or men. In an effort to create longer-acting chemical delivery, vaginal inserts or sponges that provide sustained release of spermicidal agents have been marketed. Reports of such devices are not positive, with complaints of difficulty of use and interference with intercourse. Vaginal rings that release spermicides rather than steroids have been tested, but contraceptive results have not been satisfactory.

Diaphragm. The diaphragm is a flexible spring ring with latex rubber stretched over it, inserted and held in the vagina by wedging it behind the pubic bone. It should be used with a jelly or cream spermicide and fitted very carefully to be effective; however, it is highly effective if used properly.

Cervical Cap. The cervical cap blocks only the cervix, is held in place by suction, and can supposedly be left in place from the end of one to the beginning of the next menstruation. However, blockage to uterine secretions may predispose to the development of toxic shock syndrome. Inserting and removing the cap are more difficult than with the diaphragm. It is used much less often than the diaphragm and study of its effectiveness is not extensive.

Emergent Forms of Contraception

Prostaglandins. Another form of biochemical control of conception is the use of prostaglandins (PG), long-chain fatty acids that are produced in many tissues and act as local hormones. These substances are believed to have their major actions by terminating pregnancy through interfering with uterine blood flow or stimulating the uterine smooth muscle, which interferes with implantation of the blastocyst.[8] They may also destroy the corpus luteum, essential for sustaining early pregnancy. Indeed PG can induce abortion, at least if given within the first 8 weeks. Routes of administration include oral tablets, intramuscular injections, or vaginal suppositories. The major side-effects are vomiting, nausea, and diarrhea.

Antagonists to LHRH. Antagonists to luteinizing hormone releasing hormone (LHRH), the hormone from the hypothalamus that stimulates the release of FSH and LH from the pituitary, has been found to inhibit ovulation. It is known that LHRH is necessary for maintenance of testicular function and spermatogenesis, follicular maturation, ovulation, and implantation. *Agonist analogs of LHRH* are more potent than LHRH and paradoxically have an inhibitory effect on reproductive function. The mode of action seems to be to cause inappropriate LH levels so that the midcycle surge, critical to ovulation, is missed and ovulation is inhibited. They may also prevent normal corpus luteal action and endometrial priming for implantation. They could possibly be used as a "once-a-month" contraceptive although the time of administration is critical. Presently they can be given subcutaneously, intramuscularly, intranasally, sublingually, rectally, and intravaginally. Major side-effects have so far not been a problem.[8]

Birth Control Vaccines. Birth control vaccines are in an early stage of development. The idea behind vaccines is to cause a pregnancy-specific molecule to be recognized as an antigen so that antibodies are produced. If pregnancy occurs, such a reaction interferes with support of the pregnancy. Antigens being investigated are female derived such as selected placental hormones (*e.g.,* human chorionic gonadotropin) or male antigens derived from the sperm. One difficulty with this method is reversibility; otherwise such a method could create permanent contraception, that is, sterility.

Coitus-Inhibiting Methods

Coitus Interruptus. Coitus interruptus is a method in which the penis is withdrawn from the vagina immediately before ejaculation. It is practiced in some cultures but is usually ineffective as a long-term means of birth control.

Rhythm Method. The rhythm method is based on the estimation of fertile vs. infertile times in the menstrual cycle and abstinence from intercourse during the fertile time. This method assumes that ovulation occurs only once during the cycle, roughly in the middle, that the ovum remains viable for 2 to 3 days, and that sperm remain viable for not more than 72 hours, which is the average case according to research. Discipline is required to engage in intercourse only from days 1 through 8 and from 17 through 28 in a typical 28-day cycle. Cycles are variable, however, and observations of cyclical changes in body temperature and cervical mucus (see earlier section on infertility) can help improve the efficacy of this method. The efficacies of either of the methods just mentioned are not considered high and therefore are considered inadequate as a general birth control method.

Assessment

Requests for birth control advice is a common reason for women presenting themselves at physician's offices, women's clinics, and family planning centers. Matching the method to the person as appropriately as possible is of obvious concern. Many factors may influence the acceptance or rejection of a certain method including age of each partner, religion, culture, intelligence, motivation, attitudes toward body, knowledge level, frequency of intercourse, family planning goals, menstrual disorders, and general health status.

A *general history and physical examination* with a particular emphasis on the pelvic examination and gynecological history are absolute prerequisites to prescribing a birth control method. The most common methods considered are oral contraceptives, barrier methods, and IUDs. Birth control pills are generally considered to be one of the, if not the, most effective methods of contraception. However strong contraindications include cardiovascular disease, high blood pressure, liver diseases, estrogen-related tumors (*e.g.,* breast, uterine, liver), endogenous depression, and combinations of risk factors. Relative risk factors include epilepsy, diabetes, gallbladder disease, asthma, scanty menstrual flow, varicose veins, sickle cell anemia, high plasma lipids, smoking, migraine headaches, and age over 35 years.[11] Although the incidence of serious side-effects is not high, they can be fatal. The risk of myocardial infarction in pill users is about three to four times that of controls and if the woman is a heavy smoker, the risk rises dramatically. Increased tendency to high blood pressure, subarachnoid hemorrhage, thromboembolism, cerebral vascular disorders, migraine, depression, and liver and gallbladder disease have been noted.[8] Follow-up health assessment is warranted on a regular basis. The older a woman is, the more closely she should be monitored for side-effects.

The barrier methods are generally considered highly safe but use requires high motivation, handling of the genitalia, and expert fitting. There is more potential for failure to contraception due to inadequate application of the method than with birth control pills. The use of vaginal creams, jellies, and foams may be offensive to certain people. However, this method should be presented as a possible alternative to more invasive methods for couples that are well-educated and motivated.

Health Teaching for Contraception

Oral Contraceptives. For birth control pills, emphasis is on beginning the pills on the first day of the menstrual cycle (*i.e.,* the first day of bleeding) and the necessity of taking the pills every day. The woman should understand the basic components of the pill she is taking, how it works, and the side-effects that may occur. Some formulations involve taking pills for 3 weeks and then suspending intake until the next period starts, whereas others involve taking pills every day of the cycle by packaging inert pills so that the habit of taking a pill every day is not broken. The first follow-up after drug initiation should ideally be in 6 months after commencing the method. Assessment of weight, blood pressure, and liver size is important. Additionally, investigations may include blood lipid levels, glucose tolerance, and liver function. A woman should immediately stop taking the pills and report to her physician if any shortness of breath, chest pain, severe pain in the calf of the legs, severe headache, sudden loss or blurring of vision, or flashing lights occurs.[15] If possible, a woman should stop taking oral contraceptives 4 to 6 weeks before any major surgery.

Barrier Methods. In the case of barrier methods, fitting of a diaphragm or cervical cap must be done by a professional. A woman must then be instructed on how and when to insert, remove, and care for the device. Normally, the woman is taught to place 4 ml to 5 ml of spermicide on the concave disc, to then squeeze the ring from the opposite side, spread the labia with one hand, and insert the diaphragm with the other hand. Once in the vagina the ring is pushed firmly behind the pubic bone and the forefinger is used to check that the dome covers the cervix. It can be inserted up to 2 hours before intercourse and should be left in for at least 6 hours. If inserted longer than 2 hours before intercourse, an application of spermicidal cream or foam into the vagina must be made. Emphasis on insertion of jellies, creams, or foams close to the time of intercourse and repetitively for repeated intercourse is warranted. The diaphragm when removed can be washed with mild soap, dried, and kept in a protective container. It should be inspected regularly for integrity. Repeat fitting should be done following pregnancy, pelvic surgery, or significant weight change (loss or gain of 10 lb).

An IUD is placed high in the uterine cavity under aseptic technique. Amenorrhea more than 2 weeks beyond the usual menstrual time and any indication of infection (*e.g.,* fever, discharge, pain, tenderness) should be reported. The likelihood of some cramping and heavier bleeding for the first two to three menstrual cycles should be mentioned. There may be some discomfort at the time of insertion and some bleeding following. Nothing should be inserted in the vagina for at least 2 days. A woman should be taught to check the toilet for possible expulsion for 48 hours postinsertion and to feel for the indicator string or thread left protruding through the cervix at least once a week. Insertion is recommended toward the end of the menstrual flow or at the time of ovulation.[11,15]

Evaluation

Nursing interventions for contraception largely involve health teaching so that patients understand the mode of action, methods of applying the contraceptives, effectiveness, side-effects, risks, and benefits of the means chosen. The choice of contraceptive should correspond to attitudes and beliefs about fertility, family planning goals, general health status, and lifestyle. Motivation to use the method diligently and prevent unwanted pregnancies should be assessed.

Sterilization and Abortion

Sterilization has become one of the most often used forms of birth control in the world. This is due, at least in part, to a worldwide concern with overpopulation and the desire of people to limit the size of their families.[20] With the development of safe and effective procedures for sterilizing women or men, it has become an increasingly popular choice for couples who want no or no more children and who see a long period of other methods as unwanted.

Female Tubal Ligation. One method of sterilization is to tie, cut, or block the fallopian tubes. Commonly, the fallopian tubes are accessed by laparoscopy (Fig. 100–1). A needle admitting air is used to enter the peritoneal cavity, followed by a laparoscope and the tubes are cauterized, or clips or bands put on. Alternately, a hysteroscopy can be done whereby a scope inside the uterus is used to visualize where the tubes enter the uterus and blockage is provoked with chemicals. A potentially reversible method is to inject liquid silicone into the tubes, which forms a plug that can be removed later. A laparotomy can also be performed by making a small incision just above the pubic hairline so as to visualize the tubes and obstruct them. Using recent techniques, the failure rate should be less than 1 percent, although any pregnancies that occur are more likely to be ectopic. Removal of the uterus (hysterectomy) or ovaries are of course ultimate methods for female sterilization but are irreversible and

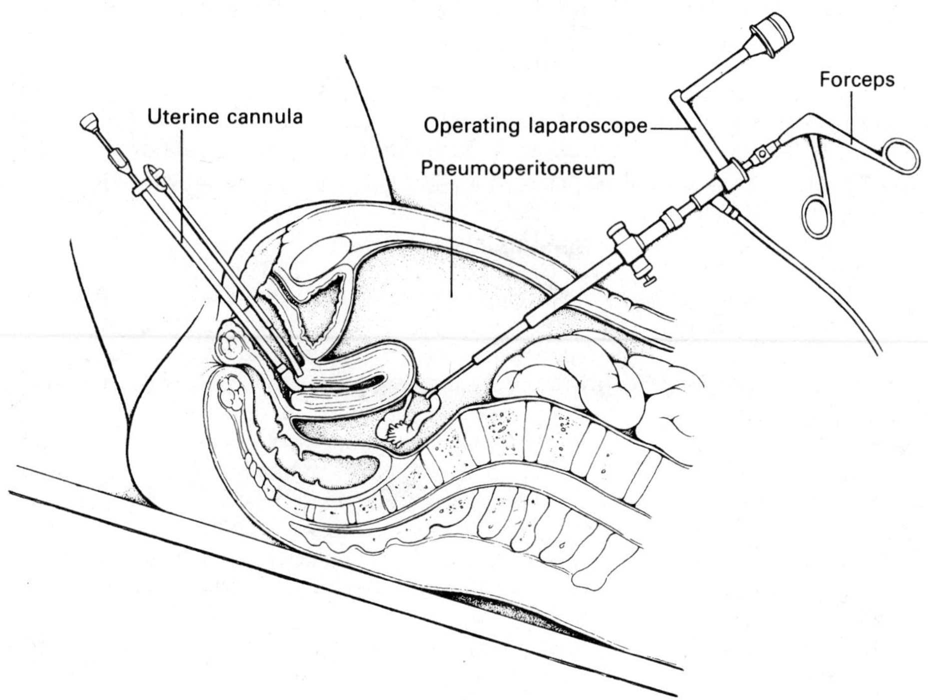

FIGURE 100–1 Tubal ligation by means of laparoscopy.

carry a risk of morbidity and mortality that is several times higher than the other conventional methods.

Vasectomy. Sterilization in men is simpler than in women as is reversal, pregnancy rates are somewhat lower, and ectopic pregnancy is not a problem. Vasectomy involves cutting the vas deferens, which carry sperm from each epididymis to the penis. It can be done as an office procedure. It is thought that occasionally the leakage of sperm from the cut ends of the vas or perhaps the absorption of degenerating sperm through the walls of the ducts may create an autoimmune response or vascular damage. The long-term effects of these outcomes are unknown.

Planned Abortion. Therapeutic abortion refers to the termination of pregnancy before 20 to 22 weeks gestation and, as a means of contraception, is extremely controversial, as is continually evidenced in the media. Recently, North American figures showed that one third of abortions were in women less than 20 years old, three quarters were in single women, nearly 60% were in women with no previous live births, and 95% were done by dilatation and suction evacuation. Abortions that are carried out within the first 10 to 12 weeks of pregnancy are associated with very low morbidity or mortality to the woman although the rate of complications increases with longer times of gestation.

Methods of planned pregnancy termination are largely determined on the basis of duration of pregnancy. In early pregnancy (up to the sixth to seventh week), *prostaglandins* can be placed in the upper vagina or in the uterus and help to expel the conceptual products by increasing smooth muscle contraction. Alternately, a catheter can be used with suction applied (*menstrual extraction*). Cervical dilatation is not necessary although paracervical anesthetic blocks may be used. Risks include the continuation of pregnancy and complications such as uterine injury and bleeding. When done by a competent health-care giver, the risks are low. Difficulties increase when the woman has never been pregnant or if she is more than 6 weeks pregnant.[5]

Beyond the early pregnancy phase, dilatation of the cervix is performed and the fetus evacuated (*vacuum curettage*). The major risk is that if done too quickly, the cervical dilatation can cause cervical damage. Sometimes laminaria tents (devices that are inserted and swell to a larger size) are placed in the cervix, 6 to 24 hours ahead of time. Ovum forceps or large suction cannulas may be needed to remove the conceptus. Complications include infection, uterine perforation, or excessive bleeding. The incidence of complications has been said to be between 2% and 8%.[5]

In the later stages, pregnancy may be terminated by *hysterotomy, dilatation and evacuation,* or the *injection of prostaglandins or saline* into the amniotic sac. Prostaglandins are directly infused into the amniotic sac and usually expulsion of the conceptus occurs within 24 hours. Because prostaglandins stimulate smooth muscle of the gastrointestinal tract as well as the uterus, nausea, vomiting, abdominal cramps, and diarrhea are common side-effects. In a saline abortion, 200 ml to 250 ml of amniotic fluid is removed and replaced with 20% saline. Uterine contractions usually begin in about 8 to 40 hours. Complications of second trimester abortions with hypertonic saline injection include infection, incomplete placental separation, excessive bleeding, and failure to abort. A major concern is hypertonic saline getting into the general circulation.[5]

Assessment

Sterilization. Voluntary surgical contraception is fast becoming a prominent method of family planning. Assessment involves good counseling to allow the patient to make a knowledgeable and confident decision. It is often possible to successfully reverse sterilization procedures, but it should be considered a permanent method. Complete and accurate information should be given about the benefits, risks, and advantages of both male and female sterilization and what to expect before, during and after surgery.[20] Benefits include being permanent, effective, and a one-time cost. Surgery has some attendant morbidity and mortality although this is not major. The decision should be made with full knowledge of alternate temporary contraceptive methods. Subjects should be encouraged to ask questions and continually feel free to change their decision prior to the process. All aspects of the procedure and its side-effects should be explained including psychological, physiological, and behavioral outcomes. Female sterilization is effective immediately, but failure rates can attend all forms of surgery. Generally accepted ranges of failure are said to be 4 to 6 per 1000 cases. A vasectomy does not make a man immediately sterile and alternate forms of contraception must be used for several weeks. Failure is also possible. Follow-up sperm counts should be done to assure success.

Planned Abortion. Assessment associated with planned abortion involves helping the woman to work through her feelings about pregnancy; suggesting alternatives to abortion and reaching the decision to abort the pregnancy of her own volition; helping her to cope with stress, ambivalence, and guilt; and helping her to understand the entire process of abortion and gaining knowledge about contraceptive methods. A menstrual, obstetrical, and general health history and a gynecological examination will be part of the process. The technique chosen for the abortion will be determined by length of gestation and general health factors.

Nursing Interventions

Sterilization procedures are frequently done in physicians' offices or clinics and require careful explanation of the procedures, the preparation required, and responses. Generally the procedure is uneventful and patients are told to report any excessive bleeding, pain, inflammation, or fever.

In any abortion situation, the safety and comfort of the woman are important factors to monitor. Meticulous explanation of each step of the procedure helps alleviate attendant anxiety. In early abortions, most women will experience only mild cramping and minimal bleeding. The setting is usually an outpatient one and the patient is sent home in 1 to 2 hours.

In a second trimester abortion, labor and delivery proceeds and safety and comfort are more crucial. During the procedure, fluid balance is monitored as are vital signs to assess for ineffective circulating volume. As the uterus contracts, pain may be experienced. Relaxation techniques may be helpful in the management of pain due to contractions. Careful perineal hygiene is important in preventing infection. Close observation for the delivery of the fetus is necessary. The cord should be clamped upon delivery and documentation of delivery of an intact placenta is critical. Bleeding should then be monitored carefully. A reassuring, caring, and supportive approach to care helps to make the experience less stressful.

Postabortion care involves assessment of physical and emotional status and the contraceptive needs of the patient. Women should be instructed to note any evidence of infection such as unusual vaginal discharge, unusual temperature elevation, pain, or bleeding. Any disorders of the menses should be reported following the abortive procedure.[16]

Evaluation

Interventions should facilitate the patient's having adequate knowledge by which to select and cope with sterilization or planned abortion with a minimum of guilt, remorse, or anxiety. A patient should feel supported during the procedure. An absence of complications, particularly infection, a stable mood state, good appetite, undisturbed sleep patterns, and motivation to resume one's life suggest adequate adjustment.

Rape-Trauma Syndrome

Women seeking health care for the results of a rape attack are usually first seen in the emergency department. It is imperative that they receive dignified, respectful, and adequate emotional and physical care. An organized medical treatment protocol, follow-up care, and referral to community agencies are important.[9] Crisis counseling immediately and over time is needed.

The amount of physical trauma is variable, although the woman may be the victim of stabbing or beating along with the rape and can require emergency care for other tissue injury. Regardless of the extent of physical injury, the emotional trauma is profound and evidence of exposure to an extremely stressful event emerges immediately and extends over a long time after the attack. There is a cluster of symptoms that rape victims experience in the acute phase of recovery. Physical ones include disorganized sleep patterns such as insomnia and terror wakenings, loss of appetite, nausea upon recall of the incident, stomach pains, and other symptoms of intense stress response. Emotional responses can involve overwhelming fears of physical injury, mutilation, or death. Feelings of degradation, shame, guilt, humiliation, blame, anger, embarrassment, and revenge have been described. Mood swings and emotional outbursts are not uncommon. Behaviorally, various responses have been described such as crying episodes with no obvious provocation, withdrawal and an overcontrolled demeanor, and fear of crowds.[9] Fears, disturbing thoughts, physical symptoms, and behavioral upsets can extend beyond the acute phase into a longer-term reorganization phase. Even though outward adjustment may seem positive, women often manifest health care problems such as nightmares, phobias, and disruption of lifestyle.

Assessment

The rape victim needs careful assessment of the extent of physical injury, and a complete physical examination for internal bleeding, broken bones, and ruptured organs is warranted in cases with extensive physical violence. A pelvic examination to document the evidence of rape is needed, describing the condition of the external genitalia and vagina. A specimen must be collected to establish coitus or ejaculation. Tests are done for gonorrhea and syphilis. A history is also taken and the possibility of pregnancy should be determined based on the menstrual cycle phase at the time of the attack.

Interventions

Any tissue injuries require appropriate medical intervention. Penicillin or other antibiotic therapy is administered to prevent sexually transmitted disease. The risk of pregnancy may be handled by giving a high-dose estrogen, usually diethylstilbestrol ("morning-after" pill), or waiting to see if pregnancy occurs and then deciding to undergo an abortion or maintain the pregnancy. The woman must have the options clearly explained and be helped to make a decision with which she is comfortable.

Dominant nursing care through this process is providing support and teaching the patient. The patient should be seen immediately and not be left in the waiting room of the emergency department or clinic. Contact with the same nurse consistently, thereby avoiding numerous questions from staff, reduces additional stressors. Explanations of each step in the medical asessment and physical examination; interpretations of the extent of injury, particularly to the genital area; and explanations of the rationale for sexually transmitted disease and pregnancy treatment are imperative. Additionally, the patient can be made aware of immediate and delayed symptom responses that can occur and be referred for counseling support. Helping the patient to determine with whom she could share this experience may help to ascertain support resources. Women all too often feel overwhelmingly denigrated, perhaps responsible for the rape, and morally stigmatized. The strength of these reactions should be assessed and, if present, even more focus placed on counseling services. Above all, the approach must be respectful with an emphasis on the positive actions the victim took to protect herself and stay alive along with plans on how to deal with ongoing recovery.[15]

Evaluation

As a result of interventions, patients will be protected against infection and pregnancy, feel supported, and feel competent in their help-seeking behaviors. Emotional stability, coping strategies, somatic complaints, and plans to utilize long-term follow-up care can be used to evaluate immediate care.

Perimenopause Transition

An important life stage for women is the transition period during which cyclic gonadal function and reproductive capability is lost (called the *climacteric*). This is a slow process and can span up to 20 years of a woman's life.[19] During this phase, many endocrinologic, biochemical, and metabolic changes occur with the formation of numerous symptoms, indicative of health status changes. The term *menopause* refers to the permanent cessation of menstruation. Perimenopause refers to the period of time prior to actual menopause when changes are already obvious biologically or clinically (*e.g.*, menstrual changes) and up to 12 months postmenstrual-period cessation. Postmenopause refers to the period of time beyond the 12 months past the last menstrual period. The common or classic symptoms of perimenopause are vasomotor symptoms, most commonly hot flashes and night sweats; emotional symptoms, such as mood changes and depression; and musculoskeletal symptoms, such as muscle aching.[18]

Natural menopause is an age-related phenomenon and believed to occur due to ovarian failure. The longevity of the ovarian cells appears to be rather precisely timed. No explanation for the programmed senescence of cells in general has been agreed upon although numerous theories of cellular aging have been advanced. Aging may involve deterioration of the nuclear material, DNA (deoxyribonucleic acid). Such errors could cause diminished protein synthesis and organ failure. Another theory is that there is a loss of some intracellular or extracellular substances that may protect against materials that are toxic to the cell, making the cells vulnerable to toxins. Another proposal is that there is an accumulation of collagen and cross-linking of collagen in the cells or an accumulation of other complex nondegradable molecules within the cells rendering them dysfunctional. A reduction in immune function occurs with aging and the development of an immunity to certain of one's own cells (autoimmunity) is a speculated cause of aging in cells. Which of these processes apply to the cellular aging of the ovaries in particular is uncertain.

With aging, the number of primordial follicles in the ovaries progessively decreases. The ovaries of a female at puberty contain an average of 380,000 primordial follicles, whereas those of a 40- to 44-year-old woman contain only 8,000.[7] THe ovaries at menopause appear shrunken, pitted, and fibrotic. The functional loss of follicles and disrupted cyclicity of the menses is accompanied by changes in the output of FSH and LH from the pituitary and in the steroid hormones from the ovaries, which have intimate feedback interactions with one another.

A consistent endocrinologic change associated with menopause is an increase in follicle-stimulating hormone (FSH), due to loss of negative feedback inhibition from estrogens and perhaps inhibin (another hormone released from the ovaries). The decline in plasma estrogens that occurs with ovarian failure is seen as a major factor in the development of clinical outcomes. Several symptom complexes are believed to be attributable to estrogen deprivation. Genitourinary atrophy, vasomotor instability (hot flashes), osteoporosis, and amenorrhea have definitely been linked to estrogen withdrawal, blood lipid changes are probably linked, and arteriosclerotic cardiovascular disease and psychosexual symptoms have a possible linkage.[7]

Assessment and Interventions

Genitourinary Atrophy. The vulva, vagina, cervix, uterus, fallopian tubes, urethra, and bladder all have large numbers of estrogen receptors and are affected by decreased circulating estrogens. In the vulvar area, there is thinning of hair on the mons and gradual shrinkage of the labia. The folds of the vaginal wall become less prominent, the color is paler, and the epithelium is easily traumatized. Vaginal secretions diminish so that intercourse may be painful or difficult because of poor lubrication. The vaginal pH rises and the alkaline environment predisposes to bacterial infections creating vaginitis. Vaginitis may in turn cause postmenopausal vaginal bleeding. The glands of the cervix atrophy, the myometrium shrinks, and the endometrium becomes thin and atrophic. The fallopian tubes decrease in motility and size. The urethra is affected by estrogen withdrawal, although the effect on the bladder is controversial.

Individuals do vary in their vulnerability to the above changes, in continued ovarian steroid production, and in rates of conversion of steroids to estrogens in peripheral tissue. In adipose tissue, liver, and specific hypothalamic nuclei, androstenedione (synthesized mainly in the adrenal glands) is converted to estrone.[7] In postmenopausal women, estrogens circulate mainly as estrone, whereas in the premenopausal phase the dominant estrogen is estradiol.

A major problem accompanying genitourinary atrophy is *tactile senory perception alteration.* This is manifested as dryness, itching, and burning of the genital tissues with dyspareunia if the atrophy is severe. Although estrogen replacement therapy may be of some help in treating the sensory complaints, cortisone or testosterone cream or other local therapy may be prescribed. Estrogens administered systemically or intravaginally can reverse the vaginal cell changes but such treatment carries with it the risks of any exogenous estrogen treatment. Women may be taught to use lubricants such as K-Y jelly during intercourse to prevent discomfort. Some women have reported that vitamin E supplements over time have alleviated the dryness of vaginal tissues.[6]

It is thought that an active sexual life can prevent some of the vaginal atrophy associated with aging. The supporting tissue of the vagina and other pelvic organs may be subject to estrogen withdrawal atrophy, leading to uterine prolapse, rectocele, and cystocele, although many other factors are influential such as parity, mode of delivery, and genetic predisposition. Perineal exercises such as the Kegel exercises may help by improving muscle tone. Maintenance of strong supporting tissues in the perineum helps to maintain good bladder emptying as well. Problems with bladder function are probably more a result of aging in general rather than estrogen withdrawal, although estrogen treatment is frequently helpful in alleviating urinary frequency, dysuria, nocturia, urgency, and stress incontinence due to pelvic relaxation.[7]

Vasomotor Instability (Hot Flashes). A sensory perceptual alteration in temperature is also common in the perimenopause. This vasomotor symptom is called a hot flush or flash and occurs in upward of 89% of women undergoing natural menopause. A hot flash is the increase in or perception of heat located in or on a region of the body, having an origin and a spread ranging from mild to severe in intensity and lasting anywhere from half a minute to 15 minutes.[21] Hot flashes may be very bothersome and can be associated with nausea, dizziness, headache, palpitations, and diaphoresis (sweating). Recent research has shown that hot flashes may begin many years before actual menopause or menstrual cycle changes. As menopause nears, the intensity and frequency of hot flashes usually increase. Hot flashes occur most frequently between 6 and 8 AM and between 6 and 10 PM. However some women may complain of flashes only during the night or only during parts of the day. There is no truly typical pattern.[21]

Medical treatment of vasomotor instability involves estrogen replacement. This has been found to be effective in many women. However, to avoid the risks of taking exogenous estrogens, women may be taught to cope with the symptoms. It is important to stress as part of health education regarding the perimenopause that hot flashes are not a disease, are generally temporary, and that worrying about them can increase the problem. Women may be encouraged to keep a diary of their experiences and to pinpoint the triggers. This can foster a feeling of control over the experience and may be helpful in itself. However, if this exercise leads to a nonhelpful fixation on the symptoms, it should be abandoned. Women may be advised to dress in a layered fashion to remove or replace clothing easily depending on perception of temperature comfort. They should avoid hot environments, highly seasoned foods, coffee, tea, and alcohol. Thoughts and emotions can trigger hot flashes. Therefore, advice to avoid getting tense or excited and to think about other situations can be helpful. Imagining pleasurable situations or cool environments at the beginning of a flash can be helpful in averting it. These techniques may act through a generalized relaxation response. Tranquilizers or mood elevators are not usually effective. Some women report that vitamin E may be helpful.[21]

Osteoporosis. A certain amount of bone mass decline is evident with aging but when there is accelerated loss, the condition is called osteoporosis. Maximum bone density is reached between the ages of 25 and 35, but a gradual decline in bone mass occurs and is evident by the ages of 40 and 50. In women, the decrease in bone mass occurs following menopause. This is a fairly silent condition until advanced enough that fractures occur. The prevalence is difficult to determine but it is estimated that 25% of women older than 60 years have spinal compression fractures, and that forearm fractures are ten times more common in women than men by age 60.[7] Hip fractures are a significant problem in older women.

Certain factors put a woman at risk for osteoporosis. The earlier the menopause, the greater the risk; familial tendencies seem to exist, and ethnic or racial differences exist. Fewer black women develop osteoporosis than white women. This may be because black women seem to have larger muscles, and with more stress on bone due to larger muscle mass the greater is the bone mass to support it. Little research has been done but it appears that women of British, European, and Oriental descent are at greater risk for developing osteoporosis than women of African, Mediterranean, or Hispanic ancestry.[21]

Clearly, the optimum health goal is to prevent osteoporosis from developing rather than trying to treat it after it develops. There are several things that can be done to minimize the risk of developing this condition. Based on knowledge of bone metabolism, nutrition is an essential part of preventive therapy. A daily calcium intake of between 800 mg and 1400 mg (the amount found in about 1 to 1¾ qt of milk) is needed. Dairy products and green, leafy vegetables are the best sources of calcium. Interestingly, the bone density of vegetarians is greater than meat eaters. Therefore, some people would be well advised to increase their vegetable and reduce their red meat intake. Increasing the stress on bones through exercise will increase the size and strength of bone. Women who smoke tend to have an earlier menopause and alcohol impairs calcium absorption, putting women whose lifestyles include these factors at greater risk for osteoporosis.

Medical treatment most often involves prescribing estrogen, and other pharmacological preparations such as androgen, vitamin D, calcium, sodium fluoride, calcitonin, parathyroid hormone, and growth hormone have been tried in various combinations. There is presently no agreement on the most effective combination of factors for treating or preventing osteoporosis. Research has demonstrated that this condition is related to estrogen levels and that estrogen can be protective against the risk of fractures in women who have osteoporosis.[1,7]

Problems related to reproductive behaviors and function are common. Although they often do not threaten biological survival, they can profoundly interfere with a person's self-esteem and quality of life. Nursing strategies for common reproductive problems encompass symptom or sign assessment (often pain or abnormal bleeding), explanation of prescribed interventions (*e.g.,* contraception, surgical sterilization), support through difficult procedures (*e.g.,* fertility evaluation), health teaching regarding normative responses (*e.g.,* menopausal symptoms), lifestyle factors that promote or prevent abnormal function, monitoring of responses, and testing alternative symptom management techniques. Since reproductive function is inextricably related to sexuality, a caring, sensitive, respectful demeanor must pervade nurse–patient interactions to effectively implement the nursing strategies and promote reproductive health/wellness.

References

1. Cutler WB, Garcia CR: The Medical Management of Menopause and Premenopause. Philadelphia, JB Lippincott, 1984
2. Dawood, MY: Dysmenorrhea. Clin Obstet Gynecol 26(3):719–727, 1983
3. Dawood, MY: Dysmenorrhea. Compr Ther 8(6):9–16, 1982
4. Fogel CI: The gynecologic triad: Discharge, pain and bleeding. In Fogel CI, Woods NF (eds): Health Care of Women: A Nursing Perspective, pp 220–256. St Louis, CV Mosby, 1981
5. Fogel CI: Abortion. In Fogel CI, Woods NF (eds): Health Care of Women: A Nursing Perspective, pp 220–256. St Louis, CV Mosby, 1981
6. Gelein JL, Heiple P: Aging. In Fogel CI, Woods NF (eds): Health Care of Women: A Nursing Perspective, pp 220–256. St Louis, CV Mosby, 1981
7. Hammond CB, Maxson WS: Current Concepts: Physiology of the Menopause. The Upjohn Company, 1983
8. Harper MJK: Birth Control Technologies. Austin, University of Texas Press, 1983
9. Harris C: Women and violence. In Fogel CI, Woods NF (eds): Health Care of Women: A Nursing Perspective, pp 139–145. St Louis, CV Mosby, 1981
10. Kase NG, Weingold AB (eds): Principles and Practice of Clinical Endocrinology. New York, John Wiley & Sons, 1983
11. MacKay ER, Beischer NA, Cox LW, Wood C: Illustrated Textbook of Gynaecology. Philadelphia, WB Saunders, 1983
12. Peckham BM, Shapiro S: Signs and Symptoms in Gynecology. Philadelphia, JB Lippincott, 1983
13. Romney SL, Gray MJ, Little AB et al: Gynecology and Obstetrics: The Health Care of Women, 2nd ed. New York, McGraw-Hill, 1981
14. Shangold MM: The pain of dysmenorrhea. J Am Med Wom Assoc 38(1):12–17, 1983
15. Smith ED: Women's Health Care: A Guide for Patient Education. New York, Appleton-Century-Crofts, 1981
16. Smith ED: Abortion: Health Care Perspectives. New York, Appleton-Century-Crofts, 1982
17. Speroff L, Glass R, Kase NG: Clinical Gynecologic Endocrinology and Infertility. Baltimore, Williams & Wilkins, 1978
18. Steiner M: Psychobiologic aspects of the menopause syndrome. In Buchbaum HJ (ed): The Menopause. New York, Springer-Verlag, 1982
19. Upton GV: The perimenopause physiologic correlates and clinical management. J Reprod Med 27(1):1–27, 1982
20. van Lith DAF, Keith LG, van Hall EV: New Trends in Female Sterilization. Chicago, Year Book Medical Publishers, 1983
21. Voda AM: Menopause, Me and You. A Personal Handbook for Women. Salt Lake City, College of Nursing, University of Utah, 1984
22. Woods, NF: Infertility. In Fogel CI, Woods NF (eds): Health Care of Women: A Nursing Perspective, pp 257–283. St Louis, CV Mosby, 1981
23. Woods NF, Mosi M, Derg GK: Prevalence of perimenstrual symptoms. Am J Public Health 72(11):1257–1264, 1982

Chapter 101

Infectious and Inflammatory Disorders Affecting Reproductive Function

Susan Garske Halverson
Sally K. Graham

Sexually Transmitted Diseases

Inflammatory and infectious problems of the reproductive system stem from diverse etiologies. The general groups of pathogens can be divided as follows: bacterial, viral, protozoan, fungal, and metazoal in origin. These infectious agents can cause a wide range of disease, from almost no symptoms to severe morbidity and even mortality.

Many of the problems discussed in this chapter are considered to be sexually transmissible disease, or STDs. STD is now the accepted term used in discussing any disease entity that can be transmitted through sexual intercourse or close physical contact in significant numbers. For example, hepatitis B is now recognized to be an STD.

The term venereal disease, or VD, is no longer used. As recently as the last decade it has become necessary to change the terminology from VD to STD to encompass the increasingly wide range of clinical problems now recognized to be sexually transmitted. A brief overview of this rapidly changing area of research is appropriate.

Historical Perspective

The earliest recorded evidence of STD dates back to 4000 to 5000 years ago. Hippocrates mentioned urethral discharge and luekorrhea in his works.[23] The Dark Ages and Middle Ages were influenced by the spread of Christianity. Although Christianity held some groups of women to a strict behavioral code, prostitution flourished. By the 18th and 19th centuries, syphilis and gonorrhea became recognized as two separate disease entities. The 20th century brought the first definite move toward prevention, especially during and after World War I. The use of penicillin after 1944 brought an even more organized approach to the spread and control of gonorrhea and syphilis.

After 1955, the prevalence of STD began to increase. Many factors are associated with this increase. After World War II, birth rates rapidly grew, producing the "baby boom" generation. According to Holmes, "STDs are most common during adolescence and earlier adulthood, the ages of greatest sexual activity."[19] Holmes suggests that young sexually active persons may be more susceptible to these diseases because of their not yet mature anatomy and physiology. Because of the larger percentage of the total population in the childbearing years, there is also an increase in the incidence of perinatal STD.

The changing patterns of marriage and divorce also influence the increase in STD. There is a much larger proportion of single people, either because of later marriage or increasing divorce rates. It is well documented that there is a higher occurrence of STD among those who are single, divorced, or separated than those who are married.[3]

The rates of STD have generally been higher for men than women. This may be due to the fact that women can be infected by different organisms such as *Neisseria gonorrhoeae* and *Chlamydia trachomatis* and be asymptomatic, whereas men would have a more noticeable presentation such as dysuria or urethral discharge. Thus, men would likely seek treatment sooner. There has also been an increase in homosexuality in the last 20 years. There is generally an increase in numbers of sexual partners in the male population evidenced by high rates of STD. Homosexual women have rarely been associated with STD. Between the years 1969 to 1979, the percentage of white male public clinic patients with syphilis who reported at least one male sexual partner increased from 38% to 70%.[19]

Obtaining an accurate and complete general medical history and a more specific sexual history will often be the role of the nurse. The nurse is obligated to be complete in taking this history, since sexual preferences and different sexual practices can cause or contribute to certain diseases of the reproductive system.

The nurse needs to possess knowledge of the different STDs, their clinical presentations, mode of transmission, course of disease, prevention, and treatment in order to take an adequate history. The manner in which the nurse approaches the patient is of utmost importance. Because the sexual history is of such a personal nature, the nurse needs to be aware of her areas of bias and her attitude toward sexual practices other than her own, since the accuracy of information received may be affected. Such techniques as open-ended questions, good eye contact, willingness to discuss issues, and the inclusion of the sexual history in the course of the regular history (not leaving it to the end) can all help to create a comfortable and confidential atmosphere.

Syphilis

Definition

Syphilis is a sexually transmitted disease that has been documented by historians since early recorded history. There are two theories on the origin of syphilis. The Columbian theory was based on the epidemic of syphilis seen in the 15th century in Europe, which coincided with Columbus' return to Spain from the West Indies. With Europe being at war, this was an especially conducive time for spread of this STD by the movement of troops and followers.[41] The environmental theory states that all treponematoses are variants of a single disease. The manifestation of disease is affected by the environment, especially temperature. Whether the disease is expressed as syphilis, yaws (a disabling skin and bone disease of the tropics), or pinta (a less serious skin disease of Central and South America) is dependent on modification of the treponeme.[41]

After World War II and the advent of penicillin there was a drop in the number of reported cases of syphilis. The rates remained fairly constant until 1981 when the rate was the highest since 1950 (see Figure 101–1). Approximately one third of those who have sexual intercourse with another person with syphilis will contract the disease themselves.[34]

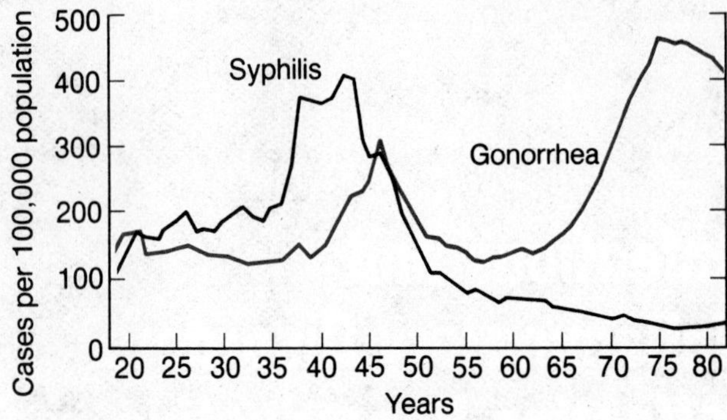

FIGURE 101–1 Rates of reported syphilis and gonorrhea in the United States, 1919–1982. (Holmes KK et al: Epidemiology of sexually transmitted diseases. Urologic Clin North Am 11(1):3–13, 1984)

Etiology

Treponema pallidum is the causative agent for syphilis. It is a member of the order Spirochaetales, which is virulent for human beings. Not visible by light microscopy because of its small size, it therefore must be identified by dark-field microscopy or electron microscopy. The organism appears to have regular tight spirals.

T. pallidum does not survive well outside its human host because it is susceptible to drying, to heat above body temperature, and to mild antiseptics. Moisture is necessary for its survival and it flourishes in the mouth and anogenital region.[9]

The body's first line of defense is the skin and mucous membranes. During sexual intercourse, the mucous membranes can be broken down and minute abrasions can allow a site for the spirochete to penetrate. The spirochete can also be passed to the fetus *in utero* by an infected mother.

By the time a patient presents with a chancre, or skin ulcer, specific antibodies can be detected in around 80% of cases. This B-cell response can be detected in the serum. The fluorescent treponemal antibody (FTA-ABS) test or the new *T. pallidum*–hemagglutinating antibody (TPHA) test are diagnostic tools.

The process by which secondary syphilis occurs in spite of the host's ability to check the primary infection is not completely understood. Three weeks to 6 months after the primary chancre has appeared the widespread rash of secondary syphilis is seen. Several reasons are the hematogenous spread of treponemes throughout the body, the establishment of lesions in the skin that may offer better growth conditions for *T. pallidum* because of reduced temperature, and the development of some degree of systemic immunity that modifies the appearance of these disseminated lesions. They otherwise would all look like chancres.[34]

In 1 to 20 years after the secondary infection the latency phase gives way to tertiary syphilis. Large granulomatous lesions (gummas) may appear in soft tissue, viscera, or trauma sites such as knees and elbows. Why syphilis reappears after such a long period of apparent host control is not completely understood.

Clinical Manifestations

Primary syphilis is manifested by the appearance of a chancre (painless hard ulcer) at the site of infection by the treponeme. The chancre begins as a macule, which then develops into a papule with an eroded surface that feels firm to palpation. It is painless unless it is secondarily infected.[24] Chancres generally appear in the genital area (on the penis in men, or on the vulva, labia, or cervix in women). But occasionally they can be found in the perianal area or around the mouth, tongue, tonsils, breasts, axilla, umbilicus, or fingers. The chancre develops in 10 to 90 days with an average of 3 weeks postcontact. Regional nontender lymphadenopathy may accompany the chancre. If untreated or unnoticed, the chancre will persist for 2 to 8 weeks and then disappear.

The differential diagnosis of primary syphilis must include herpes simplex, staphylococcal or streptococcal infections, secondary infection of an abrasion, furuncle, chancroid, granuloma inguinale, lymphogranuloma venereum, fixed drug eruption, histoplasmosis, tuberculosis, reaction to a parasite, and tumors such as squamous cell carcinoma.[24]

Six weeks to 6 months after the chancre appears, signs of *secondary syphilis* will appear in an untreated patient. This is due to the hematogenous spread of the spirochetes that have multiplied. This stage is characterized by fever, malaise, headache, sore throat, anorexia, and arthralgias. There is a papulomacular skin eruption, usually nonpruritic and painless, which can appear generalized on the body and characteristically appears on the palms and soles of the feet. Syphilis is commonly called the "great imitator" because of its many presentations. There is usually a generalized lymphadenopathy that is nontender. There can be mucous patches in the mouth, condyloma lata (moist, flat wartlike lesions that are highly infectious), "moth-eaten" alopecia, hepatitis, meningitis, periostitis, nephritis, arthritis, and myositis.

The differential diagnoses of secondary syphilis include pityriasis rosea, measles, infectious mononucleosis, erythema multiforme, leukemia, lymphoma, tinea, sarcoid, granuloma annulare, lichen planus, and other morbilliform or papulosquamous diseases.[24] If untreated, secondary syphilis will last 2 to 8 weeks and disappear and become latent.

The *third stage* of syphilis is usually divided into early latent and late latent. The early latent stage is from 0 to 5 years after the initital infection, and the late latent stage is over 5 years from initial infection. If the duration is unknown, the disease is considered to be in the late latent stage if the patient is over 30 years old or the last known negative serology was over 4 years ago.[31] Although two thirds of patients with untreated syphilis will remain latent and asymptomatic, one third may go on to develop clinical manifestations of late syphilis. These symptoms are usually divided into neurosyphilis and cardiovascular syphilis.

The central nervous system can be affected in different ways: abnormalities in the cerebrospinal fluid without symptoms, syphilitic involvement of other organs such as the aorta, syphilitic meningitis with headache, fever, stiff neck, photophobia, and acute syphilitic hydrocephalus with signs of increased intracranial pressure.

The cardiovascular system can be affected by luetic (syphilitic) aneurysm, aortic valve disease resulting in aortic regurgitation, coronary stenosis or, rarely, myocarditis.

Following the advent of penicillin, *congenital syphilis* experienced a decline. But the incidence began to rise again by 1959. Penicillin appears to be 98% effective in preventing the disease in babies born to treated mothers.[33] However, the incidence of occurrence is much higher in certain populations. The risk for congenital syphilis is high in adolescent mothers, blacks, unmarried primiparae, and those who do not seek prenatal care.

Medical Management

Primary syphilis can be established by the visualization of spirochetes of *T. pallidum* using dark-field microscopy. The spirochete is bluish white, coiled, and has three characteristic movements: watch-spring, corkscrew, and angular. Ideally three separate specimens from the lesion or chancre should be examined initially and on 3 consecutive days.[2] The treponemal test of serum exudate provides a definite diagnosis. Another treponemal test is the direct fluorescent antibody test for *T. pallidum,* or DFATP. This is an alternative to the direct dark-field examination when smears cannot be examined immediately.

Serological tests are divided into nontreponemal or nonspecific and specific treponemal antibody tests. The following are nontreponemal or reagin tests and are reported as a titer: the Veneral Disease Research Laboratory test (VDRL), the Rapid Plasma Reagin Card Test (RPRCT), and the Automated Reagin Test (ART). A VDRL is reactive in 50% to 80% of patients with primary syphilis.[25]

The more sensitive treponemal tests are the Fluorescent Treponemal Antibody-Absorption Test (FTA-ABS) and the Micro-hemagglutination Assay for *T. pallidum* (MHA-TP). The FTA-ABS is reactive in 70% to 90% of patients with primary syphilis.[24]

Syphilis is treated with penicillin 2.4 million U or with tetracycline 500 mg four times a day. Syphilis is curable at any stage of the disease. However, the later it is recognized in its course, the more permanent and nonreversible the damage can be. Permanent and irreversible damage can be avoided in congenital syphilis with an early diagnosis. Proper prenatal screening with the VDRL and the recognition of congenital syphilis at birth can assure quick treatment and avoidance of permanent problems.

Nursing Management

Assessment and Nursing Diagnosis. In order to formulate a plan, the nurse needs to consider several parameters: a thorough nursing and medical history; clinical examination; compilation of appropriate laboratory tests; age of patient; knowledge of disease entity of the patient, partner(s), and family; cultural background of the patient; and the ability of the patient to obtain and carry out the treatment and follow-up. The appropriate nursing diagnoses include knowledge deficit related to the disease and its dissemination, and potential noncompliance with treatment and follow-up monitoring related to knowledge and value conflicts.

This treatment plan will pertain to the patient with syphilis, but the general goals and interventions discussed can be applied to any patient with an infectious or inflammatory disease of the reproductive system.

Goals. The patient will learn prevention of the disease, initially and recurrently; recognize the symptoms of the disease in self and others; obtain knowledge of the pathology of the disease and how it affects the body; understand the treatment for the disease; comply with the treatment and follow-up; and maintain or improve general health and hygiene measures.

Interventions. An important nursing intervention for the management of the patient with syphilis or any other STD is education. The nurse is in a unique position to educate others about the prevention of syphilis or other STD. Nurses are instrumental in community outreach to groups such as Girl Scouts, church groups, parent groups, schools, and family education nights. Many of these organizations are focusing now on educating young people before they become sexually active.

More specifically, teaching focuses on helping young people understand acceptable alternatives to intercourse to express affection. Teaching includes the symptoms of syphilis, normal and abnormal anatomy and physiology, and how the disease is transmitted. This assists the patient in the early recognition of symptoms. The nurse discusses the latency periods of syphilis, emphasizing the serious nature of the disease if it is not treated and the groups who are at high risk. She can emphasize the concept for syphilis and any STD: the young, the homosexual, and those with multiple partners.

The treatment plan needs to be thoroughly explained to the patient and partner(s). The proper way of taking the medication must be discussed. For example, if tetracycline is used, the patient needs to take it on an empty stomach 1 hour before meals or 2 hours after meals, avoiding milk products or antacids.

The long-acting injections such as benzathine penicillin can cause muscle soreness, swelling, and potential bruising. Proper intramuscular injection technique, rotation of sites, heat therapy (sitz baths), and mild exercise are important for patient comfort and to ensure compliance.

The patient needs to be instructed regarding when to resume sexual activity. Most sources agree that 1 week after injection the patient will no longer be infectious, although with tertiary syphilis and a longer oral course of antibiotics the patient could be contagious for a longer period of time.

The importance of compliance with medications and follow-up should be stressed. After diagnosis and initial treatment a follow-up appointment is necessary in 1 to 2 weeks to determine that skin lesions are healing, that there is no secondary infection, and to clear up any questions regarding treatment or follow-up. The follow-up and treatment of sexual contacts could be the responsbility of the nurse with referral to the epidemiological department of the Public Health Department. All contacts within the last 3 to 6 months should be notified. The patient will be instructed as to the need for serological studies to determine the effectiveness of treatment. All patients being treated for syphilis should be followed with nontreponemal tests (VDRL or RPR) at 3, 6, and 12 months after treatment. If the patient has had syphilis for more than 1 year (late latent syphilis) then an additional test at 24 months is recommended.[21] Some feel that all patients treated for syphilis require a minimum 2-year follow-up. Patients with neurosyphilis may require a 3-year period of serological tests every 6 months.[9] If the titer does not become negative or has a fourfold increase after treatment, the possibilities of treatment failure, false-positive test, or reinfection must be considered.

Instruction in general health promotion and hygiene measures is certainly part of the nurse's intervention with this patient. General hygiene issues such as bathing, perineal care (front-to-back wiping), fomite transmission ("toilet-seat" myth), and cleanliness of clothes and environment can be discussed. The issues of increased risk with multiple partners, early initiation of sexual activity, and homosexuality can be discussed. Measures that can decrease the chance of STDs can be discussed such as the use of condoms, vaginal spermicides, foams and jellies, and circumcision in certain high-risk populations. The nurse plays a major role as counselor to the patient as well as educator to the general public, increasing knowledge about the STD patient and influencing patient and public attitudes.

Evaluation. These outcome criteria can be applied to the patient with any inflamatory or infectious disease of the reproductive system.

1. Establishment of primary health promotion programs, such as school programs, Girl and Boy Scout groups, parent groups, church-sponsored groups, local media campaigns, and television and radio spots
2. Continuing education and updates for health-care providers
3. Recognition of symptoms and risks by patients. Early treatment is sought by patients in the early stages of disease, representing a general level of knowledge about the disease entity. Attendance at prenatal screening, clinics, and classes by women at risk for STD, and serological screening of pregnant women results in a reduction in incidence among the general population and neonatal population, thereby reducing the risks of complication.
4. Compliance with treatment. Patients, partners, and family comply with treatment and follow-up appointments; follow-up cultures and serological tests are negative; and there is a reduction in casual and multiple sexual partners, an increased use of condoms, and absence of reinfection.
5. Attitudinal changes. On an individual level, compliance with treatment, acceptance of the disease, and the ability to verbalize concerns to the nurse are positive outcomes. On a general level, positive outcomes are the availability of health care for the indigent; availability of STD clinics; government support for family planning clinics, STD clinics, and prenatal clinics offering screening cultures and serologies; and support for research.

6. General health hygiene. On an individual level, absence of recurrence of infection in patient and partner are positive outcome criteria. On a general level, there are lower rates of infection and complications in a specific clinic or geographical area.

Gonorrhea

Definition

Since ancient times, descriptions of an infectious urethritis have been found in Egyptian, Roman, Greek and Chinese literature. Galen, a physician and prolific writer who lived around 130 AD, first named this syndrome *gonorrhea* (Greek, "flow of seed") believing that the urethral discharge was semen.[16] As previously discussed, gonorrhea and syphilis were felt to be one clinical entity until the 18th–19th century. In 1879, Neisser identified the causative organism, *Neisseria gonorrhoeae.* Today, even with modern antibiotics, gonorrhea is still a significant health problem.

Etiology

The causative agent, *Neisseria gonorrhoeae,* is a gram-negative coccus occurring in pairs; hence, a diplococcus. It is almost always sexually transmitted and infects only humans, infecting the columnar or pseudostratified epithelium of the urogenital tract. Transmission by fomites, that is, the "toilet-seat" myth, is highly unlikely although under ideal conditions, it could occur. Nonsexual close contact may account for a very small number of cases, especially in infants or prepubescent children, but the possibility of sexual abuse should be considered in those cases.

Handsfield reports that the risk of acquiring urethral infection for a man following a single episode of vaginal intercourse with an infected woman is about 20%, and increases to between 60% to 80% after four exposures.[16] The risk of a woman acquiring gonorrhea after a single exposure with an infected man has been reported to be 50%[38] and as high as 90% when uncontrolled for a number of exposures.

There are over 1 million cases of gonorrhea reported annually in the United States, which is equivalent to 443 cases per 100,000 population. It is estimated there are 1 to 1.5 million more cases annually that are not reported. The incidence of gonorrhea is partly dependent on age with 83% of cases in the United States in 1979 occurring in the 15- to 29-year-old group. Race is also a risk factor. In 1979, there were 2,819 cases/100,000 nonwhite men, compared with 240 cases/100,000 white men.[16] Other risk factors are multiple sex partners, low socioeconomic status, and marriage status, with the young single person at highest risk.

Clinical Manifestations

In the adult, mucous membranes lined by nonsquamous epithelium are most susceptible to gonococcal infection. Twenty-four to 48 hours after exposure the organism can be identified between and within epithelial cells.[16] This involvement of the mucosal tissue brings on a rapid polymorphonuclear leukocytic response and formation of exudate. If untreated, the infection can smolder for weeks or months.

In Men. The incubation period for gonorrhea in men usually ranges from 3 to 5 days but symptoms may emerge in as early as 1 day and as late as 2 weeks.[29] In men the organism penetrates the columnar epithelium of the anterior urethra and then enters the submucosa, initiating an inflammatory response. It is this response that causes the symptoms of discharge and dysuria. The infection may remain localized or may extend to the posterior urethra, seminal vesicles, or epididymis causing such problems as strictures, abscesses, and epididymitis. The infection may also disseminate by way of the blood or lymphatic systems causing distant disease such as septicemia or gonococcal arthritis. If untreated, the symptoms may disappear within 2 to 3 weeks but the man may remain infectious and a carrier of the disease.

The initial, most common indication that the inflammatory response is beginning is an uncomfortable sensation along the urethra. This may shortly be followed by some degree of dysuria and a discharge. The dysuria may only be a slight discomfort or may be described as exquisitely painful. The amount and character of the discharge also varies. Typically, it begins as a mucoid discharge that then changes to a yellow or brownish purulent discharge. The amount of discharge ranges from scanty to profuse. On clinical examination the discharge may be obvious, the meatus may be tender and swollen, and the urethra may also be tender and thickened. When the anorectal mucosa is affected, complaints range from mild or absent to rectal itching, bloody or purulent discharge, itching, or pain.[29] Symptoms from a pharyngeal infection range from absent to those common with pharyngitis.

Because the presence of symptoms is variable, with a certain percentage of infected men being asymptomatic, diagnosis is partially dependent on suspicion and a careful sexual history. The man who seeks frequent treatment for these types of symptoms or who relates a sexual history involving multiple sexual partners, birth control methods not involving condoms, and homosexual preferences should be screened carefully. Sexual contact with persons known or suspected to have gonorrhea dictates culture and treatment whether or not symptoms are present.

In Women. It is estimated that up to 80% of women infected with gonorrhea are asymptomatic and 15% of females with gonorrhea who are untreated will go on to develop some clinical signs and symptoms (see Fig. 101–2).[42]

The endocervix is the primary site of infection in women. Other sites include the urethra in 70% to 90% of cases, the periurethral (Skene's) glands and the Bartholin glands 30%, the rectum 35% to 50%, and pharynx 10% to 20%. These percentages are for coexisting endocervical infection and do not represent the sole site of infection. Disseminated gonococcal infection (DGI) can occur in 1% to 3% of patients with gonorrhea. Pelvic inflammatory disease develops in 20% of cases.[15]

The incubation period is not as well defined for women as for men, since the development of symptomatology is so varied. Most women, however, develop symptoms within 2 to

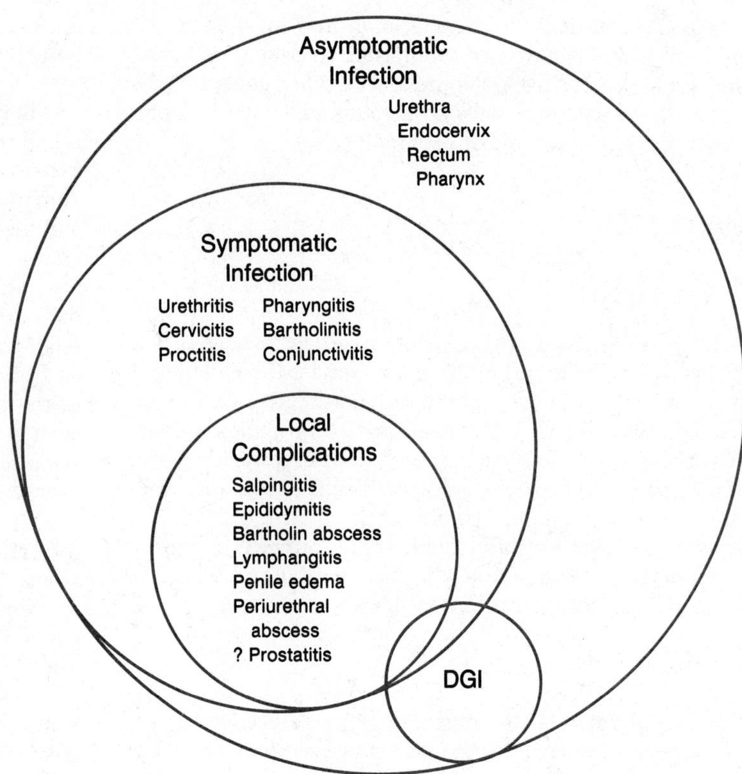

FIGURE 101–2 The clinical spectrum of gonococcal infection. (DGI = disseminated gonococcal infection.) (Holmes KK, March P, Sparling P, Weisner P [eds]: Sexually Transmitted Diseases. New York, McGraw-Hill, 1984)

30 days with an average being 10 days. The most common presenting signs are an increased purulent discharge from the vagina. This may cause concurrent vulvar pruritus; dysuria; and a change in the menstrual pattern and its frequency such as intermenstrual bleeding, menorrhagia, and lower abdominal pain. Bartholin gland involvement can cause labial swelling and pain. Anorectal involvement can cause mucopurulent anal discharge, pruritus, or more severe symptoms such as severe rectal pain, constipation, rectal bleeding, and tenesmus. Gonococcal pharyngitis can present as a sore throat. DGI has a triad of symptoms that present as fever, polyarthritis or tenosynovitis, and skin lesions that may be papular, pustular, or hemorrhagic. Pelvic inflammatory disease will be discussed in a later section of this chapter.

On physical examination, there may be no findings, or a purulent yellow exudate may be found in the endocervical canal. The cervix can be friable and bleed after being touched with a swab. Purulent exudate can also be expressed from the Skene's glands and Bartholin glands if they are affected. Proctoscopic examination can show friability of the rectal mucosa and purulent exudate if anorectal involvement is present. Gonorrheal pharyngitis can cause tonsillitis and cervical lymphadenopathy but more commonly there are no findings.

Medical Management

Diagnosis of gonococcal infection is based on the identification of *N. gonorrhoeae* by microscopy of stained smears or by culture. The Gram stain of exudate is most widely used. The gram stain is considered positive when the kidney-shaped gram-negative diplococci are seen intracellularly or near polymorphonuclear leukocytes. This simple test is both highly sensitive (90% to 95%) and specific (95% to 100%) in men, but not as sensitive in women (50% to 70%).[16] In women, a culture is obtained from the endocervix. If the history and symptoms indicate oral or rectal involvement, cultures should be taken from these sites. Serological tests are also available to detect antibodies to *N. gonorrhoeae*.

Past recommendations have advocated penicillin as the preferred initial treatment for gonorrhea. However, because current evidence shows many men also to be infected with *Chlamydia trachomatis,* which can cause posturethritis in up to two thirds of the cases, most recent recommendations involve 5 days of oral tetracycline hydrochloride four times a day. Patients who are unable to tolerate tetracycline or are unlikely to comply with that regimen maybe given tetracycline in the form of doxycycline twice a day for 5 days or penicillin G procaine intramuscularly plus probenecid orally in the clinic. Following treatment for gonorrhea the patient should return for test of cure within 3 to 7 days after completing treatment. At this time he is evaluated clinically for the presence or absence of symptoms and a culture is taken. If asymptomatic, a Gram stain of the discharge is taken to distinguish between recurrence or persistence of the gonococcal infection or presence of a nongonococcal urethritis. If the intracellular diplococci are seen on the Gram stain, the patient is treated with spectinomycin intramuscularly once. This should eradicate penicillin- or tetracycline-resistant gonococci. If nongonococcal urethritis is diagnosed, the patient is given tetracycline. In cases of probable reinfection, further patient education and counseling are indicated.

Penicillinase-producing *N. gonorrhoeae* (PPNG) was first described in 1976. The PPNG produces an enzyme that makes penicillin ineffective as a treatment.[31,42] This strain is felt to have originated in Southeast Asia and the Philippines. Because of an increase in foreign travel, new PPNG-caused infections are doubling each year and present a specical problem with treatment.[42]

With adequate treatment, the prognosis is generally good for complete recovery from uncomplicated gonorrhea. With complicated gonorrhea or disseminated disease the prognosis is more variable, depending on the speed in seeking treatment, initiation of proper treatment, compliance, and extent of disease. Follow-up cultures are necessary for all patients. If the patient was treated with tetracycline, repeat cultures should be done 4 to 5 days after the last dose, and for other regimens, 3 days after the last dose. Some authors suggest that an anorectal culture should be done in women, since 30% of treatment failures are detected only by the anorectal culture, whether or not it was done prior to treatment.[16]

Nursing Management

Assessment and Nursing Diagnosis. The general plan for care of the patient with gonorrhea is the same as discussed under syphilis and herpes genitalis—knowledge deficit and nonadherence to the treatment protocols. Potential disturbance in self-concept related to the diagnosis and follow-up may be another appropriate nursing diagnosis. The goals for the patient with gonorrhea include recognition of the manifestations of the disease and understanding of the importance of treatment and follow-up.

Interventions. The nursing role in working with patients with gonorrhea is crucial in the areas of prevention, diagnosis, and treatment. Upon initial consultation, the nurse may be the first to suspect the possibility of the existence of this problem and set in motion the process that will confirm it. A careful sexual history, as described earlier, should be taken including names and phone numbers or addresses of sexual contacts within the past 30 days. The nurse should provide information regarding the mode of transmission, signs and symptoms, medical treatment, and possible results (such as nongonococcal urethritis) following treatment. If the patient is considering self-treatment, she should explore his reasons and present information to allay any fears and hopefully persuade him to medical intervention. The nurse should be aware of the laws in her state regarding the necessity for parental notification when treating a minor for gonorrhea. Most states do not require parental consent but the fear of parental involvement may cause the young patient to avoid treatment. Gonorrhea is a disease that must be reported by the professional to the local health department and the reasons (*i.e.,* prevention and follow-up) should be explained to the patient. Depending on the type of treatment, the nurse should be aware of specific precautions and possible reactions of the involved medications and should teach the patient regarding proper administration, side-effects, and the necessity for finishing the course of home antibiotics and ensuring that the patient's partner is treated. Finally, the necessity for follow-up after finishing the treatment to verify a cure should be stressed.

Evaluation. The person with gonorrhea will recognize early manifestations of the infection and participate in the full treatment regimen and follow-up program.

Genital Herpes

Definition

Herpes (Greek, "to creep") has been a medical term for at least 25 centuries. In the 1700s, the term was used to describe conditions that we know today as cold sores and genital herpes. In the 1960s, two types of herpes simplex viruses (HSV) were noted, HSV-1 and HSV-2. It was commonly felt that HSV-1 was an "above-the-belt" infection causing cold sores, and HSV-2 was a 'below-the-belt" infection resulting from sexual transmission. Today it is known that either Type 1 or Type 2 may cause both genital herpes infections or cold sores and can be indistinguishable clinically.

The prevalence of genital herpes infections is not accurately known because clinicians are not required to report this disease to the Public Health Department. Seroepidemiological studies have found the presence of HSV antibodies in most populations of the world.[17,30] Fifty years, ago, 90% of the United States population had been infected with HSV-1 by adulthood. Today, with improved environmental sanitation and understanding of hygiene, only 50% of the population has HSV-1 antibodies by adulthood. This seropositivity is predominant in the lower socioeconomic population and represents both HSV-1 and HSV-2 infections.[10] This means that 50% of the population is fully susceptible to a genital infection when they reach adulthood and begin sexual activity. This tends to put the middle and upper socioeconomic populations at greater risk for genital herpes than the rest of the population.

Etiology

Herpes simplex virus (HSV) is a double-stranded enveloped DNA virus. It is related to several herpes group viruses known to be pathogenic in man. It is an obligate intracellular parasite. The incidence depends on the population in question and varies from 1 HSV infection for 10 gonorrheal infections to 1 HSV infection for every 2.2 gonorrheal infections.[30]

Pathology

Transmission of the virus occurs through contact with a site from which the virus is being shed (*i.e.,* mouth, oropharynx, mucosal surface, penis, vagina) with another susceptible site (all the previous sites plus cervix, conjunctivae, skin lacerations). Thus, it can be transmitted from mother to newborn through vaginal delivery, kissing in early childhood, sexual intercourse, anogenital or oral–genital contact, or autoinoculation such as scratching. The virus is very fragile and is usually killed by drying or being at room temperature. Therefore, fomite spread by towels, toilet seats, or hot tubs is highly unlikely.

The infection is associated with a local tissue necrosis, degeneration of cells, erythema, papules, vesicles, pustules, and leukocytes at the cellular level, followed by a lymphocytic response. Reepithelialization occurs when viral replication is diminished.[10] At the same time, the HSV ascends the peripheral sensory nerves and becomes inactive in the nerve ganglia. In genital infections, the virus is latent in the sacral ganglia and in oral infections, in the trigeminal ganglia. When the host is subjected to stressors such as fatigue, sun, or illness, another outbreak of the infection will occur that is usually milder than the initial outbreak. Latency can also happen after an asymptomatic infection. The reason for this latency is not completely understood.

There are currently two theories to account for reoccurrence. The ganglion-trigger theory suggests that a stimulus causes the virus to travel back down the nerve, causing an outbreak of vesicles on the skin. The second theory, the skin trigger theory, suggests that some virus is already at the skin but is eliminated by host defense mechanisms. Lesions form when the host's defenses do not suppress the virus.

Clinical Manifestations

The severity of the clinical symptoms depends on several factors such as past exposure to HSV-1 and previous episodes of genital herpes. The incubation period is 2 to 20 days with an average of 10 days before lesions occur. Most commonly, the lesions or vesicles first appear bilaterally on the labia and are usually numerous. They can also occur on the cervix 80% to 90% of the time. The lesions cause mild to severe pain, itching, burning with urination, and can be accompanied by a vaginal or urethral discharge and tender inguinal lymphadenopathy. A flulike syndrome accompanies primary herpes in 40% of men and 70% of women. Symptoms such as fever, headache, malaise, photophobia, leg ache and backache, and myalgias are common. They occur 3 to 4 days after the lesions appear. In severe cases, there can be hyperesthesias, paresthesias, or anesthesias of the perineum and back that can result in difficulty in urination and constipation.

Lesions are most painful between days 7 and 11 and then begin to subside in the second week, disappearing usually in 21 days. The patient is considered contagious until the lesions have healed.

Recurrent infections usually recur within 9 months with an average of five per year. The lesions are usually unilateral or in a cluster and there is no viremia and little adenopathy. Many patients report a prodrome of a tingling sensation at the genital site at which they subsequently develop vesicles.

Medical Management

Herpes can often be accurately diagnosed by the history and clinical picture. The ulcer is painful, which usually can differentiate it from syphilis. These two organisms can coexist, however.

A culture of cells from a lesion will offer a definitive diagnosis. Blood drawn from patients infected with HSV-1 or HSV-2 will show an elevated antibody titer for HSV. This can be inconclusive because there are different assays and they do not distinguish between HSV-1 and HSV-2. It could show the presence of a past infection but not an acute one.

The goals of treatment are decreasing a secondary infection, shortening the clinical course of the disease with attendant viral shedding and possible complications, decreasing pain, and preventing autoinfection such as HSV infection of the eye. Healing can be promoted by keeping the perineal area clean and dry. A hair dryer can be used to dry the perineum. Comfort can be promoted with sitz baths in tepid water two or three times per day. Domeboro's solution or Epsom salts applied as wet-to-dry compresses to promote drying and crusting are also appropriate. Creams, ointments, and bath powders that could prolong healing and be painful to clean should be avoided. The patient may need to urinate by holding the labia apart or even may need to urinate in bathtub filled with tepid water to avoid dysuria. The local application of ice or oral analgesics such as aspirin every 3 to 4 hours will help alleviate the discomfort. Betadine can be used as a topical antibacterial to prevent superinfection, but there have been no well-controlled studies at this time. Americaine spray and aloe vera have also been used. Acyclovir (Zovirax) ointment has been approved by the Food and Drug Administration (FDA) for use in primary genital infections. Five-percent ointment in polyethylene glycol can be applied directly to the lesions four to six times every day. This results in a decrease in the signs and symptoms of initial infection, decreased viral shedding, time for crusting and healing of lesions, and a decrease in the severity of pain and itching (see Table 101–1).

Intravenous acyclovir is approved for the treatment of primary genital herpes, 5 mg/kg/dose every 8 hours for 5 days. Intravenous therapy has the same results as topical acyclovir with the added benefit of a decreased development of new lesions after 48 hours on therapy.[30]

Acyclovir is now available for oral use as a 200-mg capsule. This preparation has been shown in double-blind placebo-controlled studies to shorten the total duration and severity of clinical symptoms (pain, adenopathy, dysuria, and malaise) and to reduce viral shedding, new lesion formation after 48 hours, and the duration of genital lesions in men and women.[7,39]

Side-effects and adverse reactions are minor and infrequent. It is suggested that patients avoid dehydration, which could cause crystallization of the drug in the kidneys.

The prognosis for patients with herpes genitalis is generally good. Although the primary infection can be very painful, recurrent infections are of much less severity and of shorter duration. Some patients never experience recurrences, some recurrences tend to be less frequent over time, and others experience recurrences on an average of five per year. Complications can occur but are rare, such as extragenital lesions (*e.g.* on buttocks or fingers, keratoconjunctivitis), aseptic meningitis, and neurological complications such as urinary retention, cervical dysplasias, neonatal infection, and psychological stress.

TABLE 101–1
Results of Controlled Therapeutic Trials of Antiviral Agents in Mucocutaneous HSV Infections in Immunocompetent Patients

Compound	*Type of HSV Infection*	*Dose and Route of Administration*	*Result*
Acyclovir	Genital	5% ointment in polyethylene glycol (PEG) 4–6 times daily	Shortened symptoms and signs of initial infection; decreased viral shedding in recurrent infections
		5 mg/kg IV every 8 hours	Shortened symptoms and signs of severe primary herpes
	Recurrent oral–labial	5% ointment in PEG 4 times daily	Decreased viral titer; no clinical effect
Ara-A (vidarabine)	Genital and oral	3% cream	Ineffective in primary or recurrent genital infection
Ara-AMP	Recurrent oral	10% cream	Ineffective
2-Deoxy-D-glucose	Genital	0.19% gel in 2% miconazole nitrate cream	Questionable
IUdR	Oral and genital	0.1–1% cream	Ineffective
	Oral and genital	5% and 20% solution in dimethyl sulfoxide (DMSO) 3 times daily	Shortens viral shedding and lesions
	Genital	30% solution in DMSO 4 times daily	Reduced viral shedding; no clinical effect; toxic
L-Lysine	Oral	500 mg twice daily orally	Ineffective in shortening course or reducing frequency of recurrences
Ribavarin	Genital	800 mg/day orally	Reduction in disease severity (?)
Phosphonoformate	Oral–labial	3% cream 6 times daily for 4 days	Shortened time of papular and vesicular stages of disease

(Adapted from Holmes KK: Lower genital tract infections in women: Cystitis/urethritis, vulvovaginitis, and cervicitis. In Holmes KK, Mardh P, Sparling PF, Wiesner PJ (eds): Sexually Transmitted Diseases, pp 557–589. New York, McGraw-Hill, 1984)

Nursing Management

Assessment and Nursing Diagnosis. As with other disease problems, the nursing management plan is formulated by considering several parameters, including the nursing history, clinical examination, appropriate laboratory tests and cultures, age of the patient, knowledge level of the patient, partner(s), and family, and the general health of the patient. The nursing management plan for the patient with genital ulcers from herpes genitalis follows the same general guidelines as for any patient with an STD. (See the management plan discussed earlier under syphilis.) The appropriate nursing diagnoses for the patient with herpes genitalis include knowledge deficit related to the recurrence and dissemintion of herpes, and potential noncompliance related to the social values and knowledge conflicts. The following pertains more specifically to herpes genitalis.

Goals. The patient will prevent the disease, initially and recurrently; recognize the symptoms and pathology of herpes genitalis; understand the importance of complying with treatment and follow-up; and maintain or improve general health and hygiene measures.

Interventions. Early education about the importance of good hygiene is appropriate. Sufficient rest, good diet, exercise, bathing, and perineal hygiene help prevent infection. The use of a condom in theory should cut down on viral spread. Abstinence during active genital lesions should be encouraged. Orogenital contact in the presence of oral lesions should be discouraged.

When an uninfected partner is pregnant or when a pregnant woman has had herpes genitalis, couples should use a condom. The importance of consistent prenatal care for the woman with herpes is extremely important. Neonatal infection is extremely serious. Primary infections in the mother result in increased spontaneous abortion, premature birth, stillborn, or if the neonate is born with the disease the death rate can be as high as 70%, and 50% of the suvivors may have neurological or ocular sequelae. The importance of viral cultures during pregnancy can avoid devastating sequelae to the infant by appropriately timed cesarean sections.

Early recognition of disease can decrease the time of infection and discomfort by using acyclovir and other palliative measures. Recognition of symptoms can assist in avoidance of sexual contact with an infected partner. Knowledge of the disease can promote more compliance with treatment. The relationship of early sexual activity and multiple partners with an increased incidence of STD and cervical cancer should be made known to the patient.

The nurse can teach the patient about the use of acyclovir and other measures. Patient compliance with treatment and follow-up help prevent complications of the disease as well as prenatal disease. Women with HSV have an increase in cervical abnormalities. There is a strong association between cervical cancer and HSV.

The nurse is a major educator of the patient with herpes or with the risk for HSV. She is particularly appropriate to deal with problems of anger, guilt, and depression or even potential suicide that can accompany the patient with herpes. Through education, the nurse can allay many fears and can reassure the patient of his ability to cope with this disease. The nurse could direct the patient to self-help groups or national agencies that have a wealth of information, pamphlets, and newsletters. One such agency is HELP (Herpetics Engaged in Living Productively), 260 Sheridan Avenue, Palo Alto, CA 94306. When appropriate, the nurse could refer the patient for mental health counseling.

Evaluation. Evaluation of the patient with herpes will include:

- Establishing early education programs about herpes genitalis
- Using condoms and spermicides by sexually active patients and pregnant women to prevent new disease
- Participating in STD clinics
- Decreasing early sexual activity or multiple partners
- Decreasing length of time of infection and neonatal infection
- Decreasing complications due to neurological involvement or self-inoculation (*e.g.*, eye infections, herpetic whitlow)
- Decreasing loss of work or school time from HSV infection
- Decreasing psychosexual problems in patients with HSV

Genital Warts (Condyloma Acuminatum)

Definition

Genital warts are considered a sexually transmitted disease. Historically, they were confused with the condyloma lata of syphilis. Genital warts are found generally among young sexually active men and women.

Because genital warts are currently not required to be reported, an accurate picture of the prevalence of this disease can only be estimated. It is generally accepted that the number of cases has been increasing.[1,28]

Condyloma acuminatum is a DNA-containing virus, belonging to the papilloma species of which there are 12 immunotypes. When an epithelial cell is infected with a papillomavirus, the cell undergoes a change. These transformed cells grow and eventually a wart develops. These cells shed the virus and new skin cells are infected, which continues the process. The virus often coexists with other STDs. Infants and young children can develop laryngeal papillomas that are transmitted by an infected mother during vaginal delivery. Genital warts can proliferate during pregnancy and resolve spontaneously without treatment. The rate at which the sexual partner of an infected patient procures the disease is close to 60%. It has a long incubation period, which can range from 2 weeks to 8 months with a 3-month average.

Clinical Manifestations

In females warts can develop first at the posterior introitus and contiguous labia. They can also spread to the vagina, cervix, vulva, perineum, urethra, and anus. In males they can be anywhere on the penis or in the urethra.

They appear as fleshy, raised masses that can be small and spiked or flat, or they can coalesce into cauliflower-shaped masses that can cover the penis or perineum. On the cervix, the wart may be flat and almost impossible to discern with the naked eye. Genital warts proliferate in a warm, moist environment and often coexist with other STDs or vaginitis. Warts are not painful but may cause some mild itching.

Medical Management

This species of human papillomavirus has not been propagated in the laboratory. Diagnosis is made by inspection of the lesions. A differential diagnosis must include condyloma lata of syphilis, sebaceous cysts, molluscum contagiosum, granuloma inguinale, benign neoplasms (*e.g.*, vulvar adenomas, endometriomas, fibromas, and lipomas), and cervical or penile carcinoma.[28]

Treatment of genital warts can be long, time-consuming, and frustrating to the patient and clinician. During pregnancy and in immunocompromised patients, genital warts can proliferate quickly and may be unresponsive to treatment.

Generally, for external warts 10% to 25% podophyllin in a compound of tincture of benzoin is applied to the wart, avoiding normal skin. This application can sting for several seconds if it comes in contact with normal tissue. This is repeated every 7 to 10 days for 3 to 4 weeks. The patient is instructed to leave it on for 4 to 6 hours unless it begins to burn and then wash it off with soap and water. Podophyllin is not without risks. There has been documented systemic toxicity such as neuropathy, coma, hepatotoxicity, and even death associated with its use. Fetal death has been described when podophyllin is applied during pregnancy. Podophyllin is known to have an oncogenic effect and is therefore contraindicated during pregnancy.

For more than a single or a few warts in the vaginal, cervical, urethral, and rectal areas other methods should be used. Fluorouracil (5-FU) has been successfully used as well as cryotherapy, electrocautery, and surgical removal.

Prognosis varies depending on the extent of the lesion, the compliance of the patient and partner, and the present condition of the patient (*e.g.*, pregnant, immunosuppressed). Genital warts tend to recur.

Nursing Management

Assessment and Nursing Diagnosis. The analysis of assessment data, goals, and interventions include the same information as previously mentioned under the earlier sections on syphilis and herpes genitalis. The appropriate nursing diagnoses for genital warts include potential body disturbance related to wart growth, knowledge deficit related to transmission and recurrence of warts, and potential health maintenance alteration related to possible infections and neoplastic changes.

Goals. The specific goal for this disease entity is that the patient will understand the prevention of transmission, that is, condom use.

Interventions. Recurrence is one of the most frustrating aspects of this disease. It takes a long time to treat and can easily reoccur. Patient compliance is necessary for success. Understanding the treatment, specifically how long to leave the podophyllin on, can help eliminate severe local irritation and burning.

Women should have other tests to rule out other concurrent infections such as *Candida albicans, Trichomonas vaginalis, Neisseria gonorrhoeae, Gardnerella vaginalis,* and *Chlamydia trachomatis.* Men should have other tests to rule out gonorrhea and nongonococcal urethritis. Homosexuals may need proctoscopy to rule out additional warts or gonorrhea. Both men and women ideally should have serological screening for syphilis.

The association between human papillomavirus infection and carcinoma of the cervix has been made. Though absolute confirmation is currently lacking, there is a strong link. The importance of yearly Pap smears and appropriate colposcopy is an area where nursing intervention and education can play an important role.

Evaluation. The patient will demonstrate understanding of the hygiene factors related to the transmission of genital warts and will understand the importance of follow-up care.

Phthirus pubis (Pubic Louse) and Scabies

Definition

Three of the species of lice can infest man: *Phthirus pubis,* the crab louse; *Pediculus humanus corporis,* the body louse; and *Pediculus humanus capitis,* the head louse. *Phthirus pubis* (pediculosis pubis, or crabs) is the cause of a common STD affecting the genital area. The cause of human scabies is a mite, *Sarcoptes scabiei.*

Pediculosis pubis and scabies are considered to be STDs, affecting adults mainly between the ages of 15 and 25. Infestations of pediculosis pubis are unusual after the age of 35. They are spread by sexual contact or close genital contact. There are, however, cases reported where infestation was acquired by toilet seats, bed linens, and clothing. Using sales figures of pediculicides, it is estimated that more than 3 million cases of pediculosis pubis are treated each year in the United States.[6] Epidemics have occurred historically in times of war, famine, and other conditions of an unsanitary environment.

Etiology

Phthirus pubis is small (1 mm to 3 mm long), round, and has three sets of legs. This blood sucking louse can grasp hair with its claws, has a wide abdomen resembling a crab under microscopy, and hence derives its popluar name "crabs." Because this louse's claws are uniquely suited to the size of hair found in the pubic area (also, groin and thighs) it is usually found there, but it can occasionally be found on the abdomen, eyebrows, and eyelashes.

The adult female lays eggs (nits) at the base of hairs and they hatch in about 7 days. The louse is dependent on human blood and regularly sucks blood from its host for survival.

The scabies mite has a rounded body, four pairs of legs, and resembles a turtle under microscopy. It burrows under the skin, laying eggs in rows that hatch and form adult mites in 10 days. The cycle is then repeated.

Clinical Manifestations

Although some patients are asymptomatic, a varying degree of sensitivity to the louse bite occurs in the individual. There may be no symptoms for 5 days at which time itching may begin accompanied by scratching, irritation, and inflammation. Occasionally fever and malaise can occur.

Immunity to the louse can occur in individuals who have been infested over long periods of time. The skin can become hard and darkly pigmented. This is known as "Vagabond's disease."

In the early stages of louse infestation there may be no clinical manifestations. The patient may complain of pubic and genital itching without any apparent cause. With a light and hand glass, the shiny, oval nits can be seen attached to the hair follicle. A small, flat fleck sometimes appearing as scabies can be the louse itself. "Blue spots" can appear in the skin as a result of the crab louse bites. There can also be superinfection from scratching.

The most outstanding symptom of scabies is intense itching, usually worse at night. The lesion is a tiny blood-tipped papule that is difficult to see. If present, the burrow is diagnostic. It appears as a thin, gray line ranging from 2 mm to 15 mm long. They are more commonly absent. The distribution of the papular pruritic rash is very important in the diagnosis. The webs and sides of fingers and toes, the anterior wrist, axillae, waist, periumbilical areas, genitalia, buttocks, and backs of knees are most commonly affected.[11,36]

Medical Management

A diagnosis is made from the patient's history of itching or sexual contact with someone with diagnosed pediculosis pubis. Definitive diagnosis is made by identification of the louse or nits under the microscope.

Treatment involves the use of a pediculicide that will kill both the adults and eggs. There are several prescription and nonprescription medications that are effective.

Some nonprescription pediculicides are RID (liquid and shampoo) and Triple-X (liquid and shampoo), containing 0.3% pyrethrins and 3.0% piperonyl butoxide. Usually a single application is enough to kill both adult lice and eggs.

Prescription medication is most commonly lindane (Kwell or Scabene), a gamma benzene hexachloride in 1% lotion as cream or shampoo. Usually 1 oz is enough for an adult. After showering, the lindane is carefully applied to affected hairy areas and left on 8 hours and then showered off. Some suggest repeating the entire process of showering, application of lindane, waiting 8 hours, and then showering again. Others suggest shampooing the lindane into affected areas and then rinsing off and drying. A single application is usually enough. Lindane is known to be a central nervous system toxin and severe reactions have occurred from its use. If the patient has extremely excoriated skin, is pregnant, or is a young child, an alternative is generally suggested. Some of these alternatives would be 6% sulfur in petrolatum, a 5% to 10% thiobendazole cream, or 10% crotamiton cream or lotion (Eurax). Reexamination is necessary after 7 days, and retreatment may be necessary if lice or eggs are observed.

All linens and clothing with which the patient has had contact for the last 2 days should be laundered in hot water. All sexual or intimate contacts should be treated. Blankets, furniture, and carpets can be sprayed with insecticides. These are not for human use. Storage of blankets, coats, and other articles for 2 weeks is usually adequate to destroy the lice because they cannot survive away from the host for longer than 10 days.

Treatment is 100% effective if done correctly. The patient may experience itching for several weeks after treatment. This is due to an allergic reaction to the nits and the bites. A topical antipruritic or anti-inflammatory cream can help. However, reinfection is a possibility and the importance of follow-up is pivotal to the success of treatment.

A diagnosis of scabies is made by a suggestive history consisting of intense itching and recent sexual contact, the distribution of the pruritic rash, and the presence of burrows. Absolute diagnosis is made by finding the mite or its eggs in the burrows or papules by taking skin scrapings and examining them under microscopy.

The treatment is the same as for pediculosis pubis except that the medication is applied from chin to toes. The prognosis is 100% cure if the treatment regimen is followed.

Nursing Management

Assessment and Nursing Diagnosis. The plan is similar to the plans previously discussed under syphilis and herpes genitalis. Nursing diagnoses include body image disturbance related to the social stigma of the diagnosis, and knowledge deficit related to the hygiene measures and the importance of treatment and follow-up.

Interventions. The general goals for the patient with lice or scabies include prevention of disease, recognition of symptoms, understanding treatment and importance of compliance and follow-up, and general health hygiene measures.

The nurse can be instrumental in the successful treatment of the patient with pediculosis pubis. Extreme tact and sensitivity in the approach and explanation of the disease and its treatment will help allay the anxiety that a patient may feel about this disease. Many patients feel "unclean" and are horrified by the diagnosis. The nurse can help ensure compliance and follow-up by establishing good rapport with the patient and contacts and encouraging communication.

Evaluation. The patient will demonstrate understanding of the diagnosis and symptoms, the treatment, and compliance with therapies. Additionally, the patient will demonstrate general health hygiene measures and will participate in follow-up care.

Chlamydial Infection

Definition

In the last 10 years, *Chlamydia trachomatis* has been recognized as causing increasing numbers of infections of the male and female genitourinary system. This organism has been shown to be possibly causing more cervicitis than *Neisseria gonorrhoeae* or herpes genitalis. A review of the family planning population in California has shown a five to seven times greater frequency for chlamydial infections than gonorrhea, where the incidence is 1% for gonorrhea and 9% for chlamydia.[44]

Etiology

Chlamydia trachomatis is an intracellular bacteria. Infection occurs when the *C. trachomatis* organisms attach to specific susceptible host cells and are ingested into the cell by phagocytosis. This occurs in 48 hours. The host cell bursts and releases more infectious particles, and the cycle starts over. The organism is transmitted sexually.[44]

The organism can infect different anatomical sites in the female genital tract causing bartholinitis, cervicitis, endometritis, acute urethral syndrome, acute salpingitis, and acute perihepatitis (Fitz-Hugh–Curtis syndrome). It can also infect newborn infants delivered vaginally, causing a conjunctivitis or a chlamydial pneumonia. The most common anatomical site in the female is the cervix.

Clinical Manifestations

Women may experience quite minor to no symptoms when infected with chlamydia. The distinctive mucopurulent cervicitis of chlamydia infection may be missed by a clinician.

There has not been a standard nomenclature for cervicitis and this leads to confusing terminology for infection. Also, there has not been a readily available and inexpensive culture for *Chlamydia,* necessitating clinicians to rely on history, symptoms, and clinical findings for a diagnosis.

The clinical manifestations of a chlamydial cervicitis may range from no symptoms to the classic symptoms of discharge, dysuria, urinary frequency, soreness, and postcoital bleeding. The male partner classically had urethral discharge and dysuria. The cervix can appear beefy red, friable to the touch (bleeds easily), and has a thick, yellow discharge from the endocervical canal.

Other special diagnostic procedures can be used to identify *Chlamydia.* These include endocervical Gram stain, cytopathology (Pap smear), colposcopy, cervical biopsy, and microbiological studies and cultures.

Medical Management

The Center for Disease Control (CDC) recommends tetracycline hydrochloride 500 mg orally four times a day for at least 7 days, with a range of 7 to 14 days, or doxycycline 100 mg twice a day for 7 days. If tetracycline cannot be used, erythromycin 500 mg four times a day for 7 days or sulfisoxazole 2 g daily for 10 to 14 days is also effective.[8]

The prognosis and recovery from chlamydial cervicitis is generally good. However, if treatment has been delayed and the infection has been allowed to smolder in the fallopian tubes, severe consequences can occur. These will be discussed more completely in the section to come covering pelvic infections.

Nursing Management

Assessment and Nursing Diagnosis. As previously discussed with other infections of the reproductive system, the nursing diagnoses for *Chlamydia* infection include recognition of the manifestations of the infection and understanding and complying with the treatment and follow-up.

Interventions. As with other STDs, other infections can coexist with *Chlamydia.* Most commonly gonorrheal and chlamydial infections can coexist in up to 60% of women.[44] This is why a tetracycline preparation is often used with a cervical infection because it is effective against both organisms.

The nurse needs to educate the patient on the importance of compliance with treatment, treatment of sexual partners, and follow-up cultures and examination.

As with all STDs, teaching the importance of the use of the condom in prevention and the risk of multiple sex partners should be part of all counseling.

Evaluation. The patient with *Chlamydia* infection will recognize the signs and symptoms of the infection, relate an understanding of the progress and dissemination of the infection, and participate in the treatment and follow-up program.

Female Genital Infections

One of the most common complaints of postpubertal female patients is vaginal discharge. Vaginal discharge can be caused by a number of different organisms and can be accompanied by symptoms such as odor, itching, or burning. However, a certain amount of discharge is normal for a woman. The nurse can educate the patient about normal discharge and cyclic variations of normal.

Bacterial Vaginitis

Definition

There is currently much controversy and ongoing research regarding the cause of bacterial vaginitis. Gardner and Dukes in 1955 documented the association between a small gram-negative bacillus that they called *Haemophilus vaginalis* and abnormal vaginal discharge in women who formerly would have been diagnosed as having "nonspecific vaginitis."[27] *Haemophilus vaginalis* was reclassified as *Corynebacterium vaginale* in 1963 because of its characteristics, which differed from *Haemophilus* classifications. In 1980 this organism was reclassified as *Gardnerella vaginalis,* a new genus, because it did not completely fit the prior classification. Most recent literature suggests that this disease is a result of the interaction between *G. vaginalis* and anaerobic microflora. Most recently an anaerobic motile curved rod has been identified in 14% of patients with *Gardnerella* vaginitis.[27]

Epidemiological studies are incomplete at this time. Up to 50% to 68% of sexually active women are infected with *G. vaginalis* at one time, but not all are symptomatic.[27] It has been found in the urethra of men, virginal women, and prepubertal girls. Although it is uncertain whether the disease is endogenous or sexually transmitted, it is generally considered a disease of sexually active women.[27]

Nonspecific vaginitis is a common problem causing an increased vaginal discharge with some itching or irritation. There can be an unpleasant odor. It is caused by bacteria that normally do not inhabit the vagina or an increased prevalence of bacteria that are normally there. A wet-slide mount is made of the vaginal secretions including a potassium hydroxide (KOH) preparation. If there is no evidence of a specific infection such as yeast, *Trichomonas,* or *Gardnerella,* then nonspecific vaginitis or vaginitis of unknown etiology is the diagnosis.

Etiology

Gardnerella is a nonmotile, nonencapsulated gram-negative to gram-variable rod. This organism causes an abnormality in vaginal secretions and rarely produces an inflammatory change of the vaginal walls; hence, the term *vaginosis.*

Clinical Manifestations

The vaginal secretions become gray, homogeneous, thin, "fishy" in odor, and normal to increased in amount. The odor may be more offensive after intercourse or during menstruation. The characteristic odor occurs because of the elevated pH (greater than 4.5) that releases amines from the anaerobic organisms. There is rarely pruritus with *Gardnerella* vaginitis, although is is not uncommon in nonspecific vaginitis.

Medical Management

Diagnosis is usually based on clinical examination and microscopy. The characteristic gray homogeneous odoriferous discharge is suggestive of *Gardnerella*-associated vaginosis. A wet mount of the secretions of a slide would show very few white blood cells, vaginal epithelial cells, and the "clue cell," which is a vaginal epithelial cell that is coated with coccobacilli, so that the cell margins become obscured. Adding a drop of 10% KOH solution to these secretions results in a release of amine or fishy odor that results from the pH of 5.0–5.5 and the presence of anaerobic organisms associated with the condition. This is called a positive sniff test, a positive KOH, or a positive amine test.

The use of a Gram stain in addition to the wet mount adds reliability. Vaginal secretions can also be cultured for confirmation. But most experienced clinicians can diagnose this disease based on clinical examination and the wet mount and KOH test, and approach 80% to 90% accuracy.

The treatment of choice is oral metronidazole (Flagyl). It is given 500 mg twice a day for 7 days and has a cure rate approaching 90% after 1 week. Ampicillin can be used 500 mg four times a day for 7 days but is usually only 50% effective. There is some variability as to the treatment of the partner. Usually, in a new diagnosis the partner would not be treated. He is instructed to abstain or wear a condom. In recurrent cases, he would be treated. Because there is evidence that metronidazole is carcinogenic in rodents and mutagenic in bacteria, it is contraindicated for pregnant women. If *G. vaginalis* is identified in an asymptomatic woman, there are differing opinions as to whether she should be treated with metronidazole because it is potentially harmful and also expensive. An alternative treatment could be boric acid vaginal suppositories. These can be made by the patient by filling a size 0 gelatin capsule with boric acid powder and inserting in the vagina at night for 1 to 2 weeks. The capsule melts and disperses the boric acid, which theoretically brings the vaginal pH down to normal range (<4.5). This brings the prevalence and concentration of the *G. vaginalis* and the anaerobic bacteria down to normal range, thereby eliminating symptoms. This latter regimen has the advantage of being cheap and available without a prescription.

The prognosis is generally good with treatment. Some women are plagued with recurrences. Intravaginal tetracycline 100 mg to 200 mg twice a day for 7 days can be used. The metronidazole can be increased to 1 g twice a day for 7 days. This can be a frustrating situation for the patient and the clinician.

Treatment for nonspecific vaginitis varies considerably. Some feel that this condition should not be treated if a causative organism cannot be identified. Others treat it with a prescription of vaginal creams or suppositories that are expensive and of questionable value. Boric acid suppositories that can be made by the patient offer symptomatic relief and sometimes can eliminate the symptoms altogether (see previous section on *Gardnerella vaginalis*). The patient is reexamined in 1 to 2 weeks if still symptomatic.

Nursing Management

Assessment and Nursing Diagnosis. The management plan follows the same general guidelines as previously discussed under syphilis and herpes genitalis. Nursing diagnoses for vaginitis include alteration in comfort related to vaginitis symptoms, and knowledge deficit regarding diagnosis, treatment, and follow-up care.

Goals. Specifically, the goals for the patient include understanding that prevention measures as well as the importance of compliance with treatment are necessary for the successful resolution of this common problem.

Interventions. The primary nursing interventions for vaginitis relate to teaching appropriate hygiene, encouraging compliance with treatment, and emphasizing the importance of follow-up care. Use of condoms or abstinence during treatment is important. Avoiding alcohol during treatment is necessary when taking metronidazole because alcohol and the drug can cause an antabuselike effect, that is, nausea and vomiting.

Evaluation. The patient will demonstrate an understanding of the importance of compliance with treatment through adherence to the therapies, modifying hygiene practices, and participating in follow-up care.

Trichomonas vaginalis

Definition

Trichomoniasis is a common sexually transmitted vaginal infection. Approximately 80% of women who are sex partners of infected men are found to be infected with *Trichomonas vaginalis,* whereas the incidence is much lower in men, especially after a 2-week period.[40] Some American investigators report symptoms in male partners of affected females to be uncommon, but European investigators report it to be a common cause of urethritis in men. The presence of *T. vaginalis* in adult female virgins is almost 0%, whereas in a prostitute population it can be as high as 75%.[40]

Etiology

The cause is a flagellated protozoan, *Trichomonas vaginalis,* which is one of three *Trichomonas* strains that parasitize humans. *T. vaginalis* is pear-shaped or ovoid with three to five flagella. Many investigators feel that various strains of *T. vaginalis* exist.[40]

Although the *Trichomonas* organism dries easily outside the body, it has been recovered from wet clothes, sponges, and toilet bowls. This nonvenereal mode of transmission is uncommon, but it is possible. Careful hygiene techniques would be helpful to eliminate fomite transmission.

Although *T. Vaginalis* has been recovered from sites such as the endocervix and fallopian tubes, it mainly affects the squamous epithelium that covers the vagina, the urethra, and Skene's glands.

Clinical Manifestation

Clinically women with *T. vaginalis* complain of an increased vaginal discharge and vulvar itching, and can have dysuria. Up to 40% of women with infections may have no complaints.[40]

During the speculum examination, the discharge can appear normal to copious in amount, homogenous in viscosity, and classically has a foamy, bubbly characteristic. The classic "strawberry" cervix caused by small hemorrhages is present in approximately 5% of all cases.

Medical Management

The diagnosis is made by visualizing the motile trichomonads on the wet-slide mount prepared from the vaginal secretions. The wet mount is prepared by mixing a drop of normal saline with a swab of vaginal secretion on a glass slide, covered with a cover slip, and examined with a microscope under 100 to 400 power. Trichomonads appear teardrop- or pear-shaped, slightly larger than a white blood cell, and have a jerky, persistent motion as they are propelled by their flagella. There is usually an increase in white blood cells on the wet mount, and there can be a mild amine odor released on the KOH preparation. Concurrent with *T. vaginalis,* there can be *Candida albicans* or *Gardnerella vaginalis.* In approximately 25% of cases, the trichomonad cannot be identified on the wet mount. There are selective culture media that can be used such as Trichosel. Trichomonads can also be see on Pap smears. It can be difficult to obtain a culture or wet mount from a male patient.

Metronidazole (Flagyl) is the treatment of choice for *T. vaginalis.* Generally 2 g is given orally in a single dose or in a divided dose of 1 g twice a day. This has been found to be very effective and ensures patient compliance. The disadvantages of this regimen are the increased frequency of nausea and other gastrointestinal reactions, occasional dark urine and, in high doses, neurotoxicity. The sexual partner is also treated whether symptomatic or not. Approximately 5% to 10% of cases fail treatment. In these cases, the treatment can be repeated or a course of 250 mg twice or three times a day for 5 to 7 days can be tried. There have been reported cases of metronidazole-resistant strains that may require high doses or intravenous doses.

Nursing Management

Assessment and Nursing Diagnosis. As with previous disorders, there are many general parameters that must be assessed. The nursing diagnoses for the patient with *T. vaginalis* include alteration in comfort related to the pain and itching of the perineal area, and knowledge deficit related to the importance of treatment and follow-up for self and partner.

Goals. The goals are the same as for syphilis and other STDs with particular emphasis on patient education so that the patient will understand the disease, recognize the symptoms, and comply with treatment and follow-up.

Interventions. Nursing interventions follow the general guidelines previously discussed for STDs. Education emphasizes prevention, one sexual partner, use of condoms, and recognition of symptoms of the the disease. During treatment, education would emphasize abstinence or the use of condoms, taking the metronidazole properly for both the patient and the partner, and avoiding alcohol for 24 hours after the last dose. Follow-up examinations are important to ensure a cure.

Evaluation. The patient will demonstrate understanding of the disease through early recognition of symptoms, compliance with treatment, and participation in follow-up care.

Candida albicans

Definition

Vaginal fungi are considered normal vaginal commensals that exist as well in the mouth and large intestine. The fungi most frequently found in the vagina are *Candida albicans* and *Torulopsis glabrata. Candida albicans,* an airborne gram-positive fungus, is responsible for approximately 80% to 95% of fungal vaginitis, whereas *T. glabrata* accounts for 3% to 16%. There are other Candida species that also have been cultured from patients with vulvovaginitis.[27]

Etiology

Candida species are considered normal inhabitants of the mouth, large intestine, and vagina. Different researchers have isolated *C. albicans* in the vaginas of up to 50% of asymptomatic sexually active females.[26, 27] Because the presence of fungus is poorly correlated with disease, *C. albicans* is considered a commensal. There is a high proportion of women with vaginal *Candida* who also have the same species in the rectum and urine.

The role of sexual transmission of vaginal fungal infections is not clear. Holmes reports that 80% of female contacts of infected men (usually having balanitis, an inflammation of the glans penis or posthitis, an inflammation of the prepuce) are carriers, whereas yeasts are isolated from 32% of women whose sexual partners are negative.[18] The prevalence of vaginal candidiasis is poorly documented but some researchers note an approximately fourfold increase from 1944 to 1976.[14]

There are other factors that correlate positively with vaginal candidiasis. There is a higher incidence of STD during the summer months. This may be due to increased perspiration, higher perineal temperatures, and increased sexual activity.[18] Other factors are pregnancy, immunosuppressive drug therapy, corticosteroids, debilitation, or other conditions that cause a compromised host.

Courses of antibiotics that affect the acid pH of the vagina or decrease the lactobacilli levels can predispose a woman to vaginal candidiasis. Penicillins, cephalosporins, and tetracyclines are much more likely to change the normal vaginal environment than erythromycin, sulfonamides, and metronidazole. In women receiving antibiotics that can predispose them to vaginal candidiasis, antifungal medications could be prescribed concurrently.

Other factors affecting the vaginal environment are oral contraceptive use, menstruation, vaginal deodorants and powders, perfumed soaps, bubble baths, wearing tight-fitting jeans or nylons, autoinfection from the bowel after a bowel movement, iron-deficiency anemia, orogenital contact, and vaginal abrasions following sexual intercourse.

Clinical Manifestations

Vaginal candidiasis presents as vulvovaginitis with the most striking characteristic being vulvar pruritis (itching). There can be marked vulvar, vaginal, and cervical erythema and edema. Vaginal discharge can be present or absent. Classically it is described as a curdy-white or cottage cheese–appearing discharge, but it can also appear very normal. There can be external dysuria and dyspareunia (painful intercourse). The perineum can have excoriations, linear fissures, or a pustular-papular dermatitis.

Medical Management

The wet mount preparation is widely used to identify the presence of fungus in the vaginal exudate. The sensitivity of the KOH preparation ranges from 19%[5] to 86%.[18] The treatment for vaginal candidiasis is antifungal agents such as the imidazoles (*e.g.*, clotrimazole, miconazole) and polyenes (*e.g.*, nystatin, Mycostatin).

These antifungal agents can be delivered in creams, tablets, or coated tampons. Clotrimazole and miconazole are most widely used in the United States. Although treatment length usually was 7 days or as long as 14 days, a 3-day treatment regimen is now showing high cure rates. Alternative therapy includes acidophilus culture or yogurt applied to the labia or as a douche (no data on efficacy), povidone-iodine preparations (to be avoided in pregnancy), gentian violet douches or local application, and vinegar douches (1 tbsp/pint of water). The most efficacious of the alternative therapies is boric acid powder in size 0 gelatin capsules (see under bacterial vaginitis section). This regimen has been reported to have up to a 92% cure rate.[46] This treatment has the added advantage of being an inexpensive treatment that can be made up by the patient or can be prescribed and dispensed by a pharmacy.

In a compliant patient, vaginal candidiasis can usually be cured with one therapeutic regimen. However, recurrent disease is unfortunately too common and can be frustrating for the patient and the clinician. Reexamination is necessary, checking on compliance, presence of new infection, reinfection, autoinoculation, poor hygiene, new sexual partner, douching away medication, or using tampons that can absorb medication. Reeducation may be necessary; changing birth control method, checking for diabetes mellitus, counseling for general health measures, and stress reduction therapy are all appropriate interventions to be considered.

Nursing Management

Assessment and Nursing Diagnosis. The nursing management plan for the patient with vulvovaginitis from a fungal overgrowth follows the same general plan previously discussed under syphilis and herpes genitalis. An additional nursing diagnosis is alteration in comfort related to the vulvar pruritus.

Goals. The goals for the patient with candidiasis include relief of discomfort from itching, compliance with treatment, and understanding the course of the infection.

Interventions. Prevention measures for candidiasis include good general and perineal health habits. Keeping the body and perineum clean and dry generally help prevent vaginitis. Daily baths, drying the perineum with a clean towel or a hair dryer, wiping from front to back after voiding or defecating, wearing cotton or cotton-crotch underwear and avoiding prolonged wearing of nylons and tight pants (to allow body perspiration to evaporate), and avoiding long-term use of antibiotics are ways of preventing candidiasis.

Sitz baths or douching with vinegar can help intense vulvar pruritus, but douching too frequently or douching with perfumed or "feminine-hygiene" products can cause vaginal epithelial breakdown and chemical irritation, resulting in further inflammation. In general, one need never douche unless specifically instructed to do so by a clinician.

Taking the antifungal medication as prescribed, even during menstruation, is necessary to ensure a cure. Instructing the patient in the use of boric acid powder in size 0 gelatin capsules inserted at night for 10 to 14 days is a very effective self-help measure that is both a treatment and prevention. Boric acid should be avoided during pregnancy because of its possible toxic effects. Clotrimazole and miconazole may be used during pregnancy.

The nurse can explore with the patient alternative ways of sexual expression other than intercourse during the treatment period. Sexual intercourse can aggravate the inflammation already present. The patient's birth control method should be considered as a potential contributing factor. Oral contraceptives can alter the vaginal environment and pH and increase the propensity for vaginal candidiasis. Some diaphragm users have an increased problem with fungal infections as well.

The sexual partner(s) is a potential source of infection and outreach should be made in order to educate and treat him. The use of a water-soluble lubricant (K-Y jelly) during intercourse can decrease vaginal excoriation.

The nurse can usually offer reassurance that vaginal candidiasis is not an STD and that it is possible for a woman to develop a yeast infection without having had intercourse. This can allay concerns, especially from an adolescent population who may be afraid to seek professional help because of the stigma attached to having an STD.

Evaluation. The patient will relate relief from the discomfort caused by the inflammation and itching, demonstrate compliance with the treatment protocol, and discuss understanding of the infection and its course.

Pelvic Inflammatory Disease

Definition

Over the past 15 to 20 years the incidence of pelvic inflammatory disease (PID) has risen along with the increase in all STDs. PID is a collective term referring to infection occurring in one or more anatomical sites in the female genital tract. More appropriately proper anatomical terms should be used in describing where the infection is, such as endometritis, parametritis, salpingitis, salpingo-ooporitis, pelvic peritonitis, and pelvic (tubal, ovarian) abscess.

Infection spreads in an upward fashion usually ascending from the cervix into the uterus and fallopian tubes. Although the mucus plug can protect a woman from ascending infection, there are times when the mucus plug is absent or not as protective, for example, during menstruation, *post partum,* postabortion, or during ovulation.

Hormone treatment can affect ascending infection. It has been demonstrated that women using oral contraceptives have significantly milder degrees of inflammation of the fallopian tubes than women using other contraceptive methods.[43] IUD users who are usually at increased risk for PID may benefit from the type of IUD that slowly releases the hormone progestin.

PID is frequently associated with sexual activity. There are incidences of iatrogenic PID, such as following an IUD insertion, abortion, or hysterosalpingogram, or with the use of an IUD. The number of sexual partners increases the likelihood of acquiring this infection to five times higher than women with one partner.[13]

Hospitalization rates in the United States from 1974 through 1981 averaged 5.3/1000 females. The risk for hospitalization for PID was greatest among women in their twenties, divorced or separated women, and nonwhite women.[49]

There is a much higher incidence of this disease in younger women. In 15- to 19-year-old females the incidence is three times that in 25- to 29-year-olds, and in 20- to 24-year-old females the incidence is two times that in 25- to 29-year-olds. Women who have had one PID are two times as likely to develop another infection as those who have never had it.[13] The second infection usually appears within 1 year of the first episode.[50]

Etiology

In the majority of cases, salpingitis or PID is usually attributable to *Chlamydia trachomatis* or *Neisseria gonorrhoeae.* Other organisms are genital mycoplasmas (such as *Mycoplasma hominis* or Ureaplasma urealyticum), aerobic bacteria (such as *Escherichia coli* and *Haemophilus influenzae*), and anaerobic bacteria (such as *Bacteroides fragilis*).

Clinical Manifestations

Inflammatory changes can be mild to severe. The fallopian tubes can be reddened and swollen and have an exudate. The inflammatory changes can advance to adhesions of the tubes and ovaries, adherence of the fimbriae, and pelvic involvement with adhesions and possible abscess formation.

The symptoms a woman experiences with PID can range from none to extreme abdominal pain, fever, and pelvic tenderness. Generally, the most common symptoms are lower abdominal pain, pain with intercourse, vaginal discharge, malaise, fever, intermenstrual or increased menstrual bleeding, and cramping. Pain is usually the main complaint. Seventy-five percent of patients with gonorrheal or chlamydial PID have vaginal discharge of recent onset. Intermenstrual or increased menstrual bleeding occurs in 40% of patients and may be due to endometritis.[14]

With gonorrheal PID the onset of symptoms is usually more rapid. Chlamydial PID is a slower, more indolent disease characterized by a longer but less severe symptomatology.

Medical Management

Diagnosis is made by a combination of history, physical examination, laboratory tests, culdocentesis, and examination of the male sexual partner. On physical examination, there will usually be abdominal tenderness, cervical motion tenderness ranging from mild to severe (positive Chandelier's sign), fundal tenderness and bilateral adnexal tenderness, and occasional adnexal mass. A temperature $>38°C$ can be present. A hematocrit, white blood cell (WBC), and sedimentation rate are beneficial when they are abnormal.[13] A Gram stain of the endocervical discharge can identify *N. gonorrhoeae* and the presence of ≥ 5 polymorphonuclear leukocytes/high-powered field.

A culdocentesis can be performed to identify purulent material from the peritoneal cavity. Laparoscopy is the most definitive diagnostic tool for PID. It is routinely used in Scandinavian countries, whereas in the United States it is used more selectively to aid in diagnosing difficult cases.

Cervical cultures can be done for *N. gonorrhoeae* and *C. trachomatis.* Culdocentesis fluid and purulent material obtained from the fallopian tubes or pelvic cavity during laparoscopy can be cultured. Ultrasonography can help detect pelvic masses and abscesses.

In the case of mild, unhospitalized PID, the patient is often started on tetracycline 500 mg four times a day for 10 days. This will cover concomitant infections of gonorrhea and *C. trachomatis.* Further treatment is addressed in the Nursing Care Plan for the Patient with Pelvic Inflammatory Disease.

The prognosis is generally good but depends on early detection, treatment, and follow-up. Sequelae are chronic pelvic pain, recurrent PID, infertility, and ectopic pregnancy.

(*Text continues on page 1518*)

NURSING CARE PLAN FOR THE PATIENT WITH PELVIC INFLAMMATORY DISEASE (PID)

NURSING DIAGNOSIS/PROBLEM 1: Alteration in comfort: pain related to infection of the internal pelvic organs manifested by pain ranging from mild to severe, fever, malaise, cramping, dysmenorrhea, and dyspareunia

GOAL 1.1: To relieve the discomfort of unpleasant and painful symptoms for the patient with PID

Nursing Interventions	Rationale	Outcome Criteria
1. Develop plan for rest with patient and family.	1. Inclusion of patient and family in development of care plan helps ensure compliance.	1. Patient will state that she feels rested.
a. Days off work b. Coverage for children c. Notify employer	a. General rest promotes quicker response to therapy.	
d. Semi-Fowler's position if hospitalized	d. Semi-Fowler's position facilitates drainage and helps avoid abscess formation.	
2. Increase fluid intake or administer IV fluids.	2. Increased fluids can reduce fever and help metabolism of drugs.	2. Patient's fever will be reduced.
3. Administer or instruct patient to administer medications ordered: a. Antipyretics (Take temperature every 4 hours and consult for fever if over 102°F orally). b. Pain medications	3 a–b. Proper use of aspirin, ibuprofen, acetaminophen, or other medications can reduce fever, pain, and cramping.	3. Patient reports relief of fever, pain, and cramps.
c. Antibiotics	c. Appropriate antimicrobial therapy taken properly will ensure eradication of infection.	
4. Instruct patient and partner about need for pelvic rest:		4. Patient will not experience dyspareunia or other pelvic pain related to noncompliance with pelvic rest.
a. No intercourse during treatment until infection cleared (minimum 10 days)	4 a. Intercourse with a pelvic infection is painful and can exacerbate symptoms and disease.	
b. No tampons during treatment	b. Any objects in vagina could exacerbate infection and risk toxic shock.	
c. No douching	c. Water under pressure can force bacteria into tubes.	
d. Showers only, no baths (not considered important by all clinicians)	d. Some clinicians feel baths could exacerbate infection.	

GOAL 1.2: To prevent the occurrence of complications by making frequent and accurate nursing assessments

Nursing Interventions	Rationale	Outcome Criteria
1. Administer general nursing care if hospitalized:		1. Patient appears comfortable:
a. Vital signs every 4 hours.	1 a. Temperature > 102°F or sudden drop in blood pressure could indicate rupture of abscess or peritonitis.	a. Seems restful. b. Vital signs are within expected limits. c. Vaginal discharge is within expected findings.
b. Check pain level every 4 hours, assessing need for pain medications.	b. Appropriately given pain medications assure patient comfort.	

(Continued)

NURSING CARE PLAN FOR THE PATIENT WITH PELVIC INFLAMMATORY DISEASE (PID) (*Continued*)

Nursing Interventions	Rationale	Outcome Criteria
c. Assist patient in turning, massage, heat pad to abdomen.	c. Generally good nursing care promotes patient comfort, anxiety reduction, and decrease in pain; promotes good circulation and healing.	
d. Check vaginal discharge for amount, color, and odor.	d. Change in discharge could indicate change in condition; *e.g.,* sudden bloody discharge could mean rupture of ectopic pregnancy.	
2. Consult with physician at earliest sign of patient deterioration; *i.e.,* temperature > 102°F, increased pain, abdominal rigidity, shock.	2. Early intervention ensures good outcome for patient; *e.g.,* as in rupture of ectopic pregnancy or rupture of abscess.	2. Patient will have early intervention when indicated by change in symptoms.

NURSING DIAGNOSIS/PROBLEM 2: Knowledge deficit related to follow-up care to ensure that treatment is appropriate and infection is gone

GOAL 2.1: To provide appropriate treatment to ensure infection cure and reduce incidence of morbidity from PID; *i.e.,* pelvic pain, infertility, abscess formation

Nursing Interventions	Rationale	Outcome Criteria
1. Instruct patient to return to clinic in 72 hours to reexamine.	1. A positive response to antimicrobial therapy should be seen in 72 hours.	1–2. Patient understands reason for follow-up and complies.
2. Instruct patient to return to clinic after completion of treatment.	2. Postantibiotic exam and cultures can determine eradication of infection or need for more treatment.	

GOAL 2.2: To provide appropriate treatment to patient's sexual partner(s) to prevent dissemination of causative organism

Nursing Interventions	Rationale	Outcome Criteria
1. Assist sexual partner(s) in getting an exam or culture and treatment.	1. Sexual partners who have symptoms of discharge or urethritis or positive cultures can reinfect females.	1–2. Sexual partner(s) comes to clinic for exam and treatment.
2. Instruct partner to return to clinic for follow-up after treatment.	2. Exam and cultures after treatment can determine eradication of infection or need for more treatment.	

NURSING DIAGNOSIS/PROBLEM 3: Knowledge deficit related to signs and symptoms of reoccurrences/complications manifested by recurrent PID and infertility

GOAL 3.1: To reduce chance of recurrent PID and subsequent pain, morbidity, and infertility

Nursing Interventions	Rationale	Outcome Criteria
1. Discuss and educate patient in appropriate birth control methods.	1. a. IUDs increase risk of PID. b. Birth control pills may reduce risk. c. Condoms help prevent STD. d. Spermicidal foams, jellies, and creams may deter some STDs.	1. Patient modifies behavior.

(*Continued*)

NURSING CARE PLAN FOR THE PATIENT WITH PELVIC INFLAMMATORY DISEASE (PID) (*Continued*)

Nursing Interventions	Rationale	Outcome Criteria
2. Discuss health risks of multiple sexual partners.		2. Patient seeks counseling and modifies behavior.
3. Determine need for counseling if appropriate (sexually active young patient, multiple sexual partners, pelvic pain, *etc.*).		
GOAL 3.2: To provide education to prevent PID from occurring, particularly in high-risk groups		
Nursing Interventions	**Rationale**	**Outcome Criteria**
1. Promote and provide early sex education in schools, Girl Scout groups, parent groups.	1. Early education and factual information lead to informed decision making regarding early sexual intercourse; also better parent/child communication.	1. Young females can make informed decisions.
2. Intervention and education of adolescent patients regarding early initiation of intercourse and risks of PID and STD.	2. PID is a disease primarily of young females.	2. Patient makes healthy decisions about early sex, use of condoms, and multiple partners.
3. Interact with patients in nonjudgmental and helpful manner, or refer to someone who can help.	3. A nonjudgmental manner promotes patient comfort level and trust of nurse.	3. Patient is able to speak openly and confidentially to nurse.

Chronic abdominal pain lasting longer than 6 months was present in 15% of women with PID in one study,[13] and up to 18.1% in another.[51] Ectopic pregnancy due to tubal blockage is much more common following PID. One half of women with an ectopic pregnancy have had PID. The risk is seven to ten times greater in women who have had PID than in women who have not.[13]

Infertility is a major consequence of PID. Weström has demonstrated the incidence of infertility after one episode to be 12%, after two episodes to be 35%, and after three episodes to be 75%. He estimates that of every 28 girls born in 1950, one is sterile at the age of 30 because of tubal infection.[13]

Nursing Management

Assessment and Nursing Diagnosis. The woman's history and physical examination must be carefully analyzed in PID. Among the expected nursing diagnoses are alteration in comfort: pain related to the infection, potential fluid volume deficit related to inadequate intake and fluid losses resulting from the elevated temperature, and knowledge deficit related to the diagnosis and potential recurrence or complications (See Nursing Care Plan for the Patient with Pelvic Inflammatory Disease.)

Goals. The goals for the woman with PID include relief from pain, intake of adequate fluid volume, and understanding of the course of the infectious process including recurrence and complications.

Interventions. During the acute stage of PID, the woman needs supportive nursing care in which her immediate needs for pain relief, adequate fluid and nutritional intake, and careful monitoring of other symptoms are met. The effect of PID on the woman's self-esteem must be considered. Because PID is often associated with sexually transmitted diseases, there may be feelings of anxiety, guilt, and fear that the woman must handle.

Because of the possibility for PID to become chronic, patient education regarding the need to complete the full course of treatment and to recognize early signs and symptoms of potential recurrence is imperative.

Evaluation. The woman with PID will relate relief of pain and discomfort, have reduction in temperature elevation along with documented adequate fluid intake, and demonstrate understanding of the infectious process through participation in the full course of treatment during the acute phase and in follow-up care to monitor for recurrence.

Toxic Shock Syndrome

Definition and Etiology

Toxic shock syndrome (TSS) is an acute febrile illness that affects menstruating women who use tampons. It is an exotoxin-mediated illness that is associated with young women but also has been reported in a variety of medical and surgical conditions not associated with menstruation. A recurrence rate of approximately 30% has been reported only in women and generally coincides with a menstrual period.[48]

Clinical Manifestations

Many symptoms have been reported, ranging from mild to severe. Some of these are malaise, myalgias, fever, vomiting, diarrhea, chills, severe hypotension, and a generalized, sunburnlike rash. The rash is followed by a sloughing of the palms and soles of the feet.

Medical Management

TSS has been associated with the presence of *Staphylococcus aureus* which has been recovered from the vaginal vault with possible microulcerations that may result from tampon use. Treatment for this potentially life-threatening illness can involve hospitalization, IV fluids, antibiotics, and management of shock.

Nursing Management

Assessment and Nursing Diagnosis. The nursing diagnoses for toxic shock are similar to those for PID. The nurse's role in the management and prevention of TSS involves education of the patient about the proper use of tampons.

Interventions. Tampons should be changed at least every 3 to 4 hours during the day, and the use of a napkin at night would be prudent. The patient who has had TSS should not wear tampons again. Avoidance of the super-absorbent tampons is important. Patient education should also include the signs and symptoms of TSS and risk factors to avoid (long-term tampon use).

Evaluation. The patient who has experienced TSS will relate her understanding regarding the proper use of tampons and discuss the early manifestations of TSS for which she will seek treatment.

Male Genital Infections

Because the male reproductive organs, like the female's, are so anatomically and functionally interrelated, any process affecting one organ has the potential to affect others. Furthermore, any disease process of the genital system may have secondary consequences such as impotence or infertility. In terms of nursing care it is important to remember not only these physiological dangers but also the anxiety raised by the threat to sexual function and masculinity.

Epididymitis

The epididymis consists of the coiled tubules carrying sperm from the testicles and participating in sperm capacitation. Epididymitis is the most common intrascrotal infection[35] and is generally associated with a chronic urinary tract infection (UTI). When associated with a UTI, the common organisms are coliform bacteria or *Pseudomonas.* Epididymitis is rare before puberty. In men under 35 years old, new studies implicate *Neisseria gonorrhoeae* and *Chlamydia trachomatis* as major causative organisms.[20] In older men, the process has been seen as a complication following prostatectomy and frequently involves coliform bacteria and *Pseudomonas.* Regardless of the cause, the process is thought to involve spread of the organism through the vas lumen from a previously established infection in the urinary tract, prostate gland, or seminal vesicles.[4]

Clinical Manifestations

The patient with epididymitis usually complains of an acute onset of scrotal swelling, pain, and tenderness, and usually an increased temperature. Clinically, the epididymis feels thickened and enlarged and is usually very tender.[32] Within a few hours of onset, the entire scrotal contents on the involved side will also be enlarged and tender. When *Chlamydia* is the causative organism, the patient may experience urethritis with an expressible discharge and relate a recent history of sexual intercourse. In severe episodes of epididymitis, scrotal edema and erythema may also be seen.

Medical Management

The patient with mild epididymitis may be managed on an outpatient basis. Moderate to severe cases are generally hospitalized because the incidence of complications is over 50%.[47] Whether admitted or not, the basic therapy is directed toward the same goals: enhancing comfort, halting the infective process, and preventing complications. Bed rest for 3 to 4 days is indicated, and the ability to manage the illness at home largely depends on the patient's willingness to comply. The scrotum is elevated and supported, and ice bags are applied to increase comfort and decrease the inflammatory response.[37] Broad-spectrum antibiotics are ordered unless there is a positive culture and sensitivities of the organism are known. When *Chlamydia* is implicated, tetracycline will be given 1.5 g intramuscularly and then followed with 500 mg four times a day for 10 days.[37] Because *Chlamydia* is sexually transmitted, the female partner should also be treated. A small percentage of patients will develop chronic epididymitis following an acute episode. Other complications include abscess, sepsis, testicular necrosis, testicular atrophy, and infection of the testicle. The long-term effects on fertility remain unknown.[47]

Orchitis

Definition and Etiology

Orchitis, or infection of the testicle, usually occurs concomitantly with epididymitis. In these cases, the process is termed *epididymo-orchitis*. Less frequently orchitis occurs as a complication of a viral infection, especially mumps. This type of orchitis rarely occurs before puberty and affects 16% to 20% of men following mumps.[35] Traumatic orchitis may follow trauma or a surgical procedure, probably due to lowered resistance of the injured tissue to infection.[29]

Clinical Manifestations

Regardless of the cause, the clinical signs and symptoms are similar. In orchitis associated with epididymitis the patient may experience a high fever and pain with radiation to the inguinal canal. He may also experience nausea and vomiting. The involved testicle is swollen and tense and the scrotal skin may be red and edematous. There is frequently an associated hydrocele.[29] It may be difficult to differentiate between epididymitis, orchitis, epididymo-orchitis, and testicular torsion due to the similarity of symptoms. Symptoms secondary to traumatic orchitis are more variable and may be acute or more insidious in onset. The patient may notice primarily a painless intrascrotal edema, which poses difficulty in distinguishing traumatic orchitis and a testicular tumor. Orchitis related to the mumps virus is also similar to acute orchitis. It generally occurs 4 to 6 days following the parotitis and subsides in 7 to 10 days.[35]

Medical Management

Treatment of orchitis is similar to that of epididymitis. Bed rest, scrotal elevation, application of ice packs, relief of pain, and antibiotics are commonly used. If a hydrocele forms, aspiration may be performed to give symptomatic relief. As mentioned, orchitis due to trauma may be difficult to differentiate from a testicular tumor. In this instance, surgical removal of the testicle is indicated to secure a diagnosis. The treatment of mumps orchitis is also similar to that of acute orchitis with an emphasis on prevention of testicular atrophy by aspirating an existing hydrocele and occasionally administration of diethylstilbestrol.[29]

Nursing Management

Assessment and Nursing Diagnosis. Alteration in comfort: pain related to the inflammation, swelling, and dysuria accompanying the infectious process is a major nursing diagnosis. Other nursing diagnoses include body image disturbance and anxiety related to embarrassment and fear of long-term implications of the illness, and knowledge deficit related to the infectious process, course of treatment, and self-care following acute care.

Goals. The goals for the man with epididymo-orchitis include relief of pain and discomfort, willingness to discuss concerns and feelings about the diagnosis and the long-term effects, and understanding of and compliance with the treatment and the follow-up monitoring.

Interventions. Accurate assessment of pain precedes the activity of relieving the pain. The immediate action is to administer medication promptly and according to the prescribed schedule. Local measures to increase comfort involve the use of a scrotal support and the application of ice packs to the scrotal area, removing them 5 to 10 minutes every hour to prevent thermal injury. When the man is allowed out of bed, continued use of a scrotal support device can be helpful in controlling pain and swelling.

Use of antibiotics requires patient education regarding the rationale for treatment, the proper administration of the medication, and the importance of completing the full course of therapy. Continuing assessment of the potential for increased infection or septic shock is imperative. Early indications of septic shock include decreased mentation, decreased blood pressure, and increased pulse.

Because there is a possibility of transmission of a communicable infection, basic principles of preventing the spread of organisms must be stressed. For gonorrheal infections, avoid contamination by urine, double-bag contaminated material, and wear gloves when in contact with urethral secretions. For mumps, respiratory isolation is the main emphasis.

Epididymo-orchitis can be a source of embarrassment and disturbed self-concept. Providing privacy at all times is an essential component of nursing. Allow the patient to express his feelings about his body and illness. Identify misconceptions he may have regarding normal function, the illness, the treatment goals, and the possible long-term effects. Including the man's partner (if appropriate) in the discussion may help to decrease fears and improve communication.

Evaluation. The man with epididymo-orchitis will express relief of pain through medication and other comfort measures, discuss feelings concerning the illness and its possible long-term effects, comply with the medication schedule, and participate in follow-up appointments.

Prostatitis

Definition and Pathophysiolgy

Prostatitis, or inflammation of the prostate gland, is usually classified into acute and chronic bacterial prostatitis and nonbacterial prostatitis. These classifications are based on the bacteriological findings and examination of prostatic secretions. As the names imply, specific bacterial organisms can be identified in the prostatic secretions in both types of bacterial prostatitis. Bacterial prostatitis is generally associated with urinary tract infection or an indwelling catheter.[29] Conversely, in nonbacterial prostatitis only evidence of inflammation, such as white blood cells, are identified in the expressed prostatic secretions.[45] It has been speculated that nonbacterial prostatitis may be caused by organisms not easily identified by current laboratory methods. Recent studies have focused on the possibility that several sexually transmitted agents, such as *Chlamydia trachomatis,* Ureaplasma urealyticum, and *Trichomonas vaginalis,* may play a role as etiologic agents in the disease.[20]

Clinical Manifestations

Diagnosis of prostatitis is made from the history and physical findings and laboratory tests. Symptoms in acute bacterial prostatitis are more dominant than those in the chronic form. The patient may complain of acute perineal and low back pain; fever; chills, dysuria; and frequency, urgency, and a decrease in the force and size of the urinary stream. Examination may reveal a tender prostate gland that may contain a tender mass or feel boggy or edematous.[12] The patient with chronic bacterial prostatitis will rarely experience a fever or major systemic symptoms but may complain of lower back pain, perineal fullness, dysuria, and may have a slight urethral discharge.[37] Symptoms of nonbacterial prostatitis may include a vague history of urinary symptoms and intermittent perineal discomfort and backache.[51]

Laboratory studies primarily involve the use of the 3–4-glass method used to localize organisms to the prostate gland. This study requires that the patient has a full bladder. The patient cleanses the glans and, if present, the foreskin. He then voids approximately 10 ml of urine into a sterile container. He continues voiding into a urinal until he has voided about half the remaining bladder urine. Then a second sterile container is placed under the meatus and he is asked to void another 10-ml specimen. If acute prostatitis is not present, he is asked to stop voiding and lean forward with a third sterile container under the meatus. Meanwhile, the physician massages the prostate gland and drops of prostatic fluid are collected. Following this, he voids again into a fourth container. The specimens are appropriately labeled and submitted for culture and sensitivity studies. Diagnosis of prostatitis is made when the prostatic or postmassage specimens contain significantly higher bacterial counts than the first two specimens.[20]

Medical Management

If considered severe, such as with urosepsis, the patient with acute bacterial prostatitis may require hospital admission and management. Cephalosporins and aminoglycosides may be used pending results of culture and sensitivity studies. Later, culture and sensitivity studies will indicate the appropriate choice of antibiotic. Usually, antibiotics are administered intravenously over a period of 10 days. With less severe manifestations, the patient may be managed on an outpatient basis. Again, the culture and senstitivity studies will dictate the appropriate antibiotic, which will be taken orally. According to the response, antibiotic treatment may be continued for 4 to 6 weeks if necessary.[12] In addition, bed rest, sedation, analgesics for relief of pain, adequate hydration, and stool softeners to prevent discomfort with defecation are indicated. Patients experiencing bladder irritation may require an anticholinergic drug. It is generally advised that urethral instrumentation and prostatic massage be avoided during the acute phase of illness.[29] However, if bladder urine retention develops, a small-caliber Foley catheter may be inserted.[37]

The treatment of chronic bacterial prostatitis is given on an outpatient basis and over a longer period of time. Antibiotics are chosen based on culture and sensitivity reports and the characteristics of the antibiotic in terms of its ability to penetrate the prostate gland. Trimethoprim sulfamethoxazole is widely used and has a cure rate of about one third.[12] The duration of antibiotic therapy varies widely and ranges from 6 weeks to 6 months. Frequent drainage of the prostate gland in order to empty the engorged acini of their inflammatory materials is recommended. This may be done by regular prostatic massage or, more preferably, increased sexual activity.[21] General recommendations include weight loss if indicated, increased exercise and fresh air, and decreased alcohol intake to promote general good health and well-being.[32] If these methods fail, some clinicians advocate attempting a transurethral resection of the prostate gland to relieve symptoms and infection.[29]

The treatment of nonbacterial prostatitis is often more frustrating. Broad-spectrum antibiotics may be tried but usually without success. With the current theory that *Chlamydia* or *Trichomonas* may be the causative organism, tetracycline or metronidazole (Flagyl) may also be used. Antispasmodics such as flavoxate, oxybutynin, and diazepam may also be tried. Some clinicians will follow the patient every week, changing the drug therapy weekly until some relief is obtained. Some patients are able to identify agents such as alcohol, caffeine, or spicy foods as exacerbating factors and are advised to avoid these.[20] Obviously, the management of this disease is frustrating for both the physician and patient and is additionally frightening for the patient as well. Reassurance that the disease is not severe, is not cancer, and is not transmissible offers great relief in itself. Additional support in the form of psychological or psychiatric therapy may be beneficial.

Nursing Management

Assessment and Nursing Diagnosis. Nursing management of the patient with prostatitis involves management of the problems associated with the acute phase of illness while hospitalized and with the less acute or chronic type if cared for at home. In the acute phase, the primary diagnoses include alteration in comfort: pain, the potential or actual treatment of sepsis and infection, and the body image disturbance related to the infection and sexuality.

Goals. The patient will relate relief of discomfort and pain, demonstrate understanding of the course of treatment for infection or sepsis, and discuss concerns related to body image and sexuality.

Interventions. The nursing assessment should be directed toward evaluating status based on these potential diagnoses and individualizing the plan accordingly. As time for discharge approaches, the nurse should begin explaining the rationale for long-term antibiotic therapy and the need to continue the antibiotic for the length of time ordered. Patients experiencing a less acute form of bacterial prostatitis or those who have chronic prostatitis should understand the need and potential benefits of frequent prostatic emptying. If a sexual partner is not available, other alternatives such as masturbation or massage should be discussed. In both chronic bacterial and nonbacterial prostatitis it is important to remember the frustration involved in a chronic, at times seemingly nonresponding and uncomfortable disease, and time should be allocated for support and ventilation of these feelings.

Evaluation. The man with prostatitis will state that he has relief from discomfort, participate in the full course of treatment for the infection, and feel comfortable discussing concerns related to his body image and sexuality.

References

1. Adler MW: Genital warts and molluscum contagiosum. Br Med J 288:213–215, January 21, 1984
2. Adler MW: Syphilis: Diagnosis and management. Br Med J 288:551–553, February 18, 1984
3. Aral SO, Holmes KK: Epidemiology of sexually transmitted diseases. In Holmes KK, Mardh P, Sparling PF, Wiesner PJ (eds): Sexually Transmitted Diseases, pp 127–141. New York, McGraw-Hill, 1984
4. Ball TP: Epididymitis. In Kaufman JJ (ed): Current Urologic Therapy, pp 357–361. Philadelphia, WB Saunders, 1980
5. Bergman JJ et al: Clinical comparison of microscopic and culture techniques in the diagnosis of *Candida* vaginitis. J Fam Pract 18(4):549–552, 1984
6. Billstein S: Human lice. In Holmes KK, Mardh P, Sparling PF, Weisner PJ (eds): Sexually Transmitted Diseases, pp 513–517. New York, McGraw-Hill, 1984
7. Bryson YJ et al: Treatment of first episodes of genital herpes simplex virus infection with oral acyclovir. New Engl J Med, pp 916–921, April 21, 1983
8. Center for Disease Control: Sexually Transmitted Diseases: Treatment Guidelines. Atlanta GA, US Dept of Health and Human Services, 1982
9. Charles D: Syphilis. Clin Obstet Gynecol 26(1):125–137, March 1983
10. Corey L: Genital herpes. In Holmes KK, Mardh P, Sparling PF, Weisner PJ (eds): Sexually Transmitted Diseases, pp. 449–474. New York, McGraw-Hill, 1984
11. Crissey JT: Scabies and pediculosis pubis. Urol Clin North Am 11(1):171–176, February 1984
12. Drach GW: Bacterial prostatitis: Diagnosis and treatment. Ariz Med 40:329–333, 1983
13. Eschenbach DA: Acute pelvic inflammatory disease. Urol Clin North Am 11(1):65–81, February 1984
14. Gardner HL: Infectious vulvovaginitis. In Monif GRF (ed): Infectious Diseases in Obstetrics and Gynecology. Philadelphia, Harper & Row, 1982
15. Handsfield HH: Gonorrhea. In Spittell JA Jr (ed): Clinical Medicine. Philadelphia, Harper & Row, 1984
16. Handsfield HH: Gonorrhea and uncomplicated gonococcal infection. In Holmes KK, Mardh P, Sparling PF, Wiesner PJ (eds): Sexually Transmitted Diseases, pp 205–220. New York, McGraw-Hill, 1984
17. Handsfield HH: Sexually transmitted diseases. Hosp Pract, pp 99–116, January 1982
18. Holmes KK: Lower genital tract infections in women: Cystitis/urethritis, vulvovaginitis, and cervicitis. In Holmes KK, Mardh P, Sparling PF, Wiesner PJ (eds): Sexually Transmitted Diseases, pp 557–589. New York, McGraw-Hill, 1984
19. Holmes KK et al: Epidemiology of sexually transmitted diseases. Urol Clin North Am 11(1):3–13, February 1984
20. Ireton RC, Berger RE: Prostatitis and epididymitis. Urol Clin North Am 11:83–93, 1984
21. Jaffe JW: Management of the reactive serology. In Holmes KK, Mardh P, Sparling PF, Wiesner PJ (eds): Sexually Transmitted Diseases, pp 313–318. New York, McGraw-Hill, 1984
22. Jick H et al: Vaginal spermicides and gonorrhea. JAMA 248(13):1619–1621, October 1, 1982
23. Kampmeier RH: Early development of knowledge of sexually transmitted diseases. In Holmes KK, Mardh P, Sparling PF, Wiesner PJ (eds): Sexually Transmitted Diseases, pp 19–29. New York, McGraw-Hill, 1984
24. Knox JM, Rudolph AH: Acquired infectious syphilis. In Holmes KK, Mardh P, Sparling PF, Wiesner PJ (eds): Sexually Transmitted Diseases, pp 305–313. New York, McGraw-Hill, 1984
25. Lang DJ: Cytomegalovirus infections. In Holmes KK, Mardh P, Sparling PF, Wiesner PJ (eds): Sexually Transmitted Diseases, pp 474–479. New York, McGraw-Hill, 1984
26. Leegaard M: The incidence of *Candida albicans* in the vagina of "healthy young women." Acta Obstet Gynecol Scand 63:85–89, 1984
27. Lossick JG: Sexually transmitted vaginitis. Urol Clin North Am 11(1):141–153, February 1984
28. Margolis S: Genital warts and molluscum contagiosum. Uro Clin North Am 11(1):163–170, Februray 1984
29. McConnell EA, Zimmerman MF: Care of Patients with Urologic Problems, pp 99–122. Philadelphia, JB Lippincott, 1983
30. Mertz G, Corey L: Genital herpes simplex virus infections in adults. Urol Clin North Am 11(1):103–119, February 1984
31. Miles PA: Sexually transmitted diseases. JOGN Nurs (Suppl) pp 102s–123s, March/April 1984
32. Murnaghan G: Chronic prostatitis. In Kaufman JJ (eds): Current Urologic Therapy, pp 285–287. Philadelphia, WB Saunders, 1980
33. Murphy FK, Patamasucon P: Congenital syphilis. In Holmes KK, Mardh P, Sparling PF, Wiesner PJ (eds): Sexually Transmitted Diseases, pp 352–374. New York, McGraw-Hill, 1984
34. Musher DM: Biology of *Treponema pallidum.* In Holmes KK, Mardh P, Sparling PF, Wiesner PJ (eds): Sexually Transmitted Diseases, pp 291–298. New York, McGraw-Hill, 1984
35. Nickel WR, Plumb RT: Other infections and inflammations of the male genitalia. In Harrison JH (ed): Campbell's Textbook of Urology, pp 682–687. Philadelphia, WB Saunders, 1978
36. Orkin M, Maibach HI: Scabies. In Holmes KK, Mardh P, Sparling PF, Wiesner PJ (eds): Sexually Transmitted Diseases. New York, McGraw-Hill, 1984
37. Paulson DF: Acute prostatitis. In Kaufman JJ (ed): Current Urologic Therapy, pp 283–286. Philadelphia, WB Saunders, 1980
38. Platt R et al: Risk of acquiring gonorrhea and prevalence of abnormal adnexal findings among women recently exposed to gonorrhea. JAMA 250:2983, 3205–3209, 1983
39. Reichman RC at al: Treatment of recurrent genital herpes simplex infections with oral acyclovir. JAMA 251(16):2103–2107, April 27, 1984
40. Rein MF, Müller M: *Trichomonas vaginalis.* In Holmes KK, Mardh P, Sparling PF, Wiesner PJ (eds): Sexually Transmitted Diseases, pp 525-536. New York, McGraw-Hill, 1984
41. Sparling PF: Natural history of syphilis.In Holmes KK, Mardh P, Sparling PF, Wiesner PJ (eds): Sexually Transmitted Diseases, pp 298–305. New York, McGraw-Hill, 1984
42. Spence MR: Gonorrhea. Clin Obstet Gynecol 25(1):111–124, March 1983
43. Svensson L et al: Contraceptives and acute salpingitis. JAMA 251(19):2553–2555, May 18, 1984
44. Sweet RL et al: Chlamydial infections in obstetrics and gynecology. Clin Obstet Gynecol 26(1):143–164, March 1983
45. Thin RN, Simmons PD: Chronic bacterial and nonbacterial prostatitis. Br J Urol 55:513–518, 1983
46. Van Slyke KK et al: Treatment of vulvovaginal candidiasis with boric acid powder. Am J Obstet Gynecol 141:145, 1981
47. Vordermark JS: The acute scrotum: Management with the use of ancillary diagnostic techniques. AUA Update Series, III, Lesson 17, pp 2–7, 1984

48. Wager GP: Toxic shock syndrome: A review. Am J Obstet Gynecol, pp 93–102, May 1, 1983
49. Washington AE et al: Hospitalizations for pelvic inflammatory disease. JAMA 251(19):2529–2533, May 18, 1984
50. Weström L, Mardh P: Salpingitis. In Holmes KK, Mardh P, Sparling PF, Wiesner PJ (eds): Sexually Transmitted Diseases, pp 615–632. New York, McGraw-Hill, 1984
51. Wyker AW: Disorders of the prostate. In Wyker AW (ed): Methods of Urology, pp 225–246. Baltimore, Williams & Wilkins, 1975

Bibliography

Adler MW: ABC of sexually transmitted diseases: A changing and growing problem. Br Med J 287:1279–1281, October 29, 1983

Adler MW: ABC of sexually transmitted diseases: Vaginal discharge–management. Br Med J 287:1611–1613, November 26, 1983

Adler MW: ABC of sexually transmitted diseases: Genital herpes. Br Med J 287:1864, December 1983

Adler MW: ABC of sexually transmitted diseases: Genital infestations. Br Med J 288:311–313, January 28, 1984

Adler MW: ABC of sexually transmitted diseases: Complications of common genital infections and infections in other sites. Br Med J 288:469–471, February 11, 1984

Adler MW: ABC of sexually transmitted diseases: Syphilis: Clinical features. Br Med J 288:468–469, February 11, 1984

Adler MW: ABC of sexually transmitted diseases: Methods of control. Br Med J 288:774–777, March 10, 1984

Alexander ER: Maternal and infant sexually transmitted diseases. Urol Clin North Am 11(1):131–139, February 1984

Amsel R et al: Nonspecific vaginitis: Diagnostic criteria and microbial and epidemiologic associations. Am J Med 74:14–22, January 1983

Baker DA: Herpesvirus. Clin Obstet Gynecol 26(1):165–172, March 1983

Brown D et al: *Gardnerella vaginalis* vaginitis: The current opinion. Reprod Med 29(5):300–305, May 1984

Brown ST: Molluscum contagiosum. In Holmes KK, Mardh P, Sparling PF, Wiesner PJ (eds): Sexually Transmitted Diseases, pp 507–512. New York, McGraw-Hill, 1984

Brown ST et al: Sensitivity and specificity of diagnostic tests for genital infection with Herpesvirus hominis. Sex Transm Dis 6:10, 1979

Brunham RC et al: Mucopurulent cervicitis: The ignored counterpart in women of urethritis in men. New Engl J Med 311 (1):1–6, July 5, 1984

Cohen L: Single dose treatment of vaginal candidosis: Comparison of clotrimazole and isoconazole. Br J Vener Dis 60:42–44, 1984

Corey L et al: Genital herpes simplex virus infections: Clinical manifestations, course, and complications. Ann Intern Med 98:958–972, 1983

Corey L et al: Intravenous acyclovir for the treatment of primary genital herpes. Ann Inter Med 98:914–921, 1983

Drusin LM: Syphilis: Clinical manifestations, diagnosis, and treatment. Urol Clin North Am 11(1):121–130, February 1984

Eschenbach DA: A guide to diagnosis and treatment of vaginal infection. Contemporary OB/Gyn 10:203–212, September 1982

Eschenbach DA: Vaginal infection. Clin Obstet Gynecol 26(1):186–202, March 1983

Handsfield HH: Recent developments in gonorrhea and pelvic inflammatory disease. J Med 14(4):281–305, 1983

Hanno PM: Priapism. AUA Update Series III, Lesson 20, pp 1–6, 1984

Hare MJ: Chlamydial infection of the lower genital tract of women. Br Med Bull 39(2):138–144, 1983

Knox GE: Cytomegalovirus: Import of sexual transmission. Clin Obstet Gynecol 26(1):173–177, March 1983

Kraus SJ: Evaluation and management of acute genital ulcers in sexually active patients. Urol Clin North Am 11(1):155–162, February 1984

Krieger JN: Biology of sexually transmitted diseases. Urol Clin North Am 11(1):15–25, February 1984

Lapides J: Fundamentals of Urology. Philadelphia, WB Saunders, 1976

Larsen SA et al: Syphilis serology and dark field microscopy. In Holmes KK, Mardh P, Sparling PF, Wiesner PJ (eds): Sexually Transmitted Diseases, pp 875–888. New York, McGraw-Hill, 1984

Lerner J: Mosby's Manual of Urologic Nursing, pp 126–129 and pp 661–669. St Louis, CV Mosby, 1982

Medical Letter: Treatment of Sexually Transmitted Diseases. Medical Letter 24:29–34, 1982

Oriel JD: Genital warts. In Holmes KK, Mardh P, Sparling PF, Wiesner PJ (eds): Sexually Transmitted Diseases, pp 496–507. New York, McGraw-Hill, 1984

Platt R et al: Risk of acquiring gonorrhea and prevalence of abnormal adnexal findings among women recently exposed to gonorrhea. JAMA 250(23): 3205–3209, December 16, 1983

Pryor JP, Hehir M: The management of priapism. Br J Urol 54:751–754, 1982

Rein MF: General principals of syphilotherapy. In Holmes KK, Mardh P, Sparling PF, Wiesner PJ (eds): Sexually Transmitted Diseases, pp 374–384. New York, McGraw-Hill, 1984

Ristuccia AM, Cunha BA: Current concepts in antimicrobial therapy of prostatitis. Urology 20:338–345, 1982

Roseman DS et al: Sexually transmitted diseases and carcinogenesis. Urol Clin North Am 11(1):27–43, February 1984

Schneider GT: Vaginal infections. Postgrad Med 73(2):255–262, February 1983

Stamm WE, Holmes KK: *Chlamydia trachomatis* infections of the adult. In Holmes KK, Mardh P, Sparling PF, Wiesner PJ (eds): Sexually Transmitted Diseases, pp 258–270. New York, McGraw-Hill, 1984

Weström L, Mardh P: Chlamydial salpingitis. Br Med Bull 39(2): 145–150, 1983

Winter CC: Priapism. In Kaufman JJ (ed): Current Urologic Therapy, pp 338–340. Philadelphia, WB Saunders, 1980

Chapter 102

Neoplastic and Non-neoplastic Disorders Affecting Reproduction

Candace Ann Walters

Although there has been a trend toward more open communication about sexuality, the possibility of illness affecting organs associated with reproduction may be overwhelming to the patient. Concerns about the course of the illness and the prescribed treatment may interfere with the emotional and physical well-being of the patient. Nurses have an important role in disseminating information and clarifying patient concerns. The nurse must promote the adoption of positive health habits and help patients discover coping mechanisms for dealing with their concerns.

In this chapter different conditions that affect the organs associated with reproduction will be explored. The conditions will be discussed based on their anatomical location. A nursing management plan will be presented to assist the patient in coping with the effects of the illness and its therapy.

Non-neoplastic Disorders of the Female Reproductive System

Atrophic Vaginitis

Definition and Etiology. Atrophic vaginitis refers to a thinning of the vaginal mucosa that is due to estrogen withdrawal. The rate of estrogen decline is an important variable in producing symptomatic atrophic vaginitis. Although commonly associated with normal menopause, atrophic vaginitis may also result from other conditions or diseases that produce a decline in estrogen levels.

Pathology. Hormonal decline in the estrogen-dependent mucosa of the vagina results in atrophy of this tissue. The vaginal mucosa becomes thinner and friable. As the glycogen-rich superficial cells atrophy, Döderlein bacilli are reduced in number and the vaginal pH becomes more alkaline. Mucus production, a function of the vaginal mucosa, is decreased along with the electrolyte content of the secretions and the elasticity of the vaginal tissues.

Clinical Manifestations. Many women with menopause-induced atrophic vaginitis do not experience symptoms, although some women notice vaginal discharge and pruritis, or vaginal dryness.[11] Sexually active women may complain of dyspareunia. Some women may complain of vaginal tenderness during a speculum examination. Occasionally, spotting will be noted after coitus or following a vaginal speculum examination including a Pap smear.

Medical Management

Diagnosis is based on the woman's history and the characteristic findings of a vaginal examination: the vaginal mucosa appears pale or pasty and thin, and the normal vaginal rugae are diminished or absent. Vaginal spotting may occur following the examination. If the woman has a history of vaginal spotting, a Pap smear is indicated. Tests may be performed on vaginal secretions to rule out the possibility of infection.

Those women without symptoms will not require any treatment for atrophic vaginitis. If vaginal dryness is the major complaint, vaginal lubricants or topical vaginal estrogen creams or suppositories may be prescribed. Constriction of the vaginal canal may be treated by the use of vaginal dilators and the recommendation of frequent coitus when possible.[11]

Nursing Management

Assessment and Nursing Diagnosis. It is important to remember that many women are asymptomatic despite having atrophic vaginitis. These women require no medical treatment. Still, because a possible knowledge deficit could affect their recognition of this condition, perimenopausal and postmenopausal women should be taught the range of symptoms associated with atrophic vaginitis. There is the potential for impaired sexual functioning, or more specifically, painful coitus related to alteration in mucus secretion of the vaginal mucous membranes. Finally, potential risks to health associated with the application of topical estrogen are of concern if the physician prescribes this medication for relief of symptoms.

Interventions. Women should be taught the symptoms of atrophic vaginitis and its etiology. Encouraging women to eat a balanced diet high in vitamins C and E may facilitate continued tissue health and repair.[12]

Evaluation. The nursing management plan is successful if perimenopausal and postmenopausal women can list the symptoms of atrophic vaginitis and relate its occurrence to estrogen withdrawal. They will be able to state actions that may facilitate continued health of the vaginal mucosa. Those women who complain of vaginal dryness or painful intercourse will be able to list alternative methods to alleviate this problem, such as the use of water-soluble vaginal lubricants. If the physician prescribes a topical estrogen compound for local vaginal application, it is important that the woman be aware of the symptoms of overdosage. These symptoms include abnormal uterine bleeding, edema, and breast tenderness.

Vaginal Fistulae

Definition. A fistula is an abnormal communication between two organs. In the reproductive system, a simple fistula is one occurrring between the vagina and the urinary tract (Fig. 102–1) or between the vagina and the rectum. When a fistula occurs between the vagina, bladder, and rectum or between the bladder, ureter, and vagina or uterus, it is classified as a mixed fistula. The descriptive name given the fistula denotes the location of the abnormal tract. Vesicovaginal fistulae are the most common type of genitourinary

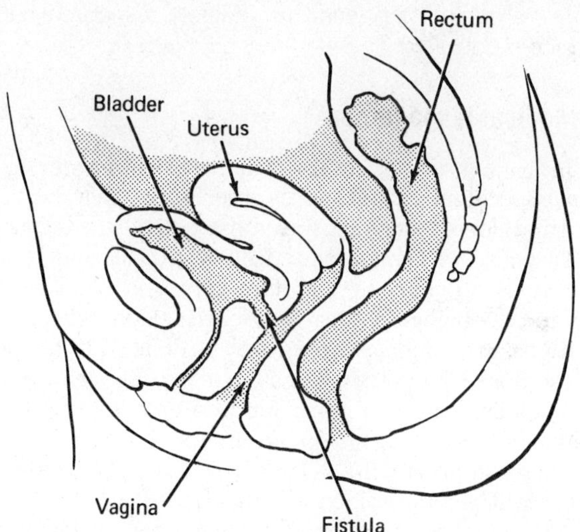

FIGURE 102–1 A fistula between the bladder and the vagina (vesicovaginal fistula)

fistulae, and rectovaginal fistulae are the most common type of intestinal–vaginal fistulae.

Etiology and Pathology. Vaginal fistulae result from conditions or therapies that injure vaginal and paravaginal structures. Illnesses that diminish the capacity of the normal healing process may contribute to the formation of fistulae. Hypertension, arteriosclerosis, diabetes, obesity, and pelvic inflammatory disease are associated with an increased risk of fistula formation. Fistulae may occur in areas of tissue destruction associated with malignant tumors or foreign bodies, for example, pessaries. Obstetrical trauma, extensive or repeated gynecological or urologic surgery, and irradiation may be complicated by the development of a vaginal fistula.

Clinical Manifestations. Symptoms of genitourinary fistulae vary with the anatomical location of the abnormal tract. A woman with a fistula between the vagina and the bladder or ureter may complain of continuous urinary leakage from the vagina both day and night. Urinary urgency generally is not associated with this condition. On the other hand, a fistula between the vagina and the urethra probably will be associated with stress incontinence or postmicturition dribbling. In contrast, symptoms associated with a fistula between the uterus and the bladder or ureter include cyclic hematuria and secondary vaginal amenorrhea. Urinary incontinence may or may not be associated with this type of fistula.

Continuous leakage of urine with a genitourinary fistula may be associated with secondary irritation and maceration of the vagina, vulva, and perineum.[12] If the fistula is large, there may be irritation of the vagina, vulva, and perineum. The pervasive odor of urine can be a prominent feature of genitourinary fistulae.

Symptoms of a rectovaginal fistula include the occasional passage of flatus or fecal material, or both through the vagina.[11] If the fistula is large, there may be irritation of the vagina, vulva, and perineum. In addition, associated odor cannot be controlled.

Medical Management

In many instances, fistulae may be visualized during a vaginal speculum examination. Large fistulae may be palpated by a gloved examining finger inserted into the vagina.[11]

Diagnosis of genitourinary fistulae is facilitated by an intravenous urogram. Cystourethroscopy and vaginoscopy or hysterosalpingography may be used to aid in the detection of a fistula. In addition, a dye test may be done. This involves the insertion of a sterile swab or tampon into the vagina prior to the administration of either intravesical methylene blue solution or intravenous indigo carmine, or both sequentially. When a genitourinary fistula is present, the vaginal swab or tampon will become stained with the dye.

After diagnosis of a fistula, a waiting period is recommended to allow sufficient time for reduction in existing edema and induration and the possibility of spontaneous healing. This time period may last from 3 months in the case of fistulae complicating surgery and up to 1 year in instances of fistulae occurring after irradiation. An indwelling urethral catheter may be inserted. Fluids may be limited and urinary antibiotics prescribed.[11] When associated edema and inflammation have diminished and revascularization and epithelialization have begun, surgical closure of the fistula can be attempted.

The transvaginal closure of a fistula is a minor procedure associated with little morbidity. A vaginal flap may be mobilized to close the fistula. Possible complications following transvaginal closure of a fistula include diminution of functional length of the vagina and stress urinary incontinence. The transvaginal approach is commonly used to treat rectovaginal fistulae, but is contraindicated in cases of a fistula located in irradiated tissue. Occasionally, a temporary colostomy or ileostomy may need to be done to allow infected tissues to heal prior to definitive therapy to close the intestinal–vaginal fistula.

Indications for a transabdominal approach to closure of a fistula include fistula diameter greater than 2 cm, multiple fistulae, a fistula affecting the ureteric orifices, recurrent fistula, vesicocervical fistulae, and poor quality of surrounding tissue, including irradiated tissue or tissue in the area of chronic infection.

In either the transvaginal or the transabdominal approach to closure of the genitourinary fistula, assurance of continuous urinary drainage is imperative. Either an indwelling urethral catheter or a suprapubic catheter, or both will be used in the postoperative period. When both the urethral and the suprapubic catheters are used, the urethral catheter may be removed after a few days. The suprapubic catheter may be left in place up to 2 weeks. This technique decreases the danger of ascending urinary tract infection and minimizes urethral irritation while assuring uninterrupted urinary drainage.

A drain is generally placed into the retroperitoneal space during surgery and removed 3 or 4 days later. Any vaginal packing will be removed within 3 days. Broad-spectrum antibiotics may be prescribed in the postoperative period. Stool softeners may be prescribed to decrease straining with stool. When food is permitted, a well-balanced diet will facilitate tissue healing. In order to further limit possible tension on the operative incisions, the woman may be cautioned to avoid vaginal intercourse for a few months after surgery.

One of the most distressing complications is the recurrence of the fistula. When this occurs despite repeated attempts to correct the problem, a urinary diversion may be necessary.

Nursing Management

Assessment and Nursing Diagnosis. Urinary continency is highly valued from the time of infancy. Constant dribbling or urine and the odor of urine are embarassing and may limit the social activities of the woman with a fistula. In addition, the constant proximity of urine to the perineal tissues may result in tissue breakdown. A few of the possible nursing diagnoses include potential for social isolation related to embarrassment associated with incontinence and odor; potential for vaginal, vulvar, and perineal irritation and maceration related to incontinence; and potential for recurrence of the fistula due to tension on suture lines and poor health of surrounding tissue.

Goals. During the preoperative period, control of incontinence and odor, promotion of health tissues, and maintenance of social relationships are the focus of nursing efforts. Promotion of adequate nutrition for healing and prevention of stress on the postoperative area are important postoperative goals.

Interventions. Nurses should teach the woman with a fistula ways to absorb urine and minimize odor. Changing of incontinence pads and frequent and careful perineal hygiene can minimize odor, prevent exacerbation of skin maceration or irritation, and promote resumption of usual activities of daily living. The woman needs to be taught to carry a small supply of extra pads for use as necessary. Encouraging the woman to maintain nutrition and hydration status during the time of waiting for maturation of the fistula and possible spontaneous closure is important. Emotional support and helping the woman to maintain patience and hope during this period is crucial.

In the postoperative period, frequent assessment of the patency of the urethral or suprapubic catheter, or both is mandatory. If continuous urinary drainage is interrupted, urine may pool and disrupt the integrity of the incision. The woman needs to know that the use of stool softeners will minimize straining with stool and prevent stress on the surgical area. Alternative methods to vaginal coitus that express caring and are acceptable to both sexual partners must be reviewed with any sexually active woman. Finally, the possibility of fistula recurrence and anticipating ways to cope with this possibility should be discussed with the woman.

Evaluation. A woman with a urinary or intestinal fistula will state acceptable ways to control incontinence and odor; perform careful perineal hygiene at least twice a day and more frequently, if necessary; maintain a level of social interactions and daily obligations acceptable to her; and prepare and consume a well-balanced daily diet, high in protein and vitamins A and C. The skin of her vulva and perineum will be pink, dry, and intact.

Postoperatively, the urinary drainage system will be patent and uninterrupted. The woman will state the rationale for the use of stool softeners and the symptoms that would necessitate consultation with the physician regarding possible discontinuation of the medication; relate the rationale for avoidance of vaginal coitus in the postoperative period; describe acceptable alternative ways to demonstrate affection and assure closeness until vaginal penetration is no longer prohibited; state that recurrence is possible; list the symptoms associated with recurrence of the fistula; describe a plan for contacting a health professional if the symptoms recur; and be continent of urine and stool.

Cystocele and Rectocele

Definition. A cystocele is a protrusion of the bladder through the pubocervical fascia into the vaginal canal. Occasionally the cystocele will protrude beyond the vaginal introitus. Different degrees of cystocele have been defined according to the amount of protrusion of the bladder. A rectocele is a protrusion of the rectum into the vaginal canal. Occasionally the rectocele will protrude beyond the vaginal introitus. (See Figure 102–2.)

Etiology. Menopause and prior childbirth are commonly associated with the development of a cystocele. Prolonged or difficult labor, or an inadequate repair of any pelvic muscle injuries associated with labor or delivery contribute to weakened pelvic muscles. Many parous women develop a cystocele or rectocele after menopause. In the older woman, lack of estrogen stimulation of the genital tract results in atrophic and weakened tissues.[29]

Any activity that involves the Valsalva maneuver may aggravate the already weakened tissues and produce or aggravate a cystocele or rectocele. Some examples of these activities include lifting heavy objects, constipation-induced straining with defecation, and protracted coughing or sneezing.[29]

Pathology. The bladder may protrude through the pubocervical fascia into the vagina due to relaxation or trauma affecting the pelvic muscles supporting the bladder and urethrovesical junction. This results in stress urinary incontinence (SUI) and risk for a urinary tract infection.

Because of relaxation or trauma affecting the perirectal fascia and pelvic muscles, the rectum may protrude through the posterior vaginal wall. Straining with stool, an action both promoting the development of a rectocele and resulting from the alteration in the rectum, may predispose to hemorrhoids along with a rectocele.

Clinical Manifestations. Women may be asymptomatic despite the presence of a moderate cystocele or rectocele.[11] When symptomatic, a woman with a cystocele and a prolapsed urethrovesical junction may complain of unplanned urination whenever her actions involve the Valsalva maneuver. She may also complain of continuous urinary dribbling due to overflow incontinence, a feeling of inadequate emptying accompanying urinary urgency and frequency, pain with urination, and other symptoms of cystitis.

In all degrees of cystocele, possible symptoms include a sensation of a lump in the vagina and a heavy, dragging sensation in the vagina following prolonged standing. Women may also experience discomfort in the lower abdomen and back. Occasionally, the woman will be forced to reduce the cystocele in order to urinate. She accomplishes this by pushing the bulging area upward and forward into the vagina with her fingers.[12] If the cystocele protrudes through the vaginal introitus, ulceration and bleeding of the exposed vaginal mucosa may occur.

With a rectocele, some women will notice a feeling of difficult or incomplete emptying of the rectum. While many women complain of constipation, some may complain of incontinence of flatus and stool.[11]

Women with a rectocele may notice a soft, bulging mass within the vagina. In some cases, the bulging mass may be visible at or beyond the vaginal introitus. Some women may find that manual reduction, or using the finger to gently push the mass backward and upward into the vagina will facilitate complete evacuation of the rectum.[29] A backache and a feeling of pressure in the pelvic area combined with a heavy, dragging sensation may be accompanying symptoms. Because hemorrhoids often accompany a rectocele, women may have a small amount of bright red bleeding with defecation.

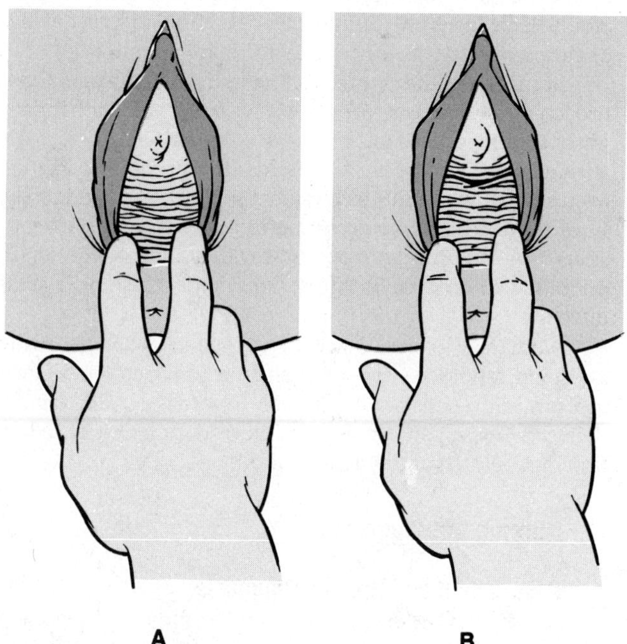

FIGURE 102–2 (*A*) A cystocele occurs when the anterior wall of the vagina and the bladder bulge or protrude into the vagina. (*B*) A rectocele occurs when the posterior wall of the vagina and the rectum protrude into the vagina.

Medical Management

A complete pelvic examination will be done to assess the extent of the cystocele or rectocele and to exclude other possible pathological causes. Because a large rectocele may spontaneously and temporarily recede when a woman is prone, the woman will be requested to bear down during the examination as though she were straining with stool.[11]

For a cystocele, the examination is frequently arranged to coincide with a time when the woman's bladder is full. A special type of speculum, the Sims' speculum, may be used as an aid in visualization of the cystocele. Because the cystocele may recede when the woman is prone, the woman may be asked to cough or perform the Valsalva maneuver during the examination in order to highlight the cystocele. For the same reason, occasionally the woman will be examined in the upright position.

Major complications associated with a cystocele include urinary tract obstruction and ascending infection. For this reason a urine specimen is necessary because of the possibility of coexisting cystitis. If the cystocele is symptomatic, either medical or surgical therapy is necessary because of the possibility of serious complication and because of the embarrassment and the interruption of the activities of daily living due to urinary symptoms. Goals of surgery include correction of the prolapse, maintenance of normal urinary patterns, and preservation of the potential for vaginal intercourse.

Surgical correction of a cystocele through the vagina is called an *anterior colporrhaphy* or an anterior repair. Through an incision in the anterior vaginal wall, the urethrovesical junction and the bladder base are repositioned and sutures are placed to strengthen the supporting fascia and related structures. Either a suprapubic or a urethral catheter will be inserted during the operation to prevent the common postoperative sequela of urinary retention.

Surgical treatment of a rectocele through a vaginal approach is called a *posterior colporrhaphy* or posterior repair. Through an incision in the posterior vaginal wall, the levator ani and superficial perineal muscles are sutured. This results in strengthening of the rectovaginal septum. Postoperatively, stool softeners may be prescribed to prevent excessive tension of the suture line associated with straining with stool. Antibiotic therapy may be prescribed to decrease the risk of infection.

Women who desire further pregnancies are generally not good candidates for successful surgical outcomes since the surgical repair can be disrupted by subsequent vaginal delivery. Obese patients may be referred for a weight reduction diet before surgery is attempted.

Nursing Management

Assessment and Nursing Diagnosis

A few relevant diagnoses related to the care of women with these conditions are potential social isolation related to embarrassment associated with urinary incontinence or alteration; potential for cystitis related to urinary retention; potential for vaginal ulceration related to tissue irritation; and potential alteration in elimination related to postoperative sequelae. For these women and women with existing rectoceles, a few of the possible nursing diagnoses include potential alteration in bowel elimination: constipation, related to exacerbation or development of a rectocele; and alteration in bowel elimination: constipation, related to fear of pain with initial postoperative bowel movement.

Interventions

Patients who are incapacitated by urinary urgency, frequency, overflow, or stress incontinence will need help to devise methods of coping with these urinary symptoms until some form of medical therapy is feasible. Some women find the use and frequent changing of sanitary napkins preferable to the use of "diapers." Some women may regulate their fluid intake to avoid times of social or other activities, but they must be cautioned about the need to maintain adequate fluid intake. Encouraging these women to discuss their concerns about incontinence is an important nursing consideration. Emotional support may help these women to resolve any feelings they may have about the threat of incontinence to their self-concept as an adult.

When symptoms of a bladder infection are present, the woman needs to understand the importance of completion of the full course of antibiotic therapy. Methods of preventing recurrence of cystitis, such as drinking fluids and making a conscious effort to urinate at least every 4 hours, should also be reviewed.

Preoperative and Postoperative Care. When surgery is recommended, the nursing management plan includes a few specialized areas in addition to the more common preoperative and postoperative strategies. The patient needs to be aware of the necessity of a urinary catheter during and after surgery. Throughout the postoperative period, intake and output will be measured. Patient education also includes teaching the function of the particular type of urinary catheter to be used. The woman must be taught that the catheter will be left in place for a few days to facilitate healing of the surgical incision and prohibit the development of urinary retention. When the catheter is removed, the possibility of urinary retention must be prevented. Catheterization may be performed immediately after the patient has voided in order to measure the volume of residual urine. By the time of discharge from the hospital, the woman should be able to completely empty her bladder with each voiding.

Health Teaching. The teaching plan for all women and particularly postpartum women includes information about Kegel exercises. The goal of these exercises is improvement or maintenance of muscle tone. Postoperatively, women need to be taught the symptoms of a recurrent cystocele as well as the symptoms of a urinary tract infection.

All multiparous and elderly women with a history of chronic constipation are at risk for the development of a rectocele and must be taught methods to promote a regular pattern of defecation of soft, formed stool. The importance of a balanced diet high in fiber and an adequate fluid intake needs to be stressed. When stool softeners are prescribed, the purpose and side-effects of the medication need to be taught. It is important to emphasize that the woman must not delay having a bowel movement when she has the urge to defecate.

After a posterior colporrhaphy, the woman may be anxious about the possibility of pain with defecation. The nurse should review the methods listed above to promote the formation of soft, formed stool. In addition, offering a pain medication prior to the first bowel movement after surgery may decrease anxiety and discomfort associated with the initial postoperative defecation.

Evaluation

A woman with a symptomatic cystocele will discuss any concerns about her self-concept related to the urinary symptoms; state a plan for control of urine in social situations; engage in her routine personal and social activities; and state the symptoms of cystitis. Postoperatively, the woman will state the purpose of the urinary catheter; after removal of the catheter, urinate clear yellow urine at least every 4 hours; indicate that she feels she has completely emptied her bladder with each voiding; describe the symptoms of cystitis and recurrent cystocele; discuss acceptable modifications of vaginal intercourse that may be used to increase the woman's pleasure when sufficient tissue healing has occurred; and perform Kegel exercises at the recommended frequency.

A woman who is at risk for developing a rectocele will pass soft, formed stool every other day or as per her routine habit; consume a well-balanced daily diet and eat meals at regular times; drink adequate amounts of fluids; state the purpose and side-effects of prescribed stool softeners; and defecate as soon as socially acceptable when she has the urge to have a bowel movement. In addition to these, postoperatively the woman will state that she passed the initial postoperative bowel movement with relative comfort; discuss the rationale for temporarily abstaining from vaginal intercourse; and describe acceptable ways for her to demonstrate caring and receive affection.

Cervical and Endometrial Polyps

Definition. Cervical polyps are benign tumors composed of normal cervical glands and stroma. In general, cervical polyps are pedunculated and protrude through the cervix.[11] Occasionally they may protrude through the vaginal introitus, Endometrial polyps are projections of the endometrium into the uterine cavity. On occasion, endometrial polyps may protrude through the vaginal introitus.[11]

Pathology. Cervical polyps are the second most common cervical lesion, with only chronic inflammation occurring more frequently.[16] Although diagnosed in women of all ages, cervical polyps are most often diagnosed in women during their reproductive years. Cervical polyps generally arise from the endocervical canal although they may arise from the ectocervix. They may be single or multiple in occurrence and are rarely larger than 2 cm in diameter. Recurrence of the polyps after removal is common.[16]

The incidence of endometrial polyps is unknown. They commonly occur in women between 30 and 59 years of age, but have been reported in women ranging in age from 12 to 81 years old.[15] Endometrial polyps are thought to be associated with estrogen activity that is excessive or unopposed by progesterone.

Clinical Manifestations. Cervical and endometrial polyps are generally asymptomatic when very small. When symptomatic, a woman with a large cervical polyp will complain of bleeding with coitus or following douching.[16] Straining with defecation may also produce slight bleeding. This bleeding may be attributed to vascular congestion within the polyp and ulceration on the tip of the polyp.[11] Symptomatic endometrial polyps are associated with nonspecific abnormal uterine bleeding. When endometrial polyps cause bleeding in a postmenopausal woman, it is important to exclude the possibility of coexisting endometrial carcinoma elsewhere in the uterus. The polyp itself is rarely cancerous.[11]

Medical Management

Smaller cervical polyps, missed by simple palpation of the cervix, will frequently be revealed by a speculum examination. Even when diagnosed, since many cervical polyps are asymptomatic and genital bleeding may be due to other more serious conditions, a Pap smear will be done and other possible causes of bleeding will be excluded.[16] Cervical polyps may be removed in an outpatient setting or on hospital admission. Recurrence of cervical polyps following their removal is common. If bleeding persists after therapy, biopsies of the cervix and endometrium will be done to rule out the presence of cancer.

On a hysterosalpingogram, an endometrial polyp may appear as an alteration in the lining of the uterus.[15] Diagnosis of the endometrial polyp is made when a curettage or scraping of the uterus is performed. In addition, endometrial polyps are frequently diagnosed at the time of a hysterectomy. Adequate treatment for the endometrial polyp is accomplished simultaneously by the diagnostic curettage or hysterectomy. If an endometrial polyp protrudes through the cervix, it is important to assure the endometrial rather than cervical origin of the polyp.

Nursing Management

Assessment and Nursing Diagnosis. One of the possible nursing diagnoses is the potential knowledge deficit leading to a disregard of abnormal vaginal bleeding.

Goals. The focus of nursing activities is assuring the prompt health evaluation and continued follow-up of women with unusual vaginal bleeding. Encouraging annual pelvic examinations and teaching the potential for recurrence of cervical polyps are important aims.

Interventions. When abnormal vaginal bleeding occurs, the nurse will counsel the woman to seek medical attention without delay. The rationale for routine complete pelvic examinations, the propensity of cervical polyps to be asymptomatic and to recur, and the possibility of a more serious cause of abnormal vaginal bleeding, form the basis of the teaching plan. Postmenopausal women, in particular, need to report any instances of vaginal bleeding. There is a risk that endometrial carcinoma also is present in the uterus of a woman with diagnosed endometrial polyps. Following cautery or curettage, the woman will be taught to expect temporary foul vaginal discharge or frank vaginal bleeding. If vaginal bleeding persists or recurs following the initial therapy, the woman will be advised to consult her gynecologist for further evaluation.

Evaluation. As a result of a successful teaching plan, the woman treated for endometrial or cervical polyps will obtain routine Pap smears and pelvic examinations; promptly report any unusual vaginal discharge or bleeding; describe the possibility of concurrent endometrial carcinoma; and continue to attend follow-up appointments as long as the health professional determines a need for continued surveillance. Postoperatively, the woman will be without any unusual vaginal discharge or bleeding and her temperature will be within the normal range.

Leiomyoma (Fibroid Tumors)

Definition. A leiomyoma is a benign uterine tumor primarily composed of dense smooth muscle cells in a whorl-like pattern within a fibrious tissue network.[15] Commonly referred to as fibroid tumors, these growths are well circumscribed and surrounded by a pseudocapsule. Some may have an associated peduncle. Leiomyomas rarely occur singly and are generally located in the uterine corpus.

Classification. The location of the tumor within the uterus forms the basis of a classification system for leiomyomas and is associated with the symptoms commonly associated with these tumors. Submucous leiomyomas are located just below the endometrium and are associated with bleeding. Submucous leiomyomas may undergo neoplastic change. Intramural leiomyomas occur within the myometrium and are often responsible for alterations in the size and contour of the uterus. Leiomyomas located immediately beneath the serosal covering of the uterus are subserous tumors. If positioned over a vein, this type of leiomyoma may cause venous rupture and result in intraperitoneal bleeding. Often located near the broad ligament, subserous leiomyomas commonly impinge on the ureters and iliac vessels.[11]

Epidemiology. Leiomyomas are the most common tumors of the female pelvis. They are most commonly diagnosed in women between 30 and 45 years of age. In the United States, a black woman is more likely to have a leiomyoma than a white woman.[11,15]

Etiology. The etiology of leiomyomas has not been fully determined. These benign uterine tumors commonly develop during the reproductive years. Growth of existing tumors may occur as a response to estrogen stimulation. Increase in the size of tumors is associated with both pregnancy and the use of birth control pills, whereas regression in size occurs with menopause.[11] Other unknown factors probably intervene in the causation of leiomyomas since they do not increase in number during pregnancy.[15]

Pathology. Many degenerative changes may occur in leiomyomas. These include hyalinization, calcification, cystic degeneration, fatty degeneration, and necrosis. These changes may be associated with events that alter blood supply to the tumor, for example, rapid growth of the tumor, pregnancy, mechanical accident, or postmenopausal atrophy.[15] Some degenerative changes such as hyalinization are asymptomatic. Others such as necrosis produce symptoms that signal the need for immediate treatment.

Overall, less than 1% of leiomyomas undergo malignant transformation to a leiomyosarcoma.[15] There is concern about the possibility of cancer in fibroid tumors developing or increasing in size after menopause.[11] Since the gross appearance of a benign leiomyoma that has undergone degenerative changes may mimic that of a leiomyosarcoma, histological verification of the nature of the tumor is necessary at the time of surgery.

Clinical Manifestations. Most leiomyomas are asymptomatic even when very large; some are symptomatic only during pregnancy. Abnormal uterine bleeding is a major characteristic of these tumors. Excessive or prolonged menstruation is common; anemia may be an associated finding. Pain often accompanies but is not characteristic of leiomyomas. A woman with a large leiomyoma may complain of a heavy, bearing-down sensation in her pelvis. Dysmenorrhea may be an associated symptom. Necrosis or inflammation of the tumor due to circulatory changes may be associated with the development of abdominal pain and tenderness.

Pressure from an enlarging fibroid tumor may result in a variety of symptoms. Women frequently seek medical attention because of an alteration in their abdominal girth or contour. Urinary frequency and urgency may result from pressure on the bladder. Urinary retention results when the tumor blocks the urethra.[11] Rarely, the tumor will press against the ureters producing hydroureter or hydronephrosis. Occasionally, constipation and painful defecation may be associated symptoms if the tumor presses against the rectum. Lower extremity edema or varicosities, or both may occur from pressure of the tumor on the iliac vessels or vena cava. Pressure on the pelvic nerves may produce pain radiating to the back and lower extremities.

Infertility may be an associated finding, although many women are able to conceive and sustain a pregnancy despite existing fibroid tumors. Leiomyomas developing during pregnancy are associated with an increased frequency of spontaneous abortion in the first trimester.[11] Premature bleeding, blockage of the birth canal, and atonic uterus may interfere with the normal progress of delivery.

Medical Management

A bimanual pelvic examination may reveal displacement of the uterus out of the pelvis and multiple, firm irregular nodules on the uterine surface. Sounding of the uterus may be done during the pelvic examination. Uterine curettage will aid in the diagnosis of submucous leiomyomas.

Treatment is conservative and consists of continued observation if the patient is asymptomatic, postmenopausal, or has multiple, small tumors. These women will be followed closely at 3- to 6-month intervals.[15] A uterine curettage will be done if abnormal uterine bleeding is the presenting symptom to rule out other possible causes of bleeding.

The type of surgery done for those women with symptoms depends in part on the age of the woman, her desire for future childbearing, the nearness of menopause, and her physical ability to tolerate surgery. Surgery will be done when the tumor is larger than a 12- to 14-week pregnancy. Uterine curettage must precede surgery whenever abnormal uterine bleeding is a symptom.

Myomectomy, the removal of the fibroid tumor only, is typically done through an abdominal incision. A single tumor or many tumors may be removed during this surgery. Myomectomy preserves childbearing potential while removing subserous, intramural, or submucous tumors. Complications of myomectomy include pelvic adhesions and bowel obstruction.

If the symptoms are severe, if there are multiple or large tumors, or if preservation of childbearing potential is not a concern, a hysterectomy is the procedure of choice. Most commonly hysterectomy is performed through an abdominal incision although it may be done through a vaginal approach if the tumors are very small and there is concurrent pelvic relaxation. In all cases, curettage of the uterus will precede the hysterectomy to rule out the presence of endometrial or cervical malignancy.[15]

Nursing Management

Assessment and Nursing Diagnosis. Assessment requires a careful history and physical examination. For the patient with leiomyoma, appropriate nursing diagnoses include alteration in comfort: pain or other discomfort related to the presence of the abnormal tissue; knowledge deficit related to abnormal bleeding, understanding the disease, and complying with treatment and follow-up care; and potential ineffective family coping: compromised, related to risk in fertility and spontaneous abortion.

Goals. The goals for the patient with leiomyoma include relief of discomfort, preventing anemia from bleeding, demonstrating understanding of the importance of follow-up care, and recognizing the possibility of unfavorable pregnancy outcomes.

Interventions. Asymptomatic women diagnosed with leiomyoma will need encouragement to attend their follow-up appointments because they may break appointments due to their overall good health. Women with leiomyomas will require close physiological follow-up and emotional support during pregnancy, labor and delivery, and the postpartum period. Those women diagnosed with asymptomatic leiomyoma will benefit from a nursing care plan aimed at symptom management.

In addition to the more common postoperative complications, after multiple myomectomy the nurse must be alert for the signs and symptoms of impending bowel obstruction. In follow-up appointments, the woman will be assessed for the possible development of adhesions. Those women who are concerned about preservation of childbearing, yet must have a hysterectomy because of the severity of associated symptoms, will need consistent emotional support. Counseling about alternative methods of building a family may be appreciated.

The nurse will recognize that careful follow-up is necessary if a postmenopausal woman diagnosed with leiomyoma receives estrogen alone. Any growth of a myoma in a postmenopausal woman may be cancerous and estrogen alone may predispose to growth of the tumor.[11] Estrogen in combination with progesterone may not have this effect.

Evaluation. The patient will state that she has relief from the discomfort associated with the tumor, or has developed methods of coping with it; have a hematocrit within normal limits and be able to carry out activities of daily living without undue fatigue; attend scheduled follow-up appointments to monitor the disorder; and recognize the potential problems associated with pregnancy and investigate family planning alternatives.

Endometriosis

Definition. Endometriosis refers to the presence and proliferation of endometrial tissue in a location distant from the uterine lining. Although a single-area ectopic implantation may exist, there are usually multiple areas of ectopic endometrial tissue.

Etiology. A variety of theories have been advanced to explain the development of endometriosis. None are proven nor individually explain all the cases of endometriosis. One theory proposes that endometrial tissue spreads between the muscle bundles of the myometrium. Another postulates spread by means of venous or lymphatic embolization. Peritoneal tissue, derived from embryonic coelomic epithelium, possibly may be capable of metaplastic change into endometrial tissue under hormonal influences or as an inflammatory response. A final theory proposes that any condition limiting the flow of menstrual fluid through the cervix may induce retrograde flow of menstrual fluid through the fallopian tubes. Endometrial cells are transported and become implanted as a result of some chemical activator secreted by the cells.[11,14]

Epidemiology. The incidence of endometriosis is not consistent throughout the world. In the United States, endometriosis is more common in white women than in black women.[11] Although it may occur at any time in a woman's life span, endometriosis generally occurs in women between 30 and 50 years of age and is unusual before 20 years of age or after menopause. Those women who delay childbirth or are unable to conceive may be at increased risk for endometriosis.

Pathology. Endometriosis is characterized by hemorrhagic spots or blood-filled cysts that are surrounded by dense adhesions.[14] The ectopic endometrial implants contain hormonally responsive glands and stroma that undergo the same changes as the uterine endometrial lining in response to the hormonal fluctuations of the menstrual cycle. Since there is no route for direct external drainage, the menstrual products remain at the site of the ectopic endometrial tissue. Eventually the ectopic menstrual products are absorbed, with fibrosis predominating as healing occurs. Pain is commonly associated with the engorged ectopic implants. Ectopic foci may occur throughout the pelvis but commonly occur on the ovary, the uterine ligaments, the rectovaginal septum, and the pelvic perineum.[11]

Clinical Manifestations. The severity of symptoms does not correlate with the extensiveness of endometriosis. Widespread endometriosis may be asymptomatic. In some cases, endometriosis is an incidental finding during gynecological surgery. Symptoms vary with the location of the ectopic endometrial tissue.

Generally, symptomatic endometriosis is characterized by pain and unusual uterine bleeding. Dysmenorrhea characteristically begins in the twenties and thirties and gradually increases in severity.[14] The pain typically starts on the first day of the menstrual period and peaks on the second or third day. Some women with extensive endometriosis may complain of a vague dull backache and cramping lower abdominal pain that worsens at the time of the menses and decreases after the onset of the menstrual flow. Dyspareunia is a common symptom in sexually active women with endometriosis, particularly if foci involve the uterosacral ligaments and the vagina.[11] Alterations in uterine bleeding are of no particular pattern; the menstrual flow may be excessive, prolonged, or frequent.

When endometrial implants occur in a tubular structure, there is discomfort as well as gradual obstruction of the tubular lumen. During the menstrual period, the stool or urine may be bloody in cases where endometriosis involves the rectum or urinary tract. A history of infertility commonly precedes the diagnosis of endometriosis.

Medical Management

Diagnosis is facilitated by a thorough patient history that may reveal characteristic symptoms of endometriosis. The patient may complain of tenderness and discomfort on vaginal examination. The health professional may be able to palpate multiple nodules, and the uterus may be fixed and retroverted on bimanual examination.[14] Laboratory values will exclude the presence of infection. Laparoscopy confirms the diagnosis and must be performed prior to the initiation of therapy. Classification systems have been devised although none have universal acceptance.[11]

An asymptomatic patient in whom an incidental diagnosis has been made may not require therapy. Mild analgesics may attenuate the slight discomfort these women experience with menstruation. For symptomatic women, therapy is planned at promoting the resolution of symptoms while conserving the woman's potential for fertility if she so desires. A young, symptomatic woman without severe symptoms or large palpable masses may be scheduled for frequent examinations if she is attempting pregnancy. If pregnancy occurs the endometriosis may be relieved as a result of decidual reaction in the endometrial foci. Other women may be offered treatment with gradually increasing doses of ovarian hormones, particularly progesterone. This hormone may be used to suppress menstruation for up to 9 months. Side-effects of progesterone therapy include weight gain, nausea, breast changes, breakthrough bleeding, an increase in vaginal discharge, and thromboembolism. Any coexisting uterine fibroids may enlarge. A history of thromboembolism is a contraindication for this type of treatment. Danazol, an antigonadotropin, has been used recently. Regression of lesions may occur within 3 to 18 months, but side-effects including hot flashes, weight gain, hirsutism, acne, and muscle enlargement may be discouraging.[14] Many infertile women with endometriosis are able to become pregnant within the first year following treatment with danazol.

If symptoms worsen, or if infertility persists more than 1 year, conservative surgery involving excision or cautery of all possible ectopic lesions and restoration of a normal pelvis will be done. In those cases where the lesion impinges on a tubular structure, surgery involves excision of the ectopic foci followed by reanastomosis. If symptoms are severe in a younger woman, hysterectomy will be done in addition to the above procedure. All or part of the ovaries will be conserved. If any endometrial implants remain, recurrence is possible due to the fluctuation of ovarian hormones. A hysterectomy with bilateral salpingo-oophorectomy will be performed for older women approaching menopause or those women who have no further desire for childbearing.

Nursing Management

Assessment and Nursing Diagnosis. Since infertility commonly precedes the diagnosis of endometriosis, a history of infertility combined with symptoms of pain and unusual bleeding needs careful analysis. The appropriate nursing diagnoses are similar to those for the patient with leiomyoma.

Interventions. Since pain is frequently associated with endometriosis, pain assessment and pain management techniques are important interventions for the nurse. Analgesics and other techniques to modify the experience of pain may be useful. For the experience of mild pain, aspirin or acetaminophen may suffice. If the pain is severe, more potent analgesics may need to be prescribed until definitive therapy can be instituted.

Because infertility associated with this disease may be permanent, much mental anguish may be experienced by the woman and her partner. They will be encouraged to express their feelings about the inability to conceive and emotional support will be offered. Alternative methods of family planning will be reviewed.

Evaluation. The patient will state that she has relief of discomfort, or has developed methods of coping with it. She will recognize the potential problems of infertility and investigate other alternatives for having a family, if that is a concern of hers.

Neoplastic Disorders of the Female Reproductive System

Cancer of the Vulva

Classification. Almost all of the histological types of cancer occurring on the vulva are squamous cell carcinoma. A small percentage of the invasive cancers are due to basal cell carcinoma. The rest are due to melanoma, sarcoma, and adenocarcinoma.[5]

Epidemiology. As with other cancers, the cause of cancer of the vulva is unknown. Vulvar cancer is a rare lesion, accounting for 3% to 4% of all primary gynecological malignancies.[22] Rarely occurring in women less than 40 years of age, invasive vulvar cancer is most commonly seen in women between 60 and 70 years of age. Women who have had cancer of the breast, cervix, urethra, or the head and neck are at increased risk of a later diagnosis of primary cancer of the vulva.[22] In part because the lesion is so rare, little is known of the epidemiology of cancer of the vulva.

Pathology. Leukoplakia is considered a precancerous change and is found in almost half of the women with cancer of the vulva.[22] More than half of the vulvar cancer lesions are located on the labia majora.[5] The labia minora, the clitoris, and Bartholin's gland are locations involved with vulvar cancer in order of decreasing frequency. Occasionally, the urethra, vagina, and anus may be involved with vulvar cancer.

Lymph node involvement is present in 30% to 40% of cases of cancer of the vulva. The inguinal nodes are commonly involved with cancer, yet their status cannot be determined by palpation alone. Pelvic lymph nodes are rarely positive if the inguinal nodes are negative. Pelvic node metastasis is a very poor prognostic sign.[5] All classifications of vulvar cancer except melanoma are thought to be spread by lymphatic embolization.[22]

Clinical Manifestations. In some instances, vulvar cancer is asymptomatic and found only on pelvic examination. The most common symptom associated with vulvar cancer is pruritis.[5] Other signs include a mass, an elevated lesion, or a sore on the vulva. An advanced vulvar tumor may be accompanied by local necrosis, infection, odor, pain, bleeding, and other drainage.

Medical Management

A complete pelvic examination will be done to assist in the evaluation of vulvar cancer. All suspicious vulvar lesions must be biopsied to establish the diagnosis of vulvar cancer. A chest x-ray study, sigmoidoscopy, and cystoscopy may be done to assess for possible metastasis.

A radical vulvectomy, the en block removal of the vulva and perineal tissues (including the labia, clitoris, prepuce, fourchette, paraurethral tissue, vestibule, and Bartholin's gland), is generally the treatment of choice for primary invasive carcinoma of the vulva. During the radical vulvectomy, drains may be placed in the wound. Postoperatively, these drains may be connected to suction to decrease the accumulation of serum in the wound and minimize the possibility of skin flap sloughs.[5] Patients may be confined to bed for 5 days. An indwelling urethral catheter will be inserted during surgery. Complications of radical vulvectomy frequently include wound sloughing and infection as well as pulmonary emboli.[5, 22]

An inguinal and femoral node dissection may be done simultaneously with the radical vulvectomy or at a later operation. Pelvic node dissection may be added to this procedure if the superficial nodes are positive. Lower extremity edema may complicate the postoperative course following retroperitoneal pelvic node dissection. The physician may prescribe low-dose heparin, prophylactic antibiotics, and well-fitting thigh-high support stockings. Use of these stockings may be recommended for as long as 6 months following surgery.[22] Teaching the woman care, application, and removal techniques of the stockings will facilitate compliance with wearing them.

Those women with positive nodes have a 5-year survival rate of 12% to 38%.[22] For all cases of vulvar cancer that are treated by radical vulvectomy and lymphadenectomy, the 5-year survival rate is between 60% and 70%.[5] The cytotoxic drug Adriamycin may be utilized alone or in combination with other chemotherapeutic drugs for patients who have advanced vulvar cancer that does not respond to surgery or irradiation.

Nursing Management

Assessment and Nursing Diagnosis. A few of the nursing diagnoses include guilt or anxiety related to delayed diagnosis of vulvar cancer; postoperative alteration in urinary elimination: difficulty in initiating or directing the stream of urine, related to postoperative edema or loss of the labia; and anxiety related to fear of pain with intercourse or the partner's reaction to the appearance of the surgical area.

Goals. Nursing activities are devised to identify feelings concerning the timing of the diagnosis of the cancer, prevent tension and contamination of the surgical incisions, promote a full and directed postoperative stream of urine, and promote a positive sexual self-concept and comfortable sexual functioning.

Interventions. Vulvar cancer is often not immediately diagnosed because the woman utilized self remedies or did not recognize the seriousness of the pruritis. Women will need emotional support if they delayed in seeking treatment because of neglect or embarrassment due to the location of the tumor. A pragmatic approach to assessment and counseling about the timing of the diagnosis may help the woman accept her health condition.

Preoperatively, a woman can expect cleansing enemas to decrease the risk of fecal contamination of the surgical area in the immediate postoperative period. Postoperatively, she will be placed on a low-residue diet for the same purpose.

The initial urge to defecate may be a time of anxiety for the woman who may fear pain. Analgesics may decrease any associated pain and assist the woman to relax during defecation. Stool softeners may be prescribed to facilitate defecation. Sitz baths may be ordered to promote healing and to assure cleanliness of the area after defecation or urination. Wound irrigations with prescribed solutions may be ordered. These may later be replaced by sitz baths followed by heat lamp application to dry the area and promote circulation. Some physicians prefer to leave the incisions exposed to the air after the initial surgical dressings are removed, whereas others prefer to continue the use of dressings throughout the postoperative period. If dressings are used they will be secured by a T binder or a perineal pad and belt.

The indwelling urethral catheter may pose a risk for urinary tract infection, but when it is removed, the woman may have difficulty voiding due to edema. When edema has decreased, the urethral catheter will be removed. Once she is able to urinate, the woman may discover difficulty in directing the stream of urine since the labia have been removed. Altering the position on the toilet and experimenting with the angle of her thighs may aid in directing the urine into the toilet.

Prescribed limitations on movement may help to minimize tension on the suture line. Assistance with turning and pillows may be necessary to maintain the necessary position.

Removal of the vulvar tissue is disfiguring and may interfere with the woman's usual sexual functioning. For some women, this may be overwhelming. Nurses should help women express any concerns they might have about threats to their self-concept, or sexual functioning due to the surgery. Some women may feel diminished by the loss of the vulva. They may fear the response of their partner to the sight of the surgical area. They may have concerns about closeness during the prescribed time period when vaginal intercourse is discouraged and about the possibility of painful vaginal intercourse after surgery. Nurses should encourage the woman to discuss her concerns with her partner. Both the woman and her partner should recognize the value of touching and caressing in expressing caring. A warm sitz bath or a mild analgesic prior to intercourse may facilitate relaxation and enjoyment of intercourse.

Evaluation. As a result of comprehensive care, the woman with vulva cancer will verbalize her concerns regarding the length of time between the occurrence of the cancer and the diagnosis of cancer. After a radical vulvectomy with inguinal or femoral node dissection, or both, the woman will have incisions that are clean and dry with well-approximated edges; state the rationale for any prescribed restriction of hip joint movement in the immediate postoperative period; request assistance with mobility in bed in the immediate postoperative period; relate or state potential methods to direct the postoperative urinary stream into the toilet; if appropriate, role play ways to appraise real or potential sexual partner's response to the surgical alterations in her anatomy; and if applicable, relate ways to facilitate comfortable vaginal intercourse that are acceptable to the woman and her sexual partner.

Cancer of the Vagina

Classification. Most of the cancers occurring in the vagina are not primary cancers. Metastasis from choriocarcinoma, and extension of cancer of the cervix or other adjacent organs (specifically the uterus, ovaries, vulva, bladder, and rectum) account for the majority of cancers occurring on the vagina.

Primary cancer of the vagina occurs very rarely. Almost all of the cases of primary vaginal cancer are epidermoid cancers. Adenocarcinoma is diagnosed in approximately 5% of elderly women with vaginal cancer, and sarcoma is even less frequent in older women. Clear cell adenocarcinoma of the vagina has been diagnosed in daughters of pregnant women who received diethylstilbestrol (DES).

Etiology and Epidemiology. Partially due to the rarity of vaginal cancer, epidemiological factors are unclear. Primarily, vaginal cancer occurs in women between the ages of 50 and 70 years old.

Adenocarcinoma of the vagina, a rare disease, has been found in young women exposed *in utero* to synthetic nonsteroidal estrogens, primarily DES. DES and other implicated nonsteroidal estrogens were prescribed for pregnant women with the objective of preventing spontaneous abortion. The daughters of these women, at a mean age of 19 years old, are at risk for certain cell changes in the vagina.[22] The majority of women exposed to DES *in utero* will have adenosis of the vagina. The incidence of adenocarcinoma of the vagina in these women is less than 0.1 percent.[4]

Pathology. In order to establish a diagnosis of vaginal cancer, the lesion must be located on the vagina without extension to either the cervix or the vulva. Most of the cases of squamous cell carcinoma are found on the upper third of the posterior vaginal wall. Most of the clear cell adenocarcinoma lesions are located on the upper third of the anterior vaginal wall.[22] However, both types may be found on any region of the vagina. An extensive primary tumor correlates with a high incidence of nodal involvement, with metastasis often occurring in the lungs.

Clinical Manifestations. The earliest symptom of vaginal cancer is abnormal vaginal bleeding associated with vaginal intercourse or vaginal speculum examination. The woman may complain of pain with intercourse. A foul vaginal discharge and pelvic pain may accompany extensive disease. When the tumor involves the rectum or bladder, pain with defecation or urination and other excretory symptoms may occur.[4]

Medical Management

Routine Pap smears aid in the diagnosis of squamous cell carcinoma of the vagina but are not as useful in cases of clear cell adenocarcinoma since it is a subepithelial lesion.[22] Therefore, all suspicious vaginal lesions should be examined and biopsied regardless of the results of cytological examination. Visualization and palpation of the entire vagina is important in diagnosing vaginal cancer because small lesions may be covered by the speculum.

In addition to a pelvic examination, physicians may order cystoscopy and sigmoidoscopy to determine whether the lesion has extended into the surrounding areas, bladder, or rectum. Biopsies of multiple sites in the vagina and on the cervix will be done.[22] Therapy for vaginal cancer is controversial over whether irradiation or surgery should be employed first.

In addition, for women who were exposed to DES *in utero,* regular pelvic examinations are recommended starting at puberty. Prophylactic resection of vaginal adenosis is controversial. Irradiation or surgery may be used to treat clear cell adenocarcinoma of the vagina. An annual chest x-ray study may be recommended to assist in the early detection of possible lung metastasis.

Nursing Management

Assessment and Nursing Diagnosis. A few of the relevant nursing diagnoses include anxiety and possibly anger related to the risk of vaginal cancer associated with prior use of DES; distress about limitation in childbearing ability related to hysterectomy or pelvic irradiation, or both; fear of painful intercourse related to vaginal incision or vaginal irradiation changes; and potential alteration in elimination related to fistula formation associated with prior irradiation of extensive vaginal lesions.

Goals. Nursing care of young women diagnosed with DES-related vaginal cancer involves promoting the resolution of feelings related to the use of the drug by the woman's mother. All premenopausal women diagnosed with vaginal cancer should be encouraged to identify their feelings about the possible effect of treatment on childbearing capability. Achieving comfortable vaginal intercourse is important for all sexually active women. Women treated with pelvic irradiation need to understand the possible complications associated with this form of therapy.

Interventions. Emotional support is necessary for both the mothers who took DES while pregnant and their daughters who are affected by *in utero* exposure to DES. Although the drug was taken to preserve a pregnancy, the mothers may have unresolved guilt over the unforeseen complication associated with the use of the medication. The daughters who were exposed to the drug *in utero* may be faced with concerns about their sexuality at an age when their developing sexuality is of prime importance. Promoting frank discussions between mother and daughter may help resolve these feelings and concerns.

Since pelvic irradiation may result in menopause, and hysterectomy precludes childbearing, premenopausal women with vaginal cancer need to be counseled about these therapy effects. Adoption and other means of acquiring children can be reviewed with women who desire to have a family at some point in the future.

Young women who were exposed *in utero* to DES should consult their physicians about the optimum frequency of routine pelvic examinations and Pap smears. Vaginal reconstruction may be offered to those women who have had surgical resections of all or part of the vagina. Teaching the technique and rationale for the prescribed use of a vaginal dilator is necessary to assure that the reconstructed vagina remains patent. Use of the vaginal dilator helps prevent closure of the new vagina. Since some women may be reluctant to insert the dilator, exploring feelings concerning insertion and use of the dilator may be helpful in assuring compliance and preventing closure of the new vagina. Tissue used to form the new vagina may not have the ability to secrete mucus. Therefore, use of water-soluble lubricants must be reviewed with the woman in order to promote comfortable vaginal intercourse.

For women with extensive vaginal lesions treated with irradiation, there is a long-term risk of fistula formation. Pragmatic counseling about reporting associated symptoms to the physician may facilitate learning. If the physician prescribes frequent chest x-rays, the nurse may counsel the patient regarding the purpose of these tests to assure compliance.

All women should be encouraged to consult their physicians whenever unusual vaginal bleeding occurs. The importance of regular pelvic examinations and Pap smears cannot be overemphasized.

Evaluation. Nursing intervention has been successful when women exposed to DES *in utero* confront their feelings about the possibility of cancer and participate in planned follow-up. All women treated for vaginal cancer should schedule and attend follow-up appointments for pelvic examinations and Pap smears at intervals prescribed by their physicians, be able to discuss their concerns about the possibility of limitations in childbearing with at least one person of their choice, and name personally acceptable aids to comfortable vaginal intercourse after vaginal reconstruction. Those women receiving irradiation for vaginal cancer will describe the symptoms of fistula formation and relate the necessity of informing their physician when any of these symptoms occur.

Cancer of the Cervix

Classification. Almost 95% of the cases of cervical cancer are due to squamous cell carcinoma. Adenocarcinoma representing malignant transformation of the columnar cells of the endocervix accounts for about 4% of the cancers occurrring on the cervix.[19] Sarcoma and malignant lymphoma rarely occur.

Epidemiology. Cancer of the cervix accounts for 6% of all cancers occurring in women. The incidence and mortality associated with invasive cervical cancer has decreased over time, whereas the incidence of carcinoma *in situ* (CIS) of the cervix has increased.

Risk factors associated with the development of cervical cancer include multiple sexual partners, the initial experience of sexual intercourse at an early age, low socioeconomic status, a large number of pregnancies, and highly stressing life changes within the previous 1 to 2 years. The association with cervical cancer of exposure of the cervix to sperm and uncircumcised male partners is controversial and not universally accepted. Cervical cancer is an infrequent development in nulliparious women and celibate women, for example, nuns.[22]

Etiology. Data from animal and human experiments implicate herpes simplex virus Type II (HSV-2) as a possible etiologic agent in the development of cervical cancer.[22] A possible role for a different virus, human papillomavirus (HPV), is also being explored.

Pathology. Almost 95% of the cases of cervical cancer occur in the squamocolumnar junction of the cervix. It is postulated that the cervix is more susceptible to carcinogens during adolescence when cellular changes similar to metaplasia occur at the squamocolumnar junction.

Certain cellular changes may precede the diagnosis of cervical cancer. Cervical dysplasia can progress through mild, moderate, and severe phases representing increasing cellular atypia and depth of epithelial penetration. At each phase of dysplasia, the lesion may regress toward normal, persist indefinitely, or progress in severity. CIS represents a cervical lesion with high malignant potential that has not yet penetrated the basement membrane of the cervical epithelium. It may follow untreated severe dysplasia, usually after a prolonged period of time. Without treatment, CIS will progress to invasive cervical cancer.

Cervical cancers are generally friable and bleed easily. They may appear as ulcerations or as cauliflowerlike growths. The principal growth mechanism of these tumors is local spread. Untreated cervical cancers will spread toward the vagina or through the endocervical canal into the uterus, or both. If the tumor extends through the vaginal wall it can penetrate the pelvic organs, particularly the bladder or rectum, or both, adjacent support structures of the reproductive organs, and the rest of the peritoneal cavity. Further extension of the tumor results in lymph node involvement. The paracervical and parametrial lymph nodes may be the first nodes involved with malignancy. The external iliac and hypogastric nodes are involved later.

Metastasis occurs in the lungs, liver, and bones, particularly the pelvic bones and vertebrae. The left supraclavicular lymph node is the most common nodal site of spread outside of the pelvis. Mediastinal nodes may also be involved with cancer.

Clinical Manifestations. Early cervical cancer can be entirely asymptomatic and be discovered only by routine Pap smear. Symptoms of advanced disease include bleeding after intercourse or between the menses, painful vaginal intercourse, and foul smelling serous or serosanguineous vaginal discharge. Fatigue and other symptoms of anemia may be present if chronic bleeding is a symptom. Pelvic pain with hematuria or rectal vaginal bleeding may occur if the cancer invades the bladder or rectum. On pelvic examination, the lesion may appear as an ulcerated area or a raised reddish lesion on the ectocervix or vaginal apex.

Medical Management

All women are encouraged to have routine Pap smears. In 1976, the American Cancer Society officially recommended screening of asymptomatic women in the general population at 3-year intervals rather than the previously accepted yearly examination. These guidelines are still controversial and do not apply to women at high risk for cervical cancer or with known cervical pathology who must consult their physician for individual recommendations for optimal frequency of Pap smears.

A Pap smear examining the ectocervix, the endocervical canal, and the pooled secretions in the vaginal fornices will assist in the diagnosis of cervical cancer. Results of the Pap smear are classed according to the degree of cellular atypia observed. The physician may recommend repeated Pap smear within a few weeks if the results are abnormal. A second abnormal Pap smear usually indicates the need for further investigation. A colposcopy, which magnifies the surface of the cervix, may be done. Biopsy will be done of any abnormal areas. A conization of the cervix will be done if the biopsy demonstrates CIS, if the lesion extends into the endocervical canal beyond visualization with the colposcope, or if no lesion is observed.

Adequate treatment for CIS may be accomplished by biopsy, cautery, conization, laser therapy, or hysterectomy. In young women desiring future pregnancy, conization followed by periodic examinations may be performed. The entire lesion as well as a surrounding margin of normal tissue must be removed for the therapy to be successful. If the lesion extends to the perimeter of the excised tissue, the possibility exists that cancer cells remain. Alternatively, CIS may be treated by a total abdominal hysterectomy. For older women, irradiation may be substituted if surgery is contraindicated or the lesions cover extensive areas of the cervix and vagina.

Diagnostic tests are done if invasive cancer is found. Cystoscopy may be ordered to check for possible involvement of the ureters and bladder. If renal function tests are abnormal, an intravenous pyelogram will be ordered. Barium enema and sigmoidoscopy may be ordered to check for rectal involvement if the cancer is extensive or if the patient is symptomatic. Lymphangiogram will demonstrate any involvement of the pelvic or periaortic lymph nodes. A computerized tomography (CT) scan of the liver may be ordered if liver function tests are abnormal. A baseline chest x-ray film will be taken. If the cancer is recurrent and the woman is a candidate for ultraradical surgery, a CT scan of the lungs will be done. Finally, an examination under anesthesia (EUA) may be scheduled to facilitate careful and complete clinical assessment of the extent of the tumor. The results of the diagnostic tests are used to describe the extent of the cancer.

Although therapy is individualized, early stage invasive cervical cancer generally is treated by radical hysterectomy with pelvic and para-aortic lymphadenectomy. Complications associated with a radical hysterectomy include fistula formation, hemorrhage, and bowel obstruction. In some instances, external or intracavitary irradiation may be administered preoperatively or postoperatively in the attempt to shrink the tumor mass or eradicate residual tumor foci remaining after surgery. External irradiation will be delivered to the pelvic field to include the common iliac nodes and the upper half of the vagina. Intracavitary irradiation involves the insertion of a device containing a radioactive material, commonly radioactive ^{137}Ce, into the vagina and sometimes the uterus. Tandem and vaginal colpostats are one way to deliver the intracavitary irradiation. Combination chemotherapy using cisplatin and 5-fluorouracil has shown some effectiveness in the treatment of advanced cervical cancer.

If cervical cancer persists despite treatment or if there is recurrent cervical cancer, the woman may be treated by ultraradical pelvic surgery, specifically pelvic exenteration. Total pelvic exenteration involves removal of the uterus, tubes, ovaries, vagina, pelvic lymph nodes, bladder, and rectum. A urinary diversion and a descending colostomy, usually a sigmoid colostomy, will be performed. If the rectum is not involved with tumor, it is possible to spare the rectum and normal bowel functioning. In this case, a colostomy is not done and the procedure is called an anterior pelvic exenteration. In a similar manner, during a posterior pelvic exenteration the bladder will be spared since it is not involved with cancer. In many cases, exenteration is performed in a woman who has had prior pelvic irradiation. For this reason, healing is sometimes delayed.

Nursing Management

Assessment and Nursing Diagnosis. Although decreasing in frequency, cervical cancer still may have a major impact among women. A few of the relevant nursing diagnoses are potential knowledge deficit related to early identification; prevention and treatment; and anxiety or depression related to the loss of the uterus and the accompanying therapies.

Goals. The goals for the women at risk for cancer of the cervix include frequent follow-up and assessment of general and gynecological health and identification of those risk factors that she can modify. For those women with cervical cancer, the goals also include acceptance of the diagnosis and effects of therapy, understanding of the importance of consistent monitoring, and resumption of previous lifestyle.

Interventions. Since there are no early symptoms of the disease and routine Pap smears are essential for the detection of early cervical alterations, women must take the responsibility for having routine Pap smears. Each woman must consult her physician regarding the optimal frequency of Pap smears for her. Nurses may counsel interested women about ways to modulate risk factors that are within the woman's control. For example, it is possible to limit the number of future sexual partners and decrease the number of significant life changes made within any time period. Women with cervical alterations such as severe dysplasia must be counseled to comply with frequent Pap smears as a method of monitoring the status of the cervix.

Nursing care for women receiving any form of therapy for cervical cancer must provide competent care for the women's physical and emotional needs. Assessment of the importance of the uterus to the woman and provision of emotional support is crucial since both the uterus and its associated functions are an integral component of the sexual self-concept of many women.

In addition to common side-effects and the nursing care associated with external irradiation, those women receiving external irradiation to the pelvis may experience changes in the bowel functioning, particularly diarrhea. Modification of fiber content in the diet, increased fluid intake, and assessment of stool consistency and frequency are nursing activities. When women are treated by total pelvic exenteration, expert nursing care is essential. This ultraradical surgery necessitates careful emotional counseling and skillful physiological monitoring. Initially, the woman may be monitored carefully in an intensive care environment. After physiological parameters are stabilized, she will return to her prior hospital room. The woman will have a colostomy, a urinary diversion, and a draining vaginal vault. Fostering acceptance of the bodily changes necessitates teaching ways to cope with the effects of surgery. Teaching approaches to help the woman incorporate her care routines into her daily life are valuable. Initial packing in the vaginal vault will be changed after a few days. When nursing assumes responsibility for packing the wound, teaching the patient self-care may begin with a description of the drainage and the purpose of the dressings. At hospital discharge, the woman must be able to perform care of the urinary diversion, colostomy, and perineal wound independently. At a later time, vaginal reconstruction may be offered.

Evaluation. The woman at risk for cancer of the cervix will participate in regular physical examination and Pap smear; and recognize those behaviors that increase her risk for cervical cancer and will modify those over which she has control. The woman who has cancer of the cervix will identify her individual concerns regarding the diagnosis and the loss of her uterus; participate in the prescribed therapies for and monitoring of the disease; and resume her previous life patterns.

Cancer of the Endometrium

Classification. More than 90% of endometrial cancers are adenocarcinomas (Fig. 102–3).[22] Adenosquamous carcinoma and, rarely, clear cell carcinoma also occur in the endometrium.

Epidemiology. Endometrial carcinoma is the most frequently occurring gynecological cancer. Primary cancer of the endometrium is diagnosed in postmenopausal women between 60 and 70 years of age.[22] While about one fourth of the cases of endometrial cancer are diagnosed before menopause, it is rare before 40 years of age. A variety of conditions have been associated with elevated risk for endometrial cancer including obesity, diabetes mellitus, hypertension, and a history of infertility. Experiencing menopause after the age of 52 and being Jewish are other factors associated with an increased risk of cancer of the endometrium.

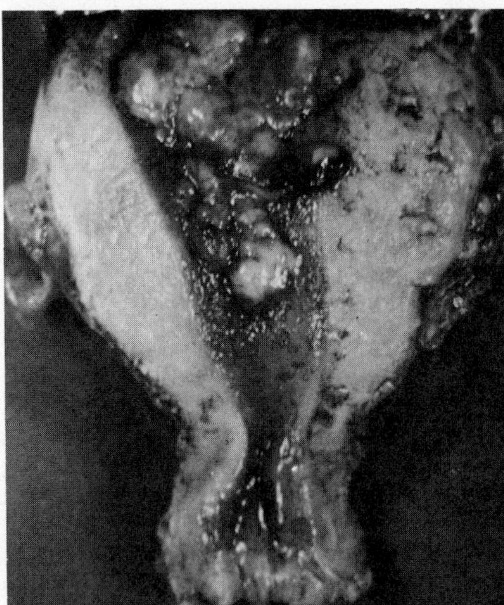

FIGURE 102–3 Adenocarcinoma of endometrium with invasion of uterine wall. (Gusberg SB, Deppe G: Malignant lesions of the corpus uteri. In Danforth DN, Dignam WJ, Hendricks CH, Maeck JVS (eds): Obstetrics and Gynecology, 4th ed, p 1096. Philadelphia, JB Lippincott, 1982)

Etiology. Although the cause of endometrial cancer is unknown, it is thought to be associated with a derangement in endogenous estrogen secretion. This type of cancer is uncommon in women who have had their ovaries removed for other reasons. The view that endometrial cancer is associated with exogenous estrogen administration is controversial.[22] Prolonged use of exogenous estrogens unopposed with progesterone may increase a woman's risk of endometrial cancer particularly if the estrogens are taken for more than 3 years.

Pathology. Adenomatous hyperplasia of the endometrium and cystic hyperplasia may be precursors of endometrial cancer in some patients. The cancers are generally found in the uterine fundus. Growth of the tumors, involving infiltration and penetration of the myometrium, is associated with enlargement of the uterus and thickening of the uterine wall.[22] Spread may occur to the broad ligament and parametrium and occasionally to the endocervix and cervix. Through hematogenous spread, metastasis may occur in the lung, bone, and brain.

Clinical Manifestations. Vaginal bleeding after the menopause, termed *postmenopausal bleeding* (PBM), is the most frequent symptom of endometrial cancer. In the perimenopausal period, menometrorrhagia, or excessive prolonged vaginal bleeding at irregular intervals, may signal endometrial cancer. Persistent irregular bleeding is a symptom of endometrial cancer in young obese women.

Medical Management

A Pap smear is not a useful screening device for endometrial cancer since the Pap smear may be positive for cancer in only 50% to 60% of cases of endometrial cancer. Therefore, a negative Pap smear does not exclude the possibility of cancer of the endometrium.

When endometrial cancer is suspected, a complete pelvic and rectal examination will be done. Because it is possible to segregate uterine tissue from endocervical tissue by means of a fractional dilation and curettage, this procedure may be done to diagnose endometrial cancer. An endometrial biopsy also may be performed. Once endometrial cancer is diagnosed, additional tests will be ordered to determine the extent of the disease.

Staging of the tumor is influenced by the size of the uterus, the depth of myometrial penetration, the presence of malignant cells in the peritoneal fluid, and the status of the pelvic and periaortic nodes.

Adequate surgical therapy for early endometrial cancer involves a total abdominal hysterectomy, bilateral salpingo-oophorectomy, and saline wash of the peritoneal cavity. Stage II endometrial cancer may be treated by a radical hysterectomy with pelvic lymph node dissection and preoperative or postoperative internal or external pelvic irradiation or by a total abdominal hysterectomy with irradiation. More extensive endometrial cancer may be treated with external irradiation or internal irradiation, or both. Chemotherapy may be used as adjuvant therapy in the more advanced stages of disease.

Nursing Management

Assessment and Nursing Diagnosis

Endometrial cancer is predominantly a problem of postmenopausal women. The nursing diagnoses may include knowledge deficit related to the significance of postmenopausal bleeding; alteration in comfort related to the surgical procedures and treatment modalities; and social isolation related to irradiation implantation.

Goals. The goals for the woman with endometrial cancer include prompt recognition and treatment of the abnormal bleeding; relief of discomfort from the therapeutic modalities; and provision of cognitive and social stimulation within the constraints of radiation safety.

Interventions

The importance of periodic gynecological evaluations cannot be overemphasized. All women with changes in their menstrual cycles must consult a health professional without delay. Postmenopausal women must seek medical attention as soon as any vaginal bleeding occurs. Individualized consultation at periodic intervals with a health professional is mandatory when a woman is taking unopposed estrogen therapy for menopausal symptoms.

Posthysterectomy Care. A total abdominal hysterectomy with a salpingo-oophorectomy is a major abdominal surgery. Some women may be confused to have postoperative vaginal bleeding despite an abdominal incision. The vaginal bleeding will taper and cease in the postoperative period. Cyclic menstrual flow will not resume. Due to manipulation of the intestines during surgery, temporary bowel atony may occur postoperatively. Auscultation of positive bowel tones must be possible before food or fluids are offered to the woman. An indwelling urethral catheter will be inserted prior to surgery. This catheter is generally removed the first day after surgery. To minimize the risk of thrombophlebitis, active range-of-motion exercise is encouraged along with early and frequent ambulation, support hose, and frequent changes of position in bed. Removal of the uterus and ovaries means the loss of childbearing ability by premenopausal women. Some women may associate the uterus with femininity and equate the loss of the uterus with a lack of femininity. Assessment of the concerns of the woman is important. Many physicians recommend resumption of vaginal intercourse beginning approximately 6 weeks after surgery for sexually active women.

Irradiation Considerations. Those women treated with intracavitary irradiation will be placed in a private room for the duration of the treatment. Consideration must be given to ways to minimize unwanted radiation exposure to visitors, nursing personnel, and to the noncancerous tissues of the woman. Isolation may be problematic for these women. Boredom may be combated by reading and quiet activities in bed.

During the time that the woman has the radiation implant in place, visitors will be restricted. No pregnant woman or individual younger than 18 years of age will be allowed to visit the woman during this time. Visitors will be encouraged not to sit on the bed. Restrictions on the visitors' distance from the bed and the duration of the visit may be imposed.

Considerations of time, distance, and shielding guide the nursing activities with these women. Nursing care must be organized so that the nurse provides for the needs of the woman yet minimizes the time spent in the woman's room. Standing at a distance from the woman while speaking with her will decrease the nurse's exposure to irradiation. Fastening the urinary drainage contained on the bed at a distance from the relative position of the radiation source will minimize the radiation exposure while the nurse periodically drains and measures the urine. In some institutions, lead shields will be placed strategically to decreased radiation exposure. Radiation badges may be used to measure the amount of exposure of the nurse over time.

The woman will be placed on strict bed rest during the time the implant is in place. Log rolling side to side is encouraged, but there may be restrictions on the degree of elevation of the head of the bed. A cleansing enema will be given to evacuate the bowel preoperatively. Antiperistaltic medications may be prescribed for routine administration as well as when the woman complains of the urge to defecate. Prevention of bowel movement during the time that the implant is in place is important. An indwelling urethral catheter will be inserted preoperatively and will remain throughout the time the implant is in place. Oral fluids will be encouraged. Pain medications will be prescribed for use if the woman complains of pain in excess of the expected pressure associated with the implant and the vaginal packing. Should the implant extend through the cervix and into the uterus, the woman will probably complain of painful uterine contractions. Frequent changing of perineal pads or blue pads will help contain drainage and prevent skin maceration. Perineal care will be provided only when necessary. A deodorizer in the room may be helpful in combating odor from any foul vaginal drainage.

It is essential that the implant be removed at the scheduled time. Since the implant is a sealed and contained source, the woman is not radioactive once the implant is removed. There is no necessity for isolation after discharge from the hospital. The woman may have a creamy or creamy pink-tinged vaginal discharge for a few months after the implant is removed. Since adhesions may form in an irradiated vagina, steps will be taken to prevent closure of the vagina. Sexually active women will be encouraged to engage in vaginal intercourse at least twice a week, beginning 3 weeks after the implant is removed. All women will be instructed in the twice weekly use of a vaginal dilator. Women will be taught to insert the dilator as deeply as is comfortable and to keep the dilator in place at least 10 minutes. Any discomfort associated with the use of the dilator will diminish as the vaginal tissues stretch. use of a water-soluble lubricant may make insertion easier. Those women engaging in sexual intercourse may increase natural vaginal secretions by lengthening the time period of foreplay. Tilting the pelvis and altering the placement of legs during intercourse may influence the depth and direction of penile entry and affect the woman's comfort and pleasure with coitus.

Cystitis, altered frequency and consistency of stool, and radiation dermatitis may occur following intracavitary irradiation. Possible long-term sequelae of intracavitary irradiation include fistula formation, and fibrosis of the ureters and small intestine.

Evaluation

The postmenopausal woman will recognize that any uterine bleeding is abnormal and will seek prompt evaluation. The woman treated for endometrial cancer will relate relief of discomfort or those mechanisms for coping with it; and if pertinent, deny excessive boredom during the time the radiation implant is in place.

Cancer of the Ovary

Classification. Approximately 90% of ovarian cancers are epithelial cancers derived from mesothelial tissue covering the surface of the ovarian capsule and lining the crypts that form following ovulation. They may be described as serous, endometroid, or mucinous. Most are of mixed cell types and are named according to the predominant type of tissue involved.

Epidemiology. One out of 80 women will develop ovarian cancer. The incidence of cancer of the ovary is high in industrialized nations except Japan. Ovarian cancer rarely occurs in the very young or very old woman. Its peak incidence occurs in women between 40 and 70 years of age. Those women with a relative high risk of ovarian cancer include pregnant women and those women using oral contraceptives. Though rare in occurrence, ovarian cancer is the fourth most common cause of cancer related death in women in the USA.[32] Women with ovarian cancer have an increased risk for subsequent development of breast cancer.

Etiology. The etiology of ovarian cancer is unknown. Exposure to talcum powder and asbestos, formerly a common contaminant of talcum powder, have been postulated as associated with the development of cancer of the ovary. There is no clear-cut evidence demonstrating an association with the use of synthetic estrogens.

Pathology. Spread of ovarian cancer to the fallopian tubes may occur. In over half of the cases of cancer of the ovary, the malignancy involves both ovaries.[32] Ovarian cancer is characterized by its propensity for spread throughout the peritoneal cavity. The liver, lung, omentum, the peritoneum, the serosal surface of the uterus, and the diaphragm are sites commonly involved in the spread of ovarian cancer. Lymphatic metastasis occurs to the periaortic and pelvic nodes. Ascites may be related to obstruction of the normal outflow of peritoneal fluid and, to a lesser extent, to increased production of transudate.

Clinical Manifestations. Early ovarian cancer is silent and without recognizable symptoms. Often, vague symptoms of abdominal discomfort and nausea are ignored. A woman with ovarian cancer may consult her physician because of vague symptoms including a feeling of abdominal fullness, rapid satiety, and a change in the way her clothes fit. The enlarging tumor mass, ascites, and altered gastrointestinal function occurring with metastasis may contribute to abdominal distention and pain. Shortness of breath signals a large tumor. Respiratory symptoms may be related to the mass of the tumor, the amount of ascitic fluid impinging on the movement of the diaphragm, or actual pleural effusion associated with metastasis.

An adnexal mass found during the pelvic examination of a perimenopausal woman or an ovary larger than 5 cm in diameter mandates further testing to determine whether this finding reflects the presence of ovarian cancer.[32]

Medical Management

Since the majority of cases of ovarian cancer are diagnosed only when the tumor is extensive, scientists are searching for tumor antigens that can be used as tumor markers. Alpha fetoprotein and human chorionic gonadotropin have the potential for assisting with the early diagnosis of initial and recurrent ovarian cancer.

When there is suspicion of ovarian cancer, a complete physical examination including a pelvic examination and a Pap smear will be performed. A negative Pap smear will not be interpreted as excluding the presence of cancer. The physician may order an abdominal ultrasound in order to visualize the tumor and direct percutaneous biopsy of suspicious areas. Some physicians may schedule a laparoscopy. CT scans of the liver, lung, abdomen and pelvis, and other diagnostic tests further clarify the extent of the tumor. A paracentesis will be done if there is increasing abdominal fullness or distention. Fluid obtained from the peritoneum either during separate paracentesis or during definitive surgery will be examined for malignant cells.

Results of these tests will be used to stage the extent of the malignancy. An exploratory laparotomy with saline washings will be performed. The fluid will be examined for malignancy. All visceral and parietal surfaces will be thoroughly examined and palpated. Any suspicious nodular areas will be biopsied. A total abdominal hysterectomy and bilateral salpingo-oopherectomy with an omentectomy will be performed at that time if these structures are involved with tumor. A bulky residual tumor, remaining after the initial surgery, is equated with a poor prognosis. Selective periaortic and pelvic lymphadenectomy also may be done. External irradiation may be recommended postoperatively.

When the ovarian cancer is extensive, cytoreduction, or removal of as much malignant tissue as possible, is performed. Following surgery, radiation therapy or chemotherapy using alkylating agents or cisplatin, or both will be administered. External irradiation or instillation of radioactive isotopes through an intraperitoneal catheter may be effective in shrinking any residual abdominal or pelvic disease.

A second exploratory laparotomy termed "second look" surgery will be done after completion of the irradiation or chemotherapy to determine whether the malignancy persists. Resection of large amounts of the tumor at this time is rarely possible. Radiation will be prescribed if there is persistent disease.

Intestinal obstruction frequently accompanies recurrent or advanced ovarian cancer. Surgical intervention is rarely possible. Instead, conservative treatment including intestinal intubation and hyperalimentation may be prescribed.

Nursing Management

Assessment and Nursing Diagnosis. Ovarian cancer is generally extensive at diagnosis and nursing care is directed toward the presenting symptoms and dysfunctions. The primary nursing diagnoses include alteration in comfort: pain, dyspnea, and vomiting, related to the extent of the tumor and ascites and anticipated grieving related to the prognosis. Other nursing diagnoses may be important depending on presenting symptoms.

Goals. The goals for the woman with ovarian cancer include relief of pain and protracted vomiting; promotion of comfortable breathing; and acceptance of the terminal nature of the disease.

Interventions. Perimenopausal and postmenopausal women who have vague symptoms of abdominal fullness, early satiety, and increasing girth must be encouraged to seek referral to a gynecologist for examination. Those having a palpable ovary on pelvic examination must also be encouraged to comply with further evaluation of this symptom.

Since ovarian cancer is generally in advanced stages at the time of diagnosis despite the woman's feeling well, emotional support and encouragement to comply with diagnostic tests that are frequently uncomfortable is an important nursing activity. As symptoms of ascites, pleural effusion, and intestinal obstruction predominate, the nurse will be involved in activities that increase the woman's comfort. Measures that decrease pain, promote unobstructed respiration, and minimize protracted vomiting will be the major thrust of the plan of care. Comfort measures and skin care are important. Pain medication will be administered, perhaps by continuous infusion.

Elevating the head of the bed or using multiple pillows under the head will assist with ease of respiration. Paracentesis may be performed to temporarily decrease the amount of ascitic fluid and facilitate movement of the diaphragm. Use of antiemetics and gastrointestinal intubation may counter vomiting associated with small bowel obstruction. For these women, hyperalimentation may be prescribed. In the terminal phase of illness, antiperistaltic medications combined with small, frequent servings of favorite foods may be sufficient nutrition.

Evaluation. The woman with ovarian cancer will state that she has an acceptable level of comfort and decreased frequency of vomiting; breathe easily for the level of activity in which she is engaging; discuss her diagnosis and prognosis with selected confidants; and prioritize her time so that she has the strength to enjoy those activities and people important to her.

Problems of the Breast

Fibrocystic Breast Disease

Definition and Etiology. Fibrocystic breast disease represents benign changes occurring in the female breast. These changes, fibrosis of the breast, cystic disease, and adenosis may occur singly or in combination.

Fibrocystic disease is the most common disorder of the female breast. As many as one half of the adult female population may be affected by this benign breast change. It generally occurs before 35 years of age, rarely beginning before adolescence or after menopause.

The cause of fibrocystic breast disease is unknown. A relative or absolute hyperestrinism may contribute to the development of fibrocystic disease. Some feel that an exaggeration of the normal hormonal stimulation occurring during the menstrual cycle is responsible for the development of fibrocystic breast disease.

Pathophysiology. Fibrosis of the breast is an overgrowth of the fibrous stroma of the breast. Periductal and lobar stroma may be obliterated by the severe breast fibrosis. This type of change is generally found unilaterally in the upper outer quadrant of the breast in women who are in their early thirties. On the other hand, cystic disease comprises stromal and epithelial hyperplasia accompanied by cystic dilation of the ducts. Generally multifocal and bilateral, it may nevertheless present as an isolated cyst. Women in the perimenopausal or postmenopausal period of life are at risk for this type of breast change. Once fibrotic or cystic changes develop in the female breast, they persist throughout life without regression.

Adenosis is a benign epithelial change generally occurring in women between 35 and 45 years of age. Marked intraductal hyperplasia without cystic dilation may result in plugging of the ductile tissue. Adenosis may be a precursor of cancer of the breast.

Clinical Manifestations. Fibrocystic breast disease is signaled by a palpable breast mass and breast pain. The pain is cyclical, appearing immediately prior to the start of the menstrual period and then disappearing until the next menstrual period. Fibrocystic breast disease produces a "lumpy" texture making discrimination of normalcy during breast self-examination (BSE) more difficult.

Medical Management

After thorough examination of both breasts, the physician may biopsy suspicious areas of the breast to assure that there is no possibility of simultaneous malignancy. Percutaneous aspiration may be performed with the obtained fluid being sent for cytological evaluation. If fluid cannot be aspirated or if the cells in the aspirant are normal, the possibility of malignancy cannot be ruled out. In this case, an incisional or excisional biopsy removing part or all of the suspicious tissue will allow evaluation of the lesion and facilitate the diagnosis.

Nursing Management

Assessment and Nursing Diagnosis. The textures of the breast in fibrocystic breast disease can be confusing to a woman doing breast self-examination. For women with fibrocystic disease, appropriate nursing diagnoses may include anxiety about breast self-examination related to a knowledge deficit about the textures of a normal and fibrocystic breast and fear that breast tenderness is related to breast cancer.

Interventions. All women must be taught the technique of breast self-examination (BSE) and be encouraged to perform BSE routinely at monthly intervals (Fig. 102–4). Careful mapping of the tissues palpated within the breast, along with a brief description of the associated textures, can help identify normal vs. abnormal alterations in the breast each month. Women with fibrocystic breast disease must consult their physicians whenever they discover a change in their breasts.

Breast pain associated with fibrocystic disease is generally described as soreness. Mild analgesics may be prescribed prior to the menstrual period to combat this pain. Some women are unnerved by the experience of breast pain and fear the possibility of breast cancer. These women should be carefully examined and then reassured that cyclic pain occurring at specific times in the menstrual cycle characterizes fibrocystic breast disease. It is debatable whether avoiding foods and beverages containing caffeine decreases

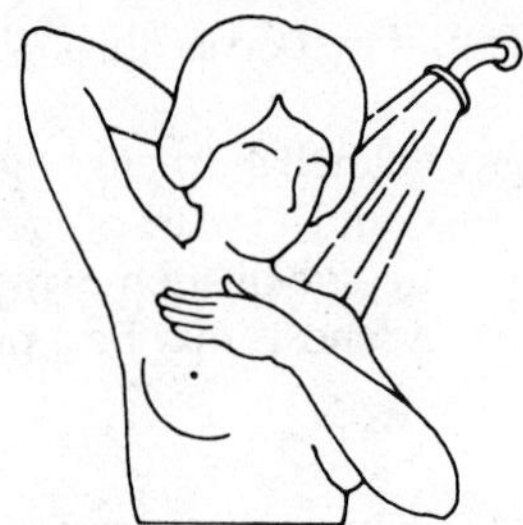

1. In the shower. Examine your breasts during bath or shower; hands glide easily over wet skin. With fingers flat, move them gently over every part of each breast. Check for any lump, hard knot, or thickening.

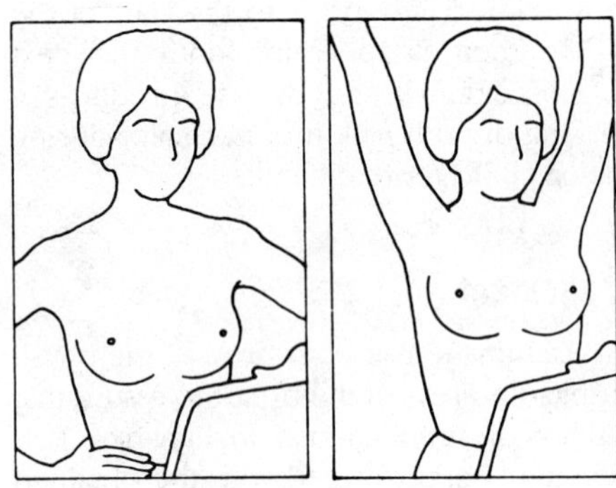

2. Before a mirror. Inspect your breasts with arms at your sides. Next, raise your arms high overhead. Look for any changes in contour of each breast—a swelling, dimpling of skin, or changes in the nipple. Then rest palms on hips and press down firmly to flex your chest muscles. Left and right breast will not match exactly—few women's breasts do. Regular inspection shows what is normal for you and will give you confidence in your examination.

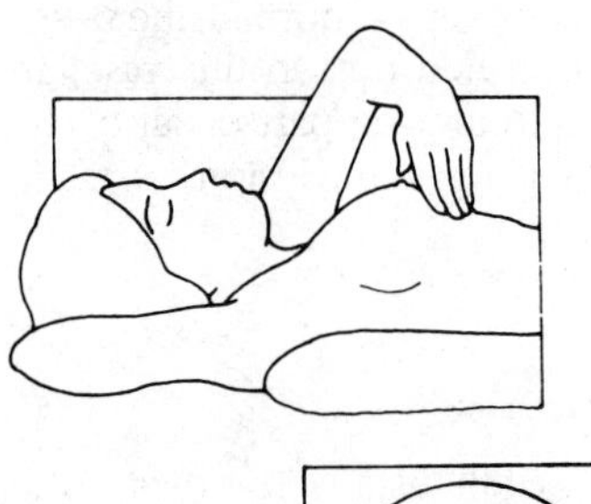

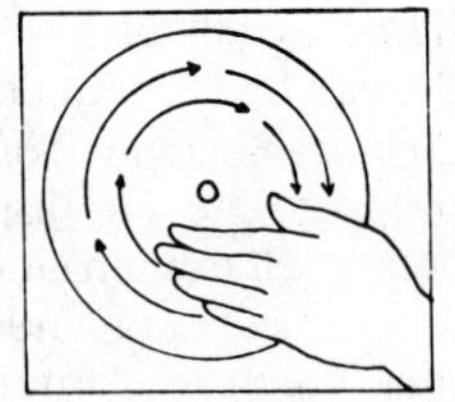

3. Lying down. To examine your right breast put a pillow or folded towel under your right shoulder. Place your right hand behind your head—this distributes breast tissue more evenly on the chest. With left hand, press gently in small circular motions around an imaginary clock face. Begin at outermost top of your right breast for 12 o'clock, then move to 1 o'clock, and so on around the circle back to 12. A ridge of firm tissue in the lower curve of each breast is normal. Then move in an inch, toward the nipple, keep circling to examine every part of your breast, including the nipple. This requires at least three more circles. Now slowly repeat the procedure on your left breast with a pillow under your left shoulder and your left hand behind your head. Notice how your breast structure feels. Finally, squeeze the nipple of each breast gently between your thumb and index finger. Any discharge, clear or bloody, should be reported to your physician immediately.

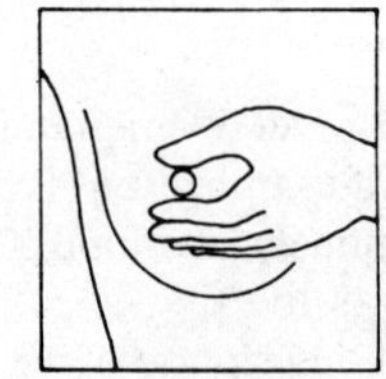

FIGURE 102–4 Self-examination of the breast. (Reprinted by permission of the American Cancer Society, Inc.)

the risk of fibrocystic breast disease. However, some women with fibrocystic disease have decreased their consumption of coffee, tea, colas, and chocolate and have reported a decrease in the "lumpy" texture of their breasts.

Evaluation. The woman will perform monthly breast self-examination; describe the textures of her breast tissue; and discuss the fact that breast tenderness is common in fibrocystic breast disease.

Cancer of the Breast

Classification and Epidemiology

Most of the cancers occurring in the breast are carcinomas and adenocarcinomas. Some sarcomas occur in the breast, whereas mixed carcinosarcomas are very rare. The most common subtype of breast cancer is infiltrating duct carcinoma.

Cancer of the breast strikes 1 in 14 women in the United States.[7] It accounts for 26% of the cancers that occur in women and 16% of the cancer deaths in women.[26] Men are susceptible to breast cancer although it is rarely diagnosed. Those men with a history of gynecomastia are at increased risk for subsequent breast cancer.

Breast cancer is more common in women who have a family history of breast cancer, particularly if the breast cancer has occurred in the woman's mother or sister. When breast cancer occurs in a familial pattern, the cancer is likely to be diagnosed before 40 years of age and to occur bilaterally. The risk of cancer of the breast also is elevated in women who have never been pregnant or those who were pregnant and delivered their first child after 30 years of age. Diagnosis of benign breast disease increases the risk of later diagnosis of breast cancer. Women with a history of cancer in one breast are at increased risk for development of breast cancer in the remaining breast.

Etiology

There is no known cause of breast cancer. In some cases, there appears to be a genetic or hereditary factor involved. Hormonal factors also may play a role. The use of estrogen for the control of menopausal symptoms may be associated with cancer of the breast. The use of birth control pills containing estrogen and progesterone has not been found to be a risk factor. Other factors that may be contributory include viral, dietary (especially a high intake of dietary fat), and immunologic factors. Irradiation of the breast, especially repeated irradiation of the breast of prepubertal girls, may increase the susceptibility to cancer. Massive doses of irradiation have been associated with the occurrence of breast cancer in some women, for example, atomic bomb survivors. The risk associated with low doses used in diagnostic radiology is unknown but felt to be small. Long-term use of reserpine for the control of hypertension may be associated with the development of breast cancer in some women. Further study in this area is necessary.

Pathophysiology

Cancer of the breast is more commonly diagnosed in the left breast than the right breast possibly because the left breast is generally larger than the right. Lesions are generally found in the upper outer quadrant of the breast possibly because relatively more glandular breast tissue is located in this area. Many breast cancers are multicentric, which may be associated with multiple routes of lymphatic spread. Bilateral cancer of the breast does occur and is more common as a sequential occurrence than as a simultaneous occurrence.

Breast cancer infiltrates into surrounding breast tissue along mammary ducts and through the lymphatics, resulting in spread of the overlying skin or deep pectoral fascia, or both. Lymphatic metastasis occurs early with the axillary lymph nodes usually being the first nodal chain affected regardless of the relative location of the cancer in the breast. Other lymph node chains, for example, the internal mammary chain, may be involved with cancer relatively early. However, it is possible for occult distant metastasis to occur in early breast cancer with or without the prior involvement of the lymph nodes with cancer. Sites of frequent metastasis are the liver, bones, pleura, adrenal glands, and the lymph nodes.

As with other cells under the influence of hormones, breast cancer cells have hormone receptors on their cell membrane or in their cytoplasm. Specimens of breast cancer obtained by biopsy are evaluated for the degree to which these receptor sites are present or absent. Receptor sites for estrogen and, to a lesser extent, for progesterone are particularly important. If the breast cancer cells have hormone receptors then the breast cancer may diminish in response to hormonal manipulations either by chemotherapy, or additive or ablative hormonal therapy. A negative receptor status usually means that hormonal manipulation will be of limited or no benefit.

Characteristics important in determining the prognosis and treatment for breast cancer include the menstrual status of the woman, that is, whether she is premenopausal, perimenopausal, or postmenopausal; the estrogen receptor status of the cancer; and the number of axillary nodes involved with cancer at the time of the initial treatment for breast cancer.[7] If the number of positive axillary nodes equals or exceeds four, the prognosis for 5-year cure is generally poor. In the absence of positive nodes, the size and grade of the tumor and the presence of any associated necrosis of the tumor are important determinants influencing prognosis.

Clinical Manifestations

The most common symptom of breast cancer is a dominant lump in the breast generally found by the patient herself. Almost 50% of the time, this lump is located in the upper outer quadrant of the breast. As the tumor grows into the overlying skin and the pectoral fascia, skin dimpling and nipple retraction may occur. An orange-peel-like texture may develop in the breast. Bleeding from the nipple may occur. Ulceration of the breast and pain are late symptoms of breast cancer. Enlargement of the axillary lymph nodes accompanies an advancing malignancy of the breast.

Medical Management

Breast cancer screening by means of mammography and a breast physical examination performed by a physician is recommended at different intervals for the general population depending on the age of the woman. Mammography is of value in screening healthy women 50 years of age or older. The American Cancer Society (ACS) guidelines do not apply to women who belong to a high-risk group or who have a suspicious breast lesion.

In addition to a general history and physical examination, a woman with symptoms of breast cancer will have a complete breast physical examination by her physician. Palpation of the axillary and intraclavicular and supraclavicular nodes is an integral part of this examination. Bilateral mammography or xeromammography will be done to delineate the characteristics of the breast mass and assess the health of the contralateral breast. In some institutions, ultrasound of the breast is also done on an experimental basis. A biopsy of the breast lesion must be done to diagnose the presence and type of cancer and determine the estrogen receptor status of the breast cancer. A chest x-ray study, complete blood count, and liver chemistry will be ordered. More extensive tests will be ordered based on the results of these examinations and the woman's symptoms.

Mastectomy. As new information becomes available, the optimum treatment of breast cancer continues to evolve.[8,9] Historically, radical mastectomy was considered optimal treatment for State I and Stage II breast cancer. As theories of the spread of cancer changed, modified radical mastectomy gained acceptance. Recent data has demonstrated superior 5-year disease-free survival rates for women with Stage I or Stage II breast cancer following tylectomy (with disease-free margins of the surgical specimen) plus external irradiation, over those associated with total mastectomy.[3] Those women with one or more positive axillary nodes received adjuvant chemotherapy. Excision of the breast mass itself surrounded by only a margin of tumor-free tissue and followed by subsequent irradiation offers the cosmetic benefit of preservation of much of the breast. Changes corresponding to fibrosis and retraction of breast tissue, such as an increase in firmness and a decrease in size of the remaining irradiated breast tissue, do occur.

A more advanced breast cancer may be treated with mastectomy followed by a variety of treatment options. Those tumors positive for estrogen receptors are more likely to respond to either form of hormonal manipulation. In addition, irradiation of the breast or combination chemotherapy, or both may be prescribed for the woman with advanced breast cancer whether or not the estrogen receptor status of the tumor is positive.

Following treatment for breast cancer, the woman will be scheduled for frequent follow-up examinations. These appointments may be scheduled at intervals of 3 to 6 months initially. In symptomatic women, serum alkaline phosphatase and transaminase determinations may be done to assess for the possibility of bone and liver metastasis. Chest x-ray films may be ordered to assess for the presence of pulmonary metastasis. A mammogram may be ordered at yearly or other intervals.

Nursing Management

Assessment and Nursing Diagnosis. Early detection of cancer of the breast is a major focus of nursing strategies. A nursing diagnosis of knowledge deficit related to performing monthly breast self-examination is of primary concern. For the woman who has breast cancer, the appropriate nursing diagnoses will vary depending on the stage and extent of the disease and the therapies used. Some of the nursing diagnoses may include disturbance in self-concept related to anatomical changes and uncertain prognosis; grieving related to the diagnosis; alteration in comfort related to the treatment modalities and the disease; alteration in family coping related to diagnosis and prognosis; and knowledge deficit related to self-care and rehabilitation following treatment.

Interventions

Breast Self-Examination. Teaching the technique of breast self-examination (BSE) to all women is of paramount importance. Utilization of the BSE certification program for BSE trainers and BSE teachers sponsored by the American Cancer Society will assist health professionals in teaching the rationale and technique of BSE.

Nurses must encourage the monthly performance of this important health habit since monthly breast self-examination assures the woman of her continued breast health status. Optimal timing of BSE for menstruating women is 3 to 5 days following the end of the menstrual period, which corresponds to the time when hormonal influences on breast tissue are minimal. Postmenopausal women are generally encouraged to designate a day of the month as the day they will routinely perform BSE each month. The method of choosing which day is at the woman's discretion as long as it assists her to remember to perform BSE.

The strategy of teaching the breast self-examination technique by means of discussion as well as an individual practice session may promote compliance with monthly BSE. Many women discover a significant lump in their breast themselves and since many women are confused by the feel of the tissues within the breast, the practice of teaching women the feeling of the glandular, ductal, fibrous, and adipose tissues composing the breast will assist in recognition of normal tissue. Demonstrating the feeling of these tissues of the breast as a part of "mapping" her breast landmarks is an integral part of the teaching process.[17] Referring to the map when doing monthly BSE will facilitate recognition of both normalcy and subtle changes within the breast. Detection of these changes promotes early consultation with a health professional and may increase the changes of diagnosing the presence of a tumor before it becomes a systemic disease.

Emotional Support. During the diagnostic period, a woman with a breast mass is frequently upset and anxious. While she undergoes diagnostic testing, she may be concerned about the possibility of cancer as well as the effects of therapy. The nurse can play a significant role in providing emotional support for the woman as she undergoes diagnostic testing. The physician will present treatment options along with the rationale for the preferred mode of therapy in the individual woman's case. It is within the nurse's domain to clarify any remaining questions that the woman may have about the proposed treatment and to discuss the woman's voiced concerns. The physical and emotional effects associated with the chosen therapy modality will guide the nursing intervention plan.

Postmastectomy Care. In addition to the common postoperative concerns, specific nursing activities are necessary for a woman who has had a mastectomy. When any type of mastectomy is performed, a tube may be placed in the surgical area to assure adequate drainage of the surgical field and to prevent hematoma formation. The nurse must monitor the vital signs and check the dressing for bleeding. Assurance of the continued and uninterrupted function of the drainage tubes placed within the surgical area is an important nursing activity. The quality and quantity of drainage will be monitored. The drainage tubes are frequently connected to some form of suction. Some physicians may prescribe periodic milking of the drains to facilitate patency of the drain.

Postoperatively, the woman should be positioned with her arm elevated on a pillow whenever possible. When the physician discontinues the drains in the surgical wound and prescribes activity for the woman's affected arm, the nurse must teach active exercises for the arm to prevent contracture of the shoulder joint and muscle shortening. When the initial surgical dressings are removed, the woman may wear a lightly padded bra. After mastectomy, the woman must practice monthly breast self-examination on the remaining breast and also palpate the operative side for changes. Some women may experience unusual sensations in the surgical area.[18] These women must understand the importance of attending all scheduled postoperative clinic follow-up appointments.

A visit from a volunteer of the Reach to Recovery program of the American Cancer Society may facilitate adjustment to surgery. Reach to Recovery volunteers are women who have had a mastectomy and subsequently received special training in counseling techniques, rehabilitation, and local resources. Not necessarily health professionals, these volunteers nonetheless provide a unique and valuable form of assistance by modeling readjustment to lifestyle following mastectomy in addition to providing information about exercises, clothing, and availability of a prosthesis.[24] Physician referral for the Reach to Recovery visit is necessary. Other types of programs are available. The Encore program of the YWCA entails a discussion group, an exercise group, and a swimming session. A physician referral is necessary prior to registration in the program. While Reach to Recovery visits are made without charge, a monetary charge is made for participation in the Encore program.

Lymphedema. Lymphedema, a complication associated with radical surgery, may occur many years following axillary dissection. Dissection of the lymph nodes draining the axilla may interfere with lymphatic drainage of the arm on the affected side. Swelling of the arm, either minimal or extensive, may follow even minor trauma to the arm. To prevent the development of lymphedema, women are taught not to keep the affected arm in a dependent position for long periods of time; to use the affected arm as much as possible; and to engage in active range-of-motion exercises with both arms. In addition, they must take precautions to prevent burns on the affected arm; prevent pressure induced by constriction, such as constrictive clothing or a tourniquet; and decrease the possibility of cuts, scratches, and irritation occurring on the affected arm to minimize the risk of infection. Additionally, there must be no blood pressure measurement, blood drawn, or injections given in the affected arm for her lifetime (see Table 102–1).

A variety of range-of-motion exercises are possible. These exercises are best performed with both arms. The physician must determine the optimal time for initiating these exercises based on the degree of healing of the surgical incision, the presence of the drainage tube, and the tension placed on the skin flaps and suture with mobility.

TABLE 102–1
Hand and Arm Precautions Following Mastectomy

Prevent Trauma to the Hand and Arm of the Affected Side:

1. Avoid burns:
   - Wear padded long gloves when reaching into a hot oven.
   - Tan sensibly and avoid sunburn.
2. Avoid cuts, scratches, and irritation:
   - No injection, blood drawing, or vaccinations in affected arm.
   - Wear thimble when sewing.
   - Promptly wash any cuts or scrapes on affected arm or hand.
   - Observe carefully for signs of infection and if present report immediately to the physician.
   - Consult with the surgeon regarding use of hormonal pills, creams, and injections.

Avoid Binding or Constricting Pressure on the Hand and Arm of the Affected Side:

- No blood pressures should be taken on affected arm.
- No constrictive jewelry should be worn on affected arm or hand.
- Carry shoulder bag or other heavy objects with the unaffected shoulder or arm.
- Wear bras with wide shoulder straps.

Breast Prostheses. Information about the availability and advantages of different types of breast prostheses is provided by the Reach to Recovery volunteers. When use of this informational source is not possible, nurses must meet this critical informational need. The contour, size, and weight of the prosthesis is crucial to prevent back pain, promote normal posture, provide a comfortable fit of the prosthesis, and assure a natural appearance when clothing is worn. A variety of types of external prostheses is available in a range of sizes, weights, and prices. Proper fit of the breast prosthesis is crucial. Some department stores have specially trained personnel to assist with fitting breast prostheses. Specialty stores catering to the needs of the woman after mastectomy are another possibility in most larger cities. Advantages vary with each type of prosthesis. Some insurance companies cover the cost of the initial prosthesis. In some states, the prosthesis may be tax deductible as a legitimate medical expense.

Breast reconstruction, by a variety of techniques, is an option for some women following mastectomy. It is realistic to expect that reconstruction will result in symmetry and a natural appearance when clothing is worn. There is generally a 4- to 6-month delay in scheduling reconstruction after a mastectomy. This waiting period allows adequate healing of the area prior to reconstruction. Breast reconstruction is covered in more detail in Chapter 97.

Attractive clothing options may be offered to help enhance the woman's personal appearance and self-esteem following mastectomy. Opaque nightgowns with gatherings at the neckline may help conceal the lack of bilateral breast protuberance. Bras must have wide shoulder straps. Women who prefer shoulder bags should be cautioned to carry the purse on the unaffected side. All new clothing must have wide armholes. A variety of attractive night wear, evening wear, and swimming suits are available for purchase or may be made with a little ingenuity. In addition, the woman must be taught comfortable ways to get into the clothing she already owns.

Radiation Considerations. External radiation and iridium needle implantation also have side-effects necessitating the teaching of coping strategies. In addition to the teaching commonly done for individuals receiving irradiation, these women must be taught the possibility of temporary esophagitis or pneumonitis following irradiation. Radiation dermatitis may be most irritating in the skin fold created by the breast lying against the rib cage. Use of deodorants and antiperspirants must be avoided during the actual treatment period.

A woman undergoing iridium implantation will be admitted to a private room in the hospital. Holding tubes will be inserted in the breast under local or general anesthesia. The radioactive source may be inserted in the tubes in the operating room or later in the patient's room as part of an afterloading procedure. The implant will remain in place 2 to 3 days depending on the dosage calculated for the individual patient. While the implant is in place the woman may engage in quiet activities such as reading. Mild pain may be combated by the use of oral narcotic analgesics. Radiation precautions concerning time and distance apply to the care of these women. Pregnant women and children are not allowed to visit while the implant is in place. See the general precautions for care of patients undergoing radioactive implantation in Chapter 19.

Chemotherapy. If a woman has positive axillary lymph nodes, then she may be placed on a regimen of adjuvant chemotherapy. Positive nodes place her at high risk for metastatic disease even though at the time of the surgery there is not other clinical sign of metastasis. At this time the nurse and patient deal not only with the physical symptoms (*e.g.*, nausea and vomiting) associated with chemotherapy but also with the acceptance of this form of therapy. If the woman is premenopausal, the chemotherapy regimen will often induce menopause. The woman must be taught the symptoms of menopause and methods of controlling menopausal symptoms.

Chemotherapy is also used for women who develop metastasis and often prolongs the life of the woman and controls some of the symptoms of a systemic cancer. Here, the patient must deal with the realization that the cancer has not been controlled by previous therapy and face the prospect of a shortened life span.

Sexuality. The nurse who is comfortable with discussing sexuality has a crucial role in helping the woman identify and cope with her concerns about possible threats to her sexual self-concept, sexual relationships, and sexual functioning resulting from the cancer and the cancer therapy. Each type of therapy for breast cancer has aspects that may threaten a woman's sexuality. All women are unique in the perceptions of and response to therapy. Care plans can be devised to facilitate coping with the patient's individual concerns about her prescribed therapy.[25]

ADLs. When metastasis causes significant difficulties in the performance of the activities of daily living (ADLs), the nurse should intervene with symptom management and suggestions for alternate methods of accomplishing tasks. The maintenance of quality in the woman's life as defined by the individual woman is the goal of nursing intervention.

Evaluation

The woman with breast cancer will demonstrate acceptance of her diagnosis through discussing it with selected confidants, proceeding with recommended therapy and resuming previous life patterns; maximize her physical appearance by use of a prosthesis and explore breast reconstruction options; state that an acceptable level of comfort is achieved; discuss mutually acceptable ways to achieve closeness with partners and family; and participate in upper extremity exercises and other activities that enhance rehabilitation.

Non-neoplastic Disorders of the Male Reproductive System

Varicocele

Definition and Etiology. The term *varicocele* refers to an abnormal twisting and dilation of the veins of the pampiniform plexus above the testes. A varicocele commonly occurs between 15 and 40 years of age.[13] Ninety percent of varicoceles occur on the left side.[27]

The mechanism responsible for the development of varicoceles may relate to venous valvular incompetence. In an older man, the sudden development of a varicocele may be a late sign of renal tumor. In this case, the varicocele occurs when the tumor invades the renal vein and obstructs the testicular vein.[1]

Pathology. Relative differences in blood flow between the left testicular vein and the left renal vein may relate to the development of incompetent valves. The effect of gravity combined with the relative frequency of incompentent venous valves in the left internal spermatic vein may predispose to dilation and pooling of blood. In some cases, testicular atrophy occurs on the affected side.[27,28]

A varicocele is frequently associated with infertility in males. This may be caused by an increase in intrascrotal temperature due to venous engorgement, an abnormal exposure of the testes to high concentrations of adrenal steroids and catecholamines due to a reflux of venous blood from the left adrenal gland, or an association of epididymal dysfunction resulting in altered spermatic motility.[27]

Despite the fact that sperm count and motility are decreased when the man is diagnosed with a varicocele, many men have been able to impregnate their partners. After surgical correction of a varicocele, the rate of fatherhood increases.

Clinical Manifestations. A man with a varicocele may note a large and prominent mass in the scrotum. Changes in position may correlate with changes in size of the mass. The mass may decrease in size when the man is recumbent, yet attain its prior size and prominence when the man stands for prolonged periods of time. Mild exercise or prolonged standing for periods greater that 30 minutes may reveal a latent varicocele.[27]

A dull ache and a heavy, dragging sensation in the scrotum are common symptoms. Occasionally, frank pain is an associated symptom. Sexual activity including masturbation may relieve the pain.[28] A history of infertility and oligospermia may be elicited.

Diagnosis. Examination of the male patient's testes and scrotum while he is standing reveals a mass of dilated veins posterior and superior to the testes that may on occasion extend to the external inguinal ring. The man may be asked to perform the Valsalva maneuver to assess its effect on the degree of dilation. When examined in the recumbent position, venous distention, and therefore the size of the mass, is decreased. Use of a Doppler ultrasound may assist in the diagnosis. A retrograde venogram will confirm the diagnosis.[27,28]

Medical and Surgical Management

A varicocele may be managed medically with a scrotal support, which relieves any associated discomfort. If the varicocele is associated with pain or unwanted infertility or if a large mass is disturbing and embarrassing to the man, surgery is the treatment of choice. Criteria for selecting those infertile men most likely to benefit from varicocelectomy include oligospermia and a marked decrease in sperm motility.[27,28]

After varicocelectomy, the sperm count improves. An improvement in seminal quality should be seen within 3 months. By 6 to 18 months after surgery, the maximal improvement in seminal quality is attained.

Following surgery, the rate of fatherhood varies from 40% to 50%. In contrast, men with a varicocele who do not have surgery have less than a 10% rate of fatherhood.[30] The preoperative size of the varicocele correlates neither with the degree of change in seminal quality nor with the pregnancy rate following surgery.

Nursing Management

Assessment and Nursing Diagnosis. The physiological changes associated with a varicocele can have profound effects on a man's self-concept and reproductive capacity. Similarly, postoperative complications, though uncommon, may be devastating. A crucial nursing diagnosis is the potential for ineffective individual and family coping related to interference with marital relationships associated with diminished reproductive ability.

Goals. The aims of nursing intervention are to assure regular performance of testicular self-examination, to identify the interference of the varicocele with fertility, and to provide postoperative comfort measures.

Interventions. Testicular self-examination (TSE) is an important way for men to assess their continued health each month. All men can learn to perform the examination technique of their testes and scrotum. Whenever a change is noted, prompt medical consultation is essential. If the man perceives the mass to be large or unsightly, his self-concept may be threatened. He may be helped by encouraging him to discuss his feelings and concerns.

For those men with a varicocele who do not elect to have surgery, a scrotal support may relieve any heavy, dragging sensation associated with the mass. Nurses can recommend purchasing two scrotal supports since one may be worn while the other one is laundered. If pain is a problem, counseling men to engage in sexual activity, if possible, may be helpful.

In the case of a couple where infertility is a major concern, examination of the man as well as the woman is always recommended. When a varicocele is diagnosed, blame should not be affixed. Rather, it may be reassuring to the couple to know that the varicocele is surgically correctable and the rate of successful pregnancies is increased after surgery. The couple will be taught to coordinate the time of maximal improvement in seminal fluid with the effort to impregnate the woman.

Wearing a scrotal support postoperatively provides support for the surgical area and decreases discomfort associated with gravity. Here again, the nurse can recommend purchasing two scrotal supports. Compromise of arterial supply to the testis and damage to the vas deferens are rare following inguinal varicocelectomy. Nevertheless, patients need to be aware of the possibility of these complications.

Evaluation. The man will perform testicular self-examination (TSE) and state the optimal frequency for the examination. Men contemplating varicocelectomy will list the complications associated with the surgery and discuss their concerns about fertility with whichever health care professional they choose. Postoperatively, the man will wear a scrotal support and acknowledge comfort in the surgical area. He will understand the purpose of frequent seminal evaluations and describe the relevance of timing of improvement in seminal fluid to the attempts to impregnate the sexual partner.

Hydrocele

Definition and Etiology. A hydrocele is a collection of fluid within the processus vaginalis (or tunica vaginalis). Hydroceles most commonly surround the testes, although they may also occur along the spermatic cord.[28]

Hydroceles are present at birth in 6% of all full-term newborn males. This condition may be due to a failure of closure or an incomplete closure of the processus vaginalis. In many cases, it may not be possible to identify the cause of hydroceles in adult males. However, the condition may be due to inflammation of the testes and epididymis, local injury, or radiotherapy. In addition, hydroceles are a frequent complication of testicular tumors.[28,30] Chronic hydroceles, generally occurring in men older than 40 years of age, are usually of unknown etiology.

Pathology. A hydrocele is an accumulation of clear yellow fluid in the processus vaginalis. Hemorrhage into the sac may occur after trauma. Occasionally, a bulky hydrocele compresses the blood supply of the affected testicle causing testicular atrophy.[28]

Clinical Manifestations. Patients with hydroceles generally notice the bulk or weight of the mass. Unless the hydrocele occurs with epididymitis, the man will not report pain. On clinical examination, the hydrocele will present itself as a tense or soft and cystic scrotal mass. If the hydrocele is enclosed in the spermatic cord, the examiner will palpate a cystic, fusiform swelling. Otherwise, a rounded, cystic intrascrotal mass that transilluminates will be diagnosed as a hydrocele. A tense hydrocele can be differentiated from a testicular tumor because testicular tumors do not transilluminate.[28]

Medical and Surgical Management

When an etiology cannot be determined, a large hydrocele may be aspirated to facilitate palpation of the testis and epididymis and rule out cancer or tuberculosis. Complications of aspiration include hemorrhage into the sac (producing a hematocele) and, rarely, infection.[28,30]

A chronic hydrocele may be treated by periodic aspiration. Aspiration may be repeated every 6 to 20 weeks. Surgery may be done if the hydrocele refills rapidly or if the man requests surgery.

Hydrocelectomy involves excision of the hydrocele sac through a scrotal incision. Indications for hydrocelectomy in the case of an acute hydrocele include patient complaints of discomfort or embarrassment due to the large bulky mass, and hematocele and complications resulting from the mass, specifically interference with testicular circulation.[28]

Nursing Management

Assessment and Nursing Diagnosis. Delay in the diagnosis of a hydrocele may relate to anxiety about the possibility of other pathological processes. The nursing diagnosis with the highest priority postoperatively is the potential extracellular fluid volume deficit from hemorrhage related to the surgery.

Goals. In relationship to the diagnosis of a hydrocele, nursing efforts are aimed at early diagnosis of the condition and prompt recognition of postoperative bleeding.

Interventions. All men need to know the rationale and technique of testicular self-examination (TSE). As part of the examination, the man should examine the scrotum every month to assure himself of his continued good health.

After hydrocelectomy or simple aspiration, assessing for signs of hemorrhage is a priority. Hemorrhage can occur internally as well as externally. A scrotal dressing will be in place for the first 24 to 48 hours postoperatively and wearing a firm scrotal support for the first few days after surgery will be helpful. Having two scrotal supports available allows one to be worn while the other is being laundered.[13]

Nursing management may include administering an oral anti-inflammatory agent during the first week after surgery. Though infection is rare following hydrocelectomy, assessing the wound for subtle signs of infection and monitoring the patient's temperature is important. Due to the anti-inflammatory medication, signs and symptoms of infection may be suppressed.

Finally, pain medications may need to be given in the postoperative period. Assessing the amount of pain and administering the appropriate medication from the alternative pain medications prescribed is an important nursing function.

Evaluation. All men will perform a testicular and scrotal examination at monthly intervals and seek prompt consultation for any perceived change in the self-examination. Before discharge, following a hydrocelectomy the male will have a clear and dry incision with well-approximated edges; have a hematocrit within normal limits; have clear mentation and a temperature within normal limits; state the name, purpose and side-effects of prescribed anti-inflammatory medications; and describe the necessity of wearing a scrotal support continuously for the first few postoperative days.

Benign Prostatic Hyperplasia

Definition. Benign prostatic hyperplasia (BPH) is a nonmalignant glandular proliferation of the prostate. Historically referred to as benign prostatic hypertrophy, BPH is the more accurate name for this disease since hyperplasia is the predominant cellular change.

Etiology and Epidemiology. The etiology of BPH is unclear. Two factors associated with the development of BPH are aging and normal testicular function. BPH is common in men over 40 years of age, with the mean age of 60 for blacks and 65 for whites. The incidence of BPH increases with increasing age from the fifth decade of life through the end of life, with more than 90% of men in their eighties having BPH.[31] There may be an increased risk for the development of prostatic cancer in men who have the nodular form of benign prostatic hyperplasia.

Pathology. In BPH, hyperplastic development of the periurethral glandular tissue in the prostate compresses the true prostatic tissue against the fibrous capsule surrounding the prostate. Local infarction and cellulitis may occur as the tissue expands within this circumscribed area. Urethral compression and urinary tract obstruction may result, although the size of the prostate does not correlate with the degree of urethral obstruction. Secondary infection from urinary retention may promote the development of renal insufficiency and hypertension.[31]

Clinical Manifestations. Symptoms of BPH result from compression of the urethra by the enlarging prostate gland and are evidenced by a decreased diameter and force of urinary stream, difficulty starting and ending the stream of urine, dribbling following micturition, a sensation of incomplete emptying of the bladder with urination, and occasionally urinary retention. As the amount of urinary retention increases, incontinence, nocturia, and frequent urinary tract infections occur.[31] When hydronephrosis and renal insufficiency occur, BUN and creatinine will be elevated and anemia may be present.

Medical Management

Rectal examination will reveal an enlarged, firm and smooth mass in the area of the prostate. Observation of the man while he is voiding will permit the examiner to assess the quality of the urinary stream. Residual catheterization after voiding will assess the amount of remaining urine and assist in determining the presence of stricture. An intravenous pyelogram with a post-voided follow-up film estimates the efficiency of micturition and documents any existing hydronephrosis and calculi. Cysturethroscopy assists in the evaluation of urethral competency at the level of the bladder neck. Cystometrics will help rule out the presence of an atonic bladder if urinary urgency and frequency are predominant symptoms. A urinalysis and culture and sensitivity of the urine will be ordered to assess for the presence of infection. Serum creatinine and BUN will be drawn to assess renal function.

Conservative therapy will be initiated whenever possible. Some men may note improvement following instrumentation associated with the above tests. Others may not experience an increase in severity of symptoms for many years. These men must be monitored periodically.

Antiandrogens, for example, progestins and flutamide, may be prescribed for some men. Subjective improvement in symptoms may occur, but objective parameters, for example, total volume of urine voided, may not change significantly. The use of flutamide has been associated with improved urinary flow rates, as well as side-effects of nipple tenderness and gynecomastia.[31] More studies of the effects of antiandrogens are necessary to evaluate their utility in the treatment of BPH.

Surgery is curative. One of four surgical techniques may be employed to relieve the symptoms of prostatism. The complete prostate and surrounding capsule may be removed by transurethral prostatectomy. Prostatectomy may also be performed by a suprapubic, retropubic, or perineal route. In a variable percentage of cases, depending in part on the type of prostatectomy performed, impotence or urinary incontinence, or both may complicate the postoperative recovery period. According to Walsh, indications for the correction of prostatism include acute urinary retention, hydronephrosis, recurrent urinary tract infection associated with a large amount of residual urine, hematuria, and patient desire for treatment due to concern about symptoms.[31]

Acute urinary retention may be precipitated by chilling, alcohol ingestion, infection, prolonged delay in micturition, and some medications including anticholinergics, antidepressants, tranquilizers, and decongestants.[31] Whenever the man is suddenly unable to urinate, an indwelling catheter will be placed. If stricture prevents insertion of the urethral catheter, a suprapubic cystostomy must be performed.

Nursing Management

Assessment and Nursing Diagnosis. Benign prostatic hyperplasia (BPH) is more common in men as they age. Nursing diagnoses include alteration in patterns of urinary elimination related to the compression of the urethra by the enlarged prostate gland; alteration in comfort: pain, related to bladder spasms following surgery; potential sexual dysfunction (impotence) related to surgical approach; and potential alteration in patterns of urinary elimination (incontinence) related to the surgical procedure.

Goals. The goals for the man with BPH include early recognition of alterations in the urinary stream, relief of discomfort in the postoperative period; and resumption of normal characteristics of urine, micturition, and sexual function.

Interventions. Because of the risk of BPH with aging, all men and particularly middle-aged and elderly men will be taught the symptoms of prostatism and be counseled to seek routine rectal examinations. Careful assessment of male nursing home residents and elderly men will aid in case finding of BPH. Men with BPH should be taught to avoid excessive alcohol intake since the diuretic effect of alcohol combined with a moderate amount of fluid may lead to an episode of acute urinary retention. Other factors contributing to the development of acute urinary retention also must be reinforced.

Some men may be embarrassed by the diagnostics tests ordered. In addition, they may be concerned about the possibility of discomfort from these tests. Pragmatic discussions about the rationale for the tests and the sensations experienced during the tests may facilitate acceptance.

In the postoperative period, assessment of the patency of urinary drainage is crucial. Bleeding and clotting may occlude urinary flow through the urethral catheter. The nurse will assess changes in color of the urine as well as patency of the drainage system. The urine will return to an amber color as bleeding decreases. If a continuous irrigation system of the urinary catheter is not used, the nurse must be prepared to manually irrigate the catheter if it becomes occluded. Depending on the surgical approach, some men will experience urinary incontinence or impotence, or both following prostatectomy. Men should be forewarned of this possibility. A gentle and loving partner may minimize the psychological effect of postoperative impotence, and a penile prosthesis may be indicated for those men who desire to achieve an erection.

Evaluation. The man who has had surgery for BPH will relate relief of discomfort in the postoperative period; have clear amber urine; be continent of urine; relate normal sexual function; and seek routine rectal examinations.

Neoplastic Disorders of the Male Reproductive System

Cancer of the Penis

Classification. Most of the malignancies occurring on the penis are squamous cell carcinoma, but basal cell carcinoma and melanoma also occur. A primary cancer of the bladder, prostate, rectum, or kidney may metastasize to the penis.[21,23]

Epidemiology. Penile cancer is relatively rare in the United States. Squamous cell carcinoma of the penis account for 4% of the malignancies and causes about 0.2% of the cancer-related deaths in men in the United States.

Penile cancer most commonly occurs from the fourth or fifth to seventh decades of life with an average age of 57 years. It rarely occurs before 40 years of age and the incidence increases with each decade past forty.[13,23]

Etiology. As with other cancers, the cause of penile cancer is not known. The occurrence of penile cancer is associated with poor personal hygiene and phimosis in an uncircumcised man. The incidence is highest in uncircumcised men or those men who are circumcised as adults. Conversely, the incidence is lowest in men who underwent neonatal circumcision, such as men of Jewish and Muslim faiths.

Pathology. Squamous cell carcinoma, the most common type of penile cancer, is generally well differentiated and is most commonly located on the glans penis or coronal sulcus. The lesion is characteristically slow growing.[6] Without treatment, the tumor generally invades the corpora, scrotum, and lower abdominal wall by direct extension but infrequently involves the urethra.

Clinical Manifestations. Patients commonly will seek medical attention for a penile mass. Characteristics of the mass may vary from a nonhealing ulceration on the penis to a luxurious warty growth. The lesions may be associated with induration or erythema, or both. Foul penile discharge is another sign associated with penile cancer. Phimosis may conceal a lesion, so that local irritation is the predominant sign.

Diagnosis. Because patients may mistake a penile lesion for a sexually transmitted disease, they may neglect seeking medical attention due to embarrassement.[10] The frequent occurrence of the lesion under the prepuce combined with phimosis may conceal the lesion until it has eroded through the prepuce and result in delayed medical diagnosis.[23] Other reasons advanced for delay in seeking medical attention include fear of penectomy and the slow growth of the lesion.

When the patient seeks medical attention, he can expect to undergo a clinical examination of the lesion that will include a rectal, bimanual, and nodal examination. These will be done to assess the extent of the tumor. A biopsy of the lesion will diagnose the classification of cancer. Other tests will be performed to assess the extent of the cancer.

Medical and Surgical Management

Prognosis parallels the state of the cancer at initial diagnosis. Surgery or radiation therapy may be offered as treatment for an early localized lesion that has not metastasized. Partial penectomy is done whenever possible. Upright micturition is preserved if a penile stump remains after adequate surgical resection. When total penectomy is necessary due to the location of the tumor, a perineal urethrostomy is created and an indwelling urethral catheter is placed during surgery. After removal of the catheter, the man must void sitting down but urinary continence is preserved.[10] When lymph nodes are positive for cancer, the prognosis is worse. Therapy for the regional lymph nodes is controversial. If the nodes are positive for cancer, an en bloc lymphadenectomy may be done. Patients undergoing lymphadenectomy may have a surgical drain placed to suction in order to decrease the pooling of lymph. Complications of this surgery include wound infection, lymphedema, seroma formation, skin flap necrosis, infection, thromboembolic disease, and hemorrhage from erosion of the inguinal vessels.[6]

Radiation therapy as definitive treatment may be offered for an early superficial lesion of the prepuce, glans, or coronal sulcus, and to those patients who refuse surgery, who are inoperable, or who have distant metastasis to decrease the tumor size and combat associated symptoms. Chemotherapy is not as effective as other forms of therapy for localized tumors.

Nursing Management

Assessment and Nursing Diagnosis. A few relevant nursing diagnoses are potential for diminishing sexual self-concept related to the penile lesion; anxiety concerning the potential threat to sexual functioning and paternity associated with diminished penile length or total penectomy; possible disturbance in sexual self-concept related to altered micturition associated with total penectomy; and potential impairment of skin integrity with disruption of the surgical incision following nodal dissection related to tension on the incision and accumulation of serous fluid.

Goals. Nursing activities are aimed at promoting the man's acceptance of the surgical alterations and promoting healing of the surgical incision following nodal dissection. Fostering development of a positive self-concept and satisfactory sexual functioning, whenever possible, are important nursing goals.

Interventions. Because phimosis may conceal the presence of a penile cancer, uncircumcised men need to know the value of penile hygiene and self-examination. Early diagnosis and treatment of the lesion is important in determining the prognosis. Symptoms of penile cancer must be reported without delay.

Since secondary infection accompanies more than 50% of lesions, odor may be a problem for these patients preoperatively. Nursing actions are aimed at controlling the odor and containing any penile discharge. In teaching dressing change techniques to the patient, hygiene is imperative. Odor and the appearance of the lesion may affect sexual desire and opportunity. The patient may be encouraged to discuss any of his voiced concerns about self-worth, masculinity, the effects of the lesion, and the proposed surgery. Common concerns of the patient include sexual adequacy, paternity, and micturition. If sufficient penile length remains after surgery, erection may be adequate for vaginal penetration. Orgasm and ejaculation are maintained. When total penectomy is done, orgasm and ejaculation can still occur in some patients, though vaginal penetration is no longer possible.[2] After total penectomy, men may avoid public restrooms since they must sit down on a toilet to urinate. Urinary continence is not affected.

After surgery, quality of care of the indwelling catheter is essential to prevent infection. The patient may have concerns about pain with removal of the catheter as well as pain with urination. The surgical drain, placed at the base of the penile shaft during total penectomy, may be connected to suction. Assessing patency of the apparatus and reporting any difficulty with the suction device is a nursing responsibility.

Before an ilioinguinal node dissection, the nurse may be involved in administering a preoperative mechanical bowel prep. After this surgery, the patient may be on bed rest with the foot of the bed elevated. During this time, measures to combat the risk of thromboembolism are very important. Elastic support stockings or ace wraps should be applied to the lower extremities. Prophylactic heparinization is controversial in this instance since it may predispose to the formation of pelvic lymphoceles. Because it is necessary to decrease suture line tension in order to promote wound healing, patients must recline with their hips flexed. Nursing personnel assist these patients to turn every 2 hours while maintaining hip flexion. A drain to suction may be placed in the surgical area. Patients may be prohibited from mobilization of the lower extremities until after the suction apparatus is discontinued. Although common after pelvic node dissection, lymphedema is a rare complication after superficial inguinal node dissection.[22]

Evaluation. As a result of sensitive and comprehensive care, all men treated for cancer of the penis will identify and discuss their concerns with at least one person of their choice. After partial penectomy, men will state that vaginal penetration and ejaculation may be possible depending on the remaining length of their penis. After total penectomy, men will state acceptable alternative methods of giving and receiving pleasure and describe how they will deal with the need to urinate if they only have access to public restrooms. Those men undergoing nodal dissection must be able to state the rationale for limitation in movement at the hip joints and use of support stockings. Postoperatively, their incision will be clear and dry with well-approximated edges.

Cancer of the Testes

Classification. Cancers of the testes are derived from either nongerminal epithelium or the germinal cells of the testes. Nongerminal epithelial cancers are sarcomas and interstitial cell tumors. Germinal cell cancers are of four types: seminomas, teratocarcinomas, embryonal carcinomas, and choriocarcinomas. Each of the germinal cell cancers may occur singly or as a mixed cellular type. About 40% of the testicular tumors are seminomas, 30% are teratocarcinomas, and 25% are embryonal carcinomas. Choriocarcinoma of the testis is rare. The cellular type as well as the extent of the tumor is important in influencing the type of therapy chosen.

Epidemiology and Etiology. Testicular cancer is one of the leading cancers occurring in young men with an average of incidence being 32 years old. It is a leading cause of cancer-related death in men in their twenties and thirties. Although the cause is unknown, the development of testicular cancer is associated with a history of undescended testes. Orchidopexy performed prior to 6 years of age is recommended to prevent later development of cancer. If performed after puberty, orchidopexy may not prevent the development of cancer.[21] A man with a history of bilateral cryptorchid testes and cancer in one testicle is at increased risk of developing cancer in the other testis. Atrophic testes is a risk factor for testicular cancer. Young men with atrophic testes must be closely monitored. Although trauma to the scrotum may occur prior to the discovery of testicular cancer, it has no relationship to the development of the cancer. The presence of a hydrocele raises the suspicion of testicular cancer since hydroceles are found in 5% to 10% of cases of testis cancer.

Pathology and Clinical Manifestations. Early testicular cancer is asymptomatic. Normal testes are smooth and uniform in consistency. Testicular cancer presents as a firm irregular area or nodule on the smooth surface of the testes. Generally painless, the cancer may be associated with mild testicular pain. Acute pain is associated with hemorrhage, necrosis, or infection within the tumor.[20] Testicular cancer is diagnosed slightly more frequently in the right testis rather than in the left one. Almost all of the solid tumors occurring in the testes are malignant. With advanced disease, metastasis occurs in the bones, lungs, liver, and cervical and mediastinal lymph nodes. Low back pain may be related to metastasis in the retroperitoneal nodes.

Medical Management

Clinical examination includes palpation of the testes and surrounding structures, transillumination of the tumor, and assessment of the abdomen for adenopathy. An intravenous pyelogram may be ordered to assess for deviation or obstruction of the ureters. An abdominal CT scan or an abdominal ultrasound will be ordered to assess for the presence of lymph node metastasis in the abdomen. Bipedal lymphangiogram may be performed. Palpation of the supraclavicular, cervical, and inguinal lymph nodes will be performed. A baseline chest x-ray study will be ordered and, rarely, a CT scan of the lung may be done to check for possible pulmonary metastasis. Radioimmunoassay of serum alpha fetoprotein and beta human chorionic gonadotropin will be done prior to and following therapy. These assays are markers of the presence of testicular cancer. Biopsy of the testis must be done through an inguinal incision in order to avoid contamination of the scrotum and its contents with malignant cells. The results of all these tests will be used to evaluate the extent of the malignancy and determine the stage of the cancer.

Assessment of serum markers must be done before and following surgical intervention. Surgery involves the removal of the testis involved with cancer through an inguinal incision. During the surgery, the cord, epididymis, and scrotum will be examined for possible spread of the tumor. In the case of seminoma, external irradiation of the para-aortic and pelvic nodes of the same side as the tumor will be done. Shielding of the contralateral testis must be done to preserve fertility. For nonseminomatous testicular cancers, bilateral retroperitoneal lymphadenectomy will be performed. Occasionally, chemotherapy will be given prior to surgery of nonseminomatous cancers or prior to irradiation of the lymph nodes in the case of seminoma, in order to shrink a large and bulky tumor mass. Chemotherapy will be administered when cancer recurs. Combination chemotherapy using cisplatin, Velban, and bleomycin has proven efficient in the treatment of testicular cancer. All men will be monitored by serum markers with abdominal CT and ultrasound at monthly intervals for the first year. Examinations will be performed every 2 months the next year since recurrence of the cancer is unusual the second year.[20]

Nursing Management

Assessment and Nursing Diagnosis. Testicular cancer is predominantly a disease of young men. Some of the nursing diagnoses that may be useful include knowledge deficit related to the importance and technique of testicular self-examination (TSE), and potential ineffective family coping: compromised related to sterility.

Goals. The goal for early detection of testicular cancer is that the man will regularly perform TSE. For the man with testicular cancer, the goal is acceptance of temporary or permanent sterility.

Interventions. Parents of newborn male infants will be cautioned to check their sons for possible undescended testes, and consult their pediatricians about the necessity for surgical correction of this disorder. It is recommended that orchidopexy be performed prior to 6 years of age.

All men must be taught the technique of TSE and be cautioned to perform TSE every month for life. They will use both their hands to palpate the smooth uniform consistency of the normal testes.

Irradiation and chemotherapy prescribed for testicular cancer may be followed by temporary or permanent sterility. Those men at risk for testicular cancer are likely to be at an age when fertility and starting a family is an important part of their lives. Anger is a common reaction to the diagnosis of testis cancer. A man with testicular cancer may be counseled to attempt sperm banking prior to the initiation of therapy. This practice is not routine, though, since many of these men are azoospermic prior to the start of therapy. Artificial insemination with pooled donor sperm may be an option for some couples desirous of having children. Adoption is another possibility, although some couples may have difficulty with the adoption process since not all adoption agency personnel are aware of the high cure rate associated with testicular cancer.

Other important toxicities commonly associated with combination chemotherapy of cisplatin, vinblastine, and bleomycin are myalgias, constipation, paralytic ileus, and severe granulocytopenia.

Evaluation. All men will perform testicular self-examination monthly. Those men with testicular cancer will discuss their understanding of their sterility in relation to the diagnosis and therapies.

Cancer of the Prostate

Classification, Epidemiology, and Etiology. The majority of cancers occurring in the prostate are adenocarcinomas. Sarcoma is rare. The median age of men with prostatic cancer is 70 years old. Cancer of the prostate is one of the most common cancers occurring in men over the age of 50. Its incidence increases with each decade of life after age 50. Black males in the United States have the highest incidence of prostatic cancer in the world. Although epidemiological studies have shown that both benign prostatic hyperplasia and cancer of the prostate occur in older men, the data is not strong enough to suggest an association between the two disease entities. It is thought that there may be an association of prostatic cancer with hormonal alterations. This form of cancer does not occur in castrated males.

Pathology and Clinical Manifestations. Prostatic cancer spreads to the seminal vesicles, bladder, urethra and the pelvic side walls. The bones and lymph nodes, for example, the iliac and hypogastric nodes, are common sites of metastatic disease. Local growth of the prostate produces obstruction of the flow of urine through the urethra. Men may complain of difficulty starting their stream of urine, dribbling, and change in the quality of the urinary stream. With advanced cancer of the prostate, urinary retention predominates and episodes of cystitis may occur. Hematuria is rare. Bone pain accompanies metastatic disease to the bone. Back pain and stiffness are common. Occasionally pathological fractures occur.

Medical Management

Rectal examination will reveal an area of firmness in the prostate that may be asymptomatic. If cancer of the prostate is suspected, transrectal or perineal needle biopsy will provide tissue for confirmation. An excretory urogram will be done to check for involvement of the bladder with tumor and for ureteral obstruction and displacement. A CT scan of the pelvis will define the presence of nodal involvement and the extent of the tumor. Bipedal lymphangiogram will further define the presence of lymph node involvement. A bone scan will detect the presence of bone metastasis. Serum alkaline phosphatase will be monitored since this enzyme is generally increased in the presence of bone metastasis. Radioimmunoassay of prostatic acid phosphatase in the bone marrow or serum will be elevated in cases of local cancer of the prostate as well as in two thirds of the cases of metastatic disease.

Adequate treatment of cancer of the prostate is accomplished by a radical prostatectomy with pelvic lymph node dissection. Radical prostatectomy may be performed through a perineal, retropubic, or transpubic route. As long as there is no ankylosis of the hips, some physicians prefer the perineal approach in elderly men since the risk of pulmonary complications is decreased. During radical prostatectomy, the prostate and capsule, the ampula, vas deferens, seminal vesicles, and bladder neck cuff will be removed. Long-term complications of this form of treatment include a variable incidence of impotence or incontinence, or both.

External irradiation of the prostate or interstitial implantation of the prostate may be done if there is evidence of local invasion by the tumor. A lymphadenectomy may be done at this time. Side-effects and complications related to irradiation include diarrhea, urinary frequency, nocturia, and spasms of the bladder neck. Some men will experience erectile impotence. Scrotal and leg edema are rare.

In order to diminish or remove the source of androgens, estrogen may be prescribed for males with extensive disease. The man's breasts may be irradiated before estrogen therapy is initiated to prevent gynecomastia. Fluid retention and dependent edema may be treated by dietary sodium restriction and diuretics. A significant risk associated with long term administration of estrogen is the development of thromboembolism. Although survival is not affected, hormonal therapy will provide relief of symptoms of metastatic disease and regression of the cancer.

Chemotherapy may be used in prostatic cancer. Cisplatin, hydroxurea, Adriamycin and 5-fluorouracil have been used sequentially. Regimens involving combinations of these and other drugs are under investigation.

Nursing Management

Assessment and Nursing Diagnosis. Cancer of the prostate commonly causes enlargement of the prostate and obstruction of the urinary stream. The appropriate nursing diagnoses would include those described under benign prostatic hyperplasia (BPH). An additional nursing diagnosis would be alteration in self-concept related to the feminizing effects of hormonal therapy.

Goals. The goals for the man with prostate cancer treated by surgery will be similar to those for BPH. An additional goal is recognition and acceptance of the diagnosis, the effects of hormonal therapy, and the need for consistent monitoring.

Interventions. All men over the age of 50 years must expect a rectal examination as part of their routine physical examinations. Because the symptoms of prostatic cancer may occur so insidiously that a man may not be aware of the changes in urinary quality, older men must be taught to be observant for subtle changes in characteristics of their urinary flow.

Concerns about sexuality are a major focus of nursing management throughout the treatment period. All of the therapies may have significant effects on the man's body image and sexual functioning. Those men experiencing erectile impotence after radical prostatectomy may by helped by surgical implantation of a penile prosthesis. Rigid, semirigid, and inflatable penile prostheses are available. Support groups for men who are impotent may be helpful.

When urinary incontinence occurs, it will threaten self-concept. Incontinence may be controlled by the application of a condom catheter connected to leg bag drainage. Assessment of the meaning of incontinence to the individual man will guide the nurse in providing support to the man experiencing this side-effect of some forms of treatment.

Feminizing effects of the hormonal manipulation can be extremely distressing. Pragmatic discussions about the possibility of these side-effects will prepare the man for their occurrence.

Evaluation. The man with cancer of the prostate will be evaluated similarly to the man with benign prostatic hyperplasia. In addition, he will discuss his concerns about the diagnosis with selected persons; relate his level of understanding regarding hormonal therapy; and participate in follow-up evaluations.

References

1. Abrams HL, Adams DF: Renal and adrenal angiography. In Harrison JH, Gittes RF, Perlmutter AD et al: Campbell's Urology, 4th ed, vol 1. Philadelphia, WB Saunders, 1979
2. Bracken RB: Cancer of the testis, penis, and urethra: The impact of therapy on sexual function. In von Eschenback AC, Rodriguez DB (eds): Sexual Rehabilitation of the Urologic Patient. Boston, GK Hall Medical Publishers, 1981
3. Fisher B, Bauer M, Margolese R, et al: Five-year results of a randomized clinical trial comparing total mastectomy and segmental mastectomy with or without radiation in the treatment of breast cancer. New Engl J Med 312:665–673, 1985
4. Frick HC: The vagina. In Holland JF, Frei E: Cancer Medicine, 2nd ed. Philadelphia, Lea & Febiger, 1982
5. Frick HC: The vulva. In Holland JF, Frei E: Cancer Medicine, 2nd ed. Philadelphia, Lea & Febiger, 1982
6. Harty JI, Catalona WJ: Carcinoma of the penis. In Javadpour N: Principles and Management of Urologic Cancer, 2nd ed. Baltimore, Williams & Wilkins, 1983
7. Hellman S, Harris JR, Canellos GP, Fisher B: Cancer of the breast. In DeVita VT, Hellman S, Rosenberg SA: Cancer Principles and Practice of Oncology. Philadelphia, JB Lippincott, 1982
8. Henderson IC, Canellos GP: Cancer of the breast—the past decade, Part I. New Engl J Med 302:17–30, 1980
9. Henderson IC, Canellos GP: Cancer of the breast—the past decade, Part II. New Engl J Med 302:78–90, 1980

10. Houston GR, Rodriguez D: Male sexuality and genitourinary cancer. In Marino LB: Cancer Nursing. St. Louis, CV Mosby, 1981
11. Jones HW, Jones GS: Novak's Textbook of Gynecology, 10th ed. Baltimore, Williams & Wilkins, 1981
12. Jones JM, Cox AR, Levy EY, Thompson CE: Women's Health Management: Guidelines for Nurse Practitioners. Reston VA, Reston Publishing, 1984
13. McConnel EA, Zimmerman MF: Care of Patients with Urologic Problems. Philadelphia, JB Lippincott, 1983
14. Merrill JA: Endometriosis. In Danforth DN (ed): Obstetrics and Gynecology, 4th ed. San Francisco, Harper & Row, 1982
15. Merril JA, Gusberg SB, Deppe G: Lesions of the corpus uteri. In Danforth DN (ed): Obstetrics and Gynecology, 4th ed. San Francisco, Harper & Row, 1982
16. Merrill JA, Gusberg SB, Deppe G, Stafl A: Lesions of the cervix uteri. In Danforth DN (ed): Obstetrics and Gynecology, 4th ed. San Francisco, Harper & Row, 1982
17. Molbo DM: Cancer. In Carnevali DL, Patrick M: Nursing Management for the Elderly. Philadelphia, JB Lippincott, 1979
18. Nail L, Jones LS, Giuffre M, Johnson JE: Sensations after mastectomy. Am J Nurs 84:1121–1124, 1984
19. Nelson JH: Uterine cervix. In Holland JF, Frei E: Cancer Medicine, 2nd ed. Philadelphia, Lea & Febiger, 1982
20. Paulson DF, Einhorn LH, Peckham MJ, Williams SD: Cancer of the testis. In Devita VT, Hellman S, Rosenberg SA: Cancer Principles and Practice of Oncology. Philadelphia, JB Lippincott, 1982
21. Paulson DF, Perez CA, Anderson T: Genito-urinary malignancies. In Devita VT, Hellman S, Rosenberg SA: Cancer Principles and Practice of Oncology. Philadelphia, JB Lippincott, 1982
22. Perez CA, Knapp RC, Young RC: Gynecologic tumors. In Devita VT, Hellman S, Rosenberg SA: Cancer Principles and Practice of Oncology. Philadelphia, JB Lippincott, 1982
23. Prout Gr, Garnick MB: Carcinoma of the penis. In Holland JF, Frei E: Cancer Medicine, 2nd ed. Philadelphia, Lea & Febiger, 1982
24. Rogers TF, Bauman LJ, Metzger L: An assessment of the reach to recovery program. CA–A Cancer Journal for Clinicians 35:116–124, 1985
25. Schwarz-Appelbaum J, Kirchner CW, Dedrick J, Jusenius K: Nursing care plans: Sexuality and treatment of breast cancer. Oncology Nursing Forum 11:16–24, 1984
26. Silverberg E: Cancer statistics, 1985. Ca–A Cancer Journal for Clinicians 35:19–35, 1985
27. Sherins RJ, Howards SS: Male infertility. In Harrison JH, Gittes RF, Perlmutter AD et al: Campbell's Urology, 4th ed, Vol 1. Philadelphia, WB Saunders, 1979
28. Smith DR: General Urology, 10th ed. Los Altos CA, Lange Medical Publications, 1981
29. Stanton SL: Clinical Gynecologic Urology. St Louis, CV Mosby, 1984
30. Stewart BH: Surgery of the scrotum and its contents. In Harrison JH, Gittes RF, Perlmutter AD et al: Campbell's Urology, 4th ed, Vol 1. Philadelphia, WB Saunders, 1979
31. Walsh PC: Benign prostatic hyperplasia. In Harrison JH, Gittes RF, Perlmutter AD et al: Campbell's Urology, 4th ed, Vol 1. Philadelphia, WB Saunders, 1979
32. Young RC, Knapp RC, Perez CA: Cancer of the Ovary.In Devita VT, Hellman S, Rosenberg SA: Cancer Principles and Practice of Oncology. Philadelphia, JB Lippincott, 1982

UNIT XIII

Nursing Management of Patients in Selected Situations

Chapter 103

Abuse of Alcohol and Other Drugs

Gaylene Bouska Altman
Janet A. Nelson
Carla A. Lee

During the last 2 decades most western countries have experienced a heightened awareness of problems of drug dependence. This is due in part to an increased use of drugs and variety of drugs abused, but it is also due to more attention being paid to the general impact on society of drug abuse. Social factors such as high unemployment and many stresses of the 20th century may contribute to this prevalence. Many drugs are abused in our society making it necessary for nurses to learn about the health problems associated with drug abuse. Any drug taken for nonmedical reasons or for a reason other then its intended purpose and prescribed dose can be a drug of abuse. This chapter addresses the issues surrounding care of patients with alcohol abuse, street drug use, and misuse of prescription drugs.

Addiction

Definitions

Drug abuse refers to any substance, taken through any route of administration, that alters the mood, the level of perception, or brain functioning. Drug abuse is the continued use of a mind-altering substance in a way that differs from generally approved medical or social practices, despite the problems caused by such use. Drug abuse may cause certain psychological and physiological changes in body requirements, creating a dependence on the drug.

Chemical dependence is a compulsive use, addiction, or habituation of a drug that is associated with a psychological or physical "need" for the drug. *Psychological dependence* is a characteristic of all drugs of abuse and connotes the user's intense desire to consume the drug in order to reach a maximum level of functioning or feeling of well-being and avoidance of pain. *Physiological dependence* connotes an altered state that occurs after the body is exposed to repeated administration of a drug. There are two important aspects to physiological dependence: tolerance and withdrawal.

- *Tolerance* is the need for higher and higher doses to achieve the same effects.
- *Withdrawal* is the appearance of certain physiological symptoms when the drug is stopped or decreased too abruptly. This requires a continued use of the drug to prevent these symptoms.

Chemical dependence is an illness characterized by a significant physiological, psychological, or social impairment. The mood-altering substances, alone or in conjunction with alcohol, are used to the point of causing damage to the individual, those around him, or both. Besides the physiological and psychological dependence on the drug, there is an unpredictability of quantities consumed and behaviors exhibited while under the influence and continued use despite adverse consequences. The basic disease process of addiction is the same regardless of which drug or drugs are being abused. The addictive disease process results in a progressive deterioration of a person's well-being, interpersonal relationships, work or school performance, and physical and spiritual health. It is becoming more difficult to identify a person who abuses only one mood-altering substance. Many chemically dependent people are polydrug abusers, meaning that they abuse two or more different mood-altering substances. Alcohol continues to be the number one drug of abuse in the United States. The abuse of drug classes other than alcohol appears to be influenced by peer group trends, availability, cost, and other variables.

The Addiction Process

It is no accident that the substances being abused are those chemicals which alter brain or central nervous system functioning, and hence the mood. Mood-altering chemicals are taken to affect one's feelings as well as one's awareness of tensions and problems.

People rarely set out to become dependent on drugs. They want to get high, feel mellow, get energy, relax, go to sleep, or talk more freely in a group. Almost all users believe that should their use of drugs ever become problematic, they would stop using them. What they fail to understand is that few people are able to abuse mood-altering substances regularly without eventually developing a psychological or physiological dependence. Furthermore, as the addiction process progresses, a system of defenses including denial, rationalization, and projection invariably develops in the user, making him the last person to realize that drug abuse is a problem.

Once the addiction has begun, various factors tend to perpetuate it. These include the addictive properties of the drugs themselves, craving, the desire to avoid withdrawal symptoms, a sense of belonging with a drug-using social group, fear, and lack of ability to cope in a "straight" world.

Factors that may motivate a person to seek help include legal problems, deteriorating physical health, feelings of disgust at one's behaviors under the influence of drugs, financial problems, and pressure from family, employers, coworkers, or concerned friends.

Alcohol Abuse

Alcohol is the number one drug of abuse in the United States today. Alcohol consumption is affected by demographic characteristics, traditions, cultural patterns, and attitudes.

Definitions of Alcoholism

There are two commonly quoted definitions of alcoholism. The American Medical Association defines alcoholism as follows: "alcoholism is a disease which is characterized by a compulsive drinking of alcohol in some form. It is an addiction to alcohol. The drinking of alcohol produces continuing or repeated problems in the patient's life."[2] Mark Keller of the Center of Alcohol Studies at Rutgers University defined alcoholism as

> a chronic disease or disorder of behavior, characterized by the repeated drinking of alcoholic beverages to an extent that exceeds the customary dietary use of ordinary compliance with the social drinking customs of the community, and that interferes with the drinker's health, interpersonal relations or economic functioning.[10]

Both definitions, although helpful, create great difficulty in identifying the alcoholic unless the person comes forward. This has led to a need to identify the patient at risk by careful screening of the problems associated with alcohol.

Metabolism of Alcohol

Ethyl alcohol (ethanol) is a sedative-hypnotic drug. If it were newly discovered today it would be classified with barbiturates, tranquilizers, and hypnotics. Ethanol is present in varying amounts in hard liquor (whiskey, gin, rum, vodka), wine, and beer. Whiskey contains approximately 43% ethyl alcohol, fortified wine 20%, table wine 12%, and beer approximately 4%. One drink (1 jigger = 1 oz) of hard liquor contains approximately the same amount of alcohol as one 4-oz glass of wine, or one 12-oz can of beer. One ounce of absolute alcohol is in 2 cans of beer, 2 glasses of wine, or 2 shots of whiskey.

Ethanol is absorbed unaltered from the gastrointestinal tract—about 80% in the intestines and the remainder from the stomach. Milk and fatty food impede absorption. It is a rapid-acting central nervous system depressant and may be detected in the blood within 5 minutes after ingestion, with the maximum concentration reached in 30 minutes to 2 hours. It is carried by the plasma to many organs of the body.[1]

Alcohol is metabolized almost exclusively in the liver with certain enzymes required. The rate of catabolic reaction is unrelated to blood concentration. It is limited by the ability of the liver to metabolize ethanol at a rate of approximately 10 ml per hour. A man of average weight can metabolize approximately one drink per hour. If the intake of ethanol exceeds the liver's ability to metabolize alcohol, by-products accumulate and may cause nausea, vomiting, hypotension, or even death if excessive amounts of ethanol are ingested.

Alcohol Intoxication

Acute intoxication can occur when alcohol is consumed. The results the person experiences are affected by the previous use of alcohol. Even 1 to 2 oz of alcohol in the uninitiated drinker can produce a decrease in inhibitions and a relaxed sensation. In general once the alcohol is consumed, time is the only factor that will affect the intoxicated state. The rate of absorption primarily depends on the concentration of alcohol in the stomach and duodenum. This concentration can be affected by the presence of food in the stomach, but once alcohol is absorbed the rate of metabolism is fixed. The faster and the more alcohol a person drinks the higher the blood alcohol levels are reached resulting in various behavior changes. Cold showers, coffee, or walking will not shorten the time of intoxication. At blood alcohol concentrations of 0.1 (100 mg/100 ml) the evidence of intoxication is definite. Many states use 0.1 to define legal intoxication levels.

Some general effects that can occur with alcohol are similar to anesthesia and sedative effects. The weight and the sex of a person are related to the amount that can be consumed before these effects are realized. Females cannot tolerate as much alcohol as males before they realize the effects of alcohol. Women also notice different levels of intoxication depending on the stage of their menstrual cycle.

Chronic alcohol consumption over long periods of time alters the sensitivity of the central nervous system, leading to tolerance. This chronic use of alcohol makes it necessary to increase the dose or blood level of alcohol in order to achieve the same desired effects or conversely a diminished effect with regular alcohol at the same amount. The repeated use of alcohol can cause tolerance to other drugs with depressant effects and the development of cross-tolerance.

Treatment of Alcoholism

There are several places for treatment of alcoholism. They include inpatient hospitalization, residential programs, halfway houses, outpatient clinics, day hospitals, and detoxification facilities.

Detoxification Programs and Specific Therapies

Hospital-based medical detoxification programs mainly use diazepam and chlordiazepoxide. These programs are for people who are severely alcohol dependent and not in good health.

Social setting programs with no inpatient care do not use medications but utilize other therapies aimed at changing the person's behavior and helping him deal with the reasons he feels it is necessary to drink alcohol. These facilities provide referral to long-term treatment. Research supports the usefulness (success) of the social setting. However success is dependent upon the patient's physical condition, nutritional status, severity of alcohol dependence, and overall medical evaluation.[15]

Specific therapies to treat alcoholism include: Alcoholics Anonymous (AA); behavior therapy, Antabuse, coping skill training, and aversion. Psychotherapy and group therapy as well as combinations of several therapies have also been used. AA is a support group. The person is assigned someone to call if he feels the need to drink. People who join admit they are alcoholics and need help. In addition to the group for persons with alcoholism, there is Al-Anon (for families of alcoholics) and Al-Ateen (for teenagers with alcoholic parents).

Behavior therapy uses social skills (how to interview, how to get a job), assertiveness training, contingency management, deep muscle relaxation, self-control training, and cognitive restructuring. Group therapy is another modality also based upon social skill training.

Coping skill training teaches new adaptive coping skills to people who engage in dysfunctional behavior. These skills include learning how to cope with people, events, and feelings that may have been the reason for drinking.

Aversion therapy is based upon Pavlov's theory of conditioning. The smell, sight, and taste of alcohol are to acquire aversive properties if repeatedly paired with noxious stimuli. Emetic aversion is more successful in stopping drinking than electric shock aversion. Research is now underway evaluatilng covert sensitization, imagined scenes of alcohol ingestion rather than actual drinking. Preliminary finds are encouraging.

Disulfiram (Antabuse) is a drug used to produce vomiting when taken with alcohol. The person must continue to take it to prevent drinking alcohol. It is useful with social skill training. It produces abstinence but doesn't get at the deeper-seated problem causing alcohol abuse.

Treatment of alcoholism is so difficult because alcoholics are a heterogeneous group. What is successful for one group may be ineffective for another. Success depends upon sex, cultural background, mental status, socioeconomic status, length of drinking, and other variables. None of the treatments are as successful as desired based upon the extent of the problem to society and the individual and his family.

There is still controversy over whether someone who has stopped drinking can ever drink again. Research indicates that moderate drinking may be possible for some people following treatment. Again it depends on many factors. The most appropriate goal for alcoholics is abstinence.[15]

Nursing Care: Screening

The identification of the alcohol-dependent individual is probably the most important step in the nursing process. Screening for the patient with alcohol abuse constitutes many social, psychological, and physiological symptoms.

Many assessment tools have been developed to evaluate drinking problems; these should be part of a routine physical examination. In general clinics and hospital settings two short forms have been used and validated for identifying the patient at risk: the Short Michigan Alcoholism Screening Test (SMAST) and the CAGE Questionnaire (Tables 103–1 and 103–2). In the SMAST, alcoholism-indicating responses are given one point each. Those scoring above 2 points are possibly alcoholic and those above 3 more probably so. If the answer to number 6 (Have you ever attended a meeting of alcoholics anonymous?) is yes, assessment should be made as to why. The CAGE test is shorter, considered reliable and a valid instrument, and can easily be incorporated into an existing health assessment form. The four questions elicit information about cutting down alcohol consumption, annoyance by criticism, guilt associated about alcohol use, and "eye openers" or early morning drinking. (The word CAGE is derived from extracting the first letter of the four ideas in the questionnaire.)

Social Symptoms

Patterns of pathological abuse are demonstrated by the patient's need for daily use of alcohol to function and an inability to cut down or stop drinking by repeated efforts. Initially alcoholics make frequent reference to alcohol and

TABLE 103–1
Short Michigan Alcoholism Screening Test

1. Do you feel you are a normal drinker? (By normal we mean you drink less than or as much as most other people.) (No)
2. Does your wife, husband, a parent, or other near relative ever worry or complain about your drinking? (Yes)
3. Do you ever feel guilty about your drinking? (Yes)
4. Do friends or relatives think you are a normal drinker? (No)
5. Are you able to stop drinking when you want to? (No)
6. Have you ever attended a meeting of Alcoholics Anonymous? (Yes)
7. Has drinking ever created problems between you and your wife, husband, a parent, or other near relative? (Yes)
8. Have you ever gotten into trouble at work because of drinking? (Yes)
9. Have you ever neglected your obligations, your family, or your work for two or more days in a row because you were drinking? (Yes)
10. Have you ever gone to anyone for help about your drinking? (Yes)
11. Have you ever been in a hospital because of drinking? (Yes)
12. Have you ever been arrested for drunken driving, driving while intoxicated, or driving under the influence of alcoholic beverages? (Yes)
13. Have you ever been arrested, even for a few hours, because of other drunken behavior? (Yes)

Alcoholism-indicating responses in parentheses.
Scoring: 0–1 points—nonalcoholic
2 points—possible alcoholic
3 points—alcoholic

(Reprinted by permission from Journal of Studies on Alcohol 36:117–126, 1975. Copyright by Journal of Studies on Alcohol, Inc., New Brunswick, N.J. 08903)

TABLE 103–2
The CAGE Questionnaire

1. Have you ever felt you should **C**ut down on your drinking?
2. Have people **A**nnoyed you by criticizing your drinking?
3. Have you ever felt bad or **G**uilty about your drinking?
4. Have you ever had a drink first thing in the morning to steady your nerves or get rid of a hang-over (**E**ye-opener)?

Scoring: 2 or 3 out of 4 answered "yes" strongly suggests alcoholism.

(Mayfield D., et al.: The American Journal of Psychiatry 131:1121, 1974. Copyright 1974, the American Psychiatric Association. Reprinted by permission.)

brag about drinking. Later, secretive use of alcohol occurs. These individuals may experience repeated periods of abstinence and then binges of excessive use. Blackout, amnesic periods for events while intoxicated, may occur. Difficulty with memory increases. Other social and occupational difficulties can occur (*e.g.,* absence from work especially on a Monday after a weekend of drinking, loss of a job, arguments and difficulties with family and friends, and difficulties with the law such as arrests for intoxicated behavior, violence while intoxicated, traffic accidents, and driving while intoxicated [DWI].

Alcoholics look for jobs that accommodate their drinking needs. Companions are picked who prefer heavy drinking.

Alcohol is used to relieve tension, anger, fatigue, depression, insomnia, and social discomfort. A person's spouse may complain about drinking behavior. The family life is further disrupted with separation or divorce. Late in the disease denial, anger, and projection are some of the main defenses. Alcoholics develop paranoid attitudes, crying episodes, depression, and finally isolate themselves until they have few or no friends. Statistics indicate that over half of suicide attempts are associated with alcohol abuse.

Family history can be helpful. Of adolescent suicides 80% are thought to come from alcoholic homes. There is also an increased likelihood that children of alcoholics will themselves become alcoholics, anywhere from one half to three fourths depending on whether one or both parents are alcoholics.

Behavioral Symptoms

Many assessment tools developed to evaluate drinking problems can be part of a routine exam. These tools are both helpful in screening for early alcoholism and for those who are willing to discuss some early concern about alcohol abuse. However, defenses of denial, guilt, and rationalization shield the middle-stage alcoholic from admitting to any problem with alcohol and the late-stage alcoholic may display a defeatist attitude. The nurse then needs to recognize many of the previously discussed changes in lifestyle and many physical clues to alcohol abuse.

The skill of the nurse in asking questions about alcohol use and the ability to observe nonverbal responses can also aid in the identification of the alcoholic. For example, patients who respond readily to questions about cigarette consumption may be vague, evasive, anxious, and avoid eye contact when asked about alcohol consumption. Questions about alcohol use can also be asked with questions about other medications used. Emphasis on the importance of knowing about alcohol consumption in relation to its effect on other drugs will at times force a patient to be more open about alcohol use. Alcohol use can be elicited as part of a diet history. Whatever the means if the patient has established secretive defenses or strong denial about alcohol use, the nurse must be an astute observer of nonverbal responses and a skilled interpreter of information elicited.

Observation of physical changes may be the only clues to alcohol abuse. Symptoms of tolerance or withdrawal are definite signs of physical dependence. Withdrawal may be noted as the development of symptoms of tremors, morning shakes, increased perspiration, or malaise after the cessation of drinking. The symptoms disappear after treatment with cross-tolerant drugs or after receiving alcohol. This reduction of symptoms may be noted after visits by family or friends.

Tolerance is present when large amounts of alcohol can be consumed without evidence of drinking. More specifically in the medical or hospital setting, tolerance is evident by a blood alcohol level of more than 100 mg% in a routine examination, more than 150 mg% without gross evidence of intoxication, more than 300 mg% at any one time or the consumption of one fifth of a gallon of whiskey or its equivalent in wine or beer for more than 1 day by an average individual. When blood alcohol levels may not be tested, the nurse should watch for cross-tolerance to other drugs. This may be noted when the patient who is receiving sedative hypnotics is initially overreactive and very sedated from these drugs. As time goes on an increasing amount of these drugs are necessary to keep the patient relaxed or sedated. Late in the course of alcoholism, tolerance decreases. Patients may complain that they "can no longer drink like they could in the past."

Psychological dependence is present in alcohol abuse. As the alcohol use becomes more dominant in the patient's existence, most activities are planned around the drinking needs and a schedule of consumption is developed. Craving for alcohol and an inability to control the amount and frequency of drinking are present. The individual may talk excessively about alcohol but eventually may become secretive and start hiding alcohol and sneaking drinks. A strong phychological dependence is definite when drinking continues despite strong medical and social containdications to continued use.

Many other less dominant but important observations can help identify the alcohol abuser. The odor of alcohol on the breath at a time of an appointment can be suggestive. Many physical changes (*e.g.,* malnutrition or general debilitation) may lead one to suspect alcohol abuse. Cigarette burns or other burns on the hands or chest indicate probable intoxication while smoking. Constant flushed face, vascular engorgement of the face, and ecchymoses on the lower extremities, arms, and chest are suggestive of alcohol abuse. Sleeplessness and noctural diaphoresis may indicate withdrawal symptoms during the night.

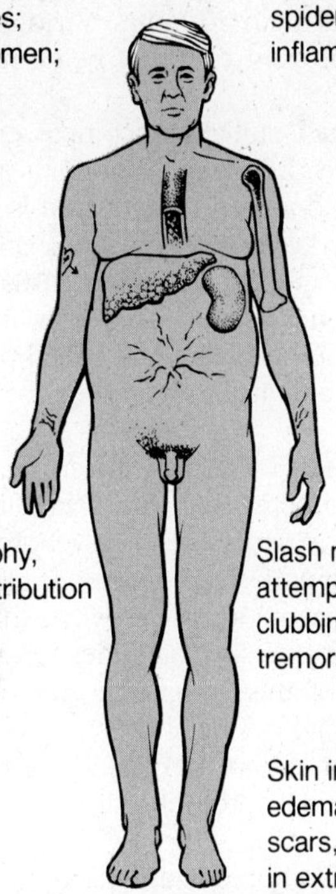

FIGURE 103–1 Clinical findings suggestive of alcoholism: appearance older than stated age; thinness, especially in the extremities, while abdomen may be enlarged; skin color pale, ruddy, dirty gray or yellow; scratch marks from generalized pruritis; unsteady gait; slapping walk. In the early stages the above findings may be present only to a minor extent and may be clues to the early recognition of alcoholism.

Physical Symptoms

Signs and symptoms associated with the deterioration of certain body systems can be an indication to alcoholism. Especially important are neurological changes and liver changes. Cirrhosis and pancreatitis in the absence of cholelithiasis and many neurological degenerative diseases are commonly associated with alcoholism. Double vision should be a potential clue for alcohol abuse. Hyperreflexia or, if drinking, hyporeflexia may be indicative of alcohol abuse with permanent hyporeflexia as a residuum of alcoholic polyneuritis. See Figure 103–1.

Anemia is a common occurrence in alcoholism. Unexplained tachycardia or cardiac arrhythmias may indicate alcohol abuse. A frequency of infection or a slow healing process are possible clues. Any woman who delivers a child born with the effect of alcohol should be recognized as an alcohol abuser. Adults who also have the fetal alcohol effects may be identified.

Several tests may be abnormal in the presence of alcoholism. As previously mentioned, a high blood alcohol level with very little intoxicated effect demonstrates tolerance. Some indirect laboratory results associated with alcoholism are hypoglycemia, hypochloremic alkalosis, low magnesium, elevated lactic acid, decreased potassium, transient increase in uric acid elevation, and increased bilirubin, an elevation in SGPT (serum glutamic-pyruvic transaminase) and SGOT (serum glutamic-oxalacetic transaminase). ECG and EEG changes also occur.

With all the above information it becomes obvious that it takes enhanced skills in screening and observation to identify the patient at risk for alcohol abuse. Knowlege of social changes, lifestyle changes, psychological changes and defenses, and physiological changes are all of importance.

Withdrawal

Symptoms of withdrawal or abstinence syndrome are definite indications of alcohol dependence. Some degree of withdrawal will occur in most individuals who chronically use alcohol. Hangovers can occur in anyone who consumes a large amount of alcohol. This does not necessarily connotate a chronic exposure to alcohol even though some authors consider this syndrome a mild withdrawal or the effects of the congeners contained in drinks.[4] The symptoms of a hangover include gastrointestinal disturbances, nausea, headache, thirst, and general lassitude and can occur anywhere from 8 to 14 hours after the drinking episode.

Withdrawal symptoms arc generally considered a hyperexcitable state or a rebound phenomenon and have been called a sympathetic storm. The onset of symptoms occurs somewhere beyond 8 hours after the last drink, and symptoms usually peak around 24 hours. Various classifications have been used, the most common being minor or major withdrawal.

Minor withdrawal initially encompasses symptoms of tremors, restlessness, insomnia, abdominal pain, anorexia, mild diaphoresis, and anxiety. The person is hyperalert and irritable, and has jerky movements. The patient may eventually experience some disorientation, visual and auditory hallucinations, and nightmares. The body temperature increases as well as the heart rate and blood pressure. There may be isolated grand mal seizures or a series of many seizures.

Delirium tremens (DTs) is characteristic of major withdrawal and can occur between the third and fifth day after the last drink. This is a severe state of psychomotor agitation, confusion, disorientation, sleeplessness, frightening hallucinations, and increased autonomic activity exhibited by fever, tachycardia, and diaphoresis. The patient may seem uncontrollable. Because of this autonomic nervous system excitability the heart rate can be above 120 beats per minute, the body temperature above 104°F, and the blood pressure elevated accompanied by profound diaphoresis. Early warning signs are the elevation of these vital signs. Patients with more severe minor withdrawal, and especially patients with seizures, may progress to major withdrawal. Patients in withdrawal can develop alkalosis, shock, fluid and electrolyte imbalance, and hypokalemia. Cardiac arrhythmias may occur, further jeopardizing an already compromised patient.

Because very little can be done to alter the course of major withdrawal, early recognition of signs and symptoms and identification of patients at risk are essential. Delirium tremens is fatal in 15% of patients and 2% to 5% of treated patients. Patients may die from uncontrolled tachycardia, heart failure, and sudden arrhythmic deaths.

Nursing Care of the Patient in Withdrawal

Persons withdrawing from alcohol are encountered in many different settings. If the patient is admitted for detoxification, the health team can be prepared for a controlled withdrawal process. However, many patients are admitted for other health reasons and the staff are not prepared or able to initially recognize the withdrawal.

Assessment. An initial assessment and history are critical. Information about the drinking episode (*e.g.,* the type and amount of beverage and duration of the drinking pattern) can offer some guidelines. The time of the last drink can help gauge when to expect the onset of symptoms. Especially important are historical data about the types of withdrawal experienced by the patient in the past, especially if they include DTs or seizures.

Medication histories are imperative, and use of anticonvulsives can indicate past seizures during withdrawal. Potential emergency conditions should be elicited. This includes a history of diabetes, chronic health problems of lung, heart, stomach, and liver. Has the patient experienced pain, bleeding, vomiting, diarrhea, difficulty with balance, double vision, periods of confusion? Has he recently fallen, or been in an auto accident or in a fight? The effects of alcohol may camouflage internal injuries.

Blood alcohol levels may offer some guidelines as to the severity of the withdrawal. Usually the greater the tolerance to alcohol the more severe the withdrawal symptoms. Drugs that are cross tolerant to alcohol (*e.g.,* antianxiety drugs and sedative hypnotic drugs) are the main indications used for the withdrawal process. After an initial therapeutic dose is established to reduce symptoms, the dosage is titrated daily so as to gradually withdraw the patient. This usually means a reduction of the drug by about 20% per day. Symptoms and vital signs are monitored closely, and the drug is administered so as to keep the heart rate somewhere below 110, the blood pressure below 150/90, and the temperature below 100°F. Hypovolemia and a history of hypertension should be ruled out.

Interventions. Nursing care includes monitoring the patient's signs and symptoms closely and providing a calm and quiet environment. The severity of tremors and diaphoresis should be monitored. Because the patient is experiencing a "sympathetic storm," any stimulation or confrontation at this time may worsen the symptoms. These patients are easily startled. Drugs are the accepted treatment; cross-tolerant drugs titrated to decreasing uses are usually used.

Some centers have avoided using drugs to treat withdrawal and have used reality orientation, a form of quiet, supportive nursing, talking the patient through relaxation techniques, and keeping the patient oriented to the environment. Family members can be helpful if trained in what to expect and how to provide comfort measures. Lighting in the room should be such to avoid shadows and hallucinations. Sudden movements, noises, strange pictures, and bright colors should be avoided. Glasses or any sharp or dangerous objects need to be removed from the room. Padding the bed is helpful. Appropriate medications and precautions should be available if seizures occur.

If DTs occur, vital signs need to be checked frequently. As the agitation increases so do the pulse, temperature, and blood pressure. Ice packs or a cooling mattress may be needed because hyperthermia may occur in the absence of an infection. Infections may become a problem. Aspiration of secretions may be encountered, further compromising the patient. Alcoholics are also prone to infection because of a poor immune response and decreased leukocytes. Circulatory collapse may occur during withdrawal and requires careful monitoring.

Fluids are required for profuse diaphoresis. The fluid status needs careful monitoring so the patient is not overhydrated in the initial stages.

Many other factors are essential to evaluate. Withdrawal without any other complications is severe alone. Many patients hospitalized for various reasons experience withdrawal because staff are not aware of the alcohol problem. It has been estimated that one third of hospitalized patients are alcohol abusers. A patient having routine surgery may go through withdrawal while in surgery because he or she stopped drinking on admission the night before surgery. A patient may be admitted to the coronary care unit for unexplained arrhythmias and then has no access to alcohol and experiences withdrawal. Many car accident victims have consumed alcohol and are admitted with multiple injuries (*e.g.*, head trauma or bleeding) and then experience withdrawal. The examples are unlimited. Care should be taken to identify the very early symptoms of withdrawal so that the patient can be treated before experiencing uncontrolled withdrawal.

Psychosocial Support and Guidance

Aside from dealing with the problem of withdrawal, how does the nurse care for this patient, especially in relation to psychological deterioration? Alcoholism is a family illness; however, many times patients have either physically or psychologically isolated themselves from their families and most relationships are superficial or are with other alcoholics. Communication can be difficult because patients are often intoxicated or experience withdrawal or denial, anger, and projection. Once the acute physiological episode is over in the hospital, the nurse may attempt to guide, not advise, this person into treatment. Anger and denial may block any attempts to refer. At times only when the patient is making a last attempt to salvage a relationship or job will he be attentive and able to confront the problem. Many will merely change lifestyles. If a single friend can be found assistance may be possible through this person. Alcoholics Anonymous can help some people; others are not ready for this move.

Many programs for treatment of alcoholism are available in the United States. These range from approaches with group therapy, psychoanalysis, and aversion therapy. The problem is how to encourage the patient for referral. The impact of alcoholism has on the individual and family must be recognized and confronted before the individual is willing to seek help. In the hospital setting patients may become frightened enough by their illness to finally seek help; this opportunity should not be overlooked. Other patients will be sent to treatment because of problems with the law. Some will finally reach "an all-time low" that triggers them to seek help. Care should be taken to avoid overzealous planning of many changes in the patient's life which are consequently doomed to failure.

Recovery from alcoholism is a lifelong process. Recurrence of problems can lead to drinking again. A supportive social network is probably one of the most important aspects of a life of sobriety.

Drug Abuse

Classification of Drugs of Abuse

The most commonly abused drugs are classified as follows:

Central nervous system depressants—drugs that produce temporary reduction of functional activity
Narcotics—drugs that selectively depress the central nervous system
Inhalants—aerosols that mainly depress the central nervous system
Stimulants—drugs that produce temporary increase in functional activity
Hallucinogens—drugs that produce temporary distortion of reality
Cannabinols—drugs that have hallucinogen properties but are usually only taken in a quantity to produce an altered state of consciousness.

These drugs are abused when they are used to exert control over one's body and central nervous system.

Exact statistical data on the number of abusers of drugs other than alcohol are difficult to determine. The abuse of both illicit drugs and of legal prescription and over-the-counter drugs occurs throughout American society. Also, many of these drugs are abused in combination or in sequence, making it nearly impossible to obtain data on the full extent of their use.

The statistics that are available, however, point to the existence of a fluctuating, pervasive public-health problem that is of vital concern to all health professionals. For instance, in 1984 prior to high school graduation, 93% of students nationwide used alcohol, 60% used marijuana, 33% used speed, 18% used hallucinogens, and 17% used cocaine. Admissions to cocaine treatment programs increased sixfold from 1975 to 1981. According to the National Institute of Drug Abuse (NIDA), 20 million Americans already have tried cocaine and four to five million are current users. The number of persons who have experienced marijuana is estimated to be 40 million, with several million who use it more frequently than on a weekly basis. The estimated number of opiate-dependent individuals has remained rather constant at 450,000 to 600,000. When drugs are abused, as with alcohol, there is more than just the concern of what the drug does to the person's body. Many social, legal, and psychological problems parallel drug misuse.

General Central Nervous System (CNS) Depressants

Alcohol is the most widely used addicting sedative drug in the United States today.

There are over 2500 sedative-hypnotic prescription drugs on the market. These drugs are commonly prescribed by physicians for sleep or to combat anxiety and tension. When they are used without close supervision, the possibility of taking increased amounts and becoming dependent is present. In street parlance the sedatives are also known as goofballs, sleepers, and downers. The barbiturates constitute the largest group of sedatives. Ninety-nine percent of illegal barbiturates come from legal pharmaceutical companies. CNS depressants are addicting and have a high tolerance level.

The different CNS depressants possess markedly different lengths of action. These are the result of physical redistribution of the drug, metabolic breakdown of the substance (usually in the liver), and excretion by the kidneys.

Drug Action

The primary action of sedative-hypnotic drugs is relaxation or depression of the central nervous system. Constant increasing doses are required to achieve the desired effect and to ward off the potentially fatal withdrawal syndrome that develops when the blood level is not maintained because of the phenomenon known as tolerance. These effects of increased use are slurred speech, disorientation, drunken behavior without the odor of alcohol, staggering, decreased control of emotions, loss of balance, irritability, and dizziness. In high doses these drugs may produce agitation, excitement, restlessness, and possibly delirium.

As a general rule, abuse of 500 mg of a barbiturate or an equivalent dose of other such drugs will result in a risk for withdrawal seizures. For the benzodiazepines, minor to moderate withdrawal symptoms can be seen with individuals taking two or three times the usual clinical dose for 16 weeks or less. The drug withdrawal syndrome is usually a mixture of possible symptoms, running a time course that tends to last 3 to 7 days for the short-acting drugs, and longer for longer-acting drugs like diazepam (Valium).

If a person is dependent on one sedative drug, any other sedative drug can be effectively substituted to maintain or exacerbate addiction. This phenomenon is known as *cross-addiction*.

Sedative-hypnotics are frequently used in combination with alcohol, opiates, cocaine, or amphetamines. These drugs dangerously potentiate the action of alcohol or poor quality heroin, reduce the anxiety and depression associated with cocaine abuse, and decrease the hyperexcitability of the amphetamine abuser.

Dangers and Side-Effects

There is always the danger of overdose associated with use of sedative-hypnotic drugs. Overdose can happen when the dependent person unknowingly continues to take more of the drug while under the influence of the drug. Overdose can also occur when the abuser inadvertently takes too large an amount of barbiturates to counteract or moderate the effects of large doses of amphetamine. Mixed with alcohol, the sedative-hypnotic drugs have a super-additive or potentiating effect which often results in death due to total depression of the respiratory mechanism.

The withdrawal syndrome that occurs when intake of the sedative-hypnotic drug is decreased drastically or stopped is as potentially harmful as the delirium tremens associated with alcohol withdrawal. It can last approximately 72 hours.

These drugs also result in an impairment of physical and mental capabilities including reduced perceptual ability, an increased distortion of surroundings, confusion, decreased alertness and concentration. Consequently, automobile accidents, self-injury from falls, and acute anxiety reactions may ensue, as well as withdrawal from those situations which require responsible and alert reactions. The suicide rate is increased with CNS depressants. High doses of the drug methaqualone result in abolititon of the person's arousal response to painful and auditory stimuli and increased feelings of indestructability.

Treatment for CNS Depressant Addiction

Withdrawal. Cessation of the physically addicting sedative-hypnotic drugs by the dependent person results in a withdrawal syndrome which is considered life threatening when left untreated or when allowed to advance in severity.

The overall goals of managing this withdrawal syndrome are to

1. Prevent seizure activity
2. Gradually detoxify the patient on decreasing doses of the sedative-hypnotic of choice
3. Prevent the onset of psychosis, delirium, or acute panic states.

With rare exception, it is recommended that detoxification and withdrawal be carried out in a hospital because of the possibility of life-endangering seizures.

Upon admission to the hospital, a comprehensive quantitative drug screen and a verified drug-taking history should be taken. Unlike alcohol withdrawal, which begins and ends rather quickly following cessation, abstinence syndrome in sedative-hypnotic barbiturates and antianxiety dependency runs a time course of 3 to 7 days for the short-acting drugs and longer for drugs like diazepam (Valium), where seizures and delirium can begin as late as day 7 or 8.[14] Withdrawal also depends upon the daily quantities consumed and the half life of the specific drugs.

Vital signs should be monitored every 3 to 4 hours for the first 3 to 5 days, then every 6 to 8 hours for the duration of the withdrawal period. A pulse of over 100 mmHg or a temperature of over 99°F should be reported.

Withdrawal from the time of onset of symptoms until the danger of seizure activity has passed lasts anywhere from 1 day to 10 days. The true physiological withdrawal syndrome will be characterized by highly increased anxiety symptoms, perceptual changes, tremor, GI upset, muscle aches, increased pulse, respiration, and temperature, labile blood pressure, drug craving, and often psychotic symptoms. With any CNS depressant, somewhere betwen 5% and perhaps 20% will develop grand mal convulsions though seldom status epilepticus. In addition, somewhere between 5% and 15% of the individuals develop an organic brain syndrome (OBS) or a hallucination/delirium state. With the barbiturates, probably at least half of the people who develop convulsions during withdrawal go on to a delirium if not treated.

Drug-hunger or pseudowithdrawal syndrome is marked only by an increase in symptoms of anxiety. It is vital that the withdrawing person be given only the scheduled doses of the sedative and not additional medication for anxiety because this only feeds the drug craving and the addiction process. These people need a great deal of reassurance and encouragement that the period of withdrawal is transitory, that they are safe, and that they are not "going crazy" as they so often believe they are.

Controlled sedative-hypnotic withdrawal is then achieved by either substituting another sedative-hypnotic or using the sedative-hypnotic of abuse and gradually reducing the dosage.

Overdose. Sedative-hypnotic overdose is a major cause of accidental and intentional suicide. It may occur when large doses are taken repeatedly over a short period of time, when a mixture of long- and short-acting sedative-hypnotics are taken, when alcohol is ingested with sedative hypnotics, or when sedative hypnotics are unknowingly used as filler or potentiation of other drugs, such as heroin.

The overdose patient will often be comatose, have pale, cyanotic skin, have depressed urine output, and may be in shock—vital signs will include a weak, rapid, or slow weak pulse, slow or rapid and shallow or Cheyne-Stokes respirations, low blood pressure, and temperature may be lowered several degrees.

Maintenance of respiratory function is the primary immediate goal. Other life-preserving measures must be implemented such as correction of circulatory depression by means of intravenous infusions of solutions, plasma expanders, and vasopressor agents. Concurrent efforts are made to promote rapid removal of the drug from the body by either aspiration of gastric contents, stimulating forced diuresis, or, as a critical or last resort measure, peritoneal dialysis or hemodialysis. Additional supportive measures are necessary to prevent the hazards of immobility when a comatose patient is admitted.

Respiratory complications are common sequelae of sedative-hypnotic overdose especially if the patient is comatose for a long time or in poor health. Severe bullous lesions of the skin are a complication of barbiturate overdose.

After the acute episode of withdrawal or overdose is over and physiological stability has been regained, the person should continue to receive long-term professional help for the drug dependence.

Narcotics

The term narcotic drugs refers to the opiates and other analgesics. The major opiates include natural substances, such as opium, morphine, and codeine; semisynthetic drugs derived from the basic poppy products including heroin, hydromorphone (Dilaudid), and oxycodone (Percodan) and synthetic analgesics, such as propoxyphene (Darvon), meperidine (Demerol), methadone (Dolophine), diphenoxylate (Lomotil), and pentazocine (Talwin).

Drug Action

In general, the opiates are considered to selectively depress the central nervous system. Intake of opium, ingested or inhaled, results in a euphoric feeling, the elimination of pain, distorted sense of time, and feelings of self-confidence. The duration of the effects of morphine and heroin is approximately 4 to 6 hours.

The drugs undergo similar metabolism by the body but differ in their degree of oral absorption. Heroin is rapidly converted by the body into morphine, with detoxification occurring primarily in the liver, and the metabolites are then excreted through the urine and bile. Over 90% of the excretion of doses of these drugs (with the exception of very long-acting substances such as methadone) occurs within the first 24 hours, although metabolites can be seen for 48 hours or more.

After or during intravenous injection, the user experiences an immediate "rush" subjectively described as a body orgasm (in the stomach, intestines, or all over). A euphoric high follows the rush in which the person may experience drowsiness, slurred speech, impaired muscular coordination, depressed reflexes, and cessation of pain. The heart rate slows, appetite and respiration are depressed, pupils are constricted as are the smooth muscle fibers, and gastrointestinal secretions are decreased. An additional action specific to the synthetic narcotic meperidine is the dilation of pupils.

Abuse of the synthetic narcotic methadone is widespread. The effects of methadone are similar to morphine but develop more slowly and last longer. While methadone is being used, it will block or prohibit the action of any other opiate taken subsequently while the methadone is active in the body. It is this blocking action that provides the rationale for methadone maintenance programs for heroin dependence.

Side-Effects

Tolerance to increasing doses of most opiates develops rapidly, particularly the more potent analgesics like heroin and morphine, but the changes in organ sensitivity develop unevenly. Almost all the opiates exhibit cross-tolerance to other members of the class. Narcotic-dependent persons can take larger doses which, if taken by a nonuser, would most likely result in death. Physical dependence also develops rapidly and increases as the dose increases. Decrease or cessation of narcotic intake results in a withdrawal syndrome that is not generally fatal but is marked by influenza-like symptoms of diarrhea, cramps, "chills with goose-flesh," vomiting, and nausea. The physical withdrawal reinforces the compulsion to continue taking the drug. There is also a strong psychological or emotional dependence on the euphoric, pleasurable effects of narcotics which is rapidly created. The user feels an increasing compulsion to continue taking the drug in order to reproduce the desired sensations.

The major adverse effects include overdose that occurs when the user knowingly or unknowingly "mainlines" a quantity of heroin that is significantly more potent than the customary supply. Also, increased incidence of constipation, menstrual irregularities and temporary sterility in female addicts, decreased interest in sexual activities, diet, hygiene, and preventive health care, abscesses at injection sites, and high incidence of tetanus, hepatitis, endocarditis, septicemia, pulmonary complications, and AIDS can occur with narcotics dependence. Thus, although there is little or no evidence that narcotics directly cause damage to the organ systems of the body, the patterns of abuse can induce serious physical adverse effects.

Treatment for Dependence on Narcotics

Withdrawal. The current treatment of withdrawal from narcotics may focus specifically on the management of withdrawal symptoms, or the use of methadone as either a detoxification agent or as a drug for long-term maintenance therapy.

Withdrawal symptoms associated with narcotic dependence are usually not considered life threatening unlike the abstinence syndromes for alcohol and the sedative-hypnotics in which seizure activity can occur. Many narcotic addicts withdraw unassisted several times during their abusing years without serious harm resulting. The psychological fears and anxiety generated by impending withdrawal are often more disturbing to the abuser than the actual physical abstinence symptoms. The psychological fear and discomfort created by the possibility of withdrawal are one of the major reasons for relapse.

The onset of narcotic withdrawal usually begins at the time of the next scheduled drug dose, ranging from 4 to 6 hours for heroin to a day or more for methadone. Within 12 hours of the last dose, there is usually the beginning of physical discomfort, characterized by tearing of the eyes, a runny nose, sweating, and yawning. Within 12 to 14 hours, and peaking on the second or third day, the patient moves into a restless sleep. Over the same peak period occurring 36 to 48 hours after the last dose of morphine and 24 to 72 hours after the last dose of heroin, the classic symptoms of dilated pupils, loss of appetite, gooseflesh, back pain, and tremor appear. This is followed by insomnia, incessant yawning, flulike symptoms including GI upset, chills, flushing, weakness, muscle spasm, abdominal pain, and ejaculation. This acute phase of withdrawal decreases after the peak and usually disappears in a week or so. The psychological craving and irritability may continue, and the protracted abstinence consisting of physiological as well as behaviorally mediated aspects, goes on for many months. The risk of death from acute withdrawal is low and exists primarily for the debilitated, malnourished person whose withdrawal symptoms become prolonged and result in acute weight loss, dehydration, and fluid and electrolyte imbalances.

Following detoxification, the narcotic-dependent person must continue with long-term treatment for the dependency. When rehabilitation, counseling, long-term treatment, and follow-up care are not followed through, relapse rates may run as high as 95% 6 months or less following detoxification.[5]

Narcotic Detoxification. Approaches to detoxification include methadone and/or narcotic antagonists. In a controlled withdrawal regimen, the initial dose of methadone may be fixed or calculated on the dosage of narcotic used per day. The initial dose is usually maintained for 1 or 2 days followed by controlled reduction in dose averaging 5 mg/day.[1] Detoxification can then be completed in approximately 4 to 10 days.

Methadone detoxification is used less frequently than methadone maintenance in which methadone is substituted for the opiate(s) of abuse. After the maintenance dose has been reached, the effects of the opiate(s) are blocked if taken while taking methadone.

Methadone hydrochloride is usually given once daily orally in orange juice or in an orange-flavored liquid to mask both its bitter taste and the amount of the dose. Over a 3- to 4-week period persons are slowly brought up to their maintenance dose. Several times a week or daily, supervised urine specimens are required of participants. These specimens are analyzed to determine if the person has taken opiates or other chemicals of abuse. Evidence that the person has taken such drugs may result in dismissal from the program.

The largest criticism of methadone maintenance is that it does not solve the primary problem of the dependence on a narcotic. It merely substitutes a legal drug for an illegal one and the addiction process continues.

The most prominent of the physical side-effects reported by those on methadone maintenance include sleep disturbances, increased perspiration, constipation, muscle cramps, and sexual dysfunction, including impotence. Withdrawal from methadone takes longer than withdrawal from heroin and may have greater discomfort associated with it.

In recent years, modest success has been obtained by the use of certain narcotic antagonists with persons who have previously been withdrawn. It is hypothesized that the narcotic antagonists prevent the narcotics from reaching specific receptor sites in the brain so that should the narcotic be taken following the ingestion of an antagonist, it would have no effect. The long-acting antagonist, naltrexone, is the antagonist of choice and appears to be most useful in those persons strongly motivated to an abstinent lifestyle.

Overdose. Heroin overdose results when abusers (1) inject an excessively potent amount of the drug, believing that their body can tolerate it; (2) decrease their habit and then inject too potent a dose; or (3) inject an excessive amount for other reasons (*e.g.*, suicide).

The cardinal symptoms of heroin overdose are pinpoint pupils and respiratory depression, which may include shallow, gasping breathing, irregular respiration with periods of apnea, tachypnea, dyspnea, or orthopnea. The skin will be either pale or bluish, depending on the depth of respiratory difficulty. Areflexia, hypotension, and bradycardia are common. The finding of a strong pulse and heartbeat, in the presence of the other diagnostic evidence can be deceptive because it may herald a terminal arrhythmia. Evidence of recent needle tracts on the extremities, in the groin area, or under the tongue can also confirm the diagnosis.

Although heroin overdose requires immediate inteventio n to prevent death, it requires less complex treatment than barbiturate overdose because of the availability of narcotic antagonists. So, following the establishment of a patent, unobstructed airway, intravenous administration of specific narcotic antagonists is necessitated. The narcotic antagonists should be used with caution because excessive amounts can result in intensified respiratory depression or can precipitate the onset of rapid, acute withdrawal symptoms. The patient will usually respond immediately after the drug is injected. If after responding the patient then lapses into coma, the antagonist can be given again. The patient who does not respond to two injections of the narcotic antagonist should be examined carefully for traumatic injury or metabolically induced coma. The patient should not be left unattended even though he or she may appear alert and oriented after the injection(s).

The major pulmonary complication of heroin overdose is acute pulmonary edema secondary to the severe respiratory depression. Often the pulmonary edema will improve substantially after respiratory assistance and the administration of narcotic antagonists.

Inhalants

Aerosols, commercial solvents, and anesthetics make up the category known as the inhalants. Inhalants are volatile chemical substances that produce altered states of consciousness and varying degress of inebriation when inhaled. They are considered to be central nervous system depressants.

Abused aerosols include preparations containing freon, insecticides, hair sprays, and deodorants. Commercial solvents include airplane glue, paint thinner, lacquer, plastic cements, leaded gasoline, nail polish remover, cleaning fluid, lighter fluid, and typewriter correction fluid. These solvents contain varying amounts and combinations of toluene, naphtha, acetone, benzene, carbon tetrachloride, xylene, and other volatile substances. Inhalation of glue vapors is considered to be one of the most physically damaging form of drug abuse.[5] Chloroform, nitrous oxide, and ether are the most commonly abused anesthetics.

Drug Action

Initial responses to inhalation of these volatile substances are similar to those experienced with alcohol intoxication: slurred speech, decreased coordination and feelings of inhibition, dizziness, ataxia, diplopia, tinnitis, and perhaps hallucinations, euphoria, muscle spasms, behavioral and personality changes, and impaired perception and judgment. As the effects wear off, the user generally feels drowsy, depressed or stuporous, sometimes nauseated, and may lapse into a period of unconsciousness. When the effects of the drug have worn off, the user generally does not remember all the events or sensations that took place during the experience.

Over time, psychological dependence on volatile substances does occur as does tolerance. Physical dependence on the inhalants has not been clearly demonstrated as there is not substantiated evidence of a withdrawal syndrome following cessation of use.

Side-Effects

The severity of the adverse effects resulting from abuse of volatile substances is related to the substances used, its strength, the amount inhaled, and the use of other drugs. Overdose is most common with glue and gasoline and can be attributed to miscalculation of tolerance by the user, suffocation that occurs when the user becomes unconscious while the plastic bag used to concentrate the glue vapors is still over the head, and the simultaneous intake of other central nervous system depressants, especially alcohol.

Evidence of serious and sometimes permanent damage to certain organ systems and cellular function has been associated with abuse of the inhalants. Damaged lung tissue, bone marrow depression, and damage to the liver, kidneys, and spleen may result. Gasoline abuse may result in lead poisoning. Severe burn injury may result if inhalants are used near combustion sources such as lighters, sparks, or matches. Use of freon products may result in sudden death due to cardiac arrhythmia. Accidents are a high risk when the person under the influence of inhalants attempts to drive or operate machinery.

Treatment for Dependence on Inhalants

To date, there has been no definite demonstration of physical dependence or withdrawal syndrome associated with the abuse of inhalants. Treatment focuses on emergency intervention in an overdose situation and long-term addiction treatment. Specific treatment interventions for inhalant overdose are essentially the same as those for barbiturate overdose. In addition, the overdosed person may benefit from the inhalation of a combination of 95% oxygen and 5% carbon dioxide or fresh air. Intense physiological support measures are necessary to prevent total respiratory collapse.

Stimulants

The major stimulants of abuse are the amphetamines, cocaine, and several nonamphetamine stimulant drugs. Nicotine and caffeine will not be addressed here, despite increasing evidence that nicotine has more addictive potential than alcohol or heroin.

Amphetamines

Amphetamines are synthetic chemicals that stimulate the central nervous system (CNS) by increasing the metabolic processes and general body responses such as tachycardia, pupil dilation, restlessness, and dry mouth. They are intended for weight control, narcolepsy, and minor mental depression.

When taken orally, the amphetamines produce increased alertness, wakefulness, feelings of well-being, suppressed appetite, increased sensory perception, a pleasant feeling of euphoria, and suppression of fatigue. When the drug is injected intravenously, the user experiences a "rush"—a rapid, intense, euphoric feeling. With increased doses the effects are exaggerated. The user feels energetic, becomes hyperactive, doesn't eat or sleep, becomes talkative, irritable, disoriented, tense, develops increased size of pupils, loses weight and sometimes eventually becomes depressed. The "speed freak" often uses the drug in binges that can last for a week or more. The drug is repeatedly injected to maintain the high level of hyperexcitation until the physical exhaustion, a depleted drug supply, or the adverse effects of the experience end the binge. Repeated use of stimulants can cause paranoia and disorganized thought.

There has been a debate about whether actual physical withdrawal can be expected with stimulants; however most investigators and clinicians feel that such a syndrome exists and that physical dependence does occur. A psychological dependence does evolve in which a strong desire to take the drug and an emotional dependence on the effects of the drug are developed.

Tolerance, the need for increasingly large doses of the drug to achieve the desired effects, is characteristic of amphetamine abuse. However, reverse tolerance can also be noted where some users show increasing effect of repeated doses, perhaps related to a CNS process similar to enhanced cellular sensitivity. Cross-tolerance exists between most stimulant drugs.

Nonamphetamines

There are several nonamphetamine drugs which generally act on the central nervous system in the same way as the amphetamines. These include methylphenidate (Ritalin), diethylpropion (Tenuate, Apisate), and phenmetrazine (Preludin), to name a few. They are injected, sniffed, or taken orally. Many of these drugs are secured by prescription from physicians and subsequently abused. Psychological dependence on the "high," feelings of euphoria, or feelings of well-being occur with abuse of these drugs.

Cocaine. Cocaine, known as "coke" and "girl" on the streets, is one of the most common central nervous system stimulants known. It is a short-acting, white crystalline powder. It is generally sniffed up the nose, smoked in its pure alkaloid freebase form, applied to the genitals, or injected in the vein or into the skin. Users experience euphoria, loss of sense of time, and overconfidence in mental and physical capabilities. Some heavy cocaine abusers inject it as frequently as 10- to 45-minute intervals for days because the intense high dissipates so quickly. After the run or binge comes the "crash" when the user becomes depressed and irritable.

It is now well known that unremitting use of cocaine can lead to a dysfunctional mental state, hallucinations, dilated pupils, increased heart rate and blood pressure, and with acute overdose, brain seizures. Users may have rough breathing, pant, and stop breathing for periods of 10 to 60 seconds. Cocaine users are at risk for cardiac and respiratory arrest. Without cocaine, the abuser can suffer symptoms of paranoia, restlessness, interrupted sleep patterns, and hallucinations and become disoriented. It is still not known whether these are true withdrawal signs or signs of absence.[9]

Such instantaneous, intense stimulation may be anxiety-producing to the user, and the user may combine the cocaine with morphine—a "speedball." When individuals speedball, the risk for acute overdose reactions increases, either because of the stimulant effect of the cocaine or the depressant effect of the narcotic. The dominant effect usually depends on which drug is injected in greater proportions. Generally when cocaine is taken in large doses morphine does not obscure hyperactivity, seizures, and hypertension.

Unlike the amphetamines, it is not clear whether tolerance to cocaine is developed with continued, chronic abuse. There is considerable danger of overdosage which can produce cocaine-induced seizures and often fatal cardiac arrhythmias. In addition, use of cocaine has been associated with toxic cardiovascular reactions including tachycardia, hypertension, ventricular arrhythmias, and death.[13] Most of these deaths have been associated with injection or smoking the freebase form of cocaine. There has also been a substantial increase in death associated with the snorting of cocaine.[6] Cocaine may cause an abnormal contraction of the arteries that lead to the heart, or cause the heart to become oxygen-starved leading to heart attack.[16]

Characteristically cocaine or amphetamine-dependent persons experience psychosis following chronic or binge use. Qualitatively, the cocaine psychosis is similar to the amphetamine psychosis but shorter in duration. Stimulant psychosis consists of paranoia, suspiciousness, delusions of persecution, visual, tactile, and auditory hallucinations, and occasional uncharacteristic aggression and violent behavior in a patient who is alert and oriented.

The person dependent on stimulants also characteristically experiences intense anxiety or fear, paranoia, depression, excitement, or hallucinations when the immediate effects wear off.

Treatment for Dependence on Stimulants

Treatment for stimulant dependence is based on the abrupt cessation of intake. Detoxification is not physically dangerous as there is no known physiologically life-threatening abstinence syndrome. Psychological and physical reactions to cessation of use do occur and are characterized by depression, anxiety, fatigue, lethargy, general malaise, and at times, suicidal ideations. These symptoms begin to resolve after approximately 1 week.

Withdrawal. The person withdrawing from stimulant drugs usually benefits from a quiet environment, supportive care, reality orientation, and continued protective observation. Rarely is medication needed although low doses of a sedative may be prescribed during the detoxification period when the patient is extremely agitated, debilitated, and unable to tolerate prolonged central nervous system stimulation.

It is recommended that a comprehensive serum drug screen be run prior to the administration of a sedative drug to rule out the possibility that the person has ingested a barbiturate or other central nervous system depressants. Use of antidepressants during stimulant withdrawal is not recommended. In some cases, inducing vomiting or conducting gastric lavage may be effective due to the delayed emptying time of oral amphetamines into the gastrointestinal tract.

Cocaine is a stimulant with more severe consequences than other drugs in this category. The conscious patient who is extremely agitated and violent may be experiencing hallucinations or delusions of persecution. Ideally the patient should be settled in a large, open, quiet area, given much reassurance, and not left unattended because of the possibility of panic and suicidal ideations. Stimulant psychoses, including cocaine psychosis, may be managed with the short-term use of haloperidol (Haldol). If this regimen does not succeed, hospitalization and higher doses of Haldol may be indicated. The goal of nursing care at this stage consists of careful, continual monitoring until the patient returns to baseline.

Toxicity. The most common cocaine emergency is toxicity. As the toxicity progresses, central nervous system effects may develop including psychosis, grand mal seizures, hyperthermia, cardiac dysrhythmia such as ventricular fibrillation, and respiratory dysfunction including Cheyne-Stokes breathing. The patient may go into coma. The psychoses associated with cocaine toxicity can mimic acute paranoid schizophrenia and cocaine toxicity must be considered a possibility in a person exhibiting mania who has no psychiatric history.

Physical findings that may indicate chronic cocaine use include ulcerated or perforated nasal septum, recurrent nosebleeds, chronic rhinitis and sinusitis, flat needle track scars or ecchymoses along veins, infected abscesses and cellulitis, one long fingernail used for scooping up the drug, drug paraphernalia, bite marks on the lips and tongue secondary to nonfatal convulsions, and traumatic injuries resulting from falls during a convulsion.

Overdose. Overdose is most likely in intravenous use, freebasing, and "body packing" in which the user swallows wrapped packets of cocaine to escape detection. "Street cocaine" is usually composed on 80% to 90% cutting agents of sugars and lidocaine, procaine, or tetracaine. Lidocaine itself can cause overdose and can be fatal with intravenous injection of 250 to 1,000 mg.

Cocaine can be fatal even in the absence of toxicity. Cocaine tachycardia may induce myocardial infarction in the user by causing an abnormal contraction of the arteries that feed blood to the heart or cause the heart to become oxygen starved. Cocaine may also cause intracerebral hemorrhage due to increased pressure in the user with hypertension.

Acute massive overdose of cocaine can produce hypertensive crises, cardiac arrhythmias, status epilepticus, and hyperthermia. There does not exist an antidote or antagonist to cocaine, so the sequelae must be treated as they arise. Cocaine's half-life is only about 60 minutes. Consequently, many symptoms of cocaine poisoning will have occurred before the user reaches the emergency room.

Emergency nursing begins with cardiorespiratory system support. Hypertensive crisis may be controlled with nitroprusside or phentolamine infusion, and severe tachycardia and supraventricular arrhythmias with propanolol. The administration of such medications should be done only by physicians who are very experienced in their use.[14]

Hyperthermia requires aggressive and rapid treatment using a hypothermia blanket, ice packs, or an ice water sponge bath and fans. Treatment is discontinued once rectal temperature is reduced to 38 to 39°C (101–102°F).

Hallucinogens

This class includes LSD, PCP, mushrooms, mescaline, psilocybin, peyote, and similar drugs. Commonly reported effects include increased sensory awareness, alteration of perception, distortion of body image, a subjective feeling of enhanced mental or spiritual awarenes, euphoria, a turning of thoughts inward, and a decreased ability to tell the difference between oneself and one's surroundings. This group tends to produce adrenalinelike or adrenergic effects including dilated pupils, a flushed face, a fine tremor, increased blood pressure, elevations in blood sugar, and an increase in body temperature. Visual hallucinations are another effect produced by these drugs. LSD users have been described as having a "wild look."

Drug Action

The hallucinogens exert effects at relatively low doses. They differ in length of action, with the "high" from LSD lasting as long as 6 to 12 hours and most others acting for 2 to 4 hours. These drugs are well-absorbed orally, exert effects at relatively low doses, and the rate of metabolism tends to parallel the length of action, with the half-life for LSD being approximately 3 hours.[14]

Physical dependence does not appear to occur with hallucinogen abuse. Withdrawal symptoms have not been reported following cessation of intake. Psychological dependence on the pleasurable, mind-expanding, awareness-stimulating effects of the drug does occur. Tolerance also develops quickly, and a person who has developed tolerance to one hallucinogen will have a cross-tolerance to the other hallucinogens. Tolerance is short-lived; within 4 days to a week of abstinence from the hallucinogens, the person becomes susceptible once again to its effects at smaller doses.[5] Cross-tolerance exists between most of the hallucinogens, including LSD, mescaline, and psilocybin.

Side-Effects

The adverse effects of being under the influence of the hallucinogens include acute anxiety and panic during the experience which may inadvertently result in physical injury, and feelings of superhuman powers which may be detrimental if the person acts on this belief. As long as 20 months or more after an LSD experience, a person may undergo a repeat of the trip known as a flashback. This flashback phenomenon occurs spontaneously, without warning, and can induce feelings of panic or fear of losing one's mind. Also, paranoia and depressed feelings can continue for up to 3 or 4 days following a "trip."[5] Reactions can include isolation, violence, poor judgment, and suicide attempts.

Treatment for Dependence on Hallucinogens

Treatment of persons who abuse hallucinogens focuses on treating adverse reactions of the drugs and long-term therapeutic approaches to deal with the basic addiction process.

The first intervention in teatment of the "bad trip" phenomenon is to establish a quiet, secure, light environment. The caregiver should be calm, display an attitude of caring, and establish communication with the person using a normal or low tone of voice. When possible, it is most beneficial to have someone with the patient at all times to provide continuous verbal orientation to person and place, assuring the patient's safety, emphasizing that what the person is experiencing is drug-related only and not reality and clarifying for the user that the experience is transitory.

Discussion of the experience also can act as the catalyst for the drug-oriented perceptions into acceptable channels. The caregiver can also provide anticipatory guidance about the probable course of the trip such as to expect alternating periods of awareness and confusion as the drug effects wear off. As the trip reaches its conclusion, periods of awareness grow longer and more frequent, and the trip passes.

Phenothiazines have been effective in controlling the LSD bad trip but can intensify and prolong a negative hallucinogen experience when given to persons who have taken other psychedelic drugs. The phenothiazines are believed to bind PCP and are contraindicated in management of a PCP episode. Short-acting sedatives may be used in such cases. Chemical agents are merely an adjunct to the interpersonal support which is so vital to uncomplicated resolution.

PCP intoxication is difficult to diagnose because it can present clinically as mania, depression, and schizophrenia—it has no classical presentation. PCP toxicity or overdose is characterized by the combination of a comalike state, open eyes, decreased pain perception, periods of excitation and hostility, body rigidity, and unresponsiveness. Symptoms of overdose can be life threatening. Hypertensive crises respond to beta blockade with propanolol; seizure activity usually yields to intravenous benzodiazepines; ECT or vigorous cooling is effective for hyperthermia.

Cannabinols: Marijuana and Hashish

Marijuana is perhaps second only to alcohol as the most widely used of the drugs described here. The most active ingredient in marijuana and hashish is delta-9-tetrahydrocannabinol (THC). While this drug is usually called a hallucinogen, at the doses most frequently taken the predominant effects are euphoria and an altered state of consciousness with no frank hallucinations. The drug can be ingested through smoking, eating, and (rarely) intravenous injection.

Drug Action and Effects

When it is smoked, the peak plasma level is reached within 10 to 30 minutes, with intoxication lasting between 2 and 8 hours, depending upon the dose. When ingested, the onset is seen in 30 to 60 minutes, a peak blood level in 2 to 3 hours, with effects lasting up to 8 hours.

Toleration of increasing doses of the drug does occur with high-dose chronic intake through both metabolic and pharmacodynamic mechanisms. There is also a cross-tolerance to alcohol.

The severity of the withdrawal syndrome upon cessation of use parallels the amount and length of exposure to the drug. The symptoms of withdrawal include irritability, restlessness, decreased appetite, insomnia, sweating, nausea and vomiting, and diarrhea.

Side-Effects

The changes in mood seen with THC depend not only on the amount and potency of the drug but also on the setting in which the substance is used and the user's expectation of what will happen. The user usually experiences euphoria, a sense of relaxation and sleepiness, increased sexual arousal, hunger, decreased sense of time, and decreased social interaction. The user develops problems with short-term memory and with carrying out multiple-step tasks. Intoxication may be associated with suspiciousness or paranoia along with some loss of insight. Prolonged use may cause personality changes.

If intoxication occurs during a high state of stress, the user may show increased irritability, aggression, and antagonism. At higher doses, frank hallucinations may occur, usually visual in type, and sometimes accompanied by paranoid delusions. As with other toxic reactions, this can be associated with confusion, disorientation, and panic.

The physiological problems that accompany moderate intoxication include fine shakes or tremors, a slight decrease in body temperature, a decrease in muscle strength and balance, a decreased level of motor coordination, dry mouth, increased appetite, and bloodshot eyes. Some users experience nausea, headache, nystagmus and mild lowered blood pressure. THC may also precipitate seizures in epileptics.[14]

Treatment of Cannabinol-Related Problems

The vast majority of individuals presenting with marijuana-related problems show either panic or toxic reactions involving high levels of anxiety or confusion. The treatment of both these states is identical.

The clinical presentation includes an exaggeration of the usual marijuana effects including the feeling of anxiety, the fear of losing control or going crazy, and the fear of physical illness. Treatment is predicated on careful diagnosis, ruling out the involvement of other drugs and preexisting psychopathology, and gentle reassurance.

A physical examination is necessary to rule out preexisting psychopathology and other drugs of intoxication. A brief history should be obtained to establish the dose taken and the individual's prior drug experience. It is helpful to collaborate with the patient's family or friends if possible.

The patient should be placed in a quiet room and given constant reassurance that problems will clear in the next 4 to 8 hours; the patient's friends should be allowed to "talk him down." It should be recalled that the level of intoxication may fluctuate over the next 5 hours or so, as active drug is released from the tissues.

No specific drug type should be used to treat every panic or toxic reaction. If, however, the anxiety cannot be controlled in any other manner, the drugs of choice would be antianxiety medications, such as chlordiazepoxide (Librium), 10 to 50 mg orally which may be repeated in an hour, if needed.

Nursing Management of the Chemical-Dependent Patient

Assessment

Much of the nursing assessment of the drug abuser parallels that of the alcoholic patient. Many of the situations are acute and impede the nurse's actual recording of assessment data. In noncrisis situations, use of assessment data as the foundation of the nursing care plan ensures continuity of care and individualized nursing interventions.

A unique challenge is presented for the nurse working on a general medical-surgical nursing unit who comes in contact with the unidentified drug abuser admitted for a secondary diagnosis or for an elective or emergency survival procedure.

Pregnant drug-dependent women also represent challenging problems. Labor and delivery for the narcotic- or sedative-hypnotic-dependent mother can become complicated if the drug abuse history is not known. Also, the neonate can experience withdrawal symptoms within a short time after birth necessitating prompt and knowledgeable nursing assessment and intervention.

Self-denial is one of the hallmarks of the disease of chemical dependency. The drug-addicted person who is hospitalized for a secondary diagnosis or surgical procedure is unlikely to volunteer the information that he or she is drug-dependent. There are signs and symptoms of drug dependence that can be identified by the nurse.

The nurse should look for puncture sites, scar tissue over veins, and needle tracks at all major, visible vein sites. Careful inspection of clothing may reveal drugs or paraphernalia. The nurse should also examine the patient's skin for evidence of abscesses and open areas.

The drug abuser often neglects personal health care and maintenance. The nurse can check the patient's weight distribution, muscular development or wasting, and mouth for evidence of vitamin deficiency. Fluid and nutritional status may be evidenced by dryness, flaking, and cracking of the skin and dulled hair. Poor dental health, unhealed sores, cuts, and multiple bruises also suggest poor nutritional status. Dulled or jaundiced skin color, decreased tone, and lack of resiliency indicate hepatic dysfunction. Respiratory congestion and incidence of sores and infection of injection sites should be noted.

Patients with an extremely high or low tolerance to

medication as well as those who focus on somatic complaints and ask for medication "like clockwork" require assessment for drug dependence. Also, patients who report "allergies" to many drugs of a drug family with the exception of one or two, or patients who specify which drugs are most effective need further assessment for the possibility of drug dependence.

Whenever possible, the nurse's assessment process should include validation of the patient's drug history or the nurse's findings by questioning the patient's family or friends (Table 103–3).

Interventions

The nurse's next goal is to assist the abuser in making a commitment to continued assessment and treatment of the addiction(s). This process begins by offering realistic, honest, direct, goal-oriented encouragement in a hopeful, nonjudgmental manner. It is inappropriate to provide false reassurance that the patient will easily overcome dependence. It is much more helpful and therapeutic to suggest short-term accomplishable goals such as aiming for acceptance into a treatment program, then focus on each day of treatment that leads to abstinence, then focus on each day of drug-free life.

When feasible, the nurse may arrange to have a recovering addict from a self-help group or a counselor from a treatment program visit the patient. The recovering addict/counselor can use a realistic, no-nonsense approach and use his or her personal insight into the dynamics of chemical dependency to succeed where health professionals may fail. Also, the recovering addict/counselor serves as an example that recovery from the disease is possible.

Whenever possible, the nurse with or without assistance from other members of the health-care team should make arrangements for the dependent person to be transferred directly from the hospital to the treatment program despite promises from the patient that he will not use chemicals. An unbroken continuity of care is crucial to the abuser who is not yet capable of resisting drug/alcohol use. Drug/alcohol abusers who are discharged from the hospital, returned to their environments, and not quickly admitted to long-term treatment programs most always resume chemical-abusing behavior.

It is essential that the nurse interact with the dependent patient in a nonjudgmental, honest, direct, open, and accepting manner. It is not therapeutic to try to use manipulative behaviors or ask indirect "trick" questions in communicating with the dependent patient. Not only is this nonprofessional, but the addict will see through the dishonesty and there will be little chance of a trusting therapeutic relationship developing.

Nursing Diagnosis. Table 103–4 summarizes much of the information previously discussed in relation to specific

(*Text continues on page 1575*)

TABLE 103–3
Nursing Assessment of the Drug Abuser

Type of Assessment	*Focus of Assessment*
Physical	Signs and symptoms indicative of overdose Signs and symptoms indicative of withdrawal Identification of physical complications Extent and type of drug/alcohol dependence Nutritional and hygenic status
Psychological	Orientation and level of consciousness Validation of drug history (by questioning person, family, friends) Determination of motivation for treatment Prior treatment history
Social	Determination of sources of support • Family and friends • Employment and financial status • Living accommodations
Alcohol/drug history	When alcohol and drug abuse first began How patterns of use have changed with time What combinations of drugs have been used in the past and most recently Time, kind, and amount of last use Current patterns of usage Any previous history of withdrawal syndrome following cessation of intake Any nutritional, physical, or psychiatric concerns Any previous inpatient or outpatient treatment, or attendance at a self-help group Any previous psychiatric, psychological, or medical attention

(After Burkhalter P: Nursing Care of the Alcoholic and Drug Abuser. New York, McGraw-Hill, 1975)

TABLE 103–4
Summary of Effects of Drugs of Abuse and Nursing Care

Drug Classification	*Drugs Type/Example*	*Street Names*	*Medical Use*	*Administration*	*Approximate Effect*	*Effects Sought by Users and Side-effects*	*Effect of Overdose*	*Withdrawal Characteristics*	*Nursing Care*
CNS Depressant	*Barbiturates* Seconal, Amytal, Nembutal, Butisol, Tuinal, Phenobarbital	Sleepers, downers, goofballs, redbirds, yellow jackets, heavens, red devils, barbs	Anesthetic, anticonvulsant, sedative, hypnotic	Oral, IV, or IM	1–16 hr	Euphoria, relaxed inhibition, relief of anxiety, sleep, prevention of withdrawal symptoms Impaired emotional control, judgment and coordination, slurred speech, disorientation, drunken behavior	Irritability, weight loss, psychosis, shallow respiration, cold and clammy skin, weak and rapid pulse, coma, death from overdose, convulsions or death from abrupt withdrawal especially with barbiturates and alcohol	Anxiety, instability, agitation, impaired cognitive function, insomnia, diaphoresis, abdominal pain, nausea and vomiting, diarrhea, hypertension or hypotension. Increased temperature, convulsion and delirium. Acute brain syndrome.	1. Assess symptoms and stage of withdrawal and report to physician. 2. Monitor vital signs frequently; monitor signs and symptoms for complications. 3. Provide safety from injury. Provide a calm, quiet, environment, free from abrupt stimuli. Observe and take precautions for seizures. 4. Titrate prescribed medications to suppress withdrawal symptoms. 5. Observe for insomnia and nightmares and provide reassurance to promote sleep. 6. Provide a sense of reality orientation, sense of security and general health.
	Sedatives: chloral hydrate (Noctal, Somnos), Doriden, meprobamate (Equanil, Miltown, Meprospan)		Sedative, hypnotic						
	Minor tranquilizers: benzodiazepines (Librium, Valium, Serax, Xanax)		Antianxiety, anticonvulsant, sedative						
	Other depressants: Placidyl, Noludar, Dormate, Valmid								
	Alcohol								

Narcotics	*Synthetic non-opiates:* meperidine (Demerol, Pethidine) methadone (Dolophine) *Opiates:* morphine, codeine, opium (paragoric, Dover's powder), Heroin *Other narcotics:* Dilaudid, Percodan, Leritine, Numorphan	Snow, stuff, H, dreamer, scag, smack	Mainly analgesic *Other uses* paregoric: antidiarrheal Codeine and some other narcotics: antitussive Methadone: heroin substitute heroin: no medical use	Oral, IM, IV; injected under skin (skin popping) smoked, sniffed	3–24 hr	Euphoria, relief from pain, prevention of withdrawal: slow and shallow respirations, constricted pupils, nausea, drowsiness, clammy skin. Excessive itching, constipation, loss of sexual desires, infection of injection sites; impaired intellectual functioning and coordination.	Stupor and coma, depressed respirations, slow pulse, unresponsive pupils, convulsions; death from cardiovascular and respiratory failure.	Watery eyes, runny nose, yawning, loss of appetite, irritability, tremors, panic or depression, goose bumps, chills and sweating, abdominal pain, muscle cramps, spasms, hypertension, tachycardia, tachypnea, craving for drugs	1. Observe for signs and symptoms of withdrawal and report to the physician. 2. Monitor vital signs frequently and observe for complications. 3. Titrate medications as prescribed for signs and symptoms. 4. Provide safety and protection. Provide a sense of security and promote general health.
Inhalants	*Glue sniffing:* Ampilare glue, Aeropolo, gasoline, amyl nitrate, nitrous oxide		None, but causes CNS depression	Inhaled	1–3 hr	Euphoria, intoxication, relaxed inhibitions, rhinorrhea, excessive lacrimation, poor muscle coordination, dreamy. Impaired perception and judgment.	Violent behavior, nystagmus. Direct damage to lungs. May cause permanent damage to central nervous system and liver. Death through suffocation or choking.	Not clearly defined. More acute signs and symptoms are those of overdose. These drugs may also be used in combination with other drugs.	1. Emergency care for respiratory difficulties and damage. 2. Assess neurological changes. 3. Provide a safe environment. 4. Provide orientation as neurological symptoms decrease. 5. Implement nursing measures as they relate to presenting signs and symptoms.
Stimulants	*Amphetamines:* Dexedrine, Benzedrine, Desoxyn, Biphetamine *Phemetrazine:* Preludin *Methylphenidate:* Ritalin *Other stimulants:* Voranil, Pondimin, Plegine, Didrex, Ionamin, Bacarate	Pep pills, uppers, speed, crystals, dexies	Weight control, narcolepsy, hyperkinesis Weight control Hyperkenesis Weight control	Oral	2–4 hr	Euphoria, increased alertness, feeling of increased irritation and activity excitation, loss of appetite, dilated pupils, increased pulse rate and blood pressure, increased temperature, insomnia, giggling, silliness, loss of weight	Agitation, hypertension, tachycardia, extreme fatigue, shakiness, tremors, restless, aggressive behavior. Confused thinking, hallucinations, psychosis, convulsions and possible death	Apathy, paranoia, depression, possible suicide behavior, long periods of sleep or insomnia, irritability, disorientation, assaultive behavior. Tachycardia, hypertension. Oversensitive to stimuli.	1. Observe for signs and symptoms of withdrawal and report to physician. 2. Provide safe environment and protect patient according to stage of paranoia, depression and suicide tendencies. 3. Monitor vital signs frequently during withdrawal. 4. Medicate as prescribed to suppress agitation and prevent exhaustion. 5. Provide a quiet environment and a sense of security. 6. Provide measures for sleep, nutrition.

(*Continued*)

TABLE 103–4
Summary of Effects of Drugs of Abuse and Nursing Care[11,12] (Continued)

Drug Classification	*Drug Type/Example*	*Street Names*	*Medical Use*	*Administration*	*Approximate Effect*	*Effects Sought by Users and Side-effects*	*Effect of Overdose*	*Withdrawal Characteristics*	*Nursing Care*
Hallucinogens	*Synthetic:* D-Lysergic (LSD) Dimethyl-tryptamine (DMT) 4 methyl-2 (STP, Dom), PCP (Sen-nylan), psilocybin-psilocyn (mush-room), mescaline (cactus).	Acid, trips, cubes, sugar, bid-D Business man's special Serenity, tran-quility, peace	None: PCP used as veterinary anesthetic	Primary oral, some injected or inhaled	LSD: 10–12 hr STP: 6–8 hr Mescaline: 12–24 hr	Insight, exhil-aration, in-creased energy, distortion of senses, illusions and hallucina-tions	Longer, more intensive "trips," loss of reality orientation, psychosis, severe hallucinations, incoherent speech, periods of uncon-trolled crying, depres-sion or panic, homo-cidal tendencies, accidental deaths, sweaty hands and feet, vomiting, exhaus-tion. Increases present mental illness, long-lasting effects, flash-backs, possible deaths	Not clearly de-fined. Fear, panic, severe apprehen-sion. Perceptual distortion, hallu-cinations. Hyper-activity, di-aphoresis, tachycardia.	1. Staff or friend shall stay with the patient constantly. 2. Protect the patient from hurting self because sud-den behavior changes may occur. 3. Monitor vital signs fre-quently. 4. Provide a quiet, calm, sub-dued environment. 5. Provide reality orientation and divert to pleasant ex-perience. 6. Avoid depressant drugs. 7. Assess general health and provide nursing measures to improve state.
Cannabinols	Marijuana Hashish Hashish Oil	Joints, pot, grass, reefers Hash	None	Smoked or swallowed	Great variation, can act as stimu-lant or depres-sant in 1–2 hr	Euphoria, re-laxed inhibition, escape, in-creased percep-tion, increased appetite, craving for sweets, dis-oriented behav-ior (*e.g.*, time and space). Im-paired memory, judgment and problem solving, bronchitis.	Fatigue, paranoia, possible psychosis, acute panic or hallu-cinations, mood swings.	Not clearly de-fined. Hyper-activity, insomnia, and decreased appetite in some patients.	Usually these patients are not in the hospital unless this drug has been used with other drugs. Some nursing mea-sures may be necessary if the increase in hyperactivity and appetite changes are severe. Observation is necessary to observe for other drug-related changes.

* Cocaine is designated as a narcotic under the U.S. Controlled Substances Act.
(Adapted from Langer JH: Drugs of abuse. Drug Enforcement (Special Issue) 2:70, 1975 and Murray RB, Huels-Koetten MW (eds): Psychiatric/Mental Health Nursing. Englewood Cliffs, NJ: Prentice Hall, 1983)

drugs. After the drug abuser is identified assessment of specific problems associated with the type of drug may offer guidelines of care. The formulation of the nursing diagnosis of "drug usage out of control" may be made upon the determination of psychological and/or physical compulsion, loss of predictability of usage and of control, and continued use of a drug(s) in spite of adverse consequences resulting in one or more areas of that person's life.

Recovery and Rehabilitation

Recovery from drug dependence is a life-long process at times interrupted by relapse. Immediate patient-care goals include the nurse assisting the patient to withdraw from the drug(s) without medical complication, to return to a stable state of physical health, and to seek further specialized chemical-dependency treatment.

Depending upon the drugs involved and the person's physical and psychological condition, withdrawal may be done on either an inpatient or outpatient basis. It is generally more effective to choose an inpatient setting to withdraw a person who is receiving little support from his or her social setting.

Detoxification is the easiest part of the person's recovery process. The more difficult part is facilitating the person's development of a new way of living in which drugs are no longer considered a viable choice.

The goals of rehabilitation include abstinence from addictive substances, admission that chemicals have been problematic for them in numerous ways, self-awareness of emotional/mental/spiritual strengths and weaknesses, development of realistic problem-solving techniques and healthy coping mechanisms, and family involvement in their own rehabilitation process. Long-term treatment for the family members affected by the disease is as essential as treatment for the individual.

Longer-term patient-care goals include assisting the person to maintain abstinence from all drugs with addictive potential following completion of the specialized treatment program, developing a well-balanced, stable life situation with nonabusing support systems and satisfactory employment, and to restructure patterns of living so that life is no longer centered around drugs.

Statistics on "success" are not available because it is very difficult to define success. The success rates appear to improve when the person is treated early in the progression of the chemical dependency, and the prognosis worsens the longer the disease is allowed to progress.

Summary

Recovery from drug dependence is a lifelong process. It is imperative that the nurse determine his or her own feelings and values concerning drug dependence. Observe for the social and environmental barriers to the patient's progress as well as his or her individual strengths and weaknesses. Do not become discouraged if progress is not made quickly and if occasional relapses occur. Nurses should learn to depend upon specialized chemical dependency caregivers to work as part of a multidisciplinary team to help facilitate the patient's recovery process.

References

1. Altman GB: Combating alcoholic withdrawal the sensible way—recognition and prevention. In Kennedy M, Pfeifer GM (eds): Current Practice in Nursing Care of the Adult: Issues and Concepts. St Louis, CV Mosby, 1979
2. American Medical Association: Manual on Alcoholism. MOP 185 9801:468-32E-25, 1968
3. Aniline O, Allen RE: Most PCP intoxication is missed. Cont Ed, p 367–371, April 1983
4. Begleiter H (ed): Biological Effects of Alcohol Advances in Experimental Medicine and Biology, vol 126. New York, Plenum Press, 1978
5. Burkhalter P: Nursing Care of the Alcoholic and Drug Abuser. New York, McGraw-Hill, 1975
6. Coleman DL, Ross T, Naughton J: Myocardial ischemia and infarction related to recreational cocaine use. West J Med 126, May 1982
7. Estes NJ, Heinemann ME: Alcoholism: Development, Consequences and Intervention. St Louis, CV Mosby, 1982
8. Estes ND, Smith-Dijulio K, Heinemann ME: Nursing Diagnosis of the Alcoholic Person. St Louis, CV Mosby, 1980
9. Gay GR: Clinical mangaement of acute and chronic cocaine poisoning. Annals of Emergency Medicine 11:562–572, 1982
10. Keller M: Problems with alcohol: A historical perspective. In Filstead WJ, Rossi JJ, Keller M (eds): Alcohol and Alcohol Problems: New Thinking and New Directions. Cambridge, MA, Ballinger, 1976
11. Langer JH: Drugs of Abuse. Drug Enforcement (Special Issue) 2:70, 1975
12. Murray RB, Wilson-Huelskoetter M: Psychiatric/Mental Health Nursing, p 459–504. Englewood Cliffs, NJ: Prentice-Hall, 1983
13. Ray O: Drugs, Society, and Human Behavior, 2nd ed. St Louis, CV Mosby, 1978
14. Schuckit MA: Alcoholism and other psychiatric disorders. Hosp Community Psychiatry 34(11):1022–1027, 1983
15. Secretary of Health and Human Services. Alcohol and Health. 5th Report to Congressw, USDHH, PHS, NIADA. December 1983.
16. Weinstock CP: Cocaine addict therapy dilemma. Medical Tribune 25(31):1–17, 1984

Chapter **104**

Multiple Trauma

Mary P. Farley

Trauma refers to an injury or wound that is either accidentally or intentionally produced and results in a threat to life or potential for long-term impairment. It is the leading killer of young people in the United States.

Although there are single organ system injuries that pose a severe threat to life, such as head injuries, a combination of injuries of lesser individual severity can be of equal or greater magnitude. Multiple trauma refers to multiple injuries sustained by a patient which may singularly, or in combination, be a threat to life or function.

Trauma is a disease of the young and previously healthy. Accidents are the leading cause of death of people between the ages of 1 and 38 in the United States. It is surpassed only by cardiovascular disease and cancer as the cause of death for all age groups. In 1982 there were 165,000 deaths from trauma in the United States.[36] This respresents one out of every 10 deaths or about 15 deaths every hour.[9] For every person who dies two people will be left with permanent disability. Statistics from the Department of Health and Human Services indicate that the death rate from motor-vehicle accidents, homicides, and suicides has risen 50% since 1976 for Americans between 15 and 24 years of age. Young Americans are reported to die of violent causes at a rate 50% higher than their contemporaries in other industrialized societies, and that rate has increased in the last 10 years.[36] More males than females are involved in serious accidents but the pattern may change as women increase their mobility and enter more hazardous jobs.

Trauma victims occupy 12% of all hospital beds and take up about 19 million hospital days per year, more than all the heart disease patients and four times the number occupied by cancer patients. In 1981 the cost of death and disability including lost wages, medical expenses, and indirect work expenses amounted to $87 billion.[37] This figure seems unbelievable until one considers that the majority of trauma patients are young and are depriving society of their most productive work years. These patients also require enormous amounts of resources for their acute and long-term care. Expensive technology is required in field care, acute care institutions and rehabilitation centers as well as many work hours by highly trained personnel. In addition to the economic costs there are emotional impacts on the patient, friends, and families that are immeasurable in the aggregate. The cost of watching a loved one suffer pain, disfigurement, or long-term impairment is high and disrupts family, career, and social patterns.

Causes of Trauma

Motor-vehicle accidents are the most prevalent cause of accidental death. About 5% to 10% of all motor-vehicle accidents result in multiple or critical injuries. Twenty-five people died from traumatic causes in the United States for every soldier killed during the course of the Vietnam War, ten of these were traffic accident victims. Twice as many males as females are involved in fatal car crashes.[9] There are ethnic as well as gender variations in the etiology of traumatic death. Forty percent of young whites die from traffic accidents. Approximately the same percentage of young urban black deaths are caused by homicide. Suicide, homicide, falls, home, recreational and industrial accidents, burns, and drownings follow traffic accidents in decreasing order of causation of death according to the National Center for Health Statistics.[36] Many of these deaths are related to substance abuse.

Between 50% and 60% of the fatal motor-vehicle accidents are caused by drunk drivers according to the Insurance Institute for Highway Safety. Pedestrians who are killed by motor vehicles are often either hit by drunk drivers or intoxicated themselves. Alcohol also is implicated in 42% of adult deaths in nonhighway-related accidents.[9] The proportion of deaths related to drug use, recreational or prescriptive, is not known.

Trauma Classification Systems

Traumatic injury is variously classified. Cause of injury, injuring agent, mechanism of injury, recipient of injury, and severity of injury schemes are frequently used for gathering statistical data, for triaging patients to appropriate treatment centers, and for prognostic purposes. Such classification schemes are necessary for planning and evaluating patient care as well as identifying methods for prevention of accidents and prevention of deaths that could occur from inadequate treatment.

Cause of injury is usually described as the precipitating event such as a motor-vehicle accident, fall, assault, explosion, falling or collapsing object, or fire. The injuring agent is then described in order to give the physician and the statistician an index of extent of the forces involved.

Injuring agents in motor vehicle accidents are usually cars, trucks, buses, or motorcycles. Airplanes, tractors, snowmobiles, and boats may be classified separately. Agents of injury in assaults would include guns, knives, or blunt objects. The recipient of injury in a motor-vehicle accident may be a driver, passenger, or pedestrian. Mechanisms of injury in trauma are then described as blunt, penetrating, or crushing; and as thermal, electrical, chemical, or radiation in burn trauma.

Descriptions of the accident gathered from bystanders or rescue personnel are of vital importance to the receiving physician. Levels of suspicion for patterns of injury and severity of injury are triggered by the history of the event. It is necessary to describe how far the patient fell or was thrown, whether the auto accident collision was head on, from the side, or from the rear. The make of the gun and distance the victim was from the muzzle or the type of knife will often help the surgeon looking for internal injuries.

Field rescue personnel trained in extrication techniques, rendering of first aid, and rapid dispatch of victims to appropriate treatment facilities have been shown to decrease mortality. The success of field cardiopulmonary resuscitation for heart attack victims and the control of battle casualties demonstrated in Vietnam by highly skilled medical corpsmen who treated, triaged, and rapidly evacuated the injured has helped spur the development of a system for trauma care.

Emergency Medical Systems

During the past two decades trauma care systems have been studied and networks for rescue and treatment have been implemented in many areas. The systems vary in organizational structure from urban to rural areas and from state to state. The response system is constructed with consideration of geographical area, population density, and available resources of equipment and personnel. Most systems have some form of radio communication capacity for dispatching emergency personnel to the scene of the accident and for communicating with local health-care providers. The basic standards of training and certification for paraprofessional emergency medical technicians, who may be volunteers or full-time employees, are specified by state laws.

There are currently three levels of certification based on assessment and treatment skills. Emergency Medical Technician-Ambulance certification requires training in driving, extrication, cardiopulmonary resuscitation, basic airway management, and splinting and bandaging skills. The Emergency Medical Technician-Intermediate also must be able to perform advanced airway management and to administer intravenous fluids. Paramedics, the highest level of certification, are trained in all of the former procedures and in addition are trained to monitor and treat cardiac arrhythmias with medications and defibrillation.[6] In addition to developing the capacity to rescue and treat patients at the scene of the accident and enroute to the hospital there is a developing categorization of hospitals based on their ability and experience in treating patients with various levels of injury.

Trauma Center Categorization

Several studies have demonstrated increased survival rates when patients are referred to institutions with large case loads of victims.[14,15,18,19,40–42] These institutions have greater experience in treating trauma victims with severe injuries and have the staff and equipment necessary for comprehensive therapy ready on a 24-hour basis. Based on these studies and recognizing the enormous expenses involved in comprehensive trauma care, the American College of Surgeons Committee on Trauma in 1979 published recommendations for patient referral to designated trauma centers based on the hospital's capacity to treat various levels of injury severity. They further defined the staff and equipment necessary for designation as a trauma center. Level I is the highest classification and requires more facilities and a team of health-care experts. In 1980 the Committee further defined the categories of injury severity that would benefit from treatment at centers with higher categorization. The purpose of the recommendations is to get the trauma patient to the right hospital in the shortest amount of time in order to increase survival and decrease long-term impairment from trauma.[6]

There is considerable debate among physicians, other health-care providers, and interested groups as to the appropriateness of these recommendations, and this debate will continue for some time. Transferring patients from the scene of an accident to a nonproximal medical facility is controversial for several reasons. It delays some definitive treatment that might be provided at local hospitals. There are also ecomonic costs in transportation and loss of revenue to local health-care providers. Families are also uprooted from their support systems in order to follow their family members to distant locations.

Severity Indices

A further objection to transporting patients to distant facilities was the lack of agreement on identification of patients at greatest risk during field resuscitation. The total extent of injury cannot be determined until various diagnostic procedures and observation during the operative procedure or in the intensive care unit are obtained.

Trauma Score. The Trauma Severity Index Conference of 1980 recommended the adoption of the "Trauma Score" as an appropriate classification of minor and major injury that could reasonably and reliably be collected at the accident scene.[10] It is based on life-threatening injuries which result in compromised airways, inadequate breathing patterns, insufficient circulatory status, and depressed levels of consciousness.

The five categories that form the basis of the Trauma Score are respiratory rate, respiratory effort, systolic blood pressure, capillary return rate, and the Glasgow Coma Score. Each category is given a score from high value (no deficit) to zero (significant threat to life).

The sum of the scores from the five categories is used to identify the overall risk to the patient. The Glasgow Coma Score has been modified by grouping of point scores into ranges of minor to critical threat to life of depressed consciousness. (See Table 104–1.) The Trauma Score is currently recommended for determining significant threat to life and triaging of victims to the appropriate medical facility, although other indices are being considered.[21,29]

Triage. The word *triage* means to sort. It refers to the process of separating minor or major injury at the scene of the injury and in the emergency room. Triaging is separating persons who require immediate care from those who can wait for aid and selecting the destination of referral. In the best circumstances triage personnel should rapidly identify those persons with the greatest injuries, provide them with the appropriate level of resuscitation, and dispatch them to the hospital most equipped to help them.

Injury Severity Score. While the Trauma Score is used to immediately identify which patients are at greatest risk at the scene of an accident, other indices are used for hospital evaluation of injury severity, level of risk to life and physical impairment, and qualilty of care needed by the trauma patient. Such indices are necessary if the system for care of trauma patients is to continue to improve.

Baker's method of quantifying injury severity is based on anatomical disruption of organs and prolonged physical impairment. It is the most commonly used index of severity utilized to compare patients who do not have the same injuries but have injuries of the same level of severity. It can be used to measure the severity of injuries in persons with multiple injuries, which considered separately do not invariably result in death but which when added together represent severe threat to life. Its strengths are in comparison of outcome of treatment between different groups of patients with various doses of traumatic injury between institutions and with various treatment approaches.[7,8] Its weakness is that it is cumbersome and not applicable until x-ray films, operative procedures, and prolonged periods of observation are obtained.

Baker divides the body into six anatomical regions: head and neck, face, chest, abdomen, extremities and pelvis and general (integument). The score then rates the injury according to severity (based on threat to life or impairment):

1 = minor
2 = moderate
3 = severe, not life-threatening
4 = serious, life-threatening, survival probable
5 = critical, survival uncertain[7]

According to a mathematical formula, the three highest scores, from three separate body regions, are squared and summed resulting in an Injury Severity Score for multiple trauma.

The scoring system can be used regardless of injuring agent or mechanism of injury. It correlates with expected length of stay, receipt of surgery, and impairment. It is prognostic for groups of patients, (not the individual patient) for morbidity and mortality from multiple trauma and is frequently used for retrospective studies of quality of care in trauma patients.

These studies have shown a positive association between patient survival, high levels of injury severity, and higher levels of hospital classification.[28,41] Time from the traumatic event to definitive therapy has been shown to be a critical factor in the outcome of severely injured patients. It is obviously easier to get patients to institutions better equipped and more experienced in trauma care in major metropolitan areas than in rural areas. Recognizing this fact has led to development of educational programs for physicians, nurses, and emergency technicians in life-saving techniques and utilization of criteria for transfer to trauma centers such as the Trauma Score and the Injury Severity Score.

Cause of Death

If death is plotted against time after injury there are three peaks in the resulting graph. The first peak is called *immediate death* which occurs in seconds to minutes from time of injury. Deaths during this period are usually due to lacerations of the brain, brain stem, high spinal cord, heart, aorta, or other large vessels. Only a few of these patients could be saved even in urban areas with rapid emergency response.

The second death peak, *early death,* occurs within minutes to a few hours after injury. This period is referred to as the "golden time" when optimal care can make the differ-

TABLE 104–1
The Trauma Score

	Rate	*Points*	*Score*
A. Respiratory			
Number of respirations in 15 seconds; multiply by four	10–24	____4	
	25–35	____3	
	>35	____2	
	<10	____1	
	0	____0	A. ________
B. Respiratory Effort			
Shallow—markedly decreased chest movement or air exchange			
Retractive—use of accessory muscles or intercostal muscle retraction	Normal	____1	
	Shallow or/ retractive	____0	B. ________
C. Systolic Blood Pressure			
Systolic cuff pressure, either arm—auscultate or palpate	>90	____4	
	70–90	____3	
	50–69	____2	
	<50	____1	
	0	____0	C. ________
D. Capillary Refill			
Normal—forehead or lip mucosa color refill in 2 seconds	Normal	____2	
Delayed—more than 2 seconds capillary refill	Delayed	____1	
None	None	____0	D. ________

E. Glasgow Coma Scale

		Total GCS Points	Score
1. Eye opening			
Spontaneous	____4		
To voice	____3	14–15	____5 (minor)
To pain	____2		
None	____1	11–13	____4 (moderate)
2. Verbal response			
Oriented	____5	8–10	____3 (severe, not life threatening)
Confused	____4		
Inappropriate words	____3		
Incomprehensible words	____2	5–7	____2 (severe, life threatening)
None	____1		
3. Motor response			
Obeys command	____6	3–4	____1 (critical, survival uncertain)
Purposeful movement (pain)	____5		
Withdrawal (pain)	____4		
Flexion (pain)	____3		E. ________
Extension (pain)	____2		
None	____1		
Total GSC Points (1 + 2 + 3)	____		

TRAUMA SCORE ________
(Total points A + B + C + D + E)

(Adapted from Panel: Current Status of Trauma Severity Indices. Trunkey DD (Moderator). J Trauma 23(2):185–201, 1983)

ence in morbidity and mortality of the critically injured. Deaths occurring during this period are usually due to subdural and epidural hematomas, hemopneumothorax, ruptured spleens, lacerations of the liver, fractured femur, or multiple injuries associated with significant blood loss. Such injuries include those patients with uncontrolled hemorrhage from open, bleeding wounds or fractures, severe maxillofacial injuries, severe neck and upper respiratory tract injuries, unstable chest injuries, pelvic fractures, blunt abdominal trauma with hypotension and/or wounds penetrating the abdomen, and injuries of the head or spinal cord producing prolonged loss of consciousness, abnormal posturing, lateralizing signs, or paralysis.

The third death peak, *late death,* occurs several days or weeks after the injury. In almost 80% of these cases the cause of death is either infection or multiple organ failure.[5,36]

The most common cause of death in patients with penetrating wounds is hemorrhage, followed by infection or pulmonary failure. Blunt trauma carries a higher mortality rate and over half of the deaths are caused by head injury. Pulmonary failure and infection are the next greatest risks to life. Inadequate resuscitation without establishing adequate oxygenation or fluid status may aggravate these head and other injuries and contribute to the subsequent causes of mortality.[12]

Injuries ranked in terms of severity are those that endanger the airway, breathing, cardiovascular stability, or neurological status. Thus, chest injury or upper airway obstruction has the highest priority for treatment followed in order by hemorrhage, head trauma with deteriorating level of consciousness, abdominal injury, and multiple fractures.

Emergency Management of Trauma Injuries

First Aid: Field Resuscitation

The cardinal rule of intervention is, "Do no further harm."

Initial injury assessment always requires attention to the ABCs: airway, breathing, and circulation (Fig. 104–1). Injuries to the spinal column must always be considered before moving a trauma victim. Careful observation of the patient at the accident site may lead to early recognition of occult injury. Questions to ask are:

What happened?

In what position was the patient found and are there obvious signs of angulation of the neck, spine, or extremities?

Is there obvious bleeding, abrasion, contusion, or pain on movement?

Depressed levels of consciousness are common in trauma victims due to head injury, hypotension, hypoxia, or intoxication. Rescue personnel and emergency room staffs must always assume a cervical spine fracture in any patient with an injury above the clavicle. Spinal, thoracic, and abdominal visceral injuries are assumed to be present until ruled out in all unconscious patients.

Priorities of Care. An extensive review of resuscitation is beyond the scope of this chapter.[9,25] The following list briefly explains first aid at the scene of the accident (It must be remembered that evaluation and treatment occur simultaneously.):

1. Move patient from danger only when the risk of further injury outweighs the risk of moving the patient.
2. Establish an airway, usually by elevating the jaw (remember the patient may have a neck injury). Remove foreign material from the mouth and throat.
3. Institute artificial respiration. Use airway adjuncts, such as oral pharyngeal, nasopharyngeal, or bag-mask devices, if available.
4. Start external cardiac compression if indicated.
5. Control hemorrhage, usually with direct pressure over wound or at pressure points of major pulses.
6. Splint spine and extremity injuries.
7. Cover open wounds with sterile or clean cloths, occlusive dressings if there is a sucking chest wound (tape, Saran wrap, or Vaseline gauze).
8. Transport as soon as possible. Prevent hypothermia.
9. Provide a history of the accident and baseline vital sign status to the receiving institution.
10. Administer supplemental oxygen as soon as possible.

Airway Compromise

Airway management is the first priority in any patient who has signs of actual or potential respiratory distress. Failure to provide a patent airway deprives tissues of oxygen which may aggravate head injuries, or further damage ischemic organs such as the kidney, liver, and heart.

Etiology. Obstruction of airways is caused by the tongue, blood, loose teeth, vomitus, or other foreign bodies as well as swelling from facial or neck injuries. Fractured jaws or direct injury to the trachea or larynx can cause severe airway compromise.

Assessment. Observation for stridor, intercostal retractions, nasal flaring, or tracheal tug should alert the clinician to impending airway obstruction.

Management. Restoration of the airway may be accomplished by removing debris from the mouth or oral pharynx and lifting the chin. Hyperextension or flexion of the neck should be avoided due to the possibility of cervical spine fractures. Availability of such adjuncts as oral or nasopharyngeal airways, esophageal airways, and endotracheal tubes will secure most airways but must be used with caution by trained personnel. Surgical entry into the trachea with needles or incisional cricothyrotomy may be necessary. Tracheostomies are avoided in emergency situations and performed only as a last resort.

Complications. Inadequate airways result in hypoxia and decreased ability to deliver oxygen to the tissues. Failure to clear debris can result in aspiration and lead to pulmonary compromise from infection or obstructed bronchi.

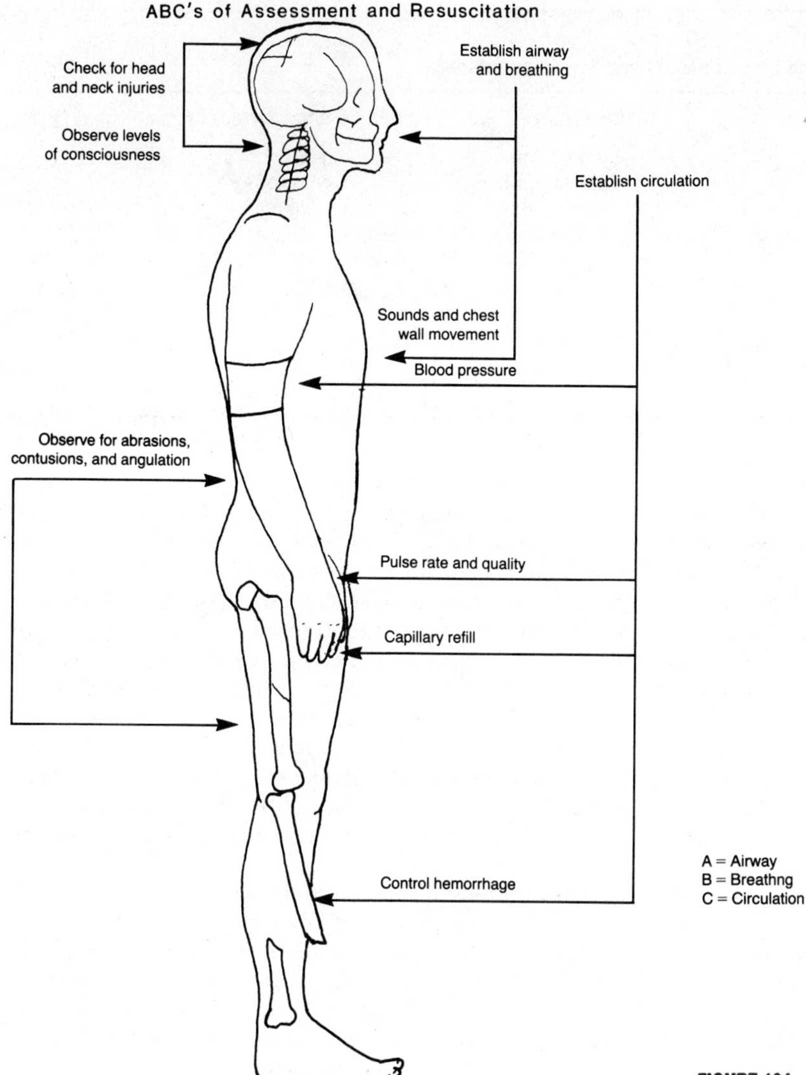

FIGURE 104–1 ABCs of assessment and resuscitation.

Compromise of the Respiratory System: Pulmonary Contusion, Pneumothorax, and Hemothorax

Blunt or crush injuries can lead to pulmonary contusion with or without fracture of the ribs. Bony fragments from ribs or penetrating injuries result in puncture of lung tissue and lead to formation of hemo- or pneumothorax, resulting in decreased surface area for gas exchange. A tension pneumothorax may develop when air in the pleural space has no means of escape from the chest cavity. The lung on the affected side collapses. As the mass of air expands it causes shifting of the mediastinum, and impairment of the remaining lung. (See Chapters 31 and 32.)

A deficit in the chest wall may cause either a tension or simple pneumothorax. Flail chest results from two or more adjacent ribs being fractured in two places causing a floating segment of the chest wall and inadequate chest wall expansion. Penetrating objects can lacerate either bronchus or trachea and result in pneumothorax.

Assessment. Exposure of the chest will demonstrate tachypnea, asymmetry of chest wall movement or paradoxical movement. Sucking chest wounds, deviated trachea, and distended neck veins are symptoms of pneumothorax. Auscultation may reveal unequal or absent breath sounds which are further clues of pneumothorax. X-ray films will delineate areas of hemo- or pneumothorax as well as evidence of pulmonary contusion, tension pneumothorax, and mediastinal air indicating a ruptured bronchus. Hemoptysis is another indication of injured lower airways. Arterial blood gases will confirm alterations in gas exchange with decreased oxygen content and altered carbon dioxide levels. (See Table 104–2 for signs and symptoms of hypoxemia relating to the circulatory and central nervous system.)

Management. Treatment is directed at restoring alveolar oxygen levels, re-expanding the collapsed lung seg-

TABLE 104–2
Signs and Symptoms of Airway and Breathing Difficulty

Respiratory	*Circulatory*	*Central Nervous System*
Tachypnea	Hypotension	Agitation
Cyanosis	Cardiac dysrhythmias	Confusion
Stridor	Tachycardia	Disorientation
Intercostal retraction	Bradycardia	Combativeness
Nasal flaring	Premature beats	
Tracheal tug	Atrial	
Sucking chest wounds	Ventricular	
Unequal or absent breath sounds by auscultation	Chest pain	
Deviated trachea		

ments, and evacuating space-occupying blood from the chest cavity. Oxygen therapy is started as soon as possible preferably by inserting an endotracheal tube and instituting mechanical ventilation by bag or ventilator. Chest tubes inserted into the pleural space will decompress both pneumo- and hemothorax and when connected to suction will provide continuous evacuation of air or blood. A tension pneumothorax may require decompression with a large bore needle or one-way valve device while chest tubes are being assembled. Insertion of a 14-gauge needle into the second intercostal space in the anterior midclavicular line will buy time until a chest tube can be inserted. An open chest wound can be covered with a sterile dressing taped on three sides to provide the one-way-valve effect of occluding the wound on inspiration and allowing air escape on expiration. Operative procedures may be required to treat major anatomical defects. Long-term ventilator support with the addition of positive end expiratory pressure (PEEP) may be required for large flail segments and extensive pulmonary contusions. (See Chapters 31 and 32.) Obtaining and interpreting arterial blood gases as well as monitoring lung sounds, follow-up chest x-ray films, and quality and quantity of chest tube output are indicated for post-emergency management of compromised respiratory status.

Complications. Hypoxemia and resulting anaerobic metabolism can result in tissue damage, infection, delayed wound healing, and inability to restore organ function.[22] Aspiration of stomach contents can cause additional injury to lung tissue. Airways should be protected by decompression of the stomach as soon as possible.

Compromise of Circulatory Status: Hemorrhage, Cardiac Tamponade, Shock

Hemorrhage from ruptured or torn vessels, resulting in either external or internal loss of blood, and fluid shifts, resulting from cell membrane dysfunction, leads to intravascular volume depletion. Significant blood loss can occur from both penetrating and blunt injury to organs, fractured bones, and lacerations of areas of high vascularity such as the face and scalp. Internal bleeding into the peritoneal or thoracic cavities, the retroperitoneal space, and intravascular or subcutaneous areas can account for massive blood losses. (See Chapters 21 and 31.)

A direct blow to the anterior chest, such as a steering wheel injury, can cause compression of the heart between the sternum and vertebra and result in cardiac contusion or tears in the descending thoracic aorta. Most patients with rupture of the aorta will die immediately at the scene of the accident. If the adventitia and fibrous sheath that surround the aorta maintain some continuity of the vessel a hematoma will form and limit the blood loss. It has been estimated that 20% of patients with thoracic aortic injuries will survive to emergency room admission and can be saved with prompt diagnosis and treatment.

Injury to the heart muscle from contusion or ischemia can result in irregular heart rhythms and decreased stroke volume. Cardiac tamponade (blood in the pericardium) can result from injury to the heart muscle itself or vessel injury leading to decreased capacity for ventricular filling and cardiac output. If intravascular volume is sufficiently depleted or cardiac function is compromised the patient will experience inadequate tissue perfusion and shock.

Shock. Shock is defined as inadequate organ perfusion. It is clinically defined as a systolic blood pressure less than 80 to 90 mm Hg in combination with tachycardia, altered state of consciousness, decreased pulse pressure, prolonged capillary blanch time, and decreased urine output. These parameters must be assessed in addition to blood pressure measurement as compensatory mechanisms may prevent the fall of systolic pressure until the young patient has lost 3 to 4 units of blood. (See Table 104–3.)

Once shock is identified, treatment is directed at determining the cause and restoring perfusion with adequately oxygenated blood. All types of shock as defined by Blalock may be present in the trauma patient—hypovolemic, cardiogenic, neurogenic, and septic shock. The most common cause is hypovolemia. *Cardiogenic shock* can be present and must be considered especially in older patients who may have had myocardial infarctions or have long-standing heart disease, those who have a serious cardiac arrhythmia, or those patients at risk for cardiac tamponade or tension pneumothorax. *Neurogenic shock* results from injury to the spinal cord and reticular activating system. The rule in trauma care is that isolated head injury does not cause shock and all other

TABLE 104–3
Signs and Symptoms of Hemorrhage

	Class I	*Class II*	*Class III*	*Class IV*
Blood loss (% BV)*	Up to 15%	20%–25%	30%–35%	40%–50%
Blood loss (ml)†	Up to 750 ml	750–1500 ml	1500–2000 ml	2000 or more
Pathophysiology	Little change	Decreased perfusion of nonvital organs (skin, muscle, fat)	Decreased perfusion of vitral organs (gut, kidneys, liver)	Decreased perfusion of heart and brain
Pulse rate	<100	>100	>120	140 or more
Pulse quality	Normal	Normal	Decrease in volume	Weak to imperceptual cardiac arrhythmias
Systolic blood pressure	Normal	Normal	Decreased‡	Decreased
Pulse pressure§	Normal or increased	Decreased	Decreased	Decreased
Skin temperature	Normal	Cool	Cool	Cold
Capillary refill	Normal	Prolonged‖	Prolonged	Prolonged
Respiratory rate	14–20	20–30	30–40	>35
CNS–mental status	Slightly anxious	Mildly anxious	Anxious and confused	Confused, lethargic, comatose
Urine output (ml/hr)	30–35 ml	25–30 ml	5–15 ml	Negligible
Fluid replacement requirements (Use 3:1 rule)	Crystalloid	Crystalloid	Crystalloid and blood	Crystalloid and blood

* % BV = Percent Blood Volume.
† Assume a 70-kg man.
‡ This is the smallest amount of blood which consistently causes a drop in BP/s in uncomplicated cases.
§ Difference between systolic and diastolic pressures
‖ Greater than 2 seconds
Adapted from Siskind J: Handling hemorrhage wisely. Nursing 84 14(1):34–41, 1984 and Shires TG: Principles and management of hemorrhagic shock. Care of the Trauma Patient. New York, McGraw-Hill, 1979

causes must be ruled out. *Septic shock* is possible but rare unless the patient's arrival in the emergency facility is delayed, usually by several hours.[33] Neck vein distension may help in the differential diagnosis of the cause of shock. If the neck veins are distended suspicion of cardiogenic shock is indicated. If neck veins are flat then hypovolemia is more likely the cause.[9]

Blood Loss Estimates. Blood loss in the trauma patient is hard to estimate. There may be significant losses from external hemorrhage at the scene that cannot be quantified as well as ongoing internal losses. There may be as much as a 30% blood loss before significant changes in supine blood pressure are detected. (See Table 104–3.) The circulating blood volume in a normal healthy adult is about 7.5% of ideal body weight. A 30% blood loss in a 70-kg man, (155 lb) is 1500 ml. This represents a class III hemorrhage according to the Committee on Trauma of the American College of Surgeons (Table 104–3). It is further defined as moderate blood loss in the trauma patient. Mild blood loss is estimated at 10% to 20% of blood volume; moderate at 20% to 40% and severe blood loss at greater than 40% of circulating volume.[34,36] Early detection of patients at risk for these levels of blood loss require observation of subtle signs.

Assessment

Evaluation of circulatory status in primary injury surveys is directed at establishing the presence of peripheral pulses, evaluating skin color and capillary blanch time, and obtaining a blood pressure if possible while looking for obvious or probable causes of blood loss. The pulse should be evaluated for quality, rate, and regularity. Blood pressure measurements are time consuming and a waste of time in the absence of femoral or carotid pulses. A faint but palpable radial pulse indicates reduced circulating volume or cardiac compromise but perfusion is present. Documentation of the site at which the pulse is obtained is helpful in evaluating the severity of circulatory compromise. Presence of radial pulses establishes less compromise than positive femoral or carotid pulses. As the distance from the heart increases it is harder to palpate pulses in patients with severe hypovolemic or cardiac dysfunction.

Blood pressure and pulses should be checked in both arms upon admission of the patient. Asymmetry of blood pressure or pulse in the upper extremities may indicate vascular damage. In the presence of fractures of the clavicle, sternum, or upper ribs unexplained shock may indicate aortic injury. Inequality of left and right arm blood pressure may be the first diagnostic clue. Confirmation of mediastinal widening and displacement of the trachea, esophagus, aorta, and lungs by x-ray films determines the need for arteriography and a thoracic exploration in surgery.

A normal blood pressure and pulse rate does not rule out serious injury in the trauma patient. The stress response has been discussed in Chapter 7. Briefly, whenever the body suffers trauma the sympathetic nervous system is activated. The release of catecholamines, epinephrine, and norepinephrine causes an increase in heart rate and stroke volume as well as vasoconstriction of the least essential vascular beds. This results in pale, cool, and diaphoretic skin, dilated pupils, and maintenance of relatively normal systolic blood pressure, especially in young trauma patients in the early stages of hemorrhage. Cardiac output cannot be easily maintained by many elderly patients as they may be unable to increase their stroke volume or to respond to catecholamine release due to long-standing cardiac disease or the intake of prescribed medications for control of hypertension. Compensatory mechanisms will also fail in the younger patients as the vascular compartment empties.

The earliest indication of impending shock is often restlessness and agitation. The pulse of bleeding patients becomes rapid and weak. Respirations may be shallow and rapid. The skin is cool and clammy, and capillary blanch time is prolonged. Blood pressure decreases as shock progresses, and the pulse pressure (the difference between systolic and diastolic pressure) narrows as diastolic pressure is maintained by norepinephrine. Mental status deteriorates as the brain is deprived of blood supply, and urinary output diminishes as blood is shunted to the heart and brain.

Management

Treatment of circulatory compromise is aimed at restoring adequate intravascular volume, optimizing cardiac function, replacing third space losses, and supporting organs which suffered ischemia.

Electrocardiographic (ECG) monitoring should be instituted upon the patient's arrival in the emergency room. A twelve-lead tracing and cardiac enzymes should also be obtained prior to the operative procedure. If cardiac contusion is suspected, serial ECG and cardiac enzymes are ordered and evaluated for 3 days postinjury.

Hemorrhage Control. Control of external hemorrhage can usually be managed by applying direct pressure to the bleeding site or over proximal arterial pressure points. The use of tourniquets should be avoided as they can produce anaerobic metabolism, may increase blood loss, and can cause ischemic limbs if they are forgotten. Internal hemorrhage is harder to evaluate and control. It requires surgical intervention and stabilization of orthopedic injuries. The use of pneumatic splints and anti-shock garments may delay deleterious effects from internal hemorrhage during transportation and initiation of fluid resuscitation.[27,30]

Fluid Replacement. Fluid resuscitation from hemorrhagic shock can be a challenge. Efforts are first directed at placing reliable intravenous lines, administering oxygen, and assessing the response to therapy by continuous monitoring of vital signs while other diagnostic procedures are being performed. Placement of two or more large-bore (14 or 16 gauge) catheters in the upper extremities is preferred. The danger of thrombophlebitis and possible pulmonary emboli contraindicates IV placement in lower extremities. Intravenous lines in the lower legs are also difficult for anesthesiologists to reach during operative procedures. However in the event of massive chest trauma with disruption of the superior vena cava, such placement is reasonable. Cutdowns to gain venous access are also recommended in preference to placement of central lines. The insertion of central venous lines by the subclavian, internal, or external jugular vein is sometimes necessary when extreme vasoconstriction and hypovolemia are present. In general these lines should be placed for monitoring of central venous pressure because they don't allow flow as fast as peripheral lines.

Observation of response to rapid fluid replacement is a necessity. Patients must be continuously observed, and all recordings must be documented. Because large volumes of crystalloid and blood replacement will be required (300 ml for every 100 ml of blood lost), the patient's temperature must be protected. Cold fluid from a shelf and banked blood may need to be warmed to prevent hypothermic complications when large volumes are administered rapidly.

Renal Function. A urinary catheter is indicated for assessment of renal function and adequacy of fluid resuscitation. Because trauma patients are at risk of renal failure from decreased kidney perfusion as well as precipitation of hemoglobin or myoglobin in the renal tubules it should be placed as soon as damage to the urethra is ruled out. Urine output should be monitored every 15 to 30 minutes. An initial specimen is sent for analysis. Urine volumes of at least 30 to 40 ml/hour are desired. In patients with major crush injuries, higher output may be desired to minimize renal tubular damage from myoglobin molecules. High urine volumes, in the absence of glucosuria or diuretics, may indicate overhydration, and the rate of fluid administration will need to be reevaluated. Dyes used for angiographic studies of vascular injuries are osmotic particles and may cause diuresis from a still depleted vascular compartment. Oliguria is usually due to inadequate volume replacement, but kinks or blood clots in the catheter should be considered.

Nasogastric Decompression. A nasogastric tube should be placed as soon as possible to decompress the stomach and check for blood in the drainage. Blood is shunted away from the splanchnic bed as a compensating mechanism in shock whichs results in ileus. Ileus in combination with depressed levels of consciousness due to head injury or alcohol predisposes patients to vomiting and aspiration. Nasogastric tubes must be placed through the mouth when there is any indication of basilar skull fracture, such as cerebral spinal fluid draining from the nose or ears.

Central Venous Pressure. Central venous pressure (CVP) measurements should be obtained in all patients requiring rapid fluid resuscitation. The normal range is 5 to 12 cm H_2O when the manometer is placed at the level of the right atrium. (See Chapters 34, 35, 38.) The zero level should be marked on the patient's chest so that all measurements will be obtained from the same reference point. It is important to remember that all connections should be secured with tape to prevent inadvertent disconnection and subsequent air embolus or blood loss.

The CVP can be a reliable approximation of the efficiency of the right ventricle in handling venous return, and is an index of blood volume if myocardial function and vascular tone are normal. Because vascular tone is altered by vasoconstriction in shock a single CVP recording cannot determine volume status. Serial measurements of the response to fluid boluses are more valuable. A minimal rise in an initially low CVP with fluid replacement indicates the need for further volume. If the CVP declines with volume it suggests ongoing fluid loss and the need for additional replacement. An abrupt or persistent elevation indicates that volume replacement is adequate or that myocardial function is compromised.[33]

Cardiac Tamponade and Tension Pneumothorax. Two conditions which can exist in trauma patients and cause inadequate myocardial function are cardiac tamponade and tension pneumothorax.

Cardiac tamponade is a result of bleeding into the pericardial sac which causes decreased filling of the ventricles from restricted cardiac movement. Although tamponade is more common in penetrating cardiac injuries, blunt trauma can also cause bleeding from the heart or great vessels. Beck's triad of symptoms consisting of elevated venous pressure, decline in arterial pressure, and distant heart sounds may be difficult to detect in a noisy emergency room or hypovolemic patient. The neck vein distention may be absent due to severe hemorrhage, and pulsus paradoxus, weakening of the pulse on inspiration, may be undetectable. Pericardiocentesis, insertion of a needle into the pericardial sac, will relieve the immediate problem, but surgical intevention is required.

A *tension pneumothorax* develops when air enters the thoracic cavity either from the lung or through the chest wall and has no means of escape. It causes complete collapse of the affected lung and as it enlarges the mediastinum and trachea are displaced to the opposite side resulting in decreased venous return and compression of the good lung. The result is decreased cardiac filling and further respiratory compromise. It is most often caused by blunt chest trauma and requires immediate release of the pressure buildup either with flutter valve insertion (one-way escape for air into the atmosphere) or insertion of a large-caliber needle. Definitive treatment requires the placement of chest tubes and connection to a suction device. Tracheal deviation, respiratory distress, unilateral absence of breath sounds, distended neck veins, elevated CVP, and cyanosis are the common indicators.

Other Measures. Electrocardiogram monitoring for rate and arrhythmias should be instituted immediately in all trauma patients. Control of external bleeding with pressure dressings and splinting of fractures which may be causing vascular damage should be ongoing while diagnostic procedures progress. Gentle handling in examining wounds and moving the patient is necessary to prevent disruption of clot formation and to prevent further stress response release of catecholamines from pain.

Sources of internal blood loss are investigated through chest x-ray films looking for hemothorax; abdominal x-ray films looking for fractured pelvis; vaginal and rectal examination followed by urinary catheter placement looking for blood from kidney or bladder trauma; and peritoneal lavage looking for free blood in the peritoneal cavity indicating a ruptured viscus. In peritoneal lavage, lactated Ringer's solution is infused through a catheter into the peritoneum and then allowed to drain by gravity back into the IV bag. The fluid return is examined for blood by visual inspection and laboratory analysis of RBC, WBC, bile, amylase, and bacteria. Positive results indicate the need for exploratory laparotomy as does penetrating injury into the peritoneum.

During the surgical procedures there may be continued hemorrhage, fluid shifts, acid–base imbalances, and prolonged operative time requiring multiple blood sampling for monitoring of volume status and cardiorespiratory status. Arterial lines and pulmonary artery catheters are placed in the operating room or the intensive care unit in patients with severe multisystem disease. Refer to Chapters 34 and 38 for use of hemodynamic lines.

The goals of therapy are to minimize ongoing losses and replenish intravascular and extravascular fluid without overloading the patient, and to restore organ perfusion and preserve function while preventing further harm secondary to treatment. Stabilization of volume status commonly takes a period of 24 hours and may be longer in patients who have continued venous oozing or fluid shifts from injured cell membranes.

Complications

The short-term consequence of not recognizing and resuscitating patients from circulatory impairment is death. There are also profound long-term consequences. Head injuries that result in prolonged hypoxia from lack of adequate oxygenation due to inadequate respirations or inadequate intravascular volume have a poorer outcome. Lack of adequate resuscitation may predispose the patient to cardiac damage, acid–base derangements, delayed wound healing with poor cosmetic results, severe pulmonary complications, renal failure, infection, and sepsis. There may be loss of viable tissue or limbs, or death from multiple organ failure.[17,22]

Compromise of the Nervous System: Head, Neck, and Spinal Injuries

Blunt trauma from falls, blows to the head or neck, or falling objects results in contusion, tearing of blood vessels, or fractures of the bony structures of the head and spinal column. Penetration from bullets or sharp objects causes open wounds as well as vessel and tissue destruction. The initial injury is often compounded by complications such as shock, hypoxia, edema, or infection. Flexion or hyperextension forces from automobile accidents, falls, and during accidents as well as gunshot wounds can result in cervical spine fractures with cord contusion or laceration, leading to edema or nerve compression resulting in partial or complete motor and sensory nerve loss. (Specifics of pathophysiology of neurological trauma are discussed in Chapters 63 and 69.)

Assessment. Evaluation of traumatic injuries starts with observation at the scene of the accident. A bullseye fracture of the windshield or obvious angulation of the neck denotes a head injury until ruled out. Rear end collisions predispose to whiplash injuries. Any injury above the clavicle should raise suspicions of associated head injuries. Any head injury with unconsciousness should alert the clinician to possible cervical spine damage. Serous fluid from the nose or ears is cerebral fluid from a basilar skull fracture until proven otherwise. Observation of a ring forming outside of blood on filter paper or linen (the ring test) and the presence of glucose in the fluid confirm the diagnosis.

Baseline evaluation of level of consciousness and level of motor function starts at the scene of the accident. Observation for deterioration should continue at 15-minute intervals.

The full armamentarium of neurological diagnostics is used to detect injury and direct definitive therapy in neurological trauma. Nothing replaces the suspicious observation of an expert clinician. Changes in mental status are often attributable to other causes, including selected myocardial cell necrosis from CNS insult, but are the first sign of rising intracranial pressure. Pupil size and symmetry are clues to changes in intracranial pressure, although isolated eye injuries may cause anisocoria. Observation of respiratory pattern will clue the observer to look for cerebral lesions. Observation of sensory levels and muscle strength should be documented before induction of anesthesia to rule out peripheral nerve injuries as well as cord lesions.

The radiology unit should be located near the emergency room. Head and cervical spine x-ray films are priorities in the diagnostic work-up of multiple trauma. The patient must be immobilized until these injuries are ruled out and delay in obtaining the x-ray films can interfere with other procedures. Angiography and computed tomography (CT) scans are helpful when access to them is convenient.

Management. In no other body system does this maxim "Do no further harm," apply with greater impact. Head injuries are variously reported to be the cause of death in 50% to 80% of all traumatic deaths.[9,15,23,28,40] Saving a patient in a vegetative state or one suffering from other sequelae of brain and spinal cord injury can be devastating to the patient, the family, and the staff who must provide care.

Establishment of adequate airways, respiration, and intravascular volume are vital to good neurological outcome. Adequate tissue perfusion must be restored without volume overload which requires monitoring of vital signs, ABGs, neurological status, and intracranial pressure. Attempts to control cerebral edema include the use of isotonic fluids, prevention of hypoxemia and hypercarbia, head elevation, a quiet environment, and avoiding occlusion of jugular venous return such as that caused by extreme neck rotation or constricting tape from endotracheal tube stabilization. The spinal cord must be maintained in good alignment with traction and careful turning protocols on special beds. The neck should be protected with immobilizing collars until fractures are stable and swelling has resolved. Provision of emotional and psychological support for the patient and family must be vigilantly attended to.

A careful balancing of therapy to restore cerebral perfusion and optimize oxygenation of brain tissue requires clinical decision making by a highly observant nurse. The spacing of procedures that are observed to alter levels of consciousness or increase intracranial pressure may contribute to control of intracranial pressure which may result in higher levels of function in the brain-injured patient. It has been observed that, after the initial injury and surgical intervention, nursing procedures and respiratory therapy affect intracranial pressure more than any other factors. The use of steroids to control cerebral swelling is controversial. Some investigators have questioned whether these low-dose steroids have contributed to the incidence of infection and sepsis.[17] Utilization of PEEP (positive end expiratory pressure) to optimize oxygenation in the lung may cause alterations in intracranial pressure and the risk–benefit ratio in the individual patient must be evaluated.

Complications. Swelling from tissue damage and iatrogenic causes leads to further impairment of nervous tissue. Infection and pneumonia can result from open wounds, inadequate respiratory toilet, and lack of appropriate antibacterial agents. Skin breakdown, malnutrition, and contractures can prolong or prohibit recovery from neurologic injury.

Compromise of the Face and Scalp: Facial Lacerations and Fractures

Blows or blasts to the face or head resulting in lacerations or fractures can cause actual or potential threat to airways and various degrees of hemorrhage. Dashboard or windshield injuries are the most common agents. Maxillofacial fractures can cause significant bleeding, airway obstruction, and cosmetic deformities. Patients, especially children, can bleed to shock levels from scalp lacerations. Basilar skull fractures are associated with cerebrospinal fluid leaks and have potential for serious infective complications.

Assessment. Change in facial contour, loose teeth, bleeding, and bruising are indications of injury. Palpation and x-ray film confirm the diagnosis. Scalp lacerations are usually obvious but blood and debris may be embedded under matted, coagulated bloody hair.

Management. Prevention of airway obstruction and shock from swelling and bleeding is the highest priority. Realignment of bones and reimplantation of teeth for optimal cosmetic results are indicated when other more life-threatening injuries are stabilized. Antibiotic therapy is usually instituted with cerebral spinal fluid (CSF) leak or open jaw fractures. Plastic closure of facial lacerations will minimize disfiguring scar formation.

Complications. Shock and airway obstruction are potential threats to life. Meningitis can occur with CSF leaks. Poor cosmetic results can result from bony malalignment or inadequate suturing techniques. Functional disability can result from improper jaw alignment or loss of teeth.

Compromise of the Gastrointestinal System: Abdominal Organ Injury

Motor-vehicle accidents with steering wheel and seat belt injuries followed by falls and blows cause blunt injury to the abdominal contents and result in organ laceration or fracture. The spleen, liver, diaphragm, and bowel are most commonly injured. Penetrating trauma from gun shot wounds, stab wounds, or explosions can result in severe hemorrhagic conditions, especially when those bullets which ricochet off bones cause multiple perforations in the bowel or with hollow nose bullets which explode on impact. Spillage of gastrointestinal contents can expose the patient to severe infection, and large third-space losses. If the esophagus is disrupted mediastinitis can result. Retroperitoneal hemorrhage from duodenal injury or rectal injury can be a focus for infection as well as blood loss. Injury to the associated organs, the spleen, liver, and pancreas, can cause severe hemorrhage, disruption of the immune system, and endocrine dysfunction. Major blood vessels can also be lacerated especially by penetrating trauma.

Assessment. Observation of injury patterns such as contusions and abrasions in conjunction with a history of the accident will lead to abdominal operative exploration in the presence of significant hypotension. Inspection of entry and exit wounds will indicate the probable trajectory of bullet wounds. However because the diaphragm can ascend to the fifth intercostal space during expiration any penetrating wound below the nipples indicates concern for abdominal organ damage. Stab wounds may or may not cause hemorrhage or organ damage. Signs of peritoneal irritation including abdominal tenderness, guarding, rigidity, and absence of bowel tones are indications for exploratory laparotomy. Blunt trauma can present with similar signs, but patients are often unable to cooperate in the examination due to decreased levels of consciousness from associated head injuries, hypotension, drugs, or alcohol. A flat plate of the abdomen examining the kidney, ureters, and bladder (KUB) scans for pelvic fractures and irregular gas patterns from displacement of bowel by expanding hematomas. The presence of ileus and hypotension indicates the need for peritoneal lavage and/or CAT scan. Positive signs of blood in the peritoneum dictate the performance of an exploratory laparotomy. It is of little importance to know which organ is injured but very important to know that an organ injury is causing significant bleeding.

Management. Restoration and maintenance of intravascular volume with surgical intervention and replacement of shed blood and third-space losses are the objective of therapy. Balanced salt solutions and blood replacement are indicated for all class III and IV hemorrhages. Surgical intervention for exploration of injury, resection of devitalized tissue, and reconstruction or bypass of injured bowel or vessels is the definitive therapy for significant organ trauma. Prevention of infection with appropriate antibiotic coverage and nutritional support is a priority with abdominal injuries. Wound care to prevent infection and loss of skin integrity from drainage or diversional ostomies becomes a primary nursing challenge in many patients. This requires not only knowledge of dressing techniques but management skills in decompression devices such as nasogastric tubes, ostomy appliances, hemovacs, and other devices. Monitoring of wound drainage quality and quantity can help in preventing complications of gastrointestinal trauma. Skill in delivery of tube feedings, parenteral nutrition, and control of infection or diarrhea from these therapies is a nursing responsibility. Prevention of stress ulcers in patients who experience shock, sepsis, or periods of prolonged deprivation of enteral nutrition is indicated.

Complications. Shock from hypovolemia or sepsis is an ongoing threat to these patients. Local infections and abscess formation can delay wound healing, cause malnutrition, and result in unattractive scars, as well as prolong the period of ileus and predispose to adhesions which could result in subsequent bowel obstruction. Delayed wound healing from inadequate nutritional support or an infective process can lead to wound dehiscence, evisceration, or fistula formation which will require further surgical procedures in already debilitated patients.

Losses from draining wounds and decompression devices have a potential for causing severe imbalances in acid–base status, intravascular volume, electrolytes, and protein wasting. Protection of the skin from excoriation can be a major logistical problem as abrasive enzymes leak from bowel or pancreatic wounds. Isolation of clean from contaminated wounds of the same abdomen requires creativity in wound dressing techniques. (See Chapter 84.)

Injuries of the Genitourinary System: Kidney and Related Injuries

Injury to the kidney, ureter, bladder, or reproductive organs is seldom an isolated injury. Injuries to the pelvis from blunt trauma are associated with bladder disruption (especially in a person with a full bladder) and urethral trauma in male patients. Penetrating injury from gunshot wounds or blunt and crush injuries can cause kidney laceration, fracture, or contusions. Reproductive organ injury of both males and females is seen in association with blunt trauma especially with forces strong enough to cause pelvic fractures.

Assessment. Blood at the urethral meatus and hematuria (blood in the urine) are the cardinal signs of genitourinary tract injury. All patients with blood at the external meatus must have a urethrogram prior to insertion of a urinary catheter. The presence of hematuria indicates the need for an intravenous pyelogram (IVP) and cystogram. Usually an IVP can be obtained by injecting the dye prior to taking a flat plate of the abdomen. The procedure also helps to identify ureteral injuries. The cystogram is used to identify bladder trauma. Renal arteriograms are also indicated in some patients. Rectal and vaginal exams are part of the physical examination of the trauma patient and will usually identify organ damage. Peritoneal lavage is used for confirmation.

Management. Prevention of exsanguinating hemorrhage and reestablishment of the urinary system are priorities of care. Urinary extravasation can lead to absess formation, peritonitis, and sepsis. The kidney is a vascular organ and blood loss is potentially significant. Operative procedures are directed at hemostasis and reconstruction, but nephrectomy may be necessary. The bladder is surgically repaired and maintenance of urinary drainage is assured with either a suprapubic or urethral catheter or both. Continuous monitoring of urinary flow and observation for signs of infection or skin loss at local wound sites or from drained organs are important aspects of patient care. (See Chapter 57.)

Complications. Urinary tract infection and calculi as well as disfigurement from urinary diversion can be long-term sequelae. Allergic reactions and hypovolemia caused by osmotic diuresis from contrast media used for x-ray film visualization can complicate the diagnostic phase. Sterility and impotence can occur with major reproductive organ injury with psychological sequelae from altered sexuality.

Musculoskeletal Injury

Etiology. Falls, crushing injuries, violence, and motor-vehicle accidents exert forces sufficient to fracture, dislocate, subluxate, or sprain bones and supporting ligaments and contuse surrounding soft tissue. Either partial or complete amputations of extremities occur with sufficient blunt forces or from sharp dissection such as chain saw or drag injuries. Orthopedic injuries always occur with soft tissue damage either integumentary, muscle, tendon, or organ. (See Chapter 88.)

Assessment. With the exception of partial or full amputation and open bleeding fractures, musculoskeletal injuries receive low priority in the initial management. The spinal column must be stabilized, and hemorrhage must be controlled through direct pressure and splinting. Bleeding from concealed fracture sites can be severe and may be the principle cause of shock. (See Table 104–3.)

Knowledge of the position in which the patient was found, whether there was bleeding or pooling of blood, any obvious deformity or dislocation as well as spontaneous movement of extremities will help in evaluating the extent of injury and risk of blood loss, obvious or occult, from musculoskeletal injury. Deformities such as shortening or angulation, swelling or bruising or muscle spasm identify occult fracture or muscle injury. Extremities are at risk from loss of blood supply, open wounds contaminated with debris from the site, and bleeding into closed compartments which can further occlude blood supply. Lack of sensation, movement, and circulation of extremities will alert the clinician to the possiblility of limb ischemia or nerve damage. X-ray films are required to define the extent of most injuries.

Management. Table 104–4 illustrates the life-threatening nature of these injuries. The objective of care is to prevent exsanguination, debride devitalized and contaminated tissue, prevent further damage, and restore as much function as possible. Restoring alignment and splinting, casting, external traction, or internal fixation procedures may take hours in the operative suite and require more that one surgical procedure.

TABLE 104–4
Estimates of Blood Loss from Fractures (in Adults)

Area of the Body	*Blood Loss (ml)*
Arm	
Humerus	1000–2000
Elbow	500–1500
Forearm	500–1000
Spine or ribs	1000–2000
Pelvis	1500–4500
Hip	1500–2500
Leg	
Femur	1000–2000
Knee	1000–1500
Tibia	500–1500
Ankle	500–1500

(Modified from Clark R, Badger FG, Seritt S: Modern Trends in Accident Surgery and Medicine. London, Butterworth, 1959 and Iverson LD, Clawson DK: Manual of Acute Orthopaedic Therapeutics. Boston, Little, Brown, & Co, 1977)

Gentle handling and turning are indicated to prevent further damage to tendons and disruptions of blood clots. Pelvic fractures can continue to bleed into the retroperitoneum for prolonged periods. Gentle log rolling may decrease the extent of the bleed. Tight bandages and casts can impair circulation and result in limb loss. Close monitoring of capillary refill, pain or tingling sensations, movement, and skin color should continue until swelling subsides. Open fracture sites as well as other wounds must be observed for signs of local infections. Antibiotics are usually started immediately with open fractures and continued for at least 48 hours after surgical procedures. Immobility is a major problem in caring for patients with multiple fractures because of both pain and the immobilization devices used to stabilize fractures. Nursing care is directed at preventing the complications of immobility while preserving optimum joint and muscle function.

Complications. As with all traumatic wounds tetanus can be a severe threat to the nonimmunized patient, and prophylaxis must an early intervention (Table 104-5).

Dyspnea and respiratory impairment may be caused by pain, tight body casts, or positioning on fractured ribs as well as fat embolism. Phlebitis, contractures, decubitus ulcers, compartmental syndrome, and infection at wound or pin insertion sites, in hematomas or systemically can result from these injuries. Delayed or nonunion of fractures can occur with infection, poor circulation, or improper immobilization necessitating repeat operative procedures and possible loss of function or extremity.

TABLE 104–5
Tetanus Prophylaxis in Adult Trauma

History of Tetanus Immunization (Doses)	Clean, Minor Wounds		Tetanus-Prone Wounds*	
	TD	TIG	TD	TIG†
Uncertain	Yes	No	Yes	Yes
0–1	Yes	No	Yes	Yes
2	Yes	No	Yes	No‡
3 or more	No§	No	No‖	No

TD = Tetanus and diphtheria toxoid; TIG = Tetanus immune globulin, human

* Any wound in which soil, feces, or foreign bodies are found even if apparently insignificant requires tetanus prevention. Compound fractures, puncture wounds, gunshot wounds, burns, wounds more than 24 hours old or from dirty needles require special caution. If history is not possible or is unreliable then a booster of tetanus toxoid must be given as well as passive immunization with antitetanus globulin.[4]

† When TD and TIG are given concurrently separate syringes and separate sites should be used.

‡ Unless wound is more than 24 hours old.

§ Unless more than 10 years old since last dose.

‖ Unless more than 5 years since last dose.

(Adapted from American College of Surgeons Committee on Trauma Early Care of the Injured Patient, p 39. Philadelphia, WB Saunders, 1976)

Rehabilitation from trauma, particularly orthopedic trauma must begin as soon as possible after the patient is stabilized. Body alignment in the position of function as well as passive and active range of motion depending upon the patient's capacity must be maintained. Both functional and psychological status depend upon support of the patient's independent function whenever possible.[20,39]

Morbidity and Mortality

Organ Failure

With the increased rate of immediate survival in multiple trauma patients resulting from emergency medical systems, advances in the treatment of shock, and early surgical intervention more patients are surviving for prolonged periods in intensive care units only to succumb to organ failure. Organs fail to respond to treatment or deteriorate from complications resulting from prolonged shock, multiple blood transfusions, sepsis, and inadequate nutritional support. The lung is the organ most commonly associated with single organ failure as well as with failure of other systems including renal failure, coagulation abnormalities, liver failure, gastrointestinal bleeding from stress ulceration, and heart failure.[17] Predisposing factors for organ failure are inadequate treatment of shock, pre-existing medical conditions in the elderly, contaminated wounds, and altered host resistance to infection associated with severe trauma.[3,24]

If patients are to have decreased morbidity rates and increased long-term survival then early interventions directed at stabilizing the endocrine and metabolic responses to trauma as well as defending the immunologic system from the effects of stress, infection, and malnutrition must be instituted.

Infection

All traumatic wounds are considered contaminated. Sources of contamination are: exogenous from soil, clothing, foreign bodies, and contaminated environments to which the wound is exposed at the time of injury or during treatment; endogenous from perforation of the genitourinary tract, gastrointestinal tract, and respiratory tracts; nosocomial, resulting from widespread use of antibiotics and invasive diagnostic or supportive procedures such as urinary catheters and other tube placement as well as indwelling intravenous lines used for fluid delivery and monitoring.

Wound infections may be localized or cause systemic sepsis. Infection is the outcome of several factors and is best expressed by the equation

$$\text{Infection} = \frac{\text{Number of Bacteria} \times \text{Virulence of Organism}}{\text{Host Resistance}}$$

The number of bacteria present is dependent both on initial injuries and exposure of the wound to infectious environments both in and out of the hospital. Virulence of organisms is determined by the type of bacteria as well as the nature, location, duration, and circulatory supply of the wound. Host resistance is affected by pre-existing medical conditions, reestablishment of local blood supply, appropriate antibiotic coverage, removal of devitalized tissue, and immunocompetence of the patient. Wound healing and resilience of the patient to bacterial invasion are often dependent on nutritional status.[4]

Nutritional Deficiency

Late mortality from trauma is primarily due to sepsis and multiple organ failure. Early and aggressive nutritional support can increase the metabolic response to injury, provide protein for wound healing and immune responses, as well as provide protection from muscle wasting and depletion of the body's energy supplies.

Maintenance of cardiovascular stability and replacement of volume losses from injury and third spacing of fluids preclude starting nutritional regimens earlier than 2 to 3 days post injury. Previously well-nourished individuals can usually tolerate 3 to 5 days of semistarvation during the hypermetabolic stage following trauma. Those patients who are likely to have prolonged stress responses (longer than 1 week) may benefit from supplementation at an earlier time and may include patients with multiple system injury, sepsis, and burns.[1] Delay in feeding patients can lead to catastrophic consequences, and institution of nutritional support must be evaluated on an individual basis. Patients with multiple fractures may have metabolic energy expenditure 25% greater than their resting metabolic rates. Patients with major infections have elevations of 50% and major burns have increases of 50% to 125% above normal resting energy comsumption. Fever alone can increase energy expenditure by 10% to 13% for each degree of fever Celsius.[3,26,33]

Determination of the route of nutritional support will depend on the functional state of the gastrointestinal tract, the degree of stress and hypermetabolism, and the relative risk of feeding complications. Patients are commonly endotracheally intubated and may have prolonged ileus, therefore they are prohibited from oral intake and may not tolerate supplemental tube feedings. Feeding by the gastrointestinal route is the method of choice both for cost containment and delivery of nutrients to the gastrointestinal mucosa and portal system. Tube placement in the duodenum or jejunum can diminish the risk of aspiration from enteral feeding products but the volume of infused solutions must be controlled in order to avoid overdistension of these areas. Concentrations of tube feedings must be titrated to obtain adequate protein-calorie concentrations and avoid diarrhea which may result from too rapid adminstration or high osmotic loads. Diarrhea if uncontrolled will result in inefficient nutritional support, loss of fluid and electrolytes, and may contaminate wounds or excoriate skin.

Multisystem-injured patients commonly require either peripheral or central intravenous hyperalimentation with the addition of fat emulsions for prolonged periods of time. These nutrient-rich intravenous solutions further expose the patient to the risk of infection and septicemia unless they are administered under strict aseptic techniques (see Chapter 80). In addition to monitoring patients for infection, either local (at the catheter insertion site) or systemic, the patient must be monitored for hyperglycemia and glucosuria which may result in osmotic diuresis and altered serum levels of electrolytes, trace minerals, and vitamins.[1] The addition of these tubes, pumps, and protection of central intravenous lines from disconnection further contribute to immobilizing appliances attached to the patient and contribute to their environmental hazards.

Environmental Hazards

The trauma patient is immobilized by tubes, drains, intravenous lines, traction, casts, dressings, respirators, and pain and is often physically restrained to prevent accidental removal of life support lines. Mentation may be clouded by altered physiologic status, pain, or drugs, as well as the psychological sequela of an altered body image. Intensive care units are noisy environments filled with blips from monitoring screens, noise from pumps, light, respirators, and alarm systems, as well as noise from other patients and staff. Normal sleep patterns and circadian rhythms of food intake and elimination are disrupted. The cumulative effect of these environmental factors on the patient's stress response is unknown. The patient's experience of emotional pain from helplessness, fear, and separation from significant others is added to physical pain. The energy requirements of coping in such an environment may be substantial not only for the patient but for the family.

Family members alternately feel shock, fright, helplessness, anger, and guilt. Families are frequently dealing with past as well as present and future relationships with the patient in addition to trying to cope with their own displacement from familiar environments. Significant others are often at risk themselves for health deterioration and injury. Nurses must direct attention not only to assessment of the patient but to the family and the environment in order to deliver optimal care to the multiple trauma patient.[31,32,35]

Nursing Management

General Principles of Care

The outcome of trauma care is dependent upon establishing and maintaining effective airways and ventilation, restoring adequate circulatory volume and tissue oxygenation with optimal cardiac function, identifying and controlling the sources of blood loss, and providing the patient with protection from infection, malnutrition, pain, exhaustion, the hazards of immobility, and threat to self-concept.

Priorities of care change as the patient progresses from immediate resuscitation to operating room, to intensive care and acute care units and on to the various stages of rehabilitation. Concern at each stage for prevention of complications is imperative for optimal patient outcome. It requires a team of cooperative, trained, and dedicated practitioners. Because there are multiple disciplines involved, communication skills and documentation must be ongoing. The team consists of a surgeon, multiple medical and surgical specialists, clinical nurse specialists and staff nurses, respiratory therapists, physical therapists, dieticians, pharmacists, social workers, and psychiatrists. Nurses must use a holistic approach to anticipate and intervene to prevent complications and preserve the patient's physical and emotional energy.

Nursing assessment of the multiple trauma patient is aimed at gathering data to identify problems that require either medical or nursing intervention. Interventions are prioritized to meet both short- and long-term goals of preserving life and restoring organ function. The distinction between nursing and medical procedures is often blurred in critical care areas. By virtue of their special training, and under covering medical orders, nurses perform designated medical procedures in the absence of a physician. Individual institutions vary as to specific tasks that are delegated to the nursing staff. The emphasis in this section will be directed toward those tasks that have primarily a nursing focus.

Nursing has several levels of care to deliver to the multiple trauma patient.

- The first is anticipating or having an index of suspicion of the risk a patient has for developing a problem.
- The second level involves obtaining a data base that will provide early detection of, or validation of, an actual problem.
- The third is providing therapy for an acute problem which prevents further deterioration and restores

physiologic or psychologic balance. The interventions are also aimed at preventing complications that are not an inevitable consequence of injury.

- The fourth level deals with anticipating problems that will interfere with rehabilitation and minimizing their impact if possible.

Ideally these levels of care are delivered concurrently.

Because the multiple trauma patient may be in a potential life and death situation priorities must be established that put physiologic stability above psychological or potential rehabilitation problems. While lifesaving measures have the highest priority, comfort and support of the patient and the family should not be considered of lesser importance. Both short-term and long-term goals should include these considerations whenever possible.

Assessment: Nursing Data Base

Nursing data base is derived from obtaining vital signs, a head-to-toe physical assessment, physiologic measurements such as central venous pressure, pulmonary artery and intracranial pressure measurements, interpretation of laboratory data, assessment of quantity and quality of drainage or secretions, and information obtained from the patient or the family members.

Vital Signs

A patient who is not breathing and has no palpable carotid pulse requires immediate cardiopulmonary resuscitation (see Chapter 35). Obtaining data regarding the ABCs (airway, breathing, circulation) is of the highest priority in any injured patient.

Airways are assessed by noting chest wall movement, inspecting for foreign bodies or obstruction by the tongue, and listening for noisy respirations. Breathing patterns are inspected for rate, depth, and symmetry of chest wall movement. Observation of agitation and use of accessory muscles for breathing or tracheal deviation demonstrates ineffective breathing patterns. Quality of the carotid pulse, the rate, amplitude, and rhythm indicate both cardiac function and quality of intravascular volume. Signs of hemorrhage, blood pressure, skin temperature, color, and capillary refill give further evidence of adequacy of tissue perfusion.

The level of consciousness is determined by the response of the patient to stimuli, pupillary response, and motor function. Assess whether the person responds to noise and touch, only to painful stimuli, or does not respond. Unconsciousness may be due to anoxia, hypotension, or brain injury. Shock or respiratory insufficiency can lead to loss of consciousness with widely dilated, equal pupils which do not respond to light. Observations of spontaneous movement, posture, and the patient's verbal responses are basic assessment parameters. Pupils should be observed for position, size, reactivity to light, and equality.

After assessing the patient for adequacy of vital functions, the nurse should start a thorough head-to-toe assessment. Assessment includes observation, palpation, auscultation, and questioning the patient regarding sensation and pain.

Pain Assessment

Pain resulting from trauma may indicate soft tissue injury, fractures, or organ damage. Numbness, tingling, and pain also result from tissue anoxia due to obstructed blood flow. All patient complaints should be carefully evaluated and documented. Note the location, severity, descriptive terms, and causes of pain on the patient record. A useful method for assessment of discomfort is the use of the PQRST mnemonic.[9]

P: provoking factors that make the pain worse, or relieve it.

Q: quality of the pain. Note the terms used to describe pain as dull, sharp, crushing, burning.

R: region or radiation of the pain. Where does the pain start and where does it radiate?

S: severity of the pain in relation to a scale of one to ten, where one is no pain and ten is the worst pain imaginable.

T: time. How long has the pain been present? Is it intermittent or constant. If it is intermittent is there an identifiable cycle such as chest wall movement that would help to localize the source?

Decreased sensation may result from injury to peripheral nerves or the spinal column as well as head injury. Note patient complaints or absence of complaints carefully. Loss of sensation in association with loss of movement, in the absence of obvious local injury or malposition, should alert the examiner to possible spinal fractures. Peripheral nerves may have been damaged by fractures, lacerations, penetrating objects, or dislocations. Numbness, tingling, burning, or decreased sensation may result from these injuries in the extremities.

Physical Assessment

The head-to-toe examination starts with observation of the head (face and scalp) and neck. Assessment of the airway and pupils is the first step. The ears, mouth, and nose are inspected for bleeding, drainage, and foreign materials. The cervical spine is gently palpated for pain and deformity without moving the head. The scalp is observed and gently palpated for bleeding, lacerations, bruising, and depressions. The jaw alignment, loose teeth, and pain on movement should be noted. The patient should be asked about sensations in the neck region. Stiffness, tenderness, or pain on movement indicate the need for a supporting collar and immobilization. Neck vein distension, soft tissue trauma, and position of the trachea are carefully observed.

The chest and spine are then examined before moving the patient. Chest wall movements are observed for expansion, symmetry, and rate. The clavicles are observed for deformity and gently palpated for pain. Any external abrasions, contusions, or penetration of the chest wall should be noted before palpating the ribs for fractures. Slipping the hand carefully under the patient and palpating the spine for point tenderness is completed before moving the patient. Stabilization of the patient's spine on a backboard, if any suspicion of spinal injury exists, should be maintained until all possibility of spinal fractures are ruled out by x-ray examination.

Abdominal and pelvic assessment starts with observation of the patient's posture. Knees drawn up toward the abdomen or a fetal position may indicate organ trauma. The pelvis is palpated for pain by gently applying pressure to the pelvic bones. The patient should be asked to localize and describe pain while the abdomen is examined for external signs of injury. Signs of distention, rigidity, or pain are to be noted.

The extremities are observed for external signs of injury and malposition. If the patient has no obvious signs of injury and no complaints of pain, he or she should be asked to move each limb separately. Testing for sensation and the presence as well as the strength of peripheral pulses should be done.

After the basic examination is completed more extensive diagnostic procedures will be carried out and will require nursing staff assistance and interpretation.

Management of the Airway and Breathing

The most immediate threat to the respiratory system is an actual or potential ineffective airway. After an airway has been established the patient may continue to have ineffective breathing patterns due to injury to the chest wall or parenchymal tissue. Later sequelae of injury may ocur when fluid accumulates in the interstitial or intra-alveolar space from fluid overload or infective processes which can result in impaired gas exchange. Pulmonary edema, pneumonia, and adult respiratory distress syndrome (ARDS) are conditions of this sort. "Late" is a relative time reference which may refer to hours or days or weeks depending upon the patient's injuries, response to therapy, and underlying health status prior to injury.

Assessment and Nursing Diagnoses

Compromise of airways and breathing is displayed by the efforts made by the patient to breathe. The person with hypoxia will be dyspneic and perhaps cyanotic. Neck muscles will be prominent, and there will be decreased air moving in and out of the mouth. Nasal flaring and intercostal rib retractions may be present. In partial airway obstruction wheezing, stridor, or gurgling will be heard. A rule to remember is that noisy breathing is obstructed beathing. As the level of oxygen in the blood falls the skin becomes pale and then cyanotic. Color changes can be observed in lips, mucous membranes, and nail beds. Anoxia will affect the level of consciousness as the patient who at first was agitated becomes more obtunded and pupils dilate with inadequate oxygenation of the brain and accumulating carbon dioxide.

Ineffective breathing patterns are manifested by shallow chest wall excursion, asymmetric movement, and decreased or absent breath sounds on auscultation. Presence of fluid in the lung parenchyma will be demonstrated by noisy respirations, rales, and rhonchi on auscultation. Interpretation of blood gases will reveal decreased oxygen content and alteration in acid–base status.

Ineffective Airway Clearance

Actual or potential ineffective airway clearance may occur in the immediate post-traumatic period and in the recovery phase. Airways may be obstructed internally by material in the pharynx or conducting airways or externally from soft tissue swelling. Depressed levels of consciousness from head injury, intoxication, hypoxia, and hypotension result in inefficient gag and cough reflexes. Altered chest wall mechanics from fractured ribs and inadequate muscle strength from debilitation may result in ineffective coughing. Swelling of the lower facial region or neck indicate a potential for obstruction of the pharynx or trachea.

Nursing Data Base

Observation for decreased or absent chest wall movement, flaring of the nares, or straining neck and intercostal muscles on inspiratory effort may be manifestations of an obstructed airway. Signs of vomitus, loose teeth, dentures, or blood in the mouth indicate impending obstruction. Abrasions, lacerations, or bruising of the lower facial structures and neck or a displaced jaw may indicate potential swelling. Palpation for air flow from the patient's nose or mouth and listening for gurgling or crowing will confirm the diagnosis. Ask the patient to talk and swallow. If the patient is unable to manage his or her own saliva the nurse must be alerted to the possibility of impending obstruction (see Table 104–2).

Interventions

The first step in treating a patient who is not breathing or is working hard at breathing is to position him in a manner that ensures an adequate airway. If a neck fracture is suspected, the jaw should be pulled forward while the neck is held in a midline, stable position. If no trauma is suspected the neck may be extended by placing one hand on the forehead and the other hand under the neck and tilting the head back. Foreign material should be removed from the mouth and pharynx with a tonsil tip suction. If the patient is mentally obtunded or comatose he or she should be prepared for endotracheal intubation and a nasogastric tube is inserted. An oral airway properly placed will secure the tongue from relaxing into the posterior pharynx and facilitate suctioning of the mouth. The head and neck of the patient must be maintained in a midline position until cervical fractures are ruled out. Patients cannot be positioned on their side or have their heads raised until x-ray films have been interpreted.

Oxygen is administered by nasal cannula or mask as soon as the airway is cleared. If the patient requires intubation both lungs are auscultated immediately after the tube is placed to eliminate the possibility of right main stem bronchus intubation, which would allow ventilation only of the right lung. The x-ray department should be alerted of the need for a film to verify the position of the tube. The tube is secured with tape while lightly restraining the patient's hands to avoid inadvertent extubation by an anxious or agitated patient. An arterial blood gas is obtained after establishing oxygen flow rates or ventilator settings.

If respiratory distress continues, associated chest injuries can be suspected. All lung fields should be auscultated to identify further respiratory compromise.

Evaluation

Observation of adequate chest wall excursion with spontaneous efforts or on the respirator indicates a patent airway. Decreased noise of respiration and decreased agitation demonstrate improvement in the ability to ventilate. Absence of intercostal or nasal flaring are further positive indications.

Ineffective Breathing Patterns

Ineffective breathing patterns may continue in spite of restoration of adequate airways. Hemothorax, pneumothorax, or flail chest may result in an inability to maintain an adequate tidal volume for adequate gas exchange. Labored and shallow breathing, abnormal chest wall movement, and diminished or absent breath sounds may be manifestations of these injuries

Nursing Data Base

Observation of asymmetric chest wall movement or paradoxical movement of part of the chest wall are signs of these injuries. The patient may be short of breath, tachypneic, or tachycardic. Gentle palpation and percussion will reveal hyperresonance over the affected side or absence of chest movement. Auscultation demonstrates decreased or absent breath sounds with grating of bone fragments producing crepitus over the fracture site. A crunching sound with each heart beat caused by mediastinal air accumulation, Hamman's sign, may be heard. A sucking sound on inspiration with deviation of the trachea from the midline, neck vein enlargement with hypotension, and distant heartsounds may indicate the presence of a tension pneumothorax.

If the patient is being ventilated with a respirator pneumothorax can be suspected if the patient complains of a sudden sharp chest pain, becomes suddenly agitated, tachypneic, tachycardic, or hypotensive. Other signs of internal pressure-induced pneumothorax, barotrauma, include continuous pressure alarm response on the ventilator and rising pressure requirements for unchanged tidal volume delivery. Subcutaneous emphysema, crackling of air in the skin on palpation, is usually a delayed sign.

Interventions

Detection of decreased breath sounds, prevention of hypoxemia and cardiac compromise, and minimization of further accumulation of pressure in the thoracic cage are nursing goals. Stabilization of the chest wall to prevent further damage to underlying lung tissue from flail segments is a goal shared by both nurses and physicians as it may require intubation and internal fixation from respirator support.

Stabilizing Chest Wall. Auscultate lungs for diminished or absent breath sounds. Prepare for chest tube placement by assembling large bore chest tubes and preparing the suction devices with appropriate water seal chambers. (See Chapter 27.) Administer oxygen and reassure the patient. Place an occlusive dressing over sucking chest wounds. Be prepared to remove it if the dressing converts the open wound into a tension pneumothorax due to air entrapment in the thorax. Splint the flailing segment with manual pressure or place an intravenous bag or sandbag over the area. If the patient is intubated assist his or her respiratory efforts with positive pressure ventilation delivered by anesthesia bag or a respirator. Obtain chest x-ray films to verify the presence of a hemo- or pneumothorax and to verify chest tube placement after insertion. Assure patency of or insert intravenous lines and administer fluids to maintain blood pressure as ordered. Measure and record the quality of chest tube drainage of either air or blood. If immediate return of blood is large, obtain blood for type and cross match as ordered. Obtain and interpret arterial blood gases.

Pain Relief. Relief of pain due to fractured ribs is difficult to accomplish in the multiple trauma patient. Until associated injuries are ruled out narcotics are usually contraindicated in the emergency room. A patient's reports of pain are vitally important in physical examinations. Patients are often more comfortable in a semi-Fowler's or Fowler's position but this too may be contraindicated until spinal fractures are ruled out. If the patient can be turned, position him or her with the flail segment down or tilted off of the posterior rib fractures. Patients who can't be medicated and can't be positioned more comfortably may be relieved by splinting their chests with pillows and by verbal reassurances. In the intensive care unit the patient's level of pain and response to pain control should be assessed frequently.

Achievement of pain control will enhance the patient's ability to breathe on his own and clear his own secretions, which may either prevent the need for intubation or shorten endotracheal intubation time. Intercostal nerve blocks can be very effective in relieving pain from fractured ribs. Patients should be monitored for hypotension following the procedure.

Chest Tube Patency. Chest tube patency must be assessed frequently. Quality of the drainage, air, blood, or both, should be recorded as well as quantity. Lung expansion is dependent upon drainage of the thoracic cavity and prevention of reaccumulation of the mass in the chest. Chest tube connections must be secure, and frequent auscultation of breath sounds is required. Tubing should be checked to make sure there are no kinks especially when the patient is placed on the side.

Evaluation

Verification of lung expansion requires a chest x-ray film, and results should be recorded on the nursing notes as obtained. Presence of breath sounds in both lung fields, symmetric chest wall movement, decreased respiratory and pulse rates and improvement in arterial blood gases signify improved pulmonary mechanics.

Support of the trauma patient with supplemental oxygen

and respirators may be prolonged due to damage of the lung tissue itself (parenchymal damage).

Impaired Gas Exchange

Impaired gas exchange due to atelectasis, pulmonary contusion, aspiration of gastric contents, fat emboli from bone fractures, fluid overload, or pneumonias results in decreased surface area for gas exchange. Multiple blood transfusions, near drowning, and systemic sepsis in addition to the above mentioned pathologies may result in the development of adult respiratory distress syndrome (ARDS, wet lung) and severe threat to the life of the patient several days after injury. (See Chapter 32.) The symptoms arise from inability to adequately oxygenate tissues.

Nursing Data Base

Manifestations of impending or actual gas exchange compromise include: observation of increased work of breathing, tachypnea resulting in respiratory alkalosis, hypoxemia manifested by increased heart rate, agitation and decreased oxygen measurement on blood gas analysis. X-ray films will show pulmonary infiltrates. Auscultation of the lungs will demonstrate rales and rhonchi, especially in the presence of a pneumonia.

The classic sign of ARDS is a lowered arterial oxygen tension which does not respond to increasing concentrations of inspired oxygen. Pulmonary shunt calculations are a more accurate measure of the difficulty encountered by oxygen in crossing the alveolar-capillary membranes. Pulmonary shunt calculations are often performed by nurses by obtaining arterial blood specimens and measuring the difference between alveolar and arterial oxygen gradients. Decreasing lung compliance (stretchability of lung tissue) is another symptom of ARDS and is calculated by nurses or respiratory therapists if the patient is on a respirator. (See Chapter 32.)

Interventions

Assist the patient to clear pulmonary secretions. If the patient can be moved position him or her in a high Fowler's position and splint the chest with pillows while the patient is coughing in order to obtain maximum force. Pain control is of primary importance if patients are expected to take deep breaths and cough or use incentive spirometers effectively. More commonly these patients will be intubated and on respirator support. They will require careful suctioning technique to prevent hypoxemia and suprainfection from contaminated catheters.

Control and monitoring of oxygen delivery and its effectiveness are nursing responsibilities. Obtaining and evaluating arterial blood gases, as ordered, are indicated to achieve optimal arterial oxygen tension with the lowest possible delivered oxygen flow. Patients may require treatment with positive end expiratory pressure (PEEP) and must be carefully monitored for possible hypotension from increased resistance to blood flow returning to the heart as well as barotrauma from increased intrathoracic pressures.

Careful titration of intravenous fluid is necessary to prevent further damage to the pulmonary interstitial space. Antibiotics are prescribed in the presence of positive sputum cultures and should be given in a minimal amount of fluid to those patients who have interstitial edema.

Sputum specimens are commonly obtained daily or on a 3-day cycle for culture and sensitivity analysis on all intubated patients. Reports should be analyzed and conveyed to the physician as soon as they are available. Diuretics and corticosteroids are often ordered for these patients and their use necessitates careful evaluation of laboratory values.

Titration of intravascular volume against the effects of the disease process and of respirator consequences often requires the use of hemodynamic monitoring with pulmonary artery catheters. Obtaining and recording these measurements every 1 to 2 hours in association with other vital signs facilitates decision making about volume replacement.

Evaluation

Institutions and physicians vary as to the level of acceptable arterial oxygen tension they prefer in their patients. In general an oxygen tension of 60 to 70 torr while receiving an inspired oxygen concentration of 40% or less is an acceptable value. Improved compliance of the lung is demonstrated by decreasing pressure requirements to deliver tidal volumes as measured by peak pressure manometers on the respirator. Clear breath sounds and decreased bacterial load of sputum culture reports demonstrate clearance of pneumonia processes. Clearance of the chest x-ray and improvement of arterial oxygen tension with decreasing levels of PEEP and decreasing oxygen concentrations demonstrate resolution of ARDS.

Management of the Circulatory System: Alteration in Tissue Perfusion

Multiple trauma patients are at risk for both short-term and long-term dysfunction of the circulatory system. Loss of blood from the intravasular compartment decreases tissue perfusion and oxygen-carrying capacity. The heart muscle may be injured from ischemia or the direct injury causing contusion or lacerations. The blood vessels may be torn or lacerated by the initial injury or obstructed by swelling from blood or fluid accumulation in closed compartments. Sepsis resulting from bacterial contamination in combination with prolonged hypoperfusion and hypoxemic episodes may contribute to extended periods of cardiovascular instability. Formation of hematomas from blood loss into localized areas not only deprives the tissue of immediate blood supply but contributes to pressure in closed compartments of limbs and potentiates tissue ischemia as well as being a nutrient-rich culture media for bacterial growth.

Alteration in tissue perfusion resulting from intravascular volume loss, fluid shifts secondary to altered cell membranes and soft tissue trauma, or ineffective pumping of the heart muscle is a sequela of traumatic injury. Arrhythmias or restriction of stroke volume from incomplete filling or emptying of the ventricles in the presence of pericardial tamponade or mediastinal structure shift from tension pneumothorax result in inadequate perfusion pressure. Injury to the great vessels can result in impedance to ventricular emptying as well as decreased flow to distal organs. The symptoms of inadequate tissue perfusion are related to inadequate organ function (see Table 104–3).

The lungs, liver, kidney, brain, and heart are of immediate concern, but long-term sequelae of inadequate perfusion will affect all body systems. Tissue hypoxia will result in metabolic and respiratory acidosis, increasing myocardial ischemia and arrhythmias, renal failure, cerebral edema from prolonged anoxia, delayed wound healing, and predisposition to skin breakdown or loss of extremities. Ischemia to the reticular activating system of the liver predisposes the patient to systemic sepsis. ARDS and disseminated intravascular coagulation (DIC) are commonly seen in patients with prolonged periods of inadequate tissue perfusion.

Nursing Data Base

The nursing data base is obtained from physical assessment of the patient's vital signs and assessing organ function. Obtaining and interpreting laboratory values supplement the physical exam. The patient serves as his or her own control in analyzing the degree of dysfunction. Blood pressure and pulse amplitude should be compared in both arms to rule out vascular injury to the thoracic aorta or from dislocated fractures or swelling which can cause restricted blood flow in the limbs. Thorough documentation allows comparison of the patient status in response to therapy.

Goals. Short-term nursing goals include: restoring tissue and organ function; providing fluid and blood replacement without overloading the cardiovascular system; controlling external bleeding and assisting with identification of internal sources of blood loss; and correction of acid–base disorders. Long-term goals include support of the insulted organs and early detection of complications such as infection, ARDS, and DIC.

Interventions

Continuous monitoring of vital signs including level of consciousness, urinary output, central venous pressure, or pulmonary artery pressures, if available, as well as ECG monitoring is required. Instituting intravenous fluid replacement followed by assessment of the patient's response every 10 to 15 minutes is started in the emergency room. Place at least two large bore IV catheters in nonaffected extremities and draw blood from the same venous stick if possible. Obtain blood specimens for baseline electrolytes, hematocrit and white blood count, liver and cardiac enzyme profiles, and amylase and creatinine determinations. Blood lactate levels are also ordered in some institutions. Additional blood tubes are necessary for typing and cross matching if blood transfusions are needed. Baseline arterial blood gases should be obtained. Administer lactated Ringer's solution rapidly, and check patient's blood pressure, urine output, and central venous pressure every 15 minutes. With severe exsanguinating hemorrhage, uncrossmatched blood may be given, but type-specific blood is preferable as soon as it becomes available. Some institutions will use normal saline, colloids, or other volume expanders in preference to uncrossmatched blood or Ringer's solution.

Administration of supplemental oxygen and early ventilatory support are indicated even in patients who are breathing spontaneously. The oxygen therapy will supplement the decreased oxygen-carrying capacity of the blood. Metabolic acidosis resulting from anaerobic metabolism is usually treated by administering fluid, but bicarbonate may need to be administered in extreme acidosis. Treatment of cardiac dysrhythmias should be instituted promptly while obtaining ECG strips for nursing documentation of indications for therapy.

Providing emotional support and explanations to both the patient and the family should be a priority in nursing management. Patients are often anxious and confused and will be subjected to some painful and embarrassing procedures. Narcotics will probably be withheld until the patient stabilizes. Verbal reassurance and a calm demeanor may be the only comfort measures the nurse can provide until assessment procedures are completed.

If the family is present make sure they are kept informed about the patient's progress and allow them to visit for short intervals whenever possible. Explanations of procedures will help to relieve both the patient's and the family's anxiety. Gentle handling of fractured limbs and wound sites will assist blood clotting and convey concern about patient comfort.

Evaluation

Indications of adequate tissue perfusion include: blood pressure restoration to 90 torr systolic or greater with decreasing heart rate, improved level of consciousness, and urine output of 30 to 50 ml/hr. Central venous pressure measurements from 5 to 15 cm of H_2O with improved color of skin and capillary refill time of less than 1 to 2 seconds further indicate adequate circulation. Periodic laboratory analysis should be evaluated for a stable or improving hematocrit, a value of 30 mg% is usually considered acceptable. ABG analysis demonstrating control of metabolic acidosis, by return of arterial pH to the 7.35 to 7.45 range, is further confirmation. Electrolytes and coagulation studies should also be returning to normal limits. Ionized calcium levels may be drawn if several units of blood have been transfused, and calcium may be given if the level is abnormally low in order to enhance clotting. Normal ionized calcium varies with the method of measurement, serum values are 1.00 to 4.50 whereas whole blood measurements are 2.32 to 2.54 mEq/liter.

Maintenance of the cardiovascular system continues to be a priority in the period of recuperation. Actual or potential fluid volume deficits can occur until cell membranes have regained their integrity and organ function is stabilized. The formation of hematomas in limb or body compartments may decrease their local blood flow and are good culture media for bacteria. Decreased cardiac output can occur from volume shifts out of the vascular space or from overload as fluid is mobilized in the postoperative period. Septic complications from prolonged tissue ischemia or from infected hematomas alter vascular resistance and cardiac function.

Management of the Neurological System: Self-Care Deficit

Injury to the neurological system can include primary head injury or secondary injury from prolonged hypoxia or low blood flow to the brain. The spinal cord or peripheral nerves may be damaged from displaced fractures, stretching of nerves, or compression. These injuries can result in alterations of thought processes, self-care deficits, and potential for injury.

Self-care deficit due to altered levels of consciousness or lack of musculoskeletal control secondary to trauma results in an inability to perform activities of daily living. (Specifics of spinal cord and head injuries are discussed in Chapters 65 and 69.)

Nursing Data Base

The nursing data base is obtained from monitoring the patient for orientation to time, place, person, and situation, and observing the patient for deficits in movement or sensation which indicate nerve tract damage.

Neurological examination includes assessing the level of consciousness, usually with the Glasgow Coma Scale, monitoring cranial nerve function, and assessing response to stimuli.

Goals. Short-term goals are aimed at preventing further injury from loss of protective mechanisms and early detection of increased intracranial pressure. Long-term goals are to maintain normal body alignment, prevent further injury, and facilitate early rehabilitation.

Interventions

Assess the patient's level of consciousness, using the coma scale every 15 minutes, until the patient is stable. Report any deterioration of two points or more to the physician immediately. Pupillary size and contour should be assessed at least hourly. Test the cranial nerves to determine the patient's ability to blink, cough, and swallow and to protect his own airway. Motor function should be assessed to ensure adequate chest wall movement for respiration and to compare limb strength from the baseline status and from right to left side. Deterioration in muscle movement may indicate increased intracranial pressure or compromise of peripheral nerves and should be reported to the physician. Obtain and evaluate blood gases in the early post-injury period to assess adequacy of oxygenation and absence of hypercapnia which can potentiate neurological injury. Protect the patient from self-injury due to agitation by padding bedrails or wrapping limbs in protective foam coverings cut from eggcrate mattresses.

The patient's skin and limbs should also be protected from abrasions and contractures which can occur with prolonged bedrest. Frequent turning and massage to prevent decubitus formation and the use of splints to maintain extremity alignment will facilitate rehabilitation. Management of bowel and bladder function should be instituted early in the course of postoperative therapy. The rehabilitation team should be consulted as soon as possible in order to minimize delay in recovery of these systems. Assessment of the patient's nutritional status will aid in providing early support for the metabolic needs of the brain as well as other body systems.

Patients may be monitored with intracranial pressure recording devices for several days post injury. These devices must be accurately calibrated and maintained with sterile technique. They are helpful in assessing the response of the patient to nursing interventions such as suctioning, turning, and positioning. If medications such as steroids or osmotic diuretics are given, laboratory specimens must be obtained and evaluated by the nurse at prescribed intervals. Evaluation of urine specific gravity is also indicated in the head-injured patient every four hours or on a more frequent basis. Alterations in respiratory patterns may indicate deteriorating neurological status. Primary shortness of breath or pain may also contribute to irregular respiratory rhythm. Because of the importance of oxygen to the brain's metabolism, any change in the patient's level of consciousness or respiratory pattern should alert the nurse to check for adequate oxygenation with physical assessment and blood gas analysis if indicated.

Patients and families are often extremely distressed by the helplessness and behavior changes that occur with neurological dysfunction. They need careful explanations and support from the nursing staff for their grieving behavior.

Evaluation

Evaluation of self-care competence is dependent upon the extent of the initial injury and the absence of secondary injury. Adequate oxygenation, with saturations equal to or greater than 90%, hypocapnia to 25 to 35 torr, and normal or slightly elevated arterial blood pH and slight hyperosmolity, aids in the prevention of secondary increases in intracranial pressure. Intracranial pressure should be maintained at levels less than 15 to 20 torr. Absence of contractures, bruising, or decubiti are criteria for evaluating the protection of the musculoskeletal and integumentary systems. Extensive retraining or rehabilitation departments or inpatient facilities may be required before the final outcome can be determined.

Management of the Gastrointestinal System

Disruption of the gastrointestinal tract and associated organs from traumatic injury can result in severe blood loss and fluid shifts in the immediate post-injury period leading to fluid volume deficits. Tissue swelling from manipulation during surgical procedures and altered cell membrane function can potentiate this problem in the postoperative period. Large amounts of fluid can be sequestered in the abdomen and result in potential skin and wound complications as well as impaired mobility. Decompression of the stomach and intestine can result in fluid and electrolyte losses and acid–base abnormalities. Prolonged ileus, or the need to rest the intestines as suture lines heal, in the presence of a hypermetabolic state post injury can result in nutritional deficits and potential for stress ulcer formation. Wounds and drain sites are potential foci for infection and skin breakdown from wound drainage. Fecal contamination from bowel spillage can predispose the patient to peritonitis or sepsis. Abdominal incisions can be very painful. Patients may have decreased ability to cough and deep breathe without adequate pain control, especially if the wound is close to the diaphragm.

Alteration in Gastrointestinal Function and Potential Alteration in Skin Integrity

Interventions

Place a nasogastric tube and aspirate the stomach contents during initial resuscitation efforts. Prepare for diagnostic evaluation of the abdomen by alerting the x-ray department of an impending CT scan or assemble supplies for peritoneal lavage. If lavage is performed, send specimens of dialysate return to the laboratory for analysis of red and white blood cell count, amylase, bilirubin, and bacteria. Cleanse abdominal wounds and cover with sterile dressings. If the intestine is exposed, saline-moistened dressings should be used to prevent dehydration necrosis of the intestinal mucosa.

Care of the Surgical Wound. Postoperatively the surgical dressings should be inspected for drainage every hour to 2 hours for the first day. Drains and drainage devices should be recorded on the nursing records. Notation should be made regarding the type of device and the location of the area being drained. The quality as well as quantity of drainage should be recorded at least once a shift. Wounds should be assessed on a regular schedule, at least once a day. If the wound edges have not been approximated dressings should be changed more frequently, usually at least once a shift. Wounds, which are considered contaminated from bowel spillage, are often left open for a few days and then closed by secondary intention after the threat of local infection is past. Dressings applied to abdominal incisions should be applied with sterile technique and an attempt should be made to isolate multiple incisions from cross contamination of drainage. Dressings should be applied to contain drainage with a minimum of occlusion to air flow. Exposed fat requires special handling in order to minimize further trauma and to avoid dehydration, as the tissues contain little endogenous water content. Wound margins should be assessed for signs of inflammatory or infective processes. Redness, swelling or induration of surrounding tissues, temperature, and tenderness should be noted and reported to the physician. The color, smell, and quantity of drainage should be serially assessed with each dressing change. (See Chapters 93 and 95.)

Patients should be aggessively medicated before dressing changes. Thorough explanations and avoidance of jerking movements when removing old dressings can avoid further tissue damage. A minimal amount of adhesive tape should be used on the patient's skin. Many patients develop allergies to the adhesive especially when surface epidermal tissue is abraided from tape removal and tape is reapplied over the raw skin. Some institutions have adhesive remover fluid available. Using remover on the skin while gently removing the tape will decrease pain and anxiety from routine dressing changes.

Pain Relief. Evaluation of patient's pain response and decisions regarding pain control can be a major challenge in multiple trauma patients. Patients may not be able to verbalize pain and anxiety because of endotracheal tubes or altered levels of consciousness. Whenever possible, alternate methods for communication should be supplied to intubated patients. Writing pads and pencils, word boards, or symbols, in the patient's language, can be made available for communicating comfort needs. Observation of patient's body posture, level of agitation, facial expressions, and heart or respiratory rates, gives important clues for detection of anxiety and discomfort. Patient response to pain-relieving medications should be assessed and recorded including the type of analgesic used, the frequency, amount, and route. Patient positioning and diversional activities are important interventions in relief of discomfort.

Stress Ulcers. Prevention of stress ulcer formation is enhanced by alleviating discomfort and sparing the patient from prolonged wound healing, which requires increased metabolic injury. The gastric mucosa can be protected from acidic damage by aspiration of stomach contents, when ileus is present, maintaining adequate blood pressure to avoid ischemic damage, and control of gastric pH. Titration of stomach acid to a pH of 5 or greater with antacids through a nasogastric tube decreases the incidence of gastric bleeding. If volume of gastric acid production is a problem the use of medications that block secretions, such as cimetidine, will decrease the loss of acid from gastric suction that contributes to acid–base disorders as well as provide additional protecion from ulcer formation.

Nutritional Support. Feeding by way of the GI tract should be started as soon as possible. In patients who are unable to tolerate enteral nutrition, hyperalimentation is given parenterally after 5 to 7 days post injury in most multiple trauma patients. Enteral nutrition is thought to be more effective and is much less expensive. Tube feedings are started as soon as GI motility returns and suture lines are felt to be secure in intubated or obtunded patients. Control of the rate of delivery and protection from aspiration are nursing responsibilities. Presence of bowel sounds, assurance of correct tube placement, and absence of gastric residuals greater than 50 to 100 ml of the delivered hourly volume, with head elevation to 30 degrees or more, are usually sufficient to protect the patient from aspiration. The patient must also be monitored for tolerance of the feeding by monitoring urine for high glucose loads and osmotic diuresis that may result from glucose intolerance. Uncontrolled diarrhea from tube feedings can lead to fluid and electrolyte depletion, inadequate nutrition, and skin excoriation.

Evaluation

Resolution of gastrointestinal disruption is demonstrated by normalization of bowel sounds, tolerance of enteral feeding, and weight maintenance. Wound healing and decreased discomfort from incision sites, as verbalized by the patient or demonstrated by their affect, reflect resolution of these secondary problems associated with gastrointestinal trauma.

Management of the Genitourinary System: Alteration in Urinary Elimination

Injury to the kidneys, ureter, or bladder can occur with both blunt and penetrating injury. More commonly, the genitourinary system is at risk from the sequela of hypotension, end products of cell brakdown, and infection. Alterations in patterns of urinary elimination as well as fluid volume and acid–base problems can result from injury to the excretory organs or from the sequela of multiple system injury.

Nursing Data Base

Laboratory analysis and patient vital signs are used to monitor renal function. Hourly urine is monitored for quantity and quality as determined by specific gravity and analysis of sugar, acetone, and protein with bedside dipsticks at least every 4 to 8 hours. Blood and serum osmolality, creatinine, blood urea nitrogen, and serum electrolytes are indices of renal function. Daily weights are obtained and used to supplement intake and output records. Urine is periodically studied for hemoglobin and myoglobin content. Signs of renal failure are evidenced by edema, neck vein distention, gallop rhythms on auscultation of the heart, and by rales in the lungs. Heart rate, blood pressure, and central venous or pulmonary artery pressures may also be elevated.

Goals. Nursing goals include: detection and prevention of renal compromise secondary to low volume status; maintenence of adequate urine output; and prevention of infection from indwelling urinary catheters.

Interventions

Monitor the urinary output, daily weight, and intake and output at frequent intervals. All routes of intake (oral, nasogastric, intravenous, irrigations, and line patency fluids) must be accounted for. Intravenous piggyback medications, which may raise the total intavenous fluid far in excess of the patient's daily fluid orders must be totaled and carefully monitored. Drainage from decompression tubes, drains, and dressings accounts for output as well as urinary catheter totals. Monitoring the patient's temperature every 2 to 4 hours will give evidence for increased insensible fluid loss, as well as early indications of infection. Observing the patient's laboratory values and administering supplemental electrolytes, as ordered, are nursing responsibilities. Obtaining routine urine cultures on a 3- or 4-day schedule is usually indicated with prolonged urinary catheterization in a critically ill patient. Observation of cloudy or discolored urine should be noted on a per shift basis. Daily catheter care and maintenance of a closed drainage system are basic interventions for prevention of infection.

In the presence of evidence of renal compromise the physician should be notified immediately. Either high or low output renal failure will dictate alteration of intravenous fluid orders, additives and consideration of the nephrotoxicity potential of antibiotics.

Evaluation

Evaluation of urinary system restoration is demonstrated by stability of the cardiovascular system and flow of adequate urine. Urine output should be geater than 30 ml/hour and of good quality; specific gravity 1.005 to 1.030, clear and amber to yellow in color, and free of casts, red or white cells, or bacteria. Serum creatinine and BUN levels should remain within normal range.

Management of Musculoskeletal Injuries

Injury to the musculoskeletal system includes both soft tissue injury and injury to the bony skeleton. Soft tissue injury may be evidenced in either open or closed wounds. Open wounds result from bullets and other penetrating objects, abrasions, incisions, lacerations, or avulsions. Closed wounds include injury to underlying tissue or organs.

The nursing diagnoses that result from these injuries include impairment of skin integrity, potential alteration in tissue perfusion, fluid volume deficits, alteration in comfort, and impaired mobility.

Alteration in Skin Integrity

Nursing Data Base

Abrasions involve only a partial thickness of the skin being scraped off and result in bleeding and potential for infection. *Lacerations* are usually jagged cuts through skin and may extend to deeper tissue. A knife may produce a sharp, straight cut which is termed an *incision*. Both lacerations and incisions may be superficial or extend into muscles, tendons, or organs depending on the force behind the injuring object. *Avulsions* occur when the full thickness of the skin is torn loose and may involve the underlying subcutaneous tissue. The most common sites for avulsion are the scalp or extremities. *Puncture wounds* are produced by penetrating, sharp, narrow pointed objects. These wounds are particularly prone to infectious consequences such as tetanus. (See Table 104–5 for tetanus prophylaxis.) Bullets, knives, sticks, or glass can result in puncture wounds which may deeply penetrate the body. The impaling object should be left in place until operative procedures can be performed.

Bleeding can be controlled by applying pressure at blood vessel pressure points. Nursing documentation of the location, description, and extent of the wounds starts when the initial head-to-toe assessment is done. A description of the injuring object as well as the duration of the wound should be obtained as soon as possible. All traumatic wounds are considered to be contaminated and the longer the wound is open before treatment, the more likely it is to become infected.

Interventions

Generally open wounds are treated by controlling the bleeding, cleansing with copious amounts of sterile saline, and perhaps administering antimicrobial agents. If they are deep they are irrigated. After removal of debris and devitalized tissue, wounds are sutured or closed by butterfly adhesive strips to approximate the skin edges and facilitate wound healing. If the wound is considered grossly contaminated it may be left open and further debrided and cleansed in the operating room. Exposed tendons, blood vessels, and abdominal viscera should be covered with a moist saline dressing and covered occlusively to keep the tissues from drying. Dehydration can lead to necrosis in these tissues.

Contusions result from blunt objects impacting the tissue. Blood vessels are injured and edema forms giving the skin a reddish or black and blue appearance. The area is usually painful and may be warm to the touch. Application of ice may be comforting to the patient but should be avoided if the patient is hypotensive or hypothermic. If lacerations are sutured in the emergency room, hairy areas of the skin should be shaved 1/4 to 1/2 inch surrounding the wound. The skin should be cleansed with antimicrobials before sutures are placed. A topical antibiotic and dry sterile dressings are then applied.

Evaluation

Control of bleeding, thorough removal of foreign material, and documentation of infection prophylaxis are the evaluative measures for wound care in the emergency room upon discharge to the operating room. Continued wound approximation and progressive signs of wound healing without signs of infection are evidence of appropriate wound care in the recuperative phase.

Injury to the skeleton may result in fractures or dislocations of the bones, torn ligaments, or muscle injury. Initial care is directed at identification of the injury and prevention of further damage.

Injury to the Bony Skeleton

Nursing Data Base

Pain localized over a bone or near a joint should be considered a possible fracture until this is ruled out. Abnormal angulation may indicate a dislocation or a fracture. In a compound fracture there will be obvious breaks in the skin, and the bone may or may not be protruding. In the presence of a fracture the patient usually guards an extremity from movement due to pain, but altered levels of consciousness due to the accident or to alcohol may blunt the pain response. The ability to move an extremity does not rule out the possibility of an underlying fracture. Bruising, puncture wounds over the course of a long bone, shortening of an extremity, or displacement of a joint indicate a possible fracture. Point tenderness along the spine, jaw, or pelvis may signal underlying bony defect. Fractures in the arms or legs may be demonstrated by pallor and parasthesia of the hands and toes due to pinching of nerves or blood vessels by bone fragments. Color, temperature, sensation, and circulation of the extremity should be observed. Peripheral pulses should be noted and documented. Particular care should be taken with dislocated shoulders and elbows due to the potential damage to vessels in these areas. Drainage from facial and skull fractures should be assessed for presence of glucose which may indicate a potential basilar skull fracture. Hematoma formation, especially in the retroperitoneal area, should be noted as the patient can lose significant amounts of blood into these fracture sites. (See Table 104–4.) The bleeding in combination with soft tissue swelling can pose a threat to tissue perfusion and can be a source of infection in the postoperative period. Fat emboli are potential complications in the postoperative period.

Goals. Short-term goals include detection of fractures, stabilization of the affected extremity, and prevention of ischemia to the limb. Long-term goals include pain control, preservation of function, and prevention of contractures or infection.

Interventions

Assist in obtaining quality x-ray examinations. Apply splints as indicated and watch for signs of decreased tissue perfusion due to constriction. Check color, sensation, and movement every 1 to 2 hours. Report numbness, pain, pallor, or absence of pulse immediately. Maintain the prescribed amount of traction, and watch for pressure sores which may develop from these devices. Protect wet casts from pressure which could cause compression of the underlying tissue if it dries in an indented position. Edges of the casts should be assessed for sharp or crumbling edges and padded to prevent abrasion of the underlying skin in the recovery phase. Pins or wires used for fixation should be assessed at their entry sites for redness, drainage, or maceration and should be cleansed frequently to prevent bacterial contamination.

As soon as possible patients should be tilted, turned, or ambulated with assistance. The use of special tilt or roto-beds is becoming more frequent in the care of these patients. The beds enhance the nurse's ability to maintain traction and prevent pulmonary complications but may contribute to sensory alteration unless the nursing staff pays particular attention to careful explanations and frequently orients the patient.

Passive range of motion exercises as ordered and prevention of disuse muscular atrophy are carried out in consultation with orthopedic and rehabilitation teams. Prevention of skin breakdown with massage and care of orthopedic devices will prevent delay of independent mobility. When bed rest is no longer required, activity tolerance must be assessed as reflected by the patient's pulse, shortness of breath, complaints of fatigue, and stability. Physical support from several nurses may be required in early ambulatory efforts, but the patient should be encouraged to bear some of his or her own weight for the sake of increasing exercise tolerance and preventing bone decalcification.

Control of the patient's pain is vitally important if he or she is to benefit from these attempts at independence. Because of the psychological as well as physiological benefits to be derived, both frequent and adequate pain control measures are indicated.

Evaluation

Evaluation of restoration of musculoskeletal function for bony defects is based on observation of adequate joint movement, prevention of skin breakdown, and function of the weight-bearing muscles.

Psychosocial Concerns: Anxiety

The interrelationship of physiological and psychological stressors becomes more evident all the time. If attainment of optimal outcomes for the patient and their significant others is to be achieved, these stressors must be dealt with concurrently. The response of these individuals will depend upon basic personality traits, usual methods of coping, perceptions of the illness and the therapeutic regimes, the environmental attitudes displayed by the staff, and the setting.

Nursing Data Base

Information is derived from questioning the patient or significant others, observation of behaviors, and assessment of the environment. Symptoms include alteration in thought processes with demonstration of distortion of reality. Anxiety may be manifested by tachycardia, hyperventilation, or extreme agitation. Dysfunctional grieving of significant others may be manifested by lack of self-care, disturbance in their sleep patterns, and, occasionally, substance abuse.

Interventions

Frequently assess patient comfort measures, including pain medication regimen, positioning, and bed placement. Provide verbal reassurance, information, and clarification of the physical status of the patient as well as the rationale of treatments. Allow and encourage the presence of significant others in delivery of care whenever possible. Promote a balance of sensory stimuli, and avoid extremes of noise, constant lighting, or uninterrupted care delivery. Promote periods of rest between procedures. Orient the patient and family to the routines of the unit. Reassure the family members that inappropriate behaviors or thought processes on the part of the patient are often transient and reflect physiological derangements, strange environments, or medication effects. Determine the perception of the patient's condition held by family members. Tell the patient it is normal to be angry. Acknowledge and accept the verbalizations of anger, denial, or grief directed at the staff, between family members, or between the patient and family. Recognize that anger and hostility may indicate fear and anxiety or may be justified by circumstances that can be changed. Slight acts of omission or commission on the part of the staff can provoke a great deal of anger on the part of a person who feels powerless, depersonalized, and who has an altered body image. Alteration in family roles is disturbing to both adults and children and may occur as a consequence of the injury or be transient during the acute phase of the illness.

Sometimes something as simple as a photograph of the patient and family will help establish a dialogue between the family members and the staff. Conferences with the nursing staff and the family members can help clarify mutual concerns. Using clinical nurse specialists, social workers, or psychiatric consultants during these sessions can enhance the communication of feelings and aid in problem solving.

Evaluation

Evaluation of decreased anxiety in the patient and the family is based on observation of behaviors. Decrease in level of agitation and increasing periods of rest and sleep may indicate control of pain and confidence in the staff's attitude about caring for the patient as an individual. Family members may verbalize their awareness of nursing staff support and identify other sources of support—their friends, church, or community. The patient and family may begin to make specific plans for the rehabilitation phase and start identifying strategies for achieving these goals. Interests other than the daily visit to the hospital or the daily plan of care for the patient become subjects of conversation between the staff or between the patient and family members.

Summary

Nursing care of the multiple trauma patient encompasses a holistic approach to the needs of the patient, significant others, the environment of care, and society at large. It requires a team approach of health-care professionals to plan and carry out the comprehensive care needed. Appreciation of the factors involved in the etiology and prevention of accidental injury direct the formation of a clinical knowledge base as well as informed citizenship.[36] Trauma nurses must continually find methods of upgrading their knowledge and skills. Mutual support and consultation among nurses caring for trauma victims are necessary to provide optimal care for patients and their families. Trauma care involves aspects of nursing from acute care through rehabilitation.

References

1. Abbot WC, Eichenique MM, Bistrian BR, et al: Nutritional care of the trauma patient. Surg Gynecol and Obstet 157:585–597, 1983
2. Abels LF: Nutrition and elimination. In Abels LF (ed): Mosby's Manual of Critical Care, chap 14. St. Louis, CV Mosby, 1979
3. Alexander JW, Ogle CK, Stinnett JD, et al: A sequential, prospective analysis of immunologic abnormalities and infection following severe thermal injury. Ann Surg 188:809–815, 1979
4. American College of Surgeons Committee on Trauma: Early Care of the Injured Patient, pp 39–40. Philadelphia, WB Saunders, 1972 (Revised 1980)
5. American College of Surgeons Committee on Trauma: Field Categorization of Trauma Patients and Hospital Trauma Index. Bull Am Coll Surg 65:28–33, 1980
6. American College of Surgeons Committee on Trauma: Hospital Resources for Optimal Care of the Injured Patient. Bulletin ACS 43–48, August 1979, Appendices February 1980, 9–35 (Revised 68(10):11–21, 1983)
7. American Medical Association Committee on the Medical Aspects of Automotive Safety: Rating the Severity of Tissue Damage: The Abbreviated Scale, 1976 (Revised 1980)
8. Baker SP, O'Neil B, Haddon W, et al: The injury severity score: A method for describing patients with multiple injuries and evaluating emergency care. J Trauma 14:187–196, 1974
9. Budassi SA, Barber J: Multiple trauma: An overview. In Mosby's Manual of Emergency Care: Practices and Procedures, 2nd ed. St. Louis, CV Mosby, 1984
10. Champion HR, Sacco WJ, Carnacco AJ, et al: Trauma score. Crit Care Med 9:672–676, 1981
11. Champion HR, Sacco WJ, Hunt TK: Trauma severity scoring to predict mortality. World J Surg 7:4–11, 1983
12. Charters AC, Stewart N: The management of trauma. In Kinney M (ed): AACN's Clinical Reference for Critical Care Nursing, p 795–819. New York, McGraw-Hill, 1981
13. Clark R, Badger FG, Sevitt S: Modern Trends in Accident Surgery and Medicine. London, Butterworth, 1959
14. Detmer DE, Moylan JA, Rose J, et al: Regional categorization and quality of care in major trauma. J Trauma 17:592–599, 1977
15. Dove DB, Stahl WM, DelGuercio, LRM: A five-year review of deaths following urban trauma. J Trauma 20:760–766, 1980
16. Eggold R: Editorial: Trauma care regionalization: A necessity. J Trauma 23(3):260–262, 1983
17. Faist E, Baue AE, Dittmer H, et al: Multiple organ failure in polytrauma patients. J Trauma 23(9):775–787, 1983
18. Foley RW, Lawrence SH, Pilcher DB, et al: Abdominal injuries in automobile accidents: Review of care of fatally injured patients. J Trauma 17:611–615, 1977
19. Gertner HR, Baker SP, Rutherford RB, et al: Evaluation of the management of vehicular fatalities secondary to abdominal injury. J Trauma, 12:425–431, 1972
20. Gordon DL, Reinstein L: Rehabilitation of the trauma patient. Am Surg 223–227, 1979
21. Gormican SP: CRAMS scale: Field triage of trauma victims. Ann Emerg Med 11(3):132–135, 1982
22. Gump FE: Trauma and hemorrhage. Surg Clin North Am 63(2):305–314, 1983
23. Iverson LD, Clawson DK: Manual of Acute Orthopaedic Therapeutics. Boston, Little, Brown, & Co, 1977
24. MacLean LD, Meakins JL, Taguchi K, et al: Host resistance in sepsis and trauma. Ann Surg 182:207–213, 1975
25. Mann JK, Oakes AR (ed): Post-Trauma Care, Critical Care Nursing of the Multi-Injured Patient: Am Assoc Critical-Care Nurses, p 114–139. Philadelphia, WB Saunders, 1980
26. Mayer T, Matlak ME, Johnson DG, et al: The modified injury severity scale in pediatric multiple trauma patients. J Ped Surg 15(6):719–726, 1980
27. McSwain NE: Pneumatic trousers and the management of shock. J Trauma 17:719–724, 1977
28. Moylan JA, Detmer DE, Rose J, et al: Evaluation of the quality of hospital care for major trauma. J Trauma 16:517–523, 1976
29. Panel: Current status of trauma severity indices, Trunkey DD (moderator). J Trauma 23(2):185–201, 1983
30. Pelligra R, Sandberg EC: Control of intractable abdominal bleeding by extermal counterpressure. JAMA 241(7):708–713, 1979
31. Roberts SL: Behavioral Concepts and the Critically Ill Patient. New Jersey, Prentice-Hall, 1976
32. Rodgers CD: Needs of relatives of cardiac surgery patients during the critical care phase. Focus on Critical Care 10(5):50–55, 1983
33. Shires TG (ed): Care of the Trauma Patient, 2nd ed. New York, McGraw-Hill, 1979
34. Siskind J: Handling hemorrhage wisely. Nursing 84 14(1):34–41, 1984
35. Strawn JM (ed): Topics in Clinical Nursing 5(3), October 1983
36. Trunkey DD: Tauma. Sci Am 249(2):28–35, 1983
37. Trunkey DD: The value of trauma centers. Bulletin American College of Surgeons 67(11):5–7, 1982
38. Trunkey DD: Overview of trauma. Surg Clin North Am 62:3, 1982
39. Turner P: Caring for emotional needs of orthopedic trauma patients. AORN 36(4):566–570, 1982
40. Van Wagoner FH: Died in hospital: A three year study of deaths following trauma. J Trauma 1:401–408, 1961
41. West J: Impact of regionalization: The Orange County experience. Arch Surg, 1983
42. West J, Trunkey DDG, Lim RC, et al: Systems of trauma care: A study of two counties. Arch Surg 114:445–460, 1979

Bibliography

Ballinger WF, Rutherford RB, Zuidema GD: The Management of Trauma. Philadelphia, WB Saunders, 1979

Committee on Injury Scaling: The Abbreviated Injury Scale. Park Ridge, IL, American Association for Automotive Medicine, 1980

Ellerby S: Fluid and blood component therapy in the critically ill and injured. Contemporary Issues in Critical Care Nursing, New York, Churchill-Livingstone, 1981

Guyton A: Textbook of Medical Physiology, 6th ed. Philadelphia, WB Saunders, 1981

McElroy CR, Eie K: The prehospital care system. Top Emerg Med 1:4, 1980

McKoy C, Bell MJ: Preventable traumatic deaths in children. J Ped Surg 18(4):505–508, 1983

Meislin HW: Priorities in multiple trauma. Topics in Emerg Med 1(1), May 1979

Mofenson HC, Wheatley GM: Prevention of childhood injuries. Pediatr Ann 12(10):716–719, 1983

Oaks A: Trauma: Twentieth century epidemic. Heart & Lung 8(5):918–922, 1979

Zschoche DA: Mosby's Comprehensive Review of Critical Care, 2nd ed. St. Louis, CV Mosby, 1981

INDEX

The letter *f* after a page number indicates a figure; *t* following a page number indicates tabular material.

T cell
cytotoxic, 194, 194f
definition of, 188, 188f
differentiation of, 196
helper, 194, 194f
protective reactions of, 196. *See also* immune response, cell-mediated
response of, measurement of, 200
suppressor, 194, 194f
types of, 194–196, 194f, 195t